D0842525

CHILDREN
AND THEIR FAMILIES

THE CONTINUUM OF NURSING CARE

THIRD EDITION

Vicky R. Bowden, DNSc, RN
Professor, School of Nursing
Vice Provost for Undergraduate Programs
Azusa Pacific University
Azusa, California

Cindy Smith Greenberg, DNSc, RN, CPNP, FAAN
Professor
Director, School of Nursing
California State University, Fullerton
Fullerton, California

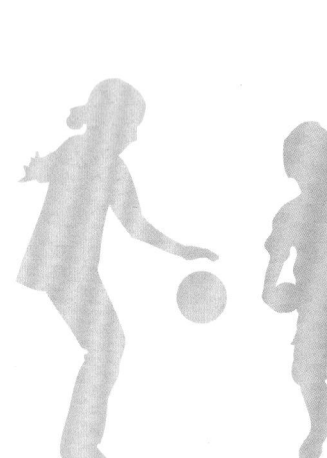

Wolters Kluwer | Lippincott Williams & Wilkins
Health

Philadelphia · Baltimore · New York · London
Buenos Aires · Hong Kong · Sydney · Tokyo

Acquisitions Editor: Patrick Barbera
Product Development Editor: Linda G. Francis
Production Product Manager: Priscilla Crater
Development Editor: Elizabeth Connolly
Design Coordinator: Holly Reid McLaughlin
Manufacturing Coordinator: Karin Duffield
Production Services: Absolute Service, Inc.

3rd Edition

9 8 7 6 5 4 3 2 1

Printed in China

Library of Congress Cataloging-in-Publication Data

Bowden, Vicky R., author.
  Children and their families : the continuum of nursing care / Vicky R. Bowden, Cindy Smith Greenberg. — 3rd edition.
    p. ; cm.
  Includes bibliographical references and index.
    ISBN 978-1-4511-8786-1 (hardback)
  I. Greenberg, Cindy Smith, author. II. Title.
  [DNLM: 1. Pediatric Nursing--methods. 2. Adolescent. 3. Child. 4. Family Health. 5. Family Relations. WY 159]
  RJ245
  618.92'00231—dc23
                                                                                        2013026513

Care has been taken to confirm the accuracy of the information presented and to describe generally accepted practices. However, the authors, editors, and publisher are not responsible for errors or omissions or for any consequences from application of the information in this book and make no warranty, expressed or implied, with respect to the currency, completeness, or accuracy of the contents of the publication. Application of this information in a particular situation remains the professional responsibility of the practitioner; the clinical treatments described and recommended may not be considered absolute and universal recommendations.

The authors, editors, and publisher have exerted every effort to ensure that drug selection and dosage set forth in this text are in accordance with the current recommendations and practice at the time of publication. However, in view of ongoing research, changes in government regulations, and the constant flow of information relating to drug therapy and drug reactions, the reader is urged to check the package insert for each drug for any change in indications and dosage and for added warnings and precautions. This is particularly important when the recommended agent is a new or infrequently employed drug.

Some drugs and medical devices presented in this publication have Food and Drug Administration (FDA) clearance for limited use in restricted research settings. It is the responsibility of the healthcare provider to ascertain the FDA status of each drug or device planned for use in his or her clinical practice.

LWW.COM

"A friend is one that knows you as you are,
understands where you have been,
accepts what you have become,
and still, gently allows you to grow."
— William Shakespeare

Our friendship with one another has grown over the years, and respect deepened as we (Vicky and Cindy)
have shared work, life changes, laughter, and many late night emails. We are blessed.

With thanks, we dedicate this edition of our text to the family members and friends who love and support us
in all of our professional endeavors, and who remind us to find balance between work and play.

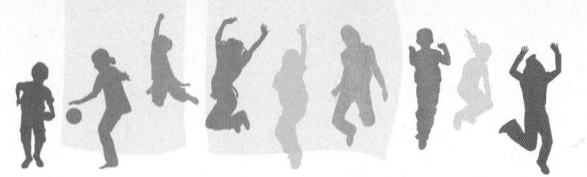

Acknowledgments

This third edition of *Children and Their Families* represents the combined assistance of contributors, Lippincott Williams & Wilkins editors, friends, and family members to support our efforts to update and enhance this text. The book has evolved and contains not just the words of the most recent contributors but also the cumulative expertise of many nursing colleagues, who provided thoughtful insights on ways to improve the text. We are grateful to our colleagues and students, especially those at Azusa Pacific University and California State University, Fullerton, who provided us with information to ensure the content was relevant, practical, and current. Special recognition goes to Margaret Brady, PhD, RN, CPNP-PC and Catherine Goodhue, MN, RN, CPNP—knowledgeable colleagues who were always willing to share their expertise and support.

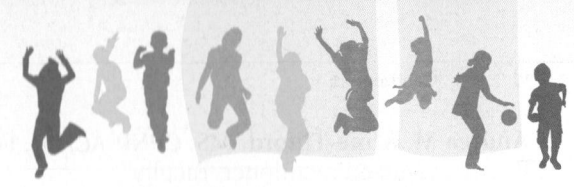

Contributors

Kathleen Adlard, MN, RN, CCNS, CPON
Clinical Nurse Specialist
Hyundai Cancer Institute
CHOC Children's Hospital
Orange, California
Chapter 22: The Child With a Malignancy

Diane Altounji, MSN, CPHON
Registered Nurse IV
Children's Hospital Los Angeles
Los Angeles, California
Chapter 22: The Child With a Malignancy

Jan Bazner-Chandler, MSN, RN, CPNP
Assistant Professor
Azusa Pacific University
Azusa, California
Chapter 20: The Child With Altered Musculoskeletal Status

Sharon Bergeron, BSN, RN, CPON
Research Educator
Hyundai Cancer Institute
CHOC Children's Hospital
Orange, California
Chapter 22: The Child With a Malignancy

Vicky R. Bowden, DNSc, RN
Professor, School of Nursing
Vice Provost for Undergraduate Programs
Azusa Pacific University
Azusa, California
Chapter 4: Infancy (Newborn to 11 Months)
Chapter 5: Early Childhood (1 to 4 Years)
Chapter 26: The Child With Altered Endocrine Status
Chapter 28: The Child With Altered Sensory Status

Margaret A. Brady, PhD, RN, CPNP-PC
Professor, California State University, Long Beach
School of Nursing, Long Beach, California
Professor/Codirector, Pediatric Nurse Practitioner
  Program
Azusa Pacific University, Azusa, California
Chapter 8: Health Assessment and Well-Child Care
Chapter 9: Pharmacologic Management

Lucinda M. Brown, MSN, RN, CNS
Clinical Nurse Specialist
Hospital Operations/General Pediatrics
Dayton Children's Hospital
Dayton, Ohio
Chapter 11: Acute Illness as a Challenge to Health Maintenance

Robin M. Clifton-Koeppel, MS, RNC-NIC, CNS, CPNP
Neonatal Clinical Nurse Specialist
Pediatric Nurse Practitioner
University of California, Irvine Medical Center
Orange, California
Chapter 14: The Neonate With Altered Health Status

Deanna Critchfield, MSN, CPNP-AC, CCRN
Advanced Practice Registered Nurse
Tampa General Hospital Pediatric Intensive Care
Tampa, Florida
Chapter 15: The Child With Altered Cardiovascular Status

Eileen K. Fry-Bowers, PhD, JD, RN, CPNP
Associate Professor, School of Nursing
Associate Director, Institute for Health Policy
  and Leadership
Loma Linda University
Loma Linda, California
Chapter 2: Advocating for Children and Families

Catherine J. Goodhue, MN, RN, CPNP
Research Program Manager
Division of Pediatric Surgery
Children's Hospital Los Angeles
Los Angeles, California
Chapter 6: Middle Childhood (5 to 10 Years)
Chapter 7: Adolescence (11 to 21 Years)
Chapter 27: The Child With an Inborn Error of Metabolism

Cindy Smith Greenberg, DNSc, RN, CPNP, FAAN
Professor
Director, School of Nursing
California State University, Fullerton
Fullerton, California
Chapter 9: Pharmacologic Management
Chapter 10: Pain Management
Chapter 17: The Child With Altered Fluid and Electrolyte Status

Lorna Kendrick, PhD, APRN, BC
Professor
California Baptist College
Riverside, California
Chapter 29: The Child With Mental Health Challenges

Kristi M. Klee, DNP, CPN
Pediatric Clinical Nurse Specialist
Seattle Children's Hospital
Seattle, Washington
Chapter 19: The Child With Altered Genitourinary Status

Andrea M. Kline-Tilford, MS, CPNP-AC/PC, FCCM
Pediatric Nurse Practitioner, Faculty
Rush University College of Nursing
Chicago, Illinois
Chapter 16: The Child With Altered Respiratory Status

Laura L. Kubin, PhD, RN, CPN, CHES
Assistant Professor
Texas Woman's University
Dallas, Texas
Chapter 1: The Child Developing Within the Family

Carlee Lehna, PHD, APRN-BC
Associate Professor
University of Louisville School of Nursing
Louisville, Kentucky
Chapter 25: The Child With Altered Skin Integrity

Rosita Y. Maley, MN, RN, CCRN
Anderson, South Carolina
*Chapter 15: The Child With Altered Cardiovascular
Status*

Mary Lou Manning, PhD, CRNP, CIC
Associate Professor
Thomas Jefferson University
Jefferson School of Nursing
Philadelphia, Pennsylvania
Chapter 24: The Child With an Infectious Disease

Kimberly Haus McIltrot, DNP, CPNP, CWOCN
Pediatric Nurse Practitioner and Wound Ostomy
    Continence Nurse
Pediatric Surgery
Johns Hopkins Children's Center
Baltimore, Maryland
*Chapter 18: The Child With Altered Gastrointestinal
Status*

Suzan Miller-Hoover, DNP, RN, CCNS, CCRN
Pediatric Clinical Nurse Specialist
Rady Children's Hospital San Diego
San Diego, California
Chapter 31: Pediatric Emergencies

Sharon E. Rose, MN, PhD, ARNP
University of Phoenix, Central Florida Campus
Maitland, Florida
Pediatric Nurse Practitioner
Doherty and Associates
Spring Hill, Florida
Chapter 28: The Child With Altered Sensory Status

Ruth K. Rosenblum, DNP, RN, PNP-BC
Assistant Professor
Doctor of Nursing Practice Program Coordinator
San Jose State University
San Jose, California
Chapter 21: The Child With Altered Neurologic Status
*Chapter 30: The Child With a Developmental or
    Learning Disorder*

Rita Secola, PhD, RN, CPON
Patient Care Services Director
Hematology Oncology Service Line
Children's Hospital Los Angeles
Los Angeles, California
Chapter 22: The Child With a Malignancy

Janice Selekman, DNSc, RN, NCSN, FNASN
Professor
University of Delaware
Newark, Delaware
*Chapter 12: Chronic Conditions as a Challenge
    to Health Maintenance*

Lori J. Silao, MN, RN, NNP-BC, PhDc
Adjunct Faculty
Azusa Pacific University School of Nursing
Azusa, California
*Chapter 3: Principles and Physiologic Basis
    of Growth and Development*

Heather C. Soistmann, MS, RN, CPN, CPHON
Staff Nurse, Clinical Scholar
Children's Hospital Colorado
Denver, Colorado
Chapter 23: The Child With Altered Hematologic Status

Lauren Sorce, MSN, RN, CPNP-AC/PC, FCCM
Pediatric Nurse Practitioner, Critical Care
Advanced Practice Nurse Manager, Pediatric Critical Care
Ann & Robert H. Lurie Children's Hospital of Chicago
Chicago, Illinois
Chapter 16: The Child With Altered Respiratory Status

Nancy Ann Varni, MS, RN, CPNP, MBA
Nurse Practitioner, Endocrinology
CHOC Children's Hospital
Orange, California
Chapter 26: The Child With Altered Endocrine Status

Kristi Westphaln, MSN, RN, CPNP-PC
Trauma Program Nurse Practitioner
Division of Pediatric Surgery
Children's Hospital Los Angeles
Los Angeles, California
Chapter 7: Adolescence (11 to 21 Years)

Shirley A. Wiggins, PhD, RN
Associate Professor of Nursing
University of Nebraska Medical Center College
    of Nursing
Lincoln, Nebraska
Chapter 10: Pain Management

Karla D. Wilson, MSN, RN, FNP-C, CPON
Nurse Practitioner
City of Hope National Medical Center
Duarte, California
Chapter 13: Palliative Care

Lindsay E. Wilson, MSN, RN, CPNP
Pediatric Nurse Practitioner
Johns Hopkins Children's Center
Baltimore, Maryland
Chapter 18: The Child With Altered Gastrointestinal Status

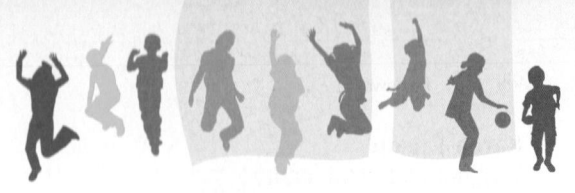

Reviewers

Michelle Ollada Alipio, BSN, RN
Credentialed School Nurse
Tustin Unified School District
Tustin, California

Chris L. Algren, EdD, MSN, RN
Associate Dean, Nursing
Executive Director, School of Nursing & Partners
  in Nursing
Belmont University
Nashville, Tennessee

Marty L. Bachman, PhD, RN
Chair/Program Director of Nursing
Front Range Community College, Larimer Campus
Fort Collins, Colorado

Janet Banks
Texas A&M University–Corpus Christi
Corpus Christi, Texas

Cheri Barber
Thomas Jefferson University
East Norriton, Pennsylvania

Margaret A. Brady, PhD, RN, CPNP-PC
Professor, California State University, Long Beach
Professor/Codirector, Pediatric Nurse Practitioner
  Program
Azusa Pacific University
Azusa, California

Jo Bunten, MSN, RN
Clinical University
Peoria, Illinois

Dawn R. Bunting, MSN, RN, CRRN
Professor
Capital Community College
Hartford, Connecticut

Jane Cerruti Dellert, PhD, RN, PNP-BC, CPNP
Assistant Professor
Seton Hall University
South Orange, New Jersey

Ellen Christian
Professor
University of Massachusetts, Dartmouth
Dartmouth, Massachusetts

Normajean Colby, PhD, RN, CPN
Faculty
Widener University
Chester, Pennsylvania

Kay J. Cowen, MSN, RNC
Clinical Associate Professor
UNCG School of Nursing
Greensboro, North Carolina

Janet Cozad
Biola University
Costa Mesa, California

Rebekah J. Damazo, MSN, RN, PNP
Professor/Pediatric Nurse Practitioner/Simulation
  Project Coordinator
California State University
Chico, California

Nancy Danou, MSN, RN, CPN
Associate Professor
Viterbo University
La Crosse, Wisconsin

Terry Delpier, DNP, RN, CPNP
Professor
Northern Michigan University
Marquette, Michigan

Laurie E. Doerner, MSN, RN
Assistant Professor
Oral Roberts University
Tulsa, Oklahoma

Lori Doll-Speck, PhD, RN, CNE
Associate Professor
Mercy College of Northwest Ohio
Toledo, Ohio

Elizabeth E. Duckham, MS, RN, CRNP, CCRC
Clinical Instructor
University of Maryland
Baltimore, Maryland

Cynthia A. Dyson, MSN, RN, BC, CNE
Assistant Professor
Charleston Southern University
Charleston, South Carolina

Carmen Susan Escoto-Lloyd
California State University, Los Angeles
Los Angeles, California

Karen Faison
Virginia State University
Petersburg, Virginia

Sherry D. Ferki, MSN, RN
Pediatric Clinical Instructor, Adjunct Faculty
Old Dominion University
Norfolk, Virginia

Dawn Lee Garzon, PhD, CPNP-BC
Assistant Professor
University of Missouri–St. Louis
St. Louis, Missouri

Kathy Ham
Southeast Missouri State University
Sikeston, Missouri

Robert Hanks, PhD, RN, FNP
Assistant Clinical Professor
The University of Texas at Arlington
Arlington, Texas

Debra K. Hearington, MS, RN, PNP-BC
Clinical Assistant Professor, School of Nursing
Virginia Commonwealth University
Richmond, Virginia

Mary T. Hickey, EdD, MSN, WHNP-C
Assistant Professor
Adelphi University
Garden City, New York

Janet S. Hickman, EdD, RN
Interim Dean/Professor
West Chester University
West Chester, Pennsylvania

Carolyn Hoffman
University of Louisville
Louisville, Kentucky

Veronica S. Hudson, MSN, DNP, RN-C
Clinical Nurse Administrator
University of South Alabama Children's & Women's
  Hospital
Mobile, Alabama

Janet Ihlenfeld
D'Youville College
Buffalo, New York

Carmen Irby
Henderson State University
Arkadelphia, Arkansas

Sharon Isenhour Sarvey, PhD, RN
Associate Professor
East Carolina University
Greenville, North Carolina

Sheri Lynn Jacobson, MS, RN, APRN, ANP
Assistant Professor
Winston-Salem State University
Winston-Salem, North Carolina

Dzifa Johnson
Alcorn State University
Alcorn State, Mississippi

Wendee L. Johnson, MSN, RN
Clinical Associate Professor
Arizona State University
Phoenix, Arizona

Lorie H. Judson, PhD, RN
Associate Director/Associate Professor
California State University, Los Angeles
Los Angeles, California

Mary C. Kishman, PhD, RN
Associate Professor
College of Mount St. Joseph
Cincinnati, Ohio

Mary A. Kisting, MS, RN
Clinical Nurse Specialist
Sparrow Regional Children's Center
Lansing, Michigan

Mary Lou LaComb-Davis, MSN, RN, CPNP
Nursing Faculty
George Mason University
Fairfax, Virginia

Patti Luttrell, MS, RN
Assistant Professor
Grand Canyon University
Phoenix, Arizona

Janice S. McRorie, MSN, RN
Faculty
Queens University of Charlotte
Charlotte, North Carolina

Michele Mendes, PhD, RN, CPN
Assistant Professor
Connell School of Nursing
Chestnut Hill, Massachusetts

Marlene Mercer, MN, RN
Assistant Professor
Dalhousie University
Halifax, Nova Scotia, Canada

Diane Montgomery, PhD, RN, CPNP
Associate Professor
Texas Woman's University
Houston, Texas

Amy Nagorski Johnson, PhD, RNC
Professor
University of Delaware
Newark, Delaware

Reviewers ix

Anna Nguyen, MS, RN, CPN
Assistant Professor
Oklahoma State University
Oklahoma City, Oklahoma

Lee Anne Nichols, PhD, RN
Associate Professor
University of Tulsa
Tulsa, Oklahoma

Maureen E. O'Brien, PhD, RN, PCNS-BC
Clinical Associate Professor
Coordinator, Advanced Practice Nursing of Children
    MSN Options
Marquette University
Milwaukee, Wisconsin

Kathy Olsen
Pocatello, Idaho

Eileen O'Shea, DNP, RN
Assistant Professor
Fairfield University
Fairfield, Connecticut

Denise Pellegrin
Nicholls State University
Houma, Louisiana

Deborah Persell
Arkansas State University
Jonesboro, Arkansas

Patricia M. Prechter, MSN, EdD, RN
Professor and Chair, Department of Nursing
    and Allied Health
Associate Vice President and Dean for Academic
    Affairs
Our Lady of Holy Cross College
New Orleans, Louisiana

Patricia Price Lea, PhD, MSN, MSEd, RNC
Associate Professor
North Carolina Agricultural and Technical State
    University
Greensboro, North Carolina

Paula C. Pritchard, PhD, RN
Interim Dean
Bethune-Cookman University
Daytona Beach, Florida

Susan Schultz, MSN, RN, ACNS-BC
Assistant Clinical Professor
Angelo State University
San Angelo, Texas

Carol Smith
The University of Akron
Akron, Ohio

Kathleen Stephenson, MS, MA, RN
Associate Professor
University of Alaska Anchorage
Anchorage, Alaska

Kathy Thornton, PhD, RN
Assistant Professor
Georgia Southern University
Statesboro, Georgia

Theresa Turick-Gibson, MA, RN-BC, PNP-BC
Professor
Hartwick College
Oneonta, New York

Aimee C. Vael, DNP, RN, FNP-BC
Family Nurse Practitioner
Warm Springs Family Practice
Warm Spring, Georgia

Lynn Waits
Georgia College & State University
Milledgeville, Georgia

Bonnie K. Webster, MS, RN, BC
Assistant Professor
University of Texas Medical Branch
Galveston, Texas

Shirley A. Wiggins, PhD, RN
Assistant Professor of Nursing
University of Nebraska Medical Center College
    of Nursing
Lincoln, Nebraska

Karen Wilkinson, MN, RN, ARNP
Nurse Practitioner
LiveSTRONG Survivorship Center of Excellence
    Network
Seattle's Children
Seattle, Washington

Kay Williams
Jacksonville State University
Jacksonville, Alabama

Angela F. Wood, PhD, RNC
Associate Professor
Carson-Newman College
Jefferson City, Tennessee

Michele Woodbeck, MS, RN
Professor
Hudson Valley Community College
Troy, New York

Elizabeth Zweighaft, MEd, MA, RN
Associate Dean/Assistant Professor
Felician College
Lodi, New Jersey

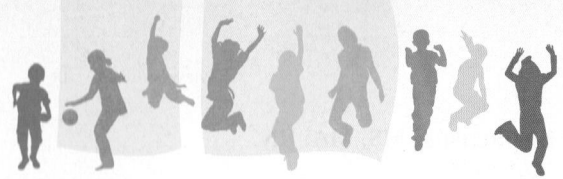

Preface

Children and Their Families: The Continuum of Nursing Care is a comprehensive textbook about children's health care that can be used by both students and nurses in a variety of clinical practice settings. In developing this textbook, our goal was to provide the student and practicing nurse with the knowledge base that would enable them to make critical assessments and judgments regarding the child and his or her family in a variety of settings across the continuum of care. Today's pediatric nurse must be well versed in the numerous social, psychological, spiritual, and physical challenges facing youth and experts in managing complex acute and chronic conditions unique to children and adolescents.

CONTINUUM OF CARE

Nurses caring for children do so in a continuum of care that encompasses ambulatory care, hospital care, primary care, rehabilitative services, case management, school health services, and community health services. Nursing faculty have recognized the extension of health care services to a multitude of community-based settings and have intentionally changed the nursing curriculum to reflect the need to broaden the scope of student learning experiences to encompass all arenas in which the child's health needs may emerge. This textbook reflects this focus, addressing the care of children in a variety of settings—from the home to schools to the medical center. In addition, this textbook thoroughly covers health promotion, surveillance, and maintenance needs of children from infancy through adolescence. It is recognized that every encounter between the nurse and the family is a teaching encounter. The duration of the nurse–family relationship provides many opportunities for the nurse to equip the family with strategies to address their current health care needs. In addition, the nurse can act in a proactive manner to give anticipatory guidance that can assist family members as they work to promote their child's growth and development.

FOCUS ON NURSING CARE

This book's interdisciplinary perspective highlights the role of the nurse working with all members of the health care team to meet the needs of children and their families. Nurses have a primary responsibility to oversee and coordinate the multiplicity of health care services provided to the child and family.

The dynamics of who implements a specific intervention is influenced by nursing practice acts and by the guidelines established by individual health care organizations. In the context of the interdisciplinary team approach, this textbook highlights the unique role of the nurse by articulating the Nursing Plan of Care. These charts summarize the nursing diagnoses, as approved by the North American Nursing Diagnosis Association, and outcomes that are consistently applicable to defined populations of children with specific health challenges. In addition, specific nursing interventions are featured in charts throughout the text. Nineteen nursing interventions classifications (NICs) have been incorporated into this textbook to further delineate the definitive nursing activities that have been identified in research and practice as essential in helping the child and family address or resolve the child's actual or potential health care problem.

ORGANIZATION OF THE TEXT

This textbook has been divided in to three units:

- Unit 1, Family-Centered Care Throughout the Family Life Cycle
- Unit 2, Maintaining Health Across the Continuum of Care
- Unit 3, Managing Health Challenges

The first two units contain Chapters 1 through 13. These chapters present theories, developmental concepts, and principles of pediatric nursing practice that are germane to each encounter with a child and his or her family regardless of their specific health care concern. These chapters provide a wealth of current knowledge that the student or nurse can use to identify and analyze the needs of a child and his or her family and to provide targeted anticipatory guidance.

Unit 3 builds on the content developed in the first two units to present the health care challenges most commonly encountered in the pediatric population. A deliberate effort was made to present the health care challenges that reflect pathologies of a particular body system in a single chapter. Thus, the reader looking for information about a specific disease or condition is able to locate the content in an efficient and logical manner.

The content in Chapters 14 to 31 is presented in a consistent format to assist the reader in reviewing the assessment, diagnosis, and treatment interventions specific to a particular body system. These chapters are structured as follows:

- Developmental and Biologic Variances
- Assessment of the Child With an Alteration in _____
- Focused Health History
- Focused Physical Assessment
- Diagnostic Criteria for Evaluating Alterations in _____

- Treatment Modalities
- Nursing Plan of Care for the Child With Altered _____

Each chapter begins with a review of important developmental and biologic variances, which explain the differences seen in children compared with adults. The "Assessment" section discusses the focused health history, the focused physical assessment, and the diagnostic tests and procedures that help the clinician determine the presence of an alteration in a particular body system. Also included is a summary of the common treatment modalities used by the interdisciplinary team to manage children facing these health challenges. The nursing plan of care draws on the information from the "Assessment" and "Treatment Modalities" sections to articulate the relevant nursing diagnoses, targeted interventions, and expected outcomes that will help the child and the child's family deal with the condition or situation.

Following this introductory content, the specific conditions—or "health challenges"—commonly seen in children are presented. The discussion of each condition begins with information on incidence, etiology, and pathophysiology. Assessment data, diagnostic test results, and nursing diagnoses unique to the particular condition under discussion are presented. As needed, the reader should refer back to the chapter's introductory section to augment his or her understanding of the general assessment and diagnostic criteria for conditions of the subject body system. The discussion of each condition concludes with presentation of the interdisciplinary care considerations specific to community settings such as the home, school, and daycare facility.

RECURRING FEATURES

A variety of pedagogic features have been incorporated into this textbook to highlight key aspects of care and to aid in identifying key information. In addition, more than 400 color photographs and drawings are included to illustrate key points.

NURSING PLAN OF CARE

These charts summarize the nursing diagnoses that are consistently applicable to defined populations of children with specific health challenges. Interventions to address the identified nursing diagnoses and expected outcomes of care are identified. If a clinical condition presents with a unique challenge that has not been adequately defined in the Nursing Diagnoses and Outcomes chart, then more specific nursing diagnoses and outcomes for that particular area of concern are listed where appropriate.

TRADITION OR SCIENCE

These features explore various areas in health care to determine whether current practice is based on tradition, historical patterns of care, or science or the best available credible evidence. These features pose a clinical question (e.g., Why are vital signs taken every 4 hours?) and then provides a response.

NURSING INTERVENTIONS

To categorize and describe specific nursing activities in more detail, Nursing Intervention Classifications relevant to the pediatric population have been selected from Bulechek, Butcher, Dochterman, and Wagner's *Nursing Interventions Classification* (6th ed.) (Mosby, 2013).

This textbook also includes nursing intervention charts developed by the authors to provide a more in-depth description of particular nursing care activities. These charts delineate specific nursing care responsibilities that can be initiated to ensure the child with a specific condition receives optimal care whether in an acute or community care setting.

TEACHING INTERVENTION PLAN

The Teaching Intervention Plans present an interdisciplinary plan focused on an aspect of care involving patient and/or family education. In each Teaching Intervention Plan, nursing diagnoses and child and family outcomes define the problem and the desired goals.

DEVELOPMENTAL CONSIDERATIONS

Appearing throughout the text where appropriate, these charts highlight important psychosocial, teaching, physiologic, or pathophysiologic differences between children and adults or between children of various age groups.

CLINICAL JUDGMENT

These features provide a self-check for the reader in evaluating his or her critical thinking skills. Each begins with a clinical situation, or vignette, followed by five questions that include

1. Question regarding an assessment of the situation
2. Question in which the student must classify or group related data into patterns
3. Question in which the student must draw a conclusion or differentiate information
4. Question regarding the interventions that should now be carried out based on the answers to the three previous questions
5. Question regarding evaluating the outcomes; evaluating what they should see as outcomes; or, if they do not see certain outcomes, then what referrals or further action should be taken

These questions are then answered based on the preceding vignette.

EVIDENCE-BASED CLINICAL PRACTICE GUIDELINES

This new feature presents links to evidence-based practice guidelines on selected topics. A brief description explains the purpose of the guideline and a URL is provided to ensure easy access for more in-depth review by the reader.

COMMUNITY CARE

These charts present special teaching or clinical information to assist the nurse working with the family in community settings.

INTERNATIONAL CONTENT

Evidence-based practice guidelines that have been developed and accepted by the international health care community are presented throughout the text. Health care resources that can be accessed by all national and international readers are presented on thePoint.

DEVELOPMENTAL AND BIOLOGIC VARIANCES DRAWINGS

Throughout Chapters 14 to 31, these features highlight important developmental and biologic variances to further refine the reader's knowledge of age-appropriate assessment and intervention criteria.

FOCUSED HEALTH HISTORY CHART

Throughout Chapters 14 to 31, this chart summarizes specific health history information the nurse needs to know to assess disorders in a particular body system.

FOCUSED PHYSICAL ASSESSMENT CHART

Throughout Chapters 14 to 31, these charts highlight or summarize assessment findings, identifying what would be considered abnormal findings.

TESTS AND PROCEDURES TABLE

Throughout Chapters 14 to 31, these tables describe the tests and procedures used most often in the assessment and diagnosis of conditions affecting a particular system or diagnostic group. Each one highlights the health care responsibilities associated with assisting the child in undergoing the test or procedure.

IN-TEXT HIGHLIGHTS

In addition to the aforementioned special features, four in-text features highlight key information:

1. **KidKare** provides ideas for directing care to meet a child's unique needs.
2. **Alert!** highlights indicators of imminent emergencies or factors to consider that indicate the need for immediate action by the health care provider.
3. **Cross-Cultural Care** indicates how cultural, ethnic, or religious practices may influence the perception of a condition, the course of the condition, or the treatment plan.
4. **caREminder** is a brief reminder of an aspect of care that is especially important for the nurse to remember to ensure safe care.

RESOURCES FOR STUDENTS

Valuable learning tools for students are available on thePoint; see inside front cover for instructions.

WATCH AND LEARN VIDEOS

A special icon throughout the book directs students to the free video clips that demonstrate important concepts related to child health nursing. These clips can be viewed on thePoint.

NCLEX-STYLE REVIEW QUESTIONS

NCLEX-style review questions that correspond with each book chapter help students review important concepts and practices for the NCLEX. These are provided on thePoint.

KEY TERMS

A list of terms considered essential to the chapter's understanding is presented in the Supplemental Resources file for each chapter on thePoint. Each term appears in the textbook in boldface type, with the definition included in text.

SUMMARY OF KEY CONCEPTS

Key concepts provide a quick review of essential chapter elements. Presented in the Supplemental Resources file for each chapter on thePoint, these bulleted lists help the student focus on important aspects of the chapter.

RESOURCES AND BIBLIOGRAPHY

A list of resources that includes organizations, hotlines, and computer resources are provided in the Supplemental Resources file for each chapter on thePoint. These lists enable the reader to access additional sources of information and explore topics of interest. The bibliography also offers articles and texts for more extensive review.

CARE PATHS

Care Paths were selected as clinical tools to present the interdisciplinary plan of care for children with selected diseases and conditions discussed in the text. Although we recognize the need for students to learn and articulate the traditional nursing care plan, we also recognize that in the health care arena, the focus is on interdisciplinary collaboration. This agenda is articulated in a plan of care that reflects all of the components of the care for a "typical" child with a particular diagnosis. Nursing diagnoses are incorporated in each care path to establish the areas of concern that need to be addressed by the health care team. For each nursing diagnosis, patient outcomes are identified as goals to be achieved over a defined time period. The care categories delineate the health care interventions to be performed in each identified time interval to enable achievement of the patient outcomes.

The student using this textbook is likely to already have benefited from the concepts presented in a nursing fundamentals course and a medical–surgical nursing course. This textbook aims to build on that knowledge and further the student's understanding of collaborative practice and the clinical tools that have been adapted in practice settings to reflect the interdisciplinary care. Through the use of these tools, the student has the opportunity to gain more knowledge about achieving patient outcomes, which in turn will have an effect on the child's length of stay and the optimal use of resources. These issues are defining the delivery of health care and thus must be vital components of any education program for the health professional.

MEDICATION ADMINISTRATION

Medication administration tables are presented on thePoint. These tables summarize information about commonly used medications.

PROCEDURES

Step-by-step instructions are presented on thePoint in a clear, concise format to facilitate performance of selected procedures that are commonly encountered when caring for children. Procedures are based on the best credible evidence available.

SUPPLEMENTAL INFORMATION

Additional information, including disease coverage or specific nursing care information, is also provided on thePoint when appropriate.

SPANISH–ENGLISH GLOSSARY

A Spanish–English Glossary lists words commonly encountered or needed in the nurse's practice.

RESOURCES FOR INSTRUCTORS

Tools to assist you with teaching your course are available on thePoint at http://thepoint.lww.com/Activate:

- An extensive collection of materials is provided for each book chapter: Prelecture Quizzes and Answers, which are quick, knowledge-based assessments that allow you to check students' reading; PowerPoint presentations, which provide an easy way for you to integrate the textbook with your students' classroom experience, either via slide shows or handouts; Guided Lecture Notes that walk you through the chapters, objective by objective, and provide you with corresponding PowerPoint slide numbers; Discussion Topics (and suggested answers), which can be used as conversation starters and are organized by learning objective; and Assignments (and suggested answers), which include group, written, clinical, and Web assignments.
- An Image Bank lets you use the photographs and illustrations from this textbook in your PowerPoint slides or as you see fit in your course.
- A sample syllabus provides guidance for structuring your pediatric nursing course.
- The Test Generator lets you put together exclusive new tests from a bank containing at least 550 questions to help you in assessing your students' understanding of the material. These questions are formatted to match the NCLEX, so your students can have practice in preparing for this important examination.

Vicky R. Bowden
Cindy Smith Greenberg

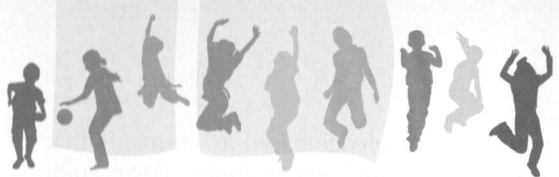

Contents

UNIT I

Family-Centered Care Throughout the Family Life Cycle

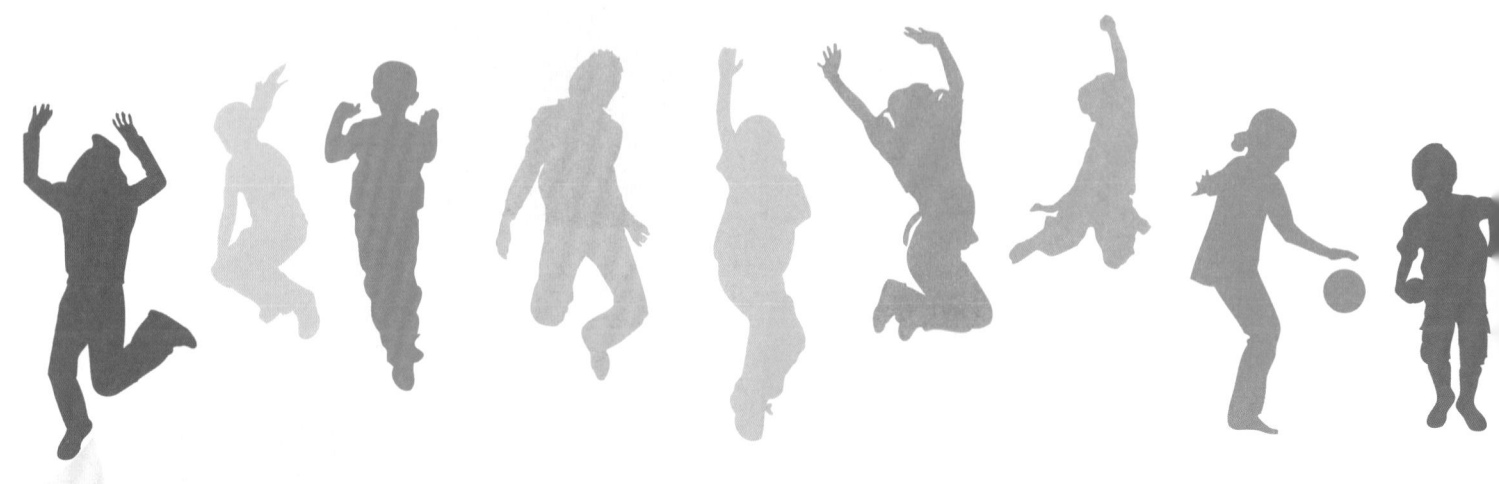

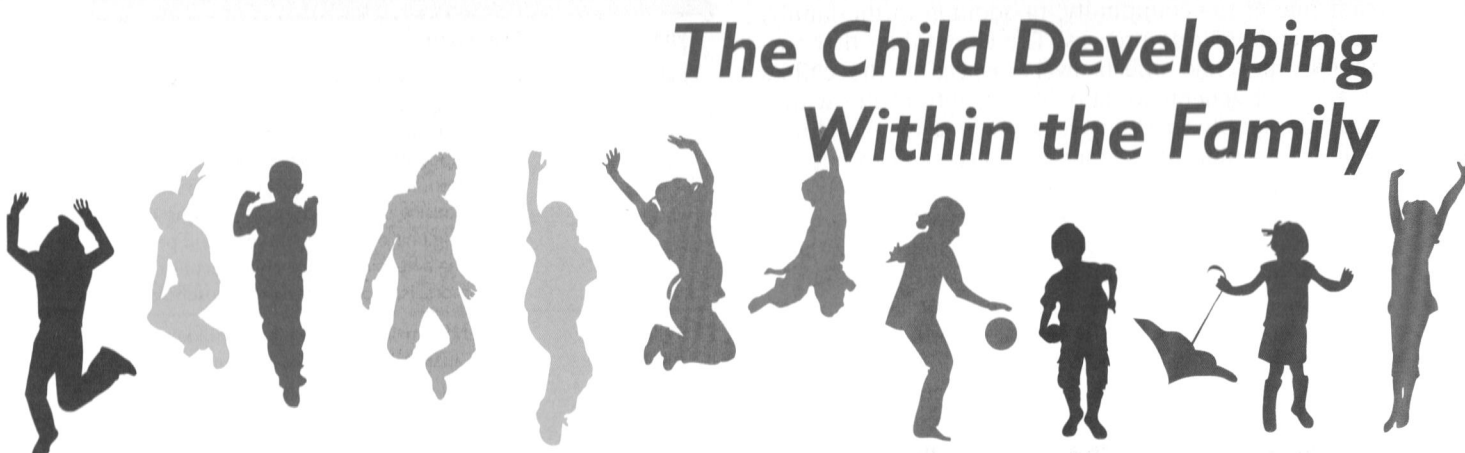

CHAPTER 1

The Child Developing Within the Family

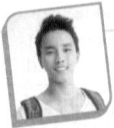

CASE HISTORY

The Tran family consists of Tung Tran, the father; Loan Pham, the mother; Ashley Tran, a 16-year-old daughter; and George, a 14-year-old son. They have just moved to a new home in the same section of town where they had been living for the past 17 years. Prior to the move, the family had been living with Loan's mother and father after immigrating to the United States from Vietnam. Loan's mother died 3 years ago and Loan's father died last year. Loan's youngest sister, Ha, also lived in the home. Loan has two other sisters. Both are married and live down the street.

The family moved so they could open a Vietnamese restaurant. The new home is above the restaurant. Tung speaks English fairly well, but Loan only speaks a few words. The family members communicate with each other in Vietnamese in the home. At home, Ashley is called Chi Lon, which means "oldest sister."

The family is strict Roman Catholic and attends church every Sunday as a group. The religious influence is apparent in their home, with crucifixes, statues, and pictures of religious figures throughout the home.

The Tran children were born in the United States. Tung and Loan have very high expectations of their children. Both children are expected to maintain an A average in school. Ashley is a B to B+-average student. The parents are upset with the amount of time that Ashley spends socializing with her friends, most of whom are not Vietnamese. Her parents also are concerned about how Ashley dresses and the amount of makeup she wears. Ashley is upset because she feels that her parents don't understand. Ashley also never uses her Vietnamese name when she is with her friends.

George maintains an A average and is very interested in mathematics, hoping to become an engineer in the future. George has several friends, many of whom are Vietnamese and share his interest in mathematics.

George is brought to the emergency department after sustaining first- and second-degree burns to his hands and forearms while helping out his father in the restaurant kitchen. Loan, Ashley, and Loan's sister Ha have accompanied George.

CHAPTER OBJECTIVES

1 Select strategies to integrate elements of family-centered care into patient care practices.

2 Discuss selected family theories, describing their strengths, limitations, and application to nursing practice.

3 Explain the family life cycle model as a framework for viewing family development across the life span.

4 Describe different family structures.

5 Describe the functions and roles of family members within the family.

6 Examine the impact of selected family issues on the family system.

7 Examine the cultural and religious influences that can affect child health care.

See thePoint for a list of Key Terms.

An African proverb states, "It takes a village to raise a child." These few, simple words emphasize the significant role of the community, in addition to the family, in the child-rearing process. The community that surrounds the child affects every aspect of the child's health and general welfare. The quality of life within this community has the greatest effect on the child's ability to achieve developmental tasks and to become a functional member of society. For some children, this community is a close-knit group that consists of one or both parents, step-parents, and siblings. For others, the community constellation may include an extended multigenerational familial group of grandparents, aunts, uncles, and cousins. In some societies, the family unit extends well beyond the child's biologic parents to include friends and family members bound closely together as a group that fosters communal or tribal living and joint accountability for the rearing of children. Variances in the structure of the family reflect changes in societal values and an openness and appreciation for greater diversity in the family structure.

 QUESTION: Using the U.S. Census terminology, how would you describe the Tran family?

The multiplicity of family configurations in today's society creates a challenge in adhering to a single definition of the term *family*. In the most recent U.S. Census, terminology was used to define both family and nonfamily households to provide mechanisms to ensure inclusiveness in the population count (Table 1-1). The traditional description of a nuclear family is no longer representative of the family units in our society. Because of the many different family configurations, it is no longer possible to define the family in strict terms of the composition of its members or within the context of its previously defined functions. Therefore, broader definitions have been used to conceptualize the family without the boundaries previously respected by the law and by societal sanctions (Chart 1-1). Bozett (1987) suggested that the most workable definition of the family is this: The family is who the patient says it is. This definition frees the nurse from value judgments about the importance of certain familial ties within a given family and allows practices and policies to be instituted that are in the best interest of the child.

caREminder

Although many definitions of family do not fit those stipulated by the law or many religious institutions, when the health and well-being of a loved one is at risk, legal and religious boundaries cannot serve as the sole inclusion criteria for family-centered health care interventions. At the same time, the nurse's actions cannot overlook the familial connections that are legally sanctioned and need to be recognized when the health care issues related to a child are in question.

TABLE 1-1 U.S. Census Bureau Definitions of the Family

Type	Definition
Household	Consists of all the people who occupy a housing unit. A household includes the related family members and all the unrelated people, if any, such as lodgers, foster children, wards, or employees who share the housing unit. A person living alone in a housing unit or a group of unrelated people sharing a housing unit, such as partners or roomers, is also counted as a household.
Family household	Household maintained by a householder who is in a family and includes any unrelated people who may be residing there. The number of households equals the number of families.
Household, nonfamily	Consists of a householder living alone (a one-person household) or where the householder shares the home exclusively with people to whom he or she is not related.
Children	Sons and daughters, including stepchildren, and adopted children of the householder.
Family Group	Two or more people (not necessarily including a householder) residing together and related by birth, marriage, or adoption.

From U.S. Census Bureau. (2012a). *Current population survey: Definitions.* Retrieved from http://www.census.gov/cps/about/cpsdef.html

CHART 1-1 Definitions of the Family

Whomever the patient says it is (Bozett, 1987).

Family refers to two or more individuals who depend on one another for emotional, physical, and economic support. The members of the family are self-defined (Hanson et al., 2005).

The family is a group of individuals with a continuing legal, genetic, and/or emotional relationship. Society relies on the family group to provide for the economic and protective needs of individuals, especially children and the elderly (American Academy of Family Physicians [AAFP], 2012).

Group of two people or more (one of whom is the householder) related by birth, marriage, or adoption and residing together (U.S. Census Bureau, 2012a).

Two or more persons who are related in any way—biologically, legally, or emotionally. Patients and families define their families (Institute for Patient- and Family-Centered Care [IPFCC], 2010).

Any group of people living together in a household...the variations of family structures and definition are almost endless, but they have certain qualities in common: Family members share their lives emotionally and together fulfill the multiple responsibilities of family life. Family is the child's primary source of strength and support (American Academy of Pediatrics [AAP], 2012a).

However one chooses to define the child's family, there is no doubt that families in today's society are faced with complex financial, environmental, and interpersonal challenges as they try to nurture, develop, and socialize their children. These challenges can create stress and often a sense of crisis within the family unit. As the family responds to normal concerns and unusual developmental and situational crises, the children learn adaptive and nonadaptive behaviors to cope with the stressors of life. In response, some children may develop physical illnesses, psychological symptoms, destructive and disruptive behaviors, depression, or anxiety, all of which can lead to social and academic difficulties when children are unable to cope with stress successfully.

Yet, for many others, the family can protect children from the negative outcomes associated with stress by teaching them appropriate mechanisms for coping with the challenges related to the transitions and changes that accompany the childhood years. It is within the context of the family that the child learns about relationships and behaviors that promote healthy interactions with others. Therefore, to begin to understand the child, it is important first to understand the family and its functions, roles, and structure. Such an understanding is fundamental to providing quality health care.

To this end, this chapter begins with a discussion of **family-centered care (FCC)**. FCC is a philosophy of care that permeates all interactions between families and health care providers. This philosophy places a high value on the contributions made by the family members in relation to their health care needs. As providers of FCC services, it is essential that nurses understand the complex structure of the family. This chapter reviews several theories that explain how families develop and interact; describes the types of families most prevalent in today's society; and explores the impact of divorce, remarriage, and single parenting on these families. Family roles, family function, and the healthy family unit are also presented.

ANSWER: The Tran family would be described as a family household (one with at least two members related by birth, marriage, or adoption, one of whom is the householder) and includes children (the sons and daughters by birth, stepchildren, and adopted children of the householder, regardless of the child's age or marital status).

FAMILY-CENTERED CARE

To understand the role of the pediatric nurse, it is important first to clarify both whom the nurse serves and the philosophy of care that drives pediatric health care practices. Pediatric services are concerned with the health of newborns, infants, children, adolescents, and young adults through 21 years of age (National Association of Pediatric Nurse Practitioners & Society of Pediatric Nurses, 2008). All health care professionals are recognizing that care of the child extends to care of the family and its needs in relation to optimizing the growth and development of the child. The child is an integral entity within the family. The child cannot be viewed as separate and apart from the group of individuals who play such an influential role in molding the child's behavior, emotions, and understanding of the world. Thus, the focus of pediatric nursing is on the child *and* the family. The philosophy of care that has been adopted in pediatric health care is aptly called *family-centered care* (Chart 1-2).

FCC is a philosophy of care that acknowledges the importance of the family unit as the fundamental focus of all health care interventions. This model of care recognizes the *collaborative* relationship between the family and the professional care provider in the pursuit of being responsive to the priorities and needs of families when they seek health care (IPFCC, 2010). The concept of FCC is not new; in fact, it is as old as, if not older than, most of the health professions. In days past, health care providers were family members. Kin served in the roles of medicine man or woman, nurturer, counselor, and even social worker. However, when health care moved to the hospital setting, individuals became separated from the family, and the focus of care concentrated on the individual alone. In addition, as previously stated, societal changes have made it increasingly difficult to define the family. These factors have added to the challenge of moving from a conceptual acceptance of FCC

CHART 1-2 Definitions of Family-Centered Care

- FCC is an approach to health care that shapes health care policies, programs, facility design, and day-to-day interactions among patients, families, physicians, and other health care professionals. FCC in pediatrics is based on the understanding that the family is the child's primary source of strength and support and that the child's and family's perspectives and information are important in clinical decision making (AAP, 2012b).

- Patient- and family-centered care is an approach to the planning, delivery, and evaluation of health care that is grounded in mutually beneficial partnerships among health care providers, patients, and families. Patient- and family-centered practitioners recognize the vital role that families play in ensuring the health and well-being of infants, children, adolescents, and family members of all ages (IPFCC, 2010).

- Family-centered practice recognizes the strengths of family relationships and builds on these strengths to achieve optimal outcomes (U.S. Department of Health & Human Services, n.d.).

- FCC is an approach to the planning, delivery, and evaluation of health care whose cornerstone is active participation between families and professionals. FCC helps support the family's relationship with the child's health care providers and recognizes the importance of the family's customs and values in the child's care (Health Resources and Services Administration, 2008).

- FCC assures the health and well-being of children and their families through a respectful family–professional partnership. It honors the strengths, cultures, traditions, and expertise that everyone brings to this relationship. FCC is the standard of practice which results in high-quality services (National Center for Family Professional Partnerships, 2012).

to reality-based methods of providing care that focus on both the child and the family.

Several significant documents have had a great impact on the acceptance of a family-centered approach to health care. The concept was introduced with the publication of two documents in 1987 that defined the elements of a family-centered approach to health care. The first was a report on children with special needs issued by Surgeon General C. Everett Koop (U.S. Department of Health & Human Services, 1987). The second was a document published by the Association for the Care of Children's Health (ACCH), *Family-Centered Care for Children with Special Healthcare Needs* (Shelton et al., 1987). Since then, federal legislation has supported the principles and practices of family-centered health care through such laws as the Individuals with Disabilities Education Act (IDEA), the Individuals with Disabilities Education Improvement Act, and the Developmental Disabilities Assistance and Bill of Rights Act. In 1992, the Institute for Patient- and Family-Centered Care was established as an organization to support the integration and development of FCC around the world. Although FCC began as a concept applied to pediatric health care, FCC concepts are now being applied to all health care arenas and across both pediatric and adult populations.

ELEMENTS OF FAMILY-CENTERED CARE

FCC is best understood by extracting and explaining the elements and principles of this philosophy of care that work together to move an individual or an institution toward providing a family-centered approach (Chart 1-3).

CHART 1-3   Key Elements and Principles of Family-Centered Care

Key Elements

Respect

Dignity

Collaboration

Communication (information sharing)

Participation (empowering the family, making decisions together)

Core Principles

Honoring diversity

Recognizing and building on strengths

Supporting choices

Ensuring flexibility in practices

Providing support

Trust

Willingness to negotiate

From American Academy of Pediatrics. (2012b). *Family life.* Retrieved from http://www.healthychildren.org/English/family-life/family-dynamics/pages/The-Perfect-Family.aspx; Institute for Patient- and Family-Centered Care. (2010). *Frequently asked questions.* Retrieved from http://www.ipfcc.org/faq.html; National Center for Family Professional Partnerships. (2012). *Family-centered care.* Retrieved from http://www.fv-ncfpp.org/quality-health-care1/family-centered-care.

In pediatric health care, the elements of FCC recognize each family's uniqueness; acknowledge the influence of the family as a constant in the child's life; and emphasize the importance of providing services that demonstrate the value of collaboration among the health care provider, the child, and the family. FCC is based on the premise that a positive adjustment to a child's level of health and well-being requires the involvement of the whole family (AAP, 2012c; Coyne et al., 2011; IPFCC, 2010; National Center for Family Professional Partnerships, 2012).

Despite the ongoing validation of the importance of FCC, actualizing FCC practices remains problematic. Technology, economic trends toward downsizing services and staffing, and the presence of a more culturally diverse population of patients are challenges to implementing FCC. Nurses struggle to find the time and energy to reach beyond the procedural boundaries of their work to meet family needs. Barriers have been created by complex organizational structures and policies that can separate the child from the family. In addition, family role stress, negotiation failures, and power struggles are issues that affect the collaborative relationship between the family and the health care providers and often impede FCC (Lotze et al., 2010).

A growing body of research has further noted the lack of congruence between family needs as perceived by the patient and the family and the same needs as perceived by members of the health care team (Agency for Healthcare Research and Quality, 2011). Violence in the health care setting has produced additional challenges to providing FCC. Concerns regarding infant or child security have tightened visitor policies and have forced hospitals to place more monitors on the children's activities and whereabouts in the hospital. A family-centered approach usually supports liberal visitation of family members for both young and old, yet it is recognized that the increased number of visitors can lead to increased confusion and security risks within a clinical facility. In addition, there is a concern that increased infection rates and spread of contagious diseases accompanies liberal visitation policies. Certainly, these concerns are valid. They can be addressed by security and infection control screening measures that are aimed at safeguarding the child while still supporting FCC.

FAMILY-CENTERED CARE INTERVENTIONS AND STRATEGIES

FCC is a philosophy of care that must be translated into action. The relevance to the child and the family goes unnoticed unless active measures are taken to ensure that family-centered practices are integrated into every aspect of the health care arena. Nursing diagnoses can be formulated from the family assessment to articulate the problems identified for a family encountering a situational or developmental crisis (Nursing Plan of Care 1-1). The interdisciplinary team can use these diagnoses to guide interventions to promote family integrity in the presence of developmental and situational issues faced by the family and its members. From

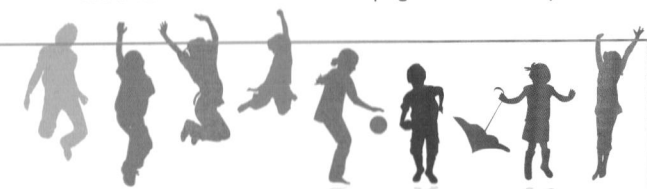

NURSING PLAN OF CARE 1-1:

The Family Encountering Situational or Developmental Crises

Nursing Diagnosis: Readiness for enhanced family coping related to situational or developmental crisis

Interventions/Rationale

- Assess family member's perception of the crisis/current event, including precipitants of the crisis, past and present coping skills and their effectiveness, strengths and abilities of family members to meet demands of the crisis, potential sources of additional stress, and available support systems.

    Provides baseline information about individual family member's understanding of the current situation. Assists in determining whether all members have a realistic and shared perception of the events and intervening variables. Provides an opportunity for expression of thoughts and feelings. Family members may be unaware of differences in individual perspectives about the current crisis.

- Assist in identification of new coping skills, personal/family strengths and abilities, and support systems that will assist the family to resume a state of functioning comparable with or better than that experienced during the precrisis state.

    During the crisis state, past methods of coping may not be satisfactory to meet the current situation. Recommendations for new coping and problem-solving strategies can provide renewed hope and encouragement to family members.

- Facilitate family discussion as members evaluate roles, sources of family conflict, family strengths, and other related family issues.

    Uses therapeutic relationships established between the nurse and the family to share feelings in a nonthreatening manner. Determines areas of dissatisfaction and/or conflict and whether family members want to resolve these issues and move to more productive ways of interacting with one another.

- Assist family to develop a chosen course of action, including formulating a time frame for implementation and criteria to determine whether plan has been effective.

    Helps family members establish new goals that are different from their current manner of functioning and are directed toward a more competent way of handling current stressors.

Expected Outcomes

- Family members share a realistic perception of the event and can discuss the impact of the current crisis on themselves and the family as a unit.

- Family members develop adaptive responses by changing responsibilities to meet the demands of the situation, using strengths of family members to enhance coping, and selecting new strategies to manage stress caused by the current situation.
- Family members identify support systems to assist them and participate in mobilizing those systems.
- Family members identify potential sources of additional stress and make efforts to reduce or eliminate additional stressors.

Nursing Diagnosis: Readiness for enhanced parenting related to developmental and situational challenges of child rearing (e.g., child's illness, adolescent/parent conflicts)

Interventions/Rationale

- Assess parent's knowledge and understanding of the physical, psychological, social, and spiritual needs of their child.

    Identifies if parents have a realistic understanding of developmentally appropriate norms for child and the unique attributes of their child that impact their child's behavior.

- Teach normal physiologic, emotional, and behavioral characteristics of children.

    Assist parents to better understand and promote the physical, psychological, social, and spiritual growth and development of their child.

- Allow parents to express their feelings about their diminished capacity to perform usual parenting roles and to use parenting skills to meet demands of the current crisis situation.

    Facilitates expression of parental feelings. Helps parents to identify frustrations and specifically identify areas of concern in their interactions with their children and with other persons sharing parenting responsibilities for the child.

- Assist parents to identify strategies to enhance parenting (e.g., ways to communicate more effectively with the child, discipline techniques, and techniques to manage parent–child conflict). Refer parents to a support group or parenting classes, as appropriate.

    Provides concrete strategies to improve parent–child communication, manage the child's behavior, and use conflict for enhancing mutual understanding. Provides an opportunity for parents to learn new parenting skills in a nonthreatening environment with parents facing similar issues.

Expected Outcomes

- Parents express knowledge of their child's developmental needs and are able to meet the developmental needs of their children.

(Continued)

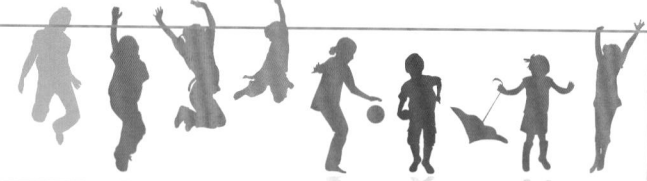

NURSING PLAN OF CARE 1-1:

The Family Encountering Situational or
Developmental Crises *(Continued)*

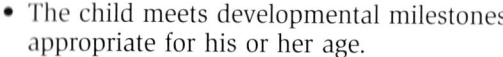

- The child meets developmental milestones appropriate for his or her age.
- Parents convey love, warmth, and acceptance to their child.
- Parents express confidence in their ability to meet the infant's or child's needs.
- Parents recognize when assistance is needed and seek help from others to manage the infant, child, or adolescent.

Nursing Diagnosis: Readiness for enhanced spiritual well-being related to managing current stress and improving family/individual coping

Interventions/Rationale

- Assess family members' feelings about usual and current religious and spiritual beliefs (see Table 8-3 in Chapter 8 for an assessment tool).
  Provides baseline data to evaluate spiritual well-being.
- Assist family members to identify barriers and attitudes that hinder growth and self-discovery. Assist family members to identify factors that may enhance growth and self-discovery.
  Exploring both growth barriers and facilitators identifies beliefs and practices that can be used to cope with current stressors. Open discussion with family members encourages self-revelation that may enhance understanding of spiritual stagnation or distress.
- Encourage participation in activities that enhance spiritual connection with a greater power

(e.g., prayer; attending worship services; listening to spiritual music; reading the Bible or Koran; reading spiritual articles or books; listening to inspirational speakers on tape, radio, or television).
  Religious practices provide many individuals a connection with a greater power. Sharing these experiences with other family members may strengthen the family unit and relationships with one another.
- Teach methods of guided imagery, relaxation, meditation, and use of silence.
  These activities can assist individuals to call on their inner strength to focus on finding comfort, strength, and hope in their life.
- Refer family for pastoral care, to a spiritual caregiver, support group, mutual self-help group, or other spiritually based program, as appropriate.
  Provides additional sources of spiritual guidance and support for the family members. Enhances personal understanding of spiritual issues through contact with mentors/leaders who have strong spiritual/religious values, knowledge, and practices.

Expected Outcomes

- Family members identify areas of spiritual ambivalence and conflict resulting from current situation.
- Family members seek appropriate support persons to assist in overcoming spiritual distress.
- Family members use strategies to ease spiritual discomfort and facilitate growth in their capacity to connect harmoniously with their inner strength and with a greater power.

legislation supporting family-centered practices to an interdisciplinary team focused on the needs of the entire family, the elements of FCC care can be operationalized through a variety of unique strategies (Nursing Interventions 1-1). These family-centered strategies need to continue to be described in the health care literature, noting exactly which strategies have been truly effective in meeting family needs (AAP, 2012c). In the same manner, nurses need to continue to *assess* family needs, *document* how FCC has been implemented, *define* factors that facilitate or hinder FCC, and *record* the cost-effectiveness of FCC. Additionally, both Coyne et al. (2011) and Harrison (2010) identified that in order for nurses to provide quality FCC, they need institutional, administrative, and interdisciplinary support.

FCC interventions recognize the importance of families in facilitating the growth of their children, especially children with special health care needs. The needs and resources of each family member and the degree to which the family wants to become involved differ with

each family. Yet, the goals remain the same: to optimize the family's ability to interact, intervene, and nurture the child during times of both physical and psychological stress. Through interdisciplinary interventions that provide education and knowledge to the family, parents and others can be empowered to make informed decisions about their child's care (AAP, 2012a; IPFCC, 2012).

Implementation of FCC interventions and ongoing ways to support FCC have been consistently documented over time to elicit positive feelings from health care staff and reports of increased parent and child satisfaction (Kendall & Tallon, 2011; Lotze et al., 2010). Family anxiety is often reduced as the family's understanding of and involvement in the child's health care activities are promoted through these interventions.

THE MEDICAL HOME

The focus on FCC has led to a national imperative to ensure that people of all ages have a place they identify as their "medical home." A **medical home** is

NURSING INTERVENTIONS I-I

Strategies to Enhance Family-Centered Care

- Change visiting policies to promote the presence of the family at the bedside.
- Establish family support groups, placing invitations to attend meetings on each child's bed.
- Develop activities or programs to support the family as they make the transition from one unit to another (e.g., from the pediatric intensive care unit to the pediatric floor).
- Be sure there is an adequate number of sleeping cots for parents.
- Establish a sibling hospital visiting policy.
- Encourage family visiting in the postanesthesia room.
- Use parent questionnaires to better understand family needs.
- Involve parents in playroom activities.
- Develop mechanisms to support regular contact between the child and out-of-town parents.
- Establish a parent committee or family advisory council to advise the hospital on issues of importance.
- Create a parent information board containing community resources and information pamphlets.
- Create a parent information and orientation program to familiarize parents with the hospital.
- Provide a brief parent welcome and orientation program.
- Incorporate the family in interdisciplinary conferences regarding the child's care.
- Use preoperative videos and tours to ease the child's and family's fear about the pre- and post-operative processes.
- Establish programs to support the infant or child's transition to home after a lengthy hospitalization.
- Encourage parents to chart the child's progress.
- Contract with parents to provide care for periods of time during the day.
- Provide the family with a copy of the child's care path.
- Coordinate and record all of the child's daily activities on a large calendar that is visible to everyone.
- Provide a parking discount for parents.
- Establish volunteer child care services for siblings while parents visit the sick child.
- Call parents with reports of the child's progress or send notes from the child for those hospitalized for a long period of time.
- Recognize and integrate ethnic, racial, and cultural activities as appropriate into the clinical setting (e.g., foods, play items, pictures on the wall).
- Aim for diversity in health care staff.
- Encourage families to bring in culturally significant items such as foods and healing and religious symbols.
- Encourage all family members to participate in home care activities.
- In the acute care setting, provide support services such as laundry and kitchen facilities to families experiencing long hospitalizations.
- Provide activities such as picnics, movies, and special events for children and their families to interact with other families who have children with the same chronic or acute condition.

more than a building, house or hospital, or a specific health care team the person sees on a regular basis. The concept of a medical home is also an approach to providing health care services in a high-quality and cost-effective manner (AAP, 2008). The AAP first defined this concept in 1992 and later refined the interpretation of the concept and the operational definition (AAP, 2008). According to the AAP, the term *medical home* represents a concept in which health care to children is accessible, continuous, comprehensive, family centered, coordinated, compassionate, and culturally effective (AAP, 2007, 2008). Well-trained physicians and health care professionals who focus on providing primary care and managing all aspects of the child's health needs deliver such care. The concept encourages a partnership between the physician (health care team) and the child and his or her family that promotes mutual trust and respect. Through identification of a medical home for every child, it is expected that health care costs can be reduced and be more effective as the family interacts with a care provider well acquainted with the unique characteristics and needs of the child (Evidence-Based Clinical Practice Guidelines 1-1).

As part of the medical home concept, care is family centered and can be provided in various locations such

EVIDENCE-BASED CLINICAL PRACTICE GUIDELINES 1-1

Developing and Implementing a Medical Home

American Academy of Family Physicians, American Academy of Pediatrics, American College of Physicians, & American Osteopathic Association. (2011). *Guidelines for patient-centered medical home (PCMH) recognition and accreditation programs.* Retrieved from

http://www.medicalhomeinfo.org/downloads/pdfs/Guidelines-PCMHRecogAccredPrograms.pdf

Guidelines released by four primary care physician societies—the AAFP, the AAP, the American College of Physicians (ACP), and the American Osteopathic Association (AOA)—and endorsed by 19 additional physician organizations. The guidelines describe the characteristics of a patient-centered medical home (PCMH), including a personal physician in a physician-directed, team-based medical practice; whole person orientation; coordinated and/or integrated care; quality and safety; and enhanced access.

American Academy of Pediatrics. (2002). The medical home. *Pediatrics, 110*(1), 184–186. Retrieved from

http://www.ftc.gov/bc/healthcare/hcd/docs/corwinmedicalhome.pdf

Policy to provide overview of desirable characteristics in a medical home.

National Center for Medical Home Implementation

http://www.medicalhomeinfo.org

Resources for health professionals, families, and those interested in creating a medical home for children and youth.

National Committee for Quality Assurance. (2011). *Patient-centered medical home.* Retrieved from

http://www.ncqa.org/tabid/631/Default.aspx

Set of standards that describe clear and specific criteria for establishing a medical home.

Medical Group Management Association. (2011). *Patient-centered medical home guidelines: A tool to compare national programs.* Retrieved from

http://www.mgma.com/Books/Patient-Centered-Medical-Home-Guidelines/

Free tool that provides a comparison of how four national organizations that provide PCMH accreditation, certification, achievement, and recognition meet the PCMH guidelines.

as the physician's office, hospital outpatient clinics, and school-based clinics (Clinical Judgment 1-1). The key component in any venue is that care is provided and coordinated by a designated physician who has established a health partnership with the family (AAP, 2007, 2008).

FAMILY THEORIES

This section presents an overview of some of the theoretical approaches that have contributed to nursing practice and our understanding of how families cope with the challenges and stressors of everyday life. These theoretical frameworks include family systems, developmental, family stress and coping, structural–functional, and interactional approaches. Two important graphic models, the family life spiral and the double ABCX model, have emerged from these theories. Health care professionals can use these models to assess family needs and dynamics and from these assessments can develop a plan of care to support family needs. (See thePoint for Supplemental Information for various family assessment tools.)

FAMILY SYSTEMS APPROACH

Viewing the family as a system is a modification of general systems theory as described by von Bertalanffy in 1968. A system is defined as a goal-directed unit made up of interdependent, interacting parts that endure over a period of time (Friedman et al., 2003). There are both open and closed systems. An open system is one that receives input from the surrounding environment. That is, the system shares information, materials, and energy with its environment. The functional goal of the system is to ensure survival, continuity, and growth of its components (Friedman et al., 2003). The open system depends on the interactions with the surrounding environment to achieve growth and change. In contrast, the closed system does not receive input from the environment. In a closed system, the units depend wholly on the relationships within the system itself for sustenance, growth, and change. Therefore, the capacity for growth and change over time is limited. In this context, the family is viewed as a complex open system consisting of two or more persons tied together by mutual interactions, goals, and needs. Each member of the family influences and is influenced by every other family member as well as by the environments with which the family members come into contact. The interrelationships within the family system are so intricately tied together that change by any one person invariably results in changes in all family members. For instance, a woman who loses her job will have reverberations on other family members as the family deals with issues such as loss of income, stress associated with the job loss, and a separation from daily social contacts.

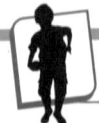

CLINICAL JUDGMENT 1-1

Promoting an Interdisciplinary Approach to Family-Centered Care

Matthew is a nurse working on a pediatric unit in a community medical center. During the past several months, he has become concerned regarding the readmission rates of several school-aged children with asthma. In particular, he believes that management of the children's asthma in the home and school has not been effective. In addition, he has noted that the children are missing many days of school because of the frequency of readmissions and the extended length of their stay in the hospital. The physicians who manage these children are members of a private practice group who take turns monitoring the children's progress when they are hospitalized. Parents have verbalized that when their child is hospitalized, they do not understand the plan of care and feel the care is fragmented.

Questions

1. In this situation, what are some of the problems you can identify?
2. Who are the members of the interdisciplinary team caring for the children with asthma?
3. What barriers exist to providing an interdisciplinary family-centered approach for the care of these children?
4. What interventions could Matthew initiate to improve patient care and enhance communication among the members of the interdisciplinary team?
5. How could Matthew determine whether any of these interventions were successful in improving the care provided to this group of children?

Answers

1. High readmission rate of children with asthma, potential ineffective home and/or school management of these children, difficulties in communication and coordination of care among members of the interdisciplinary team, parent frustration regarding health care services, and lack of parental involvement in approach to care
2. The members of the physician group, including nurses at the physicians' office; the care providers at the medical center, including nurses and the respiratory therapist; the child and the child's family; the child's teacher; and the school nurse
3. Lack of coordination and communication among team members, variety of sites in which health care is provided to the child, and no identified mechanisms to reduce the number of readmissions
4. Plan a meeting with representatives from the family, nursing unit, physician group, and school to discuss and analyze the problems; devise a communication mechanism that assists all members of the team in understanding the needs and plan of care for each child; provide education to school personnel regarding the management of children with asthma; and provide information to families on expected educational outcomes for children with asthma
5. Parents verbalize improved satisfaction with health care services, readmission rate decreases because of more preventive actions instituted by school personnel and parents, and children attend more days of school

As a unit, the family has boundaries that separate it from other systems. These boundaries act to filter or translate information that comes in to and flows out of the system. Boundaries consist of the rules, sanctions, communication patterns, attitudes, and values that bind family members together and guide their beliefs and practices. The family unit belongs to the many other systems that impinge on its boundaries. It also determines its own degree of interaction with other systems. As an open system, the family is capable of being influenced by and having an impact on the systems adjoining the boundaries. These adjoining systems include other families, the child's school system, the parent's work system, and the community in which the family lives. The interchange with other systems may include sharing of information, physical contact, shared responsibility, mutual goals, shared territory, and common language. For the family to exist as a system among other systems, a certain amount of exchange must take place. However, among families, there are varied degrees of openness, depending on the specific reaction of the family to change from the outside. The family with a high degree of openness provides for change. Change is welcomed and is considered normal and desirable. Furthermore, communication and rules within the family are related, and individual self-worth is of primary importance. A family that has little exchange with the environment is one that resists change. A closed-unit family depends on edict and law and order and operates through force, both physical and psychological. Self-worth is secondary to power and performance.

The family is a homeostatic system. This implies that as the family is undergoing a process of continual growth and change, the unit strives to maintain a sense of balance or equilibrium. Parson and Bales (1955) referred to this as the "steady state" of an "ongoing system." The family reacts to change in its steady state by attempts to reestablish equilibrium. Adaptation within the family refers to the ability of its members to modify their behavior toward each other and the outer world as the situation demands. As mentioned in the previous example, any disruption in the function of one family member results in a compensatory change in the functions of all other family members. Therefore, to restore equilibrium, all members of the system must be involved in the adaptation process.

Family systems theory is consistent with many nursing theories and conceptual models that incorporate concepts from von Bertalanffy's systems approach. Examples include theories developed by Martha Rogers, Dorothea Orem, Myra Levine, and Sister Callista Roy. Family systems theory allows the nurse to examine both external and internal factors that may influence family adaptation to health crises. Family systems theory helps us to understand why an issue that arises with one family member (mother loses job) can affect all other family members (tension between spouses, loss of family income to make house payment or pay college tuition). When a child has a health-related problem, the nurse needs to consider how this one issue reverberates and affects other family members.

Olson Circumplex Model

One of the most widely used models to describe the family that uses a systems framework is the Olson Circumplex Model. The circumplex model builds on family developmental theory and systems theory to hypothesize that families change as they deal with normal transitions in the family life cycle (Olson, 1988). These changes can and should be beneficial to the maintenance and improvement of the family system as the family transforms in composition, role structure, and role functioning. According to this model, the goal of the family system is to accommodate developmental and situational change and stress, while at the same time preserving its integrity and organizational cohesion. A variety of family coping strategies are used to help the family accommodate and adapt successfully to internal and external stressors. It is believed that the effects of these coping activities can be measured in terms of the family's level of cohesion, flexibility, and communication. **Family cohesion** addresses the degree of emotional bonding that family members have toward one another. **Family flexibility** is the amount of change in the family's leadership, role relationships, and relationship rules. **Family communication** is a facilitating dimension; it helps families make changes in the cohesion and flexibility dimensions (Olson, 1994, 2003). It is hypothesized that the central or balanced levels of cohesion and flexibility make for optimal family functioning. The extremes of cohesion (disengaged or enmeshed) and the extremes of flexibility (chaotic or rigid) are generally viewed as problematic to families (Olson, 1988). The family that is evaluated as "too" close and the family that is "too" rigid in its expectations of family members are examples of environments that are considered harmful because they do not allow and encourage individual growth within the family unit. It has been

hypothesized that families with balanced levels of flexibility and cohesion have more positive communication skills than extreme families. In addition, positive family communication enables balanced families to change their levels of flexibility and cohesion more easily than families on the extremes. Thus, positive communication skills enhance family adaptation to situational and developmental stressors (Galvin & Brommel, 1986; Olson, 1988).

Levels of family functioning change over time and as the family passes through different developmental stages. It is hypothesized that families with the balanced levels of flexibility and cohesion generally function more adequately across the family life cycle than families with extreme levels (Olson, 1988). Being balanced signifies that the family system can operate at the extremes for short periods of time, and when appropriate, because of situational and developmental stressors. In these families, extremes are tolerated and even expected; yet, the balanced family does not operate continually in that fashion. On the other hand, extreme family types tend to function only at the extremes and strongly discourage any deviation from this pattern of functioning by individual members (Olson, 1988, 2003).

During health care crises, the balanced family is more likely to adapt and change to meet the needs of the situation. The crisis may draw family members closer to one another; yet, as the event passes, family members are able to regain their independence and use their experiences to help them grow as individuals.

DEVELOPMENTAL APPROACH

The developmental framework focuses on examining the longitudinal career of the family—that is, how the family develops and changes over time. The developmental approach may also be called the **family life cycle** or the **family career**. The central theme of the developmental approach is that the family is a unit that changes over time as a result of the physical and psychosocial transitions of both adult and child members. Nurses need to be aware of these expected, normative changes and be able to provide families with anticipatory guidance as they transition through developmental changes within their family system.

Family Life Cycle

QUESTION: Would you expect the positions, roles, and norms of the Tran family to be the same as in your family?

Duvall (1962) was among the first to divide the family life cycle into eight stages with developmental tasks at each stage. These stages were based on the criteria of (1) major change in family size, (2) the developmental stage of the oldest child, and (3) the work status of the primary wage earner. These stages are

1. Couple without children
2. Oldest child younger than 30 months old
3. Oldest child from 2½ to 6 years old

4. Oldest child from 6 to 13 years old
5. Oldest child from 13 to 20 years old
6. When the first child leaves until the last child is gone
7. Empty nest to retirement
8. Retirement to death of one or both spouses

McGoldrick and Carter (2003) describe the family life cycle as a six-stage framework that commences with the separation of the young adult from their family of origin:

1. Between families: young adulthood
2. The joining of families in marriage: the young couple
3. Families with young children
4. Families with adolescents
5. Families at midlife: launching children and moving on
6. The family in later life

Several other authors have delineated stages of the family life cycle, primarily adding stages to Duvall's model to account for the childless couple and to add more detailed transitions in the elderly couple. (See thePoint Supplemental Information for various theorists' views of the developmental stages of the family.)

Each developmental stage is separated from the next by the amount of **family transition** that is required by a particular life event. For example, moving from a family unit of two adults to the addition of a newborn child signifies tremendous changes in family roles, family finances, and family allocation of time in specific home activities. Thus, the family without children is acknowledged to be at a different developmental stage than the family that is expecting the arrival of its first child. These family transitions are considered "normal," and they have implications for individual members who must critically assess their own well-being and alter their role functions and expectations to meet the changing developmental tasks of the family over the life course. Just as the child, adolescent, and adult need to accomplish individual developmental tasks or milestones, the family must also move through predictable transitions for optimal family growth and development. Milestones of individual development such as starting school, reaching adolescence, marriage, the birth of a new baby, and retirement often serve as the normal transitions that affect the entire family. Unexpected events or paranormative transitions are events that do not occur in every family, such as illness, disability, miscarriage, change in socioeconomic status, or divorce, and can result in crises within the family. These events or transitions can change the developmental course for all family members, altering the natural movement of the family through its life cycle.

The developmental theories are based on the assumption that the family is a semiclosed social system made up of interacting personalities (Hill, 1971). Using principles from systems theory, it can be said that the interrelationships within this system are so intricately tied together that change in any one part invariably results in change in the entire system (Friedman et al., 2003). In the family, each member has specific positions, roles, and normative expectations to fulfill at various points along the family life cycle. **Position** refers to the location of the family member in the family structure, such as husband–father or wife–mother. **Role** is defined as a "set of behaviors of an occupant of a particular social position" (Friedman et al., 2003, p. 322). Examples include the roles of breadwinner, disciplinarian, and student. **Norms** are the role behavioral expectations commonly shared by family members, such as an expectation that all family members will share in chores around the home. According to developmental theory, it is assumed that family members change their positions, roles, and norms at various stages in the family cycle to accommodate the addition and emancipation of children and to maintain family stability.

CROSS-CULTURAL CARE

It should be noted that family positions, roles, and norms often vary greatly from family to family and from culture to culture. Although it is not possible to identify the numerous variations of these concepts within all families, social scientists have observed dominant family configurations and family activities that are identified as normative for certain populations.

Within the developmental approach, the family is not homeostatic and cannot simply exist to maintain equilibrium. Rather, the family is an interactive system that should demonstrate fluidity and adaptability as members grow, mature, and leave the household. It is expected that the bonds of cohesion and unity will change within the family system, depending on the developmental stage of the family and the individual needs of its members. At different stages in the family life cycle, patterns of togetherness and independence emerge and exist in direct relationship to the psychosocial crises and the developmental goals of family members (Olson, 1988). With the changes in family configuration and organization, there are family life events, or transitions, that may be marked by feelings of tension, anxiety, uncertainty, and loss. Stages in the family life cycle are therefore viewed as critical periods of role change in which members are called to adjust, reorganize, consolidate, and adapt to meet the changing needs of maturing individuals in the family unit. The ability of the family to adapt, reorganize, and move to the next stage requires changes in boundaries and roles within the family. The family's ability to move through the crisis facilitates its development. If the crisis is not handled adequately, old tensions or new conflicts arise. Family therapy is often necessary when families are overwhelmed or caught in a particular stage. Therapy is then directed toward moving the family into the next developmental stage. Nurses can use developmental theory to determine the types of stressors a family may be facing at each developmental stage. For instance, anticipatory guidance can be given to the family with children who are entering their teenage years regarding changing family rules as the adolescent seeks more independence.

Family developmental theory has historically addressed the family from a traditional, two-parent view of family life. Its use can be limited, given the diversity of family forms found in today's society. It does not take into consideration couples who choose not to marry or couples who choose not to have children, because this theory uses children as markers for movement from one stage to the next. Some theorists have developed variations of the traditional family developmental stages for the divorced or remarried family in an attempt to depict the additional stages through which these families are required to move (presented later in this chapter). Other theorists have embraced the concept of critical role transitions to explain differences in the sequencing of stages and a family's approach to a new stage. Other approaches developed to better explain the changing dynamics of the family unit include the family life spiral and the changing life cycle.

> ANSWER: The Tran family positions, roles, and norms may be similar in some areas and yet different in others. For example, Tung, the father, is the primary breadwinner. Loan, the mother, is the caregiver of the house. The children are expected to achieve high grades in school. In addition, like most adolescents, Ashley is attempting to exert her independence, which in turn causes some conflict with her parents.

Family Life Spiral

The family life spiral is a developmental model devised by Combrinck-Graham (1990) that incorporates overlapping developmental tasks of the individual members of each generation in the family (Fig. 1-1). For example, Erikson's (1963) stage of "generativity" of the adult leads to childbearing and raising children. The midlife crisis of the adult usually occurs at the period in which the family unit is also dealing with the turmoil

of adolescence and the retirement of the grandparents. How a person works through individual developmental tasks has a profound effect on the others who are also trying to move into the next stage of their development. Combrinck-Graham conceptualized that the family oscillates from periods of closeness, or a **centripetal family atmosphere**, to periods of differentiation, or a **centrifugal family atmosphere**. The child requires constant care and nurturing, whereas the adolescent is moving toward independence. Centripetal forces lead to marriage, sexual intimacy, and childbearing. Centrifugal forces lead to adolescence, retirement, and preparation for death. The family moves between these two forces throughout the family life spiral. The nurse can use this model to identify the life stages of the family members and the impact they have on the family. For instance, the couple caring for a teenager with cystic fibrosis may also be caring for elderly parents while also trying to manage successful and busy careers.

Changing Life Cycle

Rankin (1989) developed a framework that describes the tasks and transitions commonly seen in the family as it develops over time: emerging family, solidifying family, reconstituting family, and contracting family. (See thePoint Supplemental Information for additional descriptions of the developmental tasks and their characteristics.)

The *emerging family* is one that is concerned with the task of becoming a family unit. According to the traditional life cycle, this is the stage of beginning families and childbearing families. In this framework, emerging families include opposite- or same-sex partners living together with a nonformalized bond. Common, expected transitions encountered by these families include changes in personal relationships, changes in family relationships, and changes in role status. The new couple

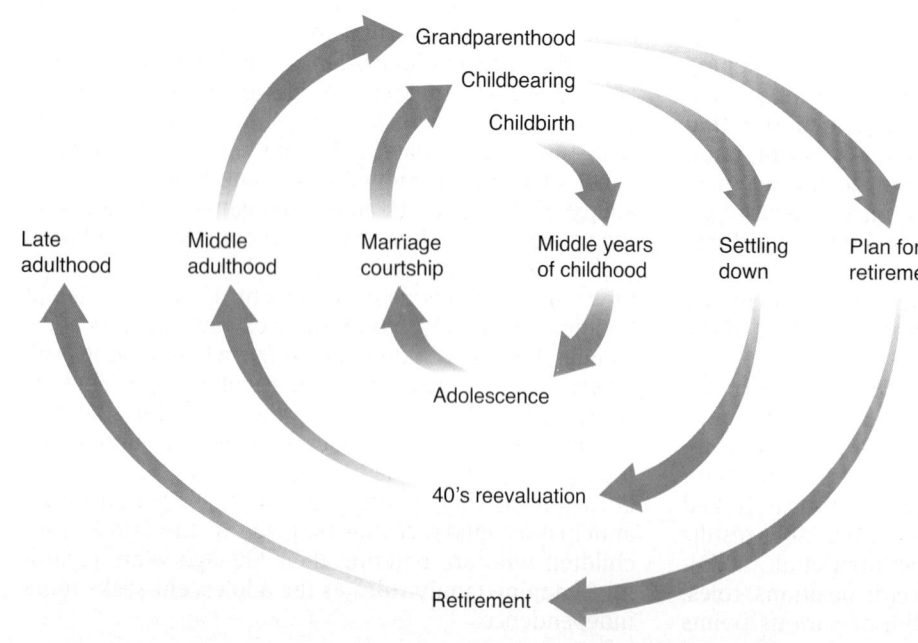

Figure 1-1 The family life spiral shows the overlapping developmental tasks of family members from different generations. Redrawn from Combrinck-Graham, L. (1985). A developmental model for family systems. *Family Process, 24*(2), 139–150. Reprinted with permission.

must establish new roles in their relationship with each other and in their relationship with their families of origin. They must also decide whether to move into a parental role. The transition to parenthood is often challenging for the traditional family as well as the non-traditional family. Decisions need to be made to define the role each parent will play in the development of the child.

The *solidifying family* is the family with the primary tasks of stabilizing the bond between the parents and socializing the children. This stage corresponds to the traditional life cycle stages of families with preschool, school-aged, and adolescent children. Common transitions that occur in these families require increasingly flexible boundaries to account for the developing independence of children and adolescents.

The *reconstituting family* is one that occurs because of changes in the relationship of its members, such as divorce, death, or separation. The members need to adapt to the loss of the previous family form and adapt to a new type of family, whether it be a single-parent family or a new step-parent family.

The *contracting family* is one that is involved in the launching and release of children to environments separate from the family. Common transitions encountered in this family type are the changes in the relationships between the children and the new roles that come with these relationships, if children are a part of the family. Adaptation to the loss of an adult partner through divorce or death and the changes that come with retirement, such as decreased income and increased leisure time, are also common transitions.

FAMILY STRESS AND COPING FRAMEWORKS

Family stress and coping theories evaluate the impact of acute, unanticipated, and severe external events on the family system. In addition, these theories are used to describe the effects of chronic, persistent stressors that may bring long-term hardships to the family. The family experiences normative and non-normative challenges that may undermine family functioning. The challenge for the health care team is to help family members optimize their resources and coping behaviors for managing the multiple stressors that can affect family life. The child's family may be a source of stress; but, more important, the family should be a resource or refuge that protects the child from the negative effects that are associated with stress (Patterson, 2002). Stress and coping theories can be used to better understand the alterations in family dynamics during times of stress. Crisis theory, the ABCX model, and the Family Adjustment and Adaptation Response (FAAR) model, described in the following sections, are examples of models that can be applied to families facing illness, loss, and grief. A criticism of the stress and coping models has been their inability to explain children's stress-coping processes. The models are typically based on using adult-level cognitive and emotional processes to deal with stressful situations. There exists a definitive need for the development or modification of a stress-coping theory specific for children.

caREminder

Children's stressors are not the same as adult stressors. Many of the stressors affecting children are related to situations with parents, teachers, and other family members that are outside the child's control. The stressors children deal with may not be amenable to change by the children themselves; adult assistance is often necessary.

Crisis Theory

A **crisis** is defined as a disruption of psychological homeostasis that occurs when a person faces an obstacle to important life goals that is, for a time, insurmountable through the use of customary methods of problem solving. A period of disorganization ensues, as does a period of upset, during which many different abortive attempts at a solution are made.

A crisis is generally self-limiting, lasting 4 to 6 weeks. During that time, the individual or family experiences four developmental phases (Lewis & Roberts, 2001). First, there is an increase in tension as the stimulus (crisis event) continues and more discomfort is felt. This is followed by unsuccessful attempts to cope with the situation, leading to more feelings of discomfort and a state of disequilibrium (second stage). The increase in tension causes the individual or family to move into the third stage, during which internal and external resources (balancing factors) are mobilized and emergency problem-solving methods are tried. One of two scenarios can occur during the fourth stage. In the first, the problem continues and cannot be solved or avoided, and stress and tension increase, leading to major disorganization. Alternatively, the problem is solved and equilibrium is restored to the family. Certain balancing factors influence the return to equilibrium at any time during the various stages of the crisis. These balancing factors include having a realistic perception of the event, adequate situational support, and adequate coping mechanisms.

Crisis intervention therapy occurs when nurses use measures to enhance these balancing factors and to assist families to return to a state of equilibrium. Crisis intervention is intended to assist the individual or family to resolve the immediate crisis and to restore equilibrium to at least the precrisis level. Crisis intervention is not an appropriate intervention method to use with a family that has a history of dysfunction and problems related to coping with stressors. These families need to be referred to more intense, long-term therapy and counseling provided by an advanced practice nurse or specialist in counseling or psychiatry.

When using crisis intervention, the nurse should view the family as previously healthy and able to cope with day-to-day stressors. At the point of crisis, the overwhelming nature of the situation may temporarily paralyze the family. If interventions are not used, damage to family functioning could be permanent. The time frame for nursing intervention is limited because of the self-limiting period of the crisis event. For instance, in the case of a child who is hospitalized after a motor vehicle accident, the nursing assessment would focus on the event that precipitated the crisis and on the problems that have arisen as a result of the crisis. The accident may have been caused by a lack of parental supervision. Now that the child is hospitalized, the parents may be at the bedside all the time, leaving other children at home unattended. A teaching program may be needed to review and institute child safety issues with the family. The nurse must act in an assertive manner with the family, assuming the role of teacher, consultant, change agent, or counselor, as needed.

Crisis intervention is a helpful short-term approach that works nicely within the context of the brief encounters the nurse may have with the child and his or her family. Using this approach, however, the nurse may fail to recognize more serious, long-standing problems in the family. Optimizing communication among the family's health care providers, whether they be in the clinic, the school, or the acute care setting, can assist in providing an accurate assessment of the family members' coping abilities and the eventual resolution of the crisis (Clinical Judgment 1-2).

ABCX and Double ABCX Models

Hill (1949) was the first to conceptualize a model that describes the processes a family undergoes when a stressor event occurs. The ABCX model describes the "precrisis variables that account for family differences in adaptation to a crisis" (Mederer & Hill, 1983, p. 45): A (the stressor event) interacting with B (the family's crisis-meeting resources) interacting with C (the perception the family has of the event) produces X (the crisis).

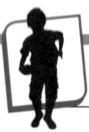

CLINICAL JUDGMENT 1-2

A Family in Crisis

Becky is a 16-year-old girl who attends public school. She is brought to the nurse's office by her friend Anna. Becky looks pale and sullen and has an unkempt appearance. Although the nurse has not seen Becky recently, she is shocked by her appearance and affect. Becky has always been particular about her appearance and has done well in her classes. A quick review of her student file reveals that she is now getting Ds in four of six classes. Anna tells the nurse that Becky is having family problems. After some discussion with Becky, the nurse learns that Becky is 3 months pregnant. Becky is afraid to tell her parents and her brothers. Her parents are separated right now, and Becky thinks they have enough problems of their own. She states that she does not love the baby's father and she thinks she is too young to be a mother.

Questions

1. To assist Becky to work through this crisis, what further data should the nurse collect?

2. What developmental characteristics of adolescents may have contributed to this current situation?

3. What roles has Becky had in her family? If she were to keep the child, how would those roles change?

4. What three interventions could the nurse use at this time with Becky?

5. Becky and the nurse agree to meet again the following week. How can the nurse determine whether Becky and her family are working through this crisis?

Answers

1. Determine whether Becky has a clear understanding of what has occurred and whether she knows the full range of choices available to her at this time. Determine the level of support Becky may have from friends, family, and the baby's father. Determine how Becky and her family have coped with problems in the past.

2. Egocentrism; focus on body image; lack of cognitive maturity; belief that although she was engaged in sexual activities, *she* would never get pregnant

3. Becky has had the roles of student, sibling, and daughter. If she keeps the child, she will take on the roles of mother and provider. Becky's family will also have additional roles, such as grandparents and providers.

4. Encourage Becky to speak with her family, offer to meet with Becky and her family, put Becky into contact with a support group that deals with teenage pregnancy, refer Becky to a physician if she has not already seen one, provide Becky with information about her choices, give Becky information about nutrition and personal care

5. Becky's affect and appearance are improved, Becky says that she has spoken with her parents, Becky arranges for her parents to meet with the nurse, Becky articulates what her choices are in this situation regarding the baby

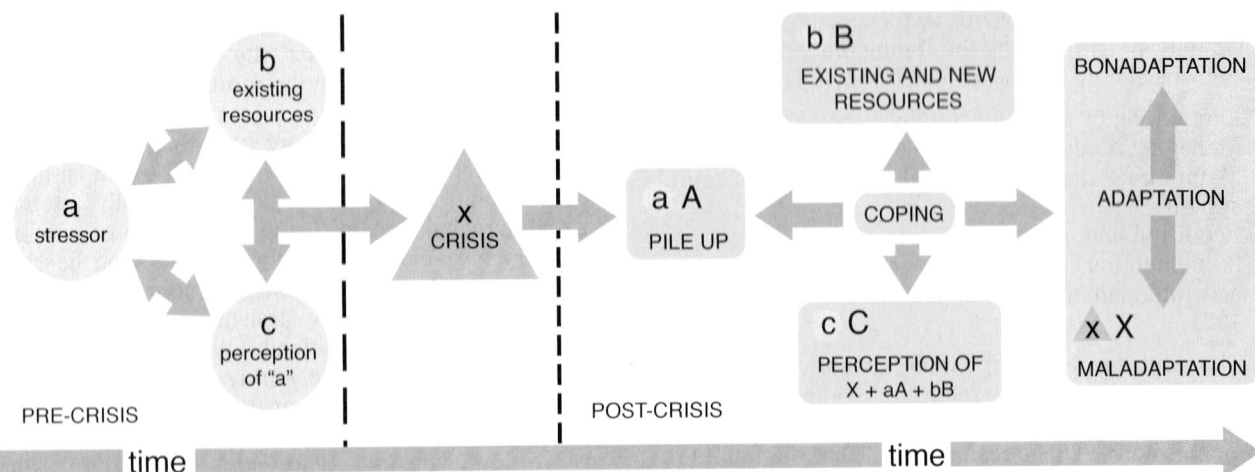

Figure 1-2 The double ABCX model shows how stressors can affect the family over time. Redrawn from McCubbin, H., & Patterson, J. (1983). The family stress process: The double ABCX model of adjustment and adaptation. In H. McCubbin, M. Sussman, & J. Patterson (Eds.), *Social stress and the family*. New York, NY: Haworth Press. Reprinted with permission.

McCubbin and Patterson (1983) expanded this model and added four factors that are believed to influence the family's adaptation over time. Their double ABCX model also includes postcrisis behaviors and explains how a family adapts to crises over time (Fig. 1-2).

The double ABCX model can be useful for health care professionals in their attempts to better understand families who are responding to a medical crisis among the family members. On the basis of the model, several actions can be used by the health care team to assist the family in achieving a high degree of adaptation to the current crisis (see Nursing Plan of Care 1-1).

The model has some weaknesses and may not be the ideal theory to apply to every family. Specifically, the double ABCX model has been criticized for its presentation of a crisis as an event-specific stressor, with commentators recognizing that most stressors in family life are not related to a single event. However, the nature of health care issues is such that one can often mark a crisis situation as the period during which a trauma or critical diagnosis involving a family member was made.

During the precrisis time period in the double ABCX model, *the stressor* (or *A factor*) is a life event or transition that affects the family unit that produces, or has the potential to produce, change in the family social system (McCubbin & Patterson, 1983). Family values, boundaries, goals, roles, and interaction patterns are just a few areas of the family life that may change.

The *B factor* includes the family's resources for meeting the demands of the crisis. Families that are adaptable and capable of making modifications in their actions are able to resist the crisis. Four types of resources used by families are family members' personal resources, the family's internal resources, social support, and coping (Mederer & Hill, 1983).

The *C factor* refers to how the family perceives the stressor and its hardships. This is the subjective meaning that family members place on how they feel they are affected by the stressor. Family values, cultural influences, and previous experiences in dealing with change all affect the perception of the current event.

The A, B, and C factors interact to produce the *X factor*, or crisis event. This event is a family stress or stressor characterized by the inability of the family to restore stability.

During the *postcrisis period*, ongoing variables may affect adaptation to stress. These variables include

- Additional life stressors and strains that affect family adaptation
- The critical resources the family uses over time
- The changing definitions the family associates with the stress events
- The coping strategies the family may use
- The eventual outcomes of the family (McCubbin & Patterson, 1983)

Recognizing that families seldom deal with one stressor at a time, during the postcrisis period, the *aA factor* refers to the pileup of stressors. This pileup can occur particularly in the aftermath of a major change in the family, such as a death or divorce. Additional stressors may emerge from individual family members, the family system, or the community in which the family and its members are a part.

In response to the crisis, the family calls on existing resources and expanded family resources to meet the demands and needs of the crisis; this is the *bB factor*. The *cC factor* is the perception that family members have about the total crisis situation and is influenced by the family's belief about what caused the original crisis, the presence of additional stressors, and the old and new resources the family is using to cope with the current situation. Families that are able to redefine the crisis situation as a "challenge" or an "opportunity for growth" are those that are more likely to adapt.

In the model, *coping* is a bridging concept wherein resources, perception, and behavioral responses interact as families try to adapt and achieve a balance within the family system. During the coping process, the family may focus energy on one or more of the following areas:

- Eliminating or avoiding stressors and strains
- Managing hardships associated with the situation
- Maintaining the integrity and morale of the family system
- Acquiring new resources
- Implementing structural changes within the family to accommodate new demands (McCubbin & Patterson, 1983)

The *xX factor* reflects the interplay between all previous factors. The goal is to reduce or to eliminate disruptions within the family system and to restore a sense of homeostasis. This does not mean that the family returns to its precrisis state of existence; rather, through the crisis process, the family makes changes in roles, relationships, and responsibilities that are reflected in this "new" family system. Failure to resolve the crisis or to allow the crisis to facilitate change and growth in the family system results in maladaptation.

Family Adjustment and Adaptation Response Model

QUESTION: How would you categorize the demands on the Tran family related to Ashley's socializing and schoolwork?

The FAAR model is a framework that allows nurses to assess a family's level of stress based on the demands the members face and their capabilities for meeting those demands. Using this model, family adaptation to stress (crises) depends on maintaining a balance between demands and capabilities. **Demands** are the sources of stress and can cause tension for an individual or family unit. Demands can emerge from individual members, the family unit as a whole, or the community. The three major types of demands are *stressors*, *strains*, and *hassles*. *Stressors* are either normative events (e.g., getting married) or non-normative events (e.g., a tornado) that happen at a discrete time and produce or call for a change in individual or family functioning. The death of a family member, an acute illness, parents divorcing, and the birth of a child are examples of stressors that may affect the family. *Strains* are ongoing tensions resulting from prior stressors or from enacting life's roles. The parent who feels overloaded in caring for a new baby, who is unable to pay bills after a marital separation, or who is unable to care for an elderly parent are examples of strains on the family. Daily *hassles* are the minor upsets that can throw off one's schedule and sense of well-being. For instance, losing your car keys, getting a call that your child is ill at school, and running out of diapers are hassles that add to the stress factor in a family (Patterson, 1988, 1995, 2002).

Families never deal with a single demand at one time. Often, the health care professional intervenes solely on the basis of the major stressor affecting the family (an acute illness) when, in fact, the strains and hassles a family is coping with may be more difficult to manage than the stressor alone.

The mediators of stress are called **capabilities**. The FAAR model emphasizes two types of capabilities: *resources* and *coping behaviors*. The family attempts to maintain balance by using both types of capabilities to meet demands (stressors, strains, and hassles). Resources are both tangible (e.g., money, health care services, extended family assistance) and intangible (e.g., self-esteem, family flexibility, and safe neighborhoods). Resources for the family may come from the individual, the family unit, or the community.

Coping is what families do to manage stress and restore family balance (Patterson, 1995, 2002). Families that rely on diverse coping strategies are more successful at achieving a balance in family functioning. Coping behaviors are learned. Children need to be taught how to manage demands and experiment with new behaviors to cope with the variety of demands that affect their development. Pediatric nurses can provide families with strategies for children to adapt to multiple demands and to assist children in determining priorities or ways to eliminate some demands. Nursing personnel should be aware of the multitude of stresses faced by children in today's society, including family issues, age-related fears, and school and extracurricular demands. Many of these issues are discussed in Chapters 4 through 7.

The FAAR model also illustrates that the meaning the family attributes to the situation is a critical factor in achieving a balance in family functioning. The family's shared meanings include members' perceptions about a *specific stressful event*, their *identity as a family*, and their *view of the world* or worldview (Patterson, 1995, 2002).

The outcome of the family's effort to achieve balanced functioning is called either family adjustment or family adaptation. **Family adjustment** is associated with achieving stability in relation to relatively minor demands (e.g., child breaks out with chickenpox). **Family adaptation** is required when more intense or complex demands are made on the family (e.g., newborn child is diagnosed with cerebral palsy). A crisis or state of disequilibrium occurs when family members cannot adjust by using their repertoire of capabilities in relation to the demands they are facing. Family adaptation occurs when, in the presence of a crisis, the family restores homeostasis by acquiring new resources and coping behaviors, reduces the demands it faces, and/or changes the meanings and perceptions associated with the situation (Patterson, 1995, 2002).

Nurses can promote family adjustment and adaptation by focusing on family strengths and teaching family members about their own capabilities. The interdisciplinary team can use the FAAR model to understand the family's complex issues and intervene in ways that encourage family members to discover the best solutions to meet their needs and the circumstances of the situation.

STRUCTURAL–FUNCTIONAL APPROACH

The structural–functional approach focuses on the relationships between family members and how well the family performs its functions. **Structure** refers to how the family is organized, the manner in which members and their roles are arranged, and how members relate to each other. The structure of the family includes the form it may take, such as a single-parent family, stepfamily, or nuclear family. In addition, the manner in which members relate to one another can be examined in reference to such areas as their communication patterns, the family power structure, and the family roles. The family structure serves to facilitate the achievement of family functions.

Function refers to the outcomes or consequences of the family structure—that is, the goals of the family that are important to its members and to society. In other words, what the family does, or the reason for its existence, is said to be its function. There are five family functions said to be most germane to assessing the family (Friedman et al., 2003): affective function, reproductive function, economic function, health care function, and socialization and social placement function (Chart 1-4).

CHART 1-4   Functions of the Family

Affective function: provides for the emotional support of its members through love, encouragement, intimacy, and acceptance. Children from families who rate high on measures of affective support have higher self-esteem, are better able to cope with stress, and have fewer behavior problems.

Reproductive function: provides for the continuation of society as well as the family

Economic function: requires the parents or adult family members to provide the economic resources to meet the financial needs of the family. Poverty and having insufficient resources are the best predictors of poor health outcomes for children.

Health care function: requires parent or adult family members to provide food, clothing, shelter, and adequate health care for all family members

Socialization and social placement function: is met when adult members take the responsibility of raising their children to be functional members of society. This occurs through effective parenting; education; and instillation of the family's culture, values, and religion. Parental involvement in the child's school and education has been associated both with better academic performance and improved social maturity.

The structural–functional model has been criticized for its static view of the family and its focus on individual members. The importance of family growth and changes over time is not emphasized as they are in the developmental and systems theories. The structural–functional model is effective for nurses who are assessing families confronted by a critical event. The model allows nurses to evaluate the impact of an event (e.g., a critical illness) on the family structure. When a change in the family structure alters the family's ability to function, it is appropriate for the health care team to intervene. Interventions include reinforcing, modifying, or changing the family's structure to help it meet the demands of the new situation. Nurses should respect and encourage adaptive coping mechanisms and counsel family members as needed to help them gain additional coping skills. Families should be encouraged to use their existing supports to meet their needs, modifying the family structure and redistributing responsibilities as necessary to account for the impact of the crisis on individual members.

INTERACTIONAL APPROACH

The focus of the interactional approach is on the way in which family members relate to one another. Viewing the family as a set of interacting personalities, this approach highlights internal family dynamics. The processes that are evaluated in the family include role-playing, communication patterns, decision making, coping patterns, and socialization processes (Friedman et al., 2003). The framework makes no attempt to view the family in relation to its interactions with external social environments; rather, the focus of this approach is solely on the internal dynamics of the family.

In the interactional approach, a **symbol** is defined as a stimulus that has a learned meaning and value for an individual. For instance, silence may be an interactional symbol. In some families, silence from a parent may indicate to all family members that this individual is thoughtfully considering his or her course of action and chooses to be silent until he or she has formulated a plan of action. In another family, silence by a parent may indicate anger and hostility—the proverbial "silent treatment." Silence, as the interactional symbol, is thus understood and interpreted differently between these two families. People learn about symbols through their interactions with other people and, during this process, come to have shared meanings and values regarding these symbols. How family members respond to a situation is determined by the value and meaning each family member and the family as a whole have assigned to aspects (or symbols) of the event.

The interactional approach can be useful to the nurse who wishes to focus attention on how the family functions as its members interact between and among themselves. As the family is affected by a crisis, this model is helpful in identifying and isolating potential or real sources of difficulty among family members as they cope with a new situation. Family members may encounter problems because they do not share the values and meanings of symbols surrounding a particular event. Therefore, members can feel alienated, misunderstood, and in conflict with others who do not understand their feelings and actions.

The interactional approach can be limiting because it does not take into context the interactions between the family and external social systems. Using this model, the family is considered to be a self-contained unit; interactions with other social organizations or individuals outside the family are not analyzed in terms of their impact on family interactions.

FAMILY STRUCTURE

> QUESTION: What type of family structure does the Tran family currently demonstrate? Is this structure different from the structure they had when they first came to the United States?

The types of family structures the nurse caring for children may encounter in practice has never been more diverse. Common family structures now include nuclear, dual-career, extended, single-parent, binuclear, blended, gay or lesbian, and communal families. However, the type of family to which a child belongs is less important than the relationships developed or the level of cohesion within that family. Regardless of the family structure, children need to feel that their family is an acceptable family form to feel secure and to feel free of prejudicial thinking from others.

The traditional nuclear family—two parents, two or more children, with one parent who stays at home with the children—is a family structure that no longer describes the typical family due to the diversity and complexity of our contemporary lifestyles. The *postmodern* **permeable** *family* (dual-earner families, adoptive families, single-parent families, blended families, and the like), is more fluid, flexible, and vulnerable to pressures from outside and within the family (Center for Youth Studies, 2012). Several trends in society have significantly altered the composition of the traditional family home, including

- Increase in divorce
- Increase in number of mothers employed outside the home
- Lower birth rate coupled with higher life expectancy
- Number of adults choosing to remain single and never marry or to remain unmarried after divorce or the death of a spouse
- Number of adults delaying marriage and childbearing until later years
- Gay and lesbian couples entering into long-term partnerships or marriages
- Use of technology-driven methods to conceive (e.g., in vitro fertilization, insemination)

Census data reveal that the number of alternative family forms has increased, as has the number of families in these categories. Nonrelatives raising children

and relatives raising children make up a large portion of family compositions. Single-parent families and stepfamilies are two of the fastest growing family compositions. The number of children being raised by relatives (not parents) and nonrelatives has increased (Annie E. Casey Foundation, 2012; Federal Interagency Forum on Child and Family Statistics, 2007, 2011; U.S. Census Bureau, 2011a, 2011c).

NUCLEAR FAMILY

The **nuclear family**, once considered the traditional family in many industrial societies, consists of a married couple and their immediate biologic children. In the United States, married-couple households with biologic children decreased from 77% of all households in 1980 to 23% in 2003 but has had a resurgence back up to 66% in 2010 (Federal Interagency Forum on Child and Family Statistics, 2007, 2011). Asian families have the greatest percentage of married-couple households (86%), followed by non-Hispanic white families (75%), Hispanic families (61%), and African American families (35%) (Federal Interagency Forum on Child and Family Statistics, 2011; U.S. Census Bureau, 2011b).

The nuclear family faces many challenges. At one time, the extended family (see discussion later in this section) was more the traditional norm. This structure allowed a greater distribution of responsibilities among family members. These responsibilities included working to obtain finances to manage family needs, child rearing, and maintaining the home and family daily needs. The trend toward more nuclear family constellations placed these responsibilities solely on two adults. Stressful economic circumstances, juggling multiple jobs, the strains of parenting, and the need to maintain a cohesive partnership all place tremendous stress on the nuclear family. Although the financial standard of living may be higher in a nuclear family than in other family structures, stress levels are often high when extended family members are not available to assist in providing economic support and child care support.

To balance the needs of the family with the internal and external stressors affecting family life, several strategies are being used to "extend" the nuclear family. Many families hire individuals to clean their home and maintain the yard. Couples may live in close proximity to their parents, with parents providing child care or babysitting services. Many parents are making more concerted efforts to share parenting responsibilities rather than rely primarily on the mother to serve as the child care provider, transporter, and disciplinarian. It has been argued that there is little federal support for the nuclear family, and activists are working toward tax laws and access to services that will support the nuclear family rather than be an additional source of stress.

> ANSWER: Currently, the Tran family structure is that of a traditional nuclear family—that is, two parents and two or more children, with one parent at home with the children.

DUAL-CAREER FAMILY

A variation of the traditional nuclear family is the **dual-career family**, also known as the *dual-earner family*. In this type of family, both parents have decided to work either for economic reasons or for personal satisfaction. This type of family is becoming more prevalent, with 60% of all nuclear families having both parents working outside the home (U.S. Department of Labor, 2012). When circumstances change, one parent may choose to stay at home to care for the children while the other parent is employed. Dual-career families are faced with challenges as they struggle to maintain the family. Parents in these families must perform at least four jobs: two market jobs for pay and two unpaid jobs in the family. The unpaid job is considered "family work" and includes household chores and child care tasks performed by the family to function effectively (Fig. 1-3). Although family work was once considered a woman's responsibility, dual-career families have been forced to redefine and renegotiate roles and tasks within the family to be functional. With both parents working, child care and the completion of household chores have become important issues for the family.

The dual-career family must often find affordable child care services to take care of their children's needs when the parents are not available. Some dual-career families deal with this situation by arranging alternating work schedules. That is, while one parent works during the day, the other is at home. In the evening, the "day worker" parent returns home to watch the children while the other parent goes to work. Although this situation eliminates the high cost of child care and maximizes parental contact with the children, it can place stress on the parent relationship because spousal contact is sacrificed.

During the past several years, little attention has been given to the nuclear family or dual-career family and the struggle that these families face in trying to maintain and promote the nuclear family. As more and more legislation and other support systems have arisen to support the nontraditional family, nuclear families may feel as though they are struggling against governmental, economic, and societal reform to maintain the strength of this type of family system. More research is needed to evaluate challenges to families that choose to maintain the nuclear family structure.

EXTENDED FAMILY

Another more traditional family unit is the extended family. The **extended family** consists of several generations of the family, including the immediate nuclear family; grandparents; and other relatives such as aunts, uncles, and cousins. Although every nuclear family is part of an extended family unit, few nuclear families elect to live and share resources with members of their extended family. In the past, the rural and agrarian focus of society promoted, and often required, multigenerational families to cohabitate and share their resources. It was not uncommon for adult children, their spouses, and their children to live with their older parents. The family as a whole engaged in one common occupation, such as farming. Thus, family members of all age ranges lived and worked together, benefiting from the sharing of resources and responsibilities.

As society changed to a more mobile, industrialized focus, so, too, has the extended family separated and restructured into smaller family units. In some communities and cultural groups, cohabitation of extended family members continues to be highly valued. However, in many cases, the nuclear family forms its own household and members seek a living pursuing their own unique areas of interest, separate from extended family members. Many nuclear families continue to rely on members of their extended families as business partners, child care providers, and caregivers of the elderly (Fig. 1-4). In addition, extended family members enjoy

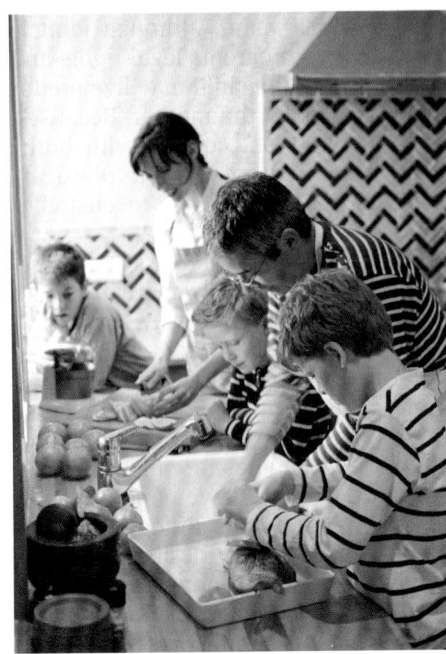

Figure 1-3 In dual-career families, both parents work and share family care duties.

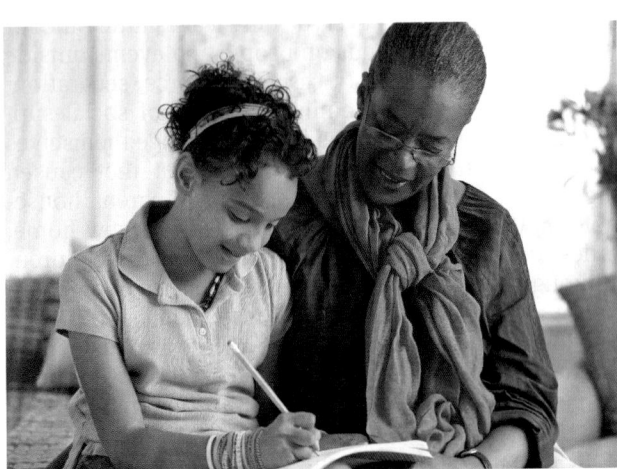

Figure 1-4 Grandparents may assume care of grandchildren to offer additional support to families.

socializing together and sharing special family events. In times of stress and crisis, extended family members are likely to offer many resources to support the family, even when long distances may separate the households.

ANSWER: When the Trans first arrived in the United States, they lived with Loan's parents and her sister. This is considered an extended family structure.

SINGLE-PARENT FAMILY

During the past three decades, one of the most dramatic changes in family configurations has been the shift toward more single-parent families or attenuated families. Single parenting occurs when one parent manages the affairs of a family without a partner. Often, a single-parent family is formed when the nuclear family unit dissolves through divorce, separation, abandonment, or death of a spouse. A shift from two-parent to one-parent families has also been noted as a result of several demographic trends, including increased proportion of births to unmarried women who conceive either by natural or medically supported methods (e.g., in vitro fertilization), delay of marriage increasing the likelihood of a nonmarital birth, single persons agreeing to raise another family member's child, and a loosening of legal restraints on adoption by single parents (U.S. Census Bureau, 2011b).

The single-parent family is likely to encounter several challenges because of economic, social, and personal restraints. Economically, single-parent families often have to adjust to a lower level of income. Divorced single mothers typically have financial and social advantages over never-married single mothers because, as a population, they are typically older, have more education, have higher incomes, and may have an economic source from their ex-spouse to aide in child-rearing expenses (U.S. Census Bureau, 2011c).

Sources of social support for the single-parent family may also be lacking. The single parent may find it difficult to maintain social relationships as a result of time and economic restraints. Balancing the family, the job, and the details of everyday life leaves little time for the single parent to focus on people and events outside the home. In addition, in cases of divorce, separation, or spousal death, the family's network of social support may erode as previous friends distance themselves from the restructured family. The event that caused the family to restructure into a single-parent household may also lead to the family seeking a new home, a new community, and a new school for the children. Although the single parent may feel a sense of independence and renewal in making these changes, the child may be overwhelmed by a sense of loss and instability.

The personal or emotional challenges of a single-parent household affect both child and parent. For instance, in the case of divorce or parental separation, a major shift in family dynamics may occur as the family becomes oriented to a single parent serving as the sole (or primary) authority and provider. If the single parent brings a new partner into the home, other relational adjustments must be made. Children from single-mother households are at increased risk for difficulties, including social impairment, psychiatric problems, and low math scores in school. Single-mother families also have higher rates of family dysfunction, maternal depression, and lower social support (Lipman et al., 2002).

Single parents are called on to provide most of the emotional support and sustenance for their children. There may be few volunteers to give the parent a break from the stream of decisions or to serve as the disciplinarian, chauffeur, or cook. The single parent may have to overcome feelings of inadequacy, guilt, anxiety, grief, or loneliness that accompany any major life event, loss, or transition. In some cases, the single-parent family must accomplish most of the same developmental tasks as two-parent families but without all the resources. For some single parents, extended family members provide an essential support structure to assist in child care, transportation for weekly activities, and ongoing emotional support.

To serve the single-parent family better, specific family concerns can be addressed by demonstrating a sense of empathy, giving credence to the family's problems, and providing specific strategies for intervening therapeutically when necessary (Nursing Interventions 1-2).

BINUCLEAR FAMILY

Ahrons and Rodgers (1987) coined the term **binuclear family** to refer to the familial structure of joint custody families. Coparenting, or the binuclear family, occurs when the child is a member of two families, after remarriage of one or both parents. The responsibility of raising and parenting the child is still considered a joint venture between the two families. Joint physical custody gives both parents legal rights and responsibilities while granting the children equal time with both parents. On the other hand, although joint legal custody can also give both parents legal rights and responsibilities for the child, the child may live predominantly with one parent, usually the mother. Because the child can benefit from frequent contact with both parents, the judicial courts recognize joint physical custody arrangements as a good answer to custody disputes (Table 1-2).

Research has shown that a father's continued involvement with his children is associated with a positive outcome for the children (Allen & Daly, 2007; U.S. Department of Health & Human Services, 2006). Research also indicates that marital conflict is a more important predictor of child adjustment than the divorce itself or the parental conflict that may exist after the divorce. In other words, children in homes in which there is parental conflict are more likely to have conduct disorders, antisocial behavior, depression, difficulty with peers, and academic problems. Children of divorced families have been shown to experience more adjustment and academic problems than children in never-divorced families. However, if parental conflict is ongoing in the home, this, too, can negatively affect the child's adjustment (U.S. Department of Health & Human Services, 2006).

NURSING INTERVENTIONS 1-2

Concerns and Interventions for the Single-Parent Family

Concern	Nursing Interventions
Parent feels helpless and overwhelmed	Encourage parent to • Work through his or her own emotions • Practice good health habits • Keep in touch with family members and friends • Socialize with other adults
The single parent feels uncertain regarding parenting and child management practices	Provide parent with information regarding normal growth and development and predictable effects of divorce or death on children.
Child exhibits behavioral problems	Teach parent to provide consistent discipline. Encourage parent to allow children to express their concerns regarding the change in the family.
Child takes on a parent helper role	Determine whether the child is still able to have his or her needs met.
Child becomes the parent's companion and confidante	Encourage the parent to seek other sources of emotional support.
Issues related to the absent parent	Openly discuss issues regarding the absent parent with all family members.
Introduction of a new adult into the household	Assist the parent to prepare the child ahead of time for the entry of a new family member. Discourage the parent from casually and frequently having partners of the opposite sex stay the night or move in. Assist family members to define clearly the roles and responsibilities the new adult will have in the household and in regard to child rearing.
Making ends meet	Encourage the parent to record income and expenses and keep a budget. Encourage the parent to plan shopping trips, using lists to avoid purchasing nonessential items.
Managing home responsibilities	Encourage the parent to teach the children to do many tasks on their own. Assist family members to list and divide housework with an assignment for each family member.

TABLE 1-2   Joint Custody: Pros and Cons

Pros	Cons
• Maintains parent–child relationships • Increases the likelihood child support will be paid • Gives parents a sense of involvement with children; maintains active participation in the parental role • Allows continued involvement of extended family members such as grandparents, aunts, and uncles • Decreases the load of the single parent, resulting in higher quality parenting	• Expects parents who cannot agree during the marriage to make joint decisions after the divorce • Has physical impact on the child who must move from one parent's house to the other parent's house on a daily or weekly basis • May require parents to reside within the same community • Children may be involved in lengthy judicial processes to acquire joint custody

Children in joint custody relationships have been shown to have fewer adjustment problems than those where only one parent has legal custody of the child (Bauserman, 2002).

BLENDED FAMILY

With the growing rate of divorce and remarriage, more and more children are either part of or know someone who is in a stepfamily. A remarried family consists of a husband and wife maintaining a household, with or without children in the home, and one or both of the spouses have previously been in a marital relationship. The **blended family** or stepfamily is a remarried family with a child younger than 18 years of age who is the biologic child of one of the parents and was born before the remarriage.

The transitions that accompany remarriage and the formation of the stepfamily present a variety of stressors for the parents and children involved. Schnitzer and Ewigman (2008) reported that young children living in homes with step or foster parents were at increased risk of fatal unintentional injury related to maltreatment. Even in the most adaptive of families, several developmental issues must be addressed and resolved if the stepfamily is to create its own new identity (Table 1-3). The time it takes to create a new sense of family varies for each family system and is almost always longer than the adults expect. For young children and preschoolers, this process takes at least 18 to 24 months; with older children, it may take as long as 5 to 7 years (Goldenberg & Goldenberg, 2008; Pryor, 2008).

The concerns of the children and adults involved may emerge in several different ways (Developmental Considerations 1-1). In addition to the stress of a new marital relationship, the step-parent often experiences difficulties with parenting of stepchildren, adjusting to the children's personalities and habits, and gaining acceptance (Goldenberg & Goldenberg, 2008; Pryor, 2008). Other stresses experienced by step-parents include relationships with former spouses, adjustment to the new roles of step-parents, and unrealistic expectations in the transition to the new role. This transition is also stressful for the children. Children often react to remarriage by experiencing feelings of anger, anxiety, and depression. Children may also respond to a blended family with a deeper sense of happiness and security. If the previous home environment was affected by a high level of marital discord, changing to a more harmonious family environment may assist in reducing stress for the child. In addition, the blended home may create a more secure financial environment for the child (Pryor, 2008).

GAY OR LESBIAN FAMILY

The gay or lesbian family is another nontraditional family that is becoming more prevalent (Nursing Interventions 1-3). The gay or lesbian family can include committed relationships with same-sex partners, a single lesbian or gay adult rearing a child, and extended families involving several close homosexual and/or heterosexual friends. Many gay and lesbian couples choose to formalize their relationship with some type

TABLE 1-3 Developmental Issues in Remarried Families	
Primary Concerns	**Developmental Issues**
Entering the New Relationship	
• Recovery from loss of first marriage (adequate "emotional divorce")	• Recommitment to marriage and to forming a family with readiness to deal with the complexity and ambiguity
Conceptualizing and Planning a New Marriage and Family	
• Accepting one's own fears and those of new spouse and children about remarriage and forming a stepfamily • Accepting need for time and patience for adjustment to complexity and ambiguity of multiple new roles • Boundaries: space, time, membership, and authority • Affective issues: guilt, loyalty conflicts, desire for mutuality, unresolvable past hurts	• Work on openness in the new relationships to avoid pseudomutuality • Plan for maintenance of cooperative coparental relationships with ex-spouses • Plan to help children deal with fears, loyalty conflicts, and membership in two systems • Realignment of relationships with extended family to include new spouse and children • Plan maintenance of connections for children with extended family of ex-spouse(s)
Remarriage and Reconstitution of Family	
• Final resolution of attachment to previous spouse and ideal of "intact" family • Acceptance of a different model of family with permeable boundaries	• Restructuring family boundaries to allow for inclusion of new spouse–step-parent • Realignment of relationships throughout subsystems to permit interweaving of several systems • Making room for relationships of all children with biologic (noncustodial) parents and other extended family • Sharing memories and histories to enhance stepfamily integration

Adapted from McGoldrick, M., & Carter, E. (1982). The family cycle. In F. Walsh (Ed.), *Normal family processes* (p. 192). New York, NY: Guilford Press; McGoldrick, M., & Carter, E. (2003). The family cycle. In F. Walsh (Ed.), *Normal family processes* (pp. 375–398). New York, NY: Guilford Press.

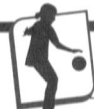

DEVELOPMENTAL CONSIDERATIONS 1-1

Child's Response to Divorce and Stepfamily

	Responses	Health Care Interventions
Early childhood	• Clinging to parents • Regressive behaviors such as thumb-sucking and bed-wetting • Belief that their angry thoughts or behaviors led to family disruption (magical thinking) • Belief that they can magically reunite the family	• Reassure children that they are not responsible for the dissolution of their parents' marriage. • Include children in family discussions using simple terms. • Praise children for age-appropriate behaviors. • Read age-appropriate books to children about stepfamily situations.
Middle childhood	• Anger about their powerlessness to stop dissolution of the family • Imagining that they caused the marital breakup • Wishing their parents were together and fantasizing that if they are "good," "bad," or "sick," the parents will come together to help • Acting out anger and guilt by having tantrums, fighting with siblings or classmates, developing psychosomatic symptoms, becoming accident prone, failing in schoolwork, or trying to break up the new marriage • Acting "angelic" and, in doing so, hiding their true feelings	• Accept the children's feelings. • Do not force the children to understand the perspective of adults. • Reassure the children they are not responsible for the dissolution of their parents' marriage. Encourage the children to communicate with parents and step-parents. • Help the children put feelings into words rather than negative behaviors.
Adolescence	• Sexual tensions such as trying to deal with their own identity and sexuality in the presence of step-siblings or a step-parent of the opposite sex • Loss of status of being "in charge" as they make way for the new head of the household • Acting out in a negative way toward the step-parent as a result of divided loyalties • Angered by step-parent who does not view them as mature • Reluctance to become part of the step-family because of the developmental drive for independence and autonomy	• Have the family adopt a dress code and make appropriate bedroom arrangements. • Allow adolescents to maintain their independence and integrate at their own pace. • Encourage step-parents to make clear to the adolescent that they are not a replacement for a deceased or absent parent. • Emphasize that the adolescent must act in a respectful, if not warm, manner toward the step-parent. • Encourage the adolescent to communicate with parents and step-parents.

(Continued)

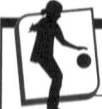

DEVELOPMENTAL CONSIDERATIONS 1-1

Child's Response to Divorce and Stepfamily (*Continued*)

	Responses	Health Care Interventions
Parents	• Conflict with new spouse with regard to loyalty to their own children, which predates loyalty to their new spouse • Inability to form solid bond with new spouse because to do so would seem like a betrayal to their relationship with their children • New spouse may feel like an outsider in an established household • Sense of failure and resentment when feelings of love do not happen immediately • Conflict regarding dissimilar parenting styles	• Listen to the parents' concerns. • Provide anticipatory guidance and direct parents to sources of information that provide realistic information about step-family life. • Reassure parents that a strong relationship with one another is not a betrayal of their biologic children. • Encourage the biologic parent to require respect from his or her children toward the new partner as these new relationships develop between the children. • Encourage the biologic parent to maintain or become the enforcer of rules for his or her children while the step-parent supports the biologic parent in the discipline process. • Encourage the formation of the "parenting coalition" for raising the children. This means that all parents and step-parents cooperate in the parenting experience. • Encourage the new spouse to accept that he or she does not have to try to be an "instant parent." • Recommend that the parents take a parenting course together. • Direct parents to support groups.

of ceremony and/or legal commitment. Legal sanction of same-sex marriages varies by state and country.

Increasing numbers of gay and lesbian adults are choosing to become parents. Gay men and lesbians can become parents in a variety of ways. Lesbians can have biologic children through insemination from a known or unknown donor or heterosexual intercourse. Gay men can have biologic children through the use of a surrogate mother. Gay and lesbian adults can also become parents through adoption, foster parenting, and coparenting. Because some gay men and lesbians have children from a previous heterosexual relationship, new homosexual relationships may result in blended or reconstituted families.

Contrary to common misconceptions, children of gay and lesbian parents do not differ from children of heterosexual parents in terms of psychological health and social relationships. Children raised by gay men and lesbians are no more likely to be gay or straight than those raised in heterosexual families (Goldenberg & Goldenberg, 2008). Studies have shown that children raised in two-parent homes, regardless of gender, are better adjusted than children raised in single-parent

homes (Grusec & Hastings, 2007). A common concern is that children of gay and lesbian families will experience the same prejudice that their parents have had to endure. Although prejudice may still occur, studies have found that children of lesbians and gay men are more aware of the diversity in our society and are better prepared to handle the ignorance and bias of homophobia.

COMMUNAL FAMILY

A **communal family** can be defined as any group of adults (with or without children), most of whom are unrelated by blood or marriage, who live together primarily for the sake of some ideologic goal for which a collective household is deemed essential (Aidala & Zablocki, 1991). Current financial burdens have spurred a recent resurgence in shared or communal living arrangements (Burris, 2009; Zaslow, 2002). Communal living came of age during the late 1960s, with many individuals joining during times of major social and cultural disjuncture. People join communes to be surrounded by individuals who share common beliefs and practices; in many cases, these are religious beliefs.

NURSING INTERVENTIONS 1-3

Working With Gay and Lesbian Families

- Examine your own attitudes and beliefs toward homosexuality and gay and lesbian parenting.
- Become better informed about the research and misconceptions regarding gay parenting.
- Be supportive of the diversity of family forms in today's society.
- *Ask questions such as, Whom do you include in your family? Who helps raise your child(ren)?*
- Convey acceptance through the use of gender-neutral terms such as parent or family member when gathering a family history.
- *Use terms such as* family member *or* significant other *rather than* husband *or* wife.
- Do not assume all parents are heterosexual. Do not assume that an absent parent is of a different gender.
- *Ask questions such as, Who else is in your household? Who else is taking care of your child? Do you have a significant other?*
- Use books, pamphlets, magazines, and posters in the health care setting that show a diversity of family structures.

- Acknowledge parents who are a couple, jointly parenting, and treat them as such. However, inquire about legal arrangements regarding medical consent.
- Ask parents whether they would like information about their family structure shared with other health care providers so that they do not have to reexplain their family arrangements continually.
- Provide anticipatory guidance to the parents regarding developmentally appropriate discussions with their child about his or her origin, concepts of a variety of loving relationships, sexuality, sexual behavior, and dealing with harassment and stigmatization.
- Become an advocate for change in social policy and attitudes. Homophobia can lead to decreased self-esteem in children of these functional, caring families.

Principles that guide communal living include collective ownership; the absence of private property accumulation by individual members; and the collective responsibility for all material, cultural, educational, and health needs of the family.

Some communal groups have been described as cults that adhere to a set of beliefs or standards that are viewed as deviant by the general society. A charismatic individual is often the source of governance for these communes. Interactions between commune members and outsiders are often discouraged. Thus, health care practices may be neglected or overlooked because commune members rely on internal resources to deal with illness and health promotion issues.

A polygamous family, also referred to as a *plural family,* is a form of the communal family. The polygamous family consists of one wife with multiple husbands and children or one husband with multiple wives and children. Among polygamous families, the latter configuration is predominant. In the United States and Canada, polygamy is prohibited. However, polygamy continues to be practiced in some areas of the world such as Africa and South Asia (among Muslims).

FAMILY FUNCTIONS

The basic unit in our society is the family. Friedman et al. (2003, p. 4) stated, "The purpose of the family is mediation. The family has to mediate the needs and demands of the family member with those of society." The family, then, is a medium for the transmission of societal values. From a developmental viewpoint, the primary function of the family is to support the development of its members by meeting basic needs, such as food and shelter; carrying out developmental tasks for individual growth and family growth through the life cycle; and adapting to hazardous events such as illness and death. From a systems point of view, the main function of family members is to support one another. Another viewpoint is that the family has several primary functions: to provide material support and supervision (e.g., food, clothing, shelter, safety, health care), to provide affective and cognitive support, to socialize children, and to provide education. From a structural–functional perspective, the family has affective, reproductive, economic, health care, and socialization functions (see Chart 1-4).

These functions not only meet the needs of the family but, in doing so, also meet the needs of the individual and the society. At times, the family may have difficulty performing some of these functions. For example, providing financially for the family is difficult when a primary wage earner is laid off from work. He or she might also have lost the family medical insurance, making it difficult to provide for adequate health care. When these challenges occur, it is important for the nurse to help the family identify additional resources to meet their functional needs.

FAMILY ROLES

Family roles and family functions are closely related. Roles are the set of behaviors of an occupant of a particular social position. The family determines the role each family member should play to carry out the functions of the family. Roles within the family can be formal or informal. Formal roles are those that must be fulfilled for the family to function smoothly. Parents take on many roles, such as providing the financial resources necessary for family needs (breadwinner), taking care of the home (homemaker), and raising the children. Similarly, children's roles might include taking care of siblings (babysitter) (Fig. 1-5), playing with siblings (playmate), and participating in school (student).

When family members are unable to fulfill their formal roles, other family members and friends need to take on these roles to keep the family functioning. This can lead to role overload for the family members and friends stepping in. For example, after a divorce, the single parent must take on all the roles previously shared with the second parent. In addition, the older child might have to add the responsibility of taking care of siblings while the single parent is working to fulfill the family's financial needs. In some cases, families choose to pay others to complete jobs that may previously have been a part of their responsibility in the home (e.g., housekeeper, daycare provider, gardener). Pediatric nurses need to assess the roles each family member plays to ensure that role overload does not occur and that the functions of the family are fulfilled. Referral to social work and community resources may provide the family with access to support for services such as transportation, child care, family counseling, and financial assistance.

Compared with formal roles, informal roles in the family are less explicit. Informal roles are the roles family members play to meet the emotional needs of the family and to help maintain the family's equilibrium. These roles change with the circumstances encountered by the family. Some informal roles include serving as the mediator between family members, providing comic relief, and helping family members compromise on an issue. Identification of the family members' informal roles can assist the pediatric nurse in assessing the coping mechanisms of the family. For instance, it is easy to assume that the family "jester" is unconcerned about a particular family issue, when in reality his or her light-hearted approach may mask emotional pain and serve as a method to help ease family tension during conflict.

HEALTHY FAMILY PROCESSES

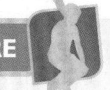 QUESTION: What areas would you need to assess to determine whether Tung and Loan Tran are engaging in healthy family interactions?

What makes a family a healthy family? What strengths, coping skills, or other characteristics are found in families that are able to adapt and reorganize when faced with the normal transitions and the unexpected transitions that accompany the family life cycle?

Many researchers believe that a healthy family starts with the quality of the relationship between family members. Healthy family processes are characterized by openness, fondness and admiration, a sense of togetherness, and resiliency in the face of chaos and stress. In the healthy family, honest differences can become opportunities to develop new understandings rather than sources of struggles and fights. The healthy family believes that family members are not adversaries; they are friends and collaborate together to meet each other's needs. Healthy families allow individuals to err or disagree without the threat of isolation. Healthy families believe that human encounters can usually be rewarding. Trust and cooperation with one another are key components of family interactions. The healthy family is optimistic and hopeful even when human situations are bad. Healthy families participate in and contribute to the community around them.

Olson (2003) has stated that healthy families are able to balance their level of togetherness versus separateness. Members are able to experience independence from the family while remaining connected to the family unit. The physical and emotional boundaries of the family allow for sharing of family space and time together. At the same time, private space is respected. Members are encouraged to participate in friendships outside the family and to share those friendships with the family.

CROSS-CULTURAL CARE

In some ethnic groups (e.g., Hispanic, Southeast Asian) or religious groups (e.g., Amish, Mormon), it may be expected that family members have a higher level of togetherness, and independence and separateness is discouraged. This should not be considered dysfunctional if all family members wish the family to be this way. Cultural beliefs are a central part of the family's character and must be considered when evaluating family dynamics.

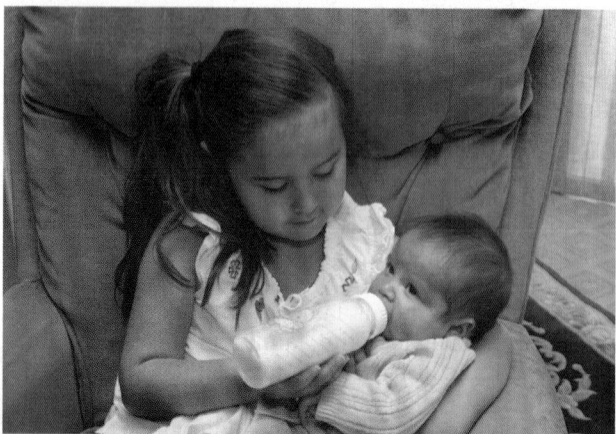

Figure 1-5 Siblings can play important roles in the family.

Olson (2003) further asserted that the healthy family has positive communication skills that help the family to balance their levels of flexibility and cohesion in the presence of situational stress or developmental change. Rules exist to guide expectations of family members, yet these rules can be changed when necessary to adapt to family stressors.

Healthy families are characterized by parents who have the knowledge, ability, and resources to adjust their child-rearing strategies and goals in view of the unique characteristics of the child, their own strengths and weaknesses as parents, and the social and familial context in which interactions take place. Parenting goals are clear and support the well-being and survival of the child. It has been noted that family rituals, characterized by routines and celebrations, are an integral part of a stable family. Routines are an important aspect of family life to consider when families encounter illness and hospitalizations that may disrupt the family's patterns.

caREminder

Encourage families to maintain and incorporate as many of their family rituals as possible into the new care routines they establish when a child may be ill or hospitalized for a lengthy period.

It is important for the nurse to recognize the characteristics of both healthy and dysfunctional families and to institute a plan of care that is based on the unique characteristics of each family. Crises related to changes in the health status of a family member will affect families in different ways. The healthy family is more likely to be adaptive to change, although still in need of resources (family, financial, social) to strengthen them as they adjust to situational and developmental stressors. Other families may need more support from the health care system, in the form of counseling and financial and community referrals, to establish a functional level of coping.

ANSWER: To determine whether the Trans are engaging in healthy family processes, you need to assess such characteristics as the degree of respect they hold for individual choice and autonomy, their negotiating skills, their ability to share positive feelings, and their ability to be resilient and adaptive to change even in their current stressful circumstances.

SPECIAL FAMILY ISSUES

The preceding sections provided an overview of typical family structures and roles. Within these family structures, issues may arise that alter family dynamics. A blended family may choose to adopt a child, a divorce may lead to custody of the children by the grandparents, or incarceration of a single parent may necessitate placing the children in foster care. The following section discusses selected family issues and their impact on the family system—namely, adoption, foster care, multiple births, divorce, grandparent families, adolescent parent families, and homeless families.

ADOPTION

Adoption is a means to provide a child with security and to meet the child's developmental needs by legally transferring ongoing parental responsibilities from the birth parents (or the state, if the child has no relations) to the adoptive parents. Through the adoption process, a new family system is created (Fig. 1-6). Emotional, social, and physical ties may, however, continue to bind the child to his or her biologic family. For example, even if adoption takes place during infancy and the birth parents choose to sever contact with the child, the child may wish to reopen relationships with the birth parents as he or she matures. The ties to the family of origin may never be severed completely.

Adults choose to become adoptive parents for many reasons. Traditionally, adoptive parents are couples who are unable to conceive their own biologic children but still wish to raise a child. Adoption also occurs when couples decide to add children to their family for a variety of religious, moral, or personal reasons independent of fertility. Declining social and legal barriers to single-parent adoption and gay and lesbian partner adoptions have also led to an increase in the number of unmarried women and men choosing adoption as a way to start their family.

Domestically, there has been a decline in the number of infants available for adoption as a result of contraception, declining pregnancy rates, abortion, and more single women (including teenagers) keeping and raising their children (Adoption Statistics, 2005). There has been an increase in the number of children with special needs available for adoption as a result of parental abuse (including prenatal substance abuse), neglect, and abandonment or as a result of parental death. Special needs children also include certain minorities, children older than 6 years of age, children with chronic illnesses or psychological problems, and children who must be adopted with a sibling. Families considering adopting a special needs child must spend time critically evaluating their resources and ability to meet the challenges of these special children. Many families assess that they have both financial and personal resources to support the child with special needs and actively pursue adoption of children who can benefit from their loving home environment.

An increasing number of American families are selecting to adopt children from foreign countries. Since 2005, the top five countries from which children were adopted internationally were China, Ethiopia, Russia, South Korea, and Guatemala (U.S. Department of State, 2011). Children adopted from overseas often come from high-risk backgrounds and locations where they have lived under conditions unlike those found in the United States. Recognizing the special needs of the child who is adopted internationally, health care providers should assist prospective parents in preparing for the challenges associated with integrating that child into the family (Chart 1-5) (Smit, 2010).

The transition to parenthood for the adoptive parent(s) does not come without its share of challenges. For instance, the unanticipated crisis of infertility places

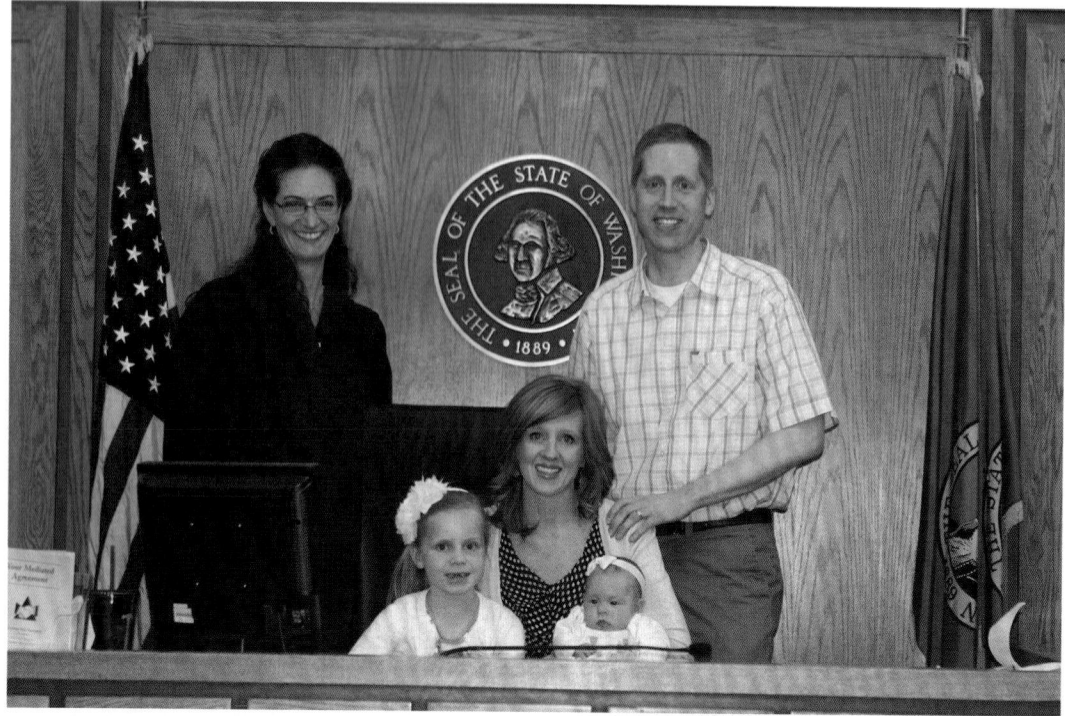

Figure 1-6 This family included the older sibling in the final court session to grant adoption approval for her new baby sister.

CHART 1-5   Issues Related to International Adoptions

Issues

- Child comes from high-risk background where poverty is common and there is limited access to prenatal care.
- Child lived in an institution (baby home, hospital, or orphanage) prior to adoption.
- Child lacked nutritional food, shelter, clothing, and health care.
- Child presents with behavioral abnormalities, attachment difficulties, conduct disorder, or either extremely aggressive or extremely passive behaviors.
- Child presents with developmental delays.
- Child is easily overwhelmed by new environment.
- Child lacked a consistent caregiver.
- Child experiences difficulty forming attachments.

Strategies to Support the Child and His or Her Adoptive Family

- Preadoptive consultations with an international adoption specialist can help ascertain whether the referred child is one the family feels adequate to parent.
- Complete physical, developmental, and emotional evaluation to determine areas of concern
- Screening the child for infectious diseases acquired in the country of origin (e.g., tuberculosis, hepatitis B, HIV, hepatitis C, syphilis, and gastrointestinal pathogens) and specific

diseases not previously screened (e.g., phenylketonuria and sickle cell anemia). Previous screenings should not be considered reliable.

- Review of immunization records. If documentation is lacking, the child should be considered unimmunized and receive the full series of immunizations.
- Completing developmental testing to compare chronologic age-appropriate norms with the child's abilities
- Seeking comprehensive health care support for behavioral issues that arise
- Adjust parenting expectations to the child's developmental, rather than chronologic, age
- Providing remedial activities specific to the delay
- Expecting that some delays may not be reversible and may indicate a lifelong physical or cognitive impairment
- Minimizing contact with friends and family until the child has an increased level of comfort with the parents
- Minimizing sensory overload and providing opportunities to gradually master new sights, sounds, smells, and textures
- Spending time with the child, teaching them how to play
- Ensuring parents serve as a consistent and reliable source of giving and receiving of affection
- Providing opportunities for the child to develop a balance between a sense of independence and reliance

the couple and the individuals at risk for psychological problems. Infertile couples often describe feelings of guilt, unworthiness, decreased self-esteem, depression, decreased marital sexual relations, and marital discord (Cousineau & Domar, 2007; Deka & Sarma, 2010). Successful transition to adoptive parenthood requires the couple to mourn and resolve issues related to their infertility. Single people who adopt may feel they must constantly justify to others why they chose adoption and why they feel secure in the knowledge that they can provide a supportive environment for raising a child.

Although the overall adoption process can be quite long, the suddenness of learning that a child is available for adoption and the quick transition to bringing that child home may not allow the parent-to-be much time to prepare emotionally or physically for the actual presence of the wished-for child. After the adoption, parents may have idealized expectations about the child's behavior that are not realized. For example, the child may not be as compliant as the parent had anticipated. If information about the birth parents was unclear and contact with the birth parents is not possible (e.g., in a *closed adoption*), adoptive parents may worry about genetic and hereditary traits that may emerge in the child. In an *open adoption*, birth parents and adoptive parents maintain a degree of ongoing communication. The adoptive parents may initially perceive the openness as a threat to their skills and confidence in establishing a new family structure.

A particular challenge to the adoptive parents is how the child, and how outsiders, may react to the adoption. The "adoptee's" understanding of the adoption changes as the child develops (Developmental Considerations 1-2). As they mature, children should be given every opportunity to learn more about their biologic parents if this is their desire. Children who avoid talking about or thinking about adoptive issues are at risk for emotional problems and identity confusion (Singer, 2010). Parents are encouraged to answer questions honestly and to consider the child's age and level of comprehension when answering questions. As children grow, it is natural for them to want to hear their adoption story and to learn more about their birth parents.

People outside the immediate family may express curiosity about the adoption simply because the child looks different from the adoptive parents. In answering these queries, it is important to respect the child's right to privacy regarding the details of the adoption and the birth parents (Singer, 2010).

It is important for the nurse to be aware of these potential concerns and to help the family focus on its strengths and resources during the transition period of the adoption process. Parenting classes specifically for adoptive parents can assist the family in adjusting to their new roles. These classes should cover the physical aspects of child care and the emotional aspects of adoption while allowing time for sharing so that adoptive parents can gain support and insights from one another. In addition, after the child has joined the family, a comprehensive medical evaluation should be completed to identify medical needs. This type of evaluation can help identify acute and chronic medical problems, vision and hearing loss, developmental delays, and behavioral and emotional concerns (Singer, 2010).

FOSTER CARE

Foster care, also known as *home care*, is a child welfare service in which children are placed in homes away from their parents in an effort to ensure their emotional and physical well-being. The foster placement system exists to protect children who are abused, neglected, or abandoned, or whose parents or primary caregivers are unable to fulfill their parenting obligations because of illness, emotional problems, or a host of other reasons. The placement into foster care by parents may have been voluntary. In many cases, children are reunited with their parents when the family has demonstrated that interventions to improve the individual, home, or family problems have been instituted. The child in foster care may be placed with relatives, in **kinship care** (care by family relatives), in nonrelative family foster care, or in residential group care (Children's Bureau, 2012). Foster parents receive training prior to the placement of children in their home, with additional training given if the placement will be for special needs children.

Children placed in foster care often enter the new living situation at risk for emotional, developmental, physical, and behavioral problems (Jee et al., 2010; Leve et al., 2012). Several factors contribute to the increased number of problems that foster children may experience. The interplay of factors that led the child to foster care placement is a key issue to consider. The child may have come from an abusive home situation or may have been considered to have such severe behavioral problems that the parents felt incapable of caring for the child. Children placed in foster care may have medical problems. Ideally, the child should have a medical exam within 24 to 48 hours of removal from the home. Comprehensive medical, dental, and visual examinations are recommended within 30 days. These examinations should include a mental health evaluation, developmental testing, and an educational assessment (Botash, 2012). Ongoing monitoring of the child should be conducted every 6 months during the first year of placement and yearly thereafter.

ALERT   *Children in foster care have a disproportionately higher incidence of pediatric acute and chronic conditions. Careful evaluation is needed to determine whether the child has been receiving regular and ongoing treatment for these conditions. It is not uncommon for children to arrive in protective care services without their inhalers or medications for such conditions as seizures and attention-deficit/hyperactivity disorder (ADHD).*

The foster child may experience difficulties related to the transitions from one home or placement setting to another. It may not be easy for the child to establish a trusting relationship with foster caregivers. The child must learn to be

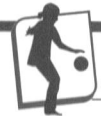

DEVELOPMENTAL CONSIDERATIONS 1-2

Issues Related to Adoption

Age	Issues	Family Interventions
Infancy	• Separation from interim caregivers and introduction of new adult caregivers • Disruption of care routines	• If possible, the adoptive family should take a parental leave from work to become acquainted with the child. • Provide as much consistency as possible regarding who will be caring for the child (including daycare providers and babysitters). • Follow infant's previous caregiving routines as much as possible, introducing changes as tolerated by the child. • Allow the infant to keep treasured security objects such as a blanket or stuffed animal.
Early childhood	• "Where did I come from?" • Generally accepting of being adopted • Want reassurance that they are loved • Introduction into a new home	• Tell the child he or she is adopted. • Use books to discuss adoption. • Use the family photo album to depict the child's story of adoption. • Answer questions about the child's birth parents honestly, yet in very simple, positive terms. • Establish behavioral expectations for the child and family routines as soon as possible to help the child define his or her new boundaries.
Middle childhood	• "Why was I adopted when most people are not?" • Worried that their value as a person is less because they are adopted • Aware that they have lost someone who played an extremely important role in their life • Imagine birth parents as rich, famous, and more attractive than adoptive parents • Adoptive parents may view child's questions about birth parents as a rejection of them • Concerns about being different from adoptive family	• Review the child's adoption story with him or her. • Assure the child that he or she is a loved and welcome member of the family. • Share letters and pictures of the birth parents with the child, if desired. • Reveal who the birth parents are, if desired. • The health care provider can reassure parents that the child's questioning is part of the normal development sequence. • Openly acknowledge any racial difference between the child and the adoptive parents. Assist adopted children to learn more about the country of their birth and their ethnic heritage.
Adolescence	• Task of developing an identity and discovering how they are different and how they are connected to "their" family • Concerns about physical appearance, traits, and family illnesses of their birth family • Interest in meeting parents • May have idealized picture of birth parents	• Give the child more information about his or her birth parents if it is available. • Provide the child with pictures and information about traits and family illnesses if possible. • Allow the adolescent to meet his or her birth parents. • If the identity of birth parents is unknown, encourage the adolescent to wait until young adulthood to begin a search for his or her parents.

flexible and to adjust to new standards for discipline and "house rules." The child may be placed in a new school where it takes time for teachers to address any special educational needs. Health care may be discontinuous because foster children often have frequent changes in primary care providers. Abuse and neglect can occur in the foster care setting. Each of these conditions is an issue that may negatively affect the foster child's health and well-being.

Foster care is intended to serve as a therapeutic and healing intervention to assist children and families in crisis. Nurses are in a position to support the positive adaptation of the child and the promotion of the child's general health and welfare. Every effort should be made to provide consistent health care, or a medical home, to the child to avoid discontinuation of necessary services and exacerbation of chronic problems (see thePoint for Supplemental Information). The nurse should be attuned to problems voiced by the child or the foster parents with regard to the foster care experience. Appropriate referrals can be made if the foster parents are not equipped to manage serious problems. Physical and behavioral markers of child maltreatment should be assessed, with appropriate interventions to remove the child from the foster

care setting if justified. The health care professional can serve as an advocate for the child in foster care, assisting in monitoring behavioral problems and general health concerns and determining the child's ability to meet developmental norms. In addition, between the ages of 18 and 21 years, adolescents "age out" of foster care and are expected to transition to independence. Lack of financial resources, poor access to health care, and few stable family connections may place these adolescents at risk for poor physical and mental health, unemployment, potential poverty status, homelessness, and incarceration. It is essential for the health care team to identify and assess the needs of these youths and to implement an individualized transition plan, with referrals, to ensure that ongoing physical, emotional, and financial needs are met (Botash, 2012; Lopez & Allen, 2007).

MULTIPLE BIRTHS

Seeing a family with twins, triplets, or even quadruplets can cause a great deal of interest among casual observers. Strangers sometimes stop the family to ask questions about the children's personalities and the parents' ability to tell their children apart (Fig. 1-7). Multiple

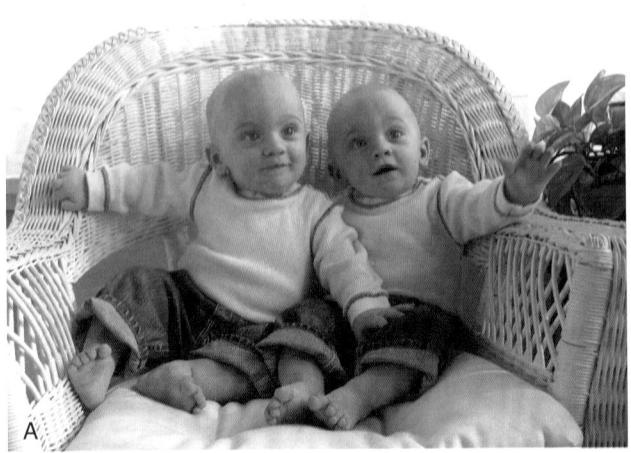
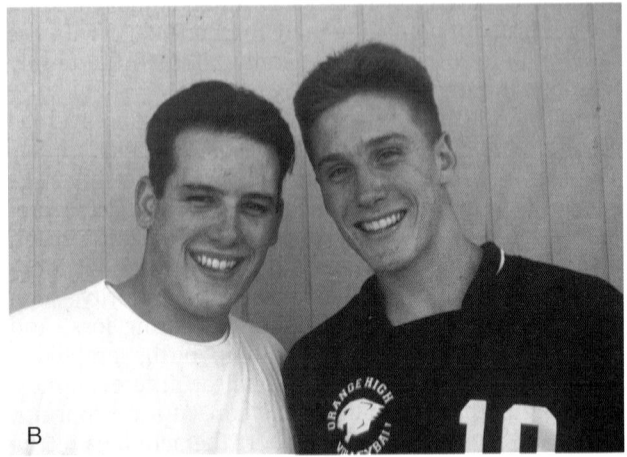

Figure 1-7 (A and B) Identical versus fraternal: characteristics of twins.

Identical Twins	Fraternal Twins
Monozygotic (Mz)	Dizygotic (Dz)
Fertilization of single ovum by single spermatozoa	Fertilization of two separate ova by two separate spermatozoa (possibly not from the same sexual partner)
Same implantation site, one placenta, one chorion, two amnions	Separate implantation site, two placentas, two chorions, two amnions (placentas have been known to fuse)
Same gender	Same or different gender
Same genetic blueprint and physical characteristics	Different genetic blueprint and physical characteristics
High similarity in behaviors that are governed by heredity	Lower rate of similarity for behaviors influenced by heredity
30% of twin births	70% of twin births
Tendency not influenced by familial patterns, maternal age, parity, or ethnicity; may be some relation to therapy for infertility	Tendency affected by familial maternal pattern of inheritance, advanced maternal age, increased parity, more frequent in blacks, increased levels of follicle-stimulating hormone and luteinizing hormone, pregnancy within 1 month of stopping oral contraceptive use, use of infertility drugs (clomiphene citrate and Pergonal), and in vitro fertilization

births such as twins, triplets, quadruplets, and quintuplets may be the result of one zygote (identical), several zygotes (fraternal), or a combination thereof (some of the children are identical and some are fraternal). In the United States, approximately 3% of babies in this country are born in sets of two, three, or more (March of Dimes Foundation, 2012).

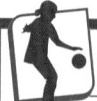

CROSS-CULTURAL CARE

The incidence of dizygotic (fraternal) twins is positively influenced by ethnicity and socioeconomic class. Dizygotic twins are more likely to occur in the African American population and are least likely to occur in the Asian population (Fletcher & Rosencrantz, 2012).

All childbearing families experience similar developmental tasks. For instance, the new infant must be integrated into the family, parents must learn new skills and reallocate tasks, grandparents must adapt to a new role, and parents must nurture and maintain their bonds of intimacy in a new context. For the parents of multiple children, these tasks are often complicated by the necessity of managing more than one child with the same amount of support generally afforded the family with one infant.

Multiple births are frequently preterm. The average gestation time for twin pregnancies is 37 weeks, triplets average 33 weeks' gestation, and quadruplets average 28 weeks (Fletcher & Rosencrantz, 2012). These preterm infants may require lengthy hospitalizations and medical treatment. They are also at high risk for long-term complications related to their prematurity, such as intellectual disability, vision and hearing loss, and cerebral palsy. Siblings in multiple births are likely to be discharged from the hospital at different times, requiring parents to manage the care of a newborn at home and to monitor and support the activities of the remaining hospitalized infant(s).

The family of multiples can expect to undergo many lifestyle changes and have many concerns related to the care of their children (Developmental Considerations 1-3). The mother of multiples is generally homebound after the birth for a longer period of time than a mother who delivered one child. Living space—including size of the car, bedroom, and play areas—and storage places for child-related supplies and equipment are often found to be inadequate. The physical and emotional energy to support the marital relationship and the relationship with older siblings can also be tested.

Equally challenging for the parents of multiples is the task of developing an attachment to and relationship with each child as a unique personality. To promote individuation, parents are encouraged to select different-sounding names for the children and to use individual names when referring to them. The children should not be dressed alike all the time and, as they grow, should be encouraged to select clothes that reflect their personalities. Parents are encouraged to

DEVELOPMENTAL CONSIDERATIONS 1-3

Concerns of Parents With Multiples

Infancy
- Efficient organization of household responsibilities
- Time management skills
- Obtaining, maintaining, and storing a stock of baby equipment and supplies (cribs, high chairs, diapers, wipes, formula, baby food)
- Ability to breastfeed or bottle-feed babies simultaneously
- Developing same feeding and sleep schedule for all infants
- Ability to respond to babies as separate individuals

Early Childhood
- Delays of verbal and motor skills
- Providing adult stimulation
- Providing activities separate from other siblings
- Providing discipline and praise in a consistent and fair manner based on each child's behavior
- Comparing one child with another in terms of behavior
- Higher incidence of delayed toilet training

Middle Childhood and Adolescence
- Entry into school and separation into different classrooms
- Individualizing educational process to meet each child's learning needs
- Discouraging excessive comparisons by teachers and peers
- Promoting independent goals, activities, and peer relationships

Ongoing
- Stress management
- Financial concerns
- Neglecting sibling needs
- Parental self-care needs and personal time
- Parental relations
- Frequent transmission of childhood illnesses among siblings
- Treatment of complications resulting from preterm birth

spend quality time with each child separately. Praise and discipline should be merited individually. Siblings should be encouraged to develop their own toy preferences, friendships, special activities, and hobbies. Others who come into contact with the children should be encouraged to treat them as individuals and expect them to think and behave differently. Several organizations, newsletters, and computer resources are available to connect these special families with others facing the same circumstances (see thePoint for Organizations).

DIVORCE

Most children do not want their parents to get a divorce. Nevertheless, many marriages end in divorce and most of those marriages involve children. In 2011, more than 11% of men and 13.5% of women older than 15 years of age were either divorced or separated (U.S. Census Bureau, 2011a). This is an increase from 3.5% of males and 5.7% of females in the same age population in 1970. The steady increase in the divorce rate has affected parents of all age groups, particularly young adults. Many families involved in a divorce have children in the infant and young child age groups. Today, more than half of school-aged children will have spent a substantial part of their youth living in a single-parent family or a stepfamily (Sandas & Siegel, 2012). Because the incidence of divorce is higher in second marriages, children who have coped with one divorce are at risk for experiencing the crisis of divorce a second time. An increasing number of divorced parents are now choosing to cohabitate with someone, forming unmarried partner households.

When divorce occurs, families must go through additional phases in the family life cycle to restabilize and address developmental concerns (McGoldrick & Carter, 2003) (Table 1-4). The frequency with which divorce occurs has forced family theorists to reevaluate the application of the family life cycle model. The impact of divorce affects families differently depending on the stage of the family life cycle at the time of the divorce and on other factors such as culture, religion, and support structures. For instance, if divorce occurs after the children have reached adulthood and left the home, issues regarding custodial arrangements and the economic consequences of the divorce for the children do not need to be discussed.

The impact of divorce also affects children differently depending on their developmental age, gender, and the degree of conflict between the parents (Developmental Considerations 1-4). It has been found that most children experience a period of emotional distress after the divorce. Many children do not receive clear communication about parental separation and thus feel confused and hurt by the changes in their family (Lansford, 2009). Studies have indicated that children from divorced families experience a higher degree of emotional distress, inability to commit to relationships, and greater acting-out behaviors and academic failure during adolescence. Parenting practices during the postdivorce period may be affected by a disproportionate increase in the number of stressors and strains related to residential relocation, economic hardship, changes in employment, and changes in school for the children (Lansford, 2009). Nursing interventions with families who are experiencing a divorce are aimed at helping the family move through each phase of the divorced family's life cycle,

TABLE 1-4   The Family Life Cycle When Divorce Occurs

Stage	Emotional Process of Transition	Developmental Issues
Divorce		
Deciding to divorce	• Accepting inability to resolve marital tensions sufficiently to continue relationship	• Accepting one's own part in the failure of the marriage
Planning the breakup of the system	• Supporting viable arrangements for all parts of the system	• Working cooperatively on problems of custody, visitation, and finances • Dealing with extended family about the divorce
Separation	• Being willing to sustain a cooperative coparental relationship and joint financial support of children • Working on resolution of attachment to spouse	• Mourning loss of nuclear family • Restructuring marital and parent–child relationships and finances; adapting to living apart • Realigning relationships with extended family; staying connected with spouse's extended family
Divorce	• Continuing to work on emotional divorce: overcoming hurt, anger, guilt, and so forth	• Retrieving hopes, dreams, and expectations from the marriage
Postdivorce		
Single-parent (custodial household or primary residence)	• Being willing to maintain financial responsibilities, continue parental contact with ex-spouse, and support contact of children with ex-spouse and his or her family	• Making flexible visitation arrangements with ex-spouse and his or her family • Rebuilding own financial resources • Rebuilding own social network
Single-parent (noncustodial)	• Being willing to maintain parental contact with ex-spouse and support custodial parent's relationship with children	• Finding ways to continue effective parenting relationship with children • Maintaining financial responsibilities to ex-spouse and children • Rebuilding own social network

From McGoldrick, M., & Carter, E. (2003). The family cycle. In F. Walsh (Ed.), *Normal family processes* (p. 192). New York, NY: Guilford Press. Reprinted with permission.

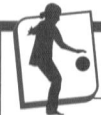

DEVELOPMENTAL CONSIDERATIONS 1-4

Impact of Divorce on the Child

Erikson's Developmental State	Family Reactions	Nursing Interventions
Trust versus mistrust in infants younger than 1 year of age	• Little impact unless infant's basic needs are not being met	• Encourage consistency in caregiving: feeding, bathing, comforting. • Encourage frequent contact of absent parent to establish bonding.
Autonomy versus shame and doubt in children 1–3 years old	• Self-blame for the divorce • Regressive behaviors • Sleep disturbances • Anger	• Educate parents on regression as a normal response to stress in this age group. • Have parents confer and agree how to handle disciplinary issues.
Initiative versus guilt in children 3–6 years old	• Self-blame for the divorce • Aggressive fantasies • Regressive behavior • Sleep disturbances • Tantrums • Bowel and bladder difficulties • Clinging • Fears of abandonment	• Encourage consistency and stability in the new family form. • Encourage new schedule or routine for daily activities and visitation. • Develop consistent patterns of joining and separating from the child. • Continue contact with noncustodial parent. • If contact with noncustodial parent is unavailable, encourage contact with grandparent or other relative. • Encourage consistent disciplinary actions.
Industry versus inferiority in children 6–12 years old	• Responsibility for divorce • Fantasies about parental reconciliation • Sadness • Fearfulness • Loyalty conflicts • Declining school performance • Depression • Anger toward one or both parents	• Provide regular opportunities for children to talk about their feelings. • Avoid blaming and speaking in a derogatory manner about either parent (children will want to choose sides). • Support children's continuing relationship with both parents. • Offer reassurance. • Empathize with children's feelings.
Identity versus role confusion in children 12–18 years old	• Engagement in self-destructive behavior: substance abuse, truancy, sexual promiscuity, eating disorders, suicide • Declining school performance • Feeling of responsibility for taking care of and nurturing their parents • Depression • Anger • Sleeper effects (seems to have no impact on the child until later events bring out true feelings), especially in females • Worries about own future • Questioning of ability to maintain relationships • Vulnerability regarding gender identity as a result of the absence of the same-sex parent	• Avoid seeking companionship from adolescents. • Provide opportunities for open discussion. • Offer appropriate support, including other family members, friends, church groups, and peer support groups. • Encourage involvement in classes that teach alternative ways to handle disagreements and to manage anger. • Encourage noncustodial parent to engage in activities with adolescents (e.g., "boys' time together"). • If noncustodial parent is not available, seek out another same-sex family member or adult friend to spend time with the adolescent.

helping parents build on the preexisting strengths and support systems, and finding ways to minimize the impact of the divorce on the children as much as possible.

Nurses in schools, clinics, and hospital settings frequently come in to contact with children who are struggling with the emotional fallout of their parents' divorce. Withdrawal, depression, somatic complaints, poor academic achievement, and destructive behaviors are but a few of the responses the nurse may encounter in working with children of divorce. The health care team can serve as an advocate for the child, rallying support systems in the school, the community, and the child's home to provide mechanisms for the child to adjust to the changes in his or her world. Community Care 1-1 highlights common difficulties that can be anticipated in divorce situations with suggestions for ways to support the child and the family when these scenarios occur.

GRANDPARENT FAMILIES

Grandfamilies—the name given to identify the increasing numbers of homes in which grandparents serve as the primary carers of their grandchildren. In the United States, it is estimated that 5.8 million children are living in homes with their grandparents as their primary care providers. Although grandparent-maintained families can be found in all cultural groups regardless of socioeconomic level, children raised by their grandparents are more likely to be African American or Hispanic, younger than age 5 years, and living in southern states (U.S. Census Bureau, 2011b). Grandparents living with grandchildren in grandparent-maintained households are more likely to be in the labor force and are most likely to have incomes below the poverty level (American Academy of Child and Adolescent Psychiatry, 2012; U.S. Census Bureau, 2011b).

Grandparents become the caregivers of their offspring's children for a variety of reasons. The primary reason has been associated with the negative consequences of parental drug or alcohol abuse and, more recently, with the increased numbers of unmarried teenage mothers and fathers (American Academy of Child and Adolescent Psychiatry, 2012). These consequences include poverty, homelessness, exposures to HIV and AIDS, and child abuse and neglect. Other reasons grandparents may become caregivers include death, mental illness, or incarceration of one or both parents. Under any of these conditions, the grandparents may become caregivers through informal arrangements made among family members or through formal arrangements made by the child welfare system (e.g., kinship care). When legal or physical custody of the child is removed from the birth parents, many grandparents accept responsibility for their grandchildren rather than allow the children to be placed in a nonrelative foster care home.

Health care professionals need to be aware of the impact this new family constellation has on the child, the grandparents, and other affected family members. For the younger grandparent, caring for grandchildren may come as an addition to their current parenting role. They may still have young children of their own residing in their household. The addition of more children may lead to financial, emotional, and marital stress. Aunts and uncles (who are still children themselves) may resent the intrusion of the new family members.

Grandparents who are older usually do not expect to take on a parenting role again. At this point in their lives, they may have been looking forward to their retirement years, when they would be freed from the responsibilities of child rearing. Although they may be financially secure and in good physical condition, raising grandchildren leads to increased physical, emotional, and economic vulnerability of the grandparents (Park, 2009; Williams, 2011). Decreasing energy levels, higher incidence of illness, and the many symptoms of aging are all factors that compete against the growing needs of active young children and rebellious teenagers. In addition, many children placed with grandparents have physical and emotional problems as a result of the parent's problems that led to this alternative caregiving situation. Extra medical and financial resources may be needed to support these children. Both the physical health and the financial health of the retired grandparent can be quickly depleted by the constant demands of a medically fragile child.

Raising grandchildren leads to major changes in at least three relationships the grandparent has formed. First, the grandparents may no longer be like their peers. The grandparent may experience feelings of social isolation from friends whose interests and activities are no longer the same. These friends may be traveling or volunteering their time to a service organization, whereas the "new parent" grandparent must worry about getting children off to school and to other social events.

The grandparents' role is also changed with respect to the relationship they have with the child's parents. Feelings of anger and resentment may exist as they are forced to take on the responsibilities of parenting. In addition, it may be difficult for the grandparents to witness the deterioration of their own child, who is addicted to drugs, for example, and thus is unable even to care adequately for himself or herself. For some of these grandparents, caring for their grandchildren may relieve some personal stress because they now know the children are in a safe and secure environment in their home.

Last, the grandparents' relationship with the grandchild is altered by their new role as parents. Typically, grandparents can be permissive and generous with their grandchildren. However, in the parenting role, the grandparent now becomes the disciplinarian, and the birth parent (who may come by for occasional visits) may become the more fun-loving adult figure.

Nurses are in a unique position to advocate for the health of children being raised by grandparents. The National Association of Pediatric Nurse Practitioners (2008b) recommends strategies for nurses to support these families, including assessing the situation, screening the children and grandparents, coordinating services, and offering resources. Along with the strains, there can also be many rewarding aspects of caregiving for both the grandparents and their grandchildren. Much joy and love can be shared in these new relationships. For some grandparents, it is

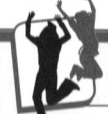

COMMUNITY CARE 1-1

Challenging Situations for the Divorced Family

Children's Adjustment to the Divorce Does Not Meet Parents' Expectations

Child's Response
- As the child gets older, divorce issues that were previously "resolved" seem to reappear and become problematic again for the child.

Anticipatory Guidance
- Assist parents to understand the lengthy process of grief and adjustment within the context of the child's developmental age.
- Revisit issues about the divorce as the child transitions to a new developmental stage.
- Allow the child to talk with health care providers about his or her feelings.

Child Is Displeased With the Visiting Schedule

Child's Response
- Child starts refusing to go to parent's house.
- Child verbalizes anger about the schedule.

Anticipatory Guidance
- Encourage the child to participate in visiting schedule negotiations.
- Revisit the negotiations on a regular basis to allow for changes in the child's schedule based on school and extracurricular activities.

Phone Calls to the Absent Parent Are Viewed as Disruptive and Disturbing

Child's Response
- Child becomes visibly emotionally distressed during calls.

Anticipatory Guidance
- Set up a mutually agreeable schedule for when and how the child can contact the absent parent.
- Avoid emotionally charged times for calls like bedtime or dinnertime.

Transitions and Handoffs Are Traumatic

Child's Response
- Child acts out and becomes very tearful, angry, or depressed.

Anticipatory Guidance
- Minimize the number of weekly transitions from one household to another.
- Return the child to some neutral place after an overnight or weekend stay (e.g., school or daycare center).
- Allow the children to contact the parent they are not with during a time period agreeable to both parents.

Divorce Contract Binds Children, Setting Limits on Their Time, Flexibility, and Personal Freedoms as They Move Between Two Households

Child's Response
- Child feels angry and hostile about divorce agreements.
- Child feels powerless to modify or influence the divorce agreement that affects his or her daily life.

Anticipatory Guidance
- Give the child a shortened version of agreement to read and review.
- Ask for the child's input on negotiations of time when possible.

Parents Argue About Money and Expenditures in the Presence of Children

Child's Response
- Child feels pressure to minimize parent expenses.
- Children feel unwanted because they know they "cost too much."

Anticipatory Guidance
- Encourage parents to hold such discussions away from children.
- Encourage parents to have a mediator discuss with them issues regarding child expenses.

Parents Are Dating and Having Sexual Relationships With Other Partners

Child's Response
- Children are unsettled by demonstrations of affection and physical contact between their parent and another adult.
- Children may mimic parental behaviors in inappropriate ways.

Anticipatory Guidance
- Parents should attempt to confine their social and sexual explorations to the nights and weekends when their children are away.

Child Refuses to Spend Time With One Parent

Child's Response

- This may be an attempt to get the rebuffed parent to come back home or pay more support, or may be an attempt by older children to display more independence.
- Child may be avoiding some activity or circumstance at the other house.

Anticipatory Guidance

- Encourage the child to discuss what is going on at the other home and why contact is being avoided.
- Analyze the visiting schedule with the child and determine whether there is conflict with the child's other activities.
- Determine whether a parent is giving out a message that visiting the other parent is not important to them.

Children Have Increased Household Responsibilities

Child's Response

- Child may feel overburdened.
- Child may volunteer to do more, yet this creates a situation of overdependence on the child.

Anticipatory Guidance

- Child should not become the disciplinarian of other children in the household.

---

an opportunity to enjoy parenting the second time around with more confidence and self-assurance. For the grandchildren, being raised in a safe and secure environment is an immeasurable benefit of this new family constellation.

Nurses can serve as a resource to grandparent caregivers to connect them with information and services that can assist them in their parenting responsibilities (Nursing Interventions 1-4). Access to support groups and individual or family counseling has been found to be beneficial in helping grandparents deal with the stressors they may experience. In 1993, the American Association of Retired Persons (AARP) established the Grandparent Information Center to provide information and resources for grandparents who are raising their grandchildren. For the names and addresses of this

and other resources for grandparents, see thePoint for Organizations.

ADOLESCENT PARENT FAMILIES

In 2010, the overwhelming majority of teenage births were to unmarried young women (88%, teens aged 15 to 19 years) (Child Trends DataBank, 2012). To work effectively with adolescent parents and their children, pediatric nurses need to be aware of the strengths and weaknesses of these families. Teen parents experience difficulties that often include low job status and educational achievement, increased likelihood of living in poverty, less partner involvement, and more time depending on welfare, all of which lead to higher stress and depression. The children of teenage parents are

---

NURSING INTERVENTIONS I-4

Ways to Support Grandparents as Caregivers

- Provide grandparents with information about their state's policies on financial assistance available to kinship caregivers.
- Direct caregivers to apply for Aid to Families with Dependent Children benefits if eligible.
- Ensure that grandparents have the same visiting and rooming-in privileges granted to parents in inpatient health care settings.
- Provide parenting classes for updating child care skills.
- Provide education of the special needs of their grandchild who may be medically fragile or who had prenatal exposure to drugs.

- Encourage grandparents not to neglect their own health care needs.
- Provide transitional care through the use of home nursing visits for newborns or the child with special needs who is discharged to the grandparents' home.
- Refer grandparents to support groups and individual or family counseling when needed.
- Refer grandparents to legal aid agencies or law firms that can assist them in working their way through the complexities of the child welfare system.

at risk because of such factors as poor prenatal care, nonstimulating environments, lack of preventive health care, poor nutrition, possible low social support, and inadequate supervision (Child Trends DataBank, 2012).

Despite these difficulties, many adolescent parents become independent and successful in their parental roles. Their strengths often include physical health as well as energy to care for an active child, optimism and idealism about the future, strong support groups made up of peers and extended family, and the developmental readiness for change and advancement. Although teenage parents tend to be more impatient with their children and have low levels of verbal interaction, they typically demonstrate considerable warmth and love toward their children. Nurses need to build on the strengths of these adolescents to increase their chances for success while assisting them in overcoming some of the difficulties associated with being a teenage parent. In terms of health outcomes, children of adolescent parents are at high risk for delays in cognitive development, poor academic achievement, and behavioral problems (Child Trends DataBank, 2012). Support from their families, peers, and health care professionals can help these adolescent families achieve success.

When most teens are struggling to gain independence from their families of origin, the teenage parent is often forced to rely on their family even more for social and economic support. Many of these parents choose to stay at home or to live together with their family members to finish high school. If this is the case, communication between the grandparents and the teenage parents regarding the parenting responsibilities for the new infant is essential. Grandparents need to provide support for the adolescent without taking over the teenager's parenting role. If the grandparents become the primary care providers for the new infant, the adolescent may fail to develop their own parenting skills. Consistent parenting and discipline practices are important in fostering the

development of the young child. Adolescent parents may have high developmental expectations of their child. Expectations that are too high, especially with regard to obedience, can lead to the parent's frustration and may put the child at high risk for abuse. This has profound implications for pediatric nurses. Providing education to adolescent parents on the normal occurrence of developmental milestones as well as appropriate disciplinary techniques is an essential task for the nurse (Fig. 1-8).

HOMELESS FAMILIES

A homeless person has been defined as an individual who lacks a fixed, regular, and adequate nighttime residence, or a person who resides in a shelter, welfare hotel, transitional program, or place not ordinarily used as regular sleeping accommodations (e.g., cars, abandoned buildings) (National Coalition for the Homeless, 2009). According to one study, approximately 3 million people (1.3 million of them children) are likely to experience homelessness in a given year (National Law Center on Homelessness and Poverty, 2012). Youth younger than 18 years of age account for 39% of the homeless population (National Law Center on Homelessness and Poverty, 2012). Unaccompanied youth account for 5% of the urban homeless population, a marked increase from 3% in 1998 (National Coalition for the Homeless, 2009), with a growing number of adolescents running away from home or being thrown out of their home as a result of conflict with their parents about substance use, violent behavior, and actions related to their choice of sexual orientation and sexual behavior (Rew et al., 2005).

Homelessness has an impact on the health and welfare of children and their families. The pediatric nurse and school nurse need to be aware of the special health needs of children in homeless families. Children younger than 5 years of age make up 42% of the homeless children in

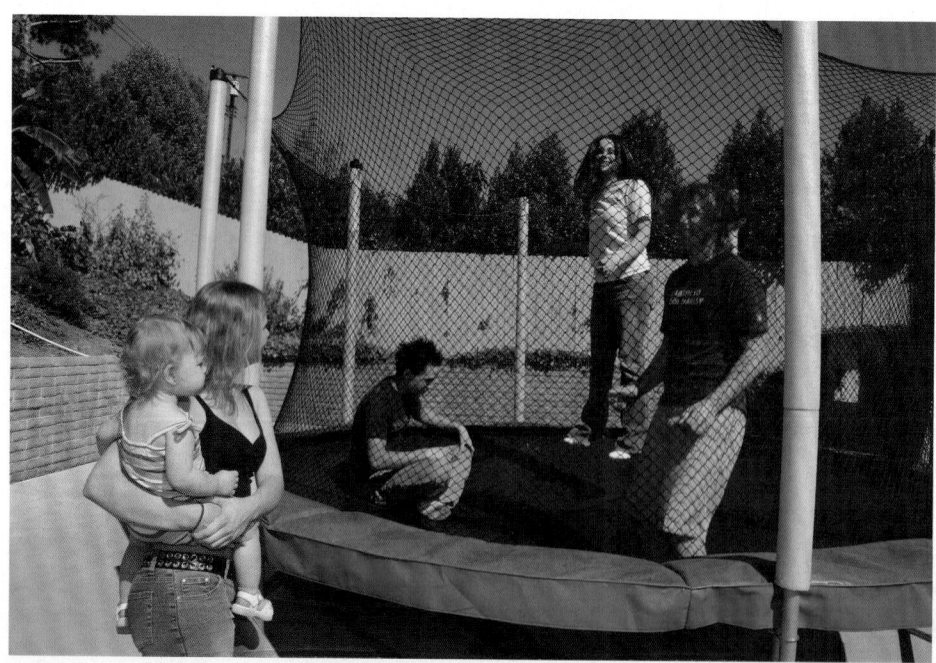

Figure 1-8 Adolescent parents face many challenges as they balance child-rearing activities with their own personal and social needs.

the United States (National Law Center on Homelessness and Poverty, 2012). Infants in homeless families are at higher risk for low birth weight and prenatal drug exposure, and older children are at higher risk for malnutrition and physical delay leading to developmental and behavioral problems such as aggression, dependency, sleep disorders, and speech difficulties. Many of these children receive inadequate or delayed health care, including immunizations and well-child or ill-child services. In addition, children of homeless families live in environments such as crowded shelters where they are exposed to other children and adults with contagious diseases. School-aged children have been noted to show more psychiatric symptoms such as depression, suicidal tendencies, anxiety, and poor school performance. School-aged children also have been noted to have a fear of being stigmatized as poor and living in a shelter (Samuels & Shinn, 2010). These findings demonstrate the need for programs to meet the physical, medical, developmental, emotional, and educational needs of these at-risk families to prevent negative outcomes for child development and socialization (Clinical Judgment 1-3).

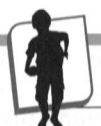

CLINICAL JUDGMENT 1-3

The Homeless Family With a Hospitalized Child

Cassie is a 12-month-old white female. She was admitted to the hospital after being seen by a nurse practitioner at a nursing center on the grounds of a homeless shelter. The nurse practitioner had seen the patient on two prior occasions 1 month apart.

Cassie has lost weight during the past 2 months despite the education on nutrition and feeding that was provided to the family. After the initial evaluation, Cassie was diagnosed with nonorganic failure to thrive.

Questions

1. What information and observations should be included in the nutritional assessment of the child?

2. Optimally, what members of the health care team should participate in the interdisciplinary care of the child with nonorganic failure to thrive?

3. What are the essential components of the discharge plan for Cassie and her family?

4. When a meal tray is brought for Cassie, you note that she gets very little of the food. Instead, the mother tells you Cassie would not eat so she finished eating her meal. What interventions should you take with Cassie and her mother?

5. What criteria should be met by Cassie and her family prior to discharge?

Answers

1. Growth parameters: length, weight, head circumference, child's general appearance, feeding schedule, description of daily nutritional intake, interactions between child and parent during feeding, availability of food and/or competition for limited food among family members, current community services the family is using to access food (e.g., Special Supplemental Nutrition Program for Women, Infants and Children [WIC], food stamps), interaction, the feeding relationship

2. Physician: conduct a medical evaluation

   Nurse: assess child–parent interactions during feeding times and coordinate care of interdisciplinary team and discharge planning

   Dietitian: assess nutritional intake and develop a meal plan to include required nutritional intake

   Occupational therapist: conduct a developmental assessment including oral–motor feeding skills

   Social worker/psychologist: assess the family resources and support systems, assist with obtaining necessary resources

3. Develop a feeding strategy with family input and concerns. Contact services that will enable the family to meet the nutritional, emotional, and developmental needs of Cassie. These services may include WIC, food stamps, a local food bank, long-term housing assistance, a parenting program with a nutritional component, and possibly supervision by a representative from the Department of Children's Services/Child Protective Services.

4. Remain present when Cassie is fed. Determine whether Cassie is truly not eating and assess the need to change the type of food offered to her. Review with the mother the importance of Cassie obtaining nutritious food. Discuss with the social worker the possibility of obtaining free meal trays for the parents while Cassie is hospitalized.

5. Cassie has demonstrated a weight gain and interest in eating. The family demonstrates understanding of the feeding plan and strategies to enhance their daughter's nutritional intake. Services that will enable the family to have access to food and shelter have been arranged.

Pediatric nurses in multiple settings such as schools, communities, and clinics should be able to identify the children and families at risk and begin to act as an advocate for the family. School nurses can act as catalysts in the school system to influence negative attitudes about homelessness and to eliminate the stigma associated with being a homeless child or "shelter kid." The nurse should be aware of community resources available for the family, such as public health and education programs, mental health services, free clinics, and shelters (Samuels & Shinn, 2010). Chapter 2 provides a thorough description of many programs that can benefit the homeless family. In addition, the nurse should be aware of the perceived barriers to obtaining well-child care for these families. These barriers include unfamiliarity with health care providers, waiting for appointments and waiting during appointments, and the cost of transportation and/or parking. The nurse can collaborate with members of the health care team to ensure that families understand the medical benefits available to them and the steps they must take to access these services. Educational materials and scheduled meetings at homeless care centers to discuss health care issues can be provided as a means to provide knowledge of the health care system to homeless families.

CULTURAL AND RELIGIOUS INFLUENCES ON THE FAMILY

The cultural composition of North America is changing, with an increase in the number and diversity of minority groups. According to the U.S. Census Bureau (2012b) population estimates for 2010, there were 308.7 million persons in the United States (a 9.7% increase since 2000), 75% of whom were white (not Hispanic or Latino), 14% were black, 5.6% were Asian, 16% were Hispanic or Latino (accounting for more than half the growth in total population between 2000 and 2010), 1.7% were Alaska Native or American Indian, and 0.4% were Native Hawaiian or Pacific Islander (U.S. Census Bureau, 2011d). To adapt to this diversity, health care professionals need to adopt a transcultural and pluralistic perspective to work with families with diverse ethnic, religious, and cultural beliefs.

CULTURAL AND RELIGIOUS CONCEPTS

QUESTION: What examples do you see in the case study that suggest that the Tran family has become acculturated??

University of Minnesota Center for Advanced Research on Language Acquisition (2012, para. 1) defines **culture** as "the shared patterns of behaviors and interactions, cognitive constructs, and affective understanding that are learned through a process of socialization." Cultural groups can be distinguished by such characteristics as mode of dress, food preferences, values, politics, language, and health care practices. **Ethnicity** refers to a common social and cultural heritage of a group that is

passed on from one generation to the next. A shared ethnicity is thought to create a sense of identity for a group (Giger, 2013). **Race** refers to the biophysiologic characteristics of a population group that make it different from others. Not every person in the population group has all the characteristics, but, in general, the population group as a whole can be distinguished by these characteristics. **Biculturality** occurs when a person crosses two cultures, lifestyles, and sets of beliefs. For instance, this might occur when an African American child is adopted by a white, North American couple or when a child is born to an Asian woman and a Hispanic man. During childhood, the cultural values and beliefs of the couple are transmitted to the child; as the child matures, the parents encourage the child to learn more about the unique cultural beliefs of each of their parents. The adolescent grows to understand that he or she is a product of the unique blend of two cultures. **Acculturation** is the process in which a cultural group adapts to or learns how to take on the behaviors of another cultural group. Complete acculturation usually never occurs and is not even necessarily desirable. **Multiculturality** is the concept that although cultural differences exist, there are also many similarities and areas of common ground between cultural groups that have immigrated to the United States.

In addition to the cultural similarities and variances among families, it is important to consider the spiritual or religious factors that motivate individual and family beliefs and actions. Spiritual and religious beliefs can directly or indirectly influence the health of children and families. **Religion** can be defined as an organized system of commonly held beliefs, rituals, and observances in the worship of God or gods. **Spirituality** is often defined as the basic quality in all humans that involves a belief in something greater than the self and a faith that positively affirms life. Spirituality most often refers to personal beliefs, transcendent experiences, and principles (Andrews & Boyle, 2011). In essence, one can be spiritual without belonging to an organized religion.

ANSWER: Some examples of acculturation by the Tran family include the father learning to speak English, Ashley's desire not to be called by her Vietnamese name outside the home, and Ashley's association with her friends, most of whom are not Vietnamese. Ashley's dress and use of makeup also may reflect her adoption of her social group's culture.

CULTURALLY SENSITIVE HEALTH CARE

It is important for health care professionals to be aware of their own cultural beliefs that affect the health care they provide to others. The AAP (2004, p. 1677) defines culturally effective health care as "the delivery of care within the context of appropriate physician knowledge, understanding and appreciation of all cultural distinctions leading to optimal health outcomes." Professionals should become knowledgeable about the cultural groups represented in their client populations.

To provide culturally competent care, it is important to have an understanding of, and respect for, the beliefs and priorities of the families they are serving. Cultural competence begins by developing a knowledge base about other cultures and by developing strategies to communicate and intervene in ways that support the cultural beliefs and values of others. In some instances, individuals may restrict their view of other groups and be unable to accept the beliefs and behaviors of other cultural groups, or they may be unaware of the different cultural beliefs guiding a family's health decisions (AAP, 2012a; Andrews & Boyle, 2011). Thus, miscommunication and cultural conflict may occur. Stereotyped assumptions about a child or parent based on their physical traits may not fully indicate the different racial and ethnic backgrounds of family members. Optimal health care support of families can be given by recognizing variances between families and ensuring their unique cultural beliefs are incorporated into care delivery practices (Tradition or Science 1-1).

TRADITION OR SCIENCE 1-1

Evidence-Based Practice

Do racial and ethnic disparities still exist in regard to treatment of illness in children within various health care settings?

Mounting evidence indicates that a person's race can significantly influence the treatment he or she receives and access to care (Benz et al., 2011; Borders et al., 2004; Tashior, 2005). A landmark 2003 report published by the National Academy of Sciences searched published studies for the preceding 10 years to identify documented racial and ethnic differences in health care. Some notable discrepancies in pediatric care include less access to kidney transplants for African American patients compared with whites; fewer psychotropic medications provided to African American youths compared with white youths; fewer prescriptions provided to African American and Hispanic children; an increase in charges for diagnostic testing; an increase in length of stay for non–English-speaking families; and parental reports of worse care provided to African American, Native American, and non–English-speaking Hispanic and Asian parents (Smedley et al., 2003; Tashior, 2005). *Healthy People 2020* includes goals to achieve health equity, eliminate disparities, and improve the health of all groups (U.S. Department of Health & Human Services, Office of Minority Health, 2010). The efforts to reduce disparities have focused on improving the overall health of all populations, with particular focus on underserved and vulnerable populations. In addition, efforts are being made to improve the quality of health care services and to close the care gaps for underserved populations. Health reform activities, providing a diverse health care workforce, and ensuring health care providers are culturally competent are steps that have been identified as decreasing health care disparities (Bahls, 2011). More research to further understand and eliminate health disparities is warranted.

HEALTH BELIEFS AND PRACTICES OF CULTURALLY DIVERSE FAMILIES

When examining the health and illness beliefs and practices of a different cultural group, it is important to remember that this information is general and not universal (Andrews & Boyle, 2011). It cannot be applied to every individual in that cultural group. The traditional belief systems of a group are adapted and modified through interactions with other cultures and through the socialization that has taken place within the context of the family (acculturation). Differences within a race, culture, or ethnic group are related to variables such as the social context of the family, the economic class, kinship ties, and geographic location of the family. The goal of the nurse is to acknowledge cultural differences while underscoring similarities and belonging. Knowledge of traditional beliefs provides a *framework* for the health care professional to begin to assess and intervene in a manner that is safe and effective. As the nurse collects data about the specific cultural and religious practices of a child and his or her family, care can be further modified to ensure optimum outcomes. The U.S. Census Bureau uses incidence, prevalence, and mortality rates of common illnesses to calculate and report racial and ethnic disparities. Although this practice is helpful to identify those at risk for certain health conditions, caution also needs to be taken because health care providers that rely too heavily on the "conventional wisdom" of "race-equals-risk" diagnosis may blind themselves to alternative explanations for the health problems of the individual (Tashior, 2005). Discussions of cultural beliefs regarding grief and loss are presented in Chapter 13, and details regarding response to pain are presented in Chapter 10.

ALERT *A cultural or spiritual practice may have the potential of interfering with the welfare and safety of a child. For instance, a child who is not fed animal products may be at risk for nutritional deficiencies such as vitamin B_{12}, calcium, iron, vitamin D, and zinc. Cultural and spiritual practices should be assessed carefully and sensitively to ensure the child's physical and developmental needs are not being inadvertently compromised.*

CULTURAL AND SPIRITUAL ASSESSMENT

Health and illness are perceived differently from culture to culture, and these perceptions affect the way a person responds to the health care environment and treatment modalities. Obtaining a person's view and cultural context of health and illness is an integral component of the health assessment process. Understanding cultural perspectives can help the nurse anticipate and be aware of why families make certain health decisions. Knowledge of a cultural group's characteristics serves as an indicator of the family's background, but it is the nurse's responsibility to clarify the characteristics that the family or individuals have chosen to identify and integrate into their lifestyle. The nurse should have some generalizations about the specific culture to which the family belongs and, by assessing and communicating with the family, the nurse should be able to clarify what does and does not apply to the family. This interaction enables the nurse to learn about the family's values, beliefs, and attitudes toward health that influence behavior (Andrews & Boyle, 2011; Mueller, 2010). A continual assessment of the family's perceptions of health care should be incorporated into ongoing discussions with the family. These data can provide useful information that can help the nurse to modify the plan of care and to illuminate areas of patient teaching.

Just as it is important for the nurse not to make care decisions based solely on a family's ethnic heritage, it is equally important for the nurse not to make assumptions on the basis of the family's religious affiliation. Individuals and families may have a certain religious affiliation without adhering to all of the religion's beliefs and practices. Nurses tend to ignore the spiritual needs of the child and family because they feel they do not know enough about the particular religion to be of any assistance. The nurse should assess the role of religion and spirituality in the family and understand the influence of religion/spirituality as a potential coping mechanism for the family (Morton & Fontaine, 2009). The role of the nurse is to show the family and the child a willingness to listen and care for them spiritually and to intervene in a manner that supports the family's spiritual needs. When nurses do not know the practices of a particular religion, every attempt should be made to discuss with the family their spiritual needs and to develop a plan of care that meets those needs. Studies indicate that nurses are actively involved in providing spiritual support in the form of activities such as prayer, home visitation with prayer, providing privacy and a safe place for family members to express their beliefs, and providing words of healing and encouragement (Morton & Fontaine, 2009).

CROSS-CULTURAL CARE

Rhee (2005) examined race- and ethnic-specific prevalence for 10 symptoms in American youth. White youths reported the highest frequency of headaches, musculoskeletal pain, and dizziness. Black youths more commonly reported feeling hot, having chest pain, having cold sweats, and having urinary symptoms. Musculoskeletal pain was more likely in families with higher income; chest pain, cold sweat, feeling hot, and urinary symptoms were reported by those with lower family incomes. Clearly, each racial/ethnic group of adolescents had its own particular tendency to certain physical symptoms. This information can be used to help guide symptom assessment and early diagnosis of physical problems when adolescents are evaluated by nurses in school or outpatient clinical settings.

HEALTH CARE IMPLICATIONS

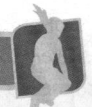 QUESTION: When caring for George Tran in the emergency department, what would you do to ensure the delivery of culturally competent care?

Cultural and religious beliefs and practices of the family can be expected to affect the management of the ill child. The nurse needs to determine whether these practices and beliefs are beneficial for the child. When possible, these beliefs need to be incorporated into the nursing care plan. When these beliefs and practices are detrimental to the health and welfare of the child, compromises need to be made to respect the family's beliefs and still maintain the health of the child. When a compromise is not possible, a legal intervention may be necessary to ensure that care is provided that is in the best interest of the child's health.

CROSS-CULTURAL CARE

When working with families, the nurse needs to encourage the use of benign or neutral folk practices while discouraging practices or remedies that have a detrimental effect on the child. It is important to share with the family the ill effects some healing practices can have on the child.

Some religious institutions offer rituals or beliefs that might help an individual prevent illness; some offer support should an illness occur. Many religions offer direction on social, moral, and dietary requirements to prevent illness. For example, the Mormon religion, as part of its belief system, discourages smoking, excessive alcohol use, and illicit drug use. Many religious institutions have rituals related to having and raising children. Childbearing is an example of an event that is affected by many religious and cultural beliefs and practices. Orthodox Jewish women believe that producing children fulfills the measure of their creation and shows obedience to the ancient rabbinical law to multiply and replenish the earth. Male circumcision is another practice with which religious rituals are associated. For example, the Brit Milah is a Jewish religious male circumcision ceremony practiced on the eighth day of life by a trained *mohel*. These are just a few examples of child-rearing practices that are influenced by religious beliefs that should be considered and incorporated into FCC practices.

Beliefs about health and illness can often affect a family's ability to comply with western medicine and nursing care. In the health care setting, providers can promote culturally competent care through interventions that bridge or link the health care system with the child and family who are responding from a different cultural context. The nurse must use knowledge of traditional cultural and religious practices as a framework within which to assess the patient and build a plan of care. The health care plan that has the most success is the one that demonstrates an appreciation for the cultural variations and similarities of each family.

ANSWER: When caring for George, you need to realize that as the oldest son, he is the one eventually to inherit the family's worth. When communicating with him, be aware that he may wish to avoid any confrontations with health care professionals and might answer questions with information he thinks you want to hear. In addition, he may avoid eye contact (eye contact is considered rude in his culture). Also, do not use your hand or finger when motioning to him because this is considered an insult, and do not touch his head. The head is considered sacred in his culture because it is where one's consciousness lies. Moreover, support any wishes that the family may have related to the use of a shaman or healer for possible remedies and spiritual healing ceremonies.

See thePoint for a summary of Key Concepts.

REFERENCES

Adoption Statistics. (2005). *Adoption statistics: Placing children*. Retrieved from http://statistics.adoption.com/information/adoption -statistics-placing-children.html

Agency for Healthcare Research and Quality. (2011). *National healthcare disparities report, 2011*. Retrieved from http://www.ahrq.gov /qual/nhdr11/chap5.htm

Ahrons, C., & Rodgers, R. (1987). *Divorced families: A multidisciplinary developmental view*. New York, NY: W. W. Norton.

Aidala, A., & Zablocki, B. (1991). The communes of the 1970's: Who joined and why? *Marriage and Family Review, 17*(1–2), 86–116.

Allen, S., & Daly, K. (2007). *The effects of father involvement: An updated research summary of the evidence inventory*. Retrieved from http:// fira.ca/cms/documents/29/Effects_of_Father_Involvement.pdf

American Academy of Child and Adolescent Psychiatry. (2012). *Grandparents raising grandchildren*. Retrieved from http://aacap.org /page.ww?name = Grandparents + Raising + Grandchildren&sectio n = Facts + for + Families

American Academy of Family Physicians. (2012). *Family, definition of*. Retrieved from http://www.aafp.org/online/en/home/policy /policies/f/familydefinitionof.html

American Academy of Pediatrics. (2004). Ensuring culturally effective pediatric care: Implications for education and health policy. *Pediatrics, 114*(6), 1677–1685.

American Academy of Pediatrics. (2007). Role of the medical home in family-centered early intervention services. *Pediatrics, 120*, 1153–1158.

American Academy of Pediatrics. (2008). *What is a family-centered medical home?* Retrieved from http://www.medicalhomeinfo.org

American Academy of Pediatrics. (2012a). *Culturally effective care toolkit: Medical education*. Retrieved from http://www.aap.org/en-us /professional-resources/practice-support/Patient-Management /Pages/Culturally-Effective-Care-Toolkit-Medical-Education.aspx

American Academy of Pediatrics. (2012b). *Family life*. Retrieved from http://www.healthychildren.org/English/family-life/family -dynamics/pages/The-Perfect-Family.aspx

American Academy of Pediatrics. (2012c). Patient and family-centered care and the pediatrician's role. *Pediatrics, 129*(2), 394–404.

Andrews, W. M., & Boyle, J. S. (2011). *Transcultural concepts in nursing care* (6th ed.). New York, NY: Lippincott Williams & Wilkins.

Annie E. Casey Foundation. (2012). *Children in single parent families by race*. Retrieved from http://datacenter.kidscount.org/data /acrossstates/Rankings.aspx?loct = 2&by = a&order = a&ind = 107& dtm = 431&ch = a&tf = 133

Bahls, C. (2011). Health policy brief: Achieving equity in health. *Health Affairs, 31*(11), 1–6.

Bauserman, R. (2002). Child adjustment in joint-custody versus sole-custody arrangements: A meta-analytic review. *Journal of Family Psychology, 16*(1), 91–102.

Benz, J., Espinosa, O., Welsh, V. et al. (2011). Awareness of racial and ethnic health disparities has improved only modestly over a decade, *Health Affairs, 30*(10), 1860–1867.

Borders, T., Brannon-Goedeke, A., Arif, A. et al. (2004). Parents' reports of children's medical care access: Are there Mexican-American versus non-Hispanic white disparities? *Medical Care, 42*(9), 884–892.

Botash, A. S. (2012). *Foster care: Health concerns of children in foster care*. Retrieved from http://childabusemd.com/foster/health -concerns.shtml

Bozett, F. W. (1987). Family nursing and life-threatening illness. In M. Leahey & L. M. Wright (Eds.), *Families and life-threatening illness* (pp. 2–25). Spring House, PA: Springhouse.

Burris, L. (2009). *Economy's slump makes communal living a possibility*. Retrieved from http://voices.yahoo.com/economys-slump -makes-communal-living-possibility-2475695.html?cat = 3

Center for Youth Studies. (2012). *Welcome to the family center*. Retrieved from http://www.centerforyouth.org/resource_centers/family_center

Child Trends DataBank. (2012). *Teen births*. Retrieved from http:// www.childtrendsdatabank.org/?q = node/52

Children's Bureau. (2012). *Foster care statistics 2011*. Retrieved from http://www.childwelfare.gov/pubs/factsheets/foster.pdf#Page = 11&view = Fit

Combrinck-Graham, L. (1990). Developments in family systems theory and research. *Journal of the American Academy of Child and Adolescent Psychiatry, 29*(4), 501–512.

Cousineau, J. M., & Domar, A. D. (2007). Psychological impact of infertility. *Best Practice and Research Clinical Obstetrics and Gynecology, 21*(2), 293–308.

Coyne, I., O'Neill, C., Murphy, M. et al. (2011). What does family-centered care mean to nurses and how do they think it could be enhanced in practice. *Journal of Advanced Nursing, 67*(12), 2561–2573.

Deka, P. K., & Sarma, S. (2010). Psychological aspects of infertility. *British Journal of Medical Practitioners, 3*(3), a336–a339.

Duvall, E. M. (1962). *Family development*. Chicago, IL: Lippincott Williams & Wilkins.

Erikson, E. (1963). *Childhood and society*. New York, NY: W. W. Norton.

Federal Interagency Forum on Child and Family Statistics. (2007). *America's children: Key national indicators of well-being, 2007*. Retrieved from http://www.childstats.gov/pdf/ac2007/ac_07.pdf

Federal Interagency Forum on Child and Family Statistics. (2011). *America's children: Key national indicators of well-being, 2011*. Retrieved from http://www.childstats.gov/pdf/ac2011/ac_11.pdf

Fletcher, G. E., & Rosencrantz, T. (2012). *Multiple births*. Retrieved from http://emedicine.medscape.com/article/977234-overview

Friedman, M., Bowden, V., & Jones, E. (2003). *Family nursing: Theory and practice* (3rd ed.). Upper Saddle River, NJ: Prentice Hall.

Galvin, K., & Brommel, B. (1986). *Family communication: Cohesion and change*. Glenview, IL: Scott, Foresman and Company.

Giger, J. N. (2013). *Transcultural nursing: Assessment and intervention*. St. Louis, MO: Mosby.

Goldenberg, H., & Goldenberg, I. (2008). *Family therapy: An overview* (7th ed.). Belmont, CA: Thomson Brooks/Cole.

Grusec, J. E., & Hastings, P. D. (2007). *Handbook of socialization: Theory and research*. New York, NY: Guilford Press.

Hanson, S., Gedaly-Duff, V., & Kaakinew, J. (2005). *Family health care nursing: Theory, practice and research*. Philadelphia, PA: F. A. Davis.

Harrison, T. M. (2010). Family-centered pediatric nursing care: State of the science. *Journal of Pediatric Nursing, 25*, 335–343.

Health Resources and Services Administration. (2008). *Family-centered care*. Retrieved from http://mchb.hrsa.gov/cshcn05/nf/6family /intro.htm

Hill, R. (1949). *Families under stress.* New York, NY: Harper & Row.

Hill, R. (1971). Modern systems theory and the family: A confrontation. *Social Science Information, 10,* 7–26.

Institute for Patient- and Family-Centered Care. (2010). *Frequently asked questions.* Retrieved from http://www.ipfcc.org/faq.html

Institute for Patient- and Family-Centered Care. (2012). *Clinicians.* Retrieved from http://www.ipfcc.org/advance/clinician.html

Jee, S. H., Conn, A. M., Szilagyi, P. G. et al. (2010). Identification of social-emotional problems among young children in foster care. *Journal of Child Psychology and Psychiatry.*

Kendall, G. E., & Tallon, M. (2011). Commentary on Shields (2010) models of care: Questioning family-centered care. *Journal of Clinical Nursing, 20*(11), 1788–1790.

Lansford, J. E. (2009). Parental divorce and children's adjustment. *Perspectives on Psychological Science, 4*(2), 140–152.

Leve, L. D., Harold, G. T., Chamberlain, P. et al. (2012). Practitioner review: Children in foster care—vulnerabilities and evidence-based interventions that promote resilience processes. *Journal of Child Psychology and Psychiatry.* Advance online publication.

Lewis, S., & Roberts, A. (2001). Crisis assessment tools: The good, the bad, and the available. *Brief Treatment & Crisis Intervention, 1*(1), 17–28.

Lipman, E., Boyle, M., Dooley, M. et al. (2002). Child well-being in single-mother families. *Journal of the American Academy of Child and Adolescent Psychiatry, 41*(1), 75–82.

Lopez, P., & Allen, P. (2007). Addressing the health needs of adolescents transitioning out of foster care. *Pediatric Nursing, 33,* 345–355.

Lotze, G. M., Bellin, M. H., & Oswald, D. P. (2010). Advancing family-centered services in healthcare: Opportunities and challenges family-centered care for children with special health care needs: Are we moving forward? *Journal of Family Social Work, 13*(2), 100–113.

March of Dimes Foundation. (2012). *Multiples: Twins, triplets and beyond.* Retrieved from http://www.marchofdimes.com/pregnancy/trying_multiples.html

McCubbin, H., & Patterson, J. (1983). Family transitions: Adaptation to stress. In H. McCubbin & C. Figley (Eds.), *Stress and the family: Vol. 1. Coping with normative transitions* (pp. 5–25). New York, NY: Brunner/Mazel.

McGoldrick, M., & Carter, E. (2003). The family cycle. In F. Walsh (Ed.), *Normal family processes* (pp. 375–398). New York, NY: Guilford Press.

Mederer, H., & Hill, R. (1983). Critical transitions over the family life span: Theory and research. In H. McCubbin, M. Sussman, & J. Patterson (Eds.), *Social stress and the family: Advances and developments in family stress theory and research* (pp. 39–60). New York, NY: Haworth Press.

Morton, P. G., & Fontaine, D. K. (2009). *Critical care nursing: A holistic approach* (9th ed.). Philadelphia, PA: Lippincott Williams & Wilkins.

Mueller, C. R. (2010). Spirituality in children: Understanding and developing interventions. *Pediatric Nursing, 36*(4), 197–203, 208.

National Association of Pediatric Nurse Practitioners. (2008b). NAPNAP position statement on supporting grandparents raising grandchildren. *Journal of Pediatric Health Care, 22*(3), e3–e4.

National Association of Pediatric Nurse Practitioners & Society of Pediatric Nurses. (2008). *Pediatric nursing scope and standards of practice.* Silver Spring, MD: American Nurses Association.

National Center for Family Professional Partnerships. (2012). *Family-centered care.* Retrieved from http://www.fv-ncfpp.org/quality-health-care1/family-centered-care

National Coalition for the Homeless. (2009). *Who is homeless?* Retrieved from http://www.nationalhomeless.org/factsheets/who.html

National Law Center on Homelessness and Poverty. (2012). *Program: Children and youth.* Retrieved from http://www.nlchp.org/program.cfm?prog=2

Olson, D. (1988). Family assessment and intervention: The circumplex model of family systems. *Journal of Psychotherapy and the Family, 4*(1/2), 7–49.

Olson, D. (1994). Curvilinearity survives: The world is not flat. *Family Process, 33,* 471–478.

Olson, D. H. (2003). Circumplex model of marital and family systems. In F. Walsh (Ed.), *Normal family processes* (pp. 514–548). New York, NY: Guilford Press.

Park, H. H. (2009). Factors associated with the psychological health of grandparents as primary caregivers: An analysis of gender differences. *Journal of Intergenerational Relationships, 7*(2/3), 191–208.

Parson, T., & Bales, R. F. (1955). *Family socialization and interaction process.* New York, NY: Free Press.

Patterson, J. M. (1988). Families experiencing stress: The family adjustment and adaptation response model. *Family Systems Medicine, 5,* 202–237.

Patterson, J. M. (1995). Promoting resilience in families experiencing stress. *Pediatric Clinics of North America, 42*(1), 47–63.

Patterson, J. M. (2002). Integrating family resilience and family stress theory. *Journal of Marriage and Family, 64*(2), 349–360.

Pryor, J. (2008). *International handbook of stepfamilies: Policy and practice in legal, research, and clinical environments.* Hoboken, NJ: John Wiley & Sons.

Rankin, S. (1989). Family transitions, expected and unexpected. In C. Gillis, B. Highley, B. Roberts et al. (Eds.), *Toward a science in family nursing* (pp. 173–186). Menlo Park, CA: Addison-Wesley.

Rew, L., Whittaker, T., Taylor-Seehafer, M. et al. (2005). Sexual health risks and protective resources in gay, lesbian, bisexual, and heterosexual homeless youth. *Journal of Specialist in Pediatric Nursing, 10*(1), 11–19.

Rhee, H. (2005). Racial/ethnic differences in adolescents' physical symptoms. *Journal of Pediatric Nursing, 20*(3), 153–162.

Samuels, J., & Shinn, M. (2010). *Homeless children: Update on research, policy, programs, and opportunities.* Retrieved from http://aspe.hhs.gov/hsp/10/HomelessChildrenRoundtable/index.shtml

Sandas, I., & Siegel, C. (2012). Separation, divorce, and blended families. Retrieved from http://www.netplaces.com/parenting-kids-with-anxiety/parenting-and-anxiety/separation-divorce-and-blended-families.htm

Schnitzer, P. G., & Ewigman, B. G. (2008). Household composition and fatal unintentional injuries related to child maltreatment. *Journal of Nursing Scholarship, 40*(1), 91–97.

Shelton, T., Jeppson, E., & Johnson, B. (1987). *Family-centered care for children with special health care needs.* Washington, DC: Association for the Care of Children's Health.

Singer, E. (2010). The 'W.I.S.E. Up!' Tool: Empowering adopted children to cope with questions and comments about adoption. *Pediatric Nursing, 36*(4), 209–212.

Smedley, B., Stith, A., & Nelson, A. (Eds.). (2003). *Unequal treatment: Confronting racial and ethnic disparities in health care.* Washington, DC: The National Academies Press.

Smit, E. M. (2010). International adoption families: A unique health care journey. *Pediatric Nursing, 36*(5), 253–258.

Tashior, C. (2005). The meaning of race in health care and research: Part 1: The impact of history. *Pediatrics, 31*(3), 208–209.

University of Minnesota Center for Advanced Research on Language Acquisition. (2012). *What is culture?* Retrieved from http://www.carla.umn.edu/culture/definitions.html

U.S. Census Bureau. (2011a). *America's families and living arrangements: 2011: Table A1.* Retrieved from http://www.census.gov/hhes/families/data/cps2011.html

U.S. Census Bureau. (2011b). *Living arrangements of children: 2009.* Retrieved from http://www.census.gov/prod/2011pubs/p70-126.pdf

U.S. Census Bureau. (2011c). *Same-sex couple households.* Retrieved from http://www.census.gov/prod/2011pubs/acsbr10-03.pdf

U.S. Census Bureau. (2011d). *2010 census briefs.* Retrieved from http://www.census.gov/2010census/data/

U.S. Census Bureau. (2012a). *Current population survey: Definitions.* Retrieved from http://www.census.gov/cps/about/cpsdef.html

U.S. Census Bureau. (2012b). *Households and families: 2010*. Retrieved from http://www.census.gov/prod/cen2010/briefs/c2010br-14.pdf

U.S. Department of Health & Human Services. (1987). *Surgeon General's report: Children with special health care needs*. (DHHS Publication No. HRS/D/MC 87-2). Washington, DC: U.S. Government Printing Office.

U.S. Department of Health & Human Services. (2006). *The importance of fathers in the healthy development of children*. Retrieved from http://www.childwelfare.gov/pubs/usermanuals/fatherhood/chaptertwo.cfm

U.S. Department of Health & Human Services. (n.d.). *Family-centered practice*. Retrieved from http://www.childwelfare.gov/admin/glossary/glossaryf.cfm

U.S. Department of Health & Human Services, Office of Minority Health. (2010). *National partnership for action to end health disparities*. Retrieved from http://www.minorityhealth.hhs.gov/npa/templates/browse.aspx?&lvl=2&lvlid=34

U.S. Department of Labor. (2012). *Employment characteristics of families summary*. Retrieved from http://www.bls.gov/news.release/famee.nr0.htm

U.S. Department of State. (2011). *Intercountry adoption: Statistics*. Retrieved from http://adoption.state.gov/about_us/statistics.php

von Bertalanffy, L. (1968). *General systems theory*. London, United Kingdom: Penguin Press.

Williams, M. N. (2011). The changing roles of grandparents raising grandchildren. *The Journal of Human Behavior in the Social Environment, 21*(8), 948–962.

Zaslow, J. (2002). *Families: Communal living: Single moms unite*. Retrieved from http://www.time.com/time/magazine/article/0,9171,1002240,00.html

See thePoint for additional resources.

CHAPTER 2

Advocating for Children and Families

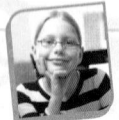

CASE HISTORY

Lindsay Jenkins is a 8½-year-old girl with type 1 diabetes mellitus. Her case history begins in Chapter 12 with her diagnosis and initial treatment for T1DM, and her treatment is continued in the Chapter 26 case history. She is the only child of Jean and Tom Jenkins. Next year, she will attend school. She has been wearing an insulin pump for the past 6 months and the regulation of her diabetes is going well. Lindsay must check her blood sugar regularly to calculate the amount of insulin the pump will deliver. She does not use separate lancets; the lancet is contained within a case and withdraws after use. In her elementary school, Lindsay is allowed to test her blood sugar in the classroom and, if she needs a snack, she is allowed to eat in the classroom as well. Her parents are concerned about her class and recess schedule: Will Lindsay be allowed to have a snack if she needs to and will she be allowed to check her blood sugar in a classroom?

There are several laws to protect children with diabetes and other chronic conditions, yet there remain great variations in practice. The right to manage medical chronic conditions at school is based on Section 504 of the Rehabilitation Act of 1973, the Americans with Disabilities Act of 1990, and the Individuals with Disabilities Education Act (IDEA) of 1990. Under these laws, diabetes is considered a disability, and schools that receive federal funding are not to discriminate against a child who has diabetes or any chronic condition. They can, however, refuse to grant a request for accommodations that are not thoroughly documented, and they can refuse to allow blood glucose testing in the classroom. States vary in their regulations of who can administer glucagons during an episode of severe hypoglycemia. A few states have additional legislation to protect children with disabilities; many school districts, however, have their own individual interpretation of the federal laws. Some schools have not allowed children to have a snack in the classroom and many have not allowed the children to test their blood sugar. Some school regulations require a student to leave class, go to the school nurse's office, wait for the school nurse, and test in the office with the nurse present.

Lindsay is a conscientious student and is anxious enough about the changes and demands of school without having to leave a classroom during instructional time. Lindsay has also experienced very low blood sugars right after exertion in her physical education classes. Going to the nurse's office and waiting to see the nurse to test her blood sugar would place Lindsay at risk for a hypoglycemic seizure. Lindsay's parents are meeting with the school administrator to discuss blood sugar testing in the classroom, to make sure Lindsay's 504 Plan is on file, and to determine whether she should also have any updates made to her individualized education program (IEP) plan. Lindsay's endocrinologist has a pediatric nurse practitioner (PNP) who works closely with the families. The PNP is a member of the National Association of Pediatric Nurse Practitioners (NAPNAP) who has been working with the state professional nursing organization to monitor the bills coming through the state legislature. Recently, a neighboring state debated legislature that would prevent classroom blood sugar testing.

Tom and Jean are supporters of the American Diabetes Association, which is a nonprofit organization that provides research, information, and advocacy. They are also members of Children with Diabetes, which lobbies on behalf of families of children with diabetes.

As you read this chapter, consider the Jenkins family and determine whether the following objectives are applicable to them.

CHAPTER OBJECTIVES

1 Review various factors and issues in the sociopolitical and medical arenas that affect the care of children and their families.

2 Describe selected strategies that nurses, parents, and the community can use to promote health maintenance in children.

3 Identify public, private, and community-based programs that provide health care resources for children and their families.

4 Describe ethical principles that may affect the care of children and their families in either standard clinical or research settings.

5 Review and contrast the legal rights of children, emancipated minors, and parents.

6 List safety and documentation strategies unique to caring for children who are involved in research studies.

7 State the educational programs available to support children with special health care and learning needs.

See thePoint for a list of Key Terms.

The challenges in providing care to children are many as we allocate scarce human, financial, and social resources to meet the health needs of children and their families. Despite numerous social, medical, and legal achievements made to secure the health and welfare of the young, the health status of children around the world remains in jeopardy. This chapter covers some of the challenges to children's health and strategies for enhancing future care through advocacy activities, attention to ethical concerns, legislation, and health care research.

MAJOR THREATS TO CHILDREN'S HEALTH

QUESTION: Is Lindsay's experience with diabetes applicable to many other children? Is it a condition influenced by poverty and education?

The state of children's health in the United States is evaluated by specific determinants, measures of health status, and use of health care services. Determinants of health generally include such factors as age, poverty, race, and ethnicity; the built environment; health insurance coverage; health behaviors; and risk factors. Measures of health status for children include, but are not limited to, prevalence of asthmatic episodes, chronic health conditions, and causes of mortality. The health of individuals living in North America continues to improve overall, with substantial advances in research, health care, public health programs, and health education. However, much room for improvement remains.

In this century, we have witnessed changing patterns in childhood illnesses. For example, many childhood infectious diseases, such as mumps and measles, have all but disappeared in North America because of the emphasis placed on immunization against certain preventable diseases. However, today, the prevalence of chronic diseases is increasing. The incidence of overweight and obesity in young children and teens is increasing rapidly. The "Youth Risk Behavior Surveillance—United States, 2011" data reported that, nationwide, 15.2% of high school students were overweight (≥85th but <95th percentile for body mass index [BMI]) and 13% were obese (≥95th percentile for BMI) (Centers for Disease Control and Prevention, 2012). The number of overweight children, coupled with the decline in physical activity in Americans of all ages, is extremely worrisome from a public health perspective because overweight and obesity are known risk factors for many chronic diseases and disabilities such as cardiovascular disease, type 2 diabetes, and hypertension.

Poverty continues to be a risk factor for parents' rating their children as either in fair or poor health. In 2010, more than one in five children were classified as poor, with 35% of Hispanic children and 39.1% of black children living in poverty. Non-Hispanic black children between the ages of 3 and 10 years experienced higher asthma attack prevalence rates than did non-Hispanic white or Hispanic children in this same age category (National Center for Health Statistics, 2012). Likewise, racial and ethnic factors are associated with substantial disparities in infant mortality rates.

Some positive changes in health outcomes have been noted. In 2010, the birthrate for teen mothers (aged 15 to 19 years) fell to a record low, dropping 44% from 1991 through 2010 (Hamilton & Vetura, 2012). Additionally, in 2008, the teenage abortion rate was 17.8 abortions per 1,000 women, which is 59% lower than its peak of 43.5 abortions per 1,000 women in 1988 (Kost & Henshaw, 2012).

Health behaviors and risk factors play an important role in health outcomes. Nursing Interventions 2-1 lists selected risk behaviors that affect children's health and ways in which the nurse can intervene to minimize these risks. Measures of morbidity and mortality are additional gauges of the status of children's health. Mortality trends that are of great concern in pediatrics are infant mortality and unintentional injury rates (Fig. 2-1). For example, infant mortality has increased as a result of the numbers of infants born weighing less than 750 g. Although decreasing, unintentional injury continues to be the leading cause of death among all children aged 1 to 14 years. In a worrisome trend, however, between 1970 and 2008, the percentage of child deaths due to homicide increased from 2% to 9% among 1- to 4-year-olds and from 2% to 6% among 5- to 14-year-olds. National data also continue to reflect substantial disparities in mortality rates among racial and ethnic groups (Singh, 2010).

Health care coverage is also an important risk factor. In 2010, 90% of children had health insurance coverage at least some time during the year, but approximately 7.3 million (10% of all children) lacked coverage during this time (Federal Interagency Forum on Child and

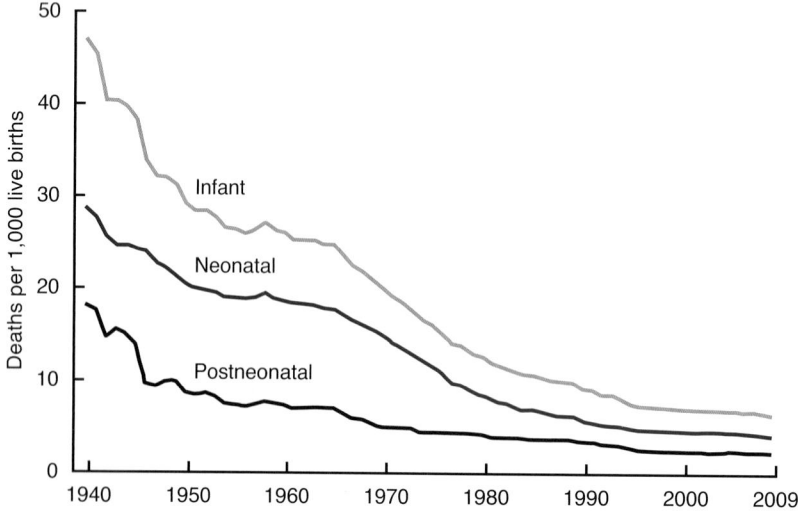

NOTE: Rates are infant (under 1 year), neonatal (under 28 days), and postneonatal (28 days–11 months) deaths per 1,000 live births in specified group.

A

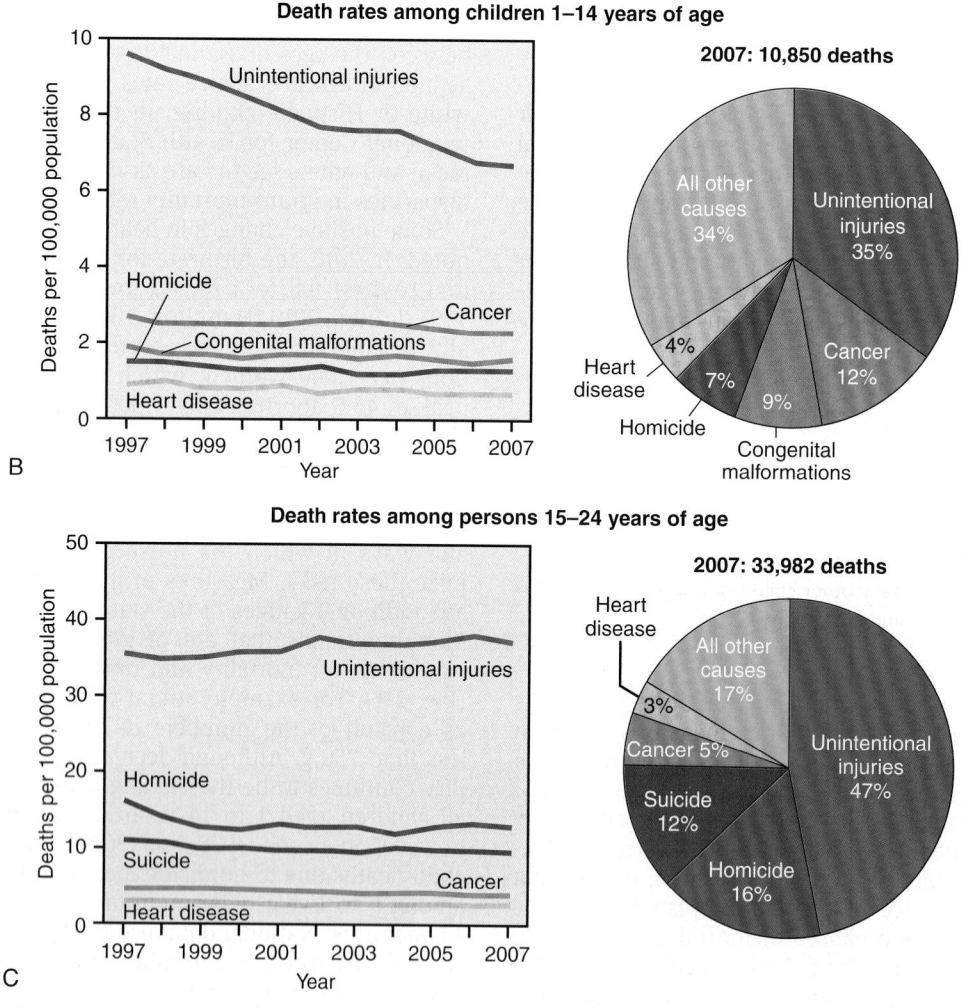

B

C

Figure 2-1 (A) Infant, neonatal, and postneonatal mortality rates: United States, 1940–2009. Rates are infant (younger than 1 year of age), neonatal (younger than 28 days of age), and postneonatal (28 days to 11 months of age) deaths per 1,000 live births in specified group. From CDC/NCHS, National Vital Statistic System, Mortality. Retrieved from http://www.cdc.gov/nchs/data/nvsr/nvsr60/nvsr60_03.pdf. (B) Death rates for leading causes of death among children 1 to 14 years of age: United States, 1997–2007. From Xu, J. Q., Kochanek, K. D., Murphy, S. L. et al. (2010). Deaths: Final data for 2007. *National Vital Statistics Reports, 58*(19), 1–136. Retrieved from http://www.cdc.gov/nchs/data/nvsr/nvsr58/nvsr58_19.pdf. (C) Death rates for leading causes of death among persons 15–24 years of age: United States, 1997–2007. From Xu, J. Q., Kochanek, K. D., Murphy, S. L. et al. (2010). Deaths: Final data for 2007. *National Vital Statistics Reports, 58*(19), 1–136. Retrieved from http://www.cdc.gov/nchs/data/nvsr/nvsr58/nvsr58_19.pdf.

NURSING INTERVENTIONS 2-1

Risk Behaviors in Children

Selected Risk Behaviors*	Examples of Nursing Interventions and Advocacy Activities
<ul><li>Cigarette smoking</li><li>Smoking during pregnancy</li><li>Use of seat belt: "rarely" or "never use"</li><li>Rode with driver who had been drinking alcohol</li><li>Texted or emailed while driving</li><li>Bullied on school property or electronically bullied</li><li>Physical inactivity</li><li>Obesity</li><li>Use of illicit drugs</li><li>Episodic heavy drinking</li><li>Carried a gun 1 day or more during the past 30 days</li><li>Injured in a physical fight during the past 12 months</li><li>Feelings of sadness or hopelessness during past 12 months almost every day for 2 weeks or more</li></ul>	<ul><li>Educate parents to start discussion of issues before those behaviors become a risk.</li><li>Encourage parents to discuss family values.</li><li>Advocate for school policies and legislation to promote health behaviors (e.g., requiring recess time, nutritional lunches at school).</li><li>Establish support groups for students needing additional support managing their stress.</li><li>Provide school programs that advocate abstaining from alcohol use and substance use.</li><li>Establish no-tolerance policies for bullying within schools and other youth-oriented venues.</li><li>Establish youth advocacy programs to train and empower students in seeking solutions</li></ul>

*Based on 2010 statistics as reported by the National Center for Health Statistics. (2010). *Health, United States, 2010 With special feature on death and dying.* Hyattsville, MD: U.S. Department of Health & Human Services, Centers for Disease Control and Prevention. Retrieved from http://www.cdc.gov/nchs/data/hus/hus10.pdf; Centers for Disease Control and Prevention. (2012). Youth risk behavior surveillance—United States, 2011. *Morbidity and Mortality Weekly Report, 61*(SS04), 1–162.

Family Statistics, 2012). Latino children were much less likely than other children to have insurance, with only 84% possessing coverage compared with 93% of non-Latino white children, 91% of Asian children, and 89% of black children (Child Trends DataBank, 2010). Uninsured children are nearly 10 times as likely as insured children to lack a usual source of health care. A report by Kenney et al. (2012) estimates "7.3 million children were uninsured on an average day in 2008, of whom 4.7 million (65%) were eligible for Medicaid or Children's Health Insurance Program (CHIP) but not enrolled" (p. 1920). Among poor children, Medicaid coverage is highest for black children (77%), followed by Latino children (72%), Asian children (68%), and non-Hispanic white children (67%) (Child Trends DataBank, 2010).

ANSWER: New cases of type 1 diabetes are diagnosed in approximately 19.0 per 100,000 youths younger than age 20 years each year. Non-Hispanic white youths have the highest incidence rate of all ethnic groups (National Diabetes Information Clearinghouse, 2011). Poverty and education have no influence on the likelihood of a child being diagnosed with this type of diabetes. However, these factors may affect ongoing management of the child's condition if the family lacks an understanding of effective management or lacks the funds and access to a medical home to ensure ongoing care for the child's chronic condition.

CHILD HEALTH INITIATIVES AND MAJOR CHILD ADVOCACY GROUPS

Data about the status of children's health provide ample evidence that the status of children's health issues must continue to be a focus of public concern. Pediatric nurses need to be familiar with three key health initiatives—*Healthy People 2020, Bright Futures in Practice,* and the *Guidelines for Adolescent Preventive Services (GAPS)*—that serve as standards to judge whether outcomes demonstrate if goals for improving child health have been achieved (see thePoint for Evidence-Based Practice Guidelines).

Healthy People 2020 is a key national initiative that has identified areas that need improvement and provides benchmarks to indicate success. Areas identified include immunization rates; injury and violence prevention; maternal, infant, and child care; and physical activity and fitness. Clinical preventive service guidelines from birth through adolescence have been developed by a variety of health care organizations. The American Academy of Pediatrics' *Bright Futures* initiative is a national health promotion and disease prevention initiative that addresses children's needs within the context of the family and community. The initiative's many publications and tools are used to strengthen the connections between state and local programs, pediatric primary care, families, and communities (see http://www.brightfutures .org/). In addition, the American Medical Association, Department of Adolescent Health (1992) *GAPS* provides a comprehensive set of recommendations that provide a framework for organizing and providing preventive health services during annual health visits between the ages 11 and 21 years (see http://www.ama-assn.org//resources/doc/ad-hlth/gapsmono.pdf).

Several key national child advocacy groups also serve as watchdogs for promoting child health. These groups include the Children's Hospital Association, the Children's Defense Fund, the World Health Organization's and the United Nations Children's Funds, and the Annie E. Casey Foundation (Kids Count Data Book). For more information and websites for these and other advocacy groups, see Organizations on thePoint.

Three national pediatric nursing organizations serve the professional needs of nurses working with children and their families: the National Association of School Nurses (NASN), the Society of Pediatric Nurses (SPN), and the National Association of Pediatric Nurse Practitioners (NAPNAP) (see thePoint for Organizations). These professional nursing organizations have advocacy groups within their membership that support local and national efforts on behalf of children. The NASN promotes programs to improve the health and education success of children. The SPN has several position statements regarding advocacy issues such as promoting literacy, preventing violence against children, and pediatric injury prevention. The Keep Your Child/Yourself Safe and Sound (KySS) program and the Healthy Eating and Activity Together (HEAT) initiatives are examples of nationally based work undertaken by NAPNAP. These two initiatives focus on nurses' role in the prevention and early identification of psychosocial morbidities and obesity issues.

ADVOCATES FOR CHILDREN'S HEALTH CARE ISSUES

An **advocate** acts to safeguard and to advance the interests of other persons—in this case, the child and family—as a means to help meet their health care needs. Advocacy can take a number of forms, from calling an agency on behalf of a child, to writing letters to legislators to improve their understanding of an issue, to working to change agency policy to better meet the needs of the families it serves. If parents need assistance beyond what the nurse can offer, they can be referred to local protection and advocacy agencies.

A variety of strategies exist to improve child health: from seeking additional funding for key programs so they can serve more children, to creating healthier and more supportive communities, to directing families to services and teaching, and supporting them as they advocate for themselves and their children. The potential roles for nurses are limitless. In caring for children and families, look for any opportunity to improve health for all children.

NURSES' ROLE

QUESTION: How does the PNP who works with the pediatric endocrinologist serve as an advocate for the Jenkins family?

Nurses serve in myriad ways to improve child health and to serve as an advocate for children and their families. Effectively teaching children about resources, self-care, and other health promotion activities is a key role for nurses (Fig. 2-2). Because the intended audience may be children or adults, those with low literacy skills, or those who speak a language other than English, teaching strategies must effectively meet the needs of many types of learners.

An important role for nurses in relation to public health programs and third-party payers is that of child advocate. Not all service systems are child friendly, easy to access, or understandable to those outside the program. Eligibility criteria can be confusing, the application process complicated, or the services offered inadequate.

Another key role for nurses is that of care coordinator or case manager. In this capacity, the nurse attempts to improve access to needed care and reduces gaps or

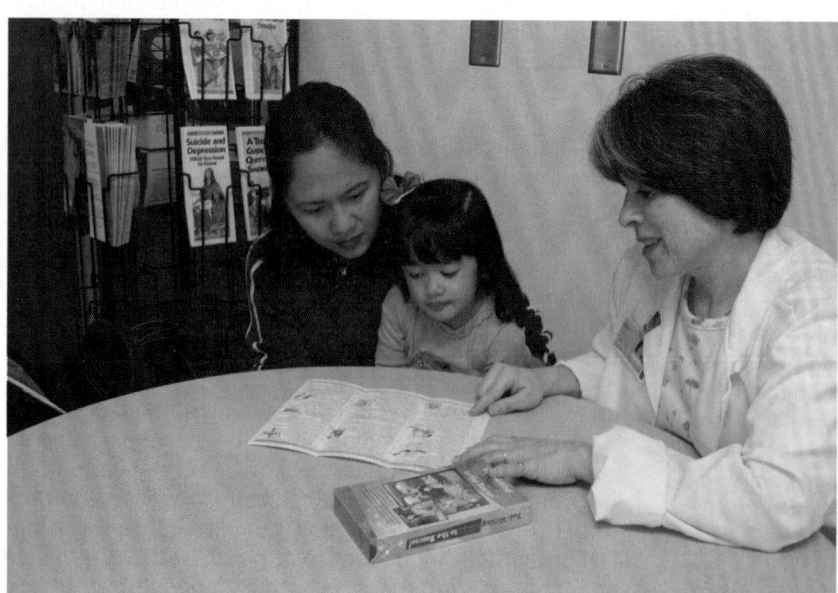

Figure 2-2 Family members must be provided the information they need to promote optimum health and to prevent illness.

duplication in services by developing and implementing an appropriate plan of care. During the care coordination process, nurses assist and collaborate with the child and family to determine their strengths and needs. They then jointly establish goals and develop a plan of care. The plan explicitly states who will do what and when, specifying the person who will assume accountability for each action item. The child and family are periodically reevaluated to determine the appropriateness of the plan and the need for any revision. The case is closed when the child has been transferred to another agency or is no longer in need of services. Case closure is a key element of care coordination, not merely the end. Children and families should be told how and under what circumstances they may reenter the service system. If they are no longer receiving services because they are ineligible, nurses should make every effort to refer them to a program that may be able to serve them.

In addition to working directly with children, nurses may work toward improving child health by developing programs or policies needed to better meet the needs of children and families. Community Care 2-1 summarizes

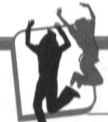

COMMUNITY CARE 2-1

Community Health Care Services for Children and Their Families

Location	Services Provided by the Nurse or Advanced Practice Nurse
Schools School nurse services School-based clinics	Preventive care Primary care Coordination of services (case management) Participation in Individualized Education Programs (IEPs) Child and family advocacy Child and family teaching Consultation to teachers and administrators Program development
Homes Home health care Hospice care Public health care services	Direct patient care Assessments of the home environment Care planning Coordination of services (case management) Child and family teaching Consultation with other health professionals Program development
Community-Based Facilities Skilled nursing facilities Community nursing centers Extended care facilities Shelters Daycare and respite facilities Community clinics Mobile clinics	Direct patient care Environmental assessments Care planning Coordination of services (case management) Child and family teaching Consultation with other health professionals Program development
Specialty Camps For children with medical conditions, disabilities, or special needs	Preventive care Primary care Direct patient care Child and family teaching Consultation with camp staff Program development Environmental assessment First aid and injury education Outdoor safety education

the many interventions the nurse can use to support community health needs. Opportunities to work in the community are available through public health agencies, hospitals, and community-based programs.

Because delivering community-based services often involves more than one agency, the nurse must be especially sensitive to issues of confidentiality. In particular, nurses need to be aware of the effect of the Health Insurance Portability and Accountability Act of 1996 (HIPAA), which required states to reform their health insurance markets to ensure that individuals with preexisting conditions that meet certain criteria could not be excluded from health insurance plans (Anderson et al., 2007). In addition, regulations were put in place to protect patients' privacy in health care settings, including hospitals, doctors' offices, and clinics. This regulatory atmosphere complicates nursing practice because nurses are often called upon to share information as part of their work on behalf of children and their families. Agencies and facilities serving children and families have their own HIPAA guidelines with which the nurse needs to become familiar.

> **ANSWER:** Assisting the family with the forms and paperwork required by the school helps to create a situation in which Lindsay's blood sugar is well managed during school hours. This assistance is a type of advocacy and it has a great impact on Lindsay's current and long-term health. Another example of advocacy is being a member of NAPNAP.

PARENTS' ROLE

> **QUESTION:** How are Lindsay's parents acting as an advocate for their daughter?

The family is the basic system in which health behavior and care are organized, secured, and performed. In most families, the parents or guardians act as advocates for their child and provide health promotion and health prevention care as well as primary management of care when the child is sick. Parents and guardians have the prime responsibility for initiating and coordinating services rendered by health professionals. Because parents have primary responsibility for meeting the health needs of their children, strategies to improve child health must be family centered and appropriately adapted to meet the cultural, language, and learning needs of families. Health practices and the use of health care services vary tremendously from family to family. Assess for the diversity in health care practices and incorporate these family differences into the collaborative plan of care with the family. Encourage parents to take responsibility for learning about resources for their family members and following up when referrals have been offered to them. Likewise, encourage parents to ask questions and challenge information that appears to be incorrect or otherwise limits access to needed services. Nurses can be very helpful in teaching parents to advocate for themselves and their children effectively.

> **ANSWER:** Lindsay's parents are being effective advocates for their daughter by meeting the administrators of the new school prior to school starting and by documenting their daughter's needs. They have also joined two organizations that advocate for children with diabetes.

COMMUNITY'S ROLE

> **QUESTION:** How have some states been an advocate for children?

Communities can help improve the health of children and families by ensuring that resources are available, appropriate, and accessible. For families of children with special health care needs, communities should also ensure access to community activities and resources and should nurture children's participation in them.

To ensure the most comprehensive array of resources for their members, communities should undertake periodic assessments to identify service demands that are not being met and to identify assets and resources in communities that may be mobilized to meet community health needs. Nurses are well positioned to take part in these assessments because they are often involved in multiple facets of community life and are in contact with diverse members of the community in schools, public health clinics, private offices, hospitals, home health agencies, and other local programs where they become aware of unmet needs and available resources.

After an assessment is completed and strengths and deficiencies are identified, communities can develop multiagency collaboratives to meet the needs of community members. Nurses can be involved in this effort to ensure easy entry to needed care and seamless transitions from one program to another; they may also identify gaps and duplications in services. Nurses may participate in community planning meetings to develop strategies for providing services. Participation may also involve seeking funding for proposals by writing grants or making presentations to community groups.

Communities should offer support to children and their families through tangible services such as self-help groups, counseling, food banks, and homeless shelters. Communities should also develop strategies to enhance access to services that already exist. Strategies may involve such ideas as providing free or low-cost local transportation, providing low-cost child care, or collocating services to make one or more programs available at the same site. Improving access may also involve working with individual programs to increase "family friendliness" with extended hours, bilingual or bicultural workers, printed materials in easy-to-read formats, and a clear and simplified application process.

Within the community, employers can also use strategies to improve the health of their employees' children and the community in which they are located. To ease the burden on families to provide health care, employers can provide health insurance, family leave to care for ill family members, and other flexible benefit arrangements to meet individual families' needs. In addition, employers can establish information and referral services for their employees and the community at large to encourage effective use of existing services.

> ANSWER: A few states have enacted legislation beyond the federal laws to protect children with disabilities.

HEALTH CARE DELIVERY RESOURCES FOR CHILDREN AND THEIR FAMILIES

Nurses who provide care to children and families must be knowledgeable about the community and public health resources available to children and their families for several reasons. First, a working knowledge of these programs lets the nurse make appropriate referrals for services to meet specific needs. Second, by knowing how to access the programs and by knowing the services that are offered, the nurse can educate families to apply for appropriate services efficiently and effectively. Applying for public services can be a difficult task because not all service systems are child friendly. If families know which services are available, what to expect, and what paperwork to bring to appointments, they may be more likely to access and use these services. Third, by being aware of the individual programs and the service systems available, the nurse can help coordinate resources and provide referrals in a way that avoids gaps, duplication, and confusion. Fourth, by knowing about these programs, the nurse can help redirect the family if family members receive inaccurate or confusing information or cannot access services for other reasons. Finally, by understanding the service systems and their strengths and limitations, the nurse can advocate with policy makers to improve and ensure adequate funding for care. This section describes the public and private programs that provide financial aid, health services, and educational resources for children in the United States.

PUBLIC PROGRAMS FOR COMMUNITY CARE SERVICES

Many publicly funded health programs serve children and families (see thePoint for Organizations). Some programs serve selected clients, such as those who meet certain income or diagnostic eligibility criteria; others are available to all who apply (Clinical Judgment 2-1).

Programs and agencies that serve children and families, including those with special needs, are constantly in flux. Legislation changes the eligibility, services, and funding for these programs, often from year to year. The programs described in this chapter are, for the most part, susceptible to legislative change and may look different in the future. To be effective in planning, providing, and directing care for children and families, nurses must be aware of these changes and their effects. Self-education can be achieved in a number of ways, including membership in professional organizations;

attendance at conferences; regular review of newsletters, journals, and newspapers; participation in advisory boards; and contact with legislators.

When working within a particular community, establish relationships with professionals from other agencies who may also serve the same clients. The school nurse, for instance, develops relationships with professionals from the local health department clinics; the office of Women, Infants, and Children (WIC); the Head Start program; regional centers; and others to understand the programs fully and to facilitate access to services. In this way, the school nurse serves children more effectively through enhanced collaboration and coordination.

Obtain in-depth information about commonly used programs and services. If you routinely refer families to the WIC program, for instance, these children will be better served if you have a working knowledge of services provided, eligibility requirements, application procedures, waiting periods, any costs involved, and the address and telephone number of the local office. Simply giving a family an agency name and telephone number is not enough to promote access to services. Public agencies often welcome health care visitors from other programs and the community, thereby providing firsthand knowledge about services. Through appropriate referrals to community health programs, you can help ensure the health of the child as well as the entire family (Teaching Intervention Plan 2-1).

Nurses are integral to the success of community health care programs. Many nurses perform outreach services to identify eligible families and encourage participation. Nurses may also serve as program administrators, overseeing operations, ensuring the quality of care offered by various providers, and training providers and their staff in program specifics. Some nurses serve children directly by providing primary care as nurse practitioners or work in supportive and facilitative roles by providing immunizations, teaching patients and families, and coordinating services through case management. Through their numerous contacts with families, nurses are in a position to work toward increasing the number of children receiving these valuable services.

Medicaid

Medicaid is a form of health insurance for low-income and disabled individuals. Established in 1965 as Title XIX of the Social Security Act, Medicaid is a federal **entitlement program** (i.e., an open-ended program that serves all eligible individuals entitled to the service, with no budgetary cap). It is financed by federal and state funds and is administered by the states. Presently, the federal government pays from 50% to 74% of each state's medical assistance payments. Importantly, states are not mandated to participate in the program, but all states do. If a state chooses to participate in Medicaid, it must follow certain federal rules. Medicaid is not a direct provider of service; rather, it provides compensation for health care services. Federal guidelines define the scope of basic services, the extent of coverage, and

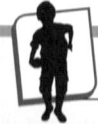

CLINICAL JUDGMENT 2-1

The Child With Multiple Special Needs

Mrs. Thompson has recently moved to the area and is beginning prenatal care in a family practice clinic for low-income families. With her for today's visit is her 2-year-old daughter who is not yet walking, appears small for her age, and has visible dental caries. At the end of Mrs. Thompson's prenatal visit, you ask to speak with her regarding her daughter.

Questions

1. What information do you want to elicit from Mrs. Thompson about her daughter?
2. When Mrs. Thompson answers your questions, which information may be particularly relevant?
3. What are the current possible problems for this child?
4. What interventions or referrals are appropriate for the child and family?
5. What factors would indicate that this child is receiving appropriate services to meet her needs?

Answers

1. What are Mrs. Thompson's perceptions about her daughter? Does she have any concerns about her health or development? Does she have a regular health care provider for her child? Has she received services from any agency or program in the past? What is her daughter's general health and developmental history?
2. A history of health problems or developmental delays, her mother's affirmation or denial that potential health or developmental problems exist, her history of past service use
3. Dental caries, possible developmental delay, possible poor nutritional status, possible lack of appropriate immunizations and other preventive health care
4. Depending on need and current service use, referrals to a pediatric primary health care provider, the local early intervention program, WIC, a pediatric dentist, the local social services agency to apply for food stamps, Medicaid, and Temporary Assistance for Needy Families (TANF), as needed. If special needs are identified, additional referrals may be necessary.
5. The child has an ongoing source of preventive and primary health care; she is enrolled in an early intervention program for assessment, monitoring, and intervention as needed; she receives WIC food coupons to meet her nutritional needs; she receives regular dental care, her mother has received information about preventing dental caries, and the child has had a health supervision visit and is current on her immunizations. She and her family are receiving TANF, Medicaid, and food stamps if determined to be eligible. Additionally, her mother receives WIC coupons as well to promote good nutrition during pregnancy.

TIP 2-1: A TEACHING INTERVENTION PLAN for the Family Accessing Needed Services

Nursing Diagnosis and Family Outcomes

- Readiness for enhanced family coping: Potential for growth related to self-actualization of needs
  Outcomes: Family will successfully receive services to meet child and family needs.
  Family members will verbalize feelings of personal growth.

Guidance for Families

- Assist the family in identifying strengths and needs.
- Identify resources in the community that may be available to meet child and family needs. If none appear to be available, call closely related programs and agencies to ask for referrals or information about needed services.
- Contact prospective agencies to determine services available, eligibility criteria, application procedures (including what the family should bring to apply), location, transportation routes, and any other information specific to the program.
- Present the information to the family. Identify benefits to be gained as a result of program participation.
- Ask the family to help identify impediments to follow-up or use of services so that these obstacles can be minimized whenever possible (e.g., "Is there anything you can think of that will keep you from applying for WIC services?").
- Some agencies and programs allow person-to-person referrals. If this is the case and families request or require this kind of assistance, seek parents' consent and then contact a key individual at the referral agency.
- Advise families to maintain a file of all correspondence, appointment notices, and so on, and to request the name of the individual whenever contact with the agency is made.

certain administrative requirements. The states administer the program and determine income eligibility criteria, specific services to be covered, and payment levels and methods. States may offer optional services beyond those required by federal statute. Because Medicaid is a state-based program, families must be residents of the state in which they apply for services.

Currently, to qualify for Medicaid, individuals must meet both financial eligibility criteria and categorical criteria (i.e., belong to one of the following groups: children, parents, pregnant women, people with disabilities, or seniors). The Patient Protection and Affordable Care Act (PPACA) of 2010 significantly expands Medicaid eligibility. Beginning in 2014, the PPACA establishes a minimum Medicaid coverage threshold for children aged 6 to 19 years and parents with incomes up to 133% of the federal poverty level (FPL). A special deduction to income equal to five percentage points of the FPL raises the effective eligibility level to 138% FPL (Kaiser Family Foundation, 2010). To determine the FPL for any given year, consult the U.S. Department of Health & Human Services website's poverty guidelines (see thePoint for Organizations). These figures are updated annually, and the website includes instructions for using the guidelines. Because programs calculate financial eligibility in different ways, counting certain income and disregarding other income, it is always best to refer a child and family to a program that might be helpful to them and allow program administrators, such as those for Medicaid, to determine eligibility.

Importantly, Medicaid expansion under PPACA also includes non–Medicare eligible adults younger than the age of 65 years without dependent children who are not presently eligible for Medicaid. Children now covered by the CHIP (see the following text) between 100% and 133% FPL will be transitioned to Medicaid. With this expansion, PPACA provides for full federal financing of the Medicaid expansion for the first 3 years, declining to 90% by 2020 and thereafter. In June 2012, in a case known as the *National Federation of Independent Business v. Sebelius* (2012), the United States Supreme Court ruled mandatory Medicaid expansion to be unduly coercive to the states and therefore unconstitutional. As a result, the practical effect is that the Medicaid expansion provision of the PPACA is optional for the states. States that do not implement the PPACA Medicaid expansion but continue to participate in Medicaid must continue to comply with all other provisions of the existing program. Further, states must maintain Medicaid eligibility rules for children that were in place in early 2010 for children until 2019.

Of particular relevance to community-based nurses is the ability to use Medicaid as a source of payment for home or extended care or school-based health services. Because long-term hospitalization can negatively affect a child's growth and development and the entire family's well-being, the option of home care for a seriously ill or disabled child is very important. Through home- and community-based waivers, authorized under the Omnibus Budget Reconciliation Act of 1981 (OBRA 81) and the Tax Equity and Fiscal Responsibility Act of 1982 (TEFRA), state governments can coordinate medical and support services to children living at home, thus avoiding costly institutional care. Eligibility criteria for these programs are broader than Medicaid standards. Thus, more children and families may be served. In addition, individual states may offer expanded medical services and respite care, and under PPACA, states can apply for grants to provide in-home services to at-risk families with children up to kindergarten entry age.

CROSS-CULTURAL CARE

To be eligible to receive Medicaid, an individual must be a citizen or lawfully admitted to the United States. Income-eligible children can qualify if they were born in this country even if their parents are not citizens or reside in this country without appropriate legal documentation. Immigrant children lawfully residing in the United States may also qualify for Medicaid in some states. There are provisions for undocumented children to receive Medicaid for medical emergencies and prenatal care and delivery.

Families may apply for Medicaid at their local welfare offices or at "out-stationed" sites in federally qualified health centers and disproportionate share hospitals (i.e., hospitals that receive extra federal funding to care for large numbers of clients receiving Medicaid). Some states allow a mail-in application for specific Medicaid subpopulations such as pregnant women and children. Waits in welfare offices can be long, and the application process itself can be difficult. These facts may discourage some families from seeking much-needed assistance. Fear of being reported to immigration authorities, or the stigma associated with the receipt of welfare, may discourage families as well (Stuber & Kronebusch, 2004). Importantly, PPACA requires states to establish a state-administered website through which all individuals can apply for Medicaid, the CHIP, or new state-based exchanges through which individuals can purchase coverage and premium and cost-sharing credits are available to individuals and families with income levels between 133% and 400% FPL (Kaiser Family Foundation, 2010). Because children frequently move across insurance programs, it is essential to coordinate resources to support seamless services to children.

The current trend in Medicaid is to encourage recipients to enroll in managed care programs to help contain program costs. In a managed care system, a defined package of services is offered for a preset monthly fee (a premium) paid by Medicaid. The Balanced Budget Act of 1997 altered the structure of the Medicaid program considerably, expanding states' discretion in administering the program and allowing states to require that most Medicaid beneficiaries enroll in managed care programs, most often health maintenance organizations (HMOs).

Each Medicaid recipient enrolled in a managed care program chooses a primary care provider who coordinates and oversees the delivery of health care services to that client. This approach should result in increased access to preventive and primary care and decreased fragmentation of care, especially for low-income individuals who previously had poor access to providers. It is also expected to decrease the use of inappropriate sources of health care, such as emergency departments used for primary care. However, because the managed care plan receives one preset monthly amount to provide all care, the provider may be reluctant to make referrals to expensive specialists or to use high-cost diagnostic tests. The health plan or provider group also may impose financial disincentives to refer.

Although Medicaid provides tremendous benefits to eligible recipients, it has several shortcomings, even with expansion under PPACA. Because of eligibility requirements, the program serves only a portion of those who need it, and eligible individuals whose income increases only modestly may see their benefits cut. These potential cuts are a particular problem for children with special health care needs, for whom ongoing care is vital. Additionally, the near poor or working poor who are uninsured may not qualify for Medicaid but may still have difficulty purchasing health care insurance through exchanges even with premium assistance and cost-sharing credits. Historically, some providers have been unwilling to accept Medicaid because of low reimbursement rates, especially in certain areas—a circumstance that may result in lack of care and inappropriate use of emergency departments. Dentists and mental health providers have particularly low participation rates in serving children eligible for Medicaid services (Kaiser Commission on Medicaid and the Uninsured, 2005). Under PPACA, reimbursement rates for primary care services will increase, but whether this will improve availability of such services for the Medicaid population remains unknown.

Early and Periodic Screening, Diagnostic, and Treatment Program

A very important component of Medicaid for children is the Early and Periodic Screening, Diagnostic, and Treatment (EPSDT) program. This separately mandated program serves Medicaid-eligible individuals younger than age 21 years. As noted earlier, under PPACA, children whose family incomes are between 100% and 133% FPL will be transitioned to Medicaid and, as a result, gain access to EPSDT. As with the basic Medicaid program, providers are reimbursed for services; the EPSDT program is not a direct-service program.

The EPSDT program was enacted through a 1967 amendment to the Social Security Act as a mandatory service under Medicaid. It was established as a federally financed, state-administered program with the goal of ensuring that children enrolled in Medicaid receive a basic set of comprehensive services to promote health and to identify and treat health problems at early stages.

The mission of the EPSDT program is to prevent unnecessary childhood illness, disability, and death by offering prevention services and to identify problems before they become serious. Under the EPSDT program, children receive a variety of comprehensive health services as described in Chart 2-1. States must help children receive these services by informing eligible families about the program, helping families make appointments,

---

| CHART 2-1 | Early and Periodic Screening, Diagnostic, and Treatment Required Services |

Comprehensive health and developmental history (including physical and mental health and nutritional status)

Comprehensive unclothed physical examination with appropriate follow-up care

Vision and hearing service with appropriate follow-up care

Immunizations

Appropriate laboratory tests including blood lead level and radiographic services

Comprehensive preventive, restorative, and emergency dental care

Health education

Anticipatory guidance

Any medically necessary treatment for identified conditions

Pregnancy care including pregnancy testing; medical care, nutritional assessments, and psychosocial assessments; counseling on hazards of tobacco, drug, and alcohol use; vitamins; childbirth education and parent training; and family planning services

---

arranging transportation, providing services in a timely fashion, and ensuring an adequate supply of providers. EPSDT services may be provided by physicians, nurse practitioners, and physician assistants in clinics, schools, hospitals, health departments, and Head Start programs.

caREminder

Adolescents, too often overlooked, are eligible to receive EPSDT benefits and should be encouraged to do so. Developmentally appropriate examinations and anticipatory guidance to prevent sexually transmitted diseases, pregnancy, and drug and alcohol use are components of the program. The examinations may be used as camp or sports physicals to allow teenagers the opportunity to participate in these activities.

Children's Health Insurance Program

The Balanced Budget Act of 1997 authorized the State Children's Health Insurance Program (S-CHIP) as Title XXI of the Social Security Act. In February 2009, the program was reauthorized under the Children's Health Insurance Program Reauthorization Act of 2009 (CHIPRA); in 2010, PPACA further modified the program, now known simply as "CHIP." Like Medicaid, CHIP is a state–federal partnership in which the federal government contributes a percentage of the funding and each state provides the balance. Initially, the purpose of this program was to expand health insurance to children whose families made too much money to qualify for Medicaid but who could not afford to purchase health insurance. As a result of the original legislation, states had three options: to expand their Medicaid eligibility to include children of families with higher incomes, to establish a separate health insurance program for higher income families, or to use a combination of these two approaches to achieve the goal of insuring more children. CHIPRA reauthorized the program through 2013, provided additional funding and programmatic options for states to promote efficient and effective strategies to identify, enroll, and retain health coverage for uninsured children who are eligible for Medicaid or CHIP but who are not enrolled. The legislation also required the development of standards by which states can measure the quality of care that children are receiving. The PPACA extends CHIP through 2015, maintains CHIP eligibility standards in place as of early 2010 through 2019, and provides additional federal funding to the states.

Service delivery varies from state to state, but many states use a managed care model for the CHIP program to provide cost-effective and comprehensive services. The benefit package may be less comprehensive than that of Medicaid but includes health, dental, and vision coverage and must be equal to the federal employees' health insurance plan, the state employees' health insurance plan, or that of the largest commercial HMO in a state. States may require that families pay a part of the cost through modest premiums or copayments. Copayments for preventive services are not permitted, nor can Native American/Alaskan native children who are members of a recognized tribe be charged any copayments.

Nurses can help to reduce the number of uninsured children by being aware of the various public insurance programs and the services they provide, knowing how to refer families to programs, and assisting them in applying. Activities such as follow-up phone calls and educational programs may help to increase awareness and to improve enrollment in public insurance programs. Many of the nation's uninsured children are eligible for a publicly funded program; however, their parents may be unaware of the program or do not think they would qualify. Promoting and ensuring the health of children through adequate insurance is the responsibility of all nurses.

caREminder

Because each state varies in how it provides CHIP coverage and how it determines who is eligible for the program, nurses need to become familiar with the CHIP program in the state in which they work to provide families with accurate information.

Special Supplemental Food Program for Women, Infants, and Children

WIC provides nutritious food, health education, and links to health care resources to pregnant and lactating women, infants younger than 1 year of age, and children up to age 5 years who are at risk for nutritional problems. Since its inception in 1974, the WIC program has expanded to serve more families and provide other activities such as outreach. The program is funded by the Food and Nutrition Service of the U.S. Department of Agriculture and is administered through grants to states and then to local health and human services organizations. Some states offer additional financial support to the program. Eligibility for the program is based on financial need and a demonstrated risk for the development or presence of a nutrition-related health problem, such as iron-deficiency anemia. The program is not an entitlement—that is, it is not required to serve everyone who is eligible—and it operates within a fixed budget determined each year by Congress. As a result, not all eligible families can be served. Pregnant and lactating women and infants up to age 1 year receive priority, followed by children up to age 5 years. Almost all pregnant women with a family income at or below 185% of the FPL qualify for WIC.

WIC provides coupons that families use to purchase specific foods meant to provide certain key nutrients, such as protein; iron; calcium; and vitamins A, C, and D. Typically, such foods include infant formula, cheese, eggs, iron-fortified baby and regular cereals, fruit juice, beans, and peanut butter. The coupons can be used at most grocery stores, although some agencies distribute food directly (Fig. 2-3).

caREminder

Some mothers may feel self-conscious using WIC coupons, feeling that others view them in a negative light. Frequent reminders and support by the nurse about the importance of good nutrition during pregnancy and infancy may help mothers refocus on the importance and necessity of this program.

WIC includes an educational component. Each family meets with a nutritionist to assess and discuss specific needs. In addition, classes are held periodically on nutrition-related topics and such topics as breastfeeding, car seat use, and immunizations. WIC staff members recognize that breast milk is the preferred form of infant nutrition and therefore promote breastfeeding through educational programs, one-on-one and group support, and breast pump loaner programs.

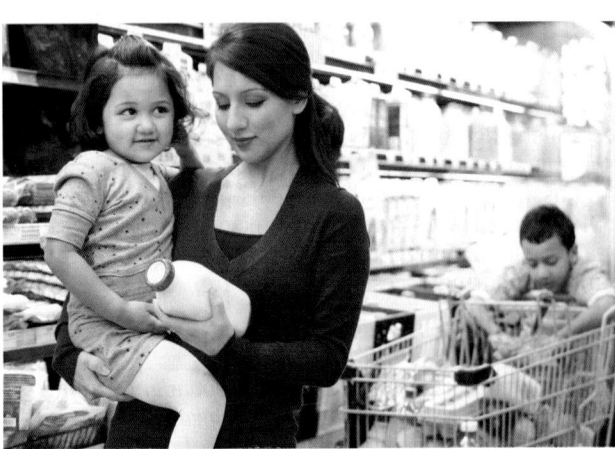

Figure 2-3 WIC provides coupons so eligible recipients can purchase healthy food items for their families.

WIC provides important links to health care providers, social services, and other public programs (such as Medicaid) to ensure that all children receive appropriate care. Some WIC offices are freestanding. Many are located in health department clinics so that families can access many services in one location. The program also includes outreach and, in certain areas, transportation to WIC offices.

Supplemental Security Income for the Aged, Blind, and Disabled

Supplemental Security Income (SSI) is a program that provides monthly payments to income-eligible individuals who are older than age 65 years, blind, or disabled. Payments vary based on income, living arrangements, and other factors. The money can be used as income or to purchase services not otherwise available, including caregiving assistance. For parents of a disabled child, the money also can pay for incidental expenses related to health care, such as parking or child care, or can help compensate for the loss of income resulting from the need to care for the child.

The program was enacted as part of the Social Security Amendments of 1972. The federal government provides matching funds to the states, which determine income eligibility guidelines and payment levels. In most states, families receiving SSI also receive Medicaid and may receive food stamps. In some states, the food stamp allotment is included in the monthly SSI payment.

A child who is a citizen or a lawful permanent resident of the United States is eligible for SSI benefits even if the parents are neither. The child also must meet certain income eligibility criteria based on the family's income and resources. Finally, the child must be medically eligible.

Children may be determined to be disabled because of physical, mental, or developmental disorders. An appeals process exists for children found to be ineligible for SSI benefits. Parents may initiate this process if they feel a determination has been made erroneously. If they file an appeal, the child may be required to see a medical provider with whom the family is unfamiliar, chosen by the Social Security Administration (SSA) to offer an additional opinion about the child's eligibility. This examination is provided at no cost to the family.

Nurses play an important role in ensuring that all potentially eligible children are referred to the SSI program. Because supportive documentation is needed to establish eligibility, nurses may help families gather and submit appropriate records and may provide support and assistance during the appeals process. Because the SSI program is an important link to Medicaid in most states, establishing eligibility for SSI can be very important in ensuring access to health care.

caREminder

Instruct families to save all correspondence from the SSA as well as copies of any documentation sent to the agency in case additional or duplicate information is needed.

Maternal and Child Health Services Block Grant

The Maternal and Child Health Services Block Grant (Title V of the Social Security Act), originally enacted in 1935, provides federal funds to the states for preventive, primary, and specialty care for pregnant women, mothers, infants, children, and adolescents. In this federal–state partnership, the states contribute a minimum of $3 for each $4 of federal money received. Currently, Title V includes three components: the maternal and child health (MCH) program, the Children with Special Health Care Needs (CSHCN) program (formerly the Crippled Children's Services program), and two discretionary grant programs—Special Projects of Regional and National Significance (SPRANS) and Community Integrated Service Systems (CISS). SPRANS projects include grants for MCH research and training, genetic disease services, hemophilia services, and other projects to improve MCH. SPRANS programs provide grants through a competitive process to health departments, universities, and other community agencies for research, training, genetic disease education, testing, counseling, referral and follow-up, regionalized hemophilia care, and innovative demonstration projects. CISS grants support home visiting programs, projects to increase the numbers of obstetricians and pediatricians who serve poor children, integrated MCH delivery systems, pregnancy services, and services for children with special health care needs.

The states must use the block grant funds to develop an MCH system that ensures comprehensive, coordinated services to improve the health of all mothers and children. They must direct these services to low-income families and those with poor access to services. Chart 2-2 defines states' goals for the MCH block grant funds. They may carry out this mandate by providing services

---

CHART 2-2   States' Goals for the Use of Maternal Child Health Block Grant Funds

- To provide and ensure access to quality MCH services for mothers and children (especially those with low income or limited availability to services)

- To reduce the incidences of infant mortality, preventable disease, and handicapping conditions in children; to reduce the need for inpatient and long-term care; to increase the number of children appropriately immunized; to increase the number of low-income children receiving health assessments and follow-up diagnostic and treatment services; to provide prenatal, delivery, and postpartum care to at-risk women; and to promote the health of children by providing preventive and primary care to low-income children

- To provide rehabilitation services for blind and disabled individuals younger than age 16 years receiving benefits under Title XVI (SSI) when those services are not provided by Medicaid

- To provide and promote family-centered, community-based care (including care coordination services) to children with special health care needs and their families and to facilitate the development of community-based systems of services for such children and their families directly or by promoting access to services through program development, coordination, or oversight. Individual states may establish their own priorities and use the money to provide MCH services within the state according to local, regional, and statewide needs.

At the state level, MCH services are managed through the state health agency. Services are usually delivered by local health departments. Private physicians, hospital-based clinics, community health centers, and school-based clinics may also be involved in MCH service delivery through grants, contracts, or reimbursement to independent community agencies and providers. The organizational structure, staff responsibilities, and specific programs and services vary from state to state. To avoid duplication and to ensure effectiveness, states must coordinate and integrate services with other programs, including health (such as the EPSDT program), social services, child nutrition (such as WIC), and education at the state and local levels.

People are often confused about Title V and Medicaid. Title V provides money to states, which determine how it will be used to improve the health of *all* women and children, especially those at high risk or living in poverty. It requires the states to develop systems that ensure access to high-quality care. Unlike Medicaid, Title V is not an entitlement program; rather, it provides a set level of funding to each state as determined by Congress. Medicaid is a form of health insurance for low-income, disabled, and elderly persons that focuses on primary acute and long-term care and only *reimburses* for services. Title V programs, in contrast, may provide services directly (for instance, in a community prenatal clinic) or may be used to plan for a comprehensive service system in a community. In fact, a family may visit a prenatal clinic established with Title V funds but may pay for the clinic's services with Medicaid.

Nurses play various important roles in MCH programs. For instance, in a maternity care program that uses Title V funds, nurses may serve as nurse midwives or nurse practitioners delivering primary care (Fig. 2-4). They may also be involved in delivering clinic, patient education, case management, or care coordination services. Within a CSHCN program, nurses may be responsible for a range of services, from case finding to determining family eligibility, developing plans of care, making referrals, coordinating services, and providing patient care. In a number of states, the director of the CSHCN program is a nurse.

Temporary Assistance for Needy Families

TANF is an assistance program developed in 1997 as a successor to the Aid to Families with Dependent Children (AFDC) program to provide cash assistance to indigent American families with dependent children. The program aims to provide assistance to needy families so that the children can be cared for in their own homes or in the homes of relatives. The program has commonly been known in the past as "welfare." In the current TANF program, there is a maximum of 60 months of benefits within one's lifetime and there is a component that requires recipients to attempt to find employment. Failure to participate in work requirements can result in a reduction or termination of benefits to the family. Unmarried minor parents have to live with a responsible adult or guardian. Paternity of children must be established to receive benefits. As with other assistance programs, it is important for the pediatric nurse to be aware of resources and refer families to such services as appropriate.

Community and Migrant Health Centers

Authorized by Title II of the Public Health Service Act, Community and Migrant Health Centers (C/MHCs) are federally funded, comprehensive primary care clinics, usually located in medically underserved areas. The program was established in 1965 and is administered by the Bureau of Primary Health Care, U.S. Public Health Service. C/MHCs provide basic preventive and primary care; ancillary services such as laboratory tests, radiographs, and pharmacy; and related services such as health education, transportation, translation, and referrals of families to other programs such as WIC and Medicaid. Each facility is governed by a board, with board members who are users of the clinic services. A major component of these clinics is MCH services, which are designed to decrease infant mortality rates and to improve the health of mothers and children, especially those from low-income families.

Nurses function in a variety of roles in these clinics. They may provide direct services such as primary care, core public health functions, traditional clinic support, patient and family teaching, and case management, and they may be involved in clinic administration. Nurse midwives and nurse practitioners play a substantial role in delivering primary care, improving access, and helping to control costs. Because a center may offer a wide range of services, from prenatal to pediatric to adult care, the nurse can draw on expertise from a variety of areas. Also, because the center may provide preventive and primary care to all members of a particular family, the nurse may get to know the entire family and be able to affect the family's overall health and well-being positively.

To refer children and coordinate care properly, nurses who work outside C/MHCs should know the system, the location of local clinics, the services they offer, and procedures for accessing services.

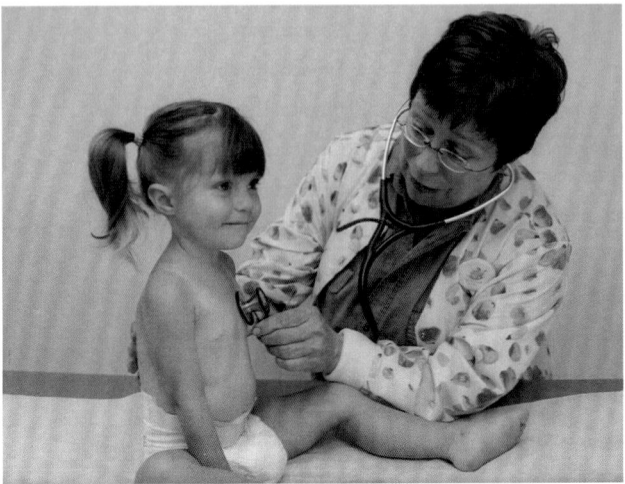

Figure 2-4 Using Title V funds, nurse practitioners can provide child health care to eligible families.

Americans With Disabilities Act

The Americans with Disabilities Act of 1990 consists of civil rights laws that prohibit discrimination based on disability. The Act defines disability as a physical or mental impairment that substantially limits a major life activity. The determination of whether any particular condition is considered a disability is made on a case-by-case basis. Certain specific conditions are excluded as disabilities, such as current substance abuse and transsexuality. These laws affect the care of children and adolescents in several ways. For instance, the law requires that no individual may be discriminated against on the basis of disability with regard to the full and equal enjoyment of public goods, services, facilities, or accommodations. Children and others with disabilities must have access to buildings with stairs and be able to ride on amusement park rides similar to nondisabled children. In addition, the law helps adolescents seeking employment because it ensures that people with disabilities are not discriminated against as they apply for jobs and receive the benefits and privileges of employment. The law also states public transportation systems, such as public transit buses, must be accessible to individuals with disabilities. Nurses can work with families to ensure the rights of their children under this law are being maintained, especially in the children's school and other places where the children participate in extracurricular activities.

EDUCATION PROGRAMS FOR CHILDREN WITH SPECIAL HEALTH CARE NEEDS

Many nurses play a critical role in providing health services in schools and early intervention programs for children with special health care needs and their families. Nurses who do not work in these areas must understand the types of services offered and know which children may be eligible to receive them to be able to refer families and coordinate services. This section describes the key education and early intervention legislation focusing on children with special needs. It also discusses how the nurse may assist in providing services. Chapter 13 supplies additional information about the ways these programs can support the needs of chronically ill children.

 QUESTION: In which of the following programs is Lindsay eligible and participating?

The Education for All Handicapped Children Act

Public Law 94-142, the Education for All Handicapped Children Act, was enacted in 1975 and became effective in 1977. This law represented an educational bill of rights for handicapped children. It required free, appropriate, and individualized education in the least-restrictive environment for individuals 6 to 21 years of age and mandated procedural protections to ensure that these requirements were met. The Education for All Handicapped Children Act Amendment of 1986 (Public Law 99-457) mandated early intervention services for 3- to 5-year-olds (previously an optional service to be provided at states' discretion) through comprehensive, coordinated, and interdisciplinary statewide programs. In addition, it required each state to develop a plan to serve children from birth through 2 years who are at risk for developmental disabilities. The law provided financial assistance to states to develop and implement the plan, to facilitate coordination of payments for early intervention services, and to provide for quality services. Agencies under this federal mandate included those dealing with education, health, human services, developmental disabilities, mental health, public welfare, children, and youth through an interagency coordinating council. Table 2-1 describes which children must be served, professionals who may be involved, and which services may be provided.

TABLE 2–1	Education for All Handicapped Children Act (Public Law 99–457*) and the Individuals With Disabilities Education Improvement Act (Public Law 108–446†)	
Who Will Be Served	**Who May Provide Services**	**Services That May Be Provided**
Child with a delay in physical, cognitive, language and speech, psychosocial, and/or self-help skills	Nurses	Assessments
	Physicians	Speech therapy
Child with a known physical or mental condition resulting in developmental delay (e.g., Down syndrome)	Special educators	Physical therapy
	Speech–language professionals (pathologists and audiologists)	Occupational therapy
Child at risk for developmental delay (this may be a biologic or environmental risk such as perinatal maternal substance abuse)		Infant stimulation
	Occupational and physical therapists	Counseling
	Psychologists	Home visits
	Social workers	Case management
	Nutritionists	Psychological services
		Health services
		Special education
		Family training

*1986.
†2004.

The law also requires that care be provided in a family-centered manner, with active participation of family members in developing the plan, choosing providers, and designating a service coordinator (see Chapter 1 for a discussion of family-centered care). It requires the development of an Individualized Family Service Plan (IFSP) for each child served. This is an interdisciplinary plan developed to determine the specific health outcomes sought for a child and the services and support that will be provided to the child and the family to help the child meet these outcomes. Specific components of an IFSP plan are described in Chart 2-3.

Nurses help identify appropriate infants, young children, and families and assist them in accessing needed early-intervention services through appropriate referrals, education about potential services, and follow-up. Children who are prospects for early intervention may be identified in neonatal or pediatric intensive care units, general pediatric units or newborn nurseries, outpatient clinics, physicians' offices, or anywhere else the nurse has contact with children and families. During the course of a truly family-centered approach to delivering care, the nurse may even identify siblings of children already in the program or children of adult patients who may benefit from early intervention services.

Within the early intervention service system, nurses play a variety of important roles while working in schools, agencies for children with special health care needs, regional centers for the developmentally disabled, home health agencies, private case management companies, or outpatient clinics. Nurses may be involved in interdisciplinary assessments, serve as case managers, provide education and support to families as they work their way through the system, or provide direct service as defined in the IFSP.

The Individuals With Disabilities Education Improvement Act

The IDEA was the primary federal program that authorized state and local aid for special education and related services for children with disabilities. The legislation was reauthorized in 2004 and is now called the Individuals with Disabilities Education Improvement Act (IDEIA). This law changed the name of special needs students from "handicapped children" to "children with disabilities." This law also established the right of adolescent students to receive further education or employment as early as age 16 years. The law also required special education to begin as early as 3 years old. Under IDEIA, educational services are to be offered to students with disabilities from the time they are young children until the time they received a stable job (Slavin, 2006).

Another component of the law requires an IEP plan for all children receiving services. An *IEP* is the individualized education program to be provided for the child with a disability and the written documentation that describes this educational program, which has been mutually decided by the school, parents, and child (when appropriate). The IEP must be child centered and must address the long-term developmental needs of the child. The law outlines many procedural requirements for determining eligibility and maintaining ongoing assessments of children and their educational outcomes. Individual states have guidelines indicating time frames within which the steps of the IEP must take place. In addition, an appeals process exists to allow parents an avenue for resolving conflicts with school or other professionals about the plan. Typically, the family approaches the school principal or the district's special education unit to request changes to the IEP or to request an appeal. All requests should be in writing, and the parents should keep a copy for their reference.

caREminder

Parents/legal guardians must be notified of IEP meetings. They may bring additional support persons of their choosing, such as child advocates, lawyers, psychologists, friends, and relatives. Parents must sign a form indicating they have been informed about the IEP. They do not have to agree with the plan details and they may request or appeal for changes.

Encourage parents to be actively involved in the IEP process, which includes assessments, plan development, referrals, and periodic reevaluation (see Teaching Intervention Plan 30-1). Nurses may be involved in the IEP process in a variety of ways. They may inform team members about the child's health care needs, help interpret complicated medical reports, be involved in making referrals or recommendations, and may also provide support to families through appropriate advocacy (Fig. 2-5). Although these tasks are most likely carried out by the school nurse, they may also be performed by a child's home health care, hospital, or clinic-based nurse, or one involved in providing transition for the child from another program, because parents are allowed to invite additional professionals to the IEP meetings.

CHART 2-3 **Components of the Individualized Family Service Plan**

Statement of family's concerns about their child *at this time*

Assessment of family strength and needs

Present level of development (physical, cognitive, communicative, socio-emotional, and adaptive)

Major outcomes for the child and family

Specific services needed to meet needs, including frequency, intensity, and method of delivery

Dates for initiating and completing the services

Any modifications of outcomes or services needed

Identification of a case manager

Transition plan (to other services providers)

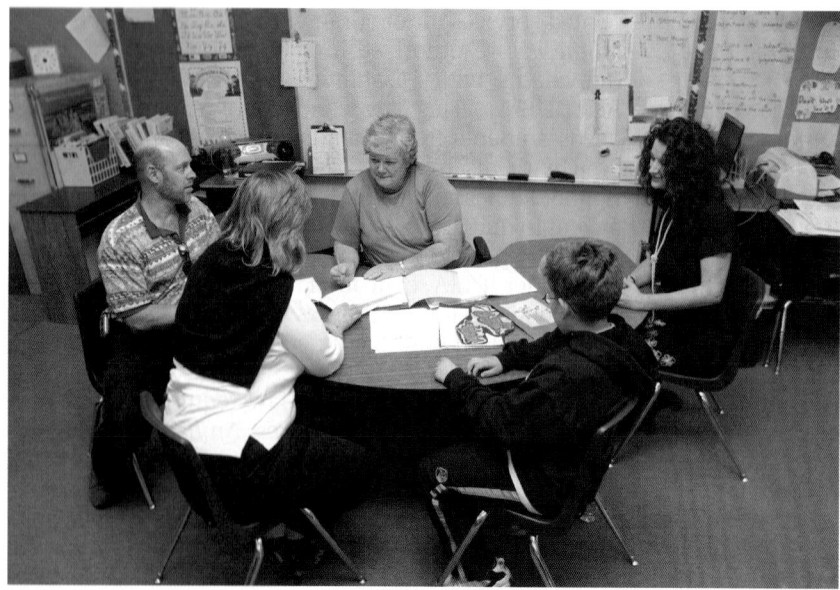

Figure 2-5 The nurse plays an active role in initiating and implementing IEPs in the school.

Section 504 of the Rehabilitation Act of 1973

Another avenue exists to obtain assistance in school settings for children with special health care needs. Section 504 of the Rehabilitation Act of 1973 assures students with disabilities the right to a free public education with other students without disabilities as appropriate and to the maximum extent possible. Students with chronic medical conditions who are in a regular education program can receive reasonable accommodations to assist them with their special health care needs while attending school. For example, students with type 1 diabetes are entitled to reasonable accommodations to test their blood glucose levels and to inject insulin. Parents, teachers, physicians, or school nurses can request a 504 Plan for students with disabilities that restrict one or more major life activities, such as caring for one's self, performing manual tasks, walking, seeing, hearing, speaking, breathing, working, and learning. The school must then meet with the parents to discuss the situation and to determine what must be done to integrate the child's health needs into the educational program (see Teaching Intervention Plan 30-1).

> **ANSWER:** Lindsay has a 504 Plan with her school and an IEP plan. The 504 Plan entitles her to manage her diabetes at school. The IEP plan is related to educational challenges of a child with a chronic condition.

Head Start

Another program that serves preschoolers, including those with special health care needs, is the Head Start program. Head Start, begun in 1965 by the U.S. Office of Economic Opportunity, is funded by the federal U.S. Department of Health & Human Services, Administration on Children, Youth and Families. It is a child development program aimed at preparing low-income preschoolers for school entry by including child development, school readiness, health, nutrition services, and linkages to other social services in its program focus. Early Head Start is a program similar to Head Start that targets low-income pregnant women and children, from birth to 3 years of age, and their parents. Early Head Start programs are not as well funded as Head Start nor are they as widely available.

Substantial health, educational, and social benefits have been noted among children who have participated in the program (Silverstein et al., 2003). The program is locally administered by community-based, nonprofit organizations; Native American tribes; and school systems (Administration for Children and Families, 2011).

The Head Start program has four major components: health (including medical, dental, mental health, and nutrition services), education, parent involvement, and social services. The health component includes examinations; immunizations; health education for children, families, and staff; and meals and snacks that meet at least one third of the daily nutritional needs of the children. In addition, referrals to health care providers are made. Health services and health education are often provided by an on-site nurse. Each child participating in Head Start is required to have a physical examination, which is oftentimes performed by a nurse practitioner.

The education component is designed to meet a preschooler's individual learning needs, such as an introduction to the concepts of numbers and letters. Additionally, it meets the ethnic and cultural needs of the communities it serves by, for instance, providing bilingual teachers. Parents are encouraged to be actively involved in the program by helping in the classroom, serving on advisory committees, and attending parent education programs. The social services component offers families referrals to other programs and resources.

Head Start is required to provide services to children with special health care needs. Ten percent of its enrollment must be available to these children. Head Start programs may coordinate services with other programs— such as the developmental disabilities, early intervention, and mental health systems—or public school special education to meet the special needs of individual students.

Nurses are often involved in Head Start programs by serving on advisory boards and by providing direct services to children. In addition, nurses may serve as consultants, providing health education programs to staff, children, and parents, or may be involved in assisting program staff to develop strategies to address prevalent health problems, such as childhood obesity or asthma.

No Child Left Behind Act

The No Child Left Behind (NCLB) Act of 2001 is legislation designed to ensure that every child in the United States receives a proper education. Congress passed the NCLB Act in January 2002, which aims to increase the performance of primary and secondary schools in the United States by holding states, school districts, schools, and educators more accountable for the success of each student. NCLB requires states to have annual standardized tests given to at least 95% of all students. The tests are designed to assess the adequate yearly progress of students in reading and math. These standardized tests must be given to students once a year in grades 3 through 8 and once in grades 10 through 12. NCLB requires annual reports to be sent to parents that include graduation rates, teacher information, and test assessments broken down by subgroups. NCLB has negative sanctions for schools that fail to meet adequate yearly progress standards. After 2 years, a failing school must provide paid busing and school choice to students; after 5 years of failing, a school will be taken over and managed completely by state authorities. This act promotes an increased emphasis on reading, especially for young children. NCLB also provides more flexibility to parents in choosing which school their children will attend (Essex, 2006). Even though this act was not specifically aimed at students with special education needs, the concept of "leaving no one behind" means that students with disabilities are able to benefit greatly from the measures in this legislation (Zipkin, 2007). Implementation of NCLB has been challenging and reform in the future is likely.

PRIVATE PROGRAMS FOR COMMUNITY CARE SERVICES

QUESTION: Which private program do you think provides a summer camp for children with diabetes?

A wide range of community-based services, from preventive, primary, and specialty care to respite and long-term care, are available to children and families. Children may receive health and related services in schools, clinics, day-care programs, camps, homeless shelters, and other locations in which nurses are often key to service delivery.

In addition to publicly funded programs previously described, a number of charitable and nonprofit organizations exist to serve children with special needs and

their families. Groups such as the Muscular Dystrophy Association, the American Cancer Society, Easter Seals, and others may provide direct assistance to families in the form of transportation, equipment, or special camps for children. They may also aid families by providing educational materials geared toward children and adults. Often, services are offered for free or at a minimal cost. Many of these organizations also provide written resource materials or courses and conferences for professionals and fund research activities (see thePoint for Organizations).

The Internet has given professionals and families alike the opportunity to search for additional resources to help them care for their children who are developing typically as well as those with special health care needs. Although not all families have access to the Internet in their homes, public and school libraries and family resource centers (FRCs) have computers available for public use and often have paid or volunteer staff available to assist families in seeking information. When referring families to the Internet for information, warn them that some information may not be appropriate to their particular child or situation and that consultation with their health care provider can help clarify the quality and appropriateness of the information they find.

A resource often not known to nurses but of tremendous benefit to families is the FRC. FRCs are located in communities within schools, hospitals, public health departments, clinics, and other public agencies. They provide information and support to families of children with special needs and help to educate families about their child's condition and the system of care. They are often staffed by parent volunteers or parent professionals. In addition to providing information, they can often link families with other families for parent-to-parent support. Family Voices is a grassroots advocacy organization for families and providers of children with special health care needs (see thePoint for Organizations). With chapters in each state, they are often able to assist families in locating resources, including their local FRC.

Nurses should identify resources within children's communities and become familiar with the eligibility requirements and services offered. In addition, nurses can support the work of these groups by sitting on advisory committees, volunteering within organizations, or supporting fundraising efforts.

ANSWER: Each summer, Lindsay attends a camp sponsored by the American Diabetes Association. In Chapter 12, "Chronic Conditions as a Challenge to Health Maintenance," you can see the effect summer camp has on Lindsay and her family.

ETHICAL ISSUES IN THE CARE OF CHILDREN

Nurses are frequently called upon to advocate for children about ethical issues related to the care of children. Nurses may find themselves in situations that require

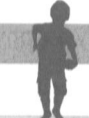

EVIDENCE-BASED CLINICAL PRACTICE GUIDELINES 2-1

Ethical Guidelines Impacting the Care of Children and Their Families

Schenk, K., & Williamson, J. (2005). *Ethical approaches to gathering information from children and adolescents in international settings: Guidelines and resources.* Washington, DC: The Population Council. Retrieved from

http://www.popcouncil.org/pdfs/horizons/childrenethics.pdf

Practical guidance on collecting information from and about young people in regard to such issues as HIV and AIDS. This applies equally well to gathering information from young people to address other health and social welfare conditions and difficult circumstances, such as those who have experienced abuse, trafficking, or displacement.

National Association for the Education of Young Children. (2005). *Code of ethical conduct and statement of commitment.* Retrieved from

http://www.naeyc.org/files/naeyc/file/positions/PSETH05.pdf

Guidelines for responsible behavior and to set forth a common basis for resolving the principal ethical dilemmas encountered in early childhood care and education.

Society for Research in Child Development. (2007). *Ethical standards in research.* Retrieved from

http://www.srcd.org/about-us/ethical-standards-research

Sixteen principles to govern practices by researchers when children are used as research subjects.

United Nations. (1959). *Declaration of the Rights of the Child.* Retrieved from

http://www.un.org/cyberschoolbus/humanrights/resources/child.asp

Declaration of the rights and freedoms that should be afforded every child.

U.S. Department of Health & Human Services, Office for Human Research Protections. (2006). *Special protections for children as research subjects.* Retrieved from

http://www.hhs.gov/ohrp/policy/populations/children.html

Regulatory requirements that must be provided for children involved in research.

ethical decision making related to concerns of informed consent, parental permission, and child assent as well as the challenging treatment issues encountered in the care of critically, chronically, or terminally ill children. Evidence-Based Clinical Practice Guidelines 2-1 provides a summary of best practices the nurse and other care providers can employ to ensure the ethical rights of children and their families are protected when providing health care, conducting research, and collecting information.

Ethical decision making should not be a unilateral process pursued solely by one health care professional. The values of the patient and family must be ascertained and considered, and nursing input is important and often sought. Every institution has an **institutional ethics committee (IEC)**, which is required by The Joint Commission. The IEC should always be consulted in difficult or unusual cases when conflict and lack of agreement exists between parents and physicians or among the professional staff regarding the course of action that is in the best interest of the child. The purpose of having an IEC is to educate health care professionals, patients, and families about ethical issues and to provide individual case consultation and recommendations based on an ethical analysis of the relevant facts and feelings of all parties. The IEC's deliberation may shed new light on the situation, help with conflict resolution, and enhance communication between health care providers and parents; it may also provide

needed guidance about whether to continue life-sustaining medical treatment (LSMT) or to transition from a "cure" to a "care" treatment focus.

DECISION MAKING AND INFORMED CONSENT

Informed consent is a legal condition whereby a person is said to have given consent based on an appreciation and understanding of the facts and implications of an action. Adults have the right to self-determination for medical care after consultation with a physician or other health care provider, and their voluntary and informed decisions generally focus on personal preferences and values. Until children reach the age of majority or are *legally emancipated* (see the "Rights of Emancipated Minors" section later in this chapter), they lack the legal empowerment and often the decisional capacity (the ability to reason, deliberate, and analyze the elements in decision making) to make medical decisions on their own. The age at which a child or adolescent can legally exercise voluntary and informed consent for treatment without parental permission varies from state to state and also depends on the medical condition. For example, treatment for sexually transmitted infections, family planning, and drug or alcohol abuse may not require parental consent, depending on state statutes.

The principles of informed consent for research participation are discussed in detail in the research section

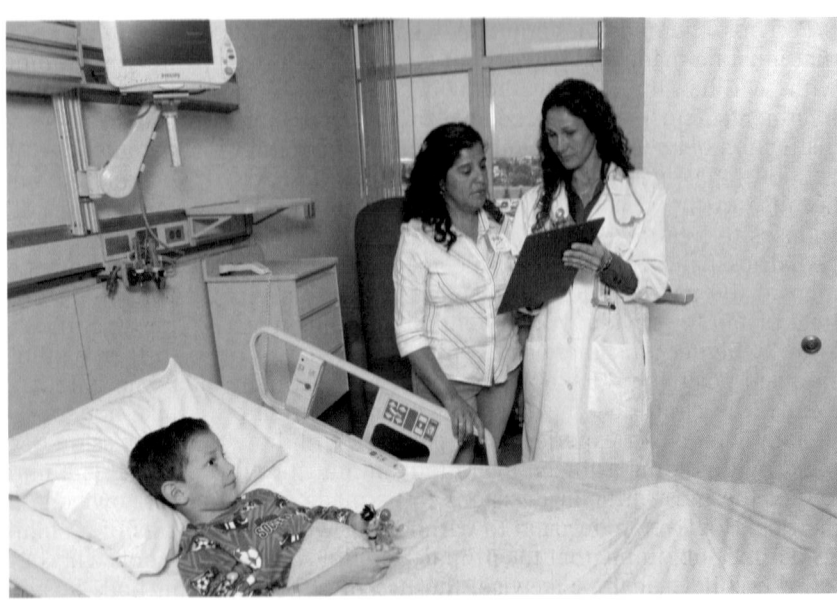

Figure 2-6 Obtaining informed consent from a child's responsible parent is essential before any procedure. A signed form, however, does not mean that full disclosure has occurred.

of this chapter. The key ethical issues related to informed consent for treatment have similarities to those required for research participation: Consent must be voluntary and based on shared information about the risks and benefits of the treatment. Furthermore, the parent must understand the information and be cognitively and mentally competent to make the decision (Fig. 2-6).

Nurses are in a position to alert physicians or others if they determine that the parent or child does not comprehend or lacks the decision-making capacity to give voluntary informed consent or **assent** (i.e., agreement to participate in a procedure or in research). A situation could also arise in which the nurse believes the physician has unduly coerced parents in their treatment decision. Such intentional or unintentional action violates ethical principles of conduct, and the nurse is obliged to intervene and disclose any concerns to the health care administration or IEC. Other ethical problems can arise when dissension occurs between parents or when the wishes of parents conflict with those of an older child or teen. Respect for a child's developing capacity for autonomy and self-determination requires that the child's wishes be considered and that the child agree with the decision being made.

After the parents and the child have been informed of the treatment options, after all health care options are considered, and after the wishes of the parents and child are known, the underlying ethical principle that must guide the overall decision-making process is to determine what is in the best interest of the child. Parents do not have the sole right to determine whether their decision is in the child's best interest, and the child does not have the sole right to dissent if the intervention is deemed essential to his or her welfare. For older children to give their assent, they need help to understand their condition and what they can expect as the outcome of treatment. In addition, the child must be cognitively able to comprehend this information, not feel pressured into a decision, and must willingly agree to the proposed intervention. For example, if a

16-year-old girl tells the nurse that she does not want to undergo the final stage of plastic surgery to repair a cleft lip deformity and her parents have signed the consent, the nurse would participate as an advocate for the child, voicing the child's desire to not have the surgery.

SANCTITY AND QUALITY OF LIFE

Life is sacred; thus, health care professionals must always act in a manner that respects the **sanctity of life**. Likewise, their actions must focus on doing what is in the child's best interest to achieve an acceptable **quality of life**. These two concepts are closely linked and provide the foundations for much of the decision making in challenging ethical situations. The health care provider is obligated to focus on these two basic principles. LSMTs are interventions—such as organ transplantation, ventilator therapy, dialysis, and use of vasoactive medications—that prolong life or alter substantially the expected progression toward death. They can also include other less dramatic interventions, such as use of antibiotics, chemotherapy, or artificially provided nutrition and hydration.

For children with life-threatening or terminal conditions, medical treatment should only be used if the benefits outweigh the burden on the child undergoing such therapies. This is often an emotionally challenging time, when the focus of care of the critically ill child or the child with a terminal illness changes from cure to care. However, this change in no way implies that the child's life is less sacred. It just signals a change of emphasis to palliative care, in which pain and other symptom control is paramount (see Chapters 10 and 13). Indeed, this change from cure to "quality care," with symptom management as the primary focus of the treatment plan, only reinforces the focus on life with dignity rather than technologically sustained life. The distinction between certain LSMTs and palliative care measures can be difficult to make, and at times, LSMTs and palliative care measures are integrated as part of the care treatment plan.

Perhaps the most emotionally charged decisions that must be made and carried out are those that deal with withholding and withdrawing life-sustaining treatments. Most ethicists believe there is no moral distinction between withholding or withdrawing interventions that are not medically indicated. However, because of the uncertainty inherent in children's responses to treatments, most professionals working in pediatrics believe it is preferable to withdraw treatment if the patient does not respond rather than not treat or fail to provide an intervention and thus never know whether this individual child might have responded positively. However, withdrawing treatment, even if the child does not respond, is often an emotionally wrenching experience for parents. Withdrawing or withholding artificial hydration and nutrition is one of the most difficult decisions to be made in pediatrics. However, a decision to withhold or withdraw LSMT does not imply that the primary intent is to hasten the child's death. Likewise, the use of adequate sedation and analgesia to relieve rapidly progressive symptoms of pain and dyspnea is not assisted suicide or a choice to end life but is rather a commitment to relieve symptoms that detract from the child's quality of life.

Sanctity of life is also an important factor in treating newborns with disabilities and with special health care needs. Federal regulations specifically prohibit withholding medically beneficial treatment from newborns with disabilities except under specified conditions: permanent unconsciousness, "futile" treatment, and "virtually futile" interventions that are excessively burdensome for the infant. In a similar vein, ethical issues of fetal well-being and treatments arise with debate about the appropriate balance between maternal and fetal interests. For instance, when a pregnant woman refuses needed medical or surgical intervention that will affect the health of her fetus or her behavior negatively affects the well-being of her fetus, warning flags are raised. The key ethical questions to be considered regarding interventions are whether the intervention has proven benefits; whether the harm to the fetus is certain, substantial, and irrevocable; and whether the risk to the mother is negligible. Such situations may require consultation with the IEC. Issues related to problematic behaviors generally revolve around use of illicit drugs and alcohol and their harmful effect on the fetus. These cases are very difficult to resolve successfully, whether the course of action is inside or outside the legal system.

DO NOT RESUSCITATE OR DO NOT ATTEMPT RESUSCITATION ORDERS

A decision not to attempt cardiopulmonary resuscitation (do not resuscitate or DNR) is one aspect of limiting LSMT. Review hospital, health care agency, or school policies on pediatric DNRs to determine the conditions and protocol that must be followed before a DNR order can be initiated and to find out how often it must be reviewed and renewed. The presence of a DNR order does not mean that other interventions are to be withdrawn or withheld. Basic care such as suctioning, oxygen administration, and medication administration must continue unless ordered otherwise. A DNR order should be discussed in a quiet setting that respects the parents' need for privacy and in a way that allows the parents the opportunity to ask questions. Seeking permission for a DNR order is an undeniable signal to the parent that the health care team believes further lifesaving measures are not in the best interests of the child. For parents to agree to such an order often requires time for quiet thought to reflect on the decision to forgo any further painful or invasive treatments for their child. Some parents may acquiesce right away, others may take hours or days to agree, and some may never give permission despite knowing the futility of further treatment. The nurse's role is to remain empathetic and to acknowledge the parents' feelings. The wishes of parents of a child with a life-threatening or terminal condition who have agreed to a DNR should be respected in both hospital and out-of-hospital settings, such as the child's school. For more in-depth discussion of the nurse's role in obtaining a DNR and other issues in end-of-life care, see Chapter 13, "Palliative Care."

GENETIC AND TECHNOLOGIC ADVANCES, INNOVATIVE THERAPY, AND OTHER PRACTICES

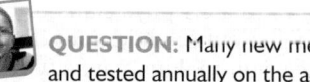 **QUESTION:** Many new medications are developed and tested annually on the adult population before being federally approved for widespread public use. The efficacy of these same medications on children can rarely be extrapolated from the research that applied to adults. What are the ethical concerns associated with pediatric pharmacologic research?

Routine screenings and genetic testing are examples of genetic and technologic advances that present ethical concerns for the pediatric population. Screening is the search for asymptomatic illness and can be done for the purpose of diagnosis, treatment, counseling, or research. Routine fetal monitoring is an example of screening for the purpose of intervention if fetal problems are identified. Likewise, genetic testing can be done to diagnose inherited conditions or to screen prospective parents to determine whether they are carriers. The exponential growth in genetic knowledge has benefited many individuals while at the same time producing challenges. Newborn blood screening panels present an opportunity for early identification and treatment of conditions known to benefit from treatment. However, genetic screening for other conditions poses ethical questions about costs, benefits, and risks. The sensitivity, specificity, and predictive value of a screening program are important considerations. For example, knowledge of a late-onset disorder may have limited benefit, could increase emotional stress, and may potentially result in denial of insurance coverage because it is a preexisting condition.

Ethical issues have arisen when determining whether certain screening should be voluntary ("opt in"), routine with the ability to "opt out" or refuse, or mandatory. Nurses often educate parents about screening tests and explain why these tests are in the best interests of their children. Nurses may also find themselves in situations in which parents need their help and understanding when struggling to decide when, and sometimes whether, to tell a child that he or she may have a late-onset genetic disease or be a carrier of a medical condition. The International Society of Nurses in Genetics (ISONG) provides substantial information to assist nurses who may encounter challenges regarding genetic screening, such as informed decision making or matters of privacy and confidentiality. Additionally, ISONG advocates for the protection of genetic information and privacy rights of families (see http://www.isong.org/index.php).

Innovative therapy is not considered to be research; however, by its very nature, it can present ethical concerns. Such therapy is defined as new and unproved interventions that are performed with no intent to gather new information, as would be done during a research investigation. Innovations in health care practices include a wide range of new diagnostic or therapeutic methods that are aimed at improving health outcomes beyond those of existing methods but that have not yet been fully assessed for safety and/or efficacy. Innovative therapies vary widely from minor variations of existing methods, or extensions of existing methods, to new indications, to completely novel technologies (National Health and Medical Research Council, 2007). Unlike research studies, innovative interventions lack specific designs and strict sampling and procedural protocols and therefore are not subject to research regulations. However, because less oversight is required, the potential to cause harm is greater, and some believe that clinicians are morally obliged to submit their innovative therapies for formal or peer review (Al Eyadhy & Razack, 2008).

The use of "off-label" medications in pediatrics is also a practice that has generated much ethical debate. Because children are not participants in the research trials for most marketed medications, many drugs currently are not labeled for use in children. This means that no pediatric-specific dosing, administration, or adverse effect information is available on the label packaging or in any product information available from the manufacturer.

ALERT *Nurses administering off-label medications to children must be alert for potential adverse reactions.*

An ill child could possibly benefit from off-label use of a medication, however, and many consider it inappropriate to deny the child an opportunity to receive the drug if it might prove therapeutic when medications approved for pediatric use have proved ineffective. Off-label use of medications thus is a common practice.

The U.S. Food and Drug Administration (FDA) Modernization Act of 1997, reauthorized in January 2002 and extended through 2007 as the Best Pharmaceuticals for Children Act (BPCA), called for increased pediatric drug research and labeling. In addition, under the Pediatric Research Equity Act of 2007 (PREA), the FDA can require pediatric studies for new drugs if the FDA determines that the drug is likely to be used in a substantial number of pediatric patients or if the drug provides a meaningful benefit to pediatric patients over existing therapeutics. Subsequently, pediatric-specific dosing information is increasingly available on medications in the pediatric population.

ANSWER: Ethical concerns related to pediatric pharmacologic research include informed consent, ensuring safety of the child, and ensuring pediatric participants and their families do not feel coerced by companies to participate in the research.

LEGAL ISSUES IN THE CARE OF CHILDREN

The health and welfare of children are highly influenced by the legal rights of children and their parents. Nurses must be aware of these legal issues and must follow legislative guidelines and statutes in the implementation and delivery of child health care programs.

RIGHTS OF CHILDREN

 QUESTION: Which laws protect Lindsay's rights while she is attending public school?

In this century, it is recognized that children have rights, and these rights should be maintained and valued in all societies around the world. It is expected that the family will be the primary resource for ensuring that these rights are met. The reality of this goal may not exist in all countries; therefore, agencies such as the United Nations and the World Health Organization actively engage in operations to protect children and to ensure their rights. Chart 2-4 presents the rights of children as identified in a hallmark document created by the United Nations. These rights form the core beliefs and values that are inherent to ensure a bright future for all children.

The rights of children related to health care that are inherent in the delivery of optimal nursing caring to children can also be articulated (Chart 2-5). Children have the right to be free from abuse and exploitation. It is also the right of the child that, within the context of the family, the child should receive food, shelter, protection, and health care management.

Federal laws about education and school health services also protect children and youth with disabilities. These laws are discussed in detail later in this chapter. Two important federal mandates address rights of the

CHART 2-4   The Rights and Needs of Children

Rights	The *Right* to . . .
Social	Life and optimal survival and development; best possible health and access to health care, education, play, and family life that is in the best interests of the child; social inclusion of the special needs child to the fullest extent possible
Economic	An adequate standard of living for proper development; protection from economic exploitation
Cultural	Respect for language, culture, and religion; abolishment of traditional practices that negatively interfere with children's health
Protective	Promotion of the child's best interests; protection from sexual exploitation, violence, child abuse and neglect, armed conflict, and harmful drugs; not to be separated from the parents unless it is in the child's best interests
Civil and political	Be heard and taken seriously; privacy; freedom from violence, torture, or cruel and inhuman treatment; nondiscrimination
Physical needs	Shelter, health care, water, food, adequate clothing, sanitation, protection from environmental pollutants

Based on American Academy of Pediatrics. (2006). *Highlights of the UN Convention on the Rights of the Child: Module 2: A course for health professionals. Children's rights and child health.* Retrieved from http://www2.aap.org/commpeds/resources/childrensrights.htm

CHART 2-5   Sample Charter of Children's Rights

Charter of Children's Rights

As a child who is seeking or receiving health care in this health care facility, I have the right to

- Receive the best possible care and treatment
- Be involved in decisions related to me based on my developmental capabilities
- Be listened to respectfully and have my thoughts, views, and feelings taken seriously
- Be given information about my treatment in a way that I will understand
- Ask for advice and be treated in an emotionally supportive manner
- Not be touched unless I have been asked for and given my permission
- Be treated in a respectful manner
- Expect confidentiality in my health care and respect for my privacy
- Receive equal treatment and care that has no bearing on my gender, religion, race, ethnicity, abilities or disability, or parents' level of income
- Be nurtured and protected in promoting my health and well-being
- Be protected from all forms of violence and abuse

individual: the Family Educational Rights and Privacy Act (FERPA) and the HIPAA. FERPA allows parents the right to access their child's education records and prohibits the release of student-specific information, such as student health records, to others. HIPAA addresses confidentiality of health records and information.

Nurses must be advocates, championing the rights of children in all aspects of a child's life. The nurse must be the voice for those who cannot speak for themselves and must be strong for those who cannot yet defend themselves. The invisibility of children in arenas of power and politics and traditions and attitudes that are not child friendly must not be tolerated. In fact, one of the most serious ethical problems facing this nation's health care system is inequality of access to care and the lack of basic health care coverage that many children still experience.

ANSWER: The right to manage medical chronic conditions at school is based on Section 504 of the Rehabilitation Act of 1973; the Americans with Disabilities Act of 1990, amended in 2008; the IDEA of 1990, amended in 1997; and the IDEIA of 2004.

RIGHTS OF EMANCIPATED MINORS

Emancipation is the process by which an individual becomes liberated from the authority and control of another person. In pediatric care, this term refers to the emancipation of a child from the authority and control of parents or other guardians. The emancipation process for a child who is a *minor* (younger than age 18 years, the age of majority) is governed by individual state laws. Most states have a specific code that lists both the specific situations and the legal proceedings necessary to secure a declaration of emancipation. Conditions that state law may require before approving a declaration of emancipation may include that the minor be at least 14 years of age, willingly lives separate and apart from parents or guardians with their consent or acquiescence, demonstrates an ability to manage financial affairs, and has a source of income other than criminal activity. A valid marriage or service in the armed forces usually qualifies as acceptable conditions for a declaration of emancipation. If all conditions for emancipation as specified in state code are satisfied, the minor then obtains full rights as an adult. When a court proceeding is needed because of a special condition or circumstances not identified in state code, the decision to grant emancipation generally takes into account both the maturity of the minor and his or her need to secure adult status. A minor who is recognized as emancipated by state-mandated criteria can consent to medical, dental, or psychiatric care without parental knowledge, consent, or liability.

RIGHTS OF PARENTS

The rights of parents or guardians in decision making are based on acting in the best interest of the child in matters of life issues and health and on the emerging independence of that child as he or she grows and develops. Thus, an older child's or adolescent's need for autonomy and developing capacity for self-determination are factors that must be considered, along with the rights of parents to make decisions for their child or to impose a certain lifestyle. In addition to legal obligations as the child's guardian until the age of majority or legal emancipation, parental roles and authority have additional dimensions determined by social, cultural, and religious views. Parents' rights relevant to child health issues include the right to give consent (or permission) to treatment; to provide direction and guidance to their child; to be assured of the privacy and confidentiality of health information; and to raise their child according to their own religion, culture, and philosophic convictions. As health care providers, nurses must respect these parental rights unless such rights are legally terminated or evidence exists of a need to seek immediate legal suspension of parental rights.

Parents are granted wide discretion in determining how their child is to be raised. However, sometimes, parents do not make decisions that are in the best interest of their child, deliberately injure their child, or act in ways that put the child in harm's way. All states have laws that define child maltreatment—physical, sexual, or emotional abuse or neglect. Health care providers are responsible for reporting suspected child maltreatment even in those circumstances when parents assert that they were acting in the best interests of their child.

If parents of a child are married to each other or have jointly adopted a child, they both have parental responsibility for the health, education, and welfare of the child and the right to make medical and educational decisions. In the case of parents who have never married, the mother has parental responsibility for the child. Unmarried fathers can get legal responsibility for their children in a number of legally sanctioned ways. Nurses are often involved in caring for children whose parents or grandparents are entwined in custody issues. Various types of custody arrangements exist, such as legal custody and decision-making authority, physical custody, sole custody and decision-making authority, and joint custody and decision-making authority. Promptly and clearly identifying legal rights regarding visitation and ability to make medical decisions is important to avoid turmoil in care and unnecessary emotional trauma for the hospitalized child.

Guardians are adults who are legally responsible for protecting the well-being and interests of their ward who is usually a minor. In most cases, parents are "guardians" for their child. The guardian is charged with the legal responsibly for the care and management of the child and for the minor child's estate. *Legal guardians*, on the other hand, may be appointed by the courts or designated in legal documents by the parents upon their death. Legal guardians are under the supervision of the court and are required to appear in court to give periodic updates about the child and the status of the child's estate. A *guardian ad litem* is a unique type of guardian in a relationship that has been created by a court order only for the duration of a legal action. Courts appoint these special representatives for infants, minors, and mentally incompetent persons, all of whom generally need help protecting their rights in court. Court-appointed guardians are most often assigned in divorce cases, child neglect and abuse cases, paternity suits, contested inheritances, and so forth, and are usually attorneys.

The protection of legal rights comes under the auspices of the courts. The rights to health and education are generally viewed as entitlements for children. However, how this entitlement to health and education is defined and implemented is open to debate. Parents are responsible for ensuring that their child is able to grow and develop in as healthy and productive a manner as possible. Only when parental choices put a child at substantial risk for harm does the moral focus turn to what is best for the child rather than the parental right to choose a particular course of action for their child. In such cases, a court order may be necessary for medical and surgical treatments. For example, the parents of a preterm infant who needs a blood transfusion may refuse because of religious convictions (e.g., Jehovah's Witnesses), or parents may refuse chemotherapy for a child newly diagnosed with leukemia because they do not believe in pharmacologic intervention (e.g., Christian Scientists).

When confronted with such challenges, the pediatric nurse should consult their IEC to determine appropriate course of action for each particular situation.

RESEARCH ISSUES IN THE CARE OF CHILDREN

Nurses can take on a variety of key leadership roles in research, including principal investigator and data collector. However, all nurses are responsible for protecting human rights and monitoring safety when their patients are involved in research studies or clinical research trials. This responsibility starts from the time patients are recruited into a study and sign the appropriate permission forms and lasts until the termination of the investigation.

The focus of research is to generate new knowledge. Because research is not part of standard health care and participation is voluntary, certain safeguards must be in place in health care settings for the protection of human research subjects. Ensuring safety is particularly pertinent for children (who are considered vulnerable subjects) and their families. The potential for physical or nonphysical injury is an inherent risk for any research participant, only much more so for children. Physical injury can be related to the use of investigational devices, experimental procedures, or medications. Nonphysical injury can take many forms, such as loss of confidentiality, psychological distress, emotional vulnerability, or social embarrassment.

Nurses caring for children and their families must know the rules, regulations, and guidelines that define research risk. Any research project conducted or supported by federal agencies must comply with Title 45 of the Code of Federal Regulations Part 46, Protection of Human Subjects, known as *the Common Rule* (U.S. Department of Health & Human Services, 2009). The Common Rule specifies that federally funded research projects must be carefully reviewed by an **institutional review board (IRB)** to ensure the safety and welfare of individuals participating in U.S. Department of Health & Human Services–sponsored research. In a health care facility, the IRB is a committee of health care providers, scientists, and community members that ensures that all research projects are conducted ethically. The IRB is charged with evaluating the scientific merit of the study, determining and weighing the risks and benefits of participation, and protecting subjects' rights. The U.S. Department of Health & Human Services Office for Human Research Protections (OHRP) (2006) has guidelines titled *Special Protections for Children as Research Subjects*. The OHRP is a particularly useful source of information for nurses working with children (see thePoint for Organizations).

Because children are considered vulnerable subjects, the pediatric nurse needs to monitor vigilantly for any deviations in any research protocol, to document and report possible adverse events, and to report any other safety concerns to the appropriate groups, including the health care agency's IRB. If deemed necessary, a nurse can also report concerns to the OHRP, U.S. Department of Health & Human Services. Such reports are confidential, and the nurse is covered by whistle-blower protection (Thomas, 2005).

ETHICAL CONDUCT OF RESEARCH

Several principles govern the ethical conduct of research. These include respect for persons, beneficence, justice, maintaining confidentiality, and securing informed consent.

Respect for Persons

Respect for persons requires that the subject is able to volunteer independently and autonomously to participate in a study. Because infants and children do not have this ability, parents must consent on behalf of their children. In addition, cognitively intact children older than the age of 7 years should always be asked to give their assent. If the child **dissents** (i.e., does not agree to be a research subject), his or her wishes must be respected. Factors inherent in respect for persons are the way children and parents are contacted and recruited for participation and the issues surrounding the consent process.

Beneficence

Beneficence implies doing "good" and avoiding harm. Thus, it requires weighing the benefits and risks associated with participation in a study. Some research studies have no direct benefit to the subject but will benefit society, whereas others result in advantageous or positive outcomes for subjects. Typically, minimal risk is considered to be the probability or likelihood of harm or discomfort (physical or nonphysical) no greater than what occurs during ordinary daily life or during routine physical or psychological examinations or tests (Thomas, 2005). Research involving children can be categorized into four risk categories: minimal risk (also called *nontherapeutic research*), greater than minimal risk but likely to confer direct benefit, greater than minimal risk with no direct benefit, and any other type of research study not falling into the previous three categories. Research on children involving any risk that exceeds minimal risk expectations must be heavily scrutinized. Other review processes are conducted (in addition to securing parental permission, child assent, or both) when a research study is judged to represent more than a minor increase over minimal risk but offers hope that knowledge gained from the study will improve the health and welfare of children (Kim, 2004). In such circumstances, if the study is federally funded, the researcher must apply to the U.S. Department of Health & Human Services for special permission.

Justice

Justice focuses on the distribution of burden and benefits among the population of interest. Who is to assume the burdens and risks of participation, and who benefits from the knowledge gained? Pediatric subjects must be selected fairly and without exploiting a group that will not benefit from the study's outcomes. For example, infants in an underdeveloped country cannot be selected by a pharmaceutical company for use in testing high-risk vaccines or medications.

The use of incentives as recruitment tools for children, parents, or both to participate in research is also an important ethical issue. Pediatric subjects should not be offered incentives that are clearly not equivalent to the care or services provided to nonparticipants. The types of incentives offered by the investigator to parents and children can influence their decision about whether to participate. Incentives can range from intangible rewards, such as altruistic feelings of helping society, to reimbursement for "services" such as time and effort, to financial reimbursement for expenses. Using incentives to motivate or encourage subjects to join a study is not inherently unethical. However, when children and families are financially or emotionally vulnerable, recruitment incentives can place them at greater than usual risk if they believe the goods or services offered through participation in the research study are things they need (Rice & Broome, 2004). Examples of vulnerability include a family living in poverty who will receive significant payment for "services" if the child enters a drug study and offering gift certificates for large amounts of money or expensive computer equipment to disadvantaged children. Therefore, incentives such as financial reimbursement for expenses or wage payment for time, effort, or burden must be scrutinized carefully for their ethical implications. The duration of the study, its burden on participants, out-of-pocket expenses for transportation, and institutional rules are some of the aspects considered when determining the type and amount of incentives.

caREminder

The overriding principle that should guide the use of incentives is that neither parents nor the child should profit financially from enrolling in a research study.

Confidentiality

When conducting or participating in research, it must be clear to what extent confidential information about subjects and research data will be protected to safeguard the subject's identity. Parents and children must be fully informed regarding what will be done to protect their identities and to avoid sensitive issues such as embarrassment, stigmatization, or prejudicial treatment. A discussion of confidentially is typically part of the informed consent process and often outlines certain security strategies that the investigator will use, such as using subject code numbers or separating identifying data from research data. Exceptions to confidentiality must be identified in advance of a parent's or child's agreement to become a research subject (e.g., when mandated reportable conditions, such as child maltreatment or sexually transmitted diseases, are uncovered during the research study).

Informed Consent

Informed consent is a central concept in ensuring patient safety and maintaining ethical practices during the research process. Numerous elements must be addressed as part of the informed consent process. Chart 2-6 lists critical information that must be addressed as part of informed consent. Much of this information appears on the consent form and serves

---

CHART 2-6	**Informed Consent: Critical Information Needed to Protect Infants and Children as Research Subjects**

Basic Issues

The Parent, Child, or Both Should Know

- That what they are agreeing to participate in is research and not part of standard care
- Why the study is needed
- Who the investigator is and how to contact him or her
- What the time commitment will be
- If there are any costs that will be incurred by them to participate
- If applicable, how a study intervention differs from routine care
- Whether they will have access to study findings
- That they can ask questions about the research at any time before, during, or after the research process
- Whether they will receive compensation and, if so, what will it be
- Whom to contact in the agency if they have questions or concerns about human subject research participation

Issues Related to Beneficence

The Parent, Child, or Both Should Know

- Risks—physical and/or nonphysical—that are associated with participation in the research and actions that can be taken to reduce risks
- Potential adverse effects and what will be done (e.g., treatment, who will cover costs) if they occur
- Expected benefits—direct and indirect—associated with participation

Issues Related to Confidentiality

The Parent, Child, or Both Should Be

- Fully informed regarding the extent of confidentiality
- Made aware of strategies used to safeguard their identities
- Told who has access to their names, identifying information, or data
- Told of any circumstances that would necessitate revealing their identities or study information to others (e.g., mandatory reporting)

Refusal Rights

The Parent, Child, or Both Should Be

- Told they can refuse to participate and that such refusal will not alter their standard care
- Aware that they can withdraw from the study at any time without prejudice
- Aware that they can refuse to answer any question

This listing is not meant to be all inclusive. Other items may need to be noted in an informed consent, depending on the type of research study.

as legal documentation that the parent and child were appropriately informed. In most circumstances, the consent form must be signed, and a copy must be given to the parent or child.

Be aware of factors that may place undue pressure on parents or children in their decision to participate in research. Examples that bear special attention include situations in which the individual providing care is one who recruits and acquires consent from the subject and those in which financial inducements may be considered excessive in light of the family's circumstances. Families may also think (albeit incorrectly) that participation in the research will improve the care their child receives. Similarly, parents of terminally or critically ill children may agree to have their child participate in experimental research interventions out of feelings of distress or despair when all other conventional treatment options have failed. Such situations require special attention by health care professionals. One safeguard that may be required is to require a waiting period (even as brief as 24 hours) before a final decision to participate can be made rather than allow parents to make quick decisions based solely on feelings of despair.

See thePoint for a summary of Key Concepts.

REFERENCES

Administration for Children and Families. (2011). *About Head Start*. Retrieved from http://eclkc.ohs.acf.hhs.gov/hslc/hs/about

Al Eyadhy, A., & Razack, S. (2008). The ethics of using innovative therapies in the care of children. *Paediatrics & Child Health, 13*(3), 181–184.

American Medical Association, Department of Adolescent Health. (1992). *Guidelines for adolescent preventive services*. Chicago, IL: Author.

Americans with Disabilities Act of 1990, Pub. L. No. 101-336, § 2, 104 Stat. 328 (1991).

Anderson, R. M., Rice, T. H., & Kominski, G. F. (2007). *Changing the US health care system* (3rd ed.). San Francisco, CA: Jossey-Bass.

Balanced Budget Act of 1997, Pub. L. No. 105-33, 111 Stat. 251 (1997).

Centers for Disease Control and Prevention. (2012). Youth risk behavior surveillance—United States, 2011. *Morbidity and Mortality Weekly Report, 61*(SS04), 1–162.

Child Trends DataBank. (2010). *Health care coverage*. Retrieved from http://www.childtrendsdatabank.org/?q = node/297

Children's Health Insurance Program Reauthorization Act of 2009, Pub. L. No. 111-3, 123 Stat. 8 (2009).

Education for All Handicapped Children Act, Pub. L. No. 94-142, 89 Stat. 773 (1975).

Essex, N. (2006). *What every teacher should know about No Child Left Behind*. Boston, MA: Pearson Education.

Federal Interagency Forum on Child and Family Statistics. (2012). *America's children in brief: Key national indicators of well-being, 2012*. Retrieved from http://www.childstats.gov/americaschildren/index.asp

Food and Drug Administration Modernization Act of 1997, Pub. L. No. 105-115, 111 Stat. 2296 (1997).

Hamilton, B. E., & Vetura, S. J. (2012). *Birth rates for U.S. teenagers reach historic lows for all age and ethnic groups* (NCHS Data Brief No. 89). Hyattsville, MD: National Center for Health Statistics.

Individuals with Disabilities Education Act of 1990, Pub. L. No. 101-476, 104 Stat. 1142 (1990).

Individuals with Disabilities Education Improvement Act, Pub. L. 108-446, 118 Stat. 2647 (2004).

Kaiser Commission on Medicaid and the Uninsured. (2005). *Early and periodic screening, diagnostic, and treatment services*. Retrieved from http://www.kff.org/Medicaid/upload/Early-and-periodic-Screening -Diagnostic-and-Treatment-Services-Fact-Sheet.pdf

Kaiser Family Foundation. (2010). *Medicaid and children's health insurance program provisions in the new health reform law*. Retrieved from http://www.kff.org/healthreform/upload/7952-03.pdf

Kenney, G., Lynch, V., Cook, A. et al. (2012). Who and where are the children yet to enroll in Medicaid and the children's health insurance program? *Health Affairs, 29*(10), 1920–1929.

Kim, A. E. (2004). Protection of child human subjects. *Journal of Wound, Ostomy, and Continence Nursing, 3*(4), 161–167.

Kost, K., & Henshaw, S. (2012). *U.S. teenage pregnancies, births and abortions: National trends by age, race and ethnicity*. New York, NY: Author. Retrieved from http://www.guttmacher.org/pubs/USTPtrends08.pdf

National Center for Health Statistics. (2012). *Health, United States, 2011: With special feature on socioeconomic status and health*. Hyattsville, MD: National Center for Health Statistics, Department of Health & Human Services, Centers for Disease Control and Prevention.

National Diabetes Information Clearinghouse. (2011). *National diabetes statistics, 2011*. Retrieved from http://diabetes.niddk.nih.gov /dm/pubs/statistics/#d_allages

National Federation of Independent Business v. Sebelius, 132 S. Ct. 2566, 2640 (2012).

National Health and Medical Research Council. (2007). *National statement on ethical conduct in human research*. Retrieved from http:// www.nhmrc.gov.au/_files_nhmrc/publications/attachments /e72.pdf

No Child Left Behind Act of 2001, Pub. L. No. 107-110, 115 Stat 1425 (2002).

Patient Protection and Affordable Care Act, Pub. L. No. 111-148, 124 Stat. 119 (2010).

Rehabilitation Act of 1973, Pub. L. 93-112, 87 Stat. 355 (1973).

Rice, M., & Broome, M. E. (2004). Incentives for children in research. *Journal of Nursing Scholarship, 36*(2), 167–172.

Silverstein, M., Grossman, D. C., Koepsell, T. D. et al. (2003). Pediatricians' reported practices regarding early education and head start referral. *Pediatrics, 111*(6), 1351–1357.

Singh, G. K. (2010). *Child mortality in the United States, 1935–2007: Large racial and socioeconomic disparities have persisted over time*. A 75th anniversary publication. Health Resources and Services Administration, Maternal and Child Health Bureau. Rockville, MD: U.S. Department of Health & Human Services.

Slavin, R. (2006). *Educational psychology* (8th ed.). Boston, MA: Allyn & Bacon.

Stuber, J., & Kronebusch, K. (2004). Stigma and other determinants of participation in TANF and Medicaid. *Journal of Policy Analysis and Management, 23*(3), 509–530.

Thomas, K. A. (2005). Safety: When infants and parents are research subjects. *Journal of Prenatal Neonatal Nursing, 19*, 52–58.

U.S. Department of Health & Human Services. (2009). *Code of Federal Regulations, Title 45, Public Welfare, Part 46, Protection of Human Subjects*. Retrieved from http://www.hhs.gov/ohrp/humansubjects /guidance/45cfr46.html

U.S. Department of Health & Human Services, Office for Human Research Protections. (2006). *Special protections for children as research subjects*. Retrieved from http://www.hhs.gov/ohrp/policy /populations/children.html

Zipkin, A. (2007). *Special education legislation: A synopsis of federal and state policies*. Retrieved from http://sitemaker.umich.edu/356 .zipkin/home

See thePoint for additional resources.

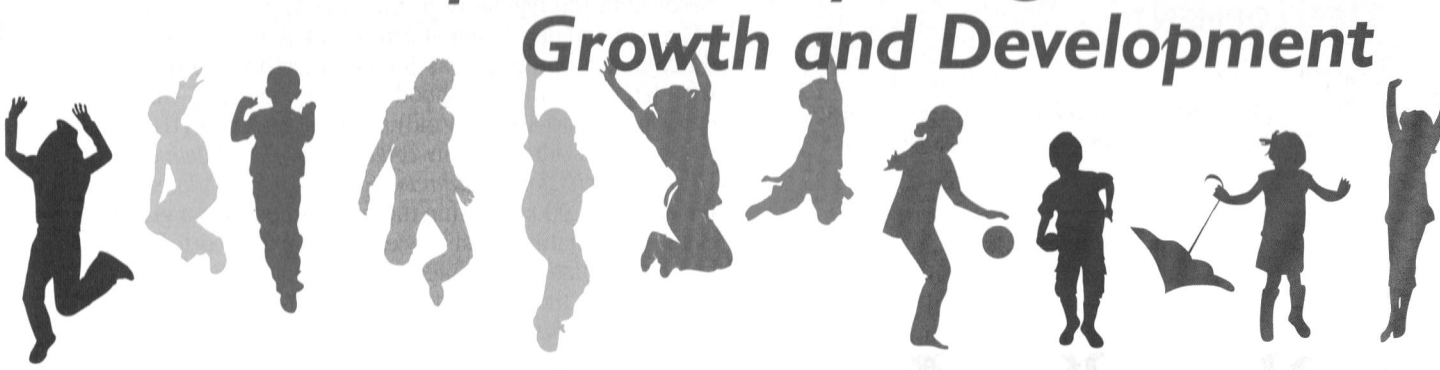

CHAPTER 3

Principles and Physiologic Basis of Growth and Development

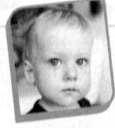 **CASE HISTORY**

Joellen Rollins, who is in the last trimester of her third pregnancy, and her husband Chris are the parents of two children: Selena, a 5-year-old girl who will be entering kindergarten in the fall, and 2½-year-old James. Selena was born at 39 weeks' gestation via vaginal birth and experienced no problems. James was born vaginally at 32 weeks' gestation as a result of the abrupt onset of preterm labor that could not be halted. James weighed 3 lb, 5 oz at birth and was 18 in. long. He spent a short time in the neonatal intensive care unit for evaluation. During his stay there, he developed some respiratory distress requiring the use of oxygen therapy. Since that time, he has not experienced any further significant respiratory problems other than two upper respiratory infections.

James is an extremely curious and active child. He is constantly "getting into things." He seems to shift his attention quickly from one thing to another and gets sidetracked easily. During the past few weeks, he has started toilet training, which has been somewhat problematic. He has had beginning success with bowel training but has had little success with bladder control.

"He's always on the go and never wants to stop what he's doing," says his mother. Moreover, when his parents ask him to do something, such as use the potty or put his toys away, he responds with a definitive "No!" Running and playing outside are his favorite things to do. His parents do report that he is a bit clumsy sometimes. There have been several instances when he has fallen, but James only experienced some bruising, cuts, and scrapes. "It's a miracle he hasn't broken anything," remarks his father.

During the past couple of months, James has started throwing temper tantrums. During some of these tantrums, James holds his breath until he collapses, at which time he begins to breathe spontaneously. Joellen and Chris have tried various methods to get James to stop his tantrums, but they have been unsuccessful.

CHAPTER OBJECTIVES

1 Explain principles fundamental to understanding the growth and development processes of children.

2 Examine the biologic and environmental factors that can influence the growth and developmental processes in children.

3 Describe the development of the body systems in children from birth through adolescence.

4 Articulate selected theories that describe the psychosocial, cognitive, interpersonal, sexual, and moral development of children from birth through adolescence.

5 Choose strategies the nurse can use to institute the process of developmental surveillance.

See thePoint for a list of Key Terms.

Human growth and development is sustained through change. Changes in the physical body occur as tissues form, structures enlarge, and organs and muscles achieve their full degree of strength and function. Developmental changes occur in the individual as cognitive, language, and social skills are achieved. Developmental theories help to explain the multitude of factors that shape our personalities and the processes that affect our growth.

PRINCIPLES OF GROWTH AND DEVELOPMENT

QUESTION: What would you expect to discover about James's growth, considering his history as a preterm newborn?

The study of human growth and development provides explanations of the similarities and differences among us that blend to create our individual physical and social self. To understand the basic principles of growth and development, it is important to understand how these and related terms are defined.

Growth refers to changes in size and function of the whole body or any part of the body. These are quantitative changes that can be measured by assessing changes in weight, length, height, and functional output. **Development** refers to the qualitative changes that are seen as an individual acquires new skills. Language and thought processes, the capacity to develop social relationships, and the emergence of a unique personality are all products of human development. Developmental assessment tools, cognitive abilities tests, and psychological assessments can measure changes over time in these areas. **Maturation** refers to those aspects of development that are genetically influenced. For instance, toilet training, riding a bike, and reading are skills that cannot be achieved until maturation of neurologic and muscular functions has taken place. Interaction with the environment has little influence on maturational changes.

The individuality of a child's growth and development is highly influenced by factors such as heredity, the environment, nutrition, sensory stimulation, and affection. Growth is systematic and occurs in a sequential pattern. Although each person emerges at birth as a unique individual, basic patterns and trends are predictable in the growth and development of all humans in all societies. Because of the regularity of the growth processes, stages of growth and development can be differentiated. This text differentiates the stages as infancy (newborn through 11 months old), early childhood (1 to 4 years old), middle childhood (5 to 10 years old), and adolescence (11 to 21 years old) as identified in *Bright Futures: Guidelines for Health Supervision of Infants, Children, and Adolescents* (Hagan et al., 2008). Within these stages, particular growth events and maturational processes are expected to occur, and differentiation and integration of growth tasks evolve. For instance, the child learning to extend his or her arm aimlessly eventually learns to grasp an object purposefully, bring that object to the mouth, transfer the object to another hand, and throw the object when requested.

Although growth is a systematic process, body systems vary in their rates of development. For example, the cardiovascular and respiratory systems, although not fully mature at birth, must carry out functions essential for the viability of life outside the womb. In addition, these systems are necessary for the progressive maturation of other organs to complete their development. The lymphatic and genital systems are examples of two systems with rates and patterns of growth that occur over an extended period of time and influence the body at a later point in life.

When evaluating a child's growth, it is important to assess the child's patterns of growth over several months or years rather than base an entire assessment on a single evaluation of the child at a particular time. The terms *normal* or *average* have been used to describe the predictable patterns of growth and development that have been studied and are known to occur within a certain time frame. From this normal or average pattern, each child can be viewed as a *variation of the theme* (Fig. 3-1).

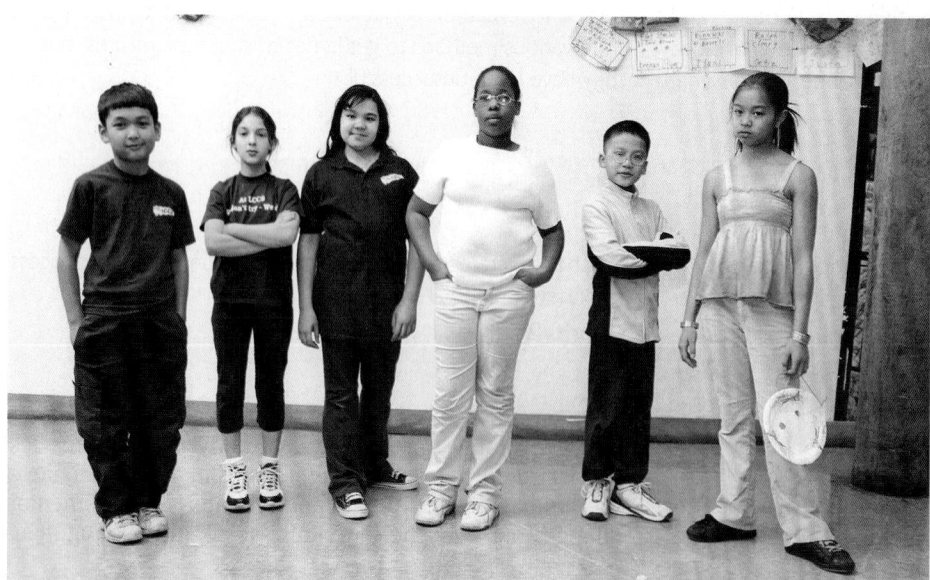

Figure 3-1 Although these children are all in fifth grade, developmental differences are significant with respect to their height, shape, and body proportions.

caREminder

Although two children are raised in the same family, and may even be identical twins, the interactions and experiences each child encounters will be different. Therefore, two children can be expected to respond differently based on their past experiences, stage of development, current disposition, and genetic potential.

That is, given certain expected growth or developmental norms, each child as an individual may grow and mature faster or slower while still demonstrating adherence to a consistent and predictable pattern of growth and development. For example, one child might be at the 90th percentile of height for his or her age, whereas another is at the 25th percentile for the same age. One child may learn to read sooner than another child. Each individual's growth and development trajectory, however, is influenced by environmental factors such as nutrition and sensory stimulation. If these environmental factors are strongly affecting the child either negatively or positively, growth and development patterns may be altered. For instance, the child who is acutely malnourished will demonstrate delays in both physical growth and psychosocial development. However, early identification and intervention can prevent potentially irreversible outcomes. Often, with intervention, the child can undergo a **catch-up period** during which growth and development occurs, bringing the child back to his or her own trajectory (Tradition or Science 3-1).

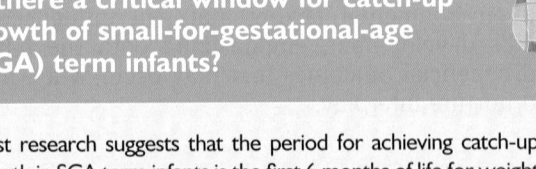

TRADITION OR SCIENCE 3-1

Evidence-Based Practice

Is there a critical window for catch-up growth of small-for-gestational-age (SGA) term infants?

Most research suggests that the period for achieving catch-up growth in SGA term infants is the first 6 months of life for weight and the first 9 months of life for length. This is the period when breast milk or formula intake would be a predominant part of the infant's diet. Fewtrell et al. (2001) found that when SGA infants were fed nutrient-enriched formula during this critical growth period, they sustained greater gains in body length and head circumference up to 18 months of age compared with infants who received standard formula. Most recently, insulin resistance has been noted as a potential adverse outcome of the failure to achieve catch-up growth. Han et al. (2010) performed a study that demonstrated if catch-up growth was not achieved within 3 months, insulin resistance resulted. The study further suggests that if the catch-up growth is not completed in the recognized 6-month period, insulin resistance may be a significant issue later in childhood, leading to obesity. It is evident that the critical period for affecting the growth trajectory in SGA infants includes the early postnatal period, and that nutritional interventions can influence the growth trajectory and sustain the gains in growth beyond the period of intervention.

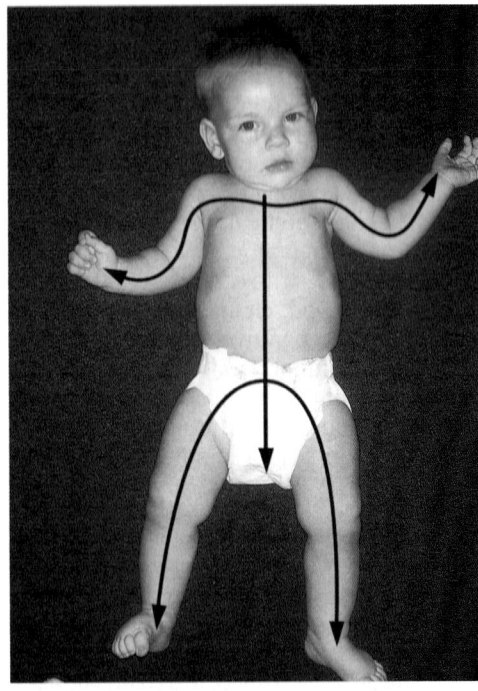

Figure 3-2 The child's pattern of growth is in a head-to-toe direction, or *cephalocaudal*, and in an inward-to-outward pattern called *proximodistal*.

The child's development of skills and functions proceeds from the simple to the complex and from the general to the specific. A young child, for example, does not progress straight from learning to talk to learning to write. Instead, several other developmental achievements must take place, each building on the previous accomplishment, to achieve a more specific and higher level skill. Development progresses in a head-to-toe, or **cephalocaudal**, fashion and in a **proximodistal**, or midline to the periphery, progression (Fig. 3-2). For example, the infant who learns to lift his or her head and then sit, crawl, walk, and run is developing in a cephalocaudal manner. The child who demonstrates random total body movements and then develops the use of a specific limb and then the use of individual fingers to grasp a small object is developing in a proximodistal progression. Knowledge of progressive traits helps the nurse to predict the sequential patterns of development. With this knowledge, the nurse can provide anticipatory guidance to parents to enhance the child's achievement of developmental skills.

As the child grows and matures, some **critical periods** are known to exist. These time periods refer to points in which the individual is highly sensitive or ready for certain actions. During a critical period, the child is vulnerable to positive and negative stimuli that can enhance or defer the achievement of a skill or function. For instance, infants who are born deaf vocalize as all infants do during the first year of life. However, by 1 year of age, the child who is deaf will likely cease these vocalizations and will not progress to other audible verbalizations without active intervention by the caregivers. Research regarding critical periods continues to accumulate, providing valuable information regarding times to ensure that opportunities are given for children to acquire specific skills and knowledge.

All humans have an inherent desire to learn and grow. Abraham Maslow called this *self-actualization*, and Carl Rogers called it *directional growth*. Children are constantly exploring their environment and testing parameters to seek new information and to acquire new skills. Factors such as illness, sensory deprivation, and physical and mental abuse can negatively affect the child's ability to focus on these inherent desires and to demonstrate progressive developmental achievements. Development is a lifelong process. As the child moves through adolescence toward adulthood, changes will continue to occur in the psychosocial, cognitive, physical, and emotional domains of the individual. Evidence-Based Clinical Practice Guidelines 3-1 highlights documents that summarize growth and developmental patterns in children and may serve as useful resources for families and caregivers.

> **ANSWER:** All newborns, regardless of their gestational age at birth, experience growth and development in a cephalocaudal fashion and proximodistal progression. Each newborn is individual in his or her growth, with some growing and maturing faster or slower than others. However, all newborns demonstrate adherence to a consistent and predictable pattern of growth and development. James's preterm status and exposure to environmental factors, such as increased nutritional needs and possible sensory overload and deprivation from his stay in the neonatal intensive care unit, may have affected his growth and development, necessitating a catch-up period to help bring him back to his trajectory.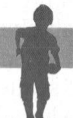

FACTORS INFLUENCING DEVELOPMENT

The research contributions of psychologists, epidemiologists, and others interested in human development have made it increasingly evident that no single factor can explain the intricacies of growth and change from infancy to old age. Rather, there are multiple biologic and environmental factors, and these are so interrelated that it is often difficult to attribute an individual's behavior or growth pattern to any specific origin. *Biologic factors* are those agents that affect patterns of development by primarily influencing the basic building blocks of the human organism—genes, chromosomes, cell division, and human reproduction. Physical traits are determined through genetic factors. However, emotional and behavioral patterns might also be influenced by genetic and hereditary factors; for instance, attention-deficit/hyperactivity disorder (ADHD) is strongly linked to genetic (biologic) factors. *Environmental factors* are the psychological, social, and ecologic influences that affect the child's development. Factors such as parenting practices, interactions with peers, and frequent hospitalizations are examples of the psychological and social factors that influence individual development. Exposure to hazardous agents, poverty, and poor nutritional intake are examples of ecologic factors that affect development. For example, a child's access to adequate calcium intake and the amount of fluoride in local drinking water can have an impact on the development of strong bones and teeth. Ongoing research aims to analyze the ways in which nature (represented by genetics and heredity) combines with nurture (represented by a person's environment) to produce a given outcome. In addition, research is aimed at focusing on interventions that will mitigate the effects of persistent health disparities associated with poverty, discrimination, or maltreatment to optimize the child's lifelong health and development (Engle et al., 2011; Shonkoff & Garner, 2012; Walker et al., 2011). Nurses play an important role in educating families about the biologic and environmental factors that will influence their child's development, emphasizing both the harmful and beneficial outcomes that may occur when nature and nurture interplay.

EVIDENCE-BASED CLINICAL PRACTICE GUIDELINES 3-1
Childhood Growth and Development Guidelines

Hagan, J. F., Shaw, J. S., & Duncan, P. M. (Eds.). (2008). *Bright futures: Guidelines for health supervision of infants, children, and adolescents* (3rd ed.). Elk Grove Village, IL: American Academy of Pediatrics. Retrieved from

http://brightfutures.aap.org/pdfs/guidelines_pdf/1-bf-introduction.pdf

Detailed description of well-child care that includes expected developmental parameters for newborns through adolescence.

Centers for Disease Control and Prevention. (2012). *Developmental milestones*. Retrieved from

http://www.cdc.gov/ncbddd/actearly/milestones/index.html

Provides milestone checklists and summary of developmental screening tools.

State of Washington, Office of Superintendent of Public Instruction. (2012). *Early learning and development guidelines*. Retrieved from

http://k12.wa.us/EarlyLearning/guidelines.aspx

Presents what children can do and learn from birth through third grade.

BIOLOGIC FACTORS

From the moment of conception, the role of genetics and heredity has a tremendous influence on the biologic growth and development of the fetus. These influences continue throughout childhood as the individual matures physically, interpersonally, and socially. Other biologic influences on development are the child's gender and his or her race and ethnicity.

Genetics and Heredity

Genetics examines the physical and chemical properties of the molecules that govern the structure and function of every cell in the body. These molecules, or genes, influence who the child is and who he or she will become. The child's genes and chromosomes carry specialized codes that have instructions to determine the child's sex, eye color, height, predisposition for certain illnesses, and even the triggers that make all the metabolic pathways work correctly. Scientists are also investigating the role of genetics on the presence of certain behavioral traits, such as homosexuality, depression, addictive behaviors, and violent behaviors (Burt, 2005; N. Fox et al., 2005; Hariri, 2009; Mann & Currier, 2010; Middeldorp et al., 2006; Riemann et al., 2012; Saudino, 2005).

Heredity is the process by which living things transmit genetic codes that specify certain patterns of growth and organization to their offspring. The primary patterns of inheritance are dominant inheritance, recessive inheritance, and X-linked inheritance (Fig. 3-3) (see Table 14-1). These patterns of inheritance influence the transmission of traits such as eye and hair color and the appearance of genetic defects. Several conditions in children can be attributed to genetic abnormalities. (Table 14-2 presents selected genetic aberrations, their clinical features, and health care interventions.)

Through the use of genetic screening techniques such as amniocentesis, chorionic villus sampling, and genetic counseling, many chromosomal aberrations and other disorders can be detected before conception or in the developing fetus (see Chapter 14 for further discussion of these diagnostic tests). Through genetic testing, human DNA, RNA, chromosomes, proteins, and certain metabolites are examined to detect inheritable disease-related genotypes, mutations, phenotypes, or karyotypes. Genomic-based research includes investigation to analyze how behavior and environment affect susceptibility to certain disorders; how specific molecular changes influence disease susceptibility; and how social, ethical, and cultural factors influence genomic health. The National Human Genome Research Institute (www.genome.gov) serves as an international resource about genomics research and issues related to genetics. Genetic testing is done for both clinical diagnostic purposes and for predictive purposes. When a child appears with certain physical characteristics or symptomology that may be indicative of a clinical condition, genetic testing may be used as a diagnostic tool. For instance, the parents of a child born with a meconium ileus may be asked to consent to genotyping to determine whether the meconium ileus is related to the presence of cystic fibrosis. **Predictive genetic testing**, however, is considered more controversial by health care providers. Predictive testing may be completed on children who are considered presymptomatic for a specific disease (i.e., if the child has this particular genotype, he or she will likely develop the disease) or predispositional for a specific disease (i.e., if the child has a particular genotype, he or she is at increased risk for developing a particular condition, but not all will). Predictive genetic testing can be completed to determine whether a child is at presymptomatic risk for Duchenne muscular dystrophy or Huntington disease, for example. Predictive testing can also be used to determine whether a child is at a predispositional risk for the development of type 1 diabetes in childhood or breast cancer as an adult (Tradition or Science 3-2) (see thePoint for Evidence-Based Practice Guidelines).

Gender

During the early stages of conception, the child's gender is determined when the sex chromosomes of the parents are joined. There are two X chromosomes in females and one X and one Y chromosome in males. The child's gender affects myriad physical, personal, and social factors related to the child's growth and development. Internal and external sex-specific biologic differences are present at birth and continue to be demonstrated throughout the course of the person's life. The most obvious biologic difference is the presence of either male or female genitalia. Other physical traits influenced by gender include hair distribution, height, and body physique. Overall health and longevity are also influenced by gender. Some diseases are noted to be more prevalent in one gender than another. For example, scoliosis is more prevalent in females, whereas hemophilia, muscular dystrophy, and color blindness are more common in males. Females, in general, have a longer life span than males. In addition, premature female infants have a higher survival rate than do premature male infants.

Gender identification is the process by which children learn and acquire the attitudes and behaviors that are attributed to feminine and masculine roles in their culture. This process continues throughout the course of the child's development. Gender identification is considered to be influenced by both biologic (gender determined at conception) and environmental factors. Gender-based interactions with family members and peers, activities, personal–social attributes, and societal values interplay to influence the way in which children perceive themselves as gender typed.

Race and Ethnicity

The child's race and ethnicity influence patterns of growth and development in both obvious and subtle ways. **Race** refers to the biophysiologic characteristics of a population group that make it different from others. Race has a genetic/hereditary influence on development. Easily visible are the influences of race on physical attributes such as skin color, hair color, body

Dominant Inheritance

One affected parent has a single gene (D) that dominates its normal counterpart (n).

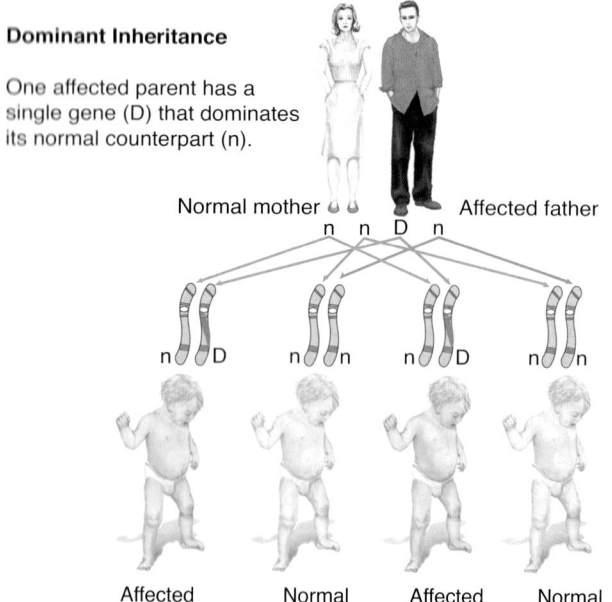

A. Each child has a 50% chance of inheriting either the D or the n from the affected parent.

Recessive Inheritance

Both parents, usually unaffected, carry a normal gene (N) that takes precedence over its recessive counterpart (r).

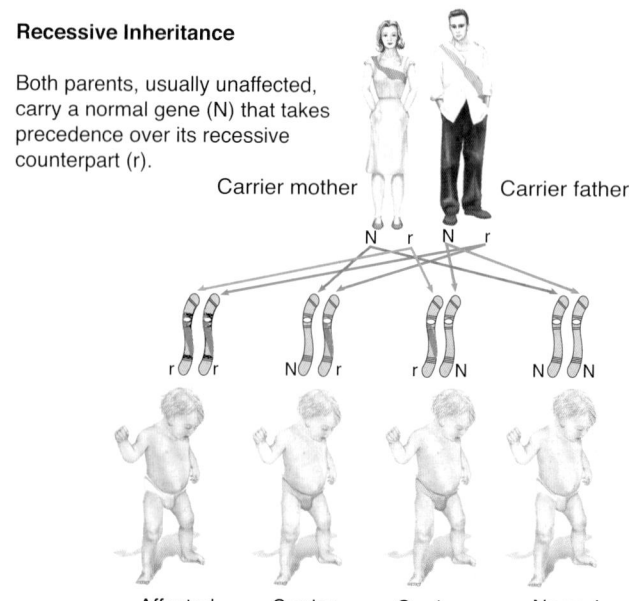

B. Each child has a 25% chance of inheriting two r genes, which may cause a serious birth defect; a 25% chance of inheriting two Ns, and thus being unaffected; and a 50% chance of being a carrier, like both parents.

X-Linked Inheritance

In the most common form of this pattern, the female sex chromosome of an unaffected mother carries one faulty gene (X) and one normal gene (x). The father has a normal male x and y chromosome complement.

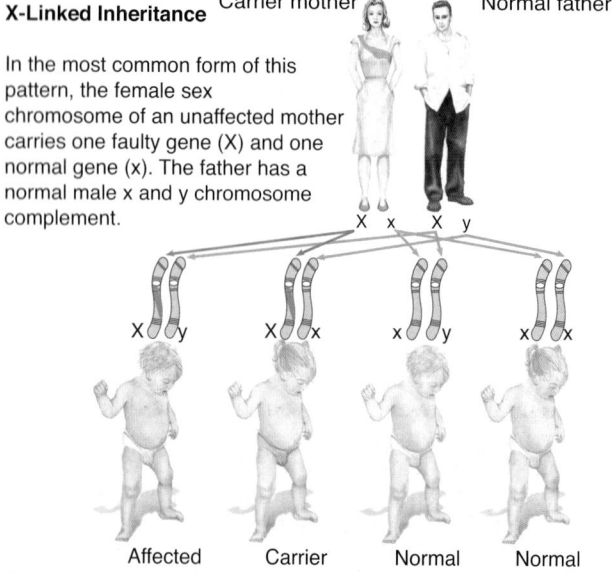

C. Each male child has a 50% chance of inheriting the faulty X and the disorder, and 50% chance of inheriting the normal x and y. Each female child has a 50% chance of inheriting the faulty X, and thus to be a carrier like the mother, and a 50% chance of *not* inheriting the faulty X.

Figure 3-3 Patterns of inheritance. (A) Dominant inheritance. (B) Recessive inheritance. (C) X-linked inheritance.

size, and physique. It is known that the incidence of specific malformations varies among population groups (Chart 3-1). In addition, certain physical variations and minor abnormalities may be considered normal findings among children of the same race. For instance, epicanthal folds, which are the vertical folds of skin that partially or completely cover the inner canthi of the eye and may indicate Down syndrome, glycogen storage disease, or renal agenesis, are normally seen in Asian children and in some non-Asian children. Similarly, lordosis, or an excessive backward concavity of the spine, is commonly seen as a normal finding in African American females. A careful review of family history can assist in determining whether specific clinical features should be further evaluated using genetic testing and other diagnostic tests to determine the presence

More Inquiry Needed

TRADITION OR SCIENCE 3-2

Should predictive genetic testing be completed on an asymptomatic child for whom there is no medical treatment during childhood that can change the course of the disease? And should results of genetic testing be shared with the child?

Rapid advances in clinical genetics have given rise to a variety of ethical concerns for clinicians and the families they serve. The research evidence remains inconclusive regarding the potential harms and benefits of both testing and disclosure, with little focus on the impact on children. Benefits of predictive testing can include the relief from uncertainty, knowing current or potential offspring's risk for the specific disease, relief from self-monitoring if the results are negative, and a greater ability to plan for the future (Hung & Carey, 2012; Ingles et al., 2011; Lerman et al., 2002; Williams et al., 1999). Hamilton et al. (2005) report that positive disease findings do not necessarily then equate to open disclosure to all family members. Rather, they found that adults tested for Huntington disease or hereditary breast and ovarian cancer chose to disclose their findings to family members selectively, and the timing of disclosure was influenced by the disease and the person's perceived need to prepare. Disclosure of test results appeared to be a complex process of selecting which family members to include in the telling, the content of the information shared, and the style used to share the information. More research is indicated to determine both the harm and benefit of predictive testing, specifically on children, and the process of disclosing this information to family members, particularly children who are extremely vulnerable to the negative consequences this information may have on their lives.

of an actual clinical condition. Likewise, carrier testing can be offered to couples who are planning pregnancy to determine whether their racial characteristics will enhance the risk of having a child affected by a specific genetic disease.

A child's **ethnicity** refers to the common social and cultural values, mores, and traditions that are passed on from one generation to the next and that create a sense of identity among members of the ethnic group. Ethnicity infers an environmental influence on growth and development of the child. Ethnicity may influence personal mannerisms, social interactions, responses to pain, and the development of one's self-concept. Race and ethnicity are another example of two closely intertwined variables that emphasize how both nature and nurture influence the way in which children grow and develop.

CHART 3-1   Common Malformations and Diseases Found in Children of Different Population Groups

Disease	Population Group
Cystic fibrosis	Northwestern European
Phenylketonuria	Northwestern European
Sickle cell anemia	African and Mediterranean
Tay-Sachs disease	Ashkenazi Jewish
Gaucher disease	Ashkenazi Jewish
Clubfoot	Polynesian
Cleft lip and palate	Chinese
Neural tube defects	White
Postaxial polydactyly	African
Ellis-van Creveld syndrome	Amish Mennonite
Thalassemia	Quebec, northern New Brunswick regions
Umbilical hernias	African
Adrenogenital syndrome	Eskimo
Glucose-6-phosphate dehydrogenase (G6PD) deficiency	African and Chinese

ENVIRONMENTAL FACTORS

Throughout the child's life span, several environmental factors can impede or enhance physical, behavioral, and emotional growth (Table 3-1). Childhood illnesses, trauma, and nutritional deprivation are examples of factors that may affect the child's long-term health status.

Physically healthy children who have limited early social, educational, and environmental experiences are also "at risk" for developmental delays. Children who experience the negative environmental influences of parental deprivation, abusive family relationships, or limited social contacts with other children their age will have difficulty achieving developmental norms unless early intervention is provided to alter their developmental trajectory. Other vulnerable children include teenage mothers, children who live in poverty, and children who are hospitalized frequently.

As the child grows, good nutritional practices and health surveillance activities can promote optimum development. On the other hand, environmental factors such as physical trauma, ongoing exposures to chemicals, communicable diseases, and the outcomes of natural disasters are all factors that can dramatically change the growth and developmental patterns of a previously healthy child. Trauma and illness can impair physical growth and can cause the child to regress developmentally. These regressive actions and behaviors might be permanent if critical functions of the body have been affected. For example, a child who was involved in a motor vehicle accident might only be able to walk with an assistive device.

TABLE 3-1   Examples of Environmental Factors That Affect Growth and Development

Type of Exposure	Possible Teratogenic Effects
Pharmaceutical Teratogens	
• Thalidomide	• Musculoskeletal deformities
• Androgenic hormones	• Pseudohermaphroditism
• Folic acid antagonists	• Various skeletal and systemic disorders
• Nicotine (smoking)	• Low birth weight, prematurity
• Alcohol	• Fetal alcohol syndrome, SGA
• Illicit drugs (e.g., marijuana, cocaine, heroin, lysergic acid diethylamide [LSD])	• Intrauterine growth retardation, prematurity, limb abnormalities, chromosomal abnormalities, malformations of the central nervous system
• Tetracycline	• Tooth enamel staining, defective tooth formation, growth inhibition of long bones
Infectious Teratogens	
• Rubella virus	• Deafness, congenital heart disease, microcephaly, hepatosplenomegaly, intellectual disabilities, fetal death
• Cytomegalovirus	• Mental/motor retardation, microcephaly
• *Toxoplasma gondii*	• Microcephaly, hydrocephaly, chorioretinitis, anemia
Family Influences	
• Violence in the home	• Physical and emotional trauma
• Poor diet	• Malnutrition
• Birth order, family size, spacing between children	• May impact academic achievement and acquisition of language skills
Community/Environmental Influences	
• Secondhand smoke	• Premature death and disease in children
	• Increased risk for sudden infant death syndrome (SIDS), acute respiratory problems, ear infections, and more severe asthma
• Air pollution	• Increased respiratory infections, development of lung disease; pollutants trigger asthmatic episodes
• Pesticides	• Death of embryo, development of cancer
• Industrial wastes	• Birth defects
• Degradation products of pesticides and industrial wastes	• Mutagenicity, carcinogenicity
• Radiation exposure	• Malformations of fetus
	• Development of cancer
• Poor housing	• Increased incidence of illnesses
• Lack of access to health care	• Increased morbidity and increased illness

caREminder

Although some children may be developmentally disadvantaged because of alterations caused by a genetic condition or illness acquired later in life, opportunities to maximize the children's potential can come through the psychosocial, familial, and community assets that enhance development. These include positive relationships developed within the family system, exposure to a wide variety of learning opportunities, and a community that supports the child and the family socially and politically.

Exposure to Teratogens

A number of drugs, chemicals, and maternal illnesses have been linked to birth defects in children. Agents that can disrupt fetal growth and produce birth defects are called **teratogens**. The effects of prenatal exposure to teratogens depend on the characteristics of the chemical agent, maternal and fetal physiology, placental factors, and the time during fetal development in which the exposure took place. Figure 3-4 presents a schematic illustration of critical periods in prenatal development during which the fetus is highly sensitive to teratogens. It is well known that by the fifth week of embryonic development, virtually all chemical agents and drugs will cross the placenta. Many of these agents will have no harmful effects on the growing fetus. Others, such as alcohol, thalidomide, heroin, antidepressants, and cocaine, are known to have direct and predictable negative effects on fetal development. At the same time, it is not always easy to predict why some teratogenic agents may affect one fetus more severely than another. For instance, a pregnant woman who carefully watches her diet and exercises regularly yet continues to consume alcohol during her pregnancy may, or may not, deliver a healthy child. Intervening variables such as the mother's general health, nutritional status, exercise habits, anxiety level, and prenatal care are factors that may compound the effects of teratogens on the developing fetus. Research regarding the correlations between teratogens and other intervening variables is continuing in an effort to determine both the short- and long-term effects of these elements on the growing fetus.

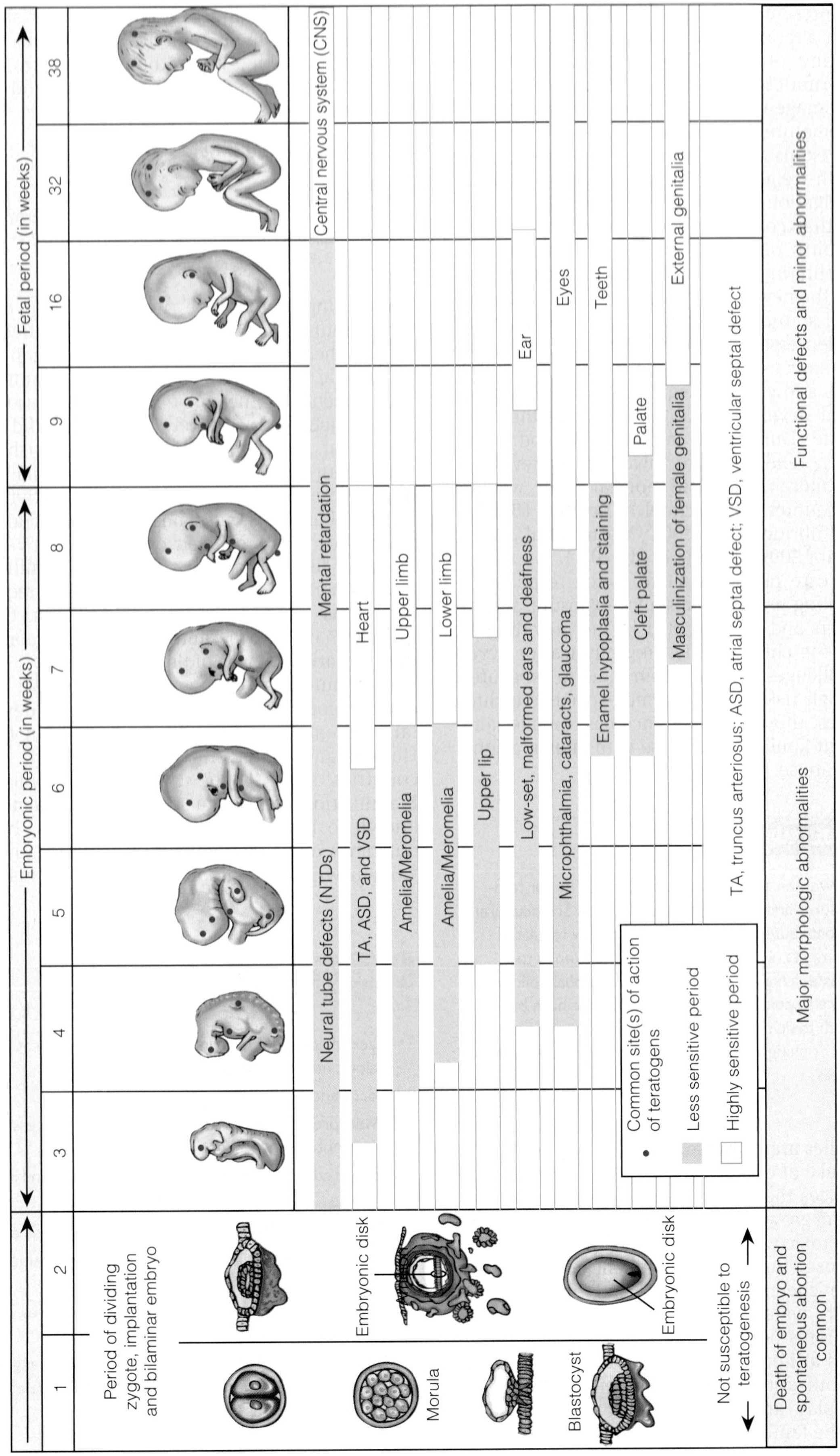

Figure 3-4 Fetal development and relative sensitivity to teratogenesis. From Moore, K., & Persaud, T. (1998). *The developing human* (6th ed.). Philadelphia, PA: W. B. Saunders. Used with permission.

Table 3-1 presents examples of the teratogens associated with alterations in growth and development. Although many of these agents can cause visible physical deformities in a child, a number of the agents also cause damage to a child's neurologic function or lead to a premature delivery. The long-term sequelae for children exposed to teratogens in utero and for very low-birth-weight survivors is a topic of considerable investigation at this time. For example, it has been noted that cocaine-exposed infants are at risk for adverse birth outcomes such as prematurity and retarded intrauterine growth. In addition, health problems beyond the newborn period that have been noted include small stature, hypertonia, poor motor performance, and depressed interactive abilities (Richardson et al., 2011; Shankaran et al., 2011; Singer et al., 2004). Children with a low birth weight are more susceptible to illness and developmental delay during the early months of life. During the middle childhood years, these children tend to score lower on achievement tests than children who had normal birth weights and may encounter more school difficulties (Breslau et al., 2011; Kilbride et al., 2004; Moster et al., 2008; Pritchard et al., 2009; Roberts et al., 2011).

All health care providers share in the responsibilities of preventing prenatal substance exposure, screening for mothers and children at risk, and providing for the needs of the child experiencing physical or developmental challenges resulting from in utero exposures. Families at high risk for teratogenic exposures include young families, those with low incomes, mobile families, immigrant families, and those with known alcohol or substance abuse.

CROSS-CULTURAL CARE

Low-income women are at a disproportionate risk for teratogenic exposures and their detrimental effects. Sociocultural factors that contribute to this risk include poorly regulated work environments, a higher probability of proximity to hazardous waste, a higher prevalence of nutritional deficiencies, adherence to culturally based practices that have been associated with toxic exposures (e.g., use of pottery for cooking), and drinking water from spent chemical tanks and from local wells.

Many families are unaware of the risk factors associated with intake of certain medications, fluids, and dietary substances that contain agents that are harmful to the fetus and growing child. Elements in the environment such as toxic wastes, secondhand smoke, and radiation also pose a threat to development (see Table 3-1). Exposures to chemical, biologic, and physical hazards in the air, water, soil, and food present ongoing risks to children's health. Children can be exposed to these hazards at home, at school, and in the community throughout critical stages of their development. Nurses can play an instrumental role in providing guidance to the family related to environmental health hazards that can affect children. Nurses should also integrate assessment of living conditions, including sources of drinking water, dietary practices, and environmental hazards, in routine perinatal and well-child health care visits.

Nutritional Deficiencies

 QUESTION: How might James's preterm status at birth have affected his nutritional status?

Maintaining appropriate nutrition from conception throughout the life span can positively affect an individual's health and quality of life. Nutrition is needed to provide the body with energy to perform several vital functions. Energy is needed for basal metabolism, which keeps the body functioning and maintains body heat. Nutrition is needed to replenish the body with energy lost from excreta, from normal processes of growth and development, and from activity requirements. Nutrition is also needed by the body systems when they are threatened or weakened by disease to maintain function and to support the healing process. It is important to note that nutritional requirements change as the body grows and develops. Chapters 4 through 7 discuss the nutritional requirements of children at various stages of development.

Poor nutrition (eating too much or too few nutrients) accounts for several health and developmental problems seen in children throughout the world. Hunger and malnutrition exists even in developed countries such as the United States and Canada. Malnutrition can be caused by several factors and is known to have adverse and, sometimes, irreversible outcomes on the growing child (Chart 3-2). Pregnant women who are malnourished are at a high risk for

| CHART 3-2 | Factors That May Cause Malnutrition |

- Lack of adequate food intake to provide the protein and caloric needs of the body
- Social and cultural differences in food habits
- Widespread ease and availability of highly processed and often nutritionally inadequate foods
- Lack of adequate nutrition education in schools and in the home
- Complacency regarding food habits
- Overeating of foods that do not meet the needs of the body
- Presence of a condition that causes higher nutritional needs (e.g., injury and the healing process)
- The presence of disease or illness that interferes with the ingestion, digestion, and absorption of food.
- Failure to adjust nutritional intake based on changing levels of activity and rest and on periods of higher metabolic demands (e.g., puberty)

miscarriages, stillbirths, and premature delivery. If the newborn is carried to term, he or she may be poorly nourished and SGA. It has been demonstrated that iron deficiency in utero or during the first 2 years of life can cause permanent damage to brain cell function and diminished cognitive functioning as demonstrated by lowered scores on developmental, learning, and school achievement tests (Black, 2012; Congdon et al., 2012).

Marasmus is a condition that affects infants who are severely malnourished. A child with marasmus looks emaciated and has a weakened heart and low resistance to infection. Body weight may decrease to less than 80% of the child's normal weight for his or her length. The child may appear fretful, irritable, and voraciously hungry. *Kwashiorkor* is a condition found in children who receive diets low in protein after weaning from breast milk or formula. These children appear listless, apathetic, and inactive. As a result of their protein deficiency, their legs and abdomen appear edematous. These children are also very susceptible to illness.

In the growing child, inadequate nutrition has been associated with lowered intelligence, poor mental health, increased susceptibility to childhood illnesses, stunted physical growth, and alterations in emotional development (Alaimo et al., 2001; Brands et al., 2012; McAfee et al., 2012). For many children, poor nutrition may be one of several variables affecting their overall well-being. Poor housing, poor sanitation, little or no medical care, poor child care practices, and limited educational opportunities for the child can all interact to affect the child's growth and development. Malnutrition, however, is more common in children who are experiencing other aspects of poverty. Thus, it becomes difficult to isolate the singular effects of poor nutrition on the child's growth and development when so many other intervening factors exist.

The early introduction of solids in infancy can cause malnutrition. Studies have shown that infants who are consistently given solid foods during the first 3 to 4 months of life have poor nutrition from excessive caloric intake (Baker et al., 2004; Gidding et al., 2006; Ong et al., 2006). Early introduction of solids interferes with formula feeding and breastfeeding, may trigger allergies, increases the chance of the infant choking, and can lead to overfeeding. Early solid food introduction may also lead to increased risk of obesity in preschool-aged children (Huh et al., 2011).

Malnutrition can also be seen in the child who comes to school each day without having had breakfast. This child may have difficulty concentrating and being attentive in school. In the older child, malnutrition is observed in teenagers who exist on fast-food or junk food diets. Teens who are left to prepare their own meals may not consistently make nutritious selections.

In addition, adolescents coping with anorexia and bulimia are at a very high risk for nutritional deficits, which affect growth and development (see Chapter 29 for a discussion of these two disorders). Hair loss,

amenorrhea (cessation of the menstrual cycle), sleep disturbances, bradycardia, cold intolerance, dry skin, and constipation are just a few of the physiologic manifestations of anorexia and bulimia. Preoccupation with food, an obsession with food rituals, and altered family and interpersonal relationships are some of the behavioral manifestations of these illnesses.

ANSWER: James, like other preterm newborns, was probably nutritionally at risk because the nutritional stores established during the last trimester were not achieved. Immaturity of his digestive system and sucking and swallowing reflexes would also most likely interfere with his ability to ingest adequate nutrition. Moreover, his energy expenditure increased as a result of his increased respiratory effort secondary to respiratory distress, causing the need for additional calories.

Family Influences on Growth and Development

The family and the environment within the home are considered the primary arena in which the child will thrive and grow. The relationships and interactions established within the context of the family serve as patterns or blueprints for the child's developing social relations and personal life skills that will impact his or her interactions outside of the home. It is within the family that the child learns about gender and social roles, self-acceptance, and self-control, for example. Within the family milieu, the child learns ways of interacting with others to meet his or her personal goals and needs.

Several family variables will influence the development of the child. These include the family structure, family functioning, and family role modeling (discussed in Chapter 1). Family conditions that place the child at risk for school performance problems include divorce, parental unemployment, single-parent households, and violence within the home. The influences of relocation, discipline, travel, play, family finances, and loss of a parent are among the many variables that affect the child as he or she interacts within the family constellation over the course of time.

Genetically, siblings are similar; they share the same parents and the same home environment, yet their experiences in the family can be different enough to create very individual and unique personal qualities. Factors that are attributed to the development of these differences include birth order, the age gap between siblings, gender, family size, childhood illnesses, temperament, sibling behavior, and parenting behavior. Parenting behaviors and child-rearing practices are important factors in determining how children will develop. The quality of interactions among the child, the parents, and the siblings influences the relationships that the child will have with others outside the home. Some of the differences between siblings can be attributed to the functioning of the emotional unit at the time each child was born. The variables that affect this emotional unit include the anxiety in the family at the time of each child's birth, characteristics of the child that trigger certain processes in the family, the intensity and direction of relationships, and how the parents relate emotionally to their extended family.

Violence within the family may also affect the child's development. *Family violence* is defined as a crime committed against someone by a family member or a relative. Types of violence that can occur in the family include child abuse (emotional or physical), sexual assault, spousal abuse, and elder abuse. Although many cases are detected and reported to the police, it is believed that more than 40% of cases are not reported to police or health care officials (Hamby et al. 2011). A child may be either the direct recipient of violence or a witness to family violence. The child who is a direct recipient of violence will suffer from physical and psychological traumas that impair normal growth and development. These issues are discussed in more detail in Chapter 29. The child who is a witness to family violence may not have impaired growth but will suffer psychological injury that may greatly affect his or her development. Children affected by family violence are at risk for low self-esteem, inability to maintain a relationship, inability to engage in healthy sexual relations as an adult, and posttraumatic stress disorder (Herrenkohl & Herrenkohl, 2007; Lewis et al., 2010; Margolin & Vickerman, 2007; McDonald et al., 2007; Moylan et al., 2010).

The relationship between the home environment and health also involves housing and neighborhood factors. Poor housing is one of the leading causes of morbidity and mortality among children in the United States (Quinn et al., 2010). In the past, health problems associated with poor housing have included tuberculosis and typhus. Today, conditions such as asthma and lead poisoning, unintentional injuries from home accidents, and neighborhood violence can severely affect the growth and development of children.

Community Influences on Growth and Development

The community encompasses all the influences provided by interaction with daycare providers, peers, school officials, religious leaders, and social acquaintances. These interactions take place within the context of a social culture that provides boundaries for acceptable and unacceptable patterns of behavior. Role expectations, gender stereotyping, and age-specific norms must be evaluated within the parameters of the community milieu at a given point in time. For instance, encouraging adolescent girls to marry and bear children might be a socially expected developmental task in some communities. However, in the United States, this practice is generally not encouraged because the adolescent female is not considered to be ready emotionally, physically, or cognitively to accept parenting responsibilities.

Public priorities and the mass media can have profound effects on children. The political and societal issues that have affected child rearing and child health care practices are discussed in Chapter 2. These include the funding and provision of mandated health services for children identified as "at risk" and the legislation that ensures that the rights of all children are protected. Public priorities are often reflected by the mass media, which in turn can influence a child's perception of socially acceptable behaviors and expectations. Research suggests that there may be a causal relationship between television violence and violence in real life. Researchers have noted both psychological and physiologic changes in children who view violence on television and from violent video games (American Academy of Pediatrics, 2009). A more thorough discussion of the influences of the media and suggestions regarding how family members and health care providers can monitor and modify these influences are presented in Chapters 4 and 7.

DEVELOPMENT OF THE BODY SYSTEMS

As a child grows, the most profound changes noted by the casual observer lie in the physical development of the child's body. External and internal body structures and functions will undergo changes that are influenced by the child's gender and age, the child's nutritional status, the presence or absence of disease, and the individual genetic attributes of a particular child.

DEVELOPMENT OF THE FETUS

The origin and development of the organ systems begin during the embryonic and fetal periods. A review of the changes that occur during these periods provides information about the origins of body structures and highlights critical periods of fetal growth when congenital malformations can occur.

Embryonic Period

By the time a pregnant woman has missed her menstrual period, the embryo developing within her has implanted in the uterus, uteroplacental circulation has begun, and a primitive neural tube and blood vessels have been formed. This is the *embryo stage*, extending from implantation until the end of the second month.

During this period, the embryonic disk is composed of three layers that develop into the major organs and tissues. The ectoderm is the rudimentary formation for the nervous system, skin, hair, nails, and sensory organs. The endoderm develops into the mucous membranes of the mouth and anus; bladder and urethra; endocrine glands such as the thyroid, parathyroid, and thymus glands; tonsils; respiratory tract; and lining of the gastrointestinal system. Major components of the musculoskeletal, genitourinary, reproductive, and cardiac systems arise from the mesoderm. Tendons, muscles, cartilage, bones, connective tissue, kidneys, ureters, heart, circulatory system, blood cells, and all reproductive organs are mesodermic.

During the fourth through the eighth week, growth of the cranial and caudal ends, and the budding of arms and legs produce a humanlike shape from the mass of embryonic tissue.

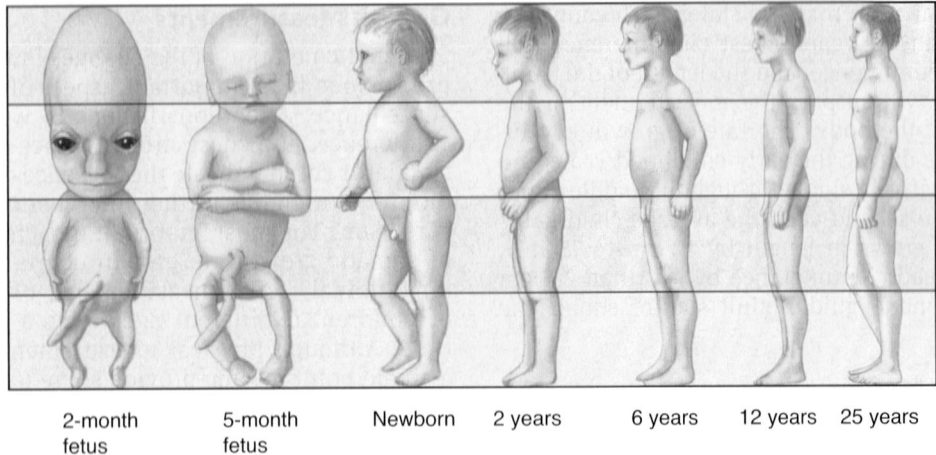

2-month   5-month   Newborn   2 years   6 years   12 years   25 years
fetus   fetus

Figure 3-5 Changes in body proportion from the second fetal month to adulthood. Adapted from Robbins, W., Brodey S., Hogan, A. et al. (1928). *Growth*. New Haven, CT: Yale University Press. Used with permission.

Fetal Period

At 9 weeks of gestation, the *fetal period* begins. During the ensuing weeks, growth of the fetus follows certain predictable patterns (see Fig. 3-4). Although cushioned and protected in the mother's womb, the fetus remains susceptible to the influences of many teratogens that can permanently alter the structure and function of various body systems. Organs that are formed from the same layer of the embryonic disk are often affected by the same teratogen. For instance, the heart and kidneys are both formed from the mesoderm. Therefore, if one of these organs is malformed, an assessment should be completed to evaluate whether the other organ arising from the same layer has also been malformed. Some teratogens are so harmful that the fetus may no longer be viable. Spontaneous abortions (miscarriages) that occur during the first trimester may result from these negative outcomes. When a teratogen affects the fetus later during the gestational period, the effects may be noted at birth when the infant presents with physical or functional impairments.

By the 10th week, the face of the fetus is recognizably human. External genitalia are clearly distinguishable by the 12th week. At this time, ultrasound evaluation of the fetus can be used to help reveal the child's sex to the expectant parents. By the 20th to the 24th week, primitive alveoli have formed and surfactant production has begun in the lungs. If birth occurs from this point on, viability of the fetus is possible. By the third trimester, structural development is complete, but functional development of the systems continues.

CHANGES IN GENERAL BODY GROWTH

From the shape of an oval body to the distinctive features of a human fetus, the child in utero grows in weight and length in a progressive and predictable pattern that continues throughout the childhood years. Failure to grow or growth retardation in utero is termed *intrauterine growth retardation*. Depending on the point in pregnancy when intrauterine growth retardation appears, early delivery of the infant by cesarean section may be completed. During the eighth month, subcutaneous fat is deposited. This fat changes the wrinkled appearance of the fetus to that of a soft, cuddly infant. The fat also aids in thermoregulation. By the third trimester, fetal weight will triple and length will double as the body stores of protein, fat, iron, and calcium increase.

Growth During Infancy

The child's body proportions undergo many changes before adult proportions are achieved (Fig. 3-5). The newborn's head is approximately one fourth of his or her total body length, and the legs are about one third of the body length. The newborn appears top heavy, with short lower extremities.

After an initial small loss of weight, most newborns regain their birth weight within 10 days of delivery. Weight gain during early infancy is approximately 20 g (0.67 oz) per day. This gain decreases to about 15 g (0.5 oz) per day during the middle and latter half of the first year. Infants double their birth weight by 5 months, although some may double their birth weight by 4 months or earlier. Should this occur, evaluation of the child's nutritional status is warranted. Birth weight is usually tripled by the first birthday. The infant's length increases about 50% during the first year. The crown-to-rump length, or sitting height, measures the same as the head circumference. Head circumference is equivalent to chest circumference during infancy. Almost no variation in head circumference parameters has been found as a result of racial, national, or geographic standards. However, head circumference varies significantly in relation to body weight. Median head circumference at 1 year of age is approximately 12 cm (4.75 in.) larger than at birth.

Growth During Childhood

 QUESTION: James, at 2 years of age, weighed 34 lb and was 35 in. in height. What would you expect his adult stature to be?

As cephalocaudal and proximodistal growth continues during the childhood years, chest circumference will exceed head circumference, and the length of the trunk and extremities will surpass the measurement of the upper portion of the body. The rate of growth continues to decelerate during the early childhood years and then remains relatively stable throughout middle childhood. During the second year, the average child gains 2.5 kg (5.5 lb), grows in length by 12 cm (4.75 in.), and increases head circumference by less than 2.5 cm (1 in.). As a general guide, adult stature equals the following:

Boys: 2 × height at age 2 years = adult height
      5 × weight at age 2 years = adult weight
Girls: 2 × height at 1½ years = adult height
      5 × weight at 1½ years = adult weight

From ages 3 to 7 years, the average child gains 2 kg (4.5 lb) in weight and 7 cm (2.75 in.) in length per year. During the school years (ages 6 to 12 years), the average weight gain is 3 kg (6.5 lb) per year and the average change in stature is an increase of 6 cm (2.25 in.) per year. Accelerated growth changes that are characteristic of the pubertal period may occur as early as 10 years of age in girls and around 12 years of age in boys.

ANSWER: Using the formula as a general guide, James's expected adult stature would be

Adult height = 35 × 2 in. = 70 in., or 5 ft 10 in.

Adult weight = 5 × 34 lb = 170 lb.

Adolescent Growth

Before puberty, growth in stature predominates in the lower extremities, whereas during puberty, truncal growth predominates. The distal extremities reach adult size before the proximal extremities, thus the common complaint among preadolescents that their feet are too big. In association with the hormonal, physical, and emotional changes that occur during puberty, the adolescent experiences a period of growth acceleration. Age at onset, peak, and termination vary considerably from one person to another. Females tend to experience the growth spurt and other pubertal changes approximately 2 years ahead of males. Therefore, although previous to this period the mean height of girls was less than that of boys, the girls catch up and surpass boys in stature during early adolescence (ages 11 to 13 years). Girls achieve mature stature sooner than boys. The male growth spurt, although slower to begin, is of a longer duration. By the completion of the adolescent years, boys will surpass girls in height. During adolescence, boys gain at least 10 cm (4 in.) in height and girls about 8 cm (3 in.). A small amount of growth in stature may occur after age 18 years, especially in boys. By the end of adolescence, mature stature is about 3.4 times birth length and mature body weight is about 20 times birth weight, unless the individual is obese or underweight.

Growth Measurements

Systematic notation of the changes in the child's body proportions is an important aspect of developmental surveillance. Alterations in length, weight, head circumference, and chest circumference from normative standards could indicate the presence of a clinical condition that requires further intervention by the health care team. The most important tools in the evaluation of somatic growth are growth charts constructed by longitudinal, serial measurements of large numbers of children at different ages over a brief period of time. Although physical measurements of a child at a single point in time provide some useful clinical information, serial measurements over months or years provide the most accurate record of the infant's or child's overall general pattern of growth. The physical measurements most often used in assessing children are height and weight; in infants and young children through age 2 years, head circumference is used. All these measurements should be made with care and with the use of a consistent technique. Chapter 8 contains a complete description of the methods to obtain weight, height, length, and head circumference measurements.

The periodic measurement of physical growth may elicit certain findings that should alert the health care provider to the existence of a health problem (Table 3-2). Because of the potential for measurement error, a single significant alteration in height, weight, or head circumference parameters should not cause alarm. The child who shows a significant change in growth parameters should be monitored closely.

TABLE 3-2	Causes of Variations in Growth Patterns	
Increase or Accelerated	**Decrease or Arrested**
Weight	
Excessive intake	Nutritional deficits
Pregnancy	Failure to thrive
Use of corticosteroids	Chronic conditions
Clinical conditions (e.g.,	(e.g., cystic fibrosis, cancer,
acquired hypothyroidism,	celiac disease, congenital
Cushing syndrome)	heart disease)
Infants of diabetic mothers	Child abuse (neglect)
Height/Length	
Endocrine conditions	Presence of scoliosis
(e.g., hyperthyroidism,	Endocrine disorder
precocious puberty,	(e.g., acquired
pituitary gigantism)	hypothyroidism, Cushing
Klinefelter syndrome	syndrome, delayed puberty,
Chromosomal abnormalities	Turner syndrome)
(e.g., XXX syndrome	
in girls)	
Marfan syndrome	
Head Circumference	
Macrocephaly	Microcephaly
Hydrocephalus	Craniostenosis
Head trauma	

More frequent growth assessments by the care provider than the normal schedule for a healthy child may be warranted.

MUSCULOSKELETAL DEVELOPMENT

> **QUESTION:** James is a very active child. His parents report that he is a bit clumsy at times, which has resulted in some falls. However, he has only experienced some bruising, cuts, and scrapes. How would you explain why these falls haven't resulted in any broken bones?

Growth and changes in the musculoskeletal system begin at conception and continue throughout life. Muscular activity is among the primary functions first achieved by the developing fetus. During the fourth to eighth months of gestation, the precursors of skeletal muscle and vertebrae (somites) appear. The back of the forming fetus is bent so the head nearly touches the tail. This tail begins to involute by the eighth week. The presence of arm and leg buds and rudimentary eyes, ears, and nose can be noted. Ossification begins around the eighth week, and the fetus assumes a humanlike appearance. Fingers, toes, elbows, knees, arms, and legs have all developed. Facial features can now be seen. The first muscle contractions occur, soon followed by lateral flexion movements.

By the end of the first trimester, the fetus can move its arms and legs independently of the trunk. By the 17th week, the grasp reflex is present and the fetus can be observed, on ultrasound evaluation, sucking the thumb. By midgestation, the fetus can move its arms and legs just as the newborn can and, when the mother has periods of rest, is likely to demonstrate a full range of movement inside the womb. This fluttering sensation is called *quickening*. Fetal movements continue in strength and frequency throughout the rest of the pregnancy. By the 29th week, the fetus can kick, suck, and turn, changing positions as needed to find a position of comfort. During the last 2 months of gestation, further refinement of the musculoskeletal system occurs. Creases develop in the soles of the feet and an increase in ear cartilage formation occurs. The neonate at rest will assume the position similar to that maintained in utero. The feet curve inward, the spine is in a rounded position, and the arms remain flexed and close to the body.

The skeleton of the infant and young child is largely made up of preosseous cartilage and physes. The bones are flexible and have a high porosity. The young child's bones can absorb a great deal of energy before breaking and may even bow rather than fracture when a trauma occurs. The young child has an active growth plate at the end of the long bones known as the *physeal* or *epiphyseal plate*. Longitudinal growth and alignment of the long bones takes place at the growth plate through the process of endochondral ossification. During this process, cartilage becomes ossified, turning it into bone. This process continues until skeletal maturity is complete in adolescence. At that time, an increase in androgenic hormones produced during puberty causes the growth plate to gradually stop functioning.

> **ANSWER:** James is a young child and, as such, his bones are flexible and porous. Bones at this age can sustain a large amount of force or energy before a fracture occurs.

The mature newborn most often assumes a flexed position of the extremities. It is believed that this flexion pattern is induced by the position of the infant in utero. In infants who are in breech position in utero, flexor positioning of the lower extremities is often absent. The premature infant also demonstrates less motor tone than the term neonate.

The full-term newborn demonstrates increased resistance against gradual stretching (tonic myotactic reflexes) in almost all flexor and in many of the extensor muscles. This can be demonstrated by extending the lower arm of the awake neonate. When released, the arm will recoil to its flexed position. Similarly, a newborn in the standing position has a stepping motion as he or she alternately flexes and extends the lower extremities. This involuntary reflex disappears at about 6 weeks of age, later replaced by voluntary stepping motions attempted between 8 months and 1 year of age. The demonstration of hypotonia (frog legs) or scissoring with spasticity would be indications that abnormalities in the infant's muscle tone are present.

As the child grows and is physically active, muscular strength and agility will increase. Low muscle tone (hypotonia) might be seen in children with hypothyroidism, Down syndrome, or a neurologic problem. During puberty, there is an increase in both total body fat and fat-free mass (FFM). Muscle tone and muscle mass increase. Strength training (also called *resistance training*) can be implemented to enhance further muscle strength, size, and power. However, gains in these areas are lost after 6 weeks if resistance training is discontinued (American Academy of Pediatrics, 2008).

NEUROLOGIC MATURATION

The neurologic and sensory organs are among the first systems to develop. Functioning of these systems is necessary for the functioning and development of other body systems. The brain and spinal cord begin to form during the first month of gestation as a longitudinal neural plate and neural groove that lengthens into a tube with two protrusions at the upper end for the brain. The upper portion will dilate and form the brain; the remaining portion of the tube will form the spinal cord.

At 8 weeks, the nerves still do not have any anatomic or physiologic connections with either smooth or striated muscle. The embryo is floating freely in the amniotic fluid, with little purposeful movement noted. Flexing of the trunk and head extension movements can be elicited in response to tactile stimulation. The hemispheres of the brain become recognizable, and cerebellar development is visible.

During the 12th to 14th week, the neuromuscular system matures, spreading caudad. By the end of the fourth month, the frontal, temporal, parietal, and occipital lobes may be distinguished. Until about the sixth month of gestation, fetal behavior is largely controlled by spinal mechanisms. As maturation continues, the medulla and lower brain centers participate in the control of specific reflexive movements. The cerebral cortex has no influence on behavior until some time after birth. During the seventh month, there is a period of rapid brain growth. Multiplication and expansion of brain function are at a peak, and the cerebral cortex is undergoing additional refinement.

At birth, brain stem functions and spinal cord reflexes are present. The autonomic nervous system is intact but immature, and the sympathetic nervous system, which innervates the heart, is still incomplete. Functions of the cerebral cortex, such as cognition and fine motor skills, are also incomplete. As a result of this immaturity, the infant is able to have cardiorespiratory function and to use reflex movements but is unable to thermoregulate efficiently or to have coordinated gross and fine motor movements.

The infant's brain weighs 25% of its adult mature weight (300 to 350 g). By 1 year of age, brain weight has doubled and is about two-thirds the weight of the adult brain. Brain growth continues until approximately 6 years of age, when it reaches 90% of the adult weight. The increase in size during the early years is primarily the result of an increase in nerve fibers and the development of nerve tracts. At birth, the infant's cranium is not normally fused, allowing for the skull to compress during the birthing process so the head can pass through the narrow birth canal. The sutures of the newborn's skull are easily palpable, with final closure of the cranium not complete until 16 to 18 months of age. The presence of two fontanels provides a gauge to the processes of cranial fusion. The posterior fontanel will close at 6 to 8 weeks of age, with the anterior fontanel closing at 16 to 18 months of age.

Neurologic development continues, with myelinization and maturation of the neural system becoming complete around age 2 years. The development of muscle tone, the extinction of reflexes, and the achievement of gross and fine motor skills reflect the continued maturation of the nervous system.

Children are born with all their neurons formed; however, the connections between these neurons proliferate and branch after birth, reaching a peak count by 3 years of age. Half of these synapses are lost by age 15 years. This suggests that there are more synapses than are needed for humans to function and that in the brain, there is selective "pruning" of unused synapses and strengthening of those that are used to foster environmental adaptation. Thus, a child's early experiences may affect the development of the neural network (S. Fox et al., 2010). The growth of the neuron network permits greater management over large and small muscles that control body movements. Refinement of neural pathways permits the child to have better control and coordination over specific body parts.

Reflexes

Reflexive movements that are characteristic of newborn behavior begin to appear in utero by the end of the first trimester. Among the first of the reflexes to appear is the Babinski toe sign (extension of the large toe, with fanning of the small toes on stimulation of the sole of the foot), with later appearance of the swallowing and sucking reflexes.

Reflexive movements of the newborn are indicative of the motor behavior control exerted by the newborn's spinal cord and medulla. Each reflex requires a specific sensory stimulus to generate the stereotyped motor response. As the child matures, motor control expands to different levels of the nervous system. Therefore, many of the reflexes present at birth will normally disappear around the fourth month of age and cannot be elicited by sensory stimulation. These include the Moro reflex, the rooting reflex, and the palmar grasp reflex. Absence of these reflexes or persistence of these reflexes past the period they would normally disappear may indicate severe problems of the central nervous system.

Gross Motor Development

The acquisition of gross motor skills precedes the development of fine motor skills. Both processes occur in a cephalocaudal fashion, with head control preceding arm and hand control followed by leg and foot control. All the extremities move randomly at birth without visible coordination occurring for several months. Movements are symmetric, with no preference shown before 1 year of age for handedness or hemisphere dominance.

The acquisition of gross motor milestones varies from child to child. Although it can be predicted that particular milestones will be achieved by a certain ages, latitude in the exact month the milestone is attained cannot be predicted. Concerns are raised when a milestone that should have been achieved is obviously not yet attained. Further evaluation of the child for developmental delays may be warranted.

Head Control

The newborn has very little head control, and marked head lag is normal. When the newborn is pulled by the arms into a semi-Fowler position, the head will be hyperextended and will lag behind the alignment of the rest of the body. In the prone position, the infant has the ability to lift the head slightly and move it from side to side. When placed in a sitting position, the infant's head will drop forward onto the chest. Although the infant will attempt to right the head in the correct position, this only serves to make the head flop from one side to another.

At approximately 2 months of age, the infant demonstrates slight head lag and is able to hold the head up reasonably well when held in an upright position. In the prone position, the child can turn the head from side to

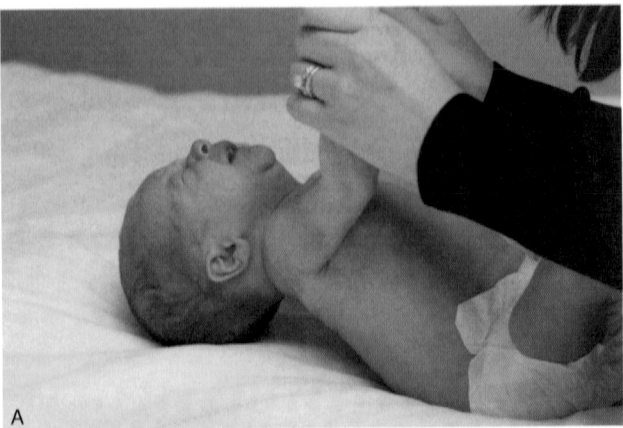

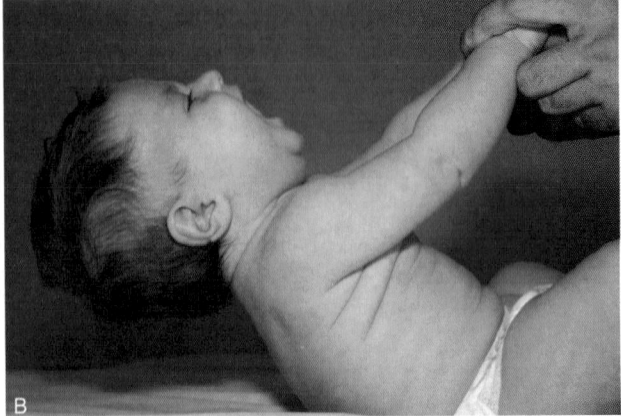

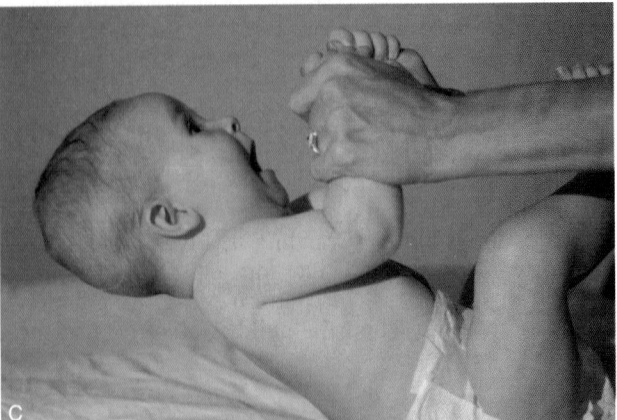

Figure 3-6 (A) The newborn has marked head lag when pulled from a lying to a sitting position. (B) The 2-month-old demonstrates slight head lag. (C) By age 6 months, no head lag is present.

side and can hold the head erect for 20 to 30 seconds at a 45-degree angle.

Between the third and fourth months, the infant achieves the ability to hold the head at 90 degrees and head lag becomes minimal. By the sixth month, head control is usually well established, as is evidenced by the lack of head lag. When prone, the infant lifts the head and upper abdomen off a surface by bearing weight on the arms. Figures 3-6 and 3-7 illustrate the development of head control during infancy.

Rolling Over

The newborn is not capable of purposefully rolling the body from one side to the other. Between 4 and 5 months of age, the infant learns to roll from front to back, then from back to front between ages 5 and 6 months. After infants can roll 360 degrees, they can then learn to pull to a sitting position and eventually learn to roll from the back to a knee–chest position to a standing position in one fluid movement.

Sitting Up

The development of head control must precede the ability to sit. The newborn infant lacks substantial head control, and the entire back is uniformly rounded; these features prohibit a sitting posture. At 2 months of age, the infant still requires adult assistance to maintain a sitting position (Fig. 3-8). Therefore, to be upright, the infant must be supported in an angled seat that provides

full head, back, and posterior support. Between 5 and 6 months of age, the spinal column has straightened enough and head control is sufficient to allow the infant to sit in a tripod position (see Fig. 3-8). The legs are extended in a wide V-based fashion, and the hands are used to provide support and stability. By 8 months of age, the infant can sit upright for long periods of time (see Fig. 3-8). The child can also easily change from a lying to a sitting position and vice versa.

Locomotion

> **QUESTION:** James is 2½ years old. Developmentally, what should James be able to accomplish at this stage related to his gait and ability to get around?

The development of locomotion involves several different but related capabilities. The child must be able to bear weight; use the arms to support, push, and raise the body; and use the legs to propel the body forward in a coordinated fashion. As the child grows, coordination and balance will be refined, permitting the child to learn to run, skip, hop, and jump.

The very young infant is unable and unwilling to bear weight on the legs (Fig. 3-9). Around 6 months of age, the infant can bear weight fairly well when pulled to a standing position. Although the infant can use the

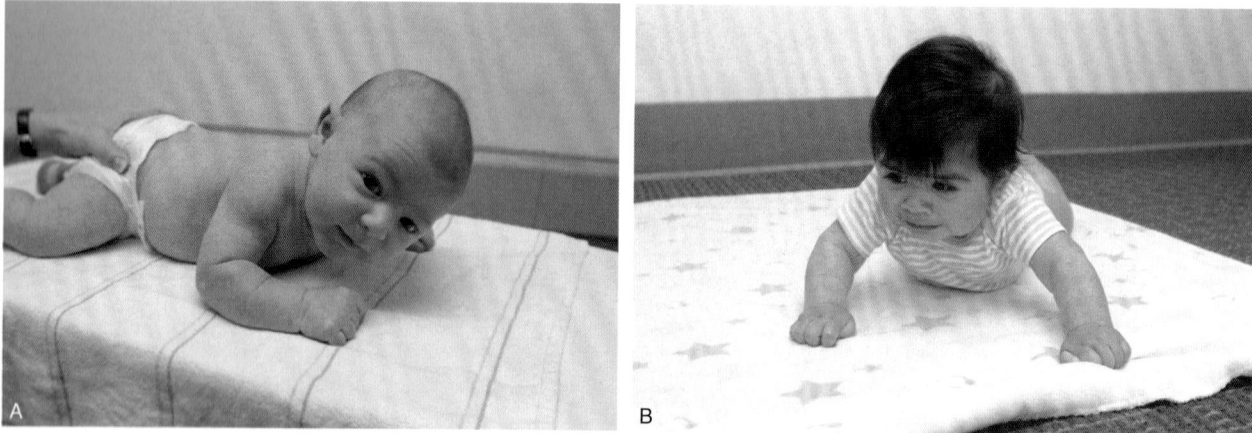

Figure 3-7 (A) The newborn is barely able to lift his head while lying prone. (B) By age 6 months, the infant easily lifts the head, chest, and upper abdomen and can bear weight on the hands.

arms to lift the upper chest off a flat surface, no attempt is yet made to use the arms to pull or push the body. Some infants may begin crawling as early as 7 months of age; other children may not initiate these movements for a few more months. Crawling involves moving the body forward using the arms and legs while keeping the belly on the floor. This pattern of movement progresses to creeping when the child is able to raise the belly off the floor and support his or her body weight with the hands and knees. The child can usually maneuver from the sitting position to the creeping position easily (Fig. 3-10). At 9 months of age, the child may also be able to pull into a standing position by holding on to something. The infant may continue to creep and pull to a standing position for quite some time without displaying further interest in walking. Creeping is a

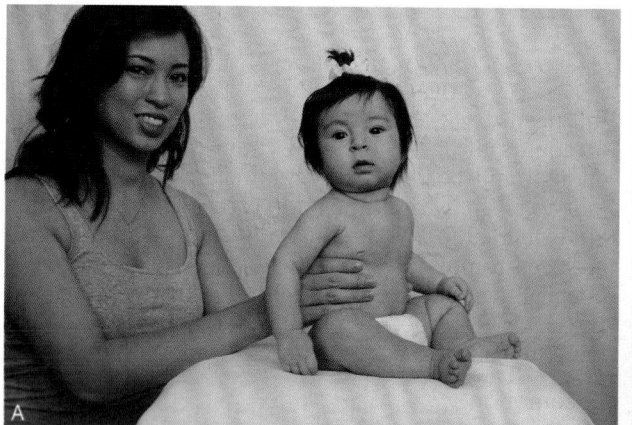

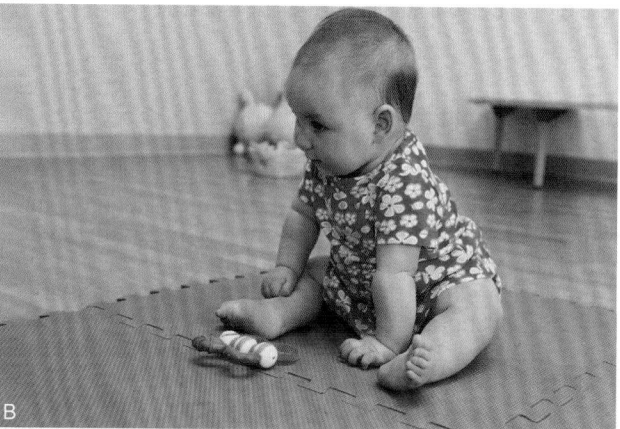

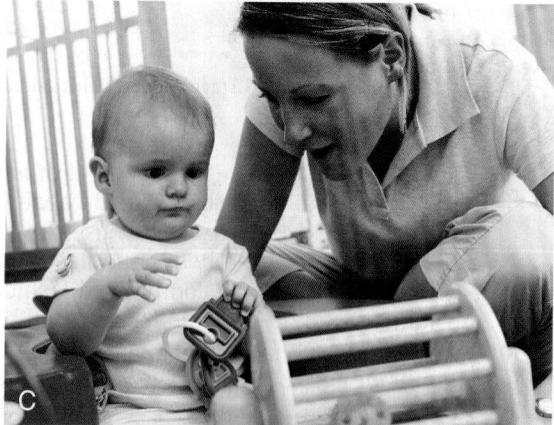

Figure 3-8 (A) At age 2 months, the infant needs assistance to maintain an upright position. (B) At age 6 months, the infant can sit alone in the tripod position, using the hands for support and stability. (C) By age 8 months, the infant can sit without support and can focus on play activities.

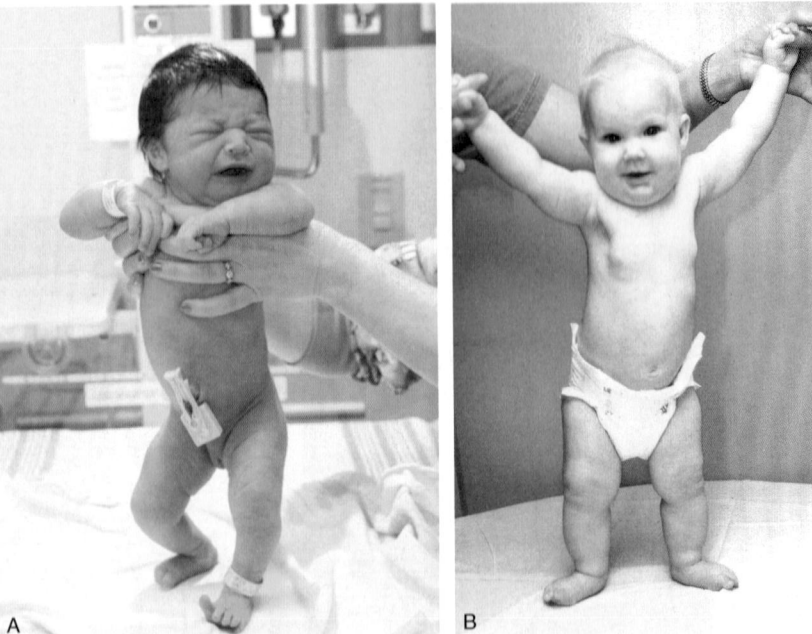

Figure 3-9 (A) The newborn is unable to bear weight on the legs. (B) By age 6 months, the infant bears full weight on the legs.

A

B

very efficient method of locomotion. Even when walking is well established during the second year, it is not uncommon for the child to use the hands and knees to move from one place to the next, especially if the child has been playing on the floor.

After the child is able to pull into a standing position, he or she next learns to stand independently and bend the knees to change from a crouching position to a standing position (Fig. 3-11). The cautious child is likely to stay close to a support mechanism (such as a piece of furniture) as he or she learns how to maneuver upright. Most likely, the first steps will be taken as the child moves from one piece of furniture to the next

or from the support of one parent's arms to those of another. Some infants may begin walking as early as 10 months of age. Ninety-five percent of children walk independently by 18 months of age (Fig. 3-12). Within 15 months of the initiation of independent walking, the child's gait will be mature. Until that time, the walk is wide based, marked by frequent stumbling. During the initial stages of learning to walk, the young child maintains the arms flexed and close to the sides of the body. The line of the body while ambulating has a forward lunge to it. As the child becomes steadier on the feet, a more upright position is assumed and the arms relax and move freely as the child walks.

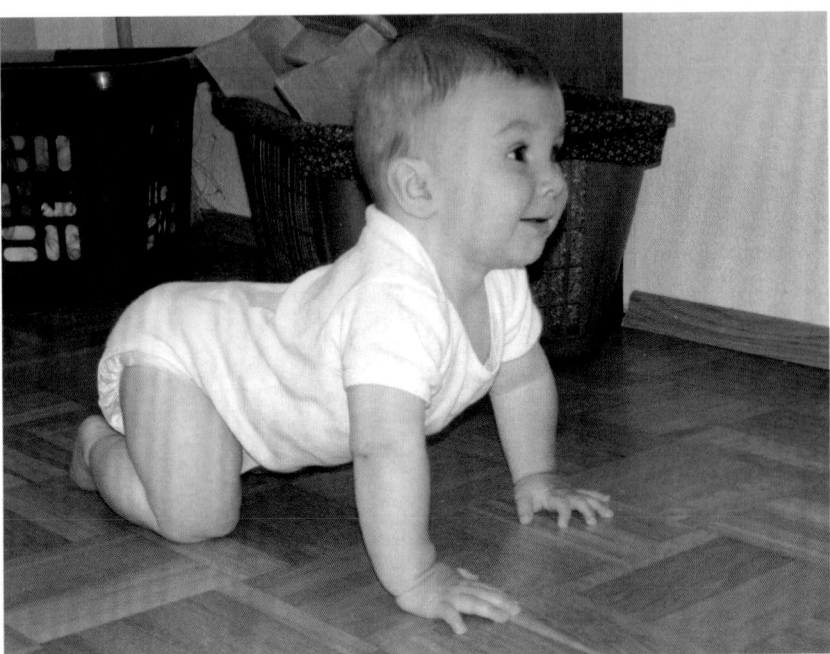

Figure 3-10 At 9 months of age, the infant is able to maneuver into a position for crawling in which the arms and knees bear weight.

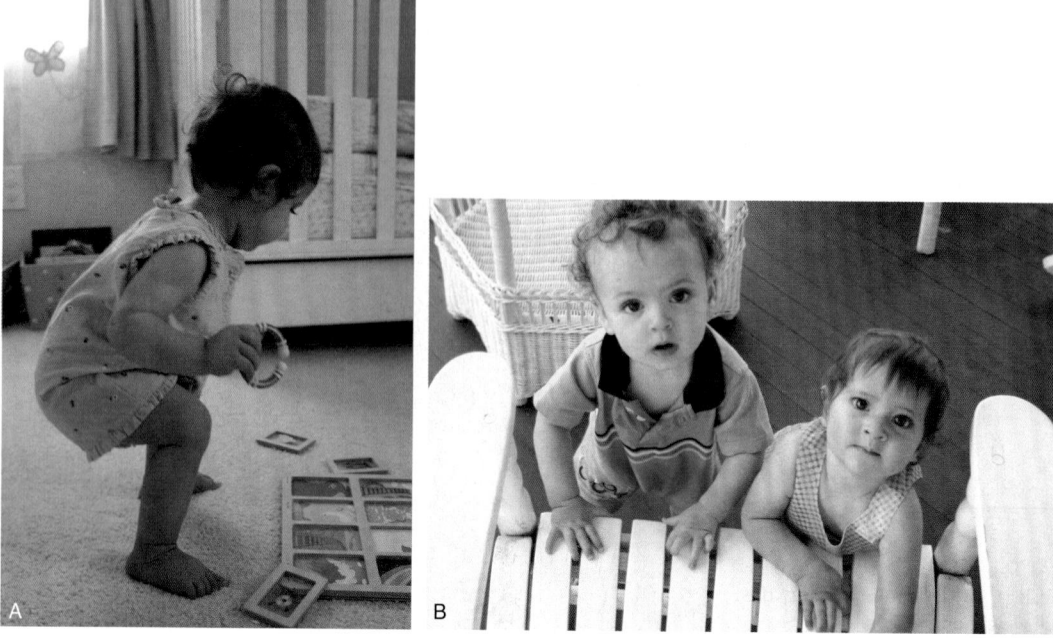

Figure 3-11 (A) By 1 year of age, the child is able to stand independently from a crouched position and (B) cruises along furniture.

By 2 years of age, the pace of the child's gait has steadily improved such that running can be accomplished without stumbling. Most 2-year-olds can kick a ball, climb well, and maneuver up and down stairs one at a time. A 3-year-old may go up and down the stairs using alternating feet, can stand on one foot momentarily, and can ride a tricycle (Fig. 3-13). Locomotion continues as the 4-year-old learns to hop and walk down the stairs on alternating feet. The arms, no longer needed to propel the body, can now throw a ball overhead and swing a bat. By 5 years of age, the child may ride a bike (with training wheels) and learn to skip (Fig. 3-14). The school-aged child can stand on one foot for 10 seconds and will learn to jump rope (Fig. 3-15).

After the child enters school, many opportunities to learn new locomotion skills are presented through participation in organized games and sports activities (Fig. 3-16). Refinement of gross motor skills such as balancing, throwing, and complex combined activities (run–turn–jump–throw) continue through adolescence. As the child experiences growth changes during puberty, clumsy movements may be noted. The rapidity

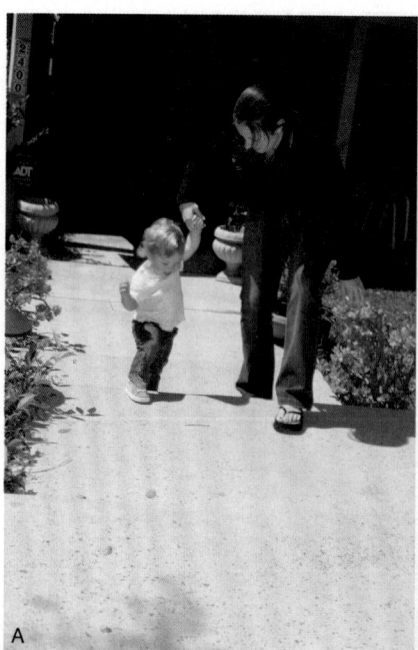
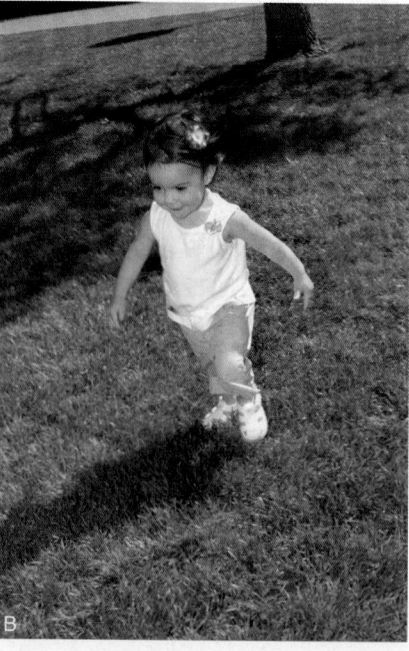

Figure 3-12 (A) At 13 months of age, the child walks and toddles quickly. (B) By 15 months of age, the child can run with arms extended outward.

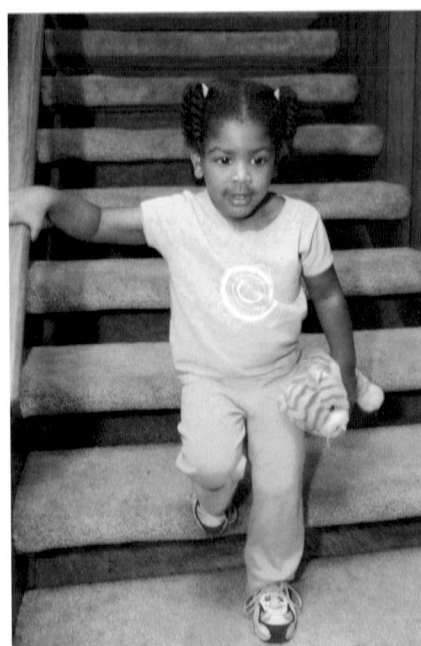

Figure 3-13 The 4-year-old child is able to walk stairs independently.

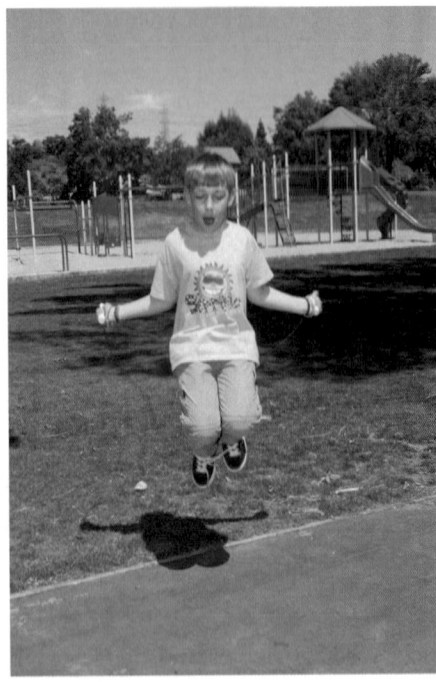

Figure 3-15 The 10-year-old can easily jump rope.

of physical changes in height, in length of extremities, and in distribution of body weight may affect the adolescent's perception of body image and proportion, requiring some mental adjustments to develop a sense of comfort with his or her changing shape. Summary tables of gross motor accomplishments of children of all ages are presented in Chapters 4 through 7.

ANSWER: By 2 years of age, the child should be well established with walking. His gait should be fairly smooth and he should be able to run easily without stumbling. James should also be able to kick a ball, climb, and go up and down stairs one foot at a time. As he approaches the age of 3 years, he should begin demonstrating the ability to go up and down stairs while alternating his feet, to stand on one foot for a short time, and even to begin to ride a tricycle.

Fine Motor Development

The newborn has very little control over fine motor movement. Actions made with the hands consist of broad sweeping actions and bringing the hand to the mouth. Objects placed in the newborn's hand will be involuntarily grasped and then dropped without notice by the infant. During the second month, the child's ability to hold an object improves. During the ensuing months, the ability to reach and grasp progresses from the gross hand control of the palmar grasp to a more refined ability to grasp smaller objects using the thumb and forefinger in a pincer grasp (Fig. 3-17). The pincer grasp begins to emerge around the eighth to ninth month. With mastery of the pincer grasp, the infant can learn to hold a cup with handles, pick up small pieces of food, and crudely hold a spoon. By 1 year of age, use

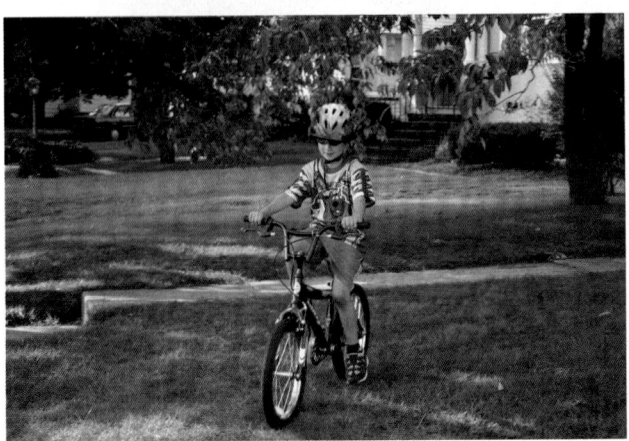

Figure 3-14 The 5-year-old is able to ride a bike.

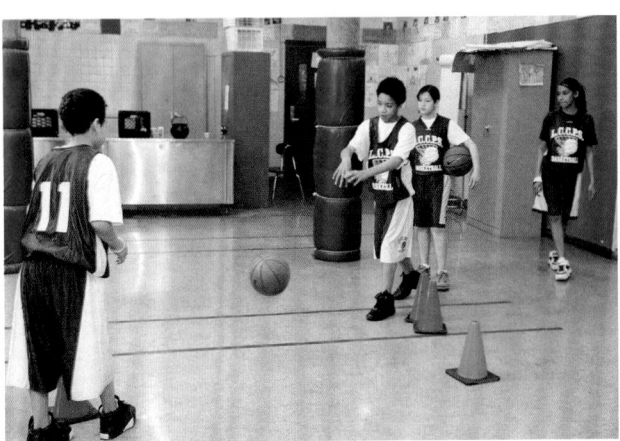

Figure 3-16 The middle school student uses multiple locomotion skills to play basketball.

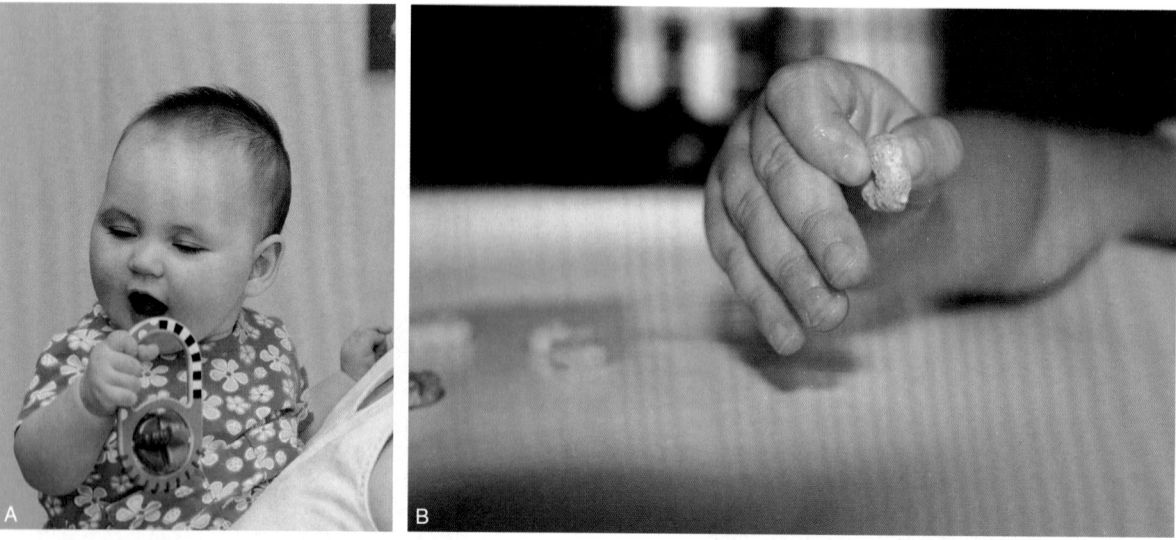

Figure 3-17 (A) Palmar grasp. The infant uses the entire hand to grasp an object. (B) Pincer grasp. The young child uses the thumb and index finger to pick up small objects.

of the pincer grasp is well established, as is the ability to transfer objects from hand to hand and hold multiple objects in a hand.

Refinement of fine motor skills continues throughout childhood (Fig. 3-18). By age 2 years, many children can hold a crayon and color using a vertical stroking motion. The pages of a book can be turned by the child and a tower of six blocks can be built. During the third year, the child uses fine motor skills to copy a circle and a cross and to build using very small blocks. The 3-year-old may be able to use scissors, and the ability to color becomes more refined (the child is able to

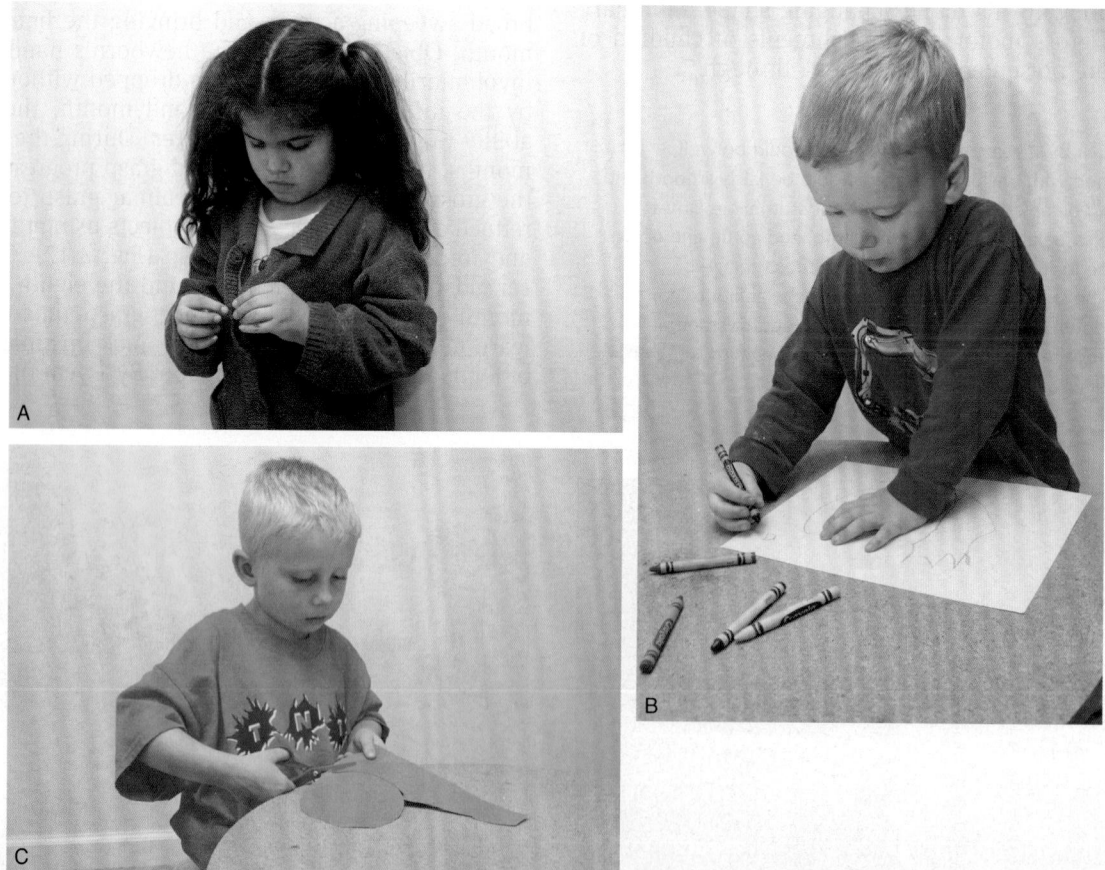

Figure 3-18 The child progressively achieves mastery of fine motor skills and cognitive abilities, such as buttoning clothes (A), holding a crayon (B), and using scissors (C).

color within certain borders). The 5-year-old is taught to write letters and draws a person with body parts.

During middle childhood, writing skills improve. The child advances to cursive writing. Fine motor coordination is enhanced by such activities as building models, sewing, playing a musical instrument, and painting. Fine motor work generally requires focused periods of concentration to complete (Fig. 3-19). Girls often demonstrate more interest in these quiet, intense activities than do boys. Middle childhood is an opportune time to introduce typing skills, which can be transferred to activities on the computer. Both boys and girls are likely to show interest in technology because these skills are being used more extensively in the classroom (Fig. 3-20). Summary tables of the fine motor accomplishments of children of all ages are presented in Chapters 4 through 7.

SENSORY ORGAN DEVELOPMENT

QUESTION: Approximately how many teeth would you expect James to have at his current age?

Sensory development begins during gestation and continues throughout the childhood years. Development of body structures (the eye, ear, nose, and mouth) impacts the sensory processes of seeing, hearing, smelling, and tasting. In healthy children, interaction with the environment improves these senses and helps the brain to establish neuronal pathways for transmission of input from these senses into voluntary and involuntary responses on the part of the child.

Eyes

At the end of the first trimester, the eyes are set far to the side of the head and the neural connections to the eyes begin to develop. Eyebrows and eyelashes do not form until the sixth month. A thin membrane keeps the eyes fused until the end of the 28th week when the eyes begin to open and the pupils respond to light.

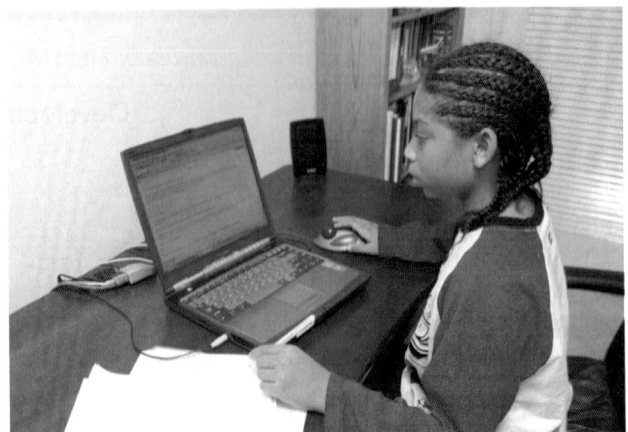

Figure 3-20 Use of the computer also involves the integration of fine motor and cognitive skills.

Visual function at birth is limited, improving rapidly during the next few years as the structure develops (Developmental Considerations 3-1). The blink reflex is present in normal newborns. Tear glands begin to secrete within the first 2 weeks of life, and the infant may experience problems with mucus plugging the tear duct. Transient strabismus is a normal finding during the first few months. By 5 to 6 weeks of age, the infant is able to fixate on an object and follow a bright light or toy. At 3 to 4 months of age, the infant is able to reach for objects at varying distances. The ability to fuse two retinal images together in the brain begins to mature at about 9 months of age but is not fully mature until around age 6 years. The macula will mature by the end of the first year. Also, by the end of the first year, mature adult functioning of eye muscles will be attained. Visual acuity, approximately 20/400 at birth, will not reach 20/20 until the child is about 4 years of age. Full maturation of the visual system and its oculomotor apparatus is almost completed by age 5 to 7 years. A discussion of conditions that can alter vision is presented in Chapter 28.

Ears

Ear formation begins around the fifth week in utero and remains susceptible to teratogenic influences until approximately the 16th week. These teratogens include ototoxic drugs, radiation, and infection. By the end of the first trimester, ear formation is complete and the ears are located in the appropriate position relative to other facial structures. In children younger than 3 years of age, the ear canal is directed upward. In the older child, the ear canal is directed downward and forward. The ears of the term neonate lay flat against the head and are well formed with firm cartilage. The top of the ear is in alignment with the inner and outer canthi of the eyes. Low-set and/or posteriorly rotated ears may indicate the presence of a chromosomal aberration.

The fetus responds to sounds as early as the 26th week of gestation. The newborn is capable of sound discrimination at birth and will fix his or her gaze on the source of the mother's voice, in preference to other human voices, within 12 hours of birth. The

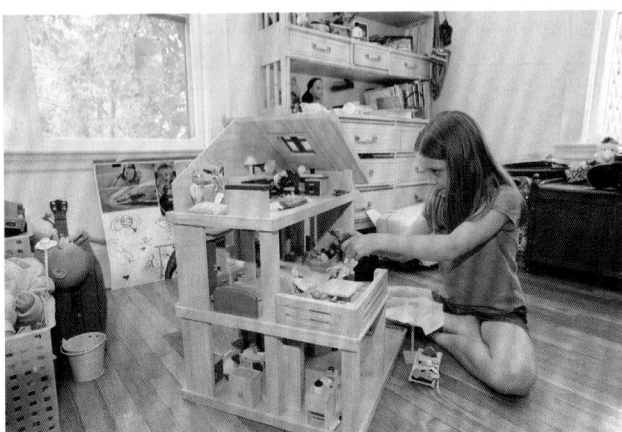

Figure 3-19 During the school years, the child uses fine motor and cognitive skills to play. The child often becomes engrossed in these quiet, independent activities.

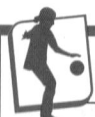

DEVELOPMENTAL CONSIDERATIONS 3-1

Development of Vision

Birth to 2 Weeks Old
Central acuity is 20/400.
Nystagmus is present.
Alertness is noted to visual stimulus 8–12 in. from eyes.
Pupils begin to enlarge.
Tear glands begin to secrete.

2–4 Weeks Old
Head and eye follow objects up to 90-degree arc.
Very little attention is given to stimuli beyond 2 ft.
Blinking is evident at approaching objects.

6–12 Weeks Old
Alertness is noted to moving objects, although convergence and following are jerky and inexact.
Head and eyes follow object through 180-degree arc.
Fascination is evident for bright objects.
Tear glands begin to display response to emotion.
Newborn regards own hands.
Visual–motor coordination begins.

16–20 Weeks Old
Central acuity is 20/200.
Interest is shown in stimuli more than 3 ft away.

20–28 Weeks Old
Color preference for bright reds and yellows develops.
Ciliary muscle function begins.
Accommodation and convergence reflexes begin.
Hand–eye coordination begins to develop.
True blinking appears.
Ultimate color of the iris can be determined.

36–44 Weeks Old
Central acuity exceeds 20/100.
Depth perception is developing.

Visual regard for object, with movement of the eyes horizontally and vertically to follow the object, is present.

1 Year Old
Pupils have enlarged to midposition and their diameter continues to increase.
Cornea is adult size (12 mm).
Central acuity is 20/50.
Fusion is present, although of poor quality and readily interrupted.
Ability to discriminate geometric forms is present.
Infant stacks blocks and can place peg in small round hole.

2 Years Old
Central acuity ranges from 20/30 to 20/40.

3 Years Old
Central acuity ranges from 20/30 to 20/40.
Convergence is smoother.
Amblyopia can occur from disuse.
Attention span is fair.
Fixation on small pictures or toys is approximately 50 seconds.
Afterimages can be described by the child.

4 Years Old
Acuity is nearly 20/20–20/30.
Child is distinguishing letters and shapes.
Lacrimal glands are fully developed.

6 Years Old
Central acuity is established.
Physiologic hyperopia decreases.
Gross attention span is approximately 20 minutes.
Detailed attention span is approximately 2 minutes.
Color shading can be differentiated.

Data from Johnson, T., Moore, W., & Jeffries, J. (Eds.). (1978). *Children are different.* Columbus, OH: Ross Laboratories.

---

neonate responds more readily to high-pitched sound and is startled by loud noises. Mucus in the eustachian tube or vernix caseosa in the external ear canal may limit hearing at birth but resolves quickly.

During the first few months, the infant begins to cease activity when sound is presented at a conversational level. By 5 to 6 months of age, the infant is able to localize and begins to imitate selected sounds vocalized by an adult. During 7 to 12 months of age, the infant is able to localize to sound presented in any plane and responds to his or her name even when spoken quietly. After the first birthday, the child is able to point to familiar objects or people when asked. By 18 months of age, the child can hear and follow a simple command without gestures or other visual cues. At this point, children who have difficulty attaining language milestones must be evaluated for hearing loss (see "Language Development" section later in this chapter for more information regarding language milestones). Developmental Considerations 3-2 further describes the development of hearing.

Congenital hearing loss is strongly linked to genetic influences. Profound hearing loss is present in 1 of every 1,000 to 2,000 newborn infants (Kochhar et al., 2007). The cause of congenital deafness can be genetic

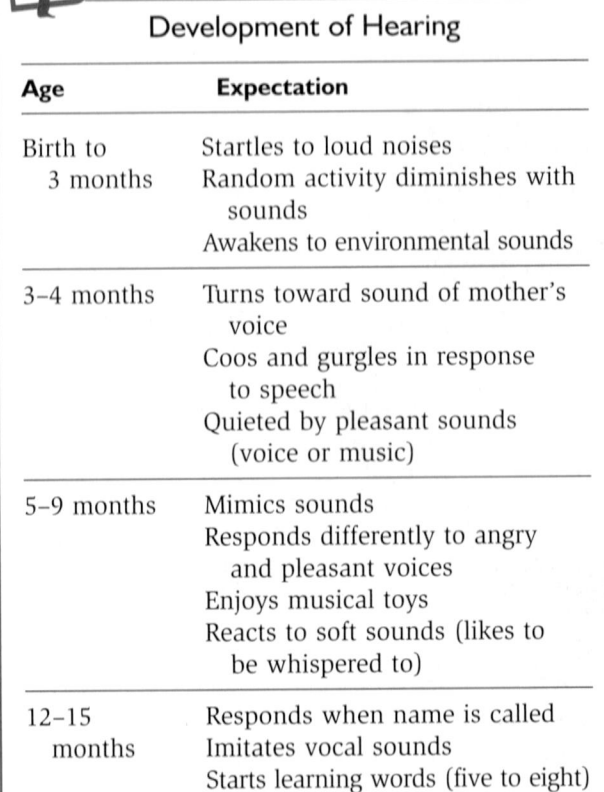

DEVELOPMENTAL CONSIDERATIONS 3-2

Development of Hearing

Age	Expectation
Birth to 3 months	Startles to loud noises Random activity diminishes with sounds Awakens to environmental sounds
3–4 months	Turns toward sound of mother's voice Coos and gurgles in response to speech Quieted by pleasant sounds (voice or music)
5–9 months	Mimics sounds Responds differently to angry and pleasant voices Enjoys musical toys Reacts to soft sounds (likes to be whispered to)
12–15 months	Responds when name is called Imitates vocal sounds Starts learning words (five to eight)

or can be acquired from intrauterine conditions such as infections (cytomegalovirus, rubella, syphilis) or anomalies. Hearing loss is greater in premature children who have corresponding postnatal complications (e.g., poor Apgar score, need for mechanical ventilation, hyperbilirubinemia). Permanent partial hearing loss is associated with bacterial meningitis, severe otitis media, certain infectious diseases (mumps, measles, Epstein-Barr virus), the use of ototoxic drugs, and head trauma. A thorough discussion of hearing disorders in children is provided in Chapter 28.

Nose

The structure of the nose may influence smell only in the sense that a blockage or malformation may impair the ability to smell. The nose of the newborn should be placed midline on the face. A malformed or misshapen nose may occur in the presence of chromosomal problems, choanal atresia, or perforation or deviation of the septum. Infants have a small nasal bridge and are obligate nose breathers until 1 month of age.

The newborn will react to strong odors such as ammonia and fresh onion. Infants are able to detect the smell of their mother's breast milk as early as 6 to 10 days after birth. The ability to smell and differentiate smells continues to improve as the child matures. Discrimination of smell is influenced by the child's attentiveness to this particular sense. For instance, the child whose temperament style is characterized by a low threshold to stimulus is likely to be highly sensitive to smells in the environment.

Mouth

Formation of the palate occurs during the seventh and eighth weeks of gestation, at which time the fetus is sensitive to teratogens that can affect development of the oral cavity. The most common abnormalities seen are cleft lip and cleft palate. Cleft lip is a result of incomplete fusion of embryonic structures surrounding the primitive oral cavity. Cleft palate represents failure of the primary and secondary palatine plates to fuse.

In healthy newborns, the hard and soft palates are intact, the uvula is midline, the tongue moves freely in the mouth, and lips and lip movement are symmetric. The oral cavity and structures within it continue to grow in proportion to other facial structures as the child matures.

Tooth formation begins at approximately the seventh week in utero, with the differentiation of specialized oral epithelial cells. Calcification of teeth begins at 4 months' gestation and is not completed until young adulthood. Eruption of teeth occurs at about the sixth month of life. Some children may experience the appearance of the first tooth before this time; in others, this does not occur until the latter months of the first year. There are 20 deciduous teeth, with eruption completed by age 2½ years. The first permanent molar and lower incisor teeth erupt around age 6 years and most are present by age 12 years (Fig. 3-21).

ANSWER: James, who is 2½ years old, should have a complete set of deciduous teeth (20) at this time.

The tonsils, located in the pharyngeal cavity, are part of the lymphatic system. Tonsillar tissue is usually not evident in the newborn. The tonsils in young children are generally larger than in adults, usually extending beyond the palatine arch until the age of 11 or 12 years.

The sense of taste is immature in newborns, although they can distinguish among sugar, lemon, salt, and quinine. Sensitivity to strong tastes becomes heightened at 2 to 3 months of age. At this time, the taste buds are maturing and they are more widely distributed on the tongue than are those of older infants. The sense of taste is not fully developed until approximately 2 years of age.

ORGAN DEVELOPMENT

During the third and fourth weeks of gestation, the main organs begin to form in a cephalocaudal direction. By the eighth week, basic organ development is complete. Although the organs are in place and functioning in a primitive fashion, the organs will not be able to work to sustain life until about the 20th week of fetal development. Further functional development of many organs continues with the transition of the fetus to extrauterine life. In addition, other functional

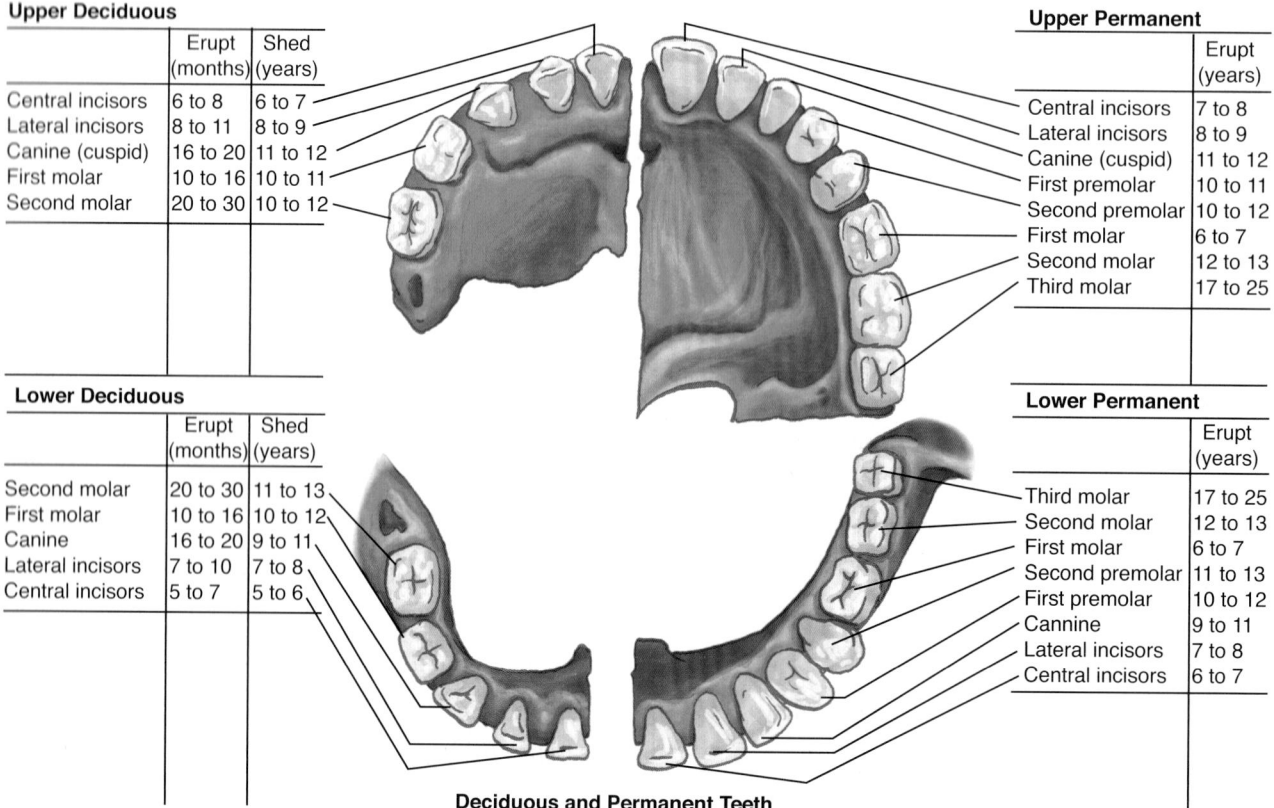

Upper Deciduous

	Erupt (months)	Shed (years)
Central incisors	6 to 8	6 to 7
Lateral incisors	8 to 11	8 to 9
Canine (cuspid)	16 to 20	11 to 12
First molar	10 to 16	10 to 11
Second molar	20 to 30	10 to 12

Upper Permanent

	Erupt (years)
Central incisors	7 to 8
Lateral incisors	8 to 9
Canine (cuspid)	11 to 12
First premolar	10 to 11
Second premolar	10 to 12
First molar	6 to 7
Second molar	12 to 13
Third molar	17 to 25

Lower Deciduous

	Erupt (months)	Shed (years)
Second molar	20 to 30	11 to 13
First molar	10 to 16	10 to 12
Canine	16 to 20	9 to 11
Lateral incisors	7 to 10	7 to 8
Central incisors	5 to 7	5 to 6

Lower Permanent

	Erupt (years)
Third molar	17 to 25
Second molar	12 to 13
First molar	6 to 7
Second premolar	11 to 13
First premolar	10 to 12
Cannine	9 to 11
Lateral incisors	7 to 8
Central incisors	6 to 7

Deciduous and Permanent Teeth

Figure 3-21 Sequence of eruption of primary (deciduous) and secondary (permanent) teeth. From Ibsen, O & Phelan, J. (1996). *Oral pathology for the dental hygienist*. Philadelphia, PA: W. B. Saunders. Reprinted with permission.

and structural changes continue as the child physically grows and matures during the ensuing years.

Skin

The back and the arms of the developing fetus are covered with fine hair called *lanugo*. This hair begins to form at 16 weeks, covers the fetus in utero, and begins to recede around the 36th week. Presence of lanugo will most likely be noted on the infant born prematurely and, to some degree, on the full-term baby. As the infant continues to mature outside the womb, lanugo continues to recede.

Another protective covering that can be found on the developing fetus is the *vernix caseosa*. This cheeselike coating on the skin develops around the 24th week, remaining until the fetus is full term. On delivery, the newborn may have varying amounts of vernix caseosa. The substance can be easily washed off the infant's skin during the first bath.

The newborn's skin is soft and smooth and has a translucent appearance. For light-skinned infants, superficial vessels are prominent, giving the skin a red color. Sweat and sebaceous glands are present in the newborn but do not become functional until 2 months of age; some do not become functional until the onset of puberty. During adolescence, considerable development of sweat and sebaceous glands is evident and associated with the development of acne vulgaris and body odor. More information regarding acne and other skin conditions that are common during childhood and adolescence, such as dermatitis, acne, and sunburn, is provided in Chapter 25.

During the first year, there is an increase in subcutaneous fat. When the child becomes ambulatory, the proportion of subcutaneous fat begins to diminish. By age 3 years, most children have a leaner appearance than has been noticed in previous years. During puberty, subcutaneous fat becomes more abundant in certain body areas, especially in females.

The fingernails and toenails began forming at the end of the first trimester. At birth, nail beds are fully formed on the normal newborn. Infants born prematurely have incomplete formation of their nails.

Cardiovascular System

Formation of the heart begins by the 16th day of gestation. Blood cells join to the yolk sac's wall, and the system of blood vessels and a single heart tube begins to take shape. The heart appears as a bulge on the anterior surface of the developing fetus. By the sixth or seventh week, the septum and then the valves begin to develop. The rhythmic beat of the heart has begun by the eighth week and can be heard with a stethoscope by the 16th week, beating at 120 to 160 bpm. Fetal circulation develops slowly, providing blood to the brain, liver, heart, and kidneys. At birth, changes in circulation occur that allow the heart and lungs to work in a coordinated effort to sustain circulation that previously was supported by the placenta (discussed in more detail in Chapter 15).

At birth, the heart of the normal infant is simply a smaller version of the adult heart with a few minor variations. Cardiac output in the newborn is initially 400 mL/kg/min, dropping to 200 mL/kg/min by adolescence. In the infant, cardiac output is a function of heart rate and not stroke volume. In the young child, the heart rate is usually higher and the stroke volume is lower than in adults. Therefore, when the body requires higher cardiac output, the young child compensates by a correlated increase in heart rate (i.e., tachycardia). During periods of sleep or persistent vagal stimulation (by suctioning, defecation, or feeding), transient decreased heart rate (i.e., bradycardia) can occur in infants and is generally well tolerated.

The mass of the right ventricle approximates that of the left ventricle in the newborn as a result of the pressure and volume work performed by the right ventricle in utero. During the next several months, the left ventricle increases in mass more rapidly than the right ventricle as it works to pump both systemically. Eventually, the left ventricle is predominant, as seen in the adult heart.

The foramen ovale closes in the normal newborn soon after birth as a result of changes in interatrial pressure. The ductus arteriosus, which generally closes within 18 hours of birth, is not gone anatomically until approximately 2 weeks of age.

During infancy, the heart is placed more horizontally and has a larger diameter in relation to the diameter of the total chest than is apparent in the adult. The apex of the heart is one or two intercostal spaces higher than in the adult. Therefore, the apical pulse, or point of maximum impulse (PMI), is auscultated at the fourth intercostal space in children younger than 7 years of age and in the fifth intercostal space in the child older than 7 years of age. The PMI becomes more lateral as the child grows and as heart diameter decreases in relation to chest diameter.

Healthy, premature infants are prone to having a high frequency of arrhythmias. This is most likely the result of the immaturity of the autonomic nervous system. Sinus arrhythmias are a normal finding in infants, although they would be considered an abnormal finding in the older child and adolescent. Innocent systolic murmurs are common in infants and young children. Diastolic murmurs at any age are considered pathologic.

The child's heart continues to grow through puberty. Heart growth is closely associated with somatic growth, including increases in body weight, FFM, and height during adolescence. FFM is an important determinant of heart size and heart growth for both boys and girls. An increase in the amount of aerobic fitness, presumably attributable to improvements in cardiac function, also affects heart growth in boys (Janz et al., 2000).

During fetal development, the main site of hematopoiesis is the liver. By birth, hematopoietic activity will primarily occur in the bone marrow. During early childhood years, most of the child's bones contain hematopoietic activity. As the child matures, this tissue in the long bones is gradually replaced with fat. During periods of extreme hematopoietic stress, the long bones can resume active blood production. During later childhood and into adulthood, the pelvis, sternum, ribs, vertebrae, skull, clavicles, and scapulae are the main production sites for blood.

Respiratory System

The respiratory and digestive systems begin formation at the same time and form as a single tube. By the fourth week, separation of the two systems begins and lung buds appear. The lung buds may be seated deep in the abdomen until the diaphragm closes during the seventh week, thus dividing the thoracic cavity from the abdominal cavity. If incomplete closures occur, diaphragmatic hernias with abdominal organ contents extending into the thoracic cavity may be evident at birth. In this case, respiration would be compromised.

Formation of the sinuses begins during the third month of gestation. Until the ages of 2 to 3 years, the child's sinuses remain very small and poorly developed.

Surfactant is produced by the lungs during the sixth month of gestation. This substance is necessary for postnatal lung expansion. Production of surfactant continues through the 28th week, and the alveoli are formed at this time. Viability of the fetus outside the womb is possible after the alveoli are formed and some surfactant is produced. In the womb, the fetus has respiratory movements, although no actual breathing is taking place.

At birth, the most dramatic respiratory changes take place when the infant draws his or her first breath. The intake of oxygen pushes amniotic fluid out of the alveoli, allowing for the expansion of the pulmonary bed. Approximately 50 million alveoli are present at birth, and 250 million more are added by 2 years of age, at which time most alveolar formation is complete (de Jong et al., 2003).

The infant and young child's respiratory system is notably different from that of the older child and adult. During the childhood years, changes in the structure and function of the respiratory system occur. The alveoli and airways grow, changing in size and configuration. The child has fewer alveoli than the adult. The collateral pathways of ventilation are not completely developed during infancy; therefore, airway obstruction can have more severe effects in the young child. By later childhood and adolescence, the terminal airways are larger and collateral ventilation is improved. The infant's sternum and ribs are primarily cartilaginous, resulting in a soft chest wall. The ribs are horizontally oriented, and intercostal muscles are poorly developed at this time. This is in contrast to the adult's rib cage, which is more rigid with more vertically angled bones.

The adult uses his or her accessory muscles to aid in the respiratory process. Poor development of these muscles requires the infant and young child to be more dependent on diaphragmatic function to contribute to the movement of the chest wall during respiration.

Infants are obligate nose breathers for approximately 1 month after birth. The cartilage in the infant's larynx is very soft and can be easily compressed if the child's neck is flexed or hyperextended. The narrowest part of the child's airway is the cricoid cartilage, and, as a whole, the larynx is proportionately smaller in diameter and straighter than the larynx in the older child and adult.

Gastrointestinal System

After the digestive system separates from the respiratory system, it begins a period of rapid growth. Because the abdominal cavity is small, from the 6th to the 10th week in utero, a part of the abdominal contents (herniation of the mid gut) will extend into the base of the umbilical cord. As the abdominal cavity grows, the intestines should move back into the abdomen. This occurs around the 10th to 12th week. Failure to do so leads to a variety of disorders, including omphalocele (a condition in which the child is born with the intestines outside the abdominal cavity) and susceptibility to intussusception and bowel obstruction.

During the second month of fetal life, the intestines begin to produce meconium as a result of fetal metabolism. The pancreas develops during the 12th week. The development of the swallowing reflex at 16 weeks allows the fetus to swallow amniotic fluid. If the fetus becomes stressed, hypoxia can cause vagal stimulation, an increase in bowel motility, and a lack of sphincter tone. The meconium may leave the bowel and move into the amniotic fluid, making it likely that the fetus will swallow some of the meconium. This is not a problem until the point of delivery, when the newborn is ready to take his or her first breaths. Further aspiration of the meconium into the newborn's respiratory passages can cause deleterious effects if not noted and treated upon delivery of the newborn.

The terminal segment of the anal canal, the anus, arises from a pit invagination of the skin. The anus is supplied by somatic sensory nerves and is sensitive to touch, even at birth. As myelinization of the spinal cord becomes complete and the musculature of the anus develops more fully, the child will develop voluntary control over defecation. This generally occurs between 2 and 5 years of age.

At birth, the child's gastrointestinal system remains immature and will not maintain full maturity until approximately 2 years of age. During the first 3 to 4 months of life, the sucking reflex and the extrusion reflex are present. The extrusion reflex protects the infant from ingesting food substances that the gastrointestinal system is too immature to digest. The production of saliva in large enough quantities to begin the process of digestion in the oral cavity does not occur until approximately age 4 months. The infant is prone to frequent spit-ups after feeding as a result of the immature muscle tone of the lower esophageal sphincter. Intestinal peristalsis is faster in young children, with emptying times of 2½ to 3 hours in the newborn, extending to 3 to 6 hours in older infants and children. Faster gastric emptying time affects the ability of the digestive tract to break down and absorb the child's oral intake. For instance, it is not uncommon for the older infant to eat corn and then defecate corn that has undergone no physical changes in appearance after having traveled through the digestive system. The frequent output of undigested food particles is further influenced by the gastrocolic reflex, which rapidly moves contents toward the colon. The newborn's stomach capacity is 10 to 20 mL, increasing to 100 to 200 mL in a 1-month-old; 360 mL in a 12-month-old; 1,500 mL in an adolescent; and 2,000 to 3,000 mL in an adult.

The infant's stomach is round and lies horizontally until about 2 years of age, when the angle becomes more vertical and upright. The intestines undergo a growth spurt when the child is 1 to 3 years of age and again in the later teen years. The liver is generally palpable 1 to 2 cm below the right costal margin during the first year of life. The spleen is normally palpable 1 to 2 cm below the left costal margin during the first few weeks of life. Thereafter, the ability to palpate these organs becomes more difficult as the trunk elongates and the child acquires additional subcutaneous fat.

The diameter of the abdomen is larger than the diameter of the chest in children younger than the age of 4 years and often has a "potbellied" appearance in both sitting and standing positions, resulting from poorly developed abdominal musculature (Fig. 3-22). A superficial venous pattern is readily visible on the infant's abdomen, remaining observable until adolescence. The omentum is poorly developed in early childhood, and thus localization of intra-abdominal infection or an inflammatory reaction is less likely to occur than in the older child and adolescent.

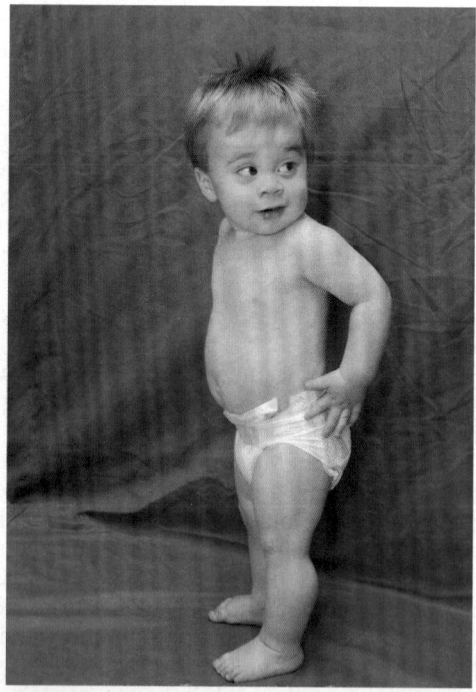

Figure 3-22 The young child's physique is characterized by a potbellied, bow-legged appearance.

Genitourinary System

At 4 weeks of gestation, the kidneys are present in a rudimentary form. Urine forms between the 11th and 12th weeks of development. In utero, the placenta serves as a pseudokidney, regulating fetal fluid and electrolyte balance. The kidneys do not function independently until after birth.

During the first 1 to 2 years of life, the kidneys reach full functional maturity. Until maturity is reached, the infant is more predisposed than older children to dehydration during periods of fluid loss such as those caused by diarrhea, fever, fluid restrictions, and reduced fluid intake. During the early years, renal blood flow is slow, the reabsorption of amino acids is limited, autoregulation is not fully developed, and the ability to concentrate urine is minimal. As the kidneys mature and develop systemically, there is increased cardiac output, increased plasma proteins, and renal function improves.

The newborn's bladder capacity is approximately 30 mL, increasing to 150 mL at age 3 years, 270 mL at age 7 years, and up to 600 to 800 mL in the adult. Although the kidneys do not reach maximal size until ages 35 to 40 years, the kidneys of infants and children have a larger diameter compared with the size of the abdominal cavity present in the adult. The child's kidneys are more vulnerable to trauma because of their size in proportion to the abdomen and because they are less protected by the ribs and have less fat padding.

Genitalia Development and Pubertal Changes

External genitalia are present at 8 weeks, the beginning of the fetal stage. However, the ability to distinguish between male and female genitalia is not possible until further formation takes place. During early embryonic development, male and female genital structures are similar. It is during the third month that primitive urogenital structures enlarge and fuse to form the male's penis and scrotum or shrink and have minimal fusion to form the female's labia and clitoris. These external changes can be detected on ultrasound. The internal sex organs are also developing at this time. The male's testes do not descend into the scrotum until about 36 weeks' gestation. An indirect hernia is produced if the tube that precedes the descent of the testes fails to close.

At birth, the external female genitalia have increased pigmentation because of hormonal influences. The clitoris and labia majora are likely to be edematous. Both the edema and increased pigmentation recede within the next month. The scrotum of the full-term male is pink or dark brown, depending on the child's complexion, and rugae are present. Both testes should be descended. Penile erections occur when the penis is stimulated or when the infant is voiding. The foreskin on the penis is not retractable if the child is not circumcised. The foreskin remains adherent until approximately age 3 years.

Both female and male reproductive organs remain relatively unchanged until early adolescence. The beginning of puberty marks the onset of significant changes in the development of the gonads, reproductive organs,

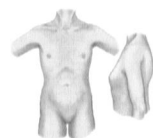

Stage I
Breasts: Preadolescent; elevation of the papilla only
Pubic hair: None

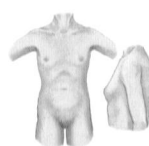

Stage II
Breasts: Breast budding (thelarche); small mound formed by elevation of the breast and papilla, with enlargement of the areolar diameter
Pubic hair: Sparse growth of long, downy pubic hair over mons veneris or labia majora; may occur with breast budding or several weeks or months later (pubarche)

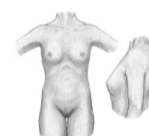

Stage III
Breasts: Further enlargement of breast tissue and areola with no separation of their contours
Pubic hair: Increased amount of hair and changes in the character of the hair (darker, coarser, and curlier); spread sparsely over the junction pubes

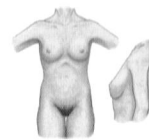

Stage IV
Breasts: Double contour form: projection of areola and papilla form a secondary mound on top of breast tissue
Pubic hair: Adult appearance but less area covered; no spread to medial aspects of thighs

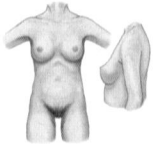

Stage V
Breasts: Larger, more mature breast with single contour form
Pubic hair: Adult distribution and quantity, with spread to medial aspect of thighs

Figure 3-23 Tanner staging. Development of secondary sex characteristics in girls.

and secondary sex characteristics. The length of time pubertal changes require and the age at which they begin vary from person to person. In general, puberty begins earlier in females (as early as age 10 years) and is of a shorter duration than for males.

Pubertal events are characterized by several other physical changes in addition to those that affect reproductive organs. Skeletal growth and body composition changes occur, increased strength and endurance are attained, and anatomic and biochemical alterations in the central nervous system and the endocrine system are seen. Figures 3-23 and 3-24 summarize the typical progression of female and male development during puberty (also called *Tanner staging*). Early or delayed onset of pubertal signs is a cause for concern because either can indicate endocrine dysfunction and can be a source of personal distress for the child (Clinical Judgment 3-1).

Endocrine and Metabolic Functions

The thyroid, thymus, and pancreas develop around the 12th week of gestation. Endocrine functions are immature at birth. For example, infants have a high metabolic rate that correlates with higher glucose needs. However, the infant also has low glycogen stores; therefore, the

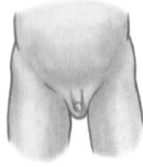

Stage I
Penis: Childhood size and proportion
Testes and scrotum: Childhood size and proportion
Pubic hair: None

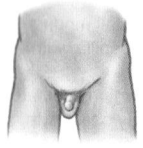

Stage II
Penis: Slight or no enlargement
Testes and scrotum: Enlargement; scrotal skin reddens, changes in texture
Pubic hair: Sparse growth of long, downy pubic hair mainly at the base of penis

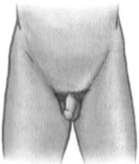

Stage III
Penis: Enlargement, particularly in length
Testes and scrotum: Further enlargement
Pubic hair: Darker, coarser, curlier hair spread sparsely over the pubic symphysis

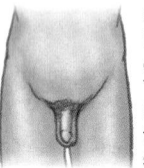

Stage IV
Penis: Further enlargement in length and breadth, with development of the glans
Testes and scrotum: Further enlargement
Pubic hair: Coarser, curlier hair; greater area covered than stage III, but still less than an adult, with no spread to thighs

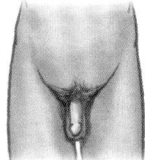

Stage V
Penis: Adult in size and shape
Testes and scrotum: Adult in size and shape
Pubic hair: Adult distribution and quantity, with spread to thighs but not to abdomen

Figure 3-24 Tanner staging. Development of secondary sex characteristics in boys.

child can become rapidly hypoglycemic during periods of stress. During adolescence, these processes change. Under stress, the adult generally becomes hyperglycemic because epinephrine and glycogen secretion stimulate glycogen breakdown, resulting in an increased blood glucose level.

Stress in the infant also stimulates the secretion of growth hormone, which then increases calcium deposition in the bone, causing hypocalcemia. The infant has immature regulation of growth hormone production. Thus, in cases of severe stress, the infant needs to be monitored for hypocalcemia.

Metabolic functions are established in utero as genetic information is transferred to the developing cells. At birth, metabolic functions should be intact and functioning. Mutational events in utero can lead to the development of biochemical disorders that affect the child's metabolic function. The affected genes result in either a structurally altered enzyme that is not capable of normal catalytic activity or causes an inhibition of enzyme synthesis. In most cases, the neonate appears normal at birth; however, signs and symptoms develop rapidly as the infant's metabolic functions begin to respond to the intake of human milk or formula and the demands of extrauterine life.

Some metabolic alterations do not make themselves known until later childhood. Rarely do problems in metabolic function appear as late as adulthood. The inborn errors of metabolism most commonly seen in the pediatric population are discussed in Chapter 27.

Many endocrine disorders are detected during adolescence because of early pubertal onset or a delay in pubertal onset. In addition, a variety of autoimmune endocrine disorders may appear during normal onset of puberty, including Hashimoto thyroiditis, Graves disease, autoimmune hypoparathyroidism, Addison disease, and type 1 diabetes. With the exception of type 1 diabetes, autoimmune disorders rarely occur before adolescence. Endocrine disorders are discussed in more detail in Chapter 26.

Immune Functions

The lymphoid system performs the same function in children as in adults; however, the maturity of the system varies at different ages. For instance, the fetus passively acquires antibodies from the mother during the sixth month of gestation. Immunoglobulins G, A, and M (IgG, IgA, IgM) are almost completely derived by transfer to the developing fetus from the mother. This allows temporary protection against diseases such as measles, mumps, poliomyelitis, and rubella. At birth, the infant has the immunologic reactivity to respond to a large variety of antigens. At the same time, this exogenous source of immunoglobulins suppresses the infant's own ability to synthesize the immunoglobulins. Therefore, as maternal stores in the infant catabolize, the child experiences a period during which immunoglobulin levels are low because the child's own system is not fully activated to create the antibodies that are needed. This usually occurs around the sixth month. Adult levels of IgM are attained at approximately 1 year of age, with levels of IgG reached at 5 years of age and those of IgA acquired at 10 years of age.

Several other factors make the infant and young child more at risk for infection. The newborn's immune system is not as efficient as that of an adult. Cell-mediated immunity is less well developed than in the adult; as a result, recovery from congenital infections may be delayed and the effects of the condition more devastating for the newborn.

Lymph nodes in children have the same distribution patterns as adults. However, the nodes are more predominant in the child until the time of puberty. The amount of lymphoid tissue is considerable during infancy and continues to increase at a steady rate until after puberty. During early childhood, lymphoid tissue responds to infection by excessive swelling and hyperplasia. These clinical signs may persist long after the primary infection has diminished. The lymph nodes can harbor infection, posing a liability for the child. Swelling of the lymph nodes and spleen can lead to other health care problems because swollen nodes can block the airway. A swollen and enlarged spleen is more at risk for traumatic injury because the child's abdominal structures have little subcutaneous fat to protect the internal organs from injury.

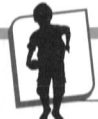

Assessment of Changes During Puberty

Tom Yee is a nurse and a father of a 12-year-old who plays on a junior high soccer team. Mr. Yee was asked to talk to the team about ways to stay healthy during their adolescent years. After the presentation, Mr. Yee asks if there are any questions. One boy shouts out, "How come my bratty little sister is now taller that I am?" Another boy interjects, "Yeah! My 11-year-old sister is starting to get a big chest too!"

Questions
1. From the comments of the boys, what do you think is at the heart of their concerns?
2. For this preadolescent age group, what are some of the topics Mr. Yee should have covered in his "keeping healthy" presentation?
3. Should Mr. Yee start a discussion about the physical and reproductive changes that occur during puberty at this time?
4. How should Mr. Yee intervene to address the concerns of these boys?
5. What are some of the physical changes Mr. Yee should tell them will occur during puberty?

Answers
1. They see other kids around them going through lots of physical changes and they are concerned if they are abnormal or if they, too, will be growing bigger and taller.
2. Nutrition, sports safety, car safety, the hazards of smoking and substance use
3. Mr. Yee can discuss some of the physical changes that will occur during puberty. However, a detailed discussion of male and female reproduction and changes in the reproductive system would not be appropriate at this time because of the setting (not because of their age). Do plan another session to discuss these other topics.
4. Briefly discuss the physical changes between boys and girls that are occurring in this age group, determine whether there is a need for another presentation that would provide more detailed information about adolescent sexuality, obtain consent from parents to have a second presentation, and ask fathers to attend with their sons.
5. Pubertal changes begin in girls as early as age 10 years. Boys develop secondary sex characteristics later and may not begin these changes for up to 2 years after girls. This development in boys includes an increase in height. Physique will change with more muscle mass added. Genitalia will enlarge and the shape will change. Hair growth will increase in certain body areas such as under the arms and in the pubic area. The hairline on the forehead may recede a little, the voice will deepen, and acne may begin to appear.

THEORIES OF DEVELOPMENT

QUESTION: James is developing a personality. What stage of personality development is James in according to Freud's theory? According to Erikson's theory? What is the major area of focus for the child with each theory? Provide examples about James to illustrate these areas.

The previous section reviewed the physical growth and development of the child. A variety of theories have been developed and tested to explain other aspects of the child's development, including personality, cognitive–intellectual, behavioral, social, language, gender identification, moral, and spiritual development.

PERSONALITY DEVELOPMENT

Understanding personality development has been strongly influenced by the *psychoanalytic perspective*, which asserts that children move through a series of stages in which they confront conflicts between biologic drives and social expectations (Berk, 2011). The most widely influential psychoanalytic theorists have been Sigmund Freud and Erik Erikson. Other theorists such as Jung, Adler, Horney, and Sullivan have also contributed to an understanding of personality development (see thePoint for Supplemental Information). Their nonstage theories uniformly disagree with Freudian theory regarding the factors that motivate the development of different personality types.

Knowledge of the various types of temperament inherent in each person also helps in understanding a child's personality. This section reviews the theory of temperament and the influence temperament has on the child's interactions with others.

Understanding the psychoanalytic theories assists nurses to identify needs and concerns of children at specific ages. Understanding theories about temperament helps explain unique differences in children as they deal with day-to-day experiences as well as stressors caused by change. The theories are useful in nursing practice when evaluating a child's response to hospitalization and the stressors related to the presence of chronic or acute illness.

Freud's Theory

The work of Sigmund Freud provides the most familiar psychoanalytic theories. Freud believed that humans are driven by a need to resolve certain biologically determined drives that center around sexual urges. Although Freud did not believe that children experienced adult sexual feelings, he did believe that children had certain sensual and pleasurable urges that they acted on through their behaviors and in their interactions with others. The sexual instinct is called *eros*. The energy created by the sexual instinct is called *libido*. According to Freud's theory, beginning with the newborn, the developing human is focused on a core need to satisfy a sensual drive (Table 3-3).

During each stage of development, a different region of the body becomes the focus of sensual pleasure. The goal of the child is to proceed through each stage without trauma so that he or she will emerge as a "well-adjusted" adult. Freud believed that trauma in any given stage would result in some *fixation* or alteration in psychosexual development. Each stage builds on the next. As the focus of sensual pleasure shifts from one body region to another, the child must be willing to let go of the previous focus and to move on to another stage of development. If conflict has occurred at a certain stage, resolution of that sensual pleasure may not be complete and the child may be reluctant to move on to the next stage. Even if the child does move onward, psychosocial adjustment may be impaired, with fixations becoming apparent as the child continues to mature.

Freud's childhood stages were derived entirely from his experiences with adults. His theory was built on his work with neurotic personalities who sought psychiatric treatment. His theories have been criticized for his views on male supremacy and gender differences. Critics of Freud's work posit that many of the sexual conflicts he believed were developmental are more likely attributable to the responses of children growing up under the mores and values of late-19th-century European society. Freud's theory also did not take into account any cultural differences among individuals. Although the areas of body focus seem appropriately correlated to the behaviors seen in children of specific age groups (sucking during infancy, gaining bowel control during early childhood), focus on these body parts can also be attributed to the natural acquisition of, and expected changes in, the functional abilities of these body structures. Freud's theories provide insight regarding how families can manage their children's sexual and aggressive drives as they mature.

> **ANSWER:** Based on Freud's theory, James is in the anal stage, which encompasses the ages of 1–3 years. The major focus of this stage is on gaining mastery in using the anal muscles. This is illustrated by attempts at toilet training.

Erikson's Theory

Erikson's theory of personality development is based on the *epigenetic principle*. This principle asserts that personality develops according to predetermined steps that are maturational and set by the growing person's readiness to be a part of a widening social radius. The critical steps are turning points, or moments of decision between progress and regression, integration, and retardation (Erikson, 1963). Erikson called these steps the *eight stages of man* (Table 3-4). Each stage is denoted by an emphasis on two opposing possible outcomes. During each stage, the individual is presented with a crisis. If a particular crisis is handled well, then a positive outcome prevails. If the crisis is not handled well, a negative outcome results. The theory also asserts that each psychosocial stage is related

TABLE 3-3 Freud's Stages of Psychosexual Development		
Stage and Body Area of Focus	**Description**	**Results of Trauma or Fixation**
Oral, birth to 1 year old (mouth)	Enjoys sucking; chewing; biting on things such as mother's breast, rubber nipple, thumb, blanket, or bottle	Oral fixations such as nail biting, cigarette smoking, gum chewing, excessive eating
Anal, 1–3 years old (anus)	Libido centered on gaining mastery in using anal muscles; toilet training accomplished at this time	Anal fixations such as parsimony, orderliness, punctiliousness, obstinacy, possessiveness; difficulty controlling anger, aggressive feelings, and impulses
Phallic, 3–6 years old (genitalia: penis, clitoris, and vagina)	Resolution of the Oedipus and Electra complex; sex roles and moral development take place	Boy will remain overly attached to his mother, fearing father may castrate him; may resent father and authority figures; girl will remain overly attached to father and have "penis envy," wishing to be a man
Latency, 6–12 years old (sex drives repressed; no area of focus)	Nonsexual urges; children focus on learning to control their impulses and find appropriate outlets for their drives; energies shift to physical and intellectual activities	Prolonged or exaggerated Oedipus or Electra complex
Genital, 12 years old to adulthood (genitalia)	Interest in peers as sexual partners; task is to learn mature patterns of heterosexual behavior	Failure to develop mature, acceptable methods of obtaining sexual gratification

TABLE 3-4   Erikson's Psychosocial Stages of Development

Stage	Characteristics	Outcomes
Trust versus mistrust, birth to 1 year old	Caregiver responds in warm, caring manner to child's needs to create trusting environment. If care is inconsistent and unreliable, mistrust develops.	*Trust:* hope, tolerates frustration, can delay gratification, sense of trust *Mistrust:* suspicion, withdrawal, focus on negative aspect of people's behavior
Autonomy versus shame and doubt, 1–3 years old	Child practices and attains new physical skills, developing autonomy. If not allowed to do things he or she can do, or pushed into doing something when not ready, child may develop sense of shame or doubt.	*Autonomy:* will, self-control, positive self-esteem, self-confidence *Shame:* compulsion, impulsivity
Initiative versus guilt, 3–6 years old	Initiative is demonstrated when the child is able to formulate a plan of action and carry it out. Believes that desires and actions are basically sound. If the child is punished for expressing his or her desires, then child will develop a sense of guilt.	*Initiative:* purpose, enjoys accomplishments, self-starters *Guilt:* inhibition, afraid to accept new challenges, guilt over one's actions
Industry versus inferiority, 6–12 years old	Child acquires skills such as reading, writing, mathematics, and social skills. Through acquisition of these skills, the child develops a sense of industry. If always compared with others, or made to believe he or she is inadequate, child will develop a sense of inferiority.	*Industry:* competence, enjoys learning about new things, perseverance, takes criticism well *Inferiority:* inadequacy, inferiority, gives up easily
Identity versus role confusion, 12–19 years old	The adolescent investigates and identifies alternatives regarding his or her vocational and personal future. Premature choices, or the inability to make these choices, will lead to role confusion.	*Identity:* fidelity, confidence in self-identity, optimism, control of one's destiny *Role confusion:* diffidence, defiance, socially unacceptable identity, sense of purposelessness
Intimacy versus isolation, 19–25 years old	Love relationships are developed. Fear of intimate relationships will lead to a sense of isolation.	*Intimacy:* love, development of deep interpersonal relationships *Isolation:* exclusivity, avoidance of commitment, avoidance of relationships
Generativity versus stagnation, 25–50 years old	Parenting, nurturing others, and fulfilling civic responsibilities are the tasks. The adult finds ways to be productive and to be of help to others to grow personally.	*Generativity:* care, concern for future generations of the society, desire to help others *Stagnation:* stagnated, rejection of others, self-indulgence, self-absorbed, highly critical of others
Ego integrity versus despair, age 50 years and older	Reflection on one's life and one's achievements. A sense of pride or despair is developed regarding the accomplishments in life that have been made or were lost.	*Positive:* wisdom, self-satisfaction *Negative:* disdain, disgust, bitterness concerning lost opportunities

to all others and is impacted by the outcomes of the previous stage. Thus, each stage lays the foundation for negotiating the challenges of the stages that follow (Erikson, 1963).

Erikson emphasizes that the effects of culture, socialization, and the historic moment will affect identity development. Therefore, his theory cannot be used as a blueprint to describe a single personality type. Children from different cultures develop and achieve the developmental tasks through a variety of socially acceptable mechanisms. For instance, achieving the outcome of industry in U.S. society is somewhat dependent on successfully completing formal academic milestones, whereas in other societies, the ability to farm or to catch animals for food is evidence of industry during middle childhood. Erikson's theory has been criticized for being overly broad and general and for being difficult to evaluate in an experimental setting.

ANSWER: According to Erikson's theory, James is in the stage of autonomy versus shame and doubt. The major focus of this stage is practicing and attaining new skills to develop autonomy. This is illustrated by James's negativism (saying no to everything) and by his temper tantrums. His negativism is a way for him to develop his identity as a separate person. His temper tantrums are a way for him to cope when he becomes overwhelmed with tasks or things that he is unable to complete or a way to make his feelings known.

Temperament

The child's characteristic way of thinking, responding, and behaving is referred to as the child's *temperament*. Temperament is considered to be an intrinsic personality factor—that is, children are born predisposed to respond to their environment in very different ways. Temperament influences the child's characteristic way of behaving and interacting with his or her environment.

Table 3-5 presents 10 temperament categories. Individual temperament characteristics are apparent within the first few months of life and are easily identified by the end of the first year. Three temperamental styles or groups form combinations of the 10 categories of temperament characteristics:

1. The *easy child* is characterized by flexibility, a positive approach to new stimuli, adaptability to change, and a predominately positive mood.

TABLE 3-5 Temperament Categories

Category	Definition	Examples of Characteristic Behaviors
Activity level	Amount of physical energy that drives the child in most situations; includes proportion of active and inactive periods	Low activity; moves at a slower pace; prefers inactive pastimes such as coloring or playing quietly with toys High activity; full of energy; fidgety when asked to sit still; restless on days when has to stay inside; tends to be impulsive (acting before thinking)
Self-control	Ability to delay actions or demands	Patient; demonstrates good self-control Impulsive; demonstrates poor self-control
Rhythmicity or regularity	Predictability or unpredictability of the child's biologic patterns such as sleep, hunger, and elimination	Very rhythmic, regular sleep patterns; will get tired at almost the same time each day; will have a bowel movement every morning around the same time Arrhythmic, irregular sleep patterns; gets tired at different times each day; bowel movements not predictable
Initial response	Typical initial response of the child to a new stimulus such as a new food, toy, person, or situation	Approachable; jumps right in to new situations without hesitation Withdrawn; holds back in a new situation until feels comfortable
Adaptability	Tolerance of change; ease with which gets used to new or changed situations	Very adaptable; tends to be compliant, cooperative, and go with the flow Slowly adapts; tends to be stubborn, strong willed, or headstrong
Sensory threshold	Level of stimulation that evokes a response; how sensitive a child is in each sense (touch, pain, hearing, smell, and vision)	High threshold; does not seem to be sensitive to environmental stimuli that affect the senses (e.g., will be able to wear most any clothes, even those that are tight fitting because of high threshold to touch) Low threshold; highly sensitive to stimuli that affect the senses (e.g., always likes to smell things and may refuse to wear certain clothes because they feel "funny")
Intensity of reaction	Amount of energy used to express emotions and actions	Low intensity; expresses emotions quietly and in a low-keyed fashion High intensity; tends to be loud and dramatic when expressing emotions
Predominant mood	General quality of mood; amount of pleasant, joyful, and friendly behavior compared with amount of unpleasant and unfriendly behavior	Positive mood; views the world through rose-colored glasses; tends to miss negative and notice positive things Negative mood; tends to miss positive and notice negative things
Distractibility/concentration	Degree to which extraneous environmental stimuli can be distracting and interfere with ongoing behavior	Low distractibility; gets caught up in what he or she is paying attention to and may not notice the things going on in the environment High distractibility; tends to shift attention quickly and often, may get easily sidetracked when trying to complete a task
Attention span and persistence	Length of time an activity is pursued along with the child's capacity to continue the activity despite obstacles	High persistence; tends to stick with difficult tasks and may not give up even when a task is well beyond his or her skill level Low persistence; tends to become frustrated and may quickly ask for help, get angry, or simply give up on a difficult task.

From Chess, S. (1990). Studies in temperament: A paradigm in psychosocial research. *Yale Journal of Biology and Medicine, 63,* 313–324; Chess, S., & Thomas, A. (1985). Temperamental differences: A critical concept in child health care. *Pediatric Nursing, 11,* 167–171; Chess, S., & Thomas, A. (1986). *Temperament in clinical practice.* New York, NY: Guilford; Thomas, A., & Chess, S. (1977). *Temperament and development.* New York, NY: Brunner-Mazel; Turecki, S., & Tonner, L. (2000). *The difficult child: Expanded and revised edition.* New York, NY: Bantam.

2. The *difficult child* is characterized by irregularity in biologic functions, negative approach to new stimuli, slow adaptability, and intense mood expressions that are usually negative.

3. The *slow-to-warm-up child* is characterized by a combination of behaviors that are marked by withdrawal tendencies to new situations, slow adaptability, and negative mood expressions of low intensity. Less irregularity is noted in biologic functions. This child is often labeled "shy" (Chess, 1990; Chess & Thomas, 1985).

Temperament is believed to have a major impact on behavior and development. The child's temperament influences the dynamic interactions between the child and other people in his or her environment, particularly parents, other family members, teachers, and peers. To explain the healthy or pathologic interactions between the child and the environment, a model of "goodness of fit" and "poorness of fit" was developed by Chess and Thomas (1986). Goodness of fit occurs when the environmental expectations and demands of parents and others are consonant, or in harmony, with the child's temperamental characteristics. When goodness of fit is present, healthy functioning and development can occur. Conversely, poorness of fit is characterized by dissonance between environmental demands and the child's capabilities and temperament style. Poorness of fit is likely to lead to the development of behavior problems and poor parent–child interaction patterns. Thus, difficulties can arise when the child's temperament is in conflict with the parent's own behavioral style. For instance, an active child may be quite a challenge for family members who are more low key, and a child who has erratic patterns for eating and sleeping may be a behavioral challenge to the grandparents who are very time oriented and orderly in their daily activities (Turecki & Tonner, 2000).

All the temperament styles may enhance positive or negative development and behavior. More important than the child's particular temperament characteristics, however, is the presence of a good fit in the interactions of the child with the environment. Parents often think that their biologic children should be born with many of their own behavioral characteristics and with a similar disposition. Parents may desire to learn about their child's temperamental characteristics so that they can be more accepting of the unique qualities in their child. Understanding temperament is important for parents: in providing guidance toward the proper parenting techniques and how to discipline and in understanding how it affects the parent's view of the child and themselves as parents. Several intervention programs have been developed to help family members who want to learn to better understand and manage their child's temperament (Gross et al., 2009; Medoff-Cooper, 1995; Melvin, 1995; O'Connor et al., 2012; Wallace, 1995). The first goal of a temperament-based intervention program is to help the families understand the unique characteristics of the child. Standardized temperament questionnaires are usually used to assist in this process. Next, family members are taught how temperament is related to behavior. Last, the family members are assisted in developing strategies to manage their child based on the child's temperament. When the families verbalize frustration with the child's behavior, the nurse can offer guidance to families that will foster the child's development and enhance interactions.

COGNITIVE–INTELLECTUAL DEVELOPMENT

Cognitive theories of development explore how an individual comes to think, to perceive, to process, and to understand information about himself or herself and the environment. Some of the approaches evaluate cognition in relation to the child's specific developmental age (Elkind, 1967; Piaget, 1926), whereas others focus on explaining the processes of cognition that occur regardless of age-specific considerations in terms of the individual's talents or intelligences (Gardner, 1993, 2006).

Piaget's Theory

Since the 1930s, Jean Piaget has been a leader in the exploration of cognitive development. He outlined a complex four-stage theory to explain the assimilation and accommodation of information. *Assimilation* refers to the process of taking in information from the environment and incorporating this into one's existing knowledge structure, or *schema*. When this information changes the person's existing schema to include the new information, this process is called *accommodation*. Each stage is characterized by a different way of thinking or of assimilating and accommodating information. Progress through each stage is gradual and orderly, varying in pace from child to child (Piaget, 1926). Piaget's stages of cognitive development are summarized in Table 3-6. Piaget coined many terms to explain the concepts in his theory. Definitions of these terms are found on thePoint Supplemental Information.

The original work of Piaget has been criticized for its weak scientific approach. Piaget used his own two children as subjects to develop his theory. His experiments were not controlled. He presented the children with a problem and observed how they reasoned and how they tried to solve that problem. Therefore, he may have underestimated the influence of formal learning on the development of cognitive processes. Piaget was able to articulate the sequences of development that lead a child to the point of adult understanding of such concepts as mathematics, time, and space. His theory does point to the importance of active experience in a child's development. Families are encouraged to seek activities and to provide play experiences for their children that give them the opportunity to solve problems and reason in a logical manner. Piaget's theories are of particular importance to health care personnel to better understand how children think about health-related events (Clinical Judgment 3-2). The nurse who is able to articulate the developmental differences in the cognitive abilities of children is better able to implement the nursing process in an age-appropriate, individualized manner.

TABLE 3-6 Piaget's Stages of Cognitive Development	
Stage	**Characteristics**
Sensorimotor, Birth to 2 Years Old	
Substage 1: use of reflexes, birth to 1 month old	Reflex responses to external stimuli Random body movements Genuinely intelligent behavior absent
Substage 2: primary circular reactions, 1–4 months old	Active effort to reproduce behavior that was first performed by chance Accidentally acquired behavior becomes a new sensorimotor habit
Substage 3: secondary circular reactions, 4–8 months old	Greater awareness of environment Increased interest in results of actions Understanding causality by recognizing that certain actions have certain results Dim awareness of before and after Achievement of hand–eye coordination Beginning development of object permanence
Substage 4: coordination of secondary circular reactions, 8–12 months old	Solution of simple problems possible Demonstration of anticipatory behavior More highly developed object permanence
Substage 5: tertiary circular reactions, 12–18 months old	Rudimentary trial and error activities present Beginning of reasoning Evident object permanence
Substage 6: invention of new meanings through deduction, 18–24 months old	Well-developed understanding of the nature of objects Understanding of the basic concept of causality Well-developed object permanence View of self as separate from others Ability to use symbols mentally
Preoperational, 2–7 Years Old	
Substage 1: preconceptual stage, 2–4 years old	Formation of symbolic thought Egocentrism in thoughts, feelings, and experiences Egocentrism in perception of objects and events Display of deferred imitation Understanding of instructions literally
Substage 2: perceptual or intuitive stage, 4–7 years old	Appearance of prelogical reasoning Judgment of experiences and objects by outside appearances and results Ability to concentrate on only one characteristic of an object at a time (centration) Use of words to express thoughts Demonstration of illogical reasoning (transductive reasoning) Play becomes more socialized
Concrete Operations, 7–11 Years Old	Acquisition of conceptual skills that permit logical manipulation of symbols Thinking is still limited by reliance on what is observed, on tangible concrete events or objects Ability to shift attention from one perceptual attribute to another (decentration) Ability to reverse thinking (reversibility) Acquisition of conservation skills Enjoyment in collecting and classifying objects Ability to appreciate a joke
Formal Operations, 11 Years Old to Death	Ability to manipulate abstract and unobservable concepts logically Use of scientific approach to solve problems Ability to conceive the distant future concretely and to set realistic long-term goals Ability to solve complex verbal problems

Elkind's Theory

Piagetian theory has been analyzed and expanded by numerous individuals. Psychologist David Elkind focused some of his work on explaining the nature of egocentrism in children. Egocentrism refers to the lack of differentiation in some area of interaction. At each stage in development, this lack of differentiation takes a unique form and is manifested in unique ways (Elkind, 1967, 1986). Children view reality quite differently at different age levels. Children's view of reality can be distorted to the degree that egocentric thought affects their behavior and actions. During infancy, the child experiences a lack of differentiation between the object and the "experiences of the object" (Elkind, 1967).

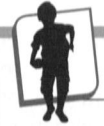

Assessment of Cognitive and Psychosocial Development

Jordan (age 7 years) and Daniel (age 4 years) are brothers admitted to the hospital as a result of injuries obtained in a motor vehicle accident. They share a hospital room. They will be discharged later in the day after teaching has been completed regarding care of their wounds. As you enter the room, they are yelling at each other, fighting over which television show to watch. The parents left to eat breakfast. Jordan has a set of small blocks on his bedside table; Daniel has six small race cars on the bed beside him. An unopened model for a plane is located at the end of Daniel's bed.

Questions

1. Based on your quick assessment of the situation, what will be the focus of your interactions with the boys today?

2. According to their ages, what stages of cognitive and psychosocial development would you place the boys in as a beginning point for your assessment?

3. Do you think the boys are acting in an age-appropriate fashion?

4. After you get the boys to calm down, you tell them that you will be teaching them how to care for their injuries at home. What aspects of care would be appropriate to teach each boy?

5. When the boys are being discharged, how would you determine whether your teaching was effective?

Answers

1. Providing age-appropriate diversionary activities, explaining the rules of conduct while in the hospital, providing discharge teaching regarding wound care

2. Jordan: middle childhood, latency stage (Freud), industry versus inferiority (Erikson), concrete operations (Piaget); Daniel: early childhood, phallic stage (Freud), initiative versus guilt (Erikson), preoperational stage (Piaget)

3. Yes. Sibling fighting would be expected at these ages. The toys they are playing with are appropriate for their age. The airplane model is too advanced for Daniel's level of fine motor skills; however, this is probably why it remains unopened on his bed.

4. Teach the boys separately because your approach needs to be different with each child. Daniel should be taught first. Terminology needs to be very simple. He can assist in his care by taking off the tape, opening packages, and helping to put the new dressing back on the wound. He can practice these activities on a doll. These activities promote feelings of accomplishment within Daniel's developmental skill level. Jordan can watch Daniel but should be asked not to intervene. When it is Jordan's turn, Jordan can participate by gathering the necessary equipment, removing the bandage, completing the first cleaning of the wound (parents do the second), and placing a new bandage on his wound. He should also clean up after the task is finished.

5. Jordan is able to tell his parents what they will need to clean his wounds and can demonstrate on a doll how to complete the dressing change. Daniel states he is the helper. His job is to be still and help his parent change his bandage.

The young child is unable to differentiate between words and their referents and to differentiate between self-created play, dream symbols, and reality. As the child matures, middle childhood is characterized by an inability to differentiate between mental constructs and perceptual givens. Adolescents are able to conceptualize the thoughts of both themselves and others; however, they are unable to differentiate between what others are thinking about and their own mental preoccupation (Elkind, 1967, 1984).

A primary focus of Elkind's work has been on adolescent thinking. Because of the emerging ability to think abstractly, adolescents become preoccupied with ideologic issues (social, political, and religious). Concepts like metaphor and simile can be grasped as well as contradictions in belief systems. On the other hand, the egocentrism of adolescence creates a situation in which the adolescent does not make totally rational choices because he or she is so caught up and consumed by thoughts of self and self-needs.

Elkind described four behaviors that typify adolescent egocentric thought processes. *Pseudostupidity* occurs when the adolescent asks apparently "dumb" questions, indicating difficulty reconciling concrete and formal operations. For instance, a trumpet player who has a band concert that evening may ask the band director if he needs to take his instrument. The *imaginary audience* is characterized by super self-consciousness. For example, an adolescent may believe that everybody is watching him and evaluating his actions and behaviors. In a sense, he believes he is onstage and everyone is focused on his activity. What he fails to perceive is that all adolescents have the same sense of super self-consciousness; thus, as individuals, they are all focused on their own actions and what others may think, and they spend little time concerned about the actions of others. *Personal fable* occurs because the adolescent thinks he or she is more special than anyone else and not subject to the natural laws. For example, an adolescent's friend gets pregnant; despite this, the adolescent continues having unprotected sexual relations, believing that she will never get pregnant. Last, the adolescent is characterized by *apparent hypocrisy*. The adolescent expresses an idea and believes that such expression is the same as having worked for and achieved an action. Or, the adolescent will claim a certain ideology and yet take actions that are in direct contrast to his or her stated beliefs. For example, the adolescent will criticize the horrible conditions caused by environmental pollutants and then will drop trash from the window of a car. No correlation is made between expressed ideologies and practical action.

Gardner's Theory

Students of psychology and education have embraced a theory of **multiple intelligences** developed by Dr. Howard Gardner. This theory addresses the concept that humans possess different talents, or multiple capacities, ranging from musical intelligence to the intelligence involved in understanding oneself (Table 3-7) (Gardner, 1993, 2006).

Gardner's theory specifically challenges the prevalent notion that intelligence is tied to the ability to provide succinct answers in a speedy fashion to problems primarily involving linguistic and logical skills (Gardner, 1993, 2006). In particular, the theory of multiple intelligences steps beyond the definitions of cognitive development asserted by theorists such as Jean Piaget. Gardner believes that Piaget and others have measured and developed their theories based primarily on a single dimension of cognition: the development of logical–mathematical intelligence. Multiple intelligences theory takes a more pluralistic view, recognizing that there are many different and discrete facets of cognition. Gardner's theory acknowledges that different people have different cognitive strengths and contrasting cognitive styles (Gardner, 1993, 2006). His theory challenges the dependence on the linguistic mode of instruction used by most educators and educational systems as the primary and most effective manner in which to help children learn. Gardner believes that all the intelligences are unevenly distributed, coexist, and can change over time. The responsibility of educators is to capitalize on the student's individual intellectual strengths.

The theory of multiple intelligences stems from the premise that there is a natural developmental trajectory of learning that begins with *raw patterning ability*. The "raw" intelligence is predominant during the first year of life. In subsequent stages, the intelligences are grasped through a *symbol system*. These symbols include learning sentences through stories, learning music through singing and playing songs, and experiencing body–kinesthetic development through dance (Fig. 3-25). Children demonstrate their abilities in the various intelligences through their grasp of the various symbol systems. As development progresses, each intelligence with its accompanying symbol system is represented in a *notational system*. For instance, mathematics, reading, musical notation, and mapping are second-order notational systems. The marks on the paper come to stand for symbols. In our culture, mastery of these symbols is typically acquired in a formal educational system. During adolescence and adulthood, the mastery of an intelligence is expressed through vocational and professional pursuits.

TABLE 3-7 Gardner's The Eight Intelligences	
Intelligence	**Application**
Linguistic: the gift of language	Poets, authors, writers
Logical–mathematical: problem-solving abilities	Mathematicians, accountants, cashiers, scientists
Spatial: ability to form a mental model of a spatial world and be able to maneuver and operate using that model	Sailors, engineers, surgeons, sculptors, painters
Musical: ability to play an instrument, sing, create music	Musicians, composers
Body–kinesthetic: ability to solve problems or to fashion products using one's whole body or parts of the body	Dancers, athletes, surgeons, craftspeople
Naturalist: ability to distinguish between different kinds of plants and animals	Zoologists, botanists, microbiologists
Interpersonal: ability to understand other people, what motivates them, how they work, how to cooperate with them	Salespeople, teachers, politicians, clinicians, religious leaders
Intrapersonal: capacity to form an accurate understanding of oneself and be able to use that understanding to operate effectively in life; allows one to understand and work with oneself	Evidence in any life experiences in which it is clear that the person truly understands his or her feelings and emotions and uses this knowledge to understand and guide personal behavior

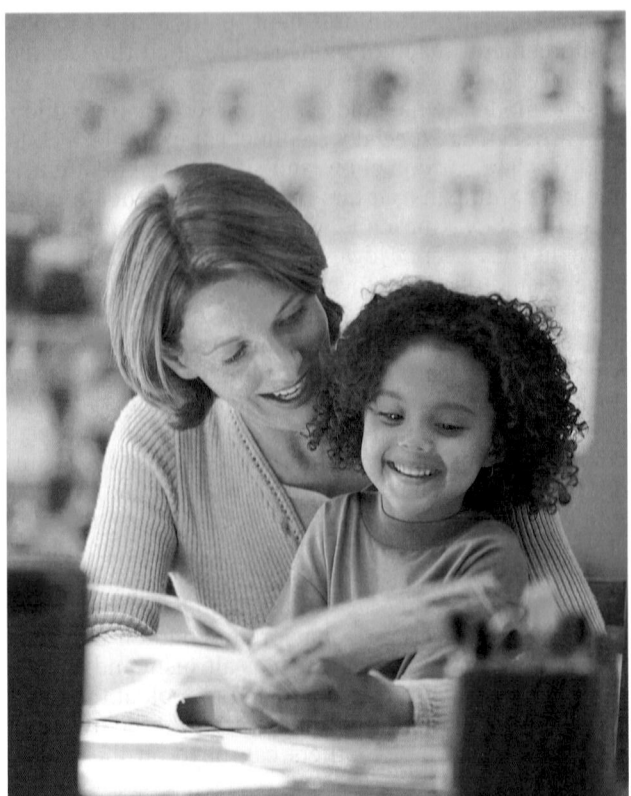

Figure 3-25 Multiple intelligence theory asserts that a young child's interest in certain activities and skills should be nurtured because this may represent a high level of intelligence in that area.

In each of the intelligence domains, it is possible to have *at-promise individuals*. These are people who are highly endowed with the core abilities and skills of that intelligence. For example, Babe Ruth, the famous baseball player, was outstanding in body–kinesthetic intelligence. With each intelligence, the particular developmental trajectory of an individual "at promise" varies. For instance, some young children with mathematical or musical intelligence are able to perform at, or near, adult-level expectations. In contrast, the interpersonal and intrapersonal intelligences appear to develop more gradually, and child prodigies in these areas are rare. In addition, mature performance in one area does not imply mature performance in another area.

Knowledge of these intelligence categories can be used by families, teachers, and health care professionals to provide activities to enhance development of the child's intelligences. The family can assist children in their choice of activities and assist adolescents in their choice of careers within the context of their dominant intelligence. Teachers and the educational system can create individual-centered schools where student profiles, goals, and interests are matched to particular curricula and particular styles of teaching and learning.

BEHAVIORAL DEVELOPMENT

Behaviorism is structured on the interactions that occur between a child and his or her environment, which in turn determines the behavior of the child.

Behaviorists believe that the roots of a person's behavior are tied to his or her experiences. If experience (the environment) is altered, then behavior change follows. This approach has been very successful in modifying the behaviors of some people in certain circumstances. The two most prevalent behavioral techniques are classical conditioning, developed by Pavlov and Watson, and operant conditioning, developed by Skinner. These behavioral theories have been criticized for their mechanical approach to human interactions. The effects of the consciousness and thought processes on individual action are not well accounted for by these theories. Human behavior is afforded little qualitative difference from the behavior and expected responses in animals. These theories are well tested in the laboratory setting, with an emphasis on the effects of the environment on human behavior. However, translation of these findings to real-life settings, where other mental processes may come into play, demonstrates that classical and operant conditionings can only partially explain a person's behavior.

Classical Conditioning Theories

Classical conditioning was first introduced by Ivan Pavlov and was further explored by John Watson. The approach to learning involves pairing a neutral stimulus with an unconditioned stimulus to elicit an unconditioned response. This process is continued until the neutral stimulus is able to elicit a response without being paired with the original stimulus. The stimulus that elicits the response before conditioning is called the *unconditioned stimulus*. The subsequent response is the *unconditioned response*. The *conditioned stimulus* is a neutral stimulus that, when paired with the unconditioned stimulus, eventually elicits the desired response by itself. The learned response is the *conditioned response*. In a similar circumstance, the individual learns stimulus generalization—that is, to apply the association of a certain behavior with a stimulus to circumstances that feature similar stimuli. The individual eventually learns *discrimination* (the process of differentiating among stimuli) and *extinction* (the weakening and disappearance of a learned response).

Classical conditioning has been thoroughly evaluated in laboratory settings in which the environment and exposure to stimuli can be highly monitored. It is a useful theory in understanding acquired emotional responses in children (e.g., unusual fears about dogs). The theory does not take into account the higher mental capacities of humans to use thinking and information-processing abilities to determine response patterns.

Operant Conditioning Theory

> **QUESTION:** Joellen and Chris describe the various methods they have used to control and stop James's temper tantrums. They report using different types of rewards if he does not have a tantrum. They have offered him special snacks, toys, or extra playtime, all without much success. Explain what is happening using Skinner's theory.

Operant conditioning holds that behaviors are repeated or are reduced in frequency based on the environmental consequences of reinforcement or punishment. B. F. Skinner popularized this concept of *stimulus–response learning*. In operant conditioning, the child's behavior is followed by a negative or positive reinforcer that decreases or increases the likelihood of that behavior being repeated. A *positive reinforcer* is a pleasant stimulus that follows a behavior and that increases the frequency of that behavior. For instance, giving a child a piece of candy each time he sits still during a haircut is a positive reinforcer that rewards the child and encourages him to sit still the next time he has a haircut because the child anticipates receiving more candy. A *negative reinforcer* is when an unpleasant stimulus is removed after a behavior has occurred and results in an increase in frequency of that behavior. For instance, a parent tells the child it is time for a bath (the unpleasant stimulus). The child throws a temper tantrum. The parent then allows the child to not take the bath. Each time the child throws a tantrum and gets out of doing something he or she perceives is unpleasant, the child is negatively reinforced to continue to use tantrums as a means to get out of doing something. *Punishment* is the process by which an unpleasant stimulus is introduced after a response has been made and the response decreases. The child who receives a spanking for biting a sibling would be expected not to repeat the biting behavior. Skinner and his associates also believed that behavior could be shaped. *Shaping* is the process in which a new behavior is acquired by taking a known behavior and continually reinforcing it to bring it closer and closer to the desired behavior. These principles have been applied successfully as behavior modification techniques to change parenting responses to a child's actions and vice versa.

ANSWER: Joellen's and Chris's actions are acting as positive reinforcers of James's behavior. They are using something pleasant, something that James enjoys, thereby encouraging him to continue the tantrums. James is learning that if he has a tantrum, he will get something good.

SOCIAL LEARNING THEORIES

The social learning theories explain human behavior based on the processes of imitation, observation learning, and reinforcement. The primary developers of social learning theory are Albert Bandura and Robert Sears. Although the behavioral theories stress the importance of structuring stimuli and reinforcements to create certain behavioral responses, social learning theorists acknowledge that a child does not have to be reinforced or punished to change his or her behavior. Children learn by observing and imitating. They watch and monitor the consequences of the behavior of others. Therefore, others, especially parents, siblings, and peers, serve as models for the child's behavior. Simply observing another person may be sufficient to lead to a learned response. Reinforcement, particularly parental reinforcement, may not be needed to elicit the learned response.

Role models who hold a high status in the child's eyes are seen as especially credible. For example, a child may watch a cartoon show and see characters interacting and fighting in a certain manner. If he is not familiar with the show, the child will most likely not imitate what he has seen. However, when the child goes to daycare and observes several of the other children pretending to be the same cartoon characters, he will be more inclined to imitate the behaviors of his respected friends. Social learning theories are helpful in explaining the powerful influence that social groups and the media can have on children's behavior. Although parents may choose not to exhibit or to expose their children to certain behaviors in the home, children may be influenced by modeling what is occurring in their play group or by other influential adults, such as grandparents or family friends.

Social learning theories are useful to help understand the presence of certain behaviors in children that may be learned from modeling, such as altruism and aggression. Parents should be encouraged to look at the models in their children's environment and to be aware of the powerful influence others can have on the child's behavior.

LANGUAGE DEVELOPMENT

Although the word *infant* means "without language," language acquisition is rooted in infancy through the many verbal and nonverbal exchanges children have with their caregivers. Language is the symbol system used for the storage and exchange of information and is a basic tool used for interpersonal relationships. It is also a primary indicator of a child's developmental level. For example, speech acquisition is tied to the achievement of other physiologic and social factors such as neurologic maturation, musculoskeletal development, and the innate desire to communicate with others. The child's ability to read and write are manifestations of language development. The presence of a speech or language disorder can have a profound effect on the child's ability to develop social relations, attain success in school, and feel confident when communicating with others (see Chapter 28 for a complete discussion of communication disorders). Although language development proceeds in certain predictable patterns, some children learn to speak sooner than others their age, whereas some children may acquire language much later. Albert Einstein and Winston Churchill are two famous individuals who are known to have been slow to speak in childhood.

Symbol Systems of Language

Language is conveyed through the use of three different symbol systems. One is *auditory expressive language*, the utterances of sound and, eventually, words. The earliest forms of auditory expressive language include open vowel sounds such as crying, cooing, and gurgling. By 5 months of age, laughing and the use of monosyllabic utterances, such as "ba" and "ga," appear. Humans also use *auditory receptive language*, which is the ability to listen and comprehend. The auditory receptive language skills of the young child are much more extensive than his or her auditory expressive language system. As early as the 26th week of gestation, fetuses can respond to sound. Development of auditory expressive and auditory receptive language skills are summarized in Developmental Considerations 3-3. It is important for family members to understand that if they use simple, clear language when speaking to a young child, effective communication can take place even if the child is not yet speaking.

caREminder

Health care providers need to be careful about the topics they discuss in the presence of a young child. The child may comprehend several of the key points of the dialogue yet may misinterpret their full meaning based on limited cognitive development.

Language is also conveyed *visually*. Gestures and hand signals are used to convey a broad scope of expressive meaning. The American Sign Language system is based on visual language skills. Prelinguistic visual milestones begin with the newborn who attends to language with alert visual fixation. As the child acquires verbal language skills, he or she will be using a broad scope of visual language skills to communicate with others. For instance, the social smile indicates that the child is happy or pleased with the actions of another person. The young child learns to wave bye-bye, blow a kiss, and point to the ground when he or she wants out of a high chair. The child points to objects he or she wants and screams if the parent does not understand this communication. Deaf infants exposed to American Sign Language use their visual and receptive language skills to acquire language that parallels the stages of oral language development in the hearing child. Sign language is also promoted for use with hearing infants. The combination of the visual language with verbal language is encouraged to facilitate infant–parent communication.

Factors That Influence Language Development

Girls are generally more advanced than boys in verbal acquisition. The speech control center of the brain is located in the dominant cerebral hemisphere, which, for most individuals, is on the left side. During infancy and early childhood, girls demonstrate advanced development of their left cerebral hemisphere, which accelerates verbal fluency. Firstborn and only children may have more advanced language skills than children who are born later. This is because younger siblings may not receive as much direct verbal input from adults as the firstborn child. In addition, the linguistic input from older siblings is not as optimal as that received from an adult in regard to learning correct language rules and structure.

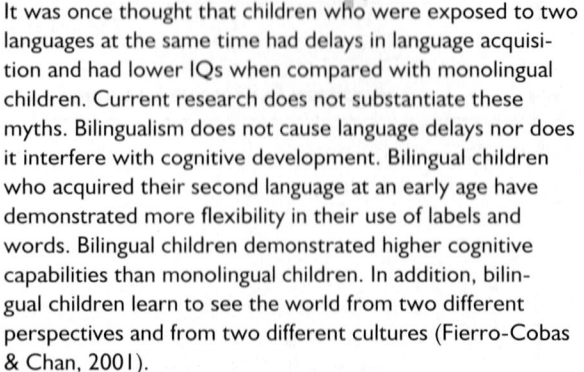

CROSS-CULTURAL CARE

It was once thought that children who were exposed to two languages at the same time had delays in language acquisition and had lower IQs when compared with monolingual children. Current research does not substantiate these myths. Bilingualism does not cause language delays nor does it interfere with cognitive development. Bilingual children who acquired their second language at an early age have demonstrated more flexibility in their use of labels and words. Bilingual children demonstrated higher cognitive capabilities than monolingual children. In addition, bilingual children learn to see the world from two different perspectives and from two different cultures (Fierro-Cobas & Chan, 2001).

A primary influence on impaired auditory expressive language development is the presence of hearing loss (discussed earlier in this chapter). Hearing loss can be congenital or acquired. Mild to moderate transient hearing loss can also be associated with otitis media with effusion.

ALERT   *Otitis media is the second most common disease of childhood (Waseem, 2013). The child who experiences an increased incidence of this disorder should be evaluated for hearing loss, and delays in speech development should be monitored carefully as the child's clinical condition improves. If speech development remains delayed or impaired, referral to a speech therapist is warranted.*

The presence of a developmental disorder may affect language acquisition. For instance, children who are mentally retarded have language delay in all areas: auditory expressive, auditory receptive, and visual. The child with a developmental language disorder will have variable degrees of expressive and receptive language impairment. Visual language skills are usually normal. Children who are autistic display delayed and deviant language.

GENDER IDENTIFICATION AND SEXUAL DEVELOPMENT

A child's gender identification and sexual development are influenced by biologic, social, and psychological factors. The biologic factors include the child's chromosomal sex, the external sexual organs, and the internal reproductive structures. Biologic problems can occur in which a child's gender is difficult to determine at birth because of the presence of ambiguous genitalia or chromosomal abnormalities. In these cases, the sexual identification that is assigned and the subsequent style of child rearing may not be consistent with the hormonal and structural factors that were present at birth. Gender identity disorder

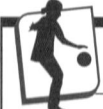

DEVELOPMENTAL CONSIDERATIONS 3-3

Development of Language

Age	Auditory Expressive Language	Auditory Receptive Language	Visual Language
Newborn	Cooing Crying	Responds to vocal stimuli by eye widening or changes in respiratory rate or suck rate	Gives alert visual fixation to caregiver's verbal stimuli Links mother's voice with her face and when crying is comforted by her voice
4–5 months	Laughing Monosyllables (ba, ga) Razzing	Turns head to locate source of a voice or bell	Social smile Visual localization of auditory stimuli (turning to a voice or a bell)
6–8 months	Polysyllabic babbling (lalalala)	Attends selectively to his or her own name when uttered by an adult Responds to tones of voice	Attends to common gesture games like patty-cake and peek-a-boo
9–12 months	Sporadically utters "mama" and "dada," then learns to spontaneously say "mama" and "dada" and label the correct parent Shakes head "no"	Comprehends the words "no" and "stop" Listens selectively to familiar words	Reciprocates and initiates gesture games Waves bye-bye Expresses desires by pointing to object and making sounds or crying
12 months	Says one or two words other than "mama" or "dada" Begins to acquire one word per week	Responds to one-step commands (give it to me) unaccompanied by a gestural cue Can bring familiar object from another room on request	Uses index finger pointing and single-word naming to signify desired object
18–24 months	Uses 10–20 words	Has receptive vocabulary of more than 100 words	Points to body parts
24 months	Acquires one or more new words per day Has vocabulary of 50 words Begins to produce jargon and two-word phrases ("me down") Begin to use pronouns Speech is one-half intelligible	Can follow simple novel two-step commands (put your shoes away, then go sit down) Name simple objects on command Has receptive vocabulary of more than 300 words	Points to objects on command
30 months	Beginning of telegraphic speech—three- to five-word sentences containing a recognizable subject and predicate but lacking conjunctions, articles, the verb "to be," and other small connecting words ("Me want bear.")	Points to objects described by use (give me the one we drink with) Follows prepositional commands (put the napkin under the cup)	Uses fingers to count one–two

Age	Auditory Expressive Language	Auditory Receptive Language	Visual Language
3 years	Acquires several new words a day Uses three- to four-word sentences Uses regular plurals Uses pronouns (I, me, you) Can count three objects Can tell age, sex, and full name Speech is three-fourths intelligible	Has receptive vocabulary of 800 words Knows function of common objects Understands spatial relationships (on, in, under)	Uses fingers to count or show age
4 years	Speaks four- to five-word sentences Can tell a story Uses past tense Names one color Can count four objects Speech is completely intelligible Normal dysfluency (stuttering)	Understands same/different	Begins to make letters and numbers
5–6 years	Speaks sentences of more than five words Uses future tense Names four colors Can count 10 or more objects Dysfluencies resolve Uses nouns, plurals, possessives Narrative has cause-and-effect sequence	Recalls part of a story Follows three-part commands Receptive language between 1,500 and 2,000 words Able to follow three- and four-step commands Understands "where," "when," and "why"	Matches identical shapes or figures Discriminates left versus right Copies square, circle, and cross Begins to write words Begins to read
7–9 years	Uses temporal prepositions (before, after) Uses past and future tenses Narrative has proper sequence	Understands passive verb forms (the cat was hit by a car)	No reversals of "b" and "d" persist Sight word vocabulary increases
10–12 years	Changes style of language (formal versus informal) to fit different contexts and different listeners (parents versus peers)	Understands multiple meanings of words Knows meanings of figurative language (simile, metaphor, analogy)	Attempts three-dimensional shapes in artwork Copies complex shapes and figures Begins to understand maps and geography Good sight word vocabulary
13 years	Complex sentence structure Can speak and write about abstract concepts	Understands linguistic explanations of abstract concepts Understands how to "play on words" (Call me a cab. Okay, hi cab)	Understands architectural plans Understands complex spatial relationships Uses and creates maps and schematic drawings

is a condition in which persons experience persistent discomfort with their assigned gender (gender determined at conception) and feel more comfortable identifying themselves as belonging to another gender.

Gender identification and awareness of one's sexuality begin in early childhood. The foundation for this process has already been laid with the development of trust and consistency of need fulfillment obtained during infancy. As the child's cognitive processes and language skills increase, opportunities arise that reinforce gender identification. The child quickly learns to imitate gender behavior and to pretend to be mommy or daddy. The child learns to name and to draw body parts. Body orifices are explored, and questions about the mother's or father's body may arise. Encourage families to use correct terminology when referring to body parts and not to overreact if the child is seen exploring his or her body parts.

During early childhood, parents may note a definite focus by the child on his or her genitalia and private parts. Name-calling using words associated with the genitalia or the elimination processes is common. The child continues to explore the body through masturbation and exploration of other children's genitalia. Parents should be teaching about personal privacy and the social appropriateness of actions. Facts about reproduction should be given.

caREminder

Children in early childhood should be taught about who can, and under what conditions someone can, touch their genitalia or private parts and what to do if someone touches them inappropriately.

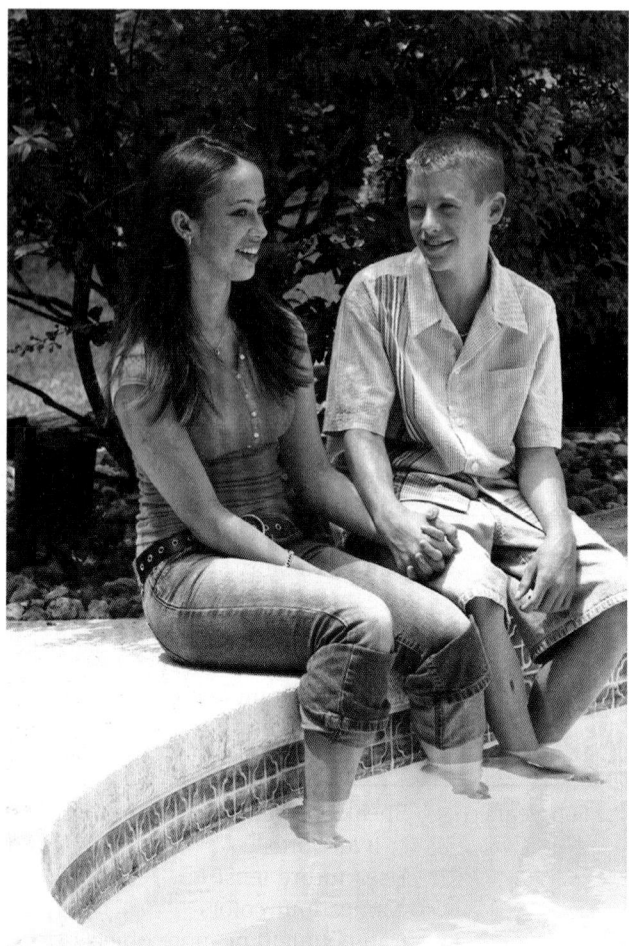

Figure 3-26 During adolescence, emerging sexuality is expressed in the development of intimate relationships.

The middle childhood years mark a change from focusing primarily on the parents for gender identification toward a focus on peers for identity development. Children at this age may engage in kissing, hugging, and other forms of physical contact with members of the opposite sex. Expressions of sexuality are primarily a response of cognitive and emotional factors rather than physical desire. The child develops close relationships with boys and girls in his or her age group. Within the context of these relationships, sexual stereotyping and role playing is reinforced. Parents and other significant adults should offer basic information about the changes that occur in the body with adolescence. In addition, discussions regarding reproduction and sexual activity should take place. Both the school-aged child and the adolescent will seek out this information from other sources to answer their queries. These other sources may provide inaccurate and misleading information.

The adolescent experiences tremendous changes in his or her sexual development as he or she deals with the physical maturation of the sexual organs (see the section on "Genitalia Development and Pubertal Changes" earlier in this chapter). Throughout puberty, the adolescent explores the changes in his or her body and the way it functions. Physical sexual desire may emerge, or

responses to physical stimuli may be associated more with the need for emotional gratification rather than physical needs (Fig. 3-26). During this period, adults should encourage the adolescent to express his or her feelings regarding his or her changing body and corresponding emotions. Parents can assist in clarifying values and in making decisions regarding gender-related activities. Information regarding sexually transmitted diseases, contraception, and pregnancy should be readily available for the adolescent. Many health care providers are directing their efforts toward encouraging adolescents to delay the start of intercourse. Early initiation of sexual activity has been associated with more risky behaviors (e.g., sex without use of contraception methods, multiple partners) and is thus more likely to result in elevated risks of sexually transmitted diseases and unplanned pregnancies (Ma et al., 2009).

MORAL DEVELOPMENT

Moral development is thought to be significantly correlated with intellectual reasoning and age. Psychologists differ in their beliefs regarding how a child's moral reasoning and subsequent moral behaviors develop.

Theoretical Perspectives of Moral Development

Proponents of Freudian psychology believe that it is the *superego*, the inner conscience of the child, that influences moral behavior. According to this theory, the child seeks to identify and internalize the ideals and values of adults around them, creating an ego ideal. The child's conscience will cause a sense of guilt when misbehavior occurs. Thus, morality is an outcome of the ego ideal and the conscience acting together to regulate thoughts and actions within the superego.

The behaviorist perspective is that moral behavior is learned like any other behavior. Sharing, giving, lying, and stealing are actions that are reinforced (positively or negatively) by authority figures and are therefore incorporated into the child's repertoire of acceptable behaviors. Social learning theorists add that these actions are influenced by watching and imitating others. None of these theories has been widely accepted as a way to explain all the variations found in moral development.

Cognitive developmental theories are used most frequently to explain the processes of moral reasoning—that is, how individuals gain their ideas about right and wrong, justice and injustice. Piaget outlined two stages of moral development. In the first stage, *moral realism*, rules are viewed as sacred, literal, and inflexible. Justice is whatever the law or authority commands. Children in this stage cannot take into account the view of other people and can think of only one thing, or aspect of a thing, at a time. Children will evaluate their own acts based on the consequences and the desire to avoid punishment, not the intent or motivation.

At ages 7 to 8 years, interaction with peers begins to be influenced by a sense of give and take. "Fairness" becomes a prominent issue. The second stage, called *moral relativism*, emerges around age 11 or 12 years. During this stage, children learn to evaluate the intentions of others before judging their answers as right or wrong. Thinking is no longer egocentric. Motives and circumstances can be taken into account when making a moral judgment. Rules are more flexible and can be elaborated and applied to several different situations and scenarios.

The sequence of moral development can be more fully understood by evaluating the works of Lawrence Kohlberg and Carol Gilligan.

Kohlberg's Theory

Kohlberg (1981) identified three levels of moral reasoning, with two stages at each level (Table 3-8). Kohlberg's theory has been the most widely tested and successfully applied to many cultures. In this stage theory, sequential development must occur to attain the next higher stage of moral reasoning. Levels of development correlate with the reasoning behind moral decisions, not the

---

TABLE 3-8   Kohlberg's Six Stages of Moral Reasoning

Stage	Moral Outlook	Reasons for Moral Actions
Preconventional Morality		
Stage 1: punishment and obedience orientation	Avoid breaking rules	Avoidance of punishment
Stage 2: instrumental relativist orientation	Right actions satisfy one's own needs and only sometimes the needs of others	Desire to serve one's own interests in a world where everyone has his own interests If you help others, they will owe you something, which is a debt to be collected later
Conventional Morality		
Stage 3: interpersonal concordance of "good boy–nice girl" orientation	Good behavior is that which pleases or helps others and is approved by them	Need to see oneself as a good person Belief in the Golden Rule Desire to maintain rules and follow authority to support stereotypical good behavior Need to gain approval of others
Stage 4: law and order orientation	Orientation toward authority, fixed rules, and the maintenance of the social order	Need to do one's duty and to show respect for authority and the social order
Postconventional Morality		
Stage 5: social contract legalistic orientation	Aware that people hold a variety of values and opinions, although there are also rights and rules that have been constitutionally and democratically agreed on	Obligation to law because of one's social contract with society Good is done because it serves the greatest number of people
Stage 6: universal ethical principle orientation	Self-chosen ethical principles based on abstract principles are the foundation for action; laws or social agreements are considered valid because they are consistent with one's ethical principles	A belief and commitment to the validity of universal moral principles Desire to uphold abstract principles that define right behavior for self Unjust laws may be broken when they conflict with broad moral principles

decisions or acts themselves. The higher stages of reasoning place an emphasis on justice, individual rights, and the rights of others.

Gilligan's Theory

Gilligan (1982) has challenged Kohlberg's view, asserting instead that women have a different orientation to moral questions. Gilligan feels that females view moral questions in terms of how the issues affect interpersonal relationships, whereas the male emphasis is on individual rights and self-fulfillment. Gilligan does not believe that Kohlberg's model reflects these gender-based responses to morality. In her view, the differences in moral reasoning can be traced to the differences in child-rearing practices of boys and girls. Boys are more likely to be encouraged to be independent, assertive, and achievement oriented. Duty and fairness are highly emphasized. In contrast, girls are more likely to be encouraged to nurture, to take responsibility for others, and to learn to be sensitive and caring. Moral decisions can cause internal conflict between the female's perception of her personal needs and the needs of others. In many cases, a female's decisions are made to maintain or solidify the relationship with others rather than assert her individual rights. Gilligan developed a model of the development of moral reasoning with three levels and two transitional stages to explain how feminine moral development is neither deviant nor arrested, but simply different (Table 3-9).

SPIRITUAL DEVELOPMENT

QUESTION: Joellen and Chris have recently developed strong religious ties to a community church and they ask how they can best foster spiritual development for James. What suggestions would you give based on James's current stage of faith development?

The spiritual dimension of the child encompasses the need to find satisfactory answers to the meaning of life, illness, and death. Although the need to find meaning and purpose for one's life does not generally begin to develop until early adolescence, all children experience a need for love, relatedness, and forgiveness. Throughout the child's life, questions regarding birth, suffering, death, hope, and forgiveness will be introduced and explored within the context of everyday experiences. The child's approach and response to these inquiries will be based on his or her corresponding level of cognitive and moral development.

Little research has been completed regarding spiritual development in children. It is known that faith, or the confidence or trust in a higher power, person, or thing, can be a driving force supporting the child and family through difficult times. Faith is most often associated with religious belief and the attitudes, observances of tenets, and values that are a part of a particular religious group. Fowler (1974) identified stages in the development of faith in children and

TABLE 3-9 Gilligan's Stages of the Ethic of Care

Stage	Description
Stage 1: preconventional	Egocentric perspective describes a great concern for self and a lack of awareness of other's needs. Being moral is surviving by being submissive to authority and the moral sanctions imposed by society.
Transition is from selfishness to responsibility to others.	
Stage 2: conventional care	There is a lack of distinction between what others want and what is right. The right, or moral, action is whatever pleases others best. Being moral involves not hurting others, with no thought of the hurt to self that might be done.
Transition from goodness to truth that he or she is a person, too.	
Stage 3: postconventional	The needs of self and others become integrated. Moral actions take into account equally self-beliefs as well as other's beliefs.

adults. Interventions can be provided that help the child meet his or her spiritual needs at those stages (Nursing Interventions 3-1). These include encouraging children to read stories regarding faith and religious figures, encouraging the use of prayer, and promoting activities with other children that have a religious or spiritual focus (Fig. 3-27). Chapter 13 contains further discussion regarding meeting the spiritual needs of children experiencing grief and loss.

ANSWER: James is in stage 1 of faith development, the intuitive–projective stage. Joellen and Chris would be the primary providers of faith to James. Suggest that they model religious gestures and behaviors so that he can learn them. Also encourage them to read faith and religious stories to him and help him learn prayers (simple ones that he can master, thereby promoting a sense of autonomy as well). Suggest that the parents engage in prayer with James as a role-modeling behavior. In addition, recommend that they participate in religious and faith activities with other families, especially those with children who are the same age as James.

DEVELOPMENTAL SURVEILLANCE

Developmental, behavioral, and emotional problems can be difficult to detect in young children. Accurate assessments of the child's growth and development may be hindered by infrequent access to the child to establish a developmental baseline assessment and

NURSING INTERVENTIONS 3-1

Nursing in the Stages of Faith Development

Stage and Description	Nursing Interventions
Stage 0: Undifferentiated, Infancy	
Feelings of trust, warmth, security, mistrust, and shame are incorporated into the child's conceptual ideas about himself or herself and his or her caregiver. These feelings are the foundation for subsequent faith development.	Focus is on supporting caregivers. Reassure parents about the adequacy of their parenting skills. Reassure parents that a child's illness is not a result of supernatural powers punishing them. Provide for trust and security needs of infant in parents' absence.
Stage I: Intuitive–Projective, Early Childhood	
Parents and other significant others provide primary knowledge of faith. Child learns to imitate religious gestures and behaviors. Egocentrism and magical thinking affect perceptions of transcendental beings. Child does not understand differences between natural and supernatural.	Minimize magical beliefs that are negative and destructive by focusing on reality. Help child to realize illness is not a result of "being bad." Promote the continuance of religious rituals during illness and crises.
Stage II: Mythical–Literal, Middle Childhood	
Learns to distinguish religious fact from fantasy. Is heavily influenced by attitudes of family and authority figures such as priest, minister, or rabbi. Uses fantasies to explain events or facts that cannot be understood. Begins to learn to differentiate between natural and supernatural. Faith beliefs are concrete and literal. God is perceived as having human qualities and characteristics. Is able to articulate his or her faith.	Clarify magical and fantastical beliefs through teaching. Explain all events and procedures that are unfamiliar in the health care setting. Promote use of prayer and other religious rituals. Allow child to talk about his or her faith.
Stage III: Synthetic–Convention, Early Adolescence	
Begins to reflect on and question religious beliefs and practices as exposed to more varied opinions. Relies on authority figures for answers to questions of faith. Begins to perceive God as a spirit and understand spiritual component of others. More clearly understands differences between natural and supernatural.	Assure child that illness is not a result of punishment by a supernatural being. Clarify conflicting and confusing information to the child. Encourage visits by respected authority figures. Promote incorporation of religious rituals and articles into hospital environment as desired by the child.
Stage IV: Individuating–Reflexive, Adolescence	
Seeks to come to terms with own beliefs and personalize them. In the process, may reject previous religious training, revert to a previous stage of religious belief and practices, or adopt some other extreme hedonistic attitude. Faith is a blended application of self-expression and beliefs and practices learned in the past.	Provide open and accepting attitude of child's beliefs. Engage in active listing as child "tries out" his or her emerging belief system. Offer support of authority figures, although these may be rejected at this time. Encourage use of religious rituals and articles as the child feels comfortable doing so.

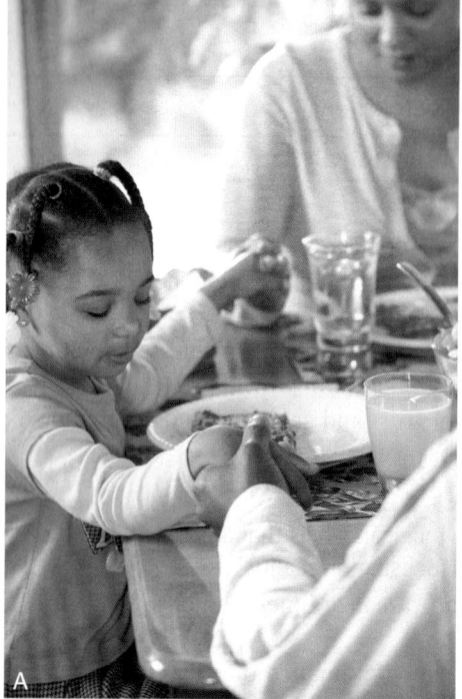
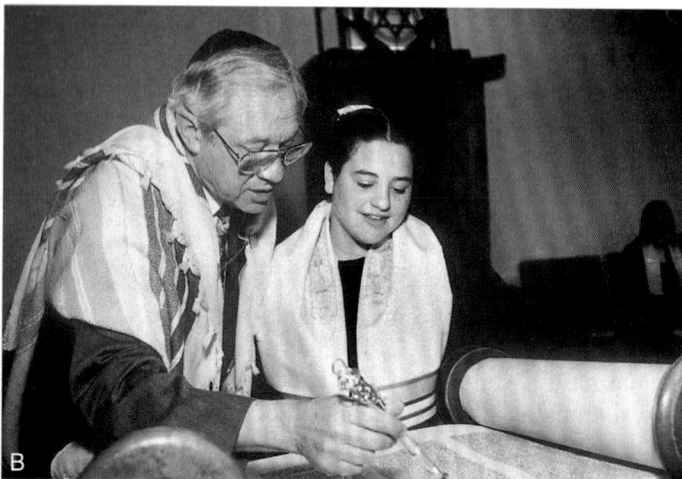

Figure 3-27 (A) The preschool child might participate in religious rituals without having a full understanding of their meaning. (B) Religious practices and traditions guide adolescents in developing their own concept of spirituality. Courtesy of Lou Metzger.

to evaluate progress over time. Many problems may present very subtly. Therefore, the uncooperative child may elicit inconclusive or false-positive findings when attempts at direct assessment are being made by the practitioner. In addition, parents may not have accurate knowledge of the developmental milestones that their child should be achieving at any given point in time.

The astute health care practitioner can use every contact with the child as an opportunity to apply **developmental surveillance**, the active and intentional evaluation of the child and the family to identify those who may be at risk for developmental variation. Developmental surveillance is a flexible, continuous process in which both informal and formal assessment techniques are used to evaluate the child's developmental progress from birth onward. The developmental surveillance process should use parental concerns and informal clinical observation of the child as the basis for early detection of developmental delays. Additionally, nurses providing direct patient care should have knowledge of the clinical conditions (i.e., low birth weight, birth asphyxia, infection) and the behaviors (i.e., irritability, head positioning, abnormal reflexes) that make the child at risk for the presence of developmental problems (Hertz, 2005). Figure 3-28 depicts the process that should be used to apply developmental surveillance techniques and to determine when to administer formal screening tests. Chapter 8 presents a summary of parental information and health care provider observations that can be elicited during contacts with the child and the family as part of the developmental surveillance process.

DEVELOPMENTAL ASSESSMENT

Valid assessment of children requires a perspective that encompasses quantitative as well as qualitative changes of developmental processes. Use of developmental screening tests has constituted the major approach to identification of children with developmental problems. Accurate screening contributes to parental well-being, helps distribute limited diagnostic services and health care dollars in an effective manner, and helps ensure that those children who need intervention are identified as early as possible.

A variety of developmental screening tests are available to help the health care provider assess children suspected of delayed development. Nurses and other health care professionals should be aware that a developmental screening test evaluates a child's development only at the current time, much like a snapshot captures the child's image at a certain point in time. A common misconception is that a developmental screening test can identify all children who will later be "normal" and all those who will later exhibit delays in development. Attempting to predict later normal development on the basis of the results of a developmental screen is dangerous because an array of environmental factors may subsequently intervene, influencing a child's development. Individual variations from developmental norms may be transient and may indicate the need for more comprehensive evaluation. However, if a child exhibits major developmental delays early in life, predicting later developmental problems can be made with a somewhat greater degree of confidence, underscoring the importance of early intervention for children with developmental problems.

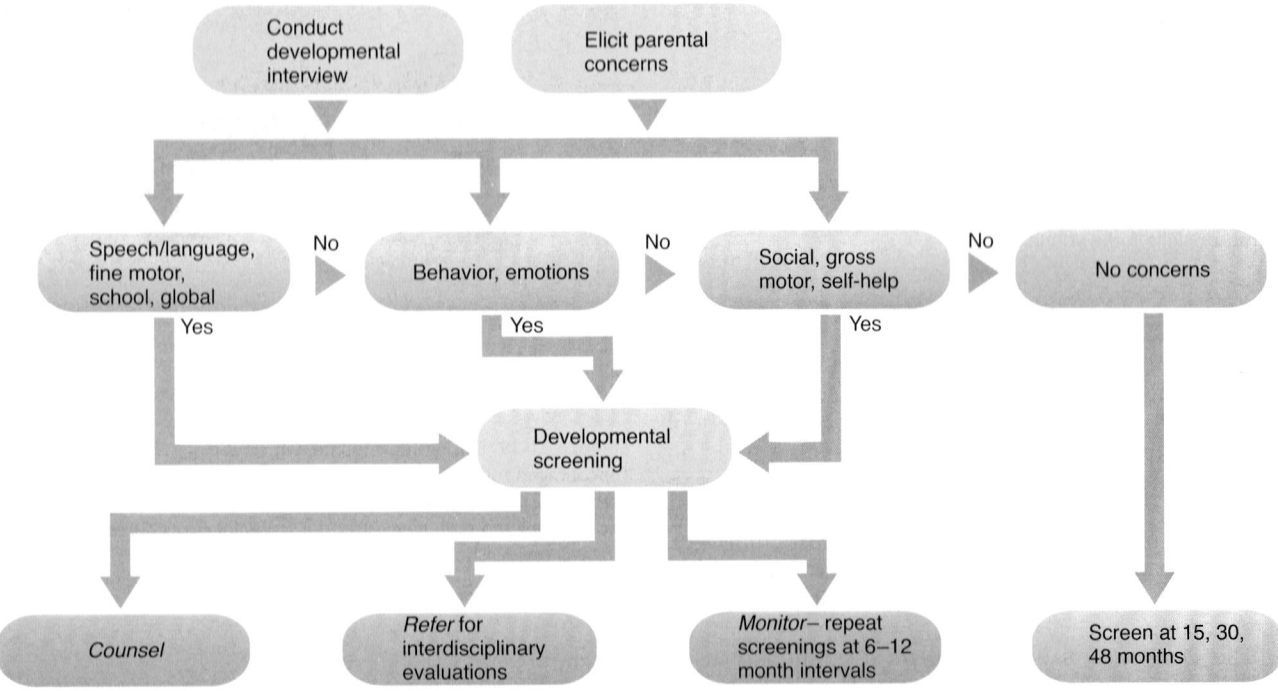

Figure 3-28 Developmental surveillance: the decision-making process.

Developmental screening should be performed routinely on children to evaluate achievement of developmental milestones. Nursing Interventions 3-2 presents a set of guidelines that should be used during all screening procedures. Well-child health care visits are an opportune time to complete the screening. Hospitalized children can be assessed before discharge when they are likely to feel more like participating in the assessment. School and camp nurses may wish to use a screening tool if they suspect delays in a child's development or if a teacher or caregiver shares concerns regarding an aspect of the child's development.

For parents, the data collected during such a screening provide information that can be used to guide activities with the child. If areas exist in which the child falls below age-specific achievements, instructions can be provided to assist the parents to enhance their child's skills in that area. Often, a child may demonstrate a specific delay simply because that task has not been emphasized in the home environment.

NURSING INTERVENTIONS 3-2

Guidelines for Developmental Screening

- Screening instruments should only be used by those trained to administer the assessment.
- Screening tools should be reliable and valid.
- Developmental screening is best conducted in an environment that is familiar and free from other distractions for the child.
- The results of developmental screening will be more valid if the tasks are familiar and relevant to the child.
- Screening instruments should only be used for a specified purpose.
- Developmental screening should involve input from the child's primary caregiver. Parents, regardless of their education, are able to provide predictive information about their children.
- Screening should be used on a pass/fail basis only with a failed developmental screening leading to further assessment.
- Screening measures must be culturally sensitive. For non–English-speaking families, use screening kits published in multiple languages.
- Developmental screening should take place periodically, and as warranted, based on the parent's concerns.
- Developmental screening is one method to determine the need for more in-depth evaluation of the child.

CROSS-CULTURAL CARE

Culture may highly influence a child's developmental achievements. For instance, in cultural environments in which fine motor skills are emphasized, delays in the area of gross motor development may be typical for that population. This is attributed to a cultural emphasis on development of fine motor skills in the young child.

Screening Tools

When a child has marked developmental problems, a screening tool can be used to gather baseline data and can serve as a measure of future progress. A variety of resources to locate developmental screening tools on the Web are presented on thePoint. These tools can be used by the health care provider to assess normal achievements or specific tasks for a particular age. The tools are all considered to be valid and reliable and vary in the amount of training required to administer them.

The Denver II is one of the most commonly used developmental screening instruments by trained health care personnel. A parent-answered prescreening form is also available, called the Denver Prescreening Developmental Questionnaire (PDQ-II). The Denver II provides an overall assessment of development that can be administered in a 15- to 20-minute period by individuals who have received training in the test administration and interpretation processes (Fig. 3-29). The PDQ-II consists of 150 questions from the Denver II. Parents are asked to answer a subset of these questions based on their child's age.

caREminder

If the child is ill, developmental screening may not provide an accurate assessment of the child's skills and abilities. The child's weakness, anxiety, and physical restrictions could affect the outcome of the assessment. For instance, if a child has an intravenous line in his or her dominant right hand, then testing of fine motor skills may not accurately reflect the child's dexterity.

Developmental screening tests like the Denver II and the PDQ-II have value as an aid in developmental surveillance when used in combination with parental concerns, child observations, immunizations, and anticipatory guidance to promote the child's growth and development.

As a result of developmental screening, if a developmental delay is assessed, the child should be referred to a specialist for more in-depth assessment and diagnosis. Pediatric nurses are in a prime position to screen for developmental problems. With appropriate training and practice, they can easily and effectively use the Denver II and PDQ-II in their practice.

See thePoint for a summary of Key Concepts.

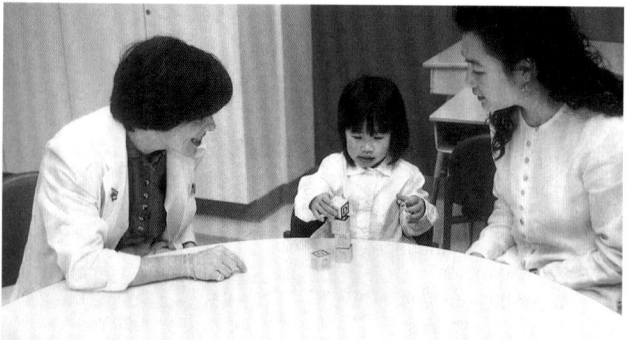

Figure 3-29 During developmental screening tests, parents are encouraged to stay near the child to promote a sense of comfort and security. Parents are instructed not to prompt the child or to ask questions during the screening. After the screening procedures, the evaluator will review the results with the parents.

REFERENCES

Alaimo, K., Olson, C., & Frongillo, E. (2001). Food insufficiency and American school-aged children's cognitive, academic, and psychosocial development. *Pediatrics, 108*, 44–53.

American Academy of Pediatrics. (2008). Strength training by children and adolescents. *Pediatrics, 121*(4), 835–840.

American Academy of Pediatrics. (2009). Media violence. *Pediatrics, 124*(5), 1495–1503.

Baker, J., Michaelsen, K., Rasmussen, K. et al. (2004). Maternal prepregnant body mass index, duration of and timing of complementary food introduction are associated with infant weight gain. *American Journal of Clinical Nutrition, 80*, 1579–1588.

Berk, L. (2011). *Infants, children, and adolescents.* Boston, MA: Pearson Education.

Black, M. (2012). Integrated strategies needed to prevent iron deficiency and to promote early child development. *Journal of Trace Elements in Medicine and Biology, 26*(2–3), 120-123.

Brands, B., Egan, B., Gyorei, E. et al. (2012). A qualitative interview study on effects of diet on children's mental state and performance. Evaluation of perceptions, attitudes, and beliefs of parents in four European countries. *Appetite, 58*(2), 739–746.

Breslau, N., Breslau, J., Miller, E. et al. (2011). Behavior problems at ages 6 and 11 and high school academic achievement: Longitudinal latent variable modeling. *Psychiatry Research, 185*(3), 433–437.

Burt, S. (2005). How are parent–child conflict and childhood externalizing symptoms related over time? Results from a genetically informative cross-lagged study. *Development and Psychopathology, 17*(1), 145–165.

Chess, S. (1990). Studies in temperament: A paradigm in psychosocial research. *Yale Journal of Biology and Medicine, 63*, 313–324.

Chess, S., & Thomas, A. (1985). Temperamental differences: A critical concept in child health care. *Pediatric Nursing, 11*, 167–171.

Chess, S., & Thomas, A. (1986). *Temperament in clinical practice.* New York, NY: Guilford.

Congdon, E., Westerlund, A., Algarin, C. et al. (2012). Iron deficiency in infancy is associated with altered neural correlates of recognition memory at 10 years. *The Journal of Pediatrics, 160*(6), 1027–1033.

de Jong, P. A., Nakano, Y., Lequin, M. H. et al. (2003). Estimation of lung growth using computed tomography. *The European Respiratory Journal, 22*(2), 235–238.

Elkind, D. (1967). Egocentrism in adolescence. *Child Development, 38*, 1025–1034.

Elkind, D. (1984). Teenage thinking: Implications for health care. *Pediatric Nursing, 10*, 383–385.

Elkind, D. (1986). David Elkind discusses parental pressures. *Pediatric Nursing, 12*, 417–418.

Engle, P. L., Fernald, L. C., Alderman, H. et al. (2011). Strategies for reducing inequalities and improving developmental outcomes for young children in low-income and middle-income countries. *Lancet, 378*(9799), 1339–1353.

Erikson, E. (1963). *Childhood and society.* New York, NY: W. W. Norton.

Fewtrell, M. S., Morley, R., Abbott, R. A., et al. (2001). Catch-up growth in small-for-gestational-age term infants: A randomized trial. *American Journal of Clinical Nutrition, 74*, 516–523.

Fierro-Cobas, V., & Chan, E. (2001). Language development in bilingual children: A primer for pediatricians. *Contemporary Pediatrics, 18*(7), 79–98.

Fowler, J. (1974). Toward a developmental perspective on faith. *Religious Education, 69*, 207–219.

Fox, N., Nichols, K., Henderson, H. et al. (2005). Evidence for a gene–environment interaction in predicting behavioral inhibition in middle childhood. *Psychological Science, 16*(12), 921–926.

Fox, S., Levitt, P., & Nelson, C., III. (2010). How the timing and quality of early experiences influence the development of brain architecture. *Child Development, 81*(1), 28–40.

Gardner, H. (1993). *Multiple intelligences: The theory in practice.* New York, NY: Basic Books.

Gardner, H. (2006). *Multiple intelligences: New horizons in theory and practice.* New York, NY: Perseus Book Group.

Gidding, S., Dennison, B., Birch, L. et al. (2006). Dietary recommendations for children and adolescents: A guide for practitioners. *Pediatrics, 117*(2), 544–559.

Gilligan, C. (1982). *In a different voice.* Cambridge, MA: Harvard University Press.

Gross, D., Garvey, C., Julian, W. et al. (2009). Efficacy of the Chicago parent program with low-income African American and Latino parents of young children. *Prevention Science, 10*(1), 54–65.

Hagan, J. F., Shaw, J. S., & Duncan, P. M. (Eds.). (2008). *Bright futures: Guidelines for health supervision of infants, children, and adolescents* (3rd ed.). Elk Grove Village, IL: American Academy of Pediatrics.

Hamby, S., Finkelhor, D., Turner, H. et al. (2011). Children's exposure to intimate partner violence and other family violence. *National Survey of Children's Exposure to Violence, U.S. Department of Justice.* Retrieved from https://www.ncjrs.gov/pdffiles1/ojjdp/232272.pdf

Hamilton, R., Bowers, B., & Williams, J. (2005). Disclosing genetic tests results to family members. *Journal of Nursing Scholarship, 37*(1), 18–24.

Han, T., Wang, X., Cui, Y. et al. (2010). No weight catch-up growth of SGA infants is associated with insulin resistance in the early postnatal period. *International Journal of Pediatrics.* Advance online publication.

Hariri, A. (2009). The neurobiology of individual differences in complex behavioral traits. *Annual Review of Neuroscience, 32*, 225–247.

Herrenkohl, T., & Herrenkohl, R. (2007). Examining the overlap and prediction of multiple forms of child maltreatment, stressors, and socioeconomic status: A longitudinal analysis of youth outcomes. *Journal of Family Violence, 22*(7), 553–562.

Hertz, D. (2005). *Care of the newborn.* Philadelphia, PA: Lippincott Williams & Wilkins.

Huh, S., Rifas-Shiman, S., Taveras, E. et al. (2011). Timing of solid food introduction and risk of obesity in preschool-aged children. *Pediatrics, 127*(3), 544–551.

Hung, I., & Carey, J. (2012). Presymptomatic genetic testing: Shifting the emphasis from reaction to prevention. In D. H. Best & J. J. Swensen (Eds.), *Molecular genetics and personalized medicine.* New York, NY: Springer Science + Business Media.

Ingles, J., Zodgekar, P., Yeates, L. et al. (2011). Guidelines for genetic testing of inherited cardiac disorders. *Heart, Lung and Circulation, 20*(11), 681–687.

Janz, K., Dawson, J., & Mahoney, L. (2000). Predicting heart growth during puberty: The Muscatine study. *Pediatrics, 105*, e63.

Kilbride, H., Thorstad, K., & Daily, D. (2004). Preschool outcome of less than 801-gram preterm infants compared with full-term siblings. *Pediatrics, 113*, 742–747.

Kochhar, A., Hildebrand, M., & Smith, R. (2007). Clinical aspects of hereditary hearing loss. *Genetics in Medicine, 9*(7), 393–408.

Kohlberg, L. (1981). *The philosophy of moral development: Moral stages and the idea of justice.* New York, NY: Harper & Row.

Lerman, C., Croyle, R., Tercyak, K. et al. (2002). Genetic testing: Psychological aspects and implications. *Journal of Consulting and Clinical Psychology, 70*, 784–797.

Lewis, T., Kotch, J., Thompson, R. et al. (2010). Witnessed violence and youth behavior problems: A multi-informant study. *American Journal of Orthopsychiatry, 80*(4), 443–450.

Ma, Q., Ono-Kihara, M., Cong, L. et al. (2009). Early initiation of sexual activity: A risk factor for sexually transmitted diseases, HIV infection, and unwanted pregnancy among university students in China. *BMC Public Health, 9*, 111. Retrieved from http://www.biomedcentral.com/content/pdf/1471-2458-9-111.pdf

Mann, J., & Currier, D. (2010). Stress, genetics, and epigenetic effects on the neurobiology of suicidal behavior and depression. *European Psychiatry, 25*(5), 268–171.

Margolin, G., & Vickerman, K. (2007). Posttraumatic stress in children and adolescents exposed to family violence: I. Overview and issues. *Professional Psychology: Research and Practice, 38*(6), 613–619.

McAfee, A., Mulhern, M., McSorley, E. et al. (2012). Intakes and adequacy of potentially important nutrients for cognitive development among 5-year-old children in the Seychelles child development and nutrition study. *Public Health Nutrition, 15*(9), 1670–1677.

McDonald, R., Jouriles, E., Briggs-Gowan, M. et al. (2007). Violence toward a family member, angry adult conflict, and child adjustment difficulties: Relations in families with 1- to 3-year-old children. *Journal of Family Psychology, 21*(2), 176–184.

Medoff-Cooper, B. (1995). Infant temperament: Implications for parenting from birth through 1 year. *Journal of Pediatric Nursing, 10*, 141–145.

Melvin, N. (1995). Children's temperament: Intervention for parents. *Journal of Pediatric Nursing, 10*, 152–159.

Middeldorp, C. M., Wray, N. R., Andrews, G. et al. (2006). Sex differences in symptoms of depression in unrelated individuals and opposite-sex twin and sibling pairs. *Twin Research and Human Genetics, 9*(5), 632–636.

Moster, D., Lie, R., & Markestad, T. (2008). Long-term medical and social consequences of preterm birth. *The New England Journal of Medicine, 359*, 262–273.

Moylan, C., Herrenkohl, T. I., Sousa, C. et al. (2010). The effects of child abuse and exposure to domestic violence on adolescent internalizing and externalizing behavior problems. *Journal of Family Violence, 25*(1), 53–63.

O'Connor, E., Rodriguez, E., Cappella, E. et al. (2012). Child disruptive behavior and parenting efficacy: A comparison of the effects of two models of insights. *Journal of Community Psychology, 40*(5), 555–572.

Ong, K., Emmett, P., Noble, S. et al. (2006). Dietary energy intake at the age of 4 months predicts postnatal weight gain and childhood body mass index. *Pediatrics, 117*, 503–508.

Piaget, J. (1926). *The language of the child.* New York, NY: Harcourt.

Pritchard, V., Clark, C., Liberty, K. et al. (2009). Early school-based learning difficulties in children born very preterm. *Early Human Development, 85*(4), 215–224.

Quinn, K., Kaufman, J., Siddiqi, A. et al. (2010). Stress and the city: Housing stressors are associated with respiratory health among low socioeconomic status Chicago children. *Journal of Urban Health, 87*(4), 688–702.

Riemann, R., Kandler, C., & Bleidorn, W. (2012). Behavioral genetic analyses of parent twin relationship quality. *Personality and Individual Differences, 53*(4), 398–404.

Richardson, G., Goldschmidt, L., Leech, S. et al. (2011). Prenatal cocaine exposure: Effects on mother- and teacher-rated behavior problems and growth in school-age children. *Neurotoxicology and Teratology*, *33*(1), 69–77.

Roberts, G., Lim, J., Doyle, L. et al. (2011). High rates of school readiness difficulties at 5 years of age in very preterm infants compared with term controls. *Journal of Developmental and Behavioral Pediatrics*, *32*(2), 117–124.

Saudino, K. (2005). Behavioral genetics and child temperament. *Journal of Developmental and Behavioral Pediatrics*, *26*(3), 214–223.

Shankaran, S., Das, A., Bauer, C. et al. (2011). Prenatal cocaine exposure and small-for-gestational-age status: Effects on growth at 6 years of age. *Neurotoxicology and Teratology*, *33*(5), 575–581.

Shonkoff, J. P., & Garner, A. S. (2012). The lifelong effects of early childhood adversity and toxic stress. *Pediatrics*, *129*(1), e232–e246.

Singer, L., Minnes, S., Short, E. et al. (2004). Cognitive outcomes of preschool children with prenatal cocaine exposure. *Journal of the American Medical Association*, *291*, 2448–2456.

Turecki, S., & Tonner, L. (2000). *The difficult child: Expanded and revised edition*. New York, NY: Bantam.

Walker, S. P., Wachs, T. D., Grantham-McGregor, S. M. et al. (2011). Inequality in early childhood: Risk and protective factors for early child development. *Lancet*, *378*(9799), 1325–1338.

Wallace, M. (1995). Temperament and the hospitalized child. *Journal of Pediatric Nursing*, *10*, 173–180.

Waseem, K. (2013). *Otitis media*. Available from http://emedicine.medscape.com/article/994656-overview

Williams, J., Schutte, D., Evers, C. et al. (1999). Adults seeking presymptomatic gene testing for Huntington's disease. *Journal of Nursing Scholarship*, *31*(2), 109–114.

See the**Point** for additional resources.

Infancy (Newborn to 11 Months)

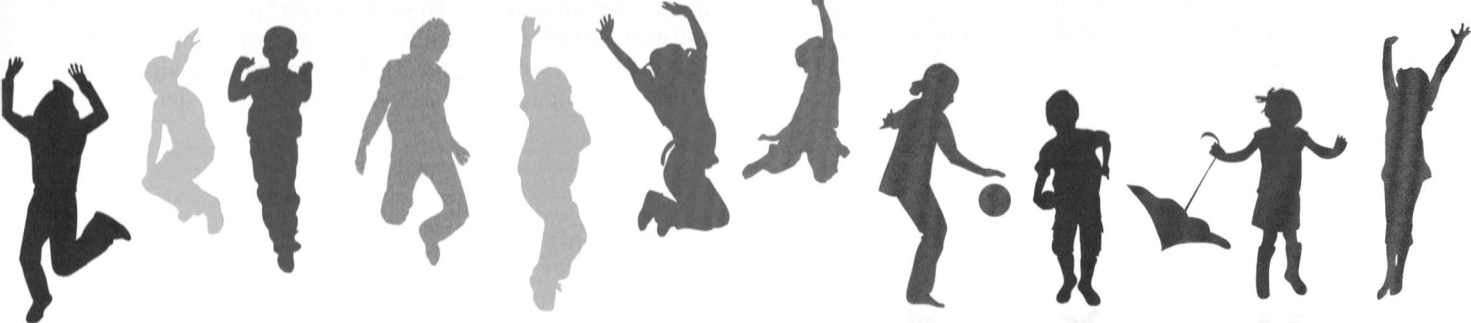

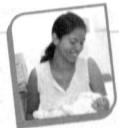

CASE HISTORY

Lela Diaz is such a different baby than her older brother. Claudia and Ignacio Diaz have a preschool-aged son, José, who, as a baby, ate like a little barracuda and then slept like a rock. Lela is proving to be much more difficult, even for an experienced mother like Claudia. Claudia breastfed her son and did not anticipate any difficulties breastfeeding her second child. Lela "did not nurse" well in the hospital, but Claudia was not too concerned. Then Claudia's breasts became engorged and she did not know what to do. Lela was also confused by the hard "marble statue" –like breasts. Claudia's hospital discharge instructions included a telephone number to call with any questions. The nurse instructs her to try showering first to see if the warm water sprayed on her breasts would help stimulate a letdown and soften the breasts. This does help, and Lela begins to show more interest in feeding.

When Lela turns 6 months old, Claudia finds a part-time job working the night shift at a nearby hotel. Claudia and Ignacio are pleased that this arrangement will increase their income but not require them to find daycare. Ignacio is certain that

Lela will sleep through the night, because at 6 months, José slept through the night. Claudia will not work two nights in a row and will nap when the children nap. Claudia is a little worried, however, because Lela is not like her brother. José started taking a bottle without a fuss while still breastfeeding when he was just a few months old. If it was food, he wanted it! Lela would rather starve than accept a plastic nipple. The first night Claudia goes to work, Lela keeps her father up half the night. She refuses a bottle; she refuses a cup. Ignacio works long hours with machinery and it is not safe for him to work without sleep. They decide to ask Claudia's mother, Selma, to come stay with them for a while.

Claudia and Ignacio do not have health insurance. Their children receive their immunizations at a free community clinic. At Lela's 8-month visit, after clarifying that Lela is taking little supplemental food and is primarily breastfeeding, a hematocrit and hemoglobin count is obtained that shows that Lela is mildly anemic. The nurse at the health department encourages Claudia to give Lela more iron-rich foods and more solid food. Claudia tries to explain that Lela does not like new foods.

CHAPTER OBJECTIVES

1 Describe developmental milestones for neonates and infants and state measures to enhance meeting these milestones.

2 Discuss the needs of the infant related to hygiene, personal care, nutrition, elimination, and safety.

3 Select age-appropriate interventions to promote healthy personal and social development of the infant.

4 Select interventions to promote illness and injury prevention for the infant and the family.

See the Point for a list of Key Terms.

A primary goal of the health care community is to collaborate with families to promote children's growth, development, adaptation, and functioning. Most parents invest considerable time, personal resources, and finances to meet their children's needs. Many parents seek child-rearing knowledge and assistance from health care professionals and others who work with children. Health care personnel must serve as an accessible support to parents as they strive to nurture, protect, and socialize their children. The interdisciplinary health care team plays a critical role in promoting healthy development. This chapter builds on the information presented in Chapter 3, "Principles and Physiologic Basis of Growth and Development," to describe issues related to promoting healthy development of the neonate and infant. Evaluation and treatment of acute disorders commonly seen in the neonatal and infant population are described in Chapters 14 through 31. Chart 4-1 summarizes the location in the text of many of these conditions. In addition, Chapter 14 is devoted to conditions that affect the neonate with altered health status.

DEVELOPMENTAL ASSESSMENT AND SURVEILLANCE

Parents of a healthy infant are likely to visit their health care provider more often during the infant's first year than at any other time during the child's life unless an acute condition arises. These repeated contacts provide the nurse ample opportunity to complete developmental surveillance (see Chapter 3). **Developmental surveillance** encompasses all activities related to detecting

CHART 4-1	Quick Reference to Conditions Common During Infancy
Condition	**Chapter**
Anorectal malformations	18: The Child With Altered Gastrointestinal Status
Apnea of infancy	16: The Child With Altered Respiratory Status
Atopic dermatitis (eczema)	25: The Child With Altered Skin Integrity
Biliary atresia	18: The Child With Altered Gastrointestinal Status
Bronchiolitis	16: The Child With Altered Respiratory Status
Cleft lip and cleft palate	16: The Child With Altered Respiratory Status
Colic	18: The Child With Altered Gastrointestinal Status
Common cold (nasopharyngitis)	16: The Child With Altered Respiratory Status
Congenital clubfoot	20: The Child With Altered Musculoskeletal Status
Congenital heart disease	20: The Child With Altered Musculoskeletal Status
Craniostenosis	21: The Child With Altered Neurologic Status
Croup	16: The Child With Altered Respiratory Status
Dehydration	17: The Child With Altered Fluid and Electrolyte Status
Developmental dysplasia of the hip	20: The Child With Altered Musculoskeletal Status
Diaper dermatitis	25: The Child With Altered Skin Integrity
Diarrhea	18: The Child With Altered Gastrointestinal Status
Epispadias	19: The Child With Altered Genitourinary Status
Esophageal atresia and tracheoesophageal fistula	16: The Child With Altered Respiratory Status
Fetal alcohol syndrome	14: The Neonate With Altered Health Status
Fever	31: Pediatric Emergencies
Gastroesophageal reflux (GER)	18: The Child With Altered Gastrointestinal Status
Gastroschisis	18: The Child With Altered Gastrointestinal Status
Hernias	18: The Child With Altered Gastrointestinal Status
Hydrocephalus	21: The Child With Altered Neurologic Status
Hypospadias	19: The Child With Altered Genitourinary Status
Metatarsus adductus	20: The Child With Altered Musculoskeletal Status
Microcephaly	21: The Child With Altered Neurologic Status
Neonatal pain	10: Pain Management
Neonatal skin lesions	25: The Child With Altered Skin Integrity
Obstructive uropathy	19: The Child With Altered Genitourinary Status
Omphalocele	18: The Child With Altered Gastrointestinal Status
Otitis media	28: The Child With Altered Sensory Status
Sepsis	14: The Neonate With Altered Health Status
Short bowel syndrome	18: The Child With Altered Gastrointestinal Status
Spina bifida	21: The Child With Altered Neurologic Status
Sudden infant death syndrome (SIDS)	31: Pediatric Emergencies

developmental problems and promoting healthy development. Techniques such as directly observing the child, eliciting parental concerns, and completing developmental screening are used to identify infants who may be at risk for developmental delay. Each encounter with the family is an opportunity to provide guidance and education about the infant's needs. *Bright Futures: Guidelines for Health Supervision of Infants, Children, and Adolescents* (Hagan et al., 2008) provides the most comprehensive set of principles, strategies, and tools that can be used by health care providers to guide teaching, health promotion activities, and developmental surveillance. The information provided in Chapters 4 through 7 of this text is consistent with information provided in these comprehensive, national guidelines.

Developmental Considerations 4-1 summarizes the developmental milestones that are accomplished during the infant's first year. This information provides the nurse with direction for specific trigger questions to ask the parents. Simply asking an open-ended question such as "How is your child developing?" is not effective (Lagerberg, 2005). Most parents would respond positively even if they lacked the information about which developmental milestones their child should be reaching at any given time. The nurse can also use knowledge of developmental milestones to summarize the developmental achievements that the family should promote and expect to see as the infant matures. Family members can then help the infant achieve these milestones.

When a child is hospitalized, continue to provide an environment for the infant that is both developmentally appropriate and family centered. Nursing Interventions Classification 4-1 summarizes the nursing activities associated with developmentally appropriate care of the neonate and infant.

Infancy is divided into three stages:

- Early infancy (birth to age 6 months)
- Middle infancy (ages 6 to 9 months)
- Late infancy (ages 9 to 12 months) (Holt et al., 2011)

Health care visits for the infant are scheduled within the first week after birth and at 1, 2, 4, 6, 9, and 12 months of age (Fig. 4-1) (Hagan et al., 2008). A primary focus of illness prevention is to encourage parents to pay attention to the recommended schedule of health care visits for their infant and to ensure that these visits are scheduled and attended. Screenings for vision and hearing occur at each visit. Growth parameter assessment is also a key element of each health visit. Developmental Considerations 4-2 provides a more detailed description of the changes in weight, height, and head circumference that should be seen as the infant grows. Chapter 8 also covers the specific immunizations and routine diagnostic tests that are completed throughout the childhood years.

Regular, periodic assessment by the same health care provider can help detect developmental problems early. Frequent visits with a primary health care provider also help to establish a trusting relationship between the family and the health care team. Therefore, when problems do arise, the family is likely to feel more comfortable seeking advice and support from the health care team.

To learn more about this topic, you can view the Watch and Learn video *Developmental Considerations in Caring for Children: Infants* on thePoint.

HYGIENE AND PERSONAL CARE

Caring for an infant entails bathing and skin care as well as monitoring thumb-sucking and pacifier use (oral care), sleep habits, and clothing. Becoming a parent does not automatically make an individual competent to perform infant care tasks. The pediatric nurse must have a thorough understanding of infant care needs and the ability to teach and demonstrate these skills to new parents.

BATHING

The infant does not need daily bathing the first few weeks of life. Washing the baby more than two to three times a week can dry out his or her skin. The diaper area must be kept meticulously clean to avoid diaper rash, but, until the cord falls off, the infant should receive sponge baths only. Before starting the bath, collect all the articles needed, including a basin of lukewarm water, two to three towels, a washcloth, mild soap, baby shampoo, lotion (optional), a fresh diaper, and clean clothes.

For the sponge bath, place the infant on a padded flat area near a sink or on a changing table. During the bath, expose only the parts of the body that are being cleansed to avoid chilling the infant. Begin the bath by cleaning the eyes from the inner area to the outer area, rinsing the cloth, and proceeding to the rest of the face. Clean the perineal area last. Dry each body part before moving on to wash another part of the body. Wash and dry all body creases carefully, particularly the folds in the neck and perineal area. These areas are particularly prone to rashes because they are warm and moist. Wash the infant's hair with a very mild, tear-free baby shampoo immediately after washing the face and neck.

To prevent infection and improper healing, do not submerge the cord area in water until the stump has fallen off, usually 7 to 10 days after birth (Tradition or Science 4-1). After the stump has fallen off, tub bathing may begin in a sink or plastic tub. Line the basin with a towel to reduce slipping and to make the surface more comfortable for the infant. Fill the basin with about 2 in. of water that is warm, not hot, to the inside of the wrist or elbow (Fig. 4-2). The first few baths should be brief, with the child monitored carefully for chilling. If the infant protests too much, sponge baths can be continued for 1 or 2 weeks before trying tub bathing again.

Parents should use bath time as bonding time by talking, cooing, and singing to their infant. The bath should be unhurried and nonstressful. If the infant is enjoying the experience, extra playtime in the water should be permitted.

When the infant is able to sit upright without much support, bathing can move from the plastic tub or sink to the bathtub. A tub ring or tub seat can be used to

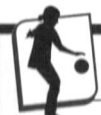

DEVELOPMENTAL CONSIDERATIONS 4-1

Milestones of the Infant (Newborn to 11 Months)

Physical Development

Newborn
10% loss of birth weight in first 3–4 days of life
73% of body weight is fluid
Head circumference is 70% of adult size
Needs to consume 120 cal/kg of weight per day
Sleeps 20–22 hr/day, with brief waking periods of 2–3 hours
Feeds every 2½–5 hours

2–4 Months
Posterior fontanel closes
Obligate (preferential) nose breathers (until about 5 months)
Begins drooling

5–6 Months
Doubles birth weight
Teeth may begin to erupt
Moves food to back of mouth and swallows during spoon feedings
Sleeps through the night for up to 8 hours
Goes 4–5 hours between feedings
Has two to four naps per day

7–9 Months
Begins teething with lower central incisors, followed by two upper incisors
Mashes food with jaws
Sleeps 14–16 hr/day, including naps

10–11 Months
Sleeps 14–16 hr/day and still naps
Stops drooling
Grows about 0.5 in./month

Sexual

All infants
Oral stage oral gratification and sucking needs (Freud)

10 Months
Begins sexual identity

Language

Newborn
Alerting
Social smile

2–3 Months
Laughs and squeals
Coos
Utters single vowel sounds such as "ah" and "eh"

4 Months
Utters two-syllable vowel sounds
Includes consonant sounds such as "m" and "b"

Produces belly laughs
Orients to voices of others

5 Months
Razzing
Intersperses vowel and consonant sounds

6 Months
Babbles
Uses about 12 speech sounds

7 Months
Makes "talking sounds" in response to caregiver while others are talking
Coos and squeals
Vocalizes up to four different syllables

8–10 Months
Uses "dada" and "mama" in nonspecific way
Responds to own name (receptive language skills develop first)
Babbles to produce consonant sounds
Vocalizes to toys

10–11 Months
Imitates speech sounds
Understands name and "no"
Understands "bye" and "pat-a-cake"
Imitates definite speech sounds
Uses jargon
Communicates by pointing to objects and by using gestures
Responds to simple verbal requests

Vision

Newborn
Fixates on human face and demonstrates preference
Blink reflex present

2 Months
Follows to midline
Produces rears
Visual acuity is hyperoptic

4 Months
Follows objects to 180 degrees

5 Months
Visual acuity 20/200
Recognizes feeding bottle

6 Months
Inspects hands
Fixates on objects 3 ft away
Strabismus no longer within normal limits
Develops hand–eye coordination

8 Months
Has permanent eye color
Depth perception developing

10 Months
Tilts head backward to see up

Hearing
Newborn
Startles to loud noises
Prefers high-pitched voices
Quieted by low-pitched noises
Responds to human voice over other noises
Auditory behavior is reflexive; generalized body movement (blinking or crying)
Recognizes certain sounds, ignores others; attends to quiet sounds more than loud ones—these are learned rather than reflexive behaviors
Turns to voice (quiet listening)

5 Months
Orients to bell (looks to side)
Stops crying in response to music

7 Months
Orients to bell (looks to side, then up)

10 Months
Localizes sound from above or below
Orients to bell (turns directly to bell)

Gross Motor
Newborn
Turns head when prone but cannot support head
Adjusts posture when held at shoulder
May squirm to corner or edge of crib when prone
Arm and leg movement are reflexive

6 Weeks to 2 Months
Holds head up 45–90 degrees when prone
May hold head steady when in supported sitting position

3 Months
Rolls over from back to side
Holds head erect and steady

4 Months
When supported, sits with rounded back and bended knees
May bear weight on legs when assisted to stand
Head lag disappears when pulled to sitting position

5 Months
Pulls to sitting position
Rolls from back to stomach
Sits alone momentarily
Shows unilateral reaching

6 Months
Sits without support
May creep an inch forward or backward

Moves from place to place by rolling
Begins drinking from a cup

7 Months
Stands while holding on
Early stepping movements
Begins to crawl or hitch
Raises head spontaneously when supine

8 Months
Pulls to standing position
Raises self to sitting position
Palmar grasp disappears

9 Months
Walks with help
Crawls, creeps, or hitches when permitted
Sits down
Holds own bottle
Drinks from cup or glass

10 Months
Continues walking skill development with help
Stands alone
May climb up and down stairs
Sits without support
Recovers balance
Changes from prone to sitting position

11 Months
May walk alone
Begins to stoop and recover
Pushes toys
"Cruises"

Fine Motor
Newborn
Follows to and slightly past midline

2–3 Months
Keeps hands open predominately
Reflex grasp replaced by voluntary grasping
Grasps objects such as rattle in open hand
May bring hands together at midline

4 Months
Uses ulnar–palmar prehension with a cube
Reaches for objects
Hands predominantly open

5 Months
Attempts to "catch" dangling objects with two hands
Begins using forefinger and thumb in pincer grasp (opposable thumb-prehension)
Retains two cubes
Recovers rattle
Reaches for and grasps objects

6–7 Months
Can grasp at will
Holds and manipulates objects

(Continued)

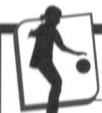

DEVELOPMENTAL CONSIDERATIONS 4-1

Milestones of the Infant (Newborn to 11 Months) *(Continued)*

Scoops pellet
Transfers from hand to hand
Demonstrates inferior pincer
Bangs objects together
Can release objects

8–9 Months
Combines spoons or cubes at midline
Retains two of three cubes offered
Achieves neat pincer grasp of pellet
Feeds self finger foods using only one hand
Releases objects at will
Rings bell
Holds bottle and places nipple in mouth when desired

10–11 Months
Plays "pat-a-cake" (a midline skill)
Puts several objects in a container
Holds crayon adaptively
Bangs two cubes together
Looks for hidden object (object permanency) (Piaget)
Achieves neat pincer grasp

Play
All infants
Engages in solitary play
May be imitative
Explores and manipulates

5–7 Months
Resists toy pull
Picks up tiny objects
Plays "peek-a-boo"
Works to get toy that is out of reach

8–9 Months
Plays "pat-a-cake"
Recognizes self in mirror

10–11 Months
Plays ball
Achieves object permanence (searches for dropped objects)

Cognitive
Newborn
Substage 1 (Piaget)
Practice of reflexes and reflex-like actions

1–3 Months
Substage II: Purposeful (Piaget)
Reproduces reflex actions

4–7 Months
Substage III: Objects (Piaget)
Oriented and imitative actions

Accidental actions are repeated
Develops habits
Responds negatively to removal of a toy

8–11 Months
Substage IV: (Piaget)
Coordination, intentional goal direction, and achievement
Experiments with object permanence
Imitates and models behavior
No concept of death
Enjoys "peek-a-boo" game
Attempts to flee from unpleasant events
Recognizes anticipatory signs
Repeats actions that elicit response from others
Dislikes restrictions
Shakes head for "no"
Appears interested in picture book

Social
Newborn
Regards face and establishes eye contact

1–2 Months
Smiles responsively
Enjoys cuddling and motion

3 Months
Smiles spontaneously

4–5 Months
Smiles at mirror image
Shows interest in siblings
Invites social interactions by smiling

6 Months
Exhibits stranger anxiety
Extends arms to be held

7–9 Months
Waves hands

10–11 Months
Demonstrates emotions of fear, anger, affection
Can indicate desires without crying
Offers object to a familiar adult
Talks to mirror

Interpersonal
0–3 Months
Self-absorbed, egocentric

4–18 Months
Symbiotic phase—mother seen as an extension of child's body and needs and vice versa

6–10 Months
Exhibits stranger anxiety
Waves arms and legs when frustrated

8–24 Months
Exhibits separation anxiety
Exhibits trust versus mistrust (Erikson)

Emotional
Newborn to 3 Months
Feeling regulated and interested in the world
Sensitive to parent's joyful interest in him or her

3–7 Months
Forming attachments
Highly specialized interest in the human world

4–10 Months
Purposeful communication
Can connect small units of feelings into simple patterns
Purposeful expression of wants and needs
Fluctuates easily between laughing and crying

10–18 Months
Complex sense of self
Communication is truly interactive, enabling young child to tune into parent and to appropriately build on parent's response

Moral
All Infants
Moral
Stage I: Preconventional level (Kahlberg)
May be disciplined by withdrawal of stimuli (e.g., food or toy) and may experience injury related to consequences of actions; however, makes no cognitive connection between these events and does not distinguish right from wrong
No moral concepts or rules exist

Spiritual
All Infants
Stage 0: Undifferentiated (Fowler)
Not capable of formulating or communicating any conceptual ideas about self or environment
Feelings of trust: sets foundation for subsequent development of faith

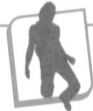

NIC 4-1 NURSING INTERVENTIONS CLASSIFICATION: Infant Care

Definition: Provision of developmentally appropriate family-centered care to the child under 1 year of age

Activities:
Encourage consistent assignment of professional caregivers.
Monitor infant's height and weight.
Monitor intake and output.
Incorporate parent preferences for bathing, when possible.
Change diapers.
Feed infant foods that are developmentally appropriate.
Provide opportunities for nonnutritive sucking.
Keep side rails of crib up when not caring for infant.
Remove small items from crib (e.g. syringe covers and alcohol wipes).
Monitor safety of infant's environment.
Provide developmentally-appropriate, safe toys and activities for infant.
Provide information to parents about child development and child rearing.
Provide visual, auditory, tactile, and kinetic stimulation during play.
Structure play and care around infant's temperament.
Talk to infant while giving care.
Encourage parents to participate in care activities (e.g. bathing, feeding, medication administration, or dressing changes).
Instruct parents to perform special care for infant
Reinforce parent's skill in performing special care for infant.
Inform parents about infant's progress.

Involve parent in the decision-making process, providing support throughout process.
Explain rationale for treatments, procedures to parents.
Give parents the option of being present for procedures or returning upon its completion.
Apply restraints when indicated and monitor throughout use.
Comfort infant through rocking, holding, cuddling, swaddling.
Monitor infant for signs of pain, including kicking, legs drawn up, steady crying, and difficulty consoling.
Use pain management strategies (e.g. distraction, parent's involvement, positioning, swaddling, or environmental manipulation).
Explain to parents that regression is normal during times of stress, such as illness or hospitalization.
Comfort infant when experiencing separation anxiety.
Encourage family to visit and stay overnight in hospital.
Provide emotional and spiritual support to parent (e.g. be available to listen, assist with maintaining or creating coping strategies or referral).
Maintain infant's daily routine during hospitalization, when possible.
Provide quiet, uninterrupted environment during nap time and nighttime.

From Bulechek, G. M., Butcher, H. K., Dochterman, J. M. et al. (Eds.). (2013). *Nursing interventions classifications (NIC)* (6th ed.). St. Louis, MO: Mosby. Used with permission.

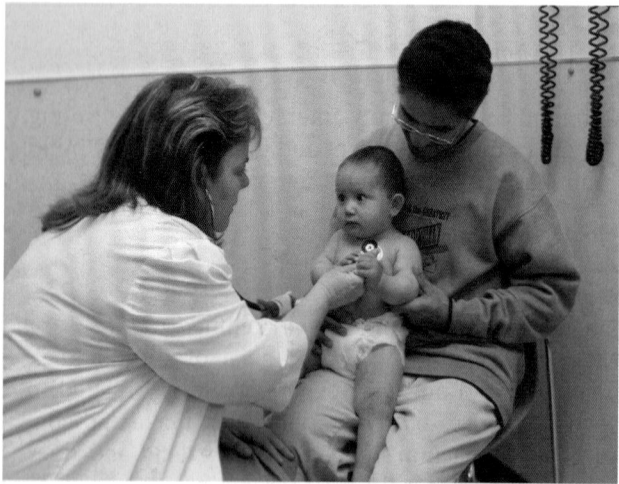

Figure 4-1 Routine visits to the health care provider ensure the infant is evaluated for achievement of age-appropriate physical and developmental milestones.

stabilize the infant as he or she plays in the bath. The older infant is likely to begin moving around quite a bit in the bathtub. The water level should remain low enough so that if the older infant were to lie on his or her abdomen in the tub, his or her face would not easily be immersed in the water. Injuries in the bath resulting from slips, trips, and falls are the most common type of childhood bathtub-related injuries, especially for children aged 4 years and younger (Mao et al., 2009.). Such injuries can be prevented by using a slip-resistant bathtub surface in all tubs and ensuring that young children are supervised at all times while they are in the bathtub.

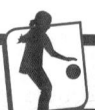

DEVELOPMENTAL CONSIDERATIONS 4-2

Normal Expected Increases in Weight, Height, and Head Circumference During Infancy

Weight Gain (Average Weekly Increase)

0–3 months	210 g (8 oz)
3–6 months	140 g (5 oz)
6–12 months	85–105 g (3–4 oz)

Height (Average Monthly Increase)

0–3 months	3.5 cm (1.4 in.)
3–6 months	2.0 cm (0.8 in.)
6–12 months	1.2–1.5 cm (0.5–0.6 in.)

Head Circumference (Average Monthly Increase)

0–3 months	2 cm (0.8 in.)
3–6 months	1 cm (0.4 in.)
6–12 months	0.5 cm (0.2 in.)

TRADITION OR SCIENCE 4-1

How should parents clean the umbilical cord stump and surrounding area?

Using alcohol to wipe the umbilical cord stump and surrounding area has been the most popular method for cleansing the site until the stump falls off. This method is no longer recommended for preterm or term infants because evidence has proved that using alcohol delays stump drying time and increases the opportunity for infection at the site. Shorter cord separation time has been noted when the cord is allowed to dry naturally. Alcohol may also destroy normal flora present around the umbilical cord, thus delaying separation time and increasing the risk of infection. Alcohol use is also more costly than natural drying (Dore et al., 1998; Evens et al., 2004; Medves & O'Brien, 1997; Zupan et al., 2004). Mullany et al. (2003) and El Arifeen et al. (2012) suggest that in developing countries, there are significant differences in resource availability, social customs, environmental cleanliness, and bacteriologic profiles that influence the increased number of umbilical cord infections seen in these countries. In developing countries, more research is needed to investigate the role of topical antimicrobials and/or other cord care regimens (e.g., use of alcohol, chlorhexidine) on infections during the neonatal period. For example, El Arifeen et al found that a single cleansing of the newborn's umbilical cord with 4% chlorhexidine reduced the infant's risk of infection and death in the first weeks of life by as much as 20%. A study by Liu et al. (2012) comparing use of alcohol, natural drying, and salicylic sugar powder on umbilical cord separation time showed the salicylic sugar powder group had the lowest rates of colonization and the shortest cord separation time of the three groups. This finding is consistent with the work by Pezzati et al. (2002) and Pezzati et al. (2003) who found that salicylic sugar powder was effective to reduce cord separation time and prevent umbilical cord infection in neonates in developing countries.

caREminder

Never leave an infant alone or just accompanied by a young child during a bath whether in a tub of water or on a counter. Instruct parents to decrease any interruptions by ensuring they are not inclined to answer their phone, text messages, or a doorbell. If a sibling screams and is demanding attention, the infant in the tub should be wrapped up and taken by the parent when responding to a situation.

SKIN CARE

Infants have relatively fragile and sensitive skin but do not generally need any lotions or talcum. Many parents like to use lotions because it gives them an opportunity to massage their infant, increasing the sense of bonding

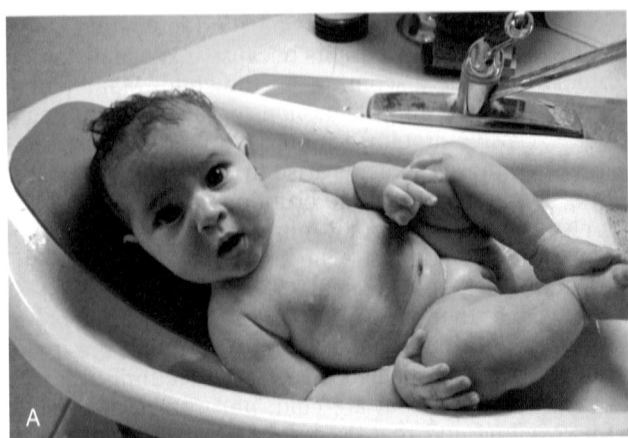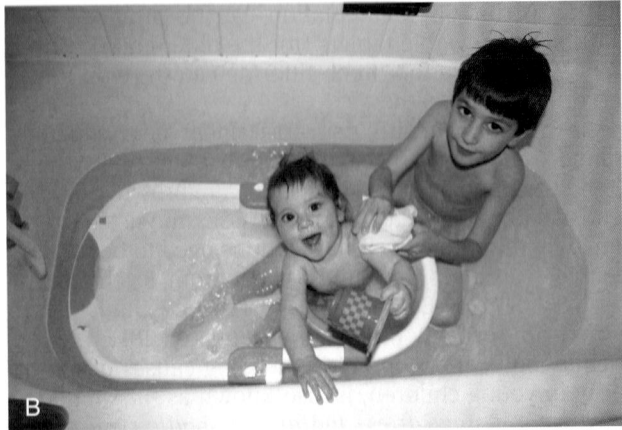

Figure 4-2 (A) Placing the younger infant in a small tub makes bath time fun and comforting. The tub should be filled with about 2 in. of warm water and placed securely. (B) Later, a baby tub can be used in the bathtub so the older infant can enjoy sitting up and splashing in the water. The bath ring holds the baby securely in place. Older siblings can join the fun and help wash the baby.

and togetherness. If lotions or powders are used, they should be hypoallergenic. Lotions should be put on the parent's hands first to warm the cream before applying it to the infant's skin. Powder should always be placed on the hand first to reduce the amount of powder in the air and to prevent the infant from inhaling it. In general, use of powder is not recommended (or needed) because of the risk that the infant will inspire it during application.

The skin acts as a tough barrier to chemicals and organisms. It is protected by the oily and minimally acidic secretions of the sebaceous glands called the **acid mantle**, which make the acid level of the skin pH 4.5 to 5. Too much bathing can disrupt the acid mantle. Several normal alterations in the infant's skin, which require no treatment, can be noted during the first few months. Erythema toxicum, a rash of red splotches with yellowish white bumps in their center, commonly appears only during the first few days after birth. Sucking blisters, which look like water blisters and are most commonly found on the hands, wrist, and forearm, are seen on newborns who have sucked a body part in utero. Milia are tiny white or yellow spots on the cheeks, nose, or chin caused by immature sweat and oil glands. These spots usually disappear within the first 2 to 3 weeks of life. Newborn acne, which is pimples on the cheeks, chin, and forehead, is caused by maternal hormones still circulating in the infant that stimulate the sebaceous glands. It usually disappears within the first few months of life. Parents should not treat the acne except by washing the infant's face two to three times per day with water. Chapter 25 presents a detailed description of both normal and abnormal skin lesions commonly seen in infants and children. Parents will often need reassurance that certain marks present at birth such as "stork bites"—flat, pink lesions located on the nape of the neck—are benign and will recede.

The infant should not be overexposed to the sun because infant's skin is quite sensitive and can be burned easily. The best sun protection for infants younger than 6 months of age is to dress them in lightweight long pants and long-sleeved shirts and keep them out of direct sunlight. To prevent eye damage, infants should also wear a hat with a brim and sunglasses designed to block at least 99% of the sun's rays.

A L E R T *Because the ingredients in sunscreen lotions may cause an allergic skin reaction, sunscreen should not be applied to infants younger than 6 months of age. If used for children 6 months to 1 year of age, sunscreen should be applied sparingly to small areas of skin, such as the face and the backs of the hands. After 1 year of age, sunscreen should always be applied before the child plays in the sun (see Chapter 25 for more information regarding application of sunscreen).*

ORAL CARE

Oral health depends on regular oral care. Performing good oral hygiene at least twice daily prevents oral infections, soothes the gums, and comforts the child while the teething process is occurring. From the time of infancy, the mouth should be cleaned at least twice a day. Gum care should be started soon after birth. The infant's erupting teeth can be brushed with a soft toothbrush or rubbed lightly with the corner of a soft washcloth. This practice accustoms the infant to the daily ritual of dental hygiene (American Academy of Pediatric Dentistry, 2011a).

Fluoride is important for tooth protection and growth. It is generally provided in sufficient amounts through the community water supply at an optimum level of 1 part per million (ppm). For children 6 months of age to 3 years, if community water is not fluoridated or is fluoride deficient (<0.6 ppm), the health care provider can prescribe fluoride supplementation after determining all other dietary sources of fluoride exposure (American Academy of Pediatric Dentistry, 2007a,

2007b, 2011b). Supplementation can be provided via solution or chewable tablets (for the older child). Children who receive too much fluoride can develop mottled or speckled teeth.

The first oral health risk assessment is conducted around 6 months of age—the approximate time when the first tooth comes in. The health care provider or the dentist will perform a caries risk assessment to determine whether proactive interventions need to be implemented to protect the child further from tooth decay (see thePoint for Evidence-Based Practice Guidelines) (American Academy of Pediatric Dentistry, 2011b). Early childhood caries, one of the leading causes of tooth decay in young children, is also known as *nursing bottle caries*, *nursing caries*, and *nursing bottle syndrome*. Early childhood caries occur when carbohydrates in formula, breast milk, and fruit juice are allowed to remain on the teeth for a prolonged period. Strongly encourage parents not to put the child to bed with a bottle at any time. The incidence of both dental caries and otitis media are elevated in children who are allowed to go to bed with a bottle of milk or juice and when frequent between-meal consumption of sugar-containing drinks and snacks occurs. Prevention is the key to good dental health.

The American Academy of Pediatric Dentistry recommends that a dental home for the infant be established by 12 months of age. The first visit to the dentist includes a thorough medical (infant) and dental (parent) histories and an oral examination of the child. The visit includes providing age-appropriate toothbrushing demonstration and counseling the parents about oral hygiene, nonnutritive habits, speech and language development, diet, oral injury prevention, and fluoride supplementation. All scheduled health care visits to primary health care providers (e.g., those at age 6 months, 9 months, and so on) should include oral assessment and health teaching to promote optimum oral health during infancy (American Academy of Pediatric Dentistry, 2011a).

Teething

QUESTION: At her 8-month visit, Lela does not have any teeth. Claudia asks the nurse whether this is normal because José got his first tooth at 6 months of age. What would you tell Claudia?

The first teeth, usually the lower central incisors, erupt between 6 and 10 months of age, although this event may not occur until the child is 1 year old. The next teeth to appear are the four upper incisors (central first, then lateral), which are evident at between 8 and 13 months of age, followed by the two lower lateral incisors, and then the first four molars (both upper and lower; see Fig. 3-14) (Hagan et al., 2008). By the time the child is 1 year old, approximately 10 teeth will have erupted. This is an average number; some children will have more and some children will be just starting to develop teeth.

Teething can be one of the most difficult and exasperating times for new parents because it is usually associated with some discomfort for the child. Many parents believe that teething elicits signs of illness, including fever, excessive drooling, and crankiness. In most cases, however, these problems arise from other sources. Rubbing the gums where the eruptions are occurring with a clean finger for about 2 minutes reduces the swelling and provides comfort. The use of topical anesthetics or analgesics is not usually very helpful because saliva washes them away quickly or the infant may touch the area with the tongue, thereby numbing the tongue rather than the affected area. Some teething rings can be chilled; rings that are cold, not frozen, also reduce the swelling and the discomfort of teething (Fig. 4-3). Alcohol spirits (such as whiskey) should never be used on the gums.

ALERT   *The use of over-the-counter topical anesthetics is discouraged because of the potential toxicity of the products to the infant (American Academy of Pediatric Dentistry, 2011a). Many of these products contain benzocaine and can lead to a condition called methemoglobinemia, in which the amount of oxygen carried through the bloodstream is reduced. Symptoms of this condition include pale gray- or blue-colored skin, lips, or nail beds; increased heart rate; shortness of breath; and confusion.*

Teething biscuits and small bagels are also good for teething infants, depending on the infant's age. The infant should not be given anything that cannot be chewed easily or that could break off into large pieces

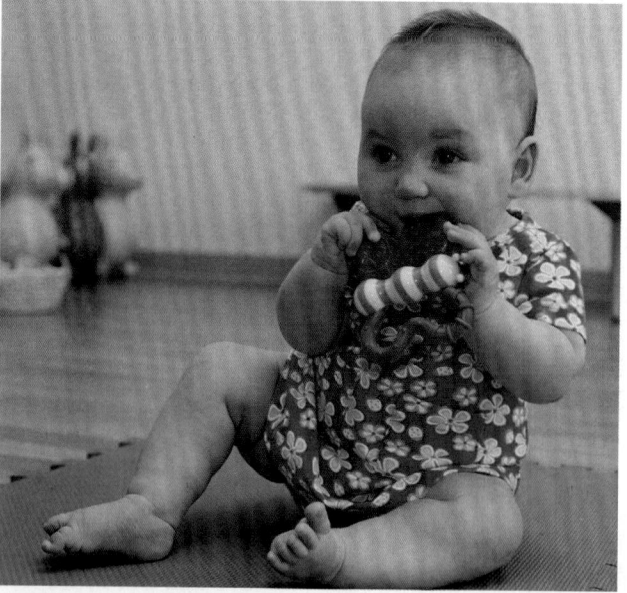

Figure 4-3 A cold teething ring can help soothe a baby's discomfort from swollen, inflamed gums during teething.

and cause choking. Many health care providers recommend a mild analgesic, such as acetaminophen, for discomfort from teething.

> *ANSWER:* The order in which teeth come in is much more predictable than the age at which a baby's teeth will arrive. A few infants are born with teeth and others don't have a tooth until after their first birthday.

Nonnutritive Sucking

Nonnutritive sucking refers to the repetitive actions of sucking and swallowing, followed by breathing, that is not used for oral ingestion of fluids (feeding) by an infant. Nonnutritive sucking may occur while the infant is at the mother's breast, when the infant sucks on a bottle nipple without ingesting fluid, or when the infant sucks parts of their hand or a pacifier. In utero, sucking and swallowing are present by 28 weeks, although not fully coordinated until about 32 to 34 weeks of gestation (Pinelli & Symington, 2005). Nonnutritive sucking supports important physiologic processes for the infant. Through sucking, vagal innervation of the oral mucosa stimulates secretion of enzymes and hormones (e.g., lingual lipase, gastrin, insulin, and motilin) that facilitate digestion (Pinelli & Symington, 2005). As a clinical intervention, nonnutritive sucking has been used to promote digestion when an infant is being fed using gastric feedings; as a means to promote gastrointestinal readiness to tolerate feedings in premature infants; and as a method to promote nipple feedings in children who have immature coordination of sucking and swallowing or who, because of prematurity, have not experienced nipple feedings. In addition, infants receive a great deal of comfort and gratification through nonnutritive sucking. For some infants, the urge to suck is very strong, particularly when they are hungry, tired, or stressed, and the child may soon learn that a hand or finger in the mouth provides a calming effect. Parents may satisfy the infant's need for oral stimulation during times of distress by offering a **pacifier** whenever the infant cries. The infant receives a great deal of comfort and gratification through nonnutritive sucking. Nonnutritive sucking reaches its height at 15 to 18 months of age. Nonnutritive sucking can result in long-term dental problems; thus, professional evaluation for children who continue to display persistent nonnutritive sucking beyond the age 3 years is recommended (American Academy of Pediatric Dentistry, 2006).

The infant is ultimately the one who selects the form of nonnutritive sucking he or she prefers. The thumb is readily available to the infant. To get a finger or hand to the mouth, the child does not have to have good hand–eye coordination or the use of palmar and pincer grasp, which would be needed to pick up a pacifier. The thumb tends to be dirty; wash the child's hands with water before nap time to ensure that the thumb is clean. When soap and water are not available, cleansing wipes can be used to clean the child's hands. Although cleansing wipes are alcohol based

and contain perfume, it is better for the thumb to be clean. Weaning the child from the thumb is generally more difficult than weaning the child from the pacifier because parents cannot regulate the presence of the thumb. If an older child is unable to break the habit of thumb-sucking, a dentist may suggest using an intraoral appliance that interferes with putting the finger or thumb in the mouth. Such devices have been successful in stopping thumb-sucking in preschool- and school-aged children.

Pacifiers, also known by the terms *dummy* (British), *soother* (Canadian), or *binky* (American), are rubber or plastic nipples given to the infant to suck on. Pacifiers come in a variety of shapes. If the infant is bottle-feeding, the shape of the pacifier should be similar to the shape of the nipple used during feedings.

caREminder

Nipples intended for use with baby feeding bottles should never be used as pacifiers because they can be aspirated when not attached to a bottle base.

Pacifier use has been associated with an overall decline in breastfeeding duration, although the specific cause of this decline is not known (Callaghan et al., 2005; Howard et al., 1999; Nelson et al., 2005). Some authors recommend restricting or avoiding pacifier use until breastfeeding is well established, usually between 4 and 6 weeks of age (Cornelius et al., 2008).

Pacifier use has also been associated with a reduced risk of SIDS, and the American Academy of Pediatrics (AAP, 2005b) recommends pacifier use after 4 weeks of age for the prevention of SIDS (Cornelius et al., 2008), although the mechanism by which pacifiers reduce the risk of SIDS is unknown (Callaghan et al., 2005; Li et al., 2005; Mitchell et al., 2006). Last, pacifier use has been associated with a higher risk of otitis media, thus pacifier use during the second 6 months of life should be reduced (AAP, 2004a; Marter & Agruss, 2007). In all of these issues, it is evident that the findings are inconclusive and conflicting with regard to when pacifiers should be introduced and discontinued.

During the early months, an adult must put the pacifier in the infant's mouth. As the infant matures, he or she will be able to find the pacifier in the crib and place it in his or her own mouth. Pacifiers can be just as dirty as thumbs. Pacifier clips can be used to attach the pacifier to the infant's shirt and to prevent the pacifier from constantly falling on the ground. Weaning from the pacifier, as with weaning from the bottle, can start with restricting pacifier use to sleep time.

SLEEP

> **QUESTION:** Claudia is concerned because Lela has a bald spot on the back of her head. What questions would you ask Claudia? What suggestions would you make about sleep positions?

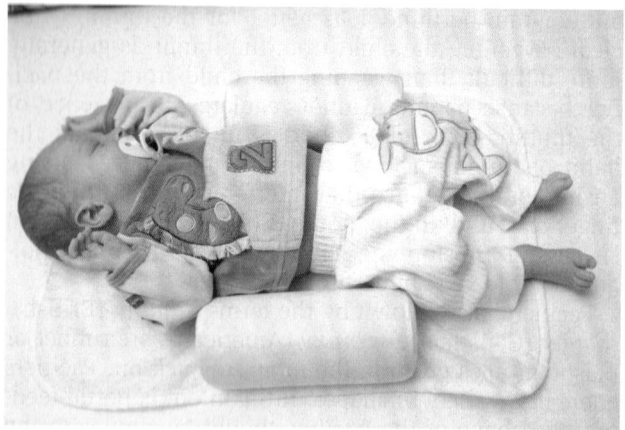

Figure 4-4 Infants should be placed on their back to sleep. A pillow or bedroll can be used to keep the baby in place.

The AAP (2005b) recommends that all infants should be placed to sleep on their backs (supine), on a firm sleep surface, without soft objects, a pillow, or other bedding materials, because sleeping in the prone position has been linked to SIDS (Fig. 4-4). There is no evidence that bumper pads or other devices that attach to the crib slats to protect against injury are beneficial and, in fact, have a potential for causing suffocation, entrapment, and strangulation. These products, along with loose bedding, heavy quilts, stuffed animals, and toys, should not be used in the infant's sleeping environment (AAP, 2011). Sitting devices such as car seats, strollers, swings, and infant carriers are not recommended for routine sleep. In particular, infants younger than 4 months of age are at risk because they may assume body positions that may lead to suffocation and airway obstruction (AAP, 2011). Infants should never be left alone on a bed.

The terms *cosleeping*, *cobedding*, and *bed-sharing* are often used to indicate an infant sharing a bed or sleeping environment. Cosleeping refers to the diverse ways in which infants may sleep in close social and/or physical contact with a caregiver (usually the mother). This definition includes an infant sleeping alongside a parent on a mattress, futon, or floor bedding as well as unsafe practices such as sharing a sofa or recliner (Academy of Breastfeeding Medicine, 2008). In some parts of the world, cosleeping may provide a means to protect the infant from environmental hazards. Cobedding refers to the placement of two or more multiple-birth infants in the same crib, bed, or incubator. An increasing number of multiple-birth infants are presenting in neonatal intensive care units. Cobedding multiple siblings is considered a way to replicate the intrauterine environment and ease extrauterine transition. There is insufficient evidence to either support or reject this practice by health care personnel in a supervised clinical setting (National Association of Neonatal Nurses, 2011). If instituted, the nursing unit should have clear protocols and ensure evaluation of the infants is completed to ensure the child's safety and physiologic stability.

Bed sharing, defined as sharing a bed with a parent or another child on a regular basis, is a form of cosleeping that is generally not recommended. This practice may increase the risk of infant suffocation. The infant may be brought into the bed for comforting or feeding; however, the child should be returned to his or her own bed before the adult goes back to sleep.

During the first month of life, the average sleeping time for an infant is 16 to 20 hours. Some infants sleep as little as 10 hours a day; others sleep as much as 23 hours a day. Not surprisingly, the infant who sleeps very little tends to grow into the child who sleeps very little and eventually into the adult who requires little sleep. As the child develops during the first year, hours spent sleeping decrease to an average of 14¼ per day at 6 months and 13¾ per day by 1 year of age (Davis et al., 2004; Moore, 2009).

For many parents, a primary goal within the first few months is to have the infant achieve a pattern of sleeping for a 7- to 8-hour period through the night. For the tired and bleary-eyed parent, this extended sleep pattern is a welcome developmental milestone. To achieve this goal, hunger metabolism and sleep–wake cycles must first be stabilized. From birth through the eighth week, the daily routine for most infants is a continual repeat of a 2¼- to 3-hour cycle that starts with the beginning of one feeding and ends with the beginning of the next feeding. Within this cycle, the parent should promote a daytime pattern of eating, followed by wake time, and followed by a nap time of approximately 1¼ hours. During the late evening and nighttime hours, the cycle should consist only of eating and sleeping activities. Between the third and fourth months, the infant will extend the nighttime sleep to 10 to 12 hours, continuing this pattern for the rest of the first year.

Concurrently, daytime naps increase in duration to approximately 2 hours; the infant subsequently drops the number of naps and feedings per day, thereby elongating the periods of wakefulness. The number of naps required decreases from six to eight naps a day for a newborn to three to four naps a day at age 3 months and to two naps at age 6 months. The need for both a morning and afternoon nap, lasting about 2 hours each, continues until the child is approximately 16 months of age.

Parents can follow several guidelines that help foster good sleep habits in children at an early age. The most important guideline is to adhere to the recommended cycle of eating, wake time, and nap time—in that order. Often, the first two activities are reversed, however, creating a situation in which the infant must have a bottle or be breastfed to go to sleep. It is important for an infant to learn how to self-soothe by thumb-sucking, rooting around in bed, head shaking, or listening to soft music or the sound of a parent's voice. Cuddling the infant and then placing the infant in the crib, continuing to talk or sing until the infant falls asleep, teaches the infant how to self-soothe and fall asleep without a bottle or breast (Mindell & Owens, 2009). Learning to identify "sleep signals" and responding to these signals will also ensure that the infant gets needed rests (Moore, 2009). Sleep signals include

- Crying, fussing, whining, whimpering without any obvious cause
- Loss of attention, loss of interest in previous activity
- Facial expression and eye contact aversion that indicates social disengagement
- Eye rubbing, yawning
- Loss of coordination or repeatedly dropping objects in a short interval of time

Two types of sleep occur: active and quiet (Developmental Considerations 4-3). Active sleep, also known as *rapid eye movement* (*REM*) *sleep*, is light sleep during which the infant may cry out or fuss. Waking the infant during this time is easy, but, if left alone, the infant can find that a blanket, pacifier, or thumb is quieting. Swaddling and nesting are also helpful; some infants like to sleep tightly swaddled, whereas others prefer to sleep

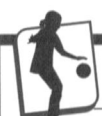

DEVELOPMENTAL CONSIDERATIONS 4-3

Infant States

The states of arousal that are not optimal times for interacting with infants are

1. **Quiet or active sleep**
2. **Drowsy**
   - Opens and closes eyes
   - Eyes glazed, with a heavy-lidded look
   - Delayed responsiveness
   - May occur when arousing from a sleep state
3. **Crying**
   - Irregular respirations
   - Facial grimaces
   - Cries
   - Color changes
   - Sensitive to stimuli and may respond with crying
   - Uses self-consoling behaviors

The states of arousal that are better times for interacting with infants are

1. **Quiet alert (this awake state is the best time for the family to interact with infants)**
   - Minimal body activity
   - Regular respirations
   - Face has a bright, shiny look
   - Eyes wide and bright
   - Most attentive to stimuli
2. **Active alert**
   - Much body activity
   - Irregular respirations
   - Facial movement
   - Eyes open, but not bright
   - Fussiness that may indicate need for a change in stimuli, feeding, or consoling

loosely swaddled. Some infants have difficulty settling back down if they awaken during the night. If the infant is older than 4 months of age, parents should not respond immediately to fussing but should wait about 10 minutes to allow the infant to settle down on his or her own. By 3 months of age, the amount of quiet sleep time nearly doubles. If the infant takes long naps during the day and wakes frequently at night, naps can be shortened to help the child be more tired at night. Deal with reasons for nighttime waking as quickly as possible, lovingly, but without sustained cuddling, which may encourage the infant to repeat the activity.

ANSWER: Ask what position Lela sleeps in and when or whether she spends time on her abdomen or on her side. Commend Claudia for using the back as the primary sleeping position and reinforce that this is the safest position. Lela is old enough now to spend more of her awake time on her abdomen. This will help her bald spot and will give her upper body a workout as she pushes up.

CLOTHING

QUESTION: Lela arrives on a lovely spring day for her 8-month visit at the health department in an outfit, a sweater, and wrapped in a blanket. What would you suggest to Claudia?

Clothing should be loose enough to prevent constricting the child's extremities. Clothing that is tight around the neck, arms, or legs, in addition to being uncomfortable, is a potential safety hazard. Garments with "feet" should be checked periodically for loose threads that could constrict the toes. Encourage parents and friends to buy big sizes and to limit the amount of clothes sized for infants 3 months and younger. Clothing should be durable, easily washable, and machine dryable. Washing instructions located on the clothing should be followed to maintain the safety and integrity of the garment (e.g., flame-retardant chemicals are removed if garments are washed with soap and not detergent). Items with snap openers down the legs make dressing and diaper changing much easier (Fig. 4-5). Oval (rather than round) necks are easier to fit over the large, round heads of infants. All sleepwear should be flame retardant.

A common misconception is that infants need to be kept warmer than adults. Parents often overdress infants, making them overheated, uncomfortable, and fussy. In the winter, several layers of clothing are warmer than a single, heavy layer; dress the infant in one more layer than the mother wears in the same environment. One exception is hats, which infants should wear regardless of the season. During the winter, hats minimize heat loss (90% of heat loss occurs through the uncovered head); during the summer, they prevent sunburn and overheating. Shoes are not necessary until the infant begins to walk outside and needs foot protection. Socks will keep the feet warm during the winter. When

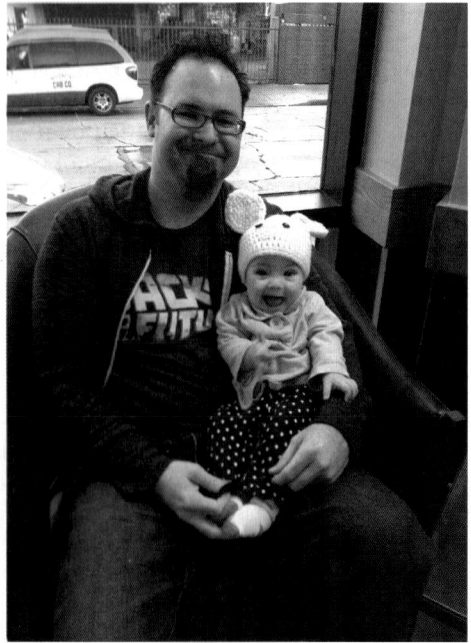

Figure 4-5 Disposable diapers make it easy to place the diaper on the infant. Specially made disposable diapers can be worn by the infant or young child in the water.

the infant begins to wear shoes, try them on with the infant bearing weight to ensure they are soft and flexible and fit the foot well. A good shoe fits the toe area well and allows at least half the width of the thumbnail between the longest toe and the end of the shoe.

> **ANSWER:** Reinforce that Lela is comfortable wearing the same number of layers that Claudia is wearing. Many parents worry that the infant needs additional protection from the elements when going out. Suggest that a hat would protect Lela from wind and sun but would not overheat her.

NUTRITION

The infant has unique dietary needs related to physiologic development and the nonnutritive benefits associated with sucking and eating. The energy content of food is called its **kilocalorie (kcal) value**. Estimated energy requirements are based on basic body metabolism, growth, and activity. The average kilocalorie requirements for children up to age 1 year are presented in Table 4-1 (Burns et al., 2013; Butte et al., 2004). Infant nutrition can be provided by breast milk or commercially produced infant formulas. Parents should not offer low-iron milks (e.g., cow, goat, soy) to their child until the child is at least 12 months old. Cow's or goat's milk can contribute to anemia because both are deficient in iron. Infants should also never receive low-fat or nonfat milk because these milks do not have the fat, calories, or iron needed to support the rapid growth and development that occurs at this age. By the time the infant is 1 year old, his or her body is physiologically ready to digest whole milk because the gastrointestinal tract is more mature and allergic reactions are less likely.

Bottle-fed infants, like breastfed infants, should not need supplemental water during the first 6 months, unless the child has a fever or diarrhea or the weather is very hot. Supplemental vitamins and minerals are generally not necessary for the first 6 months. After the sixth month, fluoride supplements are recommended if local water supplies are not fluoridated or if the infant is given cereals in which fluoridated water is not added.

Whether breastfed or bottle-fed, the infant will want to feed about every 2 hours for the first 2 to 3 weeks, taking about 2 to 3 oz each time. During the first month of life, infants should be awakened to eat if they sleep for more than 4 hours. During the second month, the infant usually develops a more sustained schedule, lasting 4 hours between feedings and taking 3 to 6 oz. This stage lasts until 3 to 4 months of age. At 4 to 5 months of age, the infant will take about 4 to 7 oz of formula or breast milk at each feeding. By 5 to 6 months of age, the infant is usually taking 6 to 8 oz per feeding. When the infant is able to go longer than 4 hours between feedings, one of the nighttime feedings should be eliminated. Some infants do so naturally as they increase the length of time they sleep at night. Other infants may get into a habit of waking frequently in the night to be fed. In this case, when the infant awakes and indicates he or she wants to be fed, the infant should be patted and calmed or should be offered a pacifier rather than feeding. After a few

TABLE 4-1	Nutritional Needs of Infants		
Age	**Breast Milk or Formula**	**Solid Foods**	**Total Caloric Needs**
Newborn to 3 months	1–6 oz every 2–4 hours (intake varies with age and weight)	No solid foods should be introduced.	(89 × weight [kg] −100) + 175
4–6 months	6–8 oz every 4½–6 hours	Introduce solid foods beginning with cereal products. Breastfed infants can be sustained on mother's milk alone.	(89 × weight [kg] −100) + 56
7–11 months	6–8 oz every 6–8 hours (with a maximum of 32 oz per day)	Introduce solid foods. Introduce the cup. Offer finger foods.	(89 × weight [kg] −100) + 22

nights of not receiving a midnight feeding, the infant may awaken but will learn not to expect food and thus will go back to sleep.

Prior to initiating feeding, the infant should be awake. Feeding should not be initiated every time the infant cries. Rather, hunger cues such as an infant that is awake and tossing about, sucking fists or fingers, and vigorous crying not soothed by a diaper change or comforting measures would indicate that the child should be fed. A sleepy child should not be fed. If the infant appears to be constantly drowsy or lethargic, not awakening every 3 to 4 hours to eat, infant alertness can be increased by loosening the infant's clothes, rubbing the infant's hands or feet, and talking to the infant. Persistent lethargy is of great concern and would warrant immediate medical attention.

CHALLENGES WITH PROVIDING NUTRITION TO THE INFANT

Some infants may be more challenging to feed as a result of poor suck, decreased motor postural control, GER, or the presence of cleft lip or palate. Nursing Interventions 4-1 presents strategies to deal with the challenging feeder (see thePoint Evidence-Based Practice Guidelines for more information on feeding children with cleft lip and/or palate).

Allergic proctocolitis (APC) is a condition in infants in the first year of life when they develop an allergy to breast milk, formula, cow's milk, or a specific food. Common gastrointestinal presentations of APC include vomiting, diarrhea, bloody stools, and anemia. Respiratory symptoms may also occur and include rhinitis, coughing, and wheezing. Other signs and symptoms include fussiness, eczema, and prolonged crying. In breastfed infants, APC is caused by food proteins derived from maternal diet and transferred through lactation. A maternal cow-free milk diet often leads to resolution of the infant's symptoms. The mother should continue taking her daily vitamins and a calcium supplementation during the maternal elimination diet. The elimination diet trial for any food or food group continues for a minimum of 2 weeks and up to 4 weeks, although in most cases, the breastfed infant will show resolution of symptoms within 72 to 96 hours of the diet change (Academy of Breastfeeding Medicine, 2011; Lucarelli et al., 2011). Treatment for formula or milk allergy is to switch the infant to a protein hydrolysate formula such as Nutramigen, Alimentum, or Pregestimil. The protein in these formulas has been broken down into amino acids. Health care providers may recommend a soy-based formula first, although 50% of infants with cow's milk sensitivity are also sensitive to soy (Sicherer, 2003). Food allergies are most often triggered by proteins introduced into the infant's diet (milk products, egg, fish, rice). Most symptoms will diminish when the causal proteins are removed from the child's diet (Boné et al., 2009). Most infant food allergies resolve by 3 years of age.

BREASTFEEDING

QUESTION: Lela is a sleepy newborn and is not showing much interest in establishing her nursing skills. This is a new problem for Claudia because her older son José was born ravenous. Review Teaching Intervention Plan 4-1. What are strategies to share with Claudia that will help wake up Lela and encourage her to breastfeed?

Human milk provides optimal nutritional support for a newborn and has recognized prebiotic and anti-inflammatory effects that enhance biological wellness for the child. Ingestion of human milk is known to aid the newborn's immature immune system to protect against gastrointestinal and nonenteric infections (Kim & Froh, 2012). Breastfeeding is the feeding method most encouraged by health care providers today, resulting from the nutritional composition of the milk, the additional immunity it provides the infant in the form of antibodies, and the fact that it has the most easily digestible form of protein. Human milk is readily available, inexpensive, and encourages bonding between the mother and infant. Ideally, the decision to breastfeed should be made before the child's birth. The AAP (2005a) recommends breastfeeding exclusively (no supplemental formulas or baby foods) for approximately the first 6 months and supports continuing breastfeeding after foods are introduced to serve as the child's milk source for the entire first year as long as it is mutually desired by the infant and the mother. Research indicates that breastfed children have a lower risk of being overweight or obese in adolescence and adult life than formula-fed children (Arenz et al., 2004; Owen et al., 2005; United States Breastfeeding Committee, 2010).

caREminder

If the infant is hospitalized, expressed human milk is the first choice for supplemental feeding. The feedings can be provided via a supplemental nursing device at the breast or a cup, spoon, dropper, syringe, or bottle (Academy of Breastfeeding Medicine, 2009).

Difficulties can arise when the mother does not have the support or instruction she needs when first attempting to breastfeed. She may not have adequate knowledge to prevent problems such as sore nipples and engorgement or know the correct interventions to implement when a problem does occur (see Teaching Intervention Plan 4-1). In her frustration, she may give up trying to breastfeed. The nurse plays an important role in providing the mother with the education she needs to breastfeed successfully (Fig. 4-6). Community resources such as the La Leche League are also available for mothers who experience difficulty with breastfeeding. Before the infant is discharged from the hospital or birthing center, provide the family with a list of resources that can be used if the need arises (see thePoint for Organizations and Evidence-Based Practice Guidelines).

NURSING INTERVENTIONS 4-1

Strategies for Dealing With the Challenging Feeder

Problem	Strategy	Rationale
Poor suck	1. Assess if nipple is correct if bottle-fed: too hard, too big, or flow too slow. 2. Assess infant state: • If infant is sleepy, talk with the baby, change diaper, gently massage infant awake. • If infant is highly irritable, move to a quiet, dimly lit room. 3. Assess parent's anxiety level. Reassure parent frequently. Provide information materials (booklets, videos). Provide counseling support as needed. 4. Assess infant's hunger level.	1. Infant may be working too hard to initiate flow or unable to handle amount of flow. 2. Infant may be too sleepy to suck well or may be overstimulated and cannot focus on eating. 3. Anxious parents may transfer anxiety to infant, and infant will not suck well. 4. An overly hungry or satiated infant will not suck well.
Decreased motor postural control (e.g., children with cerebral palsy and neurodisabilities)	1. Ensure child is in upright position with good head–trunk alignment. 2. Use chin–tuck head posture (head is upright and midline with neck flexion so that the chin is directed slightly downward and inward).	1. Alignment and stability of oral structures for feeding and swallowing may be compromised by abnormal or weak muscle tone.
Gastroesophageal reflux (GER)	1. Assess if and how much infant regurgitates after feedings. 2. Elevate infant's head after every feeding. 3. Monitor amount of formula or breast milk the infant is taking. 4. Ensure the head of the infant is elevated while feeding.	1. A wet burp occasionally after feeding is normal, but if amount of fluid is significant, projectile, or the occurrence is regular, the baby may have reflux. 2. GER is commonly seen in premature infants. Can be caused by positioning, formula intolerance, or medical conditions. Proper positioning may decrease incidence. 3. It may be necessary to limit amount taken at any one feeding. 4. Proper position can prevent reflux.
Cleft lip or palate	1. Assess extent of cleft lip or palate. If breastfeeding is not possible, modification of a nipple may be needed. 2. Monitor weight gain carefully in an infant with cleft lip or palate. 3. Feed slowly, evaluating child's ability to suck and swallow using modified nipple.	1. An infant with only a cleft lip may successfully breastfeed, if the mother prefers. If the child also has a cleft palate, breastfeeding may not be possible because of the inability to produce effective suction to extract the breast milk. 2. Ensures good nutrition and hydration. 3. Monitors for potential aspiration during feedings.

From Bowden, V., & Greenberg, C. (2012). *Pediatric nursing procedures* (3rd ed.). Philadelphia, PA: Lippincott Williams & Wilkins. Used with permission.

TIP 4-1: A TEACHING INTERVENTION PLAN to Prevent Breastfeeding Problems

Nursing Diagnosis and Family Outcomes

- Readiness for enhanced breastfeeding related to adequate knowledge and skills
  Outcomes: Mother expresses physical and psychological comfort with breastfeeding.
  Mother reports she is able to effectively initiate actions to relieve breastfeeding problems when they occur.
  Neonate feeds successfully on both breasts and appears to be satisfied after feeding.

Prevention and Intervention Measures

Painful Nipples

Prevention

- Avoid soaps, oils, lotions, or self-prescribed treatments.
- Position infant properly at breast, ensuring that entire areola is grasped.
- Hold the breast with the thumb above the areola and fingers and palm underneath it and gently compress the breast and direct it into the infant's mouth; a scissors grasp may also be used, compressing the areola between two fingers and supporting the breast to facilitate the infant's ability to grasp the areola properly.
- Apply small amount of breast milk to areola after a feeding and let it dry.
- Change nursing pads frequently; plastic-backed pads trap moisture and should be avoided.
- Expose nipples to air as much as possible; use of hair dryer on low setting may be helpful.

Interventions

- Nurse infant on less affected breast first and affected breast second
- Ensure proper positioning of infant at breast with entire areola grasped.
- Allow letdown reflex before putting infant to breast.
- Take aspirin or acetaminophen 30 minutes before a feeding to relieve excessive discomfort.
- Apply ice to nipples after feeding to decrease discomfort.

Engorgement or Mastitis

Prevention

- Frequent nursing (every 2–4 hours) on both breasts to promote complete emptying of ducts.
- Provide proper support of breasts with well-fitting nursing bra worn 24 hours a day.
- Divide feeding time relatively evenly between both breasts.
- Alternate from feeding to feeding the breast that infant nurses at first.

Interventions

- Manually express milk before putting infant to breast to nurse.
- Apply warm compresses or take a warm shower 10–15 minutes before feeding.
- If breasts are severely engorged, use cold compresses to decrease vascularity after a feeding.
- Massage breasts to promote emptying.
- If discomfort is excessive, consider taking aspirin or acetaminophen 30 minutes before feeding.
- Treat mastitis with antibiotics per health care provider presentation.

Letdown Reflex

Prevention

- Encourage infant to nurse at both breasts.
- Observe infant to see if he or she is swallowing every few sucks at the start of the feeding.
- Expose the opposite breast while nursing and see if milk flows from it as infant sucks.
- Slide a finger into the corner of the infant's mouth, breaking his or her suction to see if there is flow from that breast.

Interventions

- Relax. Sit in a comfortable chair with good support for your back and arms.
- Listen to soothing music.
- Minimize distractions by finding a quiet corner.
- Gently massage the breast.
- Apply warmth to breast. Take a warm shower.
- Avoid alcohol, illegal drugs, and smoking because all contain substances that can interfere with letdown and affect the contents of breast milk.

Latching-On

Prevention

- Verify if the infant is attaching to the nipple properly. Proper latching-on involves the infant taking the whole breast in his or her mouth, jaws closing around the areola, gums forming a circular seal, and creation of a vacuum effect; as the tongue strokes upward pressing the nipple against the palate, the milk ducts are emptied.
- Avoid bottles or pacifiers until breastfeeding is well established.

Interventions

- Ensure infant's tongue is down with the nipple directly on top of it during the feeding.
- Make sure infant is awake and alert when feeding; unwrap infant from blankets as needed.
- If nipples are partially inverted, use a nipple shield to draw out the nipple.
- Sprinkle glucose water on nipple before feeding. When the infant opens his or her mouth and tastes the glucose, the mouth can be directed and attached to the nipple in the correct fashion.

(Continued)

TIP 4-1: A TEACHING INTERVENTION PLAN to Prevent Breastfeeding Problems (Continued)

Inadequate Milk Supply

Interventions
- Encourage nursing at both breasts six to eight times daily.
- Encourage adequate rest, nutrition, and fluids.
- Avoid use of supplemental formula feedings until breastfeeding is well established (usually 3–4 weeks after delivery)

Fussy or Gassy Infant

Prevention
- Choose diet with care. What a mother eats and drinks may have some impact on breast milk volume and nutritional content.

- Drink caffeinated beverages only in moderation.
- Eliminate foods that appear to irritate the child's gastrointestinal system.

Contact Health Care Provider if
- Mother has a fever
- Infant refuses to eat
- Infant remains fussy and irritable during 2-hour time increments between feedings
- Infant is difficult to arouse or appears listless
- Infant has less than five to six wet diapers a day

The newborn's first feeding optimally occurs in the delivery room. The first "milk" that is let down is **colostrum**, a substance that is produced for several days until the mother starts producing milk. Colostrum contains more protein, salt, and antibodies than regular milk but less fat and calories. The newborn is fed when hungry, usually 10 to 12 times per 24 hours. Because of extracellular fluid, meconium loss, and limited initial food intake, infants can lose up to 10% of their birth weight but should start to regain weight by 2 weeks of age.

During the first few days of life, the infant will urinate about three to four times per day and produce stool one to two times per day. As the mother's milk supply increases, the infant will urinate and defecate more frequently. By the end of the first 2 weeks, the infant will create about six to eight wet cloth diapers or five to six wet disposable diapers and three to four stools per day (Holt et al., 2011).

ANSWER: The first important tactic to teach Claudia is to be watchful of Lela's sleep–wake cycles. Ideally, Lela will be with Claudia throughout the day so that Claudia can become attuned to the more subtle signs of wakefulness. Claudia will have to watch for Lela's wakefulness because she is not demanding to be fed. Ways to enhance her wakefulness include unwrapping her, gently washing her face with tepid water, and gentle stroking. It is important that nurses do not assume a mother who has successfully breastfed one child has all the information needed to succeed with a different child.

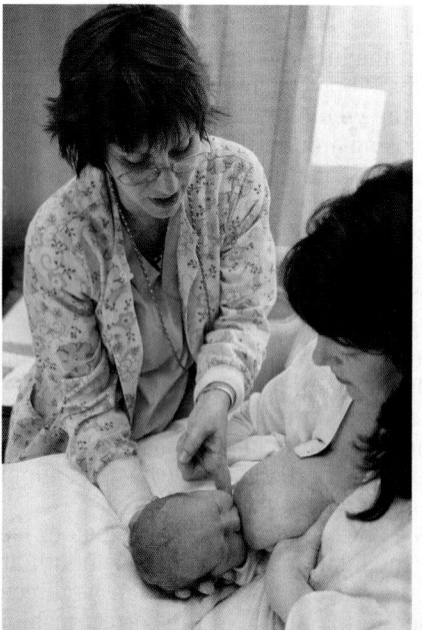

Figure 4-6 The nurse can promote a positive experience by demonstrating breastfeeding techniques and encouraging the mother.

Positioning

Proper positioning during breastfeeding enables the newborn to latch on properly and effectively and promotes the mother's comfort during feeding. Poor positioning can lead to sore nipples and a frustrated and hungry infant who is not able to suckle and get enough milk. The newborn should have the entire areola in his or her mouth, not just the nipple (Fig. 4-7).

Three comfortable positions can be used to achieve this goal: side lying, seated or cradle, and football. In the side-lying position, the mother lies on her side in the recumbent position. Pillows can be used to support the mother's back. The infant is placed in a side-lying position, cradled in the mother's arm, with the infant's mouth parallel to the mother's nipple and the feet toward the mother's waist.

In the seated or cradle position, which many mothers prefer, the mother sits upright with the infant cradled across her abdomen in a stomach-to-stomach alignment with the infant's mouth at nipple level. The mother's back and arms should be supported by a pillow under her knees (if she sits in bed) or a stool for her feet (if she sits in a chair).

The football hold is a variation on the seated position. While sitting, the mother cradles the infant's body

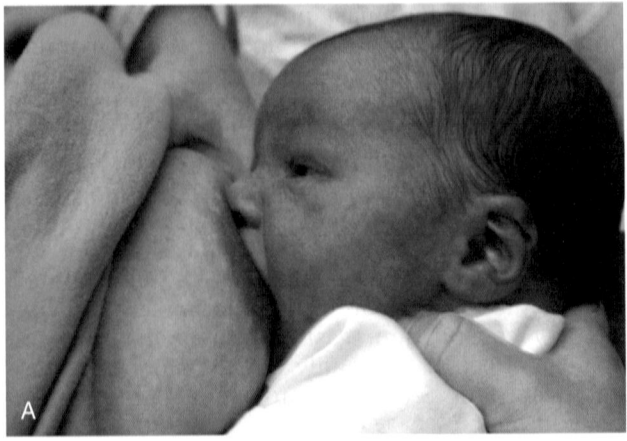

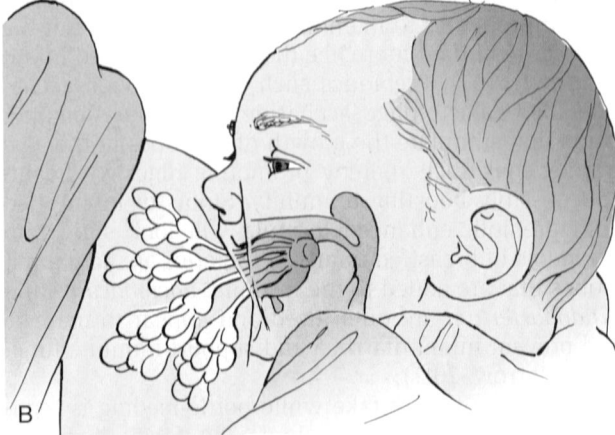

Figure 4-7 (A) A newborn with all of the nipple and areola in the mouth. (B) Diagram of newborn on breast correctly compressing milk ducts.

so that the infant is positioned at the mother's side with the feet extending toward her back. A pillow or blanket can be used to support the infant as the mother uses her arm and hand to support the baby's head and neck. This technique is often used when twins are nursed simultaneously.

Fathers may feel left out of the feeding process. One way to encourage the father's participation is to have him be the "helper." He can get the child and change the diaper if needed while the mother finds a comfortable position. He can burp the child at the end of the feeding and continue to snuggle the child. He can also participate when the infant is older by offering the infant water between feedings.

Breastfeeding Routine

The mother should nurse the infant for 20 to 30 minutes each feeding, starting with 10 minutes on the first breast, burping the infant well, and then alternating to the second breast. The infant will be much more energetic nursing from the first breast and will empty it faster than the second, so it is important with each feeding to alternate which breast the newborn nurses from first. If the infant becomes sleepy after nursing on the first breast, stimulation with a diaper change, burping, or talking may be necessary so the infant will be

alert enough to finish nursing on the second breast. To help a mother remember which breast should begin the next feeding, she can place a safety pin on the bra strap on that side. The mother can also wear a ring that she switches from hand to hand to remind her which side to start the next feeding.

Breastfed newborns do not routinely need water between feedings. Ingestion of water may unintentionally decrease milk production because the infant will not feel as hungry and will not nurse as vigorously. The well-nourished breastfed infant does not need supplemental vitamins or minerals. However, iron supplements should be started at 4 to 6 months of age for infants who are exclusively breastfed because during this period, fetal iron stores are depleted. If the infant is not regularly receiving any iron-fortified formula or iron-fortified cereal, then oral iron supplements such as ferrous sulfate may be needed. Vitamin D supplementation (400 International Units per day) is recommended for all breastfed infants to prevent vitamin D deficiency rickets (Wagner & Greer, 2008).

caREminder

Oral ferrous sulfate (an iron supplement) can stain the teeth and will cause the infant's stools to be dark green or black. Advise parents to rinse the infant's mouth with a small amount of water after administering the iron supplement and to be aware that the color of their child's stool will change as a result of the iron intake.

Pumping the Breast

If the mother must be away from the infant during feeding times because of work or other activities, she may elect to pump her breasts to provide milk for her child in her absence. Special bottle nipples are available to make the transition to bottlefeeding much smoother and to avoid nipple confusion. To prepare for returning to work, she should start pumping her breasts about 2 weeks beforehand. The ideal time to begin pumping is between the infant's first two feedings of the day. The volume of a mother's milk production diminishes during the day, so pumping early in the day will enable her to produce a good amount. Pumping can be completed at the workplace as long as the mother has time to pump (10 to 30 minutes, one to four times per day), privacy, and a place to refrigerate the milk. Many women find breast pumps easier to use than expressing breast milk by hand. Many different pumps are available, and a certified lactation consultant can assist the mother in making a choice. A mother who needs to use a breast pump should do so regularly to stimulate her milk supply.

Storing Breast Milk

Expressed breast milk can be stored safely at room temperature for 3 to 4 hours and up to 6 to 8 hours under clean conditions (60° to 85° F or 16° to 19° C); refrigerated for 72 hours, optimally, and up to 5 to 8 days under clean conditions (39° F or ≤4° C); and stored in the freezer for 6 months, optimally, and up to 12 months is acceptable (0° F or −17° C) (Academy of Breastfeeding Medicine, 2010; Bowden & Greenberg, 2012). Freezing the milk does not harm its nutritional content, but it does destroy some of the antibodies. To ensure clean conditions, breast milk should be stored in clean plastic or glass containers with tight or screw caps to prevent leakage of the milk. If disposable bags are used, the milk should be double-bagged to prevent punctures or splits and should be closed tightly with a twist tie or rubber band. In the freezer, breast milk in a plastic bag should be stored in a rigid, sealed container to reduce the possibility of freezer burn. Place the container in the back of the freezer to decrease temperature variations caused by frequent opening and closing of the freezer. When cooled, newly expressed breast milk can be added to an existing container of frozen breast milk and placed back in the freezer (see thePoint for Evidence-Based Practice Guidelines for additional information on storage and handling of human milk).

To thaw the milk, sit the container at room temperature, move the container to the refrigerator for several hours, or place the container under warm water until it has reached room temperature. Before use, shake the container of breast milk to mix the layers that have separated. The thawed milk should not be left out at room temperature for more than a few hours. By 24 hours after thawing, its ability to inhibit bacterial growth is diminished and thus the milk is not recommended for use.

> **ALERT**   *Never microwave human milk for defrosting or warming. Resultant "hot spots" from the microwave within the milk increases risk of burning the infant. Immunoglobulin A and other anti-infective properties are also reduced when microwaving.*

BOTTLEFEEDING

> **QUESTION:** Claudia is beginning to work at night. This is a time that Lela usually sleeps and only occasionally wakes to nurse a little bit. Claudia would like her to accept an occasional bottle just in case she wakes up. So far, when Claudia tries to give Lela a bottle, she grimaces, gags, and refuses to drink. What suggestions can you give Claudia?

The choice of expressing breast milk or using formula is up to the mother. She may not be able to pump at her place of work or, because of the environment, may not be able to relax enough to let her milk down. Using formula is a supplemental alternative that can be highly successful. As with breast milk, formula will meet the nutritional needs of the infant for the first 4 to 6 months of life (see Table 4-1).

Commercial formulas provide easily digestible protein; calories for energy; and fat, iron, vitamins, and minerals necessary for growth and development. Most formulas are cow's milk based. It is important to discuss with the parents the type of formula to use (see thePoint for Supplemental Information: Common Formulas for Infants and Young Children). Most infants are started on an iron-fortified formula that provides 20 kcal/oz. Low-iron formulas are not recommended for healthy infants because most infants tolerate the regular iron-fortified formulas well without any constipation, gastrointestinal disturbances, or toxic effect. If the family has a history of lactose intolerance, the health care provider may recommend a soy formula.

Infant formulas may include the addition of prebiotics and probiotics to maintain the intestinal flora of the formula-fed infant more like that of the breastfed infant (Morrow, 2011). Prebiotics such as fructo-oligosaccharide and galacto-oligosaccharide are dietary components that stimulate the growth of microbes in the gastrointestinal tract, thereby promoting digestive health and possibly boosting immunity. Stools of infants fed with prebiotic-enhanced formula will look similar to the stools of breastfed infants. Probiotics are actual microbes that are added to the formula. *Lactobacillus* and *Bifidobacterium* are often used and appear to manage and prevent infant diarrhea and support immune function (Morrow, 2011).

Controlling fluid intake while bottle-feeding is regulated by the softness of the nipple, the size of the nipple hole, and the size of the bottle. For the term newborn, three primary types of nipples are available commercially. The regular nipple is elongated and teat shaped. The NUK nipple has a wide, flat tip that fits below the hard palate. The Playtex nipple is short and has a square shape. For the premature newborn, premature or special care nipples are available, but these types are not recommended even if the infant has a weak suck. Use of these nipples does not develop the muscles needed to suck, and infants using these nipples have a greater risk for aspiration.

The breastfeeding mother may elect to introduce the bottle for supplemental feedings when she is at work or engaged in other activities that take her away from the infant during feedings. The best time to introduce the bottle for supplemental feedings to the breastfed child is at 3 to 4 weeks of age. The mother can begin offering the infant a bottle to replace one or more of the feedings from the breast. These bottles can contain breast milk, water, or formula (perhaps just 1 or 2 oz at first). Use a 4-oz bottle so as not to encourage overfeeding. As the child grows, if the child exhibits signs of hunger after consuming the 4-oz bottle, it may be time to move to a larger bottle (Institute of Medicine [IOM], 2011). It may take several tries for the infant to accept a rubber nipple, particularly if the infant has never been exposed to a pacifier. After the infant has accepted the bottle, a bottle should be offered at least once a week to maintain the infant's skill in using the nipple.

KidKare If the infant has been breastfed and balks at taking the bottle, have someone other than the mother offer the bottle (an ideal way for the father to become involved). Also, try bottle-feeding when the infant is sleepy, distracted, or very hungry. Use expressed breast milk at first because the infant is used to the taste, and spread a little on the rubber nipple. Experiment with different-shaped nipples, and warm the nipple to about body temperature. If the problem seems to be getting the infant to accept an alternate caregiver, have the alternate caregiver use the same perfume as the mother or use a receiving blanket the mother has used so the infant smells the same scents as when mother is feeding him or her.

ANSWER: The first step in helping Lela accept an occasional bottle is assessment. What type of bottle and nipple is Claudia trying? What type of liquid is in the bottle? Is it always Claudia offering the bottle? Many infants have an exaggerated gag reflex, and the elongated-type nipple may trigger her gag reflex. Suggest the Playtex nipple. If Lela does not like change, suggest using expressed breast milk warmed to body temperature. If Claudia does not have any expressed breast milk, the powdered formula mixed with warm, sterile water is a closer consistency to breast milk than the prepared formulas. Suggest that Selma or Ignacio offer the bottle and that Claudia be out of sight. Make "bottle time" a part of the daily routine so that it becomes more familiar to Lela, even if she does not really drink from it initially.

Preparing Formula

Many of the commercial formulas come premade and ready to feed and simply have to be poured into a sterilized bottle. To provide formula to the infant, select glass bottles or plastic bottles or sippy cups that do not contain bisphenol A in their composition.

ALERT *Bisphenol A has been commonly used to make clear polycarbonate plastic for products such as baby bottles, sippy cups, and baby food containers. When exposed to hot liquids, the bisphenol leaches out of the plastic into the formula in the bottle. Although not labeled as such, many plastic baby bottles are made from polycarbonate plastic containing bisphenol A (Environment California Research & Policy Center, 2012). Many countries have banned use of this substance to make baby bottles and sippy cups.*

Concentrated or powdered formulas should be prepared by carefully following the manufacturer's directions. Bottles and nipples should be cleaned after each feeding using a bottle sterilizer. Electric steam sterilizers are available, as are models that can be used in microwaves. Bottles and nipples can also be sterilized by boiling them in water for 10 minutes. Cold water sterilization is commercially available and consists of tablets dissolved in a prescribed amount of water to form a solution that is effective against bacteria.

ALERT *Instruct parents not to alter the composition of the formula by adding more or less water than directed in the instructions. Overdiluted formulas can cause water intoxication and lead to malnutrition. Feeding a too-concentrated formula can cause renal problems.*

Formula should not be prepared any more than 24 hours in advance and, after it is prepared, should be refrigerated. Discard any refrigerated formula left over after 24 hours because of the potential for bacterial growth. For feeding, the temperature of the formula should be room or body temperature, although some infants do not mind cold (from the refrigerator) formula, particularly in hot weather. Formula should not be heated in a microwave oven because doing so often heats formula unevenly and could make portions of the formula exceptionally hot and cause burns. To ensure that the formula is not too hot for the infant, shake the bottle to mix the formula and test the temperature by shaking a few drops onto the inside of the wrist. Formula should feel cool to warm.

Positioning

Positioning is as important in bottlefeeding as it is in breastfeeding. The infant's head should be elevated, and the infant should be held close to the mother in a semi-Fowler position. The bottle should be tilted so the formula fills the nipple. The nipple is placed on top of the tongue. The hole in the nipple should allow the milk to drop slowly from the bottle rather than streaming out or having to be squeezed out. Frequently during and after the feeding, the infant should be burped. The infant will burp up a little air and possibly a little formula, a very common event known as a *wet burp*. As long as the volume returned is small and the burp occurs only when air is passing the vocal cords, it is normal. Vomiting large amounts of formula immediately after feeding, or projectile vomiting, is not normal and requires referral to the health care provider. Table 18-1 describes abnormal emesis and stool associated with health concerns that must be addressed by the health care provider.

Bottles should never be "propped"—that is, the infant should not be laid down with a bottle positioned on a pillow or blanket to hold the bottle to the baby's mouth. When the infant is fed by propping the bottle, risk for aspiration of the formula is substantial and potential for developing otitis media is increased because milk pools in the eustachian tubes and contributes to bacterial growth. Furthermore, this method does not encourage maternal

> **CHART 4-2**   **Assessing Readiness to Begin Introduction of Solid Foods to the Infant**
>
> The tongue-thrust reflex is extinguished.
>
> Drooling is present.
>
> Infant is able to sit fairly upright.
>
> The suck–swallow reflex is present.
>
> Infant demonstrates sensory readiness cues (mouthing of toys and objects).
>
> Infant is easily distracted from the bottle or breastfeeding.
>
> Infant birth weight is doubled and infant weighs about 13 lb.
>
> Infant demonstrates an interest in table food (e.g., reaching for food or eating utensils, protesting when he or she sees others eat food).

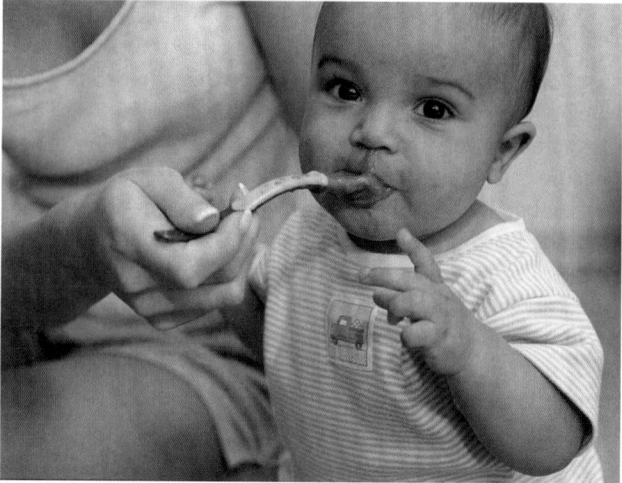

Figure 4-8 At about 4 to 6 months of age, solid foods are often introduced. The infant soon learns to manipulate the tongue and comes to enjoy this new way of eating.

bonding with the infant and may cause the child to become uninterested in feeding (Holt et al., 2011).

STARTING SOLID FOODS

By 4 to 6 months of age, the infant should be developmentally ready for the introduction of solid foods (Holt et al., 2011). The infant's chronologic age is not as meaningful as whether the infant has developed the skills necessary to handle spoon-feeding (Chart 4-2).

Introducing the Spoon

During the first attempts to feed with a spoon, food with a semiliquid consistency allows the infant to use the suck and swallow reflexes while adjusting to this new food delivery method. Introducing the spoon may cause the infant to turn away, spit out food, or bat it away with the hands; but, given patience and perseverance, the infant will eventually accept the spoon. Do not introduce the spoon when the infant is extremely hungry, tired, or ill. The best time to start solids is at the noon or early-evening feeding when the infant is not sleepy and may be more interested in a new activity. An infant spoon, coated with a pliable plastic and properly sized for the infant's mouth, is used because it feels softer than metal. If a coated spoon is not available, any spoon smaller than a teaspoon will work (Fig. 4-8).

Progression of Food Introduction

> **QUESTION:** At 8 months, Lela can sit well and has sufficient fine motors skills to pick up small objects. Lela does not like to be fed. She turns her head, makes a face, and then spits out the baby food. José, her older brother, would open his mouth like a baby bird and let Claudia spoon the food in. Claudia does not know what to do. She is tired from working three nightshifts a week in addition to caring for the children and their home and has just let Lela continue breastfeeding. What can you suggest to Claudia?

The first solid food should be rice cereal mixed with a little breast milk or formula. Rice cereal is very bland, easily digestible, and rarely causes allergic reactions. Do not mix cereals in the bottle with the formula or breast milk for the infant to drink. These approaches merely increase the calories ingested without enabling the infant to learn the process of meal taking or experience the various consistencies of solid foods, thus placing the infant at risk for obesity. When introducing rice cereal, give a small amount of breast milk or formula to drink before offering the cereal mixed with formula or breast milk. Place a small amount of cereal toward the middle or back of the tongue. The infant most likely will not know what to do with the cereal and may spit it out or make a face. Most of the first feedings will not be swallowed; rather, the food usually ends up all over the child. After the infant grows accustomed to the cereal and has no difficulty swallowing, the amount offered can be increased. After about a week, if feeding is going well, another type of cereal can be introduced. After a careful assessment of family allergies has been done, introduce rice, oats, barley, and wheat—in that order. Before adding another type of solid food, wait 7 days to rule out allergies. Wheat cereals cause the highest rate of allergic reactions in infants.

Cereal products can sustain the child's need for solid food up until age 6 months. After cereals, other solid foods are introduced as the child's nutritional needs increase. These foods are introduced very slowly, no more than one per week, again to watch for allergic reactions. The order of introduction should be vegetables, then fruits, and then meats, each pureed and of a very thin consistency. As teeth erupt and the child gains skills in swallowing and chewing, the texture of the food can be varied and can become thicker and chunkier. Avoid foods that are easily aspirated or choked on. To reduce the risk of choking or other accident, the infant should always be supervised by an adult while eating. At 6 months of age, solid foods are served two to three times per day at family mealtimes. By 9 months of age, the infant is offered solid foods three to four times a day. It may take 15 to 20 attempts before an infant accepts a particular kind of food (Holt et al., 2011).

caREminder

> *When an infant is hospitalized, it is important to assess which foods the child already eats and to avoid introducing new foods during the illness. Every effort must be made to ensure that an allergic reaction to a food is not triggered during an illness, because then ascertaining the true cause of symptoms, such as a rash, vomiting, or diarrhea, is difficult.*

Certain foods are avoided until late in the first year because they are considered major allergens or because the infant's gastrointestinal system is not adequately mature. These foods include eggs, corn syrup solids, citrus fruits and juices, tomatoes, strawberries, seafood, spices, and chocolate. When introducing vegetables such as peas, beans, or beets, finding some green or red particles in the stool is common for the first day or so after the food is first given. Because the intestinal tract has not totally matured, it must adapt to a new food, and some of it may be passed undigested.

ALERT   *To prevent botulism, do not give the infant honey or foods with a low acid content, such as home-canned fruits and vegetables, until after the child's first birthday.*

ANSWER: One suggestion when introducing solids is to encourage Claudia to allow Lela to feed herself. It is very messy at first, but some children have a very strong independent streak and will not be passively fed. Encourage her to put food directly on the tray or find a bowl that will stay on the high chair tray and have a large bib and a spoon that Lela can hold herself. She should start with iron-fortified rice cereal and then progress to vegetables.

Introducing the Cup

At 6 months of age, use of the cup to drink fluids can be started. Instead of giving a bottle, place a small amount of formula or breast milk in a cup (about one-quarter full at first) to help the child become accustomed to and proficient at using a cup. Cups with specialized covers can be used to prevent spills and to regulate the amount of fluid that flows. Handles on the cups enable the infant to grasp the cup easily and stably bring it to the mouth.

With the introduction of the cup comes the introduction of fruit juices (Tradition or Science 4-2). The amount of juice is limited to 4 to 6 oz per day so as not

---

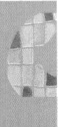

Evidence-Based Practice   **TRADITION OR SCIENCE 4-2**

Fruit juice often is recommended as a source of vitamin C and an extra source of water for healthy infants and children, but does this recommendation hold water?

Fruit juices taste good and children enjoy the flavor. Fruit juice is a natural source of vitamins; contains no fat or cholesterol; and, unless pulp is included, contains no fiber (Baker, 2007). One hundred percent fruit juices are the second largest source of energy in the diet of 2–3-year-old children (Reedy & Krebs-Smith, 2010). The AAP, Committee on Nutrition (2001) and the IOM (2011) have concluded that fruit juice offers no nutritional value for children younger than 6 months of age nor any nutritional benefits over those of whole fruit for infants older than 6 months of age and children. Excessive juice consumption may be associated with malnutrition, diarrhea, flatulence, abdominal distention, and tooth decay (AAP, Committee on Nutrition, 2001). In children aged 2–5 years, excessive fruit juice consumption has been associated with obesity and short stature (Dennison et al., 1997; Faith et al., 2006). Therefore, infants younger than 6 months of age should only be provided breast milk or infant formula. Juice should not be put in baby bottles or easily transportable covered cups that enable the child to consume these fluids easily throughout the day. Infants should not be given juice at bedtime. Children aged 1–6 years should limit daily juice consumption to 4–6 oz (120–180 mL), and children 7–18 years of age should consume no more than 8–12 oz (240–360 mL) daily (IOM, 2011).

---

to suppress the child's desire to have breast milk or formula. The first fruit juice is usually low in acidity and may be diluted to half strength with water. Low-acidity juices include apple and white grape juices. Orange, grapefruit, and pineapple juices should be avoided until the infant's bowel is more mature (Hagan et al., 2008).

When the infant is able to drink a sufficient amount of fluids from a cup, it is an opportune time for weaning from the bottle or breast. The breastfed infant who is comfortable using the cup can be weaned directly from breast to cup. Although the infant may tolerate weaning from the breast well, the mother may become depressed as she stops producing milk and feel that she is no longer "needed" for her nutritional support. Supporting the mother through this time is essential because these feelings may severely affect her relationship with the infant.

A bottle-feeding infant can be weaned by changing the fluid put in the bottle. Formula should be offered only in the cup, and only water should be offered in the bottle. The infant will be attracted to the cup because it contains the more palatable liquid. Weaning can also be completed gradually by eliminating all except the nighttime bottle. If the bottle is not in sight and not accessible during the day, the infant quickly learns that the bottle will be offered only at bedtime.

Preventing Obesity

Overfeeding or offering the wrong type of foods, especially high-calorie foods, may cause excessive weight gain, leading to obesity-associated medical problems. Research studies report a significant association between infant size and childhood and adult obesity (Eriksson et al., 2003). Infants and children younger than 2 years of age are at risk for overweight if their growth measurements are between the 84.1st and 97.7th percentiles on the World Health Organization (WHO) growth charts and as overweight if their measurements exceed the 97.7th percentile on the Centers for Disease Control and Prevention (CDC) charts (IOM, 2011). Measurements for length and weight are taken at every well-child visit (see Chapter 8). Although historically, much attention has been placed on assessment of malnutrition or failure to thrive, in developed countries, a greater risk has emerged for excess weight for length. The well-child visit includes observations about the parent's weight and weight of other children in the family. The obesity status of parents of young children is a predictor of whether a child will be obese (Hoppin & Taveras, 2004; Polhamus et al., 2005). The well-child visit also includes discussion of family dietary and exercise habits, the infant's activity state and exposure to daily physical activity, and age-appropriate caloric intake and healthy food choices. The child's length and weight measurement should be shared with the parents to help them better understand their child's growth patterns and when risk of overweight is of concern (National Association of Pediatric Nurse Practitioners, 2006). Evidence-Based Clinical Practice Guidelines 4-1 provides several national recommendations and actions for health care providers to help prevent childhood obesity.

ELIMINATION

QUESTION: Lela did not have a diaper rash until meat was introduced into her diet. Her stools immediately changed color and odor. If the stool is in contact with her skin for only a few minutes, it turns pink. Fortunately, the strong odor alerts the parents that Lela needs a diaper change. What can you recommend to the family in response to this change in Lela's stools?

If the infant was delivered without complications and did not pass meconium while still in utero (see Chapter 14), the first bowel movement after birth is to pass the meconium. **Meconium** is a sticky, thick, greenish black, tarry stool made up of epithelial cells, salts, bile, and mucus and usually is without a strong odor. This stool appears within the first 24 hours and may persist for up to 3 days.

The stools of the breastfed infant are usually yellow and very soft to thick liquid in consistency with little or no unpleasant smell. Breastfed infants pass less stool than bottle-fed infants do. The bottle-fed infant produces stools that can vary from pale yellow-brown and almost liquid to greenish brown and pasty. When the infant starts eating solid foods, the stools take on a consistency determined by the food ingested. The newborn generally has a bowel movement every time he or she is fed, but if the infant does not have a bowel movement for several days, this pattern, too, is normal. As the infant develops, normal elimination patterns become more rhythmic and individualized; some infants have two or three bowel movements a day, some have only one. Infants usually bear down, grunt, and appear to strain when having a bowel movement. This behavior is not necessarily a sign of difficulty.

The infant's first urination occurs within the first 24 hours of life. Production of urine is 200 to 300 mL/day, increasing as the infant matures, which can translate into six to eight diapers per day. Healthy urine is clear, colorless to very pale yellow, and does not have a strong odor. If an infant is dehydrated, there will be no wet diaper for several hours; the urine may appear darker in color and smell stronger than normal, indicating that it is concentrated. Although concentration of the urine is not the only indication of dehydration, be alert to the possibility and check other potential signs.

ANSWER: Changes in diet will result in changes in an infant's stool. Infants may initially lack the ability to digest new foods completely. The Diaz family is on the right track in that they change Lela immediately. A barrier cream on her buttocks could also help protect her skin.

Constipation

Constipation is when an infant produces very hard stools or no stool within the normal schedule. Hard stools are more common with formula feeding, with initiation of solid foods, and during illness. Constipation is usually caused by a change in the amount of water or fluids the infant receives while eating solids or by a lack of water ingested when ill. Also, if the weather is very hot, the child may need extra water to supply enough water in the stool.

When constipation occurs, offering low-acid fruit juices (such as apple or white grape juice) to infants younger than 4 months of age up to twice a day can be very effective. Continuing fruit juices beyond this treatment period is not recommended. Enemas and suppositories are not recommended for small infants. If the child is taking solids, increasing the amount of high-fiber baby foods such as cereals, prunes, and peaches may assist in elimination; bananas and carrots should be avoided because they may increase constipation (see Chapter 18 for more information on constipation and diarrhea).

Diarrhea

Although infants normally have very soft to liquid stools, they should not have frequent and extremely watery stools. Diarrhea is usually a sign of illness or intolerance to a specific food or type of formula. Monitoring the infant closely during diarrhea is important because frequent, watery stools can lead to dehydration (see Chapter 17). The infant must continue to ingest formula or human milk to correct the fluid loss. Breastfed and bottle-fed infants may need extra water (or electrolyte solutions) between

EVIDENCE-BASED CLINICAL PRACTICE GUIDELINES 4-1
Preventing and Managing Childhood Obesity

Daníelsdóttir, S., Burgard, D., & Oliver-Pyatt, W. (2009). *AED guidelines for childhood obesity prevention programs.* Retrieved from

http://www.aedweb.org/AM/Template.cfm?Section = Advocacy&Template = /CM/ContentDisplay.cfm&ContentID = 1659

Guidelines for school- and community-based interventions addressing rising weights in youth.

Association of State and Territorial Health Officials & National Institute for Health Care Management Foundation. (2007). *Childhood obesity: Harnessing the power of public and private partnerships.* Arlington, VA: Association of State and Territorial Health Officials. Retrieved from

http://www.nihcm.org/pdf/FINAL_report_CDC_CO.pdf

Report describing collaborations between state health agencies and private health plans to address childhood obesity.

Holt, K., Wooldridge, N., Story, M. et al. (Eds.). (2011). *Bright futures in practice: Nutrition* (3rd ed.). Elk Grove, IL: American Academy of Pediatrics. Retrieved from

http://www.brightfutures.org/nutrition/

A nutrition guide emphasizing prevention and early recognition of nutrition concerns and provides developmentally appropriate nutrition supervision guidelines for infancy through adolescence.

Centers for Disease Control and Prevention. (2011). *Nutrition, physical activity, & obesity: School health guidelines to promote healthy eating and physical activity.* Retrieved from

http://www.cdc.gov/healthyyouth/npao/strategies.htm

Nine guidelines for developing, implementing, and evaluating school-based healthy eating and physical activity policies and practices for students.

American Academy of Pediatrics. *(2012). Obesity guidelines, policy statements, and reports.* Retrieved from

http://www2.aap.org/obesity/policystatements.html

Website that shares AAP's policies on obesity assessment, prevention, and treatment.

Institute of Medicine. (2011). *Early childhood obesity prevention: Recommendations and potential actions.* Retrieved from

http://www.iom.edu/ ~ /media/Files/Report%20Files/2011/Early-Childhood-Obesity-Prevention
-Policies/Young%20Child%20Obesity%202011%20Recommendations.pdf

Policy recommendations and potential actions for implementations designed to prevent obesity in infancy and early childhood by promoting healthy environments for young children.

National Association of Pediatric Nurse Practitioners. (2006). Healthy eating and activity together (HEAT) clinical practice guideline. *Journal of Pediatric Health Care, 20*(6 Suppl.), 1–64. Retrieved from

http://www.napnap.org/Docs/HEAT%20One%20Pager%20%20%202-20-06.pdf

Guidelines for nurse practitioners designed to develop the family's ability to achieve the ideal balance between nutrition and physical activity, address the issue of childhood overweight, and ensure that children acquire healthy lifestyle habits that will keep them fit.

National Institute for Health and Clinical Excellence. (2006). *Obesity: Guidance on the prevention, identification, assessment and management of overweight and obesity in adults and children.* Retrieved from

http://www.nice.org.uk/nicemedia/pdf/CG43NICEGuideline.pdf

National guidance on the prevention, identification, assessment and management of overweight and obesity in adults and children in England and Wales.

United States Breastfeeding Committee. (2010). *Statement on breastfeeding as a critical strategy of obesity prevention.* Retrieved from

http://www.usbreastfeeding.org/Portals/0/Position-Statements/Obesity-Statement-Rev-2010-USBC.pdf

Recommendation for breastfeeding as a primary prevention strategy to reduce overweight and obesity.

feedings. When a formula intolerance is suspected, the infant should be given clear liquids for 4 to 6 hours and then be offered a soy-based or a protein hydrolysate formula (AAP, 2004b). Parents should contact the health care provider immediately if the infant refuses to accept the bottle or the breast, cries without tears, does not have a wet diaper for more than 8 hours, has a dry mouth, or if any blood is seen in the stools. The infant with diarrhea also is at risk for diaper rash. Meticulous perineal care, frequent diaper changes, and a barrier agent should be used to prevent skin breakdown (see Chapter 25 for a detailed description of diaper dermatitis).

PERSONAL AND SOCIAL DEVELOPMENT

The maturing infant is not capable of seeking activities that will provide optimal sensory and developmental stimulation; he or she depends on adults to provide meaningful activities that will stimulate development while promoting trust and security. Parents do not automatically understand all of the infant's needs nor do they necessarily have the tools to readily meet those needs. The health care provider's responsibility is to provide parents education to augment their knowledge base and to ensure an optimal environment in which the infant can learn and grow.

TEMPERAMENT

Temperament is defined as the combination of intellectual, emotional, ethical, and physical characteristics of an individual. It is the natural inborn style of behavior of each individual. Every infant has his or her own set of temperament traits or characteristics (Turecki, 2003). The nine categories or descriptors of temperament traits include activity level, distractibility, intensity, regularity, persistence, sensory threshold, approach/ withdrawal, adaptability, and mood (see Chapter 3). All children display some range or degree of each of the temperament traits; by assessing these traits, the clinician and parent can better understand how to establish an environment that is comforting to the child.

Brazelton (1992) identified three types of infant temperaments: the average child, the quiet child, and the active child. Each temperamental category represents a totally normal developmental type with specific characteristics. These characteristics often are strictly parents' perceptions of what the child is like, and many parents link the personality type to use of drugs during delivery or to parenting skills.

The average child is usually easygoing and is predictable in responses to environmental stimulations. The quiet child is unusually quiet and does not cry as much as the average child yet does not appear developmentally delayed in any way. The active child can often be referred to as a "difficult" child (Fig. 4-9). These are the children that even as infants are restless, are irritable, cry inconsolably, and often have unpredictable schedules for feeding and sleeping (Turecki, 2003).

COLIC

Crying is a normal part of the infant's development, with increased periods of crying starting about 2 weeks of age and continuing until about 3 to 4 months of age. This period has been labeled "The Period of Purple Crying" and is considered developmentally appropriate. Infants commonly have a regular "fussy" period during the day (usually around 6 pm to midnight), but if the crying does not stop and continues for more than 3 hours or the infant appears inconsolable, often pulling

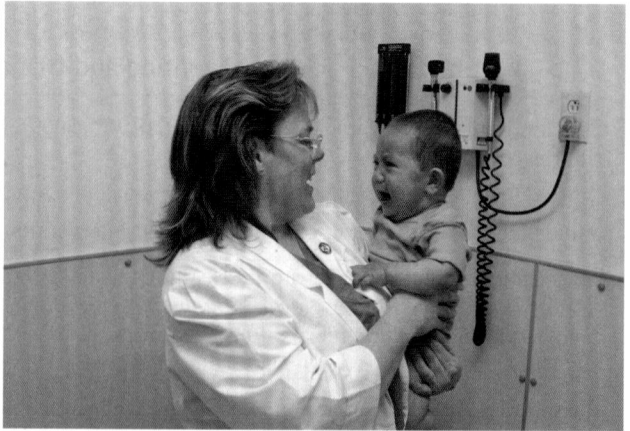

Figure 4-9 The infant with an "active" temperament may be irritable and cry inconsolably.

up the legs and passing gas, this "fussiness" may reflect **colic** (gastrointestinal pain). In breastfed infants, colic sometimes is a reaction to something the mother has eaten. In other infants, colic may result from sensitivity to milk or milk products. Breastfed infants are just as likely to have colic as those who are bottle-fed (Clifford et al., 2002). Colic may indicate a medical problem, but this circumstance is very rare. Episodes generally peak at about 6 weeks of age and stop at about 3 months of age (Neu & Robinson, 2003; Nield & Kamat, 2003).

Several interventions can reduce this problem. These interventions are directed toward creating a soothing and restful environment for the infant (Developmental Considerations 4-4) (Neu & Robinson, 2003; Nield & Kamat, 2003). Colic can also be caused by food intolerance, in which case changes in maternal and infant diet can be effective in reducing symptoms.

Behavioral interventions, reduction of stimuli, and the use of sucrose pacifiers have also demonstrated effectiveness in reducing colic symptoms (The Joanna Briggs

---

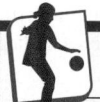

DEVELOPMENTAL CONSIDERATIONS 4-4

The REST Regimen for Managing the Child With Colic

- **R**egulating the infant's state by preventing over-arousal calms the infant. Infant states should be learned by parents and modulated (see Developmental Considerations 4-3).
- **E**nvironmental cues such as light and dark, noise and quiet, help to synchronize the infant's behavior.
- **S**tructure and repetition make events reassuringly predictable for the infant.
- **T**ouch (chest to chest or skin to skin) soothes the child and diminishes stimulation.

Institute, 2008). Behavioral strategies include using a baby carrier to keep the infant close to the body and in motion, placing the infant near a steady rhythmic sound such as a vacuum cleaner or clothes dryer, or taking the infant for a car ride in their car seat. Laying the infant on his or her stomach across the parent's knees, with a pacifier, while rocking often helps relieve any discomfort. Cuddling and rocking the infant is often helpful. Rocking with a motorized swing or cradle often enables the infant to relax and go to sleep. Vibrating chair seats are also helpful. Warm baths may also relax and soothe, creating a more comfortable state and helping to induce sleep. Decreasing stimulation, both tactile and auditory, has demonstrated effectiveness in some children, as has the use of sucrose solution (usually placed on a pacifier) (The Joanna Briggs Institute, 2008). The sucrose solution has been shown to only be effective for a short duration of time (less than 30 minutes).

Dietary modifications for the treatment of infant colic have been proposed and should be employed if a possible allergic origin is believed to be the cause of the colic. If the mother is breastfeeding, a low-allergen maternal diet is suggested and should include elimination from her diet of any foods that produce gas (e.g., cabbage, onions, broccoli) and a reduction of caffeine intake. She should also complete a 2-week trial to eliminate milk products from her diet, particularly if there is a family history of milk intolerance or other allergies (The Joanna Briggs Institute, 2008). If the infant is bottle-feeding, a low-allergen formula can be tried for a recommended period of at least 2 weeks. The use of partially hydrolysated whey protein formulas with prebiotic oligosaccharides and probiotics has been associated with a significant decrease in infant crying and may be considered on a trial (2 week) basis to determine if the formula change reduces the child's colic (Critch, 2011; Jakobsson et al., 2000; Lucassen et al., 2000; Savino & Tarasco, 2010). Use of extensively hydrolyzed whey or casein formulas is costly and not very palatable for most children. These formulas should be reserved for children with severe infantile colic or those who have atopic symptoms such as wheezing, eczema, allergic rhinitis, and GER (Savino & Tarasco, 2010). Soy protein formulas have not been shown to be effective and should not be provided to any child during the first 6 months of life (Agostoni et al., 2006). Usually, colic caused by food intolerance will improve within the 2-week period, indicating that the maternal or infant dietary changes should be continued to reduce the colic symptoms. Although simethicone drops (0.3 mL three times daily) may be recommended, research does not indicate that they are effective (Danielsson & Hwang, 1985; Garrison & Christakis, 2000; Metcalf, et al., 1994; Savino & Tarasco, 2010). Dicyclomine, an anticholinergic agent, has been shown to have some efficacy in reducing colic; however, its use is contraindicated in children younger than 6 months of age because of adverse side effects such as seizures and difficulty breathing (Savino & Tarasco, 2010). It is important for the parents to occasionally get away from an incessantly crying infant just to clear their minds and manage their own increasing stress related to the child's continuous crying. Resources to help parents manage their child's periods of crying are located at http://www.purplecrying.info. A trusted sitter or friend can stay with the child for a few hours at least once each week. If this respite is not available, the parents can alternate caregiving activities to give each other a breather. Parents should also be given support and empathy as they cope with this stressful experience.

RELATIONSHIPS

An infant's first relationships are with his or her family. Through these relationships, the infant learns how to interact with others.

Parent–Child Attachment

Attachment is the emotional bond that creates an important foundation for the relationship between the parent and the infant. Attachment encourages protectiveness and the development of trust and empathy between the parent and child. Health care professionals must do as much as possible to encourage attachment, especially if a mother or father does not immediately bond with the infant, as can occur after a particularly difficult delivery.

Certain identifiable behaviors—eye-to-eye contact, physical contact, and communication—indicate that attachment is occurring. The nurse should be concerned if the parent avoids eye contact and physical contact with the infant or if, when contact is unavoidable, the infant is not held close to the parent's body. By 3 weeks of age, the infant responds to the mother by cooing, making eye contact, sucking, pupil dilation, or face brightening. These behaviors tell the nurse that attachment is occurring normally. Some of these behaviors may be difficult to observe, particularly if birth was by cesarean section and the mother is recovering from anesthesia or if cultural practices do not allow certain behaviors. Attachment may be delayed if the parent has medical problems or is ill or if the infant is removed from the mother immediately after birth because of illness or frailty. Family discord or an ineffective support system can also contribute to poor or inadequate attachment.

To promote attachment, the mother/father and infant should have time together as soon as possible, during which the parents can cuddle, talk to, and examine the infant. Ideally, this attachment will occur within the first hour after delivery, but it can occur later without any problem. If the infant is in an intensive care unit, the parents should be allowed to view the infant and touch or stroke the infant's hand or foot.

After the infant is born, many fathers feel left out and not needed for feeding (particularly with breastfed infants) or other care. Many fathers want to achieve closeness to the baby but often feel this closeness is not possible because the mother–infant bond is so strong (Nystrom & Ohrling, 2004). Marital intimacy and support from their partner have been demonstrated as two predictors of positive father–infant attachment (Yu et al., 2012). Fathers can and should become involved with all aspects of the infant's care and cuddling.

Fathers, like mothers, need private time to bond with the infant. Inviting fathers to participate in the care of the infant and providing quality time with their partner and the child will facilitate father–infant attachment.

Sibling Adjustment to the Newborn

QUESTION: When Lela was about a month old, Claudia placed her in an infant seat on the floor in the living room where José was watching television. While in the kitchen a moment later, Claudia heard a thump and then a wail. She ran into the living room. José was sitting on the couch staring hard at the television and Lela was tipped over but still belted in her infant seat, crying. Claudia asked José, "How did your sister fall over?" José answered, "I pushed her!" How would you recommend that Claudia approach this situation

How a child experiences a mother's pregnancy and subsequent arrival of a new sibling is affected by three factors:

1. The child's state of emotional and social development
2. The child's cognitive abilities, such as the child's ability to reason and solve problems
3. The child's level of separation and independence from the mother

Some degree of stress resulting from the birth of a younger sibling can be expected. The degree of stress or upset after the birth does not predict the quality of future sibling relationships. Many older children demonstrate substantial developmental gains after the birth of younger siblings. For instance, the child who reverts to thumb-sucking may also begin to start dressing himself or herself. Siblings spaced about 2 years apart are likely to experience the greatest degree of stress with the arrival of a new brother or sister because they must deal with increased separation from the mother at a time when they find separation and the decreased or lack of attention especially difficult. In addition, a very young sibling may not have the cognitive and verbal skills to express complex emotions.

There is no "best time" to tell siblings about the pregnancy and impending birth. The timing depends on the age of the older children. Young children (younger than 6 years of age) do not need much lead time because they are not able to measure time in terms of weeks or months. The beginning of the second trimester is a good time to share the news with children, or it can be done at the point when the mother's protruding abdomen is evident to the child. School-aged children should hear the news as soon as the family plans to tell friends and other family members. Older siblings should learn the news before it is shared with grandparents or others so that they do not accidentally hear the information from someone besides the parents.

The news of the pregnancy may not be greeted with joy by the older sibling. The older child may struggle with the new role and worry about the changes that will occur in the family. Providing loving support and developmentally appropriate discussions can help the child to adapt to the changes.

The older child may also feel frustrated because he or she has already noted changes in the home environment during the mother's pregnancy. Many physical and psychological changes occur to the mother during pregnancy. Although the mother may feel physically well, the child may be deprived of the mother's attention as she focuses inward on her pregnancy and the fetus. The normal physiologic changes of pregnancy may cause the mother to be more tired, irritable, and moody. In addition, as her abdomen grows, it may be increasingly more difficult to pick up and carry younger siblings or even to sit with them on her lap.

The arrival of the new family member affects all aspects of family life and all relationships in the family. Not only are the parents welcoming a new child into the home but other children will also welcome and need to adjust to a new brother or sister. Having a sibling has been described as the single most beneficial way in which children can learn how to relate and interact appropriately with others (Fig. 4-10). During the pregnancy and after the arrival of the infant, the sibling needs to continue to feel loved, wanted, and valued. This need is important regardless of the child's age or the way he or she may show his or her feelings. To promote successful sibling relationships, a parent should know that the effect on the older child begins during the pregnancy and will continue through the first several months after the newborn's arrival at home. Teaching Intervention Plan 4-2 summarizes several interventions that can help to alleviate sibling jealousy and promote bonding between siblings (see also discussion in Chapter 5).

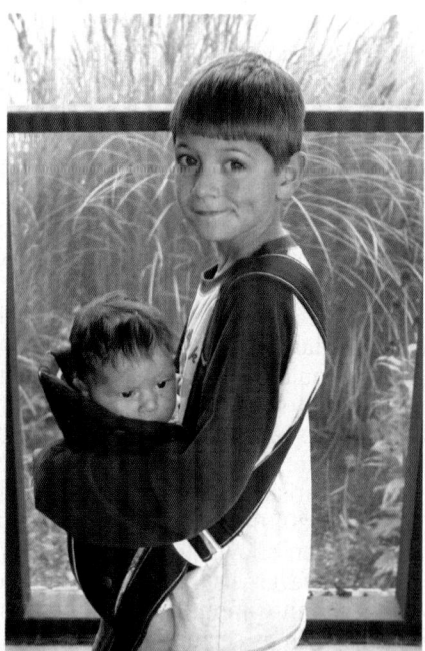

Figure 4-10 Children learn to relate and interact appropriately with others through the sibling relationship. This older brother likes to hold, cuddle, and protect his newborn sister. A positive sibling bond is being established.

TIP 4-2: A TEACHING INTERVENTION PLAN to Prepare Siblings for the Arrival of the Newborn

Nursing Diagnosis and Family Outcomes

- Interrupted family process related to addition of new members
  Outcomes: Family members will voice realistic expectation of sibling's behavior and reaction to the newborn.
  Sibling will experience feelings of support, love, and nurturance from parents.
  Sibling will participate in activities to prepare for the arrival of the newborn.
  Sibling will participate in age-appropriate care activities and social interactions with the newborn.

Guidance for Family Members

Involve the Sibling in the Pregnancy

Activities for the Child
- Have the sibling attend a doctor's appointment with the mother. If possible, allow the child to be present during the ultrasound examination.
- Let the sibling feel the fetus's movements.
- Visit friends who have a newborn in their home. Discuss what it will be like to have "our baby" at home.
- See if the hospital provides sibling classes in which the older child can learn about newborns.
- Read books together about what happens during pregnancy and what it is like to be a big brother or sister.
- Male and female toddlers and preschoolers can benefit from having a doll to teach siblings about the care of the newborn and to allow the child expression of his or her feelings regarding the arrival of the sibling.

Preparation for the Newcomer
- Encourage the older child to help prepare and decorate the infant's room. Let the sibling be involved in selecting and purchasing clothes for the newborn.
- Encourage the older child to help select the newborn's name.
- Place a picture of the older sibling in the newborn's room.
- Let the older sibling pick the outfit the newborn will wear home from the hospital.

Avoid Pursuing New Developmental Challenges

Change in the Child's Environment and Routines
- Changes in the older child's environment or routine should be made several months before the birth so that the child will not feel pushed out or shoved aside for the newborn.
- If the child will be starting a new daycare or nursery school, do this well in advance of the delivery.
- Do not make any demands for new skills such as toilet training and bottle weaning during the months just preceding the delivery. Even if the child appears ready, wait until after he or she has adjusted to the arrival of the newcomer.

Increase Father's Participation
- Have the father get more involved in the daily activities of the child. The sibling will better tolerate less motherly attention during the mother's hospitalization and after the newborn's arrival if the father or another significant family member has become more involved in the child's care.

The Time of Delivery

Siblings at the Birth
- Some hospitals and birthing centers permit siblings to be included in the birthing process. These children must be prepared in advance for the sights and sounds they will encounter.
- An adult who is emotionally close to the child should be assigned the responsibility of monitoring the child during the birthing process.
- In general, studies have shown that children younger than the age of 4 years have difficulty attending the birth. At these ages, they are still quite dependent on their mother for emotional support and can become overly concerned and distressed by the mother's physical exertion during the birthing process.

Care of the Sibling Left at Home
- Tell the child where the mother is going and who will care for the child while the mother is in the hospital. Optimally, the child should know the "babysitter" well and the sitter should have been thoroughly prepared to step in at any time.
- Prepare in advance written instructions of the older children's routines for the babysitter to follow.
- Encourage the father, grandparents, or special friends to take the child on a special outing while the mother is in the hospital.

Visiting Mother in the Hospital
- Try to have the older child visit the mother each day.
- If the older sibling cannot visit, send along a picture of mother and baby.
- Call the older children daily from the hospital.
- Take a special gift to the hospital to give to the older child as a present from his or her new sibling.

Welcoming the Newborn Home
- Have the older sibling come to the hospital and join the new family on the trip home.
- When entering the home, spend the first moment with the older sibling. Let someone else carry the newborn into the house and get the newborn settled.
- Do not give the sibling the impression of always being tired and haggard. The child may think that the mother was hurt by the newborn's birth.

(Continued)

TIP 4-2: A TEACHING INTERVENTION PLAN to Prepare Siblings for the Arrival of the Newborn (*Continued*)

- Have a special party to welcome the infant home. Some suggest doing this 1 week after the newborn comes home. Give the sibling "gifts" from the newborn. Have a cake and make it a real celebration.
- Refer to the newborn "our baby" or "your brother or sister."
- Ask visitors to give some extra attention to the older sibling.
- Allow the older sibling to unwrap the newborn's gifts.

Promoting Positive Sibling Encounters

Encourage Interactions
- Encourage the older sibling to touch and play with the newborn in the presence of an adult. Allow him or her to hold the infant while sitting in a chair or the ground.
- Encourage the sibling to talk or to tell stories to the newborn.
- Teach the sibling to attract the newborn's attention with bright toys.
- Teach the sibling when the best times are to interact with the newborn. This depends on the newborn's states of arousal.

Parents' Reactions
- At certain times, the older child's need for parental support may be more important than the needs of the newborn.
- Let the sibling play a game of "pretend baby" if his or her desire to be a baby is apparent. A few minutes of being treated like a baby is generally enough because the child must understand that being the baby means no going outside to play or walking or eating snacks or other "big boy or girl" activities.
- Do not always tell the older sibling to "be quiet" because of the newborn. Most newborns will learn to sleep through all sorts of noises. Constant silencing of the older child can cause resentment.
- Intervene promptly if the older sibling shows aggressive behavior toward the newborn, such as physical or verbal attacks.

- Teach civil behaviors. Promote sharing, respect for property, and the right to privacy. Teach children to be loyal to one another regardless of the anger they may feel at times.
- Avoid comparing and labeling the siblings.

Enlisting the Older Sibling as a Helper
- As the older child feels comfortable, let him or her help wash or feed the newborn or find toys or the pacifier for the newborn. Emphasize how much the newborn "likes" the older sibling and how it makes the newborn happy to have his or her brother or sister help.
- On the other hand, do not expect the older sibling to shoulder adult responsibilities.

Regressive Behaviors
- Do not criticize the older sibling if he or she begins or display regressive behaviors such as thumb-sucking or bed-wetting. Rather, praise and reward grown-up behaviors in siblings. Be tolerant of regressive behaviors and realize that these symptoms will resolve over time.
- If the child is old enough, encourage him or her to talk about his or her feelings about the newborn.
- Explain why the "rules" or what are considered acceptable behaviors are not the same for every child in the family.

Providing the Older Sibling With Extra Attention
- Try to give at least 30 minutes a day of special time or "our time" with just the mother and the older child.
- In the evening, have the father or another family relative or close friend participate in a special activity with the older sibling each day while mother is feeding the newborn.
- Spend some time with the older sibling looking through his or her baby album.

ANSWER: As the nurse talking to Claudia, there are several points to make. One is that Claudia must reinforce to José that we never, ever hurt our baby. The other is that this is not a good time for spanking. Spanking at this time reinforces the notion that the adult is bigger and can hurt José; therefore, José is bigger and can hurt the baby. Another issue is that José is resenting Lela and may need a little more attention at this time. Reading to a young child while nursing the baby is a good way to reduce jealousy over the time mommy is spending snuggled with that new baby. Review Teaching Intervention Plan 4-2 for other ideas to help a sibling accept a new baby.

When an Infant Cannot Come Home From the Hospital Immediately

The newborn may experience health problems that require a hospital stay after the mother has been discharged. During the pregnancy, older siblings have been told that their mother would go to the hospital and then *mother and baby* would come home from the hospital. The siblings may have difficulty understanding why the newborn cannot come home.

Parents need to provide age-appropriate explanations regarding why the baby needs to be cared for at the hospital by the doctors and nurses. If hospital policy allows, siblings should be encouraged to visit the newborn.

If the infant is in a newborn intensive care unit, older children may only be allowed to look through a window at their younger sibling. If the newborn is on a ventilator, parents need to determine whether the older sibling will do well seeing the newborn with all of that equipment. In all cases, children should be prepared by their parents for all that they might see in the hospital.

The older sibling can be given pictures of the newborn. If the sibling does visit the newborn in the hospital, a picture of the family can be taped to the baby's bassinet or incubator. The sibling can be told that the newborn likes to look at the family and is excited about coming home.

Notes can be written from the newborn to the sibling, and the sibling can write notes or color pictures to be given to the newborn. The older sibling can be given updates about the infant's progress. If the newborn is not doing well, the sibling should be told. The older child will see the parent's stress and be concerned.

When an Infant Has a Noticeable Physical Defect

If the infant looks or acts differently than other newborns, siblings must be prepared for these differences. The parents should openly discuss how "our baby" is different. Consider the sibling's developmental age when answering the questions he or she may have about why the newborn is different and how this difference may have occurred. Books about "special" babies and "special" children are available to be read to older children. Although the parents may be experiencing grief or a sense of loss, the sibling may not have had expectations about what the newborn would be like. Children can be very tolerant and accepting of how others look. The sibling's reaction to the newborn will most likely reflect the parents' reactions. Modeling a gentle approach and a loving acceptance of the infant will highly influence the sibling's acceptance of the "special" child. Chapter 12 presents more in-depth information about the special needs child.

PLAY

During the first few weeks of life, neither the newborn nor the exhausted parent is very interested in playtime. During periods of wakefulness, the newborn is bonding with the new parents, eating, and developing a sense of the surrounding environment. At this time, the infant is very egocentric; everything revolves around him or her. Ideal play activities should be adjusted to the infant's age and should promote development and movement.

At 1 month of age, brightly colored objects hung overhead, and musical mobiles, perhaps with high-contrast black-and-white motifs, are good "toys." Being able to watch himself or herself in a mirror or watch other people's faces is an activity that will absorb an infant's attention. Encourage the parents to talk to the infant frequently from a distance of about 12 to 15 in. from the infant's face so the infant can focus on their faces. By 4 months of age, infants prefer bright colors to pale colors and human faces to any other patterns (Casby, 2003) (Fig. 4-11).

During the early months, activities that include cuddling, rocking, massaging, and singing are the most nurturing for the infant. The infant is extraordinarily

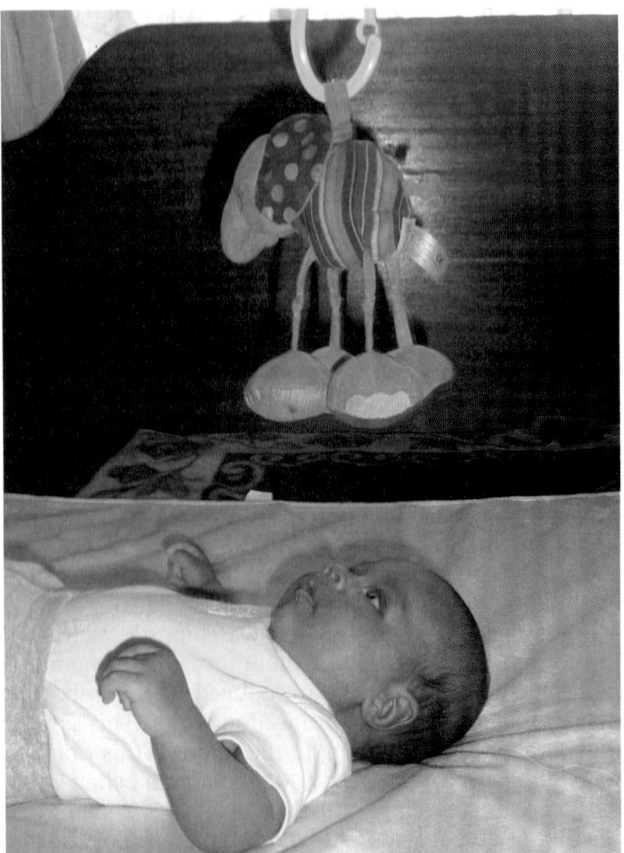

Figure 4-11 The bright colors of a toy provide visual stimulation for the infant.

sensitive to touch and movement. An infant carrier that keeps the infant close to the carrier's body is an excellent method of providing soothing movement. The newborn is also very responsive to sound. A very fussy newborn may quiet by just hearing soft music or a parent's voice. The infant should also be given the opportunity to have "floor time" or "tummy time" when awake to help strengthen abdominal and arm muscles (Fig. 4-12). The infant is placed supine or prone on a blanket on the floor, preferably a carpeted area, where he or she is

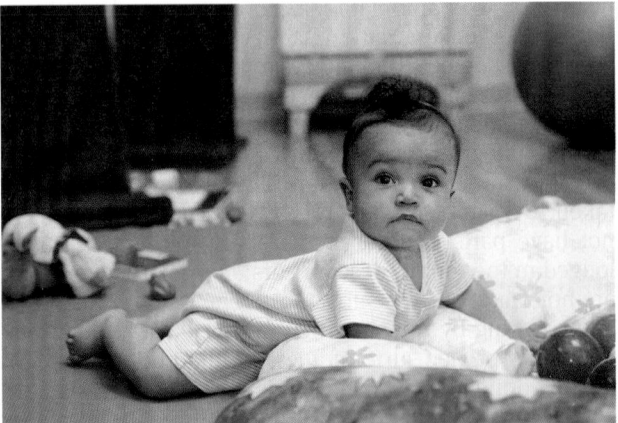

Figure 4-12 During floor time, an infant should be placed on the abdomen and allowed to move the body freely.

free to move all body parts without being confined by an infant seat or car seat. Placing the child on his or her abdomen is especially important in giving the infant an opportunity to develop head control as he or she lifts the head up and off the blanket. Toys placed close to the child aid in stimulating eye movement and gross motor movement as the child attempts to reach the toys. Parents are encouraged to join the infant on the ground and thereby increase child–parent interaction time. In addition, use cribs, car seats, and high chairs for their primary purpose only (i.e., sleeping, traveling) and limit the use of strollers, swings, and bouncer seats in favor of holding the child or using an infant carrier that holds the infant close to the body while allowing movement of the arms and legs (IOM, 2011; Koren et al., 2010; Patrick et al., 2001).

As the infant matures and developmental milestones progress, he or she will become more sociable, interacting more with surroundings. At about 3 months of age, the child begins to reach for toys and attempt to grasp (a skill that does not mature until about age 6 months). The infant loves sitting up and watching the activities in the environment. Mobiles and mirrors can be continued, "busy boxes" can be introduced to the crib, and play gyms can be used during floor time. This is also a good age to start reading to the infant if this practice has not been started already. Many parents believe they can increase the child's intelligence if they encourage reading at an early age. Although popular books foster this belief, research is not yet conclusive.

By 6 months of age, the infant is able to grasp large toys, loves to play peek-a-boo, likes to listen to stories, and usually loves water and water play. In the bath, the infant loves to pour the water in and out of cups, swatting and dunking floating objects, squirting sponges, and so on. Imitation and repetition skills are becoming more defined, and the infant loves games that enable copying what is being done (e.g., making funny faces or noises, clapping, laughing) and repeats it over and over. This is a special time for the infant and parent. The infant experimenting with the environment by banging pots and pans may be annoying, but the 6-month-old is fascinated with the sounds produced.

At 8 to 9 months of age, the infant's manual dexterity is improving and he or she is now able to use his or her hands to manipulate large objects, turn large book pages, and shake a rattle (Fig. 4-13). A large box set up with lots of objects (not always toys) is ideal. The objects can be items such as balls, oatmeal boxes, plastic margarine containers, wooden spoons, and old plastic bowls. During this time, the infant loves to imitate the activities of parents and older children (Fig. 4-14). Care must be taken to ensure that play objects are not too small; do not have parts that can come apart and can be easily lodged in the throat, nose, or ears; lack sharp edges; and are not made of toxic substances. The infant is also usually crawling by now and may be very fast and curious about his or her surroundings. "Childproofing," if not already done, is now an absolute necessity (Hagan et al., 2008; Patrick et al., 2001). **Childproofing** is the process by which the parent or other caregivers screen the child's environment for safety hazards (e.g., stairs, small items

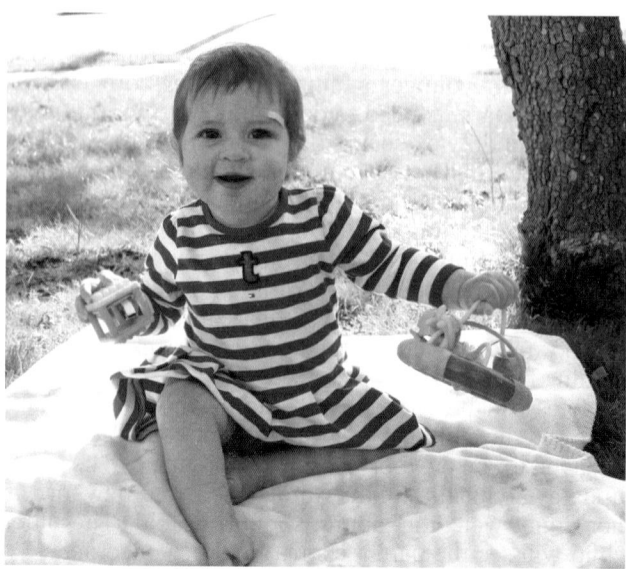

Figure 4-13 This 8-month-old child enjoys picking up and manipulating blocks and other fun toys.

that could choke the child) and use measures to eliminate these hazards to protect the child from injury.

By 1 year of age, the infant has developed enough motor control to coordinate both hands at the same time, which enables him or her to bang things together and operate simple mechanisms. The infant loves to sit in a high chair and drop items to the floor. The infant may seem to be doing this to be mischievous but in fact is discovering gravity and is amazed that the objects always move in the same direction and that objects of different types, sizes, textures, and shapes all do the same thing—hit the floor. This is usually a favorite game. The infant's manual dexterity has matured enough to pick up small objects from a plate, table, or off the floor.

Daycare and Babysitters

Daycare services provide care for the child, in exchange for financial reimbursement, when the parents are not available to do so because they are required to attend work or school. Most parents would agree that selecting

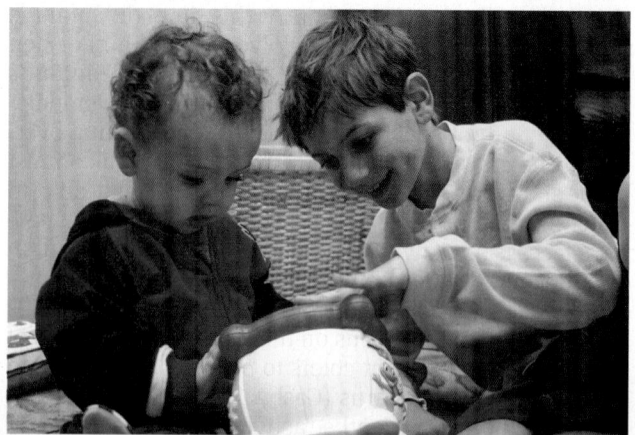

Figure 4-14 This 10-month-old child imitates the actions of the older child as they play with the drum together.

a safe and competent daycare facility is a very difficult, stressful task. They must consider such issues as the distance of the center from the parents' place of employment or from the child's home, the hours that daycare services are provided, the numbers and ages of other children being served, and the cost of the services provided (Youngblood & Carter, 2004). Opinions and research findings vary regarding the positive and negative outcomes of placing children in daycare services. Children placed in daycare early in life and for more than 30 hours per week have been noted to be at increased risk for stress-related behavioral problems. On the other hand, children in daycare centers have been noted to have higher language and early school achievement. Factors that influence any outcomes for the child include quality of the child care, number of children in the environment, parenting behaviors, and social interactions among the children at the center (Bradley & Vandell, 2007).

Types of Daycare Services

There are two basic types of daycare services: in-home care and center-based care. In-home care refers to services provided in the child's home, the home of a parent, or the home of one of the children within the daycare group. Care providers may live in the home with the family, come to the child's home, or have the children come to their home. Care provided through in-home arrangements may be offered by personnel who are authorized by a state licensing board, in which case the licensing board defines the number and ages of children who can be cared for at any one time. In addition, the board establishes certain environmental and safety criteria to which the caregiver must adhere. In-home daycare can also be provided by individuals who are not licensed, such as family members, friends, babysitters, or au pairs.

Center-based care is provided in a licensed daycare facility that may be privately owned, federally funded, or associated with a neighborhood project or workplace facility. In these settings, six or more children receive care for several hours a day. The ratio of adults to children is determined by the state for licensed daycare centers and licensed family daycare homes. All ages of children may be served, with children of similar ages generally grouped together.

Choosing a Daycare Provider

Selecting a daycare provider is one of the more complex tasks facing new parents. The considerations that must be addressed when choosing a child care provider are location, hours of service, cost, religious or cultural beliefs, and characteristics of the individual care provider. Are both parents working full time, or is this a single-parent family? Is it better to have the child care provider closer to a workplace or closer to home? How much can the family afford for child care? After these questions are answered, parents must choose in-home or center-based care (see thePoint Types of Daycare Providers: Advantages and Disadvantages).

When parents decide to use an in-home provider, they need to advertise and interview prospective care providers, unless they use an agency placement service. In either case, interviews should be conducted face to face, preferably with the child available to ascertain the potential care provider's interaction and the child's acceptance of the care provider. A list of interview questions is provided in Community Care 4-1 as a guideline to help new parents decide what to evaluate when selecting a daycare setting.

Choosing a Babysitter

Selecting the infant's first babysitter can be a difficult and sometimes scary task. This person may be a teenager within the neighborhood, a relative, or a close friend. Many of the guidelines covered earlier for hiring a daycare provider can be used to choose a good babysitter. Parents should leave the babysitter a list of emergency phone numbers and the name and phone number of the nearest available neighbor in case an emergency arises. Parents should notify the sitter where they will be, how they can be contacted, and how long they will be gone. Separation anxiety is common for a child around 9 months of age. Parents should not attempt to sneak out the door when the sitter arrives to avoid a crying scene with the infant. The child needs to learn that the parents may leave, but they will come back. Creating some ritual behaviors surrounding the parents' good-bye is preferable to having the child worry that his or her parents will simply disappear whenever a certain individual comes to the home. Inform the sitter of the child's routines (e.g., bedtime, favorite book, comforting toy). Set clear guidelines with regard to handling emergency situations and disciplinary methods. Last, ensure the sitter is aware of the "house rules" regarding their personal activities while in the home (e.g., phone calls, viewing television, restrictions on other guests in the home). Babysitters.com is an excellent resource for tips for parents and babysitters and sitter profiles and report cards across the nation.

Daycare for Sick or Medically Fragile Children

When the infant or child is sick, the parent may be unable to stay home with that child. Yet, few daycare providers appreciate having the sick child brought to them with the potential of infecting other children. To assist parents in coping with this type of situation, daycare centers for sick children have emerged. Some of these centers may have a "spots" room, where they accept children with rashes, fevers, and other potentially contagious diseases as well as children recuperating from surgeries or with noncontagious illness. It is wise to investigate the availability of such services before they are needed because centers often have a registration fee and a processing procedure that must take place before placing the child.

For those infants and young children with disabilities or long-term medical conditions requiring specialized care, daycare centers for the medically fragile child may be available. Because these children need nursing care; developmental stimulation; physical, occupational, or speech therapy; and special feeding or routine care, the staff consists of registered nurses and other allied health care personnel, along with childhood educators. Admission to these programs is generally reserved for children who cannot be served by other "regular" daycare programs, preschools, or specialized health care services.

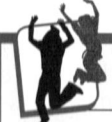

COMMUNITY CARE 4-1

Interview Questions and Tour Tips for Evaluating Daycare Options

Administration and Operations
- Is the program licensed or registered?
- What are the hours?
- Is the location convenient?
- What is the cost (or, for in home, what is the rate)?
- What days of the year is service not provided? Is tuition paid for these days?
- What meals will be provided and at what times?
- Will the child leave the facility on field trips or other excursions with the care provider?
- Are unannounced visits okay?
- How does the center communicate with the parents regarding activities, the child's progress, and any problems?
- Request at least two references from parents with a similar-aged child.

Staffing
- What is the ratio of staff to child?
- What is the education of the staff?
- How often does the staff turn over?

Tour the facility to observe
- Interaction among the children and the teachers. Are teachers truly familiar with the children, knowing each child's likes and dislikes and personality? How do they handle discipline? Do they interact with the children on their level eye to eye?
- Toys and activities. Are there enough? Are they age appropriate? Are the teachers using the instruments creatively?

- Characteristics of the environment. Is it friendly or sterile? Is it cluttered or clean (perhaps too clean and neat)? Are there indications in view of the children's activities (e.g., paintings, crafts, writing)? Are the infants all in swings or cribs or on the floor with toys and gyms?

Cleanliness
- What are the cleaning protocols for toys and equipment?
- What products are used?
- Are the diaper-changing areas clean?
- Do the staff wash their hands after changing diapers or wiping up messes?
- Are the eating areas clean?

Safety
- Are all the outlets covered?
- Are stairs covered with carpet?
- Are gates in place where necessary?
- Is the facility well lit?

Food
- Is it nutritious?
- Is the amount appropriate?
- Do the meals include age-appropriate foods?
- Is all food in the kitchen covered?
- Request a sample menu.

ALERT   *In any daycare environment, parents must address concerns about the potential for neglect or abuse. If a child's personality suddenly changes and no other outside causes (e.g., recent move, divorce, death of a family member) are apparent, a look at the child care provider may be indicated. Clinging behavior, excessive crying when dropping a child off with the care provider, or more subtle signs such as a child not looking at an adult in the face, weight loss, refusing to eat, a sad and worried look, withdrawal, and inability to be comforted are potentially signs of neglect or abuse.*

INJURY AND ILLNESS PREVENTION

One of the first priorities of new parents is to babyproof or childproof the home to prevent injury or even death. Although most parents think of babyproofing after the infant is crawling, it is never too early to start thinking of safety in cribs, car seats, and the newborn's immediate environment whether in the home or outdoors (Community Care 4-2).

HOME SAFETY

To prepare the home environment, start with general home safety issues. Ideally, all parents should know CPR and first aid and should make emergency plans for accidents and fires, including escape route planning. Emergency numbers should be posted near the

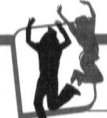

COMMUNITY CARE 4-2

Injury Prevention Guidelines for the Family With an Infant

Home Safety

- Ensure that the crib is safe. The slats should be no more than 2⅜ in. apart, and the mattress should be firm and fit snugly. As the child learns to sit and stand, the mattress should be lowered.
- Do not use soft bedding or soft toys.
- Put the infant to sleep on his or her back to reduce the risk of SIDs.
- Do not drink hot liquids or smoke while holding the infant.
- Keep all poisonous substances, cleaning agents, health and beauty supplies, medicines, and home improvement materials in a locked safe place out of sight and reach of the infant.
- Use safety locks on cabinets.
- Keep sharp objects (e.g., scissors, knives) out of reach.
- Get down on the floor and check for hazards at the infant's eye level.
- Place plastic plugs in electrical sockets.
- Do not leave heavy objects or containers of hot liquids on tables with tablecloths that the infant may pull down.
- Install gates at the top and bottom of stairs.
- Place safety devices on windows and make sure screens are secure.
- Avoid dangling electrical and drapery cords.
- Install/check smoke alarms.
- Avoid "choke" foods (e.g., nuts, carrot sticks, large pieces of fruits or vegetables).

Play Safety

- Keep toys with small parts or other small objects out of infant's reach.
- Do not use baby walkers at any age.
- Do not give the infant plastic bags, latex balloons, or small objects such as marbles.
- Teach siblings which of their toys are unsafe for the infant to play with.

Water Safety

- Set hot water thermostat at less than 120° F (48.9° C).
- Test the temperature of the bath water with your wrist to make sure it is not too hot for the infant.

- Never leave the infant alone in a tub of water or on high places; always keep a hand on the baby.
- Empty buckets, tubs, or small pools immediately after use.
- Ensure that swimming pools are enclosed by a four-sided fence with a self-closing, self-latching gate.

Car Safety

- Use an infant seat that is properly secured at all times.
- Place the car seat in the back seat of the car, facing backward toward the backrest of the car.
- Never place baby in front seat with a passenger air bag.

Safety With Others

- Never leave the infant alone or with a young sibling or pet.
- Keep the infant away from cigarette smoke. Do not allow people to smoke around the infant.
- Use babysitters who have received cardiopulmonary resuscitation (CPR) training.
- Provide the babysitter with a list of emergency phone numbers, the home address and phone number, your location, and how you can be reached.
- Keep food for animals out of child's reach. Do not let the child approach an animal that is eating.
- Never shake the baby.

Outdoor Safety

- Avoid overexposure to the sun.
- Use straps in strollers to contain the child.
- Do not allow the child to be outdoors unattended.

Emergency Preparation

- Keep own address and phone number posted near the phone.
- Keep list of emergency numbers (doctor, hospital, nearest neighbor, poison control center) near the phone.
- Learn first aid and infant CPR.
- Know signs of illness: fever >100.4° F (38° C), seizure, rash, unusual irritability, lethargy, failure to eat, vomiting, diarrhea, dehydration, or jaundice.

Adapted from Green, M., & Palfrey, J. (Eds.). (2002). Bright *futures: Guidelines for supervision of infants, children, and adolescents* (2nd ed., text rev.). Arlington, VA: National Center of Education in Maternal and Child Health.

telephone along with the address and phone number of the residence. This information is helpful to the parent who, in times of emergency, may temporarily be unable to recall his or her own address and phone number.

Smoke alarms should be installed on every level of the home, and carbon monoxide detectors are recommended near sleeping quarters (or elsewhere according to the manufacturer's directions). Every home should be equipped with a working flashlight in case of electrical failure, and a fire extinguisher should be kept near the kitchen.

Water heaters should be turned down to 120° F (48.9° C) to prevent scalding the child's skin. The cords of lamps and appliances should be shortened and covered or hidden out of the child's view to prevent the child from chewing them or getting them wrapped around the neck. Electrical outlets should be covered to prevent the child from inserting keys or other metal objects in the outlet, possibly resulting in electric shock and burns on the child. Windows should have locks and screens that are securely attached to keep the child from falling out the window. The window cords should be rolled up or placed out of reach with the use of rubber bands or twist ties so the child does not become entangled in the cords, causing suffocation. As the infant begins to crawl, safety gates should be installed to prevent entrance up or down stairs and in rooms with computer or office equipment.

Two areas that are especially hazardous are the kitchen and the bathroom because of the types of activities and equipment that are available. Babyproof locks should be installed on all kitchen cabinets. One or two cabinets can be left open if they contain items for the child to play with, such as plastic bowls, spoons, and pan lids. All sharp scissors and knives should be kept in drawers or cupboards with childproof latches. When cooking, pot handles should be turned away from the front of the range so the child cannot grab them and pull hot liquids off the stove onto himself or herself. All cleaning supplies should be placed up high, out of reach, or kept in a childproof cupboard to prevent the child from ingesting them.

In the bathroom, the toilet lid should be kept lowered to prevent drowning. Safety latches are available to prevent the child from opening the lid. Medications and toiletries should not be kept out where a child could get to them. Nonskid strips installed in the bathtub help prevent falls. A cushioned cover on the faucet will keep the child from being injured by the faucet. When bathing the infant or child, parents must never leave the child unattended.

The infant spends a lot of time unsupervised in his or her bedroom, so the nursery must be inspected carefully for any hazards. Encourage the parents to get down on their hands and knees and see the environment from the perspective of the child. All potential hazards must be removed from this level. Next, other areas of the child's environment must be evaluated for safety. Crib mobiles and monitors should be out of reach. The infant should never be left unattended on a changing table, even if strapped in place, because of the danger of falling.

Crib Safety

Safety should be addressed even before the infant is born when the parents-to-be are beginning to purchase the equipment an infant will use. Cribs are usually the first item that is either purchased or obtained through a friend or family. All cribs manufactured since 1973 in the United States are required to meet stringent federal regulations for safety to prevent infant entrapment and suffocation. If a crib is borrowed or purchased secondhand, the following checklist should be used: the side slats should be no less than 2⅜ in. apart, decorative cutouts should be avoided, and the mattress must fit snugly on all sides. The crib should have not have side rails that move up or down because these were banned for manufacturing, sale, or resale in 2010 by the Consumer Product Safety. No bumper pads, pillows, or fluffy blankets should be in the crib because they increase the danger of suffocation. The mattress should be firm, not soft, and no pillow is needed for an infant. If an older crib is obtained that has been painted, the paint should be stripped off (not sanded) because the paint may be lead based and, if inhaled, could cause lead poisoning. The crib should be repainted with high-quality enamel paint. Some new parents are opting for cribs with mesh sides rather than wooden ones

PLAY SAFETY

All children need toys to learn from and to help them meet developmental milestones. Toys are the tools of play for children. But, as with any tool, they must be appropriate for the job, and they must be safe. Toys must match the child's age and development. Manufacturer's guidelines may help, but the parents know whether their child is mature and skilled enough for a particular toy.

caREminder

Many children's toys are made of plastic that contain bisphenol A, a toxic substance that can lead to impaired brain development in exposed infants and children. Encourage parents to buy wooden toys or those labeled "PVC-free" (Environment California Research & Policy Center, 2012).

Rattles should be at least 1⅝ in. in diameter to prevent them from becoming lodged in the child's throat. All toys should be well constructed, with no loose pieces that can be removed and potentially swallowed or aspirated. This precaution is particularly important with stuffed animals or dolls because some have eyes or noses that can be pulled off and possibly swallowed. Small toys should be avoided until the child is at least 3 years old. A small cylinder, approximately the size of a child's throat, has been developed to assist parents and health care professionals in determining what toy or toy part is too small. If the object can fit into the cylinder, do not allow the child to play with the object (see thePoint for Organizations).

Balloons, although they are fun to look at and part of many birthday parties, should not be blown up or played with by children younger than 5 years old. If a balloon pops, be sure all the pieces are collected, because a crawling infant can pick up a loose piece and choke on or aspirate it. Latex balloons should not be used around children because many children are allergic to latex and they could choke on an uninflated balloon. Mylar balloons are considered safe for children.

Toys must be inspected periodically to be sure they remain in good condition; if they become broken or overly worn, they should be repaired or discarded. Projectile toys should be avoided, as should toys that produce loud noises. Noise levels at or about 100 dB (the sound of a typical cap gun at close range) can damage an infant's hearing. A quick clue to a safe toy is to look for the letters *ASTM*, which indicate that the product meets the national safety standards for the American Society for Testing and Materials.

WATER SAFETY

Drowning remains a leading cause of death in the pediatric population. Although many parents may not consider drowning a risk during the neonatal and infant periods, drowning can easily occur if the infant is left unattended in the bathtub or wanders into areas with easy access to swimming pools or hot tubs. Many parents respond to this safety hazard by enrolling their child in a swimming program specially designed to introduce infants and young children to the joy and risks of being in and around water (Tradition or Science 4-3). These programs cannot be used as a substitute for common water safety practices (e.g., the child must never be left alone in the tub, pools must be enclosed by a fence).

Water safety also includes ensuring the hot water temperature used in the home is set less than 120° F (48.9° C) to prevent burns and scalding of the infant during bath time.

CAR SAFETY

Talk with parents about temperatures inside their car. A temperature that is comfortable for the parent would be appropriate for the infant. Parents must ensure that the sun is not shining in the infant's eyes or directly on the infant. They must never leave the infant in the car alone even to run into the store quickly. To help protect the infant, parents should observe traffic rules more carefully and be watchful for reckless drivers.

Car Seat Safety

QUESTION: Lela will use the crib that the Diaz family bought new for José, and the home has been babyproofed. They have a convertible car seat, but José does not yet meet state requirements for weight, height, or age to move to a booster seat, so he is still using it. What could you recommend to this family?

Most hospitals will not discharge an infant home unless there is a car seat available to transport the child. Many acute care facilities have a car seat loan program or other means to provide car seats to those who are unable to purchase their own. Car seats that were manufactured before January 1981 should not be used because more stringent safety standards were implemented at that time (Fig. 4-15). Parents should look at all types of car seats and decide on one that fits their usage style and the size of their car (Community Care 4-3). Car seat laws vary from state to state and between the United States and Canada. Parents should review state laws to determine the specific legal requirements. Some states require car seats until age 4 years; others up until 8 years of age. States may also have a weight or height requirement that supersedes the age requirement—that is, a child who meets the age requirement but does not meet the height or weight requirement must continue to be restrained in a car seat.

The AAP (2011) recommends all infants and young children ride in a rear-facing car seat until 2 years of age or until they reach the highest weight or height allowed, as indicated by the manufacturer of the car seat. Children should continue to use a forward facing car seat until they are at least 4 years of age. In general, after the child is taller than 57 in. and is between the ages of 8 and 12 years, the regular automobile seat with a lap belt and shoulder harness may be used. Some states have enacted booster seat laws to protect children up to 8 years old. Belt-positioning booster seats cannot be used safely with lap-only belts.

TRADITION OR SCIENCE 4-3
Evidence-Based Practice

Do aquatic programs for young children help prevent drowning in their age group?

No research has demonstrated an association between aquatic programs for infants and young children and a decreased risk of drowning. Parents should not feel secure that their child is safe from drowning and water injury after the child has participated in an aquatic program. Children are not generally ready developmentally for formal swimming lessons until after their fourth birthday (AAP, Committee on Sports Medicine and Fitness & Committee on Injury and Poison Prevention, 2000; American Red Cross Advisory Council on First Aid, Aquatics, Safety, and Preparedness, 2009).

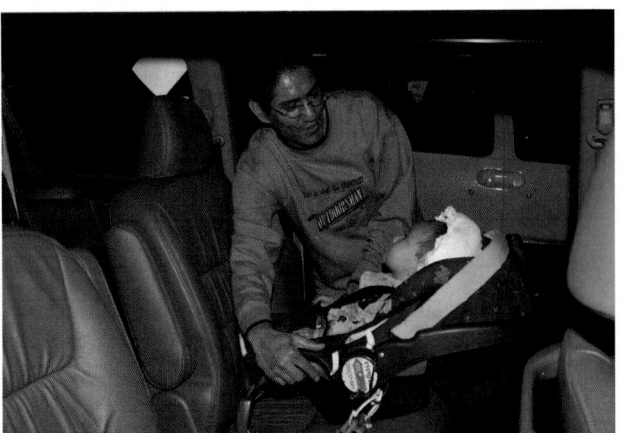

Figure 4-15 Infants should be restrained in a car seat in a rear-facing position in the backseat of the car.

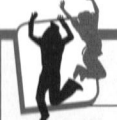

COMMUNITY CARE 4-3

Car Seat Recommendations

Birth–12 months

Children under age 1 should always ride in a rear-facing car seat. There are different types of rear-facing car seats: Infant-only seats can only be used rear-facing. Convertible and 3-in-1 car seats typically have higher height and weight limits for the rear-facing position, allowing the child to be kept rear-facing for a longer period of time.

1–3 years

The child should be kept rear-facing as long as possible. It's the best way to keep him or her safe. The child should remain in a rear-facing car seat until reaching the top height or weight limit allowed by the car seat's manufacturer. Once the child outgrows the rear-facing car seat, he or she is ready to travel in a forward-facing car seat with a harness.

4–7 years

The child should be kept in a forward-facing car seat with a harness until reaching the top height or weight limit allowed by the car seat's manufacturer. Once the child outgrows the forward-facing car seat with a harness, it's time to travel in a booster seat, but still in the back seat.

8–12 years

The child should be kept in a booster seat until he or she is big enough to fit in a seat belt properly. For a seat belt to fit properly, the lap belt must lie snugly across the upper thighs, not the stomach. The shoulder belt should lie snug across the shoulder and chest and not cross the neck or face. Remember: the child should still ride in the back seat because it's safer there.

Information from: National Highway Traffic Safety Administration (http://www.safercar.gov/parents/RightSeat.htm).

Caution parents to always follow the manufacturer's directions regarding installation and proper use.

caREminder

Car seats should ideally be placed in the center of the backseat of the automobile because this location prevents injury injured by rapid inflation of airbags during a collision and from a side impact accident No child younger than 12 years old should be in the front passenger seat because the airbag deployment, in the event of an accident, would cause injury or death.

ANSWER: The Diaz family needs two car seats. The hospital nurses caring for the Diaz family should give Ignacio the resources for community loan programs before the day of discharge. Almost all communities have car seat loan programs.

OUTDOOR SAFETY

Outside areas must be policed with the same rigorous attention to safety afforded in the home. Playgrounds can provide a tremendous opportunity for children to explore and expand their physical capabilities. Risks can be minimized if the equipment is kept in good condition and the area is appropriately designed. The area must be arranged to allow enough room between equipment to prevent collision with other equipment or interference with other play areas. The equipment should be placed far enough away from off-limit areas such as trafficked streets and railroad tracks, and it should be in good condition (e.g., no broken pieces, rusted or exposed bolts, or splinters). A soft, shock-absorbing material under the equipment (at least 6 in. of sand, mulch, or bark or rubberized matting) is required by many building codes. The area must be well maintained, with no overgrown bushes interfering with the equipment. Overgrown grass or an abundance of leaves can cause slippery areas. Cleanliness must be maintained, with no broken glass or trash accessible to children who are prone to putting foreign objects in their mouth. These guidelines can be applied to both public and home playgrounds. Home playgrounds may have additional issues to be assessed, such as whether they are fenced, what kind of vegetation is being grown around the yard (poisonous or not), whether pesticides or herbicides have been used in proximity to the play environment, and whether there are animals in the neighborhood that might present a hazard to children playing in the yard.

See thePoint for a summary of Key Concepts.

REFERENCES

Academy of Breastfeeding Medicine. (2008). ABM clinical protocol #6: Guideline on co-sleeping and breastfeeding. *Breastfeeding Medicine, 3*, 38–43. Retrieved from http://www.bfmed.org/Media/Files/Protocols/Protocol_6.pdf

Academy of Breastfeeding Medicine. (2009). ABM clinical protocol #3: Hospital guidelines for the use of supplementary feedings in the healthy term breastfed neonate. *Breastfeeding Medicine*, 3, 175–182.

Academy of Breastfeeding Medicine. (2010). ABM clinical protocol #8: Human milk storage information for home use for healthy full-term infants. *Breastfeeding Medicine*, 5(3), 127–130.

Academy of Breastfeeding Medicine. (2011). ABM clinical protocol #24: Allergic proctocolitis in the exclusively breastfed infant. *Breastfeeding Medicine*, 6(6), 435–440.

Agostoni, C., Axelsson, I., Goulet, O. et al. (2006). Soy protein infant formulae and follow-on formulae: A commentary by the ESPGHAN committee on nutrition. *Journal of Pediatric Gastroenterology*, 42, 353–361.

American Academy of Pediatric Dentistry. (2006). *Policy on oral habits.* Retrieved from http://www.aapd.org/media/Policies_Guidelines /P_OralHabits.pdf

American Academy of Pediatric Dentistry. (2007a). *Guideline on fluoride therapy.* Retrieved from http://www.aapd.org/media/Policies _Guidelines/G_FluorideTherapy.pdf

American Academy of Pediatric Dentistry. (2007b). *Policy on the use of fluoride.* Retrieved from http://www.aapd.org/media/Policies _Guidelines/P_FluorideUse.pdf

American Academy of Pediatric Dentistry. (2011a). *Guideline on infant oral health care.* Retrieved from http://www.aapd.org /media/Policies_Guidelines/G_InfantOralHealthCare.pdf

American Academy of Pediatric Dentistry. (2011b). *Guideline on caries-risk assessment and management for infants, children, and adolescents.* Retrieved from http://www.aapd.org/media/Policies _Guidelines/G_CariesRiskAssessment.pdf

American Academy of Pediatrics. (2004a). Diagnosis and management of acute otitis media. *Pediatrics*, 113, 1451–1465.

American Academy of Pediatrics. (2004b). *Pediatric nutrition handbook* (5th ed.). Elk Grove, IL: Author.

American Academy of Pediatrics. (2005a). Breast-feeding and the use of human milk. *Pediatrics*, 115, 496–506.

American Academy of Pediatrics. (2005b). The changing concept of sudden infant death syndrome: Diagnostic coding shifts, controversies regarding the sleeping environment and new variables to consider in reducing risk. *Pediatrics*, 116, 1245–1255.

American Academy of Pediatrics. (2011). SIDS and other sleep-related infant deaths: Expansion of recommendations for a safe infant sleeping environment. *Pediatrics*, 128(5), 1030–1039.

American Academy of Pediatrics, Committee on Nutrition. (2001). The use and misuse of fruit juice in pediatrics. *Pediatrics*, 107, 1210–1213.

American Academy of Pediatrics, Committee on Sports Medicine and Fitness & Committee on Injury and Poison Prevention. (2000). Swimming programs for infants and toddlers. *Pediatrics*, 105, 868–870.

American Red Cross Advisory Council on First Aid, Aquatics, Safety, and Preparedness. (2009). *ACFASP advisory: Minimum age for swimming lessons.* Retrieved from http://www.instructorscorner.org /media/resources/SAC/Min%20Age%20for%20Swim%20less.pdf

Arenz, S., Rudkerl, R., Koletzko, B. et al. (2004). Breastfeeding and childhood obesity: A systematic review. *International Journal of Related Metabolic Disorders*, 28, 1247–1256.

Baker, S. (2007). Counseling parents on feeding children. *Current Opinion in Clinical Nutrition and Metabolic Care*, 10, 355–359.

Boné, J., Claver, A., Guallar, I. et al. (2009). Allergic proctocolitis, food-induced enterocolitis: Immune mechanisms, diagnosis and treatment. *Allergol Immunopathol*, 37(1), 36–42.

Bowden, V., & Greenberg, C. (2012). *Pediatric nursing procedures* (3rd ed.). Philadelphia, PA: Lippincott Williams & Wilkins.

Bradley, R., & Vandell, D. (2007). Child care and well-being of children. *Archives of Pediatrics & Adolescent Medicine*, 161, 669–676.

Brazelton, T. B. (1992). *Touchpoints.* New York, NY: Harper Collins.

Burns, C. E., Dunn, A. M., Brady, M. A. et al. (Eds.). (2013). *Pediatric primary care* (5th ed.). Philadelphia, PA: W. B. Saunders.

Butte, N., Cobb, K. Dwyer, J. et al. (2004). The start healthy feeding guidelines for infants and toddlers. *Journal of the American Dietetic Association*, 104, 442–454.

Callaghan, A., Kendall, G., Lock, C. et al. (2005). Association between pacifier use and breast-feeding, sudden infant death syndrome, infection and dental malocclusion. *International Journal of Evidence-Based Healthcare*, 3, 147–167.

Casby, M. (2003). The development of play in infants, toddlers, and young children. *Communication Disorders Quarterly*, 24(4), 163–174.

Clifford, T., Campbell, M., Speechley, K. et al. (2002). Empirical evidence of the absence of an association with source of early nutrition. *Archives of Pediatrics & Adolescent Medicine*, 156(11), 1123–1128.

Cornelius, A., D'Auria, J., & Wise, L. (2008). Pacifier use: A systematic review of selected parental web sites. *Journal of Pediatric Health Care*, 22, 159–165.

Critch, J. (2011). Infantile colic: Is there a role for dietary interventions? *Paediatric Child Health*, 16(1), 47–49.

Danielsson, B., & Hwang, C. (1985). Treatment of infantile colic with surface active substance (simethicone). *Acta Paediatrica Scandinavia*, 74(3), 446–450.

Davis, K., Parker, K., & Montgomery, G. (2004). Sleep in infants and young children: Part one: Normal sleep. *Journal of Pediatric Healthcare*, 18(2), 65–71.

Dennison, B., Rockwell, H., & Baker, S. (1997). Excess fruit juice consumption by preschool-aged children is associated with short stature and obesity. *Pediatrics*, 99, 15–22.

Dore, S., Buchan, D., Coulas, S. et al. (1998). Alcohol versus natural drying for newborn cord care. *Journal of Obstetric, Gynecologic, and Neonatal Nursing*, 27, 621–627.

El Arifeen, S. Mullany, L., Shah, R. et al. (2012). The effect of cord cleansing with chlorhexidine on neonatal mortality in rural Bangladesh: A community-based, cluster-randomised trial. *Lancet*, 379(9820), 1022–1028.

Environment California Research & Policy Center. (2012). *New test results reveal BPA in baby foods, canned foods.* Retrieved from http://environmentamerica.org/news/mee/new-test-results -reveal-bpa-baby-food-canned-foods

Eriksson, J., Forsen, T., Osmond, C. et al. (2003). Obesity from cradle to grave. *International Journal of Obesity & Related Metabolic Disorders: Journal of the International Association for the Study of Obesity*, 27(6), 722–727.

Evens, K., George, J., Angst, D. et al. (2004). Does umbilical cord care in preterm infants influence cord bacterial colonization or detachment? *Journal of Perinatology*, 24, 100–104.

Faith, M., Dennison, B., Edmunds, L. et al. (2006). Fruit juice intake predicts increased adiposity gain in children from low-income families: Weight status-by-environment interaction. *Pediatrics*, 118, 2066–2075.

Garrison, M., & Christakis, D. (2000). A systematic review of treatments for infant colic. *Pediatrics*, 106, 184–190.

Hagan, J. F., Shaw, J. S., & Duncan, P. M. (Eds.). (2008). *Bright futures: Guidelines for health supervision of infants, children, and adolescents* (3rd ed.). Elk Grove Village, IL: American Academy of Pediatrics.

Holt, K., Wooldridge, N., Story, M. et al. (Eds.). (2011). *Bright futures in practice: Nutrition* (3rd ed.). Elk Grove, IL: American Academy of Pediatrics.

Hoppin, A., & Taveras, E. (2004). *Assessment and management of childhood and adolescent obesity.* Retrieved from http://www.medscape .org/viewprogram/3221

Howard, C., Howard, F., Lamphear, B. et al. (1999). The effects of early pacifier use on breast-feeding duration. *Pediatrics*, 103(3), e33.

Institute of Medicine. (2011). *Early childhood obesity prevention policies.* Washington, DC: The National Academies Press.

Jakobsson, I., Lothe, L., Dey, D. et al. (2000). Effectiveness of casein hydrolysate feedings in infants with colic. *Acta Paediatrica*, 89(1), 18–21.

Kim, J., & Froh, B. (2012). What nurses need to know regarding nutritional and immunobiological properties of human milk. *Journal of Obsteteric, Gynecological and Neonatal Nursing, 41*(1), 122–137.

Koren, A., Reece, S., Kahn-D'angelo, L. et al. (2010). Parental information and behaviors and provider practices related to tummy time and back to sleep. *Journal of Pediatric Health Care, 24*(4), 222–230.

Lagerberg, D. (2005). Parental assessment of developmental delay in children: Some limitations and hazards. *Acta Paediatrica, 94*(8), 1006–1008.

Li, D., Willinger, M., Petitti, D. et al. (2005). Use of a dummy (pacifier) during sleep and risk of sudden infant death syndrome (SIDS): Population based case–control study. *British Medical Journal, 332*, 18–22.

Liu, M. F., Lee, T. Y., Kuo, Y. L. et al. (2012). Comparative effects of using alcohol, natural drying, and salicylic sugar powder on umbilical stump detachment of neonates. *Journal of Perinatal & Neonatal Nursing, 26*(3), 269–274.

Lucarelli, S., Nardo, G., Lastrucci, G. et al. (2011). Allergic proctocolitis refractory to maternal hypoallergenic diet in exclusively breastfed infants: A clinical observation. *BMC Gastroenterology, 11*, 82. Retrieved from http://www.biomedcentral.com/1471-230X/11/82

Lucassen, P. L., Assendelft, W. J., van Eijk, J. T. et al. (2000). Infantile colic: Crying time reduction with a whey hydrolysate: A double-blind, randomized, placebo-controlled trial. *Pediatrics, 106*(6), 1349–1354.

Mao, S., McKenzie, L., Xiang, H. et al. (2009). Injuries associated with bathtubs and showers among children in the United States. *Pediatrics, 124*(2), 541–547.

Marter, A., & Agruss, J. (2007). Pacifiers: An update on use and misuse. *Journal for Specialists in Pediatric Nursing, 12*, 278–285.

Medves, J., & O'Brien, B. (1997). Cleaning solutions and bacterial colonization in promoting healing and early separation of the umbilical cord in healthy newborns. *Revue Canadienne de Sante Publique, 88*(6), 380–382.

Metcalf, T., Irons, T., Sher, L. et al. (1994). Simethicone in the treatment of infantile colic: A randomized placebo-controlled, multicenter trial. *Pediatrics, 94*(1), 29–34.

Mindell, J., & Owens, J. (2009). *A clinical guide to pediatric sleep: Diagnosis and management of sleep problems.* Philadelphia, PA: Lippincott Williams & Wilkins.

Mitchell, E., Blair, P., & L'Hoir, M. (2006). Should pacifiers be recommended to prevent sudden infant death syndrome? *Pediatrics, 117*, 1755–1758.

Moore, P. (2009). Infant sleep: Answers to common questions from parents. *Consultant for Pediatricians, 8*(3), 81–86.

Morrow, A. (2011). Infant feeding in the 21st century. *Journal of Pediatric Health Care, 25*(3), 195–197.

Mullany, L., Darmstadt, G., & Tielsch, J. (2003). Role of antimicrobial applications to the umbilical cord in neonates to prevent bacterial colonization and infection: A review of the evidence. *Pediatric Infectious Disease Journal, 22*, 996–1002.

National Association of Neonatal Nurses. (2011). Cobedding of twins or higher-order multiples. Retrieved from http://www.nann.org/pdf/Cobedding08F.pdf

National Association of Pediatric Nurse Practitioners. (2006). Healthy eating and activity together (HEAT) clinical practice guideline. *Journal of Pediatric Health Care, 20*(6 Suppl.), 1–64.

Nelson, E. A., Yu, L., & Williams, S. (2005). International child care practices study: Breast-feeding and pacifier use. *Journal of Human Lactation, 21*(3), 289–295.

Neu, M., & Robinson, J. (2003). Infants with colic: Their childhood characteristics. *Journal of Pediatric Nursing, 18*(1), 12–20.

Nield, L., & Kamat, D. (2003). Infant colic: What works—What doesn't. *Consultant for Pediatricians, 2*(6), 230–234.

Nystrom, K., & Ohrling, K. (2004). Parenthood experiences during the child's first year: Literature review. *Journal of Advanced Nursing, 46*(3), 319–330.

Owen, C., Martin, R., Whicup, P. et al. (2005). Effects of infant feeding on the risk of obesity across the life course: A quantitative review of published evidence. *Pediatrics, 115*, 1367–1377.

Patrick, K., Spear, B., Holt, K. et al. (Eds.). (2001). *Bright futures in practice: Physical activity.* Arlington, VA: National Center for Education in Maternal and Child Health.

Pezzati, M., Biagioli, E., Martelli, E. et al. (2002). The effect of eight different cord-care regimens on cord separation time and other outcomes. *Biology of the Neonate, 81*(1), 38–44.

Pezzati, M., Rossi, S., Tronchin, M. et al. (2003). Umbilical cord care in premature infants: The effect of two different cord-care regimens (salicylic sugar powder vs chlorhexidine) on cord separation time and other outcomes. *Pediatrics, 112*(4), e275.

Pinelli, J., & Symington, A. (2005). Non-nutritive sucking for promoting physiologic stability and nutrition in preterm infants. *Cochrane Database of Systematic Reviews*, (4), CD001071.

Polhamus, B., Thompson, D., Benton-Davis, S. et al. (2005). *Overweight children and adolescents: Recommendations for screening, assessment and management.* Retrieved from http://www.medscape.org/viewarticle/461385

Reedy, J., & Krebs-Smith, S. (2010). Dietary sources of energy, solid fats, and added sugars among children and adolescents in the United States. *Journal of the American Dietetic Association, 110*(10), 1477–1484.

Savino, F., & Tarasco, V. (2010). New treatments in colic. *Current Opinion in Pediatrics, 22*, 791–797.

Sicherer, S. (2003). Clinical aspects of gastrointestinal food allergy in childhood. *Pediatrics, 111*(Suppl.), 1609–1616.

The Joanna Briggs Institute. (2008). The effectiveness of interventions for infant colic. *Best Practice: Evidence-based Practice Information Sheets for Health Professionals, 12*(6), 1–4. Retrieved from http://connect.jbiconnectplus.org/ViewSourceFile.aspx?0=444

Turecki, S. (2003). The behavioral complaint: Symptoms of a psychiatric disorder or a matter of temperament. *Contemporary Pediatrics, 20*(8), 111–119.

United States Breastfeeding Committee. (2010). *Statement on breastfeeding as a critical strategy for obesity prevention.* Washington, DC: Author. Retrieved from http://www.napnap.org/Files/USBCObesity-Statement-Rev-2010-USBC.pdf

Wagner, C., & Greer, F. (2008). Prevention of rickets and vitamin D deficiency in infants, children, and adolescents. *Pediatrics, 122*(1), 1142–1152.

Youngblood, L., & Carter, C. (2004). Counseling parents on infant day care: How to do it effectively. *Contemporary Pediatrics, 21*(8), 54–72.

Yu, C., Hung, C., Chan, T. et al. (2012). Prenatal predictors for father-infant attachment after childbirth. *Journal of Clinical Nursing, 21*(11–12), 1577–1583.

Zupan J., Garner P., & Omari, A. (2004). Topical umbilical cord care at birth. *Cochrane Database of Systematic Reviews*, (3), CD001057.

See thePoint for additional resources.

CHAPTER 5

Early Childhood (1 to 4 Years)

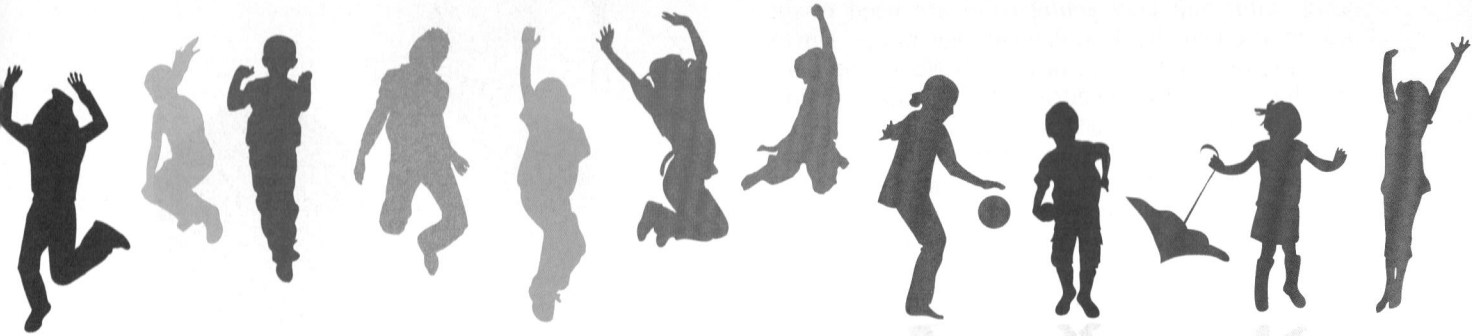

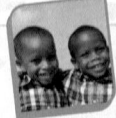

CASE HISTORY

B. J. and J. D. are 2½-year-old fraternal twins in an African American family. They have an older sister, Shawanda, who is 6 years old. All three children live with their mother. Their parents, James and Lanese Johnson, divorced about a year ago. Now, their father visits on the weekends. He takes Shawanda and the twins out to do special things, but he does not keep the three of them overnight. Lanese's mother lives in the same town and comes over to watch the kids. The family consensus is that the twins are exhausting!

The boys are big for their age, sturdy, and strong. They are very physically active and love to run, climb, and tumble. When Shawanda was their age, she loved to scribble with crayons and paint at the easel at daycare, but these activities only hold the boys' attention for a few minutes, and then it is back to exploring and practicing their gross motor skills. Shawanda also began speaking much earlier than the twins. She said many words clearly by the time she turned 2 years old. The twins, on the other hand, babble and seem to understand each other, but even their mother is not sure what they are saying.

The twins have recently moved into low toddler beds because they kept escaping from their cribs. One evening before the transition, Lanese put them both in their cribs and went to take her shower. When she got out of the shower, she heard a noise in the kitchen. When she walked into the kitchen, she found that the twins had both gotten out of their cribs and pushed a chair over to the kitchen counter. J. D. was on the counter handing down a box of breakfast cereal from the top of the refrigerator to B. J.

B. J. and J. D. have very different preferences in food. B. J. loves colorful food, especially red. He will eat tomatoes, strawberries, and watermelon. J. D. is fixated on macaroni and cheese. Every time he climbs in his booster seat, he bellows, "Roni!" Lanese is trying to use "roni" as dessert; if J. D. eats his other food, he can have "roni." The boys are using a sippy cup at meals. At their 24-month appointment, the pediatrician strongly urged Lanese to get the boys off the bottle completely, but especially at night.

Lanese is a little frustrated at the twins' lack of interest in toilet learning. When Shawanda turned 2 years old, she wanted to wear pretty panties and thus learned to use the toilet easily. The boys don't seem to notice or care if they are wet, whether in big boy pants or in diapers.

Lanese went to high school with the nurse in her pediatrician's office and is comfortable calling her for advice about the twins.

CHAPTER OBJECTIVES

1 State the developmental surveillance and milestone concerns of children aged 1 to 4 years.

2 Discuss nutrition, elimination, hygiene, and personal care needs during the early childhood years.

3 Select age-appropriate interventions to promote healthy personal and social development of the child aged 1 to 4 years.

4 Select interventions to promote illness and injury prevention for the young child and the family.

See the**Point** for a list of Key Terms.

Bright Futures defines early childhood as the period from 1 to 4 years of age (Hagan et al., 2008). The term *toddler* is also used to describe children from 12 months old to the third birthday and the term *preschooler* is often used to describe the child from 3 to 5 years of age. In this chapter, the terms *toddler*, *young child*, and *very young child* are used to discuss children in the 1 to 4 years age range. During this time, the child's rate of growth slows compared with the growth that occurred during infancy; however, many physical and developmental changes can still be expected. The child starts to walk and talk and begins to test boundaries and assert some independence. Language acquisition accelerates, and the young child is able to express desires more clearly, and sometimes in a rather loud and theatric manner. The young child has seemingly endless energy to explore the world, make new friends, and test new skills. Families must respond by being ever diligent about the child's safety, ensuring that the young child begins to develop a sense of caution and control. This chapter reviews the unique needs of early childhood, the guidelines for effective child-rearing practices, and the nurse's role in promoting healthy and safe growth and development. View the Watch and Learn videos, Developmental Considerations in Caring for Children: Toddlers and Developmental Considerations in Caring for Children: Preschoolers, for more information about growth and development during young childhood.

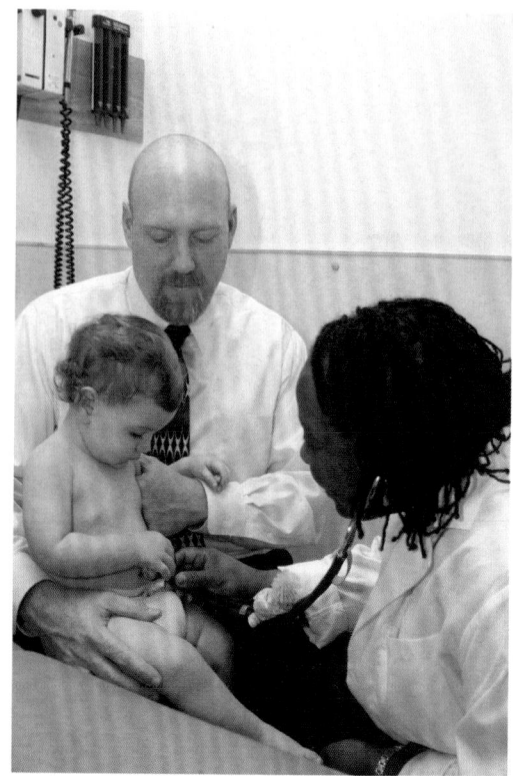

Figure 5-1 During the health examination, a young child may sit on a family member's lap to help him or her feel more safe and secure.

DEVELOPMENTAL ASSESSMENT AND SURVEILLANCE

Developmental changes during early childhood are more subtle than those that occur during infancy but are just as important for health care providers to monitor on an ongoing basis. Toddlers refine skills that have already been acquired during infancy and develop new skills that foster their curious and active personalities. As with toddlers, developmental changes during the preschool years are more subtle than those that occur during infancy but should be considered just as important. Preschoolers refine abilities, acquire new skills, become bigger and stronger, increase communication skills, and grow socially and emotionally. Speech development and the ability to communicate are especially important during this time. Developmental assessment and surveillance remain an important part of the nurse's role, especially because the number of well-child visits decreases during early childhood compared with infancy (Fig. 5-1).

Developmental Considerations 5-1 summarizes the developmental milestones that are accomplished during early childhood. This information provides the nurse with direction for specific trigger questions to ask the family to determine the child's developmental progress. Questions about how the child communicates

and comprehends instructions, how the child crawls or walks, and whether the child is toilet trained should be as open-ended as possible to elicit more information. Missing or delayed milestones must be identified so that the child can be referred to early intervention or early education services, if appropriate. State and local early childhood education services for children ages 3 to 5 years are widely available to support early identification of delays so that interventions may start before kindergarten. The nurse plays a role in teaching the family about growth and development so that they can become partners with health care team providers in identifying developmental delays and in identifying medical, genetic, and environmental factors that place the child at risk for developmental delays.

Health supervision visits to the health care provider should be scheduled at 12, 15, and 18 months of age and at 2, 3, and 4 years of age. Vision and hearing testing and screening for anemia are especially important during these years (see Chapters 8 and 28). The nurse also participates in screening the child for oral health, communicable diseases, learning disabilities, and child abuse. Selective screening of at-risk children may be needed for lead poisoning, tuberculosis, and dyslipidemia (elevation of plasma cholesterol). Chart 5-1 presents a quick reference overview for many of the conditions and illnesses that may affect the child aged 1 to 4 years.

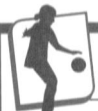

DEVELOPMENTAL CONSIDERATIONS 5-1

Milestones of Early Childhood (1–4 Years Old)

Physical

12 Months Old
Head circumference equals chest circumference
Birth weight triples to 20 lb
Height increases 3 in./year for the next 7 years
Weight increases 4–6 lb/year

18–24 Months Old
Has 10–14 temporary teeth
Anterior fontanel closes
Cuspids and first and second molars appear
Toilet learning may be initiated
Chest circumference exceeds head circumference

24 Months Old
Has 16 temporary teeth
Average weight is 30 lb
Height reaches approximately half of adult height
Toilet learning may begin; voluntary control of anal and urethral sphincters occurs
Average of 10–14 hours of sleep, including afternoon naps

36 Months Old
Nighttime control of bowel and bladder may be achieved
Weight increases 4–6 lb/year
Height increases 3 in./year

Sexual

1–4 Years Old
Anal stage (Freud)
Sensual pleasure shifts to anal and urethral areas
Identifies with male/female sex roles

3 Years Old
Knows own gender

Language

12–18 Months Old
Beginning of spoken language; may occur at same time as walking, although concentration on one or the other may occur
Recognizes nouns that stand for objects
Uses gestures to make needs known
Develops 3–20 words
Uses telegraphic speech; uses noun and verb to convey meaning
Uses words that may be quite inconsistent

18 Months to 2 Years Old
Follows directions
Points to nose, hair, eye, and so forth, on demand
Comprehends "give me that" when accompanied by a gesture

2 Years Old
Has a 50-word expressive vocabulary
Has a 300-word receptive vocabulary
Gives first and last name
Demonstrates progressive comprehension of speech
Talks without trying to convey ideas

3–4 Years Old
Has a 900- to 1,500-word vocabulary
Uses complete sentences of three to four words
Talks incessantly
Asks many questions

Vision

18 Months Old
Displays interest in pictures

2 Years Old
Identifies forms
Has 20/40 vision

3 years Old
Has 20/30 vision

Gross Motor

12–18 Months Old
Walks well
Throws ball
Stoops and recovers
Walks up stairs with help
Begins to run
Walks sideways and backward for 10 ft
Stands on one foot with help
Sits down from standing by self
Falls frequently, often used as a way of sitting down
Rolls large ball on floor

18 Months to 2 Years Old
Kicks ball forward
Throws overhand
Walks down stairs, one at a time, with help
Climbs
Sits self in a small chair

2–3 Years Old
Jumps and runs well
Jumps from bottom step
Jumps in place
Balances on one foot for 1 second
Walks on a straight line
Walks on tiptoes
Broad jumps 4–14 in.
Can pick up objects on floor without losing balance

3–4 Years Old
Rides tricycle

(Continued)

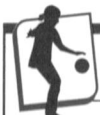

DEVELOPMENTAL CONSIDERATIONS 5-1

Milestones of Early Childhood (1–4 Years Old) *(Continued)*

Fine Motor

12–18 Months Old

Scribbles spontaneously

Builds tower of two blocks, then four blocks

Dumps raisins from container after demonstration, then spontaneously

May untie shoes

Uses opposable thumb well (prehension)

Shows preference for one hand or the other

Turns pages in a book

Uses spoon with frequent spills when getting food to mouth

18 Months to 2 Years Old

May remove articles of clothing

Holds pencil well enough for scribbling

Builds tower of four cubes

Imitates drawing a vertical line within 30 degrees

Turns doorknobs within reach

3–4 Years Old

Unbuttons large buttons

Builds tower of six to eight cubes

Can use a paintbrush

Imitates scribble

Copies a circle

Begins to wash and dry hands

Drinks from a cup

Can begin brushing teeth one to two times a day

Can take off socks and other easy-to-manipulate clothing

Snaps large snaps

Zips large zippers with help

Twists caps off bottles

Places simple shapes in correct holes

Will disassemble objects

Play

1–2 Years Old

Engages in parallel play

Imitates adult roles

Imitates housework

Will do simple household tasks

2–3 Years Old

Engages in parallel and associative play

Uses colors

Begins to play interactive games, such as tag

Plays with sand, clay, puzzles

Plays fantasy and make-believe

Plays action/ritualistic games such as tag or hide-and-seek

Cognitive

12–18 Months Old (Preoperational and Sensorimotor: Piaget)

Uses imitation to discover new ways of acting

Experiments to discover how objects behave and how they can be manipulated

18 Months to 2 Years Old (Sensorimotor: Piaget)

Concept of object permanency is fully achieved

Symbolic plane

Has a limited concept of time (no "tomorrow")

Is very egocentric

Talks to stuffed animals

Has imaginary playmates

Has a premature sense of cause/effect

Demonstrates goal-directed behavior

Believes death is reversible—a temporary restriction, departure, or sleep

Bedtime becomes very ritualistic

2–4 Years Old (Preoperational: Piaget)

Forms symbolic thought

Is egocentric in thoughts, feelings, and experiences

Understands instructions literally

Imitates others' behavior at later time

Social

12–18 Months Old

Responds to limit setting

18 Months to 4 Years Old

Attempts to please parents and conform to their expectations

Aware of family relationships and roles

Interpersonal

1–4 Years Old (Autonomy vs. Shame and Doubt: Erikson)

Differentiates between "good mother/bad mother" to "good me/bad me" or "not me"

Swings from love to hate

3–4 Years Old

Self-concept begins

Egocentric in thought and behavior

Emotional

1–2 Years Old

Shares emotions based on immediate needs (e.g., crying, screaming)

Learns how emotional reactions affect behavior of others

3–4 Years Old

Uses symbolic communication to convey ideas in terms of complex intentions

Explores different emotions in pretend play

Can communicate and comprehend emotions of self and others

Moral/Spiritual

1–4 Years Old

Moral: Stage 2: Preconventional Level (Kohlberg)

Detects concepts of fairness and sharing

Has an instrumental–relationistic orientation

Satisfies own needs

Is at a conventional level, beginning "good girl/nice boy"

Demonstrates approval-seeking behavior coupled with a desire to please

Spiritual: Stage 1: Intuitive/Projective (Fowler)

Learns to imitate the religious affect and behavior of parents

Mimics religious gestures, although does not comprehend meaning

Formulates own conceptions and explanations of faith and belief

Cannot separate feelings from intellect

Formulates imagined descriptions of God (angel—friend child can communicate with)

HYGIENE AND PERSONAL CARE

Children ages 1 to 4 years are still too young to manage their own hygiene and personal care needs. However, their inquisitive nature will ensure that they want to actively engage in learning new skills related to bathing, brushing their teeth, toileting, and dressing. The family will need to curb their child's enthusiasm and exploration only to the extent that a safe environment for learning is provided at all times. Young children should not complete hygiene and personal care activities beyond the watchful eyes or outside the reach of their family or caregivers. Adolescent siblings may help to monitor the activities of the young child; however, siblings of younger ages should not be given the responsibility for monitoring the safety of the child because their own lack of knowledge and experience will most likely prevent them from being able to anticipate hazards and prevent injury.

BATHING

The young child's increased activity level necessitates bathing daily or every other day. Bath water should be between 98.6° F or 37° C and 100.4° F or 38° C.

CHART 5-1 Quick Reference to Conditions Common During Early Childhood (1–4 Years Old)

Condition	Chapter
Autism	30: The Child With a Developmental or Learning Disorder
Breath-holding spells	21: The Child With Altered Neurologic Status
Bronchiolitis	16: The Child With Altered Respiratory Status
Child abuse	29: The Child With Mental Health Challenges
Cognitive challenge	30: The Child With a Developmental or Learning Disorder
Common cold (nasopharyngitis)	16: The Child With Altered Respiratory Status
Communicable diseases	24: The Child With an Infectious Disease
Conjunctivitis	28: The Child With Altered Sensory Status
Constipation	18: The Child With Altered Gastrointestinal Status
Croup	16: The Child With Altered Respiratory Status
Epiglottitis	16: The Child With Altered Respiratory Status
Hemolytic uremic syndrome	19: The Child With Altered Genitourinary Status
Intussusception	18: The Child With Altered Gastrointestinal Status
Laryngotracheobronchitis	16: The Child With Altered Respiratory Status
Lead poisoning	31: Pediatric Emergencies
Meningitis	21: The Child With Altered Neurologic Status
Munchausen syndrome by proxy	29: The Child With Mental Health Challenges
Nephrotic syndrome	19: The Child With Altered Genitourinary Status
Poisoning	31: Pediatric Emergencies
Premature thelarche	26: The Child With Altered Endocrine Status

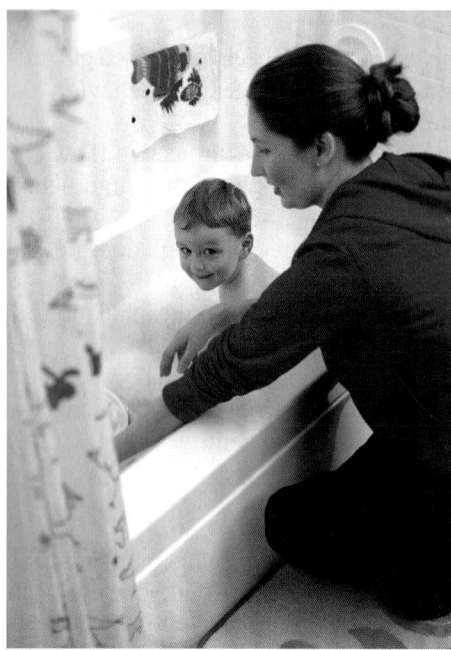

Figure 5-2 Bath time can be an enjoyable experience for the child, but safety is always a priority. Adults should closely monitor the child throughout the bath.

Wash the child's hair two to three times per week with a mild shampoo. Assess the child's scalp for scaly and crusty skin (seborrheic dermatitis) and the presence of lice or scabies. A good time to bathe the child is after eating, either after breakfast or in the evening. During the meal, the child may have spread food in the hair as well as all over his or her clothing. By the evening, the child is fairly dirty from a full day of play. Evening bath time provides an opportunity for cleansing and a way to relax the child in preparation for bedtime (Fig. 5-2).

A young child usually views bath time as another opportunity for play. However, some children may have fears associated with bathing, such as being afraid of being sucked down the drain. In this case, do not drain the tub until the child is out of the room. Use nonskid mats or gripping tape on the bottom of the tub to prevent the child from slipping. Provide plastic bath toys of appropriate size and without removable parts for water play. During rinsing of the hair, a washcloth placed over the child's eyes can prevent the shampoo from irritating the eyes. Bubble baths should be avoided to prevent urethral irritation and possible development of cystitis.

ALERT *The young child should never be left alone or be monitored by young siblings while bathing. Placing a young sibling in the bathtub with the child while the parent leaves the room does not guarantee the safety of either child (see Fig. 5-2).*

The young child is becoming more self-aware of body parts and spends time in the bath exploring his or her naked body and enjoying the unencumbered feeling of being without clothing. Young children usually have discovered their genitalia and may touch themselves frequently when the diaper or underpants are removed (Hagan et al., 2008). The child should not be punished for exploring the body in this fashion because such exploration is a normal part of development. Ask the parents in a nonjudgmental manner how they feel about this behavior and how they react to it. If the family is uncomfortable with this behavior, explain that it is normal and common among most children this age (see further discussion later in the chapter).

During bath time, caregivers should observe the condition of the child's skin and examine the symmetry of body parts. Any unusual findings should be reported to a health care provider. When examining a child, note especially bruises or other unusual marks around the genitalia and buttocks area. These marks may be signs of physical or sexual abuse.

ORAL CARE

QUESTION: Lanese calls the nurse at the pediatrician's office. She is frustrated with the struggle of putting the boys to bed. "Why can't I give them a bottle of milk to lie down with?" she asks. If you were the nurse in the office, what information could you share with her?

In early childhood, the child gains a full set of 20 primary teeth (see Fig. 3-21). While the teeth continue to erupt, the child may experience discomfort similar to that experienced during infancy when the teeth started to come in. Chewing food brings comfort to the child's gums, just as biting on a teething ring did for the infant. Drooling may increase when teeth are erupting.

It is recommended that the first oral examination occur at the eruption of the first tooth and no later than 12 months of age (American Academy of Pediatric Dentistry [AAPD], 2009). The dentist checks the child's mouth for placement of the teeth, notes any problems with initial eruption of the teeth, assesses the size of the jaw for future molars, and gives recommendations for follow-up visits and fluoride treatments. Also, the dentist educates the family about dental care, including toothbrushing technique and dietary guidelines to prevent caries. The first trip to the dentist should be a nonthreatening experience. Pediatric dentists are very sensitive to the needs and fears of children and usually go very slowly, allowing the child to become familiar with the equipment and procedures.

KidKare Children's books that have stories about trips to both the doctor and the dentist are good tools to help the child prepare for the visit. After the visit, the books can be read again to compare the child's experience with that discussed in the story and allow the child to verbalize feelings about the visit.

Many types of toothpaste have been developed just for children, made with appealing colors and flavors. A potential problem with these toothpastes is that the flavors are so good that the child wants to swallow the paste or eat the paste off the brush rather than brush with it. The effectiveness of fluoride in the toothpaste used by children and adolescents has been reviewed (Tradition or Science 5-1). The AAPD (2012a) recommends a "smear" of fluoridated toothpaste in children younger than 2 years of age and a "pea-size" amount of fluoridated toothpaste be used on children aged 2 to 5 years. Toothpaste should be kept out of reach so that the child does not try to eat the paste directly from the tube.

Help young children brush their teeth using a child-sized soft toothbrush and a pea-sized amount of toothpaste. Young children do not possess the manual dexterity needed to brush their own teeth effectively. Although the parent still must assume complete responsibility for dental hygiene, encouraging the

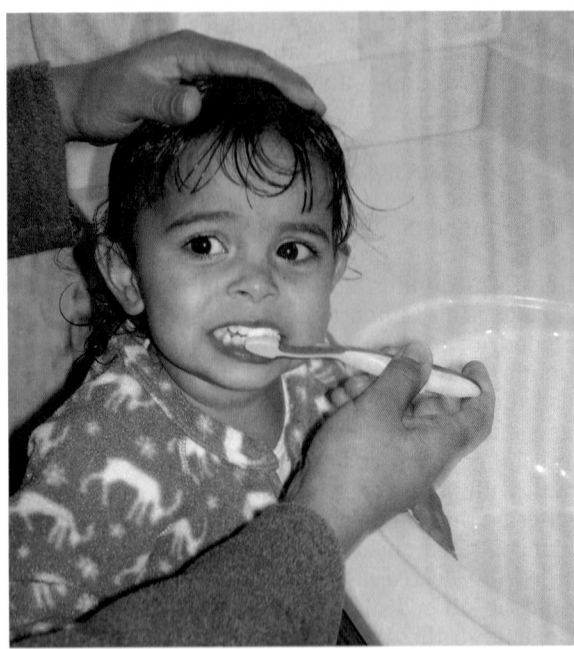

Figure 5-3 To promote good oral hygiene, encourage the child to brush his or her teeth once in the morning and once in the evening.

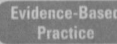

TRADITION OR SCIENCE 5-1

Is fluoride in toothpaste good for children?

When young children brush their teeth, it is not uncommon for them to swallow some, if not all, of the toothpaste they use when brushing. Despite parental supervision, it's challenging for the child to remember to spit out the paste, and not swallow it, on a frequent basis. There is concern that the use of fluoride toothpaste that contains 1,000–1,500 ppm of fluoride may cause enamel fluorosis of the teeth. With fluorosis, the teeth begin to appear marred by discoloration or brown markings; over time, the enamel may be pitted, rough, and hard to clean.

Because of these concerns, many manufacturers have made available a low fluoride children's or pediatric toothpaste that contains less than 600 ppm fluoride. Although this level of fluoride helps to reduce the problem of enamel fluorosis, it does not serve to prevent caries in children. Systematic reviews have revealed that there are benefits of using fluoride toothpaste in preventing caries in children and adolescents compared with placebo, but this result was only statistically significant at fluoride concentrations of 1,000 ppm and above; with higher fluoride concentration, the preventative effect of the fluoride toothpaste is enhanced (Rasines, 2010; Walsh et al., 2010).

It is clear then that achieving an appropriate fluoride level in toothpaste for preventing cavities places the young child at risk for fluorosis. However, the benefits associated with preventing caries outweigh the risk for developing fluorosis. The AAPD (2012a) recommends using standard fluoridated toothpaste (1,000 ppm), having the family caregiver carefully monitor the amount of toothpaste used by the child at each brushing (a pea-size amount for children aged 2–5 years), and encouraging the child to spit frequently during brushing and rinse thoroughly at the end in order to minimize fluoride ingestion.

child to participate in this routine develops good habits (Fig. 5-3). A good starting point is to brush in front of a mirror or allow the child to sit with his or her head in the parent's lap so the parent can brush the child's teeth and then have the child "brush" the parent's teeth. The easiest technique to teach at this age is the horizontal brushing technique. As the child matures, a more sophisticated up-and-down technique can be taught. The child's teeth should be brushed at least twice daily. After the child has had the opportunity to brush, the parent should finish brushing to ensure that all areas of the mouth are cleansed. Flossing may be introduced at this time, although the child does not have the manual dexterity to accomplish flossing and thus needs a parent's assistance.

Even in communities with fluoridated water, dentists may recommend fluoride treatments or fluoride supplements according to the level of fluoride in the drinking water and the amount of water the child ingests each day. Water sources that should be evaluated include municipal water supplies, wells, and commercial and home-system processed water (Holt et al., 2011). If community water is not fluoridated or is fluoride deficient (<0.3 ppm), the health care provider can prescribe fluoride supplementation, treating the child until approximately 3 years of age (AAPD, 2009, 2012b). Supplementation can be provided via solution or chewable tablets (for the older child). Monitor the use of fluoride supplements because excessive ingestion of fluoride can cause **fluorosis**, a condition characterized by staining of the teeth. Also monitor young children to prevent them from swallowing excessive amounts of fluoridated toothpaste.

If the enamel of a child's tooth is impaired, the dentist may recommend coating the child's teeth with a plastic occlusal sealant to prevent tooth decay. Although the procedure is entirely painless, it does require the child's cooperation; thus, attempting to coat the teeth of a young child may not be successful.

Early childhood caries (see Chapter 4) continue to be a concern at this age. When a child is put to bed with milk or juice in a bottle or sippy cup and does not rinse the teeth, the sugars in the milk or juice settle on the teeth for the night and promote development of caries. Discuss this concern with the family and remind them of the risk. Monitoring the amount of sweets that the child eats is also important. Fresh fruits and vegetables are good for healthy teeth, but candy is a real culprit in tooth decay. If children do eat sweets, they should brush their teeth immediately afterward to remove the sugars and prevent them from remaining in the mouth. If brushing is not feasible, they can at least rinse the mouth with plain water.

Offering the child a low-cariogenic diet, which is low in concentrated sugars and high-carbohydrate snacks, will help to decrease the incidence of cavities. Sweets should be offered after a meal because they are less cariogenic to the teeth if eaten then than if eaten between meals. Cleaning a child's teeth after sweets are eaten at the end of the meal is easier (and more likely to be done) than trying to brush them both after meals and after snacks. Foods that are hard and sticky are more cariogenic because they stay in the mouth and coat the teeth longer than soft, nonsticky foods. Eating a piece of hard candy is more damaging to the teeth than eating a candy bar. Advise the family which foods are healthiest for the teeth so that they can incorporate those suggestions into the child's diet.

> *ANSWER:* Make sure Lanese understands that when children fall asleep with milk in their mouth, the sugars in the milk sit on the teeth and eat away at the teeth. Ask if she has ever seen young children with rotten teeth. Explain that this is usually from falling asleep with a bottle and is called *early childhood caries*.

SLEEP

The active and exuberant young child requires adequate sleep each day. The exact amount and pattern of a child's daily sleep varies based on temperament, activity levels, and overall health. The 1- to 3-year-old spends approximately 12 to 14 hours per day sleeping. This time is slowly tapered to 11 to 13 hours a day for the 3- to 5-year-old. Around the age of 4 years, many children discontinue the afternoon nap. Children 1 to 4 years of age should sleep through the night without any need for a nighttime feeding. There is no "magic hour" at which the child should be placed in bed for the night. Eight o'clock in the evening is a reasonable time that allows family caregivers to have some time to themselves before they retire for the evening. Most adults gauge bedtime based on their own routines: Adults who like to retire very late often enjoy having their children stay awake until 10 or 11 PM. When the parents must rise early to take the children to daycare,

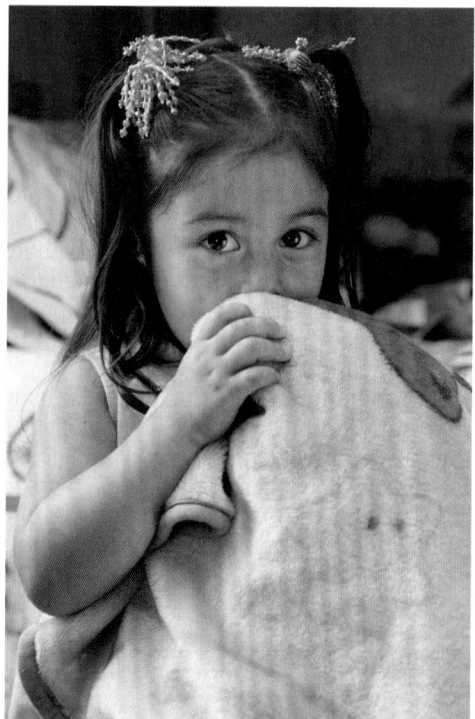

Figure 5-4 This young child finds security and comfort in her favorite blanket.

however, managing a late night–early morning schedule deprives the child of some much-needed hours of sleep. Families need to help the child establish good sleep hygiene at an early age. Sleep hygiene includes a regular sleep schedule, healthy sleep habits, an environment conducive to sleep, and physiologic practices conducive to sleep (e.g., the timing of activities such as exercise and engaging in media related activities) (Moore, 2012). Young children need a bedtime routine such as bathing, reading a story, getting a kiss goodnight, having a favorite toy or security object such as a blanket or teddy bear placed next to them, and then having the main lights turned off. Rowdy play should be avoided close to bedtime because it tends to excite the child and makes it more difficult to get the child to bed, let alone to sleep. Many children like a night-light. A routine enables children to know what will happen next and gives them a sense of security. After the routine is established, the child is less resistant to bedtime (Fig. 5-4).

Sleep Disturbances

Disturbances of sleep impact approximately 30% of all children (Moore, 2012). These disturbances may lead to emotional, cognitive, behavioral, and physical problems for the young child. Poor sleep has also been associated with health issues, such as obesity, in children and adolescents (Arens & Muzumdar, 2010). Sleep disturbances may be related to poor sleep hygiene (previously described), night terrors, nightmares, and pathophysiologic or primary insomnia (Moore, 2012). The child with persistent sleep problems should be referred to a health care provider, with an interdisciplinary approach to assessment and management of care to assist the child and his or her family.

It is not uncommon for young children to have night terrors or nightmares. **Night terrors** occur during the early hours of sleep. The child does not fully awaken and rarely remembers the night terror in the morning. For night terrors, instruct the family to let these episodes take their course while providing a safe environment and making sure the child does not harm himself or herself in any way. They should not interact with the child because the child will not have any understanding of who or what is around him or her. Because full consciousness has not been reached, the child may interpret a helpful action as a harmful one and may strike out or hurt himself or herself during the process.

Nightmares occur during the second half of sleep. The child awakes afraid, has difficulty falling back to sleep, and usually remembers the episode in the morning (Richardson, 2006). Nightmares are common during early childhood because of the child's active imagination and increased dream state. Although an occasional nightmare is normal, an increase in the number of nightmares can be a response to stress or to the child being anxious about something. Other triggers can be a change in normal routine, such as moving, starting a new school, or a death or divorce in the family. Nightmares may also be a response to a violent or scary movie, television show, video or online game, or story.

When the child has an occasional nightmare, the family should reassure the child that it was just a dream and was not real. Giving lots of hugs and words of reassurance can be supportive. The child may want the parent to search the room to ensure that there are no monsters about. Advise the family to wait until the next morning to talk about the details of the dream, at which time the child should be calmer. The parent should try to determine whether there was a specific event or stressor that may have triggered the nightmare. To help decrease nightmares, families should also avoid having the child engage in media related activities in the hour before bedtime, avoid telling scary bedtime stories, let the child sleep with a night-light, and examine how to decrease perceived stress in the child's life.

Naps

Naps continue to be an essential component of the young child's daily routine. Until about the 16th month of age, the child generally takes two naps a day—one in the morning and one in the afternoon—each of which lasts about 2 hours. Between the 16th and 20th month of age, the morning nap is usually eliminated, leaving one afternoon nap that lasts 1 to 3 hours. All children are different. Some might still want and need an afternoon nap, whereas others just need an afternoon rest period to reenergize. Many children resist ceasing all play activities, but after quiet time has been imposed, these same children are often the first to fall asleep. For the child who will not sleep, an extended period of quiet activity, such as looking at books, can be beneficial as a structured period of rest before the busy activities of the

evening, when all the family members gather at home. Nap time should be set at a consistent time each day. The afternoon nap will benefit the child most when taken after lunch and when completed before 3 or 4 PM. This allows at least 3 hours between the nap and evening bedtime. Naps taken later in the afternoon and extending past 4 PM might cause problems when the child is then unable to fall asleep at the regular bedtime hour (Mindell & Owens, 2009). In many daycare centers and preschools, the afternoon nap period is continued because a great number of children can still benefit from a scheduled period of rest in the middle of the day. During this time, many preschoolers do not actually sleep but are encouraged to remain on a mat or blanket, quietly playing, to develop the ability to relax or unwind from the tension of the day's activities.

CLOTHING

During early childhood, the child begins to participate in dressing and undressing. Participation may begin with the child simply lifting a foot to have a shoe put on or learning to slip an arm in a sleeve hole. By age 3 years, the child is able to undress without assistance (except for removing shoes) and may be able to put on most simple pieces of clothing (Fig. 5-5). Clothes should be easy for the child to put on (e.g., shirts with large neck openings and pants made of stretchy fabrics). Velcro closures on shoes and clothes are easier for the young child than buttons, zippers, snaps, and shoelaces. Items that close in the back should be avoided. Also avoid clothes with drawstrings because drawstrings can get

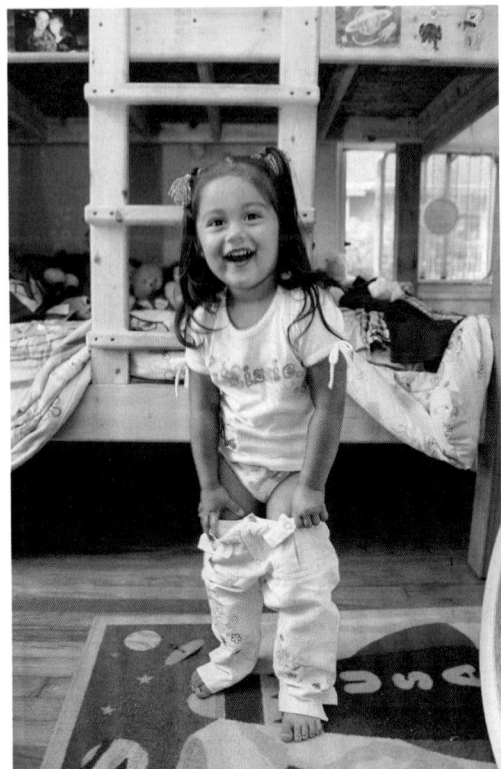

Figure 5-5 This young child is proud of her ability to dress herself.

caught on furniture or playground equipment and can lead to strangulation. When drawstrings are present in pants, jackets, and hoods, they should be cut out. Sleepwear should be flame retardant.

The child often chooses clothes based on visual appeal, regardless of whether the socks match or if layering a skirt over pants looks appropriate. Family members can support and encourage the child's participation in the selection of his or her daily clothing choices, with adults ensuring that the clothes are appropriate for the weather and activity variables that will impact the child's movement, comfort, and safety. The order in which clothing is put on is very confusing to young children, so the caregiver can help the child by placing the clothes out in the order in which they are to be put on. Shoes need to be fitted correctly and checked periodically for fit. At this age, the child may grow out of shoes faster than any other clothing item. Shoes are needed to prevent injury and provide warmth. However, wearing no shoes should also be encouraged. Allowing a child to walk barefoot on a variety of (safe) surfaces promotes proper development of ligaments and muscles and helps the child learn correct balance. Providing the child with warm, loose fitting, nonslip socks or booties will help keep the feet warm.

TOILET LEARNING

 QUESTION: Lanese calls the nurse about toilet learning. "Shawanda was so good about pee-peeing in the potty, but those boys don't care if they wear a wet diaper for hours." Review Nursing Interventions 5-1. What pertinent information can you share with Lanese?

As the child approaches the second birthday, the family may start thinking about toilet learning (Fig. 5-6). *Toilet learning* is the term used to describe the process in which the child is involved in his or her own learning about how to control his or her body functions and use the toilet. *Toilet training* has been the term most commonly

associated with these practices; however, this term implies a more adult-directed process based on adult expectations and attitudes of developmental milestones that must be achieved on a certain timeline. The key to toilet learning is the readiness of the child. Caregivers usually find that the older child (2 to 3 years old) is more interested in pursuing toilet learning.

The stages of toilet learning (Hayward, 2013) are described as

Stage 1: *Toilet Play*
- Pretends to toilet, usually with clothes on
- Observes others going to the bathroom
- Shows an interest in the toilet

Stage 2: *Toilet Practice*
- Practices flushing
- Practices pulling pants up and down
- Practices getting on and off the toilet
- Practices squatting and standing
- Practices handwashing
- Responds correctly when asked if diaper is wet or dry, clean or dirty

Stage 3: *Toilet Learning*
- Shows interest in wearing "real" underwear
- Feels the need to urinate by showing gestures, is verbal, or uses facial expressions
- Hold urine for longer periods of time
- Acquires the desire to be clean
- Has words for using the toilet and tells you when he or she has to go
- Can pull pants up and down for themselves
- Stands and sits well on his or her own
- Shows signs of pushing and concentration when he or she is ready for a bowel movement
- Tells you he or she is soiled or wet and needs to be changed

Stage 4: *Independent Toileting*
- Completes tasks of toileting independently, although will require some assistance wiping after bowel movement

Toilet learning may occur at the age of 2 years but more commonly is seen at 2½ to 3 years of age (Graham & Uphold, 2003). Daytime control is usually achieved before nighttime control. Bowel control is usually completely achieved by age 3 years. Even after toilet learning has been successful, accidents are common. Predictors of early completion of toilet learning noted by researchers include early initiation, female gender, non-white race, and single-parent families (Wald et al., 2009). Bed-wetting (nocturnal enuresis) and constipation are common problems in this age group. Bed-wetting is seen more frequently in boys and those who are deep sleepers. If a child continues to wet the bed after age 7 years, or if infection or anatomic abnormalities are suspected, referral to a health care provider is needed (Hagan et al., 2008). Constipation can make toilet learning more difficult, or it may be the result of resistance to toilet learning by the child. Studies gauging the frequency of constipation in children have found varying perceptions by parents based on the geographic location and cultural background of

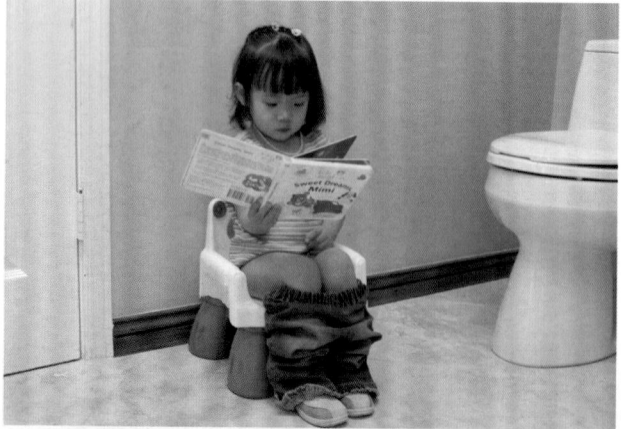

Figure 5-6 The young child might be encouraged to sit on the potty chair by using books to keep her still.

the family (Wald et al., 2009). See Chapter 18 for more information about constipation; Chapter 19 provides for information about enuresis. If parents are concerned about their child's bladder and bowel routines or unusual changes in these routines, they should contact their health care provider.

Strategies to promote successful toilet learning are presented in Nursing Interventions 5-1. When the child is learning to use the toilet, it is important to ensure good hygiene. Ensure the child washes his or her hands after all toilet attempts (whether or not successful). Teach young girls to wipe from front to back to prevent

NURSING INTERVENTIONS 5-1

Promoting Toilet Learning

To support toilet learning, encourage family members and caregivers to:

Communication
- Explain to the child you will be taking him or her to the toilet and what will happen.
- Give encouragement and positive reinforcement for trying to use the toilet.
- Let the child be in charge of as much of the process as possible. Tell him or her to let you know when he or she has to go.
- Use appropriate vocabulary for body parts and functions.
- Give simple answers to questions without making the child feel embarrassed or ashamed for asking.
- Use positive encouraging phrases like "You did it," "Way to go," "Good for you," etc.
- Ask the child gently if he or she needs to use the toilet throughout the day.
- Cue children as adults toilet, "I'll be back, my body tells me I have to use the toilet."
- Underreact to accidents and approach accidents as opportunities for the child to learn how to clean up and get dressed. Be warm and supportive and refrain from shaming, threatening, or punishing the child for having an accident.
- Avoid using words like "dirty," "naughty," or "stinky." These negative terms can make the child feel ashamed and self-conscious.

Toilet Use
- Encourage the child to sit on the toilet for the amount of time for a short period of time. Do not insist a child remain on the toilet longer than 5–7 minutes. The child may develop an association of unpleasantness with the bathroom.
- Turn on the water to use as a stimulus to urinate during early toilet learning.
- Provide a potty chair for learning and/or a step stool to use the toilet. Let the child use whichever

he or she prefers. Remember, he or she needs to feel comfortable.
- Give the child a book to read to relax while sitting on the toilet or save special books for the child to read just for when he or she is sitting on the toilet.
- Talk about the items in the bathroom and what they do (e.g., toilet, sink, soap dispenser, toilet paper).

Role Modeling and Anticipatory Guidance
- Let the child watch a parent or sibling urinate to help him or her visually learn.
- Read books with the child about toilet learning.
- Make up a song as encouragement.
- Pretend to be something or dance while going into the bathroom (e.g., bird, lion, airplane).
- Begin a routine of handwashing after each visit to the toilet.
- Postpone toilet learning if the child does not seem to catch on or does not seem interested.
- Monitor the child's fluid intake, especially before bedtime.
- Focus on the progress.
- Avoid using food or other treats as a bribe or taking away privileges.
- Avoid comparing the child to other children and their progress in toilet learning.

Clothing
- Introduce the child to underwear and show him or her yours.
- Let the child pick out "real" underwear. He or she may have a favorite character like Barbie, Dora, Batman, Spiderman, Bob the Builder, etc.
- Dress the child in easy-to-remove clothing so as to avoid getting clothes wet or having to change his or her clothes frequently. Sweatpants are the best.
- Change the child's clothes as soon as possible if they become wet or soiled.

Information used with permission from Hayward, K. (2013). *The four stages of toilet learning*. Retrieved from http://www.niu.edu/ccc /resources/ToiletTraining2.pdf bacteria form the anus to be transferred to the vaginal area. Assist the child to wipe the anal area as needed to ensure cleanliness; when accidents occur, ensure the child's clothing is changed as soon as possible.

> **ANSWER:** Determining the child's physical readiness for toilet learning includes the child's recognition that he or she has just voided or defecated. Determining the psychosocial readiness includes the child expressing an interest in toilet learning. To prevent Lanese from becoming overly frustrated, it is important that she understands that children are ready for toilet learning at different ages, and the boys just might not be ready yet. The nurse's role is to share the signs of readiness with the parent.

NUTRITION

> **QUESTION:** Lanese wants to know whether it is normal for the boys to have such strong opinions about their food. Give an example of an appropriate response. How can you further assess the boys' eating habits, and what information can you share that may improve the boys' nutritional intake and eating habits?

By the first birthday, the young child should have already started eating solid food. Because the rapid growth rate of infancy has slowed, the young child needs fewer calories per day (1,100 to 1,550 cal/day) than needed in infancy. After gaining 3 to 4 lb every 2 to 3 months during the first year, the child now gains an average of 4.5 to 6.5 lb per year and grows 2.5 to 3.5 in. per year (Patrick et al., 2001).

Introduce the child to a schedule revolving around three meals per day, with snacks midmorning and midafternoon. The young child's stomach is small, so frequent, small meals are appropriate. The diet should consist of the five basic food groups, with a variety of foods with different textures and tastes. The U.S. Department of Agriculture (USDA) recommends the use of an easy-to-follow food guide icon called MyPlate as a template for helping families select nutritious meals for children (Fig. 5-7).

Before the age of 2 years, fat is needed for brain development and should not be restricted unless the child has an underlying medical condition, such as diabetes. Avoid "diet" food and drinks (e.g., nonfat milk, diet soda). After the age of 2 years, high-fat foods should be gradually restricted so that by 5 years of age, the child is consuming no more than 30% to 35% of his or her daily calories from fat (Gidding et al., 2006).

Because the family and other caregivers choose which foods to feed the child and role-model food practices, teaching about nutritious foods is an important role for nurses. For example, one study found that mothers who consumed more than 12 fl oz of soft drinks per day were nearly four times as likely to have a child with poor dietary intake and high average intakes of milk, fruit juice, and sweetened beverages (Hoerr et al., 2006). Teach the

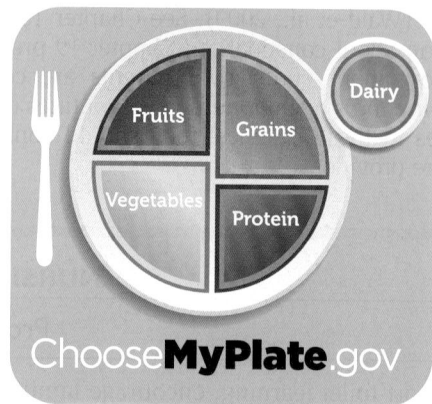

Figure 5-7 MyPlate illustrates the proportions of the five food groups that are considered the building blocks for a healthy diet.

family that young children should have the same foods that the rest of the family is eating but in portions about one fourth of the amount an adult would be served. Foods offered to the child should be of high nutrient density so that the child develops good eating habits. Good eating habits and food preferences developed early will help prevent chronic health conditions such as type 2 diabetes, heart disease, and obesity, which result in part from poor eating habits. Avoid fruit drinks, flavored milk, and sodas; encourage drinking water for thirst. Heavily spiced or salted foods should be avoided because young children may not find them palatable.

A 1- to 2-year-old has not yet mastered the use of the spoon or fork; therefore, finger foods are highly recommended. A plastic mat placed underneath a high chair and use of bibs help contain some of the mess the child makes as hands are used to experiment with food and attempts are begun to use the spoon. By 18 months of age, the child has enough control over the hands and fingers to navigate food to the mouth consistently using a spoon (Carruth et al., 2004) (Fig. 5-8). Child-sized utensils are offered for use to the 3- and 4-year-old, such as chunky handled spoons and forks that fit his or her hands; allow the child to feed himself or herself. Age-appropriate foods include those that enable the preschooler to perfect these newly developed skills. Finger foods such as diced fruit, steamed diced vegetables, shredded cheese, or cereals are ideal for the young child. Foods should be mashed or cut into small pieces to prevent choking.

caREminder

To prevent a young child from choking, never give small, hard foods such as peanuts or hard candies. Even soft, small foods such as grapes could be a hazard. For example, steamed or cooked carrots and hot dogs should be cut in half lengthwise and then quartered to prevent choking.

Young children are at risk for choking because of the small size of their airways, poor chewing ability, and a tendency to put things in the mouth. To prevent choking, adults should stay with a child who is eating

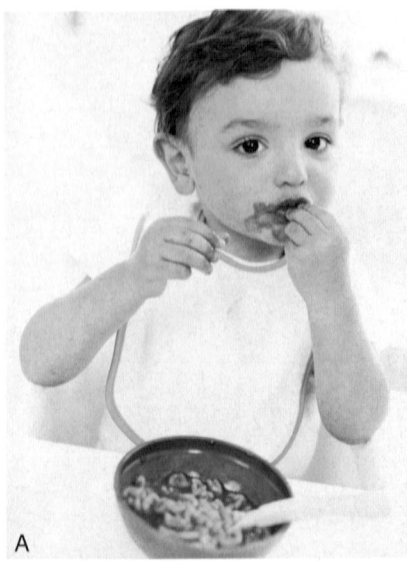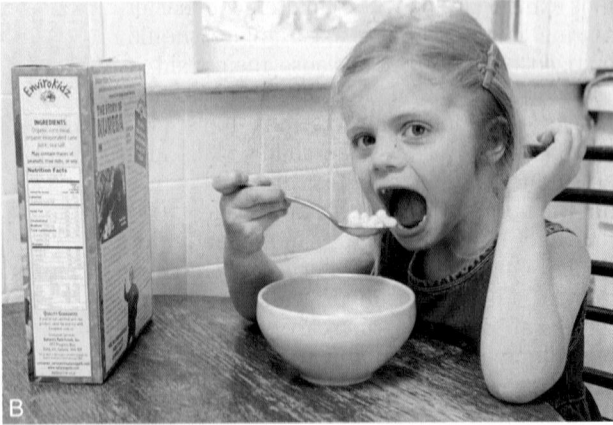

Figure 5-8 (A) This young child enjoys feeding himself. Self-feeding allows the child to investigate the different textures and tastes of foods. (B) As the child matures, she develops the manual dexterity to handle utensils.

to help monitor how much food is placed in the mouth at one time. The young child should always sit while eating and not be allowed to walk or run while chewing food. In addition, keeping children calm at mealtime can minimize the risk of choking caused by overexcitement.

At 1 year of age, the child can begin drinking whole cow's milk instead of formula or breast milk. Some mothers may continue breastfeeding to provide some or all of the child's nutritional requirements for milk. A young child should receive at least two servings of milk and other dairy products a day and take milk primarily from a cup. More than 16 oz of milk per day will interfere with the amount of solid food that a child can eat and can also contribute to iron-deficiency anemia. During young childhood, iron-rich foods (e.g., meats, fish, and poultry), iron-fortified cereals, and foods that contain vitamin C should be consumed to enhance iron absorption (Holt et al., 2011). Iron supplements may also be needed to ensure that the child is receiving adequate iron.

ALERT *Instruct the family to store iron supplements out of reach of children and to reinforce that they are medicine, not candy, because some preparations look like candy.*

Mealtimes can become a power struggle between caregivers and the young child. Reassure caregivers that young children go through periods during which they are very particular about food. **Food jags**, periods when a child will eat only a few foods, may occur. Young children also begin to be attracted by the color, smell, and shape of food. Foods that look like or smell like other foods they enjoy are most likely to be eaten. Never force a child to eat. Children may resist trying new foods, and 10 to 15 attempts may be necessary before a child will

try a new food. When introducing a new food, the caregiver can encourage the child to taste it or combine a new food with an old favorite. Adults should not assume that initial refusal of a new food represents a permanent dislike and thus label the child as a picky eater. The child will have personal likes and dislikes, as all individuals do, but these may change. The food should be offered again in a few days; if the child is not forced to eat it, often it will be accepted. If the child consistently refuses a particular food or food group, one can become creative. For instance, if the child refuses to eat raw apples, steaming, baking, or grating them onto a plate with a dip are alternative ways to serve the snack. Do not negotiate what the child eats, reward the child with treats, or threaten punishment. Mealtimes should be nonstressful but not "play" times. Family mealtimes enable the parents to role-model healthy eating behaviors and also promote social interaction (Gidding et al., 2006). Children and adolescents who have three or more shared family meals per week are more likely to be within a normal weight range and have healthy dietary and eating patterns (Hammons & Fiese, 2011). Meals or snacks, therefore, should not be eaten while watching television or as a solitary dining experience.

ANSWER: When Lanese asks about the boys' food preferences, you might respond, "It is common for young children to choose a taste or a color of food for a time." Assess specific information by asking, "What do the boys eat during a typical day?" Another tactic is to ask, "What did the boys have yesterday for each meal and snacks?" Young children need small quantities of all the food groups. Be sure that Lanese has an understanding of MyPlate and that she is offering the boys a variety of foods at each meal. Reassure her that it is okay for J. D. to have a small serving of macaroni and cheese often if he is also eating fruits, vegetables, and meats.

PHYSICAL FITNESS

Activities for the young child are selected based on emerging cognitive, linguistic, and fine and gross motor skills. Many variations exist regarding when children will master these skills during the preschool years. Families should not be discouraged or concerned because their child is not reading or coloring within the lines like another child of the same age. Developmental screening tools (see Chapter 3) can be used to assess the child's skills and to provide reassurance to the family that the child is performing within the normal range for his or her age.

At 1 year of age, mastery of gross motor activities takes precedence. One of the major accomplishments of the second year of life is learning to walk. By 2 years of age, the child is able to walk, run, carry several large objects while walking, and go up and down stairs. This accomplishment occurs over several months, beginning with the child placing the feet far apart for a wide base of support and using the hands and arms for balance. Toddlers often "cruise" furniture, using tables, sofas, and chairs as crutches to assist with their balancing act. Falls are frequent at this stage, and the family must be aware of sharp table edges that may cause injury to the child and of small wrinkles in carpets or rugs that could cause the child to fall. As gross motor skills become more developed, the child will be interested in a riding a tricycle, kicking a ball, and playing running games.

Fine motor skills are also being perfected. At 1 year of age, using a pincer grasp to pick up small items (between thumb and forefinger) is still very difficult. As the child matures during the second year, these fine motor skills become easier. The child's fine motor skills are developed enough to color with crayons, turn pages in books, and operate small toys that produce action or sounds. Because attention spans are still short, young children need a wide variety of objects to play with and touch; they prefer objects that make noise in response to playing and touching them. Filling containers with objects and dumping them out, stacking blocks and knocking them over, scribbling, and painting are favorite activities at this age (Fig. 5-9). Games that also teach spatial concepts such as under, in, over, and so on, help the child develop skills. The cause-and-effect mechanisms of mechanical toys give 2-year-olds a sense of accomplishment; something happens because they cause it to happen. All toys still need to meet the appropriate safety standards.

PLAY

Play is critical to the child's social and emotional development, helping the child to learn to get along well with others. Although there may seem to be a push to increase academics in early childhood education settings, the value of play in developing the child's ability to communicate and enhance other developmental skills should not be overlooked (Ashiabi, 2007). Play activities enhance the child's cognitive development (e.g., understanding cause and effect, problem solving), self-expression in the creative arts (e.g., music, art, drama), fine and gross motor development (e.g., hand–eye coordination, large muscle coordination), language development

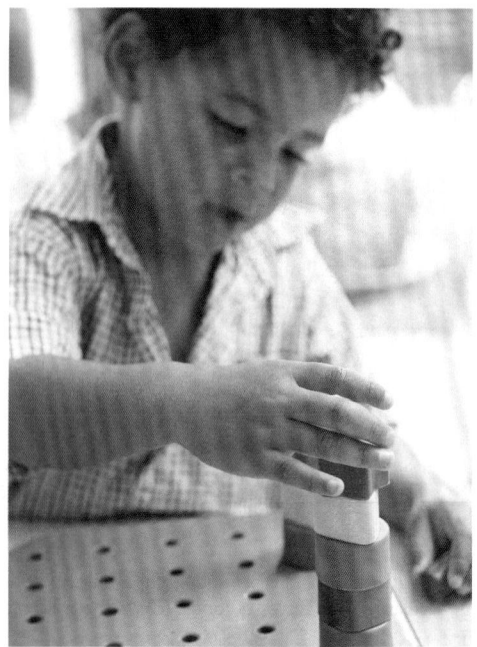

Figure 5-9 Activities such as stacking blocks help the young child refine their fine motor skills.

(e.g., communication, vocal play), sensory awareness, and social–emotional development (Moore, 2011).

The play interactions of an infant occur primarily between the adult family members and the infant. As the infant matures into early childhood and becomes more social, play interaction with peers evolves into several different types of play styles (Fig. 5-10). **Onlooker play** is when the child observes the actions of other children and does not attempt to interact with them. **Solitary play** is when a child plays alone, absorbed in an activity and uninterested in the play of other children. **Parallel play** occurs when children play with similar toys, beside other children, but are not influenced by other children's play activities. The child may have an identical toy but may play with it in a different manner. **Associative play** occurs when children are playing together in a group without organization or leadership; however, they may share materials or follow one another. For example, two children draw pictures, share paper and crayons, and discuss what they are drawing, but neither suggests that they draw the same thing. When the play is organized, with a leader–follower type of relationship established, it is considered **cooperative play**.

The young child participates in onlooker, solitary, and parallel play. Piaget described the development of play as two stages: **Practice play** occurs between the ages of 2 and 18 months. This is followed by **symbolic play**, which occurs between the ages of 18 months and 4 years. During the practice play period, the infant or young child engages in a variety of sensorimotor activities such as using the hands to repeatedly push, knock, or bat at an object. As time passes, the child tries out the same patterns of action on different objects, begins to define objects by their use, and begins to relate one object to another (Casby, 2003). During the period of

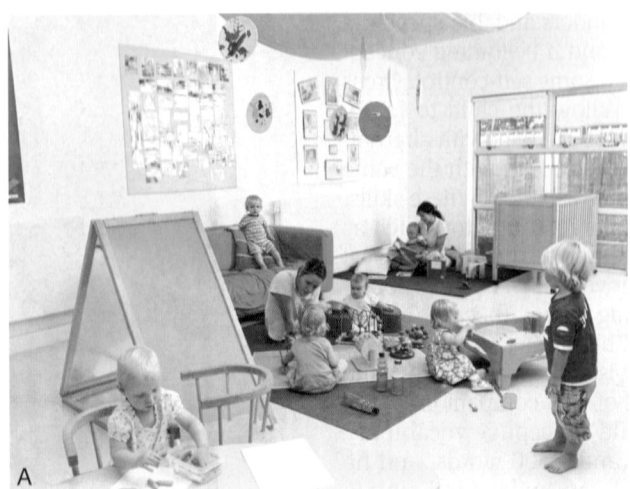

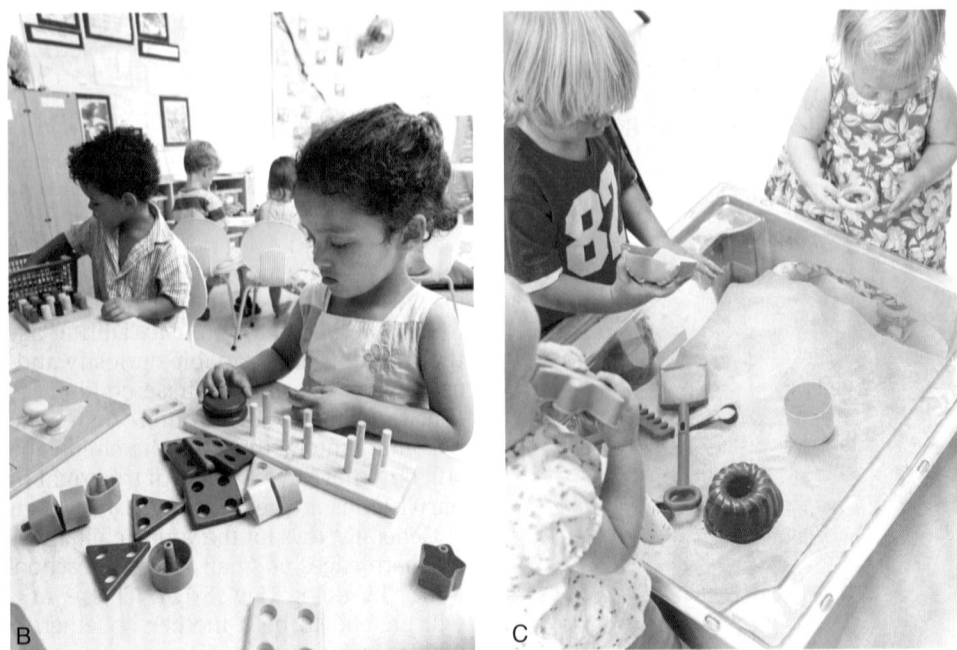

Figure 5-10 (A) Young children (e.g., the boy in the red shirt) participate in onlooker play. (B) During parallel play, children may play side by side but do not influence each other's play activities. (C) During associative play, children play together, although there is no specific organization to, nor leader guiding, their activities.

symbolic play, the child transitions from sensorimotor schemes to mental operations. During this type of play, children apply a familiar action pattern they have previously applied to themselves to other people and objects. For example, the child may take food and feed the parent. As symbolic play progresses, the child begins to demonstrate the ability to anticipate outcomes and to adapt actions accordingly (Casby, 2003).

Play activities may occur both indoors and outdoors, with the ideal "playground" including products and designs that provide opportunities for children with physical, cognitive, social–emotional, communicative, and sensory disabilities to engage in play with their peers (Moore, 2011). In addition, play opportunities should include age-mixed play, that is, play that involves children of various ages. Gray (2011) asserts that children learn more from older playmates than they can from same-age peers.

In age-mixed settings, older peers are allowed to role-model positive behaviors to younger children and practice nurturing and leadership skills. Younger children often help to inspire the imagination and creativity of older friends and can learn new skills from those in their age-mixed group.

KidKare Childress (2011) reviewed studies that involved the play of preschool children with disabilities. The author noted that play interactions affected both the parent and the child and provided positive contributions to the child's language, cognitive, and social development, affecting joint attention, toy manipulation, and child verbalizations. Encourage parents to use play to engage their special needs child, learn more about his or her unique skills and abilities, and provide more positive experiences during daily caregiving interventions that may often seem mundane or stressful.

By age 3 years, the child has understandable speech, a vocabulary of about 900 words, and a beginning concept of time. He or she has also learned some self-control. Gross motor skills have developed to allow the child to jump, kick a ball, ride a tricycle, and walk up stairs with alternating steps, although the child may still lead with the same foot to come down stairs. Play must expand on these skills. The child should have a tricycle; large, sturdy toys such as big blocks; active toys like a pounding bench; and musical toys that encourage rhythmic movement. The preschooler also likes show-and-tell, guessing games (because his or her memory is improving), and big-pieced jigsaw puzzles (Fig. 5-11). At age 3 years, play is still egocentric, but the child is becoming more tolerant of play companions.

By the age of 4 years, the child's receptive vocabulary has expanded to between 900 and 1,500 words, and he or she uses full sentences and can understand simple analogies. The child is now able to jump on one foot, skip, walk down the stairs with alternating feet, and throw a ball overhand. The preschooler is able to use scissors well, and fine manual dexterity is improving. Construction toys, jigsaw puzzles, memory games, and

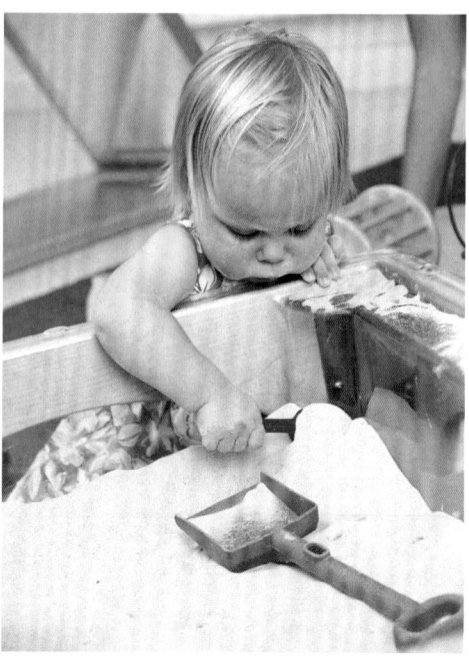

Figure 5-12 Young children are encouraged to use gross and fine motor skills in their play activity. This little worker is busy digging in sand.

fantasy play are favorites. The child will tell secrets and exaggerate stories. Children at this age love to listen to audible books and music. During ages 3 to 4 years, the child has an insatiable curiosity and will constantly ask "why" questions. These children are developing a sense of their world around them. Their play is now becoming interactive, and the child can obey limits but still does not have a sense of true right or wrong. Imaginary friends are very common among children this age.

Generally, toys for the young child must be sturdy, with no sharp edges or small pieces. Preschoolers learn many things by doing (Fig. 5-12). This is an age when they will pretend to be a mother or father, doctor or nurse, which is why pretend play and dress-up are so important. They have a lot of energy and, as their manual dexterity improves, they need large balls to bounce and tricycles to ride. Electric toys should be avoided unless they are battery operated and used under adult supervision only.

caREminder

Toys should always be chosen according to the child's age and size and should be checked often to be sure that they have not become broken or developed a dangerous, sharp edge. Children should not be allowed to place toys in their mouth nor should they run with toys that are large, easily breakable, or have sharp, accentuated borders or ends.

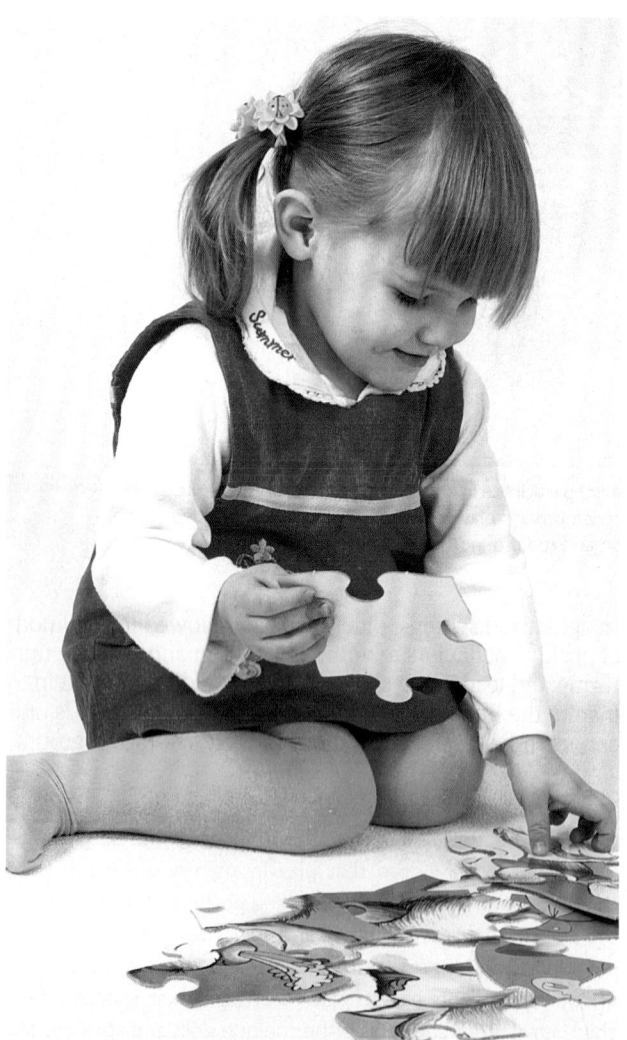

Figure 5-11 This young child enjoys playing with puzzles as she learns simple sequences and develops fine motor skills and good eye–hand coordination.

Exposing the child to a wide variety of interactions (playing alone, in peer groups, or with older children or adults), locations for play (home, friend's home, parks, libraries), and activities (structured, group, quiet, spontaneous) is beneficial. Because young children are very active, caregivers must be sure to provide enough physical space for play. Tactile exploration is important. Water tables,

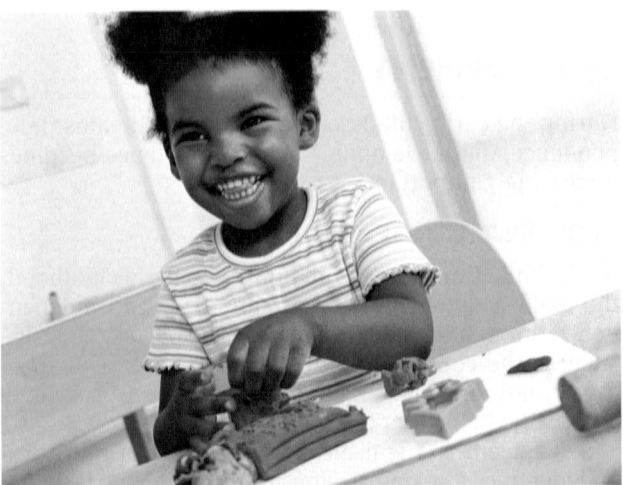

Figure 5-13 Playing with modeling clay allows for hands-on learning and tactile exploration.

sand, soap bubbles, and clay provide excellent opportunities for the child to explore different textures and to develop creativity (Fig. 5-13). Safety must always be considered, and toys must be appropriate, with no sharp edges.

Developing a healthy exercise habit during the child's early years to improve general well-being throughout life and to help prevent obesity is important. Caregivers should promote daily activity such as walking, running, riding a tricycle or bicycle, or playing with a ball (Fig. 5-14). Organized activities provided by qualified and experienced teachers, such as tumbling, gymnastics, and dancing, are recommended because these activities enhance balance and coordination (Patrick et al., 2001). Encourage the family to set an example by being active and encouraging parent–child activities.

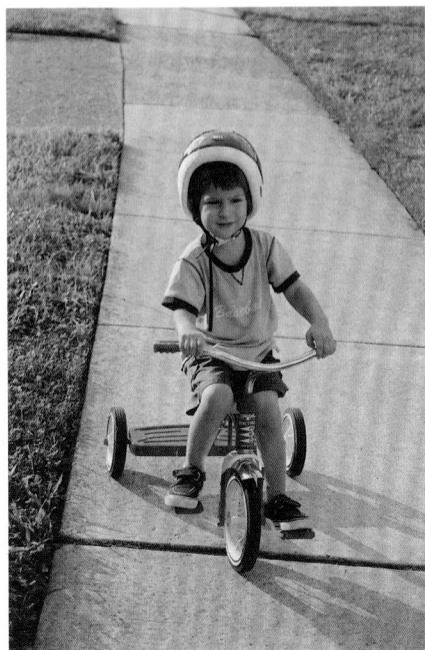

Figure 5-14 Young children love outdoor physical play, such as riding a tricycle. The child should always wear a proper safety helmet when riding a bike.

MEDIA USE

Many of today's television and other media-related programs are not appropriate for younger viewers (Shelov & Altmann, 2009). Young children believe that everything they see on TV or online is real. They may develop a distorted view of how to deal with problems because their favorite cartoon character uses violence as a method to cope with anger and frustration. Cartoons can contain much more violence than adult programming. Television and other media viewing can contribute to many psychological and physical problems because it lessens the child's creative ability and can undermine the capacity for independent thinking. Children who watch a great deal of television and engage in computer or internet gaming are also more likely than others to become obese (Shelov & Altmann, 2009). Tradition or Science 5-2 explores the impact of television on young children.

Evidence-Based Practice

TRADITION OR SCIENCE 5-2

Does television viewing have a negative impact on young children?

Providing the child (aged 1–12 years) with time during the day to watch television is one method to help the child calm down and allow caregivers time to attend to their personal activities. The deleterious effects of television viewing include weight gain, exposure to violence, and the development of attentional problems. Several studies have found a relationship in young children between television viewing and weight gain over time. That is, the more television that is viewed by the child, the greater the increase in body mass index (Jago et al., 2005; Proctor et al., 2003; Robinson, 1999; Saelens et al., 2002; van Zutphen et al., 2007). Christakis et al. (2004) found that the more television children viewed at young ages, the more likely they are to have attention problems at age 7 years. This finding has been debated by Miller et al. (2007), who also found a correlation between television exposure and attention-deficit/hyperactivity disorder (ADHD), yet could not conclude whether levels of television viewing were the cause or result of ADHD symptoms. Children watching greater amounts of television (more than 6 hours per week) have also been reported to have higher levels of violent behavior, higher levels of post-traumatic stress syndrome (after watching traumatic life events on television), and are more likely to engage in risk-taking behaviors than children who watch less television (Bernstein et al., 2007; Singer et al., 1998). Yet, these studies also question whether children with preexisting psychological or behavioral problems tend to watch more television than children without these problems.

In both Australia and the United States, it is recommended that television viewing should be discouraged in children younger than 2 years of age and should be limited to 1–2 hours per day for older children (AAP, 2011; Commonwealth of Australia, Department of Health and Ageing, 2004). More interactive activities, such as reading stories, talking, and singing, are encouraged to promote appropriate brain development. It is recognized that children's and adolescents' TV viewing time is influenced by family rules limiting the time spent watching TV and by family TV viewing (Barradas et al., 2007; Yalcin et al., 2002). Because of this, it is important to set rules to limit television viewing, monitor what is being viewed, and have adults role-model good television-viewing behaviors.

The American Academy of Pediatrics (AAP, 2011) advocates avoiding all forms of television and other entertainment media for children younger than age 2 years. Adults are encouraged to provide "media free" zones in the house where the child may play without the diversion of the television or other media device. Banning television and other forms of media completely from a child's life is quite difficult, but adults should monitor the child's media use carefully, including the amount of time spent with various media (e.g., television, computer, phones, gaming devices) and the content. Electronic monitors can be used to limit a child's TV watching. These monitors are installed between the TV set and the cable input or the antenna to prevent unauthorized watching. As a general rule, for children and teens, 1 to 2 hours of quality media viewing per day should be the limit (AAP, 2011). The caregiver should watch with the child to explain that commercials are advertisements, not a part of the program, and to talk with the child about the program and its message. This practice helps the child develop critical viewing skills and enables better choices about media programming when the child is older (Developmental Considerations 5-2). Early media exposure and watching for prolonged periods contributes to attention problems by 7 years of age (Christakis et al., 2004).

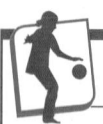

DEVELOPMENTAL CONSIDERATIONS 5-2

Guidelines for Media Viewing

- Advise families to limit children's media viewing time to no more than 1–2 hours per day.
- Encourage parents to control which shows their children watch.
- Encourage families to watch the media with their children, especially if the children are viewing a new show.
- If children are allowed to watch media while caregivers prepare a meal, shower, or engage in other activities during which play activities cannot be adequately supervised, encourage the family to select age-appropriate shows for the child to view.
- Advise families and daycare providers to familiarize themselves with high-quality, low-cost videotapes and DVDs, which are available from the library or for purchase.
- Caution families not to assume that shows and movies produced by a major "family" entertainment company are appropriate for children of all age levels. Fighting scenes or death of a mother or father may be very disturbing for the young child.
- Encourage families to provide feedback to the networks regarding the quality of programming for children.

PERSONAL AND SOCIAL DEVELOPMENT

During the early childhood years, the child gains independence, and developing social competence becomes increasingly important.

PERSONALITY DEVELOPMENT

As the child transitions from infancy to early childhood, the child acquires a sense of autonomy and independence through the mastery of various specialized tasks, such as the control of bodily functions, refinement of motor and language skills, and acquisition of socially acceptable behaviors (Fig. 5-15).

Self-esteem is a realistic, positive sense of self-worth and identity. Developing self-esteem is a lifelong task that begins at birth but is truly fostered during early childhood (see Developmental Considerations 5-1). Young children love to pretend they are adults and do appear very grown up at times. Their self-esteem is strongly tied to learning new skills. They are developing an awareness of their own skills and interests. As young children become more self-aware and aware of peers, the family may hear them express a lot of dissatisfaction with their own achievements. They may want their drawing to look like another child's drawing or to look like a "real" flower. The family can nourish feelings of self-esteem by praising the child's achievements, showing respect and support to the child, allowing the child to make decisions, listening to the child, and spending time with the child. The family needs to be a coach to the child rather than just a cheerleader who merely praises accomplishments. A coach uses praise to instill feelings of self-worth and teaches the skills the child needs by reinforcing specific actions ("You did such a good job setting the table by putting the napkins and forks in exactly the right place!").

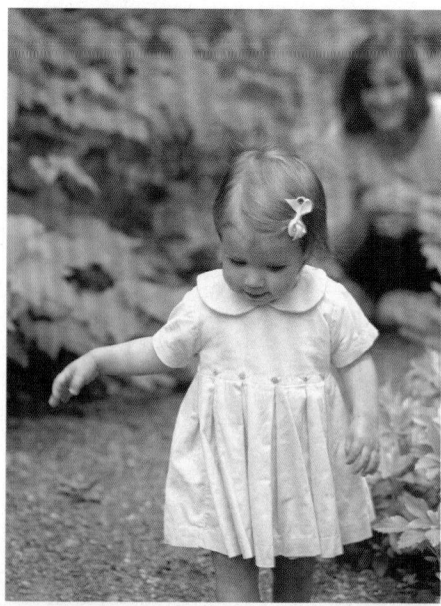

Figure 5-15 Young children enjoy being outside with their family, exploring the world.

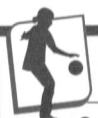

DEVELOPMENTAL CONSIDERATIONS 5-3

Strategies for Enhancing Self-Esteem

- Help the child build a healthy relationship with peers because children are sensitive to evaluation of peers.
- Treat the child with respect. Ask the child's views and opinions, and respond seriously.
- Use physical contact to communicate feelings of love and acceptance.
- Talk to the child, using the child's name frequently; give hugs, smile, and use eye contact.
- Applaud unsuccessful attempts as well as successes.
- Develop a positive, nurturing environment.
- Do not belittle the child.
- Use positive reinforcement whenever possible, and avoid negative criticism.
- Include the child in activities that interest the adult.

Building self-esteem in a child is quite challenging because the child can display a lot of negativism. This negativism is expressed through the tendency to say no to most questions. The child also acts on the impulse of the moment and may not completely understand what the caregiver wants. Nonetheless, positive comments should outweigh criticisms. Keep the rules to a minimum, if possible.

Another way to foster self-esteem is to provide opportunities for the child to make choices and decisions, thus allowing the child some control over his or her life. Children should then be given encouragement and positive feedback (when appropriate) for the decisions they have made. The child should be allowed to begin to establish self-discipline so that he or she understands logical consequences and can make appropriate choices. The family should help the child learn how to deal with mistakes and failures so the child will not avoid attempting new things. Spending a few minutes each day talking with the child about the events of the day, praising the child for accomplishments (with specific examples), or providing an environment where the child can play without being restrained by "no," "don't touch," and so on, will do much to foster healthy self-esteem (Developmental Considerations 5-3).

TEMPERAMENT

How the young child adapts to life's new challenges and meets developmental milestones may be determined by the child's temperament. An "easy" child with high adaptability will accept new activities and experiences easily. A "difficult" child is the exact opposite, will not make these transitions easily and may be very loud and vocal regarding these changes. The "slow-to-warm-up"

child initially will react with some negativity but will respond more positively with repeated exposures (see Chapters 3 and 4 for more information on temperament).

The young child becomes frustrated easily and wants to do as much as possible for himself or herself as part of asserting independence. Getting mad and temper tantrums are a common way of dealing with this frustration. Expressing anger is a normative experience for the child as he or she develops and learns to manage and regulate his or her expressions. In young children, there exists a continuum of *temper loss*. Temper loss refers to the "pattern and modulation of expressions of overt anger, including both temper tantrums and regulation of angry mood" (Wakschlag et al., 2012, p. 1099). This continuum ranges from normative misbehaviors to problem indicators. Normative expressions of anger include temper tantrums in the presence of one's parents and tantrums when frustrated, angry, or upset. Indicators that more severe emotional and behavioral problems may exist include temper tantrums with aggressive behavior, tantrums lasting more than 5 minutes, tantrums happening with nonparental adults, or tantrums happening "out of the blue" (Wakschlag et al., 2012). In these cases, the parent should seek professional intervention to better assess the child's behavior and intervene to manage these behaviors.

Temper tantrums occur occasionally in most young children, with only approximately 10% of children having daily tantrums (Wakschlag et al., 2012). During a tantrum, young children may throw themselves on the floor, kick their feet, and scream. Some children will hold their breath or bang their heads. If the child holds his or her breath until he or she faints, this behavior (although it is not pleasant to watch) does not cause any permanent damage. As the oxygen level decreases and the carbon dioxide level rises, respiration is stimulated. Head banging can cause permanent injury, however, so children who have this kind of tantrum need to be protected by being held so they cannot bang their heads; further referral to a health care provider is also warranted to ensure the child's expressions of anger are within a normative range. Tantrums may not have stopped by the time the child is 3 years old, but by the time the child is 5 years old, tantrums should be rare.

When dealing with the child's expression of anger and temper tantrums, it is important to remain calm. The best technique is to avert the tantrum altogether, if at all possible (Developmental Considerations 5-4). If tantrums are dealt with in a controlled manner, they may actually diminish over time. Humor is sometimes effective at redirecting the tantrum. A funny face or a joke may distract the child.

RELATIONSHIPS

Close relational bonds continue to exist between family members and the young child. One of the child's greatest fears is separation from family members. The family provides safety and security to the young child as he or she explores his or her expanding world. Young

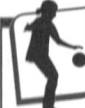

DEVELOPMENTAL CONSIDERATIONS 5-4

Managing A Child's Anger

- Childproof the home to reduce the number of times the family must say no to the child's actions and activities.
- Allow the young children to make frequent, small choices, providing clearly defined, acceptable parameters.
- Evaluate the child's temperament and the changes that occur in temperament throughout the course of the day. Plan activities accordingly.
- Make sure *no* really means "no" and not "well, maybe." Even if the child protests vehemently, the caregiver should not back down from his or her stand; otherwise, the child learns that if he or she protests enough, mom or dad will give in.
- When a tantrum has started, caregivers should
  - Ignore the child's behavior
  - Stand about 5 ft away from the child and keep doing the activity they were previously engaged in or leave the room, as long as the child is safe
  - Do not speak to the child and avoid eye contact until the child has calmed down
  - Move objects out of the way or move the child, if necessary, to prevent injury
  - Do not let the child hurt himself or herself or others
- After the angry outburst or temper tantrum, discuss the child's behavior with him or her in a calm, neutral tone. Discuss ways the child can get "in control" and manage his or her feelings of anger in ways that are not harmful to himself or herself or others.

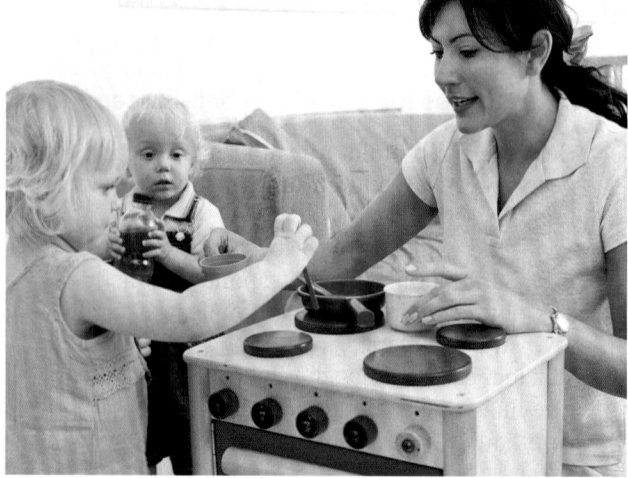

Figure 5-16 Cognitive development is promoted by allowing the child an opportunity to observe and imitate. Cooking is a favorite adult role to mimic.

children mimic parents' actions, doing so because they want parental approval and they want to be like mom or dad (Fig. 5-16).

During early childhood, it is not uncommon for the child to be introduced to a new brother or sister. Giving a new older brother or sister the support needed is important during this time, when much family attention is going to the new sibling. **Sibling rivalry**, the feelings of jealousy and resentment when someone new joins the family, is very normal (see Teaching Intervention Plan 4-2). It commonly occurs at this age because of the change in the child's routine and general changes in the environment.

When the young child does something that causes the newborn to cry, many parents discipline the older child and comfort the infant. This reaction may lead to further jealousy on the part of the child. A better reaction is to investigate the reason behind the action and talk to the preschooler about alternatives. If the child

acted out of jealousy, the parents need to look at the type of time they are spending with each child. One parent could spend quality time with the older child while the other parent cares for the newborn. When the children are old enough to play together, they should be allowed to work out differences themselves. Parents who do not take sides but instead help the children to work out their differences can turn sibling rivalry into a positive advantage (Shelov & Altmann, 2009).

Young children who are involved in a newborn's care adapt better than those who are not and thus have fewer feelings of sibling rivalry. During this time, it is wise not to introduce any new developmental tasks such as toilet learning, weaning from a nighttime bottle, or changing from a crib to a toddler bed. Encourage parents to spend extra alone time with the child to decrease sibling rivalry. The older child is used to having all of his or her time spent with the parents and will miss this greatly.

Friendships with other children are developed during early childhood; however, these friendships are not expressed in the same manner as those developed by older children and adolescents. Friends enable children to learn from what other children do and to note how other children's actions affect the environment and the people in the environment. Young children have short attention spans and thus are likely not to carry a grudge when a friend has mistreated them or ignored them. Young children are most likely to seek friendship without constraints of ethnicity, age, or gender. Friendships are a means to have a playmate and to learn how to socialize in a manner that is acceptable to other children and adults.

By the age of 3 years, the child is less egocentric than before and will actively engage in interaction with other children. Preschoolers play interactively rather than side by side. During this time, children may also start to develop friendships; by the age of 4 years, they will have a very active social life and possibly even "best" friends. Friendships are easily established but may vary in expression; for example, periods of laughter and joy may be followed by episodes of aggression and arguing. Children want to please friends and show off to them. These friendships are often based on frequency of contact with one another. That is, at this age, it would not be expected that the child would initiate a request to see or play with another child, as would happen in middle childhood. Preschoolers will find friends or make friends in whatever circumstance they find themselves to ensure that they have a playmate.

Around age 3 years, children are cognitively involved with fantasy and will drift from reality to fantasy often. At times, they may have imaginary friends. After the child turns 4 years old, he or she focuses more on reality. Children at this age can distinguish that they are not a superhero or storybook princess.

LANGUAGE DEVELOPMENT

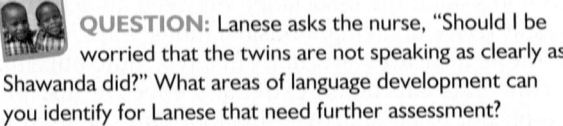

> **QUESTION:** Lanese asks the nurse, "Should I be worried that the twins are not speaking as clearly as Shawanda did?" What areas of language development can you identify for Lanese that need further assessment?

A major accomplishment affecting a young child's social development is the acquisition of language. By the end of the first year, the child has a vocabulary of about 50 words and is using pronouns; by the time the child is 3 years old, he or she has a vocabulary of hundreds of words, speaks sentences of two and three words, understands most of what is said, and can follow short, easy directions. Now family members may find that they need to spell out words that they would rather the child not hear (e.g., "Should we buy some C-A-N-D-Y?"). The child is increasingly responsive and attentive to conversations, so songs, music, and nursery rhymes are good games. Children enjoy examining pictures in books and having stories read to them (Fig. 5-17). These activities promote *early literacy* (early introduction of behaviors that foster eventual acquisition of reading and writing skills). Early literacy is discussed later in this chapter, including age-appropriate methods to encourage early literacy behaviors. Memory games, matching games, hide-and-seek, pretend games, and "Simon Says" are great fun to the child, who is the center of attention.

> *ANSWER:* Further assessment of the boys' language development is important. Determine whether the boys have had their hearing tested. Altered hearing can impair the development of clear speech. Also determine the actual level of the boys' language development. How large is their vocabulary? Are they combining words and using phrases? Share with Lanese that if the boys have had their hearing tested and their vocabulary is continuing to grow, it may be that they are putting their energy into their physical skills at this time, and language skills will catch up. Note to follow up on the boys' language skills the next time they are in the office.

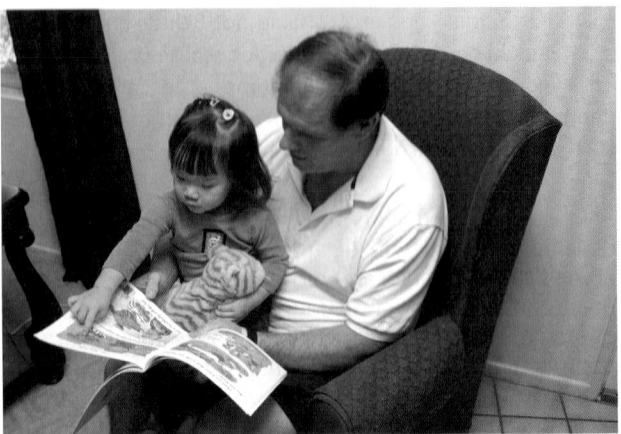

Figure 5-17 The young child enjoys examining pictures in books and listening as stories are read.

FEARS

The most common fears in early childhood are fear of separation from the family and fear of loud noises. Fears are common in children of all ages, and they change as the child matures and obtains a more concrete level of cognitive ability. For some fears, such as the fear of dogs or the fear of falling, there is a triggering event. Because of the limited cognitive understanding of the child, some fears that surface are irrational because the child does not have enough information to self-reassure and thus allay the fears (Chart 5-2).

The young child is still learning to differentiate between reality and fantasy. Because of very vivid imaginations, 3- and 4-year-olds can have some strong fears. These fears may be of real objects (e.g., dogs) as well as imaginary things (e.g., monsters in the dark). Three-year-olds have visual fears associated with burglars and people with deformities, scars, and masks. Children 4 years of age and older have more auditory fears, such as imaginary creatures and sounds heard in the dark. When a child experiences a fear, the family must take it seriously, comfort the child, and then discuss the fear with the child.

CHART 5-2   Common Fears of the Young Child

- Abandonment or separation from family members
- Animals
- Bath/toilet
- Becoming lost
- Costumed characters (e.g., Easter Bunny, Santa Claus)
- Dark
- Falling
- Nightmares (monsters)
- Noises (e.g., loud noises associated with another fearful event)
- Strangers

KidKare The family should not belittle the fear and should never use it as a threat because doing so could exacerbate the fear. Sometimes, the caregiver may need to use concrete actions to remove an imaginary fear, such as "monster proofing" the bedroom.

Most childhood fears are a perfectly normal part of development and will disappear as the child matures. Some situations, such as a move to a new house, divorce, death in the family, or a serious accident or illness, may exacerbate a child's fears. Reading books about scary situations may help a child regain control and understand that the situation is not to be feared. Another common technique to deal with a child's fears is **desensitization**, during which a fear is conquered by approaching it little by little. For example, a fear of water can be conquered by playing with water in a basin, then in a sink, then from the side of the tub (always with adult supervision) until enough confidence is obtained to get into the tub. If a fear becomes a phobia, then the health care team must be consulted. Emphasize to families that providing reassurance and comfort will help children face fears.

Regression, a change from current behaviors to past developmental levels of behavior, may occur in young children in response to sibling rivalry, fears, or stress. For example, a child who has achieved toilet learning may have accidents or refuse to use the toilet. Caution families to ignore the regressed behavior, praise the correct behavior, and not introduce new expectations during this time.

SEXUALITY

The young child develops an emerging awareness of his or her body. Caregivers may find young children examining each other's genitalia or laughing about a "bathroom" joke. Masturbation (deliberate self-stimulation that results in self-comfort or sexual arousal) also begins at this age. Many caregivers are alarmed to find their young children engaged in such activities. An adult may be shocked to discover a 3-year-old child masturbating, but such actions should not be handled in a punitive manner. Reprimanding the child or forbidding these actions could lead to unwanted consequences later because such reactions will produce guilt and remorse. Therefore, caregivers should strive to present a casual response.

Children at this age have normal curiosity about their bodies. Questions asked should be answered simply and honestly. Young children have active imaginations, and if they are told not to ask such questions, they will come up with their own answers, which may not be totally accurate. The adult should investigate the actual intention behind the question. Most have heard the old joke in which the child asks where he or she came from, and the parents go into a long detailed explanation of childbirth, only to discover that the child wanted to know the town where he or she was born. Adults must not let their own biases or prejudices influence their answers. A 3-year-old girl is very curious about the "thing" that the 3-year-old boy has that she does not; the 3-year-old boy is just as mystified that the girl can urinate without having a penis. When children ask about sexual issues, families should use the correct terms for all body parts, including genitalia. This is also a good time to introduce the idea that certain body parts are private and should not be touched by strangers (Hagan et al., 2008).

DISCIPLINE AND LIMIT SETTING

Limits are needed to define acceptable behaviors during early childhood. These limits will be tested in many ways. At the age of 3 years, the child is unable to verbalize many feelings and easily becomes frustrated. The child exhibits frustration by acting out or perhaps by hitting. A child welcomes the setting of limits because it defines expected boundaries of behavior. When boundaries are crossed, caregivers must take disciplinary action. **Positive redirection**—verbally guiding the child toward the accepted behavior—may be effective. Establishing a consistent routine is helpful in preventing children from becoming frustrated because they are unprepared to move to a new activity. When a child misbehaves, demonstrating natural or logical consequences helps the child understand the association between an action and its result (Developmental Considerations 5-5).

If these measures are not effective, time-outs may be. Time-outs can be an extremely effective disciplinary tool, but to be effective, this tool must be used appropriately. A child should not stay in a time-out until he or she does what the caregiver wants done. Rather, time-outs should be used to teach the child how to regain self-control and calm down (Fig. 5-18). Therefore, a time-out is appropriate when a preschooler hits or screams but is not appropriate when he or she will not pick up his or her toys. A time-out should be timed appropriately. The time-out should occur at the time

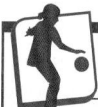

DEVELOPMENTAL CONSIDERATIONS 5-5

Strategies for Effective Discipline

- Set realistic limits.
- Be consistent with consequences.
- Do not be overly negative.
- Use positive redirection whenever possible, distracting the child toward a more positive action.
- Selectively ignore situations if the behavior is not a major issue; ignore it, but compliment and reward the more positive behavior.
- Use time-outs when appropriate (when the child is 18–24 months old): 1 minute of time out for each year of age. Time-outs should be used to allow both the adult and the child cooling off time.
- The use of corporal punishment (spanking, hitting) reinforces violent behavior and may confuse the child.
- Role-model appropriate behaviors and ensure older children in the family role-model appropriate behaviors.

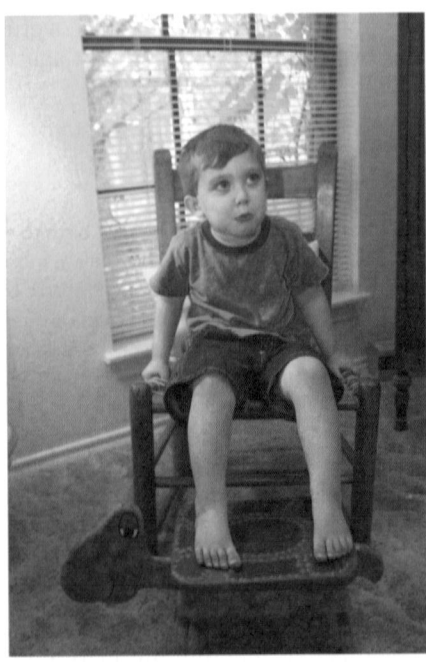

Figure 5-18 The *time-out* is a disciplinary measure used to remove a child from an activity; this allows him or her to calm down and consider what behavior was wrong.

the offense happened to ensure the child relates the offense (the behavioral problem) to the time-out period. Brief time-outs are more effective than very long ones because a long time-out enables the child to redirect attention from calming down to being resentful. The maximum time-out duration should be 1 minute for each year of age, but it may be necessary to start with much shorter time-outs. A time-out should end as soon as the child is calm. Time-outs do not have to occur in the child's room; any location where the child is removed from activity and has an opportunity to become calm will do. The nurse or caregiver must explain to the child why the child is receiving the time-out.

Caregivers should pick their battles. If the issue is not life endangering, unsafe, or amoral, let it go (e.g., allow the child to wear one red shoe and one blue shoe). Do not allow the child to become overtired, which often causes many more arguments than necessary. Never argue with a child; doing so brings the adult down to the child's level. The child is too young to say, "I've had a really busy day and need to relax for a while." Allow the young child times when they can learn how to occupy themselves for short periods of quiet time. Alerting children to transition times is very important. Many daycare settings use songs to let young children know that it is time to clean up and start doing something different. Caregivers can use a similar technique by giving children 5-minute notices that a new activity is about to start. Giving young children attractive options also helps with transition. A choice between just leaving and going home to something the child enjoys (e.g., a bath, play with the pet) is much easier to negotiate than a flat demand, but caregivers should not overnegotiate; pleading and expecting the child to understand and

agree are unrealistic. Sometimes, even when caregivers have negotiated, have not allowed the child to become overly tired, and have offered appealing options, the child is still uncooperative and needs to be gently but physically moved to the next task or place.

Families may not realize that a child younger than 18 months of age is unable to make a connection between unacceptable behavior and being spanked; they experience only the pain. The AAP (2013) and the American Psychological Association (Smith, 2012) have actively advocated against use of severe or injurious physical punishment (including spanking). These professional organizations share concerns that spanking children increases the chance of physical injury to the child. In addition, spanking models aggressive behavior and has not been proved any more effective than other disciplinary strategies at producing long-term changes in the child's behavior (Tradition or Science 5-3). Young children start to make the connection between behavior and consequences. Encourage caregivers to

Evidence-Based Practice   TRADITION OR SCIENCE 5-3

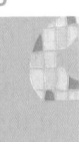

Does spanking, used as a disciplinary measure on children, have any association with behavioral problems later in the child's life?

Several researchers have noted that spanking, slapping, pushing, grabbing, and shoving children as a form of punishment is associated with higher levels of aggressive behavior and mental disorders in children at later ages. Slade and Wissow (2004) used a sample of 1,966 children who were younger than 2 years of age to evaluate spanking frequency and other characteristics. Approximately 4 years later, these children were evaluated for behavioral problems in school using family reports and documented visits by the parent with a school administrator. Among white non-Hispanic children, but not among black and Hispanic children, spanking frequency before age 2 years was significantly and positively associated with behavior problems at school age. This finding was further supported in a study by Taylor et al. (2010) examining the spanking behaviors of 2,500 mothers of 3-year-old children. Among their findings was that frequent spanking at age 3 years increased the odds of higher levels of aggression at age 5 years. Afifi et al. (2012) examined whether harsh physical punishment was linked to mental disorders even in the absence of more severe child maltreatment (e.g., physical abuse, sexual abuse). They found that harsh physical punishment of children was associated with increased odds of mood disorders, anxiety disorders, alcohol and drug abuse, and several personality disorders later in life. Researchers found 2%–7% of mental disorders were attributable to physical punishment. These findings suggest that children are vulnerable to emotional trauma and stress as a result of harsh acts of discipline. Children are believed to be too young to receive and understand harsh punishment and to modulate their expressions of those same behaviors in relationships with others. Adults can use others forms of discipline such as natural consequences, time-out, and withholding privileges to help regulate a child's behavior.

communicate the rules to the child, and the consequences for breaking them, consistently. Make sure the child knows a rule before being punished for breaking it (see Developmental Considerations 5-5).

SCHOOLING AND CHILD CARE

Early childhood education programs include preschools, daycare centers, Head Start programs, nursery schools, prekindergarten programs, and other early childhood learning programs. In 2010, approximately 64% of children aged 3 to 5 years in the United States attended some form of an early childhood education program (National Center for Education Statistics, 2012). The documented benefits of early childhood education, especially for at-risk children, include better language and cognitive skills during the first few years of elementary school than those children who did not attend similar education programs. In addition, children who have attended early childhood education programs tend to score higher on math and reading tests and are less likely to repeat a grade, drop out of school, need special education or remedial services, or get into trouble with the law in the future. Studies show these children also tend to complete more years of education and are more likely to attend a 4-year college (Karoly et al., 2005; Reynolds et al., 2011).

If the child has never attended out-of-home daycare, the initial strategy is to allow the child to adjust to the transition from home to center so that he or she is comfortable with a few hours of separation and observes group activities and the learning process. Monitoring the child's behavior when he or she starts preschool is important because some children may be too young to adapt to a very structured environment and may show signs of stress. To make good-byes easier, the family should develop a morning routine, prepare as much as possible the night before, and avoid rushing in the morning. Rushing tends to cause stress for the family, and the child feels the tension and may become upset when the family member leaves, thinking that he or she did something wrong. When the parent or family caregiver and child arrive at the center, the parent can spend a few minutes to settle the child in, perhaps by reading a book or starting a group activity. The ultimate good-bye should be short; the parent should not linger as if unsure whether to leave. If it is the first time the child and parent have been separated, a few days of adjustment may be necessary. The parent might stay longer at the center the first day and decrease the length of stay each day. When the day is over, the parent should not be surprised if the child appears preoccupied and ignores him or her; alternately, the child might burst into tears because he or she really missed the parent.

Early education programs are designed to offer the building blocks to prepare for learning in kindergarten and to provide an opportunity to develop and build age-appropriate developmental skills and abilities. Early education programs can be extremely important to the child's overall development because the child receives stimulation in areas that are not ordinarily addressed in the home environment. These programs

are also valuable as a resource for discovering potential learning disabilities at a very early age (Shelov & Altmann, 2009).

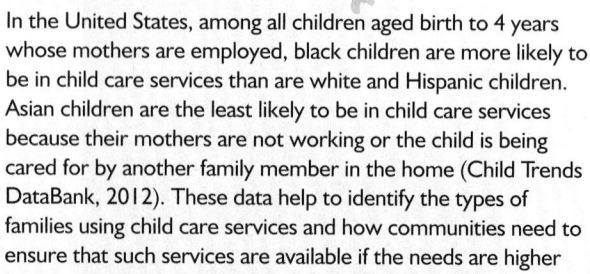

CROSS-CULTURAL CARE

In the United States, among all children aged birth to 4 years whose mothers are employed, black children are more likely to be in child care services than are white and Hispanic children. Asian children are the least likely to be in child care services because their mothers are not working or the child is being cared for by another family member in the home (Child Trends DataBank, 2012). These data help to identify the types of families using child care services and how communities need to ensure that such services are available if the needs are higher for these services based on the families in their community.

A good early education program encourages children to gain independence and self-confidence and to develop interpersonal skills (Fig. 5-19). The program should have the resources to identify any learning disorders. If a special need has already been identified, the preschool should have the appropriate resources in place to implement necessary interventions. Many community programs are not equipped to accommodate special

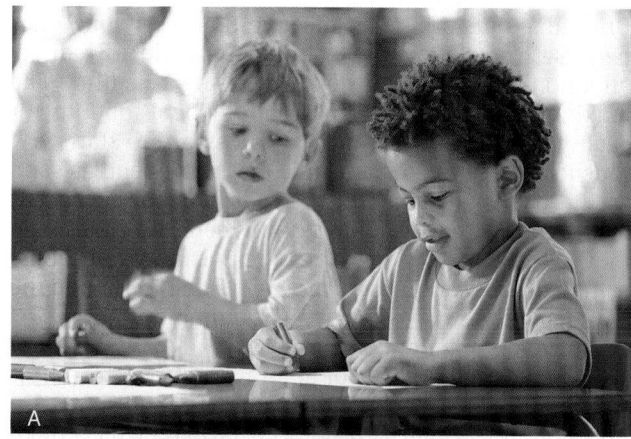

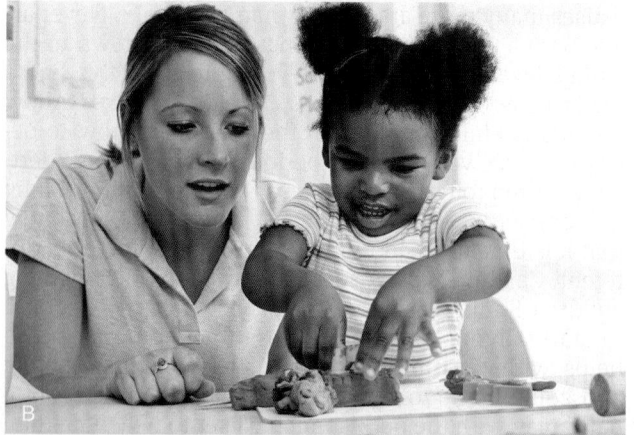

Figure 5-19 (A and B) In the preschool setting, children are exposed to a variety of activities to enhance development of multiple types of intelligence.

needs students, and parents should speak with the director for advice and referral.

Many of the questions that are asked when a daycare center is chosen are the same questions that must be asked when a formal preschool or other type of education program is chosen (see Chapter 4). Location, hours the center is open, numbers and ages of the other children, cost, and the "instructional" capacities of the program are all aspects of the program that need to be evaluated.

Early education programs have relatively small class sizes, about 10 children or fewer per one adult, and the "teacher" or aides should have experience with early childhood development or education. In many states, this experience is mandated by daycare or preschool regulations. Advise the family to investigate disciplinary methods used and be sure they are in line with home discipline techniques. The entire center and grounds should be childproofed and under adult supervision at all times. Encourage family caregivers to visit the center whenever they like and be suspicious of centers that have very strict visiting procedures.

Investigate health care issues such as what happens when a child becomes ill at the center and what the center's policies are for accepting children with apparent illness. Policies regarding infectious diseases should be strict and should emphasize handwashing by both staff and children. Child-sized sinks should be available, and toilet-trained children should be expected to wash their hands after using the restroom. If children attend who are still in diapers, the center should have a separate diaper station that is cleaned with disinfectant after each use.

The family must agree with the overall theory of the program. Although some children thrive in a structured environment, many need opportunities to socialize, learn to control emotions, and explore their own ideas. Encourage families to investigate all available programs to find the type that may be the most suitable for their child.

Promoting Early Literacy

Engaging in **early literacy** activities, which promote learning to read and write, is important during early childhood (Fig. 5-20). Early literacy does not mean

teaching young children to read before they start kindergarten. Doing so would not be developmentally appropriate, and such activities can be counterproductive if they create a situation in which the child associates reading with failure and parental disappointment. Rather, early literacy emphasizes pairing the enjoyment of books with the child's emerging developmental skills (e.g., hand–eye coordination, language acquisition). These activities will promote early familiarity and comfort with the skills that are used later to teach reading and writing. In the past, it was believed that children should learn all reading and writing skills when they entered elementary schools. The formal instruction to these skills would begin at this time, and beginning these processes earlier in the child's development was unnecessary. Language skills were thought to develop first, followed by reading and then writing. It is now known that language, reading, and writing skills develop at the same time and are intimately linked. Literacy development is a continuous developmental process that begins during the first years of life, using real-life settings and positive interactions with people and literacy materials.

Children who are not read to while they are growing up and who have little exposure to books are at increased risk for reading failure as they enter and progress through elementary school. The Early Childhood Longitudinal Study found that children whose family members read to them at least three times a week were almost twice as likely to score in the top 25% on measures of reading proficiency than children who were read to fewer than three times a week. Children who were read to three times a week as they entered kindergarten demonstrated increased mastery of letter–sound relationships at the beginning and end of words, sight–word recognition skills, and understanding words in context (National Institute for Literacy, 2006).

CROSS-CULTURAL CARE

Research indicates that ethnic disparities exist in regard to adults in the home reading to their children. For example, black and Hispanic parents are less likely to read to their children than white parents, and Spanish-speaking families have fewer books in their home and are more likely to never read to their children when compared to non–Spanish-speaking families (Sappenfield & Rosenberg, 2011). These disparities may be due to lack of time in the home for reading, discomfort by the parents in reading English, a perception that reading is not a leisure activity, a view that reading will begin when the child enters school, or a lack of resources to acquire age-appropriate books.

Provide families with information about age-appropriate reading materials and the developmental skills that are enhanced through early literacy activities (Developmental Considerations 5-6). Many health care facilities are taking an active role in literacy promotion by providing reading materials for children in the waiting areas and by distributing free books (Tradition or Science 5-4).

Ask about the child's language skills and whether family members are reading to their young child. If the

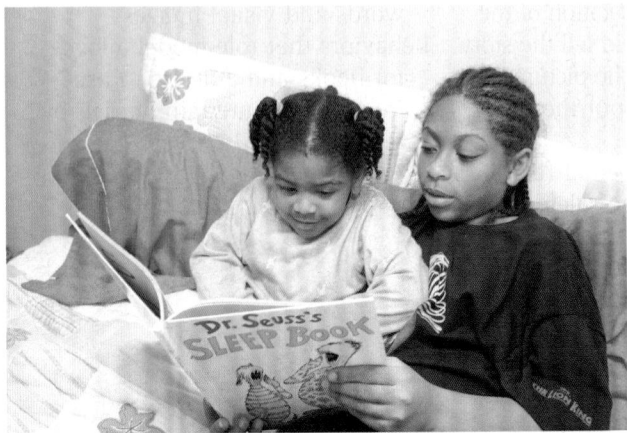

Figure 5-20 When an older sibling reads to a younger sibling, both children increase their literacy skills.

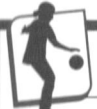

DEVELOPMENTAL CONSIDERATIONS 5-6

Promoting Early Literacy

Age	Types of Reading Materials	Caregiver Activities	Skills You Are Promoting
6–12 months	Small, hand-sized, board books with pictures of faces and only a few words per page	Read aloud to the child. Hold the book so that the child can see the words and pictures.	Physical manipulation or handling of books Behaviors related to how children pay attention to and interact with pictures in books, such as gazing at pictures or laughing at a favorite picture Hand–eye coordination as the child learns to point to specific objects in the books
12 months to 2 years	Small board books with pictures of family life, animals, and common household items Simple stories with rhymes and repetition that concentrate on particular sounds	Same as above Follow the words with a finger to show how to read from left to right or assist the child to follow the words with a finger. Repeat reading the same book, letting the child finish familiar sentences and pointing to the words that the child can "read" as the child says the words. Ask questions while reading about the pictures, the story, and the words, such as, "Show me the horse." "Where is the cow?" "Can you find the letter 'c'? The letter 'r'?" Sound out letters and talk about the story, making predictions about what will happen next.	Physical manipulation or handling of books Behaviors, such as pointing to pictures of familiar objects, that show recognition of and a beginning understanding of pictures in books Picture and story comprehension behaviors that show a child's understanding of pictures and events in a book, such as imitating an action seen in a picture or talking about the events in a story Behaviors that include children's verbal interactions with books and their increasing understanding of print in books, such as imitating reading or running fingers along printed words
3–6 years	Alphabet and number books Alphabet and number books that the child and caregiver make to read together Books that are well written and illustrated for young children	Do "picture walks" before starting to read aloud. Review the pictures in the book and discuss the meaning or interpretation of the picture. Let the child tell the story just by looking at the pictures. Take time to talk about the book and concepts. Buy books with the child (e.g., from stores, garage sales, book clubs). Help the child to start building a personal library. Get the child a library card and make frequent trips to the library. Let the child see other family members reading. Invite the child to sit beside adults and read a book while they are also reading.	Same as above Behaviors that show an emerging association between written words and visual images Behaviors that role-model a love for books and a desire to use free time to entertain oneself by reading

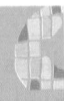

TRADITION OR SCIENCE 5-4

Evidence-Based Practice

Do clinic- and or hospital-based literacy promotion programs positively affect literacy skills in young children?

Several institutions have used programs to educate families about the importance of reading to their young children. The interventions in these programs have included providing handouts about early literacy, ensuring that primary health care providers are trained to assess for literacy activities in the home and able to provide strategies to enhance literacy activities, and ensuring that each child leaves the health visit with a developmentally appropriate book (Golova et al., 1999; High et al., 2000; McCall, 2005; Silverstein et al., 2005). Results of these interventions included significant increases over time in the frequency with which parents read to their children, an increase in the number of parents who read to their children, and an increase in children's personal libraries at home. Participating families had children who ranged in age from 5 months to 6 years, and most families were identified as low income. A study by Nagamine et al. (2001) that used a literacy intervention program in the emergency department was not associated with any measurable changes in family literacy behaviors. This environment is likely not the most effective place to promote literacy, given concerns over the child's immediate medical needs, parents' information overload at the time, or both.

Clearly, health care providers can positively affect early childhood literacy by providing parent education and the resources (e.g., actual books) for parents to implement reading activities with their child. Books can be purchased at low cost by the facility or donated by volunteer groups interested in supporting literacy programs.

adults' ability to read is limited or access to books in the appropriate language for the family is lacking, the child may be in an environment that does not foster early literacy. Adult family members may feel uncomfortable and perhaps may be unwilling to try to "read" with the child, given their own lack of literacy skills. Adults in this situation still can be encouraged to share books with children by examining the pictures and telling stories about the pictures. If an adult express a desire to improve his or her own literacy skills, provide referrals to adult or family literacy programs. Help families understand that the child greatly enjoys the attention associated with sharing books and will benefit in later years from this early exposure to reading materials.

PREVENTING INJURY AND ILLNESS

Injuries pose a major threat to health during early childhood. Unintentional injuries are the leading cause of death for children aged 1 to 4 years (Centers for Disease Control and Prevention, 2010). The child's inquisitive nature and expanding motor and developmental abilities combine to increase the risk. Although young children experience most injuries in and around their own homes, families need to be informed of the potential for injury at

homes of relatives and friends that they visit. The leading causes of unintentional injury in early childhood include motor vehicle/traffic accidents, falls, drowning, fires and burn injuries, poisoning, and unintentional suffocation (Centers for Disease Control and Prevention, 2010).

QUESTION: Lanese asks, "Ever since the boys could get out of their cribs, they occasionally surprise me by getting into mischief when I think they are in bed. What can I do about the boys roaming around when I think they have gone to sleep?" What suggestions can you offer to Lanese to help prevent injury to the twins?

Even if the home has already been babyproofed, it is now time to childproof the environment based on the unique developmental abilities of this age group. See Community Care 5-1 for a review of injury prevention guidelines. **Childproofing** the house helps keep the child safe and removes temptations and the need for the family to restrict activities and access to parts of the home. Childproofing involves adults actively searching the indoor and outdoor environment of the home and other areas where the child may frequently spend time (e.g., daycare provider's home, house of worship) to ensure that the area is safe for the child in relation to age-related safety concerns. This precaution keeps the environment "explorable," prevents conflicts, and enables the child to expand on skills that need mastering (e.g., fine and gross motor skills). In addition, when grandparents, babysitters, or other friends are in the home to watch the child, safety issues must be reviewed. Although parents may have a complete understanding of the hazards in the environment that trigger the child's curiosity, other adults may not be as well informed or maintain the same degree of vigilance regarding the child's safety.

Automobile accidents are a leading cause of death in this age group as a result of children who are not properly restrained in car seats and unsafe driving practices around areas in which small children are present. Advise the family to check whether car seats and other restraints (see Chapter 4) still fit the growing child properly. All states and Canadian provinces require young children to be restrained in a front-facing car seat when the vehicle is in motion (Fig. 5-21). The car seat should be placed in the backseat. All harness straps on child safety seats should be fastened snugly to the body so the child cannot slip out. The seat's base is attached to the vehicle using the car's LATCH system (lower anchors and tethers for children) for car's manufactured since 2002 or by using a lap belt in older car models (Fig. 5-22). Transition from a car seat to a belt-positioning booster seat should be made if the child weighs more than 40 lb (Hagan et al., 2008). The child should never be placed in the front seat of a vehicle with passenger airbags. The adult should not start the car until everyone (including the driver) is buckled up. If the child unbuckles during the car ride, the driver should pull over and stop the car until the child is rerestrained.

Children ages 5 years and younger have the highest drowning death rate (two times greater than other age groups), with 84% of these drownings occurring in the home pool (Safe Kids Worldwide, 2011). Drownings often

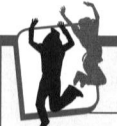

COMMUNITY CARE 5-1

Injury Prevention Guidelines for the Family During Early Childhood (1–4 Years Old)

Home Safety

Get down on the floor and check for safety hazards the child may encounter as he or she begins walking.

Test smoke detectors to ensure that they work properly. Change batteries twice yearly.

Do not leave heavy objects or containers of hot liquids on tables with tablecloths that the child may pull down.

Place safety locks on cupboards and toilet seats.

Use doorknob covers and childproof locks on all doors, sliding doors, and windows. Make sure screens are secure.

Turn pan handles toward the back of the stove. Place knives, scissors, and sharp objects toward the back of counters, cabinets, and drawers.

Keep the child away from hot stoves, fireplaces, irons, curling irons, and space heaters.

Ensure that heavy furniture, such as televisions, bookshelves, and dressers, are secure so that the child may not reach out or climb on them and pull them over.

Ensure that all electric wires, outlets, and appliances are inaccessible or protected.

Keep all poisonous substances, cleaning agents, alcohol, health and beauty supplies, medicines, and home improvement materials in a locked, safe place out of sight and reach. Never store poisonous substances in empty jars or soda bottles. Keep the number of the local poison control center near every telephone in the house and on available cell phones.

Ensure that houseplants are not toxic, in case of accidental consumption by the child.

Keep cigarettes, lighters, matches, and alcohol out of the child's sight and reach.

Use safety gates at the top and bottom of stairs. Supervise the child closely when he or she is on stairs.

Tie blind and drapery cords out of the child's reach.

Avoid placing furniture the child can climb on near windows and balconies.

Ensure that guns, if they are in the home, are locked up and that ammunition is stored and locked separately. A trigger lock is an additional important precaution.

Move the crib mattress to the lowest rung and ensure that the sides are up when the child is in it in order to prevent climbing out of the crib. Note that newer cribs no longer have rails that are able to slide up and down.

Play Safety

Keep plastic bags, latex balloons, and small objects such as marbles away from the child.

Teach older siblings which of their toys are unsafe for the younger child to play with.

Discard toys with sharp edges or broken pieces. Ensure that all toys selected are approved by the manufacturer for that child's age group.

Confine the child's outdoor play to areas with fences and gates, especially at a child care facility, unless he or she is under close supervision.

Ensure that playgrounds are safe. Check for impact- or energy-absorbing surfaces under playground equipment. Make sure playground equipment is not more than 3 ft tall and not made of pressure-treated wood.

Water Safety

Ensure that the water heater is set at less than 120° F or 48.9° C.

Test the bath water temperature with your wrist to make sure it is not hot before bathing your child.

Supervise the child constantly whenever he or she is around water, buckets, the toilet, or the bathtub.

Empty buckets, tubs, or small pools immediately after use.

Ensure that swimming pools are enclosed by a four-sided fence with a self-closing, self-latching gate.

Ensure that the child wears a life vest if boating.

Use flotation devices on the child when he or she is in the pool or hot tub. Note that inflatable flotation devices or "knowing how to swim" do not make a child safe in the water.

Keep U.S. Coast Guard–approved life jackets and preservers and a shepherd's crook at the poolside.

Car Safety

Ensure the car seat being used is appropriate for the child's size and age. Make sure it is properly secured at all times. The car seat should be in the rear-facing position in the backseat of the car until the child reaches the highest weight or height allowed for rear-facing seats, then the child can be placed in a front-facing seat appropriate for his or her height and weight.

Never leave the child alone in the car or in the house.

Safety With Others

Do not leave young siblings alone to supervise the child (e.g., in the bathtub or in the house).

Keep the infant away from cigarette smoke. Do not allow people to smoke around the child.

Choose caregivers carefully. Discuss with them their attitudes about behavior in relation to discipline. Prohibit corporal punishment.

Teach the child to use caution when approaching animals, especially if the animals are unknown or eating.

Teach the child not to talk to strangers.

Outdoor Safety

Put sunscreen on the child before he or she goes out to play.

Keep the child away from moving machinery, lawn mowers, overhead garage doors, driveways, and streets.

Ensure that a child riding in a seat on an adult's bicycle is wearing a helmet. Wear a helmet yourself.

Supervise the child whenever he or she is outside. Know where your child is at all times. A child aged 1–4 years is too young to be roaming the neighborhood alone.

Teach the child pedestrian safety skills.

Do not allow the child to be left unsupervised in or around vehicles.

Emergency Preparation

Keep your address and phone number posted near the phone.

Keep a list of emergency numbers (doctor, hospital, nearest neighbor, poison control center) near the phone.

Enroll in a child cardiopulmonary resuscitation (CPR) course.

Discuss with the health care professional what to do for falls, cuts, puncture wounds, bites, bumps on the head, bleeding, and broken bones.

Adapted from Hagan, J. F., Shaw, J. S., & Duncan, P. M. (Eds.). (2008). *Bright futures: Guidelines for health supervision of infants, children, and adolescents* (3rd ed.). Elk Grove Village, IL: American Academy of Pediatrics.

occur because secure fencing is not in place to separate the pool from easy access by the child. In addition, drowning can occur when supervising adults are preoccupied and not closely attending to children playing in the water. Concern for young children is especially important when the pool is occupied by large groups of children. Although teaching young children to swim helps, children should never be around water without adult supervision (Fig. 5-23), and all pools should be surrounded by a fence at least 5 ft high. Swimming in partially covered pools should be avoided because the child may become trapped underneath the cover. When an aboveground pool is not in use, the stairs should be removed. Local codes usually require a latched and locked gate to gain access to a pool. When boating, every person in the craft is required to have a flotation device and to be wearing it at all times.

Young children have thinner and much more sensitive skin than adults do. When a young child will be out in the sun for a prolonged period, broad-spectrum sunscreen that protects against both UVA and UVB rays with a sun protection factor of at least 15 to 30 should be applied frequently and liberally. If the weather is hot, children should be sure to drink plenty of fluids because they tend to become dehydrated easily.

Fire-related injuries in the home can be prevented by installation of smoke detectors/alarms on every level of the home and in every sleeping area. In addition, keeping matches, lighters, and other heat sources out of the reach of young children will help prevent needless injuries or death from home fires.

Suffocation is the fourth leading cause of unintentional deaths in early childhood. Suffocation can occur if the child is allowed to sleep with adults, in a water

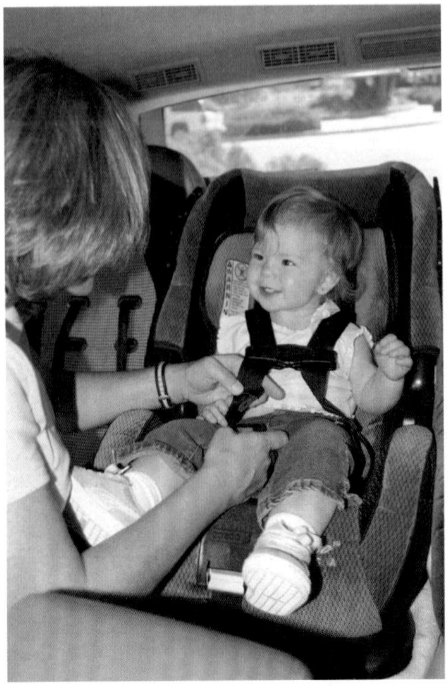

Figure 5-21 All young children must be placed in the backseat of a car, strapped into a front-facing car seat.

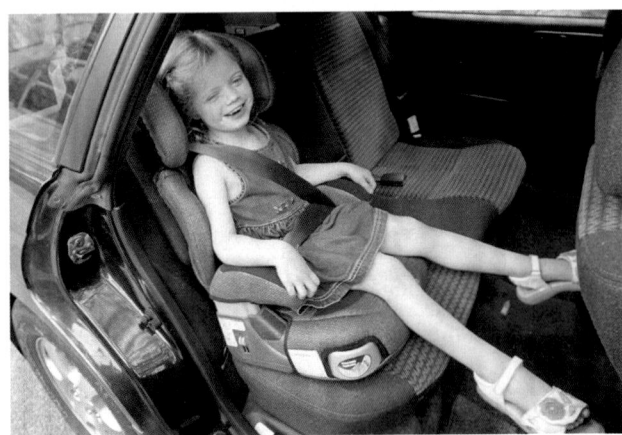

Figure 5-22 Many injuries resulting from motor vehicle accidents can be prevented by proper use of car restraints.

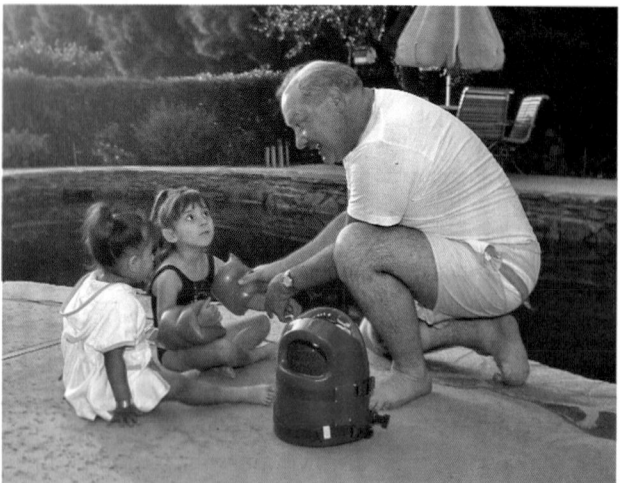

Figure 5-23 Assist the young child to wear safety equipment while swimming, and ensure the child is accompanied by an adult when in or around a pool or other swimming area.

bed, or in a bed where too much space exists between the mattress and the crib or bed slats (this space should not be more than the width of two adult fingers). Suffocation can also occur if a child becomes locked in a cabinet, toy chest, or car trunk and has no means to escape and get fresh air. Strangulation can occur from drapery and miniblind cords, hood cords, drawstrings on clothes, and hammocks, to name a few examples.

Encourage family members to remain vigilant about hazards in the home, the school, and the child's play area that may be a source of injury. The child's increasing vocabulary and overall comprehension can be misinterpreted as an ability to make choices to prevent self-harm. The young child's curiosity and inquisitiveness are likely to result in high-risk behavior. The child does not recognize the activity (e.g., playing near a pool) as high risk, but such activity unmonitored by caregivers can have dire consequences for the child. Provide anticipatory guidance to families regarding the unintentional injuries that may occur in the home. Encourage families to use Internet sites such as those discussed in Evidence-Based Clinical Practice Guidelines 5-1 to review the variety of measures that can be used in their home to protect their child.

ANSWER: In response to Lanese's concerns, you might say, "You are right to be worried. When children this age get up and out of their rooms unsupervised, it is dangerous. You might want to consider a doorknob cover for the inside of their bedroom door so they cannot let themselves out. You could also try putting the baby monitor back in their rooms so that you can hear them if they are awake and 'plotting.' You also should go through your home and double-check that there are no products under the sink or in the medicine cabinet that they can get to."

See the Point for a summary of Key Concepts.

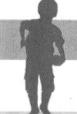

EVIDENCE-BASED CLINICAL PRACTICE GUIDELINES 5-1
Child Safety Information

Hagan, J. F., Shaw, J. S., & Duncan, P. M. (Eds.). (2008). *Bright futures: Guidelines for health supervision of infants, children, and adolescents* (3rd ed.). Elk Grove Village, IL: American Academy of Pediatrics. Retrieved from

http://www.brightfutures.org/

Health professional guidelines and parent resources provide anticipatory guidance on a wide variety of safety issues applicable to each developmental stage.

Children's Safety Network

http://www.childrenssafetynetwork.org/

National resource center that collects, collates, and disseminates information related to the prevention of childhood injuries and violence.

National Child Safety Council

http://www.nationalchildsafetycouncil.org/

National nonprofit organization dedicated to providing education and educational materials to prevent childhood injury and violence.

Project ChildSafe

http://www.projectchildsafe.org/

Provides information about child firearm injury and safety curriculum to prevent firearm injury.

Safe Kids Worldwide

http://www.safekids.org/

Worldwide resource that provides position statements, fact sheets, and the latest news about preventable child injury and critical child injury risks.

REFERENCES

Afifi, T., Mota, N., Dasiewicz, P. et al. (2012). Physical punishment and mental disorders: Results from a nationally representative US sample. *Pediatrics, 130*(2), 184–192.

American Academy of Pediatric Dentistry. (2009). *Guideline on periodicity of examination, preventive dental services, anticipatory guidance/counseling, and oral treatment for infants, children, and adolescents.* Retrieved from http://www.aapd.org/media/Policies _Guidelines/G_Periodicity.pdf

American Academy of Pediatric Dentistry. (2012a). *Guideline on fluoride therapy.* Retrieved from http://www.aapd.org/media/Policies _Guidelines/G_FluorideTherapy.pdf

American Academy of Pediatric Dentistry. (2012b). *Policy on the use of fluoride.* Retrieved from http://www.aapd.org/media/Policies _Guidelines/P_FluorideUse.pdf

American Academy of Pediatrics. (2011). Media use by children younger than 2 years. Policy statement. *Pediatrics, 128*(5), 1040–1045.

American Academy of Pediatrics. (2013). *Disciplining your child.* Retrieved from http://www.healthychildren.org/English/family-life /family-dynamics/communication-discipline/pages/Disciplining -Your-Child.aspx?nfstatus = 401&nftoken = 00000000-0000-0000 -0000-000000000000&nfstatusdescription = ERROR % 3a + No + local + token

Arens, R., & Muzumdar, H. (2010). Childhood obesity and obstructive sleep apnea syndrome. *Journal of Applied Physiology, 108*(2), 436–444.

Ashiabi, G. (2007). Play in the preschool classroom: Its socioemotional significance and the teacher's role in play. *Early Childhood Education Journal, 35,* 199–207.

Barradas, D., Fulton, J., Blanck, H. et al. (2007). Parental influences on youth television viewing. *Journal of Pediatrics, 151,* 369–373, 373.e1–373.e4.

Bernstein, K., Ahern, J., Tracy, M. et al. (2007). Television watching and the risk of incident probable posttraumatic stress disorder: A prospective evaluation. *Journal of Nervous & Mental Disease, 195*(1), 41–47.

Carruth, B., Ziegler, P., Gordon, A. et al. (2004). Developmental milestones and self-feeding behaviors in infants and toddlers. *Journal of the American Dietetic Association, 104*(Suppl. 1), 51–56.

Casby, M. (2003). The development of play in infants, toddlers and young children. *Communication Disorders Quarterly, 24*(4), 163–174.

Centers for Disease Control and Prevention. (2010). *Ten leading causes of death and injury.* Retrieved from http://www.cdc.gov /injury/wisqars/LeadingCauses.html

Child Trends DataBank. (2012). *Child care.* Retrieved from http:// www.childtrendsdatabank.org/alphalist?q = node/97

Childress, D. (2011). Play behaviors of parents and their young children with disabilities. *Topics in Early Childhood Education, 31*(2), 112–120.

Christakis, D., Zimmerman, F., DiGiuseppe, D. et al. (2004). Early television exposure and subsequent attentional problems in children. *Pediatrics, 113*(4), 708–713.

Commonwealth of Australia, Department of Health and Ageing. (2004). *Australia's physical activity recommendations for 5–12 year olds.* Canberra, Australia: Department of Health and Ageing.

Gidding, S. S., Dennison, B. A., Birch, L. L. et al. (2006). Dietary recommendations for children and adolescents: A guide for practitioners. *Pediatrics, 117*(2), 544–559.

Golova, N., Alario, A. J., Vivier, P. M. et al. (1999). Literacy promotion for Hispanic families in a primary care setting: A randomized control trial. *Pediatrics, 103,* 993–997.

Graham, M. V., & Uphold, C. R. (2003). *Clinical guidelines in child health* (3rd ed.). Gainesville, FL: Barmarrae Books.

Gray, P. (2011). The special value of children's age-mixed play. *The American Journal of Play, 3*(4), 500–522.

Hagan, J. F., Shaw, J. S., & Duncan, P. M. (Eds.). (2008). *Bright futures: Guidelines for health supervision of infants, children, and adolescents* (3rd ed.). Elk Grove Village, IL: American Academy of Pediatrics.

Hammons, A., & Fiese, B. (2011). Is frequency of shared family meals related to the nutritional health of children and adolescents? *Pediatrics, 127*(6), e1565–e1574.

Hayward, K. (2013). *The four stages of toilet learning.* Retrieved from http://www.niu.edu/ccc/resources/ToiletTraining2.pdf

High, P., LaGasse, L., Becker, S. et al. (2000). Literacy promotion in primary care pediatrics: Can we make a difference? *Pediatrics, 105*(4), 927–934.

Hoerr, S., Lee, S., Schiffman, R. et al. (2006). Beverage consumption of mother–toddler dyads in families with limited incomes. *Journal of Pediatric Nursing, 21,* 403–411.

Holt, K., Wooldridge, N., Story, M. et al. (Eds.). (2011). *Bright futures in practice: Nutrition* (3rd ed.). Elk Grove Village, IL: American Academy of Pediatrics.

Jago, R., Baranowski, T., Baranowski, J. C. et al. (2005). BMI from 3 to 6 y of age is predicted by TV viewing and physical activity, not diet. *International Journal of Obesity, 29,* 557–564.

Karoly, L., Kilburn, M. R., & Cannon, J. (2005). *Early childhood interventions: Proven results, future promises.* Santa Monica, CA: Rand.

McCall, K. (2005). Early literacy reading program: Three-year analysis. *Journal of Pediatric Nursing, 20*(3), 225–226.

Miller, C., Marks, D., Miller, S. et al. (2007). Brief report: Television viewing and risk for attention problems in preschool children. *Journal of Pediatric Psychology, 32*(4), 448–452.

Mindell, J., & Owens, J. (2009). *A clinical guide to pediatric sleep: Diagnosis and management of sleep problems.* Philadelphia, PA: Lippincott Williams & Wilkins.

Moore, L. (2011). Playground play: Educational and Inclusive. *Exceptional Parent, 41*(11), 22–24.

Moore, M. (2012). Behavioral sleep problems in children and adolescents. *Journal of Clinical Psychology in Medical Settings, 19*(1), 77–83.

Nagamine, W., Ishida, J., Williams, D. et al. (2001). Child literacy promotion in the emergency department. *Pediatric Emergency Care, 17*(1), 19–21.

National Center for Education Statistics. (2012). *Fast facts: Preprimary education enrollment.* Retrieved from http://nces.ed.gov/fastfacts /display.asp?id = 516

National Institute for Literacy. (2006). *The effect of family literacy interventions on children's acquisition of reading.* Portsmouth, NH: RMC Research. Retrieved from http://www.nifl.gov/partnershipfor reading/publications/html/lit_interventions/

Patrick, K., Spear, B., Holt, K. et al. (Eds.). (2001). *Bright futures in practice: Physical activity.* Arlington, VA: National Center for Education in Maternal and Child Health.

Proctor, M. H., Moore, L. L., Gao, D. et al. (2003). Television viewing and change in body fat from preschool to early adolescence: The Framingham Children's Study. *International Journal of Obesity, 27,* 827–833.

Rasines, G. (2010). Fluoride toothpaste prevents caries in children and adolescents at fluoride concentrations of 1000 ppm and above. *Evidence Based Dentistry, 11*(1), 6–7.

Reynolds, A., Temple, J., Ou, S. et al. (2011). School-based early childhood education and age-28 well-being: Effects by timing, dosage, and subgroups. *Science, 333*(6040), 360–364.

Richardson, B. (2006). *Practice guidelines for pediatric nurse practitioners.* St. Louis, MO: Mosby.

Robinson, T. N. (1999). Reducing children's television viewing to prevent obesity: A randomized controlled trial. *Journal of the American Medical Association, 282,* 1561–1567.

Saelens, B., Sallis, J., Nader, P. et al. (2002). Home environmental influences on children's television watching from early to middle childhood. *Journal of Developmental and Behavioral Pediatrics, 23*(3), 127–132.

Safe Kids Worldwide. (2011). *Drowning prevention fact sheet.* Retrieved from http://www.safekids.org/our-work/research/fact -sheets/drowning-prevention-fact-sheet.html

Sappenfield, O., & Rosenberg, K. (2011, October). *Racial/ethnic disparities in adults reading to two year old children: A population-based study.* Paper presented at the Oregon Public Health Association annual meeting, Corvallis, OR.

Shelov, S., & Altmann, T. (2009). *The American Academy of Pediatrics: Caring for your baby and young child, birth to age 5.* New York, NY: Bantam Books.

Silverstein, M., Iverson, L., & Lozano, P. (2005). An English-language clinic-based literacy program is effective for a multilingual population. *Pediatrics, 109*(5), e76.

Singer, M., Slovak, K., Frierson, T. et al. (1998). Viewing preferences, symptoms of psychological trauma, and violent behaviors among children who watch television. *Journal of the American Academy of Child & Adolescent Psychiatry, 37*(10), 1041–1048.

Slade, E., & Wissow, L. (2004). Spanking in early childhood and later behavior problems: A prospective study of infants and young toddlers. *Pediatrics, 113*(5), 1321–1330.

Smith, B. (2012). *The case against spanking.* Retrieved from http://www.apa.org/monitor/2012/04/spanking.aspx

Taylor, C., Manganello, J., Lee, S. et al. (2010). Mothers' spanking of 3-year-old children and subsequent risk of children's aggressive behavior. *Pediatrics, 125*(5), e1057–e1065.

van Zutphen, M., Bell, A., Kremer, P. et al. (2007). Association between the family environment and television viewing in Australian children. *Journal of Paediatrics & Child Health, 43*(6), 458–463.

Wakschlag, L., Choi, S., Carter, A. et al. (2012). Defining the developmental parameters of temper loss in early childhood: Implications for developmental psychopathology. *Journal of Child Psychology and Psychiatry, 53*(11), 1099–1108.

Wald, E., Di Lorenzo, C., Cipriani, L. et al. (2009). Bowel habits and toilet training in a diverse population of children. *Journal of Pediatric Gastroenterology & Nutrition, 48*(3), 294–298.

Walsh, T., Worthington, H., Glenny, A. et al. (2010). Fluoride toothpastes of different concentrations for preventing dental caries in children and adolescents. *Cochrane Database of Systematic Reviews,* (1), CD007868.

Yalcin, S., Tu Rul, B., Nacar, N. et al. (2002). Factors that affect television viewing time in preschool and primary schoolchildren. *Pediatrics International, 44*(6), 622–627.

See thePoint for additional resources.

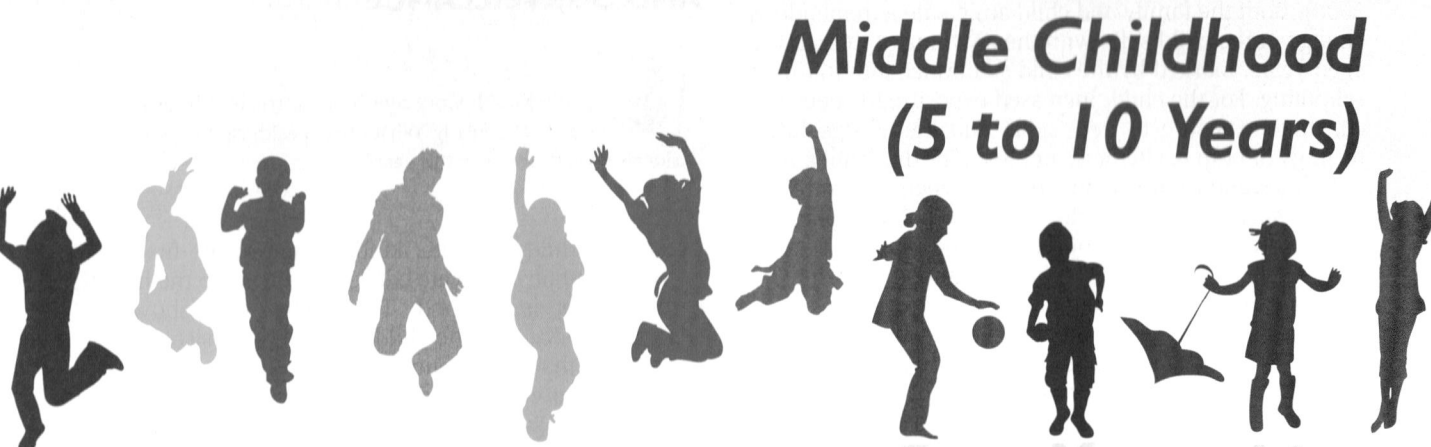

CHAPTER 6

Middle Childhood (5 to 10 Years)

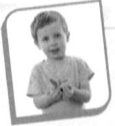

CASE HISTORY

Cory Whitworth is the youngest of six children. He just turned 5 years old and is ready to start kindergarten. He has never attended preschool or daycare. His parents, John and Wendy Whitworth, have four boys and two girls between the ages of 5 and 20 years. The oldest three boys are each about a year and a half apart. The second sister, Clarissa, is 3 years younger than Cathy. Then there is a 6-year space between Clarissa and Cory, the youngest of the family. Cory has significant household status as the baby of the family. They are members of the Church of Jesus Christ of Latter-day Saints.

Cory did not receive the hepatitis B vaccine as an infant. In the state in which he lives, hepatitis A and B vaccinations are mandatory for kindergarten attendance; therefore, Wendy has several appointments scheduled during the spring and summer with their pediatric health care provider. At the spring appointment, the pediatric health care provider verifies Cory's weight and height and asks Wendy about Cory's eating habits, dental hygiene, and sleep patterns. According to the Centers for Disease Control and Prevention (CDC) growth chart, his stature for age is greater than 97% and his weight for age is less than the 25th percentile. Wendy describes a typical day and relates what Cory eats throughout the day. Wendy states, "Cory is not a good eater; he won't eat meat, for instance. He won't eat most of the food that the rest of the family eats, so I prepare special meals for him that he eats at the breakfast bar. He doesn't like to eat unless I am eating with him or I feed him. But I do give him a nutritional shake almost every day." When asked about Cory's oral hygiene, Wendy replies that she brushes Cory's teeth every morning and evening and that he has seen a dentist. The pediatric health care provider also asks about Cory's sleeping habits. Wendy answers, "We just converted the study into Cory's room. He has a bed that looks like a blue race car. He never takes a nap now, and he usually sleeps through the night. He typically falls asleep in the living room while the older kids are watching TV. I let him stay up because that is about the only time the whole family is together."

CHAPTER OBJECTIVES

1 State the developmental surveillance concerns and milestone accomplishments of middle childhood.

2 Discuss the abilities achieved during middle childhood related to managing hygiene and personal care.

3 Describe the nutritional requirements to promote optimum growth during middle childhood.

4 Discuss the importance of engaging the child in physical activity with regard to developing lifelong health patterns of behavior.

5 Select age-appropriate interventions to promote healthy personal and social development of the child.

6 Describe strategies to help the child be successful in school.

7 Select interventions to prevent illness and injury among children aged 5 to 10 years and their families.

See thePoint for a list of Key Terms.

Middle childhood, also referred to as the *school-aged years*, is designated as ages 5 to 10 years (Hagan et al., 2008). Both the family and child anticipate a tremendous change in the child's life with the dawning of the school-aged years, marked by the child's entrance into full-time schooling. For the child, increased exposure to peers and constant exposure to new skills and knowledge bring feelings of both excitement and fear. For the family, new schedules and routines must be developed to ensure the child's success as he or she learns to balance physical needs with the demands of schoolwork, homework, and extracurricular activities. Middle childhood represents a time of tremendous developmental changes.

During this time of the child's development, the child's primary role is that of student, with the goal of gaining grade-level mastery of established educational standards. The family's primary role is to serve as advocate for the child as he or she interacts with the school and community. Optimally, family and home serve as secure environments for children to renew and refresh themselves each day and are places of solace where children's sense of self can be bolstered and individually encouraged. This chapter addresses various practical aspects of development during middle childhood.

DEVELOPMENTAL ASSESSMENT AND SURVEILLANCE

 QUESTION: Cory sees his pediatric health care provider regularly. What other health care professionals should Cory see this year?

Before the child can enter kindergarten or the first year of formal public or private education, a visit to the health care provider is required. The family must show the school evidence that the child has had a physical examination and that all immunizations are up to date. States and countries vary regarding which vaccinations are required prior to school entrance. Some include tuberculosis screening in these requirements (Hagan et al., 2008).

During the middle childhood years, health care visits are recommended every 2 years to complete developmental assessments and to screen for conditions common to this age group (Chart 6-1). Health visits include blood pressure screening; vision and hearing screening; and assessment for height, weight, and body mass

CHART 6-1	Quick Reference to Conditions Common During Middle Childhood

Condition	Chapter
Allergic rhinitis	16: The Child With Altered Respiratory Status
Appendicitis	18: The Child With Altered Gastrointestinal Status
Asthma	16: The Child With Altered Respiratory Status
Attention-deficit/hyperactivity disorder (ADHD)	29: The Child With Mental Health Challenges
Celiac disease	18: The Child With Altered Gastrointestinal Status
Childhood depression	29: The Child With Mental Health Challenges
Childhood schizophrenia	29: The Child With Mental Health Challenges
Cognitive challenge	30: The Child With a Developmental or Learning Disorder
Common cold (nasopharyngitis)	16: The Child With Altered Respiratory Status
Contact dermatitis	25: The Child With Altered Skin Integrity
Diabetes	26: The Child With Altered Endocrine Status
Encopresis	18: The Child With Altered Gastrointestinal Status
Enuresis	19: The Child With Altered Genitourinary Status
Epistasis	31: Pediatric Emergencies
Functional abdominal pain and irritable bowel syndrome	18: The Child With Altered Gastrointestinal Status
Growth hormone deficiency	26: The Child With Altered Endocrine Status
Hypertension	15: The Child with Altered Cardiovascular Status
Learning disorders	30: The Child With a Developmental or Learning Disorder
Pediculosis	25: The Child With Altered Skin Integrity
Pharyngitis	16: The Child With Altered Respiratory Status
Precocious puberty	26: The Child With Altered Endocrine Status
Scabies	25: The Child With Altered Skin Integrity
School phobia	29: The Child With Mental Health Challenges
Tonsillitis	16: The Child With Altered Respiratory Status
Tuberculosis	24: The Child With an Infectious Disease

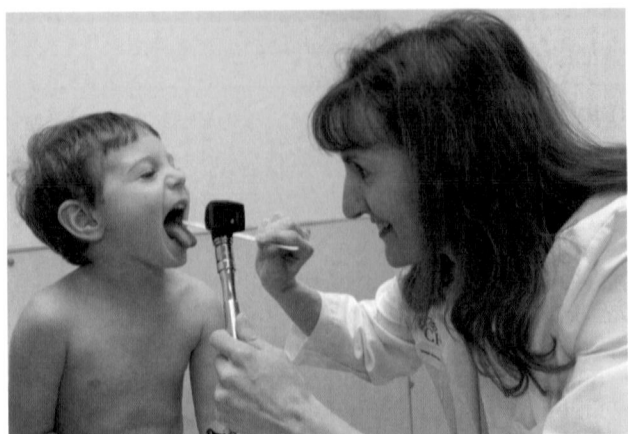

Figure 6-1 The school-aged child is likely to willingly cooperate during health care screening examinations.

indices (BMIs) that would alert the health care provider to childhood obesity (Fig. 6-1). Scoliosis screening begins around 8 years of age. Issues discussed during health visits with children and the family include nutrition and eating behaviors, oral health, parent–child relationships, school concerns, media use and access to the Internet, violence, and environmental exposures that may be unhealthy for the child (e.g., smoke, sun, play equipment) (Hagan et al., 2008).

An essential component of the health visit is assessing acquisition of developmental milestones. Developmental Considerations 6-1 presents a summary of the developmental milestones that are accomplished during middle childhood. This information is useful to provide the pediatric health care provider with direction for specific trigger questions that can be asked of the family to determine the child's developmental progress. Trigger questions should also include school performance as well as the usual concerns regarding general developmental issues.

ANSWER: All school-aged children should be examined by a dentist every year and an ophthalmologist every few years. Cory should visit a dentist to examine his teeth and identify any dental caries. He should also visit an ophthalmologist to examine his eyes and check his vision prior to entering school.

HYGIENE AND PERSONAL CARE

Preparing for school each day provides the opportunity for the child to develop good hygiene and personal care habits that include oral care, choosing appropriate clothing based on environmental conditions, ensuring adequate sleep, and making healthy food choices. The child is still too young and not knowledgeable enough to make decisions about these issues totally independent of family supervision. The child will certainly challenge the families' authority and respective "house rules" about

bedtime, snack choices, and clothing choices. As children move through middle childhood, they are cognitively able to understand and appreciate these rules and the ways that these rules affect their personal health. As children move into adolescence, teachers, peers, and the media will have increasing influence on their behaviors. Ongoing family guidance provided during middle childhood can help children in their decision-making processes.

ORAL CARE

QUESTION: Because of the emerging independence seen in children during middle childhood, many activities of daily living may be performed solely by the child, jointly by the family and child, or solely by the family. How would you assess the extent of Cory's autonomy and his development of health maintenance behaviors? How do you respond to Wendy's information?

By the time the child is 5 years old, some of the permanent teeth may start to erupt, and preventive care at an early age will forestall any problems. The number one dental problem in middle childhood is caries. Because some of the cavities are in the primary teeth, which will be lost, families may assume that it is nothing to worry about (U.S. Preventive Services Task Force, 2004). However, premature loss of primary teeth may cause other primary teeth to shift and not allow the permanent teeth room to come in later. Until the age of 7 years, children may need assistance brushing their teeth. Children who develop good oral hygiene habits do not run the risk of developing dental caries and other problems that cause premature tooth loss (Fig. 6-2). The best method of preventive care is to foster good dental hygiene habits at an early age.

A child-sized, soft-bristled toothbrush with a dab of fluoride toothpaste is recommended. Caution the family not to overuse fluoride toothpaste because the child may swallow it in amounts that can cause dental fluorosis, a condition that produces staining on the permanent teeth. For many years, dentists recommended only brushing up and down; now, any direction of brushing is considered fine as long as each tooth is thoroughly brushed from the gum line to the crown and plaque is removed daily. Children usually concentrate on the front teeth because they can see them easily and forget about the teeth in the back. Family oversight is needed to be sure those overlooked teeth are brushed as carefully.

Children should have their teeth checked by a dentist and cleaned by a dental hygienist twice a year. Chapter 3 describes the sequence in which the primary (deciduous) and secondary (permanent) teeth erupt (see Fig. 3-21). Eruption of secondary teeth, which begins around age 6 years, is not associated with the same amount of fussiness or discomfort as the eruption of primary teeth. If a primary tooth is lost before the permanent tooth erupts, the family should consult the dentist to determine whether a space retainer is needed to keep the teeth in

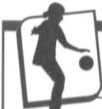

DEVELOPMENTAL CONSIDERATIONS 6-1

Milestones of Middle Childhood (5–10 Years Old)

Physical Development

- Girls: by age 11 years have achieved 90% of adult height and 50% of adult weight
- Boys: at age 12 years have achieved 80% of adult height and 50% of adult weight

All School-Aged Children
- Acceleration of growth of long bones
- Beginning of Tanner stages of prepubertal development

5–9 Years Old
- Sleep 10–12 hr/day
- Gain 3–5 lb/year
- Have 10–11 permanent teeth
- Arms grow longer in proportion to body

10 Years Old
- Sleep 8–10 hr/day
- Need 1,600–2,600 cal/day
- 12-year molars erupt

Sexual Development
- Girls: some have menarche as early as 10 years of age

All School-Aged Children
- Normal interest in same-sex relationships
- Interest in heterosexual relationships more pronounced in later school-aged years
- Latency years; sex drives repressed (Freud)

Language Development
All School-Aged Children
- By 5 years of age, have vocabulary of 1,500–2,000 words
- Know coin exchange

Vision Development
All School-Aged Children
- Have 20/20 vision

Gross Motor Development
6 Years Old
- Walk a straight line heel to toe
- Balances on each foot for 6 seconds

8 Years Old
- Crouch on tiptoes
- Put right or left foot forward on command

9–10 Years Old
- Balance on one leg with eyes closed
- Catch tennis ball with one hand

Fine Motor Development
All School-Aged Children
- Continually refine and improve previously learned skills

- Move more gracefully
- Bathe unassisted
- Use tools

Play Development
All School-Aged Children
- Engage in cooperative "team" play
- Engage in skill play (jump rope, skating)
- Enjoy testing, model building, exploration
- Collect things and classify them as hobbies
- Play board games
- Read for pleasure
- Become engrossed easily in long hours of media use

Cognitive Development
All School-Aged Children
Concrete Operations (Piaget)
- Gain ability to reason
- Grasp concept of reversibility
- Classify objects according to their characteristics
- Understand concept of conservation
- Understand concept of relativism
- Can place self in another's situation
- Understand serialization, master the ordinal number line; can group and sort/place in logical order
- Develop fundamental skills of reading, writing, and grammar
- Understand concept of reciprocity
- Understand concept of identity
- Gain greater ability to calculate distances and use directions
- Tell time
- Acquire decentration; able to focus on many aspects of experience

10 Years Old
- Capable of abstract and deductive reasoning
- Consider death irreversible, but capricious
- Use external/internal physiologic explanations

Social Development
All School-Aged Children
- Initiate social participation in school, neighborhood, and scouting groups
- Begin to manage cooperative and competitive relationships

Interpersonal Development
All School-Aged Children
- Gain independence within family
- Learn to self-regulate behavior
- Navigate issues of industry versus inferiority (Erikson)

Emotional Development

All School-Aged Children

- Use coping behaviors (strategies): avoidant coping, active coping, avoidant–active coping

Moral/Spiritual Development

All School-Aged Children

Moral—Stage 4: Conventional (Kohlberg)

- Concerned with authority figures, fixed rules in moral decisions
- Concerned with obligation to duty
- Understand that a bad act breaks a rule or does harm
- May interpret accidents or misfortunes as punishment
- Develop a conscience and sense of values

Spiritual—Stage 2: Mythical/Literal (Fowler)

- Distinguish religious fact from fantasy
- Respect and rely on authoritative figures such as parents, priest, rabbi
- Influenced by attitude of peers toward faith
- Have monomythic attitude; use fantasies to explain events or facts they do not understand
- Learn to differentiate between natural and supernatural
- Perceive God in anthropomorphic imagery, with human qualities
- Describe God in a way that implies formation of a reciprocal relationship

appropriate alignment until the permanent tooth erupts (Casamassimo & Holt, 2004).

Early orthodontic intervention may mean less extensive treatment later because young teeth are easier to move. Early treatment may also reduce the risk of relapse. If a child needs orthodontic intervention, the child must adhere to the care regimen that is needed for the braces (e.g., keeping them clean, wearing retainers). Selecting an orthodontist who is knowledgeable and will establish a good rapport with the child and family is essential because treatment will include dental visits every 4 to 6 weeks for a 2- to 4-year treatment period (Fig. 6-3).

ANSWER: Wendy has already stated that she brushes Cory's teeth. Follow up with another question to determine whether Cory is learning to brush his own teeth. An example of a response to Wendy is, "Brushing his teeth twice a day is excellent. Since he is now 5 years old, he should start brushing the front teeth and you can still make sure the molars are brushed." With the family, as well as with children, it is more effective and less a matter of personal opinion to say "Now it is time . . . " rather than "I think you should . . . "

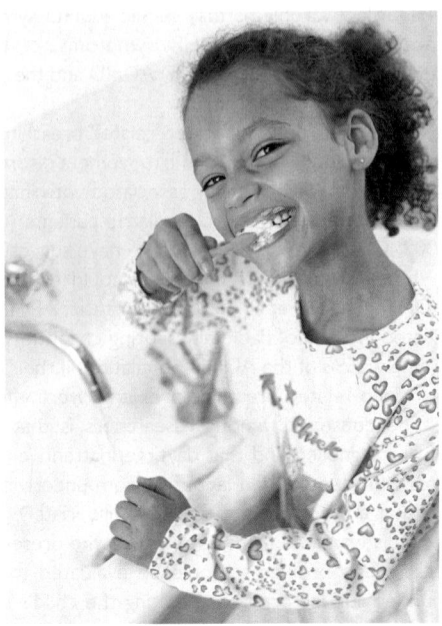

Figure 6-2 The school-aged child needs encouragement to brush after meals and at bedtime as part of a good dental hygiene program.

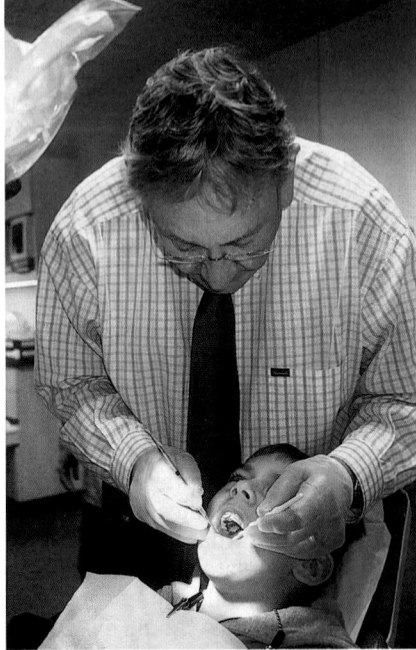

Figure 6-3 Orthodontics may be initiated in middle childhood to prevent malocclusion of the permanent teeth.

SLEEP

QUESTION: How would you elicit more information regarding Cory's sleep habits? How could you respond to Wendy's information about Cory falling asleep in front of the television?

On average, children spend 8 to 10 hours per night sleeping, although sleep duration can vary considerably and still be considered normal. The amount of time the child sleeps may vary with the day of the week (school day vs. weekend) and time of the year (school year vs. vacation). During vacations and weekends, the child is likely to sleep longer because the child's schedule is not dictated by school start times. Most children experience two awakenings per night, and approximately 20% to 41% of children experience substantial sleep problems (Carno et al., 2003).

Chronic sleep loss is a recognized problem in children and adolescents (Matricciani et al., 2012; Mindell et al., 2011). Sleep problems in childhood can negatively impact daytime neuropsychological functioning (Beebe, 2012). The most common sleep disturbances at this age can be traced to several origins: general behavioral problems, separation anxiety, desire to have special time with a parent without sibling interruptions, or an altered sleep cycle that may need some adjustment (e.g., the child may go to bed too late or may have a different bedtime at one parent's home than at the other parent's home). Some other causes of sleep disturbances can be nightmares, fear of the dark, night terrors, or sleepwalking. Health factors such as chronic cough, snoring, chronic rhinitis, and eczema also contribute to sleep problems during middle childhood (Desager et al., 2005). Although the child may not waken in the night from these problems, the child may be less alert in the morning. Children who have difficulty with initiating sleep or staying asleep may also have subsequent problems in school as a result of the cumulative patterns of disordered sleep (Tradition or Science 6-1).

Most sleep disturbances are of limited duration and resolve without intervention (Hoban, 2004). If a child continues to have sleep disturbances, a health care provider should be consulted to recommend interventions. A recent report surveying pediatric providers in a large network showed that only 3.7% of patients were diagnosed with an International Classification of Diseases Ninth Revision (ICD-9) diagnosis for a sleep disorder. This prevalence rate is lower than previous reports (Meltzer et al., 2010). It is important that pediatric health care providers incorporate questions about sleep and possible sleep disorders in their assessment of the child's well-being. Medical interventions may be needed if the sleep disturbance is related to a health problem (e.g., snoring related to enlarged tonsils).

A consistent bedtime will help ensure that the child gets adequate sleep. Families should encourage children to have a consistent bedtime routine that may include quiet reading time and time for nonstressful family talk. Homework should be stopped early enough to allow the child to have some quiet time to relax before slumber. Use of media should end early in the evening. A well-darkened room can also facilitate good sleep. Keeping pets away from the room may also be helpful, especially if the pets are likely to jump on and off of the child's bed during the night and thus awaken the child.

ANSWER: To elicit more information regarding Cory's sleep habits, follow an open-ended question with specific questions. You could ask, "What time does Cory usually fall asleep and when does he wake up?" Although Cory may be getting enough sleep, Wendy's answer alerts the pediatric health care provider to ask more questions about TV viewing and other media usage. Although many Americans fall asleep in front of the television, sleep experts strongly discourage this practice. Explain that being able to fall asleep by himself in his own bed is a learned skill for Cory, just like riding a bike is a learned skill.

More Inquiry Needed   TRADITION OR SCIENCE 6-1

Do most children with ongoing sleep problems have ADHD?

An estimated 25%–50% of children with ADHD experience problems with sleep, particularly in initiating and maintaining sleep. At one point, restless and disturbed sleep was a part of the *Diagnostic and Statistical Manual of Mental Disorders Fourth Edition* (*DSM-IV*) diagnostic criteria for ADHD. These problems, subsequently considered nonspecific criteria, have been eliminated as defining characteristics of the condition. A review by Yoon et al. (2012) describes the complexity associated with defining the relationship between sleep disorders and ADHD. Sleep problems may mimic ADHD symptoms, may exacerbate underlying ADHD symptoms, or may be associated with or be exacerbated by ADHD and the psychotropic medications used to treat it.

Researchers have found that sleep-related breathing disorders (including snoring), periodic limb movement disorder, and restless legs syndrome are highly associated with inattention and hyperactivity among general pediatric patients (Chervin et al., 2002; Chervin et al., 1997). Some have suggested that treating these causal effects effectively could eliminate the child's ADHD. Chervin et al. (2002) suggest that ADHD could be eliminated in 81% of habitually snoring children (which is approximately 25% of the ADHD population) if their snoring and other sleep-related breathing problems were effectively treated. The consensus among researchers is that ADHD may be overdiagnosed and that daytime inattentiveness and attentional difficulties may in fact arise from underlying sleep disorders that are not being managed appropriately. Further investigation is warranted, and every child who presents with ADHD and sleep problems should be evaluated to ensure that no underlying factor is accentuating the child's sleeping problems (Yoon et al., 2012).

NUTRITION

QUESTION: What information and strategies could you share with Wendy that might affect Cory's eating behaviors and nutritional intake?

By middle childhood, the child's diet should be a healthy combination of foods as shown in the U.S. Department of Agriculture (USDA, n.d.) food guide called MyPlate (see Fig. 5-7). The amount of food and caloric intake that the child eats is still not equivalent to the amounts in an adult portion (Chart 6-2). Because this is the age when most food preferences are determined, the family should offer the child a wide variety of foods. Family food habits influence children the most during this time.

For a child eating a well-balanced diet, the American Academy of Pediatrics (AAP) does not recommend the use of vitamin supplements. All the nutrients a child needs should come from the food eaten. The most recent recommendation for this age group (Holt et al., 2011) is to introduce a low-fat diet (less than 30% of calories should come from fat). This measure helps the child start a lifelong habit of healthy eating.

This is an ideal age at which to encourage children to help prepare meals (Fig. 6-4). Adult supervision is needed when the child is 5 to 8 years old, but by the time the child is 12 years old, the child should be able to prepare a simple meal without assistance. Allowing children to prepare their own school lunches encourages them to make choices of foods that they will eat and not discard or trade.

SCHOOL LUNCH PROGRAMS

As the child enters school and begins eating lunch there, monitoring what the child is eating away from home becomes difficult. Many children participate in a school lunch program or may "brown bag" their lunch from home. If the child brings a lunch from home, it should be varied, with interesting, tasty foods that the child likes. School cafeteria lunches have been a focus of media scrutiny because of a belief that they do not offer enough healthy choices for children. The National School Lunch Program recently updated its meal pattern and nutrition standards according to the *Dietary Guidelines for Americans*; this was dictated by the Healthy, Hunger-Free Kids Act of 2010 and commenced in the 2012–2013 school year in the United States. The Healthy, Hunger-Free Kids Act stipulates that more fruits, vegetables, and whole grains are incorporated into the school menu. There are also specific calorie limits as well as reductions in sodium content of the meals (USDA, 2012). One of the disadvantages of school lunch programs is that the children may pass up the school lunch altogether if it is not appealing and buy a "vending machine lunch" or trade with friends, making nonnutritious choices. One of the successful strategies offered by schools today is to teach children about healthy food at an early grade level and to elicit their help in making appropriate menu choices (Fig. 6-5).

CHART 6-2   Nutritional Recommendations During Middle Childhood

Calories per Day Age	Not Active	Active
Females 5–6 years	1,200	1,600
Females 7 years	1,200	1,800
Females 8–9 years	1,400	1,800
Females 10 years	1,400	2,000
Males 5 years	1,200	1,600
Males 6–7 years	1,400	1,800
Males 8 years	1,400	2,000
Males 9 years	1,600	2,000
Males 10 years	1,600	2,200

Food Group Recommendations

Grains

- Make half your grains whole.
- Eat at least 5–6 oz equivalents of whole grain cereals, breads, crackers, rice, or pasta every day.

Vegetables (One half of your plate, along with fruit)

- Vary vegetable intake.
- Eat more dark-green vegetables such as broccoli and spinach.
- Eat more orange vegetables such as carrots and sweet potatoes.
- Eat more dry beans and peas such as pinto beans, kidney beans, and lentils.
- Eat 1½–2 cups daily.

Fruits (One half of your plate, along with vegetables)

- Eat a variety of fruit.
- Choose fresh, frozen, canned, or dried fruit.
- Go easy on fruit juices and drink only 100% fruit juice.
- Eat 1–1½ cups daily.

Dairy

- Choose low-fat or fat-free milk, yogurt, and other milk products.
- Eat or drink 2½–3 cups daily.

Protein Foods

- Choose low-fat or lean meats and poultry.
- Eat meat that is baked, broiled, or grilled; stay away from fried meats.
- Choose varieties of protein sources; eat fish, soy products, beans, nuts, eggs, peas, and seeds.
- Eat 4–5 oz equivalents daily.
- Eat fish twice a week.

Oils (not a food group, but oils contain essential nutrients)

- Make most of your fat sources from fish, nuts, and vegetable oils.
- Limit solid fats (e.g., butter, margarine, lard).
- Keep intake of saturated fats, trans fats, and sodium low.
- Limit to 4–5 teaspoons daily.

From U.S. Department of Agriculture. (n.d.). *MyPlate information.* Retrieved from http://www.choosemyplate.gov; U.S. Department of Agriculture & U.S. Department of Health & Human Services. (2010). *Dietary guidelines for Americans 2010.* Retrieved from http://www.health.gov/dietaryguidelines/dga2010/DietaryGuidelines2010.pdf

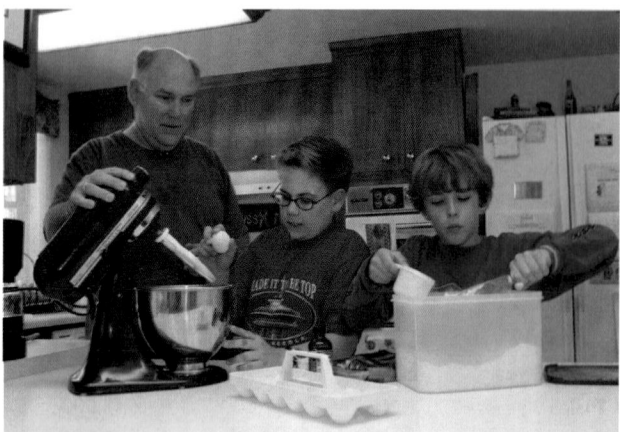

Figure 6-4 Learning to cook can be an enjoyable activity for the school-aged child.

A primary role of the nurse is to work with school programs to ensure that healthy foods are being provided. For instance, the AAP (2004) endorses a policy that restricts the sale of soft drinks in schools. The nurse can use this policy as a springboard to implement school-wide change to ensure that sweetened, carbonated, and caffeinated drinks are eliminated on school campuses and are replaced with real fruit and vegetable juices, water, and low-fat white or flavored milk. The nurse must also campaign for an ongoing plan to ensure that physical activity is a part of each child's daily school schedule. Last, every campaign to support good nutrition and daily physical activity must include families and their children as active members of the learning community. Programs implemented without a

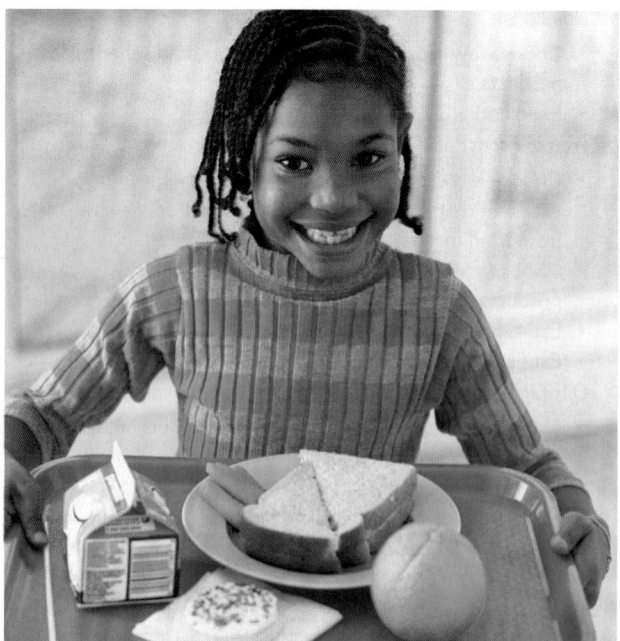

Figure 6-5 School lunches should provide a balanced, nutritious midday meal for the child. Lunchtime provides both an opportunity for physical renewal and social exchange with friends.

family-centered approach are doomed to fail when the child's home life and school life are disconnected.

> **ANSWER:** Eating is a significant part of a family culture and is difficult to change. Wendy is feeding six children, three of whom are athletic teenage boys. Their nutritional needs and their schedules are different from Cory's. In addition, Cory and Wendy are perpetuating Cory's baby status. Although there are many changes that can be recommended, it may be most effective to suggest one or two at a time. Give Wendy specific examples of appropriate meals for Cory that include small portions of a variety of foods. Strongly encourage Wendy to stop feeding Cory separately from the older children. Suggest that Wendy tell the family, "Now that Cory will be starting school, it is time for him to join the older children at the table and feed himself."

OBESITY

Obesity is the epidemic of the childhood years. Since 1971, the proportion of overweight children has more than doubled for children aged 6 through 11 years and has more than tripled among children aged 12 through 19 years. According to the CDC (n.d.b), the percentage of U.S. obese children aged 6 to 11 years in 2010 was approximately 18%, having increased from 7% in 1980. Obesity is defined as BMI greater than or equal to the 95th percentile of children with same BMI-for-age and sex percentile (CDC, n.d.a) (see Chapter 7 for more information about obesity). A number of health risks are associated with obesity in childhood, including type 2 diabetes, obstructive sleep apnea, hypertension, fatty liver disease, hypercholesterolemia, joint problems, and risk of psychological problems (CDC, n.d.a).

Inherited factors may play a role in obesity, but the rapid increase in obesity rates during the past 20 years indicates that changes in behavior are a more likely cause. Food convenience, large intake of sodas and juices, decreased physical activity, and a hurried lifestyle contribute to the epidemic. Guide families in assisting their children to make correct choices of healthy foods and to stay away from excessive salt or sugar consumption. The AAP also endorses the role of recess at school, not to replace physical education, but as a complement (AAP, 2013). Nursing Interventions 6-1 summarizes some of the recommendations for evaluating and treating childhood obesity. Several organizations have developed position statements and extensive materials to assist practitioners to use strategies to prevent, screen, and treat pediatric overweight and obesity (see Evidence-Based Clinical Practice Guidelines 4-1).

PHYSICAL FITNESS

The AAP (2006) recommends that health care providers actively promote physical fitness in children. Physical fitness programs help to start behavioral habits that will enable a child to become a healthy and fit adult. School-aged children should be encouraged to participate in 60 minutes of vigorous physical activity daily. Exercise should consist of activities that the child enjoys which

NURSING INTERVENTIONS 6-1

Recommendations for Assessment and Treatment of Obesity

Assessment

- Screen children for overweight by checking BMI at every health care encounter.
- Rule out secondary causes of obesity (e.g., genetic causes, endocrine causes).
- Assess for psychological causes of obesity.
- Assess for complications of obesity, such as obstructive sleep apnea, type 2 diabetes, and slipped capital femoral epiphysis.
- Assess family readiness for change.

Treatment

- Provide family education about medical complications (e.g., hypertension, dyslipidemia, heart disease, and diabetes) and psychosocial complications (e.g., depression, poor self-esteem) related to obesity.

- Involve the entire family in developing and implementing the program.
- Emphasize long-term permanent changes, not rapid weight loss or short-term diets.
- Support family activities that promote having everyone exercise moderately 60 minutes daily.
- Encourage a low-fat, low-cholesterol, reduced-sugar diet appropriate for the age and weight of family members. Encourage dietary practices that foster moderation rather than overconsumption.
- Encourage meal planning; discourage skipping meals.
- Counsel the family to avoid using food as a punishment or reward.

---

can be incorporated easily into the child's routine and could be continued into adulthood. These activities can include bicycling, walking, running, or swimming.

Team sports such as baseball, basketball, soccer, or football enable the child to develop group play skills. For children from 5 to 8 years old, team sports that are loosely structured and not too aggressively focused toward winning are good options. From ages 8 to 10 years, trying a variety of sports, both team and individual, is a good way for a child to find something that he or she enjoys (Fig. 6-6). Organized sports programs should not replace regular physical activity but rather should serve as complementary activities to enhance the child's physical abilities, knowledge of team skills, and knowledge of new sports.

Children will not benefit from sports unless they are suited for the sport in both age and temperament. The

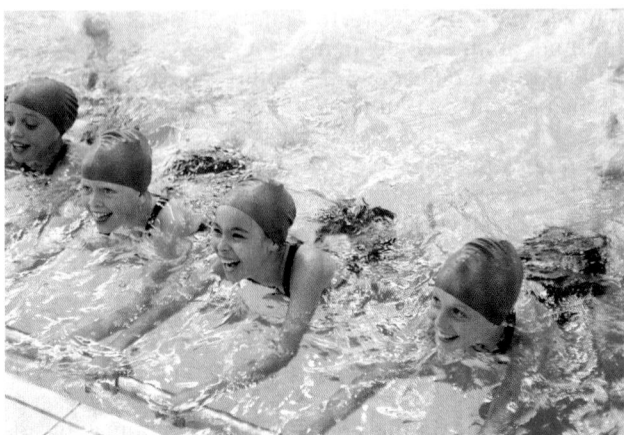

Figure 6-6 Girls and boys enjoy participating in team sports and can benefit from physical activity.

family needs to work hard to find the right sport for the child and make the experience a positive one. A family should not be as concerned with who won the game as with how the game was played and whether everyone had a good time. Praising the child's efforts and not giving tips on how the child could have done something better or differently is more positive and is what the child needs at this age. The child should be allowed to quit a sport he or she does not care for or finds too difficult. Many families believe that doing so allows the child to become a "quitter," but a bad experience with a coach or someone else on the team can cause permanent repercussions, and the child may never again participate in a sport.

Physical fitness activities also place the child at risk for injury. Most injuries occur as a result of falls, being struck by an object, collisions, and overexertion during unorganized or informal sports activities. Most injuries during team events occur during practices rather than during games. Death from a sports injury is rare; the leading cause of death from a sports-related injury is a brain injury. Most head injuries sustained during sports or recreational activities occur during bicycling, skateboarding, or skating incidents.

Children need to be monitored during physical activities to ensure they are incorporating proper body mechanics and safety precautions. When learning a new sport, children should always be supervised and given instruction regarding proper use of sport equipment, rules regarding body contact with other children, and safety precautions that must be used during participation in the sport. Chapter 7 presents a discussion about sport activities and the adolescent and suggests ways to prevent sports injury (see Community Care 7-1 and Developmental Considerations 7-4).

AGE-APPROPRIATE ACTIVITIES

By the time the child reaches age 5 years, vocabulary is about 1,500 to 2,000 words, and speech is almost 100% understood, even by strangers. He or she has developed very good balance and coordination. This child can hop and skip on alternate feet, throw and catch a ball, dress himself or herself, and complete total self-care. Pretend play, playing with puppets, and dressing up in clothes are added to the list of favorite games. This is the age when the child starts to mimic his or her parents and behave in a gender-specific fashion (Fig. 6-7).

"Play" in the traditional sense has become a declining focus of activity during middle childhood. Indoor and outdoor recreation is being replaced by use of media, including television, computer play, video games, and other social media. Recreational activity (recess and physical education classes) at elementary schools has been minimized by the elimination of trained physical education teachers from the school staff and by the increased focus on mandated testing in the educational system. Increased homework affects children's ability to get out and play, as do the busy schedules of children and families as they race from one planned activity to another (Ginsburg, 2007). Children need time to play, however, because play helps them to develop cognitively, socially, physically, and emotionally.

Middle childhood is characterized by play that embodies the need for rules and structure. This need for rituals and rules translates well into team sports and other activities that have rules and structure. The group the child participates with may actually develop very rigid and outlandish rules for some group games. This is also the time that many children enjoy being part

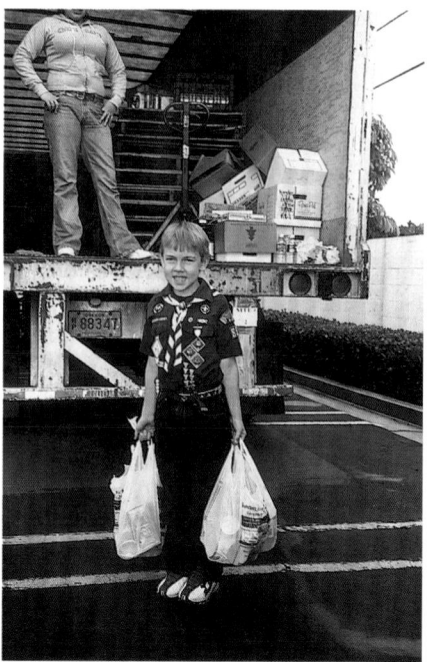

Figure 6-8 Scouting groups can expose the child to community service activities. This young scout is participating in a community canned food drive.

of a social group, such as Girl Scouts or Boy Scouts, which has a structured set of guidelines for behavior and achievements. These groups provide many opportunities for activities such as camping, making crafts, completing service projects, and participating in fundraising promotions (Fig. 6-8).

Team play is a more complex version of group play and is an ideal model for children to learn the importance of being a team player and achieving goals set for the team, not just the individual. They also learn how to handle competition and work cooperatively in a group to achieve a common goal—skills that later can be transferred to other situations. Through these accomplishments, they develop self-esteem, physical skills, and improved manual dexterity.

Another focus of the ritualistic behavior common at this age is collecting and hobbies. The school-aged child may develop the desire to collect all sorts of matching and nonmatching items (Fig. 6-9A). School-aged children have developed the ability to concentrate and participate in self-initiated quiet activities that challenge their cognitive skills, such as reading or playing computer and board games (Fig. 6-9B, C). This is an ideal age to introduce musical instrument instruction. The child has the manual dexterity, attention span, and the rule rigidity to make this experience a positive one (Fig. 6-9D).

One type of play activity that must be approached cautiously during middle childhood is the use of trampolines at home, school, and recreation centers. The AAP (2012) does not recommend trampoline use except when used in a structured training program with adequate coaching and supervision with safety measures. Fortunately, the rate of injury from trampoline use has

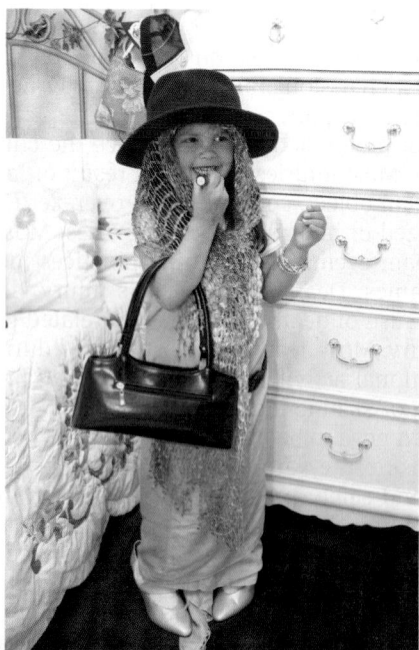

Figure 6-7 Dressing up and pretending to be different real and make-believe characters is fun for children. Here, this little girl enjoys dressing up as "Mommy."

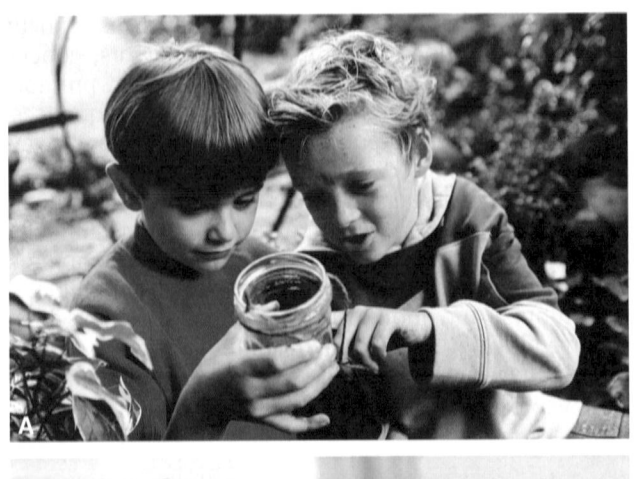
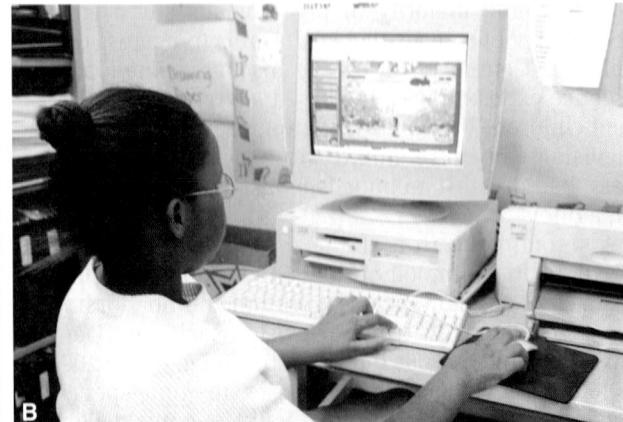
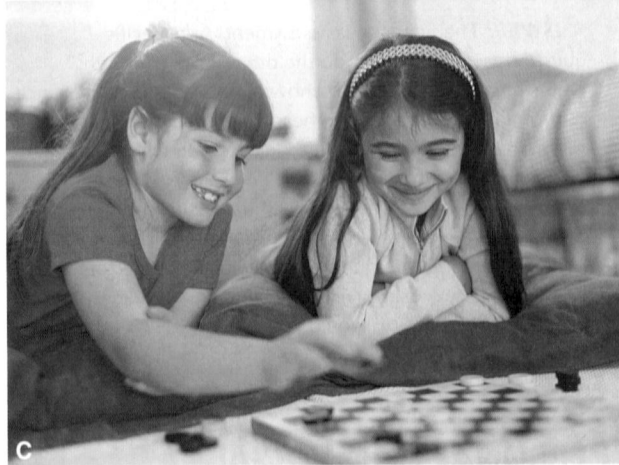
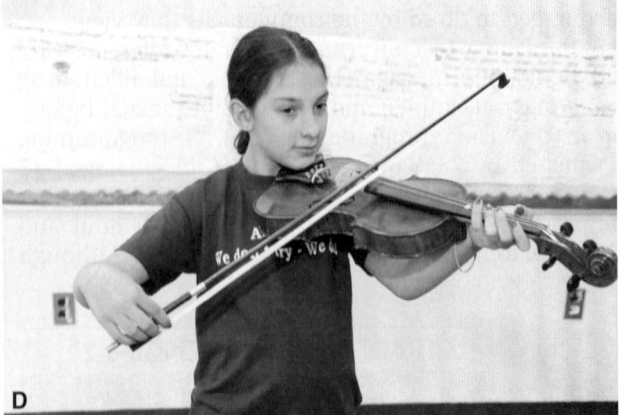

Figure 6-9 The refinement of fine motor and cognitive skills allows the child to enjoy many new activities. (A) The ability to classify objects increases the child's interest in collecting insects, rocks, stickers, or anything that strikes his or her fancy. (B) Computer games and research require the ability to read, add, think critically, and manipulate the mouse and keyboard. (C) Board games can be used to sharpen the child's cognitive skills. (D) With increased dexterity and higher level thinking, the child can learn the complexities of playing an instrument.

decreased since 2004. In 2009, there were 3,041 reported cases of trampoline injuries, which is a decrease from 3,277 reported injuries in 2004 (AAP, 2012).

Musculoskeletal injuries are the most common trampoline injuries, but more serious injuries can occur, including head and neck injuries (AAP, 2012). Home trampoline use should be discouraged; if home trampolines are used, families should ensure that their homeowners insurance covers trampoline injuries, only one person is allowed to use the trampoline at a time, and jumping is supervised. At present, there isn't sufficient data regarding trampoline park safety, so health care providers should inform families that park guidelines may differ from AAP guidelines, and children may be at increased risk for injury (AAP, 2012).

MEDIA USE

QUESTION: Wendy has mentioned that Cory watches TV or plays in the room with the TV on while Cory's teenage brothers are watching TV. Wendy states she doesn't think Cory is paying much attention to what is on the TV. What do you think is appropriate to say to Wendy?

Media use by children and adolescents has increasingly displaced other activities in the child's life, such as reading, exercising, and playing with friends. The average child or adolescent watches an average of 3 to 4 hours of television a day (Kaiser Family Foundation, 2010). With TV shows now available on demand through various portable devices, viewing of shows and movies has increased over the past 5 years (Kaiser Family Foundation, 2010). Including TV content, computers, video games, movies, music/audio, and print, youth spend over 7 hours each day 7 days a week using media (Kaiser Family Foundation, 2010). These statistics are in sharp contrast to the number of minutes daily that a child spends in meaningful conversation with his or her parents (3.5 min/day) (TV-Turnoff Network, 2005).

Media use by school-aged children raises several concerns. The first relates to the content, which increasingly emphasizes violence (Tradition or Science 6-2). The AAP Council on Communications and Media states that nearly two thirds of all programs contain violence and that children's shows contain the most violence. In these shows, violence is often glamorized, and the perpetrators of crime and violence go unpunished. A study by Gentile, Obert et al. (2004) found that the overwhelming majority of pediatricians surveyed believe that violence in the media affects aggression in children. Gentile et al. (2011) also associated media violence exposure with increased aggression in school-aged children. Viewing frightening or violent scenes on television can cause children to experience unrealistic fears, bad dreams, anxious feelings, and the fear of being alone.

A second concern is the relation between television viewing and childhood obesity. Studies have concluded that a child's weight increases with the number of hours he or she spends watching television each day (Dennison & Edmunds, 2008; Jordan, 2007; Singh et al., 2008). As television viewing time increases, the time spent exercising and engaging in other active pursuits declines. Additionally, while children watch television, they frequently snack on high-calorie and high-fat foods or are encouraged to do so by the commercials they view.

A third area of concern is the many references to, and depictions of, cigarette, alcohol, and illicit drug use; dangerous stunts; and irresponsible sexual behavior in television programming. MTV's programming is watched by 73% of boys and 78% of girls aged 12 to 19 years. An analysis of MTV coverage noted that the programs averaged 13 sexual scenes per hour and 32 uses of foul language (LifeSiteNews, 2005). Although no recent studies substantiate the effect of this exposure on actual childhood or adolescent behaviors, concern remains that this highly influential medium promotes risky behaviors with little emphasis on consequences.

Media use has potential benefits for children if viewing/use is monitored and exposure time is balanced with other family and personal activities (see Developmental Considerations 5-2). Essential guidelines for families to follow include limiting total media time, removing televisions and personal handheld devices from children's bedrooms, and monitoring the types of shows being viewed (AAP, 2009). When families set rules limiting media use, those children have decreased rates of media use (Kaiser Family Foundation, 2010).

ANSWER: The first step is assessment. Ask specific questions such as, "What do the other children watch?" Determine whether it is TV shows or movies. The difference is twofold: exposure to commercials and length of programming. Sometimes it is difficult to initiate a conversation when you perceive that your values are different than those of the client family. Approach the subject in a factual and nonjudgmental way. An example of an appropriate statement is, "The health care community has studied a number of issues related to TV exposure, including violent behavior, attention problems, and obesity. Would you like more information about television viewing and children?"

Evidence-Based Practice
TRADITION OR SCIENCE 6-2

Do violent games increase children's aggressive behaviors?

Recent data indicate that boys spend an average of 13 hr/week and girls spend an average of 5 hr/week playing violent video games (Gentile, Lynch et al., 2004). Twenty-two percent of 8–11-year-olds own M-rated (mature) video games, with boys more than two times as likely as girls to obtain them (Gentile, 2009). Most video games include violence, even between cartoon characters. Playing a lot of violent video games has been associated with having aggressive thoughts, feelings, and behaviors. Anderson et al. (2008) explored violent video game playing and aggression in children in Japan and the United States. They found that playing violent video games at a young age was a predictor of physical aggression later on (Anderson et al., 2008). Playing video games has been associated with attention problems (Swing et al., 2010). Playing video games is also related to children being less willing to be caring and helpful toward peers. These effects are seen as often among nonaggressive children as among children with documented aggressive tendencies (Anderson et al., 2003; Anderson & Bushman, 2001; Gentile, Obert et al., 2004; Robinson et al., 2001). Gentile (2009) found that 8% of video game users, in a sample of 1,178 children in the United States, had pathologic patterns of play; the youth in this sample ranged from 8 to 18 years of age. Those categorized as "pathologic" had poorer school grades and had comorbidity with attentional problems (Gentile, 2009). Children are in a critical period for learning and developing healthy ways to relate to other people and to resolve conflicts peacefully, and playing violent video games has been demonstrated to have harmful effects on children's social relationships.

PERSONAL AND SOCIAL DEVELOPMENT

The social environment of the school provides opportunities for children to develop personally and to begin to discriminate who they are as unique individuals. Social relations with peers can be quite challenging as the child learns to form bonds of friendship and learns the nuances of gender relations. Adults play an important part in the child's development of self. Teachers role-model behaviors that affect the choices that school-aged children make in their own behavior. Family support, play, and encouragement have been shown to be an important factor in increasing the resiliency of school-aged children and adolescents (Ginsburg, 2007).

PERSONALITY AND TEMPERAMENT

As described in Chapters 4 and 5, the temperament of the child—whether "easy," "difficult," or "slow to warm up"—helps to determine how a child adjusts to the environment and influences his or her personality. The difficult child is usually the child who is most challenging to live with. The nurse may need to assist the family in determining good strategies to use when dealing with a difficult child. The nurse can coach the family to remain neutral or objective in emotional situations and to not take the child's behavior personally. Families need to learn to anticipate high-risk situations and to strategize how to deal with them effectively to avoid potential disasters. Families may need to consider their own temperaments when dealing with children (i.e., whether their temperament is difficult, "high maintenance," or easy). Effective parenting entails recognizing both the child's unique temperament and one's own and considering how they interact. Parenting goals should include strategies to manage parental expectations, help the child be successful, and enhance positive developmental outcomes. Health care providers may find it necessary to counsel families to adjust their behavior and expectations to allow their children to succeed in ways appropriate to their unique temperaments (McClowry, 2002; Shelov & Altmann, 2009).

Middle childhood is a period when individuality is being sought and children begin to develop their own sense of personhood. Children seek to determine how they "fit" into their families and to decipher their roles in the school environment and in relationships with peers. A stimulating environment in which children can invent, create, experiment, and "grow" will assist in building self-confidence. As children approach their teen years, they are likely to seek more independence in decision making. Youths may push to gain more responsibility and have opportunities to achieve more autonomy. Interactions with adults can help build children's sense of self-esteem and self-worth and enhance their understanding of personal success. Children may often challenge the rules and limits set by families, finding many faults in their parents and other family members. A common statement may be "you're not my boss" or "you can't make me" as children test their limits and boundaries. Setting fair, firm, consistent limits is the most successful strategy. This is a critical stage during which the child needs mature, compassionate adults as role models because these adults can be a positive influence on the child's future life.

RELATIONSHIPS

During middle childhood, making friends and sustaining those relationships is one of the most important social accomplishments. The school-aged child is able to form complex relationships, and communication has developed to a point that the child can share feelings with friends and family (Fig. 6-10). A child may develop a "best" friend, usually someone who complements him or her and with whom he or she can feel completely comfortable. As the child moves to more independent activities, the family needs to understand that it is necessary for the child to differentiate himself or herself from parents and siblings. Help the family develop a good relationship with the child by serving as a "sounding board," by listening to the child as he or she works through various concerns and issues, and by ensuring that even with the most hectic schedule, the adult is available to talk and listen to the child.

Bullying is aggressive behavior carried out repeatedly and over time, with one or more children targeting someone perceived as less powerful. Bullying is a common experience for many children. At least half of all children have been bullied at some time in their lives, and more than 10% are bullied on a regular basis (Chart 6-3). Children who are bullied tend to be insecure and cautious, have low self-esteem, and lack social skills and friends, all of which makes them easy targets. Boys tend to be more involved in bullying others than girls (Nansel et al., 2001).

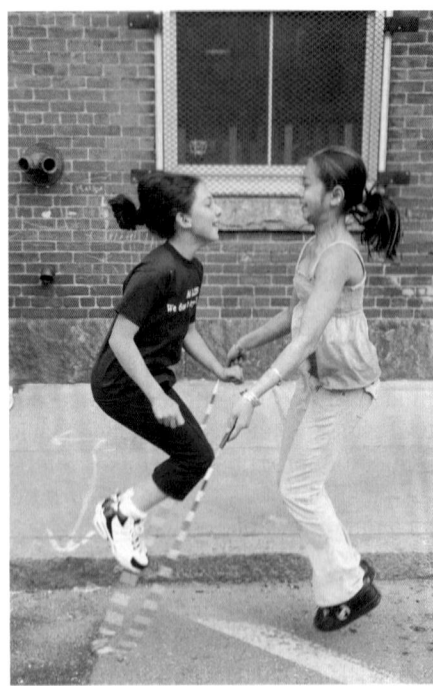

Figure 6-10 In middle childhood, same-gender activities are customary.

CHART 6-3   **Manifestations of Bullying**

Physical Bullying

- Actions that cause physical injury (hitting, punching, kicking, tripping)
- Taking items that belong to the bullied youth (money, lunch, homework)
- Damaging the belongings of others
- Engaging in extortion
- Inappropriate grabbing at youths and pulling at their clothes (snapping the bra, pulling down pants)

Verbal Bullying

- Teasing
- Name calling, insults, threats
- Spreading rumors about the youth or his or her family
- Humiliating the youth in front of peers

Nonverbal or Emotional Bullying

- Intimidation through gestures
- Social exclusion, shunning

Cyber Bullying

- Sending insulting messages by e-mail, text messaging, or instant messaging
- Sending threatening messages by e-mail, text messaging, or instant messaging
- Posting insults or threats on Web-based community sites or pages

Bullying by Proxy

- Coercing others to steal from or bully a victim

Information from Selekman, J., & Vessey, J. (2004). Bullying: It isn't what it used to be. *Pediatric Nursing, 30,* 246–249.

NURSING INTERVENTIONS 6-2

Roles for Health Care Professionals in Bullying Prevention and Intervention

- Assess for signs of bullying behaviors and victimization. To limit adverse influences on children, intervene early in situations of peer bullying.
- Engage youths in discussions about solutions to bullying, encouraging youth-led dialogue and support groups.
- Assist families in responding to signs of bullying and in identifying support and resources for those involved with and affected by bullying behaviors.
- Recommend appropriate treatment, referral, and management protocols for children who exhibit antisocial and deviant behaviors.

- Partner with schools to implement comprehensive bullying prevention programs.
- Oversee implementation of anti-bullying policies and practices, including "safe school" policies that specifically address bullying behaviors.
- Promote training and continuing education in strategies to prevent bullying.
- Participate in political action to increase resources to prevent bullying and to ensure sustained funds for programs aimed at intervention and prevention.

Many children who are bullied have psychosomatic complaints—such as headaches, stomachaches, dizziness, sleeping problems, anxiety, and abdominal pain—and feel unhappy (Sansone & Sansone, 2008). These children are at higher risk than others for depression and poor psychosocial adjustment (Due et al., 2005; Fekkes et al., 2004; Liu & Graves, 2011; Sansone & Sansone, 2008). They often come from homes where aggressive measures are used to handle discipline and difficult situations (Selekman & Vessey, 2004).

Counsel families who think their child might be a victim of bullying to discuss this possibility with the child's teacher or school counselor (Nursing Interventions 6-2). Encourage the child not to fight back but to walk away from the situation or seek help from someone he or she trusts. Some children need psychological counseling to avoid long-term emotional consequences of bullying.

FEARS

The most common fears identified during middle childhood are still some of the same fears experienced during early childhood, such as a fear of darkness, separation, and injury. Some newer fears that are now expressed have to do with failure at school and with peer relationships (not being liked, fear of being bullied) and fears related to increasing violent events in schools and the community. Some fears (e.g., darkness, separation) are a normal part of childhood, and most will subside on their own. Some may persist as ongoing stressors for the child, whereas others may develop into phobias. Changes in children's stressors have emerged during the past 30 years. In the 1970s, children reported worrying about such issues as being poor, bad dreams, getting into trouble, and family fighting. Today, children report that their biggest stressors include

- Fighting among family members
- Homework
- Liking someone or girlfriend–boyfriend issues
- Playing sports and games
- Having too many things to do (Ryan-Wenger et al., 2005)

Another fear that has gained attention over the past couple of decades is the fear of disasters, both manmade (e.g., terrorism, war, and mass violence/shootings) and natural (e.g., severe weather events). Because media coverage of such events is readily and continually available, children can be frequently exposed to the event. Children can be encouraged to discuss the event and how they feel. In the aftermath of a disaster, either manmade or natural, the child will pick up on emotional cues from his or her family (Davidhizar & Shearer, 2002; Rowe & Liddle, 2008); the child's responses also depend on his or her developmental level. Families may be overwhelmed by the event and may not recognize the signs and symptoms of distress in the child (AAP, 2005). Some common reactions include behavioral changes, changes in school performance, withdrawal, and nightmares (National Association of School Psychologists, n.d.). Nurses can intervene to help the child and family cope with the child's fears (Nursing Interventions 6-3).

caREminder

The child's fears may be based on real-life trauma and threats the child has received. The family and child need to determine the rationale for the specific fear. For instance, if the child has fear of a specific classmate, further investigation is warranted to determine whether the child has been a target of harassment and bullying. If the child is afraid of a particular adult, exploration of the child's relationship with that adult is warranted to ensure that the child has not experienced any abuse from that adult.

Many families may seek professional assistance to determine whether a fear has become a persistent stressor or a phobia (a fear that reaches abnormal proportions and becomes irrational). Nurses can assist families in dealing with their children's fears and stressors; by helping them to understand which fears and stressors

NURSING INTERVENTIONS 6-3

Helping Children Affected by Disasters (Manmade and Natural)

- Limit the child's exposure to media surrounding the event.
- Reassure the child that he or she is safe.
- Acknowledge the child's feelings.

- Be honest about the event.
- Encourage prompt return to normal routines.
- Promote and reinforce positive coping skills.
- Recognize symptoms of persistent distress.

Information from National Association of Pediatric Nurse Practitioners. (n.d.b). *Suggestions for helping children, teens, and their families cope with disasters and traumatic events*. Retrieved from http://www.napnap.org/Docs/CopingHandoutUpdated.pdf; National Association of School Psychologists. (n.d.). *Helping children after a natural disaster: Information for parents and teachers*. Retrieved from http://www.nasponline.org/resources/crisis_safety/naturaldisaster_ho.aspx

are normal at each age; and by encouraging them to use sympathy, empathy, and open communication to allow their children to express their concerns. The children should never be ridiculed, told they "worry too much," or be forced to "be brave" because these techniques could cause the fears and personal stress to increase, rather than diminish, and ultimately manifest as true phobias or physical symptomology (e.g., headaches, stomachaches, or skin disorders).

SEXUALITY

> QUESTION: Throughout the course of the spring and summer health care appointments, you notice that whenever Cory is nervous, he holds his penis. Wendy asks, "I have three other sons, but Cory touches his penis more than any of my other boys. What do you recommend?" What would you say to Wendy?

During middle childhood, the child's curiosity about his or her sexuality is greater than has been previously displayed. This is a critical time for discussions to begin about sexual development. These discussions should include sex's social implications as well as the biologic factors associated with sex. It is important that families be involved in delivering the information about sexuality and sharing their values about sex. Families may be uncomfortable discussing certain aspects of sexuality with their children and may seek the health care provider's advice about how to answer the questions presented to them. Sex education in the school environment varies in each state, although most states offer classes in the fifth or sixth grade. If families have established open lines of communication about sex from an early age, children will find it easier to approach them with questions and will not be as likely to ask peers, who may misinform them. Encourage families to use correct terminology for the sexual organs and to provide simple but honest explanations of the functions of the body parts and the actions that cause pregnancy.

Families and health care providers are encouraged to discuss sexuality and to integrate sexuality education as part of the ongoing discussions held with the child or adolescent about relationships (see Chapter 7). Families sharing their attitudes, values, and beliefs strongly influences children's and adolescents' behavior. Nurses might help provide developmentally appropriate material. School programs vary considerably in the information provided. Nurses might help the family be aware of the community's school policies regarding sexuality education. Children might share information with the health care provider regarding sexual activity or sexual concerns that they are hesitant to discuss with their family. The child may require counseling to prevent pregnancy and acquiring sexually transmitted infections. In all discussions with the child, encourage open discourse between the family and the child, providing all parties with accurate information about sexuality while supporting parental values.

> ANSWER: A favorite piece of advice recommends teaching a child that touching private parts in public is like picking your nose in public: We just don't do it! Do not try to make it a moral issue; keep it an issue of manners. When Cory touches himself in public, have Wendy tell him, "Not here, Cory."

SCHOOLING AND CHILD CARE

The biggest transition for every child and his or her family during middle childhood is the entrance into a full-time formal education environment. Whether families choose to homeschool their children or have their children attend private or public schools, the children must now adapt to new rules, learn to concentrate for extended periods of time, and adjust to the varying personalities of other children in the classroom. Evidence-Based Clinical Practice Guidelines 6-1 provides references to assist families as they prepare their child for entry into school.

School Readiness

Child Trends DataBank. (2012). *Early school readiness.* Retrieved from

http://www.childtrendsdatabank.org/?q = node/291

Statistics and trends of factors that are known to impact school readiness.

Head Start (2012)

http://eclkc.ohs.acf.hhs.gov/hslc

A federal program for children from birth to 5 years of age from low-income families that aims to improve their cognitive, social, and emotional development. The website provides guidelines for school readiness as well as policies and regulations aimed at improving language, learning, and development in children.

National School Readiness Indicators Initiative. (2005). *National School Readiness Indicators Initiative Report.* Retrieved from

http://www.gettingready.org/matriarch/

A multistate initiative that developed state-level sets of indicators for school readiness for children from birth through age 8 years. The initiatives can be used to inform public policy decisions and track progress in meeting key goals for young children.

Woodrow Wilson School of Public and International Affairs at Princeton University and the Brookings Institution. (2005). School readiness: Closing racial and ethnic gaps. *Future of Children* (15)1. Retrieved from

http://futureofchildren.org/futureofchildren/publications/docs/15_01_FullJournal.pdf

Issue of the journal *Future of Children*, which focuses on racial and ethnic *differences* in school readiness, as opposed to *levels* of readiness. Evaluates impacts on readiness for school, such as low birth weight, genetics, parenting, socioeconomic resources, and health disparities.

PREPARATION FOR SCHOOL

> **QUESTION:** Wendy indicates that Cory expresses a lot of ambivalence about school. One day he seems very excited; the next day he says he won't go. What would you tell Wendy?

Kindergarten is the child's first "real" school experience (Fig. 6-11). Kindergarten is either a half day or a full day. The kindergarten is usually centered in the elementary school and focuses on social skills and elementary academics. Before the child enters kindergarten, many school districts require testing to assess the child's readiness or to determine whether the child has the skills necessary to succeed.

Families can prepare their children by talking to them about kindergarten. They can explain how it will differ from the preschool experience, with new children to meet and different activities. The children will have more independence and more responsibilities (Shelov & Altmann, 2009). The teacher will expect the children to have more self-control, particularly if they have attended preschool.

Even for children who have attended preschool, kindergarten is a big step. The family may approach the health care provider to determine whether the child is "ready" for kindergarten. No formal statewide definition of **school readiness** exists other than an age of eligibility requirement. In most states, children are allowed to enter kindergarten in the fall of the school year if they have turned or will turn 5 years old by a certain preestablished date. Cutoff dates vary by state (Saluja et al., 2000).

In addition to meeting the age requirements for school, a child should be able to play well with others; be toilet trained; have fine manual dexterity adequate to use a crayon or fasten buttons; be able to sit quietly and listen to a story; and have enough memory skills to memorize his or her name, address, and phone number (Shelov & Altmann, 2009). Most states do not promote

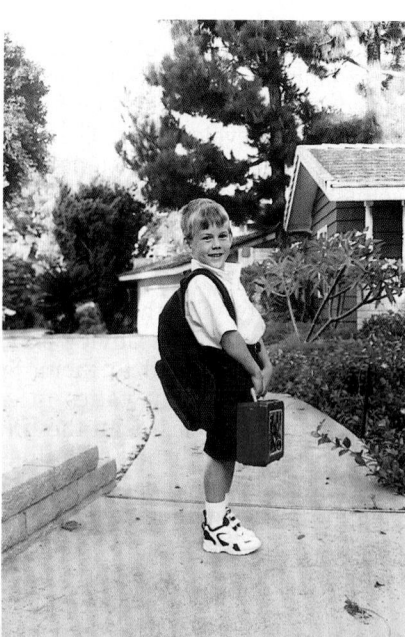

Figure 6-11 For the first day of kindergarten, this child has been prepared with a new backpack and clothes.

readiness testing; however, at the local level, districts may conduct screening/assessments. These data can be used by schools to assist in the preparation for the diversity of children entering the school (High, 2008).

> *ANSWER:* Once again, it is best to get more information before giving advice. Ask, "What worries you most?" Is Wendy more concerned about separation from her or is she worried about his readiness for kindergarten? Cory has an August birthday and therefore will probably be one of the youngest in his class. The nurse could perform a developmental assessment screening to give Wendy an idea of his developmental level. The nurse could also remind Wendy that school personnel can conduct assessments to determine Cory's readiness for school.

SCHOOL

The best teacher that a child can have is his or her family. A family can do many things at home to enhance a child's learning skills for school, such as allowing the child to assist in the kitchen to learn fractions (e.g., using ¼ cup, ½ cup); giving the child the opportunity to add and subtract the money in a wallet or coin purse; and encouraging the child to read an article from a child's magazine, a recipe, or a billboard to enhance reading skills.

After the child has started school and is attending on a regular basis, each new year should be approached with positive feelings. Families should not allow any negative experiences from a previous school year or from their own personal background to influence the child's expectations of the new year.

Promotion to the next school grade level requires that the child attains grade-specific learning goals (Fig. 6-12).

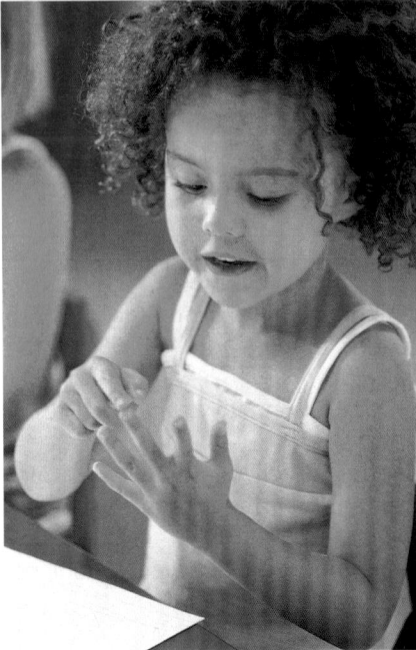

Figure 6-12 Specific learning goals during middle childhood include counting, sequencing, recognizing letters and simple words, and basic writing. Math and reading skills emerge during this period as well.

If these goals are not attained, the child may have to repeat the grade. Although research shows that attempts to relate future success to repeating a school grade are problematic and that retention may reduce the chances of graduation by as much as 50%, the process continues to be widely used and even mandated by some states. Strategic intervention before the end of the year would be a better alternative; however, most schools still follow an industrial model, and the shift to meeting individual needs has not yet been fully supported by the funding sources.

CROSS-CULTURAL CARE

Academic achievement gaps exist between white children and black and Hispanic children. The cause of these achievement gaps cannot be attributed to a single factor. Rather, studies indicate a variety of factors including socioeconomic status of the family, low-quality neighborhoods, children raised by single or teen parents, parental level of education, and parental involvement in the child's education. Although programs to help minimize achievement gaps must be multimodal in their approach, reducing racial and ethnic differences in family income has been shown to diminish achievement gaps and warrants more emphasis and political support (Duncan & Magnuson, 2005).

Homeschooling

Homeschooling, where the family educates the child in the home environment, is becoming increasingly popular. According to the National Center for Education Statistics, there were approximately 1.5 million homeschooled children in the United States in 2007, representing 2.9% of the schooled child population. This is an increase from the 1.1 million children homeschooled in 2003. In the United States, white students were more commonly homeschooled than black, Hispanic, or other racial/ethnic groups. While the majority of homeschooled children receive all of the education in the home, some also attend a traditional school for a portion of their educational day (National Center for Education Statistics [NCED], n.d.).

Families choose to homeschool their children for different reasons, including religious and academic reasons (Isenberg, 2007). Another reason is the assured safety of the child (Homeschool Companion, n.d.). Some children may have special needs or health problems (NCED, n.d.). Regardless of the motive for homeschooling, there may be a concern about the socialization of the child. Many homeschooled households become members of homeschooled online groups and participate in playdates and fieldtrips with other homeschooled children. The nurse should inquire about the child's social situation and address any issues that may arise.

The Gifted Child

Although families may be aware that their child attains some developmental milestones unusually early or possesses extraordinary capabilities (e.g., early advanced language development, unusually retentive memories), it is usually the school system that identifies a child as being potentially gifted. The definition of "gifted" varies with each source. Initially, simply a high IQ (top 1%)

was thought adequate to define a child as gifted. More recently, the definition has been expanded to include three areas: an above-average intelligence, a high level of creativity, and a high level of task commitment.

Gifted children may experience social challenges. Many children who have been identified as gifted have difficulties relating with peers because of the contrast between their chronologic age and their intelligence. Also, siblings who are not gifted often feel inferior to their gifted brother or sister. Occasionally, academic or behavioral problems may be attributed to boredom with the school curriculum.

Schools often provide testing for such children and offer special programs to enhance learning capabilities and expand areas of potential. Families and teachers can find gifted children challenging to deal with because they often have a habit of questioning traditional facts and conclusions and have an insatiable curiosity that can be irritating to authority figures. Although gifted children need to be challenged in their areas of excellence, they also should be offered the basic instruction that all children receive, although possibly to an accelerated degree (Community Care 6-1).

The Child With a Learning Disorder

Children who fail to reach academic or behavioral standards appropriate to their grade level may be recognized by the school or their families as needing some additional attention to ensure success. Chapter 30 provides an in-depth discussion of those conditions referred to as *intellectual disability, cognitive disability, cognitive deficit, intellectual deficiency,* and *mental retardation.* Most schools have screening procedures in place, often called *student study teams,* to bring together all people involved with the child in a problem-solving meeting. This team approach ensures that all perspectives are considered and allows for input from all involved parties. Student study teams frequently bring together the child's teacher, the school resource specialist, the school psychologist, the school speech therapist, a

school administrator, and, of course, the family. The first time a student study team meeting is held for a child, all team members contribute input to determine the child's current performance level and the kinds of support that have already been provided.

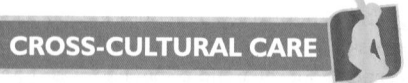
CROSS-CULTURAL CARE

Approximately 7%–8% of all school-aged children are identified with a learning disability. Boys are more likely to be identified than girls as having a learning disability. There are no significant differences in the rate of learning disabilities by race, ethnicity, or parent's level of education. Children who are uninsured and receive public assistance are more likely to be identified as having a learning disability (Child Trends DataBank, 2012).

Potential solutions can include suggesting that the parents seek medical or psychological attention for the child or that the school provide academic and psychological testing to determine whether a learning disability is present. Many times, learning disabilities are identified by looking for discrepancies between academic performance (current level of performance) and IQ score (innate ability). Additionally, schools may give behavior assessments to determine whether evidence exists for ADHD. Schools do not make medical diagnoses, however, and are required to respond only to issues that affect student learning.

If testing is determined to be appropriate, the family is offered this option, and the process begins. Schools have 15 days to respond to a family's request for assessment and must complete the testing and report back to family within 60 working days. At the posttest meeting, results from all the tests are reviewed to determine whether the child meets the qualifications for special programs. Potential outcomes of this meeting include several possible conclusions: the child is delayed but within normal developmental limits, so

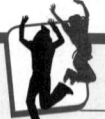

COMMUNITY CARE 6-1

Responsibilities of the Health Care Team to Gifted Children and Their Families

- Assess for achievement of normal developmental milestones and identify indicators of developmental precocity.
- Identify resources within the community to help evaluate gifted children.
- Help children and families understand the concept of giftedness.
- Help families prevent creating excessive vulnerability or privilege in the identified child.
- Help the family deal with siblings of the identified child who may feel inferior and less appreciated than the gifted child.
- Help the family avoid overstimulation of the child or the desire to push the child into too many activities.
- Advocate for appropriate educational resources in the school system.
- Help identify gifted children who may have behavioral and learning problems that require intervention.
- Foster communication between school personnel and the family.

no further action is required; the child has ADHD-like symptoms that affect his or her functioning in the classroom, so the opportunity to develop Section 504 of the Rehabilitation Act of 1973 modification plan is offered; or the child has a learning disability, so placement in a special education program is offered. If services are deemed appropriate, the family has the right either to take advantage of the programs offered or to decline services; therefore, the decision about how to proceed also takes into account the family's desires. Chapter 2 provides a thorough discussion of the educational programs available for children with special needs; Teaching Intervention Plan 30-1 provides guidance to help parents advocate for the educational needs of a child with a developmental or learning disorder.

Learning-disabled children are typically placed in a special resource program because federal guidelines require placing all children in the "least restrictive" educational environment. As a result of federal directives, many students with conditions such as Asperger syndrome, autism, and even Down syndrome may now be included in the regular education program as "full-inclusion" students. These children create severe burdens on the public education system, which by federal law must provide a "free and appropriate education" to each child. See Chapters 2, 12, and 30 for more information regarding programs for children with chronic conditions or learning disorders who may benefit from special educational programs provided through the public school system.

Homework

Homework includes those activities assigned by the teacher to be completed outside of the classroom as a strategy to further increase the knowledge and improve the skills and abilities of the child. Homework usually starts at the first-grade level at about 15 to 30 minutes several times per week, increasing to up to 2 hours each night by the time the child is in high school. The time required to complete assignments varies based on the child's ability to focus on the task, the child's comprehension of the assignment, and the presence of any learning disorder. Homework should not be a power struggle between the family and the child. Families need to allow the child to complete the homework with assistance and support. Good homework habits should be developed at an early age, and the child should have a specific time, place, and tools to complete the assignments. The decision regarding where and when a child does homework must be determined by family dynamics. Some children do best by doing the homework immediately after school, whereas others have too many distractions at that time and do better when they do homework after dinner. Both are acceptable, as long as the child develops the habit of completing the homework (Paulu, 2004) (Fig. 6-13).

Families may seek advice from the health care provider if the child experiences school problems, particularly incomplete homework. The health care provider should encourage the family to allow the child to suffer the natural consequences of not doing homework.

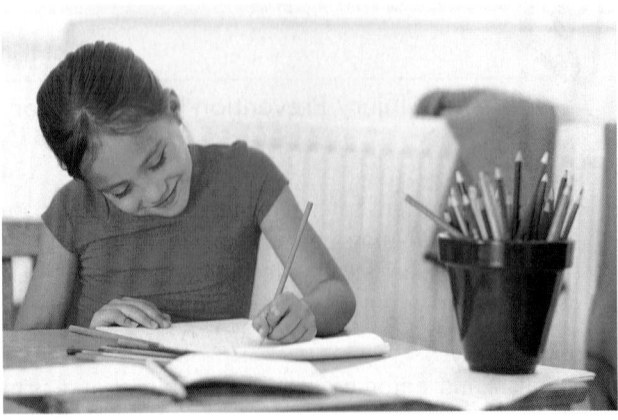

Figure 6-13 The child attending school is encouraged to establish homework routines. A quiet place without distractions helps the child focus.

Rather than engaging in a power struggle, the family can be supportive and open and show interest but should not insist the homework be completed perfectly, do the homework themselves, argue with the child about homework, or criticize the child about homework. Encourage the family to meet with school personnel regarding the problems of homework and to work with the school and coordinate with the teacher to delineate the responsibilities of the school and the child.

After-School Care

A family is often somewhat relieved when a child starts school on a full-day schedule. If the parent has not been working, now may be an opportunity to return to work, although usually, school is 5 to 6 hours long, not the 8 to 10 hours that a parent needs for work and commuting. Until children are 12 or 13 years old, they should continue to have some after-school care. Latch-key kids (children who are unsupervised at home after school at an early age) are common in today's society. Most children younger than 13 years of age do not have the maturity to make decisions in an emergency. Some children as young as 8 years old may have the skills needed to make these decisions, but legal authorities usually do not allow a family to leave the child in an unstructured environment until the age of at least 12 or 13 years. Children who are allowed to be home after school by themselves may develop fears or anxieties because they feel isolated and lonely. Nurses should be aware of the resources in the community that assist families in locating programs to care for children after school. The nurse may also help families to develop rules for children to follow when they must stay at home alone, such as locking doors, never opening the door to strangers, and having a neighbor or close friend available by phone if a question or problem arises (Community Care 6-2). Children should be taught how to use the telephone, and a list of emergency phone numbers should be posted next to the telephone, including the home address and telephone number, because a child can easily forget his or her own address and phone number in an emergency.

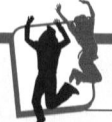

COMMUNITY CARE 6-2

Injury Prevention Guidelines for the Family During Middle Childhood

General Safety

Reinforce important safety considerations. Anticipate that the child may make errors in judgment because he or she is trying to imitate peers.

Anticipate providing less supervision.

Home Safety

Establish and enforce consistent, explicit, and firm rules for safe behavior.

Test smoke detectors to ensure that they work properly. Change batteries twice yearly with the time change.

Lock up poisons, matches, and electric tools.

Ensure that guns, if in the home, are locked up and that ammunition is stored (and locked up) separately. A trigger lock is an additional important precaution.

Reinforce the child safety rules for the home, including what to do when home alone. Remind the child not to answer the door or to invite visitors into the house when no adult is present.

Discuss telephone rules. Keep emergency phone numbers available for easy use.

Discuss what to do in case of fire or other emergencies. Conduct fire drills at home.

Activity Safety

Reinforce sports safety with the child, including the need to wear protective sports gear.

Reinforce child safety rules for bicycles, including use of proper traffic signals.

Teach the child to avoid high noise levels, especially when using music headsets.

Ensure that the child wears a bicycle helmet when riding a bicycle.

Water Safety

Ensure that home and neighborhood swimming pools are enclosed by a four-sided fence with a self-closing, self-latching gate. Children should be supervised by an adult whenever they are in or around water.

Teach the child how to swim.

Reinforce safety rules for swimming pools.

Car Safety

Based on the child's age and size, ensure that the child uses appropriate restraint and seat belt devices in the car at all times.

Prohibit children from sitting in the front seats of cars with passenger air bag devices.

Safety With Others

Keep the child away from cigarette smoke. Do not allow smoking in the home.

Teach the child safety rules regarding interacting with strangers. Ensure that the child's school curriculum has information on how to deal with strangers.

Ensure that the child is supervised before and after school in a safe environment.

Outdoor Safety

Teach the child to put on sunscreen (sun protection factor [SPF] 15 or 30) before he or she goes outside for long periods.

Reinforce the child's knowledge of neighborhood safety skills.

Do not allow the child to operate a power lawn mower or motorized farm equipment.

Emergency Preparation

Keep your address and phone number posted near the phone.

Keep list of emergency numbers (doctor, hospital, nearest neighbor, poison control center) near the phone.

Learn first aid and cardiopulmonary resuscitation (CPR) techniques.

Adapted from Hagan, J. F., Shaw, J. S., & Duncan, P. M. (Eds.). (2008). *Bright futures: Guidelines for health supervision of infants, children, and adolescents* (3rd ed.). Elk Grove Village, IL: American Academy of Pediatrics.

When families are looking for a babysitter, they must take care to select the appropriate individual to provide care for the child at home. They should interview caregivers and ask appropriate questions about their approach to discipline, general child-rearing beliefs, activities considered appropriate for the child, and so on. The ideal candidate should have local references and should be a person with whom the parents feel they can develop an open relationship.

PREVENTING INJURY AND ILLNESS

As the child's independence increases, the potential for accidents is also increased. A high incidence of accidents occurs while children are at school playing with friends (Fig. 6-14). Children do not yet have the maturity to accurately judge speeds or distances and may also accept dares to play unsafe "games" with matches or loaded firearms. Most of these accidents are preventable, and

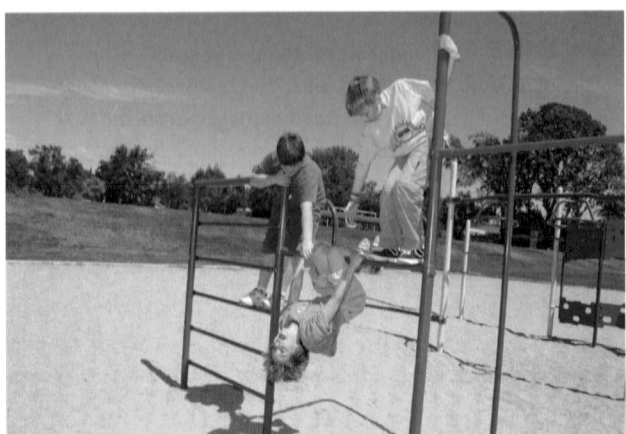

Figure 6-14 Injuries on playground equipment can occur when children do not follow safety precautions and are allowed to play unsupervised.

with a little forethought, the child will not be at risk for death or injuries with lifelong consequences.

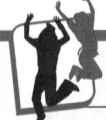 **KidKare** Many children want cell phones. Although the family may be hesitant to purchase one for the child, the device may serve as a safety support for the family. Features such as limited minutes and usage requirements can enable families to use cell phones to keep tabs on their children while limiting others' access to the child. Educate families that children who have cell phones still require monitoring by their family regarding where they are going and with whom. Remind children that having a cell phone does not mean that they no longer have to follow family safety rules.

By implementing simple routines and enforcing rules, children can be kept reasonably safe. Teach families to lock the car doors at all times and remind them that a child should never be allowed to be alone in the car. Educate families to use the appropriate type of car seat or booster seat and consistently enforce the rule that seat belts always be worn when the child is in the car (Community Care 6-3). The safest place for a child younger than 13 years is in the backseat. Only older children should be in the front seat of a vehicle with a passenger airbag (AAP, 2011). States and provinces vary in car safety requirements for children. Most states have laws that require a child to be placed in a booster seat until certain age, height, or weight requirements are met. Prior to providing information to the family, review your state or province laws to ensure that you give accurate information.

Crossing the street may also be a challenge for the 5- to 10-year-old who is still unable to judge the speed of an oncoming car or its distance from the intersection. Adult supervision should be used until the child is older than 10 years of age. The bicycle is one of the most popular "toys" during middle childhood. Mastering the skill of riding a two-wheeled bicycle means independence, a mode of independent transportation, and freedom. Because bicycles can pose serious risks to safety, a child must learn the rules of the road and abide by them (Clinical Judgment 6-1). Most of the accidents between bicycles and automobiles are caused when a child does not obey the rules and darts out in front of a car or rides against traffic.

COMMUNITY CARE 6-3

Belt Safety for Children from the American Academy of Pediatrics

Ensure that lap and shoulder seat belts fit properly.
- The shoulder belt lies across the middle of the chest and shoulder, not the neck or throat.
- The lap belt is low and snug across the thighs, not the stomach.
- The child is tall enough to sit against the vehicle seat back with his or her legs bent without slouching and can stay in this position comfortably throughout the trip.

Use a booster seat until the adult seat belt fits correctly.
- Seat belts are made for adults.
- The child should reach about 4 ft 9 in. in height and be between 8 and 12 years of age before quitting the use of a booster seat.

Use seat belts as intended by the manufacturer.
- Do not tuck the shoulder belt under the child's arm or behind the back.
- If there is only a lap belt, make sure it is snug and low on the child's thighs, not across the stomach.
- When purchasing a new or used car, try to get a lap and shoulder belt installed in the car by a dealer.
- Do not allow children or other passengers to share seat belts. All passengers must have their own car safety seats or seat belts.
- Do not use seat belt adjuster products that attach to the seat belt but are not part of the original belt. These products actually interfere with proper fit of the lap and shoulder belt.

Data from American Academy of Pediatrics. (2011). Child passenger safety. *Pediatrics, 127,* 788–793; American Academy of Pediatrics. (2013). *Car safety seats: A guide for families.* Retrieved from http://patiented.aap.org/content.aspx?aid = 6042

A properly fitted bicycle helmet that can absorb the impact of a crash should be worn at all times the child is on a bicycle (Community Care 6-4). A helmet should be worn squarely on top of the head, covering the top of the forehead. If it is tipped back, it will not protect the forehead. The helmet fits well if it does not move around on the head or slide down over the wearer's eyes when pushed or pulled. The chin strap should be adjusted to fit snugly (AAP, 2001a, 2011).

 ALERT *A helmet worn during a serious fall or accident is no longer fit for use. The helmet has served its purpose and may have been damaged in such a way that it will not be able to provide adequate protection in another crash. If any uncertainty exists about whether a helmet is still usable, throw the helmet away and replace it with a new one.*

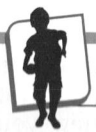

CLINICAL JUDGMENT 6-1

An Injury at School

The bike rodeo at the elementary school brings about 75 fifth and sixth graders together to learn about bike safety. The children bring their bikes from home, and with assistance from a local bike shop, they learn a few tips on bike maintenance. Police officers are on hand to teach bike safety and to monitor the children as they complete a bicycle obstacle course. Although the event has not officially started, fifth grader Ernie has been brought to the nurse's station with severe lacerations to his arms and knees. He fell off of his bike while on his way to school. You have seen him in your office several times related to complaints of a stomachache. He is a shy boy, new to the school, and is easily upset when things do not go his way.

Questions

1. What is your first assessment priority?
2. What are the issues you need to consider as you manage Ernie's injuries?
3. Although there was a lot of blood, the wounds will not require stitches. You are able to cleanse and bandage the wounds at your office. As you talk with Ernie, you learn that he was injured while trying to race away from some boys who were teasing him. You also note that Ernie is wearing shorts and has no bike helmet with him. What additional issues do you need to address with Ernie?
4. How would you proceed with Ernie after his injuries have been assessed?
5. As the bike rodeo event begins and the day progresses, how would you determine that Ernie is benefiting from the activities and is feeling better?

Answers

1. Assess Ernie's injuries to his legs and arms. Complete a neurologic assessment and brief head-to-toe assessment to ensure he has not sustained injury elsewhere and that there is no change in level of consciousness.
2. Evaluate the wounds to determine whether more extensive care is required in a more comprehensively equipped setting. Review Ernie's medical record to ensure he has no bleeding issues and to determine his immunization status.
3. During the time you are caring for Ernie, explore why he does not have a helmet and whether he knows what other clothes he can wear to protect his body while biking. You would also want to elicit from Ernie his perception of the exchange he had with the other boys who caused him to have the accident.
4. Contact Ernie's family to let them know what happened. Ask permission to administer Tylenol if needed for pain and swelling at the site. Walk Ernie back to the event area. Ernie would benefit from having a "friend" paired with him for the activities. You might ask another boy to be Ernie's "special friend" for the day and be sure to include him in activities as the day progresses. Introduce Ernie to the police officers and determine whether he can get a "loaner" helmet for the day. Ask a particular officer to keep an eye on Ernie and request that if there is some way to involve him in a special task that would make him feel important, to please do so.
5. Periodically check on Ernie to ensure the dressing is dry and intact and he is free from pain. Use these contacts to further note his general affect and his interactions with other children. Later in the week, make contact with Ernie to assess his wounds and to ask him about the bike rodeo and how the day went for him. Follow up with teachers regarding the concerns you have about Ernie and his "fitting in" at school.

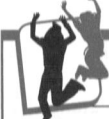

COMMUNITY CARE 6-4

Promoting Helmet Use

- Establish the habit of wearing helmets at an early age, even before children are riding tricycles in public areas.
- Allow children to help choose their helmets, selecting a design and a fit that is comfortable to them.
- Instruct the family to be role models by wearing helmets themselves.
- Explain to children why they need to protect their heads.

- Use the media to show examples of professional athletes wearing helmets (e.g., skateboarders, race car drivers).
- Give children special treats when they remember to wear their helmets.
- Encourage children's friends to wear helmets. Have extra helmets available so that wearing helmets becomes a house rule that everyone can follow.
- Do not let children ride without wearing a helmet. Be consistent in enforcing this rule.

Many communities do not require helmets even though helmet use can reduce the risk of head injury (Clements, 2005). Helmets also should be worn when a child is using a skateboard, scooter, or roller skates/blades. In addition, the child should have protective knee and elbow pads as well as wrist guards to prevent serious injury during falls off the skateboard or skates/blades. When purchasing a bicycle or skates/blades for a child, the family should also purchase a proper-fitting helmet with a Consumer Product Safety Commission sticker (Fig. 6-15). The child needs to start learning the laws of the road. Children who ride bikes should understand that it is necessary to follow the same types of traffic laws that cars do and to go with the flow of traffic, signal when stopping or turning, and obey stop signs and stoplights. Light-colored or reflective

clothing is recommended when riding at dusk. Cyclists should be encouraged to ride on paths as much as possible and to avoid the streets.

Although the number one cause of death in middle childhood is accidental injury, the third most common cause of death is drowning (Safe Kids USA, 2011). Spa-related injuries and deaths also occur in this age group (Safe Kids USA, 2011). The AAP (2010) recommends enclosures for inflatable portable pools and supports swimming lessons for children (in most cases) aged 4 years and older. As families see the child mature, their confidence in allowing the child more independence may increase to the point that they overestimate the child's survival skills. Children must have adult supervision whenever they are around water. Swimming instruction from a qualified instructor is important but should not take the place of adult supervision. Specific rules should be strongly enforced whenever a child is to be around water, such as never swim alone, do not dive unless the depth of the water is known, and wear a personal flotation device when riding in a boat.

School-aged children are often fascinated by guns, but children should never be allowed access to firearms. Even with instruction, they are not mature enough to handle a potentially lethal weapon. A loaded gun should never be kept in a car or a home. The gun should be kept unloaded and the ammunition should be stored in another location under lock and key. Even with all these precautions, many children are allowed access to firearms through friends or family members. The family must discuss with their children tactics to use if they are approached by a friend with a gun or encounter a gun in another home or at school. They should be encouraged to stay away from it, not to touch it, and to report it to an adult. In television and movies, handgun violence does not appear as devastating as it actually is, which may mislead children about inherent dangers. Frequent discussions with children about what is observed on television and comparisons with real life will help them understand that guns are not toys and must remain with adults.

See thePoint for a summary of Key Concepts.

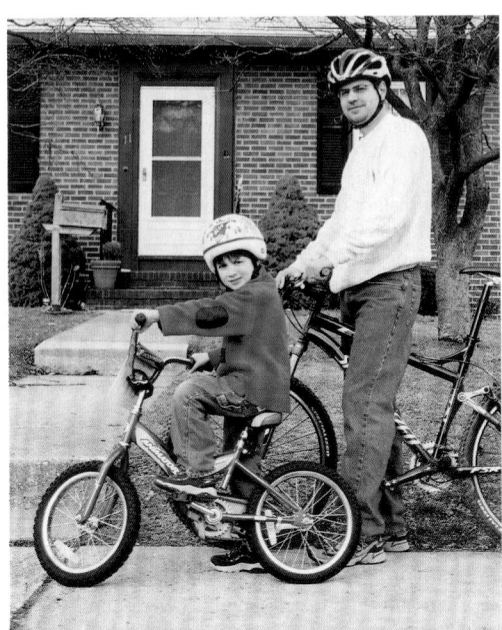

Figure 6-15 Helmets are an important aspect of bike safety. Parents can be role models for their children by also wearing bike helmets.

REFERENCES

American Academy of Pediatrics. (2001a). Bicycle helmets. *Pediatrics*, *108*, 1030–1032.

American Academy of Pediatrics. (2004). Soft drinks in schools. *Pediatrics*, *113*, 152–154.

American Academy of Pediatrics. (2005). Psychosocial implications of disaster or terrorism on children: A guide for the pediatrician. *Pediatrics*, *116*(3), 787–795.

American Academy of Pediatrics. (2006). Active healthy living: Prevention of childhood obesity through increased physical activity. *Pediatrics*, *117*, 1834–1842.

American Academy of Pediatrics. (2009). Impact of music, music lyrics, and music videos on children and youth. *Pediatrics*, *124*, 1488–1494.

American Academy of Pediatrics. (2010). Prevention of drowning. *Pediatrics*, *126*, 178–185.

American Academy of Pediatrics. (2011). Child passenger safety. *Pediatrics*, *127*, 788–793.

American Academy of Pediatrics. (2012). Trampoline safety in childhood and adolescence. *Pediatrics*, *130*, 774–779.

American Academy of Pediatrics. (2013). The crucial role of recess in school. *Pediatrics*, *131*, 183–188.

Anderson, C., Berkowitz, L., Donnerstein, E. et al. (2003). The influence of media violence on youth. *Psychological Science in the Public Interest*, *4*, 81–110.

Anderson, C., & Bushman, B. (2001). Effects of violent games on aggressive behavior, aggressive cognition, aggressive affect, physiological arousal, and prosocial behavior: A meta-analytic review of the science literature. *Psychological Science*, *12*, 353–359.

Anderson, C. A., Sakamoto, A., Gentile, D. A. et al. (2008). Longitudinal effects of violent video games on aggression in Japan and the United States. *Pediatrics*, *122*(5), 1067–1072.

Beebe, D. W. (2012). A brief primer on sleep for pediatric and child clinical neuropsychologists. *Child Neuropsychology: A Journal on Normal and Abnormal Development in Childhood and Adolescence*, *18*(4), 313–338.

Carno, M., Hoffman, L., Carcillo, J. et al. (2003). Developmental stages of sleep from birth to adolescence, common childhood sleep disorders: Overview and nursing implications. *Journal of Pediatric Nursing*, *18*, 274–283.

Casamassimo, P., & Holt, K. (2004). *Bright futures in practice: Oral health: Pocket guide*. Arlington, VA: National Center for Education in Maternal and Child Health.

Centers for Disease Control and Prevention (n.d.a). *Basics about childhood obesity*. Retrieved from http://www.cdc.gov/obesity/childhood/basics.html

Centers for Disease Control and Prevention. (n.d.b). *Childhood obesity facts*. Retrieved from http://www.cdc.gov/healthyyouth/obesity/facts.htm

Chervin, R., Archbold, K., Dillon, J. et al. (2002). Associations between symptoms of inattention, hyperactivity, restless legs, and periodic leg movements. *Sleep*, *25*(2), 213–218.

Chervin, R., Dillon, J., Bassetti, C. et al. (1997). Symptoms of sleep disorders, inattention, and hyperactivity in children. *Sleep*, *20*(12), 1185–1192.

Child Trends DataBank. (2012). *Learning disabilities*. Retrieved from http://www.childtrendsdatabank.org/alphalist?q = node/90

Clements, J. (2005). Promoting the use of bicycle helmets during the primary care visit. *Journal of the American Academy of Nurse Practitioners*, *17*(9), 350–354.

Davidhizar, R., & Shearer, R. (2002). Helping children cope with public disasters. *The American Journal of Nursing*, *102*(3), 26–33.

Dennison, B. A., & Edmunds, L. S. (2008). The role of television in childhood obesity. *Progressive Pediatric Cardiology*, *25*(2), 191–197.

Desager, K., Nelen, V., Weyler, J. et al. (2005). Sleep disturbance and daytime symptoms in wheezing school-aged children. *Journal of Sleep Research*, *14*(1), 77–82.

Due, P., Holstein, B. E., Lynch, J. et al. (2005). Bullying and symptoms among school-aged children: International comparative cross sectional study in 28 countries. *European Journal of Public Health*, *15*(2), 128–132.

Duncan, G., & Magnuson, K. (2005). Can family socioeconomic resources account for racial and ethnic test score gaps? *Future of Children*, *15*(1), 35–48.

Fekkes, M., Pijpers, F. I., & Verloove-Vanhorick, S. P. (2004). Bullying behavior and associations with psychosomatic complaints and depression in victims. *Journal of Pediatrics*, *144*, 17–22.

Gentile, D. (2009). Pathological video-game use among youth ages 8 to 18: A national study. *Psychological Science*, *20*(5), 594–602.

Gentile, D. A., Coyne, S., & Walsh, D. A. (2011). Media violence, physical aggression, and relational aggression in school age children: A short-term longitudinal study. *Aggressive Behavior*, *37*, 193–206.

Gentile, D., Lynch, P., Linder, J. et al. (2004). The effects of violent video game habits on adolescent aggressive attitudes and behaviors. *Journal of Adolescence*, *27*(1), 5–22.

Gentile, D. A., Obert, C., Sherwood, N. E. et al. (2004). Well-child exams in the video age: Pediatricians and the American Academy of Pediatrics guidelines for children's media use. *Pediatrics*, *114*(5), 1235–1241.

Ginsburg, K. R. (2007). The importance of play in promoting healthy child development and maintaining strong parent-child bonds. *Pediatrics*, *119*, 182–191.

Hagan, J. F., Shaw, J. S., & Duncan, P. M. (Eds.). (2008). *Bright futures: Guidelines for health supervision of infants, children, and adolescents* (3rd ed.). Elk Grove Village, IL: American Academy of Pediatrics.

High, P. C. (2008). School readiness. *Pediatrics*, *121*, e1008–e1015.

Hoban, T. (2004). Sleep and its disorders in children. *Seminars in Neurology*, *24*(3), 327–340.

Holt, K., Wooldridge, N., Story, M. et al. (Eds.). (2011). *Bright futures in practice: Nutrition* (3rd ed.). Elk Grove Village, IL: American Academy of Pediatrics.

Homeschool Companion. (n.d.). *Pros and cons of homeschooling*. Retrieved from http://www.homeschool-companion.com/pros-and-cons-of-homeschooling.html

Isenberg, E. J. (2007). What have we learned about homeschooling? *Peabody Journal of Education*, *82*(2–3), 387–409.

Jordan, A. B. (2007). Heavy television viewing and childhood obesity. *Journal of Children and Media*, *1*(9), 45–54.

Kaiser Family Foundation. (2010). *Generation M²: Media in the lives of 8- to 18-year-olds*. Retrieved from http://www.kff.org/entmedia/upload/8010.pdf

LifeSiteNews. (2005). *MTV watched by majority of young teens exposes children to 9 sexual scenes per hour*. Retrieved from http://www.lifesite.net/ldn/2005/feb/05020202.html

Liu, J., & Graves, N. (2011). Childhood bullying: A review of constructs, concepts, and nursing implications. *Public Health Nursing*, *28*(6), 556–568.

Matricciani, L. A., Olds, T. S., Blunden, S. et al. (2012). Never enough sleep: A brief history of sleep recommendations for children. *Pediatrics*, *129*(3), 548–556.

Meltzer, L. J., Johnson, C., Crosette, J. et al. (2010). Prevalence of diagnosed sleep disorders in pediatric primary care practices. *Pediatrics*, *125*, e1410–e1418.

McClowry, S. (2002). The temperament profiles of school-age children. *Journal of Pediatric Nursing*, *17*(1), 3–10.

Mindell, J. A., Owens, J., Alves, R. et al. (2011). Give children and adolescents the gift of a good night's sleep: A call to action. *Sleep Medicine*, *12*(3), 203–204.

Nansel, T., Overpeck, M., Illa, R. et al. (2001). Bullying behaviors among US youth. *Journal of the American Medical Association*, *285*, 2094–2100.

National Association of School Psychologists. (n.d.). *Helping children after a natural disaster: Information for parents and teachers*. Retrieved from http://www.nasponline.org/resources/crisis_safety/naturaldisaster_ho.aspx

National Center for Education Statistics. (n.d.). *Fast facts: Homeschooling*. Retrieved from http://www.nces.ed.gov/fastfacts/display.asp?id = 91

Paulu, N. (2004). *Helping your child with homework*. Retrieved from http://www.kidsource.com/kidsource/content/homework.html

Robinson, T., Wilde, M., Navracruz, L. et al. (2001). Effects of reducing children's television and video game use on aggressive behavior: A randomized control trial. *Archives of Pediatric Adolescent Medicine, 155*, 17–23.

Rowe, C. L., & Liddle, H. A. (2008). When the levee breaks: Treating adolescents and families in the aftermath of hurricane Katrina. *Journal of Marital and Family Therapy, 34*(2), 132–148.

Ryan-Wenger, N., Sharrer, V., & Campbell, K. (2005). Changes in children's stressors over the past 30 years. *Pediatric Nursing, 31*, 282–291.

Safe Kids USA. (2011). *Drowning and water-related safety*. Retrieved from http://www.safekids.org/our-work/research/fact-sheets

Saluja, G., Scott-Little, C., & Clifford, R. (2000). Readiness for school: A survey of state policies and definitions. *Early Childhood Research & Practice, 2*(2), 1–19.

Sansone, R. A., & Sansone, L. A. (2008). Bully victims: Psychological and somatic aftermaths. *Psychiatry, 5*, 62–64.

Selekman, J., & Vessey, J. (2004). Bullying: It isn't what it used to be. *Pediatric Nursing, 30*, 246–249.

Shelov, S., & Altmann, T. (2009). *The American Academy of Pediatrics: Caring for your baby and young child, birth to age 5*. New York, NY: Bantam Books.

Singh, G. K., Kogan, M. D., Van Dyck, P. C. et al. (2008). Racial/ethnic, socioeconomic, and behavioral determinants of childhood and adolescent obesity in the United States: Analyzing independent and joint associations. *Annals of Epidemiology, 18*(9), 682–695.

Swing, E. L., Gentile, D. A., Anderson, C. A. et al. (2010). Television and video game exposure and the development of attention problems. *Pediatrics, 126*(2), 215–221.

TV-Turnoff Network. (2005). *Facts and figures about our TV habit*. Retrieved from http://www.tvturnoff.org

U.S. Department of Agriculture. (2012). *National School Lunch Program*. Retrieved from http://www.fns.usda.gov/cnd/Lunch/AboutLunch/NSLPFactSheet.pdf

U.S. Department of Agriculture. (n.d.). *MyPlate information*. Retrieved from http://www.choosemyplate.gov

U.S. Preventive Services Task Force. (2004). Prevention of dental caries in preschool children: Recommendations and rationale statement. *The American Journal for Nurse Practitioners, 8*(11), 29–35.

Yoon, S. Y., Jain, U., & Shapiro, C. (2012). Sleep in attention-deficit/hyperactivity disorder in children and adults: past, present, and future. *Sleep Medicine Reviews, 16*, 371–388.

See thePoint for additional resources.

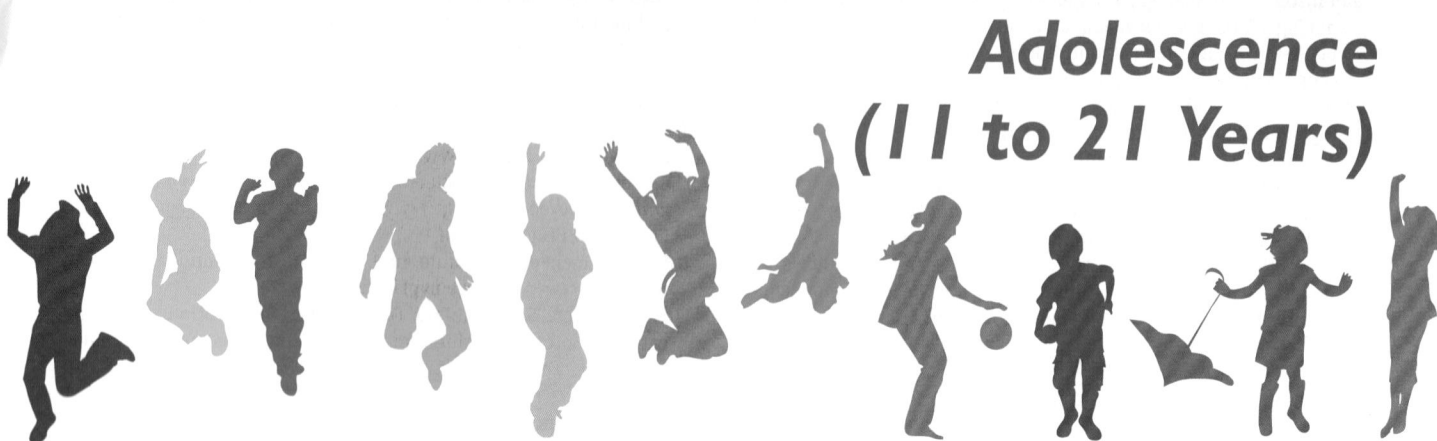

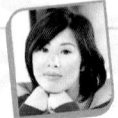

CHAPTER 7

Adolescence (11 to 21 Years)

CASE HISTORY

Ashley Tran is a 16-year-old Vietnamese American attending public high school in her junior year. She is the oldest child in her family, and at home she is called *Chi Lon* (which means "oldest sister" in Vietnamese). She has a younger brother, George. Both children were born in the United States. Her father, Tung Tran, and her mother, Loan Pham, were both born in Vietnam and immigrated to the United States. Her father now speaks English fairly well, but her mother does not. Her mother has three sisters who live nearby. Ashley is closest to her Aunt Ha, her mother's youngest sister who attended high school in the United States. Ashley's grandparents on her mother's side are deceased, and her paternal grandparents are still in Vietnam. Everyone in their family is Roman Catholic.

Ashley's parents have very high academic and professional expectations for their daughter. She is expected to attend to her studies and bring home all As; her parents would like her to be a doctor. Ashley, however, is more of a B student. She does try hard; she just doesn't care that much. And she definitely does not want to be a doctor. Her brother George, on the other hand, is a very conscientious student and very bright. Ashley's parents frequently ask why she is not doing as well in school as her brother.

Ashley is also expected to date only young Vietnamese men. However, Ashley has a boyfriend, Eric, who is not Vietnamese. Eric is a senior at Ashley's school. In order to see Eric outside of school, Ashley lies about where she is going. Eric doesn't really understand why they cannot just tell her parents, but Ashley is adamant that her parents would not understand. Eric and Ashley have had occasional, unplanned sexual intercourse without protection. Eric has urged Ashley to get on "the pill," but Ashley insists that "good Catholic girls" don't do that, and they must not have intercourse again.

Ashley is very thin and complains that she is not sleeping well. Her conflict with her parents has reached such a level of tension that she is avoiding meals at home. She is aware she is disappointing her parents, but at the same time she feels that their wishes and expectations are unreasonable. One evening, Ashley's parents discover she has lied to them in order to see Eric, and they have an extensive argument. That same week, Ashley's report card comes home from school. Ashley thinks her parents do not understand what it is like to be a teenager in the United States today, and she talks to her Aunt Ha about moving in with her.

When Ashley does not feel well at school, she visits the school nurse.

CHAPTER OBJECTIVES

1 State the age-appropriate developmental milestones of the adolescent years.

2 Distinguish components of developmental surveillance unique to the adolescent population.

3 Discuss the concerns of the adolescent related to hygiene and personal care.

4 Describe challenges to maintaining optimum nutrition in the adolescent years.

5 Describe activities that promote physical fitness in adolescents.

6 Select age-appropriate interventions to promote healthy personal and social development of the adolescent.

7 Select interventions to promote illness and injury prevention for the adolescent and the family.

See thePoint for a list of Key Terms.

The **adolescent** years begin with the onset of physiologically normal **puberty** (the sequence of events by which a child becomes a young adult) and end when an adult identity and behavior are accepted. This stage of development corresponds roughly to the period between the ages of 11 and 21 years (Hagan et al., 2008). The patient population seen by pediatric health care providers includes all children from birth through age 21 years and, in some cases, may extend beyond the age of 21 years (American Academy of Pediatrics [AAP], 2011a; National Association of Pediatric Nurse Practitioners, 2008). Clearly, those providing health care to adolescents must allow sufficient flexibility in defining this age span to encompass special situations, such as the emancipated minor (see Chapter 2) or the young person with a chronic condition that causes delayed development, prolonged dependency, or a need for continuity of health care services for pediatric acquired chronic conditions.

Adolescence is a critical growth period for young people, during which they form their own identities, develop independence from their families, and prepare to become members of society. Protective nurturing factors that can strengthen adolescents and help them resist problem behaviors include individual, family, peer, and environmental influences. Risk factors that may limit adolescents' success vary widely and include such factors as poverty, a history of mental illness in the family, use of alcohol and other substances, and lack of parental supervision and guidance. The health care provider plays an important role in promoting factors that will assist the adolescent to be resilient when facing daily challenges associated with school, family issues, and peers (Evidence-Based Clinical Practice Guidelines 7-1). This chapter reviews issues related to promoting healthy lifestyles of adolescents.

DEVELOPMENTAL ASSESSMENT AND SURVEILLANCE

Developmental Considerations 7-1 presents a summary of the developmental milestones that are accomplished during adolescence. This information can provide the nurse with direction for specific trigger questions to ask the family or child to determine the adolescent's developmental progress. Variances in attainment of developmental milestones will be affected by physical change related to the onset of puberty and by influences from family, school, and social (peer) groups. Trigger questions will elicit information about social and sexual activities and school and vocational performance as well as health maintenance activities for this age. During the adolescent years, annual health care visits are recommended to complete developmental assessments and to screen for conditions common to the adolescent years (Chart 7-1). The physical examination includes assessment of blood pressure, height, weight, body mass index (BMI), skin (acne, piercings, tattoos, abuse, and so forth), breast examination, pelvic examination, testicular examination, and inspection for sexual maturity. Health screening of the adolescent includes several assessments not incorporated in health visits of younger children. Some of these assessments are completed based on the risk assessment screening criteria. Scoliosis screening, alcohol or drug use screening, evaluating anemia in the young girl with a heavy menstrual bleeding, tuberculosis screening, and testing for sexually transmitted infections (STIs) and cervical dysplasia in all sexually active young people are essential components of surveillance and screening in this age group (Hagan et al., 2008).

EVIDENCE-BASED CLINICAL PRACTICE GUIDELINES 7-1
Adolescent Health Care Guidelines

The American Congress of Obstetricians and Gynecologists. (2013). *Adolescent health care*. Retrieved from
http://www.acog.org/About_ACOG/ACOG_Departments/Adolescent_Health_Care

Guidelines for adolescent health care related to topics such as growth and development, contraception, immunizations, and reporting sexual abuse.

American Medical Association. (2013). *Promoting adolescent health*. Retrieved from
http://www.ama-assn.org/ama/pub/physician-resources/public-health/promoting-healthy-lifestyles/adolescent-health.page?

Materials and resources related to promoting healthy adolescent lifestyles. Topics include guidelines for health care providers about suicide, alcohol use, violence prevention, and health care disparities.

Centers for Disease Control and Prevention. (2008). *Youth physical activity guidelines toolkit*. Retrieved from
http://www.cdc.gov/healthyyouth/physicalactivity/guidelines.htm

Physical activity guidelines for children aged 6–17 years.

U.S. Preventive Services Task Force. (2013). *Child and adolescent recommendations*. Retrieved from
http://www.uspreventiveservicestaskforce.org/tfchildcat.htm

Variety of evidence-based recommendations specific to management of care for physical, mental, and emotional conditions impacting children and adolescents.

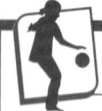

DEVELOPMENTAL CONSIDERATIONS 7-1

Milestones of the Adolescent Years

Physical
- Full height not attained until age 20–24 years, when epiphyseal plates close
- Marked increase in muscle mass in males related to increased androgen production (up to 20 times greater than previous levels)
- Muscle mass two times greater in males than in females by age 17 years, resulting in strength two to four times greater in males
- Adult cardiovascular rhythms achieved by age 16 years
- Nutritional needs greater than at other times of life:
  - Pregrowth spurt, 1,500–2,400 cal/day; pubertal girls, 2,000–2,500 cal/day; pubertal boys, 2,500–3,000 cal/day
  - Male basal metabolic rate about 10% greater at end of adolescence than that of females
- By 12 years of age, have all permanent teeth except second and third molars
- Girls: by age 11 years have achieved 90% of adult height and 50% of adult weight
- Boys: at age 12 years have achieved 80% of adult height and 50% of adult weight

Sexual Development
Genital stage (Freud)
- Learning appropriate outlets for sexual drives
- Female attains menarche at age 10–15 years
- Usually cannot reproduce for 1–2 years after menarche because of anovulation
- Early use of oral contraceptives limits potential height
- Male attains puberty between 12 and 16 years
- Tanner stages I–V usually attained between early and late adolescence

Approximate sequence of appearance of sexual characteristics in adolescence:

Female Secondary Sexual Characteristics
11–12 Years Old
- Breast tissues around and under nipples begin to grow
- Growth spurt may begin
- Internal and external organs continue growing (vagina, uterus, breasts, ovaries)
- Pubic hair becomes darker, coarser, and curlier

12–13 Years Old
- Underarm hair growth
- Onset of menstruation (average age 12.8 years and approximately 2 years after breasts start growing)
- Pregnancy is now possible

13–14 Years Old
- Underpants may be wet at times with a clear mucus; flow is often heavier in teen years and will continue naturally during adulthood, especially with ovulation and sexual arousal

14–15 Years Old
- Most of growth spurt complete (height)

15–16 Years Old
- Acne
- Voice deepens, although not as much as males'

16–17 Years Old
- Full height achieved

Male Secondary Sexual Characteristics
11 Years Old
- Testes become larger
- Scrotal skin becomes redder and coarser

11–12 Years Old
- Prostate begins functioning
- Penis begins to lengthen

12–13 Years Old
- Pubic hair grows
- May experience wet dreams, spontaneous erections, ejaculations (about 1 year after testes begin to grow)
- Growth spurt may begin

13–14 Years Old
- Rapid growth of the penis, especially enlargement occurring about 1 year after testes begin to grow
- Testes color deepens
- Two thirds of boys may experience slight growth of their breast tissue, which generally subsides within 1 year but may last 3 years

14–15 Years Old
- Underarm hair
- Mustache begins as fine hair starting at outside lip edges about 2 years after pubic hair starts to grow
- Voice change begins

15–16 Years Old
- Majority of growth spurt complete (height)

16–17 Years Old
- Chest and shoulders fill out
- Facial and body hair becomes heavier
- Acne

21 Years Old
- Full height achieved

Play
- Group/peer activities such as sports, academic teams
- Seeks parental/adult "limit setting"
- Thrill-seeking behaviors

Cognitive
- Pseudostupidity: asks "dumb" questions (Elkind)
- Difficulty reconciling concrete and formal operations
- Imaginary audience: super self-consciousness; believes everybody is watching and evaluating (Elkind)
- Personal fable: belief of being special and not subject to rational laws (Elkind)
- Apparent hypocrisy: act of expressing an idea tantamount to working for and attaining it (Elkind)
- Formal operations (Piaget)
- Abstraction and hypothetical/deductive reasoning (Piaget)
- Adaptability and flexibility
- Thinking in abstract terms
- Use of abstract symbols
- Conclusions drawn from set of observations
- Development of hypotheses and testing of them
- Considerations of abstract, theoretical, and philosophical matters
- Problem solving
- Ability to comprehend purely abstract or symbolic content
- Ability to solve math and logic problems
- Comprehension of value and belief systems in the philosophical, moral, and political realms
- Reality versus possibility views only one arrangement of the possible
- Combinational reasoning
- Propositional thinking
- Hypothetic–deductive reasoning
- Death is irreversible, universal, personal, but distant
- Uses natural, physiologic, and theologic explanations of death

Social
- Capable of sharing self with others to foster intimate relationship
- Inability to form intimate relationships may lead to sense of isolation

Interpersonal
- Identity versus role confusion (Erikson)

Moral/Spiritual
Moral
Stage 4: Conventional (12–16 Years Old [Kohlberg])
- Fixed rules in moral decisions
- Obligation to do no harm and to do duty

Stage 5: Postconventional (16 Years Old [Kohlberg])
- Social contracts understood and formulated
- Laws recognized as changeable
- Correct actions depend on standards and individual rights

Stage 6: Adulthood (Kohlberg)
- Abstract moral principles govern behavior
- Morality is easily separated from legality
- Orientation is based on universal, ethical orientation
- Able to apply situational ethics

Spiritual
Stage 3: Synthetic/Invention (Preadolescent [Fowler])
- Reflections and questioning of religious beliefs as gains more contact with people whose values and beliefs are different
- Seeking to resolve moral conflicts by appealing to outside authority figures rather than using own inner resources
- Learning to distinguish more clearly between supernatural versus natural
- Perceiving God as a spirit
- Beginning to understand spiritual component of individuals

Stage 4: Individuating/Reflexive (Adolescent [Fowler])
- Seeking to establish and maintain balance regarding religious/spiritual questions and beliefs; adapting "devil-may-care" attitude or going to other extreme and joining zealous religious group, or may suspend effort to resolve conflict

A primary goal of developmental surveillance is to promote adolescent self-advocacy—that is, to assist the adolescent in seeking out, evaluating, and using information to promote his or her own health. Prepare adolescents for self-advocacy by teaching the adolescent to ask for information and to make decisions about his or her own care by encouraging health promotion activities and by providing the adolescent with age-appropriate and correct health care information (Nursing Interventions Classification 7-1). Older adolescents may no longer be living at home. Family promotion to maintain regular health care visits and medical insurance coverage may be absent. Both factors may affect the health promotion and prevention activities of the adolescent.

caREminder

Adolescents report that they desire to receive health care from competent professionals who demonstrate warmth and compassion and communicate in a straightforward, understandable fashion. Concerns about confidentiality can be a major barrier to health care for the adolescent (AAP, Committee on Adolescence, 2008). The health care provider who interacts in a sensitive manner, providing respect and compassion, is likely to develop a strong relationship with the adolescent, which will provide a foundation for promoting ongoing access to preventive health care.

CHART 7-1   Quick Reference to Conditions Common During Adolescence

Condition	Chapter
Acne	25: The Child With Altered Skin Integrity
Alcohol and substance abuse	29: The Child With Mental Health Challenges
Anorexia/bulimia	29: The Child With Mental Health Challenges
Depression	29: The Child With Mental Health Challenges
Diabetes mellitus	26: The Child With Altered Endocrine Status
Eye injuries	28: The Child With Altered Sensory Status
Hepatitis	24: The Child With an Infectious Disease
HIV	24: The Child With an Infectious Disease
Hypertension	15: The Child With Altered Cardiovascular Status
Obesity	6: Middle Childhood (5 to 10 Years)
	7: Adolescence (11 to 21 Years)
STIs	7: Adolescence (11 to 21 Years)
	24: The Child With an Infectious Disease
Sports-related injuries	20: The Child With Altered Musculoskeletal Status
Sunburn	25: The Child With Altered Skin Integrity
Testicular torsion	19: The Child With Altered Genitourinary Status

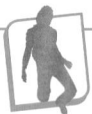

NIC 7-1 NURSING INTERVENTIONS CLASSIFICATION: Developmental Enhancement: Adolescent

Definition: Facilitating optimal physical, cognitive, social, and emotional growth of individuals during the transition from childhood to adulthood

Activities:

Build a trusting relationship with adolescent and adolescent caregiver(s)

Encourage adolescent to be actively involved in decisions regarding his/her own health care

Discuss normal developmental milestones and associated behaviors with adolescent and caregiver(s)

Screen for health problems relevant to the adolescent and/or suggested by patient history (e.g., anemia, hypertension, hearing and vision disorders, hyperlipidemia, oral health problems, abnormal sexual maturation, abnormal physical growth, body image disturbances, eating disorders, poor nutrition, alcohol, tobacco or drug use, unhealthy sexual behavior, infectious disease, poor self-concept, low self-esteem, depression, difficult relationships, abuse, learning problems, or work problems)

Provide appropriate immunizations (e.g., measles, mumps, rubella, diphtheria, tetanus, hepatitis B, hepatitis A, human papilloma virus, meningococcal meningitis)

Provide health counseling and guidance to adolescent and adolescent's caregiver(s)

Promote personal hygiene and grooming

Encourage participation in safe exercise on a regular basis

Promote a healthy diet

Facilitate development of sexual identity

Encourage responsible sexual behavior

Provide contraceptives with instruction for use, if needed

Promote avoidance of alcohol, tobacco, and drugs

Promote vehicle safety

Facilitate decision-making ability

Enhance communication skills

Enhance assertiveness skills

Facilitate a sense of responsibility for self and others

Encourage nonviolent responses to conflict resolution

Encourage adolescents to set goals

Encourage development and maintenance of social relationships

Encourage participation in school, extracurricular, and community activities

Enhance parental effectiveness of adolescents

Refer for counseling, as needed

From Bulechek, G. M., Butcher, H. K., Dochterman, J. M. et al. (Eds.). (2013). *Nursing interventions classifications (NIC)* (6th ed.). St. Louis, MO: Mosby. Used with permission.

Health care providers also play an important role in helping families better understand and support their teenagers during these challenging years. Family education includes information about the normal characteristics of adolescents, strategies to assist adolescents to manage changes in their life, and methods to manage family conflict (Nursing Interventions Classification 7-2).

Puberty encompasses the changes following gonadarche (sexual maturation) and adrenarche (maturation of the cortex of the adrenal glands). Puberty is considered "an interconnected suite of changes with wide variations in the sequence and timing of its components" (Patton & Viner, 2007, p. 369). Biologic changes include the maturation of the growth hormone insulin-like growth factor and thyroid axes. These lead to a pubertal growth spurt; maturation of many organ systems; and changes in blood lipids, hematologic indices, and enzyme systems (Patton & Viner, 2007). The onset of puberty occurs in boys at about 13 to 15 years of age and in girls as early as 9 to 16 years of age. During this period, the child may become very modest and self-conscious. Adults must avoid even "good-natured" teasing because it may cause embarrassment as the child becomes extremely sensitive about his or her body image.

As the adolescent reaches puberty, many physical changes occur. In females, the earliest sign is usually thelarche, or the development of breast tissue, followed by the development of pubic hair, and then the ultimate hallmark of late puberty, **menarche**, the first menstruation. Menarche usually occurs at about 12 years of age,

---

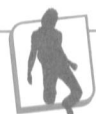

NIC 7-2 NURSING INTERVENTIONS CLASSIFICATIONS: Parent Education: Adolescent

Definition: Assisting parents to understand and help their adolescent children

Activities:

Ask parents to describe the characteristics of their adolescent child

Discuss parent–child relationship during earlier, school-aged years

Understand the relationship between the parent's behavior and child's age-appropriate goals

Identify personal factors that impact on the success of the educational program (e.g., cultural values, presence of any negative experiences with social service providers, language barriers, time commitment, scheduling issues, travel, and general lack of interest)

Identify the presence of family stressors (e.g., parental depression, drug addiction, alcoholism, low literacy, limited education, domestic violence, marital conflict, blending of families after divorce, and excessive punishment of children)

Discuss disciplining of parents themselves when they were adolescents

Instruct parent on normal physiologic, emotional, and cognitive characteristics of adolescents

Identify developmental tasks or goals of the adolescent period of life

Identify defense mechanisms used most commonly by adolescents, such as denial and intellectualization

Address the effects of adolescent cognitive development on information processing

Address the effects of adolescent cognitive development on decision making

Have parents describe methods of discipline used before adolescent years and their feelings of success with these measures

Provide online resources, books, and literature designed to teach parents about teen parenting

Describe the importance of power/control issues for both parents and adolescents during adolescent years

Instruct parents about essential communication skills that will increase their ability to empathize with their adolescent and assist their adolescent to solve problems

Instruct parents about methods of communicating their love to adolescents

Explore parallels between school-aged dependency on parents and adolescent dependency on peer groups

Reinforce normalcy of adolescent vacillation between desire for independence and regression to dependence

Discuss effects of adolescent separation from parents on spousal relationships

Share strategies for managing adolescent's perception of parental rejection

Facilitate expression of parental feelings

Assist parents to identify reasons for their responses to adolescents

Identify avenues to assist adolescent to manage anger

Instruct parents how to use conflict for mutual understanding and family growth

Role-play strategies for managing family conflict

Discuss with parents issues over which they will accept compromise and issues over which they cannot compromise

Discuss necessity and legitimacy of limit setting for adolescents

Address strategies for limit setting for adolescents

Instruct parents to use reality and consequences to manage adolescent behavior

Refer parents to support group or parenting classes, as appropriate

From Bulechek, G. M., Butcher, H. K., Dochterman, J. M. et al. (Eds.). (2013). *Nursing interventions classifications (NIC)* (6th ed.). St. Louis, MO: Mosby. Used with permission.

although menarche at any time within the range of 9 to 16 years of age is considered normal. This event is a symbolic achievement of womanhood in a young girl's life, and it should be accompanied by open discussion and accurate information about the normal changes the body undergoes. Girls will have questions about exercise, hygiene, sanitary protection, and pain. Encourage the family to be supportive and understanding of the changes, both physical and emotional, that their daughter is experiencing.

In males, the earliest sign of puberty is testicular enlargement, followed by some penile growth and the development of pubic hair. Boys experience their voices "cracking" as the larynx and vocal cords grow to their full size and the voice becomes deeper and more resonant. Boys also experience growth spurts and possibly "wet dreams" or spontaneous erections. Neither the spontaneous erections nor the wet dreams (nocturnal seminal emissions) mean that the child is sexually active or having overactive sexual thoughts. The family may need to be instructed that these occurrences are spontaneous and that the child is not doing anything to cause them.

During the 2 years following the onset of puberty, both boys and girls usually experience a growth spurt of 3 to 4 in. Body composition changes include an increase in total body fat and fat-free mass, with a greater increase in fat-free mass in boys than in girls (Carswell & Stafford, 2008). **Tanner staging** is a method used to determine the adolescent's stage of growth according to established parameters of sexual maturity (see Figs. 3-23 and 3-24).

Although many adolescents are physically mature, research indicates that brain growth continues during the adolescent years, extending well into the 20s. Therefore, when interacting with a physically mature adolescent, it is easy to treat the individual as a young adult, when in fact, thinking patterns, processing abilities, and reactions to stressful stimuli are not the same as those in the mature adult brain. For instance, the last part of the brain to mature is the prefrontal cortex, which is responsible for rational, executive brain functions. When this frontal section is not fully developed, adolescents use the temporal lobe to interpret and act on emotional stimuli. This immature brain function means they are likely to behave more impulsively, misread emotional cues, and lack emotional insight (Herrman, 2005). In addition, hormones are believed to affect brain development and behavior. Increased dopamine and decreased serotonin levels are known to lead to a desire for novel, risky, and intense stimuli (Wallis, 2004). Although much research still is needed to explore the relationship between changing hormone levels, brain development, and adolescent behavior, health care providers must remember to intervene with teens as teens and not as young adults. As Herrman (2005, p. 147) states, "Understanding of the cognitive abilities of teens, which may be constrained by physiological function, is integral in creating individually based, developmentally appropriate strategies."

HYGIENE AND PERSONAL CARE

Most families feel that by the adolescent years, they have provided their children with the skills to manage personal hygiene (bathing, hair, teeth), dress themselves, and make good choices when balancing day and nighttime activities. Not surprisingly, these same families are befuddled by the 13-year-old who stays up until midnight, then complains of being "so tired" the next day; the 15-year-old who wears one set of clothes when leaving the house, only to change into another set at school; and the 17-year-old who insists on two to three showers a day. During the time teenagers are developing pubic hair, the males are also developing some chest hair, and both sexes are developing axillary hair. This is a time to discuss the use of deodorants and regular bathing schedules. Shaving or other hair removal practices can also be discussed at this time.

Hygiene and personal care can become sources of family arguments as the adolescent develops his or her own style of personal care. Families need to maintain their rules and boundaries regarding aspects of personal care, while at the same time providing adolescents the latitude to develop their own personal care standards and daily patterns (Fig. 7-1).

ACNE

A common occurrence during the adolescent years is the appearance of acne vulgaris or common acne. Acne vulgaris is an inflammation of the sebaceous glands and

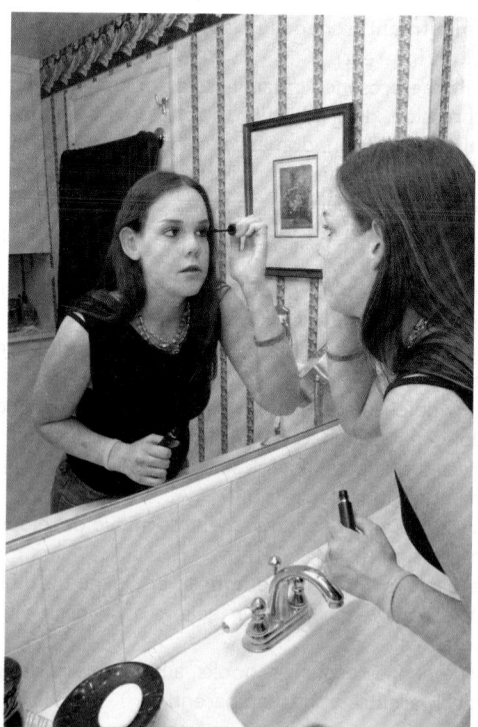

Figure 7-1 Adolescents can be very concerned about personal appearance.

hair follicles of the skin, characterized by comedones, papules, and pustules. Cysts and nodules may develop, and scarring is a common occurrence. Acne appears in both males and females but more predominantly in males. It usually occurs on the face, neck, back, and upper chest. Although it may last into adulthood, it is usually most severe during adolescence. Chapter 25 discusses care management for the adolescent with acne. The presence of acne can be very distressing and can affect self-esteem. Pharmacologic, nutritional, and skin care interventions can be implemented to help treat acne vulgaris.

BODY SHAVING

Body hair removal has been practiced for years by both adolescents and adults. Traditionally, hair removal includes facial hair for men and leg and underarm hair for women. Removal of hair on other parts of the body has become more popular in recent years and is being seen more often in the adolescent population. The extent of hair removal may be localized (e.g., the pubic area) or may encompass all areas of the body, including head, chest, arms, and legs.

Shaving is not without health concerns; shaving may increase the risk of folliculitis, an infection of the hair follicle, caused by *Staphylococcus aureus*. Adolescents should be taught not to share razors; blood-borne pathogens and infectious agents can be transferred when shaving supplies are shared. In addition, shaving in any area can cause skin irritation and increases the skin's exposure to ultraviolet rays. Discuss safe shaving practices with the adolescent and ensure that any rashes or reddened areas that develop on the skin are evaluated by a health care provider. Topical or oral antibiotics may be needed. Skin irritation can be minimized by applying soothing ointments (prescribed by the health care provider), wearing loose clothing, and ensuring that good skin care practices are maintained.

TATTOOING, BODY PIERCING, AND BRANDING

The ancient practices of tattooing and piercing are visible in 5,200-year-old mummies, ancient Mayans, Egyptian Pharaohs, and remain popular with modern day adolescents (McGuinness, 2006). Some studies suggest that between 10% and 15% of adolescents have a tattoo, and more than 25% of adolescents have at least one piercing (Carroll et al., 2002; Martel & Anderson, 2002; Sweeney, 2006). Tattoos and piercings are featured in a myriad of body locations. The three most frequent sites for piercings include the ear cartilage, tongue/mouth, and the navel (McGuinness, 2006). Other sites for piercings include the nose, nipples, and genitals (foreskin, penis, scrotum, clitoris, perineum, and labia). Branding is another form of body art created by the scarification process from a third-degree burn to the skin. After the burn heals, a design of scar tissue is left behind on the skin surface.

Adolescents make deliberate decisions to engage in body ornamentation for the purposes of self-expression,

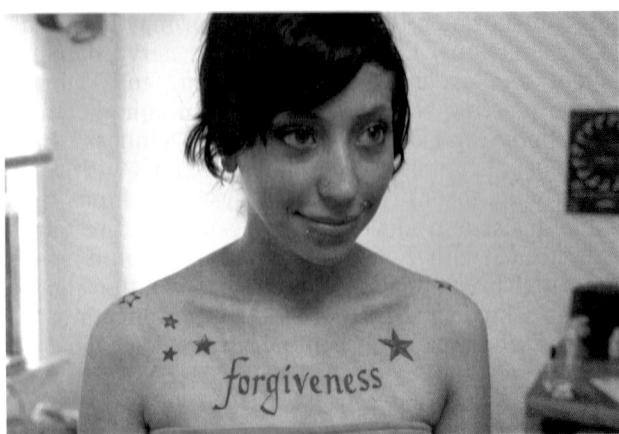

Figure 7-2 Having multiple piercings and tattoos can lead to certain health risks.

self-awareness, sexual expression, or to exert a sense of independence (Armstrong et al., 2006; Elkind, 2001; Gold et al., 2005) (Fig. 7-2). Tattoos and piercings may also be used to commemorate special occasions or to signify gang affiliation, religious beliefs, or membership in a fraternity/sorority (McGuinness, 2006). A survey found that the top adolescent-identified reasons for obtaining a body piercing included admiration for the piercing, desire to be fashionable, and hope to glean extra attention as a result of the piercing (Gold et al., 2005). Sixty-nine percent of pierced adolescents stated that the desire to rebel against their parents also influenced their decision to obtain a piercing (McGuinness, 2006).

Health care providers must be cognizant of both legal and medical implications associated with tattooing and body piercings in adolescents younger than 18 years of age; laws pertaining to the parent/guardian consent for these procedures vary by state. Forty-five states prevent minors from getting tattoos without parental/guardian consent, and 38 states prohibit both tattooing and body piercings without consent (National Conference of State Legislatures, 2012). Because parents are not always in favor of consenting for the adolescent to obtain a tattoo or piercing, the incidence of tattoo parties and use of do-your-own (DYO) kits has increased. These methods provide adolescents with an easy, low-cost, and unregulated method for self-tattooing (Griffith, 2012). Encourage the adolescent to seek the expertise of a trained technician, doctor, or nurse to have piercings, tattooing, or branding performed. Although states vary in their approaches to licensing these technicians, the Association of Professional Piercers and the Alliance of Professional Tattooists (see thePoint for Organizations) have developed safety rules for individuals who provide piercings and tattoos. Branding has not yet been regulated.

Adolescents may not be aware that tattoos, body piercings, and brandings have the potential for many complications. They can be painful, may result in infections or blood-borne diseases, or may trigger allergic reactions. Excessive bleeding, nerve damage, keloid and/or granuloma formation, and damage to the piercing site are also potential complications from body ornamentation procedures (Juhas & English, 2013; Levin et al., 2005). Adolescents with some underlying diseases, such as systemic lupus and sarcoidosis, may develop new lesions at the tattoo site; those with heart valve disease should speak with their cardiologist before having a tattoo placed (Juhas & English, 2013). The risk of complications increases when an adolescent performs his or her own procedure.

 KidKare Before getting a piercing or a tattoo, adolescents should verify with their health care provider that their tetanus shot is current.

Posttattoo care includes wearing a bandage over the area for the first 2 to 13 hours. The site needs to be washed gently with mild soap and warm water, patted dry, and allowed to air-dry for 10 minutes. Apply Polysporin, Bacitracin, or A&D ointment sparingly a few times each day for 3 to 14 days. Use of petroleum jelly will drain the color from the tattoo, and use of alcohol will interfere with healing. The tattooed area should not be soaked in water or shaved until healing is complete. The goal of posttattoo care is to prevent scab formation and allergic reaction.

ALERT   *Because tattoos are associated with risk for blood-borne diseases, the American Red Cross requires a person to wait 1 year after getting a tattoo before donating blood.*

Healing time for piercings varies from 1 to 6 months, based on the location of the piercing. If adolescents tire of their piercings, the jewelry can be removed and the pierced opening will close. Some scarring may remain. If an allergic reaction occurs, the piercing should be removed. A comprehensive teaching plan that can be implemented when an adolescent chooses to have a piercing can be found on thePoint Supplemental Information: Teaching Intervention Plan.

Branding aftercare involves cleaning the area with soap and water and applying a bandage until the wound is healed.

BODY MODIFICATION

Adolescents are becoming increasingly more interested in body modification surgery—that is, plastic surgery as a means to change body appearance. Perceived or real physical defects may be the driving motivation for an adolescent, who is trying to establish self-image and adjust socially, to change his or her body appearance. These body image concerns can erode self-esteem and have severe consequences on an adolescent's development.

As the adolescent explores surgery options, learning what the adolescent wants and what he or she perceives the plastic surgery may have to offer is essential. Ensure that adolescents have realistic goals and that the outcomes are something that the adolescent wants, not something the family or another influential person wants for them. When educating adolescents, ensure that they understand the part of the body that will be involved and how that body part may change as the body matures. As with tattoos and body piercings, the adolescent must have parental or legal guardian consent and be fully aware of associated risks before undergoing the surgery.

ORAL CARE

By the time the child has reached adolescence, ensure that twice-a-year dental checkups have been established as well as good oral hygiene habits. By 12 years of age, most, if not all, of the primary teeth have been shed. Eruption of permanent teeth is generally completed between the ages of 11 and 13 years, except for the wisdom teeth, which do not complete eruption until between the ages of 17 and 21 years. Orthodontics may be needed for oral malocclusions or to improve aesthetic appearance of the teeth. If the adolescent has orthodontic appliances, reinforce the need to provide enhanced dental hygiene because such appliances increase the opportunity for dental caries if dental hygiene is poor. The incidence of dental caries usually declines as the child matures; however, the risk of gingivitis and caries can increase during adolescence resulting from such factors as poor oral hygiene, frequent exposure to natural and refined sugar in the adolescent diet, immature enamel present on newly erupted teeth, and erosion of the dental enamel from eating disorders such as bulimia (Hagan et al., 2008).

Many of the high-risk behaviors that adolescents participate in can affect oral health. For instance, adolescents who use smokeless tobacco are at risk of developing gingivitis, gum recession, stained teeth, or halitosis. Substance use can affect soft and hard tissues of the oral cavity and lead to oral cancer. Oral piercings can cause local infections in the oral cavity, tooth fractures, and hemorrhage. Sexual activities can lead to oral infections and trauma (Hagan et al., 2008).

SLEEP

 QUESTION: Ashley frequently complains that she is tired and does not sleep well. If you were the school nurse, what might you further assess related to Ashley's sleep pattern?

The adolescent needs about 8½ to 10 hours of sleep per night. Sleep patterns exhibit a normal phase delay, with a shift occurring from the early bedtime hours and early rising of childhood to late-night slumber and (when given the opportunity) late-morning rising of adolescence (Amos & D'Andrea, 2012). With the increase in social and school activities, athletics, homework requirements, increased accessibility to and use of personal electronic devices, and possibly work activities, it is particularly important to ensure that the adolescent receives enough sleep at night. A recent study by Calamaro et al. (2009) found that the majority of adolescents sampled used a form of technology and most multitasked with various technology-based activities in the evening. Many of these adolescents also consumed caffeinated drinks; those who multitasked the most also drank the most caffeinated beverages. The survey also found that 33% of the adolescents fall asleep at school. Between 25% and 40% of adolescents complain of sleep problems, with at least 4% diagnosed as having clinically relevant **insomnia** disorder (inability to sleep) (Mindell & Meltzer, 2008; Wolfson & Carskadon, 2005). Families and health care professionals need to be alert to abnormal sleep patterns because they could indicate some other underlying problem, such as sleep apnea, drug abuse, or depression. Adolescents should be sleeping uninterrupted through the night, without nightmares or sleepwalking. If any of these aberrations are present, the teen should be seen by a health care provider to determine whether an underlying cause exists.

Insufficient sleep has been linked to impaired daytime functioning, depressed mood, and poor school performance (Beebe, 2011; Amos & D'Andrea, 2012). The challenge confronting many adolescents is that they are not behaviorally or psychologically ready to sleep until 11 PM or later. Many schools start classes too early for the adolescent to get adequate sleep given this late bedtime. School start times generally range between 7:30 and 8:15 AM. In the late 1990s, high schools in Minneapolis changed their start times from 7:15 to 8:40 AM. Attendance, enrollment, grades, and sleep patterns were evaluated before and after the change for the 18,000 high school students affected by this change. Significant results of the later school start time included improved attendance rates, slight improvements in grades, and student reports of getting more sleep (Wahlstrom, 2002). Other studies have confirmed that early school start times are associated with daytime sleepiness, dozing in class, attention difficulties, and poorer academic performance (Baroni et al., 2004; Wahlstrom, 2002).

Clearly, many factors affect the amount of sleep an adolescent receives each night. Creative changes in scheduling school, extracurricular practice times (which often start before school), late-evening activities (including work), and homework and limiting the use of various technology devices are strategies that families and school officials can use to assist teenagers to get the daily rest they need.

ANSWER: Further assess Ashley's sleep habits, and also consider the possibility that she may be sleeping poorly because of underlying depression or anxiety. Given the tension between Ashley and her parents, it is a possibility that these emotions are affecting her sleep.

NUTRITION

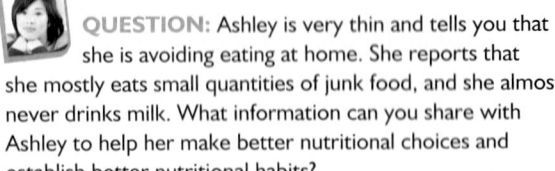

QUESTION: Ashley is very thin and tells you that she is avoiding eating at home. She reports that she mostly eats small quantities of junk food, and she almost never drinks milk. What information can you share with Ashley to help her make better nutritional choices and establish better nutritional habits?

The growth rate during adolescence is second only to the rate during infancy. Typically, the adolescent's weight doubles and height increases by about 25%. Heredity, nutrition, and general health influence the adolescent's eventual stature.

Adolescents are growing quickly and use enormous amounts of energy. This internal blast furnace keeps them hungry most of the time, and as they test their independence, food choices may be one of the areas of conflict between adolescents and families. Allowing the adolescent to make some choices is important so that food does not become a battleground. Many adolescents do not eat a good breakfast or even skip breakfast because they tend to be in a hurry in the morning or believe that it is not important. A nutritious breakfast gives the adolescent energy for a good day at school or to accomplish athletics before school. Ensure the adolescent is receiving a balanced diet based on the U.S. Department of Agriculture (n.d.) *MyPlate* (see Chapters 5 and 6), with a caloric intake of 1,500 to 2,400 calories, although some athletes may need substantially more. Dietary strategies for adolescents include the following approaches (Gidding et al., 2006; Hagan et al., 2008):

- Balance calorie intake with physical activity.
- Ensure daily physical activity lasting 60 minutes or longer.
- Eat fruits and vegetables liberally; limit juice intake.
- Use vegetable oils and margarines low in saturated fats and trans fatty acids.
- Eat whole grain products (bread, cereals, and pastas).
- Reduce intake of sugar-sweetened beverages (e.g., sodas) and foods.
- Drink nonfat or low-fat milk.
- Reduce salt intake.
- Eat more legumes and tofu instead of meats.
- Limit snacking during sedentary activity.
- Take a supplemental daily vitamin.
- Eat breakfast daily.
- Eat fish twice a week.

In addition, several nutrients may need to be added to the adolescent's diet, including folate, iron, and calcium. Folate is recommended for all female adolescents who are capable of becoming pregnant to reduce the risk of giving birth to a child with a neural tube defect. A total of 400 μg folate per day should be ingested from fortified foods and/or a supplement (Hagan et al., 2008).

Rapid growth during the adolescent years leads to an increased need for iron. Females have an increased need and also are at risk for iron-deficiency anemia as a result of blood loss through menstruation. Boys (and to some extent girls) require increased iron to manufacture myoglobin for expanding muscle mass and hemoglobin for expanding blood volume (Hagan et al., 2008). The recommended iron intakes for adolescents are

- Age 9 to 13 years (females and males): 8 mg/day
- Age 14 to 18 years (females): 15 mg/day
- Age 14 to 18 years (males): 11 mg/day

Calcium intake also needs to be increased as a result of the bone mass development that occurs during adolescence. Dietary requirements are as follows:

- Age 9 to 18 years: 1,300 mg/day
- Age 19 years and older: 1,000 mg/day

Overeating comes naturally for adolescents pressured by peers to participate in activities that involve food consumption and is driven by the media to consume fast-food products. Media and peer pressure may also contribute to the development of anorexia nervosa or bulimia. Both of these conditions are psychological illnesses that present physical symptoms. For further discussion, see Chapter 29: The Child With Mental Health Challenges. Family role-modeling of good nutritional habits is essential. Continuing to plan for regular family mealtime will promote social interaction and role-model food-related behaviors for the teen.

ANSWER: Share with Ashley the *MyPlate* icon, keeping in mind that the number of servings identified may seem like a lot to her. To further assess what Ashley is eating, you could ask her to keep a food diary for several days to a week. Encourage Ashley that making better food choices will also make her feel better. Review her food diary with her and, in particular, encourage her to think of fruits and vegetables that she could substitute for the processed snack she is currently eating. For example, apples are a great "to go" food. If Ashley is not drinking milk, discuss alternative sources for vitamin D and calcium. Be sure to follow up with Ashley. Your concern at this stressful time is very therapeutic.

DIETARY SUPPLEMENTS

A recent evaluation of U.S. data found that 25.7% of adolescents use dietary supplements, typically multivitamins and multiminerals (Picciano et al., 2007). Dietary supplements are products intended to supplement the diet that contain one or more of the following dietary ingredients: a vitamin, mineral, amino acid, herb, or other botanical; a dietary substance for use to supplement the diet by increasing the total dietary intake; or a concentrate, metabolite, constituent, extract, or combination of any ingredient just mentioned (Dorsch & Bell, 2005). Dietary substances are ingested in the form of a capsule, powder, softgel, or gelcap and are not represented as a conventional food or as a sole item of a meal or the individual's diet. Adolescents may choose to use these supplements to maintain or improve their health, increase energy, build muscle, increase or decrease weight, supplement an adequate dietary intake, or help healing during an illness or injury.

Energy drinks and sports drinks are widely consumed by adolescents. Sports drinks are flavored beverages that contain carbohydrates, minerals, electrolytes, vitamins, and other nutrients (AAP, Committee on Nutrition & the Council on Sports Medicine and Fitness, 2011). Energy drinks are beverages that promise to deliver a burst of energy when consumed and are among the most popular type of dietary supplement consumed by adolescents. The drinks contain caffeine, sugar, and other ingredients such as ginseng, taurine, guarana, and B-complex vitamins. Sale of these beverages has been aimed at students, athletes, and active individuals aged 21 to 35 years. However, younger individuals are consuming these products to give them stamina, physical endurance, mental alertness, and an overall sense of well-being. Seifert et al. (2011) found that 30% to 50% of adolescents and young adults consume energy drinks. Energy drinks have many adverse effects, especially when taken after exercise or when mixed with alcohol. Adolescents with certain underlying diseases, including cardiac conditions, diabetes, seizures, and behavioral problems, as well as those taking certain medications may experience higher incidences of adverse events (Seifert et al., 2011). Deleterious effects include insomnia, headaches, nervousness, nosebleeds, vomiting, seizures, heart arrhythmias, and even death (Braganza & Larkin, 2007; Seifert et al., 2011).

ALERT   *Sports drinks have a specific and limited use by child and adolescent athletes. "These drinks should only be used when there is a need for more rapid replenishment of carbohydrates and/or electrolytes in combination with water during periods of prolonged, vigorous sports participation or other intense physical activity" (AAP, Committee on Nutrition & the Council on Sports Medicine and Fitness, 2011 p. 1188).*

Most dietary supplements, although safe and effective for adult populations, may have adverse side effects for adolescents, and the actual effectiveness of these supplements on adolescents is unknown (Dorsch & Bell, 2005; Seifert et al., 2011). The safety, purity, potency, and efficacy of dietary supplements have not been regulated. Given this information, caution adolescents about dietary supplement use, and encourage healthy dietary intake instead of using products to supplement the vitamins and other health ingredients found in the recommended *MyPlate* foods.

OBESITY

Obesity (BMI greater than or equal to 95th percentile) is of great concern during adolescence; the incidence of adolescent obesity has tripled over the past 30 years (Centers for Disease Control and Prevention [CDC], n.d.a). Preserving self-esteem is crucial for teens, and obesity carries with it a stigma in today's society. Adolescents with a BMI that is at or above the 85th percentile and below the 95th percentile for age and gender are classified as *overweight*; those above the 95th percentile for age and gender are classified as **obese** (U.S. Preventive Services Task Force, 2010). BMI categories for children and adolescents are age and sex specific and do not correspond precisely to adult BMI categories. The prevalence of overweight 12- to 19-year olds was 18% in 2010 (CDC, n.d.a). The primary comorbidities include type 2 diabetes, hyperlipidemia, hypertension, metabolic syndrome, hepatic steatosis, obstructive sleep apnea, asthma, and orthopedic complications (Fennoy, 2010). Causes of adolescent obesity include lack of physical activity, frequent screen time, and high consumption of fat calories (Regber et al., 2007; Stewart & Gahagan, 2012).

Intervention plans for both preventing and treating adolescent obesity must include dietary adjustments, regular physical activity, and behavioral changes. Childhood and adolescent obesity is considered an epidemic. Adolescents must work in collaboration with the health care team, parents, school, and the community to implement the strategies that will help them successfully manage their weight and take advantage of opportunities for engaging in physical activity.

Bariatric surgery is showing promise as a treatment option for adolescents aged 13 years and older who meet stringent criteria. The criteria are based on the BMI (>35 or 40) and associated comorbidities as well as the severity of the comorbidities. The severely obese adolescent should be treated by a multidisciplinary team at an experienced center equipped to meet the teen's special needs (Hsia et al., 2012; Michalsky et al., 2011).

PHYSICAL FITNESS

If physical fitness has been introduced at an early age, and if families are positive role models, the adolescent most likely exercises regularly through competitive or individual sports. Many adolescents still are not as physically active as they should be. Encourage adolescents to develop a habit of exercising. The positive benefits of physical activity for the adolescent include

- Fostering a feeling of accomplishment
- Reducing the risk of certain diseases (e.g., coronary heart disease, diabetes mellitus)
- Promoting mental health
- Assisting in achieving healthy body weight and composition, reducing the risk of obesity
- Promoting a healthy lifestyle throughout life

Provide the adolescent with many opportunities to engage in physical activity while in school and through community organizations. In these venues, a positive approach to physical activity is essential (Community Care 7-1).

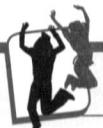

COMMUNITY CARE 7-1

Components of an Adolescent's Physical Fitness Program

Goal: Develop a Positive Attitude About Fitness
- Enjoy participating in physical activities.
- Recognize positive outcomes of regular physical activity.
- Feel competent when participating in physical activity.
- Have positive role models for physical activity.
- Select activities that reflect individual needs and interests and that can be continued into adulthood.
- Incorporate physical activity into daily life.

Goal: Participate in Physical Activity on a Regular Basis
- Be physically active every day or nearly every day through planned activities within the context of the family, school, or community.
- Engage in moderate physical activities (e.g., brisk walk) or shorter, more intense activity (e.g., basketball) daily for 60 minutes.
- Participate in a variety of noncompetitive sports (e.g., skating, biking).
- Participate in competitive, organized sports as desired.

Goal: Meet Age-Appropriate Nutritional Requirements
- Practice healthy eating behaviors that help achieve healthy body weight and composition and provide sufficient energy to engage in physical activity.

- Abstain from using alcohol, tobacco, drugs, and ergogenic aids.

Goal: Engage in Cooperative and Team-Building Experiences
- Engage in physical activities with family members.
- Seek opportunities for team sports, ensuring that all players are given equal opportunity for participation and skill building.

Goal: Prevent Injury
- Ensure the use of appropriate safety equipment (e.g., helmet, knee pads, wrist guards) during physical activity.
- Ensure appropriate supervision during physical activity (e.g., monitoring during use of weights or gymnastic equipment).
- Ensure that the environment is safe for the indoor or outdoor activity selected (e.g., bike paths, well-maintained recreation centers).
- Monitor pacing of activity to avoid injury from overexertion.
- Reduce exposure to the sun by appropriate use of sunscreen, clothing, and hats to protect the skin.

Information from Patrick, K., Spear, B., Holt, K. et al. (Eds.). (2001). *Bright futures in practice: Physical activity*. Arlington, VA: National Center for Education in Maternal and Child Health.

Hazards can occur from rough physical contact while engaging in a sport, from predisposing health issues of participating adolescents, from environmental factors (e.g., rain, lightning), and from malfunctioning equipment. The physical and social environment in the school and community should encourage participation in physical activity in a safe setting under the supervision of adults trained in physical education, health education, and safety standards for athletes (AAP, Committee on Sports Medicine and Fitness & Committee on School Health, 2004; Patrick et al., 2001) (Fig. 7-3).

Enjoyment of the particular activity appears to enhance the motivation to participate in that activity. The adolescent with a medical condition need not necessarily be restricted from sports participation. Sickle cell disease, HIV infection, and diabetes are examples of chronic conditions that should not prohibit participation in sports activities. In contrast, youths with fever or carditis are considered to be at too high of a cardiopulmonary risk to participate in sports activities. The American Academy of Pediatrics (Rice, 2008) provides recommendations for sports participation for more than 35 medical conditions. In general, for most chronic health conditions, the American Academy of Pediatrics (Rice, 2008) supports participation by affected children and adolescents in sports activities.

Adolescents need to develop their coordination and are still gaining muscle strength. Female adolescents stop increasing muscle strength at the time of their first menses, but males continue to increase their strength until they reach adulthood. A safe and structured regimen of daily physical activity will enhance coordination and normal adolescent development. However, physical and physiologic changes in the growing adolescent also place the youth at high risk for injury when engaging in physical activity. **Strength training**, the use of resistance methods to increase muscle ability to exert or resist force, is popular among adolescents and is often required in sports training programs. Strength training can be beneficial for adolescents to improve sports performance, rehabilitate after injury, prevent injuries, and enhance long-term health.

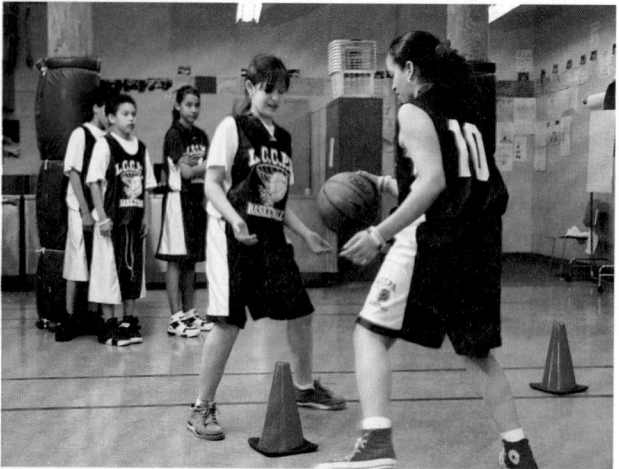

Figure 7-3 Basketball is an example of an activity that promotes physical fitness and helps the adolescent learn to work with others in a small group.

TRADITION OR SCIENCE 7-1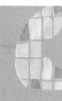

Are any potential dangers associated with backpack use in children and adolescents?

Using a backpack is an effective method of carrying school supplies, particularly in an era when lockers have been banned from many campuses. Research has concluded that when children or adolescents carry more than 10% of their body weight, they experience kyphotic postures that diminish lung capacity. Backpacks that weigh more than 15% of body weight are too heavy for a child or adolescent to maintain a standing posture. Carrying a backpack by only one strap changes posture and gait. Over a prolonged period, children may experience back pain, exacerbation of functional scoliosis, and stress on the spine and surrounding muscles (Chansirinukor et al., 2001; Chow et al., 2005; Grimmer et al., 1999; Kistner et al., 2013; Lai & Jones, 2001; Navuluri & Navuluri, 2006; Pascoe et al., 1997; Rateau, 2004; Sheir-Neiss et al., 2003). Girls experience more back pain and pathology than boys (Rodriguez-Oviedo et al., 2012). To prevent injury, it is recommended that backpacks be weighed and that children and adolescents carry no more than 10% of their total body weight (Kistner et al., 2013). Adolescents should be made aware of their posture and should be discouraged from leaning forward to correct for the heavy weight in their backpacks. Both shoulder straps should always be used when carrying the pack; incorporating hip or pelvic straps may further eliminate back strain. Weight in the pack should be evenly distributed. Backpacks on wheels are an excellent alternative to a conventional backpack (Brackley & Stevenson, 2004; Rateau, 2004).

No detrimental effects have been documented on cardiovascular health or linear growth of adolescents participating in weight lifting (AAP, 2008). Strength training may cause injury, however, when improper lifting techniques are used, too much weight is lifted, or lifts are improperly supervised. Adolescents should avoid competitive weight lifting, power lifting, body building, and maximal lifts until they have reached full skeletal and physical maturity (AAP, 2008) (Tradition or Science 7-1).

PERSONAL AND SOCIAL DEVELOPMENT

The emerging identity of the adolescent is strongly affected by family and peer relationships. Families will want to continue to monitor the youth's choice of friends, including those associations developed at school and social venues (e.g., church, sports teams) and through online communications.

TEMPERAMENT

 QUESTION: Which aspects of Ashley's behavior might be affected by the conflict of cultural norms between Ashley and her parents?

Temperament has been defined as the inherent way a person responds to environmental stimuli (see Chapter 3). Although temperaments are evident from infancy, the clash of temperaments between the child and that of his or her family may seem to be at its greatest state of disconnect during the adolescent years. The "fit" between the adolescent's temperament and the parenting style is further challenged by the adolescent's need to distance himself or herself from his or her parents emotionally, intellectually, and physically. As children progress through the adolescent years, they challenge parental norms by testing behavior limits and by testing parents' beliefs and values. Families can easily perceive that the child is "out of control." Young adolescents demonstrate a need to be separate from parents by establishing same-sex peer groups. These young adolescents vacillate from being clingy and infantile at one moment to being distinctly uncomfortable in the presence of their parents in the next. During middle adolescence, the adolescent may spend more time ignoring adult authority and become much more reliant on peer relationships. During this period, the adolescent might choose a stance directly opposite that of his or her parents and use peer support to back these ideas. Mood swings, a common occurrence during the early adolescent period, tend to smooth out during the middle adolescent period, when the teen will become more introspective. By late adolescence, emotions smooth out and become more consistent. The adolescent who has navigated successfully through early and middle adolescence usually comes to appreciate his or her parents' values and may even ask and receive advice from his or her parents (Radzik et al., 2008).

Successful adaptation during the adolescent years does not depend on the presence or absence of certain temperament styles. Families and children need to understand and accept that adolescents will at times be sullen, verbally defiant, moody, and oppositional. These behaviors are normal expressions of adolescents striving to separate from their families. To alleviate familial anxiety and to assist in reducing hostilities in the home, educate the family about normal adolescent separation behavior. Further assistance can be given through counseling and support groups to seek a better fit between the parenting style and the adolescent's temperament and to develop strategies to help both family and adolescent traverse the stages of normal development.

CROSS-CULTURAL CARE

A conflict of cultural norms may create situations in which parents consider a youth to be out of control (i.e., oppositional, exhibiting conduct and behavioral problems). Immigrant parents from a traditional, patriarchal parenting style may believe their adolescent is out of control when the teen is behaving in a fashion typical of adolescents in today's American society.

ANSWER: The conflict with Ashley's parents affects many aspects of her health. Consider the following questions: Do you think the additional stress from cultural conflicts is affecting Ashley's sleep and nutritional behaviors? Do you think there might be a relationship between Ashley's desire to fit in American culture and her sexual behaviors with her boyfriend, Eric?

RELATIONSHIPS

Adolescence is the time when individuals establish an identity for themselves outside of the family. Adolescents use their friends to elicit responses to their ideas and actions as they evolve into adults. During the early part of adolescence, teenagers are usually preoccupied with what is physically happening to their bodies. They use peer groups to stabilize themselves emotionally while entering puberty. Young adolescents usually have one very "best" friend of the same sex. Families are still important to them, even though they are trying to separate from the family.

As they enter middle adolescence, making friends becomes easier because they develop a greater repertoire of social skills and have expanded social opportunities through school and extracurricular activities. Adolescents use peers for the validation and approval they sought from their families during earlier years. Peer relationships are extremely important because the group forms formal and informal standards that adolescents use to measure themselves (Fig. 7-4). Middle adolescence is usually the low point in adolescent–parent relationships as adolescents push for independence and separation. Major conflicts may erupt as adolescents detach themselves from parental bonds.

By late adolescence, they are less dependent on peer groups and develop more individual relationships, including romantic or intimate relationships. The emancipation from the parental bond is complete, and the older adolescent tends to have far less conflict with the family.

Despite the changing dynamics between parent and child during adolescence, research indicates that adolescents who perceive that at least one parent cares

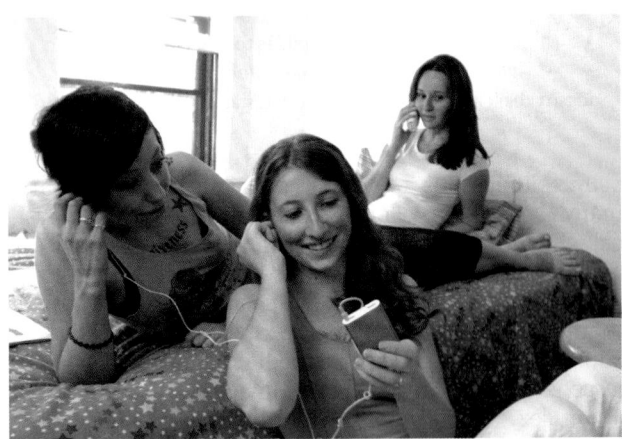

Figure 7-4 Adolescents develop relationships with their peers that provide a source of support and companionship.

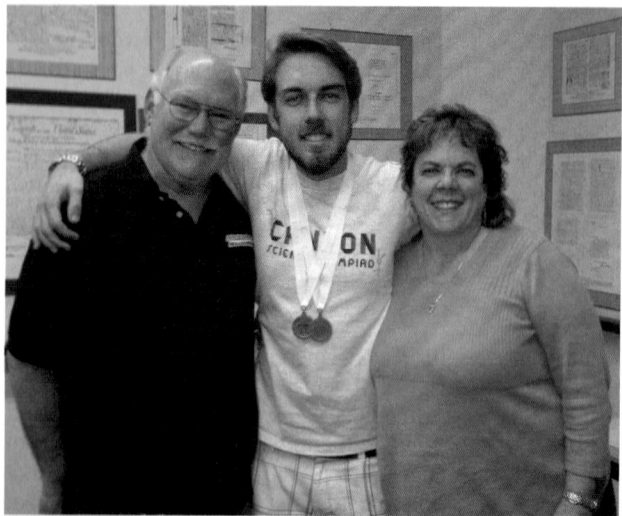

Figure 7-5 Relationships between the adolescent and his parents can continue to thrive when the adolescent feels supported, valued, and appreciated for his unique abilities.

about them and loves them are less likely to participate in risk-taking behaviors. Positive parenting behaviors have been associated with young adulthood resiliency (Johnson et al., 2011). Parental presence and monitoring (i.e., at least one parent is home at specific times, such as before or after school, at dinnertime, or at bedtime) is perceived by adolescents as evidence that a parent cares about them (Fig.7-5). The perception that school achievement is important to the parent is another factor that reassures adolescents they are loved (Devore & Ginsburg, 2005; Loewenson & Blum, 2001). Parenting practices and parent–child relationships have a profound effect on adolescent development. Although health care providers continue to emphasize good nutrition and exercise, adequate sleep, and a balance of work and play to maintain adolescent health, the protective effects of good parenting should not be overlooked. The parent–adolescent relationship must be fostered to promote optimal adolescent health and resiliency.

SEXUALITY

> QUESTION: Ashley confides to you that she and Eric have had unplanned and unprotected sex, but she doesn't think it will happen again. What should you say to Ashley?

Self-exploration is a normal part of adolescence and many adolescents voice questions about the physical changes that their bodies are going through. As adolescents enter puberty, nurses should share correct information regarding the physical changes that will occur and what are normal sexual desires during the adolescent years. Because of media influence, many adolescents have an idealized body image or misinformation about sex. Accurate information is often provided by a school health education course, but many adolescents may have additional inquiries about certain issues that they may be reluctant to discuss in a classroom setting.

Due to discomfort or a lack of information, many families may refrain from discussing any sexual information with their adolescent. There are many strategies that nurses can use to promote and enhance communication in the family. Encourage families to maintain open lines of communication so the adolescent can feel comfortable in approaching the parent with problems or questions. Active listening is an important component in communicating with adolescents about potentially uncomfortable topics; it is critical that families listen to their adolescents rather than lecture to them. Families can also share their values about sexual activity to help provide guidance. If the family identifies a knowledge deficit regarding sexual activity, nurses can help provide accurate information or resources (Salmon, 2010).

Initiation of sexual activity may begin during the latter school-aged years. Early initiation of sexual activity is most likely to occur in children with learning challenges or low academic achievement, behavioral or emotional problems (including mental health and substance abuse), low-income families, a history of physical and/or sexual abuse, family environments with marital discord, and households with low levels of parental supervision (AAP, Committee on Psychosocial Aspects of Child and Family Health & Committee on Adolescence, 2001; Madkour et al., 2010). Parental supervision has been demonstrated to have a significant effect on the initiation of early sexual activities. Adolescents who participated in family activities including mealtimes and who had positive relationships with their parents were less likely to engage in sexual activity (Pearson et al., 2006). Early initiation of sexual activity is a concern because sexual activity before age 15 years is also associated with other high-risk behaviors, including intercourse with multiple partners, intercourse with strangers, sexual activity associated with alcohol consumption, and unprotected sexual activities (AAP, Committee on Psychosocial Aspects of Child and Family Health & Committee on Adolescence, 2001).

As school-age children transition into adolescence, they begin to develop sexual orientation and gender identity. The American Academy of Pediatrics (Frankowski, 2004) defines sexual orientation as the pattern of physical and emotional attraction toward other persons. Sexual orientation is fostered via thoughts, fantasies, behaviors, and experiences; adolescents may start to gravitate toward a heterosexual, homosexual, or bisexual orientation (Frankowski, 2004; Auslander et al., 2005; Selekman, 2007). Gender identity and roles are also explored, and adolescents will continue to develop a sense of maleness or femaleness. Gender identity typically correlates to anatomic sex; transgender adolescents identify their gender as different than that of their biologic sex (Frankowski, 2004). The adolescent typically achieves a consolidated sexual identity during later adolescence and is more comfortable in developing opposite-sex relationships that have no sexual elements to them (Tradition or Science 7-2).

Sexuality is a complicated, yet important topic for nurses to approach with the adolescent. Many adolescent sexual behaviors may be exploratory or reflect peer pressure; therefore, it is important to avoid making assumptions regarding the sexual orientation of any adolescent. Non-heterosexual adolescents may be at increased risk

TRADITION OR SCIENCE 7-2

Does viewing television with sexual content affect adolescent sexual behavior?

The AAP conducted a longitudinal survey of 1,762 youths aged 12–17 years about their viewing habits, sexual knowledge, attitudes, and behaviors. Adolescents who viewed sexual content more often were more likely than others to initiate intercourse and to progress to more advanced, noncoital sexual activities. Those who watched the greatest amounts of sexual content were twice as likely to initiate intercourse than those who watched the least. Exposure to talk about sex (only) was associated with the same risks as programs depicting sexual behavior (Collins et al., 2004). Similar findings were made by Brown et al. (2006) in a longitudinal study of 1,017 black and white adolescents. The teens' *sexual media diet* (SMD) was first evaluated when they were 12–14 years old. Two years later, the assessment was repeated. White adolescents with the highest SMD scores were 2.2 times more likely to have had sexual intercourse at the ages of 14–16 years than those with the lowest SMD scores. Sexual activity by black adolescents was found to be more influenced by parents' expectations and their friends' sexual behavior than by their SMD score. Clearly, exposure to sexual content in music, movies, television, and magazines may be a factor that strongly influences initiation of sexual activity in the adolescent population.

Another study explored whether adolescents viewing TV programs with higher levels on sexual content had an association with regret following first sexual initiation. The researchers found that males who watched television programs with higher levels of sexual content were more likely to have feelings of regret. They did not find this association with females (Martino et al., 2009).

The RAND Corporation (2008) found a link between watching TV programs with large quantities of sexual content and adolescent pregnancy rates; they estimate that adolescents who watch TV programs with high levels of sexual content were twice as likely to become pregnant than those who watched programs with lower sexual content. It is important for families to monitor the programming watched by their adolescents.

romantic relationships, and those who report frequent alcohol or drug use (Siebenbruner et al., 2007).

With appropriate information regarding prevention of STIs and pregnancy, the adolescent might choose to delay sexual activity. However, education does not always mean that he or she will choose abstinence. Peer pressure and self-esteem often influence adolescents' actions more so than scientific evidence or education. The nurse interacting with the adolescent, either in the physician's office or in the school, is often the professional who explains the adolescent's responsibilities regarding sexual intercourse. Pregnancy and STIs are potential health risks for the adolescent engaging in sexual activity. These health risks are discussed later in the chapter.

Relationships where adolescents pair off into couples can be helpful in developing both behavioral and emotional autonomy; however, "hook up" behaviors are also prevalent in this population (Fig. 7-6). Adults tend to perceive the language of hook up to imply a meeting rather than a sexual encounter; the family may not speak with their adolescent about this phenomenon. *Hooking up* is a term commonly used by adolescents to describe engaging in sexual behaviors without the intent to pursue an emotional relationship. Multiple studies suggest that hooking up is prevalent among college students, with as many as 70% to 85% of students sharing that they engaged in at least one hook up encounter during their college experience. Twenty-eight percent of adolescents in grades 7 to 12 will experience a hook up. Substance use, truancy, and behavioral problems have been identified as associated components within the adolescent hook up phenomenon (Fortunato et al., 2010).

Increased Internet and social media use have implications on adolescent sexual behaviors. Many adolescents now have access to free online dating sites and their smart phones provide instant messaging, texting, and emailing. Sexually explicit texting, or "sexting," has been an increasing problem as teens have increased accessibility to mobile technology. Rice et al. (2012) found that approximately 15% of Southern California adolescents with cell phones engaged in sexting; families need to be aware of this issue because multiple risk-taking behaviors are associated with sexting.

for decreased self-esteem, feelings of isolation, physical/verbal assault, psychosocial problems, substance abuse, and increased stress/anxiety (Frankowski, 2004). Assist the adolescent to understand both the physical and psychosocial dimensions of his or her sexual development (Nursing Interventions Classification 7-3) and provide appropriate screening for high-risk populations. Avoid labeling, use open communication, use gender-neutral language, provide accurate information, and be accepting while communicating with adolescents about sexuality.

As the sexual identity of an adolescent emerges, sexual desires change and evolve. The adolescent may choose to become sexually active. The type and depth of their relationships may vary, but as the adolescent experiences his or her first "love," sexual activity becomes more likely. Increased sexual activity has been found to be more likely in adolescents who look more physically mature, those who have engaged in multiple

ANSWER: As important as the information you share is the attitude with which it is given. It must be nonjudgmental. State that you understand the conflict she is facing. Adolescents often perceive that they are the only ones who have ever had these feelings or experiences. Rather than using text as references (e.g., "Adolescents often . . . "), it is effective to personalize advice: "Another student told me that she did not realize how strong sexual feelings can be and that she used to really struggle because she believed good girls don't need birth control or protection from sexually transmitted infections." Emphasize to Ashley that it is important to have a plan that would protect her from pregnancy and STIs. Share current information regarding STIs in adolescents, and give Ashley information to review on her own. Emphasize her adult role in taking responsibility for her health and behavior. Strongly recommend that she find a health care provider whom she likes and trusts who can provide complete sexual health services.

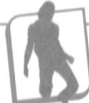

NIC 7-3 NURSING INTERVENTIONS CLASSIFICATION: Teaching Sexuality

Definition: Assisting individuals to understand physical and psychosocial dimensions of sexual growth and development

Activities:

Create an accepting, nonjudgmental atmosphere

Explain human anatomy and physiology of the male and female bodies

Explain the anatomy and physiology of human reproduction

Discuss signs of fertility (related to ovulation and the menstrual cycle)

Explain emotional development during childhood and adolescence

Facilitate communication between the child, adolescent, and parent

Support parents' role as the primary sexuality educator of their children

Educate parents on sexual growth and development through the life span

Provide parents with a bibliography of sexuality education materials

Discuss what values are, how we obtain them, and their effect on our choices in life

Facilitate the child's and adolescent's awareness of family, peer, societal, and media influence on values

Use appropriate questions to assist the child and adolescent to reflect on what is important personally

Discuss peer and social pressures on sexual activity

Explore the meaning of sexual roles

Discuss sexual behavior and appropriate ways to express one's feelings and needs

Inform children and adolescents of the benefits to postponing sexual activity

Educate children and adolescents on the negative consequences of early childbearing (e.g., poverty and loss of education and career opportunities)

Teach children and adolescents about sexually transmitted infections and AIDS

Promote responsibility for sexual behavior

Discuss benefits of abstinence

Inform children and adolescents about effective contraceptives

Instruct accessibility of contraceptives and how to obtain them

Assist adolescents in choosing an appropriate contraceptive, as appropriate

Facilitate role playing when decision-making and assertive communication skills may be practiced to resist peer and social pressures of sexual activity

Enhance self-esteem through peer role modeling and role playing

From Bulechek, G. M., Butcher, H. K., Dochterman, J. M. et al. (Eds.). (2013). *Nursing interventions classifications (NIC)* (6th ed.). St. Louis, MO: Mosby. Used with permission.

SCHOOL

QUESTION: Identify aspects of Ashley's case study that lead you to believe that the pressure Ashley feels to perform well in school is affecting her health. Do you think it is appropriate for Ashley to be assessed for depression?

School for the adolescent is very important. It is a center for socialization as well as learning (Fig. 7-7). Homeschooling is discussed in Chapter 6. Middle school is sometimes intimidating for the student coming from an elementary school and, likewise, can also be overwhelming for the student moving to high school from middle school. Many schools prepare students with orientation days and visits before admission to the next

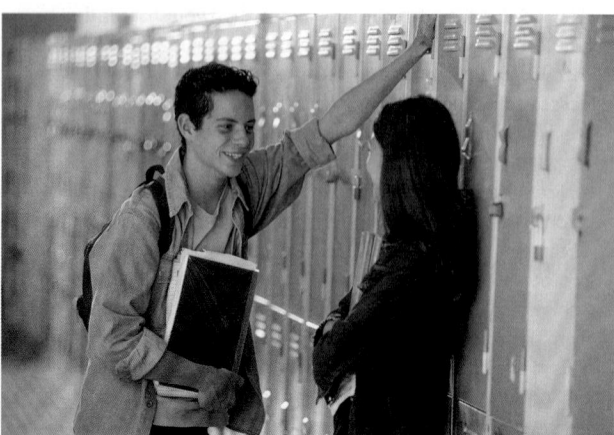

Figure 7-6 Dating becomes an important aspect of adolescent life.

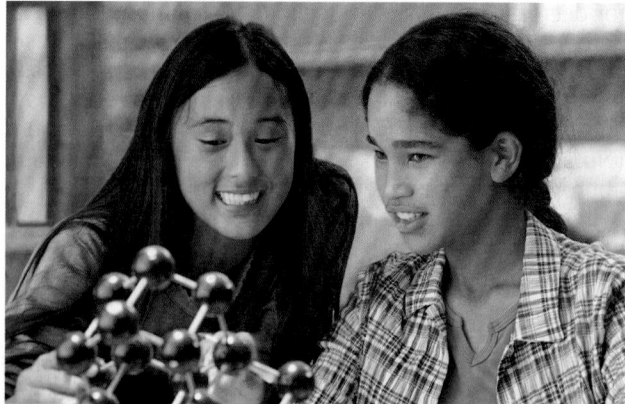

Figure 7-7 School is the center of learning and socialization for many adolescents. School classes, clubs, sports, and activities help shape the adolescent's identity.

school (middle or high school). Middle school prepares the adolescent for high school, and the high school is responsible for counseling the student to prepare for higher learning or vocational training. High school today is usually not the end of formal education. Most students are at least encouraged to apply to colleges. Sometimes, adolescents feel a great deal of pressure to achieve high academic or athletic accomplishments, and this pressure can produce bouts of depression. When persistent depressive moods interfere with the adolescent's normal functioning, encourage the family to seek health care assistance (see Chapter 29).

Homework may also be an issue for the adolescent because in middle school, high school, and college, homework is usually more intense than in lower grades (Clinical Judgment 7-1). Families are often not as involved with homework as they were when the child was in lower elementary school grades. Basic study habits should have been developed at an early age and may just need to be reinforced. Arrangements for homework, such as when and where it will be done and the consequences that will occur if it is not completed, should be worked out at the beginning of the school year. Nagging, threats, and bribery do not appear to be effective with teenagers; occasional monitoring and negotiations usually produce better results.

As adolescents consider the next stage of their academic career, the family and school officials can provide guidance in completing applications and testing for college entrance. Many adolescents may choose not to pursue further academic studies at this point in their life. Career counseling can benefit both college-bound and work-bound adolescents. Whatever choices adolescents make for their post–high school years, ensuring that their choices reflect their unique skills and talents is important.

ANSWER: The case history states that Ashley is avoiding meals at home, is very thin, and is not sleeping well. These indicate that the stress she is feeling both from pressure to perform well in school and the conflict with her parents is affecting her health. Yes, Ashley has several symptoms of depression, and it warrants further assessment.

MEDIA USE

With the explosion of technology over the past several years, children and adolescents have increasing access to the Internet through a variety of devices, including cellular phones, smart phones, tablets, laptops, and gaming consoles. The Internet is used in many positive ways, such as for completing school projects, personal entertainment, and connecting with friends through social media venues and instant messaging. Text messaging and face time on cellular phones and smart phones is another way for adolescents to stay connected. However, there are still risks to this pervasive access to the Internet, including access to inappropriate sexual content; exposure to false information;

potential victimization through profile posting or sharing personal information on social networking sites, in chat rooms, or through "phishing"; "friending" people they don't actually know; unintentional downloading of viruses through spam messages; exposure to or participation in sexting; being a victim of or a participant in cyberbullying; and potential damage to the teen's image for posting inappropriate photos or texts which can circulate forever (National Center for Missing & Exploited Children, 2011). The prevalence of electronic media devices in today's society has now made rules, such as keeping the television out of the bedroom and keeping the computer located in a common area of the home, virtually obsolete. In addition, time spent sedentary with media is time that adolescents are not engaged in physical activity. Because adolescents commonly consume snacks and sodas while using media devices, media use has contributed to the epidemic of adolescent obesity.

A recent Kaiser Family Foundation study found that children and adolescents, ages 8 to 18 years, spend an average of 7 hours and 38 minutes daily using media; because many of them multitask, they actually have a total daily media exposure of 10 hours and 45 minutes. Mobile devices are responsible for 20% of the media use (2 hours and 7 minutes). Approximately two thirds of those surveyed (66%) have their own cellular phone and 76% have an iPod or other type of MP3 player. This study also categorized them as "heavy users" (>16 hr/day), "moderate users" (3 to 16 hr/day), and "light users" (<3 hr/day) of media and found that almost one half of the heavy users have fair or poor grades; only 23% of light media users report fair or poor grades. Heavy media users also report lower levels of personal contentment. The highest levels of media use were reported in adolescents ages 11 to 14 years, Black youth, and Hispanic youth (Kaiser Family Foundation, 2010).

A survey of adolescents by Common Sense Media (2012) focused on social media use and found that 90% have used a form of social media. Seventy-five percent report having a profile on a social networking site, most commonly Facebook (68%); 22% report having a Twitter account. Adolescents with a social network profile report that social media use has a positive impact versus a negative impact on their emotional well-being; only 4% report feeling worse about themselves. Almost half of the adolescents still favor talking to friends in person. Adolescents also report the desire to "unplug" from social media (43% strongly agree or somewhat agree), and 41% describe themselves as addicted to phones. Adolescents also recognize that their parents and friends are attached to these devices and find it frustrating (Common Sense Media, 2012).

The AAP has issued a policy statement on the impact of social media on youth and families. The AAP, while recognizing the positive attributes of social media use, also points out some risks including cyberbullying and online harassment, sexting, and privacy concerns. Some families may not be aware of

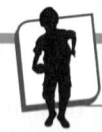

The Student Failing in School

Brock is a 17-year-old junior in high school who has come to the school health office because he fell asleep in class and injured his head when he (and his desk) fell over, hitting a nearby table. The teacher accompanies Brock to the office and shares with you his concerns regarding this seemingly minor injury. He has noticed that Brock has been falling asleep a lot in his afternoon class and that his grades have deteriorated considerably. Once a very reliable student, Brock is now inconsistent in completing homework, and his test scores have declined.

After Brock leaves the office, you review his school file. You note that, indeed, his A average has dropped to a C average during the past school year. You casually ask other teachers how Brock is performing in their classes, and their answers reveal a consistent pattern of tardiness, falling asleep in class, and apathy about school performance. The teaching staff agree that a meeting with Brock and his parents might be helpful to determine the cause for these dramatic changes in Brock's academic performance.

Brock is informed of the meeting and becomes very angry, demanding, "Why can't you guys just leave me alone? I'm passing in all of my classes, so what's the big deal?" Brock's mother is surprised that a meeting has been called because she is unaware of any problems with Brock's school performance. She is able to come to the meeting if it is scheduled late in the afternoon. She works nights and needs to sleep during the day. She reports that Brock's father will not be present because he is in the military and was deployed overseas 4 months ago.

Questions

1. What questions would you ask Brock at the meeting about his activities?

2. What are the presenting issues that you would share with Brock to support the concerns regarding his declining academic performance and his increased fatigue?

3. During the discussion with Brock, he reveals that he has taken on a part-time job that his mother did not know about. How would you proceed at this point?

4. The meeting yields several concerns regarding how Brock spends his time outside of school. How should you proceed with Brock and his mother?

5. What additional support can you provide this family as Brock makes a plan to refocus on his school activities?

Answers

1. Ask Brock to describe a typical week's schedule, detailing where and how he spends his time. Ask Brock specific questions about extracurricular activities, work, girlfriend, and peer group activities. Determine whether Brock has been involved in substance use and if he is receiving adequate nutrition. Determine his sleeping patterns. Ask Brock what he considers to be stressors in his life at this time.

2. Fatigue, decline in academic performance, tardiness.

3. Give Brock the opportunity to tell his mother about the job and the reason he chose to take it without her knowledge or permission. Provide support for both parties should the discussion become loud or hostile.

4. Brock has shared that he is playing on the school baseball team, and he leaves practice 3 or 4 days a week to go to his job until 11 PM. His mother works a 12-hour shift from 7 PM until 7 AM; thus, she had no idea he was not at home during these hours. He has been lying to her about where he is and what he has been doing. When she has called him on his cell phone, he always answered and said he was doing homework and had eaten dinner. Brock felt he had to work because he needed extra money to pay for his school activities but did not want to burden his mother. All members at the meeting need to develop a plan of action to support Brock's primary role—that of a student—while seeking means to assist the family if they are in financial crisis.

5. Brock and his mother may benefit from counseling because they are dealing with issues of loss (father's absence), trust (Brock's lying), and stress and need to discuss these issues at length. Brock must consider quitting his job or reducing the number of hours he works each week. He must also develop a plan with his parents and teachers to ensure his accountability in completing schoolwork. If his grades continue to drop, he should be prohibited from participating in extracurricular sports. Ensuring that Brock understands this consequence and the potential harm he may incur from lack of sleep and poor nutrition (e.g., work injury, falling asleep while driving) may help him understand why such concern exists about the demands he has been placing on his time.

the law or may choose not to enforce it: 13 years of age is the minimum age for signing up/having a profile on a social media site (Facebook and MySpace). It is important for families to supervise the online activities of their children and to be cognizant of their own knowledge deficits related to social media use (O'Keeffe et al., 2011).

Cyberbullying has evolved with the rise in cell phone/smart phone and computer use among adolescents. This type of bullying uses "communication technology to harass, intimidate, threaten, or otherwise harm others" (Patchin & Hinduja, 2010, p. 615). Almost 10% of adolescents, grades 6 to 10, report having been cyberbullied, and 8.3% of adolescents, grades 6 to 10, report having cyberbullied somebody (Mitchell, 2010). The Youth Risk Behavior Survey (YRBS) found that 16.2% of those surveyed had been cyberbullied (CDC, 2012f). Cyberbullying has been linked to low self-esteem (Patchin & Hinduja, 2010).

Sexting, "sending sexual images and sometimes sexual texts via cell phone and other electronic devices" (Mitchell et al., 2012, p. 14), has gained attention over the past several years. Because adolescents may have different concepts of sexting, it can be difficult to make accurate estimates. Only 1% of adolescents surveyed have sexted content that might violate child pornography laws. However, when more broadly defined as sexually suggestive material versus explicit images, 9.6% of adolescents have sexted (Mitchell et al., 2012).

Finally, online gaming addiction has been recognized in adolescents. These virtual worlds allow a player to create a character; the adolescent then spends many hours as this character in the virtual world. It is a time-consuming activity, and teens may forgo schoolwork or sleep to play. They may isolate themselves from family and friends and may act out if limits are put on the gaming. Families need to recognize when the adolescent becomes addicted and seek treatment (Young, 2009).

Supervising Internet and media use is primarily a parental responsibility (Fig. 7-8). As with the use of other electronic media (television, music players, tablets, smart phones/cell phones, and handheld gaming devices), the adolescent will pursue these activities for endless hours, given the opportunity. Parental supervision is a key factor in maintaining safe use of all electronic media. The family must first establish criteria for use of the computer/media devices, including when, where, and why they will be used (Developmental Considerations 7-2). Specific hours of the day can be selected for use in addition to delineating the amount of time allowed. Encourage adolescents and their families to communicate about privacy issues, the appropriateness of the media, and the financial risks associated with Internet use. Families can use contracts with their adolescents but must enforce the predetermined consequences if the contract is broken.

Media devices and Internet use have tremendous benefits in terms of education, communication, and recreation. Providing media device use rules will

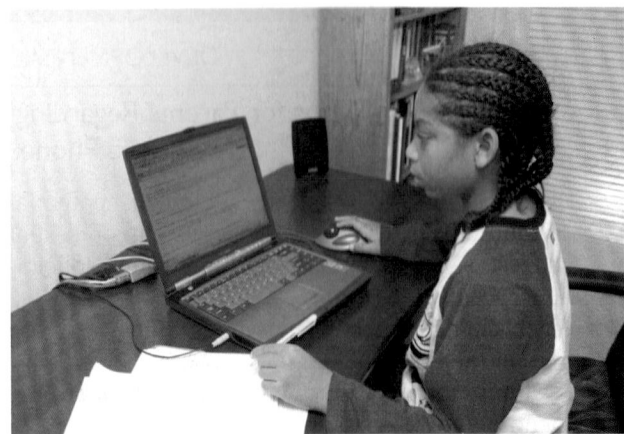

Figure 7-8 Computer use should be monitored by parents to ensure the adolescent is safely accessing the Internet.

give adolescents guidance in using these devices as a tool to benefit their education and relationships with others (Developmental Considerations 7-3). Diligent monitoring by parents will assist in maintaining the adolescent's safety and will promote opportunities for ongoing discussion of information gleaned from Internet sites.

WORK

In today's American society, it has become common for adolescents to hold part-time jobs during nonschool hours. The time spent in these part-time jobs can vary from a few weekend hours to daily work hours. July tends to be the peak in youth employment. The U.S. Department of Labor (2012) reported that 50.2% of 16- to 24-year-olds were employed in July 2012. This is a slight increase from July 2011 when 48.8% of 16- to 24-year-olds were employed. The leisure and hospitality sector employed 26% of them, and the retail trade industry employed 19% in 2012.

Both positive and negative consequences have been associated with adolescents participating in paid work experiences. Personal benefits include raising self-esteem, building personal responsibility, and developing teamwork. Of greater concern are the negative health consequences for adolescents that can arise from work conditions, including insufficient sleep from working too many hours, lack of exercise, interference with schoolwork, and time away from family and friends. In the work setting, adolescents can be exposed to multiple hazards, use dangerous equipment (despite regulations prohibiting such actions), and work long hours during the school week.

Adolescents have the highest incidence of work-related injuries than any other workforce age group because of a number of factors, including lack of training, minimal supervision, performing tasks outside of their job descriptions, and using equipment designed for adults (Sudhinaraset & Blum, 2010). Adolescent workers report a lack of consistent job training and adult supervision on the job (Runyan

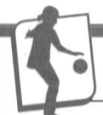

DEVELOPMENTAL CONSIDERATIONS 7-2

Tips for Parents Regarding Child and Adolescent Internet, Mobile Phone, and Texting Safety

- Discuss with the child or adolescent potential online dangers (e.g., access to violent or sexual images, sexual victimization, unwanted solicitations, scams, predators).
- Teach child/teen not to post identifying information on the Internet.
- Set limits for how much time the child/teen can spend online.
- Keep the computer in a common area of the house.
- Avoid, if possible, Internet use in the child/teen's bedroom.
- Use parental controls and/or blocking software provided by your Internet service provider.
- Discuss with the child/teen purchasing "in app" products.
- Discuss with the child/teen about using any location services (e.g., Global Positioning System [GPS]) on his or her device(s).

- Periodically review the child/teen's computer, emails, and messages. You should have all of the teen's passwords.
- Spend time with your child/teen online. Know his or her favorite sites as well as his or her online friends. Ensure your media use skills are current.
- Know who your child/teen texts and emails and monitor his or her access to the Internet and texting/messaging.
- Watch for unexplained changes in the child/teen's behavior.
- Seek assistance from law enforcement immediately if you think a predator may be targeting your child/teen.

Information from U.S. Department of Justice. (n.d.a). *Internet, mobile phones, and texting safety tips for parents.* Retrieved from http://www.justice.gov/usao/mn/downloads/PSC%20Elementary%20Safety%20Tips%20Parents.pdf

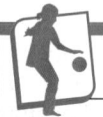

DEVELOPMENTAL CONSIDERATIONS 7-3

Internet, Mobile Phone, and Texting Safety Tips for Children and Adolescents

- Never post personal information online (name, age, birth date, address, telephone number, or school information).
- Never post your picture or pictures of your family online (they can be copied or changed or used to find you).
- Never send any inappropriate photo or message by email or text.
- Never post your plans and/or activities in a chat room or on your personal website/social media site.
- Never communicate with anyone who has made you afraid or uncomfortable. Tell your family or a trusted adult if someone makes you afraid or uncomfortable online.
- Never join an online group or game without talking to your parents.

- Never meet with someone you met online without first telling your parents/guardian.
- Never post hurtful or inappropriate messages. If someone posts something hurtful or inappropriate, tell a teacher, parent, or adult. Do not respond.
- Never click on any link that you do not know and you are not sure is legitimate.
- Never buy any "apps" or make "in app" purchases without talking to your parents/guardian.
- Never enable any location services without talking to your parents/guardian.
- Remember that people can lie online. Someone might say she is a 12-year-old girl but in reality be an older man wanting to harm you.
- Save any messages that upset you, and show them to your parents/guardian.
- Tell your passwords to your parents/guardian.

Information from the U.S. Department of Justice. (n.d.b). *Internet, mobile phones, and texting safety tips for kids.* Retrieved from http://blogs.justice.gov/main/files/2012/08/PSC-Elementary-Safety-Tips-KidsParents-2.pdf et al., 2007). They may also be unaware of their rights as employees.

In 2009, work-related injuries killed 27 adolescents younger than 18 years of age. Between 1998 and 2007, there were approximately 795,000 nonfatal young worker injuries annually treated in emergency departments (EDs) in the United States. The rate of ED-treated work injuries in adolescents is nearly two times higher than the rate for workers ages 25 years and older (CDC, n.d.b). Work has been associated with musculoskeletal pain in adolescents and increases in worker compensation claims in this age group (Breslin et al., 2003; Feldman et al., 2002). However, a recent study concluded that adolescents had an increased risk of open wounds, and older workers had an increased risk for injuries to bones, nerves, and spinal cord (P. Smith et al., 2013). Healthy People 2020 includes an objective to reduce the rate of injuries by adolescents aged 15 to 19 years treated in EDs by 10% by 2020 (CDC, n.d.b).

Nurses can assist the adolescent in making wise decisions regarding work activities. Apprise the adolescent of the laws that govern work rules for them (U.S. Department of Health & Human Services, 1997). Furthermore, discussions with families can yield information regarding whether work has affected adolescents' grades, attitudes, or behavior. Encourage families to limit work hours and have the adolescent maintain a schedule that allows 8 to 9 hours of sleep a night while also accommodating work and school.

PREVENTING INJURY AND ILLNESS

The thrill-seeking, invincible-seeming, fun-loving attributes that characterize adolescence may also place the adolescent at higher risk for sustaining injuries. Many adolescents may engage in high-risk activities without considering the immediate and long-term consequences of these behaviors. Unfortunately, unintentional injuries remain the leading cause of death within the adolescent population (CDC, 2012d). Guidelines for preventing injury and violence serve as the template for ongoing discussions between adolescents and health care providers to promote healthy growth and development during the adolescent years (Community Care 7-2). In addition, the health care provider should be vigilant with regard to adolescents' emotional and mental state of health. Chapter 29 provides a thorough review of mental health conditions that may affect adolescents, including depression and suicide.

DRIVING

Learning to drive and acquiring a driver's license are true rites of passage during the adolescent years. Yet, these accomplishments that best illustrate the adolescent's independence and maturity can also clearly demonstrate the ongoing need to temper independence with caution. Encourage the adolescent to participate in a driver's education course to learn the basic skills of driving (Fig. 7-9). In some states, these courses are required to be completed when adolescents have their driver's permit and prior to receiving their license. States vary on regulations regarding who may accompany the adolescent driver in the car, night driving, and use of electronic equipment (e.g., cell phones, smart phones, tablets, MP3 players) while driving. Encourage families to familiarize themselves with the driving laws in their state and to model good driving behaviors to their adolescent. Speak frankly with the adolescent about use of safety belts and the risks (both legal and physical) of driving while under the influence of alcohol or drugs.

The leading cause of death among adolescents continues to be motor vehicle collisions (CDC, 2012c), and distracted driving (talking on a cellular phone, text messaging, accessing Internet on portable devices) appears to contribute to fatal crashes (Wilson & Stimpson, 2010). Almost thirty three percent (32.8%) of adolescents indicated they had emailed or texted while driving a car at least once during the 30 days before the YRBS (CDC, 2012f). Males were more likely than females to be involved in a fatal crash caused by distracted driving (Wilson & Stimpson, 2010). A number of states have bans on distracted driving.

A recent survey indicated that 7.7% of teens never or rarely wear a seatbelt as a car passenger. Teens also indicated that in the 30 days prior to the YRBS, 8.2% had driven a car under the influence of alcohol (CDC, 2012f). Again, education and parental modeling continue to be important.

ALERT *Children younger than 16 years of age should not drive or ride an all-terrain vehicle because they do not yet have the physical coordination and mental judgment to handle these types of vehicles (Hagan et al., 2008).*

SPORTS INJURIES

More than 7.5 million adolescents participate in organized sports programs across the United States (Halstead, 2010). Although such programs provide enjoyment, teach teamwork, and promote camaraderie, they also place the adolescent at risk for physical injury (Mickalide & Hansen, 2012; Monroe et al., 2011). Sports injuries account for approximately 2 million injuries among adolescents and necessitate 500,000 medical visits and 30,000 hospitalizations annually (Darrow et al., 2009). The cost of hospitalizations due to sports injuries in children and adolescents ranges from $113 to $133 million annually (Safe Kids Worldwide, 2011). Most organized sports–related injuries (62%) occur during practices rather than games (CDC, 2006; Monroe et al., 2010; Safe Kids Worldwide, 2011).

Football, basketball, and cycling are associated with the greatest number of ED visits (Monroe et al., 2010). Contact sports with the highest fatality rates include baseball (highest), basketball, football, soccer, and

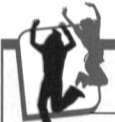

COMMUNITY CARE 7-2

Injury and Violence Prevention Guidelines for the Adolescent

Home Safety

- Check smoke and carbon monoxide detectors to ensure that they are working properly; change batteries twice yearly with the time change.
- Discuss safety rules for the home, including those about visitors; use of the telephone, computer, and other devices; and what to do in case of fire or other emergencies. Conduct fire drills at home.

Activity Safety

- Wear protective sports gear.
- Wear appropriate protective gear at work, and follow job safety procedures.
- Avoid high noise levels, especially when using music headsets.
- Always wear a helmet when riding a motorcycle, an all-terrain vehicle, or a bicycle. Even with a helmet, motorcycles and all-terrain vehicles are very dangerous.
- Discuss concussion safety and do not return to play until symptoms have resolved.

Water Safety

- Learn how to swim.
- Do not swim alone.
- Do not drink alcohol while boating or swimming.

Car Safety

- Wear a seat belt in the car at all times.
- If you are driving, insist that your passengers wear seat belts.
- Follow the speed limit and traffic rules.
- Do not drink alcohol and drive. Plan to have a designated driver if drinking.

- Prevent distracted driving: do not text message, talk on the phone, or email while driving.

Outdoor Safety

- Protect yourself from skin cancer by applying sunscreen before you go outside for long periods.
- Do not use tanning salons.
- Use insect repellant to prevent insect-borne diseases.

Emergency Preparation

- Make sure your address and phone number are posted near a phone at your house.
- Know where the list of emergency numbers (doctor, hospital, nearest neighbor, poison control center) is kept in your home.
- Know how to contact your parents in case of an emergency. Keep their work phone numbers in your purse, wallet, school notebook, or mobile device.
- Keep a cell phone or some loose change with you at all times so that you can make an emergency call if needed.

Violence Prevention

- Do not carry or use a weapon of any kind.
- Develop skills in conflict resolution, negotiation, and dealing with anger constructively.
- Learn techniques to protect yourself from physical, emotional, and sexual abuse, including rape by either strangers or acquaintances.
- Seek help if you are physically or sexually abused or fear that you are in danger.

Adapted from Hagan, J. F., Shaw, J. S., & Duncan P. M. (Eds.). (2008). *Bright futures: Guidelines for health supervision of infants, children, and adolescents* (3rd ed.). Elk Grove Village, IL: American Academy of Pediatrics; Gardner, H. G. (2007). Office-based counseling for unintentional injury prevention. *Pediatrics, 119*(1), 202–206; Halstead, M. E. (2010). Contact sports for young athletes: Keys to safety. *Pediatric Annals, 39*(5), 275–278.

---

gymnastics (Halstead, 2010). The most common types of sports-related injuries include sprains, strains, overuse syndromes, and growth plate injuries; the most commonly injured regions of the body include the ankle, knee, hand, wrist, elbow, shin and calf, head, neck, and clavicle (Franklin & Weiss, 2012; Safe Kids Worldwide, 2011). Concussions remain on the forefront among sports-related injuries in adolescents. Of an estimated 3.8 million sports-related concussions occurring annually, 60% to 65% occur in the pediatric population (Grady, 2010; Halstead, 2010). Sports that are reported to be responsible for most of the

concussion-based ED visits include football, soccer, basketball, and cycling (Grady, 2010). It is important to note, however, that there is a wide array of variability among adolescent concussion rates by gender and type of sport (Marar et al., 2012). Eye injuries are also commonly seen in adolescents playing baseball, softball, and basketball (Pollard et al., 2012). The primary factors that influence the high rate of sports-related injuries include:

- Lack of safety precautions implemented during practices and games (e.g., safe environment, safe equipment, use of protective gear)

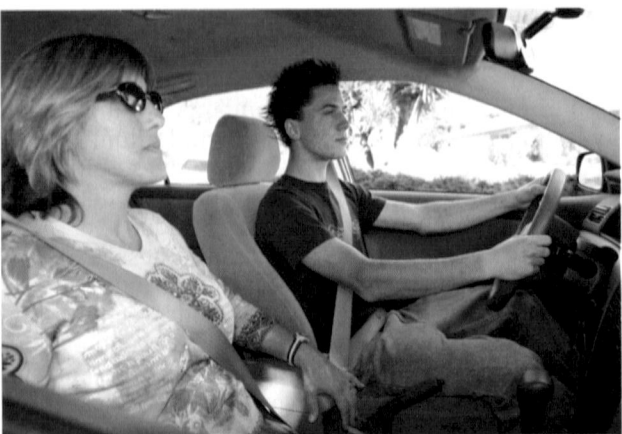

Figure 7-9 Driving safety education is one part of the injury and illness prevention plan for the adolescent population.

- Poor health of the athlete as a result of obesity, improper nutrition and fluid intake, or use of ergogenic aids
- Long practice periods, with increasing intensity and shorter rest periods, causing repetitive stress without adequate recovery time
- Anatomic and physiologic changes of growth (especially during puberty)

The young athletes have several physical and physiologic differences that place them at higher risk for injury when compared with adult athletes (Developmental Considerations 7-4). Both short- and long-term sequelae can result from improper attention to these differences when designing sports training programs. In addition, lack of attention to the general safety, nutrition, and health practices of adolescents participating in sports activities can have deleterious effects on their well-being. These negative effects include severe dyspnea, syncope, cramps, heat syncope, heat exhaustion, heat stroke, dehydration, bone injury, and mental stress (Darrow et al., 2009; Halstead, 2010).

Nurses providing care for adolescents should be aware of weight gain and weight loss methods being used by them and sports that have a greater risk of unhealthy weight management practices. Typically, athletes in sports that put the adolescent's body on display, such as gymnastics, ice-skating, swimming, and dance, are at risk. Sports in which the athlete must weigh in before competing, such as wrestling, also put the athlete at risk. Adolescents might engage in unhealthy weight control practices (both weight loss and weight gain methods) as a means to improve performance, improve appearance, or meet weight expectations of the sport. These practices may occur during the sports season only or year-round.

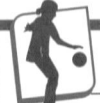

DEVELOPMENTAL CONSIDERATIONS 7-4

Physical and Physiologic Attributes of Young Athletes That Make Them Vulnerable to Sports-Related Injuries

Attribute	Implications
Large body surface area-to-mass ratio	Absorbs heat more quickly when the ambient temperature exceeds skin temperature
Larger head compared with rest of body	Greater likelihood of head injury
Smaller body size than adults, with more variation in size even within same age groups	Protective gear may not be appropriately sized
Physes (growth plates) still open	Possibility of damage to plates with certain activities (e.g., weight lifting); damage to plates can lead to early closure
Cartilage still developing	More susceptible to overuse injuries
Motor skills have not reached full maturity and mastery of complex motor skills not complete; during puberty, coordination and balance decline	Coordination and response time diminished when injury risk is evident
Higher threshold before beginning to sweat; lower sweat volume	More likely to sustain heat injuries
Produce more heat relative to body mass for the same exercise completed by an adult	Predisposed to dehydration and heat illness

caREminder

Although young male athletes are often encouraged to "bulk up" and increase their body mass, female athletes are often encouraged to maintain a low body weight. Female athletes are at risk for developing eating disorders, amenorrhea, and osteoporosis (contributing to stress fractures) (Nazem & Ackerman, 2012). This clinical problem is called the female athlete triad, and all young women engaged in intense physical activity are at risk. It is important to screen female athletes for the triad because of the associated short- and long-term risks (Deimel & Dunlap, 2012). All adolescent athletes should be carefully monitored and counseled as necessary to ensure that dietary extremes are not used to enhance their competitive edge.

Weight loss methods include food restriction; vomiting; overexercising; voluntary dehydration; and use of over-the-counter and prescribed substances such as diet pills, nicotine, and stimulants. Voluntary dehydration practices are said to include fluid restriction; spitting; and the use of laxatives, diuretics, rubber suits, steams baths, and saunas to dehydrate the body and produce the desired weight loss (AAP, Committee on Sports Medicine and Fitness, 2005).

Gaining weight might also be a goal of some athletes. Sports such as football, rugby, and weight lifting encourage weight gain to enhance body composition. Supplements or anabolic steroids may be used to gain weight and improve physique. In most cases, these substances have unproved value and are potentially harmful to the adolescent (Lorang et al., 2011; D. V. Smith & McCambridge, 2009) (Table 7-1). The use

TABLE 7-1   Ergogenic Aids Used by Young Athletes

Type	Use	Comments
Dietary supplements (e.g., protein, creatine, nucleic acid, and amino acid components)	Vitamin, mineral, herb, other botanical, or amino acid used to supplement the total dietary intake. May produce brief explosive power or muscle strength that may enhance competitive results. Promoted as producing weight loss and enhancing athletic and school performance and physical appearance.	Readily available without prescription or parental consent. Marketed as "safe" and endorsed by professional athletes who are compensated for their endorsement. Long-term health consequences of use are unknown. Supplements do not increase endurance; incremental gain in power is only 5%–7%. High osmotic load of these products can increase risks of dehydration and heat-related illness.
Caffeine	Stimulant effective in endurance sports because of effect on central nervous system, fatty acid metabolism, and muscle contraction.	Readily available and widely used. Limited performance enhancement benefits when weighed against potential for serious complications. Powerful diuretic that places athlete at risk for dehydration and sudden death from heat-related illness.
Diuretics (e.g., furosemide, hydrochlorothiazide)	Induce rapid weight loss for a short time.	Causes diuresis and substantial electrolyte abnormalities, which can lead to fatal cardiac arrhythmia. Can cause syncope from orthostatic hypertension.
Ephedra	Used to reduce weight in weight-categorized sports. Used to reduce total body fat and improve fat-free mass to enhance physique for purely cosmetic purposes.	Often added to dietary supplements. Sale of ephedra and ephedra-containing products is banned except as U.S. Food and Drug Administration approved. High morbidity and mortality rates associated with youth use related to heat-related injury and cardiac arrhythmias.
Methamphetamines	Stimulant that can substantially improve athletic performance.	Increased availability seen as major concern. Rate of cardiac-related sudden death from arrhythmias is high. Youths treated with this substance for attention-deficit/hyperactivity disorder (ADHD) are at high risk for heat-related injury and should refrain from combining ADHD medication with other stimulant products.
Androgenic–anabolic steroids	Produces increased levels of testosterone. Increases muscle mass and strength. Effects also include increased facial and body hair, deepened voice, acne, and psychological lability (testosterone rage).	Cardiac-related sudden death, most commonly related to cardiomyopathy, structural anomalies of the coronary arteries, direct trauma to the chest, or infectious myocarditis.
Blood doping	Enhance competitive edge through use of autologous blood transfusions and/or erythropoietin. Increases hematocrit above level of 60% when erythropoietin is used.	Used more by older athletes. Complication is hyperviscosity syndrome, which may result in stroke, increased rate of heat-related morbidity and mortality, and increased risk of renal damage.

Data from Gardiner, P., Dvorkin, L., & Kemper, K. (2004). Supplement use growing among children and adolescents. *Pediatric Annals, 33*(4), 227–232; Griesemer, B. (2003). Ergogenic aids elevate health risks in young athletes. *Pediatric Annals, 32*(11), 733–737; Metzl, J. (2002). Performance-enhancing drug use in the young athlete. *Pediatric Annals, 31*(1), 27–32.

of androgenic–anabolic steroids by adolescents is of primary concern. Athletes and others abuse anabolic steroids to enhance athletic performance and improve physical appearance. Taken orally or injected, anabolic steroids are typically ingested in cycles of weeks or months (*cycling*) rather than on a continual basis (AAP, 2008; National Institute on Drug Abuse, 2012a). Cycling involves taking multiple doses of steroids over a specific period of time, stopping for a period, and starting again. In addition, the adolescent will often combine several different types of steroids to maximize their effectiveness while minimizing negative effects (*stacking*) (National Institute on Drug Abuse, 2012a). Use of anabolic steroids among adolescents is reported to be 3.6% (CDC, 2012f); another survey found only 1.4% of surveyed adolescents had used anabolic steroids but the researchers felt the rate was underreported (Lorang et al., 2011). However, the side effects of these substances place these adolescents at risk for serious health problems, some of which may be irreversible. These side effects include liver and kidney tumors, high blood pressure, high cholesterol levels, jaundice, cancer, and premature skeletal maturation (National Institute on Drug Abuse, 2007; D. V. Smith & McCambridge, 2009). Careful monitoring of athletes' weight, eating patterns, hydration practices, heat illnesses, and general health are important to ensure that adolescents are not at risk for injury. Recognizing the signs and symptoms of an eating disorder (see Chapter 29), with prompt referral for medical, nutritional, and psychological intervention, is an important responsibility of the health care provider. A key AAP recommendation focuses on the need to provide individual, family, and team counseling to promote healthy weight gain and weight loss practices. Such counseling should review optimal growth parameters for the adolescent, discuss both healthy and unhealthy practices for weight gain and loss, and discuss measures to prevent dehydration, overhydration, and related injury attributable to improper dietary practices.

TOBACCO, ALCOHOL, AND SUBSTANCE USE

One of the foremost concerns regarding adolescents is preventing the use of drugs and alcohol. Tobacco and alcohol use symbolize adult status to the adolescent, and parental warnings can be perceived as a mechanism to block the adolescent from achieving independence. Education about drugs and alcohol has a strong effect on adolescent attitudes. The best time to start this education is when the child is elementary school-aged; if it is reinforced during adolescence, it is even more effective. Positive parental role-modeling is one of the best ways to prevent drug and alcohol use among adolescents. For example, several studies have shown that parental provision of alcohol, home alcohol accessibility, and the lack of parental alcohol-specific rules increase the initiation and use of alcohol by adolescents (Komro et al., 2007; van der Vorst et al., 2007; van der Vorst et al., 2005).

Tobacco Use

Despite regulatory efforts to restrict advertising of tobacco products and banning the sale of tobacco products to those younger than 18 years of age, the current rate of adolescents who report using cigarettes one or more times during the past 30 days is 18.1%, whereas 7.7% for smokeless tobacco. Males were more likely to use tobacco than females (CDC, 2012f). The media has an impact on smoking; it has been shown that adolescents who view movies with smoking actors and actresses are more likely to start smoking (U.S. Surgeon General, 2012).

Smoking and other forms of tobacco use affect every organ system in the body and are major causes of cancer, heart disease, stroke, chronic obstructive pulmonary disease, and fetal damage. More than 5 million deaths occur worldwide each year as a result of tobacco use (CDC, 2012b). For many years, tobacco companies have asserted that smoking tobacco is not addictive and does not cause cancer, lung disease, or other terminal conditions. These claims have been repeatedly refuted by the medical profession and shared in numerous educational campaigns with children and adolescents. The U.S. Surgeon General (2012) indicates that approximately 90% of smokers begin smoking by age 18 years; preventive efforts should begin in the early adolescent years. Although many adolescents understand the risks associated with smoking tobacco, they may be uninformed about the hazards associated with smokeless tobacco. The two types of smokeless tobacco, snuff and chewing tobacco, contain 28 carcinogens. The nicotine delivered by smokeless tobacco use is three to four times higher per dose than smoking a cigarette and stays in the bloodstream for a longer time, thus it leads to nicotine addiction just as cigarette smoking does. Smokeless tobacco use increases significantly the user's risk of cancer of the lip, tongue, cheeks, gums, and the floor and roof of the mouth.

Even though the long-term consequences of tobacco products are known, adolescents appear to have little concern about the outcomes that might occur 20 or 30 years from now. Peer pressure and the belief that tobacco use is enjoyable are the most influential factors among adolescents who initiate use of tobacco substances. In families who communicate well with their adolescents about smoking, the adolescents are less likely to smoke; perceived family support is also related to decreased likelihood of smoking (Harakeh et al., 2010). The selection of non-smoking friends is also influenced by parenting; adolescents who feel that parents challenge their autonomy are more likely to choose friends who smoke (Mercken et al., 2013).

Nurses should assess for tobacco and smokeless tobacco use. Ask adolescents whether they or their friends have ever tried or used tobacco products. Assess the oral mucosa for oral leukoplakia (white mouth lesions that can become cancerous). Determine whether the adolescent has any respiratory condition, such as asthma, that may be exacerbated by tobacco use. Provide education about the health risks of tobacco products and how to quit. Adolescents also need to know that smokeless tobacco is not a safer alternative to ciga-rette smoking and that cancers can develop in as few as 6 to 7 years. Excellent references for nurses work-ing with adolescents include the National Institute of Dental and Craniofacial Research, Office on Smoking and Health at the CDC, the National Spit Tobacco Edu-cation Program, the American Cancer Society, and the American Academy of Family Physicians (see thePoint for Organizations).

Alcohol Use

Underage drinking affects adolescent health risk behav-iors and has the potential for addiction. In a national study, 38.7% of high school students report having one or more drinks of alcohol during the previous 30 days. In the same study, 21.9% of students report engaging in more heavy use of alcohol as defined by five or more drinks of alcohol in a row, within a couple of hours within the past 30 days. Twenty-one and a half percent of the students stated that they had their first drink of alcohol (other than sips) before the age of 13 years. Fortunately, these numbers have decreased since 2005 (CDC, 2012f).

Parental alcohol use rules and modeling appear to be the most effective methods of establishing appropriate standards regarding drinking (Komro et al., 2007; van der Vorst et al., 2007; van der Vorst et al., 2005; Ward & Snow, 2011). Many parents do not take drinking as seriously as drug abuse, perceiving it as the "lesser of two evils" because alcohol is a legal substance. Many adolescents actually obtain their alcohol from their par-ents, either directly or indirectly (Komro et al., 2007; Ward & Snow, 2011). Adolescents report that the rea-sons they engage in occasional or regular drinking include the pleasures derived from the effects of alcohol and the social interactions associated with the drinking activities and the thrill of risk taking. Boredom is also a motivating factor (McIntosh et al., 2008). Children who begin to drink at an early age have also been shown to have similar personality characteristics that make them more likely to start drinking. These characteris-tics include those who are hyperactive, disruptive, and aggressive as well as those who are depressed, with-drawn, or anxious. Tolerance to alcohol may be directly linked to genetics. Thus, being a child of an alcoholic or having several family members who are alcoholics may place the adolescent at increased risk for alcohol abuse (AAP, Committee on Substance Abuse, 2010).

The negative effects of alcohol can be especially dev-astating when adolescents mix drinking and driving. Approximately 8% of high school students state they have been drunk while driving, and 24% report they have ridden in a vehicle operated by someone who had been drinking alcohol (CDC, 2012f). The leading causes of adolescent death are automobile accidents, homi-cides, and suicides; alcohol is a major factor in all three (AAP, Committee on Substance Abuse, 2010).

Adolescents generally consume five or more drinks at a time; this is called *binge drinking*. Approximately 22% of teens reported binge drinking on one or more days in the 30 days prior to the survey (CDC, 2012f).

Approximately 40% of adults who began drinking before the age of 12 years report having signs of alcohol de-pendence (AAP, Committee on Substance Abuse, 2010). There are four stages of becoming dependent on alcohol:

1. Experimental stage: when the adolescent tries out alcohol and likes its effect
2. Seeking-out stage: when the adolescent seeks out opportunities to drink
3. Dependency stage: when the alcohol-induced high becomes top priority for the adolescent
4. Addiction stage: when the adolescent needs alcohol just to feel "normal"

Alcohol dependence is difficult to treat but cannot be ignored. Adolescents who engage in ongoing alcohol consumption are at high risk for injury while inebri-ated. Alcohol consumption impairs judgment and the ability to make sound decisions. In addition, underage alcohol use increases the risks of carrying out or being the victim of physical or sexual assault and increases the likelihood of engaging in risky sexual activity that may lead to pregnancy or STIs (CDC, 2012a). Profes-sional intervention and programs developed to treat alcoholic adolescents can be of assistance. During health care encounters, observe the adolescent for potential alcohol abuse. Common signs to indicate physiologic dependence or withdrawal include craving alcohol, compulsive alcohol-seeking behaviors, tremulousness, agitation, weight loss, headaches, and changes in men-tal status. Ask adolescents about their use of alcohol and their activities with friends who may be drinking. Talk with adolescents about alcohol use and teach them the hazards of underage drinking. Assist the adolescent to make good decisions about alcohol use, including seeking ways to resist consuming alcohol when offered by friends or at parties. Discuss with families the strong influence they impart on their adolescent's decision to consume alcohol. Ensure that family rules have been communicated to the adolescent, and encourage par-ents not to purchase or offer alcohol to their underaged child. Last, assist school officials and teachers to create a school environment that does not tolerate alcohol use and that encourages students to have a positive sense of attachment to school (e.g., active engagement in academics and social activities, attachment to teachers, respect for school rules).

Illicit Drug Use

The use of alcohol and tobacco products by adoles-cents may be followed or accompanied by the use of illicit drugs. Marijuana is the most commonly used il-licit drug, with 39.9% of high school students stat-ing they have used marijuana one or more times. In contrast, other substances have less reported use by high school students: cocaine, 6.8%; inhalants, 11.4%; heroin, 2.9%; methamphetamines, 3.8%; and Ecstasy, 8.2% (CDC, 2012f). Synthetic marijuana (K2 or Spice) was used by 11.4% of 12th graders, which is of concern (National Institute on Drug Abuse, 2012c). Nearly 21% (20.7%) of adolescents also reported using prescrip-tion drugs without a doctor's prescription. Of primary concern to school nurses, school officials, and parents is that 25.6% of high school students state they have been offered, sold, or given an illegal drug on school property by someone during the past 12 months (CDC, 2012f).

Clubbing and raves are also a concern; adolescents have died from use of "club drugs," which include Ecstasy, gamma-hydroxybutyric acid (GHB), ketamine, and Rohypnol. Fortunately, there has been a decrease in adolescent use of these drugs in the past several years. A 2012 survey showed that 1.5% of surveyed 12th graders used Rohypnol or ketamine and 1.4% used GHB. (Johnston et al., 2013). Bath salts are a newer designer drug; bath salt exposure is highest in the 20- to 29-year age group, and use declined in 2012 (Wood, 2013).

Ingestion of hand sanitizer, containing 60% ethyl alcohol, has also been reported. Currently, there is very little information available about the incidence, but cases have been reported by ED physicians and toxicologists (Woo & Hanley, 2013).

caREminder

Nonmedical use of prescription stimulants (such as methylphenidate, which is used for the treatment of ADHD) is seen in approximately 2% of the adolescent population. These substances are used to stay awake longer to party, study, or drink more. Problems associated with taking someone else's medication may include cardiovascular effects; insomnia; psychosis; precipitation or worsening of other disorders; and potential promotion of, or worsening of, substance abuse. Assessment of adolescent substance use should include the abuse of prescription stimulants (AAP, The Council on Communications and Media, 2010; Aria & Wish, 2006; Setlik et al., 2009).

Clearly, health care providers need to meet the goal of diminishing adolescent substance use (including alcohol and tobacco) through several different avenues. Nurses can collaborate with schools to foster environments in which offering, sharing, and using substances of all kinds is not tolerated. Additionally, adolescents need to be given resources and strategies to say no to an offer of an illicit drug. Education that includes parental involvement is essential. Because adolescents are affected by social cues, it is also important to integrate systems such as athletics and school as well as positive peer relationships in treatment (National Institute on Drug Abuse, 2012b). Interventions include improved enforcement of drunk-driving laws to decrease motor vehicle injury, providing needle and syringe exchange programs to prevent HIV infection, and serving alcohol in shatter-resistant glasses to prevent alcohol-related injuries. If an adolescent is suspected of using some type of substance, the nurse may be among the first to identify the problem by putting together the pieces of history, activity, and physical signs and symptoms (Chart 7-2). If a potential overdose occurs, the adolescent must seek medical treatment as soon as possible because to delay may be fatal. Long-term management

CHART 7-2 Warning Signs of Substance Use

Reddened eyes
Pinpoint pupils
Runny or stuffy nose (constant)
Gastrointestinal upset (diarrhea)
Weight loss or gain; change in eating habits
Signs of needle tracks
Loss of coordination
Tremors
Unusual sleep patterns
Diminished academic performance
Withdrawal from friends, activities, and family
Rapid mood swings
History of bizarre behavior
Depression or agitation
Hallucinations or disorientation
Smell of smoke

is more complex and requires physical and psychological support systems for both the adolescent and the family. Referrals for adolescents to engage in substance abuse treatment may come from the criminal justice system, self-referral, school counselors and nurses, community organizations, family members, and other health care providers. Chapter 29 provides an in-depth discussion of substance abuse, including assessment and interdisciplinary interventions to assist the adolescent with these addictions.

VIOLENCE

Problem behaviors in adolescents include engaging in fighting and initiating other acts of violence on other youths and individuals. These acts of violence can include bullying, abusive relationships, and gang activity. The YRBS indicates that 32.8% of adolescents report taking part in a fight, and 3.9% of adolescents report they have been injured by someone else and required treatment from a health care provider (CDC, 2012f). Bullying (discussed in Chapter 6) can be considered a gateway problem behavior that may lead to further acts of violence. Bullying includes when a student or group of students says or does mean things to another boy or girl or when a child is teased repeatedly in a way he or she does not like. Some argue that bullying, gossiping, stealing another's boyfriend/girlfriend, and name-calling or other types of verbal abuse are also forms of violence (Bartlett et al., 2007; Srabstein et al., 2006).

Adolescents are also at risk for violence from involvement in relationships that are physically and/or emotionally abusive. Approximately 10% to 25% of high school students encounter violence within dating relationships, suggesting that 1 in 11 adolescents are victims of dating violence (Kervin & Obinna, 2010; Khubchandani et al., 2012). Chapter 29 discusses abuse, including sexual abuse.

A number of intervention programs aimed at preventing adolescent violence and recognizing adolescents at risk for violent behavior have been initiated across the country. The most effective programs combine strategies that address both individual risks and environmental conditions (Kervin & Obinna, 2010). Approaches aimed at building individual competencies, providing parent effectiveness training, improving the social climate of the school, and effecting changes in type and level of involvement in peer groups have shown to be effective strategies in promoting violence prevention and awareness (Kervin & Obinna, 2010). For example, dating violence prevention programs are recommended at the middle school level to help these young adolescents to manage relationships before they become abusive and violent. Programs aimed at high school and college students focus more on intervention, promoting nonviolent conflict resolution, and healthy partner behaviors (Khubchandani et al., 2012).

Youth gangs exist all over the country, in cities large and small, and are major contributors to the rate of violent crimes seen among adolescents. Gangs are not new to the United States; they have been around since the 18th century. As of 2009, at least 28,100 gangs were active in the United States, with more than 731,000 active gang members (U.S. Department of Justice, 2011). Easy access to guns makes today's gangs especially dangerous.

Gangs come in all sizes: very large, with subdivisions; and very small, with just a few members. If a group or clique meets the three following criteria, according to experts, it can be defined as a **gang**:

1. There is distinct group recognition by the members (e.g., use of signs, colors).
2. The group is identified by the community as a gang.
3. The group is involved in some illegal activities and has a negative reputation within the community.

Usually, gangs develop from a group of adolescents who share a common neighborhood, school, or interest. Traditionally, gang members were exclusively male, but now, a gang might recruit female members as well. Most common, recruits are from the inner city, the poor, and they are adolescents with low self-esteem, gathering together for mutual support and understanding. Usually, these adolescents have little family support (U.S. Department of Justice, 2005). The feelings of poor self-esteem are negated by being accepted by a group that has "power" (and money). Gangs group together adolescents of similar cultural backgrounds and usually exclude anyone who is not the same. Gang association has been highly correlated to an increase in violent behavior by adolescent members. Gangs use violence in retaliation for real or perceived disrespect. Gang members might carry weapons and use those weapons for illegal activity, including violence against others. Arrest, prison, injury, and possibly death are all very likely outcomes of gang membership.

Unfortunately, health care providers usually do not see gang members until they arrive in the ED after a violent confrontation. The professional should not sugarcoat the possibilities of what will occur if the adolescent joins a gang or remains in a gang. Getting out of gangs can be very difficult, however. Many ex-gang members state that the easiest way is just to "fade" away by not attending the activities as often, and not being part of the crowd. After a while, the gang member is "forgotten."

Education is one of the best tools to prevent adolescents from joining gangs. The health care professional can talk to the adolescent about alternatives to a gang lifestyle and can assist him or her in finding nongang role models. Group counseling with the family may assist in the development of a stronger family relationship. Programs can be offered to keep the adolescents busy after school, perhaps allowing them to develop other peer relationships outside of gangs, within sports, art, music, and so on. Adolescents can be encouraged to plan their future.

HEALTH RISKS FROM SEXUAL ACTIVITY

Once an adolescent makes the decision to become sexually active, it is important for health care providers to promote awareness of the many potential consequences surrounding unprotected sexual intercourse. Two of the most important consequences of unprotected sexual activities include pregnancy and STIs.

Pregnancy

 QUESTION: Is Ashley at risk for an unplanned pregnancy? What health information should a nurse share with Ashley to help her prevent a pregnancy?

During the past decade, the incidence of adolescent pregnancy has decreased, along with the percentage of high school students who report having participated in sexual intercourse. The YRBS (CDC, 2012f) reports that less than half of 9th to 12th graders had sexual intercourse (47.4%). Approximately 6% (6.2%) of the youth surveyed had intercourse before age 13 years; this rate remains unchanged since 2005. In 2005, it was reported that the percentage of students having intercourse before age 13 years had decreased in boys from 12.7% in 1995 to 8.8%. For girls, the percentage decline was 4.9% in 1995 to 3.7% in 2005 (Hagan et al., 2008). Currently, 9% of males and 3.4% of females report engaging in sexual intercourse before age 13 years (CDC, 2012e). In 2011, 329,797 births were reported to mothers aged 15 to 19 years (CDC, n.d.c). Although the incidence of teenage pregnancy has decreased overall, the rate varies with racial/ethnic background. Data based on the National Center for Health Statistics (Hamilton & Ventura, 2012) show the overall teen pregnancy rate from 2009 to 2010 is 34.3 per 1,000 females between the ages of 15 and 19 years. The rate has dropped significantly (44%) from 1991 through 2010.

Adolescents who become pregnant are at risk for not completing high school, holding low-income jobs, becoming victims of intimate partner violence, living in poverty, and becoming pregnant again during the adolescent years (Pinzon et al., 2012). Children of single adolescent mothers are at greater risk than children of adult mothers for health problems associated with prematurity, displaying lower levels of cognitive development during infancy and lower academic achievement. A particularly vulnerable group is girls who become sexually active before age 14 years. The younger a girl is when she has sexual intercourse for the first time, the more likely her partner is 4 years or more older than her, the less likely she is to use contraception, and the more likely she is to have an unintended pregnancy (Pinzon et al., 2012).

Current data indicate that 45.6% of adolescent females and 49.2% of adolescent males have had sexual intercourse by age 18 years (CDC, 2012e). Among sexually active teenagers, 15.1% of females and 10.6% of males reported not using any form of birth control during their most recent sexual encounter (CDC, 2012e). Adolescent pregnancy, although it is primarily unplanned, may also be planned. Eighteen percent of surveyed adolescents indicated their pregnancy was planned (Raneri & Wiemann, 2007) (see Chapter 1 for more discussion about single parenting).

Teaching safe sex practices is an essential component of adolescent health care. Comprehensive sexual education—education that promotes abstinence but includes information about contraception, condoms, and STIs—has been effective in both delaying the age of sexual intercourse and increasing the use of contraception and condoms to protect from STIs. Adolescent decision making about using protection during intercourse is a complex fabric of many threads, including socioeconomic conditions, psychological factors, race, peer relationships, and family values (Clinical Judgment 7-2).

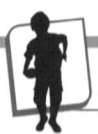

CLINICAL JUDGMENT 7-2

The Sleepy Adolescent

Sixteen-year-old Rochelle and her mother are meeting with the school nurse and the school counselor. The meeting was called by the school staff because Rochelle has been having trouble staying awake in class. Her mother is equally concerned because Rochelle struggles to get up in the morning and "spends way too much time in the bathroom getting ready." In the evening when Rochelle is supposed to be helping her mother prepare dinner, Rochelle can be found napping on the couch. Rochelle is thin and pale. During the interview, she appears sullen and does not speak unless asked a specific question. When queried, she agrees that she has been rather tired the past 3 weeks. Further questions from the nurse elicit that her last menstrual cycle was about 4 weeks ago. She denies having sexual activity. She admits to having nausea every morning and has been unwilling to eat breakfast for fear of throwing up.

Questions

1. What additional questions would you ask Rochelle at this time?
2. What are the presenting symptoms that you would share with Rochelle that would indicate she could be pregnant?
3. During your private discussion with Rochelle, she shares information about her sexual activity. How would you proceed at this point?
4. The diagnostic test confirms pregnancy. How should you proceed with Rochelle and her mother?
5. Rochelle decides to tell her mother. What additional support can you provide this family?

Answers

1. With the mother out of the room, ask Rochelle if there is any possibility she may be pregnant. Ask her about her dating practices and sexual activity. Ask about relationships with parents.
2. Nausea, fatigue, missed periods, and, if revealed by Rochelle, participating in sexual activity
3. Explain that a urine test can rule out or confirm the possibility of pregnancy. Gain Rochelle's consent for this test.
4. Encourage Rochelle to tell her mother, but inform her that, according to state statutes, her pregnancy status is confidential, as are all related decisions. Discuss pregnancy options with Rochelle. Encourage her to be tested for HIV and other STIs.
5. Be present during the discussion between Rochelle and her mother. Answer questions and provide information on options. Arrange for counseling. Arrange a follow-up appointment to further discuss options and provide disclosure of HIV and STI results.

The form of **contraception** (pregnancy prevention) most commonly used among adolescents is condoms, followed by low-dose oral contraceptive pills (OCPs). Condoms offer protection from STIs, but their effectiveness in preventing pregnancy is directly related to the consistency and correctness of use. The effectiveness of condoms ranges from 85% effective with "typical" use to 97% with "perfect" use. Adolescents do not require a health care provider to obtain condoms. Through a health care provider, a number of contraceptives are available (Table 7-2). OCPs are commonly used, but alternative means of hormonal contraception are available. Depo-Provera is an injectable progestin that is given every 12 weeks. Ortho-Evra is a combination hormone transdermal patch that is applied weekly for 3 weeks; during the fourth week a patch is not used. NuvaRing is a flexible ring worn in the vagina for 3 weeks that releases combination hormones; the ring is removed during the fourth week. All of these hormonal methods of contraception have very high effectiveness rates and are appropriate for adolescents. Prescription barrier methods, including the diaphragm, the FemCap, and Lea's Shield, are also available. A barrier method may be preferable to the hormone methods if the adolescent is only participating in sexual intercourse occasionally. The AAP (2012)

TABLE 7-2   Contraception Methods

Method	Health Care Considerations
Abstinence	Peer pressure may change desire to maintain abstinence. Ongoing assessment and information about birth control methods should be provided should the adolescent choose to engage in sexual activity. Failure rate: 0%
OCPs	Some medications can decrease the efficacy of birth control pills. During use of rifampin, penicillin, tetracycline, phenobarbital, and other drugs, women need an alternative/additional method of protection. Birth control pills can potentiate the action of some antianxiety, antidepressant, and asthma medications. Women who are currently taking any type of antianxiety, antidepressant, asthma, or antibiotic drug need to inform their health care providers and use an additional method of protection. Failure rate: 5% (OWH) and 9% (CDC)
Condoms (both male and female)	Educate about proper application and removal from male penis. Should not be used if partner is allergic to latex. Female condom can be inserted up to 8 hours prior to intercourse. Both condoms are intended for one-time-only use, and the male and female condom should not be used in conjunction with one another. Failure rate, male condom: 11%–16% (OWH) and 9% (CDC) Failure rate, female condom: 20% (OWH) and 9% (CDC)
Spermicides	Needs to be placed high in vagina to make contact with cervix. Application should be no more than 1 hour prior to intercourse. Failure rate: 30% (OWH) and 28% (CDC)
Norplant	Return to fertility is prompt after removal. May be left in place for as long as 5 years, then must be removed and replaced. Failure rate: <1% (OWH) and 0.05% (CDC)
Depo-Provera	May be a delay in fertility for up to 18 months after discontinuance. Injection must be given within first 5 days of menstrual cycle, or an additional method of protection must be used. Failure rate: <1% (OWH) and 6% (CDC)
Rhythm method	Patient needs to be aware of potential fertile days of cycle. Physical, psychological, nutritional, and health state may affect cycle and alter cycle observations. Failure rate: 25% (OWH) and 24% (CDC)
Withdrawal	Patient needs to be aware that there is high risk for pregnancy and high risk for STIs using this method. Failure rate: 15%–24% (PP)
"Morning-after" pill (combination of estrogen and progestin with ethinyl estradiol)	Menstruation can be expected 7–9 days posttreatment. Not intended as a method of family planning. Failure rate: 1% (OWH)

Information from OWH – U.S. Department of Health & Human Services, Office on Women's Health. (2011). *Birth control methods fact sheet.* Retrieved from http://womenshealth.gov/publications/our-publications/fact-sheet/birth-control-methods.cfm
CDC – Centers for Disease Control and Prevention. (2013). *Contraception: How effective are birth control methods?* Retrieved from http://www.cdc.gov/reproductivehealth/unintendedpregnancy/contraception.htm
PP – Planned Parenthood. (n.d.). *Comparing effectiveness of birth control methods.* Retrieved from http://www.plannedparenthood.org/health-topics/birth-control/birth-control-effectiveness-chart-22710.htm

recommends a dual method contraception use (e.g., condoms and hormonal contraception) or abstinence. Several methods of contraception that are used by adults are not appropriate for adolescents. An obvious method is sterilization, which is permanent. It is recommended that withdrawal before ejaculation is not appropriate for adolescents because it requires experience and self-control over ejaculation. It also has a low effectiveness rate as a result of leaking of seminal fluid prior to ejaculation. Fertility awareness–based methods or "rhythm" methods are not recommended for adolescents because they require mature, trusting, and cooperative partnerships to be effective. The fourth method that is not appropriate for most adolescents is an intrauterine device (IUD), which is only recommended after the birth of a child.

The AAP recently published its updated policy statement on emergency contraception. This method of contraception involves the administration of oral contraception (progestin-only or combined estrogen/progestin, or a progesterone agonist/antagonist) within 120 hours of un- or underprotected intercourse. Adolescents younger than 17 years of age typically require a prescription, but adolescents 17 years of age and older, female and male, do not. Pediatric health care providers are required to educate and provide emergency contraception (AAP, Committee on Adolescence, 2012).

ANSWER: Ashley is at risk for becoming pregnant because she is participating in unprotected sexual intercourse. She is also denying her responsibility to protect herself from pregnancy and STIs. Nurses working with adolescent girls cannot separate pregnancy and STIs because they are both an inherent risk of sexual activity. Nurses should ensure that the adolescent has an understanding of her own body: her anatomy and the physiology of ovulation, menstruation, and conception. The most effective methods of birth control do not protect her against STIs. Ashley needs protection from both. The most effective methods of birth control that are advocated for adolescents are the pill, the patch (Ortho-Evra), the shot (Depo Provera), and the ring (NuvaRing).

Whether a pregnancy is planned or unplanned, the goals of the health care provider include helping the adolescent have a healthy pregnancy and ensuring that the child has a healthy future (Fig. 7-10). Pregnant adolescents should be directed toward specific health care providers for specific health care concerns, childbirth and child-rearing classes, and government resources such as Women, Infants, and Children (WIC) programs (see Chapter 2). In addition, contraceptive counseling should be reinforced, or if not previously introduced, then initiated during pregnancy and continued after pregnancy. Use of both long-acting contraceptives and condoms should be encouraged. Ongoing health care interventions supported by the AAP and other organizations aimed at supporting adolescent parents and their children are presented in Community Care 7-3 (Pinzon et al., 2012).

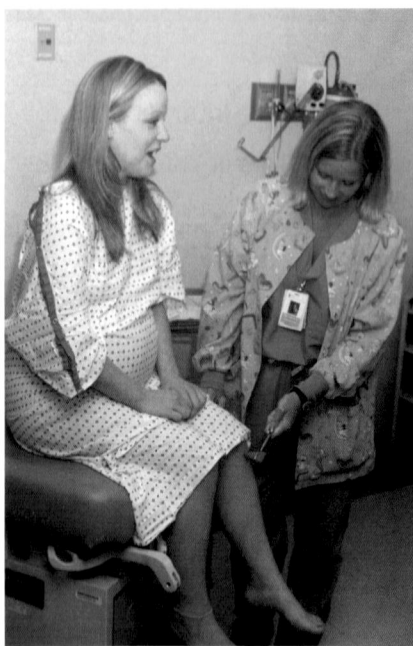

Figure 7-10 The pregnant adolescent should be encouraged to receive prenatal care and childbirth/child-rearing education.

Sexually Transmitted Infections

QUESTION: Is Ashley at risk for an STI? What health information should a nurse share with Ashley to prevent her from contracting an STI?

Adolescents are at greater risk for STIs than adults, and one in four sexually active adolescents acquires an STI each year. The rates of STIs in the United States are significantly higher than any other developed nation. Undiagnosed and untreated STIs can leave an adolescent girl infertile; approximately 24,000 women become infertile annually (CDC, 2011a). Although safe sex is promoted in various ways and taught in schools, adolescents continue to contract STIs and/or become pregnant (Fantasia & Fontenot, 2011).

Common STIs include vaginosis, chlamydia, gonorrhea, hepatitis, herpes, and genital warts/human papilloma virus (HPV). Perhaps the most common STI among sexually active adolescents is genital HPV, commonly known as *genital warts*. HPV is usually transient, has no symptoms, and self-resolves. However, in a small percentage of women, HPV leads to cervical cancer. Although HPV is considered the cause of cervical cancer, approximately 1 in 1,000 women with HPV will develop cervical cancer (CDC, 2013). According to data from the CDC Sexually Transmitted Disease Surveillance, rates of *Chlamydia* and gonorrhea infection are highest in the 15- to 24-year-old age range. Minorities continue to remain at disproportionate risk, with African Americans demonstrating higher rates of infection for *Chlamydia* and gonorrhea. Adolescents are also at risk for HIV infection (CDC, 2011b).

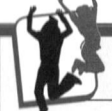

COMMUNITY CARE 7-3

Interventions for Adolescent Parents and Their Children

- Ensure that adolescent parents and their children have a "medical home" (see Chapter 2).
- Connect families with community resources (e.g., WIC, Early and Periodic Screening, Diagnosis, and Treatment [EPSDT] program) (see Chapter 2).
- Promote breastfeeding.
- Provide contraceptive use counseling.
- Emphasize the importance of completing high school.
- Encourage continuation of healthy lifestyles, including abstinence from alcohol, cigarettes, and substance use.
- Assess risk for domestic violence during and after pregnancy.

- Encourage adolescents to serve as primary caregivers for their children, even if other family members are available to assist.
- Encourage joint participation of both the mother and father (if present) in the child's care.
- Provide developmentally appropriate parenting information on infant care, infant development, child discipline, and child safety.
- Attend to adolescents' developmental needs, providing education and support systems as needed.
- Provide positive reinforcement, praising adolescents' successes with their children and with personal accomplishments.

The most effective way to prevent STI is abstinence; the second most effective method is condom use. Condoms have been proven to be effective against many STIs. They decrease the risk of heterosexually transmitted HIV by 80% and are also successful in preventing HPV infection, chlamydiasis, gonorrhea, and other STIs (Williams & Fortenberry, 2013). The HPV vaccine is available to males and females ages 9 to 26 years. Public health STI prevention efforts have not gone unnoticed; a national sample of 14- to 17-year-old male and female adolescents reported 70% to 80% condom use during last incidence of vaginal intercourse (Williams & Fortenberry, 2013). Also reassuring is another study demonstrating that 60% of sexually active adolescent females are using other modes of oral or injectable contraceptives (Williams & Fortenberry, 2013). Despite these reassuring statistics, adolescents remain at risk for health disparities related to STIs.

In addition to anatomic, educational, and behavioral risks for STIs, adolescents have less access to health care services (AAP, Committee on Adolescence, 2008). In a large collaborative survey completed by the Kaiser Family Foundation (2001) and *Seventeen* magazine, about half the adolescents (aged 12 to 17 years) identified that they did want more information about sexual health. Among adolescents aged 15 to 17 years who had engaged in sexual intercourse, only 6 of 10 had seen a health care provider. Reasons identified for decreased use of health care services include lack of health care coverage; one in four adolescents lack health care coverage. Other barriers include transportation, lack of confidentiality, and state laws regarding parental consent. Poverty, cultural traditions, and sexual violence are also factors that diminish the individual's ability to protect against STIs. Nurses can play a key role in assessing and educating the adolescent regarding the transmission of STIs (AAP, Committee on Adolescence, 2008). In addition, screening for STIs plays an important role

in STI prevention. The screening process provides an opportunity for the health care provider to dispel myths about STI transmission, promote products to prevent transmission, and teach skills for refusing unwanted sex or negotiating safer sex (Fantasia & Fontenot, 2011; Fortenberry, 2005).

ANSWER: Ashley is at risk for contracting an STI. The nurse should share with Ashley that the most effective protection from an STI is abstinence. Ashley must decide if she truly does not want to have intercourse with Eric again or if she just doesn't want to admit to herself she is sexually active. Either way, she needs to communicate with Eric. The most effective form of protection for sexually active adolescents is using a condom. Using two methods of protection against STIs and unwanted pregnancy (e.g., a condom and the pill—*the double-dutch approach*) is a very effective approach and would be appropriate for Ashley.

See thePoint for a summary of Key Concepts.

REFERENCES

American Academy of Pediatrics. (1998, reaffirmed 2011a). Age limits of pediatrics. *Pediatrics, 81,* 736. Reaffirmed 2011.

American Academy of Pediatrics. (2005, reaffirmed 2008). Use of performance-enhancing substances. *Pediatrics, 115,* 1103–1106.

American Academy of Pediatrics. (2008). Strength training by children and adolescents. *Pediatrics, 121*(4), 835–840.

American Academy of Pediatrics, Committee on Adolescence. (2008). Achieving quality health services for adolescents. *Pediatrics, 121*(6), 1263–1270.

American Academy of Pediatrics, Committee on Adolescence. (2012). Emergency contraception. *Pediatrics, 130,* 1174–1182.

American Academy of Pediatrics, Committee on Nutrition & the Council on Sports Medicine and Fitness. (2011). Sports drinks and energy drinks for children and adolescents: Are they appropriate? *Pediatrics, 127*(6), 1182–1189.

American Academy of Pediatrics, Committee on Psychosocial Aspects of Child and Family Health & Committee on Adolescence. (2001). Sexuality education for children and adolescents. *Pediatrics, 108*, 498–502.

American Academy of Pediatrics, Committee on Sports Medicine and Fitness. (2005). Promotion of healthy weight-control practices in young athletes. *Pediatrics, 116*(6), 1557–1564.

American Academy of Pediatrics, Committee on Sports Medicine and Fitness & Committee on School Health. (2000, reaffirmed 2004). Physical fitness and activity in schools. *Pediatrics, 105*(5), 1156–1157.

American Academy of Pediatrics, Committee on Substance Abuse. (2010). Alcohol use by youth and adolescents: A pediatric concern. *Pediatrics, 125*, 1078–1087.

American Academy of Pediatrics, The Council on Communications and Media. (2010). Children, adolescents, substance abuse, and the media. *Pediatrics, 126*, 791–799.

Amos, L. B., & D'Andrea, L. A. (2012). The sleepy teenager: Waking up to the unique sleep needs of adolescents. *Contemporary Pediatrics, 10*, 34–45.

Armstrong, M., Caliendo, C., & Roberts, A. (2006). Genital piercings: What is known and what people with genital piercings tell us. *Urologic Nursing, 26*(3), 173–179.

Auslander, B., Rosenthal, S., & Blythe, M. (2005). Sexual development and behaviors of adolescents. *Pediatric Annals, 34*(1), 785–793.

Bartlett, R., Holditch-Davis, D., & Belyea, M. (2007). Problem behaviors among adolescents. *Pediatric Nursing, 33*(1), 13–18.

Baroni, E., Naku, K., Spaulding, N. et al. (2004). Sleep habits and daytime functioning in students attending early versus late starting middle schools. *Sleep, 27*, A396–A397.

Beebe, D. W. (2011). Cognitive, behavioral, and functional consequences of inadequate sleep in children and adolescents. *Pediatric Clinics of North America, 58*(3), 649–665.

Brackley, H., & Stevenson, J. (2004). Are children's backpack weight limits enough?: A critical review of the relevant literature. *Spine, 29*, 2184–2190.

Braganza, S., & Larkin, M. (2007). Riding high on energy drinks. *Contemporary Pediatrics, 24*(5), 61–73.

Breslin, C., Koehoon, M., Smith, P. et al. (2003). Age related differences in work injuries and permanent impairment: A comparison among adolescents, young adults, and adults. *Occupational and Environmental Medicine, 60*(9), e10.

Brown, J., L'Engle, K., Pardum, C. et al. (2006). Sexy media matter: Exposure to sexual content in music, movies, television, and magazines predicts black and white adolescents' sexual behavior. *Pediatrics, 117*(4), 1018–1027.

Calamaro, C. J., Mason, T. B., & Ratcliffe, S. J. (2009). Adolescents living the 24/7 lifestyle: Effects of caffeine and technology on sleep duration and daytime functioning. *Pediatrics, 123*(6), e1005–e1010.

Carroll, S., Riffenburgh, R., Roberts, T. et al. (2002). Tattoos and body piercings as indicators of adolescent risk-taking behaviors. *Pediatrics, 109*(6), 1021–1027.

Carswell, J. M., & Stafford, D. E. (2008). Normal physical growth and development. In L. S. Neinstein, C. Gordon, D. Katzman et al. (Eds.), *Adolescent health care: A practical guide* (5th ed.). Philadelphia, PA: Lippincott Williams & Wilkins.

Centers for Disease Control and Prevention. (2006). *Sports-related injuries among high school athletes—United States 2005–2006 school year*. Retrieved from http://www.cdc.gov/mmwr/preview/mmwrhtml/mm5538a1.htm

Centers for Disease Control and Prevention. (2011a). *CDC fact sheet: STD trends in the United States: 2011 national data for chlamydia, gonorrhea, and syphilis*. Retrieved from http://www.cdc.gov/std/stats11/trends-2011.pdf

Centers for Disease Control and Prevention. (2011b). *HIV among youth*. Retrieved from http://www.cdc.gov/hiv/pdf/library_factsheet_HIV-amongYouth.pdf

Centers for Disease Control and Prevention. (2012a). *Fact sheets—Underage drinking*. Retrieved from http://www.cdc.gov/alcohol/fact-sheets/underage-drinking.htm

Centers for Disease Control and Prevention. (2012b). *Smoking and tobacco use: Fact sheet*. Retrieved from http://www.cdc.gov/tobacco/data_statistics/fact_sheets/youth_data/tobacco_use/index.htm

Centers for Disease Control and Prevention. (2012c). *Teen drivers: Fact sheet*. Retrieved from http://www.cdc.gov/motorvehicle-safety/teen_drivers/teendrivers_factsheet.html

Centers for Disease Control and Prevention. (2012d). Vital signs: Unintentional injury deaths among persons aged 0–19 years—United States, 2000–2009. *Morbidity and Mortality Weekly Report, 61*(15), 270–276.

Centers for Disease Control and Prevention. (2012e). *Youth Risk Behavior Surveillance System: Selected 2011 national health risk behaviors and health outcomes by sex*. Retrieved from http://www.cdc.gov/healthyyouth/yrbs/pdf/us_disparitysex_yrbs.pdf

Centers for Disease Control and Prevention. (2012f). *Youth Risk Behavior Surveillance System: 2011 national overview*. Retrieved from http://www.cdc.gov/healthyyouth/yrbs/pdf/us_overview_yrbs.pdf

Centers for Disease Control and Prevention. (2013). *Sexually transmitted diseases: Genital HPV infection—fact sheet*. Retrieved from http://www.cdc.gov/std/HPV/STDFact-HPV.htm#a5

Centers for Disease Control and Prevention. (n.d.a). *Basics about childhood obesity*. Retrieved from http://www.cdc.gov/obesity/childhood/basics.html

Centers for Disease Control and Prevention. (n.d.b). *Young worker safety and health*. Retrieved from http://www.cdc.gov/niosh/topics/youth/

Centers for Disease Control and Prevention. (n.d.c). *Teen pregnancy: The importance of prevention*. Retrieved from http://www.cdc.gov/TeenPregnancy/index.htm

Chansirinukor, W., Wilson, W., Grimmer, K. et al. (2001). Effects of backpacks on students: Measurement of cervical and shoulder posture. *Australian Journal of Physiotherapy, 47*, 110–116.

Chow, D., Kwok, M., Cheng, J. et al. (2005). The effect of backpack weight on the standing posture and balance of schoolgirls with adolescent idiopathic scoliosis and normal controls. *Gait Posture, 24*, 173–181.

Collins, R., Elliott, M., Berry, S. et al. (2004). Watching sex on television predicts adolescent initiation of sexual behavior. *Pediatrics, 114*(3), e280–e289.

Common Sense Media. (2012). *Social media, social life: how teens view their digital lives*. Retrieved from http://www.commonsensemedia.org/sites/default/files/research/socialmediasociallife-final-061812.pdf

Darrow, C. J., Collins, C. L., Yard, E. E. et al. (2009). Epidemiology of severe injuries among United States high school athletes: 2005–2007. *American Journal of Sports Medicine, 37*, 1798–1805.

Deimel, J. F., & Dunlap, B. J. (2012). The female athlete triad. *Clinical Sports Medicine, 31*(2), 247–254.

DeVore, E., & Ginsburg, K. (2005). The protective effects of good parenting on adolescents. *Current Opinion in Pediatrics, 17*, 460–465.

Dorsch, K., & Bell, A. (2005). Dietary supplement use in adolescents. *Current Opinions in Pediatrics, 17*, 653–657.

Elkind, D. (2001). Why today's adolescents behave differently from those of earlier generations. *Pediatric Annals, 30*(2), 97–102.

Fantasia, H. C., & Fontenot, H. B. (2011). The sexual safety of adolescents. *Journal of Obstetric, Gynecologic, and Neonatal Nursing, 40*, 217–224.

Feldman, D., Shrier, I., Rossignol, M. et al. (2002). Work is a risk factor for adolescent musculoskeletal pain. *Journal of Occupational and Environmental Medicine, 44*, 956–961.

Fennoy, I. (2010). Metabolic and respiratory comorbidities of childhood obesity. *Pediatric Annals, 39*(3), 140–146.

Fortenberry, J. (2005). Sexually transmitted infections. *Pediatric Annals, 34*(10), 803–810.

Fortunato, L., Young, A. M., Boyd, C. J. et al. (2010). Hook-up sexual experiences and problem behaviors in adolescents. *Journal of Child and Adolescent Substance Abuse, 19,* 261–278.

Franklin, C. C., & Weiss, J. M. (2012). Stopping sports injuries in kids: An overview of the last year in publications. *Current Opinions in Pediatrics, 24*(1), 64–67.

Frankowski, B. L. & Committee on Adolescence. (2004). Sexual orientation and adolescents. *Pediatrics, 113*(6), 1827–1832.

Gold, M., Schorzman, C., Murray, P. et al. (2005). Body piercing practices and attitudes among urban adolescents. *Journal of Adolescent Health, 36,* 352.e15–352.e21.

Grady, M. F. (2012). Concussion in the adolescent athlete. *Current Problems in Pediatric Adolescent Health Care, 40*(7), 154–169.

Gidding, S., Dennison, B., Birch, L. et al. (2006). Dietary recommendations for children and adolescents: A guide for practitioners. *Pediatrics, 117*(2), 544–559.

Griffith, R. (2012). Time to repeal the Tattooing of Minors Act 1969. *British Journal of Nursing, 21*(18), 1102–1103.

Grimmer, K., Williams, M., & Gill, T. (1999). The association between adolescent head-on-neck posture, backpack weight, and anthropometric features. *Spine, 24,* 2262–2267.

Hagan, J. F., Shaw, J. S., & Duncan, P. M. (Eds.). (2008). *Bright futures: Guidelines for health supervision of infants, children, and adolescents* (3rd ed.). Elk Grove Village, IL: American Academy of Pediatrics.

Halstead, M. E. (2010). Contact sports for young athletes: Keys to safety. *Pediatric Annals, 39*(5), 275–278.

Hamilton, B. E., & Ventura, S. J. (2012). *Birth rates for U.S. teenagers reach historic lows for all age and ethnic groups* (NCHS Data Brief No. 89). Hyattsville, MD: National Center for Health Statistics. Retrieved from http://www.cdc.gov/nchs/data/databriefs/db89.pdf

Harakeh, Z., Scholte, R. H., Vermulst, A. A. et al. (2010). The relations between parents' smoking, general parenting, parental smoking communication, and adolescents' smoking. *Journal of Research on Adolescence, 20*(1), 140–165.

Herrman, J. (2005). The teen brain as a work in progress: Implications for pediatric nurses. *Pediatric Nursing, 31*(2), 144–148.

Hsia, D. S., Fallon, S. C., & Brandt, M. L. (2012). Adolescent bariatric surgery. *Archives of Pediatric and Adolescent Medicine, 166*(8), 757–766.

Johnson, J. G., Liu, L., & Cohen, P. (2011). Parenting behaviours associated with the development of adaptive and maladaptive offspring personality traits. *Canadian Journal of Psychiatry, 56*(8), 447–456.

Juhas, E., & English, J. C. (2013). Tattoo-associated complications. *Journal of Pediatric and Adolescent Gynecology, 26*(2), 125–129..

Kaiser Family Foundation. (2001). *Sexually transmitted diseases.* Retrieved from http://kff.org/state-category/health-status/sexually-transmitted-diseases/

Kaiser Family Foundation. (2010). *Generation M2: Media in the lives of 8- to 18-year-olds.* Retrieved from http://www.kff.org/entmedia/upload/8010.pdf

Kervin, K., & Obinna, J. (2010). Youth action strategies in the primary prevention of teen dating violence. *Journal of Family Social Work, 13,* 262–374.

Khubchandani, J., Price, J. H., Thompson, A. et al. (2012). Adolescent dating violence: A national assessment of school counselors' perceptions and practices, *Pediatrics, 130*(2), 202–210.

Kistner, F., Fiebert, I., Roach, K. et al. (2013). Postural compensations and subjective complaints due to backpack loads and wear time in schoolchildren. *Pediatric Physical Therapy, 25,* 15–24.

Komro, K., Maldonado-Molina, M., Tobler, A. et al. (2007). Effects of home access and availability of alcohol on young adolescents' alcohol use. *Addiction, 102,* 1597–1608.

Lai, J., & Jones, A. (2001). The effect of shoulder girdle loading by a school bag on lung volumes in Chinese primary school children. *Early Human Development, 62,* 79–86.

Levin, L., Zadik, Y., & Becker, T. (2005). Oral and dental complications of intra-oral piercing. *Dental Traumatology, 21,* 341–343.

Loewenson, P., & Blum, R. (2001). The resilient adolescent: Implications for the pediatrician. *Pediatric Annals, 30*(2), 76–80.

Lorang, M., Callahan, B., Cummins, K. M. et al. (2011). Anabolic androgenic steroid use in teens: Prevalence, demographics, and perception of effects. *Journal of Child & Adolescent Substance Abuse, 20,* 358–369.

Madkour, A. S., Farhat, T., Halpern, C. T. et al. (2010). Early adolescent sexual initiation and physical/psychological symptoms: A comparative analysis of five nations. *Journal of Youth and Adolescence, 39,* 1211–1225.

Marar, M., McIlvain, N. M., Fields, S. K. et al. (2012). Epidemiology of concussions among United States high school athletes in 20 sports. *American Journal of Sports Medicine, 40,* 747–755.

Martel, S., & Anderson, J. (2002). Decorating the "human canvas": Body art and your patients. *Contemporary Pediatrics, 19*(8), 86–101.

Martino, S. C., Collins, R. L., Elliott, M. N. et al. (2009). It's better on TV: Does television set teenagers up for regret following sexual initiation? *Perspectives on Sexual and Reproductive Health, 41*(2), 92–100.

McGuinness, T. M. (2006). Teens and body art. *Journal of Psychosocial Nursing, 44*(4), 13–16.

McIntosh, J., MacDonald, F., & McKeganey, N. (2008). Pre-teenage children's experiences with alcohol. *Children & Society, 22*(1), 3–15.

Mercken, L., Sleddens, E. F., de Vries, H. et al. (2013). Choosing adolescent smokers as friends: The role of parenting and parental smoking. *Journal of Adolescence, 36,* 383–392.

Michalsky, M., Kramer, R. E., Fullmer, M. A. et al. (2011). Developing criteria for pediatric/adolescent bariatric surgery programs. *Pediatrics, 128*(Suppl. 2), s65–s70.

Mickalide, A. D., & Hansen, L. M. (2012). *Coaching our kids to fewer injuries: A report on youth sports safety.* Retrieved from http://www.safekids.org/sites/default/files/documents/ResearchReports/Coaching%20Our%20Kids%20to%20Fewer%20Injuries%20A%20Report%20on%20Youth%20Sports%20Safety%20-%20April%202012.pdf

Mindell, J. A., & Meltzer, J. J. (2008). Behavioural sleep disorders in children and adolescents. *Annals Academy of Medicine Singapore, 37,* 722–728.

Mitchell, K. (2010). Remaining safe and avoiding dangers online: A social media Q&A with Kimberly Mitchell. *The Prevention Researcher, 17*(Suppl.), 7–9.

Mitchell, K. J., Finkelhor, D., Jones, L. M. et al. (2012). Prevalence and characteristics of youth sexting: A national study. *Pediatrics, 129*(1), 13–20.

Monroe, K. W., Thrash, C., Sorrentino, A. et al. (2011). Most common sports-related injuries in a pediatric emergency department. *Clinical Pediatrics, 50*(1), 17–20.

National Association of Pediatric Nurse Practitioners. (2008). NAPNAP position statement on age parameters for pediatric nurse practitioner practice. *Journal of Pediatric Health Care, 22,* e1–e2.

National Center for Missing & Exploited Children. (2011). *Keeping kids safer on the Internet: Tips for parents and guardians.* Retrieved from http://www.missingkids.com/en_US/publications/NC168.pdf

National Conference of State Legislatures. (2012). *Tattoos and body piercings for minors.* Retrieved from http://www.ncsl.org/issues-research/health/tattooing-and-body-piercing.aspx

National Institute on Drug Abuse. (2012a). *Drug facts: Anabolic steroids.* Retrieved from http://www.drugabuse.gov/sites/default/files/drugfactssteroids.pdf

National Institute on Drug Abuse. (2012b). *Principles of drug addiction treatment: A research-based guide* (3rd ed.). Washington, DC: National Institutes of Health, Department of Health & Human Services. Retrieved from http://www.drugabuse.gov/publications/principles-drug-addiction-treatment

National Institute on Drug Abuse. (2012c). *Drug facts: high school and youth trends*. Retrieved from http://www.drugabuse.gov/sites/default/files/nationwide_0.pdf

Navuluri, N., & Navuluri, R. (2006). Study on the relationship between backpack use and back and neck pain among adolescents. *Nursing and Health Sciences, 8*, 208–215.

Nazem, T. G., & Ackerman, K. E. (2012). The female athlete triad. *Sports Health, 4*(4), 302–311.

O'Keeffe, G. S., Clarke-Pearon, K., & Council on Communications and Media. The impact of social media on children, adolescents, and families. *Pediatrics, 127*, 800–804.

Pascoe, D., Pascoe, D., Wang, Y. et al. (1997). The influence of carrying book bags on gait cycle and posture of youths. *Ergonomics, 40*, 631–641.

Patchin, J. W. & Hinduja, S. (2010). Cyberbullying and self-esteem. *Journal of School Health, 80*(12), 614–621.

Patrick, K., Spear, B., Holt, K. et al. (Eds.). (2001). *Bright futures in practice: Physical activity*. Arlington, VA: National Center for Education in Maternal and Child Health.

Patton, G., & Viner, R. (2007). Pubertal changes in health. *Lancet, 369*, 1130–1137.

Pearson, J., Muller, C., & Frisco, M. L. (2006). Parental involvement, family structure, and adolescent sexual decision making. *Sociological Perspectives, 49*(1), 67–90.

Picciano, M. F., Dwyer, J. T., Radimer, K. L. et al. (2007). Dietary supplement use among infants, children, and adolescents in the United States, 1999–2002. *Archives of Pediatric and Adolescent Medicine, 161*(10), 978–985.

Pinzon, J. L., Jones, V. F., & Committee on Adolescence and Committee on Early Childhood. (2012). Care of adolescent parents and their children. *Pediatrics, 130*(6), e1743–e1756.

Pollard, K. A., Xiang, H., & Smith, G. A. (2012). Pediatric eye injuries treated in US emergency departments, 1990–2009. *Clinical Pediatrics, 51*, 374–381.

RAND Corporation. (2008). *Exposure to sex on TV may increase the chance of teen pregnancy: Fact sheet*. Retrieved from http://www.rand.org/pubs/research_briefs/RB9398/index1.html

Radzik, M., Sherer, S., & Neinstein, L. S. (2008). Psychosocial development in normal adolescents. In L. S. Neinstein, C. Gordon, D. Katzman et al. (Eds.), *Adolescent health care: A practical guide* (5th ed.). Philadelphia, PA: Lippincott Williams & Wilkins.

Raneri, L., & Wiemann, C. (2007). Social ecological predictors of repeat adolescent pregnancy. *Perspectives on Sexual and Reproductive Health, 39*(1), 39–47.

Rateau, M. (2004). Use of backpacks in children and adolescents: A potential contributor of back pain. *Orthopaedic Nursing, 23*(2), 101–105.

Regber, S., Berg-Kelly, K., & Marild, S. (2007). Parenting styles and treatment of adolescents with obesity. *Pediatric Nursing, 33*(1), 21–28.

Rice, E., Rhoades, H., Winetrobe, H. et al. (2012). Sexually explicit cell phone messaging associated with sexual risk in adolescents. *Pediatrics, 130*(4), 667–673.

Rice, S.G. (2008). Medical conditions affecting sports participation. *Pediatrics, 121*(4), 841–848.

Rodriguez-Oviedo, P., Ruano-Ravina, A., Perez-Rios, M. et al. (2012). School children's backpacks, back pain and back pathologies. *Archives of Diseases in Children, 97*, 730–732.

Runyan, C., Schulman, M., Dal Santo, J. et al. (2007). Work-related hazards and workplace safety of US adolescents employed in the retail and service sectors. *Pediatrics, 119*(3), 526–534.

Safe Kids Worldwide. (2011). *Sports and recreation safety*. Retrieved from http://www.safekids.org/assets/docs/ourwork/research/2011-sports-fact-sheet.pdf

Salmon, M. (2010). Family matters. *Mental Health Today, 4*, 12–13.

Seifert, S. M., Schaechter, J. L., Hershorin, E. R. et al. (2011). Health effects of energy drinks on children, adolescents, and young adults. *Pediatrics, 127*(3), 511–528.

Selekman, J. (2007). Homosexuality in children and/or their parents. *Pediatric Nursing, 33*, 453–457.

Setlik, J., Bond, G. R., & Ho, M. (2009). Adolescent prescription ADHD medication abuse is rising along with prescriptions for these medications. *Pediatrics, 124*, 875–880.

Sheir-Neiss, G., Kruse, R., Rahman, T. et al. (2003). The association of backpack use and back pain in adolescents. *Spine, 28*, 922–930.

Siebenbruner, J., Zimmer-Gembeck, M., & Egeland, B. (2007). Sexual partners and contraceptive use: A 16-year prospective study predicting abstinence and risk behavior. *Journal of Research on Adolescence, 17*(1), 179–206.

Smith, D. V., & McCambridge, T. M. (2009). Performance-enhancing substances in teens. *Contemporary Pediatrics, 26*(2), 36–45.

Smith, P., Bielecky, A., Mustard, C. et al. (2013). The relationship between age and work injury in British Columbia: Examining differences across time and nature of injury. *Journal of Occupational Health*. Advance online publication.

Srabstein, J., McCarter, R., Shao, C. et al. (2006). Morbidities associated with bullying behaviors in adolescents. School based study of American adolescents. *International Journal of Adolescent Med Health, 18*(4), 587–596.

Stewart, L., & Gahagan, A. (2012). Managing and preventing obesity in teenagers. *Practice Nursing, 23*(5), 252–256.

Sudhinaraset, M., & Blum, R. W. (2010). The unique developmental considerations of youth-related work injuries. *International Journal of Occupational and Environmental Health, 16*, 216–222.

Sweeney, S. (2006). Tattoos: A review of tattoo practices and potential treatment options for removal. *Current Opinion in Pediatrics, 18*, 391–395.

U.S. Department of Agriculture. (n.d.). *MyPlate*. Retrieved from http://www.choosemyplate.gov

U.S. Department of Health & Human Services. (1997). *Are you a working teen?* (NIOSH Publication No. 97-132). Washington, DC: National Institute for Occupational Safety and Health.

U.S. Department of Justice. (2005). *Drugs and gangs fast facts*. Retrieved from http://www.usdoj.gov/ndic/pubs11/13157/index.htm

U.S. Department of Justice. (2011). *Highlights of the 2009 National Youth Gang Survey*. Retrieved from https://www.ncjrs.gov/pdffiles1/ojjdp/233581.pdf

U.S. Department of Labor. (2012). *Employment and unemployment among youth—summer 2012*. Retrieved from http://www.bls.gov/news.release/pdf/youth.pdf

U.S. Preventive Services Task Force. (2010). Screening for obesity in children and adolescents: US preventive services task force recommendation statement. *Pediatrics, 125*(2), 361–367.

U.S. Surgeon General Report. (2012). *Preventing tobacco use among youths and young adults: Fact sheet*. Retrieved from http://www.surgeongeneral.gov/library/reports/preventing-youth-tobacco-use/factsheet.html

van der Vorst, H., Engels, R., Dekovic, M. et al. (2007). Alcohol-specific rules, personality and adolescents' alcohol use: A longitudinal person–environment study. *Addiction, 102*, 1064–1075.

van der Vorst, H., Engels, R., Meeus, W. et al. (2005). The role of alcohol-specific socialization in adolescents' drinking behavior. *Addiction, 100*, 1464–1476.

Wahlstrom, K. (2002). Changing times: Findings from the first longitudinal study of later high school start times. *NASSP Bulletin, 86*(633), 3–21.

Wallis, C. (2004, May 10). What makes teens tick? *Time*, pp. 55–65.

Ward, B. M., & Snow, P. C. (2011). Factors affecting parental supply of alcohol to underage adolescents. *Drug and Alcohol Review, 30*, 338–343.

Williams, R. L., & Fortenberry, J. D. (2013). Dual use of long-acting reversible contraceptives and condoms among adolescents. *Journal of Adolescent Health, 52*, s29–s34.

Wilson, F. A., & Stimpson, J. P. (2010). Trends in fatalities from distracted driving in the United States, 1999 to 2008. *American Journal of Public Health, 100*(11), 2213–2219.

Wolfson, A., & Carskadon, M. (2005). Survey of factors influencing high school start times. *NASSP Bulletin, 89,* 1–16.

Woo, T. M., & Hanley, J. R. (2013). "How high do they look?": Identification and treatment of common ingestions in adolescents. *Journal of Pediatric Health Care, 27*(2), 135–144.

Wood, K. E. (2013). Exposure to bath salts and synthetic tetrahydrocannabinol from 2009 to 2012 in the United States. *Journal of Pediatrics,* Advance online publication.

Young, K. (2009). Understanding online gaming addiction and treatment issues for adolescents. *The American Journal of Family Therapy, 37,* 355–372.

See thePoint for additional resources.

UNIT 2

Maintaining Health Across the Continuum of Care

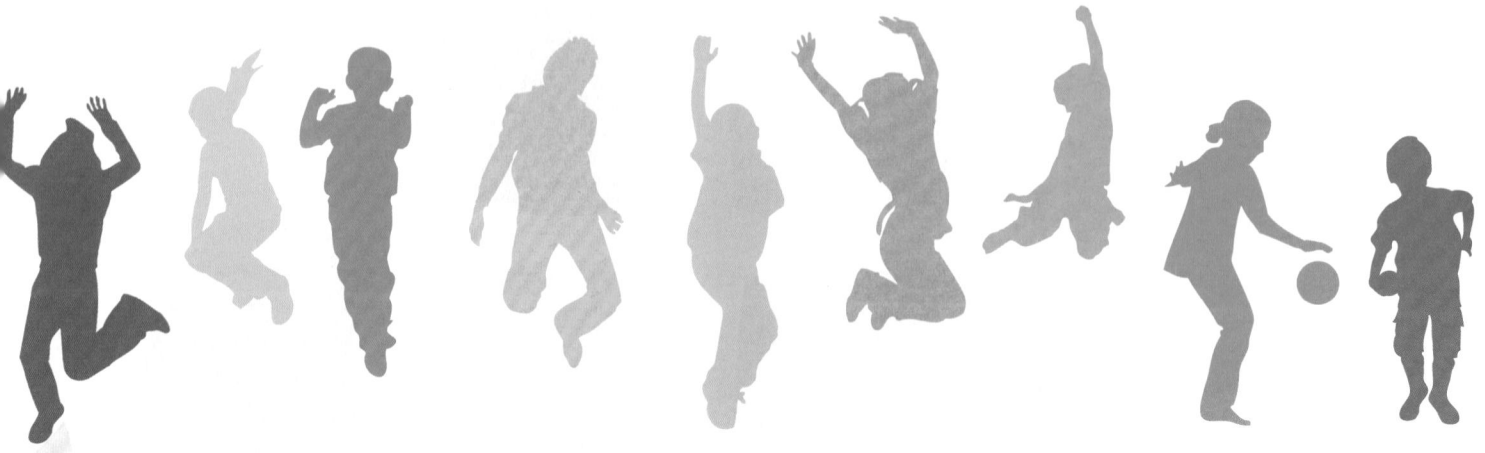

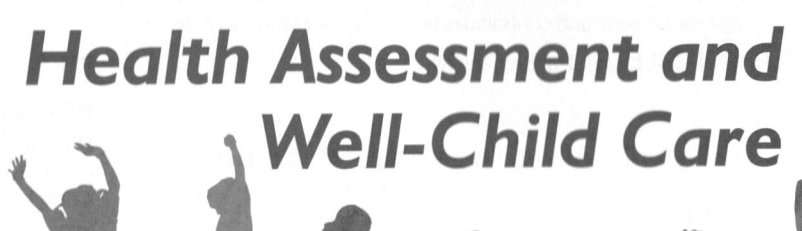

Health Assessment and Well-Child Care

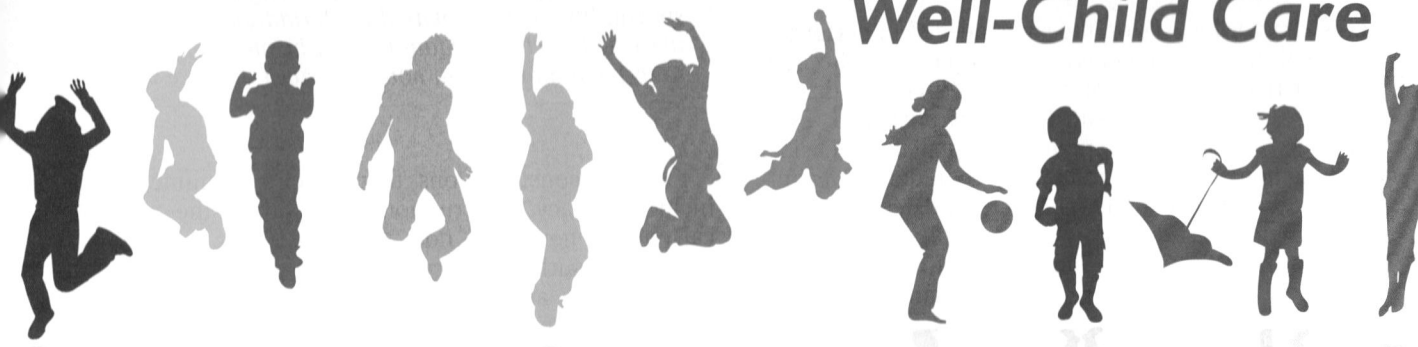

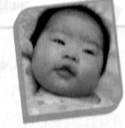

CASE HISTORY

Recall Lindsay Jenkins from Chapter 2. Her aunt and uncle are adopting a baby from Korea and the baby is arriving soon. Sally and Mark Jenkins have been trying to have children for the past 12 years and have decided to adopt. They are working with an adoption agency that specializes in Korean adoptions. They fly to Los Angeles to meet their new daughter and promptly return home. The flight home is a blur. Stephanie, their daughter, has black-button eyes and spiky black hair with a tendency to stand straight up at the crown of her head. She stares at her parents as if to say, "Who are you strange people?"

Sally is so excited to have a baby at last. She wants to do everything right. The agency requires the baby to be seen by their pediatrician within 48 hours. The first visit is not for immunizations or uncomfortable interventions but rather an opportunity for a health care provider to conduct the first

physical examination and to answer the parents' questions. The day after they return home with Stephanie, both Mark and Sally take Stephanie to visit Ms. King, the nurse practitioner.

The day of her appointment, Stephanie is 4 months 10 days old. She weighs 14 lb 3 oz, is 24 in. long, and her head circumference is 16 in. Her medical record from Korea shows that she was delivered vaginally and without difficulty. She received the diphtheria and tetanus toxoids and acellular pertussis (DTaP) vaccine at 2 months and at 4 months of age. She also received the liquid oral polio vaccine (OPV) at 2 months and at 4 months of age. Her record indicates that her mother was hepatitis B surface antigen (HBsAg) negative; there is no record of Stephanie receiving a hepatitis B (HepB) vaccine. The adoption agency recommends that all infants from Korea begin the HepB vaccination series upon arrival in the United States.

CHAPTER OBJECTIVES

1 Discuss the key components that comprise the pediatric health assessment from infancy through adolescence and the information queried or discussed in each component (e.g., reason for seeking care, past medical history, social history).

2 Elicit a pediatric health history pertinent to either the health supervision needs or illness-related problems of children from birth through adolescence.

3 Discuss key approaches to interviewing the child and the family based on developmental considerations, psychosocial/emotional considerations, and level of acuity of illness.

4 Perform a basic physical examination on a child that reflects knowledge of the developmental differences in the various body systems from birth through adolescence.

5 Identify how the physical examination process may need to be altered based on developmental considerations.

6 Differentiate normal from abnormal findings obtained while either taking historical information or performing the physical examination.

7 Discuss anticipatory guidance issues, health promotion topics, and routine health supervision screenings (e.g., speech and language assessment) that are covered during health surveillance visits of children of each age group.

8 Select age-appropriate teaching techniques to relay anticipatory guidance and disease prevention information.

9 Describe the levels of prevention that are used as primary approaches to pediatric health teaching.

10 List the childhood immunizations and the schedule of administration for routine vaccines and identify the side effects associated with, and contraindications to, each of the vaccines.

See thePoint for a list of Key Terms.

This chapter focuses on the steps needed to perform a complete health assessment of children from the neonatal period through adolescence. An in-depth discussion of the pediatric health history is presented, as is an overview of the comprehensive pediatric physical examination. Tips on examination techniques and communication with parents, children, and teenagers are also provided. The various components of well-child care and health supervision are identified, including childhood immunizations and anticipatory guidance issues. Subsequent chapters of the text contain more specific information about each body system and expand on the information found in this chapter.

Developing skills in both history taking and physical examination techniques requires that the nurse has a solid knowledge base regarding physical growth and normal developmental milestones. In addition, the nurse must be an astute listener, an inquisitive interviewer, and an observant clinician with the ability to differentiate normal from abnormal findings.

HEALTH ASSESSMENT FROM INFANCY THROUGH ADOLESCENCE

Health assessment includes obtaining a health history and performing a physical examination. The health history is a critical component of the assessment that assists the health professional in determining which areas of the physical examination merit additional attention.

COMMUNICATION SKILLS

Developing good communication skills is essential for a successful health assessment—in both obtaining a health history and performing a physical examination—and requires a conscientious and concerted effort. Astute communication skills are particularly important when working with children. Young children are nonverbal, and older children may not have the cognitive ability to put into words or to understand the importance of directly communicating their concerns. Adolescents may also be limited by their cognitive abilities; they may think the examiner will know or ask about issues that are pressing for them.

The nurse must be able to receive and send information while concentrating on both verbal and nonverbal messages that are being exchanged. Psychosocial factors related to the ability to communicate successfully include the ability to be empathetic, to be an active listener (i.e., listening to what is said, or not said, and how it is said), and to convey respect. An awareness of cultural and diversity issues such as cultural communication patterns, health beliefs and practices, and specific cultural values is another important factor, as is attending to the parent's or child's nonverbal cues.

caREminder

When asking about sensitive issues (e.g., sexuality, spirituality), explain why the information is needed. The child, or family, may be more willing to respond and give an honest answer.

External considerations that affect communication include privacy, interruptions, comfort in the physical environment, and note taking or using electronic devices. Ensuring privacy, arranging a setting so that conversations are not overheard by others, allows for more open communication. If interviewing must be done at a hospital bedside, create a sense of privacy by pulling bedside curtains to partition the area and asking visitors (nonparents) to step out of the room. Interruptions break the flow of communication and are distracting; therefore, discourage unnecessary interruptions and ask not to be disturbed except for an emergency. Ensure a comfortable room temperature, adequate lighting, and a quiet setting. If the nurse stands during the interview, the message conveyed is that of the need for haste; therefore, make sure there is a place for the child or parent and examiner to sit and see each other.

Model open, nonjudgmental, and respectful communication. When interviewing children and adolescents about their symptoms or health care issues, consider the child's or teen's developmental stage and his or her cognitive ability. Keep note taking to a minimum so attention can be focused on who is speaking and what is being said. Avoid focusing solely on inputting data into a computer program by frequently pausing and seeking eye contact with the child and family member. Clarify what has been said, and summarize the information given by the child or parent. Specific communication techniques for conducting a health history are presented in Nursing Interventions 8-1. Familiarity with a child and family can sometimes result in failure to actively listen or communicate as effectively by taking issues for granted.

HEALTH HISTORY

QUESTION: How do you anticipate Sally Jenkins will respond to the routine questions of a health history? What tactics can the nurse use to make Sally less anxious?

The complete health history is divided into component parts that are addressed in a systematic fashion (Chart 8-1). Information required from a complete health history can be obtained through either a direct interview alone or through a combination of direct interview and a health questionnaire. If a questionnaire is used, verify that the informant can both read and write and that the questionnaire is at an appropriate level of understanding.

NURSING INTERVENTIONS 8-1

Communication Techniques for Conducting a Health History

- Introduce yourself, give your title, and state the purpose of the interview.
- Ask the parent/caregiver and child how they wish to be addressed.
- Use open-ended questions as much as possible; follow with closed or direct questions when specific information is needed.
- Ask one question at a time and use language that the adult and child understand.
- Use encouraging statements to promote parent/child participation such as "Tell me more." "What other concerns or issues should we discuss?"
- Include older children and teens in the discussion and ask questions of them as appropriate.
- Ask for clarification if confused by the person's choice of words or explanation.
- Summarize to ensure that you correctly understand what was said.
- Close the interview by giving the parent/caregiver and child an opportunity to reflect to determine whether any additional information should be shared.

CROSS-CULTURAL CARE

Seek the services of an interpreter who is fluent in the language of the informant and preferably trained to perform interpreter duties whenever the historian and interviewer are not fluent in the same language. Asking a sibling to interpret for the parent may be perceived by the parent as a sign of disrespect. Parents also may be reluctant to disclose information about a genetic problem or sexual issue if their child is interpreting for them. If the family's first language is not that of the examiner, assess the child's language skills in the language spoken at home. Sometimes, it will be necessary to have the parent give the child instructions in the language with which the child is most comfortable. An individual who is familiar with both a specific language and culture is referred to as a *cultural broker*. The use of a cultural broker is preferred in instances when there is a language or cultural barrier.

For school-aged children, the parent may provide information, but also direct questions to the child as appropriate. Give the young adolescent (aged 11 to 14 years) the choice of whether the parent is present during the interview and examination but always allow time to talk alone with the adolescent. Interview the older adolescent alone. Address issues of confidentiality with both the adolescent and the parent; tell them that what each one says in confidence will not be discussed with the other unless the information is something that the individual agrees to share. Issues of confidentiality generally center on sexual activity, birth control, and feelings about oneself or the parent–child relationship. Tell the adolescent at the start of the interview that thoughts about harming oneself or others cannot be kept confidential. Encourage and promote positive communication between parent and adolescent.

Many adolescents are afraid to ask questions and are grateful when a sensitive topic is broached by the nurse. Phrasing questions in a nonthreatening way is a useful technique. For example, instead of asking a direct question about smoking, say, "Some teens your age tell me that they have tried smoking. Is this something you might have tried?" Remembering the acronym HEEADDSSS provides an easy prompt about key topics to discuss with all adolescents (Chart 8-2). To start, ask the teens what they are good at. Help them to identify their strengths. Teens who get a positive message about what is right with them are often more open to working on behaviors they could improve on.

CHART 8-1   Components of a Comprehensive Pediatric History

Identifying or biographic data

Reason for seeking care (chief complaint or health supervision visit)

History of the present illness, if applicable

Past medical history
  Prenatal, birth, and neonatal history
  Hospitalizations, accidents, surgical procedures, ingestions, injuries, and emergency department visits
  Previous illnesses (serious or chronic and childhood infectious diseases)
  Current medications: prescription, over the counter, and complementary/alternative
  Allergies (food, medication, animals, insect bites, or environmental triggers) and type of reaction
  Immunizations
  Nutrition and feeding practices
  Growth and developmental milestones
  Habits and behaviors: safety, physical activity, sleep patterns
Family health history; including a genogram
Social and environmental history
Spiritual history
Sexual history (adolescent)
Review of systems

CHART 8-2   Adolescent History

H—home/family life and involvement, exposure to violence (in the home or community, as a victim or witness), presence of a support system (profile of parents, friends, and others)

E—educational performance, employment, vocational development, future plans

E—exercise and eating behaviors and practices; amount and type of exercise; type and amount of intake, paying close attention to nutritional risk factors for eating disorders; overweight and underweight

A—activities with families and peers, including sports, after-school involvement, risk-taking behaviors (safety concerns, such as driving under the influence, drag-racing cars, hitchhiking, high-risk sex)

D—drugs (alcohol, tobacco, and other street drugs) tried and used, onset, duration, frequency, type

D—depression

S—suicidal thoughts and suicide attempts

S—sexual history

S—safety practices (e.g., use of bike helmets and safety protection equipment during sport activities)

Females

- *Menarche/menses:* age at onset; duration, quantity of flow, and frequency of menses; last menstrual period; any problems with dysmenorrhea
- *Sexual activity:* sexual behaviors and practices (include questions ranging from self-masturbation, kissing, necking, petting, and oral copulation to intercourse); if applicable, frequency of sexual coitus and age at start; sexual orientation (males, females, bisexual); number of sexual partners; issues of date rape, prior sexual molestation, assault, or prostitution
- *Contraceptive history:* understanding of various types of contraceptives for females and males; knowledge about condoms to prevent pregnancy and sexually transmitted infections

(STIs), consistency of condom use or other methods of birth control, whether she and her partner discuss using a method of birth control; current and past use of contraceptives

- *Obstetric and gynecologic history:* number of pregnancies, past gynecologic procedures or illnesses (pelvic inflammatory disease)
- *History of STIs:* type, dates, and treatment; STI history in partner; any current signs or symptoms
- *Body image:* perceptions about her body and sexual identity
- *Anticipatory guidance:* preparation for her emerging sexual development
- *Partner:* involvement and commitment to family planning
- *Other:* personal concerns or issues

Males

- *Spermarche:* age of first ejaculation
- *Sexual activity:* sexual behaviors and practices (include questions ranging from self-masturbation, kissing, necking, petting, and oral copulation to intercourse); if applicable, frequency of sexual coitus and age at start; sexual orientation (females, males, bisexual); number of sexual partners; prior sexual molestation, assault, or prostitution
- *Contraceptive history:* knowledge about condoms to prevent pregnancy and STIs, consistency of condom use or other methods of birth control, whether he and his partners discuss using a method of birth control, male responsibility if he fathers a child
- *History of STIs:* type, dates, and treatment; STI history in partner; any current signs or symptoms
- *Body image:* perceptions of his body and sexual identity
- *Anticipatory guidance:* preparation for his emerging sexual development
- *Partner:* involvement and commitment to family planning
- *Other:* personal concerns or issues

The nurse must be aware of the potential for cultural and spiritual dynamics and subtleties. These may influence who answers questions, how the child and family relate, how questions are interpreted, what information is shared with the health care team, and understanding of the importance of information being requested, which are essential to accurate data collection (Tables 8-1 and 8-3).

ANSWER: Many of the routine questions covered in the pediatric health history may be topics about which Sally has no information. The fact that she knows very little may make her feel anxious and inadequate. One tactic would be to say, "Share everything you know about Stephanie." This approach would allow Sally to discover she does have newfound knowledge about Stephanie.

Identifying or Biographic Data

To begin the health history, obtain the child's name, nickname, birth date, sex, and the identity of the person providing the information. If an interpreter is present,

include the name of this individual as well. If appropriate, record a statement about the validity and reliability of the information in the written notes about the health history. For instance, if the informant provides only vague details or inconsistent information, this should be noted. The informant may not be able to provide a complete health history for various reasons, including foster care, adoption, or death of parents. In such situations, note as "information not known by informant."

caREminder

Even if the informant is a parent, he or she may not be knowledgeable regarding the child or the child's current condition. (e.g., a noncustodial parent). Remain nonjudgmental and obtain as much information as possible.

Reason for Seeking Care (Chief Complaint)

After obtaining the child's biographic data, determine the reason for the child's visit. This section typically is designated as either the *reason for seeking care* or

TABLE 8-1	Components of a Cultural Assessment
Attribute	**Assessment Questions**
Ethnic or racial identity	• Does your child identify as belonging to a specific ethnic or racial group? If yes, which? • Do both parents identify with the same group?
Acculturation	• Where was your child born? Where were both parents born? If outside the country, how long have you been in the country and where have you lived previously? • How much is your family immersed in the dominant culture versus your ethnic culture? • Does your family's home have adornments (art, religious objects) primarily from your family's ethnic background?
Language	• What language is spoken in the home and by whom? • What language is preferred when speaking with those outside the family? • Are you able to understand and speak the dominant language (e.g., English)? • Is an interpreter needed? • Do you have concerns about reading or understanding the instructions on medicine containers?
Religion	• Do you have a religion to which you ascribe? • How much does your family participate in religious-based activities? • Are there any religious practices that you want to continue if in the hospital?
Ethnic group affiliation	• Is shopping done within the family's neighborhood with access to ethnic food choices? • What are the characteristics of the family's social networks? • Are most activities (school, shopping, recreation) performed within the ethnic group?
Community affiliation	• What are the characteristics of your family's neighborhood? Is it ethnically diverse? • Does your family feel accepted or discriminated against in the community? • Is the health care team doing anything that makes your family or child uncomfortable?
Family interactions	• How are decisions made in your family? Who makes important decisions? • How is affection demonstrated in your family? • When do children require disciplining and how is this done?
Traditions	• What do we need to know about your family's traditions to provide health care? • What are your family's dietary habits? • Are there foods or fluids that you think will help you stay healthy or get better (e.g., hot or cold beverages or foods)? • Are there any foods or fluids that you should not have or that might make you sick? • Are there special clothing or dressing preferences that you have based on your ethnic customs?
Health care practices	• Are there practices that help your child stay healthy such as herbs, vitamins, specific foods, jewelry/medals, or lotions? • How long has the problem been present? (Try to get specific times, not just "long time" or "short," because time orientation may vary among cultural groups.) • What has been done to help the child get better? Have any herbs, medicines, or other treatments been given? • Have you used any folk practices? Has the child been treated by a religious or community leader or healer? What is that person called? • Are there any medicines or treatments that you think might help? • Are there restrictions on the gender of the health care provider?

Adapted from Friedman, M. (1990). Transcultural family nursing. Application to Latino and black families. *Journal of Pediatric Nursing, 5,* 214–222.

chief complaint. These terms are used in situations when symptoms or signs of illness are the focus of the encounter. Parents and children may find the phrase "reason for seeking health care" easier to understand, especially if they do not view a symptom or clinical finding as a "complaint." In either case, record the description of the complaint or concern in the parent's, caregiver's, or child's own words. Put this statement in quotation marks; it represents the person's spontaneous response to a simple, open-ended question such as "What brings you here today?" "What seems to be the matter?" or "What concerns you about your child?"

If a symptom or problem is identified, include the duration of this concern in the statement (e.g., "My baby's been throwing up for 2 days.") Be sure to include the child, as appropriate, during history taking. The child's perception of the reason for the visit may differ from the caregiver's and may add information to the chief complaint.

A comprehensive health history is often completed during an initial health supervision visit. Although a parent may be bringing the child in for a health supervision visit, the parent often has a concern about his or her child that needs to be addressed.

History of the Current Illness

Obtaining a history of the child's current illness directs the physical examination and guides the nurse's overall assessment of the child's health. When gathering data, be sure to determine the onset, duration, and nature of each symptom; any precipitating or related factors; and any relief measures or remedies taken. At the end, the nurse should possess data that describe the chronology of the problem and any other associated manifestations plus the exclusion of other possible pertinent symptoms (i.e., negative findings). Investigate eight factors for each symptom identified (Table 8-2). Some use the mnemonic OPPQRST as a guide. The letters stand for onset (O), palliative or what helps relieve the symptom (P), provoking factor (P), quality (Q), region or radiating (R), severity (S), and timing for frequency and duration (T).

Past Medical History

Determining a child's past medical history is another important component of the overall assessment. This section of the history is a profile of the child's past illnesses, childhood infectious diseases, health care, health promotion activities, growth and development, injuries, surgeries, emergency department visits, and hospitalizations. The information obtained provides additional clues regarding past events that may have influenced the current problem or situation.

Prenatal, Birth, and Neonatal History

Determine the duration of gestation and aspects of the pregnancy, labor, and delivery. When did the mother obtain prenatal care? Did she experience any prenatal vaginal bleeding, premature contractions, or other problems? Was the child born in the hospital or at home? Was it a vaginal delivery, or, if it was a cesarean section delivery, for what reason? Did the mother consume alcohol, use drugs, or smoke during her pregnancy? Was the mother screened for Group B *Streptococcus*, HIV, and HepB? Ask about the infant's birth weight, length, Apgar score, and newborn screening test results, if known. Also ask whether the child was born prematurely and whether the infant went home with the mother after birth or if any complications, such as ABO incompatibility or hyperbilirubinemia, occurred. Ask questions about length of hospital stay for premature infants, the need for assisted ventilation, and whether any diagnostic tests were done such as lumbar punctures, blood cultures, or imaging studies.

Hospitalizations, Emergency Department Visits, Accidents, Surgical Procedures, Ingestions, and Injuries

Ask the parent about any hospitalizations, emergency department visits, accidents and injuries, surgical procedures, radiographic or diagnostic imaging studies, or poison ingestion. Include the date of the event or approximate age of the child at the time of the event. Have the parent describe the reason for these medical encounters or events and any related long-term issues.

TABLE 8-2	Symptom Assessment
Factor	**Assessment Questions**
Location	For symptoms such as pain, rash, lesions, or paresthesia, inquire about the specific body location or locations; whether the symptom is localized or generalized; and, for pain, whether it is deep or superficial or radiates.
Quality or character	Assess the character or quality of the symptom by asking the historian to describe the symptom. For example, is the pain dull, sharp, aching, burning, stinging, or throbbing? Is the rash a bright red or pink, bumpy, blistery, or flat? Does the child's cough sound like a bark or a whooping noise? Is the symptom getting better, worsening, or staying about the same?
Quantity and severity	Ask questions about the amount and severity or intensity of the symptom: • When the infant vomits, estimate how much formula or breast milk is vomited—a tablespoonful or 2–3 oz? • With heavy menstrual bleeding, does the teen completely saturate a pad? • How often must the pad or tampon be changed? Rate the intensity of the pain using a developmentally appropriate tool (e.g., face scale or numeric rating scale) or the intensity of itching using a 0- to 5-point scale, with 0 point being no itching and 5 points the worst itching you have ever had. Questioning about the effect that the symptom or illness has on the child's activity level (e.g., playing, school attendance, sleeping, and eating) is a useful method to help determine the severity of the problem.
Timing	Timing or temporal relationship of a symptom relates to its onset, duration, when it occurs, and frequency as well as precipitating factors. Try to determine the exact date or time that the symptom appeared and how long it lasted. Were there any periods when the symptom abated (i.e., was it intermittent or steady)? Timing can also be related to the quality or intensity of the symptom. Ask if there are any precipitating factors or any variations in the intensity or quality of the symptoms related to time of day, night, or month.
Setting	The setting in which the symptom appeared is often relevant. For example, is the child's stomachache present only during math class at school?
Aggravating or relieving factors	Ask about factors that may seem to make the symptom better or worse. Does the pain subside if the child does not put weight on the leg? What medication or alternate therapies has the adolescent tried for menstrual cramps and have they helped relieve the cramping?
Perceptions of the child and parent	How the parent/caregiver and child perceive the symptom alerts the nurse to areas of potential anxiety. For instance, parents of a child who has frequent epistaxis may be concerned about leukemia.
Associated factors or symptoms	Query the child about associated factors or symptoms that might be present and not mentioned by the historian. A review of systems related to the symptom is done at this point in the health history. Many health care professionals do the total review of systems here rather than after the family health or disease history.

Previous Illnesses

Ask about serious or chronic health conditions or prior life-threatening illness or childhood infectious diseases. Seek information about the age at presentation and age at diagnosis as well as treatments given.

Current Medications

Determine all current medications, including prescription, over-the-counter, and complementary medications, that the child is taking or has recently taken. Include the name and dosage as well as the method and duration of administration and the presence of any side effects. It is also important to ask about the use of complementary and alternative therapies or folk remedies. Determine when the last dose of a medication was given and the parent's understanding of the indications and dosing requirements for all medications.

Allergies

Note any known allergies. If the child has a history of asthma, allergic rhinitis or conjunctivitis, or atopic skin disease, note age of onset. Ask the parent to describe the type (e.g., if present, characteristics of rash, urticaria, wheezing, or angioedema) and severity of symptoms and how the child was treated. Also inquire about any steps the parent or child takes to avoid the allergen (e.g., foods, medications, animals, insect bites, or environmental triggers) or use of prophylactic treatments.

Immunizations

Review the child's immunization record. Ask the parent whether any untoward reactions occurred related to an immunization. If so, have him or her describe what happened. List the date of the last tuberculin skin test as well.

Nutrition and Feeding Practices

To calculate an infant's caloric intake, ask the parent about the frequency of breastfeeding or the type and amount of formula given during the past 24 hours. If warranted, question the parent about how he or she prepares the formula (i.e., preparation of powdered formula). As solids are introduced, determine what is being offered, how much, and how frequently. Also, determine whether the younger child is still feeding from a bottle or has switched to a cup. For the older child, ask about whole or reduced-fat milk intake during a 24-hour period and the number, portion size, and type of foods eaten each day (i.e., description of typical breakfast, lunch, dinner, and snacks). You might also use the U.S. Department of Agriculture MyPlate visual image (available at http://www.choosemyplate.gov/) as a questioning guideline about the types of foods consumed and portion sizes. A 3-day or 1-week food diary is useful if a nutritional disorder is suspected. See Chapters 4 to 7 for additional discussion about nutritional assessment for different age groups. Other feeding issues to address include problem areas for the breastfed and formula-fed baby (e.g., propping of bottle, taking a bottle to bed at night, breastfeeding difficulties). For toddlers and younger children, nutritional problems may be a result of snacking on food with empty calories, excessive soft drink consumption, self-feeding, food jags, and skipping meals. Inquiring about feeding practices such as eating in front of a television, fast food consumption, and the presence or lack of family meals can provide important information that is related to poor nutritional choices and eating patterns.

Growth and Developmental Milestones

> QUESTION: What are the fine motor and gross motor skills appropriate for a 4-month-old child like Stephanie?

Growth parameters are best assessed by measuring height, weight, and head circumference and calculating the body mass index (BMI) (see the section on "Physical Examination" later in this chapter). Seek evidence of the attainment of developmental milestones by performing an appraisal of key developmental areas: fine and gross motor, language, personal, social, psychosocial, and cognitive (see Chapter 3). For infants and young children, ask about age at which the milestone was achieved.

The nurse may want to use a quick checklist for this assessment that details developmental milestones for the various age groups; refer to Chapters 4 to 7 for summary tables and to *Bright Futures: Guidelines for Health Supervision of Infants, Children, and Adolescents* (Hagan et al., 2008).

For the school-aged child and adolescent, inquire about school performance (grades) and the child's socialization with peers (e.g., "What do you do after school?" "What hobbies or recreational activities interest you?"). The nurse can ask how the child is doing in each subject and whether the child is in an age-appropriate grade or in any special programs in school. Assess the ability to form friendships with peers and inquire about problem areas such as being bullied or having "bad" grades. For the adolescent, issues related to sexual development and identity emerge as major areas.

> ANSWER: Stephanie's fine motor skills should include reaching for items and grasping. Her gross motor skills should show good head control and perhaps rolling over. She should smile spontaneously, squeal, laugh, and turn toward a voice.

Habits and Behaviors

A child's habits and behaviors should also be discussed during the health history. Does the child have any unusual rituals or behaviors? Address discipline practices. For young children, gather information about toileting and temperament. Ask the older child or teenager privately about gang involvement, tobacco and drug use, alcohol consumption (Chapter 29 further discusses substance abuse), and sexual activities or practices. Be sure to ask adolescents about feelings of sadness or depression.

Obtain and update information about safety awareness and injury prevention strategies specific to each developmental stage or age for all children. Identify health promotion practices or behaviors that promote safety. These include use of car seats and restraints and protective sport equipment (e.g., bicycle helmets), use of sun protection, poison control measures, smoke and carbon monoxide detection devices, and removal of firearms from the home (see Chapters 4 to 7).

Note the amount and type of physical activity. Sleep is critical to growth, health, and recovery from illnesses or injuries. Seek information about the amount of sleep and address sleep issues such as nightmares, night terrors, or difficulty getting to sleep for frequent nights.

Family Health History

To get a more detailed picture of a child's health history, it is important to ask about the child's family health history. Obtain information about the age and health or cause of death of the child's closest family members. The use of a genogram outlining three generations of biologic relatives to diagram relationships and to identify family health problems readily provides data in a visual fashion (Fig. 8-1). Inquire about any family history of heart disease (age of onset), sudden death, high blood pressure, kidney disease, diabetes, allergies, or asthma; any genetically inherited diseases, intellectual disabilities, congenital anomalies, or illnesses; seizures; learning disabilities; and alcoholism. In addition, it is also important to ask about whether there is anyone else in the family with symptoms similar to the child's presenting problems.

Social and Environmental History

The family unit and support system are important factors in health promotion and disease prevention. Determine family cohesiveness and interpersonal relationships by seeking information about who lives with the child, who is the primary caregiver, and whether the family has a support system to help with child care or in times of need. If the biologic parents are separated or divorced, inquire about involvement of the out-of-home parent. Family living arrangements, home environment, and economic status have implications for health care planning and management. Address questions in a sensitive manner and with an explanation given to the family about the importance of the nurse knowing these issues to facilitate the care of their child.

Seek information about the safety of the home setting and community and any environmental hazards or risk factors (e.g., If the home has iron bars on the windows, can the bars be released in case of fire? If the child has access to a swimming pool, do the family members know cardiopulmonary resuscitation? Is radon or the use of pesticides an issue? Does the family live in a high crime or gang area?).

Sexual History

Questions that are part of the sexual history are found in Chart 8-2. Sexuality of the child is an issue that parents dwell on—even from the time of conception, but especially in adolescence (age 11–21) (see Chapters 3 to 7). Educating parents about the stages of sexual development and stressing that sexual development is a normal and healthy component of human growth are important messages to convey to both parent and child.

Spiritual Assessment

Spiritual and religious beliefs are often a central uniting force in family life. A spiritual assessment provides information about the family's belief system and its values.

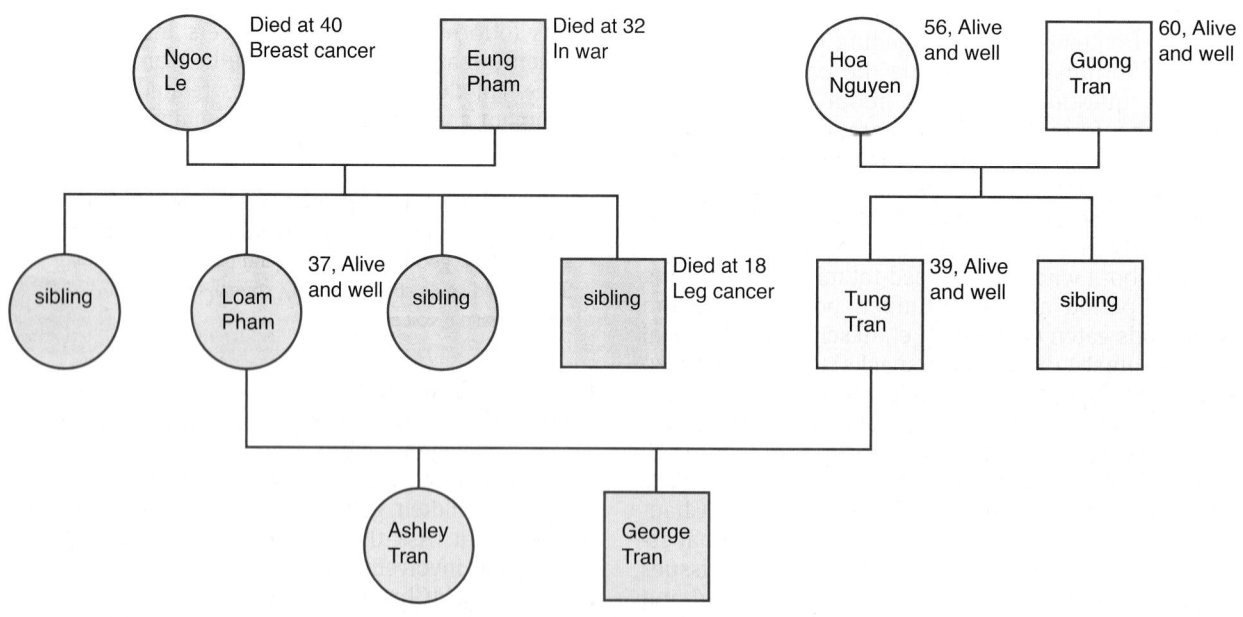

Figure 8-1 A genogram provides a pictorial overview of family health challenges and can assist in detecting disease trends or risks. Shown here is a genogram of the Tran family mentioned in Chapter 1. Note the inherited pattern of tumor-type cancers. The possibility of the genetic predisposition to cancer (the p53 mutation) may become evident with a genogram. The Tran family shows the incidence of multigenerational tumors and death at a young age. Circles represent females; squares represent males.

Questions should focus on obtaining general information about religious and spiritual beliefs (e.g., family roles and relations, rituals, dietary or other restrictions, membership in a religious or spiritual group, and medical treatment or procedures that may or may not be permitted). Questioning that focuses on the family's or child's inner resources and identity seeks to elicit information about the role of faith or spirituality in the lives of the family members and what brings joy, hope, and comfort. Interconnectedness looks at how family members show their love and support for each other. Asking questions about what gives life meaning or purpose provides the health care provider with information as to the values and beliefs that guide health behaviors and decision making. Table 8-3 provides examples of questions that are fundamental components of a spiritual assessment.

Review of Systems

The review of systems evaluates the past and present health states of each body system, is a double-check to determine whether significant data were omitted, and also allows the nurse to determine health promotion needs. Ask about specific signs and symptoms for each body system and also query about health promotion activities related to a particular body system.

Each health challenge chapter in this text (Chapters 14 to 30) discusses alterations in a body system and includes a section called "Focused Health History." This section discusses pertinent information to obtain for a review of that particular body system.

PHYSICAL EXAMINATION

QUESTION: Today's examination is to be basically noninvasive to determine the status of Stephanie's health and to allow Stephanie and her parents to get to know the physician, nurse practitioner, and office nurses. This is Stephanie's first physical examination in the United States. What are three components of a physical examination usually done at birth to rule out congenital malformations?

After obtaining a child's health history, it is important to perform a complete physical assessment. The usual approach to the physical examination of infants and young children is to start with the chest and work downward and then finish with the head and neck. The traditional sequence in preschool and older children starts with inspection of the head and works downward (head to toe). The usual sequence may need to be altered based on such factors as the child's developmental age, individual comfort level, and presenting symptoms, but the important point is to eventually cover all aspects of the examination.

caREminder

Wait until the end of the examination to perform the more intrusive procedures that are likely to distress the young child, such as inspection of the mouth and otoscopic examination of the ears.

TABLE 8-3	Components of a Spiritual Assessment
Attribute	**Assessment Questions**
Values, relatedness	• What do you value most in life? With whom do you enjoy spending time? • What brings you strength, comfort, joy, and hope?
Sources of support	• Do you use specific practices that help you cope? • Is there someone or something that you find especially helpful to you? • Who provides support for you in times of stress?
Meaning	• What is the meaning or purpose of life? • What is the meaning and purpose of suffering? • Do you feel that your current situation has a specific meaning or purpose? • In what ways will this illness affect your life's goals?
Beliefs	• What are your spiritual beliefs about a higher being, birth, death, bad things that happen, health, and illness? • What events in your life have affected your spiritual beliefs? • Do other family members share your spiritual beliefs and practices? • How can we incorporate your spiritual beliefs into your child's health care?
Affiliation	• Do you identify with a specific religion? • To what extent does your family participate in worship or related activities? • Does your child attend religious school?
Practices	• Describe the spiritual activities (e.g., prayer, scripture reading, meditation, communing with nature) that play an important part in your family life. • Do you have spiritual beliefs that relate to your daily habits and activities? • What are the spiritual practices that your child ascribes to? • Would blood product use or organ donation be proper given your religious beliefs? • Would limiting or withdrawing medical care be proper given your beliefs? • Are there specific practices relating to end of life to which you ascribe?
Dietary/dress practices	• Do your beliefs influence or prescribe your dietary or dress practices? What are they?

When examining infants, be sure that the infant is always able to view the parent. Approach toddlers and preschoolers gradually and keep them close to the parent. Modesty is an issue that surfaces with some preschool children but takes on heightened importance to school-aged children. Make every effort to provide appropriate covering and to expose only the area to be examined. Perform hand hygiene before beginning the examination and don gloves to examine the genital and rectal areas. Warm hands before palpation. Warm a cold stethoscope by rubbing it in the hands and rub the head of the stethoscope with an alcohol pad before use. Follow safety measures and have all needed equipment readily available. Allow time for the child or adolescent to ask questions and to clarify what, if any, physical findings are found. Developmental Considerations 8-1 identifies age-appropriate approaches to the physical examination.

ANSWER: It is known that Stephanie tolerates her diet well and is voiding and producing stool without difficulty. However, it is still important to examine her mouth to check the hard and soft palates for notches, clefts, and unusual arches. The incidence of cleft palate disorders is highest in Asian populations. Listening to heart sounds to determine whether there is a murmur and examining her hips for any hip joint instability are also important components of today's physical examination to rule out any congenital problems.

Vital Signs

QUESTION: How would a nurse obtain accurate vital signs on the 4-month-old Stephanie?

Begin the physical examination by measuring the child's vital signs: respiration, pulse, blood pressure, and temperature (see thePoint for Procedures and Supplemental Information). Always compare findings with normal ranges for the child's age (see Appendix B). Pain is often considered the fifth vital sign (see Chapter 10 for assessment of pain).

KidKare Choose your words carefully when explaining actions to a young child. Avoid saying, for example, "I'm going to take your pulse now." The child may think that you are going to actually remove something from his or her body. A better phrase would be, "I'm going to count how fast your heart beats."

Respiration

Measure the child's respiratory rate first before you conduct other procedures that may affect the rate. Count the number of breaths the child takes for a full minute. An accurate respiratory rate is an essential piece of information for any child with a respiratory or cardiac problem.

Pulse

Assess the apical pulse rate for 1 full minute to detect possible alterations in rhythm, preferably when the child is quiet; if the child is crying or fussy, note this. Document the child's activity during pulse assessment. Variations in heart rate generally are much more dramatic in children than in adults; a heart rate outside the normal range for age may be a subtle sign of a cardiac problem, especially in an infant. Assess for factors known to affect heart rate and quality, including medication, activity, hyperthermia or hypothermia, hypoxia, apprehension, pain, increased intracranial pressure, hypovolemia, and hemorrhage.

Blood Pressure

Measuring blood pressure is a routine part of physical assessment in children older than age 3 years and in younger children who have symptoms that warrant investigation (e.g., pulse strength difference between upper and lower extremities). Various devices can be used to measure blood pressure, including mercury-gravity or aneroid sphygmomanometers and electronic devices that use oscillometric or Doppler techniques. Use a properly sized cuff for accurate readings.

Temperature

Normal body temperature is roughly 98.6° F (37° C) measured orally. Body temperature can be influenced by many non–illness-related factors. Exercise, crying, and environmental heat can increase temperature (e.g., an infant swaddled in blankets). In contrast, exposure to cold air can lower body temperature, as can vasodilating and anesthetic agents. Diurnal variations in body temperature also occur. Body temperature is generally lowest between 1 and 4 AM and is highest between 4 and 6 PM. Axillary temperatures are taken in infants and in young children who are unable to hold a thermometer in their mouth. Tympanic and temporal thermometers can be used as appropriate.

ANSWER: While Stephanie is calm and held by Sally, count her respirations for a full minute without touching her. The quality of her breath sounds will be evaluated later. Just touching her with a stethoscope will increase her respiratory rate. With a warmed and sanitized stethoscope (the head cleaned with an alcohol swab), listen to the apical pulse for a full minute. Obtain an axillary temperature while Stephanie remains on her mom's lap. A blood pressure in all four extremities can be obtained at a later visit.

Anthropometric Measurements

QUESTION: Plot Stephanie's height, weight, and head circumference on the growth chart for girls, birth to 36 months of age, and then calculate her percentiles. What would you expect to see? BMI should be plotted in children beginning at 2 years of age.

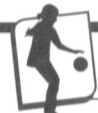

DEVELOPMENTAL CONSIDERATIONS 8-1

Physical Examination From Infancy Through Adolescence

Infancy

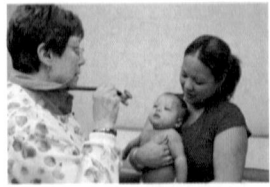

Examine an infant in a parent's lap or on the examination table if the infant is quiet. Leave the diaper on and wrap the young infant in a blanket to maintain warmth and security. Explore comforting measures, such as a having the mother feed the infant or using a pacifier if the infant becomes fussy. Talk softly and establish eye contact. Avoid sudden, startling movements. Parents can help with the ear examination by having the older infant rest his or her head against their shoulders. Use the pediatric head of the stethoscope when auscultating in small infants.

Early childhood

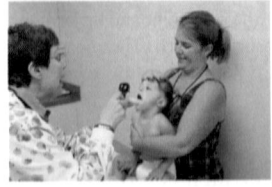

It is best to examine the young child while he or she is sitting in a parent's lap. Examiner and parent sit opposite each other with knees touching to use knees as an examination surface. Use play techniques to gain attention and distract child with stories. Let child handle equipment but be mindful of safety issues. If the child is uncooperative, quickly perform what has to be done. Call the child by name and praise him or her frequently.

Early childhood

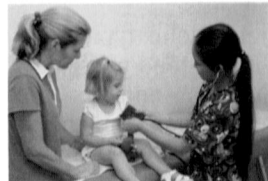

Give the preschooler the choice of either sitting on a parent's lap or sitting on the examination table. Tell the parent to stay close to and within eye contact of the child. Explain procedures in simple terms that the child understands. For instance, when taking vital signs, use simple words to explain what is being done: "I need to see how warm your body is" or "I want to hear how fast and strong your heart is." Be careful when using the word "take" with very young children. For example, it would be best to explain how it feels for the child when taking blood pressure. Say, "I need to see how your heart is working and have to give your arm a big hug" rather than "I need to take your blood pressure." This may be misinterpreted by the child as taking something away. Interact with the child, allow the child to safely handle equipment, and encourage the child to talk about himself or herself. Modesty concerns start to emerge. Be sure to tell the child when it is important not to move by saying, "Your job is to stay still so I can see how well your legs move."

Middle childhood

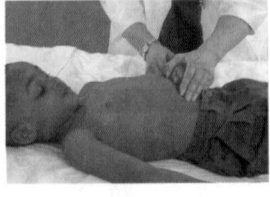

Allow the older school-aged child the choice of whether to have a parent present. Be cognizant of need for privacy and modesty concerns. Explain procedures and equipment (e.g., allow child to listen to own heart). Teach about body function while examining. Focus on dialoguing and interacting with the child. Common issues are ticklishness when palpating and hesitancy to allow genitalia to be checked. To reduce ticklishness when palpating the abdomen, place the child's hand under your hand, have the child bend at the knees, or use a stethoscope to apply pressure to palpate. These are also useful techniques to use if the child is complaining of abdominal pain and is fearful of having his or her abdomen palpated. Provide for covering of genitalia and be matter of fact with the child about examining the genitalia (i.e., explain that you look at all children's private parts to be sure that everything is fine). This is also an opportunity to teach about approaching sexual development.

Adolescence

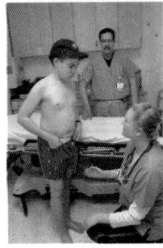

Allow the adolescent to undress in private before the physical examination. Explain what is being done and why in terms that are easy for the adolescent to understand. Actively talk with the adolescent during the examination and frequently emphasize normal findings (e.g., "Your ears are fine," "Your eyes are great"). Ask the adolescent questions about sexual changes and let him or her know that these changes are normal and expected. When examining the genitalia of an adolescent of the opposite sex or if a male examines the breasts of a female, it is common and standard practice to always have someone present who is of the same sex as the adolescent being examined.

Obtaining accurate anthropometric measurements (measurements of the body such as height, weight, head circumference) provides valuable information about how a child is growing (see thePoint for Procedures). The Centers for Disease Control and Prevention (CDC) recommends that health care providers in the United States use the World Health Organization (WHO) growth standards to monitor growth for infants and children 0 to 2 years of age and the CDC growth charts for children aged 2 years and older (Grummer-Strawn et al., 2010) (see Appendix A). When plotted on a growth chart, height/length, weight, BMI, and head circumference allow comparison with other children of the same age and sex and reveal the child's own pattern of growth. Standard growth charts are age (birth to 36 months and 2 to 20 years) and gender specific. When the CDC growth charts were revised, data on low-birth-weight infants were included but not data on very-low-birth-weight infants (VLBW) (<1,500 g). Alternate charts are available to assess the growth of VLBW infants and can be used to compare a VLBW infant's growth to other VLBW infants (e.g., the Infant Health and Development Program charts).

Growth charts for children with specific conditions have been compiled (e.g., Down syndrome, Turner syndrome, cerebral palsy, achondroplasia). These charts are useful for comparing a child with other children with similar diagnoses; however, because the charts are based on small numbers of children, they should not be used alone. Plot the child's measurements on both the CDC growth charts and the specialty charts.

> **ANSWER:** Stephanie's weight is in the 75th percentile and her height and head circumference are in the 50th percentile. Stephanie's appearance confirms that she is chubby, with dimpled wrists and knees. This provides a starting point to track Stephanie's own growth curve.

Height

For infants and young children up to age 24 months, length measurement is best done by placing the vertex of the infant's head at the top of a flat measuring board and the soles of the feet firmly against the footboard (Fig. 8-2). Be sure to extend the hips and knees fully for accurate measurement.

For children older than age 2 years, a wall-mounted stadiometer provides the most accurate standing height measurement. Place the movable measuring rod on the topmost part of the child's head while he or she is standing without shoes and with the heels, buttocks, and shoulders just touching the wall. Instruct the child to look straight ahead without tilting the head. In some older children who are unable to stand independently (e.g., wheelchair bound), upper body height is measured using adaptive equipment.

Weight

Verify that the scale is calibrated correctly before measuring a child's weight. Weigh an infant, who should be nude, on an infant scale, placing your hands close to the body to prevent the child from falling off the scale (Fig. 8-3). Change the protective paper on the scale with

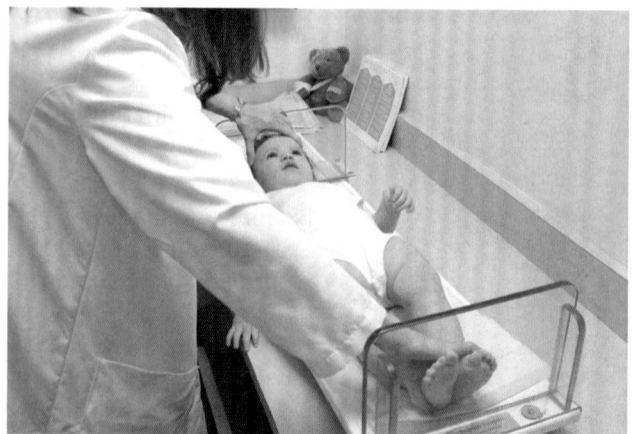

Figure 8-2 To obtain an accurate height measurement, the examiner ensures that the infant's head is against the end point and his or her hips and legs are fully extended on the measuring board. The measurement scale is calibrated from the head end point (e.g., in this example, the scale starts at 1 in.).

each use; disinfect the scale per facility policy. Use the same scale, when possible, to weigh an infant returning for assessment of weight gain or loss.

If a child is old enough to stand alone, typically after age 2 years, weigh the child on a stand-up scale; the child can wear underpants or an examination gown. If a very young child is scared to stand on the scale alone, weigh both the parent and the child and then subtract the parent's weight.

BMI measurement is useful in determining whether a child is overweight or underweight. Calculate BMI for children beginning at age 2 years as follows:

$$BMI = \left(\frac{\text{Weight in kilograms}}{(\text{Height in centimeters}) \times (\text{Height in centimeters})} \right) \times 10,000$$

or

$$BMI = \left(\frac{\text{Weight in pounds}}{(\text{Height in inches}) \times (\text{Height in inches})} \right) \times 703$$

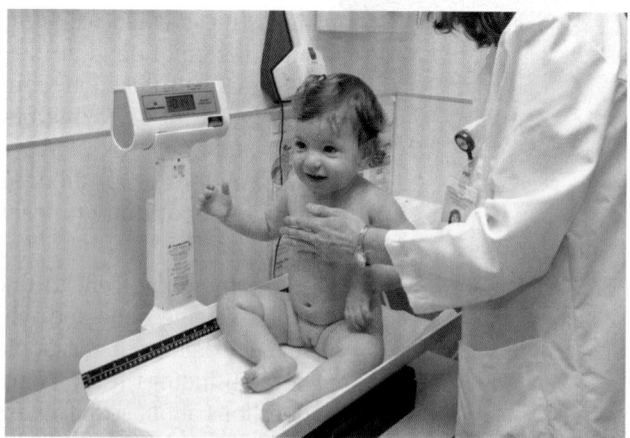

Figure 8-3 Older infants are usually more cooperative with being weighed when allowed to sit on the scale. Note the close proximity of the nurse's hands for safety.

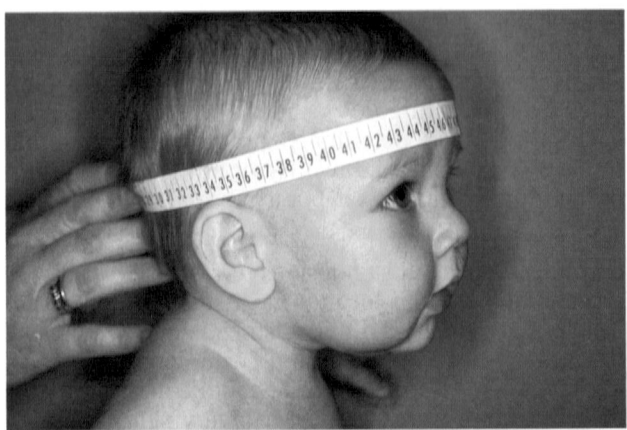

Figure 8-4 Head circumference is measured by wrapping the paper tape over the eyebrows and around the occipital prominence.

After calculating, plot the child's BMI measurement for age on the appropriate gender-based grid (see Appendix A). There are computer software programs that perform the calculation automatically. The CDC has a program to calculate BMI percentage for children and adolescents (CDC, 2012a). A child with a BMI measurement between the 85th and the 95th percentile is considered overweight; a measurement higher than the 95th percentile is obese. A child with a BMI lower than the 5th percentile is considered underweight.

Head Circumference

At every well-child visit up to age 2 years, measure head circumference (occipitofrontal circumference) by wrapping a paper tape measure around the maximum occipitofrontal circumference (Fig. 8-4). Take two separate readings; the measures should agree within 0.2 cm. If there is a difference of more than 0.2 cm, remeasure and record the average of the two measures in closest agreement to avoid error in obtaining this critical measurement (Maternal and Child Health Bureau, n.d.).

General Appearance

The child's general appearance is an important indicator of wellness or the severity of an illness. In a complete physical examination, record the child's general appearance prior to the physical assessment of the individual body systems. These observations represent the examiner's subjective impression of the child's overall state of health based on the physical examination and the time spent interviewing the child, parent, or both. Note whether the child appears sick or well, functions at a developmentally appropriate level for age, and appears well nourished and hydrated.

In addition, other relevant indicators include the child's state of hygiene in terms of body odor, general grooming, and cleanliness as well as the condition of the child's clothing. The child's behavior, interactions with others, overall personality, and activity level are important to observe. For infants and young children who are ill, the type of cry or voice (e.g., hoarse, husky, weak, or high pitched) is an important clinical assessment. Likewise, altered state of consciousness, coma, apathy,

restlessness, delirium, and irritability are descriptors that, if present, should be reported as part of the initial impression. Note any unusual postures, positions, or body movements as well as facial expressions (e.g., frozen watchfulness [hypervigilant and fearful], grimaces of pain, or avoidance of eye-to-eye contact) because these often are important assessment clues.

Integumentary System

Physical assessment of the integumentary system (the skin, hair, and nails) involves careful observation and, at times, palpation. A well-illuminated room or natural daylight is essential for accurate assessment. Room temperature is an important consideration because cold-induced cyanosis or flushing with heat can alter physical findings, especially in the newborn and young infant. Removal of nail coloring and cosmetics may be needed. Observe the entire body surface; otherwise, lesions or rashes under clothing can be missed. Maintaining modesty is always an important consideration.

Skin

Assess the skin for color, texture and moisture, temperature, and turgor. Unusual and distinctive odors can be caused by metabolic disease, poor hygiene, or infection.

CROSS-CULTURAL CARE

A child's skin color and pigmentation are influenced by racial characteristics. For example, Asian children often have a natural yellow tone to the skin that is not a result of increased bilirubin. African American children may have a bluish tinge to their gums, buccal cavity, borders of the tongue, and nail beds. Cyanosis in African American children may be difficult to detect because of their darker skin pigmentation.

Color

Changes in skin coloring that are important to note are pallor, cyanosis, erythema, plethora, ecchymoses, petechiae, and jaundice. Pallor (paleness) or an ash-gray color can be caused by anemia, syncope, shock, or lack of exposure to sunlight and is best observed in the face, mouth, conjunctivae, or nail beds.

Cyanosis occurs when reduced (deoxygenated) hemoglobin present in the blood results in a bluish skin tone. Peripheral cyanosis often results from cold or anxiety and is the result of temporary vasoconstriction; central cyanosis involves the lips, mouth, and trunk and indicates reduced oxygen-carrying capacity of the blood. Central cyanosis indicates cardiovascular, respiratory, and hematologic diseases.

Erythema, or redness of the skin, can result from many factors, including local inflammation, infection, hypothermia or hyperthermia, alcohol, blushing, allergy, or other dermatoses. Mongolian spots are a common, benign finding in young infants. They are typically found on the shoulders, buttocks, or lower back and are common in darker skinned ethnic groups (e.g., African American and East Indian descent). They appear blue or blue gray, range in size from 2 to 8 cm, and fade over the years.

Plethora is another term used to describe redness of the skin, especially the cheeks and lips, and is caused by an increased number of red blood cells. The increased production of red blood cells is a compensatory mechanism from chronic hypoxia.

Ecchymoses are large, diffuse areas of black and blue color caused by bleeding into the skin and commonly result from injury. Location and pattern of bruising may reveal cases of potential child abuse. In contrast, petechiae are small (<3 mm), distinct, pinpoint hemorrhages into the skin or mucous membranes often seen with blood disorders or systemic infection.

Jaundice is a yellowish pigmentation resulting from depositions of bile pigment in the skin, sclerae, and mucous membranes. Jaundice is indicative of hepatic disease and severe infections in infants. In contrast, carotenemia is a yellowish discoloration of the skin from deposits of carotene caused by excess ingestion of yellow and orange vegetables. Carotenemia is typically seen in the palms, soles, and face; the sclerae and mucous membranes are not involved.

Pressing the skin or nail bed causes a whitening appearance that provides contrast to assess color changes. Pressing the skin with a glass slide to produce a blanching effect helps in the assessment of jaundice (yellow remains), pallor (the color change in the skin is slight), and petechiae (lesions remain).

Texture and Moisture

Assess skin texture and moisture using inspection and palpation. Children's skin is normally smooth, soft, and slightly dry to the touch. Note any variations such as scars, keloids, excessive dryness, or dermatitis.

Temperature

Assess temperature by palpating the skin with the back of the hand, comparing both symmetric parts and the lower and upper extremities of the body for degree of warmth or coolness.

Turgor

Assess skin turgor, or elasticity, by grasping a fold of skin on the upper arm or abdomen between the fingers and quickly releasing the tissue (Fig. 8-5). Skin that

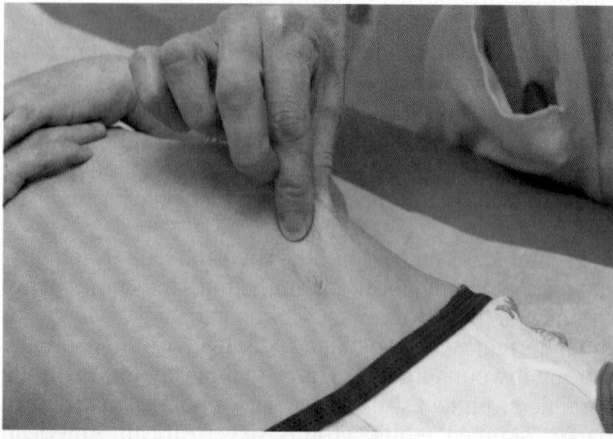

Figure 8-5 To assess skin turgor, the examiner grasps a fold of skin on the child's abdomen and quickly releases it.

immediately returns to place without residual marks has good turgor or adequate hydration. Skin that only slowly returns to place (tents) or retains marks indicates decreased turgor and poor hydration. The presence of edema is determined by pressing the thumb into any area that looks swollen or puffy; if the imprint of the thumb remains, edema is present.

Skin Lesions or Rashes

Carefully inspect all skin lesions or rashes; wear gloves to palpate. Note the location, size, distribution of the lesions over the body, and distinguishing features of the primary or secondary lesion, including color, shape, raised, craterlike or flat, hard or soft if a mass, and exudate (common primary and secondary skin lesions in children and adolescents are described in Chapter 25). Viral, bacterial, and fungal skin infections often have characteristic skin patterns and physical findings that aid in their diagnosis. Using a body diagram to sketch lesions or indicate their distribution is helpful in recording physical findings. Note any warmth or scratch marks. The dermatoglyphics, or skin patterns, of the hands and feet may indicate a genetic condition (e.g., presence of simian crease with trisomy 21).

Hair and Nails

Inspect the scalp for lesions, crusting, or scaling and the hair for distribution, color, texture, amount, and quality. In children, scalp hair is normally shiny, silky, and strong. Unusual hairiness anywhere in the body, hairlines that extend to midforehead, or tufts of hair on the skin over the spine or sacrum represent deviations from normal. Similarly, white locks of hair; loss of hair (alopecia); and dry, brittle hair (suggestive of nutritional deficiency or thyroid disorder) are important clinical findings. In newborns, lanugo (the soft, downy hair that covers the infant) is normal, as is the presence of pubic and axillary hair in the adolescent. White ova (nits) attached to the hair shafts indicate pediculosis.

Assessment of the nails involves inspection for color, shape, and texture. The nails are normally pink, convex, smooth, and hard but flexible. Two significant deviations in nail shape to note are clubbing, in which the base of the nail becomes enlarged and swollen, and spoon nails (koilonychia), in which the nail assumes a concave curve. Clubbing is associated with chronic hypoxia; spoon nails are sometimes noted in a patient with iron-deficiency anemia. Also look for nail biting or picking, pits, grooves, lines, brittleness, or signs of infection or injury. Assessment of hair and nails is also discussed in Chapter 25.

Head and Neck

Observe the head for size, shape, and symmetry from different angles and palpate for signs of fractures or swelling. The shape of a newborn or infant's head can be influenced by unusual positioning in utero, oligohydramnios (deficiency of amniotic fluid), amount of pushing during labor, positioning after birth, genetic disorders, or congenital anomalies. Palpate the suture lines and fontanels of the infant to check for overriding sutures and flat, depressed, or bulging fontanels.

The anterior fontanel measures 4 to 5 cm at its widest, and it normally closes at around age 7 to 18 months. The posterior fontanel may be closed at birth and, if open, should close around age 2 months. If still open at birth, the posterior fontanel should measure less than 1 cm at its widest part. Slight pulsations may be noted when palpating the anterior fontanel. In palpation of the newborn's skull, it may indent and then spring back; this is a normal finding called *craniotabes*.

Note head posture and control in the infant, which is a sign of developmental maturation. By the age of 2 months, slight head lag is present; by 3 to 4 months of age, head lag should be minimal. Head measurements from the most prominent point of the occiput around the head just above the eyebrows and pinna are measured serially until age 24 months and later if there is a concern.

Ask the older child to look up, down, and sideways to assess range of motion, limitations of movement, or pain. Inspect the face for symmetric appearance, proportions, and movement of facial structures. Palpate the sinuses of children and, if warranted, percuss, depending on the stage of sinus development.

The major structures of the neck are the trachea, which is normally midline, and the thyroid, located at the base of the neck. Inspect the neck for symmetry, shape, any swelling, webbing (seen in females with Turner syndrome), or venous distention. Assess for full range of motion. Palpate the trachea with the thumb and index finger on opposite sides to detect any deviations. The thyroid gland is not normally palpable in children. To palpate for an enlarged thyroid, the examiner should stand behind the child and place the fingers over the gland at the base of the neck and then ask the child to swallow. Infants and young children have short necks, making thyroid palpation difficult. Laying the infant or young child supine across the parent's lap may facilitate palpation for an enlarged thyroid.

Eyes

Assessing the eyes requires examining the external and internal structures and testing for visual acuity.

External Structures

Assessment of the external eye involves inspection for position, placement, size, symmetry, color, and movement. The distance between the inner canthi of the eyes determines whether the eyes are wide set (hypertelorism) or close set (hypotelorism); wide- or close-set spacing between the pupils of the eyes can be a normal variant or associated with a genetic condition. There are interpupillary growth curves that can be used to determine the interpupillary distance percentile for age and whether the distance is outside the range of normal. Genetic texts, such as *Smith's Recognizable Patterns of Human Malformation* (Jones, 2005), should be consulted if questions arise about interpupillary distance. (See Chapter 28 for illustrations of eye structures, eye placement, and epicanthal folds.)

Inspect the eyelids when assessing the external structures of the eyes. When the eyelids are open, their placement should be somewhere between the upper border of the iris and the upper border of the pupil. Ptosis refers to lids that droop and cover the pupil; sunset eyes are a condition in which the sclera (the white, opaque covering of the eye) is apparent between the upper lid and the iris. Both ptosis and sunset eyes are abnormal findings. Incorrect positioning of the eyelids includes entropion, lids that roll abnormally inward, and ectropion, lids that roll abnormally outward and expose conjunctiva. Note the palpebral fissures (the opening between the upper and lower eyelids). They should be symmetric, equal in width, and straight across. Slanted palpebral fissures are seen both in children of Asian descent and in children with chromosomal syndromes (e.g., trisomy 21). Inspect the inner canthus of the eye and note any redness or edema.

Note discoloration of the eyelids, change in size such as seen with edema, lesions (e.g., blocked sebaceous glands or salmon patch, as seen in newborns and young infants), and movement problems. Note excessive tearing or discharge. In young infants, inspect for any swelling of the nasolacrimal sac area and, if present, palpate the area for tenderness. The eyebrows are normally symmetric in both shape and movement and do not meet in the midline. Look for any unusual loss of hair. Inspect the eyelashes for outward curve and any debris, nits, or loss of lashes.

Inspect the edges and lining of the eyelids, also known as the *palpebral conjunctiva*, for signs of inflammation (blepharitis) or lesions (stye or chalazion). The palpebral conjunctivae are normally pink and glossy and can be inspected easily by gently pulling the lower lid downward while the child looks up. To inspect the lining of the upper lid, either hold the lashes and pull downward and forward while the child looks down, or roll the upper eyelid over a cotton-tipped applicator. The bulbar conjunctiva is transparent; however, dilation of its blood vessels results in redness (conjunctivitis). An overgrowth of conjunctival tissue (pterygium) can occur, spreading over the cornea.

Inspect the sclera for any changes in coloring, including a yellow tint resulting from jaundice, a bluish tint that may be associated with osteogenesis imperfecta, or black marks that are frequently a normal finding in dark-skinned people or may be associated with an embedded foreign body. The newborn's sclera is usually blue at birth, resulting from the thin choroid, and typically changes to white between 3 and 6 months of age. The pupils should be round, clear, and equal. Inspect them for size, equality, and movement. To test their response to light, darken the room for easier observation and separately shine light directly into the pupil of each eye. The pupils should respond with brisk constriction. The opposite eye should also show a consensual reflex movement (constriction) to the light. To test for accommodation, the child should look at a penlight that is held at a distance and then is quickly brought toward the midline of the child's nose. The normal responses are pupillary constriction and convergence of the axes of the eyes. The pupils should constrict as the object comes near. Normal pupillary findings can be noted as PERRLA: pupils equal, round, react to light, and accommodation.

Note the color, shape, and size of the iris. Lack of coloring (mild-to-complete absence) in the iris and a pinkish glow are seen in albinism. Black-and-white spots on the iris are termed *Brushfield spots* and are noted both in children with trisomy 21 and in normal children. Shapes that deviate from the characteristic roundness of the iris are important findings. A cleft or notch of the outer edge of the iris is termed a *coloboma*. Note any signs of inflammation. The cornea covers the iris and the pupil, and it should be clear and transparent.

Extraocular Muscles

Assessment of extraocular muscle function involves testing for normal range of eye muscle movement and discerning any abnormal movements, such as strabismus and nystagmus. Two key methods to assess extraocular function and binocular vision (using both eyes for vision) are the corneal light reflex test, also known as the *Hirschberg test*, and the cover test.

To test the corneal light reflex, shine a penlight into the eye from a distance of about 16 in. The light should shine symmetrically in the middle of both pupils. An asymmetric corneal light reflex is a sign of strabismus (see Chapter 28).

Investigate any malalignment (unequal or uncentered sites of reflection) for muscle imbalance. A tendency to have strabismus or intermittent crossing of eyes either inward or outward is normal during the first 6 months of life. The cover test can detect either a phoria (tendency to deviate from alignment) or trophia (overt malalignment); perform it at both near and far gazes. While the child is gazing at a near object (13 in.) and then again at a far object (20 ft), one eye is covered and then uncovered. Movement of the uncovered eye indicates malalignment. The examiner should uncover the occluded eye and observe whether the occluded eye moves; normally, the eyes remain fixated. In the alternating cover–uncover test, the occluder is moved from one eye to another while the child is fixating on an object. Movement noted in the eyes during the covering or uncovering is an attempt to reestablish fixation and indicates muscle malalignment (Burns et al., 2012).

Elicit nystagmus, or rapid, oscillating, jerky eye movements, by instructing the child to follow an object held about 12 in. away through the six cardinal fields of gaze (i.e., movements in the left and right lateral, left and right inferior, and left and right lateral superior). A few beats of nystagmus are normal only if present in the far lateral gaze.

Ophthalmoscopic Examination

The ophthalmoscopic examination is a specialized skill that involves practice and a cooperative child. It allows visualization of the interior structures of the eye through the use of light and lenses.

To see the various eye structures, it is best to perform this examination in a darkened room. Examine the child's right eye using the examiner's right eye and right hand and the child's left eye with the examiner using the left eye and left hand. Set the diopter reading at +8 to +2. First, examine the eye from a distance of 10 to 12 in., moving inward at an angle until the child's face is reached and changing the dial of the ophthalmoscope as needed to focus. The pupil reveals a red glow if the lens and cornea are transparent and the retina is normal. In newborns and young infants, the red reflex appears lighter; in darker skinned individuals, the red reflex often appears darker. While slowly moving inward, adjust the diopter setting to see the fundus clearly. If the examiner and the child have normal vision, a reading of 0 diopter results in a sharp focus of the fundus. Moving the diopters compensates for nearsighted or farsighted eyes in the child. If the examiner with normal vision must use red diopter lenses to focus the fundus, the child is nearsighted; if black diopter lenses are needed to focus the fundus, the child is farsighted. If an examiner is myopic and takes off correctives glasses to do the exam, the focusing wheel will have to be adjusted toward the red lenses to correct for the examiner's myopia to see objects clearly.

The optic disk appears creamy white, yellow-orange, to pinkish; is round or oval; and normally has clear margins. In newborns, the disk has a pale appearance. Arteries are smaller and brighter than veins and have a thin stripe of light down the middle. The macula is similar in size to the optic disk and is located to the temporal side of the disk. The macula is somewhat darker than the rest of the fundus. The fovea centralis, the area of almost perfect vision, appears as a tiny, white, glistening dot in the center of the macula and is sensitive to light.

Visual Acuity

Testing for visual acuity in young infants is generally done by testing certain reflexes and attending behaviors. Normal visual milestones are presented in Chapter 3. Test light perception by observing whether the infant blinks and has pupillary constriction in response to a bright light. An examiner should be able to elicit certain attending behaviors in a newborn or infant when an object is placed in the line of vision. These responses are age dependent. At age 3 months, an infant should be able to fixate and attempt to follow an object such as a toy, penlight, or face; by 5 months of age, the infant should follow these targets through all fields of gaze. Commonly used letter or symbol vision tests include the Allen picture cards for children aged 2 to 3 years; use of the LEA Symbols is preferred but the Snellen E chart can be used for children aged 3 to 6 years; and the standard Snellen or Sloan alphabet chart is used as soon as the child knows the alphabet. Instrument-based vision screening—photoscreening or handheld autorefraction—can also be used to test acuity in young children (6 months to 5 years of age) and in those with disabilities who are unable to cooperate with routine vision screening techniques. However, it requires a highly trained clinician and the instrument is expensive.

Color deficiency (or colorblindness) is tested using the Ishihara and Richmond pseudoisochromatic plates (formerly the Hardy-Rand-Ritter plates). Used respectively for school-aged children and preschoolers, these tests ask the child to look at pseudoisochromatic plates and identify the numbers or the symbols hidden by certain confusion colors. Failure to recognize the number or symbol against the color field is diagnostic.

Ears

Assessing the ears requires examining the external and internal structures and testing for hearing acuity.

External Structures

Inspect the external ear first for placement and position. The top of the pinna (cartilaginous portion of the ear) should meet or cross an imaginary horizontal line drawn from the inner eye to the occiput, and the pinna should angle no more than 10 degrees from a line drawn perpendicular from the imaginary horizontal line. Low-set or obliquely set ears are associated with chromosomal disorders and genitourinary abnormalities. Ears are typically extended slightly from the head; however, the newborn's ears are flat against the head. Inspect the mastoid area and palpate behind the ear; redness and swelling of this area and a protruding pinna are associated with mastoiditis.

Inspect the structures of the external ear including the helix, tragus, concha, and lobule for abnormalities in shape or structure; tenderness on movement is abnormal. Note any skin tags, nodules, sinus tracts, or pits in the skin found around the pinna. Note any discharge from the aural canal. Discharge from the external canal can be cerumen (soft, yellow-brown) or a result of external otitis (yellow or greenish discharge).

Internal Structures

The otoscope is used to visualize the canal and internal structures of the middle ear and is held in the inverted position, like a pencil, so that the examiner's little finger rests on the child's head and the otoscope moves with the child. Use the largest speculum that can fit into the ear canal to maximize the visual area. The position in which the child is examined varies with the child's age and ability to stay still. The infant's head often needs to be stabilized, for example, with the mother holding the infant next to her body and the child's head turned to one side and mother's hand stabilizing the head. To straighten the ear canal in children younger than 3 years of age, pull the pinna down and back or out (Fig. 8-6A). For children older than 3 years of age who have undergone anatomic changes, the pinna is pulled up and back to the 10-o'clock position (Fig. 8-6B). Individual variations may require manipulating the earlobe in a slightly different direction than the usual practice. Insert the speculum into the auditory meatus slowly and carefully and inspect the canal. Normally, the canal is pink with small hairs. Note any lesions, discharge, or foreign bodies in the canal.

Inspect the tympanic membrane for color and landmarks. The color is normally translucent, light pearly pink, or gray. Erythema can be a normal finding if the infant or child is crying or has a fever; however, marked erythema is associated with infection (otitis media). Serous otitis media can present as dull yellow or gray. Likewise, bubbles (circles or rings) behind the tympanic membrane indicate the presence of fluid. Perforations leave scarring and an ash-gray color. When assessing landmarks, think of the tympanic membrane as a clock. The cone of light or light reflex is seen around the 5- to 7-o'clock position. The umbo (tip of the malleus) is normally found at the center of the clock and is seen as a small, round, opaque spot. The manubrium (long process of the malleus) is the white line extending from the umbo upward to a knoblike protuberance (the short process of the malleus) around the 1-o'clock position.

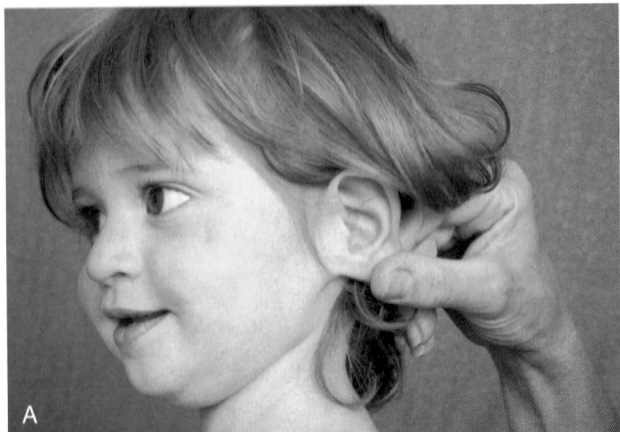

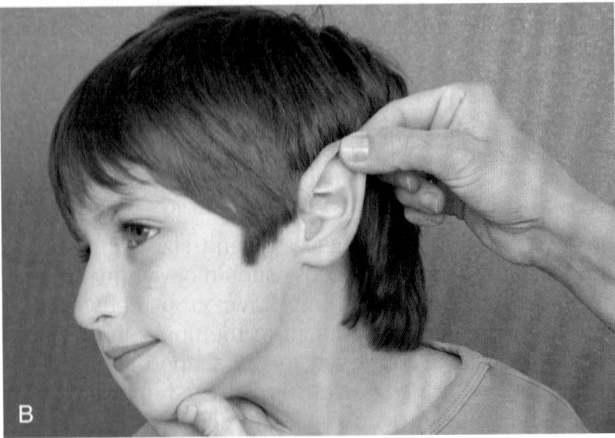

Figure 8-6 Ear examination. (A) In children younger than age 3 years, the pinna is pulled down and back to straighten the ear canal and visualize the tympanic membrane. (B) In children older than age 3 years, the pinna is pulled up and back.

Fluid behind the tympanic membrane causes bulging that distorts or obliterates the appearance of the landmarks. Negative pressure in the middle ear causes retraction of the tympanic membrane with abnormally prominent landmarks.

Compliance or mobility of the tympanic membrane can be evaluated by tympanometry testing or pneumatic otoscopy, which can be used to detect otitis media. During pneumatic otoscopy, the examiner exerts pressure against the tympanic membrane by creating a seal with the speculum and using a bulb attachment to puff air into the canal (Fig. 8-7). It is normal for the tympanic membrane to move when this is done. A tympanometer can be used to measure movement of the tympanic membrane by applying -400 to $+100$ mm H_2O pressure to the ear canal. The tympanogram reading provides valuable information. Tympanometry testing is not done in infants younger than 7 months of age because of hypercompliant ear canal.

Hearing Acuity

An assessment of hearing acuity can be performed by play audiometry in specialized settings or by audiometry using earphones in children aged 4 years and older. Other more sophisticated tests, such as evoked otoacoustic emissions and brain stem auditory-evoked response, may be performed for an infant or a child at

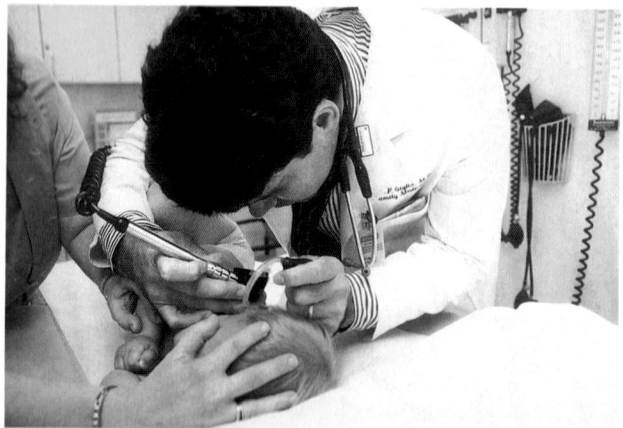

Figure 8-7 A pneumatic otoscope is used to evaluate mobility of the tympanic membrane. Note the mother helping to restrain and position the infant.

TABLE 8-4	Guide to Tonsillar Size
Scale	**Tonsillar Position**
I+	Just visible
2+	Halfway between the tonsillar pillars and the uvula
3+	Touching the uvula
4+	Touching each other

risk for hearing loss (see Chapter 28 for further information about auditory testing).

Face and Nose

Observe the face for symmetry, spacing, size of structures, and facial expression. The nose should be symmetric and midline to an imaginary line drawn from between the eyes to the center of the notch in the upper lip. Genetic differences can be observed in the shape of the bridge of the nose with a characteristic flattened appearance in Asian and some African American children. Inspect the external nares for patency, discharge, flaring, horizontal nasal creases, and any lesions. To check for patency in newborns, block one nostril and at the same time close the infant's mouth; observe whether the infant continues to breathe smoothly. Use a penlight or an otoscope to visualize the internal nasal cavity by pushing the tip of the child's nose upward while the neck is tilted backward.

For a closer inspection of the mucous lining of the inferior and middle turbinates, insert a nasal speculum gently into each nostril. Note the color, consistency, and integrity of the nasal membranes and septum as well as the septal alignment. The mucosa is normally pink, and the septum should be midline. Mucosal membranes that are pale, grayish, boggy (spongy texture; as seen with allergic rhinitis), bright red (which may be seen with upper respiratory infection, or nasal medications and substance abuse), or excoriated (digital injury as in nose-picking and snorted substance abuse) are noteworthy.

Note the amount, color, and texture of any nasal discharge. Watery discharge associated with crying is normal. In contrast, a thin, clear discharge is seen with allergies and sinusitis (either clear or mucopurulent rhinorrhea). Purulent discharge indicates either a viral or a bacterial infectious process. The finding of unilateral nasal discharge is significant as is the presence of polyps (soft overgrowths of gray mucosa).

Mouth and Throat

Assessment of the mouth and throat begins at the lips. They should be pink, firm, symmetric, and moist, with no lesions or excoriations. A thin upper lip (thin vermilion border) with a hypoplastic long or smooth philtrum is associated with fetal alcohol syndrome (see Fig. 14-12). The buccal mucosa, gingivae, tongue, and palate are normally pink, firm, smooth, glistening, and moist. However, the normal appearance of the gums, tongue margins, and buccal cavity may be a bluish color in African American children. Note the presence of texture changes, increased size (hyperplasia), furrows in or limited movement of the tongue, or any unusual odor (halitosis). Palpate for notches, clefts, or unusual arches in the hard palate. Any lesions, swelling, excoriations, or bleeding in these structures is abnormal. If the tip of the tongue cannot touch the roof of the mouth, the child has a tight frenulum, which is rare. While observing the teeth, one can assess for number; hygiene; and the presence of malocclusion, caries, or staining (see Fig. 3-21). The uvula should be midline and move upward when a gag reflex is elicited.

The tonsils normally undergo hypertrophy during early childhood, followed by gradual shrinkage beginning around age 10 years. The tonsils are normally the same color as the surrounding buccal mucosa and often have crypts on their surface (see Chapter 16). Increased redness or tonsillar exudate indicates infection. Table 8-4 provides a guide for assessing tonsil size.

The use of a tongue blade to view the oral cavity is helpful if a clear view of the buccal mucosa is not obtained. The tongue blade can be slipped between the inner cheeks and the gumline. If the child is frightened by the tongue blade, an examiner can obtain a clear view of the back of the mouth in other ways. For the infant or young child, inspect the mouth when the child cries. Tilting the young child's head backward and asking the child to say "ahhh" often enables a clear view of the tonsils, uvula, and oropharynx.

ALERT   *Never insert a tongue blade in the mouth of a child who exhibits signs or symptoms of epiglottitis because this may cause respiratory arrest.*

Thorax and Lungs

Begin assessment of the thorax and lungs with inspection of chest configuration, movement, and symmetry. Record any abnormalities such as unusual roundness (barrel shape), protuberant or depressed sternum, unusual knobbing of the rib cage, or asymmetric movement including retractions and their locations above the clavicles, suprasternal, substernal, and/or intercostal areas (Fig. 8-8). The abdomen and chest should move together in a synchronous fashion, but chest movement

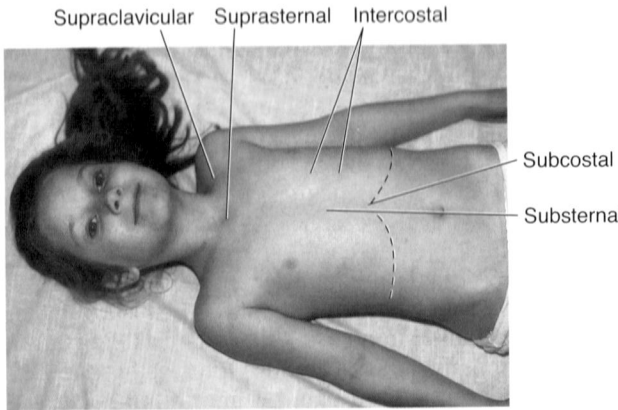

Figure 8-8 Possible sites of retractions.

associated with breathing varies with age. Abdominal or diaphragmatic breathing is characteristic of young children. In children older than 7 years of age, particularly females, thoracic respirations are predominant.

Note the rate, depth, quality, and regularity of respiration as well as the ratio of the inspiratory to expiratory phase of breathing. Respiratory rate is influenced by age and disease status.

Listen for audible signs of impaired respiratory efforts, such as stridor, barky or staccato cough, audible wheeze, snoring, or grunting. Palpate the chest for tactile fremitus (a vibratory sensation). Percussion can be helpful in the older child to determine dullness, resonance, or tympany because it can sometimes provide additional information. However, auscultation of the lungs is always necessary for evaluating the child's respiratory status. Use the diaphragm of the stethoscope to auscultate the lung fields (front, back, and axillary areas) by systematically and symmetrically (comparing one side with another) listening for breath sounds as the child takes a deep breath in and blows out. Pretending to blow out the light of an otoscope or penlight is a useful game that encourages deep breathing in younger children.

Breath sounds are classified as vesicular, bronchovesicular, or bronchotubular depending on the sound's loudness and duration during inspiration versus expiration. These breath sounds are normally heard in a distinct area of the chest but become abnormal findings when absent or heard in noncharacteristic locations. See Table 8-5 for characteristics of normal breath sounds. Atypical sounds include crackles or rales (discontinuous, soft popping, or interrupted explosive sounds), which can be coarse, medium, or fine; rhonchi (continuous snoring or low-pitched sound);

friction rubs; or wheezing (continuous, musical, high-pitched sound) (see Focused Physical Assessment 16-2). Absent or diminished breath sounds in any area are also pathologic and indicate obstruction.

caREminder

In infants and young children, lack of subcutaneous fat and smaller distances between structures may make breath sounds readily transmitted across lung fields. Keep this in mind when assessing the presence, location, and nature of breath sounds in infants and young children. To detect transmitted sounds from the upper airways, place the diaphragm next to the child's mouth or nose to determine whether what is heard in the lung fields is just like the sound as heard near the mouth or nose. Referred sounds are loudest near their origin.

Cardiovascular System

Observe the child for signs of cyanosis, edema (peripheral, sacral, or periorbital), mottled skin, clubbing of the nail bed, distended neck veins, or squatting posture because these can all be signs of cardiovascular malfunction. Inspection of the chest in infants and young children with thin chest walls often reveals a cardiac pulsation—the apical impulse (AI), which is generally the point of maximal impulse (PMI)—which is a normal finding. In contrast, any visible pulsation of the chest caused by a heave or lift of the ventricle, a sustained forceful thrusting of the ventricles during systole, is an abnormal finding. Use the fingers to determine the AI, the apex beat, or the PMI (area of most intense pulsation, which may or may not be the AI).

The location of the apical pulse or PMI varies with age. In children younger than age 7 years, the PMI is found in the fourth intercostal space. For children younger than 4 years of age, the PMI is to the left of the midclavicular line (MCL) and is midclavicular between ages 4 and 6 years. In children older than 7 years of age, it is located to the right of the MCL and is found in the fifth intercostal space (Fig. 8-9).

Use the ball of the hand to palpate for the presence of a thrill, a vibratory sensation that feels like the belly of a purring cat. Thrills are pathologic findings. Use the fingertips to detect pulsations on the chest. Percussion of the heart has limited usefulness in the examination of children because of their small chest wall size and aversion to the chest being percussed.

TABLE 8-5	Characteristics of Normal Breath Sounds		
Sound	Quality	Relationship of Inspiration (I) to Expiration (E)	Normal Location
Vesicular	Soft, swishing	I is longer, louder, and higher pitched than E (I > E)	Throughout lung field
Bronchovesicular	Louder and higher pitched than vesicular; mixed	I and E are equal (I = E)	Over manubrium and upper intrascapular region where trachea and bronchi bifurcate
Bronchotubular	Tubular, harsh, hollow	I is short; E is long (I < E)	Over trachea

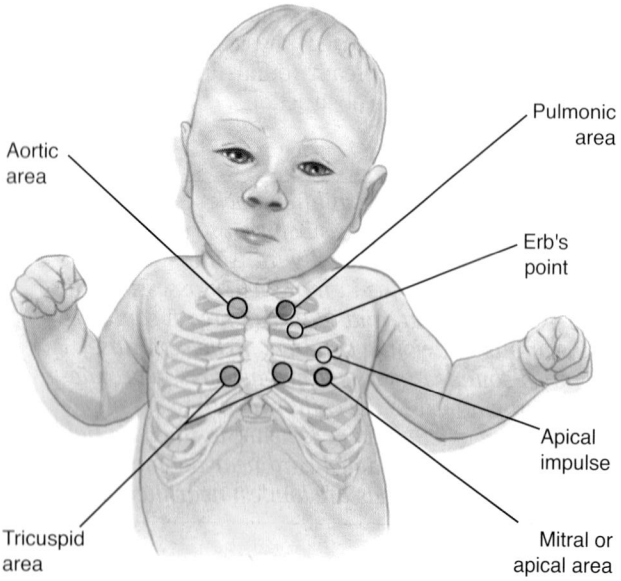

Figure 8-9 Location of the AI in a child younger than age 7 years and normal locations of heart sounds.

Heart Sounds

Auscultation of heart sounds is an essential assessment skill when examining the cardiovascular system. Heart sounds are produced by the opening and closing of the valves and by vibrations of blood against the walls of the heart and its vessels. Table 8-6 lists the sites of cardiac auscultation and provides descriptions of various heart sounds. Use the stethoscope's bell to detect low-pitched heart sounds; use the diaphragm to detect high-pitched heart sounds.

Begin auscultation at the second right intercostal area, where the closure of the aortic valve is best heard. Move to the second left intercostal space to best hear the sound of the pulmonic valve closing. Because the second heart sound (S_2) represents closure of both the aortic and pulmonic valves together, the aortic and pulmonic areas are the sites where the S_2 is heard loudest. The sound made by the closing of these two valves can sometimes be heard as a split sound during inspiration. A normal physiologic split sound of S_2 can often be heard in the pulmonic area. The aortic valve closes slightly before the pulmonic valve; the sound made by the closure of the aortic valve is normally louder than the pulmonic sound. Inspiration affects the timing of these two valve closures. Therefore, a normal

physiologic split is accentuated with inspiration and fades out with expiration. A fixed split S_2 that does not vary with respiration is abnormal.

Next, while carefully listening, inch down the left sternum to Erb's point at the second and third left intercostal spaces close to the sternum. Here, S_1 and S_2 are of equal intensity. S_1 is heard loudest at the tricuspid and mitral or apical areas. The tricuspid area is at the fifth right and left intercostal spaces close to the sternum and represents the area where closure of the tricuspid valve is best heard. The mitral area is located at the third to fourth intercostal space and lateral to the left MCL in infants and at the fifth intercostal space left MCL in children around age 7 years. Mitral valve closure is heard best at the mitral area.

Two additional heart sounds, S_3 and S_4, warrant consideration. S_3 is a normal sound produced by vibrations during ventricular filling. It is often a difficult sound for unskilled examiners to detect. S_4, although an abnormal sound in older adults, can be a normal finding in some children and young adults. S_3 and S_4 are best auscultated with the infant or child lying on his or her left side.

When listening to the heart, evaluate the rate, rhythm, quality, and intensity of the heart sounds. S_1 and S_2 should be clear and distinct sounds. In addition, their intensity should be consistent with expectations at a particular auscultatory site. The rate should be synchronous with the radial pulse and consistent with the norms for cardiac rate by age of the infant or child. Fever, exercise, and anemia increase cardiac rate and the S_1 intensity.

caREminder

Many young children have periods of sinus arrhythmia in which the heart rate increases with inspiration and decreases with expiration. This common finding is considered a variant of normal if the arrhythmia disappears during breath holding.

Murmurs

Murmurs are blowing or swooshing sounds caused by turbulent blood flow in the chambers of the heart or its vessel. Infants and children often have innocent or functional murmurs that must be differentiated from serious organic murmurs. Innocent murmurs are frequently heard in young children and are nonpathologic. A child's thin chest wall is believed to transmit these sounds easily. Functional murmurs are caused by conditions

TABLE 8-6 Differentiation of Heart Sounds by Site, Location, and Characteristics

Cardiac Auscultatory Site	Location	Characteristics
Aortic area	Second right intercostal space	S_2 heard louder than S_1; S_2 is "dubb" sound
Pulmonic area	Second left intercostal space	S_2 split heard best
Erb's point	Second and third intercostal space	S_1 and S_2 equal loudness; common site of innocent murmurs
Tricuspid area	Fifth right and left intercostal space	S_1 heard as louder sound than S_2; S_1 is "lubb" sound
Mitral or apical area	Third to fourth intercostal space and lateral to the left MCL (in infants); fifth intercostal space, left MCL (around age 7 years)	S_1 heard loudest; S_1 is synchronous with carotid pulse

TABLE 8-7 Grading Scale for Classification of Heart Murmurs by Intensity

Grade	Characteristics
I	Soft and difficult to hear
II	Soft but easily heard
III	Loud; no associated thrill
IV	Loud with an associated thrill
V	Loud and audible with edge of the stethoscope; thrill present
VI	Very loud and heard with stethoscope off the chest; thrill present

CHART 8-3 Characteristics of Innocent Heart Murmurs

- Soft sounding
- Short duration
- Occurring during systole
- Vibratory and of medium pitch
- Heard best at the left lower sternal or midsternal border
- No radiating
- Not associated with physical findings of cardiac pathology

such as fever and anemia that lead to increased blood turbulence. When these conditions are corrected, the murmur disappears. Organic murmurs are associated with pathology of the chambers, valves, or vessels.

When a murmur is detected, note the following information:

- *Location:* where it is heard the best and whether it is heard in other auscultatory areas (i.e., Does it radiate? To where?)
- *Timing:* when the murmur occurs—during S_1, which represents ventricular systole; during S_2, which represents diastole; or throughout the entire cardiac cycle
- *Intensity:* soft, loud, very loud (Table 8-7 provides a grading scale)
- *Pitch:* low, medium, or high

- *Variation with position:* heard when sitting, standing, supine, or squatting
- *Quality:* describe the sound using terms such as *musical*, *blowing*, *harsh*, or *rumbling*

Innocent murmurs of childhood differ from pathologic murmurs (Chart 8-3; Table 8-8). Auscultate with the child in at least two positions—supine, sitting, or lying on the left side—and use both the bell and diaphragm of the stethoscope. Innocent murmurs often disappear with a change of position.

Vasculature

Assessment of the vascular system involves palpation of the peripheral arteries for equality, rate, and rhythm. Palpate the radial, femoral, popliteal, and dorsalis pedis pulses to determine blood flow for vascular integrity. To assess these pulses in infants, move from lighter to

TABLE 8-8 Location and Characteristics of Benign Heart Murmurs in Children

Typical Age	Name	Description and Location	Comments
Newborn	Closing ductus	Transient, soft, ejection Upper left sternal border	Closes functionally at birth, structurally within about 7 days of age
Common in newborns to 1 year of age	Peripheral pulmonary flow murmur (or neonatal peripheral pulmonary stenosis [PPS])	Gr I–II/VI Soft, midcycle, ejectile, systolic To left of upper left sternal border and in lung fields and axillae	Especially heard in preterm infants Disappears at about 6 months of age
Common in children 2–6 years of age	Still murmur	Gr I–III/VI, musical, vibratory Early and midsystolic Mid/lower left sternal border	Can occur in infants to adolescents From blood flowing across aortic valve Decreased intensity when standing Frequently also a carotid bruit Heard with fever or anemia
Common in children 2–8 years of age	Venous hum	Gr I–II/VI Soft, hollow, continuous Louder in upright position Under clavicle Does not radiate	Can occur at any age but more common in this age Can be eliminated by maneuvers
Normal in infants and children younger than age 6 years	Carotid bruit	Gr I–III/VI Systolic ejection; musical Neck over the carotid artery	Soft, high-pitched sound
Typically in children 8–14 years of age	Pulmonary flow murmur	Gr I– II/VI Rough quality Early to midsystolic Upper left sternal border Normal P2	Can occur at any age but more common in adolescents with thin chest walls Softer in upright position; decrease/disappear with Valsalva maneuver

Gr, grades; P2, pulmonic second sound.

deeper palpation as necessary; use one or two fingers for the femoral pulses midway between the iliac crest and the symphysis pubis. Flexing the knee is helpful in palpating the popliteal pulse. Palpate for the dorsalis pedis along the upper medial aspect of the foot (Fig. 8-10).

Breasts

As part of the assessment of the thorax, after assessing the lungs and cardiovascular systems, assess the breasts. Observe the position of the nipples and note the presence and location of any supernumerary nipples. Identify and record the Tanner stage of female breast development as a measure of the acquisition of secondary sexual characteristics. Transitory breast enlargement in neonates is common and is caused by a maternal hormone effect. Gynecomastia in young children and male teenagers needs evaluation. Palpate the breasts

for masses. If masses are felt, note their location, size, shape, consistency, and mobility along with whether they are discrete masses or tender to the touch.

Teach adolescent females how to properly conduct monthly breast self-examination (BSE). The American Cancer Society recommends that women begin monthly BSE at age 20. The American Cancer Society has educational materials on BSE available for distribution by calling their local 1-800 phone number.

Abdomen

Begin the abdominal assessment by inspecting the contour and the skin covering the abdomen, generally while the child is in the supine position or resting flat in the parent's lap. Look for any unusual shapes, asymmetry, or tenseness that could denote organomegaly, ascites, inguinal or femoral bulging, malnutrition, or tumor.

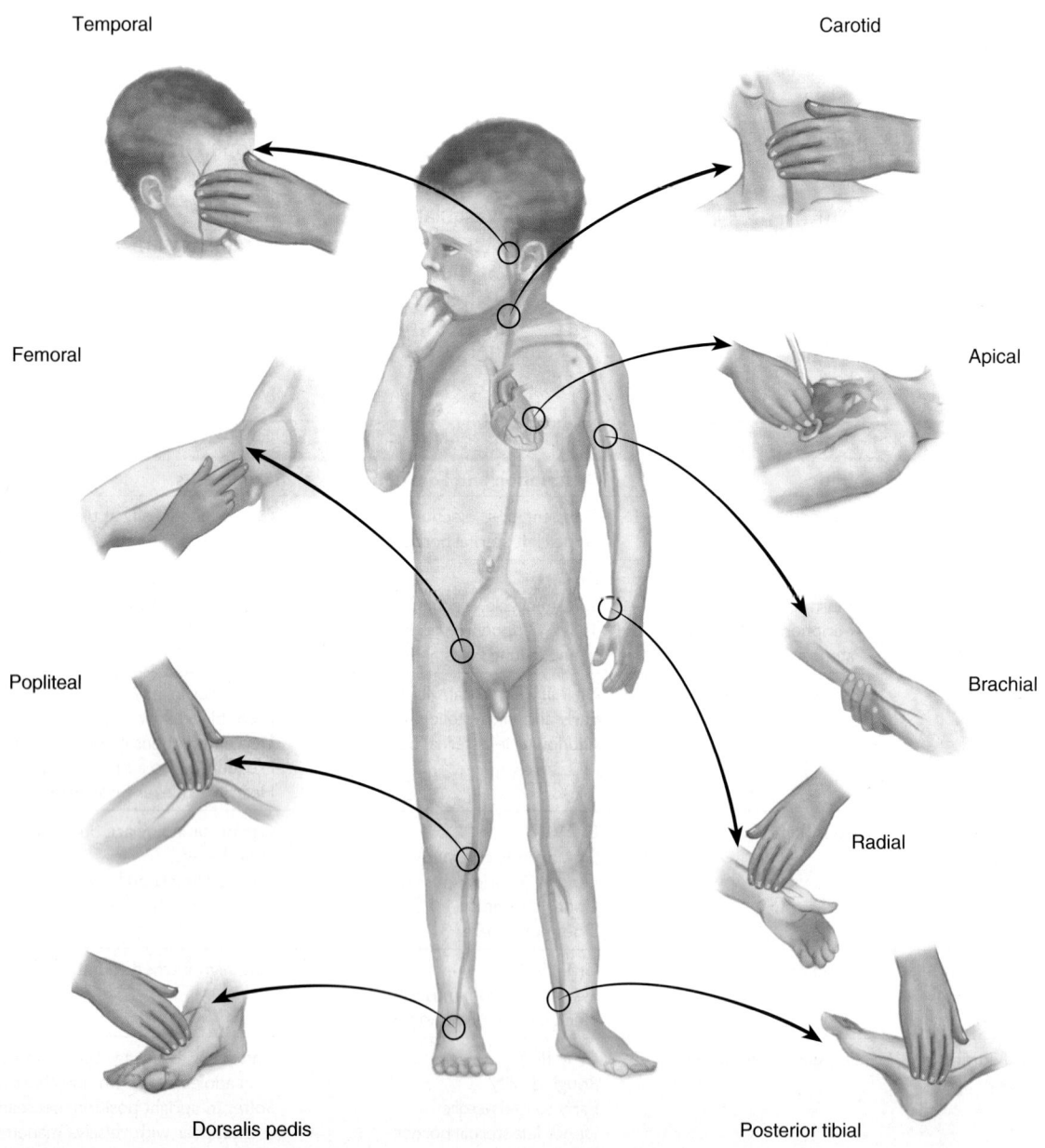

Temporal

Carotid

Femoral

Apical

Popliteal

Brachial

Radial

Dorsalis pedis

Posterior tibial

Figure 8-10 Locations of peripheral pulses.

A potbellied or prominent abdomen is a normal characteristic of infants and children until puberty. Note skin markings such as distended veins, striae, or bruises. Detection of unusual movements (e.g., peristaltic waves or abdominal respirations in children younger than age 7 years, or pulsations) can indicate gastrointestinal or pulmonary problems. In newborns and young children, inspect the umbilicus for discharge, fistulas, or signs of inflammation and palpate for herniation. Note any midline protrusion from the xiphoid process to the umbilicus as an indication of diastasis recti abdominis.

Next, perform auscultation of the abdomen for bowel sounds or bruits (murmurs) in a systematic fashion by firmly pressing the stethoscope and listening to all four (right and left, upper and lower) quadrants of the abdomen. Normally, bowel sounds are heard every 10 to 30 seconds and indicate peristaltic movement. Various pitches and frequencies of bowel sounds can indicate problems such as diarrhea or obstruction (heard as high-pitched, tinkling sounds); absent bowel sounds may indicate that peristalsis is not occurring.

caREminder

Always listen for bowel sounds before palpation to determine what the baseline sounds are because palpation can stimulate peristalsis. Gently stroking the abdomen with one's fingers can help elicit bowel sounds. Listen for at least 5 minutes before determining that bowel sounds are absent or not heard.

Because of the small size of a young child's abdomen, percussion to determine areas of dullness, flatness, or tympany has limited clinical usefulness, but it can assist the examiner in assessing for liver enlargement.

Finally, palpate the abdomen, ensuring that hands and fingers are warm. Both superficial and deep palpations are useful in assessing pain and abnormal enlargement (organomegaly) or determining the presence of a mass. With a crying infant, put one hand behind the infant's legs and bend them at the knees while at the same time gently palpating the abdomen with the index finger of the other hand when the infant exhales with each cry. Check for tenting of the abdominal skin by pinching the skin together to see if it forms a fold; tenting indicates severe dehydration.

If a child complains of abdominal pain, always palpate the area of identified pain last. Perform deep palpation by either placing one hand on top of the other or by placing one hand to support the child's corresponding back structures and using the other hand to palpate the anterior structures.

If an inflamed appendix is suspected, identify pain resulting from peritoneal irritation in the appendix region by performing the following tests with the child in a supine position: the iliopsoas, obturator, and Rovsing sign (rebound tenderness). The iliopsoas test is performed by pushing down on the child's lower thigh as the child raises his or her leg. Look for the obturator sign by picking up the child's ankle in one hand and holding the knee with the opposite hand while flexing the hip and knee

90 degrees and rotating the leg internally and externally. If either elicits pain, it suggests irritation of the respective muscle, psoas, or obturator by the inflamed appendix. To test for Rovsing sign, press deeply and evenly in the left lower quadrant and quickly withdraw pressure. If pain is elicited in the right lower quadrant during left-sided pressure or with quick release of pressure, the test is positive. In addition to these three tests, ask the older child to jump up and down to elicit whether there is peritoneal irritation; a child with appendicitis typically jumps only once and stops because of pain.

 KidKare To help with young children who are ticklish, ask them to bend their knees to relax the abdominal muscles and distract them by having them tell a story.

To palpate the liver, start in the right lower quadrant by using two to three fingers and work up. In infants and young children, the liver edge is often palpable 1 to 2 cm below the right costal margin and feels firm and smooth. The tip of the spleen is sometimes palpable during inspiration in infants and young children as a soft, thumb-shaped mass about 1 to 2 cm below the left costal margin. Any enlargement greater than 2 cm is abnormal and needs referral. Kidneys are normally difficult to palpate beyond the neonatal period unless enlarged. Sometimes, the tip of the right kidney can be a normal finding in the neonate. Palpate for a femoral hernia by placing the index finger on the femoral pulse and the middle and ring fingers just medially on the skin over the area where a femoral hernia occurs. To check for an inguinal hernia in a young male child, the examiner's smallest finger should be gently slid into the external inguinal canal at the base of each testicle while asking the child to cough or laugh to determine whether bowel is present.

Lymphatic System

Assessment of the lymphatic system involves palpation with the fingertips in a gentle but firm circular motion to detect lymph node enlargement (Fig. 8-11). If enlarged lymph nodes are felt, note their size, color of the overlying skin, location, temperature, consistency, mobility, and whether tenderness is present. Assess for nodes in the areas anterior and posterior to the sternocleidomastoid muscle by having the child's head bent slightly forward and turned toward the side being examined while sliding one's fingers against this muscle. Palpate the preauricular, mastoid, submandibular, and supraclavicular areas. To assess for the presence of axillary nodes, hold the child's arm in a slightly abducted position at the sides while palpating this area. For the inguinal area, the child should be in a supine position. Refer back to the abdominal section for assessment of the spleen.

External Genitalia

Assess the external genitalia using a matter-of-fact manner, with respect for issues of privacy and modesty. This is particularly important when examining an adolescent. Note assessment of sexual maturation using Tanner staging of sexual development for males and females as outlined in Chapter 3.

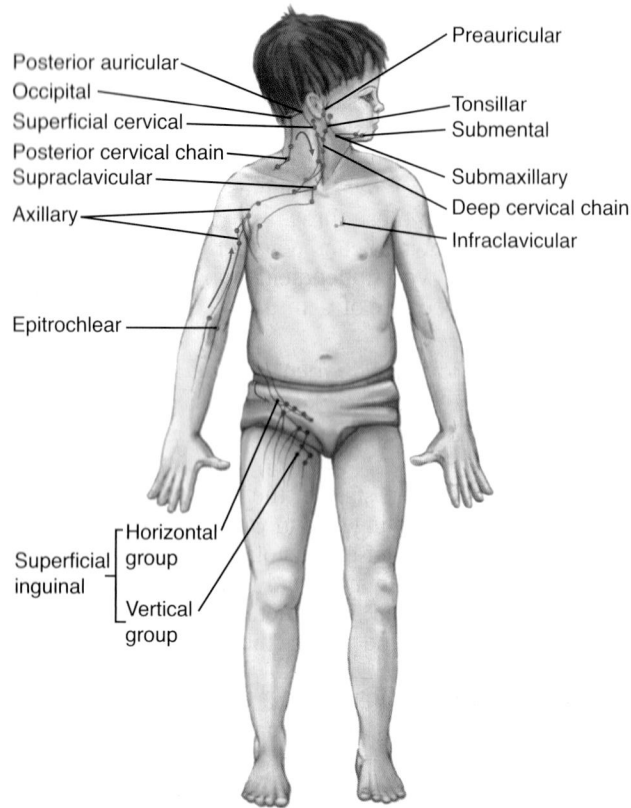

Figure 8-11 Superficial lymph nodes and lymph drainage.

KidKare Tell the child that you need to look at his or her genital area as part of the examination. Starting around age 2 to 3 years, give a brief explanation to the child that indicates the purpose of the examination (e.g., making sure the whole body is healthy, or that everything is fine with his or her private parts). Before beginning the examination, ask the parent to tell his or her child that "to know that all is fine or to see if there is a problem, it is OK for the nurse to touch your private parts." The wording of this explanation will vary depending on the presenting problem and age of the child.

Male Genitalia

To assess the male genitalia, inspect the penis for size, color, masses, and the presence of any skin lesions or discharge. Note whether the child is circumcised and, if not, whether the foreskin retracts easily. The foreskin is normally adherent in infants and young males until approximately age 3 years.

ALERT *Never forcefully retract the foreskin. This can cause paraphimosis (where the foreskin cannot be returned back over the tip of the penis and may impair blood drainage) or lead to phimosis later in life.*

Inspect the meatus for shape (slitlike), placement, and whether ulceration or discharge is present. If pubic hair is present, describe its distribution, quantity, and quality using Tanner staging. Pubic lice or nits are a significant finding. The strength and steadiness of the urinary stream are important to assess if there are questions about obstruction of flow. Also, ballooning of the foreskin in an uncircumcised male with voiding is associated with significant phimosis and should be referred to a urologist.

Inspect the scrotal sac for color, size, and symmetry and presence of rugae, masses, and lesions. The left scrotum commonly hangs lower than the right. To palpate the testes in an infant or young male, hold the thumb and index finger of one hand over the inguinal canal area to prevent the testes from retracting (the cremasteric reflex) while at the same time palpating with the other hand (Fig. 8-12). If the testes cannot be felt, have the child sit cross-legged or stand and palpate again. If they still cannot be felt, feel the inguinal canal and, if the testes are present there, try to milk them down the canal and into the sac. Cold, excitement, touch, and stimulation can stimulate the cremasteric reflex, causing the testes to ascend temporarily. Normally, the testes are smooth, equal in size, and oval; the size of the testes depends on the stage of sexual development. Note any masses, swelling, tenderness, or asymmetry and, if present, refer to a physician or nurse practitioner. Teach adolescent males how to perform testicular self-examination.

Female Genitalia

Inspection of the external female genitalia requires that the examiner be able to view the external genitalia and the vestibule (the area between the labia minora). Wear gloves and place the child's legs in a frog-leg (soles of the feet touching) position. The adolescent female may be more comfortable if her legs are placed in stirrups. The appearance of the external genitalia depends on the child's stage of sexual maturation. Observe the labia majora, labia minora, and the clitoris area for size, color, skin lesions, and masses. Note the presence of pubic hair and the appropriate Tanner stage. Refer a

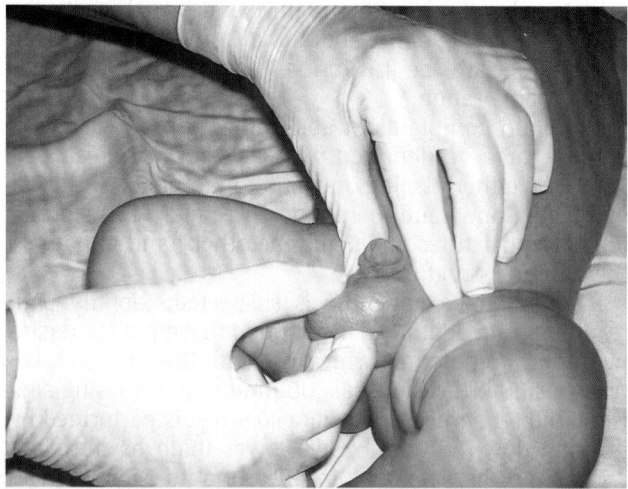

Figure 8-12 To palpate the testes in a young male, the examiner blocks the inguinal canal to prevent the testes from retracting into it.

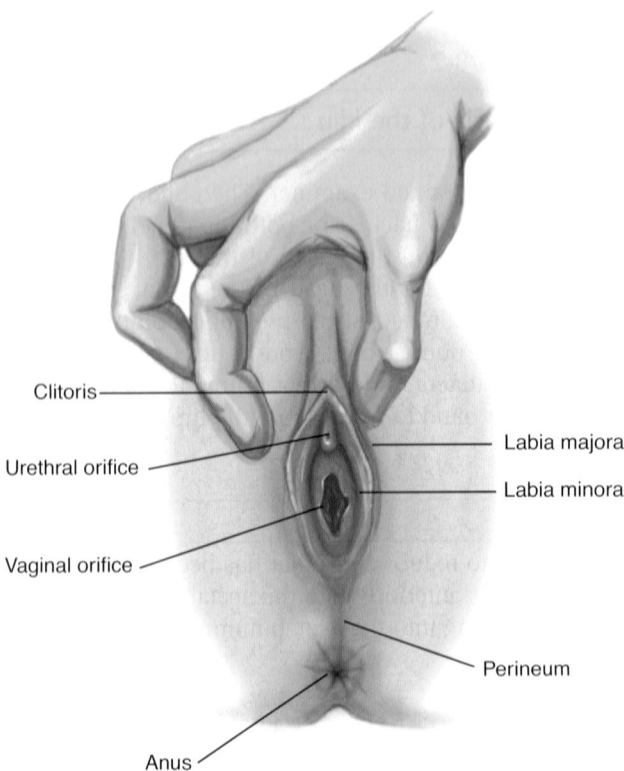

Clitoris

Urethral orifice

Vaginal orifice

Labia majora

Labia minora

Perineum

Anus

Figure 8-13 Normal female genitalia.

child with pubic hair before age 8 years for an endocrinologic evaluation.

Gentle upward and lateral traction of the labia majora allows a thorough inspection of the vestibule area, including the urethral meatus, vaginal opening, and hymen as well as the fossa and posterior fourchette (Fig. 8-13). Note any unusual redness, discharge, edema, scarring, tears, or lesions. The female genitalia is responsive to estrogen. Maternal estrogen is responsible for the redundant hymen and prominent labia seen in the young infant. Likewise, the effect of endogenous estrogen during puberty again changes the appearance of the labia and the hymenal tissue (which becomes flowery and pale pink).

Ambiguous genitalia and fused labia in infants are abnormal findings and indicate significant pathology. Minor labial adhesions are a common problem seen in young children and are treated only if there is interference with urinary or vaginal drainage. Treatment consists of application of estrogen-containing cream and good hygiene until separation occurs, followed by long-term use of petrolatum to the area. The speculum examination requires special training and is not discussed in this textbook.

Anus

Although the anus is a part of the gastrointestinal system, it is inspected while examining the external genitalia. Inspection of the anus can be performed in the supine position with the child's legs up and knees bent or in the knee–chest, prone, or side-lying recumbent position depending on the age of the child. Observe the anus for tone by scratching the anal area and noticing

the "wink" response (anal reflex). Note any unusual laxity that is not associated with the presence of stool in the ampulla. Gentle traction allows for a closer view of the anal folds or rugae, which should have a wrinkled appearance. Record the location of anal tags, scars, fissures, hemorrhoids, or lesions. Also note perianal rashes, hyperpigmentation, or rectal prolapse.

Musculoskeletal System

The musculoskeletal system is subject to tremendous changes from infancy through adolescence. For example, joint range of motion changes with age. The normal arc of motion is greatest in infancy and declines as the child matures. Therefore, the examiner must be familiar with normal physiologic findings seen in the musculoskeletal system throughout the child's development.

Assessment involves observing the infant for general body configuration and spontaneous and symmetric movements of the extremities. Position will vary (supine, prone, standing with support) depending on which section of the musculoskeletal system is being examined. Inspect the back and the neck for full range of motion. Look for obvious deformities or any unusual findings, such as a sacral dimple, extra digit, metatarsus adductus, or congenital torticollis. Palpate the clavicles, limbs, back, and neck for signs of tenderness, swelling, masses, or deformities; assess range of motion in all joints. Assess muscle strength by picking up the infant with hands under the infant's axillae. Normal infants wedge their body against the examiner's hands. Evaluate the hips for developmental dysplasia of the hip by determining the presence of key positive signs. The two techniques that are used to identify hip joint instability in newborns and young infants are the Ortolani and Barlow maneuvers (Nursing Interventions 8-2).

> **ALERT** *Never repeatedly manipulate a hip that is reducible or able to be dislocated. Doing so may cause vascular compromise.*

As the infant matures and acquires greater musculoskeletal skills and control, additional features are included in the examination. It is important to ensure that clothing does not obstruct the examiner's view and the child is not wearing shoes, which can interfere with gait analysis and assessment for limb length discrepancy. The child should wear only underwear at this point in the examination.

To begin, observe the standing child from the front, back, and side to assess body configuration, posture, symmetry, and proportions and to detect any physical deformities. Have the child walk slowly, without shoes, away from and then toward the nurse, and then walk on his or her heels and toes. Assess for gait asymmetry, irregularity, or weakness such as occurs in lower limb discrepancy or cerebral palsy. The gait of a young child is normally wide spaced but is symmetric. In contrast, a painful (antalgic) gait has a shortened stance phase, and a child with intoeing walks with one foot or both turned inward.

NURSING INTERVENTIONS 8-2

Assessment for Developmental Dysplasia of the Hip

Manual examination of an infant hip should only be performed by a trained examiner. The child should be lying supine and as relaxed as possible. Allowing the infant to suck on a pacifier or bottle may help to keep the child calm. Stand at the foot of the infant. First, place your thumbs on the inside of the infant's thighs. Place the middle finger down the outside of the infant's thigh, feeling for the head of the femur with the fingers. The hip and knee should be flexed. Both hips are grasped simultaneously to provide stability for the examination, but each should be examined independently. When in doubt about what is felt, stabilize the infant's pelvis with the thumb of one hand over the pelvis and the fingers under the sacrum. To examine an infant's left hip, use the left hand to stabilize the pelvis and the right hand to manipulate the hip. The reverse is done for the right hip.

Technique	Positive Findings in the Neonatal Period
Ortolani maneuver	To perform this maneuver, which attempts to reduce a hip that has been dislocated, abduct the hip and lift the head of the femur anteriorly into the acetabulum. If the hip is reducible, it may be felt or heard moving into the acetabulum. The examiner feels a palpable "clunk."

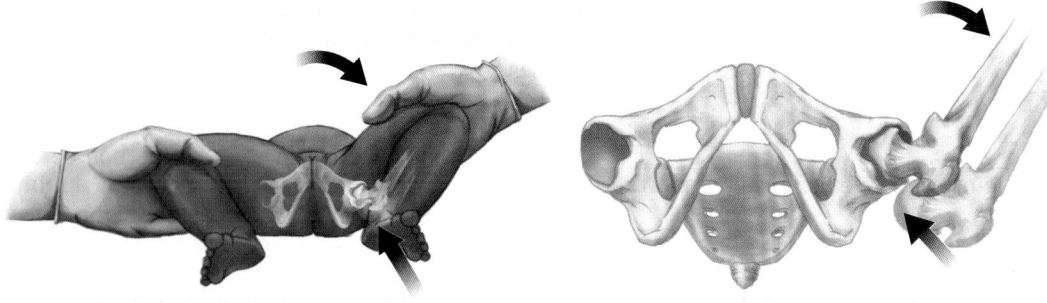

Barlow maneuver	To perform this maneuver, which attempts to dislocate an unstable hip, adduct the hip (bring 10–20 degrees past midline) and apply a gentle posterior force with the palm to the knee. If the hip is able to be dislocated, it can usually be felt slipping out of the acetabulum.

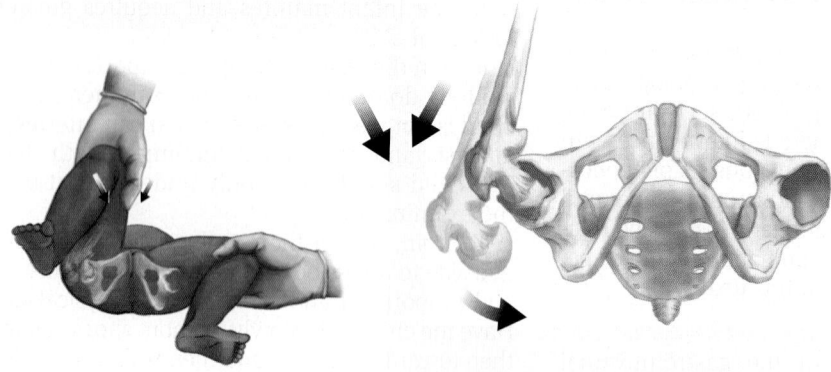

Technique	Positive Findings in the Neonatal Period
Abduction	Limited abduction of the hips

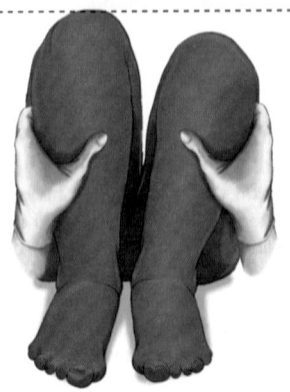

Allis sign   Compare leg lengths by placing the infant in the supine position, flex them at the knees, and compare their heights.

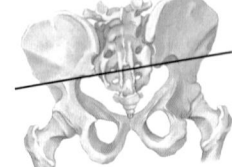

Trendelenburg gait   When the child bears weight on the dislocated side, the unaffected side of the pelvis drops.

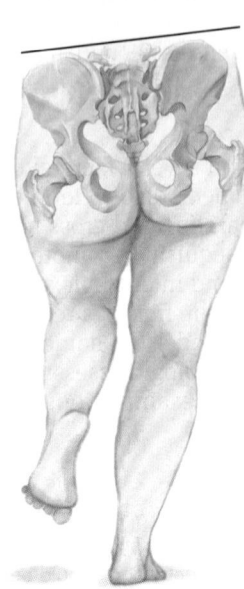

After observing the child walk, assess the pelvis and back. Place your hands on the iliac crests of the standing child to observe whether they are level or whether there is leg length discrepancy. Have the child bend one knee and raise that leg. Observe whether the pelvis remains level. If not, and the opposite side tilts downward, this suggests dislocation of the contralateral hip.

Assess range of motion in the neck and the joints of the upper and lower limbs; assess the joints for heat, tenderness, and swelling. Muscle strength and tone are determined by having the child push his or her head or limb against the examiner's resisting hand.

Screen children for idiopathic scoliosis (puberty onset) beginning at age 8 to 9 years (see Chapter 20 for more information). Observe the child from the front and back; there should be no differences in shoulder height, scapular prominence, flank crease, and pelvis symmetry. Tell the child to slowly bend forward holding the hands with palms together or arms hanging freely while the examiner sits level with and facing the child. The child should bend at the waist to 90 degrees of straight back flexion with legs straight, ankles together, and hands not touching the floor. Each level of the spine is observed. A "rib hump" is an abnormal finding suggestive of scoliosis.

Inspect the lumbosacral area for signs of overlying skin, hairy patches, hyperpigmented areas, or dimpling. These can be signs of spina bifida occulta. With the child sitting or standing, assess the neck for flexion, hyperextension, and rotation from side to side.

Next, inspect the lower extremities. There is a normal range of findings of the lower extremities based on developmental considerations. A "bowlegged" (genu varum) appearance, for example, is caused by lateral bowing of the tibia and is normal in the toddler years until 1 year after the child starts walking. A "knock-kneed" (genu valgum) appearance is a common finding between 3 and 4 years of age and may persist until 7 years of age or slightly longer. To help determine whether the child's stance is physiologic or pathologic (outside the range of normal), measure the space between the knees or the medial malleoli. In genu varum, the space between the knees when the medial malleoli are together is more than 5 cm (2 in.). Genu valgum is indicated when the knees are together and the space between the medial malleoli is greater than 7.5 cm (3 in.). Spacings greater than these measures are abnormal and are indications for referral.

Inspect the foot next. Until about age 3 years, children look flatfooted because the fat pad conceals the longitudinal arch, and greater joint laxity is common in infants and young children. Ask children who look flatfooted after 6 years of age to stand on their toes; this position should reveal the longitudinal arch. Observe the gait for pigeon toe or intoeing, which can result from rotational problems originating at the foot–ankle, leg–knee, femur–hip, acetabulum, or a combination of these sites (Burns et al., 2012). To determine hip involvement, have the child lie in the prone position with the knees flexed at 90 degrees. The degree of medial and lateral rotation can then be determined. There are specific guides to determine normal angles for specific ages that can be found in advanced practice nursing or

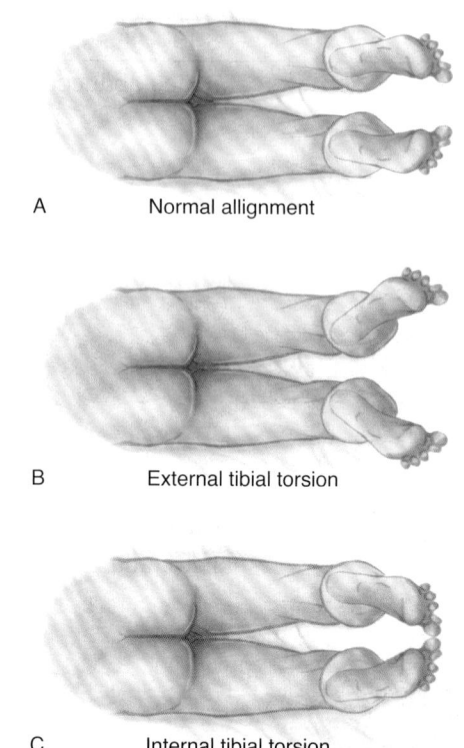

A   Normal allignment

B   External tibial torsion

C   Internal tibial torsion

Figure 8-14 Thigh–foot angle. Position the child lying on his or her stomach, with the knees close together and flexed; compare the long axis of the foot (picture an imaginary line drawn down the center of the foot from the heel to between the second and third toes) with the long axis of the thigh (femur). (A) Normal alignment: slight external rotation. (B) External tibial torsion: excessive outward rotation. (C) Internal tibial torsion: inward rotation of the foot with a negative angle.

medical texts (see Burns et al., 2012 and Marcdante et al., 2011, respectively). The thigh–foot angle can also be measured to help in the assessment (Fig. 8-14). Assess metatarsus adductus by drawing an imaginary line bisecting the hindfoot to the toes. The line should pass through the second toe or between the second and third toes (Burns et al., 2012).

Neurologic System

Neurologic assessment focuses on several factors: mental status or behavior, achievement of developmental milestones (cognitive–perceptual, fine and gross motor, personal–social, and language acquisition), motor and sensory functions, deep tendon and infant reflexes, and cranial nerve function. Although the findings related to the nervous system are reported under the name of the neurologic system, the actual neurologic assessment is integrated throughout the physical examination.

Behavior and Development

QUESTION: Sally is anxious to know what Stephanie should be doing at her age and what she will do next. Which developmental screening tool would be appropriate to assess Stephanie?

Behavioral assessment of the child is important and should occur during both the health history and the physical assessment. While taking a history and performing the physical examination, assess the child's state of consciousness and look for clues of neurologic problems, such as hyperirritability, restlessness, hyporeactivity, tics, or unusual repetitive behaviors as well as indicators of alterations in level of consciousness. The Glasgow Coma Scale adapted for pediatrics (see Table 21-1) is an objective measurement of consciousness and is a useful tool if a problem is suspected. Also assess the older child's mood and intensity as part of your neurologic assessment. A sad affect may indicate depression. It is important to obtain the parents' perspective about their child's behavior and any changes in behavior that have been noted.

To assess developmental milestones in infants and children, determine whether the child has mastered certain tasks (see Chapters 4 to 7). Standardized tests such as the Brazelton Neonatal Behavioral Assessment Scale, the Denver II, the Early Language Milestone Scale, the Ages and Stages Questionnaire or the Child Development Inventory, and the Clinical Linguistic and Auditory Milestone Scale are useful screening tests. The child may be referred for other more sophisticated testing if problems are found at the screening level.

ANSWER: The Ages and Stages Questionnaire would be a useful screening assessment tool and a fun way for Sally to see Stephanie's skills.

Motor and Sensory Function

 QUESTION: Describe the reflexes that Stephanie should display. Which infant reflexes should she not display?

Motor functioning is included as part of the musculoskeletal examination. The development of motor skills is age related, with a cephalocaudal progression of development (e.g., the child must have head control to sit and sits before he or she walks). In infancy, look for the presence or absence of specific infant reflexes (Table 8-9). Handedness, the preferential use of one hand over the other, typically does not occur until 3 to 4 years of age. Hand preference that occurs prior to 18 months of age may indicate weakness on the other side or a neurologic problem. In the older child, observe the child's level of activity and movement. Test muscle strength and symmetry by having the child squeeze your fingers, press the soles of his or her feet against your hands, and push his or her arms and legs against your hands. Assess the range of motion of all joints.

Several tests of cerebellar functioning can be performed with an older child. Have the child hop, skip, jump, and walk heel to toe. Ask the child to extend an arm and then touch a finger to the nose with eyes open and then shut. Inability to successfully perform these functions may indicate a cerebellar tumor. Similarly, have the child stand and rub the heel of one foot down the shin of the other leg with eyes open and closed. While the child is standing with heels together, have the child close his or her eyes, ask the child to stand still with arms at the side, and note whether the child leans or falls to one side; this is an abnormal finding known as *Romberg sign*.

Additional tests may elicit "soft" neurologic signs of abnormality on select motor or sensory tests. Minimal choreoathetoid (involuntary purposeless and uncontrollable) movements in the fingers of an extended arm in a child younger than age 4 years is one example of a soft neurologic sign. Another example is mirror movement of the fingers of the child's opposite hand when he or she is asked to perform a finger-to-thumb movement with one hand. These findings are called *soft* because they may or may not indicate an abnormality. Furthermore, their significance as an indication of a neurologic disorder should be interpreted cautiously because their significance is a matter of controversy and because these signs may disappear as the child ages. In contrast, hard neurologic signs such as spasticity or hypotonia strongly indicate underlying neurologic pathology.

Sensory functioning includes vision, hearing, and peripheral sensation. Vision and hearing are assessed as part of the evaluation of cranial nerves and also through separate auditory and visual testing (see Chapter 28 for more information). Assess peripheral discrimination in a child old enough to cooperate by having the child close his or her eyes then touch different parts of the body with either a pin or cotton ball or a warm or cold object. Ask the child to identify which object is being used. Again, with the child's eyes closed, touch different parts of the body at the same time and ask the child to tell what body part is being touched.

Assessment of cranial nerve function is outlined in Table 8-10. Some of the techniques used to assess individual cranial nerves are age dependent (e.g., an infant will not follow commands). If a neurologic problem or symptom is present, a complete neurologic examination is needed. Otherwise, a screening examination is usually done, including assessment of the head. (See Figure 21-7 for locations of cranial sutures.)

Reflexes

The neurologic system undergoes dramatic growth and maturation during the infancy period. The presence and disappearance of primitive infant reflexes occur in a specific sequence (see Table 8-9). Therefore, the absence or persistence of these reflexes is cause for alarm; these reflexes are important considerations in the assessment of a child during the first year of development. The Moro, grasp, tonic neck, and parachute are the most important primitive reflexes. Their presence or absence during specific periods of development or an abnormal reflex response can signal a central nervous system disorder.

Testing deep tendon reflexes is a routine part of the neurologic examination. Reflex testing can be done with a reflex hammer or the side of the hand. The usual deep tendon reflexes that are tested include the biceps, triceps,

TABLE 8-9 Assessment of Infant Reflexes

Reflex	How to Test	Usual Response	Abnormal Findings/Age at Disappearance or Appearance
Newborn Reflexes			
Babinski sign	Stroke sole of foot along lateral edge from heel upward.	Toes fan, dorsiflexion of big toe	Persistence beyond age 24 months
Crawling	Place infant on abdomen.	Crawling movements with arms and legs	Asymmetric movements
Dance or stepping	Hold infant with feet lightly touching firm surface.	Feet move up and down	Persistence beyond age 4–8 weeks
Extrusion	Touch tip of infant's tongue.	Tongue extends out	Persistence beyond age 4 months
Galant	Stroke lateral side of spine from shoulder to buttocks.	Back moves to side being stroked	Persistence beyond age 4–8 weeks
Moro	Place infant in semiupright position; let head fall backward with immediate resupport with the examiner's hands.	Symmetric abduction and extension of arms, flexion of thumb, followed by flexion and adduction of upper limbs	Persistence beyond age 4 months; asymmetric or absent response
Palmar grasp	Place finger or object in infant's open palm.	Infant's fingers curve around finger or object and resist its removal	Absence or persistence beyond age 10 months
Rooting	Stroke corner of infant's mouth.	Infant opens mouth and turns head to side being stroked	Absence or depressed; normally disappears by age 3–4 months when awake

TABLE 8-9   Assessment of Infant Reflexes *(Continued)*

Reflex	How to Test	Usual Response	Abnormal Findings/Age at Disappearance or Appearance
Startle	Clap hands loudly.	Infant extends and flexes arms quickly	Absence or persistence beyond age 4 months
Sucking	Place nipple 3–4 cm into the infant's mouth.	Infant begins sucking	Absence or depressed; normally disappears at age 3–4 months when awake
Later Reflexes			
Parachute	Suspend the infant by the trunk and suddenly flex body forward.	Infant spontaneously extends arms, hands, and fingers	Normally appears by age 6–8 months, remains throughout life
Tonic neck	Turn infant's head quickly to one side when supine.	Extension of arm and leg on side that head is turned with flexion in opposite limbs	If locked in the "fencer's position"; normal from age 2–6 months

brachioradialis, quadriceps (patellar), and the Achilles tendon (Table 8-11). Tap the area over the tendon and look for either extension or flexion. Often, children must be distracted to elicit the appropriate reflexes because prior tensing of muscles, such as occurs with anxiety or fear, can alter results (Fig. 8-15). To test for the plantar response, lightly stroke the lateral side of the sole of the foot and across the ball of the foot with an upward motion. The normal response is plantar flexion of the toes and sometimes the whole foot (note in Table 8-9 that a normal response in an infant is dorsiflexion of the great toe and fanning of the toes). If meningeal irritation is suspected, test for the presence of the Kernig or Brudzinski sign. The Kernig sign (inability to extend the legs fully when lying supine) and the Brudzinski sign (flexion of the hips,

resistance, pain, crying when the neck is flexed from a supine position) are associated with meningeal irritation.

Commonly tested superficial reflexes are the abdominal, cremasteric, and anal reflexes. Test the abdominal reflex by stroking the abdominal skin with the handle of a reflex hammer or with a wooden applicator tip, moving from the side toward the midline in all four quadrants. The umbilicus moves toward the stroking. This reflex may not be present in infants younger than age 6 months. Elicit the cremasteric reflex by gently stroking the inner aspect of the thigh of the male in a downward direction. Elevation of the testis on that side is the normal response. Test the anal reflex by stroking the perianal skin and observing a brisk contracture of the anal sphincter (the "anal wink").

Table 8-10 Assessment of Cranial Nerve Function

Cranial Nerve	Assessment of Function
I Olfactory	Not routinely tested. Have child close eyes, occlude one nostril at a time, and ask him or her to identify various common aromatic scents (e.g., vanilla, orange, peanut butter, peppermint).
II Optic	Test for visual fields and visual acuity; funduscopic examination.
III Oculomotor	Check pupil size and reactivity. Have child follow the light in the six cardinal positions of gaze and raise eyebrows. Observe position and symmetry of eyelids when open.
IV Trochlear	Have child move eyes downward and inward.
V Trigeminal	Palpate jaw and temple muscles for symmetry and strength as child bites down (motor function). Test for corneal reflex by lightly touching the cornea with a wisp of cotton. Have the child close both eyes and determine whether the child can tell when the forehead, cheeks, and chin are touched with a cotton wisp (sensory function).
VI Abducens	Check for ability of the eyes to move laterally.
VII Facial	Have the child smile, lift eyebrows, or show his or her teeth (motor function). For an infant, observe for facial symmetry when crying. Ask child to identify various tastes of substances (e.g., sugar, salt, or lemon juice) placed on the anterior two thirds of the tongue with an applicator. This test evaluates sensory function and is not routinely done.
VIII Acoustic	Test hearing. Clap hands from behind (not next to ear so air movement is felt) to see if infant responds; whisper to child from behind so he or she does not see your lips moving. (See Chapter 28 for more information on audiometry and other selected hearing tests.)
IX Glossopharyngeal	Test the child's ability to identify the taste of various substances (see cranial nerve VII) placed on the posterior of the tongue. This test is not routinely done. Phonation and swallowing are tests of motor function.
X Vagus	Elicit gag reflex by placing a tongue blade to the posterior palate; check ability to swallow, and note hoarseness. Check that uvula is midline and the soft palate rises when the child says "ahhh."
XI Accessory	To determine strength, have child shrug shoulders while pressure is applied by the examiner's hands. Similarly, tell the child to try to turn his or her head to the side while the examiner places a hand against the face to resist this movement.
XII Hypoglossal	Ask child to stick out his or her tongue and move it in all directions. Place a tongue blade against the side of the child's tongue and ask the child to move it away.

TABLE 8-11 Assessment of Deep Tendon Reflexes

Deep Tendon Reflex	Method of Testing	Normal Finding
Biceps	Flex the forearm, place your thumb over antecubital space, and tap with reflex hammer.	Slight flexion of forearm
Triceps	Abduct arm and support forearm with your hand, child's forearm hangs free; or hold child's wrist over his or her chest to flex arm at elbow. Tap directly above elbow.	Partial extension of forearm
Brachioradialis	Place child's arm and hand in relaxed position with arm flexed and palm down. Tap the radius about 1 in. (2.5 cm) above wrist.	Flexion of forearm and palm turns upward
Quadriceps	Have child's legs flexed at the knees and dangling. Tap midline just below the patella. Distract an older child by asking him or her to lock the fingers of the hands tightly together and try to pull them apart. Tap while the child is busy doing this task.	Partial extension of the lower leg
Achilles	Use same position as for quadriceps testing or, in supine position, flex knee and support that leg on the other leg. Lightly support foot in your hand in dorsiflexion and tap Achilles tendon.	Foot plantar flexes (downward)

A 4-point scale is typically used to grade the level of response: 4+, hyperactive, very brisk; 3+, brisker than average; 2+, average; 1+, diminished; and 0, no response. If the child tenses the muscle and tendon group to be tested, the deep tendon reflex is difficult to elicit.

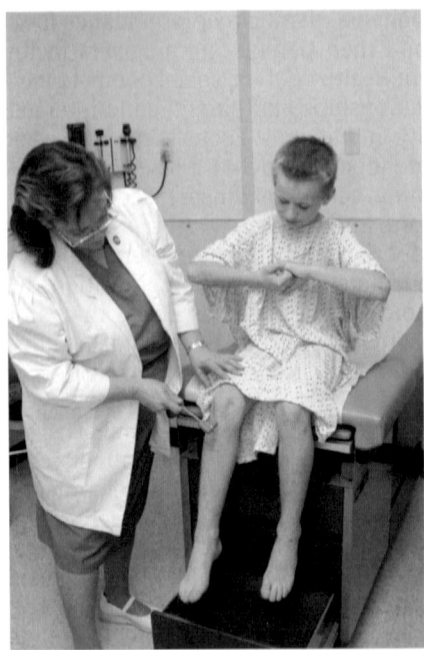

Figure 8-15 To facilitate evaluation of deep tendon reflexes in a child's lower extremities, the nurse distracts the child by asking him to lock his fingers together and then try to pull his hands apart.

ANSWER: One assessment of a young infant's neurologic well-being is the presence and absence of specific primitive reflexes. Stephanie, at 4 months of age, should still demonstrate a positive Babinski sign and a palmar grasp, and the tonic neck reflex should be extinguishing. She should no longer demonstrate the stepping reflex, Galant sign, Moro response, or a rooting reflex. Share with the parents these outward signs that indicate the formidable inward neurologic development that takes place during these early months.

DATABASE AND INTERPRETATION

Knowledge and skills of pediatric health assessment develop over time and with practice. The history plays a critical role in understanding issues influencing the child's health and well-being and in directing the physical examination. Techniques of physical examination are often easier to develop than the assessments important to accurate history taking.

Having conducted a health history and performed a physical examination, the nurse has a database from which to derive a plan of action. As additional data are received, modifications in the assessment and plan can be made.

WELL-CHILD CARE

Data obtained from a comprehensive health history, together with clinical findings based on a complete physical examination, form the framework for assessing the health care needs of the child and family. Well-child care encompasses health assessment and management

of symptoms commonly seen in minor illnesses. It also involves effective health teaching of children and their families.

HEALTH SURVEILLANCE VISITS

QUESTION: Stephanie is adjusting to a new family, a new community, and a new environment. How should her health supervision visits be scheduled based on the special needs of a child adopted from a foreign county and the needs of her new parents?

In providing health supervision for today's children, the health care professional must recognize that physical well-being, mental health, cognitive development, new psychosocial morbidities, and social efficacy are influenced by socioeconomic variables, behavior factors, family and cultural considerations, environment, education, access to health care, and the availability and quality of community resources. As such, health supervision should be done in a primary health care setting—a medical home—that is "accessible, continuous, comprehensive, family-centered, coordinated, compassionate and culturally sensitive" (Long et al., 2012, p. 88). The medical home is also referred to as the health home.

Guidelines developed for health surveillance of infants, children, and adolescents are based on the beliefs that health supervision is as follows:

- A longitudinal process that promotes a partnership and shared agenda between the health care professional, the child, and the family
- Personalized to fit the individual
- Contextual (i.e., views the child in the context of the family and the community)
- Supportive of the child's self-esteem, sense of competence, emotional health, and mastery
- Focused on the strengths as well as the problems and issues of the family and community
- Part of a seamless system that includes community-based health, education, and human services
- Complementary to health promotion and disease prevention efforts in the family, the school, the community, and the media (Hagan et al., 2008)

Effective health promotion and prevention has greater implications for infants, children, adolescents, and their parents or caregivers than with any other population group. Pediatric health supervision involves promoting health, preventing mortality and morbidity, and enhancing development and maturation. Prevention requires both an orderly and routine schedule of activities, based on knowledge of predictable physical and psychosocial development (attainment of developmental milestones), as well as recognition and prevention of disease as a constant, ongoing process rather than an episodic one.

Guidelines for health supervision visits have been developed by the American Academy of Pediatrics (AAP) and are part of their Bright Futures program.

Each health promotion visit with a health care provider should include screening procedures and health promotion and disease prevention strategies, primarily the use of immunization and the physical examination (Evidence-Based Clinical Practice Guidelines 8-1). Focus discussion on the history and assessment parameters and provide anticipatory guidance based on the child's physical and developmental stage (e.g., at each visit, measure length/height and weight and assess development; measure head circumference at every visit until the child is 2 years old; screen for autism at 18 and 24 months of age). If a scheduled well-child care visit is used to address an identified health problem, then the well-child care visit should be rescheduled.

ANSWER: Stephanie needs to receive several immunizations to catch up to the recommended schedule. Sally and her husband will benefit from frequent visits to reassure her and educate them about the health of their new daughter. One recommendation would be monthly visits between now and Stephanie's 8-month appointment, progressing to every other month until she is 1 year old.

ANTICIPATORY GUIDANCE

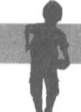

QUESTION: What is an example of anticipatory guidance appropriate for a 4-month-old child?

The components of anticipatory guidance for children of all ages and their parents or caregivers include discussions about healthy habits, social competence (including family relationships and parent–child interactions), and community interactions. Focus these discussions on age-appropriate topics in each of these areas (e.g., weaning, toilet training, school readiness); see Chapters 4 through 7 for specific information.

Issues about healthy habits center on lifestyle choices, injury and violence prevention, nutrition and healthy eating choices and practices (e.g., the family meal), physical activity, oral health, mental health (issues of self-esteem, depression, anger, and suicide), and sexuality education.

Social competence discussions emphasize the need for teaching family and societal rules about resolving conflict; age-appropriate discipline; developmentally appropriate behaviors; praise and encouraging expression of feelings; the ability to show respect for and communicate in a positive manner with siblings, peers, parents, and individuals in authority positions; showing affection; positive role modeling by parents; inquiring about school-related progress and career choices for teenagers; and allowing opportunities for socialization and achieving developmental milestones.

Community interaction discussions acquaint parents and caregivers with available community resources that are family and child focused, such as parent and community support groups, early intervention programs for at-risk children, community and after-school activities

---

EVIDENCE-BASED CLINICAL PRACTICE GUIDELINES 8-1
Preventive Services for Children

Wilkinson, J., Bass, C., Diem, S. et al. (2012). *Institute for Clinical Systems Improvement. Health care guideline: Preventive services for children and adolescents*. Retrieved from

https://www.icsi.org/_asset/x1mnv1/PrevServKids-Interactive0912.pdf

Provides guidelines for health care providers to assess the need for, and recommend, preventive services to average-risk asymptomatic children under age 18 years.

Michigan Quality Improvement Consortium. (2011). *Routine preventive services for infants and children (birth–24 months)*. Southfield, MI: Michigan Quality Improvement Consortium. Retrieved from

https://www.icsi.org/_asset/x1mnv1/PrevServKids-Interactive0912.pdf

---

Michigan Quality Improvement Consortium. (2011). *Routine preventive services for children and adolescents (ages 2–21)*. Southfield, MI: Michigan Quality Improvement Consortium. Retrieved from

http://www.mqic.org/pdf/mqic_routine_preventive_services_for_children_and_adolescents_ages_2_to_21_cpg.pdf

Provides guidelines for health care providers to offer parents education and counseling regarding routine preventive services (immunizations, nutrition, physical activity, dental health, violence/child abuse, mental health, substance abuse, coping skills, safety and injury prevention, sudden infant death syndrome [SIDS], STIs, mental health, substance abuse,) for infants and children at ages birth to 24 months and ages 2–21 years.

American Academy of Pediatric Dentistry. (2009). *Guideline on periodicity of examination, preventive dental services, anticipatory guidance/counseling and oral treatment for infants, children, and adolescents*. Chicago, IL: Author. Retrieved from

http://www.aapd.org/media/policies_guidelines/g_periodicity.pdf

Provides guidelines for health care providers to offer anticipatory guidance and preventive counseling for preventive oral health interventions for infants, children, and adolescents.

for children and teenagers, and child care resources and guidelines. The need for financial assistance, Medicaid, food, housing, and transportation are also items to address during social needs and family situation discussions.

The nurse needs to assume a proactive role in discussing anticipatory guidance issues with children and their families. Emphasizing and teaching about the value of a healthy lifestyle and behaviors is the responsibility of all members of the health care team. Every health care encounter is an opportunity for health teaching that should not be overlooked. A pediatric or adolescent health assessment is never complete if anticipatory guidance issues are not identified and addressed, whether through discussion, providing written literature, or stressing the need for a follow-up health surveillance visit. During these visits, the health care provider acts as a motivator by partnering with the child and parent to identify what the child or parent believes can be accomplished, given the family's unique situation, values, and beliefs, to change toward more healthful practices or reduce risky behaviors.

The nurse's role in managing common pediatric illnesses involves planning and delivering treatments and medications, evaluating the effectiveness of therapies, teaching patients and their families, assessing the urgency of a situation (see Chapter 31), and giving feedback to physicians and other health care professionals. Specific disease management is covered throughout this text (Table 8-12).

When instructing family members on home management, be cognizant of factors that affect teaching effectiveness (Chart 8-4). Help the family by solving problems that address factors that might influence successful home management. Take time to practice procedures or administration of medications with the parent or child, and plan for return demonstrations to assess competency level (see Chapter 9). The parent or child, depending on his or her age, needs specific information about signs and symptoms that indicate a worsening or an improvement in the child's condition. Finally, access to a telephone and an emergency plan of action if the child's condition suddenly worsens are important considerations for planning home management care.

The nurse plays a key role in promoting health maintenance behaviors in children and their families. Active listening and watchful observation during the history and physical examination and effective teaching techniques optimize the nurse's effectiveness in fulfilling this role.

ANSWER: If Stephanie is not rolling over now, she will be soon. Parents often become accustomed to placing the baby down for a few minutes without anticipating the baby rolling off. This new skill enables the infant to roll from changing tables, beds, or couches in a few seconds and makes him or her vulnerable to trauma from falls. Sally, as a new caregiver, should establish the habit of never taking her hand off Stephanie on a surface from which she could fall.

CHART 8-4 Factors That Influence Teaching on Home Management

- *The family's financial resources:* if they have money or insurance coverage for expensive medications or treatments (e.g., prepacked oatmeal bath for a rash is fairly expensive; for families with limited resources, cornstarch may be suggested as an alternative)
- *Comprehension of information given:* the need to deliver education and instructions in the native language and/or the need for interpreter services; the degree of complexity of the information that must be given and followed (e.g., a cognitively delayed parent may need repeated educational sessions or may not be able to cognitively process and follow through with a home treatment plan). Literacy level (the ability to read, write, and follow written instructions) may influence comprehension if written materials are used.
- *Home environment:* safety factors, sanitation, physical surroundings
- *Lifestyles:* work commitments of parents and schooling considerations
- *Previous skill levels and available equipment:* for example, do they have a thermometer? Do they know how to use it?
- *Social network:* to assist with other children or provide needed relief for parents
- *Willingness to perform the required treatment:* in other words, emotional readiness and stability
- *Access to home health care resources:* for example, a visiting nurse or respiratory therapist

---

TABLE 8-12 Common Childhood Symptoms of Illness

Symptom	Chapter
Runny nose, cough, sore throat, wheezing	16: The Child With Altered Respiratory Status
Earache	28: The Child With Altered Sensory Status
Rash/itching	25: The Child With Altered Skin Integrity
	24: The Child With an Infectious Disease
Abdominal pain, nausea, vomiting, diarrhea	18: The Child With Altered Gastrointestinal Status
	17: The Child With Altered Fluid and Electrolyte Status
Headache, seizure	21: The Child With Altered Neurologic Status
Limp, fractures	20: The Child With Altered Musculoskeletal Status
Fever	31: Pediatric Emergencies
Anemia	23: The Child With Altered Hematologic Status
Dysuria, frequency	19: The Child With Altered Genitourinary Status

LEVELS OF PREVENTION

> **QUESTION:** What primary and secondary prevention topics are indicated for Stephanie at her age and given her recent adoption?

Health is more than the absence of disease. Being healthy is being whole in mind, body, and spirit. Many of the conditions that affect health—food, shelter, education, income, sustainable resources, peace, social justice, and equity—are not readily amenable to intervention through the health care system. Nonetheless, children and their families are entitled to broad-based health education services and health care that promote healthy lifestyles and prevent illness.

CROSS-CULTURAL CARE

In developing countries, overpopulation, poor sanitation, contaminated water, malnutrition, and inadequate housing present major threats to health. In developed countries, major health problems are more likely to be lifestyle related and the result of accidents, alcohol and substance abuse, tobacco use, violence, or environmental pollution. Poverty is a linking factor and threatens health in all societies. Another threat is the escalating problem of obesity in children, which is now viewed as a significant pediatric health issue with implications for children worldwide.

Child health has improved remarkably in the United States since the beginning of the 20th century. This progress has resulted from a combination of social and economic changes, advances in therapeutic medicine and surgery, and implementation of public health measures, such as immunization programs aimed at the prevention of specific childhood diseases. Today, health care is more prevention focused than ever.

The objectives set forth in the Healthy People 2020 report (U.S. Department of Health & Human Services, 2010) establish a health care agenda in which preventive strategies for social and medical problems are identified in addition to treatment. Preventive health care is viewed as part of a continuum of intervention that includes primary, secondary, and tertiary levels.

Prevention efforts can be targeted at the individual child, the family, or the community. Preventive strategies can decrease the probability that low- or medium-risk children will develop particular diseases or conditions and subsequently enter high-risk categories of disease states or impaired health status. Therefore, children at low or medium risk benefit the most from participation in prevention programs.

Primary Prevention

Primary prevention is directed at recognizing susceptibility to disease and protecting against disability by using strategies to prevent disease or disability from occurring. Primary prevention efforts often target those individuals at increased risk. The use of immunizations is an excellent example of primary prevention. Other examples of primary prevention include chlorination and fluoridation of water, applying dental sealants to prevent tooth decay, and anticipatory guidance given to parents and family members of young children about the need to keep chemicals out of their child's reach.

Secondary Prevention

Secondary prevention is directed at early identification of risk factors for specific diseases and the initiation of early detection and intervention to prevent the development of such diseases. Because of the increased awareness of specific factors known to be antecedents of childhood illnesses and disabilities, the care of children is becoming more focused on prevention. Many secondary prevention efforts are the result of government or social agency initiatives. Examples of secondary prevention strategies include state-mandated neonatal screening for specific congenital and inherited metabolic disorders such as phenylketonuria and congenital hypothyroidism, hearing and vision screening in schools, and special screening programs for genetic diseases in at-risk populations. An early intervention program with youths at risk for violence is an example of a secondary prevention strategy aimed at youth when they are most likely to be addressed successfully before becoming entrenched in a pattern of violent behaviors.

Tertiary Prevention

Tertiary prevention is the avoidance of complications and additional disability for those children with known diseases, disabilities, or medical conditions (special needs children). Tertiary prevention focuses on eliminating, reducing, or halting the progression and/or severity of a disability associated with existing disease states. Rehabilitation services to restore functionality and self-sufficiency are key elements in tertiary prevention practices. An example of tertiary prevention is the provision of chest physiotherapy to a child with cystic fibrosis. Clinical practice guidelines for children with chronic diseases or conditions such as diabetes, juvenile arthritis, and asthma emphasize tertiary prevention strategies aimed at improving the quality of the child's life and would be considered efforts aimed at prevention of further disability.

Nurse's Role

Nurses play important roles in protecting children's health at all three levels of prevention. As health care continues to move from acute care settings to the home, short-stay centers, child care centers, schools, and school-linked services, nurses have opportunities to provide direct clinical prevention services (e.g., immunizations), coordinate services as case managers, provide leadership in the development and implementation of community-based prevention strategies, and continue to advocate at local, state, and national levels for greater awareness of children's health issues and service needs. Nurses have the opportunity to protect and promote children's health by supporting the development and implementation of policies and legislation that will best serve this vulnerable population.

> ANSWER: Immunization is a form of primary prevention. Stephanie's immunization schedule will need to be compared with the recommended schedule, and any doses that are missing will be given. A form of secondary prevention includes performing a newborn metabolic screening. Stephanie will receive a purified protein derivative test to determine whether she has been exposed to tuberculosis. Because this is an international adoption, Stephanie's parents need information about her unique health supervision needs. The AAP has an excellent brochure, *A Healthy Beginning: Important Information for Parents of Internationally Adopted Children*, which identifies and explains the rationale for these special health supervision needs.

IMMUNIZATION

The widespread use of immunization remains one of the most significant advances in pediatrics, altering the morbidity and reducing mortality associated with once common and feared childhood diseases. The use of vaccines has repeatedly proved to be the most cost-effective way of eliminating preventable diseases.

Despite this historical success, we are currently experiencing unacceptably low rates of immunization as a result of complacency and fears of harmful consequences. In 2011, the estimated rate of coverage with recommended vaccines (four or more doses of DTaP; three or more of inactivated poliovirus vaccine [IPV]; one or more of measles, mumps, and rubella [MMR]; three or four of *Haemophilus influenzae* type B [Hib]; three or more of HepB; one or more of varicella; and four or more pneumococcal conjugate vaccine [PCV]) in children aged 19 to 35 months was 68.5% (±1.3%), as reported in the U.S. immunization survey (CDC, 2012g). For select diseases, high rates of coverage are needed to provide protection to the general population—a concept known as *herd immunity* (see thePoint for Supplemental Information). The reporting of over 27,000 cases of pertussis in 2010 and sporadic outbreaks of imported measles represent worrisome evidence of the need to remain vigilant (CDC, 2012d, 2012f). Reasons for low immunization rates include failure of health care providers to use every encounter as a chance to vaccinate, failure to administer vaccines to vulnerable children on time, unnecessary delays in vaccine administration based on misinformation about contraindications, and the erroneous beliefs held by some parents that the diseases are no longer a threat or that vaccines are responsible for various conditions such as autism.

Vaccine failures and waning immunity also contribute to the inability to eradicate some diseases. The resurgence of measles in college-aged students in the 1980s led to further study of the vaccine's immunogenic properties and identification of the need for a booster vaccination when the levels of protection begin to fall around the age of 12 years. Tetanus is another example of a vaccine given in infancy that needs to be boosted around age 12 years, every 10 years thereafter, and at times of injury. Breakthrough cases of varicella occurred after only one vaccine, and a second booster dose is now recommended for all children. The use of DTaP is being critically analyzed as to reports of possible waning pertussis immunity as compared to immunity provided with the whole-cell pertussis vaccine.

Recommended Childhood Immunization Schedule

> QUESTION: What would be an appropriate immunization schedule for Stephanie for the next 6 months?

Routine childhood immunization is an integral part of health maintenance for children. In the United States, the Advisory Committee on Immunization Practices (ACIP) of the CDC, the AAP Committee on Infectious Diseases, and the American Academy of Family Physicians (AAFP) share the responsibility for establishing recommendations for the administration of vaccines in the public and private sectors. Delay in providing recommended immunizations at recommended times can put the child at risk for acquiring serious disease. To ensure that all children are adequately protected, health care providers are encouraged to follow the recommended routine and catch-up immunization schedules and administration guidelines from the ACIP, AAP, and AAFP (see Appendix C). New guidelines come out yearly, typically in January, and are available on the CDC and AAP websites. The WHO provides guidelines for immunization practices for the rest of the world because many developing countries do not have the infrastructure to generate national guidelines.

The pediatric nurse needs to be familiar with issues regarding childhood immunizations (Nursing Interventions 8-3). Vaccine research is ongoing, and recommendations for their use often change as new data emerges about vaccines and the level of and persistence of the immunity they confer. New combination vaccines are being tested and, if proven to be safe and effective as well as affordable, will help to reduce the number of injections needed. Chart 8-5 presents resources for current information regarding immunization practices in the United States.

The recommended age for beginning primary immunization of infants is at birth (see Appendix C). Children who began primary immunization at the recommended age but did not complete the immunization series according to the recommended schedule should receive only the missed doses rather than beginning the series again. Information regarding the recommended immunization schedule for infants, children, and teens who start late or are behind schedule is found in Appendix C. Immunization schedules contain information about the minimum age for a first dose of a vaccine, the minimum interval between doses, and whether a particular

NURSING INTERVENTIONS 8-3

Immunization Management

Educate parents and family members about vaccine-preventable diseases and potential sequelae.

Educate parents and family members about recommended immunizations for children (see Chart 8-5 for resources): reasons and benefits of use, side effects, and adverse reactions; if the family will be traveling or has been exposed, include information about vaccinations such as typhoid fever, cholera, and rabies.

Follow the CDC, AAP, and AAFP guidelines for immunization schedule and administration.

Encourage parent(s) and caregivers to remain up to date with their adult vaccine schedule because adults can be a source of illness to their child.

Give families a copy of the Vaccine Information Statements (VIS) available from the CDC.

Obtain informed consent prior to administering vaccine.

Administer immunizations simultaneously as separate or combined injections when possible (see Tradition or Science 8-1).

Document vaccination information such as manufacturer, lot number, expiration date, site, etc.

Identify contraindications for administering immunizations (e.g., history of severe anaphylactic reaction to a vaccine or vaccine component, encephalopathy, or brain or serious nervous system disease within 7 days after a dose of DTaP)

Follow vaccine storage requirements and special administration guidelines (e.g., give within the specified time after reconstitution, do not expose to light, keep at established refrigeration temperature).

Assist families who cannot afford vaccines to identify providers who participate in Vaccines for Children (VFC), a federal program to provide vaccines at no charge to VFC providers.

Inform family of comfort measures that can be helpful after vaccine administration to child (see Nursing Interventions 8-4).

Observe patient for adverse reactions, particularly syncope, for 15 minutes after vaccine administration.

Report adverse events that occur following vaccination to the Vaccine Adverse Event Reporting System (VAERS).

Provide parents with a copy of their child's updated immunization record and encourage enrollment in state-supported immunization registry

---

CHART 8-5 Resources for Immunization Practices in the United States

Allied Vaccine Group (www.vaccine.org)

AAP Childhood Immunization Support Program (www.cispimmunize.org)

CDC National Immunization Program (NIP) (www.cdc.gov/vaccines and http://www.cdc.gov/vaccines/parents/index.html

Immunization Action Coalition (IAC) (www.vaccineinformation.org)

IAC—Administering Vaccines: Dose, Route, Site, and Needle Size (www.immunize.org/catg.d/p3085.pdf)

Morbidity and Mortality Weekly Report (MMWR), a newsletter issued weekly by the CDC

National Network for Immunization Information (www.immunizationinfo.org)

Package inserts accompanying the vaccines

Recommendations of the ACIP of the CDC

The Red Book: Report of the Committee on Infectious Disease, published regularly by the AAP

The CDC *Epidemiology and Prevention of Vaccine-Preventable Diseases* "The Pink Book": Course Textbook (12th ed.), May 2012 (http://www.cdc.gov/vaccines/ [search for Pink Book])

vaccine is needed at all (e.g., PCV and Hib are not given to children aged 7 years or older because these diseases do not pose the health risk that they do in young infants and children).

CROSS-CULTURAL CARE

Children adopted from abroad may not be properly immunized before their arrival in the United States. Immunizations should begin immediately, according to the recommendations listed in Appendix C. Immunization status of refugee or immigrant children should also be reviewed upon arrival in the United States, and deficiencies should be addressed.

Educating and reminding family members about the importance of keeping their child up to date with vaccines is an important role of the pediatric nurse. A discussion of each of the immunizations recommended from infancy through adolescence follows, including information about schedule, common side effects, and other considerations.

ANSWER: The recommended schedule of immunizations for Stephanie for the next 6 months can be found by reviewing the CDC Recommendation for Immunizations for Infants and Young Children found in Appendix C.

Diphtheria–Tetanus–Acellular Pertussis Vaccines

Diphtheria and tetanus are rare diseases in the United States. Those infected are usually elderly people who have not received tetanus and diphtheria toxoids vaccine (Td) boosters in the previous 10 years. Serologic tests indicate that naturally **acquired immunity** (see thePoint for Supplemental Information) to tetanus and diphtheria toxin does not occur in the United States. Universal vaccination with boosters (Td) at 10-year intervals after their adolescent tetanus toxoid, reduced diphtheria toxoid, and acellular pertussis vaccines (Tdap) booster dose is necessary to provide continued protection. Pertussis is commonly known as *whooping cough* because of the high-pitched inspiratory whooping sound heard in children with this disease. It is an acute, highly communicable infectious disease with significant mortality in infants younger than 1 month of age. Diphtheria is an acute infection of the upper respiratory tract, the trachea, or both and is associated with membranous obstruction of the upper airway.

The DTaP vaccine is a combination of diphtheria and tetanus toxoid and acellular pertussis given as a series of five injections. It is an inactivated vaccine. During the first year of life, three doses of DTaP are recommended—at ages 2, 4, and 6 months—with a fourth dose given between 15 and 18 months of age. The fifth dose of DTaP is recommended between 4 and 6 years of age and serves as a booster at primary school entry. Multiple doses of DTaP vaccine are necessary to provide adequate and lasting immunity.

Antibody titers decrease over time; therefore, immunity is boosted with recommended administration of a single dose of Tdap (the adolescent preparation that has a much lower dose of acellular pertussis and diphtheria) at ages 11 to 12 years with subsequent regular Td (tetanus and a much lower dose of diphtheria toxoid) every 10 years thereafter. A Tdap booster dose is also recommended for 13- to 18-year-old children who have not received Td (catch-up immunization). Because of recent national outbreaks in pertussis, especially in the 13 and 14 year old group, studies are underway investigating how long vaccine protection lasts with DTaP and Tdap with possible implications for future vaccine recommendations (CDC 2012d, 2012e, 2012f). Parents, child care providers, and grandparents who have close contact with infants less than 12 months of age should be vaccinated with Tdap to prevent the spread of pertussis to vulnerable infants.

The vaccine is injected intramuscularly in either the vastus lateralis or the deltoid muscle, depending on the child's muscle mass. In 1% to 3% of children, there may be tenderness, redness, or swelling at the site of the injection and fever that usually presents within the first 48 hours (Burns et al., 2012) (Nursing Interventions 8-4). Rarely, a child may spike a temperature of 105° F (40.6° C) or higher after DTaP immunization, have nonstop crying for more than 3 hours, or have seizures. Other extremely rare occurrences include serious allergic reaction, coma, lowered consciousness, or permanent brain damage. It is difficult to know whether these extremely rare conditions are related to vaccine administration or just coincidental problems.

The only true contraindications to immunization are a history of severe anaphylactic reaction to a vaccine or vaccine component, encephalopathy, or brain or serious nervous system disease within 7 days after a dose of DTaP. The current DTaP has a significantly lower probability of vaccine-associated reactions than

---

NURSING INTERVENTIONS 8-4

Potential Reactions Associated With Immunization

Potential Reaction	Interventions
Pain with injection	Apply topical anesthetics (e.g., EMLA, LMX4, vapocoolant) at the injection sites, giving enough time for the anesthetic to have the desired effect (see Chapter 10).
	Administer oral sucrose for infants up to 3 months of age.
	Encourage parents to hold a young child during injection.
	Use distractions such as bubbles, blowing on pinwheels, and reading stories to reduce attention to pain and potentially relax the muscle. Encourage teens to use headsets to listen to music.
Localized redness or tenderness (a potential side effect of any immunization given intramuscularly or subcutaneously)	Ice packs for the first 24 hours, followed by warm compresses if the inflammation persists, can help with symptomatic relief. Routine use of acetaminophen before and after vaccine administration is no longer recommended. Its use should be determined case by case based on the Prymula et al. (2009) study that demonstrated decreased antibody response with routine acetaminophen use. This topic is still under study.
Fever	Acetaminophen as needed
Myalgia	Acetaminophen as needed

the previous version. Systemic reactions (anaphylaxis, anaphylactic shock, encephalopathy, or encephalitis) may occur up to 7 days after administration of DTaP; most reactions occur within 72 hours.

There are no documented cases of central nervous system injury or death associated with DTaP administration. Generally, immunizations should not be given to a child with serious illness. Exercising this precaution avoids adding the risk of complicating an existing illness or confusing symptoms of the illness with a side effect of the vaccine. Most DTaP reactions occur with the fourth or fifth dose.

caREminder

Signs and symptoms that may warrant careful consideration about administration of subsequent vaccination with DTaP include convulsions, with or without fever, occurring within 3 days after vaccination and the following events occurring within 48 hours of vaccination: fever 105° F (40.6° C) or higher that is not attributed to another cause; collapse or shocklike state; and persistent, inconsolable crying lasting 3 hours or more.

Haemophilus Influenzae Type B Vaccine

Hib is the most virulent of the six strains of *H. influenzae*. In past years, it was the leading cause of invasive diseases, including bacterial meningitis. The Hib vaccine has proved to be a major safeguard for the health of young infants and children.

Three conjugate vaccines and two combination vaccines are licensed for use in infants in the United States: PRP-OMP (PedvaxHIB), PRP-T (ActHIB), and PRP-T (Hiberix). It is important to know the manufacturer guidelines because each of these conjugate vaccines have unique instructions regarding administration (number of doses needed, age criteria, etc.). For example, infants given PRP-OMP (PedvaxHIB) at ages 2 and 4 months do not require a third dose at age 6 months. However, PRP-T requires three doses at ages 2, 4, and 6 months. Both of these vaccines require a final booster dose recommended between 12 and 15 months of age. In contrast, Hiberix is only given as a booster dose to children 12 months to 4 years of age.

Two combination vaccines are licensed for children: DTaP-IPV/Hib (Pentacel) and HepB-Hib (Comvax) (CDC, 2012c). Again, it is critical to follow the manufacturer's guidelines. See Appendix C for information about use of these two vaccines.

Hib vaccine is an inactivated vaccine administered intramuscularly in either the vastus lateralis or the deltoid muscle, depending on the muscle mass. The Hib vaccines are major weapons in the prevention of childhood bacterial meningitis and epiglottitis; their use brought about a dramatic decline in the incidence of all types of invasive infections resulting from Hib. The number of Hib doses that the child receives depends on the age at which the vaccine was first given. Aside from a slight fever and soreness at the injection site, no other side effects are commonly associated with this vaccine (see Nursing Interventions 8-4).

Hepatitis B Vaccine

Hepatitis B virus (HBV) is a potentially fatal viral infection, frequently culminating in cirrhosis or liver cancer during adulthood. HBV infection can occur perinatally or any other time during childhood. HepB vaccine is given in a series of three intramuscular doses. The AAP and the CDC recommend administration of HepB vaccine to all infants at birth. The three-dose schedule of HepB vaccination for infants born to HBsAg-negative mothers is dose 1 at birth; dose 2 one month after dose 1; and dose 3 at 6 to 18 months of age. Routine testing of infants to determine the presence of anti-HBsAg is not recommended except in infants whose mothers tested positive during pregnancy. If medically stable, a child born prematurely should receive the full dose of each vaccine at the appropriate chronologic age.

Approximately 95% of infants and 90% of adults who receive three injections develop immunity to the virus (CDC, 2012c). Universal vaccination of all infants is recommended, and adolescents who have not previously received three doses of HepB vaccine should initiate or complete the series by 11 to 12 years of age. No follow-up antibody testing is needed for infants born to HBsAg-negative mothers.

Infants born to HBsAg-positive mothers should receive HepB vaccine and HepB immune globulin (0.5 mL) within 12 hours of birth, in addition to completing the series of three vaccines. Administration of HepB vaccine and HepB immune globulin within 24 hours after birth is 85% to 95% effective in the prevention of both acute and chronic HepB infection. Within 1 to 2 months of the last dose of vaccine and between the ages of 9 to 18 months, these infants should be tested to determine whether they are immune. If they are not immune and are anti-HBs antigen and HBsAg negative, additional vaccinations are given along with repeated testing for the presence of protective antibodies (CDC, 2012c).

Two recombinant DNA HepB vaccines are available in the United States. The most common side effect observed after vaccination has been soreness at the injection site (see Nursing Interventions 8-4). Rarely, anaphylaxis or anaphylactic shock may occur within 7 days. Comvax is a combination HepB-Hib vaccine that can be used after 6 weeks of age.

Measles–Mumps–Rubella Vaccine

Before the advent of the current vaccine, measles and rubella were common childhood diseases associated with a characteristic exanthem. Measles was associated with significant morbidity and death. Rubella, on the other hand, was a mild disease for children but resulted in devastating sequelae for the fetus of a pregnant woman, especially during her first trimester. Mumps is characterized by swelling of the parotid glands and has associated secondary complications, although they are less severe and less frequently seen than with measles.

MMR vaccines may cause an allergic reaction because they contain minute amounts of neomycin, and the measles and mumps vaccine components are derived from chick embryo tissue cultures, which may contain allergenic substances (such as gelatin). Studies have demonstrated that serious allergic reactions in individuals with egg allergies are "extremely low." Routine skin testing prior to administration of MMR is not recommended for egg-allergic children nor is the use of special protocols (CDC, 2012c).

MMR vaccine should be administered between ages 12 and 15 months, with a second dose at either age 4 to 6 years or 11 to 12 years to provide lasting immunity to measles. A minimal interval of 4 weeks between doses is recommended. The vaccine should not be administered to infants younger than age 12 months because persisting maternal antibodies can interfere with the immune response. Because rubella presents a high risk to a developing fetus, the goal of rubella immunization is protection of unborn children rather than the recipient of the immunization. Vaccination of pregnant women with MMR is contraindicated.

MMR is a live attenuated vaccine and is administered by subcutaneous injection. Because of the risk of a diminished immune response or tissue damage, intramuscular injection is not recommended. Occasional soreness, redness, or swelling at the site of the injection can result after vaccination (see Nursing Interventions 8-4). Occasionally, 5 to 12 days after the first dose, there may be a rash, fever, generalized lymphadenopathy, or a seizure related to a high fever. At 1 to 3 weeks after the first dose, there may be joint pain, stiffness, or swelling lasting up to 3 days. Systemic reactions (anaphylaxis, anaphylactic shock, encephalopathy, or encephalitis) rarely occur after MMR administration.

MMRV is a combination vaccine with varicella. It is licensed for use with children from 12 months until their 13th birthday. Studies of children aged 12 to 23 months comparing the use of MMRV combination vaccine with separate injections of MMR and varicella vaccines given at the same time showed a 21.5% incidence of fever of ≥102° F between 5 and 12 days after vaccination for MMRV versus a 14.9% incidence for the separate MMR/varicella injections. Likewise, the incidence of seizures was also compared in this age group and time frame and revealed one additional febrile seizure per 2,300 to 2,600 children for the MMRV vaccine (CDC, 2012c).

Inactivated Poliovirus Vaccine

QUESTION: Stephanie received the OPV in Korea; the vaccine is no longer given in the United States. Does this present a problem for Stephanie? What questions can you anticipate that Sally may have regarding this immunization?

Poliovirus is an enterovirus with three serotypes that caused a range of diseases from asymptomatic illness to lower motor neuron paralysis. In 2000, the enhanced injectable inactivated poliovirus vaccine (eIPV) for subcutaneous administration became the vaccine of choice to provide protection against polio, replacing the trivalent polio vaccine (OPV) because of its associated risk of vaccine-acquired polio. The OPV is no longer distributed in the United States. The inactivated vaccine is highly immunogenic and, after three doses, induces immunity equal to or greater than that of the OPV. There have been no documented cases of vaccine-associated polio paralysis with the use of the inactive vaccine. The vaccine is given intramuscularly in the vastus lateralis with a primary series of three doses at 2, 4, and 6 to 18 months of age; and a booster at 4 to 6 years. Local inflammation is the most common side effect. Serious reactions to IPV have not been documented; allergic reaction may occur in those allergic to streptomycin, polymyxin B, and neomycin.

ANSWER: The OPV that Stephanie received in Korea has an extremely slight risk of sequelae. Stephanie has had no reaction to the OPV and will now receive the IPV in the United States; therefore, she is at no additional risk at this point. Sally may have questions regarding the risks associated with the vaccine, and you can reassure her that there have been no cases of paralysis associated with the IPV.

Varicella-Zoster Vaccine

Chickenpox, the primary infection caused by the varicella-zoster virus, is an extremely contagious type of herpesvirus. It is generally considered a benign, self-limited infection in the usually healthy child. However, chickenpox has a high financial impact and inflicts harm in certain populations, particularly neonates and immunocompromised children.

Varicella vaccine (Varivax; a live, attenuated varicella-zoster virus vaccine) is recommended for administration in children at 12 to 18 months of age with a second dose at 4 to 6 years or in any child aged 18 months or older who has not been immunized and has no history of chickenpox. The second dose is given at least 3 months after the first in children younger than age 13 years; for those older than 13 years of age, doses should be administered at least 4 weeks apart. The vaccine is given subcutaneously in the upper arm or anterolateral thigh. Local reactions of pain, erythema, and swelling occur in approximately 19% of children (CDC, 2012c).

The Varivax vaccine is well tolerated, with a small percentage of children experiencing mild fever and/or rash development generally within 3 weeks after immunization. Lesions, often located on the face, chest, and back, usually resemble mosquito bites and can last a few days. Other adverse reactions include pain at the site of injection and fever, as with other vaccines. Transmission of varicella vaccine virus is an uncommon event. Nevertheless, if the child develops lesions, teach parents to avoid close association with immunocompromised individuals, pregnant women without history of or immunity to varicella, and newborn infants of such mothers.

> **ALERT** *Varivax is contraindicated in individuals with a history of hypersensitivity to any component of the vaccine, including gelatin; individuals with a history of anaphylactoid reaction to neomycin; females who are pregnant; and individuals who are immunosuppressed, have cellular deficiencies, or received blood products within the past 5 months.*

Hepatitis A Vaccine

Hepatitis A causes a viral primary infection in the liver that is most often nonsymptomatic in infants and young children. Children between 12 and 23 months of age should receive the vaccine. Havrix and Vaqta are approved for intramuscular administration in the deltoid in a series of two doses. The second dose of Havrix is given 6 to 12 months after the first dose. The second dose of Vaqta is administered 6 to 18 months after the first dose. Muscle soreness and slight redness are the most common side effects (see Nursing Interventions 8-4).

Pneumococcal 13-Valent Conjugate Vaccine and Pneumococcal Polysaccharide Vaccine

Streptococcus pneumoniae continues to be the leading cause of bacteremia, bacterial pneumonia, and meningitis in children and is a common cause of otitis media. Children younger than 2 years of age are particularly vulnerable because of their decreased ability to produce antibodies against polysaccharide antigens and the frequency of colonization in this age group. Therefore, immunization of infants with the 13-valent PCV, Prevnar, can prevent *S. pneumoniae* disease and its complications. It is an inactivated vaccine that significantly reduces invasive disease associated with serotypes (both in the vaccine and other serotypes not included) and is greater than 90% effective in eliminating invasive disease (CDC, 2012c).

A four-dose series (at 2, 4, 6, and 12 to 15 months of age) is recommended. Dosing needs for infants and children who start later vary with age of the child (see Appendix C). Doses are administered intramuscularly in the vastus lateralis. The PCV is a safe and effective vaccine. Fever can occur within 7 days of any dose in about 24% to 35% of children but is typically not a high fever. Redness and tenderness at the injection site occur in a small percentage of children and typically are more common with the fourth dose (CDC, 2012c) (see Nursing Interventions 8-4).

For children aged 2 years or older with chronic illnesses associated with an increased risk of pneumococcal disease, vaccination with a 23-valent pneumococcal polysaccharide vaccine (PPSV23) is recommended. High-risk conditions include functional or anatomic asplenia, cochlear implants, chronic disorders of the pulmonary system, cardiovascular diseases, nephrotic syndrome or renal failure, diabetes mellitus, chronic liver diseases, immunosuppressive conditions, chemotherapy with alkylating agents, antimetabolites, or long-term systemic corticosteroids. The vaccine is given either intramuscularly or subcutaneously. Revaccination is recommended for children at highest risk for severe pneumococcal infection, including those likely to have a rapid decline in their serum antibody concentration. The second dose should be given 5 or more years after initial vaccination. Highest risk children are defined as those with functional or anatomic asplenia, immunosuppression, transplant, chronic renal failure, or nephrotic syndrome. Local reactions are the most common adverse event (CDC, 2012c).

Influenza Vaccine

Human influenza is very contagious, and the highest illness attack rate is in children. There are two licensed influenza vaccines: trivalent inactivated (TIV) and live attenuated (LAIV). These vaccines should ideally be given in the months of September, October, and November, before the influenza season begins, so the individual has sufficient time to build up immunity. The vaccine formulation is changed each year based on the flu strains predicted to be most prevalent. Both vaccines are grown in chicken eggs and contain residual egg protein; therefore, individuals with a history of hypersensitivity, especially anaphylactic reactions, to eggs or to a previous dose of influenza vaccine must be cleared by an allergist and then closely monitored if the vaccine is administered. In 2011, the ACIP amended their guidelines allowing persons with egg allergy involving only urticaria without other symptoms to receive TIV (CDC, 2012c).

The TIV is given intramuscularly or intradermal. The intramuscular preparation is recommended as an annual vaccination for children 6 to 23 months of age. Fluzone intradermal is not given to children; it is given only to those between the ages of 18 and 64 years. The CDC ACIP recommends annual influenza vaccination for all persons aged 6 months or older. It is an especially critical immunization for children with chronic cardiopulmonary disease (hemodynamically significant heart disease), rheumatoid arthritis, Kawasaki syndrome, metabolic diseases, renal failure, hemoglobinopathies, immunosuppression, or long-term aspirin therapy. Children younger than 8 years of age should receive two doses at least 1 month apart if they are first-time vaccine recipients. Certain children aged 6 months to 8 years, regardless if they have received influenza vaccine before, may also need a series of two immunizations in subsequent years; refer to ACIP guidelines for recommendations related to special need situations and children and when vaccine supplies are limited.

Soreness at the injection site can occur with the TIV and typically lasts only 1 to 2 days. Young children who have not had a prior influenza vaccine can experience fever, malaise, and myalgia occurring in less than 1% of TIV recipients (see Nursing Interventions 8-4).

The LAIV is recommended for healthy people aged 2 to 49 years and is administered intranasally. The LAIV has better efficacy than the TIV in young children

(Belshe et al., 2007; CDC, 2012c). Because those who receive the LAIV can shed vaccine virus for up to 3 weeks after receiving the vaccine, the TIV is the preferred vaccine if a child is in contact with a severely immunocompromised person. LAIV is contraindicated in children and adolescents receiving aspirin-containing therapy because of the association of Reye syndrome with aspirin and wild-type influenza infection. Other children who should receive TIV, not LAIV, include those who are immunosuppressed or those with asthma, a recent wheezing episode, chronic pulmonary or cardiovascular conditions, metabolic or renal diseases, and hemoglobinopathy (CDC, 2012c).

Reactions to the LAIV can include nasal congestion or rhinorrhea, headache, fever, vomiting, abdominal pain, and myalgia; these reactions are more commonly seen after the first dose. Acetaminophen, rest, and adequate hydration may be helpful. The LAIV should not be given if a child has congestion that would impede spraying. This intranasal vaccine comes in a prefilled nasal sprayer (0.2 mL), with 0.1 mL sprayed into each nostril immediately after thawing. There is no need to repeat the dose if the recipient sneezes after administration. Two doses administered at least 4 weeks apart are required for children 2 through 8 years of age who are receiving influenza vaccine for the first time. Always refer to the current ACIP guidelines for immunizing children 2 to 8 years of age. Similar to TIV recommendations, those with LAIV who previously received influenza vaccine may be recommended to receive a second dose in a subsequent year.

Meningococcal Vaccine

Neisseria meningitides is associated with acute and potentially severe invasive infections. It is the leading cause of bacterial meningitis in children and a common etiologic agent linked to sepsis and focal infections in children and young adults. Its polysaccharide capsule helps bacteria to resist phagocytosis and lysis.

There are two types of meningococcal vaccines currently licensed: meningococcal polysaccharide vaccine (MPSV4) and quadrivalent meningococcal conjugate vaccine (MCV4). MPSV4 vaccine is no longer routinely administered. Menactra and Menveo are licensed MCV4 vaccines given intramuscularly between the ages of 2 and 55 years. Both MCV4 vaccines offer protection against meningococcal groups A, C, Y, and W-135. The major difference between these two MCV4 vaccines is Menactra is conjugated to diphtheria toxoid; Menveo is conjugated to CRM$_{197}$.

Routine immunization with MCV4 vaccine should begin at age 11 or 12 years with a booster dose at 16 years of age. Recommendations for catch-up vaccination can be found on the CDC and AAP websites. Refer to the ACIP guidelines for immunization guidelines for younger children at risk for invasive meningococcal disease; these children receive a two-dose primary series with boostering guidelines. Children who received meningococcal vaccination before 7 years of age and continue to be at high risk should be revaccinated 3 years after their first dose. Revaccination is recommended for children at high risk who were vaccinated at 7 years

of age or older every 5 years after their previous dose (CDC, 2012c).

There are no recommendations for a booster dose except in the case of high-risk individuals. Local pain, headache, and fatigue are the most commonly reported side effects, occurring in a small percentage of children.

In 2012, U.S. Food and Drug Administration (FDA) approval was given for MenHibrix, the first vaccine licensed for infant immunizations providing protection again serotypes C and Y and the combination vaccine Hib-MenCY-TT (MenHibrix) that also contains protection against meningococcal groups C and Y. In late fall 2012, the ACIP recommended the use of HibMenCY in infants at high risk for meningococcal disease with a 2, 4, 6, and 12 to 15 months of age schedule. High-risk infants include those with persistent complement pathway deficiencies and anatomic or functional asplenia, including infants with sickle cell disease (CDC, 2012b).

Rotavirus Vaccine

Rotavirus (RV) is the primary cause of severe diarrhea in young children worldwide. RV vaccines are live-attenuated oral agents. There are two currently in use: RV5 (RotaTeq) and RV1 (Rotarix). Routine immunization is recommended for infants unless contraindications are known (e.g., severe combined immunodeficiency or severe allergy to latex). RV immunization should be postponed in infants with acute, moderate, or severe gastroenteritis until their condition improves. Dosage guidelines vary by manufacturer product and age at first administration (see Appendix C). Doses are generally administered at 2, 4, and possibly 6 months of age. Adverse events associated with vaccine administration include diarrhea, vomiting, nasopharyngitis, otitis media, and bronchospasm.

Human Papillomavirus Vaccine

Human papillomavirus (HPV) is a highly prevalent cause of STI that can cause cervical and anal cancer. There are two recombinant HPV vaccines approved for use in females, both effectively prevent cervical cancer and precancers. HPV4 (Gardasil) is effective against HPV types 6, 11, 16, and 18 and also prevents genital warts. HPV2 (Cervarix) is effective against HPV types 16 and 18. HPV4 is approved for females and males from 9 through 26 years of age; HPV2 is approved for females starting at age 10 years through 25 years.

The HPV series is given intramuscularly over a 6-month period, with the second and third doses given 2 and 6 months after the first dose. The ACIP recommends routine vaccination of females starting at 11 or 12 years of age with either HPV4 or HPV2; the minimum age is 9 years. The goal is to vaccinate girls before initiation of any sexual activity, not only vaginal intercourse. Oral HPV infection is strongly associated with oropharyngeal cancer (D'Souza et al., 2007). Routine vaccination of males with HPV4 should also begin at 11 to 12 years of age but can begin as early as 9 years of age.

Local pain, swelling, and erythema are the most commonly reported side effects; fever and nausea are reported less frequently. Syncopal episodes after HPV administration have been reported; however, their frequency is no greater than that which occurs after other adolescent vaccine administrations. To avoid this problem, have the adolescent sit during administration and for a short time afterward.

Considerations, Precautions, and Contraindications for Immunization

Strict attention to proper vaccine storage as well as administration protocol (e.g., exposure to light or limitations in length of time vaccine can be out or mixed before administered) is essential to ensure vaccine effectiveness. In medical offices, use a thermometer to maintain a daily temperature log.

Simultaneous administration of routine vaccines at different anatomic sites is safe (Tradition or Science 8-1). Not all brands of a specific vaccine are interchangeable. Always check the manufacturer's guidelines. For example, when immunizing against pertussis, the use of a vaccine from a single manufacturer is preferred. However, in a situation where the manufacturer of the previous dose is unknown or the manufacturer's product is not available, the rule is simple: Use any product; do not miss the opportunity to immunize the child.

Fears and lack of knowledge regarding contraindications to immunization can needlessly interfere with a child's protection against life-threatening, but preventable, disease. Awareness of the reasons for withholding immunizations, both for the child's safety in minimizing adverse reactions and in achieving maximum benefit, is important for the pediatric nurse (Tradition or Science 8-2).

Low-grade fever and minor respiratory infections are *not* contraindications for vaccination. The only true contraindications to immunization are a history of severe anaphylactic reaction to a vaccine or vaccine component or encephalopathy within 7 days after a dose of DTaP. Any adverse vaccine event must be reported in the VAERS. The Vaccine Injury Compensation Program provides a system of no-fault compensation associated with the administration of specified vaccinations. A guide discussing contraindications to childhood vaccinations is available at no charge from the CDC.

Evidence-Based Practice

TRADITION OR SCIENCE 8-1

Is simultaneous administration of routine vaccines safe?

Multiple studies have demonstrated the safety, reactogenicity, and immunogenicity of routine childhood vaccines when administered simultaneously as separate or combined injections (Heininger, 2007; Klein et al., 2012; Lim et al., 2011; Pichichero et al., 2007; Zepp et al., 2007). Separate but simultaneous injections of recommended childhood vaccines improve immunization rates and are cost-effective by eliminating multiple office visits; combined vaccines achieve these goals plus minimize distress to infants, which can be easier for parents.

Evidence-Based Practice

TRADITION OR SCIENCE 8-2

Is there a link between the MMR vaccine and autistic spectrum disorder (ASD)?

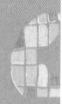

Some parents refuse to vaccinate based on an unsubstantiated correlation between the MMR vaccine and ASD; the topic has been amplified by inaccurate postings on the Internet. A link between the MMR vaccine and ASD was initially proposed by Wakefield et al. (1998) based on a sample of 12 children. This stance was later retracted by 10 of the authors, noting that no causal link was established between the MMR vaccine and ASD (Murch et al., 2004). Wakefield was discredited for his fraudulent research paper (Editors of the Lancet, 2010).

A steady increase in children with ASD has been noted, but with no change in the rate of increase when the MMR vaccine was introduced in the study population (Mäkelä et al., 2002; Taylor et al., 2002). The seeming increase in cases of ASD may be attributed to a broader definition of the concept of ASD and increased detection. Many studies and a comprehensive analysis of the body of research on this subject have demonstrated a lack of correlation between MMR vaccination and ASD (Demicheli et al., 2012; Madsen et al., 2002; Smeeth et al., 2004). In fact, the incidence of ASD continued to increase when MMR was withdrawn (Honda et al., 2005) and when thimerosal was removed from vaccines (Schechter & Grether, 2008).

The evidence is convincing that there is no correlation between the MMR vaccine and ASD.

---

caREminder

High fevers and severe illness are reasons to delay immunization, but only until the child has recovered from the acute stage of the illness to avoid adding the risk of adverse side effects from the vaccine to a child who is already ill or confusing symptoms of the illness with a side effect of the vaccine. Minor illnesses such as a cold, otitis media, or mild diarrhea without fever are not contraindications to immunization.

Vaccines derived from live viruses are generally not administered to any child with an altered immune system because severe vaccine-induced illness may result. MMR and varicella vaccination are contraindicated in children with immunodeficiency or therapeutic immunosuppression. This includes children on high-dose, long-term steroid therapy (>14 days) for at least 1 month until after discontinuing steroids. There are similar warnings about the need to delay immunizations for a specified period of time for children receiving immunoglobulin and blood products. However, MMR is recommended for all asymptomatic HIV-infected persons and should be considered for all symptomatic HIV-infected persons because of the severity of the illness if an HIV-positive individual were to contract measles. Immunization with MMR or varicella is generally deferred during pregnancy.

⚠ ALERT   *As with any medication, rare severe systemic reactions such as anaphylaxis or generalized urticaria are possible after vaccine administration. Because of the potential for anaphylaxis with the administration of a vaccine, observe any patient receiving a vaccine for several minutes after the vaccine is given for signs of immediate allergic/anaphylactic reaction.*

Strategies for Improving Immunization Status

Education remains the most important tool in increasing immunization rates in this country and the world. Do not assume that the general public understands and accepts the premises for routine childhood immunizations. It is important to assess the parent's or caregiver's level of knowledge about immunizations and the diseases they prevent. Remember that changes in the recommended schedules of immunization can also be confusing to parents. They may not understand that certain vaccine-preventable diseases, such as measles and varicella, are highly contagious and that unimmunized children are at risk if exposed to such diseases should an outbreak occur. New parents may not know the recommended times for the various vaccinations or the number of doses needed for full protection. Inform parents that combination vaccines are safe and reduce the number of injections that the child will receive, which is an important consideration. As always, provide opportunities for parents to ask questions.

Without a doubt, the risk from disease is always greater than the risk from vaccine for all individuals for whom vaccines are not contraindicated. Obtain informed consent before vaccinations are given. Many providers use immunization sheets (e.g., those available through the CDC) to provide information about the vaccines and their known side effects.

Explain the risks and benefits of immunization; it is the caregiver's responsibility to decide whether the child should be immunized (Clinical Judgment 8-1).

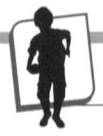

CLINICAL JUDGMENT 8-1

An Unimmunized Young Child

Jason is a 15-month-old who was brought into the clinic by his mother because he has a cold, has been very fussy, and has been pulling at his ears. He has not been to your clinic before.

Questions
1. What other information should the nurse obtain?
2. What are the major issues that must be addressed at this visit?
3. Is Jason too sick to receive immunizations today?
4. Which immunizations should Jason receive today?
5. What should Jason's mother be taught about potential reactions to the vaccines?

Answers
1. The history of present illness:
   How long has Jason been sick? (3 days)
   Has he had a fever? (He has felt pretty warm but not hot.)
   What, if anything, has been done to treat him? Has it helped? (no treatment)
   Is anyone else sick at home? (brothers have colds)
   Review of systems
   Past medical history
   Birth history
   Previous illnesses (colds; diarrhea; no injuries or serious or chronic illnesses)
   Current medications (none)
   Allergies (none known)
   Immunization status (received the HepB vaccine in hospital at birth; none since)
   Growth and development
   Family and social history
   Physical examination (normal except bilateral mucoid discharge from nares and bulging, erythematous tympanic membranes; axillary temperature of 99.4° F [37.4° C])
2. Upper respiratory tract infection and bilateral otitis media; vaccine-hesitant parents.
3. No. He does not have a high fever or serious illness.
4. HepB (second dose), DTaP, IPV, MMR, Hib, varicella, pneumococcal, hepatitis A
5. The use of acetaminophen should be decided on a case-by-case basis.
   Application of ice at injection site, if needed, for 24 hours, and then warm compresses
   Immunization-specific reactions (e.g., soreness at site, rash)
   Notification of health care provider of fever more than 105° F (40.6° C), seizure, persistent and inconsolable crying lasting 3 hours or more, or collapse or shocklike state
   Importance of continuing immunization series

Laws in most states require certain immunizations before school entry. Parents may decline immunizations on religious or, in some states, ideologic grounds. However, in the event of an epidemic, the health of the greater community takes precedence over the rights of the unimmunized individual. For instance, if a case of polio were to occur in a school setting, unimmunized children could be excluded from school for a specified period of time. If available, use state or regional immunization registries to help track and improve the delivery of vaccines.

The general public in the United States has no firsthand experience with most vaccine-preventable illnesses because many have been virtually eliminated as a result of routine childhood immunization practices. The phenomenon of "out of sight, out of mind" is operational; the longer it has been since a disease was prevalent, the harder it is to convince people that there is still a threat. Pediatric nurses must educate parents and caregivers about the need to vaccinate to ensure a healthy start and a healthy tomorrow for children. The CDC and the AAP have resources on their websites focusing on parental refusal to vaccinate and addressing concerns of vaccine-hesitant parents.

See thePoint for a summary of Key Concepts.

REFERENCES

Belshe, R. B., Edwards, K. M., Vesikari, T. et al. (2007). Live attenuated versus inactivated influenza vaccine in infants and young children. *New England Journal of Medicine, 356*, 685–696.

Burns, C. E., Dunn, A. M., Brady, M. A. et al. (Eds.). (2012). *Pediatric primary care* (5th ed.). Philadelphia, PA: W. B. Saunders.

Centers for Disease Control and Prevention. (2012a). *BMI percentile calculator for child and teen English version.* Retrieved from http://apps.nccd.cdc.gov/dnpabmi/

Centers for Disease Control and Prevention. (2012b). *CDC Advisory Committee on Immunization Practices recommends HibMenCY for infants at increased risk for meningococcal disease.* Retrieved from http://www.cdc.gov/media/releases/2012/a1024_HibMenCY.html

Centers for Disease Control and Prevention. (2012c). *Epidemiology and Prevention of Vaccine-Preventable Diseases:* The Pink Book: Course Textbook (12th ed.). Retrieved from http://www.cdc.gov/vaccines/pubs/pinkbook/index.html

Centers for Disease Control and Prevention. (2012d). National, state, and local area vaccination coverage among children aged 19–35 months—United States, 2011. *Morbidity and Mortality Weekly Report, 61*(35), 689–696.

Centers for Disease Control and Prevention. (2012e). Pertussis epidemic—Washington, 2012. *Morbidity and Mortality Weekly Report, 61*(28), 517–522.

Centers for Disease Control and Prevention. (2012f). *Press briefing transcript. Pertussis epidemic in Washington State—2012 Telebriefing.* Retrieved from http://www.cdc.gov/media/releases/2012/t0719_pertussis_epidemic.html

Centers for Disease Control and Prevention. (2012g). Summary of notifiable diseases: United States, 2010. *Morbidity and Mortality Weekly Report, 59*(53), 2–111.

Demicheli, V., Rivetti, A., Debalini, M. G. et al. (2012). Vaccines for measles, mumps and rubella in children. *Cochrane Database of Systematic Reviews,* (2), CD004407.

D'Souza, G., Kreimer, A. R., Viscidi, R. et al. (2007). Case-control study of human papillomavirus and oropharyngeal cancer. *New England Journal of Medicine, 356*, 1944–1956.

Editors of the Lancet. (2010). Retraction—Ileal-lymphoid-nodular hyperplasia, non-pervasive developmental disorder in children. *Lancet, 375*(9713), 445.

Grummer-Strawn, L. M., Reinold, C., & Krebs, N. F. (2010). Use of World Health Organization and CDC growth charts for children aged 0–59 months in the United States. *Morbidity and Mortality Weekly* Report, *59*(RR-9), 1–15.

Hagan, J. F., Shaw, J. S., & Duncan, P. M. (Eds.). (2008). *Bright futures: Guidelines for health supervision of infants, children, and adolescents* (3rd ed.). Elk Grove Village, IL: American Academy of Pediatrics.

Heininger, U. (2007). Booster immunization with a hexavalent diphtheria, tetanus, acellular pertussis, hepatitis B, inactivated poliovirus vaccine and *Haemophilus influenzae* type b conjugate combination vaccine in the second year of life: Safety, immunogenicity and persistence of antibody responses. *Vaccine, 25*(6), 1055–1063.

Honda, H., Shimizu, Y., & Rutter, M. (2005). No effect of MMR withdrawal on the incidence of autism: A total population study. *Journal of Child Psychology and Psychiatry, 46*(6), 572–579.

Jones, K. (2005). *Smith's recognizable patterns of human malformation* (6th ed.). Philadelphia, PA: Elsevier/Saunders.

Klein, N. P., Weston, W. M., Kuriyakose, S. et al. (2012). An open-label, randomized, multi-center study of the immunogenicity and safety of DTaP-IPV (Kinrix™) co-administered with MMR vaccine with or without varicella vaccine in healthy pre-school age children. *Vaccine, 30*(3), 668–674.

Lim, F. S., Phua, K. B., Lee, B. W. et al. (2011). Safety and reactogenicity of DTPa-HBV-IPV/Hib and DTPa-IPV/I-Hib vaccines in a postmarketing surveillance setting. *Southeast Asian Journal of Tropical Medicine and Public Health, 42*(1), 138–147.

Long, W. E., Bauchner, H., Sege, R. D. et al. (2012). The value of the medical home for children without special health care needs. *Pediatrics, 129*(1), 87–98.

Madsen, K. M., Hviid, A., Vestergaard, M. et al. (2002). A population-based study of measles, mumps, and rubella vaccination and autism. *New England Journal of Medicine, 347*, 1477–1482.

Mäkelä, A., Nuorti, J. P., & Peltola, H. (2002). Neurologic disorders after measles–mumps–rubella vaccination. *Pediatrics, 110*, 957–963.

Marcdante, K. J., Kliegman, R. M., Jenson, H. B. et al. (Eds.). (2011). *Nelson essentials of pediatrics* (6th ed.). Philadelphia, PA: Saunders Elsevier.

Maternal and Child Health Bureau. (n.d.). *Accurately weighing & measuring: Technique.* Retrieved from http://depts.washington.edu/growth/module5/text/contents.htm

Murch, S. H., Anthony, A., Casson, D. H. et al. (2004). Retraction of an interpretation. *Lancet, 363*, 750.

Pichichero, M. E., Bernstein, H., Blatter, M. M. et al. (2007). Immunogenicity and safety of a combination diphtheria, tetanus toxoid, acellular pertussis, hepatitis B, and inactivated poliovirus vaccine coadministered with a 7-valent pneumococcal conjugate vaccine and a *Haemophilus influenzae* type b conjugate vaccine. *Journal of Pediatrics, 151*, 43–49.

Prymula, R., Siegrist, C. A., Chlibek, R. et al. (2009). Effect of prophylactic paracetamol administration at time of vaccination on febrile reactions and antibody responses in children: Two open-label randomized controlled trails. *Lancet, 374*(9698), 1339–1350.

Schechter, R., & Grether, J. K. (2008). Continuing increases in autism reported to California's developmental services system: Mercury in retrograde. *Archives of General Psychiatry, 65*, 19–24.

Smeeth, L., Cook, C., Fombonne, E. et al. (2004). MMR vaccination and pervasive developmental disorders: A case–control study. *Lancet, 364*(9438), 963–969.

Taylor, B., Miller, E., Lingam, R. et al. (2002). Measles, mumps, and rubella vaccination and bowel problems or developmental regression in children with autism: Population study. *British Medical Journal, 324,* 393–396.

U.S. Department of Health & Human Services. (2010). *Healthy people: Developing healthy people 2020.* Retrieved from http://healthy people.gov/2020/

Wakefield, A. J., Murch, S. H., Anthony, A. et al. (1998). Ileal–lymphoid–nodular hyperplasia, non-specific colitis, and pervasive developmental disorder in children. *Lancet, 351,* 637–641.

Zepp, F., Behre, U., Kindler, K. et al. (2007). Immunogenicity and safety of a tetravalent measles–mumps–rubella–varicella vaccine co-administered with a booster dose of a combined diphtheria–tetanus–acellular pertussis–hepatitis B–inactivated poliovirus–*Haemophilus influenzae* type b conjugate vaccine in healthy children aged 12–23 months. *European Journal of Pediatrics, 166,* 857–864.

See thePoint for additional resources.

CHAPTER 9

Pharmacologic Management

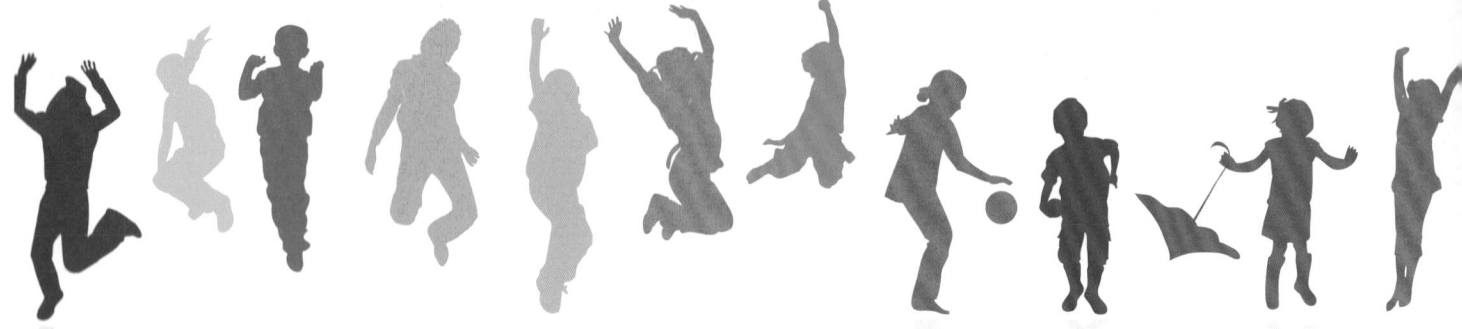

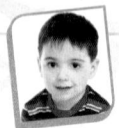

CASE HISTORY

José Diaz is 4½ years old. He has been very congested with a cold for the past several days. Now he is irritable, whiney, and pulling on his left ear. His mother, Claudia, is concerned because José has asthma, and often, a viral or bacterial infection will trigger a flare-up. Sure enough, José wakes up in the night coughing incessantly and wheezing. After a nebulizer treatment of albuterol, José's coughing subsides enough for him to sleep, but he is still wheezing. The next morning, Claudia takes him to the pediatrician who gives Claudia a written prescription for Prelone, a liquid glucocorticoid. Claudia has had experience with this medicine before and knows that José will retch it right back up and then resist taking the medication. Claudia is uncomfortable confronting the physician and asks the nurse what other type of medicine she could give José.

José's regular medications include a morning and evening nebulizer treatment with albuterol and fluticasone (or inhaled corticosteroid). His asthma is also exacerbated by allergic triggers. He weighs 40 lb.

CHAPTER OBJECTIVES

1 Discuss age-based variations in pharmacokinetics and pharmacodynamics.
2 Describe safety measures to reduce the risk of error in administering medications to children.
3 Explain developmentally appropriate techniques to administer medications via different routes to children.
4 Discuss key principles regarding parental and patient education when medications are prescribed for children and adolescents.

See thePoint for a list of Key Terms.

Medication administration is one of the most challenging and critical aspects of pediatric nursing. Unlike the adult "one-dose-fits-all" principle, dosing for children must be individualized. Medication administration to children must focus on age-related developmental considerations because the pharmacokinetic and pharmacodynamic drug effects are less predictable in children, especially in neonates and young infants. This is because of their much smaller size and immature organ systems. Consequently, safe administration of the right dose to the right patient

at the right time through the right route is a critical issue. Children are at highest risk for medication errors resulting from increased potential of mathematical errors in calculating dosages or drawing up medications and are more vulnerable to potential side effects and overdose. Ensuring safe administration of medication is a multidisciplinary responsibility that involves the nurse, physician, and pharmacist who all serve to check and balance each other.

DEVELOPMENTAL CONSIDERATIONS IN PHARMACOKINETICS AND PHARMACODYNAMICS

QUESTION: The correct dosage for prednisolone is 1–2 mg/kg/day. Given José's weight and a twice-daily order, how many milligrams per dose should José receive?

PHARMACOKINETICS

Pharmacokinetics involves the action of the body on a drug or how a pharmacologic agent or drug moves through the body over time. Pharmacokinetics involves the absorption, distribution, metabolism, and elimination of drugs as well as their protein-binding ability, half-life, bioavailability, and time to peak concentration. A child's size and age are key factors that affect the ability of his or her key organ systems to handle the absorption, distribution, metabolism, and elimination of drugs. For example, the capacity of the neonate's enzyme network to metabolize drugs ranges from 10% to 40% of that of the adult. Renal elimination of drugs in the neonate is also less efficient and takes several years to reach adult capacity. Liver function reaches adult capacity and exceeds it within the first several months of age. Because a child's age is one of the most influential variables in understanding the pharmacokinetic functions of absorption, distribution, metabolism, and elimination and excretion of drugs, different dosages are required for neonates (preterm and term), infants, and young children (Chart 9-1). Thus, pharmacokinetic principles are significant consideration in predicting dosage requirements. All four pharmacokinetic functions are important considerations in the choice of medications and the selection of safe dosages for a child.

caREminder

Some children metabolize drugs rapidly. Periods of rapid growth may lead to subtherapeutic drug levels, and some drugs may have paradoxical effects in children. Also, preverbal children cannot describe symptoms associated with side effects. Therefore, the nurse must closely monitor children for desired effects, toxic effects, and side effects of drugs and must educate parents and children about these drug-related issues.

Body weight or body surface is a key factor that must be considered in calculating dosages for a child. **Body surface area** (BSA) is the measured or calculated surface of a human body—the area covered by skin. As the child increases in weight and organ system maturity and his or her metabolic rate changes, larger and sometimes smaller amounts of drugs (depending on the balance

---

CHART 9-1   Developmental Pharmacokinetics

Factors That Affect Absorption of Drugs

1. Gastrointestinal
   Gastric pH is high in neonates, with adult values by 2 years of age. Acidic drugs are more bioavailable; basic drugs have decreased bioavailability.
   Gastric and intestinal motility (transit time) is decreased in neonates and infants but increased in older infants and children.
   The bile acid pool and biliary function are diminished in the newborn and reach full capacity during the first several months of life.

2. Rectal
   Only select drugs are suitable for rectal administration. In addition, length of exposure to the rectal mucosa affects absorption.

3. Intramuscular
   Variable in the pediatric age group secondary to (1) blood flow and vasomotor instabilities, (2) insufficient muscle tone and contraction, and (3) decreased muscle oxygenation.

4. Topical/transdermal
   Decreased with increased thickness of the stratum corneum and directly related to skin hydration.
   Neonates and infants have increased skin permeability, allowing greater penetration of medication and a greater surface area-to-body weight ratio with potential for toxicity.

5. Intraocular
   The membranes of infants and neonates are particularly thin; ophthalmic eye medications can cause systemic effects in infants and young children.

Factors That Affect Distribution

1. Neonates have a higher proportion of total body water that rapidly reduces during the first year of life. Adult values are gradually reached by 12 years of age. This factor is an important consideration related to the water solubility of a drug.
2. Children have a lower proportion of body fat than do adults, so lower doses of lipophilic drugs (e.g., digoxin) are required.
3. Protein binding of drugs is age dependent. Total protein concentration at birth is only 80% of adult values, which leads to more free or active drug circulation and potential for toxicity.
4. Fetal albumin in the newborn period has limited drug-binding ability.
5. An immature blood–brain barrier during the newborn period can lead to higher concentrations of drugs in the brain than at other ages.

Factors That Affect Metabolism

1. The newborn's enzymatic microsomal system is less effective.
2. Liver maturation varies among individuals; each liver enzyme becomes functional at a different rate.

Factors That Affect Elimination

1. Glomerular filtration and tubular secretion are reduced at birth.
2. There is gradual increase in renal function, with adult values reached after the first 1–2 years of life.

between growth and distribution in body tissues and drug metabolism) are needed to maintain therapeutic drug levels (e.g., the nurse may administer 25 mg of a drug to a 1-year-old child vs. 100 mg of the same drug to a 10-year-old child). In pediatrics, there are no standard amounts of a drug given per age; rather, dosage is based on weight using an established amount or dosage range of the drug per body weight (e.g., 10 mg/kg/day for children older than 1 month of age or 100 to 200 mg/kg/day). Dosages must be calculated using either BSA or weight per kilogram until the child reaches an adult weight (see the later section, "Prescribing the Correct Dose") because the child's size is a critical factor in the absorption, distribution, metabolism, and elimination of drugs. The child's size must be taken into consideration so as not to overwhelm the body's organ systems that are responsible for these functions.

A mother who is breastfeeding and taking medications requires careful evaluation because her infant may be exposed to harmful drugs through the ingestion of breast milk. Certain medications are contraindicated with breastfeeding because of their adverse effect on the developing infant (e.g., methotrexate). Other medications may be taken by the mother with instructions about how soon before or after breastfeeding the mother can take the drug; instructions to take the drug before the infant's longest sleep period; or, if necessary, instructions on the need to temporarily withhold breastfeeding. Hale's (2012) *Medications and Mothers' Milk* is an excellent resource on this topic.

It is also important to consider herbal supplements taken by breastfeeding mothers. They may have one or two main ingredients but can contain many other chemicals that may not be identified on the label. Mothers, therefore, may assume that herbs are natural and thus safe when breastfeeding. However, certain herbs can be very harmful to infants (e.g., buckthorn berry, coltsfoot leaf). The Organization of Teratology Information Services has information on medications and herbal agents in its databases (see thePoint for Organizations). Be aware of these issues when caring for an infant who is breastfeeding and educate mothers about the use of medications and herbal teas or supplements. The same caution exists about giving herbal supplements or complementary medications or agents to infants or children of any age. Their use should be approved by the primary care provider.

> **ANSWER:** First, convert José's weight from pounds to kilograms. Forty pounds divided by 2.2 is equivalent to 18 kg. José's dose would be 18–36 mg/day divided in two doses. The physician's order is for 15 mg twice a day. This fits within the desired 9–18 mg per dose.

PHARMACODYNAMICS

Pharmacodynamics refers to the actions of the drug on the body or how a drug produces physiologic and biochemical changes at the cellular, tissue, and organ levels. It involves the dose-response relationship influencing time of peak action and the onset and duration of action. For example,

ceftazidime works by binding to penicillin-binding proteins on the cell walls of susceptible microbes to inhibit bacterial cell wall synthesis. Furosemide is a sulfonamide "loop" diuretic and acts on the loop of Henle and proximal and distal renal tubules. Thus, the action of a drug, or its pharmacodynamics, is another important consideration in selecting the drug of choice to use in pharmacotherapy.

Liver enzymes are not mature in infants, so when drugs are metabolized via hepatic enzyme systems, clearance may be delayed with a prolonged drug half-life. Therefore, infants are more sensitive than older children and adults to the same concentration of certain medications, such as opioid analgesics and benzodiazepines. Because of differences in pharmacodynamics, acetaminophen is less toxic to children who have greater stores of glutathione than adults.

THE SIX RIGHTS

Administering medications to children can be challenging and even hazardous. Children's immature systems for metabolizing drugs and their smaller size put them at risk for adverse consequences of medication administration. In addition, their cognitive processing may limit their understanding that medications are needed to help them recover or maintain their health. Meticulous attention to the six rights of medication administration will help ensure accurate medication administration in the least emotionally traumatic manner.

The six rights that follow are guidelines to facilitate safe administration of the correct medication:

1. The right medication
2. The right dose
3. The right patient
4. The right route
5. The right time
6. The right approach

Documentation of assessments (with medications, this includes assessment for side effects) and interventions is always important; some consider documentation the seventh "right."

THE RIGHT MEDICATION

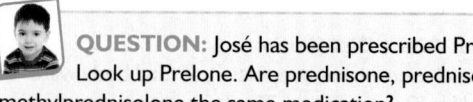

> **QUESTION:** José has been prescribed Prelone. Look up Prelone. Are prednisone, prednisolone, and methylprednisolone the same medication?

Selection of a medication is based on the child's need for pharmacologic therapy and the ability of the child's body to handle the drug (i.e., to absorb, distribute, metabolize, and eliminate the drug). Many medications prescribed for children do not have U.S. Food and Drug Administration (FDA) approval for use in children; this practice is known as *off-label use*. Prescribers use pediatric pharmacologic reference sources to prescribe these off-label medications and ask pediatric nurses to administer these medications. With the enactment of the FDA's Pediatric Studies Rule in 1998, new drugs that seek FDA approval and are likely to be used in children must include labeling information for pediatric use.

The nurse's responsibility in administering the right medication should be viewed as a multistep process. To administer the right medication, the nurse must

1. Know the medication to be administered—its indication for use, action, contraindications, side effects, and special nursing considerations (e.g., take a 1-minute apical pulse before administering digoxin).
2. Understand the connection between the patient's condition, illness, or disease and the use of a particular medication. If such a link is not present, clarify the medication order.
3. Select the correct medication from the patient's medication drawer or from medications sent to the unit from the pharmacy.
4. Verify the medication label with the patient's medication administration record; a triple verification of labels with the medication administration record can help to prevent medication identification errors. Check the label when first obtaining the drug, when preparing the dose, and when returning the container to the patient's medication box or discarding it.

This process is absolutely necessary to ensure that every child receives the correct medication. The nurse must know the indications for the medication prescribed and its potential side effects and must be knowledgeable about the child's medical illness, disease, or condition so that if an unusual, unlikely, or contraindicated medication is prescribed for a pediatric patient, the nurse can clarify the order. For example, an order to give trimethoprim-sulfamethoxazole (Bactrim) to a child with a known sulfa allergy should alert the nurse to address this issue with the practitioner who prescribed the medication. It is also important to ensure that all allergies to medication are clearly visible on the patient chart, all order forms, and on the medication administration record.

The nurse must also properly identify the medication sent from the pharmacy or the medication taken from the patient's personal supply, as ordered, with the patient's medication administration record. Check the expiration date. Do not use expired medications; return them to the pharmacy and order a replacement medication.

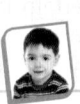
ANSWER: All three medications are glucocorticoids; however, the dosage for an equivalent effect is very different.

THE RIGHT DOSE

QUESTION: If a medication is so foul tasting that the child gags and spits the medicine back up, how do you determine the dose you have given?

There are two considerations in dosing: prescribing the correct dose for the child and dispensing the correct dose for the child.

Key points to remember when determining the right dose include the following:

• Pediatric dosages are calculated based on weight in kilograms or BSA.
• Adult dose reference ranges rather than kilogram dosing may be used in children who weigh more than 50 kg (with some providers using 40 kg as the cutoff point).
• Always double-check math calculations, particularly when preparing a medication that is not supplied as an exact dose. Double-checking mathematical calculations helps to prevent mathematical errors and makes it more likely that the correct amount of medication (a portion of the amount supplied) is given to the patient.
• Compare calculations with the actual order to verify that it is within the recommended range.

Prescribing the Correct Dose

In pediatrics, dosages are calculated using body weight or BSA. To verify the right dose using body weight, look up the established standard dose from a pediatric reference and multiply this number by the child's weight in kilograms to determine whether the dose ordered is correct. For example, if the reference dose is 10 to 20 mg/kg/24 hr divided every 6 hours and the child's weight is 10 kg, the child should receive 100 to 200 mg/24 hr or 25 to 50 mg every 6 hours.

A reverse calculation can also be done starting with the original order. For example, the order says to give 25 mg every 6 hours for a child weighing 10 kg. Multiply 25 mg by 4 (every 6 hours is four times a day) to find the total daily dose, which in this case is 100 mg/24 hr. Divide the 100 mg/24 hr by the patient's weight to obtain the milligrams per kilogram per 24 hours. Thus, 100 mg/10 kg comes out to 10 mg/kg/24 hr. Look up the reference range for the drug and compare the two. In this case, the reference range is 10 to 20 mg/kg/24 hr; hence, the dose that was ordered (100 mg/24 hr) is within the established reference range.

BSA is the most accurate measure for dosing medications for children; it is primarily used when calculating doses of cancer chemotherapeutic drugs. Infants have more BSA than would be expected from their weight because the ratio of BSA to weight varies inversely with length. To verify the right dose using BSA, the child's height and weight are needed. First, determine the correct dose from a pediatric reference and then use a **nomogram** (Fig. 9-1)—a graphic calculating tool, usually containing three parallel lines scaled for related variables so that when a straight line connects values of any two, the value may be read directly from the third at the point intersected by the line—which computes the relationship between height and weight, to obtain the child's BSA.

ALERT   *The nomogram includes both pounds and kilograms; make sure the correct scale is used. If the weight is measured in kilograms but graphed in pounds, the resulting BSA will be incorrect.*

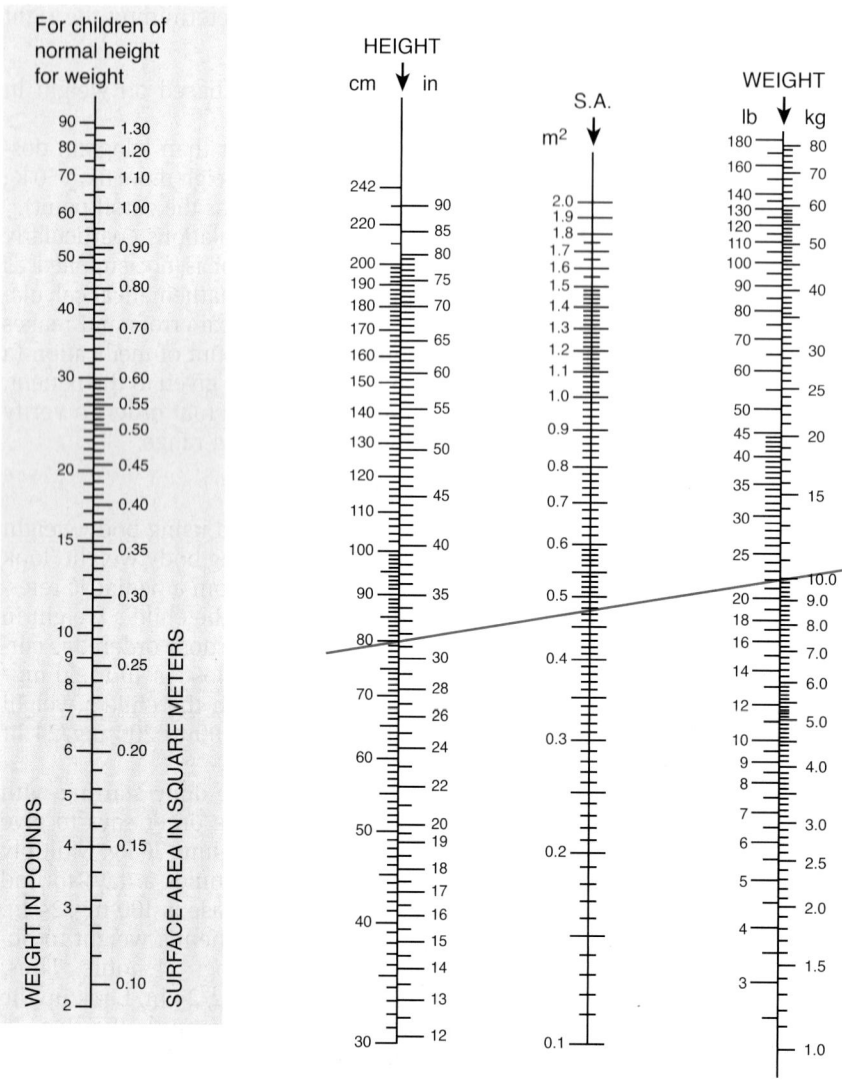

For children of normal height for weight

WEIGHT IN POUNDS

SURFACE AREA IN SQUARE METERS

HEIGHT

cm ↓ in

S.A.

m²

WEIGHT

lb ↓ kg

Figure 9-1 Nomogram for estimation of BSA. If the child is of average size, use the shaded box on the left to find the weight (on left) and then the corresponding surface area (on right). In the nomogram on the right, the child's surface area is indicated where a straight line that intersects the height and weight levels intersects the surface area (S.A.) column. In this example, the intersecting line indicates a child who is 80 cm tall and weighs 10 kg; the BSA is 0.47 m².

An alternative to using the nomogram to calculate BSA is Mosteller's formula: BSA equals the square root of weight (measured in kilograms) times height (measured in centimeters) divided by 3,600.

$$\text{SA (m}^2) = \sqrt{\frac{\text{Weight(kg)} \times \text{height(cm)}}{3600}}$$

After you have verified the correct dose from a pediatric reference and you know the child's BSA, you can determine whether the correct dose has been ordered. To do this, multiply the dose given in the pediatric reference by the child's BSA. For example, if the reference recommends 100 mg/m²/24 hr divided every 12 hours and the child's BSA is 0.5 m², the child should receive 50 mg/24 hr or 25 mg/12 hr. If the actual order reads 25 mg/12 hr (50 mg/24 hr), the dose ordered is within the established reference range.

When looking up reference ranges for dosing, verify the maximum amount of the medication that should be given either per dose or per 24 hours. Maximum dosage is important, especially in the overweight child. For example,

if the body weight of a child weighing 100 kg were used to determine a drug dose, the amount of drug ordered would likely exceed the liver's capacity to metabolize the drug or the renal system's ability to safely eliminate the drug. Often, adult range of dosing is used as the drug reference for children who weigh more than 50 kg.

Although most drugs are dosed by weight, there are certain factors that may also influence dosing in children. For example, age-related metabolic changes and organ dysfunction may be factors, in addition to weight, that are considered when determining an appropriate dose of a medication for an individual child. Therefore, monitor drug levels and physiologic parameters of children with kidney, liver, or heart failure. Likewise, closely monitor preterm and young infants for untoward (or adverse) drug effects.

ALERT *The nurse is responsible for knowing whether the prescribed dose of medication is within a safe dosage range. If the prescribed dose is incorrect, notify the prescribing practitioner immediately.*

Dispensing the Correct Dose

Before administering a medication to a child, nurses are often called on to draw up an individualized dose from either a multidose container or a single-dose container that contains more medication than needed. It is important, therefore, to set up equations in a consistent fashion when drawing up an individualized medication. For example, if a multidose container is labeled as cephalexin (Keflex) 250 mg/5 mL and the ordered amount is 200 mg of oral suspension, set up the equation as follows: 250 mg/5 mL = 200 mg/x mL. To calculate the value of x, cross multiply so that $250x = 1,000$; then divide 1,000 by 250 so that $x = 4$. This tells you that 4 mL must be drawn up to obtain the necessary 200 mg cephalexin. Similarly, an oral syringe containing 15 mg/mL ranitidine syrup may be sent from the pharmacy. If the order calls for 10 mg ranitidine syrup orally, set up the equation as 15 mg/1 mL = 10 mg/x mL to calculate that the nurse would draw up 0.67 mL. This is the proportion method of calculation.

Nurses can also use a formula method of calculation that labels each component of the medication calculation in the equation as either dose ordered (D), dose on hand (H), and quantity (Q) of the dose on hand. The formula to solve is dose ordered divided by dose on hand times quantity equals the desired amount of medication to be given. The equation reads

$$\frac{D}{H} \times Q = \text{Amount of medication to be given}$$

For example, if the order calls for 10 mg ranitidine syrup orally and you have 15 mg/mL ranitidine syrup, set up the equation as:

$$\frac{10 \text{ mg}}{15 \text{ mg}} \times 1 \text{ mL} = 0.67 \text{ mL}$$

Administering intravenous (IV) medications is often challenging in pediatrics, especially if the nurse must prepare a drug that comes as a powdered medication. The final volume is not always equal to the initial fluid volume used; the powder may also add volume. The nurse must first dilute the powdered medication with sterile normal saline or water, then determine the final concentration of the medication, and then calculate how much fluid is needed to obtain the ordered amount of medication. For example, a child is to receive 225 mg ampicillin IV, and a 250-mg vial is sent from the pharmacy. The vial says to use 1.8 mL sterile diluent with a resulting final volume of 2 mL. The resulting solution is 250 mg/2 mL. The nurse sets up a math proportion and calculates that 1.8 mL of the final volume is needed to obtain 225 mg ampicillin (225 mg/x mL = 250 mg/2 mL).

Infusion times are also important considerations for maintaining blood levels of the drug or to prevent adverse reactions. Use only recommended infusion times to deliver IV medications. Infusion times (e.g., 5, 20, 30, 60 minutes) and required fluid volume dilutions for medications are based on established concentration levels necessary to deliver IV medications; consult a reference source for dilutions and infusion times. The IV rate for infusion is calculated and the volume to be infused is entered into the pump computer together with the rate of infusion, which is based on an hourly rate. Thus, if 20 mL is to be infused over 30 minutes, the IV pump is programed to deliver 20 mL (volume to be infused) at a programmed rate of 40 mL/hr. The pump signals at 30 minutes when the 20 mL infusion is completed.

ANSWER: Usually, the decision to readminister the dose depends on the toxicity of the drug (e.g., digoxin has a narrow therapeutic range, whereas cephalexin has a broad therapeutic range), absorption rate of the drug, and amount of time between administration and vomiting. Generally, if it is less than about 5 minutes, readminister the medication; if it is more than that, do not readminister unless it is certain that the child did not get the dose. Readminister only once per dose. However, certain high-alert medications with narrow therapeutic ranges are not routinely readministered even if the vomiting occurred less than 5 minutes after administration. Rather, the nurse should consult with the physician about the appropriateness of readministration. If it is known that a child will vomit or fight a particular medication, then a change in medication may be the solution.

THE RIGHT PATIENT

All children who have been admitted to a health care facility should be identified by an identification (ID) band attached to their body and not according to the bed they are in. Accurate identification serves two purposes:

1. To reliably identify the individual as the person for whom the service or treatment is intended
2. To match the service or treatment to that individual

For administration of medication and other services or treatments, The Joint Commission adopted a two-identifier requirement to ensure reliable identification of patients as a safety goal. Acceptable identifiers can include two of the following on a wristband: the individual's name, date of birth, assigned ID number, telephone number, or other person-specific identifier. Bar coding with two or more person-specific identifiers is also being used. Take the patient's medication administration record to the bedside to perform your double-identifier check. Verify the medication about to be delivered by checking the medication label with the child's ID band.

If the child does not have an ID band in place, the nurse must first verify the identity of the child before administering any medication. A parent should identify a baby or a younger child. Ask an older child his or her name and date of birth or other identifier.

ALERT *Use extra caution when there are children with the same last names on the unit or when the parent of the child does not speak English. Charts may be confused and orders may be written for the wrong patient. Check allergy wristbands to verify that the child does not have an identified allergic reaction to the medication about to be administered.*

THE RIGHT ROUTE

QUESTION: Prednisolone is available in an IV and an oral form. If José worsens and is admitted to the hospital, could his medication be administered at the same dose intravenously?

The route of administration affects the absorption, effectiveness, and the speed of action of medications. For example, based on efficacy studies, certain childhood immunizations are administered intramuscularly (IM), whereas others are given subcutaneously (SubQ). The nurse, therefore, must be familiar with the various routes of administrations for all childhood vaccines. Medications given via differing routes—IV, IM, SubQ, oral, or rectal route—or prescribed as inhaled or intranasal agents will have differing peaks and durations of action. Morphine sulfate administered IV rather than SubQ as ordered could severely compromise a child's respiratory status because the IV route results in faster absorption of the medication. Similarly, medications given through a jejunostomy tube rather than a gastrostomy tube will have different absorption rates because of the different motility rates in various sections of the gastrointestinal tract. Inhaled corticosteroids are not used as "a rescue medication" when systemic steroids are needed during an asthma exacerbation.

Incorrect administration techniques can also be problematic. Faulty administration of SubQ insulin can result in lipodystrophy. Application of a thick layer of topical cortisone medication can result in increased steroid absorption resulting in striae of the skin, and too rapid IV infusion of vancomycin can result in red man syndrome (an anaphylactic-like reaction causing an erythematous, maculopapular rash and intense flushing of the skin; patients may also experience dizziness, headache, chills, chest pain, and respiratory difficulties). Therefore, careful attention to proper administration technique and vigilance in monitoring for adverse reactions are critical nursing responsibilities.

To reduce the chance that the medication is administered via the wrong route, colored syringes (e.g., amber colored) may be used as an added safeguard to help differentiate oral medications from IV medications that are dispensed in clear syringes from the pharmacy. For IV drugs, routinely label all infusion lines to be sure that the right drug is inserted into the right infusion line. Use extra caution for patients with multiple IV infusion lines and gastric infusion devices so that gastric medications are not incorrectly injected into IV and arterial lines.

ANSWER: José's medication probably could not be administered at the same dose intravenously. Prednisolone is available in an IV form; however, the most commonly used IV steroid agents for status asthmaticus is methylprednisolone IV administered at 0.5–1.0 mg/kg/6 hr.

THE RIGHT TIME

Medications given at the wrong intervals can affect therapeutic blood levels. The use of military time helps to reduce the problem of medications being given at incorrect times. Each institution may have its own policy about scheduled times (e.g., once, twice, three, or four times per day) for medication. The general rule of practice is to administer a medication within the time frame of a half hour before or after the scheduled time period. Adhering to scheduled medication times is particularly important for medications that must be given every 4, 6, or 8 hours around the clock to maintain therapeutic drugs levels for optimum drug effectiveness.

There are certain situations in which the pediatric nurse must be particularly alert to timing issues. If drug blood levels are ordered at specific times to coincide with administration of certain medications at specific times, the nurse is responsible for administering the medication at the required time and notifying the laboratory of the time that the blood sample must be collected. Determining peaks and troughs of drugs is an important part of the management plan for certain medications.

Some medications should be given with meals, just before meals, on an empty stomach, or at a specified time (e.g., 2 hours after meals or at 8 AM, 3 PM, and 9 PM). Therefore, timing of these drugs is an important issue. For example, drug absorption can be altered if a certain drug is given with food, or a drug may need to be given before meals to promote effective gastrointestinal functioning. A daily dose of steroids, for example, is often given in the early morning to mimic the normal physiologic response of the body. Thus, the nurse must be knowledgeable about the medications being administered and their mechanism of action.

caREminder

Timing is often important when administering oral medications to infants. Because many young infants are fed on demand, the nurse may need to adapt the medication schedule for certain drugs based on the infant's feeding pattern.

THE RIGHT APPROACH

QUESTION: Describe the "right approach" for a child in early childhood. How is it different from that for an infant or a child in middle childhood?

Often, individuals are less attuned to the sixth right of administering medications to children. The right approach—how one addresses the child and the task at hand and considers the emotional status and developmental level of the child—is especially important when administering medication to children because of their varying cognitive levels, inability to recognize cause and effect ("I get the medicine now and it makes me feel better in a little while"), and lack of abstract thought. One's approach to the child, age-appropriate explanations, and administration techniques often affect the success of administering the medication to the child in the least emotionally traumatic manner possible (Developmental Considerations 9-1).

ANSWER: Infants cannot anticipate an unpleasant taste. Position the infant upright and present a pleasant- or neutral-tasting substance to ensure that the child is awake and swallowing. Give the medication slowly enough to allow the child to swallow and prevent any risk of aspirating, and give a pleasant-tasting "chaser." Four-year-old children are very different. They remember bad tastes and smells. The smell and memory of the taste may be enough to induce retching without even tasting the medication. An aversion to the artificial fruit-flavored syrup may make the oral suspensions even more noxious. Four-year-olds can put up amazing resistance and can also understand the necessity of taking a medicine (e.g., "You need to take this medicine to make it easier to breathe"). Successful administration requires eliciting some degree of cooperation on the part of the child. Practicing atraumatic nursing care also means not overpowering children but instead gaining their cooperation and being sensitive to their emotional needs. Give them other options. Do not rule out suggesting a tablet form of a medication in place of an unpleasant-tasting drug. A prednisone tablet is very small. The child may accept a crushed pill in pudding or even swallow half a small pill on a slice of banana. However, certain oral medications including, but not limited to, enteric-coated pills, extended-release products, and sublingual medication should not be crushed or altered.

AVOIDING COMMON ERRORS IN MEDICATION ADMINISTRATION

Medication administration involves a series of steps: calculating and prescribing a drug, transcribing the medication order, dispensing the drug, and delivering the drug to the patient. Errors in administration can involve mistakes at any one or more of these steps. Likewise, an error can involve a mistake by a single health care care provider or multiple providers. Knowledge of common problems associated with each of these steps is important to avoid a drug error.

PRESCRIBING AND TRANSCRIPTION ERRORS

QUESTION: Given the plethora of corticosteroids, what are some possible errors in transcribing these medications?

Medication errors related to prescribing and transcription are generally grouped into four categories: poor handwriting, decimal errors, misused abbreviations, and incorrect calculations. Many health care agencies have adopted electronic medication records, which eliminate the problem of incorrect interpretation of handwriting.

However, to avoid a transcription error in situations when typed medication orders are not common practice, the nurse and pharmacist must carefully interpret handwritten medication orders and clarify all medication orders that are not clearly written.

Decimal errors, the most common error in pediatric medication calculation, can be avoided by never placing a decimal and a zero after a whole number (called the *trailing zero*) because the decimal point might not be read correctly (e.g., 4.0 mL might be read as 40 mL; write 4 mL). Place a zero (called the *leading zero*) before fractions that are less than one (e.g., write 0.6 mL, not .6 mL, which might be confused with 6 mL if the decimal is inadvertently missed). Put a space between the number and its unit for easier readability.

Use abbreviations sparingly. For instance, do not use the abbreviations q.d., q.o.d., IU, or u. Instead, write out "every day," "every other day," "International Unit," or "unit." It is recommended that the Latin abbreviations for the eyes and ears not be used; instead, write out right or left and ear or eye. Avoid other dangerous abbreviations including μg (write mcg instead), H.S. (write out half strength or at bedtime), S.C. or S.Q. (write SubQ or subQ), and c.c. (write mL). In addition, because they are easily confused with one another, always write out morphine sulfate and magnesium sulfate; do not use abbreviated drug names. Urge prescribers to write out instructions rather than using abbreviations.

Look-alike and soundalike (similar) drugs can also be a cause of error. Carefully look at the spelling of the drug and note its correct pronunciation. The vaccines Tdap and DTaP are not the same vaccines. High-alert medications deserve special precautions and should never be hurriedly administered.

Ask for clarification of medication doses that are not within the pediatric reference range. The individual who ordered the medication may have made a mathematical error or used an incorrect weight when calculating the amount of medication that was needed. Use caution when interpreting large doses more than 1,000. Commas should be used for dosing units at or above 1,000 or words such as 100 thousand or 1 million should be used to avoid errors.

Important points for the nurse to remember to decrease prescribing and transcription errors include the following:

- Clarify medication orders that are poorly handwritten.
- Pay strict attention to the rules about when a leading zero is necessary and not using a trailing zero.
- Use abbreviations sparingly, and only use approved abbreviations.
- Double-check all math calculations.
- Verify with the pharmacist or prescriber unusually large volumes or dosage units for a single-patient dose.
- When a parent, caregiver, or patient questions the administration of a drug, listen to the concerns, answer questions, and recheck the medication dose and/or call the prescribing provider if appropriate.
- When anything about a medication or its administration is unusual, ask questions. A single question may prevent a medication error

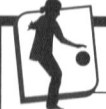

DEVELOPMENTAL CONSIDERATIONS 9-1

Medication Administration

Age Group/Developmental Group	Tips/Guidelines
All ages	• Solicit the parent's involvement in medication administration as appropriate. • Some oral medications are extremely difficult for a child to take because of palatability issues. In such instances, the medication may need to be mixed with food or a liquid to disguise its taste. Some pills may be crushed and mixed in small amounts of apple-sauce, chocolate syrup, ice cream, or pudding to disguise their taste. Do not crush enteric-coated pills. • Preschoolers and older children may wish to suck on an ice pop or ice prior to oral medications to numb the tongue and reduce unpleasant tastes. • Offer choice of fluid after oral medication administration, as appropriate, to reduce taste of medication. • Whenever possible, take the child to the treatment room for painful procedures such as IV insertion and injections. Do not perform painful procedures at the child's bedside or in the playroom to maintain these as safe havens for the child. • If possible, give medications IV rather than IM or SubQ to avoid pain and intrusion. • Never lie to a child that an injection will not hurt. Use a topical anesthetic whenever possible before injections to decrease pain.
Infancy	• Unless contraindicated, hold the infant in an upright position while delivering oral medication. • An infant who has just been fed and is sleeping deeply may not want to suck. Try to administer medications either before a feeding or when the infant is not sleeping deeply after a feeding. • Place oral medication in a *small* amount of pleasant-tasting, nonessential food (e.g., not formula, cereal) if an infant can eat from a spoon. Check compatibility of the medication with the substance mixed in (e.g., Viracept has a very bitter taste when mixed with acidic juices and should be mixed with milk). Remember that the more liquid the medication is mixed with, the greater the volume the child must take. • If the infant cannot eat from a spoon, place oral medication in a nipple that is not attached to a bottle. • If the infant refuses to take oral medication, place it in a syringe and squirt it inside the mouth, toward the back of the jaw. Then rub the submandibular area bilaterally to elicit swallowing. • Very strong–tasting medications may cause an infant to gasp and increase the risk of aspiration. Prepare the infant that something to swallow is coming in his or her mouth; introduce a nipple, then give a small amount of juice (or other diluent), then juice with the medication. • For difficult-to-feed infants or those with respiratory difficulties, administer oral medication slowly. The infant may need to rest between short spurts of medication administration. • Praise an older infant for compliance. Comfort after administration.

Age Group/Developmental Group	Tips/Guidelines
Early childhood	• Explain in simple terms the reason for the medications, such as "This will help you get well" or "This will make your tummy ache go away." • Use administration approaches used with infant, with the exclusion of the nipple. In the stage of initiative, older children in this age group may think it is fun to use an oral syringe. Assist or supervise children as they push the syringe plunger to get the medication into their mouth. • Offer realistic choices that will allow the older child in this age group some control over the situation (e.g., "Would you like to take your medicine with water or juice?" "Do you want your IV in your right hand or your left hand?") • An older child may want to suck on ice pop to numb the tongue before taking unpleasant-tasting medications. • Provide distraction. • Permit expression of anger. • Provide preparation through play. • If the child is not able to cooperate in taking oral medications, situate the child on your lap with his or her legs in between your legs. Place one of the child's arms behind your back and hold the other arm in your nondominant hand while administering the medication with your free hand. This is often a two-person procedure, especially if the child spits out the medication. • In a two-person procedure, have one person hold the child in his or her lap as described previously while the other person places the fingers of one hand around the child's cheek and slowly instills the oral medication from a syringe into the side of the child's mouth with the other hand. After a small amount is instilled, press the child's cheeks together until he or she swallows the medication; repeat this maneuver until medication administration is complete. • After the medication has been administered, praise the child for his or her efforts. • Have another person available to help the child hold still to ensure safety during injections. Place a Band-Aid on an injection site, because older children of this age fear their blood will "run out of the hole." Allow the child to assist in placement. Comfort after injection.
Middle childhood	• Give concrete explanations of the purpose of the medication using drawings and diagrams of targeted body parts. • Some children may hide their medication and pretend they have taken it; be alert for this. • Give as much choice as possible regarding administration. • The child may want to suck on an ice pop to numb the tongue before taking unpleasant-tasting medications. • Allow independence from the parent in the process of medication administration.
Adolescence	• Use approaches suggested for the school-aged child. • Depending on the maturity of the adolescent, use more abstract rationales for medication. • Educate adolescents about safe self-medication.

ANSWER: The variety of corticosteroid compounds and dosages, including very similar-sounding names, increases the risk of a prescription or transcription error. The nurse should verify that the prescribed dose is appropriate for the prescribed medication.

DISPENSING AND ADMINISTRATION ERRORS

The pharmacist or the nurse may be involved in dispensing errors. Math errors may be made in calculating portions of medication to draw up to obtain an exact dose. If the nurse makes a math error, the amount of medication that is to be drawn up is incorrectly identified. In some situations, the amount to be drawn up is correctly calculated; however, the amount drawn up is not the amount calculated. Double checking calculation should be a routine practice in nursing.

Two registered nurses should check high-alert medications (drugs that have a high risk of causing harm when an error occurs) such as insulin, digoxin, opioids, drugs used for sedation, heparin infusions, and chemotherapeutic agents before they are administered. Review the original order for these medications and verify that the dose of the drug that was ordered is the amount that has been drawn up to administer to the child. For digoxin and chemotherapeutic agents, verify from the original order that, based on a reference range for the dosing and the patient's weight or BSA, the correct dose was ordered. Chemotherapeutic agents are typically administered only by nurses certified to deliver these agents.

Smart pumps (computerized IV infusion pumps) are a major advance in medication safety and can help reduce medication administration errors. Such enhanced IV pumps contain dynamic software that is programmed to ensure that the first five rights of medication administration are maintained (the sixth right, approach, cannot be ensured by technology). There are currently two types of smart pumps. The technology in type 1 pumps allows the nurse to identify the drug, its concentration, and solution, which provides a safety guardrail. Type 2 pumps contain the same technology found in type 1 pumps, with the addition of built-in bar code readers to identify bar-coded drug labels as well as to confirm unique patient identification information and record the bar-coded ID badge of the nurse. Remember, however, that technology is not a replacement for sound nursing judgment. Sometimes, the nurse will start to administer a medication and the parent or child may question why the medication is being given. They may even refuse to take the medication because of concerns about, or prior adverse reactions to, a drug. Always listen to their concerns, because the prescribing provider may have made a mistake or may be unaware of prior adverse reactions or that the child has a contraindication to the medication.

Compatibility of medications mixed in a syringe or administered in IV tubing may also be an issue. Certain drugs are incompatible if mixed together in a syringe, administered in the same IV line without first flushing the tubing, or if given with certain solutions (e.g., lipid or parental nutrition). The nurse must consult a drug compatibility chart when administering IV medications or mixing medications in a syringe. Vaccines that are manufactured as single-dose agents are never to be mixed (e.g., a single dose of measles, mumps, rubella, and varicella vaccine cannot be mixed in the same syringe with a single dose of hepatitis A vaccine; however, manufactured combination vaccines are to be given as one injection).

ALERT *To decrease dispensing and administration errors:*
- *Double-check math calculations and amounts that are drawn up for dispensing.*
- *Use a two-nurse system to verify doses and amounts drawn up for high-alert medications.*
- *When a parent or patient questions whether a medication should be administered, answer questions and, if appropriate, double-check the medication order and/or call the prescriber to discuss the concern expressed by the patient or parent.*

REPORTING ADVERSE DRUG REACTIONS AND MEDICATION ERRORS

It is important to complete appropriate agency forms if an adverse drug reaction or medication error occurs. In the case of an adverse drug reaction, identify the patient's symptoms and notify the prescriber and pharmacist. Discontinue use of the medication until instructed to do otherwise. Likewise, if a medication error is made, notify the prescriber and pharmacist immediately. Monitor the child for adverse reactions.

ADMINISTERING MEDICATION TO CHILDREN

Successful medication administration must focus on safety and age-appropriate behavioral and developmental considerations. All health professionals are responsible for administering safe dosages and monitoring for toxic effects and side effects of drugs. The nurse must know how to calculate therapeutic dosages to determine whether they are safe to administer and what toxic effects and side effects are associated with the drugs being administered. Follow general safety measures to reduce the occurrence of adverse events (Nursing Interventions 9-1).

Medication administration reflects one of the finer points of the art of pediatric nursing. The resistance of the infant, young child, or preschooler to swallowing foul-tasting or smelly medications can be dramatic in its display and time consuming for the nurse. Assess the child's cognitive level. Parents often like to know the name of the medication that their child is receiving.

NURSING INTERVENTIONS 9-1

Safety Tips for Medication Administration

- Never leave medications at the child's bedside unless permitted by institution policy.
- When checking medication labels, pay close attention to the spelling of the medication because many drugs have similar names.
- Perform hand hygiene before preparing medications.
- Prepare medications in a quiet, well-lit area.
- Avoid distractions when drawing up and administering medications. Some hospitals require nurses wear a medication vest or sash as a signal to others to not distract the nurse during medication preparation and/or administration.
- Check drugs for discoloration or unusual precipitates.
- Use a calculator to check drug doses and calculate doses twice.
- Do not give a drug that another nurse has prepared.
- If medications are prepared in a syringe beforehand, label the syringe with the name of the drug, its concentration, date and time drawn, and your initials.
- Remember to remove syringes (and needle if used) from the child's bedside and place in an appropriate sharps box.
- For liquid oral medications, use an oral syringe or medication cup to ensure accurate dosage measurement. Teach parents that use of a household teaspoon or tablespoon may result in dosage error because they are inaccurate.
- Remember to remove caps from oral syringes before administering medications and discard in a proper receptacle. Caps left at a child's bedside or when left in place (which then pop off while administering the medication orally) may be aspirated.
- Be aware of drug incompatibilities with other medications or fluids. This is especially important when administering multiple IV medications or when the patient is receiving parenteral nutrition or lipids.
- There should be a health care prescriber's order if the nurse is to administer medication brought in from home. The pharmacist should identify the medication.

- Check the time interval between medication administrations for all PRN (as needed) drugs to ensure that enough time has elapsed.
- Label external medications "for external use only" and store separately from other medications.
- Record IV fluid amounts used to deliver IV medications in the patient's intake and output record.
- Be especially careful when administering high-alert medications such as antineoplastic drugs, digoxin, insulin, or opioids. Medications delivered by the parenteral route also demand vigilance both in preparation and while infusing.
- Use vials of sterile water or normal saline for injection as a one-time injection solution and not as multiple-dose vials.
- Be aware of potential drug–drug and drug–food interactions.
- Monitor results of drug levels when ordered.
- Obtain a careful drug allergy history and, if applicable, be sure that an allergy alert is posted on the patient's chart and that the patient wears an allergy alert bracelet.
- Check with the pharmacist or current drug manual before crushing tablets to ensure that crushing is not contraindicated.
- Administer enteral medications through oral or catheter-tipped syringes only. Use the largest syringe size that is practical; larger syringes generate fewer pounds per square inch than smaller syringes, thus reducing the potential of tube rupture. Do not use Luer-Lok–tipped syringes to avoid inadvertent IV or IM administration of medication because needles cannot be attached to oral or catheter-tipped syringes. It is desirable to flush with water or saline after medication administration to infuse the medication. When determining the amount of flush solution, consider the child's fluid status (e.g., potential for fluid overload), gastric or intestinal tube size, institutional policy, and manufacturer recommendation. It is important to verify compatibility of medications when multiple medications are administered at one time (to avoid clogging the tube).

Explain to the child (or parent, when applicable) the reason that a medication is being given and any procedure that is necessary for the administration of the medication, using explanations that are simple and appropriate to the child's cognitive level. A child may cooperate more readily with a procedure if the proper explanation has been made. Soliciting the aid of the parents can be especially useful because they may have already developed a method of medication administration that is acceptable to the child. Do not deceive the child about the fact that you are administering medication (e.g., by pretending that you are giving the child something good to eat). Similarly, do not use the medication as a reward or punishment. Guidelines for administering medication by age group are presented in Developmental Considerations 9-1.

ROUTES OF ADMINISTRATION

Some of the more common routes of medication administration include oral, IV, IM, rectal, otic, ophthalmic, and topical and are discussed in the following paragraphs. Administration of inhaled medication is discussed in Chapter 16 and intrathecal medication is discussed in Chapter 22. For information on enteral, nasal, and subcutaneous administration, see thePoint for Procedures on Medication Administration.

Administering Oral Medication

QUESTION: Describe different techniques and measuring devices to give liquid medications. Which would be most appropriate for a 4-year-old?

The oral route should be used to administer medications whenever possible (see thePoint for Procedures on Medication Administration). The gastrointestinal tract provides a vast absorptive area for medications, and administration by this route is less invasive, thus less traumatic, than IM or IV injection.

Children, however, have a natural aversion to foul-tasting and smelly substances. They may cry and refuse to take medication administered orally or may try to spit out the dose if it tastes or smells bad. When administering oral medication, never mix it with the infant's formula or necessary food source (e.g., cereal) or with the child's favorite food. Doing so may lead to the dislike of that food as well as to a distrust of the caregiver. Similarly, distrust may result if the child is told that the medication tastes good or desirable. The overall objective of administering oral medications is to administer the entire dose to the child while creating the least aversion to the medication as possible

KidKare When possible, offer the child a choice of drink after distasteful medications (unless contraindicated). Older children can suck the medication from a syringe, pinch their nose, or drink through a straw to decrease the input of odor, which adds to the unpleasantness of some oral medications.

A complication associated with administering oral medications is aspiration. Positioning and strategies noted in Developmental Considerations 9-1 will reduce this risk. Proper positions for administering oral medication to an infant and young child are shown in Figure 9-2.

ANSWER: A cooperative 4-year-old could take an oral medication in a small medication cup. With an uncooperative child, spills are less likely with the syringe. A standard syringe may be used to draw up a liquid medication; however, errors involving the route of administration have led to manufacturers producing syringes specifically for oral medication. The hub is off-center so that they look different from a standard syringe. Spoons with measured increments in the handle are commonly given to parents by pharmacies but are infrequently used in hospitals. Small plastic measuring cups are accurate for larger volumes (e.g., more than 15 mL).

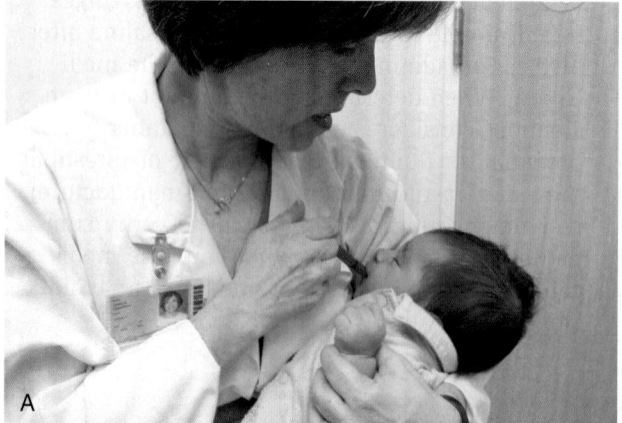
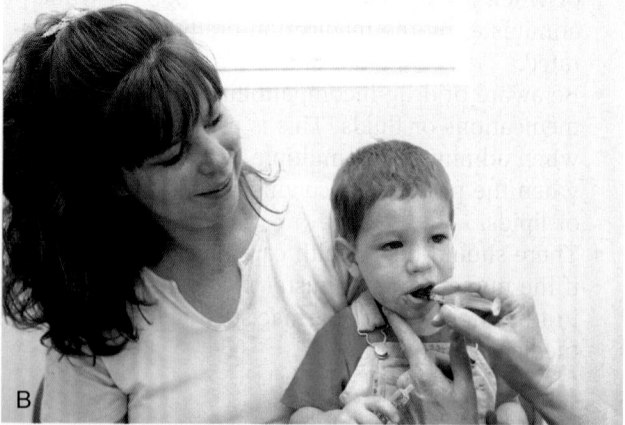

Figure 9-2 (A) Administering oral medication to an infant. Note how the right-hand-dominant nurse can control the infant's movements by holding the infant's left arm (the infant's right arm is tucked under the nurse's left arm) and tucking the infant's head in the crook of her arm. The nurse can then use her right hand to administer the medication. (B) Administering oral medication to a young child. With the child sitting on the parent's lap, place the syringe on the side of the tongue and slowly drip the medication into the child's mouth.

Administering Intravenous Medication

QUESTION: If José's respiratory condition warranted hospital admission, José could receive his systemic glucocorticoid intravenously. What is a concern of administering IV glucocorticoids to young children?

The IV route provides direct access into the vascular system. For this reason, it is an ideal route to use when drugs must be delivered rapidly, when high serum concentrations of a drug must be maintained, or when reliable absorption is necessary. For the child with established IV access, administration of medications via this route can be performed in a manner that is relatively nonthreatening to the child. See Chapter 17 for a discussion of venous access and IV therapy and thePoint for Procedures on Medication Administration, including Heparin Lock/Flush, Peripheral Catheters, Peripherally Inserted Central Catheters, Totally Implantable Devices, and Tunneled Catheters.

To minimize adverse effects associated with high serum drug levels (e.g., nephrotoxicity, ototoxicity) and to avoid venous irritation from concentrated solutions, IV medications are usually diluted. Young children may develop fluid overload from the extra 50 mL of fluid commonly given to administer medication "piggybacks" to adults. Most institutions have specific policies on diluting drugs and administering diluted drugs. IV medications can be delivered in various ways, depending on the drug (e.g., pain medications or diuretics may be given IV push, whereas antibiotics are often given over 30 to 60 minutes) and the child's fluid status (e.g., infants cannot handle large fluid volumes; children with renal, cardiac, or other problems may require fluid restriction).

caREminder

Some medications are very irritating to the veins (e.g., nafcillin sodium and phenytoin). Giving them over a longer period or in more fluid can help minimize this irritation.

IV medications can be given directly into the IV tubing (IV push) or via volume control chamber or syringe pump. Medications given IV push immediately enter the vascular system with almost instantaneous effects (Fig. 9–3). IV push medications are usually administered over a few minutes and necessitate small amounts of extra IV fluids. Syringe pumps are used to deliver medication with minimal amounts of excess fluid required (Fig. 9-4). Low-volume tubing can be used to minimize the amount of drug wasted in the tubing. The pump is set to administer the drug over the predetermined period. For children who can tolerate extra fluid volume, IV medications can be administered via small volume IV bags (piggyback). A volume control chamber (e.g., buretrol) is sometimes used. The drug is diluted in a specific amount of fluid in the volume control chamber, taking into account how much fluid the drug must be diluted in, the child's IV flow rate, and the fluid volume in the tubing. After the volume control chamber is empty, the drug remains in the IV tubing. Therefore,

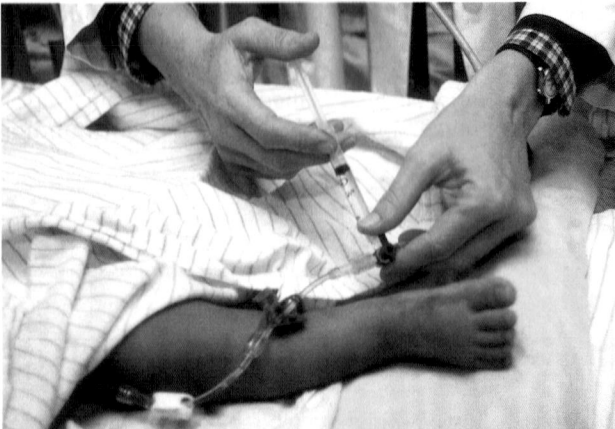

Figure 9-3 Medications administered via IV push enter the vascular system immediately.

it is necessary to know how much fluid the tubing holds (commonly 15 to 20 mL) so at least that amount can be given to flush the medication through the tubing into the vein. Tag the volume control chamber with tape or a designated sticker so that everyone is aware that a medication or flush is infusing. Some medications are given via syringe in a "B" or medication port of an IV pump. After the delivery of the B port medication, the tubing is cleared of medication via IV solutions delivered in the IV main port line. The principle of clearing or flushing tubing after the delivery of IV medication always remains the same regardless of how the IV medication is delivered (i.e., as a push, via a buretrol, in a B port, or through an infusion pump).

ALERT   *Include the extra fluid given to administer IV medications and flush the tubing in the calculation of the child's total fluid intake, particularly in young children who may not be able to handle the extra fluid or those with unstable fluid balance.*

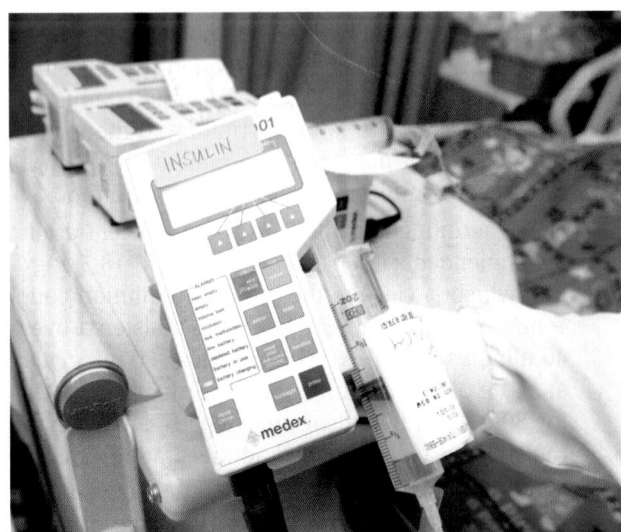

Figure 9-4 Syringe pump used to administer IV medication. Proper labeling assists in identifying when medications have been added to infusions.

IV medication can also be given via continuous drip. Standardizing IV infusion concentrations can reduce the number of medication errors.

Adverse effects of IV medication administration include extravasation of the drug into surrounding tissue, resulting in temporary or permanent damage, and reaction to the drug, including side effects and anaphylaxis. The nurse must intervene to minimize these hazards (Clinical Judgment 9-1). Before administering an IV medication, check the site to ascertain

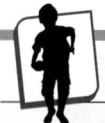

CLINICAL JUDGMENT 9-1

Intravenous Medication Administration

Ari is a 12-year-old boy who has been hospitalized for the past 4 days with staphylococcal pneumonia. His current weight is 38 kg. As part of his treatment, he is receiving IV fluid at 125 mL/hr and nafcillin 1,200 mg/4 hr via peripheral IV. The reference source says that nafcillin must be diluted 10–20 mg/mL and given over 30–60 minutes. Ari has had his IV restarted four times since admission and complains bitterly that the IV site burns during nafcillin administration. You review his chart and find that the nafcillin has been given in 65 mL of fluid followed by 15 mL to flush the IV tubing, then 45 mL to maintain his 125 mL/hr IV rate.

Questions

1. The recommended dose of nafcillin is 100–200 mg/kg/24 hr given every 4–6 hours. Is Ari's dose within the suggested range?

2. What factors concerning Ari's IV may indicate a problem?

3. Is the nafcillin being diluted in the best way to manage this situation?

4. How will you dilute the nafcillin based on Ari's current IV rate?

5. What will indicate that the more prolonged administration of a less concentrated solution has addressed the problem? If nafcillin administration remains problematic, what are alternatives for you to consider or address with the rest of the health care team?

Answers

1. Yes:

$$38 \text{ kg} \times 100 \text{ mg} = 3,800 \text{ mg/24 hr}$$
$$= 633.3 \text{ mg/4 hr}$$
$$38 \text{ kg} \times 200 \text{ mg} = 7,600 \text{ mg/24 hr}$$
$$= 1,266.7 \text{ mg/4 hr}$$

Ari is receiving 1,200 mg/4 hr, almost 190 mg/kg/24 hr.

2. Ari's IV has been restarted on an average of once every 24 hours, which is too frequent. In this situation, it may indicate that the nafcillin is injuring the veins. Nafcillin is very irritating to the veins, but when well managed, the patient should not be very uncomfortable during administration.

3. No, it is diluted in the maximum concentration recommended (1,200 mg ÷ 65 mL = 18.5 mg/mL, which is close to the maximum dilution concentration), and the nafcillin is administered over 40 minutes (65 mL + 15 mL flush = 80 mL given at a rate of 125 mL/hr = 2 mL/min = 40 minutes for 80 mL), a period of time slightly longer than the shortest recommended administration time of 30 minutes.

4. Infuse the nafcillin over a longer period of time (60 minutes), diluted in more fluid. Subtract the 15 mL of fluid needed to flush the medication through the tubing to find out the amount of fluid left for that hour in which to dilute the nafcillin: 125 − 15 = 110 mL to dilute the 1,200 mg nafcillin. 1,200 mg − 110 mL = 10.9 mg nafcillin/mL. This concentration is closer to the recommended minimal dilution of 10 mg/mL and should be less irritating to the vein than the previously administered 18.5 mg/mL.

5. Effective management may be indicated by maintenance of one peripheral IV site for 72 hours and the nafcillin not burning upon administration. If the problem continues, dilute the nafcillin in even more fluid, either manipulating the IV rate to end up with the same fluid balance (e.g., giving 150 mL the hour the nafcillin is administered and then 100 mL the next hour) or, if Ari can tolerate the extra fluid, increasing the fluid amount for the hour the nafcillin is administered. Consult with the clinical pharmacist. The length of time over which the nafcillin is administered should not be increased beyond 60 minutes because this may affect serum drug levels and administration of other medications he is receiving. It may be appropriate to insert a PICC line (peripherally inserted central catheter).

that the IV fluid has not infiltrated the tissue. Medications given intravenously enter the vascular system quickly. Anaphylaxis or toxic side effects (e.g., respiratory or cardiac depression) may manifest immediately or after a period of time. Know the medication's potential side effects and adverse reactions, monitor the child for these, and teach the child and family to notify the health professional if these or any other unusual signs or symptoms appear. Check your institution's policy on which drugs must be administered by a physician and which must be verified for accuracy by another nurse.

As noted previously, many medications are incompatible with other drugs, diluents, and IV solutions. Check a reference source for compatibilities, flush well between administration of incompatible drugs, or give via different IV access. Do not mix medications or give medications in the same line when administering blood products.

> ANSWER: Glucocorticoids are not irritating to the vein; for that reason, they would not need to be diluted or given especially slowly. José is big enough and does not have any cardiovascular complications that would create fluid restrictions. IV administration of a medication allows for a rapid increase in serum levels of a medication. A side effect of high-dose glucocorticoid administration is mania and psychosis. For José, his parents, and the nurses, administering the medication while preventing dramatic increases in serum level is a concern.

Administering Intramuscular Medication

When using the principles of atraumatic care, administration of medications via the IM route should be rare. Children fear invasive procedures, needles, and shots. Using an IM injection to deliver pain medication in itself causes pain and, frequently, psychological distress in the child. Most drugs, including pain medications and antibiotics, can be given orally or intravenously. The rectal route may be psychologically traumatic but should not be physically painful.

If a medication is ordered IM, advocate for the child. Consider whether the medication can be given via another less traumatic route, such as orally or rectally. If the child has an IV line, can that route be used to administer the drug? If the drug is to be given routinely, it is probably less traumatic to insert an IV line than to give repeated injections. Check with the pharmacist and/or prescriber to change the route of administration, if appropriate. If a medication must be administered IM, use a topical anesthetic (e.g., EMLA, LMX4, vapocoolant) prior to giving the injection.

Prior to administering an IM injection, evaluate the child's size, muscle development, motor capabilities, and diagnosis (see thePoint for Procedures on Medication Administration). These factors help determine the most appropriate site for injection (Fig. 9-5). For example, a child must have been walking for at least a year before the dorsogluteal site is used. Even then, the muscle is small, poorly developed, and close to the

sciatic nerve, which is relatively large in young children. Therefore, the ventrogluteal or vastus lateralis site is a safer choice in an infant. If multiple injections are necessary, rotate injection sites.

> **KidKare** Tell the child it is all right to make noise or cry out during the injection. His or her job is to try not to move the extremity.

Volume of fluid to be injected and needle size must also be considered when administering IM injections. The maximum volume that the muscle will accommodate depends on muscle size; thus, it varies with age of the child and the site used. Needle gauge and length also vary depending on the muscle mass. Generally, a 25-gauge needle is used for neonates, a 23 gauge for infants, and 20- to 22-gauge needles for older children.

Complications associated with giving IM injections in children include intra-arterial or IV injection, nerve injury, muscle fibrosis or contracture, and infection at the injection site. IM injections may also not be deposited in the muscle. A study of obese adults demonstrated that injection at the dorso- and ventrogluteal sites would be deposited in subcutaneous tissue (Zaybak et al., 2007). If it is necessary to use this route, give meticulous attention to proper technique, and note location to avoid complications.

Administering Rectal Medication

The rectal route is not the preferred route because of potential emotional trauma to the child and unpredictable absorption in the colon. Absorption can be further affected by the presence of stool in the colon and rectum. However, the rectal route may be the best choice for a child who cannot tolerate oral medication and in whom a parenteral route is not available (see thePoint for Procedures on Medication Administration).

Avoid cutting rectal suppositories if possible. If the suppository must be cut to obtain the ordered dose, then it must be cut lengthwise. Cutting a suppository lengthwise helps absorption at the required rate. The drug may not be dispersed evenly within the suppository.

Position the child in a left lateral position with the right leg flexed or in the knee–chest position to expose the anus and help relax the external sphincter for ease of insertion. Remove the suppository packaging and lubricate the suppository with a water-soluble lubricating jelly. Gently insert the apex of the suppository (pointed end) past the internal anal sphincter to prevent expulsion (Bradshaw & Price, 2007). In an infant or young child, insert the suppository with the little finger. The index finger can be used for older children.

> **KidKare** Instruct the child to pant like a puppy because this provides distraction and relaxes the anal sphincter.

Hold the child's buttocks together until the child relaxes or loses the urge to push. If the child has a stool

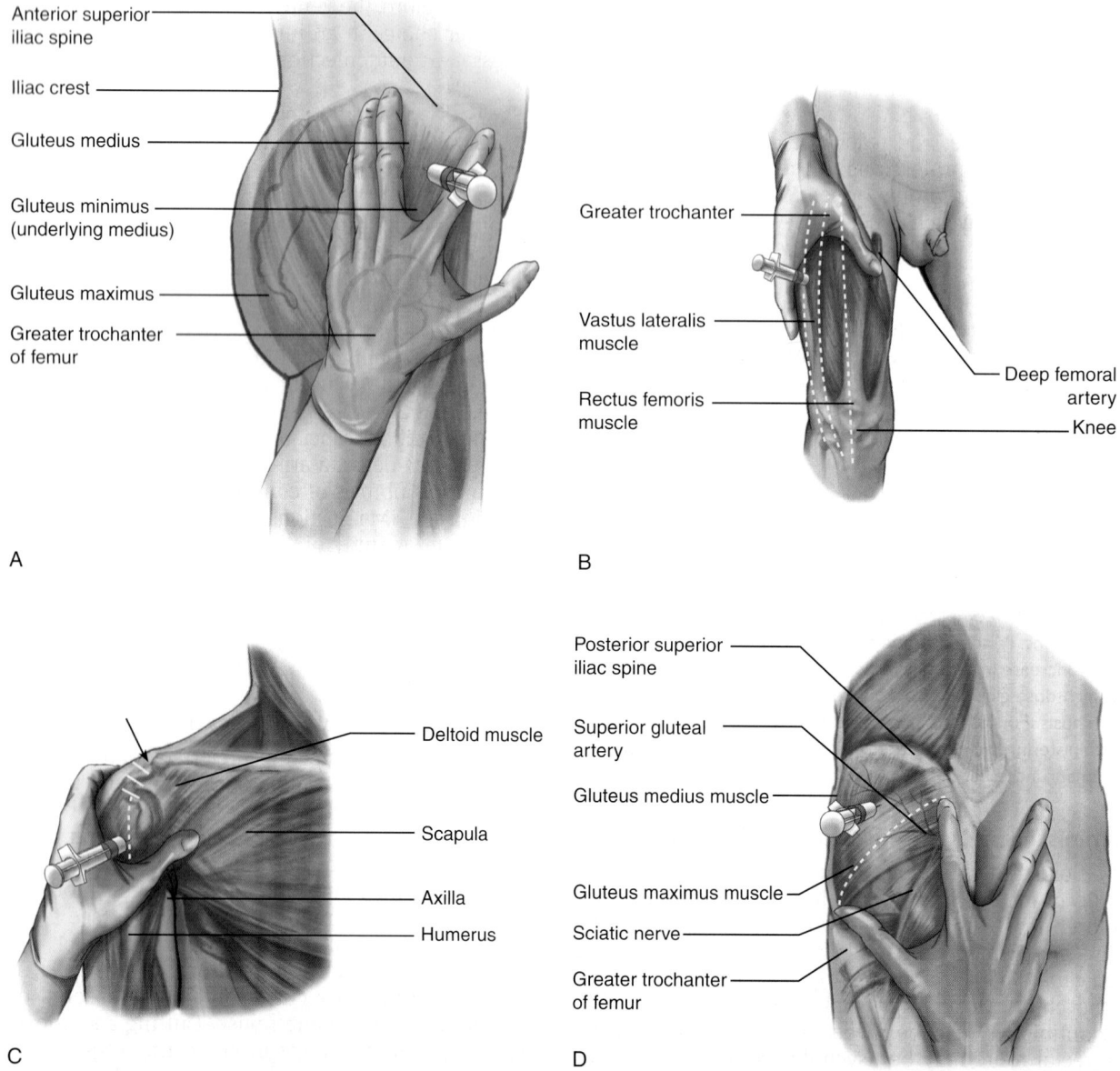

Anterior superior iliac spine

Iliac crest

Gluteus medius

Gluteus minimus (underlying medius)

Gluteus maximus

Greater trochanter of femur

A

Greater trochanter

Vastus lateralis muscle

Rectus femoris muscle

Deep femoral artery

Knee

B

Deltoid muscle

Scapula

Axilla

Humerus

C

Posterior superior iliac spine

Superior gluteal artery

Gluteus medius muscle

Gluteus maximus muscle

Sciatic nerve

Greater trochanter of femur

D

Figure 9-5 IM injection sites in children. (A) Ventrogluteal: Use the hand opposite the side for injection to locate landmarks (e.g., to give in child's left hip, use your right hand to locate landmarks). Locate by placing your palm on the greater trochanter, index finger on the anterior superior iliac spine, and middle finger on the posterior edge of the iliac spine. Inject into center of V formed by index and middle fingers. (B) Vastus lateralis: Palpate greater trochanter and knee. Divide into thirds; site is in middle third. Draw two imaginary lines from greater trochanter to knee: one midanteriorly and one midlaterally. Injection site is located between these lines in midlateral anterior thigh. (C) Deltoid: Identify lower edge of acromion process and point on arm in line with axilla. Site is one to three finger breadths (depending on size of child) below acromion process and just above axilla. Inject into middeltoid region. (D) Dorsogluteal: Locate posterior superior iliac spine and the greater trochanter; imagine a line between the two. Inject in the upper outer region above this line into the gluteus medius muscle.

within 30 minutes, examine the stool for the presence of the suppository.

Administering Otic Medication

Do not administer otic medication if the medicine is cold. Cold medication may cause discomfort and produce vomiting or vertigo in the child. If kept in the refrigerator, allow the medication to come to room temperature before administration. Warm the solution by

gently rotating the bottle in your hands before administration (see thePoint for Procedures on Medication Administration).

Have the child lie in a supine position with his or her head turned to the appropriate side. For children younger than 3 years of age, pull the earlobe down and back; for older children, pull the pinna up and back (Fig. 9-6). Administer the ordered amount of drops into the ear canal, holding the dropper a half inch above the ear canal and

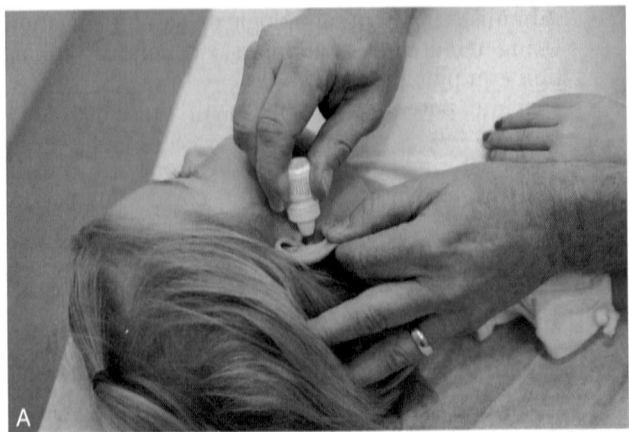 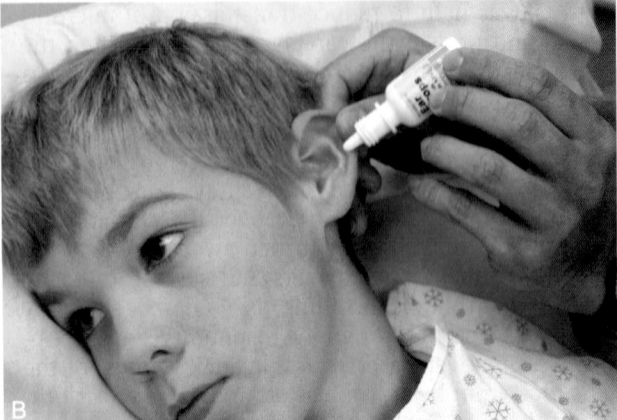

Figure 9-6 Positioning for administering ear drops. (A) In the child younger than 3 years of age, the pinna is pulled down and back. (B) In the child older than 3 years of age, the pinna is pulled up and back.

being careful not to touch the dropper to the ear to prevent contamination of the dropper with microorganisms. Gently massage the tragus (area anterior to the ear canal) unless contraindicated because of pain. Have the child remain in the supine position with the head turned for 2 to 3 minutes. Insert a small cotton ball into the entrance of the ear canal to prevent the medication from leaking out into the external ear.

Administering Ophthalmic Medication

Bring medication to room temperature before administration to avoid unnecessary discomfort during administration (see thePoint for Procedures on Medication Administration). If it is not room temperature, warm eyedrops by holding the vial between the hands until warm. Assess the eyes for debris, and cleanse them with a cotton ball soaked with normal saline if necessary. Move from the inner canthus of the eyelid to the outer canthus. Use only one sweep of the eye with each cotton ball to prevent contamination.

Position the child supine in bed, or another flat surface, looking up. Restrain the uncooperative child for administration. Rest your dominant hand against the child's forehead. With the other hand, pull down the lower eyelid to expose the conjunctival sac. This positioning prevents poking the child in the eye with the dropper or medication tube and allows for correct placement of the medication.

With the eyedropper, instill the correct amount of drops into the conjunctival sac, being careful not to touch the dropper to the eye to prevent contamination of the dropper or bottle. An alternate method of administration is to have the child close his or her eyes and tip the head backward. Place the medication drops on the inner canthus of the eye and instruct the child to open the eyes.

If administering ointment, place a thin ribbon of ointment along the entire conjunctival sac from the inner canthus to the outer canthus. Twist the ointment tube at the end to dislodge the ointment from the tube. Have the child keep his or her eyes closed for up to 1 minute after administration.

Ophthalmic medication should not be shared. Teach families that each family member must have his or her own medication to prevent cross-contamination.

Administering Topical Medication

Medications are given topically through the skin (transdermally) and are absorbed because of the skin's relatively rich blood supply (see thePoint for Procedures on Medication Administration). Because skin thickness and blood flow to the skin vary with age, the potential for toxic effects of the drug must be considered. Children have a larger BSA and a thinner layer of cutaneous and subcutaneous tissue, so there is an increased risk for systemic absorption and effects through topical application.

Assess the child's skin integrity before administration of topical medication. Observe for cleanliness and clean off dirt and excess lotions as needed. Do not apply topical medication to skin with open lesions unless ordered.

Cleanse the skin as ordered or per reference manual recommendations before application of the medication. Use a basin of warm water and a washcloth only. If an open wound is present, use gauze instead of a washcloth. Dry skin well after washing. Some medications require cleansing all old medication off the skin before applying new medication. Other medications require applying new sterile medication over the old medication without cleansing the area.

Apply topical medication to the site. Use the correct amount as ordered and the administration technique for the type of topical medication (see also Chapter 25).

caREminder

An excessive amount of medication may result in irritation of the skin and adverse systemic effects. Unintentional absorption through mucous membranes can result in systemic toxicity.

Administer gels, ointments, pastes, lotions, and creams using cotton swabs, tongue blades, or gloved hands. Gloves help to reduce transmission of microorganisms and protect the caregiver from absorbing the medication through his or her hands. If a powder is ordered, sprinkle it over the site; ensure that the child's head is turned away so that none is inhaled. If a spray is ordered, check with a reference source or the manufacturer's recommendations; most sprays must be shaken before administration. Spray over the site and ensure that the child's head is turned away to reduce the potential of inhalation. Powders and sprays are easily inhaled, which may cause lung tissue damage or may increase absorption through the respiratory system. Apply a dressing over the site, if indicated, to prevent the medication from being rubbed off and to protect clothing and the site. Occlusive dressings may increase absorption of the medication and should not be used with topical steroids.

Apply transdermal and topical systemic medication patches to a flat area of the skin; they are self-adhesive. Flat areas help the medication remain in contact with the skin, promoting even absorption. Rotate application sites to reduce skin irritation. Do not cut medication patches to fit area or reduce dose because cutting alters the dose administered. The medication may not be distributed evenly on the patch, and one cannot predict the amount of medication left on the patch.

EDUCATION ABOUT PHARMACOLOGIC AGENTS

Before children are discharged from a health care setting, family members and older children should have a basic understanding about all medications that are to be taken at home, including over-the-counter medications. Education should include the information presented in Teaching Intervention Plan 9-1.

Assess the ability to pay for prescription and over-the-counter medications, if this could be an issue, and provide information about resources available to help obtain needed medications. Assess if the child will take the form of medication prescribed (e.g., the child only tolerates liquid medications and the pill form was prescribed). Assess if the family has proper storage for medications (e.g., if receiving drugs that need to be refrigerated, do they have a refrigerator?).

Also assess the ability of a parent to administer a medication or for the child to self-administer a medication before discharge from the health care setting. Return demonstrations are an important evaluation tool to assess safe administration of medication. Situations that would require return demonstrations include

- Administering oral medications to infants and young children
- Measuring small amounts or exact doses using a syringe. Although consumers were more likely to obtain a correct dose with a syringe over a dosing cup, one-third measured inaccurately with a syringe (Sobhani et al., 2008)
- Giving injections or delivering medications through special tubing (e.g., nasogastric, gastrostomy, or jejunostomy tubes)

- Administering ophthalmologic or nasal medications
- Using metered-dose inhalers, spacers, or inhalation equipment
- Teaching parents or patients with limited cognitive abilities
- Administering multiple medications (to ensure that the correct dose and the correct medication are given as directed)

ADMINISTERING MEDICATION IN SCHOOL, CAMP, OR CHILD CARE SETTINGS

 QUESTION: What are some issues that might arise related to administering medications to José after he starts kindergarten?

Nurses who administer medications to children in non-medical settings, such as schools, camps, or child care settings, should have a written protocol that outlines the agency's regulations on administering medications. See Chart 9-2 for key elements that should be addressed in such a protocol.

School districts often allow nonnursing staff to administer medications to children under the training and supervision of a nurse. In such instances, the nurse is responsible for the training of those who will be administering medications and the ongoing supervision of these individuals. Documentation of such training and supervision is important.

The family or health care provider may request that over-the-counter medications be administered to children in nonmedical settings. Once again, the agency should have a protocol in place to handle these requests. Often, statements from both the parent and physician are required. In such instances, each child's over-the-counter medication should be labeled with the child's first and last name as well as the name and phone number of the physician who recommended the medication. Note the current date and date of expiration. Identify instructions regarding dosing and frequency as well as indications for when to notify the parent or physician that the child is not responding as anticipated.

ANSWER: José will need to have a copy of his prescription, an inhaler and spacer, and directions on their use at the school for any possible acute asthmatic episodes.

VERBAL ORDERS

All health care agencies should have a policy and protocol about nurses taking verbal orders for administration of medication. This should be a practice that is done only in emergency or unusual circumstances. The nurse who takes such orders should listen to what the prescriber says, write the order down, and then read the order back to the prescriber.

TIP 9-1: A TEACHING INTERVENTION PLAN for Medication Management at Home

Nursing Diagnosis and Family Outcome

- Deficient knowledge: Correct techniques for medication management
  Outcome: Child and family will appropriately store, administer, and monitor for side effects of medications.

Interventions

Teach the child and family the following about medications:

Medication-Specific Issues

- The reason the drug is being given, how much should be taken, and the frequency of administration. Make sure that the parent and older child know the name of the medication.
- Specific instructions about taking an "as-necessary" drug or a drug that is to be taken under specific circumstances (e.g., a drug used for fever control or medications to be taken as part of a rescue plan for a child whose asthma symptoms are worsening). Cover when, how often, and how long to take as-necessary drugs.
- Signs and symptoms that indicate that the drug is effective or not effective (e.g., fever subsides or child remains febrile)
- Signs and symptoms of medication adverse reactions, side effects, or toxicities
- Possible drug interactions with other medications or foods
- Storage issues, if applicable (such as the need for refrigeration or to keep at room temperature, avoid direct sunlight)
- Monitoring issues (such as peak flow or blood glucose levels), if applicable
- Pregnancy risk factors of a drug for specific drugs prescribed for female teenagers
- Tips about administering "difficult-to-take" drugs (e.g., offering an ice pop or ice to numb the tongue prior to unpalatable medications)
- Written individualized medication information (essential). If the parent cannot read, provide pictures (e.g., a picture of a medication measuring spoon with the numbers written in and an arrow pointing to the amount to be administered; if the medication is to be taken twice a day, a picture of the child sitting up in bed smiling and stretching with the sun up and one of the child lying in bed with eyes closed and the moon in the sky).

Herbs

- Signs and symptoms of herbal adverse reactions, side effects, or toxicities

- Caution about the use of alternate or complementary therapies and the need to discuss these with a health care provider before their use because they may contain dangerous elements such as iodine and heavy metals.

Storage

- Store all medications out of children's reach, in a locked cupboard, if possible.
- Never remove medication labels.
- When medication is no longer needed, safely dispose of it at your pharmacy, community household hazardous waste center (check if they accept medications), or place unused drugs in sealed bag/container (crush solid drugs, mix with water) with undesirable substance (kitty litter, coffee grounds) and dispose in trash.
- Check all medications once a year and discard all leftover, outdated, or unlabeled medications.
- Follow storage instructions as directed (e.g., refrigerate medication if label indicates; do not freeze).

Administration

- Follow label instructions or administer as indicated by your health care practitioner or pharmacist.
- Give most medications on an empty stomach for better absorption; for exceptions (e.g., erythromycin), read and follow label instructions.
- Use oral syringes or medication measuring spoons to measure doses; household teaspoons are not accurate for medication measurement.
- Do not tell a child that medication is "candy."
- If needed, mix in small amounts of nonessential foods (e.g., applesauce, jelly), not in favorite or staple foods.
- If child immediately vomits the entire dose, readminister recommended dose unless instructed not to do so (e.g., digoxin).
- If child vomits more than 1 hour after a dose was administered, wait and give the next scheduled dose.
- Give the entire course of antibiotics even if the child's condition improves, unless otherwise instructed.
- Never give medications prescribed for someone else even if the illnesses seem similar.

Contact the Health Care Provider if

- Child vomits more than one dose of the medication
- Symptoms of illness that the medication is to treat do not improve
- Child's condition appears worse or changes occur, such as a rash or trouble breathing

CHART 9-2   Key Elements for Protocol on Administration of Medicines in a Nonmedical Setting

- The child's first and last names are on the container.
- Medication is prescribed by a licensed health professional; the name, address, and phone number of the health professional who ordered the medication appear on the container.
- Medication is in the original package or container.
- The date the prescription was filled and the date it expires appear on the container.
- Medication is in a childproof container.
- A statement from the health care provider indicates the name of the drug, the diagnosis or reason the medication is needed, and whether any serious reactions might occur or an alert for the nurse about the possibility of a serious drug reaction.
- A policy about self-administration of medication (e.g., the use of inhalers or an EpiPen) should be identified for children who are capable of self-administration, exhibit responsible behaviors, and are in need of speedy access to their medication.
- Information about security and proper storage of medications should be identified in the agency's protocol.
- Nonmedical agencies generally require a written request from the child's parent or guardian asking them to administer the medication per the health care provider's specific instruction.

RESOURCES FOR SAFE MEDICATION PRACTICES

The Institute for Safe Medication Practices is an excellent resource that provides education about adverse drug events and their prevention. All health care providers should be familiar with the national safety goals identified by The Joint Commission that pertain to medication preparation and administration to pediatric patients. A useful source of information about complementary and alternative agents is the National Center for Complementary and Alternative Medicine. Pediatric nurses should be familiar with current reference handbooks that focus on pediatric and neonatal patients and should have them readily available. Many hospitals subscribe to Micromedex, an online program that contains current information about pharmacologic agents.

See thePoint for a summary of Key Concepts.

REFERENCES

Bradshaw, A., & Price, L. (2007). Rectal suppository insertion: The reliability of the evidence as a basis for nursing practice. *Journal of Clinical Nursing*, 16(1), 98–103.

Hale, T. W. (2012). *Medications and mothers' milk* (15th ed.). Amarillo, TX: Hale.

Sobhani, P., Christopherson, J., Ambrose, P. J. et al. (2008). Accuracy of oral liquid measuring devices: Comparison of dosing cup and oral dosing syringe. *Annals of Pharmacotherapy*, 42(1), 46–52.

Zaybak, A., Güneş, U. Y., Tamsel, S. et al. (2007). Does obesity prevent the needle from reaching muscle in intramuscular injections? *Journal of Advanced Nursing*, 58(6), 552–556.

See thePoint for additional resources.

CHAPTER 10

Pain Management

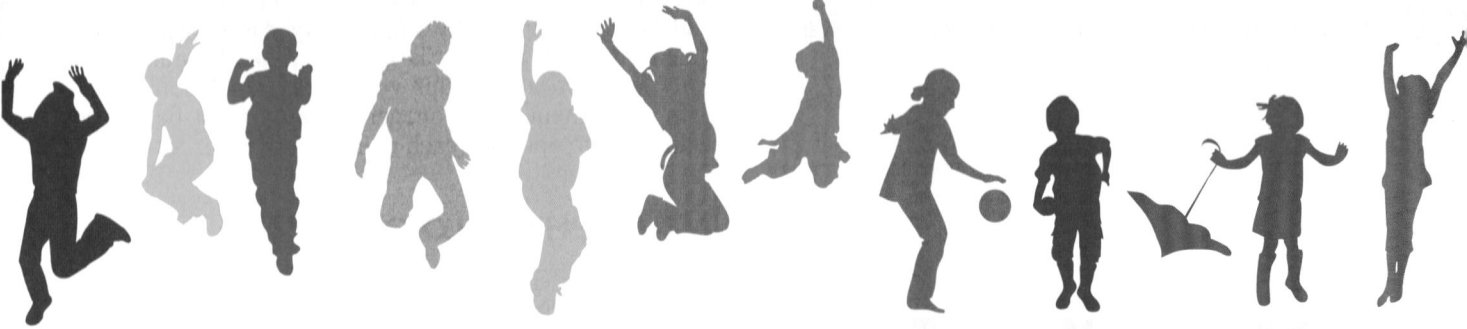

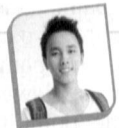

CASE HISTORY

The Tran family was introduced in Chapter 1, with Ashley, the older sister; the parents, Loan Pham and Tung Tran; and George, the younger brother. In this case study, George is struggling with metastatic cancer that originated from osteogenic sarcoma in his right leg. George is currently at home. He had limb salvage surgery several months ago, with chemotherapy both before and after the surgery, but the cancer continues to spread. It had metastasized to his lungs prior to diagnosis. He has some respiratory distress with mild exertion, and he tires very easily. The health care team and his family are managing his pain, and their goal is to keep George pain free.

George is taking a long-acting opioid, MS Contin, every 12 hours, morning and evening, and a nonsteroidal anti-inflammatory drug (NSAID), ibuprofen, two tablets four times a day, with meals and at bedtime. He also has an order for immediate-release morphine sulfate if the pain breaks through his long-acting opioid and NSAID regimen. This sometimes occurs when he has an active day. George is on adult doses of his pain medication. He weighed more than 50 kg at the time of diagnosis but weighs less than that at this time.

George demonstrated in the hospital and at home that he is reluctant to admit when he is in pain. He told the nurses that "it made him feel like a baby" to complain about pain because in Vietnamese culture, pain is considered part of living. His home care nurse came up with the idea of establishing a database in George's computer for him to enter his pain rating and any descriptions of pain and other symptoms at regular intervals throughout the day. The database follows the comprehensive pain assessment guidelines of the National Comprehensive Cancer Network Clinical Practice Guidelines. It includes the intensity of the pain, which George evaluates on a 10-point scale. It also includes whether the pain occurs at rest or with activity, the location of the pain, and the quality of the pain. George and the home health nurse review this database weekly and then send it to the nurse practitioner who works with George's oncologist. This system of pain evaluation works well for all those involved. George prefers documenting his symptoms privately on the computer, and the health care team has richer data from which to develop George's pharmacologic pain management interventions.

George has also developed a number of strategies to help him cope with pain—most effective for him is distraction. When he had pain before his diagnosis, he found video games distracted him. Video games still are engrossing for George, and the more his life in the video game is at stake, the greater the distraction. When his friends come over and play group combat video games, he can block out his pain and his altered body image. He also enjoys reading and doing online coursework offered by the "virtual high school." His parents continue to be proud of his academic achievements. When he is very tired, he will put on headphones and listen to music favorites. As you read the following objectives, apply them to George Tran and the management of his pain.

CHAPTER OBJECTIVES

1 Explain the physiologic mechanisms that lead to the sensation of pain.

2 Identify factors that may intensify or modulate the pain experience.

3 Discuss the assessment techniques and tools used to evaluate pain in children.

4 Describe pharmacologic interventions used to manage pain in children.

5 Describe biobehavioral nursing interventions to control pain and anxiety in children.

6 Contrast manifestations of chronic pain and acute pain and how management strategies for children in special pain situations may differ.

7 Discuss the role of the nurse on the interdisciplinary pain team.

See thePoint for a list of Key Terms.

Pain is a warning that alerts us to injury and illness. When a child experiences pain, we are obligated as health care providers to intervene and prevent further pain. The bedside nurse can relieve a child's pain or be the final obstacle that leaves the child to suffer.

Until fairly recently, the notion that children do not experience pain, or feel it less intensely than adults do, was unfortunately widespread in the medical community. The literature before 1970 is virtually devoid of information about children's pain. Advances in science and consumer demands have encouraged changes in how children's pain is recognized and treated. The explosion of knowledge in this field has expanded our knowledge of the phenomenon of pain and the implications for assessing and treating children. Application of this knowledge, however, remains deficient in clinical practice, with the result that pain in children continues to be undertreated (American Academy of Pediatrics [AAP] Committee on Fetus and Newborn et al., 2006; Groenewald et al., 2012; Kozlowski et al., in press).

Pain has deleterious effects. It must be recognized and treated. A significant number, up to 96%, of children report experiencing pain (A. van Dijk et al., 2006), and neonates are subjected to many painful and stressful procedures, the majority without analgesia (Carbajal et al., 2008). Almost all of the 2,181,000 children 15 years of age and younger who were discharged from hospitals in 2007 underwent procedures, operationalized as surgeries, invasive procedures, and therapeutic treatments (e.g., injection of chemotherapy) (M. J. Hall et al., 2010). Less than one third of hospitalized children undergoing painful procedures have documented pain management interventions (Stevens et al., 2011). Pain and discomfort are most frequently mentioned as the worst aspects of hospitalization and the most in need of improvement (E. M. Taylor et al., 2008). An estimated 20% to 35% of children have chronic pain (American Pain Society [APS], 2012; King et al., 2011). To improve the treatment of children's pain, the health care team must make a consistent effort to ensure that comfort is a priority for all patients.

Each child's experience of pain depends on existing pathology and individual characteristics such as physiology, developmental level, temperament, coping styles, and previous experiences. Knowledge of pain physiology and of developmentally appropriate assessment and management techniques is necessary for the nurse to care and advocate for this vulnerable population. The pain assessment and management plan must be individualized to optimize each child's pain relief.

NEUROPHYSIOLOGY OF PAIN

Pain is a highly complex, dynamic, and subjective process. Acute pain elicits a reflexive withdrawal, with physiologic, metabolic, and behavioral responses. In contrast, an individual tends to adapt to persistent or chronic pain. Thus, the response to pain may be attenuated, but chronic pain is just as valid and debilitating to the child as acute pain.

Historically, pain impulse transmission was viewed as a predictable response pattern, from one point to another. However, research indicates that the portion of the nervous system that responds to pain is "plastic"—changeable and variable between and within individuals, even to the same stimuli at different times (Fitzgerald & Walker, 2009). Many factors influence how the stimulus is transmitted, what path it takes, how it changes (or is modulated) along the way, and how the person perceives it. The basic mechanisms of pain impulse transmission in children are similar to those in adults.

NOCICEPTIVE AND NEUROPATHIC PAIN

The four levels of **nociception** (the activity produced in the nervous system by noxious, potentially tissue-damaging, stimuli)—transduction, transmission, perception, and modulation—are briefly summarized in Chart 10-1. Numerous reviews offer a more in-depth study of the pathophysiology of pain (Godfrey, 2005; Harvey & Dickenson, 2008; R. R. Myers & Shubayev, 2011; Renn & Dorsey, 2005; Woolf, 2004).

Neuropathic pain refers to conditions associated with injury or dysfunction of the peripheral, central, or autonomic nervous system (ANS) or abnormal processing of sensory input. Defining clinical characteristics of neuropathic pain are **dysesthesia** (impaired sensitivity to touch, such as paresthesia and cutaneous hypesthesia), **hyperalgesia** (excessive sensation from pain), **allodynia** (nonpainful stimuli, such as light touch, is perceived as painful), motor abnormalities, and autonomic disturbances. Chronic nociceptive pain may also alter the excitability of the peripheral and central nervous systems (CNS), resulting in sustained or recurrent pain with neuropathic qualities.

DEVELOPMENTAL PATTERNS

Neuroanatomic and neuroendocrine components of the pain pathway are sufficiently developed in the neonate to allow the transmission and perception of pain (Badr et al., 2010) (Developmental Considerations 10-1).

CHART 10-1   Levels of Nociception

Transduction

- Tissue injury from trauma, surgery, or disease releases chemical mediators, such as prostaglandins, bradykinin, serotonin, norepinephrine, substance P, and histamine, which cause pain at the periphery and facilitate movement of pain impulses along peripheral nerves. Primary afferent fibers, most commonly A delta and C fibers, when excited by mechanical, thermal, or chemical stimuli, depolarize and transmit information about noxious stimuli from the periphery to the dorsal horn of the spinal cord (see Fig. 10-1).

- Pain can be controlled at this level of nociception with NSAIDs, local anesthetics, and some anticonvulsants. NSAIDs relieve pain by interfering with the production of prostaglandins. Local anesthetics and some anticonvulsants block sodium channels, thereby preventing conduction of the action potential of primary afferent fibers.

Transmission

- All incoming information related to pain crosses the dorsal horn of the spinal cord on its entry into the CNS. Neurotransmitters (adenosine triphosphate, glutamate, substance P) continue the pain impulse from the peripheral nociceptors to the dorsal horn neurons. The signals are transmitted through the CNS to the brain stem, thalamus, and the cerebral cortex.

- Exogenous and endogenous opioids block the release of some neurotransmitters, including substance P, by binding to opioid receptors at the spinal level. Chronic pain, such as neuropathic pain, is treated by preventing glutamate and aspartate from binding with N-methyl-D-aspartate (NMDA) receptors at the spinal level. Dextromethorphan, ketamine, and methadone are believed to relieve pain by acting as NMDA antagonists.

Perception

- At this level of nociception, the person becomes conscious of the pain. Several central structures are involved in pain perception; no single "pain center" exists. The reticular system is believed to warn the individual to recognize pain and initiate an autonomic response. The somatosensory cortex provides recognition of the location and quality of the pain. The limbic system initiates the emotional and behavioral response to pain. Cognitive and behavioral techniques, such as distraction and guided imagery, modify pain perception by directing the cortical structures to attend to competing information.

Modulation

- The CNS rapidly sends descending messages back through the dorsal horn, thus inhibiting the transmission of noxious stimuli. Neurotransmitters such as endorphins, enkephalins, serotonin, norepinephrine, gamma-aminobutyric acid, and neurotensin modulate pain. Baclofen and antidepressants (e.g., the tricyclics and some selective serotonin reuptake inhibitors) are used to modulate chronic pain at this level of nociception.

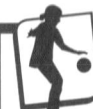

DEVELOPMENTAL CONSIDERATIONS 10-1

Pain Conduction and Perception in the Young Child

Conduction	Myelination in process: A delta nerves with varying degrees of myelin with possibly slower conduction velocity offset by shorter distances the impulse has to travel; C fibers also conducting impulses
Nerves in skin with increased density at birth, increasing sensitivity to stimuli
Newborns possibly deficient in neurotransmitters that inhibit pain impulse transmission
Perception of pain	Age dependent; possible inability to verbalize pain in terms that adults understand
Possible increased intensity of pain experience as a result of lack of control or unfamiliar situations
Limited repertoire of coping methods
View of pain as punishment
Inability to understand cause and effect (medicine makes pain go away)

Although infants may not remember painful experiences as distinct, actual events, the functional structures for long-term memory—specifically, the integrity of the limbic system and diencephalons—are well developed in newborns (Ponder, 2002). These early painful experiences may be stored as procedural memory: not accessible to conscious recall. This possibility would explain why the infant who experiences a heel stick withdraws from subsequent swabbing of the heel with an alcohol wipe, seemingly in response to the memory of a previous painful procedure.

Ample evidence indicates that both term and preterm neonates have the capacity to experience and remember pain much like older children and adults do (Fig. 10-1). In fact, one important difference in the nociceptive pathways of newborns *increases* their vulnerability to pain. Mechanisms that inhibit pain impulse transmission, neurotransmitters, and receptors are not mature in the neonate (Fitzgerald & Walker, 2009).

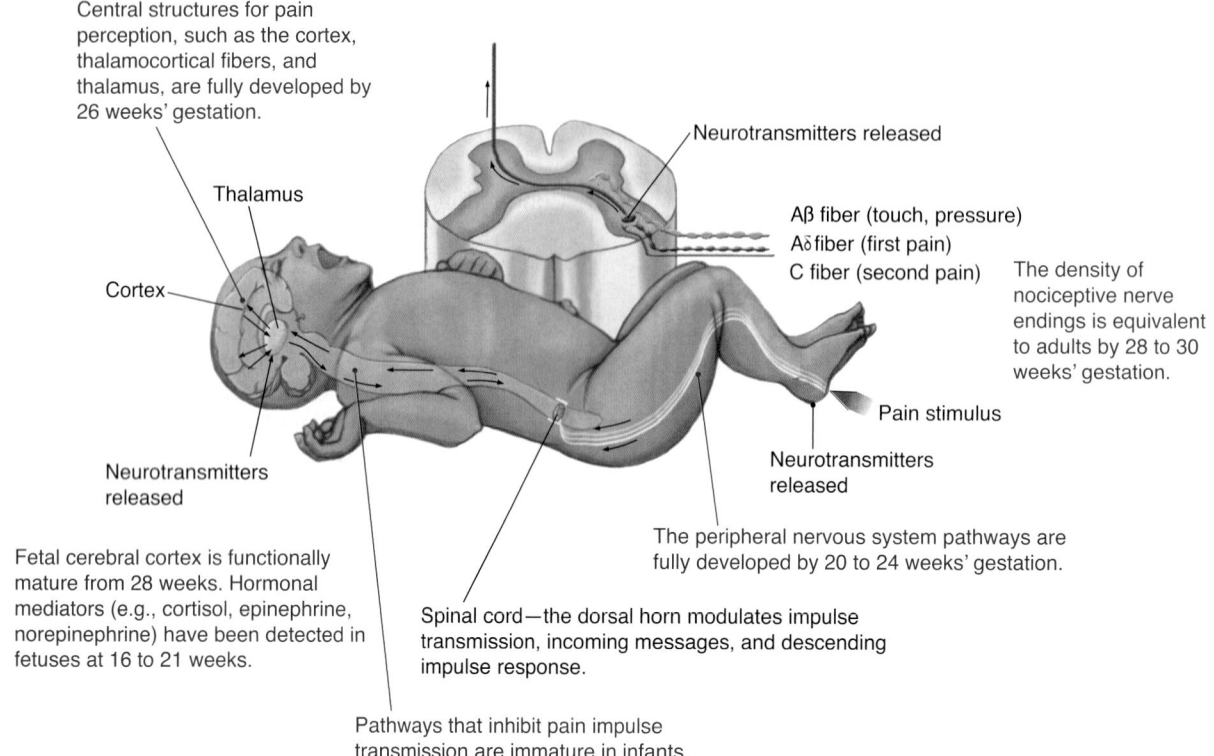

Central structures for pain perception, such as the cortex, thalamocortical fibers, and thalamus, are fully developed by 26 weeks' gestation.

Thalamus

Cortex

Neurotransmitters released

Neurotransmitters released

Aβ fiber (touch, pressure)
Aδ fiber (first pain)
C fiber (second pain)

The density of nociceptive nerve endings is equivalent to adults by 28 to 30 weeks' gestation.

Pain stimulus

Neurotransmitters released

The peripheral nervous system pathways are fully developed by 20 to 24 weeks' gestation.

Fetal cerebral cortex is functionally mature from 28 weeks. Hormonal mediators (e.g., cortisol, epinephrine, norepinephrine) have been detected in fetuses at 16 to 21 weeks.

Spinal cord—the dorsal horn modulates impulse transmission, incoming messages, and descending impulse response.

Pathways that inhibit pain impulse transmission are immature in infants.

Figure 10-1 Transmission of pain impulse in an infant.

Therefore, neonates likely feel even more pain with the same stimulus than an older child or adult would experience. Tissue injury in infants has long-term effects, altering response in later life (Schmelzle-Lubiecki et al., 2007).

caREminder

The nervous system of a young child is still developing and malleable. Early pain experiences may permanently alter how the child processes and reacts to future painful stimuli. Limit painful procedures such as suctioning, needle sticks, and tape removal to those that are absolutely necessary. Monitor environmental stimuli (such as lights, noise) because these contribute to sensory input that may increase pain in the neonate. Ensure that pharmacologic, biobehavioral, and environmental (dimming lights, reducing noise—lowering voices and volume on phones, do not bang items on the top of the isolette) interventions are consistently used to prevent or optimally reduce the pain of every necessary procedure.

FACTORS THAT INFLUENCE THE PAIN EXPERIENCE

Perception of pain results from the integration of physiologic and psychosocial factors inherent in the pain experience. The multiple factors that influence

children's pain experiences do not operate in isolation. They are listed separately for ease of discussion, but all contribute in varying degrees to the overall pain experience. Considering them when providing care and remembering that children react individually, given their unique characteristics and situation, is important.

TYPE OF PAIN EXPERIENCE

 QUESTION: Based on his history, what are George's experiences with acute and chronic pain?

Children may experience pain acutely, possibly as the result of a therapeutic procedure or brief illness or condition, or chronically.

Acute Pain

Acute pain is a common adverse stimulus that occurs as the result of injury, surgery, or illness. The severity of the physical damage and physiologic response may play a role in the child's overall perception of pain. The acute pain experience generally resolves as the body heals.

Although pain can be beneficial as a warning to avoid further injury, the effects of pain are generally deleterious. Pain, in children of any age, evokes a negative physiologic, metabolic, and behavioral stress response. Unrelieved acute pain can lead to impaired mobility; anorexia, causing poor nutritional intake; delayed wound healing; anxiety and irritability; somatic symptoms;

sleep disturbances; avoidance; developmental regression; and increased parental distress. Untreated pain affects length of convalescence and hospitalization. Pain can have a considerable effect on morbidity and mortality. For example, premature infants undergoing cardiac surgery who received relatively light anesthesia had more postoperative complications and mortality than those given deeper anesthesia (Anand et al., 1987).

Procedural pain is a specific type of acute pain related to care. Children's health care experiences often involve painful procedures, specifically the pain of needles for shots and blood sampling.

caREminder

Procedures that may seem minor to an adult may be remembered by a child as a terrible experience, which may influence the child's reaction to subsequent procedures and health care experiences.

Pain is a major source of iatrogenic stress in prematurely born infants. Stabilizing premature infants and delivering lifesaving care to them frequently subjects them to stressful, invasive, and painful procedures. On average, these fragile newborns endure 10 painful procedures per day. Whereas about 34% of these procedures were performed while the infant was receiving analgesia for other reasons, almost 80% were performed without analgesia specifically administered for the procedure (Carbajal et al., 2008). There is a lack of recognition about the need for pain control and a lack of knowledge about the long-term consequences of untreated pain in this population (Anand et al., 2006).

Unstable vital signs, particularly blood pressure, as a result of pain may result in additional complications, such as intraventricular hemorrhage, in the premature infant. The physiologic effects of pain result in a catabolic state, which has the potential to be especially damaging to infants and young children, who have higher metabolic rates and less nutritional reserves than adults. Medical and developmental outcomes can be improved by attending to early signs of stress while delivering care and attempting to minimize stressful episodes (AAP Committee on Fetus and Newborn et al., 2006).

Chronic Pain

Acute pain may develop into chronic pain if the pain experience extends beyond the normal trajectory of healing for the amount of tissue damage sustained. Although neurochemical, neuroanatomic, and neurophysiologic changes accompany some chronic pain syndromes, lack of objective indicators for pain, despite subjective or behavioral expressions of pain, characterizes chronic pain pathology.

Chronic pain is pain that persists beyond the expected healing time, arbitrarily defined as longer than 3 to 6 months (APS, 2012). Chronic pain may be persistent, recurrent, or both and can be experienced as fluctuations in pain severity, quality, regularity, and predictability.

The most common types of chronic pain conditions are headaches, abdominal pain, and musculoskeletal pain (APS, 2012). Biologic, psychological, developmental, and sociocultural factors affect the severity of children's chronic pain experiences and any associated functional disabilities. Chronic pain experiences during childhood may increase the risk for chronic pain during adulthood (Walker et al., 2010).

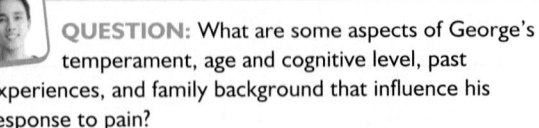

ANSWER: George experienced severe acute pain and both mild procedural pain and severe pain for short intervals when he was hospitalized for his right leg limb salvage procedure. He experienced the usual procedures: intravenous (IV) insertion, lab blood draws, and also the surgery. George also experienced chronic pain in a more mild form before the diagnosis of the osteogenic sarcoma, and now he experiences the chronic pain of metastatic cancer.

CHILD CHARACTERISTICS

Characteristics of the child—such as age and cognitive level, previous pain experience, temperament and coping style, gender, and ethnic and cultural background—influence the interpretation of and response to acute, chronic, and procedural pain. These characteristics cannot be changed, but their influences must be understood by the nurse to better care for the child experiencing pain.

QUESTION: What are some aspects of George's temperament, age and cognitive level, past experiences, and family background that influence his response to pain?

Age and Cognitive Level

Age and cognitive ability influence how a child defines and understands pain (Developmental Considerations 10-2). As the child's age and level of cognitive development increase, the child's understanding of pain, coping strategies, and the effect of pain also increases.

Children's ability to communicate their pain and describe the experience reflects their maturity. Children younger than 8 years of age display more behavioral distress than older children when subjected to painful procedures (Dahlquist et al., 1994; Humphrey et al., 1992). School-aged children and adolescents rank the word *pain* to indicate greater pain intensity than the words *hurt* and *ache*, respectively (LaFleur & Raway, 1999). A child's language of pain also reflects previous pain experiences, ethnic and cultural background, and, specifically, the words and expressions used by family members and peers. Children, families, and providers who have different linguistic backgrounds face additional challenges in discussing pain (Isaacs et al., 2011).

 KidKare Find out what words the child uses to describe pain and use these terms during interactions with the child.

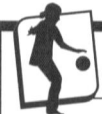

DEVELOPMENTAL CONSIDERATIONS 10-2

Cognitive Level Effect on the Pain Experience

Remember that developmental gains build on each other and that children often regress when stressed. The behaviors that were achieved most recently are the first lost.

Infancy
Lacks words for pain
Has memory for painful events
Responds to parent's anxiety

Early Childhood
1-2 years
Responds differently according to temperament (difficult, easy, and so forth)
Uses words for pain (e.g., owie, boo-boo, hurt)
Is egocentric; needs autonomy, sense of control

3-5 years
Has language to express pain
Mixes fact and fiction; has magical thinking
Lacks cause-and-effect thinking
Has beginning concept of time (medicine will start working when the television show is over)
Fears bodily injury or mutilation
Thinks the more blood there is, the worse the injury must be

Uses delays to put off treatments
Does better if allowed to handle equipment and see how it works
Needs some control over situation

Middle Childhood
Fears body mutilation
Has logical reasoning but needs to relate abstractions to concrete things
Beginning to understand cause and effect
Can delay gratification
Understands time
Relies less on parent and more on self-initiated coping resources

Adolescence
Understands abstractions
Needs to maintain self-esteem, control
Benefits from practice of biobehavioral techniques beforehand to maintain control
Feels invincible, so may not adhere to treatment or medication regimens
Thinks that the nurse knows when pain medication is needed, so may not request analgesics

---

Children are believed to judge pain severity and unpleasantness by comparing the pain with previous sensations (McGrath & Hillier, 2003). Younger school-aged children tend to select the extremes of Likert-type pain rating scales regardless of the number of rating choices (Chambers & Johnston, 2002), whereas reports from adolescents reflect a greater variation. Older children generally develop a wider frame of reference as they encounter more diverse pain experiences. Therefore, a child who has experienced pain before may be better able to describe it than a child who has not.

Research comparing children's expectations of pain with their actual pain experiences indicates that younger children are less accurate than older children in predicting their procedural pain intensity. Also, children who expect more pain tend to report more postoperative pain than others do (Cheng et al., 2003).

Previous Pain Experience

Past experience with pain also affects pain perception. Infants who have experienced painful procedures display a more intense behavioral response to subsequent procedures (Holsti et al., 2005; Von Baeyer et al., 2004). Repeated painful events in infants born at or less than 28 weeks' gestational age was associated with lower cortisol response to stress and lower facial reactivity to pain (Grunau et al., 2005). Older children who were exposed to painful procedures as

neonates demonstrate a lower pain threshold, which suggests that this behavioral response persists (Buskila et al., 2003; Hermann et al., 2006; McClain & Kain, 2005).

In addition to past exposure to pain, the nature of a child's pain experience affects the child's subsequent response. Fear and anxiety may intensify the perception of pain (Kain et al., 2006; Kleiber et al., 2007), especially if previous experiences have been negative. It may be challenging for the young child to differentiate his or her fears from sensory pain and other symptoms (Wennstrom & Bergh, 2008). Children with a history of negative pain experiences are likely to experience distress during subsequent painful events (Dahlquist et al., 1986; Kleiber et al., 2001). It is the quality, not the quantity, of previous procedures that is related to the distress.

caREminder

Optimizing pharmacologic and biobehavioral strategies to prevent pain, anxiety, and distress during the first procedure will help to relieve pain during subsequent pain experiences.

Temperament and Coping Styles

Temperament has been described as innate personality that predisposes the child to react with a certain behavioral response style (Thomas & Chess, 1977). It is a relatively stable trait and correlates with the child's response to pain. "Difficult" (poorly adaptable) children are more prone to display distress behaviors than "easy" (adaptable to new situations) children (Rocha et al., 2003). More intense children also tended to receive more postoperative pain medications (Helgadóttir & Wilson, 2004). Temperament has not been shown to influence the actual intensity of the pain experience, but it does seem to influence children's expression of pain behaviors.

Anxiety amplifies the pain experience. Many of the cognitive–behavioral techniques for pain reduction (relaxation, deep breathing, distraction, hypnosis) work because they reduce anxiety and fear and increase the child's sense of control or mastery over the situation (Schurman et al., 2010). Children who feel a sense of control and are actively involved in their situations respond with more adaptive behaviors. For example, the child who helps remove bandages often tolerates a painful dressing change better than one who is restrained and must endure the procedure passively.

Coping style, the strategies a child uses to cope with stressors, is another individual characteristic influencing pain. Examples of different coping styles are information seeking, approaching, or attending to the pain versus avoiding, distracting, or focusing attention away from the painful stimuli (Fig. 10-2). In an experimental pain situation, matching coping style with intervention (e.g., distraction or focusing on the pain in a nondistressing manner) results in better pain outcomes for older children; for younger children, distraction was more effective (Piira et al., 2006). This suggests that children may need different coping strategies based on age and coping style. Children with chronic pain may benefit from learning to use a variety of coping styles (active and passive) depending on the severity of their pain and other individualized factors (M. J. Mitchell et al., 2007).

Gender

Studies have demonstrated that gender may influence a child's response to pain. Boys may be more stoic, underestimate their pain, and report a greater perceived ability to control and reduce pain, whereas girls were more likely to exhibit behavioral distress, overestimate, and use more affect-laden words to describe their pain experiences (C. D. Myers et al., 2006; Sallfors et al., 2003). Perception of pain has been found to decrease for boys from grades 3 to 9, but prevalence of complaints, especially headaches, increases for girls (Sundblad et al., 2007). A substantial increase in chronic pain prevalence is observed in girls during early adolescence (Fendrich et al., 2007; Perquin et al., 2000), and females are more likely to report continuing pain (Martin et al., 2006). Children from 6 to 17 years of age with advanced cancer described few differences in the ability to report pain based on gender, age, or ethnicity (Van Cleve et al., 2012). Differences in pain scores between boys and girls may be a reflection of culture, with female children demonstrating a greater willingness to report pain (Kozlowski et al., in press).

Gender differences in coping strategies have been found, but there was no difference in coping efficacy (Lynch et al., 2007). Girls used more social support seeking and positive statements, whereas boys used more behavioral distraction techniques (Keogh & Eccleston, 2006; Lynch et al., 2007). A quality improvement project in a pediatric intensive care unit (PICU) identified that boys significantly decreased their pain ratings using mental imagery; however, the pain rating scores for the girls did not demonstrate the same significant decline (Kline et al., 2010).

Gender variation may result from societal norms and expectations reinforced much earlier in children's lives. For example, parents of young children report that their boys are less sensitive than girls to common bumps, bruises, and pains. Daycare workers are more likely to provide physical comfort to girls hurt on the playground than to boys. Gender-related differences thus may be influenced by ethnic, cultural, and societal expectations and customs. Health care providers are not immune to these societal biases of pain expression and must take care that they do not affect treatment.

Ethnicity and Cultural Background

Research in adults indicates that ethnic differences in pain sensitivity and tolerance exist and may contribute to ethnic disparity in the experience and treatment of clinical pain (Green et al., 2003; Im et al., 2007). Biologic, psychological, and sociocultural factors; cultural or ethnic background; and social setting all influence pain perception, communication, tolerance, response, coping strategies, treatments, and effectiveness of these treatments. Culture shapes an individual's subjective experience of pain and teaches behavioral responses to pain through modeling, direct explanations, instruction, and observation. Culture acquisition begins in infancy and continues into adulthood. Yet, individuals within an ethnic or cultural group must not be stereotyped as having a particular set of pain beliefs and behaviors. Intracultural variation results from individual experiences, education, and current circumstances.

Few studies have examined cultural effects of children's perceptions and communication about pain. A systematic review of 15 studies comparing pediatric pain outcomes associated with procedural experiences suggested that cultural factors, including pain behavior, are associated with children's pain experiences

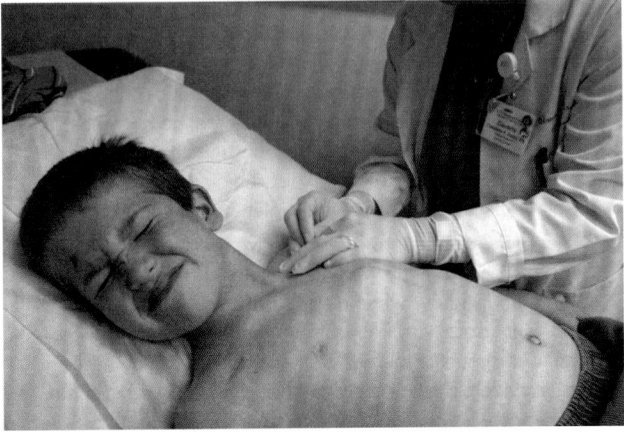

Figure 10-2 Some children prefer to look away from painful stimuli, like this child who is having his implanted port accessed.

(Kristjánsdóttir et al., 2012). Research regarding validity and reliability of pain scales indicates that behavioral pain scales are less reliable than self-report pain scales for children of different cultural backgrounds. These findings suggest that differences in children's behavior during painful procedures may reflect cultural influences. No differences in the sensation of pain have been reported, but there are differences in pain-related behavior. A retrospective study with six different ethnic groups examined preoperative outcomes of adolescents with idiopathic scoliosis in which Caucasian children reported significantly more pain than Japanese or Korean children (Morse et al., 2012). The researchers suggested the need to examine ethnic differences related to pain and other functional outcomes.

Genetic and cultural factors influence variability in individual response to pain treatments. Genetic factors may alter the absorption, distribution, metabolism, excretion, or action of medications.

CROSS-CULTURAL CARE

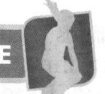

Data reports from the U.S. Food and Drug Administration (2012) suggest that certain ethnic groups have DNA variations that make the enzyme needed to metabolize codeine more active in certain ethnic groups, including African/Ethiopian children (29%), compared to Caucasian (3.6%) and Asian children (1.2%). Diet and herbal remedies can alter drug metabolism, but children and parents may not divulge the use of alternative therapies to relieve pain to a traditional health care provider.

PARENTAL INFLUENCE

Because children are legal minors, their health care rights are assumed by their parents. Parents and legal guardians access and secure treatment for children in pain. Therefore, the parents' perceptions, expectations, beliefs, and treatment concerns influence children's pain experiences. Explore the parents' cultural beliefs about pain. Supplying information about pain management and discussing parents' concerns may be effective for updating parents' knowledge and ensuring the parental participation necessary to provide optimal pain relief for children (Franck et al., 2012; Kain et al., 2007).

The meaning given to a child's pain may be a parental barrier to providing effective pain relief. Parents of children who died of cancer reported that their children died in pain (Heath et al., 2010; Jalmsell et al., 2006). Yet, families and children with cancer expected the child would suffer with symptoms, like pain (Ameringer et al., 2006; Woodgate & Degner, 2003). They believed it was necessary for the child to continue to fight these symptoms because fighting the symptoms was more tangible and less frightening than fighting the cancer.

Results of research into the accuracy and value of parents' assessment of children's pain have been mixed. Parents' predictions of children's pain and distress correlate with children's actual behaviors (Kankkunen et al., 2004) and the child's self-report (Baxt et al., 2004; Zisk et al., 2007). Some studies indicate better correlation between parent and child pain ratings than

between those of health care providers and children (Garcia-Munitis et al., 2006); other studies indicate that parents under- or overestimate their child's postsurgical pain (Voepel-Lewis et al., 2005), whereas still others found strong correlations between children's, parent's, and nurses' ratings of the child's pain (Brahmbhatt et al., 2012). Parents' pain estimations for their children improve when the parents are provided with actual assessment tools (Kankkunen et al., 2009; Solodiuk et al., 2010). Pain ratings of child and parent and of child and nurse demonstrate a moderate relationship. Therefore parents' and nurses' ratings of a child's pain should be considered estimates, not self-reports (Zhou et al., 2008).

Parents report that their children experience more pain than they had expected after the day of surgery. Unsatisfactory discharge information, inability to comply with discharge instructions resulting from fatigue, lack of trust in children's self-reports of pain, and fear of addiction from pain medications were significant barriers to parents' ability to manage their children's pain after surgery (Kankkunen et al., 2004; Kankkunen et al., 2003).

Parental satisfaction with children's pain management reflects not the amount of pain children experience after surgery but whether parents receive enough information and feel that their expectations have been met (Melnyk et al., 2004; Pöder et al., 2010). Poor communication between health care providers and parents as well as low expectations for pain relief continue to be barriers to effective pain management (Kankkunen et al., 2003). Parents are hesitant to voice their concerns about their child's pain because they do not want to be perceived as difficult or as challenging the nurses' expertise (J. Simons et al., 2001). Therefore, nurses must open the lines of communication and encourage dialogue about children's pain if relief is to be achieved.

ANSWER: George has always been a child with an easy temperament and, despite a rich history of pain experiences, he seldom exhibits pain behaviors. This makes it challenging for his home health nurse and his worried mother to reassure themselves that his pain is well managed. Contributing to George's reluctance to admit pain is his desire to be seen as an adult and a man.

George has had many and varied pain experiences. His most intense pain experiences, both physical and emotional, were during his hospitalization for his limb salvage surgery. He copes well with chronic pain at home, but as is explored in Chapter 13 with regard to palliative care, he becomes very anxious and distressed at the idea of hospitalization. He has developed several strategies of distraction that are effective for him—particularly active and violent video games.

George's medications are to be given on a routine basis. George works directly with his home health nurse, and he and his family know when his pills are to be taken. One important strategy to keep George as pain free as possible is clear communication between the family and the health care providers. Having a home health nurse who can speak Vietnamese would help George's mother appreciate a routine pain medication schedule.

INFLUENCE OF HEALTH CARE PROFESSIONALS AND SYSTEMS

> **QUESTION:** How has George's oncologist's decision to use hospice care in the home affected George's pain management?

Assessment and treatment decisions made by the health care team affect the adequacy of pain management. Children are often assessed inappropriately, undermedicated, and, consequently, pain management is suboptimal (Fortier et al., 2009). Barriers to effective pain management are numerous and result from complex interactions among patients, their families, health care professionals, and health care systems (Czarnecki et al., 2011).

All health care providers, including nurses, contribute to ineffective pain management (Twycross, 2010; Twycross & Collins, in press). Nurses do not consistently assess infants and children with developmentally appropriate, valid, and reliable pain intensity scales (Broome & Huth, 2003). Nurses also often believe that children overreport their pain (Vincent, 2005). Patient, family, nurse, and physician communication regarding pain may be incomplete and ineffective (Van Niekerk & Martin, 2003). Physicians tend to order inadequate amounts and, occasionally, inaccurate doses of pain medications to be given on an as-needed (PRN) basis (Czarnecki et al., 2011). Given these PRN orders, nurses tend to undermedicate by administering dosages less often than prescribed (Shrestha-Ranjit & Manias, 2010). Nurses also tend to choose the lowest opioid dose or administer nonopioid analgesics instead of opioids. These errors may be based on inadequate or inappropriate knowledge, attitudes, and beliefs about pain assessment and pain management for children (Twycross, 2010). The priority nurses place on pain influences clinical practice and how well patients' pain relief needs are met.

caREminder

Pain management is a major facet of nursing care. Its central role must be recognized as a priority, and adequate time must be allotted to assess and manage pain appropriately.

> **ANSWER:** George is receiving home health care through an adult hospice organization that is accustomed to patients in severe and chronic pain and therefore is less likely to be undermedicated.

ASSESSING PAIN IN CHILDREN

> **QUESTION:** Evaluate George's assessment tool according to the following information. Is it standardized? Is it adequately assessing all aspects of his pain?

Standardizing the pain assessment techniques used within a health care organization to include only valid, reliable, and developmentally appropriate tools facilitates efforts to communicate and document pain experiences effectively. Inconsistent techniques make it difficult to assess effectiveness of pain management. Nurses must carefully examine the needs of the setting and the patient before selecting the tools to assess pain in children. Because fear and anxiety influence the pain experience, these should also be assessed. Some instruments have beginning psychometric adequacy to assess fear or anxiety (Foster & Park, 2012).

In 1968, McCaffery, a nurse, defined pain as "whatever the experiencing person says it is, existing whenever he says it does" (p. 95). Based on this definition and our understanding of pain, patients' subjective reports are considered the gold standard for pain assessment. Unfortunately, many children are unable to state where they hurt, how much they hurt, or even if they hurt. The infant or child's signs of pain may be misinterpreted for other causes of stress or irritability. Keeping in mind that pain is defined by the International Association for the Study of Pain (1979, p. 249) as "an unpleasant sensory and emotional experience associated with actual or potential tissue damage or described in terms of such damage," one should be highly suspicious of tissue damage if children report pain, act as though they are in pain, or any other reason exists to indicate that a child may have tissue damage.

An initial pain assessment should determine pain location, onset, duration, pattern, quality, intensity, and aggravating and alleviating factors (Nursing Interventions 10-1). (See also the**Point** for Procedures.) Children as young as 2 years of age can indicate where they hurt, although their verbal descriptors may be nonspecific. For example, if the child has a limited vocabulary, "My tummy hurts" may actually indicate chest pain. The onset of pain provides key information to determine its potential cause. The quality of pain helps distinguish nociceptive, somatic, and visceral pain from neuropathic pain. This distinction is important for developing an effective pain management plan. Information about aggravating and alleviating factors helps to define the functional limitations of the child's pain. Alleviating factors that have been successful in the past should be included in the child's individualized treatment plan.

Valid, reliable, and clinically sensitive pain assessment tools are available to estimate the intensity of pain for children from birth through adolescence. Pain assessment techniques can be classified as subjective reports, behavioral observations, or physiologic monitoring. Assessments that use a combination of methods may provide the most accurate appraisal of the child's pain-related distress. Composite pain measures use more than one parameter to assess the pain experience (Table 10-1). Typically, behavioral and physiologic indicators are used to assess pain in infants. For older children, self-report and behavioral or physiologic indicators are used.

A proposed hierarchy of assessment techniques can guide nurses in determining the presence and intensity of patients' pain (Manworren et al., 2004). Ranked in

NURSING INTERVENTIONS 10-1

Pain History Questions for Verbal Children and Their Family*

1. What words do you use for pain? (Use these terms when conducting the interview.)
2. When did the pain start? (*onset*) Have you felt this pain before? If so, when, and what do you think caused it?
3. How long have you been feeling this pain? (*duration*)
4. How often does the pain occur? (*frequency*) Is it all the time (*continuous pattern*) or just happens now and then (*intermittent*)? Is there a certain time of day it occurs?
5. Where is the pain? (*location*) Does it go to (*radiate to*) other places? Point to the areas with one finger or use body outline tools to identify the site. Do you hurt anywhere else?
6. How severe is the pain? (*intensity*) Use this tool (e.g., 0- to 10-point rating scale, visual analog scale [VAS], poker chip tool, faces scale) to quantify intensity.

7. What does the pain feel like? (*quality*) Describe it— for instance, pinching, burning, stabbing, dull, aching, sharp, throbbing. "Like an elephant stomped on it." (Be careful not to lead the child to provide a quality indicator that is inconsistent with their actual pain experience. Instead, encourage children to use their imagination to help you understand how the pain feels.)
8. Does anything make the pain worse? Better? What pain relief methods have you tried? What works best? What would you do/not do again (medications and nonpharmacologic or behavioral interventions)?
9. How does the pain affect you? Can you put the pain out of your mind and carry on normal activities of daily living? Or does the pain keep you from doing things you want to do?

*Encourage the family to supplement the child's self-report with their observations or provide key information to define these factors for infants and younger children.

TABLE 10-1   Multidimensional Tools for Pain Assessment

Tool	Parameters	Comments
Premature Infant Pain Profile (PIPP) (Stevens et al., 1996) Age: preterm and full-term neonates	Gestational age, behavioral state, heart rate, oxygen saturation, brow bulge, eye squeeze, nasolabial furrow	Assessment of procedural and postoperative pain and determination of the efficacy of nonpharmacologic interventions
CRIES (Krechel & Bildner, 1995) Age: term newborns	Crying Requires oxygen administration Increased heart rate and blood pressure Expression Sleeplessness	Valid and reliable assessment of postoperative pain; easy to use
Neonatal Infant Pain Scale (Lawrence et al., 1993) Age: preterm to 6 weeks	Six behaviors: facial expression, cry, breathing patterns, arms, legs, state of arousal	Easy to use clinically for acute pain; needs further testing for more ongoing pain (e.g., postoperative)
Children's Hospital of Eastern Ontario Pain Scale (CHEOPS) (McGrath et al., 1985) Age: 1–7 years	Six categories: crying, facial expression, verbalizations, torso activity, if/how child touches wound, leg position	Tested in acute postoperative pain; insensitive to pain of longer duration; easy to learn; time considerations in that many behaviors are evaluated across the six categories
COMFORT Scale (Ambuel et al., 1992; Johansson & Kokinsky, 2009; M. van Dijk et al., 2001) Age: 0–3 years	Eight dimensions: alertness, calmness, respiratory response or crying, movement, mean arterial pressure, heart rate, muscle tone, facial expression	Valid and reliable as a measure of distress (Ambuel et al., 1992; Wielenga et al., 2004) and pain (Bear & Ward-Smith, 2006; Caljouw et al., 2007; Johansson & Kokinsky, 2009; M. van Dijk et al., 2000); scale may be valid without the physiologic indicators (Carnevale & Razack, 2002; M. van Dijk et al., 2005)

order by their importance and reliability for assessing pain are self-report, presence of pathology or a condition associated with pain, behavior, proxy ratings, and, last, physiologic indicators of pain. Also consider events that influence the pain experience, obtain a pain history, and discuss expectations for pain relief with both the child and the family.

After the initial assessment, reassessment of pain should include at least location of pain and pain intensity. Conduct reassessments at routine intervals and at appropriate intervals after interventions are implemented (e.g., 15 minutes after IV administration of medications, 60 minutes after oral medications are given, 30 minutes after changing position).

Ideally, when a child has surgery, the child and family should be told before the procedure how pain will be assessed. This practice provides an opportunity to introduce and practice assessment under less stressful conditions. It also provides information regarding the child's baseline pain level. If the child is unable to accurately demonstrate the assessment method, another standard pain assessment tool may be introduced. Once an acceptable method is chosen, use this one consistently.

ANSWER: George's nurse is using a standardized comprehensive tool that measures intensity by self-report, location and quality of the pain, and whether the pain occurred at rest or with activity. Yes, it meets the recommended criteria. For more information, see the National Comprehensive Cancer Network website (www.nccn.org/professionals).

SELF-REPORT STRATEGIES

Pain is a subjective experience. Thus, self-report of pain is a critical component of a thorough pain assessment. Children as young as 18 months of age may indicate "ow," "ouch," and "hurt" (Stanford et al., 2005). Subjective reports of pain intensity may be solicited through the use of verbalizations or other nonverbal self-report tools (Table 10-2 and Figs. 10-3 to 10-7).

Use of the same self-report tool improves communication. The child, family, and health care team will be confused if, for example, at different times, a 6-point scale (0 being no pain, and 5 the most pain you could have) is used and at other times an 11-point scale (0 being no pain, and 10 the most pain) or other method of pain assessment is used. In this example, a pain intensity rating of 5 points could indicate either moderate or severe pain, depending on the tool used.

Developmentally appropriate pain intensity scales can be used to obtain a self-report from children as young as 3 years of age (Zempsky & Schechter, 2003). Although even younger children may be able to indicate that they are in pain and say where it hurts, pain intensity rating requires the child to understand certain abstract concepts.

Communicating children's self-report of pain requires assessment tools that are appropriate for ethnicity as well as age (Tradition or Science 10-1). Avoid

stereotyping, but be aware that cultural factors influence a child's behavioral response to pain.

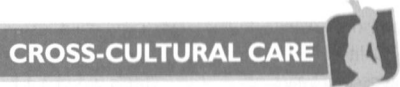

CROSS-CULTURAL CARE

Chinese characters are read vertically downward and from right to left. Thus, horizontally oriented scales are probably less appropriate for this population. Vertically oriented VASs give more reliable results (Aun et al., 1986).

BEHAVIORAL OBSERVATIONS

In the absence of self-report of pain, behavioral observations may be used. Cry patterns, facial expressions, and body movements have been investigated as behavioral measures of infant pain (Developmental Considerations 10-3). Published pain assessment tools that have demonstrated acceptable reliability and validity include observation of multiple behaviors to assess pain (Table 10-3). Behavioral signs of pain are more consistent for short, sharp, procedural pain than for longer lasting pain, such as postoperative pain (Gaffney et al., 2003). Neonates experiencing persistent pain may exhibit symptoms of energy conservation versus the usual behavioral signs and symptoms of acute pain (AAP Committee on Fetus and Newborn et al., 2006).

Crying is one of the most widely accepted indicators of pain in infants. Accordingly, cry is often included as one dimension of valid and reliable behavioral pain scales. Amount or duration of crying has been used as an indicator of pain intensity. The cry of an infant generally evokes a response from the care provider. A pain cry is high pitched, tense, and irregular (Beacham, 2004). Cry characteristics differentiate cries of pain from cries indicating hunger, frustration, or fright. Unfortunately, clinicians interpret these cry characteristics inconsistently. Therefore, nurses must also use contextual cues to determine the stimulus that elicits an infant's cry.

Facial expressions indicate response to painful stimuli. A fairly consistent facial response to pain in infants includes several specific facial muscle actions. The overall expression is a frown or grimace, with eyes squeezed tightly shut, brows lowered together and bulging, nasolabial furrow, open square mouth with tight mouth stretch, taut cupped tongue, and chin quiver (Grunau & Craig, 1987) (Fig. 10-8). These characteristics are less pronounced and are therefore difficult to see in premature infants because their facial musculature is poorly developed and in ventilated infants, who have tubes and tape obstructing part of their face. In these situations, the three facial actions—brow bulge, tightly closed eyes, and nasolabial furrow—are sufficient to identify pain.

By 4 years of age, children have learned to control their facial expressions and may mask facial indications of pain (Gaffney et al., 2003). Closed eyes (95%), frown (78%), and clenched jaw (41%) were facial indications of pain exhibited by children 8 to 17 years of age at least once during a 3-day postoperative pain study (Tesler et al., 1998). These facial expressions did not correlate

TABLE 10-2   Self-Report Methods for Pain Assessment

Method	Description	Comments
Direct questioning: measures pain location, intensity, quality Age: children as young as 2–3 years	Ask the child, using his or her word for pain, if he or she has pain, how the pain feels, where it is, when it occurs, and what helps relieve it.	Verbalizations by the child are the best marker of the subjective experience of pain; in nonverbal children, parents should be questioned.
Finger Span Scale (Merkel, 2002): measures pain intensity Age: children as young as 2–3 years	Ask the child how much he or she hurts. The thumb and index finger are close together, almost touching, for a small amount of pain but are spread wide to indicate a lot of pain.	This method is difficult to document but is a reliable method of communicating pain intensity.
Numeric Rating Scale: measures pain intensity Age: most children older than 7 years	Ask the child to rate pain on a 0- to 5-point or 0- to 10-point scale (0 being no pain, 10 being the worst pain you could have).	The child must understand numeric value, seriation, and greater than and less than. Define each number to ensure that the child's understanding is consistent with yours. Advantages to using a numeric rating scale are that it requires no equipment and is quick to administer.
VAS (see Fig. 10-3): measures pain intensity Age: most children older than 7 years	A single horizontal or vertical line, typically 10 cm long, is anchored by descriptors of pain at each end, such as "absent" to "severe." The child marks the line at any point on the continuum to indicate pain intensity	Sometimes this scale is constructed with marks at equal intervals (a true VAS contains no markings between the anchors), which adds a numeric dimension to the tool. It can be a vertical or horizontal scale. See Shields et al. (2003) for predictors of a child's ability to use a VAS.
FACES (see Fig. 10-4 for one example) (Bieri et al., 1990; Bosenberg et al., 2003; Hicks et al., 2001; Hunter et al., 2000; D. Wong & Baker, 1988): measures pain intensity Age: children as young as 3 years	This scale consists of cartoon drawings or pictures ranging from no pain to the worst possible pain. The child chooses the picture that is most like how he or she is feeling at that time.	This scale is quick to administer and does not require verbal responses. Several different valid and reliable versions exist. Scales with smiling "no pain" face at the beginning produce significantly higher ratings than scales with neutral "no pain" faces (Chambers et al., 2005).
Oucher (see Fig. 10-5) (original Caucasian version developed by Beyer et al. [1992] and Yeh [2005]): measures pain intensity Age: photographs as young as 3 years; generally, school-aged and older children can use the numeric scale	Six photographs depict a young child's facial expression, from no hurt to the biggest hurt you could ever have. Children point to the picture that most closely approximates their own level of discomfort. This method also uses a numeric 0- to 100-point scale.	Four versions have been developed to accommodate cultural bias: Caucasian, African American, Hispanic, and Asian. To use the numeric scale, the child must be able to understand sequencing and numeric value (i.e., be able to count to 100 by ones).
Poker chip tool (see Fig. 10-6) (Hester, 1979): measures pain intensity Age: 4½–13 years	Four red poker chips represent "pieces of hurt." The child chooses chips from 0 (no hurt) up to 4 chips (most hurt you could have).	This tool is good for preschool children. It is concrete, simple to use, and resembles a toy, so it is nonthreatening. It is easy to carry and disinfect, and it provides a nonverbal response (useful for intubated patients or when language barrier exists).
Body outline tool (see Fig. 10-7) (Eland & Anderson, 1977; Savedra et al., 1989; Van Cleve & Savedra, 1993): shows location of pain and measures intensity (if colors are ranked) Age: 4 years or younger	This is a line drawing of a child's body, unclothed, nongender specific, front and back. The child marks an X or colors the painful area. Colors can be ranked in order of increasing pain intensity before coloring.	Young children may reverse right and left sides and front and back of body. Validate responses and color choices with the child.
Adolescent Pediatric Pain Tool (APPT) (Savedra et al., 1993): shows location of pain and measures intensity and quality Age: 8–17 years	This tool consists of a front and back body outline, a 100-mm word–graphic rating scale, and a pain descriptor list.	This tool evaluates three components of pain, so the child should be able to provide a more precise description than a method that evaluates only one component.

TABLE 10-2	Self-Report Methods for Pain Assessment *(Continued)*		
Method	**Description**	**Comments**	
Pain diary: evaluates various aspects of the pain experience; used to assess chronic and recurrent pain Age: children who can write and record events	The child records events preceding pain onset, precipitating factors, severity, activity level, and events out of the ordinary that occurred. The child may also record medications or psychological techniques used.	This tool is inexpensive to use. Information is recorded shortly after it happens, so it should not be subject to recollection distortion. The child is actively involved in managing pain, which contributes to a sense of control. Information obtained is not as structured as in other methods, so you may obtain superfluous data. This tool is subject to the child's biases.	
Varni/Thompson Pediatric Pain Questionnaire (Varni et al., 1987): measures pain intensity and quality; identifies location, sensory, affective, and evaluative aspects of pain perception; used to assess chronic and recurrent pain Age: 8 years or younger	This tool has forms for the child, adolescent, and parent that use a combination of (1) VAS, (2) color-coded scale and body outline, (3) pain descriptors to circle, and (4) questions about family history and socioenvironmental influences.	This tool provides a detailed history of pain.	

All responses require careful validation with the child.
Recommended ages are for cognitive rather than the chronologic age of the individual.

with children's self-report of pain. Facial expression as a method to assess pain for the school-aged population is not considered a precise measure for documenting the presence of pain (Schiavenato, 2008).

Gross body movements observed in children with pain include those consistent with fighting off the pain, such as kicking, squirming, arching, or behaviors consistent with protecting or limiting further pain, such as withdrawal from painful stimuli, guarding, or limiting movement.

Individual behavioral responses to pain are complex and unique to the individual child and painful stimulus. For example, young children may use physical activity or sleep as a coping strategy to avoid or manage pain. Sleep may indicate pain, comfort, or exhaustion. The child may have been experiencing pain, obtained relief, and is finally able to sleep; alternately, sleep may be interrupted by pain. There is a greater burden on the child and family when pain is associated with multiple symptoms including altered sleep, fatigue, and nausea (Miller et al., 2011). Children may also sleep because of exhaustion, despite continued pain.

caREminder

Do not assume that a sleeping child has obtained adequate pain relief.

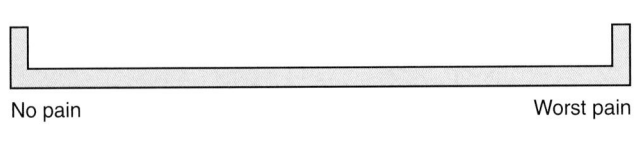

No pain   Worst pain

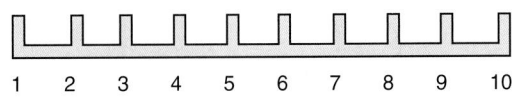

1   2   3   4   5   6   7   8   9   10

Figure 10-3 Visual analog scale (VAS). It is a true VAS only if it has a 10-cm line (top) and a numeric pain scale (bottom).

Emotions such as anxiety may manifest as distress. Tools that assess distress may not evaluate behaviors that are pain specific, but distress can intensify the pain experience and should be addressed. Often, psychological interventions (e.g., preparation, distraction, imagery) are effective in reducing distress.

PHYSIOLOGIC PARAMETERS

Several physiologic parameters have been investigated as pain indices. They include heart rate, blood pressure, transcutaneous oxygen ($TcPO_2$) levels, palmar sweating, and hormone levels. Most are thought to reflect a global response to stress; they give an indication of physiologic status but are not necessarily specific to pain. Changes in physiologic parameters may reflect anxiety, fear, or anger. Therefore, these indices may be more valid pain indicators in young infants (whose pain may not be influenced by fear, anger, or anxiety).

Autonomic Arousal

Pain is a stressor that activates the compensatory mechanisms of the ANS. The ANS has two branches: the sympathetic nervous system (SNS) and the parasympathetic nervous system (PNS). SNS stimulation produces the "fight-or-flight" response, which results in tachycardia, peripheral vasoconstriction, diaphoresis, pupil dilation, and increased secretion of catecholamines as well as adrenocortical, thyroid, and pancreatic hormones.

Painful stimuli produce other signs of autonomic arousal. Research yields conflicting results, however, possibly because of differences in measurement, populations, and pain situations. Respiratory rate, systolic blood pressure, $TcPO_2$ level, heart rate, and intracranial pressure have been found to increase with painful stimuli (Johnston et al., 2003). Conversely, decreased heart rate, respiratory rate, oxygen saturation, and $TcPO_2$ levels have also been noted in response to pain (Foster et al., 2003; Logan et al., 2002). These variations underscore the possibility that vital sign

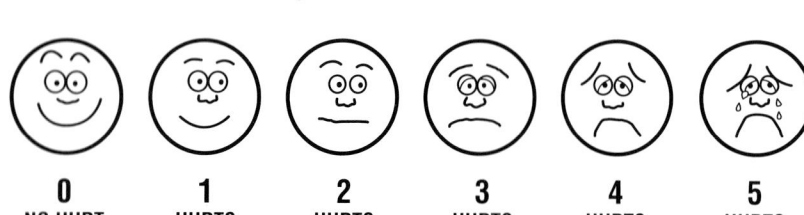

0	1	2	3	4	5
NO HURT	HURTS LITTLE BIT	HURTS LITTLE MORE	HURTS EVEN MORE	HURTS WHOLE LOT	HURTS WORST

Figure 10-4 FACES pain rating scale. From Hockenberry, M. J., & Wilson, D. (2009). *Wong's essentials of pediatric nursing* (8th ed.). St. Louis, MO: Mosby. Used with permission.

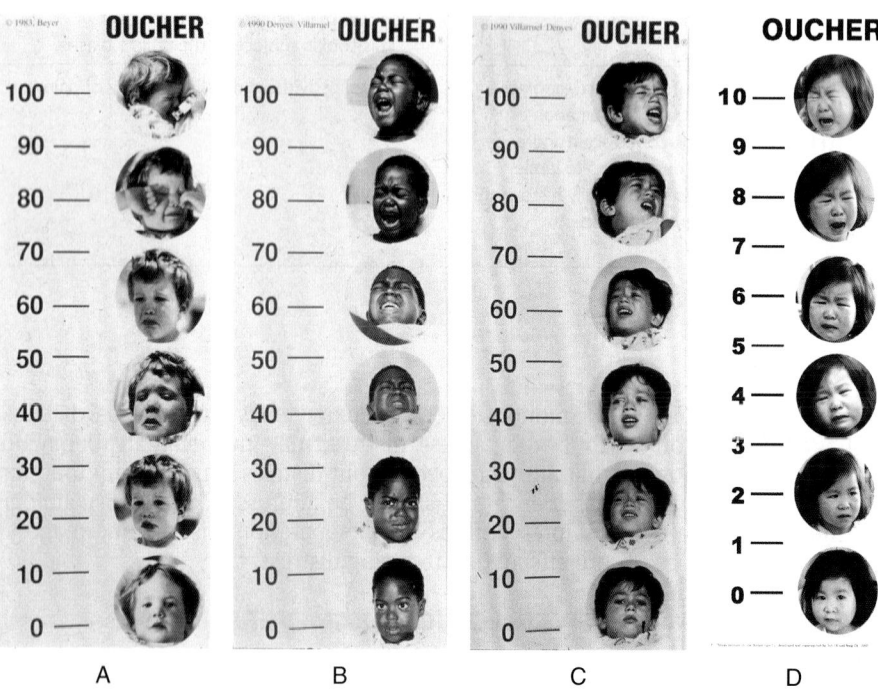

Figure 10-5 The Oucher pain assessment tool. (A) The Caucasian version. Developed and copyrighted in 1983 by Judith E. Beyer, PhD, RN (University of Missouri-Kansas City School of Nursing), USA. (B) The African American version. Developed and copyrighted in 1990 by Mary J. Denyes, PhD, RN (Wayne State University) and Antonia M. Villarruel, PhD, RN (University of Michigan), USA. Cornelia P. Porter, PhD, RN and Charlotta Marshall, RN, MSN, contributed to the development of this scale. (C) The Hispanic version. Developed and copyrighted in 1990 by Antonia M. Villarruel, PhD, RN (University of Michigan) and Mary J. Denyes, PhD, RN (Wayne State University), USA. (D) The Asian version. Developed and copyrighted in 2003 by C. H. Yeh and C. H. Wang (Chang Gung University), Taiwan, Republic of China.

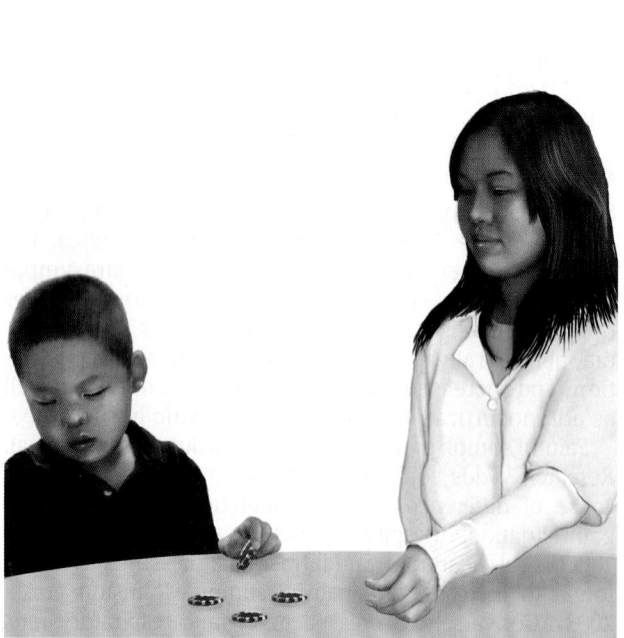

Figure 10-6 Poker chip tool. Here, the nurse asks the child to identify the number of chips that indicate the degree of hurt.

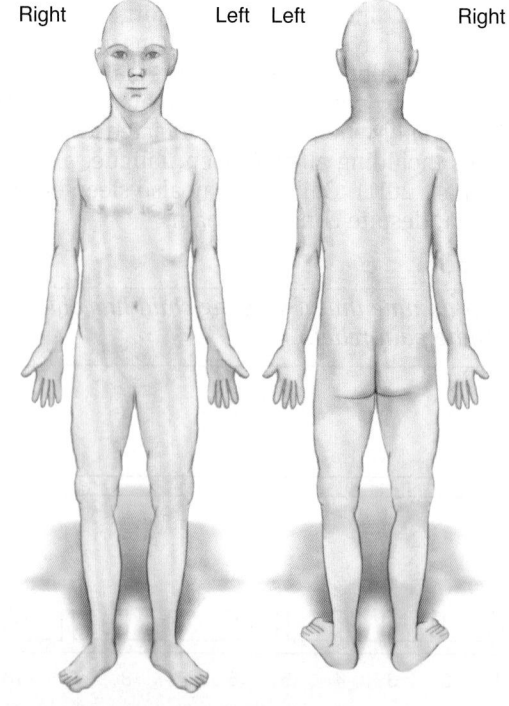

Figure 10-7 Body outline pain assessment tool.

TRADITION OR SCIENCE 10-1

Does a child's cultural background influence pain expression?

Children's cultural background may affect pain expression, but the same assessment tools are used in all populations. Initial studies of the reliability and validity of these tools included primarily white children. Although translations of assessment tools are available, few tools have been validated for cultural fitness (Van Cleve et al., 2001). Some diversity is emerging. African American, Hispanic, and Asian versions of the Oucher pain intensity scale have been developed, and their reliability and validity has been demonstrated (Beyer et al., 1992; Beyer & Knott, 1998; Yeh, 2005). Luffy and Grove (2003) found that the FACES and African American Oucher scales are valid and reliable tools for measuring pain in African American children and that the FACES scale was the most preferred. Gharaibeh and Abu-Saad (2002) found the poker chip, the FACES, and the word description scales to be valid and reliable for pain assessment with Jordanian children, but females preferred using the poker chip tool and males preferred the FACES scale. A translated version of the APPT has been tested in Spanish-speaking children of at least two different sociocultural backgrounds and has demonstrated initial validity and reliability (Van Cleve et al., 2001). The Face, Legs, Activity, Cry, Consolability (FLACC) Scale and Faces Pain Scale-Revised (FPS-R) were cross-culturally adapted into Brazilian Portuguese for use in Brazilian children and adolescents with cancer (Silva & Thuler, 2008). More studies of pain assessment tools are needed to document preferences and the reliability and validity of tests in children of various ethnicities.

In addition to influences on pain expression, children's culture may increase their risk of having their pain undertreated (Kristjánsdóttir et al., 2012). English-speaking Hispanic parents had more misconceptions about pain medications than English-speaking Caucasian or Spanish-speaking Hispanic parents (Fortier et al., 2011).

changes may merely reflect physiologic stress. Therefore, when assessing vital signs, consider how they are related and how other factors—such as the child's situation, body position, fear and anxiety, behavior, and any medications given—may affect the parameters being evaluated.

Dilated pupils, another sign of autonomic arousal, may also be found in response to pain. Pupil size can be used as a component of pain assessment and to determine adequacy of treatment (e.g., small or decreased pupil size may indicate that the interventions were effective, and dilated pupils may signal untreated pain).

Hormonal and Metabolic Responses

Neuroendocrine hormone response is closely correlated with immune system response. Psychological and physical stress depresses immune responsiveness, an effect associated with an increased incidence of infections. Secretion of catecholamines, growth hormones, beta-endorphins, glucagon, cortisol, and other corticosteroids has been shown to increase in infants during minor procedures, such as endotracheal suctioning, and routine nursing care and in those given inadequate anesthesia during surgery. These infants experienced significantly more postoperative mortality and morbidity than infants given appropriate pain management (R. W. Hall & Anand, 2005). Hormonal and metabolic responses are quite variable, however, and none has been shown to be a definitive measure of pain. In the current state of technologic development, measuring hormonal response is invasive and expensive, and results are not immediately available so assessment of this is not appropriate for clinical decisions regarding pain management.

DEVELOPMENTAL FACTORS IN PAIN ASSESSMENT

Children manifest pain differently depending on their developmental stage. Nurses must know how to assess pain appropriately in children of all chronologic and developmental ages.

Solicit parental input to increase accuracy of the assessment. The parent knows the child's normal behaviors and can be invaluable in detecting and interpreting changes that may indicate pain. These assessments are susceptible to the parent's interpretations and biases, so a degree of subjectivity is inevitable. Parental appraisal of the child's pain may be influenced by the parent's own anxiety. Therefore, use parental judgment as an adjunct to, not instead of, the child's self-reports (Zhou et al., 2008; Zisk et al., 2007). The parent is also a good resource when assessing the child's usual coping style, which later affects decisions about interventions. Teaching parents about the cues children use to signal pain and the strategies they use to manage it can further add to the precision of the assessment process (Pöder et al., 2010).

Preterm Infants

Nurses' judgment of pain in newborns is influenced by the vigor of the baby's response. Because the preterm infant and the extremely ill child's response to pain is less robust than that of a term infant or healthier child, the health care team must recognize subtle pain cues (Fig. 10-9). Preterm infants often become limp, flaccid, or listless. Health care providers should take preventive measures to help support the infant during painful and stressful procedures (Fig. 10-10). The cry of a premature or medically compromised infant is higher pitched than that of a healthy term infant and has more characteristics that arouse a caregiver. This finding may be related to the inability of preterm infants to demonstrate the strong grimace and vigorous body movements that term infants display (Badr et al., 2010).

Distinguishing between agitation and pain is difficult, particularly in preterm infants, who may show more physiologic instability in response to these stressors (Ramelet, 1999). Behaviors of agitation and pain are related and may resemble each other, but interventions are different, although some overlap. To distinguish between pain and agitation, assess the infant in terms of the nature of the painful stimuli, the environment, and behaviors (Table 10-4).

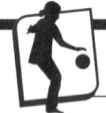

DEVELOPMENTAL CONSIDERATIONS 10-3

Pain Indicators in Preverbal Children*

Verbalizations

Preterm infant: Cry: less frequently heard in response to painful stimuli than in term infant; has more characteristics that arouse listener; higher pitched, often of shorter duration

Term infant: Cry: high pitched, tense, irregular, arouses the listener

Early childhood: Cry, pet terms for pain (e.g., owie, boo-boo)

Facial Expression

Preterm infant: Weaker grimace than in term infant

Term infant: Pain grimace (eyes tightly closed, brows lowered and drawn together, deepened furrow between nose and outer corner of lip [see Fig. 10-8])

Early childhood: Grimace, clenched teeth, tightly shut lips or biting lips, wide-open eyes, wrinkled forehead

Body Movement

Preterm infant: Less vigorous movements than term infant; often limp, flaccid, or listless

Term infant: Withdrawal of limb, rigid, guarded, flaccid

Early childhood: Self-limited movement, flexed or rigid extremities, guarding of painful area, restless (flailing, kicking, rolling head side to side, frequent position changes), touching or pointing to painful area, aggressive actions (biting, hitting, pushing caregiver)

Physiologic Changes

In an unstable child, you may just see greater instability:
- Variability in heart rate, respiratory rate, shallow respirations
- Increased intracranial pressure
- Decreased oxygen saturation
- Increased or decreased blood pressure
- Dilated pupils
- Diaphoresis

Behavior

Infants: Change in sleep patterns, may sleep more or less than usual; irritable, cannot be comforted; avoids eye contact

Early childhood: Same behaviors as in infants, plus changes in activity level, anger, self-consolation (e.g., "rub my tummy," rubbing own tummy)

Parental Input

How do the parents perceive their child's level of comfort? Is this typical behavior? What are the changes? Does anything help alleviate the pain?

*The context in which the painful event is experienced affects the response. For example, an infant in a deep sleep often responds less vigorously to stimuli; severely ill children often move less vigorously and vary more (greater changes, wider ranges) in physiologic parameters.

TABLE 10-3   Behavioral Tools for Pain Assessment

Tool	Behaviors	Comments
FLACC (Malviya et al., 2006; Merkel et al., 1997; Voepel-Lewis et al., 2002; Voepel-Lewis et al., 2010; Willis et al., 2003) Age: 0–19 years	Face Legs Activity Cry Consolability	Developed for use postanesthesia, but ease of use led to validity testing across all clinical acute care settings
Gauvain-Piquard Rating Scale (Gauvain-Piquard et al., 1991; Gauvain-Piquard et al., 1987) Age: 2–6 years	15 behaviors in three categories: pain items, psychomotor atonia, anxiety items	Evaluates cancer pain intensity of longer duration, thus rates behaviors at times other than during procedures; depression closely associated with pain; variability in scores suggests scale discriminates between pain levels
Behavioural Observational Pain Scale (BOPS) (Hesselgard et al., 2007) Age: 1–7 years	Three indicators: facial expression, verbalization, and body position	Simpler to use than CHEOPS; validated in postoperative children
Parents' Postoperative Pain Measure (Chambers et al., 2003; Finley et al., 2003) Age: 2–12 years	15-item behavioral checklist including items such as complain, cry, play, not do things normally does, act more worried, act more quiet, less energy, less eating	Reliable and valid; designed specifically for parents to use at home postoperatively

This is not an all-inclusive listing. Responses should be evaluated in a situational context (stimuli, pain event) and validated with self-report or physiologic parameters as appropriate.

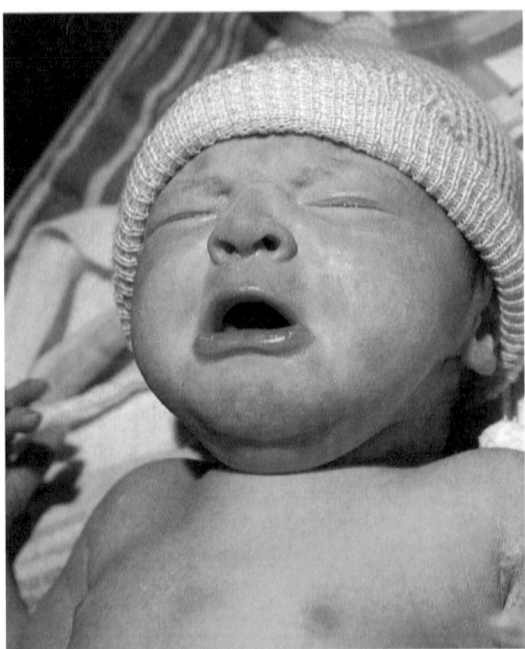

Figure 10-8 Facial expression of pain in an infant, with forcefully closed eyes, lowered brows, deepened furrow between nose and outer corner of lip, and square mouth with cupped tongue.

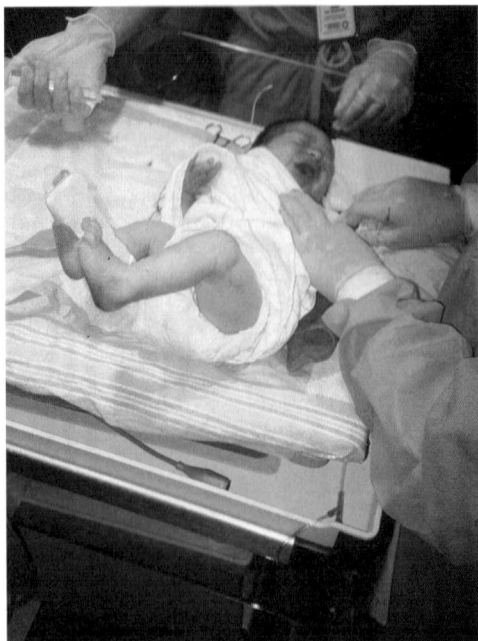

Figure 10-9 Lack of physical boundaries adds to the disorganization (inability to stay in control and filter out extraneous stimuli) of this baby showing stress cues of crying, finger extension and splaying, and some leg extension.

caREminder

The nurse is in a key position to assess for cues that indicate stress (e.g., gaze aversion, hiccups, yawning, flaccid posture) and physiologic instability (vital sign changes) resulting from pain. Implement interventions as appropriate for the situation—for example, allowing rest periods for the infant to regroup or stopping the procedure, giving pain medication, and providing physical boundaries and support.

Infancy

Crying is one way that an infant communicates to others. Although crying is a subjective measure, it is a valid method of assessing an infant's distress and must be recognized and responded to. When assessing the infant's behavior, consider environmental factors (see Table 10-4) and determine how long the infant has been crying to arrive at appropriate interpretations and actions. Rely on behavioral observations and physiologic monitoring and maintain a high index of suspicion that pain is present.

An infant's state influences the behavioral response to pain. Infants in deep sleep states are less likely to demonstrate as robust a response to pain as active, awake infants. Consider this difference when assessing infants for pain.

caREminder

If an infant is not responding vigorously, do not assume that the infant is not in pain. The infant may be in a sound sleep state or too weak to respond.

Early Childhood

Young children may not understand the word pain but can report "hurt," "owie," or "boo-boo." Even older children and adolescents may use different words for pain that reflect different intensities; these words, therefore, may have to be further defined by the child in pain. The young child may be able to indicate where the pain is but not be able to describe its intensity. If children are having difficulty localizing the pain, it may be helpful to tell them to point to their pain (using their term for it) with just one finger or have them show you where they would need a bandage placed.

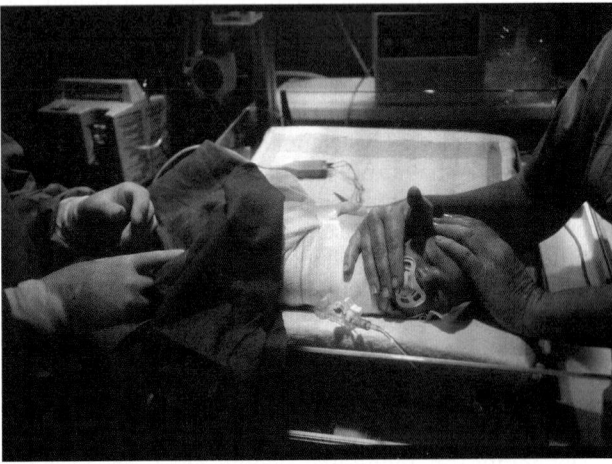

Figure 10-10 Appropriate management of a baby undergoing a painful procedure includes pharmacologic interventions, physical support, and containment.

TABLE 10-4   Is It Pain or Agitation?

Environmental Factors

May exacerbate perceived pain intensity or precipitate agitation:

- *Recent occurrence or presence of any stimulus presumed to be painful:* Overt and covert, such as incision pain, fracture, otitis media, postextubation edema
- *Routine care* is a stressor for sick and compromised infants who have a greater degree of autonomic instability; plan care to allow undisturbed time and deliver care in a developmentally supportive manner; assessment should include considering basic infant care issues (e.g., time since last feeding, dry diaper).
- *Noise and light levels:* Low levels contribute to an atmosphere of calm; high levels may have no effect on an infant in pain or may exacerbate the intensity of pain expression; high levels further disorganize an agitated infant and escalate the situation.
- *Caretaker* who does not routinely care for the child will not be as sensitive to the infant's subtle cues, particularly of agitation, and may not as readily calm the child or know what is most effective in doing so.
- *Lack of physical boundaries:* Well-defined boundaries (blankets, nests, buntings, something to push against to feel contained and keep extremities from flailing) assist an infant to stay organized; boundaries are particularly important for preterm infants, who do better with loose wrapping, whereas a term infant may need to be tightly swaddled.

Behavioral Cue	Pain	Agitation
Cry	Greater intensity, high pitched, tense, sudden, loud	Whining, tends to be more annoying than alerting to the caretaker
Facial expression	Pain facies, grimace; preterm show weaker response	Frowning, may look more "wild eyed," out of control
Activity	Tensed muscles, flexed extremities, may swipe at painful area; preterm may be limp, listless	Random movements of head and flailing extremities, hypertonic, arched posture
Sleep	Altered patterns	More regular patterns, agitated during awake state
Arousal	Greater intensity, wider fluctuations in vital signs, shallow breathing	Vital signs more stable, see decompensation as agitation is prolonged

These are generalizations; each infant is unique in response to situations and behaviors and must be evaluated individually.

Middle Childhood

School-aged children begin to communicate pain in terms that adults use. They are able to communicate effectively and generate excellent descriptors of pain such as squeezing, stabbing, and burning. Most can list things that aggravate and help alleviate their pain.

Self-report is considered the most reliable gauge of pain, so asking the child about the pain experience should provide the most accurate method of assessment. This approach avoids the problem that arises when the amount of pain the patient reports does not match the overt behavioral demonstration (Clinical Judgment 10-1). Recognize the potential for the child to regress with illness, pain, and hospitalization and consider this when selecting assessment methods. If the child is functioning at a less sophisticated developmental level, choose assessment methods that are appropriate for this lower level.

School-aged children and adolescents may show fewer overt behaviors in response to pain than younger children (Gaffney et al., 2003). School-aged children and adolescents may try to rest quietly when in pain. Observed body movements might be lying still, rigid, or curled in a fetal position; guarding or touching the painful area; and clenching fists. Children in these age groups may also be irritable, angry, sad, depressed, restless, withdrawn, and aggressive; sleep patterns may change.

Depending on individual coping style, school-aged children and adolescents may want to look at what is causing the pain (attend to the pain) or may look away and try to distract themselves from it.

Adolescence

 QUESTION: Does George's pain management plan acknowledge his desire to be in control?

The expanding cognitive abilities of adolescents should enable them to understand abstractions and describe pain in adult terms. Adolescents may not state that they are experiencing pain, however, because they think the nurse knows that they are in pain and will do something (e.g., giving medications) if and when it can be done. Adolescents may also be afraid to say they are in pain because their peers or family will consider them to be "babies." Remaining in control is particularly important to adolescents, and they may reflect this need by suppressing overt behaviors that indicate pain. In addition, adolescents may not report pain because of fear that they will be restricted from participating in social activities (Ameringer, 2010). This behavior does not mean that they are not experiencing pain. Fear of addiction is another factor that may prevent children, adolescents, and parents from expressing pain or accepting medications.

ANSWER: Yes. Allowing George to privately document his pain experience, take his medications at regular intervals, and select his NSAID all give him control over his situation.

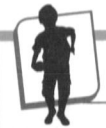

A School-Aged Child in Pain

Carmen is a 7-year-old girl, weighing 25 kg, who was hit by a car while riding her bike yesterday. Her left femur is fractured and she is in traction; an IV catheter is in place. Her mother is staying with her. When she was admitted, both Carmen and her mother were taught how to use the FACES scale to rate pain. Carmen has orders for acetaminophen with hydrocodone elixir (2.5 mg codeine/167.5 mg acetaminophen/5 mL) 5 mg every 4 hours orally PRN for pain; ibuprofen 200 mg every 4 hours orally PRN for pain; morphine sulfate 2 mg every 2 hours IV PRN for severe pain. Carmen received acetaminophen with hydrocodone elixir 2 hours ago. When you go in to take her vital signs, she rates her leg pain as FACE 1 of the 0–5 FACES, her heart rate is 80 bpm, her respiratory rate is 22 breaths/min, and her blood pressure is 106/64 mm Hg. She cries or moans frequently and is lying rigid.

Questions

1. Do you think Carmen is in pain?
2. What behaviors indicate that she is or is not in pain?
3. What would you do to treat Carmen's pain? When would you reevaluate Carmen's pain?
4. The next time Carmen's pain is reassessed, she picks FACE 4 of the 0–5 FACES. What would you do at this time?
5. When you evaluate Carmen 1 hour later, she picks FACE 2 of the 0–5 FACES, and she cries with movement but is engrossed in the television show she is watching. What should you do?

Answers

1. Yes.
2. Nonverbal cues that indicate that she is having pain are crying and unwillingness to move.
3. Medicate with ibuprofen. Plan to give the PRN ibuprofen around the clock because it is particularly effective for musculoskeletal pain. Carmen's subjective rating of her pain is FACE 1 of the 0–5 FACES, which indicates a small amount of pain. This subjective rating of pain is incongruent with objective findings; therefore, review how to use the FACES pain scale and verify Carmen's understanding of how to use the tool. Reassess in 1 hour.
4. Give morphine at 2 mg IV.
5. She seems more comfortable but is still rating mild to moderate pain. It has been 3 hours since she received the acetaminophen with hydrocodone elixir, so administer again and plan to alternate the elixir and ibuprofen every 2 hours, and give the morphine for breakthrough pain. Consider contacting the health care prescriber for an order for Valium or another muscle relaxant if Carmen has muscle spasms that contribute to her pain.

KidKare Explain that opioid use for moderate to severe pain will not lead to addiction, which is actually a psychological craving for a drug. Physical dependence can be managed by tapering the dosage. Discuss the difference between "good drugs" and "bad drugs"; emphasize that "say no to drugs" does not apply to analgesics given for pain and monitored by the health care team.

Pain, when combined with the other adolescent stressors of rapid physical and psychological change, may cause an adolescent to regress. Regression impairs coping abilities, and the adolescent may not function at the level at which he or she did previously. Recognize the potential for regression when selecting assessment methods. If an adolescent is functioning at a less sophisticated developmental level, choose assessment methods that are appropriate for this lower level.

Children With Communicative Impairment

Children may be unable to communicate their pain as a result of physical (e.g., cerebral palsy, coma) or cognitive impediments. The child with disability still has the capability to experience both acute and chronic pain, although the child may lack the ability to communicate about pain effectively.

Parents provide valuable information in recognizing and assessing pain in children with cognitive impairments (Burkitt et al., 2011; R. B. Davies, 2010; Ely et al., 2012; Herr et al., 2011), although they may overestimate their child's pain during the early postoperative period (Voepel-Lewis et al., 2005). Parents report unique behaviors and behavior clusters used by their children to express pain (Chen-Lim et al., 2012; Hunt et al., 2003).

If the child has cognitive deficits, use tools for pain assessment that are appropriate for that child's developmental level. Do not use chronologic age as a basis for pain assessment. When the child is unable cognitively to communicate pain, assessment methods used for infants may be used (e.g., crying, moaning, refusal to move, decreased appetite, irritability, sleep disturbance). Tools to provide a more objective measure of pain in this population have been developed (Table 10-5). Regardless of the tool, use the child's typical behaviors when pain free as a baseline to evaluate for pain and response to treatment. Use the method the child usually uses to communicate (e.g., pictures, letter board, shaking head, blinking eyes, specific words for pain). Clinical practice recommendations are established for the nursing assessment of pain in patients who are unable to self-report

TABLE 10-5   Tools for Pain Assessment of Children With Impaired Communication

Tool	Parameters* and Scoring	Comments
Non-communicating Children's Pain Checklist–Revised (NCCPC-R) (Breau, McGrath et al., 2002) Age: 3–18 years	Seven categories of 30 behaviors: vocal, eating/sleeping, social, facial expression of pain, activity, body/limbs, physiologic; 30 behaviors scored how often observed (0, not at all; 1, just a little; 2, fairly often; 3, very often); scores summed to create total scores (0–90 points)	Demonstrated reliability and validity; length of administration (approximately 10 minutes) may limit clinical use; score of 57 points or more is indicative of pain
Non-communicating Children's Pain Checklist–Postoperative Version (NCCPC-PV) (Breau, Finley et al., 2002) Age: 3–19 years	Six categories of 27 behaviors: vocal, social, facial expression of pain, activity, body/limbs, physiologic; scored how often observed (0, not at all; 1, just a little; 2, fairly often; 3, very often); scores summed to create total scores (0–81 points)	Reliable and valid for assessment of postoperative pain of children with severe intellectual disabilities; length of administration (approximately 10 minutes) may limit clinical use; score of 11 points or more indicates at least moderate pain
Checklist Pain Behavior (CPG) (Duivenvoorden et al., 2006; Terstegen et al., 2003) Age: 2–19 years	10 items: tense face; grimace; deeper nasolabial furrow; looking sad, almost in tears; eyes squeezed; panics/panic attack; cries softly; moaning/groaning; penetrating sounds of restlessness; tears	Items discriminate between "absence of pain" and "presence of pain"
Pain Indicator for Communicatively Impaired Children (PICIC) (Stallard et al., 2002) Age: not indicated; in study, mean age of 10.1 years (standard deviation, 4.9 years)	Six behaviors: crying, screaming, distressed face, tense body, difficulty in consoling, flinching	Presence of one or more of these cues correctly identified almost 75% of those considered to be in pain, whereas their absence identified 94% not in pain; a distressed-looking or "screwed-up" face is the strongest individual predictor of the presence of pain
Revised FLACC (Malviya et al., 2006; Voepel-Lewis et al., 2010) Age: 4–19 years	Face Legs Activity Cry Consolability; allows for individualization of the tool via open-ended descriptors in each category, which is scored from 0 to 2 points with a total of 0–10 points	Demonstrated reliability and validity; expanded original FLACC descriptors in Legs and Activity including verbal outbursts, tremors, increased spasticity, jerking movements, and respiratory pattern changes such as breath holding and grunting; scores suggest pain intensity of mild (0–3 points), moderate (4–6 points), severe (7–10 points)
Paediatric Pain Profile (PPP) (Hunt et al., 2004; Hunt et al., 2007) Age: 1–18 years	20 items: cheerful, sociable, withdrawn, cried/moaned, hard to comfort, bit self/banged head, difficult feeding, sleep disturbance, frowned, grimaced/screwed up face, looked frightened, ground teeth, restless, spasmed, drew legs up, touched particular areas, resisted being moved, pulled away, twisted and turned/writhed or arched back, involuntary movements; items scored 0–3 points	Demonstrated reliability and validity; short, takes 2–3 minutes to complete; a score of 14 points or more suggests significant pain
Individualized Numeric Rating Scale (Solodiuk & Curley, 2003; Solodiuk et al., 2010)	10-point numeric rating scale with word anchors and parent pain cues	Convergent validity

*Items are given as representations of the concept and may not represent exact wording from tool. Although scores on some tools may suggest increasing pain intensity, if pain is present, it must be treated regardless of the intensity. Use cutoff scores in conjunction with other assessments to guide nursing interventions.

(Herr et al., 2011). The American Society for Pain Management Nursing has established a position statement that guides assessment of pain in populations who are unable to self-report, including preverbal infants, very young children, and children with intellectual disabilities. The recommended clinical practice for pain assessment with infants and children includes the use of a hierarchy of pain assessment approaches, including (1) obtaining self-report whenever possible, (2) searching for possible causes of pain and observing patient behavior, (3) obtaining parental proxy report of pain, and (4) initiating an analgesic trial (Herr et al., 2011).

MANAGING PAIN IN CHILDREN

> **QUESTION:** Which diagnosis in Nursing Plan of Care 10-1 is most applicable to George? What would be a measurable outcome specifically for George to evaluate the expected outcome in Nursing Plan of Care 10-1?

The role of the health care team in pain management is to listen to the child and family, provide relevant education, maintain continuity of care, strive for the best pain assessment, and intervene appropriately. Core principles of acute pain management have been developed to ensure safe and effective pain management in the health care setting (American Society for Pain Management Nursing et al., 2009). Inadequate pain management results in needless physical and psychological suffering.

> **A L E R T**   *Maintain a high index of suspicion regarding the presence of pain, and advocate actively for pain relief on behalf of the child. Children of all ages experience pain, and when the presence of pain is suspected, interventions must be implemented. Consider severe, unrelenting pain a medical emergency, and immediately implement pharmacologic interventions as ordered.*

To make appropriate management decisions, consider the individual child, the child's condition, and the type and intensity of the child's pain. The most successful pain management strategy is a dynamic, proactive approach (Nursing Interventions 10-2). This approach involves maintaining control of the pain with around-the-clock management. Interventions can be classified as pharmacologic or biobehavioral (nonpharmacologic). These methods should be used in conjunction to augment their individual effects.

Nursing diagnoses applicable to the child in pain are based on assessment findings. Identifying them may seem simple, but psychological aspects of pain must also be considered. Discuss the expectations of the child and family regarding pain relief. Do they expect that the child will achieve complete pain relief? Is their expectation realistic in the specific situation? Do they expect that pain will be relieved enough so that the child can participate in certain activities? Realistic goals should be mutually decided upon by the child, family, and health care team to avoid misunderstanding and mismanagement of the pain. Appropriate management techniques are determined based on the identified diagnoses (Nursing Plan of Care 10-1).

> **ANSWER:** An appropriate diagnosis is chronic pain related to effects of condition. The expected outcome is that the child will perform activities of daily living and developmentally appropriate activities. For George, time spent on his online high school courses each day would be a measure of his ability to concentrate on an enjoyable and developmentally appropriate activity.

PHARMACOLOGIC PAIN MANAGEMENT

Drug therapies are the essential interventions for treating pain and are thus an important component of managing both acute and chronic pain. Nurses play a key role in administering analgesics and monitoring for efficacy and side effects of these pain-relieving medications. A thorough understanding of nociception and pain pathways; accurate assessment of type and intensity of pain; knowledge of drug pharmacokinetics; and education of patients, families, and other health team

---

NURSING INTERVENTIONS 10-2

ABCDEs of Pain Management

Assessment is multidimensional and is more than just a pain intensity score.

Believe that the child has pain if the history supports it or the child reports it (either by behavior or words).

Communication is clear, concise, and patient focused.

Do something/intervene. Interventions should consider the child's developmental age and the type and intensity of pain.

Evaluate the effectiveness of interventions; go back to assessment.

NURSING PLAN OF CARE 10-1

The Child in Pain

Nursing Diagnosis: Acute pain related to effects of condition, treatment, injury

Interventions/Rationale

- Assess pain initially, every 2–4 hours, and as necessary (see Nursing Interventions 10-1); observe nonverbal cues such as posture, breathing patterns, movement, and facial expression; ask about the family's perception of child's comfort level. Use information from family regarding child's usual behavior when in pain to assess level of pain.

  Provides baseline assessment and collects information to develop pain management plan. Changes noted on subsequent assessments provide information about whether pain management is adequate. The family knows their child's behaviors best and are excellent resources regarding their child's behavior. A child's pain response is influenced by developmental age, condition causing pain, previous experience with pain, culture, and family's responses to pain.

- Allow child to express feelings of pain; offer comfort and supportive measures.

  Conveys the uniqueness of the child and the experience; may reassure the child and family and reduce anxiety.

- Teach child and family about condition, prognosis, medications, and treatment plan.

  Provides a knowledge base on which the child and family can make informed decisions.

- Encourage family to participate in care to the extent they feel comfortable doing so. Provide the family with concrete information about what they can do to help the child (e.g., read a story, help the child with coping strategies such as deep breathing).

  Teaching family empowers them and helps them feel that they have skills to support their child. Children seek parental comfort and may be more receptive to comfort measures provided by the parent.

- Administer medications (nonopioids, opioids, and coanalgesics) as ordered before pain escalates; evaluate effectiveness at appropriate interval, at least within 1 hour. When IV opioids are given, administer slowly over 5 minutes and observe for changes in respiratory patterns; reassure child and family that addiction is not a concern (see Nursing Interventions 10-3).

  Pharmacologic strategies are the mainstay of pain management. Reassessment gives information about effectiveness of interventions and the need to alter them. Pain is easier to manage when it is less severe.

- Assess the effect of discomfort on the child's sleep. Help child and family to make a realistic and integrated schedule of activities, rest and sleep, exercise, and stress management. Organize care (e.g., medicate before activities, provide uninterrupted opportunities to rest and sleep).

  Active involvement increases child's and family's sense of control, which may decrease stress and anxiety (which lower pain threshold). A proactive, preventative approach to pain management prevents pain from escalating; escalated pain is harder to control and alleviate. Decreasing pain enhances sleep.

- Control environmental factors such as room temperature, noise, and light.

  Noxious environmental factors may reduce pain tolerance.

- Provide a pleasant, relaxed atmosphere for eating and activities.

  Unpleasant sights and odors can stimulate the vomiting center or pain center in the brain.

- Provide psychological support (see Nursing Interventions 10-4). Explain all procedures to child in a developmentally appropriate manner (see Nursing Interventions 10-5).

  May decrease stress, fear, and anxiety, which lower pain threshold and can alter pain perception and interfere with the child's ability to express pain.

- Identify, teach, and model coping behaviors that are effective for the child; encourage the child and family to practice these strategies (see Nursing Interventions 10-6 and 10-7).

  Coping strategies that the child can use are most effective in altering or reducing pain perception; many require practice to increase effectiveness.

- Implement biobehavioral strategies such as positioning, distraction, imagery, music, back rubs, and relaxation techniques.

  Biobehavioral measures can decrease pain and discomfort and augment the therapeutic effects of medications by modifying physiologic reactions to pain; they increase a sense of control and help the child cope.

- Evaluate adequacy of pain management (see Nursing Interventions 10-10).

  Provides information about effectiveness of management and enables prompt revision of management plan if it is not achieving desired outcomes.

Expected Outcome

- Child will remain free of pain. If pain cannot be alleviated, it will be reduced to an acceptable level, as defined by the child, family, and health care provider.

Nursing Diagnosis: Chronic pain related to effects of condition; altered pain processing

Interventions/Rationale

- See previous interventions as for acute pain and Nursing Interventions 10-9.
- Evaluate current management regimen. Explore the need for opioids, nonopioids, and coanalgesics and biobehavioral measures. Ensure around-the-clock dosing.

  Using nonopioids, even if they are not effective alone, can reduce the dosage of an opioid required to effectively manage pain. Combining classes of analgesics enhances the effectiveness of each and may achieve pain relief with lower dosages of each single drug. Around-the-clock dosing helps prevent the pain from escalating and becoming more difficult to manage.

- Encourage the child to participate in developmentally appropriate activities and adhere to behavioral expectations and discipline based on family norms, home responsibilities such as chores, and school attendance.

  These activities are normalizing for children; they help children to regain or achieve appropriate developmental tasks, decrease attention to pain behaviors (while making sure that pain control is as good as possible), and emphasize a productive role.

Expected Outcome

- Child will perform activities of daily living and developmentally appropriate activities with minimal interference from pain and medication side effects.

Nursing Diagnosis: Anxiety related to effects of pain, lack of control over pain

Interventions/Rationale

- Assess child and family for behaviors that reflect anxiety.

  Children and family frequently experience anxiety when faced with pain. Increased anxiety levels can increase pain perception and interfere with use of coping strategies.

- Encourage child and family to learn about child's condition and treatment plan. Explain all procedures to child in developmentally appropriate terms.

  Provides knowledge base on which to make informed decisions and may decrease anxiety.

- Organize care to provide a pace that the child and family can cope with and develop plan in conjunction with child and family. Provide predictability for the child (e.g., perform procedures at a consistent time and place each day, wear a specific object that signifies procedure time, maintain "safe" areas and times).

  Predictability reduces anxiety. A pace that the child and family can accommodate provides them time to recover and maintain optimal coping

strategies. Anxiety decreases coping abilities, thus increasing pain perception.

- Plan experiences that the child can control, manipulate, and succeed in to decrease anxiety arising from feelings of powerlessness (e.g., encourage child, as age appropriate, to participate in decisions regarding care and schedule, such as which dressings to remove first, how fast to remove them). Allow child to assist with dressing changes (e.g., removing old dressing, holding tape); encourage child to apply dressing to doll or stuffed animal.

  Gives control and choice to the child, which may reduce pain perception.

- Assist child to assume a position of comfort; use biobehavioral approaches for comfort (e.g., back rubs, distraction with toys and games, imagery, soothing music, relaxation, controlled breathing).

  Biobehavioral methods to relax may reduce pain perception.

- Project a calm, unhurried attitude while performing procedures.

  Staff (and family) attitudes and actions such as abruptness, rushing, and irritation increase a child's level of anxiety and decrease ability to cope.

- Listen and provide emotional support.

  Children and families who feel that they have been heard and their concerns are being addressed may be less anxious.

- Prepare the child for procedures or consequences of pain in a developmentally appropriate manner (see Nursing Interventions 10-5). Emphasize that painful procedures are not punishment.

  Child's cognitive abilities influence understanding of pain and use of coping strategies.

- Maintain sensitivity toward families who are battling with feelings of anxiety and may be angry with health care providers. Consider mental health referral when applicable.

  Provides a therapeutic environment.

Expected Outcomes

- Child will not demonstrate behaviors of, or verbalize, anxiety. Increased feelings of control will prepare child for painful situations and procedures. Child's pain will be controlled at acceptable levels.

Nursing Diagnosis: Deficient knowledge: Causes of pain and interventions

Interventions/Rationale

- Explain all procedures to child in age- and culturally appropriate terms. Emphasize that painful procedures are not punishment.

  Ability to cope is influenced by knowledge, realistic expectations, and ability to control and manage pain.

(Continued)

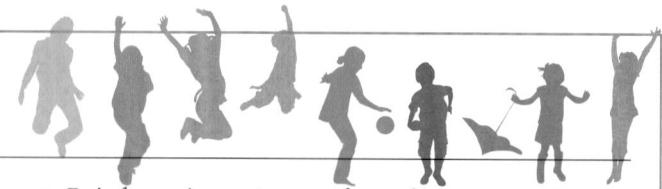

NURSING PLAN OF CARE 10-1

The Child in Pain (*Continued*)

- Answer questions in a nonthreatening manner. Provide concise and honest information at child's level of understanding.

  Understanding the plan of care can help the child adhere to the plan.
- Give child and family verbal and written instructions regarding list of medications, dosages, schedule, possible side effects, how to avoid or manage them, and when to report them to the physician or clinic. Also tell them where and how to obtain refills.

  If a knowledge deficit exists, families cannot appropriately maintain the child's level of functioning or avoid complications.
- Have child and family demonstrate biobehavioral strategies to manage pain.

  Allows for validation that child and family are performing technique appropriately and that technique is effective.

- Reinforce importance of regular communication and follow-up appointments with health care provider. Provide contact information of health care provider to consult for follow-up care.

  Routine communication enables health care provider to detect adverse trends promptly and to implement interventions to address them. Drug therapy requires frequent assessments to monitor the drug's effectiveness and side effects.

Expected Outcomes

- Child and family will receive developmentally and culturally appropriate explanations of pain and pain management.
- Child and family will understand pain mechanisms and know what they can do to relieve pain.

---

members are essential to effective pain relief. When there is reason to suspect that a child might be in pain, a trial of an analgesic is appropriate.

Categories of Medications

Medications used for pain management are classified into three categories, depending on their mechanism of action:

1. Nonopioid analgesics generally work at the site of injury to inhibit prostaglandin synthesis, thus decreasing pain.
2. Opioid analgesics, previously known as *narcotic analgesics*, relieve pain by binding to the opioid receptors in the CNS, blocking the release of substance P, and preventing the pain impulse from crossing the neuronal synaptic cleft.
3. Coanalgesics have a primary indication other than pain relief, but they can also provide analgesia in certain painful conditions. This category tends to be a catch-all grouping of medications that includes anticonvulsants, antidepressants, and anesthetics (i.e., coanalgesics are any medications other than nonopioids or opioids that are used to treat pain).

These three categories of medications are typically used in combination to attack pain in a variety of ways at various points on the nociceptive pathway. By combining these analgesics, less of each individual medication is required to relieve pain, and the potential for side effects is less than it would be with single-agent therapy. This approach is called *balanced* or *multimodal analgesia*. Be familiar with concepts important

to treatment with analgesics, such as ceiling effect, titration, tolerance, equianalgesia, and physical and psychological dependence (see thePoint for Supplemental Information).

Nonopioid Analgesics

Nonopioid analgesics are indicated for mild to moderate pain or for use in conjunction with opioids for moderate to severe pain to augment and decrease opioid requirements. They work well for musculoskeletal pain. Nonopioids differ from opioids in that they are antipyretic, have a ceiling effect, and do not produce tolerance or physical or psychological dependence. Nonopioid analgesics include acetaminophen and NSAIDs (see thePoint for Supplemental Information). They differ from each other in chemical structure, so if one drug is not effective, another nonopioid should be tried. The most commonly used nonopioids—over-the-counter acetaminophen and ibuprofen—are safe and effective for relieving children's pain.

ALERT *The overall incidence of side effects with acetaminophen is low in comparison with that for NSAIDs. However, unbridled use of acetaminophen can result in liver toxicity. Caution children and families about this potential threat, and caution them that a child may inadvertently receive too much acetaminophen because it is included in many common over-the-counter remedies for treating symptoms of pain, flu, and the common cold.*

Opioid Analgesics

Opioid analgesics are indicated for moderate to severe pain that is not relieved with nonopioids. Opioids differ from nonopioids in that they do not have an antipyretic effect or a ceiling of analgesia. Therefore, opioids will not mask fever, and opioid doses can be titrated upward until pain is relieved or intolerable side effects develop (Nursing Interventions 10-3). Several opioids are available in low-dose preparations combined with nonopioids. Because of nonopioid ceiling of analgesia and potential for toxicity at higher doses, the nonopioid component limits titration of these combination drugs.

The different opioid drugs are classified, according to their receptor binding properties, as agonists, partial agonists, agonists–antagonists, or antagonists (see thePoint for Supplemental Information). Opioid analgesics include centrally and peripherally acting mu-agonist opioids.

Morphine, codeine, hydrocodone, oxycodone, and hydromorphone belong to a class of chemicals called *phenanthrenes*. Methadone is a synthetic opioid chemically classified as a benzomorphan derivative. Fentanyl and meperidine are considered phenylpiperidine derivatives. Although allergic reactions to opioids are rare, allergic reactions to one opioid in a class indicates allergy to all opioids in that class. Choosing an opioid from another class may limit the patient's risk of a subsequent allergic reaction.

Physical dependence on opioids develops in as little as 7 days of continuous use. Symptoms of opioid withdrawal, also known as *opioid abstinence syndrome*, include anxiety, irritability, chills, hot flashes, salivation, tearing, rhinorrhea, diaphoresis, piloerection, nausea, vomiting, diarrhea, abdominal cramps, and insomnia. Infants may also demonstrate increased crying; poor feeding (but ravenous sucking); and increased muscle tone, tremors, and jitteriness. To decrease the risk of opioid withdrawal, the dose should be gradually decreased (10% to 20% per day) or the time between doses gradually increased; do not simply eliminate doses (APS, 2008).

ALERT *Use caution with children who may have developed physical dependence. Use of antagonists (naloxone) or mixed agonist–antagonists to reverse side effects may precipitate sudden withdrawal.*

If withdrawal symptoms are present, ensure a quiet, darkened environment; handle an infant as little as possible; ask older children what their needs are; and provide comfort measures (offer pacifier, swaddle infants; apply cool cloth to forehead for older children). Sedatives may be used to manage symptoms of withdrawal. Use a scoring method similar to one developed for neonatal abstinence syndrome (for infants born to opioid-addicted mothers; see Chapter 14) to help to keep monitoring and tracking of opioid weaning consistent.

Coanalgesics

Coanalgesics include medications such as tricyclic antidepressants, selective serotonin reuptake inhibitors, anticonvulsants, benzodiazepines, and local anesthetics. These drugs play a role in pain management by potentiating the effects of analgesics, treating the side effects of analgesics, or exerting an analgesic effect of their own (see thePoint for Supplemental Information). Most drugs in this category are not labeled for pediatric use.

NURSING INTERVENTIONS 10-3

Opioid Side Effects

Common Opioid Side Effects	Interventions
Nausea and vomiting	Administer nonsedating antiemetic, phenothiazine antiemetic, or antihistamine as ordered.
Pruritus	Administer an antihistamine as ordered; apply cool compresses to the site.
Sedation	Assess level of consciousness; for chronic therapy, add stimulant as ordered (e.g., caffeine, dextroamphetamine, methylphenidate).
Respiratory depression (especially with IV, epidural, high doses)	Assess level of sedation, respiratory rate, depth, and assess SaO_2. Have resuscitation equipment and naloxone available. Sedation always precedes respiratory depression, so monitor sedated children closely.
Constipation	Assess bowel sounds, administer a stimulating laxative and a stool softener, encourage ambulation, and increase fluid and fiber intake.
Urinary retention	Monitor intake and output, apply a warm compress over the bladder, have the child ambulate if possible. May require catheterization.

Treatment of side effects also depends on the specific situation and whether they interfere with activities of daily living. For example, sedation may be desired during the immediate postoperative period but not desired for the patient with cancer.

caREminder

Painful procedures should not be performed without the addition of analgesic drugs.

Scheduling for Analgesic Administration

Pain is best managed by a proactive, preemptive approach. Anticipating and treating pain is much more effective and humane than trying to manage pain after it is present. Although PRN (*pro re nada*, which means *as needed*, *as necessary*) analgesic dosing may be appropriate for periodic pain such as an occasional headache, treating constant pain such as pain from diseases, surgery, and trauma demands a pain management strategy that provides pain relief for a longer duration than one dose of an analgesic can provide. PRN administration of pain medication tends to propagate a pain cycle with peaks (side effects like sedation) and troughs (pain) of drug action. If pain is present or anticipated for most of the day, medications must be scheduled and administered around the clock, with additional doses of analgesics available for prompt relief of breakthrough pain. Analgesic schedules should take into account the duration of action and half-life of the specific drug.

The effect of nonopioid medications is optimized by administering these nonsedating analgesics to opioid-naive patients and by providing opioids for breakthrough pain. If, despite the use of scheduled nonopioids, a child continues to have pain, the management plan should progress to also provide opioids on a scheduled basis. When sustained-release or long-acting opioid analgesics are administered, additional quick-acting opioid preparations may be needed as a rescue dose during breakthrough pain episodes.

Route of Administration

 QUESTION: If George's morphine dose were changed to IV, would the dose remain the same?

Route of analgesic administration will determine the rate of drug absorption and, therefore, the time and duration of analgesic effect. Dose is also route dependent. First-pass metabolism through the liver leaves only a small fraction of the drug available to relieve pain. If a route circumvents first-pass metabolism, the required dose of the analgesic is substantially lower than when the same drug is administered by a route that requires first-pass metabolism. For example, the IV route circumvents first-pass metabolism, so the recommended starting dose in a child for morphine by the IV route is 0.1 mg/kg, whereas the starting dose for morphine by the oral route to achieve equianalgesia is 0.3 mg/kg.

Oral Administration

If the child is able to take medications orally, and pain can be controlled, the oral route is preferred for analgesic administration. The oral route is convenient, and relatively steady blood levels of drug can be achieved to ensure steady and consistent pain control, with few peaks and valleys of pain and side effects. Oral analgesics are typically less expensive and come in a variety of formulations (e.g., liquids, suspensions, chewable tablets, pills, extended-release capsules) to increase palatability.

Disadvantages of the oral route are delayed onset of action (typically 45 minutes) and delayed peak drug effect (typically 1 to 2 hours), which make this route less than optimal for severe pain of sudden onset. Children may be particularly vulnerable to undertreatment by this route because they may refuse oral medications that have a noxious taste. Children also have difficulty understanding the need to take a medication regularly to prevent recurrence of pain because they do not anticipate that the medication will wear off and that delay in taking it will delay its effects.

Intramuscular Administration

Injections are not recommended for administering analgesics and are specifically considered unacceptable for administering pain medications to children (APS, 2008). Children may not report or may deny pain in order to avoid an intramuscular injection. Painful administration makes this route inconsistent with the goal of analgesic therapy.

Other disadvantages of this route are the wide fluctuations in drug absorption, delayed peak effect (30 to 60 minutes), and rapid falloff of action. Injections also pose the potential risk of sterile abscess formation and fibrosis of the muscle and soft tissue. A rarely mentioned disadvantage is nurses' dissatisfaction with their role in administering medications by this route.

Intravenous Administration

IV administration circumvents first-pass metabolism and therefore provides a rapid onset of action. This route is most effective when treating unpredictable, severe pain of sudden onset. Initially, IV bolus doses of opioids are titrated to provide effective pain relief. This route is the preferred route of analgesic administration for patients who are unable to tolerate oral medications.

Continuous IV infusions of opioids provide a steady blood level and may be indicated for opioid-tolerant patients with persistent painful conditions. The APS (2008) warns, however, that administering continuous opioid infusions to opioid-naive patients (either as a sole infusion or as a background infusion with patient-controlled analgesia [PCA]) may increase the incidence and severity of adverse side effects without improving the quality of analgesia. The implementation of IV bolus morphine monitoring guidelines has been successful in detecting respiratory depression in the pediatric setting (Ellis et al., 2011). Additional safety monitoring is enhanced when nurses implement such guidelines into practice.

ANSWER: George's dose would need to decrease if it were given intravenously instead of orally by as much as one third because of the first-pass effect.

Subcutaneous Administration

The subcutaneous route circumvents first-pass metabolism, but absorption is slow. Although subcutaneous administration of opioids is considered an alternative to the IV or oral route for providing steady-state analgesia, the need to use a needle to provide bolus doses or continuous infusions by this route makes it less acceptable for children.

Transdermal Administration

Local anesthetics and lipophilic opioids have been formulated to permit transdermal absorption. Although manufactured specialty local anesthetic creams provide onset of anesthetic action in 10 to 60 minutes after application, transdermal opioids have a delayed onset of action (12 to 16 hours) and are therefore not indicated for acute pain management. Only a few pain medications are available as transdermal formulations, and even fewer can be obtained at doses appropriate for children. However, this formulation provides a nonpainful route of analgesic administration.

Transmucosal Administration

The sublingual (under the tongue), buccal (between the teeth and cheek), and intranasal routes can be grouped as transmucosal medication administration techniques. With these techniques, drugs are absorbed into the venous blood, bypassing first-pass metabolism to achieve rapid onset of effect. Children may be less receptive to the sublingual and buccal routes of administration because these analgesics have a noxious taste. Administration of analgesics by the intranasal route may cause a burning sensation on the nasal mucosa in addition to the unpleasant taste. Even with these disadvantages, children may prefer these routes over injections. The intranasal route is a safe and effective method of pain management for children in a variety of clinical areas (Mudd, 2011).

Rectal Administration

Although the rectal route is also considered an alternative to IV or oral administration, it is not well accepted by children older than 2 years of age. Drug absorption varies and is less predictable after rectal administration. Drug absorption by the rectal route depends on rectal content, irritation, drug retention, and amount of drug absorbed directly into the systemic circulation versus the amount that is exposed to first-pass metabolism. Consider, for example, the difference in pediatric rectal and oral doses of acetaminophen. Although oral acetaminophen is dosed at 10 to 15 mg/kg to achieve an analgesic blood level, rectal doses of 40 to 60 mg/kg may be required. Pain scores have not been shown to be significantly different when these two routes of administration were compared (Owczarzak & Haddad, 2006; van der Marel et al., 2001), although the rectal route may provide longer analgesia for moderately painful procedures (Capici et al., 2008).

Regional Analgesia

This route encompasses a variety of techniques, including peripheral nerve blocks and intrathecal and epidural infusions. The use of regional anesthetic techniques is becoming more common for pain management after pediatric urologic, orthopedic, and general surgical procedures as well as for the relief of pain from sickle cell disease and cancer. Regional analgesia is typically administered and managed by an anesthesiologist and can be quite effective in managing pain.

Peripheral Nerve Blocks

Peripheral nerve blocks can be used for procedures or injuries (femoral nerve block for fractured femur), for surgery with or without anesthesia (dorsal penile nerve or caudal block for circumcision), or to manage postoperative pain (ilioinguinal block for herniorrhaphy). Circumcision is a frequently performed and painful procedure that has clear evidence of the benefit of the use of the dorsal penile nerve block (Brady-Fryer et al., 2009). Potential contraindications to these techniques include anatomic abnormalities, bleeding disorders, allergies to local anesthetics, and infection at the puncture site (McCamant, 2006). Disposable local anesthetic infusion pumps have been developed to extend peripheral nerve blockade for a limited time after hospital discharge.

Intraspinal Administration

The intraspinal routes provide profound analgesia with minimal systemic side effects. Intraspinal most commonly refers to the *epidural* route, in which medication is infused into the epidural space (the space outside the dura); the *intrathecal* route (medication infused into the cerebrospinal fluid in the space surrounding the spinal cord) may be used to manage longer term pain syndromes. Analgesia is achieved at much smaller doses than required for systemic administration of opioids because intraspinal opioids bind directly to the receptors on the dorsal horn of the spinal cord (APS, 2008). Opioids administered by the epidural route are also largely absorbed systemically by the epidural venous plexus. Therefore, intrathecal doses are considerably smaller than epidural doses, which in turn are substantially smaller than IV or oral doses. For example, 0.1 mg intrathecal morphine is equianalgesic to 1 mg epidural morphine, which is equianalgesic to 10 mg IV or 30 mg oral morphine (APS, 2008).

Epidural analgesia is the most commonly used regional anesthetic technique for intra- and postoperative pain management for children requiring urologic, orthopedic, and general surgical procedures below the nipples (T4 dermatosomal level). It works by blocking nociceptive impulses from entering the CNS. Use of this technology to relieve pain from sickle cell vaso-occlusive crisis and cancer is increasing.

The biggest advantage of epidural analgesia is profound pain relief. Analgesia is achieved through epidural infusions with or without patient-controlled epidural boluses of local anesthetics, opioids, and coanalgesics such as clonidine. Epidural analgesia decreases morbidity and mortality associated with acute pain by decreasing pulmonary and cardiovascular complications, improving ventilatory function, and decreasing pain with movement.

Disadvantages of the epidural route are primarily drug related. Local anesthetics provide analgesia with minimal risk of causing sedation or respiratory depression. Local anesthetics administered by the epidural route can, however, cause hypotension and bradycardia by blocking the SNS and causing arterial and venous vasodilation. This hemodynamic response is age dependent and rarely occurs in children younger than 8 years of age. Epidural local anesthetics can also cause apnea in the fully conscious patient by blocking the motor efferents to the muscles involved in respiration. Another disadvantage of epidural local anesthetics is the potential for motor blockades that, although rarely life threatening, limit patient mobility.

Hydrophilic opioids, such as hydromorphone or morphine, administered by the epidural route remain in the cerebrospinal fluid longer than lipophilic opioids do, thus providing longer duration of analgesia. Unfortunately, the hydrophilic opioids also have an increased risk for rostral spread, which increases the risk for sedation and respiratory depression.

Epidural catheters can be placed in children of all ages. Although the caudal, lumbar, and thoracic approaches are all used, the caudal approach is used most frequently because it is the easiest to access in infants and young children (Samol et al., 2012). To achieve analgesia at the thoracic level from the caudal approach, the catheter is threaded up the epidural space. Unlike adults, infants and children are usually heavily sedated or anesthetized for catheter placement.

Epidural placement is contraindicated in patients with acquired or congenital bleeding disorders because of the risk for epidural hemorrhage. Inability to place the catheter, infection at the site of catheter placement, and hemodynamic instability are other relative contraindications for epidural analgesia. Complications of epidural catheter placement include postdural puncture headache, neurologic sequelae (cauda equina syndrome), pain at the catheter site, and backache.

caREminder

Physiologic monitors can alert the nurse to respiratory events, but they must be used in addition to frequent, skilled patient assessments. In addition to monitoring for effective analgesia, routinely assess for level of consciousness, respiratory effort, cardiac function, and level of sensation, especially if local anesthetics and hydrophilic opioids are given.

Patient-Controlled Analgesia

PCA is a technique that enables patients to administer their own opioid bolus doses by a computer-controlled infusion pump. The pump is most commonly connected to an IV, but PCA is also used epidurally. The PCA pump is programmed, as ordered, to deliver a patient-controlled dose at an interval not more frequent than the ordered "lockout" period. Thus, the child can activate the pump and self-administer small, frequent bolus doses of opioid to optimize pain relief through a rapid response system. Medication can be administered as a patient-demanded bolus only or in addition to a continuous infusion. PCA use and prescriptions vary depending on the child's diagnosis; type of pain; previous hospital experiences; history of opioid tolerance or naiveté; and the recommendations, standards, or practices of individual institutions or prescribers.

The advantage of using PCA as part of a pain management plan is that it adjusts for the patient's individual variation in pharmacokinetics and pharmacodynamics. Also, the push-button device is easy to use and concrete, something the child can touch and hold. For some patients, particularly adolescents, PCA gives them a sense of control over their pain. PCA technology avoids the need for the child to ask, beg, or bargain for analgesic administration. After two decades of use in children, this technology is considered safe and effective.

One of the most important disadvantages is that anyone can push the PCA button—the nurse, the family member, the friend, or the 2-year-old sibling who is incapable of understanding the connection between pushing the button and opioid administration or the potential dangers. *PCA by proxy* is the term used when an unauthorized person activates the dosing mechanism. Teach family and visitors not to push the button for the child. Although the total amount of opioid that can be administered is preset, someone else pushing the button bypasses one of the built-in safety features of the system, which is that an oversedated patient cannot self-administer medication. **Authorized agent–controlled analgesia (AACA)** is a mechanism for pain management in which one individual is authorized and educated to activate the PCA mechanism in response to the patient's pain when the patient is unable to do so (Wuhrman et al., 2007). This method is appropriate for children too young to self-administer medication, those unable cognitively to understand the concept (e.g., developmentally delayed children), and those physically unable to manipulate the button (e.g., children with cerebral palsy). The authorized agent may be the child's nurse, family member, or significant other. Guidelines for AACA should clearly delineate the conditions under which the practice shall be implemented and should outline monitoring procedures to ensure safe use of AACA. Nurse-controlled analgesia (NCA) allows the nurse to administer the programmed analgesic and has been established as safe (Verghese & Hannallah, 2010). Parent-proxy PCA has also been found to be as safe as NCA and standard PCA (Anghelescu et al., 2012). It is essential to teach the parent who is designated to act as the proxy the basic concept of PCA, side effects associated with opioids, and simple methods of pain assessment, including indicators of pain and oversedation.

Another important disadvantage of PCA is that the child must continuously titrate and therefore attend to the pain to keep it under control. PCA is not a panacea; opioid side effects still occur and may discourage the child from achieving optimal pain relief. A general recommendation is that children older than 5 years of age have the cognitive ability to use PCA (Wuhrman et al., 2007). Rather than following a strict age cutoff

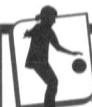

DEVELOPMENTAL CONSIDERATIONS 10-4

Criteria That Indicate a Child's Suitability for Patient-Controlled Analgesia

- Able to activate the device. A child with physical limitations may need a device that is adapted with the help of a biomedical engineer or occupational therapist.
- Able to quantify pain. The child needs to activate the pump when pain is starting or increasing so that treatment is not delayed until pain is severe or intolerable.
- Unable to tolerate oral analgesics. Oral analgesics provide a longer duration of pain relief, so a child who can tolerate this formulation does not need to frequently request analgesia or activate a system to deliver it.
- Understands the relation between pushing the button and receiving medication.
- Understands the machine's safety mechanisms.
- Reports unsatisfactory pain relief with current regimen. The child and family must understand that the PCA is not a panacea, merely an alternate way to relieve pain. If the child's pain is not effectively relieved with PCA, other methods of controlling pain should be considered.

for PCA use, evaluate a child's appropriateness for PCA (Developmental Considerations 10-4).

Assess for appropriate and effective use of PCA by reviewing hourly PCA attempts and injections data. Although most PCA pumps provide immediate feedback (by a signal) to the child that the button has been depressed, it takes a few minutes for the child to experience pain relief, and the child may interpret the delay as a sign that the pump does not work. Determine whether the child has made more attempts than injections. Does he or she push the button repeatedly to get only one dose? Does the child demand PCA frequently? Is hourly lockout reached or is the button pushed several times every hour? How hard does the child have to work to maintain comfort? Is the child able to rest and sleep? Does the child report that pain is well controlled? What is the child's pain intensity score?

With this additional assessment, the nurse can determine whether the child understands the machine and whether PCA is appropriate for relieving the child's pain. This assessment also alerts the nurse to any need to provide additional education to the child and family to optimize PCA use. However, assessment may also indicate that other methods of pain control would provide more effective pain relief to this individual child.

Dose

QUESTION: Why does it matter whether George weighs more or less than 50 kg?

Analgesic doses required to relieve pain vary by child, route, drug, frequency, and administration techniques. Individual patient factors known to affect dose variability include type, cause, and severity of pain; ethnic and gender-related responses to analgesics; concomitant administration of other medications; past pain experiences; and previous opioid tolerance (APS, 2008).

Recommended doses of analgesics and coanalgesics that have a ceiling of effect generally reflect the dose required to achieve therapeutic analgesic blood levels, whereas recommended doses of opioids and coanalgesics that lack a ceiling of effect are considered initial dosages. These recommended doses are based on empiric evidence and clinical experience and must be titrated to achieve optimal analgesia while minimizing analgesic-related side effects.

Initial analgesic dose recommendations vary by age and weight. In adults, research suggests that weight does not correlate with analgesic requirements for pain relief. Yet for children, initial analgesic doses are recommended in milligrams (or micrograms) per kilogram of the child's body weight. These recommendations are approximate, and the prescriber should order doses based on clinical circumstances.

Give special consideration to children on both ends of the age and weight spectrum. Children who weigh more than 50 kg should be started at adult dose recommendations. Calculating doses by milligrams per kilogram in these children results in doses that exceed initial adult recommendations; therefore, this approach puts them at increased risk of overdose. Special consideration should also be given to the smaller and younger child. The pharmacokinetics and clinical effects of opioid analgesics for infants and children older than 6 months of age are similar to those in adults (APS, 2008). Younger infants and neonates have slower drug clearance and longer elimination half-lives. Therefore, for preterm and term infants younger than 6 months of age, initial recommended pediatric opioid analgesic doses should be reduced to one-quarter to one-third the recommended starting dose for older children (APS, 2008).

Special dose considerations are required for children with disease processes that affect drug metabolism, elimination, and the severity of analgesic side effects. Closely monitor children with liver, renal, pulmonary, cardiac, or neuromuscular diseases when opioids are administered and as doses are titrated to achieve pain relief. Infants and children with comorbid conditions may also require reduced analgesic doses and longer intervals between doses to adjust for their altered pharmacokinetics and their response to analgesics.

Opioid analgesics are frequently prescribed as *range orders*, such as hydrocodone/acetaminophen one to two tablets orally every 4 hours or morphine 2 to 4 mg IV every 2 hours PRN for pain. To ensure that opioids are administered consistently by all nurses who care for a patient, The Joint Commission requires health care organizations to specify required elements of range orders. The American Society for Pain Management Nursing and the APS (Gordon et al., 2004) recognize that range orders provide for flexibility and safe dose adjustments, enabling nurses to respond promptly to a patient's unique and varied analgesic needs. To interpret range orders, complete a thorough pain assessment, assess the child's current clinical status, and consider the child's prior exposure and response to ordered or similar medications and concomitant administration of other drugs. Evaluate the child's response to each dose. Document and communicate assessments and interventions to facilitate safe and consistent treatment.

Children who report decreasing pain relief from previously effective doses of opioids may be experiencing tolerance to the analgesic effects of the opioid and may, therefore, require a different dosage or another drug. The Joint Commission has guidelines for processes to be implemented for added safety for opioid use in hospital settings (The Joint Commission, 2012).

caREminder

When converting the opioid-tolerant child to another opioid, equianalgesic tables provide an approximate point to dose from. Evaluate the child's clinical response to the new analgesic dose and titrate the dose to provide optimal pain relief.

ANSWER: Children who weigh less than 50 kg are traditionally given pediatric dosages according to weight. George, however, is still close to 50 kg and his pain is relieved by the adult dose.

Child and Family Education Regarding Pharmacologic Management

Explore child and family preferences for pharmacologic pain management and address any knowledge deficits that may be barriers to achieving optimal pain relief. A thorough pain history provides information about what has been successful and unsuccessful in the past. Previously successful interventions provide an excellent basis for a pain management plan. However, past medication use may not apply to the patient's current situation. Take such opportunities to educate the patient and the family about the pharmacologic options and the benefits of a balanced approach to pain relief.

Frequently cited patient and family barriers to using pharmacologic interventions are pain tolerance, pain expectations, and fears of opioid analgesics. Stoicism is highly valued by society. Patients and family expect pain from surgery, trauma, cancer, and common health care procedures. They may not be aware of pain's deleterious effects and may fear analgesics; these fears might cause them to choose pain over pain relief. Fears that using opioid analgesics will lead to addiction, respiratory depression, and death may deter children and families from allowing these medications to be included in the pain management plan. The horrors of drug abuse and addiction are publicized in the media but are also familiar to families from personal experiences and community awareness efforts, especially school campaigns. Inform patients and families about pain relief strategies and the harmful effects of pain. Review ordered analgesics, specifically drug, route, dose, and frequency. Encourage the child and family to report onset of pain and unrelieved pain so that interventions can be provided promptly and the pain management plan can be adjusted to optimize analgesic interventions. Assure the child and family that reports of pain will be taken seriously and that pain relief is an important part of the child's treatment plan.

Openly discuss addiction and substance abuse with patients and families. Reassure them that opioid addiction is rare when these analgesics are prescribed for pain control. Remind them that addiction is defined by compulsive drug use, impaired control over drug use, craving, diminished recognition of significant problems associated with drug use, and a dysfunctional emotional response of continued use of drugs despite harm (American Society of Addiction Medicine, 2011). Educate patients and families about monitoring that is used to detect potential respiratory depression. Assure them that the goal of opioid treatment is to balance pain relief and analgesic side effects to achieve optimal pain management.

BIOBEHAVIORAL STRATEGIES AND COMFORT INTERVENTIONS

Nonpharmacologic therapies for pain management, or comfort measures, traditionally have been considered solely a nursing responsibility. These biobehavioral interventions are now common and often are termed *complementary, alternative,* or *integrative therapies.* These interventions are not alternatives to analgesics, however. Regardless of the term used to characterize these strategies, they should be provided in addition to, not instead of, pharmacologic therapies (Clinical Judgment 10-2).

Biobehavioral interventions provide coping strategies that may help to reduce pain perception and increase comfort. For example, cognitive–behavioral interventions may alter perception of the pain being experienced. Depending on the individual child and situation, biobehavioral interventions, used alone or in various combinations, may prove effective in reducing the physiologic, behavioral, and subjective expressions of anxiety, fear, and discomfort associated with pain. They also help the child maintain control. Unfortunately, their effectiveness among children is highly variable, with limited research available to support effectiveness. Also, some techniques require time to be learned and implemented. Moreover, a role model or coach knowledgeable in the technique or its performance may be unavailable at the time pain relief is needed. Always consider the child's developmental level, individual needs, and pain experience when selecting these techniques.

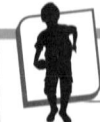

CLINICAL JUDGMENT 10-2

An Infant in Pain

Diep is a 3-kg, 1-week-old patient 20 hours after major abdominal surgery. Vital signs are heart rate, 166 bpm; respiratory rate, 50 breaths/min and shallow; and oxygen saturation, 90%. She has slept for brief periods since surgery and has a high-pitched cry that is more intense after repositioning. She keeps her eyes closed most of the time and is not interested in her environment. She has had 0.1 mg morphine IV every 4 hours since surgery.

Questions

1. Is Diep's pain being relieved by the doses of IV morphine?
2. What behaviors indicate that Diep is in pain?
3. Is Diep receiving adequate analgesia for her level of pain?
4. What should you do to better manage Diep's pain?
5. When should you reevaluate Diep's pain level, and what will indicate that your interventions have been effective?

Answers

1. No.
2. Shallow respirations; intense, high-pitched cry; sleep pattern disturbance; lack of socialization
3. Pain behaviors indicate that Diep is not receiving adequate analgesia with the morphine dose administered.
4. Add a nonopioid such as acetaminophen or NSAID if not contraindicated by current clinical condition (poor urine output, potential for bleeding). Both dose and frequency of morphine could be increased, but slow titration is required in neonates because their livers are immature, increasing the potential for drug accumulation. Reevaluate pain status. Implement biobehavioral interventions such as positioning: place firm boundaries around her, blanket rolls or parent's (nurse's) hands, to help her feel more secure; swaddle; offer pacifier or sucrose. Monitor for respiratory depression. Diep is at high risk for respiratory depression, but opioids are not contraindicated.
5. Evaluate about 60 minutes after analgesics and nonpharmacologic interventions. Effective interventions will be demonstrated by decreased amount and intensity of crying. Possibly may see increased interest in environment but, given the stress of recent surgery and altered sleep patterns for the past 20 hours, would anticipate catch-up sleep to occur with longer periods of deep sleep.

Parental Involvement

Parents and children want to be together during painful procedures (Franck et al., 2012). Professional health care organizations have begun to recognize the importance and value of the parental presence during invasive procedures (AAP & APS, 2001; American Association of Critical Care Nurses, 2010; Emergency Nurses Association [ENA], 2010a; Morrison et al., 2010). Parents who are knowledgeable about what is going to happen and about specific things they can do to facilitate pain management generally feel less helpless, are less anxious, and are better able to support their children. A parent's sensitive response to a child's reaction can promote the child's coping skills (Curry et al., 2012).

Treatment of children's pain by parents generally is suboptimal. The Parents' Postoperative Pain Measure, a validated pain assessment tool specifically designed to help parents quantify their children's pain at home after surgery, and explicit written instructions that supplement verbal discharge directions may guide parents to provide better pain management (Finley et al., 2003;

Kankkunen et al., 2003). Parents may inadvertently encourage pain behaviors in children with chronic or recurrent pain conditions by rewarding the child with special privileges or relieving them of responsibilities, such as school attendance and chores, because of their pain (Bursch et al., 2003). Strategies that reduce parental anxiety have been associated with decreases in children's reports of pain and their pain behaviors (AAP & APS, 2001; C. Taylor et al., 2011). Parents who are prepared can support pain management interventions for their child through their presence (Rennick et al., 2011). Therefore, carefully prepare parents for what will happen during a procedure, and detail how they can coach the child to cope (Teaching Intervention Plan 10-1).

The child may display more distress behaviors when the parent is present. Providing the child with developmentally inappropriate amounts of control, lack of parental attention to the child, providing praise and apologies to the child rather than focusing on distraction and coping skills, and level of parental distraction coaching may elicit these distress responses (Kleiber & McCarthy, 1999; McCarthy et al., 2010). Health care

TIP 10-1: A TEACHING INTERVENTION PLAN for Parents of a Child Undergoing a Painful Procedure

Nursing Diagnosis and Family Outcomes

- Deficient knowledge: Supporting the child undergoing a procedure

  Outcomes: Family will support the child during procedure.

  Parents and other family members will discuss interventions they can implement to support the child during a procedure.

Interventions

Include the parents when teaching the child about the procedure.

Speak with the parents after teaching, not in the child's presence:
  - Clarify interpretations of what was taught.
  - Correct misconceptions.
  - Discuss how the child may respond before, during, and after the procedure.

Discuss how parents can help the child cope. Give concrete, specific, and developmentally appropriate suggestions for how they can assist their child:
  - Hold the child's hand.
  - Speak in a low, soothing tone; maintain eye contact with the child.

- Touch other parts of the child's body, depending on the child's preference (using firm touch, pressure, stroking).
- Keep the child informed of the procedure's progress, if doing so is consistent with the child's coping style (e.g., "It's half over now").
- Coach the child during use of previously practiced relaxation techniques (e.g., deep breathing, counting).
- Use distraction (e.g., blow bubbles, read stories).
- Use positive reinforcement of desired behaviors (e.g., "You are breathing so deeply;" "You are holding your hand so still") rather than apologizing (e.g., do not say "I'm so sorry they are hurting you" or "I'm sorry you have to go through this").
- Avoid threats, such as painful procedures (e.g., injections), in an attempt to get the child to behave.

---

providers and parents should focus on the child and reinforce coping and distraction strategies to reduce distress during painful procedures.

Cognitive–Behavioral Interventions

The goal of cognitive–behavioral interventions is to teach patients to identify, evaluate, and change sensory and thought patterns to facilitate coping behaviors (Gerik, 2005). Cognitive–behavioral interventions are effective for facilitating cooperation with medical procedures, modifying pain behaviors, decreasing psychological disability, reducing pain, lessening reliance on analgesics, and enhancing self-efficacy and pain coping (Landier & Tse, 2010). Cognitive–behavioral plans involve providing developmentally appropriate information, including sensory information, and encouraging active participation in mind–body strategies, also known as a *coping plan*, to avert attention from pain and to modify behaviors that may initiate or exacerbate the pain. General principles of psychological care should not be overlooked (Nursing Interventions 10-4).

Specific cognitive–behavioral interventions include task analysis, distraction, relaxation, biofeedback, and hypnosis. These strategies have been used successfully with children who have pain from procedures, major surgery, sickle cell disease, cancer, headaches, fibromyalgia, and rheumatoid arthritis (Accardi & Milling, 2009; Carter & Threlkeld, 2012; Landier & Tse, 2010;

McCarthy et al., 2010; Sieberg et al., 2012). Children older than 8 to 9 years of age benefit from cognitive strategies, such as relaxation techniques, that they can initiate and maintain themselves. Younger children benefit from being coached in distraction, imagery, and hypnosis. The effectiveness of information and coping strategies varies by age among adolescents (LaMontagne et al., 2003).

Advantages of using cognitive–behavioral interventions are that they are generally independent nursing actions that are noninvasive, can be used in many situations, and provide the child and family with some control over the pain. These techniques may require time and practice and may not achieve the desired results when first used.

Providing Information and Task Analysis

Ideally, preparation is done before the child is in pain. When a painful event happens under emergency conditions, preparation occurs almost concurrently.

Provide children and families with concrete, objective information about painful diseases and before surgeries and other medical procedures (Nursing Interventions 10-5). Be honest if pain is anticipated.

Break down complex procedures into specific steps, and reinforce coping strategies for each distinct task. Model, or demonstrate, coping behaviors. Detail parents' coaching role and reinforce the need to emphasize

NURSING INTERVENTIONS 10-4

Providing Psychological Support for the Child in Pain

- Encourage use of previously learned coping skills; remember that children regress when stressed.
- Perform painful procedures in designated areas, *not* in the child's room or playroom.
- Do not talk over the child; talk to the child or leave the vicinity.
- Reinforce that pain is not a punishment for misdeeds.
- Be honest; clarify communication.
- Ask the child, "What do you think will help you in this situation?" and "What can I do to help?"
- Give the child control whenever possible (within reasonable limits), let the child remove a dressing,

- help set up for a finger stick, or prepare a site by wiping with alcohol.
- Suggest actions the child *can* do ("hold your leg still") rather than actions that the child cannot do ("do not move your leg").
- Have the child and parents practice appropriate coping actions before they will be needed; give positive reinforcement for desired behaviors.
- Use the power of suggestion to help increase the efficacy of any strategy (e.g., "When you go on an imaginary trip, the lumbar puncture seems to be over faster" or "This cold massage can make your leg feel better").

the coping plan rather than praising the child or apologizing for the pain.

Encourage the child to take an active role in managing situations. Feeling in control of a situation may reduce anxiety. The child might help remove a dressing, pick the site in which to insert an IV line, or arrange a schedule for the day (given that certain events must occur).

KidKare Give sensory information such as "This may feel like it is pinching, stinging, poking, cold" or "You might not feel much of anything; tell me what it feels like for you." Tell the child it may hurt but that there are things that can be done to help make it not so bad.

Distraction

QUESTION: George is receiving an around-the-clock medication regimen; however, if he experiences breakthrough pain, he is able to distract himself effectively with action life-and-death video games. Do you think other teenage boys would also find these a successful distraction from pain?

A goal of distraction interventions is to divert the child's attention away from the pain through controlled, purposeful behaviors (Tradition or Science 10-2). A variety of distractors have been tested with children for painful procedures: party noisemakers and bubble blowers, kaleidoscopes, nonprocedural talking and listening to stories, humor and jokes, music, puppetry, counting, pop-up books, videos, and video games (Fig. 10-11). The distractor must be unique and powerful enough to hold the child's attention,

leaving fewer attentional resources available to focus on distressing and painful stimuli (Carlson et al., 2000). This finding has inspired the use of virtual reality devices and the development of pain reduction programs tailored to specialized patient populations (Das et al., 2005; Gershon et al., 2004; Schmitt et al., 2011; Wint et al., 2002).

Distraction techniques should be developmentally appropriate and tailored to the child's preferences. If distraction is successful, remember that the child will display fewer overt signs of distress even if pain is not reduced. Therefore, distraction techniques should be used with pharmacologic interventions if the situation warrants.

ANSWER: Action video games have demonstrated a unique ability to engross teenagers' attention. Therefore, they are likely to be applicable to other teenagers.

Relaxation

Relaxation eases pain by decreasing stress, reducing muscle tension, inducing feelings of control, changing autonomic reactivity, and providing distraction. Relaxation alone is effective in treating children's migraines and other headaches (Eccleston et al., 2012). However, no data indicate that relaxation alone is effective in lessening chronic, cancer, surgical, or procedural pain; therefore, it should be combined with analgesics, distraction, imagery, or hypnosis.

Relaxation training teaches children awareness of and control over physiologic and muscular reactions to anxiety. Children should learn and practice relaxation techniques with a coach before using them. Under stressful conditions, a support person may be needed to guide the child in relaxation techniques.

NURSING INTERVENTIONS 10-5

Helping the Child Cope With Planned Painful Events

Before the Procedure

- Be honest and specific about what will happen, if doing so is consistent with the child's coping method.
- Give information as appropriate to the child's developmental level and previous experiences. The older the child, the more details should be included with rationales for actions and the further in advance of the event the child should be told.
  - Infant: as the procedure is carried out
  - Age 1–3: immediately before the procedure (does not understand the rationale for a painful procedure)
  - Age 4–7: up to a day in advance (unable to reason beyond the immediate event because understanding of cause and effect does not emerge until early school age)
  - Age 8 and older: several days in advance (gives the child time to think about what methods they can use to cope in the situation).
- Give procedural information:
  - What is to be done and why
  - Where the procedure will occur (treatment room, operating room)
  - How the child will get to where the procedure will be performed
  - What equipment will be used
  - Who will be in the room
  - Who will do the procedure
  - How long it will take
- Show the child the room and let him or her manipulate equipment when possible.
- Give sensory information:
  - What the room will look like
  - Sounds the child may hear (e.g., beeping from the pulse oximeter, buzzing alarms, machinery moving)

- Smells to expect
- How it will feel (e.g., hard table, cold antiseptic, pressure, pinch)
- Elicit and answer questions. Discuss what the child thinks will happen, how they usually respond to similar situations, and things they might do to cope with this one.
- Prepare room and equipment before bringing child to room; seeing things being set up or delays in performing procedure heighten anxiety.

During the Procedure

- Administer analgesics and anesthetics to prevent and relieve the pain of the procedure.
- Implement biobehavioral interventions:
  - Ensure that favorite objects (blanket, stuffed animal) are present.
  - Minimize extraneous noise; move noisy machines, mute alarms; speak quietly in a low tone.
  - Avoid sudden, jarring movements.
  - Position the child for comfort within restrictions for the procedure.
  - Tell the child what you are doing, if doing so is consistent with the child's coping method.

After the Procedure

- Give a clear signal when procedure is finished (pick up, sit up, "It's done now").
- Review the experience with child and family (play therapy).
- Clarify perceptions.
- Reinforce or reward positive coping behaviors.
- Discuss alternatives for future success.

KidKare When teaching relaxation techniques, keep the environment quiet. Enhance relaxation by telling children to feel their bodies sinking into the furniture. Instruct them to wipe their minds clean, like a whiteboard, thinking of nothing but the words that you are telling them. Speak in a calm, low, measured tone.

Deep breathing and tension–relaxation (alternately tensing and relaxing specific muscle groups) are two common relaxation techniques used in clinical practice. One deep breathing method is to have the child slowly take five deep breaths in through the nose and slowly exhale through pursed lips. Monitor for hyperventilation when implementing these breathing techniques. Consider instructing the child using a PCA pump to use

this technique after pushing the PCA button. If the pain is not relieved after taking 100 deep breaths, the child should push the PCA button again.

Another breathing method is to have the child count from 1 to 10, saying the number with each exhalation, and gently inhaling through a slightly open mouth. This sequence can be repeated until the child experiences calm. "Blowing the pain away" can be particularly effective with younger children. At the first sign of pain, children are taught to take a breath and blow out as hard as they can. Doing so helps them to maintain control by acting upon the aversive stimulus rather than letting it overwhelm them.

Muscle relaxation can be taught in a variety of ways. A descriptive way to help children learn what tenseness and relaxation feels like is to tell them, "Hold your arms [legs] out very straight, tense or squeeze your muscles

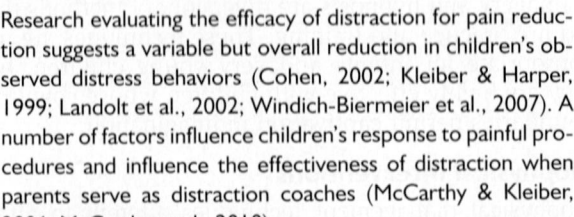

TRADITION OR SCIENCE 10-2

Evidence-Based Practice

Is distraction effective in reducing pain?

Research evaluating the efficacy of distraction for pain reduction suggests a variable but overall reduction in children's observed distress behaviors (Cohen, 2002; Kleiber & Harper, 1999; Landolt et al., 2002; Windich-Biermeier et al., 2007). A number of factors influence children's response to painful procedures and influence the effectiveness of distraction when parents serve as distraction coaches (McCarthy & Kleiber, 2006; McCarthy et al., 2010).

Infants exposed to movie distraction displayed fewer distress behaviors than infants not exposed (Cohen et al., 2006). Virtual reality games have been effective in reducing children's self-reported pain during procedures (Aminabadi et al., 2012; Das et al., 2005; Gershon et al., 2004; Schmitt et al., 2011; Wolitsky et al., 2005). A meta-analysis that included 28 randomized controlled trials with 1,951 children found that distraction, as well as hypnosis, was effective in reducing self-reported pain in children undergoing needle-related procedures. Combined cognitive–behavioral interventions reduced observer-reported and behavioral measures of child distress (Chambers et al., 2009; Uman et al., 2006). Another meta-analysis of 19 studies with a total sample of 535 children concluded that distraction reduced distress behavior and self-reported pain (Kleiber & Harper, 1999). School-aged children report that distraction is helpful in managing pain (Sng et al., 2013). Research demonstrates that distraction is effective in reducing pain behaviors. Distraction should not be used as a replacement for pharmacologic management if the situation warrants such.

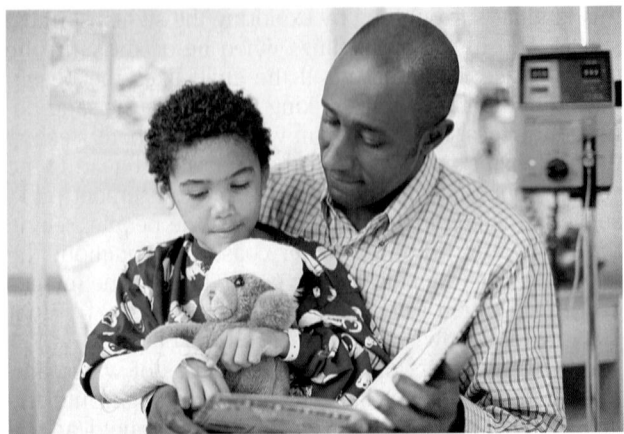

Figure 10-11 A child using distraction for pain management.

of physiologic functions. This visual feedback enables children to recognize and alter physiologic functions, such as muscle tension, skin temperature, and heart rate, by using their body's responses, like a video game controller. The child is instructed to use mental imagery to increase or decrease reactivity in the system being monitored. Reinforcement occurs when the child is able to effect change in the desired direction, thus strengthening self-control over the physiologic function. Use of biofeedback requires specialized training and equipment. This technique has been effective in reducing and relieving pain from migraines and recurrent headaches, complex regional pain syndrome, and sickle cell disease (Goddard, 2011; Kropp et al., 2013; Myrvik et al., 2012).

Imagery and Hypnosis

Imagery is a method of distraction and can also enhance relaxation. Children are actively involved in creating vivid, visual daydreams, picturing themselves engrossed in a pleasant situation or visualizing creative ways to decrease their body's pain, such as pain switches or magic gloves (Kuttner, 1986) (Nursing Interventions 10-6). Imagery and hypnosis have been shown to reduce pain from procedures, cancer, surgery, migraine, and functional abdominal pain (Butler et al., 2005; Gottsegen, 2011; Kline et al., 2010; Kohen, 2010; Landier & Tse, 2010; Pölkki et al., 2008).

Imagery begins with achieving a relaxed state. Guide the child to choose a favorite place. Cue the child to experience

until the count of 10 [count from 1 to 10], now let go." Or "Breathe in and hold it. Feel the tightness in your chest. Breathe out all at once and feel the tension leaving your body completely." Another method of muscle relaxation is to start with the feet and work gradually up the body. For example, "Feel your feet relaxing, sinking into the mattress. They are very heavy. Now feel your calves sinking further down, very relaxed," and so on.

Biofeedback Training

Biofeedback is another technique for teaching relaxation. Computer programs provide a visual depiction

---

NURSING INTERVENTIONS 10-6

Imagery: The Pain Switch and Magic Glove

Coach the child in using imagery to help "block" the traveling of pain messages. The *pain switch* controls the area of pain (e.g., leg, arm, abdomen) and the child visualizes turning the pain switch off to that area so that messages cannot travel, much as a light switch controls electricity. Color can also be incorporated into the imagery. Have the child picture a color—for example, red when pain can travel or is present, black when the switch is turned off.

A *magic glove* can be "put" on the hand, finger by finger, to diminish the pain associated with venipuncture or finger stick. A magic blanket might be used in areas where a glove would not work, such as the back or abdomen. The hands are extremely sensitive parts of the body. One can take the magic glove and hold it over other parts of the body (e.g., over the cheek before dental work) to induce numbness or decrease pain.

this familiar surrounding by exploring the sights, sounds, smells, and his or her feelings when he or she is in the special place. For example, if the child likes the beach, have him or her imagine walking and feeling the sand between the toes, feeling the sun warming the body, feeling the cool water on his or her feet or knees, and hearing the waves lapping at the shoreline. For an amusement park, suggest smelling the popcorn, hearing the people, seeing the lights, and riding the roller coaster. Throughout the experience, let the child be the guide. Prompt the images of "What do you see, hear, smell, feel, or taste?" "What are you doing now?" or "Where are you going?"

Be aware of fears the child has, such as of water, animals, or activities, so that they are not brought into the imagery, making it a negative experience. Do not lead the child; let the child become immersed in his or her personal image and take command of the experience. It is important to remember that imagery-induced relaxation may not be lasting and repetition is essential (Pölkki et al., 2008).

Hypnosis is an altered state of consciousness, an intensified trance, in which concentration is focused and absorbed and attention is intensified, yet the child is physically relaxed. Peripheral awareness is reduced, but social cues are heightened (Butler et al., 2005). The child dissociates from immediate physical surroundings and experiences, allowing perceptions and sensations to be modified or enhanced. Hypnosis is effective in reducing pain, but not in alleviating pain, so analgesics are also required. A hypnotic state must be induced under the supervision of an experienced practitioner.

Imagery and hypnosis are diversionary methods that require practice and training. These techniques are not appropriate for infants and very young children, but they are highly effective with children whose cognitive boundaries permit captivation in imagination.

Biophysical Interventions

Biophysical management techniques attempt to affect physiologic responses directly during painful experiences. Biophysical strategies used to reduce pain in older children and adolescents are generally contraindicated in high-risk neonates because of the physiologic response that is evoked, which may cause deleterious vital sign changes and make the infant more susceptible to intraventricular hemorrhage. Strategies appropriate for older children include cutaneous stimulation, acupuncture and acupressure, and transcutaneous nerve stimulation. Nursing Interventions 10-7 and Tradition or Science 10-3 provide developmentally appropriate biophysical interventions for preterm and high-risk infants.

NURSING INTERVENTIONS 10-7

Biobehavioral Pain Management and Comfort Strategies for Infants

Using several methods can enhance soothing. Monitor infants for cues indicating stress (e.g., gaze aversion, hiccups, finger splaying [rigid extension and separation of fingers], yawning, fussing, becoming limp, going into a sleep state or "shutting down," bradycardia) and implement or withdraw interventions on the basis of the infant's response. Ability to comfort is a function of the child's unique response, the pain situation, the interventions implemented, and the caretaker's sensitivity in reading the baby's cues.

- Environmental stimuli: Dim lights, decrease noise.
- Supportive boundaries: Use blankets or bunting; adult hands surround infant, containing the child but not moving.
- Swaddling: Tightly wrap in blanket with extremities flexed and hands uncovered to facilitate hand-to-mouth behavior; tight wrapping provides too much stimuli for preterm infants who should be loosely wrapped with boundaries to push against, which gives a feeling of containment and security.
- Positioning: Decrease muscle tension and pulling on painful area, limit movement—for example, support legs in a flexed position if there is an abdominal incision or elevate extremity.
- Hand-to-mouth behaviors: Encourage.
- Sucking: Offer pacifier, thumb, or fingers.

- Sweet solutions: Encourage breastfeeding or give oral sucrose solution or glucose or coat a pacifier with the solution and let the infant suck on it 2 minutes prior to and during painful procedures (may decrease pain perception); remove the pacifier when the procedure is completed and infant is calm.
- Auditory stimuli: Use uterine sounds, instrumental music, humming, or parent's voice (more effective with older infant); make sure not to overstimulate the child.
- Holding: Support parent with proper armrests, footrests, or pillows so the parent is comfortable.
- Rocking: Use rhythmic, continuous, horizontal motions (the person holding the child stands and gently turns trunk side to side, with feet stationary, so that the child moves in the horizontal plane).
- Touch: Use firm pressure or stroking; preterm infants do better with firm touch on their head or heels, not the trunk.
- Visual stimuli: This is more effective with an older infant. Use parent's face, pictures, or mobiles.
- Recovery periods: If infant is showing signs of stress, stop procedures when possible and allow infant to reorganize; implement other comfort measures to augment those already in use.

TRADITION OR SCIENCE 10-3

Are nonnutritive sucking and sweetened solutions effective in reducing pain behaviors in infants?

Sucking during painful stimuli such as circumcision, in addition to other analgesia such as dorsal penile nerve blocks (South et al., 2005); heel stick (Akman et al., 2002; Blass & Watt, 1999); and eye examinations (A. Mitchell et al., 2004) attenuates pain distress behaviors and has a pacifying effect for preterm infants and newborns. Sucking a pacifier at a rate of at least 30 sucks per minute provides an analgesic effect (Blass & Watt, 1999). No short-term negative effects of nonnutritive sucking have been identified; data on long-term effects are not available (Pinelli et al., 2002).

One of the most widely studied biobehavioral interventions for neonatal procedural analgesia is the use of sweet-tasting substances. Studies in rats demonstrated raised pain thresholds with the use of sucrose and reversal of these effects by an opioid antagonist (Blass et al., 1987). Thus, it was hypothesized that sucrose, and perhaps other sweetened solutions, have analgesic properties that are mediated through opioid pathways.

Reduced cry times and pain scores have been demonstrated in preterm and term infants given varied concentrations and amounts of sucrose and glucose solutions (Akcam & Ormeci, 2004; Akman et al., 2002; Gradin et al., 2002; Greenberg, 2002; A. Mitchell et al., 2004; A. Mitchell & Waltman, 2003; Razmus et al., 2004; Reis et al., 2003; Taddio et al., 2003). Sucrose and glucose are effective for providing analgesia during procedures with as little as 0.05–2 mL 7.5%–50% concentration (Kassab et al., 2012; Okan et al., 2007; Wong et al., 2003). Repeated use of sucrose for procedural pain in preterm infants is effective and safe (Stevens et al., 2005). Sucrose and glucose are easy-to-use methods of pain relief for infants. The analgesic effect of these sweetened solutions fades as children age. Future research is needed to identify when and why these analgesic properties vanish.

Similar analgesic effects have been noted with breastfeeding in healthy newborns (Efe & Ozer, 2007; Gray et al., 2002; Shah et al., 2012) and late preterm infants (Simonse et al., 2012). The sweet milk or the skin-to-skin contact may be the key to the success of this intervention. Kangaroo care, in which the preterm neonate is placed in skin-to-skin contact with a parent, has also been shown to decrease physiologic measures (Ludington-Hoe et al., 2005) and objective pain scores after heel lancing (Johnston et al., 2003). Maternal holding is more analgesic than nonmaternal holding (Phillips et al., 2005).

Researchers have tried to differentiate the benefits from nonnutritive sucking and sucrose but have concluded that a combined approach that includes skin to skin contact, swaddling, and rocking is best for relieving the pain of heel sticks and other painful procedures (Akman et al., 2002; Greenberg, 2002; Liaw et al., 2012; A. Mitchell et al., 2004; Riddell et al., 2011). There is a need for ongoing research of both single and combined pharmacologic and nonpharmacologic interventions that provide evidence for decision making related to the optimal management of infant pain (Yamada et al., 2008). Nurses must recognize the differences in nonpharmacologic approaches needed between the neonate and older infant (Riddell et al., 2011).

Positioning

Swaddling and holding are comforting and help infants and small children achieve a more relaxed state (Riddell et al., 2011). Facilitated tucking (in which the caregiver places a hand on the infant's head and feet while providing flexion and containment), swaddling, and other positional interventions serve to limit excessive, uncontrolled movements that may exacerbate pain. They also provide physical boundaries that may assist infants in organizing themselves. Infants older than 3 to 6 months of age often fight against swaddling, which may intensify anxiety and pain. The amount of comfort derived from being held is a function of the individual child's personality and situation. Multiple interventions should be used to manage procedural pain in neonates, including both pharmacologic and nonpharmacologic approaches (Johnston et al., 2011).

Proper positioning and splinting provides support for and decreases muscle tension over painful areas (Fig. 10-12). The child's situation dictates appropriate actions. Pressure on an incision may exacerbate pain but might be helpful when a child with an abdominal incision has to cough and breathe deeply; pressure may reduce abdominal pain caused by gas; or elevation of a swollen extremity may decrease swelling and thus pain.

During procedures, positioning for comfort (a secure, parental-hugging hold and close physical contact) has not been demonstrated to be more effective at reducing pain, fear, and distress scores than traditional procedure positioning (laying the child down and restraining him or her) (Cavender et al., 2004), although upright positioning during IV starts reduces distress scores (Sparks et al., 2007).

Cutaneous Stimulation

Cutaneous stimulation is often applied over the painful area. This technique may not be possible in some situations, such as with an extremely painful area, altered skin integrity, or with a cast or dressing in place. When direct cutaneous stimulation is not feasible, alternative sites may be used, including sites adjacent to the painful area, between the pain and the brain, or the contralateral site. Use caution when applying cutaneous

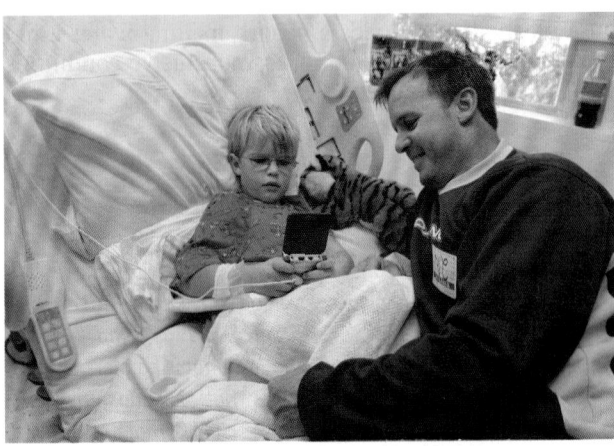

Figure 10-12 Children will often assume a position of comfort to alleviate pain, such as with this child who flexes his knees after abdominal surgery. Distraction with electronic games and parental presence may also help reduce pain perception.

strategies in preterm infants to avoid physiologic instability and damaging their more friable skin.

Massage improves circulation, loosens tight joints, decreases stress hormone levels, promotes relaxation and sleep, and can help in pain relief. In adults, massage has been shown to reduce surgical and cancer pain when used as an adjunct to analgesics (Anderson & Cutshall, 2007; Toth et al., 2013; Wang & Keck, 2004). Massage may be done on the total body or localized to the back, extremities, or painful area (use alternative sites if massage directly applied to the painful site is not tolerated). Use a firm movement to massage, particularly with ticklish children. Gentle massage of the leg for 2 minutes prior to heel stick may decrease pain response in preterm infants (Jain et al., 2006).

Healing or *therapeutic touch* is another cutaneous intervention that may relieve pain. Studies suggest it may be beneficial for pain (Bardia et al., 2006; Engebretson & Wardell, 2007; J. Wong et al., 2013).

Thermal cutaneous therapies involve application of heat or cold. Heat acts through conduction or convection to increase blood flow to skin and superficial organs but decreases blood flow to underlying muscles, which promotes muscle relaxation. Thermoreceptors in the skin are activated by heat. These receptors generate nerve signals that block nociception in the spinal cord. Heating devices appropriate for thermal application include hot packs; hot water bottles; warm, moist compresses; heating pads; chemical gel packs; and warm baths. Muscle temperature should reach at least 40° C (104° F) to achieve optimal biophysical effect (McCarberg & O'Connor, 2004). Heat is most effective in relieving pain from inflammation and spasm.

Cold causes vasoconstriction and local hypoesthesia, reducing swelling and muscle spasm. Wrap ice, ice packs, and chemical gel packs to protect the skin from direct contact, and apply for no more than 15 minutes at a time. Ice massage is effective for injection pain; headaches; toothaches; or brief, painful procedures. Ice massage may be done using an ice cube. Another convenient method is to fill a paper cup with water and freeze it; the water expands over the cup edges, and the cup is held at the bottom for the massage. Use circular or back-and-forth motions. Have the child lie on a plastic-backed pad to absorb melting water. Cold therapy is contraindicated in vaso-occlusive conditions such as sickle cell disease.

ALERT *Heat and cold applications are not recommended for use on infants, who are more prone to thermal injury because of their skin structure. These interventions should also be avoided in children with conditions that alter skin sensations, such as spina bifida, or nonverbal children who are unable to alert care providers of temperature extremes that may cause tissue injury. Stop thermal therapies if the child complains or if blanching or redness occurs; monitor skin integrity. Do not use on sleeping children.*

Acupuncture and Acupressure

The premise underlying acupuncture and acupressure is that pain is relieved by strategically placing needles (acupuncture) or pressure (acupressure) to restore the flow of chi (qi) through the 12 meridians of the body. Few studies have investigated the effectiveness of acupuncture or acupressure for children (Jindal & Mansky, 2008; Landgren et al., 2010). Studies in adults indicate that acupuncture reduces the pain of dental restoration, sickle cell disease, low back pain, dysmenorrhea, and migraine headaches.

Transcutaneous Electrical Nerve Stimulation

Transcutaneous electrical nerve stimulation (TENS) is a method by which a small electrical current is applied to the skin by conductive pads attached to a battery-operated generator. Parameters such as amplitude (amount of energy applied to skin), rate (number of times the nerve is stimulated per second), and pulse width (depth of stimulation) can be variably set depending on the effect desired. Electrodes are placed around the painful region or along peripheral nerve routes, acupuncture or trigger points, or at spinal segments. The mechanism of action is thought to be through stimulation of large-diameter cutaneous nerve fibers that inhibits nociceptive responses at the spinal cord and descending pathway. Low-frequency and high-frequency TENS also lead to the release of endogenous opioids. TENS is contraindicated in patients with allergy to the conduction gel, loss of sensation, or pacemakers or defibrillators as well as over the uterus during pregnancy and for stimulation over the anterior neck (Boensch, 2011). Although clinical evidence indicates TENS is effective at relieving pain, few studies have been done with children.

When used at conventional settings, TENS causes a tingling, buzzing sensation. This sensation, coupled with being unfamiliar with the machine, may produce fear in the child. Demonstrate use of the equipment on a family member and then suggest the child try it on a nonpainful area. When the child appears comfortable with the machine, suggest using TENS for a painful area.

MANAGEMENT OF SPECIAL PAIN SITUATIONS

Managing procedural or chronic pain requires some of the same management strategies as acute pain, but additional techniques are important to consider. Other special situations include managing pain in the emergency department and at home.

Procedural Pain

Managing procedural pain requires considering not only the type of procedure and the anticipated intensity and duration of pain but also the meaning of the event, the coping style and temperament of the child, the child's pain history, and the family's ability to minimize the child's distress and provide comfort during the procedure. Limit the number of painful procedures to only those that are absolutely necessary. Painful procedures should be performed in the least painful manner and performed or supervised by the most skilled clinical personnel (AAP & APS, 2001). Use behavioral coping strategies and local anesthetics whenever possible. To help reduce fear and anxiety, which may increase perception of pain, prepare the child and family for the procedure (see Nursing Interventions 10-5). To help decrease anxiety and increase comfort, address basic comfort measures such as hunger (if food and fluids are not restricted prior to the procedure) and thermal regulation; have the child void prior to the procedure. Children have considerable pain and fear of procedures involving needles. The health care team can advocate for the child by adopting evidence-based guidelines to manage procedural pediatric pain related to use of needles (ENA, 2010b).

Local Anesthetics

Local anesthetics can alleviate procedural pain (e.g., from lumbar puncture, venipuncture, or wound repair). Local anesthetics can be delivered in a number of different formulations. The topical (transdermal) route can be used to give medications painlessly or to reduce the pain of local infiltration. The onset of anesthesia of these local anesthetic solutions is between 2 and 60 minutes, varying by product and technique. Topical anesthetics should be applied when needles are to be used (e.g., IV insertion, lumbar puncture, bone marrow aspiration, laceration repair).

Apply skin anesthetics such as lidocaine–prilocaine, liposomal lidocaine, or amethocaine to intact skin before a procedure (Tradition or Science 10-4; Fig. 10-13). Properly timing administration can be accomplished by organizing nursing care or having the child or family apply the agent on an outpatient basis.

Local anesthetics can be injected subcutaneously with a small needle into the skin around the area to be manipulated. Do this 5 to 10 minutes before the procedure and test the area for insensitivity before beginning the procedure. Arguments against using locals are that the "caine" stings for about 30 seconds after injection and the child is subjected to an additional injection. The small needle used for infiltration of the tissue with lidocaine most commonly causes less pain, however, than when the area is manipulated without the benefit of the local anesthetic.

caREminder

The stinging sensation caused by lidocaine can be reduced by buffering the solution (9 parts lidocaine to 1 part sodium bicarbonate), which raises the pH of the solution.

Dermal anesthetics are intended for application to broken skin such as laceration repair, where they can reach dermal structures, blood vessels, and nerve endings. In contrast to skin anesthetics, these agents (e.g., lidocaine, adrenaline, and tetracaine; lidocaine-epinephrine; tetracaine–phenylephrine) do not penetrate the dermis well. Follow the manufacturer's directions for use of the agent; some are not recommended for use on mucous membranes or body parts supplied by end arteries, such as the fingers or toes, because of the potential risk of ischemia from the vasoconstrictive effects of epinephrine. Apply agents to the wound 10 to 30 minutes prior to suturing. Look for blanching of the wound bed to assess effectiveness.

Evidence-Based Practice

TRADITION OR SCIENCE 10-4

Which topical agents are most effective in reducing procedure-associated pain?

Lidocaine–prilocaine cream (e.g., EMLA [eutectic mixture of local anesthetics]) and lidocaine dispersed in liposomes (e.g., LMX4, Maxilene) have been demonstrated to be equally effective for topical anesthesia (Kleiber et al., 2002; Koh et al., 2004). Liposomal lidocaine is more effective than placebo (Taddio et al., 2005). Lidocaine–prilocaine requires covering with an occlusive dressing for 60 minutes prior to the procedure, whereas liposomal lidocaine does not require occlusion and provides skin anesthesia within 30 minutes. Liposomal lidocaine also produces few adverse skin reactions (Poonai et al., 2012; Taddio et al., 2005). Amethocaine (tetracaine), which requires occlusion for 30–45 minutes, is as effective as lidocaine–prilocaine (O'Brien et al., 2005) if not superior in reducing pain (Lander et al., 2006). In infants, topical tetracaine has not been demonstrated to reduce pain associated with venipuncture (Lemyre et al., 2007) or with peripherally inserted central catheter (PICC) insertion (Ballantyne et al., 2003). Pretreating the skin with laser may reduce the time required to achieve anesthesia with transdermal agents (Koh et al., 2007; Singer et al., 2006).

The efficacy of injected buffered lidocaine and liposomal lidocaine are comparable (Luhmann et al., 2004). Needle-free jet injection systems can also be used to deliver lidocaine and prevent pain upon venipuncture better than placebo (Migdal et al., 2005) or lidocaine–prilocaine cream (Jimenez et al., 2006). Jet injection systems achieve a more rapid onset of action (2–3 minutes) than creams (Migdal et al., 2005). However, they are not pain free and they are more expensive than needles (Lysakowski et al., 2003); depending on facility charges, costs may be comparable with topical creams.

An advantage of skin refrigerants is their rapid onset of action, but they are equally effective as other topical agents such as amethocaine (E. H. Davies & Molloy, 2006; Soueid & Richard, 2007), lidocaine–prilocaine (Reis & Holubkov, 1997), placebo (Costello et al., 2006), or no intervention (Costello et al., 2006; Soueid & Richard, 2007). Applying an ice bag for 3 minutes prior to venipuncture reduced subjective and behavioral pain responses in school-aged children (Movahedi et al., 2006). Systematic reviews found insufficient evidence for or against use of skin cooling for pain reduction (Taddio et al., 2010).

Evidence varies on the efficacy of lidocaine–prilocaine cream versus iontophoresis. Galinkin et al. (2002) found that they are comparable; others found that lidocaine–prilocaine cream provides better analgesia (Moppett et al., 2004; Squire et al., 2000). Although erythema, pruritus, and tingling occurred in the iontophoresis group, pain scores and time required for adequate anesthesia were less than in the EMLA group (Squire et al., 2000).

Regardless of the use of topical agents, some children still report high pain levels, which may be influenced by genetics. Children reporting higher pain were younger, more active, had higher state and trait anxiety, and possessed a specific genotype (Kleiber et al., 2007).

(Continued)

TRADITION OR SCIENCE 10-4

Which topical agents are most effective in reducing procedure-associated pain? (Continued)

The agent and method of topical analgesia is situation specific. Factors to consider when selecting local anesthetic agents for clinical use include efficacy, ease of use (factoring in time and technical requirements), minimal side effects, and cost. Walsh and Bartfield (2006) found that parents are willing to spend both time and money to reduce the pain of their child's IV catheter placement. The ENA (2010b) describes guidelines for needle-related procedural pain in pediatric patients, including biobehavioral, anesthetic, and other nonpharmacologic interventions such as pacifiers and sucrose. These guidelines can be adapted for all settings where pediatric procedures are implemented.

Iontophoresis of lidocaine uses an electric field to drive local anesthetics across intact skin. Iontophoresis provides analgesia in 10 to 25 minutes, depending on the amount of electric current used. The grounding electrode often causes a tingling sensation that children may not like. Place the medication electrode on the child and the grounding electrode on a family member and maintain skin-to-skin contact between the family member and child.

ALERT   *Do not use iontophoresis on body parts supplied by end arteries. If the child complains of undue burning or pain during treatment, pause the treatment and inspect the site under the electrode. Stop the iontophoresis if excessive irritation is present or discomfort persists.*

Vapocoolant sprays or skin refrigerants (e.g., Frigiderm, Ethyl Chloride, Pain Ease) cool the skin, which may decrease the number of pain impulses being transmitted. Spray the refrigerant for a few seconds onto the cleansed and prepared site immediately before needle insertion. It can also be sprayed onto a cotton ball. The cotton ball is then applied to the injection site, using forceps, for 15 seconds.

Sedation

Sedation is a depressed state of consciousness induced by the use of medications. It is generally used for painful procedures such as bone marrow aspiration, lumbar puncture, laceration repair, and fractures but may be used for nonpainful procedures such as magnetic resonance imaging or computed tomography. When sedation is planned, nothing is given by mouth for 2 hours before the procedure. Clear liquids may be consumed up to 2 hours before the procedure; breast milk may be consumed up to 4 hours before the procedure; infant formula, nonhuman milk, and light foods may be consumed up to 6 hours before the procedure (American Society of Anesthesiologists, 2011).

ALERT   *When sedation is induced, one member of the health care team, proficient in pediatric basic life support, must continually monitor the child, with this being the member's only responsibility. Moderate sedation can readily progress to deep sedation, rendering the child unable to maintain protective reflexes and a patent airway. Standards for the care of children undergoing sedation have been described and include protocols for safety from the levels of minimal sedation through general anesthesia (Etzel-Hardman, 2011).*

Personnel competent to perform pediatric advanced life support, particularly airway management and intubation, and equipment for resuscitation must be readily available. Continuously monitor the child's oxygen saturation and heart rate; the use of capnography is encouraged (AAP et al., 2006). Document vital signs such as heart rate, respiratory rate, blood pressure, oxygen saturation, and level of consciousness at least every 5 minutes (Nursing Interventions 10-8).

Chronic Pain

Pain that persists a month beyond the usual expected disease or injury course is considered chronic. In contrast to acute pain, chronic pain does not have a biologically protective function. Some causes of chronic pain in children are cancer, sickle cell disease, juvenile rheumatoid arthritis, and recurrent pains (headache, abdominal and limb pain). Distinguishing between acute and chronic pain is important because assessment and management differ.

Impact on the Child

QUESTION: It may not be possible to isolate the effect of chronic pain from the limb salvage procedure and the effect of metastatic disease, but what are some of the most significant changes in George's life?

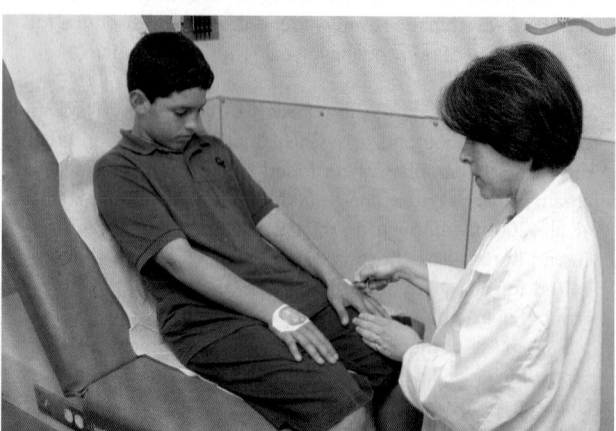

Figure 10-13 EMLA cream reduces the pain of IV catheter insertion and reduces the child's distress. Cover two potential sites in case the first stick is unsuccessful.

NURSING INTERVENTIONS 10-8

Child Undergoing Procedural Sedation

- Ensure availability of appropriately sized resuscitation equipment and opioid receptor antagonist (naloxone) and benzodiazepine receptor antagonist (flumazenil), as appropriate. Administer as ordered or per institution protocol.
- Review child's health history. Note and inform prescriber of conditions that would make the child more vulnerable to the effects of sedating medications (e.g., hepatic, renal, or cardiovascular dysfunction). Ask about medication and latex allergies.
- Obtain information about medications that the child is taking.
- Elicit history of previous sedation.
- Verify that the child has fasted for the ordered length of time.
- Teach the child and family about the effects of sedation.
- Assess the child's level of consciousness and protective reflexes before sedation.
- Obtain baseline heart rate, respiratory rate, blood pressure, oxygen saturation, and carbon dioxide level, as appropriate.
- Place an IV catheter, as appropriate.
- Administer medications per prescriber's order or institution protocol.
- Monitor the child's heart rate, respiratory rate, blood pressure, oxygen saturation, carbon dioxide level, and level of consciousness and responsiveness per institution protocol.

- Monitor the child's electrocardiogram, as appropriate.
- Monitor the child for adverse effects of medication, including excessive somnolence, respiratory depression, hypercarbia, hypoxemia, apnea, arrhythmias, and agitation.
- Position the child as appropriate for the procedure and ensure a patent airway.
- Provide airway and respiratory support (airway positioning, supplemental oxygen, bag–mask ventilations) if indicated.
- Evaluate whether the child meets discharge criteria: sufficient recovery from the effects of medications and return to baseline level of functioning (stable cardiovascular function and airway patency, can be aroused, can talk and follow directions as age appropriate, has age-appropriate motor skills [e.g., infant can sit, older child can walk], and has an adequate state of hydration). Evaluate children with disabilities for return to their baseline status.
- Give families written discharge instructions.
- Document all medications and fluids administered (dose, route, time), vital signs, monitoring devices used (continuous pulse oximetry), untoward or significant reactions and actions taken, child's response, and discharge instructions given.

The effects of chronic pain on the child may include sleep disturbances, exhaustion, irritability, mood disturbances, and depression. These effects are probably related to depletion of serotonin and endorphins. Many children respond to chronic pain by regressing to earlier developmental stages. Another reaction may be an increased response to minor injuries. For example, an exaggerated response would occur when a child bumps his or her knee and then reports that it hurts horribly and cries for 20 minutes.

The primary task of childhood is achievement of developmental milestones such as socialization and self-differentiation. Chronic pain may delay acquisition of normal skills. For example, an infant may experience feeding problems or motor development delays related to limitation of movement. A school-aged child may experience withdrawal or delay in achieving self-care skills or socialization skills involving school or peer involvement (Developmental Considerations 10-5). The primary goal for managing chronic pain is to improve both functional abilities of the child and quality of life (APS, 2012).

The extent to which pain affects a child depends on the interplay between physical limitations caused by the pain and the degree to which physical and emotional factors interfere with activities of daily living. Children may restrict themselves to activities that are easy for them, not trying new activities that could promote a sense of success and accomplishment and enable them to acquire new skills. Achievement of milestones may also be delayed because the family is overprotective and may limit the child's experiences for fear they may exacerbate the pain.

ANSWER: The greatest change for George is that he no longer attends school. He and his family have countered that loss by enrolling George in online high school courses as a means of achieving his developmental goals.

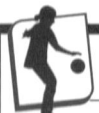

DEVELOPMENTAL CONSIDERATIONS 10-5

Potential Effects of Chronic Pain

Children of all ages respond to ongoing pain by regression to earlier stages of development.

Infancy
Withdrawal or difficulties in social interactions
Feeding problems
Sleep pattern disturbances
Motor development delays related to limitation of movement

Early Childhood
Withdrawal, aggression
Motor lags
Loss of recently achieved developmental milestones (e.g., toileting, motor skills)

Middle Childhood
Withdrawal, aggression, out-of-control behaviors, depression
Delay in achieving self-care skills
Delay in achieving socialization skills (school and peer involvement)

Adolescence
Alteration in body image and peer relationships
Withdrawal, oppositional behavior, depression
May affect achievement of independent self-care skills

Effect on the Family

QUESTION: Who do you think is especially vulnerable in the Tran family?

Negative repercussions are usually seen in the family system when a member suffers from chronic pain. In addition to those of the patient, the needs of the family must be recognized and addressed. The ongoing nature of the child's suffering may result in exhaustion and ensuing irritability. Parental employment may be jeopardized by the time and energy demands imposed by the situation. Other financial problems may occur because of expenditures related to the pain.

Siblings of the child in pain may feel neglected because of the increased attention focused on the child experiencing pain. Marital difficulties may be caused by the prolonged stress on the family system. The parents may feel inadequate because they feel they are unable to help their child or prevent their child's suffering. This feeling of inadequacy can manifest itself as anger: directed inward as depression, directed at each other, or, not uncommonly, directed at health care providers. Feelings of inadequacy may also be manifested as controlling

behaviors by the parents, such as stating that only a certain nurse can take care of the child. Remember that the parent is generally acting out of concern for the child and may use control as a coping strategy. Be sensitive to the parent's needs, recognizing that the parent knows the child better than other members of the health care team.

caREminder

Involve the family as fully as they wish to participate in health care decisions concerning management of their child. If a parent's controlling behaviors are interfering with the treatment regimen, convene a care conference to reevaluate the treatment plan and rationales for decisions and maintain a consistent approach by the health care team.

Children experiencing chronic pain may find that others discredit their complaints or label them as psychosomatic. Assessment and management of these children require astute perception and a holistic approach, embracing the philosophy that the health team is working *with* the family in achieving the desired outcomes.

ANSWER: George's sister, Ashley, is particularly vulnerable. She has a previous history of depression (see Chapter 29), which may resurface with her family and brother's suffering.

Assessment of Chronic Pain

QUESTION: Assess and evaluate George's pain management assessment and treatment plan.

When pain is chronic, the methods and tools used for acute pain may assist in the assessment process. Often, because persistent pain results in adaptation, one does not see the more dramatic response behaviors that are seen with acute pain. Therefore, depending primarily on physiologic indices such as vital sign changes, which have since stabilized, may prevent the nurse from recognizing many instances of pain (Chart 10-2). The initial response to chronic pain can result in behavior and school problems before a diagnosis is even made. A common marker of the dysfunction caused by the pain is school avoidance (not attending school regularly).

Patients with neuropathic pain typically describe the quality of their pain with terms such as *burning, shocking, stabbing, shooting, tingling,* or *like pins and needles.* These sensations persist despite healing of an injury or surgical site and in the absence of physical signs of injury or tissue damage. Physical symptoms of nervous system dysfunction that may provide objective evidence of the neuropathic origins of the child's reports of pain include motor abnormalities such as spasms, tremors, weakness, and atrophy as well as symptoms of autonomic dysregulation such as cyanosis, erythema, mottling, swelling, and poor capillary refill of the painful area.

CHART 10-2 **Signs and Symptoms of Chronic Pain in Children**

- Stable vital signs
- Altered muscular movement leading to misused, tense muscles, which leads to decreased movement, which leads to altered sensory input
- Disrupted sleep causing the child to tire readily and be more irritable, with decreased ability to concentrate
- Developmental regression
- Change in eating patterns
- Behavior or school problems
- Withdrawal from peer group activity
- Depression
- Aggression

they are believed. When the child is monitored for a time, health care providers may feel comfortable that they know the situation and become biased in their assessments and conclusions.

ALERT   *A new disease or advancing pathology may have occurred since the last visit. This possibility should not be overlooked as a potential cause of pain. Complaints of increased or different pain must be investigated.*

Children with chronic pain present their own unique assessment challenges. It is beneficial to use tools that use a variety of methods to provide a comprehensive pain assessment (see Table 10-2). Pain symptom diaries may provide useful information, particularly when assessing chronic pain. Identify the reason for collecting information so the child can focus the narrative. For example, if the aim is to identify the etiology of recurrent pain, the child should record events preceding pain onset, precipitating factors, and so forth. If the goal is to evaluate effectiveness of ongoing management, the child may record medications or psychological techniques used, record activity level, and rate the intensity at specified intervals during the day. Family, teachers, and health care team members need to remember that the body adapts to pain that is ongoing and that the child therefore may not demonstrate behaviors that are typical of acute pain. This should help avoid a common assumption that the child is not experiencing pain and is exaggerating the pain ratings.

Assessment of chronic pain should include a routine health history that encompasses aspects of the child's pain and functional ability. Elicit a description of a typical day. Identify difficult activities (e.g., comfortably positioning an infant for feeding, dressing self for a school-aged child), those that exacerbate pain (no nap for a young child, participation in sports for an adolescent), and activities that reduce the pain (position, distraction, medications). Keeping a symptom diary may help identify proactive steps to avoid exacerbating the pain. Also obtain a diet history because chronic pain may cause loss of appetite. Evaluate aspects of family functioning, such as parental mental health, stressors in the family, other siblings with the same disease, pain that started after a grandparent died of cancer, and perceptions such as that relatives have migraines and they "are genetic, so nothing can be done."

Complete a thorough physical examination. This step serves a dual purpose. The first is to evaluate the child's baseline status. The second is to assure the child and family that the child's pain is being taken seriously and

Management of Chronic Pain

Help the family to establish realistic goals and set priorities. The goals should not be too basic or easy because the child needs to be challenged; however, they should not be so difficult that they cause frustration.

Many of the techniques previously discussed apply to the management of chronic pain in children. Obviously, strategies are influenced by the origin and type of pain. Pathology should be addressed and treated. The focus in acute pain is on rest, symptomatic treatment, and avoiding stress. The focus shifts from chronic pain to helping the child regain or achieve appropriate developmental tasks, decreasing attention to pain behaviors (while making sure that pain control is as good as possible), and emphasizing a productive role.

Children with chronic pain benefit from an interdisciplinary approach that combines behavioral, biophysical, and pharmacologic strategies. Interventions are planned on the basis of assessment findings, goals, and priorities of the family (Nursing Interventions 10-9). Family members should reward positive behavior—that is, praise the child for performing activities of daily living even when having pain. Less attention should be paid to complaining after it is determined that complaints are not caused by new or different pain.

The child should resume self-care and activity to the fullest extent possible. Strongly encourage school attendance because it is a normalizing activity. If the child has missed school for a time, address school reintegration (see Chapter 12). Ensure that the teacher is educated, with parental permission to ensure privacy, about the biopsychosocial etiology of the pain. Teachers who attribute pain to physical causes respond more positively to the child than if they believe it is a psychological cause (Logan et al., 2007).

Treatment of neuropathic pain is extremely difficult. Multiple pharmacologic agents, such as antidepressants, anticonvulsants, local anesthetics, and opioids, may be prescribed to reduce neuropathic pain intensity. Psychologic, cognitive behavioral, and physical therapies are also used to restore function and provide coping strategies for children living with neuropathic pain.

Reassess pain and reevaluate the treatment program on a routine basis. The benefit of an interdisciplinary approach can be realized by using the strengths of different team members; the nurse should be a contact person for the family and coordinate team member

NURSING INTERVENTIONS 10-9

Chronic Pain

- Believe that the child has pain.
- Help the child and family establish realistic goals and work toward these goals steadily, with small steps. Reinforce the fact that overexertion is usually counterproductive.
- Provide environmental manipulation:
  - Coordinate with physical therapy to evaluate need for and providing adaptive aids, such as a cane or slip-on shoes, or adding a railing to the stairway.
  - Evaluate the effect of different positions to promote comfort and functional activity.
  - Rearrange the daily schedule to provide more time for difficult activities or to allow the child to perform them in the morning, when fatigue may be less of an issue.
  - Schedule rest periods and promote uninterrupted sleep.
- Optimize nutritional intake.

- Teach stress reduction techniques: biofeedback, exercise, relaxation.
- Implement biophysical interventions: TENS, cutaneous stimulation, nerve blocks.
- Provide pharmacologic interventions:
  - The oral route is preferable for chronic pain.
  - Medicate to provide pain relief or at least so child can participate in normal activities.
  - Single-drug therapy may be tried, but complex pain problems often require combinations of drugs (acetaminophen, NSAIDs, antidepressants, anticonvulsants, benzodiazepines, opioids).
  - Individualize schedule and promote around-the-clock dosing, with additional dosing available for breakthrough pain.
  - Watch for signs of withdrawal when discontinuing medications. Reduce dosage slowly to avoid withdrawal and acute exacerbation of pain; wean from sedatives first.

activities. This role may involve coordinating with the health care prescriber and pharmacist for medication schedule, dose, or drug changes; the psychologist for behavioral and coping strategies; the physical therapist for functional activity and strength training; the nutritionist for diet modifications; or the social worker for family support issues (Clinical Judgment 10-3).

ANSWER: Although George's condition is chronic, it is also progressive with increasing disability and increasing pain. His treatment plan, supported by the National Comprehensive Cancer Network Clinical Practice Guidelines, offers regular assessment and continuous treatment.

Pain in the Emergency Department

Children frequently present to the emergency department in pain. Airway, breathing, and circulation (ABC) must be addressed first. If defibrillation is not necessary, consider *D* a reminder to assess and treat discomfort. Severe pain is considered an emergency in itself and requires immediate attention after the ABC have been evaluated and stabilized.

The child in the emergency department may experience pain resulting from pathology, from diagnostic or therapeutic procedures, or from some combination of these sources. If painful procedures are necessary, prepare the child before the procedure when possible. When interventions must be done on an emergent basis, explain what is being done as it is happening.

Position the child securely for procedures. Children are routinely restrained without sedation or analgesia for painful procedures, something that would be unthinkable with an adult. If a child is unable to follow directions and allow a procedure to proceed safely with analgesia alone, the child should be sedated.

KidKare Tell children what they *can* do ("Squeeze your mommy's hand as hard as this hurts." "Count to 10." "Make your arm like a noodle.") instead of what they *cannot* do ("Don't tense up your arm.").

Use a topical anesthetic for venipunctures, lumbar punctures, laceration repairs, urinary catheterization, and other painful procedures. IV opioids or sedation should be used for more painful procedures. Children undergoing sedation in the emergency department should be assumed to have full stomachs.

Address pain management early to avoid escalating the pain and the child's and family's distress. Always provide psychological support and use biobehavioral techniques when possible. In the emergency department, drugs are usually given to control pain because of time constraints and the amount of pain experienced.

Children in shock should not be given opioids until hemodynamic stability is achieved. If severe pain is present in a child with potential hemodynamic compromise, small doses of short-acting opioids may be given repeatedly (e.g., morphine or fentanyl every 5 minutes). Headache associated with head injuries often can be managed with nonopioid analgesics. These agents are

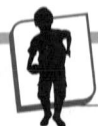

CLINICAL JUDGMENT 10-3

An Adolescent in Pain

Charles is a 14-year-old with hemophilia who weighs 50 kg. He is well known to your clinic because he has a history of multiple bleeding episodes. He is not receiving routine medication, only factor XIII for acute bleeding episodes. He comes in today limping and complaining of joint pain at 8 points on a 10-point scale. Charles greets all the nurses with a hug and smile but seems much less cheerful than normal. Vital signs are normal for age.

Questions

1. What more would you ask Charles about his current complaints?

2. Charles indicates that this pain is primarily in his left knee and ankle, although all lower extremity joints are painful intermittently. This pattern has been present for about 7 months, becoming increasingly painful until reaching its present level about 2 weeks ago. He has lost 2 kg since last weighed 6 months ago and is not sleeping well ("I can't get comfortable"). He misses at least 1 day of school a week, and his grades are dropping. He still swims but can't ride his bike to school anymore. On the basis of this history, what are your concerns?

3. What is his current problem?

4. How should Charles's pain be managed?

5. When and how will you reevaluate Charles?

Answers

1. History of current pain complaint: Did he hurt himself recently? Does he think it is an acute bleed? Where is the pain? What does it feel like? How long has it been present? Is it always at this level or is it intermittent? Is pain interfering with activities of daily living, including eating and sleeping, school attendance and performance, and with activities that he enjoys (swimming, bike riding, and roping)? If pain is interfering, to what extent? Does anything help relieve the pain?

2. The pain is affecting Charles's quality of life as evidenced by sleeping and eating disturbances; it is also interfering with school, socialization, and, potentially, his ability to achieve independence and self-care skills.

3. Chronic arthritic pain from previous bleeding episodes

4. Start oral acetaminophen and an opioid around the clock. Advocate for a physical therapy consultation. Discuss biobehavioral methods of pain relief such as cutaneous stimulation (cold) and cognitive–behavioral methods (progressive muscle relaxation, meditation, guided imagery, self-hypnosis). Have Charles select one to learn and use until his next appointment. Have Charles keep a symptom diary.

5. Reevaluate in 1 week. Charles should call the clinic sooner if the pain worsens or is not less than 4 out of 10 points in 2 days (Charles's goal). At this time, review his symptom diary. Ask if Charles is satisfied with his pain management plan. Develop a plan to wean from the opioid if Charles has not already reduced his dosage. Is the behavioral technique working? Does he like it? Does he want to learn another?

---

preferable because opioids may mask signs of changing neurologic status. If opioids are required, use small amounts that do not affect level of consciousness. Aggressive pain management is required for children with burns. Opioids combined with nonopioids should be given as soon as possible. Dressing the wounds and applying cold compresses aid in pain relief. Fractures can be extremely painful; short-acting IV opioids should be given. Ibuprofen or acetaminophen with codeine and application of cold may be effective for less severe fracture pain. Pain resulting from minor injuries may be managed with acetaminophen, ibuprofen, or another NSAID as age appropriate or a weak opioid such as codeine. Reevaluate pain intensity and efficacy of interventions frequently, at least every time vital signs are taken.

Community Care: Managing Pain at Home

The majority of children who experience pain are not seen in the health care setting. Well-child care can include anticipatory guidance for managing minor pain at home. Ice, massage, bandages, rest, distraction, or other biobehavioral interventions may be quite effective. Acetaminophen or ibuprofen, particularly effective for musculoskeletal pain, may be given.

ALERT *Aspirin use is thought to be associated with an increased risk of Reye syndrome and should not be given, particularly when a viral infection is present, unless ordered by a health care provider.*

Aspirin may be used to manage chronic inflammatory disease such as juvenile rheumatoid arthritis. Teach the child and family to consult the health care provider if pain is accompanied by signs of systemic disease.

Always give written instructions to children being discharged from a health care setting and their family. Instructions should include intensity of pain to expect with the condition or procedure, how long the pain might last, and how to use a developmentally appropriate assessment tool—preferably a method that was used in the health care setting—to assess pain level. Rank interventions in order of what to try first or what to do for certain pain levels (e.g., if pain is severe, give the opioid; if mild, give acetaminophen). Include activity restrictions, if any (e.g., after sedation, the child requires close supervision for at least 8 hours and should participate in no potentially dangerous activities such as bathing, using tools, bike riding, skating, or using playground equipment). Teach the family to evaluate the effectiveness of interventions. If medications are used, emphasize that regular dosing is most effective. Describe side effects of medications, ways to prevent them, and what to do if they occur (e.g., if receiving opioids, increase fluid and fiber intake to decrease constipation). Also, provide the number of the person to call if pain management is inadequate. Research suggests that parents need to be engaged in active decision making with their health care providers in order to enhance their understanding of the pain management information (Tait et al., 2008).

ENSURING EFFECTIVE OUTCOMES OF PAIN MANAGEMENT

For the child experiencing mild to moderate pain, biobehavioral interventions alone may adequately manage the pain. For moderate to severe pain, use of medications coupled with appropriate biobehavioral strategies best support the child. Pharmacologic management of pain can be achieved using a single drug or combinations. Dose must be titrated; schedule, route, and drug combinations must be optimal. Side effects must be anticipated and managed. The adequacy of pain management must be evaluated on a routine basis (Nursing Interventions 10-10).

THE INTERDISCIPLINARY PAIN TEAM

Effective management of pain in children requires the efforts of many individuals sharing their expertise. These experts include nurses, pediatricians, anesthesiologists, pharmacists, psychologists, physical therapists, social workers, child life workers, and others. Some centers

---

NURSING INTERVENTIONS 10-10

Checklist for Assessing Adequacy of Pain Management in Children

Pharmacologic Strategies

- Have the child and parents been asked about their previous experiences with pain and their preferences for use of analgesics?
- Do the child or family have reservations about the use of opioids for pain treatment?
- Is the child being adequately assessed at appropriate intervals?
- Are analgesics ordered for prevention and relief of pain?
- Is the analgesic strong enough for the pain expected or the pain being experienced?
- Is the timing of drug administration appropriate for the pain expected or experienced?
- Is the route of administration appropriate for the child?
- Is the child adequately monitored for the occurrence of side effects?
- Are side effects appropriately managed?
- Has the analgesic regimen provided adequate comfort and satisfaction from the perspective of the child and family?

Biobehavioral and Nonpharmacologic Strategies

- Have the child and family been asked about their experience with and preferences for a given strategy?
- Is the strategy appropriate for the child's developmental level, condition, and type of pain?
- Is the timing of the strategy sufficient to optimize its effects?
- Is the strategy used with, rather than instead of, analgesics?
- Is the strategy adequately effective in preventing or alleviating the child's pain?
- Are the child and family satisfied with the strategy for prevention or relief of pain?
- Are the treatable sources of emotional distress for the child being addressed?

Adapted from American Pain Society. (2008). *Principles of analgesic use in the treatment of acute pain and cancer pain* (6th ed.). Glenview, IL: Author.

are large enough to support a specific pediatric pain program. Such a program is optimal because pain management is an expanding field of research and practice patterns change with new knowledge. Some centers incorporate the pediatric population into the general pain program. Others rely on individuals with knowledge in the field.

NURSE'S ROLE IN PAIN MANAGEMENT

Nurses contribute substantially to managing pain in children and should take a lead role as part of the interdisciplinary team. Assess pain during initial patient contact and routinely when assessing vital signs. Work with the family to set realistic goals and a plan for action. For example, Ashley will walk to the end of the hall. She will take her pain medication 30 minutes before this walk and use cold packs. Reevaluate the interventions and goals at appropriate intervals.

The nurse is pivotal in ensuring the effectiveness of medications and helps to educate the other health care team members who write the orders. To ensure that medications are optimally effective, be familiar with mechanism of action, peak and duration of action, and side effects. Plan care on the basis of this information. Prevent pain when possible, observe for effectiveness of and tolerance to medications, and schedule to keep pain intensity at a minimal level. Around-the-clock management is imperative.

The nurse must advocate for the child. Advocacy may involve convincing the family that opioids are appropriate for the situation or consulting with the prescriber regarding an ineffective medication regimen. Health care team members need to collaborate to promote effective communication and to decrease the amount of frustration that may be involved in this process (Nursing Interventions 10-11). Nurses have assumed leadership roles in pain management through pain relief nurse programs and nursing-directed pain management services (Chen-Lim et al., 2012; Jeffs et al., 2011; McCleary et al., 2004).

DOCUMENTATION

However pain is managed, the plan must be clear, consistent, and well documented so that all team members can work efficiently together. An effective way to achieve these goals is to use interdisciplinary protocols for pain management. Standards for pain management have been developed by various organizations, such as the APS, AAP, Oncology Nursing Society, Agency for Healthcare Research and Quality (AHRQ), and the World Health Organization. Protocols should include institution- or unit-specific guidelines for pain assessment for children of various ages. These guidelines should outline the specific behaviors to be included, tools to be used, frequency of assessments, interventions, and documentation requirements. Including psychosocial and developmental issues is particularly critical if the team cares for adults as well as children and the physician members are not pediatricians. Child life specialists can be particularly valuable in this situation, providing biobehavioral pain management such as relaxation, distraction, and procedural preparedness.

Assessment of pain by nurses is performed most consistently when pain is viewed as the fifth vital sign. To

---

NURSING INTERVENTIONS 10-11

Optimizing Pain Management

- Make sure that the currently ordered regimen has been followed and used to the fullest extent (highest doses, most frequent intervals) possible.
- Keep the focus on the child (not "what you ordered is not working" or "I cannot stand his crying anymore").
- Believe that everyone is trying to provide excellent patient care.
- Offer objective physiologic and behavioral evidence of pain, not vague statements ("He has slept fitfully for no longer than 20 minutes at a time; he lies stiffly in bed, grimaces and cries when moved; he is consolable with a pacifier but not for longer than 2 minutes" vs. "He appears to be in pain"). Knowing the prescriber's criteria for pain indicators is a benefit; the patient report can address these criteria (e.g., if the prescriber believes that all young children are irritable and cry after surgery because they are in a strange environment but takes vital sign changes as valid, emphasize vital sign changes).

- State current management regimen, both pharmacologic and biobehavioral (e.g., morphine at 1 mg IV is ordered every 2 hours, it was last given 90 minutes ago, his mother is holding him and his favorite video is on).
- Ask the prescriber or pharmacist for management suggestions. If the prescriber has no suggestions or is reluctant to change the regimen, reiterate your assessment that the child is experiencing pain and your suggestion for management ("What about increasing the morphine to 1.5 mg or adding an NSAID?").
- Be persistent in advocating for the child, do not get angry, and remember everyone is working toward the same goal.

facilitate consistent documentation of pain assessments, the child's flow sheet should include a designated area next to the vital sign recordings for this purpose. Management of more complex pain problems, rapidly changing regimens, or weaning from opioids may best be documented on a separate pain flow sheet. Other issues that should be addressed by the pain team or person responsible for pain management in the institution are quality improvement and outcome monitoring; home care needs, community resources, and school integration; and research use or implementation of clinical research.

Assessment and management of pain in children are challenging. We must continue to meet this challenge; the comfort and well-being of children depend on it.

See the Point for a summary of Key Concepts.

REFERENCES

Accardi, M. C., & Milling, L. S. (2009). The effectiveness of hypnosis for reducing procedure-related pain in children and adolescents: A comprehensive methodological review. *Journal of Behavioral Medicine*, 32(4), 328–339.

Akcam, M., & Ormeci, A. R. (2004). Oral hypertonic glucose spray: A practical alternative for analgesia in newborn. *Acta Paediatrica*, 93, 1330–1333.

Akman, I., Ozek, E., Bilgen, R. et al. (2002). Sweet solutions and pacifiers for pain relief in newborn infants. *Journal of Pain*, 3, 199–202.

Ambuel, B., Hamlett, K., Marx, C. et al. (1992). Assessing distress in pediatric intensive care environments: The COMFORT Scale. *Journal of Pediatric Psychology*, 17, 95–109.

American Academy of Pediatrics, American Academy of Pediatric Dentistry, Coté, C. J. et al. (2006). Guidelines for monitoring and management of pediatric patients during and after sedation for diagnostic and therapeutic procedures: An update. *Pediatrics*, 118(6), 2587–2602.

American Academy of Pediatrics & American Pain Society. (2001). The assessment and management of acute pain in infants, children and adolescents. *Pediatrics*, 108(3), 793–797.

American Academy of Pediatrics Committee on Fetus and Newborn, American Academy of Pediatrics Section on Surgery, & Canadian Paediatric Society Fetus and Newborn Committee. (2006). Prevention and management of pain in the neonate: An update. *Pediatrics*, 118(5), 2231–2241.

American Association of Critical Care Nurses. (2010). *Practice alert: Family presence during resuscitation and invasive procedures*. Retrieved from http://www.aacn.org/wd/practice/docs/practice alerts/family%20presence%2004-2010%20final.pdf

American Pain Society. (2008). *Principles of analgesic use in the treatment of acute pain and cancer pain* (6th ed.). Glenview, IL: Author.

American Pain Society. (2012). *Assessment and management of children with chronic pain. A position statement from the American Pain Society*. Glenview, IL: Author. Retrieved from http://www .americanpainsociety.org/uploads/pdfs/aps12-pcp.pdf

American Society for Pain Management Nursing, Emergency Nurses Association, American College of Emergency Physicians et al. (2009) *Optimizing the treatment of pain in patients with acute presentations*. Retrieved from http://www.aspmn.org/Organization/ documents/OptimizingPositionPaper.pdf

American Society of Addiction Medicine. (2011). *Public policy statement: Definition of addiction*. Chevy Chase, MD: Author.

American Society of Anesthesiologists. (2011). Practice guidelines for preoperative fasting and the use of pharmacologic agents to reduce the risk of pulmonary aspiration: Application to healthy patients undergoing elective procedures. *Anesthesiology*, 114, 495–511.

Ameringer, S. (2010). Barriers to pain management among adolescents with cancer. *Pain Management Nursing*, 11(4), 224–233.

Ameringer, S., Serlin, R. C., Hughes, S. H. et al. (2006). Concerns about pain management among adolescents with cancer: Developing the Adolescent Barriers Questionnaire. *Journal of Pediatric Oncology Nursing*, 23(4), 220–232.

Aminabadi, N. A., Erfanparast, L., Sohrabi, A. et al. (2012). The impact of virtual reality distraction on pain and anxiety during dental treatment in 4-6 year-old children: A randomized controlled clinical trial. *Dental Research Dental Clinics Dental Prospects*, 6(4), 117–124.

Anand, K. J. S., Aranda, J. V., Berde, C. B. et al. (2006). Summary proceedings from the Neonatal Pain Control Group. *Pediatrics*, 117(3), S9–S22.

Anand, K. J., Sippell, W. G., & Aynsley-Green, A. (1987). Randomised trial of fentanyl anaesthesia in preterm babies undergoing surgery: Effects on the stress response. *Lancet*, 1(8524), 62–66.

Anderson, P. G., & Cutshall, S. M. (2007). Massage therapy: A comfort intervention for cardiac surgery patients. *Clinical Nurse Specialist*, 21(3), 161–165.

Anghelescu, D. L., Faughnan, L. G., Oakes, L. L. et al. (2012). Parent-controlled PCA for pain management in pediatric oncology: Is it safe? *Journal of Pediatric Hematology/Oncology*, 34(6), 416–420.

Aun, C., Lam, Y. M., & Collett, B. (1986). Evaluation of the use of visual analogue scale in Chinese patients. *Pain*, 25, 215–221.

Badr, L. K., Abdallah, B., Hawari, M. et al. (2010). Determinants of premature infant pain responses to heel sticks. *Pediatric Nursing*, 36(3), 129–135.

Ballantyne, M., McNair, C., Ung, E. et al. (2003). A randomized controlled trial evaluating the efficacy of tetracaine gel for pain relief from peripherally inserted central catheters in infants. *Advances in Neonatal Care*, 3, 297–307.

Bardia, A., Barton, D. L., Prokop, L. J. et al. (2006). Efficacy of complementary and alternative medicine therapies in relieving cancer pain: A systematic review. *Journal of Clinical Oncology*, 24, 5457–5464.

Baxt, C., Kassam-Adams, N., Nance, M. L. et al. (2004). Assessment of pain after injury in the pediatric patient: Child and parent perceptions. *Journal of Pediatric Surgery*, 39, 979–983.

Beacham, P. S. (2004). Behavioral and physiological indicators of procedural and postoperative pain in high-risk infants. *Journal of Obstetric, Gynecologic, and Neonatal Nursing*, 33, 246–255.

Bear, L. A., & Ward-Smith, P. (2006). Interrater reliability of the COMFORT Scale. *Pediatric Nursing*, 32, 427–434.

Beyer, J., Denyes, M., & Villarruel, A. (1992). The creation, validation, and continuing development of the Oucher: A measure of pain intensity in children. *Journal of Pediatric Nursing*, 7, 335–346.

Beyer, J., & Knott, C. (1998). Construct validity estimation for the African-American and Hispanic versions of the Oucher Scale. *Journal of Pediatric Nursing*, 13, 20–31.

Bieri, D., Reeve, R. A., Champion, G. D. et al. (1990). The Faces Pain Scale for the self-assessment of the severity of pain experienced by children: Initial validation and preliminary investigation for ratio scale properties. *Pain*, 41, 139–150.

Blass, E., Fitzgerald, E., & Kehoe, P. (1987). Interactions between sucrose, pain and isolation distress. *Pharmacology Biochemistry and Behavior*, 26, 483–489.

Blass, E. M., & Watt, L. B. (1999). Suckling- and sucrose-induced analgesia in human newborns. *Pain*, 83, 611–623.

Boensch, S. (2011). Stimulation-produced analgesia: TENS, acupuncture and alternative techniques. *Anaesthesia & Intensive Care Medicine*, 12(1), 28–30.

Bosenberg, A., Thomas, J., Lopez, T. et al. (2003). Validation of a six-graded faces scale for evaluation of postoperative pain in children. *Paediatric Anaesthesia*, 13(8), 708–713.

Brady-Fryer, B., Wieve, N., & Lander, J. A. (2009). Pain relief for neonatal circumcision. *Cochrane Database of Systematic Reviews*, (4), CD004217.

Brahmbhatt, A., Adeloye, T., Ercole, A. et al. (2012). Assessment of post-operative pain in children: Who knows best? *Pediatric Reports*, 4(1), e10.

Breau, L. M., Finley, G. A., McGrath, P. J. et al. (2002). Validation of the non-communicating children's pain checklist–postoperative version (NCCPC-PV). *Anesthesiology, 96*, 528–535.

Breau, L. M., McGrath, P. J., Camfield, C. S. et al. (2002). Psychometric properties of the non-communicating children's pain checklist–revised. *Pain, 99*, 349–357.

Broome, M. E., & Huth, M. M. (2003). Nursing management of the child in pain. In N. L. Schechter, C. B. Berde, & M. Yaster (Eds.), *Pain in infants, children, and adolescents* (2nd ed., pp. 417–433). Philadelphia, PA: Lippincott Williams & Wilkins.

Burkitt, C. C., Breau, L. M., & Zabaliz, M. (2011). Parental assessment of pain coping in individuals with intellectual and developmental disabilities. *Research in Developmental Disabilities, 32*, 1564–1571.

Bursch, B., Joseph, M. H., & Zeltzer, L. K. (2003). Pain-associated disability syndrome. In N. L. Schechter, C. B. Berde, & M. Yaster (Eds.), *Pain in infants, children, and adolescents* (2nd ed., pp. 841–848). Philadelphia, PA: Lippincott Williams & Wilkins.

Buskila, D., Neumann, L., Zmora, E. et al. (2003). Pain sensitivity in prematurely born adolescents. *Archives of Pediatrics & Adolescent Medicine, 157*, 1079–1082.

Butler, L. S., Symons, B. K., Henderson, S. L. et al. (2005). Hypnosis reduces distress and duration of an invasive medical procedure for children. *Pediatrics, 115*, 77–85.

Caljouw, M. A. A., Kloos, M. A. C., Olivier, M. Y. et al. (2007). Measurement of pain in premature infants with a gestational age between 28 to 37 weeks: Validation of the adopted COMFORT Scale. *Journal of Neonatal Nursing, 13*, 13–18.

Capici, F., Ingelmo, P. M., Davidson, A. et al. (2008). Randomized controlled trial of duration of analgesia following intravenous or rectal acetaminophen after adenotonsillectomy in children. *British Journal of Anaesthesia, 100*(2), 251–255.

Carbajal, R., Rousset, A., Danan, C. et al. (2008). Epidemiology and treatment of painful procedures in neonates in intensive care units. *Journal of the American Medical Association, 300*(1), 60–70.

Carlson, K. L., Broome, M., & Vessey, J. A. (2000). Using distraction to reduce reported pain, fear, and behavioral distress in children and adolescents: A multisite study. *Journal of the Society of Pediatric Nurses, 5*(2), 75–85.

Carnevale, R. A., & Razack, S. (2002). An item analysis of the COMFORT scale in a pediatric intensive care unit. *Pediatric Journal of Critical Care Medicine, 3*, 177–180.

Carter, B. D., & Threlkeld, B. M. (2012). Psychosocial perspectives in the treatment of pediatric chronic pain. *Pediatric Rheumatology, 10*, 15.

Cavender, K., Goff, M. D., Hollon, E. C. et al. (2004). Parent's positioning and distracting children during venipuncture. *Journal of Holistic Nursing, 22*(1), 32–56.

Chambers, C. T., Finley, G. A., McGrath, P. J. et al. (2003). The parents' postoperative pain measure: Replication and extension to 2-6-year-old children. *Pain, 105*, 437–443.

Chambers, C. T., Hardial, J., Craig, K. D. et al. (2005). Faces scales for the measurement of postoperative pain intensity in children following minor surgery. *Clinical Journal of Pain, 21*, 277–285.

Chambers, C. T., & Johnston, C. (2002). Developmental differences in children's use of rating scales. *Journal of Pediatric Psychology, 27*, 27–36.

Chambers, C. T., Taddio, A., Uman, L. S. et al. (2009). Psychological interventions for reducing pain and distress during routine childhood immunizations: A systematic review. *Clinical Therapeutics, 31*(Suppl. 2), S77–S103.

Chen-Lim, M. L., Zarnowsky, C., Green, R. et al. (2012). Optimizing the assessment of pain in children who are cognitively impaired through the quality improvement process. *Journal of Pediatric Nursing, 27*(6), 750–759.

Cheng, S. F., Foster, R. L., & Hester, N. O. (2003). A review of factors predicting children's pain experiences. *Issues in Comprehensive Pediatric Nursing, 26*, 203–216.

Cohen, L. (2002). Reducing infant immunization distress through distraction. *Health Psychology, 21*, 207–211.

Cohen, L. L., MacLaren, J. E., Fortson, B. L. et al. (2006). Randomized clinical trial of distraction for infant immunization pain. *Pain, 125*, 165–171.

Costello, M., Ramundo, M., Christopher, N. C. et al. (2006). Ethyl vinyl chloride vapocoolant spray fails to decrease pain associated with intra venous cannulation in children. *Clinical Pediatrics, 45*, 628–632.

Curry, D. M., Brown, C., & Wrona, S. (2012). Effectiveness of oral sucrose for pain management in infants during immunizations. *Pain Management Nursing, 13*(3), 139–149.

Czarnecki, M., Simon, K., Thompson, J. J. et al. (2011). Barriers to pediatric pain management: A nursing perspective. *Pain Management Nursing, 12*(3), 154–162.

Dahlquist, L. M., Gil, K. M., Armstrong, F. D. et al. (1986). Preparing children for medical examinations: The importance of previous medical experience. *Health Psychology, 5*, 249–259.

Dahlquist, L. M., Power, T. G., Cox, C. N. et al. (1994). Parenting and child distress during cancer procedures: A multidimensional assessment. *Children's Health Care, 23*, 149–166.

Das, D. A., Grimmer, K. A., Sparnon, A. L. et al. (2005). The efficacy of playing a virtual reality game in modulating pain for children with acute burn injuries: A randomized controlled trial. *BMC Pediatrics, 5*(1), 1.

Davies, E. H., & Molloy, A. (2006). Comparison of ethyl chloride spray with topical anaesthetic in children experiencing venepuncture. *Paediatric Nursing, 18*, 39–43.

Davies, R. B. (2010). Pain in children with Down syndrome: Assessment and intervention by parents. *Pain Management Nursing, 11*(4), 259–267.

Duivenvoorden, H. J., Tibboel, D., Koot, H. M. et al. (2006). Pain assessment in profound cognitive impaired children using the Checklist Pain Behavior: Is item reduction valid? *Pain, 126*, 147–154.

Eccleston, C., Palermo, T. M., Williams, A. C. et al. (2012). Psychological therapies for the management of chronic and recurrent pain in children and adolescents. *Cochrane Database of Systematic Reviews*, (12), CD003968.

Efe, E., & Ozer, Z. C. (2007). The use of breast-feeding for pain relief during neonatal immunization injections. *Applied Nursing Research, 20*, 10–16.

Eland, J. M., & Anderson, J. E. (1977). The experience of pain in children. In A. K. Jacox (Ed.), *Pain: A sourcebook for nurses and other health professionals* (pp. 453–476). Boston, MA: Little, Brown.

Ellis, J., Lamontagne, C., Pascuet, E. et al. (2011). Improved practices for safe administration of intravenous bolus morphine in a pediatric setting. *Pain Management Nursing, 12*(3), 146–153.

Ely, E., Chen-Lim, M. L., Zarnowsky, C. et al. (2012). Finding the evidence to change practice for assessing pain in children who are cognitively impaired. *Journal of Pediatric Nursing, 27*(4), 402–410.

Emergency Nurses Association. (2010a). *Emergency nursing resource: Family presence during invasive procedures and resuscitation in the emergency department.* Des Plaines, IL: Author. Retrieved from http://www.ena.org/IENR/CPG/Documents/Family PresenceCPG.pdf

Emergency Nurses Association. (2010b). *Emergency nursing resource: Needle-related procedural pain in pediatric patients in the emergency department.* Des Plaines, IL: Author. Retrieved from http://www.ena.org/IENR/CPG/Documents/PedPainManagement CPG.pdf

Engebretson, J., & Wardell, D. (2007). Energy-based modalities. *Nursing Clinics of North America, 42*, 243–259.

Etzel-Hardman, D. (2011). Pediatric sedation and distraction. *Journal of Pediatric Nursing, 26*(2), 172–173.

Fendrich, K., Vennemann, M., Pfaffenrath, V. et al. (2007). Headache prevalence among adolescents: The German DMKG Headache Study. *Cephalalgia, 27*, 347–354.

Finley, G. A., Chambers, C. T., McGrath, P. J. et al. (2003). Construct validity of the Parents' Postoperative Pain Measure. *The Clinical Journal of Pain, 19*, 329–334.

Fitzgerald, M., & Walker, S. M. (2009). Infant pain management: A developmental neurobiological approach. *Nature Clinical Practice. Neurology, 5*(1), 35–50.

Fortier, M. A., MacLaren, J. E., Martin, S. R. et al. (2009). Pediatric pain after ambulatory surgery: Where's the medication? *Pediatrics, 124*(4), e588–e595.

Fortier, M. A., Martin, S. R., Kain, D. I. et al. (2011). Parental attitudes regarding analgesic use for children: Differences in ethnicity and language. *Journal of Pediatric Surgery, 46*(11), 2140–2145.

Foster, R. L., & Park, J. (2012). An integrative review of literature examining psychometric properties of instruments measuring anxiety or fear in hospitalized children. *Pain Management Nursing, 13*(2), 94–106.

Foster, R. L., Yucha, C. B., Zuk, J. et al. (2003). Physiologic correlates of comfort in healthy children. *Pain Management Nursing, 4*(1), 23–30.

Franck, L. S., Oulton, K., & Bruce, E. (2012). Parental involvement in neonatal pain management: An empirical and conceptual update. *Journal of Nursing Scholarship, 44*(1), 45–53.

Gaffney, A., McGrath, P. J., & Dick, B. (2003). Measuring pain in children: Developmental and instrumental issues. In N. L. Schechter, C. B. Berde, & M. Yaster (Eds.), *Pain in infants, children, and adolescents* (2nd ed., pp. 241–264). Philadelphia, PA: Lippincott Williams & Wilkins.

Galinkin, J. L., Rose, J. B., Harris, K. et al. (2002). Lidocaine iontophoresis versus eutectic mixture of local anesthetics (EMLA) for IV placement in children. *Anesthesia & Analgesia, 94*, 1484–1488.

Garcia-Munitis, P., Bandeira, M., Pistorio, A. et al. (2006). Level of agreement between children, parents, and physicians in rating pain intensity in juvenile idiopathic arthritis. *Arthritis and Rheumatism, 55*, 177–183.

Gauvain-Piquard, A., Rodary, C., Francois, P. et al. (1991). Validity assessment of DEGR Scale for observational rating of 2–6-year-old child pain. *Journal of Pain and Symptom Management, 6*, 171.

Gauvain-Piquard, A., Rodary, C., Rezvani, A. et al. (1987). Pain in children aged 2–6 years: A new observational rating scale elaborated in a pediatric oncology unit preliminary report. *Pain, 31*, 177–188.

Gerik, S. M. (2005). Pain management in children: Developmental considerations and mind–body therapies. *Southern Medical Journal, 98*, 295–302.

Gershon, J., Zimand, E., Pickering, M. et al. (2004). A pilot and feasibility study of virtual reality as a distraction for children with cancer. *Journal of the American Academy of Child and Adolescent Psychiatry, 43*, 1243–1249.

Gharaibeh, M., & Abu-Saad, H. (2002). Cultural validation of pediatric pain assessment tools: Jordanian perspective. *Journal of Transcultural Nursing, 13*, 12–18.

Goddard, J. M. (2011). Chronic pain in children and young people. *Current Opinion in Supportive and Palliative Care, 5*(2), 158–163.

Godfrey, H. (2005). Understanding pain, part 1: Physiology of pain. *British Journal of Nursing, 14*, 846–852.

Gordon, D. B., Dahl, J., Phillips, P. et al. (2004). The use of "as-needed" range orders for opioid analgesics in the management of acute pain: A consensus statement of the American Society for Pain Management Nursing and the American Pain Society. *Pain Management Nursing, 5*(2), 53–58.

Gottsegen, D. (2011). Hypnosis for functional abdominal pain. *American Journal of Clinical Hypnosis, 54*(1), 56–69.

Gradin, M., Eriksson, M., Schollin, J. et al. (2002). Pain reduction at venipuncture in newborns: Oral glucose compared with local anesthetic cream. *Pediatrics, 110*, 1053–1058.

Gray, L., Miller, L. W., Philipp, B. L. et al. (2002). Breastfeeding is analgesic in healthy newborns. *Pediatrics, 109*, 590–593.

Green, C. R., Anderson, K. O., Baker, T. A. et al. (2003). The unequal burden of pain: Confronting racial and ethnic disparities in pain. *Pain Medicine, 4*, 277–294.

Greenberg, C. S. (2002). A sugar-coated pacifier reduces procedural pain in newborns. *Pediatric Nursing, 22*, 271–277.

Groenewald, C. B., Rabbitts, J. A., Schroeder, E. R. et al. (2012). Prevalence of moderate-severe pain in hospitalized children. *Paediatric Anaesthesia, 22*(7), 661–668.

Grunau, R., & Craig, K. (1987). Pain expression in neonates: Facial action and cry. *Pain, 28*, 395–410.

Grunau, R. E., Holsti, L., Haley, D. W. et al. (2005). Neonatal procedural pain exposure predicts lower cortisol and behavioral reactivity in preterm infants in the NICU. *Pain, 113*, 293–300.

Hall, R. W., & Anand, K. J. S. (2005). Short-and long-term impact of neonatal pain and stress: More than an ouchie. *Neonatal Reviews, 6*, 369.

Hall, M. J., DeFrances, C. J., Williams, S. N. et al. (2010). *National Hospital Discharge Survey: 2007 Summary* (National Health Statistics Reports, No. 29). Hyattsville, MD: National Center for Health Statistics.

Harvey, V. L., & Dickenson, A. H. (2008). Mechanisms of pain in nonmalignant disease. *Current Opinion in Supportive and Palliative Care, 2*(2), 133–139.

Heath, J. A., Clarke, N. E., Donath, S. M. et al. (2010). Symptoms and suffering at the end of life in children with cancer: An Australian perspective. *Medical Journal of Australia 192*(2), 71–75.

Helgadóttir, H. L., & Wilson, M. E. (2004). Temperament and pain in 3 to 7-year-old children undergoing tonsillectomy. *Journal of Pediatric Nursing, 19*, 204–213.

Hermann, C., Hohmeister, J., Demirakça, S. et al. (2006). Long-term alteration of pain sensitivity in school-aged children with early pain experiences. *Pain, 125*, 278–285.

Herr, K., Coyne, P. J., McCaffery, M. et al. (2011). Pain assessment in the patient unable to self-report: Position statement with clinical practice recommendations. *Pain Management Nursing, 12*(4), 230–250.

Hesselgard, K., Larsson, S., Romner, B. et al. (2007). Validity and reliability of the Behavioural Observational Pain Scale for postoperative pain measurement in children 1–7 years of age. *Pediatric Critical Care Medicine, 8*, 102–108.

Hester, N. O. (1979). The preoperational child's reaction to immunization. *Nursing Research, 28*, 250–255.

Hicks, C. L., von Baeyer, C. L., Spafford, P. A. et al. (2001). The Faces scale-revised: Toward a common metric in pediatric pain measurement. *Pain, 93*, 173–183.

Holsti, L., Grunau, R. E., Oberlander, T. F. et al. (2005). Prior pain induces heightened motor responses during clustered care in preterm infants in the NICU. *Early Human Development, 81*(3), 293–302.

Humphrey, G. B., Boon, C. M., van Linden van den Heuvell, G. F. et al. (1992). The occurrence of high levels of acute behavioral distress in children and adolescents undergoing routine venipunctures. *Pediatrics, 90*, 87–91.

Hunt, A., Goldman, A., Seers, N. et al. (2004). Clinical validation of the paediatric pain profile. *Developmental Medicine & Child Neurology, 46*, 9–18.

Hunt, A., Mastroyannopoulou, K., Goldman, A. et al. (2003). Not knowing: The problem of pain in children with severe neurological impairment. *International Journal of Nursing Studies, 40*, 171–183.

Hunt, A., Wisbeach, A., Seers, K. et al. (2007). Development of the Paediatric Pain Profile: Role of video analysis and saliva cortisol in validating a tool to assess pain in children with severe neurological disability. *Journal of Pain and Symptom Management, 33*, 276–289.

Hunter, M., McDowell, L., Hennessy, R. et al. (2000). An evaluation of the faces pain scale with young children. *Journal of Pain and Symptom Management, 20*, 122–129.

Im, E.-O., Chee, W., Guevara, E. et al. (2007). Gender and ethnic differences in cancer pain experience: A multiethnic survey in the United States. *Nursing Research, 56*, 296–306.

International Association for the Study of Pain. (1979). Pain terms: A list with definitions and notes on usage. *Pain, 6,* 249.

Isaacs, T., Laurier, M. D., Turner, C. D. et al. (2011). Identifying second language speech tasks and ability levels for successful nurse oral interaction with patients in a linguistic minority setting: An instrument development project. *Health Communication, 26*(6), 560–570.

Jain, S., Kumar, P., & McMillan, D. D. (2006). Prior leg massage decreases pain responses to heel stick in preterm babies. *Journal of Paediatrics and Child Health, 42,* 505–508.

Jalmsell, L., Kreicbergs, U., Onelöv, E. et al. (2006). Symptoms affecting children with malignancies during the last month of life: A nationwide follow-up. *Pediatrics, 117,* 1314–1320.

Jeffs, D., Wright, C., Scott, A. et al. (2011). Soft on sticks an evidence-based practice approach to reduce childen's needlestick pain. *Journal of Nursing Care Quality, 26*(3), 208–215.

Jimenez, N., Bradford, H., Seidel, K. D. et al. (2006). A comparison of a needle-free injection system for local anesthesia versus EMLA for intravenous catheter insertion in the pediatric patient. *Anesthesia & Analgesia, 102,* 411–414.

Jindal, V., & Mansky, P. J. (2008). Safety and efficacy of acupuncture in children: A review of the evidence. *Journal of Pediatric Hematology/Oncology, 30*(6), 431–442.

Johansson, M., & Kokinsky, E. (2009). The COMFORT behavioural scale and the modified FLACC scale in paediatric intensive care. *Nursing in Critical Care, 14*(3), 122–130.

Johnston, C. C., Fernandes, A. M., & Campbell-Yeo, M. (2011). Pain in neonates is different. *Pain, 152,* s65–s73.

Johnston, C. C., Stevens, B. J., Pinelli, J. et al. (2003). Kangaroo care is effective in diminishing pain response in preterm neonates. *Archives of Pediatrics & Adolescent Medicine, 157,* 1084–1088.

Kain, Z. N., Caldwell-Andrews, A. A., Mayes, L. C. et al. (2007). Family-centered preparation for surgery improves peripoperative outcomes in children: A randomized controlled trial. *Anesthesiology, 106,* 65–74.

Kain, Z. N., Mayes, L. C., Caldwell-Andrews, A. A. et al. (2006). Preoperative anxiety, postoperative pain, and behavioral recovery in young children undergoing surgery. *Pediatrics, 118,* 651–658.

Kankkunen, P., Pietila, A. M., & Vehviläinen-Julkunen, K. (2004). Families' and children's postoperative pain: Literature review. *Journal of Pediatric Nursing 19,* 133–139.

Kankkunen, P., Vehviläinen-Julkunen, K., Pietila, A. M. et al. (2003). Is the sufficiency of discharge instructions related to children's postoperative pain at home after day surgery? *Scandinavian Journal of Caring Science, 17,* 365–372.

Kankkunen, P., Vehviläinen-Julkunen, K., Pietilä, A. M. et al. (2009). Promoting children's pharmacological post-operative pain alleviation at home. *Pediatric Nursing, 35*(5), 298–302.

Kassab, M. I., Roydhouse, J. K., Fowler, C. et al. (2012). The effectiveness of glucose in reducing needle-related procedural pain in infants. *Journal of Pediatric Nursing, 27*(1), 3–17.

Keogh, E., & Eccleston, C. (2006). Sex differences in adolescent chronic pain and pain-related coping. *Pain, 123,* 275–284.

King, S., Chambers, C. T., Hugeut, A. et al. (2011). The epidemiology of chronic pain in children and adolescents revisited: A systematic review. *Pain, 152*(12), 2729–2738.

Kleiber, C., Craft-Rosenberg, M., & Harper, D. C. (2001). Parents as distraction coaches during I.V. insertion: A randomized study. *Journal of Pain and Symptom Management, 22,* 851–861.

Kleiber, C., & Harper, D. C. (1999). Effects of distraction on children's pain and distress during medical procedures: A meta-analysis. *Nursing Research, 48,* 44–49.

Kleiber, C., & McCarthy, A. M. (1999). Parent behavior and child distress during urethral catheterization. *Journal of the Society of Pediatric Nurses, 4,* 95–104.

Kleiber, C., Schutte, D. L., McCarthy, A. M. et al. (2007). Predictors of topical anesthetic effectiveness in children. *The Journal of Pain, 8,* 168–174.

Kleiber, C., Sorenson, M., Whiteside, K. et al. (2002). Topical anesthetics for intravenous insertion in children: A randomized equivalency study. *Pediatrics, 110,* 758–761.

Kline, W. H., Turnbull, A., Labruna, V. E. et al. (2010). Enhancing pain management in the PICU by teaching guided mental imagery: A quality-improvement project. *Journal of Pediatrics Psychology, 35*(1), 25-31.

Koh, J. L., Harrison, D., Myers, R. et al. (2004). A randomized, double-blind comparison study of EMLA and ELA-Max for topical anesthesia in children undergoing intravenous insertion. *Paediatric Anaesthesia, 14,* 977–982.

Koh, J. L., Harrison, D., Swanson, V. et al. (2007). A comparison of laser-assisted drug delivery at two output energies for enhancing the delivery of topically applied LMX-4 cream prior to venipuncture. *Anesthesia and Analgesia, 104,* 847–849.

Kohen, D. P. (2010). Long-term follow-up of self-hypnosis training for recurrent headaches: What the children say. *International Journal of Clinical and Experimental Hypnosis, 58*(4), 417–432.

Kozlowski, L. J., Kost-Byerly, S., Colantuoni, E. et al. (in press). Pain prevalence, intensity, assessment and management in a hospitalized pediatric population. *Pain Management Nursing.*

Krechel, S. W., & Bildner, J. (1995). CRIES: A new neonatal postoperative pain measurement score: Initial testing of validity and reliability. *Paediatric Anaesthesia, 5,* 53–61.

Kristjánsdóttir, O., Unruh, A. M., McAlpine, L. et al. (2012). A systematic review of cross-cultural comparison studies of child, parent, and health professional outcomes associated with pediatric medical procedures. *Journal of Pain, 13*(3), 207–219.

Kropp, P., Meyer, B., Landgrad, M. et al. (2013). Headache in children: Update on biobehavioral treatments. *Neuropediatrics, 44*(1), 20–24.

Kuttner, L. (1986). *No fears, no tears: Children with cancer coping with pain* [Videotape]. Vancouver, Canada: Canadian Cancer Society.

LaFleur, C. J., & Raway, B. (1999). School-age child and adolescent perception of the pain intensity associated with three word descriptors. *Pediatric Nursing, 25,* 45–55.

LaMontagne, L., Hepworth, J. T., Cohen, F. et al. (2003). Cognitive–behavioral intervention affects adolescents' anxiety and pain following spinal fusion surgery. *Nursing Research, 52,* 183–190.

Lander, J. A., Weltman, B. J., & So, S. S. (2006). EMLA and amethocaine for reduction of children's pain associated with needle insertion. *The Cochrane Database of Systematic Reviews,* (3), CD004236.

Landgren, K., Kvorning, N., & Hallström, I. (2010). Acupuncture reduces crying in infants with infantile colic: A randomised, controlled, blind clinical study. *Acupuncture in Medicine, 24*(4), 174–179.

Landier, W., & Tse, A. M. (2010). Use of complementary and alternative medical interventions for the management of procedure-related pain, anxiety, and distress in pediatric oncology: An integrative review. *Journal of Pediatric Nursing, 25*(6), 566–579.

Landolt, M. A., Marti, D., Widmer, J. et al. (2002). Does cartoon movie decrease children's pain behavior? *Journal of Burn Care & Rehabilitation, 23*(1), 61–65.

Lawrence, J., Alcock, D., McGrath, P. et al. (1993). The development of a tool to assess neonatal pain. *Neonatal Network, 12,* 59–66.

Lemyre, B., Hogan, D. L., Gaboury, I. et al. (2007). How effective is tetracaine 4% gel, before a venipuncture, in reducing procedural pain in infants: A randomized double-blind placebo controlled trial. *BMC Pediatrics, 7,* 7. Retrieved from http://www.biomedcentral.com/1471-2431/7/7

Liaw, J. J., Yang, L., Wang, K.-W. K. et al. (2012). Non-nutritive sucking and facilitated tucking relieve preterm infant pain during heel-stick procedures: A prospective, randomised controlled crossover trial. *International Journal of Nursing Studies, 49*(3), 300–309.

Logan, D. E., Catanese, S. P., Coakley, R. M. et al. (2007). Chronic pain in the classroom: Teachers' attributions about the causes of chronic pain. *Journal of School Health, 77*(5), 248–256.

Logan, H. L., Sheffield, D., Lutgendorf, S. et al. (2002). Predictors of pain during invasive medical procedures. *The Journal of Pain, 3*, 211–217.

Ludington-Hoe, S. M., Hosseini, R., & Torowicz, D. L. (2005). Skin-to-skin contact (kangaroo care) analgesia for preterm infant heel stick. *AACN Clinical Issues, 16*, 373–387.

Luffy, R., & Grove, S. K. (2003). Examining the validity, reliability, and preference of three pediatric pain measurement tools in African-American children. *Pediatric Nursing, 29*, 54–59.

Luhmann, J., Jurt, S., Shootman, M. et al. (2004). A comparison of buffered lidocaine versus ELA-Max before peripheral intravenous catheter insertions in children. *Pediatrics, 113*, e217–e220.

Lynch, A. M., Kashikar-Zuck, S., Goldschneider, K. R. et al. (2007). Sex and age differences in coping styles among children with chronic pain. *Journal of Pain and Symptom Management, 33*, 208–216.

Lysakowski, C., Dumont, L., Tramer, M. R. et al. (2003). A needle-free jet-injection system with lidocaine for peripheral intravenous cannula insertion: A randomized controlled trial with cost-effectiveness analysis. *Anesthesia & Analgesia, 96*, 215–219.

Malviya, S., Voepel-Lewis, T., Burke, C. et al. (2006). The revised FLACC observational pain tool: Improved reliability and validity for pain assessment in children with cognitive impairment. *Paediatric Anaesthesia, 16*(3), 258–265.

Manworren, R. C. B., Paulos, C. L., & Pop, R. (2004). Treating children for acute agitation in the PACU: Differentiating pain and emergence delirium. *Journal of Perianesthesia Nursing, 19*, 183–193.

Martin, A. L., McGrath, P. A., Brown, S. C. et al. (2006). Children with chronic pain: Impact of sex and age on long-term outcomes. *Pain, 128*, 13–19.

McCaffery, M. (1968). *Nursing practice theories related to cognition, bodily pain, and man–environment interactions.* Los Angeles, CA: UCLA Students Store.

McCamant, K. L. (2006). Peripheral nerve blocks: Understanding the nurse's role. *Journal of PeriAnesthesia Nursing, 21*, 16–26.

McCarberg, B., & O'Connor, A. (2004). A new look at heat treatment for pain disorders: Part 1. *APS Bulletin, 4*, 10–11.

McCarthy, A. M., & Kleiber, C. (2006). A conceptual model of factors influencing children's responses to a painful procedure when parents are distraction coaches. *Journal of Pediatric Nursing, 21*, 88–98.

McCarthy, A. M., Kleiber, C., Hanrahan, K. et al. (2010). Factors explaining children's responses to intravenous needle insertions. *Nursing Research, 59*(6), 407–416.

McClain, B. C., & Kain, Z. N. (2005). Procedural pain in neonates: The new millennium. *Pediatrics, 115*, 1073–1075.

McCleary, L., Ellis, J. A., & Rowley, B. (2004). Evaluation of the pain resource nurse role: A resource for improving pediatric pain management. *Pain Management Nursing, 5*(1), 29–36.

McGrath, P. A. & Hillier, L. (2003). Modifying the psychologic factors that intensify children's pain and prolong disability. In N. L. Schechter, C. G. Berde, & M. Yaster (Eds.), *Pain in infants, children, and adolescents* (2nd ed., pp. 85–104). Philadelphia, PA: Lippincott Williams & Wilkins.

McGrath, P. J., Johnson, G., Goodman, J. et al. (1985). CHEOPS: A behavioral scale for rating postoperative pain in children. In H. L. Fields, R. Dubner, & F. Cervero (Eds.), *Advances in pain research and therapy* (pp. 395–402). New York, NY: Raven Press.

Melnyk, B. M., Small, L., & Carno, M. (2004). The effectiveness of parent-focused interventions in improving coping/mental health outcomes of critically ill children and their parents: An evidence base to guide clinical practice. *Pediatric Nursing, 30*, 143–148.

Merkel, S. (2002). Pain assessment in infants and young children: The finger span scale provides an estimate of pain intensity in young children. *American Journal of Nursing, 102*(11), 55–56.

Merkel, S. I., Voepel-Lewis, T., Shayevitz, J. R. et al. (1997). The FLACC: A behavioral scale for scoring postoperative pain in young children. *Pediatric Nursing, 23*, 293–297.

Migdal, M., Chudzynska-Pomianowska, E., Vause, E. et al. (2005). Rapid, needle-free delivery of lidocaine for reducing the pain of venipuncture among pediatric subjects. *Pediatrics, 115*, e393–e398.

Miller, E., Jacob, E., Hockenberry, M. J. (2011). Nausea, pain fatigue, and multiple symptoms in hospitalized children with cancer. *Oncology Nursing Forum, 38*(5), e382–e393.

Mitchell, M. J., Lemanek, K., Palermo, T. M. et al. (2007). Parent perspectives on pain management, coping, and family functioning in pediatric sickle cell disease. *Clinical Pediatrics, 46*, 311–319.

Mitchell, A., Stevens, B., Mungan, N. et al. (2004). Analgesic effects of oral sucrose and pacifier during eye examinations for retinopathy of prematurity. *Pain Management Nursing, 5*, 160–168.

Mitchell, A., & Waltman, P. A. (2003). Oral sucrose and pain relief of preterm infants. *Pain Management Nursing, 4*, 62–69.

Moppett, I. K., Szypula, K., & Yeoman, P. M. (2004). Comparison of EMLA and lidocaine iontophoresis for cannulation analgesia. *European Journal of Anaesthesiology, 21*, 210–213.

Morrison, L. J., Kierzek, G., Diekema, D. S. et al. (2010). 2010 American Heart Association guidelines for cardiopulmonary resuscitation and emergency cardiovascular care. Part 3: Ethics. *Circulation, 122*(18), S665–S675.

Morse, L. J., Kawakami, N., Lenke, L. G. et al. (2012). Culture and ethnicity influence outcomes of the scoliosis research society instrument in adolescent idiopathic scoliosis. *Spine, 37*(12), 1072–1076.

Movahedi, A. F., Rostami, S., Salsali, M. et al. (2006). Effect of local refrigeration prior to venipuncture on pain related responses in school age children. *Australian Journal of Advanced Nursing, 24*, 51–55.

Mudd, S. (2011). Intranasal fentanyl for pain management in children: A systematic review of the literature. *Journal of Pediatric Health Care, 25*(5), 316–322.

Myers, R. R., & Shubayev, V. I. (2011). The ology of neuropathy: An integrative review of the role of neuroinflammation and TNF-α axonal transport in neuropathic pain. *Journal of the Peripheral Nervous System, 16*(4), 277–286.

Myers, C. D., Tsao, J. C., Glover, D. A. et al. (2006). Sex, gender, and age: Contributions to laboratory pain responding in children and adolescents. *Journal of Pain, 7*, 556–564.

Myrvik, M. P., Campbell, A. D., & Butcher, J. L. (2012). Single-session biofeedback-assisted relaxation training in children with sickle cell disease. *Journal of Pediatric Hematology/Oncology, 34*(5), 340–343.

O'Brien, L., Taddio, A., Lyszkiewicz, D. A. et al. (2005). A critical review of the topical local anesthetic amethocaine (Ametop) for pediatric pain. *Paediatric Drugs, 7*, 41–54.

Okan, F., Coban, A., Ince, Z. et al. (2007). Analgesia in preterm newborns: The comparative effects of sucrose and glucose. *European Journal of Pediatrics, 166*(10), 1017–1024.

Owczarzak, V., & Haddad, J. (2006). Comparison of oral versus rectal administration of acetaminophen with codeine in postoperative pediatric adenotonsillectomy patients. *Laryngoscope, 116*, 1485–1488.

Perquin, C. W., Hazebroek-Kampschreur, A. A., Hunfeld, J. A. et al. (2000). Pain in children and adolescents: A common experience, *Pain, 87*, 51–58.

Phillips, R. M., Chantry, C. J., & Gallagher, M. P. (2005). Analgesic effects of breast-feeding or pacifier use with maternal holding in term infants. *Ambulatory Pediatrics, 5*, 359–364.

Piira, T., Hayes, B., Goodenough, B. et al. (2006). Effects of attentional direction, age, and coping style on cold–pressor pain in children. *Behaviour Research and Therapy, 44*, 835–848.

Pinelli, J., Symington, A., & Ciliska, D. (2002). Nonnutritive sucking in high-risk infants: Benign intervention or legitimate therapy? *Journal of Obstetric, Gynecologic, & Neonatal Nursing, 31*, 582–591.

Pöder, U., Ljungman, G., & von Essen, L. (2010). Parents' perceptions of their children's cancer-related symptoms during treatment: A prospective, longitudinal study. *Journal of Pain and Symptom Management, 40*(5), 661–670.

Pölkki, T., Pietilä, A., Vehviläinen-Julkunen, K. et al. (2008). Imagery-induced relaxation in children's postoperative pain relief: A randomized pilot study. *Journal of Pediatric Nursing, 23*(3), 217–224.

Ponder, B. L. (2002). Effects of pain in the human neonate. *American Journal of Electroneurodiagnostic Technology, 42*, 210–223.

Poonai, N., Alawi, K., Rieder, M. et al. (2012). A comparison of amethocaine and liposomal lidocaine cream as a pain reliever before venipuncture in children. *Pediatric Emergency Care, 28*(2), 104–108.

Ramelet, A. (1999). Assessment of pain and agitation in critically ill infants. *Australian Critical Care, 120*, 92–96.

Razmus, I. S., Dalton, M. E., & Wilson, D. (2004). Pain management for newborn circumcision. *Pediatric Nursing, 30*, 414–417, 427.

Reis, E. C., & Holubkov, R. (1997). Vapocoolant spray is equally effective as EMLA cream in reducing immunization pain in school-aged children. *Pediatrics, 100*(6), e5.

Reis, E. C., Roth, E. K., Syphan, J. L. et al. (2003). Effective pain reduction for multiple immunization injections in young infants. *Archives of Pediatrics & Adolescent Medicine, 157*, 1115–1120.

Renn, C., & Dorsey, S. G. (2005). The physiology and processing of pain: A review. *AACN Clinical Issues: Advanced Practice in Acute and Critical Care, 16*, 277–290.

Rennick, J. E., Lambert, S., Cilderhose, J. et al. (2011). Mothers' experiences of a touch and talk nursing intervention to optimize pain management in the PICU: A qualitative descriptive study. *Intensive and Critical Care Nursing, 27*(3), 151–157.

Riddell, R. R. P., Racine, N. M., Turcotte, K. et al. (2011). Non-pharmacological management of infant and young child procedural pain. *Cochrane Database of Systematic Reviews*, (10), CD006275.

Rocha, E. M., Prkachin, K. M., Beaumont, S. L. et al. (2003). Pain reactivity and somatization in kindergarten age children. *Journal of Pediatric Psychology, 28*(1), 47–57.

Sallfors, C., Hallberg, L. R., & Fasth, A. (2003). Gender and age differences in pain, coping and health status among children with chronic arthritis. *Clinical and Experimental Rheumatology, 21*, 785–793.

Samol, N. B., Furstein, J. S., & Moore, D. L. (2012). Regional anesthesia and pain management for the pediatric patient. *International Anesthesiology Clinics, 50*(4), 83–95.

Savedra, M. C., Holzemer, W. L., Tesler, M. D. et al. (1993). Assessment of postoperative pain in children and adolescents using the Adolescent Pediatric Pain Tool. *Nursing Research, 42*, 5–9.

Savedra, M. C., Tesler, M. D., Holzemer, W. L. et al. (1989). Pain location: Validity and reliability of body outline markings by hospitalized children and adolescents. *Research in Nursing & Health, 12*, 307–314.

Schiavenato, M. (2008). Facial expression and pain assessment in the pediatric patient: The primal face of pain. *Journal for Specialists in Pediatric Nursing, 13*(2), 89–97.

Schmelzle-Lubiecki, B. M., Campbell, K. A., Howard, R. H. et al. (2007). Long-term consequences of early infant injury and trauma upon somatosensory processing. *European Journal of Pain, 11*, 799–809.

Schmitt, Y. S., Hoffman, H. G., Blough, D. K. et al. (2011). A randomized, controlled trial of immersive virtual reality analgesia during physical therapy for pediatric burns. *Burns, 37*(1), 61–68.

Schurman, J. V., Wu, Y. P., Grayson, P. et al. (2010). A pilot study to assess the efficacy of biofeedback-assisted relaxation train as an adjunct treatment for pediatric functional dyspepsia associated with duodenal eosinophilia. *Journal of Pediatric Psychology, 35*(8), 837–847.

Shah, P. S., Herbozo, C., Aliwalas, L. L. et al. (2012). Breastfeeding or breast milk for procedural pain in neonates. *Cochrane Database of Systematic Reviews*, (12), CD004950.

Shields, B. J., Palermo, T. M., Powers, J. D. et al. (2003). Predictors of a child's ability to use a visual analogue scale. *Child Care Health Development, 29*, 281–290.

Shrestha-Ranjit, J. M., & Manias, E. (2010). Pain assessment and management practices in children following surgery of the lower limb. *Journal of Clinical Nursing, 19*(1–2), 118–128.

Sieberg, C. B., Huguet, A., von Baeyer, C. L. et al. (2012). Psychological interventions for headache in children and adolescents. *Canadian Journal of Neurological Sciences, 39*(1), 26–34.

Silva, F. C., & Thuler, L. C. (2008). Cross-cultural adaptation and translation of two pain assessment tools in children and adolescents. *Jornal de Pediatria, 84*(4), 344–349.

Simons, J., Franck, L., & Roberson, E. (2001). Parent involvement in children's pain care: Views of parents and nurses. *Journal of Advanced Nursing, 36*, 591–600.

Simons, S. H. P., & Tibboel, D. (2006). Pain perception development and maturation. *Seminars in Fetal and Neonatal Medicine, 11*(4), 227–231.

Simonse, E., Mulder, P. G., & van Beek, R. H. (2012). Analgesic effect of breast milk versus sucrose for analgesia during heel lance in late preterm infants. *Pediatrics, 129*(4), 657–663.

Singer, A. J., Weeks, R., & Regev, R. (2006). Laser-assisted anesthesia reduces the pain of venous cannulation in children and adults: A randomized controlled trial. *Academic Emergency Medicine, 13*, 623–628.

Sng, Q. W., Taylor, B., Liam, J. L. et al. (2013). Postoperative pain management experiences among school-aged children: A qualitative study. *Journal of Clinical Nursing, 22*(7–8), 958–968.

Solodiuk, J., & Curley, M. A. Q. (2003). Pain assessment in nonverbal children with severe cognitive impairments: The individualized numeric rating scale (INRS). *Journal of Pediatric Nursing, 18*, 295–299.

Solodiuk, J. D., Scott-Sutherland, J., Meyers, M. et al. (2010). Validation of the individualized numeric rating scale (INRS): A pain assessment tool for nonverbal children with intellectual disability. *Pain, 150*(2), 231–236.

Soueid, A., & Richard, B. (2007). Ethyl chloride as a cryoanalgesic in pediatrics for venipuncture. *Pediatric Emergency Care, 23*, 380–383.

South, M. M., Strauss, R. A., South, A. P. et al. (2005). The use of non-nutritive sucking to decrease the physiologic pain response during neonatal circumcision: A randomized controlled trial. *American Journal of Obstetrics and Gynecology, 193*, 537–542.

Sparks, L. A., Setlik, J., & Luhman, J. (2007). Parental holding and positioning to decrease IV distress in young children: A randomized controlled trial. *Journal of Pediatric Nursing, 22*(6), 440–447.

Squire, S. J., Kirchhoff, K. T., & Hissong, K. (2000). Comparing two methods of topical anesthesia used before intravenous cannulation in pediatric patients. *Journal of Pediatric Health Care, 14*(2), 68–72.

Stallard, P., Williams, L., Velleman, R. et al. (2002). The development and evaluation of the pain indicator of communicatively impaired children. *Pain, 98*, 145–149.

Stanford, E. A., Chambers, C. T., & Craig, K. D. (2005). A normative analysis of the development of pain-related vocabulary in children. *Pain, 114*, 278–284.

Stevens, B., Abbott, L. K., Yamada, J. et al. (2011). Epidemiology and management of painful procedures in children in Canadian hospitals. *CMAJ: Canadian Medical Association Journal, 183*(7), E403–E410.

Stevens, B., Johnston, C. C., Petryshen, P. et al. (1996). Premature infant pain profile: Development and initial validation. *Clinical Journal of Pain, 12*, 13–22.

Stevens, B., Yamada, J., Beyene, J. et al. (2005). Consistent management of repeated procedural pain with sucrose in preterm neonates: Is it effective and safe for repeated use over time? *The Clinical Journal of Pain, 21*, 543–548.

Sundblad, G. M. B., Saartok, T., & Engström, L.-M. T. (2007). Prevalence and co-occurrence of self-rated pain and perceived health in school-children: Age and gender differences. *European Journal of Pain, 11*, 171–180.

Taddio, A., Appleton, M., Bortolussi, R. et al. (2010). Reducing the pain of childhood vaccination: An evidence-based clinical practice guideline. *CMAJ: Canadian Medical Association Journal, 182*(18), E843–E855.

Taddio, A., Shah, V., Shah, P. et al. (2003). B-endorphin concentration after administration of sucrose in preterm infants. *Archives of Pediatrics & Adolescent Medicine, 157*, 1071–1074.

Taddio, A., Soin, H. K., Schuh, S. et al. (2005). Liposomal lidocaine to improve procedural success rates and reduce procedural pain among children: A randomized controlled trial. *Canadian Medical Association Journal, 172*, 1691–1695.

Tait, A. R., Boepel-Lewis, T., Snyder, R. M. et al.(2008). Parents' understanding of information regarding their child's postoperative pain management. *Clinical Journal of Pain, 24*(7), 572–577.

Taylor, E. M., Boyer, K., & Campbell, F. A. (2008). Pain in hospitalized children: A prospective cross-sectional survey of pain prevalence, intensity, assessment and management in a Canadian pediatric teaching hospital. *Pain Research and Management, 13*(1), 25–32.

Taylor, C., Sellick, K., & Greenwood, K. (2011). The influence of adult behaviors on child coping during venipuncture: A sequential analysis. *Research in Nursing and Health, 32*(2), 116–131.

Terstegen, C., Koot, H. M., de Boer, J. B. et al. (2003). Measuring pain in children with cognitive impairment: Pain response to surgical procedures. *Pain, 103*(1–2), 187–198.

Tesler, M. D., Holzemer, W. L., & Savedra, M. C. (1998). Pain behaviors: Postsurgical responses of children and adolescents. *Journal of Pediatric Nursing, 13*(1), 41–47.

The Joint Commission. (2012). Safe use of opioids in hospitals. *The Joint Commission Sentinel Event Alert, 49*, 1–5.

Thomas, A., & Chess, S. (1977). *Temperament and development.* New York, NY: Brunner/Mazel.

Toth, M., Marcantonio, E. R., Davis, R. B. et al. (2013). Massage therapy for patients with metastatic cancer: A pilot randomized controlled trial. *Journal of Alternative and Complementary Medicine.* Advance online publication.

Twycross, A. (2010). Managing pain in children: Where to from here? *Journal of Clinical Nursing, 19*(15–16), 2090–2099.

Twycross, A., & Collins, S. (in press). Nurses' views about the barriers and facilitators to effective management of pediatric pain. *Pain Management Nursing.*

Uman, L. S., Chambers, C. T., McGrath, P. J. et al. (2006). Psychological interventions for needle-related procedural pain and distress in children and adolescents. *Cochrane Database of Systematic Reviews,* (4), CD005179.

U.S. Food and Drug Administration. (2012). *FDA drug safety communication: Codeine use in certain children after tonsillectomy and/or adenoidectomy may lead to rare, but life-threatening adverse events or death.* Retrieved from http://www.fda.gov/Drugs/DrugSafety/ucm313631.htm

Van Cleve, L., Muñoz, C., Bossert, E. A. et al. (2001). Children's and adolescents' pain language in Spanish: Translation of a measure. *Pain Management Nursing, 2*, 110–118.

Van Cleve, L., Muñoz, C. E., Savedra, M. et al. (2012). Symptoms in children with advanced cancer: Child and nurse reports. *Cancer Nursing, 35*(2), 115–125.

Van Cleve, L. J., & Savedra, M. C. (1993). Pain location: Validity and reliability of body outline markings by 4 to 7-year-old children who are hospitalized. *Pediatric Nursing, 19*, 217–220.

van der Marel, C. D., van Lingen, R. A., Plueim, M. A. L. et al. (2001). Analgesic efficacy of rectal versus oral acetaminophen in children after major craniofacial surgery. *Clinical Pharmacology & Therapeutics, 70*, 82–90.

van Dijk, A., McGrath, P. A., Pickett, W. et al. (2006). Pain prevain nine- to 13-year-old school children. *Pain Research & Management, 11*(4), 234–240.

van Dijk, M., de Boer, J. B., Koot, H. M. et al. (2000). The reliability and validity of the COMFORT Scale as a postoperative pain instruin 0 to 3-year-old infants. *Pain, 84*, 367–377.

van Dijk, M., de Boer, J. B., Koot, H. M. et al. (2001). The association between physiological and behavioral pain measures in 0–3-year-old infants after major surgery. *Journal of Pain and Symptom Management, 22*, 600–608.

van Dijk, M., Peters, J., van Deventer, P. et al. (2005). The COMFORT behavior scale: A tool for assessing pain and sedation in infants. *American Journal of Nursing, 105*(1), 33–36.

Van Niekerk, L. M., & Martin, F. (2003). The impact of the nurse–physician relationship on barriers encountered by nurses during pain management. *Pain Management Nursing, 4*, 3–10.

Varni, J., Thompson, K., & Hanson, V. (1987). The Varni/Thompson pediatric pain questionnaire. I. Chronic musculoskeletal pain in juvenile rheumatoid arthritis. *Pain, 28*, 27–38.

Verghese, S. T., & Hannallah, R. S. (2010). Acute pain management in children. *Journal of Pain Research, 15*(3), 105–123.

Vincent, C. V. H. (2005). Nurses' knowledge, attitudes, and practices: Regarding children's pain. *MCN. The American Journal of Maternal Child Nursing, 30*, 177–183.

Voepel-Lewis, T., Malviya, S., & Tait, A. R. (2005). Validity of parent ratings as proxy measures of pain in children with cognitive impairment. *Pain Management Nursing, 6*, 168–174.

Voepel-Lewis, T., Merkel, S., Tait, A. R. et al. (2002). The reliability and validity of the face, legs, activity, cry, consolability observational tool as a measure of pain in children with cognitive impairment. *Anesthesia & Analgesia, 95*(5), 1224–1229.

Voepel-Lewis, T., Zanotti, J., Dammeyer, J. A. et al. (2010). Reliability and validity of the face, legs, activity, cry, consolability behavioral tool in assessing acute pain in critically ill patients. *American Journal of Critical Care Nurses, 19*(1), 55–61.

Von Baeyer, C. L., Marche, T. A., Rocha, E. M. et al. (2004). Children's memory for pain: Overview and implications for practice. *The Journal of Pain, 5*, 241–249.

Walker, L. S., Dengler-Crish, C. M., Rippel, S. et al. (2010). Functional abdominal pain in childhood and adolescence increases risk for chronic pain in adulthood. *Pain, 150*(3), 568–572.

Walsh, B. M., & Bartfield, J. M. (2006). Survey of parental willingness to pay and willingness to stay for "painless" intravenous catheter placement. *Pediatric Emergency Care, 22*, 699–703.

Wang, H. L., & Keck, J. F. (2004). Foot and hand massage as an intervention for postoperative pain. *Pain Management Nursing, 5*, 59–65.

Wennstrom, B., & Bergh, I. (2008). Bodily and verbal expressions of postoperative symptoms in 3- to 6-year-old-boys. *Journal of Pediatric Nursing, 23*(1),65–76.

Wielenga, J. M., De Vos, R., de Leeuw, R. et al. (2004). COMFORT Scale: A reliable and valid method to measure the amount of stress of ventilated preterm infants. *Neonatal Network, 23*(2), 39–44.

Willis, M. H. W., Merkel, S. I., Voepel-Lewis, T. et al. (2003). FLACC behavioral pain assessment scale: A comparison with the child's self-report. *Pediatric Nursing, 29*, 195–198.

Windich-Biermeier, A., Sjoberg, I., Dale, J. C. et al. (2007). Effects of distraction on pain, fear, and distress during venous port access and venipuncture in children and adolescents with cancer. *Journal of Pediatric Oncology Nursing, 24*, 8–19.

Wint, S. S., Eshelman, D., Steele, J. et al. (2002). Effects of distraction using virtual reality glasses during lumbar punctures in adolescents with cancer. *Oncology Nursing Forum, 29*(1), E8–E15.

Wolitsky, K., Fiyush, R., Zimand, E. et al. (2005). Effectiveness of virtual reality distraction during a painful medical procedure in pediatric oncology patients. *Psychology & Health, 20*, 817–824.

Wong, D., & Baker, C. (1988). Pain in children: Comparison of assessment scales. *Pediatric Nursing, 14*, 9–17.

Wong, J., Ghiasuddin, A., Kimata, C. et al. (2013). The impact of healing touch on pediatric oncology patients. *Integrative Cancer Therapy, 12*(1), 25–30.

Wong, C. M., McIntosh, N., Menon, G. et al. (2003). The pain (and stress) in infants in a neonatal intensive care unit. In N. L. Schechter, C. B. Berde, & M. Yaster (Eds.), *Pain in infants, children, and adolescents* (2nd ed., pp. 669–692). Philadelphia, PA: Lippincott Williams & Wilkins.

Woodgate, R. L., & Degner, L. F. (2003). Expectations and beliefs about children's cancer symptoms: Perspectives of children with cancer and their families. *Oncology Nursing Forum, 30*, 479–491.

Woolf, C. J. (2004). Pain: Moving from symptom control toward mechanism-specific pharmacologic management. *Annals of Internal Medicine, 140*, 441–451.

Wuhrman, E., Cooney, M. F., Dunwoody, C. J. et al. (2007). Authorized and unauthorized ("PCA by proxy") dosing of analgesic infusion pumps: Position statement with clinical practice recommendations. *Pain Management Nursing, 8*(1), 4–11.

Yamada, J., Stinson, J., Lamba, J. et al. (2008). A review of systematic reviews on pain interventions in hospitalized infants. *Pain Research Management, 13*(5), 413–419.

Yeh, C. H. (2005). Development and validation of the Asian version of the Oucher: A pain intensity scale for children. *Journal of Pain, 6*, 526–534.

Zempsky, W. T., & Schechter, N. L. (2003). What's new in the management of pain in children? *Pediatrics in Review, 24*, 337–348.

Zhou, H., Roberts, P., & Horgan, I. (2008). Association between self-report pain ratings of child and parent, child and nurse and parent and nurse dyads: Meta-analysis. *Journal of Advanced Nursing, 63*(4), 334–342.

Zisk, R. Y., Grey, M., Medoff-Cooper, B. et al. (2007). Accuracy of parental–global impression of children's acute pain. *Pain Management Nursing, 8*, 72–76.

See thePoint for additional resources.

CHAPTER 11

Acute Illness as a Challenge to Health Maintenance

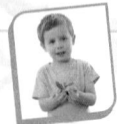

CASE HISTORY

Remember the Whitworth family and Cory Whitworth in Chapter 6? Cory has never been a good eater, but during the past few days, he has refused to eat at all and has had a fever off and on, although he is still drinking. This morning, he seemed more comfortable and playful, so Wendy sent him off to kindergarten. The school called when he began crying and guarding his abdomen. Wendy took him directly to the pediatrician's office; however, after an initial physical examination, the pediatrician sent them to the nearest hospital with a pediatric facility to determine whether appendicitis was the cause of the intense abdominal pain.

In the emergency room, it is determined that Cory has a perforated appendix and will require emergency surgery and hospitalization with intravenous (IV) antibiotics. Although the Whitworths have had children in the emergency room for various cuts and breaks, this is the first time one of their children has needed surgery. When Wendy hears the words *emergency surgery* and *hospitalization*, she becomes extremely anxious and overwhelmed. She feels as if she cannot absorb any more information. The Whitworth family had just changed insurance carriers, and not only is the new insurance card not in Wendy's wallet but she is also not sure of the name of the new insurance company. Her husband is out of town today and tomorrow. When she tries to reach him, she finds that his cell phone is turned off for a meeting. Her oldest son, Ken, attends community college on the far end of town, so she calls her second son, Collin, at high school to help her by going home to get the insurance card and bringing it to the hospital.

CHAPTER OBJECTIVES

1 Facilitate care during acute illness to minimize stress for the child and family.

2 Discuss the impact of hospitalization on the child's and family's coping and adaptation responses.

3 Select nursing interventions to provide basic care needs for the child during an episode of acute illness.

4 Discuss interventions that provide psychosocial support to the family during hospitalization.

5 Describe nursing care of the child having surgery.

6 Identify factors that prepare the child and family for a smooth transition from the acute care environment to a community setting.

See thePoint for a list of Key Terms.

Acute illnesses or conditions are those in which changes occur relatively rapidly, reach a certain level of acuity, and then subside. Chronic conditions, in contrast, are present for a prolonged period of time, potentially never resolving. An acute illness is a threat to a child and his or her family characterized by suddenness, severity, and disruption of the normal patterns of everyday life. Acute illness encompasses the minor illnesses that are frequent in childhood (e.g., viral respiratory infections, gastroenteritis, fractures, trauma) and those of a more serious nature (e.g., meningitis, congenital heart disease, appendicitis). The critical nature of the illness and the uncertainty regarding its outcomes challenge the child's emotional well-being and the integrity of the family system.

An acute illness is generally unexpected and may be the result of a traumatic event such as poisoning or injury. For some children, however, the acute illness may be an exacerbation of a chronic condition or the terminal stages of a life-threatening condition and, therefore, an "expected" part of the disease process. Regardless of the precipitating illness, admission to the acute care setting is stressful for all children and their families. Stress and family disruption can be reduced by implementing care based on the developmental and physiologic needs of the child and family and by considering the environment, security issues, and specific care needs of the child.

THE ACUTE CARE EXPERIENCE

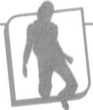 QUESTION: How would family-centered care benefit the Whitworth family? Who should be allowed to stay with Cory, and who should be allowed to visit Cory at the hospital?

The hospitalization of a child is stressful for both the child and the family. An acutely ill child and his or her parents often experience removal from their familiar environment, restricted visiting hours for other family members (e.g., grandparents, siblings) and friends, disruption in routines, a lack of recognition of parents as the primary caregivers who know the child best, and a disruption of their role in planning the child's care. Families may incur financial hardship as parents lose time from work and have expenses such as travel, parking, meals, and babysitters for their other children. Increased parental anxiety and stress have a negative effect on the child's outcomes (Melnyk et al., 2006).

Recognizing that illness and hospitalization are stressful events for families, the **family-centered care** approach has become the philosophical underpinning for the care of children and their families (see Chapter 1). As a partnership between health care providers, patients, and families, the family-centered care model emphasizes dignity, respect, open communication, collaboration, and the restoration of control to individuals and families. Parents want an interactive relationship with health care providers that offers information about their child's care and also demonstrates compassion and sensitivity to the parent's and child's needs (Fisher & Broome, 2011).

Family-centered care encourages liberal 24-hour visitation policies, sibling involvement in hospitalization, pet visitation policies, family conferences to promote shared decision making, assisting families to use support systems, and family education with regard to the care of the child. Family presence during health care procedures typically decreases anxiety for the child and the parents. Family presence, even during resuscitation, is supported by many professional organizations (Fullbrook et al., 2007; Henderson & Knapp, 2006) (Nursing Interventions Classification 11-1).

NIC 11-1 NURSING INTERVENTIONS CLASSIFICATION: Family Presence Facilitation

Definition: Facilitation of the family's presence in support of an individual undergoing resuscitation and/or invasive procedures

Activities:

Introduce yourself to the staff treating the patient and family

Determine suitability of the physical location for family presence

Obtain consensus from the staff for the family's presence and the timing of the family's presence

Apprise the treatment team of the family's emotional reaction to the patient's condition, as appropriate

Obtain information concerning the patient's status, response to treatment, identified needs

Introduce yourself and other members of the support team to the family and patient.

Communicate information concerning the patient's current status in a timely manner

Assure family that best care possible is being given to the patient

Use the patient's name when speaking to the family

Determine the patient's and the family's emotional, physical, psychosocial, and spiritual support needs and initiate measures to meet those needs, as necessary

Determine the psychological burden of prognosis for family

Foster realistic hope, as appropriate

Advocate for family, as appropriate

Prepare the family, ensuring they have been informed about what to expect, what they will see, hear, and/or smell

Inform the family of behavior expectations and limits

Provide a dedicated staff person to assure that family members are never left unattended at the bedside

Accompany the family to and from the treatment or resuscitation area, announce their presence to the treatment staff each time the family enters the treatment area

Provide information and explanations of the interventions, medical/nursing jargon, and expectations of the patient's response to treatment

Escort the family from the bedside if requested by the staff providing direct care

Provide the opportunity for the family to ask questions and to see, touch, and speak to the patient prior to transfers

Assist the patient or family members in making telephone calls, as needed

Offer and provide comfort measures and support, including appropriate referrals, as needed

Participate in the evaluation of the staff's and own emotional needs

Assist in identifying need for critical incident stress debriefing, individual defusing of events, etc., as appropriate

Participate, initiate, and/or coordinate family bereavement follow-up at established intervals, as appropriate

From Bulechek, G. M., Butcher, H. K., Dochterman, J. M. et al. (Eds.). (2013). *Nursing interventions classifications (NIC)* (6th ed.). St. Louis, MO: Mosby. Used with permission.

It is essential to include the family as an integral member of the health care team. Research demonstrated that parents wanted to actively participate in their child's care but were limited by nurses' willingness to communicate and negotiate shared care (Corlett & Twycross, 2006). Parents' primary motive for being with the child is to provide emotional support; they are willing to help with care but experience ambiguous boundaries between parents' and nurses' roles (Coyne & Cowley, 2007). An expectation that parents are continually present to provide all care can increase parents' stress. Assess parents' desire for involvement and explicitly negotiate boundaries of care. Obtain family input in developing the plan of care for the child and family.

Children also want to be involved in their care and decision making (Coyne, 2008; Moore & Kirk, 2010). Give the children as much control as they desire and as is developmentally appropriate. **Atraumatic care** is provision of care in a manner that minimizes the emotional and physical threat to the child. Regardless of the setting in which care is delivered, implement principles of atraumatic care (Nursing Interventions 11-1) to help minimize the negative effects that may result from interactions with the health care setting.

> *ANSWER:* A benefit of family-centered care for the Whitworth family would include having a family member stay at the bedside and actively participate in Cory's care throughout the hospitalization. Cory's family should be allowed to identify those individuals whose presence and support will promote family coping. For example, open visitation by friends and family members facilitates support of Cory and his family. However, it is important that Cory still has periods to rest and have optimal sleep. All the members of the family as well as preidentified members of their church should be allowed to visit Cory.

THE ACUTE CARE ENVIRONMENT

The acute care environment encompasses various settings including inpatient units, outpatient clinics, pediatric emergency rooms, same-day surgery centers, pediatric rehabilitation units, and palliative care units. For a discussion of specific care settings, see thePoint for Supplemental Information: Care Delivery Settings for Children. No matter the setting, the acute care environment is typically busy and full of unexpected and often unpleasant events for the child. Anxiety, fear, pain, discomfort, surprise, fatigue, frustration, mistrust, and anger are common experiences for the child and the family. Nurses must be sensitive to these experiences and develop a plan of care that enhances family function and reduces the stressors associated with interaction in the acute care setting. Room design, including waiting rooms, should address comfort, education and information needs, facilitation of social interaction, and privacy needs. Play area design should be appropriate to the ages and physical conditions of the children served. Excessive noise levels can

have negative psychophysiologic effects (Macedo et al., 2009) and disrupt sleep patterns (Salandin et al., 2011; Stremler et al., 2007). Privacy and noise reduction are important factors in all designs, particularly treatment rooms, so that children are not frightened by what they see and hear in other rooms. The latter guideline holds true especially for emergency departments, which can be chaotic and consequently terrifying for children (Fig. 11-1).

Skilled interventions critical to caring for the child and family in the acute care setting include

- Facilitating entry into the acute care setting
- Integrating age-appropriate principles of growth and development in all care
- Supervising or implementing routine care and procedures in a nonthreatening way
- Maintaining, to the extent possible, the child's daily routines
- Maintaining safety
- Responding to the unique psychosocial needs of the child and family
- Addressing the needs of the child undergoing surgery
- Implementing effective discharge

NURSING CARE OF THE CHILD AND FAMILY DURING THE ADMISSION PROCESS

> *QUESTION:* Cory and his family had very rapid transitions: from pediatrician's office, to emergency room, to surgical suite, and then to the pediatric care unit. He did not have the benefit of a hospital tour nor have his parents had a child hospitalized before. How would you individualize nursing care during admission for the Whitworth family? For whom is the admission process most stressful?

The admission process is the beginning of the relationship between the child, the family, and the health care staff. It assumes great importance because a positive first impression serves as a basis for establishing a trusting and supportive relationship among the health care team, the child, and the family, which generally leads to improved outcomes (Nursing Interventions 11-2).

With the increase in technology and use of bedside computers, some facilities have adopted a "bedside admission process" that bypasses the admitting department (Fig. 11-2). This allows direct access to the pediatric setting where developmentally appropriate communication techniques are the standard of care and can help relieve fears and anxiety associated with an unfamiliar environment.

PREPARING THE CHILD AND FAMILY FOR ADMISSION: HOSPITAL TOURS

To meet the developmental needs of prospective patients and their families, they should have an opportunity to tour the acute care setting before hospital admission or

NURSING INTERVENTIONS 11-1

Delivering Atraumatic Care

Aspect of Care	Interventions
Psychological	Always explain what is happening to the child—in his or her terms, not in adult or medical terms. Do not go into a lot of detail; keep it simple, direct, and honest. Do not tell the child it is not going to hurt if it is, but do not dwell on the pain factor. The use of topical anesthesia and medications assists in obtaining the cooperation of the child in the procedure. Ask the child to draw a picture of what is going to happen; you may find many misconceptions as well as opportunities for discussion. Keep the parents involved as much as possible in nurturing and supporting the child; do not isolate the child from the parent. The parent's absence may be more traumatic to the child than the procedure. It is important to discuss the concept of parent and family presence during procedures as a part of the admission process. Decisions that the family makes regarding presence or absence during procedures need to be respected and communicated as part of the plan of care.
Environment	Keep the child's environment as nonthreatening as possible. Interpret the surroundings from the child's point of view. What does that large machine look like? Possibly a monster? Are there all types of implements out that cause pain or look scary? Is the room very sterile with no friendly items around? The machines can be draped with sheets or put in other areas; the implements can be put away. To soften the area and to distract the child from any potential procedures, add pictures (even hand drawn) of rainbows, butterflies, or flowers or add a stuffed animal.
Restraints	Use restraints as minimally as possible and use the least restrictive one that provides safety (e.g., start with mittens first before a full arm restraint). Attempt, at first, to distract the child by playing games or with toys, singing songs, reading stories, or telling silly jokes. If the IV is in the child's right hand and the child is right handed, both the nurse and the child should draw left handed and make designs, "silly" pictures, or play board games that only require one hand. If it is absolutely necessary to restrain a child, allow periods of freedom while supervised (e.g., during bath or meals).
Pain	Medicate freely. Do not withhold medication after surgery because the infant or child is not crying. Look for other signs of distress: pallor, furrowed brow, grimaces, shallow and rapid breathing, withdrawal of limb or area in pain, or thrashing around. Obtain the child's subjective rating of pain if possible. Always ask the family and child, if age appropriate, the types of painful procedures that they have experienced and what words the child uses for pain. It is also helpful to know what strategies to use to relieve the pain (i.e. certain positions, comfort items, and methods of distraction).
Surgery	Prepare child prior to hospitalization, if possible, with a visit to see the environment, play with the items to be used to gain familiarity (blood pressure cuff, masks [both surgical and anesthesia], IV equipment, etc.), and have the schedule explained. Once a child is admitted, it may be helpful, based on the child's developmental age and personality, to again show him or her the equipment that may be used during a procedure. It is not necessary to show the child equipment that he or she won't remember because of being sedated or anesthetized. Have the child draw pictures and tell a story about the experience to get a better idea of the child's true impressions.
Suturing	Use topical anesthesia prior to injecting the area with an intradermal anesthetic. Use as fine a needle as possible (30 gauge if possible). Cover the wounds with as small a dressing as possible and decrease the size of the dressings as the wound improves. A child may correlate the size of the dressing with the severity of the wound.

(Continued)

NURSING INTERVENTIONS 11-1

Delivering Atraumatic Care *(Continued)*

Blood drawing	Draw blood as infrequently as possible. Attempt to draw as few specimens as possible for the maximum amount of tests. When doing heel sticks on infants, use a nontraumatic lancet such as a Tenderfoot rather than a regular lancet or a scalpel blade. When doing venous draws, apply a topical anesthetic in enough time prior to the draw to allow for sufficient anesthesia. Use sucrose analgesia prior to blood draws, IVs, and injections in babies under the age of 12 months (Harrison et al., 2010)
IVs	Prior to the insertion, use a topical anesthetic. Attempt to place the IV in a location where the child or infant will not need a lot of restraints or arm boards. If this is not possible, use padded or air-filled arm boards of the appropriate size and with a non-threatening look (e.g., colorful covers with pediatric designs) to provide extra cushioning. Allow the older child to become familiar with the IV equipment by using tubing for play or creative endeavors. Soften the impact of IV poles and pumps by attaching pictures of animals, butterflies, or rainbows or by adding stuffed animals to them.
Injections	Advocate for the child; ask if medications can be administered via a less traumatic route. Use the appropriate length and bore needle. Administer medication in the largest muscle mass possible, as deep as possible. Use a topical anesthetic in enough time prior to injection to provide local anesthesia. If medication is very irritating, mix with a small amount of lidocaine, unless it is contraindicated.

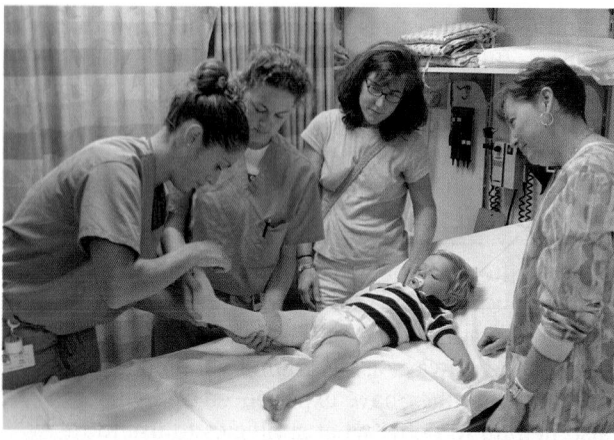

Figure 11-1 A child may be overwhelmed by the sights, sounds, and bustle of the emergency room. A parent's presence can help the child cope with this unfamiliar, sometimes frightening environment.

surgery (Chart 11-1). A successful preoperative tour can create a positive impression of the surgical experience and defuse a potentially threatening event for the child and family. It lets the child and family meet the care providers and other staff members and become accustomed to the environment. This is particularly useful for children in early childhood who may be especially frightened by hospitalization and are old enough to benefit from the desensitization effects of a preadmission program (Fig. 11-3).

Most children undergoing surgery desire comprehensive information about their surgery and postoperative pain (Fortier et al., 2009). If an older child is especially anxious about surgery, the facility may arrange for a tour through an operating room (OR) that is not in use, a preoperative area, and a postanesthesia care unit (PACU). If the child is to be admitted to intensive care unit (ICU) after surgery, a tour of this area may be warranted. Presurgery tours are essential for major,

NURSING INTERVENTIONS 11-2

Guidelines for the Admission Experience

- Ensure that the child knows why he or she is coming to the hospital.
- Incorporate parents' feedback regarding methods or tools that have helped the child adjust to past experiences.
- Encourage use of familiar, comforting toys and belongings during the admission.

- Explain in age-appropriate terms the steps to the admission process (admission, laboratory work, patient unit, etc.).
- Use multisensory mechanisms for education, such as play materials, books, and videos that illustrate aspects of hospitalization.

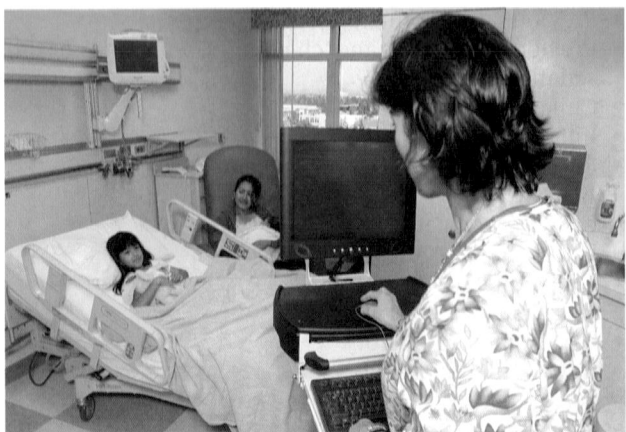

Figure 11-2 Bedside admitting can be easier and less stressful for the child and family.

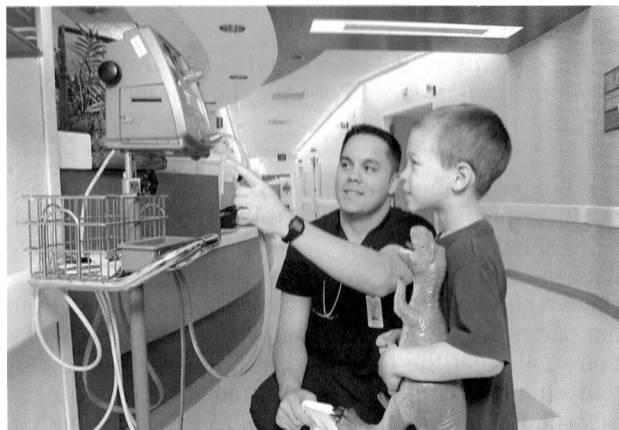

Figure 11-3 A hospital tour familiarizes the child with the new environment.

elective surgical procedures such as insertion of spinal instrumentation for scoliosis. Make the tour more child friendly by using a large doll or stuffed animal to help demonstrate machinery that the child will encounter. A child may be reassured to see a teddy bear on the operating table "have a special sleep for surgery" and then "wake up" to be hugged. Explain the purposes of hospital pajamas, masks, caps, shoe covers, and gloves and let the child try them on. Let the child hear the beeps of an electrocardiograph (ECG) machine and feel

the stickiness of the ECG pads, place a pulse oximeter probe on the child's fingers or toes, put a blood pressure cuff on the child, or let the child listen to his or her own heartbeat through a stethoscope.

If the facility cannot provide tours of the OR, substitute with photographs, a slide show, or a video presentation of a tour. Many facilities are implementing virtual preoperative tours available online prior to surgery (Tourigney et al., 2011). No matter what form the tour takes, presenting a certificate to each child upon completion of the tour gives the child a concrete reminder of his or her experience.

Some facilities have taken the hospital tour to the local community. In this outreach program, health care personnel use a video and discussion to present the hospital tour to schools and other community organizations.

CONDUCTING AN ADMISSION ASSESSMENT

Obtain physiologic and psychosocial data during the admission assessment. The data collected about the child and family allows the nurse to develop an individualized plan of care. Ideally, perform the assessment when the child's primary caregiver is present. The caregiver is able to give historical information about the child's health status, such as childhood illnesses and immunizations. The assessment can be initiated via a phone call placed 1 to 2 weeks prior to surgery. Basic information such as cultural needs, religious preferences, and language barriers can be identified prior to the day of admission. Psychosocial assessments of younger children, especially during infancy and early childhood, cannot be completed without the assistance of a parent. The exception to this is the adolescent whose privacy and confidentiality needs may preclude the presence of a family member. However, family members can provide great insight into any age child.

Communicate with the caregiver in a context of respect for their role as the person most knowledgeable about the child, whether this individual is the parent, grandparent, or other legal guardian. Recognizing this, the term *parent* used in this chapter refers to all primary caregivers.

CHART 11-1   Guidelines for Conducting a Hospital Tour

- Determine whether a preadmission tour would benefit or frighten the child.
- Keep groups small—about 10 children per group.
- Conduct the tour for 20–30 minutes, depending on the children's attention span. The nurse or child life specialist conducting the tour should have time dedicated for the tour with no interruptions.
- Encourage parents to join the tour.
- When unable to actually tour the site (e.g., emergency on unit, presenting at a school), use an indirect method of presenting the hospital tour, such as a puppet, film, or slide show.
- Present the tour and explanations at the child's developmental level.
- Avoid dwelling on unpleasant or threatening events or intrusive procedures.
- Give the children and parents an opportunity to ask questions.
- Give the children an opportunity for therapeutic play, using dolls and hospital equipment.
- Give the children something to take home to remind them of the hospital tour, such as a coloring book, mask, or head cover.
- Encourage parents to discuss the tour afterward with the child and to clarify any concerns he or she may have about the hospital.

caREminder

The objective of the assessment is to learn the information needed to provide the best possible care for the child.

If the parent understands the objective of the assessment, to provide the best possible care for the child, he or she will most likely be more willing to cooperate with the assessment. Provide as much privacy as possible, with minimal noise or stimulation. Learning from the parent about how the child copes with new situations and what the child has been told about the current situation is important in planning how to approach the child. In addition, approaching the child with a communication style that matches developmental age is a key ingredient in completing an assessment that is most productive for the nurse and least frightening for the child (Developmental Considerations 11-1).

Most acute care settings have standardized forms for the admission assessment. These forms can cue the nurse to elicit all the important information in the most efficient manner possible. The tool's design helps the nurse better understand the child's physiologic and developmental needs as well as the social, spiritual, and cultural practices that might be affected by hospitalization. The tool must be comprehensive and useful to serve as a sufficient mechanism for determining the child's condition upon admission and should cover key assessment areas of the child's history, including

- Present illness or reason for seeking health care
- Birth history
- Previous health challenges
- Previous surgeries and challenges with anesthesia/sedation
- Childhood illnesses
- Immunizations
- Recent exposure to communicable diseases
- Allergies
- Current medications
- Pain history (acute and chronic)
- Nutritional assessment
- Elimination patterns
- Family medical history
- Environmental history
- Social history
- Growth and developmental history

At a minimum, the admission assessment should also include a general head-to-toe physical assessment of

- Skin, head, eyes, ears, nose, and throat
- Neurologic system
- Cardiovascular and respiratory systems
- Gastrointestinal system
- Genitourinary/reproductive system
- Musculoskeletal system

Based on this general examination, establish priorities for more in-depth assessment in a particular area. For example, if an infant has no bowel sounds, the need for further immediate assessment and intervention becomes the priority of the examination. The documentation of findings, reporting of variances from the norm to appropriate personnel, and the development of a plan of care are also key ingredients of admission care.

DEVELOPMENTAL CONSIDERATIONS 11-1

Communicating With Children

Stage	Guidelines for Communication
Infancy	Allow the infant to keep the parent in view. Rely on the parent to interpret the infant's nonverbal cues. Use pacifiers and blankets for security.
Early childhood	Be concrete in verbal descriptions. Use visual aids such as puppets and dolls. Allow the child to handle instruments before you use them, when possible. Demonstrate the use of an instrument on a parent prior to using it on the child. Provide opportunities to ask questions. Encourage the parents to be present for interactions. Respect emerging sense of modesty.
Middle childhood	Allow time for composure and privacy. Use teaching aids such as dolls and diagrams. Provide explanations of equipment function.
Adolescence	Provide assurance of privacy and confidentiality. Provide some time away from the parent. Respect the adolescent's privacy and opinions by not prying or being judgmental. Although the adolescent is capable of abstraction, do not overestimate this capability. Provide diagrams and models to ensure comprehension.

ANSWER: The admission process is most stressful for Wendy. She has never had a child hospitalized before, her husband is out of town, and her only immediate family support is her high school–aged son. Remember that stress decreases problem-solving abilities. Wendy's anxiety level and sense of being overwhelmed may affect her ability to answer extensive questions regarding Cory's history. The nurse should focus on the questions most pertinent to the surgery first (e.g., "Does Cory have any allergies?" and "When did he last eat or drink?"). Cory is sedated and prepared for surgery as soon as it is determined that the appendix has ruptured. Much of the physical assessment will be done without his awareness. Also, permission to use the extended support of their family and church will help to decrease some of the stress inherent in Cory's emergency hospital admission. Prompt the family with concrete examples: "Do you have a religious affiliation?" "Is there someone in your church that you should contact?" "Would you like to speak with our chaplain at the hospital?" "Do you have any other family or friends that you want to make aware that Cory is in the hospital?"

NURSING CARE OF THE CHILD AND FAMILY DURING HOSPITALIZATION

Soon after admission to an acute care setting, the child and family encounter routines related to that setting. These routines include procedures that are part of the child's diagnostic evaluation and treatment as well as care that affects activities of daily living (ADLs). The most common routines include hygiene, safety, routine procedures, medication administration, and infection control. Each of these provides an intrusion into the child's and family's privacy because they represent and mandate a departure from the family's way of life at home. Continuity between home life and hospital life is often difficult to achieve; nonetheless, an admission assessment that reveals as much as possible about home routines, likes, dislikes, coping mechanisms, favorite toys, and activities can help the nurse assist the child and family in bridging the gap between home and hospital routines (Fig. 11-4). Many routines from the home environment (including various ADLs, sleep patterns, and nutrition habits) can be transferred, or adapted with minor changes, to the hospital environment.

PROMOTING ACTIVITIES OF DAILY LIVING

QUESTION: For the Whitworth family, what are the steps you would take to delineate the role of family members and the role of the nurse regarding Cory's ADLs?

Perhaps the hospital routines that are most disruptive to home patterns are those regarding ADLs. Bathing, oral care, dressing, and toileting are such basic functions that the ways in which one performs them are taken for granted. Having an acute illness changes the way in which these basic functions are performed as a result of the child's physical condition and restrictions caused by treatment devices.

ADLs are determined by culture as well as by family practices, rituals, and individual preferences. By assessing them thoroughly during admission, the nurse can enhance desired patient outcomes. This is true because much greater cooperation is achieved if care delivery mimics as closely as possible what was done at home. Communicating the child's and family's preferences to all involved care providers is a key part of developing an interdisciplinary plan of care for the child.

ANSWER: As soon as the child is stabilized, set aside time to meet with the parents for a care conference. The time taken is very worthwhile and saves time and emotional energy throughout the course of the stay. Ask the parents what aspects of Cory's care they would like to provide. Systematically go through specific examples of ADLs (e.g., "Would you like the nurses to give Cory his bath or is that something you prefer to do?").

Bathing

Safety and privacy are the greatest concerns in bathing. Infants through preschoolers should never be left alone when bathing. Infants who can sit alone may be bathed in a tub under constant supervision. Young children also need to be bathed, but they can help. Preschoolers can be more independent with bathing but still need assistance. Children of these ages are more comfortable if a parent or grandparent helps them with their bath, especially after they reach the stage of stranger anxiety, which begins around age 6 to 8 months. Middle childhood–aged children can bathe themselves, especially after age 8 years, barring developmental or physical disabilities, but may not be as thorough as they should. During middle childhood, children who have the physical strength to bathe alone are not at risk for accidents while bathing, unlike infants and those in early childhood. However, assess developmental

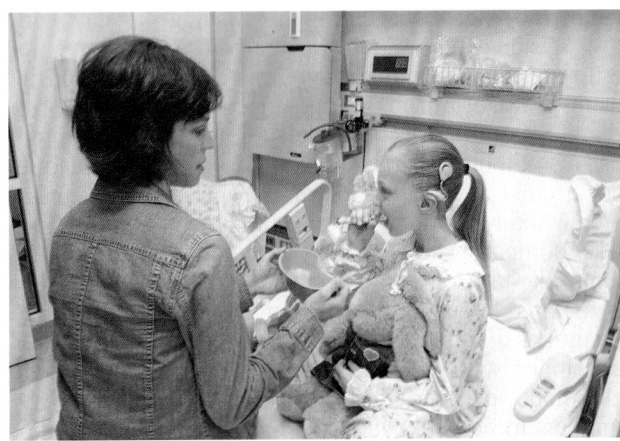

Figure 11-4 Having familiar objects and maintaining home routines normalizes the environment and helps the child cope with hospitalization.

capacities before making this professional judgment. Developmentally delayed children of all ages may require constant supervision during the bath. Adolescents are often preoccupied with hygiene, and the primary concern becomes having the "space" and time to carry out the desired hygiene rituals in the most private, autonomous way possible. For patients who are too ill to get into a tub or shower, the bed bath becomes a necessity. Prepackaged single-use disposable baths reduce adult patient agitation and nursing time over basin and soap and are cost-effective (Larson et al., 2004); more research is needed with children.

Frequency and timing of bathing are often culturally determined. Respect habits within the confines of standards acceptable for infection control and scheduling. Some children are accustomed to bathing in the morning, whereas others prefer to bathe before bed. If the child is fairly independent, arranging for a shower or bath before bedtime may greatly increase their personal satisfaction. A bath every day is not necessary, provided that the patient is clean enough for infection control; however, cleanse face, hands, and perineal area daily.

CROSS-CULTURAL CARE

Not all cultures use the same types of products for bathing and hair care. Checking with the parents for assistance and asking them to bring in supplies is helpful. Bathing and hair care may be left to willing family members as long as it does not jeopardize patient safety.

For children hospitalized for longer than a few days, periodic hair washing is necessary. Wash an infant's hair daily or every other day to prevent cradle cap. Older children typically need one or two shampoos per week.

Oral Care

Providing oral care for children is a necessary and challenging aspect of hygiene. Young children often do not like to have their teeth brushed and thus resist. Children younger than the age of 8 years need assistance with mouth care. Although it is important to permit preschool-aged children to begin brushing their own teeth, they need one thorough brushing per day with the assistance of an adult. Infants whose teeth have not erupted still need mouth care; this can be provided by using a washcloth or sponge-tipped applicators to rub the gums and oral cavity. After the teeth have erupted, use a soft toothbrush and dental floss to remove plaque. For a child at high risk of caries, such as living in an area without fluoridated water, a minute amount of fluoride toothpaste can be used. Children in early childhood often like to use a familiar brush, although supervision is required to ensure that the child does not ingest large quantities of fluoridated toothpaste and continue to need assistance with brushing and flossing. During middle childhood, children can brush their teeth but need reminders to be attentive to the back surfaces of the molars. After they demonstrate an ability to spit and not swallow, a fluoride mouth rinse is recommended at least

once a day, especially at the night cleaning. Adolescents are usually sensitive about halitosis and how their teeth look, so they are usually compliant with brushing. Some may need to be reminded about flossing and the use of fluoride mouth rinse (Blevins, 2011).

Children who have been treated with certain types of immunosuppressive or chemotherapeutic agents may experience stomatitis. Oral care for these children is key in minimizing the occurrence of infection and/or severity of the condition (see Chapter 22).

Dressing

Some hospitalized children are too sick to dress in anything other than a gown or pajamas. If this is not the case, parents may wish to select outfits for the infant or young child to wear that are more attractive and warmer than the hospital gown. Older children may feel like donning clothes from home. Encourage the child to choose the clothes to wear. This may be especially important to adolescents, whose chief developmental concerns are body image and personal appearance.

Toileting

Many children regress developmentally during hospitalization. Young children who have just begun to master toilet training may revert to diapers. No interventions usually are needed. When children return home, they usually resume their former developmental level. If a child has recently been toilet trained, make a concerted effort to assist the child in maintaining continence. It is important that family members understand that regression is a normal part of hospitalization for children and that previously mastered developmental tasks will be regained upon discharge. The key guideline in toileting is to ensure the patient's privacy and dignity no matter what the age. Adolescents may be particularly embarrassed by the use of a bedpan, especially in a shared room. Male patients of school age and older may be embarrassed by assisted toileting from female nurses, particularly with regard to the use of urinals. Being direct and matter of fact and allowing as much privacy as possible are the preferred interventions in these situations. Keeping toileting implements, such as urinals and bedpans, out of sight when not in use and keeping bedside commodes emptied, clean, and stored as covertly as possible are also common sense interventions related to toileting. Promptly answering the call light promotes trust that assistance is available when needed. This decreases the sense of humiliation and anxiety.

Sleep

The hospital environment is notorious for promoting sleep pattern disturbances. Sleep is necessary to maintain and promote health. Sleep deprivation, however, has deleterious effects on the immune system and can impair healing. Because deep sleep is necessary to growth hormone secretion (Morris et al., 2012), sleep pattern disturbances are a serious concern for care providers in pediatric hospitals.

In the hospital, sleep pattern disturbances can result from three basic types of sources: physiologic, psychological, and environmental. Physiologic factors can include diseases that cause pain, such as juvenile rheumatoid arthritis, and medications that decrease rapid eye movement sleep, such as barbiturates, opiate derivatives, and benzodiazepines. Psychological factors include separation anxiety, which may be the most prevalent cause of sleep disturbance, along with having a preexisting stressor such as a dysfunctional family. The hospital environment also has many factors that can precipitate sleep pattern disturbance; these include noise (such as monitors and alarms), too much light, and treatments and assessments that frequently wake the child (L. Meltzer et al., 2012).

Assessment of home preferences and routines for sleeping is a step toward eliminating sleep pattern disturbance in the hospital. Determining the child's bedtime, sleep duration, bedtime rituals, and nap pattern helps the nurse develop a plan of care that prevents sleep pattern disturbance (Developmental Considerations 11-2; Nursing Interventions 11-3). Model measures to reduce the risk of sudden infant death syndrome, such as placing infants supine for sleep; do not use soft objects or soft bedding in the crib (American Academy

of Pediatrics, Task Force on Sudden Infant Death Syndrome, 2011).

caREminder

Arrange medication schedules, whenever possible, so they do not interrupt a child's sleep. Plan schedules for weighing and acquiring vital signs to coincide with sleep patterns. Weighing is typically performed in the morning upon awakening, prior to feedings. Frequency of assessment of vital signs is determined based on the child's condition; obtain assessments prior to putting the child to sleep, and schedule periods of uninterrupted sleep.

Nutrition

Nutrition can become a major challenge in the care of the hospitalized child. Interruption of personal preferences, habits, or family and cultural practices along with malaise from illness can decrease the child's appetite. Certain medications and treatments can interfere with a child's appetite (e.g., methylphenidate [Ritalin] can

---

DEVELOPMENTAL CONSIDERATIONS 11-2

Sleep Promotion in Hospitalized Children

Developmental Stage	Developmental Guideline
All ages	Post a daily schedule at the child's bedside; include nap times and bedtime. Establish a light–dark cycle if the room has no window. Eliminate noxious stimuli (see Nursing Interventions 11-3). Synchronize hospital routines with the child's normal routines. Treat the child's pain.
Infancy	Provide a sense of security for the infant by rocking and holding during the evening; adhere to home bedtime rituals, such as taking a bottle while rocking. Swaddle a younger infant. Play a familiar lullaby using a musical toy. Place supine for sleep and "back to sleep."
Early childhood	Adhere to home bedtime rituals, such as reading a story, having a snack, and brushing teeth. Use transitional objects from home such as toys, blankets, and clothes. If the parents cannot be present, encourage them to leave pictures of themselves and the family or tape-recorded stories. Arrange telephone calls to family at bedtime.
Middle childhood	Allow the child to express fears of separation through imaginary play with puppets or dolls or through drawings or writing stories. Adhere to bedtime rituals. Arrange telephone calls to family at bedtime.
Adolescence	Enforce mutually agreed upon bedtime. Encourage quiet activity in the hour before bedtime: relaxing music, reading, television. Give back rub. Maintain home bedtime rituals.

NURSING INTERVENTIONS 11-3

Eliminating Noxious Stimuli

- Coordinate care to decrease noise.
- Place noisy equipment away from the head of the bed.
- Keep alarms turned low and promptly respond to them; it is important that monitor alarms are of an appropriate volume so that staff can hear them in order to respond quickly during an emergency.
- Guard against loud talking, laughing, and music.
- Decrease volume on overhead paging system or use cell phones to minimize overhead paging.

- Provide acoustic design measures in the building (e.g., carpet, padded trash can lids, acoustic ceiling tile).
- Cycle light to maintain day and night differentiation.
- Control bright light through dimmed lighting.
- Replace white light with soft yellow lighting.
- Turn off overhead lighting when possible; use direct light at individual bedside as needed; use flashlights to check on children.
- Drape isolettes/cribs to prevent bright light.
- Shield child's eyes and ears.
- Evaluate benefit of providing soft music with a low pitch and slow tempo to promote relaxation.

suppress a child's appetite) and sense of taste (e.g., chemotherapeutic agents and clarithromycin [Biaxin] can result in a metallic aftertaste). Consider all these factors when planning care. Work with the dietitian to determine the optimal diet within the bounds of a prescribed diet. Select developmentally appropriate foods (see Chapters 4 to 7), with input from parents and children who are old enough. Foods may also be brought in by family members, assuming they meet the child's nutritional needs and any dietary restrictions. Make provisions for appropriate storage and refrigeration of this food. Many facilities now have unit-based dietary staff and kitchens so that children can order on demand foods that appeal to them at each meal.

CROSS-CULTURAL CARE

The child may be accustomed to having certain staple foods at every meal. Accommodating these preferences may improve the child's intake as well as satisfaction with care.

MAINTAINING SAFETY

Providing a safe environment for children in the hospital is a particular challenge for the following reasons:

- Children are at risk for unintentional injury.
- Continuous visualization of the child may not always be possible.
- The environment is potentially harmful (equipment, toxic substances).

The challenge to providing a safe environment for a child while in the hospital is to maintain a developmentally appropriate approach. As the child matures, the safety risks and precautions change (Developmental Considerations 11-3). General safety principles include proper identification of the child and treatment to be performed and engineering controls that contribute to overall environmental safety.

Patient Identification

Nurses are responsible for many aspects of care that require impeccable attention to correct patient identification. Examples include administering medications or blood products, obtaining blood samples, performing and preparing children for a variety of medical and surgical procedures, and transporting children to and from various departments. Under any of these circumstances, the consequences of mistaken identity can range from mere embarrassment to personal and professional tragedy. Accurate identification serves two purposes: to reliably identify the individual as the person for whom the service or treatment is intended, and to match the service or treatment to that individual. It is not permissible to use a bed number or only verbally verify the child's name (e.g., "Are you Johnny?") before implementing medical procedures. Verifying the child's identity with two identifiers (e.g., name, date of birth, medical record number) and matching the service about to be performed (by checking the medication label, laboratory requisition, medical record) to the individual is a vital part of every nursing procedure. This is especially pertinent when dealing with preverbal infants or with children whose communicative abilities have been precluded by delayed development or impaired by illness or medical treatment. Document that these precautions have been taken. For example, record the identification bracelet number of a neonate and later note matching it with the birth record and the mother's matching name band. Regulatory agencies such as The Joint Commission and the Centers for Medicare & Medicaid Services (CMS) have standards related to patient identification (see thePoint for more information).

Accurate identification of the child in the acute care setting is aided by placement of an identification (ID) band on the child's wrist or ankle upon admission (Nursing Interventions 11-4). If the child has any known allergies, identify these in a similar manner. This is often done with a separate, brightly colored band placed on the same extremity as the ID band.

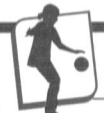

DEVELOPMENTAL CONSIDERATIONS 11-3

Ensuring Child Safety in the Acute Care Setting

Developmental Stage	Age-Specific Activities and Risks	Guidelines During Hospitalization
Infancy	*Activities:* Rolls over Creeps Crawls Pulls to stand Walks *Risks:* Suffocation Falls Choking Drowning	Keep the side rails up on the crib at all times. Always leave infant in a secure environment, such as a crib with side rails up or strapped in a stroller with wheels locked. Do not leave in prone position or propped with pillows. Do not use pillows or soft bedding. Do not allow parents to sleep while holding or rocking infant. Do not leave with bottle propped. Put a net or Plexiglass dome over crib after age 6 months. Never leave unattended near water, in stroller, or in high chair. Avoid wearing removable jewelry when caring for an infant. Do not leave small medical objects in bed or within reach of child
Early childhood	*Activities:* Walks Explores environment Put objects in mouth Feeds self Continues to perfect gross and fine motor skills *Risks:* Falls Burns Suffocation Poisoning Electrical shock from uncovered outlets Drowning Choking	Keep sharp objects out of reach. Keep out of reach any small, hard objects, such as buttons or coins, or balloons that could be aspirated. Keep medication and toxic substances out of reach. Ensure that the crib is covered and side rails are up. Evaluate motor skills for safety of using a large bed; keep side rails up when the child is in bed. Do not leave the child unattended near water. Do not leave the child unattended when not secured, such as unbelted in a stroller or wheelchair. Supervise feeding. Avoid foods that present a choking hazard, such as whole grapes, hot dogs, peanuts.
Middle childhood	*Activities:* Continues to refine fine motor skills Participates in gross motor activities such as sports *Risks:* Falls	Keep side rails up when the child is in bed; if parents/child do not wish this, obtain consent for release. Ensure that child understands mobility limitations. Supervise play activities to minimize risk taking that could lead to falls or other injuries. Discuss stranger safety as age appropriate to hospital setting.
Adolescence	*Activities:* Demonstrates thrill-seeking behaviors Has a preoccupation with body image *Risks:* Substance abuse Noncompliance with medical regimen that affects body image (e.g., not wearing splints)	Provide adolescent-oriented activity rooms that promote age-appropriate activities geared to interest, expression of feelings, and peer interactions. Discuss safety as appropriate to child's treatment, hospital setting, and safety off the unit.

NURSING INTERVENTIONS 11-4

Pediatric Identification Strategies

- Ensure the presence of a name band in locations where direct physical care is provided (e.g., the emergency department, day surgery unit, or an inpatient setting). In the emergency department, the child's parent or caregiver may verify the child's name and date of birth. Place ID bands on the child as soon as possible to assist in accurate identification for all clinicians.
- Always verify the child's identification before performing any nursing procedure. Younger children may answer to any name. Older children may think it is funny to "switch" and trick the nurse. Identification verification requires two separate identifiers (e.g., name, date of birth, medical record number) to identify the child and match the service to be performed with that child.
- Identify and double-check the organ, extremity, or side of the body to be treated with other health team members, taking time-out prior to treatment initiation to deliberately verify patient identity and the service to be performed. The procedure site (if applicable) is marked by the practitioner performing the procedure.
- Double-check crib and wrist tags before removing or returning infants to crib or room.
- Be aware of more than one child with the same name. This occurs frequently in newborn nurs-

eries prior to the infant acquiring a first name. Patients who have duplicate names should have an alert noted on either the paper chart or via the electronic medical record.
- Be aware of the child's whereabouts, on or off the unit.
- Check both ID bands from the delivery setting to match names and numbers in the case of handing a newborn to a mother. It is not realistic to expect newly delivered mothers to recognize their newborns, especially if they are exhausted, sick, or under the influence of mind-impairing medication.
- Ask the mother to keep her own ID band on her wrist when a newborn must remain hospitalized after the mother's discharge. Such ID bands are not removable without cutting them off, and any such handling of the ID band will be readily noticeable.
- Take immediately accessible photographs (digital, Polaroid) of the parents (especially the mother) and infant together in the event of an expected prolonged hospitalization of the newborn. Keep one for the chart, and give parents the other one. Have the parent bring his or her ID band at the time of discharge.

caREminder

If ID or allergy bands are removed (e.g., for IV placement in that extremity), replace them immediately.

Engineering Controls

General engineering controls that enhance environmental (electrical and mechanical) safety contribute to the child's overall safety. These include physical adjuncts such as cribs, side rails, immobilizers, and safe modes of transport. Close monitoring can prevent the child from getting into dangerous situations.

Cribs

Cribs are typically used for infants and young children. Ensure that the crib sides are locked at the highest level when the child is unattended. When providing care to an infant or young child in a crib with the side down, stand next to the child to prevent him or her from rolling off the crib. If you must turn your back or reach for something, always keep one hand on the child's trunk to prevent him or her from falling (Fig. 11-5).

Covers for cribs such as Plexiglass domes, plastic, or netting are commonly used in the pediatric setting. Use them when the child is old enough to pull to stand and thus could conceivably fall out of the crib (Fig. 11-6).

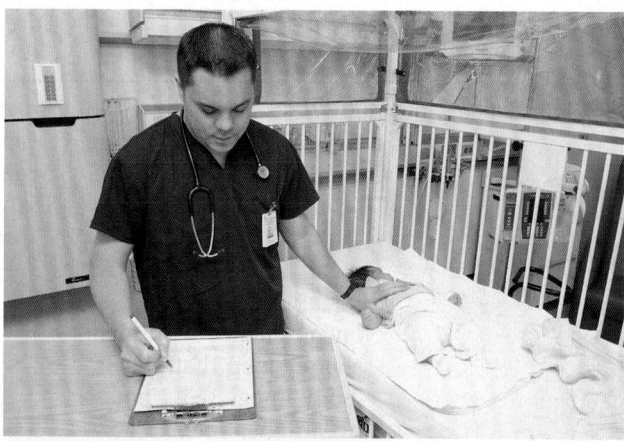

Figure 11-5 Safety is always a priority. Keep at least one hand on the infant at all times when not properly secured.

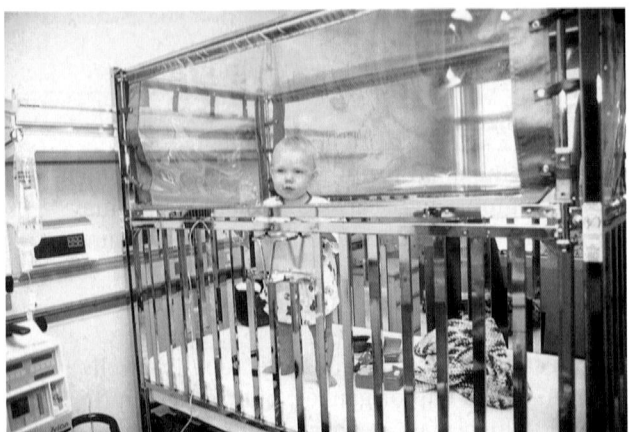

Figure 11-6 A crib cover can be used to restrain a child who is old enough to stand up.

Side Rails

Side rails are commonly used in the hospital to prevent the patient from falling out of bed. Because side rails vary in design, learn how to operate them in that particular setting. Ensure that they are locked in place when leaving the bedside and know how to lower them quickly in an emergency.

Immobilizers

The terms *restraint, immobilization, clinical holding,* and *holding* are often used interchangeably in pediatrics (Brenner, 2007), but there is a distinction between restraining a patient for behavioral reasons and for reducing risk of interfering with treatments. Behavioral health care reasons for restraint are to protect the patient or others from injury because of violent or aggressive behavior (The Joint Commission, 2011). Because restraints to protect surgical and treatment sites are not considered restraint by The Joint Commission (although some state regulations do), the term *immobilization* will be used to indicate actions used to restrict activity as part of the treatment plan (e.g., traction); to prevent interfering with tubes, dressings, or healing tissue (e.g., elbow immobilizers); or to facilitate administration of medications or treatments.

The Joint Commission plays a leadership role in ensuring that hospitals are protecting consumer rights through the appropriate use of restraints. In 2011, The Joint Commission released standards that require that arm, leg, or jacket restraints be checked periodically for neurovascular integrity and general safety and that this assessment information be documented in the patient's chart. Hospital policy dictates the frequency of assessment, but assessment must be performed at least every 15 minutes in behavioral health care settings. Release immobilization devices, when able (e.g., elbow immobilizers), and restraints at least every 2 hours; document assessment of the child's overall status, including hygiene, elimination, and nutrition. A licensed independent practitioner's order stating the reason for the restraint, type of restraint, and duration of restraint is required and must be rewritten every 24 hours.

A serious infringement of patients' rights is the use of restraints for punishment. Never use a restraint to discipline a child or place them in "time-out." Time-outs are used to help the child regain self-control of behavior. The use of restraints imposes an external control rather than allowing the child to develop internal control.

Nurses report using physical restraint to promote inactivity or immobility, to prevent interference with tubes or dressings, to prevent touching or scratching healing tissue, to facilitate administration of medications or treatments, to prevent children from getting out of bed or into dangerous places, or to protect staff from combativeness (Snyder, 2004). Nurses often use these devices because they *think* the child will interfere with treatment (Snyder, 2004).

❗ ALERT   *Because use of restraints and immobilization can result in complications such as falls, incontinence, and pressure sore formation, it is prudent to minimize use of these while still providing a safe environment and preventing disruption of medical treatments (Nursing Interventions 11-5). Exhaust all alternatives to immobilization (e.g., distraction, parental or staff presence) before using any restraint, and implement the least restrictive methods first.*

Limb Immobilizers

Limb immobilizers are used when children could harm themselves if not immobilized, and they are used to prevent treatment interference, such as ensuring the integrity of IV sites, catheters, endotracheal tubes, feeding tubes, and surgical sites and dressings. Many commercial immobilizers are available; most include a soft sponge to protect circulation.

❗ ALERT   *When immobilizing limbs, ensure that the immobilizer cannot tighten around the extremity. Use padding to protect circulation, and fasten it in a way that prevents impaired circulation. Never tie immobilizers to bed side rails because raising or lowering of the rail could injure the immobilized limb.*

Elbow Immobilizers

Elbow immobilizers are sometimes used to prevent the child from reaching the face to do harm. They prevent elbow flexion but leave the hands free for play and exploration (Fig. 11-7). They may be needed after cleft lip and palate repair or to prevent pulling out oral or nasal feeding tubes.

Mummy Immobilization

Mummy immobilization is useful when performing procedures for which the infant or young child must remain still. With appropriate teaching, it may be used by a parent who must perform procedures with the child at home, such as changing tracheostomy tubes or

NURSING INTERVENTIONS 11-5

Alternatives to Using Immobilization

- Increase supervision of child by parents, family, friends, volunteers, or nurses.
- Have windows to increase ability to observe the child when not physically in the same room.
- Actively listen to the child.
- Ask the parent the most effective methods of obtaining compliance from and distracting the child.
- Take the child to the nurses' station or playroom, unless contraindicated by the child's condition.
- Provide activities to distract the child and to promote expression of feelings such as anger or aggression.

- Prepare the child for procedures as developmentally appropriate because a prepared child may maintain better control and need less restraint.
- Hold the child's hand or foot; simple touch may comfort the child and help remind them to "hold still."
- Protect and cover the site (e.g., tape IVs well, cover with a cup or gauze); put clothes on the child, which make it physically more difficult to pull out a tube or disrupt a wound.
- Ensure that the child's hygiene, nutrition, toileting, and comfort needs are met.
- Minimize environmental stimuli if they trigger the child's loss of control.

performing wound care. Place the child on the diagonal of a blanket with the feet and head at opposite corners. Wrap the sides over the child's chest and secure the feet by tucking the lower corner over them (see Fig. 11-7).

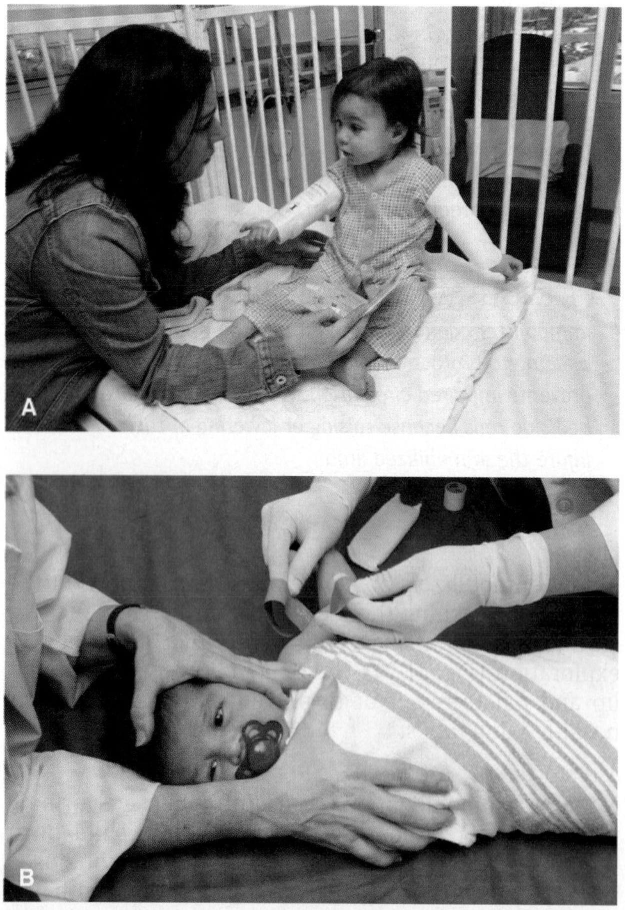

Figure 11-7 Two types of restraints. (A) Elbow restraint. (B) Mummy restraint.

Tape can be used to hold the folds in place. Papoose boards (manufactured boards with canvas flaps that attach in place by Velcro to secure the child during procedures) may also be used.

Safety Belts

Always use safety belts when young children are placed in infant seats, swings, or high chairs. A strap should be secured to the chair that runs between the child's legs up to the belt to prevent the child from sliding down and injuring himself or herself.

Transports

During transport or transfer of the child, several actions can increase safety. It is unsafe to carry a child for a long distance because of the risk of tripping, slipping, falling, or fatiguing. Walking for a distance is not an appropriate option for sick children. Use transport devices, such as wheelchairs and stretchers, to transport children from the pediatric unit to other areas of the hospital, such as radiology or the laboratory. Use a crib-type stretcher with side rails covering the entire length for infants and young children requiring stretcher transport. Never leave a pediatric patient alone when being transported. Also, have ready, easy access to the child's head at all times should vomiting or respiratory distress occur. When the child is being transferred in or out of a stretcher or wheelchair, lock the wheels in place to prevent falls. Always secure the safety straps or "seat belts" on wheelchairs, strollers, and wagons.

Falls

Families expect that children will be safe when they are hospitalized. However, falls do occur. They may occur because of being dropped by staff or families, slipping or tripping, or falling from a bed or chair. Younger children, because of developmental changes, have an increased incidence of falling as they gain motor skills and command of their environment. It is essential that facilities use pediatric fall prevention protocols. These protocols include implementing a standardized assessment tool (Ryan-Wenger et al., 2010), initiating interventions to prevent falls, and educating families about fall risk both in the hospital and at home. Specific interventions are discussed in the preceding sections related to cribs, side rails, immobilizers, and transports.

Latex Allergies

The acute care setting poses a hazard for those who are allergic to latex because the environment contains many products that contain latex as well as airborne latex allergens (particularly from powdered latex gloves). Those with increased exposure to latex are at highest risk of developing latex allergy. Early reports of latex sensitivity were from patients with myelomeningocele. It is now recognized that patients who have undergone multiple surgeries and those with a history of atopy are also at high risk for developing latex allergy (Yeh et al., 2012) (Tradition or Science 11-1).

The most common allergic reaction to latex is a delayed hypersensitivity presenting as contact dermatitis (Yeh et al., 2012). A less common but more serious reaction is an immediate response that presents as urticaria, rhinoconjunctivitis, bronchospasm, and anaphylaxis. Maintain a high index of suspicion regarding latex allergy because its symptoms are difficult to distinguish from other allergic reactions or causes.

The best treatment for latex allergy is identification of high-risk populations and minimizing latex exposure in these children. Latex is found in many products used both in the home and in the health care setting, such as tubing in blood pressure cuffs and stethoscopes, pulse oximeter probes, bulb syringes, catheters, disposable diapers, and some toys (see thePoint for Supplemental Information: Examples of Latex Items in Medical and Community Environments). Make latex-free substitutions when possible. The Spina Bifida Association of America maintains a current list of latex-safe alternatives (see thePoint for Organizations).

Label the medical and dental charts of children at high risk for, or identified with, latex allergy. Notify the child's school or child care center to have nonlatex gloves and an EpiPen available, and notify health care providers in an emergency.

In the acute care setting, latex avoidance is particularly important because many products contain latex. Initiate latex precautions and teach the child and family about latex-containing products. In addition to using latex-free products such as latex-free IV tubing and injection ports, carefully administer medications to prevent latex exposure. It is questionable whether syringes with rubber stoppers on the plunger may leak latex into the medication. Therefore, draw up medications immediately before administration.

Schedule the high-risk child going to surgery as the first case of the day to minimize exposure to airborne latex. Notify the anesthesia care practitioner of the latex allergy. With early identification of children at risk for developing latex allergy and meticulous attention to latex avoidance, latex allergy and the resultant deleterious effects may be minimized.

Visitor Identification and Management

Despite how busy any pediatric setting may become, the nurse must be aware of every individual on the premises and also of visitors' or callers' relationships to specific children. Be aware of strangers on the unit and those asking questions about the children. The possibility of unauthorized adults trying to obtain information about a child's condition, or even of kidnapping and abduction, is very real. This is especially true in large and busy settings where visitor flow is difficult to control. Many facilities now have locked units, and visitors are given passes which open the unit doors. It is a challenge at times to promote an open but safe visitation process.

All visitors should receive prior parental permission; however, this is not the reality in most practice settings, especially with short-stay admissions. Determine information about visitor restrictions with the initial admission assessment. This alerts the nursing staff to situations in which custody issues may arise or in which there are restraining orders preventing specific individuals from seeing certain children. Most facilities allow families to opt out of the hospital admission directory and will respect families who request limited visitation by other family members or friends.

Most of the missing children in the United States are abducted by one of their own parents (Finkelhor & Ormrod, 2002). Some of these abductions occur when the family is experiencing unusual circumstances, such as hospitalization for an acute illness. Proper patient and visitor identification policies, along with a well-planned and structured infant and child security program within the hospital setting, can prevent child abductions and provide a safe environment for the acutely ill child.

Evidence-Based Practice

TRADITION OR SCIENCE 11-1

Is latex allergy more prevalent in children who are exposed to medical procedures? What are the risk factors?

Studies demonstrate a high incidence of latex allergy in children exposed to medical procedures, including those with spina bifida, esophageal atresia, urogenital disorders (Cremer et al., 2007; Yeh et al., 2012), chronic renal failure (Dehlink et al., 2004), hematologic and oncologic disease (Bostanci et al., 2003), and those requiring home ventilation (Nakamura et al., 2000). Sparta et al. (2004) found a positive correlation between the number of operations and latex sensitivity, whereas Hourihane et al. (2002) found that a previous operation increased the odds of latex sensitization 13 times, whereas multiple operations had a less marked effect. Spina bifida has a disease-associated propensity for latex sensitization (Ausili et al., 2007). More inquiry is needed to identify children most at risk, the factors involved, and how much latex exposure may result in sensitization.

Infant and Child Security

Crime and violence against children have drawn much attention at the national level in recent years. Several cases of kidnapping of children from hospitals and nurseries have occurred. Gang violence has become a concern in the pediatric setting as younger and younger children are victims of gang crimes in urban settings and are hospitalized with injuries. Security measures to protect these victims from further retaliation have become necessary.

The safety and protection of patients and others must be secured in the acute care setting. A good security program combines several approaches. The facility must develop and adhere to policies that safeguard children; educate and promote teamwork by all staff, parents, and visitors; and provide physical and electronic security measures (Rabun, 2005).

Security policies vary according to setting. Most units that deal with newborns have strict policies regarding infant, mother, and father ID banding; saving cord blood; obtaining footprints and photographs of the infant shortly after birth; and identifying the person to whom the infant is discharged. Pediatric units must have similar policies in place (Chart 11-2). The institution should post and enforce the policy that parents are not allowed to leave children unattended in waiting rooms.

All staff, parents, and visitors must be familiar with security policies and adhere to them. Staff should be informed of the policies during orientation and should inform parents and children (as appropriate) during the child's admission to the facility. Everyone must be alert for suspicious behavior and report it immediately. Abductors often do not target a specific child but plan carefully, visit the facility, and seize the opportunity to take a child when it presents itself. The more obstacles a potential abductor encounters, the greater the chance to prevent the abduction (Teaching Intervention Plan 11-1). Teamwork is essential both to deter a potential abductor and to ensure rapid response if

an abduction occurs. Critical incident response policies must be in place to ensure a rapid, coordinated response when an incident occurs. A rapid response increases the chance that the child will be found. Most facilities actually practice abduction scenarios so that

CHART 11-2 Sample Security Policies for a Pediatric Unit

- All staff must wear the institution's photo ID above the waist; consider adding some other identification to indicate those who are allowed to transport the child.
- All staff are to monitor and report any suspicious behavior by visitors (e.g., visiting "just to see" infants, questioning the facility's procedures or physical layout, carrying a large package off the unit, taking hospital lab coats or scrubs).
- Keep staff locker rooms locked; do not let visitors borrow scrubs or lab coats.
- Do not post any child's name outside the door of their room.
- All visitors must enter and exit through an access-controlled corridor.
- Parents or visitors must wear an ID wristband or show a photo ID.
- Question anyone transporting a child without displaying the proper identification, either the institution's photo ID or an authorized ID band for that child.
- Upon admission, assess for high-risk children (e.g., custody issues, child abuse).
- At admission, footprint and photograph infants and perform and document a complete physical examination.
- Assign infants to rooms close to the nurses' station, not near stairwells or exits; keep infants in line-of-sight supervision.
- Transport children via appropriate mechanism (bassinet, wheelchair, gurney); *never* carry the child in the halls.
- Transport only one child at a time.

TIP 11-1: A TEACHING INTERVENTION PLAN for Parents to Deter Child Abduction From a Hospital

Nursing Diagnosis and Family Outcomes

- Ineffective protection related to child's age and vulnerability in acute care setting
  Outcomes: Family will be knowledgeable about and comply with safety policies.
  Child will not be abducted from health care facility.

Interventions

Educate the Parents
- Never let your child be taken from the room by anyone without a proper ID photo badge.
- Do not hesitate to question staff regarding their identity and the reason for taking the child.
- Stay with your child if possible.
- Do not give out personal information, such as your address, to anyone without him or her having a legitimate reason for needing it.
- Become familiar with hospital personnel who work on the unit; meet the nurse assigned to care for your child.
- Report suspicious behavior immediately.
- Observe the facility's policies regarding security, safety, and visitation.

staff members are knowledgeable when an actual situation occurs.

Physical and environmental controls can play a key role in preventing abduction. Carefully screen visitors who are allowed to gain entry to the facility's inpatient area, as noted earlier. In cases of individual need for increased protection, use visitor restrictions that designate who may and may not visit the child. In newborn nurseries, arrange visitation hours that permit viewing without physical access to the infants. Ensure that identifying data, such as mother's full name, are not displayed on the crib card or where visitors could view it. The abductor may attempt to take the child from the home. Measures such as surveillance cameras and door alarms increase environmental security.

ALERT *Specific photo IDs should be mandatory for personnel allowed to transport children. This policy makes it readily apparent when an unauthorized person is moving the child.*

Health care facilities are also increasing their security staff. Emergency rooms are improving security by having armed personnel on guard at all times and limiting access through the use of locked doors that, with the exception of employees, can be entered only with permission. These constraints may seem excessive and annoying to the patients and families if they do not understand the reasons for them. Review the rationale for implementing security precautions; all staff should reinforce and comply with these precautions.

PERFORMING ROUTINE PROCEDURES

Performing procedures, including specimen collection, on children can be time consuming at best. At worst, it can be frustrating or even impossible without taking extreme measures, such as using restraints. Small children are afraid of procedures and often are very unwilling to cooperate. Knowing not only how to minimize trauma to the child and parent but also how to perform the task requires skill. Explain the purpose of, steps to, and outcomes expected from the procedure to the child and parent. This requires knowing the major fears of the child's age group, understanding the best time to give information as determined by the child's developmental level, providing preparation at that time, and addressing fears by using language or props that the child can understand. Therefore, perform a developmental assessment of the child and intervene to promote coping and to preempt pain (see Chapter 10).

Use honest, understandable language when talking to children about pain and procedures. Ambiguity or unfamiliarity with language is a problem in early childhood, but older children are also subject to misunderstanding, especially if ambiguous or unfamiliar terms are used (Table 11-1). Include explanations about what will happen and why, what the effects

will be, and how the child can help during the procedure. Choose vivid language and sensory information for preparations, such as color, sound, size, or shape. Avoid jargon, fantasy, and ambiguity when asked if a procedure is going to hurt. Do not be dishonest about the outcome or the pain involved; try to describe it as well as possible.

A systematic review of the research indicates that parental participation during procedures may not have an impact on child distress, but it is not detrimental (Piira et al., 2005). It may be that children are more likely to express distress to a parent or that benefits such as fewer post procedure effects are not captured in the research. Parents who were present either had less distress and higher satisfaction or were no different from absent parents (Piira et al., 2005).

In addition to preparing the child and family, successful procedure performance also depends on knowledge of age-dependent variances and proper equipment selection and use (Nursing Interventions 11-6). Considerations for and techniques of medication administration to children are discussed in Chapter 9.

MAINTAINING INFECTION CONTROL

Infection control is an increasingly important focus in health care settings. Hepatitis B, hepatitis C, and HIV are the most common risks to health care workers (Kuruuzum et al., 2008). The spread of these diseases and others, such as drug-resistant tuberculosis, has increased the need for facilities to provide exposure control plans and workplace and engineering controls that protect patients, visitors, and health care workers. It is essential to follow all hospital guidelines and policies designed to prevent the spread of infection.

Standard Precautions

The control of potential infections is of critical importance in pediatric care because nosocomial infections are significant contributors to morbidity and mortality in young hospitalized patients (Auriti et al., 2010). The most effective way to minimize exposure to and transmission of pathogens is by following standard precautions.

caREminder

Handle all body fluid using standard precautions, regardless of whether it has been tested and identified as containing contagions. This includes wearing gloves to change diapers.

The overriding goal of infection control programs is the protection of all patients and staff at all times from infectious disease. Although health care providers can be infected by contact with patients, patients are more susceptible to infection. This is because hospitalization is more likely to occur when the general state of health is impaired and the ability of the immune system to ward off infection is likely compromised. Furthermore, many patients experience invasive procedures, which allow a port of entry for exogenous bacteria to enter the

TABLE 11-1   Language Considerations for Children

Potentially Ambiguous	Clearer
The doctor will give you some "dye." *To make me die.*	"The doctor will put some medicine in the tube that will help her be able to see your more clearly."
Dressing, dressing change *Why are they going to undress me? Do I have to change my clothes? Will I be naked?*	"Bandages; clean new bandages."
Stool collection *Why do they want to collect little chairs?*	Use child's familiar term, such as *poop, BM,* or *doody.*
Urine *You're in?*	Use child's familiar term, such as *pee.*
Shot *Are they mad at me? When people get shot, they're really badly hurt. Are they trying to hurt me?*	"Medicine through a (small, tiny) needle."
CAT scan *Will there be cats? Or something that scratches?*	Describe in simple terms. If child is old enough to understand, explain what the letters of the common name stand for.
PICU *Pick you?*	Describe in simple terms. If child is old enough to understand, explain what the letters of the common name stand for.
ICU *I see you?*	Describe in simple terms. If child is old enough to understand, explain what the letters of the common name stand for.
IV *Ivy?*	Describe in simple terms. If child is old enough to understand, explain what the letters of the common name stand for.
Stretcher *Stretch her? Stretch who? Why?*	"Bed on wheels."
Special, funny *It doesn't look/feel special to me.*	"Odd, different, unusual, strange."
Gas, sleeping gas *Is someone going to pour gasoline into the mask?*	"Medicine, called anesthesia. It is a kind of air you will breathe through a mask like this to help you sleep during your operation so you won't feel anything. It is a different kind of sleep." Explain differences.
Put you to sleep *Like my cat was put to sleep? It never came back.*	"Medicine, called anesthesia. It is a kind of air you will breathe through a mask like this to help you sleep during your operation so you won't feel anything. It is a different kind of sleep." Explain differences.
Move you to the floor *Why are they going to put me on the ground?*	"Unit; ward." Explain why the child is being transferred and where.
Or to the (treatment room) table *People aren't supposed to get up on tables.*	"A narrow bed."
Take a picture (radiographs, computed tomography [CT], and magnetic resonance imaging [MRI] machines are far larger than a familiar camera, move differently, and don't yield a familiar end product).	"A picture of the inside of you." Describe appearance, sounds, and movement of the equipment.
Flush your IV *Flush it down the toilet?*	Explain in simple terms, "Put some water in your IV tube."
Potentially Unfamiliar	**Concrete Explanation**
Take your vitals	"Measure your temperature; see how warm your body is; see how fast and strong your heart is working." Nothing is "taken" from the child.
Electrode, leads	"Sticky like a Band-Aid, with a small wet spot in the center and small strings that attach to the snap" (monitor electrodes) "Paste like wet sand, with strings with tiny metal cups that stick to the paste" (EEG electrodes) "The paste washes off easily afterward; the strings go into a box that will make a picture of how your heart (or brain) is working." Show child electrodes and leads before using. Let child handle them and apply them to a doll or to self.

TABLE 11-1 Language Considerations for Children (*Continued*)

Potentially Unfamiliar	Concrete Explanation
Intravenous, IV	"Medicine that works best when it goes right into a vein" (IV). "It's the quickest way to help you get better." First, ask the child if he or she knows what a vein is and why some medicine is OK to take by mouth and others work best in a vein. Explain concept of initials if child is old enough.
Hang your (IV) medication	"Bring in new medicine in a bag and attach it to the little tube already in your arm. The needle goes into the tube, not into your arm, so you won't feel it."
NPO	"Nothing to eat. Your stomach needs to be empty." Explain why. "You can eat and drink again as soon as . . ." Explain with concrete descriptions.
Anesthesia	"The doctor will give you medicine; you may hear it called *anesthesia*. It will help you go into a very deep sleep. You will not feel anything at all. The doctors know just the right amount of medicine to give you so you will stay asleep through your whole operation. When the operation is over, the doctor stops giving you that medicine and helps you wake up."
Incision	"Small opening." Follow with discussion of how cuts and scrapes received while playing have healed in the past.

Hard Impact	Softer Impact
This part will hurt.	"It [Your _____] may feel [or feel very] sore, achy, scratchy, tight, snug, full, or . . . [other descriptive term]."
The medicine will burn.	"Some children say they feel a very warm feeling."
The room will be very cold.	"Some children say they feel very cool."
The medicine will taste (or smell) bad.	"The medicine may taste (or smell) different than anything you have tasted before. After you take it, will you tell me how it was for you?"
Cut, open you up, slice, make a hole	"The doctor will make a small opening." Use concrete comparisons, such as "your little finger" or "a paper clip" if the opening will indeed be small.
As big as . . . (e.g., size of an incision or of a catheter)	"Smaller than"
As long as . . . (e.g., for duration of a procedure)	"For less time than it takes you to . . . "
As much as . . .	"Less than . . . "
You will have to say good-bye to your parents.	"That will be the time when you say 'See you later' to your parents."
Lots of children feel sick to their stomachs and throw up when they wake up.	"Your stomach has also been asleep and resting. It may need time to wake up. As your stomach wakes up, you will slowly be able to drink and then eat food again. Some children say they feel sick while their stomachs wake up; other children say they feel fine."
You will have a sore throat when you wake up.	"Your throat may feel very dry when you wake up."
You are angry/scared/sad. That was very hard for you.	"How was that for you? Was it the way you thought it would be? Or harder or easier? Is there something else we should tell people about this?"

From Gaynard, L., Wolfer, J., Goldberger, J. et al. (1998). *Psychosocial care of children in hospitals: A clinical practice manual* (pp. 62–65). Rockville, MD: Child Life Council. Adapted with permission.

body. To reduce the spread of microorganisms by direct contact with patients, perform hand hygiene before *and* after contact with each child.

Appropriately disinfect patient care materials between children, or use single-use disposable equipment to reduce the spread of microorganisms by indirect contact. Instruct children and employees to cover their nose and mouth when sneezing and coughing, using disposable tissues if possible, and then perform hand hygiene to reduce airborne contamination.

When following standard precautions, health care personnel wear gloves and other personal protective equipment, as needed, for protection from contact with blood and other body fluids. Perform hand hygiene after gloves are removed. Change gloves between patients and remove before contact with objects such as the telephone or a pen.

Strict adherence to standard precautions can become another stressor for the child and family in the acute care setting. Children and families may be approached by personnel wearing protective devices, such as gowns, masks, and goggles. Parents may be required to wear this personal protective equipment when caring for their children.

NURSING INTERVENTIONS 11-6

Procedures

Procedure	Variances	Nursing Considerations
All	Children understand and react to situations based on cognitive maturity; gear teaching and support to cognitive level. Developmentally appropriate support helps child maintain control.	Prepare for procedure as developmentally appropriate. Give choices as appropriate. Offer coping strategies (e.g., pacifier for infant, distraction for young child). Teach parents techniques to support child during procedure (e.g., distraction). Have another staff member available to hold/assist as needed. Do not perform procedures in the child's bed if possible, or the playroom; keep these safe areas. After the procedure, provide comfort measures and positive reinforcement. See Chapter 10 for considerations for painful procedures.
Blood specimen collection	Small total blood volume in young children increases risk of anemia and fluid volume deficit with frequent blood draws. Most laboratories can analyze values based on a small amount of blood. Infant's skin is thinner, does not provide a good barrier to toxic agents, and is susceptible to damage.	Use a topical anesthetic on site prior to nonurgent blood draws. Use a bandage to prevent bleeding after specimen collection, especially in preschoolers. In neonates and children requiring frequent blood sampling, maintain ongoing tally of the amount of blood extracted (in cubic centimeters). Collect minimal amount of blood required to perform laboratory analysis. In infants (<2 months), cleanse antiseptics from skin afterward.
Venipuncture	Common sites are veins on dorsum of hand, antecubital flexor surface of foot, and wrist (very sensitive area).	Help child maintain control of situation; if appropriate, offer choice of sites and have child help cleanse site. If unable to obtain venous access after two or three attempts, have another practitioner do the puncture. After procedure, apply pressure to site until bleeding stops, then cover as appropriate (e.g., no tape for premature infant, bandage for preschooler).
Capillary puncture 	Can use medial and lateral aspects of the heel up to about 18 months of age; do not puncture posterior curvature to avoid striking the calcaneus. Use side of finger in older children.	Choose site carefully (check landmarks). Warm the extremity prior to drawing blood; wet a disposable diaper with warm water and wrap around the foot or hand. Do not squeeze extremity excessively when drawing blood (causes cells to hemolyze so may obtain false high K^+ level).
Urine specimen collection	Language used by the nurse may be misunderstood by the child.	Use child's words such as *pee-pee* to make request.

Procedure	Variances	Nursing Considerations
	Adolescent may be unable to void on request or may be reluctant to have test completed because of concerns over body image, body functions, and privacy or suspicion that specimen is requested for drug testing. Urine may be aspirated from cotton balls for small-volume tests such as specific gravity, pH, or glucose; disposable diapers with absorbent gel are difficult to aspirate from and yield inaccurate results.	Provide privacy for older child and adolescent. Clean area or teach child/parent correct cleaning method for clean-catch specimen. Provide potty chair or urine collector in toilet for preschool- or school-aged child. Explain to adolescent why test is needed. Offer child something to drink; most infants void shortly after feeding. Too much fluid may dilute the specific gravity of the urine. Place cotton balls near the urethra inside the diaper to squeeze out urine for small volume testing; do not aspirate urine from diaper. Run water in sink to trigger urge to void.
Urine bag 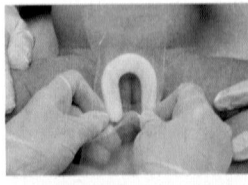 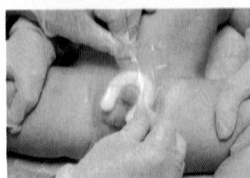	Lack of bowel/bladder control does not allow young children to voluntarily cooperate with specimen collection. Use urine bag to collect urine for larger amounts (e.g., routine urinalysis).	Clean and dry perineal skin. Apply chemical adhesive (e.g., tincture of benzoin) to help maintain seal (do not use on premature infants, neonates). To place on female, position lower half of adhesive on bag on perineum first, then press on adhesive up toward symphysis. To place on male, insert penis and scrotum into bag opening; adhesive adheres to perineum and symphysis. Ensure bag does not cover anus to reduce contamination. Cut a hole in the diaper and pull the urine bag through the opening; thus, when the child voids, it is easily visible and the bag can be removed immediately.
Urine catheterization	Swelling of the labia in female neonates, resulting from maternal hormones, makes it difficult to visualize urethral opening; may have excess tissue overlying opening. Choose urinary catheter size depending on child's age. Use of shorter length urinary catheters, not feeding tubes, and basing length of insertion on sex and age and first appearance of urine flow	Have second person maintain child in frog-leg position. Use thumb and forefinger to spread labia. Exert slight pressure up and out to reveal urethral opening in female. Apply sterile lubricant, using specific adapter containing 2% Xylocaine around meatus and into urethral meatus. Have extra catheter ready; if the first is contaminated or inadvertently placed in vagina, leave it in place and put the second catheter in other opening (urethra). Insert indwelling catheters to the hub of the catheter and do not inflate balloon until urine is seen; after balloon inflation, pull catheter back to seat at bladder base. If indwelling catheter or urine bag with drainage tubing is used, ensure collection tubing is out of young child's reach and out of view.

(Continued)

NURSING INTERVENTIONS 11-6

Procedures (Continued)

Procedure	Variances	Nursing Considerations
Stool collection	May be particularly embarrassing for school-aged child and adolescent.	Know the words the child uses for stool. With non–toilet-trained child, scrape stool from a diaper using tongue blade and place in stool collection cup. Ask toilet-trained child to use a potty chair or place a collection container in the toilet. Provide privacy.
Sputum specimen collection	Infants/young children will not cough productively on command; must use suctioning to obtain specimen.	Do not exceed 80–100 mm Hg suction pressure. Limit suctioning time to 10 seconds.
Nasogastric/orogastric tube placement	The young child cannot cooperate by swallowing during tube insertion.	Use an age-related, height-based equation (ARHB) or nose-ear-mid-umbilicus (NEMU) measurement (Cirgin Ellett et al., 2012; Cirgin Ellett et al., 2011). Measure tip of tube from child's nose to earlobe to midumbilicus. Mark level on tube with tape, lubricate tip with water or soluble lubricant, and quickly insert. In young child, may need to angle tube toward occiput rather than up. Do not exert pressure on nares when taping tube to cheek.

See thePoint for information on the following procedures: Blood Drawing from Peripheral Sites: Heel Stick and Finger Stick; Urine Collection: Routine Voided; Urinary Catheterization: Insertion and Removal; Enteral Tube Placement and Management: Naso-/Orogastric Tubes

Furthermore, infection control measures may impede family and cultural practices. Some families may want to store food in the room. Others may want to keep plants, flowers, or small pets (e.g., fish). These items can harbor bacteria or act as vectors for insect infestations. To compound the problem, some families may belong to cultures that do not adhere to the germ theory of disease; they may not adhere to western standards of hygiene related to handwashing and food storage practices. In such cases, the nurse is challenged to educate the family in such a manner as to promote their compliance with infection control standards as well as their satisfaction with the acute care experience.

Isolation

Isolation refers to protecting the child and others from infectious agents. This may be done in a variety of ways, depending on the disease. Whatever isolation technique is required, the child usually must be sequestered from the environment at large. For example, the child may be confined to a private room, may need to keep a draining wound covered, or may need to wear a mask when leaving the room. Children in isolation may be sequestered from others in the environment. Such measures can be frightening for the child and annoying and cumbersome for families. Sequestration can impair the child emotionally and socially. Young children and preschoolers cannot fully understand these processes and hence have greater difficulty coping during periods of required isolation. Provide developmentally appropriate diversional activities for the child to enhance coping.

The intervention of, perhaps, greatest importance for promoting effective coping of the isolated child is educating the family. The family who understands the reason for isolation can become the nurse's ally in finding ways to make the experience more acceptable to the child. Families are often the best source for learning what the child fears, which activities he or she prefers, and which measures he or she finds most comforting. Social isolation is an unpleasant experience usually accompanied by depression, fatigue, frustration, and anger. Therefore, minimizing the impact of isolation is an important challenge for the nurse. Additional tips for minimizing social isolation include the following:

- Discuss with the parents and significant others the importance of visiting their child.
- Include parents in the process of explaining the isolation to the child when developmentally appropriate.
- Encourage parents to provide pictures and videos of family, friends, and pets.
- Provide access to a telephone or online social networks for children with medical conditions.
- Arrange for the child life specialist to visit the child for therapeutic play.

EDUCATING THE CHILD AND FAMILY

Education is an integral component of nursing care and a standard of professional practice. To promote positive patient outcomes, the nurse must adopt education strategies that enhance learning readiness and facilitate effective learning. The process of patient teaching resembles the nursing process. Teaching begins with an assessment of the problem and of readiness to learn. It then progresses to development of a plan, implementation of the plan, and evaluation of the plan's effectiveness.

Learning needs are affected by many factors, including prior experience with illness, cultural background, language skills, educational level, and developmental level. During the admission assessment, determine the factors that may influence learning and establish a rapport. Throughout the initial interview, collect data about the child's physical and psychosocial needs. Then analyze the data to determine whether the child and family understand the situation. Identifying knowledge deficits upon admission enables the nurse to plan teaching strategies that address the family's learning needs and promote coping.

caREminder

Every contact with the child and family is a teaching opportunity. After evaluating readiness to learn, barriers to learning, and preferred learning methods, present content at an appropriate level (e.g., if they are anxious, present simple, focused information; if they are asking appropriate questions, proceed to more complex topics). Issues taught may range from specific care of the child to anticipatory guidance and health promotion.

PROMOTING COPING: THE CHILD

To provide support to children and help them cope with their experiences, one must first understand how children typically respond to hospitalization.

Child's Response to Hospitalization

Children tend to respond to hospitalization with emotional upset. Seminal work by Prugh et al. (1953) revealed how children react negatively to the stress of hospitalization with separation anxiety, loss of control, and fears. Since then, hospitalization has changed with higher acuity, shorter stays, and increased parental involvement. Still, negative consequences, such as aggression, hyperactivity, anxiety, depression, posttraumatic distress, and somatization, are common (Davydow et al., 2010; Melnyk et al., 2007; B. L. Murray et al., 2007; Nelson & Gold, 2012). Be aware of the threat that hospitalization poses to normal development, and intervene to reduce the risk.

Separation Anxiety

Hospitalized children between the ages of 6 months and 4 years are at the greatest risk for separation anxiety. Older children are still at risk, but increasing cognitive abilities and concept of time help them cope. Classic work by Robertson (1958), who expanded on the work of John Bowlby, describes the phases through which young children progress when separated from their parents:

- *Protest:* In this phase, lasting hours to days, the child searches for the lost parent, angrily protests, cries frequently, and rejects hospital staff. When the parent returns, the child readily goes to him or her.
- *Despair:* In this phase, the child becomes more sad and apathetic, mourning the lost parent; however, he or she cries less and searches the environment less. The child makes few demands on the environment and those within it. When the parent returns, the child may not readily approach him or her or may cling to the parent.
- *Denial:* In this phase, the child becomes cheerful, interested in the environment and new persons, and seemingly unaware of the lost parent. The child is friendly with staff and begins to develop superficial relationships. When the parent returns, the child typically ignores them as a coping mechanism to avoid further emotional pain. Bowlby called this stage *detachment.* This stage is more common to long-term separation. With rooming-in of parents, hospitalization rarely progresses to this stage. Because the child becomes increasingly "easier" to work with, it may be mistakenly interpreted that the child is coping effectively. Children who progress to denial, however, suffer long-term impaired parental relationships and impaired trust, which can lead to problems in establishing close relationships, attention deficits, self-centeredness, and decreased intellectual functioning. Therefore, the pediatric nurse must develop interventions that reduce separation anxiety (Developmental Considerations 11-4).

Separation anxiety is not unique to younger children. Although preschoolers exhibit fewer symptoms of restlessness, hyperactivity, and irritability, they do exhibit more somatic symptoms such as vomiting, urinary frequency, diarrhea, and dizziness (Clinical Judgment 11-1).

School-aged children manifest anxiety but exhibit fewer panic reactions than younger children. Children of this age have a concept of time and understand that parents need to leave and that they will return. In addition, school-aged children are separated from their

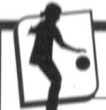

DEVELOPMENTAL CONSIDERATIONS 11-4

Minimizing Separation Anxiety and Loss of Control

Stage	Stressor	Intervention
Infancy	Separation	Promote rooming-in of parents. Play peek-a-boo to promote mastery of the separation experience. Seek volunteer support for holding and stimulating the infant in the parent's absence. Provide tactile, auditory, and visual stimulation such as mobiles over the crib, cuddly toys, musical toys, or tape recordings. Minimize the number of caretakers; have consistent nurse assigned to care for the infant.
	Loss of control	Provide comfort measures such as pacifier, holding, rocking, talking in a soothing voice, and cuddling. Heparin lock IV when possible. Use a crib with a canopy to allow freedom of movement in the crib. Alter the environment by using infant seat, buggy, or stroller and bringing the infant to playroom or nursing station when possible. Provide toys, such as stuffed animals, mirrors, and mobiles.
Early childhood	Separation	Encourage rooming-in of parents. Teach parents to assess symptoms of stress, such as protest and withdrawal. Encourage parents to provide comfort measures. Play hide-and-seek with the child to promote mastery of the separation experience. Use doll play to demonstrate that parents will return. Give the child time frames for when parent will return: "After *Sesame Street* is over."
	Loss of control	Have parents bring in "transitional objects" from home to promote familiarity with the environment (e.g., favorite toys, clothes, tapes of family members' voices, photographs of family members and pets). Promote home rituals, such as feeding and bedtime rituals. Promote dietary practices similar to those at home. Encourage autonomy by giving choices when possible, such as with toys or games. Take the child to the playroom. Provide opportunities for medical and therapeutic play. Teach the parents that regression is a typical response to hospitalization and will usually resolve when the child returns home. Be truthful with the child.
Middle childhood	Separation	Promote communication with siblings and friends. Maintain normalcy by encouraging the child to do homework from school. Be available to talk to the child. Be supportive when the child expresses feelings of loneliness. Take the child to the playroom. Explain to the parents the importance of frequent visits. Rooming-in may not be necessary for older school-aged child.
	Loss of control	Provide opportunities to discuss the medical situation. Encourage the child to discuss his or her understanding. Provide explanations of the medical situation using diagrams, equipment, and concrete explanations. Allow opportunities for the child to achieve the developmental goal of "industry" by helping with tasks. Promote choices in care, if possible.

Stage	Stressor	Intervention
Adolescence	Separation	Promote peer interactions.
		Promote parent visitation. Teach parents the importance of the adolescent's need for control.
		Provide activities, such as "rap sessions," dances, and makeup sessions.
	Loss of control	Develop the plan of care with the adolescent.
		Respect the adolescent's need for independence. Offer choices in routines, if possible.
		Allow for privacy.
		Be open and forthright about the medical situation. Allow time to discuss this with the adolescent.

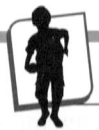

CLINICAL JUDGMENT 11-1

Separation Anxiety

Cory never attended daycare, preschool, or a Mothers' Morning Out program. He began attending kindergarten this fall, which was a difficult separation at first but recently has become easier. Wendy and Cory are still in the emergency room when Wendy's older son brings in the health insurance card. Wendy is asked to take the card to the admissions desk. When Wendy steps out of the room, Cory begins to scream, "Stay! Stay!" and kick, despite the presence of his older brother. Wendy returns and sends the older brother to the desk with the card.

Questions

1. What is your assessment of Cory's behavior and his mother's response?
2. Which phase of separation anxiety is Cory manifesting?
3. Cory is 5 years old; will the nursing staff and family feel he is behaving appropriately?
4. What information should the nurse share with Cory's family to help them understand Cory's strong feelings about separating from his mother?
5. Which of Cory's behaviors will the nursing staff on the pediatric floor use to evaluate the effects of hospitalization and separation on Cory?

Answers

1. Cory is having separation anxiety. Separating from a parent can be viewed as a learned skill. In the familiar setting of kindergarten, Cory is able to separate calmly; in unfamiliar circumstances, he regresses and displays separation anxiety. Wendy responds by staying and relieving Cory's anxiety.
2. Cory is demonstrating the "protest" phase of separation. In most hospitalized children today, separations are short and the protest phase is the most commonly seen behavior.
3. The staff in the emergency room, especially if they do not work exclusively with children, may feel that Cory is not "being a big boy." They may very well make their judgments known to Wendy. Cory's family is not surprised by his behavior; in the past, Cory has been very vocal in his refusal to separate.
4. It is important that Wendy understands that a strong protest is indicative of a strong attachment and trust relationship. It will also be helpful to Wendy to explain the signs of the "despair" phase, especially the possibility that Cory may be angry and not greet her joyfully on her return.
5. The desired outcome is that Cory has minimal episodes of despair and anxiety. Cory's rudimentary skills of separating and trusting a parent, particularly his mother, to return should be supported and encouraged. Initially, short absences are helpful in establishing trust. Some children respond well to a security object (e.g., a blanket or stuffed animal). Children who do not have a previous attachment to an object may benefit from keeping something belonging to the parent until the parent returns.

friends and school, which play a major part in their psychosocial development. A school-aged child's anxiety is related to fear of the unknown or the unexplained, and his or her coping mechanisms usually include denial and rationalization.

The adolescent suffers separation anxiety when separated from peers rather than parents, but it is still crucial that he or she is confident in the family's personal commitment. The adolescent's efforts to maintain peer contact may break hospital rules. For example, the adolescent may leave the hospital without permission, leave the unit after hours to meet peers in the lobby, use the telephone excessively (to the exclusion of participating in the hospital regimen), or refuse hospital treatments that are viewed as disfiguring or displeasing to peers.

To help prevent separation anxiety while a child is in the hospital, it is important to minimize separation of the child from support systems. Encourage open visitation and provide parents with the environment (e.g., sleep space, showers) and support (e.g., information, equipment) to facilitate their role as a member of the team caring for their child. Encourage friends and schoolmates to send cards and videos and to visit when appropriate. Bringing in transitional objects, such as pictures of families and friends, to put in the room can help to decrease the separation anxiety that may be felt.

Loss of Control

Hospitalized children commonly experience loss of control (Basso, 2010; Forsner et al., 2009; Ullán et al., 2012; Wilson et al., 2010). Unlike separation anxiety, which decreases as the child ages, control issues persist because the child is removed from the normal environment. Young children and preschoolers are at highest risk for loss of control. The young child has just gained the ability to explore the environment. Developmental milestones such as potty training and the ability to feed oneself may be initiated or mastered. Hospitalization may interfere with the young child's search for autonomy. A broken leg that is immobilized or a peripheral IV line in the dominant hand may place limitations on the child who can ambulate or feed himself or herself. A previously potty-trained young child who is limited to bed rest and receiving IV fluids may regress to voiding in the bed. This loss of control can be very stressful for the patient. Nurses can help alleviate this stress by allowing choices whenever possible. If the young child is being potty trained at home, continue with the routine when hospitalized. Allow the child to feed and dress himself or herself as much as possible. Keep the child on the home schedule, and provide positive reinforcement when the child accomplishes tasks on his or her own.

Fears

Children's fears are developmentally based (see Chapters 4 to 7). Children older than 4 years of age identify pain and discomfort as the worst aspects of hospitalization (Lindeke et al., 2006).

Many fears are actualized in the hospital: separation, loss of control, unfamiliar environment, body mutilation, and painful events (Coyne, 2006; Forsner et al., 2009; H. Meltzer et al., 2008; Salmela et al., 2011). Provide developmentally appropriate explanations to counter unrealistic fears, and intervene to minimize trauma caused by those fears that are real. Encourage parental presence during procedures or in the PACU, allow choices and have the child make decisions whenever possible, and use topical anesthetics to reduce pain from needle sticks (Developmental Considerations 11-5; see also Chart 5-2).

Strategies for Enhanced Coping of the Child

 QUESTION: After the surgery, Cory will remain in the hospital for about a week. He will have an abdominal incision with a drain and will receive IV antibiotics. What aspects of the following programs would be beneficial to Cory?

The nurse must support the child in developing effective coping behaviors while in the hospital. Outcomes that may be a goal for the hospitalized child and family include the following:

- Family will exhibit adequate internal levels of cooperation to organize daily family activities during hospitalization.
- Family will verbalize the need for hospitalization and adopt strategies for maintaining relationship with hospitalized child during hospitalization.
- Family will articulate an optimistic, but realistic, definition of the situation by discharge.
- Family will recognize and use resources by discharge.
- Child/family will be knowledgeable regarding the disease process and necessary medical intervention during hospitalization and after discharge.
- Child/family will be knowledgeable about and understand the rationale for hospital routines.
- Child will use developmentally effective coping strategies:
  - Engage in play or discussion to decrease fear of procedures
  - Feel a sense of trust and security in relation to parental support
  - Obtain sleep and rest necessary for achieving wellness
- Child/family will practice developmentally appropriate coping strategies.
- Child will gain age-appropriate mastery of environment through play and establishment of routines that mimic home environment to the extent possible.
- Child/family will perform ADLs in new environment.

Children use many different strategies to cope with the stress of illness, such as information seeking, social support, emotional behaviors, information limiting or avoiding, and physical exercise. This reinforces the need for individualized intervention. Children appreciate nurses who have a positive affect; treat them as individuals; manage pain; provide advocacy, entertainment, and support; and meet basic needs (Schmidt et al., 2007).

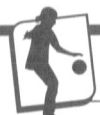

DEVELOPMENTAL CONSIDERATIONS 11-5

Fears Experienced by Hospitalized Children*

Developmental Stage/Fears	Interventions

Infancy
  Loud noises
  Sudden movements
  Loss of physical or emotional support
  Strangers
	Talk to in soft, soothing tones
	Handle with firm, confident movements
	Swaddle
	Have parents hold infant, perform care
	Keep parents in sight
	Maintain consistent caregivers
	Post sign with infant's behavioral cues

Early childhood
  Dark
  Some machines (animistic thinking)
  Body mutilation
  Unknown
  Supernatural
	Mimic home routines as feasible
	Maintain consistent routines
	Use a dim light for sleep
	Let child approach and handle equipment safely
	Explain what is going to happen
	Keep parents in sight
	Reassure that taking specimens will not mutilate them
	Use bandages after intrusive procedures

Middle childhood
  Bodily injury, pain
  Unfamiliar environments
  Death
	Explain the environment and what will be happening
	Maintain routines, post schedule
	Reassure that taking specimens will not mutilate them
	Have them tell you why they are sick

Adolescence
  Body disfigurement
  Pain and discomfort
  Loss of physical abilities
  Death
	Explain the environment, treatments, expected outcomes
	Have them tell you about their illness
	Ask about concerns, clarify perceptions

*Separation and loss of control are issues in all stages (see Developmental Considerations 11-4).

Preparation helps a child to cope (Brewer et al., 2006; Frisch et al., 2010; Wennström et al., 2008). When teaching, be alert to the child's cues indicating how much information is desired and prepare the child based on this. To promote coping, teach the child strategies that can reduce stress, such as relaxation, imagery, distraction, and positive self-talk (see Chapter 10 for further discussion of these techniques). Parent involvement also helps the child cope (Melnyk et al., 2006).

Art

Children often reveal their fears and concerns through drawing. What children draw and how they draw it may be significant (Clatworthy et al., 1999). For example, very large things may imply aggressive tendencies (often, the health care team or equipment, such as needles, is large); tiny things (the child in bed) may imply feelings of insignificance or inferiority. Based on knowledge of growth and development, the nurse can use drawings as an effective method of assessment and as vehicle for communication with the child. When identifying the child's concerns and perceptions, the nurse can correct misconceptions and support coping skills. (Use drawings for psychotherapy only if you have the appropriate training.) Supply drawing materials that are familiar to the child, are nonthreatening, and which may support coping through distraction. Most children draw without prompting; some ask for guidance about what to draw. A broad, nondirective response may help elicit issues of concern to the child (e.g., "Why don't you draw what it will be like after surgery?" or "Why don't you draw what you are thinking of right now?"). Remember, however, that not every drawing has therapeutic significance—a picture may just be a picture.

Music

Music can also be used to promote coping (Klassen et al., 2008; Liu et al., 2007; Whitehead-Pleaux et al., 2007). The child can select the music, giving him or her control over the situation and providing a familiar milieu and distraction (Fig. 11-8). Honor the child's preference, although music that has a slow tempo (60 to 72 bpm) with a soft tone; soft to moderate volume; notes that are close on the musical scale; and a smooth, consistent rhythm is more sedating (Stouffer et al., 2007).

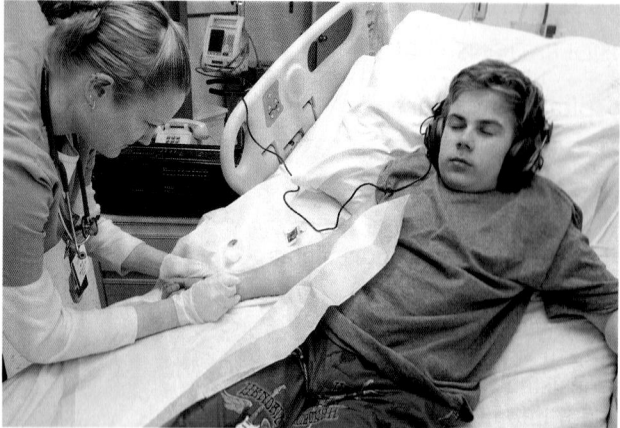

Figure 11-8 This adolescent listens to soothing music to promote relaxation and coping during stressful procedures.

Play

Play is a mechanism through which children cope, learn, test new ideas, and test newly acquired psychomotor skills. It is the medium through which children grow and develop. Play also provides children with a sense of control. In the acute care setting, children might engage in normative or therapeutic play. Normative play is activity in which children spontaneously engage and from which they derive pleasure. Therapeutic play is activity directed by the nurse to promote emotional and physical well-being, such as playing with medical equipment during hospitalization.

Therapeutic Play

Therapeutic play can be used to promote coping by helping children work through hospital experiences (H. C. W. Li, 2007; W. H. Li et al., 2011). This may be effective for a number of reasons: it provides the child with information, the child feels a sense of control and mastery when able to manipulate the equipment and play situation, and the nurse or child life specialist can use the session to model effective coping behaviors. Unlike normative play, therapeutic play is goal directed. Nevertheless, both types of play should be provided in the hospital.

Although the terms often are used interchangeably, therapeutic play is different from play therapy. Play therapy is play that helps a child express and work through emotional or psychological issues. It is usually considered a form of psychotherapy that is supervised by a professional educated in play therapy methods. Play therapy may be directed by the therapist or by the child with the therapist guiding the session. Nurses and child life specialists most commonly guide children during therapeutic play sessions.

Conduct therapeutic play sessions in a protected, nonthreatening environment (Nursing Interventions Classification 11-2). Do not allow treatments, doctors, or other distressing interruptions during the play session. Be accepting of the child's play behaviors and avoid expressing approval or disapproval.

Therapeutic play includes instructional play (Fig. 11-9), emotional outlet play, and physiologically enhancing play (Fig. 11-10). Gear these types of play to the child's physical, emotional, and cognitive abilities (Chart 11-3). The nurse must incorporate play into the plan of care and value this time as essential to the child's development and emotional well-being. Do not force the child to play, however, if he or she is not emotionally or physically ready.

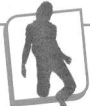

NIC 11-2 NURSING INTERVENTIONS CLASSIFICATION: Therapeutic Play

Definition: Purposeful and directive use of toys or other materials to assist children in communicating their perception and knowledge of their world and to help in gaining mastery of their environment

Activities:

Provide a quiet environment that is free from interruptions

Provide sufficient time to allow for effective play

Structure play session to facilitate desired outcome

Communicate the purpose of play session to child and parent

Discuss play activities with family

Set limits for therapeutic play session

Provide safe play equipment

Provide developmentally appropriate play equipment

Provide play equipment that stimulates creative, expressive play

Provide play equipment that stimulates role playing

Provide real or simulated hospital operating room medical equipment to encourage expression of knowledge and feelings about hospitalization, treatments, or illness

Supervise therapeutic play sessions

Encourage child to manipulate play equipment

Encourage child to share feelings, knowledge, and perceptions

Validate child's feelings expressed during the play session

Communicate acceptance of feelings, both positive and negative, expressed through play

Observe the child's use of play equipment

Monitor child's reactions and anxiety level throughout play session

Identify child's misconceptions or fears through comments made during (hospital role) play session

Continue play sessions on a regular basis to establish trust and reduce fear of unfamiliar equipment or treatments, as appropriate

Record observations made during play session

From Bulechek, G. M., Butcher, H. K., Dochterman, J. M. et al. (Eds.). (2013). *Nursing interventions classifications (NIC)* (6th ed.). St. Louis, MO: Mosby. Used with permission.

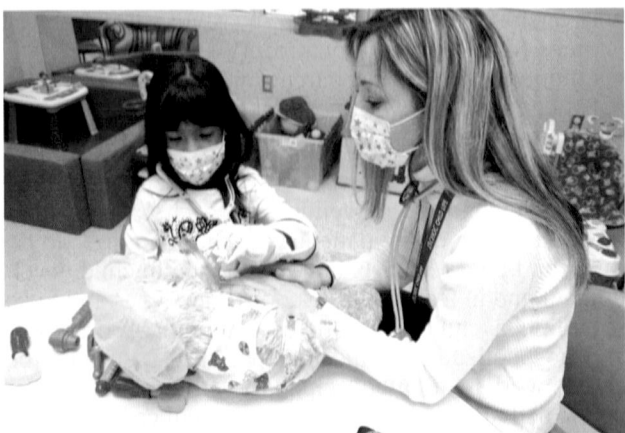

Figure 11-9 Instructional play can help prepare a child for surgery.

The Hospital Playroom

The hospital playroom should be a distinctive area equipped to meet the unique cultural and age-appropriate developmental needs of the population being served (Fig. 11-11). Children and families should be encouraged to engage in activities in the hospital playroom and should always feel welcome to enter.

caREminder

Do not perform any uncomfortable or painful procedures (such as an injection) in the playroom itself to promote the child's perception that, within the confines of this room, he or she is safe from intrusion and discomfort as much as possible.

To prevent the spread of infection in the playroom, follow standard precautions. Ensure that body fluids are not spread in the playroom. If a child's infectious secretions cannot be safely contained, do not permit that child in the playroom. To help minimize spread of infection, wash toys with soap and water or a 10% hypochlorite (chlorine bleach) solution after use. Also, follow the facility's

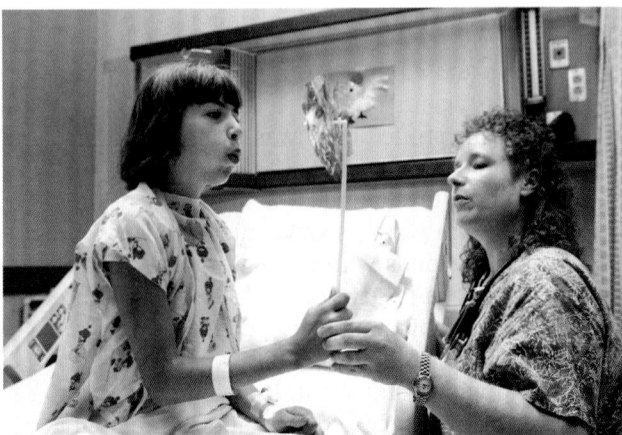

Figure 11-10 This example of physiology-enhancing play encourages deep breathing after surgery by using a pinwheel.

CHART 11-3   Materials and Methods for Use in Play

Instructional Play

Purpose: To prepare the child for procedures or to learn about his or her disease

- Dolls or stuffed animals dressed as doctors, nurses, children, and family members
- Hospital gowns and pajamas
- ID bracelets
- Surgical hats, masks, and booties
- Stethoscopes
- Blood pressure cuff, thermometers, and tape
- Large syringes without needles
- Bandages and dressing materials
- Equipment such as an IV pole, stretcher, and bed
- Oxygen masks
- Wash basin and towels
- Laboratory coats
- "Good Patient" stickers

Therapeutic Play

Purpose: To allow the child to express anxiety or articulate fears about his or her disease or hospitalization

- Punching bags
- Paints and crayons
- Inflatable bopper clowns
- Pegboard and hammers
- Dress-up clothes
- Puppets
- Blank books for writing stories or poetry
- Interactive video games
- Opportunities to play "doctor and nurse"
- Games such as peek-a-boo, hide-and-seek
- Sessions for telling "hospital stories"
- "Rap" groups
- Skits
- Song-writing sessions
- Water play
- Aggression play toys, such as blocks, clay, Play-Doh, punch pillows, squirt guns, and tin cans

Physiology-Enhancing Play

Purpose: To allow the child to improve his or her physical health

- Lung expansion—straw blowing, tuned bottle blowing, blowing bubbles, blowing up and popping paper bags, pinwheel spinning, kazoo or woodwind instrument playing
- Pain management—reading stories, pop-up books, telling jokes, playing musical tapes, playing video games
- Improve range of motion/muscle strength—leave toys just out of reach, take a doll on an airplane ride, arm wrestle, reach to hang up decorations, throw bean bags

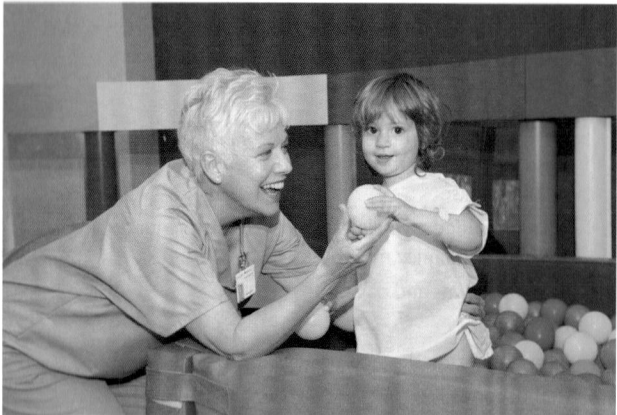

Figure 11-11 It is important to provide safe, age-appropriate activities in the hospital playroom.

guidelines for infection control in the playroom (Nursing Interventions 11-7). Effective control is enhanced by consistent adherence to the policy. Toys brought from home can be contaminated with potentially dangerous bacteria and may provide unnecessary risks for nosocomial infection (Fleming & Randle, 2006), cleanse these toys appropriately to prevent the spread of infections through toys.

Child Life Programs

Child life programs are designed to minimize stress for children and families during hospitalization and to promote the hospitalized child's continued growth and development; they are an essential component of quality pediatric care (American Academy of Pediatrics, 2006). To help the child cope successfully with hospitalization, child life programs organize interventions in the following categories:

- Preparation for hospitalization, procedures, and surgery
- Play
- Diversional activities during invasive, painful procedures (e.g., lumbar punctures, IV starts)
- Emotional support for parents and siblings
- Patient advocacy with hospital staff
- Promotion of family-centered environment

The child life specialist is responsible for designing and implementing interventions in each category that meet the needs of the patients and their families. To do this, child life specialists must be trained in child development and in techniques to address anxieties and fears regarding a child's condition, impending procedures, and hospitalization. Child life specialists also must be able to work in an interdisciplinary setting so that therapeutic activities incorporate all aspects of care.

Because child life specialists are one of the few health care professionals who do not cause the child pain or discomfort, this specialist is often the one with whom the hospitalized child feels most comfortable. The child life specialist may become the primary health care professional to whom the child expresses feelings of anxiety, fears, and anger (Koller & Goldman, 2012).

For school-aged children with hospitalizations lasting more than a few days, a teacher may be provided through the local school district or the child life program. Teachers provide programmed instruction and assist children in keeping current in the homework they would be completing if they were in school with other children.

Pet Therapy

Pet visitation or animal-assisted therapy involves the touching, holding, or cuddling of animals to promote therapeutic results (Fig. 11-12). Pet visits distract children from the confines of their illness. Children can openly display affection and joy toward the pet. Pet visits also give children an opportunity to learn about animals. Organizations exist that provide trained animals expressly for this purpose. The animals need to be well cared for, with careful veterinary support and

---

NURSING INTERVENTIONS 11-7

Infection Control for Recreational Activities in the Acute Care Setting

All personnel and visitors must perform hand hygiene
- Upon entering and leaving the unit
- When serving food to patients
- After assisting patients with toileting or diapering
- After blowing or wiping a patient's or own nose
- After removing gloves used for handling body fluids
- When leaving an isolation area or handling articles from that area
- When leaving the toilet

Prevent toys and equipment from becoming vectors for infectious agents by
- Not allowing stuffed or unwashable toys in the playroom
- Scrubbing all toys handled by infectious or drooling patients in warm, soapy water and rinsing for at least 30 seconds with manual friction; spray with disinfectant; leave on surface for amount of time specified by manufacturer; rinse with water
- Wiping all nonsubmersible toys with cloth saturated with disinfectant, leave on surface for amount of time specified by manufacturer, wipe with water-moistened cloth

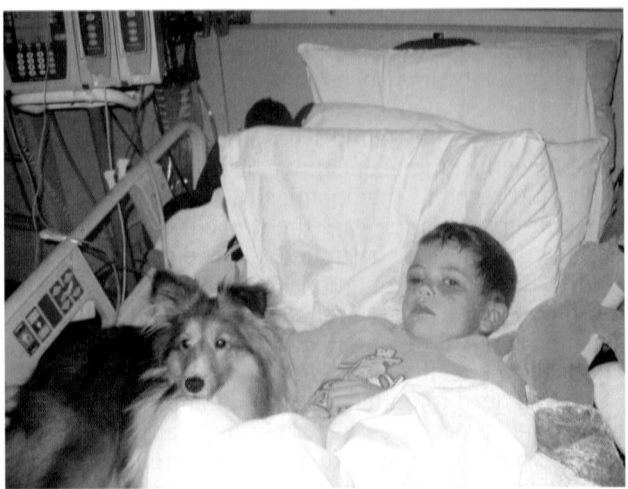

Figure 11-12 Pet visits can help reduce the stress of hospitalization for a child.

health screening (Chart 11-4). With the proper screening, the child's own animal may visit (Hemsworth & Pizer, 2006). When developing such a program, however, key points must be addressed, such as assessing for potential allergies; the child's acceptance of animals; and protocols for animal screening, grooming, and training. If pet visitation is not possible, videos of the child's pet may provide some comfort to the child while in the hospital.

> *ANSWER:* Therapeutic play and normative play will be important for Cory. The suddenness of his illness may be best understood through reenacting similar events in imaginative play—for example, a toy ambulance rushing someone to the hospital. A doll with an incision and drain may help decrease anxiety about his incision. Normative play will be an essential outlet for a 5-year-old boy accustomed to active play with four athletic brothers.

PROMOTING COPING: THE FAMILY

Family coping is just as important as the child's coping during acute illness. Hospitalization of a seriously

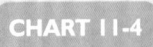
- Establish a mechanism for screening and approval of animals.
- Obtain parent's consent for the child to participate in the pet program.
- Ensure that the choice of animals complies with state and local health department regulations.
- Identify designated areas for animal visitation.
- Identify key personnel who will manage animals on location in the facility.
- Consult with the infectious disease or immunology department to determine patient restrictions regarding pet visitation.

ill child can precipitate a crisis for the family. Family coping skills are important factors to consider during a child's acute illness and hospitalization because families who face serious illness in a child (or family member) are at risk for psychosocial maladjustment (Melnyk et al., 2006). Families who use effective coping skills tend to adjust to the child's hospitalization and do much better. Therefore, assess the family's coping skills, promote the use of effective skills, and teach additional skills if needed.

Family's Response to Hospitalization

Family members are typically affected by hospitalization based on their relationship to the child and their role in the family. Parents may exhibit responses that include stress, fear, anxiety, helplessness, anger, uncertainty, guilt, and a sense of having no control (Coyne & Cowley, 2007; Hopia et al., 2005). The parents' coping abilities may be reduced by financial, emotional, or physical stressors; the severity of the child's condition; and the need to care for their other children as well as the hospitalized child (Diaz-Caneja et al., 2005). Assess the parents' response and provide intervention and support to help the family cope with the acute hospitalization of a child.

Siblings' coping skills can be affected by misperceptions about the sick child's condition and feelings of loss, parent neglect, isolation, or loneliness (Rozdilsky, 2005; Wilkins & Woodgate, 2006). The sibling may exhibit anxiety, depression, or acting-out behaviors. Difficulty in school and altered roles within the family may be apparent for the affected sibling. To practice family-centered care, the nurse must understand the effects of hospitalization on the patient and family and intervene to promote effective coping by all family members.

Strategies for Enhanced Parental Coping

Building a supportive relationship, communicating effectively, and encouraging parental involvement in the care of the ill child are integral to the implementation of family-centered care.

Rapport and Communication

> *QUESTION:* What communication techniques would you use to support the Whitworth family? How would you assess the coping skills of the Whitworth family? What are some examples of specific questions to ask that promote family coping?

Rapport between parents and nurse results in more individualized care for the child. The degree of rapport is influenced by the nurse's knowledge of the child and the parent's knowledge of the nurse. The nurse's demonstration of interest in learning about the child as a person and the child's condition is important in establishing rapport.

Communication, or sharing of information, is the cornerstone of building a trusting, supportive relationship with a family. Successful coping depends on timely information delivered in a coordinated, knowledgeable manner. Effective, empathic communication can help children and families cope, adapt to challenging situations, and lead to improved outcomes (Levetown, 2008).

Communication and building a trusting relationship begin during the admission assessment. Ask the child and family why they have come to the acute care setting and what their expectations are of the health care team, then share information about what the family may expect during their visit. Assessment and sharing of expectations should occur during the prehospital visit or at the time of admission to the acute care setting. If this exchange does not occur in a timely fashion, the family's trust of the hospital staff can be undermined.

Throughout the acute care experience, assessing an individual's readiness for communication becomes a key component of effective communication, which is integral to providing support to the child and family. Parents and children are involved in a stressful situation, so determining the level at which they can participate is a vital skill (e.g., if they are anxious, discuss only simple, basic concepts or allow them to discuss what is distressing them before progressing to other topics).

Receptivity to feedback from the child or family is key in this determination. Some families use maladaptive coping mechanisms such as anger, criticizing the care delivered, and demanding special treatment to deal with the stress of a child's hospitalization. The nurse must recognize the maladaptive behavior, interpret it as such, and respond therapeutically. For example, when a parent criticizes the care the nurse delivers, the parent may be angry or frustrated. Defending oneself may lead to further confrontation. Conversely, acknowledging the emotion (e.g., "You sound like you are angry. Tell me about it.") might address the parent's issues and lead to effective problem solving.

Parents need to understand and be informed of treatments and procedures in terms they can understand. Having staff communicate with the parent and child when providing care helps to create a sense of comfort and reassurance. Talk directly to the child as well as the parent. Inadequate communication and excluding the child of middle childhood and older reduces trust of the child (Kelsey et al., 2007). Interventions for facilitating communication between parents and staff are presented in Nursing Interventions 11-8.

NURSING INTERVENTIONS 11-8

Facilitating Communication With Parents of Acutely Ill Children

- Use active listening techniques:
  Convey an unhurried demeanor and minimize interruptions.
  Position self at same level when communicating (e.g., sit down).
  Be aware of nonverbal messages conveyed in body stance and voice inflection.
  Consider cultural background of parents when using some techniques (e.g., maintaining eye contact is considered disrespectful in many Asian cultures).
  Clarify what you think you heard (e.g., "You are angry because the doctors did not talk with you this morning.").
  Encourage and accept expression of feelings (use statements such as "This is a difficult time for you.").
  Reflect parents' statements (e.g., "You feel guilty because you didn't call the doctor sooner.").
  Ask the parents specific questions about their needs (e.g., "Do you need to go get something to eat? I will sit with Sandy while you are gone.").
  Do not take anger personally.
- Provide information:
  Give honest, accurate information.
  Use short, simple explanations.

Be tactful in stating information but do not try to minimize the seriousness of a situation.
  Avoid letting long periods of time pass without giving information, especially in critical situations, even if it is only to tell the parents that the child's condition has not changed and what is being done to support the child.
  Volunteer information freely and in a timely manner to promote trust.
  Teach and reinforce knowledge of disease process, treatments, and how parents can support their child.
- Be consistent:
  Give same information over time and by different health team members.
  Minimize the number of health team members interacting with the parents.
- Reinforce importance of the parent's role:
  Acknowledge parents' expertise in knowing their child.
  Encourage and provide opportunities for parents to provide physical care for the child; parents may need to be shown how they can do this (e.g., demonstrate how to bathe a child with an IV).
  Ensure parent involvement in care conferences.

ANSWER: Cory and his family had very little time for communication and to absorb information as they went from pediatrician to emergency room to surgical suite. The nurses will need to give consistent and concise answers and be active listeners. Remember that Cory's parents may need to hear the same information several times to absorb it. Questions such as "Is there someone to help you with your other children while Cory is in the hospital?" or "Is there someone you can call to support you?" may be helpful to promote family coping.

Parental Visitation and Participation

QUESTION: Wendy has not left the hospital or slept since Cory's admission. What might you say to help Wendy? Based on Wendy's previous answers, identify extended support networks available to Wendy. What do you think is a beneficial pattern of visitation and family participation for the Whitworth family?

Parental involvement helps reduce the child's anxiety, promote parent coping, and improve satisfaction with care (Fig. 11-13). Family-centered care reflects the importance of parental involvement. True family-centered care views parents as partners in care, not as visitors.

Include the parent as an active participant in developing the plan of care. Parents have varying expectations of their role in caring for their hospitalized child (Power & Franck, 2008). For example, one parent may regard a nurse's action as a relinquishment of parental control. Another parent may see parental participation in the child's care as a shirking of the nurse's duty. Assess the parents' needs and preferences for participation in care when planning interventions. Also, discuss the health care team's expectations regarding parent participation in the child's care with the parent at the onset of the hospital stay.

Today, most facilities that care for children have 24-hour open visitation for parents and grandparents. This policy encourages parents and grandparents to participate in their child's care and to room-in when possible. Although evidence demonstrates the importance of liberal visitation policies (Tradition or Science 11-2), they can also be a source of conflict between the family and the health care team members. The health care providers might have concerns about increased physiologic stress on the child, interference with ability to provide care, and physical and emotional exhaustion of the family members. Conflicts might also arise over who may visit the child, the number of visitors, visiting hours, and inconsistent enforcement of the policies (Griffin, 2003). Guidelines that define how the hospital can meet the family's visitation needs can serve as a useful communication tool. Guidelines can also maintain infection control and safety standards and enhance the family's satisfaction with the facility.

If parents cannot be present to support the child in person, do not assume they do not care or are "bad" parents. Encourage parent visitation in the child's care to the extent possible, and encourage the participation of significant others. If parents are reluctant to visit because the child cries and protests when they leave, explain that this is a normal response to separation. If parents are absent as a result of work, sibling care, or other responsibilities, reinforce that the child will be attended to in their absence. Provide the family with the name and telephone number of a contact person knowledgeable about the child; the nurse can also initiate regular telephone contact with the family. When appropriate, assist the child in calling home. Assisting the family with logistics (e.g., handouts regarding hospital visitation policies and support services; transportation, meal, and lodging assistance) may help to increase visitation.

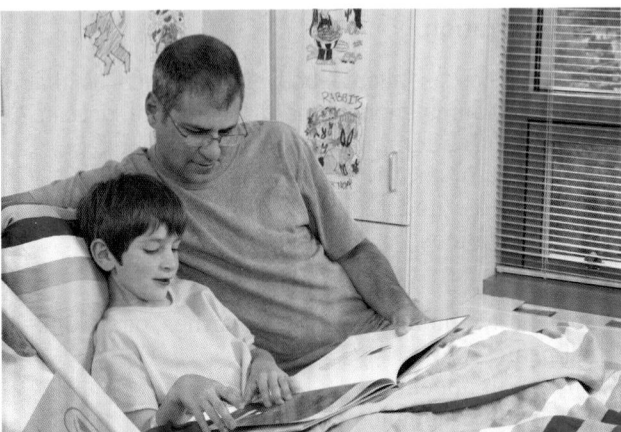

Figure 11-13 Visitation helps reduce the child and parent's anxiety and improve coping.

Evidence-Based Practice

TRADITION OR SCIENCE 11-2

Should open visitation in acute care facilities be allowed?

The presence of family and friends at the bedside has been shown to decrease stress and provide reassurance to the child and parent (Board, 2005; Smith et al., 2007). Parents want to protect their child (Dudley & Carr, 2004) and view their participation as essential for the child's emotional welfare (Coyne, 1995). Chinese parents view participation as an unconditional aspect of being a parent (Lam et al., 2006). Family presence allows for increased opportunity for education and communication with the health care team. Although in some cases, exhaustion of family members may occur, studies have shown that open visitation often allows family members to relax and be less anxious during times they are not with the patient (Berwick & Kotagal, 2004). Open visitation was not found to increase infection in an adult ICU (Adams et al., 2011). Using principles of family-centered care in the implementation of visitation policies that give guidelines, not rules, and recognizing first that the family is the constant in the child's life and, second, that hospitals must be flexible in their visitation policies best meets the needs of children and families.

For a family who does not have a mobile phone, assisting the family in obtaining a temporary pager may also enhance coping and satisfaction for children and families. Treatment of acute illness frequently involves waiting, which exacerbates anxiety and frustration. Having a pager may enable the child and family to leave the clinic or child's room to go to the cafeteria or playroom and return when paged. Having a pager also lets the parents run errands, eat, or just leave the room while the child sleeps, knowing they can be paged when the child awakens. In addition, share the unit phone number and encourage the parent to call and speak to the nurse at any time when they are away from the hospital. These options allow the family choices that increase their control and promote coping.

ANSWER: Assessment of Wendy's coping includes asking her, "What will be the hardest aspect of this hospitalization?" Wendy identifies separation from her children as the most stressful aspect of the hospitalization. Parents need to know they are welcome to stay with their child as much as they would like. Sometimes, parents may need to be given "permission" to go home. An example of what to say is, "You are welcome to stay as long as you like, but it is important that you take care of yourself too. Under what conditions could you go home and relax and sleep?" It is very easy for the entire focus to be on the child who is sick. You can also assist this family to identify a combination of family, church, and neighborhood support to decrease the entire family's level of anxiety and enhance their coping with this hospitalization. You can encourage the Whitworth family to work out a schedule whereby there is always one member of the family with Cory. John and Wendy can plan to take turns spending the night. Wendy's older children are in school, so she can spend the school hours at the hospital with Cory.

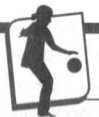

Strategies for Enhanced Sibling Coping

QUESTION: How would you assess the coping and the needs of Cory's siblings? What is an example of a question you could ask Wendy about her other children? What questions could you ask Cory's siblings? Prior to Cory's hospitalization, his siblings each had an assigned afternoon to watch Cory. What do you think might be a beneficial pattern of visitation for Cory's older brothers?

Family-centered care also addresses the needs of siblings. Assess each sibling for risk factors that affect coping and signs of stress and ineffective coping (Developmental Considerations 11-6). Children who perceive more changes in their parents' behavior and negative interpersonal effects on their lives often experience more adjustment problems (J. S. Murray, 2002; Simon, 1993). Siblings often may feel neglected or jealous of the attention that is being given to the ill sibling. The nurse can help facilitate the sibling's understanding of the illness. Child life therapists, social workers, and psychiatrists might also help the sibling cope, especially in the case of life-threatening or terminal illnesses.

KidKare Ask the siblings how they think things are different since the child has been sick or in the hospital. Early identification of those children at high risk for ineffective coping enables the nurse to arrange intervention and to follow up with the primary health care provider.

Parent perceptions of the effects of illness on the siblings have not been found to correlate with siblings' self-report; therefore, it is more accurate to obtain information directly from the sibling (Houtzager et al., 2005).

DEVELOPMENTAL CONSIDERATIONS 11-6

Sibling Coping With Hospitalization

Risk Factors in the Sibling
- Sibling is undergoing stress in other areas, such as school or peer relationships.
- Sibling had a poor relationship with the parents or the ill child before the illness began.
- Sibling has not developed effective coping skills as part of general life strategies.
- Sibling is cared for outside of own home.
- There is an increased change in the parents' behavior.

Risk Factors in the Ill Child
- Ill child is developmentally delayed.
- Ill child has multiple disabilities.
- Ill child has chronic or genetically transmitted disorder.

- Ill child has an altered body image, such as that caused by amputation, burns, disfigurement, or scars.
- Ill child has a terminal condition.
- Ill child is in an ICU.
- Ill child is undergoing prolonged or repeated hospitalizations.

Signs of Stress
- Somatic symptoms—vomiting, diarrhea, or abdominal pain
- Change in appetite
- Change in academic performance
- Change in temperament—irritability, nervousness, sorrow, difficulty concentrating

On the basis of assessment findings, implement interventions to promote sibling coping (Nursing Interventions Classification 11-3). Siblings who received education about the patient's hospitalization, illness or injury, and treatment demonstrated less anxiety than siblings who received no intervention (Gursky, 2007). Psychological interventions can be effective in reducing psychological maladjustment and improve medical knowledge (Prchal & Landolt, 2009). Encourage parents to include siblings in activities and conversations, inform them about what is happening, and teach them about their sibling's condition. Ideally, the routine for the siblings is disturbed as little as possible and they are able to play with their friends as before.

Encourage parents to have the sibling visit (Fig. 11-14). Sibling visitation helps normalize hospitalization for the patient, especially for a child with a condition that requires a prolonged stay. For prolonged hospitalizations, videophones can play a key role in supplementing sibling visitation to promote increased contact among siblings on an ongoing basis. Sibling visitation also helps the sibling adapt to the situation. It dispels misconceptions the sibling may have about the hospitalized child, such as

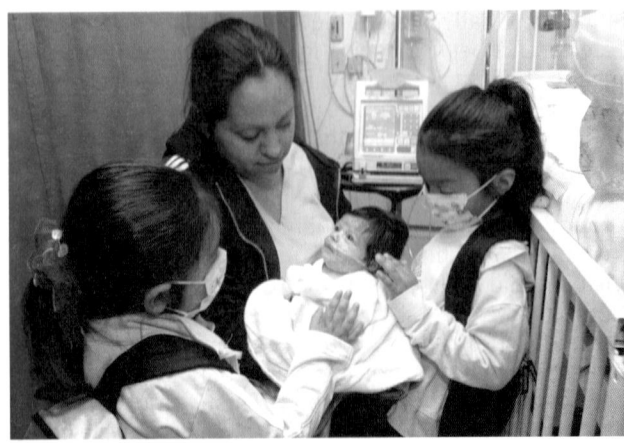

Figure 11-14 Sibling visitation helps normalize the hospital experience for the ill child and helps the sibling to cope with the situation as well.

things are "worse" than reported or the child is dead. It helps reduce separation anxiety of siblings when parents spend time at the hospital. Sibling visitation also provides opportunities for nurses to intervene directly, educate, allay fears, and promote a realistic understanding of the

---

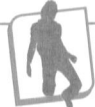

NIC 11-3 NURSING INTERVENTIONS CLASSIFICATION: Sibling Support

Definition: Assisting a sibling to cope with a brother or sister's illness/chronic condition/disability

Activities:

Explore what sibling knows about brother or sister

Appraise stress in sibling related to condition of affected brother or sister

Appraise sibling's coping with illness/disability of brother or sister

Facilitate family members' awareness of sibling's feelings

Provide information about common sibling responses and what other family members can do to help

Perform sibling advocacy role (e.g., in case of life-threatening situations when anxiety is high and parents or other family members are unable to perform that role)

Recognize that each sibling responds differently

Encourage parents or other family members to provide honest information to sibling

Encourage parents to arrange for care of young sibling in their own home, if possible

Assist sibling to maintain and/or modify usual routines and activities of daily living, as necessary

Promote communication between well sibling and affected brother or sister

Value each child individually, avoiding comparisons

Help child to see differences/similarities between self and sibling with special needs

Encourage sibling to visit affected brother or sister

Explain to visiting sibling what is being done in care of affected brother or sister

Encourage well sibling to participate in care of the affected brother or sister, as appropriate

Teach well sibling ways to interact with affected sister/brother

Permit siblings to settle own difficulties

Recognize and respect sibling who may not be emotionally ready to visit an affected brother or sister

Respect well sibling's reluctance to be with or to include child with special needs in activities

Encourage maintenance of parental or family interactional patterns

Assist parents to be fair in terms of discipline, resources, and attention

Assist sibling to clarify and explore concerns

Use drawings, puppetry, and dramatic play to see how younger sibling perceives events

Clarify sibling concern for contracting the illness of the affected child, and develop strategies for coping with concern

Teach pathology of disease to sibling, according to developmental stage and learning style

Use concrete substitutes for sibling who is unable to visit affected brother or sister (e.g., pictures and videos)

Explain to young siblings that they are not the cause of illness

Teach sibling strategies for meeting own emotional and developmental needs

Praise siblings when they have been patient, have sacrificed, or have been particularly helpful

Acknowledge the personal strengths siblings have and their abilities to cope with stress successfully

Provide referral to peer sibling group, as appropriate

Provide community resource referrals to sibling, as necessary

Communicate situation to the school nurse to promote support for younger sibling, in accord with parental wishes

From Bulechek, G. M., Butcher, H. K., Dochterman, J. M. et al. (Eds.). (2013). *Nursing interventions classifications (NIC)* (6th ed.). St. Louis, MO: Mosby. Used with permission.

situation. Finally, it eases the strain on parents who often face conflict between being in the hospital and supervising the children at home. Some hospitals have developed special play areas in the hospital for siblings. These areas allow the sibling to visit the patient and provide a safe and developmentally appropriate environment to play in while the parents are with the patient.

Reduce chaos by controlling the hours for sibling visitation and limiting the number of persons who visit a child at any one time. Although sibling visitation has not been shown to be related to greater cross infection (Rozdilsky, 2005), screening siblings for infectious symptoms or exposures may protect vulnerable patients and their visitors. This type of screening can limit potential exposures to varicella, measles, and respiratory syncytial virus. A sibling visitation policy provides a consistent approach that the staff can follow and present to families (Nursing Interventions 11-9).

ANSWER: A question the nurse could ask Wendy is, "What time of day is it most important for you to be home with your other children?" This type of question turns Wendy's focus to her family, "gives permission" to leave Cory, and validates the needs of the other family members. Although Cory's siblings are teenagers and preteens, they continue to have needs of their own. The nurse should include them in the assessment of family coping, such as asking them, "What has been the hardest part of having Cory in the hospital?" They may have questions about Cory's experience, appendicitis, and his surgery. They may be reluctant to voice their concern that this could happen to them, but they are probably thinking it. Continuing the siblings' visitation pattern normalizes Cory's afternoon routine.

Support Groups

Parents usually find it helpful to discuss concerns about their ill child with other parents who have similar experiences (Buarque et al., 2006; Danino & Shechtman, 2012; Hurst, 2006). To facilitate this, the nurse can introduce parents to each other or refer them to a specific support group. Many types of support groups exist, ranging from disease-specific support groups, to support groups for siblings and grandparents, and online support groups.

The unit-based support group is a particular type of support group. It is especially useful during hospitalization because it can provide a brief escape from the stress of the hospital environment. In this support group, parents can discuss their immediate concerns about hospitalization. The presence of other parents makes it easier to discuss issues that they may have difficulty addressing individually with a staff member. These support groups are usually led by a professional such as a nurse, child life specialist, or social worker. The group leader must have an understanding of group theory and excellent communication skills.

Having a hospital staff member lead the group helps parents solve problems that they identify in the group, such as displeasure with routines or concern over a child's behavior. In a support group for an infant special care unit, for example, the group may be led by the unit-based social worker and a translator to provide a means for families, as needed, to better understand hospitalization and vent their frustrations with it. Each week, a member of a different discipline attends the support group so parents can discuss specific questions with that representative. This type of group helps parents feel like part of the team.

NURSING INTERVENTIONS 11-9

Sibling Visitation

- Find out if a sibling would like to visit. Respect the child's feelings.
- Establish specific times for sibling visitation, preferably times when siblings will be out of school and when many procedures are not being carried out. Screen siblings every 24 hours to identify symptoms of communicable disease, such as rash, runny nose, or cough; many institutions have a standard form. Teach the family about sibling screening policy. Indicate clearance of sibling for visitation on the unit.
- Explore the visiting child's understanding and provide age-appropriate information before the child comes to the unit. Visual aids can familiarize children with what they will see.

- If visiting children must wear isolation clothing, allow them to dress in gowns, gloves, and masks and role-play before the visit.
- Ask parents if they want help responding to sibling's questions, concerns, anger, frustrations, or fears during the visit.
- Control the environment to make it as familiar and nonthreatening to the visiting sibling as possible.
- Use drapes or dividers to provide privacy and shield the visiting sibling from confusing or disturbing sights.
- Avoid interrupting the visit for intrusive procedures or examinations.
- Be sure the sibling is always accompanied by another family member.
- Ensure that the sibling performs hand hygiene upon entering and leaving room.

NURSING CARE OF THE CHILD UNDERGOING SURGERY

Surgery is a frequent reason for children to interface with the acute care setting. Although it may be unexpected, most admissions to the hospital for surgery are planned. Thus, families and children anticipate their entry into the acute care setting. Coordinated care and preparation of the child and family for their surgical experience can decrease the stress and anxiety associated with a sick child. See Evidence-Based Clinical Practice Guidelines 11-1.

PREOPERATIVE CARE

Preparation of the child and family for surgery can be a highly specific process, tailored to the child's needs and developmental status, and to the procedure required. In many facilities, the nurse is a primary source of information for the child and family. The nurse may need to clarify information and misconceptions or counsel the child and family as the emotional impact of the need for surgery is understood.

caREminder

Clarify family understanding by routinely reviewing discussions the family has had with the surgeon, anesthesiologist, and other members of the health care team.

Teaching

 QUESTION: How much preoperative teaching is appropriate for Cory and his mother?

Preoperative anxiety has been identified as a universal phenomenon and can be expected to affect young children as well as older patients. Children's anxiety is related to their parents' anxiety (Kain et al., 2006). A goal of preparing children and families for surgery is to minimize the impact of the unexpected and to endeavor to make the unknown known in a nonthreatening manner. By doing so, the anxiety of facing the unfamiliar can be reduced. Adequate preparation may also bolster feelings of control. Preparation for procedures by providing adequate information can positively influence children's coping and the outcome of their hospitalization (Brewer et al., 2006).

Individualize preoperative teaching strategies based on the child and family's developmental level, anxiety level, previous experiences, and whether the surgery is done emergently or as a planned event (Developmental Considerations 11-7). Keeping in mind that children usually regress when stressed and that high anxiety levels interfere with information processing, present information in simple terms and provide sensory descriptions (e.g., what the child will feel, see, taste, smell, or hear). Ask the child what he or she knows about the surgery and what he or she wants to know. Explain the expected sequence of events

---

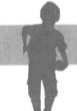 **EVIDENCE-BASED CLINICAL PRACTICE GUIDELINES 11-1**

Caring for the Child Undergoing Surgery or Procedures

Cincinnati Children's Hospital Medical Center

http://www.cincinnatichildrens.org/service/j/anderson-center/evidence-based-care/bests/

Source for Best Evidence Statements (BESts) such as Preoperative Education: Timing of Patient/Family Preoperative Education and its Relationship to Retention of Information

---

Koller, D. (2007). *Child Life Council evidence-based practice statement: Preparing children and adolescents for medical procedures.* Retrieved from

http://www.childlife.org/files/EBPPreparationStatement-Complete.pdf

The statement from child life specialists details the importance of group preparation of pediatric surgical patients and their families.

American Academy of Pediatrics & American Academy of Pediatric Dentistry. (2006). *Guideline for monitoring and management of pediatric patients during and after sedation for diagnostic and therapeutic procedures.* Retrieved from

http://www.aapd.org/media/Policies_Guidelines/G_Sedation.pdf

A review of the guidelines for monitoring and providing management of pediatric surgery patients undergoing sedation and anesthesia.

Institute for Clinical Systems Improvement (ICSI). *Preoperative evaluation.* Retrieved from

https://www.icsi.org/_asset/7y87p4/Preop.pdf

Provides guidelines for evaluation for elective, non-high-risk operative procedures.

Institute for Clinical Systems Improvement (ICSI). *Non-OR procedural safety.* Retrieved from

https://www.icsi.org/_asset/1hht9h/NonOR-Interactive0912.pdf

Provides guidelines for safe site procedural safety for invasive procedures performed outside of the OR.

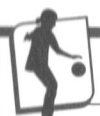

DEVELOPMENTAL CONSIDERATIONS 11-7

Preparation of the Child for Surgery

Infancy

Avoid making changes in an infant's routine prior to surgery (e.g., starting to introduce solids or changing sleeping schedules).

Infants who are used to being around a variety of people will be less cranky in the unfamiliar environment of the acute care setting.

Place familiar items in bed with the child, such as a music box or stuffed animal.

Early Childhood

Provide detailed information to parents; give simple and brief information to the child.

Allow time to play and space for exploration.

Encourage contact with security object.

Use imitation.

Dispel misconceptions.

Reinforce that there will be parental presence.

Middle Childhood

Give more detailed explanation.

Reinforce peer involvement.

Introduce to hospital units and equipment.

Dispel myths.

Respect privacy; reduce exposure of body.

Provide simple reading materials.

Adolescence

Encourage peer interaction and telephone access, when possible.

Emphasize positive attributes; consider body image changes.

Use reading materials/videos/CDs.

Explain all activities; include patient in all decisions.

Respect need for privacy and allow for private teaching.

All Age Groups

Provide diversional activities when stable (videos, CDs, TV, books, toys).

---

and what will happen. Considering the literal, concrete thinking in early childhood, use simple, brief language. Children during middle childhood are in the psychosocial stage of industry versus inferiority and have an increased ability to process information. Speak directly to the child and actively engage him or her (e.g., selecting a scented anesthesia mask); explain activities (e.g., "The purpose of the belt on the stretcher is to prevent you from falling, not to tie you down."). During adolescence, as the capacity for abstract thinking develops, ensure that the level of information and detail matches the adolescent's ability and needs by periodically asking what his or her understanding is and if he or she wants different information.

Help identify appropriate coping strategies; demonstrate relaxation methods, distraction, and deep-breathing techniques so that the child can practice them in advance and they may be sufficiently useful for the child to maintain control (see Chapter 10 for a discussion of these techniques). Use a peer model to demonstrate coping skills.

caREminder

Build on the previous experiences of the child when presenting new information. For example, if the child has been hospitalized before, explore what the child remembers of the experience and use that information in presenting the new information. Written material alone is not effective (MacLaren & Kain, 2007). Use videos, tours, pictures, manipulation of medical equipment, or role playing to increase the effectiveness of the information and to help allay fears and correct misconceptions.

Provide opportunities for the child and family to express emotions, fears, and anxieties and to ask questions. Evaluate understanding and clarify misperceptions. When surgery is planned, prepare children younger than 6 years of age no more than a week in advance; prepare children older than 6 years of age at least 5 days in advance (MacLaren & Kain, 2007), which gives them time to incorporate the information and practice coping techniques. When surgery is done on an emergent basis, condense teaching and present essential information, perhaps just as events are occurring.

ANSWER: Cory and his family had very little time for preoperative teaching. Before surgery, the nurses should give consistent and concise information and be active listeners. Expect that Cory's parents may need to hear the same information several times to absorb it.

Consents

During admission, the family is generally required to sign a bewildering array of forms, most of which contain a large amount of material in relatively small type. One of these forms requiring signature is a general consent form, which is required before any patient is admitted. The amount of information provided to the family at this time varies greatly depending on the facility or the person who asks the family to sign.

Informed consent is the standard for all patients who are admitted to the hospital or undergo medical procedures. When the patient is a child, it is particularly important to keep the parents informed so that they can make treatment decisions for their child based on the most complete information available. The explanations should be comprehensive and should describe the potential benefits and risks of each procedure or regimen (see Chapter 2 for more information on consent and assent).

The parent or legal guardian is asked to sign a consent form for any specific procedure to be performed whenever possible. In an emergency, when a delay in obtaining consent is likely to lead to loss of the patient's life or significant functioning, the physician can authorize an emergency procedure. The institution should have a clear written policy for these cases.

Generally, the procedural or surgical consent form is more detailed than the general consent form required for hospital admission. These specific authorizations are used in obtaining informed consent. Informed consent is based on the concept that the child, parent, or guardian has the right to receive details and information about the child's health as well as the expected risks and benefits of the specific procedures and alternative methods of treatment. The informed consent form gives the child and family clear explanations in language that they can comprehend. Based on this information, the family can weigh the implications, analyze expected outcomes, consider alternatives, and then decide to approve or refuse the procedure based on the child's best interests. Informed consent requires the physician and family to collaborate with respect to health care.

Preoperative Assessment

 QUESTION: Based on the case studies featuring Cory, can you identify any preoperative risks that Cory may have?

One of the nurse's principal responsibilities when caring for a child before surgery is the preoperative assessment of the child and family. The goal is to identify those factors that might put the child at risk for adverse perioperative outcomes and inform the parents of the potential risks.

Children have a higher incidence of perioperative cardiac arrest and mortality than adults (Braz et al., 2006). The most common causes of anesthesia-related cardiac arrest in children are respiratory then cardiovascular (Bharti et al., 2009). Risks for perioperative critical incidents include higher American Society of Anesthesiologists status (American Society of Anesthesiologists physical status classification), age (infants), and emergency surgery (Bharti et al., 2009).

Assess for preexisting respiratory and cardiovascular disease, prematurity, neuromuscular disease, and chronic steroid therapy because these children are at increased risk for perioperative complications. Also, consider the child's age, developmental level, surgical procedure to be performed, presurgical preparation, and the psychological status of the child and family. Identifying the factors that may influence a child's surgery and recovery aid the nurse in developing and implementing strategies to facilitate the most positive outcome.

Because children have a higher incidence of respiratory events, evaluate for a history of a recent upper or lower respiratory infection that might cause potential respiratory complications. In some cases, the surgery may be postponed, especially if endotracheal intubation is necessary. Use of a face mask or laryngeal mask airway to administer anesthesia, instead of a tracheal tube, can decrease the child's incidence of respiratory adverse events (Becke, 2012). The decision to proceed with surgery rests with the surgical team; if postponed, a delay of 4 to 6 weeks is typical (Burd et al., 2006).

Children with asthma are at risk for perioperative complications, most often bronchospasm (Dones et al., 2012). To decrease the incidence of respiratory complications, corticosteroids such as prednisone and a beta-agonist may be administered prior to surgery.

Premature infants are at increased risk for developing postoperative apnea during the first 6 months of life (Walther-Larsen & Rasmussen, 2006). Although the use of regional anesthesia in this high-risk group has been shown to decrease the risk of apnea, continuously monitor these infants for complications for 12 hours postoperatively. Administration of caffeine decreases the incidence of postoperative apnea in this high-risk group (Walther-Larsen & Rasmussen, 2006). In addition, infants with bronchopulmonary dysplasia are at risk for hypoxemia and right heart failure and will also require admission to a pediatric intensive care unit (PICU) for close observation postoperatively.

Because innocent heart murmurs are common in children, a heart murmur may be detected during the presurgical assessment (see Chapter 8 for discussion of innocent murmurs). It is important to identify children with cardiac anomalies prior to anesthesia because of the changes in vascular resistance that occur, potentially altering intracardiac shunts. If signs of a potentially pathologic murmur are detected, then further follow-up with a cardiologist is warranted. In the child with a known cardiac anomaly, obtain details of the type of defect, previous surgeries, and current status and notify the anesthesia care provider prior to surgery. Antibiotic prophylaxis to prevent bacterial endocarditis may be ordered.

Children with neuromuscular disorders may be at risk for increased intracranial pressure as a result of cerebral vasodilation during induction. Impaired airway function and decreased reflexes postoperatively may be present in children with preexisting neuromuscular weakness such as muscular dystrophy. Children receiving anticonvulsants should have therapeutic drug levels checked preoperatively to avoid perioperative complications related to nontherapeutic drug levels.

Patients with sickle cell anemia are at increased risk for postoperative complications related to general anesthesia. Preoperatively, assess the type of sickle crises, date of most recent crisis, and organ involvement. Transfusion and hydration may be indicated preoperatively to prevent sickling related to hypoxia, hypothermia, and hypovolemia and hypoperfusion states that can occur during the perioperative and postoperative periods.

Routine preoperative laboratory testing is not recommended; it should be individualized (Ireland, 2006). A hematocrit level is typically obtained in infants younger than 1 year of age, in menstruating girls, or in those with chronic conditions; pregnancy testing of menarcheal females is controversial (Burd et al., 2006). A type and crossmatch for packed red blood cells in case of the need for a blood transfusion may be indicated. Obtain the laboratory results 24 to 48 hours before surgery and ensure that the values are available in the medical record. The parents and patient should be counseled on potential complications and informed of the reason for the testing.

caREminder

Review the laboratory test results during the presurgical assessment and notify the surgeon of abnormal findings. A decision will be made whether to cancel the surgery.

ANSWER: No surgical risks were identified during Cory's preoperative assessment. However, his radiographs identified previously undiagnosed scoliosis. Cory's mother and older brother also have scolioss.

Preoperative Fasting

Surgical patients must remain on NPO (nothing by mouth) status for a minimum time before scheduled surgery. This practice is based on the need for the patient to have a relatively empty stomach, which reduces the risk of aspiration if vomiting occurs after anesthesia administration. Allowing the child to drink *clear* fluids until 2 hours prior to the operation does not result in any increased gastric volume (Brady et al., 2009). Withholding fluids and solids can often result in a fussy; agitated; and possibly dehydrated, hypoglycemic child. In light of this finding, the standardized order of "NPO after midnight" is increasingly being replaced with shorter, more individualized time frames (Crenshaw, 2011). The American Society of Anesthesiologists (2011) recommends the following NPO guidelines: 6 hours for a light meal of solids and nonhuman milk such as formula, 4 hours for breast milk, and 2 hours for clear liquids. Patients undergoing emergency surgery may not have the opportunity to be NPO for the recommended time frame. In these cases, the risk of aspiration must be assessed against the need for surgery.

caREminder

To avoid misunderstanding and potential delay or cancellation of surgery, give specific written instructions regarding fasting to the family.

The NPO guidelines apply to healthy children (Community Care 11-1). The anesthesiologist orders the specific time period the child is to remain NPO. Children who are at higher risk of aspiration include those with delayed gastric emptying, esophageal reflux, obesity, pregnancy, a tenuous airway, systemic disease, previous vomiting during induction, and emergency surgery. Except when surgery is unanticipated, high-risk patients generally have food withheld for 12 hours and clear fluids withheld for 8 hours. An IV line may be started to avoid dehydration.

Skin Preparation

Because skin ordinarily sustains a wide variety of potentially infectious bacteria and other microorganisms, many sanction skin cleansing prior to surgery to reduce surgical site infections (SSIs). The rationale is that mechanical scrubbing with an antimicrobial soap solution removes microbes, flakes of dead skin cells, oils, and other debris that foster the growth of the bacteria. Even with the most thorough skin cleansing, however, live human skin can never be completely "sterilized" of all microorganisms.

To reduce SSIs, some facilities aspire to achieve such a progressive reduction of bacteria that children are instructed to begin antimicrobial skin preparation before admission to the hospital for elective procedures. However, there is conflicting research about whether preoperative washing more effectively reduces SSIs over no washing, and research does not demonstrate that chlorhexidine is more effective than other cleansers (Webster & Osborne, 2012).

The evidence is inconclusive as to whether hair removal reduces SSIs (Tanner et al., 2011). Regardless, hair removal is rarely deemed necessary in prepubescent children because they have scant amounts of body hair. If hair removal is necessary, it is completed with the goal of preserving skin integrity. Clippers are associated with fewer SSIs than a razor (Tanner et al., 2011). Razors, although able to remove hair closer to the root than clippers, are more apt to produce microscopic abrasions and nicks in the skin that serve as a port of entry and thus a potential source of infection. Therefore, use clippers if hair removal is indicated. Because many individuals are sensitive to depilatories, their use requires testing on a patch of skin 24 hours prior to use. Children, in particular, because of their skin structure, develop adverse reactions to depilatories; therefore, their use is rarely indicated. There is insufficient evidence to determine the optimal time for hair removal (Tanner et al., 2011). However, although it prolongs anesthesia time, hair removal after the child is anesthetized reduces anxiety in the child and minimizes scratches and nicks because the risk for the child making sudden movements is eliminated.

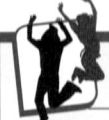

COMMUNITY CARE 11-1

Preoperative Fasting Instructions

- Normal meals and snacks may be eaten until bedtime on the evening before the day of surgery.
- A light meal of dry toast may be eaten up to 6 hours before the start of surgery.
- Clear fluids may be ingested until 2 hours before the start of surgery. Clear fluids are fluids you can see through such as water, apple juice, cranberry juice, Jell-O, ginger ale, and so forth. Fluids that should *not* be ingested include milk, orange juice, and other fluids that contain particulate matter and are not clear.
- Infants who receive formula should finish their last feeding 6 hours before the start of surgery. Like older children, they may drink *clear* fluids up to 2 hours before the start of surgery.

- Infants who are breastfed may nurse until 4 hours before they are scheduled for surgery.
- Exceptions to these rules may be made by the anesthesiologist, taking into account the health status and special considerations of the individual child.
- If the child must take any oral medication, generally, it may be taken with a small sip of water. Medications that are important to continue include antibiotics, anticonvulsants, bronchodilators, and other drugs ordered by the surgeon or anesthesiologist. Inform the health care team of these and any other medications that your child is currently taking.
- Gum chewing in children old enough to safely chew gum, when NPO up to the time that sedatives are administered, enhances comfort (Poultion, 2012).

This is an example of information the nurse may provide to the patient and family before surgery. Specific instructions may vary; check your facility's protocol.

Ensure removal of body-piercing jewelry before surgery because electrical burns can occur with electrocauterization. The skin tract may close with temporary removal, so a nonmetallic spacer may be substituted.

Surgical Suite

QUESTION: Given Cory's behavior in the emergency department, would you advocate his mother's presence prior to anesthesia and in the PACU?

Just prior to transporting the child to the OR, one last assessment is performed. Most facilities have a form that must be completed that covers standard assessment parameters (Table 11-2).

To eliminate wrong site, wrong procedure, wrong person surgery, perform a preoperative verification process and time-out before the start of any surgical or invasive procedure (The Joint Commission, 2010). Prior to moving the child into the room where the procedure will be done, mark the site according to institutional protocol. The parent or whoever has authority to provide informed consent for the child should participate in the site-marking process. A final verification process or time-out involving active communication of all team members must occur in the location where the procedure is to be performed. This verifies the correct patient, correct procedure, and correct site.

Some facilities may allow parents to be present during the initial administration of anesthesia in a designated "anesthesia induction area" or preoperative holding area (Fig. 11-15). A few facilities allow parents to be present when the initial anesthesia takes place in the sterile environment of an OR. These practices attempt to address the child's fear and separation anxiety and cultivate a smoother induction because preoperative anxiety can negatively impact postoperative recovery, with possibly long-term effects (Ahmed et al., 2011). The evidence does not demonstrate that parental presence alleviates the child's or parents' anxiety; premedication with midazolam has demonstrated effectiveness (Chundamala et al., 2009). Some legal and other concerns may argue against parents in the OR. For one, parents may not fully comprehend the OR routine and may interpret an unremarkable event or comment as malevolent circumstance. Another concern is the reaction of a "civilian" in the OR and the possibility that an unpredictable reaction (such as fainting) may occur. These concerns may have some basis but may be addressed with proper screening of the child, parent, and situation and with adequate preparation.

To determine the appropriateness of parental presence during induction, consider the child's developmental level, age, willingness to cooperate, previous hospital experiences, and level of anxiety. Behavioral characteristics are better predictors of the child's anxiety than anxiety ratings, and pediatric anesthesiologists are better at predicting a child's anxiety than parents (Berghmans et al., 2012; MacLaren et al., 2010). Parents' desire to be present must also be considered. Prepare the parent who wishes to be present for how the OR will look, the sequence of events, how the child may react (e.g., eyes rolling back, drooling, involuntary movements), and specific actions they can do to support the child (e.g., sitting next to him or her, maintaining physical contact, talking to the child). A preoperative information audiovisual aid can help reduce parental anxiety (Berghmans et al., 2012). This can be

TABLE 11-2   Pediatric Presurgical Check

Aspect of Care	Nursing Action	Rationale/Considerations
Identification verification	Verify that ID band matches with patient/family statement and chart documentation.	The ID band functions as a safety measure so that the proper patient receives the correct surgery.
Preoperative workup within hospital parameters (often 72 hours)	Check that laboratory values are in the chart. Assess laboratory values for relationship to normalcy and identify any values that lie outside normal ranges.	Pay special attention to potentially significant outliers that may indicate change in patient status or electrolyte imbalance.
Consents completed: general consent, surgical consent	Confirm that all required consent forms are fully filled out, with dates, proper procedure identified, and witness.	Lack of properly signed consents can result in litigation and refusal of reimbursement to the institution.
Surgical attire	Dress child per facility's policy regarding perioperative attire.	Some facilities allow children to wear underwear to the OR to reduce anxiety.
Family notification	Verify that the family/guardian is informed regarding location of surgical waiting room, anticipated length of surgery, and areas to obtain amenities such as coffee and refreshments.	Concerned family members generally want to remain nearby when possible so they may be notified regarding the ongoing status or outcome of surgery as soon as possible.
Allergy status	Prominently note known or suspected allergies in the chart.	Ask patient or family members about any allergies, including episodes of hives and food or medication allergy.
Familial history of problems with anesthesia	Elicit family history of reaction to anesthesia.	Intolerance or adverse reactions to anesthesia can be life threatening and may be hereditary.
Vital signs	Chart current vital signs; identify any unusual trends or values outside the norm.	Unusual patterns or change in vital signs may indicate change in patient status.
Body weight and height	Document current height and weight.	Height and weight are the primary parameters used to determine drug dosages, blood volume, and fluid requirements.
Urine	Encourage child to void prior to surgery, and document; note any changes or unusual appearance in urine.	The opportunity to void in the OR may be limited, and the child will receive generous amounts of IV fluids intraoperatively.
NPO status	Keep the child NPO as ordered; inform family of underlying rationale.	Stomach contents may be aspirated during intubation. Anesthesia may reduce gastric motility as well as cause nausea and vomiting.
Removal of foreign objects or personal belongings	Check for and ask the child about the possible presence of hair pins, jewelry, and so forth. Remove these prior to transport to the OR. If items (e.g., a ring) are not removable, notify the OR nurse of their presence so that any hazard that these may produce can be minimized.	Metal or other materials may be a risk factor for burns from the cautery used in surgery or from pressure sores during prolonged surgery. Check even infants for earrings; older children may have other body areas pierced, such as umbilicus.
Removal of prostheses	Remove contact lenses, eyeglasses, and orthodontic appliances prior to transport to the OR. Note any exceptions.	Items such as contact lenses and orthodontic appliances are commonly encountered in the preadolescent and adolescent population.
Nail bed assessment	Remove any nail polish from fingers and toes prior to transport to the OR.	Nail polish can obscure the ability to accurately assess for oxygenation and capillary refill.
Dentition	Examine the mouth and inquire about potentially loose teeth. If identified, note and report to the OR nurse or anesthetist.	Children intermittently loosen their primary teeth, which can pose a hazard should the child be intubated.
Preoperative medication	Administer any prescribed medications prior to transport to OR. If intramuscular medications are ordered, check with anesthesia care practitioner to give via different route.	Light sedation is often desirable to allay anxiety associated with surgery. Administer medication with enough time to achieve desired effect and monitor the patient for any adverse reactions.
Operative site preparation	Comply with facility standards for skin preparation for cleansing or hair removal of operative site skin.	The skin at the operative site should be as free of oil and debris as possible to reduce risk of infection.

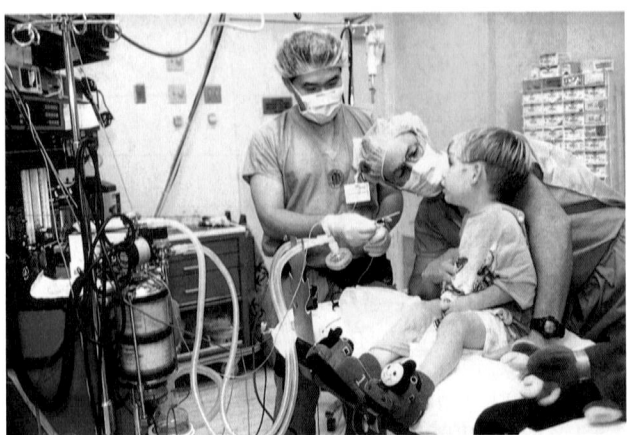

Figure 11-15 A parent's presence in the preoperative area can help reduce the child's separation anxiety. The child must be prepared for the parent's appearance in OR garb.

an emotional experience for the parent; provide support before and after the induction.

When the facility does not permit parents into the OR, the anesthesiologist may administer sedation (e.g., midazolam, ketamine) either nasally or orally to the child in the preoperative holding area. These agents relax the child and create an amnesiac effect so that the child separates from the parent and remembers little about it. Preoperative sedation may reduce preoperative anxiety, but, because of amnesic properties, children may be anxious postoperatively because they do not realize the surgery is completed. Some studies note postoperative negative behaviors with midazolam premedication (Wright et al., 2007); others noted it to be protective (Karling et al., 2007). Midazolam may be most beneficial for anxious children who are not rated by parents to have an impulsive temperament (Wright et al., 2007).

ANSWER: Nurses should advocate and facilitate Wendy's presence in the preoperative setting during the initial administration of anesthesia and also in the PACU. Cory has demonstrated strong separation anxiety and this family has had a very rapid sequence of frightening events. The nurses in both areas can help this family gain an understanding of the situation, decrease the sense of loss of control, and establish a pattern of positive and helpful relationships throughout the acute care experience.

POSTANESTHESIA CARE

After surgery, most patients are taken to the PACU (also called the *recovery room*) or the ICU. This unit provides resources and skilled nursing personnel to closely monitor the child who is emerging or recovering from the effects of the anesthesia. Intensive surveillance and immediate effective intervention are essential because the surgical patient is physiologically unstable as a result of the anesthesia.

The Child's Response to Surgery

Children differ from adults in their response to surgery in several ways (Nursing Interventions 11-10). For example, children are at greater risk of surgical hypothermia than adults; this is caused by four factors. First, the mechanism responsible for thermoregulation is immature and developing, as are most of the child's physical systems. Second, a child is prone to increased heat loss from the body because there is relatively little subcutaneous tissue. Third, a child has a relatively large proportion of body surface area to body weight, which further facilitates heat loss. Fourth, a child loses more heat through respiration than the adult. The ability to achieve and maintain optimal body temperature is inversely proportional to age; that is, the younger the child, the more likely he or she is to have difficulty maintaining body temperature.

Postoperatively, children can suffer many of the same sequelae as adults. They may suffer headache, especially after receiving an inhalational agent. Nausea and vomiting are common, particularly in children who have undergone strabismus surgery, have a surgery duration longer than 30 minutes, are older than 3 years of age, or have a history of postoperative nausea and vomiting (in the child or relatives—mother, father, or siblings) (Kranke et al., 2007). Postoperative bleeding, dizziness, vertigo, loss of appetite, muscle soreness and pain, and sore throat, even after surgery that did not involve endotracheal intubation, are also prevalent. At times during the postoperative period, the child's normal movements may need to be restricted to ensure safety or to keep IV lines or nasogastric tubes in place (see earlier section on "Engineering Controls").

Monitor for signs of malignant hyperthermia: tachypnea, tachycardia, and chaotic dysrhythmias. Later signs are increased temperature, muscle rigidity, hyperkalemia, hypercalcemia, and myoglobinuria. Malignant hyperthermia is an inherited syndrome in which succinylcholine and inhalation agents trigger a fulminant hypermetabolic state.

Visitation in the Postanesthesia Care Unit

The presence of a parent or other trusted family member in the PACU provides invaluable support and can reduce the hospitalized child's sense of isolation and separation anxiety. Thus, many PACUs encourage one parent to visit at the bedside when the child is physiologically stable. At times, facilities may restrict parental visitation, especially when the child is not fully recovered from the effects of anesthesia or when patient acuity level requires a high level of technical interventions.

SAME-DAY SURGERY

For many types of surgeries and patients, outpatient procedures can be performed safely and efficiently. The major disadvantage of same-day surgery is the abbreviated contact with health care providers. Provide thorough postoperative assessment and interventions to compensate for this shortened time for patient and family interactions. It is not mandatory that the child ingest and retain fluids (Awad & Chung, 2006). Letting the child choose whether

NURSING INTERVENTIONS 11-10

Postanesthesia Concerns for the Pediatric Patient

Aspect of Care	Reasons for Concerns	Interventions
Airway management	Laryngospasm after extubation	Position the child to maintain airway; head midline, may need to displace mandible anteriorly, open mouth.
		Administer 100% oxygen via positive pressure ventilation if laryngospasm occurs.
		Anesthesia care practitioner may administer a dose of succinylcholine.
		Assist with reintubation, if needed.
	Postintubation croup	Provide humidified mist to child.
		Give racemic epinephrine treatment via aerosol nebulizer as ordered.
		Give corticosteroids before extubation, if ordered.
		If croup persists longer than 2–4 hours, expect to hospitalize the child overnight for observation.
	Apnea	Use a cardiac monitor, apnea monitor, and pulse oximeter to monitor the child's status.
		Provide assisted ventilation as necessary.
	Airway complications caused by bleeding after nasopharyngeal surgery	Keep appropriate pediatric resuscitative equipment available at the bedside.
		Assess the oral and nasal cavities for bright-red blood.
		Observe for excessive swallowing.
		Monitor for changes in vital signs.
		Provide fluid resuscitation.
		Elevate the head of the bed.
		Apply an ice pack to neck or nose.
		Keep the child as quiet as possible.
		Do not remove clots.
		Administer pain medications as needed.
	Aspiration	Suction the mouth, pharynx, and trachea if vomiting or excessive accumulation of secretions occurs.
		Administer oxygen.
		Position the child prone or on the side.
	Delayed return to consciousness	Before extubation, assess child's muscular strength, respiratory effort, airway protection, and eye opening.
		Identify any residual effects of drugs.
Fluid maintenance	Preexisting volume depletion resulting from illness	Closely monitor intake and output. Urine output should average 1–2 mL/kg/hr.
	NPO status before surgery	Establish and protect venous access.
	Fluid imbalance resulting from child's higher basal metabolic rate (than adults) and greater body surface area; during illness, trauma, or stress, the child's extracellular fluid is easily depleted	Administer maintenance fluids that are hypotonic and contain glucose.
	Although child has relatively greater fluid demands than the adult, actual amount of fluids required is small.	Prevent fluid overload by administering all fluids, blood, and blood products with a volumetric infusion pump.

Aspect of Care	Reasons for Concerns	Interventions
	Accelerated hypoglycemic reactions caused by fluid loss and stress of illness and surgery	Monitor for symptoms of hypoglycemia; check blood glucose if symptoms present.
	External loss of fluid from vomiting, diarrhea, and nasogastric suctioning	Administer isotonic replacement fluids.
	Postoperative hemorrhage resulting from bleeding of an open vessel, continuous third-spacing fluid shift, or coagulopathy	Monitor circulatory status by assessing vital signs, urine output, central venous pressure, and pulmonary artery pressure. Give blood or blood products as ordered.
Seizures	Risk factors, such as previous history of seizures; intracranial injury, hemorrhage, or tumor; increased intracranial pressure; or metabolic or nutritional disorders that may result in electrolyte imbalances, such as hypoglycemia, hypocalcemia, and hyponatremia	Assess the child for predisposing factors that increase risk for seizures. Treat seizures promptly with diazepam or lorazepam as ordered. Ensure that the child's airway is maintained. Provide additional respiratory support after drug therapy begins. Keep resuscitation equipment immediately available. Prepare the child for a complete diagnostic workup as needed to determine the cause of the seizure.
Thermoregulation	High ratio of body surface area to body mass and large head in relation to body size, thus loses heat readily	Use warming lights and warming blankets; increase the room temperature. Warm IV fluids.
	Hypothermia with increased risk of apnea, hypoventilation, hypotension, hypoglycemia, and metabolic acidosis (in neonates)	Wrap the child's head and extremities to preserve body heat. Administer supplemental oxygen. Use pulse oximetry to monitor the adequacy of oxygen therapy.
	Cool OR	
	Postoperative shivering, which can increase oxygen requirements by 400%–500%	Treat shivering with small dose of IV meperidine as ordered, or place heat on the child's skin.
	Hypothermia causes slowed recovery from anesthetic agents and may delay elimination of muscle relaxants	Frequently assess the child's temperature to evaluate the effectiveness of warming measures.
	Heat loss via vasodilation, lack of muscle tone, and inhibition of temperature regulation caused by general anesthesia and neuromuscular block	
Emergence delirium	Increased prevalence in children and young adults	Involve the parents in recovery by having them hold, reassure, and comfort the child.

(Continued)

NURSING INTERVENTIONS 11-10

Postanesthesia Concerns for the Pediatric Patient *(Continued)*

Aspect of Care	Reasons for Concerns	Interventions
	May be exacerbated by hypoxia, nausea, dizziness, inability to move, pain, fear, anxiety, full bladder, hypotension, gastric distention, and pharmacologic agents or postoperative medications	Immediately rule out hypoxia as the cause. Give opioids to treat pain. Catheterize the bladder if warranted. Use a soft, soothing voice and light touch to calm the child. Protect the child from self-injury by padding the bed or crib rails. Relax physical restraints if they cause the child to fight harder. Secure all venous access devices, tubes, drains, and dressings.
Emergency resuscitation	Equipment too large for the child. Immediate need for pediatric dosages of resuscitation medications	Use equipment specifically designed for pediatric patients. Organize resuscitation equipment for pediatric patients on a cart, including defibrillator paddles, intraosseous and IV needles, and oxygen equipment. Ensure that the staff is competent in using pediatric equipment. Keep essential resuscitation medications immediately available in pediatric dosages. Ensure that the child's age and weight are easily retrieved from the medical record. Keep pediatric emergency drug dosage calculation cards handy.

to drink reduces the incidence of vomiting immediately postoperatively (Schreiner et al., 1992; Tabaee et al., 2006) (Chart 11 5; Teaching Intervention Plan 11-2).

PREPARING FOR DISCHARGE FROM AN ACUTE CARE SETTING

QUESTION: What are some aspects of discharge preparation that Cory's family will need to know before Cory's discharge?

A common philosophy is that "discharge planning begins on the day of admission." Upon admission, assess the child's and parent's readiness to learn, barriers to learning, and learning preferences. Because patients are now discharged earlier and often require home care, discharge may be complex and require more family preparation, including education, skill development, and supply acquisition. To prepare families for discharge in the limited time available, use every interaction with the patient and family, formal and informal, as an opportunity to assess, teach, and evaluate learning. To increase effectiveness, make the teaching individualized, meaningful, and family focused. A casual conversation can turn into a teaching and learning opportunity. For example, when entering

---

CHART 11-5 Discharge Criteria for Same-Day Surgery Patients

Child must

- Have vital signs stable, similar to preoperative baseline vital signs, with no signs of respiratory distress
- Have no signs of complications as related to anesthesia or specific to type of operation (e.g., no excessive bleeding from wound; minimal nausea, vomiting, dizziness)
- Have pain well controlled
- Regain preoperative cognitive functioning; may still be very sleepy and need assistance with motor functions
- Have parents state understanding of postoperative care, signs of complications, and when to call health care provider and be given written instructions and prescriptions as indicated

---

TIP 11-2: A TEACHING INTERVENTION PLAN for the Child After Same-Day Surgery

Nursing Diagnoses and Family Outcomes

- Deficient knowledge: Postoperative care, expected postoperative course, signs of complications
  Outcome: Child/family will verbalize and demonstrate appropriate postoperative care and state signs of complications.
- Acute pain related to effects of surgery
  Outcome: Child will have pain adequately managed and verbalize or display minimal pain behaviors.
- Risk for infection related to effects of invasive procedures, break in skin integrity
  Outcome: Child will not develop infection.

Interventions

Educate the Child and Family

- *Activity restrictions:* Usually restrict to quiet activities for 24 hours because of effects of anesthesia; no unsupervised activities for 24 hours that require coordination (e.g., stair climbing, sports), then as appropriate to the procedure (e.g., when myringotomy tubes are placed, child must wear earplugs when in water, such as during bathing and swimming)
- *Intake:* Clear liquids, then increase as tolerated or as specific to procedure (e.g., posttonsillectomy soft foods); how to tell if drinking enough: if voiding once every 8 hours, intake is probably sufficient; tips to promote fluid intake: popsicles, serve fluid in small cups, encourage a few sips with every television commercial
- *Voiding:* If the child has not voided prior to discharge, notify the health care provider if the child does not void within 8 hours after discharge
- *Incision/wound care:* If appropriate, whether to change dressing; amount and type of drainage expected; any special site care; elevation, ice, cleansing
- *Pain management:* How to assess as age and child appropriate; pharmacologic and nonpharmacologic management strategies with potential side effects of drugs and actions to minimize these (e.g., drink plenty of fluids with codeine to counter constipating effects)
- *Proper use of any equipment* (e.g., crutches)

Contact Healthcare Provider if

- *Signs of complications pertinent to procedure:* Excessive bleeding; acute onset, excessive, or poorly controlled pain; unable to tolerate oral fluids; insufficient urine output; altered motor or cognitive functioning, lethargic, unable to arouse

---

the room to administer an oral medication, the mother may ask what medication you are giving. This inquiry offers the opportunity for the nurse to teach the parents about the child's current medications and potential discharge medications. Parents are often "information overloaded" at admission and discharge. Recognizing and using teaching opportunities throughout the hospitalization will result in more successful discharge teaching.

All teaching must be in collaboration with and communicated to other members of the health care team. A documentation system, such as an interdisciplinary patient-teaching tool, enhances communication among the health care team on the child's progress toward reaching discharge teaching goals.

Include follow-up care during discharge preparation. Because hospital stays are relatively brief, follow-up appointments or arrangements are crucial to the patient's health and safety. Follow-up appointments are used to periodically assess the child's progress toward wellness or adaptation. Assist with arrangements for schooling; outpatient therapies; home health referrals; and in-home equipment, supplies, services, and medications as indicated (see Chapter 12 for more discussion).

Follow-up after discharge helps parents obtain more information regarding care of their child and provides support to parents in reassuming (or assuming) their role as primary caregiver. Support after discharge may be more effective because parents may be less anxious, better able to assimilate information, and have had an opportunity to identify specific questions and issues. Postdischarge follow-up can be performed through a telephone call or a home visit, if needed.

ANSWER: For Cory's family, preparation for discharge will include demonstrating competence and confidence in their ability to care for his surgical incision, discussing Cory's diet and appropriate foods for him to eat, and scheduling his follow-up appointment with the pediatric surgeon.

PROLONGED HOSPITALIZATION

Advances in technology have made it possible for many children to survive critical illness who years ago would have died. Some of these children are acutely ill for a period of time, and although their health status stabilizes, they continue to have care needs that necessitate hospitalization. These children may remain in the hospital for many months, or even years. To a child and his or her family, the hospital environment can be confusing and overstimulating. Periods of rest are often broken by painful events and procedures. The hospital certainly is not an environment that is conducive to normal parenting or achievement of tasks that promote growth and development in the child. Also, incorporation of the family's cultural mores is hampered during prolonged hospitalization because exposure to the foods, language, and traditions of the culture are usually limited.

EFFECT ON THE CHILD

Growing up in the hospital may lead to delayed development of psychosocial skills. Prolonged hospitalization may interfere with the development of trust and attachment (Freund et al., 2005). This is of particular concern in infants, who may not form a primary attachment with parents as a result of multiple caretakers meeting the child's needs in often inconsistent ways. It is important to have consistent caretakers who all follow a consistent plan, maintain the child's routine, and set consistent limits on behavior. Develop a plan jointly with the parents, health team, and child if he or she is old enough to participate in the discussion.

Early developmental intervention to prevent the negative effects of prolonged hospitalization is preferable. Encourage developmentally appropriate tasks, even though they may take longer to perform. For example, a young child needs to learn to feed himself and a preschooler needs to dress herself. Performing tasks for themselves fosters a sense of control, which often is difficult to achieve in the hospital. This bolsters self-esteem and socialization skills. It is also important to create personal space for the child, even if it is only a small area, which also helps develop a sense of control. Help the child identify acceptable outlets for expressing negative feelings such as gross motor activity, pounding toys, or words to use. Take infants to the playroom; provide school for older children; children of any age benefit from trips outside. Remember to treat the child as a child, not as a disease.

EFFECT ON PARENTING

Prolonged hospitalization imposes different parenting demands than those in the home. Initially, parents need to deal with the child's illness and uncertainty regarding the outcome (see Chapter 12 for a discussion of chronic conditions). Parents may feel that their role is less important because the health care team has the technologic expertise to care for the child's physical needs.

Implement interventions to strengthen the parent–child bond. Identify a few key staff members for the family to communicate with. This enables these staff members to become familiar with the family's needs and strengths and how to best support them. If parents are unable to stay with the child, minimize interruptions when they do visit. Encourage them to perform normal parenting tasks (e.g., providing physical care, promoting acquisition of developmental tasks, setting limits) and reinforce how important they are to their child. Offer information freely to make parents feel they

are an integral part of the child's care. There will be times when parents cope better than at other times; negotiate with them about how involved they want to be in the child's care. When hospitalization is prolonged, families often become close to each other and close to the nursing staff, sharing information about themselves and their child.

caREminder

Keep information confidential. If families want to share information with the families of other patients, it is the parents' prerogative.

Financial concerns often become more of an issue with prolonged hospitalization. Initially, parents may have been given a paid leave from work. After a period of time, they may need to return to work to maintain insurance benefits and income. They may feel powerless and guilty because they must work and thus cannot be with the child as much as they would like. Parents may feel stuck in a position, unable to change jobs because of preexisting condition exclusions on much-needed insurance. All these factors may make the parent less able to support the child during his or her hospitalization.

CARE CONFERENCES

Patient care conferences are useful in the coordination of care for children with prolonged hospitalization. A care conference is a meeting that is set up before the discharge of a medically complex patient. The social worker or case manager usually assembles the health care team members to meet to discuss the physiologic and psychosocial needs of the child and family during the hospitalization through discharge. The nurse plays a vital role in providing information to the health care team regarding the child's course of illness and future needs. Care conferences should include all members of the health care team involved in the child's care (e.g., parents, nurses, social workers, medical staff, nutrition counselors, child life specialists, pharmacists). This interdisciplinary team approach helps to promote understanding and trust between the family and health care team. Focus the conference on the needs of the child and family and how they can be met. Debrief the family after the meeting to ensure their understanding of the discussion and future steps. The advantages to the implementation of care conferences include

- Promoting clear, effective communication between the family and members of the health care team
- Facilitating collaboration between the family and health care team
- Facilitating the identification of priorities and development of a comprehensive plan of care to address psychosocial, physical, and developmental needs of the hospitalized child and family
- Ensuring adequate preparation for discharge and transition to home

DISCHARGE

After a prolonged hospitalization, discharge presents a greater challenge than normal. The child must adjust, or readjust, to the home environment, with resulting changes in lifestyle. Parents often need to change their schedule and demands of care. Family routines and dynamics will change with the introduction or reintroduction of the child who has been hospitalized. Siblings may need to adjust to changing behavioral expectations, household chores, and routines.

The child and family benefit from a period of transition prior to the actual discharge. Assess what will be needed in the setting the child will be going to; not all children may be able to be discharged home. Determine what equipment, schooling, therapy, respite care, home care, and transportation will need to be arranged (see Chapter 12). Have the parents assume total care of the child in the hospital for 24 hours to gain familiarity and comfort with the process while still having medical support close by.

Remember to talk to the child about the planned discharge. When medically stable, the child may be able to leave the hospital for brief periods of time. These home passes may help the child and family adjust to the change. When the child returns to the hospital, talk concretely about how it was—what he or she did, ate, or saw; sleeping arrangements; and so forth. This will make the impending discharge more real to the child and help ease the transition.

Acute illness and hospitalization of a child are stressors that jeopardize the emotional and physical well-being of the child and threaten family cohesiveness; prolonged hospitalization exacerbates the situation. Using developmentally and culturally appropriate approaches to provide information and emotional support while addressing the child's physiologic needs in the most atraumatic manner possible, the interdisciplinary team can minimize the negative consequences of acute illness and hospitalization.

See thePoint for a summary of Key Concepts.

REFERENCES

Adams, S., Herrera, A., Miller, L. et al. (2011). Visitation in the intensive care unit: Impact on infection prevention and control. *Critical Care Nursing Quarterly*, 34(1), 3–10.

Ahmed, M. I., Farrell, M. A., Parrish, K. et al. (2011). Preoperative anxiety in children risk factors and non-pharmacological management. *Middle East Journal of Anesthesiology*, 21(2), 153–164.

American Academy of Pediatrics. (2006). Child life services. *Pediatrics*, 118(4), 1757–1763.

American Academy of Pediatrics, Task Force on Sudden Infant Death Syndrome. (2011). SIDS and other sleep-related infant deaths: Expansion of recommendations for a safe infant sleeping environment. *Pediatrics*, 128(5), 1030–1039.

American Society of Anesthesiologists. (2011). Practice guidelines for preoperative fasting and the use of pharmacologic agents to reduce the risk of pulmonary aspiration: Application to healthy patients undergoing elective procedures: An updated report by the American Society of Anesthesiologists Committee on Standards and Practice Parameters. *Anesthesiology*, 114(3), 495–511.

Auriti, C., Ronchetti, M. P., Pezzotti, P. et al. (2010). Determinants of nosocomial infection in 6 neonatal intensive care units: An Italian multicenter prospective cohort study. *Infection Control and Hospital Epidemiology*, 1(9), 926–933.

Ausili, E., Tabacco, F., Focarelli, B. et al. (2007). Prevalence of latex allergy in spina bifida: Genetic and environmental risk factors. *European Review for Medical and Pharmacological Sciences*, 11(3), 149–153.

Awad, I. T., & Chung, F. (2006). Factors affecting recovery and discharge following ambulatory surgery. *Canadian Journal of Anaesthesia*, 53(9), 858–872.

Basso, R. (2010). Expressive arts in pediatric orientation groups. *Journal of Pediatric Nursing*, 25(6), 482–489.

Becke, K. (2012). Anesthesia in children with a cold. *Current Opinion in Anaesthesiology*, 25(3), 333–339.

Berghmans, J., Weber, F., van Akoleyen, C. et al. (2012). Audiovisual aid viewing immediately before pediatric induction moderates the accompanying parents' anxiety. *Paediatric Anaesthesiology*, 22(4), 386–392.

Berwick, D. M., & Kotagal, M. (2004). Restricted visiting hours in the ICUs: Time to change. *Journal of the American Medical Association*, 292(6), 736–737.

Bharti, N., Batra, Y. K., & Kaur, H. (2009). Paediatric perioperative cardiac arrest and its mortality: Database of a 60-month period from a tertiary care paediatric centre. *European Journal of Anaesthesiology*, 26(6), 490–495.

Blevins, J. (2011). Oral health care for hospitalized children. *Pediatric Nursing*, 37(5), 229–235.

Board, R. (2005). School-age children's perceptions of their PICU hospitalization. *Pediatric Nursing*, 31, 166–175.

Bostanci, I., Yilmaz, R., Dallar, Y. et al. (2003). Latex sensitivity in hematologic and oncologic non-atopic pediatric patients. *Pediatric Asthma, Allergy & Immunology*, 16, 117–120.

Brady, M. C., Kinn, S., Ness, V. et al. (2009). Preoperative fasting for preventing perioperative complications in children. *Cochrane Database of Systematic Reviews*, (4), CD005285.

Braz, L. G., Braz, J. R. C., Módolo, N. S. P. et al. (2006). Perioperative cardiac arrest and its mortality in children: A 9-year survey in a Brazilian tertiary teaching hospital. *Pediatric Anesthesia*, 16, 860–866.

Brenner, M. (2007). Child restraint in the acute setting of pediatric nursing: An extraordinarily stressful event. *Issues in Comprehensive Pediatric Nursing*, 30, 29–37.

Brewer, S., Gleditsch, S. L., Syblik, D. et al. (2006). Pediatric anxiety: Child life intervention in day surgery. *Journal of Pediatric Nursing*, 21, 13–22.

Buarque, V., Lima, C., Scott, R. P. et al. (2006). The influence of support groups on the family of risk newborns and on neonatal unit workers. *Jornal de Pediatria*, 82(4), 295–301.

Burd, R. S., Mellender, S. J., & Tobias, J. D. (2006). Neonatal and childhood perioperative considerations. *Surgical Clinics of North America*, 86, 227–247.

Chundamala, J., Wright, J. G., & Kemp, S. M. (2009). An evidence-based review of parental presence during anesthesia induction and parent/child anxiety. *Canadian Journal of Anaesthesia*, 56(1), 57–70.

Cirgin Ellett, M. L., Cohen, M. D., Perkins, S. M. et al. (2012). Comparing methods of determining insertion length for placing gastric tubes in children 1 month to 17 years of age. *Journal for Specialists in Pediatric Nursing*, 17(1), 19–32.

Cirgin Ellett, M. L., Cohen, M. D., Perkins, S. M. et al. (2011). Predicting the insertion length for gastric tube placement in neonates. *Journal of Obstetric, Gynecologic, and Neonatal Nursing*, 40(4), 412–421.

Clatworthy, S., Simon, K., & Tiedeman, M. E. (1999). Child drawing: Hospital—An instrument designed to measure the emotional status of hospitalized school-aged children. *Journal of Pediatric Nursing*, 14(1), 2–9.

Corlett, J., & Twycross, A. (2006). Negotiation of parental roles within family-centred care: A review of the research. *Journal of Clinical Nursing*, 15, 1308–1316.

Coyne, I. T. (1995). Partnership in care: Parents' views of participation in their hospitalized child's care. *Journal of Clinical Nursing*, 4, 71–79.

Coyne, I. (2006). Children's experiences of hospitalization. *Journal of Child Health Care*, 10, 326–336.

Coyne, I. (2008). Children's participation in consultations and decision-making at health service level: A review of the literature. *International Journal of Nursing Studies*, 45(11), 1682–1689.

Coyne, I., & Cowley, S. (2007). Challenging the philosophy of partnership with parents: A grounded theory study. *Internal Journal of Nursing Studies*, 44(6), 893–904.

Cremer, R., Lorbacher, M., Hering, F. et al. (2007). Natural rubber latex sensitisation and allergy in patients with spina bifida, urogenital disorders and oesophageal atresia compared with a normal paediatric population. *European Journal of Pediatric Surgery*, 17, 194–198.

Crenshaw, J. (2011) Preoperative fasting: Will the evidence ever be put into practice? *The American Journal of Nursing*, 111(10), 39–43.

Danino, M., & Shechtman, Z. (2012). Superiority of group counseling to individual coaching for parents of children with learning disabilities. *Psychotherapy Research*, 22(5), 592–603.

Davydow, D. S., Richardson, L. P., Zatzick, D. F. et al. (2010). Psychiatric morbidity in pediatric critical illness survivors: A comprehensive review of the literature. *Archives of Pediatrics & Adolescent Medicine*, 164(4), 377–385.

Dehlink, E., Prandstetter, C., Eiwegger, T. et al. (2004). Increased prevalence of latex sensitization among children with chronic renal failure. *Allergy*, 59, 734–738.

Diaz-Caneja, A., Gledhill, J., Weaver, T. et al. (2005). A child's admission to hospital: A qualitative study examining the experiences of parents. *Intensive Care Medicine*, 31(9), 1248–1254.

Dones, F., Foresta, G., & Russotto, V. (2012). Update on perioperative management of the child with asthma. *Pediatric Reports*, 4(2), e19.

Dudley, S. A., & Carr, J. M. (2004). Vigilance: The experience of parents staying at the bedside of hospitalized children. *Journal of Pediatric Nursing*, 19, 267–275.

Finkelhor, D., & Ormrod, R. (2002). *Kidnapping of juveniles: Patterns from NIBRS*. OJJDP Bulletin. Washington, DC: U.S. Department of Justice, Office of Justice Programs, Office of Juvenile Justice and Delinquency Prevention.

Fisher, M., & Broome, M. (2011). Parent-provider communication during hospitalization. *Journal of Pediatric Nursing*, 26(1), 58–69.

Fleming, K., & Randle, J. (2006). Toys: Friend or foe? A study of infection risk in a paediatric intensive care unit. *Paediatric Nursing*, 18(4), 14–18.

Forsner, M., Jansson, L., & Söderberg, A. (2009). Afraid of medical care school-aged children;s narratives about medical fear. *Journal of Pediatric Nursing*, 24(6), 519–528.

Fortier, M. A., Chorney, J. M., Rony, R. Y. et al. (2009). Children's desire for perioperative information. *Anesthesia and Analgesia*, 109(4), 1085–1090.

Freund, P. J., Boone, H. A., Barlow, J. H. et al. (2005). Healthcare and early intervention collaborative supports for families and young children. *Infants & Young Children*, 18, 25–36.

Frisch, A. M., Johnson, A., Timmons, S. et al. (2010). Nurse practitioner role in preparing families for pediatric outpatient surgery. *Pediatric Nursing*, 36(1), 41–47.

Fullbrook, P., Latour, J., Albarran, J. et al. (2007). The presence of family members during cardiopulmonary resuscitation: European Federation of Critical Care Nursing Associations, European Society of Paediatric and Neonatal Intensive Care and European Society of Cardiology Council on Cardiovascular Nursing and Allied Professions joint position statement. *Nursing in Critical Care*, 12(5), 250–252.

Griffin, T. (2003). Facing challenges of family centered care I: Conflicts over visitation. *Pediatric Nursing*, 29(2), 135–137.

Gursky, B. (2007). The effect of educational interventions with siblings of hospitalized children. *Journal of Developmental and Behavioral Pediatrics*, 28(5), 392–398.

Harrison, D., Bueno, M., Yamada, J. et al. (2010). Analgesic effects of sweet-tasting solutions for infants: Current state of equipoise. *Pediatrics*, 126, 894–902.

Hemsworth, S., & Pizer, B. (2006). Pet ownership in immuno-compromised children: A review of the literature and survey of existing guidelines. *European Journal of Oncology Nursing*, 10(2), 117–127.

Henderson, D. P., & Knapp, J. F. (2006). Report of the national consensus conference on family presence during pediatric cardiopulmonary resuscitation and procedures. *Journal of Emergency Nursing*, 32(1), 23–29.

Hopia, H., Tomlinson, P. S., Paavilainen, E. et al. (2005). Child in hospital: Family experiences and expectations of how nurses can promote family health. *Journal of Clinical Nursing*, 14, 212–222.

Hourihane, J. O., Allard, J. M., Wade, A. M. et al. (2002). Impact of repeated surgical procedures on the incidence and prevalence of latex allergy: A prospective study of 1263 children. *Journal of Pediatrics*, 40, 479–482.

Houtzager, B. A., Grootenhuis, M. A., Caron, H. N. et al. (2005). Sibling self-report, parental proxies, and quality of life: The importance of multiple informants for siblings of a critically ill child. *Pediatric Hematology and Oncology*, 22, 25–40.

Hurst, I. (2006). One size does not fit all: Parents' evaluations of a support program in a newborn intensive care nursery. *Journal of Perinatal and Neonatal Nursing*, 20, 252–261.

Ireland, D. (2006). Unique concerns of the pediatric surgical patient: Pre-, intra-, and postoperatively. *Nursing Clinics of North America*, 41, 265–298.

Kain, Z. N., Caldwell-Andrews, A. A., Maranets, I. et al. (2006). Predicting which child–parent pair will benefit from parental presence during induction of anesthesia: A decision-making approach. *Anesthesia and Analgesia*, 102(1), 81–84.

Karling, M., Stenlund, H., & Hägglöf, B. (2007). Child behaviour after anaesthesia: Associated risk factors. *Acta Paediatrica*, 96, 740–747.

Kelsey, J., Abelson-Mitchell, N., & Skirton, H. (2007). Perceptions of young people about decision making in the acute healthcare environment. *Paediatric Nursing*, 19(6), 14–18.

Klassen, J. A., Liang, Y., Tjosvold, L. et al. (2008). Music for pain and anxiety in children undergoing medical procedures: A systematic review of randomized controlled trials. *Ambulatory Pediatrics*, 8(2), 117–128.

Koller, D., & Goldman, R. D. (2012). Distraction techniques for children undergoing procedures: A critical review of pediatric research. *Journal of Pediatric Nursing*, 27(6), 652–681.

Kranke, P., Eberhart, L. H., Toker, H. et al. (2007). A prospective evaluation of the POVOC score for the prediction of postoperative vomiting in children. *Anesthesia & Analgesia*, 105(6), 1592–1597.

Kuruuzum, Z., Yapar, N., Avkan-Oguz, V. et al. (2008). Risk of infection in health care workers following occupational exposure to a noninfectious or unknown source. *American Journal of Infection Control*, 36(10), e27–e31.

Lam, L. W., Chang, A. M., & Morrissey, J. (2006). Parents' experiences of participation in the care of hospitalised children: A qualitative study. *International Journal of Nursing Studies*, 43, 535–545.

Larson, E., Ciliberti, T., Chantler, C. et al. (2004). Comparison of traditional and disposable bed baths in critically ill patients. *American Journal of Critical Care*, 13(3), 235–241.

Levetown, M. (2008). Communicating with children and families: From everyday interactions to skill in conveying distressing information. *Pediatrics*, 121(5), e1441–e1460.

Li, H. C. W. (2007). Evaluating the effectiveness of preoperative interventions: The appropriateness of using the children's emotional manifestation scale. *Journal of Clinical Nursing*, 16(10), 1919–1926.

Li, W. H., Chung, J. O., & Ho, E. K. (2011). The effectiveness of therapeutic play, using virtual reality computer games, in promoting the psychological well-being of children hospitalised with cancer. *Journal of Clinical Nursing, 20*(15–16), 2135–2143.

Lindeke, L., Nakai, M., & Johnson, L. (2006). Capturing children's voices for quality improvement. *MCN. The American Journal of Maternal Child Nursing, 31*, 290–295.

Liu, R. W., Mehta, P., Fortuna, S. et al. (2007). A randomized prospective study of music therapy for reducing anxiety during cast room procedures. *Journal of Pediatric Orthopedics, 27*(7), 831–833.

Macedo, I. S. C., Mateus, D. C., Costa, E. D. M. et al. (2009). Noise assessment in intensive care units. *Brazilian Journal of Otorhinolaryngology, 75*(6), 844–846.

MacLaren, J., & Kain, Z. N. (2007). Pediatric preoperative preparation: A call for evidence-based practice. *Pediatric Anesthesia, 17*, 1019–1020.

MacLaren, J. E., Thompson, C., Weinberg, M. et al., (2010). Prediction of preoperative anxiety in children: Who is most accurate? *Anesthesia and Analgesia, 108*(6), 1777–1782.

Melnyk, B. M., Crean, H. F., Feinstein, N. F. et al. (2007). Testing the theoretical framework of the COPE program for mothers of critically ill children: An integrative model of young children's posthospital adjustment behaviors. *Journal of Pediatric Psychology, 32*(4), 463–474.

Melnyk, B. M., Feinstein, N., & Fairbanks, E. (2006). Two decades of evidence to support implementation of the COPE program as standard practice with parents of young unexpectedly hospitalized/critically ill children and premature infants. *Pediatric Nursing, 32*(5), 475–481.

Meltzer, H., Vostanis, P., Dogra, N. et al. (2008). Children's specific fears. *Child: Care, Health and Development, 35*(6), 781–789.

Meltzer, L., Davis, K., & Mindell, J. (2012). Patient and parent sleep in a children's hospital. *Pediatric Nursing, 38*(2), 64–71.

Moore, L., & Kirk, S. (2010). A literature review of children's and young people's participation in decisions relating to health care. *Journal of Clinical Nursing, 19*(15–16), 2215–2225.

Morris, C. J., Aeschbach, D., & Scheer, F. A. J. L. (2012). Circadian system, sleep and endocrinology. *Molecular and Cellular Endocrinology, 349*(1), 91–104.

Murray, B. L., Kenardy, J. A., & Spence, S. H. (2007). Brief report: Children's responses to trauma- and nontrauma-related hospital admission: A comparison study. *Journal of Pediatric Psychology, 33*(4), 435–440.

Murray, J. S. (2002). A qualitative exploration of psychosocial support for siblings of children with cancer. *Journal of Pediatric Nursing, 17*(5), 327–337.

Nakamura, C. T., Ferdman, R. M., Keens, T. G. et al. (2000). Latex allergy in children on home mechanical ventilation. *Chest, 118*, 1000–1003.

Nelson, L. P., & Gold, J. I. (2012). Posttraumatic stress disorder in children and their parents following admission to the pediatric intensive care unit: A review. *Pediatric Critical Care Medicine, 13*(3), 338–347.

Piira, T., Sugiura, T., Champion, G. D. et al. (2005). The role of parental presence in the context of children's medical procedures: A systematic review. *Child: Care, Health and Development, 31*, 233–243.

Poultion, T. J. (2012). Gum chewing during pre-anesthetic fasting. *Paediatric Anaesthesia, 22*(3), 288–296.

Power, N., & Franck, L. (2008). Parent participation in the care of hospitalized children: A systematic review. *Journal of Advanced Nursing, 62*(6), 622–641.

Prchal, A., & Landolt, M. A. (2009). Psychological interventions with siblings of pediatric cancer patients: A systematic review. *Psychooncology, 18*(12), 1241–1251.

Prugh, D., Staub, E., Sands, H. et al. (1953). A study of the emotional reactions of children and families to hospitalization and illness. *American Journal of Orthopsychiatry, 23*(1), 80–106.

Rabun, J. B. (2005). *For healthcare professionals: Guidelines on prevention of and response to infant abductions* (8th ed.). Arlington,

VA: National Center for Missing and Exploited Children. Retrieved from http://www.missingkids.com/en_US/publications/NC05.pdf

Robertson, J. (1958). *Young children in hospitals.* London, United Kingdom: Tavistock.

Rozdilsky, J. R. (2005). Enhancing sibling presence in pediatric ICU. *Critical Care Nursing Clinics of North America, 17*, 451–461.

Ryan-Wenger, N., Kimchi-Woods, J., Erbaugh, M. et al. (2010). Challenges and conundrums in the validation of pediatric falls risk assessment tools. *Pediatric Nursing, 38*(3), 159–167.

Salandin, A., Arnold, J., & Kornadt, O. (2011). Noise in an intensive care unit. *Journal of the Acoustical Society of America, 130*(6), 3754–3760.

Salmela, M., Aronen, E. T., & Salanterä, S. (2011). The experience of hospital-related fears of 4- to 6-year old children. *Child: Care, Health and Development, 37*(5), 719–726.

Schmidt, C., Bernaix, L., Koski, A. et al (2007). Hospitalized children's perceptions of nurses and nurse behaviors. *MCN. The American Journal of Maternal Child Nursing, 32*, 336–342.

Schreiner, M. S., Nicolson, S. C., Martin, T. et al. (1992). Should children drink before discharge from day surgery? *Anesthesiology, 76*(4), 528–533.

Simon, K. (1993). Perceived stress of nonhospitalized children during the hospitalization of a sibling. *Journal of Pediatric Nursing, 8*, 298–304.

Smith, A., Hefley, G. C., & Anand, K. J. (2007). Parent bed spaces in the PICU: Effect on parental stress. *Pediatric Nursing, 33*, 215–221.

Snyder, B. S. (2004). Preventing treatment interference: Nurses' and parents' intervention strategies. *Pediatric Nursing, 30*(1), 31–40.

Sparta, G., Kemper, M. J., Gerber, A. C. et al. (2004). Latex allergy in children with urological malformation and chronic renal failure. *Journal of Urology, 171*, 1647–1649.

Stouffer, J. W., Shirk, B. J., & Polomano, R. C. (2007). Practice guidelines for music interventions with hospitalized pediatric patients. *Journal of Pediatric Nursing, 22*, 448–456.

Stremler, R., Wong, L., & Parshuram, C. (2007). Practices and provisions for parents sleeping overnight with a hospitalized child. *Journal of Pediatric Psychology, 33*(3), 292–297.

Tabaee, A., Lin, J. W., Duipton, V. et al. (2006). The role of oral fluid intake following adeno-tonsillectomy. *International Journal of Pediatric Otorhinolaryngology, 70*(7), 1159–1164.

Tanner, J., Norrie, P., & Melen, K. (2011). Preoperative hair removal to reduce surgical site infection. *Cochrane Database of Systematic Reviews,*(11), CD004122.

The Joint Commission. (2010). *Universal protocol for preventing wrong site, wrong procedure, wrong person surgery.* Retrieved from http://www.jointcommission.org

The Joint Commission. (2011). *Hospital accreditation standards.* Oakbrook Terrace, IL: Author.

Tourigney, J., Clendinneng, J., Chartrand, J. et al. (2011). Evaluation of a virtual tour for children undergoing same-day surgery and their parents. *Pediatric Nursing, 37*(4), 177–183.

Ullán, A. M., Belver, M. H., Serrano, I. et al. (2012). Perspectives of youths and adults improve the care of hospitalized adolescents in Spain. *Journal of Pediatric Health Care, 26*(3), 182–192.

Walther-Larsen, S., & Rasmussen, L. S. (2006). The former preterm infant and risk of post-operative apnoea: Recommendations for management. *Acta Anaesthesiologica Scandinavica, 50*(7), 888–893.

Webster, J., & Osborne, S. (2012). Preoperative bathing or showering with skin antiseptics to prevent surgical site infection. *Cochrane Database of Systematic Reviews,* (9), CD004985.

Wennström, B., Hallberg, L. R., & Bergh, I. (2008). Use of perioperative dialogues with children undergoing day surgery. *Journal of Advanced Nursing, 62*(1), 96–106.

Whitehead-Pleaux, A. M., Zebrowski, N., Baryza, M. J. et al. (2007). Exploring the effects of music therapy on pediatric pain: Phase 1. *Journal of Music Therapy, 44*, 217–241.

Wilkins, K. L., & Woodgate, R. L. (2006). Transition: A conceptual analysis in the context of siblings of children with cancer. *Journal of Pediatric Nursing, 21*, 256–265.

Wilson, M. E., Megel, M. E., Enenbach, L. et al. (2010). The voices of children: Stories about hospitalization. *Journal of Pediatric Health Care, 24*(2), 95–102.

Wright, K. D., Stewart, S. H., Finely, G. A. et al. (2007). Prevention and intervention strategies to alleviate preoperative anxiety in children: A critical review. *Behavior Modification, 31*(1), 52–79.

Yeh, W. S., Kiohara, P. R., Soares, I. S. et al. (2012). Prevalence of sensitivity signals to latex in meningomyelocele patients undergoing multiple surgical procedures. *Revista Brasileira de Anestesiologia, 62*(1), 56–62.

See the Point for additional resources.

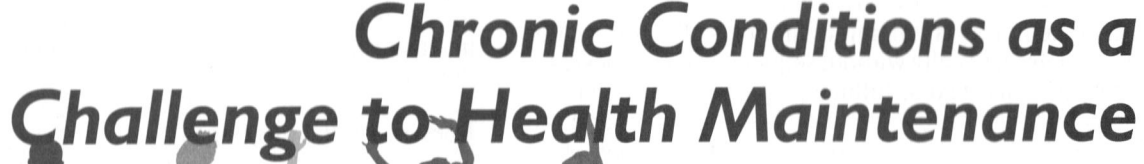

CHAPTER 12

Chronic Conditions as a Challenge to Health Maintenance

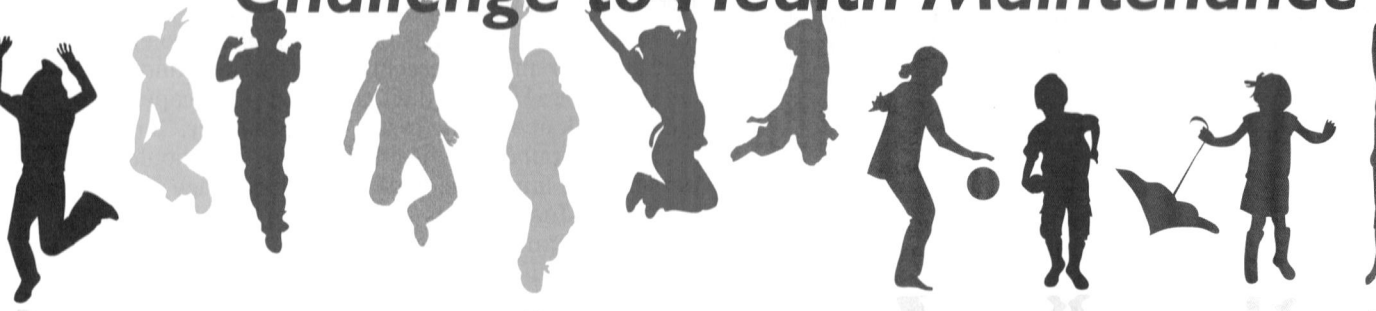

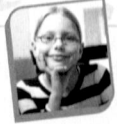

CASE HISTORY

Lindsay Jenkins went to the doctor with her father, Tom, on the Monday after her family returned from Thanksgiving with her grandmother and relatives. She had been unusually thirsty for days now and was often excusing herself to use the restroom. On Sunday evening, she vomited. Her grandmother and aunts had commented on how thin she looked. Her pediatrician had her urine tested for ketones, took her history, and diagnosed her with type 1 diabetes. Lindsay was admitted to the hospital. Lindsay's mother, Jean, had left town that morning on business.

When Tom called his wife to tell her they had to go to the hospital, Jean was devastated. "It was almost like hearing that she was dying. I just kept thinking, 'Why couldn't it be me and not my child?' I joined them at the hospital the next day, but I felt so guilty for not being there when they first heard the diagnosis. Lindsay's blood sugar was still running very high when I arrived at the hospital and Lindsay said hateful things to me. I know now how belligerent and out

of character she can be when her blood sugar is high, but at that time it just added stress to the situation. I remember thinking that she could never be in anyone else's care again and that we would never again have a night away."

"The first year of having a child with diabetes takes over your life. Every meal focuses on the numbers: the number of carbohydrates, the blood sugar numbers, and the amount of insulin. Tom and I attended classes given by diabetes educators, nutritionists, and insulin pump manufacturers. The first time she was away from us was at a weekend camp run by a local diabetes association. The kids swam, played games, and had a camp experience while the camp doctors and nurses managed their insulin and intake. I don't think I slept but about an hour that first night. I was so anxious to know that Lindsay was all right. But I am so glad she went. It proved to me that she could be okay without my constant vigilance, and she has gone to diabetes camp every summer since then."

CHAPTER OBJECTIVES

1 Define chronic condition.

2 Discuss the broad spectrum of disorders that can be defined as chronic conditions; discuss reasons for the disparity in determining the prevalence of children with chronic conditions.

3 Analyze the impact of chronic conditions on children and families.

4 Understand interventions to promote health and normalization for children with chronic conditions and their families.

5 Discuss issues related to having a child with a chronic condition.

6 Contrast pediatric rehabilitation and habilitation with adult rehabilitation.

7 Delineate nursing interventions and strategies to assist the child in gaining independence during the rehabilitative and habilitative processes.

8 Discuss the impact of having a chronic condition on the child/adolescent.

9 Discuss the advocacy role of the nurse related to the laws protecting children and adolescents with chronic conditions.

10 Describe nursing strategies to improve the transition from pediatric settings to adult services.

See thePoint for a list of Key Terms.

UNDERSTANDING CHRONIC CONDITIONS

An acute illness is temporary and episodic; it is treated and resolves, usually without sequelae. Acute illnesses—such as otitis media, influenza, gastroenteritis, lacerations, or appendicitis—typically last a few days or a few weeks. Sometimes the recovery may take longer, such as for pneumonia or a fractured bone. Many conditions, however, can last for years and sometimes for a lifetime; these conditions are termed *chronic conditions*. The definition of a **chronic condition** is one that lasts at least 6 months and requires long-term monitoring and management to control the symptoms and to impact the course of the disease. It includes physical, cognitive, psychological, and social disorders that can range from mild (such as some allergies or learning disabilities) to significant impairments (such as autism or cerebral palsy [CP]) (van der Lee et al., 2007). Chronic conditions are usually caused by irreversible pathologic alterations. Although some chronic conditions may alternate between periods of **remission** (times when no symptoms are evident) and **exacerbation** (times of acute symptomatology related to the condition), the condition still persists.

TERMINOLOGY RELATED TO CHRONICITY

 QUESTION: Which of the terms related to chronicity most accurately describes Lindsay?

There are multiple terms that are used to refer to certain conditions and the children who have those conditions. This section attempts to differentiate and define this terminology as well as provide guidance about appropriate use.

Chronic Condition Versus Chronic Illness

Some confusion exists regarding the difference between the terms *chronic illness* and *chronic condition*. Although all chronic illnesses fit the definition of a chronic condition, very few chronic conditions can be defined as chronic illnesses. A **chronic illness** "implies being sick and needing to recover" (Selekman et al., 2013, p. 701). In other words, the individual is perceived as being sick and not in a state of wellness and is treated as though he or she is not well. An example of a chronic illness is cancer, for which the goal is remission of symptoms. Often, the health care community begins to use the term *cured* after 5 years without symptoms, although it is used with caution.

The vast majority of chronic conditions, however, are *not* chronic illnesses. Conditions such as Down syndrome, myelomeningocele, CP, cystic fibrosis (CF), asthma, diabetes, sickle cell disease, blindness, and attention-deficit/hyperactivity disorder (ADHD) are all chronic conditions, not chronic illnesses. Although children with such conditions might be ill during a period of exacerbation, their chronic condition is always present;

it is *not* an illness from which they can recover. They should not be treated as being ill, except perhaps during periods of exacerbation (Selekman et al., 2013). Therefore, it is strongly recommended that nurses and families use the term *chronic condition* rather than chronic illness.

Person-First Language

Since the 1990s, there has been an emphasis to ensure that children and adolescents with chronic conditions are not referred to "as" their condition. It is inappropriate to speak about "the cystic," "the diabetic," or "the asthmatic"; rather, the health care provider should use **person-first language**. This type of language focuses on the fact that patients are people first and foremost, and they happen to have a chronic condition. Thus, we refer to "the adolescent with asthma," "the child with diabetes," or "the infant with CF." This allows the health care team to focus first on the child or adolescent as a person rather than on the child's disorder. As one adolescent stated to a health care provider, "I am *not* my condition and my condition is *not* who I am. Just because I have a chronic condition, do not treat me like I am sick."

Disability and Related Terms

Numerous terms are used to refer to the population of children and adolescents with chronic conditions. These terms include *disabled*, *children with special health care needs*, *handicapped*, *compromised*, *impaired*, and *technology dependent*.

The term **disability** has at least two official definitions: an educational definition according to the Individuals with Disabilities Education Improvement Act (IDEIA, 2004) and a broader definition as detailed in the Americans with Disabilities Act (ADA, 1990). The IDEIA definition of disability is characterized by disorders that will qualify a student for special education and related services (e.g., autism, intellectual disabilities, speech and language impairment, and traumatic brain injury).

The ADA definition of disability focuses on key life functions that are expected of a child of a particular age (Chart 12-1). This law states that a person with a disability is one who has a physical or mental impairment that substantially limits a major life activity *or* has a record of such impairments *or* is regarded as having such an impairment (ADA, 1990). ADA includes the same disabilities noted in IDEIA and expands the list to include those with chronic contagious and noncontagious diseases, including tuberculosis, HIV, CP, epilepsy, muscular dystrophy, multiple sclerosis, drug addiction, and alcoholism (ADA, 1990). Major life activities include the ability to care for one's self, perform manual tasks, walk, see, hear, speak, breathe, learn, or work.

These definitions will have a significant effect on who will qualify for various services. There are also multiple chronic conditions that are not listed in these definitions. A discussion of the broad spectrum of chronic conditions appears later in this chapter.

CHART 12-1 **Definition of a Child With a Disability**

A child with a disability means a child with "mental retardation, hearing impairments (including deafness), speech or language impairments, visual impairments (including blindness), serious emotional disturbance . . . , orthopedic impairments, autism, traumatic brain injury, other health impairments, or specific learning disabilities; and who, by reason thereof, needs special education and related services" (IDEIA, 2004).

For children who are between the ages of 3 and 9 years, the phrase *child with a disability* "may, at the discretion of the State and the local education agency, include a child experiencing developmental delays, as defined by the State and as measured by appropriate diagnostic instruments and procedures, in 1 or more of the following areas: physical development; cognitive development; communication development; social or emotional development; or adaptive development; and who, by reason thereof, needs special education and related services" (IDEIA, 2004).

Developmental Disability

When a disability has an impact on the development of a child, it is called a **developmental disability**. The U.S. Department of Health & Human Services [USDHHS], Administration for Children and Families (2000) defines developmental disabilities as

> Severe, life-long disabilities attributable to mental and/or physical impairments which manifest themselves before the age of 22 years and are likely to continue indefinitely. They result in substantial limitations in three or more of the following areas: self-care, comprehension and language, skills (receptive and expressive language), learning mobility, self-direction, capacity for independent living, economic self-sufficiency, ability to function independently without coordinated services (continuous need for individually planned and coordinated services). (SECTION 102. DEFINITIONS. [42 USC 15002])

Frequently, children younger than 5 years of age with symptoms suggesting these conditions are referred to as *having developmental delays* rather than *disabilities* (Moeschler & Shevell, 2006). This might be because of the concern by health care providers about labeling a child with a condition that might disappear as the child matures or because of the difficulty in making an accurate diagnosis in a young child. A delay implies a maturational lag and being slower in achieving developmental tasks than children of the same age. There is, however, no clear differentiation between a developmental delay and a developmental disability, and neither of these general terms provides guidance to the health care team in planning care.

Children With Special Health Care Needs

Children with chronic conditions also are often referred to as **children with special health care needs**. The American Academy of Pediatrics uses the definition of the federal Maternal and Child Health Bureau's Division of Services for Children with Special Health Care Needs, which states, "Children with special health care needs are those who have or are at increased risk for a chronic physical, developmental, behavioral, or emotional condition and who also require health and related services of a type or amount beyond that required by children generally" (Bernstein, as cited in Hagan et al., 2008, p. xxii).

In essence, this population uses and needs health care and related services more than the general pediatric population. The definition focuses on the need for services and the concept of risk instead of an identified medical condition or functional impairment. The risks can be classified as biologic risks (i.e., premature birth, genetic and chromosomal abnormalities, trauma, and HIV) or environmental risks (i.e., social and economic factors, abuse, neglect, and air pollutants) (Selekman et al., 2013).

Terms to Avoid

There are many terms that are used interchangeably to refer to children with chronic conditions; however, some terms have a more negative connotation and should be avoided. For instance, the term *handicap* should be avoided. A **handicap** is a limitation imposed on the individual by environmental demands and is related to the individual's ability to adapt or adjust to those demands (Selekman et al., 2013). In other words, one is not born with a handicap; a handicap is imposed on someone by society. Telling a child that he or she cannot do something because of a chronic condition, preventing a child access to places and opportunities, treating a child differently, using derogatory labels to describe a child (e.g., *retarded* or *crippled*), and not allowing a child to strive for and reach developmental milestones all play a part in developing a handicap. It should be noted, however, that the term *handicap* was once very acceptable and was used in a number of federal laws.

Another phrase that should be avoided in referring to children is **technology dependent**. This phrase is most commonly used to describe children who require respiratory or feeding tube equipment. However, the use of this phrase puts an emphasis on the technology rather than on the child, thus impersonalizing the child. It is interesting to note that this term is never used to refer to children who wear glasses, hearing aids, insulin pumps, or braces.

When children with chronic conditions are referred to as **compromised children** or **impaired**, it implies that they are less than whole and had to settle for less. Although families may *feel* they have had to compromise their hopes and dreams for the reality of their situation, the children are *not* compromised as human beings (Selekman et al., 2013).

Nursing education promotes the individuality of each person and stresses the holistic nature of a person's being. It encourages support of the wellness components and treating individuals with respect. Emphasis has always been placed on promoting the self-esteem and self-worth of children, especially those

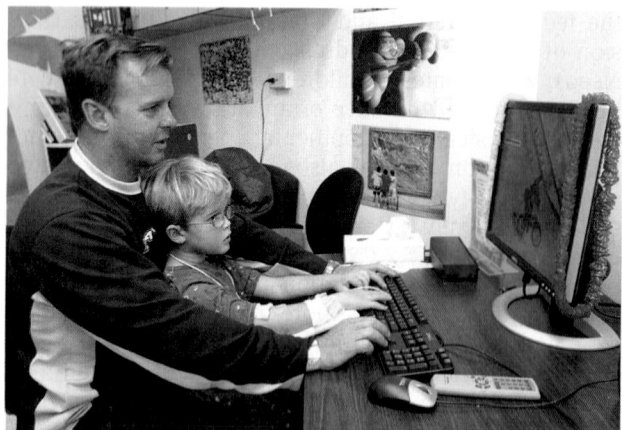

Figure 12-1 Sick or well, the focus should be on promoting the child's strengths and providing opportunities for enhancing developmental milestones.

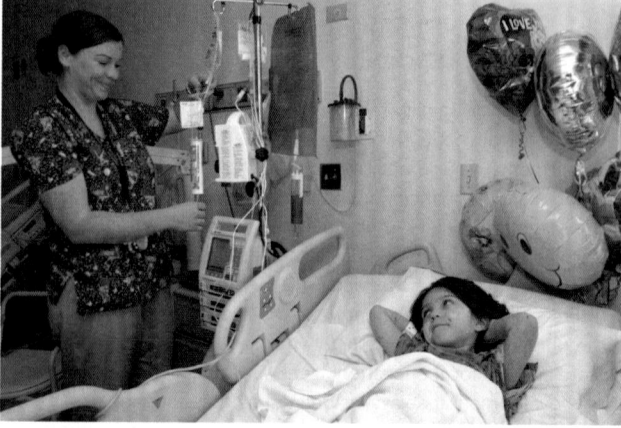

Figure 12-2 The child who is frequently hospitalized develops a warm rapport with the nursing staff. Developing a trusting relationship is important in helping the child feel secure.

with a chronic health concern. Therefore, it is essential to focus on children's wellness, their strengths, and their potential rather than their limitations and technology (Fig. 12-1).

ANSWER: Lindsay is a child with a chronic illness that is also a chronic condition. Lindsay is not a child with a developmental delay nor does she meet the ADA definition of disability because she does not have a physical or mental impairment that substantially limits a major life activity. Lindsay is a child with special health care needs. She will need access to medical care and services more than other children.

THE SPECTRUM OF CHRONIC CONDITIONS

Chronic conditions take many forms in children and adolescents, and these forms might change as the child ages or may even change from day to day. Some chronic conditions are genetic or congenital (e.g., Down syndrome or being born without a body part), some are acquired (e.g., traumatic brain injury, traumatic physical injury, or HIV disease), and some are idiopathic with no known cause. Some conditions are caused by high-risk behaviors that the parents engaged in prior to conception or during the pregnancy. Others are the result of conditions of the mother during the pregnancy (e.g., maternal infections). Some genetic conditions are obvious at birth (e.g., Down syndrome) and some are not (e.g., sickle cell disease or CF).

Some conditions affect only one organ system (e.g., clubfeet or blindness) and some affect multiple organ systems (e.g., CF, which affects the pulmonary, pancreatic/gastrointestinal, reproductive, and electrolyte systems). Some conditions progress during childhood, often causing death (e.g., muscular dystrophy); some are static (e.g., epilepsy and CP); and some alternate between periods of remission and periods of exacerbation (e.g., inflammatory bowel disease and asthma). Some will result in a shortened life span (e.g., CF and muscular dystrophy) and others will have no effect on the life span (e.g., deafness or blindness).

Some conditions, or the treatments for them, put the affected individuals at risk for serious complications. For example, those with sickle cell disease are at a higher risk for stroke, those treated for cancer may be at risk for secondary cancers, and individuals with corrected myelomeningocele have a higher risk for latex allergy. Some chronic conditions may result in numerous hospitalizations during exacerbations or disease progression, whereas those with other conditions may never set foot in a hospital (Fig. 12-2).

Some chronic conditions result in little or no impact on the child and family (e.g., the need to wear glasses or to take a daily medication for a condition such as hypothyroidism); some have significant impact on the child's development and his or her potential for eventual independence as well as on the family (e.g., having both a severe intellectual disability and CP). In such cases "habilitative" and rehabilitative services may be needed for the child. It should be noted that the ability to cope with and adjust to the chronic condition is not necessarily related to the severity of the condition. This concept is covered later in this chapter.

Some chronic conditions are secondary to, or complications of, another risk factor. Premature birth is a high risk factor for numerous long-term health problems. Gestational age plus the impact of social factors and medical comorbidities (i.e., infections, central nervous system [CNS] bleeds, and ineffective lung function) increase the likelihood of CP, intellectual and developmental disabilities, visual impairment, and neurodevelopmental deficits (Kelly, 2010) (Tradition or Science 12-1).

The vast majority of chronic conditions present in a mild or minor form, resulting in minimal negative impact on the child's ability to engage in the usual childhood activities, perform regular school work, and achieve independence (Allen, 2010). All chronic conditions have an impact on the family and on the child. Most also have an impact on the schools and the community. It is

TRADITION OR SCIENCE 12-1

What will be the long-term sequelae of fetal surgery on development and on the way chronic conditions present?

Intrauterine fetal surgery implemented to correct or treat selected conditions in utero has demonstrated a degree of success. Increased perinatal survival has been noted in conditions such as congenital cystic adenomatoid malformation, extralobar pulmonary sequestration, sacrococcygeal teratoma, urinary tract obstruction, twin–twin transfusion syndrome, and myelomeningocele when treated in utero. Other conditions such as congenital diaphragmatic hernia and congenital heart disease have shown mixed results in regard to the effectiveness of the intrauterine surgery on overall survival rates compared to those infants who had postnatal surgery for their condition. In addition, even though survival rates may be improved in many conditions, long-term complications or residual disease may still be present (UnitedHealthCare, 2012; Walsh et al., 2011). The relative newness of these procedures and the ongoing advances in the operative procedures indicate that this is a case where more inquiry and investigation are needed to determine the long-term benefits of fetal surgery to correct or treat acute and chronic conditions in children. In addition, research is needed to determine if there are specific conditions within the fetus (i.e., gestational age, overall health of the fetus, characteristics of the disease) that would indicate a higher degree of infant mortality and fewer postnatal complications.

essential for the pediatric nurse to understand the spectrum of chronicity and to be able to support the family and the child through the experience.

THE PREVALENCE OF CHRONIC CONDITIONS

The numbers used in the professional literature to indicate the prevalence of chronic conditions in the pediatric population are confusing and contradictory. In essence, they depend on the definition used for disability and what constitutes a chronic condition. The prevalence of chronic conditions has increased since the 1990s, with estimates of 12.8% in 1994 and 26.6% in 2006 (Van Cleave et al., 2010). The Federal Interagency Forum on Child and Family Statistics (2009) states that 14% of children have special health care needs. Adolescents have a higher prevalence of chronic conditions than younger children (41.8% vs. 20.2%) and males are affected more than females (59.3% vs. 40.7%) (USDHHS, Health Resources and Services Administration, 2011). Another statistic used approximates 18% of school-aged children have a functional disability that requires interventions (Nielsen et al., 2012) This means that approximately one in four children and adolescents has a chronic condition that should be considered when completing health assessments, setting goals and planning for care, and delivering care. Almost all of these children will ultimately attend school.

PSYCHOLOGICAL ADJUSTMENT TO A CHILD WITH A CHRONIC CONDITION

In addition to having a solid knowledge of the physiologic components of chronic conditions affecting children and adolescents, pediatric nurses need a keen understanding of family dynamics as well as child and adult psychology. Having a child with a chronic condition adds additional challenges and stressors to a family's life.

Although there is a variable amount of adjustment and coping with the ongoing demands of having a child with a chronic condition, there are specific times when stress has a greater chance of being at a high level for families of a child with a chronic condition. These times include

- The period before the diagnosis is made
- The time surrounding getting a diagnosis
- The period when the family is adjusting to the ongoing care demands of the child
- Times of exacerbations requiring hospitalization and deterioration of the child's condition

Be aware of the potential stressors that could interfere with the psychological health of the family and take measures to facilitate and support successful coping and psychological health.

BEFORE THE DIAGNOSIS

Some children are born with physical signs that are visible and clearly fit a pattern for an immediate diagnosis, even while in the delivery room. Down syndrome and many congenital anomalies are examples. Myelomeningocele is obvious at birth, and a diagnosis can be made on day 1 of life. How the health care team responds to the parents in the delivery room and in the postpartum area can result in an aura that "something is very wrong with your baby."

Still, other conditions appear with such diffuse symptomology, such as asthma, CF, sickle cell disease, cancer, and autism, that identifying whether a pathologic problem exists might be difficult to discern and often takes years for the condition to develop and be accurately diagnosed. Parents of children with chronic conditions might sense that something is wrong with their child, sometimes years before a diagnosis is made. The symptoms might be subtle but of sufficient concern to the parents, yet the parents might delay seeking a medical evaluation as a result of fear of the unknown, lack of confidence in their assessment skills, and concern that they will be labeled as *overly concerned* by the health care provider. They might first try a variety of home remedies or a change in behavior or dietary management. They might also compare their child with their friends' children or with their other children to note any differences.

Many families carefully consider how they will present their child's problem to the health care provider because they want to be sure their complaint is seen as legitimate. One strategy families often take is to wait until the child's next routine visit to bring up any noted problems. This might be detrimental if the problem, such as new-onset diabetes or acute asthma, is progressing rapidly. Another strategy is to seek help on a different issue that they know will get attention. The caregiver then asks the health care provider to check out the symptoms that have been actually causing them concern. To elicit this information in a way that will help the family feel comfortable, it might be helpful to ask the following question at each health care encounter: "What are your concerns or questions today about his [her] development [or body function]?"

Some health care providers might not explore the family's concerns and the signs that they describe to determine whether there is any credibility to them, often as a result of time constraints or failure to focus on anything other than the cause of the visit. They might tell the family that they worry too much and that they, the family members, are just anxious (Clinical Judgment 12-1). Nurses and physicians should take every parental concern seriously and be sure to check out all problems noted; then the appropriate education and support can be provided. Friction might also develop between the family members as one expresses concern and the other sees nothing wrong.

THE DIAGNOSIS

QUESTION: Identify the emotions expressed by Tom and Jean upon Lindsay's diagnosis. What could you do? What could you say to help support this family at the time of diagnosis?

Families will often need assistance coping with the process of diagnosing a chronic condition, the diagnosis itself, and the impact of the diagnosis on the child's future. Waiting for a diagnosis certainly can be very stressful for families. Painful testing; uncertainty about the outcomes; uncertainty about the interruption in work, school, and home schedules; and not knowing how to provide treatment for a child who does not feel well all result in stress responses by family members. For some families, however, receiving a diagnosis is a relief and a validation that their child does, in fact, have a real problem. There might also be relief if family members know that the problem can be managed with minimum inconvenience and if the condition will not interfere with the child's life span or cognitive functioning.

Parental Response

Because individuals handle stress differently, be prepared for family members to respond to their child's diagnosis with a variety of behaviors, including crying, anger, and silence. They might ask, "Why did this happen?" "Why my family?" "Why this child?" They may express anger with comments such as, "I knew something was wrong with him, but nobody believed me." They might express guilt with comments such

as, "I should have picked up on the symptoms earlier" or "I should have insisted that those tests were done or insisted that we have a second opinion somewhere else." Reinforce to the family members that these are normal reactions to the shock of finding out that their child has a chronic condition. Family members might be in a state of disbelief or denial when told of the diagnosis.

With a diagnosis of a chronic condition, parents may mourn the loss of the dreamed-for child and their life as they planned it to be (Gordon, 2009). These initial feelings might be followed by despair, depression, frustration, and confusion. Parents may have concerns for the child's future, grieve for the perceived changes the diagnosis may have on the family's quality of life, and may question their effectiveness as parents, which may affect their self-esteem and their confidence in their parenting skills. Nursing interventions for various emotional responses family members might have after a child is diagnosed with a chronic condition are presented in Nursing Interventions 12-1.

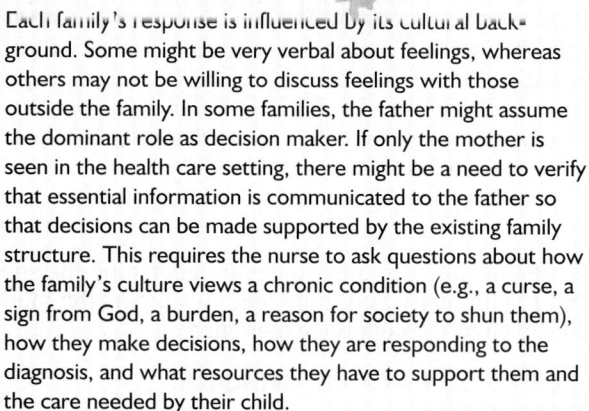

CROSS-CULTURAL CARE

Each family's response is influenced by its cultural background. Some might be very verbal about feelings, whereas others may not be willing to discuss feelings with those outside the family. In some families, the father might assume the dominant role as decision maker. If only the mother is seen in the health care setting, there might be a need to verify that essential information is communicated to the father so that decisions can be made supported by the existing family structure. This requires the nurse to ask questions about how the family's culture views a chronic condition (e.g., a curse, a sign from God, a burden, a reason for society to shun them), how they make decisions, how they are responding to the diagnosis, and what resources they have to support them and the care needed by their child.

Preparing for Discharge

Provide specific information about a child's chronic condition in a written format, at the reading level and in the language of the family. Be prepared for the family members to ask the same questions over and over as information is assimilated. The nurse should also allow the family members to vent their feelings, including anger and sadness. It is important to remember that families usually do not initially comprehend all the information given to them nor do they react to or cope with the news of their child's diagnosis at the same rate or in the same way (Teaching Intervention Plan 12-1). Do not presume that family members who have advanced educational degrees or health care backgrounds have a greater understanding; continually evaluate the family's ability "to understand, process, and act on information" (Juhlmann, 2010, p. 249).

For the infant or child who is hospitalized during the time of diagnosis, it is important for the pediatric nurse to be a role model for parents, showing them how to interact with and care for their child.

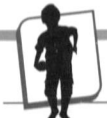

The Child With a Learning Disability

Danyael was diagnosed with specific learning disabilities at age 10 years and with inattentive ADHD as an adolescent. She had gastroesophageal reflux as an infant. As a young child, she had no interest in having books read to her. She socialized well but did not appear to be interested in the environment around her. She did not show interest in watching television. She learned to read at grade level, but by fourth grade, it was determined that she did not comprehend most of what she read. Although rote learning, such as spelling, was at grade level, all other subjects were below level. Danyael was repeatedly told she didn't pay enough attention to her studies or to directions; she was kept in from recess to redo work that wasn't considered neat enough.

Danyael was a second child to a mother who knew child development but did not know her legal rights. The mother expressed her concerns repeatedly to the pediatrician and teachers. She sought second opinions without receiving a diagnosis. The mother arranged tutoring twice a week, but Danyael continued to receive failing grades on tests that measured understanding, even though she had repeated the information accurately to the tutor. Finally, without being informed of her rights under IDEIA, Danyael's mother took her daughter for a private comprehensive psychological assessment, although this cost was beyond her means. It was this evaluation that resulted in a diagnosis of learning disabilities. However, it was another 2½ years before the elementary school acknowledged the disabilities because no one relayed the test result to the school psychologist. The school continued to give Danyael failing grades on exams and to tell her mother she worried too much. Danyael was passed from grade to grade, but her grades were poor. Her self-esteem was low and her mother felt like an ineffective parent.

As the new nurse at Danyael's high school, you have met Danyael, having seen her a few times in your office for minor maladies. You have been reviewing her file and realize she has not had an individualized education program (IEP) developed.

Questions

1. What could have been done to assist the family and the child in the past?
2. How were the repeated failures affecting Danyael's self-esteem?
3. What could have been done to assist Danyael until a diagnosis was made?
4. Who should have been an advocate for this family?
5. How can you, as the pediatric nurse, help the family to differentiate normal alterations in growth and development from pathologic and abnormal conditions?

Answers

1. When the mother first had concerns, she should have been encouraged to keep a list of the behaviors that concerned her or a log of her child's behaviors. As her concerns were presented to teachers and school administrators, she should have been provided information on IDEIA and informed of her right to have her child tested at no cost in the school system.
2. Repeated school failures can further diminish academic performance as the child learns to "give up." The child's self-esteem during school-age years is greatly tied to mastery of new concepts. When children receive constant negative reinforcement in regard to their learning, self-esteem is bound to suffer.
3. Provide alternative learning strategies and document to see what works and what does not. Identify her strengths and promote them. Learn from the family what measures they implement at home to help her achieve and incorporate the same techniques in the classroom.
4. If symptoms are identified at age 3 years or younger, advocate for an evaluation by the state's early intervention team. After the child reaches age 3 years, the public school system, including the school nurse, is obligated to serve as an advocate to ensure the child is provided additional resources to enhance learning when a learning disorder is identified. The nurse in the pediatrician's office should also have acted as an advocate for this child.
5. Provide information on developmental parameters to assist the family to recognize the ranges of what is considered "normal" in both physical and cognitive parameters.

NURSING INTERVENTIONS 12-1

Supporting the Emotional Responses of Family Members

Emotion	Examples	Problematic Examples	Nursing Interventions	Outcomes
Grief	Despair, remorse	Withdrawal; unrelenting sadness	Validate feelings Offer support Help the family re-establish structure in life	Family members begin to integrate fact that child has chronic condition into how they view the child in a positive way
Denial	Forgetting Overcompensation Disbelief	Interference with treatment Distrust	Reflect back statements Clarify feelings Offer feedback Help family members recognize that responses are normal	Family members begin to make appropriate plans for future Family members ask questions that show understanding of condition
Guilt	Self-blame	Spousal blame Continual self-recrimination	Give information Explore ideas about why child has condition	Self-blame comments subside Projection of blame onto others decreases Coping with realistic guilt
Anger	Aggression Hostility	Acts helpless Interferes with treatment plan	Include family members when developing treatment plan Remain nondefensive Engage in stress-relieving practices, i.e., yoga or journaling	Family members begin to actively participate in planning care Family members accurately and constructively direct anger
Fear	Anxiety Self-doubt Disoriented	Hypochondriacal Panic attacks Avoidance	Have family members participate in development and implementation of treatment plan Point out parental competence Repeat instructions, if needed Provide reading literature by other families who have experienced the same condition	Family members initiate discussion of new treatment approaches Family members carry out needed treatments
Loneliness	Quiet Isolated	Marital discord Job difficulties	Assist in establishing contact with potential support persons/groups Help family re-establish or develop social connections	Family contacts support group and goes to meetings Family reports social activities that give them enjoyment

Information from Gordon, J. (2009). An evidence-based approach for supporting parents experiencing chronic sorrow. *Pediatric Nursing, 35*(2), 115–119; Johnston, C., & Marder, L. (1994). Parenting the child with a chronic condition: An emotional experience. *Pediatric Nursing, 20*, 611–614.

TIP 12-1: A TEACHING INTERVENTION PLAN for Family Members in the Initial Period After Diagnosis of a Child's Chronic Condition

Nursing Diagnosis and Family Outcomes

- Deficient knowledge: Condition and family members' role in the treatment plan

  Outcomes: Family members will be given instruction geared toward their learning style, level of understanding, and knowledge deficits.

  Family will be able to implement essential care for the child.

Instructional Interventions

Verify Cause of Knowledge Deficit. For Example:
- Excessive anxiety
- Fear of condition
- Illiteracy
- Impaired communication
- Lack of prior teaching
- English is their second language
- Misinterpretation of information
- Unwillingness to learn

Assess Baseline Knowledge or Experience With the Chronic Condition
- What have the family members already been taught?
- Does the family know anyone else with this condition?
- What have they heard about children with this condition?
- Is there any aspect of the child's care that is of particular concern to them?

Assess Family Structure, Function, and Usual Patterns as They Impact Care
- Who will be providing care to the child?
- Who will be backup for care?
- Where is the child when not with the family?
- What does the family need to know to care for the child safely at home?
- Will any family routines be affected by the presence of the chronic condition?
- What will be the child's involvement in his or her care, based on age and cognitive development?
- What will be the siblings' involvement in the child's care, based on age and cognitive development?
- How are siblings and friends affected by the presence of the child's chronic condition?
- What does the parent want to learn first?

Design Teaching Plan Based on Family Assessment
- Involve all caregivers and significant family members.
- Adapt teaching plan to accommodate the usual patterns of family or help the family members change these patterns.

- Begin with essential skills needed for the child's safe care and move on to those needed for long-term care and in-depth understanding of the child's condition and needs.

Present Content Using Standard Teaching Principles
- Use language best comprehended by the parent (e.g., English, Spanish, Creole).
- Use vocabulary understood by parents while teaching them medical language that they may hear in the future.
- Use a variety of teaching techniques to meet unique learning styles.

  Discussion

  Direct demonstration

  Video/audio

  Books

  Practice equipment

  Computer programs

  Meetings with other families and children with the condition
- Encourage questions.
- Explore question for possible concerns not evident in questions.
- Be alert for information overload.
- Allow practice and return demonstration of skills.
- Provide source of backup for later questions.

  Home nursing visits

  Phone calls from care provider

  Support group

  Written material

Educate for Future
- Expand natural parenting skills to promote development despite presence of chronic condition.
- Learn how the child can continue prior activities or activities can be adapted to accommodate limitations of condition.
- Learn to find new knowledge on own.

  Support groups

  Reading

  Electronic support groups
- Learn to question and collaborate with health care providers.
- Learn to evaluate accuracy of information provided.
- Learn to educate staff and other caregivers about child's unique needs.
- Prepare for change in care brought on by progression or improvement of condition, developmental changes of child/caregivers, and need for child to increase self-care.

Continue to educate the family and the child about both normal child care and the special care needed based on the child's special needs while serving as a support person as well. It is especially important to point out all the positive attributes of the child and the things this child is doing that are perfectly normal for his or her age. Recommending that family members and the child (if appropriate) keep a pad of paper nearby to record their questions as they occur may help caregivers feel more organized in their thoughts when the medical specialist or others providing care for their child come into the room. This exercise can be continued at home; parents can keep a list of questions and bring them with them when they meet with their health care provider.

In addition to answering parent questions, discharge teaching should prepare the family to anticipate and deal with specific changes in the child's health status at home. Families should be able to make informed decisions, have enough basic self-care skills to survive until their next teaching or health-related visit, and recognize problems and know how to respond. See the Watch & Learn video: Care of the Hospitalized Child: Parent and Family Participation.

When teaching important skills, be sure to ask the families to do a demonstration of the skill they have just learned. It is helpful to have the parent demonstrate the skill again on the first office visit after discharge to ensure accuracy and provide an opportunity for the parent to ask questions. This is also a prime opportunity for the nurse to praise the families for what they have learned and the quality care they are providing to their child. Remind them to focus on the normalcy of their child as well. Be careful not to take over the care from the family. Sometimes, health care professionals can make families feel inadequate by doing the care quickly and competently and not including the family in bedside discussions with other health care professionals (Fig. 12-3). This may make some families more fearful of demonstrating the skill and they may avoid their child more.

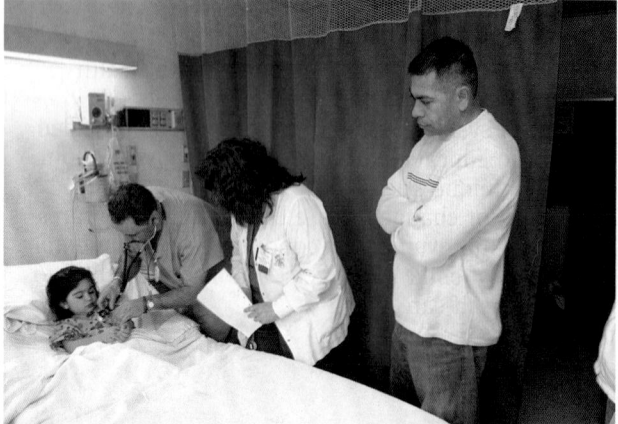

Figure 12-3 Early after the diagnosis, the family may not be comfortable participating in assessment and care planning discussions, especially if the health care provider makes no effort to include them.

> **ANSWER:** Two emotions stand out in this case study: grief and guilt. Review Nursing Interventions 12-1. One of the most important things you can do is to physically be there; give your presence. Take the time to sit down and be at eye level. Ask the parents, "How are you doing?" Maintain eye contact and really listen. Let them know they are not alone, that most other families also have these feelings at first but that it does get better. Draw their attention back to Lindsay, who is responding well physically to the management of her blood sugars and accepting this new aspect of who she is. She is tall for her age, she loves animals, and she has diabetes.

Whom to Tell

Parents might have concerns about sharing their child's diagnosis with family, friends, and others who might have contact with their child for fear that the stigma or label will interfere with their child's future opportunities or will reflect poorly on them as parents. This is especially true for conditions that affect a child's neurologic or mental health status. Help provide the family with information booklets and fact sheets that they can hand out to others to explain the condition and educate them about the child's limitations, if any, or needed accommodations. They can be empowered to request that individuals not use certain pejorative terms around them or their child, such as *retard* or *cripple*. It can be explained that these are the terms that result in handicaps and they do not want their child growing up believing they are handicapped.

Family members are often hesitant to inform the school that their child has a diagnosed chronic condition. Reinforce that by withholding information about the diagnosis from those who need to know in the health care community and in the school, they and their child will be denied multiple resources and services they might need. In other words, "no diagnosis, no service." This will affect the support services they can receive for the care they provide their child as well as the accommodations that might be needed to meet the child's academic needs.

ONGOING CARE DEMANDS

The primary goals for the child's plan of care is to normalize the family's and the child's lives as much as possible and to promote the optimal health of the child. How a family views the child's chronic condition might dictate how they react to and guide the child's care and development. The child who is viewed as sick, fragile, and vulnerable might be treated differently than the child who is viewed and treated as a "normal child who happens to have a chronic condition." Unfortunately, family members sometimes respond to their child with a chronic condition as if he or she could die at any moment, even though the child might live for decades. This might result in the family being overprotective of the child. For instance, families of children with a chronic condition might not engage in sufficient discipline and might spoil their children by allowing them anything

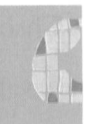

Evidence-Based Practice

TRADITION OR SCIENCE 12-2

Do health care providers have an understanding of the challenges of parenting a child with a chronic condition?

The research literature is rich with studies evaluating parental response to the care and management of children with a chronic condition. One example is a metasynthesis completed by Coffey (2006), which reviewed 11 qualitative studies with a focus on parenting a child with a chronic illness. The studies included data from both mothers and fathers. Parents shared how worry is a bona fide part of everyday life and how often they felt overwhelmed by the care the child requires every day. Mothers have been identified as the primary caregiver who often experiences exhaustion as they "carry the burden" of caring for their chronically ill child. Parents describe a loss of freedom and a loss of support systems because they are not able to leave their home on a regular basis because of their care obligations. Parents feel their role is that of an advocate for their child. They realize they must take charge, and they want their experience and knowledge of their child's care recognized.

Responses of single or "lone" parents to managing the complexities of life with a chronically ill child are discussed infrequently in the literature (Brown et al., 2008). These parents may face additional challenges caused by fewer financial resources, less support from other family members, and less flexibility to manage changes in the family schedule associated with illness or hospitalization. Single parenting is increasing in our society and it is important that research among children with chronic conditions encompass the concerns of those from all family types, including those headed by single parents, adolescent parents, and gay/lesbian couples.

The need for nurses and other health care professionals to provide ongoing support and community resources for parents of chronically ill children is evident. Coffey (2006) suggests that future research needs to focus more on understanding the role of the nurse in support of this group of parents.

loss of privacy resulting from the need for many support services and personnel in the home; and strains in spousal relationships, sibling responsibilities, and friendships (Allen, 2010). Families describe frustrations with the health, social service, and educational systems; want a system that treats their child as a whole person as opposed to disciplines claiming only a piece; and desire one professional to be the key coordinator in their child's care (Elias & Murphy, 2012; Simkiss, 2011). Families investigate the Internet, ask for advice from professionals, and seek practical tips from other families regarding medical management; health promotion and exercise; toilet training strategies; sexuality issues; financial assistance; vocational counseling; sources for dental treatment, respite care, and child daycare; management of behavioral problems and discipline practices; support groups; and so forth. Despite these pressing issues, many family members demonstrate unconditional love, an absolute devotion to their children's care, commitment to their futures, and hopes for good quality of life (Fig. 12-4).

There are four major responsibilities for families caring for a child with a chronic condition. These include

- Managing the condition
- Identifying, accessing, and coordinating community resources
- Maintaining the family unit
- Maintaining self (Sullivan-Bolyai et al., 2003)

The pediatric nurse can play a major role in the first two responsibilities and should be an advocate and a family support for the last two.

Managing the Condition

Managing a child's chronic condition is often easier for the families when they feel knowledgeable about the condition, competent in the skills needed to care for the condition, aware of which symptoms indicate problems and which do not, and supported by the health care community should they have a problem. The documents highlighted in Evidence-Based Clinical Practice

they wish. At the other end of the spectrum, families might neglect or abuse the child with a chronic condition by failing to keep medical appointments and failing to follow the plan of care (Telfair et al., 2005). Parents might also give up control altogether and choose to place their child in an institution, which in some cases might be the best option for the family (Elias & Murphy, 2012) (Tradition or Science 12-2).

Families have reported enormous amounts of stress, emotional turmoil, and sometimes grieving if full return of function is not achieved. Sometimes, these emotions intensify because they may feel less support at home than in the controlled hospital environment. It may take months for family members to feel comfortable handling the technical aspects of their child's care (Allen, 2010). Multiple stressors have been reported in families caring for children with special health care needs, such as social isolation; financial and employment strains;

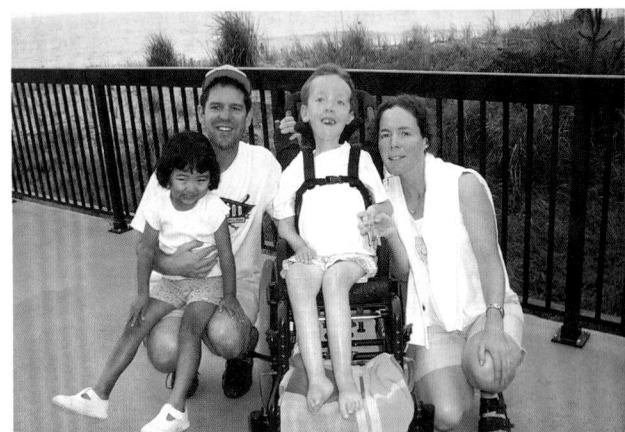

Figure 12-4 Jack Freedman, a 10-year-old with spinal muscular atrophy enjoys traveling and making family memories. When diagnosed as an infant, his family was told he would not live for more than a year.

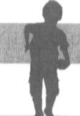

EVIDENCE-BASED CLINICAL PRACTICE GUIDELINES 12-1

Care of the Child With a Chronic Condition

Elias, E. R., & Murphy, N. A. (2012). Home care of children and youth with complex health care needs and technology dependencies. *Pediatrics, 129*(5), 996–1005. Retrieved from

http://pediatrics.aappublications.org/content/early/2012/04/25/peds.2012-0606.abstract

Report that presents an approach to discharging the child with complex medical needs and technology dependencies from hospital to home. Also addresses the ongoing needs of the child and family in the home environment.

The Future of Children. (2012). *Children with Disabilities 22*(1). Retrieved from

http://www.futureofchildren.org/futureofchildren/publications/journals/journal_details/index.xml?journalid = 77

Entire issue explores issues surrounding children with disabilities, including prevalence, treatment, consequences, and medical and home care needs.

Murphey, D., Cooper, M., & Moore, K. A. (2012). *Children with disabilities: State-level data from the American Community Survey.* Retrieved from

http://www.childtrends.org/Files/Child_Trends-2012_10_01_RB_ChildDisabilities.pdf

Report provides survey data from United States regarding incidence of children identified as having at least one disability by a responsible adult in the household.

Chronic Care: Self-Management Guideline Team, Cincinnati Children's Hospital Medical Center. (2007). *Evidence-based care guideline for chronic care: Self-management.* Retrieved from

http://www.cincinnatichildrens.org/assets/0/78/1067/2709/2777/2793/9199/a8b6f19b-e8fe-476e-9ee1-6b51a7112e28.pdf

Recommendations for self-management by families of children with chronic conditions in order to improve health outcomes.

National Heart, Lung, and Blood Institute. (n.d.). *Students with chronic illnesses: Guidance for families, schools, and students.* Retrieved from

http://www.nhlbi.nih.gov/health/public/lung/asthma/guidfam.pdf

Guidelines for families, school administrators, and students regarding how to promote health and welfare of child with a chronic condition.

Guidelines 12-1 can serve as resources for articulating the care needs of the child with a chronic condition. Teaching families about their child's chronic condition is not something that is done only once; rather, parent and family teaching should be an ongoing process. A home visit might be helpful early during the child's care. In addition to teaching the needed skills, it is also helpful to assist the family to develop care routines; to coordinate the care in a way that allows for periods of rest, without treatments, for both the family and the child; and to determine a method of remembering when to do tasks and in what manner.

However, families might feel overwhelmed by the technical skill expectations and knowledge needed to manage their child's chronic condition, especially when equipment fails or does not work properly, their child refuses to participate in the skill, or their child's condition deteriorates. These situations might make families feel like they have failed their child in that they are unable to provide for their child's needs and cure what ails them. There might be times when the stress is too much for the family; stress might result from the physical stress of caring for a child who is growing bigger and whose condition depends on technology or the psychological stress that accompanies this care. Family members must be supported in being able to acknowledge when they need help. They should have a list of resource people they can contact when they have concerns about technology, symptoms, or stress responses (Elias & Murphy, 2012; Simkiss, 2011).

Families and caregivers must learn all the basic principles of body mechanics to provide safe care to the child and to protect themselves from injury. Interventions are especially needed when the child gets too heavy for the families to handle safely or if they express that the child's behaviors have become too embarrassing for them to go out in public or too aggressive and potentially dangerous for the child to be around others. Evaluation is the key to ensuring that home care interventions have been effective. For instance, just because the nurse has made a referral or had the family participate in a teaching session does not mean that the problem has been resolved. One nurse practitioner mother, whose adolescent was finally diagnosed as having ADHD at age 13 years and who had unsuccessfully advocated for the school system to meet her child's needs, made the following comment: "Every time I send my child out into the world, the world sends him back." This should remind us that the diagnosis is just the beginning of helping the family, school, and community make accommodations so that the child and family can be successful in their adaptation.

Identifying, Accessing, and Coordinating Community Resources

Families might also be overwhelmed by the large number of "others" who are needed to help in the child's care. The interdisciplinary team might include physical therapists, occupational therapists, speech therapists, nutrition therapists, respiratory therapists, pain managers, intravenous (IV) therapists, psychologists, social service members, home care service members, durable equipment suppliers, school personnel, and many others. The pediatric nurse can be instrumental in ensuring that a case manager is assigned to coordinate all these individuals to avoid overlap of services, to ensure consistency in the messages and treatments needed, to limit the number of health care visits needed each month by arranging for the family to see multiple specialists at the same time, to limit the number of health care providers coming to the home, and to attempt to promote some semblance of normalcy in the family's life. The case manager can also be responsible for assisting the family in identifying, accessing, and coordinating community resources, especially related to financial assistance and planning for emergencies, such as equipment failure, power failure, and medical emergencies. Knowing that the team is communicating and working together decreases family stress and lets the family know that the team is focused on what is best for the child and family.

The ongoing assessment of learning needs of the family and child, even when they appear quite knowledgeable, is a part of each health care encounter to ensure family members are properly maintaining their child's treatment plan. It is essential to remember that as the child grows, procedures may have to be performed differently and may have to be retaught to accommodate any necessary changes. An example is percussion and postural drainage. This procedure is often performed one way for a young child with CF and performed differently as the child enters school and as the child reaches puberty.

Maintaining the Family Unit

 QUESTION: What was the impact of the American Diabetes Association precamp weekend on the Jenkins family, particularly the mother?

It can be very stressful for families living with a child who needs continuous health-related interventions. The stress that results often causes families to focus primarily on their child's condition, treatments, and the time involved. For example, families with a child on a ventilator or tracheostomy tube may fear not hearing their child's need for suctioning; those with a child with type 1 diabetes might become rigid about intake and maintaining tight control of the blood sugar in an attempt to stave off long-term sequelae. Focusing solely on a child's condition, however, shifts the focus away from the fact that the child also has normal developmental needs. Ensure that every health-related visit and hospitalization promotes what is normal for age regarding the child and the progress that the child has made toward achieving developmental tasks (Chart 12-2).

CHART 12-2 **Family Interview Questions on Impact of Condition on Child and Family**

- How do you think your child's condition has affected him or her and your family?
- Tell me about your child and school.
  Explore:
  Transportation concerns
  Academic achievement
  Reactions of classmates and teachers
  Participation in field trips and other special activities
- Describe your child's ability to dress and toilet himself or herself.
  Explore:
  Concerns about appearance
  Detail regarding self-care abilities
- Tell me about disciplining your child. How does this compare with discipline for your other children?
- Tell me about your child's friendships.
  Explore:
  Rejections by previous friends
  Having friends over
- What does your child do for fun?
  Explore:
  Previous favorite pastimes
  Group activities
- What are concerns you have about your child as you think about the future?

Accept the family with the reactions and coping mechanisms (both effective and ineffective) they bring to the situation. A coping mechanism should not be judged as good or bad based on the nurse's personal value system. Do not presume that families will be at a particular point in their response to coping with their child's chronic condition simply because the child's problem was just diagnosed or has been present for years. Although multiple stressors can interfere with the coping process, research studies have supported the idea that families can adjust quite well and are often satisfied with their family life; they did not perceive the chronic condition to be a dominant factor of their lives (Allen, 2010).

Although it is common for health care providers to ask families how they are coping in the months after diagnosis, they often forget to do so 1, 5, and 10 years later. Ask families how they are coping, especially as the child enters different stages of development. It may be one thing to cope with a young child with Down syndrome, but it is completely different for the family to cope with an adolescent with Down syndrome. Needs change and the challenges they present also change. Some of the more common nursing diagnoses and outcomes for families of a child with a chronic condition are in Nursing Plan of Care 12-1.

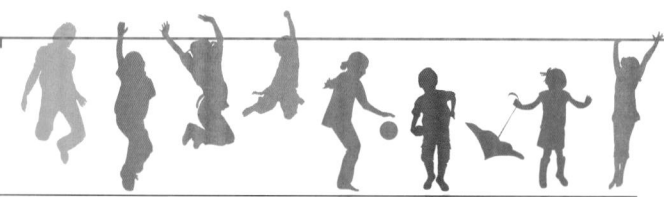

NURSING PLAN OF CARE 12-1:

The Family Members and Caregivers of a Child With a Chronic Condition

Nursing Diagnosis: Deficient knowledge: New and complex treatment regimen and/or home care needs

Interventions/Rationale

- Assess family's knowledge of child's condition and care needs.
  Assists in focusing teaching to family's needs.
- Teach the family to manage child's condition (e.g., treatments and symptoms to report to health care provider).
  Appropriate management facilitates optimal outcomes.
- Use developmentally appropriate methods to teach child and family about the condition.
  Knowledge facilitates appropriate management of condition and enhances the successful transition to home management.
- Provide multiple sources of family/child education including videos, reading material, and hands-on demonstration.
  Providing multiple methods of teaching is the best way to present new material to adult learners.
- Demonstrate required care; provide opportunity for return demonstration.
  Helps the child and family master care needs.
- Teach child/family to identify and report symptoms that indicate a change in the child's condition and/or a deleterious side effect of medication or other treatments.
  Allows for prevention or early detection of problems and early intervention.
- Provide opportunities to room-in whenever possible.
  Rooming-in gives the family caregivers a chance to be the primary care providers for their child, to work with the actual equipment they will have in the home, and to give the medications. The care is provided with support as needed from the nursing staff.

Expected Outcome

- Family/caregiver identifies and demonstrates all home care treatment skills.

Nursing Diagnosis: Ineffective family therapeutic regimen management related to lack of education, support, or physical ability to carry out plan of care; complexity, cost, side effects; knowledge deficit about how to implement regimen; failure to accept seriousness of problem or benefits of regimen; fear of being different; lack of continuity of care

Interventions/Rationale

- Assess family's knowledge of child's condition and care needs.
  Assists in focusing teaching based on family needs.

- Instruct family members about signs of infection and changes from expected response. Stress the need to contact the physician if these occur.
  Child/family cannot manage program if a knowledge deficit exists.
- Provide family with information regarding medications child is receiving. Discuss which of these may be continued upon discharge or when exacerbation of condition has passed.
  Ensures family has accurate knowledge to manage child's condition.
- Complete a nutritional assessment. Develop a plan to modify the family diet if needed to meet the child's current health needs.
  Ensures family has accurate knowledge to manage child's condition.
- Help family/caregivers learn new care activities.
  Throughout the course of the child's life, the family will need to make adjustments in the plan of care for the child to account for developmental changes and changes in the child's condition.
- Evaluate the need for education of others who will be in contact with child (e.g., babysitters, schoolteachers, neighbors). Assist parents in providing information as needed.
  Support systems are important to give the family relief time to build on their strengths.
- Verify that modifications in the home environment have been made. Confirm that home care is referral complete (e.g., equipment delivered to home, family knows how to use it, and it is appropriate to that home).
  Equipment to manage the child's care and modifications to the home environment may be suggested that improve quality of care for the child and make care processes easier for the family.
- Provide families with access to supplies as necessary. Provide them with information on available support/financial resources (e.g., local public health department, regional centers).
  Access to support systems/resources may help the family manage the care for the child.
- Teach family to manage the child's condition.
  Appropriate management facilitates optimal outcomes.
- Provide plans of care to the child's school nurse. Ensure additional equipment (i.e., inhalers, spacers, catheters, medication) is ordered to be used in the school setting.
  Enhancing communication with the school nurse ensures continuity of the plan of care while the child is in school and enhances communication between the health care provider and the school nurse.

Expected Outcome
- Family will successfully manage the child's care needs and will identify sources of support to help in managing the child's condition.

Nursing Diagnosis: Powerlessness related to lack of ability to control progression of condition; inability to communicate with health care provider

Interventions/Rationale
- Assess the family's stress levels, coping mechanisms, and support systems.

  Knowledge of stressors and support can be used to assist families to build on their strengths.
- Encourage family discussion of feelings and acknowledge their normalcy.

  Venting of feelings may help decrease anxiety and feelings of powerlessness and may validate that what the family is feeling is a normal part of coping and adaptation.
- Involve the family in caring for the child.

  Helps the family maintain control and reinforces the family member's ability to provide adequate care
- Support family members' competence in assessing the child's behavioral cues and responses.

  Reinforces caregiving role and the family members' ability to meet the child's needs.

Expected Outcomes
- Family will verbalize feelings of powerlessness and the impact it has on the family.
- Family will identify positive coping strategies to deal with child's chronic condition.

Nursing Diagnosis: Risk for caregiver role strain related to multiple care needs of child; no other caregivers

Interventions/Rationale
- Provide ongoing access to all members of interdisciplinary team for diagnosis and treatment of condition. Use these contact opportunities to evaluate caregiver's coping experiences.

  The goal of the interdisciplinary team is to support the family as they manage the child's condition and successfully integrate that care into daily family life. Early identification of caregiver role strain can elicit evaluation of the situation and interventions to decrease stress.
- Refer to home care agency/nursing, respite care, and daycare services for continued care of complex problems.

  Provides relief and assistance in managing complex care of the child. Provides opportunities for family members to be away from the child to pursue their own interests.
- Collaborate with interdisciplinary team (social worker, physician, school nurse, etc.) to develop a plan for the child to participate in family, school, and social activities to his or her maximum capacity.

  Provides additional support system for the family to ensure the child's successful adaptation at home and school.
- Explore siblings' knowledge of condition and family's expectations of siblings.

  Unrealistic expectations may be placed on siblings to manage home environment and/or care for chronically ill child.
- Discuss past and present coping mechanisms. Assist to identify effective and ineffective coping mechanisms.

  Identification of coping mechanisms can provide guidance for selection of appropriate methods.
- Instruct in use of relaxation techniques (e.g., deep breathing, meditation, journaling, hot baths).

  Practicing the methods may help in using them when faced with a stressful situation.
- Identify causative or contributing factors to stress.

  Identifies the stresses that are exceeding the resources of the family.
- Allow the family members to discuss their feelings.

  Venting one's feelings may help in decreasing frustrations.
- Discuss the effects of the current schedule on caregiver (e.g., physical health, emotional status, and relationships).

  Successful coping depends on the ability of identified resources and self-care. Burnout is associated with exhaustion—physical and emotional.
- Initiate referrals and health teaching; assess family resources and support systems.

  Referrals can provide respite care and sharing of responsibilities and provide a view that others can help and are competent.
- Encourage caregiver to participate in support groups.

  Support groups can provide mutual support, anticipatory guidance, and education.
- Provide positive encouragement to the caregiver.

  Being appreciated and encouraged can decrease feelings of strain.

Expected Outcomes
- Families will identify and use other caregivers for the child.
- Families will take time away from the child to meet their own needs.
- Caregivers will verbalize their need to maintain social relationships outside of those that focus on the child with a chronic condition.

(Continued)

NURSING PLAN OF CARE 12-1:

The Family Members and Caregivers of a Child With a Chronic Condition (Continued)

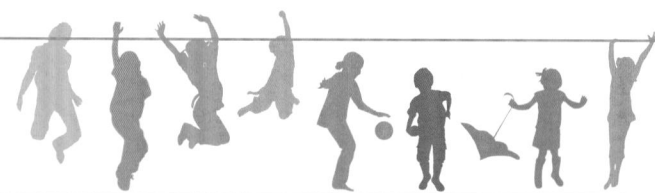

Nursing Diagnosis: Disturbed sleep pattern related to physical care needs of child

Interventions/Rationale

- Evaluate family member's ability to get appropriate sleep/rest. Assist in determining whether current sleep/rest patterns meet individual caregiver needs.

  Establish baseline data to explore whether this is an ongoing concern or of a temporary nature resulting from exacerbation of the child's condition.

- Develop a plan to provide the caregiver with uninterrupted sleep. This may include use of night care providers and giving family caregivers permission to go home at night from the hospital.

  Provides strategies for temporary and potential long-term relief of sleeplessness.

Expected Outcome

- Caregivers will identify own sleep needs and develop strategies to meet them.

Nursing Diagnosis: Readiness for enhanced family processes related to need for family to work together to accomplish tasks and to develop new ways to meet needs of individual members

Interventions/Rationale

- Offer emotional support as child/family goes through periods of adjustment/grief/mourning.

  A child with a chronic condition poses challenges that require adjustments in the daily life of the whole family. Families can draw upon previous coping strategies and support systems to help them maintain homeostasis.

- Allow families to be the expert on care of the child; give acknowledgment and positive reinforcement to efforts to provide a stimulating, healthy environment.

  Positively affirms role of each family member in care of the child.

- Provide time for family members to discuss concerns and problems; find out how long a specific approach has been used and how the approach works and does not work.

  Examines family resources and provides mechanisms to offer alterative coping strategies as needed.

- Support family competence in assessing the child's needs and in caring for the child.

  Reinforces new behavior and bolsters the family's feelings of competence.

- Encourage participation and cooperation in care, reward all efforts, and give choice and control over situation as appropriate.

  Minimizes perception of powerlessness. Maximizes personal responsibility of child/family for daily care.

Expected Outcomes

- Families will cope with demands imposed by the child's chronic condition, develop new coping strategies to manage demands and to promote family functioning, and feel a sense of achievement that they were able to do so.

Nursing Diagnosis: Grieving related to anticipated shortened life expectancy of child resulting from chronic condition; change in family life plan as envisioned prior to child's diagnosis

Interventions/Rationale

- Elicit parental and sibling concerns about child's condition and future implications of that condition on child and family.

  The fear of death may be present and may arise each time the child experiences a serious exacerbation of clinical signs.

- Identify for the family members feelings they may have at any point; assure them that in most cases, those feelings are a normal part of grieving.

  Family members will go through grieving process as they adjust to the loss of "the perfect child" and adapt to the impact the child's condition may have on quality and longevity of the child's life.

- Provide strategies to enhance coping (e.g., use of support groups, use of spiritual supports, increased knowledge of child's condition).

  Enhances family knowledge base and provides repertoire of strategies to cope as family deals with ongoing demands of child's condition. The child and family may need additional support services to effectively grieve and cope with the child's condition and to learn to manage home care.

- Promote child/family decision making (e.g., include family members in conferences, encourage them to be advocates for child).

  Regular updates on the child's status assist family in the decision-making process.

- Recognize that each family member will cope differently and at his or her own pace. Respect differences in coping strategies and assist all family members in dealing with differences.

  Responses may vary from acceptance to anger, withdrawal, and depression.

Expected Outcome

- The family members will progress through the grieving process in an adaptive manner.

Maintaining Family/Caregiver Health

It is not uncommon for caregivers to neglect their own physical needs in their love and dedication to the child. Help families recognize their physical needs and find realistic ways to have those needs met. Encourage parents to accept offers of help from friends or family members to watch siblings, bring meals, or assist in providing care to the child. Suggest that home caregivers nap or rest when the child is resting. Ensure that the care needs of the child can be met by more than one competent individual in the household, thereby allowing caregivers time to pursue their own activities and interests. If needed, families may choose to pursue respite care services (discussed later in the chapter) as a means to allow the caregivers an opportunity to take a trip or have a weekend away from the child who requires a great deal of care.

Impact on the Parents' Relationship With One Another

Because each parent copes with a child's chronic condition in his or her own way, some parents might find it difficult to share their feelings with their partner, especially when one partner is not yet ready to deal with the issues. The increased isolation from one's support system may cause stress on the relationship, especially if one partner goes to work each day or stays away from home for longer periods of time. Isolation may also occur when frequent hospitalizations of the child occur, thus requiring a parent to remain with the child, away from the partner, in the hospital setting. Parent support groups might prove helpful. It is important to encourage the couple to find time for themselves.

Impact on Grandparents and Others

Parents who have been informed that their child has a chronic condition generally expect that they will be supported and assisted by the child's grandparents, aunts, uncles, and other family members. For many, this is the case. However, this is not always the case for others. Some extended family members live too far away or are unable to assist their children for physical or psychological reasons; others express fear in the required knowledge and skills and may avoid caring for the child. They might feed into the guilt felt by the parents by relating the condition to something the parent did during their adolescence or their pregnancy. Occasionally, extended family members will blame the condition on one specific parent, especially if they had never approved of that person and the marital relationship. In addition to losing emotional support, long distances from family members may mean the parent might be losing a source of respite care. This is also true when close friends or family of the parents begin to shy away from visiting because of fears of what to say and how to help.

Birth of Subsequent Children

The birth of subsequent children can cause anxiety for parents until it can be determined whether the newest child has the same chronic condition as an older child. Parents might need additional assurances that the subsequent child is healthy, even if there are no signs of a problem. Some have had all their children born before the first one is diagnosed, and then they find that others have the same condition. Parents will then need additional support. Remember that each child is an individual and no two children present with the same condition in the exact same way. Parents who have more than one child with a particular condition need to be provided with this information so that the subsequent children are not compared with the sibling.

There might be moments of discomfort for parents when the younger children surpass the older child with a chronic condition in motor or academic skills. This is an ideal time to discuss the limitations of the older child with the younger child and to promote sensitivity in not making fun of or causing embarrassment because of the differences that may exist.

Impact on Siblings

An increasing amount of research has been done on the healthy siblings of children with chronic conditions. The research is inconsistent regarding the outcomes for these healthy siblings, but more recent studies show a positive sibling adjustment (Nielsen et al., 2012). The degree of adjustment difficulty in healthy siblings appears to be related to the degree of disruption of family life that occurs because of the affected child's condition as well as the family's resources to cope with the effects of the disruption. Coping difficulties were seen in the healthy siblings' sleeping and eating patterns.

Healthy siblings need information regarding their sibling's condition; this information needs to be age appropriate and presented frequently during the healthy child's life span. Healthy siblings can also be encouraged to participate in the care provided to their sibling with a chronic condition (Fig. 12-5). Siblings should have the

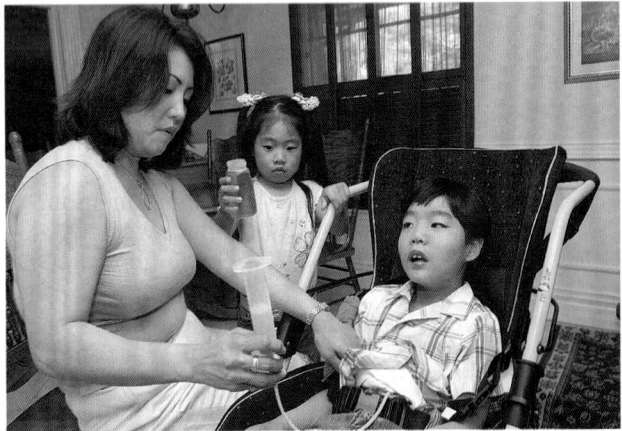

Figure 12-5 Siblings need to be fully informed about their sibling's care needs and condition and be allowed to participate in care activities as much as they wish to and in age-appropriate ways.

opportunity to meet with the health care provider or with groups of other siblings in similar situations in order to talk about their feelings and experiences (Nielsen et al., 2012). In addition, healthy siblings may be asked to take on additional household responsibilities. Parents should discuss with their children that these added responsibilities should be viewed as a sign of trust and maturity rather than a chore. Parents need to be sure to praise their nonaffected children for their assistance.

Some healthy siblings may be jealous of the attention given to the affected child and may therefore engage in attention-seeking or acting-out behaviors; some may complain of symptoms that are psychosomatic in nature. Sometimes, children may be embarrassed by a sibling with a chronic condition; other times, they may feel the need to defend their sibling from rude remarks and bullying. Because there is typically a decrease in social activities and family outings in families with a child who depends on a great deal of technology, efforts should be made to ensure that the healthy siblings are given special time outside the home, both with significant adults and with peers. Above all, healthy siblings need to feel free to share their feelings, to be provided with education about the sibling's condition, and to be assured that they will not "catch it" or develop it. This education should be ongoing and not just at the time of diagnosis and discharge.

In some areas, there are support groups for healthy siblings of children with chronic conditions. See Teaching Intervention Plan 12-2 for various interventions for siblings of a child with a chronic condition.

In some cases, siblings have the same condition, especially if they are genetically caused. In one respect, this may enhance the siblings' feelings of normalcy because they are each undergoing testing and treatments. However, in the case in which one child dies, siblings with the same condition may experience great fear as they approach the age at which their sibling passed away. For example, in one family of four children, all but the oldest had CF. These three siblings assisted each other with percussion and postural drainage and shared equipment. The oldest child, who was unaffected by CF, required years of psychological support during her adolescence. She felt guilty for not having the condition and felt different from the rest of the family. The health care team assisted her in recognizing and dealing with her conflicting emotions. The oldest girl with CF died at age 16; when the next sister reached that age, she became depressed and afraid of dying. It was helpful for staff to point out that she was healthier than her sister, with a big difference being that she had begun menstruation and her sister never had (Clinical Judgment 12-2).

TIP 12-2: A TEACHING INTERVENTION PLAN for the Sibling of a Child With a Chronic Condition

Nursing Diagnosis and Family Outcomes

- Deficient knowledge: Condition and the effect it will have on the affected sibling, the family, and themselves
  Outcomes: Sibling will understand the reason actions related to the chronic condition are being taken.
  Sibling will identify how he or she can participate in the child's care.

Instructional Interventions

Verify Baseline Knowledge
- What have they been told by their sibling, parents, friends, or health care providers?
- What questions do they have about the condition, how it affects their sibling, and how it affects them?
- Do they know anyone else with this condition?
- What do they most want to learn now?

Assess Sibling's Involvement With Child With Chronic Condition
- Are they ever asked to help with care?
- What do they wish they could do? What do they wish they did not have to do?
- Are there any activities in which they would like to participate that are not allowed because of their sibling's needs?

- How are friendships affected by the presence of the sibling's chronic condition?

Design Teaching Plan Based on Sibling Assessment
- Be specific and increase detail as cognitive ability, age, and interest increase. Do not hide facts of the condition.
- Begin teaching items they are most curious and concerned about.

Present Content Using Standard Teaching Principles
- Use vocabulary understood by the child while teaching medical language that he or she may hear in the future.
- Adapt teaching approach to accommodate the sibling's cognitive and physical development (more pictures with preschoolers; pamphlets, books, and computer programs for school-aged siblings).
- Encourage questions.
- Explore questions for possible concerns not evident in questions.
- Provide source of backup for later questions.

Sibling Support Group
- Provide sibling support group.
- Encourage friendship and communication between siblings and other members of support group.

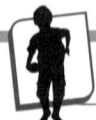

CLINICAL JUDGMENT 12-2

Sibling of a Child With a Chronic Condition

Lili and Nica are 5-year-old twin girls. Lili has spastic diplegic CP that results in the need to wear braces, use a walker, and receive assistance getting on and off the toilet. Nica has no health problems. Their parents report that sometimes, Lili says she wishes that she "had legs like Nica's," but more often, Nica says, "I wish I had cerebral palsy." Their parents report the following story during a routine health assessment for Lili and ask for your guidance in handling the situation.

One day, a piano tuner came over to check the family piano. Lili and Nica were sitting on the couch and were introduced. Lili piped up, "I have cerebral palsy, my legs aren't strong like Nica's, and I can't run to the potty myself. I wear braces because I have cerebral palsy, but I'm getting stronger, and I can walk in my walker." The piano tuner said to her, "Well, I'm sure there are lots of people to help you to the potty and to walk." To which Lili replied, seriously "Yes, that's right." Nica looked sad that she didn't have something special to tell the piano tuner. She put down the picture she had been enthusiastically working on for the last half hour and went out of the room.

Questions

1. What additional information would you try to elicit from the twins' parents before addressing their concerns? What would you look for in the twins' interactions if they were both present?

2. What are the signs that Nica may be having difficulty adapting to having a sibling with a chronic condition?

3. Do you think Nica is having a problem because her sister has a chronic condition?

4. What steps could the family take to assist and support Nica?

5. What outcomes would indicate that the twins are developing as expected?

Answers

1. Is this common behavior or does it occur only occasionally? Are there times when Nica is the one who is boasting rather than Lili? What other indications of expected sibling rivalry are present? Are there any times when it seems to occur more or less often? If Lili and Nica are both present, how do they interact with each other? Does Lili dominate the interaction, or does Nica appear to be on an even par with her sister? Why did Nica leave the room and what did she do after she left?

2. Her comments about her sister and her failure to engage in the common sibling exchange when each tries to best the other in achievements and for attention. The fact that she did not show off her drawing.

3. Without repeated observations, it is impossible to answer this question. Although the behaviors indicated that she is having difficulties and may be upset, the practitioner would need to verify this as part of a pattern.

4. Fully inform both girls of the facts about Lili's condition. Reassess the interactions of the parents with the children to see whether they are focusing more on Lili and her accomplishments and problems to the exclusion of Nica. Work with the family to develop a plan to have times at which Nica is the center of attention to balance the time Lili must be. If Nica's behavior remains negative or if she begins to actively withdraw or stop engaging in activities, refer to a family counselor.

5. Both girls continue to develop a relationship as sisters; each has opportunities to develop personal interests. Each sister may still want something that the other sister has while still being happy for who she is.

HOSPITALIZATIONS AND DETERIORATION

Having to hospitalize a child because of an exacerbation or deterioration of a condition results in added stressors for families of children with chronic conditions, especially if these visits are frequent. For example, there is the commute between home and hospital or home and work, and there are decisions that have to be made regarding time off from work and care of the other children in the family. Many parents want to be with their child each and every time they are hospitalized (Fig. 12-6). Other parents may not feel the need to be present as much as when the child was first diagnosed or as much as the parents whose child is experiencing their first hospital admission for an acute condition. Some parents may feel a loss of parental control and competence as their care responsibilities are

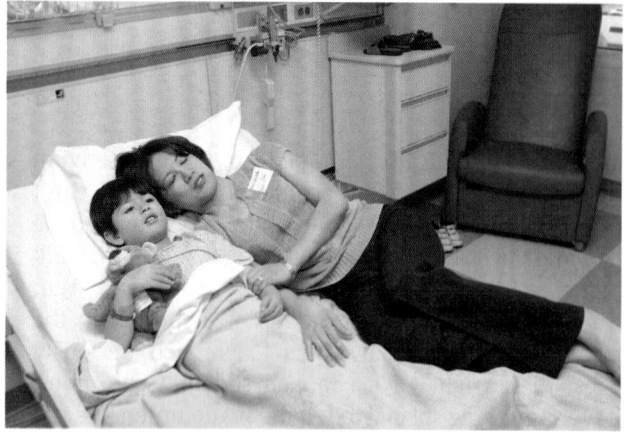

Figure 12-6 Encouraging family caregivers to stay in the hospital room with their child allows them to gradually take on responsibility for the care needs of a child requiring complex physical care when they are home.

increasingly completed by the hospital staff "as they increasingly must adapt to the hospital staff, and they may begin to lose their feeling of competence" (Lewis & Vitulano, 2003, p. 391). A significant number of hospital visits during the first 5 years of a child's life may impair the attachment between child and parent (Lewis & Vitulano, 2003). Although some parents express a significant desire to be with their child and to provide as much care as possible, just as they do at home, others see the hospitalization as a period of respite and take the time to tend to their own needs. Be careful not to misinterpret this behavior as uncaring. Rather, see it as a sign that the family trusts the nursing staff to provide quality care to their child in their absence and that they also are aware that this is an opportunity to meet their own needs and those of the other children in the family.

Staff who see children frequently in the acute care setting might become very attached to them and to their families. Regardless of how many times a child has been hospitalized, never assume that they do not need the same amount of education, support, and clarification of what is going to occur as other patients. They might experience great sadness as they see children start to deteriorate who have been in and out of the hospital for years. Those children and adolescents who are in school might miss being with their peers. Encourage the school to keep the student included, even during hospitalizations.

IMPACT OF A CHRONIC CONDITION ON A CHILD/ADOLESCENT

It is often not until preschool that young children born with chronic conditions begin to perceive differences between themselves and their peers. It is during this time that they recognize differences between male and female and differences in skin color. This is also when they might become aware that aspects of their

condition (e.g. physical immobility, breathing difficulties) make them different from their friends. To help young children cope with these differences, it is important both to acknowledge these differences and to treat them as normal. Children with chronic conditions will often perceive themselves as normal when they see that they are being treated just like other children.

The first task when working with older children and adolescents with chronic conditions is to *find out what the condition means to them*. What is their concept of the chronic condition and how do they think it affects their life? A nursing plan of care for the child with a chronic condition identifies interventions to support the child as he or she adjusts to the impact the condition has on his or her life (Nursing Plan of Care 12-2).

IMPACT ON PHYSICAL DEVELOPMENT

Consistently promote physical development for a child with a chronic condition and ensure that the child is receiving enough nutrients to support growth. This may be especially true for children who are unable to feed themselves or who are fed through alternative means as well as children and adolescents with conditions such as spastic CP, in which a great deal of motor activity requires additional nutrients. Children with neurologic and orthopedic conditions often have decreased physical activity. They might be slow to crawl and walk, or they may be confined to a wheelchair. Decreased physical activity, especially disuse, often leads to osteoporosis and osteopenia, which could put them at risk for bone fractures later in life. Rehabilitative services such as physical therapy (PT) and occupational therapy (OT) can assist in developing goals and daily exercises for the child.

caREminder

Not all children who are below targeted growth parameters have impaired growth. It is important to evaluate whether a child is following his or her own growth curve. A child in the 10th percentile at birth who remains between the 10th and 15th percentiles throughout the first years of life may be doing well, although he or she is clearly smaller than most children of the same age. Other children have conditions that make the use of the growth charts inappropriate. In a child with idiopathic scoliosis or scoliosis secondary to myelomeningocele, height may indicate very little about the child's actual development, although it can be used as part of the evaluation of the progression of the vertebral defect.

IMPACT ON ACHIEVING DEVELOPMENTAL MILESTONES

Family members of children with chronic conditions are often acutely aware of the developmental milestones typically achieved at their child's age. Although the developmental tasks are the same for children with chronic conditions, the rate of accomplishing them

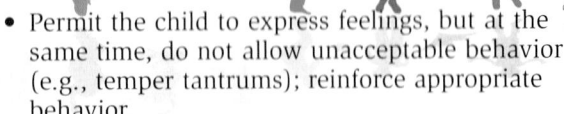

NURSING PLAN OF CARE 12-2:
The Child With a Chronic Condition

Nursing Diagnosis: Anxiety related to uncertain prognosis; actual or perceived loss of body integrity; threat to self-concept

Interventions/Rationale
- Inform the child about his or her condition and treatment in developmentally appropriate language, use age-appropriate techniques to discuss situations (e.g., drawing, telling a story, situation completion), and allow the child to cry.
  Not knowing increases the child's anxiety, even if no new information emerges. The child can recognize that the health care team is caring.
- Provide the child/family support from the facility chaplain, social worker, or the child's own support system.
  The medical staff can focus on the care of the child and the family if they are supported in coping with the situation.
- Use open-ended questions to elicit the child's and family member's thoughts and fears.
  This approach can more accurately answer the issues at hand.
- Maintain routine and consistent staff if possible.
  Predictable routines promote security.
- Instruct in use of relaxation techniques (e.g., deep breathing, meditation, journaling). Role-play adaptive coping skills and support and reinforce use.
  Practicing the methods may help in using them when faced with a stressful situation.

Expected Outcomes
- The child will verbalize feelings of anxiety.
- The child will identify and use methods to reduce feelings of anxiety.

Nursing Diagnosis: Delayed growth and development related to physical effects of the chronic condition or its treatment; decreased access to usual socialization experiences

Interventions/Rationale
- Complete a baseline developmental assessment appropriate to the child's physical and cognitive abilities. Compare with prior assessments, if available.
  Provides comparative data to determine whether delays are perceived or actual in nature. Provides data about delays that can be used as focus for future interventions.
- Discuss and promote the concept of "normalizing" experiences to promote self-sufficiency, adjustment, and mental growth.
  Promotes self-sufficiency, adjustment, and mental growth.

- Permit the child to express feelings, but at the same time, do not allow unacceptable behavior (e.g., temper tantrums); reinforce appropriate behavior.
  Promotes self-efficacy.
- Provide toys, games, equipment, educational supplies, and teaching that will enable the child to increase cognitive, social, and motor skills.
  Tailored activities facilitate the child's ability to participate and achieve milestones.
- Communicate and interact with the child in an age-appropriate fashion; maintain dignity in all interactions with the child.
  Simplifying communication may help the child process information.
- Allow and encourage family members, siblings, and nondisabled peers to visit and interact with the child.
  Consistent interaction with family diminishes normal separation anxiety and increases the child's ability to cope and may limit regressive responses.
- Foster self-worth, provide personal space so the child's belongings are accessible, and encourage the child to care for the physical environment if appropriate.
  Fosters self-efficacy, self-worth, autonomy, and responsibility.
- Promote self-esteem. Identify and recognize the child's strengths and promote these often.
  Positive self-esteem enhances positive coping and psychological adjustment.
- Arrange for the school-aged child to have normal educational experiences through hospital-based teachers or by attending his or her local school.
  Provides opportunities for growth and development and socialization.
- Encourage peer visitation if not contraindicated.
  Peers can help occupy the child's time and will decrease social isolation. Peers are important to adolescents, and interactions help them meet developmental milestones.
- Assist the family in evaluating the child's regressive responses to the illness or chronic health condition. Explain the effects of acute illness or chronic condition on a child.
  Children typically regress when ill. A chronic condition may impose restrictions that limit the child's energy or ability to engage in age-appropriate activities. Families who understand their child's responses are better able to support the child and assist the child in achieving his or her potential.

(Continued)

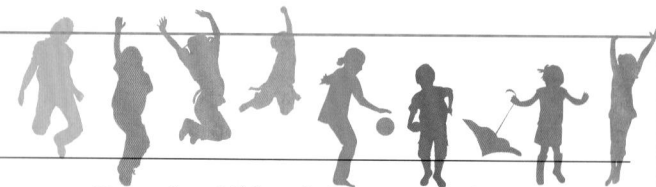

NURSING PLAN OF CARE 12-2:

The Child With a Chronic Condition *(Continued)*

- Assist the family to plan age-appropriate developmental activities for the child based on the child's capabilities.

    Will help the child master skills to achieve developmental potential.

Expected Outcomes

- The child will have growth along his or her own growth curve, optimized within the restrictions imposed by the chronic condition.
- The child will participate in developmentally appropriate socialization experiences.

Nursing Diagnosis: Disturbed body image related to being different than peers; perceiving self as sick

Interventions/Rationale

- Explore the child's perception of body image and concerns of health status. Encourage discussion concerning misconceptions, fears, the reality of public discrimination, and social stigma.

    Lack of knowledge or inaccurate perceptions may increase anxiety and result in activities that undermine the treatment plan. Knowing the child's perception enables teaching the child to address inaccurate beliefs or modification of the treatment plan to accommodate concerns.

- Actively listen while engaging in dialogue regarding feeling about self and personal appearance.

    May reveal self-perceptions and allow discussion of reality versus perception. Child may be embarrassed and feel insecure and resentful about condition and ability to participate in activities considered normal for age. Expression/ discussion of feelings may help coping and acceptance of new appearance.

- Encourage and reinforce positive self-statements. Discuss ways to highlight good feelings about self (e.g., improving grooming, hygiene).

    Reducing negative thoughts can help increase positive body image.

- Assist child to find methods to enhance physical appearance, personal comfort, and daily management of disease process.

    Promotes active adaptation to condition, with a variety of coping strategies to enhance self-esteem and promote normalization in daily life.

- Encourage families to ensure that the child's home and bedroom are age appropriate and do not resemble a mini intensive care unit (ICU).

    Promotes normalization and the "person-first" concept of being a child who happens to have a chronic condition.

- Inform parents of the importance of treating their child like any other child.

    Helps the child to feel normal and may avoid behavioral problems from lack of limits.

- Prepare the child to assume self-care responsibilities.

    Will help the child achieve developmental potential.

Expected Outcome

- The child will verbalize a positive body image.

Nursing Diagnosis: Social isolation related to lack of social skills; embarrassment, limited mobility, or decreased energy secondary to specific condition; communication barrier

Interventions/Rationale

- Determine impact of chronic condition on child's ability to participate in school activities.

    Provides evaluation of current situation to determine whether further interventions are needed.

- Contact school nurse/teacher to discuss any needed modifications in the child's activities; understand the law and the rights of the child with a chronic condition in the school environment.

    Collaboration with school officials will provide a supportive environment for the child to ensure social isolation is minimized and to promote cognitive development.

- Model and role-play appropriate social interactions.

    Observing appropriate response and productive interactions may help the child to develop a repertoire of positive responses.

- Convey that you have time to spend with the child, actively listen, and observe verbal and nonverbal communication. Verify communication.

    Can convey caring and may increase the child's trust and comfort with you.

- Collaborate with the interdisciplinary team (e.g., social worker, physician, school nurse) to develop a plan for the child to participate in family, school, and social activities to his or her maximum capacity.

    Provides an additional support system for the family to ensure the child's successful adaptation at home and school.

- Promote coping methods that deal with changes in the child's appearance (e.g., select flattering clothes, improve personal grooming and hygiene).

    Learning methods to compensate for changes in appearance can help improve child's self-esteem and improve social activity.

Expected Outcome
- The child will participate in developmentally appropriate social activities.

Nursing Diagnosis: Sexual dysfunction related to specific effect of condition or its treatment on sexual maturation; nonavailability of partners

Interventions/Rationale
- Discuss the relationship between sexual functioning and the disease process of the adolescent. Teach the importance of adhering to the medical treatment plan designed to reduce or control disease symptoms.
  Misinformation and lack of knowledge may affect adolescents' concerns and desires to seek intimate relationships.
- Provide an atmosphere of openness, understanding, and acceptance.
  Encourages the adolescent to share his or her feelings and concerns about these very sensitive issues.

Expected Outcome
- The adolescent will verbalize acceptance of and satisfaction with sexual functioning.

Nursing Diagnosis: Ineffective coping related to inability to adapt to the chronic condition; failure to restructure life after diagnosis of chronic condition

Interventions/Rationale
- Encourage the child to identify/express (e.g., verbally, through drawings, play) feelings and concerns about disease. Be an empathic listener.
  Encouraging open expression of feelings may help the child mobilize his or her emotions and validate his or her concerns.
- Identify the actual, perceived, or potential loss.
  Identification of the loss may help the child begin to grieve effectively.
- Identify the stress level of the child.
  Stress may inhibit the ability to resolve emotional issues. A therapeutic approach can be taken if there is understanding of the stress level.
- Assess coping strategies in stressful situations. Help build on previously successful coping strategies. Assist the child/family to look at alternative solutions, but avoid choosing the answer for them.
  Identifies child's/family's usual style in confronting emotional pain/loss. Adaptive coping strategies may provide some relief for the overwhelming grief.
- Provide realistic assessment of the event or situation.
  False reassurances are not helpful and may encourage dysfunctional coping strategies.
- Explain to the child/family that emotional responses to loss are appropriate and commonly experienced.

Acknowledging the loss is not a sign of weakness or loss of control. Grief is a universal experience.
- Make referrals to other professional (e.g., social workers, religious leaders) and community resources as appropriate.
  Support systems can help in the process of grieving.

Expected Outcome
- The child will successfully work through the grieving process and create a new definition of self and life goals.

Nursing Diagnosis: Hopelessness related to failing physiologic condition; prolonged pain; prolonged activity restriction; loss of something valued (ability to socialize, perform in school)

Interventions/Rationale
- Ask the child how he or she sees things, whether anything helps him or her feel better, and what might improve the situation.
  Hopelessness characterizes depression and may result in passivity and despondency.
- Use play therapy/role playing to assist the child in gaining mastery over the issues of concern.
  Provides a mechanism for the child to express self in a nonthreatening manner.
- Allow the child to make decisions concerning care. Keep decisions simple. Restrict choices so as not to overwhelm the child.
  Provides the child opportunity to have some control over his or her life.
- Engage the child in activities that match or are slightly below his or her developmental level. Provide opportunities for success; avoid activities that set the child up for failure.
  Providing positive opportunities may help the child experience the ability to solve problems. Encourage further engagement in problem solving.
- Advance to increasingly higher level tasks and praise and reinforce accomplishments.
  Allows/encourages the child to demonstrate age-appropriate behaviors and developmental tasks.
- Allow the child to make decisions concerning care (e.g., when to brush teeth, comb hair) as appropriate. Keep decisions simple. Restrict choices so as not to overwhelm child.
  Allows the child to make simple decisions regarding care.

Expected Outcomes
- The child will express feelings in age-appropriate ways.
- The child will verbalize a sense of control and a positive outlook on life.

and the methods by which they are achieved may be different. For example, young children learn to say single words. However, a nonverbal child with Down syndrome may learn to use sign language to express certain words. Both of these examples demonstrate cognitive and social development and should be applauded. The same is true for the child or adolescent who learns to use eye signals and computers to communicate.

Children who spend a significant amount of time in the hospital are also often slower in their physical and emotional development. They might have had less nurturing by a consistent caregiver and less love provided because the focus is on the physical skills needed. Children who are frequently admitted to the hospital and those who depend on technology are not as free to explore the environment and to view nature (Fig. 12-7). They interact with adults much more than with children their own age. Adolescents have less opportunity for social events, which are so important for this age group. Adolescents with chronic conditions are often treated like younger children and are not afforded greater responsibilities and independence. They should be encouraged to begin taking responsibility for their care and know their health history because this will make it easier to transition into adult health care services.

Family members might often feel discouraged that their child has not achieved a particular developmental milestone and think, "If my child didn't have_____, he [she] would be able to do _____." Many families experience recurrent and/or chronic sorrow as they watch their children struggle to achieve developmentally appropriate tasks, especially as they become more acutely aware of differences and delays between their children and healthy peers. This chronic sorrow is not continuous but rather occurs sporadically throughout the child's life (see Chapter 13 for more discussion on chronic sorrow). Although families might adapt functionally in that they do all that is needed to keep the child moving forward, they might not internally accept the situation. Encourage families of children with chronic conditions to recognize the milestones that their children *do* reach. If the first milestone is 6 months late, help the family to expect all milestones to be at least that late. If they come earlier, the family may be pleased.

IMPACT ON PSYCHOLOGICAL DEVELOPMENT

 QUESTION: Discuss the impact diabetes has on Lindsay. What aspects of her development are affected by her chronic condition?

Although most children and adolescents are successful in coping with the needs associated with their chronic condition, it has been noted that children with chronic conditions are at a slightly increased risk for psychological adjustment problems (Knafl & Santacroce, 2010; Taylor et al., 2008). In addition to the normal adjustment concerns related to childhood and adolescence, those with both chronic conditions and low self-esteem are particularly vulnerable to mental health problems (Vessey & Sullivan, 2010). There is an increase in stress on both the child and family when the onset of the condition is sudden, the course of the condition is unpredictable, there are functional limitations, and the signs of the condition are visible (Knafl & Santacroce, 2010).

Children and adolescents might have specific concerns related to their condition. For example, the adolescent with seizures may have anxiety about losing consciousness and losing control, especially in front of peers. Bowel problems might cause a child to feel discomfort in being with others as a result of the odor or possible loss of control. The stress of having a chronic condition can also be cumulative. "Cumulative risk may arise from such stresses as loss of autonomy, relative immobilization, impaired function, and disfigurement" (Lewis & Vitulano, 2003, p. 391). However, young people might also learn to use their condition and symptoms to manipulate a situation; the child with asthma might learn to use wheezing as a means of getting out of household responsibilities or activities.

How a child and family cope with the child's chronic condition can affect the child's body image and self-esteem. Children with chronic conditions should *not* be treated as if they are sick (except during exacerbations) or different. Promote a "you can do it" attitude. Remember that a child should *not* be defined as his or her condition. The fact that a child has a chronic condition should just be another component of the child's personality. A nursing goal should be to *assist them to compensate for their disabilities* (Developmental Considerations 12-1).

Children with chronic conditions often begin to feel different from their peers and, perhaps, "abnormal" when others stress the child's differences and the significant accommodations that have to be made regarding these differences. When the home is set up like a mini ICU, for example, it gives the message that the child is sick. The focus is on the illness component and the goal becomes getting the child well. Home medical

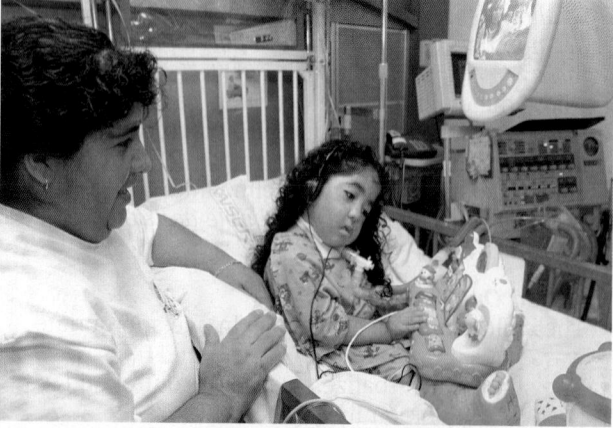

Figure 12-7 The presence of a chronic condition does not necessarily prevent the child from engaging in age-appropriate activities.

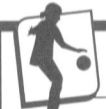

DEVELOPMENTAL CONSIDERATIONS 12-1

Potential Effects of Chronic Conditions on Development

Stage	Expected Developmental Achievements	Potential Barriers to Developmental Achievements	Strategies to Promote Development
Infancy	Sense of trust and security Sensorimotor skills Gross motor control	Family grief Altered feeding experiences Restriction of movement Hospitalization(s) Painful procedures Chronic discomfort Multiple caregivers Inconsistent routines Lack of consistent response to infant cues	Provide consistent care from a limited number of caregivers. Establish reciprocity—caregiver responds to infant's cues and infant is given opportunity to respond to caregiver's cues. Expose infant to normal range of environmental stimuli while ensuring periods without stimuli. Assist family members in the development of attachment and caregiving roles. Enroll in early intervention program if appropriate. Promote cognitive development and attainment of motor skills.
Early childhood: 1–3 years old	Autonomy and self-control Increasing gross and fine motor skills Independent activity Development of speech Cognitive and social growth Initial development of egocentric thought Normal negativism, confrontations over everyday activities, especially feeding and discipline	Negative response to anything that is restrictive Family member's desire to control all activities Limited interaction with other children and adults beyond family Family conflict between need to discipline and need to complete life-sustaining care Decreased quality and quantity of play opportunities	Teach and support development of usual parenting skills. Encourage active interactions with environment (e.g., mobility devices as needed; playing on floor; going out in neighborhood, to mall, to see family and friends). Encourage full range of play activities to develop social, fine and gross motor ability, and cognitive skills. Set limits as usual. Support family as child becomes more active and less under their complete control.
Early childhood: 4–5 years old	Initiative Egocentrism increases Beginning to understand internal body, thought processes still preoperational Still understands events only through his or her own experience with them	Medication requirements Dietary restriction Mobility restriction or inability to be mobile without assistance Need for adult supervision but need to be with peers	Promote active involvement with environment. Enroll in activities (preschool, daycare) that allow interaction with other children. Identify and correct incorrect associations between events and causes.

(Continued)

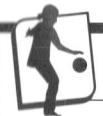

DEVELOPMENTAL CONSIDERATIONS 12-1

Potential Effects of Chronic Conditions on Development (Continued)

Stage	Expected Developmental Achievements	Potential Barriers to Developmental Achievements	Strategies to Promote Development
	Varying understanding of body function and illness	Repeated separations from family Caregiver difficulty with limit setting	Begin education about condition. Allow and encourage participation in self-care activities.
Middle childhood	Industry Sense of accomplishment/mastery from activities undertaken Begin development of independence from family Develop relationships with peers, school, play groups Refine gross and fine motor, cognitive, and social skills	Differences from peers Dependence on medical care Restriction on independence Requirements for adult monitoring Medication, dietary, activity requirements/restriction School absences Inability to fully participate in desired activities	Promote full participation in school. Explore ways to increase stamina and decrease exhaustion. Help family deal with fears related to vulnerability of child. Identify barriers to achievement and develop plan to overcome or bypass them. Educate about normal changes caused by conditions. Encourage increasing self-care. Encourage child to develop strategies to deal with negative aspects of condition.
Adolescence	Sense of identity Increased independence from family Develop problem-solving skills, abstract thought Fuller understanding of body function and condition Development of sexuality Accept changes in body image: rapid physical growth, sexual maturation Prepare for life as an adult; choice of vocation Reluctance to accept own vulnerability, leading to increased risk-taking activities	Altered body image Decreased growth Visible deformity Need for adult supervision and/or assistance with daily activities Medication and dietary requirements Possible vocational limitation Need to explain condition to others	Educate about normal changes of adolescence. Explore questions related to sexuality. Prepare for transition to adult caregivers. Explore sources of social problems. Continue education about condition and care of condition. Encourage active participation in decisions about own care. Reevaluate level of participation in own care and increase if appropriate. Integrate care requirements into daily activities.

equipment should be as inconspicuous as possible, with the room resembling a typical child's room. Children who depend on technology, especially those on ventilators, often have decreased opportunities to explore their environment, to play hide-and-seek, to catch lightning bugs, and to interact with others their age (Selekman et al., 2013). They often have a loss of privacy. Families should be encouraged to provide age-appropriate activities (Fig. 12-8). For adolescents who depend on technology, in-style clothing should be modified to accommodate the equipment to make the child feel similar to their peers.

Continue to educate the child about his or her chronic condition when the child moves to new developmental

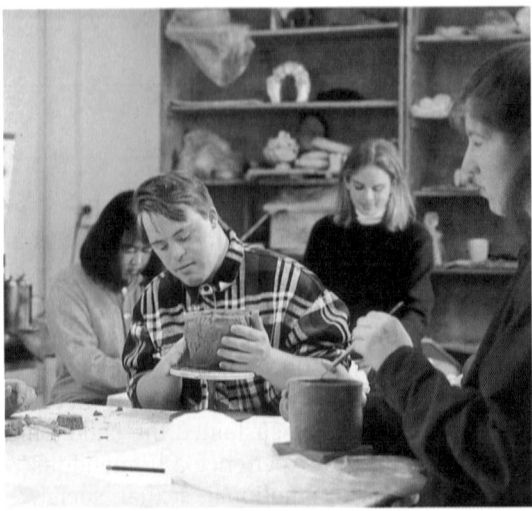

Figure 12-8 The adolescent with disabilities benefits from learning new skills and interacting with others.

stages or activities (e.g., begins school and travels on the school bus), the condition takes on a new dimension (e.g., blood sugar becomes more difficult to control through the growth spurt of puberty and adolescence), or the family changes (e.g., divorce, remarriage, birth of a child, departure of a sibling for college). As the child develops cognitively and emotionally, the need and ability to learn about his or her condition also evolves. In addition, the impact of the condition on the child, as perceived by the child, will also change. By empowering self-responsibility, the child or adolescent should feel pride in his or her accomplishments, knowledge base (that often can be used to impress one's peers), skill set, and ability to overcome obstacles. If presented in a positive way, the child's self-esteem should increase.

Specialty camps during the summer are specifically geared to children with specific chronic conditions. There are camps for those with cancer, diabetes, cognitive and neuromuscular deficits, and obesity, where the goal is to allow children to be children and to be with others who have the same condition so that the stigma is erased. Conventions for those who are deaf or of short stature also promote self-esteem and normalcy. The Special Olympics provides a forum for individuals with disabilities to compete and for which they can train during the year and receive recognition. All these forums promote self-esteem and self-respect for both the children and their families.

> *ANSWER:* Lindsay's ability to spend time with her peers and away from her parents is affected by her diabetes. Sleeping over at a friend's house becomes much more problematic. There are fewer options for children with chronic conditions who wish to attend summer day camps and overnight camps.

REHABILITATION AND HABILITATION

Children and adolescents with orthopedic and neurologic chronic conditions are often engaged in long-term rehabilitation. For adults, **rehabilitation** usually

entails trained and committed health professionals who perform a wide range of services and provide care to the patient to improve or assist with *restoring* function lost through injury or illness or learning to accommodate for functions that have been lost. The process includes patient and family support and education to help them adapt to an altered level of functional capacity and possibly altered lifestyle. Principal goals of rehabilitation are to help individuals learn lifelong management of their condition or disability, institute health maintenance and preventive strategies, return to work, and otherwise be a contributing member of society. For some children with traumatic disabilities, rehabilitation focuses on *relearning* previous skills and abilities and *returning* to the community; however, this is not the case for most children. The Association of Rehabilitation Nurses (2007) identifies its focus as "improving the quality of life for children and adolescents with disabilities and their families," to collaborate with the interdisciplinary team, and to "assist children to function at their maximum potential and become contributing members to both their families and society."

Habilitation is similar to rehabilitation because it involves the same professionals who provide services to the child and family; however, the focus is on helping the child with acquired and developmental disabilities learn *new* skills and first-time abilities to achieve his or her maximum potential (Selekman et al., 2013). Learning developmental tasks the first time are challenging enough; yet, for the child affected by a disabling condition since birth or early childhood, the skills can be even more difficult to acquire. The terms *rehabilitation* and *habilitation* are often used interchangeably, and both can occur simultaneously. For instance, the infant who is a victim of abusive head trauma (shaken baby syndrome) might be admitted to a rehabilitation unit to relearn feeding skills; therapists will also focus on new developmental tasks, such as rolling or sitting up (if the child had not yet attained that skill before his or her injury).

Rehabilitation and habilitation services for children have dramatically expanded during the past half century as a result of ongoing advances in technology and medical science, a substantial decrease in child mortality rates, and children with chronic conditions living longer, often into adulthood. The expansion of rehabilitation and habilitation services for children has also been influenced by the changing nature of hospital reimbursement, decreased lengths of hospital stays, the belief that outpatient and home care services reduce costs, patient preferences, the belief that children should live and thrive better in a natural home-like environment, and legislation that has supported the rights of individuals with disabilities (American Academy of Pediatrics, 2005).

UNIQUE FEATURES OF PEDIATRIC REHABILITATION AND HABILITATION

Rehabilitation of children differs from that of adults in several ways (Developmental Considerations 12-2). The primary difference between children and adults that

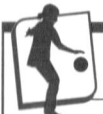

DEVELOPMENTAL CONSIDERATIONS 12-2

Differences Between Rehabilitation of the Adult and of the Child

In Adult Rehabilitation	In Pediatric Rehabilitation
The focus is on reintegrating or compensating for what is lost.	The focus is on helping the child to attain skills and abilities at a level that may have been previously unknown to the child.
The needs for rehabilitation involve suddenly acquired conditions such as trauma, stroke, and heart disease or debilitating conditions such as diabetes, arthritis, and pulmonary disease.	The needs for habilitation involve some form of chronic condition, congenital anomaly, or disabling condition acquired as a result of medical interventions that have sustained the child's life.
Physical development is complete for the most part. Emotional development and cognitive development have also reached a plateau, with growth continuing but with less variance than in the pediatric population.	The child continues to experience a tremendous amount of physical, emotional, sexual, social, and cognitive development.
The family is important as a source of support and as an adjunct to treatment.	The family must simultaneously learn to care for the child and foster the child's development as well as learn to manage their own individual and family needs.
The goal is to teach the adult to care for himself or herself.	The goal is to teach the child to care for himself or herself as appropriate for age and capabilities.
The focus is on vocational rehabilitation, teaching skills and knowledge so that the adult can perform or resume an occupation.	The focus is on educational rehabilitation, reaching the highest academic level possible while teaching the life skills that would be accomplished by any child, such as ordering food in a restaurant, receiving change from a purchase, and using public transportation. Therapeutic support services also assist in developing skills such as walking, building a block tower, combing one's hair, and learning to color.
The necessity for rehabilitation is a new concept. Before the condition that brought him or her to the point of requiring rehabilitation, the adult was able to care for himself or herself and to complete daily activities.	The child's disability is the norm. The child has a known dependence and, depending on the age at onset, is likely not to have known a life without his or her chronic condition.
Experiencing chronic pain, discomfort, or the need for treatment as a result of the condition and undergoing rehabilitation may be relatively new experiences.	The experience of chronic pain or discomfort or the need for treatment may not be new to the child. The child with a disability or a chronic condition may already have spent many years with these experiences as a result of the condition.

Information adapted from Selekman, J. (1991). Pediatric rehabilitation: From concepts to practice. *Pediatric Nursing, 17*, 11–14, 33; Selekman, J., Bochenek, J., & Lukens, M. (2013). Children with chronic conditions. In J. Selekman (Ed.), *School nursing: A comprehensive text* (pp. 700–783). Philadelphia, PA: F. A. Davis.

forms the basis for understanding all variations in rehabilitative and habilitative services is that adults have reached a level of physical and mental maturity that children have not. Children are in the midst of their growth and development, learning new skills and tasks. The child's cognitive level continues to change, as do his or her emotional, psychosocial, and sexual areas of development. Pediatric physicians, nurses, and therapists

need to apply knowledge of developmental theories and age-appropriate strategies to the treatment plan (see thePoint for Supplemental Information for additional information about members of the rehabilitation health care team). For example, the rehabilitation team working with a 15-month-old child would focus on mobility, play, and communication skills (Fig. 12-9). Toileting and dressing would not be focal points because most

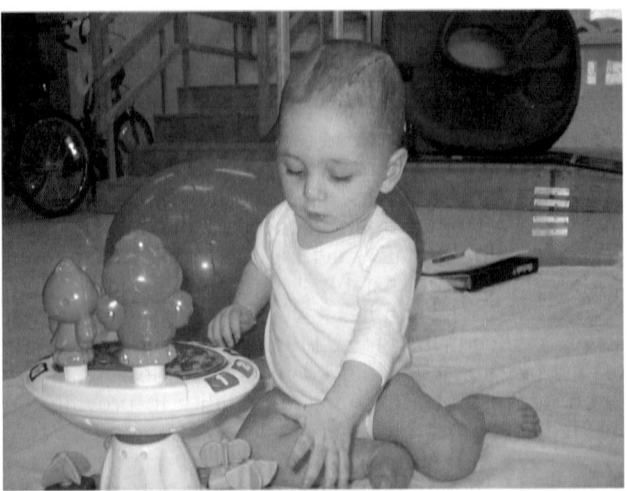

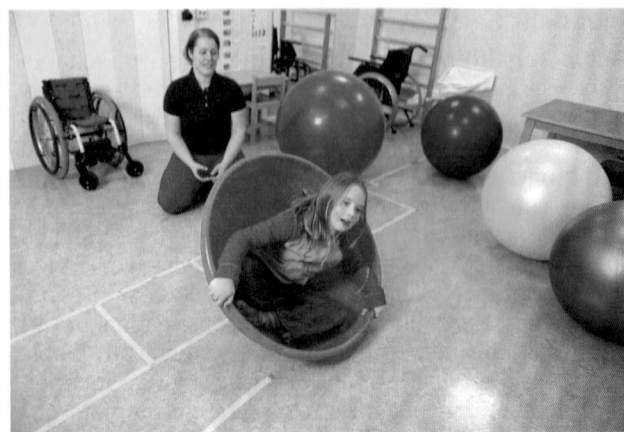

Figure 12-10 Play is the young child's motivation for participation in rehabilitation therapies.

Figure 12-9 Pediatric rehabilitation and habilitation services help the child reattain lost skills and learn new skills that are appropriate to his or her developmental age.

young children would not have mastered these skills yet. The child's learning process is affected by cognitive and developmental factors that may not have an influence on the adult's ability to learn. For example, young children and preschoolers learn through exploration, by discovering their world. If a child's environment is limited to the length of an oxygen or ventilator tube, or if experiences are limited by physical immobility, the focus of rehabilitative care would be on assisting the child to compensate for this limitation. For instance, the family may be instructed to use a more mobile oxygen tank that could be easily moved from room to room to broaden the world of the child who is oxygen dependent. Or perhaps the young child with limited physical mobility would be encouraged to explore his or her environment in a power wheelchair. Unlike an adult, the child may not be aware that there is a world full of exciting adventures and experiences beyond the scope of what can be immediately seen and touched.

The adult in rehabilitation often has a repertoire of past knowledge and experiences from which to build new adaptive skills and to learn to compensate for what he or she has lost as a result of illness or injury. However, the child may not have such a strong experiential basis on which to build. For example, a kindergartner who experiences disfiguring burns on the arms and upper chest must relearn how to hold a spoon and a drinking cup and must also acquire the new ability to write.

caREminder

Rehabilitation and habilitation programs are designed for the child to achieve greater mental, physical, and social development. The child must be rehabilitated to his or her current developmental stage and habilitated to acquire new developmental tasks that the child would be acquiring had the injury not occurred.

The adult's rehabilitation goals are to improve function, gain independence, and return to work. Many of the therapy sessions are directed with these goals in mind. Therapies can be difficult, with a grueling repetitive nature to the exercises, yet the adult can usually stay motivated by comprehending the ultimate goals. Children, on the other hand, have a different focus. The work of a child is play and learning in school. Therapists and nurses often have to incorporate fun and creative play into the therapies or treatment sessions to keep the child motivated and involved (Fig. 12-10). The goal of pediatric habilitation or rehabilitation for the school-aged child is school entry or reentry; therefore, general education (ABCs, reading, writing, and arithmetic) should also be incorporated into treatment sessions and the overall plan.

Adults most often require rehabilitation because of a sudden disability resulting from a stroke, illness, or injury. In contrast, children most commonly need rehabilitation because of a disability resulting from a chronic condition. Although conditions requiring rehabilitative and habilitative services vary widely, they often share many challenges and commonalities in the functional limitations that can affect the child. These include neurodevelopmental challenges, physical disabilities, conditions caused by genetic disorders, chronic conditions, and complex medical conditions. More complete discussions of specific disease processes can be found in Chapters 14 through 31 of this text, in which alterations in specific body systems are presented.

LEVELS AND SETTINGS OF REHABILITATIVE AND HABILITATIVE CARE

Rehabilitative and habilitative services for children fall along a continuum of health care. The choice of setting for an individual child is determined by the child's level of medical acuity, the family's insurance, and the availability of specialty pediatric rehabilitation services in the community. *Level of care* can be defined as the intensity of rehab involved. The different levels can be grouped as inpatient services and outpatient services.

Inpatient Services

Acute rehabilitation refers to the phase of rehabilitative services provided immediately after an injury, illness, or surgical procedure. Ideally, rehabilitation services such as proper positioning, bowel and bladder programs, range-of-motion (ROM) exercises, and family education should start as early as feasible. Some children begin therapies while in the pediatric or neonatal intensive care units. Early rehabilitative services can prevent secondary complications such as pressure ulcers, muscle contractures, and constipation or urinary tract infections. After the child is medically stable, therapeutic services are delivered through an inpatient (hospital setting) pediatric rehabilitation program or a center providing coordinated and integrated services with physician oversight and around-the-clock nursing care.

The pediatric **subacute rehabilitation** program focuses on rehabilitation services to children who are considered to be medically fragile, oftentimes those with technologic needs. Children transferred to subacute care generally do not require the medical intensity of acute care but are still not well enough to go home. They are admitted and receive continuous care in a subacute inpatient care facility. The pediatric nurse should be an advocate to coordinate and eliminate duplication of services. Continued patient and family teaching is emphasized, with a goal of reentry to the child's home, school, and community.

Outpatient Services

Outpatient rehabilitation provides services to children who no longer require hospitalization. Outpatient rehabilitation can consist of comprehensive programs (day rehab, where children receive intensive interdisciplinary coordinated services during the day and go home with their families at night), single service or multiple services (not program-based or coordinated, yet receiving one or multiple types of therapies, usually weekly), and community-based services (occurring in the home or school setting). Many children with congenital or special developmental health care needs never require hospitalization for rehabilitation services. Instead, these children receive periodic evaluation by a pediatric physiatrist (a physician who specializes in physical medicine and rehabilitation) or primary care provider who may prescribe therapies. Therapy services should be prescribed to meet specific goals and focus on reinforcement of adaptive techniques to optimize functional ability and independence.

Community-based rehabilitation delivers therapy services in the child's natural environment (e.g., home, school, early childhood education program, child care setting). Treatment plans are formulated by the family and community care providers, typically as part of the individualized family service plan (for children under the age of 3 years), an IEP (for ages 3 through 21 who require special education), or a 504 Accommodation Plan (for individuals who need accommodations in the school, including rehabilitation services, but do not need special education) (Selekman et al., 2013). Therapeutic services generally focus on educating the family, optimizing academic achievement, and the functioning of the child in the school setting and the community.

Children can also live in residential settings (long-term care facilities) instead of with their families. Many of these institutions have incorporated rehabilitation or habilitation programs. These residential settings are much less common than in the past but are still necessary as an alternative setting for caring for children with complex or unstable long-term physical health care needs. Some families have described the emotional strain involved when forced to make the difficult choice of having their child placed in one of these facilities, often because of a caregiver's inability to provide the needed care or for financial reasons. Many families stay involved with their children, often accompanying them to doctors' appointments and caring for them at home on weekends or holidays.

Some of these settings might also provide respite care or short-term care to provide a rest or break for the family. Occasionally, coordinated relief of caregiver responsibilities is needed in times of crisis or undue emotional or physical stress. The major emphasis during this time is on psychosocial support for the family.

ASSESSMENT OF THE CHILD WITH REHABILITATIVE AND HABILITATIVE NEEDS

Regardless of the level of care or the setting, assessment of the child with a long-term disability requires the use of standardized measurement tools and ongoing assessment information gathered by members of the rehabilitation or habilitative team (Focused Health History 12-1). Measurement tools in rehabilitative and habilitative care provide an objective measure of the child's functional abilities. They also provide information regarding the needs of the child and the family, the effectiveness of interventions, and the success of a specific rehabilitative or habilitative program. There is no tool that comprehensively addresses all the special needs of children and their families. Because no single tool provides a complete picture of a child's needs, measurement tools should not be used in isolation. Rehabilitation and habilitation teams generally find it useful to adopt two or more pediatric measurement tools, tailoring aspects of each to capture the specific needs of a particular patient population. The Functional Independence Measure for Children (WeeFIM) and Pediatric Evaluation of Disability Inventory (PEDI) are the most common tools to measure functional capabilities and performance in pediatric rehabilitation (see thePoint for Diagnostic Tools for a review of the outcome tools that can be used by the pediatric rehabilitation team).

MANAGEMENT OF FUNCTIONAL LIMITATIONS

The focus of care for the child dealing with the effects of a sudden illness, injury, or a chronic condition is to enable the child to lead a life as independent and age appropriate as possible. Achieving that goal requires that all of the child's growth and developmental needs, in addition to

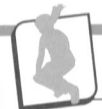

FOCUSED HEALTH HISTORY 12-1

The Child With Rehabilitation and Habilitation Needs

Current history	Primary diagnosis and associated disorders, sensory deficits, cognitive/communicative issues, motor impairments, functional limitations, safety precautions, services, and treatments Current medications *Symptoms and treatment program* • *Neurologic:* Increased or decreased responsiveness to stimuli, irritability, lethargy, decreased strength, persistence of primitive reflexes (thumb/fist posturing, symmetric tonic neck reflex, asymmetric tonic neck reflex, Moro), asymmetry, dystonic or abnormal movements, hypotonia, hypertonia, spasticity, or seizures may reflect the child's typical level of functioning. Changes from the child's normative level may indicate changing condition. • *Specific neurologic support strategies:* Environmental stimulation strategies, positioning, and ROM • *Additional system assessment based on child's condition (e.g., respiratory, elimination, musculoskeletal, skin):* Determine typical manifestation of child's specific condition. Changes from the child's normative manifestations may indicate changing condition. • *Specific support strategies: respiratory:* Ventilator care, artificial airway management, apnea monitor, bilevel positive airway pressure (BIPAP), suctioning/respiratory care procedures, oxygen, nebulizer treatments • *Specific support strategies: elimination:* Toileting program, catheterization schedule, devices used for incontinence management, bowel program • *Specific support strategies: musculoskeletal:* ROM exercises, positioning use of splints and devices • *Specific support strategies: skin integrity:* Dressing changes, sitting and turning tolerances, pressure relief methods, specialty equipment (cushions/mattresses)
Past medical history	*Prenatal history:* Maternal conditions (e.g., placental abruption, toxemia, coagulation disorders, Rh incompatibility, trauma) or maternal infections (e.g., rubella, cytomegalovirus, toxoplasmosis) and/or multiple pregnancies are associated with CP; complications of delivery *Neonatal history:* Infant's gestational age in weeks and birth weight (prematurity and low birth weight associated with CP), spontaneous breathing at birth, meconium staining, Apgar scores (5-minute Apgar score less than 7 points may be associated with asphyxia, traumatic delivery, hemorrhage, nuchal cord), neonatal intensive care unit admission and length of stay, need for assisted ventilation or oxygen, jaundice/need for bilirubin lights, seizures, drug exposure (type/presence of withdrawal), cranial bleeds, infections (bacterial meningitis, viral encephalitis associated with CP), hypoglycemic events (may be associated with neurologic insult) *Previous health challenges:* Past surgeries: gastrointestinal procedures such as fundoplication, gastronomy tube, or button (swallowing problems); orthopedic procedures such as tendon releases or bone surgeries (i.e., for CP, brain injury, muscular dystrophy); neurosurgical procedures such as rhizotomy, baclofen pump placement (CP); urinary diversion procedures such as for spina bifida, muscular dystrophy Frequent exacerbations of chronic conditions: asthma attacks, hypoglycemic episodes with diabetes, seizures, congestive heart failure, anaphylactic reactions, multiple infections from immune suppression Pain issues (related to scoliosis, hip dislocation, spasticity, contractures)

(Continued)

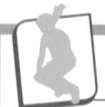

FOCUSED HEALTH HISTORY 12-1

The Child With Rehabilitation and Habilitation Needs (Continued)

Nutritional assessment	Growth patterns plotted on growth curves (head circumference, height, weight, and body mass index), food allergies *Feeding patterns:* Poor suck, difficulty swallowing, episodes of coughing, pocketing or choking during meals, increased time to eat meals, and poor intake are signs of feeding difficulties *Specific feeding strategies:* Type, consistency, texture, formula type, amount and frequency of feedings, and supplements
Family medical history	Genetic conditions, presence in other family members of symptoms similar to those for which the child is being evaluated
Social history	*Education and school:* Grade level, special education modifications, school or private therapies (type and amount), aide required in class, school nursing services required *Home:* Child and family level of coping and adaptation, support network, family knowledge of condition, family skill in performing care to prevent and manage complications, assistance and education required, child and family learning style, safety and compatibility of home environment, adequate supply of utility services, disaster plan in place, access to needed equipment, transportation services needed, financial situation, insurance, cultural viewpoints and religious beliefs affecting care, disciplinary practices
Growth and development	Late acquisition of developmental milestones and current functional level: mobility skills (rolling, sitting, crawling, standing, walking, transfers, wheelchair skills), self-care requirements (eating, grooming, dressing, personal hygiene, bladder and bowel management, language, communication, and cognitive skills), daily routine, household chores, vocational skills, life skills, recreational activities Equipment, adaptive and assistive devices used

Note: See Chapter 8 for a comprehensive health history and Chapters 14 through 30 for the focused health history of specific body systems.

the impact of the disability, be considered and addressed by the health care team. First, a focused and comprehensive health history and assessment of the child with rehabilitation or habilitation needs is performed (see Focused Health History 12-1). In addition to the child's condition, the family's ability to care for the child identifies areas requiring special attention. Then, appropriate goals can be identified with the child and family to direct the plan of care (see thePoint for Nursing Plan of Care for the Child in Rehabilitation/Habilitation). The plan of care in rehabilitation differs from that when managing a child with an acute condition. In rehabilitative services, the plan of care is for the interdisciplinary team, and interventions are communicated as goals (both short and long term) for the child and family to achieve.

As with all children, the approach to care should be guided by the child's understanding of and ability to cope with a given situation. For example, an 8-year-old with a developmental disability undergoing orthopedic surgery may not benefit from a coloring book depicting the operating room and recovery room. If his or her cognitive ability is at a 4-year-old level, it may be more beneficial to have the child handle equipment such as the face mask used by the anesthetist, trying it on a doll's face and then on his or her own face. Likewise, placing a bandage "cast" on a doll's leg helps prepare the child for what he or she will find after surgery. The child with physical impairments, regardless of his or her level of intelligence, should be afforded every opportunity to participate in self-care activities that will foster independence.

Regardless of the reason for rehabilitative and habilitative services, the basic components of the treatment program need to identify and address the child's functional limitations in the following areas: ambulation and mobility, dressing, personal hygiene, bladder and bowel management, grooming, language and communication, eating, and the use of adaptive and assistive devices.

Ambulation and Mobility

Ambulation depends on an ability to perceive one's position in space (proprioception), maintain a sense of balance, and support the body while shifting weight to move the feet in sequence. Children with hemiplegia or diplegia may learn to walk if spasticity and impaired control are not too severe. These children might be at a modified independent level requiring a device, crutches, walker, or long- or short-leg braces for stability. Children with quadriplegia, depending on the severity and type, may walk only with the assistance of a helper and a supporting device, usually for short distances. Wheelchair mobility requires a good seating system for stability and the strength either in the upper extremities to be able to reach the wheels and move them with the hands or in the lower extremity to be able to touch the floor and move the wheelchair with the feet. A power wheelchair might be considered if strength, balance, and endurance are a problem, although the controls may require adaptation. Proper seating is essential and is a particular challenge with growing children. An ill-fitting wheelchair exaggerates abnormal movement. Individuals with cognitive issues or perceptual deficits may have difficulty steering properly and safely. Therefore, safety factors to be considered include the child's level of development and judgment. The rehab nurse is always aware of how the child moves about the environment as he or she provides supervision and assistance as necessary.

Transfers are essential in many activities of daily living (getting on and off the toilet or in and out of a tub, for example). Some children with disabilities have balance issues, poor muscle control, or visual problems that impair their ability to maneuver and perform these skills. Generally, children with spastic diplegia with upper extremity function can use a slide board or pivot independently. Moderately affected children who are able to support their weight on their lower extremities and maintain balance can also pivot transfer with assistance. When an injury to the spinal cord is involved, the transferring situations are usually from one seated surface to another (e.g., bed to wheelchair, wheelchair to toilet or shower chair). Children who are more disabled may require a two-person or mechanical lift transfer. Pediatric nurses working in rehabilitation must know the type of transfer, the assistance required, and how to incorporate body mechanics in every transfer performed for the patient and their own safety.

Dressing

Dressing is a developmental milestone and a basic activity of daily living. When a child has physical limitations, the caregiver frequently fosters dependence without intending to do so. The functional abilities necessary for independence in dressing include cognitive recognition of the garments that are appropriate for the weather conditions, motor planning or sequencing of the task (underwear before pants and shoes), the ability to access clothing from storage areas, the strength to shift weight and maintain balance in a sitting or standing position while negotiating limbs into the garment, the flexibility to reach parts of the body, eye–hand coordination, and the manual dexterity to maneuver the garments and/or assistive devices. Children with disabilities benefit from nurses who know their assistance level requirements and can assist them to foster independence in this area.

Personal Hygiene

Personal hygiene, like dressing, is an activity of daily living that in our culture generally commands respectful privacy. Personal hygiene includes activities related to bathing, washing, and toileting. These activities require accessibility of bathroom fixtures. Safety in performing these activities is also a concern. Children with a mild disability may need only initial assistance in preparation and supervision, especially in areas of safety (e.g., monitoring the water temperature, placement of bath mat, and level of water in the tub or the sink). Children with a moderate disability require physical assistance in performing parts of the care. Children who have more severe functional limitations may be completely dependent or able to assist the caregiver only partially in these areas. Generally, the more dependent a child is, the more the responsibility of providing privacy falls on the caregiver (e.g., ensuring that bathing, toileting, and dressing are not done in the presence of others). Rehab nurses can be pivotal educators by ensuring privacy and by teaching modesty and sexuality when the opportunity arises during bathing or toileting an individual.

Bladder and Bowel Management

Bladder and bowel management refers to the control of urine and bowel movements. The functional skill of continence is one of the most important developmental milestones a child achieves. If not met, a child may be left behind or may have limited participation in activities—for instance, not going to preschool if continence is a prerequisite. The timing, strategies, and expectations of toilet-training practices differ widely. For children with disabilities who have physiologic, environmental, and social challenges, a team approach to their bladder and bowel management might be necessary, and generally, the nurse takes the lead. Bladder and bowel control might require the use of equipment (e.g., urinal within reach for the mobility challenged or supportive toilet seat for the child with trunk weakness), medications (e.g., laxatives, anticholinergics), or assistance (e.g., cueing the child with a brain injury to toilet before and after therapy). Another example is the child with spina bifida who needs to compensate for the loss of these functions. Routine clean, intermittent catheterizations might need to be performed by a caregiver initially but can be performed independently by the child upon reaching school age. The goal is to be independent and dry between catheterizations because urinary accidents interfere with socialization. A bowel program (such as a daily suppository to prevent fecal incontinence and embarrassment for the school-aged child) may continue to be administered by the caregiver for a longer period of time, although it ultimately will become the child's or adolescent's responsibility.

Grooming

Grooming activities include hair brushing and oral hygiene as well as shaving or makeup application in adolescence and adulthood. Although perhaps not considered as critical as dressing and personal hygiene, these activities of daily living are vitally important to the child's self-esteem. Generally, these activities require upper extremity strength, manual dexterity, and visual acuity with eye–hand coordination. The rehab nurse's contribution might be to ensure that the child performs these skills as able.

Language and Communication

Language and communication are essential functional components. Language development involves the ability to hear, to interpret, and to understand situations encountered in the environment. It also involves the ability to formulate thoughts and to interact with the environment and with other persons in it. Communication skills are essential to interacting with others. Making one's needs known in a manner that is understood by others is a basic function of all humans. Compromise of this process can be related to several conditions: cognitive deficits, sensory impairment (e.g., vision, hearing), motor impairment (e.g., dysarthria, or difficulty forming words with the structures of the mouth), or an alteration in physical structures (e.g., tracheostomy). Rehab nurses working with a child who has a communication impairment assist the team in developing a reliable yes/no system and help the child use signs, gestures, verbal language, or an alternative communication device. Augmentative or alternate communication systems provide a means to interact and facilitate meeting the child's needs. Some are very simple (picture and word boards) and others are quite sophisticated (alphabet board or technologic talking systems). Rehab nurses require patience, a familiarity of the device used by the child, and knowledge of strategies used to facilitate language or communication skills.

Eating

Eating problems may include poor control of the lips, the tongue, and the airway protective mechanisms; slow eating; and poor chewing and swallowing ability. Visual–motor problems interfere with the coordination of motions for scooping and carrying the food to the mouth. Feeding problems may also be related to a variety of other clinical problems, such as hypotonia, a weak suck, conditions resulting in decreased energy to eat (i.e., anemia or cyanotic cardiac conditions), poor coordination of swallow, tonic bite reflex, hyperactive gag reflex, exaggerated tongue thrust, drooling, aspiration, gastroesophageal reflux, and the child's inability to communicate hunger. Constipation can also affect the child's appetite. Pediatric rehab nurses are attuned to feeding and developmental issues as they provide for a safe eating environment, assist children with this skill, use alternative (nasogastric or gastric) feedings, and continuously monitor for problems.

Adaptive and Assistive Devices

To maximize the child's independence and to support the child's recovery from an injury or illness, the rehab nurse needs to know what **adaptive devices** and **assistive devices** the child uses. Adaptive and assistive devices are equipment or tools used to alter the environment and enhance functional abilities. The use of positioning devices that maintain alignment is essential in rehab. In addition, positioning the child in relation to his or her external environment can positively foster the child's function. For example, speaking to a child from above his or her line of sight fosters poor muscular alignment; speaking at eye level promotes positive alignment. Positioning toys on the right side of the bed for a child who favors his or her right side fosters continued preference and possible contracture development. Contractures may develop when muscles consistently have increased tone and remain in shortened positions for prolonged periods. Therefore, positioning the child with items of interest to the left side enhances the child's desire to turn in this direction and fosters elongation of the trunk muscles and extremities.

The use of "sidelyers" and corner seats for infants and young children promotes flexion and appropriate positioning for play and functional activities. Supportive orthotics or braces also work to reduce spasticity, maintain ROM, prevent contractures, and promote function. Orthotic devices may be used to maintain a group of muscles in a lengthened state so that function of the joint is improved.

One of the most commonly prescribed orthotics is a short leg brace called an *ankle–foot orthosis* (Fig. 12-11). This type of brace serves to correct foot drop and might further increase muscle tone in the hips, providing a more stable sitting or standing position. Correcting the child's atypical foot position may alter the position of the hips and knees when the child stands, thereby improving gait.

A variety of splints may be used to improve hand function. A common one is the resting hand splint. In this splint, the thumb is held in an abducted position with the wrist in a neutral or slightly extended position. This maintains the hand in an open position to prevent deformity and maintain function. Even with loss of fine motor control of the hand and fingers, a

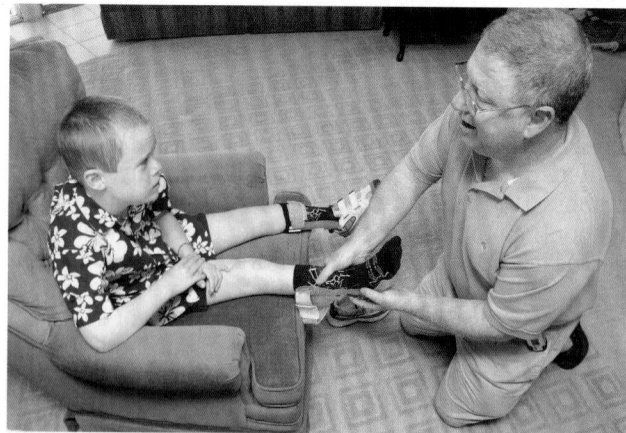

Figure 12-11 Ankle–foot orthotics provide the support needed for independent or assisted walking.

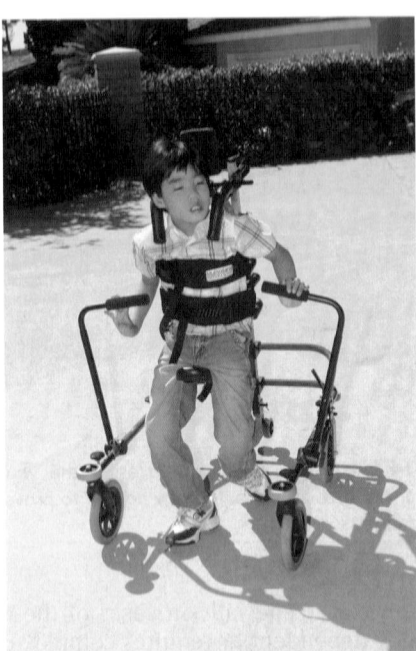

Figure 12-12 The use of a mobile prone walker helps the child to better participate in daily activities at school and at home.

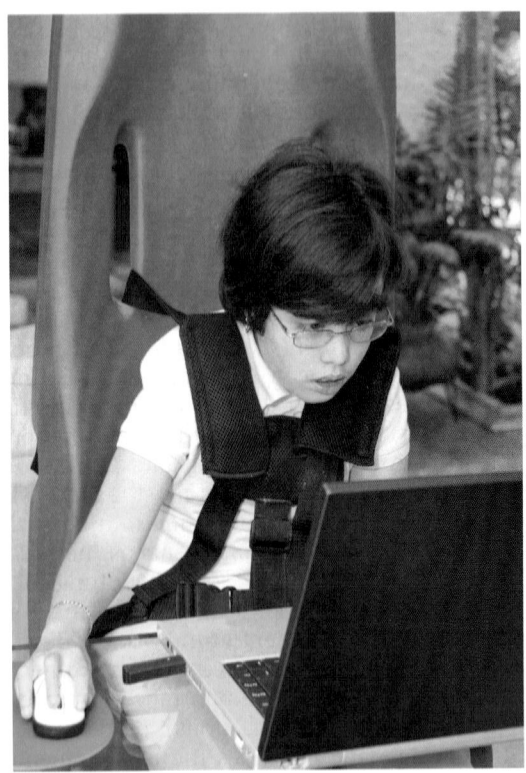

Figure 12-13 This custom-molded seating system properly positions the child so he can use the laptop computer.

functional grasp with fingers and opposing thumb is tremendously advantageous. The loss of this level of function significantly affects the child's degree of independence.

Other devices include the prone stander, which promotes skeletal alignment, preserves bone mineralization, and allows the child to participate in activities (Fig. 12-12). Standers also provide an opportunity to see the world from a different viewpoint, gaining a new perspective of life (similar to a small child who can finally see over the countertop and discover new terrain).

Scooters, tricycles, and wheelchairs provide a means of moving independently within the environment, which increases opportunities to explore, learn, have fun, and participate in social interactions. The variety of wheelchair adaptations is incredible. There are accommodating features such as headrests, custom-molded seating systems, lateral supports, and extremity supports (arm rests and leg rests) (Fig. 12-13). An array of controls for power mobility exist (e.g., sip and puff control, chin control, and joystick). Children with disabilities often enjoy the freedom of power mobility, which may allow them to leave their parent's side at the mall, keep up with their peers in the school hallways, and participate in new community activities when the environment is accessible.

It is virtually impossible to describe all the adaptive and assistive devices available—the list is endless and continuously growing as technology advances. There are low-tech feeding tools (e.g., built-up utensils, plate adaptations, and variable cup holders) for independent eating and aids for dressing and bathing. Electronic aids and adaptive switch toys allow for play and leisure, voice activation devices and environmental controls are

high-tech devices used for emergency call systems, and school aids (e.g., books on tape, large-print textbooks, page turners, and voice-activated computer programs) might enhance the child's independence and ability to learn. All these devices change the environment so the child can perform at his or her best.

COMMUNITY REENTRY AND ONGOING HEALTH CARE NEEDS

Preparing the child for discharge from the inpatient unit or rehabilitation setting to the home and community begins at admission. Determination of goals may even be set during the preadmission phase; this will guide the discharge process. Typically, the home is the primary outcome identified. Every member of the team maintains this focus during the assessment of the child and integrates it into the development of the child's plan of care. In addition to identifying the child's health status and functional ability, key assessments include the level of coping and adaptation, skill in performing the care required, and compatibility with the home environment and lifestyle. Of primary importance is whether the physical environment can accommodate the needs of the child. The team investigates potential issues during the initial interviews. Family members are asked to describe their home environment: type of community, transportation available, type of dwelling, number of stairs or rails, location and description of principal rooms in the house, and specifics regarding the supply of utility services as necessary. Services in the community are explored throughout admission. Depending on the needs of the child, a home or school visit by key rehabilitation or home care team members might be conducted before discharge. In this manner, potential obstacles to the success of community care, home care, or the rehabilitation program can be identified.

Prior to discharge, arrangements are made for family members to provide all the child's care for a specified period of time (generally 24 hours) without assistance from nursing staff. In this way, unforeseen problems or obstacles identified can be discussed and comprehensively addressed with the team prior to discharge. Pediatric nurses provide a therapeutic environment for learning to help prepare the child and family for life outside the inpatient unit. Nurses must make a conscientious effort to incorporate teaching into daily tasks; therefore, they use teachable moments as they provide care and support. For instance, when putting antiembolism stockings on an adolescent patient, the perceptive nurse informs the patient of the risk for deep vein thrombosis (DVT) resulting from puberty and from being immobile, reviews the importance of prevention (ambulation and use of medications), discusses assessment techniques, and describes the management of a DVT complication. This educational focus is paramount in daily rehabilitative care.

Another useful educational technique to help patients prepare for life in the community is to ask what-if questions. For instance, in the hospital setting, it is common to catheterize every 4 hours around the clock, and patients and families get into the routine. Question the teen about how he will manage his catheterization schedule if he is asked to go to an eight-o'clock movie. Should he just skip the catheterization or decline the invite? Or is the safer solution to catheterize early before going to the movies? These discussions regarding all aspects of care help patients and families with problem-solving and life skills.

Some of the issues that confront children with chronic conditions and their families are similar to those for adults with disabilities. These include home care needs, transportation, respite care for caregivers, and assurance that primary care needs are addressed.

HOME CARE

Most children with chronic conditions do not need home care services. Family members might have to administer medications and perform procedures (e.g., catheterization, percussion, and postural drainage) (Fig. 12-14). For some, however, home care might require both visiting nurses and aides as well as large pieces of equipment and medical supplies (Community Care 12-1). Referral to community services, initiated as early as possible, requires having a firm sense of the child's anticipated needs. Home care agencies and community providers are notified and supplied with essential information by the nurse, care manager, or social worker before discharge. At times, members of the home care and equipment companies meet with the child and the family during

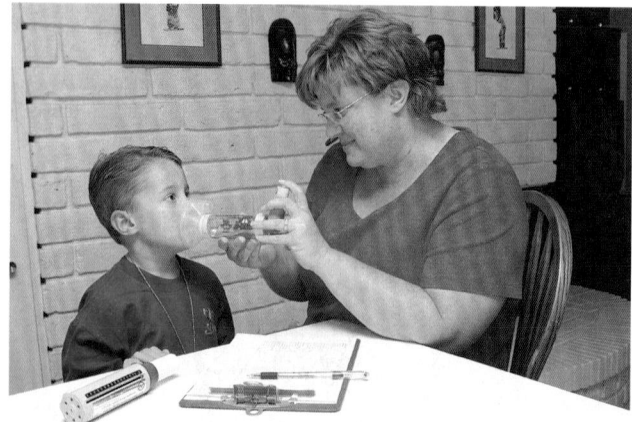

Figure 12-14 Encourage the family to assist the young child to manage his or her care at home, thereby helping to prevent the need for hospitalization.

the inpatient stay (especially in cases of the child who is technology dependent or requires complex care). The home care nurses are invited to the health care facility to learn the child's needs and to participate in the transfer process. When this is not possible, creating a video of the child's care may be a useful alternative. Patients and families are active participants in learning and should be fully informed regarding the child's ongoing care needs for a coordinated and safe discharge home. At this time, summaries of the child's progress, continued goals, and care needs are provided to the primary caregiver as well as to the community rehab care provider, primary care physician, and referrer to facilitate continuation of care across the continuum.

caREminder

When visiting the home to provide services, remember the principles of public health nursing: You are a guest in the home and the family is ultimately responsible for the child's care needs.

The rules surrounding treatment in the home need to be flexible to accommodate the family's needs. For example, many procedures that are done under sterile conditions in the hospital are often done using clean protocols in the home and school.

All equipment, supplies, and medications the child will require after discharge are delivered to the child's hospital room and should be used by the family members prior to discharge. Frequently, families will need two pieces of equipment in case one breaks (e.g., ventilators). They might need oxygen tanks, suction machines, dialysis equipment, or freezer space for clotting factors and they might need to find child-safe areas for needles and sharps containers. It is essential for families with children who require large amounts of equipment to do a home assessment. This includes ensuring that there is enough electrical power, clean running water, and cleanliness to accommodate the child's condition (Nursing Interventions 12-2).

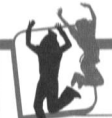

COMMUNITY CARE 12-1

Questions for Families to Ask the Home Care Agency

- Does the nurse who will be caring for my child have pediatric experience?
- Has the agency handled children with this condition before?
- If we have any problems or questions, will there be a nurse on call 24 hours a day?
- What are my options if I do not agree with the nurse who comes to my home?
- Does your agency provide other services such as case management and therapy?
- (Private duty) How often does your agency not have enough nurses to cover the number of cases? What can we do if a nurse is not available to care for our child?
- Will the nurse call and make an appointment with us for her visits or just show up?
- How will the billing be handled? Do you work directly with the insurance company?
- Will your agency arrange for the equipment that we need?
- Whom do we call if there is a problem with the equipment and/or if it needs to be repaired or replaced?
- Will your agency arrange for the medical supplies that we may need? Who reorders them?

PRIMARY CARE

Too often, children with chronic conditions do not see their primary care provider enough because they see their various specialists on a routine basis. It is essential, however, for all children and adolescents with chronic conditions to receive a physical at least every year and to ensure that their immunizations and other preventive health care initiatives are addressed by their medical home (see Chapter 1). This includes dental care and an assessment of their growth and development.

RESPITE CARE

Having a child who requires highly technical care as well as constant assistance can drain the family of its energy and can increase family stress. In addition, this situation makes it very difficult for the family to find child care providers or babysitters so that they can "go out" as a family or couple or take the other children to normal activities of childhood. Sometimes, parents might need to quit their jobs to provide the care their child needs, which can further isolate parents from peers and social support and from meeting their own life goals.

To allow families a break from this constancy of care, the pediatric nurse can encourage *respite care*. Respite care is a way to give families a break by providing temporary child care, support, and referral services. Respite care involves having qualified providers provide care for the child in either the child's home or an inpatient or respite home setting so that family members can have a break from the constant care and, instead, care for themselves or even take a vacation. Day and overnight camps may also provide respite opportunities for the family as well as a unique educational experience for the child.

Families may be eligible for respite services through Medicaid or other state-funded programs. Respite care might be arranged by social services or the hospital. The pediatric nurse can be an advocate for the family to acquire these services. Choosing a respite program requires a careful analysis of the family's needs, the available respite resources, the amount of time away desired by the family, and the unique needs of the child.

TRANSPORTATION ISSUES

Transporting equipment necessary in treating a chronic condition, such as oxygen or a wheelchair, takes strength and physical dexterity as well as a vehicle that can accommodate this equipment. This is essential to get to school, health care visits, and family outings. Without appropriate transportation, the family is restricted to the home, thus increasing the isolation and stress on the family. Social services might need to be contacted to ensure that the family has the appropriate gear to safely transport the child and all necessary equipment to health care visits. If the family relies on public transportation, they should be provided with the contact number for local services to transport them and their child.

PAIN MANAGEMENT

Some individuals with chronic conditions experience a great deal of pain. Multiple finger sticks to test for blood sugar, rheumatoid arthritis, percussion and postural drainage, and the pain from vaso-occlusive crises in sickle cell disease or from the treatments for cancer are examples of the discomfort experienced by children. Although there is a dearth of literature exploring the impact of chronic pain on children, Gold et al. (2009) validated that those who experience chronic pain during the school years also had impairments in school performance (often because of increased absences) and daily physical and emotional functioning; this was often seen in their inability to participate with their peers. Families need to be able to act as advocates for their child at times when the assessment or treatment of the condition causes the child pain or discomfort.

Help the family identify ways to minimize the pain as much as possible. One teen found that if she played the piano first thing in the morning, it helped allay the stiffness in her arthritic fingers; another used EMLA before having any blood draws for her cancer.

NURSING INTERVENTIONS 12-2

Family and Home Assessment

Expected Outcome	Intervention
Family caregivers will have adequate training and preparation to care for the child at home.	Before discharge or at the first visit, identity the family members who will actually be providing the care. Review all written instructions with the caregivers. Observe the caregivers' demonstrations of any medically related task they will be completing independently. Leave booklets with pictures and/or videos that can be used as references with the caregivers in the home. Review the care path with caregivers and make changes if needed to meet the child's and the family's needs.
Family caregivers will respond appropriately to situations that indicate potential medical problems.	Provide the family with written lists of signs and symptoms that signal potential variances from what is considered the baseline for the child. Review steps to be taken should a medical problem arise. Alert emergency services in the community to the presence of a child in the home who may need their assistance. Post important phone numbers in a prominent location in the home.
Telephone service will be available to the family.	Identify a local business or neighbor who will allow the family to use their phone in an emergency. If no phone is in the home, a cell phone can be rented through many home care companies or through local fire departments.
Basic utilities will be available to the family.	Assist the family to secure the basic utilities needed to provide for the child's needs. • Bottled water can be used if there is no running water. • Electrical generators can be rented from local utility companies. If equipment required for the child's care and electricity are not available, use battery-powered equipment. • Many local governments assist with heating costs in an emergency. Many churches stock blankets and warm clothing for families in need. • If electricity is available to the family, alert the local utility company and place the family on a priority service list. • If refrigeration is required and there is none, dry ice can be obtained from any food market at little or no cost. If dry ice is used, care must be taken not to touch it directly and not to store the medication directly on it.
The home will be a safe environment.	Assess for home safety. • If electrical equipment is needed, use a three-pronged grounded plug. Avoid extension cord use. • To avoid overheating and the risk of fire, place plywood or other wood under the electrical equipment rather than having it rest directly on carpet. • Cover knobs and buttons on all equipment with clear tape. This enables them to be checked while lessening the risk of accidentally changing the setting. • Store medications, needles, syringes, sharps, and sharps containers in a locked container. • Attach a list of all medications and their dosages to the list of emergency phone numbers. • Properly store all medications. • Unplug all equipment when not in use. • Avoid throw rugs to lessen the possibility of tripping on them.

FINANCIAL CONSTRAINTS

 QUESTION: What are the costs associated with having a child with diabetes like Lindsay?

The economics of providing health care for children with chronic conditions has a significant impact on the availability of services for children with chronic conditions. It is estimated that approximately 14% of those with special health care needs were responsible for 42% of the pediatric health care expenditures (Kogan et al., 2010). In addition, in 2006, 8.8% of families with children with special health care needs were without health insurance and 33.1% had inadequate health insurance (USDHHS, Health Resources and Services Administration, Maternal and Child Health Bureau, 2008). Resources to fund all the necessary interventions for children with chronic conditions are insufficient. This is certainly one reason why families need many advocates to help them through the insurance maze to access the services their child needs without depriving their families of their needs. In addition, all children with special health care needs should receive regular, ongoing comprehensive care within a medical home (Goldstein et al., 2010). Chapter 1 discusses the concept of medical home, an environment in which health care to children is accessible, continuous, comprehensive, family centered, coordinated, compassionate, and culturally effective.

For those families whose income precludes them from receiving Medicaid but who do not make enough to purchase private insurance, there is the State Children's Health Insurance Program (SCHIP). Looman et al. (2009) found that families of a child with special health care needs whose health care providers helped them feel like partners in the care of their child and who communicated well with other providers on the team were less likely to report financial problems. See Chapter 2 for a more complete discussion on funding options for children with chronic conditions.

ANSWER: The costs include insulin, insulin syringes, a glucometer and associated supplies, and emergency glucagon (approximately $125/month) (Mercer, 2010).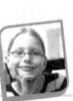

PARTICIPATION IN SCHOOL

 QUESTION: Jean and Tom quickly discovered that they needed to be strong advocates for their daughter in the school system. After discharge from the hospital, Lindsay could not attend school until the proper forms were completed. What personnel in the school environment should be informed about Lindsay's condition?

School is an important component in the lives of all children and adolescents, not only for the academic learning that occurs but also because of the social and emotional components as well. At school, children learn rules and values that build on the ones learned at home; they learn to interact with others, and they have expectations placed on them and are held to the same standards as their peers (Fig. 12-15).

Schoolteachers and staff are often un- or undereducated about many of the conditions experienced by children in their classrooms and how these conditions affect the student. They also are often unaware of the laws that provide these students with rights to an appropriate education with the needed accommodations. Typically, it is the school nurse who becomes the coordinator of the student's care while in the school setting. The school nurse interacts with the health care provider to ensure continuity of care; interacts with the family to ensure that medications and equipment are available in the school to meet the child's needs; and teaches the faculty, administrators, and other staff (e.g., maintenance staff, bus drivers, cafeteria staff) about the child's condition on a need-to-know basis to prevent problems and provide emergency care if needed. The school nurse will develop an individualized health care plan (IHP); an IHP is very similar to care plans developed in hospitals, but they are tailored specifically to the needs of students in schools. The IHP is developed solely by the school nurse for his or her use only. The school nurse will also develop an emergency action plan that will be distributed to those school personnel who have contact with the student. This plan will instruct school staff about things to avoid (i.e., allergens, sugary foods), what symptoms indicate a problem (i.e., chest pain, trouble breathing), and what to do in the event of a problem. The school nurse will work with all these individuals to educate them to the degree needed to increase their comfort level and to

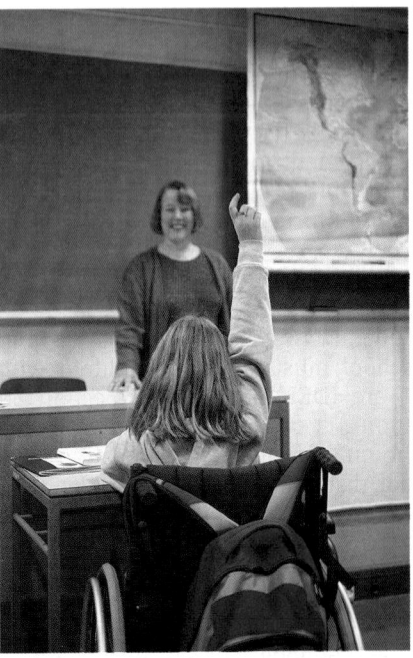

Figure 12-15 School attendance allows the child with a chronic condition to develop both socially and cognitively.

provide a safe environment for the student. The state's Nurse Practice Act guides what tasks can and cannot be delegated; nursing assessment can *never* be delegated.

Although children with chronic conditions can reap many benefits in the school environment, some problems, such as an increased incidence of teasing and bullying or difficulty making friends, might exist. These challenges are often exacerbated by the child's differences. Intervention approaches include having the child present information to the class about the condition, assigning buddies to assist the student with special health care needs, and making and enforcing school policies that do not tolerate bullying behaviors.

Children in the school whose condition relies on technology often depend on others for their care and, in some cases, rely on others to speak for them. Care needs are most common in the following areas: respiratory (requiring ventilators, tracheostomies, oxygen), nutritional support (requiring gastrostomy or nasogastric tubes, IV nutritional support), mobility (requiring wheelchairs, braces, crutches), and urinary (requiring catheterization) (Selekman et al., 2013). This requires school personnel to be familiar with the importance of the equipment, designate appropriate space to store the equipment and provide the services, and be knowledgeable about the use of these devices and how to troubleshoot when problems arise.

School staff might be fearful that children with special needs are more fragile than other children. They may be concerned about possible exposure to pathogens both from the child with a chronic condition to the class and vice versa, and they also may be concerned about the child's safety. Families may express frustration that teachers have lower expectations for their child and that their child's education will suffer. It is up to the school nurse to eliminate barriers and to make the integration process go smoothly, with **normalization** as the overall goal. Normalization involves establishing a normal pattern of living, with daily routines and participation in age-appropriate activities, including school attendance. If full integration or normalization is not possible, children with special health care needs should have specific goals (as written in an IEP or 504 Plan) to assist the student to achieve integration to as high a level as possible (Community Care 12-2). Chapter 2 provides more information about IEPs.

Federal Laws Advocating for Children With Disabilities

The two federal laws that guide the accommodations that the school must make for children with chronic conditions are IDEIA (2004) and Section 504 of the Rehabilitation Act of 1973. Children with chronic conditions who qualify for special education through their local school districts are covered by IDEIA. This law mandates a free and appropriate public education in the least restrictive environment from the age of 3 through 21 years. The goal is to educate all children regardless of their disability. The least restrictive environment means that most of these children are included in regular classrooms. In 2008, 11.16% of U.S. children aged 6 to 17 years, or almost 6 million young people, received

special education services under IDEIA (Rehabilitation Research and Training Center on Disability Statistics and Demographics, 2010). More than 10% of the 3- to 5-year-old population also received these services.

IDEIA also mandates that all children who are referred to determine their eligibility to receive special education services will receive an evaluation that is bias free. It is essential for pediatric nurses to understand this component of the law in order to be advocates for their patients. If eligible, students must receive the medical support and services necessary to stay in the school setting. This might mean tracheostomy care, insulin administration, catheterizations, tube feedings, alternative communication devices, or accessibility for a wheelchair. Nursing services are considered one of the related services to which these children must have access; others include PT, OT, speech therapy, and nutrition support services. It also includes the additional academic services as necessary so that the student can be as successful as possible.

An essential component of IDEIA is the development of an IEP for the student. The IEP is developed by an interdisciplinary team that includes the school nurse and the family. It looks like a nursing care plan with objectives, an intervention plan, and how and when the student will be evaluated to ensure that the plan is working toward meeting the objectives. One of the main objectives is **mainstreaming** the child into the regular classroom setting, which means they are integrated into the class with their peers for as much of the school day as is possible.

"Children who have disabilities are nearly three times as likely to repeat at least one grade as are children who have no disabilities" (Byrd, 2005, p. 233). It is estimated that one in five children who repeat a grade has a disability. This might be the result of issues such as increased absences because of the condition, failure of the school to carry out the IEP, or family problems. Advocacy is needed to ensure that the student does not begin a downward spiral of school failure and low self-esteem.

For those students who do not qualify for special education under IDEIA but who need accommodations to fully participate in the school environment, the Rehabilitation Act of 1973 provides the legal basis for the development of a plan. Section 504 of the Rehabilitation Act of 1973 states that no otherwise qualified individual with a disability shall be excluded from participation nor be denied the benefits of or be subjected to discrimination simply because of the disability (Clay, 2004). This section of the act is referred to as a *504 Accommodation Plan*. These accommodations might simply be an allowance for the student to carry his or her asthma inhaler or have specialized seating in the classroom, or it might include the need for wheelchair access ramps, use of the school nurse's office for specialized bathroom needs, or altering the class schedule to allow for student rest and to optimize learning.

Acquiring Vocational Skills

Vocation and employment options are a key aspect of function and development. IDEIA requires that by age 16 years, a student's IEP must include the adolescent's specific vocational goals (also see Chapter 2).

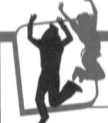

COMMUNITY CARE 12-2

Interdisciplinary School-Based Care for the Child With a Chronic Condition

Actions for the School Nurse

- Maintain IHP for every student who may need treatment at school. Include information on medications, dosages, triggers, and emergency procedures. Develop an emergency action plan if needed.
- Alert staff members about students with a history of condition likely to manifest in the classroom.
- Assist with the administration of medication in accordance with school policy.
- Monitor response to treatment using criteria appropriate to condition.
- Communicate with the family about problems at school and the student's general progress in controlling his or her condition at school.
- Advocate for the development of a 504 Accommodation Plan or an IEP, depending on the student's needs.
- Conduct inservice training on chronic conditions as needed.
- Develop a resource file for the staff to use to access additional information regarding the child's condition and community resources to assist in meeting the child's needs.
- Consult with staff to help develop appropriate school activities for student with specific conditions.
- Collaborate with the Parent–Teacher Association to offer family education programs in the school if numerous children have similar conditions or children with multiple chronic conditions have common needs.
- Collaborate with community-based treatment and support groups.

Actions for the Guidance Counselor

- Recognize that learning to cope with any chronic illness can be difficult. Teachers may notice low self-esteem, withdrawal from activities, discouragement about the steps needed to control the condition, or difficulty making up schoolwork.
- Offer special counseling with the faculty, student, and/or family to help the student handle problems more effectively.

Actions for the Physical Education Instructor and Coach

- Encourage exercise and participation in sports for students with chronic conditions that impact their ability to engage in usual physical education programs.
- Support the student's IEP or Accommodation Plan if it requires medication before exercise.
- Understand what to do if an acute episode occurs during exercise. Have the child's emergency action plan available.
- Encourage students with chronic conditions to participate actively in sports but also recognize and respect their limits. Permit less strenuous activities if a recent illness precludes full participation.
- Refer your questions about a student's ability to fully participate in physical education to the family and school nurse.

Actions for the Classroom Teacher

- Know the early warning signs of problems for specific chronic conditions (e.g., wheezing with asthma, irritability with hypoglycemia).
- Have a copy of the child's Accommodation Plan and emergency action plan in the classroom. Review it with the student and parents. Know what steps to take in case of a problem.
- Develop a clear procedure with the student and family for handling missed schoolwork.
- Understand that students with some chronic conditions may feel drowsy or tired, different from the other kids, anxious about access to medication, embarrassed about the disruption to school activities that their condition causes, and/or withdrawn.
- Help the student feel more comfortable by recognizing these feelings. Try to maintain confidentiality. Work with the student and plan education of classmates about the child's condition.
- Know the possible side effects of the child's medications and how they may impact the student's performance in the classroom. Refer any problem to the school nurse and family.
- Encourage the student with a chronic condition to participate fully in physical activities.
- Allow a student to engage in quiet activity if recovery from an acute episode precludes full participation.

The adolescent, parents, vocational counselor, educators, therapists, physician, and nurse all participate in the planning process and play a role in guiding the teen and family with idealistic and realistic objectives. Cognitive deficits and mobility limitations are the greatest factors in determining the vocational possibilities for an individual with a disability. The young adult may achieve development of skills and hopefully enter the workforce in competitive employment, supported employment, or even a sheltered workshop where they can be productive and develop a positive self-esteem.

The nurse in the school or community can help create opportunities to learn new skills, investigate adaptive hobbies, and foster talents. The nurse should also keep an open mind and ask the child with a disability, "What do you want to be when you grow up?" If the child answers, "I want to be a veterinarian," suggest that the child visit and volunteer at the local humane society, which can foster her idea of caring for animals. If the child says, "I want to be a baseball player," explain that a professional athlete needs to be physically fit to achieve this goal. Propose that the child get involved in "buddy ball" or adaptive sports now and begin incorporating a fitness program in his daily routine. Generally, children's goals are supercilious; however, with participation in the activity and time, they will usually gain a more realistic perspective and oftentimes even formulate different ideas. The most important point is to raise the question to the child with a disability that bestows an impression that he or she should be productive and work later in life.

When determining life skills and adaptation, it is also important to consider the child's ability to socialize with peers and to experience success. Recreational activities for children with disabilities may be as therapeutic in facilitating physical function as they are in teaching them alternative ways to participate in activities (Fig. 12-16). Children with disabilities can participate in athletics at a variety of levels that use leisure time, can be fun, and may promote fitness and self-esteem. Each experience brings an opportunity for the child to achieve and obtain mastery of age-appropriate developmental skills and abilities.

ANSWER: Although all of this communication is guided by the Health Insurance Portability and Accountability Act (HIPAA) laws, parents are often willing to have information about their child's condition shared with those who need to know. For example, Lindsay may experience a seizure from low blood sugar at school. Her bus driver and her teachers need to know the signs of hypoglycemia and what action to take. Lindsay's parents have granted permission to notify the parents of her classmates that Lindsay has diabetes. Consider how many elementary school events are celebrated with sugar.

PROGNOSIS AND TRANSITIONING

With advances in health care, it is estimated that 95% of children with chronic conditions reach adulthood (Bittles et al., 2002). This is a relatively new development; 40 years ago, this was not the case and many of these children died within years of diagnosis. For example, in 1960, the average age of death for a child with CF was 5 years; in 1974, it was 16 years; and in 2009, it was 35 years (Cystic Fibrosis Foundation, 2011). What has happened is that new seemingly unrelated comorbidities have occurred as the body adapts to certain conditions. For example, youth in their late teens and early adulthood who have CF are at risk for developing diabetes because of the chronic involvement of the pancreas. This type of diabetes appears to be a cross between type 1 and type 2. Individuals who have been treated for cancer are also developing conditions years after the initial treatment and "cure." These "late effects" (see Chapter 22) might be the development of other types of cancers in other locations or conditions such as learning disabilities. Another example is fractures that occur as a result of osteopenia, which can develop in individuals who are wheelchair dependent and unable to use their lower limbs.

Rather than a cure then, the focus for children with chronic conditions is on the adjustments that need to be made throughout their lives in order for them to be

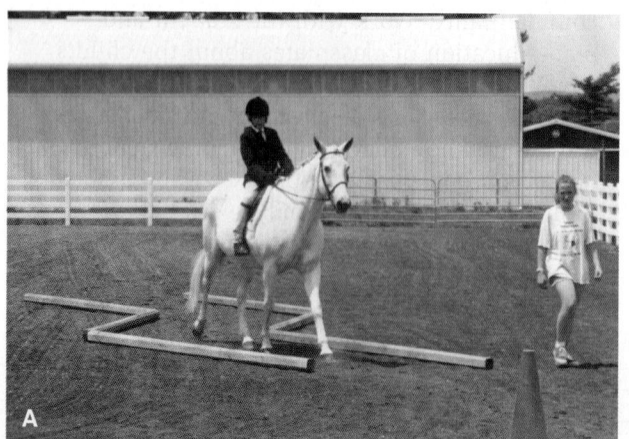
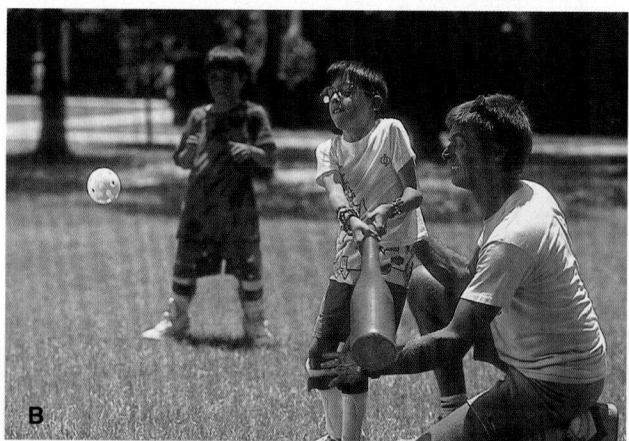

Figure 12-16 Therapeutic riding and adapted sports are rehabilitative activities that provide socialization and an opportunity to achieve.

as healthy and functional as possible. Their care needs to have a coordinated, collaborative approach that involves the family.

One of the mandates under IDEIA is to assist the adolescent to transition to further education or employment and independent living. However, all children with chronic conditions, not just those who qualify for special education, need to engage in this process. This includes transitioning from pediatric health care to adult health care services. Pediatric nurses should be assisting children and their families to prepare for eventual responsibility for their personal health care. Transitioning actually begins from the moment the child is diagnosed and/or moves from one developmental stage to another. As early as they are cognitively and physically able, children with chronic conditions should learn to perform the skills needed for their care. They should be able to record critical information (e.g., blood sugars, peak flow readings) and relate it to the health care provider (Fig. 12-17).

As children transition into preschool, initial adjustments will be needed. Parents and the children themselves should be able to identify what works and what does not. In this way, when they enter the school environment, they will be able to assist in the development of an IEP or an Accommodation Plan. IDEIA mandates that the process of adult transitioning needs to begin by at least age 16 years with career exploration activities. This transition plan must be written into their IEP, including the services needed to assist these students as they transition out of high school and into the adult world.

Preparing to transition from pediatric health care to adult health care should be part of the process. "Transition programs should enhance the youth's self-confidence, autonomy, and ability to self-advocate" (Shah & Boudos, 2012, p. 74). Students with chronic conditions need to be empowered to know about their condition, the treatments and medications they take, and the accommodations they need to be successful. They will need this information as they move to educational and work environments so that they can indicate what accommodations they need. The nurse can work with the adolescent to develop a list of the accommodations that have been helpful. This list can also be helpful to assist families who must continue to advocate for their children even into adulthood.

Some specialty centers have arrangements with specialty centers that cater to adults with specific conditions, such as sickle cell disease. They might actually set up appointments for the adult health care provider to come to the pediatric setting or for the advance practice nurse to accompany the teen to the adult center for his or her first appointment. Teens need to know what to expect and how it will differ from the "pediatric" focus of care.

Reiss and Gibson (2002) have identified the following factors as some of the components for successful transitioning: "1) the family, young adult, and provider have a future orientation; 2) transition is started early; 3) family members and health care providers foster personal and medical independence; 4) planning occurs for the future; 5) the young adult verbalizes the desire to function in the adult medical world; and 6) reimbursement for services is not interrupted" (p. 1312). Some families have difficulty relinquishing control of their child's care in order for the child to become more independent. This might require the health care team to remind families of the normalcy of letting go and the fact that their child is reaching a new stage of development. Even when the young adult is not capable of self-care, families need to recognize that they are also aging and this may be a good time to begin making plans for the future care of their child.

Transition services are not just limited to health care. They also include job planning and resources, vocational rehabilitation, health insurance coverage, family planning, and whether the condition warrants Social Security benefits. Most of the organizations that cater to young people with chronic conditions have materials that will assist in the transition. Transition is a process, not an event—it occurs over time.

"Children with chronic conditions are children first; they have the same needs as their peers, they have rights to participate fully in the school environment, and they have specific health care needs. They can enjoy full inclusion in the community and can plan for a future" (Selekman et al., 2013, p. 778). In addition to providing physical and emotional care, the pediatric nurse is their advocate to assure comprehensive and coordinated care as they transition to the home and school settings and into adulthood.

See thePoint for a summary of Key Concepts

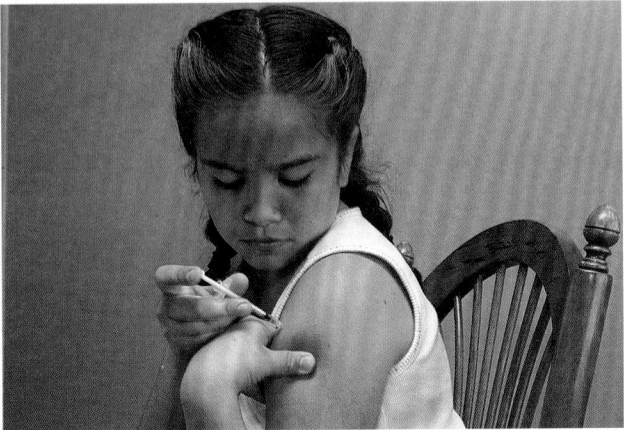

Figure 12-17 The child with a chronic condition should be encouraged to become more and more responsible for managing his or her own treatment and medications.

REFERENCES

Allen, P. J. (2010). The primary care provider and children with chronic conditions. In P. Jackson Allen, J. Vessey, & N. Schapiro (Eds.), *Primary care of the child with a chronic condition* (pp. 3–21). St. Louis, MO: Mosby.

American Academy of Pediatrics. (2005). Helping families raise children with special health care needs at home. *Pediatrics, 115*(2), 507–511.

Americans with Disabilities Act of 1990, Pub. L. No. 101-336, § 2, 104 Stat. 328 (1991).

Association of Rehabilitation Nurses. (2007). *Role description: Pediatric rehabilitation nurse.* Retrieved from http://www.rehabnurse.org/pubs/role/Role-Pediatric-Rehab-Nurse.html

Bittles, A., Petterson, B., Sullivan, S. et al. (2002). The influence of intellectual disability on life expectancy. *The Journals of Gerontology. Series A, Biological Sciences and Medical Sciences, 57*(7), 470–472.

Brown, R., Wiener, L., Kupst, M. et al. (2008). Single parenting and children with chronic illness: An understudied phenomenon. *Journal of Pediatric Psychology, 33*(4), 408–421.

Byrd, R. (2005). School failure: Assessment, intervention, and prevention in primary pediatric care. *Pediatrics in Review, 26*(7), 233–243.

Clay, D. (2004). *Helping schoolchildren with chronic health conditions.* New York, NY: The Guilford Press.

Coffey, J. (2006). Parenting a child with chronic illness: A metasynthesis. *Pediatric Nursing, 32*(1), 51–59.

Cystic Fibrosis Foundation. (2011). *Frequently asked questions.* Retrieved from http://www.cff.org/AboutCF/Faqs/

Elias, E., & Murphy, N. (2012). Home care of children and youth with complex health care needs and technology dependencies. *Pediatrics, 129*, 996–1005.

Federal Interagency Forum on Child and Family Statistics. (2009). *America's children: Key national indicators of well-being, 2009.* Washington, DC: U.S. Government Printing Office.

Gold, J., Yetwin, A., Mahrer, N. et al. (2009). Pediatric chronic pain and health-related quality of life. *Journal of Pediatric Nursing, 24*(2), 141–150.

Goldstein, K., Altman, S., & Zimmerman, A. (2010). State and federal benefits for children with special healthcare needs. *Pediatric Annals, 39*(4), 240–247.

Gordon, J. (2009). An evidence based approach for supporting parents experiencing chronic sorrow. *Pediatric Nursing, 35*(2), 115–119.

Hagan, J. F., Shaw, J. S., & Duncan, P. M. (Eds.). (2008). *Bright futures: Guidelines for health supervision of infants, children and adolescents.* Elk Grove, IL: American Academy of Pediatrics.

Individuals with Disabilities Education Improvement Act, Pub. L. No. 108-446, 118 Stat. 2647 (2004).

Juhlmann, A. (2010). Taking the little steps: Providing complex care. *Pediatric Annals, 39*(4), 248–253.

Kelly, M. (2010). Prematurity. In P. Jackson Allen, J. Vessey, & N. Schapiro (Eds.), *Primary care of the child with a chronic condition* (pp. 756–771). St. Louis, MO: Mosby.

Knafl, K., & Santacroce, S. (2010). Chronic conditions and the family. In P. Jackson Allen, J. Vessey, & N. Schapiro (Eds.), *Primary care of the child with a chronic condition* (pp. 74–89). St. Louis, MO: Mosby.

Kogan, M., Newacheck, P., Blumberg, S. et al. (2010). State variation in underinsurance among children with special health care needs in the United States. *Pediatrics, 125*(4), 673–680.

Lewis, M., & Vitulano, L. (2003). Biopsychosocial issues and risk factors in the family when the child has a chronic illness. *Child and Adolescent Clinics of North America, 12*(3), 389–399.

Looman, W., O'Conner-Von, S., Ferski, G. et al. (2009). Financial and employment problems in children with special health care needs: Implications for research and practice. *Journal of Pediatric Health Care, 23*(2), 117–129.

Mercer, A. (2010). *The cost of diabetes.* Retrieved from http://www.diabeteshealth.com/read/2010/10/09/6898/the-cost-of-diabetes/

Moeschler, J., & Shevell, M. (2006). Clinical genetic evaluation of the child with mental retardation or developmental delays. *Pediatrics, 117*(6), 2304–2316.

Nielsen, K., Mandleco, B., Roper, S. et al. (2012). Parental perceptions of sibling relationships in families rearing a child with a chronic condition. *Journal of Pediatric Nursing, 27*, 34–43.

Rehabilitation Act of 1973 (Section 504), 29 U.S.C., §794 et seq

Rehabilitation Research and Training Center on Disability Statistics and Demographics. (2010). Annual disability statistics compendium. New York, NY: Author. Retrieved from http://disabilitycompendium.org/

Reiss, J., & Gibson, R. (2002). Health care transition: Destinations unknown. *Pediatrics, 110*(6 Suppl.), 1307–1314.

Selekman, J., Bochenek, J., & Lukens, M. (2013). Children with chronic conditions. In J. Selekman (Ed.), *School nursing: A comprehensive text* (pp 700–783). Philadelphia, PA: F. A. Davis.

Shah, P., & Boudos, R. (2012). Transitions from adolescent to adult care. *Pediatric Annals, 41*(2), 73–78.

Simkiss, D. (2011). Community care of children with complex health needs. *Pediatrics and Child Health, 22*(5), 193–197.

Sullivan-Bolyai, S., Sadler, L., Knafl, K. et al. (2003). Great expectations: A position description for parents as caregivers: Part I. *Pediatric Nursing, 29*(6), 457–461.

Taylor, R., Gibson, F., & Franck, L. (2008). The experience of living with a chronic illness during adolescence: A critical review of the literature. *Journal of Clinical Nursing, 17*, 3083–3091.

Telfair, J., Alleman-Velez, P., Dickens, P. et al. (2005). Quality health care for adolescents with special health-care needs: Issues and clinical implications. *Journal of Pediatric Nursing, 20*(1), 15–24.

UnitedHealthCare. (2012). *In utero fetal surgery.* Retrieved from https://www.unitedhealthcareonline.com/ccmcontent/ProviderII/UHC/en-US/Assets/ProviderStaticFiles/ProviderStaticFilesPdf/Tools%20and%20Resources/Policies%20and%20Protocols/Medical%20Policies/Medical%20Policies/In_Utero_Fetal_Surgery.pdf

U.S. Department of Health & Human Services, Administration for Children and Families. (2000). *The Developmental Disabilities Assistance and Bill of Rights Act of 2000.* Section 102. Definitions. [42 USC 15002]. Retrieved from http://www.acf.hhs.gov/programs/aidd/resource'dd-act?page=2

U.S. Department of Health & Human Services, Health Resources and Services Administration. (2011). *Children with special healthcare needs in context: A portrait of states and the nation 2007.* Retrieved from http://www.mchb.hrsa.gov/nsch/07cshcn/

U.S. Department of Health & Human Services, Health Resources and Services Administration, Maternal and Child Health Bureau. (2008). *The national survey of children with special health care needs chartbook 2005–2006.* Rockville, MD: U.S. Department of Health & Human Services.

Van Cleave, J., Gortmaker, S., & Perrin, J. (2010). Dynamics of obesity and chronic health conditions among children and youth. *Journal of the American Medical Association, 303*(7), 623–630.

Van der Lee, J., Mokkink, L., Grootenhuis, M et al. (2007). Definition and measurement of chronic health conditions in childhood: A systematic review. *Journal of the American Medical Association, 297*, 2741–2751.

Vessey, J., & Sullivan, B. (2010). Chronic conditions and child development. In P. Jackson Allen, J. Vessey, & N. Schapiro (Eds.), *Primary care of the child with a chronic condition* (pp. 22–41). St. Louis, MO: Mosby.

Walsh, W. F., Chescheir, N. C., Gillam-Krakauer, M. et al. (2011). *Maternal-fetal surgical procedures.* Technical Brief No. 5 (AHRQ Publication No. 10[11]-EHC059-EF). Rockville, MD: Agency for Healthcare Research and Quality.

See thePoint for additional resources.

CHAPTER 13

Palliative Care

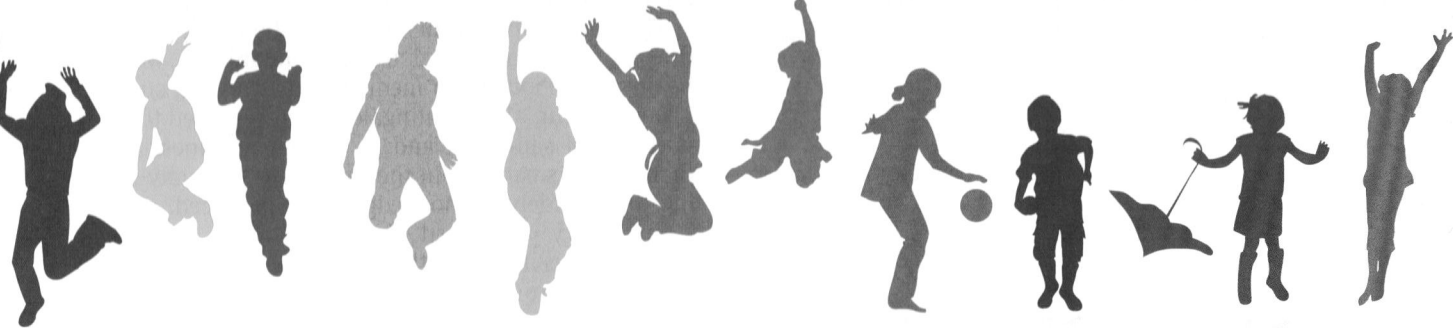

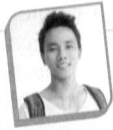

CASE HISTORY

Remember Ashley Tran (Chapter 7), George Tran (Chapter 10), and their parents Loan and Tung? George has osteogenic sarcoma (the assessment, diagnosis, and treatment are discussed in Chapter 22). At the time of diagnosis, George's cancer had already metastasized to his lungs. He received chemotherapy, followed by a limb salvage procedure. Unfortunately, the cancer has continued to spread. George spent time in the hospital at the time of his limb salvage procedure and received his chemotherapy as an outpatient. It has been 8 months since George was diagnosed; he is now 15 years old. He is noticeably thinner and weaker. He has progressive disease with significant respiratory involvement.

Initially, George tried to return to school. He found it very difficult, both physically and emotionally. He continues to have pain and weakness in the affected leg. Some days he did not have the strength to get around the school without using crutches. He discovered that the state university has an online independent study high school program, and he began taking classes online. George has a few very good friends who share his interest in computers and video games. They come over several times a week to visit George and play video games, but George does not go out very often.

A home care nurse visits George once a week and performs the skilled nursing care that is needed. George's mother, Loan, does not work outside the home. She has been providing much of his day-to-day care, although George insists on doing as much for himself as he can. A close friend of the family, who has been like an older brother to George,

spends time after school every day with George going over schoolwork or playing video games. Loan has two sisters in the area. Her youngest sister, Aunt Ha, who Ashley lived with for a time, is able to come and help often. Loan's brother died of "leg cancer" in Vietnam. Loan was only 5 years old when he died, but she remembers his funeral and she is certain he died at home.

George's condition is deteriorating. He has profound dyspnea and circumoral cyanosis with exertion. Even at rest, he has some shortness of breath, and he has a constant nonproductive cough. He is extremely thin and cannot eat much. The family faces the choice of admitting George to the hospital or trying to keep him home. Since his limb salvage procedure, George is insistent that he will not go back to the hospital. The surgery on his leg was distressing for George, and he is quite adamant that he is staying home. It upsets his parents, but he tells them, "I know that I am dying and I want to die here. I am not going back to the hospital." It is George's father, Tung, who wants George to go to the hospital and still talks about George "getting well."

Osteogenic sarcoma is a disease that affects primarily adolescents and young adults. George's oncologist sees both adolescents and adults and has a working relationship with a hospice service. It is not a pediatric hospice service, but because George is not a young child, the service is confident they could work with the Tran family. The Tran family comes to the decision to keep George home and work with the hospice service.

CHAPTER OBJECTIVES

1 Relate the sociopolitical influences on the development of palliative care services for children.

2 State the core definitions and principles of palliative care.

3 Describe models used to guide palliative care services.

4 Delineate barriers to implementation of pediatric palliative care.

5 Select strategies that enhance communication during the provision of palliative care.

6 Identify interdisciplinary measures to promote quality of life at end of life.

7 Describe interdisciplinary care interventions at the time death occurs.

8 Examine the process of grief and bereavement in the family coping with the death of a child.

9 Describe bereavement responses of children when a loved one dies.

10 Explain support measures that health care providers can implement as they grieve the loss of a pediatric patient.

See the**Point** for a list of Key Terms.

The death of a child at any age is difficult for the parents and family, which may include siblings, grandparents, aunts, uncles, and cousins. The loss can also be hard for the friends, nurses, and other health care professionals who care for the child and the child's family. An important part of the nursing management of the child with a life-threatening condition involves providing interventions to support the effects of the physical illness as well as provide for the psychosocial, spiritual, and social aspects of care related to the end of life (EOL) (Knapp et al., 2012). This chapter discusses the provision of palliative care for a child with a life-threatening condition and his or her family. Palliative care definitions and concepts are presented. Barriers to palliative care are discussed, and interdisciplinary interventions to promote palliative care are shared. When children have a terminal condition, the child and family will experience loss, grief, and, eventually, bereavement. These concepts and their impact on the child, the family, and the health care provider are reviewed. Strategies to assist the child and family cope with impending death are also reviewed.

HISTORICAL PERSPECTIVES OF PEDIATRIC PALLIATIVE CARE

Throughout the 19th century, the focus of health care was to treat symptoms and provide comfort. Pharmaceutical preparations were inadequate, and most medications were derived from locally grown herbs and plants. Health care practices were steeped in religion, mythology, and superstition. There were a limited number of physicians who had received any formal education or

training and even fewer trained nurses. Medical care was frequently provided by women in the community who developed expertise in assisting to relieve symptoms (Kalisch & Kalisch, 2003). Consequently, patients either recovered or died within a short time. Illnesses that are considered minor or insignificant today were then common causes of death.

The early 20th century brought about a change in the approach to general living standards as well as health care. Pioneers in medicine and nursing, such as Lister, Pasteur, and Nightingale, had recognized the importance of sanitation and its impact on illness more than 50 years earlier, but their theories were only starting to be widely acknowledged and practiced. As the 20th century progressed, with technologic and scientific advances including the development of a variety of medications from insulin to antibiotics, the focus began changing from treatment of symptoms and comfort care to attempts to cure (Coyle, 2010).

These advances in health care have had a ripple effect. Improved sanitation and immunizations drastically reduced the deaths from common childhood illnesses, resulting in a decrease in infant and child mortality (Coyle, 2010). In underdeveloped countries, some illnesses such as immunization-preventable infections, diarrhea, and dehydration remain frequent causes of death in children. In developed countries, the improvements in sanitation and medical care have resulted in childhood death becoming a rare occurrence for a family. In the mid-20th century, the ability to revive some people by the use of cardiopulmonary resuscitation (CPR) drastically changed attitudes related to death (Corr, 2011). By the 1970s, it became standard practice that, unless previously determined otherwise, attempts to resuscitate would be performed on all patients within the acute care setting regardless of diagnosis or potential quality of life. This has led to a blending of expectations between curable and incurable illness, such that in medical and societal views, death is considered both a personal and medical failure (Egan City & Labyak, 2010).

Thus, the death of a child has become an unusual experience. The trajectory of death has also changed. In previous centuries, when a child became ill, he or she either recovered within a short time or died within days or weeks of the onset of illness. Death usually occurred in the home environment with the child cared for by family and friends (Field & Cassel, 1997). In today's health care environment, many children with illnesses and traumas now live for months to years with the illness prior to succumbing to death (Crane, 2011). Children survive longer because of advances in early diagnosis and treatment of life-threatening conditions.

Reports indicate that approximately 7% to 10% of children in the United States have a chronic or debilitating illness (Levetown, 2000; Perrin et al., 2007). There are approximately 55,000 deaths per year in children, with half of these deaths occurring during the neonatal period (Docherty et al., 2007; Field & Behrman, 2003; Levetown et al., 2010; Schmidt, 2011). Two thirds of all infants die in the intensive care unit, and, overall, 75% to 85% of childhood deaths occur in the acute care setting (Beckstrand et al., 2010). In addition, there are approximately 900,000 birth tragedies (defined as in utero death or stillbirths) each year. Of the remaining childhood deaths, accidents are the leading cause of death in all age groups older than 1 year of age; cancer is almost always the leading cause of death by disease in all age groups (Field & Behrman, 2003; Hendrickson & McCorkle, 2008). It is estimated that 15,000 infants, children, adolescents, and young adults (up to age 24 years) die annually from the complications of a complex chronic condition. On any given day, it is estimated that 5,000 of these patients are living within the last 6 months of their lives (Feudtner et al., 2001). Today, there are approximately 3,000 hospices in the United States that provide services to children. (See thePoint for Supplemental Information for more websites related to hospice services.)

Although palliative care concepts have traditionally been applied to children with cancer, the importance of developing services for children with other life-threatening conditions has become evident (Eccleston et al., 2012). In particular, the need for palliative care arises among children with the following conditions:

- Life-threatening conditions for which treatment is available but may fail
- Conditions in which premature death is expected but long periods of intensive treatment to prolong good quality of life are anticipated (cystic fibrosis, HIV)
- Progressive conditions that may extend over many years and for which no curative treatment is available (mucopolysaccharidosis)
- Conditions with severe disability that, although not progressive, lead to extreme vulnerability and in which premature death is likely (cerebral palsy)
- Neonatal conditions in which the diagnosis of a terminal condition may be made prenatally or is evident at birth (Chaffee, 2001; Goldman, 2001; Liben & Goldman, 1998)

DEFINITION AND APPROACHES TO PEDIATRIC PALLIATIVE CARE

A simplistic definition of **palliative care** is "actions to relieve symptoms." The World Health Organization (WHO, 1998) defined palliative care as an approach that improves quality of life in patients and families facing life-threatening illnesses. The WHO definition also includes the need to provide relief of pain and other distressing symptoms as well as the need to affirm life. WHO (2009) further defines death as a normal process, which integrates physical, psychological, emotional, and spiritual needs as part of routine care. They also suggest that palliative care can be provided across any setting and be initiated early within the course of an illness. Based on these definitions, it is clear that palliative care is a component of all health care and is not provided solely as part of the dying process (Klein & Saroyan, 2011). Figure 13-1 presents a diagram that depicts the need to address palliative care at the time of diagnosis regardless of cure

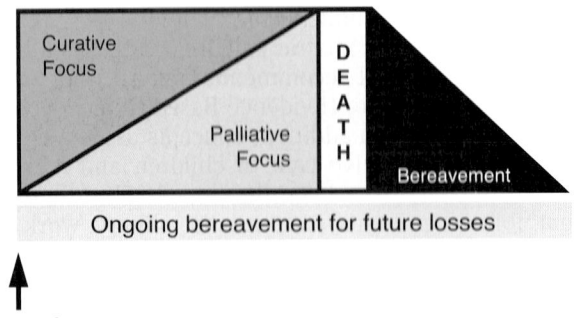

Diagnosis

Figure 13-1 The progression of palliative care interventions. Adapted from American Association of Colleges of Nursing & City of Hope National Medical Center. (2012). *End-of-life nursing education consortium-pediatric palliative care (ELNEC-PPC) faculty guide.* Duarte, CA: City of Hope.

potential. As the individual's condition deteriorates and the curative focus diminishes, the diagram illustrates the need to have an increasing emphasis on palliative care interventions. If death is the outcome, palliative care continues for surviving family members as part of bereavement care (American Association of Colleges of Nursing [AACN] & City of Hope [COH] National Medical Center, 2012).

In 2007, the Children's Hospice and Palliative Care Coalition's professional advisory committee further strengthened the definition of palliative care and its relationship to family-centered care (FCC) by including the following definition within their framework of care:

> Pediatric Palliative Care is both a philosophy of care and an organized, structured system of delivering care to children with life threatening conditions and their families. The goal of Pediatric Palliative Care is to prevent and relieve suffering and to maximize quality of life for children of all ages, and their family members/support systems. (Sumner, 2010, p. 998)

When care changes from curative intent to palliation, the focus becomes management of symptoms and promoting comfort, which requires FCC at its foundation (Ferrell & Coyle, 2010; Fochtman, 2011) (see Chapter 1 for more information on FCC). It is important to remember that the child's family may comprise biologic and nonbiologic members. In family-centered palliative care, all aspects of the child's life—including physical care, symptom management, cultural components, and spiritual components—are interlinked with the interdisciplinary team, which may encompass grandparents, siblings, friends, church members, community members, and health care team partners (Sumner, 2010). Pediatric palliative care adheres to a family-centered model that addresses the emotional needs of the child and family and demonstrates respect, clarifies goals, acknowledges their preferences and choices, and enhances open communication and shared decision making with the health care team related to their psychosocial and medical care (Durall et al., 2012; Last Acts Palliative Care Task Force, 2002).

Most recently, the care of individuals facing the EOL has received renewed attention by both health care providers and the public. Pediatric interest groups have been focusing on pediatric palliative care, resulting in the development of recommendations to improve pediatric palliative care (Evidence-Based Clinical Practice Guidelines 13-1). In addition, concepts associated with provision of palliative care to children and a variety of care models have been developed. The discussion that follows presents the interdisciplinary work that has been pursued to identify aspects of palliative care unique to the pediatric population.

INSTITUTE OF MEDICINE REPORT: *WHEN CHILDREN DIE*

 QUESTION: Which of the unique concerns of palliative care for children identified in Chart 13-1 apply to George and the Tran family?

The Institute of Medicine (IOM) is a nonprofit organization associated with the National Academy of Sciences. The organization provides science-based advice on matters of biomedical science, medicine, and health.

Three IOM reports have been instrumental in examining the state of EOL health care. These reports are *Approaching Death: Improving Care at the End of Life* (Field & Cassel, 1997), *Improving Palliative Care for Cancer* (Foley & Gelband, 2002), and *When Children Die: Improving Palliative and End-of-Life Care for Children and Their Families* (Field & Behrman, 2003).

When Children Die provides a summary of the "state of the science" of pediatric EOL care. From this report and the research conducted about pediatric palliative care, it is recognized that certain palliative care concerns are unique to or particularly evident with children (Chart 13-1). The report made major recommendations that provide clear directions to improve the quality of care to children and their families with respect to ensuring a family-centered approach; managing financial concerns; educating health care professionals; and broadening the research base for pediatric palliative, EOL, and bereavement care (Field & Behrman, 2003) (see thePoint for Evidence-Based Practice Guidelines). The IOM report clearly established that much more needs to be done to address and support the unique challenges of caring for children with life-threatening medical conditions (Carter et al., 2004).

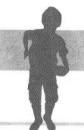

EVIDENCE-BASED CLINICAL PRACTICE GUIDELINES 13-1

Pediatric Palliative Care

American Academy of Pediatrics, Committee on Bioethics and Committee on Hospital Care. (2000). Palliative care for children. *Pediatrics*, *106*(2), 351–357. Retrieved from

http://pediatrics.aappublications.org/content/106/2/351.full

Consensus paper presenting an integrated model for providing palliative care for children living with a life-threatening or terminal condition.

Friebert, S., & Huff, S. (2009). *NHPCO's pediatric standards: A key step in advancing care for America's children.* Retrieved from

http://www.nhpco.org/resources/pediatric-hospice-and-palliative-care

Best practices in pediatric palliative and hospice care. Resources include online training, palliative care policies, and standards of practice.

International Children's Palliative Care Network. (n.d.). Retrieved from

http://www.icpcn.org.uk/

Online resources to enhance pediatric palliative care and assist palliative care providers to communicate with one another and learn from one another.

The Initiative for Pediatric Palliative Care Curriculum and Quality Improvement Tools. (2006). Retrieved from

http://ippcweb.org/quality.asp

Comprehensive, interdisciplinary curriculum that addresses knowledge, attitudes, and skills that health care professionals need in order to better serve children and families. Also includes tools and resources to monitor and improve quality of care to children with life-threatening conditions.

Field, M. J., & Behrman, R. E. (2003). *When children die: Improving palliative and end-of-life care for children and their families.* Report of the Institute of Medicine Task Force. Washington, DC: National Academy Press. Retrieved from

http://www.iom.edu/Reports/2002/When-Children-Die-Improving-Palliative-and-End-of-Life-Care-for-Children-and-Their-Families.aspx

Consensus report on the state of pediatric palliative care. Provides recommendations to improve care practices at the point of care, within the community, and nationally.

ANSWER: Each of the following concepts is applicable to the Tran family. First, the wishes of George, a 15-year-old, are counter to those of his father, an adult. The health care team will have to wrestle with the issue of who makes the decisions regarding his care—George or his father. Nurses advocate respecting the autonomy of the patient. If the family cannot come to an agreement, the health care team is faced with the ethical dilemma of respecting the autonomy of the patient or the wishes of the parent. Formal advanced directives signed by a minor, in most cases, are not recognized as binding documents. In most situations, parents have absolute authority over making health care decisions that affect the child.

Second, Ashley has suffered from clinical depression as an adolescent (see Chapter 29). She has expressed the wish that she should be the one with cancer; she should be the one to die, not her brother. Nurses will need to continue to monitor her well-being as her brother's health declines. Siblings must be considered in the care management of the pediatric patient, with special attention given by the health care team to the siblings' developmental needs (Fochtman, 2011).

Finally, the Tran family is Vietnamese American. The mother, Loan, does not speak fluent English; thus, there are language and cultural variances. The educational needs of the child and family pose considerable challenges for the health care team. Language and cultural variances, cognitive development, and family dynamics must all be considered.

CHART 13-1   Palliative Care Issues Unique to Children

- Children are not small adults. Developmental differences must be taken into account when dealing with the spectrum of pediatric patients, which ranges from neonates to adolescents. Additionally, care management of the child must change over time as the child changes developmentally (e.g., cognitively, emotionally, physically).
- A smaller number of children die compared with adults.
- A heterogeneity of illnesses affect the pediatric population. Many conditions are rare, making diagnosis, prognosis, and medical management difficult and uncertain.
- Many illnesses affecting children are familial in nature, thus more than one family member may have the same condition.
- Formal advanced directives signed by a minor are, in most cases, not recognized as binding documents. In most situations, parents have absolute authority over making health care decisions that affect the child.
- The time continuum for managing a pediatric condition can be extremely variable, with the need for palliative care extending over days, months, or even years.
- Many children lack any type of public or private health insurance.
- Siblings must be considered in the care management of the pediatric patient, with special attention given by the health care team to the siblings' developmental needs.
- The educational needs of the child and the family pose considerable challenges for the health care team.

LAST ACTS: *PRECEPTS OF PEDIATRIC PALLIATIVE CARE*

Last Acts, a former national program, was developed and supported by a grant from the Robert Wood Johnson Foundation for the purpose of establishing guidelines leading to the improvement of care and caring near the EOL for infants, children, adolescents, and their families. Representatives from the IOM as well as many pediatric nursing organizations, including the Association of Pediatric Oncology Nurses (now the Association of Pediatric Hematology/Oncology Nurses), the National Association of Neonatal Nurses, and the Society of Pediatric Nurses, were members of this task force. The work by this group was published in 2002 as the *Precepts of Palliative Care for Children, Adolescents and Their Families* (Last Acts Palliative Care Task Force, 2002). These precepts acknowledge that comprehensive management of physical, psychological, social, spiritual, and existential needs are essential in providing care for children who are born with serious medical conditions and those who develop such illnesses during a later stage of childhood or adolescence.

Last Acts further identified the core principles from which palliative care must be integrated throughout the trajectory of a child's illness. These principles include

- Respecting patient goals, preferences, and choices
- Providing comprehensive care
- Using the strength of interdisciplinary resources
- Acknowledging and addressing caregiver concerns
- Building systems that support responsible palliative care policies and regulations (see thePoint for Supplemental Information)

INTEGRATED PALLIATIVE CARE MODEL

The American Academy of Pediatrics (AAP) and others developed and support a care model in which cure-directed treatment and palliative care are integrated, allowing children to benefit from both philosophies of care (American Academy of Pediatrics [AAP], Committee on Bioethics and Committee on Hospital Care, 2000). This model is based on the belief that traditional definitions of palliative care are too narrow and rigid and may hinder children from access to palliative care services when the focus is providing those services only to those children actively dying. The integrated care model accommodates children with recurrent malignancy for whom death is a certainty as well as children with cystic fibrosis for whom premature death is often a certainty but one that is many years away. Chaffee (2001) further discusses this model in terms of developing an appropriate collaborative plan of palliative care for a child with a life-limiting illness (see thePoint for Supplemental Information). Members of the collaborative team include the family, primary care group, tertiary care group, palliative care group, community, school, and resource group. Successful collaboration depends on reciprocal communication among all groups as well as maintaining pertinence and applicability to the family circumstances. Frequent reassessment of the plan is needed as the child's illness progresses to ensure the plan is practical and is meeting the needs of the child and family (Nielson, 2012).

Kane et al. (2000) share that palliative care "involves a gradual transition from a posture of hope for a cure to a state in which patient and family embrace the possibility of death and hope for other things of importance to them, such as peace and understanding, control of pain, enriching relationships, a meaningful death, and divine concern with the fate of their loved one" (p. 168). From a biopsychosocial–spiritual model of patient care, it is asserted that the introduction of palliative and supportive care services *early during the course of a severe illness* "may serve as a bridge between a scientific, disease-oriented approach to diagnosis and treatment, and a humanistic, person-oriented form of care" (Kane et al., 2000, p. 171).

FOUR CORNERSTONES OF CLINICAL PRACTICE IN PEDIATRIC PALLIATIVE CARE

> **QUESTION:** What is one example of nursing care with the Tran family that reflects one of the cornerstones of clinical practice?

Empirical studies and anecdotal feedback from parents and families have consistently demonstrated that they are seeking a quality of care and a connection to, and genuineness from, practitioners that is all too often missing. The Initiative for Pediatric Palliative Care is an example of an interdisciplinary group that identified four cornerstones of clinical practice in pediatric palliative care:

1. Responding to the ethical claim of the child/family
2. Adopting a collaborative relational stance
3. Cultivating cultural humility
4. Developing a reflective practice

Responding to the Ethical Claim of the Child and Family

Development of these cornerstones began with the premise that the foundation for clinical practice should be grounded in what children and their families have said is important to them (Browning, 2003a). The first cornerstone presents the concept that the extreme vulnerability of the dying child and the family imposes an ethical claim on the health care providers. This is a claim that practitioners are not free to opt in or opt out of; rather, practitioners, by the nature of their caregiving role, must accept an ethical obligation to the child and his or her family.

Adopting a Collaborative Relational Stance

The second cornerstone asserts that clinical practice in pediatric palliative care is fundamentally relational, involving a "two-way" relationship with the child and the family. In this relationship, engaged practitioners must move fluidly between the position of "expert" and the position of "learner." In this relationship, children and their families are regarded as experts with regard to their own experiences.

Cultivating Cultural Humility

Cultivating cultural humility, the third cornerstone, expresses the need to reflect on one's own culture as well as the culture of the child and the family. This requires the capacity for awareness and self-critique regarding one's own culture and beliefs. Additionally, this entails efforts to understand the world from the viewpoint of the patient. This cornerstone demonstrates a commitment to understanding similarities and differences between professional values, goals, and priorities and those of the child and his or her family. In application of this cornerstone, practitioners must also recognize and understand biomedicine as a culture—one that is often new and foreign to the child and family.

Developing a Reflective Practice

Developing a reflective practice examines the question: What do I do in practice and how do I do it? Reflective practice embodies the concepts of self-awareness (values, thoughts, feelings, assumptions), practice-based learning (learning by doing), and tacit knowledge (knowing in action). As a cornerstone, this concept reflects the importance of constant evaluation of one's beliefs and how those beliefs are translated into palliative care practices.

> **ANSWER:** There are many right answers. Examples that show the collaborative relationship between nurses and the family are a good fit. This might include the nurse teaching the family how to monitor the child's pain by keeping a pain log so that they use this information to titrate the pain medication. In addition, examples that explore the ability to see this experience through the family's eyes also model one of the cornerstones.

NURSING CARE OF GRIEVING FAMILIES

To plan interventions appropriate for the child and family, a baseline assessment is completed (Focused Health History 13-1). The health care provider's attitudes, strengths, and limitations in working with children and families who have experienced loss influence the relationship with the grieving family. A structured assessment is completed in a private area, conveying an unhurried, nonjudgmental attitude. All interactions with the child and family provide opportunity for informal data collection regarding the family's grief and

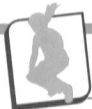

FOCUSED HEALTH HISTORY 13-1

The Grieving Family

Current history	Type of loss (e.g., death, disfigurement, material possession) Circumstances surrounding the loss Stage of acute grief or bereavement; period of time since loss
Past medical history	History of other significant losses (persons, pets, objects) and responses to them Usual patterns of coping Measures that have been used previously to comfort family members
Nutritional assessment	Changes in eating patterns
Family medical history	Review of deaths in the family, including cause, age at time of death, and unusual circumstances surrounding the death
Social history	Changes in sleeping patterns Changes in activity level Changes in interactions with friends and family members Usual support systems (family, spiritual, community) and the availability of these support systems in the current situation
Growth and development and psychological assessment	Behavioral manifestations of grieving (aggressiveness, anger, anxiety, sadness, depression, withdrawal, attention-seeking behaviors) Child's cognitive level and understanding of the concept of death Understanding of the grieving and bereavement process Sense of control in the current situation and how this affects the ability to deal with the loss

Note: See Chapter 8 for a comprehensive health history and Chapters 14 through 30 for the focused health history of specific body systems.

loss. Listen astutely to the family and answer their questions honestly.

The staff can help the family by establishing a relationship, by being present both physically and emotionally, and by continuing to focus on the family as a system (Nursing Plan of Care 13-1). Educate the family about normal grieving and encourage them to talk about the death, their reaction to it, and their feelings. Assist siblings to receive education, attention, and support. When necessary, refer the family for counseling. Often, the staff nurse caring for the dying child is in an excellent position to initiate the bereavement support process.

A study by Wolfe et al. (2008) indicates that parents are reporting better preparedness for the EOL course and decreased suffering in their children as well as substantial improvements in advance care planning. This is thought to be attributed to the increased focus during the past decade in educating health care professionals on the issues of palliative care and hospice. Caring for dying children and their bereaved families is one of the most challenging components for a nurse. Here, more than anywhere in our practice, we must be especially aware of how we deliver care and communicate to patients and their families because the messages we provide can either hinder or facilitate their choices. If we keep in mind that the ultimate outcome when caring for a child with a life-threatening or terminal condition

is to add life to the child's years, not simply add years to the child's life (AAP, Committee on Bioethics and Committee on Hospital Care, 2000), we will be able to do a great service as advocates to the children and families under our care.

BARRIERS TO PEDIATRIC PALLIATIVE CARE

There is often disparity between the way children die and the way they want to be cared for when dying. This multifactorial issue is related to barriers within the health care system concerning acceptance of the realities of life-limiting disease, access to palliative care services and hospice, communication with the family, and the understanding of death (Durall et al., 2012).

FAILURE TO ACCEPT REALITIES OF LIFE-LIMITING DISEASE

 QUESTION: Is there a family member who is struggling to admit that George is dying?

Most health care professionals report that they did not receive any specific education or training related to EOL care within their schooling and have learned by

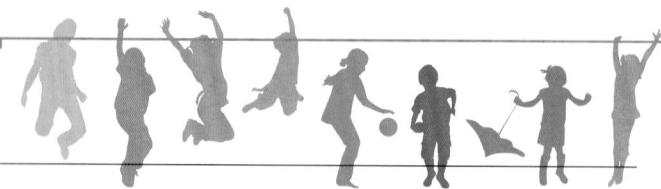

NURSING PLAN OF CARE 13-1:

For the Grieving Family After a Loss

Nursing Diagnosis: Grieving related to reaction of death of a loved one

Interventions/Rationale

- Encourage the family members to talk about feelings of anger, sadness, guilt, and frustration.
  The grief and bereavement process is the process of coping with and adapting to the loss.
- Observe for reactions to loss that may indicate dysfunction: delayed grieving, inhibited grieving, displaying various physical conditions, and no demonstration of grief.
  Responses to loss vary from person to person; however, each has the potential to respond in a fashion that indicates grieving is being suppressed. Suppression of grief can lead to physical maladies and changes in relationships with other family members.
- Provide environment that supports expression of grieving behaviors (e.g., crying, anger).
  Reinforces appropriateness of expressing grief.
- Discuss responses to grief and what to expect during the grieving process. Repeat over time with family as needed.
  The experience of grief may make it difficult for the family to take in and retain information; thus, discussions of the grief responses may need to be repeated over time.
- Help the client identify his or her own strengths for managing the loss.
  Reinforces positive, adapting grieving behaviors.
- Help family members work through their grief by encouraging individual expression and coping patterns.
  Individuals grieve and show grief differently. It is essential to affirm that grief responses will vary and to encourage family members to be supportive of these differences.

Expected Outcomes

- Family will verbalize feelings and will work through bereavement tasks.
- Family will have dysfunctional responses recognized early and will be offered psychosocial and spiritual counseling.
- Family members will go through the stages of grief in their own manner and reach resolution.

Nursing Diagnosis: Interrupted family processes related to changes in relationships and roles in the family secondary to death of a family member

Interventions/Rationale

- Assist family to openly discuss changes in the family since loss of the loved one.
  Provides recognition of how each individual perceives changes in the family dynamics.

- Assist family to develop strategies to adapt to changes in family roles and functions.
  As an open system, the family should strive to seek to adapt to the enforced changes in their family structure and all cooperate in developing meaningful ways to reestablish family cohesion and adaptation.

Expected Outcomes

- Family will remain supportive of all members.
- Family will incorporate changes in power alliances, assigned tasks, decision making, and communication patterns to accommodate for loss of family member.

Nursing Diagnosis: Spiritual distress related to crisis of the illness, suffering, or death of a child

Interventions/Rationale

- Assess for expressions of spiritual distress (e.g., lack of hope, meaning, and purpose; acceptance; love; forgiveness of self; inability to express previous state of creativity; inability to pray or participate in religious activities; refusal to interact with spiritual leaders).
  Indicate inability to integrate meaning of life and purpose in life through connecting with self, others, and creative outlets.
- Provide a list of community resources and support for emotional and spiritual needs.
  Assists family members to seek internal and external support to manage the current crisis.

Expected Outcomes

- Family will verbalize distress and will have spiritual counselors available for support.
- Family will articulate ability to find strength from spiritual support systems.

Nursing Diagnosis: Impaired social interaction related to gradual withdrawal from friends and community resources after loss of child

Interventions/Rationale

- Observe family members' interactions and potential discomfort in social situations. Assess for report of change of style or pattern of social interactions.
  Anger that others were spared the pain of the death of a child can lead to self-imposed social isolation.
- Involve family members in support groups or in social/recreational activities with families who have experienced similar loss.
  Provides support system to family in comfort of environment with others who have had a similar experience.

- Promote the sibling's participation in activities with friends and in school.
   Encourages ongoing, daily interactions with peers.

Expected Outcomes

- Family members will maintain social relationships with other family members, friends, and neighbors.
- Family members will use community resources appropriately.

Nursing Diagnosis: Chronic sorrow related to ongoing and pervasive sense of loss since death of child

Interventions/Rationale

- Determine events that may trigger recurring and pervasive sadness experienced by the family members.

Missed birthdays, family celebrations, and school-related events may enhance feelings of continual loss.

- Assist family members to develop strategies to manage feelings of depression, sadness, lethargy, and malaise.
   Chronic sorrow may intensify over time and may interfere with the person's ability to reach a high level of personal and social well-being. A repertoire of interventions to manage the feelings associated with chronic sorrow will assist the individual in the coping process.

Expected Outcomes

- Family members will establish a plan to manage trigger events that lead to chronic sorrow.
- Family members will successfully manage grief and come to resolution.

role models and trial and error (Gallagher et al., 2012). Many report that they have a great deal of discomfort in communicating bad news and prognoses with children and their families. They claim they have little formal training to assist them in decision making regarding the discussion of ending curative treatments; providing supportive care and pain management; or in addressing the psychological, social, and spiritual aspects of care (Hilden et al., 2001).

A child's death affects a family and community much differently than the death of an older person. We do not consider it natural for a child to die before the parents, and families find it hard to adjust to role changes that affect the family structure. It is difficult to ask families to abruptly switch from curative-intent therapy to comfort care. This transition could be eased if health care professionals explain early within the illness that death is a possible outcome and thus offer curative and palliative care simultaneously (Levetown et al., 2010). During the past several decades, failure to acknowledge the limitations of medicine has led to a significant increase in the initiation and maintenance of futile interventions. Inappropriate use of aggressive curative treatments can prolong the dying process and contribute to physical, emotional, and spiritual distress (Wolfe, Klar et al., 2000). Often, a family's decision making is based on limited comprehension of the actual situation because of inadequate or poor communication from the health care provider. Because many health care professionals are uncomfortable communicating bad news, the full array of options are often not made available or understood by the family (Jacobs, 2005; Levetown, 2008; Sine et al., 2001).

ANSWER: George's father, Tung, is struggling to accept that George is dying.

ACCESS TO PALLIATIVE CARE SERVICES AND HOSPICE

QUESTION: What are some of the influences that have affected the Tran family's decision to care for George at home?

Integrating palliative care services into care of children with life-threatening conditions can be challenging because often, health care providers, patients, and families view this as giving up or only a viable option if all other measures have failed (Rushton, 2004; Solomon et al., 2005). Many do not realize that palliative care can coexist with interventions aimed at cure or stabilization of disease and prolongation of life (Last Acts Palliative Care Task Force, 2002). Not all patients who are critically ill go on to die of their disease, but they can benefit from palliative care services even if they are not near the EOL (Ferrell & Coyle, 2010). If more health professionals, patients, and families understood the purpose and goals of palliative care and hospice services, usage would likely be higher.

Since the 1970s in the United States, a grassroots effort has facilitated the development of hospice programs in many communities. In essence, **hospice** is a form of health care that provides palliative care services across a variety of settings based on the philosophy that death is a natural part of the life cycle. Hospice care provides an interdisciplinary team to work with a patient and family to support them physically, emotionally, and spiritually through the latter phases of illness and the dying process by promoting a "living until you die" philosophy; the care then continues to support the family through bereavement (AACN & COH National Medical Center, 2012). According to Children's Hospice International (2003), less than 1% of children in the United States who could benefit from hospice services receive it.

The few children who receive palliative care and hospice services are usually referred late within the illness, when there is limited time to reap the full benefits of the programs. Typically, services are not fully understood by the health care provider, there is a hesitancy to acknowledge that there is no chance for cure, or there may not be accessibility to a pediatric hospice within the child's community or palliative care services within the acute care setting. Thus, acute interventions are often prolonged even when it is evident the child is in the final stages of death. Other common barriers may include institutional regulations that have restrictive visiting hours, inadequate policies for pain and symptom management, and limited FCC. Regulations related to insurance and third-party payment often do not provide for adequate financial compensation for palliative care and hospice. They may not pay for them at all within an inpatient setting and only have limited reimbursement for outpatient services, although it is speculated that appropriate palliative care and hospice interventions would actually decrease overall medical costs. A statement frequently uttered by health care providers is that "it is too early to refer to hospice." Early identification of patients for palliative care and hospice services allows time for the child and family to set and achieve goals, to develop relationships with the palliative health care team, and to benefit from supportive care services (Tradition or Science 13-1).

ANSWER: One factor affecting the Tran family's decision is George's determination to stay home. His family will do their best to respect his desires. Another family characteristic is the fact that Loan remembers her older brother's death from the same disease. She is having an easier time accepting the outcome of this disease because she has a previous experience with it, even though she was quite young.

Yet another factor is the oncologist's experience with a hospice service. The oncologist's willingness to coordinate George's care through a hospice service affects the family's ability to care for George at home.

COMMUNICATION WITH THE FAMILY

Effective communication imparts medical information, dispels myths or preconceived notions about the disease and treatment, helps the patient and family to make informed decisions about care, and ultimately improves patient outcomes and satisfaction (Levetown, 2008). An essential component of communication is to realize that it is a dynamic, ongoing process and that it is possible to deliver too much information at any one time. It is important to ask what the family knows, what they are ready to hear, and to be prepared to repeat the information over the course of time. In times of crisis or stress, concentration and understanding may be impaired as a result of overwhelming feelings of loss and helplessness. Elicit understanding by repeating what the person has said or by asking for clarification. Do not assume that what you are saying and what the patient and family are hearing is the same message (Browning, 2003b).

More Inquiry Needed

TRADITION OR SCIENCE 13-1

Do dying children receive unnecessary interventions at the EOL?

Carter et al. (2004) were interested in determining what care interventions were provided to children during the last days and hours of their lives. A retrospective chart review of 105 children who died at their institution revealed the following:

- Comfort care services were provided to 55% of children, and pain medications were given to 90% during the last 72 hours of life.
- Intubation and ventilation was done on 98% of the children, although 63% of them had that support withdrawn within the last 48 hours of life.
- Nutritional support was initiated in 96% of the children and withdrawn during the last 48 hours for 23% of them.
- Almost all the children (96%) had at least one laboratory or diagnostic test or radiographs done within the last 48 hours of life.

Carter et al. (2004) found that discussions of a life-threatening situation were documented in only 23% of the children, and only 12% of children had a do-not-resuscitate (DNR) order written, only one child was actually referred to hospice. The authors concluded that more care interventions initiated toward comfort or palliation might reduce unnecessary, nonbeneficial, and potentially burdensome tests for children at the EOL. Pierucci et al. (2001) demonstrated that when ill newborns were referred to a palliative care consultation service, there was a significant enhancement of EOL care, as evidenced by fewer days in the intensive care unit; less invasive procedures such as intubation and mechanical ventilation, radiographs, blood draws, central lines, and feeding tubes; decreased use of vasopressor and paralytic agents; and limited use of CPR. In addition, families were more frequently referred to social service and hospital chaplains for support than families who were not referred to the palliative care service. Both these studies (Carter et al., 2004; Pierucci et al., 2001) demonstrate the impact on human suffering as well as health care costs in relation to how illnesses are managed during the last days of life. Implementation of EOL care pathways, algorhythms, and standardized orders are recommended as one way to help decrease initiation of unnecessary interventions in EOL care (Bookbinder et al., 2005; Bookbinder & McHugh, 2010; Luhrs & Penrod, 2007). A comprehensive literature review of EOL pathways by Watts (2012) confirmed that the development, implementation, and influence of such pathways to improve palliative care practices remains in its infancy.

When caring for children who are dying, or for the family members after the child's death, it is important to remember that the words and actions used can have an impact on the patient's and family's entire experience of the illness and dying process in either a negative or positive manner. Sitting down to talk and maintaining eye contact with the family helps to establish that you care about what is happening to them. Say things clearly and simply, and provide definitions to medical terminology. Try to "listen with the patient's or families' ears." If you were in their situation, what words would be helpful to you to hear and how would you say them so there is a clear understanding of the intent?

Semantics are often crucial in effective communication. Telling a family that "there is nothing more that we can do for your child" is a callous and unnecessary way to tell a family that there is no more effective treatment that will cure their child. Instead, say to them, "We do not have treatment that will stop the progression of the disease [injury]. During this time, prior to death, we will focus on providing types of therapy to keep your child as comfortable as possible to enhance his [her] remaining life." A health care provider might say, "A miracle could keep your child from expiring," instead of saying, "Despite all our efforts, the disease is not responding to the treatment, and it is clear that your child is dying, as evidenced by the inability of the organs, such as the kidneys and heart, to work properly." The first statement gives false hope, and many people in our multicultural society, for whom English is often a second language, do not realize that the word "expire" is commonly used within the context of death. The second statement definitely informs the family that death is the expected outcome. The expansion of that statement is then, "What we can do now is concentrate on administering treatment that offers comfort." The focus of hope then becomes a proactive form of therapy that provides, as a goal, a dying process that enhances remaining life. The end result provides an atmosphere of care, which places the child and family in an environment that respects their relationship, promotes safety, and relieves suffering (AACN & COH National Medical Center, 2012) (Nursing Interventions 13-1).

Body language and tone of voice should provide comfort and support. Whenever talking to patients and families about distressful news, it is important not to appear rushed; sit down with them and allow time for answering questions (Mack & Grier, 2004). Another important part of communication is being able to listen in order to understand and support family preferences (Hinds et al., 2012). Allow children and their families to share their stories, their sadness, and their joys. Part of listening is also observing the nonverbal cues being exhibited by the patient and family. Children of all ages commonly express their most important feelings through play and nonverbal methods. The nurse's use of active listening measures can make a huge difference in how a family views their child's illness and last days of life.

THE CHILD'S UNDERSTANDING OF DEATH

> QUESTION: What is George's understanding of death based on his developmental level and the information provided in the case history?

Another barrier to palliative care is the child's own understanding of his or her condition, its potential outcomes, and the issues surrounding death and dying.

Families and health care providers might wish to protect the child from the realities of the situation but in doing so present a barrier to the implementation of palliative care services by not communicating fully or openly with the child about the child's condition. When children's concerns and questions about their condition and about death are not addressed, their fears will magnify (Ethier, 2009).

Communication becomes the key in helping to meet the psychological needs of the dying child. Addressing and working through unresolved issues, hidden fears, and the need for the child to make plans might decrease suffering and facilitate a more peaceful death (AACN & COH National Medical Center, 2012). Dying children are usually aware of their illness and the fact that they are dying (Kreicbergs et al., 2004). Remain alert to the child's desire to talk about death and his or her condition. This might be expressed by behavioral changes or questions about other topics because death is rarely expressed directly.

If their impending death is not discussed, children do not always initiate the discussion because they sense that doing so will make their family sad. Children can feel guilty that they caused their family's sadness and then they might try to protect their family by not talking about the things that concern them the most. Family members must be helped to understand that the child often knows that he or she is very sick and dying. Not talking about these issues actually adds to the child's burdens because he or she must then expend energy to leave this very important topic out of conversations.

caREminder

The family knows their child best, and if they feel strongly that their child should not be told of his or her impending death, the nurse should elicit their reasons. Although it is not appropriate to lie to or deceive the child, you must respect the family's wishes.

It is important to understand that a child's perception of death, its finality, irreversibility, causality, and the cessation of body function are based on developmental stage and cognitive level. It is unknown how preverbal children perceive death. Behavioral changes associated with death are primarily thought to be a response to the family's physical and emotional state (Ethier, 2009). Children in early and middle childhood interpret death as a sleep state or as a temporary trip. Their magical thinking can lead them to believe that their behavior led to someone becoming ill or leaving (dying). It is not until children reach school age that they understand that death is permanent and irreversible. Older school-aged children also begin to appreciate that death is not only inevitable but that it is also universal and that all body functions cease when death occurs. Adolescents perceive death similarly to adults; they ask about death, have concerns related to spirituality and the afterlife, and search for the meaning of why it happens

NURSING INTERVENTIONS 13-1

Unclear or Distressful Versus Helpful Communication

Unclear or Distressful	Helpful
Referring to the child as "the patient"	Referring to the child by name
"It's time to pull back."	"Let's discontinue treatments that are not providing benefit."
"Your child is stable today."	"There has been no improvement in your child's condition."
"Do you want us to do everything for your child?"	"Everything is being done to care for your child and to keep him [her] comfortable."
"There is nothing more we can do."	"We should change the goals of care."
"A miracle may turn things around."	"In my experience, I have not seen a child in this situation survive."
Avoidance	Frequent contact and communication
"You have other children to comfort you" *or* "You are young and can still have other children."	"Each child you have is a unique and special individual to you. Your other children may be a comfort for you, but they do not replace the loss of this child."
"I know how you feel."	"I am sorry that this is happening to your child and family."
"This will make you a better/stronger person."	"Would you like me to talk with other family members or be with you when you talk with them?"
Standing in the doorway or at the foot of the bed and avoiding eye contact	Sitting and facing the patient or family, in the conference room if available, and maintaining eye contact
Appearing vague or helpless	Letting your genuine concern and caring show
"If the disease had been found earlier and treatment had started sooner, maybe things would be different."	"You have done a wonderful job taking care of your child throughout his [her] life and this illness. You should be proud of what you have been able to provide your child."
"Do you want us to do CPR?"	"CPR is a method of trying to keep your child alive with machinery to keep him [her] breathing and/or medications to keep the heart beating and kidneys working. In your child's situation, it will not save his [her] life for more than possibly a few hours or days; your child will not be aware of his [her] surroundings and he [she] will still die from this disease. By not doing CPR, your child will be able to be in your arms at the time of his [her] death and will be surrounded by loved ones."

(Fochtman, 2011). Developmental Considerations 13-1 depicts children's concepts of death related to developmental stage, potential behaviors, and communication strategies they might invoke or methods an adult might use in discussing death with them.

Even if the facts of the illness are discussed openly, the child often needs help in expressing feelings such as fear of the unknown about dying or sadness about not being able to play with friends. Self-expression in writing, play, and art can facilitate the manifestations of a child's feelings. They can also present a nonthreatening method to initiate open communication with family and friends (Ethier, 2009). By examining these creative efforts and discussing them with the child, the family and nurse can help the child understand what is happening and develop needed and effective coping techniques.

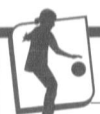

DEVELOPMENTAL CONSIDERATIONS 13-1

Children's Perceptions of Death and Associated Behaviors

Concept of Death	Behavior	Communication Issues
Infancy		
No known concept Death viewed as separation	May be clingy or irritable	Related to infant's perception of separation anxiety Need comfort from persons important to them
Early Childhood (Ages 1–4 Years)		
Does not have comprehension of death Aware someone is missing Aware of other people being "sad"	Altered sleep patterns Irritable Clingy	Similar to infants as related to separation anxiety Needs reassurance
Middle Childhood (Ages 5–10 Years)		
Knows the word *death* or *dead* but has little understanding of the meaning Sees death as temporary or reversible May feel ambivalent about absent person May develop "magical thinking," viewing themselves as the cause	Withdrawal Regression Irritable May feel confused or guilty Concerned about whether the person who has died has food, clothing, and so forth Uses imaginative play Anticipates return Has imaginary conversations with the dead	Children may parrot what they have heard others say They may be very curious and ask uninhibited or frank questions Bereaved siblings may feel that their thoughts or actions caused the death Therapeutic play is often an effective intervention to address feelings and anxieties May still have fears related to separation and need family to be close They need the opportunity to express concerns, fears, and curiosity
Early Adolescence (Ages 11–14 Years)		
Begins to understand death as irreversible Sees death as natural May begin to realize they or others might die Associates death with fear, violence, or destruction May be uncomfortable expressing feelings May have anxiety related to mutilation fears	Asks specific questions about death and death-related rituals, such as funerals, burials Curious about how the body feels after death Needs burial and closure rituals if a pet dies May use play to cope with feelings Often denies death May "act out" at school or with family	Needs to express fears about potential loss of a parent A dying child may try to "protect" family by withdrawing May choose favorite nurse as confidante May seem outwardly uncaring, although inwardly upset Siblings of ill, dying, or dead sibling may need more specific information about cause of illness or death Bereaved or dying children may have feelings of guilt related to blaming themselves for causing the illness or death

(Continued)

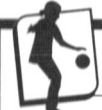

DEVELOPMENTAL CONSIDERATIONS 13-1

Children's Perceptions of Death and Associated Behaviors (Continued)

Concept of Death	Behavior	Communication Issues
Middle and Late Adolescence (Ages 15–21 Years)		
Accepts finality of death Over time, develops mature understanding of death Has fears that he or she may die May have morbid curiosity related to gruesome or violent death Becomes concerned about practical matters associated with death Denies own mortality by risk-taking behaviors Incorporates cultural rituals and attitudes to death and is interested in exploring issues related to afterlife	May feel or express sadness, loneliness, or anger May have reckless demeanor or tough, uncaring attitude Tries to act adultlike but may develop regressive behavior Often wants to touch the body after death May use rituals to decrease anxiety Often develops regressive behavior with staff or family May use creative outlets such as writing, music, or art Peer support may seem more important than family May be very concerned about body image Ill child may want to be involved with funeral planning and "putting their affairs in order"	Needs questions answered openly and in a nonjudgmental manner, especially when related to morbid curiosity Needs more detailed explanations of illness and potential causes of death Requires discussion about reckless behavior and consequences Wants opportunity to voice fears and concerns Dying adolescents have the need to discuss value of life and concerns related to dying but may find it difficult to initiate these conversations Siblings of ill or dying child may act sad or depressed or may seem oblivious to situation and become angry if their plans or activities are disrupted; often want to be at school or with friends and not at home or the hospital yet have difficulty in voicing concerns

From American Association of Colleges of Nursing & City of Hope National Medical Center. (2012). *End-of-life nursing education consortium-pediatric palliative care (ELNEC-PPC) faculty guide*. Duarte, CA: City of Hope; Brown-Hellsten, M., Hockenberry-Eaton, M., Lamb, D. et al. (2000). *End-of-life care for children*. Austin, TX: The Texas Cancer Council. Retrieved from http://www.childend oflifecare.org/frame_dyn.html?about/index.html; Ethier, A. (2009). Care of the dying child and family. In D. Tomlinson & N. E. Kline (Eds.) *Pediatric oncology nursing: Advanced clinical handbook* (pp. 576–656). Berlin, Germany: Springer.

KidKare As children deal with their impending death, they may designate who they want their treasured belongings to be given to after they die. This is a method of coping. Do not discourage such actions on the part of the child.

ANSWER: As an adolescent, George has an understanding of death that is similar to an adult's understanding. His statement in the case study, "I know I am dying and I want to die here," is evidence that George understands and accepts his impending death.

ACHIEVING QUALITY OF LIFE

QUESTION: As you read through this section, what are some aspects of George's care that must be addressed to maintain a quality of life for him as his disease progresses?

Dying is a personal experience. What one person defines as **quality of life** in the stages of his or her illness and the final phase of death may differ significantly from the next person. Ferrell and Grant (2000)

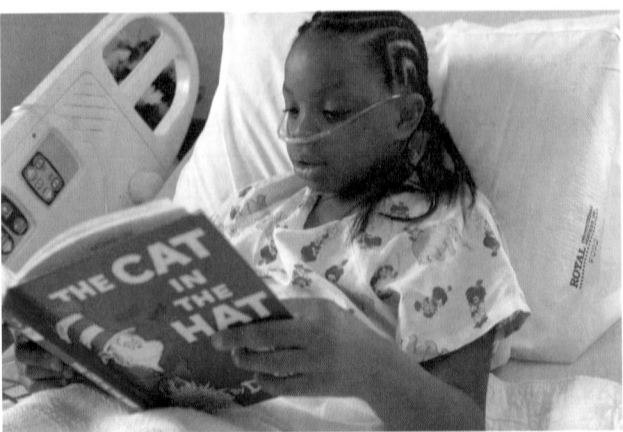

Figure 13-2 Focusing on quality of life includes providing diversional activities that consider the child's level of fatigue, ability to concentrate, and personal interests.

developed a model depicting the multiple dimensions of care as physical well-being and symptoms, psychological well-being, social well-being, and spiritual well-being. These aspects of care must be addressed to achieve quality of life for all individuals. In the situation of a child with a serious illness, the application of the model must incorporate both the child and the family caregiver's point of view because the child's quality of life is directly interwoven with the family's perspective (Field & Behrman, 2003). Although children may not be able to understand the term *quality of life*, they are able to tell you what they like and what is important to them in making their life comfortable and meaningful. Unfortunately, they are rarely asked, and their care is typically defined by those (family members and health care providers) who speak for them, often resulting in the child's desires and goals being overlooked (Fig. 13-2).

ENVIRONMENT OF CARE

The physical environment of the child receiving palliative care includes the actual bed or chair where the child spends time. Both should be comfortable and able to support the child physically. Make the child's environment amenable to the child's activities, such as sleeping, reading, playing games, or visiting with friends.

The child must be able to move within the environment to spend time with people, to spend time alone, or to spend time sleeping. What works well early during the terminal phase might not work as the disease progresses and the child's physical condition deteriorates, so make adjustments as needed to facilitate both physical and emotional comfort. At times, especially when a child is primarily confined to bed, the bed might be placed in a common room, such as the dining room or family room, to decrease isolation from the family. This might also require placing a commode in a private place near the bed if the bathroom is not easily accessible. Evaluate the environment repeatedly to ensure that it remains appropriate for the child and the family.

PHYSICAL CARE AND SYMPTOM MANAGEMENT

Acute, chronic, or debilitating illnesses lead to multiple symptoms as the disease progresses. These symptoms may cause metabolic and organic changes that affect the physical well-being of the child. Assessing and managing symptoms encompasses those services aimed at developing and implementing a plan of management for all symptoms related to the child's changing condition over time. This includes the use of formal assessment tools that are age specific for evaluating pain and other symptoms. Specific problems that need to be managed include pain, feeding, nausea and vomiting, neurologic problems, depression, anxiety, and sleep disorders (Belasco et al., 2000; Collins et al., 1998; Lambert, 2002). The nurse plays a predominant role in managing the physical symptoms of the dying child. Nursing Interventions 13-2 summarizes physical symptoms of the dying child and specific interventions that can be used by the nurse to comfort the child. The interventions are directed toward meeting physical needs and symptom management (Tradition or Science 13-2).

Pain Control

Pain or fear of pain is often the most significant concern for a patient and family and one of the most challenging to manage by health care providers (see Chapter 10 for a full review of pain pathophysiology and management). Physiologic tolerance to opioids, dealing with side effects, and determining the best route of administration must all be considered when the pain control program is developed and continually reevaluated. Fears and concerns related to side effects and addiction frequently inhibit health care providers in administering appropriate medication, and patients and family members often need to be reassured about the realities of addiction. Explain and reinforce the difference between physiologic dependence and drug addiction with drug-seeking activity. Some caregivers may fear specific drugs and may prefer alternatives to opioids. In almost all cases, the goal is to maximize the child's comfort and quality of life. Side effects of opioids are common, and anticipatory management is essential. Patient and family education regarding the use of opioids and the expected side effects and management is a critical component of nursing care. Also, it is important to reassure patients and families that it is always possible to administer appropriate doses of medications to manage pain (Van Cleve et al., 2012).

caREminder

Children who require long-term pain control often need to have opioid dosages increased periodically, possibly by 30%–50% at a time, to maintain comfort. Meperidine (Demerol) is never used for such long-term pain control because of the resultant accumulation of a toxic metabolite (normeperidine) after as few as 3 days of treatment.

NURSING INTERVENTIONS 13-2

Management of the Physical Symptoms Associated With the End of Life*

Symptom	Possible Causes	Medications	Nursing Interventions
Pain That May Be Either Acute or Chronic (refer to Chapter 10 for more specific details)			
Restlessness Irritability/crying Withdrawal Refusal to move	Disease progression Metastases Trauma Neuropathic Idiopathic	Opioids and nonopioid analgesics Adjuvant medications such as nonsteroidal anti-inflammatory drugs Anticonvulsants Antidepressants Benzodiazepines Steroids	Slow, gentle movements Quiet environment Heat or ice Massage Family presence Cuddling/reassurance Distraction Guided imagery, relaxation Art/music therapy
Neurologic			
Seizures	Brain tumor Cerebral bleeding Increased intracranial pressure Infection Metabolic disorders, fluid and electrolyte imbalances Oxygen deprivation	Anticonvulsants	Patient safety Oxygen or suctioning Monitoring of anticonvulsant levels and adjusting as indicated Reassurance
Restlessness/ agitation Delirium/ confusion	Pain Medication reaction Metabolic changes Central nervous system insult/bleeding Hypoxia Urinary retention or constipation Anxiety/worry/fear Insomnia/nightmares Spiritual distress	Assess and improve pain management Eliminate medications that may be contributing to problem Oxygen Correct electrolyte abnormalities Use antianxiolytics as indicated Add stool softeners and laxatives	Biobehavioral interventions Encourage open communication to address fears Use calm, reassuring manner and tone of voice If hospitalized, bring favorite items from home to place in child's room
Pulmonary			
Dyspnea	Anemia Pulmonary disease Pneumonia Pleural effusions Muscle weakness Lung metastases Anxiety	Oxygen Antianxiolytics Morphine Albuterol inhalation	Cool mist, fans Loose-fitting clothing Elevating head of bed Quiet environment Reassurance Treatment of underlying cause

Symptom	Possible Causes	Medications	Nursing Interventions
Slowing of respirations Agonal breathing	Progression of dying process characterized by moaning and sighing, with pauses between breaths; may continue for hours to days	Oxygen Morphine	Comfort and educate the family about the respiratory process to decrease distress Quiet, calm environment Reassurance Elevate head of bed
Cardiovascular/Circulatory			
Irregular heart rate Fatigue Temperature fluctuations Color changes Mottling Pallor Cyanosis	Anemia Decreased oxygenation Shutting down of body as dying process progresses	Antipyretics for fevers Oxygen Packed red blood cell (PRBC) transfusions if anemia is impairing quality of life and symptoms will abate when delivered	Keeping warm or cool, depending on temperature Explain color changes to family
Gastrointestinal			
Diarrhea Constipation Nausea/vomiting Anorexia	Bowel obstruction Fluid electrolyte imbalance Fecal impaction Medications Opioids Poor dietary intake Underlying disease	Stool softeners Laxatives Antidiarrheal agents Antiemetics	Small, frequent meals Nutritional supplements Aggressive bowel care regimen Perianal skin care Treating underlying cause as appropriate In some situations, a nasogastric tube may relieve bowel obstruction or a colostomy may be indicated for palliation
Renal			
Urinary incontinence Urinary retention Anuria Oliguria	Opioids Disease progression Infection Renal shutdown as death approaches	Treating urinary tract infection with antibiotics if symptomatic	Intermittent or indwelling urinary catheter Running water Warm baths Increasing fluid intake Privacy for voiding attempts Explanations to family that as death approaches, urination decreases
Musculoskeletal			
Weakness Hemiparesis Contractures	Pain Disease progression Fatigue Medication side effects Inadequate rest Prolonged immobilization Metabolic disturbances	Possibly appetite stimulant to increase caloric intake, resulting in more energy Eliminating medications causing fatigue, if possible Sleep aid	Physical therapy Range of motion Rest periods May need walker or wheelchair Modify environment to save strength (e.g., bedside commode)

(Continued)

NURSING INTERVENTIONS 13-2

Management of the Physical Symptoms Associated With the End of Life* (Continued)

Symptom	Possible Causes	Medications	Nursing Interventions
Skin			
Breakdown/ irritation Rashes Pressure ulcers Pruritus	Dehydration Malnutrition Immobility Incontinence Opioids Medication reactions	Antifungal agents Steroid creams Antihistamines for itching	Creams or ointments to dry or hydrate skin depending on assessment Thorough cleaning and drying Pat to clean or dry; avoid rubbing Barrier ointments for perianal region Massage
Hematologic			
Anemia Fatigue Thrombocytopenia Bleeding Neutropenia Infection	Anemia of chronic disease Bone marrow–based disease progression Residual effects of cancer treatment Poor diet	Blood product transfusions if they will improve quality of life Medications for treatment of infections Oxygen	Pressure to areas of bleeding (nose is the most common location) Rest Warm environment

*All suggested interventions are recommended only if they will improve quality of life. They may not be appropriate for every patient's situation.

Other Symptoms Associated With the End of Life

Nursing Interventions 13-2 provides a comprehensive discussion of symptoms that a child may experience at the EOL (AACN & COH National Medical Center, 2012). Symptoms associated with the EOL vary in severity and may wax and wane as the disease and dying process progress. As death approaches, some symptoms become more prominent, especially those related to anorexia, somnolence, and changes in breathing patterns. Individual children need help dealing with symptoms of their particular terminal illness with interventions by members of the health care team. It is crucial that the cause of each symptom is determined in order to deliver the correct treatment. For example, administering larger doses of opioids will not help abdominal pain from constipation; the only effective treatment is eliminating constipation with the use of stool softeners and laxatives. Consider treatment of specific physical problems in the dying child as part of the child's long-term care. For example, constipation commonly occurs in the child receiving opioid pain management and generally continues until the child dies. Thus, laxatives, normally given on an as-needed basis, must be administered routinely whenever someone is receiving opioids. The presence of a daily bowel movement is an indication

that the medication is working, not that it is time to stop giving the laxative.

Keep the child clean, dry, well hydrated, and physically comfortable. Excretions and secretions must be removed to prevent skin breakdown. Loss of urinary and bowel control might occur, and steps to prevent this or to clean the child are immediately used. Encourage a child who is hungry, thirsty, and capable of swallowing to eat and drink. If the child is receiving parenteral or enteral fluids, a volume sufficient to maintain full hydration is given to help make the child comfortable. Oral care is especially important when the child is not drinking or cannot brush his or her own teeth.

KidKare Even if the child does not appear to be conscious, talk to the child during care and explain what is happening and why. Talk about the weather, television programs, and other interests of the child. Post pictures from home or school around the bedside if the family desires.

Initiate provisions to prevent or eliminate symptoms whenever possible while providing for comfort. Some symptoms, such as anorexia, cause no discomfort for

TRADITION OR SCIENCE 13-2

Are parents satisfied that at the EOL, their child's pain and symptom management needs are adequately identified and treated?

Wolfe, Grier et al. (2000) identified that suffering from pain was nearly three times more likely in children whose parents reported that the primary care physician was not actively involved in providing EOL care. Treatment alleviated pain for only 27% of children and dyspnea for only 16% of the children. For all children, medical records indicated that parents were significantly more likely to report that the child had symptoms of fatigue, poor appetite, constipation, and diarrhea than did the physicians caring for the child. This suggests that EOL symptoms were not recognized nor therefore treated by the medical team. Similarly, Meyer et al. (2002) found that 25% of parents, in analyzing their child's EOL care, felt their child was not comfortable in his or her final days. Furthermore, they believed that they (the parents) had little or no control during their child's final days. More recent studies have documented that many parents are very happy with their child's overall care at the EOL yet continue to raise concerns as to whether their child's pain and other symptoms, such as anorexia and anxiety, were managed as effectively as possible (Gilmer et al., 2012; Heath et al., 2010; Hechler et al., 2008). More research is needed to ensure children receive adequate symptom management and also to determine if parental perceptions can be improved by more effective communication between the health care team and the family.

ANSWER: Physical care and symptom management, as well as pain control, will all be an important focus of nursing care and management for George. As you read on, note that the psychological support, social support, and cultural and spiritual support will also be areas that the interdisciplinary team will want to attend to with George and his family. These may be areas where nurses do not feel as confident of their skills as compared to their knowledge and skills in symptom and pain management. Nurses who work in palliative care must develop well-rounded skills to meet the needs of the families in their care.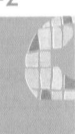

PSYCHOLOGICAL AND SOCIAL SUPPORT

Children with a life-threatening condition continue at some level to have the same emotional, social, and developmental needs as their healthy peers. Illness, regardless of the type, can impact the social structure and integrity of any family. In minor illnesses, the changes are usually temporary, but in catastrophic illnesses and death, roles are irrevocably altered. Relationships at all levels through the family—parent to parent, parent to ill child, parent to well child, sibling to sibling, parent to grandparent—are disrupted and may result in chaos, insecurity, and uncertainty. There may be adjustments in interactions with extended family, peers, and community members. Financial burdens resulting from changes in income from loss of work and nonmedical costs of care can drastically alter family lifestyle and activities. Older children might be aware of these changes and feel responsible.

All children, and especially those managing a terminal condition, need to have a degree of independence and some control in day-to-day decision making. For a young child, it might be as simple as what cup to drink out of, whereas an older child may elect to attend school, even if only for a few hours a day, to maintain some sense of normalcy. These measures are small ways in which a child can preserve some form of dignity and control of how and with whom he or she spends the last days of his or her life (Fochtman, 2011).

As the child's condition worsens, emotional responses to the realization that life is ending may include anxiety, sadness, grief, fear, depression, hopelessness, denial, guilt, and anger. In addition, the child might feel loneliness and isolation, especially if he or she is hospitalized or removed from family members and peers. Commonly, children might not express true emotions in an effort to protect friends and family or when this type of openness is outside the family norm. School-aged children and adolescents need to be involved in purposeful activity and spend time with peers. Adolescents, with their more comprehensive understanding of death and dying, often express concerns about their individuality and body image as well as concerns about the future. They expect and need honesty from adults.

An interdisciplinary team of professionals, laypersons, family members, and friends can best provide these components of care for the dying child. The role of each member of this team changes over time, especially as the focus of the care becomes the support of a

the patient, but they do cause a great deal of distress to the caregivers because they often focus on the lack of food and drink ingested by the child. It is important for them to understand that terminal dehydration and anorexia do not cause suffering in the individual who has no desire for food and water (Fochtman, 2011). When a child has reached the stage of terminal dehydration and anorexia, it is not appropriate to initiate enteral or parenteral feedings because they do not promote comfort at this point and will not sustain life. It is crucial to educate families to help them understand that these are common and natural components of the dying process.

The nurse, as an expert in providing physical care to the ill, is the essential member of the team to guide the patient and family through this stage of the dying process. The use of both pharmacologic and biobehavioral interventions is critical in the management of the patient, but the biobehavioral intercessions, in particular, offer family members an excellent opportunity to take an active role in providing comfort measures (see Chapter 10 for an extensive discussion of nonpharmacologic comfort measures). Successful use of one or more of these methods often gives the family a sense of mastery and accomplishment while enhancing the child's comfort and security.

peaceful death rather than the promotion of continued life. For the dying child, the preservation of relationships with family members, friends, and trusted health care providers and the maintenance of personal dignity can be of utmost importance.

CONTINUING IN SCHOOL

As the illness of the terminally ill child progresses, a frequent question is whether the child may continue to go to school. The answer is usually yes. School plays a very important part in a child's life. In addition to helping the child acquire knowledge, school activities promote self-esteem and allow the child to be identified as an important member of society (Wood, 2006). At school, the child can continue to gain independence and maintain some degree of control over the environment.

School provides opportunities for socialization. Encourage the child to maintain contact with peers and help peers to maintain contact with the child. Attendance at school also minimizes exclusion from school activities that are important to the child. Regardless of whether the child goes to classes regularly, the school-aged child needs to maintain academic success. Both the child and teacher must set attainable goals without the child being relieved of responsibility for learning and completing assignments. Making no academic demands can lead the child to believe that he or she has no value in life or is close to death (Tradition or Science 13-3).

Some families might be concerned about the child attending school because they see it as a potential site of physical and emotional danger. Other families want to spend more time with their child and thus they see school attendance as an impediment. Identify and discuss these issues so that the child may still attend school if he or she desires.

Teachers and school staff members need information and support for themselves (Community Care 13-1). The school nurse works with the child and family to establish the nature of the material to be discussed and the manner of its presentation. Accurate information and answers help prevent incorrect conclusions. Some children want to present this information to their peers themselves. Others want the teacher, treatment center staff, or school nurse to tell their fellow students about their loss of hair or need for a wheelchair or other assistive device.

Regardless of what the classmates and the school staff are told, prepare the child for the questions and changes in relationships that arise after returning to school. By practicing responses and role-playing possible situations, the child learns how to answer questions and to understand peer reactions. When working with students, faculty, and staff, stress the need for openness and free communication. Acknowledge and address fears. Few adults and older children are comfortable discussing or facing death, which can make them avoid the affected child. They need to learn that the child knows that he or she is sick and that avoiding opportunities to discuss the illness robs the terminally ill child of needed opportunities to share the experience. The child also wants to participate in life. Continue full and open discussion of day-to-day events.

CULTURAL AND SPIRITUAL SUPPORT

As discussed in Chapter 1, *spirituality* refers to a search for meaning in life and a relationship with the universe (Heilferty, 2004); *religious beliefs* are those formed within the context of practices and rituals shared by an organized group to establish or find a connection with a god (Davies et al., 2002). Thus, a child may or may not have a religious link with his or her spiritual being. A child's spirituality is often what allows him or her to find hope and meaning in life and provides the foundation for his or her beliefs in the afterlife.

A child who has a formal religious faith might intertwine those feelings with the spiritual self. Spirituality frequently provides the foundation of hope related to life (Ray, 2010). Impending death might challenge or diminish that hope, but with guidance, that hope can be redefined to contribute meaning to the dying process (Ersek & Cotter, 2010). Instead of attempting to redirect hope, many health care professionals try to maintain false hope by continuing to provide curative or life-prolonging treatments even when there is a minimal chance of cure. Unfortunately, what they accomplish often leads to greater suffering, diminished quality of life, isolation from family, increased morbidity, and, at times, a hastening of death (Wolfe, Klar et al., 2000).

When dealing with the grieving child and family, recognize and address cultural and religious concerns (see Table 8-2 for components of a cultural assessment and Table 8-3 for components of a spiritual assessment). Grieving and bereavement are treated differently among cultures, which influences the response of the

---

Evidence-Based Practice

TRADITION OR SCIENCE 13-3

Is school attendance valuable for the child with a terminal illness?

A study conducted in France evaluated the educational careers of 30 children with incurable cancer receiving palliative care (Bouffet et al., 1997). Forty percent of the children did not wish to attend school as they approached the last months of their lives. Reasons for the nonattendance included disease debilitation (blindness, neurologic damage) that prohibited learning; parent's belief that given the context of his or her child's disease, the attendance was "useless"; and child's own fear of attending. However, many children demonstrated a genuine desire to attend school, with increasing disability and fatigue decreasing their motivation over time. The study highlighted the importance of having the child sustain relationships with peers and his or her teachers. School attendance for the child with a terminal disease can offer the child a sense of growth and purpose in the midst of his or her declining state. Although participation in some physical activities may need to be curtailed, participation in classwork and school projects provide a natural outlet for the child's expression of self and the impact of his or her condition (Page & Page, 2011). Ongoing research is needed to continue to evaluate the impact of the terminally ill child in the classroom on other children, teachers, and parents.

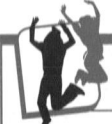

COMMUNITY CARE 13-1

Helping Teachers and Staff to Cope With Terminally Ill Children in School

Address the Staff's Personal Concerns and Attitudes Toward Terminal Illness, Death, and Dying
- Evaluate the staff's prior personal experiences with death.
- Discuss with staff the fears of working with a child who is dying.
- Discuss concerns about other students and how they are coping with having a terminally ill peer.
- Evaluate uneasiness or concerns about teacher–pupil ratio.
- Educate the staff about the child's condition and the needs of the terminally ill student.
- Encourage meaningful communication among children and among children and teaching staff.
- Encourage staff to tell the student that he or she is a valuable person and will not be forgotten.
- Work with the child and family to modify the child's instructional program in light of fatigue, absences, and effects of medications.
- Allow rest periods for the child while at school.
- Send work home on the weekend before it is assigned, so work can be done at the student's own pace.
- Hold the student to whatever academic and behavioral standards he or she is able to meet.
- Do not isolate the student from activities or peers.

Teach Ways to Protect the Child From Injury or Illness
- Teach the child not to share utensils.
- Wash hands after blowing nose and toileting.
- Ask family to keep children who are sick at home.
- Develop written instructions for emergency care of the specific child.

Develop a Plan for After the Death of a Child
- Share reactions within the class through discussions and writing.
- Correct misunderstandings about the illness and death or the student's responsibility for it.
- Encourage creative expressions of grief such as letters and memorials.
- Present information about death rituals and funerals.
- Listen to and empathize with the children; hear what they say.
- Refer students (classmates) for additional help/counseling as needed.
- Acknowledge that the bereavement process may last 6 months or more.

---

child and family. When assessing the family, it is important for the nurse to seek out such factors and to take steps to accommodate the family's wishes even if their requests are unfamiliar. If the nurse is unsure of the family's cultural beliefs or needs, ask the family to share them. It is imperative to be cognizant of differing cultural practices and beliefs and to understand behavior based on these ideas (Davies, Contro et al., 2010). It is equally important not to expect certain behaviors based on cultural influence.

CROSS-CULTURAL CARE

Nurses often offer support with a pat on the hand or the back. For Native Americans, touching is reserved for family or very close friends; therefore, touching is not an appropriate method of providing support for Native Americans. The subculture of gender may also influence the grieving patterns of Native Americans; women often openly and emotionally express their grief, whereas men may show little emotion and seek no support. These patterns, although common, are not exclusively related to gender (Nishimoto, 1996), and interventions are tailored to the individual response.

Many families draw great strength from their faith, although spiritual beliefs are not always expressed by involvement with a particular church or religion. Concepts such as hope, faith, and a sense of meaning and purpose in life are directly tied to the spiritual domain. Spirituality or religion may or may not be a source of support for the family. Some families hope for religious miracles at the time of their child's diagnosis or death. If desired, encourage family to seek their minister, priest, rabbi, imam, or members of their church for support and modify the plan of care to accommodate religious practices (Fig. 13-3).

To assess the family's spiritual beliefs, look for evidence of involvement with a religion, such as religious symbols, medals, statues, books, or music (see Chapter 8 for a discussion of spiritual assessment). These may be used to initiate discussion of spiritual strengths or needs. Many religions have specific death services or rituals; make every effort to allow for them (Chart 13-2). When death occurs, the family may wish to complete special prayers or services and death rites to prepare the body for burial.

Spiritual beliefs and cultural practices often help to define people both as individuals and as a family unit.

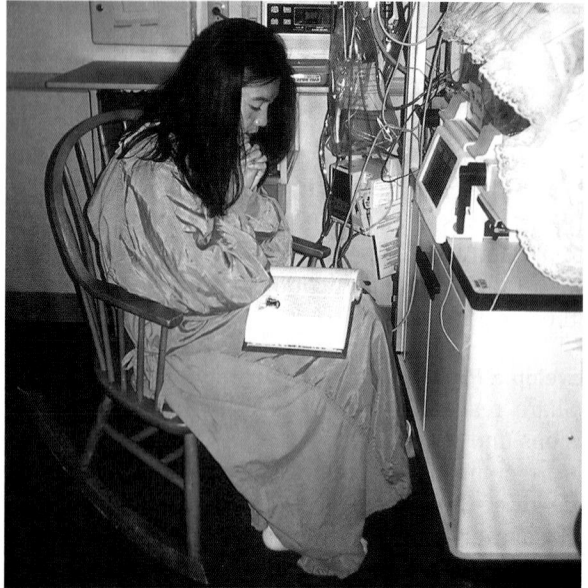

Figure 13-3 A family's religious practices, a source of spiritual support, should be incorporated into care.

Respect for and allowing adherence to their values provides comfort and strength that assists with coping during the child's illness and after his or her death (Taylor, 2010).

WHEN DEATH OCCURS

In unexpected death, family members may have no time for preplanning and preparation. Often, it is in a crisis situation in which the health care team has implemented resuscitation efforts as a result of trauma to the child or a sudden downturn in the status of a child with a terminal illness. Chapter 31 discusses pediatric resuscitation, including the value of family presence during resuscitation efforts (also see thePoint for Procedures). When death occurs unexpectedly, the family has to make decisions about the child's body, including whether an autopsy should be done and/or if organs will be donated. Because there may be limited time to contact family and support persons to help them with decision making, they may have to rely on health care providers who are essentially strangers (Sumner, 2010).

When death is expected, the decisions are related not to what to do to prevent death but to what can be done to enhance the dying process by directing interventions to minimize suffering and maximize quality of life for the patient and family. Planning can be done regarding what treatments to continue or halt. These might include such measures as allowing natural death (AND) by requesting a DNR or do-not-intubate status, eliminating antibiotics or blood transfusions if they are no longer providing a benefit, and withdrawing interventions such as ventilator support as well as having time to make decisions regarding whether death

---

Death Rituals of Different Religions

Muslim

Organ donation or transplants may be opposed. The dead must be buried intact, so autopsy is uncommon and cremation is not permitted. Grief is not shown in the dying person's presence, and impending death is hidden from the dying person. After the death, loud expressive mourning occurs. The body is wrapped in special cloth and buried in the ground.

Hindu

Hindus believe in reincarnation. Death may be seen as God's will, and believers need time for prayer readings from holy Sanskrit books. Strings (to signify a blessing) may be tied around the wrist or neck of the child. Families may want to wash the body after death, and they may not want the body to be touched by non-Hindus. Transfusions, transplants, and autopsies are permissible; cremation is preferred.

Jewish

Burial usually takes place within 24 hours of death. The body must not be mutilated, so organ donation, autopsies, embalming (which removes blood that is considered a body part), and cremation are forbidden. The body must return to the earth. The body of the deceased is never left unattended until buried.

Christian Scientists

Believers may oppose the use of drugs, blood transfusions, or other treatments. Healing is seen as spiritual renewal, so Christian Scientists may want treatment or support from another Christian Scientist. Autopsy is permitted only in cases of sudden death.

Episcopal or Catholic

Infant baptism is not mandatory but can be done if the family desires. If a priest is unavailable, family members or health care providers can baptize by pouring a small amount of water over the child's head and saying, "I baptize you in the name of the Father, the Son, and the Holy Spirit." Anointing of the sick is offered to all seriously ill patients. This sacrament is often given to those who are dying and is no longer given only if death is imminent. Donation and transplantation of organs is permitted, and believers do not think that extraordinary artificial means of sustaining life must be used.

---

will occur at home or in the acute care setting (Klein & Saroyan, 2011).

DISCONTINUING TREATMENT

A difficult aspect of the care of the terminally ill child is deciding what care to perform and what to omit. New curative treatments should not be initiated if there is no chance of cure. This is often a requirement for participation in hospice programs. However, some treatments are given for palliative as well as curative reasons (Tomlinson et al., 2011). Radiation therapy, usually given to "cure" the tumor, can also reduce its size and reduce pain. Giving antibiotics to cure the constant colonization of an indwelling urinary catheter is probably a futile effort. However, treatment of a urinary tract infection that is causing dysuria, frequency, and pain can improve the child's quality of life. A child may receive oxygen or be suctioned to promote comfort. Providing enteral or parenteral fluids can be appropriate to maintain hydration if the child is unable to drink and complains of thirst or hunger.

A decision about continuing treatment for the dying child might be necessary when the care being given is causing discomfort with no benefit to the child. Hemodynamic monitoring, insertion of central lines to administer total parenteral nutrition to meet *long-term* nutrition needs, and taking daily weights or laboratory studies are examples of interventions that are futile in most situations. The family and health care team must work together to determine when these interventions should be stopped.

caREminder

As death nears for the child, direct care activities, except for comfort measures, are omitted to allow for a more peaceful environment. Another important decision is determining what, if any, resuscitation measures will be implemented. When it is apparent that the child is close to death, usually no interventions are appropriate. Communicate the resuscitation status of the child to all those involved in the child's care, including ancillary staff.

TIME-OF-DEATH DECISIONS

Decisions made at the time of death often relate to organ donation, autopsy, and funeral arrangements. The nurse plays an instrumental role in the decision-making process with the family by facilitating contact with appropriate personnel, ensuring that the family understands the choices before them, and completing tasks to ensure that family decisions are acted on by the health care team.

Organ Donation

As previously discussed, when approaching the family about decisions that must be made at the time of death, the nurse must be sensitive to the family's cultural and ethnic background. Some interventions, such as organ donation, are not permitted in certain cultures. Discuss the subject of organ donation only after the family has been told that their child is dying and the feasibility of organ donation is confirmed (Cowl et al., 2012). It is important for the nurse to be familiar with the state and agency's protocol for identification of potential organ donors. Some states do not allow health care professionals to approach the family about organ donation and relegate these responsibilities to those identified as part of an organ donation team (generally associated with the organ donation agency).

When discussing organ donation with the family, be alert for comments that indicate that the family does not understand the process because the general public often poorly understands the concept of brain death. The family might not comprehend that the child has been pronounced dead and that equipment, such as a ventilator, is being used to maintain circulation to the organs that will be donated and not being used to preserve the child's life.

caREminder

Do not let preparation for the donor process interfere with the family's wishes to be with their child before the ventilatory support is removed. Throughout the process, the child's body is treated with respect.

Autopsy

The decision about an autopsy is often made by the medical examiner's office in unexpected death or when criminal intent is suspected, but in expected death (such as death from progression of a chronic disease), the decision is left up to the child's legal guardians. Present facts about the autopsy (Teaching Intervention Plan 13-1) with sensitivity and give the family enough time to make the decision. Most important, respect is afforded to families who forgo autopsy because of cultural or religious prohibitions. Chart 13-2 discusses some of the cultural and religious beliefs associated with death, including permitting postmortem examination of the child.

Funeral Arrangements

Funeral arrangements need to be made by the family. This is something few families are prepared to do. If local mortuaries offer free or low-cost funerals for infants and children, provide such information to the family. For the family whose child has just died, talking about a funeral may be very disturbing. A service can be a source of comfort or distress to a family member. There are often different issues for surviving family members based on their relationship to the child as well as their gender. For instance, in many cultures, it is more socially acceptable for the mothers to openly grieve. Many times, a father may feel like he cannot express his full emotions publicly. A mother is often offered more support than a father, and the father may feel "left out" or that his grief has less value than the mother's. The health care team can assist in identifying the individual needs of family members as funeral service arrangements are made. All family members can contribute to the arrangements (e.g., choosing a favorite piece of music, a poem to be read), thereby giving each member a special memory of their final farewell to their loved one (Perko, 2010).

CARE AT THE TIME OF DEATH

Each child's death is a special, albeit sad, moment. The fact that the child will die soon is often known when the child is terminally ill. It is helpful to prepare families for the physical changes that are going to occur

---

TIP 13-1: A TEACHING INTERVENTION PLAN for the Family Considering an Autopsy

Nursing Diagnosis and Family Outcome

- Deficient knowledge: Autopsy
  Outcome: The family makes an informed decision regarding performance of an autopsy.

Interventions

- Determine any religious or cultural prohibitions against and exceptions for permitting an autopsy.
- Teach the following:
  - Autopsies are not mandated unless the cause of death may be a criminal matter. Advise the family that they have a choice regarding whether an autopsy be performed.
  - Health insurance companies may not cover the cost of an autopsy.

- The autopsy may help to clarify the cause of death and/or confirm the diagnosis of the child.
- The autopsy can help the medical team to understand the disease or the impact of the injury and thus help other children.
- Alternatives to a full autopsy can include examination of specific organs only, examination of the cord and placenta, blood or tissue sampling for genetic analysis, radiographic examination, and the possibility of laparoscopic autopsy.
- The child will feel no pain.
- The child's body will be respected and there will be no obvious indication of an autopsy.
- The family will get feedback about the autopsy from their family health care provider.

From Chichester, M. (2007). Requesting perinatal autopsy: Multicultural considerations. *MCN. The American Journal of Maternal Child Nursing, 32,* 81–86; Wright, C., & Lee, R. (2004). Investigating perinatal death: A review of the options when autopsy consent is refused. *Archives of Disease in Childhood Fetal and Neonatal Edition, 89,* F285–F288.

---

during the last weeks, days, hours, and minutes of life. If the family is prepared for physical symptoms, they are less likely to panic with alterations in appearance, such as mottling and cyanosis or changes in respiratory status when moaning and agonal breathing occur. Even when death is anticipated, the reality as it occurs might seem overwhelming, and having systems of support at hand might help to ease the transition from life to death. Making advance preparations regarding which mortuary to contact might help relieve the stress of trying to make a decision after the death.

caREminder

Offer the family the opportunity to be with their child after the death and before the child receives postmortem care. Ask family members if they want someone to be with them or if they want to be alone with their child. Some families welcome the option of giving care such as the final bath. Stay with the family members if they request.

As previously discussed, during and after the death, it is important to honor cultural and religious practices. Encourage families to invite their clergy member, priest, imam, or rabbi to join them. Encouraging and allowing the family to spend as much time as they wish with the child is often one of the memories that sustains them. The child's ability to hear and understand is not always clear to caregivers, but this should not stop efforts to talk to and communicate with the child. Holding the child or assisting in caring for the child's body by bathing and dressing provides a comforting ritual for many families (Fochtman, 2011). The presence of multiple

intravenous lines, tubes, and even ventilatory support are not reasons to deny this request (Fig. 13-4).

Allow parents to determine who will attend the final visit with the child—other family members and siblings of the child, a religious leader, or friends. In cases of severe injuries, prepare the visitors for how the child looks. Prepare the child and room for the visit, although it might be beneficial to leave much of the resuscitation equipment in the room to reinforce the fact that efforts were taken to save the child.

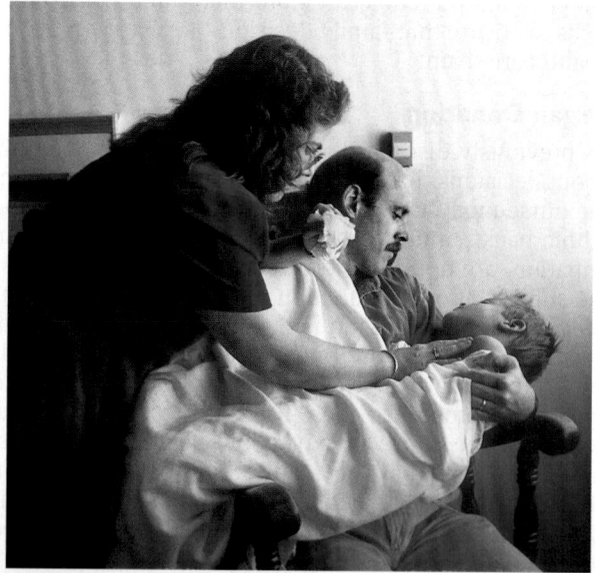

Figure 13-4 Parents' wishes to hold their dying child should be respected and facilitated.

Families who do not want to see their child after the death can be gently encouraged to do so. Even when the death was the result of severe trauma, family members who see their child have fewer fantasies about the event (Levetown et al., 2010). Offer the family members the opportunity to hold their child, and allow the length of the final visit to be determined by the needs of the individual family.

Give mementos and personal items of the child to the family, and initiate the rest of the agency's bereavement protocol or policies. Provide written information about support available for the family over the difficult months ahead.

The nurse can act as the gatekeeper who helps the family find needed privacy and facilitates communication among family members. Suggest ways for the family to discuss the events with their other children. Be prepared for the family to express grief in a variety of ways, including anger and rage, and do not take negative responses personally.

CARE OF PARENTS

Often, when death is anticipated, parents are reluctant to leave the child's bedside; supplying sleeping couches and meals in the room can be viewed as a tremendous kindness and support to the family. Within the home environment, using a child-monitoring system, such as the readily available baby or video monitors, can allow a parent to feel comfortable to leave the child's room for short periods. Using community resources such as neighbors, friends, and members of their religious community to assist with siblings, provide meals, do household chores, and generally be available for assistance can take some of the burden off of routine activities of daily living needed to keep a household functioning.

Parents are often in a state of shock. Assess parent's decision-making ability carefully. Assistance with driving home or caring for other children might be needed. Caregiver fatigue, sleep deprivation, physical exhaustion, and depression can all affect the caregiver's ability to make decisions and interact with other family members. For many caregivers, the full impact of the child's death might be delayed until they recover from the physical demands of caring for their child. Encouraging parents to regularly eat small meals and drink fluids as well as rest when the child is sleeping can help to sustain them through this time.

CARE OF SIBLINGS

Siblings of dying and dead children need care also (Trotzuk & Gray, 2012). At times, with good intentions, family members might try to protect the siblings from the reality of the dying process; however, this can inadvertently increase fears because the sibling's fantasies may be more detrimental to his or her emotional health than the actual reality of the dying process (Fochtman, 2011). Siblings often have been involved in some manner throughout their sibling's illness, thus it is important to allow siblings to participate in the final process of their brother's or sister's life as well. Many times,

siblings may wish to be present at the death, help with the physical care of the body, and plan the funeral. Studies in the 1980s demonstrated that when siblings participated in the care of their dying sibling, they had a more positive adjustment (Lauer et al., 1985; Martinson et al., 1987). If they are present in the acute care setting, inform siblings about what is happening and give them an opportunity to express their questions and fears. If children want to see their brother or sister, discuss this issue with the parents. It is generally preferable to honor this request; however, if they do not wish to see their sibling, they should never be forced to do so.

CROSS-CULTURAL CARE

In Japanese culture, there is emphasis on the importance of the family over the individual. Siblings are expected to be patient with the sick or dying child. Research by Saiki et al. (1994) found that siblings usually did not complain when attention was focused on the dying child, but in some siblings, physical or emotional problems did develop. Japanese mothers are the primary caregivers, and families are not comfortable receiving support from outside the family. Therefore, Japanese families, especially mothers, struggle to provide care on their own at the expense of their own health and the needs of siblings (Saiki et al., 1994). An appropriate intervention would be to remind parents to pay attention to the needs of siblings. Regardless of the child's cultural background, allow siblings of a child who has died to be involved to the degree that they wish to be involved. Freely and openly address their questions and concerns.

If the siblings are not present, advise family members on ways to talk to them about their brother's or sister's death. Fantasies and misunderstandings are common, and some children see themselves as responsible for the death. These ideas must be identified and dispelled. However, if the sibling is responsible—for example, after a firearm injury or fatal accident—emergency emotional support for the sibling must be initiated immediately.

Siblings may choose not to attend a funeral service or may not be present based on parental wishes. When a child is at the funeral of a family member, advise the family to have a person sit with the child to answer questions or take him or her out if he or she feels that he or she needs to leave during the service. This person should be a close friend or family member who would be comfortable with the child. Children may feel that they should cry, and they may need permission to do so. Often, children feel that they need to "be strong" at the funeral service so as not to further upset their family. Before the service, bring parents and children together to discuss expressions of grief and to prepare the children for what they may see at the funeral. These discussions will provide family members an opportunity to comfort surviving children and prepare them for the many emotions they may experience over the next days and weeks.

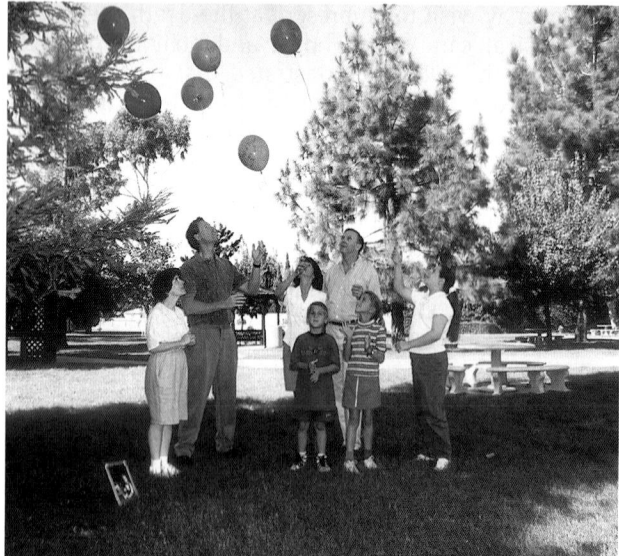

Figure 13-5 On the anniversary of a child's death, family members and friends meet to symbolically send balloons (non Mylar) up to heaven with messages inside for the deceased child.

FOLLOW-UP CARE

The health care staff and/or a bereavement coordinator play an important role in follow-up care with the family who has lost a child. Follow-up efforts can include sending a personal letter from the nursing staff to the family followed by a call within 2 weeks of the child's death, at which time additional support can be offered and referral to counseling can be made if needed. The family can be contacted at times that are likely to trigger resurgence of the grief response, such as the child's birthday, major holidays, or the anniversary of the child's death, so that additional support can be provided (Fig. 13-5). A tracking card and check sheet can be used to identify dates for follow-up interventions.

Include extended family members and friends in bereavement programs based on their degree of involvement with the person who has died and their desire to seek help in managing their grief. Persons such as out-of-state grandparents, spouses of the noncustodial parent, daycare providers, and parents of the child's friends are often not seen and are thus overlooked by the health care providers who are caring for the child and family.

Extended family and friends are often unsure of how they can help the grieving family. They fear they will do something wrong when they call or visit, so they do neither. This contributes to the isolation of the grieving family in a time of great need. Provide suggestions of helpful activities to family members (Community Care 13-2).

caREminder

Reassure friends and family that if they act genuinely and with sincerity when they are with the grieving family, what they do will rarely be wrong.

SPECIAL CONSIDERATIONS RELATED TO THE CAUSE AND PLACE OF DEATH

The cause of death (expected, unexpected, or traumatic) and place where the death occurs affects the choice of health care provider interventions and the family's response to the loss. These issues must be considered to meet the needs of the family when delivering care.

PERINATAL LOSS

Palliative care services can be integrated into the neonatal intensive care unit (NICU) and the labor and delivery areas. The need for palliative care services in these areas is very real. In 2005, as reported by the Centers for Disease Control and Prevention's National Vital Statistics Report system, more than 18,000 infants died in the first month of life, and there were 25,000 reported fetal deaths (Macdorman & Kirmeyer, 2009). In perinatal loss, a parent can experience a significant grief reaction even when a pregnancy has been brief. As the pregnancy becomes real to the parents, particularly to the mother, there can be significant investment and bonding even before the signs of pregnancy are clear to others.

Nurses in many settings care for families experiencing perinatal loss, miscarriage, stillbirth, and neonatal death. This could be in the emergency department (ED); labor and delivery, neonatal care, mother–baby, or women's units; or primary care settings in the community. The goals of care are to meet the family's medical needs, validate the loss, and teach about usual responses to the loss.

Regardless of the setting of a perinatal death, offer the parents the option of touching, fondling, or holding the deceased fetus or infant even if it is grossly malformed (Fig. 13-6). This gives parents a chance to attach to their infant. Lundqvist et al. (2002) found that the behaviors of health care professionals were directly related to that of the grieving mothers' feelings of both empowerment and powerlessness after the death of a

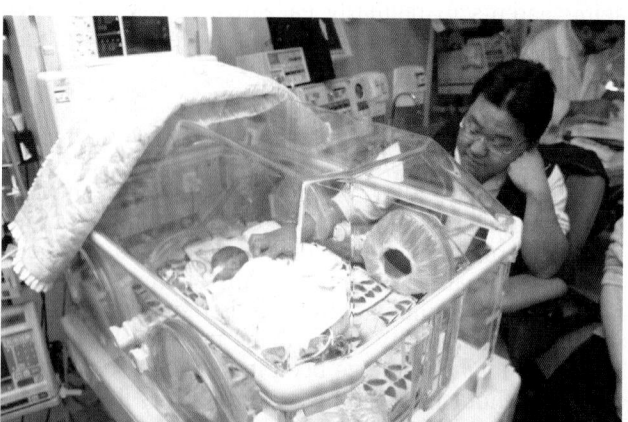

Figure 13-6 A father spends time with his dying infant.

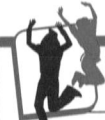

COMMUNITY CARE 13-2

Suggestions for Family and Friends After the Death of a Child

- *Be yourself.* Show your concern and sorrow in your own way. You will not be effective without natural and total sincerity.
- *Be there.* Brief telephone calls and visits say, "I care and I want to help."
- *Say, "I'm sorry."* After you have expressed your sorrow, allow the parents or family to respond. Don't be afraid of silence. Often, your caring presence is enough.
- *Touch.* A hug or a hand to hold can sometimes say more than words.
- *Find helpful activities.* Don't wait to be asked to do something. Look around for what is needed. Provide a meal, do errands, or babysit the other children.
- *Don't protect.* There are many helpful things to do, but shielding the family from the reality of the situation is not one of them. They need to make their own decisions and work through their grief.
- *Talk about the child.* Don't be afraid that mentioning the child will remind them of their grief. They haven't forgotten. They need to talk about their child. When you avoid the subject, it seems that you are saying that the child didn't exist.
- *Cry with them.* Family members and friends often feel that they must "hold up" to be supportive. This is not necessarily true. Your tears show that you care. However, if your own grief is so overwhelming that you cannot function, it is probably best to wait to interact with the parents or family until you can function.
- *Laugh with them.* It is important to recall humorous incidents and endearing qualities about the child. These memories may bring mutual smiles and laughter. Remember, though, that jokes and trivial discussions are not appropriate at this time.
- *Don't look for something positive.* There is nothing positive in the situation, and anything you try to point out as positive may be perceived by the parents or family as a lack of understanding for their pain.
- *Avoid stock responses.* Don't use such cliché phrases as, "I know how you feel." "Be thankful that . . . " "Don't cry." "It's better this way." "You have other children." "You can have other children." "It's God's will."
- *Listen with understanding.*
- *Acknowledge the family's feelings and questions.* You cannot answer these questions, so don't try. Just acknowledge their right to be angry.
- *Reassure.* It is common for those who are grieving to feel guilt and to engage in an "if only" type of exercise. Although this is normal, repeated reassurance is necessary.
- *Be patient.* Every person grieves differently and on his or her own timetable. You cannot rush the process.

---

baby. When health care providers attended to the needs of the mother by seeing the mother as an individual, seeing the situation "through the mother's eyes," and showing empathy for the mother's feelings, a sense of empowerment was established for the mother. On the other hand, an insistence on following prescriptive rules of the acute care setting rules, of feelings not being taken into account, and a fear of sharing feelings with staff who seemed distant and disconnected all led to a sense of powerlessness by the 16 mothers interviewed in this study. Parental fantasies about the infant's appearance are often worse than the reality of the anomalies or condition of the deceased infant. Seeing and holding the infant validates the existence of the infant and makes the reality of the death more clear. Clean and wrap the infant as appropriate for the gestational age in preparation for this visit, and describe the appearance of the baby to the family before the visit. Stay with the family at the beginning of the visit and then offer them time alone with the infant. Decisions about the length of this visit and the individuals who will be present are left up to the family.

ALERT   *Be cautious about allowing fathers or other family members to decide whether the mother is to see her deceased child. Offer this opportunity to the infant's mother independent of family input. If the woman is incapable of seeing the child or making the decision at the time of the infant's death, an option to visit at the morgue can be provided if the baby cannot be taken from the morgue.*

Photographs of the child can be taken, with nursing personnel preparing the child in such a way as to offer a peaceful and attractive remembrance of the child. If the family decides not to see the infant, allow the body to be kept on the unit as long as possible to allow them time to change their minds.

Immediately after the death, activate the perinatal bereavement protocol. Immediately notify bereavement team support persons (e.g., nurses, social workers, physicians, or other parents who have experienced perinatal losses) so they can visit as soon as possible after the death. *Resolve Through Sharing* is an example of a program that is used internationally to support families experiencing a perinatal loss. This program trains health care providers to serve as counselors who can intervene with families to facilitate coping with their loss.

The bereavement team members can help parents make the many decisions needed during the immediate postdelivery period. Each time parents make a decision, they are able to take control in a very difficult situation. An autopsy may be desired by the parents or required by law. For some infants, the option to donate organs may be viable.

The parents must determine how and where the infant will be buried. Requirements for burial vary from state to state, but it is usually required for all births after 20 weeks' gestation. Parents may choose to have the institution dispose of the body. If the infant is to be buried, the parents can be asked whether there is a special outfit, blanket, or other object they would like to have buried with the infant. Provide sufficient time without pressure so that a family decision may be made.

When an infant's death occurs on the perinatal unit, a decision must be made about where the mother will be placed during the immediate postdelivery period. Involve parents in this choice because it is an action that can increase their sense of control. Many agencies attempt to place a woman whose infant has died on a nonobstetric unit. Regardless of the unit where she stays, alert all staff members to her loss. The Resolve Through Sharing program recommends placing a simple card with a photo of a flower on the door to the woman's room (Fig. 13-7). The photo is a visual reminder to all personnel that a loss has occurred. This prevents inadvertent comments about the infant who has died and reminds caregivers that this woman and her family need more than the usual postpartum care.

When the perinatal death occurs in the ED, take special care to protect the family and to provide them with an opportunity to see and hold the infant. Avoid terms such as *spontaneous abortion* because the term *abortion* is more closely associated with voluntary termination of pregnancy. Be especially careful of where the fetus is placed. Putting the fetus on a cold metal tray can be very disturbing to the parents. Offer a remembrance packet to the parents. This packet may include a photograph of the child and a lock of the child's hair.

Referral to a support group and teaching about the normal reactions that follow perinatal death are essential components of the care provided to these families even if the interactions with the health care system are brief. Prepare parents for the intensity of their reactions and for the fact that they will each react differently. The loss of a fetus early during pregnancy is different from the loss of a baby in later pregnancy, and both are different from the loss of an older child or adult. The grief might focus more on what could have been rather than what was.

People's reactions to the couple's loss will also differ. Sometimes, a seemingly helpful comment can be dismissive. For example, someone might say, "Don't worry, you'll get pregnant again real soon," or "At least you have two healthy kids at home." These comments diminish the loss of that specific pregnancy. If the loss was early during the pregnancy, other family members might act as if they are ignoring the loss because they are afraid to hurt the couple by talking about it. Offer pamphlets with suggestions for the family and friends to the parents to share with their support persons. If the death occurs during a later stage of pregnancy, when many people know about the expected birth, help the parents to plan how to respond to questions about their new baby. One such response is, "Thank you for asking. I am doing well, but my baby died just after he was born."

Much of the grief work of families who have experienced a perinatal loss occurs after discharge from the acute care institution. Use of detailed perinatal loss follow-up tools assists primary care providers in community settings to thoroughly address the parents' physical and emotional status, autopsy results, and the parents' support network and ability to communicate with significant others and to give anticipatory guidance regarding grief reactions and future pregnancies. If symptoms of unresolved grief are present 12 to 18 months after the loss, make a referral for in-depth counseling.

DYING IN THE ACUTE CARE SETTING

Children who die in the acute care setting may be in the general pediatric unit, ED, critical care unit, or an operating room (OR). The principles of care are the same in all locations, but the site of death and the circumstances that bring the child to the unit can have a significant bearing on the needs of the family.

General Pediatric Unit

When a child dies on a general pediatric unit, the child is often at the terminal stage of long-term disease. Care is similar to that described for the emotional and physical care of the dying child. Encourage open visiting. Families who spend a lot of time at the hospital during the child's illness might need health care provider support and encouragement to leave the room and the unit to meet their own needs and the needs of their other children. After the child's death, the staff working with the child might also need support. Other children on the unit who knew the child frequently need help to address their grief as well.

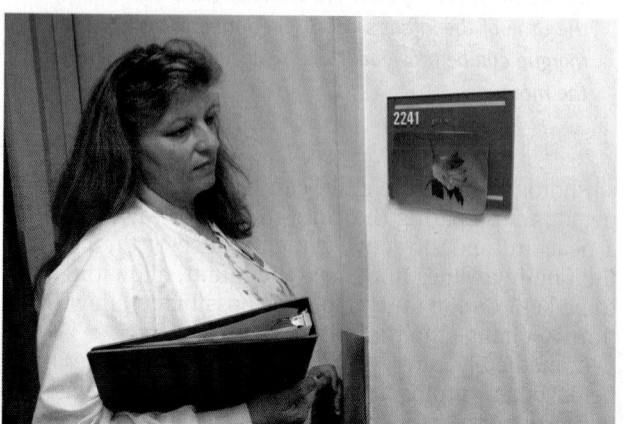

Figure 13-7 The Resolve Through Sharing purple rose on the door alerts all staff to the family's loss.

Emergency Department or Critical Care Unit

Children who die in an ED or a critical care unit are often the victims of accidental or intentional trauma. Others die because of sudden illness, such as respiratory failure, sudden infant death syndrome, or fulminating meningitis. In addition, children who have been in treatment for a chronic condition and who are admitted to an ED or critical care unit might die because of an acute crisis that does not resolve.

When the death is from trauma, other family members or friends might have been injured or killed. Determine the relationship among all victims and provide support appropriate to the situation. When one or both parents are injured or dead, the emotional support of surviving children is essential. Issues of authority for consent must be clarified. When the affected family members are in different facilities, lines of communication between family members and the health care team must be established.

When the child's death is the result of violence, steps to document the injuries, preserve evidence, and notify law enforcement authorities, if they are not already involved, are needed. Nurses must also work with social service, pastoral care, and other support personnel to initiate crisis support care for the parents and other children.

When the death is suspected to be the result of family violence, the nurse must report suspected abuse. Social workers and law enforcement authorities then have a major role in initiating child protection activities for other children and initiating action against the perpetrator. The nursing role is one of assessment, documentation, and parent and family support. The facts of the case are rarely clear when the child is first brought to the ED.

caREminder

A nonjudgmental approach to all family members is taken to avoid the damage that can be caused by the false accusation of an innocent parent.

In other cases, the child's fatal injury might occur because the parent or another person did not use appropriate safety precautions to protect the child (Clinical Judgment 13-1). Take, for example, a mother who does not clean out the drawers in the bathroom cabinet when she has her first baby; as a result, she does

---

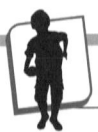

CLINICAL JUDGMENT 13-1

A Child Experiencing the Traumatic Death of a Sibling

Nine-year-old Eric G. and his 4-year-old sister Sara were playing at home while their parents worked in the garden. Eric and Sara had been carefully instructed never to play with the gun that Mr. G. kept in a cabinet over the refrigerator. Around 4 PM, Eric and Sara were searching for snacks to eat before dinner. Eric pulled a chair up to the kitchen counter and began searching the cabinets. He finally found a full bag of chips hidden in the cabinet over the refrigerator, just behind the gun. When he moved the gun, he was fascinated by how it felt and looked and brought it down "just for a minute." The gun discharged, hitting Sara in the chest. The emergency response team transported Sara to the hospital. After briefly interviewing Eric and his parents, the police helped them get to the hospital. There, Eric tells you that the policeman said he killed his sister.

Questions

1. What other data about Eric and his family should be obtained at the time of their admission?

2. What assessment finding indicates that Eric was misinterpreting comments made to him?

3. What simple tools can be used to help Eric express his feelings?

4. What immediate referrals would you make for Eric's care?

5. What types of concerns would you have about Eric's reaction to his sister's injury and possible death?

Answers

1. Who do the children live with? Which members of Eric's family provide his greatest support? Has Eric had any prior experience with such an event?

2. Eric says that the policeman said that he killed his sister, but the police officers only remember asking Eric what happened to his sister.

3. Drawing, storytelling, and reading stories that contain the themes that Eric expresses in his comments to staff and family.

4. A child life worker, social worker, psychologist, or psychiatrist should see Eric within an hour of his sister's admission.

5. Eric is likely to react strongly to any comments made in the hours and days after the accident. Even supportive comments made by caring adults may be misinterpreted by Eric. He will feel responsible for her death.

not discard the half-full bottle of antimalarial pills. Her 2-year-old girl is poisoned when she eats these pills, mistaking them for candy. Or, an aunt who decides to hold her infant nephew in the front seat rather than get the car seat from her brother's car because they were "just going down the block." She never thought they would be hit from behind, but they are, and the baby dies the next day from a ruptured spleen and liver. Such parents and family members need supportive care and might need referral to a mental health professional to resolve their guilt about their role in the child's accidental death.

When the child is admitted to the ED or critical care unit, the family assessment process must be accelerated. The nurse must determine what the family knows and expects, and then reinforce and clarify that information. Focus comments on what families want and need to know. The critically ill or injured child is often fully alert and aware of the surrounding activities despite serious injuries. Answer the child's questions and give the child opportunities to express concerns and, if age appropriate, participate in care decisions.

The family must be helped to comprehend a rapidly evolving series of events concerning their child's condition and the multiple decisions they need to make. Family members need rapid preparation for what they will see, feel, and experience. Discuss the possibility of the child's death as soon as such an outcome seems likely. Encourage questions even when they are repeated multiple times.

Ask the family whether a clergy member, either the hospital chaplain or someone from their place of worship, should be called. Respect their need to carry out specific religious rituals for the time of death. Give the family frequent updates on their child's condition. Families unfamiliar with the ED and critical care environments might need permission to approach or touch their child. They may also welcome being asked to help with simple care. This allows them to have a sense that they are caring for and comforting their child even at the time of death. When answering questions, be as direct and complete as possible, and try to not rush the family as they work to absorb the reality of the impending or actual death of their child.

Operating Room

Another possible place of death for the hospitalized child is the OR. Parents may express a need to be with their child when it becomes clear that the child will die in the OR. Individual institutions have procedures regarding such eventualities because the decision to grant a parental request to enter the OR, or to ask parents whether they want to enter the OR, must often be made quickly.

Designate one member of the OR team as the person who confirms that death is likely. Offer the parents the chance to be with their child in the OR. Other persons who can be with parents, such as the child's siblings, clergy, extended family, or friends, should be identified. Be careful not to give parents the message (verbally or nonverbally) that they *must* go into the OR.

If the parents choose to go to the OR suite, prepare them for what they will see and how the child will look. Also, prepare the OR environment and staff for the parents' visit. Visible blood on the child, the bed, or on surgical instruments should be cleaned or covered up. Have one staff member, preferably a nurse, support the parents during the visit. If possible, offer the parents a place to sit during the visit. Help the parents approach and touch their child because they may need to receive permission from the health care team to do this. Allow parents the opportunity to be present when life support is discontinued.

After the child's death, offer parents additional time to be with their child before, during, or after postmortem care is completed. At this point, movement of the child to the recovery area may be considered.

DYING IN THE COMMUNITY

 QUESTION: What is one unique and beneficial aspect of selecting hospice care for the Tran family?

Children with complex chronic conditions may die in the community instead of an acute care hospital setting (Feudtner et al., 2001). These deaths might occur in the home or in a hospice or respite care facility.

Home Care

Families have reported that providing EOL care in the home was a valuable and positive experience for the dying child and all family members. Primary benefits include the freedom for family and friends to visit at any time, less disruption to family life, ability to cater to the child's unique needs (e.g., dietary preferences), and allowing more family members to participate in the child's care and be present at the time of death. Challenges that remain when the child is at home are ensuring adequate symptom management; ensuring availability of professional support at all times of the day; watching the child physically decline; and managing the fatigue, loneliness, and fears of both the patient and family members (Collins et al., 1998; Kopecky et al., 1997; Liben & Goldman, 1998).

Kopecky et al. (1997) reviewed a home-based palliative care program for children. The sample consisted of 126 children referred from a variety of clinical areas. Of the 93 children who died, 53% died at home, 18% died in community hospitals, and 29% died in tertiary care centers. Children in the home-based program experienced fewer hospital readmissions, with an average of 80% of the child's surviving days spent at home. Additionally, when adequate support for families was in place, there were few calls and pages initiated by the patient's families. Family support in the program was offered via home visits, regular telephone calls, and a pager. The authors concluded that the home-based palliative program was effective for many children in providing adequate support to the children and their families by the team of health professionals.

Hospice Care

Another option for children who are approaching death is enrollment in a pediatric hospice program. Hospice programs all subscribe to similar standards and practices. Traditionally, the child must be in the terminal phase of illness, usually with death expected in the ensuing 4 to 6 months, and the child and family must have decided to forgo any further treatments or diagnostic efforts to sustain life. However, these standards are perceived as a barrier to access pediatric hospice services, and many states are challenging the hospice enrollment standards and are forging ahead with legislation to improve pediatric access to hospice services that removes or minimizes these barriers. In many cases of children with a chronic condition, it is impossible to determine whether or when the child is within 4 to 6 months of dying. Furthermore, the child may need ongoing treatments to sustain life even during the dying process. For example, the child with cancer may need chemotherapy or radiation even during the last months of his or her life to decrease the uncomfortable growth of a tumor and this is considered to be part of palliative care.

The initial visit of the hospice worker is usually made within 24 hours of the referral because the family's needs are usually acute and the child might be close to death. The essential components of hospice care include assistance with pain and symptom control, support for children and families, and education about the physiologic processes of death. The site where hospice services are delivered and the scope of services provided differ from hospice to hospice and even from family to family.

Many children enrolled in hospice are cared for at home. The hospice staff helps the child and family deal with pain, manage symptoms, and maintain nutrition; they do anything needed to promote the comfort of the child. Emotional support for the entire family is an essential component of hospice care both before and after the child's death. Although nurses are often in the home at the time of the death, many families choose not to call the nurse until after the death so that the family can be alone with the child. Most hospice programs continue to support the family after the child's death because the acute stage of grief can extend for 2 years after the child's death.

In some cases, the child needs to be admitted to an *inpatient hospice*. Inpatient hospice units meet the needs of families who cannot provide care in the home when the child is not a candidate for admission to an acute care or rehabilitative setting. The inpatient hospice can address the psychological and physical needs of children and their families while providing the excellent nursing and medical care needed.

ANSWER: One of the unique benefits of hospice care is the psychological support offered to the patient and family as well as the extended support that the Tran family can receive after George's death.

Respite Care

Although families are better able to maintain control and life is less disrupted when dying children are cared for at home, the family still experience stress as a result of the illness, the child's care, and their own fatigue. **Respite care** allows the family to leave the child with the assistance of a home health aide or hospice volunteer (see Chapter 12). Respite care can also be a part of the hospice program or a separate program offered to the family (Horsburgh et al., 2002). Care of these children is complex and time-consuming; respite care offers caregivers a specified period of time to seek rest and refreshment. With respite care, family members can continue to work and participate in activities that the dying child cannot attend.

Such services are provided with different options based on the family's needs. Some families report needing short-term breaks (a few hours or part of a day). Night care also may be needed to provide family members the ability to get sufficient rest. Away-from-home respite care may include nursing and symptom management for periods of several days or a week or more. Such services allow families to have vacations without the sick child. Emergency respite is also needed when a crisis occurs at the home.

GRIEF AND BEREAVEMENT

Grief is the painful, sad, and anguished feeling accompanying loss. Grief is usually thought of as a reaction to the death of a loved one; however, other losses, such as the loss of an object (e.g., long-term home), a relationship (e.g., divorce), or anything—tangible or intangible—that is highly valued, can result in a grief reaction. A family eagerly anticipating the birth of their healthy newborn will experience grief and bereavement if the child is premature, stillborn, or born with a congenital abnormality or serious illness. The unanticipated diagnosis of leukemia or diabetes in a previously healthy teenager elicits grief within the family and for the afflicted child. When grief from any type of loss is unresolved, it can reappear during an attempt to resolve the grief associated with a later loss. There are many types of grief that have different characteristics, manifestations, and responses. The nurse should be able to identify the type of grief and implement appropriate interventions based on the exhibited behaviors. Table 13-1 explains the types of grief and characteristics associated with each type.

When a person significant to a family has died, each member of the family is in need of immediate help and assistance. If family members have the needed knowledge and coping mechanisms, then immediate help assists them until their resources can be mobilized. For family members without needed resources, the nurse's role is one of educator and support person as the family is helped to move through the bereavement process to life without the loved one.

Bereavement, often called *mourning*, is the mental work following the loss, which allows adaptation to that loss. The care of the child and family facing death

TABLE 13-1   Types of Grief

Type of Grief	Definition	Characteristics
Anticipatory grief (Rando, 2000)	Anticipated and real losses associated with diagnosis, acute and chronic illnesses, and terminal illness. Experiencing anticipatory grief may provide time for preparation of loss, acceptance of loss, finishing unfinished business, life review, and resolving conflicts. For survivor, anticipatory grief provides time for preparing for life without the deceased, including preparation for role change, mastering life skills such as paying bills, and learning how to manage a checkbook.	With acute illness, chronic illness, accidents, and other changes in health, a patient may experience loss of general health, loss of functionality, loss of independence, loss of role in the family (breadwinner, caretaker), and loss of lifestyle as a result of dietary or activity restrictions. Loss of a limb or body part (breast, uterus) may cause loss of self-confidence and changes in perception about body image. Family members and significant others will also experience losses when patient is ill, including loss of role in the family, loss of relationship, loss of finances, loss of security, loss of companionship, loss of relationship, etc. AIDS can cause multiple losses over short periods of time, such as loss of a job, material possessions, body image due to changes in physical appearance, functionality, privacy (the secret is out), friends, partners, and social acceptance. With diagnosis of terminal illness, additional losses may include loss of control (choice), loss of physical and/or mental function, loss of relationships, loss of body image, loss of future, loss of dignity, or loss of life.
Uncomplicated grief	Also known as "normal" grief. Typical feelings, reactions and behaviors to a loss; grief reactions can be physical, psychological, cognitive, or behavioral. Children mourn or grieve based on their developmental level (Doka, 1989; Parkes & Prigerson, 2009; Worden, 2009).	Reactions to loss can be physical, psychological, and cognitive. Symptoms of grief in younger children: • Nervousness • Uncontrollable rages • Frequent sickness • Accident proneness • Antisocial behavior • Rebellious behavior • Hyperactivity • Nightmares • Depression • Compulsive behavior • Memories fading in and out • Excessive anger • Excessive dependency on remaining parent • Recurring dreams . . . wish-filling, denial, disguised Symptoms of grief in older children: • Difficulty in concentrating • Forgetfulness • Poor schoolwork • Insomnia or sleeping too much • Reclusiveness or social withdrawal • Antisocial behavior • Resentment of authority • Overdependence, regression • Resistance to discipline • Talk of or attempted suicide • Nightmares, symbolic dreams • Frequent sickness • Accident proneness • Overeating or undereating • Truancy • Experimentation with alcohol/drugs • Depression • Secretiveness • Sexual promiscuity • Staying away or running away from home • Compulsive behavior

TABLE 13-1　Types of Grief (*Continued*)

Type of Grief	Definition	Characteristics
Complicated grief includes		Those at risk for any of the four types of complicated grief may have experienced loss associated with • Traumatic death • Sudden, unexpected death such as heart attacks, accidents • Suicide • Homicide • Dependent relationship with deceased • Old-old person or those with chronic illnesses (survivor may have difficulty believing death actually occurred after years of remissions and exacerbations) • Death of a child • Multiple losses • Unresolved grief from prior losses • Concurrent stressor (the loss plus other stresses in life such as divorce, a move, children leaving home, other ill family members, financial issues, etc.). • History of mental illness or substance abuse • Patient's dying process was difficult including poor pain and symptom management, psychosocial and/or spiritual suffering • Poor or few support systems • No faith system, cultural traditions, religious beliefs
Chronic grief	Uncomplicated grief reactions that do not subside and continue over very long periods of time.	
Delayed grief	Uncomplicated grief reactions that are suppressed or postponed. The survivor consciously or unconsciously avoids the pain of the loss.	
Exaggerated grief	Survivor resorts to self-destructive behaviors such as suicide.	
Masked grief (Brown-Saltzman, 2006; Corless, 2010; Loney, 1998; Parkes & Prigerson, 2009; Worden, 2009)	The survivor is not aware that behaviors that interfere with normal functioning are a result of the loss.	Complicated grief reactions can include any of the normal grief reactions, but the reactions may be intensified; prolonged; last more than a year; and/or interfere with the person's psychological, social, and physiological functioning. Other complicated grief reactions may include • Severe isolation • Violent behavior • Suicidal ideation • Workaholic behavior • Severe deterioration of functional status • Symptoms of posttraumatic stress disorder • Denial beyond normal expectation • Severe or prolonged depression • Loss of interest in health and/or personal care • Severe impairment in communication, thought or motor skills • Ongoing inability to eat or sleep • Replacing loss and relationship quickly • Social withdrawal • Searching and calling out for deceased • Avoidance of reminders of the deceased • Imitating the deceased Survivors experiencing complicated grief should be referred to a grief and bereavement specialist/counselor.
Disenfranchised grief (Doka, 2002)	The grief encountered when a loss is experienced and cannot be openly acknowledged, socially sanctioned, or publicly shared. Usually, the survivor experiencing disenfranchised grief is not recognized by employers for time off for funeral/memorial service or grief; may not be recognized by biological family members and excluded from rites, rituals, and traditions for loss.	Those at risk for experiencing disenfranchised grief include partners of HIV/AIDS patients, ex-spouses, ex-partners, fiancés, friends, lovers, mistresses, coworkers, and children experiencing the death of a step-parent and others persons close to the patient but not biologic family members. The mother of a stillborn delivery may also experience disenfranchised grief because society may not acknowledge a relationship between the mother and a child who experienced death prior to birth.

From American Association of Colleges of Nursing & City of Hope National Medical Center. (2012). *End-of-life nursing education consortium-pediatric palliative care (ELNEC-PPC) faculty guide*. Duarte, CA: City of Hope. Reprinted with permission.

is not simple. Mourning is typically thought of as the outward social expression of the loss and may be dictated by cultural norms and rituals as well as the individual's personality and life experiences. Anticipatory mourning is the process of emotional preparation leading up to the time of death (Rini & Loriz, 2007). Anticipatory mourning allows family members time to begin grief work prior to the actual death of the loved one.

The death of a child affects not only the individual family members but also the family unit as a whole. Adults helping children must deal with their own grief and need to mourn while helping the child do the same. The child may be the one who is dying, or the child may be a sibling or friend of a child who has died. The loved one whom the child loses through death can be a grandparent, parent, sibling, other family member, or a friend. For the child, resolution of the experience of the loss of a loved one involves both progression through the bereavement process and achievement of normal developmental milestones. The role of the nurse includes facilitating the grieving process by assessing grief and assisting survivors to acknowledge the loss by expressing grief in their own way (Fig. 13-8).

GRIEF RESPONSES

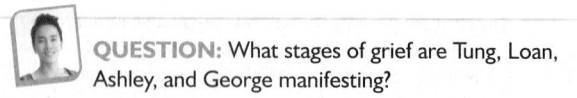

QUESTION: What stages of grief are Tung, Loan, Ashley, and George manifesting?

Grief caused by the potential or actual loss of a loved one or by an anticipated outcome results in both physiologic and emotional responses. Physiologic symptoms include waves of physical distress, such as shortness of breath, an empty feeling in the stomach or heart, physical weakness, and a loss of appetite. An inability to concentrate or sleep, a general sense of unreality, and a need to withdraw from others is also common.

Kübler-Ross (1969) described five common responses to death or anticipated death: denial and isolation, anger, bargaining, depression, and acceptance. These stages of grief or reactions to mourning explain the coping mechanisms people use to deal with losses. Although Kübler-Ross presented these mechanisms as sequential reactions, they actually occur more randomly, with individuals moving among the reactions before achieving full resolution. Not all persons experience each reaction.

Denial and Isolation

Denial and isolation are common responses to bad news, loss, or death. Denial can be overt, such as when a parent says, "The doctor told us Sammy has a very bad head injury, but with all these new machines, he will be back at school in no time." Signs of denial can also be more subtle, such as when the family attempts to go on with life as usual with no adaptation for essential disease care. At times, the denial takes the form of psychological isolation. In this case, the child or parent is able to talk about the illness or the potential or actual death, with no emotion or acknowledgment of what the death will mean.

Denial can be therapeutic if it allows individuals to distance themselves from the trauma of the diagnosis or death itself to activate coping mechanisms or to reach out for help. Prolonged denial, however, can cause missed opportunities for needed emotional care, for actual disease treatment, or for amelioration of negative symptoms.

Anger

The reaction of anger can be quite pronounced. Often, the trigger for this reaction is the loss of the person who is dying or who has died, but anger can also be triggered by the loss of the expected future. It is not unusual for displaced anger to be directed at persons who have no role or culpability in the death or loss. These persons can be health care workers, family members, friends, or anyone with whom the grieving individual interacts. Anger can be directed at family members whose children are alive and thriving, at health care providers, or at a higher power such as God. The anger can also be self-directed because of actual or perceived personal failure in preventing the loss from occurring.

caREminder

Do not take the anger of a grieving person personally. Address specific issues and correct patient care concerns if possible. Allow the angry person time to overcome this reaction and to move on in his or her grieving process.

By not overreacting to the angry person, the nurse allows continued development of the therapeutic relationship that the person needs to complete the grieving and bereavement process. To help prevent disruption of

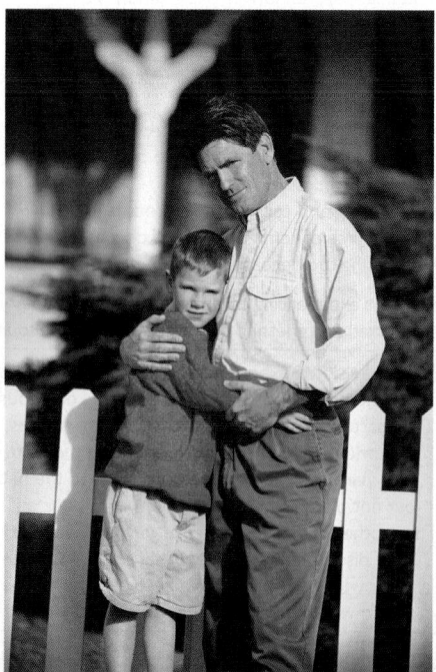

Figure 13-8 There is no script for grief and bereavement. Each family member responds to the loss of a loved one in unique way.

family relationships, teach family members that anger is a normal part of the grief reaction.

Bargaining

In bargaining, the grieving person offers some action, perhaps to a higher being, in exchange for a cure or the return of the loved one. Promising good behavior, returning to active participation in religious activities, and offering to support a special cause are all examples of bargaining. A major component of bargaining is the maintenance of hope.

Bargaining can be therapeutic and may actually help the person look to the future even when that future is not clear. On the other hand, bargaining can cause individuals to seek out alternative but ineffective treatments "just in case" they might work. These can be physically, emotionally, and financially draining on the family and may delay use of traditional, but not so promising, approaches to care.

Depression

Depression can be based on both current and prior losses as well as an anticipation of losses to come. The depressed person may be dealing with a chronic or acute illness in the family, coping with his or her own impending death, or preparing for the loss of a loved one who is dying. Expressing underlying fears and concerns helps the grieving individual move beyond the depression. Accept and support this behavior. Attempts to cheer the person up discount the real concerns and issues that the depressed person is trying to deal with.

Acceptance

Acceptance or resolution of the fact that the loss will occur or has occurred is necessary for the grieving person to move on with life. Acceptance helps the dying person peacefully move on to death. For the family of a child with an unexpected illness, acceptance helps them incorporate the diagnosis and all associated health care needs into their lifestyle and routine. This does not mean family members will no longer experience anger, isolation, bargaining, or depression as the child's condition vacillates between periods of calm and periods of exacerbation. Acceptance, in the face of impending or eventual loss, means the person can see past the current and perceive what the future will bring even if it is a future without the one they love.

ANSWER: Tung appears to be in denial, as evidenced by his statement regarding George getting well. We do not have much information on which to base the assessment of Loan, but her experience with her brother and the day-to-day care she provides George lead us to believe she is in the accepting stage of grief. Ashley is still wishing that she could take her brother's place—she is in the bargaining stage of grief. George has stated that he is dying and he is making plans for his own death. He also appears to be in the acceptance stage.

BEREAVEMENT TASKS

The grief process is rarely orderly and predictable; it typically includes a series of tasks that the survivor engages in, often referred to as *grief work* (Lindemann, 1994). Rando (2000) suggests that a person must complete six bereavement tasks, and that the process of working through these tasks facilitates adjustment to the loss. These tasks are

1. Recognizing the loss
2. Reacting to the separation
3. Recollecting and reexperiencing the deceased and the relationship
4. Relinquishing old attachments to the deceased and to the shared world
5. Readjusting to allow movement into a new world without the loved one but without forgetting the old world
6. Reinvesting in the new world

Recognizing the Loss

In recognizing the loss, a person accepts the reality of the loss. Families of a child with a chronic illness, congenital defect, or disfigurement must accept the reality that their child will not be like other children. For the family of a dying child, they must accept that their child will not recover or return and that the child will not be a part of their lives again (Rando, 2000).

During this task, ill, disabled, or disfigured children recognize that they are different from their peers. The child's level of cognitive understanding affects this perception of the loss. The dying child needs to understand what it means to be dead and what causes a person to die. Ask the child about his or her observations so that misconceptions can be corrected. Have these discussions occur as soon as possible after the diagnosis, death, or loss to avoid missed opportunities to talk and to avoid sending the message that the loss is not to be discussed. Often, the challenge is not to get the child to talk but to be sure that, when the child wants to talk, someone is there to listen.

Reacting to the Separation

Reaction to the separation has been described as experiencing pain. The grieving person must feel, identify, accept, and express the psychological reactions to the loss (Rando, 2000). This can bring out intense and painful feelings.

There is also a need to identify and mourn secondary losses that occurred with the primary loss (Rando, 2000). For the parents whose child has died, this can mean loss of the socialization they enjoyed when they served as class parents in their child's school. For the boy whose father died, this might mean there is no one to take him on the father–son camping trip. An illness can separate a child from peers and family, with frequent exacerbations of the illness and hospitalizations curtailing previously enjoyed activities.

Often, a child displays aggression, sadness, anger, or other strong emotional reactions. Address these reactions when they occur, and discuss appropriate methods to express the emotions. Most important, determine the source of the emotional reaction. Strong emotional responses frequently result from unexpressed fears and concerns or from a misunderstanding of the relationship between events.

Recollecting and Reexperiencing the Deceased and the Relationship

The next task is to review and remember realistically the relationship with the person who died or to remember how relationships were before the onset of illness or other loss. This often involves reviving and reexperiencing the feelings that come with these memories. This process allows the grieving person to acknowledge both the good memories and the unpleasant ones and prevents memorializing the person as a saint when it is not warranted (Rando, 2000). For the parents of a child who dies, this can mean realizing that the child made them angry, too, and that the surviving sibling is not their only child who could be difficult. For a child, it might mean acknowledging that not everything an older sibling did was good and that not all of the older child's behaviors should be emulated.

In cases of loss in which severe dysfunction or death of a child occurs, the sibling survivor might take on roles and attributes of the affected child. These roles can be positive, such as taking on the love of a sport, or negative, such as taking on the physical symptoms of the child's illness or a love of the reckless driving that led to the accident or subsequent death. The sibling might want to keep possessions and pictures of the affected child (when healthy) and should be given the opportunity to choose these items. The sibling might also reenact rituals or events that were a part of the previous life with the loved one. Allow the child to do so, but also address the feelings behind these activities to help the child acknowledge and deal with them.

Relinquishing Old Attachments

To go on with life without the deceased child, or with the child in an altered state and appearance, the grieving individual must give up his or her ties to the world they shared. This does not mean that he or she must dramatically change his or her life, but it does mean that he or she must acknowledge that the child is no longer a part of his or her life or that the future will be different from the one they *would* have shared (Rando, 2000). For the parents, it can mean recognizing that life no longer revolves around the activities shared with the child. For a child, it might mean accepting that the loved one will not be the person who will provide help and support as the child moves into adulthood and begins to raise a family.

Readjusting

Bereaved persons must begin to move into a new reality in which the deceased person does not have an active part (Rando, 2000). The family of a child who died might plan a vacation in the middle of the school year. A child whose best friend died of complications of cystic fibrosis might join the soccer team even though they made a pact not to do things that they could not both participate in. At the same time, treasured traditions shared with the now deceased child may be continued among other family members. Pictures of the child remain on the wall, with new photos added of current events and the family members who participated in those special moments.

Reinvesting in the New World

An active reinvestment in the new world without the loved one, or with the loved one's new limitations, is the final step. It is not enough to simply move on; the person must become involved in the world again (Rando, 2000). Parents might begin planning for other children who are wanted for themselves, not as replacements for the child who has died or who is severely ill. Siblings must continue normal physical and emotional development. A young child needs to develop autonomy and increased physical abilities, such as bladder and bowel control. The school-aged child needs to increase participation in activities in school and with peers. Continued achievement in school and other activities is also important. The adolescent needs to begin to differentiate from the family even if the death of a family member has drawn the adolescent into new and closer attachments to family members.

The time for the completion of the bereavement process is much longer than was once thought. For most individuals, the time period is 18 months. When a child has died, the time can be even longer. It is not unusual for a family member to have a resurgence of the grief reaction at certain trigger points long after the date of a death, such as when the child would have been starting high school or a first job. Grieving persons must be prepared for the occurrence of these feelings and must be helped to understand that the feelings are normal. Healing takes time and cannot be rushed.

Complicated Bereavement

Anyone who experiences a loss or the death of a loved one is at risk for dysfunctional or complicated bereavement. Complicated bereavement is present if, since the time of the loss or death, there is some compromise, distortion, or failure of one or more of the six tasks of bereavement. Such individuals are unable to accept the loss, experience the pain, or move on to a life that is different. Such mourners often try to deny, repress, or avoid aspects of the loss, including the step of relinquishing the relationship with the deceased child or other loved one (Rando, 2000).

Family members are at high risk for complicated bereavement. Individuals are also at risk if the loss was sudden or unexpected or if the relationship with the child or other family members was characterized by anger, ambivalence, or dependency. Other risk factors for complicated bereavement occur when losses are perceived as preventable, there are unaddressed loss issues from the past, there are mental health problems, or the mourner perceives a lack of support. Although research verifies that support groups may be of assistance to such individuals (Heiney et al., 1995), referral for mental health counseling might be needed for persons experiencing dysfunctional bereavement.

BEREAVEMENT RESPONSES OF THE DYING CHILD

Children who are dying react to their impending death in a multitude of ways, usually based on their cognitive and developmental level. They will have a wide range of feelings, which might include regression, anger, sadness, loneliness, isolation, and fear. Frequently, children will have wisdom beyond their years related to perceiving the seriousness of their illness and possibility of death, which might seem at times to be broader than their parents' understanding and acceptance (Davies, Limbo et al., 2010). In 1978, Bluebond-Langner published a study, the results of which remain valid in today's society. The study demonstrated how dying children became aware of their own impending death. She defined five stages of awareness:

1. The child interprets the parents' behavior as being different from when he or she has a simple illness, leading the child to the understanding that there is something seriously wrong.
2. The child sees family members crying, becomes used to the hospital, perceives that he or she is receiving special treatment, and learns about the disease and its implications.
3. The child has more knowledge about the waxing and waning of the illness as well as the purposes and implications of the treatment.
4. The child is increasingly aware of his or her differences from healthy peers and starts accepting that the disease is a permanent condition.
5. The child knows the limitations of medical care and prepares for impending death (Bluebond-Langner, 1978).

BEREAVEMENT RESPONSES WHEN A PARENT LOSES A CHILD

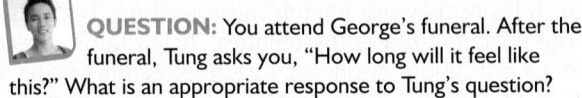

QUESTION: You attend George's funeral. After the funeral, Tung asks you, "How long will it feel like this?" What is an appropriate response to Tung's question?

The death of a child is one of the most difficult experiences that a parent can face. The child whose parent has died loses a part of his or her past, but the parent whose child has died loses a part of his or her future. Successful bereavement is facilitated when family members are helped to recognize that they will each mourn differently. Individual parents might progress through grieving differently. They might vary in both degree and display of response and speed with which they achieve resolution. Individual reactions change over time. Each person comes to the end of the acute grief reaction at a different point during the ensuing 1 to 2 years.

For some parents, the death of a child is a time of great personal growth accompanied by immeasurable pain. For others, it is a time of overwhelming sadness that does not remit for years, if ever. The time and pattern of the bereavement process for the grieving parent is much longer than for bereavement from other losses, and often there is never full resolution of the grief. With skilled care by the entire health care team, however, the parent can be helped to successfully complete the bereavement process and move on to a life without the child (Armstrong-Dailey & Zarbock, 2009; Kachoyeanos & Selder, 1993).

Although each parent reacts to the death of the child in a unique way, several patterns are seen. Parents who had ambivalent relationships with their child or were unable to help their child in the time before death report more problems with bereavement than those who had a good relationship and were able to support the child at the time of death. Parents whose child died after a chronic illness have less acute responses than those whose child died after an accident or brief illness. The ability to clearly identify the cause of death also helps parents in their time of grief. Parents who are with their child at the time of death or who see their child soon after the death are better able to realize that the child is dead. Such visits also reduce concerns about the nature and extent of the damage to the child's body and decreases fantasies about the child's death (e.g., the hope that the child is not in fact dead and will someday reappear) (Kachoyeanos & Selder, 1993).

Parental responses to the death of their child continue long after the usual 1- or 2-year grieving period common with the death of friends, grandparents, or parents when the child is an adult. Parents must undergo a life transition as they move from the old reality to a new reality: from life with their child to life after their child's death. This transition process is characterized by a sense of uncertainty and a variety of trigger events (Kachoyeanos & Selder, 1993).

Trigger events reinforce the fact that the parent's reality has changed. The first trigger event is the actual death of the child. At this time, the parents must accept the irrevocability of the death. Trigger events continue long after the child's death. Doing something that was previously done with the child, passing the site of the accident where the child died, or hearing music that the child liked are examples of events that can reactivate memories of the child and feelings about the child's death. The reality of the child's death is reinforced when special dates such as birthdays or family holidays occur. These dates can be used as special occasions to remember the child. The dates might also have been times when developmental achievements (e.g., beginning to walk, joining the Girl Scouts, graduation, marriage, or birth of a grandchild) would have taken place. Triggers are experienced by parents regardless of how old the child was at death or how much time has elapsed since the child's death (Kachoyeanos & Selder, 1993).

Parents need to structure a new reality after the child's death. This effort is apparent in many of their actions. Parents often compare themselves with others in judging how well they are doing. Talking with other parents who have lost a child and participating in support groups help the parents learn that their reactions are normal. These activities help parents learn strategies for coping with their pain and the challenges they face. They learn that they will emerge from the period of deep and painful grief (Kachoyeanos & Selder, 1993).

A frequent concern from parents is the need for reassurance that they were good parents. They may overtly ask whether they provided good care to the child or brought the child for treatment at the right time. Others seek affirmation of their parenting skills indirectly by listening to comments of those who cared for their child. Thus, a random remark while looking at pictures of the child such as "Aren't those pajamas pretty" can provide positive feedback, whereas a simple statement such as "Look at how messy that bib was" can be interpreted as a negative evaluation of the parents' ability to meet even the most basic hygienic need of their child.

Parents often have a strong desire to return to the "normal" world they knew before the child's death (Kachoyeanos & Selder, 1993). This desire might lead the parent to engage in an activity, such as suddenly taking a family vacation to a theme park with the other children, which appears inappropriate in light of the recent death. Often, such activities are undertaken with the hope that they will make the negative and painful emotions dissipate. This rarely happens.

There could be fears by the parents that they or other family members might forget the child or how the child looked when well. As a result, they engage in "presencing" by looking at pictures or videotapes in which the child appears and keeping the child's possessions for months, sometimes years. When the possessions are given away, they are given away to someone meaningful. Although keeping the possessions intact permanently might be a sign of dysfunctional grief, it is generally better for the parents to delay dismantling the child's room and disposing of the child's possessions for several months (Kachoyeanos & Selder, 1993). This allows them time to thoughtfully decide what they want to keep and what they want to give away.

ANSWER: There are many therapeutic answers. We cannot guess how long George's father will feel intense grief. Platitudes are not acceptable. One example of an appropriate response is to acknowledge his grief and say, "I can only imagine how much it must hurt."

BEREAVEMENT RESPONSES WHEN A CHILD LOSES A LOVED ONE

Children do not need to have a loved one die or to experience a great loss themselves to learn to cope with grief. As children see grief and loss around them, discuss these issues with them. This prevents development of the belief that discussion of grief and death is taboo. The loss of a pet can be a powerful learning experience. If a pet runs away, the child can be encouraged to discuss feelings about the missing animal. If the pet dies, this is a chance for the child to talk about how the pet died, why it died, and how that death makes both the adult and child feel. The child can also be introduced to the rituals that the family's culture uses to say good-bye to a dead loved one and to express grief and sadness.

Discuss causes of loss honestly, with both internal and external causes acknowledged. When the cause of a death is unknown, this uncertainty can be stated. Flowery analogies or stories may only confuse the child.

In the case of suicide, saying that the person had an illness that affected his or her thinking, causing the person to end his or her life, is a better explanation than saying that the person was unhappy or disappointed with life. For the child who was a significant part of the suicide victim's life, this explanation helps alleviate misconceptions, especially if the child thinks he or she was a cause of the person's unhappiness.

After a death, some changes in the child's life are inevitable. Behavior of adults around the child changes as they grieve. The child's daily routine may change during the acute phase surrounding the death and the funeral and because of the absence of the loved one. Help family members understand how important it is to have as few additional changes around the time of the death as possible. A safe, familiar environment and routine are essential for the child during the bereavement period. Avoid unnecessary changes in the child's daily life (e.g., changing sleeping arrangements; place of residence; and degree of contact with remaining family members, school, or daycare center).

Even the most skillful and sensitive care does not guarantee that each child will have a smooth progression through the bereavement process. However, when the child's needs and reactions are recognized and addressed, the child has the opportunity to successfully navigate the painful time after the death.

To deal with the powerful reactions experienced after the death of a loved one or the grief associated with an unexpected personal loss, children must learn to deal with strong feelings such as longing, anger, sadness, and confusion. When children display behaviors that indicate they are having these feelings, regardless of the reason, address the feelings. Teach family members to not ignore strong or negative feelings or to do things to take the child's mind off the feelings. This approach does not make the feelings, or the events that caused them, go away. When well-meaning adults seek to protect the child in this way, they deny the child the opportunity to acknowledge and then learn to cope with feelings and fears. Acknowledging strong and unpleasant feelings and helping the child work through those feelings lets the child know that the feelings are normal. The child will also develop the core skills needed to deal with such emotions throughout life.

Even very young children are aware when someone around them has died. The child senses and observes the changes without being told. All children need an opportunity to discuss the emotions that accompany their grief and to learn about the ramifications of a particular death on themselves and their family.

> **KidKare** Focus discussions about death on the child's specific questions and what is behind those questions. Exhaustive explanations and teaching sessions are usually not appropriate.

Discussions about what happens to the body after death can benefit even young children. If the child asks or indicates a desire to go to the funeral, if at all possible, grant this request. Throughout the service, ensure the child is accompanied by a trusted adult who can control his or her own grief to serve as a resource and support for the child.

> **KidKare** Give details to the child about what will happen and what will be seen at the funeral or wake. If there will be a coffin, prepare the child for how the coffin looks. If the coffin is going to be open, it is important to prepare the child for seeing the dead person. Explain that the dead person may be dressed in their favorite clothes and will look like they are asleep and, often, there might be items such as toys, books, flowers, etc., in the coffin with them. Tell the child that people might cry and be upset because they are sad that the person has died. If the child goes to the cemetery, explain to the child that the coffin might be placed in the ground and dirt shoveled in to cover it. Assure the child that it is all right if he or she wants to leave at any time during the ceremony.

Death of a Parent

A child whose parent has died needs special attention (Sutter & Reid, 2012). Because of the unique bond between the child and parent, particularly the infant and mother, the death of a parent results in both loss of self (the part that was bound to the parent) and loss of other (the parent who died). The remaining parent and other family members are also grieving, making it hard for them to meet the child's needs for consistent support and attachment. The child might worry that the surviving parent will die, too. The loss of a parent is difficult for the child. Adults often have several significant persons in their life with whom they form attachments; however, a child usually has only two significant attachments: those to each parent. The parent meets the child's physiologic and emotional needs and gradually helps the child meet those needs independently. When a parent dies, someone else must take over the missing parent's role, be it the other parent or someone else. Infants and young children need immediate and consistent replacement of this primary caregiver role.

Activities shared with the dead parent might no longer be enjoyed. For the infant or young child, this can be eating or the development of new abilities like smiling, rolling over, or toilet training. Young children

who cannot express themselves verbally may display emotions through play or other behaviors. For the older child, activities that they may have shared with the deceased parent might include assistance with homework, attending sports activities, going to the movies, or participating in special school events. The child, regardless of age, may exhibit regressive behavior for a short time. In some cases, problems might not be evident initially; they may occur at the beginning of the next developmental phase, such as the progression from school age to adolescence.

Death of a Grandparent

Depending on their relationship, involvement, and frequency of contact with the child, death of a grandparent might elicit many of the same behaviors associated with the death of a parent. In some cases, the grandparent may have been the primary caregiver of the child. In other cases, grandparents may have a lesser role in the day-to-day family constellation. In all cases, it is important to acknowledge the grandparent's death with the child and determine the child's understanding of the causes of the death and the degree to which they are feeling the loss.

Death of a Sibling

> **QUESTION:** Review Nursing Interventions 13-3. What interventions would you incorporate into a plan of care for Ashley following her brother's death?

Siblings of the deceased child need care based on their age, developmental stage, and relationship with their sibling. Do not protect siblings from all information about the child's illness or give them evasive answers to their questions about the death. During the past few years, there has been a dramatic improvement in the emotional health of siblings of children who have died. These positive changes have been attributed to alterations in how death is dealt with in American society. Death is spoken of more openly than it once was, and care for the siblings is integrated into plans of care.

Siblings of deceased children experience stress as the result of the death. This stress can impact the child's relationship with peers, making him or her more vulnerable to social difficulties in school and other community settings (Gerhardt et al., 2012). If the child was ill before the death, this stress is compounded by the changes in family structure and environment as a result of the illness. This stress can be effectively managed if the siblings are given the help and support they need during and after the acute phase of grief. Siblings need to grieve, to say good-bye. Outdoor activities, yelling, singing, play therapy, support groups, and art therapy may help the grieving child. A multidimensional home care program that addresses physical, emotional, and other needs of the family during the terminal phase of an illness is also beneficial (Fig. 13-9). Teach family members about the needs of the siblings and ways to

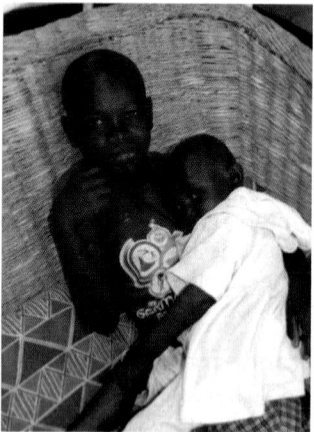

Figure 13-9 Dying at home allows siblings an opportunity to be together, sharing laughter and building memories.

help them progress through the bereavement process (Nursing Interventions 13-3).

Assure family members that the child who died was unique and their remaining children cannot, and should not, take over the life of that child. Neither current nor future children should be made into "replacement" children to compensate for the lost child. Replacement children are given the burden of assuming their own identity as well as that of the dead child.

Family members need help to understand how their actions and the home environment can positively or negatively affect the future self-concept and emotional health of surviving siblings. Children who demonstrate a positive self-concept have been made to feel special and are reported as being highly competent. Children who experience low self-concept report that they feel that they do not compare favorably with the deceased child or that another child has displaced them.

Physical and somatic complaints by siblings are not uncommon. Siblings might be frustrated at their inability to change what is happening or have feelings of guilt and anger. Often, they are living in a household of sorrow and may feel responsible for the event or think that if they had died, the parents would not be as sad. Many times, parents are so preoccupied with the care of the dying child or with their own grief that they overlook the healthy siblings. All siblings need to feel like important members of the family and need a

---

NURSING INTERVENTIONS 13-3

Helping Siblings Grieve

- Teach the sibling about the normal emotions that accompany grief and bereavement:
  - Help the sibling identify and express feelings about the child who has died.
  - Let the sibling know that feeling sad, angry, or scared is okay for adults and for children, and that crying is okay (even for boys).
  - Assess what the sibling knows and wants to know about the child's death, and provide necessary teaching.
  - Involve siblings in family discussions about the dying child and after the child's death.
  - Encourage siblings to express their feelings and thoughts in their own way through discussion, writing letters, poetry, or art.
  - Share your own memories and feelings with the sibling.
  - Allow laughter and fun times, which can occur even in the midst of great sadness.
  - Decrease the sense of abandonment by being with the sibling both physically and emotionally.
  - Consider whether the sibling relationship was positive or negative and how that has affected grieving.
  - Use physical touch as a way of reassuring and comforting the sibling.

- Reassure the sibling that it is not likely that anyone else (particularly the parents) will also die within the near future.
  - Look for evidence that the sibling is protecting other family members (e.g., by not telling them his or her fears and concerns or trying to lessen the grief of others).
- Promote normalcy in the sibling's life and routines:
  - Continue to expect the sibling to have responsibilities at home and at school.
  - Encourage the sibling's involvement with friends and peers.
  - Be aware that, if other children are added to the family at some point in time (e.g., by adoption or birth), the sibling of the child who died may feel displaced by the new addition.
- Educate family members not to
  - Give any indication that the surviving child is not "as good" as the deceased sibling
  - Indicate that the surviving child is in any way responsible for the sibling's death
  - Express a preference for or wish to have a child who, in some way (e.g., gender, ability), is like the child who died
  - Display a preference for the deceased child by comments or comparisons

responsible and caring adult to help them cope with their grief and loss.

> ANSWER: Although Ashley is cognitively an adult in her understanding of death, she will probably need continued support. Teaching her the normal emotions that accompany grief and bereavement is important. Ashley's family and culture are very stoic. She may wonder if she is the only one feeling this way or if something is wrong with her because of the intensity of her grief. It will be important for Ashley to develop new routines and a new focus. She will be graduating from high school soon; it is hoped that this can be a focus for her and her parents. Ashley, because of her experience with depression, has an established relationship with a counselor. She also has supportive relationships with the school nurse and some of her high school teachers.

Death of a Friend

Children might face death in the ranks of their peers, school staff, family, or community. The cause is often acute or chronic illness, but increasing numbers of children are exposed to death as a result of violence. Schools need to include content about death and dying in the school curriculum and have a crisis plan that can be activated quickly after a death in the school community. The school nurse plays a significant role in the development and implementation of a death education curriculum and crisis plans.

Implement educational programs about the facts of death; recognizing depression; understanding grief; and fostering effective communication between child and teacher, child and child, and child and family. Include in the discussion how to interact with a bereaved student who is returning to school, how to accept and address his or her grief, and the importance of resuming a normal relationship. Teach staff and students how to recognize students who are grieving or who are at risk for suicide. Provide detailed information on ways to help those individuals obtain assistance.

ALERT *Emphasize with students that when a friend talks about taking his or her own life, or the life of others, it is essential to share this information with a counselor, teacher, or some other trusted adult. In this case, getting the friend help is more important than keeping a secret.*

The school crisis plan should detail all needed steps from the notification of student, faculty, and staff about the death to the implementation of long-term support services. The crisis plan should be flexible enough to be used if the person who died is a student, faculty, or staff member or significant person in the community and whether death is from illness, suicide, or violence.

Policies about holding memorial services on campus and student attendance at funeral services on school

days should be developed. The plan would also include a detailed plan about how the students' and staff's emotional needs will be met on both an acute and long-term basis. A training program for staff and teachers for both the acute event and residual problems is needed. A plan to evaluate the outcome each time the plan is implemented is essential.

The suicide of a student, staff member, or community member requires special attention. Students might want to follow the example of the student who committed suicide because they desire the same attention or because it appears to be a particularly attractive way to deal with the concerns of adolescence. The death must be acknowledged and the usual grief activities completed.

A recurrence of grief reactions can occur on anniversary dates (e.g., 1 year after a bus crash that killed members of the junior class on the way to school). Remind faculty to look for signs of an increased grief response on significant occasions, such as the day the star football player would have received the district trophy if he had not died after a car accident.

Grief support groups have been found to be very helpful for school-aged and adolescent children. Sessions held at school have the advantages of being easy to attend and occurring in a setting familiar to the child. Support groups can also be based at sites where the loved one of a child was treated.

BEREAVEMENT SUPPORT FOR PEDIATRIC HEALTH CARE PROVIDERS

> QUESTION: Imagine yourself caring for a dying child. When that child dies, what support would you need?

The death of a child can be a traumatic event for the care provider (Stutzer, 2008b). This is true whether interactions with the child and family were brief or long-standing and whether the child's death was unexpected or the anticipated outcome of an illness or injury. Even the most emotionally balanced nurse can experience an acute response to the death of a child. Caring for the dying child causes increased stress because nurses often feel helpless or limited in their ability to alleviate distress for the child (Docherty et al., 2007; Papadatou et al., 2001). This might not happen with each child's death, but it does happen and it is normal. Nurses must learn to care for and support themselves and their peers when faced with the strong emotions and responses that can accompany death (Fig. 13-10).

Contrary to popular belief, one does not "get used to" working with dying children and their families (Stutzer, 2008a). Health care providers can, however, develop coping skills through education and by their personal and professional experience in caring for the dying child. Those staff that have built up a repertoire of skills can recognize their own feelings, allow time and distance for their own grieving, develop personal support mechanisms, and gain personal satisfaction in assisting children and families through the illness and

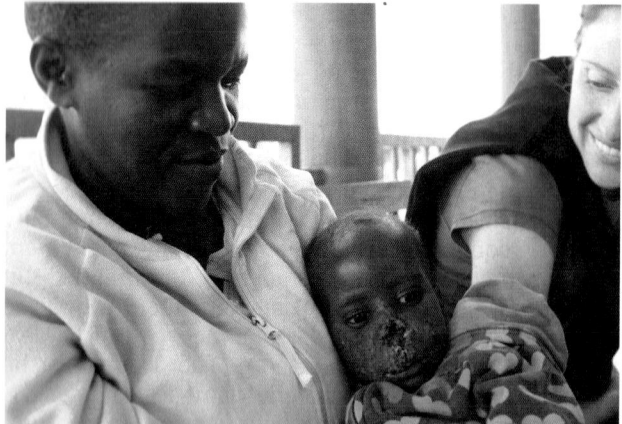

Figure 13-10 Caring for a dying child is stressful but can also be extremely rewarding.

dying process. In addition, these staff can also serve as mentors to less experienced staff by modeling skill and compassion in dealing with death as an experience-based personal growth process (Stutzer, 2008a).

Care providers have repeatedly documented that working with terminally ill children is intense and often overwhelming. Furthermore, it is recognized that a nurse's grief is different from that of a surviving family member's grief (Rashotte et al., 1997). Therefore, models of normal grief and bereavement processes used for adult family survivors are not sufficient as a framework to understand the grief responses and processes of health care providers who have cared for a child who has died.

The death of a favorite patient can be stressful and painful for nurses working with dying children (Stutzer, 2008a). Yet, nurses often report personal renewal from the experience of helping the child and family. They simultaneously grieve for the loss of the child while renewing their personal and professional commitment to the larger mission of achieving a cure for most of the children in their care. Several studies have explored the responses of health care providers to the loss of pediatric patients. One researcher described a form of "emotional tension" present in the struggles verbalized by 15 American nurses who work with terminally ill children (Kaplan, 2000). In this qualitative study, nurses voiced their struggle to balance the intense emotional feelings that exist when treating dying children with their need to be competent care providers. The nurses' emotional experiences were influenced by the relationships they had established with the child and by the child's dying process. A number of the nurses acknowledged that they hid their emotional responses when the child was doing poorly or had died, and that they experienced personal suffering when their patients were dying. They also reported that they were unable to grieve properly. They described recognizing the need to grieve and express feelings and acknowledged that doing so was an appropriate manner in which to respond to a child's death. Barriers to grieving included several work environment issues. The work environment did not integrate time or space for care providers to process emotional feelings

and reactions to the dying process and death of their patients. Instead, nurses felt that they had to hide in the bathroom to express themselves fully. Often, the nurses were asked to care for a newly diagnosed child within minutes of another patient's death without an opportunity to regroup or refocus. Kaplan (2000) believed that, in general, society does not consider the fact that these care providers have worked intensely with their patients and within the confines of their work have developed a type of relationship that results in a grief reaction. In this regard, these care providers, as well as other medical providers, are disenfranchised grievers.

Unit-based interventions and activities give all hospital personnel involved with the care of the child a chance to remember the child and express their grief (Chart 13-3). They also reinforce the fact that not all children die and that some children treated for serious or terminal illness survive and flourish. Such programs are found to be helpful by staff members by legitimizing the staff's grief experience and providing an opportunity for grief to be openly shared with colleagues.

Often, an individual nurse wants to attend the funeral or reach out to the family. This might be an essential step to help the nurse resolve his or her own grief. Families can find such expressions of caring and grief both helpful and comforting. To be most therapeutic for the family, keep the focus on the family.

caREminder

When visiting the family, avoid platitudes. Call the child by name and use direct language. For example, say, "I'm so sorry that Mary died" rather than "your child has expired." This lets the family know that you see the child as a unique, special person, and it helps the family internalize the reality of the death.

When a nurse does attend the funeral or visit the family at home, the visit should not be so brief that the family feels further abandonment and isolation.

CHART 13-3   Care for Health Care Providers Who Work With Dying Children

Plan unit-based memorial services to be held throughout the year.

Provide support sessions for staff members from all services (nursing, social work, medicine, housekeeping).

Keep a memorial book on the unit with pictures, letters, and poems about the children.

Provide critical stress debriefings after particularly difficult deaths.

Identify specific nurses who will care for the dying child and who can offer support to each other as well as to the family and the child.

Plan a yearly party with survivors.

Rotate staff members to settings where they see children who are doing well.

However, be sensitive to whether the family welcomes the visit. If a personal telephone call is made, give the family the opportunity to decline to talk. You can simply tell the family member that you were thinking of them and then ask whether it is a good time to talk.

As nurses, we might not be able to prevent a child's death, but we can have an impact on the dying process by helping to alleviate pain and suffering; facilitate coping; and provide physical and emotional support to the patient, family, and colleagues. Developing the professional maturity to recognize and use strengths can enable a nurse to provide beneficial care to dying children and their families on an ongoing basis. Knowing when to step back, gather strength, and renew oneself is an important part of the process and will help us learn from every patient.

ANSWER: Nurses who care for dying children often care for each other and must develop the ability to understand their own needs. Nurses, too, need quiet time to say good-bye to a child. Nurses will often attend a funeral together, both to support each other and to acknowledge to the family this death is a loss for them as well. To work with children who die, nurses need to develop their own spiritual concepts of life and death. It is not easy, but there is reassurance and satisfaction in knowing that you can give something few others can. One activity that is important to many nurses who work with dying children is to also spend time with healthy children.

See thePoint for a summary of Key Concepts.

REFERENCES

American Academy of Pediatrics, Committee on Bioethics and Committee on Hospital Care. (2000). Palliative care for children. *Pediatrics, 106*(2), 351–357.

American Association of Colleges of Nursing & City of Hope National Medical Center. (2012). *End-of-life nursing education consortium-pediatric palliative care (ELNEC-PPC) faculty guide*. Duarte, CA: City of Hope.

Armstrong-Dailey, A., & Zarbock, S. (2009). *Hospice care for children*. New York, NY: Oxford University Press.

Beckstrand, R. L., Rawle, N. L., Callister, L. et al. (2010). Pediatric nurses' perceptions of obstacles and supportive behaviors in end-of-life care. *American Journal of Critical Care, 19*(6), 543–552.

Belasco, J. B., Danz, P., Drill, A. et al. (2000). Supportive care: Palliative care in children, adolescents, and young adults—Model of care, interventions, and cost of care: A retrospective review. *Journal of Palliative Care, 16*(1), 39–46.

Bluebond-Langner, M. (1978). *The private words of dying children*. Princeton, NJ: Princeton University Press.

Bookbinder, M., Blank, A., Arney, E. et al. (2005). Improving end-of-life care: Development and pilot-test of a clinical pathway. *Journal of Pain Symptom Management, 29*(6), 529–543.

Bookbinder, M., & McHugh, M. (2010). Societal perspective regarding palliative care. In M. Matzo & D. Witt (Eds.), *Palliative care nursing: Quality care to the end of life* (3rd ed., pp. 75–95). New York, NY: Springer Publishing.

Bouffet, E., Zucchinelli, V., Costanzo, P. et al. (1997). Schooling as a part of palliative care in paediatric oncology. *Palliative Medicine, 11*(2), 133–139.

Brown-Saltzman, K. (2006). Transforming the grief process. In R. Carroll-Johnson, L. Gorman, & N. J. Bush (Eds.), *Psychosocial nursing care: Along the cancer continuum* (2nd ed.). Pittsburgh, PA: Oncology Nursing Press.

Browning, D. (2003a). Module 4: Responding to suffering and bereavement. Activity 2: Cornerstones of clinical practice in pediatric palliative care. In M. Solomon, D. Browning, D. Dokken et al. (Eds.), *The initiative for pediatric palliative care curriculum*. Newton, MA: Education Development Center. Retrieved from www.ippcweb.org/quality.asp

Browning, D. (2003b). To show our humanness: Relational and communicative competence in pediatric palliative care. *Bioethics Forum, 18*(3/4), 23–28.

Carter, B. S., Howenstein, M., Gilmer, M. J. et al. (2004). Circumstances surrounding the deaths of hospitalized children: Opportunities for pediatric palliative care. *Pediatrics, 114*(3), e361–e366.

Chaffee, S. (2001). Pediatric palliative care. *Primary Care Clinics in Office Practice, 28*(2), 365–390.

Children's Hospice International. (2003). *About children's hospice, palliative and end-of-life care*. Retrieved from http://www.chionline.org/resources/about.php

Collins, J. J., Stevens, M. M., & Cousens, P. (1998). Home care for the dying child. A parent's perception. *Australian Family Physician, 27*(7), 610–614.

Corless, I. B. (2010). Bereavement. In B. R. Ferrell & N. Coyle (Eds.), *Oxford textbook of palliative nursing* (3rd ed., pp. 597–612). New York, NY: Oxford University Press.

Corr, C. A. (2011). Death in modern society. In G. Hanks, N. Cherry, N. Christakis et al. (Eds.), *Oxford textbook of palliative medicine* (4th ed., pp. 31–40). New York, NY: Oxford University Press.

Cowl, A. S., Cummings, B. M., Yager, P. H. et al. (2012). Organ donation after cardiac death in children: Acceptance of a protocol by multidisciplinary staff. *American Journal of Critical Care, 21*(5), 322–327.

Coyle, N. (2010). Introduction to palliative care nursing. In B. Ferrell & N. Coyle (Eds.), *Oxford textbook of palliative nursing* (3rd ed., pp. 3–11). New York, NY: Oxford University Press.

Crane, K. (2011). Pediatric palliative care gains recognition. *Journal of the National Cancer Institute, 103*(19), 1432–1433.

Davies, B., Brenner, P., Orloff, S. et al. (2002). Addressing spirituality in pediatric hospice and palliative care. *Journal of Palliative Care, 18*(1), 59–67.

Davies, B., Contro, N., Larson, J. et al. (2010). Culturally-sensitive information-sharing in pediatric palliative care. *Pediatrics, 125*(4), e859–e865.

Davies, B., Limbo, R., & Jin, J. (2010). Grief and bereavement in pediatric palliative care. In B. R. Ferrell & N. Coyle (Eds.), *Oxford textbook of palliative nursing* (3rd ed., pp. 1081–1098). New York, NY: Oxford University Press.

Docherty, S., Miles, M., & Brandon, D. (2007). Searching for "the dying point": Provider's experiences with palliative care in pediatric acute care. *Pediatric Nursing, 33*, 335–342.

Doka, K. (1989). Grief. In R. Kastenbaum & B. Kastenbaum (Eds.), *Encyclopedia of death*. Phoenix, AZ: Oryx Press.

Doka, K. (2002). *Disenfranchised grief: New directions, challenges, and strategies for practice*. Champaign, IL: Research Press.

Durall, A., Zurakowski, D., & Wolfe, J. (2012). Barriers to conducting advance care discussions for children with life-threatening conditions. *Pediatrics, 129*(4), e975–e982.

Eccleston, C., Palermo, T. M., Fisher, E. et al. (2012). Psychological interventions for parents of children and adolescents with chronic illness. *Cochrane Database of Systematic Reviews*, (8), CD009660.

Egan City, K., & Labyak, M. (2010). Hospice palliative care for the 21st century: A model for quality end-of-life-care. In B. R. Ferrell & N. Coyle (Eds.), *Oxford textbook of palliative nursing* (3rd ed., pp. 13–52). New York, NY: Oxford University Press.

Ersek, M., & Cotter, V. (2010). The meaning of hope in the dying. In B. R. Ferrell & N. Coyle (Eds.), *Oxford textbook of palliative nursing* (3rd ed., pp. 579–596). New York, NY: Oxford University Press.

Ethier, A. (2009). Care of the dying child and family. In D. Tomlinson & N. E. Kline (Eds.), *Pediatric oncology nursing: Advanced clinical handbook* (pp. 576–656). Berlin, Germany: Springer.

Ferrell, B. R., & Coyle, N. (2010). *Oxford textbook of palliative nursing* (3rd ed.). New York, NY: Oxford University Press.

Ferrell, B. R., & Grant, M. (2000). *Quality of life model.* Duarte, CA: City of Hope.

Feudtner, C., Hays, R., Haynes, G. et al. (2001). Deaths attributed to pediatric complex chronic conditions: National trends and implications for supportive services. *Pediatrics, 107*(6), E99.

Field, M. J., & Behrman, R. E. (2003). *When children die: Improving palliative and end-of-life care for children and their families.* Report of the Institute of Medicine Task Force. Washington, DC: National Academy Press.

Field, M. J., & Cassel, C. K. (Eds.). (1997). *Approaching death: Improving care at the end of life.* Report of the Institute of Medicine Task Force. Washington, DC: National Academy Press.

Fochtman, D. (2011). Palliative care. In C. Baggott, D. Fochtman, G. Foley et al. (Eds.), *Nursing care of children and adolescents with cancer and blood disorders* (pp. 468–509). Glenview, IL: Association of Pediatric Hematology/Oncology Nurses.

Foley, K. M., & Gelband, H. (Eds.). (2002). *Improving palliative care for cancer.* Washington, DC: National Academy Press.

Gallagher, K., Cass, H., Black, R. et al. (2012). A training needs analysis of neonatal and paediatric health-care staff in a tertiary children's hospital. *International Journal of Palliative Nursing, 18*(4), 197–201.

Gerhardt, C., Fairclough, D., Grossenbacher, J. et al. (2012). Peer relationships of bereaved siblings and comparison classmates after a child's death from cancer. *Journal of Pediatric Psychology, 37*(2), 209–219.

Gilmer, M., Foster, T., Bell, C. et al. (2012). Parental perceptions of care at end of life. *The American Journal of Hospice & Palliative Care.* Advance online publication.

Goldman, A. (2001). Recent advances in palliative care. Importance of palliative care for children is being increasingly recognized. *British Medical Journal, 322*(7280), 234.

Heath, J., Clarke, N., Donath, S. et al. (2010). Symptoms and suffering at the end of life in children with cancer: An Australian perspective. *Medical Journal of Australia, 192*(2), 71–75.

Hechler, T., Blankenburg, M., Friedrichsdorf, S. et al. (2008). Parents' perspective on symptoms, quality of life, characteristics of death and end-of-life decisions for children dying from cancer. *Klinische Pädiatrie, 220*(3), 166–174.

Heilferty, C. M. (2004). Spiritual development and the dying child: The pediatric nurse practitioner's role. *Journal of Pediatric Health Care, 18,* 271–275.

Heiney, S. P., Ruffin, J., & Goon-Johnson, K. (1995). The effects of a support group on selected psychosocial outcomes of bereaved parents whose child died from cancer. *Journal of Pediatric Oncology Nursing, 12*(2), 51–61.

Hendrickson, K., & McCorkle, R. (2008). A dimensional analysis of the concept: Good death of a child with cancer. *Journal of the Association of Pediatric Oncology Nurses, 25*(3), 127–138.

Hilden, J. M., Emanuel, E. J., Fairclough, D. L. et al. (2001). Attitudes and practices among pediatric oncologists regarding end-of-life care: Results of the 1998 American Society of Clinical Oncology Survey. *Journal of Clinical Oncology, 19*(1), 205–212.

Hinds, P. S., Oakes, L. L., Hicks, J. et al. (2012). Parent-clinician communication intervention during end-of-life decision making for children with incurable cancer. *Journal of Palliative Medicine, 15*(8), 916–922.

Horsburgh, M., Trenholme, A., & Huckle, T. (2002). Paediatric respite care: A literature review from New Zealand. *Palliative Medicine, 16*(2), 99–105.

Jacobs, H. (2005). Ethics in pediatric end-of-life care: A nursing perspective. *Journal of Pediatric Nursing, 20*(5), 360–369.

Kachoyeanos, M., & Selder, F. (1993). Life transitions of parents at the unexpected death of a school-age and older child. *Journal of Pediatric Nursing, 8,* 41–49.

Kalisch, P. A., & Kalisch, B. J. (2003). *American nursing: A history.* Philadelphia, PA: Lippincott Williams & Wilkins.

Kane, J. R., Barber, R. G., Jordan, M. et al. (2000). Supportive/palliative care of children suffering from life-threatening and terminal illness. *American Journal of Hospice and Palliative Care, 17*(3), 165–172.

Kaplan, L. J. (2000). Toward a model of caregiver grief: Nurses' experiences of treating dying children. *Omega: Journal of Death and Dying, 41*(3), 187–206.

Klein, S. M., & Saroyan, J. M. (2011). Treating a child with a life-threatening condition. *Pediatric Annals, 40*(5), 259–265.

Knapp, C., Madden, V., Woodworth, L. et al. (2012). An overview of pediatric palliative care. In C. Knapp, V. Madden, & S. Fowler-Kerry (Eds.), *Pediatric palliative care: Global perspectives* (pp. 3–13). New York, NY: Springer Publishing.

Kopecky, E. A., Jacobson, S., Joshi, P. et al. (1997). Review of a home-based palliative care program for children with malignant and non-malignant diseases. *Journal of Palliative Care, 13*(4), 28–33.

Kreicbergs, U., Valdimarsodottir, U., Onelov, E. et al. (2004). Talking about death with children who have severe malignant disease. *New England Journal of Medicine, 12,* 1175–1186.

Kübler-Ross, E. (1969). *On death and dying.* New York, NY: Macmillan.

Lambert, P. (2002). Paediatrics: Part 7: Palliative care of the dying child. *World of Irish Nursing, 10*(7), 29–30.

Last Acts Palliative Care Task Force. (2002). *Precepts of palliative care for children, adolescents and their families.* Retrieved from http://www.napnap.org/Docs/PalliativecarePS_support.pdf

Lauer, M., Mulhern, R. K., Bohne, J. B. et al. (1985). Children's perceptions of their siblings' death at home or hospital: The precursors of differential adjustment. *Cancer Nursing, 8,* 21–27.

Levetown, M. (Ed.). (2000). *Compendium of pediatric palliative care.* Alexandria, VA: National Hospice and Palliative Care Organization.

Levetown, M. (2006). Pediatric care: Transitioning goals of care in the emergency department, intensive care unit, and in between. In B. R. Ferrell, & N. Coyle (Eds.), *Textbook of palliative care nursing* (pp. 925–943). New York, NY: Oxford University Press.

Levetown, M. (2008). Communicating with children and families: From everyday interactions to skill in conveying distressing information. *Pediatrics, 121*(5), e1441–e1460.

Levetown, M., Hellsten, M. B., & Jones, B. (2010). Pediatric care: Transitioning goals of care in the emergency department, intensive care unit, and in between. In B. R. Ferrell & N. Coyle (Eds.), *Oxford textbook of palliative nursing* (3rd ed., pp. 1019–1048). New York, NY: Oxford University Press.

Liben, S., & Goldman, A. (1998). Home care for children with life-threatening illness. *Journal of Palliative Care, 14*(3), 33–38.

Lindemann, E. (1994). Symptomatology and management of acute grief. *American Journal of Psychiatry, 101,* 141–148.

Loney, M. (1998). Death, dying, and grief in the face of cancer. In C. C. Burke (Ed.), *Psychosocial dimensions of oncology nursing care.* Pittsburgh, PA: Oncology Nursing Press.

Luhrs, C., & Penrod, J. (2007). End-of-life care pathways. *Current Opinions Supporting Palliative Care, 1*(3), 198–201.

Lundqvist, A., Nilstun, T., & Dykes, A. K. (2002). Both empowered and powerless: Mothers' experiences of professional care when their newborn dies. *Birth, 29*(3), 192–199.

Macdorman, M. F., & Kirmeyer, S. (2009). Fetal and perinatal mortality. *National Vital Statistics Report, 57*(8), 1–20.

Mack, J. W., & Grier, H. E. (2004). The day one talk. *Journal of Clinical Oncology, 22,* 563–566.

Martinson, I., Davies, E., & McClowery, S. (1987). The long term effects of sibling death on self-concept. *Journal of Pediatric Nursing, 2,* 277–335.

Meyer, E., Burns, J., Griffith, J. et al. (2002). Parental perspective on end-of-life care in the pediatric intensive care unit. *Critical Care Medicine, 30*(1), 226–231.

Nielson, D. (2012). Discussing death with pediatric patients: Implications for nurses. *Journal of Pediatric Nursing, 27*(5), e59–e64.

Nishimoto, P. (1996). Venturing into the unknown: Cultural beliefs about death and dying. *Oncology Nursing Forum, 23*, 889–894.

Page, R., & Page, T. (2011). *Promoting health and emotional well-being in your classroom*. Sudbury, MA: Jones and Bartlett.

Papadatou, D., Martinson, I. M., & Chung, P. M. (2001). Caring for dying children: A comparative study of nurses' experiences in Greece and Hong Kong. *Cancer Nursing, 24*(5), 402–412.

Parkes, C. M., & Prigerson, H. (2009). *Bereavement: Studies of grief in adult life* (4th ed.). New York, NY: Routledge.

Perko, K. (2010). Care as death nears. In A. E. Ethier, J. Rollins, & J. Stewart (Eds.), *Pediatric oncology palliative and end-of-life care resource* (pp. 131–134). Glenview, IL: CureSearch & Association of Pediatric Hematology/Oncology Nurses.

Perrin, J., Bloom, S., & Gortmaker, S. (2007). The increase of childhood chronic conditions in the United States. *Journal of the American Medical Association, 297*, 2755–2759.

Pierucci, R. L., Kirby, R. S., & Leuthner, S. R. (2001). End-of-life care for neonates and infants: The experience and effects of a palliative care consultation service. *Pediatrics, 108*(3), 653–660.

Rando, T. (Ed.). (2000). *Clinical dimensions of anticipatory mourning*. Champaign, IL: Research Press.

Rashotte, J., Fothergill-Bourbonnais, F., & Chamberlain, M. (1997). Pediatric intensive care nurses and their grief experiences: A phenomenological study. *Heart Lung, 26*(5), 372–386.

Ray, K. (2010). Spiritual distress. In A. E. Ethier, J. Rollins, & J. Stewart (Eds.), *Pediatric oncology palliative and end-of-life care resource* (pp. 97–103). Glenview IL: CureSearch & Association of Pediatric Hematology/Oncology Nurses.

Rini, A., & Loriz, L. (2007). Anticipatory mourning in parents with a child who dies while hospitalized. *Journal of Pediatric Nursing, 22*, 272–282.

Rushton, C. H. (2004). Ethics and palliative care in pediatrics: When should parents agree to withdraw life-sustaining therapy for children? *American Journal of Nursing, 104*(4), 54–63.

Saiki, S. C., Martinson, I. M., & Inano, M. (1994). Japanese families who have lost children to cancer: A primary study. *Journal of Pediatric Nursing, 9*, 239–250.

Schmidt, K. (2011). Pediatric palliative care: Starting a hospital-based program. *Pediatric Nursing, 37*(5), 268–274.

Sine, D., Sumner, L., Gracy, D. et al. (2001). Pediatric extubation: Pulling the tube. *Journal of Palliative Medicine, 4*(4), 519–524.

Solomon, M. Z., Sellers, D. E., Heller, K. S. et al. (2005). New and lingering controversies in pediatric end-of-life care. *Pediatrics, 116*(4), 872–883.

Stutzer, C. (2008a). Moral distress. In N. Kline, W. L. Hobbie, M. C. Hooke et al. (Eds.), *Essentials of pediatric hematology/oncology nursing: A core curriculum* (3rd ed., pp. 239–240). Glenview, IL: Association of Pediatric Hematology/Oncology Nurses.

Stutzer, C. (2008b). Professionals' grief, distress, and bereavement. In N. Kline, W. L. Hobbie, M. C. Hooke et al. (Eds.), *Essentials of pediatric hematology/oncology nursing: A core curriculum* (3rd ed., pp. 237–238). Glenview, IL: Association of Pediatric Hematology/Oncology Nurses.

Sumner, L. (2010). Pediatric hospice and palliative care. In B. R. Ferrell & N. Coyle (Eds.), *Oxford textbook of palliative nursing* (3rd ed., pp. 997–1018). New York, NY: Oxford University Press.

Sutter, C., & Reid, T. (2012). How do we talk to the children? Child life consultation to support the children of seriously ill adult inpatients. *Journal of Palliative Medicine, 15*(12), 1–7.

Taylor, E. J. (2010). Spiritual assessment. In B. R. Ferrell & N. Coyle (Eds.), *Oxford textbook of palliative nursing* (3rd ed., pp. 647–662). New York, NY: Oxford University Press.

Tomlinson, D., Bartels, U., Gammon, J. et al. (2011). Chemotherapy versus supportive care alone in pediatric palliative care for cancer: Comparing the preferences of parents and health care professionals. *Canadian Medical Association Journal, 183*(17), e1252–e1258.

Trotzuk, C., & Gray, B. (2012). Parents' dilemma: Decisions concerning end-of-life care for their child. *Journal of Pediatric Health Care, 26*(1), 57–61.

Van Cleve, L., Muñoz, C. E., Riggs, M. L. et al. (2012). Pain experience in children with advanced cancer. *Journal of Pediatric Oncology Nursing, 29*(1), 28–36.

Watts, T. (2013). End-of-life care pathways and nursing: A literature review. *Journal of Nursing Management, 21*(1), 47–57.

Wolfe, J., Grier, H. E., Klar, N. et al. (2000). Symptoms and suffering at the end of life in children with cancer. *New England Journal of Medicine, 342*(5), 326–333.

Wolfe, J., Hammel, J. F., Edwards, K. E. et al. (2008). Easing of suffering in children with cancer at the end of life: Is care changing? *Journal of Clinical Oncology, 26*(10), 1717–1723.

Wolfe, J., Klar, N., Grier, H. E. et al. (2000). Understanding prognosis among parents of children who died of cancer: Impact on treatment goals and integration of palliative care. *Journal of the American Medical Association, 284*(19), 2469–2475.

Wood, I. (2006). School. In A. Goldman, R. Hain, & S. Liben (Eds.), *Oxford textbook of palliative care for children* (pp. 128–142). Oxford, United Kingdom: Oxford University Press.

Worden, W. (2009). *Grief counseling and grief therapy: A handbook for the mental health practitioner* (4th ed.). New York, NY: Springer Publishing.

World Health Organization. (1998). *Expert commission: Cancer pain relief and palliative care*. Geneva, Switzerland: Author.

World Health Organization. (2009). *WHO definition of palliative care*. Retrieved from http://www.who.int/cancer/palliative/definition/en/

See thePoint for additional resources.

UNIT 3

Managing Health Challenges

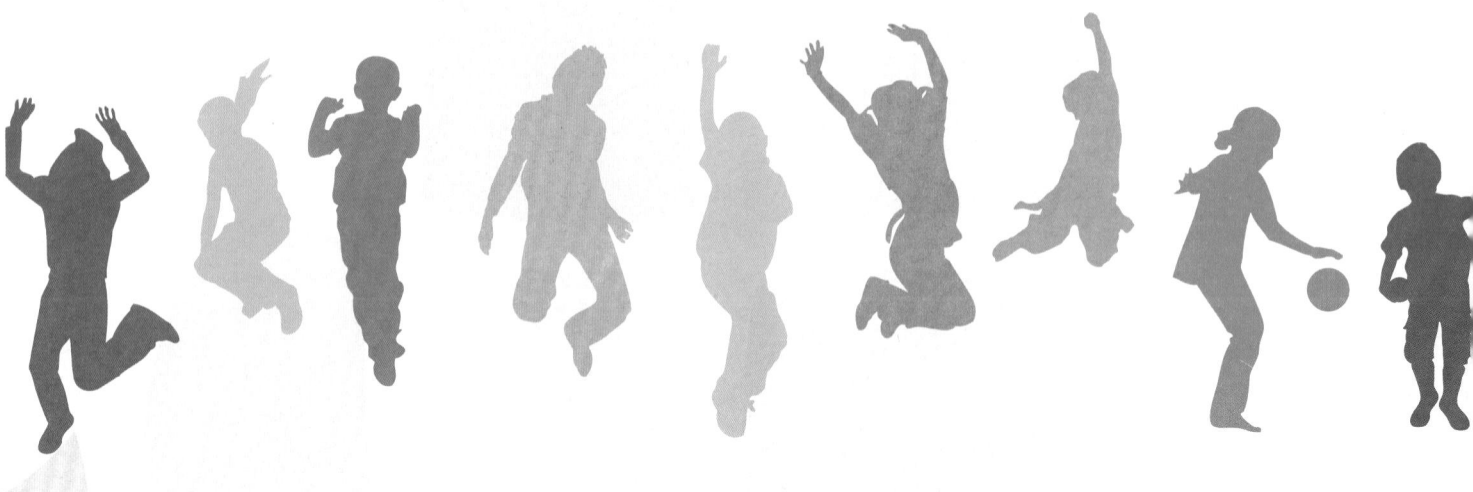

CHAPTER 14

The Neonate With Altered Health Status

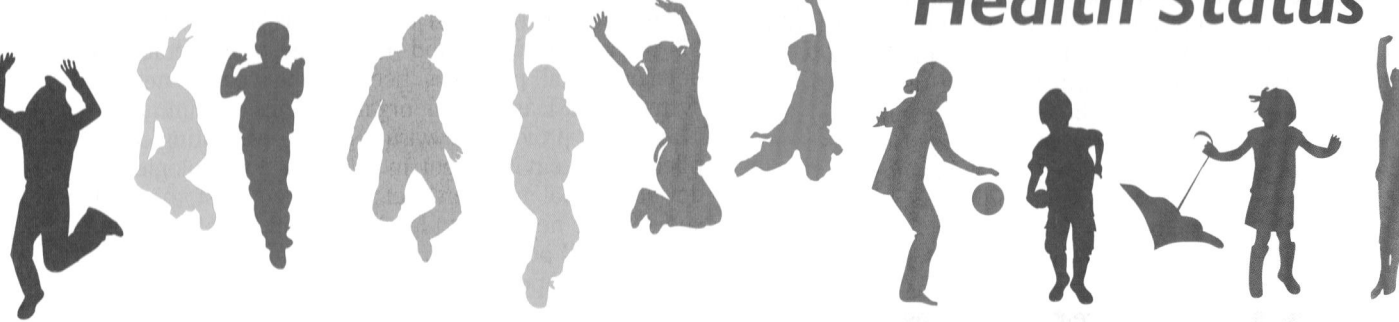

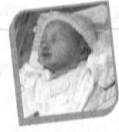

CASE HISTORY

Ben and Abby Goldman are expecting their first child. Abby has been told that she has an incompetent cervix. She miscarried her first two pregnancies and has been on bed rest since the 20th week of this pregnancy. Her membranes ruptured while she was sleeping, and, despite medical efforts to stop labor, Abby delivered Gabriella Ruth Goldman at 28 weeks' gestation.

Abby's membranes were ruptured for almost 48 hours before Gabriella was delivered, and Abby received two doses of betamethasone. Gabriella underwent a spontaneous vaginal delivery, and her Apgar scores on blow-by oxygen were a 5 at 1 minute and a 6 at 5 minutes. Her heart rate was consistently more than 100 bpm. Her respiratory effort remained irregular, and her muscle tone improved from flaccid at 1 minute to some flexion at 5 minutes. She would grimace in response to gentle stimulation at both 1 and 5 minutes. On oxygen, her central color was pink, but her extremities were cyanotic. Although she initially demonstrated irregular respiratory effort, she quickly began having periods of apnea and was not able to maintain her respiratory effort. She was intubated and placed on a ventilator. She received surfactant therapy via endotracheal

tube. A peripherally inserted central catheter (PICC) line was placed and she began a course of antibiotics.

At birth, Gabriella weighs 1,282 g, is 37 cm long, and her head circumference is 27 cm. She has lots of dark brown hair and abundant fine lanugo over her body. Without careful positioning, her arms are flaccid at her side and the pinna of her ear folds flat to her head. Her skin is pink with visible veins; the plantar surfaces of her feet are smooth, with no creases and only a few red marks; the demarcation of her breast is barely visible; and her genital area has a prominent clitoris and noticeable labia minora.

During subsequent weeks, Gabriella faces many challenges: thermoregulation problems, sepsis, hypoglycemia, patent ductus arteriosus (PDA), difficulties weaning from the vent, hyperbilirubinemia, gastrointestinal reflux, and retinopathy of prematurity (ROP). Abby and Ben are in the neonatal intensive care unit (NICU) as much as possible and want to understand what Gabriella is going through. The nurse in the NICU has to possess many skills and must be both an intensive care nurse with a nonverbal patient and a family-centered nurse who provides information and support to Gabriella's family.

CHAPTER OBJECTIVES

1 Explain the etiology, prognosis, and patient outcomes of common disorders affecting the preterm newborn.

2 Describe the pathophysiologic principles related to developmental alterations in the term newborn.

3 Describe the nursing assessment measures that help to identify developmental disorders and common problems associated with the high-risk newborn.

4 Identify appropriate uses of the New Ballard Score, the Neonatal Behavioral Assessment Scale, and the Assessment

of Preterm Infant's Behavior scale that assist the health care team in identifying developmental disorders and health care problems of high-risk newborns.

5 Discuss nursing care for a neonate with altered health status.

6 Identify evidence-based interdisciplinary interventions commonly used for each health challenge in newborns.

See thePoint for a list of Key Terms.

The neonatal period is a vulnerable time in the human life cycle. Healthy term newborns often make the transition to extrauterine life without complications and continue to thrive through the newborn period. However, some term newborns experience complications during this period.

The premature newborn faces transition to extrauterine life with immature body systems, including respiratory, cardiac, and central nervous systems. Preterm birth is the delivery of an infant prior to completing 37 weeks of pregnancy. Preterm birth is on the rise, comprising 12% of all live births in the United States; this is a 36% increase from 1980 (Martin et al., 2012). Neonatal mortality depends largely on birth weight and gestational age; those with greater weight and term gestational age have the lowest mortality rates.

Newborns demonstrate illness through insidious signs and symptoms. Astute assessment skills are needed to identify early signs of impending problems. For example, subtle changes in the newborn's breathing or feeding patterns and behavior may be the earliest signs of neonatal sepsis. Early recognition of these signs is vital to provide prompt interventions and prevent complications.

The focus of this chapter is to describe nursing assessments and outline interdisciplinary interventions used to assist and support the newborn's transition to extrauterine life and continued growth and development. This chapter will also discuss conditions that might occur in neonates such as hyperbilirubinemia, hemolytic disease of the newborn (HDN), birth injuries, and exposures as well as challenges more commonly associated with low birth weight (LBW) and preterm birth such as surfactant deficiency, chronic lung disease (CLD), necrotizing enterocolitis (NEC), and PDA.

DEVELOPMENTAL AND BIOLOGIC VARIANCES

The term and preterm newborn are different in many ways. A term newborn is born after 37 completed weeks of gestation and, as a result of complete intrauterine development, possesses the necessary physical attributes to successfully adapt to the extrauterine environment. A healthy term newborn at birth is pink (although hands and feet may remain blue for the first 24 hours) and exhibits strong muscle tone and reflexes, vigorous cry and respiratory effort, normal respiratory rate, and a normal cardiac rate and rhythm.

The preterm newborn is defined as one born before 37 weeks' gestation and is extremely vulnerable to developmental problems because the central nervous system (CNS) and other organ systems are immature. The uterus provides a warm, slightly oscillating, fluid-filled, quiet environment in which all physiologic and developmental needs are met. In stark contrast, the NICU subjects the newborn to loud and sudden noises, bright light, painful procedures, irregular patterns of handling, and rapid temperature changes, all of which may have detrimental effects on the developing immature systems of the premature newborn. The NICU environment may precipitate hypoxia as a result of needed medical and nursing procedures, leading to damage of the developing CNS and other body systems. Reducing light, noise, and temperature changes and providing periods of "hands-off" care improve the preterm infant's neurobehavior (Montirosso et al., 2012). Late preterm newborns are infants born between 34 and 36 6/7 weeks' gestation. These infants are a high-risk population because they experience more problems, such as respiratory distress, altered thermoregulation, hypoglycemia, and feeding problems than term infants. They also have increased mortality (Tomashek et al., 2007). When compared to term infants, late preterm infants have a longer length of hospital stay after birth, higher rehospitalization rate, and breastfeeding problems (McDonald et al., 2012; Medoff Cooper et al., 2012) (Evidence-Based Clinical Practice Guidelines 14-1). To identify those who may be at risk, carefully assess transitional events and the early course of late preterm infants.

The sick term newborn is less vulnerable than the premature newborn to developmental problems because the term neonate's CNS and other biologic

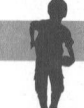

EVIDENCE-BASED CLINICAL PRACTICE GUIDELINES 14-1

Care of the Late Preterm Infant

National Perinatal Association. (2013). *Multidisciplinary guidelines for the care of late preterm infants.* Retrieved from http://www.nationalperinatal.org/lptguidelines.php

Reviews the interdisciplinary interventions necessary to optimize the outcomes and limit the morbidities of late preterm infants.

Association of Women's Health, Obstetric and Neonatal Nurses. (2010). *Assessment and care of the late preterm infant.* Retrieved from

https://www.awhonn.org/awhonn/store/productDetail.do;jsessionid=DB2BCEC64926AF0E3FCF883C3DFF86C4?productCode=LPI-2010

Provides guidelines for nursing care of the late preterm infant.

Academy of Breastfeeding Medicine. (2011). ABM clinical protocol #10: Breastfeeding the late preterm infant (34(0/7) to 36(6/7) weeks gestation). *Breastfeeding Medicine, 6*(3), 151–156. Retrieved from http://guideline.gov/content.aspx?id=34449&search=hyperbilirubinemia

This guideline outlines the methods to promote breastfeeding in the late preterm infant.

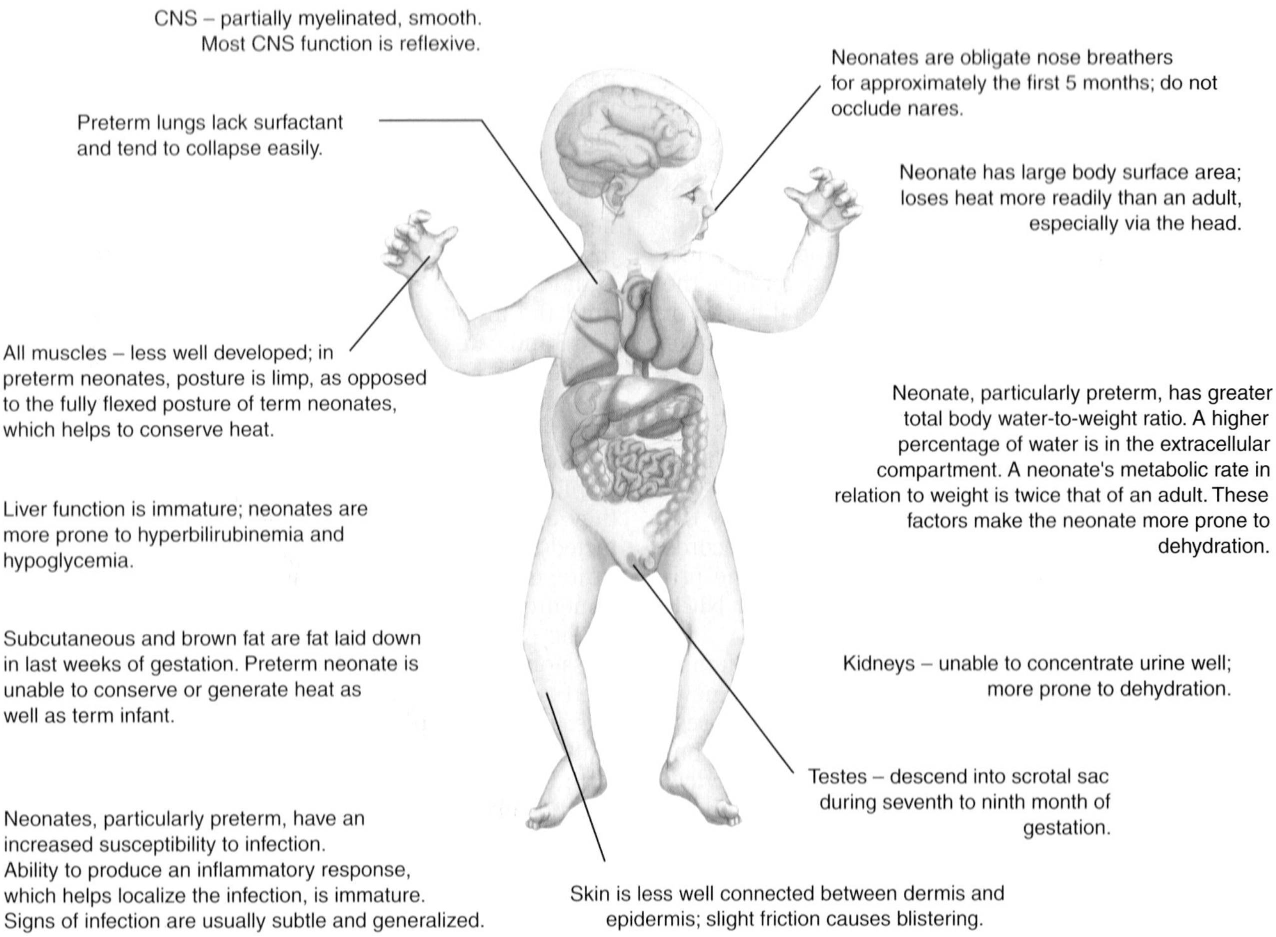

CNS – partially myelinated, smooth. Most CNS function is reflexive.

Preterm lungs lack surfactant and tend to collapse easily.

Neonates are obligate nose breathers for approximately the first 5 months; do not occlude nares.

Neonate has large body surface area; loses heat more readily than an adult, especially via the head.

All muscles – less well developed; in preterm neonates, posture is limp, as opposed to the fully flexed posture of term neonates, which helps to conserve heat.

Neonate, particularly preterm, has greater total body water-to-weight ratio. A higher percentage of water is in the extracellular compartment. A neonate's metabolic rate in relation to weight is twice that of an adult. These factors make the neonate more prone to dehydration.

Liver function is immature; neonates are more prone to hyperbilirubinemia and hypoglycemia.

Subcutaneous and brown fat are fat laid down in last weeks of gestation. Preterm neonate is unable to conserve or generate heat as well as term infant.

Kidneys – unable to concentrate urine well; more prone to dehydration.

Testes – descend into scrotal sac during seventh to ninth month of gestation.

Neonates, particularly preterm, have an increased susceptibility to infection. Ability to produce an inflammatory response, which helps localize the infection, is immature. Signs of infection are usually subtle and generalized.

Skin is less well connected between dermis and epidermis; slight friction causes blistering.

Figure 14-1 Developmental and biologic variances in the neonate.

systems (pulmonary, gastrointestinal) are more mature and organized. However, certain conditions or disease processes such as congenital anomalies, sepsis, birth injuries, and meconium aspiration can present challenges to the term newborn, leading to a stay in the NICU and potential long-term complications (Fig. 14-1).

ASSESSMENT

Infant mortality and morbidity has decreased even for the smallest of newborns, such as those born at 24 to 26 weeks' gestation. Goals include improving not only survival of the premature newborn but also neurodevelopmental outcome and reducing important morbidities such as cerebral palsy (CP), ROP, and intraventricular hemorrhage (IVH). Researchers are investigating how the NICU environment, routine handling and nursing care, and family involvement contribute to the overall outcome of the preterm newborn.

Surgery, premature body systems, and withdrawal from intrauterine drug exposure are examples of factors that may inhibit the normal progression of neurobehavioral development. Additionally, studies of the NICU environment have shown that bright lights, noise, and common procedures—such as suctioning the endotracheal tube, changing the infant's position, or assessing

vital signs—can cause deleterious changes in vital signs (Smith et al., 2011; Wachman & Lahav, 2011). Although techniques to assess and manage pain in the hospitalized infant have progressed greatly, undertreated pain continues to affect the neurobehavioral development of the newborn.

Assessing for developmental problems in the newborn involves evaluating neurologic and behavioral functioning. The neurologic examination focuses on the presence, quality, and symmetry of reflexes (see Table 8-9), such as the grasp and Moro reflexes, and the quality of muscle tone. The behavioral examination complements the neurologic examination and helps to describe the quality of behavioral performance. The combination of these two assessments is the neurobehavioral assessment that determines the newborn's behavioral capabilities, interactive qualities, and adaptations to the extrauterine environment. The nurse can use information obtained from this assessment to plan interventions that support and optimize the newborn's development.

FOCUSED HEALTH HISTORY

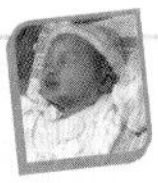

QUESTION: What are some pertinent aspects of Gabriella's history that place her at risk?

The purpose of the health history is to collect data regarding the quality of progression in the high-risk newborn's development. Whether the nurse is caring for the newborn in the regular newborn nursery, the NICU, or the family's home, specific health patterns are important to assess for all newborns. After delivery, a healthy term newborn is generally cared for in a normal nursery where the nurse focuses on establishing feedings and promoting normal function of body systems. Review the labor and delivery records to determine the presence or absence of prenatal care, general health of the mother, length of labor, and any difficulties encountered during labor, such as maternal fever or fetal distress. Note also delivery difficulties, such as the need to use vacuum extraction at the time of delivery. This information can help identify potential problems in the newborn.

In the delivery room or within the NICU, review the labor and delivery records and begin neonatal records to help identify potential problems. Focus on the primary problem of the newborn that prompted NICU admission.

In the home or at a clinic visit, ask the primary family member or caregiver for information related to the newborn's current health and developmental status. Assess the quality of the caregiver's attachment and responsiveness to the newborn's needs during the interview (Focused Health History 14-1). Obtain information related to the health of the mother during pregnancy, the quality of the labor and delivery, and the initial newborn course. This information assists the nurse to focus on specific health patterns and physical characteristics that may be altered if the pregnancy or neonatal course was difficult. Specific at-risk newborns include those who were admitted to the NICU, born prematurely, or experienced a difficult transition, as evidenced by a low Apgar score (less than 6) at 5 minutes. Responses to the nurse's health history questions can suggest developmental delays and help guide the physical examination.

ANSWER: Gabriella's gestational age is her greatest risk because she is 12 weeks premature. Her Apgar scores are objective measurements that also reflect her status. Although her heart rate was more than 100 bpm at all times, she was unable to manifest a vigorous response because of her prematurity. The length of time the membranes were ruptured also is an identifiable risk factor; rupture of membranes more than 24 hours before birth places an infant at risk for a systemic infection.

FOCUSED PHYSICAL ASSESSMENT

Physical assessment of the newborn involves inspection, observation, smell, palpation, percussion, and auscultation. Assess key parameters during the examination of all newborns (Focused Physical Assessment 14-1) (see thePoint for Supplemental Information: Growth Parameter Assessment). The purpose of the neonatal

examination is to identify existing abnormalities (congenital anomalies) and provide baseline data for comparison as the newborn adapts to the extrauterine environment. Assess the newborn at delivery, immediately upon admission to the nursery, and then frequently thereafter.

Apgar scoring (Fig. 14-2) was developed as a quick delivery suite evaluation of newborns' immediate adjustment to extrauterine life. Record the Apgar score at 1 and 5 minutes after birth and repeat every 5 minutes until the infant's condition stabilizes. A total score of 0 to 3 indicates severe distress, requiring immediate resuscitation. Scores of 4 to 6 signify moderate difficulty, and scores of 7 to 10 indicate the absence of difficulty. Many healthy newborns do not receive a score of 10 because their hands and feet remain blue (acrocyanosis) for several hours after delivery and can persist until they are 24 hours of age. The Apgar score is also affected by other factors, including the degree of prematurity, maternal sedation or analgesia, and the presence of neuromuscular disorders in the infant.

The Apgar score is a useful tool to evaluate the progression of resuscitation; however, Apgar scores are not used to determine the timing of resuscitative measures. The standard of care for neonatal resuscitation requires that assessment and intervention begin immediately at birth, not a full minute later (Perlman et al., 2010). Low Apgar scores are associated with increased mortality (Lie et al., 2010). Recent research has also demonstrated that an Apgar score less than 4 at 5 minutes of life is highly associated with the subsequent development of CP in both term and preterm infants (Lie et al., 2010).

DIAGNOSTIC CRITERIA

QUESTION: What information is missing from the case study to complete the neuromuscular maturity component of the New Ballard Score (NBS)? How many points did you assess Gabriella for the physical maturity of the NBS?

The specific diagnostic tests and procedures used to assess a newborn depend on the suspected disorder (Tests and Procedures 14-1) (for more information see thePoint for Procedures: Blood Drawing from Peripheral Sites: Heel Stick and Finger Stick). Prenatal tests commonly performed to determine fetal well-being include amniocentesis, chorionic villus sampling, fetal ultrasonography, and specific blood tests (e.g., maternal serum α-fetoprotein, triple-marker screening). Routine newborn screening for metabolic diseases is discussed in Chapter 27.

Several assessment scales are available to assist in evaluating the progression of development in the newborn. The most common are the NBS, the Neonatal Behavioral Assessment Scale (NBAS), and the Assessment of Preterm Infant's Behavior (APIB) scale.

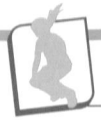

FOCUSED HEALTH HISTORY 14-1

The Neonate With Altered Health Status

Current history	Neonate's age in weeks, corrected age (age adjusted for prematurity, calculated by subtracting the number of weeks born before 40 weeks of gestation from the chronologic age) *Current medications/therapies:* Seizure medications, diuretics, sodium/potassium supplements, specialized formulas, supplements, need for apnea monitoring Symptoms of concern in the neonate: *Poor feeding patterns:* Increased time to complete feedings, poor nippling, inability to coordinate suck and swallow, frequent regurgitation, cyanosis with feedings, poor intake *Altered elimination patterns:* Fewer wet diapers, constipation, diarrhea, water-loss stools *Central nervous symptom variations:* Altered sleep/wake cycles (sleeping less than 3 hours between feeds, abrupt changes between states), hypotonia, hyperextension of head, lethargy, unresponsiveness to stimuli, irritability, unable to console, asymmetric movements of extremities, bicycling motion of lower extremities *Delayed acquisition of developmental milestones:* Not tracking, not reaching for objects, smiling late, turning over late *Poor growth:* Poor weight gain along own growth curve, poor head growth *Cardiorespiratory:* Respiratory distress (tachypnea, periodic breathing, apnea, retractions, nasal flaring, grunting, pallor, cyanosis), need for oxygen, tachycardia, bradycardia, poor peripheral pulses, capillary refill longer than 3 seconds *Problems with thermoregulation:* Hypothermia (respiratory distress, peripheral vasoconstriction, hypoglycemia, acidosis), hyperthermia (tachycardia, warm extremities, sweating) *Metabolic instability:* Symptoms of hypoglycemia (apnea, pallor, cyanosis, lethargy, hypotonia, poor suck, jitteriness, temperature instability, high-pitched cry, seizures)
Past medical history	*Birth history:* Spontaneous breathing at birth, meconium staining, prematurity, NICU admission, need for assisted ventilation, Apgar scores (5-minute Apgar score <7 may be associated with asphyxia, traumatic delivery, hemorrhage, nuchal cord), seizures, drug exposure (type/presence of withdrawal), hypoglycemic events, type of delivery, complications of delivery, maternal health, prenatal care *Infant health:* History of other illnesses and hospitalizations, whether follow-up appointments have been maintained, current immunization status and any reaction to them, any identified allergies to medications, topical agents, foods
Nutritional assessment	Adequate growth (head circumference, weight, length) plotted on growth chart, recent weight loss/gain, poor feeding, decreased activity
Family medical history	Family history of illness, genetic conditions, other premature or ill offspring
Social history	Adequate income and resources to provide food, safe home, transportation to clinic visits; adequate heat and running water in home, telephone; how family is adjusting to the birth of this infant
Growth and development	Achievement of developmental and physical milestones, response to environment, activity patterns, presence of sleep/wake periods

Note: See Chapter 8 for a comprehensive health history.

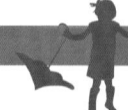

FOCUSED PHYSICAL ASSESSMENT 14-1
The Neonate With Altered Health Status

Assessment Parameter	Alterations/Clinical Significance
General appearance	Normal: spontaneous movements, flexed position, palmar grasp, lusty cry, normal muscle tone
	Frog position of legs, decreased muscle tone, weak grasp associated with prematurity
	Decreased movement, weak palmar grasp: birth asphyxia, neurologic damage
	High-pitched cry: prematurity, neurologic abnormality, drug withdrawal
	Increased muscle tone: drug exposure, birth asphyxia
	Hypotonia: neurologic damage
Integumentary system	Color
	Normal: pink; acrocyanosis during first 24 hours of life
	Central cyanosis: congenital heart disease
	White/pale: respiratory distress, hypothermia, hypovolemia, anemia, sepsis
	Mottled: acidosis, hypotension, hypothermia, shock
	Jaundice in first 24 hours of life: hemolysis, sepsis, biliary atresia
	Jaundice after first 24 hours of life: immature liver
	Plethoric, ruddy: polycythemia, hyperthermia
	Normal: mature, intact, presence of subcutaneous fat, vernix, scant lanugo, milia, erythema toxicum; capillary refill <3 seconds
	Thin, translucent blood vessels; lack of vernix, abundant lanugo: prematurity
	Lack of subcutaneous fat: prematurity, intrauterine growth retardation (IUGR)
	Petechiae: trauma, sepsis
	Edema: trauma
	Peeling skin, long fingernails and toenails: postterm
	Meconium staining: meconium aspiration, fetal distress
	Prolonged capillary refill: hypovolemia, acidosis, hypothermia
Head and neck	Normal: normocephalic, minimal head lag
	Microcephalic: TORCH syndrome/transplacental infections, congenital anomalies
	Hydrocephalic: congenital anomalies, IVH, meningomyelocele
	Encephalocele: herniated brain
	Anencephaly: absent cerebral tissue/neural tube defect
	Molding: difficult delivery, prolonged labor
	Cephalhematoma: difficult delivery, use of vacuum extraction
	Caput succedaneum: pressure on presenting part, prolonged labor
	Full anterior fontanel: increased intracranial pressure (ICP), IVH
	Sunken anterior fontanel: dehydration
	Increased head lag: hypotonia, prematurity
	Asymmetric tonic neck reflex: prematurity, neurologic dysfunction
	Decreased neck range of motion (ROM): fetal positioning
	Fractured clavicles: birth trauma
Eyes	Normal: clear, white sclera; blink reflex present; presence of red reflex; eyes in line with ears
	Sclera yellow or hemorrhage present: jaundice, birth trauma
	Absent blink reflex: neurologic damage, facial nerve paralysis
	Absent red reflex: congenital cataracts, retinoblastoma
	Low-set ears: trisomy 21

Assessment Parameter	Alterations/Clinical Significance
Ears	Normal: adequate cartilage formation
	Cartilage flattened, folded: prematurity
Nose and oral cavity	Normal: well-formed structures, intact palate and mouth structures
	Nose off midline: congenital malformation
	Nares not patent: choanal atresia
	Hard/soft palate not intact: cleft lip/palate
	Absent gag reflex: neurologic abnormalities
	Absent or weak sucking or rooting reflex: prematurity, neurologic difficulties
Thorax and lungs	Normal: symmetric chest wall; easy breathing with clear breath sounds
	Asymmetric expansion: pneumothorax, phrenic nerve damage
	Grunting, nasal flaring, retractions: surfactant deficiency/pneumonic sepsis, retained lung fluid
	Respiratory rate: 40–60 breaths/min normal; tachypneic: congenital heart disease, respiratory distress
	Rales/rhonchi/wheezing: fluid in alveoli, decreased ventilation, PDA
	Decreased breath sounds: pneumothorax, diaphragmatic hernia, surfactant deficiency, pneumonia
Cardiovascular system	Normal heart rate: 80–150 bpm (term), 120–160 bpm (preterm)
	Irregular rate: supraventricular tachycardia, congenital heart block
	Bradycardia: hypothermia, sepsis, apnea
	Tachycardia: hypovolemia, hyperthermia, anemia, acidosis, congestive heart failure
	Murmur: first 24 hours of life may be normally heard, congenital heart disease, PDA, acidosis, anemia
	Active precordium: PDA of prematurity
	Decreased pulses: congenital heart disease
	Increased pulses: PDA
Abdomen	Normal: palpate sharp edge of liver 1–2 cm below costal margin; umbilical cord with three vessels; meconium passage within 24 hours after birth
	Distention: obstruction, NEC, renal abnormality, fetal hydrops
	Scaphoid (sunken abdomen because of intestines in chest): diaphragmatic hernia
	Decreased bowel sounds: obstruction, NEC
	Hyperactive bowel sounds: hypermotility, colitis
	Tense/tender: NEC, abdominal mass
	Hepatosplenomegaly: hemolysis, sepsis
	Two-vessel cord: congenital anomalies, renal anomalies
	Bowel loops palpable: obstruction, feeding intolerance
	No stool within first 24 hours: obstruction, imperforate anus, Hirschsprung disease
	Water-loss stools: diarrhea, colitis, rotavirus, feeding intolerance
	OB+ stools: anal fissure, NEC, colitis
	Reducing substance positive: carbohydrate intolerance
	Bright-red streaks: anal fissure, colitis
	Meconium plugging: Hirschsprung disease, cystic fibrosis

(Continued)

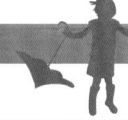

FOCUSED PHYSICAL ASSESSMENT 14-1
The Neonate With Altered Health Status *(Continued)*

Assessment Parameter	Alterations/Clinical Significance
External genitalia	Normal: well-formed, sexually differentiated structures
	Blood-tinged discharge: maternal hormones
	Ambiguous genitalia: congenital anomalies, adrenal hyperplasia
	Nonpatent anus: congenital imperforate anus
	Penis, meatus displaced to ventral surface: hypospadias
	Penis, meatus displaced to dorsal surface: epispadias
	Failure to void within first 24 hours: renal obstruction, polycystic kidneys
	Undescended testes: prematurity
	Fluid-filled scrotal sac: hydrocele
Musculoskeletal system	Normal: intact spine, normal muscle tone for gestational age
	Spine not intact: meningomyelocele
	Muscle tone as noted under general appearance
	Limited ROM in all four extremities: clavicle injury, brachial plexus injury
	More/less than 10 digits/webbing: congenital syndromes
	Buttock creases asymmetric: hip dysplasia
Growth and gestational age	Plot preterm infant growth parameters on growth charts specifically for preterm infants (accessible at http://members.shaw.ca/growthchart/). Once an infant surpasses 50 weeks of age, use the regular Centers for Disease Control and Prevention growth charts.
	Small for gestational age (SGA)/IUGR: smoking during pregnancy, poor maternal nutrition, transplacental infection, drug exposure
	Large for gestational age (LGA): diabetic mother/postterm
	NBS estimates gestational age

OB+, occult blood positive; TORCH, toxoplasmosis, other infections, rubella, cytomegalovirus, herpes simplex.

The New Ballard Score

The NBS (Ballard et al., 1991) is the most widely accepted scoring tool to assess postnatal gestational age. Using both specific neuromuscular and physical characteristics of the newborn shortly after birth, the NBS accurately estimates gestational age in neonates of various ages, from extremely premature to postterm (Fig. 14-3). The NBS may be used from birth through day 7 of life (Sasidharan et al., 2009).

After the gestational age assessment is completed, plot the weight, length, and head circumference to identify newborns in whom these measurements are **appropriate for gestational age (AGA)**, **large for gestational age (LGA)**, or **small for gestational age (SGA)**, because

Sign	0	1	2
Heart rate	Absent	Slow, < 100 beats per minute	> 100 beats per minute
Respiratory effort	Absent	Slow and irregular	Good, strong cry
Muscle tone	Flaccid	Some flexion of extremities	Active motion
Reflex irritability	None	Grimace	Cough or sneeze
Color	Pale, blue	Body pink, extremities blue	Completely pink

Figure 14-2 The Apgar scoring system evaluates the neonate's adjustment to extrauterine life at 1 and 5 minutes.

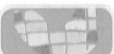 **TESTS AND PROCEDURES for Evaluating the Neonate With Altered Health Status**

Diagnostic Test or Procedure	Purpose	Findings and Indications	Health Care Provider Responsibilities
Radiograph: chest, abdominal	To examine soft tissue and bony structure; Abdominal: to diagnose free air in abdomen and evaluate bowel and other organs	Evaluate lung aeration, lung expansion, lung disease, heart size; bony structures density; intramural air indicates NEC	Shield newborn with gonad shield; protect self with lead apron; keep others 10 ft away from area. Hold newborn during procedure to ensure adequate positioning and avoid rotation.
Pulse oximetry	To measure oxygen (O_2) saturation of blood; noninvasive; measures amount of light absorbed by hemoglobin in the blood	Saturations <80% may indicate poor blood O_2 content. Saturations >100% may indicate hyperoxia.	Protect probe from phototherapy light. Ensure correlation with heart rate. Change site every 12 hours to avoid skin breakdown resulting from pressure. Test may be inaccurate in anemic patients.
Ultrasound (head, abdominal, fetal)	Evaluation of internal anatomic structures through emission of sound waves to evaluate tissue density, movement of tissue, and flow of blood	Heart defects and pulmonary artery pressures; presence of blood in ventricles, brain masses, and in fetal structures	Assist to position newborn. Sedate as needed.
Pneumogram	Twelve- to 24-hour sleep study to measure the presence of apnea, bradycardia, and desaturations	Results read by physician; presence of apnea/bradycardia indicates need for apnea monitor at home.	Ensure monitor is on and apnea/bradycardia episodes are documented on test strip.
Transcutaneous monitoring	Measurement of carbon dioxide (CO_2) and O_2 transcutaneously that correlates with blood CO_2 and O_2. Skin is heated to measure values.	Transcutaneous CO_2 values more accurate than O_2 values. High CO_2 readings may indicate hypoventilation.	Change probe site every 2–4 hours. Monitor for skin burns. Obtain blood gas sample to correlate findings.
Arterial blood gas	Analysis of arterial oxygenation, CO_2 retention, and loss or gain of buffer system acid versus base by the blood system	Normal findings: pH: 7.35 to 7.45 $PaCO_2$: 35–45 mm Hg PaO_2: 50–80 mm Hg HCO_3: 22–26 mEq/L Base excess (BE): 5 to +5 Elevated $PaCO_2$ indicates hypoventilation. Decreased PaO_2 indicates hypoxemia.	Avoid allowing air into sample. If sample obtained from heel as capillary blood gas extremity, must have good perfusion to obtain accurate results. Capillary blood values for pH and CO_2 usually correlate with arterial values; do not rely on O_2 values, which do not correlate well.
Hemoglobin/ hematocrit	To determine the amount of circulating red blood cells (hematocrit) and O_2-carrying capacity of the blood (hemoglobin)	Range for hemoglobin values is 17–19 g/dL; for hematocrit, value is 50–63%	Heel stick samples may have higher values as a result of sludging of red blood cells.
Serum glucose	To detect the presence of hyperglycemia or hypoglycemia	Normal values: Term newborn: 40–120 mg/dL Preterm newborn: 30–160 mg/dL	Do not draw sample from a central line with glucose infusing because erroneous values may result.

HCO_3, bicarbonate; $PaCO_2$, partial pressure of arterial carbon dioxide; PaO_2, partial pressure of arterial oxygen.

NAME_____   DATE/TIME OF BIRTH_____   SEX_____

HOSPITAL NO._____   DATE/TIME OF EXAM_____   BIRTH WEIGHT_____

RACE_____   AGE WHEN EXAMINED_____   LENGTH_____

APGAR SCORE: 1 MINUTE_____   5 MINUTES_____   10 MINUTES_____   HEAD CIRC._____

EXAMINER_____

SCORE
Neuromuscular ____
Physical ____
Total ____

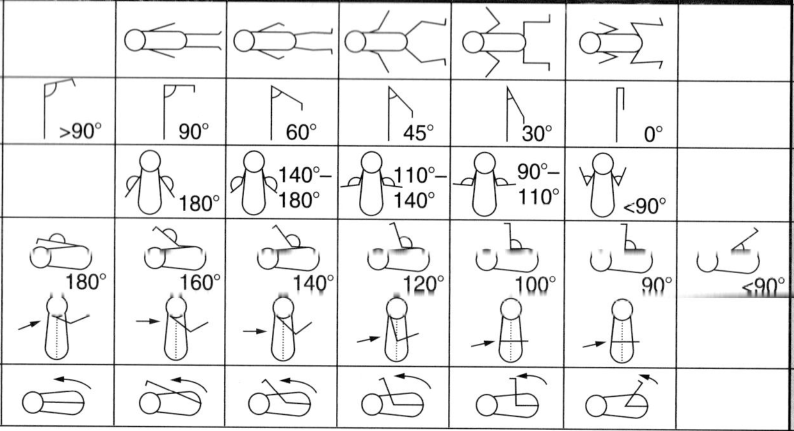

NEUROMUSCULAR MATURITY

NEUROMUSCULAR MATURITY SIGN	SCORE							RECORD SCORE HERE
	−1	0	1	2	3	4	5	
POSTURE								
SQUARE WINDOW (Wrist)	>90°	90°	60°	45°	30°	0°		
ARM RECOIL		180°	140°–180°	110°–140°	90°–110°	<90°		
POPLITEAL ANGLE	180°	160°	140°	120°	100°	90°	<90°	
SCARF SIGN								
HEEL TO EAR								
					TOTAL NEUROMUSCULAR MATURITY SCORE			

MATURITY RATING

Score	Weeks
−10	20
−5	22
0	24
5	26
10	28
15	30
20	32
25	34
30	36
35	38
40	40
45	42
50	44

PHYSICAL MATURITY

PHYSICAL MATURITY SIGN	SCORE							RECORD SCORE HERE
	−1	0	1	2	3	4	5	
SKIN	sticky, friable, transparent	gelatinous, red, translucent	smooth, pink, visible veins	superficial peeling and/or rash, few veins	cracking pale areas, rare veins	parchment, deep cracking, no vessels	leathery, cracked, wrinkled	
LANUGO	none	sparse	abundant	thinning	bald areas	mostly bald		
PLANTAR SURFACE	heel-toe 40–50 mm:−1 <40 mm:−2	>50 mm no crease	faint red marks	anterior transverse crease only	creases ant. 2/3	creases over entire sole		
BREAST	imperceptible	barely perceptible	flat areola no bud	stippled areola 1–2 mm bud	raised areola 3–4 mm bud	full areola 5–10 mm bud		
EYE-EAR	lids fused loosely: −1 tightly: −2	lids open pinna flat stays folded	sl. curved pinna; soft; slow recoil	well-curved pinna; soft but ready recoil	formed and firm instant recoil	thick cartilage, ear stiff		
GENITALS (Male)	scrotum flat, smooth	scrotum empty, faint rugae	testes in upper canal, rare rugae	testes descending, few rugae	testes down, good rugae	testes pendulous, deep rugae		
GENITALS (Female)	clitoris prominent and labia flat	prominent clitoris and small labia minora	prominent clitoris and enlarging minora	majora and minora equally prominent	majora large, minora small	majora cover clitoris and minora		
					TOTAL PHYSICAL MATURITY SCORE			

Figure 14-3 The NBS estimates gestational age based on the neonate's neuromuscular and physical maturity. From Ballard, J. L., Khoury, J. C., Wedig, K. et al. (1991). New Ballard Score, expanded to include extremely premature infants. *The Journal of Pediatrics, 119*, 417–423. Reprinted with permission.

each group has specific clinical and risk factors. Based on the intrauterine growth chart (Battaglia & Lubchenco, 1967), babies are classified as AGA if they weigh between the 10th and 90th percentiles, LGA if they weigh more than the 90th percentile, and SGA if they weigh less than the 10th percentile. Although easy to administer, the NBS may give erroneous results in cases of prematurity, neurologic disorders, and asphyxiated newborns.

Neonatal Behavioral Assessment Scale

The NBAS is a comprehensive tool used to assess the healthy full-term newborn's behavior. This tool combines evaluation of the reflexes, motor capacity, state regulation, and interactive abilities. The examiner observes the newborn through various states of sleep, arousal, and wakefulness and evaluates the interactions between the newborn and the environment. The results obtained demonstrate the newborn's ability to organize states, habituate to the external environment and stimuli, regulate motor activity, respond to reflex testing, orient to visual and auditory stimuli, interact with the caregiver, and self-console (Brazelton, 1984). The tool is also useful to demonstrate to families how their newborn responds to caregiving.

The preterm newborn may be assessed with a modified NBAS that includes both the original full-term scale and additional subscales specifically focused on the preterm newborn's behavior. The preterm newborn behaves differently from the full-term newborn. The preterm newborn may be better served if tested using the APIB, which is more discrete in its assessment of preterm neonatal functioning.

Assessment of Preterm Infant's Behavior Scale

The APIB is useful for preterm and high-risk full-term newborns up to 44 weeks' gestation. Administrating the APIB requires specialized training and an experienced clinician. The focus of this assessment is to determine how newborns cope (their competence) with the environment and the quality of their responses (Als et al., 2005). The information gained from this tool assists in assessing the infant's degree of fragility and tolerance to interactions and in determining what modifications can be made to the environment to enhance the newborn's ability to interact.

> **ANSWER:** Gabriella's neuromuscular maturity, as measured by the square window maneuver, the arm recoil, the popliteal angle, the scarf sign, and the heel-to-ear maneuver, is missing. Based on the description of Gabriella in the case study, she has 1 point for skin, 1 point for lanugo, 1 for plantar surface, 0 for breast, 1 for eye/ear, and 1 for genitals. This is a total of 5 points.

TREATMENT MODALITIES

Care for the newborn focuses on assisting the neonate in transitioning to extrauterine life and then maintaining physiologic stability, particularly thermoregulation and prevention of hypoglycemia and infection.

Newborns are more likely than any other age group to require resuscitation, and how the infant is cared for at birth may have lifelong effects. Fortunately, most newborns make the transition to extrauterine life smoothly. Very small percentages (approximately 10%) require some level of assistance. To best serve these newborns, the Neonatal Resuscitation Program trains health care professionals to skillfully perform neonatal resuscitation in an evidence-based, standardized, methodical manner (Perlman et al., 2010). It teaches integrated steps including evaluating the infant, making decisions, and taking actions based on the overall evaluation. One goal of the program is to have at least one person at every delivery whose primary responsibility is the newborn and who is able to initiate resuscitation. Additionally, either that person or another health care professional immediately available should have the skills to perform a complete resuscitation.

Most newborns respond to warming, drying, positioning, suctioning, and stimulation. Some newborns require more vigorous steps such as ventilation, chest compressions, endotracheal intubation, and administration of medications. Decisions for care are based on the newborn's overall response to previous actions.

Monitor the neonate after immediate stabilization at birth, and implement interventions as indicated to ensure adequate cardiorespiratory adaptation, thermoregulation, normoglycemia, initiation of feedings, and bonding with parents. An overriding dictate of neonatal care, especially important for premature infants with a more immature CNS and other body systems, is that care is delivered in a developmentally appropriate manner. Two treatment modalities that meet this mandate are skin-to-skin holding (kangaroo care) and developmental care.

SKIN-TO-SKIN HOLDING

Skin-to-skin holding, or kangaroo care (Fig. 14-4), is the practice of holding an infant, clothed only in a diaper, skin-to-skin against the bare chest of the father or between the breasts of the mother (Nursing Interventions Classification 14-1). Offer families the opportunity to provide skin-to-skin holding (Tradition or Science 14-1).

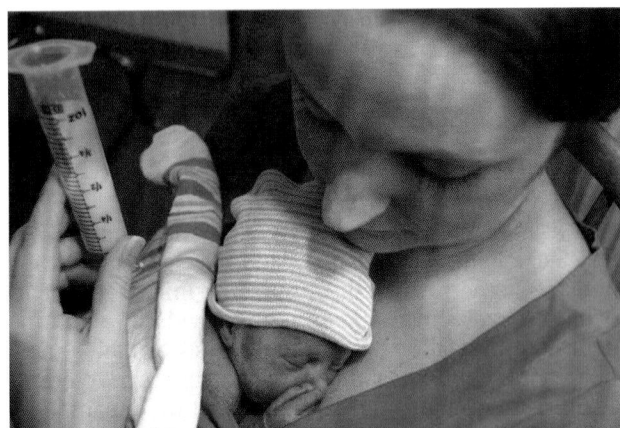

Figure 14-4 Kangaroo care involves skin-to-skin contact between parent and neonate.

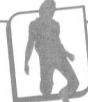

NIC 14-1 NURSING INTERVENTIONS CLASSIFICATION: Kangaroo Care

Definition: Facilitation of skin-to-skin contact between parent or other caregiver and physiologically stable preterm infant

Activities:

Explain advantages and implications of providing skin-to-skin contact with infant

Monitor parent factors influencing involvement in care (e.g. willingness, health, availability, and presence of support system)

Ensure that the infant's physiological status meets guidelines for participation in care

Prepare a quiet, private, and warm environment

Provide parent with a reclining or rocking chair

Instruct parent to wear comfortable, open-front clothing

Instruct parent how to transfer infant from incubator, warmer bed, or bassinet while managing equipment and tubing

Position diaper-clad infant in prone, upright position on parent's bare chest

Turn infant head to one side in a slightly extended position to facilitate eye contact with parent and keep airway open

Avoid forward flexion and hyperextension of infant head

Infant's hips and arms should be flexed

Secure infant and parent position (i.e. tie binding cloth around infant-parent dyad, wrap parent's clothing around infant, and place blanket over dyad)

Instruct parent how to move infant in and out of binding cloth

Encourage parent to focus on infant, rather than high technological setting and equipment

Encourage parent to gently stroke infant in prone upright position

Encourage parent to gently rock infant in prone upright position

Encourage auditory stimulation of infant

Support parent in nurturing and providing hands-on care for infant

Instruct parent to hold infant with full, encompassing hands

Encourage parent to identify infant's behavioral cues

Point out infant physiological state changes to parent

Encourage parent to sit, stand, walk, and engage in other activities of interest while providing skin-to-skin contact

Encourage postpartum mothers to ambulate every 90 minutes while providing skin-to-skin contact, to prevent thrombolytic disease

Instruct parent to decrease activity when infant shows signs of overstimulation, distress, or avoidance

Encourage parent to let the infant sleep during care

Encourage breast-feeding during care, as appropriate

Encourage parent to provide care at least 60 minutes, if possible, to avoid frequent and potentially-stressful changes

Instruct parent to gradually increase time of each skin-to-skin contact, with length eventually becoming as continuous as possible

Monitor parents' emotional reaction to and concerns regarding kangaroo care

Monitor infant's physiologic status (e.g., color, temperature, heart rate, and apnea)

Instruct parent how to monitor infant's physiological status

Support parent to continue skin-to-skin contact at home

Discontinue care if infant becomes physiologically compromised or agitated

From Bulechek, G. M., Butcher, H. K., Dochterman, J. M. et al. (Eds.). (2013). *Nursing interventions classifications (NIC)* (6th ed.). St. Louis, MO: Mosby. Used with permission.

DEVELOPMENTAL CARE

QUESTION: Looking at Nursing Interventions 14-1, what is an aspect of care that, according to the assessment given in the case study, is appropriate for Gabriella from the delivery room through discharge?

Developmental care is a philosophical approach to caring for the newborn based on the specific behavioral responses of the infant to caregiving and other activities. Sick premature infants respond to their environments differently than healthy term infants do. The focus of developmental care is to provide an environment and interaction pattern that the sick infant's neurobehavioral and physiologic organization can tolerate. Health care providers learn to interpret the meaning of infant behaviors. The nurse watches each infant for behavioral and physiologic cues and varies care based on the infant's response.

caREminder

Behaviors that indicate stress in the premature infant include facial grimace, yawning, tongue protrusion, hiccoughing, finger splaying, gaze aversion, fussing, crying, and vomiting. Physiologic stress cues include changes in heart or respiratory rates (tachycardia, bradycardia, tachypnea, apnea), grunting, gasping, cyanosis, and decreased blood oxygen levels (reflected in decreased oxygen saturation or transcutaneous carbon dioxide [TcPco$_2$] levels). The infant exhibits these signs when the environment is stressful, such as in the presence of bright lights and loud noises or when handled excessively.

To effectively deliver developmentally appropriate care, specific elements both in the NICU environment and in the individual infant are considered (Nursing Interventions 14-1). Care may be clustered (many caregiving activities provided at one time) if the infant demonstrates organized and stable behavior. Alternatively, perform only one

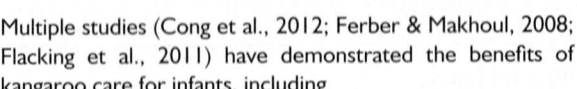

TRADITION OR SCIENCE 14-1

Is skin-to-skin holding beneficial to preterm infants?

Multiple studies (Cong et al., 2012; Ferber & Makhoul, 2008; Flacking et al., 2011) have demonstrated the benefits of kangaroo care for infants, including

- Significantly increased sleep time
- Reduced activity
- Less agitation, apnea, and bradycardia
- Improved stability of oxygen saturation
- Decreased hypothermia
- Reduced pain behaviors with painful stimuli

Mothers report improved lactation with kangaroo care (Flacking et al., 2011). Parents who participate in kangaroo care increase their comfort level in providing care and report increased fulfillment and ability to know their infants, thus promoting parental attachment.

Although meta-analysis is difficult to perform, and further research would be desirable to validate positive outcomes (Conde-Agudelo et al., 2011), overall, the evidence demonstrates that kangaroo care has clinical benefit for both infants and parents; has no apparent negative effects; and therefore should be incorporated into nursing practice.

caregiving activity (such as diapering) if the infant demonstrates decompensation (desaturation or bradycardia).

Providing developmental care is the standard of care in the NICU and permeates all interactions with the newborn (see thePoint for Procedures: Developmental Care of the Newborn). Implementing developmental care decreases the time the premature newborn is on the ventilator and on supplemental oxygen, improves short-term growth, and reduces length and cost of hospital stays (Peters et al., 2009). Individualizing care, such as offering nipple feedings when infants are in quiet awake states, results in more successful feeding—an important discharge criterion for the premature infant. Additionally, premature newborns provided with developmental care have improved neurodevelopmental outcomes to 24 months corrected age (Peters et al., 2009). Developmental care is a family-centered concept that improves both medical and developmental outcomes for premature newborns.

ANSWER: Gabriella's posture is identified as flaccid, and it is noted that her arms are not flexed. She lacks the physical strength and neuromuscular maturity to assume and maintain a flexed position. The aspect of care that will be started in the delivery room is developmentally appropriate positioning. Premature infants benefit in several ways from a flexed spine and flexed extremities as they adjust to an extrauterine environment. Developmentally appropriate positioning helps to maintain body temperature and prevents skin breakdown and cranial molding (flattening of the head). Nurses will position Gabriella to promote the development of strong flexor tone, just as she would have if she had remained in utero.

NURSING PLAN OF CARE

Although health challenges in newborns can result from various causes, the presence of any one of these challenges can create common health care needs for the newborn and family. Challenges result from immature functioning of body systems in the newborn, particularly the premature infant. The stress on family functioning processes associated with the birth of a sick infant also must be addressed. These challenges are outlined in Nursing Plan of Care 14-1.

ALTERATIONS IN NEONATAL HEALTH STATUS

Several disorders place the newborn at risk for ongoing health problems. Congenital anomalies, prematurity and LBW, birth injuries, and perinatal asphyxia are examples of conditions that require skilled nursing assessment and interventions to promote healing and optimal development. In addition, specific diseases of the newborn have different care requirements. The most common disorders are discussed in this section.

CONGENITAL ANOMALIES

Congenital anomalies are abnormalities or defects that are present at birth. Such defects are the leading cause of infant mortality in North America and Europe (Heron, 2011; Kung et al., 2008). Approximately 3% to 4% of all births involve either a minor or major congenital anomaly; however, the specific incidence varies according to the defect, the geographic area (possibly because of environmental factors or a limited gene pool), or cultural practices such as **consanguinity** (sharing blood, having a common ancestor). Mating between people who are closely related can result in an increased incidence of progeny who are homozygous for autosomal recessive traits possessed by both parents.

Anomalies are inherited through gene transmission (**genotype**: the specific genetic makeup of the individual) or are initiated by a stimulus during embryogenesis at the time when developing structures are vulnerable (**phenotype**: the specific manifestation of a trait, the observable characteristics of the person). Normal phenotypic variations occur, such as hair and eye color, height, or weight. Stimuli or **teratogens** (agents that can disrupt fetal growth and produce birth defects) that can produce phenotype anomalies include drugs, environmental toxins, radiation, infection, diet, and metabolic disorders (see Table 3-1). Defects may occur alone or in a typical pattern with other abnormalities (identified as a syndrome, association, or sequence).

Pathophysiology

The inheritance of genetic traits, abnormalities, or diseases is determined by both the type of chromosome where the gene is located (autosome or sex chromosome) and whether the gene itself is recessive or dominant. Autosomal diseases are inherited through the nonsex chromosomes (pairs 1 to 22); sex-linked diseases

NURSING INTERVENTIONS 14-1

Providing Developmentally Appropriate Care

Element	Intervention
Environment	Provide calm and soothing ambiance.
	Avoid loud, sudden noises; pad trash can lids; close isolette portholes gently; carefully place items on top of isolettes; decrease decibel level of telephones, intercoms, and overhead music.
	Lighting should be modifiable to provide adequate lighting for examinations and procedures but be able to dim for rest and to facilitate eye opening in the infant to interact with families or the environment.
Positioning	Support the infant in a flexed, tucked position either with a positioning aid (bumper, nest, blankets) for rest or with the caregiver's hands during procedures.
	Side-lying or prone positioning is best
	Change position gently while supporting the infant in a tucked position; avoid extreme limb extension.
Handling	Avoid giving too much stimulation at one time.
	Approach the infant slowly (e.g., place your hands on the infant gently for a few seconds then gently turn infant over instead of abruptly opening isolette and flipping infant on his or her back).
	Observe the infant's cues for tolerance of handling and indications to reduce or stop stimulation.
	Procedures may need to be implemented in stages, allowing the infant to recover before proceeding (e.g., pause and provide containment or a pacifier to suck on).
Self-regulation	Observe the infant for behaviors used to self-soothe (e.g., hand-to-mouth movements).
	Support self-soothing behaviors or positions of the infant.
	Post a list of the infant's stress cues, cues that indicate relaxation, and self-soothing methods of the infant.
State regulation (the newborn's ability to regulate his or her behavioral state)	Observe infant for differentiated sleep/wake cycles.
	Provide a calm, stable environment.
	Time activities to coincide with the infant's patterns (e.g., offer feedings when the infant is in a quiet, awake state).
	Swaddle to promote state regulation during stressful procedures (e.g., endotracheal tube suctioning, heel stick).
Caregiving event	Incorporate all the previous interventions into care delivery.
	Provide care when the infant is in a quiet, awake state, if medically feasible.
	Observe the infant's cues and modify care based on them.
	Talk softly to the infant (as tolerated).
	Have two health care providers perform noxious procedures: one to perform the procedure and one to support the infant with containment and promotion of self-soothing behaviors.
	Plan procedures prior to implementation; consider necessity of procedure versus physiologic cost to the infant; have all equipment readily available.

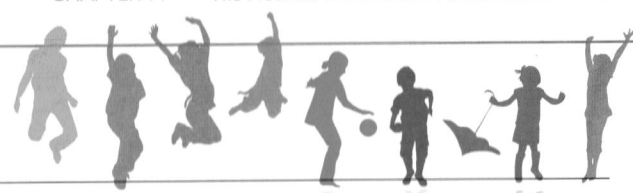

NURSING PLAN OF CARE 14-1:

The Neonate With Altered Health Status

Nursing Diagnosis: Ineffective thermoregulation related to immature skin structure, decreased amount of subcutaneous tissue, or physiologic stress

Interventions/Rationale
- Maintain external heat source whenever the isolette door must be opened for procedures.

  When the isolette door is open, heat is lost to the environment and the infant may experience cold stress. External heat source is required to prevent cold stress (see thePoint for Procedures: Warming Devices, Use of).
- During bathing, provide an external heat source.

  Bathing can induce cold stress in the preterm and term neonate. Provide an external heat source (such as a heat lamp) to minimize cold stress.
- Use radiant warmers for larger neonates who require close observation.

  Radiant heat warmers provide radiant heat with the benefit of open access to the neonate for close visual observation and nursing care. Although used also for the preterm infant, radiant heat warmers do not provide humidity and may increase insensible water losses in the preterm neonate with immature skin.

Expected Outcomes
- Neonate will be maintained within a neutral thermal environment.
- Neonate will have a stable temperature between 36.4° and 37.0° C (97.5° and 98.6° F).

Nursing Diagnosis: Risk for infection related to effects of immature immune system

Interventions/Rationale
- Strict hand hygiene is required immediately prior to touching neonate.

  Hand hygiene is the single most important intervention to prevent nosocomial infections in the NICU.
- Ensure clean preparation of expressed breast milk (EBM) and/or formula for feeding.

  Bacteria can be introduced into feedings during preparation. Bacteria in feedings can cause bloodstream infection in the at-risk neonate. Nurses preparing feedings at the bedside must ensure clean technique.
- Ensure sterile technique for all invasive procedures (endotracheal tube suctioning, central line insertion, and care).

  Sterile technique helps to prevent the introduction of bacteria during invasive procedures.

Expected Outcome
- Neonate will remain infection free.

Nursing Diagnosis: Risk for impaired skin integrity related to thin skin from immaturity

Interventions/Rationale
- Use emollients to maintain skin integrity and prevent dry, cracked skin.

  Emollients help to keep the skin intact by preventing cracking and bleeding.
- Use humidity to avoid dry, cracked skin.

  Humidity helps to reduce dry skin and keep the skin intact.
- Use tape and adhesives minimally to prevent epidermal stripping; use barrier to tape (such as pectin-based products) whenever possible.

  Tape and adhesives make a strong bond to the epidermis of the LBW neonate. Because the skin of the premature neonate is immature, when tape is removed, the epidermis remains bonded to the tape or adhesive, causing epidermal stripping. This wound provides a portal of entry for bacteria and may lead to infection.
- Remove antiseptics (povidone iodine, alcohol) as soon as possible using normal saline wipes.

  The immature skin of the preterm neonate is thin and a poor barrier to anything put on the skin. Topical antiseptics may be easily and quickly absorbed into the bloodstream. Removal with normal saline wipes is the safest way to limit absorption by the skin.

Expected Outcome
- Neonate will have intact skin.

Nursing Diagnosis: Delayed growth and development related to poor feeding and weight gain

Interventions/Rationale
- Minimize caloric loss by maintaining infant in neutral thermal environment; if in open crib, move away from window and avoid drafts. May need to limit time outside isolette to avoid cold stress and loss of calories.

  Maintaining a neutral thermal environment will limit the loss of calories from thermoregulation and will maximize growth.
- Limit nippling (bottle or breast) attempts to 30 minutes to decrease calories used for feeding intake.

  Calories are needed to nipple or breastfeed. Limiting the attempts to 30 minutes will help maximize the calories available for growth.

Expected Outcome
- Neonate will demonstrate adequate growth and feeding patterns.

(Continued)

NURSING PLAN OF CARE 14-1:

The Neonate With Altered Health Status *(Continued)*

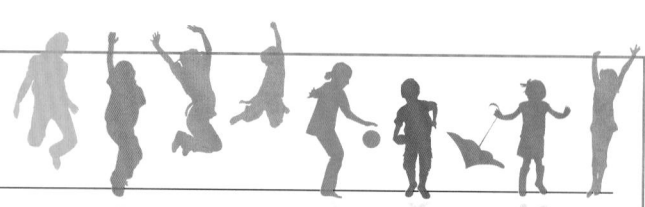

Nursing Diagnosis: Risk for impaired attachment related to effects of hospitalization, sick neonate's ability to interact with parents

Interventions/Rationale
- Explore family's understanding of neonate's condition and causative factors.
  Parents may blame themselves for causing the neonate's condition. Accurate understanding may facilitate a more realistic perspective and enable the parents to interact more positively with the infant.
- Encourage skin-to-skin care by families.
  Providing skin-to-skin care may help the family to recognize the unique role they play in their child's life and how they can contribute to the infant's care and physiologic well-being. Parents demonstrate more positive affect, touch, and adaptation to infant cues when participating in skin-to-skin care.
- Support parents' competence in assessing their infant's behavioral cues and responses.
  Reinforces parental role and the parents' ability to meet their child's needs.
- Involve parents in providing care for their infant.
  Reinforces parental role and the parents' ability to meet their child's needs.

Expected Outcomes
- Families will participate in the newborn's care, as appropriate, and will begin to verbalize positive statements regarding the newborn.
- Parent–infant attachment will occur.

Nursing Diagnosis: Interrupted family processes related to reaction to an acutely ill newborn

Interventions/Rationale
- Assess the family's stress levels, coping mechanisms, and support systems.
  Knowledge of stressors and support can be used to assist family members and build on their strengths.
- Encourage family discussion of feelings and acknowledge their normalcy.
  Venting of feelings may help decrease anxiety and validate that what they are experiencing is normal.
- Involve the family in caring for their infant.
  Helps maintain normalcy and reinforces the family's ability to provide adequate care.

Expected Outcomes
- Family will visit the newborn frequently, maintain mutual support, and seek external resources as needed.

Nursing Diagnosis: Risk for disorganized infant behavior

Interventions/Rationale
- Assess for the infant's behavioral cues that indicate stress, avoidance, approach, and regulation; deliver care accordingly.
  Each infant differs in the ability to regulate the environment and communicate needs. Reading and responding appropriately to the infant's cues demonstrates to the infant that he or she can influence the environment and contributes to the infant's physiologic stability.
- Teach the family to recognize the infant's cues and how to respond.
  Facilitates parental role attainment.
- Support the family's competence in assessing their infant's behavioral cues and responses.
  Reinforces parental role and the family's ability to meet their child's needs.
- Structure the environment to minimize stimuli. Cluster caregiving activities when possible. Monitor the neonate for stress cues when interacting and providing care.
  Minimizing stimuli may facilitate behavioral organization. Clustering care provides longer periods of uninterrupted sleep.

Expected Outcomes
- Neonate will maintain physiologic and behavioral stability.
- Neonate's behavioral cues will be recognized, and interventions will be implemented to assist infant in maintaining physiologic and behavioral stability.

Nursing Diagnosis: Deficient knowledge: Well-child care or complicated home care

Interventions/Rationale
- Provide multiple sources of family education including videos, reading material, and hands-on demonstration.
  Providing multiple methods of teaching is the best way to present new material to adult learners.
- Provide opportunities to room-in whenever possible.
  Rooming-in (staying with the infant and all required equipment in a homelike environment within the hospital; family provides all care to the infant) gives the family a chance to be the primary care providers for their infant, to work with the actual equipment they will have in the home, and to give the medications. This care is provided with support, as needed, from the NICU staff.

Expected Outcome
- Family will be able to provide competent care of the newborn after discharge.

are inherited through the X chromosome. Diseases are not inherited through the Y chromosome (Table 14-1; see Fig. 3-3).

Chromosomal aberrations are disorders caused by changes in the number or structure of chromosomes. Chromosomal aberrations do not follow the straightforward patterns of single-gene inheritance. Sometimes, an error occurs while chromosomes are being sorted during the production of the sperm or the egg; this is called *nondisjunction*. Nondisjunction can occur during meiosis I or meiosis II. During meiosis I, the error occurs when the homologous pairs both travel into the same daughter cell. The result is two daughter cells that have two copies of the chromosome and two cells that are missing that chromosome. In meiosis II, the error occurs when the sister chromatids do not separate and thus go into the same daughter cell. At fertilization, the egg (23 chromosomes) and the sperm (23 chromosomes) fuse to create a zygote, which has 46 chromosomes. If a sperm or egg, because of nondisjunction, carries an extra copy of one of the chromosomes, the reproductive cell will contain a total of 24 chromosomes, instead of 23. If this sperm or egg joins with a normal sperm or egg during fertilization, the result will be a total of 47 chromosomes instead of 46, resulting in **trisomy**. *Monosomy* occurs when there is only one copy of a chromosome that is normally present in two copies. These eggs and sperm have 22 chromosomes,

not the normal 23. When fertilized, the outcome is 45 chromosomes in total. A fetus with monosomy of the autosomes is generally less likely to survive than one with trisomy. Changes in the number of sex chromosomes (e.g., Turner syndrome, Klinefelter syndrome) cause milder effects than trisomy or monosomy.

Many other disorders are caused by the effects of multiple genes or by interactions between genes and the environment. Such inheritance is classified as multifactorial. Multifactorial disorders are difficult to analyze because they do not follow the single-gene patterns of inheritance and their genetic causes are often unclear. Examples of conditions caused by multiple genes or gene–environment interactions include neural tube defects, cleft lip and palate, pyloric stenosis, congenital heart disease, diabetes, obesity, schizophrenia, and certain types of cancer.

Not all congenital anomalies result from genetic aberrations. Prenatal exposure to teratogens may also cause congenital anomalies (see Chapter 3).

Assessment

Prenatal diagnosis of some congenital anomalies may be possible with ultrasonography, amniocentesis, or chorionic villus sampling. Obstetric factors may suggest anomalies such as polyhydramnios, which may result from a problem with swallowing (e.g., a CNS disorder such as anencephaly) or from a blockage of

TABLE 14-1	Patterns of Single-Gene Inheritance	
Pattern	**Description**	**Examples of Conditions**
Autosomal dominant	One copy of the mutated gene is capable of passing on the trait (causing disease), even though the matching gene from the other parent is normal. The mutated gene dominates the outcome of the gene pair. Typically occurs in every generation of an affected family; a vertical transmission pattern.	Familial hypercholesterolemia, achondroplasia, Marfan syndrome, retinoblastoma, neurofibromatosis I, Treacher Collins syndrome, Huntington disease
Autosomal recessive	Two copies of the mutated gene are necessary to have the trait—one inherited from the mother and one from the father. An affected child usually has unaffected parents who each carry a single copy of the mutated gene (they are *carriers* of the affected gene). Typically, disorders are not seen in every generation of an affected family; a horizontal transmission pattern. Often, the disease results in a defective enzyme in a biochemical pathway.	Cystic fibrosis, sickle cell disease, Tay-Sachs disease, congenital hypothyroidism, galactosemia, phenylketonuria, albinism
X-linked dominant	Caused by a mutated gene on the X chromosome. Very rare. Females are more frequently affected than males because daughters have 100% inheritance from fathers combined with 50% from mothers, whereas sons only have 50% from mothers. All daughters of an affected male and a normal female are affected; all sons are normal. Affected females and normal males have a risk that half the sons will be affected and half the daughters will be affected. Fathers cannot pass X-linked traits to their sons. Families with an X-linked dominant disorder often have both affected males and affected females in each generation.	Vitamin D–resistant rickets (hypophosphatemic rickets), Rett syndrome
X-linked recessive	Caused by a mutated gene on the X chromosome. Males are more frequently affected than females because females with a mutation in a gene on the X chromosome usually have a nonmutated gene on their other X chromosome that can compensate for the mutation. An affected man has two unaffected daughters who each carry one copy of the abnormal gene and two unaffected sons; an unaffected woman who carries one copy of an abnormal gene for an X-linked recessive disorder has the risk for an affected son, an unaffected daughter who carries one copy of the abnormal gene, and two unaffected children who do not have the abnormal gene. Fathers cannot pass X-linked traits to their sons. Families with an X-linked recessive disorder often have affected males, but rarely affected females, in each generation.	Color blindness, glucose-6-phosphate dehydrogenase (G6PD) deficiency, hemophilia, Duchenne muscular dystrophy, Becker muscular dystrophy, Lesch-Nyhan syndrome

the gastrointestinal tract (e.g., intestinal atresia); oligohydramnios, which may result from low urine output because of genitourinary anomalies; or IUGR (e.g., fetal alcohol syndrome [FAS], trisomy 18, maternal opioid use, maternal phenylketonuria).

Some congenital anomalies are physically obvious at birth and apparent on physical examination (e.g., cleft lip and palate). Other anomalies are more subtle, and the history, although always essential, provides important data (e.g., fragile X, in which affected boys often have delayed acquisition of developmental milestones; as they grow older, physical signs of the condition become more pronounced). See Table 14-2 for clinical features of selected congenital aberrations.

Diagnostic testing depends on the suspected aberration or anomaly. Chromosomal analysis, DNA analysis, and fluorescent in situ hybridization (FISH) may be useful in confirming a chromosomal or genetic aberration. Biochemical genetic studies (metabolic screening) involve the study of enzymes in the body to detect abnormalities, such as inborn errors of metabolism or amino acid and organic acid disorders (see Chapter 27). Testing may be done from a sample of blood, urine, spinal fluid, or other tissue.

Interdisciplinary Interventions

Treatment of congenital anomalies is based on the defects. Pathology and treatment of many defects are discussed in the chapter specific to the primary system that is affected. Many congenital anomalies result in long-term or permanent alterations in health and development (see Chapter 12) or limited life span. If genetic factors are suspected, the parents should receive genetic counseling (see Chapter 3).

Genetic counseling and prenatal diagnosis provide parents with knowledge to make informed decisions regarding the current pregnancy and its outcome or future pregnancies. If a defect is identified prenatally, parents can learn about the condition and prepare themselves to care for their affected child; if the defect is serious, parents can decide whether to terminate the pregnancy. Arrangements can also be made to deliver the infant at a facility that is prepared to care for the infant. Prenatal therapy is possible for some conditions (diaphragmatic hernia, uropathy, spina bifida, hydrocephalus) but is experimental.

When an anomaly is identified at or after birth, inform parents promptly. More extensive discussions can occur after definitive diagnosis, when more information is available and the family has had some time to process the information, although shock and grief over the loss of their "perfect" child may interfere with their ability to assimilate information. Give the family a realistic appraisal of the condition, its prognosis, and the interventions available. Encourage them to participate actively in decisions regarding their child's care. Frequent, open communication is the key in providing care that lessens the parents' feelings of helplessness and facilitates their identification with their role as parents.

Care needs, teaching, and anticipatory guidance vary based on the prognosis and associated defects. Initially, the family is often in shock and is going through the grief process. Provide a calm, nurturing environment; clear, concise information; and opportunities to hold the baby and create memories (e.g., pictures, hand or footprints). If the infant survives, routine infant care and teaching is important, in addition to any special care needs.

DISORDERS OF PREMATURITY AND LOW BIRTH WEIGHT

Low birth weight (LBW) is defined as a birth weight less than 2,500 g (5.5 lb), and **very low birth weight (VLBW)** is a birth weight less than 1,500 g (3.5 lb). **Extremely low birth weight (ELBW)** is a birth weight less than 1,000 g (2.2 lb). Every year, an estimated 15 million babies are born preterm worldwide (Blencowe et al., 2012). The national preterm birth rate (birth before 37 weeks completed gestation) in the United States has slowly declined over the past 5 years. In 2011, 11.7% of infants born in the United States were preterm, which is the lowest rate in the past decade (March of Dimes Foundation, 2012). Preterm birth is the leading cause of newborn death and the second leading cause of death in children younger than 5 years of age. LBW infants account for 8.1% of all births and VLBW infants account for 1.49% (Hamilton et al., 2012).

The causes of premature delivery remain unknown. Maternal or fetal sepsis and high-risk pregnancies, such as those with multiple gestation, abruptio placentae, and pregnancy-induced hypertension, all contribute to premature delivery. In many cases, no specific causal factor can be identified, and in some cases, there are multiple causal factors.

Prematurity and LBW were the second leading cause of infant death in 2011 (Hoyert & Xu, 2012). Racial differences exist as well, with African American infant mortality rates approximately 2.2 times the rates for white or Hispanic infants (Hoyert & Xu, 2012).

LBW without prematurity (i.e., a birth weight that is low despite a pregnancy carried to term) is considered **intrauterine growth retardation (IUGR)** and is associated with causes of poor placental circulation such as maternal hypertension, smoking during pregnancy, substance abuse, and cardiac or pulmonary problems. Often, no cause can be identified in the newborn with IUGR. Such newborns may be symmetrically growth retarded, meaning that all growth parameters are compromised, or asymmetrically growth retarded, meaning that head circumference is AGA but birth weight and other growth parameters are compromised.

When women present to the hospital in preterm labor, methods to stop labor are administered, including tocolytics. When these measures fail and preterm delivery is likely, administration of antenatal steroids decreases the incidence of IVH and respiratory distress and serves an overall protective function to the preterm newborn.

Pathophysiology

Premature newborns have a higher incidence of morbidity and mortality than term newborns. This higher incidence is likely related to LBW. Although survival

TABLE 14-2 Selected Genetic Aberrations

Condition/Incidence	Clinical Features*	Outcome/Prognosis	Interventions
Single-Gene Inheritance			
Treacher Collins syndrome (mandibulofacial dysostosis) 1/50,000 births	Downward-sloping palpebral fissures Coloboma (notch in the lower eyelids) Underdeveloped facial bones Small jaw and chin (micrognathia) Small, abnormally shaped, or absent external ears Large mouth Conductive hearing loss and cleft palate often present Normal development and intelligence	Normal life span	Supportive care as needed Maintain airway, intake Hearing aids Anticipatory support for psychological issues Speech–language therapy Reconstructive surgery
Achondroplasia (dwarfism) 1/20,000–1/ 40,000 births 80% are new mutations	Short stature (approximately 4 ft) Trunk is normal, limbs short, upper arms and thighs are more shortened than the forearms and lower legs Short fingers, space between middle and ring fingers (trident hand) Large head with prominent forehead Joint laxity Midface hypoplasia (nose flat at the bridge) Delayed motor milestones; normal intelligence	Infants who are homozygous for achondroplasia seldom live beyond a few months Unexpected infant death in 2%–5% likely from central apnea secondary to compression of arteries at the level of the foramen magnum Mortality increases in third to fourth decade of life	Track growth and head circumference using growth curves standardized for achondroplasia (Horton et al., 1978) For infants, provide firm neck and back support (no umbrella strollers) and limit uncontrolled head movement (no swings or carrying slings) Symptomatic management of frequent middle ear infections and dental crowding Anticipatory support for psychological issues Teach measures to control obesity, starting in early childhood Modify the environment to accommodate the child's short stature Dress as appropriate to age, not size Growth hormone therapy, lengthening of the limb bones, and surgery to correct bowing of the legs may be done (refer to Trotter & Hall [2005] for more information)
Marfan syndrome 1/5,000 births	Connective tissue disorder, very tall, slender, long, extremities Joint laxity Long, narrow face; arched palate; crowded teeth Pectus excavatum or carinatum Scoliosis Flat feet Myopia, glaucoma Femoral, inguinal hernias Aortic root dilation, aortic regurgitation, mitral valve prolapse	Slightly shortened life span because of cardiovascular complications Survival into the 60s	Advise against contact sports or weight lifting (may contribute to development of aortic aneurysm) Symptomatic management of complications associated with aortic dilation
Fragile X syndrome 1/4,000–1/6,000 males, 1/8,000 females	Delayed developmental milestones, learning disabilities, and cognitive defects, typically combined with behavioral problems (e.g., inattention, hyperactivity, autism) With age, physical features become more apparent—characteristic long, narrow face with jutting jaw; large ears and high forehead; enlarged testicles (macroorchidism); flat feet; unusually flexible finger joints; high-pitched, jocular speech	Usually, males are more severely affected than females Typically normal life span	Special education program with modifications in classroom environment and curriculum Speech–language therapy and occupational therapy (OT) Medication to manage hyperactivity, attention difficulties, or other behavioral problems For adolescents with mental impairment, vocational training
Lesch-Nyhan syndrome 1/380,000 births	Deficiency of the enzyme hypoxanthineguanine phosphoribosyltransferase Self-mutilation (lip and finger biting, head banging) Hypotonia Spastic muscle movements Severe gout Cognitive challenge	Death often in the second to third decade of life	Prevent self-injury: behavioral extinction techniques, reduce stress (which increases self-mutilation); restraint may be necessary Symptomatic treatment: allopurinol for gout, lithotripsy for kidney stones; baclofen or benzodiazepines may be used for spasticity

(Continued)

TABLE 14-2   Selected Genetic Aberrations *(Continued)*

Condition/Incidence	Clinical Features*	Outcome/Prognosis	Interventions
Chromosomal Aberrations			
Trisomy 21 (Down syndrome) 1/600–1/800 births; risk increases with increasing maternal age	Protruding tongue Transverse palmar crease Oblique palpebral fissure Hypotonia Hyperflexibility Variable cognitive challenge Higher incidence of congenital heart defects, digestive problems (e.g., gastroesophageal reflux disease, celiac disease), leukemia, hearing loss, hypothyroidism	Life span may be limited by associated conditions Often live beyond fifth decade; premature aging occurs	Monitor growth Chart using growth charts for typical children and for children with Down syndrome (specific growth charts available at www.growthcharts.com) (Cronk et al.,1988; Styles et al., 2002) Refer to lactation consultant (hypotonia and protruding tongue may interfere with feeding) Refer to early intervention program, full inclusion in school based on abilities Speech–language therapy and OT Teach measures to control obesity Symptomatic care for associated defects (see Van Cleve & Cohen [2006] for more information)
Trisomy 18 (Edwards syndrome) 1/4,000 births	Weak cry Classic clenched fist with the index finger overlapping the third and fourth fingers Hypoplastic nails Wide-spaced eyes Micrognathia Deformed and low-set ears Prominent occiput Clubfeet and rocker-bottom feet Cognitive challenge	Most die within the first year of life	Supportive care
Trisomy 13 (Patau syndrome) 1/8,000 births	Midline anomalies are characteristic, such as holoprosencephaly (failure of the forebrain to divide properly), cleft lip and palate Microphthalmia Ear malformations Polydactyly Apnea Cognitive challenge	Most do not survive beyond early infancy	Symptomatic care
Turner syndrome (45XO) 1/2,500 female births	Short stature Webbing of the neck Low hairline on the back of the neck Ptosis Broad chest with widely spaced nipples Lymphedema (puffiness or swelling) of the hands and feet Infertile, with failure to go through puberty Skeletal abnormalities Heart defects (coarctation of the aorta) Kidney problems Normal intelligence, mild learning problems (math; visual–spatial coordination tasks, such as mentally rotating objects in space)	Normal life span	Monitor cardiac status and blood pressure (hypertension common, resulting from coarctation or kidney problems) Teach healthy diet and physical activity to reduce obesity Anticipatory support for psychosocial issues Modify the environment to accommodate the child's short stature; dress as appropriate to age, not size Medications: growth hormone (for stature) or estrogen replacement therapy (to stimulate acquisition of secondary sexual characteristics) (refer to Frías & Davenport [2003] for more information)
XXY males (Klinefelter syndrome) (47XXY) 1/800 male births	Tall stature Before puberty, small penile length, small testes May have low levels of the hormone testosterone beginning during puberty, which may cause gynecomastia, reduced facial and body hair, and infertility Normal intelligence; mild learning and speech and language difficulties	Normal life span	Cognitive and psychosocial testing, speech–language therapy, and remedial education as indicated Testosterone therapy at onset of puberty (to promote acquisition of secondary sexual characteristics, muscle mass)

TABLE 14-2 Selected Genetic Aberrations (Continued)

Condition/Incidence	Clinical Features*	Outcome/Prognosis	Interventions
Other Genetic Causes			
CHARGE syndrome 1/8,500–1/10,000 births	**C**oloboma **H**eart defect **A**tresia, choanal **R**etarded growth and development **G**enital hypoplasia **E**ar anomalies/deafness Major criteria: Coloboma, choanal atresia Visual impairment, blindness Anomalies of external ears (absent or hypoplastic lobes, asymmetry, decreased cartilaginous folds, triangular concha) and of inner ear (ossicular malformations, chronic serious otitis), hearing loss Cranial nerve dysfunction causing asymmetric facial palsy and/or swallowing/feeding difficulties Balance, speech problems Cleft palate Tracheoesophageal fistula, esophageal atresia, omphalocele Heart defects Genital hypoplasia, typically recognized only in males (micropenis/cryptorchidism) Autism or autistic-like behaviors (possibly resulting from combined vision and hearing deficits) Developmental delay	High infant mortality If child survives 1 year, will likely survive childhood	Symptomatic care Early referral for appropriate developmental and educational services Physical therapy to facilitate mobility Provide a structured environment that allows the child to anticipate events and gain a sense of control Educational support to address multisensory impairment

*Presentations of many conditions vary widely; all features may not be present. See Chapter 30 for more interventions specific to cognitive challenge.
  Many condition-specific organizations exist; information and support from these organizations are often helpful.

rates of premature infants have been rising over the last 20 years, premature birth before 23 weeks' gestation is generally not compatible with life. In general, the younger the gestational age at birth, the higher the mortality rate. For infants born at 24 weeks, survival to discharge is 59%, increasing to 83% at 26 weeks and 95% at 30 weeks (Manktelow et al., 2013).

Although premature infants have the necessary anatomic structures, many problems occur because all body systems are extremely immature. This immaturity leads to problems with thermoregulation, surfactant deficiency, CLD, PDA, sepsis, IVH, apnea of prematurity (AOP), feeding and nutrition problems, NEC, and ROP. Each of these disorders requires different specific care in addition to the general assessment and care required for premature and LBW newborns.

Assessment

The premature newborn has physical characteristics that are different from those of term newborns (see Focused Physical Assessment 14-1). The premature newborn's posture lacks flexion, and muscle tone is decreased. This flaccidity is obvious when the very premature newborn is supine because the arms and legs remain extended. Also, the arm recoil is slow and reduced. As the newborn grows and matures, so does the strength and ability for flexion.

The skin is thin and may be transparent. Blood vessels are easily discernible. The skin can be very moist and even gelatinous. The more premature the newborn is, the thinner and more gelatinous the skin. This thin skin is a poor barrier to the elements (Developmental Considerations 14-1), and exposure to caustic agents may not only impede skin integrity but also may lead to systemic effects.

Lanugo is very fine, downy body hair that develops in utero (after about 22 weeks' gestation) and is shed during the seventh to eighth month of gestation (Fig. 14-5). As the fetus grows, lanugo is abundant and then decreases again near term.

Color is an important indicator of well-being in any newborn. Inspect the mucous membranes, including the lips and tongue, for central cyanosis. Monitor for other color abnormalities, including jaundice and ruddiness, which may indicate pathology, especially if they occur within the first 24 hours.

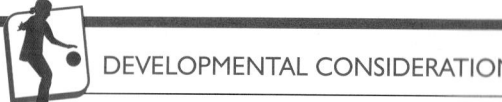

DEVELOPMENTAL CONSIDERATIONS 14-1

Factors Modifying Cutaneous Water Losses in Preterm Infants

Young gestational age TEWL increases proportionally with degree of prematurity

Increasing postnatal age TEWL decreases as infant matures

Increased ambient temperature TEWL increases as temperature increases

Increased ambient humidity TEWL decreases proportionally as humidity increases

Use of radiant warmer TEWL increases 40%–100%

Phototherapy TEWL increases by up to 50%

TEWL, transepidermal water loss.

Assess the quality and quantity of respirations; note signs of respiratory distress. Auscultate lung sounds in the axillae of the premature infant. **Periodic breathing** (clusters of breaths separated by intervals of apnea) is common in the premature newborn, and apnea may indicate sepsis, especially during the first 12 hours of life.

Observe the chest to assess movement and symmetry as well as the presence or absence of an active precordium. An active precordium is easily seen on the thin chest of a premature newborn and may indicate a PDA. Auscultate all heart borders. Note the quality and location of murmurs, which are common in the premature newborn.

The head of the premature newborn is large in proportion to the rest of the body. This disproportion reflects the cephalocaudal progression of growth. Gently palpate the anterior fontanel to assess for fullness or depression. Normally, the anterior fontanel is soft and flat. Often, the sutures of the premature head are overriding, causing a palpable ridge, especially after the first 4 to 5 days of life.

The abdomen of a premature newborn is soft and slightly rounded but not generally distended unless

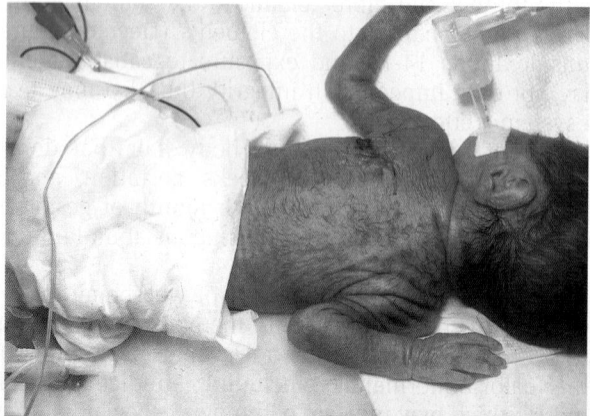

Figure 14-5 Lanugo on a premature neonate.

resuscitation at birth included bag-and-mask ventilation, which may have forced air into the stomach. Auscultate the abdomen for bowel sounds in all four quadrants. Abnormal abdominal examination findings are distention, discoloration, observable bowel loops, and absence of bowel sounds. If the premature newborn is receiving enteral nutrition, perform an abdominal examination before every feeding and measure the abdominal girth at regular intervals. Also note feeding residuals (food that is present in the stomach 3 hours after feeding), including amount and color. Stools may be tested for the presence of occult blood and reducing substance. Stools containing microscopic amounts of blood will test positive for occult blood, which may be an early sign of NEC or another feeding disorder. Stools that contain more than 0.5% sugar will test positive for reducing substance; this finding is abnormal and may indicate feeding malabsorption.

Interdisciplinary Interventions

The birth of a sick or premature infant is a stressful event for the family. Sources of stress include illness of the infant, separation of parents and other family members from their infant and each other, and a need for increased emotional and financial support (Griffin, 2006). Use a family-centered approach to provide effective support to these families in crisis by

- Establishing caring relationships with the family
- Treating the family as partners in the care of their infant
- Providing technically competent care to the infant
- Providing clear explanations to the family
- Giving the family an opportunity to see and touch their infant in the delivery room or prior to transport

Conversely, specific behaviors by nursing staff or by unit policies may increase the stress experienced by the mother and family (Obeidat et al., 2009). These behaviors include

- Restricting the mother's access to the infant
- Using negative language and demeanor (such as lecturing, ordering, short conversations, unfriendly attitude)
- Directing the mother in infant care (as opposed to teaching infant care)
- Ignoring or minimizing the mother's concern for her infant

Nurses in the NICU have a vital role in supporting families during the prolonged hospitalization of their sick newborn. Using a family-centered approach, with an empathetic and active listening demeanor, will greatly improve the mother's experience and support the family as a whole.

Community Care

In general, as immaturity increases and birth weight decreases, the likelihood of intellectual and neurologic deficits (e.g., CP, hearing and vision defects, and learning difficulties) increases. Surveillance for neurodevelopmental delays or problems, provision of early intervention and special education resources, and long-term follow-up must be provided for all newborns experiencing a major illness.

THERMOREGULATORY PROBLEMS

QUESTION: Gabriella is at risk for hypothermia for many reasons: her weight-to-surface area ratio, her lack of fat stores, and her inability to maintain a flexed position. Look carefully at Nursing Interventions 14-2. What nursing interventions would prevent or ameliorate heat loss specifically for Gabriella?

Maintaining a normal temperature is vital to the premature newborn because hypothermia leads to deleterious consequences (Chart 14-1). Term newborns respond more efficiently to hypothermia than preterm newborns. Limited ability to produce heat, coupled with many mechanisms of heat loss, make the premature newborn very susceptible to hypothermia. The term newborn is able to increase muscle activity, initiate nonshivering or chemical thermogenesis, and use brown fat stores to generate heat. The preterm newborn is unable to increase muscle activity or to assume a flexed position because of poor motor tone and limited brown fat stores. Additionally, premature newborns may be unable to initiate thermogenesis because of limited stores of fat and insufficient amounts of other chemicals such as glucose, liver enzymes, and hormones.

CHART 14-1   Thermoregulation in Preterm Infants

Predisposing factors for thermoregulatory problems:
- Lack of subcutaneous and brown fat stores
- Thin skin
- Immature CNS
- Limited ability to assume a flexed posture
- Increased surface area-to-body mass ratio

Consequences of hypothermia:
- Increased metabolic rate and oxygen demand
- Apnea
- Respiratory distress
- Cyanosis

Nonshivering thermogenesis involves the release of norepinephrine to mobilize brown fat to increase metabolic rate and generate heat. The quantity of brown fat increases with increasing gestational age. In the term newborn, brown fat is located in the axillae, between the scapulae, in the mediastinum, around the liver, and down the spine (Fig. 14-6). Use of brown fat increases

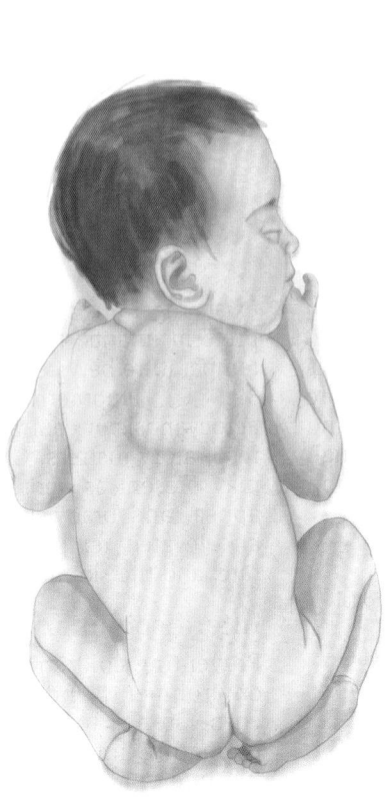

Posterior view: Suprascapular

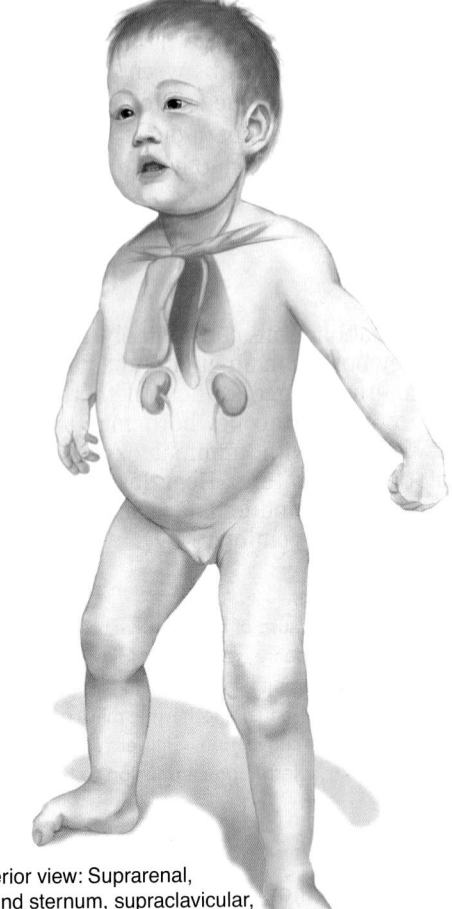

Anterior view: Suprarenal, around sternum, supraclavicular, neck region

Figure 14-6 Location of brown fat in term neonates.

NURSING INTERVENTIONS 14-2

Mechanisms of Heat Loss and Prevention Techniques

Heat Loss Mechanism	Example	Prevention Techniques
Convection: Heat loss occurring when heat is exchanged between two objects within the same environment	Loss of heat from the neonate's skin to the cooler, surrounding air. For example, cold drafts in the delivery room or nursery will lead to heat loss through convection. The premature neonate is especially vulnerable to this type of heat loss because the amount of body surface exposed is increased as a result of the lack of a flexed posture from poor muscle tone.	Warm the delivery room or nursery. Avoid drafts. Prewarm the isolette. Transport the neonate in an isolette. Use plastic sleeves on the isolette portals. Swaddle the neonate with warmed blankets.
Conduction: Loss of heat through direct contact with an object that is cooler	Placing a neonate on a cold scale or next to cool blankets	Pad the scale with a warm blanket before weighing. Use warm blankets to dry the neonate.
Evaporation: Loss of heat through conversion of water to its gaseous state	A newly delivered neonate who is wet with amniotic fluid and a neonate receiving a bath. Extremely premature neonates are very vulnerable to evaporative heat loss as a result of thin and extremely permeable skin.	Dry the neonate quickly after delivery or bathing. Warm all solutions before applying to the neonate. Administer warmed oxygen.
Radiation: Loss of heat across a gradient between two objects in the environment that are not in direct contact with each other	Loss of neonate's body heat to the surrounding, cooler incubator walls	Avoid placing the bassinet/isolette near cold walls or windows. Use a double-walled isolette. Prewarm the isolette.

the metabolic rate considerably and is initiated when the newborn is in an environment colder than the neutral thermal range. A neutral thermal environment is one in which the newborn maintains a normal core temperature with minimal oxygen consumption and calorie expenditure. Heat loss is generated through convection, conduction, evaporation, and radiation (Nursing Interventions 14-2).

ANSWER: Because of her LBW, Gabriella requires additional techniques to decrease her heat loss. These include immediately wrapping Gabriella in plastic wrap after delivery and placing her on an exothermic mattress. Then, to prevent heat loss from convection, Gabriella should be placed in an isolette upon admission to the NICU.

Assessment

Carefully monitor the temperature of the newborn to detect hypo- or hyperthermia early. Although controversy exists regarding the exact optimal body temperature for preterm infants, term infants do best with an axillary temperature between 97.2° F and 99.9° F (36.2° C and 37.7° C). Hypothermic newborns may appear pale, with acrocyanosis or central cyanosis, mottling, and signs of respiratory distress. Chronic hypothermia in newborns may present as poor weight gain, metabolic acidosis, apnea, and bradycardia. Hyperthermia presents with an elevated temperature, heart rate, and respiratory rate, and the skin may appear ruddy.

Interdisciplinary Interventions

Preventing cold stress, promoting a neutral thermal environment, and monitoring for hypothermia are cornerstones to caring for all newborns, especially premature infants (Clinical Judgment 14-1). Nursing interventions to decrease heat loss begin at delivery: Term infant and infants weighing more than 1,500 g are delivered in a warm delivery room and quickly dried to prevent evaporative heat loss. Remove the wet linen to prevent conductive heat loss.

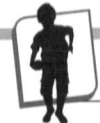

CLINICAL JUDGMENT 14-1

Preterm Infant With Hypothermia

Yolanda is an infant born at 32 weeks' gestation, who was just admitted to the NICU after a precipitous delivery in the emergency department. She was placed under the radiant warmer upon admission. Vital signs are heart rate, 160 bpm; respiratory rate, 80 breaths/min; temperature, 96.4° F (35.8° C) axillary; and weight, 2,330 g. Yolanda has nasal flaring with grunting; pulse oximeter readings are dropping into the 80s. She is pale with acrocyanosis, has a weak cry, is floppy, and shows minimal response to stimulation. Laboratory values are as follows: pH, 7.31; blood bicarbonate, 18 mEq/dL; and serum glucose, 25 mg/dL.

Questions

1. What data from the assessment are indicative of a clinical problem?
2. What are pertinent nursing diagnoses that must be considered at this time?
3. Considering Yolanda's history, which nursing diagnosis must be addressed immediately and why?
4. What nursing actions must be implemented to prevent further deterioration of Yolanda's status?
5. What parameters must be monitored carefully until Yolanda is normothermic and routinely after that?

Answers

1. Low temperature, symptoms of respiratory distress (grunting, nasal flaring, tachypnea), oxygen saturation in the 80s, pale, floppiness with minimal response to the environment. Acrocyanosis would be normal during the first hours after birth; central cyanosis would indicate a problem. An infant of 32 weeks' gestation would be hypotonic but should demonstrate limb recoil with stimulation and would respond to the environment. Abnormal laboratory values include pH and bicarbonate levels that reflect acidosis and a serum glucose value of 25 mg/dL, which indicates hypoglycemia.

2. Hypothermia

   Impaired tissue perfusion: cardiopulmonary, cerebral, gastrointestinal, peripheral, renal

   Impaired gas exchange

   Risk for infection

   Risk for disorganized infant behavior

   Risk for impaired attachment

3. Hypothermia must be addressed immediately because it will create or exacerbate other clinical problems such as respiratory distress, acidosis, and hypoglycemia. Tachypnea is caused by the increased oxygen demand from the increased metabolic rate to keep warm. Hypothermia leads to peripheral vasoconstriction, resulting in decreased tissue perfusion and subsequent hypoxia and metabolic acidosis. These lead to pulmonary vasoconstriction, which results in increased pulmonary artery pressure and right-to-left shunting of blood, worsening the hypoxia. Hypoxia may impair surfactant release, further worsening the respiratory distress and acidosis. Increased metabolism also consumes glucose, leading to hypoglycemia. Breakdown of glycogen to glucose while hypoxic generates extra lactic acid, worsening the acidosis.

4. Ensure that the temperature probe for the radiant warmer is positioned on a solid mass surface or the trunk or lower extremities, not on air-filled cavities such as the stomach or lungs. Position the probe on the surface of the infant that faces the heat source; the infant must not lie on the probe. Ensure that the warmer is on servocontrol (controlled by the infant's temperature, not manually). Position the warmer away from drafts and opening doors. Make sure that Yolanda is dry and on dry linen. If these are in place, Yolanda may require an additional heat source such as a heat lamp, warmed blankets, or artificial heat blankets. Prewarm equipment such as stethoscopes and scales.

5. Temperature 97.2°−99.1° F axillary (36.2°−37.3° C), cardiorespiratory status, arterial blood gases (pH, bicarbonate, oxygen), blood glucose

Infants who weigh less than 1,500 g require different and additional measures to reduce heat loss immediately after delivery, including placing a plastic wrap on the infant (without drying the infant) and using an exothermic mattress (Kattwinkel et al., 2010; McCall et al., 2010) (Fig. 14-7). Once in the NICU, warm the scales, stethoscopes, and blankets, and place a cap on the premature newborn's head to prevent heat loss. Other devices that may be used in the NICU to promote a neutral thermal environment

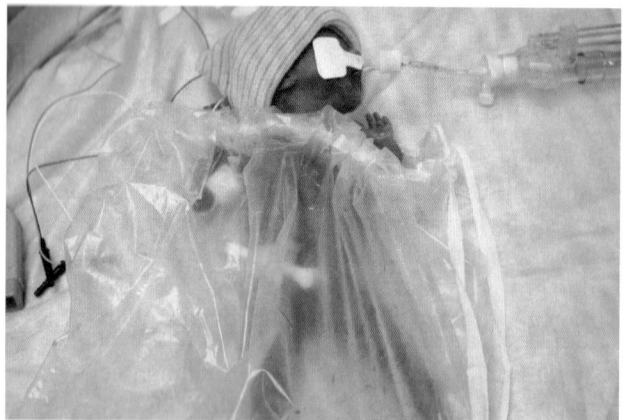

Figure 14-7 At birth, the body of an extremely preterm infant may be placed in a plastic bag to conserve heat.

include radiant warmers, isolettes, and plastic wraps (Fig. 14-8).

Closely monitor the newborn's skin and core temperatures and the isolette or ambient temperature. Apply a skin probe to continuously monitor skin temperature

in all premature newborns under a radiant warmer or in an isolette. The skin temperature is the first to decrease in cold stress. The lower left abdomen is the ideal place for a skin probe; avoid areas over brown fat and bone, such as over the liver and the spine. Secure the skin probe in place; if it is accidentally dislodged, the device may sense cooler room air, generate heat in response, and overheat the infant. Monitor the location of the probe to prevent thermoregulatory problems. Do not allow the newborn to lie on the probe, which may increase the temperature readings artificially. Monitor the newborn's core temperature by the axillary route every hour until it is stable and then every 2 to 3 hours.

 KidKare Avoid routine rectal temperatures because they may cause tissue damage and are stressful to the newborn.

Compare the isolette ambient temperature with previous measurements of ambient temperature to detect temperature instability, which is an early sign of sepsis. As the newborn's skin temperature decreases, the ambient temperature will increase accordingly,

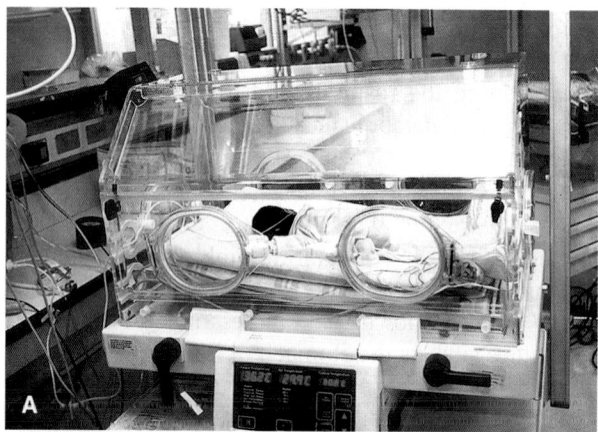
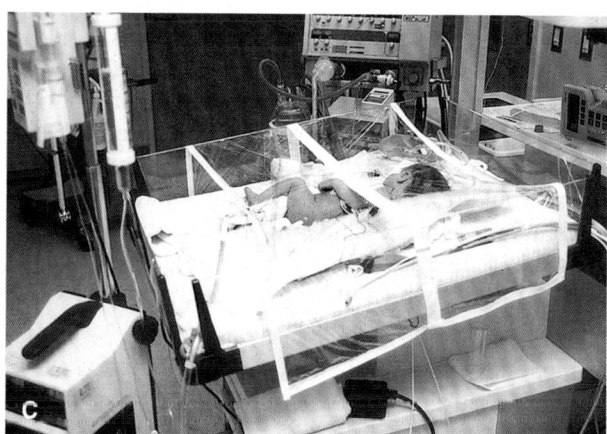
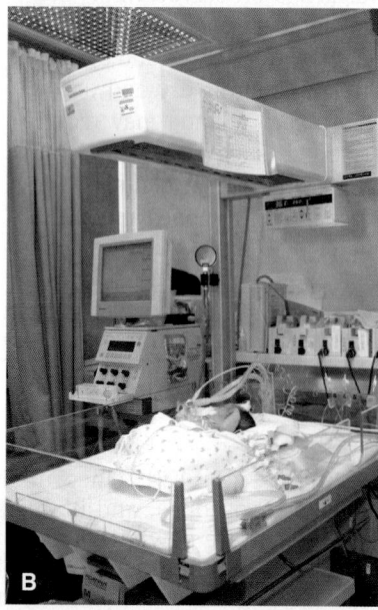
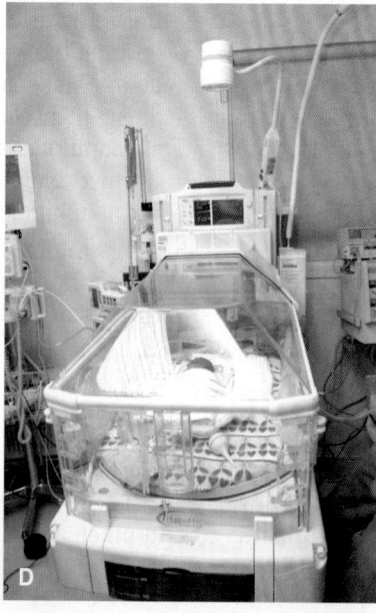

Figure 14-8 Various methods help neonates maintain thermoregulation. (A) Isolette. (B) Radiant warmer. (C) Plastic wrap. (D) Combination unit: radiant warmer and isolette.

Investigate further if any changes in ambient temperature occur.

Clustering care, if the newborn tolerates this approach, is one method to reduce heat loss and limit fluctuations in temperature. Collaborate with other members of the health care team to time procedures and examinations to limit heat losses and to provide extended sleep periods. However, remain alert to signs of stress in the newborn (as previously discussed) because some newborns are unable to handle many procedures or care activities performed at one time. Individualized care is the goal; assess the ability of the newborn to tolerate interactions and handling. If the newborn exhibits signs of stress, the nurse may need to stop and give the newborn time to recover.

Radiant Warmers

Radiant warmers provide heat quickly and efficiently and allow access to the newborn for stabilization and resuscitation measures. However, they allow for convective heat loss and an increased insensible water loss from the skin, especially in the ELBW newborn. Therefore, use radiant warmers for initial stabilization only, and move the newborn to an isolette as soon as possible.

Isolettes

An isolette provides minimal radiant and convective heat losses and allows for constant visual observation of the newborn. Use the portholes, which allow for minimal heat loss during nursing care, at all times. Avoid opening the isolette unnecessarily. Most isolettes have double walls, which serve as a buffer to radiant heat loss because the inside wall is warmed by the ambient air temperature of the isolette.

Combination Units

Combination units, such as the Giraffe OmniBed, serve as both a radiant warmer (in the open position) and an isolette (in the closed position). Often used for the very preterm newborn, these combination units provide the benefits of an isolette (with built-in humidification system) in addition to the benefits of quick and easy access to the newborn (for surgeries and other procedures).

SURFACTANT DEFICIENCY

QUESTION: Gabriella is responding well to the surfactant therapy she received. What is the role of the nurse in assessing and responding to Gabriella's changing lung compliance?

Respiratory distress, common in premature newborns, is often the presenting symptom of many diseases and problems. Respiratory distress may be caused by sepsis, hypoglycemia, hypothermia, or lung immaturity. In utero, the placenta performs respiratory functions because the fetus's lungs are filled with fluid and do not participate in air exchange. At delivery, the lungs normally become filled with air, are perfused by blood, and participate in oxygen and carbon dioxide exchange. To perform this function, the lungs must inflate properly, a process that requires the presence of surfactant.

Pathophysiology

The lungs of a premature newborn lack a phospholipid called **surfactant**, which is necessary for effective respiratory function. Surfactant acts like a detergent to reduce the surface tension of the lungs, promoting their expansion. Without surfactant, the lung collapses after every expiration and reinflates with great difficulty, requiring the newborn to generate intense pressures with every breath. Surfactant is generally produced in the lung at approximately 35 weeks' gestation, but production may be delayed by maternal complications such as diabetes.

Assessment

The diagnosis of surfactant deficiency is based on maternal history, neonatal physical examination, and laboratory and radiographic findings (Table 14-3). The newborn with surfactant deficiency displays signs of moderate to severe respiratory distress, including sternal, substernal, and intercostal retractions; grunting; and nasal flaring. Central cyanosis is common, and hypotension may be present if the newborn is severely distressed and acidotic.

Surfactant deficiency is diagnosed by chest radiograph and clinical presentation (presence of respiratory distress, carbon dioxide retention, and oxygen requirements). Although not routinely used for diagnosis, laboratory studies include a lung profile that may reveal an immature lecithin-to-sphingomyelin (L/S) ratio or the absence of phosphatidylglycerol (PG). Both these biochemical markers are examined from the amniotic fluid at the time of rupture of the membranes or a tracheal aspirate may be obtained from the newborn. Analysis of arterial or capillary blood gases may reveal respiratory acidosis from carbon dioxide retention and hypoxemia. Electrolyte levels may show dehydration, especially in the extremely premature newborn, from the increased insensible water loss that occurs through thin skin. Finally, the chest radiograph may reveal a reticulogranular or "ground-glass" pattern evenly throughout the lungs caused by massive atelectasis.

TABLE 14-3	Indicators of Surfactant Deficiency	
Maternal History/ Factors	**Physical Examination of Newborn**	**Lab/Radiographic Findings**
Premature labor Fetal gestational age <35 weeks Lack of treatment with corticosteroids Absent PG	Cyanosis Labored breathing Retractions Tachypnea Grunting Nasal flaring Poor tissue perfusion Skin mottling Hypotension	Respiratory/ metabolic acidosis Reticulogranular pattern on chest radiograph Massive atelectasis or air bronchogram

Nursing Diagnoses and Outcomes

Nursing diagnoses and outcomes generally applicable for newborns with a health challenge are presented in Nursing Plan of Care 14-1. In addition, the following nursing diagnosis and outcomes may apply for a newborn with surfactant deficiency:

Nursing Diagnosis: Impaired gas exchange related to effects of poor lung compliance and atelectasis
Outcomes:
• Infant will display blood gas levels within normal limits.
• Infant will show no signs of adverse effects from assisted ventilation or oxygen administration.

Interdisciplinary Interventions

Care of the newborn in respiratory distress caused by surfactant deficiency involves monitoring all body functions and supporting the newborn with supplemental oxygen and assisted ventilation if needed. The mainstay of treatment for surfactant deficiency is administration of exogenous surfactant. Many types of exogenous surfactant are available; all require intratracheal administration. Exogenous surfactant coats the lungs to improve ventilation and oxygenation and to reduce protein leakage that commonly accompanies surfactant deficiency. Protein leakage occurs in damaged lungs, causing pulmonary edema. Overall, the most commonly reported response after administration of surfactant is rapidly improved oxygenation and a decreased need for respiratory support.

The use of exogenous surfactant has improved initial outcomes for newborns with surfactant deficiency. Early use of surfactant has decreased the incidence of CLD, a morbidity associated with surfactant deficiency (Bahadue & Soll, 2012).

Surfactant administration may have adverse effects on the newborn. Instilling surfactant into the trachea may cause acute reduction in oxygenation by blocking large and small airways. Careful ventilation is needed to minimize this effect. When surfactant is administered,

lung compliance may suddenly increase. Because of this rapid change in lung compliance, pneumothorax can occur. Monitor ventilation requirements carefully and decrease pressures, according to the newborn's response, to avoid overdistending the lungs.

The nurse, in collaboration with respiratory therapists and the medical team, must be vigilant in monitoring chest wall expansion, improved breath sounds, and a decreased need for oxygen. Decrease the amount of supplemental oxygen according to the newborn's overall skin color and the pulse oximeter readings. The nurse has an important role in monitoring the newborn before, during, and after administration of surfactant (Nursing Interventions 14-3).

ANSWER: An infant's response to surfactant therapy can be very dramatic. The nurse must be very attentive. The change in lung compliance may mean that the inspiratory pressure previously required just to open Gabriella's "stiff lungs" is now enough to almost bounce her off the bed. Just as dramatic may be the change in oxygenation, Gabriella became noticeably pinker even as the nurse decreased the oxygen percentage delivered by the ventilator. The nurse focuses on the infant's response to the mechanical ventilation and communicates the changes or adjusts the ventilator settings, within ordered parameters, to maintain optimal ventilatory support. For example, the nurse may decrease the amount of supplemental oxygen to maintain her oxygen saturation within normal limits (88%–95%) and wean the ventilator settings to the lowest amount of pressure to minimize lung trauma. The nurse also relays and explains the changes to concerned family members (the mother is often still receiving care).

CHRONIC LUNG DISEASE

Despite surfactant replacement, noninvasive techniques of respiratory support, and improved ventilation strategies, CLD can still occur. Lung disease is the result of positive pressure ventilation (PPV) and exposure to

---

NURSING INTERVENTIONS 14-3

A Neonate Receiving Surfactant Administration

Before Surfactant Administration
• Obtain and record baseline vital signs.
• Note ventilator settings, oxygen settings, pulse oximeter readings, and transcutaneous monitor readings.

During Surfactant Administration
• Note amount instilled and neonate's response.
• Monitor vital signs continuously.
• Watch for cyanosis and improved chest wall movement.
• Increase oxygen and ventilation as needed.

After Surfactant Administration
• Avoid suctioning for at least 4 hours if possible.
• Monitor vital signs frequently.
• Carefully observe for signs of improvement, including increased oxygenation, decreased need for respiratory support, and improved chest movement.
• Wean ventilator settings as needed.

supplemental oxygen. PPV is not physiologic (negative pressure is how air enters the lung in normal breathing), and alternating lung over- and underinflation leads to ventilator-induced injury. Lung tissue that is overinflated sustains cellular disruption, which initiates the inflammatory process within the lung. Excess fluid in the lung (from the inflammatory process) leads to the need for ongoing assisted ventilation, supplemental oxygen, and diuretics (to control the fluid in the lungs).

CLD is classified as mild (oxygen requirement for 28 days), moderate (oxygen requirement at 36 weeks postmenstrual age), or severe (need for ventilation support at 36 weeks postmenstrual age). Other definitions exist; however, these three classifications assist to provide a basis for research of infants with this morbidity. The overall incidence is of CLD is 25% to 35% of infants weighing less than 1,500 g at birth. The incidence of CLD clearly increases with decreasing gestational age and need for mechanical ventilation. Infants at the edge of viability (23 to 25 weeks' gestational age) have a higher incidence of severe CLD, whereas infants of greater than 26 weeks' gestational age are more likely to develop mild CLD (Horbar et al., 2012). The cause of CLD is multifactorial (Chart 14-2).

Infants with CLD may continue to have respiratory problems throughout childhood. Those infants who require supplemental oxygen at discharge from the NICU are at an increased risk for rehospitalization for respiratory problems throughout the first 2 years of life. To prevent complications after discharge, work collaboratively with the medical team to determine the discharge plan for infants with supplemental oxygen. Teach the family methods to reduce harmful exposures in the home (e.g., pets, environmental tobacco smoke) that may exacerbate respiratory symptoms as well as use of home apnea monitoring and administration of medications.

PATENT DUCTUS ARTERIOSUS

QUESTION: Gabriella has difficulties with her ductus arteriosus relaxing, which allows additional blood flow to be diverted back to the lungs. Of the symptoms mentioned, which are the early warning signs that a PDA exists? What interventions should the nurse implement in response to these signs?

The ductus arteriosus is a fetal shunt located between the pulmonary artery and the aorta. In fetal circulation, the ductus arteriosus allows the majority of oxygenated blood from the placenta to flow directly to the systemic circulation, bypassing the lungs. After birth, the oxygen content of the blood increases, and the ductus arteriosus functionally closes in response. In PDA, the fetal shunt persists after delivery—that is, the ductus arteriosus stays open. This condition is common among preterm newborns. Because vascular resistance in the pulmonary artery is less than the systemic pressure in the aorta, persistence of a PDA leads to excessive blood volume in the pulmonary circulation, causing pulmonary edema. Diagnostic signs include the presence of congestive heart failure (a late sign), unstable blood pressures and widened pulse pressures, bounding peripheral pulses, metabolic acidosis, pulmonary edema, and an increasing need for oxygen support. A PDA is diagnosed from a bedside echocardiogram, a chest radiograph, and the presence of clinical symptoms (see Chapter 15).

Initially, treatment of PDA during the neonatal period includes fluid restriction, diuretics, and ventilator support. If the newborn remains symptomatic, medication therapy is initiated to close a PDA. Indomethacin or ibuprofen, prostaglandin inhibitors that promote ductal closure, are equally effective in closing the PDA; ibuprofen is better tolerated by the neonatal kidney but may still cause adverse effects (Giniger et al., 2007). These drugs are most effective when given during the first week of life. Side effects include elevated blood urea nitrogen and creatinine, decreased urine output, and decreased platelet function. Evaluate these values at regular intervals during treatment.

If administration of indomethacin or ibuprofen is ineffective, the premature newborn may need surgical closure of the PDA. Potential complications include phrenic nerve paralysis, lung contusions, sepsis, and ligation of the pulmonary artery. Mortality and morbidity is highest in the very sick, unstable newborn. Details of surgery and complications are discussed in Chapter 15.

ANSWER: Often, the first sign of a PDA the nurse sees is an unexplained drop in oxygen saturation on the pulse oximeter. The appropriate action is to initiate problem solving starting with Gabriella and the airway, breathing, and circulation (ABC). Is her airway open? Place a stethoscope on her chest and assess breath sounds and heart sounds. The PDA usually creates an easily identifiable "washing machine" murmur. Thus, the change in oxygenation and the presence of a murmur are two early warning signs that blood is shunting through the ductus arteriosus into the pulmonary circulation.

NEONATAL SEPSIS

QUESTION: Why is Gabriella treated as if she is septic?

Sepsis does occur in term infants and is a common complication in premature newborns because of their inability to adequately respond to infection, their exposure to bacteria from invasive devices, their thin skin, and their poor nutritional state. Additionally, sepsis may result transplacentally before birth from prolonged rupture of membranes or from direct contact with the vaginal canal during birth. Maternal or fetal sepsis may be a cause of premature delivery, which often complicates the newborn's hospital course and results in increased mortality. The premature newborn's immature immune system responds poorly to infection because limited neutrophil storage and altered neutrophil function weaken the inflammatory response.

Sepsis can kill a newborn within hours because of the infant's inability to localize infections. The nurse must be vigilant for the subtle signs of sepsis and articulate them to the other members of the health care team. Early identification and treatment of infection can prevent serious complications.

Assessment

Signs of sepsis in premature newborns are often vague, subtle, and nonspecific, making diagnosis difficult. Apnea, lethargy, temperature instability, poor feeding, respiratory distress, increasing oxygen requirements, and hyperbilirubinemia are all signs of sepsis in the newborn. Cardinal signs of sepsis include poor feeding, increased apneic spells, jaundice, temperature instability, increased oxygen requirement, and lethargy (see Chapter 24 for further discussion of sepsis). When infection is a potential problem, the physician or advanced practice nurse will initiate a specific (septic) workup that commonly includes the following:

- Complete blood count (CBC)
- Blood cultures
- Tracheal aspirate for culture
- Urine culture
- Chest radiograph
- Lumbar puncture, to determine if meningitis is present

Positive cultures plus a CBC showing an elevated or decreased white blood cell count, an increased number of immature white cells, and decreased platelets may indicate the presence of sepsis. Additional tests that may be performed on the cerebrospinal fluid to determine the presence of infection include glucose level, white blood cell count, and protein level.

Interdisciplinary Interventions

Preventing infections in the ELBW infant population is paramount because neonatal infections among this high-risk group are associated with poor neurodevelopmental and growth outcomes in early childhood (Adams-Chapman, 2012). Preventing nosocomial infection is particularly challenging in the NICU because the preterm infant has multiple tubes and lines, frequent procedures, and immature body functions (e.g., thin skin, poor response to infection). Meticulous hand hygiene is a mainstay in preventing nosocomial infections and must be followed by all health care professionals.

Because of the newborn's decreased ability to respond to infection, broad-spectrum antibiotics are initiated immediately; waiting for laboratory test results would delay treatment. The nurse's role is to assist with the diagnostic workup, including obtaining many of the blood samples. Additionally, maintain an ongoing assessment of the newborn, and document and communicate findings with the rest of the team. Sepsis in the newborn can escalate quickly, necessitating vigorous interventions such as intubation, volume resuscitation, initiation of dopamine and dobutamine drips to support cardiovascular function, and other resuscitative efforts. Each of these interventions has specific indications. For example, intubation is required when the newborn is apneic or in respiratory failure. Volume resuscitation in the form of normal saline restores intravascular volume that may be depleted as a result of capillary leak of fluid into the subcutaneous tissue. Dopamine and dobutamine are medications that are used to maintain blood pressure and to improve cardiac contractility.

caREminder

Every member of the family and health care team has a role in preventing infection. Handwashing is the number one way to prevent the transmission of nosocomial infections. All individuals must perform hand hygiene before and after handling any newborn.

Use sterile technique for all invasive procedures, such as suctioning the endotracheal tube and inserting bladder catheters. Handle central lines using sterile technique as well, because these lines are an easy portal of entry for microorganisms.

ANSWER: Gabriella will be treated from birth as if she is septic because her mother's membranes ruptured prematurely (which may be because of an infection) and the membranes were ruptured for 48 hours before her delivery (which allows plenty of time for an organism to enter the uterus). Many of the symptoms of sepsis are also symptoms of prematurity. It is impossible to know whether Gabriella is floppy because of an infection because any infant will be floppy at only 28 weeks' gestation. A CBC and blood culture are drawn prior to the administration of antibiotics, but as a result of their immature and inadequate response to infection, preterm infants are treated with broad-spectrum antibiotics quickly, without waiting for cultures to confirm the diagnosis.

INTRAVENTRICULAR HEMORRHAGE

IVH (bleeding within the ventricles in the brain) is almost exclusively a problem related to prematurity, specifically in infants of less than 28 weeks' gestation. IVH is the most common brain injury in premature infants, and its incidence is directly related to the degree of prematurity. Although the incidence of IVH has declined over the years because of advances in perinatal medicine (specifically the prenatal administration of corticosteroids), it remains at 45% for infants weighing 500 to 750 g (Ballabh, 2009), with higher rates in the presence of decreasing gestational age, PDA, and respiratory distress syndrome.

The causes of IVH are not completely understood but may involve the dynamic interaction between the hemodynamic status of the newborn and the fragility of the capillary bed. Clearly, preterm newborns with respiratory distress are at an increased risk for IVH. In addition to preterm birth, other risk factors include

- Chorioamnionitis
- Preeclampsia
- Hypotension
- Hypothermia
- Umbilical lines

Pathophysiology

Normally, the blood vessels of the brain are protected from fluctuations in blood flow through autoregulation. Autoregulation allows the arterioles to constrict and dilate despite fluctuations in systemic pressure to ensure constant blood flow to the brain. The premature newborn is unable to autoregulate because the CNS is immature and, as a result, blood flow to the brain varies. This fluctuation directly affects the flow to the germinal matrix: a temporary, highly vascularized structure located in the subependyma of the ventricular walls in the brain of premature newborns that produces precursor cells, which will later develop into neurons and glial cells for eventual migration into the cerebral cortex. The thin-walled blood vessels of this structure are easily ruptured.

PPV, hypoxia, hypotension, and rapid volume expansion can contribute to IVH. A very sick premature newborn may have hypotension from a persistent PDA and may require assisted ventilation, which increases the risk for the development of an IVH. In IVH, the blood vessels in the germinal matrix, located in the subependymal area of the ventricles, rupture and bleed into the lateral ventricle. If the hemorrhage is large, a blood clot may form within the ventricle, or blood may spread throughout the ventricular system and into brain tissue. IVH is categorized as grades I through IV (Chart 14-3) based on results of cranial ultrasonography.

CHART 14-3 Classification of Intraventricular Hemorrhage

Grade I: Germinal matrix hemorrhage only

Grade II: Germinal matrix hemorrhage with extension into the ventricles

Grade III: Germinal matrix hemorrhage with dilated ventricles

Grade IV: Intraventricular hemorrhage with extension into brain tissue

---

Prognosis for a newborn with IVH depends on the severity of the hemorrhage and the presence of associated problems, such as asphyxia and sepsis. Overall mortality for newborns with severe IVH (grades III and IV) is about 75% (Linder et al., 2003), and this rate increases if ventricular dilation and posthemorrhagic hydrocephalus develops. Newborns with grades I or II hemorrhages generally have a low incidence of long-term neurologic sequelae.

Common complications of IVH are ventricular dilation, posthemorrhagic hydrocephalus, and periventricular leukomalacia. Ventricular dilation occurs in approximately 50% of newborns with IVH; it is caused by a clot that blocks the flow of cerebrospinal fluid. Posthemorrhagic hydrocephalus results from progressive ventricular dilation and occurs in 31% of all grades III and IV IVH (Linder et al., 2003). Moderate to severe IVH has the highest incidence of developing hydrocephalus. Signs and symptoms of hydrocephalus include increasing head circumference, change in level of consciousness, apnea and bradycardia spells, and increasing need for respiratory support.

Periventricular leukomalacia is an ischemic injury to the white matter in the brain. This injury is commonly noted in newborns who die of IVH. The true incidence of periventricular leukomalacia is unknown because this complication cannot be accurately detected with bedside cranial ultrasound testing.

Assessment

Common symptoms of IVH include a sudden decrease in hematocrit, severe and sudden unexplained deterioration of vital signs, bulging fontanels, changes in activity level, and sudden lethargy. The diagnosis is confirmed by cranial ultrasonography. More than 90% of newborns with IVH bleed within the first 4 days of life, and 50% bleed within 24 hours of birth.

Nursing Diagnoses and Outcomes

Nursing diagnoses and outcomes generally applicable for newborns with a health challenge are presented in Nursing Plan of Care 14-1. In addition, the following may be applicable for a newborn with IVH:

Nursing Diagnosis: Risk for ineffective cerebral tissue perfusion related to effects of blood within the ventricle

Outcome: Newborn will maintain cerebral perfusion pressure adequate to provide oxygen and nutrients to the brain.

Interdisciplinary Interventions

Preventing IVH is the most important goal because once IVH has occurred, the damage to the CNS is irreversible. Nursing procedures such as endotracheal tube suctioning and rapid infusions of fluid can cause IVH (McLendon et al., 2003). Nurses are crucial in implementing IVH prevention techniques because many of these techniques involve the way that care is delivered to this fragile population (Nursing Interventions 14-4).

NURSING INTERVENTIONS 14-4

Reducing the Risk of Intraventricular Hemorrhage

- Optimize the peripartum management of the ELBW newborn in the delivery room (standard resuscitation team, standardized resuscitation techniques).
- Implement methods to improve temperature upon admission to the NICU, such as using the polyethylene wrap in the delivery room, preheating the isolette or combination unit, and putting a hat on the neonate's head.
- Minimize stressors using developmental care techniques: reduce environmental noise, light, and noxious stimuli; support infant in a flexed, tucked position; and avoid unnecessary procedures and routine suctioning.

- Monitor infant for stress cues and alter interventions based on these observations.
- Promote self-comforting behaviors in infant.
- Manage pain.
- Avoid tight bili masks (eye shields).
- Maintain the infant's head in a neutral, midline position as often as possible for the first 3 days of life.
- Perform vigilant monitoring of hemodynamic and respiratory status and intervene immediately to avoid rapid changes in these vital functions that may lead to IVH.
- Avoid overhydration.
- Avoid routine endotracheal or nasopharyngeal suctioning

Acute management of IVH includes support of all vital functions, including increasing ventilation pressures and supplemental oxygen to maintain normal ventilation and oxygenation, providing packed red blood cells to correct anemia caused by bleeding, and infusing volume replacement to maintain tissue perfusion. During the acute event of an IVH, monitor all vital signs carefully and frequently because the newborn's condition may be extremely unstable.

APNEA OF PREMATURITY

Apnea is defined as a cessation of respiratory air flow for 20 seconds or longer in the preterm newborn and 15 seconds or longer in the term newborn (see Chapter 16). Pathologic apnea is a pause in respiration associated with cyanosis, marked pallor, hypotonia, or bradycardia. *Apnea of prematurity* refers to apnea in newborns of less than 37 weeks' gestation; it usually presents between days 2 and 7 of life. As the premature newborn develops and matures, the incidence of apnea decreases. All newborns are periodic (irregular) breathers. However, the cessation of breathing for longer than 20 seconds is abnormal and requires intervention, regardless of gestational age. The incidence of AOP decreases as gestational age at birth increases. It is estimated that more than 50% of preterm infants experience AOP, with nearly all experiencing AOP when they weigh less than 1,000 g at birth (Finer et al., 2006).

Apnea in the newborn may be the first presenting sign of many problems. Specifically, apnea can result from sepsis, seizures, metabolic disturbances, and intrauterine drug exposure.

Pathophysiology

AOP is a result of the immaturity of the CNS, which fails to initiate breathing. The medulla oblongata, the most inferior part of the brain stem, controls respiratory drive.

As a result of prematurity, the patterned firing of the neurons in this section of the brain is altered. Additionally, premature newborns' response to hypoxemia and hypercarbia is diminished, leading to apnea. Bradycardia may follow apnea, leading to the often-used term in the NICU of *apnea–bradycardia spells* or *A/B spells*.

Assessment

Apnea that occurs in premature newborns with no underlying disease is generally categorized as AOP. The physical examination reveals a vigorous premature newborn with no signs of sepsis or metabolic disturbances. If you observe cessation of breathing, intervene as needed; report all incidences to the medical team. To initiate the appropriate treatment, it is important to investigate all potential causes of apnea. AOP is a diagnosis of exclusion, in that no specific diagnostic tests exist.

If AOP continues, and the infant is approaching discharge, a pneumocardiogram may be performed. This study continuously measures heart rate, respiratory rate, and pulse oximetry values during a specified period. This information is plotted on a graph and can clearly demonstrate the occurrence of apneic spells and any associated bradycardia and desaturation. Results from this study are used to determine the type of apnea, rule out any possible treatable cause, and determine discharge needs such as home cardiac monitoring.

Nursing Diagnoses and Outcomes

Nursing diagnoses and outcomes generally applicable for newborns with a health challenge are presented in Nursing Plan of Care 14-1. In addition, the following may be applicable for a newborn with AOP:

Nursing Diagnosis: Ineffective breathing pattern related to effects of an immature CNS

Outcomes:

• Infant's apnea and bradycardia spells will be recognized immediately and stimulation will be initiated.
• Infant will experience no adverse sequelae resulting from ineffective breathing pattern.

Interdisciplinary Interventions

Nursing interventions include close monitoring for apnea and subsequent bradycardia and appropriate documentation. During an apnea–bradycardia spell, gently stimulate the newborn by rubbing his or her back or foot to initiate breathing. If this measure is not effective, provide more vigorous stimulation, progressing to bag-and-mask ventilation as necessary (Fig. 14-9).

Documentation is extremely important and should include the following:

• Duration of apneic episode
• Lowest heart rate during the episode
• Lowest oxygen saturation
• Interventions performed

Position the newborn in the prone position to minimize the number of apneic episodes. The prone position improves oxygenation and decreases the work of breathing.

The medical team initiates pharmacotherapy if the spells are severe or frequent. Severe or frequent spells cause the body to shunt blood from nonvital organs, such as the bowel, to vital organs such as the heart and brain. Treatment is initiated to control the spells, avoid ischemic damage to the bowel, and prevent the development of NEC.

Treatment includes respiratory stimulants such as the methylxanthines (aminophylline, theophylline, and caffeine) and, when needed, doxapram to decrease the occurrence of apnea. These drugs act by stimulating the CNS and increasing alveolar ventilation. Common side effects of caffeine and theophylline are tachycardia and irritability. Additionally, oral formulations may be irritating to the gut and lead to feeding intolerance. These medications should not be given if the heart rate is more than 180 bpm. If medications are not successful, continuous positive airway pressure (CPAP) may be initiated through a nasal device to help decrease the work of breathing and improve lung compliance.

Most newborns outgrow AOP and can be successfully weaned from medications and CPAP. However, some symptomatic newborns, those with cyanotic color changes and bradycardia, require medications at discharge and home apnea monitoring. Teach the family how to correctly administer medications and monitor for side effects. Also provide teaching related to the apnea monitor and newborn cardiopulmonary resuscitation.

Community Care

Newborns discharged with home apnea monitors and medications to treat apnea need close follow-up (see thePoint for Procedures: Apnea Monitors). Nurses and respiratory therapists provide follow-up visits in the home to ensure that the family is comfortable with the home apnea monitor and with techniques for handling

Nursing Interventions in Apnea

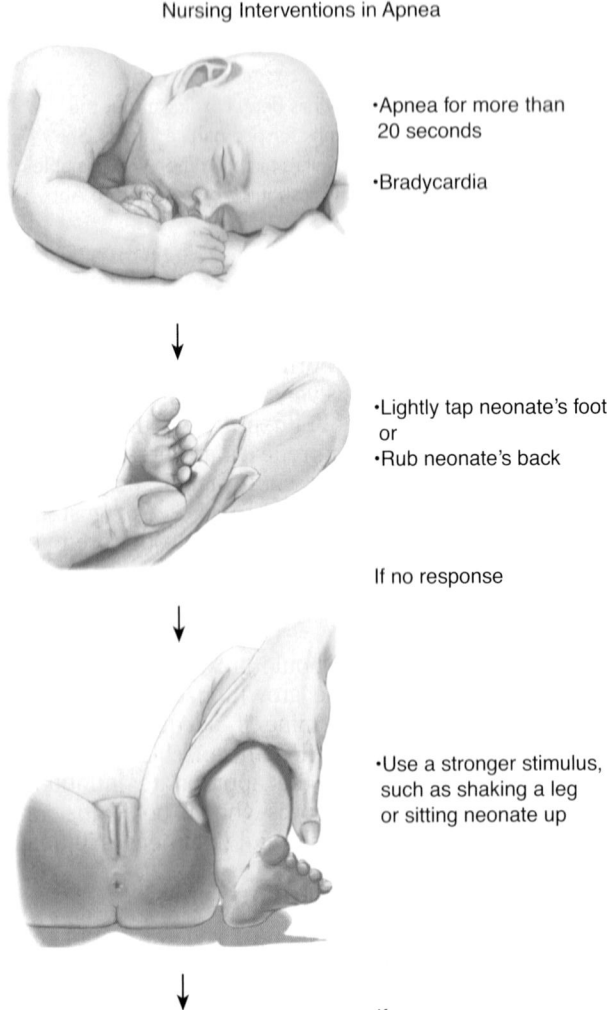

• Apnea for more than 20 seconds

• Bradycardia

• Lightly tap neonate's foot or
• Rub neonate's back

If no response

• Use a stronger stimulus, such as shaking a leg or sitting neonate up

If no response

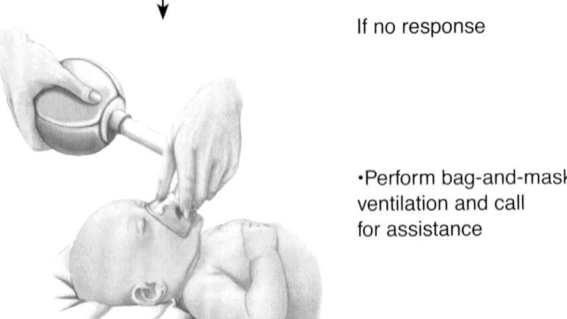

• Perform bag-and-mask ventilation and call for assistance

Figure 14-9 Nursing interventions progressively increase in invasiveness for AOP.

emergencies. Provide ongoing reinforcement of teaching at this time.

Typically, the newborn is seen in the clinic 1 to 2 weeks after discharge, depending on his or her stability. At this first clinic visit, the physician or advanced practice nurse reviews with the primary caregiver the number and severity of apneic spells and interventions required, if any. Adjustments are made to the home apnea monitor alarms as needed, and the medications are reviewed for appropriate dosing. Weaning from medications is determined by the newborn's progress and number of apneic spells.

FEEDING AND NUTRITION PROBLEMS

> **QUESTION:** Abby has been reading about the benefits of breast milk for premature infants. She asks you the day after Gabriella's birth, "When will I be able to breastfeed Gabriella?" How should you respond to Abby's question?

Premature newborns require a high caloric intake for growth, tissue repair, and development of subcutaneous fat. Premature newborns have immature gastrointestinal systems, however, and require additional specialized support to obtain nutrition and maintain growth. Although sucking reflexes are present early in development, effective and coordinated suck–swallow reflexes do not develop until 32 to 34 weeks' gestation. Therefore, providing enteral nutrition to the premature newborn is challenging.

Assessment

The premature newborn should grow along the natural progression of intrauterine growth had the pregnancy carried to term. To determine if adequate growth is occurring, plot the weight, length, and head circumference of the newborn on the appropriate intrauterine growth curve weekly. Newborns who fall below the curve are not growing appropriately, and treatment is initiated.

Nursing Diagnoses and Outcomes

Nursing diagnoses and outcomes generally applicable for newborns with a health challenge are presented in Nursing Plan of Care 14-1. In addition, the following may apply for a newborn with feeding and nutrition problems:

Nursing Diagnosis: Imbalanced nutrition: Less than body requirements related to inability to take enteral feedings and acute illness
Outcome: Newborn's caloric and nutritional needs will be met via enteral or parenteral routes.

Nursing Diagnosis: Interrupted breastfeeding related to inability or decreased ability to breastfeed and acute illness
Outcomes:
• Newborn will demonstrate normal growth as measured on the intrauterine growth curve.
• Newborn will gain weight at a rate of 15 to 30 g/day.

Interdisciplinary Interventions

Feeding and nutritional assessment are the most important interventions for nurses caring for premature newborns. Parenteral nutrition is used initially until the newborn has become stable and ready to handle enteral feeding. Parenteral nutrition includes administering solutions containing amino acids, dextrose, vitamins and minerals, and lipids through a peripheral or central venous catheter (e.g., PICC or tunneled catheter [e.g., Broviac]; see Chapter 17). Weaning from parenteral nutrition is begun slowly as enteral feedings are introduced.

caREminder

> *Often, the quality of feeding tolerance and behavior are the first clues to other problems. For example, one of the first signs of an infection in a premature newborn may be feeding intolerance.*

Signs and symptoms of feeding intolerance may include emesis, gastric residuals that are greater than 50% of the previous feeding, or bilious emesis or aspirates. Assess for these subtle changes and collaborate with other health care team members to intervene early and avoid complications.

Perform an abdominal examination before any feeding. If bowel loops, abdominal distention, or decreased bowel sounds are present, notify the medical team to determine a course of action. If the abdominal examination is normal, initiate feeding. Nursing Interventions 14-5 provides instruction for administering gavage feedings (see also thePoint for Procedures: Enteral Tube Placement and Management: Naso/Orogastric Tubes and Weighted Tubes; Feeding, Infant).

NURSING INTERVENTIONS 14-5

Administering Gavage Feedings

• Introduce a feeding tube through the mouth into the stomach.
• Aspirate slightly to measure the residual (the amount of formula left in the stomach since the previous feeding).
• If the residual is not abnormal (green, bilious, or greater than 30% of the previous feeding), administer the feeding.
• Monitor the newborn's color and ability to tolerate the process during tube insertion and

feeding administration. Provide a pacifier to encourage nonnutritive sucking during feeding.
• Apnea and bradycardia are potential side effects during tube insertion, and cyanosis may occur during the feeding. If these complications occur, immediately discontinue the feeding, clear the airway if needed, and administer supplemental oxygen.

Initially, enteral feedings are offered slowly and are termed *trophic, minimal enteral feeds* (MEFs), or *stimulation* or *stim* feeds because they are used to prime the gut for absorption. Premature newborns are fed slowly and gradually, taking up to 3 weeks to achieve complete enteral feeds. This gradual approach is needed because premature newborns commonly experience initial problems, and the instability of other body systems can make enteral feeding undesirable.

Breast milk is the enteral feeding of choice because it contains easily digested proteins, antibodies, and immunoglobulins and has a high protein content. EBM from the premature newborn's mother has both a higher protein and fat content than breast milk from a term infant's mother. If breast milk is unavailable, the infant may be fed human breast milk donated to an established human milk bank. The human milk bank screens all donors and pasteurizes the EBM. If EBM is unavailable either from the mother or the human breast milk bank, formulas specially designed for premature infants are used because they contain additional minerals, different types of fat, and extra protein to support the growth of premature newborns. Initially, formulas are introduced cautiously and are slowly increased in volume as the newborn demonstrates tolerance.

Because of their inability to suck and swallow efficiently, premature newborns are fed through intermittent or continuous gavage feedings. Intermittent bolus gavage feedings are more physiologically appropriate and may improve production of the enteric hormones required for successful feeding. Continuous gavage feedings are often better tolerated by the extremely premature newborns because of their small gastric volumes. During gavage feedings, offer the infant a pacifier to promote the association of sucking with feeding. As infants mature and achieve the ability to coordinate breathing, sucking, and swallowing, which typically occurs at about 32 to 34 weeks' gestation, oral feedings are introduced (see thePoint for Procedures: Feeding, Infant). Infants should be medically stable, able to maintain physiologic stability (maintain color and cardiorespiratory parameters and tolerate caregiving activities and environmental stimuli), and able to sustain regular breathing patterns and oxygen saturation during nonnutritive sucking. Breastfeeding is best for all infants, including the preterm infant. However, if the mother is unavailable for a feeding, the nurse offers a bottlefeeding upon the infant's cues, or readiness signs. Feeding readiness include fussiness without crying, hand-to-mouth behaviors, and rooting. Nurses can also elicit readiness signs by swaddling the infant and offering the pacifier, which may increase alertness. Infants will perform better at the bottle when a feeding is offered based upon cues. See Nursing Interventions 14-6 for information on oral feeding of the infant.

NURSING INTERVENTIONS 14-6

Feeding the Premature Infant

- Provide a quiet environment and remove distractions.
- Remain focused on the infant throughout the feeding, avoiding ongoing conversations with others.
- The infant should be in the awake, alert state for successful feeding; attempt to wake the infant with a soft voice, change the diaper, and ready the infant for the feeding experience.
- Elicit the rooting reflex by stroking the infant's lips with the nipple.
- Place the nipple in the mouth when a positive rooting response has been initiated.
- Allow infant to set the pace for feeding; if there is a pause, wait for the infant to resume sucking.
- Be alert to signs of stress (bradycardia, desaturations, behavioral stress cues) and stop the feeding if they occur to allow a rest period.
- After feeding, hold the infant in an upright position for at least 5 minutes and note behavior.

Breastfeeding the Premature Infant
- Offer skin-to-skin holding frequently (as infant tolerates) to promote suckling at the empty breast. As

feeding progresses, the infant may suckle at the full breast. This practice encourages the infant to become familiar with the natural nipple and also enhances the mother's own milk supply.
- Obtain assistance from a certified lactation consultant to assist with placing preterm infants to breast. Breast shields and different breastfeeding positions may be used to enhance the infant's efforts at the breast.
- Milk transfer (how much the infant takes from the breast) can be a concern because preterm infants have low sucking pressure. Careful monitoring of weight gain or loss, along with urine and stool output, is helpful in determining whether the infant's intake is adequate.

Bottle-Feeding the Premature Infant
- Swaddle the infant and hold in a neutral head–neck flexion (avoiding extension and excessive flexion) and in midline.
- Avoid twisting, turning the bottle in the infant's mouth, or moving the infant's jaw passively because these actions inhibit coordination of suck–swallow–breathe and only increase milk flow.

ANSWER: One response to Abby's question about breastfeeding Gabriella is: "You are absolutely right that your breast milk is the best source of nutrition for Gabriella. In fact, you should begin pumping your breasts to stimulate milk production. You need to let your body know that Gabriella needs milk, even though she is not strong enough to nurse yet. Save all the milk you express and label it with the date and time, even if it is only a little bit. We will give her the first milk you express first because it has the highest amounts of immune properties. The combination of coordinating breathing around sucking and swallowing is not easy to do; feeding is physically challenging. Somewhere between 32 and 34 weeks' gestation, premature babies are able to start nursing a little. First, Gabriella will get her fluids and calories through the IV in her arm (her PICC line). Then we will begin to give her your breast milk through a tube to her stomach, and when she gives us cues that she is ready, we will start putting her to your breast to nurse. So to answer your question, maybe in 6 weeks, maybe a little bit sooner than that. We will start giving Gabriella your breast milk as soon as it is safe for her."

NECROTIZING ENTEROCOLITIS

NEC is an acquired disease characterized by necrosis of the mucosal and submucosal layers of the gastrointestinal tract. It most commonly occurs in infants with a median gestational age of 29 weeks and in those weighing less than 1,500 g, although there are reports of it developing in term newborns (Fox & Godavitarne, 2012). Overall mortality is 22%, depending on the severity of the disease and associated problems (Fox & Godavitarne, 2012). If surgery is required, mortality rises to 40% to 51% (Kelleher et al., 2013).

Pathophysiology

The causes of NEC are not completely understood. It appears to be initiated when the body shunts blood away from vital organs (such as the bowel) during hypoxemia. This shift leads to decreased blood flow to the bowel, causing bowel wall ischemia. Bacteria then colonize the bowel and form a substrate (foundation) that allows bacterial invasion of the bowel wall.

Timing, method, and type of feeding for premature newborns and its association with NEC continue to be controversial. Clearly, infants who develop NEC have been exposed to some type of enteral substrate for bacterial growth, either EBM or formula. EBM use is associated with a lower incidence of NEC than formula use.

Assessment

NEC produces gastrointestinal and systemic signs and symptoms that must be immediately reported to the medical team, including abdominal distention; visible bowel loops; and a shiny, possibly discolored abdomen. Additionally, bilious or large feeding residuals, grossly bloody or occult-positive stools, lethargy, decreased bowel sounds, and sepsis-like symptoms occur with NEC. Sepsis-like signs are further described as temperature instability, poor perfusion, metabolic acidosis, and hypotension.

Radiograph of the abdomen reveals dilated bowel loops, ileus, or the classic sign of NEC: **pneumatosis intestinalis** (air in the bowel wall). Perforation of the bowel wall may ensue with late NEC, requiring immediate surgery.

Nursing Diagnoses and Outcomes

Nursing diagnoses and outcomes generally applicable for newborns with a health challenge are presented in Nursing Plan of Care 14-1. In addition, the following may be applicable for a newborn with NEC:

Nursing Diagnosis: Risk for ineffective gastrointestinal perfusion related to effects of hypoxic insult
Outcome: Newborn will demonstrate adequate intestinal circulation, as evidenced by tolerance to feedings or no signs of NEC.

Interdisciplinary Interventions

Nursing interventions revolve around immediate recognition of early signs of NEC, including increasing gastric residuals and abdominal distention. Perform an abdominal examination: Inspect the abdomen for the presence of loops or distention, auscultate for bowel sounds, palpate for distention, and examine the stools for presence or absence of blood. Additionally, evaluate gastric residuals for amount and color. If the residuals are bilious or greater than 30% of the previous feeding, hold the feeding and notify the medical team.

When NEC is diagnosed, assess the condition of the newborn and be alert to signs of a worsening condition, including unstable vital signs, increasing blueness of the abdomen, increasing abdominal girth, hypotension, and metabolic acidosis. A decompression gastric tube is inserted to empty the stomach and reduce the air in the intestine. Enteral feeds may not be restarted until 7 to 10 days after the initial event and are done with great caution.

Surgical intervention is initiated if bowel perforation occurs. NEC is a dynamic disease, in which segments of bowel wall worsen while others recover. The timing of surgery will dictate what is seen when the abdomen is entered. The goal is to remove the necrotic areas of the bowel and preserve as much healthy bowel as possible. One complication of surgery for NEC is short bowel syndrome, in which a large portion of the gut is removed, as a result of necrosis, and the newborn is left with minimal amounts of intestine for absorption. These newborns have long-term feeding and nutrition difficulties and may be frequently hospitalized throughout infancy and childhood. They often depend on parenteral nutrition, with associated risks of central venous line complications, sepsis, cholestasis, and liver failure. The goal of establishing enteral nutrition, facilitating intestinal adaptation through which the remaining small bowel gradually increases its absorptive capacity, is never achieved in some children.

RETINOPATHY OF PREMATURITY

ROP is a disorder affecting the retinas of extremely premature newborns. It is a pathologic fibrous process that results from injury to the developing premature retinal vasculature. ROP occurs in very premature newborns; newborns born at 34 weeks' gestation or later are unlikely to develop ROP. ROP is covered in detail in Chapter 28.

BIRTH INJURIES

Birth injuries include trauma that occurs surrounding the birth (Chart 14-4). Birth injuries such as lacerations and bruising may also occur during cesarean sections or during resuscitation. Birth trauma is estimated to occur in 25.85 per 1,000 births (Moczygemba et al., 2010).

Injuries that occur intrapartum are often related to an abnormal fetal presentation, such as breech or abnormal fetal position leading to compression fractures. Additionally, oligohydramnios (decreased amniotic fluid) may be associated with epidermal shearing of the skin caused by excessive rubbing against the uterine wall without the amniotic fluid as a cushion. The risk of nerve injury is increased with breech positions, prolonged or precipitous labor, prematurity, multiple gestation, and shoulder dystocia.

Common birth injuries are soft tissue injury, extracranial hemorrhage, fracture, and peripheral nerve injury. Soft tissue injuries include bruising, abrasions, and petechiae over the presenting part. Edema may also be present. Because each of these injuries requires different care, they are covered in detail after a general discussion of assessment and care of newborns with birth injuries.

Assessment

A complete and thorough physical examination is imperative to quickly identify birth traumas. Note any history of a difficult or prolonged labor, LGA status, or birth to a diabetic mother. Birth injury may cause reduced ROM in the extremities or asymmetric movements. The skull may have edema, petechiae,

---

| CHART 14-4 | Perinatal Events/Conditions Associated With Birth Injuries |

- Macrosomia
- Vacuum extraction
- Abnormal fetal presentation
- Oligohydramnios
- Shoulder dystocia
- LGA infant
- Precipitate labor
- Second stage of labor exceeding 60 minutes
- Vaginal breech delivery

---

or soft-tissue swelling. Skin tears and bruising suggest soft tissue injuries. Radiographs reveal any bone fractures.

Nursing Diagnoses and Outcomes

In addition to the nursing diagnoses listed in Nursing Plan of Care 14-1, the following may be applicable to the newborn with a birth injury:

Nursing Diagnosis: Acute pain related to fracture, skin breakdown, or edema
Outcome: Newborn's pain will be managed appropriately. The infant will show no signs of pain, such as increased crying or poor feeding.
Nursing Diagnosis: Risk for injury related to improper positioning of paralyzed extremity
Outcome: Newborn's affected extremity will be positioned properly. The infant will display normal joint ROM.
Nursing Diagnosis: Impaired skin integrity related to disruption of skin surface from trauma
Outcome: Newborn will show adequate wound healing.

Interdisciplinary Interventions

Most injuries, such as a fractured clavicle or caput succedaneum, need supportive care only. Other injuries need splinting and immobilization. The nurse collaborates with other health care team members, including the physician and occupational therapist, to provide needed interventions.

SOFT TISSUE INJURIES

Soft tissue injuries are generally self-limiting and require only supportive care and reassurance to the family. Scleral hemorrhages may be noted soon after birth and are a result of increased pressure on the fetal head during delivery. Edema, petechiae, and bruising also result from increased pressure on the presenting part of the fetus. Closely monitor petechiae because they also may be a symptom of a bleeding disorder or sepsis.

EXTRACRANIAL HEMORRHAGE

The descent through the birth canal can be stressful to the fetus. For successful vaginal delivery to occur, the fetal skull bones override one another to accommodate the small space of the pelvic inlet and vaginal tract. As a result, the head may undergo molding. Additionally, the obstetrician may facilitate delivery of the fetal head using vacuum extraction (application of a suction device to the fetal presenting part) to assist delivery. Vacuum extraction devices may potentially cause trauma to the fetal head, leading to edema and bleeding.

Caput succedaneum and *cephalhematoma* are the most common birth injuries; subgaleal hemorrhage (SGH) is relatively rare (Fig. 14-10). Caput succedaneum is localized scalp edema that occurs over the presenting part in a vertex delivery. The edema is often marked with bruising, petechiae, and broken skin. The edema is above the periosteum and crosses the suture

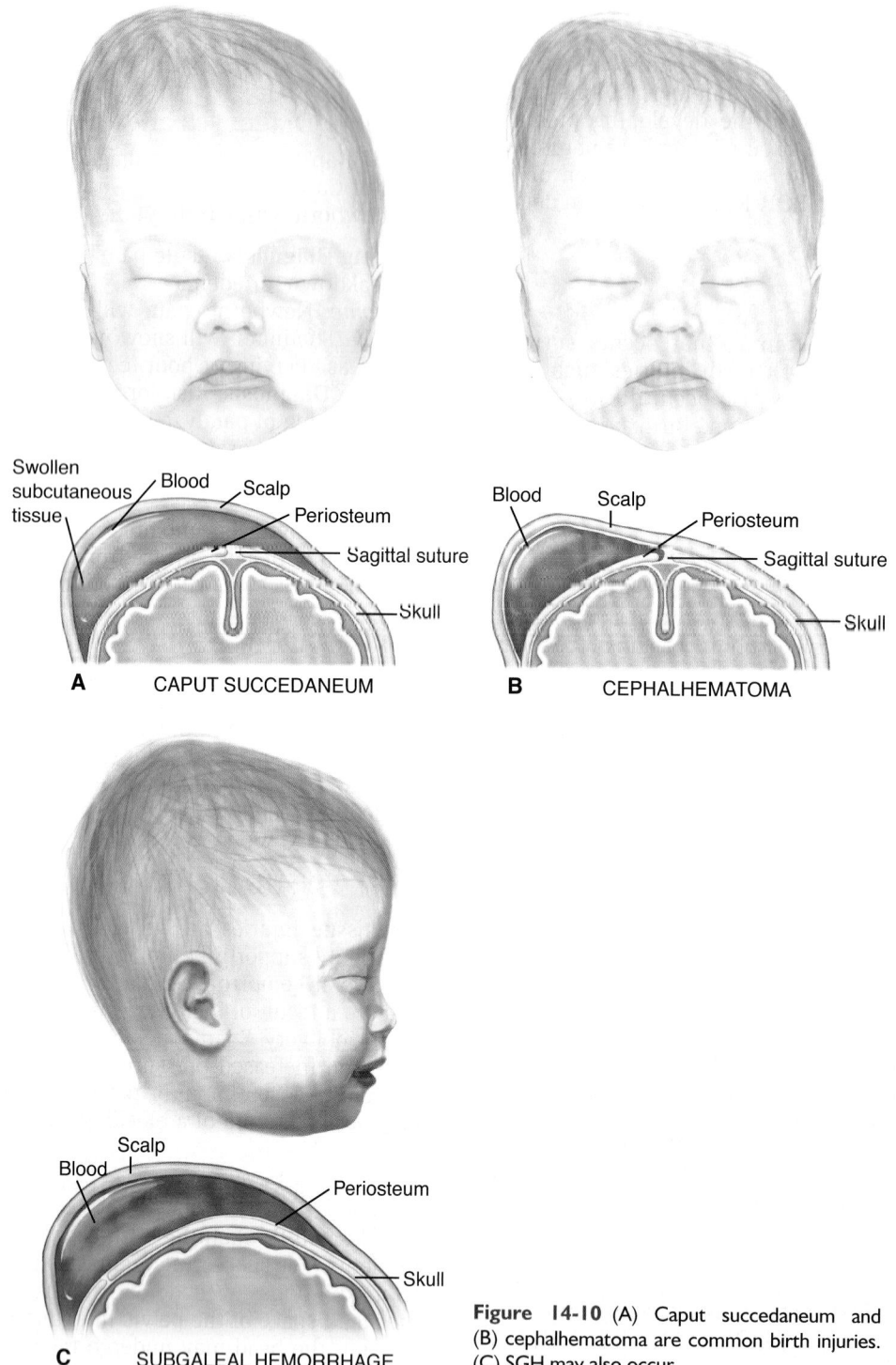

Figure 14-10 (A) Caput succedaneum and (B) cephalhematoma are common birth injuries. (C) SGH may also occur.

lines of the skull. This benign injury resolves within 2 to 3 days after birth.

Cephalhematoma is subperiosteal bleeding over the cranial bone. This type of hemorrhage commonly occurs after vacuum-assisted deliveries, prolonged and difficult labors, and primiparous births.

An SGH occurs when shearing forces rupture blood vessels that bridge the subgaleal space. The subgaleal space is a potential space (a space that is normally empty but has the capacity to hold several hundred milliliters of blood) located between the scalp and the skull. The incidence of SGH is approximately 1 in 2,500 live births (Schierholz & Walker, 2010). Vacuum-assisted deliveries substantially increase the risk for SGH. SGH is associated with considerable morbidity and mortality during the immediate postdelivery period, but the long-term outcome for survivors is good (Swanson et al., 2012). SGH presents with subtle edema that extends to the neck and behind the ear. The edema may not be present at delivery but will evolve during the next several hours. The affected area of the scalp will be boggy and fluctuating, with dependent edema. In large, very severe SGH, the ear will become edematous and pushed forward, and the eyes will become puffy. Hypovolemic shock may ensue if SGH diagnosis is delayed.

Assess for skull and scalp abnormalities, and note the location of any edema, petechiae, or bruising. Edema that crosses the suture line suggests caput succedaneum. Skull indentation is an important finding that possibly indicates an underlying fracture, and it requires further investigation, such as a radiograph. Assess for signs of increased ICP such as a full or tense anterior fontanel, irritability, poor feeding, and apnea.

A cephalhematoma differs from a caput succedaneum in that it does not cross suture lines, has little or no ecchymosis, and takes longer to resolve—as long as 2 months. Also, a cephalhematoma can continue to bleed, leading to anemia. Hyperbilirubinemia may also be a prolonged problem resulting from lysis of the blood underneath the periosteum. If this complication develops, closely monitor the serum bilirubin level to provide prompt interventions for hyperbilirubinemia, including phototherapy. On occasion, a cephalhematoma may overlie a skull fracture.

SKULL FRACTURE

Skull fractures may result from fetal skull passage through the maternal ischial spines, sacral promontory, or symphysis pubis. Normally, the fetal skull tolerates the pressure generated by birth because its incompletely ossified bone is flexible. However, a traumatic delivery may result in a skull fracture.

Skull fractures related to birth trauma can be linear or depressed. Linear skull fractures are most often present over the frontal or parietal bones and rarely occur over the occipital bone. The newborn is often asymptomatic, with only a cephalhematoma noted on physical examination. Diagnosis is made by skull radiograph. Healing takes place without intervention, and the only monitoring needed is for increased ICP, including measuring the head circumference, monitoring for a bulging or tense anterior fontanel, and noting irritable or lethargic behavior.

A depressed skull fracture appears over the parietal bone. It is evident on physical examination as a visible skull indentation. The newborn is often asymptomatic and will rarely require intervention. In rare cases, depressed skull fractures may be associated with intracranial bleeding. In these cases, the newborn may exhibit signs of increasing ICP and will require ongoing evaluation.

CLAVICULAR FRACTURE

Clavicular fractures are the most common fractures diagnosed as birth trauma. Clavicles are at risk for fracture during shoulder dystocia or in a breech delivery with arms extended. Assess carefully because the newborn is often asymptomatic or merely exhibits limited movement in the affected arm, local swelling or tenderness at the site of the fracture, and an abnormal Moro reflex. Crepitus may be noted at the fracture site as well. Crepitus is the sound made by fractured bone fragments rubbing together.

A fractured clavicle is diagnosed by physical findings and radiograph. Treatment is determined by the severity of the fracture. Generally, arm immobilization using a soft splint in a flexed position against the chest is all that is needed. Callus formation, as detected by radiograph at the fracture site, is often noted by 10 days of age and indicates healing.

Nursing interventions include periodically checking for skin breakdown, removing the splint for bathing, and teaching the family. Family education includes the correct application of the splint, frequency of skin checks, and follow-up appointments.

PERIPHERAL NERVE INJURIES

Peripheral nerve injuries result from stretching or hyperextension of nerve tissue. They generally occur during birth or traumatic or difficult delivery. Nerve damage ranges from very limited edema that resolves quickly to complete paralysis. The most common peripheral nerve injuries are facial nerve palsy and brachial plexus palsy (Fig. 14-11).

Facial nerve palsy results from prolonged pressure on the facial nerve from the maternal pelvis that causes nerve damage. Presentation of facial nerve palsy varies and ranges from inability to close the eye or open the mouth to paralysis of the lower portion of the face. The injury is apparent at birth or within a few days after birth. Most newborns recover spontaneously, with slow improvement of movement within 3 weeks.

Brachial plexus palsy results when the cervical and thoracic nerve roots are damaged as a result of excessive lateral flexion and traction on the neck. The injury is usually unilateral and occurs most frequently on the left side. Clinical presentation varies with the location and extent of damage. At birth, the newborn has decreased movement from the shoulder to the hand. *Erb–Duchenne* paralysis, the most common type, is caused by damage to the C5 and C6 nerve roots and presents as shoulder and upper arm paralysis. The arm is adducted and internally rotated and kept in the "waiter's tip" position; Moro reflex and biceps and radial reflexes are decreased or absent. *Klumpke* paralysis involves damage to the C8 to T1 nerve roots that affects the lower arm and hand. The affected arm remains flaccid, with the hand in a clawlike position. The Moro and grasp reflexes are absent. *Erb–Duchenne–Klumpke* paralysis involves damage to the entire brachial plexus that affects the hand and arm. The upper and lower arm and hand are completely paralyzed. Brachial plexus injuries have a good prognosis. With supportive care, most newborns recover.

Peripheral nerve palsies are supportively managed. Management includes immobilization with a soft splint or brace and institution of passive ROM exercises at day 10. The nurse, in collaboration with the physical

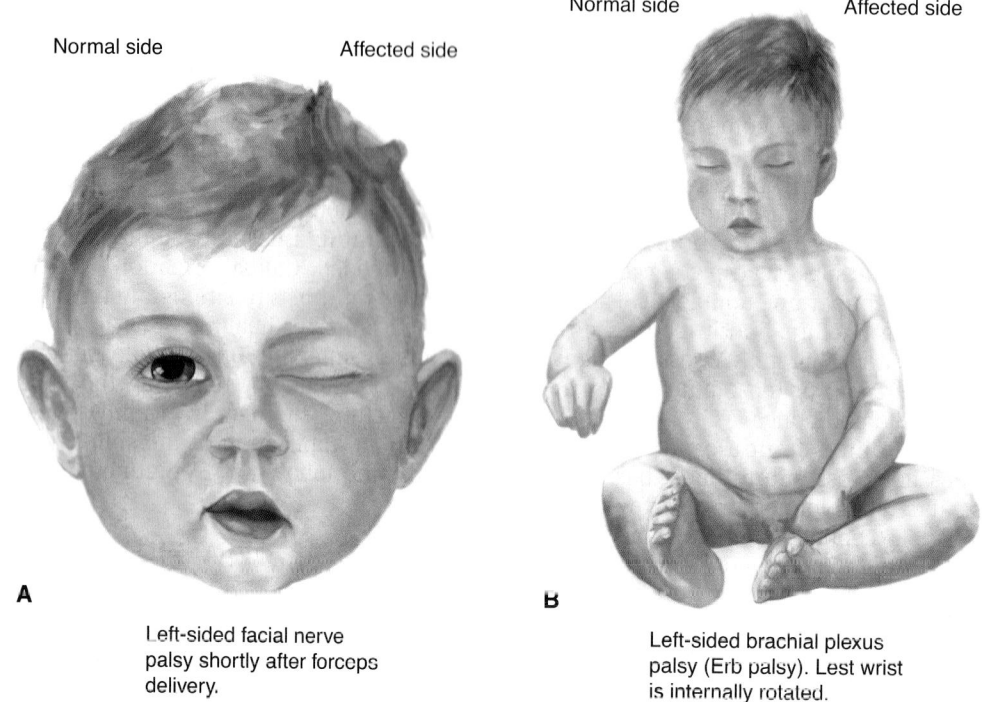

Normal side   Affected side

Normal side   Affected side

A

Left-sided facial nerve
palsy shortly after forceps
delivery.

B

Left-sided brachial plexus
palsy (Erb palsy). Lest wrist
is internally rotated.

Figure 14-11 (A) Facial nerve palsy and (B) brachial plexus palsy are common peripheral nerve injuries in neonates.

therapist, provides family education to reinforce ongoing therapy. Surgical intervention, if needed, is considered at 3 to 6 months of age (Brauer & Waters, 2007).

HYPOXIC ISCHEMIC ENCEPHALOPATHY

Because the fetus depends on a steady supply of maternal blood to deliver oxygen until the lungs take over, any interruption in that flow during birth can result in perinatal asphyxia. The incidence of perinatal asphyxia with subsequent moderate or severe hypoxic ischemic encephalopathy (HIE) is rare—less than 1 case per 1,000 live births (Becher et al., 2007). HIE is a clinical syndrome present in newborns with brain injury caused by perinatal asphyxia. Causes of perinatal asphyxia include interrupted umbilical blood flow, abruptio placentae (separation of the placenta from the uterus prior to delivery), placental insufficiency (inadequate placental perfusion), and trauma during delivery. A common cause of fetal hypoxia is umbilical cord compression during birth. The easily compressed vein in the umbilical cord interrupts blood flow to the fetus, whereas the less distensible arteries continue to pump blood into the placenta, causing fetal hypotension.

Common causes of placental insufficiency are maternal anesthesia, pregnancy-induced hypertension, and oxytocin (Pitocin) hyperstimulation that does not allow for adequate placental perfusion. The fetus responds to placental insufficiency with bradycardia and decreased variability as noted on the fetal monitor.

Trauma during delivery is another potential cause of fetal asphyxia. Cephalopelvic disproportion may lead to the fetus becoming "stuck" in the birth canal or compressing the cord while moving through the canal.

In severe cases, the clavicle is purposefully fractured to deliver the newborn quickly.

Pathophysiology

The fetus initially responds to hypoxia with tachycardia. Tachycardia increases cardiac output. Simultaneously, blood is shunted away from the kidneys and gut to the heart and brain. With worsening fetal hypoxia and acidosis, hypotension results from cardiac and respiratory failure. The heart rate may increase slightly but eventually decreases, and bradycardia ensues. These events are often recorded on the fetal monitor during labor. The fetal monitor reveals a loss of beat-to-beat variability, fetal tachycardia, then bradycardia, and poor short-term variability and late decelerations. Perinatal asphyxia is the leading cause of HIE.

Clinical and experimental studies from the 1990s demonstrated two phases of neuronal death following hypoxia. The first is an immediate neuronal death related to hypoxia of the cells with exhaustion of the energy stores within the cells. The second phase, which usually takes place within 6 hours of the initial insult, is a delayed neuronal death and includes free radical damage and progressive cell death. This second phase accounts for the final cell loss and subsequent development of encephalopathy and increased seizure activity. In term and preterm infants with evidence of intrapartum hypoxia and encephalopathy, magnetic resonance imaging (MRI) studies have demonstrated this two-phase cellular death process.

The prognosis for perinatal asphyxia and resultant HIE varies, ranging from death immediately after birth, to severe neurologic deficits, to no sequelae.

Apgar scores alone are poor predictors of the adverse neurologic sequelae of perinatal asphyxia. Therefore, combining the Apgar score with the entire clinical picture, including timing of onset and severity of seizures and neurologic examination findings, gives a better estimation of outcome.

Assessment

The initial signs of HIE appear immediately after birth. The newborn is limp, cyanotic, bradycardic, and apneic. Muscle tone, reflexes, and spontaneous movement are extremely depressed in the asphyxiated newborn and are often the last parameters to return during recovery. The intrapartum history may reveal substantial fetal distress, including prolonged bradycardia, late decelerations, and poor fetal heart rate variability.

All body systems may be affected, including the heart, kidneys, lungs, metabolic system, and the brain. The heart may show signs of damage, including poor contractility, within the first 24 hours after birth. Other clinical findings include central cyanosis, tachypnea, rales in the lower lung fields, hepatomegaly, and a systolic murmur.

Clinically important HIE almost always affects the kidneys. The effects on glomerular filtration and tubular function depend on the degree, severity, and duration of the decreased blood flow to the kidneys.

Respiratory distress—including sternal, substernal, and intercostal retractions; grunting; and nasal flaring—is common. Acute hypoglycemia and hypocalcemia are metabolic complications.

Brain damage from asphyxia is manifested by HIE that appears soon after birth and continues for 7 to 10 days. HIE may produce cerebral edema for up to 72 hours after birth and seizures for 24 to 48 hours after birth. Seizures that occur within the first 24 hours are a grave sign, often indicating poor neurologic outcome. HIE produces subtle and generalized tonic seizures as a result of CNS insult and developing cerebral edema (Table 14-4).

caREminder

To determine whether the newborn's movements are tremors or seizure activity, check for subtle signs of seizures, such as lip smacking, rapid eye movements, and tongue thrusting.

Blood tests are used to determine the presence of asphyxia. Cord blood gases are obtained from the umbilical cord immediately on delivery and demonstrate severe acidosis and hypoxemia. Hypoglycemia is not uncommon.

TABLE 14-4 Differentiating Seizures From Jitteriness		
Assessment Findings	**Seizures**	**Jitteriness**
Ceases with passive flexion	No	Yes
Activity induced	No	Yes
Associated with cyanosis or bradycardia	Yes	No
Eye deviations	Yes	No

A bedside echocardiogram demonstrates poor heart function and decreased contraction of the ventricles. Oliguria (urine output <1 mL/kg/hr) and hematuria are common, and the blood urea nitrogen and creatinine levels are elevated.

Nursing Diagnoses and Outcomes

Nursing diagnoses and outcomes generally applicable for newborns with a health challenge are listed in Nursing Plan of Care 14-1. In addition, the following may be applicable to a newborn with perinatal asphyxia:

Nursing Diagnosis: Risk for ineffective cerebral tissue perfusion related to effects of anoxia

Outcome: Newborn will show no signs of neurologic deterioration and will respond appropriately to the environment.

Interdisciplinary Interventions

Care of the asphyxiated newborn is complex. It begins at delivery and continues in the NICU. Depending on the extent of asphyxiation and sequelae, community care may be ongoing.

Delivery Team Management

The initial stabilization process is labile and often unpredictable. The neonatal team usually consists of a nurse, respiratory therapist, and physician. They must act quickly at delivery to establish an airway and begin ventilation. Other resuscitative measures include cardiac compressions, if the heart rate is very low, and emergency medications such as epinephrine administered through the endotracheal tube or through an umbilical venous catheter inserted by the resuscitation team. The nurse's role in resuscitating an asphyxiated newborn involves assessing heart rate and initiating compressions. Also, the nurse may assist the respiratory therapist in establishing and maintaining an adequate airway by stabilizing the endotracheal tube, applying PPV, and assessing for breath sounds. Quick and efficient stabilization is imperative to the newborn's survival.

Neonatal Intensive Care Unit Team Management

On the newborn's arrival to the NICU, quickly ensure the presence of a patent airway, and establish baseline vital signs. Perform a complete physical examination to detect any congenital anomalies or other complications. Evaluate the newborn's muscle tone, response to care, and reflexes to establish a baseline neurologic assessment that will be helpful for later comparison.

The nurse assists with placement of invasive lines to better monitor blood pressure and obtains specimens for laboratory tests. Closely monitor for aberrations in all laboratory values, and perform bedside glucose, hemoglobin, and hematocrit testing as ordered. Also monitor the newborn's response to treatments and assist in determining the extent of organ involvement. For example, meticulous monitoring of urine output aids in assessing renal damage. Documenting neurologic symptoms helps to determine CNS damage.

The medical team aggressively treats the newborn by promoting oxygenation, providing ventilation, and administering medications. The physician evaluates chest radiographs, serial blood gas levels, and other laboratory studies to guide treatments. The goals of treatment are to avoid hypercapnia, control seizures, and restrict IV fluids to prevent cerebral edema. Closely monitor for signs of cerebral edema and increasing ICP (Chart 14-5).

Phenobarbital is the medication of choice to control seizures. Other supportive therapies with seizures include correcting any metabolic abnormalities, ensuring an adequate airway, and promoting oxygenation and ventilation. Monitor the newborn's response to the seizure medications by noting the time that the seizures stopped, and observe for side effects. The most common side effect of phenobarbital is respiratory depression.

The family is often distressed by the unexpected events of the birth and will need reassurance and frequent updates about the newborn's condition. Explain the current treatments and, if indicated, the newborn's responses to the family. Facilitate communication with the physician. If sequelae are severe, involve the social worker as soon as possible to provide additional support to the family.

The team will need to work quickly to determine if the infant qualifies for total body cooling (TBC); if appropriate, initiate this therapy within 6 hours after birth. In multiple randomized controlled trials, TBC has been shown to improve mortality, without increasing major disability in survivors, and improve neurodevelopmental outcomes at 18 and 24 months (Jacobs et al., 2013). Therapeutic hypothermia involves TBC using a cooling mattress bed to induce hypothermia (33° to 34° C [91.4° to 93.2° F]), with the purpose of reducing the body's core temperature and, subsequently, the temperature within the brain. The goal is to begin therapeutic hypothermia within 6 hours after birth (the earlier it is initiated, the more favorable the outcome), if the newborn meets specific clinical criteria, and to continue cooling for 72 hours after birth. Although not completely understood, brain cooling provides protection to the brain through multiple pathways, including reducing cellular metabolism and energy depletion and reducing edema and excitatory transmitters.

CHART 14-5 Signs of Increasing Intracranial Pressure in the Newborn

- Increasing lethargy
- Increasing head circumference
- Tense anterior fontanel
- Widening sutures
- Apnea
- Deteriorating vital signs
- Seizures

INFANTS OF DIABETIC MOTHERS

Infants of diabetic mothers include all infants affected by abnormal maternal glucose levels, whether those levels result from gestational diabetes (abnormal glucose levels induced by pregnancy) or from preexisting maternal diabetes. Approximately 3% to 10% of all pregnancies are complicated by glucose control problems, most of which are caused by gestational diabetes (Reece et al., 2010). The infant of a diabetic mother is at risk for many problems. To decrease the risk to the newborn, the mother's blood glucose level must be assessed and properly controlled before and during pregnancy to minimize hypoglycemia and hyperglycemia. Diabetes screening should begin at 26 to 28 weeks of gestation. Common problems in infants of diabetic mothers include macrosomia (increased adipose tissue) and subsequent traumatic delivery, hypoglycemia within a short time after delivery, respiratory distress from surfactant deficiency, electrolyte disturbances, polycythemia, and congenital anomalies.

Pathophysiology

Insulin does not cross the placenta, but glucose does. The fetus increases its own production of insulin in response to the high glucose levels from the mother. This state of hyperinsulinism leads to macrosomia, increased fat accumulation, and LGA status. Because of the hyperinsulinemia, hypoglycemia occurs rapidly after delivery when the maternal supply of glucose abruptly ceases. The hyperinsulinemia can last for several days, and the infant may require IV therapy to maintain normal glucose values.

Infants of diabetic mothers have a higher incidence of respiratory distress and surfactant deficiency than other newborns. Poorly controlled maternal diabetes appears to impair fetal pulmonary maturation (Negrato et al., 2012). This association has led many obstetricians to delay delivering these infants until 37 to 38 weeks to ensure adequate lung maturity.

Hypocalcemia and hypomagnesemia are also common problems of infants of diabetic mothers, resulting from the newborn's decreased hypoparathyroid functioning. The frequency and severity of abnormal maternal blood glucose levels can contribute substantially to the likelihood of congenital abnormalities (Wender-Ozegowska et al., 2005), such as congenital heart disease, and CNS defects, such as lumbosacral agenesis.

Assessment

A maternal history of diabetes mellitus or gestational diabetes is usually present, but many mothers exhibit no history or have not obtained appropriate prenatal care. Infants of diabetic mothers have a characteristic appearance as a result of the increased subcutaneous fat: full face, smaller head circumference-to-weight ratio, and a larger weight-to-length ratio. The placenta and umbilical cord are often very large.

A complete assessment is vital to detect congenital anomalies, specifically congenital heart defects. Close observation is necessary to detect hypoglycemia, which may be asymptomatic or may be marked by lethargy, a high-pitched cry, jitteriness, and seizures. Monitor for respiratory distress and auscultate for cardiac murmurs. Evaluate hemoglobin and hematocrit results to monitor for polycythemia. A polycythemic newborn appears ruddy in color. Also monitor electrolytes for the presence of hypocalcemia; supplemental calcium may be necessary.

Because of the infant's large size, traumatic delivery and subsequent birth trauma is common. If the infant exhibits decreased movement or cries when an extremity is moved, investigate further for injury. Not all diabetic mothers are identified before delivery. Therefore, most LGA newborns are at risk for blood glucose problems; perform serial blood glucose determinations after birth.

Interdisciplinary Interventions

Monitor closely for the signs and symptoms of hypoglycemia; obtain blood glucose values every 30 to 60 minutes after birth until values stabilize, then every 2 to 4 hours for 24 hours until stability is confirmed, and initiate early feedings, as appropriate (see thePoint for Supplemental Information: Care Path: An Interdisciplinary Plan of Care for the Infant of a Diabetic Mother). Feedings are contraindicated if respiratory distress is present because of the risk of aspiration. IV fluids are initiated if feedings are withheld.

INTRAUTERINE EXPOSURES

Teratogens such as infectious agents, radiation, high temperatures, and chemicals have deleterious effects on the developing fetus. The effects often depend on dose, timing, and genetic resilience or susceptibility. Infants exposed to drugs or alcohol may suffer short-term withdrawal and long-term effects on growth and neurodevelopment. They may also be exposed to social and environmental risk factors associated with parental substance abuse.

FETAL ALCOHOL SPECTRUM DISORDERS

Ethyl alcohol ingestion by pregnant women is the most common identified cause of teratogenesis (chemically induced physical or mental anomalies) in a fetus. These anomalies fall into the category of fetal alcohol spectrum disorders (FASD), a group of disorders that includes FAS.

About 30% of pregnant women report consuming alcohol; 8% report binge drinking (four or more drinks on one occasion) (Ethen et al., 2009). Although the incidence of FAS is estimated at 0.33 to 2.2 cases per 1,000 live births in the United States and at 0.97 per 1,000 live births in the developed world (May et al., 2009), this is likely an underestimate because many newborns with FAS are not diagnosed properly.

FASD represents a continuum of structural anomalies and behavioral and neurocognitive disabilities associated with maternal prenatal chronic, heavy, or binge alcohol ingestion. The child may not have the characteristic facial features, so FASD may not be recognized until school age, when intellectual, cognitive, social, and behavioral difficulties are apparent.

Newborns most severely affected by alcohol ingestion present with FAS, a syndrome of growth deficiency and characteristic facial features associated with a strong history of prenatal maternal alcohol ingestion. Additionally, mild to moderate cognitive deficiency and delayed motor and language development are recognized early during infancy. Newborns with FAS have lower thresholds for arousal than healthy newborns and are more restless and irritable.

Pathophysiology

The active ingredient of alcohol is ethanol. Ethanol's metabolites are readily transferred across the placenta and to the fetus. Ethanol is a CNS depressant and it migrates into the fetal brain, liver, kidneys, and pancreas. The rate of fetal ethanol metabolism is half that of the adult, and the fetus relies on the placenta for ethanol clearance. This combination of circumstances produces amniotic fluid with high ethanol levels and a newborn that may appear intoxicated at birth.

Ethanol and its metabolites are teratogens, depending on the time of exposure. Weeks 3 through 8 of gestation are the most vulnerable times for toxicity because cells are dividing and organs are developing. The exact amount of maternal alcohol ingestion that causes FAS is not clear, but a "threshold level" appears to exist at which organogenesis is disrupted. This threshold is unknown, however, so the Surgeon General's Advisory on Alcohol Use in Pregnancy urges pregnant women or women who are considering becoming pregnant to abstain from alcohol use completely (Carmona, 2005).

FAS is the leading known preventable cause of cognitive challenge in developed countries. The prognosis for these newborns may be poor because the damage done to the CNS is irreversible and results in lifelong learning problems and disabilities. Approximately 70% of children with heavy prenatal alcohol exposure are neurobehaviorally affected (Mattson et al., 2013). As these children grow and develop, educational programs can help these individuals realize their potential but cannot offer a cure. Early diagnosis and interventions are important to help newborns with FAS develop into self-sufficient adults. Some will require constant supervision, whereas others may live independent lives. Academic struggles are common because adolescents with FAS have significantly lower intelligence scores and have an increased incidence of attention-deficit/ hyperactivity disorder (ADHD) (Ornoy & Ergaz, 2010).

Assessment

Diagnosis can be challenging because the physical characteristics common to newborns with FAS are general and broad, and not all newborns with FAS look or act the same. Physical manifestations of FAS range from mild to severe. Common signs of FAS include SGA status (in length, weight, or both); microcephaly; poor growth; smooth, wide philtrum; thin vermilion border (upper lip);

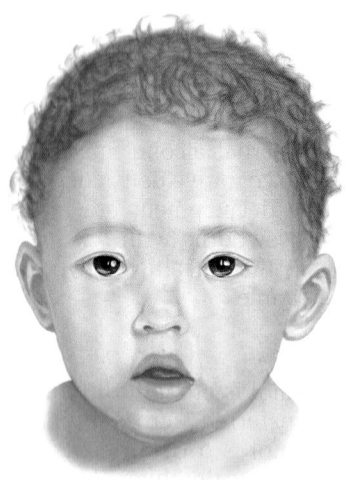

A

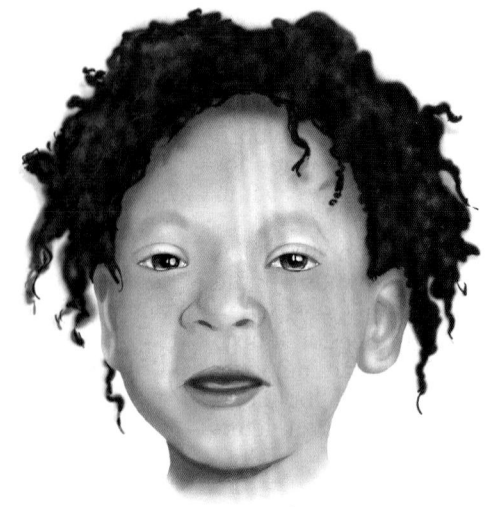

B

Figure 14-12 Typical facial characteristics of FAS include short palpebral fissures; a smooth, wide philtrum; a thin vermilion border; and micrognathia. (A) Child at age 1 month and (B) 3 years.

short palpebral fissures; low-set ears; and micrognathia (small chin) (Fig. 14-12). Additionally, congenital heart diseases, such as ventricular septal defect, atrial septal defect, and tetralogy of Fallot, are associated with prenatal alcohol exposure. Renal anomalies may also occur. The diagnosis is made by reported maternal alcohol consumption during pregnancy and the presence of a cluster of anomalies.

FAS newborns are small at birth and fail to grow normally or demonstrate appropriate catch-up growth. Head growth is often less than the 10th percentile. Facial anomalies are common and affect the midface. Other complications of FAS include irritability, poor feeding stemming from ineffective coordination of suck and swallow, and hypersensitivity to external stimuli. Newborns with FAS are less able to habituate to aversive stimuli as measured by the NBAS. Alcohol withdrawal often presents within 24 hours after birth, with tremors, irritability, and abdominal distention.

CNS effects in most children with FAS take the form of microcephaly and other brain abnormalities (Sowell et al., 2008). The most profound effect of FAS is cognitive challenges resulting in poor academic performance. Most children with FASD do not have below average intelligence and may not qualify for special education services based on basic psychological testing; specialized testing is required to document deficits in executive functioning such as planning, organization, and attention (Mattson et al., 2011).

Nursing Diagnoses and Outcomes

Nursing diagnoses and outcomes generally applicable for newborns with a health challenge are presented in Nursing Plan of Care 14-1. In addition, the following may be applicable for a newborn with FAS:

Nursing Diagnosis: Imbalanced nutrition: Less than body requirements, related to poor nippling
Outcomes:
• Newborn will ingest adequate calories and nutrients.
• Newborn will display adequate growth.

Interdisciplinary Interventions

Nursing interventions are mainly supportive during the neonatal period. To minimize CNS irritability and hypersensitivity to the environment, gear nursing interventions to maintaining a quiet environment that promotes normal wake and sleep patterns. Additionally, cluster care if the infant tolerates it, and minimize unnecessary handling.

Nutritional management is critically important for the newborn with FAS because poor feeding is common. Optimize calorie intake and promote normal suck–swallow patterns.

DISORDERS RELATED TO EXPOSURE TO STIMULANTS, OPIOIDS, OR OTHER SUBSTANCES

The incidence of substance abuse among pregnant women, including use of stimulants, opiates, inhalants, marijuana, hallucinogens, tranquilizers, and sedatives, has been reported to be 5% (Substance Abuse and Mental Health Services Administration, 2011). Prenatal drug exposure has far-reaching implications for the newborn, the family, the health care professional caring for these mothers and newborns, and society at large.

Stimulants such as cocaine and methamphetamine and opioids such as heroin are common drugs abused prenatally. Polydrug use (use of more than one drug) is common, although most users deny it when asked (Kuczkowski, 2007). Polydrug use during pregnancy results in newborns with lower birth weight, shorter length, and smaller head circumference than infants whose mothers did not use these substances during pregnancy. The fetus exposed to intrauterine drugs may exhibit **neonatal abstinence syndrome (NAS)** (withdrawal symptoms after birth). Stimulants and opioids are considered together in this section, despite their major pharmacologic differences, because many substance-using mothers are polydrug users. In addition, withdrawal symptoms may be similar.

Cocaine is a stimulant that increases dopamine release and decreases uptake of norepinephrine. When used during pregnancy, cocaine and other stimulants cause massive vasoconstriction throughout the body, including the vessels in the uterus and placenta. As a result of the increase in blood volume that occurs with pregnancy, the vasoactive effects of cocaine are enhanced. The vasoconstrictive properties of cocaine lead to preterm labor, placental insufficiency, or abruptio placentae. Additionally, cocaine's vasoconstrictive properties may decrease blood flow to the placenta and fetus, causing substantial vasoconstriction, subsequently leading to short-term hypoxic episodes in the fetus.

Cocaine has potentially teratogenic effects, and its use during pregnancy increases the risk of birth anomalies, especially during the first 3 months of gestation. Cocaine crosses the placenta quickly, and metabolites can be detected in the fetus for up to 4 days after exposure. Common birth defects associated with cocaine use include genitourinary malformations, prune-belly syndrome, limb defects, cardiovascular defects, brain lesions, and cerebral infarcts. Maternal cocaine use is associated with IUGR, including reduced head circumference. Other malformations associated with cocaine use include congenital heart disease, encephalocele, and microcephaly. Withdrawal symptoms are uncommon and are usually mild when present. Perhaps the most serious complications of cocaine use during pregnancy are the increased risks of preterm delivery and abruptio placentae. Cocaine appears to have a specific effect on birth weight, even more potent than that of tobacco use. When these substances are used during pregnancy, LBW is common.

Methamphetamine has effects similar to those of cocaine, including vasoconstrictive properties that may alter blood flow and oxygen supply to the fetus. Currently, long-term effects on the fetus from methamphetamine exposure are unknown.

Opioids are CNS depressants that produce feelings of relaxation. Codeine, heroin, methadone, and morphine are the most commonly abused opioids. Heroin is six times as potent as morphine and highly addictive. These drugs readily cross the placenta; at birth, when the maternal supply ceases, the newborn may show signs of withdrawal at 24 to 72 hours.

Heroin reduces uteroplacental blood flow and inhibits fetal growth. Combined with inadequate maternal calorie and protein intake, it produces IUGR, including poor brain growth. During pregnancy, maternal heroin use creates fetal addiction. Abrupt withdrawal from heroin during pregnancy is not recommended, however, because maternal withdrawal symptoms are detrimental to the fetus. If the mother attempts to stop using heroin or if her intake is erratic, fetal withdrawal and possibly death may occur. Often, the mother is placed on methadone maintenance during her pregnancy to avoid fetal death. Methadone is a synthetic opioid drug that works as a substitute for heroin. The benefits of methadone maintenance are that the level of drug can be maintained as a constant at an exact dose and that the drug does not exert the mood-altering effects of heroin. Methadone withdrawal can also harm the fetus.

Newborns exposed to intrauterine opioids are at high risk for child abuse as a result of their withdrawal behaviors, such as irritability and decreased sleep. These behaviors are difficult to manage, especially for a drug-abusing mother who has limited coping skills or resources. Withdrawal behaviors may last for up to 6 months. These infants are also at increased risk of neurodevelopmental problems (Hunt et al., 2008).

A majority of pregnant women treated with methadone also smoke cigarettes (Burns et al., 2007). Intrauterine exposure to opioids and nicotine increases the risk of LBW and preterm birth. The neonatal team caring for newborns prenatally exposed to tobacco and methadone can expect a slower taper of medications and prolonged, difficult withdrawal behaviors. These infants may require prolonged hospitalization because of the severity of withdrawal symptoms, although this possibility has not been demonstrated in research studies.

Assessment

Obtain a complete maternal history regarding all legal, illegal, over-the-counter, and prescription drug use to identify newborns at risk. The neonatal abstinence scoring system (Finnegan, 1985) is a tool used to assess the severity of drug withdrawal behaviors in term infants. This scoring system attempts to rate withdrawal behaviors on an objective scale. It lists 21 symptoms commonly seen in newborns during withdrawal. Score the newborn 2 hours after birth and then every 4 hours for the first 5 days of life. If the symptoms are increasing in severity, score the newborn every 2 hours. This tool was tested on term newborns, not preterm newborns.

Score newborns whose mothers are suspected drug users every 2 to 3 hours for the first 48 hours of life, regardless of the initial score. Thereafter, if the newborn scores 7 or less, complete scoring every 4 hours for 48 hours. A score of 7 or less is categorized as mild withdrawal. Use nursing judgment to avoid waking the newborn unnecessarily.

If the score is 8 or more, medication is initiated, and scoring continues for 5 days. Each scoring interval rates the newborn's behavior during the entire 2- or 4-hour interval, not just the behavior present at the time of scoring. Awaken the newborn to elicit reflexes and specified behavior.

Cocaine-exposed newborns demonstrate increased muscle tone, tremors, and prolonged retention of primitive reflexes. The cocaine-exposed newborn does not present with specific withdrawal behaviors and may only demonstrate irritability several weeks after birth. Premature delivery and associated problems are the primary challenges for the cocaine-exposed newborn (see earlier discussion of prematurity and LBW).

For opioid-exposed newborns, the prenatal and labor and delivery history may show high-risk maternal factors such as a lack of prenatal care or an admitted history of drug use. Drug-addicted pregnant mothers commonly do not obtain prenatal care or obtain it only sporadically. Labor and delivery events are also important, including the presence of meconium or fetal distress. Heroin-addicted newborns have a greater than normal incidence of meconium aspiration.

The physical examination findings and mental state of the mother are also helpful. Often, the mother admits to heroin use or to having taken illicit drugs in the past. Needle tracks from illicit drug injections are also high-risk findings. The mental status examination findings may be helpful if the mother is able to answer questions coherently.

At birth, assess gestational age to determine whether the newborn has grown appropriately in utero. Many drug-exposed newborns are SGA but have a head circumference that is proportionally large. This type of SGA is described as "head-sparing SGA."

Upon admission to the nursery, assess the newborn further. Newborns exposed to opioids display withdrawal symptoms within 2 to 6 days after delivery, when the drug blood level becomes critically low (Chart 14-6). CNS symptoms appear first, followed by gastrointestinal disturbances. The most common symptom of NAS is tremors.

The increased activity, poor feeding, irritability, increased metabolic rate, and decreased sleep typical of NAS lead to inadequate weight gain and growth. Investigate each withdrawal symptom as it appears to help rule out other causes, such as hypoglycemia or hypocalcemia. Tremors are not uncommon with other abnormalities, such as hypoglycemia, hypocalcemia, or hypomagnesemia; these conditions must be ruled out before treating for drug exposure.

At the time of admission, maternal blood work and urine samples may be sent, depending on the mother's history and presentation. Legal issues regarding such testing are determined on a state-by-state basis. Generally, if the maternal history poses a risk, the newborn's urine sample is sent to the laboratory for qualitative toxicologic assessment immediately after birth. Urine collected more than 36 hours after birth is likely to test negative for drugs. Meconium or hair samples, if available, are superior samples for toxicology screening because these samples show long-term drug exposure.

CHART 14-6 Symptoms of Opioid Withdrawal in the Neonate*

Tremors

High-pitched cry

Sneezing

Irritability

Increased muscle tone

Poor feeding

Diarrhea

Weight loss and inadequate weight gain

Decreased sleep

Poor state control

Increased sensitivity to environmental stimuli

Increased activity

*Symptoms appear gradually and progress in severity and frequency. Most symptoms appear by 3 days and can last 4 to 6 weeks or longer, depending on the drug.

Nursing Diagnoses and Outcomes

Nursing diagnoses and outcomes generally applicable for newborns with a health challenge are presented in Nursing Plan of Care 14-1. In addition, those identified in Teaching Intervention Plan 14-1 are also applicable for a newborn with intrauterine drug exposure.

Interdisciplinary Interventions

For mild withdrawal symptoms, reduce noise levels and darken the environment to assist the newborn to be calm and to sleep. Advise other health care workers not to disturb the newborn and to talk quietly while near the bedside. Provide periods of undisturbed sleep, limiting examinations and procedures.

KidKare To help calm the irritable newborn, provide boundaries in the crib with blankets, offer a pacifier, and swaddle the infant. Cluster care activities to promote longer periods of sleep and to avoid unnecessary handling.

Skin care can be a challenge in these newborns as a result of frequent, watery stools. Also, skin breakdown at the knees and nose is common from rubbing against the blankets during irritable spells. Apply barrier creams to the diaper area to prevent skin breakdown. Protect knees by using sheepskin or occlusive dressings.

Teach the family about withdrawal symptoms and treatment (see Teaching Intervention Plan 14-1). Provide this teaching objectively and clearly, avoiding causal and accusatory statements. It is vital that the family understand the withdrawal course, treatment (including medication administration), and expected behaviors. Model appropriate interactions and infant care to assist the family to learn coping and calming skills for their newborn.

Pharmacologic intervention is indicated if the score is more than 8 for three consecutive scores or if the average of three consecutive scores is 8 or more. Additionally, if the total score is 12 or more for two consecutive intervals, therapy should be initiated before the 4-hour interval has elapsed (Finnegan, 1985). Based on the neonatal abstinence score, the prescriber may initiate pharmacotherapy that helps to control the diarrhea, improve feeding behaviors, and control crying. There is limited evidence as to the best medication to use for NAS, and there is a variety of practice across NICUs. Recent recommendations include morphine and methadone because both of these medications replace what the infant is withdrawing from (Kraft & van den Anker, 2012).

Phenobarbital or clonidine may be used in combination with a narcotic, although minimal research has been completed on either of these drugs in relation to efficacy in treating opioid withdrawal in the newborn. Use of phenobarbital or clonidine may assist in controlling irritability and improving sleep patterns, especially in those infants with symptoms from polydrug exposure.

A nutritional consultation may be helpful to optimize caloric intake. A formula with 24 cal/oz may be needed to meet the metabolic needs of these newborns.

TIP 14-1: A TEACHING INTERVENTION PLAN for the Newborn With Neonatal Abstinence Syndrome

Nursing Diagnoses and Family Outcomes

- Impaired skin integrity related to frequent, loose stools
  Outcomes: Family will state reason for skin breakdown.
  Family will demonstrate appropriate cleansing and application of diaper cream.
- Sleep deprivation related to irritability
  Outcomes: Family will state importance of sleep to overall health.
  Family will demonstrate swaddling and calming techniques, darkening environment.
  Family will safely and accurately administer medications.
- Imbalanced nutrition: Less than body requirements related to increased activity and poor sleep cycles
  Outcomes: Family will feed newborn safely and efficiently.
  Family will state need for increased calories.
  Family will prepare specialized formula accurately and store it safely.
- Impaired parenting related to drug abuse and decreased resources/support
  Outcome: Family will complete needed referrals and seek and use resources.

Teach Family/Caregivers About

Medications

- Measure medication carefully and give at designated times.

- Administer medications as prescribed, and give phenobarbital in small amount of formula.
- Monitor for lethargy or increased irritability; give only what is prescribed to avoid overdose.
- Keep medications out of reach of children.

Nutrition

- Promote small, frequent feedings; use high-calorie (24 cal/oz) formula.

Special Considerations

- Promote adequate sleep by providing quiet environment, swaddling, or offering pacifier; allow prolonged periods of sleep.

Skin

- Protect diaper area with barrier creams.

Psychosocial

- Provide referrals to community resources (public health department, mental health services, addiction treatment center, food subsidy programs).
- If caregiver feels "out of control" and unable to cope, call a friend to watch infant, call health care provider, or close door and allow infant to cry.

Contact Health Care Provider if

- The infant develops water-loss stools, increase in irritability, vomiting, fever more than 100.4° F (38° C), lethargy, poor feeding, or accidental overdose.

Bottlefeeding may be ineffective, and an experienced occupational therapist may assist with nippling evaluation and interventions. Breastfeeding is not recommended for newborns of mothers with a drug history. Some drugs, especially cocaine, are passed to the infant through breast milk. Often, the newborn will need IV fluid and nutrition to maintain proper growth. Such treatment requires a longer hospitalization.

Community Care

A clinical social worker assists with the placement of the newborn if the mother is unable or unwilling to care for her newborn. Working closely with the clinical social worker is vital to provide the best home care situation for the mother and newborn. Additionally, the clinical social worker assists the mother to obtain necessary social services, parenting classes, and referrals (Clinical Judgment 14-2).

DISORDERS RELATED TO TOBACCO SMOKE

Smoking during pregnancy is a risk factor to the fetus. Approximately 15% of pregnant women smoke (Substance Abuse and Mental Health Services Administration, 2010).

Tobacco smoke reduces maternal blood oxygen levels, and nicotine readily crosses the placenta, appearing in fetal blood at levels higher than those seen in maternal serum. Mothers who smoke while pregnant are more likely to deliver preterm and deliver an infant of LBW (Dietz et al., 2010). Smoking is associated with an increased rate of term SGA delivery (Joubert et al., 2012). Smoking during pregnancy continues to be one of the most common preventable causes of infant morbidity and mortality.

Environmental tobacco smoke continues to pose a risk to newborns after delivery. Infants exposed pre- and postnatally have more crying and irritability (Johansson et al., 2008), poorer asthma control (Oh et al., 2012), and lower reading performance (Cho et al., 2013) than those not exposed. Smoking in the home is also a high risk factor for sudden infant death syndrome (Dietz et al., 2010).

Pathophysiology

The components of cigarette smoke, including nicotine and carbon monoxide, inhibit cell uptake of amino acids in the placenta. These amino acids are the building blocks of proteins that are essential for adequate fetal growth. Without these proteins, LBW may occur.

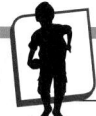

CLINICAL JUDGMENT 14-2

Infant of a Substance-Abusing Mother

Hannah is a 3-day-old term newborn who is SGA, delivered to a mother who is taking methadone and abusing heroin. Hannah is irritable and has increased muscle tone, diarrhea, frantic sucking, and vomiting.

Her vital signs are as follows: heart rate, 180 bpm; respiratory rate, 70 breaths/min; no other signs of respiratory distress; temperature, 100.6° F (38.1° C) axillary; and weight, 1,800 g.

Questions

1. What other assessment data should the nurse collect?
2. Which assessment findings are abnormal?
3. What is the cause for Hannah's symptoms?

4. What nursing interventions should initially be implemented?
5. How will the nurse know that Hannah is improving?

Answers

1. Quality of Moro reflex, presence of skin breakdown (knees, chin), number of hours spent sleeping between feedings, comparison of birth weight to current weight to determine presence of significant weight loss (>10% of birth weight), presence of tremors (while disturbed or undisturbed), nasal congestion or rhinorrhea, sweating, and mottled skin

2. Irritability, increased muscle tone, diarrhea, frantic sucking, vomiting, rapid respiratory rate, elevated temperature; weight indicates SGA

3. Hannah is experiencing NAS. After delivery, when the supply of heroin and methadone is gone, the infant responds with active withdrawal symptoms. These may occur any time after delivery but are most common within 48–72 hours. The most common symptoms include CNS irritability and gastrointestinal hypermotility. Weight

loss is a result of the hypermetabolic state in which there is increased oxygen consumption at the cellular level.

4. Initiate the Neonatal Abstinence Score Sheet to provide ongoing documentation of behaviors in an objective format. Provide a quiet and darkened environment. Swaddle with blankets and provide rhythmic rocking. Provide small, frequent, and calorie-dense feedings. Offer a pacifier. Collaborate with the medical team to initiate medications to alleviate the withdrawal symptoms. Include the family by demonstrating appropriate interventions that assist in calming the infant.

5. Neonatal Abstinence Score Sheet scores of 8 or less, daily weight gain, sleeping at least 3 hours between feedings, coordinated suck–swallow patterns with minimal spillage of formula, no vomiting or regurgitation, presence of awake/alert states, appropriate response to caregiver interactions

---

Additionally, nicotine produces vasoconstriction and may lead to reduced placental blood flow, reducing blood flow to the fetus and limiting the availability of nutrition and oxygen.

In response to this vasoconstriction and limited blood flow, the fetus increases its production of fetal red blood cells, inducing polycythemia. Although compensatory, polycythemia has inherent problems because the blood is more viscous than normal and can begin to sludge, leading to further hypoxia from blocked blood vessels.

Interdisciplinary Interventions

Nursing interventions are geared toward preventing smoking and supporting smoking cessation programs and techniques. Recognizing smoking as an addiction is an important conceptual step in truly assisting the individual with cessation. Encourage smoking cessation during pregnancy or at least reducing the number of cigarettes smoked. After birth, if the family is unwilling to stop smoking, encourage them to refrain from smoking inside the home.

NEONATAL HYPERBILIRUBINEMIA

QUESTION: On the seventh day after birth, Gabriella's unconjugated bilirubin level rises enough to require phototherapy. You discover Abby crying by Gabriella's isolette. She says to you, "I don't understand why this has happened." The cascade of hemoglobin breakdown is not easy for health care professionals to understand; it is predictably baffling to the family. How will you explain this development to Abby? Why would you indicate that for hyperbilirubinemia in the premature infant, phototherapy is the therapy of choice?

In utero, the placenta serves as the primary organ to clear bilirubin from the fetus's system. After birth, the newborn liver must take over the task of excreting bilirubin while production of bilirubin increases from excessive breakdown of red blood cells. **Hyperbilirubinemia** is defined as excessive levels of bilirubin in the blood, often caused by a pathologic process.

Jaundice is a yellowing of the skin that is one of the most common physical findings during the initial newborn period. Jaundice occurs when bilirubin is deposited into the subcutaneous tissue, and it becomes visible when the serum bilirubin levels exceed 7.0 mg/dL. Jaundice caused by normal physiologic processes occurs in 84% of all healthy term newborns (Bhutani et al., 2013), generally peaking at 3 to 5 days of life (Keren et al., 2008); it is even more frequent in infants born at less than 38 weeks' gestation (American Academy of Pediatrics, 2004).

ALERT *Jaundice that occurs within the first 24 hours of life or after 2 weeks of life signifies an abnormal physiologic process and should be followed up immediately.*

Breastfed infants have a higher incidence of jaundice than those who are not breastfed. This higher incidence may be related to the quality of suckling at the breast. Newborns who have difficulty breastfeeding may develop jaundice from dehydration and caloric deprivation. If the newborn is healthy, with no signs of other causes of jaundice, then continued, frequent breastfeeding is recommended.

Premature newborns are at risk for hyperbilirubinemia resulting from immaturity of the liver, relatively limited albumin binding sites, and, often, severe illness that requires prolonged parenteral nutrition. Premature newborns often present with elevated bilirubin levels that peak at about 1 week of life, in contrast to the term newborn, in whom levels peak at around day 4 of life. Common causes of hyperbilirubinemia in the newborn are increased bilirubin production (from increased breakdown of red blood cells), decreased excretion of bilirubin, or both (Table 14-5).

Pathophysiology

Bilirubin is the end product of the breakdown of heme, a substrate of hemoglobin. It is released into the bloodstream as red blood cells are broken down. Newborns produce bilirubin at more than twice the rate of the adult (about 6 to 8 mg/kg/day). This large bilirubin production is necessary because newborns' red blood cells have a short life span. Newborns also have a greater number of circulating red blood cells than adults, resulting in part from the naturally occurring hypoxic intrauterine environment.

In utero, bilirubin produced by the fetus crosses the placenta to maternal circulation and is excreted by the maternal liver. After delivery, the newborn begins to build up bilirubin levels that exceed the capacity of the neonatal liver (which can excrete only approximately two thirds of the circulating bilirubin). After the red blood cell has been broken down and the bilirubin is released into the bloodstream, it binds to albumin in the plasma. After all the albumin-binding sites are saturated, bilirubin circulates freely in the plasma. This freely circulating bilirubin has a high affinity for fatty tissue, such as brain tissue, and can, therefore, cause serious neurologic sequelae if allowed to remain at high levels. Hypoxia and subsequent asphyxia decrease the pH of the blood, impairing albumin's ability to bind bilirubin. Asphyxia also causes damage to other organs, such as the liver, which may impair its ability to metabolize and excrete bilirubin.

After the bilirubin reaches the liver, it is transferred from the albumin to the liver cell. In the liver, the bilirubin is transformed in the presence of the hepatocyte microsomal enzyme glucuronyl transferase and is conjugated for excretion into bile. Most of the bilirubin, approximately 95%, is excreted into bile. The bile is secreted into the intestine, and the bilirubin is expelled through the stool. Newborns may have delayed intestinal motility coupled with poor fluid intake, which leads to decreased urine and stool output, thus delaying bilirubin excretion. In this situation, the bilirubin in the stool is reabsorbed through the intestine, causing higher levels of circulating bilirubin.

There are two types of bilirubin: conjugated and unconjugated. Conjugated bilirubin has been converted in the liver to a water-soluble form that is easily excreted in the biliary tree. Unconjugated bilirubin has not been converted in the liver and is fat-soluble. Fat-soluble bilirubin has a high affinity for extravascular tissue, including fatty and brain tissue.

The newborn's liver is immature, and the large amount of bilirubin that is produced and cannot be excreted is deposited in the skin, producing jaundice. This process accounts for the jaundice occurring in healthy term newborns after 24 hours of life.

If the hyperbilirubinemia has been controlled, and the level of unconjugated bilirubin has been kept to a minimum, the prognosis for a full recovery with no sequelae is good for the term newborn (Ip et al., 2004). Conversely, if the unconjugated bilirubin level is high, bilirubin may accumulate in nervous tissue, and bilirubin

TABLE 14-5	Common Causes of Hyperbilirubinemia	
Increased Bilirubin Production	**Decreased Bilirubin Excretion**	**Increased Production and Decreased Excretion**
Hemolytic disease	Prematurity	Prematurity
Bacteremia	Bowel obstruction	Bacterial infections
Cephalhematoma	Hypothyroidism	Congenital infections
Excessive bruising	Hypoxia	
Polycythemia	Breast milk jaundice	

encephalopathy may occur. Bilirubin encephalopathy presents with jaundice, lethargy, poor feeding, arching of the back, and a high-pitched cry. Bilirubin encephalopathy occurs when bilirubin crosses the blood–brain barrier and damages the CNS. **Kernicterus**, a term often used to describe bilirubin encephalopathy, is a postmortem diagnosis involving yellow staining of brain tissue. Infants with bilirubin encephalopathy have long-term neurologic disabilities such as motor deficits (they are often unable to walk), hearing loss, and difficulty speaking; it can even lead to death.

Any newborn with a bilirubin level that meets the requirements for an exchange transfusion (in which the entire blood volume in the body is exchanged with new blood to immediately lower the bilirubin level) is at risk for hearing deficits.

Assessment

Jaundice is the first clinical manifestation seen in newborns with elevated bilirubin levels. Noting the onset of clinical jaundice is important because the appearance of jaundice before the first 24 hours of life or after the third day is abnormal and may indicate a hemolytic process, sepsis, or other abnormal condition requiring prompt intervention. Assess for jaundice in the newborn a minimum of every 8 to 12 hours.

Assess the blood types of the mother and newborn to determine whether risk factors for jaundice, such as ABO or Rh incompatibility, are present. Additionally, evaluate the obstetric history to determine whether the delivery was complicated or traumatic enough to have caused extensive bruising.

Visible jaundice tends to progress from the face downward. Guidelines to use when estimating the extent of involvement of jaundice are as follows:

- Light jaundice: appears on the face
- Slightly higher jaundice: appears on face, trunk, abdomen
- Hyperbilirubinemia: visible orange color extending to the thighs or the entire abdomen

Once visible jaundice appears, send a blood sample to the laboratory for serum bilirubin determination, or perform a transcutaneous bilirubinometry (or TcB) test; further follow-up is indicated. An infant's risk of developing significant hyperbilirubinemia may be assessed by using the infant's predischarge bilirubin level and gestational age (Bhutani et al., 2013).

caREminder

> *Assess total serum bilirubin according to the newborn's hours of age and taking into account any risk factors. Plot the total serum bilirubin and notify the physician or nurse practitioner of the results.*

The term newborn's serum bilirubin levels peak at the fifth postnatal day. Newborns with elevated levels that increase more than 5 mg/dL/day are at high risk for sequelae and require treatment for hyperbilirubinemia.

Assess the newborn's liver size, presence of bruises or petechiae, and level of activity. Newborns with a hemolytic process often have hepatosplenomegaly. Newborns with hyperbilirubinemia may have excessive extravascular blood or bruising. High levels of bilirubin may lead to lethargy and decreased tone.

Monitor the newborn's intake and amount of weight loss. A newborn who feeds poorly at the breast or is disinterested in feeding after 24 hours is at risk for developing hyperbilirubinemia. Newborns often lose weight during the first week of life, but excessive weight loss (more than 10%) may indicate dehydration, which concentrates the blood, leading to an elevated serum bilirubin level.

Anemia is rare in newborns with physiologic jaundice, but it may occur in hemolytic jaundice because of the excessive breakdown of the red blood cells. Hemolytic jaundice is an abnormal process and requires frequent assessments of severity and progression. Additionally, specific laboratory tests are ordered to determine the extent of the hemolytic process. Newborns who appear pale should have a screening hemoglobin assessment. Other clinical signs of anemia include tachycardia and hypotension.

Bilirubin encephalopathy is a particular risk for newborns with serum bilirubin levels more than 20 mg/dL. This condition may manifest in poor feeding, hypotonia, and lethargy. More severe brain damage may reveal itself in high-pitched crying, spasticity, opisthotonos, and seizures. Neurologic deficits such as deafness, altered gait, and decreased mental ability may persist.

Simply inspecting the newborn is not an effective method to determine whether jaundice is present. Blood studies, including total and direct bilirubin, Coombs tests, and blood grouping, are performed at the first sign of visible jaundice. Additionally, TcB is now available as a noninvasive method to assess jaundice. TcB uses a special device by which the jaundice levels are assessed through the skin. TcB correlates well with total serum bilirubin and can be used as an alternative to total serum bilirubin determination in the term infant with physiologic jaundice (Ip et al., 2004).

Interdisciplinary Interventions

All newborns discharged from the newborn nursery should have bilirubin levels assessed (American Academy of Pediatrics, 2004) (Evidence-Based Clinical Practice Guidelines 14-2). Additionally, all newborns should be seen by a health care provider 48 to 72 hours after discharge from the nursery to reassess the progression of jaundice, the establishment of healthy feeding routines, and weight gain or loss. Newborns with high risk factors, including poor establishment of breastfeeding, must be seen within 24 hours of discharge.

Acute assessment skills are vital to initiate early treatment for jaundice. As discussed earlier, jaundice appearing after the first 24 hours of life in a healthy term newborn is physiologic jaundice and often requires no treatment. Monitor feeding behavior (infants should nurse 8 to 12 times per day) and the number of wet

EVIDENCE-BASED CLINICAL PRACTICE GUIDELINES 14-2

Neonatal Jaundice

National Collaborating Centre for Women's and Children's Health. (2010). *Neonatal jaundice* (NICE Clinical Guideline 98). Retrieved from

http://guidance.nice.org.uk/CG98

This guideline reviews the standard of care approach to neonatal jaundice in infants of 38 weeks' gestation or older.

American Academy of Pediatrics. (2011). *Phototherapy to prevent severe neonatal hyperbilirubinemia in the newborn infant 35 or more weeks of gestation.* Retrieved from

http://pediatrics.aappublications.org/content/128/4/e1046.full.pdf + html

This guideline reviews the use of phototherapy and management of neonatal jaundice.

diapers to ensure adequate intake and output. Daily total and direct bilirubin levels may be ordered by the physician if jaundice continues to increase. Increasing lethargy, poor feeding, and decreasing output are all signs of worsening jaundice and require evaluation by a physician or nurse practitioner (see the Point for Care Path: An Interdisciplinary Plan of Care for the Infant With Hyperbilirubinemia). Hyperbilirubinemia is treated with phototherapy, exchange transfusions, or medications.

Phototherapy

Interpret bilirubin levels according to the infant's age in hours (American Academy of Pediatrics, 2004). Initiation of phototherapy is determined by the prescriber. Treatment with phototherapy involves the use of a range of bilirubin levels, rather than an absolute number, and allows the clinician to assess many clinical variables of each newborn. For example, a newborn with severe bruising from a traumatic delivery who is not breastfeeding well may need phototherapy initiated at the lower end of the range. In contrast, a healthy, vigorous breastfeeding newborn may not need phototherapy for hyperbilirubinemia until a higher level is reached. The exact level of bilirubin at which phototherapy is needed has not been determined. A combination of factors is considered when initiating treatment, including high-risk factors (excessive bruising, poor feeding), gestational age (infants at 37 weeks' gestational age or less are at increased risk), and bilirubin levels. Phototherapy works by converting bilirubin in the skin to a water-soluble form that can be excreted by the liver without conjugation. It is initiated for any form of unconjugated hyperbilirubinemia and can be used in conjunction with other treatments such as exchange transfusion. Phototherapy is most effective in treating slowly developing hyperbilirubinemia and is an adjunct treatment for the more rapidly increasing forms of hyperbilirubinemia, such as those caused by hemolytic processes. Phototherapy can be delivered by placing the newborn under fluorescent or light-emitting diodes (LEDs) phototherapy lights (Fig. 14-13) or by wrapping the neonate in a fiberoptic blanket (see the Point for Procedures: Phototherapy). Natural sunlight also aids in altering the

structure of bilirubin so that it can be excreted from the body.

Bilirubin can absorb only light of certain wavelengths. White, blue, and green lights can be used to deliver phototherapy. The differences between the colored lights are the spectral band each one emits. The blue lights have been shown to be more effective for photo-degradation because of the narrow spectral band they emit. Although blue lights are more effective, they may cause headaches in health care workers and may also obscure the newborn's color because the blue hue they emit is deceiving. Green light penetrates the skin better; however, clinical application can be difficult because the green hue can make the newborn appear sick. These lights, like the blue ones, can be unpleasant for health care providers to work with.

Phototherapy is delivered by placing the newborn un-clothed underneath the phototherapy lights to expose the skin to the light. It is the nurse's responsibility to ensure that the phototherapy light is positioned appropriately and the light intensity is evaluated. Follow the manufacturer's directions for using the lights and positioning them relative to the infant. If the light is too far away, insufficient energy is delivered to the skin, thereby reducing the efficacy of phototherapy. If the light is too close to the infant, too much energy is directed to

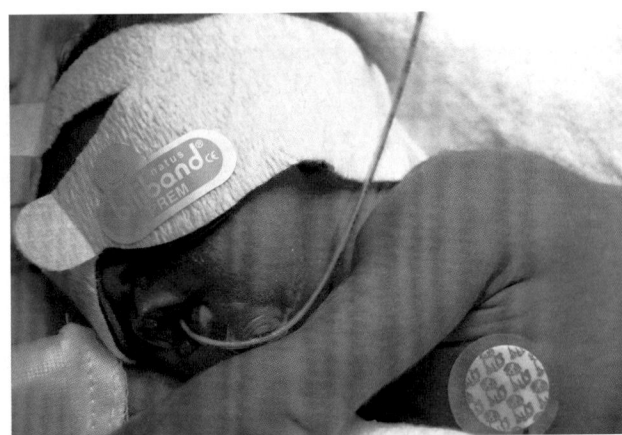

Figure 14-13 Protect the eyes and maintain a normal temperature in an infant undergoing phototherapy

the skin, potentially leading to hyperthermia; if halogen lights are used, the heat they generate increases the risk of burning the infant. If infants can maintain their temperature, place them in a bassinet with the lights as close as possible, within about 10 cm of the infant (except in the case of halogen lights) (American Academy of Pediatrics, 2004). Assess the infant's temperature in an open crib frequently (e.g., every 30 minutes for the first hour, then every 2 hours and as needed). If the infant requires an isolette to maintain temperature, position the lights as close as possible. Measure the luminosity (intensity) of the light at least once per shift by using a phototherapy meter placed at the level of the newborn while he or she is undergoing phototherapy. The purpose of measuring the intensity is to ensure a minimum level of microwatts emitted from the lights. If the level is too low, ensure that the lights are directly over the infant. If the level is still too low, obtain a new phototherapy unit to ensure maximum therapy. Standard phototherapy is 15 $\mu W/cm^2$; intensive phototherapy is 30 $\mu W/cm^2$. During phototherapy, cover the newborn's eyes to prevent microscopic injury to retinal cells. Apply and secure eye patches or phototherapy masks when phototherapy is initiated; keep them in place at all times while the newborn is under the phototherapy lights to protect the eyes from damage. When properly applied, the mask covers the eyes but does not occlude the nares.

ALERT   *Check the position of the phototherapy mask frequently to ensure it has not shifted to obstruct the nares. Also ensure that excess pressure is not applied across the nose when positioning the mask.*

The infant must remain in a crib or isolette while under the phototherapy light. Usually, this requirement limits opportunities for family–infant bonding to times when the baby is removed from the phototherapy light for feeding. During feedings, turn off the lights and remove the eye patches to provide stimulation and to inspect the eyes for drainage or edema.

The fiberoptic blanket (e.g., BiliBlanket) is also available to treat hyperbilirubinemia. This device is a bank of phototherapy lights that is flexible and is wrapped around the newborn, much like a blanket. Although not as effective as special blue lights, fiberoptic lights in the form of a blanket, in addition to bank lights, is a useful adjunct therapy when bilirubin levels are dangerously high.

When a fiberoptic blanket is used, place it below the armpits, wrapped around the torso, and secured in place so that the light cannot reach the infant's eyes. A major advantage of the fiberoptic blanket is that it permits greater opportunity for family–infant bonding. The family can pick up, hold, and feed their infant while phototherapy is in progress (Fig. 14-14). Also, the fiberoptic blanket allows greater environmental stimulation because the infant is not restricted to a specific phototherapy light location and does not need to wear eye shields.

To improve efficiency of the treatment, expose as much of the skin as possible to the light. The newborn is usually diapered to contain urine and stool. This diapering also serves to protect the reproductive organs because the side effects of phototherapy on these organs are unknown.

Monitor the newborn's temperature closely by obtaining axillary temperature measurements; hyperthermia is not uncommon. Hypothermia may also be a problem if the room has drafts, which can lead to convective heat loss.

Metabolic rate and insensible water loss may increase during phototherapy. Metabolic rate changes may be caused by hyperthermia, which is a common problem for newborns, because phototherapy lights (except for the fiberoptic lights and LEDs) emit heat. Newborns require increased calories to balance this metabolic rate and to assist with eliminating bilirubin through the intestinal tract. Reduce insensible water loss by keeping the skin temperature constant and avoiding heat. Monitor for dehydration.

Frequent feedings are also essential to prevent dehydration. Dehydration is common in newborns who have poorly established feeding patterns and lethargy.

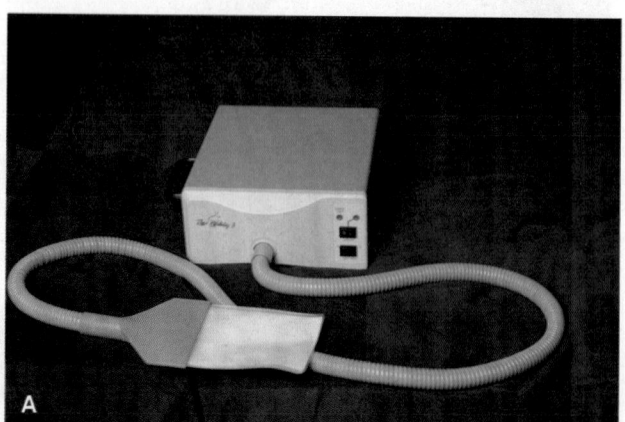 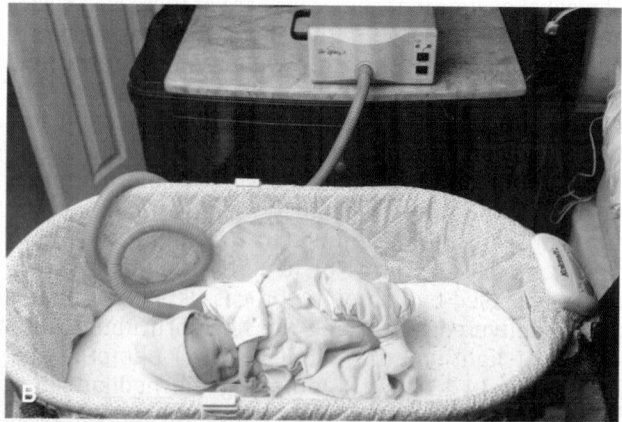

Figure 14-14 (A) Fiberoptic blanket equipment. (B) The fiberoptic blanket is wrapped around the infant to direct radiating light to the skin.

High bilirubin levels tend to make the newborn listless and lethargic, leading to poor feeding. Also, water-loss stools, commonly referred to as *bili stools*, may occur as a result of photodegradation of bilirubin. Increase breastfeeding or bottlefeeding during treatment to offset both calorie loss and dehydration.

Skin care is essential for the newborn undergoing phototherapy because the frequent water-loss stools in combination with dry skin can lead to skin breakdown. Frequent diaper changes and position changes may prevent breakdown of the skin. Lotions are generally not applied to the skin of newborns who are receiving phototherapy because of the risk of skin burns. However, avoiding lotions has not been extensively researched, and this practice may vary at institutions. It is also common for the newborn receiving phototherapy to develop a rash similar to a heat rash. This rash requires no treatment and often resolves when phototherapy treatment is discontinued.

Newborns with a high direct bilirubin level (>2.0 mg/dL) should not receive phototherapy. A high direct hyperbilirubinemia level is associated with liver disease, such as neonatal hepatitis or congenital obstructive jaundice. Although conjugated bilirubin is generally not toxic to the newborn's CNS, it must be evaluated carefully. When used in these cases, phototherapy causes "bronze baby" syndrome, producing a gray–brown discoloration of the skin and darkening of both serum and urine. These effects are benign and lessen after the phototherapy lights are removed, but they may take months to fully resolve.

Exchange Transfusion

If phototherapy is ineffective in resolving the hyperbilirubinemia, and the bilirubin level continues to increase—approaching levels at which kernicterus may occur—more drastic interventions may be required. Exchange transfusion, which involves removing the newborn's blood and replacing it with new blood, is described in more detail later in the section on "Hemolytic Disease of the Newborn" (HDN). This procedure is rarely done for newborns with physiologic jaundice and is most commonly used for severe hemolytic processes involving intractable anemia, as occurs in HDN.

Community Care

It is imperative that the family knows how to assess jaundice. Nurses are the primary educators of families with newborns and are in a pivotal role to provide vital information related to general neonatal care. Discharge teaching related to jaundice includes explaining

- What causes jaundice and its common signs and symptoms
- How to evaluate feeding and output quantities
- How to monitor for changes in activity level and skin color
- When to call the physician

Teach the family how to assess the jaundice in their newborn's skin by focusing on the progression of jaundice, which begins in the face and moves to the abdomen and lower extremities. Teach them to monitor the number of wet diapers per day to help evaluate adequate intake. Also, stress the importance of noting the newborn's activity because increasing jaundice leads to lethargy and poor feeding. Finally, encourage them to use indirect sunlight through a window to help decrease jaundice because sunlight photodegrades bilirubin from the skin, much like phototherapy.

Phototherapy can be used in the home setting with select newborns and their families. Before initiating home phototherapy, whether with the fiberoptic blanket or the traditional bank of lights, assess the newborn and the family to determine the appropriateness of home treatment. The ideal candidate is a healthy, full-term newborn with no other underlying disease or problems who has a well-established feeding pattern. The family must be willing and able to provide the phototherapy treatment and carefully monitor the newborn's skin color, feeding vigor, and activity. Detailed family training and education is a must for home phototherapy to be successful (Community Care 14-1).

ANSWER: Here is an example of an explanation you could give to Abby, a parent of a premature infant with hyperbilirubinemia: "All babies, when they are inside their mothers, have a lot of red blood cells. Because their lungs are not working, they are getting all of their oxygen from their mother, and they need more red blood cells to have enough oxygen. When they are born and the lungs begin to function, they do not need so many red blood cells, so the red blood cells start breaking down. The liver is in charge of breaking down the red blood cells, but premature babies have very immature livers. Gabriella's liver is having a hard time keeping up with the amount of red blood cells that need to be processed. When a red blood cell breaks down, bilirubin is released. The liver breaks down the bilirubin and it is excreted in stool. When the liver can't keep up, like Gabriella's right now, there is extra bilirubin circulating around that gets deposited in the skin. A little bilirubin in the skin is not harmful, but if we let the amount of circulating bilirubin get really high, it can deposit in the brain, and *that* is harmful. Fortunately, certain wavelengths of light can help break down the bilirubin and make it water soluble and easier to excrete. Gabriella is under these phototherapy lights to help her break down bilirubin. We make sure her eyes are protected from the lights and she has enough fluids—first, to make sure she does not get dehydrated and, second, to help her excrete the extra bilirubin. We make sure she is comfortable and we turn her regularly so that all of her skin is exposed to the light—just like getting an even tan."

HEMOLYTIC DISEASE OF THE NEWBORN

HDN causes destruction of erythrocytes (red blood cells) in the neonate whose blood is not compatible with the mother's blood. Because erythroblasts (immature circulating erythrocytes) appear in great numbers in the fetal blood as the body attempts to increase production of red blood cells in response to the anemia

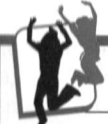

The Newborn Receiving Fiberoptic Phototherapy at Home

Home phototherapy for neonatal jaundice is a safe, cost-effective alternative to extended hospitalization when the newborn meets certain criteria. These criteria include

- No health problems other than neonatal hyperbilirubinemia
- Gestational age of more than 37 weeks
- Birth weight greater than 2,500 g
- Apgar score at 5 minutes of 7 or higher
- Age between 2 and 7 days at start of home phototherapy
- Safe home environment with grounded electric outlet
- Infant's caregiver willing and able to follow instructions for using the home phototherapy system
- Infant's caregiver willing and able to monitor key indicators of the newborn's physical state
- Infant's caregiver agreeable to allowing daily nursing assessment and drawing of necessary blood specimens

The fiberoptic system is a common means of home phototherapy and, generally, the nurse is responsible for teaching the infant's caregivers about its use. In addition, the nurse provides instruction on care of the newborn who is receiving phototherapy at home. Outcome objectives for the infant's caregivers include the following:

- Identify components of the fiberoptic system.
  - For blanket: illuminator box, cable connector, and fiberoptic blanket with disposable cover
  - For lights: light bank
- Set up fiberoptic system and be sure it is working.
  - For blanket: Wrap the newborn in the fiberoptic blanket, placing it below the armpits and securing it around the torso so that light cannot

reach the neonate's eyes and to reduce exposure of reproductive organs.
  - For lights: Apply eye shield correctly. Identify complications of eye shield applied too tightly or loosely.
- Diaper newborn to reduce exposure of reproductive organs to light.
- Monitor the newborn's body temperature.
- Monitor the newborn's output.
  - Frequency and description of voidings
  - Frequency and description of bowel movements
- Monitor newborn for signs of dehydration.
  - Decreased urine output
  - Decreased body weight
  - Decreased skin turgor
  - Dry mucous membranes
  - Sunken eyeballs
  - Sunken fontanels
  - Irritability
  - Lethargy
- Provide newborn with frequent feedings to help prevent dehydration and enhance the effectiveness of phototherapy.
- Interact with infant while phototherapy is in progress. When using the blanket, the caregiver can hold the infant. When using the light bank, turn off the lights during feedings, remove the eye shield, and hold the infant. Replace the shields and reposition the infant before reinitiating phototherapy.
- Discuss the importance of ongoing blood tests and nursing assessments for the newborn receiving phototherapy at home.
- Provide the caregiver with a telephone number to call for concerns about the newborn or the fiberoptic system during home phototherapy.

---

that occurs when erythrocytes are destroyed, HDN is also known as *erythroblastosis fetalis*.

The incidence of HDN has decreased remarkably since the 1960s, when Rh immunoprophylaxis (RhoGAM) became available. Rh immunoprophylaxis provides a means of preventing the generation of Rh isoantibodies in the mother who is Rh negative and whose baby is Rh positive.

In HDN, maternal antibodies destroy fetal erythrocytes. HDN can result from any one of a number of incompatibilities among erythrocyte antigens, the most common of which are related to the Rh factor and to the ABO blood groups. Erythrocyte antigen incompatibilities may cause the generation of maternal isoantibodies

that can subsequently enter the fetal circulation and destroy fetal erythrocytes. However, even when the blood of the newborn and that of the mother are incompatible, HDN does not necessarily occur because some mothers at risk do not actually develop and transfer isoantibodies to the neonate.

When the Rh factor is involved, the neonate's erythrocytes are Rh positive and the mother's erythrocytes are Rh negative. When the ABO blood groups are involved, the neonate's erythrocytes are positive for the A or B antigens (or both) and the mother's erythrocytes are usually negative for both of these antigens. HDN is rare when the mother possesses the A antigen and the newborn possesses the B antigen or vice versa.

Blood group incompatibility is more common than Rh factor incompatibility, but Rh factor incompatibility is more likely to result in major physical alterations for the neonate.

CROSS-CULTURAL CARE

The potential for HDN varies among racial and ethnic populations according to the extent to which the different red blood cell antigens are present or absent. For example, the possibility of HDN secondary to Rh factor incompatibility is greater among whites than among other groups because approximately 15% of the white population is Rh negative. About 5% of the black population is Rh negative; thus, this group has less potential for Rh factor incompatibility. Among Chinese, Japanese, and Native Americans, Rh factor incompatibility is unusual because Rh-negative individuals are rare in these populations.

Pathophysiology

Because HDN stemming from Rh factor incompatibility generally is more serious than that resulting from ABO incompatibility, Rh factor incompatibility is the primary focus of this discussion. Although a number of antigens are present in the Rh system, the common terms *Rh positive* and *Rh negative* refer to the D antigen. Rh-positive erythrocytes have the D antigen, whereas Rh-negative erythrocytes do not have the D antigen.

HDN develops during pregnancy when maternal anti-D antibodies cross the placenta into the fetal circulation and coat Rh-positive fetal erythrocytes. This event targets fetal erythrocytes for destruction, primarily by the reticuloendothelial cells of the spleen.

Maternal anti-D antibodies are produced after the mother is exposed to fetal Rh-positive blood. Most often, such exposure occurs through transplacental hemorrhage during pregnancy or through bleeding at the time of childbirth. Maternal anti-D antibodies remain with the mother and tend to have a greater effect on subsequent pregnancies in which the fetus is Rh positive.

In ABO incompatibility, anti-A and anti-B antibodies occur naturally in people who lack the A or B antigens. These antibodies are formed when the immune system is stimulated by the A and B matter found in food and bacteria.

The primary pathophysiologic alterations associated with HDN are anemia and hyperbilirubinemia. Anemia is a concern both before and after the birth of the affected child. It occurs when red blood cell production cannot keep pace with red blood cell destruction. Initially, the body responds by increasing red blood cell production in the bone marrow, as demonstrated by an increased reticulocyte count. Also, extramedullary sites of erythropoiesis develop in the liver and spleen. As anemia progresses, the fetus will become tachycardic as a compensatory mechanism to improve oxygen delivery to body tissues. When prolonged, this tachycardia leads to congestive heart failure and *hydrops fetalis*, a condition characterized by massive edema. Ultimately, death may occur.

Before birth, hyperbilirubinemia usually does not occur because bilirubin is removed from the fetus by the placenta. After birth, however, hyperbilirubinemia secondary to hemolysis presents as a major concern.

The prognosis for HDN has improved with the use of advanced diagnostic and therapeutic measures. In particular, intrauterine diagnosis and treatment have contributed substantially to decreasing the morbidity and mortality associated with severe HDN. The most noteworthy advance with regard to HDN has been the development of Rh immunoprophylaxis to prevent the formation of maternal anti-D antibodies, thereby preventing HDN.

Assessment

The hallmark of HDN is jaundice secondary to hyperbilirubinemia. Unlike physiologic jaundice of the neonate, jaundice associated with HDN usually appears within 24 hours of birth. In severe cases, the newborn may be jaundiced at delivery.

Manifestations of anemia may be present, depending on the neonate's ability to produce the number of red blood cells needed to compensate for the increased rate of erythrocyte destruction. Efforts to maintain a balance between production and destruction of red blood cells usually lead to some degree of hepatosplenomegaly. When balance is not achieved, the neonate becomes anemic, pale, and lethargic. These newborns are often severely ill, with congestive heart failure and severe generalized edema (hydrops fetalis), including pleural effusions and ascites.

ALERT *Severe anemia in HDN may have a delayed onset. Continue to be alert for signs of anemia in the neonate with HDN, even when such signs are not initially present.*

Laboratory manifestations of HDN during the prenatal period generally show an increasing concentration of bilirubin in the amniotic fluid and decreasing numbers of erythrocytes in the fetal blood. When the maternal pregnancy history and the maternal anti-D titer indicate that the fetus is at risk for HDN, amniocentesis and fetal blood sampling procedures may be used as early as the 18th week of gestation to identify the presence and severity of HDN.

Amniocentesis is performed to obtain a sample of amniotic fluid. The concentration of bilirubin in the fluid is measured with a spectrophotometer. The amniotic fluid's optical density at a wavelength of 450 nm is determined, and the fluid may then be classified by Liley zone (Chart 14-7). Depending on the initial optical density, amniocentesis is repeated every 1 to 4 weeks to determine whether the optical density is increasing. Severe HDN is associated with increasing optical density.

> **CHART 14-7 Liley Zone Classification of Amniotic Fluid Bilirubin Levels**
>
> Zone I: Absent or mild HDN
> Zone II: Mild to moderate HDN
> Zone III: Severe HDN

Fetal blood sampling by percutaneous umbilical sampling under ultrasound guidance provides a more accurate means of assessing HDN during the prenatal period. However, it involves considerable risk for fetal–maternal hemorrhage. Thus, it is usually reserved for the fetus whose amniotic fluid bilirubin concentration indicates severe HDN. Also, it is used when amniocentesis is contraindicated.

After birth, the primary laboratory manifestation of HDN is an elevated level of indirect (unconjugated) bilirubin. This laboratory value may be somewhat elevated during the first week of life as a result of physiologic jaundice. However, in HDN, the bilirubin level is pathologic and may increase quickly. Also, HDN is associated with a positive direct antiglobulin (direct Coombs) test, which indicates attachment of the maternal anti-D antibody to the neonate's red blood cells.

Perinatal and postnatal blood counts with HDN usually show an increase in reticulocytes and nucleated red blood cells, which are signs of increased erythrocyte production. Hemoglobin levels are decreased when anemia is present.

Nursing Diagnoses and Outcomes

Nursing diagnoses and outcomes generally applicable for newborns with a health challenge are listed in Nursing Plan of Care 14-1. Those applicable to a newborn with jaundice or hyperbilirubinemia were presented earlier. Refer to Nursing Plan of Care 23-1 for those for a child with anemia. The following nursing diagnosis and outcomes also apply to a newborn with HDN:

Nursing Diagnosis: Fear that neonate will incur chronic impairment or die as a result of HDN
Outcomes:
- Family verbalizes fears concerning potential for chronic impairment, stillbirth, or death of neonate with severe HDN.
- Family receives informational and emotional support.

Interdisciplinary Interventions

Management of the neonate with HDN requires close monitoring of the red blood cell profile and bilirubin levels. These laboratory values provide evidence of worsening anemia and hyperbilirubinemia or of improvement in response to therapeutic interventions.

Two primary interventions are associated with the management of HDN: phototherapy and exchange transfusion. Phototherapy is discussed in detail earlier in the section on "Neonatal Hyperbilirubinemia."

Exchange Transfusion

Exchange transfusion (removal of blood and replacement with new blood) is indicated for neonates with moderate to severe HDN and for those with rapidly increasing bilirubin levels. LBW and high-risk infants receive their first exchange transfusion sooner than other neonates with HDN. Exchange transfusion helps to correct both anemia and hyperbilirubinemia.

Exchange transfusion for Rh incompatibility uses donor blood that is Rh negative. With ABO incompatibility, the donor blood is group O. Using this blood type prevents infusion of red blood cells with the antigen that would attract the respective maternal antibody and be prematurely destroyed.

During exchange transfusion for HDN, 5 to 20 mL of the neonate's blood is alternately removed and replaced with donor blood. The total volume of exchange is usually twice the neonate's blood volume (about 170 mL/kg body weight). Caution is exercised to avoid fluid overload, and aseptic technique is maintained throughout exchange transfusions. Generally, exchange transfusion is done through arterial and venous umbilical catheters. Neonates at risk for HDN have moist dressings applied to the umbilical cord shortly after birth to prevent it from drying and to keep the umbilical vessels suitable for access should an exchange transfusion become necessary.

During and after an exchange transfusion, observe the neonate closely to identify and respond quickly to complications that may occur. Infants who require exchange transfusion for hemolytic disease are at increased risk of sepsis, leukocytopenia, thrombocytopenia, hypocalcemia, and hypernatremia (Smits-Wintjens et al., 2013).

- Note vital signs frequently, monitoring for arrhythmic, hypotensive, respiratory, and body temperature alterations.
- Obtain blood samples, particularly checking for hypoglycemia, electrolyte alterations, and acid–base imbalance.
- Note seizure activity that may occur secondary to hypocalcemia.
- Measure intake and output accurately, noting imbalance between these measurements.
- Note adverse reactions to blood transfused to the neonate.
- Inspect umbilical cord site, monitoring for hemorrhage.

Despite an effective exchange transfusion, "rebound" hyperbilirubinemia may occur as the concentration of tissue bilirubin equilibrates with that of serum bilirubin. Additional exchange transfusions may be required if hyperbilirubinemia continues or increases.

Recombinant erythropoietin (rEPO) has been helpful in treating infants with severe HDN-associated anemia (Manoura et al., 2007).

Treating HDN in the Unborn Child

When amniocentesis or fetal blood sampling results indicate severe HDN in the unborn child, intervention is necessary to prevent stillbirth. Induction of premature birth is likely when fetal development reaches the point at which survival outside the uterine environment can be expected, usually at a gestational age of 32 weeks or more.

When it is too early to induce premature birth, severe HDN is managed by intrauterine blood transfusion under the guidance of ultrasonography. The preferred method is by intravascular transfusion through the umbilical vein.

Rh Immunoprophylaxis

Despite the increased ability to diagnose, monitor, and treat HDN, substantial interdisciplinary interventions are directed toward preventing this disorder. Prevention by immunoprophylaxis is possible in cases of Rh factor incompatibility. Generally, Rh immunoprophylaxis is provided by giving anti-D gamma globulin within 72 hours of childbirth to mothers who are Rh negative and whose babies are Rh positive. Rh immunoprophylaxis is recommended after spontaneous and induced abortions and may be given to women who experience vaginal bleeding during the first trimester of pregnancy. Rh immunoprophylaxis may also be administered to women during pregnancy, usually during the 28th week of gestation.

Rh immunoprophylaxis is effective in most women who receive it, and, as a result, the incidence of HDN has decreased remarkably. It is important that women at risk for anti-D antibody formation be identified so that Rh immunoprophylaxis can be given in a timely manner.

Community Care

HDN is likely to provoke stress for parents and other family members. Particularly with severe HDN, there may be fear that the baby will die or live with chronic impairment. Be sensitive to the family's stress. Educate them about HDN, relay ongoing information about the baby's physical state, and provide emotional support.

The nurse and other members of the interdisciplinary health care team have a major role in the prevention and early treatment of HDN. In addition to patient care and family education, provide community education that underscores the importance of early prenatal care. Prenatal care identifies women at risk for giving birth to children with HDN and leads to monitoring of their unborn children for evidence of the disease.

Discharge planning may include instruction in and provision of care for hyperbilirubinemia and plans to monitor hemoglobin levels for anemia for 8 to 12 weeks. Folic acid and, in some cases, B_{12} supplementation may be given. Home phototherapy using the phototherapy light or, more commonly, the fiberoptic blanket is an option for newborns with HDN. Generally, this therapy continues until the serum bilirubin level decreases to less than 10 mg/dL.

NEONATAL HYPOGLYCEMIA

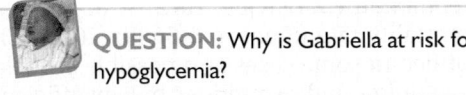

QUESTION: Why is Gabriella at risk for hypoglycemia?

The brain is glucose dependent; it must have a continual supply of glucose to function properly. The fetus receives a continuous supply of glucose from the placenta. During the third trimester, the fetus begins to store energy in preparation for delivery and the first few hours after birth. At delivery, the maternal supply of glucose ceases and the newborn initiates glycolysis, glycogenolysis, and gluconeogenesis. These processes mobilize liver glycogen to maintain normal serum glucose levels. Glucose values decrease rapidly after birth and stabilize by 3 to 4 hours of life. At this time, enteral feedings (breastfeeding or formula) are initiated to maintain normal glucose values.

The definition of hypoglycemia is controversial, and opinions vary regarding an exact safe level of glucose. A pragmatic approach has been adopted until further research evidence can better define the level of hypoglycemia that could potentially result in brain injury (Adamkin, 2011). Transient blood glucose concentration as low as 30 mg/dL is common in healthy neonates by 1 to 2 hours after birth; severe and sustained hypoglycemia in the healthy term newborn is unusual. Most healthy term newborns have the ability to withstand the stress of labor, the subsequent loss of a glucose source (with the cutting of the umbilical cord), and the brief period in which glucose supplies are limited (because of limited breast milk supply from the mother). Healthy term newborns are well-equipped with alternative fuel sources, such as fatty acids, that assist to protect the brain.

Certain newborns are at risk for hypoglycemia, however, and nurses must be vigilant in identifying these newborns and providing prompt treatment. These newborns include preterm and late preterm infants, who may be cared for in the newborn nursery; infants of diabetic mothers; infants who are LGA, SGA, or have experienced IUGR; and any newborn presenting with clinical illness (hypothermia, respiratory distress, jaundice during the first 24 hours of life, abnormal body movements).

ALERT *Serious consequences of hypoglycemia include brain damage, resulting in developmental delay and learning disabilities. Prompt assessment of newborns with risk factors can prevent such complications.*

The prognosis for infants with hypoglycemia is related to the duration and severity of the hypoglycemia as well as the underlying cause. Newborns with symptomatic and recurrent hypoglycemia are more likely to have long-term sequelae than newborns who are asymptomatic. Transient hypoglycemia is the most common type during the neonatal period; it is of short duration and rarely recurs. Major long-term sequelae of severe, prolonged hypoglycemia are neurologic, including cognitive challenge and cerebral atrophy.

Assessment

Most normal nurseries and NICUs have specific protocols for screening high-risk newborns for hypoglycemia. SGA and LGA newborns and those of diabetic mothers should

CHART 14-8 | Signs and Symptoms of Hypoglycemia in the Newborn

High-pitched cry

Apnea

Cyanosis

Irritability

Lethargy

Respiratory distress

Hypotonia

Pallor

Seizures

Tremulousness

all receive a screening glucose evaluation by capillary blood glucose methods at the bedside shortly after birth and then at regular intervals. Signs and symptoms of hypoglycemia are nonspecific and variable (Chart 14-8) and mimic many other diseases, such as sepsis. Because of the lack of obvious symptoms in some infants, maintain a high index of suspicion of hypoglycemia based on history or presence of subtle signs.

Interdisciplinary Interventions

Nursing interventions include preventing hypoglycemia and promptly identifying newborns at risk. Newborns at risk may be fed early, either at the breast or with formula. Any symptomatic newborn with blood glucose less than 40 mg/dL is treated promptly with IV glucose (Adamkin, 2011). If the newborn is unable to feed well or is in respiratory distress, IV therapy to administer glucose is initiated to maintain normal glucose levels. In severe cases of refractory hypoglycemia, corticosteroids may be administered either intravenously or intramuscularly. Corticosteroids such as hydrocortisone are used to decrease peripheral glucose use and increase gluconeogenesis.

Obtain bedside glucose measurements every 30 minutes in newborns treated for hypoglycemia until stable values are achieved, and then every hour for 3 hours to ensure stability. Assess for the presence of signs and symptoms of hypoglycemia, as mentioned earlier.

> **ANSWER:** Gabriella is at risk for hypoglycemia because of her immaturity and her lack of fat stores. Because of her prematurity, she will not immediately establish a feeding schedule as a full-term infant would. Therefore, initially, her glucose level will be tied to her IV fluids and the patency of that line.

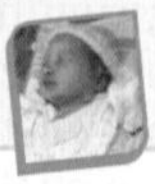

MECONIUM ASPIRATION

Meconium aspiration is a condition in which the newborn, either before or during the birth process, passes his or her first meconium stool and breathes the material into the respiratory tract with some of his or her first breaths. Meconium is a very viscous, sticky, forest-green liquid that consists of gastrointestinal secretions, bile acids, salts, mucus, pancreatic juice, cellular debris, amniotic fluid, swallowed vernix caseosa, lanugo, and blood. The substance can be found in the fetal gastrointestinal tract as early as the 16th week of gestation.

Meconium staining of the amniotic fluid (indicating that the substance was passed before birth) is seen in about 4% of deliveries prior to 37 weeks' gestation, 10% to 20% of term deliveries, and 30% to 40% of postterm deliveries (Stenson & Smith, 2012). Meconium aspiration syndrome (MAS) will develop in about 5% of these infants (Stenson & Smith, 2012). The clinical picture includes respiratory distress and radiographic findings of aspiration ("fluffy" appearance on radiograph) in an infant whose symptoms cannot otherwise be explained. The most widely accepted theory regarding the reason for the passage of meconium into the amniotic fluid suggests that it occurs with relaxation of the anal sphincter during an episode of fetal hypoxia. During intrauterine asphyxia, insufficient oxygen is transported to the fetal intestine, which relaxes anal sphincter tone and evacuates the meconium. Passage of meconium may, however, also represent a maturational event: it is rare before 37 weeks' gestation but is increasingly common in pregnancies lasting longer than 40 weeks.

Pathophysiology

Regardless of the cause, when meconium is passed into the amniotic fluid, it can be aspirated into the lungs, creating many mechanical and physiologic changes. The degree of severity of the condition is related to the viscosity of the meconium, which is usually described as thick, moderate, or thin. A large amount of thick meconium could rapidly cause complete obstruction of the upper airways, with associated hypoxia, hypercapnia, and acidosis. More commonly, diffuse particles of meconium migrate to smaller peripheral airways, causing obstruction, air trapping, and surfactant inactivation. Partial or complete mechanical obstruction results in air trapping, atelectasis, overdistended or hyperexpanded regions, and possible pneumothoraces. Obstruction is caused by a ball-and-valve effect in which air is allowed into the lung but is obstructed from exiting.

Chemical inflammation, infection, or both in the lower airways is also seen in this syndrome. Ventilation–perfusion mismatches ensue, creating hypoxia and acidosis. These factors produce pulmonary vasoconstriction and may result in persistent pulmonary hypertension of the newborn.

Historically, the diagnosis of meconium aspiration held connotations of high morbidity and mortality, especially related to poor neurologic outcomes. Today, most infants with meconium-stained amniotic fluid suffer little or no pulmonary sequelae. Of the infants who develop MAS, approximately one third require mechanical ventilation (Dargaville, 2012) with about a 2.5% to 5% mortality rate (Stenson & Smith, 2012). CP has been identified in some cases as a possible sequela of meconium staining and aspiration, but insufficient data exist to prove or refute this contention. Anoxic encephalopathy is an uncommon but tragic outcome in some instances of meconium aspiration. Several reports have documented abnormal long-term pulmonary function among children who had MAS as newborns. The most common abnormalities noted were spontaneous wheezing and exercise-induced bronchospasm, suggesting small airway injury and disease. CLD may occur when a prolonged period of mechanical ventilation is required. When severe MAS is accompanied by persistent pulmonary hypertension of the newborn, it is often fatal.

Assessment

Newborns with MAS are often term, postterm, or SGA. Symptoms range from mild respiratory distress to severe hypoxemia and respiratory failure. Infants with minimal meconium aspiration characteristically present with tachypnea and mild cyanosis. Those with more severe MAS have marked respiratory distress with cyanosis, irregular or gasping respirations, grunting, and intercostal and substernal retractions. The chest is typically hyperinflated, and the anteroposterior diameter of the thoracic cage is increased. Arterial blood gas values show evidence of severe hypoxemia, hypercapnia, and combined respiratory and metabolic acidosis. Lung sounds may be diminished.

Nursing Diagnoses and Outcomes

In addition to those discussed in Nursing Plan of Care 14-1, the following nursing diagnoses and outcomes apply to the newborn with MAS:

Nursing Diagnosis: Ineffective airway clearance related to effects of meconium in lungs
Outcome: Newborn will maintain patent airway.
Nursing Diagnosis: Impaired gas exchange related to effects of altered ventilation and perfusion of lungs
Outcome: Newborn will maintain oxygen saturation of at least 92%.

Interdisciplinary Interventions

Infants delivered through meconium-stained amniotic fluid require expert care at delivery. To prevent MAS, newborns delivered through meconium-stained amniotic fluid may receive intrapartum and nasopharyngeal suctioning to clear the airway of meconium prior to delivery of the shoulders. Routine intrapartum suctioning is no longer recommended based on current research (Perlman et al., 2010).

Newborns who are delivered through thick, particulate meconium and are not vigorous at birth are intubated, suctioned, ventilated with a resuscitation bag and 100% oxygen, and admitted immediately to the NICU, where they may be placed on mechanically assisted ventilation. Additional measures may include surfactant therapy and use of a high-frequency oscillatory ventilator. Surfactant therapy may be effective in MAS patients because the presence of meconium in the lungs produces inflammation and may deactivate the surfactant that the newborn is producing. The high-frequency oscillatory ventilator is useful in treating severe MAS. (A full discussion regarding mechanical ventilation support for MAS is beyond the scope of this chapter.)

Monitor for development of pneumothorax. Signs and symptoms of pneumothorax include bradycardia, hypotension, carbon dioxide retention, and hypoxemia. The treatment for pneumothorax includes a thoracocentesis to immediately remove the air source.

If there is no or poor medical response to the high-frequency oscillatory ventilator, surfactant therapy, or other treatments, and the newborn has signs of persistent pulmonary hypertension, inhaled nitric oxide (iNO) may be used. iNO selectively dilates the pulmonary bed, thereby increasing pulmonary blood flow. Use of iNO has substantially reduced the need for extracorporeal membrane oxygenation (ECMO) therapy. However, some infants do not respond to iNO, and ECMO support is considered.

ECMO is a highly invasive therapy involving temporary cardiopulmonary bypass (Fig. 14-15). Because of this procedure's invasiveness, ECMO candidates must meet specific criteria for treatment, including reversible disease, severe hypoxemia, persistent air leak (pneumothorax), and mortality rates greater than 80% with current therapies. The goal of ECMO therapy is to allow the lung disease to improve over a period of days by giving the lungs a "rest." ECMO therapy carries many potential complications, such as alterations in cerebral blood flow. The survival rate of newborns receiving ECMO therapy is variable and depends on the facility at which it is performed. In general, infants requiring ECMO for MAS have a 95% survival rate (Dargaville, 2012). ECMO therapy for MAS is very expensive, both financially and emotionally. Intensive nursing care (sometimes with a 2:1 or greater ratio of specialized pump technicians and nursing staff to one infant) is needed as well as specific technologic requirements. Care of the infant on ECMO therapy is similar to care of the infant undergoing cardiopulmonary bypass surgery for congenital heart defects. It is beyond the scope of this chapter to discuss such care in depth; refer to texts concerning pediatric critical care for further information.

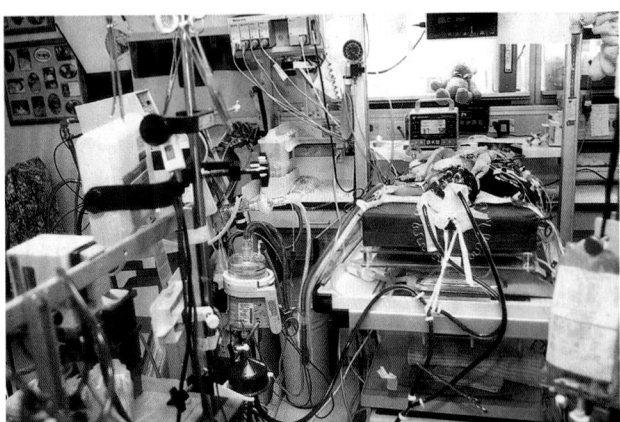

Figure 14-15 ECMO is a highly invasive therapy involving temporary cardiopulmonary bypass. Support the family in seeing the baby beneath the lines.

As in other diagnoses involving illness in the newborn, the psychosocial and emotional manifestations in parents and family members include shock, fear, anxiety, and grief over the loss of the expected perfect or "normal" infant. Mothers especially require sensitivity and honest, supportive communication regarding the infant's prognosis because they are undergoing fatigue, pain, and hormonal fluctuations immediately after childbirth.

Social service and other counseling interventions are imperative for family support. Because tertiary centers are often located many miles away from home and the usual support systems, assistance with securing food, transportation, lodging, and resources for sibling care is required.

See thePoint for a summary of Key Concepts.

REFERENCES

Adamkin, D. H. (2011). Clinical report-postnatal glucose homeostasis in the later preterm and term infants. *Pediatrics, 127*(3), 575–570.

Adams-Chapman, I. (2012). Long-term impact of infection on the preterm neonate. *Seminars in Perinatology, 36*(6), 462–470.

Als, H., Butler, S., Kosta, S. et al. (2005). The assessment of preterm infants' behavior (APIB): Furthering the understanding and measurement of neurodevelopmental competence in preterm and full-term infants. *Mental Retardation and Developmental Disabilities Research Reviews, 11*(1), 94–102.

American Academy of Pediatrics. (2004). Management of hyperbilirubinemia in the newborn infant 35 or more weeks of gestation. *Pediatrics, 114,* 297–316.

Bahadue, F. L., & Soll, R. (2012). Early versus delayed selective surfactant treatment for neonatal respiratory distress syndrome. *Cochrane Database of Systematic Reviews,* (11), CD001456.

Ballabh, P. (2009). Intraventricular hemorrhage in premature infants: Mechanism of disease. *Pediatric Research, 67*(1), 1–8.

Ballard, J. L., Khoury, J. C., Wedig, K. et al. (1991). New Ballard Score, expanded to include extremely premature infants. *The Journal of Pediatrics, 119,* 417–423.

Battaglia, F. C., & Lubchenco, L. O. (1967). A practical classification of newborn infants by weight and gestational age. *The Journal of Pediatrics, 71,* 159–163.

Becher, J., Stenson, B. J., & Lyon, A. J. (2007). Is intrapartum asphyxia preventable? *BJOG: An International Journal of Obstetrics and Gynaecology, 114,* 1442–1444.

Bhutani, V., Stark, A., Lazzeroni, L. et al. (2013). Predischarge screening for severe neonatal hyperbilirubinemia identifies infants who need phototherapy. *The Journal of Pediatrics, 162*(3), 477–482.

Blencowe, H., Cousens, S., Oestergaard, M. et al. (2012). National, regional, and worldwide estimates of preterm birth rates in the year 2010 with time trends since 1990 for selected countries: A systematic analysis and implications. *Lancet, 379*(9832), 2162–2172.

Brauer, C. A., & Waters, P. M. (2007). An economic analysis of the timing of microsurgical reconstruction in brachial plexus birth palsy. *Journal of Bone and Joint Surgery. American Volume, 89,* 970–978.

Brazelton, T. (1984). *Neonatal behavioral assessment scale* (2nd ed.). Philadelphia, PA: J. B. Lippincott.

Burns, L., Mattick, R. P., Lim, K. et al. (2007). Methadone in pregnancy: Treatment retention and neonatal outcomes. *Addiction, 102*(2), 264–270.

Carmona, R. H. (2005). *Surgeon General's advisory on alcohol use in pregnancy.* Retrieved from http://www.surgeongeneral.gov/press releases/sg02222005.html

Cho, K., Frijters, J. C., Zhang, H. et al. (2013). Prenatal exposure to nicotine and impaired reading performance. *The Journal of Pediatrics, 162*(4), 713–718.

Cong, X., Cusson, R., Walsh, S. et al. (2012). Effects of skin-to-skin contact on autonomic pain responses in preterm infants. *The Journal of Pain, 13*(7), 636–645.

Conde-Agudelo, A., Belizan, J. M., & Diaz-Rossello, J. L. (2011). Kangaroo mother care to reduce morbidity and mortality in low birthweight infants. *Cochrane Database of Systematic Reviews,* (3), CD002771.

Cronk, C., Crocker, A. C., Pueschel, S. M. et al. (1988). Growth charts for children with Down syndrome: 1 Month to 18 years of age. *Pediatrics, 81,* 102–110.

Dargaville, P. A. (2012). Respiratory support in meconium aspiration syndrome: A practical guide. *International Journal of Pediatrics, 2012,* 965159.

Dietz, P., England, L., Shapiro-Mendoza, S. et al. (2010). Infant morbidity and mortality attributable to prenatal smoking in the US. *American Journal of Preventive Medicine, 39*(1), 45–52.

Ethen, M. K, Ramadhani, T. A., Scheuerle, A. E. et al. (2009). Alcohol consumption by women before and during pregnancy. *Maternal and Child Health Journal, 13*(2), 274–285.

Ferber, S. G., & Makhoul, I. R. (2008). Neurobehavioural assessment of skin-to-skin effects on reaction to pain in preterm infants: A randomized, controlled within subject trial. *Acta Paediatrica, 97*(2), 171–176.

Finer, N. N., Higgins, R., Kattwinkel, J. et al. (2006). Summary proceedings from the Apnea-of-Prematurity Group. *Pediatrics, 117,* S47–S51.

Finnegan, L. (1985). Neonatal abstinence. *Current Therapy in Neonatal-Perinatal Medicine, 21,* 236–240.

Flacking, R., Ewald, U., & Wallin, L. (2011). Positive effect of kangaroo mother care on long-term breastfeeding in very preterm infants. *Journal of Obstetric, Gynecologic, and Neonatal Nursing, 40*(2), 190–197.

Fox, T. P., & Godavitarne, C. (2012). What really causes necrotizing enterocolitis? *ISRN Gastroenterology, 2012,* 628317.

Frías, J. L., & Davenport, M. L. (2003). Health supervision for children with Turner syndrome. *Pediatrics, 111,* 692–702.

Giniger, R. P., Buffat, C., Millet, V. et al. (2007). Renal effects of ibuprofen for the treatment of patent ductus arteriosus in premature infants. *Journal of Maternal–Fetal & Neonatal Medicine, 20,* 275–283.

Griffin, T. (2006). Family-centered care in the NICU. *Journal of Perinatal & Neonatal Nursing, 20,* 98–102.

Hamilton, D., Martin, J., & Ventura, S. (2012). Births: Preliminary data for 2011. *National Vital Statistics Reports, 61*(5), 1–18.

Heron, M. (2011). Deaths: Leading causes for 2007. *National Vital Statistics Reports, 59*(8), 1–95. Retrieved from http://www.cdc.gov /nchs/data/nvsr/nvsr59/nvsr59_08.pdf

Horbar, J. D., Carpenter, J. H., Badger, G. J. et al. (2012). Mortality and neonatal morbidity among infants 501-1500 grams from 2000–2009. *Pediatrics, 129*(6), 1019–1026.

Horton, W. A., Rotter, J. I., Rimoin, D. L. et al. (1978). Standard growth curves for achondroplasia. *The Journal of Pediatrics, 93,* 435–438.

Hoyert, D., & Xu, J. (2012). Deaths: Preliminary data for 2011. *National Vital Statistics Reports, 61*(6), 1–52.

Hunt, R. W., Tzioumi, D., Collins, E. et al. (2008). Adverse neurodevelopmental outcome of infants exposed to opiate in-utero. *Early Human Development, 84,* 29–35.

Ip, S., Chung, M., Kulig, J. et al. (2004). An evidence-based review of important issues concerning neonatal hyperbilirubinemia. *Pediatrics, 114,* e130–e153.

Jacobs, S., Hunt, R., & Tarnow-Mordi, W. (2013). Cooling for newborns with hypoxic ischaemic encephalopathy. *Cochrane Database of Systematic Reviews,* (4), CD003311.

Johansson, A., Ludvigsson, J., & Hermansson, G. (2008). Adverse health effects related to tobacco smoke exposure in a cohort of three-year olds. *Acta Paediatrica, 97*, 354–357.

Joubert, B. R., Håberg, S. E., Nilsen, R. M. et al. (2012). 450K epigenome-wide scan identifies differential DNA methylation in newborns related to maternal smoking during pregnancy. *Environmental Health Perspectives, 120*(10), 1425–1431.

Kattwinkel, J., Perlman, J. M., Aziz, K. et al. (2010). Neonatal resuscitation: 2010 American Heart Association guidelines for cardiopulmonary resuscitation and emergency cardiovascular care. *Pediatrics, 126*(5), e1400–e1413.

Kelleher, J., Mallick, H., Soltau, T. D. et al. (2013). Mortality and intestinal failure in surgical necrotizing enterocolitis. *Journal of Pediatric Surgery, 48*(3), 568–572.

Keren, R., Luan, X., Friedman, S. et al. (2008). A comparison of alternative risk-assessment strategies for predicting significant neonatal hyperbilirubinemia in term and near-term infants. *Pediatrics, 121*, e170–e179.

Kraft, W., & van den Anker, J. (2012). Pharmacologic management of the opioid neonatal abstinence syndrome. *Pediatric Clinics of North America, 59*(5), 1147–1165.

Kuczkowski, K. (2007). The effects of drug abuse on pregnancy. *Current Opinion in Obstetrics and Gynecology, 19*, 578–585.

Kung, H., Hoyert, D., Xu, J. et al. (2008). Deaths: Final data for 2005. *National Vital Statistics Reports, 56*(10), 1–120.

Lie, K., Groholt, E., & Eskild, A. (2010). Association of cerebral palsy with Apgar score in low and normal birthweight infants: Population based cohort study. *British Medical Journal, 341*, c4990.

Linder, N., Haskin, O., Levit, O. et al. (2003). Risk factors for intraventricular hemorrhage in very low birth weight premature infants: A retrospective case-control study. *Pediatrics, 111*(5), e590–e595.

Manktelow, B., Seaton, S., Field, D. et al. (2013). Population-based estimates of in-unit survival for very preterm infants. *Pediatrics, 131*(2), e425–e432.

Manoura, A., Korakaki, E., Hatzidaki, E. et al. (2007). Use of recombinant erythropoietin for the management of severe hemolytic disease of the newborn of a K0 phenotype mother. *Pediatric Hematology and Oncology, 24*, 69–73.

March of Dimes Foundation. (2012). *Premature birth report card.* Retrieved from http://www.marchofdimes.com/mission/prematurity-reportcard.aspx

Martin, J., Hamilton, B., Ventura, S. et al. (2012). Births: Final data for 2010. *National Vital Statistics Reports, 61*(1), 1–71.

Mattson, S. N., Crocker, N., & Nguyen, T. T. (2011). Fetal alcohol spectrum disorders: Neuropsychological and behavioral features. *Neuropsychology Review, 21*(2), 81–101.

Mattson, S., Roesch, S., Glass, L. et al. (2013). Further development of a neurobehavioral profile of fetal alcohol spectrum disorders. *Alcoholism, Clinical and Experimental Research, 37*(3), 517–528.

May, P., Gossage, J., Kalber, W. et al. (2009). Prevalence and epidemiologic characteristics of FASD from various research methods with an emphasis on recent in-school studies. *Developmental Disabilities Research Review, 15*(3), 176–192.

McCall, E. M., Alderdice, F. A., Halliday, H. L. et al. (2010). Interventions to prevent hypothermia at birth in preterm and/or low birthweight infants. *Cochrane Database of Systematic Reviews,* (3), CD004210.

McDonald, S. W., Benzies, K. M., Gallant, J. E. et al. (2012). A comparison between late preterm and term infants on breastfeeding and maternal mental health. *Maternal and Child Health Journal.* Advance online publication.

McLendon, D., Check, J., Carteaux, P. et al. (2003). Implementation of potentially better practices for the prevention of brain hemorrhage and ischemic brain injury in very low birth weight infants. *Pediatrics, 111*(4), 543–550.

Medoff Cooper, B., Holditch-Davis, D., Verklan, M. et al. (2012). Newborn clinical outcomes of the AWHONN late preterm infant research-based practice project. *Journal of Obstetric, Gynecologic, and Neonatal Nursing, 41*(6), 774–785.

Moczygemba, C. K., Paramsothy, P., Meikle, S. et al. (2010). Route of delivery and neonatal birth trauma. *American Journal of Obstetrics and Gynecology, 202*(4), 361e1–361e6.

Montirosso, R., Del Prete, A., Bellu, R. et al. (2012). Level of NICU quality of developmental care and neurobehavioral performance in very preterm infants. *Pediatrics, 129*, e1129.

Negrato, C. A., Mattar, R., & Gomes, M. B. (2012). Adverse pregnancy outcomes in women with diabetes. *Diabetology & Metabolic Syndrome, 4*, 41.

Obeidat, H., Bond, E., & Callister L. (2009). The parental experience of having an infant in the newborn intensive care unit. *Journal of Perinatal Education, 19*(3), 23–29.

Oh, S. S., Tcheurekdjian, H., Roth, L. A. et al. (2012). Effect of secondhand smoke on asthma control among black and Latino children. *Journal of Allergy and Clinical Immunology, 129*(6), 1478–1483.

Ornoy, A., & Ergaz, Z. (2010). Alcohol abuse in pregnant women: Effects on the fetus and newborn, mode of action and maternal treatment. *Environmental Research and Public Health, 7*(2), 364–379.

Perlman, J., Wyllie, J., Kattwinkel, J. et al. (2010). Part 11: Neonatal resuscitation: 2010 international consensus on cardiopulmonary resuscitation and emergency cardiovascular care science with treatment recommendations. *Circulation, 122*(Suppl. 16), S516–S538.

Peters, K., Rosychuk, R., Henderson, L. et al. (2009). Improvement of short- and long-term outcomes for very low birth weight infants: Edmonton NIDCAP Trial. *Pediatrics, 124*(4), 1009–1020.

Reece, E., Leguizamon, G., & Wiznitzer, A. (2010). Gestational diabetes: The need for common ground. *Obstetric Anesthesia Digest, 30*(2), 84–85.

Sasidharan, K., Dutta, S., & Narang, A. (2009). Validity of New Ballard Score until 7th day of postnatal life in moderately preterm neonates. *Archives of Disease in Childhood. Fetal and Neonatal Edition, 94*, F39–F44.

Schierholz, E., & Walker, S. R. (2010). Responding to traumatic birth subgaleal hemorrhage, assessment, and management during transport. *Advances in Neonatal Care, 10*(6), 311–315.

Smith, G., Gutovish, J., Smyser, C. et al. (2011). Neonatal intensive care unit stress is associated with brain development in preterm infants. *Annals of Neurology, 70*(4), 541–549.

Smits-Wintjens, V., Rath, M., van Zwet, E. et al. (2013). Neonatal morbidity after exchange transfusion for red cell alloimmune hemolytic disease. *Neonatology, 103*(2), 141–147.

Sowell, E. R., Mattson, S. N., Kan, E. et al. (2008). Abnormal cortical thickness and brain–behavior correlation patterns in individuals with heavy prenatal alcohol exposure. *Cerebral Cortex, 18*, 136–144.

Stenson, B. J., & Smith, C. L. (2012). Management of meconium aspiration syndrome. *Paediatrics and Child Health, 22*(12), 532–535.

Styles, M. E., Cole, T. J., Dennis, J. et al. (2002). New cross sectional stature, weight, and head circumference references for Down's syndrome in the UK and Republic of Ireland. *Archives of Disease in Childhood, 87*, 104–108.

Substance Abuse and Mental Health Services Administration. (2010). *Results from the 2009 National Survey on Drug Use and Health: Volume I. Summary of national findings* (Office of Applied Studies, NSDUH Series H-38A, HHS Publication No. SMA 10-4856Findings). Rockville, MD: Author.

Substance Abuse and Mental Health Services Administration. (2011). *Results from the 2011 National Survey on Drug Use and Health: Summary of national findings.* Rockville, MD: Author.

Swanson, A., Veldman, A., Wallace, E. et al. (2012). Subgaleal hemorrhage: Risk factors and outcomes. *Acta Obstetricia et Gynecologica Scandinavica, 91*(2), 260–263.

Tomashek, K. M., Shapiro-Mendoza, C. K., Davidoff, M. J. et al. (2007). Differences in mortality between late-preterm and term singleton infants in the United States, 1995–2002. *The Journal of Pediatrics, 151*(5), 450–456.

Trotter, T. L., & Hall, J. G. (2005). Health supervision for children with achondroplasia. *Pediatrics, 116,* 771–783.

Van Cleve, S. N., & Cohen, W. I. (2006). Part I: Clinical practice guidelines for children with Down syndrome from birth to 12 years. *Journal of Pediatric Health Care, 20,* 47–54.

Wachman, E. M., & Lahav, A. (2011). The effects of noise on preterm infants in the NICU. *Archives of Disease in Childhood. Fetal and Neonatal Edition, 96*(4), F305–F309.

Wender-Ozegowska, E., Wróblewska, K., Zawiejska, A. et al. (2005). Threshold values of maternal blood glucose in early diabetic pregnancy: Prediction of fetal malformations. *Acta Obstetricia et Gynecologica Scandinavica, 84,* 17–25.

See thePoint for additional resources.

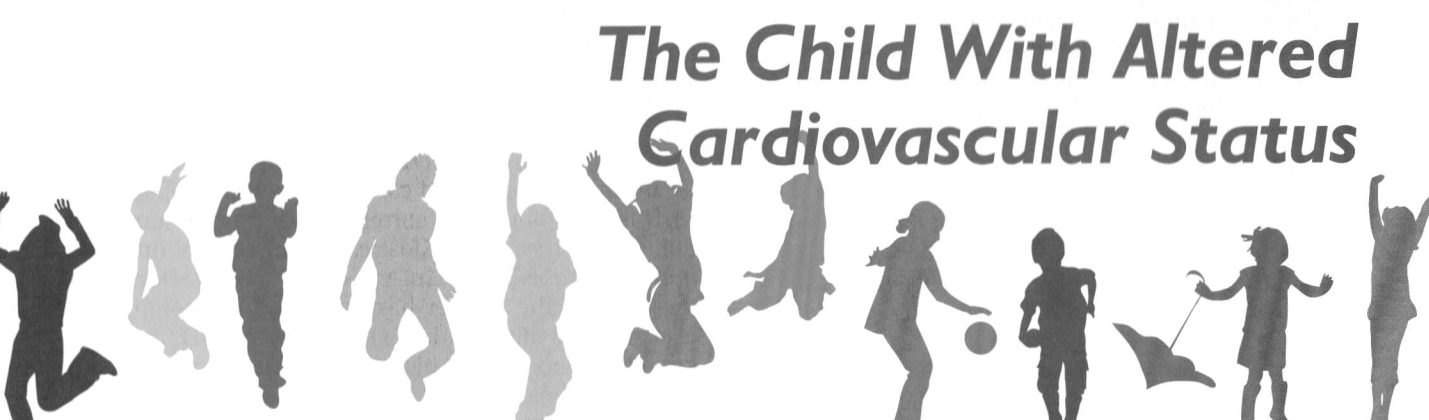

CHAPTER 15

The Child With Altered Cardiovascular Status

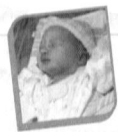

CASE HISTORY

Recall Gabriella Goldman from Chapter 14? Born prematurely, she is now 6 days old (or 29 weeks gestational age). The staff has attempted to wean Gabriella from the ventilator and supplemental oxygen with little success. She has just started receiving gavage feedings of her mother's breast milk. So far, she is tolerating her feedings. She continues to have a peripheral intravenous (IV) access for fluids and medication administration.

Late on the night shift, Gabriella's respiratory rate increases and her oxygen saturation decreases. The nurse caring for Gabriella follows the ordered parameters and increases her inspired oxygen percentage. Gabriella vomits during two of her gavage feedings; her oxygen saturation and her heart rate decrease during the most recent feeding. The morning nurse

begins a thorough assessment and notes Gabriella's breathing is moderately labored at a respiratory rate of 56 breaths/min. Her breath sounds are coarse, but she is moving air well. The nurse notices a continuous heart murmur that definitely was not there the day before. Gabriella is also receiving 5% more oxygen than she was the day before.

Gabriella's nurse notifies the nurse practitioner and anticipates a chest radiograph and echocardiogram to confirm the clinical suspicion of a patent ductus arteriosus (PDA). Gabriella's health care team discusses the merits of different treatments: fluid restriction alone, indomethacin or ibuprofen and fluid restriction, or surgery. (You may wish to read ahead to "Defects With Increased Pulmonary Blood Flow" section for a discussion of a PDA.)

CHAPTER OBJECTIVES

1 Identify genetic, environmental, maternal, and multifactorial influences on congenital heart disease.

2 Describe specific assessment skills that assist in the identification and care of the child with altered cardiovascular status.

3 Identify invasive and noninvasive diagnostic tools that help in evaluating children with suspected heart disease.

4 Describe information to include in the teaching plan when preparing a pediatric cardiac patient for a procedure.

5 List nursing interventions and potential complications during the acute and convalescent phases of postoperative care for the cardiac patient.

6 Explain the pathophysiology associated with, presentation of, and interdisciplinary interventions for the child with heart failure, cyanosis, and acquired heart disease.

7 Describe the anatomic variations associated with the more common congenital defects, and explain the hemodynamic consequences of these defects.

8 Discuss the various medical and surgical treatments of congenital heart defects, and differentiate between curative and palliative procedures.

See thePoint for a list of Key Terms.

Altered cardiovascular status in children typically occurs as one of two primary types of heart disease: congenital and acquired. Congenital heart disease (CHD) is a functional or structural disease of the heart that is present at birth, even though the illness may not manifest itself clinically until later in life. Mortality from CHD is declining in the United States, although CHD remains a major cause of death in infancy and childhood. Worldwide, CHD occurs in 9 of every 1,000 live births (van der Linde et al., 2011). It is thought that the occurrence of CHD is underestimated, as efforts to record all true cases of CHD are limited. Researchers may also have difficulty ascertaining statistics on children with CHD in rural areas, in areas with a high population of indigent families, and in underdeveloped nations. Another reason for faulty statistics may be the failure to record children with mild versions of a defect, such as mild pulmonary stenosis or mild coarctation of the aorta (COA).

Historically, many children with congenital heart defects did not survive to adulthood. Many now survive, and the number of adults with severe CHD now exceeds the number of children with CHD (Marelli et al., 2010).

caREminder

In 25% of infants with CHD, the diagnosis is not made until after discharge from the newborn nursery (Brown et al., 2006); 6 weeks is the median age at diagnosis (Mahle et al., 2009). Do not assume that the presence of a cardiac condition would already have been ruled out in the older child who presents with questionable symptoms.

The incidence of CHD is more than twice as high in preterm infants as it is in term infants (Tanner, 2005). Infants born with prenatally diagnosed CHD are more likely to have a lower birth weight and gestational age than those who are diagnosed after birth. Advances in fetal echocardiography have improved early detection of CHD and decreased neonatal morbidities associated with complex CHD, such as hypoplastic left heart syndrome (HLHS) (Levey et al., 2010). Various factors related to the incidence of CHD include genetic, environmental, maternal, and multifactorial influences. Parents of a child with CHD may express concerns that the condition will recur if they have a family history of CHD or if one of their children is affected with a congenital heart defect. Either case suggests a *genetic* influence. The likelihood that CHD will recur in a family depends on specific lesions, chromosomal issues, gender, race, and environmental factors. CHD risk to subsequent siblings of a child with CHD is approximately 2%. The risk that parents with CHD will pass on heart abnormalities to their own children is also 2%. Children who are born as part of a multiple birth have a 7.9% risk of CHD (Øyen et al., 2009). *Environmental* or teratogenic insults, such as the ingestion of drugs (recreational or

prescribed) or alcohol during pregnancy, can increase the risk of heart defects in the fetus. Toxic exposure of the mother to some drugs such as lithium carbonate, especially early during the pregnancy, is known to be associated with heart disease in the child. Aspirin products have long been implicated as teratogens in CHD, but evidence does not support this conclusion (van Gelder, 2011). *Maternal* conditions such as diabetes or lupus have caused cardiac problems in offspring. CHD is also thought to correlate with in vitro fertilization (IVF) procedures. Most cases of CHD fall into the *multifactorial* category (or caused by many factors). In these cases, the mother has no known environmental exposures or illnesses known to lead to CHD, and the family has no known history of CHD. When discussing the reasons for heart disease with family members, explain that any deaths of elderly family members from atherosclerotic heart disease are different from childhood heart disease.

Syndromes that affect other body systems can be associated with congenital heart defects. For example, Down syndrome, trisomies 13 and 18, heterotaxy syndrome (malposition of internal organs in conjunction with asplenia or polysplenia and complex CHD), and 22q11 deletion syndromes are all associated with congenital heart defects. Approximately 5% to 8% of children with CHD also have a chromosomal defect (Arabi et al., 2007).

Cardiac conditions that develop after birth are known as *acquired heart disease*. Heart disease in children occurs in all cultures and in all ethnic populations.

DEVELOPMENTAL AND BIOLOGIC VARIANCES

 QUESTION: What is the direction of blood flow through the ductus arteriosus in fetal circulation?

Developmental and biologic variances occur throughout development and can be divided into those that occur during embryologic development, those that manifest as a result of cardiovascular changes at birth, and those that occur during childhood development.

FETAL STRUCTURES AND CIRCULATION

The heart starts to form early during the first 3 weeks of embryologic development, with fetal cardiac circulation essentially developed before the eighth week. During this vulnerable stage of fetal development, congenital heart lesions can occur. The heart in the fetus begins as a simple tube that, over a short time, is transformed into a functional, complex organ. One end of the primitive linear tube eventually gives rise to the arterial system, and the opposite end becomes the venous system. As the tube widens, it folds and bulges, evolving into four separate chambers. By the end of the third week of gestation, the heart is beating; by the fourth week, the atrium and the ventricles are visible heart structures (see Chapter 3).

In fetal circulation, blood flows from the placenta through the umbilical vein, through the liver, the ductus venosus, and then into the inferior vena cava (Fig. 15-1). At the vena cava, fetal blood from the liver mixes with blood from the lower portion of the body and then drains into the right atrium. Blood from the upper portion of the body—the head, the arms, and the brain—returns to the right atrium through the superior vena cava. After blood enters the right atrium, a division occurs wherein some blood bypasses the lungs through the foramen ovale into the left side of the heart, passing through to the left atrium, the left ventricle, and then out the aorta. The rest of the blood travels through the right atrium into the right ventricle and out the pulmonary artery. A portion of this blood travels through the

lungs; the rest crosses the ductus arteriosus and flows into the descending aorta.

Fetal blood flow through the heart has more than one potential pathway. The vascular resistance in the placental, pulmonary, and systemic circulation is a major factor influencing distribution. The lowest vascular resistance is found in the placenta. In the fetus, pulmonary vascular resistance (PVR) is very high, whereas systemic vascular resistance (SVR) is lower. The fetus has a naturally hypoxic environment that acts as a vasoconstrictor on the pulmonary vascular bed, keeping resistance high. SVR is low because of the relatively large volume of flow through the placenta. These factors, combined with the areas of shunting, lead to a small volume of fetal blood circulating through the lungs.

The right ventricle in the fetus is the dominant ventricle, pumping slightly more than half of the combined

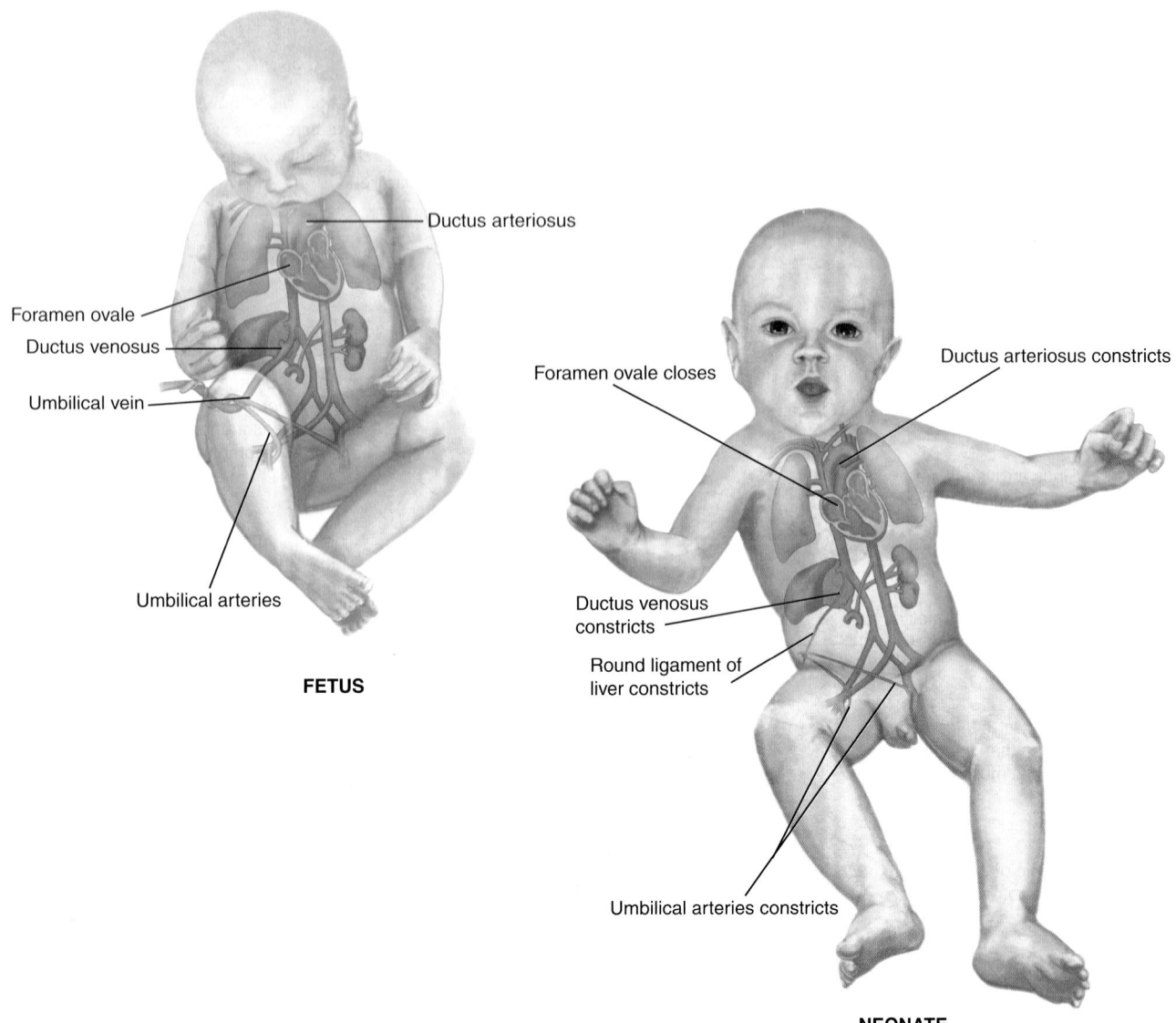

FETUS

NEONATE

Figure 15-1 Fetal circulation and changes at birth.

ventricular output. Pressures in both ventricles are equal, unlike in the adult where normal right ventricular pressure is much lower. In the adult, cardiac output is influenced by stroke volume and heart rate. In the fetus, cardiac output largely depends on heart rate because the fetus is unable to substantially increase stroke volume. A decrease in heart rate can cause a precipitous and life-threatening decrease in fetal cardiac output.

BIRTH-RELATED CHANGES

At birth, the organ responsible for oxygenation changes from the placenta to the lungs. The unique fetal circulatory structures—the placenta, the foramen ovale, and the ductus arteriosus—undergo abrupt changes at birth (see Fig. 15-1). In the fetus, the fluid-filled, not fully expanded lungs have a high PVR, making the pressure on the right side of the heart high and limiting blood flow to the lungs. At birth, alveolar oxygen tension increases, and a large volume of circulating blood shifts from placental flow to the pulmonary arteries. Together, these conditions cause vasodilation in the pulmonary vascular bed, thereby creating a lower PVR and lower right-sided heart pressure. This change in blood flow causes left atrial pressure to increase, forcing the flaplike foramen ovale to close, thereby creating higher pressures on the left side of the heart. Elevated arterial oxygenation and other factors cause shunting across the ductus arteriosus to cease. Constriction of the ductus arteriosus is generally achieved within the first few days of life. With closure of the ductus arteriosus and the foramen ovale, the two levels of circulatory shunting in the heart cease. When these anatomic shunts are no longer present, the transition to extrauterine circulation is complete.

At birth, the ventricular walls are of equal thickness. Eventually, the muscle of the left ventricle wall becomes thicker from the work of pumping blood to the systemic circulation. This developmental process explains why neonatal systemic blood pressure is low during the early days after birth—the ventricular strengthening and pressure changes are still occurring.

PEDIATRIC VARIATIONS

The structures and functioning of the cardiac system in infants and children differ from those in adults (Fig. 15-2). These normal biologic and developmental variations require a modified approach to cardiac assessment. Cardiac assessment variations are related to the natural progression of growth and development in children.

> **ANSWER:** In fetal circulation, blood flows from the right to the left through the ductus arteriosus as one of two shunts that facilitates the circulatory detour of the pulmonary vasculature.

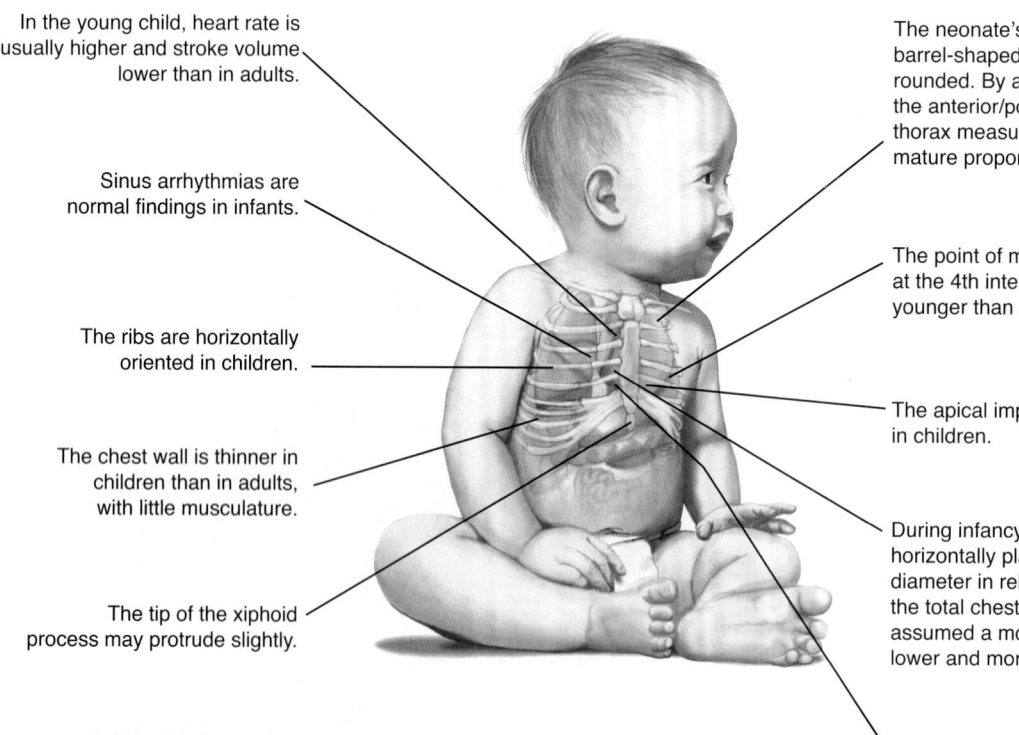

In the young child, heart rate is usually higher and stroke volume lower than in adults.

Sinus arrhythmias are normal findings in infants.

The ribs are horizontally oriented in children.

The chest wall is thinner in children than in adults, with little musculature.

The tip of the xiphoid process may protrude slightly.

The neonate's thorax is barrel-shaped; the infant's, rounded. By age 6 years, the anterior/posterior to transverse thorax measurement ratio assumes mature proportions.

The point of maximum impulse is located at the 4th intercostal space in the child younger than 4 years old.

The apical impulse may be visible in children.

During infancy the heart is more horizontally placed and has a large diameter in relation to diameter of the total chest. By age 7, the heart has assumed a more adult position that is lower and more oblique.

The neonate is unable to increase stroke volume to increase cardiac output; therefore, an increase in the neonate's cardiac output depends on heart rate.

Figure 15-2 Developmental and biologic variances in the cardiovascular system.

ASSESSMENT

Assessment for alterations in cardiovascular status includes a focused health history and focused physical assessment. The findings obtained are then supplemented with various diagnostic criteria for evaluating cardiovascular disorders.

FOCUSED HEALTH HISTORY

QUESTION: Which of the items identified in Focused Health History 15-1 apply to Gabriella?

A comprehensive pediatric evaluation must include a recording of the child's current history or chief complaint, the maternal and fetal history, the postnatal history, and the family history (Focused Health History 15-1).

For the current history, obtain information about the reason that the child and family are seeking an evaluation. For example, for a history of chest pain, note whether the pain is related to activity, the duration of the chest pain, whether the pain occurs while taking a breath, and whether the child has episodes of syncope or palpitation. For complaints of tachycardia or palpitations, note whether these episodes coincide with the ingestion of cold medications or antiasthmatic drugs. For infants, ask about feeding because some patterns of feeding behavior may indicate cardiovascular problems. Determine whether the child has attained age-appropriate developmental milestones.

Ask about the pregnancy history, including any potential maternal/fetal teratogenic event that may have influenced cardiac development. A severe infection such as measles or influenza, especially when accompanied by high temperatures during the first trimester, has the potential to alter fetal cardiac development. Note whether the mother used medications before realizing that she was pregnant. For example, teratogens associated with CHD include phenytoin, valproic acid, lithium, retinoic acid, and thalidomide.

caREminder

Phrase questions carefully during the interview to avoid inflicting feelings of guilt on the mother for actions or behaviors during her pregnancy that may have affected the child. Be aware and considerate of cultural beliefs and practices during the interview.

The fetal environment of a mother with a chronic illness such as diabetes or lupus can also cause negative outcomes on fetal development. Document any history of drug or alcohol use and the severity of abuse, if any (see Chapter 3). Evaluate the mother's nutritional status as well. This information is limited by what the mother can, or is willing to, reveal.

A family history relevant to cardiac problems and to other medical events also needs to be completed.

Family histories are sometimes obtuse or vague. A typical vague historical account from a worried parent might be, "My mother said she had a baby who died and it was blue," or "My husband says his mother lost a child as an infant but she won't talk about it." When parents start exploring their past and talking to relatives, a more complete family history may evolve. In some cases, genetic counseling may be warranted. Current family lifestyle (diet, exercise, tobacco use) should also be explored.

ANSWER: Under Current history, Gabriella is recently experiencing vomiting; under Past medical history, Gabriella has a history of premature birth.

FOCUSED PHYSICAL ASSESSMENT

QUESTION: You are the nurse on the morning shift assessing Gabriella. Organize the information gathered from your review of the case study as it relates to inspection, palpation, and auscultation. Identify what additional areas you wish to assess. What information helps to differentiate if her problems are cardiovascular, respiratory, or gastrointestinal?

Physical assessment of the cardiovascular system uses the techniques of inspection, palpation, and auscultation (Focused Physical Assessment 15-1). Assess for **cyanosis** (bluish or purplish discoloration of the skin, mucous membranes, or both). The ability to visibly assess for cyanosis depends on the degree of desaturation and the natural skin hue of the individual. The more oxygen unbound to hemoglobin there is circulating in the body, the more likely the child will appear cyanotic. Cyanosis is more easily seen in lighter skinned individuals and in natural light. In children with darker skin, cyanosis appears dark purplish black—an aubergine or eggplant color. When assessing a child with dark skin, inspect the nail beds, mucous membranes, palms of the hands, and soles of the feet. In newborns who normally have acrocyanosis (peripheral cyanosis), determining whether a child actually has clinically significant cyanosis is more difficult. Collect other data, such as whether poor feeding and tachypnea are present, to gain a more complete clinical picture of the child. Perform cardiac inspection, which can reveal information about the child's cardiac status, without waking a sleeping child or disturbing an awake child. For example, observe movement of the shirt or child's clothing to evaluate respirations and chest movement. Look for any evidence of accessory muscle use. If possible, observe the infant during feeding, noting any tiring such as with sweating or skin color changes.

Palpate the chest for the apical impulse (AI), heaves, and thrills. The AI normally is noted as a gentle, nonsustained tap. In children younger than 4 years of age, the AI is normally at the fourth intercostal space (ICS), just left

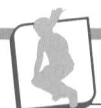

FOCUSED HEALTH HISTORY 15-1

The Child With Altered Cardiovascular Status

Current history	Chest pain: frequency, duration, relation to activity, sporadic, short lasting or persistent, with or without exertion, with or without dizziness, syncope, or palpitation Heart palpitations, tachycardia, tachypnea, dyspnea, syncope, or parents' feeling that the baby's heart races Frequent vomiting Cyanosis: worse with feeding, defecation, or activity Puffy eyelids, scrotal or lower extremity edema Irritability, weak cry, difficult to console Limited activity level, trouble keeping up with siblings Use of certain positions to ease breathing (e.g., calmer with head of bed elevated, squatting during play) Recent febrile illness, especially pharyngitis Arthralgia Use of any medications (cold medication, antiasthmatic drugs)
Past medical history	**Prenatal/Neonatal History** Maternal exposure to infections, prescription and over-the-counter medications; illicit drug or alcohol use during pregnancy; mother's history of chronic illness; history of premature birth **Previous Health Challenges** Syndrome or genetic disease that is associated with heart disease (e.g., trisomies 21, 13, 18; Turner syndrome; Marfan syndrome; fetal alcohol syndrome) Other condition that increases risk of acquired heart disease (e.g., diabetes); previous illness; history of heart palpitations, tachycardia, or syncope; or baby's heart races History of common communicable infections, particularly frequent respiratory illnesses, and ability to recover
Nutritional assessment	Intake, type, amount, and time it takes to feed Difficulty breast-feeding; if bottle-fed, duration longer than 20–30 minutes for a feeding or consuming less than 3 oz per feeding; tiring while feeding; vigorous sucking, then fatigue; need for frequent rest periods; tachypnea or diaphoresis during feedings Inadequate weight gain but normal height for age; inadequate gains in weight and linear growth Risk factors associated with acquired heart disease (e.g., high intake of saturated fats)
Family medical history	Any family history of childhood cardiac diagnosis, miscarriages, stillbirths for mother or on either grandparent's side Family history of cardiac disease occurring before age 55 years, any early (<40 years old) deaths related to cardiac disease, familial hypercholesterolemia; other siblings with similar cardiac diagnosis
Social and environmental history	Activities and amount of physical activity, sedentary lifestyle Personal use of or presence of tobacco smoke in the child's environment Drug or alcohol use
Growth and development	Delayed acquisition of developmental milestones

Note: See Chapter 8 for a comprehensive health history.

FOCUSED PHYSICAL ASSESSMENT 15-1

Cardiovascular System

Assessment Parameter	Alterations/Clinical Significance
General appearance	Fretfulness, lethargy, agitation, distress, and weakness are common with hypoxia, heart disease, and heart failure.
	Underweight and linear growth below average are common with growth retardation caused by cardiac conditions.
	Dysmorphic features associated with chromosomal aberrations are associated with heart disease (e.g., trisomies 13, 18, 21; Turner syndrome).
	Unusual positioning: Position of comfort with head elevated may indicate heart failure.
	Squatting may be a sign of hypoxia; squatting reverses a right-to-left shunt, thus getting more blood to the lungs; children with tetralogy of Fallot may squat instinctively to improve oxygenation.
	Fever may indicate bacterial illness.
Integumentary system	Observe color at rest:
	• Pallor or mottling of skin is seen in severe anemia, heart failure, and cardiogenic shock.
	• Cyanosis in mucous membranes indicates central cyanosis—seen with hypoxia and CHD.
	• Cyanosis or mottling of nail beds, palms, and soles of feet may be the result of cold or inadequate perfusion.
	• Jaundice in infants is seen with severe heart failure.
	Diaphoresis, especially with activity or feeding, may occur in children with left-to-right shunts.
	Clubbed digits (widened terminal phalanges) are a sign of chronic hypoxia.
	Dependent edema may indicate heart failure.
	Capillary refill longer than 3 seconds may indicate cardiovascular compromise or, in a cold child, vasoconstriction.
	Rash may be seen with streptococcal and Kawasaki disease.
	Scars from previous heart surgeries.
Face, nose, and oral cavity	Periorbital edema is seen in heart failure.
	Unusual facial characteristics (coarse features, widely spaced eyes, oblique palpebral fissure, low-set or malformed ears) or congenital anomalies (microcephaly, cleft lip or palate) may indicate syndromes or genetic conditions associated with heart disease.
	Nasal flaring is a sign of respiratory distress and can be secondary to heart disease.
Thorax and lungs	Observe for pulsation in chest or hyperactive precordium (apparent in normal children with thin chest walls and those with severe cardiac pathology).
	Bulging or prominence on the chest wall, especially on the left side where the apex of the heart is most commonly situated, may indicate cardiomegaly.
	Asymmetric movement of chest suggests possible paralysis of the diaphragm (can result from injury to the phrenic nerve during cardiac surgery).
	Tachypnea, even with rest, and chest retractions indicate respiratory distress, possibly resulting from heart failure.
	AI palpation, downward or lateral displacement occurs with cardiomegaly; abnormal placement also occurs in dextrocardia, pneumothorax, diaphragmatic hernia, and pectus excavatum.
	Presence of heaves or lifts indicates sustained forceful thrusting of the ventricles during systole—seen with aortic stenosis, left ventricular overload, and hypertension.
	Thrills are the result of turbulent blood flow and indicate pathology.
	Rales, rhonchi, and wheezing are seen in heart failure.

(Continued)

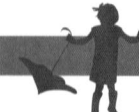

Cardiovascular System (Continued)

Assessment Parameter	Alterations/Clinical Significance
Cardiovascular system	Tachycardia in the absence of fever, crying, or stress may indicate cardiac pathology.
	Normally, no difference between femoral and brachial pulses or, in infants, between blood pressure in arms and legs; differentiation in blood pressure and pulses can be an indicator of COA.
	Weak pulses in left arm suggests obstructive lesions or heart failure.
	Bounding pulses may indicate volume overload, aortic runoff lesion, and aortic insufficiency.
	Changes in rhythm associated with respirations is a normal variant in children (sinus arrhythmia); rhythm change not associated with respirations, or irregular rhythm, may indicate pathology.
	Normally, heart sounds are louder than in adults because chest wall is thinner.
	Fixed splitting of S_2 is seen with atrial septal defect (ASD).
	Murmur (turbulence of blood flow): may or may not be present with a heart lesion, and murmurs vary with lesion; may be present with anemia; innocent murmurs common in school aged children and not associated with pathology.
	Gallops or rubs are associated with pathology.
	If murmur is present, note intensity, location, quality, and timing and whether systolic or diastolic.
Abdomen	Hepatomegaly is seen in heart failure (normally, in infants, the liver should not be palpable more than 3 cm below the right costal margin; in older children, the liver should not be palpable below the costal margin).
Neurologic system	Neurodevelopmental delays more common in children with CHD, possibly resulting from genetic syndromes, microcephaly, decreased cerebral perfusion, use of cardiopulmonary bypass, intraoperative hypothermic circulatory arrest

of the midclavicular line (MCL). In children between the ages of 4 and 7 years, the AI is at the MCL. For children older than 7 years of age, the AI is at the fifth ICS to the right of the MCL. Note any displacement of the impulse.

Also palpate the peripheral pulses for quality and equality, noting any irregularities in rate and volume between the right and left arms and legs. Assess the child's blood pressure. When taking blood pressure, the child must be in a relaxed state. If the child is stressed or fidgety, the risk of artificially high or low pressure is increased.

ALERT   *Indications of COA are weaker pulses or lower blood pressure in the lower extremities than in the upper extremities. Bounding pulses can indicate a PDA or aortic insufficiency.*

Palpate the liver borders to document evidence of hepatomegaly (enlarged liver) from right-sided heart failure. In smaller, thinner children, the liver is more easily palpable. When assessing a child, palpate the borders of the liver. If the liver is distended, chart how many centimeters below the rib cage its borders are palpable.

Cardiac auscultation is another aspect of the physical examination. Auscultation of heart sounds requires more skill than other portions of the child's physical assessment. Do not expect to hear a murmur from all children with known cardiac lesions because some malformations seldom produce abnormal heart sounds. Listen carefully and describe exactly what you hear (see Chapter 8 for more information regarding physical assessment of the cardiovascular system).

Auscultate the anterior chest as well as the lateral and posterior chest area. Note the rate and regularity of the heartbeat and the intensity and quality of the heart sound. Document any abnormality of the first and second heart sounds, such as a split heart sound, or any extra heart sounds such as murmurs, gallops, or rubs. Identify the location on the thorax where the extra heart sound is heard most distinctly. This information aids in identifying the anatomic origin of a murmur. A murmur is also graded according to its intensity (loudness), which can help identify the severity of the murmur (see Table 8-7). Further evaluation may be required to distinguish an innocent or asymptomatic murmur from one that indicates the presence of a pathologic condition. The term *innocent* indicates that the murmur represents a normal finding, with no implication that a pathologic condition or process is present. Innocent murmurs can be exacerbated by factors such as fever, anemia, anxiety, and exercise, which can accentuate an innocent murmur that normally would not be audible.

> **ANSWER:** So far, inspection reveals moderately labored breathing with a respiratory rate of 56 breaths/min. Auscultation identifies coarse breath sounds and a continuous murmur. Palpation, which has yet to be completed, would include palpation of peripheral pulses, comparing the right and left sides. Because Gabriella has vomited twice during the past 12 hours, gently palpate her abdomen before her next scheduled feeding to determine whether it is soft (as opposed to distended and rigid). Also palpate for the degree of hepatomegaly. Use the stethoscope to assess Gabriella's bowel sounds. Check her recent stool pattern. Revisit the assessment of heart sounds and determine where on her chest the murmur is loudest.
>
> It is difficult with premature infants to single out the body system experiencing difficulty. The nurse must perform a thorough and systematic assessment to accurately convey the complete picture. Gabriella's immediate change is respiratory (increased heart rate and increased oxygen requirement) and gastrointestinal (vomiting), but the presence of the murmur and the discovery of bounding pulses indicate cardiovascular involvement.

DIAGNOSTIC CRITERIA

> **QUESTION:** The nurse anticipates a portable transthoracic echocardiogram (ultrasound). Review Tests and Procedures 15-1, Evaluating Cardiovascular Status. Why is an echocardiogram the diagnostic test of choice?

Several diagnostic procedures augment information obtained from the history and physical examination of the cardiovascular system and give direction to diagnosis and management of these children. **Cardiomegaly** (enlarged heart) visualized on a chest radiograph is commonly the first piece of evidence that causes health care personnel to consider the presence of a heart defect. Commonly used tests are described in Tests and Procedures 15-1.

> **ANSWER:** In Gabriella's situation, blood flow through the ductus arteriosus is not a long-standing situation that would cause changes that could be seen by an x-ray (enlarged heart), although increased pulmonary vascular markings would likely be seen, nor is it an electrical conduction problem visible on an electrocardiogram (ECG). The echocardiogram is noninvasive, "images" the blood flow, and is ideal for diagnosing a recently symptomatic PDA in a premature infant.

TREATMENT MODALITIES

The cardiac team is composed of an interdisciplinary group of health care professionals who collaborate with the child and the family to create goals and a treatment plan.

The cardiac team includes nurses, physicians, respiratory therapists, dietitians, social workers, and other ancillary personnel. In pediatric cardiac programs, health care team members meet regularly to discuss children with cardiovascular diagnoses and determine appropriate plans of care. The treatment options available for children with cardiac disease include interventional catheterization; cardiac surgery; pacemakers; cardiac transplantation; medical management using pharmaceutical, dietary, and activity interventions; supportive care; and community care.

CARDIAC CATHETERIZATION

A cardiac catheterization suite is a specially equipped area in the hospital with an operating table, fluoroscopy cameras, hemodynamic monitoring equipment, and specialized personnel. Cardiac catheterization involves the use of catheters threaded into the heart to visualize the anatomy of the heart chambers or blood vessels and assist in treatment of the child's condition. Catheterization of the right side of the heart is completed by passing the catheter into the femoral vein and advancing it through the inferior vena cava to the right atrium, right ventricle, and pulmonary artery. If the foramen ovale is patent, or if an ASD is present, the catheter may be advanced from the right atrium into the left atrium through these openings to evaluate the left side of the heart. If there is no atrial or ventricular communication, evaluation of the left side of the heart is completed by passing a new catheter into the femoral artery and advancing it into the descending aorta, left atrium, and left ventricle.

If further anatomic clarification is needed after noninvasive imaging, if the child's history and assessment are not consistent with noninvasive imaging findings, or if the child has a very complex lesion, an *angiography* is performed. This involves rapidly injecting a radiopaque dye through the catheter at a predetermined location and recording the dye's movement, visualized by radiograph or fluoroscope, via digital recording, DVD, or film. This recording enables the health care team to replay the images later to further visualize and analyze the structure of the heart.

Many, if not most, pediatric cardiac catheterizations are interventional, performed as outpatient procedures. The use of echocardiography has reduced the need for diagnostic cardiac catheterization in all but the most complex patients. See Evidence-Based Clinical Practice Guidelines 15-1.

Interventional Catheterization

Some interventional procedures are performed urgently to save a life, whereas others may eliminate or delay surgery. Interventional catheterization can provide the child with a procedure that is associated with less physical and emotional trauma; a shorter, less expensive hospital stay than that required after surgery; and a faster recovery.

Standard interventional procedures include electrophysiologic studies with ablation, percutaneous balloon angioplasty, myocardial biopsy, atrial septostomy, placement of vascular occlusion devices, and stents and occlusion device closures.

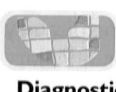

TESTS AND PROCEDURES for Evaluating Cardiovascular Status

Diagnostic Test or Procedure	Purpose	Findings and Indications	Health Care Provider Considerations
Chest radiograph	Defines silhouette of heart, shows pulmonary markings (use posterior and lateral views) Provides a baseline prior to cardiac surgery and for comparison with cardiac changes postoperatively Assesses status of noncardiac tissues (e.g., lungs, size of thymus, rib notching) that may be affected by compromised cardiac function	Heart size and shape; may detect abnormal placement, enlargement of the chambers, and cardiomegaly. Pulmonary vascular markings; increased in some CHD, decreased in right-to-left shunting. A cardiothoracic ratio of <50% is normal; >50% indicates cardiomegaly.	Advise the family that variations from normal can help in the differential diagnosis of heart disease and can enable documentation of trends, such as increasing heart size.
Pulse oximetry, transcutaneous	Identifies and monitors child's oxygen saturation level Helps the practitioner know when to wean a child off oxygen Can reduce the need for arterial blood gas testing and can assist in titrating oxygen administration	Normal values range from 94% to 100%. Values less than this range can be acceptable and expected in a cyanotic child. Typical values with CHD vary based on the lesion.	Position probe on finger, toe, earlobe, wrist, foot, or the spongy tissue between the thumb and the index finger. Observe data shown on the monitor readout, which generally include heart rate and oxygen saturation. Verify that a good arterial waveform is present and correlates with both the monitored and auscultated heart rate to ensure a more accurate reading. Be aware that an inaccurate reading is more likely if the child is moving, experiencing peripheral vasoconstriction, is cold or in shock, or if the child has low cardiac output. Set and verify alarm parameters at the beginning of each shift. If readings fall below parameters, assess the child immediately for respiratory distress.
ECG	Provides a graphic display of the electrical activity of the heart Produces data about the size and workload on the heart, assists in determining the anatomy of a defect and disturbances in conduction	Interpretation is age dependent. ECG of a normal newborn is characterized by right ventricular dominance; normal QRS deflection is negative in lead I and positive in lead aVF. After infancy, the normal QRS is positive in leads I and aVF.	For a 12-lead ECG, assist the child in lying very still for approximately 1 minute. Use distraction for children who are unwilling to cooperate. Inform the child that no electricity is involved.

Diagnostic Test or Procedure	Purpose	Findings and Indications	Health Care Provider Considerations
	Can be conducted continuously at the bedside (usually involves a three-lead system used to constantly monitor the child's heart rhythm) with multiple leads (typically a 12-lead) or via Holter monitoring (continuous ECG monitoring for 8–24 hours via electrodes attached to a small recorder carried by the ambulatory child with time, activities, and any symptoms recorded in a diary)		Although most modern multilead ECG machines print out a diagnosis at the top of the ECG strip, the diagnosis must be verified by a cardiac specialist because the machine-generated diagnosis may be inaccurate for the pediatric patient. Explain the use of leads and the need for them to adhere to the skin. During continuous bedside ECG monitoring, inspect the lead site daily and change the leads frequently. Ensure that the minimum and maximum heart rate alarm limits are set and that the alarms are functioning and activated. Teach the child and family how to keep a diary if Holter monitoring is used.
Cardiac enzymes (serum creatine kinase [CK] and lactate dehydrogenase [LDH] isoenzyme)	Assess myocardial compromise via blood specimen	Normal total CK: 70–380 International Units/L Normal total LDH: 327–874 International Units/L Levels are elevated with myocardial damage, cardiovascular injury, central nervous system damage such as cerebral infarct and periventricular hemorrhage, pulmonary infarct, necrosis of the kidney, liver damage, and ischemic rhabdomyolysis.	Keep in mind that myocardial insult can occur in infants as a result of asphyxia, tricuspid insufficiency, and papillary muscle infarcts. In children, myocardial damage causes elevations for about 7–10 days after the insult. Analyses for cardiac enzymes in infarcts need not occur immediately.
Brain natriuretic peptide	Measures an endogenous peptide hormone secreted by the cardiac ventricles in response to increased wall stress and related ventricular filling pressures via blood specimen Differentiates between acute heart failure and lung disease Monitors the effects of treatment for heart failure, cardiomyopathy	Normal: <100 pg/mL. More than 100 pg/mL is an indicator for heart failure, ventricular dysfunction, rejection in pediatric heart transplant recipients, and persistent pulmonary hypertension.	Prepare child as age appropriate for blood specimen collection.

(Continued)

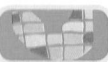

TESTS AND PROCEDURES for Evaluating Cardiovascular Status *(Continued)*

Diagnostic Test or Procedure	Purpose	Findings and Indications	Health Care Provider Considerations
ECG (transthoracic)	Uses ultrasound to show anatomic visualization of heart structure (valves, ventricles, septa, atria, vessels) Measures chamber enlargement, wall thickening, stroke volume, and blood shunting Assesses pericardial effusion Indicates function of cardiac muscle and pumping ability	Image of heart in motion can provide specific diagnosis of heart abnormalities, such as PDA and VSD, trends, and function.	Tell the child and family that the procedure is painless but that it requires child to be still for approximately 20–45 minutes. Use play therapy, books, videos, and other distraction to help minimize activity. Anticipate the need for sedation in young children. Be aware that obesity, a thick chest, or motion by the child can obstruct visualization of structures.
ECG (fetal)	Diagnoses CHD prenatally as early as 18–22 weeks	Four chambers in the heart and two great vessels: If screening identifies that the four chambers are not equal in size or the great vessels are unable to be visualized or do not arise in the correct location, refer the patient to a pediatric cardiologist.	Assess pregnant women for risk factors associated with CHD such as mothers with a family history of CHD, previous children with CHD, suspected chromosomal abnormalities (i.e., after amniocentesis), irregularities of fetal heart rates, or maternal diabetes. Anticipate change in plan for a routine delivery, such as delivering the infant in a high-risk unit and providing life-sustaining measures if required.
Transesophageal echocardiography/ pacing	Uses an esophageal probe placed to provide ultrasonic pictures of cardiovascular structures and function, especially left atrium, pulmonary value, mitral valve, and atrial septum; supplements information gathered from a standard transthoracic ECG Can be done pre- and postoperatively to evaluate lesion and repair and intraoperatively to assess the status of the surgical repairs after the child is disconnected from cardiopulmonary bypass and before the child's chest is sutured closed Aids in developing differential diagnosis of complex arrhythmias Allows stress testing of children who are unable to exercise	Can pace and capture the rhythm of the heart to treat tachyarrhythmias.	Inform child and family about the need for heavy sedation or general anesthesia for testing. Ensure the test is performed in a monitored situation. Assist with coordinating procedures, assessing and monitoring the child, administering the medications, and providing teaching.

Diagnostic Test or Procedure	Purpose	Findings and Indications	Health Care Provider Considerations
Magnetic resonance imaging	Uses a magnetic field to clarify structures of the heart, especially aortic arch and branch pulmonary arteries. Allows measurement of ejection fraction, especially of right ventricle, and regurgitant function. Builds a three-dimensional model of the heart to visualize the anatomy.	Indicated when it is difficult to obtain desired image using ECG. Can sometimes obtain enough information to avoid cardiac catheterization. Displays abnormalities in cardiac chamber contraction and abnormal patterns of blood flow in the heart and great vessels.	Explain to child and family that the test is noninvasive and there is no exposure to ionizing radiation (x-rays). Anticipate the need for sedation in young children; older children who can cooperate and hold their breath do not require sedation. Inform child that the machine makes loud humming and intermittent thumping noises; use music as a distraction. Remove all metal/magnetic items such as pins, hairpins, and metal zippers. Surgical implants, such as pacemakers, are a contraindication.

Electrophysiology Studies

Electrophysiology study procedures are used for arrhythmias that do not respond to pharmaceutical management or when it is believed that the technique will eliminate the need for pharmaceutical management. Closed-chest catheter ablation techniques have been successful in diagnosing and then treating ventricular and supraventricular tachycardias. The preparation and procedures are much like those for diagnostic cardiac catheterization, but electrophysiology studies use catheters with multipolar electrodes that map the path of the heart's electrical impulses. After the arrhythmogenic tissue is located, accessory pathways can be destroyed through thermal energy delivered via the intracardiac catheter.

Percutaneous Balloon Angioplasty and Balloon Valvuloplasty

Percutaneous balloon angioplasty and balloon valvuloplasty techniques permit a balloon-tipped catheter to be floated into a vascular area or valve that is stenotic. Pulmonary stenosis, pulmonary valve stenosis, aortic valve stenosis, and COA are common indications for percutaneous balloon dilation. Once inserted, the

EVIDENCE-BASED CLINICAL PRACTICE GUIDELINES 15-1

Pediatric Cardiac Catheterization Guidelines

Feltes, T. F., Bacha, E., Beekman, R. H., III. et al. (2011). Indications for cardiac catheterization and intervention in pediatric cardiac disease: A scientific statement from the American Heart Association. *Circulation, 123,* 2607–2652. Retrieved from

http://circ.ahajournals.org/content/123/22/2607.full.pdf + html

Report reviews evidence and provides recommendations for diagnostic catheterization and interventional treatment options.

American Academy of Pediatrics Section on Cardiology and Cardiac Surgery. (2002). Guidelines for pediatric cardiovascular centers. *Pediatrics, 109,* 544–549. Retrieved from

http://pediatrics.aappublications.org/content/109/3/544.full.pdf + html

Policy statement describes critical elements and organizational features of centers in which high-quality outcomes have the greatest likelihood of occurring.

Bashore, T. M., Balter, S., Barac, A. et al. (2012). 2012 American College of Cardiology Foundation/Society for Cardiovascular Angiography and Interventions expert consensus document on cardiac catheterization laboratory standards update: A report of the American College of Cardiology Foundation Task Force on expert consensus documents. *Journal of the American College of Radiology, 59,* 2221–2305. Retrieved from

http://content.onlinejacc.org/article.aspx?articleid = 1212373

Consensus statement discusses evolving areas of clinical practice and/or technologies that are widely available or new to the practice community.

balloon is inflated over the stenotic area to deform or rupture the site. This increases the luminal diameter by expanding the intimal lining of a vessel at the restricted area. By enlarging the vessel, these procedures decrease the pressure gradient and improve blood flow through the stenotic area.

Myocardial Biopsy

Myocardial biopsy is performed to collect a small piece of cardiac tissue for analysis. It is used to identify myocardial disease, such as cardiomyopathy, and to detect the presence and degree of rejection in cardiac transplantation.

Atrial Septostomy

Atrial septostomy is performed using either balloon (Rashkind procedure) or blade techniques. Atrial septostomy remains the standard initial palliation for infants with transposition of the great arteries (TGA). It may also be used for any lesion in which a large atrial communication is required to increase intracardiac shunting. This procedure is done in the catheterization laboratory or at the bedside. The catheter is introduced into the left atrium from the right atrium through a patent foramen ovale. Either the balloon is inflated and pulled back quickly to create a larger opening or the blade on the tip of a catheter is crossed through the opening where it incises the atrium as it crosses, thereby creating a larger opening. These techniques may sound harsh, but they can provide an effective tool in saving and improving the lives of infants.

Vascular Occlusion Devices

Various techniques have been developed to perform transcatheter vascular occlusion. A device can be implanted to embolize vessels such as the PDA. *Coil embolization* is one device used to occlude a vessel. A coiled wire is delivered through an end-hole catheter by extruding the wire out of the catheter at a predetermined location. Upon extrusion, the piece of steel coils back on itself, promotes clot formation, and acts to embolize the vessel. Soon after coil placement, fibrous tissue grows around the device, ensuring its immobility. Successful vessel closure using such devices may enable certain children to avoid surgical intervention. Coil embolization in the PDA or collateral vessel to occlude systemic flow to **pulmonary collaterals** (additional abnormally developing pulmonary vessels) may also enable some children to avoid surgery, resulting in fewer risks and less trauma.

Stainless steel *stents* may be inserted in areas of the pulmonary artery system that are stenotic. These stents are made of a stainless steel mesh, resembling a very small version of chicken wire, which is compressed into a small-diameter tube that expands when extruded into place. Through expansion, the stent effectively increases the diameter of the vessel and endothelializes into the vessel wall over time.

Occlusion Device Closures

As an alternative to surgical repair, ASDs can be closed in the catheterization laboratory with an Amplatzer septal occluder—a self-expandable, double-disk device made from wire mesh. The device is placed through the atrial septum, opened in the left atrium, and pulled against the opening to occlude the ASD. Currently, multiple other devices are under clinical investigation for use in closing ventricular septal defects (VSDs) and replacing pulmonary valves.

Precatheterization Care

Initially, ascertain whether the child has undergone catheterization before and what the child remembers about the other experience. It is not unusual for a child with complex CHD to have had multiple catheterizations. Prepare parents and the patient for cardiac catheterization before the day of the procedure, in a relaxed setting, and in an honest, open manner. Orient discussions toward deescalating anxiety in the child. Consider the age, cultural beliefs, and maturity of the child when explaining the environment and the catheterization routine and use a chronologic description of what will happen from admission to discharge (Fig. 15-3). Preparing the child and the family helps decrease anxiety and enables them to be better informed.

 KidKare During precatheterization teaching, assure the older child that the procedure will be done in the fold of the leg and that his or her genitalia will be covered. The child will probably not know where the "groin" is located or what it is; using the word *fold* or *bend* to describe the area of the leg is much clearer to the child.

Teaching can include a tour of the catheterization laboratory, recovery area, and the areas where families and friends will be waiting. This helps to alleviate anxiety about the laboratory with all its technical equipment and strange personnel. During this tour, if possible, have the child meet a staff member dressed in catheterization lab attire who will be present on the day of the study. Explain the rationale for restraints and the importance of staying in bed and keeping the affected leg immobilized after the procedure. If the child has a clear concept of time, include an explanation of how long the procedure will last. Assure the child that there is little pain or discomfort. A relaxed, informed child can develop a sense of personal control, anticipate events, and overcome misconceptions.

KidKare Encourage the child to pick out a favorite toy, doll, or blanket to keep throughout the procedure and in the recovery area.

On the day of cardiac catheterization, perform a baseline assessment, which includes an evaluation of the child's physiologic status with an emphasis on the cardiac state and peripheral extremities. Palpate lower extremity pulses and mark them with a pen for easy location. Document height and weight accurately to ensure accurate calculations of drug doses and other parameters. If a child has signs of systemic infection, such as a runny nose, fever, or skin rash, the

My care path for a cardiac catheterization

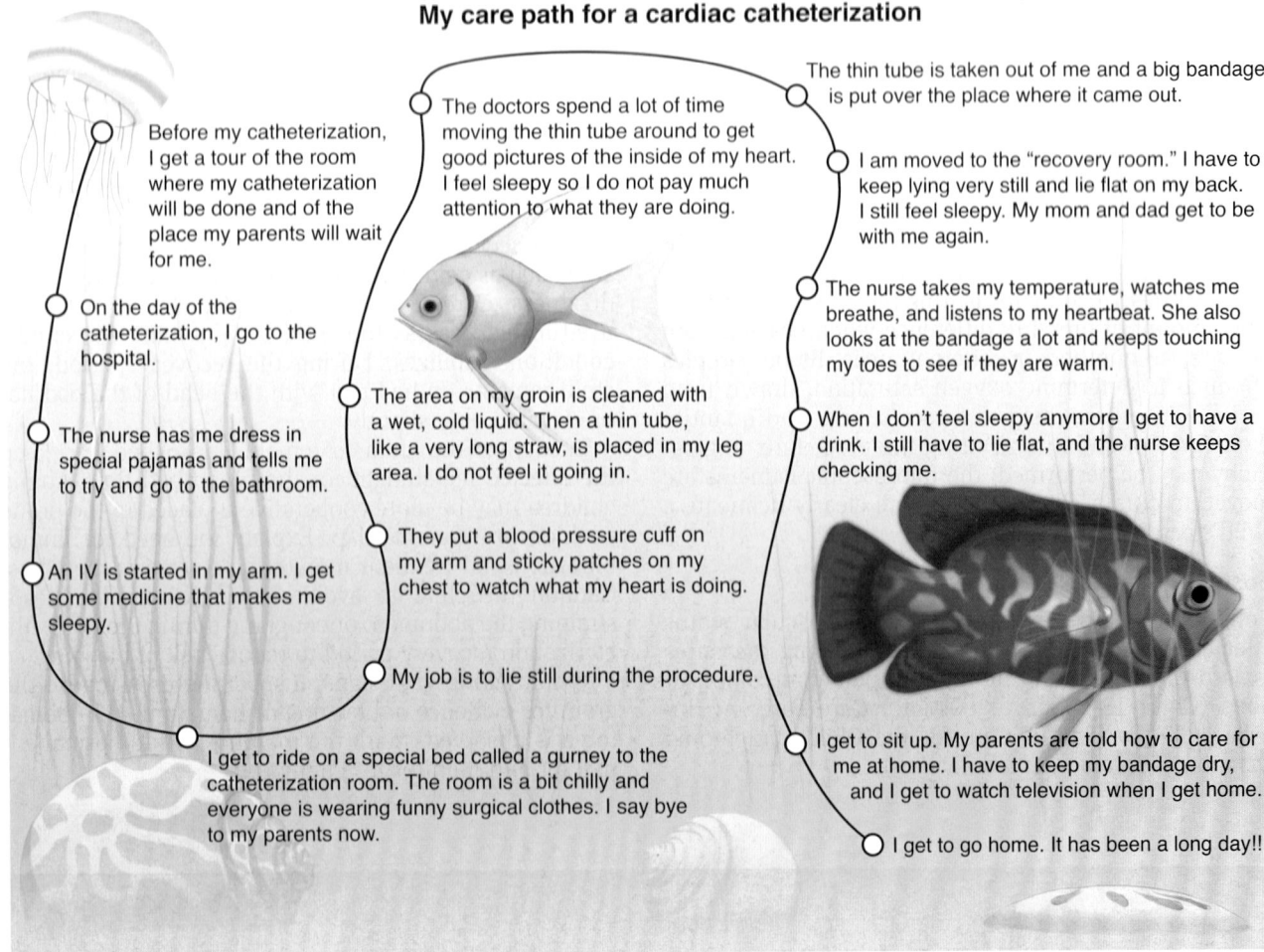

Before my catheterization, I get a tour of the room where my catheterization will be done and of the place my parents will wait for me.

On the day of the catheterization, I go to the hospital.

The nurse has me dress in special pajamas and tells me to try and go to the bathroom.

An IV is started in my arm. I get some medicine that makes me sleepy.

I get to ride on a special bed called a gurney to the catheterization room. The room is a bit chilly and everyone is wearing funny surgical clothes. I say bye to my parents now.

The doctors spend a lot of time moving the thin tube around to get good pictures of the inside of my heart. I feel sleepy so I do not pay much attention to what they are doing.

The area on my groin is cleaned with a wet, cold liquid. Then a thin tube, like a very long straw, is placed in my leg area. I do not feel it going in.

They put a blood pressure cuff on my arm and sticky patches on my chest to watch what my heart is doing.

My job is to lie still during the procedure.

The thin tube is taken out of me and a big bandage is put over the place where it came out.

I am moved to the "recovery room." I have to keep lying very still and lie flat on my back. I still feel sleepy. My mom and dad get to be with me again.

The nurse takes my temperature, watches me breathe, and listens to my heartbeat. She also looks at the bandage a lot and keeps touching my toes to see if they are warm.

When I don't feel sleepy anymore I get to have a drink. I still have to lie flat, and the nurse keeps checking me.

I get to sit up. My parents are told how to care for me at home. I have to keep my bandage dry, and I get to watch television when I get home.

I get to go home. It has been a long day!!

Figure 15-3 A care path for a child undergoing cardiac catheterization.

catheterization may be delayed. Verify that the child has had nothing to eat or drink prior to the procedure, noting when the last fluids or food were ingested. Ascertain carefully whether the child has any history of allergies because the contrast dyes used during angiography can trigger allergic reactions. Elicit information about any adverse reactions from previous catheterizations.

If venous access has not been established, a peripheral IV line is started before catheterization to provide medication access and to prevent dehydration. During the catheterization, the child's feet are not easily accessible for inspection or to assess for infiltrations; therefore, avoid placing IV lines in the feet whenever possible.

Before the catheterization, administer the prescribed sedation. The choice of medication varies depending on the institution, age of the child, and type of catheterization planned. Procedural sedation is provided for routine catheterizations. General anesthesia may be used for procedures that place the child at greater risk or for more complex interventional catheterization. Before sedation, have the toilet-trained child void, preferably before transportation to the catheterization laboratory.

After the child has been sedated, keep the child flat in bed to avoid the risk of injury resulting from altered mental status and potential complications from the catheterization process.

Care During Catheterization

During the procedure, the child receives continuous monitoring of vital functions, including blood pressure, pulse oximetry, and cardiac rhythm. Emergency drug doses that are calculated before the procedure must be readily available.

The catheterization laboratory can be quite cool. Wrap the head and extremities of small children and infants in blankets or use a mechanical warming blanket to maintain adequate body temperature. An infant's temperature must be monitored continuously by a rectal probe. After the child is positioned securely, the site for catheter insertion is prepared. Preparation usually involves cleansing the side with chlorhexidine or other antiseptic and injecting topical lidocaine over the intended puncture site.

Catheters are introduced into the cardiovascular system through the venous system to the right atrium or through the arterial system to the left side of the heart.

A percutaneous sheath is placed, usually using the groin's femoral artery, vein, or both. The sheath minimizes vessel trauma and allows various catheters to be inserted and withdrawn without creating any new insertion sites. Using fluoroscopy, the catheters are visualized as they are manipulated into different chambers and vessels (Fig. 15-4).

Accessing different areas of the heart and blood vessels enables pressure measurements and blood gas sampling in each area. The severity of an obstruction can be better described by measuring the pressure **gradient** (the amount of pressure difference when passing from one area to another) in different areas. Blood samples obtained to determine oxygen saturation, drawn from various chambers, help to locate shunts and quantify the degree of shunting. During the procedure, angiography may be performed; the fluoroscopic cameras are moved to obtain all angles that will clearly delineate a child's cardiac defects on film.

Postcatheterization Care

Continuously assess the child's cardiovascular status after cardiac catheterization. Direct nursing measures toward preventing and monitoring potential complications (Chart 15-1; see thePoint for Care Path: An Interdisciplinary Plan of Care for the Child Undergoing Diagnostic Cardiac Catheterization).

Postcatheterization assessment includes recording vital signs, checking the insertion site, monitoring and comparing catheterized extremities, and assessing the child's level of consciousness. After the procedure, assess vital signs in a similar manner as for the postoperative patient (generally, every 15 minutes until the child is awake and stable, then every half hour for 3 hours, then hourly up to 6 hours or more, as needed). When checking the child, assess for signs of hypotension such as cold, clammy skin; increased heart rate; or dizziness. Cardiac monitoring and pulse oximetry are used to help assess the child's status until the child's condition stabilizes. During the recovery period, the child remains on bed rest with the head of the bed flat or elevated only slightly.

Encourage the child to remain flat in bed and keep the affected leg straight for the prescribed time. Young children may be more cooperative if placed in the prone position in a parent's lap. Explain the need for immobilization and frequent monitoring to family members. Caution the child to avoid sitting, raising the head, straining the abdomen, or coughing during the postcatheterization recovery period to reduce risk of bleeding.

When taking vital signs, inspect the dressing on the groin for evidence of bleeding or hematoma. If a hematoma is observed, mark the margins with a permanent marker and monitor for changes.

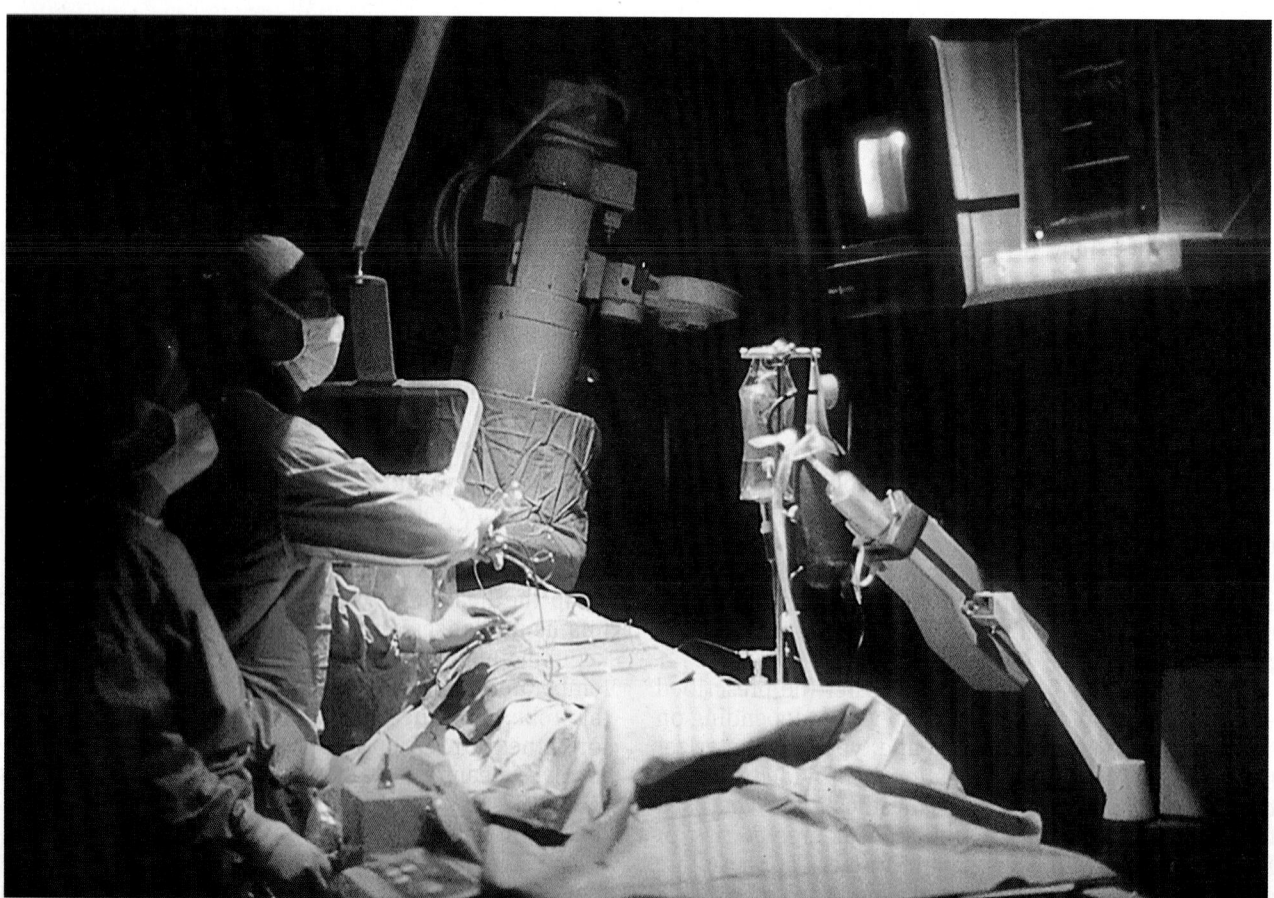

Figure 15-4 During cardiac catheterization, the child is under conscious sedation to prevent movement during the procedure. The physician introduces a catheter into the right or left femoral vessel and observes the movement and manipulation of the catheter on a monitor.

CHART 15-1   Potential Complications After Cardiac Catheterization

Complication	Description
Hemorrhage	Vessel bleeding at insertion site, decreased hematocrit
Hematoma	False aneurysm, subacute hematoma
Vomiting	Caused by anxiety, NPO (nothing by mouth) status, sedative drugs
Hypovolemia	Status, blood loss, diuretic action of dyes
Hypotension	Caused by medications, bleeding, contrast media
Arrhythmia	Transient bradycardia, premature ventricular contractions
Venous occlusion	Usually transient, from a clot, intimal tear, or herniation
Loss of pulses	Loss of pulse in catheterized extremity, usually transient, caused by vessel vasospasm, usage of larger catheters; smaller child at greater risk
Arterial thrombus	Aggregation of blood factors causing arterial occlusion
Renal damage	Clearance of contrast media, hematuria, oliguria, anuria
Pulmonary embolus	Risks greater in patient with intracardiac mixing and polycythemia from venous stasis pressure at puncture site
Fever/infection	Low grade, 4–8 hours, catheter induced (rare)
Allergic reaction	From sedatives, contrast media (rare)
Perforation	Tamponade, cardiac perforation by angiographic catheter (rare)
Arteriovenous fistula	When both the artery and vein are punctured, a communication between them shunting blood from the distal extremity
Central nervous system insult	Strokes, seizures from air embolus (rare)
Death	Highest occurrence in infants (rare)

ALERT   *Even though clot formation has occurred at the catheter insertion site, hemorrhaging could occur during the recovery period. The groin dressing must remain intact and the site must remain uncovered to enable the nurse to note any blood drainage immediately.*

With each set of vital signs, assess both lower extremities, including palpation of dorsalis pedis and posterior tibial pulses and inspection for color, temperature, and capillary refill. Also ensure that the affected leg remains immobilized. The affected foot may be cyanotic or cooler temporarily, especially if vasospasm of the vessel occurs or if the child's core temperature is also low; notify the physician if this persists longer than 2 hours.

Assess level of consciousness and initiate clear liquids after the child is fully awake and the gag reflex is intact. Encourage fluids to help the kidneys filter out the contrast dyes. Give written and verbal discharge instructions, including signs and symptoms to watch for, to children and their parents before they return home (Teaching Intervention Plan 15-1).

CARDIAC SURGERY

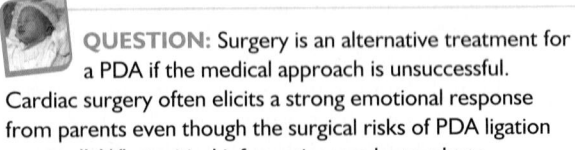

QUESTION: Surgery is an alternative treatment for a PDA if the medical approach is unsuccessful. Cardiac surgery often elicits a strong emotional response from parents even though the surgical risks of PDA ligation are small. What critical information can be taught to Gabriella's parents that may help decrease their anxiety?

Advances in pediatric cardiovascular surgery during recent decades have helped to reduce mortality and have enabled definitive repairs at an earlier age than was formerly possible. The focus of care has moved beyond merely increasing survival by a few years to enabling a greater number of children with complex CHD to live to adulthood. Cardiac surgery may be palliative or corrective.

Palliative Surgeries

Surgeries that are not curative but rather are performed for heart defects as a surgical bridge are called **palliative procedures**. These surgical interventions may allow the child's condition to become more stable and provide time for the child to grow until a more definitive surgical procedure is possible. Sometimes, palliative procedures are performed in stages to improve the long-term outcome for a particular heart defect.

Pulmonary Artery Banding

Pulmonary artery banding is provided to children who have conditions in which pulmonary blood flow to the lungs is excessive. These children cannot tolerate or are not ready for total surgical repair, yet other medical interventions have failed to manage heart failure, necessitating this procedure. Banding narrows the pulmonary artery, thereby minimizing pulmonary blood flow. Banding is performed through a lateral thoracotomy incision and placement of a Teflon tape band around the main pulmonary artery. If the band is too tight, reversal of the shunt and cyanosis may result. If the band is too loose, excess blood flow to the lungs will continue.

Shunts

For cyanotic infants, a **shunt** (an abnormal formation or artificially placed pathway through which blood flows from one area to another) is placed to increase pulmonary blood flow by creating an additional pathway for blood to reach the lungs. Some common lesions for which a shunt may be created in the neonate include pulmonary atresia, tricuspid atresia, tetralogy of Fallot, or severe pulmonary stenosis. Furthermore, a neonate or premature infant with medically unmanageable hypoxic spells or cyanosis may require shunt placement.

TIP 15-1: A TEACHING INTERVENTION PLAN for the Child Going Home After Cardiac Catheterization

Nursing Diagnosis and Family Outcomes

- Deficient knowledge: Lack of information regarding management of the child at home after a cardiac catheterization

  Outcomes: Child will have complications related to cardiac catheterization recognized early and interventions implemented.

  Child and family will express concerns and will remain calm and supportive of the child.

  Child and family will follow written discharge instructions for care of the child and the puncture site.

  Family will contact physician to make follow-up appointments and if any complications occur.

Treatment of the Child

Activity

- A child may resume normal activities, but no running, bike riding, skating, jumping, swimming, or other vigorous "roughhousing" or sports for the next 3 days.
- Children may return to school 2 days after discharge.

Catheterization Site

- Inspect the catheterization site daily for a week. Some bruising at the catheterization site is common. If there is drainage from the catheterization site, call your doctor.
- A small amount of blood on the bandage is normal. If bleeding that soaks through the bandage has occurred, hold pressure on the catheterization site until the bleeding stops and call the doctor.

Bathing

- After a catheterization, a child should avoid prolonged bathing for 2 days. A sponge bath or brief shower is permitted.

Diet

- Resume previous diet at home.

Pain

- Most children do not need any medicine for pain when at home, although a child may have some slight groin discomfort.

Behavior

- Even after a short stay in the hospital, it is possible to see temporary changes in the child's behavior (e.g., irritability, irregular sleep pattern, bad dreams, an increase in "childish ways"). It is important to be understanding while still keeping basic discipline rules.
- Because illness and hospitalization affect the whole family, you may see changes in the child's behavior at home or in school *and* changes in the behavior of siblings.

Follow-Up

- You should schedule a follow-up appointment within a week. After reviewing the catheterization procedure, the doctor will discuss the results and the plan of care with you.

Contact Health Care Provider if

- Your child has a fever higher than 101° F during the week after the heart catheterization
- The leg in which the catheterization was done becomes cooler, paler, or more numb than the other leg

---

Infants with severe cyanosis from restricted blood flow to the lungs may benefit from a systemic to pulmonary artery shunt. A *Blalock-Taussig* shunt is a procedure in which the subclavian artery is anastomosed to the pulmonary artery. Access to the vessels is through a lateral thoracotomy incision or median sternotomy. Because it is not an open-heart surgery, the shunt procedure is completed without putting the child on cardiopulmonary bypass. A modification of this procedure, known as the *modified Blalock-Taussig shunt*, is more frequently used; in this approach, a Gore-Tex tube graft is placed from the subclavian artery to the pulmonary artery. The shunt's size is selected to be large enough to maximize pulmonary flow while avoiding excessive flow and heart failure. Even children who are very small or quite ill can usually tolerate this procedure without major complications. Common problems of a Blalock-Taussig shunt procedure include thrombus or closure of the shunt, heart failure from excessive pulmonary blood flow if the shunt is too large, and hypoperfusion of the affected arm.

Slightly older children who have obstructive flow to the lungs may require a *Glenn procedure*, also called a *bidirectional Glenn shunt*. The bidirectional Glenn shunt is a palliative surgery that optimizes the child's cardiovascular status and is frequently used as a staging procedure as part of the Fontan surgery (described later in this chapter). The bidirectional Glenn shunt is an anastomosis of the superior vena cava to the pulmonary artery, which allows some blood to flow to the pulmonary system by bypassing the right side of the heart. This surgery is most commonly done through a midsternal incision.

Corrective Surgeries

The surgical trend in recent years has been toward surgical intervention early in life, often during infancy. The timing of surgeries depends on the anatomy of the lesion, the child's growth and development, any concurrent illnesses, and family needs. Parents are encouraged to schedule the surgery when other family events and sources of stress are minimal. Reasons to hasten surgery

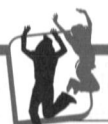

COMMUNITY CARE 15-1

Activity Recommendations for the Child With Cardiac Disease

Postcardiac Catheterization Routine

Keep the child out of school for 2 or 3 days or over a weekend.

No gym class or playground activities for 1 week.

After 1 week, the child can return to normal activities.

Postcardiac Surgical Care

Encourage fellow students to send cards and drawings to post on the wall in the intensive care unit (ICU).

Avoid situations that could induce a blunt chest trauma.

Involve the school nurse in administering midday dosages of required medications as indicated.

Keep the child out of gym classes or playground activities for 6 weeks to allow time for the sternum to heal.

Keep the child out of school 1 week after discharge from hospital.

include preventing development of aortopulmonary collateral vessels, avoiding deterioration of ventricular function, and minimizing risks of **pulmonary hypertension** (abnormally elevated blood pressures in the pulmonary artery). For children who develop irreversible pulmonary hypertension, surgery may no longer be an option. Surgery may have to be delayed because other medical conditions make the child a poor surgical candidate. Surgery may also be delayed to enable the child to grow. For example, if the child needs a valve replacement, it is to the child's advantage that surgery be delayed to allow the heart to grow larger. This delay enables placement of a larger valve, one that the child will not quickly outgrow.

Preoperative Teaching

As with any patient scheduled for surgery, the information given by the health care provider to the child and family must include an explanation of the intended surgery, complications that may occur, and a description of the medical equipment that will be used to support the child during the recovery period. Answer all questions honestly and in simple, age-appropriate terms so the child and family can comprehend them (see Chapter 11 for preparing a child for surgery; Community Care 15-1). Giving the child and family a chronologic explanation of the events that will occur from admission to discharge is helpful (Nursing Interventions 15-1). Allow the child

NURSING INTERVENTIONS 15-1

Cardiac Preoperative Teaching Topics

Chronologic Course of Events

Family blood donation

Preoperative day ICU tour

Surgical procedure

ICU stay

Convalescence

Discharge planning

Follow-up

Child's General Appearance

Monitors

Sedation/pain management

Ventilator support

Chest tubes

Arterial and IV lines

Pacemaker

Postoperative Respiratory Needs

Ventilation: tube, suctioning

Turn, cough, deep breathing, incentive spirometry

Nasotracheal suctioning

Nasal cannula, oxygen mask, or tent

Activity Progression

How to pick up child after surgery

ICU: bed rest, chair

Ambulation/playroom

Nutrition

NPO: preoperatively, ICU

IVs

How eating is advanced

Wound

Care and dressing

Sensory Stimuli

Noises, personnel

Child interactions/coping

Restraints

Pain management

and parents to absorb information and to ask questions at their own pace. The preoperative teaching period is a good time to assess family needs, interactions, and patterns of coping. Incorporate this information into the child's plan of care to ensure that the unique needs of the family are being met.

A preoperative tour of the ICU helps alleviate stress for the older child and for parents and family members who have had no prior experience with an ICU. It can be overwhelming for parents to see ventilators, monitors, and a large variety of tubes and lines entering and exiting any small child, much less their own (Fig. 15-5). During preoperative teaching, a visit with another child and his or her parents in the ICU may alleviate some of their fears.

Explain to the parents the type of chest incision that the child will have. The surgeon makes this decision based on the type of surgery that is scheduled. (All cases of *cardiopulmonary bypass* [*pump*] require separation of the sternum.) Either a midsternal or a lateral thoracotomy incision is used for cardiac surgical procedures. Some surgeons use a mammary incision for female patients. This incision enables the patient to wear a V-neck shirt or swimsuit without showing a scar.

Tell parents that predicting exactly how long tubes and lines will be required or how long their child will be in hospital after surgery is not possible. Provide general guidelines and explain that they will be given daily updates on their child's progress. For many routine surgeries, a child spends most of the hospital stay in the ICU. Typically, a child who was once quite ill achieves a particular level of stability and may progress so quickly toward being able to return home that the parents are surprised.

Many hospitals have designated blood donor systems to encourage the family to have members donate blood for the child's surgery. After the blood has been drawn, it is screened for suitability and then is designated for use during the child's surgery. Teach parents that the designated blood donation procedure usually takes at least 3 days to have the blood available for transfusion.

caREminder

Any signs of a concurrent illness, such as an ear infection, cough, runny nose, or fever, may delay surgery. Advise parents to call the physician if any signs of infection occur during the immediate preoperative period.

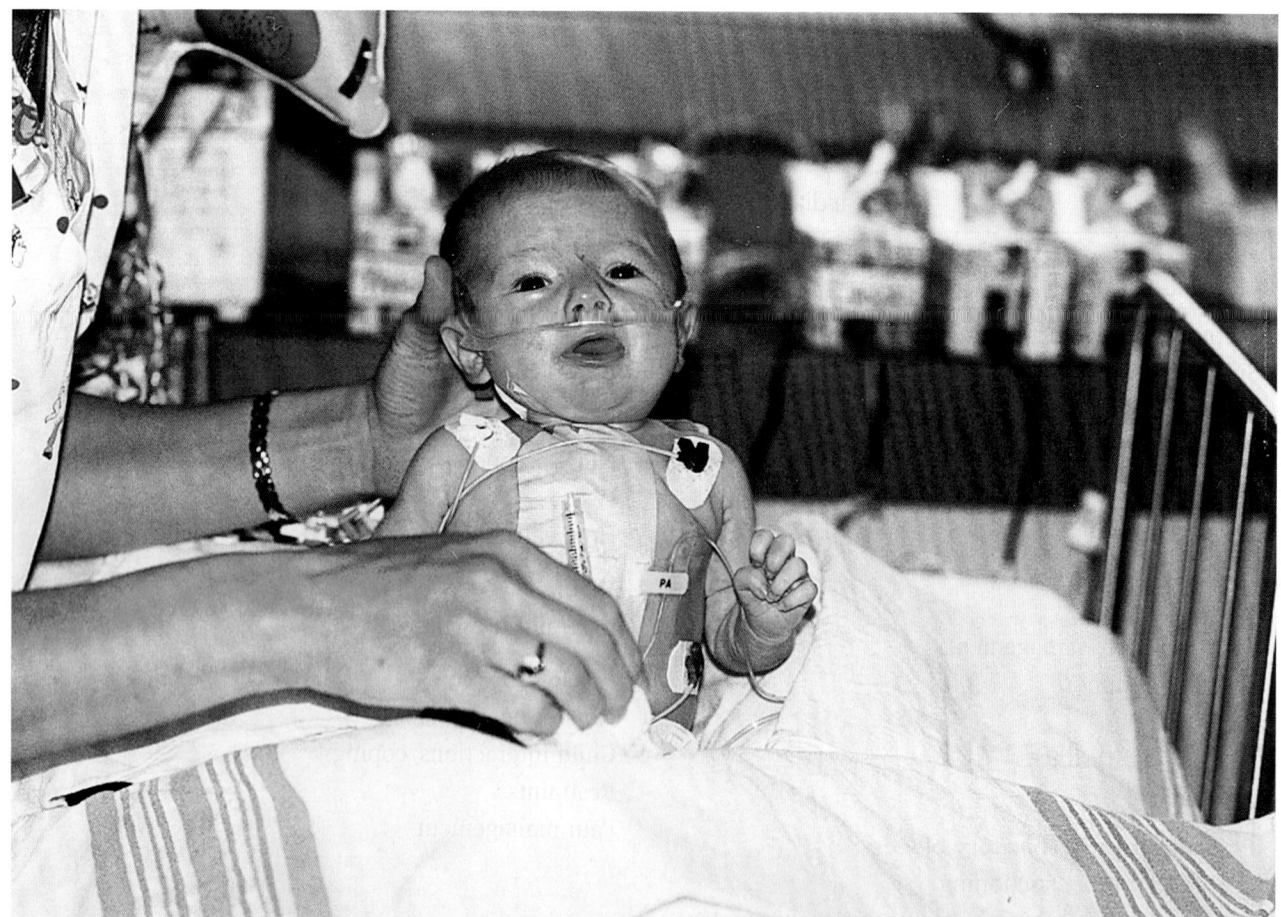

Figure 15-5 The child returning from cardiac surgery often has many wires and tubes attached to monitors, pumps, and equipment. Parents should be prepared for how the child will look after surgery. As the child's condition improves, use of the equipment is discontinued. This infant is 2 days postcardiac surgery. He is alert and attached to only a few monitoring devices and equipment.

Intraoperative Care

In the surgical suite, the child is intubated, and most of the monitoring and IV lines are placed before the chest incisions are made. Monitoring and invasive lines include ECG leads, nasogastric tube, pulse oximetry, indwelling urinary catheter, peripheral IV lines, arterial line, and a minimum of one central line with *central venous pressure* monitoring. In cardiac patients with complex conditions, the surgical team may place direct intracardiac lines, such as left atrial and pulmonary artery lines, to monitor pressures.

Cardiopulmonary Bypass

If the heart and lungs will be connected to a cardiopulmonary bypass pump to oxygenate and perfuse the body while the heart is stopped, incisions are placed midsternally by separating the skin and then splitting the sternum. The right side of the heart is cannulated, capturing venous blood before it returns to the heart. Venous blood is shunted to the pump, where it is oxygenated and circulated, and its temperature is regulated. The oxygenated blood is returned to the body through the cannula in the ascending aorta. During the time on pump, the heart is stabilized with an electrolyte solution called *cardioplegia* that helps immobilize and protect the heart during surgery. The cardiopulmonary bypass pump also reduces the body's metabolic rate and decreases oxygen demand during surgery by creating a hypothermic state.

After the cardiac surgical repairs are done, the child is rewarmed gradually until normothermia is achieved; as the child warms, the heartbeat will return. Occasionally, the surgeon may need to regulate the heart's rate and rhythm with a temporary pacemaker and wires. Before closing the chest, temporary pacing wires may be placed on the outside of the heart and passed through the chest wall. Mediastinal chest tubes are placed to evacuate any bleeding from around the heart; pleural chest tubes will reinflate the lung and drain fluid. Depending on the nature of the surgery and the monitoring needs, transthoracic central lines may be placed in the right or left atrium, the pulmonary artery, or both. These lines enable more detailed hemodynamic monitoring than that provided by a central venous pressure line alone. The sternum is closed and secured with wire. Finally, the skin is sutured shut. The chest may be left open with a Gore-Tex patch covering the area to allow for swelling of the heart. In such cases, the chest is typically closed within 24 to 48 hours after surgery.

Nonpump Cases

Surgeries that do not require entering the heart and thus can be done without cardiopulmonary bypass are termed *nonpump cases*. Examples are repairs of COA and PDA. These surgeries are usually completed using a lateral thoracotomy approach. With this approach, the pleural space is entered; therefore, chest tube placement is required before the chest is closed. Children will likely have a central line and an arterial line. Generally, nonpump cases will not have pacing wires or transthoracic lines placed.

> **ANSWER:** If Gabriella did have surgery—in addition to an explanation of the intended surgery, possible complications, and devices or tubes that will be in place during recovery—also identify when the parents can be reunited with Gabriella and how her pain will be managed.

Postoperative Care

During the acute care phase, interventions focus on stabilizing the child, minimizing complications, and facilitating recovery. Small or abrupt changes in the status of a child must be efficiently noted and acted on during the critical postoperative period.

Vital sign parameters are defined by the surgical team and may vary from those typically associated with a normally functioning heart depending on the specific needs of an individual child. For example, if the child still has intracardiac mixing after surgery, a liberalized range of oxygen saturation is considered acceptable. Continuous blood pressure monitoring is provided in the critical care unit through arterial catheters connected to a transducer and monitor. These catheters are placed in the femoral artery or the radial artery or, in neonates, the umbilical artery. Perform and record a head-to-toe assessment, concentrating on the child's cardiopulmonary status, every shift and as needed for changes in status. Cardiac assessment is performed more frequently, depending on the child's condition.

Managing Changes in Body Temperature

Hypothermia occurs during the immediate postoperative period because of core temperature cooling associated with cardiopulmonary bypass. Initiate warming measures upon arrival to the ICU. Monitor the child's temperature continuously, using bladder or nasopharyngeal probes, which more closely approximate core temperature (measured from the pulmonary artery) than a rectal probe (Maxton et al., 2004) (Nursing Plan of Care 15-1).

As the child recovers, an elevated temperature can be associated with the need for pulmonary toilet (evacuation of accumulated mucus from the lungs). Initiate cooling measures, including a cooling blanket and administration of antipyretics. After the first postoperative day, spikes in temperature are indications that blood, sputum, and urine cultures must be drawn.

Maintaining Cardiac Output

Evaluate information from hemodynamic lines, vital signs, and peripheral pulses to obtain information about the child's volume or preload status. Problems with preload can be related to excessive chest tube drainage that is causing hypovolemia or to fluid leaking into the interstitial spaces from the vascular bed. Administer volume replacement as required. A 5% albumin solution is a commonly used intravascular volume expander, unless the child is bleeding, in which case blood and other fluids are used.

Continuously evaluate the child's *afterload* (SVR) by assessing blood pressure, capillary perfusion, toe temperature, and urine output. Afterload may be increased in the vasoconstricted patient as a result of hypothermia or poor cardiac output. Vasodilators such as milrinone,

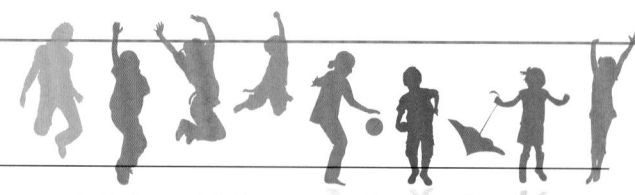

NURSING PLAN OF CARE 15-1:
The Child With Altered Cardiovascular Status

Nursing Diagnosis: Decreased cardiac output related to effects of decreased preload/hypovolemia, postoperative bleeding, increased afterload, altered myocardial contractility, arrhythmias, or cardiac defects

Interventions/Rationale

- Obtain baseline and frequent assessments of vital signs (blood pressure, heart rate, respiratory rate), cardiac rhythm (ECG monitoring), quality and strength of apical and peripheral pulses, color and warmth of the skin, and level of cyanosis (e.g., circumoral, digital, mucous membranes, clubbing). Assess for signs and symptoms of decreased cardiac output such as hypotension, edema, cool extremities, delayed capillary refill, weak peripheral pulses, mottled extremities, abnormal filling pressures, low urine output, and mental status changes. Notify health care provider immediately of major changes in child's status.
  Baseline assessments provide an index on which to compare changes. Rhythm disturbances may cause decreased cardiac output. Frequent assessment enables prompt detection of changes and interventions to address the alteration.
- Monitor intake and output, hemodynamic parameters, and laboratory values.
  Low urine output may indicate decreased kidney perfusion from decreased cardiac output. Electrolyte imbalances may contribute to decreased cardiac output.
- Administer oxygen as ordered. Monitor oxygen saturation and arterial blood gases as obtained.
  Supplemental oxygen can help increase oxygen available to the myocardium. The need for oxygen is based on the defect and may be contraindicated in a child with low pulmonary pressures who is shunting blood to the lungs at the expense of the systemic circulation.
- Administer medications, such as vasodilators, vasoconstrictors, and inotropes, as ordered to facilitate cardiac output; monitor for desired effect and side effects. Titrate medications as ordered.
  Volume replacement can improve problems caused by decreased preload. Vasodilators may reduce afterload, and inotropes may improve heart contractility, both improving cardiac output. Titrating medications helps maintain a balance between contractility, preload, and afterload.
- Implement measures to conserve child's energy expenditure: limit child's activity; provide comfort measures to reduce fretting (provide pacifier, rock, play soft music); provide small, frequent feedings; encourage quiet activities (read stories, watch TV); encourage frequent rest periods; and schedule activities to provide periods of uninterrupted sleep.

Activity restriction may reduce workload on the heart. Extended feeding events can cause unnecessary energy expenditure.

Expected Outcome

- Child will demonstrate a cardiac output adequate to maintain perfusion of body as evidenced by stable vital signs, level of consciousness within normal limits, hemodynamic stability, adequate tissue perfusion and end-organ perfusion (e.g., evidenced by urine output of 1–2 mL/kg/hr), and no signs of venous congestion.

Nursing Diagnosis: Impaired gas exchange related to effects of cardiac surgery and anesthesia, fluid shifts, hypoventilation, atelectasis, effusions, pulmonary congestion, pain, immobility, underlying congenital disease

Interventions/Rationale

- Assess quality and rate of respirations; auscultate chest for breath sounds and rubs; monitor oxygen saturation levels; draw arterial blood gases as ordered; and report diminished breath sounds, rales, rhonchi, rubs, cough, or decreased oxygen saturation retractions.
  Frequent assessment enables prompt detection of changes and interventions to address the alteration. The presence of pericardial and pleural rubs can indicate effusion.
- Monitor temperature.
  Fever can be an early indicator of atelectasis.
- Encourage coughing and deep breathing.
  Coughing and deep breathing help to expand lungs and eliminate secretions.
- Position the child upright if possible. Assist the child to ambulate after he or she is extubated and hemodynamically stable.
  Upright positioning assists in allowing maximal diaphragmatic excursion. Early ambulation helps avoid hazards of immobility such as atelectasis and pneumonia.

Expected Outcome

- Child will demonstrate adequate ventilation and gas exchange evidenced by adequate arterial blood gas results, minimal pulmonary secretions, and normal breath sounds.

Nursing Diagnosis: Risk for imbalanced fluid volume related to effects of volume overloading from myocardial dysfunction, use of diuretics, altered ratio of electrolytes from diuretic therapy, fluid administration, poor nutritional status, cardiopulmonary bypass, prolonged operative time, anesthesia, bleeding

Interventions/Rationale

- Assess vital signs and weight and check for symptoms of fluid volume deficit (e.g., weight loss, poor turgor, tachycardia) or excess (periorbital or dependent edema, bulging fontanel in infants) and heart failure (e.g., irritability, tachycardia, tachypnea, dyspnea, rales, fatigue when feeding, anorexia, periorbital or dependent edema, oliguria, hepatomegaly). Notify health care prescriber of major changes.

  Changes in these parameters may reflect alteration in fluid balance. Increased fluid volume can lead to heart failure.

- Calculate fluid requirements for the child. Evaluate whether they coincide with the order for fluid infusion and with the child's condition.

  Fluid needs are calculated based on the child's weight and condition. Children with cardiac problems often require fluid restriction.

- Monitor intake and output; frequency depends on child's status.

  Measuring intake and output provides information from which to calculate fluid balance.

- Administer fluids and medications, such as diuretics and fluids, as ordered. Monitor for desired effect and side effects.

  Fluids and medications are often necessary as mechanisms to treat symptoms and pathology, such as potassium and calcium imbalance, which are critical during the postoperative period.

- Use an infusion device (pump) to administer IV fluids.

  Infusion devices provide more accurate fluid delivery than gravity alone and may prevent inaccurate fluid volume administration.

Expected Outcomes

- Child will exhibit clear breath sounds without signs of heart failure or edema; weight will approximate the dry weight (child's weight without excess fluid).
- Child will demonstrate electrolyte laboratory values within acceptable parameters.

Nursing Diagnosis: Hypothermia (postsurgical) related to effects of cardiopulmonary bypass, immaturity of the thermoregulation centers, low cardiac output state, cool surgical suite

Interventions/Rationale

- Assess the child for any signs of cold stress such as low core or skin temperature, cold or cyanotic extremities, pallor, and metabolic acidosis. Monitor the child's temperature.

  Frequent assessment enables early detection of cold stress and interventions to reduce it.

- Maintain a neutral thermal environment. Use techniques for warming such as warming lights and warm blankets, changing the temperature setting on the ventilator, and increasing the room temperature. Cover the child's head. Keep neonates in a temperature-regulated warmer isolette or a radiant warmer bed. Warm equipment before putting it in contact with the child (e.g., stethoscopes). Warm fluids and blood products using a specially designed fluid warmer, especially if large amount of volume replacement is necessary.

  An external heat source helps warm the child and may minimize cold stress, energy expenditure, and oxygen consumption. Most body heat is lost through the head. Cold stress will cause vasoconstriction and dramatically increase SVR, stress myocardial function, and reduce cardiac output.

Expected Outcome

- Child will remain normothermic and free from complications of thermal imbalance.

Nursing Diagnosis: Risk for injury (neurologic) related to cardiopulmonary bypass, intracardiac mixing (emboli), low cardiac output, hypotension, hypoxia, electrolyte imbalances and fluid shifts, narcotics, anesthesia

Interventions/Rationale

- Assess neurologic status frequently. Check pupils; monitor for changes such as subtle alterations in behavior, in strength and equality of movement of extremities, or in vigor and coordination of suck.

  Frequent assessment enables prompt detection of changes and interventions to address the alteration.

- Monitor for seizure activity, which in an infant can manifest as staring, tremors, or sucking.

  Early detection of seizure activity enables prompt implementation of interventions.

- Administer anticonvulsant therapy as indicated and as ordered.

  Medications may be required to control seizure activity.

- Be prepared to intervene for status epilepticus (e.g., with airway protection, medications).

  Preparation enables prompt intervention.

Expected Outcomes

- Child will remain free of neurologic deficits. Seizures will be controlled with appropriate anticonvulsant therapy.

Nursing Diagnosis: Risk for infection related to pulmonary status, congenital defect, prolonged operative time, excessive postoperative bleeding, prosthetic devices, compromised nutritional status, surgical wound, use of indwelling catheters

Interventions/Rationale

- Adhere to strict hand hygiene (handwashing at sink or use of alcohol sanitizers) immediately prior to coming in contact with the child.

  Hand hygiene is the single most important intervention to prevent nosocomial infections.

(Continued)

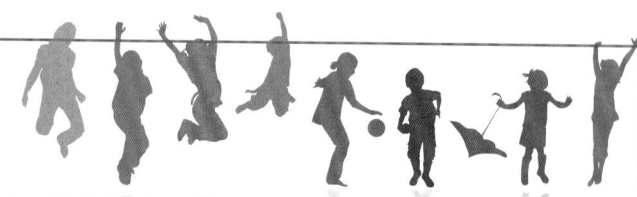

NURSING PLAN OF CARE 15-1:

The Child With Altered Cardiovascular Status (Continued)

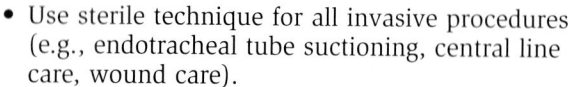

- Use sterile technique for all invasive procedures (e.g., endotracheal tube suctioning, central line care, wound care).

  Sterile technique helps to prevent the introduction of bacteria during invasive procedures.

- Implement interventions to facilitate gas exchange (e.g., respiratory treatments, chest physiotherapy, suctioning).

  Pooling of secretions and blood (as may occur with many congenital heart defects) in the lungs may result in pulmonary vascular congestion and may compromise pulmonary compliance, making the child more susceptible to respiratory infection.

- Teach child and parents to avoid contact with persons who are ill.

  Avoiding contact with ill people reduces the child's risk of exposure to communicable diseases.

- Assess for signs of infection such as fever, abnormal lab values (e.g., white blood cell count), increased respiratory secretions, crackles, and rales and intervene as indicated if present.

  Early detection and intervention may reduce progression of infection.

Expected Outcomes

- Child will be afebrile, with a white blood cell count within normal limits.
- Child will be free of any signs and symptoms of infection.

Nursing Diagnosis: Imbalanced nutrition: Less than body requirements related to effects of increased caloric need, necessity for fluid limitations, child's inability to take in adequate calories without fatigue

Interventions/Rationale

- Calculate calorie and fluid requirements for the child. Evaluate whether the calories required can be delivered within the child's fluid restrictions. Consult with a dietitian.

  Calorie and fluid needs are calculated based on the child's weight and condition. Children with cardiac problems often require fluid restriction but have increased caloric needs as a result of higher metabolic rates and body requirements for postoperative healing.

- Provide small, frequent feedings. Administer nasogastric feedings as ordered.

  Small, frequent feedings help meet the child's caloric requirements without fatiguing the child and reduce the risk of gastric distention, which compresses the diaphragm, thereby limiting lung excursion and exacerbating respiratory distress.

Nasogastric feedings may conserve energy because the child does not need to suck.

- Weigh a hospitalized child daily. Assess length and head circumference (in children younger than 3 years of age) upon admission. Track trends in growth.

  Daily weight monitoring and tracking trends provide feedback on adequacy of caloric intake, enable prompt detection of negative trends, and allow implementation of interventions to improve intake.

Expected Outcome

- Child will maintain weight and grow along own growth trajectory.

Nursing Diagnosis: Anxiety related to unfamiliar environment, equipment, people, overstimulation, diagnosis

Interventions/Rationale

- Prepare the child, as developmentally appropriate, and family for procedures. Tour the ICU preoperatively (for most school-aged children and older, with parents), talk with other patients and families, and use books and drawings. Modify the environment to reduce stimuli.

  Knowing what to expect may help reduce anxiety and distress. Overstimulation may exacerbate anxiety.

- Assess the child's anxiety level and signs of anxiety (e.g., tachycardia, tachypnea, verbalizations, lack of eye contact, withdrawal).

  Detecting anxiety allows interventions to be implemented.

- Involve parents to provide touch, distraction, comfort, and other interventions to reduce anxiety.

  Parental presence provides the child with a sense of security; parents know best what may comfort child.

Expected Outcome

- Child will demonstrate behaviors indicating decreased anxiety.

Nursing Diagnosis: Impaired parenting related to symbolic meaning of the heart, separation, lack of control and fear of the unknown, alterations in routine, overprotection of the child, financial and social constraints

Interventions/Rationale

- Allow parents to verbalize feelings; acknowledge and validate parental feelings.

  Letting the parents know that the nurse has heard what they have said fosters trust and provides support.

- Encourage parental presence in hospital and interaction with the child. Support parental competence in assessing their child's needs and in caring for their child.

    Parental support reinforces new behaviors and bolsters the parents' feelings of competence.
- Model developmentally appropriate communication and care techniques.

    Modeling demonstrates skills and behaviors that the parents can learn and adopt.
- Use support resources (e.g., social worker, child life worker, support groups) to provide parents with additional mechanisms to share feelings and learn coping strategies.

    An interdisciplinary team approach is necessary to enhance parental coping.

Expected Outcomes

- Parents will verbalize feelings regarding their child's illness.
- Parents will demonstrate appropriate bonding and attachment behaviors.

Nursing Diagnosis: Deficient knowledge: Lack of information regarding cardiovascular condition and treatment

Interventions/Rationale

- Assess child and family's knowledge of the child's condition and current management and readiness to learn.

    Assessment provides baseline information and focuses teaching topics.
- Arrange time and setting for teaching so child and family can focus on the information and skills to be learned.

    Distraction impairs ability to focus and master content and skills.
- Teach child and family about condition and management using materials and techniques appropriate for age, cultural beliefs, and literacy level. Present information that is most important to the family first. Provide verbal and written instructions; use props as indicated (e.g., syringes to measure ordered medication dosage).

    Selecting materials and information to meet the family's needs and beliefs enhances understanding of and adherence to the management plan.
- Evaluate understanding of teaching provided.

    May identify misunderstandings or topics that require further teaching.
- Assess family's ability to adhere to treatment plan; intervene as indicated.

    Child and family may understand teaching, but factors such as lack of insurance, funds, transportation, or social support may interfere with adherence to management plan.

Expected Outcomes

- Child and family will accurately discuss child's condition.
- Child and family will manage child's condition to keep child as healthy as possible and will demonstrate appropriate medication administration as indicated.

Nursing Diagnosis: Deficient knowledge: Healthy lifestyle choices

Interventions/Rationale

- Assess family's nutrition and physical activity behaviors.

    Family assessment provides baseline information and facilitates development of a plan that complements the family's lifestyle to promote healthy changes.
- Assess family's knowledge of healthy choices regarding nutrition and physical activity.

    Information about the family's knowledge level assists in focusing teaching to family's needs.
- Discuss healthy food choices and the importance of physical activity (based on the child's age) and provide specific amounts of time to target for daily physical activity. Encourage parents to provide positive reinforcement for children with desirable activities (e.g., a trip to the park vs. providing food incentives).

    Food choices and activity instruction provide information for the family to set personal goals and activities.
- Discuss the consequences of sedentary lifestyle (including excessive screen time) and unhealthy food choices.

    Lack of knowledge may contribute to negative lifestyle habits.
- Assist the family in identifying the goals for changes in lifestyle. Remain nonjudgmental, even if they do not desire change. Encourage realistic, incremental lifestyle changes.

    The family, as a unit, must desire the change. Consideration of level of motivation is important to promote positive outcomes. Short-term goals are more readily achieved, promoting self-efficacy and demonstrating measurable results.
- Encourage family members to plan daily menus and acceptable activities together.

    Involving all members of the family promotes adherence and implementation by all members.
- Assist the family to evaluate progress toward goals; revise goals and activities as indicated.

    Evaluation helps to encourage modification of goals and activities to facilitate success.

Expected Outcomes

- Family will identify the importance of healthy nutrition and physical activity levels.
- Family will demonstrate incorporation of healthy lifestyle changes.

nitroprusside, or nitroglycerin, infused intravenously, may reduce afterload. In the presence of poor cardiac function, vasoactive and **inotropic** (influences the contractility of a muscle) agents are administered intravenously and titrated to maintain adequate cardiac output. Commonly infused inotropic medications include dopamine, dobutamine, milrinone, and epinephrine.

caREminder

Peripheral vasoconstriction, assessed as cold feet and poor capillary refilling time, can be an early sign of diminished cardiac output. A thermometer probe placed on the toes can be used to monitor subtle changes in peripheral temperatures.

If diminished cardiac output is refractory to large dosages of multiple inotropic infusions, cardiac assist devices may be used. *Ventricular assist devices* are pumps used to provide critical support to a patient in severe refractory heart failure or as a bridge to transplantation. *Left ventricular assist devices* support heart function. Blood is diverted from the left heart and returned back to the aorta via a pump. *Extracorporeal membrane oxygenation* is prolonged external cardiopulmonary bypass that allows the cardiopulmonary system to rest so that reversible pathology can resolve. All support devices are invasive and are associated with a variety of complications. When the patient's cardiac function stabilizes, the child is weaned from support devices.

Minimizing Risk for Cardiac Tamponade

Cardiac tamponade occurs when a volume of fluid large enough to interfere with ventricular filling and pumping collects in the pericardial sac and critically suppresses cardiac output. It is most likely to occur during the immediate postoperative period but may also occur during later stages of recovery. Signs and symptoms of cardiac tamponade include hypotension, muffled heart sounds, decreased systemic perfusion, sudden cessation of chest tube drainage, narrowing pulse pressures, widening mediastinum on chest radiograph, and increased right and left atrial pressures. Cardiac tamponade can lead to cardiac arrest and may necessitate surgical re-exploration of the chest cavity. If this condition is not detected by early assessment, death may ensue.

Managing Arrhythmias

Arrhythmias may occur from surgical injury to the heart or fluid and electrolyte imbalances, primarily hypokalemia (see Chapter 17). Monitor and evaluate the ECG, which runs continuously; document the rhythm and any changes. If temporary pacing wires are present, they are connected to a temporary pacemaker according to hospital protocols. Antiarrhythmic agents are administered, as ordered, while the child is monitored for signs of side effects.

Managing Temporary Pacing Wires

Temporary pacing wires are placed in the heart muscle and are brought out through the chest at the end of an open heart surgical case. In general, the wires on the right side of the chest are atrial wires, and the wires on the left side of the chest are ventricular wires. This arrangement may vary, however. For example, in patients with dextrocardia (congenital growth of heart inside the right side of the chest), wires will be reversed. The wires may be connected to an external temporary pacemaker (an emergency backup pacer used only if needed) that is placed next to the child. Connection to the temporary pacemaker is usually for 48 hours or until the child is out of danger for arrhythmia. Nursing interventions related to care of the child with pacing wires are discussed in Nursing Interventions 15-2.

Maintaining Fluid and Electrolyte Balance

As a response to surgery and cardiopulmonary bypass, aldosterone and antidiuretic hormone are secreted. These hormones increase sodium and water retention and potassium excretion. During the postoperative period, excess fluid, which has settled into the interstitial

---

NURSING INTERVENTIONS 15-2

Caring for the Child With Temporary Pacing Wires

Secure wires to the child's chest, avoiding tension on the wires and preventing them from dangling so they cannot be inadvertently pulled out.

Mark the wires as either positive or ground and negative.

Attach pacemaker control boxes to the bed with a safety pin. This minimizes the risk that the pacemaker could fall on the floor when a child is held or is up in the chair.

If wires are disconnected from the pacemaker, place them in a finger cot or part of a disposable glove and tape the wires to the child's chest.

Protect pacer wires from microshock. Avoid placing any electrical equipment on the bed, such as infusion pumps or tape recorders. Remove all liquids near electrical equipment or pacing wires.

Temporary wires are pulled out at the bedside before discharge by the health care provider.

After discontinuation of pacing wires, monitor the child for signs and symptoms of cardiac decompensation.

spaces, diffuses back into the systemic system. Because of excessive total body fluids, diuretics and fluid restrictions may be necessary.

Postoperatively, assess for hydration by palpating fontanels in infants, checking mucous membranes and skin turgor, and assessing for signs of edema. Edema is most evident in the hands, feet, sacrum, and periorbital areas. Fluid restrictions are calculated, and intake is adjusted to meet limitations. When children are stable, weigh them daily and closely monitor and document intake and output. Hypotensive episodes can be treated with small IV fluid volume boluses given as ordered. When the child can tolerate oral intake, fluid limits are advanced slowly.

Monitor urine output, which is an indicator of fluid volume status and of end-organ perfusion, hourly while indwelling urinary catheters are in place. Renal failure is more likely to occur in children with heart disease associated with cyanosis and in those with periods of hypotension. Monitor the child's electrolytes as well as other pertinent laboratory values. Acid or base deficits may be related to poor pulmonary function. Acidosis is also an indicator of poor cardiac output. Hypokalemia is treated with IV bolus doses of potassium while the child is in the ICU.

Promoting Respiratory Function

Ensure that chest tubes remain patent and monitor and evaluate drainage, noting its consistency and color. Mediastinal chest tubes are discontinued after drainage subsides, which is usually by the second postoperative day. Although the procedure is quick, removing tape from dressings and skin is painful, and removal of chest tubes is uncomfortable. Medicate the child for pain well before the removal of chest tubes.

ALERT　*More than 1 mL/kg/hr chest tube drainage during the immediate postoperative period is considered excessive. If a coagulopathy is ruled out, too much bleeding may necessitate the child's return to surgery so that the surgeon can explore for potentially bleeding vessels.*

During cardiopulmonary bypass, the child's lungs are deflated, causing atelectasis. Also, cardiopulmonary bypass causes water and sodium retention and potassium depletion, so fluid settles in the interstitial spaces of the pleura, which increases body weight temporarily. Changes occur in the alveoli, and small pulmonary vessels become more permeable, resulting in interstitial pulmonary edema. This edema causes leukocyte aggregation and sequestration in the lung, creating a mild decrease in lung compliance. Moreover, sternal pain can deter a patient from coughing and taking deep breaths to reexpand the lungs.

Perform pulmonary assessment and document changes as they occur. Note the child's general appearance and color. Mild tachypnea and decreased tidal volume usually occur postoperatively. Check for signs and symptoms of impaired pulmonary function, including dyspnea, tachycardia, tachypnea, pallor, diaphoresis, adventitious breath sounds, poor cough, and use of accessory muscles. Irritability, exhaustion, and an alarmed look can also be signs of respiratory distress. Cyanosis, abnormal arterial blood gas values, and low oxygen saturation levels can be normal in children with intracardiac mixing.

Most children are extubated within 24 hours of surgery, with some, such as older children and those who are predicted to be stable, being extubated during surgery. However, critically ill postoperative patients can require ventilation for cardiopulmonary support over many days. Perform endotracheal suctioning as needed, noting the character, amount, and consistency of pulmonary secretions.

After the child has been extubated, ensure that the airway is patent and monitor for stridor or wheezing. Assess chest wall rise and expansion and respiratory rate and quality. Position infants in the "sniffing position," with the head slightly back and nose pointing up. Elevate the head of the bed to encourage lung expansion and ease the work of breathing. Administer supplemental oxygen and wean as tolerated. Perform pulmonary hygiene including coughing, deep breathing, breathing treatments, incentive spirometry, and nasotracheal suctioning. Chest physiotherapy is used to mobilize secretions and reinflate regions of atelectasis. Schedule nursing care and cluster tasks to prevent exhaustion and hypoxia. As the child tolerates it, encourage activity. Administer pain medication on a regular basis. Balance minimizing pain and maximizing alertness so the patient can produce a strong cough.

Postoperative cardiac surgical patients are at risk for developing pleural effusions. Effusions can develop from an imbalance between filtration and reabsorption of pleural fluids. Chylothorax, a condition in which a characteristic type of lymph fluid called chyle accumulates in the chest cavity, may develop. The accumulation of chyle in the chest cavity leads to difficulty breathing because the lungs cannot expand normally. Chylothorax may develop when the thoracic duct is injured during manipulation of the structures within the thoracic cavity. Chylothorax may be managed with ventilatory support, as indicated, and pleural fluid drainage. A fat-restricted diet supplemented with medium-chain triglycerides may be ordered to reduce chyle production. If so, explain the rationale for this to the child and parent and encourage the child to select appropriate foods. Somatostatin or octreotide may be given intravenously or subcutaneously. Monitor for adverse effects, including diarrhea, hypoglycemia, and hypotension.

Preventing Hemorrhage

Be alert for signs of acute bleeding, which may include increased heart rate, narrowing pulse pressures, and decreased perfusion and blood pressure. Bleeding can occur from the numerous suture lines in the heart and great vessels. Neonates with an immature liver and clotting system are at higher risk for bleeding. Cardiopulmonary bypass also traumatizes blood from the mechanical actions of the blood passing through the pump and tubing. While on bypass, the patient is fully anticoagulated (heparinized) to keep blood from clotting in the pump tubing. Anticoagulation is reversed after the surgical repairs are complete, but it can lead to clotting abnormalities postoperatively. Ensure that blood is readily available. Monitor the child's clotting factors, complete blood count, and platelets. Blood is replaced as necessary, but judiciously. Cardiac nursing units have an emergency sternotomy tray available and a protocol for reopening a chest incision in the ICU in the event of an emergency such as sudden or excessive bleeding.

Monitoring Neurologic Functioning

Neurologic insults may result from hypotensive states, hypoxia, or an embolic event. However, the causes are not always clear. Perform a neurologic examination, including level of consciousness, pupillary response, movement of extremities, and responses to stimuli. Be alert for other changes that may indicate alterations in neurologic status, such as irritability, a high-pitched cry, poor feeding, or rigidity. Subtle neurologic changes such as poor eye focusing or confusion are usually normal and transient. More severe changes include seizures, coma, and one-sided weakness.

Seizures that are related to neurologic dysfunction or electrolyte imbalances may occur. Seizures may be difficult to distinguish from normal jitteriness (see Table 14-4). Subtle signs of focal seizure activity might include chewing, eye deviation, or hypotonia. Anticonvulsant medications are administered to suppress seizure activity.

Preventing Infection

Children who are particularly debilitated pre- or postoperatively, who require prolonged ventilation, or who are undernourished are especially at risk for infection. Prophylactic antibiotics are usually administered prior to the surgical incision and for 48 hours after surgery.

Assess temperature and all dressings frequently, and change dressings based on agency policy and procedures. Document the absence or presence of redness, exudate, edema, the approximation of the chest incision, and any invasive line insertion sites. Dress and secure pacing wires to the chest and label for easy access in case of an emergency (see Nursing Interventions 15-2). Monitor white blood cell count values daily.

Managing Sedation and Pain

While a child is critically ill, sedation can be a component of hemodynamic management. Because sedation reduces SVR and PVR, it may improve cardiac performance. When a child is heavily sedated, the eyelids may not shut completely; provide eye care to prevent corneal damage.

Pain and anxiety are major issues for patients and families. After assessing for possible causes of pain and adequacy of pain control interventions, medicate the child appropriately (see Chapter 10). It is important for children to be comfortable enough to take deep breaths, cough, and be involved in activities between resting. Assess the child for signs and symptoms of pain, which include crying; restlessness; irritability; grimacing; splinting; rigid posture; and increased heart rate, respiration, or blood pressure. Position the child for comfort. Provide comfort measures such as bundling (for infants), placing the child in a particular position, or providing a pacifier. Use other noninvasive procedures to augment the effectiveness of

opioid pain medications, such as distractions like cartoons, music, favorite or new toys, or a soothing voice. Supplement opioid analgesia with acetaminophen. Administered on a regular basis, acetaminophen alleviates the general soreness of surgery, does not suppress respirations, and allows a child to be alert and interact.

Managing Nutrition

If a child is extubated; has active bowel sounds; is passing flatus; and has a soft, nondistended abdomen, the child may be ready to resume oral feeding.

Infants are started on a 5% dextrose solution or pediatric electrolyte solution. The older child is given ice chips and sips of water. When giving fluid, elevate the child's head 30 to 40 degrees; alternately, have the parent hold the child in his or her lap. Observe whether the suck–swallow reflex is normal. After the feeding, keep the child's head elevated for 30 minutes to prevent vomiting. As the child demonstrates tolerance of fluids by mouth, the volume of maintenance IV fluids is decreased. Calculate 24-hour fluid totals based on the ordered fluid limit: subtract the ordered IV therapy fluids to determine the remaining amount of fluid for oral intake per hour. Fluid limits are based on the child's "dry weight."

When the child is allowed to eat, document daily nutritional intake. Arrange a dietary consult if the child has the diagnosis of failure to thrive or demonstrates poor nutritional intake.

Feedings via a nasogastric tube may be needed for a critically ill neonate until he or she is strong enough to receive oral feedings. This process may take 1 to 2 months with the help of a feeding specialist (Woodward, 2011).

Providing Psychosocial Support

After a child is extubated and is hemodynamically stable, the child may increase activity and sit up in a chair even before most invasive lines are discontinued. When lines are removed, children may ambulate and begin to participate in activities in the playroom. Part of a nurse's postoperative interaction is to boost confidence. Children may be afraid to move and walk because of fear and pain. Providing positive reinforcement and prodding a child to increase activity may help smooth recovery from surgery.

An important nursing intervention is to lessen the negative effects of surgery on the child's physical, emotional, and social well-being. Negative behavioral changes, such as clinging behavior, fear of uniforms, depression, or regression, are normal and to be expected. Uncooperative behaviors are self-protective and are an expression of anger. A combination of medications for pain, distraction techniques, comfort measures, prodding the child to advance activities, and accepting negative behaviors may help a child cope with the pain and stress of hospitalization.

KidKare When a child is overwhelmed by multiple lines and tubes, he or she may choose one item about which to complain constantly, such as tape on an arm. The child may focus on something seemingly trivial because of the inability to fight all current stress and the lack of control over the situation. Reassure parents that this coping mechanism is normal.

Parents suffer greatly at the sight of ill children and their inability to protect them from pain. Parents usually protect and comfort their child continually in day-to-day life. Normally, a parent controls every aspect of a child's life and meets all physical and emotional needs. At home, parents decide when to feed, bathe, change, put down for naps, and plan activities. Suddenly, they are compelled to relinquish their child to strangers whom they allow to perform strange, painful, and unusual procedures in hopes of an improved future. This loss of control, although voluntary, may be overwhelming and may cause parents to feel guilty, saddened, and stressed.

Help by encouraging parents to express fears and concerns regarding their child's condition. Encourage families to participate in a child's care as often as they can and to do as much as they feel comfortable doing. Promote parents' touching and comforting of their child and allow them to hold the child as much as is practical. Explain all procedures to parents while encouraging questions and enabling them to verbalize concerns. Parents benefit from continual updates on the child's status and progression. Also, nurses are instrumental in making referrals to support systems when needed.

Community Care

Assess discharge planning needs in advance and provide follow-up referrals if necessary. Discharge teaching includes postoperative expectations and written discharge instructions (Teaching Intervention Plan 15-2). To promote recovery, parents must be comfortable with activity restrictions for discharge.

Discharge instructions must include details about immunizations. Immunizations are avoided around the time of surgery. Otherwise, despite illnesses and hospitalizations, instruct families to maintain immunizations at scheduled times.

Medical alert bracelets are not considered necessary for all children with cardiac conditions but they are recommended for children with pacemakers, heart transplants, and automatic implantable cardioverter defibrillators (AICDs) and for those receiving anticoagulant therapy. Children who have a history of seizure activity after surgery may wear bracelets, as recommended by the health care provider, until they are seizure free for a specified time.

Neurologic growth and development are frequently impaired in children with CHD. Impairment is indicated by factors such as lower IQs, difficulty with practical reasoning tasks, language delays, hypotonia, poor eye–hand coordination, gross and fine motor delays, behavioral difficulties, and personal social difficulties (Majnemer et al., 2008). Referral to programs with physical, occupational, and speech and language therapy, plus educational and psychological support, may be indicated.

PACEMAKERS

Pacemakers can be used in children who have impaired impulse formation or conduction problems and are symptomatic. Bradycardia requiring pacemaker insertion in children is of primarily two types. One type, *sick sinus syndrome*, or *sinus node dysfunction*, occurs when the heart's pacemaker functions normally but not fast enough to provide an adequate cardiac output. *Atrioventricular block*, the second category of bradycardia, occurs when the pacemaker functions appropriately but the signal is not transmitted through to the atrioventricular node and ventricles. Atrioventricular block may be caused by a congenital heart block, medications, or a heart infection or may occur as a postsurgical complication.

Most pacemakers are placed in the cardiac catheterization laboratory. In children, leads are placed on the external heart muscle of the atrium and ventricles; the generator is inserted in either the chest or abdominal space. The location of lead placement depends on the type of heart problem and size of the patient. If pacemaker placement is not successful in the cardiac catheterization laboratory, surgical placement involving a thoracotomy and abdominal incision is required. In the past, permanent pacemakers were too large to be placed in small children, but modern pacemakers are now small and lightweight enough that they have been used in infants. Provide routine postsedation or postoperative care as indicated.

Community Care

Children have their pacemakers checked regularly on an outpatient basis. A specialized computer and magnet that communicates through radiofrequency signals is placed over the pacemaker generator and is used to change settings and evaluate the pacemaker. It is a noninvasive way to check the activities of the pacemaker and battery usage.

As part of the pacemaker package, children are given a transtelephonic system to take home. This system enables them to periodically transmit ECGs to the clinic over their home telephones. The placement of a pacemaker requires long-term follow-up and future surgeries. Periodically, minor surgery is required to replace the battery in the pacemaker. Lead wires can be fractured. Replacing lead wires involves a surgery that is more extensive than just battery replacement.

Psychosocial responses to pacemaker insertion depend on the personal responses of individual families. The child may have body image disturbance or self-concept changes caused by scars, activity restrictions, and continual follow-up (see Chapter 12 for nursing interventions).

Instruct parents of children with pacemakers to have the child avoid contact sports such as gymnastics and football. In addition, children must avoid highly magnetic areas, such as magnetic resonance imaging machines. Parents also need to know that high-voltage areas, such as those near high-tension wires, can also interfere with the function of a pacemaker. Emphasize to parents that modern microwave ovens do not affect pacemakers.

CARDIAC TRANSPLANTATION

Cardiac transplantation has become an option for extending the length and quality of life of children who have exhausted available medical treatment and palliative surgeries and are no longer surviving well, as

TIP 15-2: A TEACHING INTERVENTION PLAN for the Child After Cardiac Surgery: Discharge Instructions

Nursing Diagnosis and Family Outcomes

- Deficient knowledge: Lack of information regarding postoperative care of the child at home
  Outcomes: Family will provide child with support, assistance, and encouragement to manage or master tasks related to postoperative care.
  Child, as age appropriate, and family will follow written discharge instructions, seeking assistance as needed to ensure safety and promote the well-being of the child.
  Child, as age appropriate, and family will demonstrate an understanding of the child's postoperative care needs.
  Child, as age appropriate, and family will verbalize measures to meet the child's needs.

Treatment of the Child

Medications
- Carry a list of your child's medications with you at all times (the name of each medication, the dosage, and how often it is taken).
- Always get your prescriptions filled before you run out.
- Never stop giving any medicine. Your cardiologist will determine when the medication is to be changed or stopped.
- Bring the medications and the list when you come in for your first follow-up visit.

Wound Care
- Only sponge bathe your child the first week. Do not apply lotions or powders to the incision site during the first 2 weeks after surgery.
- Keep the incision area clean and dry. If the incision area gets dirty or soiled, cleanse the area with mild soap and water.
- Do not remove Steri-Strips placed over the incision site. Occasionally, these strips become loose and fall off. Do not worry if they do.
- Observe the incision site daily for redness, swelling, or drainage.
- Be aware that tingling, itching, and numbness are normal sensations from the wound and will eventually go away.
- If there are areas of the incision that are constantly irritated by clothing or the chin rubbing, cover them with a bandage to prevent irritation and to promote faster healing.
- Keep a shirt over the incision when your child is outside to protect it from the sunlight.

Activity
- Gradually encourage the child to increase activity each day. Generally, children recover quickly and are able to participate in most of their normal activities. Activity level improves as the child recovers.
- Be aware that infants and children tend to pace themselves and will rest if they feel tired. Try to maintain a sensible balance of rest and exercise.
- Avoid lifting your child under the arms because this may cause discomfort by placing stress on the surgical site. Instead, slide your hands under your child's buttocks and support the chest when lifting.
- To allow the breast bone to heal, for 6 weeks, do not allow the child to engage in rough play or activities such as bicycling, climbing, skateboarding, or contact sports; avoid activities that would put pressure on the child's chest, such as heavy lifting, or any activity that might cause a blow to the chest.
- Try to avoid large crowds and/or people with active infections for at least 2 weeks (e.g., birthday parties, church, school, shopping malls).
- Be alert for possible clinging behavior and/or sleep disturbances initially. Use positive reassurance and assist in returning to a normal routine.

Diet
- Allow your child to return to his or her normal diet with no restrictions.

Immunizations
- Expect immunizations to be delayed, normally for 6–8 weeks after surgery.

Dental Care
- Whenever possible, delay routine dental care for 4–5 months after your child's surgery. Remember, some children with cardiac problems are required to take antibiotics for dental work to prevent an infection in the child's heart.

Discomfort
- Administer acetaminophen, unless otherwise ordered by the health care provider, for complaints of some incisional or chest discomfort after discharge.

Contact Your Health Care Provider if

You think there is a change in your child's behavior, which may or may not indicate illness. Watch for the following signs of illness:
- A change in feeding pattern
- Breathing harder or faster
- Puffiness of the hands, feet, or face, especially around the eyes
- Excessive sweating, especially evident on the forehead
- Weakness, irritability, weak cry in infant
- Cool, pale, mottled hands or feet
- Few wet diapers or poor urine output
- Temperature higher than 101° F (38.4° C)

demonstrated by disabling cardiac symptoms or limited life expectancy. The diagnosis that most often leads to cardiac transplantation in older children is cardiomyopathy. Congenital cardiac defects associated with cardiac transplantation are HLHS and other complex single-ventricle hearts. Survival after cardiac transplantation has been correlated to age at the time of transplantation and ranges from 11 to 18 years. Children younger than 1 year of age at the time of transplantation have the longest median survival rate, whereas those transplanted between 11 and 17 years of age have a median survival of 11 years (Kirk et al., 2010).

Pediatric Donors

Although the list of infants and children waiting for transplantation is shorter than that for adults, the supply of donor pediatric hearts is extremely limited. Children on the waiting list outnumber the donor heart supply. Most pediatric donors have died from sudden infant death syndrome, trauma, or birth asphyxia.

Determining when to place a child on the waiting list for an available heart is difficult. Decisions depend on the expected natural history of the particular underlying heart problem. Decisions regarding when the heart failure is terminal, coupled with the shortages of available donors, severely complicate the timing of transplantation surgeries.

For a child to be included on the waiting list, the possibility of any other systemic diseases that might rule out the viability of transplantation must be explored. Also, a psychosocial profile of the family that considers their resources and commitment to the program is developed. The depth of ethical decisions, the financial burden, the need for patient adherence to medications, and constant follow-up make the care of these children complex.

Once a child is listed with the United Network for Organ Sharing on the national computer, they can be matched with a donor based on blood type, body weight, length of time on the waiting list, and the child's medical stability.

After a heart transplant, the major challenge in caring for the child is maintaining the balance between immunosuppression and factors such as adverse medication side effects, infection, and rejection of the donor organ. For the child, side effects from, and expense of, immunosuppressive medications and constant follow-up care are generally the areas of greatest concern. For the health care practitioner, the largest issue is the balance between infection and rejection, which hinges on maintaining immunosuppression.

Rejection and Immunosuppression

Rejection occurs because of an incompatibility of cell surface antigen, which invokes a humoral and cellular immune response against the heart. Rejection of the foreign heart is attempted by all recipients' immune systems. The recipient's body never learns to accept the foreign tissue.

Management of rejection varies but traditionally has included triple-medication therapy with cyclosporine, azathioprine (Imuran), and prednisone. Triple therapy is used so that the practitioner can prescribe lower dosages of each medicine, thus decreasing overall side effects. Susceptibility to infections is a complication of all the immunosuppressive medications used today.

Cyclosporine inhibits T-cell function, but exactly how it works is unclear. Cyclosporine is the immunosuppressive drug that has increased both rate and duration of survival among transplant recipients. Side effects include tremors, gum hyperplasia, hirsutism, flushing, nephrotoxicity, seizures, and hypertension.

Azathioprine (Imuran) is a suppressor of bone marrow function that inhibits purine synthesis and metabolism. The white blood cell count of children receiving this drug is followed closely to monitor for the side effect of depressed bone marrow function. Side effects may include high blood pressure, tremors, gum hyperplasia, hirsutism, and nephrotoxicity.

Prednisone, a corticosteroid, influences the immune system through its strong anti-inflammatory action and immunologic effect. Because of the severity of side effects of prednisone, transplant recipients with mild and few rejection episodes may be weaned off prednisone therapy. Side effects of corticosteroids include poor wound healing, ulcers, growth impairment, delayed sexual maturation, glucose intolerance, increased appetite, hyperlipidemia, cushingoid appearance, acne, and sun sensitivity. The development of a cushingoid appearance manifested by excessive weight, overgrowth of hair, and moon-shaped face can be a great source of stress for a school-aged child or adolescent, necessitating close monitoring for adherence. Usually, most of the symptoms subside in those children able to tolerate lower dosages of the immunosuppressive medications.

Serial myocardial biopsies are the most reliable predictor of rejection. They are performed in children of all ages but are technically more difficult in infants. Children are also followed closely through noninvasive clinical evaluation, including echocardiography, chest x-ray, and evidence of signs and symptoms. Episodes of rejection may be managed by courses of IV steroid therapy or other strong immunosuppressive medications.

Over a life span, the long-term effects from immunosuppressive therapy on small children are unknown. Chronic usage of drugs for immunosuppression has led to renal dysfunction, malignancies, and hypertension. One important limiting factor for long-term survival of heart transplant recipients is cardiac allograft vasculopathy, which is an accelerated form of coronary artery disease. It occurs in 50% of patients during the first several years after surgery. The only definitive treatment is retransplantation.

Routine immunizations are still given to transplant recipients even though they are receiving immunosuppressive agents. However, no live viruses are used. Normal childhood infections in these children generally are well tolerated. Although transplantation has enabled many children to survive otherwise terminal diseases, it is not a panacea and is still an evolving field of care.

Psychological Stress

Children receiving heart transplants experience psychological stress, which may lead to anxiety, behavioral difficulties, depression, and other psychiatric problems.

Normalizing the child's life as much as possible by providing routine, expectations for conduct, discipline, and developmentally appropriate activities may help diminish some of the negative effects of a chronic condition (see Chapter 12).

SUPPORTIVE CARE

When parents learn that their child has the diagnosis of a heart condition, substantial psychological and social consequences affect the family. The heart is viewed by many as an extremely important organ in the body that symbolizes the emotion of love. Parents usually need time to cope with the realities of having a child with a cardiac condition.

Parents of children with a correctable cardiac lesion may be just as anxious, if not more anxious, than those of a child with a very complex congenital lesion. Many children with cardiac lesions have no outward signs of cardiac disease. Specific symptoms that would cause the parents to feel that their child has a problem may not be evident. These parents may also experience fear and guilt about putting their otherwise "perfect" child through medical interventions. The parents may accept the child's condition more easily if the practitioner can point out some measurable feature, such as the echocardiogram results and the location of the lesion, to assure them that the corrective intervention is essential. Seeing the chest radiograph of an enlarged heart with heart failure or comparing a poor growth curve may help parents appreciate and understand the existence of the heart defect.

Parental support groups or parent meetings with other families of children with CHD may be a source of support for parents, helping them to sort out the emotions and stresses of having a child diagnosed with CHD.

Parents of symptomatic children are often emotionally drained and have infrequent breaks from child care responsibilities. Babysitters are often fearful to take on the management of medication administration and the emotional burden of an ill child. Parents may be fearful of creating situations in which their child could become symptomatic. The simple activities one normally does with an infant, such as feeding, can become tedious and painstaking events. Encourage parents to take personal time, alone or as a couple, and develop respite options.

Treatment options for a child with heart disease are not always clear and usually include expensive and invasive procedures. At times, families of children with complex heart disease are required to make choices for their child that will markedly alter the course of that child's life. Financial and religious factors may influence these decisions. For example, parents may continue a job they may have otherwise quit in order to maintain their health insurance benefits or may refuse a job transfer so they can stay near a medical center where they are comfortable with the staff and facility. The needs of families in a world that can provide high-technology care are multifaceted, involving ethical, religious, financial, and emotional components.

COMMUNITY CARE

Most school-aged children with CHD are able to attend normal schools. If a child is being kept out of school, contact a social worker or the child's cardiologist to confirm that a medical need exists for the child to be denied access to school. Some parents may have inappropriate fears about the vulnerability of their child and may overprotect the child. Most children can be encouraged to participate in playground activities at their level of tolerance but should not be pressured to exercise beyond their personal limits.

Children with severe cardiac lesions that need a more sedentary lifestyle require school programs to be modified on an individual basis. Such modifications enable the child to participate at a level the child can tolerate. For instance, a nap could be substituted for recess activities. Transportation to and from school could be arranged instead of having the child walk. If a period of school is missed, it is often associated with a procedure such as surgery or cardiac catheterization. Tell parents to encourage classmates to keep in contact with the ill child, perhaps visiting the child's home and sending cards to the hospital.

Children with minor cardiac issues, or those whose lesions are repaired, generally can travel without limitations. Extreme heat and sudden climate change can stress ill children and can cause venous pooling from vasodilation. Aggressive travel itineraries may overtax the endurance level of a child with limited reserve. Children with unrepaired lesions, heart failure, cyanosis, or the propensity for sudden illness or complications need to have ready access to appropriate emergency care. After cardiac transplantation, children are not allowed to travel to underdeveloped countries, where the risk of illness from water sources and limited medical care is greater.

If the family is traveling to a large metropolitan area, the child's cardiologist usually can locate a physician in the vacation area to call if necessary. Instruct parents to carry a list of emergency contact medical personnel and medications and a short, written synopsis of the child's history.

Airplane travel or travel to areas of high altitude is restricted in children with heart disease that is associated with cyanosis, pulmonary hypertension, and severe heart failure. Higher elevations have a lower partial pressure of oxygen, which may further compromise the child's oxygen-carrying capacity. Supplemental oxygen is used if high-altitude travel is necessary. Commercial airlines will not allow families to bring their own oxygen tanks. If oxygen support is necessary, arrangements must be made in advance with the airlines and with a medical supply company at the family's destination.

Well-child care and teaching must not be overlooked when caring for a child with a cardiac defect or problem. Historically, antibiotics were provided for routine dental care and medical interventions as prophylaxis against infective endocarditis for most patients with heart lesions. The American Heart Association (Wilson et al., 2007) changed the antibiotic prophylaxis for dental procedures to include patients with cardiac conditions associated with the highest risk of adverse outcomes from endocarditis, including prosthetic cardiac valves, previous endocarditis, unrepaired CHD associated with cyanosis, 6 months' postcomplete repair of CHD disease with prosthetic material, or repaired CHD with prosthetic material and a residual defect. Antibiotic prophylaxis is not recommended for the placement, adjustment, or removal of orthodontic appliances for any cardiac patients. Antibiotic prophylaxis solely to prevent infective endocarditis is no longer recommended for any cardiac patient having a gastrointestinal or genitourinary procedure. A wallet card with the recommendations is available from the American Heart Association for the patient and family.

NURSING PLAN OF CARE

The effects of heart disease on the child and family are both acute and long term. When heart disease is suspected, the health care team acts rapidly to ensure that the child's physiologic status is as stable as possible. Nursing diagnoses during the early critical stages focus on oxygenation, cardiac output, and fluid volume concerns related to the child's specific condition (see Nursing Plan of Care 15-1).

Because the heart is vital to human existence, the presence of a cardiac condition is likely to cause considerable apprehension and fear for the parents and the family. The plan of care for the child with a cardiac condition must include interventions to help the parents cope so that they are able to deal with the facts related to their child's illness. An important role of the nurse is to assist the family in understanding the child's condition and the treatment plan.

Provide teaching and emotional support to children and their families. Prepare them for testing and procedures. Monitor the child on an ongoing basis, particularly during procedures. Protect the child from injury while also maintaining readiness for any necessary emergency support in case the child becomes hemodynamically compromised.

Most children affected with CHD or an acquired heart condition are able to lead normal lives. Nursing care that addresses alterations in development, body image, and self-esteem concerns is indicated when the child's condition is severely limiting or disabling (see Chapter 12) or the child's life span is limited (see Chapter 13). Chapter 11 discusses nursing care of the child who is hospitalized or undergoing surgery. Chapter 10 provides an in-depth discussion of pain management.

ALTERATIONS IN CARDIAC STATUS

Heart disease in children can be classified as congenital or acquired. Heart failure or cyanosis may occur as a result of heart disease regardless of the etiology. An understanding of both heart failure and cyanosis is critical to providing care to children with heart disease regardless of whether it is congenital or acquired. Both conditions will be reviewed, followed by discussion of congenital and acquired heart diseases.

HEART FAILURE

Heart failure is one of the major manifestations of cardiac disease. It is a clinical syndrome in which the heart's pumping ability is inadequate to meet the metabolic demands of the body. Heart failure is usually seen in infants, because most cardiac lesions are repaired or palliated during the first year of life. If a well child presents with heart failure beyond the first year of life, it may be the result of an acquired cardiac disease such as rheumatic fever, bacterial endocarditis, or viral cardiomyopathy. Older children may present with heart failure later in life because of the presence of a previously undiscovered lesion.

 QUESTION: Based on Gabriella's current condition, would she be at risk for developing heart failure if her PDA goes untreated? Why or why not?

Pathophysiology

Heart failure may be a result of excessive circulation to the lungs, volume and/or pressure overloading, or poor myocardial function. Heart failure can be a right- or left-sided heart problem, although children usually present in biventricular failure. Right ventricular dysfunction causes right ventricular end-diastolic pressure to increase, leading to systemic engorgement. Left ventricular dysfunction causes left ventricular end-diastolic pressure to increase, causing pulmonary venous engorgement. The ventricles dilate in response to elevated pressures.

The presence of a congenital heart defect is the most common reason for children to develop heart failure (Rossano et al., 2012). Lesions with left-to-right shunts typically result in volume overloading. For example, a child with a large VSD has shunting from the left side of the heart to the right. Because blood travels the path of least resistance, some blood crosses from the left ventricle to the right side without exiting the aorta and circulates to the lungs repeatedly, causing an extra load on the lungs. An obstructive lesion of the left heart may cause pressure overload. For example, in the case of aortic stenosis, the left ventricle is constantly pumping against a restricted valve. Depending on the stressors and severity of the stenosis, this obstruction could lead to failure of the left heart. Neonates with a severe left-sided obstruction may be without symptoms initially because their patent ductus is open; therefore, pressures may be relieved by shunting across the patent ductus. Symptoms appear as the ductus closes (Madriago & Silberbach, 2010).

Nonstructural conditions, such as a chronic heart rhythm disturbance or cardiomyopathy that is causing poor myocardial function, may also lead to heart failure. Arrhythmias that may cause heart failure include chronic supraventricular tachycardia, atrial fibrillation or flutter, and congenital heart block. Supraventricular tachycardia is the most common emergently presenting arrhythmia in the pediatric population. In dilated cardiomyopathy, the cardiac chambers are dilated and myocardial contraction is weakened, leading to heart failure.

CHART 15-2 Clinical Manifestations of Heart Failure

Systemic Venous Congestion

Weight gain

Hepatomegaly

Edema

Jugular venous distention (children)

Pulmonary Venous Congestion

Tachypnea

Dyspnea

Cough (children)

Wheezes

Rales

Retractions (infants)

Nasal flaring (infants)

Compensatory Response

Tachycardia

Cardiomegaly

Gallop murmur

Diaphoretic

Fatigue

Failure to thrive

Heart failure leads to pulmonary venous congestion, systemic venous congestion, and poor myocardial pumping (Chart 15-2). Increased pulmonary blood flow is the physiologic effect of the most common heart defects. Symptoms occur when the heart's compensatory mechanisms have exceeded the point of efficiency and cardiac output is diminished.

As the heart fails, the body uses available compensatory mechanisms in an attempt to meet the circulatory needs. Tachycardia, a compensatory response to decreased cardiac output, results from an increased release of catecholamines (epinephrine and norepinephrine) and causes rapid filling of stiff ventricles in an attempt to increase the force and rate of myocardial contraction. Tachycardia also increases oxygen consumption of the heart. Tachycardia that is too rapid decreases the heart's filling time and coronary perfusion. Although initially it has a compensatory advantage, excessive tachycardia may become destructive, ultimately impeding cardiac output (Madriago & Silberbach, 2010).

Cardiomegaly occurs as a muscular response to the need to increase cardiac output. The heart dilates to increase the myocardial fiber stretch to improve the force of contraction. Stretching and dilation are advantageous, within limits, to increase cardiac output. Beyond a certain point, however, the increased myocardial stretch results in diminished pumping efficiency and fails.

Systemic Venous Congestion (Right-Sided Failure)

Elevation of right atrial filling pressures restricts the emptying of the vena cava into the right atrium. Blood pooling in the venous circulation raises systemic venous pressures, resulting in fluid sequestration to the interstitial spaces and hepatomegaly. Blood flow to the kidneys is diminished, and the renin–angiotensin–aldosterone system is stimulated, resulting in vasoconstriction and sodium and water retention, which further compounds fluid retention and decreases urine output.

Pulmonary Venous Congestion (Left-Sided Failure)

Imbalances between filtration and reabsorption of fluid in the pulmonary capillary bed caused by increased pulmonary capillary pressures can lead to respiratory symptoms arising from pulmonary congestion.

ANSWER: Gabriella's PDA results in pulmonary volume overload as a result of her left-to-right shunt. Over time, her respiratory status will suffer further because of the pulmonary congestion, her pulmonary vasculature will be damaged because of the increased pressure within the vasculature, and her cardiac musculature will be damaged as it compensates for the increased blood volume flowing to and from the lungs, resulting in heart failure.

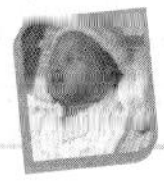

Assessment

The diagnosis of heart failure is typically based on findings from the child's history, physical assessment, and diagnostic tests. When obtaining a history, ask whether the child fatigues easily or exhibits poor exercise tolerance. Parents may report that an infant tires with feedings and is anxious, irritable, and difficult to console. Failure to thrive, growth retardation, or poor weight gain (e.g., a child who is in the bottom percentile of the growth charts for weight, despite normal height) are all suspicious signs, as are poor nutritional intake, nausea, failure to meet developmental milestones at a normal pace, and delays in gross motor skills.

During the physical assessment, note any abnormalities in the cardiac assessment. When the heart is auscultated, a gallop rhythm or extra heart sound (S_3 gallop murmur) may be heard, resulting from excessive preload and ventricular dilation. On palpation, the pulses may be weak and thready. A hyperactive precordium, noted when viewing the child's chest, may indicate cardiac enlargement.

Note weight gain and swelling of soft tissue in dependent or sensitive areas, such as the sacrum, scrotum, or eyelids, which may indicate fluid retention from right-sided heart failure. Distended neck veins (despite sitting up) and ankle edema are other areas less commonly used to assess fluid retention in children. Hepatomegaly may indicate right-sided heart failure.

Tachypnea (shallow and rapid breathing) that worsens with feeding or activity can reflect pulmonary congestion and may indicate left-sided heart failure. Grunting, nasal flaring, and/or retractions that worsen in recumbent positions are manifestations of dyspnea, or increased work of breathing.

Irritation from bronchial edema may cause a chronic, dry, hacking cough. Pulmonary obstruction, which causes edema of the bronchial mucosa from a distended airway, may cause wheezing. One of the late signs of heart failure is rales on auscultation. Rales occur from fluid settling into the alveolar spaces, causing pulmonary edema.

Diaphoresis, fatigue, and exercise intolerance are important signs. During feeding or physical activity, the infant or child with heart failure may be diaphoretic. Diaphoresis, usually seen as a cool sweat on the forehead, occurs because of an increased sympathetic response triggered by increasing cardiac output stimulating *baroreceptors* (stretch receptors that respond to changes in blood pressure) in the vessels.

Diagnostic Tests

No single diagnostic test can confirm the diagnosis of heart failure. A chest radiograph is commonly used as part of the decision-making process. A positive radiograph shows cardiomegaly and increased pulmonary vascular markings from excessive pulmonary blood flow.

Nursing Diagnoses and Outcomes

QUESTION: Which nursing diagnosis best describes Gabriella the morning of the case study?

In addition to those listed in Nursing Plan of Care 15-1, the following nursing diagnoses and outcomes may apply to the child with heart failure:

Nursing Diagnosis: Ineffective breathing pattern related to effects of excessive fluid in lung spaces, breathing difficulties from poor cardiac output, and increased respiratory rate required to compensate
Outcomes:
• Child will exhibit normal respiratory rate and will perform normal work of breathing.
• Child will demonstrate clear breath sounds and oxygen saturation within normal limits for the child.
Nursing Diagnosis: Imbalanced nutrition: Less than body requirements related to effects of increased work of feeding and increased calorie requirements
Outcomes:
• Parents will verbally demonstrate understanding of feeding techniques and child's nutritional needs.
• Child will demonstrate growth curve appropriate for age.

ANSWER: Gabriella's nursing diagnosis is *Ineffective breathing pattern related to effects of excessive fluid in lung spaces and increased respiratory rate required to compensate.* This explains why her symptoms are respiratory, but the problem is cardiovascular.

Interdisciplinary Interventions

When caring for a child with heart failure, direct interventions at conserving energy and decreasing metabolic demands on the weakened myocardium. Interventions are also directed toward removing excess accumulated fluids

so that the pump has optimal preload (circulating blood volume). If a coexisting illness such as a viral infection exacerbates symptoms of heart failure, it must be treated. To maximize oxygen-carrying capacity, if the child is cyanotic, blood products and fluids may be ordered to maintain hematocrit and blood values at normal levels.

Unstable patients in heart failure from arrhythmias require immediate IV adenosine or synchronized cardioversion. Complete heart block is rare. Emergency treatment includes medications and temporary or permanent pacemaker placement as indicated. Occasionally, these arrhythmias are detected in utero, and the fetus is treated via medications given to the mother.

Oxygen Therapy

Administer oxygen judiciously. Full oxygen saturation decreases the work of breathing by increasing arterial oxygen levels, thereby relieving respiratory distress; however, oxygen can be detrimental because it is also a pulmonary vasodilator. Pulmonary vasodilation can cause increased tachypnea and fluid retention in the lung beds and worsen oxygenation, further exacerbating heart failure in cases in which the lungs are already overloaded. Therefore, children should not automatically be given oxygen to improve their respiratory status. Oxygen can actually worsen their symptoms over time. If oxygen is administered, monitor oxygen saturation levels to keep within limits appropriate for the child (see thePoint for Procedures: Oxygen Administration).

Pharmacologic Interventions

Pharmacologic methods of treatment aim to relieve symptoms and improve the heart's pumping ability, including optimizing preload, afterload, and contractility. Improving cardiac output by manipulating preload and afterload may have a potent hemodynamic effect; monitor children closely for tolerance and negative effects.

Diuretics are medications given to lessen the workload on the heart by removing extra fluids the heart has to pump, ultimately decreasing preload. In heart failure, the renal tubular system tries to increase preload under the action of the renin–angiotensin–aldosterone system by retaining sodium and water to increase circulating volume. Diuretics are given to counteract this compensatory mechanism. Furosemide (Lasix), which inhibits electrolyte reabsorption at the loop of Henle, is the most commonly used diuretic, but it promotes loss of potassium as well as sodium. Therefore, spironolactone (Aldactone), a potassium-sparing diuretic, is used with furosemide to prevent excessive potassium loss.

ALERT   *Diminished cardiac output compromises perfusion to the kidneys, requiring close monitoring of renal function. Diuretics improve urine output but do not specifically help renal perfusion.*

Positive inotropic agents are administered to improve myocardial contractility. Digoxin (Lanoxin) is a commonly used cardiac glycoside administered orally or intravenously as a positive inotrope. It decreases the workload of the heart and improves myocardial function. Dosages are given based on the child's weight. To avoid digoxin toxicity, ensure that blood levels, obtained periodically and when symptoms occur, are within normal limits.

caREminder

Digoxin toxicity is a serious complication of therapy in any age group. Signs and symptoms of digoxin toxicity in infants and children include nausea; vomiting; anorexia; and an irregular, low apical heart rate.

Teach parents to have the telephone number of a poison control center readily available in any household should accidental ingestion or overdose of digoxin occur. Instruct parents to keep digoxin out of the reach of children at all times and to allow only those family members who have been carefully trained to administer this medication. Digoxin has a very narrow safety margin with a narrow gap between therapeutic and toxic levels.

Sympathomimetic agents—the rapidly acting catecholamines dopamine, dobutamine, and epinephrine—are positive inotropic drugs that are administered intravenously to improve myocardial contractility. These agents are used most often in critical care areas. Common side effects, particularly with increased dosages, are tachycardia and arrhythmia.

Vasodilators enhance cardiac output by decreasing afterload, as measured by reduced left ventricular end-diastolic volume and pulmonary capillary wedge pressure. Vasodilators such as nitroglycerin dilate the systemic veins, leading to lowered blood pressure and reduced venous congestion, which in turn decreases preload. They also dilate the coronary arteries, improving myocardial blood flow.

Captopril (Capoten) and enalapril (Vasotec) are angiotensin-converting enzyme inhibitors. They are used to block the conversion of angiotensin I to angiotensin II; this action results in vasodilation and increased sodium excretion. Another arterial vasodilator is sodium nitroprusside (Nipride), which also reduces afterload. The amount of medication given is titrated by slowly increasing dosages based on the child's weight, symptoms, and level of tolerance.

Energy Conservation

In the presence of impaired circulation and pulmonary congestion, limit the child's energy expenditure by promoting rest (Clinical Judgment 15-1). Rest lowers metabolic requirements and oxygen needs. Schedule nursing care so that activities are clustered and followed by long periods of undisturbed rest. Sedation may be provided for an acutely ill child with heart failure who is restless and irritable to reduce oxygen demand. For young children and older children, television and video games provide an emotional distraction and encourage inactivity. Breathing and eating are strenuous activities for infants in heart failure, leaving no extra energy for play or motion. They tend to limit their own activity by falling asleep.

Learning to sit up, to walk, and other gross motor activities require extra energy that a child with limited cardiac reserves may not have. As the child's condition allows, encourage age-appropriate play to enhance cognitive and motor development. After surgical repair, when the child is no longer in heart failure, these children tend to catch up developmentally with their peers.

Positioning

In addition to receiving excessive circulation during heart failure, the lungs also have decreased compliance, requiring more work to expand. Small children may be propped up in an infant seat, ensuring that they are not slouched over—a position that causes pressure on the diaphragm and thus limits diaphragmatic excursion. An upright position also decreases pulmonary congestion by encouraging blood to pool in dependent areas, moving fluid away from the lungs and minimizing the work of breathing.

Nutritional Interventions

Feeding issues can be perplexing. Both the increased metabolic needs of the child's overworked heart and the extra work of breathing demand extra energy. The logical deduction is to encourage an infant to eat as much as possible. The drawback is that feeding takes energy, too. In addition, feeding distends the infant's abdomen, which exerts pressure on the diaphragm, decreasing lung expansion. Feeding also increases fluid levels in the circulatory system. Fluid restriction may be used for older children, but an infant's nutritional intake depends on fluids.

Because infants with heart failure fatigue easily, feedings may take longer than with healthy children. Small and frequent feedings are better tolerated and decrease the likelihood of vomiting. Formulas with increased calories and nutritional supplements are given to meet the greater caloric requirements.

Weigh the child daily, and document intake and output meticulously to follow trends in nutritional stability and diuresis. Because scales vary, weigh the child on the same scale daily at the same time before feeding. Fluid and sodium restrictions, although common for older children, vary by age and are individualized to the child.

Community Care

Teach parents the signs and symptoms of heart failure and the parameters for when they need to notify health care providers. The term *heart failure* conjures up an image in the parents' mind of a terminal state, which frightens families. Parents associate heart failure with the heart stopping suddenly. For many children, heart failure is a condition that can be medically managed and, if caused by a congenital heart defect, corrected with surgical repair. When teaching, include an explanation of the warning signs that indicate that a child's condition is deteriorating and that medical intervention is necessary. Give parents specific guidelines on how to administer medications, the rationale for each medication, and potential adverse reactions.

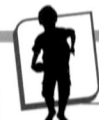

A Child's Adaptation to Restrictions of Condition

Six-year-old Jenny G. was on bed rest at home because of recurrent heart failure caused by myocarditis. Despite the fact that anything more than quiet activity made her short of breath and often worsened her failure to the degree where she would be too tired to even eat the next day, she was always sneaking out of her room and playing actively in the hall. She talked about being bored and missing all her friends and activities at school.

Jenny's teacher worked with her mother to develop a special project to be completed in conjunction with her classmates. She was put in charge of updating the classroom's dinosaur display. A giant dinosaur had been placed on a bulletin board near the front of the room. Using a collection of dinosaur cut-out books, Jenny was to get pictures of all the types of dinosaurs they discussed each day. She was also asked to practice her writing skills by putting her classmates' names on the cutout dinosaurs. To practice her arithmetic, she kept track of the number of dinosaurs she made each day and how many she sent in to her classmates by way of her friend who stopped by two or three times a week. Jenny had a great sense of pride in her accomplishment, along with quiet activity. Now that her friends have a reason to visit, they are more likely to stay to play a game after school, although they still want to play outdoors and the visits are still fairly brief. Jenny also got a 92 on her last math quiz.

Questions

1. Are these activities addressing the identified reason Jenny is not staying quiet?
2. What data from the vignette support your conclusion?
3. What other data would help confirm this conclusion?
4. What strategies would you use to promote Jenny's continued good health?
5. What outcomes would indicate that Jenny is doing well?

Answers

1. She reported feeling restless and bored and that she missed her friends from school. These activities give her something focused to accomplish each day and allow her to do the same activities as her classmates.
2. She is making the dinosaurs for the class, sending them in as requested, learning her math, and seeing her friends. She is also spending more quiet time at home as desired.
3. Her episodes of fatigue could be tracked. In addition, other physiologic parameters such as heart rate or blood pressure should indicate improvement.
4. Work with Jenny and her family to identify additional interventions such as this that can meet both her physiologic and psychosocial needs. Encourage Jenny to discuss her illness with her friends and to answer their questions.
5. Jenny is able to move back into the classroom easily with minimal loss of achievement as a result of her absence.

HEART DISEASE ASSOCIATED WITH CYANOSIS

Cyanosis is a sign of hypoxemia and is caused by circulating deoxygenated hemoglobin, as reflected in a bluish hue to the skin, nail beds, and mucous membranes.

Pathophysiology

When oxygen saturation of hemoglobin is reduced, the circulation compensates by increasing the extraction of oxygen by peripheral tissues. Reasons other than cardiac issues can cause a child to appear cyanotic. Structural changes in the lungs, such as bronchopulmonary dysplasia, pulmonary edema, pulmonary arterial venous fistulas, and some neurologic abnormalities, may cause cyanosis in a child. The nurse cannot assume that the child who appears dusky or cyanotic has a primary cardiac problem because clinical assessment of hypoxemia is notoriously unreliable.

Cyanosis in CHD results mainly from two anatomic situations. The first is that pulmonary venous blood, rather than being delivered to the systemic circulation, is being redelivered to the pulmonary circulation, increasing pulmonary blood flow, as occurs in TGA and total anomalous pulmonary venous return (TAPVR). The second is restricted pulmonary blood flow (right-to-left shunts), as occurs in pulmonary atresia and tetralogy of Fallot. The severity of cyanosis depends on the volume of pulmonary blood flow or the degree of intracardiac mixing (shunting).

Hematologic problems associated with cyanotic heart disease include polycythemia, dehydration, bleeding, clubbing of nail beds, hypoxic spells, neurologic injury, and negative developmental outcomes. Polycythemia is caused by low arterial oxygen levels that trigger erythropoietin production in the kidneys, which stimulates the bone marrow to increase red blood cell production. Polycythemia is a compensatory mechanism in which the body attempts to have more hemoglobin available to increase oxygen-carrying capacity and thereby improve oxygenation to tissues. When the hematocrit value reaches a level of 65% or more, blood viscosity increases to such a degree that there is a risk of complications such as cerebrovascular accidents or strokes. Children may also be anemic if not enough iron is present to create the excess hemoglobin.

Chronic tissue hypoxia also stimulates increased red blood cell production, creating a condition of polycythemia. This compensation increases the amount of hemoglobin available to carry oxygen to tissue.

When a child who is polycythemic from cyanosis contracts a virus, especially one that causes vomiting or diarrhea, teach parents to monitor the child closely for dehydration because the child is at greater risk for hemoconcentration.

Excessive hemoglobin limits space in the vascular bed for platelet and other coagulation factors. Therefore, children with chronic polycythemia tend to have abnormalities of hemostasis. These children may bleed postoperatively, bruise easily, or be prone to epistaxis (nosebleeds).

Clubbing is a thickening, widening, and flattening of the toenails and fingernails (Fig. 15-6). For unknown reasons, clubbing develops with chronic arterial desaturation and polycythemia. Clubbing is not seen solely in children with heart disease associated with cyanosis but may be associated with other diseases such as cirrhosis of the liver, chronic respiratory conditions, or hereditary nonspecific clubbing.

Children with tetralogy of Fallot and some other heart defects may have tetralogy or hypercyanotic spells, often called *tet spells*. These spells commonly occur when a child's heart has not yet been repaired and changes in

pulmonary outflow resistance and SVR result in sudden changes in the degree of right-to-left shunting. Hypercyanotic spells occur in young infants, most commonly at 2 to 4 months of age; may be precipitated by agitation; and are characterized by worsening cyanosis, disappearance or decrease in heart murmur intensity, hyperpnea, irritability or prolonged crying, limpness, fainting, and convulsions. These symptoms may be short lived and subtle or may last for hours. A prolonged, severe spell may end in syncope, seizures, or cardiac arrest.

ALERT *Tet spells may arise without warning or after a predictable precipitating event. To decide whether a child is having a tet spell, auscultate the heart. The intensity of the cardiac murmur decreases during a spell.*

Substantial neurologic complications are a risk of chronic cyanosis. Chronic hypoxia and underperfusion put these children at elevated risk for stroke, meningitis, and brain abscesses. Hyperviscosity of blood from polycythemia increases the chances of thromboembolic events such as thrombus, brain abscesses, and abnormal neurologic development. With modern management techniques, more children with cardiac cyanosis are candidates for early surgical repair. Early intervention may lead to fewer neurologic complications from chronic cyanosis.

Assessment

History and physical assessment of cyanosis are discussed under the general assessment section at the beginning of this chapter.

Diagnostic Tests

Clinical determination of cyanosis is made by measuring the child's hemoglobin level. A child who is severely anemic and has a large left-to-right shunt may not appear cyanotic because the hemoglobin level may be too low for the child to appear blue. Further assessment, including a complete blood count, arterial blood gases, pulse oximetry, chest radiograph, and ECG, assists in developing an accurate diagnosis.

Oxygen is used in the diagnosis of CHD. When 100% oxygen is administered to an infant with intracardiac shunting from CHD or central cyanosis, arterial blood gas measurement may show only inconsequential improvements of partial pressure of serum oxygen concentration (PaO_2). Oxygen may actually destabilize some children with severe forms of CHD. However, an infant with an underlying pulmonary problem may improve considerably with supplemental oxygen. Also, children with intracardiac mixing may worsen their cyanosis with crying and activities, whereas the child who is cyanotic for other reasons, such as bronchopulmonary dysplasia, may improve with supplemental oxygen or crying.

Normal oxygen saturation of red blood cells is 95% to 100%. Depending on the heart defect, a child might have an expected saturation level ranging from 85% to 89% or less. A PaO_2 level of 80 to 100 mm Hg can be

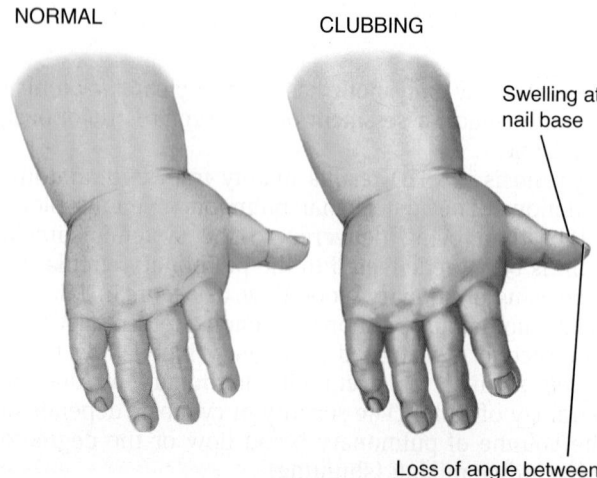

NORMAL   CLUBBING

Swelling at nail base

Loss of angle between finger and nail

Figure 15-6 Clubbing of the nails.

considered normal for a healthy child; a cyanotic child may show a PaO_2 level around 45 mm Hg. Hypoxia is defined as reduced arterial PaO_2 and reduced oxygen saturation, leading to diminished tissue oxygenation.

Interdisciplinary Interventions

Treatment of tet or hypercyanotic spells is directed toward preventing conditions that may potentiate a cyanotic response, such as dehydration or crying. When a child has a known cyanotic condition, the practitioner must respond especially aggressively and quickly to childhood illnesses that may cause dehydration (Clinical Judgment 15-2). Because a high hematocrit level carries the risk that the child's blood will become too viscous, monitor the complete blood count closely in cyanotic children. In addition, assess these children for evidence of bruising, petechiae of the skin, or epistaxis.

In treating a cyanotic spell, interventions are aimed at raising the SVR. Provide calming and comforting measures to decrease oxygen demand and hyperventilation.

Oxygen is administered as well as morphine sulfate to relax the right ventricular infundibulum, which increases pulmonary blood flow and, therefore, decreases the right-to-left shunt. During a cyanotic spell, place the child in the knee–chest position, which blocks blood flow to the legs and decreases venous return from the legs. These effects reduce left-to-right shunts, resulting in improved blood flow to the lungs. Although healthy, mobile young children may squat—and squatting is a normal position in some cultures—a cyanotic young child may occasionally squat while playing, instinctively eliciting the same effect as the knee–chest position.

Total repair of tetralogy of Fallot is commonly done before 1 year of age in the United States. Oral propranolol (Inderal) is useful in controlling spells by stabilizing the reactivity of the peripheral vasculature. During severe cyanotic spells, as the child becomes more hypoxic and pulmonary blood flow decreases, the child may develop metabolic acidosis. Acidosis necessitates immediate correction with sodium bicarbonate intravenously.

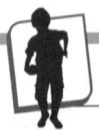

CLINICAL JUDGMENT 15-2

Dehydration in the Child With Congenital Heart Disease

Eleven-month-old Rochelle presents at the clinic with what is described as 24 hours of vomiting and diarrhea. She is cyanotic, listless, tachypneic, and has a temperature of 101.5° F (38.6° C). The mother states that her child has a heart problem.

Questions

1. What historical data would be helpful to clarify the diagnosis?
2. What are potential complications of dehydration and diarrhea particular to this child that the nurse needs to consider in her nursing care?
3. Does Rochelle need to be admitted to the hospital?
4. What would be appropriate interventions?
5. What factors would indicate that Rochelle has recovered with no ill side effect from this dehydration episode?

Answers

1. Historical data would include asking the following questions: What is the actual cardiac diagnosis for the child? Is there a history of any cardiac surgery? Is the child normally cyanotic? How do past episodes compare with the current one? What is the child's normal oxygen saturation? What medications, if any, is the child taking? How many dosages of the medications were missed? Has she been exposed to anyone with a history of vomiting and diarrhea? How many, and how large, were the stools the child had? When did she last urinate?

2. Children with heart disease that causes cyanosis may be at risk for hypercyanotic spells, and dehydration can be a triggering response. The complete blood count may be too high as a result of hemoconcentration. Also, cyanotic children are at increased risk for stroke and brain abscess.

3. Yes. Because Rochelle is listless and tachypneic, she is exhibiting clinical signs of deterioration from dehydration. Also, reasons for the vomiting and diarrhea, other than a virus, need to be ruled out.

4. Administer IV fluids, low-flow oxygen supplementation, antipyretics, and antiemetics, and begin a pulse oximetry monitor. If Rochelle was taking digoxin, a blood level should be obtained, because one symptom of an elevated or toxic digoxin level is vomiting. Notify Rochelle's pediatric cardiologist of the admission. Send stool cultures for evaluation. Routine laboratory values should include a blood culture with routine blood work (complete blood count and an electrolyte panel). Anemia and electrolyte imbalances need to be ruled out.

5. Rochelle has no vomiting or diarrhea. She is interacting playfully and tolerating oral intake, and her oxygen saturation levels on room air are at baseline.

Collateral vessels develop in children with CHDs associated with cyanosis such as pulmonary atresia. These vessels are the body's attempt to improve oxygenation. They usually arise from the thoracic aorta and supply parts of the pulmonary system. These vessels tend to be fragile and tortuous. When a surgeon is correcting lesions to improve a child's oxygenation, these vessels are problematic because they may be numerous and difficult to reach surgically. Many collaterals can be occluded in the catheterization laboratory with occlusion devices, such as coils, or ligated during surgery, if they can be reached. Taking out collateral vessels can be laborious and may require repeat procedures.

For the child with CHD, palliative surgeries may be performed to improve cardiac mixing or increase blood flow to the lungs and thereby promote growth and development. A permanent cardiac repair to remove areas of shunting and allow normal blood flow to the lungs may definitively alleviate cyanosis and diminish compensatory responses. Cardiac transplantation may become the only option for a child with worsening symptoms who has received maximum medical management and for whom there are no other surgical options.

Teach parents of a cyanotic child how to differentiate between worsening blueness and cyanotic spells. It is not surprising to see a cyanotic infant who is obese. Parents fear the child crying and turning blue, so they may continually pacify the infant with a bottle. Another fear for parents is having their child turn more cyanotic with increased activity. Most cyanotic children limit their own activity levels. They may be as active as their peers but do tend to fatigue sooner. When teaching, include a discussion of aggressively preventing dehydration to avoid an overly viscous blood volume; also, teach parents ways to prevent obesity and alternative ways to handle their concerns about activity.

CONGENITAL HEART DEFECTS

Understanding a child's precise cardiac defect is important because management and health outcomes depend on the defect. Each lesion has its own natural history of adverse effects on PVR and on ventricles, valves, or other structures. With some defects, survival and preventing complications require prompt diagnosis and treatment during early infancy, whereas with other conditions, children may grow into adulthood before becoming symptomatic. Hospitalized children with cardiac diagnoses may be in various stages of repair, undergo surgical trauma, or have inadequate or disrupted surgical repairs.

 QUESTION: Gabriella's PDA results in shunting. What are the blood flow and consequences of Gabriella's shunt?

Normally, oxygen-depleted blood drains from the venous system through the inferior and superior vena cava into the right heart. From there, blood is pumped to the lungs to pick up oxygen. The oxygen saturation of blood returning to the right heart and the pressures in the right chambers are normally low. The blood that enters the left atrium from the lungs is normally fully saturated and is pumped by the left ventricle under high pressure to the systemic circulation.

In some situations, shunting occurs. Blood pumped to the systemic circulation mixes with deoxygenated blood. This is called a *right-to-left shunt* and may cause cyanosis. Blood pumped to the systemic circulation that is not mixed with deoxygenated blood is called a *left-to-right shunt* and may cause overcirculation to the lungs, possibly resulting in heart failure. Either type of shunting can occur as a consequence of various CHDs.

ANSWER: During fetal circulation, the ductus arteriosus exists to shunt blood away from the lungs, which are not in use, and back into systemic circulation. For neonates, if the ductus arteriosus relaxes enough to permit blood flow, the higher systemic pressures and lower pulmonary pressures cause the blood flow to move in reverse of fetal circulation, flowing from the left side to the right and adding additional blood flow to the lungs.

CHDs can be classified as defects with increased pulmonary blood flow, defects with decreased pulmonary blood flow, obstructive defects, defects of the great vessels, and defects with a functional single ventricle.

Defects With Increased Pulmonary Blood Flow

Defects that increase pulmonary blood flow include PDA, ASD, VSD, and atrioventricular canal defect, also called *atrioventricular septal defect* or *endocardial cushion defect*.

PATENT DUCTUS ARTERIOSUS

PDA is the persistence of the fetal structure that connects the aorta and the pulmonary artery. It is generally at the lesser curvature of the aortic arch distal to the subclavian artery and is connected to the left or main pulmonary artery.

Pathophysiology

At birth, the newborn's lungs expand, and the right side of the heart and pulmonary artery pressures decrease. When the umbilical cord is cut, systemic pressures increase, causing arterial blood to shunt from the aorta to the pulmonary artery. Oxygenated blood normally causes the ductus to constrict and close by 6 weeks of age; failure to close leaves the infant with a PDA. If the PDA remains open, blood flows from the high pressure in the aorta to the path of least resistance through the ductus, thus causing excessive blood flow to the lungs (Fig. 15-7).

The ductus arteriosus closes by 48 hours of life in 80% of term infants and in almost 100% of term infants by 96 hours of age (Agarwal et al., 2008). Slight flow from a small PDA may not clinically overstress a heart, but the child is still at a greater risk than other children for air embolus, bacterial endocarditis, or clots. Also, if a PDA is left untreated, the rate of mortality increases with age. Over time, even a minor PDA puts the patient at risk for developing pulmonary hypertension.

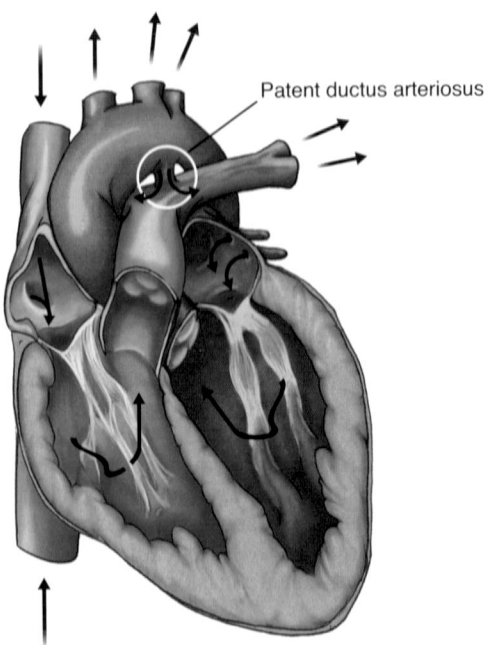

Figure 15-7 Patent ductus arteriosus.

In preterm infants, the incidence of PDA is inversely related to gestational age. The younger the infant's gestational age, the more likely the infant is to have a PDA. PDA affects 50% of infants born at 27 weeks' gestation and over 80% of infants born at 23 weeks' gestation (Hajj & Dagle, 2012). A PDA in the premature infant is not considered a congenital lesion but a situational defect because it occurs functionally as a result of the premature delivery. Premature infants with PDAs are commonly symptomatic.

Assessment

 QUESTION: Is Gabriella's presentation of symptoms typical for a preterm infant?

Assessment findings that occur in the presence of a PDA vary depending on the age of the child and the size of the shunt. In general, the larger the shunt, the greater the likelihood that the child will have symptoms of heart failure.

Obtain a thorough history. Children whose initial diagnosis is made after the infancy are often described by parents as having frequent pulmonary infections. They may be thinner than other children of the same age.

Auscultation reveals a continuous, machinery-like murmur best heard at the second and third ICSs. Peripheral pulses are bounding, from the runoff of blood (excess volume of blood) from the aorta to the pulmonary artery. These children also have widened pulse pressure. The diagnosis of PDA may be confirmed and treated through data obtained by radiograph, two-dimensional echocardiography, and color flow Doppler studies. The chest radiograph of a child diagnosed after toddlerhood may show an enlarged heart.

 ANSWER: The presence of a murmur, bounding pulses, and pulmonary symptoms of heart failure are typical in a preterm infant.

Interdisciplinary Interventions

QUESTION: Will there be any long-lasting sequelae of Gabriella's PDA after her discharge from the hospital? Does it depend on whether the ductus is closed surgically or medically?

Interventions for PDA typically involve pharmacologic therapy or surgery to close the opening. In some cases, medications are used to keep the ductus open to provide adequate circulation. Preterm infants without bleeding tendencies who have good renal function may receive orally administered indomethacin, a prostaglandin inhibitor, to encourage ductal closure. Success in closing PDAs with indomethacin varies (Malviya et al., 2008). Ibuprofen may also be used to encourage ductal closure (Tradition or Science 15-1). Term infants typically undergo transcatheter closure of the PDA in the catheterization lab.

Nonpharmacologic interventions to close the ductus are low risk. In recent years, PDAs have been successfully

---

Evidence-Based Practice   TRADITION OR SCIENCE 15-1

Is indomethacin the only medication effective in closing ductus arteriosus?

Indomethacin has been used since 1976 to close PDA, but it has renal, gastrointestinal, and cerebral side effects. Both indomethacin and ibuprofen inhibit the synthesis of prostaglandin. Studies show that ibuprofen is as effective as indomethacin in PDA closure (Neumann et al., 2012; Ohlsson et al., 2010; Thomas et al., 2005; Witoslaw et al., 2005), even in extremely preterm infants. In extremely low-birth-weight infants with gestational age ≤28 weeks, Su et al. (2008) found a PDA closure rate of 88.3% with ibuprofen versus 88.1% with indomethacin; Erdeve et al. (2012) demonstrated a rate of 83.3% with oral ibuprofen.

A factor in determining treatment is the side effect profile of the treatment. Some research trials indicate that ibuprofen may cause less adverse effects on the kidneys, gut, and brain than indomethacin but may increase the risk for chronic lung disease, whereas indomethacin may reduce the risk of severe intraventricular hemorrhage and surgical duct ligation (Ohlsson et al., 2010; Sekar & Corff, 2008). Researchers are continuing to examine the efficacy and safety of ibuprofen versus indomethacin to close PDAs.

Prophylactic treatment with ibuprofen is not recommended to prevent PDAs because it unnecessarily exposes infants to potential side effects without conferring any important short-term benefits (Ohlsson & Shah, 2011).

occluded using devices in the catheterization laboratory. If the child is not a good candidate for PDA closure in the catheterization laboratory, surgical ligation is usually done during early childhood. The procedure is a non-pump case and is accomplished through a thoracotomy incision. Potential, but rare, complications include phrenic nerve damage, diaphragmatic paralysis, laryngeal nerve damage, chylothorax, transient hypertension, and atrial flutter. As with any thoracotomy incision, the risk of chylothorax is increased. Nursing care postoperatively must include aggressive chest physiotherapy and pulmonary toilet. Ensure adequate pain management to discourage chest splinting (guarding) and encourage deep breathing.

A PDA may be protective in an infant with a cardiac lesion, such as HLHS, that depends on an open ductus arteriosus to provide adequate circulation. The PDA acts as a natural shunt, allowing blood flow to mix and bypass an obstructed area. To ensure that the PDA remains patent, these infants receive an infusion of prostaglandin E₁ (PGE_1). This substance, found throughout the body, is involved in the regulation of virtually all organ systems. Given intravenously, it is a potent dilator of the ductus arteriosus and is used for left-sided obstructive lesions to improve systemic perfusion, acid–base balance, and urine output.

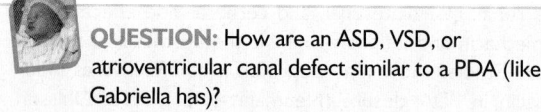

ANSWER: No, timely ligation of the ductus stops the increased pulmonary blood flow and there are seldom cardiovascular sequelae. If the ductus is ligated surgically, it will not reopen. If it is closed with medication, there exists the possibility of it reopening, but this is still usually during the neonatal course and not after discharge.

ATRIAL SEPTAL DEFECT

QUESTION: How are an ASD, VSD, or atrioventricular canal defect similar to a PDA (like Gabriella has)?

An ASD is a communication between the right and left atria through the septum that persists beyond the newborn period. There are three classifications of ASD, which are based on the actual location of the defect in the atrial septum. If the opening in the atrial septum is high in the septum, it is called a *sinus venosus* defect. Sinus venosus ASDs are the second most common ASD and are located near the junction of the superior vena cava and the right atrium. These ASDs are often associated with anomalous pulmonary venous return, which is discussed later in this chapter.

The most common ASD, an *ostium secundum* defect, is located mid septum. These ASDs are located in the fossa ovalis center of the septum and can be closed in the cardiac catheterization laboratory. *Ostium primum* defects, the third classification of ASD, are located low in the septum. These ASDs lie inferiorly to the foramen ovale in the lowest portion of the septum. Ostium primum ASDs may also be associated with a cleft in the mitral valve and mitral insufficiency.

Pathophysiology

With ASD, blood shunts from the left atrium to the right atrium because pressures are greater on the left side of the heart. This left-to-right shunt may cause the mean pressure in the right atrium and left atrium to be similar. The amount of blood that shunts across the septum is relative to the size of the defect. If the ASD is large enough, the shunt creates a burden on the right side of the heart from excess blood volume in the right heart circulation and the pulmonary bed (Fig. 15-8).

If an ASD is left unrepaired, the likelihood of right and left cardiac hypertrophy increases with time. As the atrium enlarges and stretches, the patient may have atrial arrhythmias. Chronic excessive pulmonary blood flow carries a risk of increased PVR, leading to pulmonary hypertension and an elevated risk of pulmonary emboli.

Assessment

In the fetus, the foramen ovale is naturally open; therefore, a diagnosis of ASD cannot be made in utero. Children with ASDs may be on the slender side with slight growth retardation. They may tire more easily than their peers during athletic activities. They may have a greater likelihood of repeat pulmonary infections. Because they generally lack any obvious symptoms, they are frequently identified during a physical examination only as having a murmur. If the ASD is not detected during early childhood, a child may remain asymptomatic until adulthood. ASDs are usually clearly delineated through the use of echocardiography.

Children are usually asymptomatic but in severe cases may have heart failure. If the child is symptomatic, a chest radiograph may show cardiomegaly with an

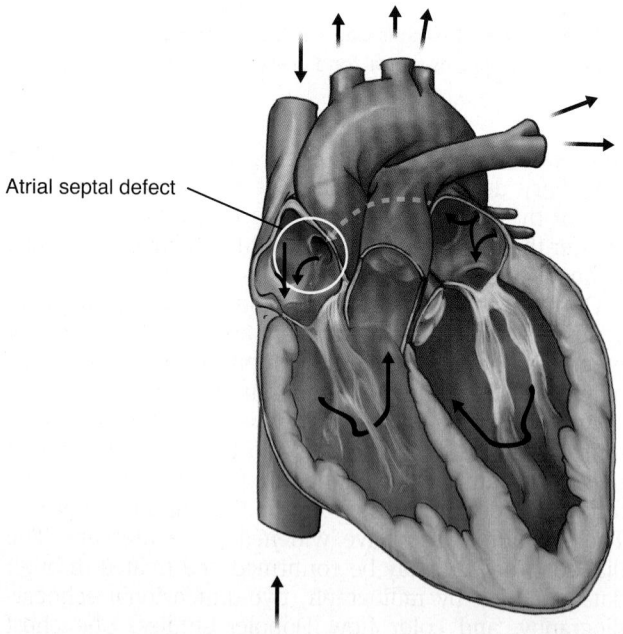

Figure 15-8 Atrial septal defect.

enlarged right atrium and right ventricle and increased pulmonary blood flow. Assess for signs of a left-to-right shunt and heart failure.

Interdisciplinary Interventions

Treatment is provided during infancy if the child has heart failure. If the child is asymptomatic, the ASD is generally closed during early childhood, usually via cardiac catheterization. Spontaneous closure of the secundum type of ASD is 87% during the first 4 years of life (Park, 2008). Sinus venosus ASDs require a patch closure, and the surgeon must avoid damage to the sinoatrial node to prevent arrhythmias. Surgical repair is completed through a median sternotomy incision, with the child on cardiopulmonary bypass, and only if closure is not possible in the cardiac catheterization laboratory. A rare surgical complication of repairing an ASD is complete heart block from suture damage that causes edema at the atrioventricular node and bundle of His. If partial anomalous venous return exists, the patch closure is placed so that it directs venous return to the left atrium with a baffle. Instead of the septum being repaired vertically, the patch angles over to envelop the oxygenated blood returning to the right atrium and directs it to the left atrium.

VENTRICULAR SEPTAL DEFECT

A VSD—the most common CHD, accounting for 15% to 20% of all cases of isolated CHD—is an opening or communication in the septum, usually the membranous portion, between the right and left ventricles (Park, 2008). A VSD may be located in multiple and various places in the septum. Physiology of a VSD depends on the size and location of the defect and the effects on PVR (Fig. 15-9).

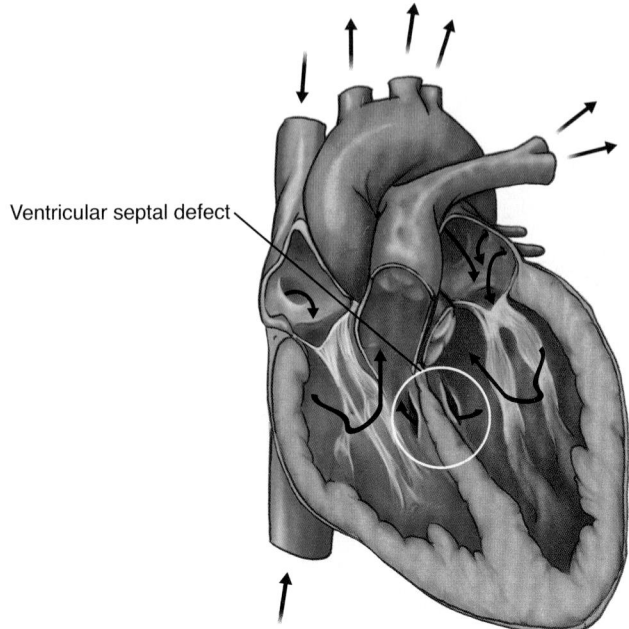

Ventricular septal defect

Figure 15-9 Ventricular septal defect.

Three types of VSDs occur: membranous, muscular, and supracristal. The most common VSD (70% to 80% of cases) is the *membranous* type, which occurs in the outflow tract of the left ventricle below the aortic valve. *Muscular* VSDs (25% of cases) are located entirely within the muscular septum. Muscular VSDs, found in approximately 5% of the population, commonly exist in multiple locations, creating a Swiss cheese effect. The overlapping holes can limit the surgeon's ability to find the VSDs. *Supracristal* VSDs occur in the infundibular septum and can result in prolapsing aortic valve cusps.

Pathophysiology

The larger the VSD, the greater the amount of shunting that occurs. Large VSDs can rob the systemic circulation of a considerable portion of blood flow. Excessive flow through the right ventricle can overwork the ventricle and overcirculate the pulmonary bed.

Repairing a VSD early in life helps prevent lung disease and heart failure. Thirty percent to 40% of membranous and muscular VSDs, particularly small ones, may decrease in size or close spontaneously within the first 6 months of life (Park, 2008). Large defects also tend to become smaller over time. Full, spontaneous defect closures are most likely to occur within the first year of life (Chang et al., 2011).

If a moderate to large VSD is left untreated, PVR will eventually increase from constant excess flow to the pulmonary bed. Over time, as PVR increases, pressures in the right and left ventricles may change, causing higher pressures in the right ventricle than the left. When this pressure change occurs, the shunt reverses. PVR exceeding systemic pressure is called *Eisenmenger complex*. Severe pulmonary hypertension may cause the condition to be inoperable. If the VSD is repaired in these circumstances, the sudden reduction of excessive blood flow to the lungs may prove fatal. Right-sided heart failure occurs because pulmonary vessels remain constricted postoperatively. The high pressure in the lungs overburdens the right ventricle, which no longer has the VSD to act as a release valve. Other defects that put patients at risk for pulmonary hypertension are atrioventricular canal defects and truncus arteriosus (described later in this chapter).

VSDs are the most common lesion to coexist with other cardiac anomalies. A VSD in combination with other lesions can have different effects on the heart. As with PDAs, depending on the specifics of the individual's combination of lesions, a VSD could be an asset that counters problems caused by another defect.

Assessment

In the presence of a small VSD, growth and development are normal, and the child lacks symptoms. To be classified as small, a VSD must be smaller than the orifice of the aortic valve so that flow across it is restricted and the blood volume shunted is limited. A large VSD is one that is larger than the orifice of the aortic valve and is unobstructed; thus, pressure can equalize between the left and right ventricles.

An infant born with a VSD may not have an audible murmur until 6 to 8 weeks after birth, when PVR decreases and heart failure can develop. Children with moderate to large VSDs are prone to having decreased exercise tolerance, repeated pulmonary infections, slowed to impaired growth and development, and heart failure. Chest radiograph results vary, depending on the amount of shunting, but can exhibit increased pulmonary vascular markings and cardiomegaly. Cyanosis and clubbing may indicate a reversed shunt caused by increased PVR. Assess for signs of a left-to-right shunt, decreased exercise tolerance, increased PVR resulting in a right-to-left shunt, and heart failure.

Interdisciplinary Interventions

Monitor children with a VSD for signs and symptoms of heart failure, poor growth and development, and poor feeding. In the presence of heart failure, standard treatment for VSD includes diuretics and digoxin (Lanoxin). Medical management includes antibiotics for prophylaxis against infective subacute bacterial endocarditis for all dental visits. The physician also may elect for surgical repair to alleviate the risk of infective endocarditis.

Infants with heart failure, failure to thrive, increasing PVR, or some combination of these factors require VSD repair. If the child is asymptomatic, repairs are scheduled early in life, most within the first 12 months of life. If the child is too small or ill for repair but is in heart failure, then palliative pulmonary artery banding is done. Most children are able to avoid this additional procedure and undergo only one surgery to complete the repair (see thePoint for Care Path: Interdisciplinary Plan of Care for the Child With Surgical Repair of a VSD).

Surgery is completed through a median sternotomy incision with the child on cardiopulmonary bypass. A stitch closure is done for small VSDs; for larger defects, a patch is sewn over each hole. At some pediatric cardiac centers, VSDs from selective cases have been closed in the catheterization laboratory, but this technique is not yet approved by the U.S. Food and Drug Administration for general care.

Although most children tolerate surgery well, complications do occur. Heart block is a potential complication because septal sutures may cause edema in close proximity to the conduction system. Postoperative echocardiography and monitoring of mixed venous gases and oxygen saturation can help determine whether any residual VSDs are left after the repair is done. Inotropic medications are generally administered to support cardiac output during the immediate postoperative period. Postoperative pulmonary hypertension is now managed successfully in many patients previously considered high risk. Management in critical care includes sedation, hyperventilation, inotropic agents for right heart failure, and PGE$_1$ to decrease PVR. New inhalation therapies that decrease pulmonary blood flow, such as nitric oxide, assist in managing pulmonary hypertension.

ATRIOVENTRICULAR CANAL DEFECT

Another type of defect that increases pulmonary blood flow is an atrioventricular canal defect, also called *atrioventricular septal defect* or *endocardial cushion defect*.

Pathophysiology

Normally, in utero, the fetal endocardial cushions grow and separate into two openings that develop into the tricuspid and mitral valves. The cushions also contribute to the development of both the atrial and ventricular septa (Park, 2008).

An atrioventricular canal consists of a large central hole, where the cushion did not develop properly, that allows blood to flow among all four chambers. Levels of shunting occur where the lower portion of the atrial septum and the upper portion of the ventricular septum do not meet in the middle (Fig. 15-10).

Along with the left-to-right shunting at the atrial and ventricular levels, varying degrees of valve insufficiency exist. Valve insufficiency results from inadequate fusion of the centrally located endocardial cushion tissue. Both the septum and the mitral and tricuspid valve leaflets are underdeveloped.

Directions and pathways of flow between chambers depend on pulmonary and systemic resistance, pressure in chambers, and compliance of chambers. Because of the free flow of blood among the chambers, children with atrioventricular canal defect are at risk for pulmonary hypertension and heart failure.

Without surgical intervention, these children generally die early in life. Their longevity depends on the size of the communication between chambers and the degree of atrioventricular valve incompetence. Early surgical correction can help prevent the development of pulmonary hypertension from excessive pulmonary blood flow.

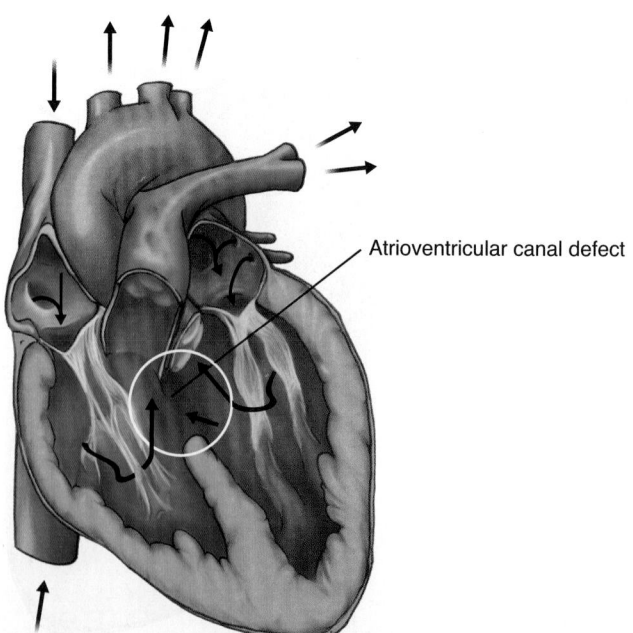

Atrioventricular canal defect

Figure 15-10 Atrioventricular canal defect.

Assessment

An atrioventricular canal defect can be diagnosed in utero by a level II fetal echocardiogram. If the defect is undiagnosed at birth, these children tend to present early in life with failure to thrive, repeated pulmonary infections, and heart failure. They may be underweight, tachypneic, and tachycardic. Varying degrees of cyanosis are present and worsen with activity. The presence of this defect is frequently associated with Down syndrome and heterotaxy syndrome.

Interdisciplinary Interventions

With an incomplete or partial atrioventricular canal, differing degrees of partial fusion of the endocardial cushion result in varied atrial and ventricular valve abnormalities. If the atrioventricular canal defect is mild, it can be treated much like an ASD.

Medical management includes controlling heart failure by using diuretics and digoxin (Lanoxin). Caloric supplements are provided to support the increased metabolic demand by providing more calories per feeding and allowing the infant to expend less energy.

If the child is asymptomatic, repairs are scheduled early in life, usually toward the end of the first year. If the child is too small or ill for surgery but is in heart failure, palliative pulmonary artery banding is done. Most children are able to avoid this additional procedure and have a complete surgical repair.

Surgical repair is done through a median sternotomy incision with the child on cardiopulmonary bypass. A Dacron patch is used to surgically close the septal defects. The mitral and tricuspid valves are reconstructed or replaced when necessary.

Complete heart block can occur as a consequence of edema after atrioventricular valve repair. Postoperatively, echocardiography is done to monitor for valvular dysfunction in the reconstructed valves. If pulmonary hypertension is present preoperatively, then you can expect instability postoperatively if the child has to do the work of breathing. Therefore, the child typically receives mechanical ventilation, being weaned from the ventilator slowly over several days.

> **ANSWER:** All three defects—an ASD, VSD, and atrioventricular canal defect—allow blood flow from the left side of the heart to the right side of the heart, resulting in increased pulmonary blood flow. If left untreated, all will result in pulmonary damage and heart failure.

Defects With Decreased Pulmonary Blood Flow

Defects with decreased pulmonary blood flow include tricuspid atresia, tetralogy of Fallot, and pulmonary atresia.

TRICUSPID ATRESIA

Tricuspid atresia is a cardiac lesion in which the tricuspid valve is missing, so no connection exists between the right atrium and the right ventricle (Fig. 15-11).

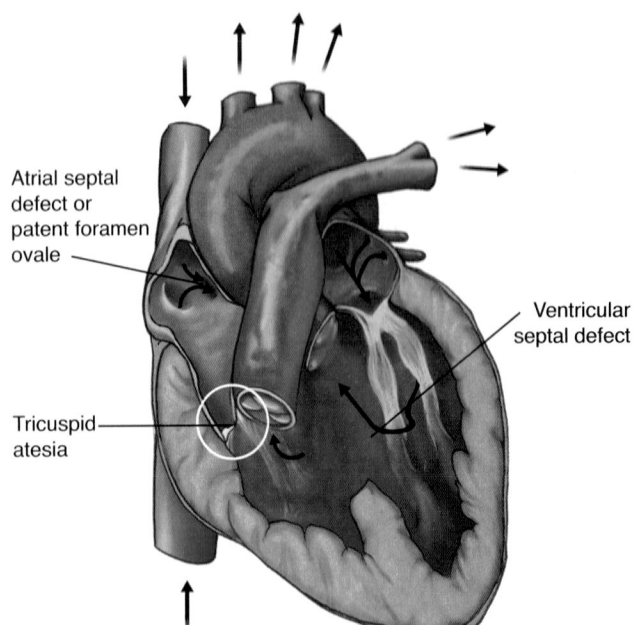

Figure 15-11 Tricuspid atresia.

Pathophysiology

In tricuspid atresia, blood cannot flow from the right atrium to the right ventricle; therefore, pulmonary blood flow is greatly reduced and depends on other shunts. The right ventricle is generally hypoplastic, and the inflow portion of the right ventricle is missing. In infants, survival depends on the presence of an associated defect, such as an ASD, VSD, or PDA, that enables some cardiac mixing. Coexisting lesions associated with tricuspid atresia might include pulmonary stenosis, TGA, COA, and hypoplastic pulmonary arteries (Park, 2008).

Without intervention, children with tricuspid atresia die early during infancy. These infants may require a shunt to increase pulmonary blood flow. Infants will likely grow and develop more slowly than the average baby because, until the completion of the staged repair, the amount of oxygen available for the body's needs is inadequate.

Assessment

Infants with tricuspid atresia are cyanotic from restricted pulmonary blood flow and can have hypoxic spells. Clinical manifestations include poor feeding and tachypnea. Chest radiograph shows a normal or slightly increased heart size with decreased pulmonary vascular markings.

Interdisciplinary Interventions

Palliation to increase pulmonary blood flow to the lungs can be provided by placing a Blalock-Taussig shunt. If the neonate has inadequate intracardiac mixing, a balloon atrial septostomy can be done to increase right-to-left shunting. Depending on the specifics of the particular lesion, some children have excessive pulmonary blood flow. In these cases, a pulmonary artery banding procedure is desirable to control heart failure by limiting the excessive pulmonary blood flow.

Surgery for tricuspid atresia requires two procedures. A hemi-Fontan or bidirectional Glenn shunt is the preparatory surgery performed first. This procedure is essentially an anastomosis (connection) of the superior vena cava to the pulmonary artery. It redirects partial venous return straight to the lungs and decreases the workload on the single ventricle by approximately 20%.

The final repair is the Fontan procedure, which enables the single usable ventricle to act as the systemic pump. All the systemic venous return is directed to the lungs and bypasses the ventricle. This redirection is accomplished through a surgical connection between the right atrium and the pulmonary artery and is known as an *intracardiac Fontan*. Some surgeons use an extracardiac Fontan, which involves the use of a Gore-Tex tube to connect the inferior vena cava directly to the right pulmonary artery. Some surgeons choose to leave a small fenestration, or opening, between the Fontan circuit and the right atrium that acts like an ASD. This opening allows a small amount of intracardiac mixing and relieves pressure in the right atrium. After the Fontan procedure, many children can experience improvements in growth and development.

TETRALOGY OF FALLOT

Tetralogy of Fallot is the name given to a commonly occurring combination of four problems with manifestations and a course that are somewhat predictable. The child with tetralogy of Fallot has

- A large VSD
- Some degree of right ventricular outflow tract obstruction or pulmonary stenosis
- An aorta that is positioned so that it overrides the ventricular septum
- A right ventricle that becomes hypertrophic from continually pumping against the obstruction (Fig. 15-12)

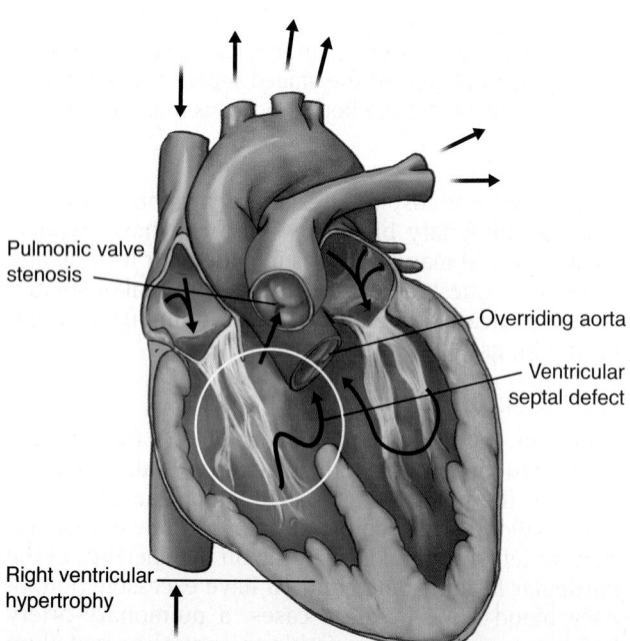

Figure 15-12 Tetralogy of Fallot.

Pulmonic valve stenosis

Overriding aorta

Ventricular septal defect

Right ventricular hypertrophy

Without treatment, most patients die by about 20 years of age. Complete repair of tetralogy of Fallot is associated with excellent survival (Jonas, 2009). Pulmonary valve replacement is frequently needed after tetralogy of Fallot repair; this replacement typically occurs during adulthood (Harrild et al., 2009).

Pathophysiology

The VSD leads to shunting, the amount of which varies depending on the amount of obstruction to right ventricular outflow and the size of the VSD. These children have diminished blood flow to the lungs and excessive blood flow to the body of poorly oxygenated blood (Park, 2008).

Children with tetralogy of Fallot have varying degrees of pulmonary stenosis, with correlating proportions of cyanosis. Cyanosis may not be obvious in the neonate, but as early months pass, infundibular pulmonary stenosis increases, which in turn increases the right-to-left shunting through the VSD. Children with tetralogy of Fallot have normal growth and development, but, if left untreated, they eventually suffer worsening cyanosis, clubbing, polycythemia, and exercise intolerance. When the secondary lesion of pulmonary stenosis is present, with the right balance, it may act as a left ventricular outflow obstruction to decrease pulmonary blood flow from excessive shunting across the VSD. This circumstance may help prevent heart failure but further complicates surgical repair of the heart.

Assessment

Assess for difficulty feeding, failure to gain weight, poor development, and symptoms of cyanosis (clubbing, dizziness, and loss of consciousness). These children are mildly cyanotic at rest and have increasing cyanosis with crying, activity, or straining (such as with a bowel movement). Children tend to limit their own activity levels relative to their level of hypoxic tolerance.

Some children with tetralogy of Fallot can be acyanotic. If, along with a large VSD, mild or moderate pulmonary stenosis is present and limits the amount of intracardiac mixing, a child may not be blue. Such children are often called *pink tets*.

A chest radiograph of the child with tetralogy of Fallot shows decreased pulmonary blood flow and a normal heart size. The heart shows a boot-shaped silhouette from right ventricular hypertrophy pushing the heart apex upward. Echocardiography can provide information that clearly defines the defect. If the coronary anatomy cannot be clearly delineated by echocardiography, a diagnostic heart catheterization is performed. Catheterization provides specific preoperative information about the direction and the amount of shunting, the coronary anatomy, and each portion of this heart defect.

Interdisciplinary Interventions

Medical management includes monitoring oxygen saturation to determine the degree of hypoxia, optimizing oxygenation, and recognizing and treating hypercyanotic spells (see the description of cyanosis and its management earlier in this chapter).

Some children require a palliative procedure to increase pulmonary blood flow. A Blalock-Taussig shunt can decrease cyanosis and eliminate tet spells. Children who may benefit from a shunt placement before total corrective surgery are those who are too ill or small for complete repair. Also, if the coronary artery crosses the right ventricular outflow tract, standard surgical repair may be ruled out. If a shunt is placed, it is removed at the time of the definitive surgical repair. At some cardiac centers, selected patients have undergone balloon dilation of the outflow tract in the cardiac catheterization laboratory to widen the pulmonary artery and increase pulmonary blood flow before surgical repair.

Surgical repair is done through a median sternotomy incision with the child on cardiopulmonary bypass. The VSD is patched in such a way as to direct blood flow to include the overriding aorta toward the left ventricle. The right ventricular outflow tract is widened by resecting the infundibular tissue and placing a patch.

Most children survive surgery without long-term problems. Possible surgical complications include bleeding, heart conduction problems, pulmonary valve regurgitation, residual VSD, and persistent right ventricular failure. Lifelong follow up is required; annual office visits may include echocardiogram and ECG as well as periodic magnetic resonance imaging, exercise testing, and Holter monitor evaluations (Cincinnati Children's Hospital Medical Center, 2010). Regular activity is encouraged and physical activity recommendations are determined by the amount of right heart pressure, right ventricular volume overload, residual shunting, presence of arrhythmias, and degree of pulmonary regurgitation (Caplan & Allen, 2011).

PULMONARY ATRESIA

Pulmonary atresia is a severe version of pulmonary stenosis. At birth, the only pulmonary blood flow is via the PDA. Without immediate medical intervention, these children have a very poor prognosis.

Pathophysiology

In pulmonary atresia, the pulmonary valve fails to develop, and the valve is imperforate. Generally, but not always, the right ventricle is also poorly developed and thus is unable to function effectively. Pulmonary atresia can occur with or without an intact ventricular septum (Fig. 15-13) (Park, 2008).

Assessment

Children with pulmonary atresia present within the first day of life with severe cyanosis and tachypnea. Assess for and report breathing difficulties, irritability, lethargy, and evidence of cyanosis.

Interdisciplinary Interventions

As with most heart lesions, antibiotics are provided for routine dental care and medical interventions as prophylaxis against infective endocarditis. Goals of care are oriented toward minimizing cyanosis. In infancy, children with pulmonary atresia undergo heart catheterization to define anatomic and physiologic features. A balloon

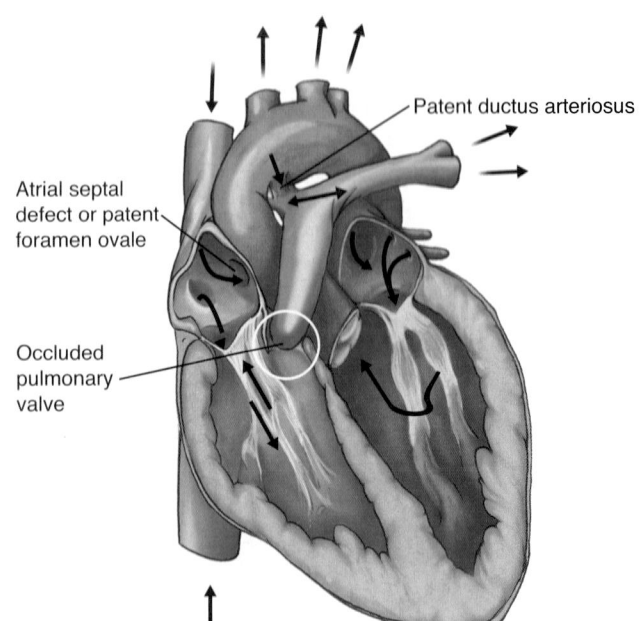

Figure 15-13 Pulmonary atresia.

atrial septostomy may be done to improve shunting across the atria. In infancy, a systemic-to-pulmonary artery shunt procedure is performed to increase pulmonary artery blood flow by creating a left-to-right shunt.

After the child has grown and is a little older, and if the right ventricle is large enough, a valved conduit is placed, using a homograft, to provide circulation from the right ventricle to the pulmonary arteries (Rastelli procedure). This surgery enables biventricular function and separates the pulmonary and systemic circulations. When the right ventricle is hypoplastic, a modified Fontan procedure is used to provide separate pulmonary and systemic circulations.

Depending on the specific dynamic of the child's pulmonary arteries, and if the right ventricle is of adequate size, some children benefit from a surgery that includes pulmonary valvulotomy and placement of a patch on the right ventricular outflow tract. This procedure opens communication between the right ventricle and pulmonary arteries. Blood passes through the right ventricle and pulmonary arteries and can stimulate growth of those areas.

Children with pulmonary atresia and poor distal pulmonary artery development may still have a poor quality of life even after multiple heart catheterizations and surgeries.

Obstructive Defects

Obstructive defects, including those defects that block the flow from the ventricles, include COA, aortic stenosis, and pulmonary stenosis.

COARCTATION OF THE AORTA

COA is a deformity that is created by localized constriction or narrowing of the aortic wall. This lesion is typically located at the junction of the aortic arch and descending aorta, distal to the origin of the left subclavian

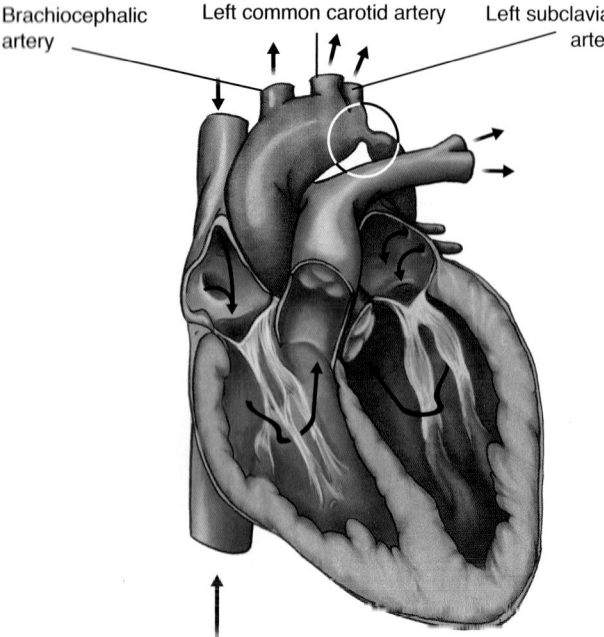

Brachiocephalic artery   Left common carotid artery   Left subclavian artery

Figure 15-14 Coarctation of the aorta.

artery (Bernstein, 2011). The COA is located in the area directly opposite of where the ductus arteriosus existed. Coarctation can be preductal (in which the area of narrowing is proximal to the ductus) or postductal (in which the obstruction is distal to the ductus). Any length of the aorta may be obstructed, but obstruction usually occurs in the upper thoracic arch (Fig. 15-14).

Pathophysiology

Narrowing of the aorta mechanically obstructs the pumping of the left ventricle, thereby putting a strain on the left ventricle. When the aorta is obstructed or narrowed, pulmonary blood flow is normal and no areas of intracardiac mixing exist, unless the child has a coexisting lesion. As blood is pumped out of the left ventricle to the aorta, some blood flows to the head and upper extremities at a high pressure. The rest of the blood meets the obstruction and is forced through the constricted area, but at a decreased flow as a result of the narrowing, traveling down the descending aorta. Therefore, upper extremity pressures are greater than normal and also greater than pressures in the lower extremities.

Children with COA develop hypertension; however, the actual mechanics of this are unclear. Normal heart function produces a pulsatile flow to the organs. When an aortic coarctation is present, organs receive a nonpulsatile flow caused by the obstructed area. It is thought that nonpulsatile renal blood flow, by causing arterial vasoconstriction, stimulates the renin–angiotensin–aldosterone system.

Assessment

As with other defects, manifestations depend on the severity of the narrowing of the aorta. Assess for decreased or absent pulses in the lower extremities.

caREminder

Measure blood pressure in all four extremities to document the pressure gradient between the upper and lower extremities, which may indicate hypertension. Promptly report any finding of a pressure gradient more than 10 mm Hg in an infant.

Infants with moderate to severe aortic narrowing can have failure to thrive and heart failure. Adolescents have upper extremity hypertension. Infants with severe coarctation may have renal shutdown and early death from heart failure if the COA is not treated. Approximately 6% of patients with COA also have other defects. Thirty percent of patients with Turner syndrome have COA (Park, 2008).

Interdisciplinary Interventions

Balloon angioplasty in the catheterization laboratory is an option for some COA lesions. These children can have excellent results while avoiding the more invasive, traumatic surgical repair. However, inadequate relief of the pressure gradient may occur, necessitating surgical repair.

When surgery is required, the aorta is cross-clamped through a posterior lateral thoracotomy incision so that the vessel can be repaired without the need for cardiopulmonary bypass. A COA can be surgically repaired in several ways, depending on the specifics of the lesion. The most common repair for COA, in patients of all ages, is the end-to-end anastomosis. Other less common methods may include patch angioplasty, Dacron conduit, or subclavian flap aortoplasty. Patch angioplasty uses a Dacron patch to widen the area of flow around the coarctation. The Dacron conduit is used as a bypass tube graft. The subclavian flap aortoplasty, done in infants, sacrifices the subclavian artery, which is used as a flap to patch the constriction of the aorta.

Monitor the child's blood pressure closely during the immediate postoperative period. The child's blood pressure is tightly controlled, being kept low, to avoid excessive pressure on the fresh suture lines of the aortic repair site. A child may have residual hypertension even after successful surgical repair. Complications, although uncommon, may include infection, hemorrhage, renal dysfunction, paralytic ileus, or spinal cord ischemia that produces paraplegia. These complications may occur from cross-clamping the aorta during the repair, which causes lack of blood flow below the aorta.

In children with complicated multiple lesions as well as COA, the coarctation is surgically repaired. This repair relieves obstruction to the heart's pumping action. Subsequently, other surgical cardiac repairs may be scheduled.

AORTIC STENOSIS

Aortic stenosis is a narrowing in the area of the aortic valve that obstructs left ventricular outflow. It can occur at the valve itself or it may be a discrete muscular area of obstruction. Three categories of aortic stenosis exist. In *valvular* aortic stenosis (the most common lesion), the valve leaflets are abnormal, with features such as a small annulus or thickened cusps. The second most common lesion is *subvalvular*, in which a fibromuscular membrane is present below the valve. This membrane can be localized or long and tubular. The least common lesion is *supravalvular*, consisting of an annular constriction in which the aortic lumen is narrowed above the valve.

Pathophysiology

Aortic stenosis may be a result of a birth defect or rheumatic fever. Rheumatic fever damages the heart valves by causing lesions on the leaflets and scar formation over time. Aortic stenosis develops as the heart attempts to overcome resistance through the stenotic area. Resistance to ejection of blood through the heart can result in left ventricular hypertrophy.

In a normal valve, no measurable gradient exists when pressures are measured before and after the valve orifice. In a stenotic valve, pressures are higher before blood passes through the stenotic valve and lower after it passes through the valve. The ascending aorta dilates from the turbulent jet of blood shooting through the constricted area (Fig. 15-15) (Park, 2008).

Stenotic aortic valves may go undetected for many years or may present early in life with severe hemodynamic changes. Stenosis and calcification of valves tend to progressively worsen with age.

Assessment

The severity of signs and symptoms associated with aortic stenosis depends on the amount of valvular deformity and blockage. Children with mild to moderate aortic stenosis are usually asymptomatic but may have exercise intolerance. Older children with aortic stenosis are at risk for exertional chest pain, easy fatigability, or syncope (Park, 2008).

Assess for symptoms of reduced cardiac output and heart failure. In severe cases, cardiac output is decreased from a poor left ventricular ejection fraction. Infants with critical aortic stenosis (obstruction of blood flow to the body, resulting in severe left ventricular failure and shock, with dependency on patency of the ductus arteriosus for blood flow to the body—a true newborn emergency) have heart failure. Symptoms in older children with severe aortic stenosis may include angina, syncope, left ventricular heart failure, dyspnea, fatigue, and palpitations; note any reports of such symptoms. Chest radiographs may show left ventricular enlargement with dilation of the ascending aorta.

Interdisciplinary Interventions

Instruct children with moderate to severe aortic stenosis to restrict exercise by avoiding sustained strenuous activity. Critically ill newborns may require management in the neonatal intensive care unit with oxygen and PGE₁. PGE₁ infusion maintains the patency of the ductus arteriosus, thus improving systemic blood flow and avoiding both acidosis and decreased perfusion to extremities and organs.

Balloon valvuloplasty can be performed in the cardiac catheterization laboratory. This procedure includes the risk of inducing aortic regurgitation, and the rate of early reintervention is high in neonates with critical aortic stenosis (Maskatia et al., 2011).

If the child is symptomatic and has severe left ventricular dilation and dysfunction, surgical repair is done through a sternal incision. The surgical procedure varies depending on the type and severity of the lesion. Valvular repair may involve an aortic valve commissurotomy (dilating the valve and incising the commissures of the valve). Potential postoperative complications include residual stenosis and aortic insufficiency.

If the risk of aortic valve insufficiency is too great, the child may require an aortic valve replacement. Delaying valve replacement, if possible, until the child is large enough to receive an adult-sized valve is advantageous. The goal is to limit the total number of valve replacement surgeries required throughout a lifetime. If the valve is replaced with a metal valve, the child must receive long-term anticoagulant therapy.

Recently, the trend in valve replacement surgery is to use a pulmonary autograft, which enables some adolescents to avoid anticoagulant therapy. The stenotic aortic valve is removed, and the patient's own pulmonary valve is transplanted in its place. The root where the patient's own pulmonary valve was located is replaced with a *homograft* valve. Homograft tissue is tissue donated from a cadaver and preserved for later surgical insertion. Because of the high pressures on the left side of the heart, it is thought that the patient's own valve will last longer in the aortic position and function better than a homograft valve. However, this approach involves more complicated surgery because two valves are replaced.

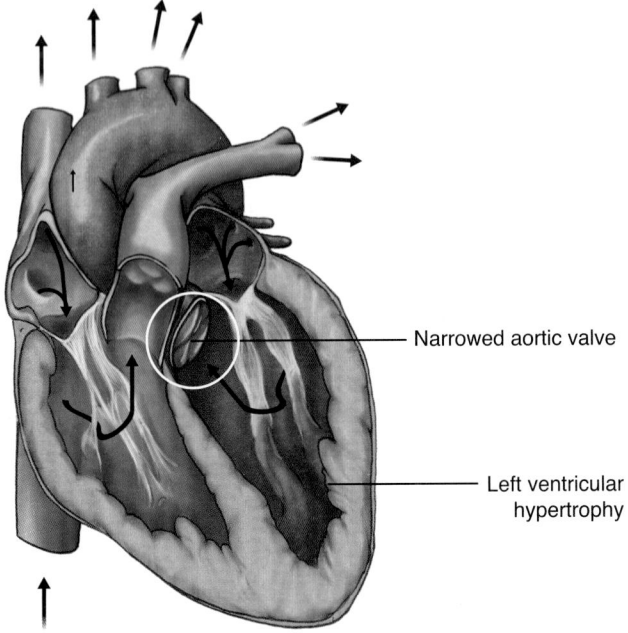

Narrowed aortic valve

Left ventricular hypertrophy

Figure 15-15 Aortic stenosis.

PULMONARY STENOSIS

Pulmonary stenosis is a narrowing at some location along the right ventricular outflow tract. Pulmonary valvular stenosis is the most common lesion producing obstruction to flow of the right ventricular systolic ejection. The cusps of the three-leafleted pulmonary valve may be thickened and fused, and the diameter of the opening varies (Fig. 15-16).

Pulmonary stenosis is classified into three types based on the location of the right ventricular outflow obstruction. *Subvalvular*, or *infundibular*, stenosis is uncommon and is located below the level of the pulmonary valve. *Supravalvular* stenosis is located in the pulmonary arteries above the pulmonary valve. This condition is often associated with congenital rubella and Williams syndrome, a genetic disorder. *Valvular* stenosis, characterized by dysplasia of the valve, makes up 90% of the cases (Park, 2008).

Pathophysiology

Pulmonary stenosis reduces blood flow to the lungs. Obstruction to the flow of the right ventricle leads to increased right ventricular pressure and right ventricular stroke volume workload. Over time, the extra workload may cause the right ventricle to fail and cause heart failure.

Assessment

Assessment findings associated with pulmonary stenosis are related to the severity of the obstruction. A child with mild stenosis may have no symptoms and thus may not require invasive interventions. Most children with pulmonary stenosis are acyanotic and have no activity restrictions.

For the child with moderate pulmonary stenosis, note how easily the child becomes fatigued and observe for evidence of exertional dyspnea. In severe cases, an infant may be cyanotic and may have signs and symptoms of heart failure; assess for these signs. These infants may need urgent surgical repair or palliation. Some patients may benefit from dilation in the cardiac catheterization laboratory. In severe cases, development of the peripheral pulmonary arteries may be affected by various areas of stenosis.

Interdisciplinary Interventions

A balloon valvuloplasty may be performed in the cardiac catheterization laboratory to dilate and rupture the deformed valve through circumferential stress. This intervention is the procedure of choice because it is less invasive than surgery, has low risks, and produces good outcomes.

Surgical repair involves pulmonary valvulotomy with resection of any muscle mass and patch widening of the pulmonary arteries as required. The surgery is completed through a sternal incision and sometimes requires the use of cardiopulmonary bypass. If the pulmonary arteries are stenotic, they may require patch widening or stent placement in the catheterization laboratory. After repair, the pulmonary valve is regurgitant, yet most patients are asymptomatic and merely require follow-up the rest of their lives.

Defects of the Great Vessels

Problems with placement or development of the blood vessels leading to or from the heart are termed *defects of the great vessels*. These include TAPVR, truncus arteriosus, and TGA.

TOTAL ANOMALOUS PULMONARY VENOUS RETURN

In newborns with TAPVR, the pulmonary veins do not return to the left atrium; instead, they abnormally return to the right side of the heart. This blood returning back to the right side of the heart can go to the systemic venous circulation first and then to the right atrium or directly to the right atrium (Fig. 15-17). Partial anomalous pulmonary venous return occurs when one or more, but not all, of the pulmonary veins drain into the venous system.

The pulmonary veins are abnormally routed in different ways. The most common type of TAPVR is called *supracardiac*, in which the pulmonary veins drain directly into the superior vena cava. Another type is called *intracardiac*, in which the pulmonary veins drain into the coronary sinuses or flow directly into the right atrium. The supracardiac and intracardiac types of TAPVR are generally nonobstructive. With *infracardiac* TAPVR, the common pulmonary vein runs below the diaphragm into the portal system. A fourth type of TAPVR is a mixed combination of the other types.

Pathophysiology

The abnormal positioning of the pulmonary veins leads to mixing of systemic and pulmonary circulations, resulting in cyanosis. The presence of an ASD is necessary

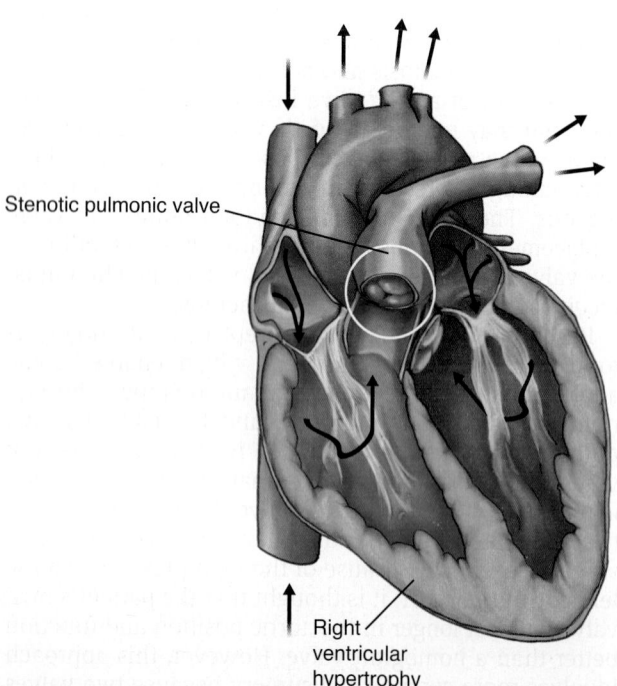

Stenotic pulmonic valve

Right ventricular hypertrophy

Figure 15-16 Pulmonic stenosis.

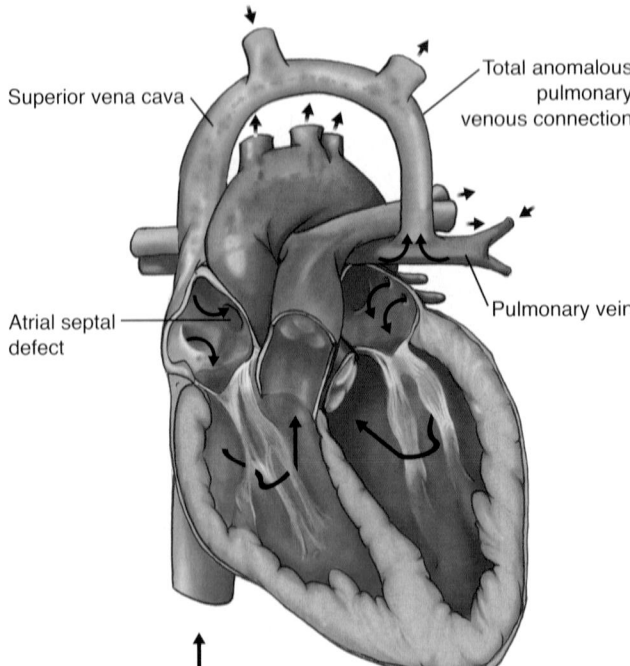

Figure 15-17 Total anomalous pulmonary venous return.

for cardiac mixing and survival. In children with TAPVR, the left atrium is relatively small from lack of blood flow and the right atrium may be distended from excessive blood flow.

Assessment

A newborn's degree of cyanosis depends on the adequacy of mixing through the foramen ovale or ASD and the extent to which flow is obstructed by the misdirected pulmonary veins themselves. Assess for signs and symptoms of cyanosis, heart failure, poor feeding, and failure to thrive. Chest radiograph shows cardiomegaly of the right atrium and right ventricle with increased pulmonary vascular markings. These children are also prone to repeat pulmonary infections.

Interdisciplinary Interventions

The clinical status of newborns with TAPVR can deteriorate quickly if the defect is left untreated. Medications to control heart failure, such as digitalis and diuretics, are administered. Some infants can benefit from a balloon atrial septostomy to encourage right-to-left shunting and improve intracardiac mixing.

Surgical repair is performed through a median sternotomy incision with the child on cardiopulmonary bypass and is done during infancy. The mortality rate depends on the location of the veins and the presence of pulmonary vein obstruction. The type of surgical correction varies depending on the location of the veins. For supracardiac lesions, the pulmonary veins are anastomosed to the left atrium, and the ASD is patched. For intracardiac TAPVR, a communication is created between the coronary sinus and the left atrium, and the

ASD is patched. For an infracardiac lesion, an anastomosis is created from the pulmonary veins and patched to the left atrium, and the pulmonary vein that extends below the diaphragm is ligated.

Children with TAPVR are sensitive to fluid volume loading because of the small left atrium. They may require a high right atrial pressure to ensure left atrial filling. Postoperative complications include atrial arrhythmias, pulmonary hypertension, and pulmonary vein obstruction.

Partial anomalous pulmonary venous return of one or more, but not all, of the pulmonary veins is repaired surgically through a median sternotomy. If the veins drain into the right atrium, many of these defects can be repaired by simply widening the ASD patch to direct flow of the anomalous pulmonary veins toward the left atrium.

TRUNCUS ARTERIOSUS

In truncus arteriosus, also known as common arterial trunk, the embryonic division of the primitive fetal truncus into the aorta and pulmonary artery fails to occur. At birth, a single large vessel, the common trunk, arises from both ventricles across a large VSD.

Four categories of truncus arteriosus exist. Type I is the most commonly occurring version of truncus, defined by a partial separation of the aorta and pulmonary artery. A short pulmonary trunk arises from the posterior aspect of the large truncus or aorta. Type II truncus occurs when two pulmonary arteries arise from the posterior aspect of the truncus. Each one is connected separately to the truncus instead of a main pulmonary artery. Therefore, no main pulmonary artery is present. Type III truncus is much like type II, except that the two pulmonary arteries arise separately from the lateral aspect of the truncus. In type IV, no pulmonary arteries exist. Only bronchial arteries arise from the descending aorta.

Pathophysiology

The opening of the common trunk has one valve with three to four leaflets. The common trunk leaves the heart and gives rise to the systemic and pulmonary circulations. Systemic and pulmonary blood mix completely (Fig. 15-18).

Assessment

Diagnosis of truncus arteriosus can be made in utero by a fetal cardiologist using echocardiography. Physical findings depend on the amount of pulmonary blood flow. The infant may exhibit cyanosis in varying degrees and signs and symptoms of heart failure; assess for these. Note any history of frequent pulmonary infections, failure to thrive, or dyspnea with feeding. Chest radiographs show marked cardiomegaly with increased pulmonary vascular markings. Without surgical intervention, most children die of heart failure within 6 to 12 months (Park, 2008).

Interdisciplinary Interventions

Medical management includes measures to control heart failure, including digoxin and diuretics. A systemic-to-pulmonary artery shunt may be helpful for infants with

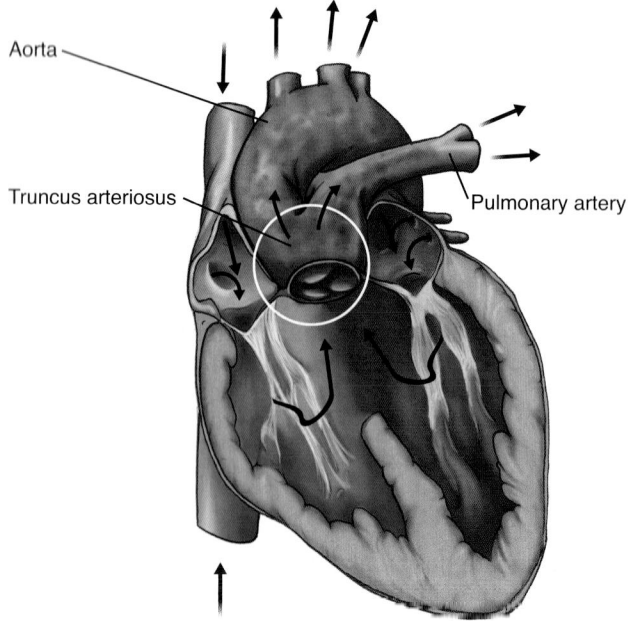

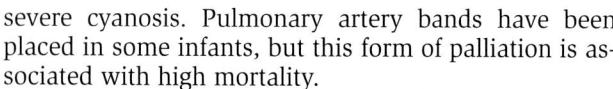

Figure 15-18 Truncus arteriosus.

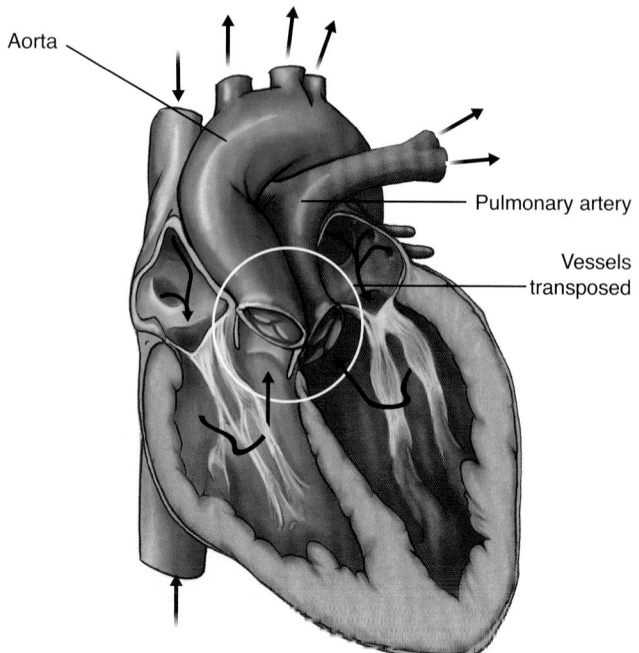

Figure 15-19 Transposition of the great arteries.

severe cyanosis. Pulmonary artery bands have been placed in some infants, but this form of palliation is associated with high mortality.

The definitive surgical repair, the Rastelli operation, involves detaching the pulmonary trunk from the truncus so the truncus can pump the systemic circulation independently. Then a prosthetic or homograft valved conduit is connected to the right ventricle to direct flow to the pulmonary arteries. The VSD is closed so that the left ventricle pumps exclusively to the aorta. Even though this surgery is complicated and associated with a high mortality rate, surgery is done during infancy because most children do not survive past that stage without repair (Russell et al., 2012).

Repeat surgeries are done throughout the child's life to replace conduits that have been outgrown or that malfunction. Potential postoperative complications include arrhythmias, pulmonary problems, and persistent heart failure. Worsening regurgitation of the imperfect truncal valve may occur over time.

TRANSPOSITION OF THE GREAT ARTERIES

TGA, also called *transposition of the great vessels*, is a malformation in which the aorta arises from the right ventricle and the pulmonary artery arises from the left ventricle (Fig. 15-19). TGA is the most common etiology for cyanotic CHD in the newborn. This lesion presents in about 5% of all patients with CHD (Bernstein, 2011).

Pathophysiology

With TGA, two parallel and separate circulations exist. One circulation system consists of the pulmonary veins traveling to the left atrium, left ventricle, pulmonary artery, and returning again to the pulmonary veins. The second system consists of blood flowing from the vena

cavae, right atrium, right ventricle, then to the aorta and back again. Patient survival depends on adequate intracardiac mixing of blood between these two circulations via a PDA, a patent foramen ovale, or a VSD. Although the prognosis is variable, the overall survival rate in uncomplicated TGA exceeds 90% (Bernstein, 2011).

Assessment

Assessment findings at birth depend on the presence of associated lesions. Diagnosis of TGA can be made in utero by a fetal cardiologist using echocardiography. Infants with TGA are cyanotic at birth, although the cyanosis may be subtle. Heart failure develops during the first weeks of life. Assess for murmurs and signs and symptoms of cyanosis. These children present with hepatomegaly, feed poorly, and develop dyspnea. During infancy, progressive acidosis and hypoxemia occur unless adequate intracardiac mixing is established.

An accurate preoperative view of the coronary artery anatomy is necessary before treatment. In most cases, anatomy can be defined with echocardiography alone; otherwise, catheterization is required. Chest radiographs show cardiomegaly with increased pulmonary vascular markings on cardiac silhouette.

Interdisciplinary Interventions

Preoperatively, IV PGE_1 might be used to keep the PDA patent and to improve systemic arterial flow in children with inadequate intracardiac mixing. A palliative balloon atrial septostomy may be performed urgently in those children without a coexisting lesion. A coexisting lesion may enable stabilization without PGE_1 infusion.

The arterial switch surgery is the surgical repair of choice for TGA and it corrects the parallel circulations.

During the arterial switch surgery, the trunks of the aorta and the pulmonary artery are dissected and reversed onto their appropriate ventricular outflow tracts. Also, the coronary arteries are reimplanted into the stump of the new aorta. This surgical repair is frequently done during the first weeks of life, and long-term survival for these children is 97% (Tobler et al., 2010). Complications include coronary artery occlusion and pulmonary artery stenosis.

Defects With a Functional Single Ventricle

In single-ventricle defects, only one of the two ventricles is of adequate functional size. Defects include HLHS and single ventricle. Tricuspid atresia, a condition associated with hypoplastic right ventricle, is discussed earlier in the chapter under "Defects With Decreased Pulmonary Blood Flow" section.

HYPOPLASTIC LEFT HEART SYNDROME

HLHS is a diagnostic label given to a syndrome in which the entire left heart did not develop normally (Fig. 15-20).

Pathophysiology

HLHS includes hypoplasia of the left ventricle, mitral atresia, aortic atresia, and hypoplasia of the ascending aorta and aortic arch. The left ventricle and mitral valve may be entirely absent or poorly developed.

HLHS is fatal without intervention, usually within the first 2 weeks of life. Historically, limited numbers of children with HLHS survive through the final surgery. However, with recent increased experience in postoperative management by large centers, survival rates have improved considerably.

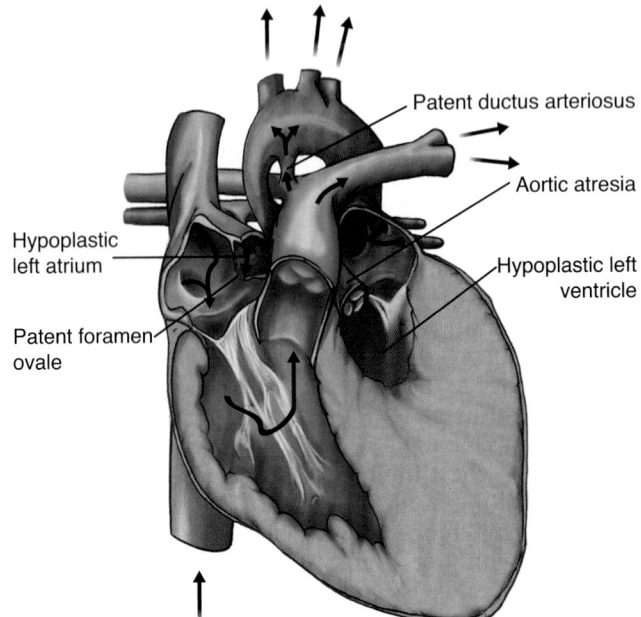

Figure 15-20 Hypoplastic left heart syndrome.

Patent ductus arteriosus

Aortic atresia

Hypoplastic left atrium

Hypoplastic left ventricle

Patent foramen ovale

Assessment

HLHS can be detected prenatally with a level II fetal echocardiogram. At birth, assess for signs and symptoms of cyanosis. However, signs and symptoms may not be readily apparent during the initial newborn period despite the severity of this condition. Chest radiographs show cardiomegaly, and generally, children with HLHS do not have an audible murmur. An echocardiogram may provide enough information so that a cardiac catheterization may not be necessary.

Interdisciplinary Interventions

Historically, infants with HLHS died because no effective treatment interventions were available. Currently, two treatment options exist: palliative surgery or cardiac transplantation. Religious backgrounds and family interactions can affect the family's decision, and some may opt for no intervention (therefore, the infant will die). The health care team must be as realistic and honest as possible in allowing parents to express their feelings and helping them to comprehend the potential implications of each choice. Each option has its own medical, emotional, and economic burdens.

If parents choose not to provide any surgical intervention, they may leave the newborn in the hospital and visit with the baby at the bedside. Others have taken a relatively stable newborn home after medical interventions have been withdrawn and have allowed the child to die with family support at home. The choice of allowing the child to die is an extraordinary situation for nurses. The nurse must provide emotional support to a family during the grieving process and help them resolve any guilt or anger over their child's cardiac defect.

If the parents choose to stabilize the newborn for surgery, interventions focus on maintaining adequate systemic perfusion and a balanced pulmonary circulation. These include keeping the ductus open with an IV infusion of PGE_1 and low-dose dopamine to maintain adequate systemic perfusion and balance the pulmonary circulation. Usually, newborns receive mechanical ventilation until stabilized. Acidosis is treated aggressively with ventilation and sodium bicarbonate, and diuretics are administered to manage heart failure. Infants should be maintained on 25% to 35% oxygen to keep the PaO_2 level in the high 30s to low 40s mm Hg. This measure helps to balance PVR and SVR.

A newborn waiting for cardiac transplantation remains hospitalized. About 16% die waiting for a heart to become available for transplantation (Guleserian et al., 2011).

Surgical palliation involves three stages in which the child receives a series of three surgical interventions. Stage I is the Norwood procedure; stage II is the hemi-Fontan or bidirectional Glenn shunt, done at about 4 months of age; and stage III is the Fontan procedure, which usually completed around 2 to 4 years of age.

In stage I, the initial palliative surgery, the Norwood procedure, is done to create an unobstructed and permanent flow from the right ventricle to the aorta. The right ventricle becomes the systemic ventricle by using the proximal pulmonary artery and patches of pericardial or homograft tissue to reconstruct the aorta. Usually, an atrial septostomy is done to encourage adequate mixing. Also, the distal main pulmonary artery is attached to a shunt between the right ventricle and the pulmonary artery or to a modified Blalock-Taussig shunt.

When the child outgrows the Norwood shunt, the child is scheduled for the next surgery. Stage II consists of the hemi-Fontan procedure or a variation of the Glenn shunt done to decrease the volume load on the right ventricle. This procedure is basically an anastomosis of the superior vena cava to the pulmonary artery and removal of the newborn shunt that was placed during the first surgery.

Stage III, the final surgery, involves the completion of the Fontan procedure, which separates the pulmonary and systemic circulations. This surgery connects venous return directly through the right atrium to the pulmonary artery. This connection leaves the systemic blood flow to be pumped by the single ventricle. Therefore, systemic flow is separated from the returning venous blood that goes directly to the lungs. A new approach for Fontan completion is to place a stent covered with a thin layer of Core Tex from the inferior vena cava to the hemi-Fontan baffle. This procedure can be performed in the catheterization laboratory and is associated with fewer postprocedure pleural effusions, lower mortality, and a shorter length of stay (Maher et al., 2004).

SINGLE VENTRICLE

The diagnosis of single ventricle denotes a condition in which both the right atrium and the left atrium empty into one ventricular chamber. The second ventricle may be a tiny chamber or may be a remnant of the one larger chamber (Fig. 15-21).

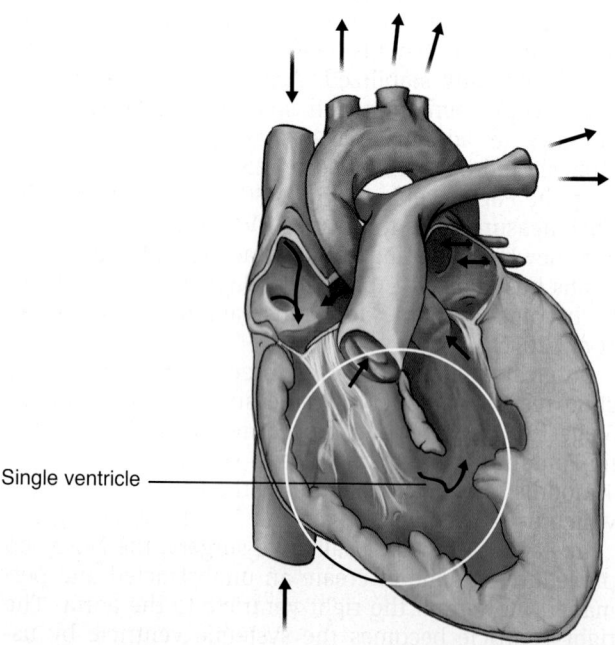

Single ventricle

Figure 15-21 Single ventricle.

Pathophysiology

Both great vessels usually come off the single ventricle, so oxygenated and deoxygenated blood are completely mixed in the chamber. Children with single ventricle also have a high incidence of heterotaxy syndrome (Park, 2008).

Assessment

Clinical manifestations vary depending on the specific combination of problems. Cyanosis, failure to thrive, and difficulty fighting pulmonary infections are common manifestations.

Interdisciplinary Interventions

Palliative surgical interventions include a Blalock-Taussig shunt if pulmonary blood flow is restricted. When medical management of heart failure is not adequate, pulmonary artery banding may be used to restrict pulmonary blood flow. If cardiac dynamics allow, many patients may benefit from a modified Fontan procedure.

ACQUIRED HEART DISEASE

Acquired heart disease refers to those disorders of the heart that are not present at birth. This category includes cardiac disorders other than anatomic defects, although some illnesses, such as arrhythmias and cardiomyopathy, can also have a congenital origin. Some acquired problems, such as arrhythmias, can develop as sequelae of CHD, surgery, or both.

ARRHYTHMIAS

Arrhythmia, sometimes called *dysrhythmia*, is a generic term for a variety of classifications of abnormal heart rhythms. Most are transient and benign and rarely require treatment. However, disturbances in rhythm occur that necessitate treatment.

Advances in care have enabled improved control and suppression of cardiac arrhythmias. Improvements in cardiac surgical techniques have promoted longer lives in children with complex heart disease. This progress, and the resulting increase in survival rates, has led to an increase in the population of patients with an increased risk for arrhythmias.

During the immediate postoperative period, children who have had cardiac surgery are at particular risk for electrolyte imbalances—particularly potassium, magnesium, and calcium—and hemodynamic changes that can precipitate arrhythmias. For example, hypovolemia, hypoxia, fever, and hypothermia may be underlying causes of arrhythmia. Anesthesia and medications may cause depression and irritability of the ventricles. Direct damage to the conduction system can occur from suture lines, dissection, and mechanical manipulation of the heart chambers. Other causes may include gastric dilation; chest trauma; sympathetic catecholamine release resulting from pain, fear, or anxiety; drug toxicity; and arrhythmogenic medications, including antiarrhythmics with proarrhythmic effects.

Sinus tachycardia is common after pediatric cardiac surgery. Other arrhythmias common in children include sinus bradycardia and supraventricular tachycardia (Chart 15-3).

CHART 15-3 **Common Pediatric Arrhythmias**

Arrhythmia	Description/Causes	Causes	Management
Sinus tachycardia	Normal configuration with rate faster than acceptable parameters for child's age Normal or abnormal depending on child's age and situation (i.e., fussy or crying infant's heart rate situationally faster than normal for the child's age but no medical intervention necessary)	Cardiac surgery Fever, sepsis Dehydration Pain, anxiety Hypotension Acidosis Anemia Drugs, catecholamines	Medical treatment rarely necessary Interventions are focused toward treating the underlying causes because sinus tachycardia is frequently a compensatory mechanism for an underlying problem.
Sinus bradycardia	Normal in configuration with rate too slow for the age of the child Common in preterm newborns	Immaturity of newborn conduction system Measures such as suctioning, feeding, or passing of a nasogastric tube resulting from increased susceptibility to stimulation of the vagus nerve (cranial nerve X) Cardiac surgery (damage to the sinoatrial node) In children without cardiac disease, may be a late sign of hemodynamic compromise	Requires immediate intervention; if left untreated, may lead to death within a short period Medications (e.g., atropine, epinephrine) Pacemaker
Supraventricular tachycardia	Most common form of symptomatic rhythm disturbance seen during the newborn period (Kothari & Skinner, 2006) Sudden burst of heart rate greater than 220 bpm in an infant and 180 bpm in a child, without variations in the pulse rate; possible compromise in cardiac output	Wolff-Parkinson-White syndrome: heart with an accessory pathway providing a reentry mechanism for impulses creating atrial tachycardia (heart structurally normal) VSDs, ASDs, and the Ebstein anomaly of the tricuspid valve	May subside spontaneously Vagal maneuvers if documented with a 12-lead ECG. To disrupt the rhythm, have the child gag, cough, or create the motion of holding one's breath as if to strain when having a bowel movement. Pacemaker (if the child has one): The rate can be increased to a rate much higher than the child's usual rate to overdrive pace the abnormal rhythm while decreasing the heart rate to normal. Cardioversion Medications: digitalis, propranolol (Inderal), verapamil, and amiodarone. IV adenosine, used to break supraventricular tachycardia, is rapid and short acting and has minimal side effects.

QUESTION: Review the case study and identify the arrhythmia Gabriella experienced during the night. What may have caused the arrhythmia?

Assessment

Identify children at risk for cardiac arrhythmias. After a rhythm disturbance occurs, the arrhythmia must be identified and its clinical significance must be evaluated. Assess the child's blood pressure, urine output, peripheral pulses, temperature of extremities, skin color, capillary refill, and level of consciousness. Arrhythmias that affect cardiac output require prompt treatment. Continuously assess and monitor the child's response to the arrhythmia and treatments. Nursing care includes ruling out potential precipitating events and considering underlying causes before intervening (Nursing Interventions Classification 15-1).

Irregularities in cardiac rhythms may be documented and diagnosed through continuous ECG monitors, 12-lead ECG, Holter monitors, transesophageal probes, and electrophysiology studies (described earlier in this chapter).

Interdisciplinary Interventions

The therapies available for children with arrhythmias include pharmacologic management and suppression, ablative therapy, implantable antiarrhythmia devices,

cardioversion, and pacemakers. The use of specific tools depends on the needs of each patient. Pacemakers are discussed earlier in the "Treatment Modalities" section of this chapter (Clinical Judgment 15-3).

Pharmacologic Interventions

Pharmacologic management is the simplest approach to controlling or suppressing arrhythmias. Drawbacks include nonadherence to the medication regimen (especially in the adolescent population), adverse effects, and failure of the medications to control the arrhythmia. The availability of a variety of drugs and advancements in pharmacotherapeutics are overshadowed by the lack of information about long-term efficacy of using antiarrhythmia medications in the growing child, with potentially toxic effects.

Radiofrequency Ablation

Arrhythmias such as supraventricular tachycardias can also be managed by radiofrequency ablation (RFA). Reasons for using ablation in children include patient choice, arrhythmia refractory to conventional medical therapy, life-threatening arrhythmia, adverse antiarrhythmic drug effect, tachycardia-induced cardiomyopathy, and impending surgery.

Currently, no consensus exists among centers or practicing pediatric electrophysiologists regarding standard indications for, or timing of, the use of RFA for

---

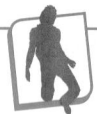

NIC 15-1 NURSING INTERVENTIONS CLASSIFICATION: Dysrhythmia Management

Definition: Preventing, recognizing, and facilitating treatment of abnormal cardiac rhythms

Activities:

Ascertain patient and family history of heart disease and dysrhythmias

Monitor for and correct oxygen deficits, acid–base imbalances, and electrolyte imbalances, which may precipitate dysrhythmias

Apply electrocardiographic (ECG) "wireless" telemetry or "hardwired" electrodes and connect to a cardiac monitor, as indicated

Ensure appropriate lead selection in relation to patient needs

Ensure proper lead placement and signal quality

Set alarm parameters on the ECG monitor

Ensure ongoing monitoring of bedside ECG by qualified individuals

Monitor ECG changes that increase risk of dysrhythmia development (e.g., arrhythmia, ST-segment, ischemia, and QT-interval monitoring

Facilitate acquisition of a 12-lead ECG, as appropriate

Note activities associated with the onset of dysrhythmias

Note frequency and duration of dysrhythmia

Monitor hemodynamic response to the dysrhythmia

Determine whether patient has chest pain or syncope associated with the dysrhythmia

Ensure ready access of emergency dysrhythmia medications

Initiate and maintain IV access, as appropriate

Administer Basic or Advanced Cardiac Life Support, if indicated

Administer prescribed IV fluids and vasoconstrictor agents, as indicated, to facilitate tissue perfusion

Assist with insertion of temporary transvenous or external pacemaker, as appropriate

Instruct patient and family about the risks associated with the dysrhythmia(s)

Prepare patient and family for diagnostic studies (e.g., cardiac catheterization or electrical physiologic studies)

Assist patient and family in understanding treatment options

Instruct patient and family about actions and side effects of prescribed medications

Instruct patient and family self-care behaviors associated with use of permanent pacemakers and AICD devices, as indicated

Instruct patient and family measures to decrease the risk of recurrence of the dysrhythmia(s)

Instruct patient and family how to access the emergency medical system

Instruct a family member CPR, as appropriate

From Bulechek, G. M., Butcher, H. K., Dochterman, J. M. et al. (Eds.). (2013). *Nursing interventions classifications (NIC)* (6th ed.). St. Louis, MO: Mosby. Used with permission.

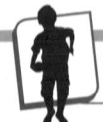

CLINICAL JUDGMENT 15-3

A Child With Altered Cardiovascular Status

Rick is a 14-year-old boy admitted to the emergency room after passing out while playing basketball with his brother in their backyard. He has a permanent cardiac pacemaker that was inserted 5 years earlier.

Now Rick is awake and complaining about having to go to the hospital. His mother states he has been easily fatigued lately.

Questions

1. During your assessment, what other information would you elicit about Rick's current illness?

2. What are reasons for syncope in a child with a permanent pacemaker?

3. What would be your initial intervention?

4. What information might be gained by placing the patient on a cardiac monitor?

5. If Rick is currently hemodynamically stable and his rhythm on the monitor is normal, what further action is required?

Answers

1. What is his underlying cardiac problem? When was his last cardiac follow-up appointment? Does he take any antiarrhythmic medications? Did he miss any dosages? What are his previous cardiac surgeries? Is this his first episode of syncope? What are his pacemaker settings? What are his heart rate and blood pressure?

2. It is important to make sure Rick has been recently for a checkup because the pacemaker battery is 5 years old and it may have reached its limits. He could be having an arrhythmia that is abnormal and faster than the pacemaker settings. He could have a cracked pacing lead, causing the pacemaker to malfunction. If he is taking antiarrhythmic medications to suppress a tachyarrhythmia and has been nonadherent in taking the medications, he could have a breakthrough arrhythmia.

3. Place Rick on the cardiac monitor to determine his current heart rhythm.

4. This will depend on the reason for his syncope. Information gained from a basic ECG will simply let you know if he is currently using his pacemaker and if his rhythm is normal at this time. It is also possible that his syncope was caused by a rhythm disturbance that occurred on exertion when playing basketball.

5. His cardiologist should be notified of his admission to the emergency room. Rick should be referred to his pacemaker clinic and placed on a 24-hour Holter monitor to determine his heart rhythm over this period of time. Also, if there was a lapse in taking his medications, teaching and behavior modification efforts should be used.

---

supraventricular tachycardia in young children. In some centers, RFA is used as a primary treatment in children aged 1 to 4 years. Complications associated with the procedure include atrioventricular block (second or third degree), ventricular perforation, pericardial effusion, emboli, brachial plexus injury, and pneumothorax. A risk of death remains associated with RFA complications, and this fact must be presented and discussed with families in relation to the mortality risk associated with supraventricular tachycardia itself. Until follow-up data on outcomes are available, health care providers should monitor children who receive RFA for subsequent arrhythmias, valve dysfunction, or myocardial dysfunction.

Implantable Device Therapy

Arrhythmias have been managed by implanting devices such as AICDs and pacemakers. AICDs are used in a select group of patients for whom ablation and medical management have not controlled the arrhythmia.

These devices are expensive, require implantation in the cardiac catheterization laboratory, and necessitate extensive follow-up. AICD is a system that senses the heart's rhythm and can provide defibrillation for ventricular tachycardia and ventricular fibrillation. The system consists of epicardial sensing leads attached to the heart to sense the rhythm, wire mesh patches on the epicardium for defibrillation, and a pulse generator placed in the chest or abdominal cavity. AICDs have had limited usage in the pediatric population. Unmanageable ventricular tachyarrhythmias have not been common in children, and the relative size of the device limits its placement in small children. Even though current use is low, the population of children who survive complex surgeries is increasing, so the population of older children who would benefit from the use of an AICD will also increase (see thePoint Supplemental Information: A Teaching Intervention Plan for the Child With an Automatic Implantable Cardiac Defibrillator: Discharge Instructions).

ANSWER: Gabriella experienced sinus bradycardia during her gavage feeding. She may have experienced stimulation of the vagus nerve as a result of the gavage feeding.

CARDIOMYOPATHY

Cardiomyopathy is a disease of the heart muscle that damages the muscle tone of the heart and reduces its ability to pump blood, resulting in heart failure. Cardiomyopathy is a leading cause of heart failure and is the most common reason for heart transplantation. Cardiomyopathy occurs in just over 1 per 100,000 children (Wilkinson et al., 2010). Incidence is significantly higher in infants younger than 1 year of age than in children aged 1 to 18 years, in black children than in white children, and in boys than in girls (Wilkinson et al., 2010).

Cardiomyopathy may be termed *ischemic* or *nonischemic*. Ischemic cardiomyopathy is a disease that is caused by ischemia to the heart. Such cases often result from coronary artery disease. Nonischemic cardiomyopathy occurs because of structural damage or malfunction of the heart muscle. Nearly all cases of pediatric cardiomyopathy are nonischemic.

Cardiomyopathy may also be termed *primary* or *secondary*. Primary cardiomyopathy is independent of other disease or is a result of unknown causes (idiopathic). Because the causes of primary cardiomyopathy are not fully understood, preventive education cannot be provided. Secondary cardiomyopathy occurs as a result of a known cause, such as heart muscle inflammation (myocarditis) caused by viral or bacterial infections. AIDS has also been associated with cardiomyopathy. Cardiomyopathy has also been associated with exposure to certain toxins, including cancer therapy with chemotherapeutic agents such as doxorubicin (Adriamycin), and certain disorders that affect the heart or other organ systems.

The clinical course for patients is quite varied. Death can be sudden (presumably from a lethal arrhythmia) or progressive, with slow deterioration of heart function and worsening symptoms of heart failure. Yet other children with the diagnosis of cardiomyopathy may have cardiac function that remains static for many years and can live a relatively active life (Nugent et al., 2005).

Pathophysiology

Cardiomyopathy in children falls into three functional classifications based on the mechanism of heart failure as systolic impairment or abnormal compliance:

1. Dilated (congestive): Cardiac dilation and enlargement of all four chambers, with progressive deterioration of cardiac output and heart failure. Decreased stroke volume and decreased cardiac output lead to systemic and pulmonary congestion, which are compensated for by increased heart rate, increased sympathetic stimulation, and dilated chambers.
2. Hypertrophic: Gross ventricular hypertrophy leading to impaired ventricular filling. Thickening of the ventricular wall narrows the ventricular cavity, restricting its ability to fill and causing abnormal stiffness of the left ventricle. Hypertrophic cardiomyopathy is most commonly noted during adolescence and early adulthood after symptoms begin to express themselves.
3. Restrictive: Impaired diastolic ventricular filling related to excessive stiffness of the ventricular walls. Secondary factors that can cause restrictive cardiomyopathy include glycogen deposits, neoplastic infiltrates, and iron deposits. Despite poor filling, contractile function is normal.

Assessment

The clinical presentation of cardiomyopathy is the same regardless of the underlying cause. Assess for a murmur and for signs and symptoms of heart failure, such as hepatomegaly, tachycardia, jugular venous distention, fatigue, dyspnea on exertion, and orthopnea. As heart function worsens, the likelihood of arrhythmias increases. Common initial symptoms include shortness of breath, dyspnea on exertion, paroxysmal nocturnal dyspnea, peripheral edema, and history of syncope or palpitation.

The chest radiograph shows four-chamber enlargement and pulmonary congestion. This pulmonary congestion can lead to pulmonary hypertension and possible pleural effusions. An echocardiogram is the main diagnostic tool; it diagnoses as well as monitors changes in the size of the heart walls and cardiac output. Myocardial biopsy is done when cardiomyopathy is suspected. The biopsy can be useful in ruling out myocarditis and some of the causes of cardiomyopathy but generally does not add to the treatment plan.

Interdisciplinary Interventions

If a specific reason (such as a carotene deficiency) for the cardiomyopathy can be found, the child may benefit from interventions directed specifically to treat the origin of the illness. Otherwise, management is aimed at extending the length and improving quality of life for the child by minimizing symptoms and complications.

Medications given vary somewhat, depending on the type of cardiomyopathy. For dilated cardiomyopathy, pharmacologic therapy is the same as that for heart failure. For hypertrophic cardiomyopathy, beta-blockers such as propranolol (Inderal) are administered to decrease outflow tract obstruction and to minimize arrhythmias. Calcium channel blockers such as verapamil or nifedipine may be used to improve diastolic filling. For restrictive cardiomyopathy, interventions include diuretics but not digoxin because systolic function is adequate. Steroids are administered to patients with known inflammatory disease. Children with cardiomyopathy are at risk for clot formation and benefit from anticoagulant medications such as aspirin or warfarin (Coumadin).

Activity restriction or bed rest is recommended to reduce the workload on the heart. As children become ill, fatigue is the limiting factor on activities. As heart functions worsen, children are subjected to increasingly frequent hospital admissions for inotropic support such as IV dobutamine.

One of the more complicated features of caring for a child with cardiomyopathy is determining the proper timing for a heart transplant (see the earlier discussion of "Cardiac Transplantation"). For a child to die prematurely, when survival with transplantation was a wanted and practicable option, is tragic. Yet the practitioner does not want to prematurely recommend transplantation for a child who could have maintained a relatively decent quality of life with cardiomyopathy.

Caregivers need to provide emotional support and strategic management of activities that are enjoyable to a child but do not overtax the heart. When increasing activity is a drain on energy reserves, appetites tend to decrease as well. Nutritional consultation and favorite foods that are nutritionally balanced can be beneficial.

LIPID ABNORMALITIES

Dyslipidemia is abnormal (decreased or elevated) concentrations of cholesterol, triglycerides, or both; hyperlipidemia is elevated concentrations of cholesterol, triglycerides, or both. The atherosclerotic process begins during childhood in association with high blood cholesterol levels (McMahan et al., 2008). Individuals with abnormal lipid profiles during childhood have a much greater chance of developing atherosclerotic disease during adulthood. Educational promotions aimed at reducing serum cholesterol levels in children have been made in the hopes of establishing good childhood health habits that will extend into adulthood and reduce adult atherosclerotic disease.

Pathophysiology

Cells require cholesterol for survival. Cholesterol is used for the synthesis of cellular membranes and steroid production. Because the body has the ability to produce cholesterol, it is impossible to completely remove cholesterol through diet restriction.

Lipoproteins are protein-coated packages that carry cholesterol and fat in the blood. Low-density lipoprotein (LDL) cholesterol is the main transporter in the plasma of cholesterol to cells and is synthesized in the liver. Because LDL deposits cholesterol on the artery walls, promoting atherosclerosis, high levels are undesirable. High-density lipoprotein (HDL) cholesterol transports cholesterol from the bloodstream to the liver for secretion in the bile. This is desirable because it removes cholesterol from the body, thus it cannot build up on artery walls. *Triglycerides* are compounds of fatty acids synthesized from carbohydrates and are the main storage fuel for energy. Triglycerides are carried on *very low-density lipoprotein* molecules. The importance of elevated triglyceride levels measured during childhood to cardiovascular risk in adulthood is unknown.

There are three forms of lipoprotein abnormalities: genetic, disease related, and environmental. Genetic causes of elevated lipoproteins are the primary form of the disease. Familial hypercholesterolemia is an autosomal dominant condition. Thus, parents with familial lipid diseases have a 50% chance of passing the condition on to their children.

Several genetic disorders in children lead to dyslipidemia. In familial *hypercholesterolemia*, faulty gene coding of LDL receptors causes ineffective LDL clearance and results in elevated plasma levels. Familial hypercholesterolemia is a rare genetic disease that does not respond well to treatment and causes young children to develop coronary artery disease. In children, *hypertriglyceridemia* causes elevated triglyceride levels and, frequently, low HDL values. Another genetic disorder of lipids is familial *hypoalphalipoproteinemia*, which causes low HDL values. These children are at risk for developing early heart disease, especially if early interventions are not taken.

During childhood, some of the secondary disease-related causes of dyslipidemia include diabetes mellitus, hypertension, hypothyroidism, liver disease, and nephrotic syndrome. During infancy, dyslipidemia is usually related to glycogen storage diseases or congenital biliary atresia. Secondary environmental causes of dyslipidemia include obesity, inactivity, smoking, steroids, oral contraceptives, and, especially, a diet high in cholesterol and fats.

Assessment

In most individuals, atherosclerosis, or hardening of the arteries, is not diagnosed until adulthood when they are already symptomatic and have substantial disease present. It can be assumed that this disease develops slowly throughout life, starting during childhood, and may be well underway by adolescence, but the child is asymptomatic.

Diagnostic Tests

Screening is recommended for children with a family history of premature cardiovascular disease or dyslipidemia; whose family history is unknown; or with risk factors for cardiovascular disease such as cigarette smoking, hypertension, obesity, or diabetes (Daniels et al., 2011). Screening should take place after the age of 2 years but no later than 10 years. If a child has values within the normal range, testing should be repeated in 3 to 5 years (Daniels et al., 2011).

A lipid profile provides valuable information about total cholesterol, total triglycerides, HDL cholesterol, and LDL cholesterol. Desirable *total cholesterol* levels are less than 170 mg/dL, borderline levels are 170 to 199 mg/dL, and high levels are ≥200 mg/dL (Expert Panel on Integrated Guidelines for Cardiovascular Health and Risk Reduction in Children and Adolescents [Expert Panel], 2011). Plasma lipids are separated via a centrifuge and are grouped based on size and density. Blood is not drawn specifically to determine LDL levels; this information is calculated based on the levels of the other three components.

For *LDL cholesterol*, a value of less than 110 mg/dL is a desirable level. Borderline levels are 110 to 129 mg/dL, and high levels are ≥130 mg/dL (Daniels et al., 2011). Individuals with high levels of LDL cholesterol are at high risk for coronary heart disease.

For *HDL cholesterol*, a value of less than 40 mg/dL is a cardiac risk factor in children and adolescents (Expert Panel, 2011). High levels of HDL are considered to shield against vessel disease.

Triglyceride levels of more than 150 mg/dL are considered abnormal (Daniels et al., 2011).

Interdisciplinary Interventions

Modification of risk factors is the goal for all children with dyslipidemia. Because there have been no lifelong studies showing the results of childhood preventive measures to lower cholesterol levels, it can only be assumed that early treatment can minimize the risk of developing coronary artery disease as an adult.

Cholesterol-reducing medications should be considered for children who are older than 8 years and who have high LDL concentrations (Daniels et al., 2011). Interventions for younger patients with elevated cholesterol readings should focus on weight reduction and increased activity in conjunction with nutritional counseling. Reduced-fat dairy products such as 2% to fat-free milk can be used for children as young as 1 year of age in the context of child's growth, appetite, intake of other sources of fat, and risk for obesity (Expert Panel, 2011).

If diet therapy and exercise alone are not successful in controlling resistant cholesterol levels, drug therapies are administered judiciously. Three bile acid–binding resins—cholestyramine resin, colesevelam, and colestipol—are the recommended drugs for pediatric patients. They work by binding bile acids in the intestines; they are excreted in the feces and therefore are not absorbed systematically. Occasionally, niacin is taken alone or as adjunct therapy with resin binders. High doses of niacin suppress production of LDL cholesterol by the liver. Liver function tests must be ordered routinely during niacin treatment because it can cause hepatic inflammation. Statins, such as lovastatin or simvastatin, may also be used in children. Generally, statins should not be started before the onset of menses in girls and before the age of 10 years in boys (Expert Panel, 2011).

Community Care

Modification of risk factors requires education about nutrition therapy and weight management. Regular physical activity and smoking cessation are also important, and pharmacotherapy may be indicated.

Nutritional education includes teaching about a diet low in total fat, cholesterol, and saturated fat for children older than 2 years of age (Tradition or Science 15-2). A recommended dietary program is one that derives 30% of energy from total fat, with 7% to 10% from saturated fat, and less than 300 mg/day of cholesterol. The remaining 20% of fat should be a combination of monosaturated and polyunsaturated fats. Intake of trans fats should be limited as much as possible (Expert Panel, 2011). Obesity education focuses on achieving a proper weight ratio for height, age, and body structure. Obese children tend to come from

---

TRADITION OR SCIENCE 15-2

Does a low-fat diet interfere with growth or nutritional adequacy in children?

Dietary fat is an important component of balanced nutrition. Dietary fat intake is particularly important in young children because it is essential for normal development, especially myelinization of the nervous system. Reducing fat intake is an important component of managing dyslipidemia in adults, but for children, some still voice concerns about long-term consequences of fat-modified, cholesterol-lowering diets on adequate nutrition and growth and about potential adverse psychological effects. Several studies have shown that fat intake is not associated with growth of young children (Boulton & Magarey, 1995; Jacobson et al., 1998; Lagstrom et al., 1999; Niinikoski et al., 1997; Shea et al., 1993). Studies have shown no adverse effect on neurologic development (Rask-Nissilä et al., 2002) or academic functioning, psychological symptoms, or family functioning (Lavigne et al., 1999). The evidence demonstrates that reduced-fat diets for children are safe. Children receiving dietary intervention are significantly more likely to make healthy food choices (Van Horn et al., 2005). Teach children and families how to eat a healthy diet and be more physically active (see Daniels et al. [2011]; Expert Panel [2011]; Gidding et al. [2006]; and Williams et al. [2002] for specific interventions).

---

obese families. In those cases, behavior modification and education have to meet the needs of the family as a whole. If an obese child is living in a family of normal-weight individuals, overeating habits may have an emotional component, and those problems, as well as dietary adjustments, must be addressed. Nutritional education has to emphasize that eating habits must change for a lifetime (see Evidence-Based Clinical Practice Guidelines 4-1).

The current culture of our society popularizes sedentary activities such as watching television, using computers, and playing video games. Maintaining cardiovascular fitness requires regular physical activity. To increase awareness, it may be helpful for a family to document the hours they spend participating in sedentary activities and compare them with the hours spent on physical activities.

Smoking habits generally begin during the adolescent years. If a teenager is diagnosed with dyslipidemia and the parents deny that the child smokes, counsel the child separately. Preemptive education of children can help alleviate the potential problem of smoking.

Through behavior modification, most individuals are able to regulate their blood cholesterol levels. A thorough understanding of dyslipidemia, risk factors, and preventive care is important. Cholesterol awareness and education is an important teaching tool in all aspects of nursing care.

HYPERTENSION

In children, high blood pressure is defined as a systolic and/or diastolic blood pressure greater than or equal to the 95th percentile for the child's age, height, and gender on three or more occasions (National High Blood Pressure Education Program Working Group on Hypertension Control in Children and Adolescents, 2004).

Currently, hypertension in children is classified into four groups (National High Blood Pressure Education Program Working Group on Hypertension Control in Children and Adolescents, 2004):

1. Normal: systolic/diastolic pressure less than 90th percentile
2. Prehypertension: more than 90th and less than 95th percentile, or blood pressure exceeding 120/80 mm Hg
3. Stage 1: blood pressure between the 95th percentile and 5 mm Hg more than the 99th percentile
4. Stage 2: blood pressure more than the 99th percentile plus 5 mm Hg

Hypertension is further classified as *primary* (essential), if no cause can be found for the elevated blood pressure, or *secondary*, if it results from other pathology such as renal disease, heart or vascular disease (PDA, COA), endocrinopathy, or central nervous system changes. If hypertension is caused by underlying pathology, that pathology should be treated to reduce the blood pressure. This discussion focuses on primary hypertension.

An estimated 2% to 19.4% of children worldwide are hypertensive (Hansen et al., 2007; Rafraf et al., 2010; Salvadori et al., 2008; Sorof et al., 2004; Stergiou et al., 2005). Another 2% have white-coat hypertension, in which blood pressure is elevated when taken in a health care setting but normal outside a clinical setting, and 3.8% have masked hypertension, in which blood pressure is normal in a health care setting but elevated when out of a clinical situation (Stergiou et al., 2005). Although primary hypertension is far more common among adults, the rate among children is rising—a trend that researchers link to the increase in childhood obesity (Rafraf et al., 2010). Familial predisposition and elevated body mass index are risk factors for primary hypertension (Robinson et al., 2005). In one study, 30% of children with a family history of essential hypertension had a diastolic blood pressure in the more than 95th percentile (Joshi et al., 2003).

Pathophysiology

When a child has high blood pressure, the heart must pump harder and the arteries are under greater strain as they carry blood. Over time, high blood pressure can damage the heart, kidneys, and brain. Hypertension puts a child at higher risk for stroke, heart attack, kidney failure, loss of vision, and atherosclerosis. Left ventricular hypertrophy is present in about 20% to 40% of hypertensive children, with obesity being the primary risk factor for left ventricular hypertrophy (Hanevold et al., 2004; National

High Blood Pressure Education Program Working Group on Hypertension Control in Children and Adolescents, 2004). Hypertensive children tend to have other medical problems such as obesity, high blood lipids, diabetes mellitus, or some combination of these factors. Childhood hypertension is a predictor for adult hypertension.

Assessment

The history, physical examination, and laboratory evaluation of hypertensive children and adolescents should include assessment for additional risk factors for other problems, particularly for cardiovascular disease. Elicit information about family history of hypertension; hyperlipidemia; diabetes; obesity; and cardiovascular, renal, or endocrine disease. Ask about the child's diet and habits (smoking, alcohol intake) and sleep history because snoring, abnormal sleep patterns, or sleep-disordered breathing may be associated with higher blood pressure (Weber et al., 2012).

For health maintenance, blood pressure should be measured

- When a child older than 3 years of age is seen in a medical setting
- In a child younger than 3 years of age with a history of a neonatal condition requiring intensive care; symptoms of hypertension, hypotension, elevated intracranial pressure, recurrent urinary tract infections, renal or cardiac disease; malignancy or transplant (solid organ, bone marrow); treatment with medications known to affect blood pressure

Auscultation is the preferred method of measuring blood pressure in children because automated devices require frequent calibration and established reference standards for children are lacking. Automated devices are acceptable when auscultation is difficult (e.g., in young children) or when frequent measurements are required. The cuff width should be 40% of the circumference of the arm as measured midway between the olecranon and acromion, and the cuff bladder length should cover 80% to 100% of the circumference of the arm. If a cuff is too small, use the next larger size. Explain to the child and family why monitoring is important, how it is done, and what equipment is used (see the**Point** for Procedures: Vital Signs: Blood Pressure).

KidKare When measuring a child's blood pressure, use language that is appropriate for the child's developmental level. For example, "I'm going to see how your heart is working. You will feel like your arm is getting a hug."

Have the child rest quietly for 5 minutes before measuring blood pressure. Use the right arm whenever possible for consistent measurement and comparison with standard norms. When deflating the cuff, note Korotkoff (K) sounds. Note K1, the onset of the beating or tapping sound, as the systolic reading (systolic blood pressure). Note K5, the disappearance of Korotkoff sounds, as the diastolic reading (diastolic blood pressure). If sounds can be heard to 0 mm Hg, repeat the measurement, using less pressure on the head of the stethoscope. If the very low K5 measurement persists, use K4, muffling of the sound, as the diastolic blood pressure (National High Blood Pressure Education Program Working Group on Hypertension Control in Children and Adolescents, 2004).

Compare the child's blood pressure with previous readings and age-appropriate norms (see Appendix B) to detect changes in status and potential pathology. Blood pressure is typically equal in the upper and lower extremities until about 6 to 9 months of age. At that time, blood pressure in the lower extremities is higher than in the upper extremities.

If the child's blood pressure is more than the 90th percentile, repeat the measurement twice at the same visit and use an average of the readings for systolic blood pressure and diastolic blood pressure (National High Blood Pressure Education Program Working Group on Hypertension Control in Children and Adolescents, 2004). If the child's blood pressure is more than or equal to the 95th percentile, repeat the measurement on at least two additional occasions to confirm the diagnosis (National High Blood Pressure Education Program Working Group on Hypertension Control in Children and Adolescents, 2004).

Clinic measurements may be unreliable for assessing a child's hypertensive status because the child may be stressed by the visit or, because blood pressure constantly fluctuates, the reading may not capture hypertensive periods. Ambulatory blood pressure monitoring, typically over 24 hours, enables more comprehensive blood pressure assessment and may be performed in children for whom more information on blood pressure patterns is needed.

Assess for signs and symptoms of hypertension, including headache, bounding pulse, visual changes, dizziness, nosebleeds, heart palpitations, and nausea. In infants and young children, the symptoms of hypertension may be irritability, excessive crying, poor feeding, or failure to gain weight. Although a child may not demonstrate symptoms, high blood pressure still puts the child at risk for long-term health problems.

Diagnostic Tests

Laboratory screening for hypertensive children also commonly includes urinalysis and culture, complete blood cell count with platelets, blood urea nitrogen, creatinine, electrolytes, fasting glucose, and lipid panel. A renal ultrasonography is performed to evaluate kidney function.

Interdisciplinary Interventions

Management of the child with hypertension involves nonpharmacologic and pharmacologic interventions. Nonpharmacologic interventions are indicated for children with blood pressure in the more than 90th percentile.

Nonpharmacologic Interventions

The first line of treatment should be family-based therapeutic lifestyle modifications that focus on diet and exercise. Encourage a diet that is high in fresh fruits and vegetables and low in salt. The National High Blood

Pressure Education Program Working Group on Hypertension Control in Children and Adolescents (2004) salt-restriction recommendations are a sodium intake of less than 1.2 g/day for 4- to 8-year-olds and 1.5 g/day for older children. Teach children and families to avoid adding salt to their food, to avoid processed foods and salty snacks such as chips and pretzels, and to review school menus for sodium content.

Physical activity is key to weight, blood pressure control, and cardiovascular fitness. The National High Blood Pressure Education Program Working Group on Hypertension Control in Children and Adolescents (2004) recommends regular, moderate aerobic activity for 30 to 60 minutes on most days and limiting sedentary activities to less than 2 hours per day. Children who have uncontrolled stage 2 hypertension should not participate in competitive sports until their blood pressure is under control.

If the child is overweight, teach methods of weight reduction. Diet therapy, as discussed earlier in "Lipid Abnormalities" section, can help with weight reduction.

Encourage children and families to practice stress reduction and relaxation techniques and to limit caffeine intake, which may also help lower blood pressure. Children with hypertension should also quit, or never start, smoking, which can worsen the long-term associated heart problems. Alcohol intake can also increase the risk for hypertension and should be discouraged.

Pharmacologic Interventions

If the child has symptomatic hypertension, established hypertensive target organ damage, or mild hypertension unimproved by 6 months of lifestyle changes, medications are indicated (National High Blood Pressure Education Program Working Group on Hypertension Control in Children and Adolescents, 2004). Angiotensin-converting enzyme inhibitors, angiotensin receptor blockers, beta-blockers, calcium channel blockers, and diuretics may be prescribed. The goal of pharmacologic therapy is to reduce blood pressure to less than the 95th percentile, unless concurrent conditions are present; if so, the goal is to reduce blood pressure to less than the 90th percentile (National High Blood Pressure Education Program Working Group on Hypertension Control in Children and Adolescents, 2004). Educate the child and family about the effects and side effects of prescribed medications, and caution them not to discontinue the medications without direction from their health care provider even if the child feels better and has no symptoms of hypertension.

Community Care

Managing hypertension requires a long-term commitment to healthy lifestyle habits. Teach and reinforce the nonpharmacologic interventions discussed here. Advocate for increased physical activity and healthy food choices at schools. Actions such as removing vending machines or replacing sodas and candy with healthier choices; pricing healthy food choices lower than unhealthy choices; and limiting sales of cookies, doughnuts, and candy as fundraisers may have a positive effect on children's intake.

Although severe hypertension is rare in children, even mild to moderate hypertension over time can damage the heart, kidneys, and blood vessels. Therefore, taking clinical measures to reduce these risks and optimize health outcomes is important.

INFECTIVE ENDOCARDITIS

Children with heart defects may develop endocarditis, a serious infection of the endocardial surface of the heart. A bloodstream infection is believed to be more likely to lodge in the heart as a complication of having CHD or, in the rare case of a child with Kawasaki disease or rheumatic heart disease, with valve dysfunction. Endocarditis can also occur in a child without any heart disease and is often associated with central indwelling venous catheters. This infection usually involves the aortic or mitral valve.

Pathophysiology

In children with CHD or valve dysfunction, bacteria or other pathogens attach to endocardial surfaces because these children have areas in their heart where the cardiac endothelium is damaged or interrupted by an abnormal flow, turbulence, or artificial materials and is therefore susceptible. Infectious organisms that are most likely to be found in a positive blood culture in the presence of endocarditis are *Staphylococcus aureus*, *Streptococcus*, and *Candida* (Hickey et al., 2009; Wilson et al., 2007). Pathogens that cause endocarditis are introduced into the bloodstream by dissemination from infected tissue or by procedures that damage mucosal surfaces. Bacteria may enter the bloodstream from the mouth after dental procedures or after an infection in the throat, ears, or chest. Indwelling vascular catheters and intestinal, urinary tract, and vaginal procedures or surgeries also are events that put the child at increased risk for endocarditis. Improved cardiac surgical repair techniques, repairing pediatric conditions at an earlier age, and giving prophylactic antibiotics have improved outcomes for patients at risk for endocarditis.

Damage to the endothelial tissue of the heart chambers or valves stimulates platelet deposition and localized thrombosis. This process eventually results in sterile clumps of platelets, fibrin, and, occasionally, red blood cells; these clumps are called *vegetations*. Invading organisms can adhere to vegetations and promote further thrombosis.

Assessment

Signs and symptoms of endocarditis can be elusive. Symptoms might include fever, decreased activity level, a new murmur or changes in an existing one, and neurologic symptoms such as seizures. Laboratory values showing decreased hemoglobin, increased sedimentation rate, and hematuria can help in making the diagnosis. Skin changes such as petechiae (minute hemorrhages from fragile capillaries) are rare in children and are probably caused by microemboli from vegetations.

Diagnostic Tests

When endocarditis is suspected, a definitive diagnosis is achieved through blood cultures drawn from two separate sites. A negative blood culture does not rule out endocarditis; it just indicates a lesser likelihood that it is present.

Routine chest radiographs, echocardiography, and transesophageal echocardiography are tools used to aid in the diagnosis of endocarditis by locating vegetation within the heart. However, negative findings (no vegetation) do not rule out endocarditis.

Interdisciplinary Interventions

If the diagnosis of bacterial endocarditis is suspected, antibiotics are administered after blood cultures are drawn. Antibiotic selection is based on culture and sensitivity results. Antibiotics are administered intravenously over a 4- to 6-week period.

The most therapeutic and cost-effective treatment of endocarditis is preventive therapy with antibiotics. The American Heart Association (Wilson et al., 2007) recommendations include oral amoxicillin for prophylaxis with some routine dental work for cardiac patients at highest risk. Clindamycin or erythromycin is taken if the patient is unable to take amoxicillin. Antibiotics should be taken 1 hour before a procedure.

Preventing endocarditis is important. Teach parents the importance of notifying any health care provider, including dentists, about the child's condition and potential need for prophylactic antibiotic therapy. The American Heart Association produces several patient education pamphlets with complete guidelines that can be given to patients who are at risk for endocarditis. Be proactive in counseling parents of high-risk children who could benefit from prophylactic antibiotics. In addition, teach the child and parents about signs and symptoms of bacterial endocarditis, including those that warrant a call to their health care providers.

KAWASAKI DISEASE

Kawasaki disease is a generalized vasculitis that is an acute, usually self-limiting, multiple-organ system disease of childhood. This disease was first described by Kawasaki (1967) as mucocutaneous lymph node syndrome. The etiology of the disease is unknown but may involve an infectious agent. Kawasaki disease occurs most frequently in Japan and in children of Japanese and Pacific Island heritage. Black and Hispanic children are at intermediate risk, and white children are at lowest risk (Newburger et al., 2004). Kawasaki disease most commonly occurs in winter and spring and affects children younger than 5 years of age (Gerding, 2011). The incidence of Kawasaki disease varies worldwide. Japan has the highest incidence at 134 per 100,000; incidence in the United States is 17.1 per 100,000 (Pinna et al., 2008).

Approximately 20% of children with Kawasaki disease develop coronary artery abnormalities, which lead to ischemia, myocardial infarction, and death in some children. Kawasaki disease is the leading cause of acquired heart disease in children (Gerding, 2011); therefore, follow-up care in community settings is an important piece in the continuum of care for this disease.

Pathophysiology

Kawasaki disease is generally regarded as a triphasic disease comprising acute, subacute, and convalescent stages. The acute phase (1 to 11 days) is characterized by progressive inflammation of the small vessels; complications may include early arthritis, uveitis, meningitis, perivasculitis, myocarditis, pericarditis, mitral insufficiency, and heart failure. During the subacute phase (11 to 21 days), inflammation of the medium-sized muscular arteries leaves the patient at risk for coronary artery aneurysm and at greatest risk for serious cardiovascular complications as well as late-onset arthritis, gallbladder hydrops, fingertip and toe desquamation, thrombocytosis, mitral insufficiency, and coronary artery thrombosis. The convalescent phase (21 to 60 days) begins as the walls of the vessels begin to heal inward. Complications of this phase may include the persistence of arthritis; aneurysms may persist and long-term scarring may form in affected vessels. The children at greatest risk for complications are children with prolonged fever (Newburger et al., 2004).

Assessment

Assess for signs and symptoms of infection and inflammation. The diagnosis is confirmed if the child has been febrile for at least 5 days and demonstrates at least four of the clinical criteria as shown in Chart 15-4. Children are often very irritable, perhaps as a result of cerebral vasculitis and aseptic meningitis.

Diagnostic Tests

Laboratory features associated with Kawasaki disease include a leukocyte count of more than 15,000 leukocytes/μL with left shift; an elevated erythrocyte sedimentation rate and C-reactive protein level of 770 mg/L; a platelet count of 500,000 to 1,000,000 platelets/mm³; and sterile pyuria (Newburger et al., 2004).

Interdisciplinary Interventions

Children with Kawasaki disease may need hospitalization for diagnostic purposes, for medical indications, or for initiation of therapy. An echocardiogram is obtained at baseline and at regular intervals throughout the disease course and convalescence to monitor myocardial and coronary artery status. Monitor the child closely for signs of heart failure, such as increased respiratory rate, increased heart rate, dyspnea, rales, and abdominal distention.

Comfort Measures

Joint pain may limit a child's mobility and may require comfort measures. Frequent oral care and a clear-liquid diet are provided to minimize mucous membrane pain. Assess mobility and consider passive range-of-motion exercise and elevating affected limbs if arthralgia develops.

Environmental modification may reduce irritability; these modifications may include dim lighting and noise control. Provide age-appropriate bed rest activities to minimize the child's activity and irritability; child life and volunteer services may be very useful in providing diversional activities.

Pharmacologic Interventions

Intravenous immunoglobulin (IVIG) is administered in conjunction with high-dose aspirin during the acute phase to reduce the risk of coronary artery abnormalities. Current recommendations indicate that a single infusion of IVIG is ideal. Therapy should be instituted within the first 10 days of illness and, whenever possible, between days 5 and 7 (Newburger et al., 2004). The high-dose aspirin in conjunction with the IVIG appears to provide an additive anti-inflammatory effect. The aspirin dose is adjusted to low-dose administration anywhere from day 3 to day 14 after administration of IVIG. Aspirin is used for its antiplatelet effects. Aspirin therapy usually continues for a minimum of 6 to 8 weeks; if coronary arterial abnormalities develop, it may be continued indefinitely (Newburger et al., 2004). Children who are on chronic aspirin therapy for its antiplatelet effect should not use ibuprofen because it antagonizes the irreversible platelet inhibition that is induced by aspirin (Newburger et al., 2004).

Monitoring of children receiving IVIG is similar to that for any patient receiving a blood product, including frequent observation for signs of allergic reaction. Particularly while high-dose aspirin therapy is delivered, be alert to signs and symptoms of bleeding caused by aspirin's anticoagulant effect, such as tarry stools, excessive bruising, altered mental status, or excessive bleeding from the gums.

Community Care

Care in the community focuses on follow-up, instruction in cardiopulmonary resuscitation (CPR) if cardiac damage has occurred, and signs of heart failure. Home

---

> **CHART 15-4 Clinical Criteria for Kawasaki Disease***
>
> - Fever that persists for 5 days or more
> - At least four of the following:
>   - Bilateral conjunctivitis (without exudate)
>   - Oral mucosal changes (dry, cracked lips and tongue; strawberry tongue; diffuse reddening of the oral and pharyngeal mucosa)
>   - Changes in the extremities (edema of the hands and feet, reddening of the palms and soles, membranous desquamation of the fingertips and toes)
>   - Erythematous rash, often in the perineal area
>   - Nonpurulent swelling of cervical lymph nodes more than or equal to 1.5 cm in diameter
>
> *Kawasaki disease can be diagnosed in children with fever for more than 5 days and less than four other features when coronary artery abnormalities are detected by two-dimensional echocardiography or angiography.

care includes teaching about potential cardiac sequelae and the importance of adhering to therapy. Teach parents to monitor the child's temperature for several days after the return home and report any fever. The family needs to understand that the disease is not spread from person to person. Except for measles and varicella vaccines, immunizations may be given at their scheduled times. To reduce the risk of Reye syndrome, which is associated with varicella or influenza infection that occurs concurrently with aspirin therapy, it is recommended that the child have an annual influenza vaccine. The health care provider may substitute another antiplatelet medication for aspirin during the first 6 weeks after varicella vaccination (Newburger et al., 2004).

caREminder

Measles and varicella vaccines should not be administered for 11 months after high-dose IVIG therapy because of the potential that neutralizing antibodies will diminish the effectiveness of live vaccines. If the child is at high risk of exposure to measles, immunization can occur earlier, with reimmunization 11 months or more after IVIG (Newburger et al., 2004).

Encourage families to obtain schoolwork for the child to do at home, and facilitate the return to school when the child is cleared by the health care provider. The school nurse needs to be alerted to any limitation or necessary follow-up. Provide written discharge instructions so that they are available for future reference.

Frequency of follow-up visits after hospitalization is based on the degree of coronary artery involvement and risk of myocardial ischemia. The child is assessed for cardiac arrhythmias, heart failure, valvular problems, and myocarditis. Serial ECGs and echocardiograms are used to assess for these conditions. All other symptoms of Kawasaki disease are self-limiting and will resolve within 6 to 8 weeks.

ACUTE RHEUMATIC FEVER

Acute rheumatic fever is a sequela of group A beta-hemolytic streptococcal respiratory infections. It is a multisystem disorder that may involve the heart, joints, central nervous system, and the skin. A latency period of about 20 days intervenes between a reported incidence of pharyngitis and the onset of symptoms of acute rheumatic fever. During the latency period, patients are asymptomatic.

The incidence of rheumatic fever in the United States has dropped dramatically during the past 50 years, decreasing from 50 per 100,000 to 0.5 per 100,000 (Gerber, 2011). Improved socioeconomic conditions in the United States have been a major factor in reducing the incidence of this disease. Additionally, aggressive treatment of streptococcal pharyngitis with antibiotics and the initiation of long-term prophylactic therapy for those children who have had a prior episode of rheumatic fever have contributed to the reduction in incidence and severity.

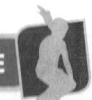

CROSS-CULTURAL CARE

Acute rheumatic fever remains prevalent in socially and economically deprived population groups in which widespread poverty and overcrowding exist. Children need to be considered at risk if their living situation is characterized by poor sanitation practices and crowding. When the child presents with a cold or any of the clinical manifestations noted in the Jones criteria, the current or past presence of a streptococcal infection must be determined.

The increased incidence of streptococcal infections during fall, winter, and early spring is associated with an increased incidence of acute rheumatic fever during these same periods. Children aged 5 to 15 years are more susceptible than others to group A streptococcal infections and therefore are also more susceptible to acute rheumatic fever. However, the condition has also been noted in older age groups where close personal quarters are maintained (e.g., the military services) (Gerber, 2011). The disease is slightly more common in girls than in boys and is now seen more in blacks than in other ethnic groups.

Recent outbreaks of rheumatic fever have not led to an overall increase in the incidence rate. Unlike previous outbreaks, in which overcrowding and poor sanitation were important predisposing conditions, the new outbreaks have occurred in middle-income and rural populations in which adverse socioeconomic conditions could not be implicated. Investigators have speculated that virulence factors associated with particular strains of group A beta-hemolytic *Streptococcus* may have played a greater role in these incidents.

Pathophysiology

Group A beta-hemolytic streptococcal infection of the respiratory tract acts as a trigger for acute rheumatic fever in predisposed individuals. Host susceptibility to acute rheumatic fever implicates immune response genes, which are present in approximately 15% of the population. The immune response triggered by colonization of the pharynx with group A streptococci consists of

- Sensitization of B lymphocytes by streptococci antigens
- Formation of immune complexes that cross-react with cardiac sarcolemma antigens
- Myocardial and valvular inflammatory response

The disease involves the heart, joints, central nervous system, skin, and subcutaneous tissues. Acute rheumatic fever is characterized by an exudative and proliferative inflammatory process of the connective tissue.

Assessment

The diagnosis of acute rheumatic fever is made by clinical criteria because no single laboratory test is diagnostic. The *Jones criteria* provide a guideline in establishing the diagnosis of acute rheumatic fever (Chart 15-5). Traditionally, two major or one major and two minor criteria (plus supporting evidence of streptococcal infection)

CHART 15-5   Jones Criteria (Revised)

Major Manifestations

Carditis

Polyarthritis (two or more joints with heat, pain, redness, and tenderness and swelling)

Sydenham chorea

Erythema marginatum (macular erythematous rash with a circinate border on trunk and extremities)

Subcutaneous nodules (nontender, movable on scalp, over joints, and spinal column)

Minor Manifestations

Polyarthralgia (pain in two or more joints without heat, swelling, and tenderness)

Fever (low grade)

Previous rheumatic or heart disease

Acute Phase

Elevated erythrocyte sedimentation rate

C reactive protein

Leukocytosis

Prolonged PR interval on ECG

---

justified the diagnosis of rheumatic fever. However, physical findings may be so subtle and transient that the child's symptoms are marginal with respect to the standards of the criteria.

Assess for regurgitant murmurs, cardiomegaly, heart failure, pericardial friction rubs, and choreas. If rheumatic fever appears likely on the basis of appropriate evaluation but does not fully meet the revised Jones criteria, a diagnosis of suspected acute rheumatic fever is appropriate, resulting from the serious consequences of missing the diagnosis.

The most serious manifestation of acute rheumatic fever is carditis. It is the only manifestation that can cause mortality during the acute stage of the illness or that may result in long-term sequelae. Rheumatic carditis affects the endocardium and the pericardium. Overall, endocarditis is the most important manifestation because it is the only finding that results in residual chronic cardiac disease. Acute rheumatic carditis has four main clinical signs:

1. Regurgitant murmur
2. Cardiomegaly
3. Heart failure
4. Pericardial friction rubs

The absence of a murmur makes the diagnosis of rheumatic carditis unlikely. Carefully and frequently examine the child for the presence of a new murmur. The most common murmur is one of mitral regurgitation and generally occurs early during the acute attack. The murmur is holosystolic, is heard best at apex, and radiates to the left axilla. The murmur also has a high-pitched, blowing quality; is unchanged by

position; and has an intensity of two or greater on a scale of six.

If the rheumatic process affects the central nervous system, the child will exhibit chorea (Sydenham chorea, chorea minor, St. Vitus' dance). The latency period for chorea is from 1 to 6 months after an upper respiratory infection. Chorea is characterized by purposeless, involuntary movements; emotional lability; and muscular incoordination. The onset of the disease is usually insidious. Initially, the child is more clumsy than usual and may have a shortened attention span, which may lead to school-related problems.

Interdisciplinary Interventions

Treatment of acute rheumatic fever must match the manifestations and severity of the attack. Supportive management of carditis includes inotropic agents, diuretics, vasodilators, and, occasionally, corticosteroids. A definitive diagnosis is essential before aspirin or corticosteroids are administered because these anti-inflammatory agents can mask other diagnoses, such as septic arthritis. Chorea is treated with sedatives and minor tranquilizers and a quiet environment as required.

Community Care

Prevention of acute rheumatic fever must be a priority for all health care providers working with children. All children older than 3 years of age with the symptoms of fever and sore throat need to be cultured for *Streptococcus*, and those with positive cultures need to be treated with penicillin. Include this preventive teaching in anticipatory guidance discussions for parents, starting when the child is of preschool age, stressing the importance of contacting the physician for sore throat and fever that lasts for 24 hours or for a rash. Also mention the importance of notifying the physician when another child with strep throat is reported in school. Most schools send notification of potential contact with such illnesses home to the parents.

See thePoint for a summary of Key Concepts.

REFERENCES

Agarwal, R., Deorari, A. K., & Paul, V. K. (2008). Patent ductus arteriosus in preterm neonates. *Indian Journal of Pediatrics*, 75(3), 277–280.

Arabi, M., Majdalani, M., Nemer, G. et al. (2007). Molecular markers of congenital heart disease. *Congenital Cardiology Today*, 5(3), 1–8.

Bernstein, D. (2011). Acyanotic heart disease: The obstructive lesions. In R. M. Kliegman, B. F. Stanton, J. W. St. Geme et al. (Eds.), *Nelson textbook of pediatrics* (19th ed., pp. 1561–1571). Philadelphia, PA: Elsevier/Saunders.

Boulton, T. J. C., & Magarey, A. M. (1995). Effects of differences in dietary fat on growth, energy and nutrient intake from infancy to eight years of age. *Acta Paediatrica*, 84(2), 146–150.

Brown, K. L., Ridout, D. A., Hoskote, A. et al. (2006). Delayed diagnosis of congenital heart disease worsens preoperative condition and outcome of surgery in neonates. Heartheart.bmj.com *Heart*, 92(9), 1298–1302.

Caplan, R., & Allen, P. J. (2011). Physical activity recommendations for adolescents with repaired tetralogy of Fallot: Review of the literature and guidelines for practitioners. *Pediatric Nursing*, 37(4), 191–199.

Chang, J.-K., Jien, W.-J., Chen, H.-J. et al. (2011). Color Doppler echocardiographic study on the incidence and natural history of early-infancy muscular ventricular septal defect. *Pediatrics & Neonatology*, 52(5), 256–260.

Cincinnati Children's Hospital Medical Center. (2010). Best evidence statement (BEST). Follow-up testing after tetralogy of Fallot repair.

Daniels, S. R., Pratt, C. A., & Hayman, L. L. (2011). Reduction of risk for cardiovascular disease in children and adolescents. *Circulation*, 124(15), 1673–1686.

Erdeve, O., Yurtturtan, S., Altug, N. et al. (2012). Oral versus intravenous ibuprofen for patent ductus arteriosus closure: A randomised controlled trial in extremely low birthweight infants. *Archives of Disease in Childhood. Fetal and Neonatal Edition*, 97(4), F279–F283.

Expert Panel on Integrated Guidelines for Cardiovascular Health and Risk Reduction in Children and Adolescents. (2011). Expert panel on integrated guidelines for cardiovascular health and risk reduction in children and adolescents: A summary report. *Pediatrics*, 128(Suppl. 5), S213–S256.

Gerber, M. A. (2011). Rheumatic fever. In R. M. Kliegman, B. F. Stanton, J. W. St. Geme et al. (Eds.), *Nelson textbook of pediatrics* (19th ed., pp. 920–925). Philadelphia, PA: Elsevier/Saunders.

Gerding, R. (2011). Kawasaki disease: A review. *Journal of Pediatric Health Care*, 25(6), 379–387.

Gidding, S. S., Dennison, B. A., Birch, L. et al. (2006). Dietary recommendations for children and adolescents: A guide for practitioners. *Pediatrics*, 117, 544–559.

Guleserian, K. J., Schechtman, K. B., Zheng, J. et al. (2011). Outcomes after listing for primary transplantation for infants with un-operated-on non-hypoplastic left heart syndrome congenital heart disease: A multi-institutional study. *Journal of Heart and Lung Transplantation*, 30(9), 1023–1032.

Hajj, H., & Dagle, J. M. (2012). Genetics of patent ductus arteriosus susceptibility and treatment. *Seminars in Perinatology*, 36(2), 98–104.

Hanevold, C., Waller, J., Daniels, S. et al. (2004). The effects of obesity, gender, and ethnic group on left ventricular hypertrophy and geometry in hypertensive children: A collaborative study of the International Pediatric Hypertension Association. *Pediatrics*, 113(2), 328–333.

Hansen, M. L., Gunn, P. W., & Kaelber, D. C. (2007). Underdiagnosis of hypertension in children and adolescents. *Journal of the American Medical Association*, 298(8), 874–879.

Harrild, D. M., Berul, C. I., Cecchin, F. et al. (2009). Pulmonary valve replacement in Tetralogy of Fallot: Impact on survival and ventricular tachycardia. *Circulation*, 119(3), 445–451.

Hickey, E. J., Jung, G., Manlhiot, C. et al. (2009). Infective endocarditis in children: Native valve preservation is frequently possible despite advanced clinical disease. *European Journal of Cardiothoracic Surgery*, 35(1), 130–135.

Jacobson, M. S., Tomopoulos, S., Williams, C. L. et al. (1998). Normal growth in high-risk hyperlipidemic children and adolescents with dietary intervention. *Preventive Medicine*, 27(6), 775–780.

Jonas, R. A. (2009). Early primary repair of tetralogy of Fallot. *Seminars in Thoracic and Cardiovascular Surgery: Pediatric Cardiac Surgery Annual*, 12(1), 39–47.

Joshi, S., Gupta, S., Tank, S. et al. (2003). Essential hypertension: Antecedents in children. *Indian Pediatrics*, 40(1), 24–29.

Kawasaki, T. (1967). Acute febrile mucocutaneous syndrome with lymphoid involvement with specific desquamation of the fingers and toes in children. *Arerugi*, 16(3), 178–222.

Kirk, R., Edwards, L. B., Yucheryavaya, A. Y. et al. (2010). The registry of the International Society for Heart and Lung Transplantation: Thirteenth official pediatric heart transplantation report-2010, *The Journal of Heart and Lung Transplantation*, 29(10), 1119–1128.

Kothari, D. S., & Skinner, J. R. (2006). Neonatal tachycardias: An update. *Archives of Disease in Childhood Fetal and Neonatal Edition*, 91(2), F136–F144.

Lagstrom, H., Seppanen, R., Jokinen, E. et al. (1999). Influence of dietary fat on the nutrient intake and growth of children from 1 to 5 y of age: The Special Turku Coronary Risk Factor Intervention Project. *American Journal of Clinical Nutrition*, 69(3), 516–523.

Lavigne, J. V., Brown, K. M., Gidding, S. et al. (1999). A cholesterol-lowering diet does not produce adverse psychological effects in children: Three-year results from the dietary intervention study in children. *Health Psychology*, 18(6), 604–613.

Levey, A., Glickstein, J. S., Kleinman, C. S. et al. (2010). The impact of prenatal diagnosis of complex congenital heart disease on neonatal outcomes. *Pediatric Cardiology*, 31(5), 587–597.

Madriago, E., & Silberbach, M. (2010). Heart failure in infants and children. *Pediatrics in Review*, 31(1), 1–4.

Maher, K., Gidding, S., Baffa, J. et al. (2004). New developments in the treatment of hypoplastic left heart syndrome. *Minerva Pediatric*, 56(1), 41–49.

Mahle, W. T., Newburger, J. W., Matherne, P. et al. (2009). Role of pulse oximetry in examining newborns for congenital heart disease: A scientific statement from the AHA and AAP. *Pediatrics*, 124(2), 823–836.

Malviya, M., Ohlsson, A., & Shah, S. (2008). Surgical versus medical treatment with cyclooxygenase inhibitors for symptomatic patent ductus arteriosus in preterm infants. *Cochrane Database of Systematic Reviews*, (1), CD003951.

Majnemer, A., Limperopoulos, C., Shevell, M. et al. (2008). Developmental and functional outcomes at school entry in children with congenital heart defects. *Journal of Pediatrics*, 153(1), 55–60.

Marelli, A., Beauchesne, L., Mital, S. et al. (2010). Canadian Cardiovascular Society 2009 Consensus Conference on the management of adults with congenital heart disease: Introduction. *Canadian Journal of Cardiology*, 26(3), e65–e69.

Maskatia, S. A., Ing, F. F., Justino, H. et al. (2011). Twenty-five year experience with balloon aortic valvuloplasty for congenital aortic stenosis, *American Journal of Cardiology*, 108(7), 1024–1028.

Maxton, F. J. C., Justin, L., & Gillies, D. (2004). Estimating core temperature in infants and children after cardiac surgery: A comparison of six methods. *Journal of Advanced Nursing*, 45(2), 214–222.

McCrindle, B. W., Urbina, E. M., Dennison, B. A. et al. (2007). Drug therapy of high-risk lipid abnormalities in children and adolescents. *Circulation*, 115(14), 1948–1967.

McMahan, C. A., Gidding, S. S., & McGill, H. C. (2008). Coronary heart disease risk factors and atherosclerosis in young people. *Journal of Clinical Lipidology*, 2(3), 118–126.

National High Blood Pressure Education Program Working Group on Hypertension Control in Children and Adolescents. (2004). The fourth report on the diagnosis, evaluation, and treatment of high blood pressure in children and adolescents. *Pediatrics*, 114, 555–576.

Neumann, R., Schulzke, S. M., & Bührer, C. (2012). Oral ibuprofen versus intravenous ibuprofen or intravenous indomethacin for the treatment of patent ductus arteriosus in preterm infants: A systematic review and meta-analysis. *Neonatology*, 102(1), 9–15.

Newburger, J. W., Takahashi, M., Gerber, M. A. et al. (2004). Diagnosis, treatment, and long-term management of Kawasaki disease: A statement for health professionals from the Committee on Rheumatic Fever, Endocarditis and Kawasaki Disease, Council on Cardiovascular Disease in the Young, American Heart Association. *Circulation*, 110(17), 2747–2771.

Niinikoski, H., Lapinleimu, H., Viikari, J. et al. (1997). Growth until 3 years of age in a prospective, randomized trial of a diet with reduced saturated fat and cholesterol. *Pediatrics*, 99(5), 687–694.

Nugent, A., Daubeney, P., Chondros, P. et al. (2005). Clinical features and outcomes of childhood hypertrophic cardiomyopathy: Results from a national population-based study. *Circulation*, 112(9), 1332–1338.

Ohlsson, A., & Shah, S. S., (2011). Ibuprofen for the prevention of patent ductus arteriosus in preterm and/or low birth weight infants. *Cochrane Database of Systematic Reviews*, (7), CD004213.

Ohlsson, A., Walia, R., & Shah, S. S. (2010). Ibuprofen for the treatment of patent ductus arteriosus in preterm and/or low birth weight infants. *Cochrane Database of Systematic Reviews*, (4), CD003481.

Øyen, N., Poulsen, G., Boyd, H. A. et al. (2009). Recurrence of congenital heart defects in families. *Circulation*, 120(4), 295–301.

Park, M. (2008). *Pediatric cardiology for practitioners* (5th ed.). St. Louis, MO: Mosby.

Pinna, G., Kafetzis, D., Tselkas, O. et al. (2008). Kawasaki disease: An overview. *Current Opinion in Infectious Diseases*, 21(3), 263–270.

Rafraf, M., Gargari, B. P., & Safaiyan, A. (2010). Prevalence of prehypertension and hypertension among adolescent high school girls in Tabriz, Iran. *Food and Nutrition Bulletin*, 31(3), 461–456.

Rask-Nissilä, L., Jokinen, E., Terho, P. et al. (2002). Effects of diet on the neurologic development of children at 5 years of age: The STRIP project. *Journal of Pediatrics*, 140(3), 328–333.

Robinson, R. F., Batisky, D. L., Hayes, J. R. et al. (2005). Significance of heritability in primary and secondary pediatric hypertension. *American Journal of Hypertension*, 18(7), 917–921.

Rossano, J. W., Kim, J. J., Decker, J. A. et al. (2012). Prevalence, morbidity, and mortality of heart failure–related hospitalizations in children in the United States: A population-based study. *Journal of Cardiac Failure*, 18(6), 459–470.

Russell, H. M., Pasquali, S. K., Jacobs, J. P. et al. (2012). Outcomes of repair of common arterial trunk with truncal valve surgery: A review of The Society of Thoracic Surgeons Congenital Heart Surgery Database. *Annals of Thoracic Surgery*, 93(1), 164–169.

Salvadori, M., Sontrop, J. M., Garg, A. X. et al. (2008). Elevated blood pressure in relation to overweight and obesity among children in a rural Canadian community. *Pediatrics*, 122(4), e821–e827.

Sekar, K. C., & Corff, K. E. (2008). Treatment of patent ductus arteriosus. Indomethacin or ibuprofen? *Journal of Perinatology*, 28(Suppl. 1), S60–S62.

Shea, S., Basch, C. E., Stein, A. D. et al. (1993). Is there a relationship between dietary fat and stature or growth in children three to five years of age? *Pediatrics*, 92(4), 579–586.

Sorof, J. M., Lai, D., Turner, J. et al. (2004). Overweight, ethnicity, and the prevalence of hypertension in school-aged children. *Pediatrics*, 113(3), 475–482.

Stergiou, G. S., Yiannes, N. J., Rarra, V. C. et al. (2005). White-coat hypertension and masked hypertension in children. *Blood Pressure Monitoring*, 10(6), 297–300.

Su, B. H., Lin, H. C., Chiu, H. Y. et al. (2008). Comparison of ibuprofen and indometacin for early-targeted treatment of patent ductus arteriosus in extremely premature infants: A randomised controlled trial. *Archives of Disease in Childhood. Fetal and Neonatal Edition*, 93(2), F94–F99.

Sun, L. C., Wang, J. K., Lin, M. T. et al. (2005). Persistent truncus arteriosus: Twenty years experience in a tertiary care center in Taiwan. *Acta Paediatrica Taiwanica*, 46(1), 6–10.

Tanner, K., Sabrine, N., & Wren, C. (2005). Cardiovascular malformations among preterm infants. *Pediatrics*, 116(6), e833–e838.

Thomas, R. L., Parker, G. C., Van Overmeire, B. et al. (2005). A meta-analysis of ibuprofen versus indomethacin for closure of patent ductus arteriosus. *European Journal of Pediatrics*, 164(3), 135–140.

Tobler, D., Williams, W. G., Jegatheeswaran, A. et al. (2010). Cardiac outcomes in young adult survivors of the arterial switch operation for transposition of the great arteries. *Journal of the American College of Cardiology*, 56(1), 58–64.

van der Linde, D., Konings, E. E. M., Slager, M. A. et al. (2011). Birth prevalence of congenital heart disease worldwide: A systematic review and meta-analysis. *Journal of the American College of Cardiology*, 58(21), 2241–2247.

van Gelder, M. M., Roeleveld, N., & Nordeng, H. (2011). Exposure to non-steroidal anti-inflammatory drugs during pregnancy and the risk of selected birth defects: A prospective cohort study. *PLoS One*, 6(7), e22174.

Van Horn, L., Obarzanek, E., Friedman, L. A. et al. (2005). Children's adaptations to a fat-reduced diet: The Dietary Intervention Study in Children (DISC). *Pediatrics*, 115(6), 1723–1733.

Weber, S. A. T., Santos, V. J. B., Semenzati, G. O. et al. (2012). Ambulatory blood pressure monitoring in children with obstructive sleep apnea and primary snoring. *International Journal of Pediatric Otorhinolaryngology*, 76(6), 787–790.

Wilkinson, J. D., Landy, D. C., Colan, S. D. et al. (2010). The pediatric cardiomyopathy registry and heart failure: Key results from the first 15 years. *Heart Failure Clinics*, 6(4), 401–413.

Williams, C., Hayman, L., Daniels, S. et al. (2002). Cardiovascular health in childhood: A statement for health professionals from the Committee on Atherosclerosis, Hypertension, and Obesity in the Young (AHOY) of the Council on Cardiovascular Disease in the Young, American Heart Association. *Circulation*, 106(1), 143–160.

Wilson, W., Taubert, K. A., Gewitz, M. et al. (2007). Prevention of infective endocarditis: Guidelines from the American Heart Association: A guideline from the American Heart Association Rheumatic Fever, Endocarditis, and Kawasaki Disease Committee, Council on Cardiovascular Disease in the Young, and the Council on Clinical Cardiology, Council on Cardiovascular Surgery and Anesthesia, and the Quality of Care and Outcomes Research Interdisciplinary Working Group. *Circulation*, 116(15), 1736–1754.

Witoslaw, B., Szymankiewicz, M., & Gadzinowski, J. (2005). Efficacy of ibuprofen for treatment of patent ductus arteriosus (PDA) in neonates <34 weeks of gestation. *Pediatric Research*, 58(2), 377.

Woodward, C. S. (2011). Keeping children with congenital heart disease healthy. *Journal of Pediatric Health Care*, 25(6), 373–378.

See thePoint for additional organizations.

CHAPTER 16

The Child With Altered Respiratory Status

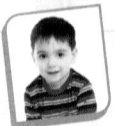

CASE HISTORY

Recall the Diaz family, who was introduced in Chapter 4, with the mother, Claudia, asking questions about the growth and development of her baby daughter Lela? In Chapter 9, the focus was on the older brother, José, who has trouble taking his asthma medication. José is 4 years old and was diagnosed with asthma this past fall, about 6 months ago. Since the time of his diagnosis, Claudia has noticed several factors that trigger his asthma, including upper respiratory tract infections, pollen, and cold air.

One evening following a warm, early-spring day, José is outside playing as the sun sets and the air cools. When he comes inside, he begins to cough. Claudia sets up his nebulizer and gives him a treatment of albuterol, which lessens his coughing. Within an hour, José is again coughing constantly and wheezing. After one hard coughing fit, José has a hard time catching his breath; he looks pale and ashen, and his wheezing is very pronounced. Claudia tells

her husband, Ignacio, that she thinks they should go to the emergency room. They leave Lela, the baby sister, with Claudia's mother, Selma, and head to the hospital.

At the hospital, the emergency department nurse observes José sitting cross-legged and leaning forward on his hands. His mouth is open and he is breathing hard with an easily audible inspiratory wheeze. He is using his subclavicular accessory muscles with each breath. His respiratory rate is 32 breaths/min, his pulse is 112 bpm, and he is afebrile. Claudia explains that he was fine; he was outside running and playing and then came in and began coughing and wheezing, and she gave him an albuterol treatment. The nurse places a pulse oximeter probe on his finger, which takes a few seconds to establish reliability but settles down, vacillating between 89% and 90%. After reporting her assessment and receiving orders, the nurse adjusts the oxygen flow to 30% and places a simple oxygen face mask on José.

CHAPTER OBJECTIVES

1 Describe the developmental and biologic variances in children's respiratory systems that predispose them to respiratory problems.

2 Describe the common alterations in health patterns within the child's respiratory system in terms of etiology, pathophysiology, clinical manifestations, and interdisciplinary interventions.

3 Describe the nursing assessment of the child with compromised respiratory function.

4 Discuss the nursing care responsibilities associated with diagnosis of respiratory difficulties in children.

5 Select evidence-based therapies for specific respiratory conditions.

6 Select nursing care interventions to support the child with an acute or chronic respiratory illness.

See thePoint for a list of Key Terms.

Respiratory conditions, both acute and chronic, are the leading causes of morbidity in children. Nurses caring for infants, children, and youth most commonly encounter children with a compromised respiratory system. Respiratory conditions during childhood can be acute or chronic, life threatening, and can present as either the primary clinical problem or a secondary complication (also called a *comorbid condition*). Infectious respiratory conditions, such as influenza and respiratory syncytial virus (RSV), are widely recognized as major causes of respiratory mortality and morbidity for young, healthy children.

Growth and maturation of the respiratory system during childhood is characterized by changes in its physiologic and anatomic features. The physiologic processes of respiratory control and gas exchange in children, although immature, are determined by respiratory mechanisms similar to those of adults. However, anatomic structural variations in the respiratory tracts of infants and young children result in substantial differences in the manifestations of respiratory disturbances as compared to adults. A key aspect of providing respiratory care in pediatric patients is recognizing these similarities and differences. Note these variations when identifying normal versus abnormal symptoms.

Assessment of the respiratory system is critical in pediatric care. Key functions of the nurse in the acute or ambulatory health care settings involve identifying changes in respiratory status and quickly instituting corrective measures, if needed. In respiratory care, developing and refining assessment skills is essential to providing age-appropriate care for children. Therefore, the skilled nurse must have an excellent working knowledge and a keen understanding of the clinical importance of these unique anatomic and physiologic features of children's respiratory systems. Because respiratory system infections are relatively common in children and are a leading etiology in respiratory morbidity, understanding how infections can affect the respiratory system is important. Knowledge of both acute and chronic respiratory conditions helps the nurse provide appropriate care throughout the child's development.

DEVELOPMENTAL AND BIOLOGIC VARIANCES

> QUESTION: Is it possible that José could "outgrow" his asthma as he gets older?

The child's respiratory system differs in many ways from that of the mature adult. The child is physically smaller and functionally immature; thus, the pediatric respiratory system has much less reserve capacity. Children are more vulnerable to respiratory illnesses and complications than adults. Infants and children develop **respiratory distress** (impaired respiratory function) and **respiratory failure** (respiratory impairment in which the partial pressure of arterial oxygen [PaO_2] falls below 60 mm Hg, carbon dioxide tension rises to more than 50 mm Hg, and the arterial pH drops to less than 7.35) much more readily than adults. Unique differences in the size, structure, and function of the respiratory system in children are shown in Figure 16-1.

This section summarizes variances in major structures and provides suggestions for modifying assessment skills and intervention techniques to provide optimal care to the child with altered respiratory status.

CENTRAL NERVOUS SYSTEM CONTROL

Respiratory rate and depth are controlled by central and peripheral chemoreceptors located in the circulatory system. Although these receptors are present at birth, fewer exist in the infant and young child than in the mature adult. Term infants and young children respond to **hypoxemia** (inadequate oxygen in the blood) and **hypercarbia** (excessive carbon dioxide in the blood) as an adult does by increasing the rate and depth of respiration to normalize blood gas concentrations of oxygen and carbon dioxide. The premature infant, however, may respond to low blood oxygen levels initially with an increased rate of respiration, followed by a slowing respiratory rate, apnea, or both. Conditions such as bronchopulmonary dysplasia (BPD), pneumonia, and bronchiolitis put premature infants at especially high risk for developing hypoxia and apnea, so nursing care must focus on careful monitoring of the infant's physical status, findings from noninvasive monitoring devices (e.g., pulse oximetry, carbon dioxide monitoring), and evaluation of blood gases.

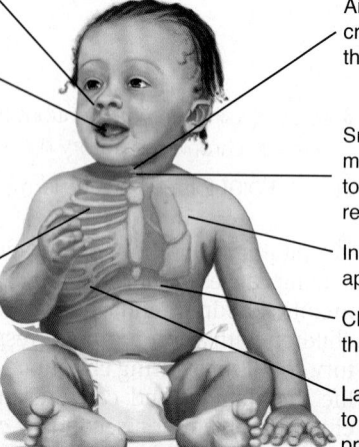

Infants up to 4-6 weeks are obligate nose breathers

The tongue is larger in proportion to the mouth, making airway obstruction more likely in unconscious child

Smaller lung capacity and underdeveloped intercostal muscles give children less pulmonary reserve

Higher respiratory rates and demand for O_2 in young child make hypoxia easy to occur

Airway is smallest at the cricoid in children younger than 8 years

Smaller, narrower airway; make children more susceptible to airway obstruction and respiratory distress

Infants and toddlers appear barrel-chested

Children rely heavily on the diaphragm for breathing

Lack of firm bony structure to ribs/chest makes child more prone to retractions when in respiratory distress

Figure 16-1 Developmental and biologic variances: respiratory.

AIRWAYS

The pediatric airway is much smaller in diameter and shorter in length than the adult airway. During childhood, the airways continue to grow in both diameter and length. For example, in newborns, the trachea is 4 cm long; it is 7 cm long in 18-month-old infants; and in adults, it is 12 cm long. Airway inflammation or a small amount of mucus can produce a critical decrease in the airway diameter and increases the resistance to airflow dramatically, leading to substantial respiratory distress or even failure (Fig. 16-2). The pediatric tongue is larger in proportion to other structures than the adult tongue and therefore causes airway obstruction more readily.

The pediatric larynx is funnel shaped because of a narrowing at the cricoid cartilage, with the narrowest portion at the level of the cricoid ring (Fig. 16-3). The cartilage surrounding the entire larynx is quite soft and can be compressed easily, subsequently causing airway occlusion when the neck is flexed or hyperextended. Maintaining an optimal neck position (sometimes called the *sniffing position*) by placing a towel under the occipital area of the head is an important nursing consideration for the pediatric patient. The right mainstem bronchus arises from the trachea at a wide angle in children (vs. the much sharper angle of the left mainstem bronchus). This wide angle allows fluid and objects to preferentially travel down the right mainstem bronchus, making this a common location for aspiration.

CHEST WALL AND RESPIRATORY MUSCLES

The cartilaginous chest wall is twice as compliant and flexible as the bony chest wall of the adult. Thus, with respiratory difficulty, children may display chest **retractions**, a visible clinical phenomenon in which the bones and cartilage structures of the chest become

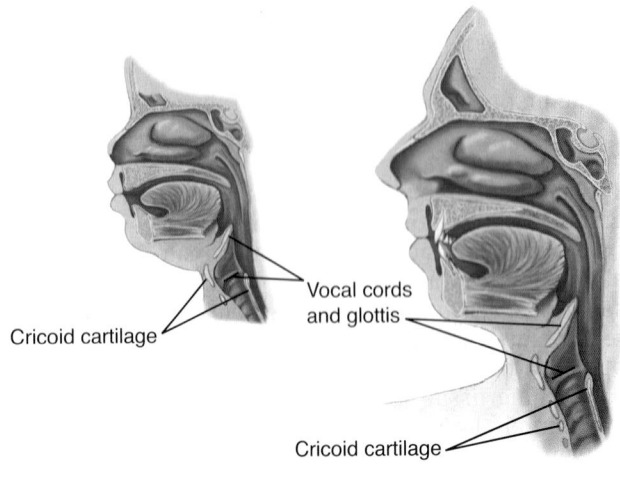

Figure 16-3 Differences in the upper airway between a child and an adult. The infant's larynx is funnel shaped, with the narrowest part of the airway at the cricoid cartilage. The adult airway is cylinder shaped, with the narrowest portion of the airway at the glottis.

more prominent with inspirations (see Fig. 8-8). Chest retractions are a result of increased work of breathing and reduce the efficiency of ventilation.

The shape of the chest and the angle of rib articulation relative to the sternum and vertebrae are other anatomic variations of the chest wall that adversely affect the mechanical efficiency of breathing in the infant and young child. Until the child reaches 7 or 8 years of age, the ribs are horizontal in orientation, in contrast to the 45-degree angle present in the older child and adult. This orientation accounts for the barrel-shaped appearance of the chest in the infant and young child. Because of this horizontal orientation of the ribs, the intercostal muscles do not have the leverage necessary to lift the ribs and aid in chest expansion during respiration. Young infants and children with diagnoses such as pneumonia must be assessed carefully and frequently for the development of respiratory fatigue and subsequent respiratory failure as a result of these anatomic variations.

The muscles responsible for efficient and effective respirations include the diaphragm, the intercostal muscles, and the muscles supporting the head and the upper and lower airways. These muscles are relatively underdeveloped in pediatric patients. They lack the tone, strength, and coordination necessary to prevent and effectively manage episodes of respiratory distress.

The diaphragm, which is the main muscle of respiration in patients of all ages, is located higher in the thorax in infants and young children and is inserted horizontally, versus obliquely, as in adults. Any condition that impedes diaphragmatic movement, such as abdominal distention caused by accumulation of air or fluid, can substantially compromise respiratory status. In addition, the intercostal muscles are underdeveloped and function only to stabilize, rather than actually lift, the chest wall. Because of these important variations in the respiratory muscles, children with neuromuscular

1 mm circumferential edema causes 50% reduction of diameter and radius, increasing pulmonary resistance by a factor of 16.

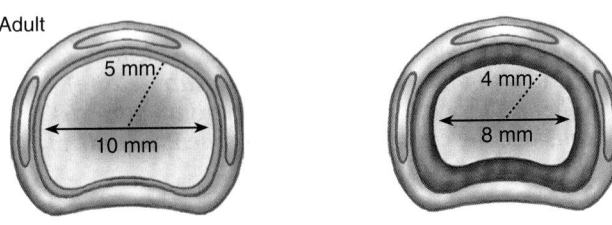

1 mm circumferential edema causes 20% reduction of diameter and radius, increasing pulmonary resistance by a factor of 2.4.

Figure 16-2 A small amount of mucus can produce significant obstruction of the pediatric airway.

weakness or paralysis secondary to disorders such as muscular dystrophy or spinal muscle atrophy syndrome may exhibit respiratory compromise or distress as one of the first presenting symptoms of their disease.

LUNG TISSUE

The ability of lung tissue to inflate and deflate increases gradually throughout childhood as the tissue grows and matures. Many factors affect lung tissue in individuals of all age groups. For example, the presence or absence of *surfactant* (a protein secreted by the alveoli to reduce surface tension) and the number and character of elastic fibers in the lung tissue can affect the ability of the lung tissue to inflate and deflate. Infants born prematurely lack surfactant, which develops relatively late during intrauterine development and contributes to the stability of the alveolar surfaces. Without surfactant, the lung tissue's ability to inflate and deflate is greatly decreased, and lack of surfactant leads to severe respiratory distress and even death.

Children also have less elastic tissue in the alveoli than adults. This variation tends to cause the alveoli to lose patency, leading to higher incidences of pulmonary edema, pneumomediastinum, and pneumothorax. Minimal elastic recoil properties cause a higher incidence of **atelectasis** (partial or complete alveolar collapse) in pediatric patients than in adults. In addition, poorly developed pathways of collateral ventilation can lead to rapid small airway obstruction and significant respiratory distress. Because of all these variations, neonates are especially susceptible to the development of pulmonary edema.

> **ANSWER:** As José gets older, larger, and stronger, his asthma symptoms may decline. He may continue to have some reactive airway disease (e.g., wheezing), but his larger airways, stronger musculature, and more mature lung tissue may result in less dramatic symptoms.

ASSESSMENT

Collecting the health history and performing the physical assessment of the child with a respiratory system disturbance is the first step in the nursing process. During the history, the child and family have an opportunity to tell their story about the illness and what prompted them to seek care from the health care team. Make the assessment a positive experience by allaying the child's fears and discomfort and establishing a relationship of trust and communication with the child and family.

FOCUSED HEALTH HISTORY

> **QUESTION:** Review Focused Health History 16-1. Analyze the information in the case study and identify the information regarding the Diaz family that is missing. Integrate any additional information you have about the Diaz family. What are some unique characteristics of the Diaz family that you will incorporate into your collection of a health history?

When taking a history, begin with the reason for the visit or hospitalization. When possible, use the child's or family's own words to document all descriptions of the child's symptoms (Focused Health History 16-1). When taking a history of a respiratory system problem, follow general history-taking guidelines (see Chapter 8) and also include questions about the environment—things that make the symptoms worse (called *triggers*)—and potential comorbid conditions or symptoms. As with general history taking, remember that clear and detailed information about the current illness, as well as other factors (environment, family), helps to formulate an initial plan of care and directs further questioning to determine the most likely diagnosis.

The child's past medical history—including birth history, previous health problems, childhood illnesses, immunizations (routine and yearly, including annual influenza vaccine and pneumococcal vaccination), and allergies—helps put the current illness into perspective. For example, a child presenting with paroxysmal coughing episodes may cause the nurse to consider foreign body aspiration (FBA), croup, bronchitis, or pneumonia, depending on the presence of other accompanying symptoms. However, if the child is not fully immunized or was never immunized against pertussis, has not been screened recently for tuberculosis, or has recently visited or lived in another country, additional possibilities for the symptoms must be considered. Focus on birth weight, gestational age, and any complications involved with the child's birth. Lungs develop in utero; therefore, premature infants, whose lungs do not have time to develop fully, may have respiratory complications throughout the life span.

Ensure that family medical history includes any inherited (e.g., genetically linked), chronic, or infectious respiratory conditions. Also include a careful environmental assessment, including where the child usually resides (home) and other places in the child's daily environment (e.g., school, child care setting, and relatives' homes). Using the environmental history, you can examine relationships between known exposures and symptoms, provide anticipatory guidance to prevent further exposure, empower families to seek information about environmental issues, and give families the knowledge and skills to advocate for their children's health and well-being.

caREminder

> *Children often spend large amounts of time away from their usual home setting (e.g., at school, relative's home, babysitter's, child care setting). When taking a history about environmental risks, consider the child's daily environment outside of the regular home setting.*

Assess nutrition and general growth and development factors. Growth impairment caused by chronic hypoxia and poor nutritional intake is sometimes the first sign of decompensation in the child with chronic respiratory problems.

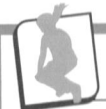

The Child With Altered Respiratory Status

Current history	Onset of respiratory distress (e.g., sudden or incremental) Chest pain with breathing Shortness of breath relative to activity level Difficulty breathing (e.g., retractions, flaring) Difficulty eating Cough (duration, onset, intermittent or continuous, paroxysmal, worse at night, production of sputum) Nasal congestion Runny nose (color of mucus) Sore throat Airway noise (barking cough, dry cough, congested cough, stridor, or wheeze) Easy fatigability Other persons in the household who are ill Allergies (animals, plants, other allergens or irritants, foods, medicines) **Current Medications** Medications (including over-the-counter medications) or complementary and alternative medical practices and home remedies related to current treatment of any current or chronic respiratory problems Supplements (e.g., vitamins) Medications (including any of those listed earlier) unrelated to current or chronic respiratory problems
Past medical history	**Prenatal/Neonatal History** Apgar score, spontaneous breathing at birth Meconium-stained amniotic fluid Prematurity Required mechanical ventilation Required continuous positive airway pressure (CPAP) Required high-flow nasal cannula Required oxygen Prenatal maternal infections (e.g., chlamydia or herpes simplex) Maternal smoking history; illicit drug use **Previous Health Challenges** History of respiratory illness such as strep throat, tonsillitis, bronchiolitis Number of colds per year including "typical course"; coughing, wheezing, or other noisy breathing associated with colds; cough worse at nighttime; post-tussive emesis History of otitis media History of tuberculosis History of respiratory diseases (e.g., asthma, cystic fibrosis [CF], BPD) History of known allergies or asthma **Immunizations** Status of current immunizations (including influenza and pneumococcal vaccines) Date of past tuberculosis test and results
Nutritional assessment	**Weight loss** Failure to gain weight between office visits Excessive weight gain Decrease in physical activity Decrease in appetite Changes in bowel patterns and appearance of feces

(Continued)

FOCUSED HEALTH HISTORY 16-1

The Child With Altered Respiratory Status (*Continued*)

Family medical history	Family history of allergies, asthma, tuberculosis, pertussis, CF Focus on sibling history of respiratory illness, allergies
Social history	Cultural (any customs that may affect treatment) Number of persons living in the household and relationship to patient Child's primary caregiver
Environmental history	Home environment (age and type of dwelling, condition of home [water damage may indicate mold exposure], sources of heating/cooling) Types of household products used (e.g., chemicals, pesticides, cleaning supplies, paint fumes, hobby supplies) Environmental exposures such as plant allergens, animal allergens (pets, rodents, insects), powders, aerosols, household irritants Outdoor air exposures (e.g., levels of air pollution in local community) Tobacco use of household members or visitors to home Family members' and caregiver's occupational exposure (clothing from work site may be a source of exposure to heavy metals or chemicals)
Growth and development	Physical milestones Developmental milestones Habits (e.g., play, sleep) School attendance and performance

Note: See Chapter 8 for a comprehensive health history.

ANSWER: The case study does not include information regarding José's birth history, immunization history, and nutritional assessment or his family, social, and environmental history. His medications are covered in more depth in the Chapter 9 case study. The Diaz family is Mexican American and, although both parents are bilingual, there may be aspects of the health history that the couple struggle to explain adequately in English and could relay with more accuracy and detail in Spanish. Carefully evaluate the need for a medical translator. It is also appropriate to ask if any cultural remedies have been used with José.

FOCUSED PHYSICAL ASSESSMENT

QUESTION: Which techniques has the nurse used to assess José? What additional information do you anticipate the nurse will identify as the physical assessment is completed?

Use the techniques of observation, inspection, auscultation, palpation, and percussion when performing a physical assessment of the respiratory system in infants, children, and adolescents. Focused Physical Assessment 16-1 summarizes possible physical assessment findings and highlights abnormalities and their implications.

Note the shape, size, and symmetry of the thoracic cavity. Notice the type and quality of breathing and the depth and regularity of respirations. In the child younger than 7 years of age, respirations are diaphragmatic and the abdomen rises with inspiration; later, the breathing becomes thoracic. Note respiratory effort and appearance of retractions, nasal flaring, and use of accessory muscles. Breathing should be quiet and nonlabored, at a respiratory rate normal for age (see Appendix B), with an inspiratory phase slightly longer than or equal to the expiratory phase. Count the respiratory rate for a full minute, ideally when the child is asleep or quiet. **Tachypnea** (rapid breathing or panting) may be observed in the presence of fever, respiratory disease, anxiety, or stress.

The color of the face, trunk, and nail beds (and the shape of the nail beds) can also provide clues to the child's respiratory status. Skin and mucous membranes should be pink. Nail beds should be pink, and the nails should be flat, with the angle between the nail and the nail base at approximately 160 degrees.

While observing respiratory status, assess also for speech patterns (shortness of breath can be seen in quick, short sentences) and activity level.

During auscultation, assess the quality and intensity of the breath sounds, noting the area of the chest where they are heard (see Table 8-5). *Vesicular* breath sounds are low-pitched, soft sounds (heard more during inspiration than during expiration) audible throughout lung field. *Bronchovesicular* breath sounds are moderately pitched,

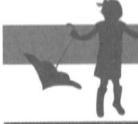

The Child With Altered Respiratory Status

Assessment Parameter	Alterations/Clinical Significance
General appearance	Fretting, lethargy, agitation, distress, or weakness is common with hypoxia.
	Presence of tachypnea, dyspnea, or orthopnea indicates respiratory compromise.
	Underweight or linear growth below average may be the result of growth retardation with chronic respiratory conditions (e.g., CF).
	Unusual positioning: Position of comfort with head elevated may indicate hypoxia; refusal to lie flat because of respiratory compromise in that position.
	Fever may indicate bacterial or viral illness.
Integumentary system (skin, hair, nail beds)	Observe color at rest.
	Cyanosis indicates inadequate oxygenation.
	Mottling of the chest may indicate severe hypoxemia.
	Mottling and cyanosis may also be related to vasoconstriction or polycythemia.
	Digital clubbing (tissue proliferation on terminal phalanx) indicates chronic hypoxemia (commonly seen in children with CF).
Head and neck	Tenderness; palpable lymph nodes may indicate infection.
Face, nose, and oral cavity	Nasal flaring (bilateral widening on respiration) is associated with the child's attempt to improve oxygenation.
	Tenderness upon palpation of sinuses indicates sinusitis.
	Exudate on the tonsillar surface, hypertrophy of tonsils, or tonsillar erythema is noted in tonsillitis.
	Erythema in back of throat is seen with sore throat.
Thorax and lungs	Observe the shape, size, and symmetry of the thoracic cavity. Palpate chest for chest expansion, tenderness, pulsations, and masses.
	A round chest in an older child usually indicates chronic lung disease.
	Observe breathing pattern, rate, and exertion:
	• Abdominal breathing in an older child may indicate a respiratory disorder or a fractured rib.
	• Prolonged expiratory phase may indicate an obstructive respiratory disorder, such as asthma.
	• Prolonged inspiratory phase may indicate an upper airway obstruction, such as croup or foreign body.
	• Retractions are associated with both obstructive and restrictive lung diseases.
	• Absent or diminished breath sounds are associated with obstruction, atelectasis, or pneumothorax.
	• Adventitious breath sounds, including rales, rhonchi, and wheezes, are associated with fluid, secretions, obstruction or narrowing of the airway, pulmonary edema, inflammation, exudate, tumors, and foreign bodies.
Cardiovascular system	Tachycardia is noted in respiratory distress.
	Capillary refill longer than 3 seconds may indicate cardiovascular compromise.
Abdomen	Distended abdomen may occur if child is breathing rapidly and swallowing air or with an acute abdominal process.

(Continued)

FOCUSED PHYSICAL ASSESSMENT 16-1

The Child With Altered Respiratory Status *(Continued)*

Assessment Parameter	Alterations/Clinical Significance
Musculoskeletal system	Pectus excavatum or pectus carinatum (asymmetric deformities of the chest) may compromise lung expansion. Severe scoliosis may compromise lung expansion.
Neurologic system (behavior and development, reflexes, motor and sensory)	Decreased sensorium may indicate hypoxia and is an ominous sign. When the child assumes the tripod position, refuses to lie down, prefers to sit upright, and leans forward, these indicate epiglottitis or acute asthma exacerbation.

harsh sounds heard over the manubrium. *Bronchotubular* breath sounds are high-pitched, hollow sounds (inspiratory sounds greater than expiratory sounds) heard over the trachea. Adventitious (abnormal) breath sounds that can be auscultated include wheezes, crackles (rales), and rhonchi (Focused Physical Assessment 16-2).

Listen for audible abnormalities including stridor and grunting. Stridor is a high-pitched, harsh, whistling sound heard on inspiration and is produced by turbulent airflow through laryngeal or tracheal obstruction. It is usually more pronounced when the child is crying or agitated. Grunting is a noise the infant may make as he or she attempts to provide self-induced positive end-expiratory pressure. By grunting, the infant closes the glottis which results in the build up of positive pressure in the airways and increased resting volume of the lung. Grunting is an attempt to increase the child's functional residual capacity and increase oxygenation.

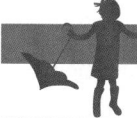

FOCUSED PHYSICAL ASSESSMENT 16-2

Adventitious Breath Sounds

Sound	Description	Pathology and Examples
Crackles		
Fine	Intermittent, high-pitched, soft popping sounds; heard late in inspiration; sound similar to hair rolling between fingers; not cleared by coughing	Fluid in alveoli (pneumonia)
Coarse	Loud, bubbling, low-pitched sounds; heard on expiration; cleared by coughing	Fluid in bronchioles and bronchi (bronchitis)
Friction rub	Superficial, coarse, low-pitched, grating sound; sounds similar to two pieces of leather rubbing together; heard on inspiration and expiration	Pleural inflammation from loss of normal lubricating fluid (pleuritis)
Rhonchus		
Sonorous	Continuous, low-pitched, moaning, vibrating sound that clears with coughing; heard throughout respiratory cycle	Air flow obstruction (mucus) in large bronchi and trachea (bronchitis, upper respiratory tract infection)
Wheezes		
Sibilant	Continuous, high-pitched, musical, hissing sound. Heard predominantly during mid to late expiration.	Air flow through narrowed passageway because of inflammation, collapse, secretions, or tumors (asthma)
Audible without stethoscope: inspiratory	Sonorous, musical sounds are heard on inspiration.	High obstruction (croup)
Audible without stethoscope: expiratory	Whistling, sighing sounds are heard on expiration.	Low obstruction (bronchial foreign body)

ALERT *Grunting is usually an ominous sign and may indicate impending respiratory failure in the infant or young child. Other clinical signs of respiratory distress and impending respiratory failure that require immediate attention include increased work of breathing (severe retractions and grunting), diminished or absent breath sounds, development of hypoventilation (apnea or gasping respirations), altered level of consciousness (lethargy or inability to be consoled by parents), poor systemic perfusion (capillary refill of more than 2 seconds, mottling, or both), tachycardia, and bradycardia (late sign).*

Palpate the chest to assess for chest expansion, tenderness, pulsations, and masses in the thoracic region. **Subcutaneous emphysema** (crepitus) is a manifestation of free air that has leaked from the respiratory system into the subcutaneous tissue, most commonly resulting from a pneumomediastinum or pneumothorax. It results in swelling and can usually be palpated over the neck, shoulders, and upper chest. It has been described as feeling the sensation of crisped rice cereal under the skin. Assess and palpate for symmetry of chest wall excursions, especially in a child in whom trauma is suspected. Trauma to the rib cage can result in fractures and a "flail chest" (asymmetric movement of the chest) with decreased movement of the affected side. The position of the trachea may deviate from the normal midline position in the presence of atelectasis and with pneumothorax, making palpation of this structure important.

Use percussion to identify areas of consolidation or other internal changes within the lung. Percuss with a gentle motion to achieve sufficient tones, keeping in mind that the pediatric patient's thinner chest wall will produce a more resonant tone. A normal percussion finding includes dullness over the heart and resonance over the lung fields. If a consolidation such as pneumonia is present, the resonance over the lungs will change to a dull sound.

ANSWER: The nurse has used inspection but not auscultation. Did you anticipate that José's breath sounds might be difficult to assess because of the loud inspiratory stridor? The nurse does not hear air moving well in the lower lobes but is not certain if the sound is masked by the stridor or if José is truly not moving air well.

DIAGNOSTIC CRITERIA

QUESTION: Of the four groups of diagnostic tests identified in the following pages, three are typically used to evaluate a child's condition with asthma. José has already had one in use: the pulse oximeter. Which diagnostic test will most fully reflect the respiratory status of José?

Four major groups of diagnostic tests and procedures used in the evaluation of the respiratory system and respiratory disorders in children include (1) measurement of lung volumes and flow rates (pulmonary function tests and peak flow measurement), (2) direct or indirect blood and body fluid analysis (e.g., arterial blood gases, pulse oximetry, capnography, fluid cultures, sweat chloride test), (3) imaging techniques (radiographs, fluoroscopy, bronchography, computed tomographic [CT] scan, scintigraphy, magnetic resonance imaging [MRI]), and (4) direct visualization of the respiratory tree (laryngoscopy, bronchoscopy). These diagnostic tests, used alone or in combination, may yield information necessary in the diagnosis and treatment of acute and chronic lung disease. Tests and Procedures 16-1 describes the purpose, findings, and indications of individual diagnostic tests as well as the specific responsibilities and considerations for the health care provider.

Measurement of arterial blood gases is considered one of the most useful diagnostic tests when a child presents with respiratory distress, impending cardiopulmonary failure, or both. Therefore, knowing normal arterial blood gas values for children is important for the nurse evaluating the child (Tests and Procedures 16-2). Pulse oximetry and apnea monitors are examples of noninvasive and portable methods to detect respiratory compromise in the pediatric patient. Pulse oximetry is primarily used in inpatient and outpatient clinical settings by health care providers (Fig. 16-4). Apnea monitors are used in both clinical and home settings as both a diagnostic tool to assess for apnea and a system to alert care providers that a child is experiencing an apneic event and intervention may be warranted (see thePoint for Procedures).

ANSWER: Pulse oximetry can read the oxygen saturation of José's hemoglobin, but it cannot detect an increase in carbon dioxide or pH changes. An arterial blood gas measurement, although invasive, obtains information that cannot be obtained readily through a noninvasive alternative.

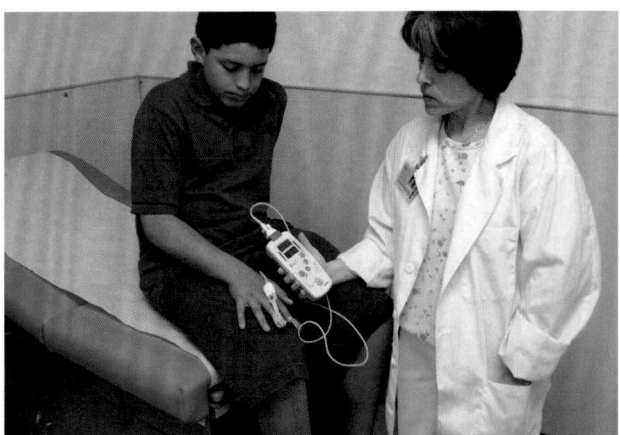

Figure 16-4 Child with a pulse oximeter. The finger probe has a red sensor light that fascinates some children.

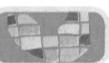

TESTS AND PROCEDURES 16-1 Evaluating Respiratory Status

Diagnostic Test or Procedure	Purpose	Findings and Indications	Health Care Provider Responsibilities
Pulmonary function tests (spirometry)	Measures airway function, lung volumes, and gas exchange. Used to determine the presence, nature, and extent of pulmonary disease. Does not indicate the cause of the dysfunction.	Abnormalities of particular measurements may occur in different diseases. Restrictive diseases cause decreased VC and TLC. Obstructive diseases may cause an increase in TLC and RV, decreased VC, and decrease in FEV_1 and forced expiratory flow between 25% and 75% VC ($FEF_{25\%-75\%}$).	Most results are effort dependent. Emphasize the need for maximum cooperation during the test to achieve valid results. Some tests require that the child's nose be clamped. Child should not eat immediately prior to examination: coughing required during the test sometimes stimulates vomiting. Test may be performed before and after bronchodilator therapy for best results.
Bronchoprovocation tests	Used as an attempt to provoke mild bronchospasm in patients in a controlled setting. Substances such as histamine and methacholine are introduced to determine whether the child's airways constrict.	Positive test is diagnostic for airway hyperresponsiveness (a characteristic feature of asthma) and can determine severity of asthma. Negative test makes a diagnosis of asthma less likely.	The morning of the test, the child should not take any asthma medications and should avoid caffeinated beverages, chocolate, extremely hot or cold environments, and exercise. The child should be free of any respiratory illnesses at time of tests. At the end of the test, a bronchodilator may be given to reverse any constriction of the airways. Test must be performed by a trained individual.
Peak flow measurement	Used to measure the greatest flow velocity during a forced expiration. Child exhales forcefully and quickly into the meter while taking maximal deep inhalation.	Peak flow rate decreases as airway obstruction increases. Values should be compared with the individual child's baseline or "personal best," not average predicted normal values.	Child must be developmentally able to follow instructions (generally older than 4 years of age). May not be appropriate if child is in severe respiratory distress. Accurate peak flow measurement is effort dependent. Child and caregivers should be instructed to keep a log of peak flow measurements when well and ill.
Arterial blood gas	Used to measure and analyze PaO_2, partial pressure of arterial carbon dioxide ($PaCO_2$), and alterations in the pH.	The $PaCO_2$ measurement indicates adequacy of ventilation. PaO_2 is used to detect altered oxygenation. pH indicates the acid/base balance. Bicarbonate (HCO_3) level indicates whether the condition is acute or chronic.	Air should not be allowed to enter the syringe with the sample; doing so can alter the results. Firm pressure should be applied to the puncture site for 5 minutes to prevent hematoma or bleeding. Arterial puncture is painful and may be associated with altered findings if child has been crying or screaming for a prolonged period.

Diagnostic Test or Procedure	Purpose	Findings and Indications	Health Care Provider Responsibilities
Pulse oximetry	Monitors arterial oxygen saturation (SaO$_2$). Can also detect and provide a digital display of the pulse rate.	SaO$_2$ can be used to estimate PaO$_2$ using the oxyhemoglobin dissociation curve. Used to evaluate respiratory function and check for hypoxemia. Healthy children have a saturation of 98%–100%.	Information enables continuous monitoring and evaluation of SaO$_2$ (see thePoint for Procedures). Accurate monitoring is diminished with significant patient/extremity movement and/or cool periphery. Children with anemia can have normal SaO$_2$ measurement but may be hypoxemic if the anemia is severe.
Apnea monitor	Used to detect pauses of breathing lasting 5–20 seconds depending on the selected alarm parameters.	May indicate child has apnea of prematurity (AOP), apnea of infancy (AOI), or an apparent life-threatening event (ALTE).	Unless otherwise ordered, the apnea monitor should be used continuously, except during bathing or at times when the infant is involved in interactive activities with the caregiver (see thePoint for Procedures).
Sputum culture/tracheal aspiration	Used to detect presence of and identify bacterial, fungal, or other respiratory pathogens.	Presence of pathogens usually indicates infection. However, samples with a variety of bacteria without predominance of one organism may represent usual flora for that child. Observe sputum for color, consistency, and odor. Color of sputum may or may not indicate infection. Infection with *Pseudomonas aeruginosa* causes the sputum to have a distinct "sweet" odor.	Specimen should be collected within 3–7 days after onset of signs and symptoms and before antimicrobial therapy is initiated, unless the culture is being completed to examine the effectiveness of therapy. The specimen should be placed in a sterile container for culture or a tube with appropriate medium. Specimen must be from bronchial tree, not just saliva from mouth. Specimens should not be frozen and should be transported as soon as possible.
Throat culture (throat swab)	Used to determine bacterial cause in pharyngitis. Reliable method to differentiate infection with group A beta-hemolytic *Streptococcus pyogenes* from infection with viral organisms.	Positive throat culture for *S. pyogenes* indicates strep throat.	Specimens should be obtained from the posterior pharynx and each tonsillar area. Any white patch or inflamed area should be cultured. Results take 24–48 hours to obtain. Special test kits are available for *S. pyogenes* that can yield results in 7 minutes.

(Continued)

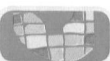 **TESTS AND PROCEDURES 16-1 Evaluating Respiratory Status** (*Continued*)

Diagnostic Test or Procedure	Purpose	Findings and Indications	Health Care Provider Responsibilities
Nasal and nasopharyngeal culture or washing	Preferred method used to detect bacterial, viral, and other respiratory pathogens because a large number of ciliated epithelial cells are essential for optimal recovery of the pathogens.	Able to detect *Bordetella pertussis, Candida albicans, Corynebacterium diphtheriae, Neisseria meningitidis, Haemophilus influenzae,* and others.	For a culture, the flexible swab should be inserted into the nare and rotated against the anterior hairs for a good specimen. For a washing, normal saline should be instilled into the nostril and then immediately suctioned with a catheter into a specimen container.
Sweat chloride test	Used in diagnosis of Cystic Fibrosis. Measures amount of sodium and chloride content in the sweat.	Sweat chloride of >60 mEq/L indicates positive test for CF. Levels of 40–60 mEq/L are elevated and may indicate presence of CF. A confirmatory test will be needed.	Test takes about an hour for enough sweat to be collected. A positive reading requires the sweat test to be performed at an approved CF center.
Lung biopsy and/or thoracentesis	A needle is inserted through an intercostal space into lung tissue to obtain a lung aspirate specimen for histology and culture.	Purulent fluid indicates infection (empyema). Presence of lymphocytes with chyle indicates chylothorax. Presence of lymphocytes may indicate malignancy, and bloody fluid may indicate hemothorax.	Bleeding and pneumothorax are potential complications.
Chest radiograph	The best initial imaging technique to detect abnormalities of the pulmonary, mediastinal, and musculoskeletal structures of the thorax.	Air or fluid in the pleural space indicates a pleural effusion or pneumothorax. Hyperinflation often implies air trapping seen in bronchiolitis or asthma. Atelectasis, infiltrates, or both may indicate pneumonia.	Determine whether adolescent female patients may be pregnant. Anteroposterior view is more appropriate for children younger than 2 years of age.
Fluoroscopy	Related to chest radiographs, but image is continuous on a computerized screen and enables continuous observation of chest movements during inspiration and expiration.	Useful in assessing diaphragmatic movement. Can detect air trapping and presence of pulsation in intrathoracic masses.	Child should be immobilized. In some cases, sedation may be required. Determine whether adolescent female patients may be pregnant. Lead shields are used to protect radiosensitive areas, such as gonads and thyroid gland.
Bronchography	Uses a contrast medium instilled directly into the tracheobronchial tree to visualize the bronchi for narrowing, obstruction, dilation, or malformation of the bronchial tree.	Provides information about the most peripheral bronchioles. Chronic distal bronchial obstruction and dilation indicate bronchiectasis.	Signed consent required. Child must be NPO (nothing by mouth) 6–12 hours before test and after test until gag reflex returns. Important to check whether child has any loose teeth prior to test. Usually performed with child under general anesthesia.

Diagnostic Test or Procedure	Purpose	Findings and Indications	Health Care Provider Responsibilities
Computed tomography (CT) scan	A sequence of radiographs that show a cross-sectional view of the thorax. Used to detect masses or locate lesions.	Presence of mediastinal mass may indicate tumor; hilar adenopathy may indicate infection with tuberculosis. May be used to obtain greater detail of lung pathology than can be noted on a plain chest radiograph.	Sedation or immobilization of child usually required. NPO 3–4 hours prior to examination because intravenous (IV) contrast media may be used to further visualize cardiac chambers and vessels.
Radionuclide scintigraphy, lung scan (V/Q scan)	A nuclear medicine scan performed to detect alterations or defects in perfusion (Q), inequalities in ventilation (V), or both.	Scintigraphy is able to detect noninfectious inflammatory diseases, presence of pulmonary emboli, pulmonary complications of HIV infection, and tumors.	Signed consent required for injection of radionuclides intravenously. Young or uncooperative child may be sedated and thus should be NPO 4 hours before procedure. If sedation is not used, it is not necessary to keep child NPO.
Magnetic resonance imaging (MRI)	Uses magnetic waves to provide two- and three-dimensional views on the transaxial, coronal, and sagittal planes.	Easily detects abnormalities of soft tissues, presence of solid masses, chest wall deformities, and vascular abnormalities.	Child must be able to cooperate and lie still; the younger child may need sedation. Any clothing with metal snaps or metal items, such as barrettes, should be removed. Presence of a pacemaker or central nervous system clip is a contraindication to MRI.
Laryngoscopy/ bronchoscopy; rigid or flexible fiberoptic	Procedure similar to insertion of an endotracheal (ET) tube used to provide direct visualization of the airways using a lighted laryngoscope.	Aids in diagnosing cause of upper airway obstructions (including foreign bodies), abnormalities in major airways, aspiration of thick mucus plugs, obtaining secretions for bronchial lavage and cultures, aspiration of thick mucus, and obtaining secretions for cultures. Flexible equipment affords more detailed visualization of mucosa; rigid equipment can remove foreign bodies from major airways.	Signed consent necessary. Suction equipment and oxygen should be ready and available at bedside. Sedation required for flexible bronchoscopy; general anesthesia required for rigid bronchoscopy.

FEV$_1$, forced expiratory volume in 1 second; RV, residual volume; TLC, total lung capacity; VC, vital capacity.

TESTS AND PROCEDURES 16-2 Pediatric Arterial Blood Gases

	pH	PaCO$_2$ (mm Hg)	PaO$_2$ (mm Hg)	HCO$_3$ (mEq/L)	Causes of Imbalance
Normal Values					
Preterm infant	7.11–7.36	27–40	55–85	21–28	
Term infant	7.35–7.45	27–41	54–95	21–28	
Child	7.35–7.45	35–45	80–100	21–28	
Abnormal Values					
Respiratory acidosis (acute alveolar hypoventilation)	<7.30	>50	WNL or <80	WNL	Chronic lung disease (chronic bronchitis, asthma), respiratory depression from drugs or anesthesia, pneumonia, respiratory distress
Respiratory alkalosis (acute alveolar hyperventilation)	>7.50	<30	WNL	WNL	Anxiety, fear, pain, improperly adjusted ventilator (overventilation), salicylate toxicity, fever, hyperventilation, hypoxia, tetany, head trauma, sepsis
Metabolic acidosis	<7.30	WNL	WNL	<21	Severe diarrhea, kidney failure, diabetic ketoacidosis, shock, burns, malnutrition, ingestion of salicylates
Metabolic alkalosis	>7.50	WNL	WNL	>28	Loss of HCO$_3$ by intestines, severe vomiting, CF, gastric suctioning, severe diarrhea, renal failure, diuretics, loss of kidneys
Respiratory acidosis with metabolic compensation (chronic alveolar hypoventilation)	WNL	>50	WNL or <80	>28	Kidneys try to retain more HCO$_3$ by increasing retention
Respiratory alkalosis with metabolic compensation (chronic alveolar hyperventilation)	WNL	<30	WNL	<22	Kidneys try to reduce HCO$_3$ by increasing excretion
Metabolic acidosis with respiratory compensation	WNL	<30	WNL	<22	Lungs try to reduce PaCO$_2$ by increasing ventilation
Metabolic alkalosis with respiratory compensation	WNL	>50	WNL	>28	Lungs try to increase PaCO$_2$ slightly by hypoventilation

PCO$_2$, partial pressure of carbon dioxide; WNL, within normal limits.

TREATMENT MODALITIES

Respiratory illnesses in children, both acute and chronic conditions, require aggressive and immediate intervention. Respiratory failure is one of the leading causes of cardiopulmonary arrest in children (American Heart Association, 2011). A thorough assessment of the child's status, followed by quick actions that support oxygenation and ventilation, can serve to avert an impending respiratory arrest. In the case of acute respiratory problems, children generally respond well and promptly to the simple administration of oxygen and medications. For children with a chronic respiratory condition, oxygen, medications, airway clearance techniques (ACTs), and nutritional support can assist them through exacerbations of the illness and provide them with the strength to maintain a high level of wellness despite their chronic conditions. Some conditions may require use of an artificial airway, mechanical ventilation, or tracheostomy.

ADMINISTRATION OF OXYGEN

> QUESTION: Consider the various modes of oxygen delivery (see Supplemental Resources on thePoint: Procedures: Oxygen Administration). Why was a simple mask used to deliver oxygen to José instead of nasal cannula?

Oxygen is indicated for the treatment of hypoxemia and can be the most dramatic, life-saving intervention for that condition. Although oxygen is important, assess patency of the airway first. Oxygen is indicated for the presence of or risk of low PaO_2 levels and is also indicated to improve oxygenation when cardiac output is low, to decrease pulmonary vascular resistance, to enhance elimination of carbon dioxide, or to accelerate removal of nitrogen from air-containing spaces such as a pneumothorax.

Oxygen can be delivered by mask (Fig. 16-5), nasal cannula, oxygen hood, oxygen tent, or via endotracheal or tracheal tube (see thePoint for Procedures). The mode of oxygen delivery used is based on the concentration or percentage of oxygen desired and on the child's ability to cooperate with therapy. To ensure patient safety, measure and monitor the concentration of inspired oxygen carefully and document response during oxygen therapy. Oxygen therapy in children should use the least amount of oxygen required to normalize PaO_2 (more than 60 to 80 mm Hg) and SaO_2 (more than 93%). When oxygen is administered through an artificial airway, such as an ET tube or a tracheostomy tube, the gas must be artificially heated and humidified.

caREminder

To decrease the risk of mucociliary dysfunction, injury to the respiratory epithelium, and thickening of secretions, children receiving oxygen therapy through an artificial airway should receive warmed, humidified oxygen.

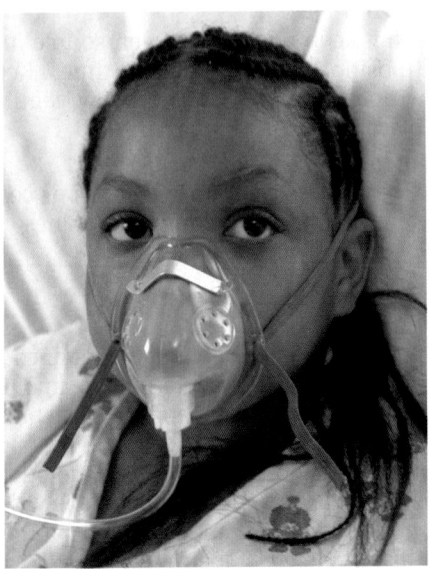

Figure 16-5 Child receiving oxygen via a face mask.

The use of oxygen therapy in the home is becoming more prevalent. Teaching Intervention Plan 16-1 describes care of the child receiving home oxygen therapy and the educational needs of the family.

> ANSWER: José is breathing primarily through his open mouth. For a nasal cannula to be an appropriate mode of delivery, the child must keep his or her mouth closed and breathe through the nose.

MEDICATIONS

Medications are an important component of treating respiratory disorders in children. Routes of administration are oral, inhaled, IV, and injectable (subcutaneous or intramuscular). Inhaled medications are used most often to increase respiratory tract absorption and to decrease systemic absorption.

Classes of Medications

The main classes of medications used for respiratory disorders include bronchodilators, corticosteroids, and leukotriene modifiers/mast cell stabilizers. Other groups of medications often used in conjunction with these include, but are not limited to, antibiotics, antivirals, mucolytics and expectorants, decongestants, antihistamines, and diuretics. The pharmaceutical agents used for a particular respiratory disorder are addressed in the discussion of the condition. Principles of inhalation therapy and aerosolized medications are addressed here.

Inhalation and Aerosol Therapy

> QUESTION: José uses a nebulizer at home. Evaluate the other methods of aerosol therapy. What supportive rationale can you offer for why this method of medication delivery is an appropriate choice for José?

Bronchodilators, corticosteroids, and mast cell stabilizer medications are delivered by inhalers or nebulizers. However, bronchodilators and corticosteroids are also available in oral and IV forms. Administering medications by inhalation is effective because the medication reaches the small airways and works directly on the lungs. Medications are nebulized or aerosolized by using compressed air or oxygen. A variety of machines (compressors) are available for use with a handheld nebulizer, often for use in the home. The handheld nebulizer has the advantages of being able to aerosolize almost any drug available in liquid form, allowing modification of dose volume and concentration and requiring minimal patient coordination. The child or infant usually uses a mask attached to the nebulizer cup, which is held over the nose and mouth. The medication is dispersed as a mist. Older children can use the mouthpiece and should be instructed to take slow, deep breaths through the mouth during the treatment (Fig. 16-6). Nebulizers are effective for most children younger than 5 years of

TIP 16-1: A TEACHING INTERVENTION PLAN for the Child on Home Oxygen Therapy via Natural Airway

Nursing Diagnoses and Family Outcomes

- Deficient knowledge: Home management with oxygen therapy
  Outcome: Parents/caregivers will verbalize the need for oxygen, care of the infant/child while receiving oxygen therapy, and safety precautions; parents/caregivers will demonstrate care of the child and use of the oxygen.
- Deficient knowledge: Risk for injury related to use of oxygen in the home and fire hazards
  Outcomes: Family shall remain free of injury, and the potential for fire or explosion shall be minimized.
  Infant/child will exhibit adequate oxygenation and ventilation, as evidenced by normal (for age and child) respiratory rate and effort and color of child.

Teach the Child/Family

Physiology and Need for Oxygen

- Discuss with parents/caregivers how oxygen enters the body and how it is used by the body. Explain the need/rationale for oxygen for their child.

Use of Oxygen

- Explain and demonstrate how to place/change the nasal cannula under the nose and over the ears, with the portion with the holes positioned under the nose, and how to attach the cannula to the flowmeter on the tank.
- Show parents/caregivers how to open the oxygen device and how to regulate the flow (depends on device being used in the home).

Physical Care

- Provide appropriate skin care on the face. Use hypoallergenic tape or skin protectant on the areas where the cannula is secured on the face.
- Provide humidity with oxygen if flow is more than 1 L/min, or instill normal saline drops to nares, as needed; oxygen can be drying to the nares.
- Provide nasopharyngeal suctioning to nares with bulb syringe or suction catheter as needed to keep nares patent and to allow adequate flow of oxygen to child.

- Do not use petroleum-based creams or ointments or oil-based products on the child (they are combustible).

Health Maintenance

- Describe and have parents/caregivers identify "normal" color and respiratory status for their infant/child.
- Teach parents/caregivers how to detect changes in color (pale, dusky, or blueness of lips/nail beds) and respiratory status (retractions, nasal flaring, accessory muscle use, and increased respiratory rate). Instruct caregivers on need to notify the health care provider if these changes are present.
- Stress importance of regular follow-up visits with health care provider.

Home Safety and Modifications

- Ensure that family has the following available in the home:
  - Notification sticker (oxygen in home) for fire department (place on front window where easily visible)
  - Fire extinguisher and label for area where oxygen is kept
  - Smoke detector
  - Battery-operated flashlight available in child's room in event of power failure
  - List of emergency numbers posted by all phones
- Do not allow smoking in the home. Post NO SMOKING signs. Do not burn incense, candles, or fires in the home. Keep the oxygen tank more than 5 ft away from the heater or any other heat sources.
- Reduce static electricity of clothes by using fabric softener.
- Keep oxygen source upright and secured in holder at all times.
- If traveling, keep portable oxygen source in upright position and secure at all times. Keep window open slightly in car to allow ventilation. Avoid places that allow smoking.

Contact the Health Care Provider if

- Child experiences respiratory distress or color changes in nail beds/mucous membranes

---

age and older children who have difficulty coordinating a metered dose inhaler (MDI).

KidKare Allow the child using a nebulizer to hold the mask up to his or her face instead of using the elastic strap around the head. When the child is getting the treatment, he or she may like to have "teddy" or "dolly" wear a mask and "get a treatment," too.

The MDI is a simple, portable, self-contained handheld canister that delivers a predetermined amount of the specified medication to the patient. Most bronchodilators, corticosteroids, and mast cell stabilizers are available in an MDI. Although MDIs have the advantage of being very portable and can provide efficient drug delivery with rapid preparation and administration time, they have the disadvantage of being difficult to coordinate

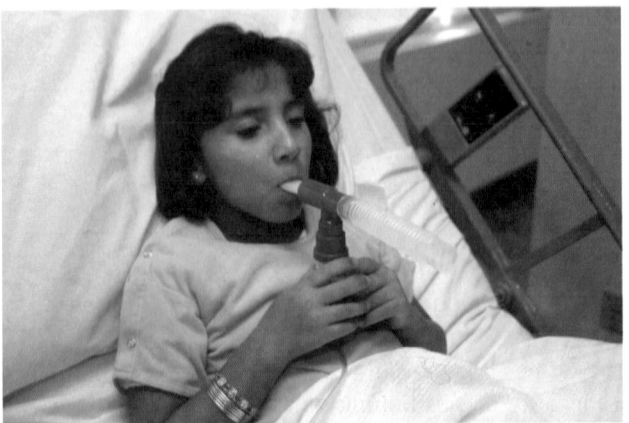

Figure 16-6 Child receiving treatment with a nebulizer.

and use correctly. A spacer device should be used with MDIs regardless of age (Fig. 16-7). Use of a spacer allows time for the medication to remain suspended and achieve smaller particle size. The spacer device may have a mouthpiece or face mask. Using spacers with mouthpieces requires coordination of breathing and drug dispersal, so spacers with masks may facilitate dosage in younger children.

Another device for inhalation is the dry powder inhaler. The dry powder inhaler, which is similar to the MDI, consists of a suspension of microfine, solid particles of drug contained in a small MDI-sized device with a mouthpiece. These medications rely on the force of the child's inhalation to propel the medication into the lower airways, making this form of medication appropriate only for older children.

A third type of device for administering inhaled medications is the breath-activated inhaler. With this device, medication is delivered as the patient initiates a breath. The child must seal his or her lips around the device before inhaling and should hold his or her breath for 10 seconds. Evaluate the child's ability to perform this technique properly before he or she uses the device on a daily basis.

If the infant or child is receiving aerosol or inhalation therapy, it is essential to assess the child's response to the

treatment. This information is used for determining the ongoing need for the medication and titration of medication frequency. Assess breath sounds and respiratory effort before and after the treatment for effectiveness. For the child receiving bronchodilators (beta-adrenergic agents), assessing the heart rate and/or jitteriness is also important because these are common side effect of these medications. If these side effects are excessive, alternate medication selection may be indicated.

caREminder

Be sure to have the child rinse their mouth and wash their face after using an inhaled corticosteroid to decrease the chance of systemic absorption and side effects related to the medications.

ANSWER: José is 4 years old. The nebulizer is very simple to use and requires no special skills. Simply breathing in and out deeply will allow the medication to work directly on the lung tissue.

AIRWAY CLEARANCE TECHNIQUES

During illness or exacerbation of chronic disease, airway clearance mechanisms may be dysfunctional, leading to retained secretions, or there may be hypersecretion of mucus in the airways. Accumulation of secretions in the airways can lead to partial or total airway obstruction. This can lead to alterations in gas exchange and ventilation, producing a favorable environment for infection. Children with conditions such as CF, BPD, bronchiectasis, or dysfunctional motility of cilia; those receiving mechanical ventilation; and those with acute problems after general anesthesia can benefit from ACTs.

Suctioning the trachea and nasopharyngeal airway is a method to enhance airway clearance by removing secretions that cannot be removed by the child's spontaneous cough. Suctioning may also be used to obtain secretions for diagnostic purposes (see thePoint for Procedures).

Traditionally, chest physical therapy (CPT) (also called *postural drainage* and *percussion*) has been the primary intervention for pulmonary conditions with hypersecretion or retained bronchial secretions. True CPT comprises four parts: postural drainage, percussion, deep breathing, and coughing (Walsh et al., 2011). In many children, only pieces of this therapy may be possible (e.g., some children may not be developmentally able to take a deep breath on command). Other ACTs include positive expiratory pressure (PEP) therapy, oscillatory PEP, high-frequency chest compression, and specialized breathing techniques such as autogenic drainage (Walsh et al., 2011). Ongoing research to match the most effective therapy with the individual will improve quality of life in this rapidly expanding area. Nursing Interventions 16-1 summarizes information on these techniques as well as traditional ACTs. Advantages and disadvantages of these techniques are also addressed, along with age indicators.

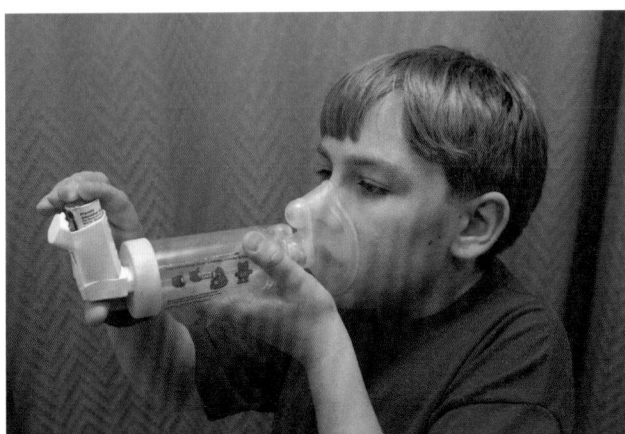

Figure 16-7 Commercial spacer device.

NURSING INTERVENTIONS 16-1

Airway Clearance Techniques

Airway Clearance Technique and Description	Benefits/Advantages	Disadvantages/Problems
Postural drainage and percussion/vibration: Mobilizes secretions by using dependent positioning, gravity, and percussion/vibration Vibration with exhalation can be used Mechanical percussor can be used (instead of cupped hands)	Gold standard Localize therapy to involved segment Can be assisted with mechanical percussor Percussion/vibration assists in loosening secretions from the walls of the bronchi to facilitate removal Used for all ages, especially infants, young children, and preschool children who may be unable to cooperate with the controlled breathing techniques	Time-consuming Requires patient repositioning during therapy May require rolls/blankets to maintain positioning during therapy Generally in each position for 1–5 minutes Difficult to apply in some settings May not be well tolerated by unstable patients Difficult to tolerate with severe gastroesophageal reflux due to increased intrathoracic and increased abdominal pressure during chest physiotherapy Head-down position contraindicated for infants because of the risk for increased gastroesophageal reflux. Modified therapy excluding head-down position may be used. Monitor oxygen saturation levels, particularly with Trendelenburg positioning, which may be poorly tolerated by children with respiratory compromise Adherence challenges
Autogenic drainage (self-drainage): Controlled method of breathing using three different lung volumes Active cycle of breathing technique: breathing technique that combines three methods: thoracic expansion exercises, breathing control, and forced expiratory techniques in a set cycle	Effective Needs no external devices Enables independence Absence of desaturation or compromise during therapy No costly equipment	Labor and time intensive to teach and learn Must be able to understand directions Child must be developmentally 12 years of age or older Not useful for infants and young children
PEP: Child breathes out 10–20 times through a flow resister, creating positive pressure in airway to about 15–20 cm H_2O during exhalation, followed by two to three "huff" coughs Cycle repeated up to 20 minutes	Enables independence Not reported to cause compromise with desaturation Can be done by children older than 3 years of age	Potential complication of pneumothorax due to increased intrathoracic pressure

Airway Clearance Technique and Description	Benefits/Advantages	Disadvantages/Problems
High-frequency chest compression: High-frequency oscillation to chest wall delivered by a vest to mobilize secretions	Enables older children to be independent Possible future application for younger children	Trial time needed to determine effectiveness before rental or purchase Patients may not tolerate the feeling from the compression Equipment must be rented or purchased Requires storage space May be uncomfortable if child has venous access device that is being used during the respiratory treatment
Exercise: Any activity that requires physical exertion, endurance, and upper body strengthening	May not cost anything May apply in many situations Socially acceptable May also improve cardiovascular fitness, self-esteem, and general health	May cost for membership to clubs or gyms; depends on climate Limited to physical ability Children with preexisting conditions such as asthma (with exercise component) may need to observe special precautions when exercising (e.g., premedicate)
Flutter valve: Small pipelike device with a metal ball rotating freely within pipe to vibrate the airway, loosening secretions and accelerates expiratory airflow to propel secretions outward Patients inhale and actively exhale through the pipe, which generates positive pressure to about 15–25 cm H_2O. Oscillations are transmitted to airways. Done for 5–15 breaths, followed by two to three huffs through flutter until lungs are clear, or for 20 minutes.	Enables independence	Requires purchase of the device Requires cooperation Requires developmental level; ability to follow directions

Determining the appropriateness of these newer interventions for a particular patient requires assessing the severity and type of lung disease, physical and developmental ability to perform the technique, and effectiveness of the particular technique. Other psychosocial factors to be considered are motivation to learn, adherence to treatment, cost, and payer or reimbursement. Ideally, these techniques should be performed 30 minutes before mealtimes as a safety measure to avoid vomiting and aspiration and to promote comfort (Fig. 16-8).

caREminder

When possible, supplemental continuous gastrostomy tube or nasogastric tube feedings should be discontinued for at least 30 minutes before postural drainage and percussion.

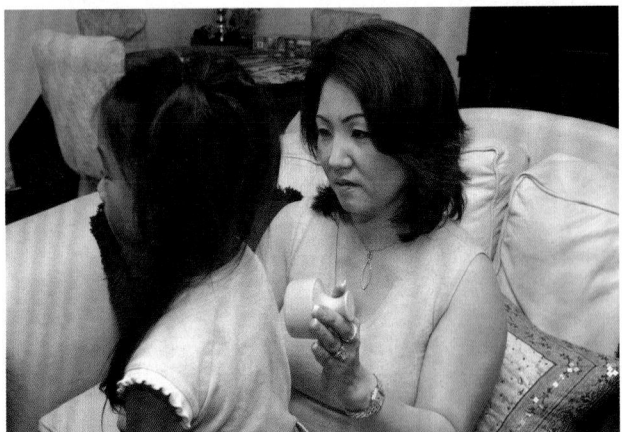

Figure 16-8 Postural drainage and percussion is used to assist with expulsion of mucus from the airway.

ARTIFICIAL AIRWAYS AND MECHANICAL VENTILATION

Noninvasive measures such as oxygen therapy and ACTs may not meet the needs of all children who require oxygenation and ventilation. When respiratory effort is increased but inadequate to maintain gas exchange because of airway obstruction, intrapulmonary pathophysiology, neuromuscular disease, or other factors, artificial or mechanical ventilation may become necessary.

Several methods are available to provide artificial ventilation. A bag-and-mask unit, or Ambu bag, is used to manually ventilate a child who has not been intubated (had an ET tube placed). Effective bag-and-mask ventilation is best provided with a self-inflating bag and a mask that fits properly over the child's nose and mouth.

To provide an open airway, extend the infant's or child's neck slightly in the sniffing position and lift the jaw (Fig. 16-9). The jaw-thrust maneuver is used in the pediatric trauma victim with possible spinal injury or in infants for whom overextending the neck can occlude the airway. Place the mask, held in your nondominant hand, over the nose and mouth to create a seal. With your dominant hand, compress the bag rhythmically and in synchrony (or slightly faster) with the child's spontaneous respiratory efforts, if present, compressing the bag only enough to make the chest rise and fall. Aggressive ventilating will lead to gastric distention. Ensure that the bag is connected to an oxygen source, with oxygen delivered at a flow rate of 10 to 15 L/min.

When prolonged artificial ventilation is needed because of respiratory failure or anesthesia, or when the airway is obstructed, intubation—placement of an artificial airway—is necessary and mechanical ventilation is provided. ET intubation is the insertion of an artificial airway (an ET tube) through either the nose (nasotracheal) or the mouth (orotracheal) into the trachea (Fig. 16-10). Another, less invasive, device for mechanical ventilation is the laryngeal mask airway, which is used most commonly in the operating room.

Mechanical ventilation replaces the work of breathing and involves inflating the lungs with compressed gas applied by either positive or negative pressure. Positive-pressure ventilators are more commonly used than negative-pressure machines. They work by creating pressure at the airway opening that is greater than the intra-alveolar pressure, thus forcing pressurized gas into the lungs. This flow of compressed gas improves gas exchange and inflation of poorly ventilated portions of the lungs. Negative-pressure machines are more cumbersome and are primarily used for long-term ventilation in persons with respiratory failure caused by neuromuscular diseases. The machine works by creating intermittent negative pressure around the thorax, causing the chest to be drawn outward and inspiration to occur. Negative-pressure machines do not require an artificial airway. Another mode of providing mechanical ventilation is called high-frequency ventilation. This machine works by delivering oxygen under high pressures at a rapidly cycling rate.

Closely monitor the respiratory and cardiovascular status of the child receiving mechanical ventilation. Many children are sedated while intubated and may have a nasogastric tube in place to decompress the

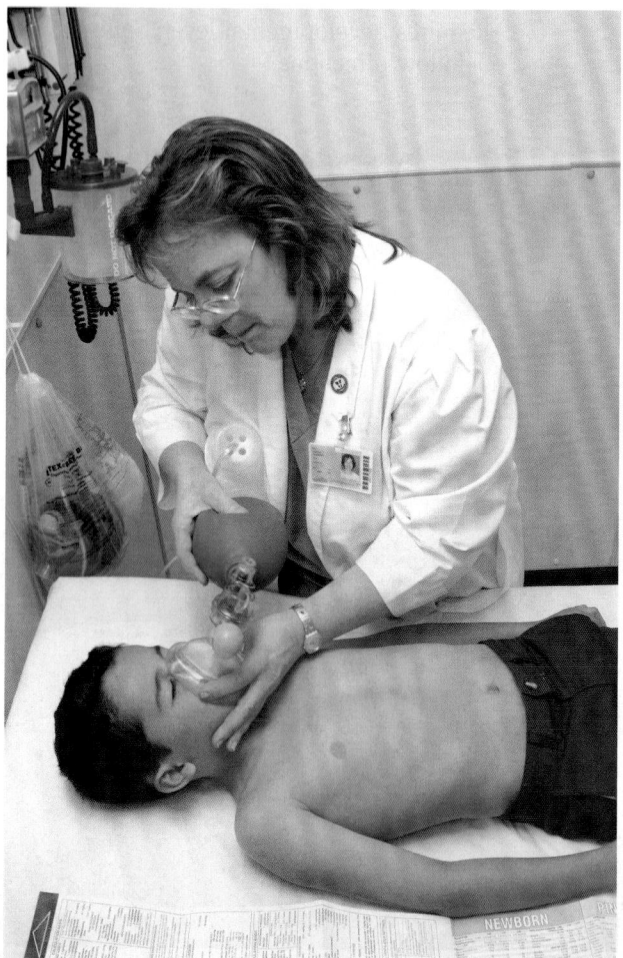

Figure 16-9 Child being ventilated using the bag-and-mask technique.

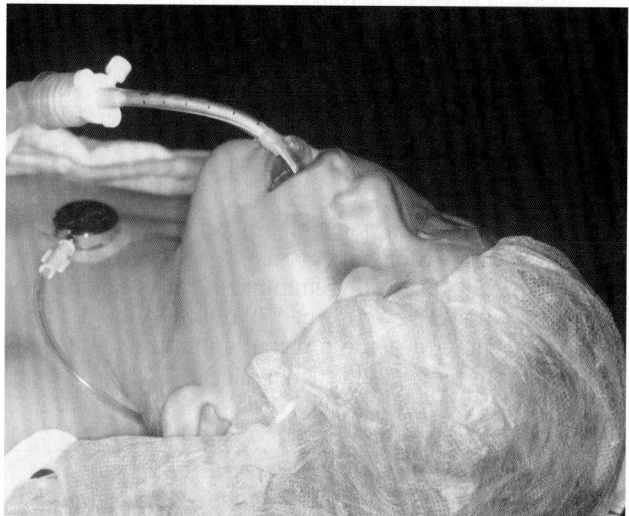

Figure 16-10 An intubated child. The tube has not yet been secured in place.

TRADITION OR SCIENCE 16-1

Does infant position affect outcomes of newborn infants receiving mechanical ventilation?

In patients of different ages undergoing mechanical ventilation, research has indicated that prone position may improve oxygenation in the short term. Prone positioning has been demonstrated to be safe for prolonged periods of time in ventilated, critically ill children; however, this short-term improvement in oxygenation has not been associated with fewer ventilator days or reduced mortality in children (Balaguer et al., 2003; Curley et al., 2005; Fineman et al., 2006). More research is needed to determine the various risks and benefits associated with different laying positions for this population of ventilated patients.

stomach (Tradition or Science 16-1). Perform suctioning based on the presence of adventitious breath sounds, increased respiratory effort or distress, or both. Chest physiotherapy may be ordered to further promote removal of secretions. Provide oral care and frequently monitor skin to ensure the ET tube is not causing skin irritation around the mouth or nares. Ensure the ventilator alarms are on and set within acceptable parameters to provide early notification of distress. Assist the family and the child, as appropriate, to understand the rationale for the use of mechanical ventilation. As appropriate, provide medications to help the child remain calm and quiet while being ventilated, which will ensure optimal respiratory outcomes.

TRACHEOSTOMY

A tracheostomy consists of the surgical placement of an artificial airway directly into the trachea below the larynx. Many conditions (congenital or acquired) that can cause upper airway obstruction, respiratory failure, or prolonged intubation in children may require placement of a tracheostomy tube. Emergencies such as epiglottitis or FBA may require a tracheostomy for more short-term management. In some clinical conditions, such as laryngotracheomalacia, subglottic stenosis, or vocal cord paralysis, the tracheostomy may be intermediate or long term until the condition is outgrown or corrected. In some cases, such as in chronic respiratory failure with long-term mechanical ventilation, the tracheostomy may be permanent.

Tracheostomy tubes are made of Silastic, silicone, or metal and are available in various sizes and lengths. The appropriate size is determined by patient age and size. Single-cannula tracheostomy tubes are most commonly used in pediatric patients because they have a smaller inner diameter and are usually made of Silastic, which conforms better than other materials to the shape of the trachea. For older children, a tracheostomy tube with an inner cannula may be used. The inner cannula is removed for cleaning, whereas the outer cannula is left in place. Additionally, some tracheostomy tubes have external cuffs. Many pediatric tubes do not have an external cuff because of the child's small airway diameter and the increased risk of trauma to the airway caused by the cuff. Because cuffless, single-cannula tracheostomy tubes are used in most children, explanation of the nursing care focuses on these topics.

While the child is hospitalized, nursing care involves preparing the child and caregivers preoperatively, providing skilled postoperative nursing care, and facilitating a successful discharge plan for home management if the tracheostomy will be intermediate or long term. Preoperatively, explain to the child and caregivers why the tracheostomy tube is needed, what the basic anatomy and physiology of the airway are, how breathing will be different, what to expect postoperatively, and how the child will look when he or she returns from surgery. If possible, allow the family to see a tracheostomy tube and supplies to help decrease anxiety about what to expect.

Focus postoperative nursing care on close observation to maintain a patent airway and to monitor for possible complications such as hemorrhage, edema, subcutaneous emphysema, pneumothorax, and accidental decannulation. Because infants and children are at greater risk for tracheostomy obstruction related to the relatively smaller airway, they should be initially managed in an intensive care or close observation unit postoperatively.

ALERT   *All children with a tracheostomy should have an extra tracheostomy tube of the same size and one that is one-half size smaller available at the bedside in case the tube in place is dislodged or becomes obstructed and cannot be cleared (Dougherty et al., 2011).*

Respiratory assessments include vital signs and examination of the child's color, respiratory rate and effort, breath sounds, and type and amount of secretions. For the first 5 to 6 days, until the tracheocutaneous tract is well formed, long sutures (stay sutures) attached to the trachea are often taped to the chest. The sutures can be used to keep the stoma open in the event of an accidental decannulation. The surgeon removes the sutures when the tract in the trachea is formed.

The airway must remain patent to prevent obstruction and possible complications. The child may require frequent suctioning for several hours immediately after the procedure because excessive and sometimes bloody secretions are common. Provide suctioning on an as-needed basis thereafter to prevent occlusion of the tracheostomy tube by secretions and mucus plugs. To prevent complications of suctioning—such as hypoxemia, hypotension, bradycardia (vasovagal responses), laryngospasm, bronchospasm, atelectasis, and trauma to the airway—gauge the suction pressure (should be 80 to 100 mm Hg); limit the time for suctioning (no longer than 4 to 5 seconds) and the number of suction passes; monitor the depth of the suction catheter (0.25 to 0.5 inch [0.635 to 1.27 cm] beyond the tip of the length of the airway); and provide manual ventilation with oxygen, rest time between suction passes, or both.

caREminder

Saline instillation with suctioning should be used with caution. Some studies have demonstrated that instilling saline before suctioning has an adverse effect on oxygen saturation, which may last up to 5 minutes (Bowden & Greenberg, 2012). Instilling saline is also believed to dislodge bacteria into the lower airway. On the other hand, recent research has shown that routine bacteria in the ET tube may be eliminated or reduced by regular saline installation (Walsh et al., 2011).

The functions of warming, filtering, and humidifying inspired air that the upper respiratory tract normally performs are bypassed in a child with a tracheostomy. Therefore, the inspired air must be humidified and warmed to maintain loose secretions, prevent occlusion of the tube by secretions, and prevent drying of the tracheal mucosa. Nursing care is directed toward maintaining appropriate humidification via a mist collar or through the mechanical ventilator. In addition, promoting adequate fluid intake to keep the child well hydrated is important. Appropriate patient hydration and airway humidification will generally keep secretions thin (Dougherty et al., 2011). To prevent infection and irritation of the skin around the tracheostomy tube, provide stoma care to keep the skin clean and dry. Keep the tracheostomy ties clean and dry and change them daily and as needed when soiled.

ALERT   *Some pediatric tracheostomy tubes have metal fibers. These tracheostomy tubes must be changed to silicone or plastic tube prior to certain tests, including MRI. If unsure about the presence of metal fibers in the tube, contact the otolaryngology provider. If the tube must be changed for a procedure, return to the original tracheostomy at the end of the procedure.*

The schedule of tracheostomy tube changes varies depending on the institution or physician preference. The first tube change usually is done by the surgeon about 5 days after the tracheotomy is performed. Subsequent tube changes are generally performed once a week in the child with a well-healed tracheostomy stoma, usually before a feeding or meal to avoid stimulation that could cause emesis.

Because many children go home with tracheostomy tubes, it has become necessary to teach parents or other primary caregivers how to care for the child at home (Fig. 16-11). Teaching Intervention Plan 16-2 outlines a teaching plan for the child who has had a tracheostomy tube placed. It is also helpful to ensure that visiting

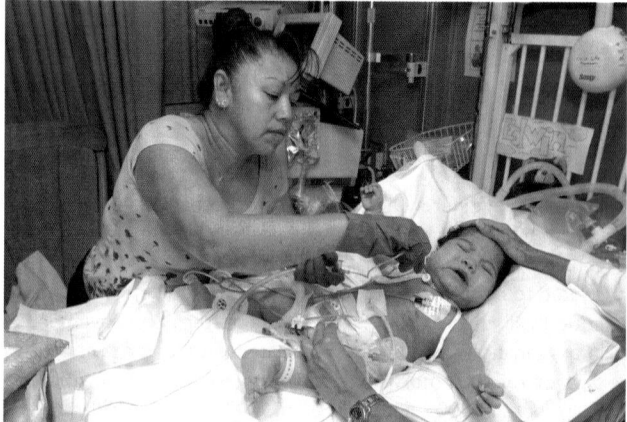

Figure 16-11 Families should be given ample opportunity to take care of the child's tracheostomy before the child is discharged.

nursing is provided after discharge to assist the family with routine care. Caregivers should be trained in cardiopulmonary resuscitation (CPR) prior to the child's home discharge. See Evidence-Based Clinical Practice Guidelines 16-1 for a list of guidelines for care of the child with a tracheostomy or ET tube.

NURSING PLAN OF CARE

QUESTION: One nursing diagnosis for José is ineffective breathing pattern related to respiratory disease process. Based on the information in the case study, what is another important nursing diagnosis?

Health promotion and disease prevention activities are essential for infants, children, and adolescents with acute and chronic respiratory conditions. These activities should focus on promoting a child's growth and development and on adequate home management. Preventive care, monitoring and early detection of symptoms, adequate management (whether at home or in the hospital), and health education are critical components of respiratory care for children. For example, sedentary lifestyles and obesity have grown to epidemic proportions in this country. Health promotion and disease prevention activities that focus on developing and encouraging healthy lifestyles can lead to improvements in overall health as well as specifically enhancing respiratory functioning. Therefore, nursing care in these areas can reduce the risk for complications, exacerbations of respiratory conditions (e.g., asthma attacks), morbidity (e.g., hospitalizations, emergency room visits, school days missed), and development of comorbid conditions related to the child's preexisting condition. It can also reduce or prevent the recurrence of respiratory illnesses.

Multiple nursing diagnoses may be used to address altered respiratory function and status (Nursing Plan of Care 16-1). For example, ineffective breathing pattern

TIP 16-2: A TEACHING INTERVENTION PLAN for the Child Receiving Home Tracheostomy Care

Nursing Diagnoses and Family Outcomes

- Deficient knowledge: Risk for injury related to management of tracheostomy
  Outcome: Family will verbalize and identify factors in handling an airway emergency with a tracheostomy.
- Deficient knowledge: Home maintenance management of tracheostomy
  Outcome: Family will identify and demonstrate all aspects of home care of the child prior to discharge.

Teach the Child/Family

Suctioning

- Identify need for suctioning, such as sound of mucus in the tracheostomy tube, breathing sounds "rattled," child is restless or appears anxious, child's color is pale or dusky, or there is difficulty feeding.
- Wash hands thoroughly before and after each suctioning procedure. Alcohol or disinfectant foam is an acceptable substitute when soap and water are not available. Nonsterile gloves should be worn for the protection of the caregiver who is not a family member or by anyone who is concerned about infection.
- Connect suction catheter to suction tubing and be careful not to touch tip of catheter. Insert the suction catheter to the predetermined depth (depending on tracheostomy tube size) and place thumb over port to apply suction. Pull back catheter while twirling catheter between thumb and index finger.
- Flush mucus from catheter with sterile saline, and repeat as necessary.
- If catheters are being reused, a regular cleaning procedure should be instituted. A common cleaning procedure follows:
  - Wash and flush used catheters with hot, soapy water.
  - Flush the catheter with 3% hydrogen peroxide (H_2O_2).
  - Soak catheters overnight in hot, soapy water.
  - Flush catheters with hot water and allow to air dry.
  - Wipe catheters with alcohol (Dougherty et al., 2011).

Stoma Care

- Perform daily site care and observe for signs of infection, skin breakdown, or complications around the tube site and the neck.
- Keep skin and stoma site clean and dry. Gently clean around the stoma using a clean gauze or cotton-tipped applicator. If the stoma is well established, a clean, wet washcloth may be used to clean the site. Wipe from the stoma outward. Use half-strength H_2O_2 to remove thicker, crusted secretions if necessary. Rinse with water after

cleaning with half-strength H_2O_2 to prevent dryness of the area. Application of a barrier cream around the stoma site may be warranted if the site is noted to be erythematous. Changes in the appearance of the stoma site should be reported to the health care provider (Dougherty et al., 2011).
- Change tracheostomy ties daily and as needed when soiled or wet.

Daily Care and Home Environment

Tracheostomy Tube Change

- Perform routine tracheostomy tube change once a week or more often as needed or as ordered by the health care provider. Ideally, routine tube changes are done with two individuals.
- Gather all supplies, wash hands thoroughly, and prepare child for procedure. Have a second person to assist with positioning of the child. Position child with neck slightly extended; may use a towel roll placed under the shoulders.
- Suction child to minimize secretions. Cut old ties while holding tracheostomy tube in place. If tracheostomy tube has a cuff, deflate it. Remove old tube from stoma and gently insert new tracheostomy tube with obturator into the stoma using a downward and forward motion following the curve of the trachea.
- Quickly remove the obturator, assess for adequacy of ventilation, and secure the tracheostomy ties. If tracheostomy tube has a cuff, inflate it with the required volume.
- Take caution when feeding the infant or child so that food or formula does not get into the tracheostomy. If this should occur, suction the tracheostomy immediately. Never prop a bottle or leave the infant or child unattended while feeding.
- Bathe the child in a tub, being sure to keep the water shallow and not allowing water to get into the tracheostomy tube. Never leave the child unattended in the tub, and do not put the child in a shower. Avoid use of talcum and baby powders on the infant or child.
- Encourage normal play both indoors and outdoors as much as possible. Avoid toys that are fuzzy or have small, removable parts. On cold and windy days outside, cover the tracheostomy with a mask or 100% cotton scarf. Avoid playing in sandboxes or in or around pools, lakes, and oceans; avoid participating in rough contact sports.
- Avoid buying clothes with high, tight necklines that may cover the tracheostomy opening.
- Do not permit smoking in the child's home or around the child.

Safety and Emergency Care

- Change or replace the tracheostomy tube immediately if accidental dislodgment or occlusion of the tube occurs.

(Continued)

TIP 16-2: A TEACHING INTERVENTION PLAN for the Child Receiving Home Tracheostomy Care (*Continued*)

- Keep all emergency telephone numbers by the telephone and a copy with the family at all times.
- Have all necessary equipment (e.g., extra tracheostomy tube with ties, suction machine, catheters, self-inflating bag) with child when traveling or going on "outings" outside the home.
- Keep flashlight handy in case of power failure, and notify electric and telephone companies that there is a child with special life-sustaining health care needs in the home.
- Keep all immunizations up to date, including annual influenza vaccination.
- Check tension on tracheostomy ties daily. Tracheostomy ties should be tight enough to allow the smallest finger to be slipped underneath the tracheostomy ties. Twill tape tracheostomy ties can stretch after being initially secured, so recheck in 1-2 hours for appropriate tightness.

- Place tracheostomy tie knots on the side of the neck to prevent skin breakdown on the back of the neck.

Contact Health Care Provider if

- Child develops fever more than 101° F (38.3° C)
- Child is having difficulty breathing or the breathing pattern changes
- Child's lips or nail beds become bluish or dusky
- Child has increase in secretions or change in color, odor, or consistency of the secretions
- Blood (greater than a teaspoon) is leaking from the tracheostomy
- There is difficulty inserting the tube with a routine tracheostomy tube change
- There is a rash, drainage, or unusual odor around the tracheostomy stoma or food or formula is coming through the tracheostomy tube

---

may be used to describe a child in respiratory distress related to an asthma exacerbation. Respiratory distress in children may also lead to comorbid problems in other body systems (e.g., cardiac, immune). In addition, many respiratory conditions are chronic. Refer back to Nursing Plan of Care 12-1 for a summary of the diagnosis and care interventions for the child with a chronic condition. The nurse's plan of care should encompass all primary and secondary effects of the child's respiratory illness.

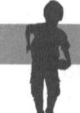

EVIDENCE-BASED CLINICAL PRACTICE GUIDELINES 16-1

Care of the Child With a Tracheostomy or Endotracheal Tube

American Association for Respiratory Care. (2010). AARC Clinical Practice Guidelines. Endotracheal suctioning of mechanically ventilated patients with artificial airways 2010. *Respiratory Care, 55*(6), 758–764. Retrieved from

http://apicwv.org/docs/1.pdf

Clinical practice guidelines on the ET suctioning of mechanically ventilated adults and children with artificial airways.

American Thoracic Society. (2000). *Care of the child with a chronic tracheostomy* Retrieved from

http://ajrccm.atsjournals.org/content/161/1/297.full

A consensus statement of the comprehensive standards of care for children with a tracheostomy.

Cincinnati Children's Hospital Medical Center. (2011). *Best evidence statement (BESt). Basic pediatric tracheostomy care.* Retrieved from

http://www.cincinnatichildrens.org/templates/cchmc2010/TemplateI.aspx?pageid = 99194

Practice standards for maintaining skin integrity, preventing accidental decannulation, and maintaining tracheostomy tube patency.

Cincinnati Children's Hospital Medical Center. (2008). *Best evidence statement (BESt). Techniques for suctioning pediatric tracheostomies.* Retrieved from

http://www.cincinnatichildrens.org/templates/cchmc2010/TemplateI.aspx?pageid = 99194

Practice guidelines for the suctioning techniques to be employed on pediatric tracheostomies.

Great Ormond Street Hospital for Children. (2012). *Tracheostomy: Care and management review.* Retrieved from

http://www.gosh.nhs.uk/health-professionals/clinical-guidelines/tracheostomy-care-and-management-review/

Interdisciplinary guidelines for care of child with tracheostomy. Includes quick reference algorithms.

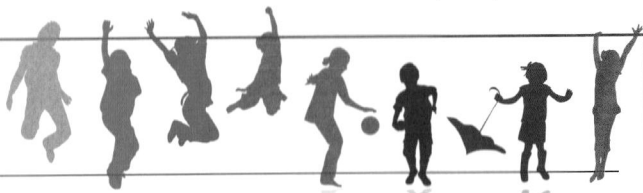

NURSING PLAN OF CARE 16-1:

Care of the Child With Altered Respiratory Status

Nursing Diagnosis: Ineffective airway clearance related to excess thick secretions, obstruction, or infection

Interventions/Rationale

- Conduct a complete respiratory assessment with each routine vital sign check and as indicated by the child's condition.

  Enables early detection and correction of abnormalities. Thick secretions increase hypoxia and will be reflected by changes in respiratory status. Colored or odorous secretions may indicate bleeding or infections.

- Encourage child to cough, especially after respiratory treatments. Teach effective cough techniques as developmentally appropriate.

  Ineffective cough may be caused by respiratory muscle fatigue, severe bronchospasm, and/or thick, tenacious secretions.

- Provide humidified oxygen as ordered.

  Decreases viscosity of secretions.

- Encourage increased fluid intake (clear liquids; avoid dairy products) if no contraindications, such as cardiac or renal disease, are present.

  Fluid intake prevents dehydration from insensible losses through mouth breathing and increased respiratory rate. Assists to decrease viscosity of secretions and increase ciliary action to remove secretions.

- Administer prescribed medications and IV fluids; monitor for response and side effects.

  IV fluids help to maintain adequate hydration. Mucolytic agents, bronchodilators, and antibiotics may be used to increase effectiveness of cough, enhance work of breathing, and treat infections that may cause thick, tenacious secretions.

Expected Outcome

- Child's airway will be free of secretions, as evidenced by normal or improved breathing, normal arterial blood gases, and/or oxygen saturation 92% or greater on pulse oximetry.

Nursing Diagnosis: Ineffective breathing pattern related to effects of respiratory disease process

Interventions/Rationale

- Conduct a complete respiratory assessment with each routine vital sign check and as indicated by the child's condition.

  Enables early detection and correction of abnormalities. Hypoxemia, hypercapnia, and hypocapnia will cause breathing pattern changes as the autonomic nervous system attempts to maintain homeostasis.

- Provide oxygen as needed to the child to maintain oxygen saturation at more than 92% or within parameters defined as child's personal best.

  Oxygen therapy may be required to increase oxygen saturation. A decrease in saturation indicates ineffective oxygenation, which in turn increases the work of breathing.

- Place child in an upright position to optimize ventilation.

  PaO_2 may increase in the prone position.

- Provide reassurance to the child to allay anxiety. Keep child as calm as possible.

  Increased restlessness and anxiety indicate insufficient oxygenation. Increased work of breathing can lead to fatigue. Energy expenditures increase the child's oxygen demands.

- Administer prescribed medications and IV fluids; monitor for response and side effects.

  Corticosteroids may help reduce bronchial inflammation, antibiotics may be used to treat infection or sepsis, and bronchodilators may be useful to enhance airway clearance.

Expected Outcomes

- Child will demonstrate an effective respiratory rate, rhythm, and effort and will experience improved gas exchange in the lungs, as evidenced by blood gases within child's normal parameters.
- Child will verbalize ability to breathe comfortably without sensations of dyspnea and related feelings of fear or anxiety resulting from shortness of breath.

Nursing Diagnosis: Impaired gas exchange related to consequences of underlying respiratory disease process

Interventions/Rationale

- Conduct a complete respiratory assessment with each routine vital sign check and as indicated by the child's condition.

  Signs of hypoxia, such as changes in level of consciousness, cyanosis, respiratory distress, ventilation (rate, quality, pattern, and depth), and vital signs indicate impaired gas exchange and compensatory efforts to manage these physiologic changes.

- Closely monitor oxygen saturation levels via pulse oximetry and arterial blood gases, and note changes.

  Pulse oximetry provides an estimate of oxygen saturation; blood gases (arterial or capillary) are objective indications of oxygenation status. Progressive hypoxemia is apparent on serial blood gases despite increased concentrations of inspired oxygen.

(Continued)

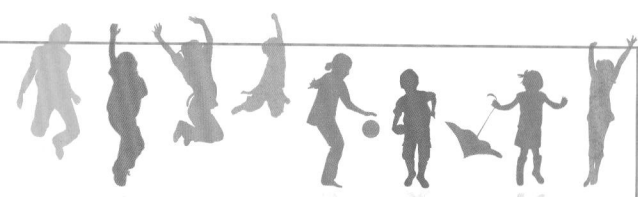

NURSING PLAN OF CARE 16-1:

Care of the Child With Altered Respiratory Status (*Continued*)

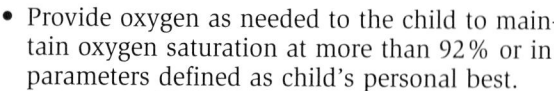

- Provide oxygen as needed to the child to maintain oxygen saturation at more than 92% or in parameters defined as child's personal best.

  Oxygen therapy may be required to increase oxygen saturation. A decrease in saturation indicates ineffective oxygenation, which may indicate that the child's condition is worsening.

- Anticipate the need for intubation and mechanical ventilation. Assist with these procedures as needed.

  Intubation is indicated in the presence of impending respiratory failure. Mechanical ventilation provides supportive care to maintain adequate oxygenation and ventilation parameters to the child.

Expected Outcomes

- Child will demonstrate improved gas exchange in the lungs, as evidenced by blood gases within child's normal parameters and an alert, responsive mental status or no further reduction in mental status.

Nursing Diagnosis: Decreased cardiac output related to consequences of respiratory distress and failure

Interventions/Rationale

- Perform a complete assessment of cardiovascular status, including vital signs, hemodynamic pressures, urine output, skin temperature, peripheral pulses, and respiratory effort.

  Decreasing cardiac output will be reflected by changes in blood pressure, decreasing strength of peripheral pulses, decreased urine output, cool extremities, and changes in ventilation that may necessitate changes in positive end-expiratory pressure.

- Administer prescribed medications and IV fluids; monitor for response and side effects.

  Inotropic agents may be used to increase cardiac output. Sedatives and analgesics are used to relieve pain and agitation. Neuromuscular blocking agents may be needed if the child is ventilated to promote synchronous breathing. IV fluids are administered to maintain fluid balance without causing edema.

Expected Outcome

- Child will demonstrate adequate cardiac output, as evidenced by strong peripheral pulses; normal vital signs; urine output greater than 2 mL/kg/hr; and warm, pink, dry skin.

Nursing Diagnosis: Risk for infection related to pooling of lung secretions, ineffective cough, and contagious nature of condition

Interventions/Rationale

- Conduct a complete assessment to monitor for respiratory infection, including auscultating breath sounds; evaluating for changes in sputum; and observing for fever, chills, increase in cough, shortness of breath, nausea, vomiting, diarrhea, and decreased appetite.

  Early assessment of signs of infection will facilitate early intervention. Bronchial breath sounds and rales may indicate pneumonia. Sputum changes, such as an increase in production, changes in consistency, and changes in color, may indicate presence of infection.

- Evaluate child's and family's understanding of techniques to prevent infection, such as careful hand hygiene, adequate rest and nutrition, avoiding contact with sick individuals, and so forth. Provide additional education as needed.

  Increased knowledge and subsequent implementation of activities to prevent infection will reduce infection risk.

- Follow standard infection control precautions during all contact with the child.

  Following standard precautions reduces the risk of transmission of microorganisms.

- Encourage child to cough and expectorate secretions frequently. Encourage strict handwashing and infection control practices for the child, family members, and all care providers.

  Retained secretions provide an environment for bacterial growth.

Expected Outcomes

- Child will be free from infection, and the parents will demonstrate adequate knowledge of risk for infection, signs/symptoms of infection, and measures to reduce infection risks.

Nursing Diagnosis: Imbalanced nutrition: Less than body requirements related to underlying chronic lung disease and increased work of breathing

Interventions/Rationale

- Assess child's nutritional status, including height, weight, body mass index percentile, diet history, child's ability to eat, and possible causes for poor appetite.

  Assessment provides baseline data to assist in determining interventions. Increased metabolic needs caused by increased work of breathing will require greater caloric intake. Work of breathing may leave little energy for other activities, including eating.

- Assist child/parents to plan well-balanced meals that incorporate child's food preferences and dietary limitations imposed by disease process (e.g., low-to-moderate fat, high-protein, high-calorie meals for the child with CF). Encourage small feedings of nutritious soft foods and liquids. Add nutritional supplements as ordered.

These measures minimize metabolic expenditures while providing nutritious high-calorie foods that are appealing and easy to digest.
- Ensure frequent oral care is provided.
   Dry mucous membranes and poor oral hygiene may contribute to decreased appetite and worsening nutritional status.

Expected Outcomes
- Child will demonstrate adequate nutritional intake for age, and caregivers will identify steps to achieve and maintain ideal body weight.

ANSWER: Because José's oxygen saturation is between 89% and 90%, another nursing diagnosis is impaired gas exchange related to underlying respiratory disease process.

ALTERATIONS IN RESPIRATORY STATUS

Respiratory conditions are among the most common maladies affecting children, ranging from those that develop in utero, such as malformations of the palate and trachea, to chronic conditions such as asthma. Respiratory health directly affects children's stamina and their ability to engage in activities in settings that are conducive to safe air exchange. The nurse plays a primary role in educating children and their families about ways to safeguard their respiratory health. In addition, the nurse plays a critical role in determining if and when a child's respiratory condition may place other children at risk for infection. Thus, the role of the nurse is to both collaborate in improving the health of children with a respiratory condition and protect the health of children who may be exposed to contagious respiratory conditions.

CONGENITAL ABNORMALITIES OF THE RESPIRATORY SYSTEM

Congenital abnormalities or malformations of the respiratory systems are fortunately rare. These disorders result in respiratory dysfunction primarily caused by airway obstructions or collapse. Congenital conditions include choanal atresia (a unilateral or bilateral bony or membranous septum between the nose and pharynx), Pierre Robin syndrome (abnormally small jaw with upper airway obstruction [resulting from tongue prolapse into the pharyngeal airway] and cleft palate; Fig. 16-12), laryngomalacia (weakness and poor tone of the larynx), and tracheomalacia (weakness and poor tone of the trachea).

These abnormalities are generally diagnosed at birth or shortly thereafter, when the child exhibits varying degrees of respiratory distress. The presence of **cyanosis**

(bluish skin color caused by inadequate oxygenation of the blood) is a key finding. The treatment is largely supportive; the primary goal of treatment is to maintain a patent airway. Surgical interventions to relieve the obstruction (such as for choanal atresia), structurally support the airway (such as for severe tracheomalacia), or the delivery of positive pressure ventilation (such as for severe trachea or laryngomalacia) may be necessary. Adequate nutritional support to promote optimal weight gain is essential. These conditions may improve with surgical intervention and/or growth and in the absence of other congenital anomalies, the prognosis for normal respiratory function is good.

Early and ongoing support and education of the family is of utmost importance. A diagnosis of a congenital anomaly creates a crisis for the family. Reinforce the concept that in most cases, the cause of the defect is unknown and not the fault of the parents. Also educate the family about appropriate positioning and feeding techniques to ensure adequate intake of formula or breast milk (either by actual breastfeeding or breast milk expressed into a bottle) and solid foods as the infant reaches the appropriate age for introducing them. Routine infant health care is administered. Parents need

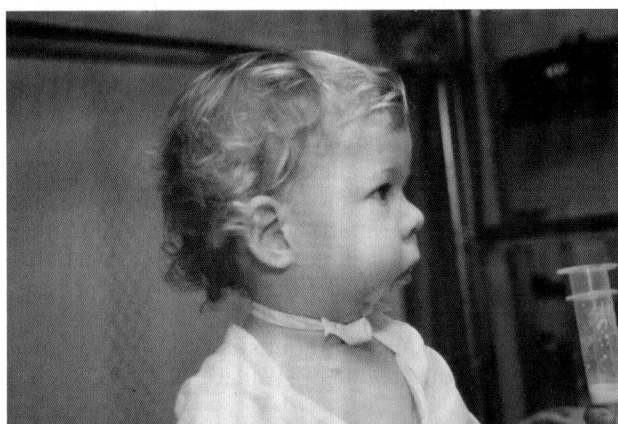

Figure 16-12 In the child with Pierre Robin syndrome, malformation of the mandible makes the chin appear recessed and restricts the tongue to a posterior position, causing easy occlusion of the airway. A tracheostomy may be necessary to maintain an open airway.

to be informed that the infant's symptoms may worsen during respiratory illnesses. If they have any concern about worsening respiratory distress, instruct them to seek assistance from their health care professional. All caregivers for the child should be instructed in CPR.

UPPER RESPIRATORY INFECTIONS AND OBSTRUCTIONS

Upper respiratory tract infections are extremely common in infants and young children. The upper respiratory tract, or upper airway, consists primarily of the nose, mouth, and oropharynx. For purposes of this book, infections of the epiglottis, larynx, and trachea are considered in the upper respiratory tract as well. Infections of this area of the respiratory system are usually viral and self-limiting. Although the respiratory tract is equipped with several natural defense mechanisms, invading organisms frequently gain access to these structures, resulting in respiratory conditions that range from mild to life threatening. When infection occurs, organisms travel freely among the structures of the upper airway, including through the eustachian tubes to the inner and middle ears. The severity of resulting illness depends on age, organism, and the integrity of the child's immune response. Some infections can lead to inflammation or obstructions of the airway; obstruction can also result from noninfectious causes. Most upper respiratory conditions are treated in the home or in ambulatory care settings.

ALLERGIC RHINITIS

QUESTION: As described in the Chapter 9 case study, José has seasonal allergies that trigger his asthma. Summarize the relationship between children with allergic rhinitis and children with asthma.

Allergic rhinitis is a condition characterized by sneezing; nasal itching; thin, watery rhinorrhea; and nasal congestion. The conjunctivae and posterior pharynx may also be involved. Allergic rhinitis may be seasonal, with symptoms that correspond to specific pollen peaks in the spring or fall, or may be perennial (year-round symptoms). Some children have perennial symptoms with additional flares during pollen seasons. Allergic rhinitis is the most common of all allergic disorders, affecting 10% to 30% of adults and nearly 40% of children (Wallace et al., 2008). Allergic rhinitis accounts for 2 million days lost from school, 28 million days of restricted activity, and a cost of more than $3.3 billion for health care provider visits annually (Hayden, 2007; Salib et al., 2008). The prognosis for allergic rhinitis is good if symptoms are controlled with treatment (Wallace et al., 2008).

Pathophysiology

Airborne allergens come into contact with mast cells and basophils at mucosal surfaces. Mast cells have immunoglobulin E (IgE) receptors on their membrane surfaces that bind to IgE in serum. Exposure to the appropriate airborne allergens cross-links the mast cell IgE receptors and triggers the release of chemical mediators. This mediator release causes an immediate reaction, which includes sneezing, itching, nasal congestion, and mucous secretion accompanied by nasal mucosal edema. Four to 12 hours later, a late-phase reaction occurs, causing a second, more prolonged period of nasal congestion.

Assessment

Diagnosis of allergic rhinitis is based on clinical history, family history, physical findings, and laboratory evaluation (skin test). Assess for complaints of nasal congestion, pruritus, clear rhinorrhea, and paroxysms of sneezing. The nasal congestion may be bilateral, unilateral, or variable and is often worse at night. Chronic rhinitis symptoms may lead to irritability and fatigue, which can cause inattentiveness and difficulty concentrating in school. Parents may tell you that their children sniff, snort, and frequently clear their throats. They may also twitch, pick or rub their nose and have episodes of repetitive sneezing. In conjunction with nasal symptoms, the eyes may itch and water. Bronchospasm with coughing, shortness of breath, or chest tightness may occur in children who also have asthma. Other symptoms may include fatigue, irritability, headache, depression, and anorexia.

A predisposition to allergic rhinitis is often familial; therefore, determining whether other family members (parents, siblings, or grandparents) have a history of hay fever or allergies can help establish the diagnosis.

On physical examination, look for certain characteristic features that distinguish allergic rhinitis from the common cold (rhinitis) (Table 16-1). The child may have bluish discoloration of the infraorbital area (called *allergic shiners*) caused by increased venous flow related to the local allergic vigor. The child may have a transverse crease across the lower third of the nose caused by rubbing the nose (called the *allergic salute*). Examination of the nasal cavity using a nasal speculum may reveal edematous mucosa, with swollen, boggy, and pale-pink to blue-gray turbinates. Nasal secretions are generally clear, watery, or white.

TABLE 16-1	Differences Between Allergic Rhinitis and the Common Cold	
Symptoms	Allergic Rhinitis	Common Cold
Family history of atopy	Yes	No
Conjunctival pruritus	Yes	No
Fever	No	Yes
Pharyngitis/laryngitis	No	Yes
Purulent secretions	No	Yes
Sinus pain	Yes	No

Microscopic examination of the nasal secretions reveals abundant eosinophils. Skin testing for sensitivity to allergens believed to contribute to the nasal symptoms may help establish specific triggers for the allergy symptoms (e.g., dust mite, cat, dog, trees, grass, or ragweed).

Interdisciplinary Interventions

The mainstay of treatment for allergic rhinitis is avoiding the offending allergens. Environmental control measures that can help relieve symptoms by limiting exposure to common indoor allergens are shown in Community Care 16-1.

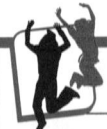

COMMUNITY CARE 16-1

Home and School Environmental Control of Allergies

Suggestions for eliminating or reducing triggers can be provided to families and may include

Home
- Do not allow smoking in the home or car; encourage smokers to always smoke outside. Refer family members who are smokers to local smoking cessation programs (e.g., American Lung Association, American Cancer Society, local smoking quitline).
- Encase mattresses, box springs, and pillows with airtight hypoallergenic covers. The child should avoid sleeping or lying on rugs or upholstered furniture. Use synthetic materials for all bedding, and wash bed linens weekly in hot water (130° F [54.4° C]). Place stuffed toys in the clothes dryer (on air fluff) at least once a week to reduce dust mites.
- Remove clutter (dust collectors) including knick-knacks, pictures, wall hangings, trophies, and stuffed toys from the child's bedroom. Wet-dust and clean the child's bedroom twice a week.
- Use shades, vertical blinds, or curtains that are washable in hot water (130° F [54.4° C]). Wash curtains every 1–2 weeks.
- Hardwood floors are preferable to carpeting. If able, remove carpeting from the child's room. If unable, vacuum twice a week with the windows open to increase ventilation and reduce dust collection. The child should be out of the room or house during vacuuming.
- Do not allow pets, particularly dogs and cats, in the child's bedroom. Wash the pet weekly. Ideally, the pet should be kept in areas of the home without carpet.
- Avoid painting or using cleaning products around the child. The child should not be in the house when these chemicals are being used. Consider using natural cleaning products like diluted white vinegar (useful in removing mold, mineral deposits, and crayon marks), baking soda (can be used as a general cleaner), and club soda (a good spot remover). Avoid perfumes, powders, aerosol sprays, and hairsprays around child.
- Clean and dust the kitchen floor and cabinets 1–2 times a week to remove cockroach allergen present in house dust (especially in apartment buildings). Keep brown paper grocery bags, cardboard boxes, and newspapers outside.
- Avoid using humidifiers in the house because they promote the growth of dust mites and can harbor fungi and molds if not cleaned properly. Ideally, the humidity level in the house should be kept at 25%–40%.
- Other strategies to reduce home environmental allergens and pollutants can be found at the U.S. Environmental Protection Agency (EPA) website (http://www.epa.gov/iaq/pubs/airclean.html).

School
- Clean chalkboards when students are not in the classroom; clean erasers outside.
- Replace paint and marker caps when they are not in use to control strong fumes.
- If possible, include non–fur-bearing pets such as fish or snakes, which are preferable in classrooms to reduce allergen exposure from furry pets. Wet-dust bookshelves weekly.
- Avoid upholstered furniture. Furniture should be made of vinyl, leather, or wood.
- Bare wood or tile floors are best. If possible, remove rugs and keep floors clean.
- Consider placing small rugs and carpets (without rubber backs) in clothes dryer (on air fluff) at least weekly to reduce dust mites and soil collection. Carpets can trap dust and soil.
- Opening windows to allow fresh air exchange is good, but check pollen and pollution levels first.
- Wet-dust fan blades and air exchange vents at least monthly.
- Clean or change window air conditioner filters at least monthly.
- Use air conditioners or a dehumidifier to keep relative classroom humidity at 35%–45%.
- Have teachers and staff avoid perfumes, scented talcum powder, and hairsprays.
- Use liquid rather than bar soap (mild or unscented) for handwashing.
- More EPA guidelines and strategies for healthy school environments can be found on the EPA website (http://www.epa.gov/schools/).

Parents of children with seasonal (pollen-induced) allergic rhinitis must be cautioned that pollen counts are highest in the morning between 5 and 10 AM. Environmental measures to reduce allergen exposure should include wet-mop dusting, closing household windows at least during the allergy season, and frequently changing ventilation filters. One may be able to further limit exposure by limiting household pets and making the home smoke free. When pets are in the home, confining the animals to carpet-free areas in the home, routine bathing of the pet (at least weekly), and placing litter boxes away from areas that supply air to the rest of the home may reduce allergens in the home (Wallace et al., 2008). Cockroaches are another significant allergen, especially in inner city populations.

Medical management involves the use of oral or intranasal antihistamines, decongestants, intranasal corticosteroids, leukotriene modifiers, mast cell stabilizers, and allergen-specific immunotherapy (Wallace et al., 2008). Antihistamines are used to block histamine from binding at its H_1 receptor site, thereby preventing the vasodilation, sneezing, and hypersecretion it causes. Decongestants may be helpful in reducing nasal obstruction through vasoconstriction, but the suitability of over-the-counter preparations for the younger child should be verified through the health care professional. Nasal corticosteroids are used to decrease inflammation in the nasal passages. For moderate to severe cases of allergic rhinitis, leukotriene modifiers and mast cell stabilizers may be used. In children with more severe symptoms, immunotherapy may be used. Immunotherapy may be administered subcutaneously and, in some cases, using the sublingual route (Park et al., 2012).

As with any medication, educate parents and children regarding the uses and side effects of these medications. Medications for rhinitis include sedating and nonsedating forms. The availability of over-the-counter cold preparations for children changes; therefore, instruct parents to read the package label carefully. Children who are not responding to oral medications as anticipated may warrant a referral to an allergist for further evaluation.

ANSWER: Although not all children who have allergic rhinitis also have asthma, a significant portion of children with asthma also have allergies. The allergies can act as a trigger for their asthma; therefore, controlling their allergic response also helps to control their asthma. What is difficult for many families is maintaining a preventative medication regime when the child does not appear sick.

SINUSITIS

Sinusitis in children is usually seen as a viral or bacterial infection in the paranasal sinus structures. Viral upper respiratory tract infections are common in children, and sinusitis can complicate as many as 6% to 8% of cases in children. Sinusitis is nearly twice as likely to complicate an upper respiratory tract infection in children who attend daycare than in those who do not. It affects nearly 1% of the pediatric population and accounts for nearly 20 million antibiotic prescriptions each year (DeMuri & Wald, 2012). Sinusitis characteristically responds well to antibiotic therapy, although prolonged courses may be required. Complications can occur as a result of local extension of the disease, such as orbital cellulitis. Intracranial infection, with associated neurologic symptoms, is also a potential sequela of sinusitis. Prompt, appropriate antibiotic therapy usually prevents the onset of these potentially life-threatening ophthalmologic and neurologic complications.

Pathophysiology

The paranasal sinuses, which encompass the ethmoid, maxillary, sphenoid, and frontal sinuses, are hollow areas in the skull beneath the turbinates in the nasopharynx. Ethmoid and maxillary sinuses are present at birth. The sphenoid sinuses are formed by 5 years of age, and frontal sinuses continue developing until adolescence (Fig. 16-13). The various functions of the sinuses include warming and humidifying inspired air, trapping inspired particles, secreting mucus, and reducing the weight of the skull.

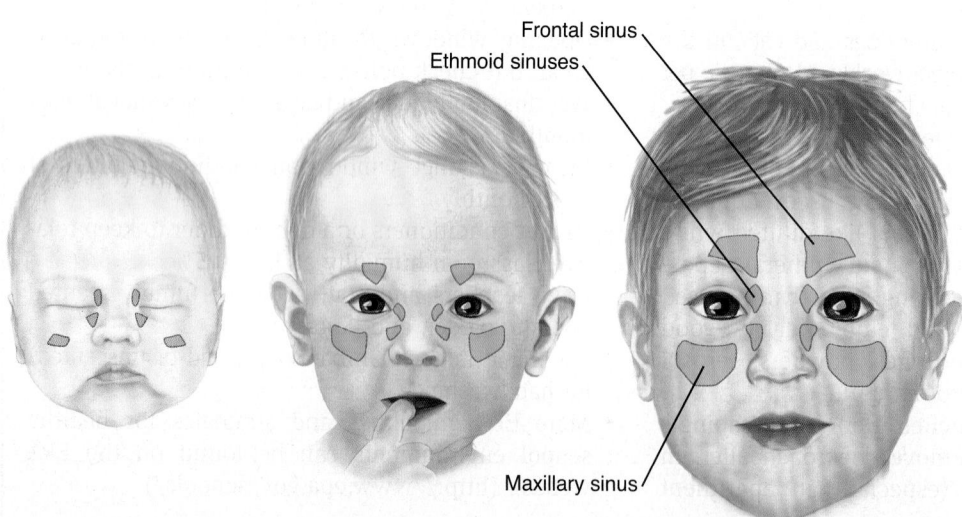

Frontal sinus
Ethmoid sinuses
Maxillary sinus

Figure 16-13 Development of the frontal, ethmoid, and maxillary sinuses.

The sinuses are prone to infection most frequently after a viral upper respiratory tract infection because the sinus cavities in children are smaller in area than in the adult. Inflammation and edema of the mucous membranes during an upper respiratory tract infection can lead quickly to obstruction of the opening to the nasopharynx. The normally sterile sinus cavity is then invaded by bacteria. Recently, *Haemophilus influenzae* has become a more common cause of acute bacterial sinusitis in children. *Streptococcus pneumoniae* has been waning as a cause of acute bacterial sinusitis (DeMuri & Wald, 2012).

Assessment

Children with sinusitis have various clinical manifestations and histories. Ask questions to elicit any evidence of common symptoms of sinusitis: nasal congestion, rhinorrhea, cough, headache, toothache, and worsening of symptoms after initial appearance of improvement in symptoms (DeMuri & Wald, 2012). The infant or younger child may exhibit fever and irritability after a viral upper respiratory tract infection. The older child may have symptoms such as purulent rhinorrhea, malodorous breath, headache, anorexia, sore throat, a feeling of fullness or pain in the face (especially over the sinuses), cough, or a disturbed sense of smell.

History of symptoms and physical examination are needed to diagnose sinusitis in children younger than 6 years of age. A positive history for sinusitis would include symptoms that last more than 10 days without evidence of improvement.

Diagnosis can be made on history and physical examination in most children. Radiographic studies (plain films, CT scan, MRI) are generally reserved for children with a normal examination when attempting to exclude the diagnosis of sinusitis or in those children in which symptoms (severe headache, seizures, abnormal intraocular motion) suggest complicated disease (orbital cellulitis, orbital abscess, subdural empyema, brain abscess, meningitis) (DeMuri & Wald, 2012).

Interdisciplinary Interventions

Symptomatic relief measures and consideration of antimicrobial therapy are the main interventions for sinusitis. Antimicrobial therapy in the treatment of sinusitis is controversial, although generally supported in the literature. If treating with an antimicrobial agent, the first-line therapy in children is amoxicillin clavulanate. Antibiotics are usually given orally for 7 to 10 days, plus an additional 7 days after the child is symptom free (DeMuri & Wald, 2012). Hospitalization for sinusitis is rarely required, although on rare occasions, children with sinusitis may develop an advanced infection or complication that requires hospitalization for more intense neurologic monitoring and parenteral antibiotic therapy. Limited data is available on the use of saline sinus rinses, although available data has not demonstrated substantial relief with their use. Glucocorticoid sinus washes have demonstrated only slight symptom relief—not significant enough to support their routine use. Decongestants and antihistamines have not demonstrated symptom improvement in children and should not

be recommended because of the risk for toxicity associated with the use of these medications (DeMuri & Wald, 2012). Encourage parents to administer additional clear liquids during the acute phase to promote hydration and sinus drainage.

ALERT *The U.S. Food and Drug Administration has recommended that over-the-counter products such as decongestants, expectorants, antihistamines, and cough suppressants not be used to treat infants and children younger than 4 years because of serious and potentially life-threatening side effects.*

NASOPHARYNGITIS AND PHARYNGITIS

Nasopharyngitis (common cold) and pharyngitis (throat infections) are among the most frequently encountered complaints in the pediatric ambulatory care setting. Contracting an infection is predominantly determined by age and exposure to infection (Tregoning & Schwarze, 2010). These inflammatory syndromes of the nasopharynx and oropharynx are attributed predominantly to infectious agents or, less commonly, to secondary involvement in systemic or noninfectious illnesses.

Pathophysiology

The nasopharynx and oropharynx consist of mucous membrane layers composed of stratified squamous epithelium; the inflammatory process is initiated in these structures by viruses or bacterial pathogens. The lymphatic drainage system is involved secondarily. Excessive drying of the mucous membranes during the winter months and passive or active smoking are other potential contributing factors because they irritate the mucous membranes and increase susceptibility to infection. The virulence of viral or bacterial pathogens depends on mucosal cell wall antigens. Viral particles are transmitted by air, by direct contact, and sometimes by food-borne transmission.

When the mucous membranes are involved, infection can spread through the lymphatic drainage system and saliva to other parts of the oral cavity and respiratory tract. The uvula and epiglottis may become inflamed. Unresolved nasopharyngitis and pharyngitis, combined with fever, decreased appetite, and reduced fluid intake, can dehydrate an infant rapidly. Complications such as otitis media, lymphadenitis, and peritonsillar abscess may also occur if the infection is not self-resolved (for viral conditions) or treated effectively with antibiotics (for bacterial infections).

Viral upper respiratory infections constitute nearly all cases of pharyngitis and nasopharyngitis. Rhinovirus, RSV, coronavirus, and adenovirus are the most common pathogens in children younger than 3 years of age; therefore, routine testing for group A beta-hemolytic streptococci (GABHS) is not recommended in the absence of known exposure (Shulman et al., 2012). Influenza, parainfluenza, Epstein-Barr virus, and Coxsackie virus A are among the more prevalent causative agents in older

TABLE 16-2	Comparison of Viral and Bacterial Pharyngitis	
	Viral Pharyngitis	**Streptococcal Pharyngitis**
Signs and symptoms	White blood cell (WBC) count usually normal Gradual onset Headache, low-grade fever Rhinitis, cough, and hoarseness common; abdominal discomfort uncommon Slightly red pharynx with moderately enlarged tonsils Absent marked cervical lymphadenopathy	WBC count elevated Abrupt onset Headache, fever up to 104° F (40° C) Common complaints are sore throat, abdominal discomfort, and trouble swallowing; headache rhinitis, cough, and hoarseness uncommon Erythema and enlargement of tonsils with white exudate on posterior pharynx and tonsils Firm, tender cervical lymph nodes present
Treatment	Symptomatic treatment only	Antibiotics to eradicate organisms, either penicillin or erythromycin for 10 days, plus symptomatic treatment
Complications	Few complications	Complications include otitis media, sinusitis, peritonsillar abscesses, acute cervical adenitis, rheumatic fever, meningitis, and acute glomerulonephritis
Duration	Usually self-limiting, lasting 5–7 days	Without antibiotics, child may be acutely ill for 2 weeks; if left untreated, group B *Streptococcus* may lead to further complications, including rheumatic fever, acute poststreptococcal glomerulonephritis

children and adolescents. Pharyngitis is most commonly attributed to GABHS in the 5- to 15-year-old child. Other etiologic agents include *Corynebacterium diphtheriae*. Infection with diphtheria was common at the turn of the century; immigrant and other nonimmunized populations in the United States remain at risk for contracting this organism today. *Mycoplasma pneumoniae* can also cause pharyngitis that is clinically indistinguishable from GABHS, most commonly in the adolescent population. Gonococcal pharyngitis may be seen in sexually active or sexually abused children. Table 16-2 compares pharyngitis caused by viral versus bacterial agents.

Assessment

Observe for the hallmark symptoms of nasopharyngitis: clear rhinorrhea, nasal stuffiness, cough (usually worse at night because of postnasal drip), generalized malaise, and irritability. Caution should be taken, however, in confusing a viral illness (rhinorrhea, cough, oral ulcers, hoarseness) with bacterial pharyngitis. Sudden onset extreme throat discomfort is the chief complaint in most cases of pharyngitis (Fig. 16-14). With GABHS, white exudate, petechiae, or both may be visible on the posterior palate and tonsils, whereas tonsillopharyngeal inflammation, high fever, scarlet fever rash, anterior cervical lymphadenopathy, nausea, vomiting, abdominal pain, and history of exposure are present with bacterial pharyngitis. Dysphagia and laryngitis may accompany either pharyngitis or nasopharyngitis.

Interdisciplinary Interventions

Current recommendations by the Infectious Diseases Society of America (Shulman et al., 2012) exist on the diagnosis and treatment of pharyngitis and nasopharyngitis.

Diagnosis should be made with rapid antigen test and/or culture. In the event of a negative rapid antigen test, a culture should be done; however, a culture is not necessary when the rapid antigen test is positive. Standard treatment for GABHS is penicillin or amoxicillin for 10 days. For those who are penicillin allergic, a cephalosporin may be used. Instruct parents to monitor carefully for signs of complications or disease progression and to seek medical attention promptly if they occur. Parents may also be advised to position the infant in an infant seat or with the head of the bed elevated for comfort and

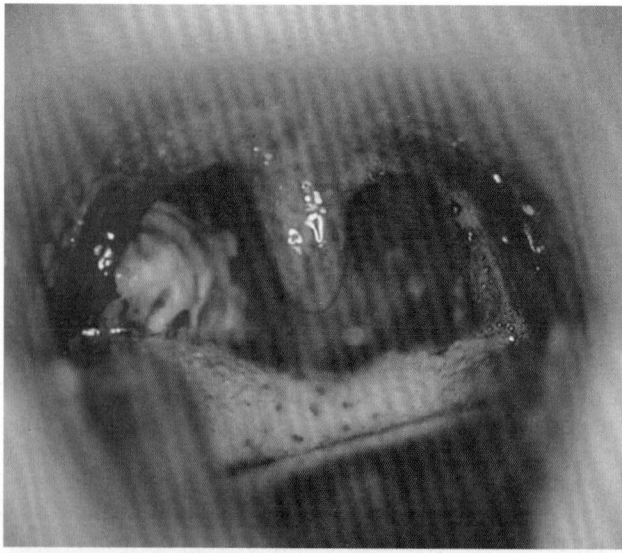

Figure 16-14 Pharyngitis. Note the redness of the pharynx, tonsillar exudate, and white strawberry tongue coating.

to facilitate drainage of nasal secretions. A bulb syringe may also be used to clear nasal passages before feedings, especially for infants, to promote feeding and nippling.

Community Care

Supportive care, including rest, nutritious foods, and cool fluids, is the primary intervention. General fever reduction methods should be used for children with temperatures higher than 101° F (38.3° C). Acetaminophen, the drug of choice for reducing fever, may be alternated with nonsteroidal anti-inflammatory drugs for temperatures. Comfort measures such as cool fluids and ice pops may be given; warm saline throat irrigations (saltwater gargle) may be comforting for the older, cooperative child. The most common carrier of infection is the human hands. Frequent handwashing by the child and caregiver is necessary to reduce the spread of the infection. Symptoms generally resolve in 5 to 7 days. Follow up testing and testing of asymptomatic household contacts is generally not recommended (Shulman et al., 2012).

TONSILLITIS

Tonsils and adenoids are important to the normal development of the body's immune system because they serve as part of the body's defense against infection. However, they may become a site of acute or chronic infection (tonsillitis). The tonsils are located on either side of the pharyngeal cavity. The palatine, or faucial, tonsils enlarge when infected and are readily seen behind the faucial pillars at the sides of the oropharynx. Adenoids are the nasopharyngeal tonsils, which are located adjacent to the palatine tonsils on the posterior wall of the nasopharynx. Tonsillar tissue increases in size during childhood as a result of acute nasopharyngeal infections that commonly occur in the school-aged child (Fig. 16-15). Tonsils reach their maximum size

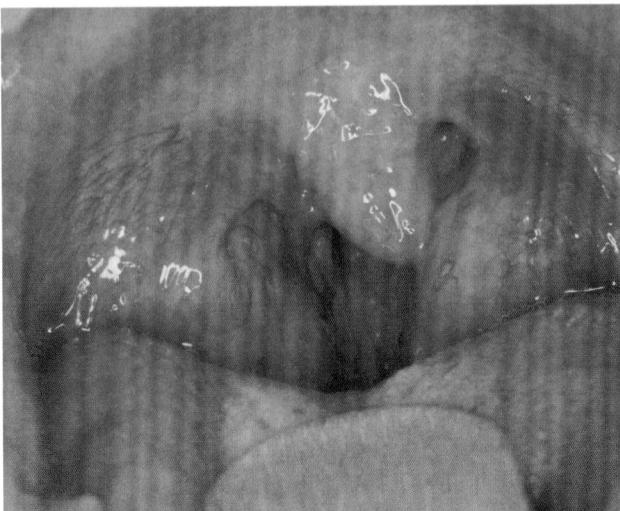

Figure 16-15 "Kissing tonsils" occur when the tonsils are so enlarged that they touch the uvula and/or each other, greatly narrowing the airway.

between 8 and 12 years of age and then begin to involute, or shrink, during puberty. Tonsillitis most often affects school-aged children; however, the condition is not limited to the pediatric population.

Pathophysiology

Repeated acute infections centered in lymphoid tissue, such as the tonsils, draw the body's defenses to that location, causing the tissue to swell. The acute infectious process inflames the tissues of the tonsils and may cause exudate to form on the tonsils. Enlarged tonsils and adenoids impinge on the pharyngeal opening of the eustachian tube, preventing it from ventilating and draining the middle ear, thus contributing to incidence of otitis media as a sequela to tonsillitis. Other symptoms include reddened pharynx and tonsils, sore throat, dysphagia, fever, and swollen lymph nodes in the neck region.

Acute tonsillar infection is thought to result largely from infection with GABHS, although other organisms can cause tonsillitis, including *H. influenzae*, pneumococcal infection, and viral agents. GABHS is particularly problematic because it cannot be identified by rapid strep test. GABHS may be obtained by throat culture, although cultures are difficult to obtain and are at times inconclusive. Children generally recover from tonsillitis, but if it is caused by GABHS that is not completely eradicated, serious sequelae, such as rheumatic fever or acute glomerulonephritis, may occur. Chronic tonsillitis is a common affliction of childhood; however, its exact incidence is unknown.

Assessment

Children with acute or chronic tonsillitis present with clinical signs and symptoms similar to those of pharyngitis. Inspect for inflammation of the tonsils and surrounding tissues, accompanied by varying degrees of soreness of the mucosa. This soreness may cause the child to refuse to eat or drink because of discomfort on swallowing. Additional clinical manifestations include exudate on the tonsillar surface, substantial erythema, recurrent or persistent sore throat, and possible obstruction to swallowing or breathing caused by hypertrophied tonsils or adenoids. Occasionally, the throat may be dry and irritated, and the breath may be offensive. If the tonsils and adenoids are hypertrophied, determine whether they are obstructing the upper airway. Children with tonsils and adenoids that cause chronic obstruction of the airway may develop respiratory distress with chronic hypoxia and, if left untreated, may develop pulmonary hypertension. These children may present as "mouth breathers" and snore during sleep and have sleep apnea. An expert in sleep medicine should evaluate a child who has chronic obstruction and snoring and/or apnea during sleep.

Hypertrophy or acute infection of the tonsils must be carefully evaluated. Many apparently enlarged tonsils are, in fact, normal in size. The misinterpretation arises from the fact that tonsils are normally larger during early childhood years than later in life. Tonsils may virtually meet in the midline in some normal, asymptomatic children, especially when the child gags. Ascertain whether hypertrophy, if present, is chronic or the result of a recent acute infection. Tonsils can increase in size tremendously with an acute infection and recede after the infection subsides.

Inspect an older child's tonsils simply by asking the child to say "aaah." If the child is unable to hold the tongue down, use a tongue blade lightly to help. Younger children consider the examination of the mouth and throat intrusive and may be uncooperative. Infants and young children whose cooperation cannot be gained will usually open their mouths during crying to allow a good view of the oropharynx. If a tongue blade is needed, use it cautiously and quickly.

Interdisciplinary Interventions

When tonsillitis is present, it is necessary to test for GABHS by culturing the tonsillar surface. A throat culture can be best obtained using the same techniques as those for inspecting the throat. Identifying the causative organism directs the antibiotic course that will be used. The recommended treatment for acute tonsillitis secondary to GABHS is usually penicillin unless a contraindication (i.e., penicillin allergy) exists. In cases of penicillin allergy, cephalosporins may be used. Antibiotics are generally administered orally or intramuscularly; the oral dose should be given for 10 days. Teach the parent that administering the complete course of antibiotic is essential because, although symptoms may subside in 24 to 72 hours, the full course is necessary to prevent complications such as rheumatic fever and glomerulonephritis.

Tonsillectomy and adenoidectomy are controversial surgical interventions for chronic tonsillitis. Recurrent throat infection (documented with positive throat cultures) has been one of the leading indications for surgery. Tonsillectomy has been documented to decrease the number of infections in children with recurrent tonsillitis; however, the number of throat infections also declines in many children who have not had tonsillectomies. As such, current recommendations do not support tonsillectomy for recurrent infections (Shulman et al., 2012). Chronic upper airway obstruction is also a major indication for surgery. Symptoms of upper airway obstruction are more prominent during sleep and include mouth breathing, heavy breathing, restlessness, loud snoring, and, in extreme cases, apnea. The child with upper airway obstruction extensive enough to warrant tonsillectomy may also exhibit sleep disturbances and enuresis. Patients with severe obstruction improve after surgery; many patients with mild to moderate symptoms improve without it. Before considering tonsillectomy, health care professionals, in collaboration with parents, should carefully document that sore throats are caused by GABHS and are frequent (more than five per year), symptomatic (fever, exudate, erythema, adenitis), and costly in terms of missed school and work days and medical expenses.

Tonsillectomy and adenoidectomy surgeries usually are performed on an outpatient basis. However, with the increase in obesity, there are increasing numbers of children with sleep-disordered breathing requiring tonsillectomy and adenoidectomy. Those children have demonstrated an increased risk of intraoperative complications during surgery and, as such, may require hospitalization postoperatively (Nafiu et al., 2009). It is imperative for the nurse to prepare the child and family for the surgery and teach both child and family the postoperative care protocol.

Observe for potential hemorrhage during the postoperative period. Small amounts of bright-red blood may be present soon after the surgery. It is normal for the child to have one emesis of old blood after the surgery and small amounts of blood-streaked mucus within the first few hours after the surgery.

caREminder

Suctioning should be avoided after a tonsillectomy or adenoidectomy. Children should avoid coughing, clearing the throat, or blowing the nose after surgery to prevent disturbing the surgical site.

If the child spits up bright-red blood frequently or has repeated emesis of old blood from the stomach or if he or she becomes tachycardic, pale, and restless, notify the surgeon immediately. Occasionally, it may be necessary for the child to return to surgery to ligate a bleeding vessel. If no bleeding occurs, ice chips and water may be given soon after surgery once the child is fully alert. Advance the diet from clear liquids to soft diet, as tolerated. Give pain medication in the form of a liquid or syrup, if available, within the first 2 hours after surgery. The child should receive pain medication as needed every 4 hours during the first 24 to 48 hours to control pain and to make swallowing fluids more comfortable.

Dehydration is a potential complication postoperatively in these children secondary to pain at the surgical site or the presence of a postoperative fever. Ensuring proper fluid intake in the face of poor oral intake and presence of fever is critical for the child to reduce the risk of dehydration. Teaching ways to provide fluids to the child is a part of the discharge teaching for the family.

Most children are discharged on the day of surgery. Children with comorbidities may require hospitalization. Teaching Intervention Plan 16-3 highlights key instructions for care of the child at home.

Community Care

The child with uncomplicated acute tonsillitis is usually managed on an ambulatory basis. The symptoms of a sore throat may be treated in the home with acetaminophen or nonsteroidal anti-inflammatory drugs, throat lozenges or hard candies, cool fluids, ice chips or ice pops, and saltwater gargles to keep the throat moist. Discourage the use of topical anesthetics sprays because their efficacy in young children is unproved and because of the risk of systemic absorption and allergic sensitization. Stress the importance of clear liquids to encourage hydration (dairy products should be avoided because they promote thickening of mucus).

TIP 16-3: A TEACHING INTERVENTION PLAN for the Child After Tonsillectomy or Adenoidectomy

---

Nursing Diagnoses and Family Outcomes

- Acute pain related to effects of surgical procedure
  Outcome: Child will demonstrate indicators of comfort and will receive adequate periods of rest.
- Deficient fluid volume related to decreased intake of fluids and loss of fluids (vomiting, secretions)
  Outcome: Child will have adequate fluid intake with minimal fluid losses.
- Deficient knowledge: Signs of postoperative complications
  Outcome: Family/caregiver verbalizes and describes home treatment and early signs of postoperative complications.

Teach the Child/Family
Home Management of the Child
- Allow the child to engage in quiet activity for the first week after surgery. The child may return to school per the surgeon's recommendation.
- Give analgesics for pain every 4–6 hours as needed. Use acetaminophen for pain relief; avoid use of ibuprofen unless directed by surgeon.

- Apply an ice collar to the child's neck, which may help with pain management.
- Be aware that halitosis is common for 1–2 weeks after surgery. Provide mouth care by using mouth rinses, instructing the child not to gargle.
- Encourage the child to drink plenty of fluids (1–1.5 qt) daily. Consider syringe feeding for infants if needed.
- Offer tepid fluids or slow-melting fluids such as ice pops or Italian ices and offer a soft diet, avoiding spicy, rough, or coarse foods for the first 7–10 days.
- Use caution with straws; utensils; and sharp, pointed toys that may be put in the mouth and injure the surgical site.
- Avoid crowds and protect the child from contact with persons who are ill.
- Emphasize the importance of the surgical follow-up appointment, usually 1–2 weeks after surgery.

Contact Health Care Provider if
- Persistent bleeding, frequent swallowing, coughing, or blood in vomitus is present
- Child complains of an earache
- Child has a fever more than 101° F (38.3° C)
- Child complains of posterior neck pain

Occasionally, the throat swelling is severe; symptoms indicate epiglottitis; or the child may become severely dehydrated and therefore require hospitalization for treatment with IV fluids, parenteral antibiotics, and emergency equipment available in case of airway obstruction.

CROUP

Croup is one of the most common acute respiratory conditions seen during early childhood (6 months to 5 years of age), with a peak in the second year of life, and the most common cause of upper airway obstruction (Everard, 2009).

Although croup is generally a benign condition resulting in minimal airway obstruction, it can be life threatening, resulting in respiratory failure. Young children are at particular risk because inflammation and narrowing in their small airways can easily result in obstruction. Croup may include inflammation of the upper airway, including the larynx, extend down to the glottis (vocal cords), and then extend further to the subglottic region and involve the trachea, bronchi, and bronchioles. When croup extends down to the bronchioles, it is called laryngotracheobronchitis (LTB). Children with spasmodic croup have inflammation of the larynx. Differentiating croup from other disease entities

such as acute epiglottitis (supraglottitis) and tracheitis is important because they have significantly different care considerations.

Infectious agents associated with LTB are usually viral and affect the subglottic region. Parainfluenza 1 and 3 account for many cases of LTB. Other viral agents associated with LTB include influenza, RSV, adenovirus, rhinovirus, human metapneumovirus, enterovirus, and, more rarely, measles virus and herpes simplex virus.

Pathophysiology

The underlying pathophysiology of LTB is inflammation and edema of the larynx, trachea, and bronchi; laryngeal muscle spasm; and production of mucus that further obstruct the airway. Inflammation in LTB narrows the subglottic region, the smallest portion of the upper airway in children, thus producing the classic symptoms of upper airway obstruction found in children with croup. Hoarseness occurs because the vocal cords swell; the barking cough is caused by inflammation of the larynx tissues.

Assessment

The incubation period for LTB is usually 2 to 6 days and is typically preceded by a mild upper respiratory infection with symptoms of rhinorrhea, mild cough, and low-grade fever. Children presenting with LTB look ill and appear to be in acute respiratory distress. Listen for hoarseness, inspiratory stridor, and the characteristic "barking" or brassy cough. Clinical signs, depending on the severity of airway obstruction, may include suprasternal, substernal, and intercostal retractions; intermittent cyanosis during coughing; and altered mental status related to hypoxia and carbon dioxide retention. A thorough respiratory assessment is important because the child with upper airway obstruction with mild hypoxia develops muscle fatigue and hypoventilation that can result in severe hypoxemia and hypercapnia. Rarely, ET intubation is necessary because of complete airway obstruction or respiratory distress.

A characteristic concern in children with LTB is parental anxiety, which is usually high. However, the degree of anxiety depends on many factors, including parental experience with previous croup episodes, lack of sleep from child's barking, and the severity of the child's respiratory distress and degree of anxiety and irritability.

Interdisciplinary Interventions

Children with croup are treated with the administration of steroids. A recent Cochrane review demonstrated effectiveness of dexamethasone or budesonide in reduction of airway edema, symptoms, need for other medications, and decreases hospitalization (Russell et al., 2011). Current data on the use of racemic epinephrine demonstrates that it does reduce symptomatology; however, the effects are short lived (Bjornson et al., 2011). Rarely, emergency measures for airway protection (ET intubation) are required. General supportive measures for the child include hydration, fever reduction measures, and maintaining a calm and reassuring atmosphere for the parents. As with any respiratory condition, hydration is an important nursing action. Encourage clear fluids, particularly fluids the child prefers, unless respiratory distress is severe, in which case the child should be NPO and should be hydrated intravenously. Give antipyretics if the child is febrile (fever higher than 101° F [38.3° C]). Ensure that parents understand the distinction between bacterial and viral illnesses so they are not distressed when antibiotics are not prescribed. LTB is generally a self-limiting illness in which children's symptoms subside in 3 to 5 days, and full recovery without complications is the norm.

Children who present with respiratory distress symptoms, such as cyanosis, and who are severely hypoxic, fatigued, in respiratory distress, or unable to drink sufficient fluids are hospitalized to receive airway support, oxygen, and IV fluids. For those children who are not in extremis, observe for any deterioration of respiratory status and monitor vital signs, including rate, rhythm, and depth of respirations; cardiac rate and rhythm; and neurologic status. Tachycardia, cardiac arrhythmias, or both may be seen with hypoxia. A decreased level of consciousness is an ominous sign for a child with respiratory distress. Ensure that equipment for intubation and tracheostomy is readily available.

Mist therapy (croup/mist tents or mist via mask or nasal cannula), widely used in the past, has questionable efficacy for treating LTB (Moore & Little, 2006). Current therapy relies on aerosol inhalation therapy with medications such as racemic epinephrine. Racemic epinephrine is believed to work via topical alpha-adrenergic stimulation, which causes mucosal vasoconstriction and leads to decreased edema in the subglottic region. Facilitate the administration of respiratory inhalation treatments at the prescribed frequency to disrupt regular feeding and sleeping patterns as little as possible.

Community Care

Two of the most important interventions are to minimize anxiety and maximize opportunities for rest. Providing a comfortable environment free from noxious stimuli lessens respiratory distress. Encourage children to engage in quiet play that provides diversion and reduces anxiety. Coloring books, watching favorite videos and DVDs, listening to music, reading stories, and doing puzzles are some examples.

Nutritional supports for children with croup are generally short term. Encourage oral intake of clear fluids, especially fluids the child prefers. Dairy products should be avoided until respiratory status is stable. When solid food is resumed, the child may find frequent, small, nutritious snacks more appealing than a full meal.

Teach parents and other caregivers about medications, respiratory inhalation treatments, and ways to assess their child's respiratory status. Although most children recover without complications, caregivers must be able to recognize and describe signs of impending respiratory failure and know how to access emergency services. A home health referral may be indicated if the parents' assessment ability is in question and the child's condition does not warrant hospitalization. The child should be afebrile and free from cough before returning to school or daycare.

During the acute phase of the illness, parental anxiety may be very high. Provide information and support, emphasizing the short-lived nature of the illness. For the child who remains at home, help the parents to mobilize their extended family and community resources to relieve them of some care responsibilities and provide them opportunities for adequate rest.

ACUTE EPIGLOTTITIS (SUPRAGLOTTITIS)

Epiglottitis is a rare, acute inflammation of the supraglottic structures, the epiglottis, and aryepiglottic folds. It characteristically does not involve the subglottic and tracheal regions. Epiglottitis constitutes one of the true pediatric emergencies. If treatment is delayed, it may rapidly progress to complete airway obstruction, cardiopulmonary arrest, and a potentially fatal outcome. When prompt diagnosis and coordinated, well-organized management occurs, the prognosis for full and uncomplicated recovery is excellent.

The incidence of epiglottitis is significantly reduced since the institution of *H. influenza* type B (HIB) vaccination in 1985. A recent study has demonstrated that the mean age for epiglottis is 44 years (Shah & Stocks, 2010); however, epiglottitis is also seen in children of all ages. Approximately one third of epiglottitis cases in children and adolescents (younger than 18 years of age) involve infants younger than 1 year of age. Epiglottitis occurs year-round but is more common during winter and early spring.

Epiglottitis most commonly results from infection of the supraglottic structures by GABHS, *S. pneumoniae*, HIB, beta-hemolytic streptococci, and, rarely, other bacteria and some viruses. The infecting organism can be isolated from the upper airway as well as from the blood. Direct invasion by the bacteria causes inflammation of the supraglottic structures, with subsequent edematous swelling of these structures and bacteremia. All patients who have the clinical picture of this disease must be managed with the same cautious approach.

Assessment

Diagnosis of epiglottitis is made primarily from clinical signs. Consider epiglottitis in any child with acute upper airway obstruction and respiratory distress, including stridor of sudden onset (developing over a few hours) accompanied by high fever (more than 102.2° F [39° C]), sore throat, hoarseness, dysphagia, and drooling. Often, these symptoms are preceded by symptoms of an upper respiratory infection. Epiglottitis seldom causes the barking cough characteristic of croup. Agitation, characterized by irritability and restlessness, is almost always present. Observe whether the child assumes the "tripod" position, the hallmark of epiglottitis—the child refuses to lie down, preferring to sit upright and lean forward, mouth open, to attain the best airway possible and to allow secretions to run out of the mouth. As the obstruction increases, cyanosis may occur, and retractions of the supraclavicular and substernal area may be present. Parents are usually very fearful and anxious as they witness and describe rapid onset of symptoms.

Never attempt direct visualization of the upper airway in any child with symptoms of epiglottitis. Direct visualization of the upper airway may precipitate complete airway obstruction and respiratory arrest. It should be attempted only by a person skilled in intubation and with all necessary equipment present at the bedside. Upon visualization, the epiglottis is cherry red, and it and the surrounding tissues are extremely swollen. The laryngeal orifice may be severely narrowed, and pooling of mucous secretions often occurs. A lateral neck radiograph may demonstrate the "thumb" sign (large, rounded soft mass below the base of the tongue); however, this diagnostic technique may be unreliable.

ALERT   *Do not use tongue blades or other instrumentation to visualize the epiglottis. Such actions can cause the epiglottis to spasm and totally occlude the airway.*

Interdisciplinary Interventions

Skilled pediatric personnel should carefully monitor children with suspected epiglottitis at all times and in a controlled medical environment (e.g., hospital room or emergency room with airway equipment appropriately sized for pediatric use). The child and the parents are usually extremely anxious, and the most important interdisciplinary intervention is keeping the child quiet and undisturbed until ET intubation is performed. Minimize episodes of crying by allowing the child, if possible, to sit upright in the parent's arms. Never force the child into a supine position because this position may cause the inflamed epiglottis to obstruct the airway, compromise diaphragmatic excursion and air movement, or enable the child to choke on swallowed secretions.

Respiratory status, including rate and depth of respirations and the presence of retractions, nasal flaring, and stridor, must be carefully monitored. Give humidified oxygen by face mask and keep the head of the bed elevated at all times. If the child does not tolerate the face mask, use any means necessary to provide humidified oxygen. Monitor SaO_2 levels using pulse oximetry. IV antibiotics must be given as soon as possible; IV line placement should be done using pain-relieving techniques to reduce anxiety. Upon strong suspicion or confirmation of the diagnosis, intubation should be performed in the operating room under general anesthesia. Intubation sometimes is not possible because of laryngospasm or severe swelling; in these cases, placement of a tracheostomy is required (see "Treatment Modalities" section earlier in the chapter).

Other important interventions include administering and monitoring sedative medication because the risk of accidental extubation is high. Mild sedation also allows the child to breathe spontaneously, making full mechanical ventilation unnecessary. Assess for possible respiratory complications, monitor body temperature, and provide adequate fluid and calorie intake. Children are ready for extubation when an air leak around the ET tube is present, signifying a reduction in edema of the epiglottis. Intubated children may be fed through an enteral tube; feedings should be stopped in preparation for extubation. Children who are not intubated must be NPO during the acute phase of the illness. Oral intake should be allowed as the child's respiratory condition is improved (Clinical Judgment 16-1).

As with any hospitalization, parental anxiety is high, especially if the child is admitted in acute respiratory distress. During this period, provide calm, factual, step-by-step information. Repeat this information as the family's stress level decreases and they are able to formulate questions. Initial information should include the course of events in the immediate future—for example, when and where the child will be intubated; where the family may wait; when they may first visit the child after airway management is accomplished; how the child will be given nutrition, hydration, and medication; and how long they should expect the child will need to remain intubated and sedated.

Recovery from epiglottitis is usually rapid, with ET extubation occurring in 2 to 3 days as the fever dissipates, the child can handle secretions, and airway

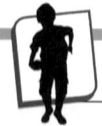

CLINICAL JUDGMENT 16-1

The Drooling Child

Jimmy, a 5-year-old child, presents in the emergency room with respiratory stridor upon inspiration and a temperature of 102.5° F (39.2° C). He is drooling and prefers to sit forward with his chin slightly protruded. His mother states that he developed the difficulty breathing "so suddenly," and both mother and child appear anxious.

Questions

1. What additional data would you collect during your initial assessment?
2. Is this an upper or lower respiratory problem?
3. What actions would your initial interventions include?
4. Is obtaining a throat culture indicated at this time? Why or why not?
5. What interventions should be implemented to maintain a patent airway in this child?

Answers

1. Heart rate, respiratory rate, work of breathing, duration of fever, and other signs of respiratory illness. Is the child voiding? When did he last eat or drink (to assess for dehydration and shock)? No visual inspection of the oral cavity is ever indicated if epiglottitis is suspected.
2. An upper respiratory problem, as distinguished by inspiratory stridor resulting from an obstruction. In this case, the obstruction is a swollen cherry-red epiglottis.
3. Interventions include maintaining an airway. Keep the child with his mother to help reduce anxiousness and allow him to remain in the tripod position because this helps maintain an open airway. Provide oxygen via mask or blow-by oxygen as the child tolerates. If respiratory distress becomes severe, immediately notify the health care prescriber and anticipate intubation.
4. A throat culture should not be obtained because manipulation of the oropharynx for visualization or when obtaining a culture may precipitate airway spasm and obstruction from the swollen epiglottis.
5. The primary therapy is to maintain the airway. Therefore, provide oxygen support via face mask or bag–valve mask ventilation as needed until the provider is ready to intubate the child.

narrowing is resolved. Reassuring and supporting the parents is key during this recovery phase because the rapid progression and critical nature of this disorder render it extremely frightening. Nurses and social workers can assist families by providing frequent, accurate education and updates on the child's condition, and allowing parental visitation or rooming-in as much as possible. Tell parents when they should expect the child to resume normal dietary habits and when discharge from the hospital is expected. Begin teaching about administration of oral antibiotics at home (to complete a 7-day course) when the IV line is discontinued.

Community Care

Urge immunization with the HIB capsular polysaccharide vaccine for the patient and all siblings of appropriate age (see Chapter 8) if they are not already immunized. Prophylaxis with rifampin by mouth is recommended for all household contacts, if at least one contact is younger than 4 years of age, regardless of immunization status. Daycare and nursery school contact groups should be managed on an individual basis. The HIB vaccine and rifampin prophylaxis can both be obtained from the county public health agency in many states.

BACTERIAL TRACHEITIS

Bacterial tracheitis is an uncommon, but potentially life-threatening, acute bacterial infection of the mucosa of the upper trachea with thick, adherent tracheal membranes. It is also called *membranous laryngotracheitis* or *membranous croup*. This rare disease may be seen in children between 3 and 8 years of age; peak incidence is in the fall and winter months because it usually follows an acute viral respiratory illness (Miranda et al., 2011). This condition is unrelated to ethnicity, gender, or socioeconomic status. Bacterial tracheitis is a serious cause of airway obstruction and can be life threatening. With early recognition and treatment, outcomes are generally very good. The most common causative organisms are *Staphylococcus aureus*, *Streptococcus pneumoniae*, *Moraxella catarrhalis*, *H. influenza*, and *Streptococcus pyogenes*; however, tracheitis can all be caused by viruses (Miranda et al., 2011; Tebruegge et al., 2009).

Assessment

The child with bacterial tracheitis usually appears quite ill and presents with a history of a prior upper respiratory tract infection, viral croup, or both, followed by a high fever, cough, and increasing inspiratory stridor unaffected by position. The trachea is inflamed and appears erythematous and edematous, with thick, tenacious, purulent secretions. Respiratory distress is a key symptom in bacterial tracheitis and requires immediate medical attention. The physician uses laryngoscopy or bronchoscopy to confirm the diagnosis. Tracheal cultures are obtained during the endoscopic procedure (Miranda et al., 2011).

Interdisciplinary Interventions

Vigorous management, including early recognition of bacterial tracheitis and prompt attention to the airway, is necessary to prevent the airway from being obstructed by the thick secretions. The child should be hospitalized, and appropriate emergency airway management equipment should be available. Younger children are likely to require intubation during treatment to maintain a patent airway due to anatomic narrowing of the airways. Antimicrobial therapies aimed at the infectious organism are critical, as are maintaining adequate gas exchange, nutrition, hydration, and fever management.

APNEA

Apnea is cessation of airflow into and out of the lungs. Apneic episodes lasting longer than 20 seconds and shorter respiratory pauses associated with cyanosis, bradycardia, **pallor** (paleness), or limpness are considered pathologic apnea. Apnea is a description of a characteristic clinical syndrome, not a specific disease process. Three general types of apnea occur:

1. *Central apnea* is an impairment of the mechanisms that control breathing, which results in absence of nasal airflow and ventilatory effort.
2. *Obstructive apnea* is usually caused by anatomic abnormalities and occurs when nasal airflow is absent despite normal or exaggerated respiratory effort. Obstructive apneas include *obstructive sleep apnea* (OSA), which is the most common type of sleep apnea.
3. *Mixed apnea* includes central and obstructive components and may require multiple treatment methods.

Although apnea can occur at any age, the premature infant is at greater risk. Normal respiratory system development is such that the lungs and respiratory center of the brain are designed to breathe and control respiration at term. Although they are capable of breathing air by 23 weeks' gestation, the lungs and respiratory center of premature infants have not fully matured, leading to disruptions in the regularity of respiration.

Apnea of prematurity is the occurrence of pathologic apnea and periodic breathing in an infant less than 37 weeks' gestation. It commonly occurs in infant less than 33 weeks' gestation and generally represents an immaturity of the respiratory control center. Short episodes of apnea lasting less than 10 seconds that are not accompanied by heart rate changes or hypoxia are generally not clinically significant. In infants with apnea lasting longer than 20 seconds or events associated with heart rate changes or hypoxia may affect long-term neurodevelopmental outcomes and should be evaluated for further treatment such as caffeine citrate (Moriette et al., 2010).

Apnea of infancy (AOI) describes episodes of breathing cessation or respiratory pauses in a previously healthy infant of at least 37 weeks' gestation.

Apparent life-threatening event (ALTE) is the current term for more severe disturbances of a frighteningly serious nature. An ALTE is defined as an event in which an infant has a convincing history of an episode of apnea that is sudden in onset; considered frightening to the observer; and is characterized by color change (cyanosis, pallor, or erythema), marked change in muscular tone (limpness, rarely stiffness), and choking, gagging, or both (Scollan-Koliopoulos & Koliopoulos, 2010; Warren et al., 2007).

Acute apneic episodes with cyanosis in term infants can have a variety of treatable causes, including seizures; infection; breath-holding spells; congenital heart disease; cardiac dysrhythmia; electrolyte imbalances; congenital central hypoventilation syndrome; brain stem compression; anemia; or exposure to alcohol, sedatives, and narcotics. ALTE can also be the result of a profound central nervous system insult or depression involving structural damage to the brain stem (as in trauma, infection, or edema) or interference with cerebral metabolic function (e.g., drug overdose, hypotension, severe hypoxia). In some cases, it may be idiopathic (Scollan-Koliopoulos & Koliopoulos, 2010). The prognosis for these infants depends on the etiology and treatment of the underlying cause.

Assessment

Apnea may present simply as a parental report of prolonged asymptomatic respiratory pauses during sleep or dramatically as a witnessed complete cessation of breathing and absence of a heart rate. Because apneic episodes, regardless of their severity, typically occur away from the view of the medical team, the significance of the event is based largely on the caregiver's recollection of the event. A single mild episode that required little or no intervention does not necessitate an extensive diagnostic evaluation or aggressive therapy and has little prognostic importance. The healthy infant who presents with a history of AOI or an ALTE, for whom the obvious treatable causes have been evaluated, presents a greater challenge in diagnosis and management.

Infants usually appear entirely normal by the time they reach medical attention after an ALTE. The most important element of assessment is, therefore, to obtain a careful history from the person who witnessed the event. Interview the witness to determine the color of the child when found (pale or cyanotic), whether the child had any respirations, and whether the child was limp. Determine whether there was evidence of vomiting. Ascertain whether the apneic episode occurred when the child was asleep or awake and when the event occurred in relation to the most recent feeding. Collaborate with other health care personnel to gain as much detail as possible about the event itself, the physical condition of the infant before and after the event, and circumstances surrounding its occurrence. Assess the reliability of the historian, and look for any signs of child abuse or neglect; also evaluate the potential for sepsis.

OSA may occur in children of any age and affects between 1.2% and 5.7% of children. OSA risk factors include obesity, adenotonsillar hypertrophy, neuromuscular diseases, and craniofacial abnormalities (American Academy of Pediatrics [AAP], 2012). Symptoms include snoring, periods of observed apnea, heavy breathing, broken or restless sleep, bad dreams, and failure to grow or thrive. Morbidities associated with OSA may include inattentiveness, developmental disorders, mood disorders, enuresis, hypertension, ventricular dysfunction, insulin resistance, or excessive daytime sleepiness (Loghmanee & Sheldon, 2010).

Screening for OSA should occur at routine child health maintenance visits (AAP, 2012). The primary diagnostic test for apnea is the polysomnographic study (PSG; or sleep study). Other diagnostic tests may include, but are not limited to, arterial or capillary blood gases (persistent acidosis indicates a severe event or a chronic metabolic disorder); complete blood counts (anemia may precipitate apnea, polycythemia reflects chronic hypoxia, elevated WBC count indicates infection); and serum electrolyte, glucose, and blood urea nitrogen levels (numerous abnormalities, such as hypocalcemia and hypoglycemia, may contribute to the development of apnea). Many health care professionals diagnose OSA based on physical examination and nocturnal pulse oximetry. If the primary care provider is unsure about the referral for a PSG, or unclear about the diagnosis, a referral to a pediatric otolaryngologist for further evaluation may be warranted (AAP, 2012).

Interdisciplinary Interventions

Optimal care of infants who have had an episode of apnea accompanied by color change or who present with an ALTE includes hospitalization for observation, monitoring by health care personnel, a thorough evaluation for possible causes, and parent training (see thePoint for Care Paths). Continuous cardiorespiratory monitoring and frequent assessment of color, breathing patterns and effort, and tone are appropriate health care interventions.

ALERT *Health care professionals should promote preventive practices to decrease the risk of sudden infant death syndrome (SIDS). Specific interventions include supine positioning for sleep, safe sleeping environments, and elimination of smoke exposure (AAP, 2011).*

The preterm infant who continues to exhibit symptomatic apnea during the hospital stay should also be evaluated carefully for hypoxia or anemia, which can cause apnea in the premature infant. In the absence of hypoxia or anemia, preterm infants who are still having clinical episodes of apnea can be discharged with home apnea and bradycardia monitoring equipment.

Agents such as theophylline, aminophylline, or caffeine are sometimes useful in decreasing the severity and frequency of apneic episodes in the infant with apnea of prematurity. These medications are central nervous system stimulants that act on the respiratory center of the brain and therefore are sometimes effective in treating central apnea only. Besides stimulating the respiratory center, these drugs also act on the kidney, heart, and skeletal and smooth muscles. Side effects include tachycardia and increased diuresis. Parents and caregivers must be taught to draw up and administer the medications and observe for toxic side effects (tachycardia, vomiting, excessive irritability). Teach them to monitor for therapeutic drug levels and to report toxic levels.

Treatment of OSA primarily focuses on tonsillectomy, adenoidectomy, or both. Other options include weight reduction, inhaled corticosteroids, or positive-pressure airway breathing (including CPAP).

Community Care

Parental anxiety is characteristically the foremost psychosocial issue challenging nurses and other members of the health care team in working with the infant and family after admission to the hospital with an apneic episode or after an ALTE. Much guidance and reassurance is needed, in conjunction with education, to increase parental confidence and problem-solving skills.

Because no specific treatment currently exists for infants with AOI or ALTE of unknown etiology, home apnea and bradycardia monitoring is the primary therapy. Ongoing therapy can be equally anxiety producing as the initial ALTE for parents and families. Home monitors serve only to alert the caregiver that an apneic episode is occurring. The parent or caregiver must then respond and act to evaluate and terminate the apneic episode. Most parents feel the need to use the monitor at all times when the infant is not being directly observed. Home apnea monitoring often adversely affects parents' ability to work, socialize, nurture their other children, and generally maintain their former life functions because of their obsessive focus on the monitor and its every nuance.

Before initiating home apnea monitoring, and while the infant is still hospitalized, conduct a thorough review of the family's living arrangements and verify that appropriate resources are present to successfully support a home apnea monitoring program. Minimum environmental requirements include electricity, a telephone in the home, and availability of caregivers trained to respond to the apnea alarm. This inpatient evaluation of the family system is crucial in determining the teaching plan and coordinating follow-up. It may be necessary to contact community resources when appropriate, according to the family's needs.

Parental education for home apnea and bradycardia monitoring includes information on monitor use, alarms, indications for help, and CPR. Parents and caregivers are also taught to keep a log or diary of all apnea and bradycardia alarms, especially those requiring any intervention. If both parents work outside the home, alternative caregivers (extended family members, daycare providers, and so on) must also receive this education (see thePoint for Care Paths). Because of the diligence required for successful home monitoring, many parents find it difficult to stop home monitoring when it is no longer required for their infant. The caregiver has learned to rely on the monitor to provide a comforting reassurance that the child is well.

FOREIGN BODY ASPIRATION

FBA remains a persistent problem and an important cause of morbidity and mortality in the pediatric age group. Foreign bodies retained in the airway can be potentially life threatening and can produce severe lung damage.

Quantifying the overall incidence of FBA is difficult because most foreign bodies aspirated into the respiratory tract are expelled immediately by spontaneous coughing and never require medical intervention. However, FBA remains a common cause of mortality and morbidity among children during the first 3 to 4 years of life.

Most episodes occur during eating or play. Commonly aspirated objects include foods such as hot dogs, peanuts, other nuts and seeds, grapes, popcorn, and carrots as well as items such as small plastic toys, marbles, buttons, earrings, and latex balloons. Factors related to a young child's physical and developmental status predispose him or her to the risk of FBA (see Chapter 3). Young children (particularly those 6 months to 2 years of age) explore the environment by putting objects in their mouth and are at highest risk for aspiration. They also have insufficient size and number of teeth to thoroughly chew foods. In addition, they may seek relief from the teething process by chewing on hard objects. Exposure to certain foods may therefore be inappropriate for a young child's cognitive and dental stage of development and may lead to choking and aspiration.

Pathophysiology

The pathophysiology of FBA varies depending on the size of the foreign body, the location of the object in the respiratory tract, and the acute or chronic nature of the condition. If an object is too large or of a shape that does not allow it to be expelled by coughing, respiratory symptoms result. Foreign bodies in the upper airway often cause a mechanical or partial obstruction that results in nonspecific respiratory signs and symptoms such as cough, wheeze, stridor, **dyspnea** (labored or difficult breathing resulting from air hunger), voice changes, cyanosis, retractions, and **hemoptysis** (coughing blood). At times, a carefully assessed history reveals an episode of coughing, choking, or breathing difficulty that can be traced back to an aspiration event; but on many occasions, the discovery of an FBA is made without ever obtaining such a history.

Assessment

The location of the foreign body is a key factor in determining the signs, symptoms, and physical assessment findings (Table 16-3). Although nearly all children who

TABLE 16-3	Locations of Foreign Body Aspirates and Associated Findings
Location of Foreign Body	**Clinical Findings**
Supraglottic	Cough, dyspnea, drooling, gagging, changes in phonation
Larynx	Cough, stridor, changes in phonation; at times, severe respiratory distress
Trachea, intrathoracic	Expiratory wheeze, inspiratory noise
Trachea, extrathoracic	Inspiratory stridor, expiratory noise
Bronchi	Cough, asymmetric breath sounds or wheeze, hyperresonance
Esophageal	Drooling, dysphagia, stridor, respiratory distress

have aspirated a foreign body exhibit a chronic cough, a history of an acute coughing episode, or both, other symptoms vary according to where in the respiratory tract the object is lodged.

Perform a respiratory assessment. The child with a foreign body that lodges in the upper airway, such as the larynx or trachea, usually presents with an acute and rather fierce onset of stridor and respiratory distress necessitating immediate intervention to dislodge the foreign body. A foreign body lodged in the bronchus may act as a ball valve, obstructing the airway perhaps partially on inspiration and completely on expiration. Wheezing localized to one side of the chest on inspiration and diminished breath sounds on expiration result. In children with an esophageal foreign body, the distended esophagus compresses the nearby trachea, thus causing respiratory distress. Physical assessment findings may reveal asymmetry of chest wall movement and wheezing or diminished breath sounds in a localized area of the lungs. If the obstruction is located in the upper airway, stridor is common.

Radiographs may be normal, may allow clear visualization of the presence of a foreign body, or may show changes directly related to the foreign body or caused by secondary inflammatory changes. Abnormalities are less likely to be noted on chest radiograph for foreign bodies located above the bifurcation of the mainstem bronchus. Lateral neck films are obtained when this location is suspected.

"Chronically" retained foreign bodies can lead to a marked inflammatory response in the respiratory tract and, possibly, death. The right mainstem bronchus is a common site for foreign body lodgment because of its angle. Airway inflammation and narrowing secondary to edema often occurs. Materials such as nuts, which contain fats, cause an especially intense inflammatory response. Recurrent infections such as lipoid pneumonia or a lung abscess may ensue. Chronic obstruction of air exchange to the alveoli could mimic obstructive emphysema on chest radiographs. Foreign bodies that have been dislodged by coughing can lead to involvement as described here in different lung segments.

Interdisciplinary Interventions

Emergency treatment for the choking child includes the use of abdominal thrusts (the Heimlich maneuver) in the child older than 1 year of age and use of back blows and chest thrusts in the infant younger than 1 year of age. Use these methods in situations in which the aspiration was witnessed or strongly suspected and the child has an ineffective cough with increasing stridor and respiratory distress or has become unconscious and apneic.

In many cases, the object is not coughed up spontaneously and is lodged farther down in the respiratory tree; therefore, the foreign body has to be removed as soon as possible to prevent further airway damage. Rigid bronchoscopy to remove the foreign body after aspiration is the most common medical intervention. This procedure is very safe and effective when carried out by an experienced physician. Rigid bronchoscopy enables removal of the object and any associated inflammatory material; it also provides a means of assessing the condition of the airway.

Nursing care responsibilities for the infant or child undergoing rigid bronchoscopy focus on preoperative preparation and postoperative monitoring. Explain the reason for the procedure to the family. IV hydration, emptying of stomach contents, and preoperative assessment of respiratory status are fundamental nursing interventions. Postoperatively, frequently assess quality and symmetry of breath sounds, vital signs, color, and respiratory effort. Atelectasis, bronchospasm, and pneumothorax all are possible postbronchoscopy complications.

Community Care

The psychosocial consequences of an FBA incident vary in intensity, depending on the severity of the event. The most dramatic scenario involves the infant or child with a complete airway obstruction who is experiencing respiratory arrest and requires immediate resuscitation. This experience is extremely terrifying for both the child and the caregivers. Asphyxiation with subsequent brain damage or even death may occur. The grief and guilt that parents and caregivers experience in this situation are tremendous and often incapacitating. Extensive support and counseling services are crucial for these families. Less severe episodes of FBA may also raise feelings of guilt or embarrassment about inadequate supervision or about not recognizing symptoms.

The most effective "therapy" for FBA is prevention. Anyone who works with children should be certified in CPR, including airway obstruction management. Education for parents and other caregivers of infants and young children regarding aspiration risk factors is an essential role for all pediatric health care providers. Information on common items aspirated, age groups especially at risk, and developmental and environmental considerations can help parents be more aware of potential dangers and take proper precautions.

Environmental factors such as a high degree of distraction during play and mealtimes and insufficient adult supervision may also contribute to FBA. Remind parents that watching television during meals can be a dangerous distraction to young children and should be avoided. Caregivers of children at play must be cautioned about being vigilant with small children to keep them from putting objects in their mouths. Visitors to the home should place purses and other personal items out of reach of the small child. Last, products containing any small, cylindrical components should bear labels discouraging use around young children and should detail the age groups particularly affected.

LOWER RESPIRATORY INFECTIONS AND OBSTRUCTIONS

Lower respiratory infections and obstructions include influenza, bronchiolitis, bronchitis, and pneumonia.

 QUESTION: Because José has a preexisting condition (asthma), he is at greater risk for respiratory infections. José will go to kindergarten next year. What information can the nurse share with Claudia to help her keep José from catching lower respiratory infections?

INFLUENZA

Influenza illnesses have been described and defined epidemiologically for centuries. Influenza viral agents were the first proved to be respiratory tract pathogens. Consequently, the terms *flu* and *influenza* are perhaps the most overused diagnostic labels for nondescript infectious conditions in both medical and lay circles. This confusion is probably increased by influenza's broad range of clinical manifestations and its wide prevalence in the community.

Influenza infection often occurs in epidemics that sweep throughout a community in a matter of 6 to 8 weeks. Thousands of individuals die from influenza infections in the United States each year. Morbidity is highest in susceptible populations, such as infants and persons older than 65 years of age. Children with preexisting conditions such as BPD, CF, asthma, and congenital respiratory conditions (e.g., Pierre Robin syndrome) are at increased risk for morbidity and mortality associated with the flu. It is imperative to recognize the elevated vulnerability of this population. The incidence of infection is highest, however, in children of school age.

Pathophysiology

The influenza viruses are large, single-stranded RNA viruses. Influenza viruses have a high affinity for epithelial cells of the respiratory tract mucosa. The virus causes a lytic infection of the respiratory epithelium with a loss of ciliary function, decreased mucus production, and desquamation of the epithelial layer. The incubation period for influenza virus can be as short as 2 to 3 days, and viral replication usually continues for 10 to 14 days after primary infection.

There are three influenza virus types, specific in their protein and antigen composition: influenza A, B, and C. Influenza A and B, and less commonly C, cause seasonal outbreaks and epidemics. Influenza A causes pandemics. Literally, hundreds of subtypes of these categories "shift" their complement of antigens on a regular basis. These mutations largely account for the ability of influenza to produce serious epidemics in populations of people who have been previously immunized or have experienced influenza infection. This regular antigenic shift makes the preparation and distribution of influenza vaccines necessary on an annual basis.

Assessment

Infections with influenza viruses may be manifested by mild, moderate, or severe clinical symptoms. Generally, a child with influenza infection has a more sudden onset of these symptoms than do children with parainfluenza, RSV, or adenovirus infections. Look for fever of sudden onset accompanied by a flushed face, dry throat and nasal mucous membranes with dry cough, sore throat, muscle pain, headache, and malaise. During the acute phase of the illness, the child may be quite ill and require hospitalization if dehydrated or if a secondary infection develops. Fever, sore throat, and headache normally subside in 3 to 5 days; other symptoms, such as fatigue and malaise, may persist for several weeks. Provide supportive interaction to parents to allay anxiety regarding progression of the illness and complications. Children are often disappointed at missing important events and activities, yet they do not have the strength to participate.

Influenza is difficult to distinguish from other respiratory illnesses in children. Most recently, commercial rapid diagnostic tests have been developed that can detect influenza viruses within 30 minutes (Schrag et al., 2006). Diagnostic tests for influenza also include viral culture, serology, rapid antigen testing, polymerase chain reaction, and immunofluorescence assay.

Interdisciplinary Interventions

Inactivated influenza vaccine is used to prevent influenza in children (see Chapter 8). The only specific contraindication for the use of this inactivated vaccine is anaphylactic hypersensitivity to eggs.

Interventions for children with influenza include supportive care to alleviate or minimize symptoms. Antiviral agents such as zanamivir and oseltamivir may also be used for influenza A or B within certain populations. These agents have shown effectiveness by reducing the influenza course by 1 to 3 days when an early diagnosis is made (Schrag et al., 2006). Administration of acetaminophen every 4 to 6 hours for fever and muscle aches is also beneficial.

ALERT *Never treat children 18 years of age or younger with aspirin or other salicylate derivatives because of the relationship among viral syndromes, aspirin, and Reye syndrome.*

Other antipyretic therapies include undressing the child with a persistent fever to permit radiant heat loss and giving tepid sponge baths.

caREminder

Do not bathe a shivering child because the child likely will shiver more and remain febrile.

Teach parents the signs and symptoms of respiratory deterioration, the signs of dehydration and ways of preventing and treating it, and the reason that aspirin administration is contraindicated in children.

Clear liquids for children and oral rehydration formulas for infants replace losses from fever, tachypnea, and vomiting. Parents should offer oral fluids in small amounts (30 to 60 mL) on a frequent basis. If the child becomes dehydrated and requires hospitalization, he or she should receive parenteral fluids. Bed rest is important and should be encouraged for the first 3 to 5 days. If the child is home, teach the parents or caregiver what to watch for, such as increased lethargy, excessive vomiting, or respiratory distress that may indicate that the child needs to be seen by a health care professional.

ALERT *Supplemental oxygen may be needed for chronically ill children with an influenza infection because of their poor respiratory reserves and increased propensity to develop hypoxemia.*

ANSWER: The nurse should share that it is important that José receive the flu vaccine each fall. Additional teaching may be needed to explain why this vaccine is unlike his other childhood immunizations and a vaccination is needed each fall. In addition, teaching José good hand hygiene techniques and emphasizing the importance of hand hygiene may help prevent him from catching influenza and other viruses.

BRONCHIOLITIS

QUESTION: How are José's symptoms different from a child with bronchiolitis or bronchitis? Examine Table 16-4 for more information.

Bronchiolitis is an acute inflammation and obstruction of the bronchioles, the smallest, most distal sections of the respiratory airway network. It generally occurs during the first 2 years of life, with a peak incidence between 2 and 6 months of age. Premature infants, immunodeficient infants, and those with underlying comorbid conditions such as BPD, CF, or congenital heart disease are extremely vulnerable to respiratory failure and other severe complications of bronchiolitis (Vicencio, 2010). However, it is now known that previously healthy infants also succumb to RSV disease (Hall et al., 2009). Many infants can be managed at home; a few require hospitalization.

TABLE 16-4	Characteristics of Acute Bronchitis, Bronchiolitis, and Asthma		
	Acute Bronchitis	**Bronchiolitis**	**Asthma**
Etiology	Viral or bacterial infection	Usually viral infection	Bronchial hyperreactivity Hereditary component Allergic component Exacerbated by infections
Pathology	Transient inflammation of lower airways from trachea to bronchi Sloughing of respiratory mucosa and mucosal congestion No decrease in airflow or gas exchange	Infectious inflammation of small bronchioles Sloughing of respiratory epithelium into airway Tissue edema and mucus production Leads to decreased airflow and decreased gas exchange	Recurrent airway inflammation in response to allergens or irritants Airflow decrease as a result of bronchoconstriction; leads to decreased gas exchange Mucus plugging occurring in the airways
Clinical symptoms	Primary symptom is cough, which may be loose and productive Low-grade fever lasts 3–5 days Rhinitis Some wheezing possible on expiration Severe hypoxia uncommon	Starts with upper airway infection of 1–3 days duration Progresses to tachypnea retractions, rales, and cough Fever Wheezing variable Severe hypoxia can occur	Episodic expiratory wheezing (sometimes inspiratory wheeze if severe) can be brief or prolonged Nonproductive cough Severe hypoxemia common
Treatment	Bronchodilators if wheezing Antibiotics for documented bacterial infection Avoidance of irritants	Oxygen therapy, if documented hypoxia Fluid support if unable to maintain adequate intake Respiratory support with bronchodilator therapy unproven Corticosteroids rarely helpful Antiviral agents, if indicated (e.g., documented influenza)	Bronchodilators and corticosteroids Respiratory support if signs of respiratory insufficiency or failure Preventive and environmental control measures Education stressing prevention and/or early detection and treatment

Pathophysiology

In bronchiolitis, the bronchioles become narrowed, and some even become totally occluded as a result of the inflammatory process, edema of the airway wall, accumulation of mucus and cellular debris, and smooth muscle spasm. It may also cause thickening of the muscular wall and destruction of ciliated cells. This narrowing of the airway lumen can profoundly decrease airflow. Impaired clearance of secretions and decreased airflow lead to bronchiolar obstruction, atelectasis, and hyperinflation, causing impaired gas exchange that results in hypoxemia. Carbon dioxide retention occurs in the severely affected infant. The illness is self-limiting and generally resolves with adequate intervention.

Acute bronchiolitis most often has a viral cause. In some areas of the United States, bronchiolitis is the most common cause for hospitalization among infants younger than 1 year of age (Vicencio, 2010). RSV, which has a high affinity for the respiratory tract mucosa, is the most common cause of bronchiolitis (Hall et al., 2009; Vicencio, 2010). This virus is highly contagious and extremely prevalent in communities during the winter and spring months. Nearly all children have been infected with RSV by the age of 2 years. RSV is transmitted by direct contact with infected secretions via hands and respiratory droplets. Adults as well as children are infected with RSV disease; thus, the source

of viral infection in an infant is usually a family member with a mild respiratory illness. Infections with other viruses, primarily adenovirus, parainfluenza, and influenza, have been associated with bronchiolitis in smaller numbers of cases. In a small percentage of infants with bronchiolitis, suprainfection with a bacterial pathogen can occur.

Assessment

Diagnosis of bronchiolitis is made by history and physical examination. Initially, it may be difficult to determine if the child has bronchiolitis, acute bronchitis, or asthma (Table 16-4). Diagnostic criteria include exposure to ill persons, seasonal timing, and upper respiratory symptoms. The infant with bronchiolitis has typically had an upper respiratory infection for 2 to 3 days. Parents report sneezing and nasal discharge initially, followed by development of a harsh, dry cough and low-grade fever. Listen for wheezing on auscultation. The infant may develop increasingly distressed breathing and tachypnea. Inquire about feeding difficulties or loss of appetite caused by nasal congestion and the increased work required to breathe.

Because a major consequence of airway obstruction is impaired gas exchange, the child with bronchiolitis has many of the signs and symptoms of hypoxia and respiratory distress, including tachypnea and increased work of breathing. Look for chest retractions; rhonchi and wheezes or crackles are generally heard in all lung fields. Check for dehydration, which can be severe because respiratory distress often prevents adequate oral fluid intake. In addition, the elevated respiratory rate causes insensible fluid loss (see Chapter 17). When the infant becomes ill during winter months, dry air may further exacerbate the condition. Hypoxia and hypercarbia result in restlessness and irritability, making the child difficult to console, even by parents.

A nasal swab may assist in an RSV diagnosis. A chest radiograph may be done if the child is hypoxic.

Interdisciplinary Interventions

The care of a child with bronchiolitis involves respiratory, pharmacologic, and nutritional support (see thePoint for Care Paths). Infants with moderate to severe respiratory distress caused by bronchiolitis or children experiencing respiratory distress with feeding difficulties are usually hospitalized. Others may require only supportive care at home.

Hospitalized infants with RSV bronchiolitis are at high risk for respiratory failure and may require mechanical ventilation during the acute phase of the illness. Clinical indications for mechanical ventilation include worsening respiratory distress with increased work of breathing, increased heart rate, poor peripheral perfusion, apnea, bradycardia, hypercarbia, and altered mental status.

Because RSV and other causative agents are shed in high titers for days after the onset of the illness, contact isolation to prevent infecting other patients, staff, and family members is strongly recommended. RSV is easily transmitted on hands, clothing, equipment, cribs, and so forth. Limiting child-to-child contact, washing toys after use, and careful handwashing are the most effective methods of preventing nosocomial infections.

Respiratory Support

Humidified oxygen should be administered to infants who demonstrate oxygen desaturation of less than 90% (Schuh, 2011). Continuous pulse oximetry is recommended for infants in acute distress. Take care to document oxygen saturations when the child is awake during quiet time, asleep, and with crying. Desaturations to less than 90% with crying are likely; therefore, close monitoring until saturations return to baseline (more than 92%) is essential. The infant should be suctioned when clinically indicated before feedings, prior to inhalation therapy, and as needed. The use of inhalation therapies (e.g., albuterol, hypertonic saline, or racemic epinephrine) may be trialed and continued if the child has a positive response to the therapy. However, routine use of these medications should not be implemented. Helium oxygen mixture may provide relief for increased work of breathing (Schuh, 2011). If a child continues to have respiratory distress, interventions with noninvasive or invasive ventilator support may be required. Chest physiotherapies have not been found to be helpful (Roqué i Figuls et al., 2012).

Pharmacologic Support

The major thrust of therapy for bronchiolitis focuses on supportive therapy. However, inhaled ribavirin, an antiviral agent, may be used in children with immunocompromise or severe cardiac disease (Schuh, 2011).

caREminder

Nurses and respiratory therapists administering ribavirin should wear a specially designed mask to prevent exposure to ribavirin particles released into the air. Although no studies link ribavirin use to defects in human embryos, it is recommended that pregnant personnel wear a mask when in the room of the child receiving ribavirin.

Bronchodilators and corticosteroids have limited effects on a child with bronchiolitis. However, this pharmacologic therapy may assist with respiratory benefits, such as ease of breathing, improved oxygenation, and increased respiratory drive. Using these medications on an individualized basis is critical to evaluate for responsiveness. These medications should not routinely be used unless a child demonstrates improvement.

Preventive therapies for bronchiolitis are used in limited populations. Children who qualify should begin to receive palivizumab immunoprophylaxis 1 month prior to the start of the anticipated RSV season.

Nutrition and Rest

Nutritional care for the infant with bronchiolitis includes supportive fluid and electrolyte replacement. Close monitoring of fluid and electrolyte status, including accurate measurement of intake and output with urine specific gravities, is essential to assess for dehydration.

caREminder

In the case of severe respiratory distress or altered mental status, the infant or child should be NPO, and fluid should be given intravenously.

Infants hospitalized with acute bronchiolitis are using all their energy to breathe. These infants are too uncomfortable to respond to the social stimuli they are accustomed to, such as interaction with siblings. Minimizing energy expenditure and oxygen consumption should remain a primary goal of therapy until oxygen saturation levels are continuously within normal limits. Soothing activities, such as play with musical toys and holding and rocking by parents, will help the infant relax. As the child's condition improves, quiet play activities may be gradually reintroduced.

Respiratory distress or air hunger creates anxiety in both infant and parents. Parents are often suffering from frustration and worry as well as being completely exhausted at the time of admission to the hospital. These parents need the opportunity to express their feelings and receive support. Nurses or social service personnel are the ideal members of the health care team to provide these interventions to the family of an ill infant.

Community Care

Caregivers play an active role in health management because most children are not hospitalized and do not require 24-hour care by the health care team. Parental or caregiver education is essential, especially if the child is not hospitalized and is cared for at home. Teach the parents to recognize the signs of increasing respiratory distress, such as grunting, retractions, pallor, and cyanosis, and state appropriate actions to take. Also instruct how to count the respiratory rate for a full minute during both sleep and awake times. Encourage parents to promote fluid intake, to measure and record the infant's oral intake during the illness, and to observe for signs of dehydration. Other issues relevant to the care of the infant with bronchiolitis in the home include positioning with the head of the bed elevated for comfort and to facilitate removal of secretions and quiet play activities as the child's energy level permits. Encourage parents to call their health care provider if they have any concerns about their infant's respiratory status. Teach families respiratory infection control measures, such as washing hands, avoiding exposure to illness, and staying current with routine immunizations. Additional preventive measures include eliminating exposure to cigarette smoke and limiting contact with crowded areas and other children (e.g., daycare).

BRONCHITIS

Bronchitis is defined as a transient inflammatory process involving the distal trachea and major bronchi. Bronchitis can be acute, chronic, or recurrent. As with most viral respiratory infections, the peak incidence is in winter and early spring. The disease appears to be more common in younger children and in males.

Pathophysiology

In the child with a competent immune system, bronchitis is most commonly caused by a virus. However, acute bronchitis caused by bacteria may occur as a secondary infection while airways are vulnerable from a prior viral attack or other insult. Although exposure to irritants such as gastric acid or passive smoke and environmental pollutants can produce acute symptoms, these insults contribute more commonly to symptoms in children with reactive airways (see the section on "Asthma").

Chronic and recurrent bronchitis in children are conditions that are not clearly understood. Viral or bacterial agents attack the airway mucosa. Pathologic changes commonly seen in chronic bronchitis in childhood include thickened bronchial walls, mucous gland hypertrophy, and chronic inflammation. The ciliated epithelium becomes damaged, mucous gland activity increases, and neutrophils infiltrate the airway wall and lumen. This process accounts for what sometimes appears to be purulent sputum in the absence of a bacterial infection. Mucociliary transport is disrupted, and this stasis contributes to secondary bacterial infection.

Chronic bronchitis in children may be a symptom of an underlying pulmonary disorder and may be an important factor in predisposing the child to chronic respiratory symptoms and lung dysfunction even into the adult years.

Assessment

Take a careful history. The onset of viral bronchitis is generally gradual, beginning with upper respiratory symptoms such as rhinitis and a minimal cough. Three to 4 days later, the cough becomes more pronounced. Note the quality of the cough; a bronchial cough begins as dry and nonproductive and progresses to become looser and more productive. Auscultation of the chest may be unremarkable during the early stages; rhonchi and wheezing may be heard as the cough progresses. Low-grade fever (<101° F [38.3° C]) is common. Young children generally swallow the mucus, often resulting in vomiting and paroxysmal coughing. During the recovery phase of the last 7 to 10 days, the cough subsides and the fever resolves. If the cough or fever persists beyond 2 weeks, suspect a secondary bacterial infection and refer the child for appropriate medical treatment.

Interdisciplinary Interventions

Treatment for acute bronchitis is largely supportive. Adequate rest and humidification of room air improve comfort. Exposure to irritants such as cigarette smoke should be strictly avoided. A productive cough is common. Therefore, the use of cough suppressants should be discouraged to enable the child to cough and expectorate. Reserve antibiotics for conditions in which a bacterial infection has been confirmed by culture. Antipyretics may be administered to help reduce the fever. Bronchodilators, such as albuterol, corticosteroids, or both, may be considered to reduce airway inflammation and constriction and to improve ease of breathing. However, there is currently no definite data supporting the routine use of these medications (Becker et al., 2011).

Comfort the child with acute bronchitis, and monitor for respiratory distress. Focus nutritional support on maintaining adequate hydration. Encourage the child to drink plenty of fluids and eat foods such as ice pops, fruit ices, broth, and gelatin to prevent dehydration. The child's appetite for foods is usually diminished, and posttussive emesis is common. Small, frequent feedings (or clear liquids if vomiting is frequent) are appropriate for the acute phase of the illness. As cough diminishes, regular diet may be gradually resumed.

Community Care

Quiet activities such as watching television, playing with puzzles, and reading books are recommended for the young child or school-aged child while recovering from bronchitis. Allowing for adequate rest is an important consideration because frequent coughing may disrupt sleep. After the first few days, when the child is feeling better, school homework should be resumed. The child may return to school when he or she receives adequate rest at night, is not coughing, and is afebrile. Normal energy level may not be restored for several days to weeks. Teach parents and caregivers that the child must be protected from passive smoke and other environmental pollutants because such conditions may lead to a repeated bronchitis episode. Dust- and allergy-proofing the home environment, especially sleeping quarters, helps prevent subsequent recurrences (see Community Care 16-1).

> *ANSWER:* Cough is one of the presenting symptoms with bronchiolitis, bronchitis, and asthma. However, José is afebrile and wheezing, which are solely symptoms of asthma.

PNEUMONIA

The term *pneumonia* describes any inflammatory condition of the lung parenchyma, resulting most frequently from infection, in which the alveoli are filled with fluid, blood cells, or both, and oxygen exchange is impaired. Pneumonia can be a primary illness (often called *community-acquired pneumonia* or CAP) or can develop as a complication of another respiratory infection or underlying illness. It is distinguished from the more common upper respiratory tract infections by the presence of lower respiratory tract signs and symptoms, such as tachypnea, rales, and associated areas of infiltration on chest radiographs.

Data from the 1970s–1980s suggests the annual incidence of pneumonia is 34 to 40 cases per 1,000 in children younger than 5 years of age; newer data is not available (Don et al., 2010). Pneumonia is a major cause of morbidity and mortality in children worldwide. Most deaths from pneumonia occur in Third World countries,

yet pneumonia also remains an important factor in morbidity in developed countries, especially among the chronically ill pediatric population.

The causes of pneumonia in children vary depending on the season and the child's age and health status. Pneumonia most likely develops when the body is unable to defend against infectious agents. Infectious agents may be viruses, bacteria (Chart 16-1), mycoplasma, fungi, chemicals, foreign substances, or various other organisms or materials. Newborn infants acquire pneumonia pathogens by several means. Transplacental infection, aspiration of organisms during passage through the birth canal, and contact with humans or contaminated equipment immediately after birth are the most common mechanisms. After 1 month of age, viruses become the most common cause of pneumonia. *S. pneumoniae* is the most common causative agent in all pediatric pneumonias (Don et al., 2010).

Children with chronic illnesses, such as asthma, BPD, or CF, often develop recurrent or persistent pneumonias because of respiratory compromise. Immunodeficiencies, congenital heart disease, neuromuscular diseases, and various hematologic and oncologic diseases are all conditions that can render the child compromised in the ability to fight pneumonias and other infections.

Not all inflammation of the lung is infectious in origin. Pneumonia can be caused by aspiration of foreign substances. Gastroesophageal reflux with aspiration, smoke inhalation, hydrocarbon ingestion, aspiration of baby talcum powder, near-drowning, and some autoimmune processes (such as pulmonary hemosiderosis) can all result in a pneumonia-like syndrome.

Pathophysiology

Although the term *pneumonia* refers to a multitude of disorders that differ widely depending on causative agent, each involves an inflammatory response. The

CHART 16-1	Common Viral and Bacterial Causes of Pneumonia	
Causative Agent	**Age**	**Season**
Viral		
RSV	Infants, young preschool	Winter
Parainfluenza viruses 1 and 2	Preschool	Fall
Parainfluenza virus 3	Infants and preschool	Spring
Influenza viruses A and B	Preschool, school age	Winter
Adenoviruses	All ages	Year-round
Bacterial		
Chlamydia pneumoniae	May be acquired during birthing process; All ages	Year-round
Mycoplasma pneumoniae	School age	Year-round, with peaks in fall and early winter
Streptococcus pneumoniae	May be acquired during birthing process; All ages	Year-round

respiratory tract is normally equipped with a variety of natural mechanisms to guard the lungs against infection. The nose filters air, the cough reflex expels objects or organisms in the laryngeal airway, and cilia in the walls of the trachea and bronchi trap small particles and remove them in mucus. When any of these defenses is impaired, pathogens invade and initiate the inflammatory response.

Viral pathogens enter the upper respiratory tract and spread through the airways. The severity of the inflammatory response and the associated pathophysiology vary. Characteristic features include loss of alveolar cell wall integrity, resulting in accumulation and stasis of fluid and mucus and smooth muscle contraction. These changes obstruct airflow and cause **ventilation–perfusion mismatch**, a condition in which the diminished alveolar–capillary gas exchange is no longer adequate for the blood supply, thus resulting in hypoxia and hypercapnia.

Bacteria are introduced into the lungs through the inhalation of infectious droplets or through the bloodstream. Alveolar involvement in bacterial pneumonia is characteristically more intense than that seen in viral infections. The alveoli can fill rapidly with proteinaceous fluid, causing ventilation–perfusion mismatch, or bacterial agents can cause necrosis of intra-alveolar septa, causing abscesses and destruction of lung architecture.

Similar processes occur in aspiration pneumonia. When gastric contents, secretions, blood, or volatile chemical compounds enter the lung, the presence of one or more of these irritants initiates the characteristic inflammatory response. Gastroesophageal reflux is associated with pneumonia when the acidic contents enter the pharynx, where, if protective mechanisms fail, it is aspirated. Baby talcum powder and other fine-particle materials inhaled into the pharynx and lower airways precipitate tissue inflammation. Hydrocarbons (organic solvents found in gasoline, furniture polish, cleaning compounds, lighter fluid, paint thinner, kerosene, and other substances) aspirated into the alveolar space dissolve surfactant lipids and impair surface tension, thereby reducing activity of surfactant. Atelectasis, alveolar cell damage, edema, granulocyte infiltration, hemorrhage, and necrosis can result. Smoke inhalation also can cause chemical irritation, depending on the source of the smoke.

Assessment

Pneumonia, regardless of etiology, is generally associated with fever, cough, increased work of breathing, dyspnea, tachypnea, crackles, and cyanosis. Nonspecific findings of vomiting and abdominal pain may also be present (Don et al., 2010).

Viral pneumonia may have a gradual onset, beginning with an upper respiratory tract infection of 3 to 4 days' duration. This initial illness may include low-grade fever and rhinorrhea, with a gradual development of cough and increasing respiratory distress. The child in respiratory distress may manifest cyanosis, grunting respirations, retractions, coarse crackles, or wheezing.

Bacterial pneumonia has a more acute pattern of onset; however, symptoms of a viral infection may suddenly worsen, indicating a bacterial superinfection. Chest pain may also be present. Fever and increased respiratory rate are hallmark manifestations of bacterial pneumonia. Check for dehydration stemming from poor oral intake and increased insensible fluid losses from fever and tachypnea. Tachycardia, hypotension, and poor perfusion may indicate sepsis and early shock.

The young child with fever, retractions, tachypnea, or grunting will be irritable and difficult to console. Hypoxia and hypercarbia result in decreased level of consciousness in a child of any age. Be ready to help parents cope with anxiety related to the often severe acute onset of respiratory symptoms.

Families of children with chronic conditions live with constant concerns regarding exposure to a potentially fatal infection and may exhibit and act on feelings of guilt and anger upon diagnosis of pneumonia. Counseling and support for these families during acute illness episodes is imperative.

Culture confirms the diagnosis of bacterial pneumonia. Common bacterial pathogens include *Streptococcus pneumoniae, H. influenzae, Staphylococcus aureus,* group B streptococci, *Chlamydia pneumoniae,* and *M. pneumoniae.* Viral causes of pneumonia should also be considered, including rhinovirus, RSV, human metapneumovirus, human bocavirus, influenza and parainfluenza viruses, and adenovirus (Don et al., 2010; Esposito et al., 2012). Chest radiographs may be used to determine the lung fields affected by the pneumonia or if additional problems exist (e.g., atelectasis, pleural effusions) in all hospitalized children. Chest radiographs are currently not recommended for children who are treated in the outpatient arena (Bradley et al., 2011).

Interdisciplinary Interventions

Interventions for pneumonia involve careful assessment of respiratory status and general supportive care (see thePoint for Care Paths). Whether a child with pneumonia requires hospitalization depends on age, general health status, and the suspected organism. Because infants readily develop respiratory distress with accompanying hypoxia, apnea, poor feeding, and dehydration, hospitalization is common.

For the hospitalized child, blood culture, complete blood count, chest radiograph, and viral testing should be done. Careful and frequent respiratory assessment—including evaluation of respiratory rate and effort, color, presence and location of retractions, breath sounds, and oxygen saturation levels—is required for the infant or child with pneumonia. Report changes in respiratory status immediately for further medical evaluation. Supplemental oxygen may be needed to keep saturation levels more than or equal to 92%. For hospitalized children, continuous pulse oximetry is indicated. Implement chest physiotherapy (percussion, vibration, and postural drainage) to facilitate clearing of secretions, with special attention paid to any identified areas of involvement or infiltration on the chest radiograph (see "Treatment Modalities" section earlier in this chapter).

Antibiotics are the mainstay of bacterial pneumonia. Use of appropriate medications is determined by culture (if available) and age. Infants younger than 3 to 6 months of age are generally hospitalized and treated with broad-spectrum antibiotics such as ampicillin. Fully immunized preschool and school-aged children with mild to moderate pneumonia should be treated with amoxicillin. If atypical pneumonia is suspected in the school-aged child or adolescent, a macrolide should be used. Any hospitalized child should be treated with ampicillin; a third-generation cephalosporin should be added if the child is unimmunized or if invasive pneumococcal strains are the suspected etiologic agent (Bradley et al., 2011). For children with moderate to severe pneumonia secondary to influenza, neuraminidase inhibitors (zanamivir and oseltamivir) therapy should be initiated to shorten the duration of illness and lessen the likelihood of household transmission (Bradley et al., 2011; K. Wang et al., 2012).

caREminder

Children in severe respiratory distress should be NPO because of the increased work of breathing and the risk of aspiration.

Fluids and medications are administered intravenously. Fever and tachypnea result in insensible fluid loss; thus, the child with pneumonia is at risk for dehydration. Intake and urine output and urine specific gravity are measured frequently, and skin turgor is assessed to monitor hydration status. Body temperature is monitored, and fevers are treated with antipyretics because a high body temperature can increase oxygen requirements and exacerbate insensible fluid loss. As respiratory status improves, the diet can be advanced from clear liquids to regular diet as tolerated. For recurrent aspiration pneumonia, suck and swallow coordination and gastroesophageal reflux may be evaluated to identify risk for aspiration before full oral feedings are resumed. If oral intake is allowed, feedings should be given with caution to avoid aspiration.

The child and family require constant information and support from all health professionals during an acute pneumonia episode. Social services may provide counseling services or referrals in the event of life-threatening or chronic illness. After the child's condition becomes more stable, parents, nurses, and child life specialists should collaborate in planning quiet, diversionary activities that are age appropriate.

Community Care

Home health support for parents who must learn to perform respiratory assessment and administer medication is an option for the older child being treated at home. Children with pneumonia are usually evaluated in an ambulatory care setting 2 to 3 weeks after treatment is completed to ensure that their respiratory symptoms are fully resolved or, if a chronic condition exists, to ensure that they are being managed effectively at home. Repeat chest radiographs may be completed to evaluate persistent symptoms or confirm complete recovery.

CHRONIC CONDITIONS OF THE RESPIRATORY SYSTEM

Chronic conditions of the respiratory system can have a serious effect on children and adolescents and may substantially alter their quality of life and physical and social development (see Chapter 12 for a more extensive discussion of the effect of chronic conditions on the child and the family). Such conditions can affect all other aspects of the child's and family's physical and emotional health and can lead to development of comorbid conditions, increased risks for morbidity, and, at times, early death. The most common chronic conditions seen in childhood and adolescence are asthma, BPD, and CF. Chronic pulmonary conditions during childhood and adolescence are characterized by periods of relative wellness interspersed with periods of acute exacerbation, often necessitating health care interventions (e.g., ambulatory care visits, emergency room visits, or hospitalization). Although no cures exist for these chronic conditions, self-care management is essential. Extensive child and family education is required related to prevention, recognition of symptoms, early and ongoing medical treatments, and optimization of self-care and home care strategies.

ASTHMA

Asthma is defined by the National Heart, Lung, and Blood Institute (2007) as follows:

A chronic inflammatory disorder of the airways in which many cells and cellular elements play a role: in particular, mast cells, eosinophils, neutrophils (especially in sudden onset, fatal exacerbations, occupational asthma, and patients who smoke), T lymphocytes, macrophages, and epithelial cells. In susceptible individuals, this inflammation causes recurrent episodes of coughing (particularly at night or early in the morning), wheezing, breathlessness, and chest tightness. These episodes are usually associated with widespread but variable airflow obstruction that is often reversible either spontaneously or with treatment. (p. 9)

Asthma is one of the most common chronic diseases of childhood in the United States. In 2009, it was estimated that 9.6% of children younger than 18 years of age carry the diagnosis of asthma. This trend has been steadily increasing (Centers for Disease Control and Prevention [CDC], 2011b). Prevalence of pediatric asthma is highest among Puerto Rican Hispanics, non-Hispanic blacks, and multiracial children (CDC, 2011a). During childhood and adolescence, pediatric asthma can have a profound effect on growth and development and on the daily lives of families. During the past few decades, assessment, management, and self-care strategies for children and adolescents with asthma have resulted in increased longevity along with an increased shift from hospital to home care. Significant advances in evidence-based management guidelines, pharmacologic products, and durable medical equipment have resulted in improved disease outcomes and quality of life for these children and their families. Comprehensive asthma management programs that address important issues such as accurate diagnosis, patient and family education, environmental control, and early treatment of asthma exacerbations have been shown to significantly improve the overall health of children with asthma (National Heart, Lung, and Blood Institute, 2007).

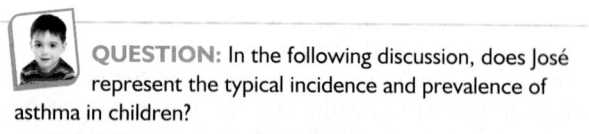

QUESTION: In the following discussion, does José represent the typical incidence and prevalence of asthma in children?

Pediatric asthma is the single largest public health burden, with more than 6.5 million children and adolescents with asthma in the United States (National Heart, Lung, and Blood Institute, 2007). Asthma is the third leading cause of hospitalization among children younger than 15 years of age. It is the leading cause of school absenteeism caused by a chronic condition and has been estimated to account for 14.4 million lost days of school annually (American Lung Association, 2012).

CROSS-CULTURAL CARE

Social disparities play a large role in pediatric asthma prevalence, morbidity, and mortality. Populations from low socioeconomic and urban, inner city areas have high rates of asthma and asthma-related morbidity and mortality. Prevalence of asthma among African American children is high (43% higher than among whites) (American Lung Association, 2011). The CDC reports asthma prevalence is highest among Puerto Rican Hispanics, non-Hispanic blacks, and multiracial children than non-Hispanic white children (Moorman et al., 2011).

ANSWER: José is Mexican American, lives in a suburban environment, and thus does not represent the prevalence of asthma among inner city African American children. However, José is typical in that he does have seasonal allergies, and his allergies are a trigger for his asthma.

Pathophysiology

The pathology of asthma is best described as a condition characterized by reversible (in most cases) changes in the airway that lead to bronchoconstriction, airway hyperresponsiveness, and airway edema. At a cellular level, mast cells in the airways release inflammatory and chemotactic mediators, such as histamine, causing smooth muscle contraction and bronchoconstriction. Increased mucous secretion by goblet cells causes epithelial damage. The increase in mucous secretion then leads to increased permeability and sensitivity to inhaled allergens, irritants, and inflammatory mediators. The result is airway edema, mucous hypersecretion and plugging, and substantial airway narrowing,

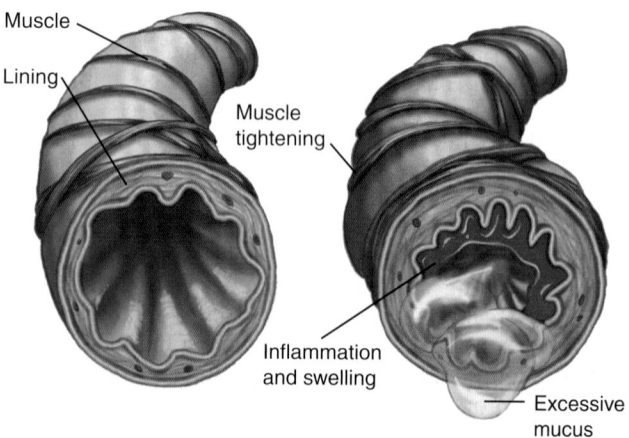

Figure 16-16 Asthmatic airway compared with a normal airway.

leading to rapid airway obstruction (Fig. 16-16). This acute reaction, called the *early asthmatic response*, generally resolves with bronchodilator treatment within 1 to 3 hours.

"Remodeling" or permanent changes in the airway may occur. Persistent changes in the airway structure, such as subbasement fibrosis, mucous hypersecretion, injury to epithelial cells, smooth muscle hypertrophy, and angiogenesis, may occur (National Heart, Lung, and Blood Institute, 2007).

The physiologic changes that occur during an acute episode contribute to the clinical findings characteristic of asthma exacerbation. Air becomes trapped behind the narrowed airways and the functional residual capacity increases, causing hyperinflation of the lungs, which can be seen on a chest radiograph. This hyperinflation helps keep the airways open that are already narrowed from bronchoconstriction, mucosal edema, and mucus. The accessory muscles of respiration help to maintain the lungs in a hyperinflated state; therefore, the child has chest retractions. Hypoxemia results from ventilation–perfusion mismatch because areas of the lung are not being well ventilated.

A key development in the study of asthma has been the recognition that a late asthmatic response also occurs. Mediator release from the mast cells causes direct migration and activation of inflammatory infiltrates, predominantly eosinophils and neutrophils, and mast cell degranulation causes the release of leukotrienes and prostaglandins, which leads to further inflammation. Airway response in the form of obstruction can occur 4 to 6 hours later and can last 24 hours or more. The late asthmatic response has a number of features characteristic of chronic asthma: reduced responsiveness to bronchodilators, increased mucous secretion, heightened airway responsiveness, and the development of airway inflammation. With the onset of the late asthmatic response, a vicious self-perpetuating cycle of asthma symptoms ensues.

The precise cause of the inflammatory response seen in asthma is yet to be discovered. Three potential causes include innate immunity, genetics, and environmental factors. Innate immunity refers to the balance between T helper (Th1)–type and Th2-type cytokine responses in early life. Numerous factors are believed to affect this balance and potentially lead to immune changes in which the Th1 immune response that fights infection is dominated by Th2 cells, leading to the expression of allergic diseases and asthma. It is hypothesized that exposure to other children, less frequent use of antibiotics, and "country living" are factors that enhance the Th1 response and lower the incidence of asthma (National Heart, Lung, and Blood Institute, 2007).

Scientific evidence exists that asthma is partly hereditary (Rance et al., 2011). **Atopy** (an increased predisposition to form antibodies on exposure to common environmental antigens) is present in most patients with asthma. Atopy is at least partially hereditary, although exposure to certain allergens early in life (e.g., pollens, animal dander) may influence the development of asthma in a child who is genetically predisposed. Food allergens, however, are rarely responsible for airway reactions in children. Although the link between asthma and atopy is not completely clear, exposure to allergens may cause airway inflammation and may lead to increased airway responsiveness.

Other factors felt to be involved in the development of airway reactivity and asthma include respiratory infections and environmental pollutants (many of which may be seasonal in nature; Tradition or Science 16-2). RSV bronchiolitis, for example, has been causally linked to enhanced airway reactivity, especially in children with a family history of atopy.

Assessment

QUESTION: The peak expiratory flow rate (PEFR) is an important assessment tool. Why would the nurse assessing José in the emergency department not obtain a PEFR?

According to National Heart, Lung, and Blood Institute (2007) guidelines, a careful history is one of most important elements in evaluating the child. Historical data can identify possible high-risk patients and

assist in planning for appropriate interventions. The key information to compile is listed in Focused Health History 16-2. The history can help to evaluate for other conditions that may present with cough, wheezing, and shortness of breath. Additionally, if the child presents with recurring episodes, the history can identify possible precipitating factors and treatments that have been effective in the past.

Suspect asthma in a child with wheezing and varying degrees of respiratory distress; for many children, a history of chronic cough (worse at night) is a classic symptom. The hallmark manifestation of asthma is the result of airway obstruction. The child may present with a worsening cough and wheezing and may complain of chest tightness or posttussive emesis (Clinical Judgment 16-2). Because of bronchospasm, airway inflammation, and mucus plugging, expiration becomes increasingly difficult and leading to air trapping. The child with a persistent asthma exacerbation may be unable or unwilling to lie flat because breathing is more difficult in this position.

The National Heart, Lung, and Blood Institute (2007) guidelines suggest using multiple measures of the child's level of current impairment (frequency and intensity of symptoms, low lung function, and limitations of daily activities) and future risk (risk of exacerbations, progressive loss of lung function, or adverse side effects from medications) to assess the child's status. Some children can be at high risk for frequent exacerbations even if they have few day-to-day effects of asthma. Some children may have early or prodromal signs and symptoms hours to days before an asthma exacerbation.

ALERT   *Pay special attention to children at high risk of asthma-related death. Children with a history of the following events are at increased risk:*
- *Prior admission to an intensive care unit (ICU) for asthma (with or without intubation)*
- *Two or more hospitalizations for asthma, three or more emergency room visits for asthma, or both, during the past year*
- *Hospitalization or emergency room visit for asthma during the past month*
- *Current use of or recent withdrawal from systemic corticosteroids*
- *History of psychiatric disease or psychosocial issues*
- *History of nonadherence to asthma treatment plan (National Heart, Lung, and Blood Institute, 2007)*

Focus the physical examination on general health, including growth and development, hydration status, and any signs of medication-related side effects.

Hypoxemia is universal in the child with moderate to severe symptoms. Monitor blood gases. In the early phases of an asthma exacerbation, a child is generally tachypneic and releasing more carbon dioxide than usual. Carbon dioxide retention is often noted when children are nearing respiratory failure and can be an

---

Evidence-Based Practice

TRADITION OR SCIENCE 16-2

Does secondhand smoke exacerbate asthma symptoms?

Environmental pollutants such as tobacco smoke have been clearly linked to asthma exacerbations in children (CDC, 2012). In children with asthma, parental (particularly maternal) smoking has been associated with increases in symptom severity and hospitalizations. Exposure rates among children are high, with approximately 60% of children aged 3–11 years in the United States exposed to secondhand smoke (CDC, 2007).

FOCUSED HEALTH HISTORY 16-2

The Child With Asthma

Nature of symptoms	Shortness of breath, wheezing, cough, chest tightness, rhinorrhea, conditions such as sinusitis, eczema
Pattern of symptoms	Frequency (daily, weekly, monthly), timing (morning vs. nighttime), onset and duration, severity, seasonal, perennial, diurnal variation, associated with physical activity
Aggravating factors or triggers	Upper respiratory infections, environmental allergens and irritants (dust mites, mold, inhalants, chemicals, pollens), secondhand smoke exposure or smoke, strong emotional expressions (crying, laughing hard), exercise, weather changes, pets, air pollution, foods or medications, menstruation cycle, stress
Typical exacerbation	Prodromal signs and symptoms, temporal progress, and usual management and response to treatment
Previous and current drug therapy	Dosage, mode of delivery, response, side effects
Development of disease	Age at onset, age at diagnosis, progress of disease, previous evaluations, treatments, and response to current management
Effect of disease	Number of emergency room visits, hospitalizations and ICU admissions in past year, school attendance and performance, activity limitations and exercise tolerance, sleep disturbances, child's growth and development, child's behavior, effect on siblings, economic impact
Living situation/environment	Presence of smokers in home, pets, housing conditions, home age, heating/air conditioning, carpeting, humidifier, cockroaches
Family and patient perception of asthma	Knowledge of and belief in chronic nature of asthma, coping styles, family support systems, capacity to recognize exacerbation, economic resources
General medical history	Presence of or history of allergic disorders (allergic rhinitis, atopic dermatitis), recurrent respiratory tract infections, birth history (early injury to lung tissue), symptoms of gastroesophageal reflux, detailed review of systems
History of allergies	History of adverse reactions to medications, food, or allergens (pollen, mold, pets)
Family medical history	History of IgE-mediated allergy in close relatives, asthma in close relatives

Note: See Chapter 8 for a comprehensive health history.

ominous sign. Hypoxemia and hypercarbia result from air trapping in the alveoli and ventilation–perfusion mismatch. A $PaCO_2$ level more than 50 mm Hg indicates ventilatory failure, unless the child has a preexisting chronic lung disease. Review chest radiograph reports. Typical chest radiograph findings in the child with extensive asthma symptoms are hyperexpansion, atelectasis, and a flattened diaphragm. Younger children are particularly prone to develop atelectasis because of their small airways and underdeveloped collateral ventilation. Infiltrates and pneumothoraces are uncommon findings.

Monitor blood pressure. Pulsus paradoxus (a decrease in systemic blood pressure with inspiration) occurs because the negative pleural pressures become more negative as a result of lung hyperinflation. A decrease of 12 mm Hg or more in systolic blood pressure with inspiration rather than with expiration indicates moderate distress. A decrease of 20 mm Hg or more occurs in severe asthma exacerbations. Pulsus paradoxus may be difficult to assess in the young child because of rapid heart and respiratory rates. In the preverbal child, also evaluate the quality of the cry (weak vs. lusty).

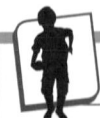

CLINICAL JUDGMENT 16-2

The Child in Respiratory Distress

Six-year-old Danielle comes to the community health clinic with her mother. The child presents with a history of onset of wheezing, shortness of breath, chest tightness, and cough that developed the previous night. Danielle is lethargic and pale, and her skin is cool and clammy. She is sitting in a tripod position; her eyes are open wide with a fearful countenance.

Questions

1. What historical data would help to clarify the diagnosis?
2. Is this an upper or lower respiratory problem?
3. Is the child in respiratory distress?
4. What would be your initial intervention?
5. How would you determine whether oxygen therapy and bronchodilators are effective in relieving the child's respiratory problems?

Answers

1. Number of similar occurrences of these respiratory signs the child has had in the past year; family history of asthma; introduction of new animals, products, or other environmental factors at home or school; occurrence of respiratory illness in other family or friends at this time
2. Lower respiratory, as distinguished by wheezing and chest tightness resulting from bronchial constriction
3. Yes. Respiratory distress occurs when there is an inadequate ability to meet the oxygenation needs of the body. Signs of respiratory distress include nasal flaring, retractions, poor chest expansion, cool extremities, poor peripheral pulses, and changes in level of consciousness.
4. Provide oxygenation to the child—100% oxygen at 6 L—given via face mask or nasal cannula. Do not have her lie down; let her assume a position of comfort.
5. The signs and symptoms of respiratory distress would be alleviated. The child would become more alert and pink and would appear calm and able to verbalize that the tightness in her chest has diminished or that she is able to breathe easier.

Diagnostic studies helpful in evaluating the child with asthma symptoms include spirometry, PEFR, pulmonary function tests, bronchoprovocation (with methacholine, histamine, cold air, or exercise), arterial blood gases, pulse oximetry, and chest radiographs (see Tests and Procedures 16-1). In addition, examination of biomarkers of inflammation is demonstrating promise as a useful tool for diagnosis and assessment of asthma. Biomarker assessment includes total and differential cell count and mediator assays of sputum, blood, urine, and exhaled air (National Heart, Lung, and Blood Institute, 2007)

Spirometry is used to obtain objective measures of lung function. During the initial assessment, spirometry helps to establish a diagnosis of asthma. Spirometry is also recommended after treatment is initiated and peak inspiratory function is stabilized, during periods of progressive or prolonged loss of asthma control, and, finally, as an assessment tool every 1 to 2 years to evaluate response to therapy. It has been suggested that children as young as 2 to 6 years of age can successfully participate in spirometry (Beydon et al., 2007).

In contrast, peak flow meters are used to measure PEFR and are designed for monitoring purposes rather than diagnostic purposes. PEFR is considered a valuable measurement in assessing asthma severity and in evaluating response to therapy. PEFR is the greatest velocity of flow that can be generated in forced expiration, starting with fully inflated lungs. Evaluate PEFR in a serial manner using a peak flow meter and compare it with the baseline or "personal best" for the individual rather than with normal values. PEFR decreases as airway obstruction and inflammation worsen (Fig. 16-17). Children younger than 5 years of age are generally not able to perform PEFR tests, and they may be too stressful for the child in severe distress, potentially worsening his or her status (see thePoint for Procedures).

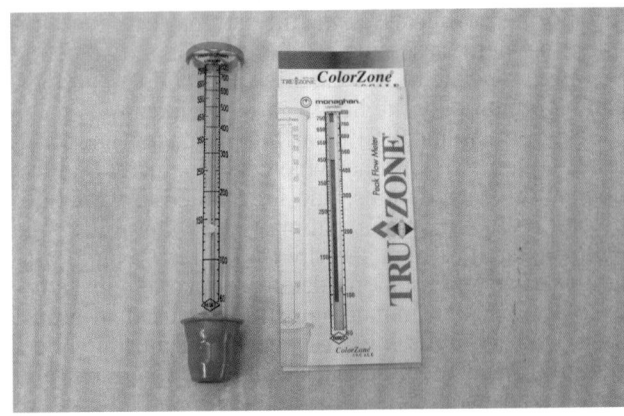

Figure 16-17 The child may use a peak flow meter and chart to monitor PEFR.

ANSWER: Two rationales support the nurse's decision not to try to obtain a PEFR: José's level of respiratory distress and his age. José is working very hard just to ventilate himself. Asking him to focus on a diagnostic procedure could precipitate a worsening of his respiratory distress. As a 4-year-old, José may be able to provide baseline PEFR values on a good day, and this may be a valuable daily activity for his caregiver to track. During a stressful event, children rely on earlier coping skills, and asking a preschooler to perform a complex task at a very stressful time is unlikely to be successful.

Interdisciplinary Interventions

The National Heart, Lung, and Blood Institute (2007, p. 4) has identified two primary goals of asthma therapy:

1. Reduce impairment (prevent chronic symptoms, require infrequent use of short-acting beta$_2$-agonist, maintain [near-] normal lung function and normal activity levels)
2. Reduce risk (prevent exacerbations, minimize need for emergency care or hospitalization, prevent loss of lung function, prevent reduced lung growth [for children], have minimal or no adverse effects of therapy)

These goals are accomplished through an interdisciplinary plan that includes assessment and monitoring, education, control of environmental factors, and careful selection of medication and delivery devices to meet the child's needs and individual circumstances. The following section discusses these care components as well as the management and treatment of exacerbations.

Assessment and Monitoring

QUESTION: Does the case study regarding José in Chapter 9 provide enough information to classify the severity of his asthma?

Assessment for purposes of diagnosis are discussed in the preceding section. This section discusses the ongoing assessment and monitoring of the child with asthma. Activities associated with assessment and monitoring include assessing the asthma severity to initiate treatment, assessing asthma control and adjusting therapy as needed, and ensuring the child is periodically monitored by the health care provider.

Severity classification of asthma is based on symptom frequency, nighttime symptoms, character and frequency of exacerbations, and lung function variability before treatment. When asthma is well controlled, the child's overall asthma severity is classified as intermittent or persistent (mild, moderate, or severe) and a stepwise approach to managing asthma is used to adjust therapy. Therapy is initiated depending on the child's age group and the assessed degree of impairment and risk. Impairment refers to the frequency and intensity of symptoms and functional limitations being experienced by the child. Risk refers to the likelihood of asthma

exacerbations, progressive decline in lung function, or risk of adverse effects of medication (National Heart, Lung, and Blood Institute, 2007). Tables 16-5 to 16-10 provide an overview, by age (0 to 4 years, 5 to 11 years, and youths 12 years and older), of the National Heart, Lung, and Blood Institute guidelines for initiating therapy and adjusting therapy. In addition, the tables provide the stepwise approach to increase therapy (stepped up) or decrease therapy (stepped down) as indicated by the child's condition.

Assessment of the child with asthma begins by classifying asthma severity. If the child is presenting with symptoms, identify the precipitating factors for the current episodic symptoms (e.g., child was exercising at school, child spent night at friend's house where cats are present). Determine whether comorbid conditions exist that may affect asthma management, such as sinusitis, obesity, or stress. Last, assess the child's knowledge and skills for self-management (National Heart, Lung, and Blood Institute, 2007).

Monitoring of the child includes an evaluation of the child's daily peak flow monitoring records and using spirometry to assess current status. Samples of peak flow monitoring charts are provided by National Heart, Lung, and Blood Institute or makers of peak flow meters and can be downloaded from the Internet.

Schedule follow-up visits for the child. The child is seen at 2- to 6-week intervals while gaining control of asthma symptoms, at 1 to 6 months after asthma control is achieved and to ensure control is maintained, and at 3-month intervals if a step-down therapy is anticipated (National Heart, Lung, and Blood Institute, 2007).

ANSWER: José is on albuterol and cromolyn sodium morning and evening. In addition, he has another recent episode of an exacerbation of his asthma. However, we still do not have a clear picture of his incidence of daytime and nighttime symptoms.

Education

QUESTION: What is the role of the nurse regarding the education about José's asthma?

A primary goal of asthma management is to ensure the child and the family have the tools and knowledge to self-monitor and manage the child's condition. Education focuses on promoting optimal physical growth and function by minimizing airway obstruction, maximizing physical function despite airway obstruction, and preventing and treating exacerbations and complications of asthma and its therapy. The child should also achieve and maintain normal psychosocial growth and function by maintaining optimal psychosocial development and maximal participation in his or her own health care. To promote optimal family functioning, these interventions are integrated into the normal daily lifestyle of the family.

TABLE 16-5 Classifying Asthma Severity and Initiating Therapy in Children

Classifying Asthma Severity and Initiating Therapy in Children

Components of Severity		Intermittent Ages 0–4	Intermittent Ages 5–11	Mild Ages 0–4	Mild Ages 5–11	Moderate Ages 0–4	Moderate Ages 5–11	Severe Ages 0–4	Severe Ages 5–11
Impairment	Symptoms	≤2 days/week	≤2 days/week	>2 days/week but not daily	>2 days/week but not daily	Daily	Daily	Throughout the day	Throughout the day
	Nighttime awakenings	0	≤2x/month	1–2x/month	3–4x/month	3–4x/month	>1x/week but not nightly	>1x/week	Often 7x/week
	Short-acting beta₂-agonist use for symptom control	≤2 days/week	≤2 days/week	>2 days/week but not daily	>2 days/week but not daily	Daily	Daily	Several times per day	Several times per day
	Interference with normal activity	None	None	Minor limitation	Minor limitation	Some limitation	Some limitation	Extremely limited	Extremely limited
	Lung Function • FEV₁ (predicted) or peak flow (personal best)	N/A	Normal FEV₁ between exacerbations; >80%	N/A	>80%	N/A	60–80%	N/A	<60%
	• FEV₁/FVC		>85%		>80%		75–80%		<75%
Risk	Exacerbations requiring oral systemic corticosteroids (consider severity and interval since last exacerbation)	0–1/year (see notes)	0–1/year (see notes)	≥2 exacerbations in 6 months requiring oral systemic corticosteroids, or ≥4 wheezing episodes/1 year lasting >1 day AND risk factors for persistent asthma	≥2x/year (see notes); Relative annual risk may be related to FEV₁				
Recommended Step for Initiating Therapy (See "Stepwise Approach for Managing Asthma" for treatment steps.) The stepwise approach is meant to assist, not replace, the clinical decisionmaking required to meet individual patient needs.		Step 1 (for both age groups)		Step 2 (for both age groups)		Step 3 and consider short course of oral systemic corticosteroids	Step 3: medium-dose ICS option and consider short course of oral systemic corticosteroids	Step 3 and consider short course of oral systemic corticosteroids	Step 3: medium-dose ICS option OR step 4 and consider short course of oral systemic corticosteroids

In 2–6 weeks, depending on severity, evaluate level of asthma control that is achieved.
- Children 0–4 years old: If no clear benefit is observed in 4–6 weeks, stop treatment and consider alternative diagnoses or adjusting therapy.
- Children 5–11 years old: Adjust therapy accordingly.

Key: FEV₁, forced expiratory volume in 1 second; FVC, forced vital capacity; ICS, inhaled corticosteroids; ICU, intensive care unit; N/A, not applicable

Notes:
- Level of severity is determined by both impairment and risk. Assess impairment domain by caregiver's recall of previous 2–4 weeks. Assign severity to the most severe category in which any feature occurs.
- Frequency and severity of exacerbations may fluctuate over time for patients in any severity category. At present, there are inadequate data to correspond frequencies of exacerbations with different levels of asthma severity. In general, more frequent and severe exacerbations (e.g., requiring urgent, unscheduled care, hospitalization, or ICU admission) indicate greater underlying disease severity. For treatment purposes, patients with ≥2 exacerbations described above may be considered the same as patients who have persistent asthma, even in the absence of impairment levels consistent with persistent asthma.
- Annual trivalent influenza vaccination recommended for children 6 months of age or older, especially in children at high risk for complications (e.g., asthma, chronic medical conditions) (AAP, 2012).

From National Heart, Lung, and Blood Institute. (2007). Guidelines for the diagnosis and management of asthma. Washington, DC: Author. Retrieved from http://www.nhlbi.nih.gov/guidelines/asthma/asthsumm.pdf

TABLE 16-6   Assessing Asthma Control and Adjusting Therapy in Children

Assessing Asthma Control and Adjusting Therapy in Children

Components of Control		Well Controlled		Not Well Controlled		Very Poorly Controlled	
		Ages 0–4	Ages 5–11	Ages 0–4	Ages 5–11	Ages 0–4	Ages 5–11
Impairment	Symptoms	≤2 days/week but not more than once on each day		>2 days/week or multiple times on ≤2 days/week		Throughout the day	
	Nighttime awakenings	None	≤1x/month	>1x/month	≥2x/month	>1x/week	≥2x/week
	Interference with normal activity	None		Some limitation		Extremely limited	
	Short-acting beta₂-agonist use for symptom control (not prevention of EIB)	≤2 days/week		>2 days/week		Several times per day	
	Lung function • FEV₁ (predicted) or peak flow personal best • FEV₁/FVC	N/A	>80% >80%	N/A	60–80% 75–80%	N/A	<60% <75%
Risk	Exacerbations requiring oral systemic corticosteroids	0–1x/year		2–3x/year	≥2x/year	>3x/year	≥2x/year
	Reduction in lung growth	N/A	Requires long-term follow-up	N/A		N/A	
	Treatment-related adverse effects	Medication side effects can vary in intensity from none to very troublesome and worrisome. The level of intensity does not correlate to specific levels of control but should be considered in the overall assessment of risk.					

Recommended Action for Treatment	Well Controlled	Not Well Controlled		Very Poorly Controlled
(See "Stepwise Approach for Managing Asthma" for treatment steps.) The stepwise approach is meant to assist, not replace, clinical decisionmaking required to meet individual patient needs.	• Maintain current step. • Regular followup every 1–6 months. • Consider step down if well controlled for at least 3 months.	Step up 1 step	Step up at least 1 step	• Consider short course of oral systemic corticosteroids, • Step up 1–2 steps

- **Before step up:**
  Review adherence to medication, inhaler technique, and environmental control.
  If alternative treatment was used, discontinue it and use preferred treatment for that step.
- Reevaluate the level of asthma control in 2–6 weeks to achieve control; every 1–6 months to maintain control.
  Children 0–4 years old: If no clear benefit is observed in 4–6 weeks, consider alternative diagnoses or adjusting therapy.
  Children 5–11 years old: Adjust therapy accordingly.
- For side effects, consider alternative treatment options.

Key: EIB, exercise-induced bronchospasm; FEV₁, forced expiratory volume in 1 second; FVC, forced vital capacity; ICU, intensive care unit; N/A, not applicable

Notes:

- The level of control is based on the most severe impairment or risk category. Assess impairment domain by patient's or caregiver's recall of previous 2–4 weeks. Symptom assessment for longer periods should reflect a global assessment, such as whether the patient's asthma is better or worse since the last visit.
- At present, there are inadequate data to correspond frequencies of exacerbations with different levels of asthma control. In general, more frequent and intense exacerbations (e.g., requiring urgent, unscheduled care, hospitalization, or ICU admission) indicate poorer disease control.

From National Heart, Lung, and Blood Institute. (2007). *Guidelines for the diagnosis and management of asthma.* Washington, DC: Author. Retrieved from http://www.nhlbi.nih.gov/guidelines/asthma/asthsumm.pdf

TABLE 16-7 Stepwise Approach for Managing Asthma Long Term in Children, 0–4 Years of Age and 5–11 Years of Age

Step up if needed (first check inhaler technique, adherence, environmental control, and comorbid conditions)

Assess control

Step down if possible (and asthma is well controlled at least 3 months)

Children 0–4 Years of Age

	Step 1	Step 2	Step 3	Step 4	Step 5	Step 6
	Intermittent Asthma	**Persistent Asthma: Daily Medication**				
		Consult with asthma specialist if step 3 care or higher is required. Consider consultation at step 2.				
Preferred	SABA PRN	Low-dose ICS	Medium-dose ICS	Medium-dose ICS + LABA or Montelukast	High-dose ICS + LABA or Montelukast	High-dose ICS + LABA or Montelukast + Oral corticosteroids
Alternative		Cromolyn or Montelukast				

Each Step: Patient Education and Environmental Control

Quick-Relief Medication
- SABA as needed for symptoms. Intensity of treatment depends on severity of symptoms. With viral respiratory symptoms: SABA q 4–6 hours up to 24 hours (longer with physician consult). Consider short course of oral systemic corticosteroids if exacerbation is severe or patient has history of previous severe exacerbations.
- Caution: Frequent use of SABA may indicate the need to step up treatment. See text for recommendations on initiating daily long-term control therapy.

Children 5–11 Years of Age

	Step 1	Step 2	Step 3	Step 4	Step 5	Step 6
	Intermittent Asthma	**Persistent Asthma: Daily Medication**				
		Consult with asthma specialist if step 4 care or higher is required. Consider consultation at step 3.				
Preferred	SABA PRN	Low-dose ICS	Low-dose ICS + LABA, LTRA, or Theophylline OR Medium-dose ICS	Medium-dose ICS + LABA	High-dose ICS + LABA	High-dose ICS + LABA + Oral corticosteroids
Alternative		Cromolyn, LTRA, Nedocromil, or Theophylline		Medium-dose ICS + LTRA or Theophylline	High-dose ICS + LTRA or Theophylline	High-dose ICS + LTRA or Theophylline + oral corticosteroids

Each Step: Patient Education, Environmental Control, and Management of Comorbidities

Steps 2–4: Consider subcutaneous allergen immunotherapy for patients who have persistent, allergic asthma.

Quick-Relief Medication
- SABA as needed for symptoms. Intensity of treatment depends on severity of symptoms: up to 3 treatments at 20-minute intervals as needed. Short course of oral systemic corticosteroids may be needed.
- Caution: Increasing use of SABA or use >2 days a week for symptom relief (not prevention of EIB) generally indicates inadequate control and the need to step up treatment.

Notes
- The stepwise approach is meant to assist, not replace, the clinical decisionmaking required to meet individual patient needs.
- If an alternative treatment is used and response is inadequate, discontinue it and use the preferred treatment before stepping up.
- If clear benefit is not observed within 4–6 weeks, and patient's/family's medication technique and adherence are satisfactory, consider adjusting therapy or an alternative diagnosis.
- Studies on children 0–4 years of age are limited. Step 2 preferred therapy is based on Evidence A. All other recommendations are based on expert opinion and extrapolation from studies in older children.
- Clinicians who administer immunotherapy should be prepared and equipped to identify and treat anaphylaxis that may occur.

Key: Alphabetical listing is used when more than one treatment option is listed within either preferred or alternative therapy. ICS, inhaled corticosteroid; LABA, inhaled long-acting beta₂-agonist; LTRA, leukotriene receptor antagonist; oral corticosteroids; oral systemic corticosteroids; SABA, inhaled short-acting beta₂-agonist

- The stepwise approach is meant to assist, not replace, the clinical decisionmaking required to meet individual patient needs.
- If an alternative treatment is used and response is inadequate, discontinue it and use the preferred treatment before stepping up.
- Theophylline is a less desirable alternative due to the need to monitor serum concentration levels.
- Steps 1 and 2 medications are based on Evidence A. Step 3 ICS and ICS plus adjunctive therapy are based on Evidence B for efficacy of each treatment and extrapolation from comparator trials in older children and adults—comparator trials are not available for this age group; steps 4–6 are based on expert opinion and extrapolation from studies in older children and adults.
- Immunotherapy for steps 2–4 is based on Evidence B for house-dust mites, animal danders, and pollens; evidence is weak or lacking for molds and cockroaches. Evidence is strongest for immunotherapy with single allergens. The role of allergy in asthma is greater in children than adults.
- Clinicians who administer immunotherapy should be prepared and equipped to identify and treat anaphylaxis that may occur.

Key: Alphabetical listing is used when more than one treatment option is listed within either preferred or alternative therapy. ICS, inhaled corticosteroid; LABA, inhaled long-acting beta₂-agonist; LTRA, leukotriene receptor antagonist; SABA, inhaled short-acting beta₂-agonist

From National Heart, Lung, and Blood Institute. (2007). Guidelines for the diagnosis and management of asthma. Washington, DC: Author. Retrieved from http://www.nhlbi.nih.gov/guidelines/asthma/asthsumm.pdf

TABLE 16-8 Classifying Asthma Severity and Initiating Treatment in Youths 12 Years of Age and Adults

Assessing severity and initiating treatment for patients who are not currently taking long-term control medications

Components of Severity		Classification of Asthma Severity ≥12 years of age				
			Intermittent	Persistent		
				Mild	Moderate	Severe
Impairment	Symptoms		≤2 days/week	>2 days/week but not daily	Daily	Throughout the day
Normal FEV₁/FVC:	Nighttime awakenings		≤2x/month	3–4x/month	>1x/week but not nightly	Often 7x/week
8–19 yr 85%	Short-acting beta₂-agonist use for symptom control (not prevention of EIB)		≤2 days/week	>2 days/week but not daily, and not more than 1x on any day	Daily	Several times per day
20–39 yr 80%	Interference with normal activity		None	Minor limitation	Some limitation	Extremely limited
40–59 yr 75%	Lung function		• Normal FEV₁ between exacerbations • FEV₁ >80% predicted • FEV₁/FVC normal	• FEV₁ >80% predicted • FEV₁/FVC normal	• FEV₁ >60% but <80% predicted • FEV₁/FVC reduced 5%	• FEV₁ <60% predicted • FEV₁/FVC reduced >5%
60–80 yr 70%						
Risk	Exacerbations requiring oral systemic corticosteroids		0–1/year (see note)	≥2/year (see note)		
				Consider severity and interval since last exacerbation. Frequency and severity may fluctuate over time for patients in any severity category. Relative annual risk of exacerbations may be related to FEV₁.		
Recommended Step for Initiating Treatment (See "Stepwise Approach for Managing Asthma" for treatment steps.)			Step 1	Step 2	Step 3 and consider short course of oral systemic corticosteroids	Step 4 or 5 and consider short course of oral systemic corticosteroids
				In 2–6 weeks, evaluate level of asthma control that is achieved and adjust therapy accordingly.		

Key: EIB, exercise-induced bronchospasm; FEV₁, forced expiratory volume in 1 second; FVC, forced vital capacity; ICU, intensive care unit

Notes:

- The stepwise approach is meant to assist, not replace, the clinical decision making required to meet individual patient needs.
- Level of severity is determined by assessment of both impairment and risk. Assess impairment domain by patient's/caregiver's recall of previous 2–4 weeks and spirometry. Assign severity to the most severe category in which any feature occurs.
- At present, there are inadequate data to correspond frequencies of exacerbations with different levels of asthma severity. In general, more frequent and intense exacerbations (e.g., requiring urgent, unscheduled care, hospitalization, or ICU admission) indicate greater underlying disease severity. For treatment purposes, patients who had ≥2 exacerbations requiring oral systemic corticosteroids in the past year may be considered the same as patients who have persistent asthma, even in the absence of impairment levels consistent with persistent asthma.
- Annual trivalent influenza vaccination recommended for children 6 months of age or older, especially in children at high risk for complications (e.g., asthma, chronic medical conditions) (AAP, 2012).

From National Heart, Lung, and Blood Institute. (2007). *Guidelines for the diagnosis and management of asthma*. Washington, DC: Author. Retrieved from http://www.nhlbi.nih.gov/guidelines/asthma/asthsumm.pdf

TABLE 16-9 Assessing Asthma Control and Adjusting Therapy in Youths ≥12 Years of Age and Adults

Components of Control		Classification of Asthma Control (≥12 years of age)		
		Well Controlled	Not Well Controlled	Very Poorly Controlled
Impairment	Symptoms	≤2 days/week	>2 days/week	Throughout the day
	Nighttime awakenings	≤2x/month	1–3x/week	≥4x/week
	Interference with normal activity	None	Some limitation	Extremely limited
	Short-acting beta₂-agonist use for symptom control (not prevention of EIB)	≤2 days/week	>2 days/week	Several times per day
	FEV₁ or peak flow	>80% predicted/personal best	60–80% predicted/personal best	<60% predicted/personal best
	Validated questionnaires ATAQ ACQ ACT	0 ≤0.75* ≥20	1–2 ≥1.5 16–19	3–4 N/A ≤15
Risk	Exacerbations requiring oral systemic corticosteroids	0–1/year	≥2/year (see note)	
			Consider severity and interval since last exacerbation	
	Progressive loss of lung function	Evaluation requires long-term followup care.		
	Treatment-related adverse effects	Medication side effects can vary in intensity from none to very troublesome and worrisome. The level of intensity does not correlate to specific levels of control but should be considered in the overall assessment of risk.		
Recommended Action for Treatment (See "Stepwise Approach for Managing Asthma" for treatment steps.)		• Maintain current step. • Regular followup at every 1–6 months to maintain control. • Consider step down if well controlled for at least 3 months.	• Step up 1 step. • Reevaluate in 2–6 weeks. • For side effects, consider alternative treatment options.	• Consider short course of oral systemic corticosteroids. • Step up 1–2 steps. • Reevaluate in 2 weeks. • For side effects, consider alternative treatment options.

*ACQ values of 0.76–1.4 are indeterminate regarding well-controlled asthma.

Key: EIB, exercise-induced bronchospasm; ICU, intensive care unit

Notes:

- The stepwise approach is meant to assist, not replace, the clinical decision making required to meet individual patient needs.
- Involve the adolescent in the development of the written asthma action plan.
- Encourage adolescents to keep a copy of the written asthma action plan with them at school and other locations frequented outside of the home (e.g., camps, family member homes).
- Encourage physical activity.
- The level of control is based on the most severe impairment or risk category. Assess impairment domain by patient's recall of previous 2–4 weeks and by spirometry/or peak flow measures. Symptom assessment for longer periods should reflect a global assessment, such as inquiring whether the patient's asthma is better or worse since the last visit.
- At present, there are inadequate data to correspond frequencies of exacerbations with different levels of asthma control. In general, more frequent and intense exacerbations (e.g., requiring urgent, unscheduled care, hospitalization, or ICU admission) indicate poorer disease control. For treatment purposes, patients who had ≥2 exacerbations requiring oral systemic corticosteroids in the past year may be considered the same as patients who have not-well-controlled asthma, even in the absence of impairment levels consistent with not-well-controlled asthma.

ATAQ = Asthma Therapy Assessment Questionnaire©
ACQ = Asthma Control Questionnaire©
ACT = Asthma Control Test™

Minimal Important
Difference: 1.0 for the ATAQ; 0.5 for the ACQ; not determined for the ACT.

Before step up in therapy:

—Review adherence to medication, inhaler technique, environmental control, and comorbid conditions.

—If an alternative treatment option was used in a step, discontinue and use the preferred treatment for that step.

From National Heart, Lung, and Blood Institute. (2007). Guidelines for the diagnosis and management of asthma. Washington, DC: Author. Retrieved from http://www.nhlbi.nih.gov/guidelines/asthma/asthsumm.pdf

TABLE 16-10 Stepwise Approach for Managing Asthma in Youths ≥12 Years of Age and Adults

Intermittent Asthma	Persistent Asthma: Daily Medication
	Consult with asthma specialist if step 4 care or higher is required. Consider consultation at step 3.

Step 1
Preferred:
SABA PRN

Step 2
Preferred:
Low-dose ICS
Alternative:
Cromolyn, LTRA, Nedocromil, or Theophylline

Step 3
Preferred:
Low-dose ICS + LABA OR Medium-dose ICS
Alternative:
Low-dose ICS + either LTRA, Theophylline, or Zileuton

Step 4
Preferred:
Medium-dose ICS + LABA
Alternative:
Medium-dose ICS + either LTRA, Theophylline, or Zileuton

Step 5
Preferred:
High-dose ICS + LABA
AND
Consider Omalizumab for patients who have allergies

Step 6
Preferred:
High-dose ICS + LABA + oral corticosteroid
AND
Consider Omalizumab for patients who have allergies

Step up if needed
(first, check adherence, environmental control, and comorbid conditions)

Assess control

Step down if possible
(and asthma is well controlled at least 3 months)

Each step: Patient education, environmental control, and management of comorbidities.
Steps 2–4: Consider subcutaneous allergen immunotherapy for patients who have allergic asthma (see notes).

Quick-Relief Medication for All Patients
- SABA as needed for symptoms. Intensity of treatment depends on severity of symptoms: up to 3 treatments at 20-minute intervals as needed. Short course of oral systemic corticosteroids may be needed.
- Use of SABA >2 days a week for symptom relief (not prevention of EIB) generally indicates inadequate control and the need to step up treatment.

Key: **Alphabetical order is used when more than one treatment option is listed within either preferred or alternative therapy.** ICS, inhaled corticosteroid; LABA, long-acting inhaled beta₂-agonist; LTRA, leukotriene receptor antagonist; SABA, inhaled short-acting beta₂-agonist

Notes:
- The stepwise approach is meant to assist, not replace, the clinical decision making required to meet individual patient needs.
- If alternative treatment is used and response is inadequate, discontinue it and use the preferred treatment before stepping up.
- Zileuton is a less desirable alternative due to limited studies as adjunctive therapy and the need to monitor liver function. Theophylline requires monitoring of serum concentration levels.
- In step 6, before oral corticosteroids are introduced, a trial of high-dose ICS + LABA + either LTRA, theophylline, or zileuton may be considered, although this approach has not been studied in clinical trials.
- Step 1, 2, and 3 preferred therapies are based on Evidence A; step 3 alternative therapy is based on Evidence A for LTRA, Evidence B for theophylline, and Evidence D for zileuton. Step 4 preferred therapy is based on Evidence B, and alternative therapy is based on Evidence B for LTRA and theophylline and Evidence D zileuton. Step 5 preferred therapy is based on Evidence B. Step 6 preferred therapy is based on (EPR—2 1997) and Evidence B for omalizumab.
- Immunotherapy for steps 2–4 is based on Evidence B for house-dust mites, animal danders, and pollens; evidence is weak or lacking for molds and cockroaches. Evidence is strongest for immunotherapy with single allergens. The role of allergy in asthma is greater in children than in adults.
- Clinicians who administer immunotherapy or omalizumab should be prepared and equipped to identify and treat anaphylaxis that may occur.
- Annual trivalent influenza vaccination recommended for children 6 months of age or older, especially in children at high risk for complications (e.g., asthma, chronic medical conditions) (AAP, 2012).

From National Heart, Lung, and Blood Institute. (2007). Guidelines for the diagnosis and management of asthma. Washington, DC: Author. Retrieved from http://www.nhlbi.nih.gov/guidelines/asthma/asthsumm.pdf

Child and family education must be an integral part of asthma care. Parents and children with asthma often have a poor or incomplete understanding of the disease and its management, and this lack of knowledge may lead to increased need for hospitalization and increased health care costs. Self-care management in children and adolescents depends on the individual's cognitive abilities, maturity, and fine and gross motor skills to manage the daily responsibilities of asthma care. Cognitive and language abilities will affect how well the child is able to perceive and communicate changes in breathing patterns. Both the family and the child should assess for asthma symptoms daily, including increased cough, wheezing, shortness of breath, or irritability, then initiate additional therapy as instructed. Beginning in the preschool years, the child should be taught to recognize changes in breathing and to communicate them to an adult. Even the ability to recognize the responsible adult in a given situation should be practiced with a preschool child. Responsibility to recognize changes in breathing patterns, to communicate these changes, and to initiate additional therapies should increase as the child matures.

Fine and gross motor abilities of children and adolescents also play a role in these assessment and self-care management strategies. For example, spirometry and peak flow measurements require fine and gross motor skills. Both require the individual to follow verbal instructions closely, hold the mouthpiece without air leakage, then fully inhale and exhale. Incorrect technique in these assessments can lead to misguided prescriptions or management plans. Children younger than 6 years old may lack the motor skills needed to perform these measures. In these cases, assessment of pulmonary function in these children must rely on other measures, such as parent or child recall of symptom history, auscultation of lung fields, assessment of respiratory effort, or pulse oximetry.

The essential components of family and patient education program are outlined in Community Care 16-2. Asthma self-management programs have been developed for various settings to promote awareness, knowledge, and treatment adherence. Several of these programs and educational brochures are available through the American Lung Association (Open Airways) or the Asthma and Allergy Foundation of America (Wee Wheezers, Power Breathing) (see thePoint for Organizations) and are presented in the National Heart, Lung, and Blood Institute (2007) document. Educational programs that focus on self-management skills help shift the often crisis-oriented nature of asthma care to one of proactive intervention and prevention.

Gear any education and materials to the child's cognitive, affective, and developmental levels. Ensure that the information given to families is also provided to schoolteachers, the school nurse, coaches, camp counselors, and other community personnel to ensure awareness of asthma, ensure continuity of treatment, and facilitate problem solving if the child has an acute episode. The importance of regular follow-up with a *consistent* health care provider cannot be overemphasized.

Progress must be closely monitored in relation to history of acute exacerbations, responses to therapy, and adherence to treatment.

ANSWER: The nurse has an obligation to provide ongoing education to the family about the disease and about the medical system. If Claudia made a good decision about when to access care in a hospital, then that should be made clear to Claudia. One of the greatest problems in the management of childhood chronic disease is the lack of continuity of care. Claudia takes her children to the health department for immunizations, to the pediatrician for problems, and now she and José have had their first visit to the hospital emergency department. The nurse can ensure the family leaves with a record of the visit so that the pediatrician can fully understand this exacerbation.

Control of Environmental Factors and Comorbid Conditions

Assessment of the environmental factors and comorbid conditions that affect asthma severity can be completed in several ways. A verbal history provided by the child and parent can determine recent exposures and a history of the symptoms associated with increasing asthma severity. An assessment of the home may reveal the presence of previously unknown or unsuspected allergens (Tradition or Science 16-3). Advise the family on ways to reduce exposure to environmental allergens within the home and community that may exacerbate asthma (see Community Care 16-1).

Skin or in vitro testing may also be used to assess sensitivity to allergens. Allergen immunotherapy may be considered for children with persistent asthma when there is clear evidence that the asthma symptoms are related to exposure to specific allergens to which the child is sensitive.

A history and treatment of comorbid symptoms may improve overall asthma control. Conditions that may adversely affect asthma control include allergic bronchopulmonary aspergillosis, gastroesophageal reflux, obesity, OSA, rhinitis, sinusitis, stress, and depression. Advise children with these conditions to seek or maintain care provided by a medical specialist to ensure that recognition and treatment of these conditions is maintained.

Medications

A stepwise approach is used to select the medication and delivery devices to meet the child's needs and presenting symptoms (see Tables 16-7 to 16-10). After a diagnosis has been made and therapy has been initiated, the child's level of asthma control is monitored daily, and therapy is adjusted accordingly. The goal of therapy is to identify the minimum amount of medication required to help the child maintain asthma control.

Medications have two primary roles in the treatment of asthma. The first role of medication use is to provide long-term control by preventing symptoms. The second role of medications is to treat acute symptoms and exacerbations.

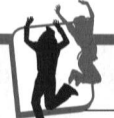

COMMUNITY CARE 16-2

Components of an Asthma Education Program

Topic	Content
Definition of asthma	Emphasize chronic nature of asthma, prognosis, and goals of therapy.
Signs and symptoms	Discuss main symptoms of an acute episode, variability of symptoms, and ways to recognize mild/prodromal symptoms. Identify symptoms that need immediate treatment.
Pathophysiology	Describe the characteristic changes that occur in the airways (inflammation, bronchospasm, mucus) and the role of medications.
Asthma triggers and avoidance of triggers	Help family/patient identify possible aggravating factors that may exacerbate asthma. Offer suggestions for home environment modification (see Community Care 16-1).
Management of asthma	Establish an asthma action plan: • Monitoring of symptoms (frequency, response to medication, or environmental triggers) • Need for preventive care and routine monitoring • Environmental controls (reduce or eliminate environmental exposures) • Medications (dose, frequency, method of delivery, actions, side effects) for each zone (green, yellow, red); encourage daily medications even when well • Importance of early treatment of asthma exacerbations
Written guidelines	Use an asthma action plan for all children: • Asthma action plan should be posted at home. • Plan should be shared with child care and school personnel.
Correct use of inhalation devices	Demonstrate correct use of MDIs, nebulizer treatments, spacing devices, and care of these devices.
Use of peak expiratory flow meter	Instruct in peak flow monitoring as indicated for • Children with at least moderate persistent asthma • Children older than 5 years of age Teach use of peak flow meter: • Instruct to keep record of readings to identify personal best (determined by recording peak flow twice daily for 2 weeks). • Instruct when to initiate or change treatment based on peak flow readings (yellow zone, 50%–80% of personal best; red zone, <50% of personal best).
Fears and misconceptions/ feelings about asthma	Respond to patient and family concerns regarding medications. Clear up any misconceptions (asthma not caused by psychological factors, deaths usually related to undertreatment of asthma, children should maintain active lives). Acknowledge negative feelings of having asthma. Refer to appropriate self-management programs/community resources.
Communication with child's school, daycare, camp, and so forth	Review importance of notifying school of child's condition, need for medication (especially rescue medications like albuterol) in school, and ability to participate in sports and physical education.

TRADITION OR SCIENCE 16-3

More Inquiry Needed

Should pets be removed from the home to prevent allergic sensitization in children?

Numerous studies have demonstrated that pet allergies are clearly associated with wheezing and bronchial hyperresponsiveness in adults. Thus, asthma has been thought to be worsened by exposure to pets. However, recent studies indicate that living with a pet early in life reduces the incidence of asthma and may have a possible protective effect. These longitudinal studies demonstrated that children exposed to pets in the home as newborns and during the first year of life had a lower incidence of asthma at ages 12–13 years than children not exposed to pets. Pet allergen exposure itself does not appear to be the protective factor; rather, endotoxin exposure from presence of the pet in the home is hypothesized to provide the protective influence. Endotoxin, a component of gram-negative bacterial cell walls, is found throughout nature. High levels of allergen exposure are also thought to induce immunologic tolerance. Clearly, more research is needed to better understand the relationship between pet exposure and asthma sensitivity. In the meantime, prospective parents need not remove pets from the home before a child's arrival (Bacharier & Strunk, 2003).

Corticosteroids are considered to be the most effective method to achieve long-term control of asthma. These anti-inflammatory agents reduce airway hyperresponsiveness, inhibit inflammatory cell migration and activation, and block late-phase reaction to allergens (National Heart, Lung, and Blood Institute, 2007). Inhaled corticosteroids are the most consistently effective at all steps of care for persistent asthma. Oral corticosteroids may be used to gain prompt control of asthma and are required for severe persistent asthma (see Tables 16-7 and 16-10).

Other medications used to gain long-term control include cromolyn sodium and nedocromil. These anti-inflammatory agents inhibit activation and release of mediators from mast cells, thus maintaining airway stability. Immunomodulators (omalizumab) is a monoclonal antibody given intramuscularly to prevent binding of IgE to the high-affinity receptors on basophils and mast cells (National Heart, Lung, and Blood Institute, 2007). This is used as an adjunctive therapy for children aged 12 years and older who have demonstrated sensitivity to specific allergens and who require a step up in care to manage their persistent asthma. Leukotriene modifiers are used for children requiring step 2 care for mild persistent asthma. These products interfere with the pathway of leukotriene mediators that are released from mast cells, eosinophils, and basophils (National Heart, Lung, and Blood Institute, 2007). Long-acting beta$_2$-agonists such as salmeterol and formoterol are bronchodilators that open the airways by relaxing smooth muscle contraction and reducing bronchospasm, thereby enhancing mucociliary clearance and decreasing vascular permeability.

Methylxanthine is a sustained-release theophylline that has some mild anti-inflammatory effects and can be used as adjunctive therapy with inhaled corticosteroids for children older than 5 years of age. For a more detailed description of these medications and their recommended use, dose, adverse effects, and care concerns, please refer to the National Heart, Lung, and Blood Institute (2007) asthma guidelines.

Medications are also used to provide quick relief for acute symptoms and exacerbations. These acute symptoms may be brought on by environmental exposures (as described earlier) or perhaps by exercise-induced bronchospasm that was not effectively managed by the medications previously described to step up or down care for long-term asthma control. Quick-relief medications include anticholinergics given via an MDI or nebulizer solution. These agents inhibit muscarinic cholinergic receptors and reduce the intrinsic vagal tone of the airways (National Heart, Lung, and Blood Institute, 2007). Short-acting beta$_2$-agonists (SABAs), such as albuterol, levalbuterol, and pirbuterol, are rapid-acting bronchodilators that open the airways by relaxing smooth muscle contraction, enhancing mucociliary clearance, and reducing bronchospasm. Systemic corticosteroids may be used in addition to SABAs for moderate and severe exacerbations to speed recovery and to prevent recurrence of the exacerbation (National Heart, Lung, and Blood Institute, 2007) (see the National Heart, Lung, and Blood Institute [2007] asthma guidelines for further information on medications to treat acute symptoms of asthma).

Determine the medications the child is using and whether any complementary and alternative medications or treatments (chiropractic medicine, acupuncture) are being used.

ALERT   *There is insufficient evidence to support recommending the use of complementary and alternative medications for treatment of allergy. Families who use herbal treatments for asthma should be cautioned about the interactions that some of the ingredients may have with their prescribed asthma medications.*

Ask to view any records the child has been keeping of his or her symptoms and/or peak flow monitoring. Advise children with moderate or severe persistent asthma to keep daily peak flow monitoring records. These tools will aid the child and family to recognize adequate and inadequate asthma control.

Watch the child using their peak flow meter and inhaler. Although the steps in this process seem easy, incorrect use of the inhaler means less medication is getting to the airways. Provide instruction materials and sample peak flow charts to the family (see thePoint for Procedures). Each health care encounter should include an assessment of asthma severity, measures to maintain control, and the child's responsiveness to the therapies initiated.

Management and Treatment of Exacerbations

> QUESTION: Based on the following information and José's condition, what do you anticipate the nurse in the emergency department will do next?

An acute or subacute episode of asthma is identified as progressive and worsening shortness of breath, cough, wheezing, and/or chest tightness. These symptoms indicate decreases in expiratory airflow and require immediate intervention. Children whose asthma has been well controlled using inhaled corticosteroids are less likely to have an exacerbation; however, all children are at risk for exacerbations. Respiratory infections, exercise-induced bronchospasm, extreme changes in weather, exposure to a known (or unknown) allergen, and stress can precipitate a worsening of asthma symptoms. Severe exacerbations can be life threatening. Act quickly to assess the degree of severity and to determine the measures already taken to relieve the child's symptoms. Use the child's written asthma plan to help the family determine how to adjust the medications. School nurses should have copies of this written plan at the child's school site. Remove allergens in the environment that may be contributing to the exacerbation, or withdraw the child from such an environment. If the child does not have a written asthma plan, or if the child continues to deteriorate despite the increased use of inhaled corticosteroids and SABAs, then management in an urgent or emergency care or hospital setting is warranted.

When the child presents in the health care setting with an acute exacerbation, assess and carefully monitor alertness, heart rate, respiratory rate, breath sounds, pulse oximetry, and PEFR (if the child is able); perform a full pulmonary assessment, including visual inspection of chest (accessory muscles), auscultation of breath sounds, and other respiratory assessments. Typically, supplemental oxygen is ordered to correct hypoxemia. Administer repetitive or continuous SABA treatments to reverse airflow obstruction rapidly. Oral systemic corticosteroids may be ordered to decrease airway inflammation if the child does not respond promptly to the SABA treatments. Usually, the child will prefer a high-Fowler position or sitting up and leaning slightly forward. Continuously monitor the child in acute distress, including comprehensive reassessments of the child's response to therapy after the first hour. For acute exacerbation that responds poorly to initial interventions, or when ongoing observation and stabilization of the child is needed, hospitalization may be indicated. If the child is becoming less alert or drowsy, this may indicate impending respiratory failure. ET intubation and assisted ventilation must be considered if steady clinical deterioration occurs despite continued intensive therapy.

> ANSWER: José's history, presentation of physical symptoms, and oxygen saturation will affect the decision regarding whether José will receive inhaled SABA by nebulizer or MDI, up to three doses during the first hour, and oral corticosteroids if needed. If José is responding to the nebulized medication and his respiratory distress is resolving, inhaled SABA will be continued every 60 minutes. This treatment will continue for 1–3 hours. If he continues in respiratory distress despite his initial treatments, oxygen will be administered. Hospitalization may be warranted for ongoing administration of oxygen, nebulized SABAs, oral or IV corticosteroids, and IV therapy.

Community Care

The National Heart, Lung, and Blood Institute (2007) asthma guidelines represent the best evidence to date regarding the assessment, monitoring, and management of asthma. The primary emphasis of these standards of care is to encourage early diagnosis and ongoing assessment by the child's medical home providers and to provide teaching and preventive measures that will ensure the child's overall health and well-being. Patient education should occur at all points of care with the child and family.

Patients often overestimate medication adherence (Elder & Mellon, 2008). Adherence to medications and therapies can also be augmented by recognizing the importance of each caregiver in the home. Acknowledging the role of various caregivers in the home is critical when managing complex and demanding chronic illnesses including asthma (Zarelli, 2009). Adherence to preventive medication therapies in asthma can be challenging. One small study has documented that rates of prescription refills are relatively low in children with persistent asthma, although better in oral montelukast than in inhaled corticosteroid medications. Rates of prescription refill have been noted to be higher within the first month after a visit to a health care provider. These findings highlight the need for ongoing patient and caregiver education and monitoring of prescription refills (Fitzpatrick et al., 2009). Adherence to asthma therapies is often better when families are able to establish a daily routine for their medications. This provides an opportunity for nurses and other health care providers to assist patients and caregivers manage their asthma, improving associated asthma morbidity and mortality (Peterson-Sweeney et al., 2010). Family routines that can positively impact asthma health are noted in Community Care 16-3. Surveillance of environmental triggers must also occur in all settings (home, school, daycare, and so forth) in which the child is likely to spend time. Review the National Heart, Lung, and Blood Institute (2007) standards thoroughly and use the information and products provided by this agency and others to help children and their families effectively manage the child's chronic condition.

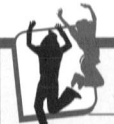

COMMUNITY CARE 16-3

Examples of Family Routines to Improve Asthma Health

Routine health care/asthma care visits (e.g., every 3 months)

Routine prescription refill (e.g., monthly or use mail order refill)

Routine location for storing preventative and rescue medications (e.g., kitchen counter)

Preventative medication (e.g., budesonide) administration with oral hygiene

Peak flow monitoring after breakfast

Routine house cleaning (e.g., weekly)

Adapted from Peterson-Sweeney, K. (2009). The relationship of household routines to morbidity outcomes in childhood asthma. *Journal for Specialists in Pediatric Nursing, 14*(1), 59–69.

BRONCHOPULMONARY DYSPLASIA

BPD, which results in chronic lung disease, is the most common complication of premature birth. Although primarily associated with preterm birth, BPD is also associated with prenatal infection and inflammation, oxygen toxicity, mechanical ventilation, patent ductus arteriosus, postnatal infection, and decreased host antioxidant defenses (Gien & Kinsella, 2011). Additionally, there is increasing literature relating genetic associations and the development of BPD (McColley & Morty, 2011; Sampath et al., 2012). The definition of BPD depends on meeting specific criteria of gestational age, oxygen, and use of positive pressure (Jobe & Bancalari, 2001). The effects of BPD may last several months to years. Although infants with BPD may have a prolonged and complicated neonatal course, the long-term pulmonary prognosis for survivors of BPD is relatively good. Between the years 1993 and 2006, the diagnosis of BPD decreased by 4.3% thought to be due to the improvement in pulmonary therapies during this time (Stroustrup & Trasande, 2010).

Pathophysiology

The pathology of BPD is complex and multifactorial. The lungs have alveolar hypoplasia with decreased alveolar complexity, variable interstitial fibroproliferation, decreased and dysmorphic capillaries, negligible airway epithelial lesions, variable smooth muscle hyperplasia, and decreased severe arterial/arteriolar vascular lesions (Coalson, 2003). Risk factors for the development of BPD include prematurity (associated with immature lung development), intrauterine exposure to inflammation, and a genetic predisposition (Groothius & Makari, 2012).

The most important underlying pathologic process in BPD is the profound alteration of lung compliance, which is reduced as a result of a combination of factors. These factors include fibrosis of the airways and marked hyperplasia of the bronchial epithelium, which occur secondary to alveolar damage, and increased fluid in the lung as a result of disruption of the alveolar–capillary membrane. Damage to the alveolar-supporting structures results in overdistension and leads to air trapping, fibrosis, airway edema, and bronchoconstriction, increasing airway resistance and decreasing compliance. Increased airway resistance increases the work of breathing, resulting in tachypnea and wheezing.

Pulmonary gas exchange is impaired by several factors. Hypoxia occurs secondary to ventilation–perfusion mismatch in the areas of alveolar collapse. Increased pulmonary vascular resistance causes intrapulmonic shunting, thus also contributing to hypoxia. Hypercarbia is common and is also caused by ventilation–perfusion mismatch as well as by hypoventilation.

Growth failure in infants with BPD is almost universal and results from increased energy expenditure and caloric needs, caused by the increased work of breathing, and high resting oxygen consumption. Growth failure and lung disease may also be complicated by gastroesophageal reflux with frequent emesis, poor oral feeding skills, and recurrent respiratory infections (Groothius & Makari, 2012).

Cor pulmonale (hypertrophy or failure of the right ventricle caused by disorders of the lungs, pulmonary vessels, or chest wall), pulmonary hypertension, systemic hypertension, and left ventricular hypertrophy are complications of BPD that result from the fibrosis and chronic hypoxia. The pulmonary vasculature of infants with cor pulmonale develops increased reactivity to hypoxia, resulting in pulmonary hypertension and left ventricular hypertrophy with congestive heart failure.

The effects of invasive positive-pressure therapy (e.g., intubation and mechanical ventilation, including high-frequency oscillatory ventilation) have been associated with an increased risk of additional lung damage (Kugelman & Durand, 2011). However, noninvasive positive-pressure therapy has had some positive outcomes.

Assessment

The clinical manifestations of BPD are a direct reflection of the pathophysiology of this disorder. Tachypnea, dyspnea, and wheezing are intermittently or chronically present, secondary to airway obstruction and increased airway resistance. Increased work of breathing, as evidenced by intercostal or substernal retractions and use of accessory muscles, is common in the infant with BPD. Infants who have been intubated for long periods may develop subglottic stenosis, which results in inspiratory stridor. Furthermore, hypoxemia and hypercapnia are chronic states that contribute to the problem. The child might turn cyanotic when crying or after a few moments without supplemental oxygen. Infants with moderate to severe BPD are frequently described as irritable and difficult to comfort. This behavior may result from hypoxia or underlying neurologic dysfunction. They may develop irregular sleep patterns as a result of frequent medical treatments, medications, and therapies. Inguinal hernias are often present, which may be a result of the continuous increase in abdominal pressure caused by high airway resistance and use of accessory respiratory muscles. These infants also have extraordinarily large insensible fluid losses because of tachypnea and excessive perspiration related to hypercarbia.

The incidence of neurologic abnormalities and developmental delay in infants with BPD varies, but these problems are known to occur in children with BPD. Infants who are born prematurely likely experience some degree of developmental delay with or without neurologic insult. Even if there is no evident damage to the neurologic system during hospitalization in the neonatal intensive care unit, children with BPD may show signs of problems when they are school age. These problems can range from vision and hearing loss to speech delays, learning disabilities, and poor attention span. Developmental delays result from long-term ventilatory support, poor nutritional status, inadequate sensory stimulation, neurologic sequelae, and decreased energy and respiratory reserves.

Nursing assessment requires close observation and awareness of BPD signs and symptoms. Take a thorough history, including the child's baseline symptoms (retractions, respiratory effort), requirements (oxygen needs), and nutritional intake. Next, complete a physical examination focusing on respiratory, cardiac, nutritional, and developmental status. An interdisciplinary team may assist in a comprehensive evaluation. Report any abnormal findings to the team and implement appropriate interventions and referrals.

Interdisciplinary Interventions

Just as the pathophysiology of BPD is multifactorial, its treatment is multifaceted. Medical management of BPD centers on preventing and minimizing hypoxia and hypercarbia, treating bronchoconstriction and airway hyperreactivity and inflammation, treating pulmonary edema, and promoting repair of chronic lung injury.

These desired ends are achieved in varying degrees by medical therapies such as supplemental oxygen, diuretics, bronchodilators, anti-inflammatory agents, and various modes of respiratory support. Pulmonary hypertension responds at least in part to oxygen, a potent pulmonary vasodilator. Low-flow supplemental oxygen is administered, at times on a long-term basis, in an attempt to prevent chronic hypoxia and subsequent complications. Tracheostomy is considered for those who require assisted ventilation for more than 3 months as a neonate or who have chronic hypercarbia and increased work of breathing.

Management of Hypoxia

The primary and most important aspect of therapy in infants with BPD is managing hypoxia. Maintaining adequate tissue oxygenation is imperative to prevent severe morbidity and potential death. Supplemental oxygen therapy is prescribed to promote growth and neurodevelopment and to prevent or control pulmonary hypertension. Administering and monitoring oxygen

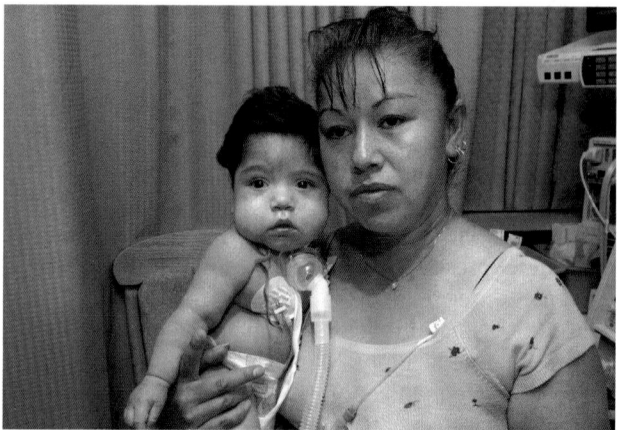

Figure 16-18 Humidified oxygen is provided to the child using a mist delivery device.

therapy is a major nursing responsibility in the care of an infant with BPD. Pulse oximetry or transcutaneous oxygen monitors are used to continuously or intermittently display oxygen saturation. SaO$_2$ levels of 92% to 95% (≥95% during feeding and sleeping), depending on severity of illness, are necessary to facilitate an improved rate of weight gain and to control pulmonary hypertension. The nurse must respond to the infant's changing oxygen needs, titrating oxygen flow to keep saturations within the prescribed parameters. Feedings, periods of increased activity, and periods of sleep are occasions when desaturations are most likely.

Tailor the mode of oxygen delivery to the specific needs of the infant. Most infants with mild to moderate BPD can tolerate a nasal oxygen cannula. Children with tracheostomies may use a tracheostomy mist collar (Fig. 16-18). Humidification is necessary for liter flow equal to or greater than 1 L/min to prevent airway irritation and mucus plugging. Monitor infants for increased oxygen demand, especially during acute illnesses, fever, stress, and periods of increased activity. Reassessment should include child's color, presence and degree of respiratory distress (report any retractions, nasal flaring, or use of accessory respiratory muscles), breath sounds, vital signs, and level of consciousness.

Other nursing interventions for the infant with BPD include administering multiple oral and inhaled pharmacologic agents, monitoring their effectiveness, and identifying possible adverse effects (Table 16-11).

Respiratory Care

Because excessive airway secretions present difficult problems for the infant or child with BPD, diligent airway clearance is needed to prevent mucus plugging and airway obstruction. Cough is often ineffective in children with BPD because of generalized debilitation. Nasopharyngeal or tracheal suctioning is needed frequently to maintain patent airways, especially during illnesses or respiratory tract infections. Chest physiotherapy may also help improve secretion clearance and lessen atelectasis. Always collaborate with respiratory therapists and parents to schedule chest physiotherapy

TABLE 16-11	Bronchopulmonary Dysplasia Medications and Side Effects	
Type of Medication	**Action**	**Possible Side Effects**
Bronchodilators		
Aminophylline Terbutaline Albuterol (inhaled)	Bronchodilators open the airways of the lungs. They work by relaxing the muscles around the airways. These medicines can be used alone or in groups.	Increased heart rate Shakiness or tremors Hyperactivity
Diuretics		
Furosemide (Lasix) Spironolactone (Aldactone) Chlorothiazide (Diuril)	Diuretics cause an increased amount of water and salt to be excreted in the urine. They also decrease the amount of fluid in the lungs.	Imbalances in potassium (hypokalemia/hyperkalemia) and calcium (hypocalcemia) Muscle cramps and irregular heart rhythm are signs that serum electrolytes must be closely monitored
Anti-Inflammatory Drugs (Corticosteroids)		
Prednisolone (oral liquid) Budesonide (Pulmicort) (inhaled)	Anti-inflammatory drugs are used in children whose wheezing is not controlled with bronchodilators. These medicines are not rescue medications. They reduce airway inflammation and are primarily used on a long-term basis to prevent wheezing and respiratory distress.	Short-term use causes little or no side effects. Longer term effects may include impaired growth and decreased ability to fight infections, although the data are mixed (Kelly et al., 2012; Stefanovic et al., 2011; T. Wang et al., 2012)

to occur 30 minutes before feedings and before rest periods if possible. Suctioning should immediately follow chest physiotherapy and be done at other times as needed.

Positioning and comforting interventions are of extreme importance in caring for the infant with BPD. Ill or premature infants who are chronically "air hungry" are extremely irritable and may be difficult to console. With the collaboration of physical and occupational therapists, develop individualized plans for the handling and activity level of these infants that accommodate their developmental level and ability to tolerate stimulation. Frequent and prolonged rest periods are necessary because of increased energy demand and sleep deprivation. Watch for signs of overstimulation in the neurologically immature child such as cyanosis, avoidance of eye contact, vomiting, diaphoresis, and falling asleep.

Nutritional Support

Because growth failure is common in the infant with BPD, providing nutritional support is a crucial, although difficult, aspect of caring for these children. Management of feedings in infants and young children with BPD has direct implications for long-term outcome because an adequate caloric intake is necessary for growth of healthy lung tissue and resolution of the disease. Yet, these infants suffer from a myriad of conditions that impair their ability to feed: gastroesophageal reflux, often with aspiration; emesis; chronic fatigue; behavioral oral aversion; and swallowing dysfunction caused by poor oral–motor development. For the healthy infant, feeding is generally viewed as a pleasant and positive experience; however, for the child with BPD, it is often perceived as a battle. It can seem that the more that nurses and parents are concerned and anxious about

nutrition and place pressure on the infant or child to eat, the less the child eats. Feeding with the infant or child with BPD can be a frustrating and challenging experience, and coordinated interdisciplinary effort is the key to successfully approaching these problems.

Begin with a nutritional assessment that includes documentation of anthropometric (precise measurement of the body includes weight, height, and head circumference) and biochemical data, dietary intake, and clinical status. Strategies in nutritional support then focus on optimizing the caloric intake to meet individual needs. Concentrating formula to provide more calories per ounce; medication to control gastroesophageal reflux; and small, frequent feedings all are appropriate for mild to moderate growth failure.

Infants with severe growth failure, or for whom the previously listed strategies are unsuccessful, should be considered for surgical placement of a gastrostomy tube or percutaneous endoscopic gastrostomy tube. This procedure may or may not be performed in conjunction with a Nissen fundoplication, depending on the severity of gastroesophageal reflux. Because parents sometimes view the need for a gastrostomy tube as a sign of their failure to feed their infant orally, the entire health care team must provide support and stress the benefits of this mode of therapy. Calorie-dense formulas can be administered with minimal risk of aspiration, in a continuous infusion if necessary, to promote optimal growth. Feeding specialists and caregivers can provide therapy to develop and refine suck and swallow coordination skills concurrently so that as the infant's growth, strength, and ability to orally feed improve, tube feedings can be slowly weaned and the frequency and amount of oral feedings can be increased (Nursing Interventions 16-2). This strategy temporarily relaxes the intense focus on eating and can transform parental anxiety into energy

---

NURSING INTERVENTIONS 16-2

How to Improve Feeding Capabilities in an Infant With Bronchopulmonary Dysplasia

- Have baby in a calm, alert state before beginning to feed.
- Position the baby in the caregiver's lap with the baby's neck in a neutral position, hips and knees at 90 degrees of flexion, both upper extremities with elbows flexed at 90 degrees, and head elevated at least 30 degrees.
- Carefully monitor physiologic parameters, especially respiratory rate. Feedings may need to be limited or postponed if the infant remains tachypneic.
- Choose a nipple that allows moderate resistance to flow without excessive energy expenditure. Standard-shaped nipples are preferred.
- Present the nipple slowly and calmly, with minimal intraoral stimulation.

- Emphasize normal total body posture during feeding. Head and neck posture can alter oral–motor patterns during sucking. Ideally, marked neck extension should be reduced to aid oral–motor control. The goal of improving head and neck positioning may need to be approached slowly to minimize stress to the infant.
- Allow baby to set the nippling pace, with rests as needed.
- Stop nippling if baby begins to sweat or cries inconsolably for 1 minute or longer; if respiratory rate or heart rate increases excessively, as determined by the provider; or if feeding takes longer than 20 minutes.

devoted to interventions such as positive oral stimulation and nonnutritive sucking during tube feedings.

In addition to services initiating while in the hospital, infants with BPD discharged to home should have a referral to early intervention program. With this, infants will be assessed for their individual level of developmental delay and therapeutic interventions will commence. Therapies received in the home through early intervention program include speech, occupational, and physical therapies. Close collaboration with the primary provider during this time will be helpful to meet the ongoing developmental needs of the infant.

Family Education and Support

Other nursing and social service interventions should focus on providing education and support. Teach parents about all aspects of BPD, especially topics related to home care. If the child is to receive oxygen, arrangements must be made for administering the oxygen (Community Care 16-4). Medication administration, feeding and nutrition, developmental interventions, chest physiotherapy, and suctioning are among the most important topics of education for the parents and family of a child with BPD. Family members are taught CPR. Teach them the symptoms that indicate the child's respiratory condition is worsening and when to seek medical attention.

Community Care

The emotional effect on parents and family of having a child with BPD is profound. The development of a chronic condition with life-threatening implications in a premature infant, followed by complex home care, is a situation so laden with stress and anxiety that it is often described by families as an "emotional roller coaster" from which they have no opportunity to escape. The

family must deal with grief and sorrow over the loss of the expected healthy child, financial demands, and social isolation.

Social isolation is a common psychosocial issue for these families. Caring for a frequently hospitalized infant with a chronic illness can absorb virtually all the parents' time and energy. They must balance time with the ill child against time with their other children and time for themselves. Family sacrifices often have to be made. Parents and older siblings may be required to adjust work, school, and recreational schedules. Social interactions are often drastically reduced because of lack of time, energy, transportation, and financial resources. In addition, clear-cut social guidelines for approaching families with chronically ill children are limited. At a time when support is most important, individuals in the family's social network may feel awkward and tend to withdraw. Assessing social support and interactions is crucial when planning care for a family with a child who has BPD.

Parent support groups facilitated by nursing or social service professionals are often successful in addressing parental anxiety and promoting positive coping. Sibling reactions and coping, financial stress, profound chronic fatigue, and uncertainty about their child's physical and intellectual future are topics many parents find comforting to discuss with others who have had similar experiences and concerns. Some families, too, are referred by social services for private counseling to address and facilitate stress management.

CYSTIC FIBROSIS

Once considered a fatal childhood disease, CF is a chronic, multisystem condition. Ongoing advances in understanding the pathophysiology of CF, particularly

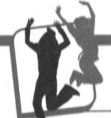

COMMUNITY CARE 16-4

Methods of Home Oxygen Delivery and the Child With Bronchopulmonary Dysplasia

Method	Advantages	Disadvantages	Special Considerations
Compressed gas in tank	Usually the least expensive system Can be used with any flow rate; continuously or intermittently (with proper flow meter)	Large tanks take much storage space Under very high pressure; if valve were broken or jarred loose, tank would behave like a high-powered rocket Heavy, cumbersome	Tanks vary in size from very large to portable (with a cart). Store all tanks with a stable base and secured against falling over. When traveling, the system should be secured in the vehicle to prevent rolling or other movement.
Liquid oxygen	Twice as much oxygen can be stored in the same amount of space as tanks Very light and portable; the most convenient system May be more cost-effective than tanks if high flow is required	Usually the most expensive system Evaporates when not being used continuously Not practical with low flow rates	Portable system is filled from a larger reservoir. When traveling, the system should be secured in the vehicle to prevent rolling or other movement.
Oxygen concentrator	Machine separates oxygen from nitrogen in the room air; never needs to be refilled Practical for rural areas or areas not routinely serviced by oxygen companies	Runs by electricity; backup system needed for power outages Noisy Increases electric bills Difficult to transport in a two-story home or outside the home	Must have grounded electrical outlet. When traveling, the system should be secured in the vehicle to prevent rolling or other movement. A portable system of compressed gas should be dispersed for emergency use and transport to clinic for illnesses.

All oxygen systems should be kept away from any open flame, combustible materials, or sources of sparks.

its genetic and molecular mechanisms, has greatly improved diagnosis and treatment and thus improved survival rates, life expectancy, and quality of life for children and adolescents with CF. The median age of survival for individuals with CF has been slowly increasing and is currently estimated to be in the late 30 years of age (Cystic Fibrosis Foundation, 2011). Intensive research has also resulted in better screening tests to detect carriers through genetic testing.

CF is a highly complex disease and requires a holistic approach to care by a trained, interdisciplinary team, including physicians, advanced practice nurses, nurses, dietitians, social workers, psychologists, and respiratory care practitioners. Coordination and communication with the child, family, and other health care providers are essential. Specialist care in a dedicated CF center has been associated with improved survival and quality of life in children. As with any chronic condition, the primary objectives of CF care for children should focus on (1) ensuring optimal care, including treatments, routine monitoring, and general pediatric preventive care; (2) facilitating access to pertinent health care resources and support; (3) assisting the family in coordinating care among specialists and primary care providers and in accessing medications, dietary supplements, and durable medical equipment; and (4) supporting quality of life and independence.

Although CF is rare overall, it is more common among white northern Europeans. It is the second most common inherited life-shortening disease of childhood. The overall prevalence of CF in the U.S. population is estimated to be 1 in 3,700 live births, with nearly 1,000 cases diagnosed annually. It affects males and females equally (American Lung Association, 2010).

Pathophysiology

CF is an autosomal recessive genetic condition. In such conditions, the risk of disease transmission is 25% if both parents carry the gene, and the chance that the child will be a carrier of the disease is 50% (see Fig. 3-3). Prenatal screening is common in women from populations that have an elevated prevalence of CF or in women with known or suspected family histories. Prenatal testing is also done when obstructed fetal bowel is detected by ultrasound because CF is associated with meconium ileus.

The gene responsible for CF is located on chromosome 7. CF results from mutations in the cystic fibrosis transmembrane regulator (CFTR), a protein that regulates chloride and sodium transport in secretory epithelial cells of the body's exocrine glands. The alteration in the CFTR protein results in abnormal ion concentration across the apical membranes of these cells. They do not release chloride, resulting in an improper salt balance. This imbalance causes the mucous secretions of the pulmonary, gastrointestinal, and reproductive systems to become thick and sticky and to block ducts in those organs. The sweat glands are also affected by blocked or abnormal transport and produce sweat with elevated sodium and chloride concentrations (Fig. 16-19).

The most CF common mutation, DF508, occurs in more than 90% of individuals with CF in the United States (Rowe et al., 2005). More than 1,000 other gene mutations of CFTR genes have been described, resulting in a large variability in severity and progression of the disease. A small number of these mutations occur with reasonable frequency, but most are rare. For example, 99% of those who are homozygous for the DF508 allele have pancreatic insufficiency, whereas only 36% of people with CF with other mutations are pancreatic insufficient (Rowe et al., 2005). Beyond the specific gene mutation, existence of modifier genes and environmental factors, including viral and bacterial pathogens, impact the progression of the disease (Bombieri et al., 2011).

Clinical consequences of CF are progressive pulmonary damage (e.g., airway obstruction, inflammation, infection, scarring), pancreatic dysfunction, liver disease that may lead to cirrhosis, gut motility problems, and elevated sweat electrolyte levels. Approximately 80% to 85% of children with CF are pancreatic insufficient, resulting in malabsorption of important nutrients, fats, and proteins. Approximately 98% of males are sterile because of blockage of the vas deferens by thick secretions or from abnormal development (atresia of the vas deferens) that prevents passage of sperm. Females can become pregnant, but the thick cervical mucus acts as a natural barrier to sperm. Although the true biologic fertility in CF remains unknown, females with normal lung function appear to experience relatively few problems with pregnancy; those with decreased lung function and chronic infection tend to have poorer pregnancy outcomes (Edenborough, 2001).

The thickened, sticky mucus of a child with CF is ineffective in removing bacteria from the body and, in fact, constitutes an ideal medium for bacterial growth.

Thus, the child with CF is especially prone to pulmonary infection. Bacterial lung infections are responsible for most morbidity and mortality among children with CF, and these infections are often caused by multiple pathogens. The most common cultured bacteria are *Pseudomonas aeruginosa*, *S. aureus*, *Burkholderia cepacia*, and *H. influenzae*. Children with CF often remain colonized with organisms such as *P. aeruginosa*, which is never eradicated from the lungs.

ALERT   *Burkholderia* cepacia *cause extremely virulent infections and have been associated with rapid deterioration of pulmonary function.* B. cepacia *has been associated with death in approximately 2% of children with mild or moderate forms of CF. To prevent spreading, children with* B. cepacia *should not have contact with CF patients.*

Children with CF often experience acute pulmonary exacerbations, many of which are caused by respiratory viruses. Infections such as RSV may result in severe pulmonary complications, particularly in infants. Exacerbations cause fatigue, decreased appetite, weight loss, increased sputum production, increased cough, hemoptysis, decreased spirometry values, and poor response to outpatient therapeutic measures such as oral antibiotics and increased pulmonary treatments at home. Treating pulmonary exacerbations requires careful monitoring, aggressive therapies, and, often, hospitalization.

Adolescents' cognitive development is normal, but secondary sexual development may be delayed, causing teens to look younger than their peers. During the adolescent years, infertility must not be assumed for either gender; teens should receive appropriate referrals for informed family planning and life decisions.

Assessment

CF is often diagnosed early in life, although children with less severe CF may not be diagnosed until later childhood. The clinical presentation of CF can be extremely varied, although the most common symptoms are very salty tasting skin; persistent cough; excessive appetite but poor weight gain; and foul-smelling, greasy, bulky stools. As people live longer with CF, other symptoms and complications may manifest themselves (Chart 16-2).

Before diagnosis, newborns often present with meconium ileus and bowel obstruction and perforation requiring surgical intervention. Young infants may be irritable and present with failure to thrive despite good appetite. Children with CF may appear physically small for their age in both linear growth and weight.

When assessing a child known to have CF, include an intensive history (by system) of current and past symptoms, changes in activity tolerance, exercise, sleep and rest disturbances, and sleep position. Although you should carefully assess all systems, the primary focus should be on the respiratory system.

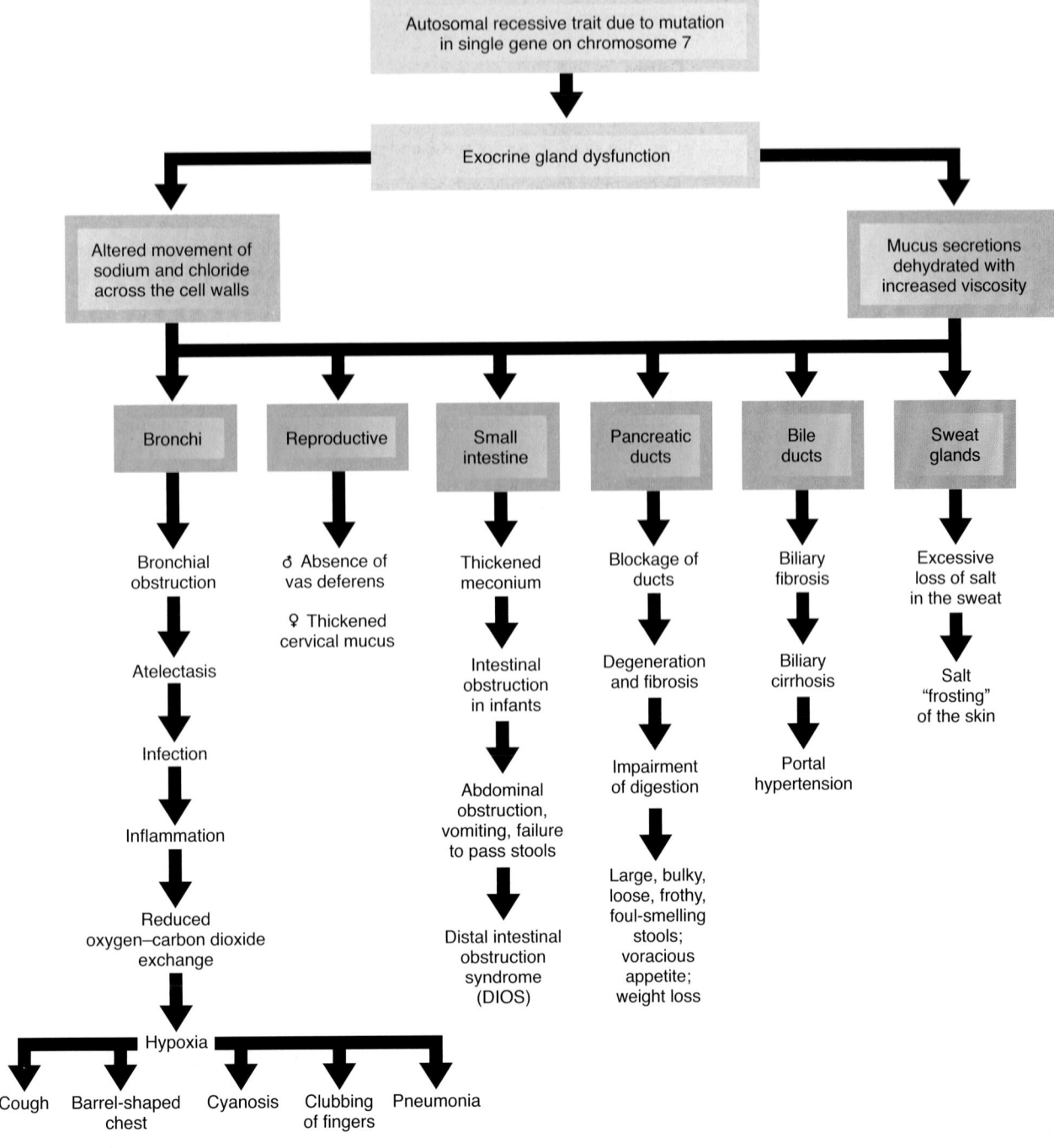

Figure 16-19 Manifestations of CF.

The respiratory assessment may reveal a barrel-shaped chest with increased anteroposterior diameter caused by hyperaeration and increased work of breathing. Another physical finding characteristic of hypoxia and common in young children with severe CF is mild to severe clubbing of the nail beds caused by chronic hypoxia. Assess oxygenation by inspecting the color of the mucous membranes, nail beds, and skin. Use pulse oximetry to monitor oxygen saturation. Assess breath sounds for equal aeration of all lung fields and for presence or absence of rales, crackles, and wheezing, particularly in the upper lobes and the right middle lobe. Assess breathing for rate, depth, effort, and use of accessory muscles. Obtain a history on sputum characteristics, including color changes, volume, viscosity, and presence or absence of blood. Also elicit history of headaches and pain, changes in breathing during activities of a typical day, and cough pattern. The characteristic cough of CF may increase during pulmonary exacerbations, can be paroxysmal, and frequently ends with posttussive emesis. The comprehensive pulmonary assessment in CF includes a comparison of the

CHART 16-2	Complications of Cystic Fibrosis	

Complications	Causes
Pulmonary	
Minor hemoptysis	Common after 10 years of age. Blood streaking is from mucosal irritation in the airway.
Major hemoptysis	Occurs more frequently with age in less than 10% of adults. Bleeding is caused by high systemic pressure of bronchial circulation when infection erodes a blood vessel.
Pneumothorax	Incidence increases with age (approximately 16%–20% of patients older than 16 years of age experience this complication). Rupture of subpleural blebs through visceral pleura. High rate of recurrence.
Nasal polyps	Occurs in 10%–25% of CF patients. Most common in older children and adolescents; etiology is unknown.
Chronic sinusitis	Occurs in more than 90% of CF patients. Etiology is thought to be from abnormal occlusion of the ducts that prevents mucus drainage; maxillary and ethmoid sinuses are most commonly involved.
Cor pulmonale	Occurs in advanced disease. Right ventricular hypertrophy, chronic hypoxemia and pulmonary hypertension, and right-sided heart failure are noted.
Pulmonary hypertrophic osteoarthropathy	Occurs in approximately 4% of older patients; etiology is unclear.
Gastrointestinal	
Diabetes	Occurs in 8%–15% of patients, with onset during adolescence. Etiology is unknown. It is postulated that insulin deficiency is secondary to fibrosis of the pancreas, which destroys the islet's architecture; usually nonketotic.
Distal intestinal obstruction syndrome equivalent (formally called *meconium ileus equivalent*)	Incidence is 10%–20% of adult CF patients. Usually occurs during adolescence or later. May be partial or complete obstruction; etiology is multifaceted. Intestinal mucoproteins may be more viscous. Enteroglucagon release results from increased undigested fats that slow transit time. A fecal mass forms at the ileocecal region and extends distally.
Cholelithiasis	Occurs in up to 12% of patients and is rarely symptomatic prior to the teenage years. Stones are usually cholesterol. Etiology results from alterations in bile lipid composition.
Liver disease	Occurs in about 4% of patients, peaking in adolescence and decreasing after 20 years of age.
Multilobar cirrhosis	Results from thickened secretions in bile ductules, causing plugging, ductular proliferation, inflammation, and cirrhosis.
Gastroesophageal reflux	Occurrence of symptoms varies. There is a transient, inappropriate relaxation of the lower esophageal sphincter. Contributing factors include positioning, cough, and increased intra-abdominal pressures versus thoracic pressure gradient.
Pancreatitis	Acute pancreatitis occurs in approximately 10% of patients. It can occur with pancreatic sufficiency. It is an inflammatory response. The exact causative mechanism is unclear.
Fibrosing colonopathy	Occurs in a small percentage of patients. Risk factors include age younger than 12 years. There is a strong association with oral pancreatic high-dose enzyme intake for more than 6 months.

Information from Brennan, A. L., Gyi, K. M., Wood, D. M. et al. (2006). Relationship between glycosylated haemoglobin and mean plasma glucose concentration in cystic fibrosis. *Journal of Cystic Fibrosis, 5,* 27–31; Kerem, E., Conway, S., Elborn, S. et al. (2005). Standards of care for patients with cystic fibrosis: A European consensus. *Journal of Cystic Fibrosis, 4,* 7–26.

current chest radiograph with baseline films and spirometry values with prior results.

On physical examination, note the child's overall size, general condition, muscle tone, and muscle mass. Some children with CF may have a protuberant abdomen. Assess the skin for bruising; old surgical scars; and indicators of adequate, excessive, or inadequate fluid balance. Assess the oral mucous membranes, especially of infants, for oral lesions, which may result from CF medications (pancreatic oral enzymes) or from thrush, a fungal superinfection that may be caused by long-term use of oral antibiotics. Thrush may also manifest as candidal vaginitis in the female adolescent or monilial diaper rash in the infant. Examine the rectal area of infants for perirectal irritation from unabsorbed supplemental pancreatic enzymes. Ask questions to elicit a history of a prolapsed rectum. Other history and symptoms that require assessment are irritability and any associated behaviors; emesis; stool pattern (frequency and characteristics); and reports of abdominal pain, discomfort, heartburn, or any combination of symptoms that may indicate gastroesophageal reflux.

The sweat test is the definitive test for CF. An elevated sweat sodium chloride level greater than 60 mEq/L is a positive diagnostic result that should be confirmed by a second test at a CF center (Cystic Fibrosis Foundation, 2011). The sweat sample is usually obtained by stimulating a small patch of sweat glands on the inner aspect of the forearm. An adequate quantity of sweat, at least 50 mg and preferably 100 mg, must be collected to ensure reliable results. Two positive sweat test results and the presence of clinical symptoms or a family history confirm the diagnosis. False-negative skin tests are associated with technical problems (failure to dry skin before collecting sweat; errors in weighing, dilution, elution, or computation) or physiologic factors (inadequate volume secondary to low sweat rate, edema) (Beauchamp & Lands, 2005). Siblings are usually tested when a diagnosis is confirmed.

Interdisciplinary Interventions

The care and treatment of CF is often complex and requires a multidisciplinary approach. Specialized CF centers that meet specific criteria and are accredited by the Cystic Fibrosis Foundation deliver quality care and maintain strict standards of practice. Although most CF centers are directed by pediatric pulmonologists, other pediatric specialists such as gastroenterologists, infectious diseases specialists, geneticists, and endocrinologists also are involved. Additional team members include nurses, advance practice nurses (nurse practitioner or clinical nurse specialist), registered dietitian, respiratory care practitioner, medical social worker, physical therapist, child life specialist, and genetic counselor. As the life expectancy for children with CF increases and more survive into adulthood, pediatric health care teams must foster a "wellness" focus and incorporate planning for adult CF care. Planning for a productive life is the norm.

The family is central to chronic disease management teams. The child should be an active member in the CF care team. Working together, the child, parents, family, and the interdisciplinary team develop individualized management plans to treat the complex needs of the child and family (see the Point for Care Paths). Although each member of the CF care team has specialized knowledge and a clearly defined role, overlap in role functions may occur, depending on the needs of the individual family. The goal of the team is to normalize the lives of the family, maintain existing pulmonary function, and prevent further pulmonary damage so the child can benefit as new treatment options become available.

CROSS-CULTURAL CARE

CF is a condition that primarily affects people of white European genetic background. The CF care team must be sensitive to cultural issues for individuals and families from varying backgrounds. Families may experience a sense of isolation within their cultural environment. Lifestyle practices within certain cultures may affect the care of an infant or child. The CF team members must work to understand these cultural differences and support choices that will support the child's health care maintenance needs. Further research is needed to examine the effects of cultural differences and practices among families on chronic disease management.

Because of the chronic pulmonary infections, activities and lifestyles for children with CF may be altered. For example, *B. cepacia* is extremely communicable among the CF population, so room isolation, limited social interactions with others with CF, and infection control measures are required during hospitalization and community events for children colonized or infected with this organism. For example, the Cystic Fibrosis Foundation has a policy that prohibits anyone with CF and *B. cepacia* from participating at Cystic Fibrosis Foundation–sponsored events. Because of the highly communicable nature of *B. cepacia*, the Cystic Fibrosis Foundation believes this policy enables people with CF who are not infected with *B. cepacia* to more safely participate in its events (Cystic Fibrosis Foundation, 2011).

Medical Management

Medical management of CF is multifaceted. Successful chronic disease management requires complete assessments and routine monitoring of treatments. Therapy for CF has shifted from crisis/exacerbation management to a proactive preventative approach to children with CF (McDonald et al., 2009). A comprehensive annual review, generally conducted at CF centers by the multidisciplinary team, should include assessments such as a full clinical examination and respiratory, nutritional, and psychosocial assessments as well as a critical review of current therapies and treatments. Clinical diagnostic tests during the annual review may include complete blood count including iron status, blood chemistries, microbial cultures, bone density examinations (to evaluate for osteoporosis secondary to poor nutritional intake), and auditory assessments (to evaluate for hearing loss as a result of ototoxic antibiotic therapy). In addition to the annual reviews, documenting overall health maintenance (immunizations, annual influenza vaccine, and adherence history) is important.

For some children with early symptoms of pulmonary exacerbations, treatment may be managed in the home setting with oral antibiotics, aggressive pulmonary therapy, and close follow-up. Hospitalization is required for children who have declining pulmonary status or active infection. Such stays are often called "tune-ups." During the tune-up period, aggressive pulmonary and nutritional therapies are instituted, along with IV antibiotics and an exercise program, and response to these therapies is evaluated. Frequency of aerosol treatments and airway clearance therapies is increased. A daily program to increase or prevent loss of endurance during hospitalization is part of the plan of care. The gastrointestinal therapies include nutritional assessment and evaluation of blood chemistries for nutritional deficits, including measurement of hematocrit, hemoglobin, albumin, prealbumin, and vitamins A and E levels (see "Nutritional Support" section).

Today, with a shift toward ambulatory services, many individuals with CF initiate their tune-ups in the hospital and complete them at home. During the hospital phase, antibiotics are administered as appropriate based on findings from sputum cultures. The shift to home care depends on factors such as severity of illness, venous access, ability and resources of the family (plumbing, electricity, telephone), time/skill to perform ACTs, and payer source (Flume et al., 2009a).

The daily medications required to maintain the baseline health include a long list of pharmaceutical agents (Table 16-12). The Cystic Fibrosis Foundation recommends continuing baseline chronic therapies to treat CF during acute exacerbations and increasing ACTs. There is currently not enough data to recommend for or against continuing inhaled antibiotics if the same medication is being administered intravenously during an exacerbation. Because the most commonly identified organism during a CF exacerbation is *P. aeruginosa*, antibiotic selection is usually targeted toward this organism. It is unclear whether there is benefit to the use of routine corticosteroid therapy during an acute exacerbation (Flume et al., 2009a).

Monitoring all therapies (with laboratory tests, pulmonary function tests, bone density studies, and radiographic studies) and coordinating the team consults are both part of the medical management of CF. Identifying new symptoms that may indicate complications is an ongoing process. Managing CF by intervening promptly when new symptoms occur contributes to improved outcomes.

Nutritional Support

Key components of the nutritional assessment in CF care are to determine baseline nutritional requirements and need for pancreatic enzyme replacement or vitamin therapy and to monitor for changing nutritional needs if comorbidities (e.g., diabetes) develop. Nutritional assessments are conducted at each encounter and hospitalization. Plot physical growth (e.g., height, body mass index) on the growth chart to monitor progress and response to therapeutic interventions. The dietitian assesses physical growth, conducts a nutritional assessment at each admission, identifies dietary requirements and goals, and initiates an overall plan to meet the child's high-caloric nutritional needs. Serum laboratory results such as albumin, prealbumin, glucose, electrolytes, and complete blood count are assessed. Levels of vitamins A and E are assessed annually, and skinfold measurements are obtained as indicated. Guidelines for administering pancreatic enzymes are provided in Nursing Interventions 16-3. Effectiveness of replacement enzymes is monitored through fecal fat studies.

Infants are usually given an elemental formula to optimize absorption. Elemental formulas are composed of simple and easily absorbed forms of carbohydrates (glucose polymers or monosaccharides), proteins (amino acids or casein hydrolysates), and fat as medium-chain triglycerides. Elemental formulas are relatively expensive, and costs may vary across individual pharmacies. Special state-funded programs may provide assistance. Infants may thrive adequately on breast milk or standard infant formula without gastrointestinal complications as long as enzymes are adjusted appropriately. The older child is managed with a high-calorie, high-protein diet, including snacks and nutritional oral supplements to boost calories and nutrition. Pancreatic enzymes are administered at each feeding, meal, and snack to optimize nutrient absorption.

If weight gain and progress toward nutritional goals are not demonstrated, alternate feeding routes are considered. Gastrostomy tubes, (such as percutaneous endoscopic gastrostomy tubes), low-profile ("button") gastrostomies,

TABLE 16-12	Pharmaceutical Agents Used in the Care of the Child With Cystic Fibrosis
Category	**Purpose**
Aerosols Bronchodilators	Relax smooth muscle/open up airways
Inhaled antibiotics	Antimicrobial, for topical lung therapy
Mucolytic enzyme	Thin/loosen mucus
Pancreatic enzymes	Increase food/nutrient absorption
Vitamins/minerals (A, D, E, K)	Fat-soluble vitamin supplement in water-miscible form; supplement overall diet
H₂ blocker	Alter gastrointestinal acidic environment; gastroesophageal reflux therapy
Prokinetic agents	Enhance gastrointestinal motility; gastroesophageal reflux therapy
Oral and IV antibiotics	Antimicrobial for *Streptococcus aureus* Antimicrobial for *Haemophilus influenzae* Antimicrobial for *Pseudomonas aeruginosa*

NURSING INTERVENTIONS 16-3

Administering Pancreatic Enzymes

Recommended dose of lipase: 1,000–3,000 lipase units/kg/meal.

- Encourage three meals and two to three snacks per day.
- Discourage eating throughout the entire day.
- Administer enzymes before or with meals (and with vitamins), with snacks, with milk and oral or bolused nutritional supplements, and before nocturnal feeds begin (and occasionally after completion, as prescribed). Usually, half the standard pancreatic lipase dose is given with snacks.
- Open capsules and mix contents with a small amount of applesauce, rice, carrots, ice cream, or other nonalkaline food. Do not crush microcapsules.

- Avoid allowing microcapsules to sit in alkaline food, which disrupts the enteric coating.
- Assess the oral mucosa and perirectal area for irritation from contact with unswallowed or unabsorbed enzymes.
- Monitor stool pattern and characteristics.
- Be alert to complaints such as bloating, flatus, abdominal pain, loose and frequent stools with steatorrhea, poor growth, or some combination of these symptoms.
- Instruct family and child not to adjust the dose.
- Instruct family and child to check the expiration dates and store enzymes in a cool place.

or jejunostomy tubes (J-tubes) are possible options (see Chapter 18). Nocturnal drip feedings through the gastrostomy tube are recommended to supplement oral intake.

Respiratory Support

A respiratory care practitioner works as part of the interprofessional team. The respiratory care practitioner instructs the families on the most effective ACT, which is individualized to the patient. In general, no one form of ACT has been documented to be superior to another. However, each patient should be evaluated individually for the most effective ACT for that child (Flume et al., 2009b).

Nursing Support

The nurse's primary role is to provide direct care. In the hospital setting, this role is central because the nurse is the person most consistently at the bedside. Coordinating care and monitoring the overall response to therapies (e.g., breathing treatments, self-care participation, activity level, elimination pattern, and appetite) provide essential information to determine progression toward clinical outcomes. The nurse also initiates and maintains IV lines for antibiotic therapy and other IV medications as needed. Measuring accurate height and weight upon admission is essential along with daily weight measurement to monitor nutritional progress. Additionally, the nurse provides emotional support for the child and parent during frequent and long hospitalizations.

The CF team nurse, usually an advanced practice registered nurse, assists in coordinating overall care, ensuring that the team functions smoothly, that roles within the team are understood, and that clinical care is properly coordinated. Important functions include assessing for the need for team and family conferences and education regarding treatment, medicines, options for venous

access, and alternate routes for nutritional supplementation; assessing for home IV antibiotic therapy and discharge readiness; providing follow-up telephone calls to the caregivers and to the schools when indicated; and ensuring continuity of care by providing care at office or clinic visits. This arrangement puts the nurse in a unique position to follow up and provide interventions from an ambulatory and an inpatient perspective. The nurse, in some centers, may be able to perform school visits and assist with school reintegration, if indicated. Early identification and preparation for procedures, including preparation for changes in level of care, are also central to the CF team nurse's role. Additionally, the CF team nurse educates the team and coordinates their involvement when a new diagnosis is made.

Social Services

The medical social worker helps caregivers and children to cope with and integrate CF into their lives. The families are helped to connect with the appropriate state and federal programs for medical care, such as Children's Medical Services (Title V); state Medicaid; Aid to Families with Dependent Children; and Supplemental Security Income for the Aged, Blind, and Disabled. The social worker also is a source of emotional support and provides appropriate referrals as needed. The social worker acknowledges that each family is unique, with individual needs and stresses. Many social workers facilitate support groups and provide parent-to-parent networking.

Physical Therapy

The physical therapist evaluates the muscles used for breathing and posture and assesses the child's ability to carry out daily activities. The physical therapist also prescribes individualized exercise programs and monitors endurance. The roles of the physical therapist and respiratory care practitioner may overlap in certain regions of the country. The child with CF is assessed on a regular basis and is provided a home exercise program.

Child Life Services

The child life specialist's focus of practice is on therapeutic play along with recreational and diversional activities. This professional helps the child cope with hospitalization, medical visits, and procedures through play and can contribute to motivational and behavioral programs to encourage children to do their treatments, drink their nutritional supplements, cooperate with therapy, and take medicines. Some child life departments may offer in-hospital school programs or assist with arrangements for in-home teachers.

Education regarding self-care and ways to integrate CF care into daily schedules is necessary to help the family foster independence and age-appropriate skills of daily living. All too often, the health care team may be so focused on the disease process that lags occur in educating families to integrate developmentally appropriate strategies as a part of the child's care. Each developmental stage merits review with the family and the patient, when age appropriate, to facilitate strategies that will allow this specialized care to be provided daily (Developmental Considerations 16-1). Caregivers must understand concepts such as offering the young child a choice of juice to take with medicines; there is no unacceptable choice and the young child maintains the "control" for mastery of that stage.

Caregivers and patients must also be kept informed regarding changes in condition and updates on expanding and newer therapies. They must be educated when new therapies are introduced for maintenance care, such as oxygen, enteral home nutrition programs, home IV antibiotic administration, home maintenance of venous access devices, administration of aerosolized antibiotics, or the use of newly prescribed medications.

Psychological Support

As part of the interdisciplinary team, psychologists provide invaluable contributions to the CF team. Despite advances in CF care and increasing lifespan of those affected with CF, it continues to be a stressful condition for both the child and family. Both preventative and reactive psychological care are needed during the spectrum of the disease process. Crucial components of the psychologist's role include evaluating the psychological effects of living with disease, providing comprehensive evaluation and intervention when difficulties occur, evaluating the patient and family's resources, and actively facilitating transitions when appropriate (e.g., high school, adult services) (Nobili et al., 2011).

Community Care

CF presents challenges, obstacles, and opportunities that can shape the child's future. For parents, child-rearing roles and responsibilities can be complicated by the increased demands and restrictions imposed by CF (e.g., constant need for daily treatments), numerous contacts with health care services, altered plans for family outings and vacations, fatigue, depression, and, possibly, financial constraints.

Children living with CF must incorporate a variety of treatments into their daily life, and these treatment demands and restrictions can often result in psychological stress and burdens for children and their families. Psychological functioning of the child and family depends on multiple factors, such as family income, family structure, parental education levels, social support, and coping styles. Thus, nurses caring for these children and families must carefully assess for developmental and psychosocial risks.

The general approach for children with CF is to normalize their daily living activities (e.g., home, school, recreational) within the child's specific limitations. Typical childhood events such as a common cold can create substantial problems for the child with CF. Thus, parents need to use strict respiratory infection prevention strategies such as handwashing, isolating the child from people with respiratory or other infections, and isolating the child from others with CF. Provide anticipatory guidance for parents and children as they seek to maintain normalcy in their daily home lives.

For the parents of an infant or child newly diagnosed with CF, the process of adjustment may be compared with the grief process. Parents often have difficulty regaining stability for 6 months to 1 year after diagnosis. Patients and their families may generally function adequately but need additional support during times of crisis. Some examples are the first hospitalization after diagnosis, the death of another child at the CF center, the transition to adult care, addition of new home therapies such as oxygen or IV antibiotics, or the first day of school.

Work closely with school personnel to develop an educational plan that will promote learning and to reduce CF-associated risks. Encourage parents to provide school personnel with information (available through local CF centers) about CF and about their child's specific needs. Parent–teacher conferences at the beginning of each school year are an effective way to provide information and establish communication to reduce the sense of difference the child may feel at school. Encourage school attendance so that the child can socialize and diversify his or her strengths to prepare for future goals. Social isolation because of sporadic school attendance can lead to other psychosocial issues, such as depression.

During adolescence, planning for the future and choosing a career are central tasks. Children must choose careers that will fulfill their ability to work despite changing conditions. Career and vocational counselors can assist in this planning process. Transitional care during the adolescent years, necessary to guarantee lifetime continuity of care, requires close cooperation between the patient's pediatric and adult CF centers. Transition to adult care usually occurs at approximately age 16 to 18 years, but the timing should be determined by the adolescent's social maturity and health status.

The CF team members work in concert with each other, the families, and the children to support a common goal.

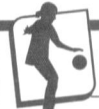

DEVELOPMENTAL CONSIDERATIONS 16-1

Self-Care Strategies for the Child With Cystic Fibrosis

Developmental Stage	Strategies
Infancy	Discuss normal developmental behaviors with parents. Respond to crying promptly (0–3 months). Respond to cues as indicated (>3 months). Establish regular routines. Incorporate special care into routines. Provide reinforcement about PD&P and comfort related to "sensorimotor stimulation." Monitor all developmental progress. Provide recommendations for home schedule/time management. Provide health care teaching: • Disease management • Discuss normal acquisition of developmental skills, especially for first-time, new parent
Early childhood	Discuss normal developmental behaviors with parents. Institute measures to promote age-appropriate behaviors. Assess and monitor feeding behaviors. Support choices for beginning of "daycare"/out-of-home care. Provide information regarding age-appropriate behavioral management. Provide information for self-care skills: • Incorporate distraction techniques for resistant behaviors. • Use games to gain cooperation. Allow child simple choices that are all acceptable. Encourage sharing of care between primary caregivers at home. Assist with integrating therapy schedules into family rituals. Teach coughing secretions "up" and into tissue. Provide information to identify basic symptoms that indicate need for health care team visit. Support exercise as part of ADLs: • Provide opportunities for therapeutic play. • Offer medications in a medicine cup. • Allow child to help gather supplies. • Encourage "blowing" activities, such as bubbles, horns, pinwheels. Provide information on disease management. Provide information for self-care skills: • Assistance with pill swallowing. • Begin PEP therapy (~4 years of age).
Middle childhood	Institute measures to promote age-appropriate behaviors. Assess understanding of • Medications • Nutrition/snacks • Respiratory treatments Provide information for self-care skills: • Assist with pill swallowing. • Allow choices with food/snack selection. Give responsibilities for simple tasks regarding therapies: • Set up nebulizer. • Prepare medications. • Clean nebulizer.

(Continued)

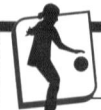

DEVELOPMENTAL CONSIDERATIONS 16-1

Self-Care Strategies for the Child With Cystic Fibrosis *(Continued)*

Developmental Stage	Strategies
	Remind child to initiate ACT time. Have child answer health team's questions. Include child in decision making. Incorporate exercise as part of ADLs: group or solo sports. Encourage use of wind instruments (horns). Coach during PEP/ACT therapy by caregiver. Discuss school performance/attendance and ways to ensure self-care at school. Provide information on disease management.
Adolescence	Institute measures to promote age-appropriate behaviors. Discuss/assess/monitor normal developmental concerns/issues. Provide information to facilitate increased self-care skills: • Self-administer medications, aerosol treatments, snack/meals, ACT. • Take inventory of medications. • Arrange for refills for medications. • Schedule clinic appointments. • Set up nocturnal/daily oxygen and check flow rate. Assess and monitor: • Understanding of disease process • Medication • Problem-solving skills • Current self-care behaviors Provide information on disease management. Encourage and facilitate with individual and caregiver: • Monitoring of self-care by caregiver from afar • Decision for when parental presence is desired at clinic • Involvement in decision making • Negotiation of schedule with special events Support exercise as part of ADLs: • Aerobic and anaerobic • Upper body strengthening • Stretching • Energy conservation techniques Provide information on education and career planning. Facilitate discussion of peer relationships/dating. Discuss transitioning plans (to adult care) and process. Initiate referrals to support choices: • Genetic counseling • Sexuality issues Provide information on insurance and health care systems.

ADLs, activities of daily living; PD&P, postural drainage and percussion.
Developed by Linda Tirabassi. Reprinted with permission of Long Beach Memorial Medical Center, Long Beach, CA.

Because of the complexities and variations of CF, many of the team's functions overlap or may be carried out differently across different centers. Supporting a family through the decision-making process of the end-of-life stage is generally a process shared by all team members but may be the primary responsibility of the clinical social worker. It is also critical for the CF team members to acknowledge the support systems of the family and to consult other professionals, such as pastoral care services or psychologists.

End-of-Life Care

Death can be difficult to predict in individuals with CF. The understanding of the situation by the patient and caregiver should be evaluated throughout the course of the disease. In the terminal stage of the disease, the focus becomes the prevention of unpleasant symptoms, including chronic pain, dyspnea, and anxiety. The patient, family, and health care team should work in concert to provide adequate comfort, analgesia, and anxiolysis. It is important for the family to understand that care does not stop in the terminal stage of disease; rather, the primary aim of management becomes comfort and symptom management. Palliative care intervention provides many benefits, including providing relief from pain, addressing spiritual needs of the patient, support to live life as normally as possible, and support for family and caregivers. Palliative care does not hasten nor prolong death. Because of the difficulty predicting end of life in CF, many patients are receiving active and palliative care modalities in concert. As a result, most patients with CF succumb to their disease in the hospital setting rather than at home. Support for family members and friends can begin prior to death and continue afterward (Sands et al., 2011).

See thePoint for a summary of Key Concepts

REFERENCES

American Academy of Pediatrics. (2011). SIDS and other sleep-related infant deaths: Expansion of recommendations for a safe infant sleeping environment. *Pediatrics*, 128(5), e1342–e1367.

American Academy of Pediatrics. (2012). Diagnosis and management of childhood obstructive sleep apnea syndrome. *Pediatrics*, 130, 576–584.

American Academy of Pediatrics Committee on Infectious Diseases. (2012). Recommendations for prevention and control of influenza in children, 2012–2013. *Pediatrics*, 130(4), 780–792.

American Heart Association. (2011). *Pediatric advanced life support. Provider manual*. Dallas, TX: Author.

American Lung Association. (2010). *State of lung disease in diverse communities: Cystic fibrosis*. Retrieved from http://www.lung.org/assets/documents/publications/solddc-chapters/cf.pdf

American Lung Association. (2011). *Trends in asthma morbidity and mortality*. Retrieved from http://www.lung.org/finding-cures/our-research/trend-reports/asthma-trend-report.pdf

American Lung Association. (2012). *Asthma: Schools*. Retrieved from http://www.lung.org/lung-disease/asthma/becoming-an-advocate/national-asthma-public-policy-agenda/schools.html

Bacharier, L. B., & Strunk, R. C. (2003). Pets and childhood asthma - how should the pediatrician respond to new information that pets may prevent asthma? *Pediatrics*, 112(4), 974–976.

Balaguer, A., Escribano, J., & Roque, M. (2003). Infant position in neonates receiving mechanical ventilation. *Cochrane Database of Systematic Reviews*, (2), CD003668.

Beauchamp, M., & Lands, L. C. (2005). Sweat-testing: A review of current technical requirements. *Pediatric Pulmonology*, 39, 507–511.

Becker, L. A., Hom, J., Villasis-Keever, M. et al. (2011). Beta2-agonists for acute bronchitis. *Cochrane Database of Systematic Reviews*, (4), CD001726.

Beydon, N., Davis, S. D., Lombardi, E. et al. (2007). An official American Thoracic Society/European Respiratory Society statement: Pulmonary function testing in preschool children. *American Journal of Respiratory Critical Care Medicine*, 175, 1304–1345.

Bjornson, C. L., Vandermeer, B., Durec, T. et al. (2011). Nebulized epinephrine for croup in children. *Cochrane Database of Systematic Reviews*, (2), CD006619.

Bombieri, C., Claustres, M., DeBeek, K. et al. (2011). Recommendations for the classification of diseases as CFTR-related disorders. *Journal of Cystic Fibrosis*, 10(Suppl. 2), S86–S102.

Bowden, V., & Greenberg, C. (2012). *Pediatric nursing procedures* (3rd ed.). Philadelphia, PA: Lippincott Williams & Wilkins.

Bradley, J. S., Byington, C. L., Shah, S. S. et al. (2011). The management of community-acquired pneumonia in infants and children older than 3 months of age: Clinical practice guidelines by the pediatric infectious diseases society and the infectious diseases society of America. *Clinical Infectious Diseases*, 53(7), e25–e76.

Centers for Disease Control and Prevention. (2007). *Secondhand smoke*. Retrieved from http://www.cdc.gov/DataStatistics/archive/second-hand-smoke.html

Centers for Disease Control and Prevention. (2011a). CDC Health Disparities and Inequalities Report—United States, 2011. *Morbidity and Mortality Weekly Report*, (60, Suppl.), 1–114.

Centers for Disease Control and Prevention. (2011b). Vital signs: Asthma prevalence, disease characteristics, and self-management education—United States, 2001–2009. *Morbidity and Mortality Weekly Report*, 60(17), 547–552.

Centers for Disease Control and Prevention. (2012). *Common asthma triggers*. Retrieved from http://www.cdc.gov/asthma/triggers.html

Coalson, J. J. (2003). Pathology of new bronchopulmonary dysplasia. *Seminars in Neonatology*, 8, 73–81.

Curley, M. A. Q., Hibberd, P. L., Fineman, L. D. et al. (2005). Effect of prone positioning on clinical outcomes in children with acute lung injury: A randomized controlled trial. *Journal of the American Medical Association*, 294(2), 229–237.

Cystic Fibrosis Foundation. (2011). *What you need to know*. Retrieved from http://www.cff.org/aboutcf/

DeMuri, G. P., & Wald, E. (2012). Acute bacterial sinusitis in children. *New England Journal of Medicine*, 367, 1128–1134.

Don, M., Canciani, M., & Korppi, M. (2010). Community acquired pneumonia in children: What's old? What's new? *Acta Paediatrica*, 99, 1602–1608.

Dougherty, J. M., Kandrak, G., Kinney, Z. et al. (2011). Pediatric tracheostomy and ventilator care. *Spring*, 42–47. Retrieved from http://http://ce.nurse.com/ce131-60/pediatric-tracheostomy-and-ventilator-care/

Edenborough, F. (2001). Women with cystic fibrosis and their potential for reproduction. *Thorax*, 56, 649–655.

Elder, M. A., & Mellon, M. (2008). Long-term inhaled corticosteroid therapy in children and adolescents with persistent asthma: Facilitating adherence to guidelines-based therapy. *The American Journal for Nurse Practitioners*, 12(11–12), 9–18.

Esposito, S., Cohen, R., Domingo, J. D. et al. (2012). Do we know when, what and for how long to treat? Antibiotic therapy for pediatric community-acquired pneumonia. *Pediatric Infectious Disease Journal*, 31(6), e78–e85.

Everard, M. L. (2009). Acute bronchiolitis and croup. *Pediatric Clinics of North America*, 56, 119–133.

Fineman, L. D., LeBrecque, M. A., Shih, M. C. et al. (2006). Prone positioning can be safely performed in critically ill infants and children. *Pediatric Critical Care Medicine*, 7(5), 413–422.

Fitzpatrick, A. M., Kir, T., Naeher, L. P. et al. (2009). Tablet and inhaled controller medication refill frequencies in children with asthma. *Journal of Pediatric Nursing*, 24(2), 81–89.

Flume, P. A., Mogayzel, P. J., Robinson, K. A. et al. (2009a). Cystic fibrosis pulmonary guidelines: Treatment of pulmonary exacerbations. *American Journal of Respiratory and Critical Care Medicine*, 180, 802–808.

Flume, P. A., Robinson, K. A., O'Sullivan, B. P. et al. (2009b). Cystic fibrosis pulmonary guidelines: Airway clearance therapies. *Respiratory Care*, 54(4), 522–537.

Gien, J., & Kinsella, J. P. (2011). Pathogenesis and treatment of bronchopulmonary dysplasia. *Current Opinion in Pediatrics*, 23, 305–313.

Goldrick, B. A., & Goetz, A. M. (2007). Pandemic influenza: What infection control professionals should know. *American Journal of Infection Control*, 35(1), 7–13.

Groothius, J. R., & Makari, D. (2012). Definition and outpatient management of the very low-birth-weight infant with bronchopulmonary dysplasia. *Advances in Therapy*, 29(4), 297–311.

Hall, C. B., Weinberg, M. D., Iwane, M. K. et al. (2009). The burden of respiratory syncytial virus infection in young children. *New England Journal of Medicine*, 360(6), 588–598.

Hayden, M. L., & Womack, C. R. (2007). Caring for patients with allergic rhinitis. *Journal of the American Academy of Nurse Practitioners*, 19(6), 290–298.

Jobe, A. H., & Bancalari, E. (2001). Bronchopulmonary dysplasia. *American Journal of Respiratory and Critical Care Medicine*, 163, 1723–1729.

Kelly, H. W., Sternberg, A. L., Lescher, R. et al. (2012). Effect of inhaled glucocorticoids in childhood on adult height. *New England Journal of Medicine*, 367(10), 904–912.

Kugelman, A., & Durand, M. (2011). A comprehensive approach to the prevention of bronchopulmonary dysplasia. *Pediatric Pulmonology*, 46, 1153–1165.

Loghmanee, D. A., & Sheldon, S. H. (2010). Pediatric obstructive sleep apnea: An update. *Pediatric Annals*, 39(12), 784–789.

McColley, S. A., & Morty, R. E. (2011). Update in pediatric lung disease. *American Journal of Respiratory and Critical Care Medicine*, 186(1), 30–34.

McDonald, C. M., Christensen, N. K., Lingard, C. et al. (2009). Nutrition knowledge and confidence levels of parents of children with cystic fibrosis. *Infant, Child, and Adolescent Nutrition*, 1(6), 325–331.

Miranda, A. D., Valdez, T. A., & Pereira, K. D. (2011). Bacterial tracheitis: A varied entity. *Pediatric Emergency Care*, 27(10), 950–953.

Moore, M., & Little, P. (2006). Humidified air inhalation for treating croup. *Cochrane Database of Systematic Reviews*, 3, CD002870.

Moorman, J., Zahran, H., Truman, B. et al. (2011). Current asthma prevalence—United States, 2006–2008. *Morbidity and Mortality Weekly Report*, 60, 84–86.

Moriette, G., Lescure, S., El Ayoubi, M. et al. (2010). Apnea of prematurity: What's new? *Archives of Pediatrics*, 17(2), 186–190.

Nafiu, O. O., Green, G. E., Walton, S. et al. (2009). Obesity and risk of peri-operative complications in children presenting for adenotonsillectomy. *International Journal of Pediatric Otorhinolaryngology*, 73, 89–95.

National Heart, Lung, and Blood Institute. (2007). *National Asthma Education and Prevention Program expert panel report 3: Guidelines for the diagnosis and management of asthma.* Retrieved from http://www.nhlbi.nih.gov/guidelines/asthma

Nobili, R. M., Duff, A. J. A., Ullrich, G. et al. (2011). Guidelines on how to manage relevant psychological aspects within a CF team: Interdisciplinary approaches. *Journal of Cystic Fibrosis*, 10(Suppl. 2), S45–S52.

Park, I. H., Hong, S. M., & Lee, H. M. (2012). Efficacy and safety of sublingual immunotherapy in Asian children. *International Journal of Otorhinolaryngology*. Advance online publication.

Peterson-Sweeney, K. (2009). The relationship of household routines to morbidity outcomes in childhood asthma. *Journal for Specialists in Pediatric Nursing*, 14(1), 59–69.

Peterson-Sweeney, K., Halterman, J. S., Conn, K. et al. (2010). The effect of family routines on care for inner city children with asthma. *Journal of Pediatric Nursing*, 25, 344–351.

Rance, K., O'Laughlen, M., & Ting, S. (2011). Improving asthma care for African American children by increasing national guideline adherence. *Journal of Pediatric Health Care*, 25(4), 235–249.

Roqué i Figuls, M., Giné-Garriga, M., Granados Rugeles, C. et al. (2012). Chest physiotherapy for acute bronchiolitis in paediatric patients between 0 and 24 months old. *Cochrane Database of Systematic Reviews*, (2), CD004873.

Rowe, S. M., Miller, S., & Sorscher, E. J. (2005). Mechanisms of disease: Cystic fibrosis. *New England Journal of Medicine*, 352, 1992–2001.

Russell, K. R., Liang, Y., O'Gorman, K. et al. (2011). Glucocorticoids for croup. *Cochrane Database of Systematic Reviews*, (1), CD001955.

Salib, R., Harries, P., Nair, S. et al. (2008). Mechanisms and mediators of nasal symptoms in non-allergic rhinitis. *Clinical & Environmental Allergy*, 38, 393–404.

Sampath, V., Garland, J. S., Le, M. et al. (2012). A *TLR5* (g.1174C > T) variant that encodes a stop codon (R392X) is associated with bronchopulmonary dysplasia. *Pediatric Pulmonology*, 47, 460–468.

Sands, D., Repetto, T., Dupont, L. J. et al. (2011). End of life care for patients with cystic fibrosis. *Journal of Cystic Fibrosis*, 10(Suppl. 2), S37–S44.

Schrag, S. J., Shay, D. K., Gershman, K. et al. (2006). Multistate surveillance for laboratory-confirmed, influenza-associated hospitalizations in children: 2003–2004. *Pediatric Infectious Disease Journal*, 25(5), 395–400.

Schuh, S. (2011). Update on management of bronchiolitis. *Current Opinion in Pediatrics*, 23, 110–114.

Scollan-Koliopoulos, M., & Koliopoulos, J. S. (2010). Evaluation and management of apparent life-threatening events in infants. *Pediatric Nursing*, 36(2), 77–83.

Shah, R. K., & Stocks, C. (2010). Epiglottitis in the United States: National trends, variances, prognosis and management. *The Laryngoscope*, 120, 1256–1262.

Shulman, S. T., Bisno, A. L., Clegg, H. W. et al. (2012). Clinical practice guideline for the diagnosis and management of group A streptococcal pharyngitis: 2012 update by the infectious diseases society of America. *Clinical Infectious Diseases*, 55(10), e86–e102.

Stefanovic, I. M., Verona, E., Cicak, B. et al. (2011). No effect of fluticasone propionate on linear growth in preschool children with asthma. *Pediatrics International*, 53(5), 672–676.

Stroustrup, A., & Trasande, L. (2010). Epidemiological characteristics and resource use in neonates with bronchopulmonary dysplasia: 1993–2006. *Pediatrics*, 126(2), e291–e297.

Tebruegge, M., Pantazidou, A., Thorburn, K. et al. (2009). Bacterial tracheitis: A multi-centre perspective. *Scandinavian Journal of Infectious Diseases*, 41, 548–557.

Tregoning, J. S., & Schwarze, J. (2010). Respiratory viral infections in infants: Causes, clinical symptoms, virology, and immunology. *Clinical Microbiology Reviews*, 23(1), 74–98.

Vicencio, A. G. (2010). Susceptibility to bronchiolitis in infancy. *Current Opinion in Pediatrics*, 22, 302–306.

Wallace, D. V., Dykewicz, M. S., Bernstein, D. L. et al. (2008). *Journal of Allergy and Clinical Immunology*, 122(2), S1–S84.

Walsh, B. K., Hood, K., & Merritt, G. (2011). Pediatric airway maintenance and clearance in the acute setting: How to stay out of trouble. *Respiratory Care*, 56(9), 1440–1444.

Wang, K., Shun-Shin, M., Gill, P. et al. (2012). Neuraminidase inhibitors for preventing and treating influenza in children (published trials only). *Cochrane Database of Systematic Reviews*, (4), CD002744.

Wang, T., Li, Y., Ye, Y. Y. et al. (2012). Effects of inhaled corticosteroids on bone age and growth and children with asthma. *Chinese Journal of Contemporary Pediatrics*, *14*(5), 359–361.

Warren, J., Biagioli, F., & Hamilton, A. (2007). Evaluation of apparent life-threatening events in infants. *American Family Physicians*, *76*(1), 124–126.

Zarelli, D. A. (2009). Role-governed behaviors of stepfathers in families with a child with chronic illness. *Journal of Pediatric Nursing*, *24*(2), 90–100.

See thePoint for additional organizations.

CHAPTER 17

The Child With Altered Fluid and Electrolyte Status

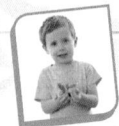

CASE HISTORY

Do you remember Cory Whitworth, the 5-year-old boy from Chapters 6 and 11? In Chapter 11, Cory was diagnosed with a perforated appendix. Upon admission to the emergency department, the nurse begins a health history. His mother reports that he has refused to eat for the past couple of days and has had a fever off and on but was still drinking some fluids. He has been drinking mostly apple juice. She has not taken his temperature with a thermometer but gauged the fever by touch. When asked about his urine output, his mother explained that Cory takes himself to the bathroom. Cory just looked at the nurse when asked how many times he went "pee-pee" yesterday. They do not have a scale at home; Cory was last weighed at the physician's office 2 months ago.

Cory is in pain. He alternates between crying and rocking. His knees are drawn up and he is holding his abdomen.

He is pale and his eyes are somewhat sunken. His lips are dry and cracked and his oral mucous membranes are dry. His vital signs are temperature, 101.8° F (38.8° C); heart rate, 108 bpm; and respiratory rate, 34 breaths/min.

Cory will have emergency surgery because of a ruptured appendix. After surgery, he will not be able to take any oral fluids or food. He may have his stomach decompressed with a nasogastric (NG) tube. (NG tube use is not routine, but it may be placed. It is important that the child and family are taught about this preoperatively.) He will rely on intravenous (IV) solution to maintain his fluid and electrolyte balance.

Consider the following objectives and apply them to Cory from initial assessment through surgical treatment of his perforated appendix.

CHAPTER OBJECTIVES

1 Discuss the physiologic principles that regulate fluid and electrolyte balance.

2 Compare total water distribution, intracellular fluid, and extracellular fluid in infants, children, and adults.

3 Review assessment parameters for a child at risk for fluid or electrolyte imbalance.

4 Identify laboratory tests used to assess fluid and electrolyte balance.

5 Calculate maintenance fluid therapy requirements and identify nursing care priorities for a child receiving intravenous fluid therapy.

6 Discuss nursing care measures for the child receiving parenteral nutrition.

7 Describe the assessment and treatment of hypertonic and hypotonic dehydration.

8 Explain the principles of acid–base balance.

9 Discuss the causes and treatment of specific electrolyte imbalances.

See thePoint for a list of Key Terms.

Water is critical to human survival. Not only is it the primary fluid within the body but it also provides a medium in which body solutes (electrolytes) are dissolved and metabolic reactions occur. Fluid and electrolyte balances can be altered as a result of a disease, injury, or therapeutic intervention that hinders the body's normal physiologic mechanisms for regulating fluid intake and output.

PRINCIPLES OF FLUID AND ELECTROLYTE BALANCE

> **QUESTION:** Has thirst been an adequate regulatory mechanism to keep Cory well hydrated prior to intervention by the health care team?

DISTRIBUTION OF FLUIDS AND ELECTROLYTES

In the human body, water is distributed in two main compartments: **intracellular fluid** (ICF), fluid located within the cells; and **extracellular fluid** (ECF), fluid located outside the cells. ECF is further divided into **intravascular fluid** (fluid within the vascular system, also called *plasma*) and **extravascular fluid** (fluid outside the blood vessels). Extravascular fluid is either **interstitial fluid** (located in the spaces between the tissue cells, such as lymph and pulmonary interstitial spaces) or **transcellular fluid** (located in spaces that are separated from plasma and interstitial fluid by cellular barriers, such as cerebrospinal fluid, synovial fluid). The cell membrane provides a barrier between the ECF and ICF; fluid moves through this barrier by osmosis. Fluid movement between the two ECF compartments occurs through filtration.

Electrolyte concentrations are not uniform; they differ between the ECF and the ICF. Fluid and electrolytes continuously move from one compartment to another. This movement is influenced and controlled by regulatory mechanisms: hydrostatic, osmotic, and oncotic pressure; passive and active transport; diffusion; and osmosis (see thePoint for Supplemental Information). To illustrate the concept of movement and transportation between compartments, consider this example: Sodium is the principal cation in ECF; potassium is the principal cation in ICF. To maintain equilibrium between sodium and potassium concentrations, water moves from ICF to ECF through passive transport mechanisms. Maintaining this equilibrium is a continuous, ongoing process.

REGULATORY MECHANISMS

Several physiologic mechanisms regulate fluid and electrolyte homeostasis in the body.

The Kidneys

The kidneys regulate fluid balance through their ability to concentrate and dilute urine. Antidiuretic hormone, a hormone produced by the hypothalamus and stored in the pituitary gland, stimulates renal reabsorption of water. When serum sodium levels are high, antidiuretic hormone is secreted and increases the permeability of the kidneys' distal tubules and collecting ducts to water, enabling the kidneys to retain more water.

The angiotensin–renin system, along with aldosterone, also assists the kidneys in regulating fluid and electrolyte homeostasis. When the kidneys detect reduced blood flow, they produce renin, which in turn stimulates production of angiotensin within the blood vessels. The angiotensin stimulates release of aldosterone, a hormone that stimulates sodium reabsorption. As a result, sodium and water reabsorption is increased in the renal tubules. This mechanism produces (1) increased blood flow to the kidney, (2) increased intravascular volume, and (3) increased blood pressure.

The Gastrointestinal Tract

The gastrointestinal tract affects the electrolyte levels of gastrointestinal secretions. Water and sodium are reabsorbed and potassium is excreted. Normally, fluid is replaced through oral fluid intake. Because of the large absorptive surface area of the gastrointestinal tract, changes in fluid and electrolyte balances can occur rapidly. Imbalances must be treated quickly and appropriately to prevent decompensation in the child's health status.

Thermoregulatory Mechanism

Insensible water loss refers to invisible, continuous, and passive water loss from the skin and lungs resulting from heat expenditure. This process is one method that the body uses to regulate temperature. No electrolytes are lost or excreted in insensible water loss.

The integumentary system, as a thermoregulatory mechanism, affects fluid and electrolyte balances. Losses of fluid, sodium, potassium, and chloride (Cl^-) occur in sweat. In contrast to insensible water loss, this process is intermittent and is more dependent on environmental temperature.

Thirst Mechanism

Most regulatory mechanisms involve the excretion of fluid and electrolytes. The exception is thirst, the impetus to ingest water. The thirst center is located in the hypothalamus; thirst is stimulated by a decrease in the intravascular volume, an increase in the osmolality of ECF, or both. As a major regulatory mechanism, thirst is unreliable. The infant and young child can experience thirst but have a limited ability to take action to meet this need. They depend on others to provide oral fluids and to appropriately regulate the type and amount of fluid intake.

> **ANSWER:** Thirst has not been an adequate regulatory mechanism as evidenced by the fact that Cory is moderately dehydrated. Despite the fact that he is old enough to communicate his thirst or even go get a cup of water, the combination of fever, abdominal pain, and anorexia he experienced was enough to allow him to become dehydrated.

DEVELOPMENTAL AND BIOLOGIC VARIANCES

Infants and children are more susceptible than adults to fluid and electrolyte imbalances (Fig. 17-1). In an infant, for example, a high basal metabolic rate makes the normal turnover rate of water and electrolytes two to three times faster than in an adult. Approximately 50% of ECF in the infant is exchanged each day. This fact makes an infant more susceptible to substantial physical changes from fluid deficit.

The amount of total body water and the proportional sizes of the ICF and ECF compartments change from infancy to adolescence (Fig. 17-2). Infants and young children have a high proportion of total body water, stemming from a high proportion of ECF and low total body fat. Total body fat increases dramatically during the first year of life, with a concurrent decrease in the amount of total body water. During the first year of life, total body water decreases to about 60% of body weight. This proportion remains fairly constant until adolescence, when characteristic sex differences occur. Normally, males have greater muscle mass and less body fat than females. Therefore, the sexually mature male has about 60% total body water, the female, about 55%.

ASSESSMENT

Disease, age, environment, and activity level all affect fluid and electrolyte status. Imbalances in fluids and electrolytes are reflected in many body systems. Thus, assessment of a child with a known or suspected fluid or electrolyte imbalance requires a multisystem evaluation.

FOCUSED HEALTH HISTORY

QUESTION: Study Focused Health History 17-1. Which of the items identified apply to Cory? Discuss those areas where gaps in the health history provided by the parent and child would be frustrating to health care workers.

Health history pertinent to fluid and electrolyte status includes current and previous illnesses, health habits, and fluid intake and output (Focused Health History 17-1).

Intake and output affect fluid and electrolyte balance profoundly. In the health history, include questions about the amount as well as the type of fluids

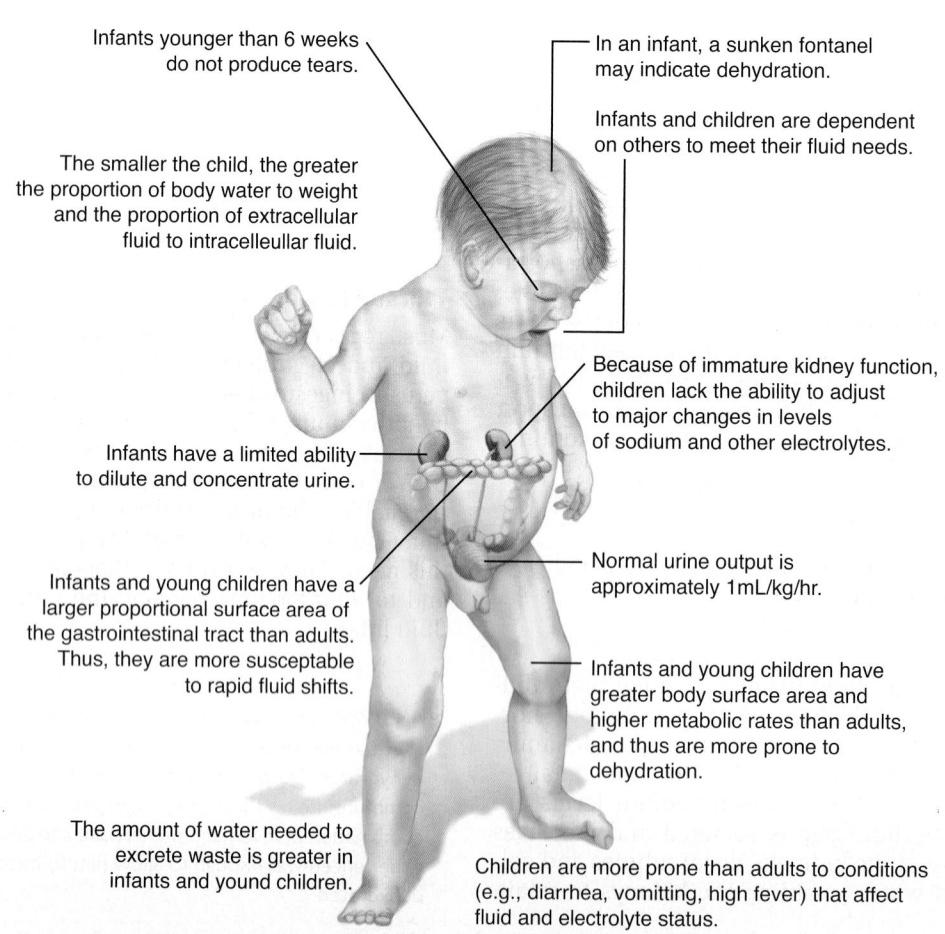

Infants younger than 6 weeks do not produce tears.

The smaller the child, the greater the proportion of body water to weight and the proportion of extracellular fluid to intracelleullar fluid.

Infants have a limited ability to dilute and concentrate urine.

Infants and young children have a larger proportional surface area of the gastrointestinal tract than adults. Thus, they are more susceptable to rapid fluid shifts.

The amount of water needed to excrete waste is greater in infants and yound children.

In an infant, a sunken fontanel may indicate dehydration.

Infants and children are dependent on others to meet their fluid needs.

Because of immature kidney function, children lack the ability to adjust to major changes in levels of sodium and other electrolytes.

Normal urine output is approximately 1mL/kg/hr.

Infants and young children have greater body surface area and higher metabolic rates than adults, and thus are more prone to dehydration.

Children are more prone than adults to conditions (e.g., diarrhea, vomitting, high fever) that affect fluid and electrolyte status.

Figure 17-1 Developmental and biologic variances: fluid and electrolyte status.

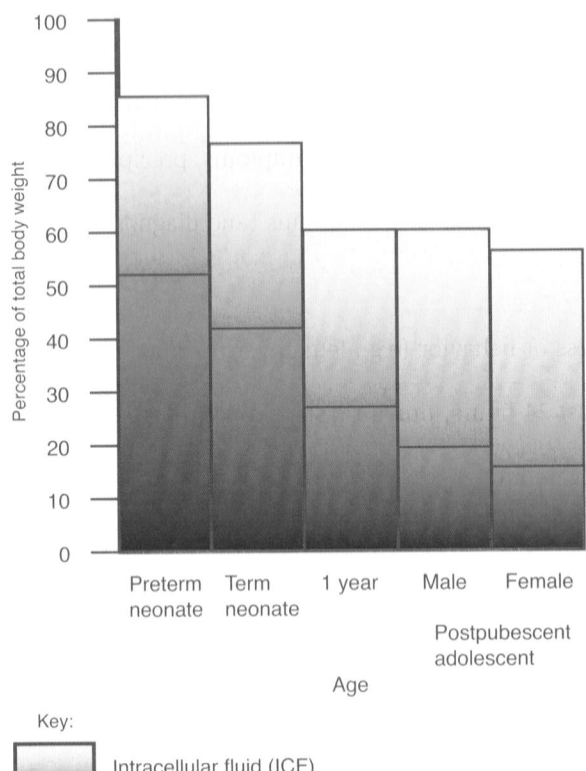

Figure 17-2 Total body water distribution by age. Note the changes in intracellular and extracellular fluid volume.

ingested. Also investigate fluid intake carefully to uncover possible causes of imbalance. For instance, feeding an infant formula prepared with too much water, either as a cost-saving measure or through error, may lead to water intoxication. Conversely, feeding formula prepared with too little water (which results in a formula with high osmolality that pulls water into the gut) can lead to dehydration and electrolyte imbalance. An older child or an adolescent with an eating disorder (i.e., anorexia or bulimia) may also have insufficient fluid intake and thus be at risk for severe, possibly life-threatening, electrolyte imbalances.

Major routes of fluid output are urine, stool, and vomiting. To assess voiding patterns, ask the parent how many wet diapers the infant or young child has each day, and ask an older child how often he or she voids.

KidKare When asking a child about output patterns, clarify the type of output using terms that the child and family use for *urine* and *stool*.

Ask about potential exposure to poisons or toxins, which can interfere with cellular function and metabolism, leading to fluid and electrolyte imbalances.

ANSWER: Children in early childhood are notoriously poor historians and this is frustrating for health care workers. They have the skills to take food and drink and go to the bathroom by themselves but not to report those activities accurately. Aspects of the Focused Health History with regard to current history that can be applied to Cory include no appetite but some drinking for 3 or more days; presence of fever, but no specific temperatures; undetermined weight loss; and undetermined number of voidings the previous day. It is to be expected that the health history from this age group is lacking specifics, and nurses should not belabor the fact and make the parents feel inadequate.

FOCUSED PHYSICAL ASSESSMENT

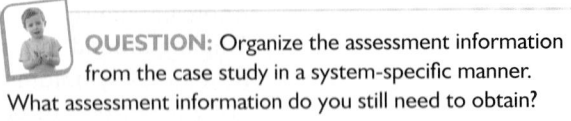

QUESTION: Organize the assessment information from the case study in a system-specific manner. What assessment information do you still need to obtain?

Physical assessment for a child with altered fluid and electrolyte status includes a general survey and a system-specific examination that focuses on level of hydration (Focused Physical Assessment 17-1). The general survey evaluates the child's appearance and level of distress. It always includes weighing the child and comparing the result with previous recent weights, if available. Any substantial fluid loss or gain will be reflected in weight changes.

Fluid deficit may compromise peripheral perfusion and cause insufficient blood flow to the brain, as reflected in changes in vital signs and level of consciousness. The child may report dizziness when standing up after lying down. Electrolyte imbalance may also cause altered vital signs and level of consciousness as well as more system-specific findings (e.g., impaired muscle function). Specific vital sign changes point to the type and degree of imbalance. For example, temperature elevation typically occurs in hypernatremia (sodium excess) because hypernatremia causes excessive fluid loss, making less water available for heat loss through sweating. Note the child's temperature. Fever, which increases metabolic rate, increases the rate of fluid loss.

ALERT *Because a child's young, healthy blood vessels normally compensate well in response to decreased fluid volume, decreased blood pressure is an ominous, late sign of fluid volume deficit.*

Skin turgor is an indication of fluid status. To evaluate skin turgor, gently lift the child's abdominal skin between the thumb and forefinger, then release. Skin that does not return to its original shape but stays raised or "tented" indicates poor turgor.

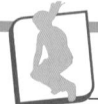

The Child With Altered Fluid and Electrolyte Status

Current history	When symptoms started and duration and nature of symptoms, precipitating factors, and home management of current illness
	Recent contact with someone who is sick; their symptoms (and diagnosis, if known)
	Recent weight change
	Fever, diaphoresis
	Change in level of consciousness or behavior (e.g., lethargy, irritability, weakness), headaches
	Number of voidings during past 24 hours; time of last void/wet diaper, urine amount, color, odor
	Stool appearance, consistency, amount
	Anorexia, nausea, vomiting, or abdominal pain
	Tingling around mouth, in fingertips, or hands (reported with hypocalcemia)
	Relation of symptoms to food ingestion
	Presence of sore throat or oral lesions that interfere with intake
	Exposure to high environmental temperatures
	All medications (e.g., diuretics, digitalis, potassium supplements), home remedies (e.g., teas, herbs), vitamins, or food supplements the child is currently receiving
	Known or possible ingestion of or exposure to poisons
Past medical history	**Prenatal/Neonatal History**
	Presence of congenital defects, especially those involving the gastrointestinal or genitourinary systems
	Previous Health Challenges
	Recurrent, chronic, or episodic illness; hospitalization or surgery and child's response
Nutritional assessment	Time the child last ate; type of food or fluid and amount ingested
	Is the child retaining food and fluid?
	Describe typical intake of food and fluid type, how prepared, frequency, and quantity; for infants or young children, include whether intake is by bottle, breast, or cup; if breastfed, note any change in mother's diet; if a commercial formula is used, note formulation (e.g., ready-to-feed, powder) and how formula is prepared (dilution amounts)
	Change in the child's appetite or oral intake; is the child complaining of thirst?
Family medical history	History of same illness in other family members (describe symptoms and any treatments)
Social and environmental history	Psychosocial: financial status, issues regarding obtaining adequate food supply, sanitation for food storage and preparation
	Child care issues: who cares for child and where (e.g., child care center, home)
	Cultural: practices that may overheat infants (e.g., wrapping in blankets even in hot temperatures), administration of home remedies that may cause fluid or electrolyte imbalance
Growth and development	Daily routines and habits: sleeping, feeding, toileting

Note: See Chapter 8 for a comprehensive health history.

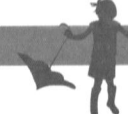

FOCUSED PHYSICAL ASSESSMENT 17-1

Altered Fluid and Electrolyte Status

Assessment Parameter	Alterations/Clinical Significance
General appearance	Level of distress associated with degree of alteration
	Weight change over time: if the child is not following growth trajectory as plotted on growth charts, weight loss or failure to gain weight may indicate malnutrition; rapid weight loss may indicate fluid volume deficit; rapid weight gain may indicate fluid volume excess
Integumentary system	Pale, ashen, mottled, or cyanotic skin, nail beds, or mucous membranes; diaphoresis; delayed capillary refill (>3 seconds); decreased skin temperature may indicate poor perfusion associated with fluid volume deficit
	Increased skin temperature may be seen with hypernatremia; also may indicate fever, which increases insensible water loss
	Dry skin and mucous membranes, poor turgor, tenting, sunken eyeballs, absence of tears associated with fluid deficit
	Doughlike feel to skin seen with hypernatremic dehydration
	Edema can be seen with fluid volume excess
	Excoriated anal and diaper area from diarrheal stools
Thorax and lungs	Change in respiratory rate and quality:
	• Slow and shallow seen with hypochloremia
	• Deep and rapid seen with moderate and severe dehydration
	• Tachypnea increases insensible water loss
	Moist breath sounds (crackles) and cough associated with fluid volume excess
Cardiovascular system	Change in pulse rate or quality:
	• Rapid, weak, thready with fluid deficit
	• Bounding pulse, neck vein distention with fluid volume excess
	Gallop rhythm with fluid volume excess
	Dysrhythmias associated with electrolyte imbalance (hyper- and hypokalemia)
	Elevated blood pressure may be seen with fluid volume excess
	Decreased blood pressure seen with fluid volume deficit
Abdomen	Abdominal distention (hypokalemia, in neonate associated with hypocalcemia)
	Hepatomegaly with fluid volume excess
	Abnormal peristaltic waves seen with pyloric stenosis, which can result in hypochloremic alkalosis
Neurologic system	Change in level of consciousness: unresponsiveness, irritability, lethargy, confusion associated with fluid volume deficit and electrolyte imbalance (sodium, calcium, magnesium, phosphate)
	Weak, high-pitched cry associated with hypernatremia
	Sunken or bulging fontanel in infant may indicate fluid deficit or excess
	Change in muscle tone: hyperreflexia (hypomagnesemia), weakness or flaccidity (hyper- and hypokalemia, hypercalcemia, hypermagnesemia); tetany or positive Chvostek sign (i.e., facial twitching as the facial nerve is tapped) (hypocalcemia)

Electrolytes play a vital role in cellular metabolism and neuromuscular function. Electrolyte imbalances may produce neurologic symptoms, muscle cramps, increased or decreased muscle tone, and hypoactive or hyperactive reflexes.

ANSWER: Organize Cory's assessment data as follows:

- Integumentary system: pale, dry lips and oral mucous membranes; sunken eyeballs
- Thorax and lungs: increased respiratory rate
- Cardiovascular: increased heart rate
- Neurologic: irritable

Also obtain vital signs, including heart and respiratory rates, blood pressure, and temperature, and obtain a weight. Checking and noting skin turgor and capillary refill can be quickly accomplished. Monitor for changes in pulse rate or quality and other vital signs and neurologic changes.

DIAGNOSTIC CRITERIA

Diagnostic tests assist in evaluating fluid and electrolyte balance in the body (Tests and Procedures 17-1). Nursing responsibilities related to diagnostic studies include obtaining specimens, accurately labeling and sending specimens to the laboratory, and following up on results. Follow-up involves evaluating results and notifying the physician or advanced practice nurse of values outside normal age-appropriate ranges.

TREATMENT MODALITIES

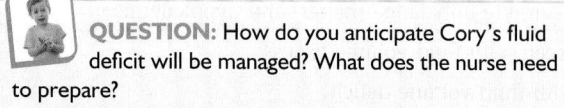

QUESTION: How do you anticipate Cory's fluid deficit will be managed? What does the nurse need to prepare?

Alterations in fluid and electrolyte balance are managed by correcting the specific imbalance (e.g., giving fluid when the child is dehydrated) and treating the underlying cause (e.g., controlling diarrhea). Whenever possible, fluid and electrolyte imbalances are treated with oral fluid ingestion. When oral fluids cannot be given, IV fluids or enteral or parenteral nutrition (PN) must be administered to meet the child's fluid, electrolyte, and nutrition needs. Enteral feeding may be possible when oral is not and is physiologically superior and preferred over parenteral feeding.

INTRAVENOUS THERAPY

IV therapy is used in clinical situations that require administration of fluids (and sometimes medications) to a child who cannot maintain a normal fluid balance by oral ingestion. The route, volume, and type of fluid administration are key factors in managing the child

receiving IV therapy. See Evidence-Based Clinical Practice Guideline 17-1 for guidelines pertinent to IV therapy.

Route of Administration

IV fluids can be given by peripheral vein, central vein, or intraosseous access. The route of fluid administration depends on the child's clinical situation, the type of fluids and medications administered, and the duration of IV fluid therapy. In addition, the potential for **infiltration** (inadvertent escape of nonvesicant fluids or medications from the IV tubing or vein into subcutaneous tissues) or **extravasation** (inadvertent escape of vesicant fluids or medications, typically chemotherapeutic agents, from the IV tubing or vein into subcutaneous tissues) must be minimized because some agents can cause tissue damage.

Peripheral Venous Access

Peripheral IV lines are used for short-term administration of fluids and medications that are isotonic and not irritants or **vesicants** (agents that produce tissue blistering). Potential sites of peripheral IV catheter placement include the scalp (in infants), dorsum of the hand, arm (including the antecubital fossa), foot, and leg. Factors considered in determining placement site include the child's age and condition, comfort, safety, measures required to position or secure the IV line, and condition of the vein (see thePoint for Procedures). In infants, for instance, the scalp veins generally are easier to cannulate than extremity veins, so they are sometimes used. Many parents find a scalp IV line in their infant quite distressing. Discuss the scalp placement procedure, including the rationale, with the parents before placing the IV line and offer to save for them any hair that is shaved from the infant.

Preferably, position the child upright for IV starts. Children in early childhood who were held upright by a parent during IV starts demonstrated lower distress, and parents were more satisfied than when the IV was started with the child in a supine position (Sparks et al., 2007). When placing IV lines in extremities, access the most distal sites first. Do not use the antecubital fossa until other sites have been exhausted. A catheter in the antecubital region, or any joint, is easily disturbed by joint flexion, and the immobilization required may cause joint stiffness and pain. Allow an older child a choice of catheter placement sites, as appropriate. If the arm is used, use the nondominant one when possible; in an ambulatory child, avoid using the feet or legs if possible.

KidKare If it is necessary to secure an IV line with an arm board, tell the child that the arm board is there to help him or her remember not to move that arm too much.

When a peripheral IV line is needed for intermittent administration of medication but is not required for continuous IV fluid administration, an IV lock may

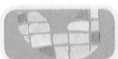 **TESTS AND PROCEDURES for Evaluating Altered Fluid and Electrolyte Status**

Diagnostic Test or Procedure	Purpose	Findings/Indications	Health Care Provider Considerations
Blood chemistry/ electrolyte analysis (Na^+, K^+, Ca^{++}, Cl^-, Mg^{++}, PO_4^-, albumin, blood urea nitrogen [BUN], creatinine)	Analyzes various chemical components of blood	Few disorders produce a single abnormality; several components are usually analyzed to detect a pattern of abnormal results that may point to a disorder. Na^+, K^+, and Cl^- help maintain osmotic pressure and acid–base balance. • Hyponatremia associated with severe diarrhea, vomiting, edema • Hypernatremia associated with dehydration • Hypokalemia associated with diarrhea, severe vomiting • Hyperkalemia associated with renal disease, massive cell damage, acidosis • Hypoproteinemia results in decreased Ca^{++} levels • Hypoalbuminemia often results in edema • Increased BUN leads to kidney disease, shock, dehydration • Decreased BUN leads to negative nitrogen balance and overhydration	Obtain specimens correctly. Get free flow of blood because, when hemolyzed, cells break, releasing potassium, resulting in elevated K^+ levels and an inaccurate analysis of actual serum K^+ values. Do not draw blood from same extremity in which an IV line is infusing. Provide psychological and physical support when specimen is obtained; use topical anesthetic when possible. Evaluate results based on patterns of findings, including child's symptoms.
Blood hemoglobin (Hgb) and hematocrit (Hct)	Measures Hgb, the main component of erythrocytes, which are the vehicle for transporting oxygen and carbon dioxide; and Hct, the concentration of erythrocytes in plasma. Hgb is important buffer in blood; helps maintain acid–base balance.	Increased Hgb and Hct lead to ECF volume decrease (decrease in blood loss) and hyperosmolar fluid imbalance. Decreased Hgb and Hct lead to ECF volume excess and hypoosmolar fluid imbalance.	Support child when obtaining specimen. Put blood in correct tube and label specimen accurately. Ensure that results are obtained in a timely manner.
Arterial blood gases	Assesses acid–base status	Based on uncompensated values: • Low pH: acidosis • High pH: alkalosis • Decreased PCO_2: respiratory alkalosis • Increased PCO_2: respiratory acidosis • Decreased bicarbonate (HCO_3^-) plus base excess: metabolic acidosis • Increased HCO_3^- plus base excess: metabolic alkalosis	Use local anesthetic; specimen collection is painful. Maintain pressure over puncture site with two fingers for minimum of 2 minutes, longer if child has bleeding problems. Expel air bubbles in syringe. Place sample on ice if not immediately analyzed.

(Continued)

 **TESTS AND PROCEDURES** for Evaluating Altered Fluid and Electrolyte Status *(Continued)*

Diagnostic Test or Procedure	Purpose	Findings/Indications	Health Care Provider Considerations
Urine specific gravity	Measures kidney's ability to dilute and concentrate urine	Normal values: neonate, 1.001–1.020; older than 1 month of age, 1.001–1.030 Low specific gravity may indicate fluid excess or kidney disease. High specific gravity may indicate fluid deficit, the presence of glucose, large amounts of protein; radiographic contrast media elevate results.	Evaluate findings in relation to age (infants do not concentrate urine well, so they usually have low readings) and confounding factors (e.g., if a child with diabetes is spilling glucose in urine, the specific gravity does not accurately reflect hydration status).
Urine osmolality	More exact measure of urine concentration than specific gravity	Normal value: 50–1,400 mOsm/kg H_2O, depending on fluid intake Normal value after 12-hour fluid restriction: >850 mOsm/kg H_2O	Evaluate findings in relation to age and confounding factors.
Urine pH	Measures acidity/alkalinity of urine; reflects ability of renal tubules to maintain normal H^+ concentration in plasma and ECF	Varies widely with kidney function, average pH = 6 Acidic urine (pH <7): high-protein diet or acidosis (e.g., diarrhea, dehydration, respiratory disease, uncontrolled diabetes) Alkaline urine (pH >7): vegetarian diets and those high in citrus fruits and dairy products; diseases associated with hyperventilation, urinary tract infection, or chronic renal failure	Obtain freshly voided specimen for most accurate results; otherwise, refrigerate specimen.
Stool analysis	Evaluates stool for consistency, color, odor, absence or presence of blood, mucus, food residue, tissue fragments, bacteria, and parasites	Diet influences color; normal brown color is the result of the breakdown of bile; if passage is rapid (e.g., diarrhea), stool may be yellow or green (normal findings in breastfed infant). Consistency may indicate amount of water loss. Characteristics may help diagnose disease—for example, diarrhea with mucus and blood (typhus, cholera, amebiasis), diarrhea with mucus and pus (ulcerative colitis, shigellosis, salmonellosis).	Obtain fresh stools to provide the most accurate results; warm stools are best for ova and parasite detection. Avoid testing stool contaminated with urine or toilet bowl water.

be used (see thePoint for Procedures). Catheter gauge, the child's diagnosis, the medication administered, the flush solution used, and the length of time between flushes are all variables that affect longevity of the IV site. The evidence is not definitive on whether to use heparin or saline solution to flush the IV lock (Tradition or Science 17-1). Follow facility-specific protocols for

maintaining IV locks, which are based on patient population and standards of practice in the community.

Central Venous Access

Central venous catheters (CVCs) are catheters that are inserted into the superior or inferior vena cava (Fig. 17-3). The umbilical vein may be used in an infant

EVIDENCE-BASED CLINICAL PRACTICE GUIDELINES 17-1

Intravenous Therapy

Infusion Nurses Society. (2011). *Infusion Nursing Standards of Practice.* Retrieved from
http://www.ins1.org/i4a/pages/index.cfm?pageID=3310

Presents specific, evidence-based guidelines on all aspects of IV therapy.

O'Grady, N. P., Alexander, M., Burns, L. A. et al. (2011). *Guidelines for the prevention of intravascular catheter-related infections, 2011.* Retrieved from
http://www.cdc.gov/hicpac/pdf/guidelines/bsi-guidelines-2011.pdf

Provides guidelines for care to prevent IV catheter–associated infections to reduce the incidence of infections associated with intravascular therapy.

Mermel, L. A., Allon, M., Bouza, E. et al. (2009). Clinical practice guidelines for the diagnosis and management of intravascular catheter-related infection: 2009 update by the Infectious Diseases Society of America.* *Clinical Infectious Diseases, 49,* 1–45. Retrieved from
http://cid.oxfordjournals.org/content/49/1/1.full.pdf+html

Provides guidelines for care of patients with IV catheter–associated infections or those at risk for such infections.

*See erratum at http://cid.oxfordjournals.org/content/50/3/457.full.pdf+html

---

Evidence-Based Practice
TRADITION OR SCIENCE 17-1

What flush solution should be used to lock peripheral IV catheters in children?

Saline flush has been demonstrated to be sufficient to maintain patency in IV lines that are larger than 24 gauge (Hanrahan et al., 1994; Randolph et al., 1998; Shah et al., 2005). When smaller than 24-gauge catheters were used, some studies found heparin more effective in maintaining patency of the line (Danek & Noris, 1992; Kleiber et al., 1993; Mudge et al., 1998; Schultz et al., 2002; Treas & Latinis-Bridges, 1992); others found no difference between heparin and saline (Arnts et al., 2011; Hanrahan et al., 2000; Heilskov et al., 1998; Kotter, 1996; Paisley et al., 1997). Cook et al. (2011) and Goldberg et al. (1999) found that saline prolonged catheter longevity for 24-gauge catheters. In studying 22- and 24-gauge catheters (the vast majority were 24 gauge), Mok et al. (2007) found no differences in catheter longevity and incidence of IV complications between saline, 1 unit heparin/mL, and 10 units heparin/mL. They suggest that catheter longevity may be the result of using a positive-pressure flush technique and not the type of solution. While the data is not consistent and is insufficient to make definitive recommendations for type of flush solution for 24-gauge catheters, the evidence is strengthening in support of use of saline.

Use preservative-free saline and heparin for neonates because neonates are not able to metabolize preservatives well. This inability may result in the accumulation of toxic amounts, a condition called *gray baby syndrome* or *gasping syndrome* that presents as metabolic acidosis, lethargy, and hypotension. The most common preservative is benzyl alcohol, an antibacterial agent that is used in many medications.

during the first few days after birth. CVCs are used in situations that require long-term venous access. They are particularly good for administering medications that are irritating to peripheral vessels, antineoplastic agents, blood and blood components, and for obtaining blood samples. They should be used to administer fluids with high dextrose concentrations (>10%), hyperosmolar solutions (>600 mOsm/L), and medications with pH of <5 or >9 (Infusion Nurses Society, 2011). Generally, CVCs are classified as nontunneled, tunneled, implanted ports, or peripherally inserted central catheters (PICCs).

Nontunneled Catheters

Nontunneled catheters are generally used for short-term central access in the acute care setting. They are placed percutaneously, usually into the femoral,

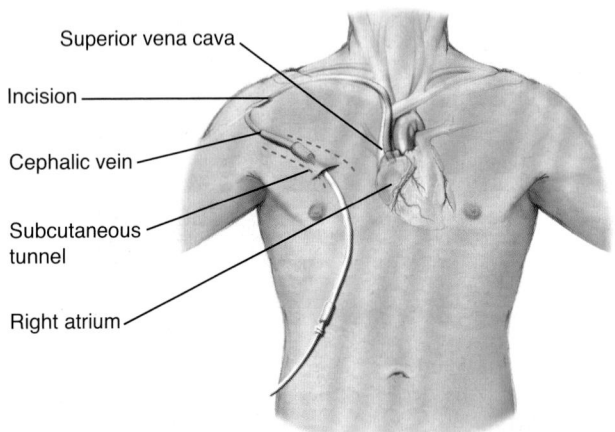

Figure 17-3 Position of a tunneled CVC in the superior vena cava. Note that the skin insertion site is a distance from the vein entry site, with the catheter being tunneled under the skin for this distance.

subclavian, or jugular vein, using local anesthesia and sedation or general anesthesia. Because of the insertion method (direct puncture into a large vein, not tunneled under the skin), nontunneled catheters carry a greater risk than tunneled catheters of becoming dislodged or infected.

Tunneled Catheters

Broviac, Hickman, and Groshong are some brand names of catheters that are *tunneled* beneath the skin for several inches (the tunnel may be shorter in infants and young children) from the skin exit site to the vein insertion point (Fig. 17-4) (see thePoint for Procedures). These catheters have a Dacron cuff situated under the skin 1 to 2 in. proximal to the exit site, which secures the catheter and reduces the risk of infection by blocking the migration of pathogens from the skin along the catheter tunnel to the central circulation. General anesthesia is required to place tunneled catheters in children. Broviac and Hickman catheters, when not used for infusion, require a heparin flush after each use or at least once daily. Check facility and manufacturer's recommendations. A Groshong catheter requires a saline flush. Participation in contact sports may be limited for a child with a tunneled catheter.

Implantable Ports

Implantable ports (e.g., Port-A-Cath, Infuse-A-Port) are surgically placed under the skin of the arm or chest and sutured to the muscle wall with the child under general anesthesia. No part of the port is external. Implantable ports have a self-sealing silicon septum (which can be palpated under the skin) enclosed in a metallic or plastic chamber. This chamber provides a reservoir that connects to a large central vein by means of a Silastic catheter. The port is accessed with deflected-tip (Huber-type), noncoring needles to prevent leakage (see thePoint for Procedures). Patients generally report that accessing the port with a needle is less traumatic than venipuncture, although some children still react negatively to the needle stick associated with port access. To make port access more

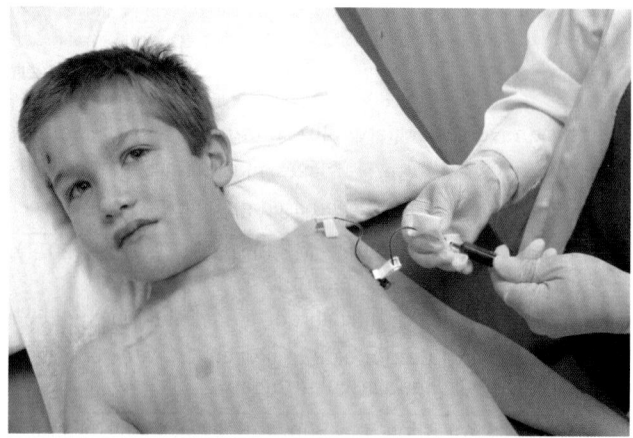
Figure 17-5 Implanted ports are accessed with special noncoring needles, and a semipermeable dressing is used when the port is accessed for continuous infusions.

tolerable, topical anesthetic can be used. To insert the needle, palpate the skin over the port to identify the septum. Needles can be left in place for a maximum of 7 days (Fig. 17-5). The port should be flushed with heparin to maintain patency. Because an implanted port is placed under the skin, it is less visible than other catheters and may affect body image less negatively, although body image may still be altered. When the site has healed after placement, the child usually has few restrictions on activity, although contact sports usually are discouraged.

Peripherally Inserted Central Catheters

A PICC line (Fig. 17-6) is inserted peripherally by means of a percutaneous puncture. It is generally inserted above the antecubital fossa into the basilic or cephalic vein and is threaded into the superior vena cava (see thePoint for Procedures). In infants, other sites may be used. A PICC line is a good choice for the child who requires antibiotic therapy for a period of weeks up to a year. Insertion is usually performed under local anesthesia combined with sedation. However, in infants,

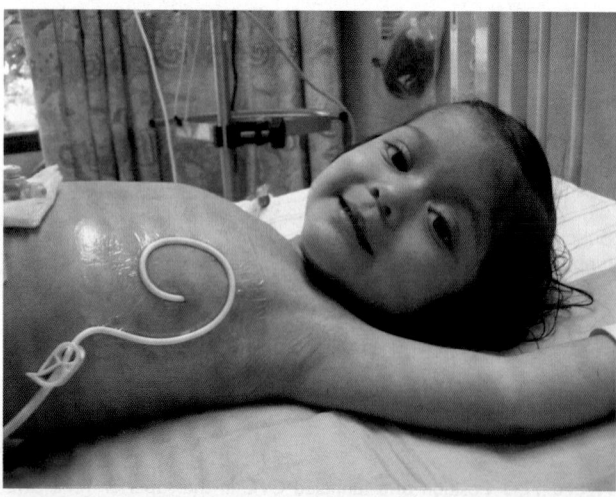
Figure 17-4 Although a tunneled CVC can be hidden under clothing, it often has a negative effect on body image.

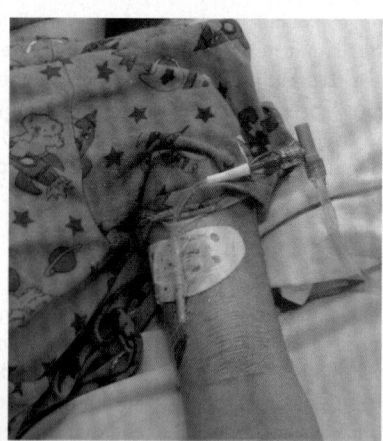
Figure 17-6 A PICC line in place. Use caution not to displace the catheter; note the securement device to assist with this.

local anesthesia often causes the vessels to constrict; thus, IV sedation and analgesia may be given before PICC insertion. A PICC line is often not sutured in place. Although Graf et al. (2006) found that complications are fewer with sutures versus tape, a review of the literature evidenced that the rate of complications was lower with use of a securement device (Frey & Schears, 2006). Use extreme caution during dressing changes to avoid displacing the catheter.

Complications of Central Venous Catheter Use

Pneumothorax, hemothorax, malposition, arrhythmias, and perforation of the central vessel are possible complications directly related to percutaneous CVC placement and presence. Malposition and catheter embolism are possible complications of PICC placement and presence.

Because of the CVC's central access and long-term use, infection is a particular concern when these catheters are used. Children are at increased risk for catheter-related infection and skin irritation (which can lead to infection) because they tend to play with the dressing or tubing, which can introduce contamination from soiled hands, vomit, or stool. Several factors are associated with an increased incidence of catheter-related bloodstream infections in children, including older patient age and multiple indications for PICC use (I. Levy et al., 2010), pediatric intensive care unit exposure, administration of PN as the indication for PICC insertion (Advani et al., 2011), and exchange of a PICC needing replacement rather than insertion at a new site (McCoy et al., 2011). Length of dwell time influences risk of infection: Some have found that risk increases at longer than 9 days (Njere et al., 2011), others suggest the risk increases at longer than 21 days (Advani et al., 2011). If central access is needed after the infant is 7 days of age, replacement of an umbilical vein catheter with a PICC may reduce risk of infection (Butler-O'Hara et al., 2012).

Thrombus formation is another risk associated with CVCs (Higgerson et al., 2011). Factors that may increase the risk of thrombosis include small vessel size compared with the catheter size, a relatively short catheter, and a long dwell time. PN may also increase risk of thrombosis (de Jonge et al., 2005).

Central Venous Catheter Site and Line Care

Meticulously follow facility protocols for CVC insertion site and line care. These protocols should detail how often to clean the site, the proper cleansing technique, how often to flush the catheter, appropriate flushing solution, how often to change tubing, and how to properly maintain a dressing. Dressings on CVCs are either transparent semipermeable membranes (e.g., Tegaderm), changed weekly unless the risk for dislodgement outweighs the benefit of changing the dressing; or gauze and tape, changed every 2 days (O'Grady et al., 2011). Implanted ports need a dressing only when accessed.

When a small-gauge CVC is in place, as is common in infants, administering blood may clot the catheter. Follow the manufacturer's recommendations for

appropriate use. When CVCs do not have infusions running, most must be flushed with heparin to maintain patency; follow facility protocol and manufacturer recommendations. If a tunneled catheter is ruptured or fractured, it can often be repaired.

Intraosseous Access

The intraosseous route provides temporary vascular access in children aged 6 years and younger in emergency situations until venous access can be obtained. A large-bore needle is placed into the bone marrow cavity, optimally in the proximal tibia (Fig. 17-7). Fluids, blood, and most medications (cytotoxic drugs should be avoided) are rapidly absorbed into the systemic circulation from this site. The marrow space can be rapidly accessed even in hypotensive children or when cardiopulmonary resuscitation is in progress. After initial fluid resuscitation, vascular access may be more readily achieved. Bone marrow obtained when the intraosseous needle is inserted can be used to assess hemoglobin, electrolyte levels, blood chemistry values, and blood gases.

Volume of Fluid Administered

Calculation of fluid and electrolyte requirements takes into consideration the child's maintenance needs, volume needed to replace ongoing abnormal losses, and volume needed to correct existing fluid deficits. The child's clinical condition is also a determining factor. For example, a child with impaired renal or cardiac function may be given less fluid to prevent fluid overload, whereas a child with major burns likely will require increased fluid intake.

Maintenance fluid therapy provides fluid and electrolytes in amounts equal to normal ongoing losses. Normal metabolism produces solutes, which must be excreted in urine, and heat, which is dissipated by insensible water loss. Therefore, fluid needs are related to metabolic rate. Weight is widely used to calculate maintenance fluid requirements. IV fluids are calculated per hour, so a quick method for estimating hourly fluid requirements is also used; note that these two methods arrive at similar, but not precisely the same, calculations (Developmental Considerations 17-1).

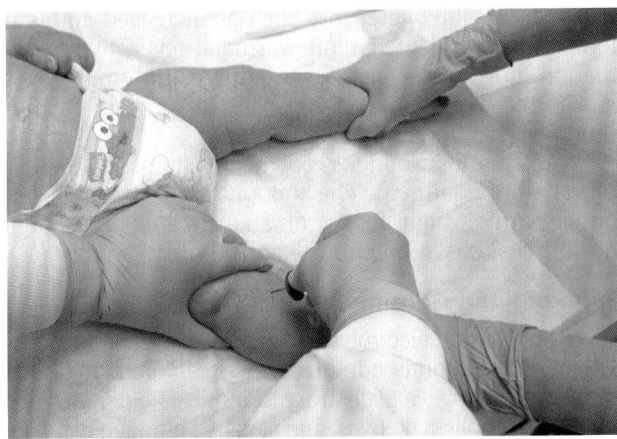

Figure 17-7 Intraosseous needle being inserted for emergency vascular access.

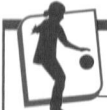

DEVELOPMENTAL CONSIDERATIONS 17-1

Maintenance Fluid and Electrolyte Requirements

Body Weight	Daily Maintenance Formula	Hourly Maintenance Formula
Maintenance Fluid Calculations		
Up to 10 kg	100 mL/kg/24 hr	4 mL/kg/hr
11–20 kg	1,000 mL + 50 mL/kg/24 hr for each additional kg over 10 kg (up to 20 kg)	40 mL/hr + 2 mL/kg/hr × (weight − 10 kg)
>20 kg	1,500 mL + 20 mL/kg/24 hr for each additional kg over 20 kg (maximum total fluids are normally 2,400 mL/24 hr)	60 mL/hour + 1 mL/kg/hr × (weight − 20 kg) (maximum rate of fluids is 100 mL/hr)
Maintenance Electrolytes		
Sodium	2–3 mEq/kg/24 hr	
Potassium	1–2 mEq/kg/24 hr	
Example: A 22-Kg Child		
	Daily Maintenance Formula	Hourly Maintenance Formula
100% maintenance	10 kg × 100 mL = 1,000 mL	
	10 kg × 50 mL = 500 mL	
	2 kg × 20 mL = 40 mL	
	Total = 1,540 mL/24 hr, or 64 mL/hr	
	Sodium = 44 − 66 mEq/24 hr	
	Potassium = 22 − 44 mEq/24 hr 2/3 = 66%	60 mL + (1 mL × 2 = 2) or 62 mL/hr
Two-thirds maintenance (e.g., for child needing fluid restricted)	1,540 × 0.66 = 1,016 mL/24 hr, or 42 mL/hr	

Abnormal losses are those that occur either in excessive amounts or by abnormal routes. Abnormal ongoing losses are calculated by measuring losses in vomitus, gastrointestinal suction, diarrhea, and excessive urine output; and considering any conditions that increase insensible water loss such as increased ambient temperature, use of radiant warmers, fever, hyperventilation, burns, or excessive sweating. Abnormal losses are corrected on an ongoing basis to prevent further fluid and electrolyte deficits.

Correcting fluid deficits replenishes fluids lost before initiation of treatment. This amount is calculated based on measured weight loss or on an estimated percentage of fluid lost based on clinical signs of dehydration.

Type of Fluid Administered

Both glucose and electrolytes should be included in maintenance IV solutions administered to children. In short-term IV therapy, 5% dextrose solutions help minimize protein catabolism, ketosis, and negative nitrogen balance, although they do not provide total caloric needs. A 10% dextrose solution is usually administered to neonates.

Glucose is metabolized rapidly, which decreases the osmolality of the solution. Decreased osmolality allows the "free water" to move rapidly to a more hypertonic space, often the brain in young children, causing cerebral edema. Electrolytes in solutions help prevent fluid from shifting out of the vascular space. A hypotonic solution (e.g., D_5 0.2 normal saline [NS]) is usually given because children need more free water than adults as a result of their higher daily fluid turnover. The optimum concentration of these components depends primarily on the child's serum electrolyte values as well as the underlying disease process.

Two basic types of IV fluid preparations are used: crystalloid and colloid (see thePoint for Supplemental Information). The type used for volume replacement depends on the nature of the loss as well as on ongoing maintenance needs. Crystalloids are solutions that equilibrate rapidly between the vascular and interstitial spaces. Colloids help maintain plasma oncotic (osmotic) pressure. Albumin is the most abundant plasma protein. Because large plasma proteins like albumin are unable to cross the capillary membrane easily, these colloids remain in the vascular space and exert osmotic force to pull fluid into the circulatory space. This dynamic serves to maintain intravascular volume.

Interdisciplinary Interventions

Prepare the child and the family to ease their anxiety and fear. Clearly describe the IV equipment, supplies, and the procedure itself to the child and family.

KidKare Allow an older child to make choices about the therapy whenever it is medically safe to do so. Permit the child to choose the extremity to be used or the timing of catheter placement to give the child some sense of control over his or her environment.

Before initiating IV fluid therapy, review the documented order to double-check that the appropriate solution and rate of infusion have been ordered. Address any questions or concerns about the documented order to the prescriber before initiating therapy.

Usually, the nurse is responsible for placing peripheral IV catheters. PICC lines are inserted by trained practitioners. Other central catheters require surgical placement. Before placement of any type of catheter, question family members and the child, if appropriate, about any specific concerns that they may have.

caREminder

When documenting catheter placement, include the exact location of the catheter, the gauge or size of the catheter, the date that the catheter is placed, number of attempts, and the name of the person who performed the placement.

After the catheter is placed, ensure a safe environment for the child during IV therapy. Secure the catheter, taking care not to obscure the insertion site (Fig. 17-8). In some cases, the child's extremity also may have to be secured to prevent the catheter from becoming dislodged.

Monitor the IV infusion carefully to ensure that the child receives the correct volume of fluid at the correct rate of infusion. Infusion pumps are usually used for IV therapy in infants and young children. Verify that the pump has free-flow protection, is set correctly, and is delivering the infusion at the rate ordered. If an infusion pump is not used, or if it malfunctions, the IV fluid can be delivered through microdrip tubing that delivers fluid at a slow rate.

Observe the child and site of IV infusion for signs of complications every hour. Potential complications include infection, infiltration of fluid into the surrounding tissue, phlebitis, and thrombophlebitis (Nursing Interventions 17-1) (see thePoint for Procedures). Air embolus is a concern, particularly with CVCs. Signs of air emboli include respiratory distress, cyanosis, tachypnea, and hypotension. To prevent air embolus, secure all tubing connections and use air-eliminating filters on tubing and IV pumps that set off an alarm when air in tubing is detected. When air is detected, clamp IV catheter or tubing to prevent further air entry. Place the child in the left lateral Trendelenburg position to try to prevent air from entering the left side of the heart and circulating through the system. Promptly aspirate air from the catheter with a syringe. If symptoms occur, notify the prescriber immediately; this may be a medical emergency. Support cardiorespiratory function; administer oxygen as ordered.

Vascular overload or electrolyte imbalance may also occur. Teach the older child, the parents, and other caregivers to observe for and report any signs of complications, particularly infiltration (Clinical Judgment 17-1).

Playing with or pulling at the catheter or tubing increases the risk of breaking the IV line, which can result in complications such as exsanguination and air embolism. Regardless of the type of venous access device used, it must be protected as developmentally appropriate (Developmental Considerations 17-2). If the child attends school or daycare, provide guidelines for catheter care for parents to give to teachers and care providers (Community Care 17-1).

Nursing responsibilities also include assessing the child's overall status and monitoring intake and output. This measure includes both IV and oral intake as well as all output. Record daily weights to assess the adequacy of fluid volume management.

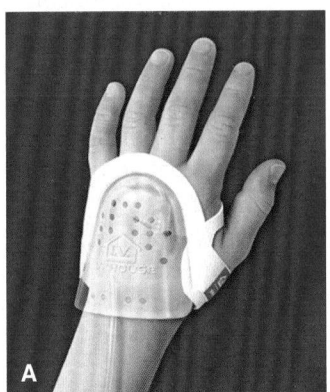
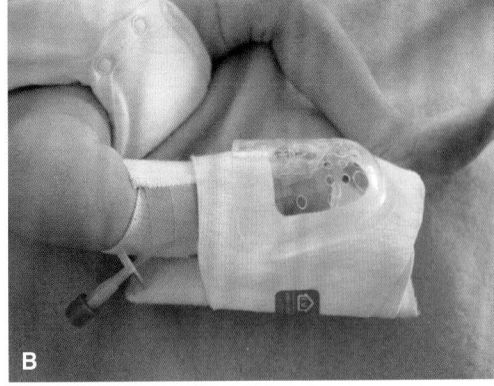

Figure 17-8 (A and B) Peripheral IV catheter in place. An IV House over the IV site secures the device and protects it from bumping or pulling.

NURSING INTERVENTIONS 17-1

Preventing and Treating Complications of Peripheral Intravenous Therapy

Complication/Signs	Nursing Interventions
Infection: Introduction of pathologic organisms locally or systemically	Perform hand hygiene before and after contact with child.
Redness at the catheter insertion site	Maintain sterility of supplies and site for IV insertion and dressing and tubing change.
Exudate from the catheter insertion site	Minimize manipulation of, or trauma to, the insertion site.
Fever	Change IV solution per protocol, usually within 24 hours.
Elevated white blood cell count	Change tubing per protocol, usually within 24–72 hours.
Catheter occlusion: Blockage of catheter usually by clotted blood or precipitates such as incompatible solutions, PN, or medications	Maintain fluid infusion rate. If catheter appears occluded, *gently* flush line (avoid exerting too much force, which may push the clot into the vascular system or rupture the vein or the catheter); use NS initially to flush. If unable to establish patency, remove IV.
Fluid will not infuse or unable to flush	
Frequent infusion occlusion or high-pressure pump alarms	
Infiltration (extravasation): Fluid leaks into subcutaneous tissues	Ensure that site, especially distal to catheter insertion, is easy to assess.
Fluid leakage around the catheter site	Monitor the area distal to catheter insertion site and dependent area for signs of complications at least every hour.
Swelling when compared with the opposite extremity	
Site cool to the touch	If complications occur, discontinue IV. Use a standard scale to document the degree of infiltration (Infusion Nurses Society, 2011). Attempt to aspirate any residual drug from the IV device (Doellman et al., 2009). Elevate the affected extremity for 24–48 hours. In older infants and children, use thermal treatments for 15–20 minutes, every 4 hours, for 24–48 hours; apply warm or cold compresses, depending on the infiltrated fluid or medication: cold for hyperosmolar fluids and DNA-binding vesicants (except mechlorethamine), dry heat for non–DNA-binding vesicants, either heat or cold for isotonic or hypotonic fluids and medications, depending on child preference (Doellman et al., 2009). Use thermal treatments for 15–20 minutes, every 4 hours, for 24–48 hours.
Decreased rate of infusion	
Tenderness, pain	
	Notify prescriber if medications have extravasated.
	Administer drugs (e.g., hyaluronidase) to neutralize or help diffuse extravasated vesicants (medications that cause tissue damage on extravasation) as ordered.
	Usually, no neutralizing drugs are given when fluid or nonvesicant medications have infiltrated. A saline washout procedure to remove extravasated solution may be used (Doellman et al., 2009).

Complication/Signs	Nursing Interventions
Phlebitis: Injury to the vein without clot Red streak along the vein Warmth along the vein, tenderness Possible edema	Dilute antibiotics in adequate amount of fluid; infuse over longest period recommended to provide better hemodilution of drug. Change insertion site routinely per facility protocol. Use a standard scale to document the degree of phlebitis (Infusion Nurses Society, 2011). Apply moist heat to site for 20 minutes several times a day. Consider a PICC if medications are irritants.
Thrombophlebitis: Injury to the vein with a clot Tenderness Edema Area warm to touch	Discontinue IV. Elevate the extremity. Monitor for signs and symptoms; notify prescriber if any develop.

ALERT *During IV fluid therapy, monitor for and promptly report signs of fluid volume overload, such as increased respiratory rate, respiratory distress, and crackles on lung auscultation. If signs of fluid volume overload occur, support the child's respiratory effort, elevate the head of the bed, and check the infusion setup for errors (e.g., inaccurate programming of the pump infusion rate).*

PARENTERAL NUTRITION

Children have enormous metabolic needs and require high amounts of energy and protein to support their continued growth. The basic purpose of IV nutritional support is to restore or maintain optimum nutritional status. IV nutrition also provides fluid to aid in the excretion of wastes and to replace insensible fluid losses. However, the parenteral method of delivering fluids, electrolytes, and calories into the central venous system bypasses the gastrointestinal tract, the central thirst

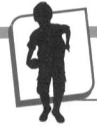

CLINICAL JUDGMENT 17-1

Child With Phlebitis

Tran is a 3-year-old who has a peripheral IV for antibiotic therapy. His current IV has been in place 2 days.

Shortly after the nurse started this antibiotic dose, Tran started crying and picking at the IV site in his left hand.

Questions
1. What assessment data regarding the IV site should the nurse collect?
2. Are any of the IV site assessment findings abnormal? If so, which ones?
3. Should the IV be taken out?
4. After discontinuing the IV in the left hand, what should be done to care for the site?
5. What is the usual course of symptom resolution with phlebitis?

Answers
1. Color of the site (redness), streaking, pallor (there is a faint red line proximal to the IV site); temperature of the surrounding skin (left wrist is warmer than right); presence of edema (left hand and wrist appear slightly more swollen than right); palpate the site (unremarkable, no fibrosis or hardened line felt)
2. Yes; a faint red line proximal to site, site warmer than opposite limb with slight edema. Tran is also complaining of pain at the site.
3. Yes.
4. Apply warm or cold compresses, depending on what seems to soothe Tran. Let Tran assume position of comfort. Monitor site for symptom resolution. Teach these interventions to the parents and child (if old enough).
5. Swelling, redness, and pain will decrease during the next 1–3 days.

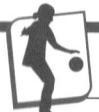

DEVELOPMENTAL CONSIDERATIONS 17-2

Safety Implications for Venous Access Devices

General Precautions	When Connected to Infusion	When Heparin or Normal Saline Locked
Maintain meticulous hand hygiene practices. When involving the child in self-care activities related to the venous access device, make sure they have completed hand hygiene. *Never* use scissors near venous access devices. For central venous access devices, keep extra clamp with child. For a tunneled catheter, after transparent dressing is applied, coil and tape catheter on top of, or to the side of, the dressing.	Use IV extension tubing to • Enable mobility related to developmental level • Keep infusion out of reach of child from crib, playpen, etc.	Peripheral IV: Verify joint/extremity mobility and that no pressure areas are present. Ensure that the catheter is secured with tape and that the slide clamp is in the closed position. Tunneled catheter: Keep clamped on designated clamp area. Access port: Keep noncoring needle extension clamped. PICC: Keep clamp on extension tubing (if present).
Only use Luer-Lock connections.	Tape connections for added security.	Secure any dangling catheter or extension tubing to avoid pulling and possible dislodgment. Secure tubing.
For infants and young children: Dressing in a "onesie" or close-fitting clothing helps protect from exploring hands. Tunnel IV tubing under clothing and away from infant.	For infants learning to walk or ambulatory young children: Tape IV tubing over shoulder and to the back to prevent repeated stepping on IV tubing and subsequent pulling at the exit site.	

Home Care

Perform hand hygiene after toileting/changing diapers, before manipulating catheter or line, and frequently. Place bottles of alcohol-based hand rub throughout home. Assess typical activities for developmental level and provide anticipatory counseling related to safety with venous access—for example, child has a PICC and typically takes Tae Kwon Do classes so alternate activity may need to be substituted; infant should be mastering crawling so tubing extension may be needed, monitor child to avoid entanglement in tubing. Child should wear medical alert bracelet. When leaving home, carry emergency kit in diaper bag or backpack along with alcohol-based hand rub, a backup smooth-edged clamp, tape, equipment to access device, card with information about type of device and its location, and contact information for child's health care provider.	Turn infusion pump control panel away from child; keep pump out of reach of child. Make sure that caregiver can hear pump alarms when not in same room (increase alarm volume, use an intercom).	

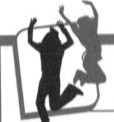

COMMUNITY CARE 17-1

Information to Give Teachers and Care Providers About Central Venous Access Devices

[*Child's name*] has a tube (catheter) in place that is used to deliver medicine into his or her bloodstream. The device should not be noticeable under most clothing. It should not interfere with most normal activities; however, this child should avoid contact sports. The catheter/tubing should be secured close to the child's body to prevent it from dangling and possibly pulling or becoming dislodged. A clear bandage over the site helps to secure the catheter. If the dressing is loose, have the school nurse or the child reinforce it with tape and notify the parent or caregiver. The child should be carrying emergency supplies to help take care of problems, such as cleaning supplies, syringes, and a clamp if the tubing does not have one on it.

Tailor information to the type of access device the child has:

- *Implantable device (port):* This device is under the skin and usually requires no additional care. If a needle is in place, with tubing attached, and any bleeding occurs from the tubing, use the clamp to compress the tubing and stop the bleeding.

- *Tunneled catheter (e.g., Broviac):* The catheter is placed in the child's chest and is well secured, but avoid manipulating the catheter and do not let children pull at it or play with it. The catheter has a cap on the end. In the unlikely event that the cap comes off or the catheter is severed and blood comes out of the catheter, use the clamp to compress the catheter.

- *PICC:* The catheter is well secured and covered with a clear bandage, but avoid manipulating the catheter and dressing and do not let children pull at them or play with them. The catheter has a cap on the end. In the unlikely event that the cap comes off or the catheter breaks, pinch the tube firmly between your fingers, fold it over on itself, and tape securely (it may be recommended not to use a clamp).

No problems are anticipated, but please contact parents if any of these problems, or other problems, occur or if you have any questions.

Ensure that parent contact information is on school and health records.

---

mechanism, and the hunger regulatory mechanism. Therefore, the gut should be used whenever possible to provide nutrition (see Chapter 18). Enteral (oral or tube) feedings, even in small amounts of 5 to 10 mL/hr, are beneficial in helping maintain gut structure, integrity, and function. Use of the gut maintains the intestinal villi (which atrophy if not stimulated) and enzyme activity and prevents breaks in the mucosal wall through which bacteria can enter the system and cause sepsis. Using the gut also helps avoid the hypermetabolic state that occurs after major stress or critical illness.

PN provides complete nutrition for children who cannot consume sufficient nutrients through the gastrointestinal tract to meet and sustain metabolic requirements. PN solutions provide protein, carbohydrates, electrolytes, vitamins, minerals, trace elements, and fats.

Good candidates for PN include children with short gut syndrome, cancer, or increased metabolic needs because of injury. Contraindications to using PN include an anticipated course of less than 5 days, the immediate postoperative period after surgery, risk that exceeds the perceived benefit, and situations in which aggressive nutritional support is not desired. A child rarely receives PN exclusively for prolonged periods, with no oral intake. Partial therapy, in which enteral intake is supplemented with PN, provides the benefit of gut stimulation while still providing adequate calories, nutrition, and fluids.

PN can be provided by peripheral or central venous access. Peripheral delivery of IV nutrition should be restricted to a maximum of 10% dextrose, and peripheral administration should be of limited duration (Infusion Nurses Society, 2011). If the final concentrations of the PN solutions exceed 10% dextrose and 5% protein, pH less than 5 or more than 9, and osmolality more than 600 mOsm/L, the solution should be administered through a CVC (Infusion Nurses Society, 2011). Concentrations higher than this frequently produce a chemical phlebitis. Peripheral PN should be limited to short-term support when the benefit exceeds the risk. In younger children, the large amounts of protein and calories needed for growth necessitate prohibitively high fluid volumes for peripheral delivery. Even with calorie supplementation with fat emulsions, the full caloric needs of smaller children usually cannot be met by peripheral PN. For these children, PN infusion through a CVC is usually required.

Daily caloric requirements are calculated along with disease-specific needs when administering PN. Caloric intake must be more than the child's maintenance requirements (which are based on body weight) to allow for growth and any necessary healing. Caloric requirements are increased in many clinical situations, including burns, sepsis, major surgery or injury, cardiac dysfunction, and chronic illness.

To balance nutrition during prolonged therapy and to prevent fatty acid deficiency, IV fat solutions (lipids) are required. The younger the child, the more quickly fatty acid deficiency can occur. If preterm infants do not receive essential fatty acids, 40% demonstrate deficiency by the third day of life, and 81% have essential fatty acids deficiency by day 7 (Farrell et al., 1988).

Fat emulsions have a low osmolarity; therefore, they may help decrease the incidence of phlebitis when administered peripherally with solutions that have high dextrose concentrations. Administration of fat emulsions has been associated with detrimental effects, however, such as decreased pulmonary diffusion and peripheral oxygenation, chronic lung disease, bilirubin toxicity, alteration in leukocyte function, sepsis, and free radical stress (Simmer & Rao, 2005). Serum triglyceride levels also must be monitored periodically in the child receiving IV fat emulsions.

Complications of Parenteral Nutrition

Possible complications of PN include all of those commonly seen in any form of IV therapy (see Nursing Interventions 17-1). Sepsis and metabolic complications such as hyperglycemia and hypoglycemia, acidosis, calcium and phosphorus abnormalities, and trace metal deficiencies may occur. Electrolyte and mineral levels, BUN, creatinine, liver enzymes, bilirubin, total protein, albumin, and a complete blood cell count are some of the values that should be monitored on a routine basis during prolonged therapy.

Liver dysfunction may also occur. Etiologies of this complication include prematurity, duration of PN, sepsis, and enteric flora/bacterial overgrowth (Rangel et al., 2012). Other complications can occur if the PN solution is infused too rapidly. These events can include respiratory distress, nausea, and electrolyte imbalances.

Interdisciplinary Interventions

Care responsibilities for a child receiving PN include those for any child receiving IV therapy: site, catheter, and tubing care; and close monitoring for signs of complications from the catheter (infiltration, occlusion, infection, phlebitis) and from the IV infusion (fluid and electrolyte imbalances, metabolic complications). Vigilantly maintain clean technique for catheter site and tubing care. Lipids provide an excellent medium for bacterial growth; thus, maintain sterile technique when preparing and administering these solutions.

Monitor the child's rate of growth by recording daily weights and evaluating growth on a standardized growth chart. Keep careful intake and output records.

caREminder

During continuous infusion, maintain a fairly constant PN infusion rate to avoid glucose overload. Never abruptly increase or decrease the infusion rate in an attempt to "even out" the infusion, unless otherwise ordered.

Monitor laboratory values according to facility protocol; note and investigate abnormal results. Monitor serum glucose level by serum laboratory values or by bedside capillary blood glucose methods because the child receiving PN is adapting to a high glucose solution. Report values out of normal range values.

Promote developmentally appropriate tasks that might be limited by restrictions imposed by long-term PN infusions (Teaching Intervention Plan 17-1). Depending on the child's needs, parents, the nurse, a child life specialist, and a physical or occupational therapist may all be involved in promoting the child's physical and emotional development.

Consider the child and family's psychological needs in both hospital and home care situations. Lack of, or restrictions on, oral intake can be very frustrating for the child and family. Many social situations have eating as a focal point; to many parents, being able to feed their child is a central facet of being a "good," nurturing parent. Use principles of therapeutic communication when dealing with the child and family.

Children receiving PN who have other medical needs may associate oral intake (stimulation) with uncomfortable procedures such as suctioning, NG or orogastric tube insertion, or endotracheal intubation and may therefore develop an aversion to oral feeding. This possibility underscores the importance of providing positive oral experiences, such as sucking on a pacifier for younger children or hard candy, if allowed, for older children. Take a proactive approach to prevent adverse psychosocial and developmental effects of prolonged restriction of oral intake during PN therapy. The child should receive a program of oral stimulation, coordinated by the occupational therapist, as well as positive tactile and social stimulation during PN infusion. The *oral stimulation program* promotes dealing with textures, tastes, and movement of food in the mouth and decreasing aversive responses to the introduction of food and may involve gum massage and oral–motor exercises to promote muscle strengthening for specific muscle groups with increased or decreased tone.

Other challenges associated with resuming oral intake are also best addressed proactively. The child receiving PN may not be hungry and may not want to eat. Parenteral nutritional support should be decreased as oral intake is increased. Monitor intake, but do not focus on how much is eaten and do not force the child to eat. Promote mealtimes as pleasant social situations. Ill children often have little control over situations; one situation in which they often can exert control is refusing to eat when allowed oral intake. Not focusing on the issue, offering as many choices as possible (e.g., type of food, where to eat, when to eat), and emphasizing control in other areas (which games to play, when to have rest periods) may help defuse the situation.

The dietitian should be involved in ensuring that PN infusions are nutritionally complete and, along with the occupational therapist, should facilitate the transition to oral intake. If the child is experiencing discomfort related to an underlying disease process, provide adequate pain relief to facilitate positive interactions during mealtime.

TIP 17–1: A TEACHING INTERVENTION PLAN for the Family With a Child Requiring Home Parenteral Nutrition

Nursing Diagnoses and Family Outcomes

- High risk of injury related to effects of ongoing PN infusion
  Outcome: Child will suffer no injury associated with PN infusion.
- Deficient knowledge: Management of PN therapy
  Outcome: Parents, caregivers, and the child, if old enough, will be knowledgeable about and appropriately manage home PN.

Teach the Child/Family

Safety Issues Regarding Child Health
- How to assess fluid balance
- Assessment for signs of electrolyte imbalance and infection

Safety Issues Regarding Child Development
- Use techniques to promote achievement of age-appropriate developmental milestones (e.g., place infant who is learning to crawl, or young child learning to walk, on the floor with enough tubing to be mobile; monitor to prevent child chewing on, pulling on, or getting entangled in tubing; closely monitor a child in early childhood who is using scissors so the catheter or tubing is not inadvertently cut; involve children in middle childhood and adolescents in their own care to promote independence; use portable infusion pumps for mobility).
- Stabilize infusion pumps and poles so they will not fall on child.
- Have plastic cover over pump controls so the child cannot change the infusion settings; turn pump face away from child so the lighted numbers are not tempting to play with (check pump settings frequently).
- Use developmentally appropriate methods to secure venous access device (see Developmental Considerations 17-2).
- Often, home PN is cyclically delivered, usually during sleep time; encourage gross motor activity during infusion-free periods; if awake during infusion, limit activities to circumscribed areas and arrange quiet activities (e.g., doing homework at the kitchen table, watching television in the family room).
- Promote mealtimes as pleasant social events; encourage the entire family to eat together.

Basic Emergency Measures
- General problem-solving techniques
- How to clamp the catheter if it breaks or becomes disconnected
- What to do if the infusion infuses too rapidly (slow infusion rate, monitor child, test blood glucose level, notify health care provider)
- Keep a list of emergency phone numbers posted by every phone in the house.
- Notify local electric and utility companies of the child's medical situation in case of a power outage.
- Pumps need to be plugged into a three-pronged outlet for grounding; an adaptor can be obtained from a hardware store if needed.

Safety Issues for Night PN Infusion
- Adapt sleeping arrangements so the parents can hear and respond to pump alarms.
- Keep the path to the child's room clear to avoid parental injury from tripping over obstacles.

Management of PN Therapy
- Review and observe return demonstration on central line site and catheter care.
- Properly store supplies (clean, dry place away from high-traffic areas [the kitchen counter is not a good place for storage]) and parenteral solutions (keep in small cardboard box in top shelf of refrigerator to avoid anything spilling on them).
- Take a small bag of supplies (syringe, heparin, tape, clamp, extra cap) when going away from home.
- Know procedure for initiating and maintaining the PN infusion (visual inspection of solution, expiration date, clean technique, managing infusion device).

Contact Health Care Provider if
- Child develops signs of fluid or electrolyte imbalance or infection
- Catheter problems occur

Home Parenteral Nutrition Therapy

Teamwork is essential to ensure that PN therapy is successful at home. Child, parent, and caregiver education is a major component of discharge planning. Address social, financial, and medical issues considering parent and caregiver limitations. If the child requires a continuing program of oral–motor stimulation, an occupational or speech therapist may teach parents what to do.

Begin parent, caregiver, and child education in the hospital as soon as the need is identified. Coordination between the hospital, the home care agency, and all caregivers is a priority when planning for discharge. Financial support is a major concern for many families. Social services personnel, the case manager, and others involved in discharge planning should help the family assess their financial and social support resources and provide assistance before deciding to discharge the child on PN. Care needs of the child with a chronic condition and home care needs are discussed in Chapter 12.

Children discharged on home PN therapy and their parents have multiple teaching needs (see Teaching Intervention Plan 17-1). Reinforce the importance of ongoing care to evaluate the effectiveness of therapy; assess the family's knowledge and ability to provide home PN safely during these visits.

ANSWER: The nurse would anticipate that Cory will receive fluids and medications via a peripheral IV for a few days. To Wendy Whitworth, this sounds like a very long time, but in the realm of venous access, it is not a long time. Cory is already in pain, distressed, and dehydrated. He may be unable to cooperate for this procedure and, as a result of his degree of dehydration, it may not be easy to start an IV on him. In the interest of atraumatic care, the emergency department nurse should coordinate with the surgery department to determine how quickly Cory might move to a presurgical area and the surgical nurse or perhaps the anesthesiologist might place the peripheral IV. Immediate appropriate actions would include assessing potential IV sites, applying topical anesthetic cream, verifying fluid orders, and preparing the IV bag and tubing.

NURSING PLAN OF CARE

QUESTION: Which nursing diagnoses listed in Nursing Plan of Care 17-1 are applicable to Cory?

Nursing diagnoses and care generally appropriate for the child with altered fluid and electrolyte status are identified in Nursing Plan of Care 17-1. Because fluid and electrolyte imbalances produce widely varying effects, additional diagnoses not listed may be appropriate for children with specific alterations.

ANSWER: The nursing diagnoses most pertinent to Cory are as follows:

- Risk for imbalanced fluid volume related to NPO (nothing by mouth) status, presence of an NG tube, inadequate fluid resuscitation or overhydration, equipment malfunction, child/parent changing infusion rate
- Imbalanced nutrition: Less than body requirements related to effects of disease process or condition (inability to ingest sufficient nutrients, inability to absorb nutrients via gastro intestinal tract)

ALTERATIONS IN FLUID AND ELECTROLYTE BALANCE

Normally, thirst mechanisms, the kidneys, and the respiratory system work together to maintain fluid and electrolyte balance. When this balance is upset, the resulting alterations can be life threatening.

FLUID IMBALANCES

The body maintains a delicate fluid balance. Excessive fluid losses or inadequate intake may result in dehydration; excess fluid volume may result in edema.

DEHYDRATION

QUESTION: Based on his history, which type of dehydration do you think Cory has?

Gastrointestinal output, in the form of diarrhea and emesis, is the most common cause of dehydration in children. Worldwide, diarrheal disease is the second leading cause of morbidity and mortality in children, causing approximately 801,000 deaths yearly (Liu et al., 2012). Among children in the United States, gastroenteritis accounts for over 1.5 million outpatient visits, 200,000 hospitalizations, and about 300 deaths yearly (Jablonski, 2012).

Pathophysiology

Dehydration occurs when fluid loss exceeds fluid intake. The primary cause can be an overall increase in fluids lost or decreased intake. Dehydration can also result when fluid shifts occur and the fluid accumulates in a space outside ICF and ECF spaces, such as the abdominal cavity (a phenomenon sometimes called *third spacing*). Because fluid moves from the intravascular space, this shift results in intravascular fluid deficit and dehydration. The body maintains equal osmolality between ICF and ECF compartments. Osmolality changes in one compartment lead to compensatory water shifts as the body attempts to restore equal osmolality among compartments.

In adults, the greatest proportion of water is stored in the intracellular space. Therefore, to be lost from the vascular volume, water must shift out of the intracellular space into the extracellular space. Children have a greater proportion of body water in the extracellular space (see Fig. 17-2), which makes it easier for water to be lost from the intravascular space. This is one of the reasons why children are more prone to dehydration than adults. Fever, increased respiratory rate, diuretics, hemorrhage, burns, and adrenal insufficiency can also lead to dehydration.

Untreated, dehydration can negatively affect circulatory blood volume. Initially, reduced blood volume results in a reduction of blood flow to the skin, muscles, and viscera and, later, to the kidneys. As plasma blood volume becomes more depleted, circulation is further compromised, resulting in reversible (and eventually irreversible) shock and death.

Classification of dehydration is made based on the child's serum sodium level: 130 to 150 mEq/L in isotonic dehydration, less than 130 mEq/L in hyponatremic (hypotonic) dehydration, and more than 150 mEq/L in hypernatremic (hypertonic) dehydration.

Isotonic dehydration occurs when sodium and water are lost in proportional amounts. The net result is a reduction in the circulating blood volume. The major fluid loss is from the ECF compartment, which, in children, is proportionally larger than the ICF compartment.

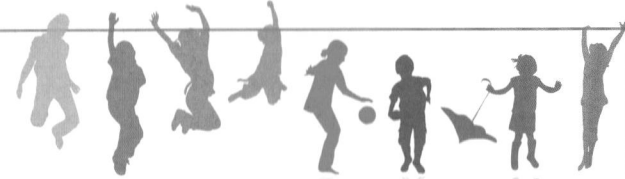

NURSING PLAN OF CARE 17-1:

The Child With Altered Fluid and Electrolyte Balance

Nursing Diagnosis: Risk for imbalanced fluid volume related to inadequate fluid resuscitation or overhydration, equipment malfunction, child/parent changing infusion rate

Interventions/Rationale

- Calculate fluid requirements for the child and evaluate whether they coincide with the order for fluid infusion and with the child's diagnosis.

  Fluid needs are calculated based on the child's weight and condition (e.g., may be decreased in children with neurologic, cardiac, or renal problems or increased in the presence of high metabolic needs or certain conditions, such as sickle cell disease).

- Use infusion device with free-flow protection to monitor flow rate; use volume control chambers per facility policy.

  Infusion devices provide more accurate fluid delivery than by gravity alone; free-flow protection helps avoid inadvertent fluid administration. Volume control chambers limit the amount of fluid available for infusion at one time.

- Keep infusion device positioned so that the child cannot change the rate or stop/start infusion.

  Reduces the chance that child will alter the ordered infusion rate.

- Assess the child, IV site, and infusion system every hour for complications; discontinue the IV as indicated and assess need for restarting the line.

  IV administration is an artificial method of delivering fluids that bypasses the body's regulatory systems, thus making it easy to under-/over-hydrate a child. Frequent assessments facilitate prompt detection and treatment of complications.

- Monitor vital signs, maintain accurate intake and output, weigh daily at the same time on the same scale in the same clothes; assess for edema (e.g., bulging fontanel, periorbital, dependent) or fluid deficit (e.g., sunken fontanel, poor skin turgor, dry mucous membranes, tachycardia).

  Changes in these parameters may reflect alteration in fluid balance.

- Explain to child/parents importance of keeping infusion constant; caution them not to regulate the IV (unless appropriate, as in care-by-parent units or teaching for home IV therapy).

Expected Outcomes

- Child will maintain normal fluid balance evidenced by normal heart rate, blood pressure, and urine output for age and weight; the infant will have a normal fontanel (not sunken or bulging); eyes will not be sunken and periorbital edema will not occur.

Nursing Diagnosis: Ineffective tissue perfusion (specify type: renal, cerebral, cardiopulmonary, gastrointestinal, peripheral) related to effects of fluid deficit, electrolyte imbalance

Interventions/Rationale

- Monitor for signs of ineffective tissue perfusion:
  - Renal: urine output less than 1 mL/kg/hr, high specific gravity ($\geq$1.030)
  - Cerebral: irritable, altered behavior, decreased level of consciousness, sluggish pupillary response
  - Cardiopulmonary: capillary refill time more than 2 seconds, weak or thready pulses
  - Gastrointestinal: decreased bowel sounds, nausea or vomiting, abdominal distention
  - Peripheral: cool, clammy, pale, mottled, or cyanotic skin

    Symptoms vary based on the system affected. Early detection facilitates prompt intervention and reduction of negative sequelae.

- Notify physician or advanced practice nurse immediately if signs of ineffective tissue perfusion are noted.

  Immediate notification facilitates initiation of treatment. Prolonged ineffective tissue perfusion leads to anaerobic metabolism, lactic acidosis, organ ischemia, and, ultimately, multiorgan system failure.

Expected Outcome

- Child will regain and maintain adequate tissue perfusion.

Nursing Diagnosis: Imbalanced nutrition: Less than body requirements related to effects of disease process or condition (inability to ingest sufficient nutrients, inability to absorb nutrients via gastrointestinal tract)

Interventions/Rationale

- Assess for factors contributing to current imbalance (presence of illness or condition; child's intake of food and fluids; how food and formula are prepared; alteration in parent child interactions, neglect, abuse).

  Allows identification of cause of problems so interventions can be targeted appropriately.

- Observe child's relationship to food. Attempt to distinguish between physical and psychological causes for inadequate intake.

  Ill children often have little control over situations. One situation in which they often can exert control is refusing to eat when allowed oral intake. Interventions will vary based on cause of inadequate intake.

(Continued)

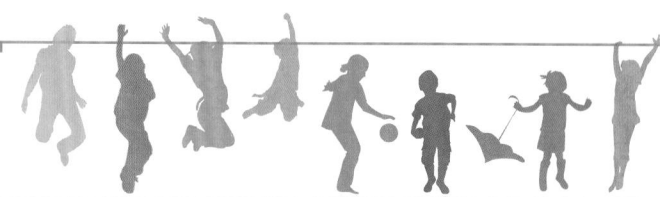

NURSING PLAN OF CARE 17-1:

The Child With Altered Fluid and Electrolyte Balance (Continued)

- Calculate child's caloric needs; obtain nutrition consult as indicated. Measure weight daily, measure height and head circumference (in children younger than 3 years of age) weekly or as indicated. Periodically plot measurements on growth chart. Record oral intake accurately, monitor intake and output, and note unusual losses (e.g., vomiting, diarrhea, increased metabolic needs).

  Regardless of the specific situation, the child needs enough protein for tissue repair; calories for energy (both carbohydrate and fat sources); and enough electrolytes, vitamins, minerals, and trace elements for normal body functioning. Children experience growth spurts, which require an increase in required nutrients. Ongoing monitoring of intake, output, and growth parameters gives an indication of whether intake is adequate to meet needs.

Expected Outcomes
- Child will take in (oral, enteral, IV) sufficient fluid and nutrients based on age and medical needs.
- Child will gain weight at a rate appropriate for his or her age and will maintain growth on own trajectory.

Nursing Diagnosis: Deficient diversional activity related to restriction/limitation of movement, weakness from disease process

Interventions/Rationale
- Take the child for walks, to the playroom, or sit in the hallway where there is activity. Have developmentally appropriate toys, games, and books in crib/at the bedside. Encourage activities that do not require use of the extremity in which an IV is present.

  Activities provide a distraction, take the child's mind off imposed limitations, and may improve coping. A lack of stimulation may result in boredom, irritability, or depression.
- Teach the child/parents how to move the IV pole, unplug the infusion pump (if battery operated) for walks, and plug it back in.

  Gives the child/parent control in a situation and knowledge to safely manipulate equipment.
- Set up study schedule and encourage keeping up with lessons from school if appropriate.

  If the child will be unable to attend school, keeping up with assignments may provide distraction and a feeling of accomplishment and may reduce anxiety related to missing schoolwork.
- Encourage peer visitation if not contraindicated.

  Peers can help occupy the child's time and provide a distraction. Peers are very important to adolescents, and interactions help them meet developmental milestones.

Expected Outcomes
- Child will be able to perform activities normal and appropriate for his or her developmental level.
- Child will verbalize no complaints of boredom nor display apathy from lack of stimulation.

Nursing Diagnosis: Deficient knowledge: Recognition and management of fluid and electrolyte imbalance and complications of therapy

Interventions/Rationale
- Discuss with the child/parents why various tests and procedures are indicated and why IV infusion is necessary. Show equipment to the child. Explain that a catheter is like a plastic noodle in their arm and that the needle is not left in.

  Understanding the rationale for interventions helps the child and parents cope with and adhere to the treatment regimen. Children fear needles; reassurance that a needle is not present may decrease anxiety.
- Teach reasons for covering the infusion site and limiting movement (e.g., to avoid touching/picking at site; immobilize the area to reduce catheter dislodgment, limit movement to avoid pulling on infusion tubing).

  The child/parents need information and teaching to deal appropriately with IV equipment, to cope with limitations of movement, and to help prevent complications.
- Explain to parents that an infant still needs to be held; teach them methods to pick up and hold their infant with an IV.

  Helps parents to overcome their fear of handling their child and to better meet the child's needs.
- Tell them to call the nurse if the IV is not infusing appropriately (e.g., not dripping; the alarm is sounding; or if the site is painful, red, swollen, cool, or warm to the touch.)

  Facilitates prompt recognition and treatment of adverse events.

Expected Outcomes
- Child and parents will demonstrate understanding of the tests and procedures performed.
- Parents will provide care to their child, including providing appropriate nutritional intake.
- Child, if old enough, and parents will recognize early symptoms of fluid and electrolyte imbalance and implement appropriate interventions.

Hyponatremic dehydration, also commonly called *hypotonic dehydration*, can result from either water retention or sodium loss. Defects in renal water excretion are almost always the cause of water retention, resulting in hyponatremia. Hypotonic dehydration can occur when sodium is lost with water but the net loss of fluid is replaced, either orally or intravenously, by hypotonic solutions. This imbalance may occur if formula is diluted with water beyond manufacturer recommendations or if fluid is replaced with electrolyte-free water. Because sodium is more abundant in the extracellular space, fluid in the intracellular space is normally hypotonic in relation to fluid in the extracellular space. In hypotonic dehydration, the ICF becomes relatively more concentrated because the sodium in the extracellular compartment is diluted. Because water follows sodium, water shifts from the ECF to the ICF compartment.

Hypernatremic dehydration is marked by elevated sodium levels in the ECF compartment. Thus, water shifts from the ICF to the ECF compartment in an effort to restore equal osmolality. This shift decreases intracellular volume substantially, but clinical signs of fluid loss are not as apparent as in other types of dehydration, even in the presence of similar fluid loss, because the shift of fluid into the extracellular space helps to maintain vascular volume.

ANSWER: Cory's dehydration is a result of inadequate oral intake in the presence of increased metabolic need from his fever. The history is not compatible with hyponatremic dehydration. He most likely has isotonic dehydration. When his sodium level returns, it can be confirmed.

Assessment

QUESTION: You have already identified the manifestations of dehydration that Cory exhibits. What is another factor that may affect your assessment?

Dehydration is classified as mild, moderate, or severe. Clinical manifestations depend on the type of dehydration, its cause, and the severity of fluid loss (Table 17-1). Infants and young children are more susceptible to dehydration and may have more severe manifestations.

Obtain a thorough history of the child's recent intake and output (see Focused Health History 17-1) and ask about potential exposures to ill persons, poisons, and hot environments. Assess peripheral perfusion as reflected in changes in vital signs and level of consciousness. Weigh the child and compare the result with previous recent weights, if available. Rapid weight loss is a sign of fluid loss. Assess for other signs of fluid deficit, such as dry mucous membranes, sunken eyeballs, lack of tears when crying (in children 6 weeks and older), sunken fontanel in infants, and poor skin turgor.

Signs and symptoms of isotonic dehydration may be similar to those of hypovolemic shock. The risk of hypotonic dehydration is increased in infants with immature renal function and in those whose oral intake after diarrhea consists of hypotonic or electrolyte-free solutions. The most common solutions erroneously used in these situations are water or sugar water. Assess for the presence of clinical signs, including poor skin turgor and signs of vascular collapse (e.g., increased heart and respiratory rates, decreased blood pressure, delayed capillary refill). Neurologic manifestations may occur as brain cells swell.

Clinical manifestations of hypertonic dehydration include a doughlike feel to the skin, lethargy, irritability, and seizures. Neurologic signs are related to the decreased intracellular volume of brain cells.

ANSWER: Cory is in acute pain. He is tachycardic and tachypneic, but this can also be a result of pain. Obtaining Cory's blood pressure may or may not be helpful. Although a decreased blood pressure is a late sign of dehydration, Cory's level of pain may be increasing a somewhat low blood pressure so that it appears normal for his age.

TABLE 17-1   Clinical Signs of Dehydration

Sign	Mild	Moderate	Severe
Loss of body weight	5%	5%–9%	>10%
Level of consciousness	Alert to restless, irritable	Restless to lethargic	Lethargic to comatose
Blood pressure	Normal	Normal; may be low when upright	Low
Heart rate	Normal	Increased	Increased
Pulse	Normal	Faint, thready	Impalpable
Mucous membranes	May be dry	Dry	Dry, parched
Eyeballs, fontanel	Normal	May be normal or sunken	Sunken
Skin turgor	May be normal	Poor	Poor, tenting
Skin temperature	Normal	Cool	Cool, mottled, cyanotic
Urine output	May be low (normal is 1 mL/kg/hr)	Low, concentrated, oliguric	Low, anuric

Diagnostic Tests

Serum sodium is evaluated to identify the type of dehydration. Serum BUN and creatinine and urine specific gravity and osmolality, which are increased in the presence of fluid volume deficit, may also be evaluated. The use of urine specific gravity may not identify dehydration (Colletti et al., 2010).

Interdisciplinary Interventions

 QUESTION: Why is oral fluid intake not appropriate for Cory?

Dehydration that causes clinical manifestations calls for prompt fluid replacement. The priority intervention is to restore and maintain intravascular volume. After volume is restored, any remaining fluid and electrolyte deficit can be corrected by administering an appropriate solution at an appropriate rate. This solution is given in addition to any normal maintenance fluids that the child needs.

Mild to moderate dehydration can be corrected with oral fluid intake. Severe dehydration may require IV fluid replacement therapy (see thePoint for Care Path). Indications for IV therapy to correct a fluid deficit include shock and impaired circulation, severe dehydration, or children suspected of having paralytic ileus (Colletti et al., 2010).

Isotonic solutions—never hypotonic solutions—should be used for initial rehydration therapy. Hypotonic fluid shifts out of the extracellular space and thus does not help restore vascular volume.

ALERT   *Using isotonic fluids is critical in children with hypernatremia because hypotonic solutions cause water to move into brain cells, causing cerebral edema, seizures, and profound neurologic sequelae. The rate of fluid replacement should also be more gradual, over 48 hours rather than 24 hours, in the case of hypertonic dehydration. When the sodium level decreases too quickly, similar fluid shifts occur in the brain.*

IV fluids should contain sodium when the serum sodium level is below normal limits. Common solutions include lactated Ringer's, NS, ½ NS, and ¼ NS (Tradition or Science 17-2). If the child is hemodynamically unstable, 20-mL/kg boluses of isotonic solutions should be given until vital signs indicate stability.

caREminder

To avoid serious cardiac sequelae associated with hyperkalemia, potassium should not be added to IV fluids until the child has voided, demonstrating adequate renal function.

TRADITION OR SCIENCE 17-2

What fluid is most appropriate as maintenance fluid?

Historically, isotonic solutions were recommended to restore volume followed by hypotonic fluids for maintenance (Holliday et al., 2007), but IV administration of hypotonic fluids has the potential to cause hyponatremia (Hanna & Saberi, 2010; Yung & Keeley, 2009). Isotonic solutions, such as NS (Choong et al., 2011; Choong et al., 2006; Moritz & Ayus, 2007; Neville et al., 2010; Neville et al., 2006) or 0.9% saline in 5% dextrose (Kannan et al., 2010), for maintenance fluid have been advocated to reduce the incidence of hyponatremia. Further research is indicated to determine the appropriate recommendation because administration of hypotonic fluids does not always explain the development of hyponatremia (Beck, 2007), and 0.45% saline, when accompanied by adequate volume expansion with isotonic fluid, was not found to result in a drop in serum sodium (Saba et al., 2011). Dextrose also must be considered, because in children with gastroenteritis and dehydration, larger amounts of IV dextrose administration were associated with fewer return visits requiring admission (J. A. Levy & Bachur, 2007). The National Patient Safety Agency (2007) and the Institute for Safe Medication Practices (2009) have issued alerts noting the risk associated with use of hypotonic IV solutions. Clinical judgment considering the child's situation is required to prescribe the correct fluid.

Therapy, whether oral or IV, should continue until

- Vital signs are stable
- Weight has stabilized
- Adequate urine volume is present
- Serum electrolytes are within normal limits
- Acidosis, if present, has been corrected

Nursing responsibilities when caring for a child with dehydration include initial assessment and ongoing monitoring. Investigate the underlying cause of the dehydration (Clinical Judgment 17-2). Assess cardiac output by measuring blood pressure with the child in both the upright and supine positions. Lower blood pressure in the upright position may indicate a decrease in ECF volume. The nurse can expect the child to exhibit tachycardia as a compensatory measure to maintain cardiac output in the presence of decreased vascular volume. Assess temperature: Increased body temperatures can lead to increased respiratory rate and a resulting increase in metabolic needs. This process can increase insensible fluid loss through skin and lungs. Administer antipyretics as ordered. Weigh daily and monitor trends.

ANSWER: Cory is NPO for surgery. His fluids will have to be administered intravenously.

A Dehydrated Infant

Ten-day-old Dan is brought to the clinic by his mother. She states that he is sleeping a lot, feeding poorly, and is very fussy when he is awake. The nurse's physical assessment findings include heart rate, 160 bpm; respiratory rate, 60 breaths/min; capillary refill, 2 seconds; skin and mucous membranes, dry; abdominal skin remains raised for 2 seconds after being pinched; fontanel, sunken; and weight, 3.5 kg.

Questions

1. What questions should the nurse ask the mother?
2. What signs and symptoms indicate dehydration?
3. What is the problem? How severe is it?
4. What interventions should be implemented?
5. What follow-up is appropriate?

Answers

1. How many wet diapers has the baby had in the past 24 hours? (three) How much stool? (no change in stooling patterns, about three per 24 hours) Any fever? (no) Is the baby breastfed or bottle-fed? If bottle-fed, what type and how is formula prepared? For any feeding method, how often does the baby eat? How much? (Dan is breastfed three to four times in 24 hours; 10 minutes each side is attempted; he latches intermittently during feeding; mother complains of sore, cracked, bleeding nipples) What did the baby weigh at birth? (3.8 kg)

2. Three wet diapers during the past 24 hours (normal is six to eight); increased heart rate, respiratory rate, delayed capillary refill, dry skin and mucous membranes, poor skin turgor, sunken fontanel, and behavior changes; only three to four feedings per 24 hours (normally, should nurse 10–12 times in 24 hours)

3. Dehydration secondary to poor feeding. Dan has lost 0.3 kg since birth. He is moderately dehydrated.

   $3.5 \div 3.8 = 0.92 = 92\%$ of birth weight = 8% weight (fluid) loss

   Dan's poor latch during breastfeeding is the major contributing factor to mother's sore, dry, cracked nipples. Candidiasis of the breast can also lead to nipple cracking, redness, and discomfort, but this possibility was ruled out.

4. The dehydration must be addressed while supporting continued breastfeeding, if possible. Assist mother to comfortable breastfeeding position then in latching Dan to breast. Observe for deep latch, suck, and swallow. Teach mother to evaluate appropriate latch (Dan is fish-mouthed, she can see and hear Dan swallow, she does not have breast pain after initial latch). Review breastfeeding techniques with mother. Instruct mother to breastfeed every 2–3 hours around the clock; supplement with formula as needed. Teach mother how to manually express milk. Manual expression can assist in achieving good latch if breasts are engorged, give reassurance that mother has plenty of milk for the baby, and expressed milk can be used as a nipple and areolar lubricant and protectant. The antibodies in breast milk can assist in healing any cracks, prevent infection, and soothe any sensitivity. Also educate mother on use of lanolin on nipples as a soothing and protective agent. Instruct parents to call health care provider if Dan does not have six to eight wet diapers in 24 hours, if lethargy increases, or if he does not eat well (if he breastfeeds poorly and then refuses supplemental formula).

5. Return to clinic tomorrow to ensure Dan has sufficient intake as evidenced by weight gain, voiding six to eight times in 24 hours, normal vital signs and capillary refill, good skin turgor, moist mucous membranes, and decreased fussiness and sleepiness. Observe feeding technique; refer to lactation consultant if problems with breastfeeding continue.

Community Care

Oral fluid replacement therapy is commonly provided in the home care setting. Commercial oral solutions (e.g., World Health Organization oral rehydration salts, Rehydralyte, Pedialyte, Infalyte) contain water, electrolytes, HCO_3 or citrate, and glucose. Glucose is necessary to facilitate transport of sodium and water across the bowel wall.

CROSS-CULTURAL CARE

Oral rehydration therapy (ORT) is commonly used, particularly in developing countries, to treat diarrheal dehydration. ORT is simpler to implement than IV rehydration and effectively treats dehydration (Hartling et al., 2006). In developed countries, IV therapy is still commonly used to treat dehydration, probably because it is readily available and established care patterns are difficult to change.

Oral rehydration should be given frequently and in small amounts (Teaching Intervention Plan 17-2). When educating parents, provide detailed, specific information about the type of fluids to give; how much to give; and how long to continue rehydration therapy.

EDEMA

Fluid movement between the vascular and interstitial compartment is regulated by hydrostatic pressure and osmotic pressure (see thePoint for Supplemental Information). Edema—abnormal accumulation of fluid in the interstitial tissues—results from an imbalance in the physiologic forces that regulate fluid movement. This imbalance either causes excess fluid to enter the interstitial fluid compartment or causes excess fluid to remain in this compartment. *Filtration* (movement of fluid across a semipermeable membrane) occurs across capillary beds and also influences the movement of fluid into the interstitium. Hypoproteinemia (low serum protein level), for instance, decreases oncotic pressure in the capillaries. Thus, because of osmotic pressure, fluid shifts out of the vascular bed and into the interstitial space, resulting in edema. In another example, increased fluid in the blood vessels causes vascular congestion. As a result, fluid leaks from the vessels, across the capillary membrane, and into the interstitial space, causing edema. Edema can be local or generalized throughout the body. Severe edema in all body tissues is known as *anasarca*.

Various conditions, such as renal dysfunction (which influences sodium reabsorption and retention), liver disease (which often causes hypoproteinemia), cerebral edema, and steroid administration, influence the formation of edema. Managing each of these conditions is more difficult in a child with coexisting cardiovascular disease because the compensatory mechanisms by which the body might respond (sympathetic nervous system activation, activation of the renin–angiotensin–aldosterone system, and ventricular hypertrophy) may already be activated to manage the cardiovascular disease.

Assessment

Excess fluid in the ECF compartment can be detected through a rapid gain in body weight. Parents may be the first to note the child's unusual weight gain by observing that his or her clothes suddenly do not fit. Weigh the child.

caREminder

One kilogram of body weight equals the weight of 1 L of water; thus, the amount of fluid gain or loss can be calculated from weight gain or loss.

Assess for edema, which, for children, usually occurs first in dependent areas (the sacrum, ankles, and feet) or in the periorbital area. Assess for other physical signs of edema, which include a bounding pulse and hepatomegaly (enlarged liver). In the presence of respiratory distress, crackles can be heard on auscultation of the lungs. Distended neck veins may be visible in an older child assessed in a supine or semi-Fowler position.

Nursing Diagnoses and Outcomes

In addition to those presented in Nursing Plan of Care 17-1, the following nursing diagnoses and outcomes may apply to the child with edema:

Nursing Diagnosis: Excess fluid volume related to effects of disease process or treatment, inability to excrete fluid, or osmolality imbalance
Outcomes:
- Child will not experience respiratory distress as evidenced by normal respiratory rate, absence of retractions or nasal flaring, and no cyanosis of nail beds and mucous membranes.
- Child will maintain baseline weight, without rapid gain from fluid excess, and will demonstrate slow, long-term weight gain along his or her growth curve.

Nursing Diagnosis: High risk for impaired skin integrity related to friable skin
Outcomes:
- Child's skin will remain intact, without any evidence of breakdown.
- Interventions will be implemented to prevent tissue breakdown at pressure sites and dependent areas.

Nursing Diagnosis: Impaired physical mobility related to restriction of normal range of motion
Outcomes:
- Child will maintain maximum range of motion while edema is present.
- Child will remain as independent as possible within the limits set by the edema.

Nursing Diagnosis: Body image disorder related to perception of the edema
Outcomes:
- Child will verbalize acceptance of his or her physical appearance.
- Child will continue to have social interactions with peers consistent with his or her age and developmental milestones.

TIP 17-2: A TEACHING INTERVENTION PLAN for Home Management of the Dehydrated Child

Nursing Diagnoses and Family Outcomes

- Deficient fluid volume related to effects of increased fluid losses or needs or of decreased intake
  Outcomes: Child will maintain vascular volume as evidenced by normal heart rate and blood pressure.
  Child's urine output will be at least 1 mL/kg/hr.
- Deficient knowledge: Management of dehydration
  Outcome: Child's parents will verbalize understanding of how to treat episodes of vomiting and diarrhea and state methods to manage fluid loss at home.

Teach the Child/Family

Detection, Prevention, and Management of Dehydration
- Signs of dehydration (decreased urine output, dry mucous membranes, lack of tears, sunken eyeballs or fontanel, change in level of consciousness)
- *Not* to use boiled skim milk or other concentrated solutions because they contain too much salt
- *Not* to use home remedies (uncarbonated soda, Jell-O, fruit juice, tea) because they usually have low sodium concentrations, which can cause hyponatremia, and have inappropriately high osmolality from excessive carbohydrates, which can exacerbate diarrhea
- Proper methods of preparing infant formula; not to overdilute formula to make more
- The importance of good handwashing technique, particularly in the presence of infectious diseases
- Components of
  - ORT to replace existing losses
  - Maintenance therapy to replace continuing losses after ORT is completed; ways to combine with adequate dietary intake

Amount of Oral Rehydrating Solution to Give
- ORT: 75 mL/kg over 4 hours
- Offer a teaspoonful every 1–2 minutes. If vomiting occurs, wait 5–10 minutes then give a teaspoonful every 2–3 minutes. Continue to repeat unless emesis consistently occurs in an amount that exceeds the intake.
- If the child wants more solution and exhibits no signs of overhydration, give more.
- Increase the amount of solution given if diarrhea or symptoms of dehydration continue.
- Decrease the amount of solution if the child appears well hydrated or periorbital edema develops.
- Continue breastfeeding throughout ORT and illness.
- For non-breastfeeding or older children, oral feedings should be resumed as soon as possible after initial rehydration.
- Stop giving ORT when hydration is normal.
- Maintenance therapy: Give the child as much fluid as he or she wants. After each diarrheal stool or emesis, give
  - <10 kg: 60–120 mL fluid
  - >10 kg: 120–240 mL fluid

Contact Health Care Provider if
- The amount or frequency of vomiting or diarrhea is increasing
- Diarrhea or vomiting does not improve after 24 hours of treatment
- Child appears worse (decreased level of consciousness, decreasing urine output, dizziness when upright, increased fever, seizures)
- Child's fluid status does not improve (no urine output within 8 hours, tongue and cheeks do not become moist, no tears with crying)
- Child refuses to eat or is unable to ingest more solution than is vomited

---

Nursing Diagnosis: Deficient knowledge: Care of the child with edema

Outcomes:
- Child and parents will demonstrate an understanding of causes of edema and of the need for any tests and procedures.
- The parents will provide care to their child, including appropriate nutrition and measures to prevent sequelae of edema such as skin breakdown.
- The child will provide self-care, as appropriate.

Interdisciplinary Interventions

Interventions for the child with edema focus on determining and treating the underlying cause. Diuretics may be administered to promote renal excretion of water and sodium and to help remove excess fluid. Diuretics are indicated in children with pulmonary edema, increased cerebral edema, generalized edema, hypertension, or renal dysfunction. If a potassium-wasting diuretic is administered, carefully monitor serum potassium levels.

Nursing care of the child with severe edema requires strict and accurate monitoring of intake and output. Note discrepancies between intake and output and discuss them with the health care team. Weigh the child each day, at the same time of day, on the same scale, and with the child wearing the same amount of clothing.

caREminder

Compare daily weight with previous measurements and note trends. If a substantial weight gain occurs, assess the child for other signs of fluid retention, such as rales or periorbital or dependent edema.

Protect edematous tissue, which is easily injured. Regularly change the position of a child with limited mobility. Use low-pressure mattresses and other devices that help reduce the pressure on dependent areas when needed. Elevating areas of localized edema promotes increased venous and lymphatic drainage of interstitial fluid. Keep the child's skin clean and dry and inspect all pressure areas for signs of breakdown at least daily.

Ensuring appropriate nutritional intake can be a challenge in the child who must receive a minimal amount of fluids but has high caloric needs. Record daily calorie counts. A dietitian can help devise meal plans that provide all necessary nutrients and are appealing to the child.

Community Care

The nurse, child life specialist, social worker, and parent can help the child deal with distortions of his or her normal body image. Body image can be a major issue to the child or adolescent with severe edema. Include on-site school personnel and the child's regular teacher in the plan of care. They may be able to provide routine, normalizing experiences for the child.

Teach parents and siblings, as appropriate, about disease management, administration of medications and side effects, skin care, positioning, and promoting appropriate nutritional intake.

ACID–BASE IMBALANCES

Regulation and maintenance of acid–base balance in body fluids is essential to the action of hormones, enzymes, and all basic physiologic functions. Normal acid–base balance is maintained through the interaction of a complex system of buffers, respiratory compensation, and the metabolic component of kidney function. When an alteration occurs, the body mobilizes these physiologic mechanisms to restore normal acid–base balance.

A buffer is a weak acid. It can facilitate a change in the pH of the blood when a stronger acid or a base is added. The body's most effective buffer is the bicarbonate–carbonic acid (HCO_3–H_2CO_3) system. Other effective buffers include proteins, hemoglobin, and phosphates.

In normal metabolism, all cells produce H_2CO_3 and metabolic acids. H_2CO_3 is excreted by the lungs in the form of carbon dioxide. Metabolic acids are excreted through the kidneys. The effectiveness of the HCO_3–H_2CO_3 buffering systems can be measured in the arterial blood gas values of pH, carbon dioxide, and HCO_3 (see Tests and Procedures 16-2 for more information on these values).

Alterations in acid–base homeostasis are classified as either metabolic or respiratory based on their cause. The imbalance is termed *respiratory* when it is primarily caused by a change in the partial pressure of carbon dioxide ($PaCO_2$) in arterial blood; imbalances resulting from all other primary changes are classified as *metabolic*. An abnormally low pH is called *acidosis*, or *acidemia*. An abnormally high pH is termed *alkalosis*, or *alkalemia*. Severe acidosis (pH <7.0) and severe alkalosis (pH >7.55 with an HCO_3 level >28 mEq/L) are life threatening if not corrected.

Respiratory compensation can be affected within minutes by any change in respiratory pattern. Any clinical condition that affects the respiratory system can also affect respiratory compensation. If a child's respiratory rate is too slow or too shallow, carbon dioxide will increase, serum pH can decrease, and acidosis may occur. If a child's respiratory rate is too rapid, carbon dioxide will decrease, serum pH may increase, and alkalosis can occur.

The renal system regulates the excretion of hydrogen ions (H^+) and HCO_3. This compensatory mechanism is a slow, long-term response that can take days to restore acid–base balance. Urine pH can be valuable in determining whether the renal compensatory mechanism is functioning. In metabolic acidosis, urine pH less than 6.0 indicates that the renal system is reabsorbing HCO_3 and excreting H^+, thus compensation is occurring. Renal compensatory mechanisms to correct acidosis help protect the cells but do not change the underlying cause of the disorder.

Acid–base disorders are common in children. The causes are varied and cover a wide range of clinical conditions and exogenous pathologic processes (Table 17-2). Arterial blood gas and serum electrolyte values are used to diagnose the imbalance's origin (metabolic or respiratory) and devise a plan of care.

Interdisciplinary Interventions

The goal of treatment for a child with an acid–base disorder is to correct the primary cause, for example, by administering insulin and fluid to a child with diabetic ketoacidosis. Most children who are acidotic and who have adequate circulation, renal function, and pulmonary function can be managed by treating the underlying cause of the acid–base imbalance. Many do not require alkali therapy such as with sodium bicarbonate.

ALERT   *It is imperative to correct any low blood pressure along with the acidosis. Together, they present a life-threatening situation. Complete collapse of the cardiovascular and respiratory systems may be imminent.*

Nursing responsibilities include monitoring the child's status and adequacy of ventilation, including vital signs (heart rate and rhythm, respiration, blood pressure, and temperature). Maintain a clear airway and ensure adequate ventilation.

caREminder

Observe the child's work of breathing and auscultate the lungs. Assess for actual air movement along with respiratory effort. Assist the child with positioning for maximum ventilation and minimum effort by elevating the head of the bed and not letting the child slouch, which interferes with diaphragmatic excursion. Administer oxygen and perform suctioning if necessary. Provide manual ventilation if the child's respiratory effort does not appear to be adequate.

TABLE 17-2   Acid–Base Imbalances

	Respiratory Acidosis	Respiratory Alkalosis	Metabolic Acidosis	Metabolic Alkalosis
Imbalance	H_2CO_3 excess; CO_2 is retained and pH decreases	H_2CO_3 deficit; not enough CO_2 is retained and pH increases	HCO_3 deficit	HCO_3 excess
Causes	Events that depress the respiratory drive or interfere with ventilation: • Pulmonary diseases (e.g., pneumonia, asthma) • Central nervous system disorders that affect the neuromuscular system (e.g., muscular dystrophy, Guillain-Barré syndrome, tumors, botulism) • Ingestion of substances (e.g., opiates, barbiturates, alcohol)	Events that can cause hyperventilation: • Hypoxia • Sepsis • Fever • Anxiety • Ingestions • Pulmonary disease (e.g., pneumonia, chronic lung disease) • Mechanical over-ventilation	Loss of base from ECF, via renal or intestinal loss, or gain of acid by ECF: • Hypovolemia • Diabetes • Congenital heart disease • Sepsis • Cold stress • Inborn errors of metabolism	H^+ loss or HCO_3 retention: • Vomiting or NG suctioning • Administration of sodium bicarbonate • Massive blood transfusion • Milk–alkali syndrome (chronic ingestion of milk and antacids containing calcium carbonate)
Signs to assess for	Respiratory distress Central nervous system depression: disorientation, coma Hypoxia: restlessness, irritability, tachycardia, arrhythmias Muscle weakness	Dizziness Numbness and paresthesias of fingers and toes Tetany Convulsions Unconsciousness	Deep, rapid breathing (Kussmaul respirations) Shortness of breath on exertion Weakness Drowsiness, stupor When pH is <7.2, cardiac contractility is reduced, thus blood pressure decreases, dysrhythmias occur, cardiovascular collapse typically follows	May be asymptomatic or show signs similar to those of dehydration Tachycardia Hypoventilation Muscle hypertonicity or tetany (alkalosis decreases blood levels of ionized calcium), progressing to convulsions Confusion, irritability, coma
Treatment	Correct underlying problem. Administer oxygen; low flow only if carbon dioxide narcosis is present. Improve ventilation, increase aeration (position to facilitate ventilation, antibiotics for respiratory infections, chest physical therapy). Administer sodium bicarbonate.	Correct underlying problem. Do not overventilate; have child focus on slowing breathing, breathe into paper bag.	Correct underlying problem. Administer sodium bicarbonate. Provide low-protein, high-calorie diet Position to facilitate ventilation.	Correct underlying problem. Administer fluid containing sodium and potassium. Avoid antacids.

If a child requires mechanical ventilation, the nurse and respiratory therapist must collaborate to evaluate ventilator settings frequently. One iatrogenic cause of respiratory alkalosis is overventilation. Frequently monitor the appropriateness of ventilator parameters, the adequacy of ventilation, and the child's response to any changes made. Compare vital signs with those obtained previously and observe for trends that indicate that the child's status is improving or deteriorating. A normal temperature should be the goal, because body temperature alterations (hypothermia and hyperthermia) increase metabolic demands and cause further deterioration of acid–base balance. Warm a child with hypothermia with blankets and an external warming source if necessary. Provide a child with hyperthermia with a light bedcover or none and lower the room temperature if possible. Antipyretics, such as acetaminophen and ibuprofen, may be ordered to decrease fever and thus decrease metabolic demands.

Monitor the child continuously for changes in level of consciousness. Closely monitor laboratory values, interpret the findings in light of the child's condition, and change the treatment regimen accordingly. Report significant changes or findings that do not fall within normal parameters for the child's age to the medical team.

Monitor intake and output. Parents and other family members who stay with the child can aid in obtaining this information. The method of fluid administration depends on the child's physical condition, level of consciousness, and age. The physician or advanced practice nurse will order IV therapy if indicated.

Community Care

Reinforce safety issues (keeping poisons out of reach; providing appropriate, balanced intake) with children and parents. Teach the family how to manage conditions such as vomiting and diarrhea that cause dehydration and can lead to metabolic alkalosis or metabolic acidosis. In children with chronic conditions such as diabetes, maintain blood glucose within acceptable ranges and adhere to treatment regimen. Help the child to manage anxiety that may lead to respiratory alkalosis.

ELECTROLYTE IMBALANCES

The body maintains a delicate balance of electrolytes, all of which contribute to homeostasis and healthy functioning. Electrolyte imbalance has many causes. More than one electrolyte imbalance may occur simultaneously. Assessing all electrolytes and addressing each imbalance is important to provide complete, comprehensive treatment (Nursing Interventions Classification 17-1).

> QUESTION: After surgery, Cory returns with an NG tube placed to decompress his stomach and remove gastric secretions. What are the two electrolytes that are affected by removing gastric secretions?

Sodium Imbalance

Sodium (Na^+) is the principal cation in ECF. Therefore, it exerts the greatest proportion of ECF osmolarity. Sodium influences distribution of body water and helps maintain acid–base balance and neuromuscular function.

HYPONATREMIA

Hyponatremia is defined as a serum sodium level less than 130 mEq/L. Clinical symptoms are more severe with a level less than 120 mEq/L.

A variety of situations can cause hyponatremia that result in either a net sodium loss or net water excess. Net sodium loss can result from increased gastrointestinal output such as diarrhea, vomiting, NG suction (a major cause of hyponatremia in children), diuretic therapy, excessive diaphoresis, and kidney disease. Net water excess can be caused by dilutional hyponatremia or sodium deprivation that results from increased water intake with decreased sodium intake, administration of hypotonic IV solutions, administration of excessively diluted formulas, or syndrome of inappropriate antidiuretic hormone secretion (see Chapter 26).

Important factors in the development of symptoms include the rate at which the sodium level declines and the duration of the low level. Severe hyponatremia that occurs rapidly over a few hours is called *water intoxication*. Neurologic consequences result from a too-rapid change in sodium balance, which causes massive fluid shifts into the cerebral space. The cranium of a child with a closed fontanel is a fixed space. Normal cerebral contents (brain, cerebrospinal fluid, blood) occupy part of that space. Shifting of excess fluid into the cerebral compartment causes cerebral edema, which can produce seizures, coma, respiratory arrest, and brain damage (see Nursing Interventions Classification 17-1).

Interdisciplinary Interventions

Treatment of hyponatremia depends on the cause. The goal is to raise the serum sodium level in a slow and controlled manner and then maintain within normal limits.

caREminder

Hyponatremia can be prevented in the child receiving IV fluids by not infusing hypotonic solutions unless their use is indicated by a documented elevated serum sodium level.

When a net loss of sodium and body water is present, oral or IV sodium and fluid replacement may be ordered. Nursing assessments and interventions are similar to those for preventing or treating hypovolemic shock in children with hyponatremic dehydration. When a net water excess is present, treatment is directed toward reducing the ECF and ICF excess. Measures may involve restricting water intake or diuretic therapy. Nursing care is similar to that for the child with fluid overload and edema.

The nurse is responsible for implementing treatment, monitoring the child's response, and providing child and family teaching. Monitor and document the child's intake, output, and fluid balance.

Community Care

If hyponatremia is caused by excessive oral fluid intake, either directly or through diluted formula, in addition to assessing the family's knowledge of fluid and nutrition, assessing the family's socioeconomic status is important. Parents experiencing financial hardship may dilute formula to make it last longer. They may not understand that prolonged feeding with overdiluted formula can harm their child. Provide education on formula preparation and delivery. Dietitians and social service case workers can also provide valuable assistance and resources to families in need.

HYPERNATREMIA

Hypernatremia is a serum sodium level exceeding 150 mEq/L. The most severe clinical manifestations of hypernatremia occur when the serum sodium level exceeds 160 mEq/L.

Hypernatremia results from insufficient fluid intake or excessive fluid loss or from excessive salt intake or insufficient sodium excretion. This may be caused by an altered thirst mechanism or an inability to respond to thirst (as may occur in infants and disabled or comatose children), increased insensible water loss, increased gastrointestinal output, excessive solute intake (e.g., from incorrectly diluted formulas, boiled skim milk), renal immaturity (e.g., in premature infants), or such disorders as diabetes insipidus or renal medullary impairment.

Children with hypernatremia are often dehydrated. Cellular dehydration results when water shifts out of

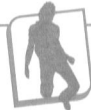

NIC 17-1 NURSING INTERVENTIONS CLASSIFICATION: Electrolyte Monitoring

Definition: Management of the patient with urinary drainage equipment

Activities:

Monitor the serum level of electrolytes

Monitor serum albumin and total protein levels, as indicated

Monitor for associated acid–base imbalances

Identify possible causes of electrolyte imbalances

Recognize and report presence of electrolyte imbalances

Monitor for fluid loss and associated loss of electrolytes, as appropriate

Monitor for Chvostek's and/or Trousseau's sign

Monitor for neurologic manifestation of electrolyte imbalance (e.g., altered sensorium and weakness)

Monitor adequacy of ventilation

Monitor serum and urine osmolality levels

Monitor EKG tracings for changes related to abnormal potassium, calcium, and magnesium levels

Note changes in peripheral sensation, such as numbness and tremors

Note muscle strength

Monitor for nausea, vomiting, and diarrhea

Identify treatments that can alter electrolyte status, such as GI suctioning, diuretics, antihypertensives, and calcium channel blockers

Monitor for underlying medical disease that can lead to electrolyte imbalance

Monitor for signs and symptoms of hypokalemia: muscular weakness, cardiac irregularities (PVC), prolonged QT interval, flattened or depressed T wave, depressed ST segment, presence of U wave, fatigue, paresthesia, decreased reflexes, anorexia, constipation, decreased GI motility, dizziness, confusion, increased sensitivity to digitalis, and depressed respirations

Monitor for signs/symptoms of hyperkalemia: irritability, restlessness, anxiety, nausea, vomiting, abdominal cramps, weakness, flaccid paralysis, circumoral numbness and tingling, tachycardia progressing to bradycardia, ventricular tachycardia/fibrillation, tall and peaked T waves, flattened P wave, broad and slurred QRS complex, and heart block progressing to asystole

Monitor for signs/symptoms of hyponatremia: disorientation, muscle twitching, nausea and vomiting, abdominal cramps, headaches, personality changes, seizures, lethargy, fatigue, withdrawal, and coma

Monitor for signs and symptoms of hypernatremia: extreme thirst; fever; dry, sticky mucous membranes; tachycardia; hypotension; lethargy; confusion; altered mentation; and seizures

Monitor for signs and symptoms of hypocalcemia: irritability, muscle tetany, Chvostek's sign (facial muscle spasm), Trousseau's sign (carpal spasm), peripheral numbness and tingling, muscle cramps, decreased cardiac output, prolonged ST segment and QT interval, bleeding, and fractures

Monitor for signs and symptoms of hypercalcemia: deep bone pain, excessive thirst, anorexia, lethargy, weakened muscles, shortened QT segment, wide T wave, widened QRS complex, and prolonged P-R interval

Monitor for signs and symptoms of hypomagnesemia: respiratory muscle depression, mental apathy, Chvostek's sign (facial muscle spasm), Trousseau's sign (carpal spasm), confusion, facial tics, spasticity, and cardiac dysrhythmias

Monitor for signs and symptoms of hypermagnesemia: muscle weakness, inability to swallow, hyporeflexia, hypotension, bradycardia, CNS depression, respiratory depression, lethargy, coma, and depression

Monitor for signs and symptoms of hypophosphatemia: bleeding tendencies, muscular weakness, paresthesia, hemolytic anemia, depressed white cell function, nausea, vomiting, anorexia, and bone demineralization

Monitor for signs and symptoms of hyperphosphatemia: tachycardia, nausea, diarrhea, abdominal cramps, muscle weakness, flaccid paralysis, and increased reflexes

Monitor for signs and symptoms of hypochloremia: hyperirritability, tetany, muscular excitability, slow respirations, and hypotension

Monitor for signs and symptoms of hyperchloremia: weakness; lethargy; deep, rapid breathing; and coma

Administer prescribed supplemental electrolytes, as appropriate

Provide diet appropriate for patient's electrolyte imbalance (e.g., potassium-rich foods or low-sodium diet)

Teach patient ways to prevent or minimize electrolyte imbalance

Instruct patient and/or family on specific dietary modifications, as appropriate

Consult physician, if signs and symptoms of fluid and/or electrolyte imbalance persist or worsen

From Bulechek, G. M., Butcher, H. K., Dochterman, J. M. et al. (Eds.). (2013). *Nursing interventions classifications (NIC)* (6th ed.). St. Louis, MO: Mosby. Used with permission.

---

the ICF, pulled by the now hyperosmolar ECF. Children with hypernatremia often do not have circulatory disturbances because of the relative increase in vascular volume that occurs as fluid is pulled from the ICF into the ECF. Neurologic manifestations result when cerebral vessels shrink and tear as cellular dehydration occurs. The outcome is often a cerebral hemorrhage. Assess for neurologic signs in children with hypernatremia that may include lethargy, irritability on stimulation, and a high-pitched cry. Irritability may be a worrisome clinical sign, possibly indicating a cerebrovascular injury.

Interdisciplinary Interventions

The primary goals in treating hypernatremia are to bring the serum sodium level down to normal and to restore adequate hydration gradually, allowing the child's body to adjust to these changes. A too-rapid change in sodium level can disrupt the cell membranes in the cerebral vessels, possibly causing cerebral hemorrhage. If fluid is replaced too rapidly, water quickly crosses into brain cells (sodium levels decrease more slowly because of the blood–brain barrier), causing swelling of the brain cells and increased intracranial pressure (see Chapter 21). To reduce the risk of increased intracranial pressure, replacement of fluid deficit in hypernatremia is done over at least 48 hours. Fluid boluses of 20 mg/kg or more may be administered to a child in shock, however (see Chapter 31).

After fluid replacement therapy is initiated, the focus shifts to determining and treating the underlying cause of hypernatremia. Obtain a complete history to help evaluate the onset of clinical symptoms. This history should include the child's normal weight and a dietary history, including the amount and types of intake and output. Record the child's daily weight and compare it with previous weights to monitor fluid balance. Monitor laboratory data and report any clinically meaningful findings to the physician or advanced practice nurse. Other nursing responsibilities may include administering prescribed IV fluids with the appropriate sodium content. If the child has altered level of consciousness, position the child upright or on his or her side to enable adequate ventilation and to decrease the risk of aspiration.

A nutrition consultation can help provide the optimum electrolyte concentration and the maximum calories for the prescribed volume of fluid intake, whether administered orally or intravenously.

Community Care

Teach children and parents to maintain adequate fluid intake, particularly when children have excessive losses as when sick (e.g., vomiting, diarrhea, fever) or in high environmental temperatures. Also educate parents to avoid excessive solute administration (e.g., dilute formula properly; do not give boiled skim milk).

Potassium Imbalance

The primary intracellular ion, potassium (K^+), plays a major role in neuromuscular excitability. The ratio of intracellular potassium to extracellular potassium is a major determinant of cell membrane resting potential. Potassium also participates in cell metabolism through its action in protein and glycogen synthesis. Potassium is absorbed from the intestines and excreted in urine, feces, and sweat.

Blood pH affects serum potassium levels. When acidosis occurs, H^+ increase in number and are distributed equally in body compartments. To maintain electroneutrality, as H^+ moves into the cell, K^+ moves out of the cell. The result is an elevated serum potassium level with a concomitant decrease in serum pH. With alkalosis, this shift is reversed, and changes in potassium levels are less pronounced.

caREminder

If acidosis persists, total body potassium may be depleted even though the serum potassium level is elevated because potassium is moving out of the ICF, where it is most abundant.

HYPOKALEMIA

Hypokalemia, defined as a serum potassium level less than 3.5 mEq/L, may be caused by inadequate potassium intake and excessive renal potassium loss, as often occurs in a child receiving diuretic therapy (many diuretics promote increased potassium excretion in the distal tubule of the kidney). In diabetes, hyperglycemia typically produces an osmotic diuresis and high urine output, resulting in potassium loss. Because the hyperglycemic child is acidotic, serum potassium levels may not decrease to reflect the total body deficit of potassium until the acidosis starts to resolve. Gastrointestinal potassium losses occur through vomiting and diarrhea. Integumentary loss of potassium occurring in sweat and burns may also occur.

Clinical manifestations of hypokalemia include general muscle dysfunction and dysrhythmias (see Nursing Interventions Classification 17-1).

Interdisciplinary Interventions

When the potassium level falls below normal values, oral or IV potassium replacement is needed to restore and maintain adequate intracellular potassium concentrations. The route and rate of potassium replacement depends on the child's serum potassium concentration and renal function. Moderate to severe hypokalemia may be treated with potassium supplements administered either orally or IV.

ALERT *Before administering a potassium supplement, ensure that the child is producing urine, which demonstrates renal function. Because potassium is excreted through the kidneys, if renal function is inadequate, potassium readily accumulates. This can lead to ventricular dysrhythmias and cardiac arrest.*

Mild hypokalemia can often be resolved with dietary modifications. A dietitian can help the child and family increase potassium content in their diet based on the child's preferences and the family's resources and finances. For instance, salt substitutes that contain potassium can provide a low-cost potassium source. Involve social services to help low-income or at-risk families identify and use community resources.

Nursing responsibilities include ongoing assessment. Because potassium influences cell membrane excitability, muscle weakness or dysfunction is often apparent. Observe the child's activity level to evaluate generalized weakness and determine whether it is progressive.

If the child is receiving a potassium-wasting diuretic or has other risk factors for hypokalemia, ask whether he or she is tired ("Can you do the things you normally do?") or ask the parents about the child's activity level. Instruct the child to tell the parent or caregiver if he or she feels tired or otherwise "different."

Also assess respiratory effort, cardiac function, and the presence or absence of bowel sounds. Report signs of compromise to the health care team. Position the child with the head of the bed elevated to optimize respiratory effort and provide manual ventilation as needed. Withhold feedings when bowel sounds are absent.

Assess the child receiving digoxin therapy for signs of digoxin toxicity because hypokalemia potentiates digoxin.

Community Care

Teach the child and parents how to administer prescribed medications and monitor for their side effects and how to avoid potentially dangerous drug interactions. For example, if the child is taking a potassium-wasting diuretic and a potassium supplement, the family needs to remind the health care provider of this regimen when changing medication (hyperkalemia can occur if the diuretic is discontinued but not the potassium supplement). Discuss with the family the benefit of obtaining all prescriptions from one pharmacy or at least informing the pharmacist of other medications or food supplements that the child is receiving. Often, the pharmacist monitors for potential drug interactions and alerts the prescriber and family if any are noted.

If the family's financial status or access to medications is an issue, they can request that the prescriber order a commercial salt substitute (potassium chloride [KCl]) rather than a more costly pharmaceutical preparation.

HYPERKALEMIA

A serum potassium level more than 5.0 mEq/L can result from various conditions. Dehydration or renal disease can impair renal excretion of potassium. Because potassium is the primary intracellular ion, damage to cells or the cell membrane (as occurs in crush injuries and burns, for instance) releases potassium from the cells into the ECF. This process may also occur with transfusion of stored blood when old, damaged red blood cells release their intracellular potassium.

Clinical manifestations of hyperkalemia vary with the severity of the imbalance (see Nursing Interventions Classification 17-1). The most serious manifestations are cardiovascular changes. Severe hyperkalemia is a life-threatening emergency that requires immediate treatment.

ALERT   *Severe dysrhythmias and cardiac arrest may result when potassium levels rise above 6.0 mEq/L.*

Interdisciplinary Interventions

Treatment of hyperkalemia must be initiated promptly to prevent serious physiologic effects. Several measures can lower a dangerously high potassium level (Nursing Interventions 17-2). During treatment, assess for rebound hypokalemia that may result

Continuously monitor electrocardiogram (ECG) waveforms for dysrhythmias. Assess vital signs, including heart rate, heart rhythm, and blood pressure, and intervene to support optimal cardiorespiratory function as needed. Have emergency equipment readily accessible.

Monitor serum potassium levels. Collect blood specimens carefully because a hemolyzed blood sample can result in falsely elevated potassium levels.

caREminder

To avoid blood cell hemolysis, warm an extremity if blood is being obtained by skin puncture. Do not excessively squeeze or milk an extremity to obtain blood. Use blood that flows easily from a skin puncture or vein and do not use excessive pressure to force blood from the syringe into the specimen collecting device.

Monitor potassium intake by calculating intake of potassium from IV fluids, medications, and foods. Many foods contain potassium. Foods low in potassium include pears, apples, pineapple, rice, green beans, and salads without tomatoes.

Ensure adequate fluid intake to help increase output of potassium in urine. Potassium is excreted through the kidneys; therefore, monitor renal function through urine output volume and related laboratory values such as BUN and creatinine levels.

Monitor for hyperkalemia in a child receiving multiple blood transfusions or a child with renal dysfunction who requires blood administration. To help prevent this complication, the freshest blood available should be transfused.

Community Care

For the child with hyperkalemia resulting from a chronic medical condition, teach the family how to manage the child's condition at home. Include other members of the health care team, such as social service case workers and the dietitian, in designing the teaching plan for the family.

Instruct the child and family to avoid foods high in potassium and assist them to make dietary modifications that fit in with the family's lifestyle and dietary habits. Teach parents to keep potassium-containing salt substitutes away from children and to avoid their use in a child with renal problems.

Calcium Imbalance

Calcium (Ca^{++}) is vital to cardiac, muscle, and nerve function and helps maintain normal cell membrane permeability. It also plays a role in the secretion of certain hormones (e.g., parathyroid hormone, calcitriol,

NURSING INTERVENTIONS 17-2

Management of Hyperkalemia

Medical Treatment Option*	Nursing Intervention
Create Chemical Antagonist to the Membrane Effects of Potassium	
Administer calcium gluconate 10% IV to temporarily stabilize the cell membrane.	Ensure that IV is not infiltrated; monitor IV closely before and during infusion because calcium extravasation causes severe tissue necrosis.
	Administer calcium slowly as ordered.
	Monitor ECG during infusion; report ECG changes or bradycardia immediately.
	If child is receiving digoxin, administer calcium slowly while monitoring for signs of digoxin toxicity because hypercalcemia potentiates digoxin toxicity.
	Monitor effectiveness of therapy (decrease in signs of hyperkalemia) and for return of negative effects resulting from hyperkalemia because effects of calcium are effective within minutes but are short lived.
Expand the ECF Volume	
Decrease, by dilution, the extracellular potassium concentration.	Administer IV fluid as ordered.
	Monitor for change in signs of hyperkalemia that indicate effectiveness of therapy.
	Monitor for signs of fluid overload.
	Calculate fluid balance and intake and output.
Increase Cellular Uptake of Potassium	
Administer insulin IV, which facilitates cellular potassium uptake; glucose is usually administered with insulin to prevent hypoglycemia.	Administer insulin and glucose as ordered.
	Monitor for signs of hypoglycemia.
	Monitor for changes in potassium levels; effects usually occur in 30 minutes and last several hours.
Administer nebulized beta-adrenergic agonists (e.g. albuterol, salbutamol).	Administer beta-adrenergic agonists as ordered.
	Monitor for changes in potassium levels; effects usually occur in 30 minutes and last 2–3 hours.
In the presence of metabolic acidosis, administer sodium bicarbonate to normalize pH and reverse the shifting of potassium out of the cell that occurs with acidosis.	Administer sodium bicarbonate as ordered.
	Monitor for return of hyperkalemia because effects may only last 1–2 hours.
Remove Potassium From the Body	
Administer potassium-wasting diuretics (e.g., furosemide) to increase renal excretion of potassium.	Administer diuretic as ordered.
	Monitor urine output.
	Monitor for signs of dehydration.
	Evaluate effectiveness of therapy based on clinical changes.
Administer a cation exchange resin (e.g., Kayexalate) that exchanges 1 mEq potassium for 1 mEq sodium; it is usually administered in a suspension with sorbitol.	Administer via NG tube or by enema as ordered.
	Maximize effect of enema by having the child retain it for 2–3 hours.
	Monitor for signs of dehydration because sorbitol creates an osmotic load that pulls water into the gut.

Medical Treatment Option*	Nursing Intervention
	Monitor for change in potassium levels, which show a maximal decrease in 3–4 hours (other treatment options are usually used as interim measures to decrease the cardiotoxic effects of excess potassium while waiting for removal techniques to have an effect).
	Monitor serum sodium and potassium levels.
	Monitor for fluid overload and hypernatremia resulting from sodium-exchanging properties of resin.
Institute peritoneal dialysis or hemodialysis.	Prepare child for dialysis as appropriate.
	Implement interventions and monitoring as specific to type of dialysis.

*Treatment choice is based on symptoms (e.g., dysrhythmias) rather than serum level.

calcitonin) and the activation of some enzymes (e.g., insulin and glucagon). Circulating calcium concentrations are maintained by interactions of vitamin D metabolism, calcitonin, and parathyroid hormone. Parathyroid hormone helps regulate calcium concentration by stimulating reabsorption of calcium from bone and glomerular filtrate.

The largest calcium stores in the body are in the bones and teeth. This calcium is not readily available for use by the body. A small amount of body calcium is found in the plasma as protein-bound calcium, bound to diffusible molecules such as phosphate and citrate, or as ionized calcium. The level of ionized calcium, the physiologically active form of calcium, is about half that of total calcium.

Serum calcium levels are affected by serum protein concentration, pH, and phosphorus. Because calcium binds to protein, hyperproteinemia may result in hypocalcemia. pH affects the physiologic availability of calcium. Acidosis causes hypercalcemia by decreasing calcium binding to serum proteins and increases the amount of calcium released from bone; alkalosis causes the opposite effect. Calcium and phosphorus normally have an inverse relation; when the level of one rises, the level of the other falls.

HYPOCALCEMIA

Defined as a total calcium concentration less than 8.8 mEq/L, hypocalcemia can result from inadequate dietary intake, vitamin D deficiency, hyperalbuminemia, renal disease, or diuretic therapy. Transfusion of blood containing citrate as an anticoagulant, particularly large or rapid infusions, may cause hypocalcemia because the citrate binds with calcium and decreases the amount of available ionized calcium. In a newborn, ingestion of cow's milk, which is high in phosphate, may lead to hypocalcemia because newborns have a relatively high rate of tubular phosphate absorption and a physiologically low glomerular filtration rate. Correcting acidosis may lead to hypocalcemia because, in an acidotic state, the calcium that moves out of the bones may be lost through urine output. Restoring normal pH causes calcium to reenter the bones, resulting in hypocalcemia.

Hypocalcemia causes increased cell membrane permeability. Thus, clinical manifestations are characterized by increased neuromuscular excitability, particularly affecting the neuromuscular and cardiovascular systems (see Nursing Interventions Classification 17-1); assess for these signs. The child may complain of numbness or tingling of the nose, ears, fingers, and toes. Laryngospasm may produce high-pitched inspiratory noises and may result in apnea. Severe hypocalcemia can cause seizures and cardiac arrest.

Interdisciplinary Interventions

Asymptomatic hypocalcemia can be treated with dietary modifications involving increased intake of foods rich in calcium, such as dairy products, bony fish (e.g., sardines), and green leafy vegetables (see Table 20-1). Calcium supplements and vitamin D may be administered. Treatment of symptomatic hypocalcemia typically includes IV administration of calcium.

ALERT   *Before administering IV calcium, ensure that the IV is correctly placed with no signs of complications. Infiltration of calcium causes severe tissue necrosis. Administer IV calcium slowly, monitor the site closely, and monitor the ECG during infusion for QRS changes and bradycardia.*

Maintain seizure precautions for a child with hypocalcemia. Ensure that emergency equipment to provide manual ventilation is readily available.

Community Care

Teach children and families which food sources are rich in calcium and encourage adequate intake of calcium and vitamin D. Ten to 15 minutes of sun exposure, without sunscreen, two to three times a week to the face, arms, or hands may also help satisfy vitamin D requirements. Instruct parents not to give cow's milk to young infants.

HYPERCALCEMIA

Hypercalcemia is defined as a total calcium level exceeding 10.8 mEq/L. Causes include increased resorption of calcium from bone resulting from a malignancy (see Chapter 22), immobility, hyperparathyroidism, or hyperthyroidism; increased gastrointestinal absorption of calcium from excessive oral intake of calcium or vitamin D; and decreased excretion of calcium resulting from renal failure or diuretic therapy. Acidotic states also cause an increase in physiologically available calcium.

Hypercalcemia decreases cell membrane permeability, with a resultant decrease in neuromuscular excitability. High calcium levels may be asymptomatic, an incidental finding when other laboratory values are obtained. Hypercalcemia may also have a nonspecific presentation such as bone pain, fatigue, or polyuria and polydipsia. Assess for ECG changes that may be present (see Nursing Interventions Classification 17-1). Assess deep tendon reflexes, which are usually hypoactive with diminished muscle tone and strength. Renal calculi and renal failure, caused by the increased excretion of calcium in urine, or pathologic fractures may occur. Decreased motility in the gastrointestinal tract may cause abdominal pain, anorexia, nausea, and vomiting.

Interdisciplinary Interventions

Hypercalcemia is often an indication of an underlying disease that requires treatment. Severe hypercalcemia is treated with aggressive hydration with NS. Generous fluid administration helps maintain vascular volume in the presence of dehydration and promotes calcium excretion, which occurs though the kidneys. After ensuring adequate hydration, diuretics are often administered to further promote diuresis. Administration of phosphate binds the calcium and can rapidly lower serum calcium levels. Medications that decrease the absorption of calcium, such as calcitonin, glucocorticoids, and IV bisphosphonates (which inhibit bone resorption of calcium), may also be administered (Lynch & Wood, 2011).

Nursing responsibilities include monitoring serum calcium levels and reporting any abnormal findings to the health care prescriber. Also assess neuromuscular and cardiac status (including ECG waveforms), maintain fluid balance, and provide parent teaching.

Monitoring fluid balance in hypercalcemia is important for several reasons. The child may be dehydrated on initial presentation or during the course of therapy, or administration of large fluid volumes may overload the vascular system. Moreover, two goals of treatment are to promote urinary calcium excretion and prevent renal damage from the deposits of calcium salts. Monitor intake and output and evaluate fluid balance as often as indicated by the child's overall status (e.g., every hour, every 12 hours, or every 24 hours). Evaluate other indicators of fluid balance (e.g., blood pressure, presence of edema or signs of dehydration, rales when auscultating breath sounds) and implement interventions as indicated. If the child's blood pressure is low or unstable, diuretics should be used with caution.

Encourage mobilization to prevent the development of hypercalcemia caused by excessive resorption of calcium from the bones. If the child must be immobilized, ensure adequate fluid intake to prevent renal damage and handle the child gently when moving to avoid fractures.

Community Care

Education is an important component of family care, particularly when the primary cause of the hypercalcemia is a chronic condition. Teach the child and family signs and symptoms of calcium imbalance and instruct them to notify their health care provider if they occur. If medications are used to manage hypercalcemia, teach the child and family about administration, side effects, and potential interactions with other medications or food.

Include teaching about food sources of calcium and the degree to which these sources must be limited. A dietitian should be involved to help the family adapt dietary restrictions to their lifestyle. Because excessive intake of vitamin D can cause hypercalcemia, instruct parents to keep vitamin supplements out of children's reach and tell them about the hazards of excessive vitamin supplementation.

Magnesium Imbalance

Magnesium (Mg^{++}) imbalance is less common than imbalances of other electrolytes, but it can be life threatening if severe. A neuromuscular depressant, magnesium, is necessary for forming soft tissue and bone and for maintaining normal cellular function and muscle and nerve activity. It is the second most abundant intracellular ion and is found in small amounts in the ECF. Normal plasma values in children are 1.5 to 2.3 mEq/L (Fenton et al., 2011; Finberg et al., 1993).

Magnesium affects cell functions through its interactions with calcium. Calcium often opposes the actions of magnesium. Magnesium is excreted primarily in urine and in small amounts through the gastrointestinal tract. Absorption occurs primarily in the upper gastrointestinal tract. Food sources of magnesium include green vegetables, whole grains, legumes, nuts, meat, and dairy products.

Besides restoring magnesium balance, treatment also focuses on correcting the primary cause of the imbalance.

Because magnesium imbalances are relatively rare compared with other electrolyte imbalances, they may be overlooked. Assess the child for conditions that may lead to imbalance as well as for electrolyte imbalances associated with hypomagnesemia (e.g., hypokalemia, hypocalcemia, hypochloremic alkalosis) and hypermagnesemia (e.g., elevated BUN and creatinine levels). Assess the child's vital signs to detect hypotension, cardiac dysrhythmias, and respiratory impairment. Also assess muscle tone and monitor serum electrolyte values.

HYPOMAGNESEMIA

Defined as a serum magnesium level less than 1.5 mEq/L, hypomagnesemia can be caused by inadequate intake (e.g., malnutrition, prolonged IV therapy without supplement), impaired absorption (e.g., in the presence of excessive calcium intake, diarrhea, vomiting, hypoparathyroidism, or bowel resection), or increased excretion (e.g., use of thiazide diuretics, aldosterone excess). Administration of citrated blood, which binds free magnesium, may also cause hypomagnesemia. Severe hypomagnesemia interferes with the release of parathyroid hormone; thus, hypomagnesemia and hypocalcemia often coexist. Parathyroid hormone stimulates absorption of magnesium in the intestines and release of calcium from bones. Hormones (e.g., calcitonin, aldosterone) that inhibit intestinal absorption of magnesium also stimulate calcium resorption into the bones.

caREminder

Hypocalcemia that does not respond to treatment may indicate a concomitant hypomagnesemia that also requires treatment.

Assess for signs and symptoms of hypomagnesemia, which can be similar to those of hypocalcemia. Manifestations of increased neuromuscular irritability (hyperactive reflexes, tetany, seizures) and impaired cardiac function (hypotension, tachycardia, ECG changes, and dysrhythmias) are of most concern.

Interdisciplinary Interventions

Mild hypomagnesemia can be corrected by increasing the child's intake of magnesium-rich foods. This diet may be supplemented by magnesium-based antacids (e.g., milk of magnesia). Moderate to severe hypomagnesemia may require IV administration of magnesium supplements. Assess renal function (which is necessary for excretion of excess magnesium) before administering these supplements to prevent iatrogenic hypermagnesemia.

IV administration of magnesium requires close monitoring. Infiltration of magnesium into the tissues can lead to necrosis and sloughing of the surrounding area. Optimally, magnesium is administered into a central vein and is infused slowly to decrease discomfort caused by vasodilation (feeling hot, flushing). Rebound hypermagnesemia may result from magnesium infusion. Assess deep tendon reflexes during infusion to detect hyporeflexia, a relatively early sign of hypermagnesemia.

Nursing care also addresses symptom management. For instance, a child with muscle spasms needs reduced environmental stimuli (e.g., low noise level, dim lighting). Handle the child gently to avoid causing additional discomfort from neuromuscular excitability.

HYPERMAGNESEMIA

Hypermagnesemia, a serum magnesium level exceeding 2.3 mEq/L, can be caused by impaired excretion (e.g., decreased renal function) or excessive intake (e.g., magnesium-containing antacids, IV supplementation, treatment of maternal eclampsia with magnesium, which crosses the placenta and can cause elevated magnesium levels in neonates). Signs and symptoms of hypermagnesemia reflect altered neuromuscular function (e.g., hyporeflexia, lethargy, respiratory depression) and cardiac function (e.g., flushing from vasodilation, bradycardia, hypotension, dysrhythmias). Assess for the presence of these manifestations.

Interdisciplinary Interventions

If hypermagnesemia is detected, promptly discontinue all medications and IV fluids containing magnesium as ordered. Severe hypermagnesemia, or hypermagnesemia in the presence of renal failure, is treated with IV administration of calcium (usually calcium gluconate in children), which blocks the neuromuscular effects of magnesium. (See the section on "Hypocalcemia" for discussion of hazards associated with IV calcium infusion.) Thiazide diuretics may be given to remove excess magnesium, and IV fluids may be given to increase urine output. Children with severe hypermagnesemia may require dialysis.

Nursing care focuses on carefully monitoring fluid balance. Fluid excess may occur because of impaired myocardial contractility arising from the effects of magnesium, because of impaired renal function, or as a result of both. Signs of fluid overload include fluid intake greater than output, increased respiratory rate, and rales.

Phosphorus Imbalance

Although it is relatively rare, phosphorus (PO_4^-) imbalance can be life threatening when severe. Phosphorus is crucial to the integrity of cells and cell membranes and plays an important role in producing energy for normal metabolic activity and growth. Most phosphorus, like calcium, is found in the bones. A small percentage is found in ECF. Children have higher serum phosphorus levels than adults because of their rapid skeletal growth. Normal serum phosphorus levels vary depending on age (see Appendix D). Renal excretion, intestinal absorption, and bone mineralization all affect serum phosphorus level. Parathyroid hormone inhibits tubular reabsorption of phosphorus and increases its excretion in urine. The excretion and retention of phosphorus is closely related to glomerular filtration and general kidney function. When renal function is impaired, the kidney retains phosphorus and serum levels become elevated.

Increased serum phosphorus levels can lead to decreased levels of serum calcium. Usually, phosphorus and calcium vary inversely because parathyroid hormone, while inhibiting absorption of phosphate, promotes calcium uptake. In a child with malabsorption or malnutrition, levels of both electrolytes are low.

As with all electrolyte imbalances, in phosphorus imbalance, identifying and treating the underlying cause of the imbalance is the ultimate goal. Phosphorus levels are monitored along with associated electrolytes, such as calcium and magnesium, and serum pH. Indicators of renal function, such as BUN and creatinine, are also monitored.

HYPOPHOSPHATEMIA

Hypophosphatemia may result from inadequate intake and impaired absorption. Inadequate phosphorus intake is particularly prevalent in preterm infants who have high phosphorus needs because of rapid growth. Hypophosphatemia caused by "refeeding syndrome" may occur after carbohydrate administration in severely malnourished children. In this syndrome, phosphate shifts intracellularly, leaving the ECF and entering the cell when glucose enters the cell. Intracellular shifting of phosphate also occurs with alkalosis and after administration of corticosteroids or insulin. Antacids containing aluminum or magnesium hydroxide bind phosphate and can decrease serum phosphate levels. Hypophosphatemia also may result from increased urinary excretion of phosphorus stemming from decreased tubular reabsorption, administration of thiazide diuretics, ECF volume expansion, or hyperparathyroidism.

Because of phosphate's role in energy production for cellular metabolism, mild hypophosphatemia may manifest as weakness and tissue hypoxia. As the deficit becomes more severe, signs and symptoms similar to those of encephalopathy (irritability, confusion, seizures, coma, paresthesia) and other manifestations may appear (see Nursing Interventions Classification 19-3). Assess for these signs and symptoms.

Interdisciplinary Interventions

Ensuring adequate phosphorus intake is the primary preventive measure in hypophosphatemia. This measure is especially important in preterm infants receiving PN or breast milk, which does not adequately meet their phosphorus needs during rapid growth. Breast milk fortifier should be given as ordered. The health care prescriber and dietitian should collaborate in writing orders for PN to ensure a balance of essential nutrients.

Treatment of mild hypophosphatemia typically involves increasing dietary phosphorus intake to restore serum phosphorus levels. Phosphorus supplements can be given orally, in the form of phosphate salts, or intravenously. The route of administration is chosen according to the cause and severity of deficit. During IV phosphorus administration, carefully monitor renal function to avoid hyperphosphatemia. Levels of other electrolytes are also monitored to detect any imbalances that may be associated with hypophosphatemia or its treatment.

Teach the child and family about treatment measures, ways to increase intake of foods high in phosphorus,

and the need to avoid phosphate-binding antacids and diuretics.

HYPERPHOSPHATEMIA

Phosphorus excess is generally not of major concern unless renal excretion of phosphorus is impaired. Hyperphosphatemia most commonly results from decreased glomerular filtration of phosphorus, such as occurs in chronic renal disease. It can also be caused by excessive phosphorus intake, occurring orally, intravenously, or from administration of phosphate-containing enemas. Hyperphosphatemia may also develop in children receiving treatment for malignancies, especially lymphoma or leukemia, who have rapid cytolysis of cells with resultant release of intracellular phosphorus.

Because of the inverse relationship between phosphorus and calcium, hypocalcemia usually develops concurrently with hyperphosphatemia. Thus, signs and symptoms of hyperphosphatemia mimic those of hypocalcemia. Assess for these signs and symptoms, which include hyperreflexia, tetany, tachycardia, nausea, abdominal cramps, and diarrhea.

Interdisciplinary Interventions

Treatment of hyperphosphatemia aims to increase phosphorus excretion and decrease phosphorus intake. Excretion is promoted by maintaining high urine output through the administration of oral and IV fluids. Dietary intake of high-phosphate foods (see Table 20-1) is reduced. Calcium carbonate and calcium acetate can be used as oral phosphate binders. Aluminum-containing antacids bind phosphorus, preventing gut absorption, and thus may be ordered. However, phosphate binders that contain aluminum have a limited role in therapy (only when serum phosphate is more than 7 mg/dL) because they cause heavy metals to accumulate in the brain and bones, causing osteomalacia and encephalopathy (Perry & Salusky, 2012). Sevelamer, lanthanum carbonate, and magnesium iron hydroxycarbonate are calcium-free phosphate binders used in adults; preliminary data suggest that these can be safely used for children (Cannata-Andía et al., 2010). Hypocalcemia should be treated concurrently. A child with severe hyperphosphatemia may need dialysis.

Monitor for electrolyte imbalances associated with hyperphosphatemia (e.g., hypocalcemia, hypomagnesemia) and assess urine output as an indicator of renal function. Institute seizure precautions to prevent injury caused by tetany. Teach the child and family about the treatment regimen and instruct them to avoid phosphate-containing foods.

ANSWER: NG suction causes both sodium and potassium loss. Cory's sodium and potassium levels will be monitored and he will receive IV fluid replacement with sodium and possibly with potassium supplement as well.

See thePoint for a summary of Key Concepts.

REFERENCES

Advani, S., Reich, N. G., Sengupta, A. et al. (2011). Central line-associated bloodstream infection in hospitalized children with peripherally inserted central venous catheters: Extending risk analyses outside the intensive care unit. *Clinical Infectious Diseases*, 52(9), 1108–1115.

Arnts, I. J. J., Heijnen, J. A., Wilbers, H. T. M. et al. (2011). Effectiveness of heparin solution versus normal saline in maintaining patency of intravenous locks in neonates: A double blind randomized controlled study. *Journal of Advanced Nursing*, 67(12), 2677–2685.

Beck, C. E. (2007). Hypotonic versus isotonic maintenance intravenous fluid therapy in hospitalized children: A systematic review. *Clinical Pediatrics*, 46, 764–770.

Butler-O'Hara, M., D'Angio, C. T., Hoey, H. et al. (2012). An evidence-based catheter bundle alters central venous catheter strategy in newborn infants. *The Journal of Pediatrics*, 160(6), 972–977.

Cannata-Andía, J. B., Rodriguez-García, M., Román-García, P. et al. (2010). New therapies: Calcimimetics, phosphate binders and vitamin D receptor activators. *Pediatric Nephrology*, 25(4), 609–616.

Choong, K., Arora, S., Cheng, J. et al. (2011). Hypotonic versus isotonic maintenance fluids after surgery for children: a randomized controlled trial. *Pediatrics*, 128(5), 857–866.

Choong, K., Kho, M. E., Menon, K. et al. (2006). Hypotonic versus isotonic saline in hospitalized children: A systematic review. *Archives of Disease in Childhood*, 91(10), 828–835.

Colletti, J. E., Brown, K. M., Sharieff, G. Q. et al. (2010). The management of children with gastroenteritis and dehydration in the emergency department. *The Journal of Emergency Medicine*, 38(5), 686–698.

Cook, L., Bellini, S., & Cusson, R. M. (2011). Heparinized saline vs normal saline for maintenance of intravenous access in neonates: An evidence-based practice change. *Advances in Neonatal Care*, 11(3), 208–215.

Danek, G., & Noris, E. (1992). Pediatric IV catheters: Efficacy of saline flush. *Pediatric Nursing*, 18(2), 111–113.

de Jonge, R. C. J., Polderman, K. H., & Gemke, R. J. B. J. (2005). Central venous catheter use in the pediatric patient: Mechanical and infectious complications. *Pediatric Critical Care Medicine*, 6, 329–339.

Doellman, D., Hadaway, L., Bowe-Geddes, L. A. et al. (2009). Infiltration and extravasation: Update on prevention and management. *Journal of Infusion Nursing*, 32(4), 203–211.

Farrell, P. M., Gutcher, G. R., Palta, M. et al. (1988). Essential fatty acid deficiency in premature infants. *American Journal of Clinical Nutrition*, 48, 220–229.

Fenton, T. R., Lyon, A. W., & Rose, M. S. (2011). Cord blood calcium, phosphate, magnesium, and alkaline phosphatase gestational age-specific reference intervals for preterm infants. *BMC Pediatrics*, 11, 76.

Finberg, L., Kravath, R., & Hellerstein, S. (1993). *Water and electrolytes in pediatrics: Physiology, pathology, and treatment* (2nd ed.). Philadelphia, PA: W. B. Saunders.

Frey, A. M., & Schears, G. J. (2006). Why are we stuck on tape and suture? A review of catheter securement devices. *Journal of Infusion Nursing*, 29(10), 34–38.

Goldberg, M., Sankaran, R., Givelichian, L. et al. (1999). Maintaining patency of peripheral intermittent infusion devices with heparinized saline and saline: A randomized double blind controlled trial in neonatal intensive care and a review of literature. *Neonatal Intensive Care*, 12(1), 18–22.

Graf, J. M., Newman, C. D., & McPherson, M. L. (2006). Sutured securement of peripherally inserted central catheters yields fewer complications in pediatric patients. *Journal of Parenteral and Enteral Nutrition*, 30(6), 532–535.

Hanna, M., & Saberi, M. S. (2010). Incidence of hyponatremia in children with gastroenteritis treated with hypotonic intravenous fluids. *Pediatric Nephrology*, 25(8), 1471–1475.

Hanrahan, K. S., Kleiber, C., & Berends, S. (2000). Saline for peripheral intravenous locks in neonates: Evaluating a change in practice. *Neonatal Network*, 19(2), 19–24.

Hanrahan, K. S., Kleiber, C., & Fagan, C. L. (1994). Evaluation of saline for IV locks in children. *Pediatric Nursing*, 20(6), 549–552.

Hartling, L., Bellemare, S., Wiebe, N. et al. (2006). Oral versus intravenous rehydration for treating dehydration due to gastroenteritis in children. *Cochrane Database of Systematic Reviews*, (3), CD004390.

Heilskov, J., Kleiber, C., Johnson, K. et al. (1998). A randomized trial of heparin and saline for maintaining intravenous locks in neonates. *Journal of the Society of Pediatric Nursing*, 3(3), 111–116.

Holliday, M. A., Ray, P. E., & Friedman, A. L. (2007). Fluid therapy for children: Facts, fashions and questions. *Archives of Disease in Childhood*, 92(6), 546–550.

Higgerson, R. A., Lawson, K. A., Christie, L. M. et al. (2011). Incidence and risk factors associated with venous thrombotic events in pediatric intensive care unit patients. *Pediatric Critical Care Medicine*, 12(6), 628–634.

Infusion Nurses Society. (2011). Infusion nursing: Standards of practice. *Journal of Infusion Nursing*, 34(1S), S1–S110.

Institute for Safe Medication Practices. (2009). Plain D5W or hypotonic saline solutions post-op could result in acute hyponatremia and death in healthy children. *Medication Safety Alert*, 14(16).

Jablonski, S. (2012). Oral rehydration of the pediatric patient with mild to moderate dehydration. *Journal of Emergency Nursing*, 38(2), 185–187.

Kannan, L., Lodha, R., Vivekanandhan, S. et al. (2010). Intravenous fluid regimen and hyponatremia among children: A randomized controlled trial. *Pediatric Nephrology*, 25(11), 2303–2309.

Kleiber, C., Hanrahan, K., Fagan, C. L. et al. (1993). Heparin vs. saline for peripheral IV locks in children. *Pediatric Nursing*, 19(4), 405–409.

Kotter, R. W. (1996). Heparin vs saline for intermittent intravenous device maintenance in neonates. *Neonatal Network*, 15(6), 43–47.

Levy, I., Bendet, M., Samra, Z. et al. (2010). Infectious complications of peripherally inserted central venous catheters in children. *The Pediatric Infectious Disease Journal*, 29(5), 426–429.

Levy, J. A., & Bachur, R. G. (2007). Intravenous dextrose during outpatient rehydration in pediatric gastroenteritis. *Academic Emergency Medicine*, 14(4), 324–330.

Liu, L., Johnson, H. L., Cousens, S. et al. (2012). Global, regional, and national causes of child mortality: An updated systematic analysis for 2010 with time trends since 2000. *Lancet*, 379(9832), 2151–2161.

Lynch, R. E., & Wood, E. G. (2011). Fluid and electrolyte issues in pediatric critical illness. In B. P. Fuhrman & J. J. Zimmerman (Eds.), *Pediatric Critical Care* (4th ed., pp. 944–962). Philadelphia, PA: Elsevier.

McCoy, M., Bedwell, S., & Noori, S. (2011). Exchange of peripherally inserted central catheters is associated with an increased risk for bloodstream infection. *American Journal of Perinatology*, 28(6), 419–424.

Mok, E., Tany Kwong, K. Y., & Chan, M. F. (2007). A randomized controlled trial for maintaining peripheral intravenous lock in children. *International Journal of Nursing Practice*, 13(1), 33–45.

Moritz, M. L., & Ayus, J. C. (2007). Hospital-acquired hyponatremia: Why are hypotonic parenteral fluids still being used? *Nature Clinical Practice, Nephrology*, 3(7), 374–382.

Mudge, B., Forcier, D., & Slattery, M. (1998). Patency of 24-gauge peripheral intermittent infusion devices: A comparison of heparin and saline solutions. *Pediatric Nursing*, 24(2), 142–146.

National Patient Safety Agency. (2007). *Reducing the risk of hyponatraemia when administering intravenous infusions to children*. Retrieved from http://www.nrls.npsa.nhs.uk/resources/?EntryId45=59809

Neville, K. A., Sandeman, D. J., Rubinstein, A. et al. (2010). Prevention of hyponatremia during maintenance intravenous fluid administration: A prospective randomized study of fluid type versus fluid rate. *Journal of Pediatrics*, 156(2), 313–319.e2.

Neville, K. A., Verge, C. F., Rosenberg, A. R. et al. (2006). Isotonic is better than hypotonic saline for intravenous rehydration of children with gastroenteritis: A prospective randomised study. *Archives of Disease in Childhood*, 9(3)1, 226–232.

Njere, I., Islam, S., Parish, D. et al. (2011). Outcome of peripherally inserted central venous catheters in surgical and medical neonates. *Journal of Pediatric Surgery*, 46(5), 946–950.

O'Grady, N. P., Alexander, M., Burns, L. A. et al. (2011). *2011 Guidelines for the prevention of intravascular catheter-related infections*. Atlanta, GA: Centers for Disease Control and Prevention.

Paisley, M. K., Stamper, M., Brown, J. et al. (1997). The use of heparin and normal saline flushes in neonatal intravenous catheters. *Pediatric Nursing*, 2(5)3, 521–524, 527.

Perry, K. W., & Salusky, I. B. (2012). Chronic kidney disease mineral and bone disorder. In F. Glorieux, J. M. Pettifor, & H. Juppner (Eds.), *Pediatric bone* (2nd ed., pp. 795–820). Philadelphia, PA: Elsevier.

Randolph, A. G., Cook, D. J., Gonzales, C. A. et al. (1998). Benefit of heparin in peripheral venous and arterial catheters: Systematic review and meta-analysis of randomised controlled trials. *British Medical Journal*, 316(7136), 969–975.

Rangel, S. J., Calkins, C. M., Cowles, R. A. et al. (2012). Enteral nutrition–associated cholestasis: An American Pediatric Surgical Association Outcomes and Clinical Trials Committee systematic review. *Journal of Pediatric Surgery*, 47(1), 225–240.

Saba, T. G., Fairbairn, J., Houghton, F. et al. (2011). A randomized controlled trial of isotonic versus hypotonic maintenance intravenous fluids in hospitalized children. *BMC Pediatrics*, 11, 82.

Schultz, A. A., Drew, D., & Hewitt, H. (2002). Comparison of normal saline and heparinized saline for patency of IV locks in neonates. *Applied Nursing Research*, 15(1), 28–34.

Shah, P. S., Ng, E., & Sinha, A. K. (2005). Heparin for prolonging peripheral intravenous catheter use in neonates. *Cochrane Database of Systematic Reviews*, (4), CD002774.

Simmer, K., & Rao, S. C. (2005). Early introduction of lipids to parenterally-fed preterm infants. *Cochrane Database of Systematic Reviews*, (2), CD005256.

Sparks, L. A., Setlik, J., & Luhman, J. (2007). Parental holding and positioning to decrease IV distress in young children: A randomized controlled trial. *Journal of Pediatric Nursing*, 22(6), 440–447.

Treas, L. S., & Latinis-Bridges, B. (1992). Efficacy of heparin in peripheral venous infusion in neonates. *Journal of Obstetric, Gynecologic, and Neonatal Nursing*, 21(3), 214–219.

Yung, M., & Keeley, S. (2009). Randomised controlled trial of intravenous maintenance fluids. *Journal of Paediatrics and Child Health*, 45(1–2), 9–14.

See the**Point** for additional organizations.

The Child With Altered Gastrointestinal Status

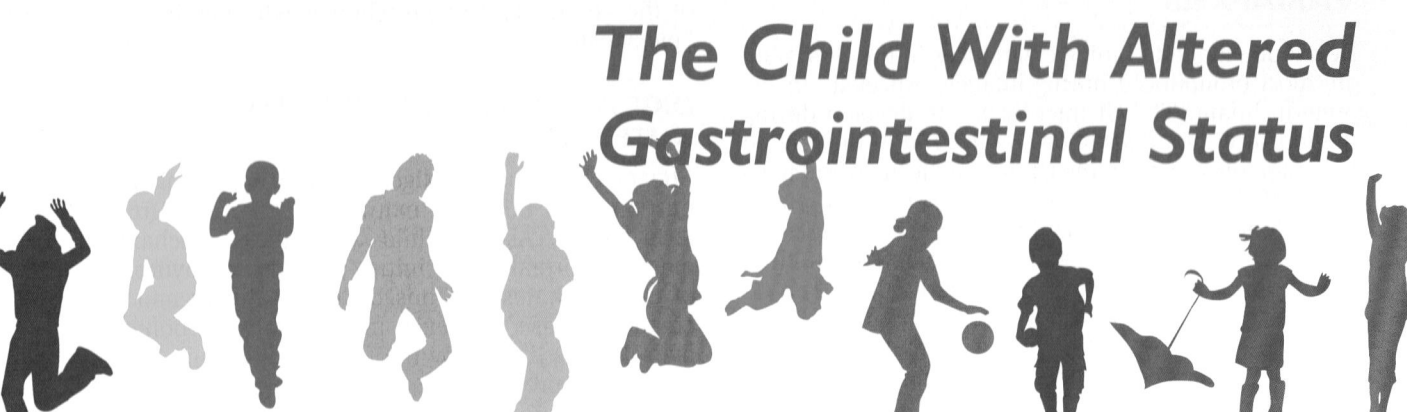

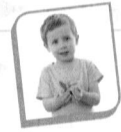

CASE HISTORY

Recall Cory Whitworth featured in Chapters 6, 11, and 17? Review the case study in Chapter 17 for more information about the history and assessment of Cory's fluids and electrolytes. Cory is a 5-year-old kindergartner who, at his last appointment, was above the 97th percentile for his height but below the 25th percentile for his weight. His history reveals that he is a poor and picky eater. During the previous several days, Cory has complained of a stomachache, has been refusing to eat, and is drinking a little. His fever has come and gone periodically. Early this morning, he seemed better, but about an hour ago, he began crying and guarding his abdomen.

The nurse in the emergency department begins examining Cory. His appearance is of a pale, thin boy in acute pain.

He is crying and holding his stomach area. His vital signs are as follows: temperature, 101.8° F; heart rate, 108 bpm; and respiratory rate, 34 breaths/min. His abdomen is flat and firm with hypoactive bowel sounds in all four quadrants. Cory allowed the nurse to listen to his abdomen with the stethoscope, but when the nurse attempts a deeper palpation, he begins to thrash and fight. The nurse obtains a blood sample for lab work and inserts a peripheral intravenous (IV) line. Cory then goes to the imaging department for an ultrasound, which is equivocal, followed by a computed tomographic (CT) scan with contrast. The diagnosis of ruptured appendix is confirmed, and Cory undergoes an appendectomy. After surgery, Cory is admitted to a pediatric surgical unit.

CHAPTER OBJECTIVES

1 Discuss components of the history and physical assessment that are important to consider when evaluating a child with an alteration in gastrointestinal status.

2 Identify specific tests and laboratory results that assist the health care team to identify alterations in gastrointestinal status.

3 Discuss diet modifications and alternative feeding methods used to treat alterations in gastrointestinal status.

4 Review the important pathophysiologic principles that help to differentiate gastrointestinal disorders.

5 Describe the interdisciplinary interventions commonly used for disorders of the gastrointestinal system.

See thePoint for a list of Key Terms.

The gastrointestinal (GI) system is a complex organ system that extends from the mouth to the anus and includes the esophagus, stomach, small and large intestines, liver, and pancreas. The primary functions of the GI system are ingestion, digestion, absorption of nutrients, and elimination of solid waste. Proper function of the GI system is essential for normal growth and for maintaining fluid and electrolyte balances. This system also plays an important role in metabolic functions, such as protein synthesis and glucose homeostasis, and in immunologic function.

Alterations in GI status may be congenital or acquired, acute or chronic, and may vary in severity from minor to life threatening. The nurse may encounter the child with altered GI status in both acute care and community settings.

DEVELOPMENTAL AND BIOLOGIC VARIANCES

Developmental and biologic variances in the GI system are most pronounced during infancy, especially in the preterm infant. The GI tract begins to develop during the fourth week of gestation. By the end of the second trimester, the organs of the GI tract are formed and have many of the structures that enable elementary physiologic function. During the third trimester, these structures become more developed and differentiated in their functions. Some functions, particularly those related to ingestion, digestion, and absorption of nutrients, are not fully developed at birth, a circumstance that accounts for the special feeding requirements of infants (Fig. 18-1).

INGESTION OF NUTRIENTS

Food intake, along with calorie and nutrient requirements, varies from infancy to childhood to adolescence. During periods of rapid growth, such as infancy and adolescence, calorie and nutrient requirements are increased, which leads to an increase in food intake. During periods of slower growth, food intake may decrease. This variation may help to explain the behavior of the young child or preschooler who has become a "picky eater."

DIGESTION AND ABSORPTION OF NUTRIENTS

The mechanisms for digesting and absorbing major nutrients are not fully mature in the premature and term infant. As the child ages, these mechanisms mature. Normally, the initial breakdown (hydrolysis) of carbohydrates depends on both salivary and pancreatic amylase. However, in the infant, carbohydrate hydrolysis is limited by the fact that although salivary amylase is present by 34 weeks' gestation, secretion of pancreatic amylase does not begin until age 4 to 6 months. Because of this delay, young infants are relatively intolerant of starches and may experience diarrhea if starchy food sources, such as cereals, are offered too early.

Lactose is the primary source of carbohydrate in breast milk and most infant formulas. Lactose is hydrolyzed in the intestinal villi by the enzyme lactase.

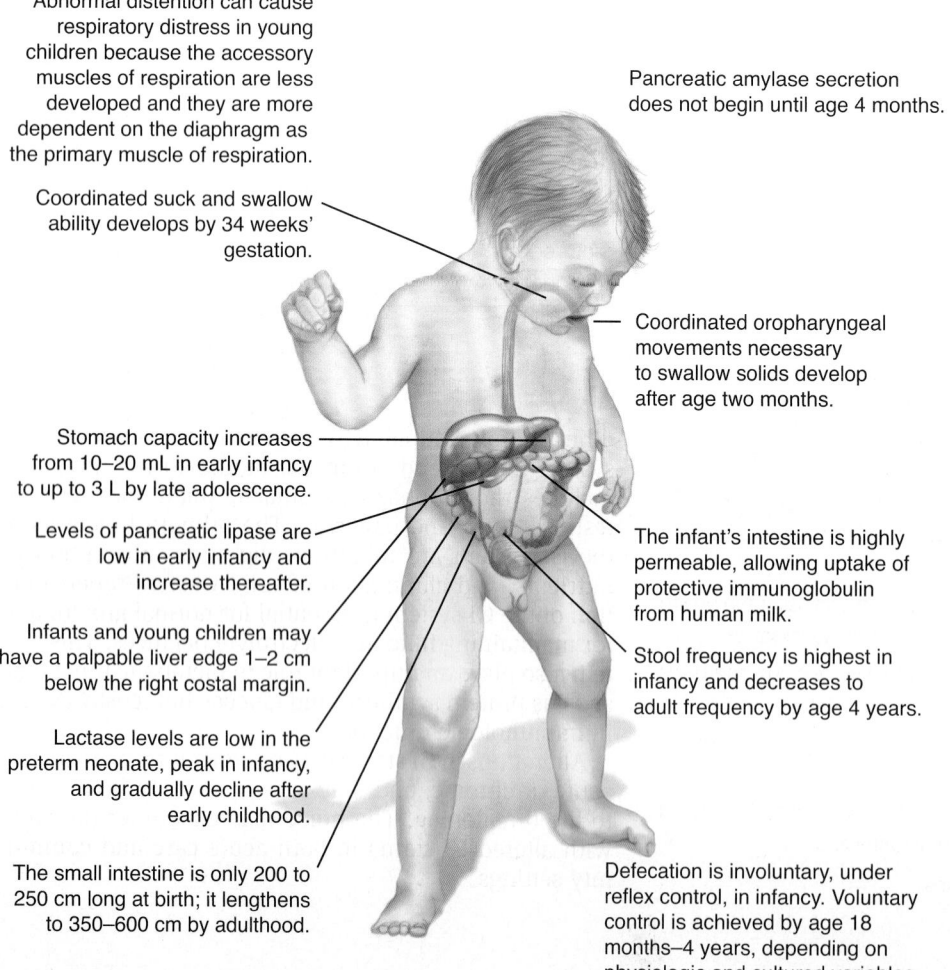

Abnormal distention can cause respiratory distress in young children because the accessory muscles of respiration are less developed and they are more dependent on the diaphragm as the primary muscle of respiration.

Coordinated suck and swallow ability develops by 34 weeks' gestation.

Stomach capacity increases from 10–20 mL in early infancy to up to 3 L by late adolescence.

Levels of pancreatic lipase are low in early infancy and increase thereafter.

Infants and young children may have a palpable liver edge 1–2 cm below the right costal margin.

Lactase levels are low in the preterm neonate, peak in infancy, and gradually decline after early childhood.

The small intestine is only 200 to 250 cm long at birth; it lengthens to 350–600 cm by adulthood.

Pancreatic amylase secretion does not begin until age 4 months.

Coordinated oropharyngeal movements necessary to swallow solids develop after age two months.

The infant's intestine is highly permeable, allowing uptake of protective immunoglobulin from human milk.

Stool frequency is highest in infancy and decreases to adult frequency by age 4 years.

Defecation is involuntary, under reflex control, in infancy. Voluntary control is achieved by age 18 months–4 years, depending on physiologic and cultured variables.

Figure 18-1 Developmental and biologic variances: GI system.

Lactase levels are highest during early infancy and begin to decline after 4 years of life, depending on ethnicity. In some individuals, lactase levels may decline to the point where lactose intolerance occurs. Therefore, school-aged children may not tolerate lactose well.

CROSS-CULTURAL CARE

Lactase deficiency and lactose malabsorption occur in 50%–80% of Hispanic people, in 60%–80% of black and Ashkenazi Jewish people, and in almost 100% of Asian and American Indian people. Approximately 20% of Hispanic, Asian, and black children younger than 5 years of age experience lactase deficiency and lactose malabsorption in contrast with Caucasian children, whose symptoms usually do not present until after this age (Heyman, 2006).

Digestion and absorption of protein is relatively efficient in the preterm and newborn infant. The infant's highly permeable intestine enables uptake of protective immunoglobulin (Ig) proteins from human milk. This same permeability allows cow's milk protein and other potential allergens to pass through the intestinal barrier into the bloodstream, making infants more susceptible to food protein allergies and GI infections.

Digestion and absorption of fat during infancy is limited by low concentrations of bile acids and low levels of pancreatic lipase, one of the enzymes responsible for breaking down ingested fats. The breastfed infant absorbs fat more efficiently than the formula-fed infant as a result of unique characteristics of the lipase in breast milk.

ELIMINATION

Normal patterns of GI elimination vary throughout the life cycle. The number and consistency of stools, as well as the ability to control elimination, changes from infancy to early childhood. Stool frequency in the infant may be highly variable. During the first 3 days of life, the infant has meconium stools that are dark green-black, thick, and sticky. The newborn may have three to seven stools per day, depending on the type and amount of feeding given. After about a month, the breastfed infant may go up to a week without any stool, without any signs of discomfort or abdominal distention because of the low residue of breast milk. The color and consistency of stool also vary. A breastfed infant's stools may have a yellow, "seedy" appearance and a somewhat runny consistency; a formula-fed infant's stools may have a yellow or brownish color and a more pasty consistency. As solid foods are introduced, stool color may be affected by the particular foods the child eats. By age 4 years, stool frequency decreases to the adult level of one or two stools per day. Stool consistency is also comparable with the adult's.

ASSESSMENT

Assessment of the child with altered GI status relies on a careful health history, physical assessment, and diagnostic tests.

FOCUSED HEALTH HISTORY

QUESTION: Review Cory's case and identify critical information that correlates with the areas identified in Focused Health History 18-1. What are other critical pieces of information the nurse should gather?

The focused health history is an important part of the overall assessment of the child with altered GI status (Focused Health History 18-1). Many GI conditions have relatively few observable physical findings, which makes the history of symptoms and factors that affect their onset and duration an important tool. Conversely, symptoms that initially appear to be of GI origin may indicate a pathologic process in another system. For example, pneumonia or urinary tract infections may present as abdominal pain.

Ask about feeding habits—for example, what the child eats, when, how often, and how foods are prepared. Also inquire about changes in appetite and fluid intake (increased, decreased, type of intake) and bowel habits (frequency, appearance, use of aids such as laxatives or enemas). Ask whether symptoms are related to meals, specific food intake, lifestyle, activity, or sleep patterns. Obtain information on the absence or presence of pain, including onset, type and characteristics of pain, location, duration, and any measures that relieve or exacerbate pain (see Chapter 10 for more information about pain).

When obtaining the history, pay careful attention to the timing and characteristics of the symptoms. Include the child in the interview as much as possible and encourage description of symptoms in familiar terms. Clarify the parent's or child's reports to avoid under- or overrepresentation of symptoms. For example, if the parent reports that the child had "a lot of diarrhea last night," ask the parent to estimate how many episodes of diarrhea the child has had during the previous 24 hours and at what times the episodes occurred. Question the parent regarding the volume of the stool output using a familiar measure such as a tablespoon, a cup, or number of saturated diapers to estimate the amount. Finally, define the characteristics of the stool, including color, consistency, presence of blood or mucus, greasiness, and presence of foul smell.

ANSWER: Cory has had a stomachache, intermittent fever, and refused to eat. In addition, the nurse should ask about Cory's most recent healthy weight and if he is on any medication. Try to determine Cory's output the previous day with regard to urine, stool, and vomiting. Ask Cory directly about his abdominal pain: "Where does it hurt most?" "Does anything make it hurt less?" "Does anything you do make it hurt more?"

FOCUSED HEALTH HISTORY 18-1

The Child With Altered Gastrointestinal Status

Current history	Recent weight loss or gain Nausea, retching, regurgitation Abdominal pain or distention, when pain occurs in relation to vomiting Bulges in abdominal or inguinal area with crying or straining Diarrhea Constipation Blood in vomitus or stool Color and characteristics of vomitus and stool Related systemic problems: fever, fatigue, urinary tract symptoms (change in color, frequency, pain), respiratory symptoms (cough, wheezing, asthma), skin lesions, rashes, pruritus, changes in hair or nails Presence of pain/discomfort/irritability Changes in sleep patterns
Past medical history	**Prenatal/Neonatal History** • History of maternal prenatal infections • Birth weight, length, gestational age • Failure to pass meconium **Previous Health Challenges** • History of GI illness, recurrent respiratory or urinary tract infection, congenital heart disease • Problems with growth, weight gain • Feeding difficulties • Formula, milk, and food allergies • Experiences with pain Status of immunization with hepatitis B vaccine Previous hospitalizations
Past surgical history	Previous surgeries and dates
Nutritional assessment	Usual diet and intake; recent change in diet, food intake • Feeding method (breast, bottle, cup, tube fed) • Method of formula preparation Systemic medications child has recently taken or is currently taking; how the medication is taken (e.g., on empty stomach; with food or fluid, with what and how much; taken in conjunction with other medications; if tablets, swallowed or crushed); any changes noted in GI tract function secondary to medication; complementary or alternative health care practices Use of vitamin, mineral supplements
Family medical history	Family history of GI conditions
Social history	Disturbed/abnormal parent–child interaction Recent changes, stressors in family, lifestyle Exposure to affected individuals (hepatitis, diarrhea) in home, daycare, school History of recent travel History of recent trauma (e.g., falling off bicycle or skateboard, car accident) or emergency room visits Presence or exposure to pets or animals Recent exposure to food prepared outside home School absences
Growth and development	Developmental milestones, especially feeding milestones

Note: See Chapter 8 for a comprehensive health history.

FOCUSED PHYSICAL ASSESSMENT

QUESTION: Based on the information you already have about Cory's physical assessment, what additional information do you anticipate finding in your physical assessment?

Physical assessment of the GI system must occur in the context of an overall comprehensive physical examination. Manifestations of altered GI function are varied and may be subtle. Children with conditions that alter intake, digestion, or absorption of nutrients may exhibit signs of growth failure or malnutrition. These children may have altered skin integrity or abnormal findings on neurologic or musculoskeletal examination. Children with conditions that result in excessive loss of fluid and electrolytes from the GI tract may present with the physical findings of acute dehydration. The child with gastroesophageal reflux disease (GERD) may present with the physical findings of pneumonia secondary to aspiration of refluxed stomach contents.

Throughout the physical assessment, keep in mind the potential relationships between the GI system and altered physical findings in other systems (Focused Physical Assessment 18-1).

FOCUSED PHYSICAL ASSESSMENT 18-1
The Gastrointestinal System

Assessment Parameter	Alterations/Possible Clinical Significance
General appearance	Change deviating from growth trajectory in weight and height; head circumference for children younger than 3 years of age: potential over- or undernutrition, acute or chronic condition
	Unwell, listless: acute or chronic illness, anemia
	Poor state of hygiene: neglect, abuse
	Obese, cachectic: possible over- or undernutrition
	Alterations in speech: cleft palate, altered motor development, undernutrition, congenital syndromes, cerebral palsy
	Flat affect: possible profound nutritional deficit
Integumentary system (skin, hair, nails)	Color: jaundice may indicate liver dysfunction or pancreatitis; pallor is a sign of blood loss or iron deficiency
	Integrity: lesions, rashes may be seen with malnutrition, diarrhea, poor hygiene, neglect, or chronic conditions
	Impaired wound healing, skin lesion can be a result of zinc deficiency, malnutrition, steroid side effects
	Turgor: tenting is present in dehydration; edema may indicate fluid volume excess or protein deficiency or hypoalbuminemia
	Hair: color changes, depigmentation; dry, coarse texture; sparse distribution; hair that is easily plucked may be signs of vitamin or protein deficits or general malnutrition
	Nails: clubbing can be present in cystic fibrosis, liver disease; splitting is seen with nutritional deficiencies
Eyes	Periorbital edema can be present with fluid volume excess or protein deficiency/hypoalbuminemia
	Jaundiced sclera often indicates elevated bilirubin levels, liver dysfunction
Ears/hearing	Structural deformities may be associated with oral or facial defects or syndromes and cleft palate
Face, nose, and oral cavity	Perioral, oral lesions may be present in malnutrition, Crohn disease, ulcerative colitis, celiac disease, immunodeficiency or suppression
	Enamel hypoplasia associated with celiac disease, cheilosis; glossitis/vitamin B_6 deficiency, vitamin B_{12} deficiency
	Fetor may indicate progressive lower bowel obstruction

(Continued)

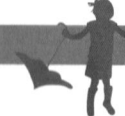

The Gastrointestinal System (Continued)

Assessment Parameter	Alterations/Possible Clinical Significance
Thorax and lungs	Increased respiratory rate associated with abdominal distention, ascites resulting from compression of the diaphragm
	Breath sounds (wheeze, rhonchi) may be associated with GERD, primary aspiration resulting from oral–motor dysfunction
Abdomen	Inspection
	• Shape, contour; presence of distention may indicate partial or total bowel obstruction, malnutrition, retained flatus, ascites; irregular contour may indicate pyloric stenosis
	• Color, discoloration; erythema associated with necrotizing enterocolitis, trauma
	• Visible peristaltic waves seen in pyloric stenosis
	• Visible mass may suggest hernia, hydrocele
	• Prominent venous pattern associated with collateral circulation resulting from presence of implanted venous access device, portal hypertension, superior vena cava syndrome
Abdomen	Inspection
	• Note presence and location of appliances, such as gastrostomy tube, colostomy, implanted venous access device
	• Note presence and location of prior surgical incisions and the corresponding surgical procedure
	Auscultation
	• Absent bowel sounds indicate postoperative ileus or ileus from other etiologies
	• High-pitched, hyperactive bowel sounds associated with obstruction
	• Vascular bruits, rushes suggest vascular abnormality
	Percussion
	• Tympanic sound of higher pitch associated with presence of excessive gas; dull sound associated with masses, fluid or solid organ elicits a dull pitch
	• Enlarged liver span may suggest biliary atresia, cholestasis, heart failure
	Palpation
	• Pain, tenderness associated with appendicitis, inflammatory bowel disease (IBD), functional abdominal pain, inflammatory process
	• Rigidity associated with peritonitis, obstruction
	Abdominal girth (circumference); compare with baseline to determine whether the abdomen distention is trending upward or decreasing in response to therapy or disease progression
	Inguinal region: bulging, more prominent with crying, straining, or laughing; possibly mild tenderness suggests the presence of hernia; bulging with acute irritability, refusal to eat, followed by bilious or feculent vomiting indicates incarcerated hernia
External genitalia and breasts (includes anus)	Anus, rectum, vagina: anus located anteriorly or presence of urine or stool in an unusual place associated with anorectal malformations
	Fissure associated with constipation
	Lesions, excoriation, inflammation associated with infection, diarrhea
	Rectal prolapse associated with cystic fibrosis, malnutrition
	Skin tags and fistulas associated with Crohn disease
	Rectovaginal fistula suggests congenital structural defects

Because GI tract function may be reflected in growth and nutritional status, accurately measuring and recording growth parameters are critical aspects of GI assessment. Measuring weight regularly is essential to evaluate the child's progress toward the goals for growth, development, and nutrition with GI dysfunction (see Chapter 8 for information on obtaining anthropometric measurements).

The abdominal examination is a major part of GI system assessment; this evaluation may present unique challenges in children. (For further discussion of techniques for physical examination, see Chapter 8.)

caREminder

The usual order of physical assessment techniques is altered during assessment of the abdomen. To obtain an accurate assessment of bowel sounds, auscultation must precede percussion and palpation.

An infant may become distressed during the examination, crying and tensing the abdominal wall. This behavior may interfere with the nurse's ability to appreciate changes in assessment parameters. Place the infant in a parent's lap during the examination to help soothe the infant and facilitate the examination. Provide comfort measures, such as a pacifier.

The older child may become frightened or ticklish during the examination. Demonstrate parts of the examination on a doll or stuffed animal to help put the child at ease and enhance cooperation. Allow the child to handle examination tools. Distract the child with toys or conversation about favorite activities. Drape the adolescent to avoid unnecessary exposure and acknowledge their privacy concerns.

During inspection, observe the color, shape, and contour of the abdomen. Note any signs of distention or asymmetry. Peristalsis may be visible in the thin, malnourished infant or in the infant with obstruction caused by pyloric stenosis. Note the presence of any hernias. A prominent venous pattern may be seen in children with cirrhosis of the liver.

Inspect GI tract secretions, such as vomitus and stool, if available. Mucus and blood may suggest infectious and inflammatory conditions. Changes in stool color, consistency, or odor can point to GI tract dysfunction (Table 18-1).

Auscultate all four abdominal quadrants to assess bowel sounds, which represent peristaltic movement of contents throughout the intestinal tract. Normal bowel sounds have a metallic, tinkling quality and may be heard every 10 to 30 seconds. The absence of bowel sounds indicates intestinal **ileus** or functional intestinal obstruction. Increased, or hyperactive, bowel sounds may be heard in acute gastroenteritis. High-pitched, hyperactive bowel sounds may indicate partial intestinal obstruction.

caREminder

Listen for a full 5 minutes in all four abdominal quadrants to establish the absence of bowel sounds.

TABLE 18-1	Abnormal Findings: Emesis and Stool
Parameter	**Finding/Potential Pathology**
Emesis	
Hematemesis	Emesis containing blood Bright-red blood indicates acute upper GI bleeding Brown, "coffee ground" blood indicates ongoing or chronic process
Bilious vomiting	Emesis containing bile Green or yellow, indicates GI obstruction
Feculent vomiting	Emesis containing stool Brown, foul smelling, indicates GI obstruction
Stool	
Hematochezia	Bright-red or maroon blood per rectum Usually associated with bleeding from lower GI tract or anal fissures
Melena	Dark, tarry stool Usually associated with bleeding passed from upper GI tract versus bright red from lower GI tract
Currant jelly stool	Stool with red blood and mucus Associated with intussusception
Steatorrhea	Fatty stools Possibly pale, bulky, malodorous, float in toilet or have an oily ring in the diaper Associated with fat malabsorption and pancreatic insufficiency, such as with cystic fibrosis
Acholic stool	Clay-colored stool Occurring with biliary atresia, biliary tract obstruction, or bile deficiencies

Use abdominal percussion to distinguish between solid organs or masses and the presence of fluid or gas in the abdominal cavity. Percuss the abdomen in all four quadrants. Tympanic, drumlike sounds are heard over air-filled organs, particularly the stomach and intestines. When the abdomen is distended, increased tympanic sounds may be heard if gas has accumulated because of an ileus or obstruction. In some cases, an infant may have increased tympanic sounds because he or she has swallowed air while feeding or crying. Flat, dull sounds on abdominal percussion may indicate an accumulation of fluid, a solid mass, or an organ such as the liver.

Measure liver size, or span, by percussing along the right midclavicular line. The normal liver span of the child varies according to age. It averages 2.6 cm at 6 months, 3 cm at 12 months, 3.5 cm at 24 months, 4.4 cm at 4 years, 5 cm at 6 years, 5.4 cm at 8 years, and 5.8 cm at 10 years.

Palpate the abdomen to assess for enlargement of solid organs and to detect the presence of masses. Also assess the character of the abdomen (soft or hard) and the presence of tenderness or pain. To promote relaxation of the abdominal muscles, have the child lie supine and flex the knees before palpating. Preschool and school-aged children in particular may be ticklish, which makes palpation difficult.

KidKare To reduce ticklishness during palpation, ask the child to place his or her hand on top of your hand and palpate or press down with you. Coach the child to breathe normally throughout the examination.

If a child is crying, you can best feel the difference between a firm and soft abdomen when palpating during the inspiratory phase of the respiratory cycle. Palpate in an area distant from the identified area of pain when abdominal pain is reported. In the case of the preverbal child or the child who has difficulty verbally identifying the exact location of the pain, observe for changes in facial expression or body posture or changes in the pitch of crying during palpation of the abdomen to assess for the location of pain.

ALERT *If you identify a mass in the area of the kidneys, do not repalpate it. If the mass is a tumor, repeated palpation can cause it to release cells that are potentially metastatic.*

In infants and young children, the edge of the liver is normally palpable 1 to 2 cm below the right costal margin in the midclavicular line. The liver edge should not be palpable in the adolescent. Enlargement of the liver, known as *hepatomegaly*, is present when the liver is palpable more than 3 cm below the right costal margin. Report any enlargement to the advanced practice nurse or physician.

Measuring abdominal girth is a fairly accurate way to monitor progressive abdominal distention in children. Use a paper tape measure to avoid the stretching that may occur with a cloth tape measure and to promote infection control. If the tape measure is not long enough, tape two together to provide sufficient length. Measure the abdomen over the umbilicus, pulling the tape measure taut but not tight (Fig. 18-2). Obtain the measurement on expiration. When ostomies, tubes, or other devices prevent measuring over the umbilicus, obtain the measurement over the same area each time to enable comparison. When taking serial measurements, mark two small lines with a marker or ballpoint pen on each side margin of the tape measure and on the right and left sides of the abdomen to indicate where to place the tape measure. If you are doing serial readings and movement causes the child discomfort, leave the tape measure in place under the child, making sure that it is smooth and not twisted.

ANSWER: You may anticipate dry mucous membranes related to decreased fluid intake. You may also anticipate that Cory identifies the right lower quadrant of his abdomen is more painful and that rebound tenderness of the abdomen is present.

DIAGNOSTIC CRITERIA

QUESTION: Based on Cory's symptoms, which tests can assist in the diagnosis of appendicitis/ruptured appendix? (Refer to Tests and Procedures 18-1.)

A wide variety of diagnostic tests and procedures are used to evaluate alterations in GI structure and function. Laboratory studies analyze blood, GI secretions, urine, and stool. Radiographic and nonradiographic

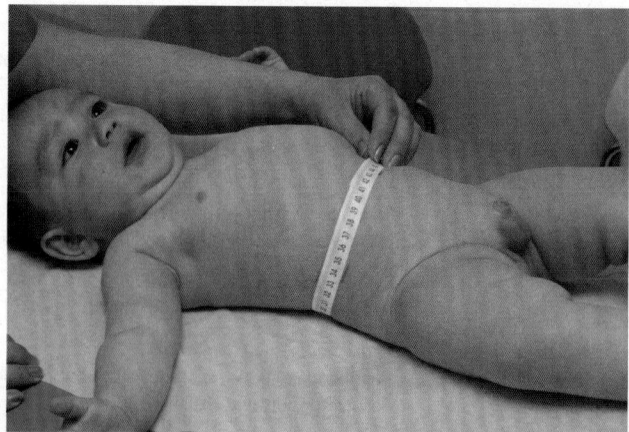

Figure 18-2 Measure abdominal girth over the umbilicus whenever possible.

 **TESTS AND PROCEDURES for Evaluating Altered Gastrointestinal Status**

Diagnostic Test or Procedure	Purpose	Findings and Indications	Health Care Provider Considerations
Imaging (Radiographic and Nonradiographic)			
Plain film abdominal radiograph; also can be ordered as KUB (kidney, ureter, and bladder)	Initial radiographic; evaluation of structures of the organs within the abdomen	Obstruction, air and fluid levels, structural changes, and calcifications	Infants and younger children may require assistance with positioning and immobilization.
Barium swallow	Radiographic evaluation of esophagus	Structural abnormalities, strictures, foreign bodies, ulcerations, varices, and motility disorders	Child must be NPO (nothing by mouth) before examination.
Upper GI series with small bowel follow-through	Radiographic evaluation of esophagus, stomach, and small intestine with contrast medium	Structural abnormalities, strictures, obstruction, ulcers, IBD, and motility disorders	Child must be NPO before examination (infants, 3–4 hours; older children, after midnight for morning test). Children who are unable or unwilling to drink contrast medium used in examination may require nasogastric (NG) administration. Younger children may require immobilization during examination. Fluids are given after the test to facilitate passage of barium. Stool may be whitish or clay colored from barium.
Barium enema	Radiographic evaluation of colon with contrast medium	Structural and functional changes; polyps	Contraindicated in patients with fulminant ulcerative colitis or suspected perforation. Test performed before upper GI studies to prevent contamination from previous contrast. Infants do not require bowel preparation. Bowel preparation for older children may include clear liquid diet, cathartics, or enema. Stool may be whitish or clay colored from barium.
Abdominal ultrasound	Visualization of size, structure of liver, gallbladder, biliary tract. Differentiation of solid organs, cysts, and fluid collections	Strictures, cysts, abscesses, tumor, gallstones, and appendicitis. Solid organs appearing as echogenic structures (consist of tissues with multiple acoustic interfaces); cysts and fluid collections echo free (echolucent or anechoic) because they lack internal reflectors	Prepare child and family by advising them that test will take 20–30 minutes. Lubricant gel, which feels wet and cold, will be used on skin over abdomen. Younger children may require assistance with positioning and immobilization.

(Continued)

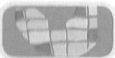

TESTS AND PROCEDURES for Evaluating Altered Gastrointestinal Status *(Continued)*

Diagnostic Test or Procedure	Purpose	Findings and Indications	Health Care Provider Considerations
CT, with or without contrast	Radiographic study that shows relationships among anatomic structures; reveals the shapes of the organs, tissue densities, outlines; shows structural alterations	Tumors, presence of intra-abdominal or hepatic abscess or cyst, and obstruction of biliary ducts	Child may be required to take oral or IV contrast material before the test. If unable to take contrast by mouth, may require NG administration. Child must lay still for 30–90 minutes during test. Often requires sedation in young children who are unable to cooperate.
Endoscopic retrograde cholangio-pancreatography	Combines endoscopy with imaging and contrast medium to identify pancreatic and biliary duct disorders; used for both diagnostic and interventional therapy; interventions include stricture dilation, stent placement, cyst drainage, and stone extraction	Structural disorders, such as duct stenosis; choledochal cyst; obstructions caused by bile duct stones	Same as preparation for upper GI endoscopy. IV access for administration of contrast medium; obtain signed consent.
Magnetic resonance cholangiopancreatography (MRCP)	Noninvasive imaging study of the biliary and pancreatic ducts	Structural disorders indicating such alterations as inflammation, cysts, congenital abnormalities	Contraindications are similar to those for magnetic resonance imaging (MRI): presence of cardiac pacemaker, ocular or cochlear implants, possibly nerve stimulating devices.
Liver biliary scan (hepatoiminodiacetic acid [HIDA] scan)	Radionuclide scan to visualize flow in the biliary ductal system, both uptake and excretion	Biliary atresia, biliary tract obstruction after liver transplant	Child is NPO before test. IV access required to administer contrast medium.
Cholangiogram, intraoperative study	A radiograph study to evaluate the biliary tract The iodine is excreted in the bile from the liver. Intraoperative cholangiogram: A needle or catheter is inserted into the gallbladder, where diluted contrast is injected to observe the extent of the biliary obstruction.	Presence and location of stones and other causes of obstruction, such as strictures; biliary atresia	Document patient allergies before procedure (contrast medium used is usually iodine based). Patients with history of iodine or seafood allergy or history of previous reaction to iodine-based contrast medium must be identified.

Endoscopic Examination

Upper GI endoscopy	Uses a fiberoptic endoscope to directly visualize the lumen and mucosal lining of the esophagus, stomach, and upper portion of the small intestine	Tissue abnormality from biopsy, upper GI bleeding, ulcers, gastritis, esophagitis, and hiatal hernias identified and evaluated	The child must be NPO before the procedure. Sedation or general anesthesia will be used depending on child's clinical risk and purpose of procedure. IV required. Monitor vital signs and oxygen saturation during the procedure and afterward until the child is fully awake. Monitor for signs of pulmonary aspiration, perforation, or bleeding.

Diagnostic Test or Procedure	Purpose	Findings and Indications	Health Care Provider Considerations
	Biopsies are acquired to substantiate diagnoses; used therapeutically to sclerose esophageal or gastric varices, evaluate hiatal hernia, remove a foreign body, dilate esophageal stricture, place a percutaneous endoscopic gastrostomy (PEG) tube or a gastrostomy–jejunostomy (G-J) tube		
Endoscopy, wireless capsule	Noninvasive evaluation of the entire small bowel through an ingestible capsule that contains a camera; two images are captured per second and are transmitted from the capsule via digital radiofrequency to a receiver that is worn on the body in a vest-type carrier. The data are then downloaded and analyzed using a special program.	Evaluation of disorders of the small bowel, such as in Crohn disease or a history of bleeding without an identified source; contrast radiographic studies are done prior to the wireless capsule to rule out impeding the forward movement of the capsule.	The child is NPO 8 hours prior to the procedure and longer as indicated. Clear liquids may be taken several hours after the initiation of the study. A light meal may be eaten 2 hours or more into the study, which is completed in 8 hours. Family need to notify physician for complaints of chest pain, dysphagia, nausea, vomiting, or fever. Family is instructed to check frequently for presence of pulsing light on the receiver device and to return to outpatient setting if pulsing stops before 6 hours. Child returns to the outpatient setting after 8 hours when study is completed. Family need to monitor the child's stool for passing of capsule after procedure is completed. Currently approved as an outpatient study. Use is limited to about age 6 years or ability to swallow the capsule, although there are reports of endoscopic placement. Limitations include inability to obtain biopsies, battery life if progression is slow because of decreased motility, and age. Adaptations are underway for use with younger children. A dissolvable capsule design without the video that can be administered prior to the video capsule to screen for potential impediment is also underway.

(Continued)

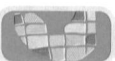 **TESTS AND PROCEDURES for Evaluating Altered Gastrointestinal Status** *(Continued)*

Diagnostic Test or Procedure	Purpose	Findings and Indications	Health Care Provider Considerations
Lower GI endoscopy (colonoscopy)	Uses a fiberoptic endoscope to directly visualize the lumen and mucosal lining of the colon and terminal ileum Used therapeutically to remove polyps Biopsies may be done in conjunction with colonoscopy. Flexible sigmoidoscopy is an examination of the sigmoid colon and rectum.	Diagnosis and evaluation of IBD, GI or rectal bleeding, and diarrhea	Bowel preparation usually required preprocedure, as determined by physician. Infants may require only clear liquids 12–24 hours before the procedure. Older children's preparation may include cathartics by mouth or NG tube or enemas. Sedation or general anesthesia is used in pediatrics. Requires an IV. Pulse oximetry monitoring. Monitor the child during and after procedure for abdominal pain, bleeding, and any change in vital signs.

Motility Studies

pH study/impedance	Traditionally, a pH probe is passed transnasally into the distal esophagus. The probe is attached to an external monitor that measures and records the intraesophageal pH. Often combined with multichannel impedance. Alternatively, an intraluminal esophageal wireless pH capsule (BRAVO capsule) is placed endoscopically. Recordings are transmitted to a pager-sized device worn by the patient or placed in a backpack.	Used to evaluate for gastroesophageal reflux (GER). Reflux of acid stomach contents will result in pH readings less than 4. The impedance catheter measures pH as well as the type and direction of the flow of the esophageal contents. It can distinguish between acid and nonacidic reflux.	The traditional pH study is usually 18–24 hours. The wireless pH study is usually a 48-hour study. The child must be NPO before the probe placement and must be off acid antagonists during the examination. pH probe placement must be maintained throughout the test. A log is kept to record sleep/wake periods, start and stop of feedings, position changes, and occurrence of any reflux symptoms (cough, choking, emesis, apnea, bradycardia, or cyanosis). Family members may participate in record keeping and should have instruction. With the wireless pH capsule, the child is instructed to take small bites of food and chew well for comfort and to avoid dislodging the capsule. The recording device must remain within 3 ft of the patient when showering and with a maximum range of 9 ft for receiving data. Caution must be taken not to drop or damage the wireless receiver.
Esophageal manometry	A long, flexible catheter with pressure transducers is passed into the esophagus orally or transnasally; intraluminal pressures of the lower esophageal sphincter (LES) and esophageal body are measured.	Motility disorders of the esophagus; used in the workup of patients with dysphagia and dysmotility	The child must be NPO before the procedure. Sedation is required for catheter placement.

Diagnostic Test or Procedure	Purpose	Findings and Indications	Health Care Provider Considerations
Gastric emptying study	Evaluates rate at which stomach empties after ingestion of radionuclide-labeled solid or liquid meal	Motility disorders of stomach	Child must be NPO before test. Prepare child and parents about the need to ingest radionuclide-labeled meal in radiology, with images taken every 15 minutes for up to 3 hours.
Colonic manometry	A flexible catheter with attached pressure transducers is inserted into the colon with the aid of a colonoscope. It measures the strength and coordination of the colonic contractions.	Diagnosis of dysmotility disorders that can result in chronic constipation or chronic pseudo-obstruction	Requires bowel preparation per prescriber. Child is sedated for placement of the catheter. Requires an IV. Monitor child for signs of rectal bleeding, abdominal distention, or perforation after procedure. During the study, the child remains in the area of the testing and is confined to the bed. Family is prepared to bring activities for distraction because the test may take 4–6 hours.
Anorectal manometry	A small catheter with a balloon is inserted into the rectum and inflated to simulate a bowel movement. The catheter is connected to a computer and a graph is produced.	Used to test function of internal and external anal sphincter; can be used to diagnose disorders of defecation and Hirschsprung disease	Usually performed without sedation; family member can remain with child. Test lasts about 45 minutes.
Biopsy			
Liver biopsy	Percutaneous needle aspiration of liver used for microscopic examination of tissue cells and structure	Used to diagnose and/or evaluate the extent of liver disease, evaluate graft function after liver transplant	Child must be NPO for biopsy. Blood prothrombin time, activated partial thromboplastin time, and platelet count are done before the procedure. Notify the physician regarding any abnormal levels. The procedure is most often done with moderate sedation or general anesthesia. Establish IV access for administration of the necessary medications. Monitor vital signs and oxygen saturation during the procedure and for 6–8 hours afterward. The child must remain positioned on the right side for 2–4 hours after the procedure. A pressure dressing is placed over the biopsy site. Observe the child for signs of bleeding, peritonitis, or pneumothorax after the procedure. Check hematocrit level 4–6 hours after the procedure.

(Continued)

 **TESTS AND PROCEDURES for Evaluating Altered Gastrointestinal Status** *(Continued)*

Diagnostic Test or Procedure	Purpose	Findings and Indications	Health Care Provider Considerations
Esophagus, stomach, intestinal biopsy	To diagnose mucosal abnormalities and evaluate response to therapy; done in conjunction with endoscopic procedure	Abnormal findings from biopsy are histologic changes, which can be caused by GERD or gastritis; infectious processes such as *Helicobacter pylori* infection Intestinal biopsy for diagnosing celiac disease, villous atrophy from infection, or malnutrition; used to confirm diagnosis in IBD Indicated to evaluate the response to therapy when symptoms persist and child does not exhibit anticipated progress toward goal	Same as for endoscopic procedures
Stool			
Occult blood (guaiac test)	To detect fecal occult blood from a GI source; a small amount of stool is applied to guaiac paper and then two drops of developing solution are placed on the reverse side. Paper will turn blue in the presence of blood.	Gastritis, IBD, peptic ulcer disease, malabsorption, chronic unexplained anemia; menstrual blood, anal fissures, and perianal skin breakdown may cause false-positive results.	Family education about collection of specimen if home testing is desired. Use standard precautions.
Stool pH	Screening test for malabsorption of sugar, using pH paper; small amount of fresh liquid stool is applied to pH paper, and resulting color is compared with pH color chart.	A pH value less than 6 indicates malabsorption.	Use standard precautions.
Reducing substances	Screens for intestinal malabsorption of sugars; a Clinitest tablet is placed in five drops of fresh liquid stool mixed with 10 drops of water. Resulting color is compared with Clinitest color chart.	A reading more than 0.5% indicates malabsorption of sugars.	Use standard precautions.
Fecal fat	A 72-hour stool collection to evaluate the ability of the GI tract to digest and absorb fat from dietary intake	Elevated levels of fat in the stool are found in patients with malabsorption syndromes, short bowel syndrome, biliary tract obstruction, and pancreatic insufficiency with cystic fibrosis.	All stools for a 72-hour period are collected in one heavy plastic screw-cap container. Specimen must stay refrigerated during collection period. A concurrent diet record may be requested. Provide instructions regarding collection procedure if home testing is desired.

Diagnostic Test or Procedure	Purpose	Findings and Indications	Health Care Provider Considerations
Stool for white blood cells (methylene blue stain)	Rapid, nonspecific screening test to detect the presence of polymorphonuclear leukocytes in the stool	Leukocytes may be present in diarrhea caused by invasive bacteria such as *Salmonella* or *Shigella* species and in ulcerative or antibiotic-associated colitis. Barium in the specimen may interfere with test results.	Collection of fresh stool specimen in clean, plastic container with a lid. Specimen is sent immediately to the lab.
Ova and parasite	To identify the presence of specific parasites in the GI tract	Presence of parasites or their eggs indicates infestation.	Special specimen container with preservative is necessary. Fresh stool specimen is placed in designated container. Test may be repeated on 3 consecutive days.
Bacterial culture	To identify presence of bacterial organisms that cause intestinal infections, commonly in children with fever and diarrhea. Other bacterial tests may be ordered that are organism specific (e.g., *Clostridium difficile*, cryptosporidium).	Presence of abnormal bacteria indicates infection. Infection with organism specific to the ordered study	Specimen should be obtained before antibiotic therapy is started. Specimen should not be mixed with urine and should be transported directly to the lab.
Rotazyme (enzyme immunoassay)	To identify presence of rotavirus	Infection with rotavirus, a common cause of vomiting and diarrhea in infants and young children during the winter months	Stool should be collected in sterile specimen container. Specimen should be refrigerated if immediate transport to lab is not available.
Alpha 1-antitrypsin	To identify protein loss in the stool	Protein-losing enteropathies and diarrheal disease	Fresh stool specimen is sent to lab in clean container.
Other			
Hydrogen breath test	Uses gas–liquid chromatography to measure amount of hydrogen exhaled after ingestion of a carbohydrate solution; usually lactose based	Used to diagnose carbohydrate malabsorption and bacterial overgrowth of the intestine Elevated levels of hydrogen may be found in the breath of patients with lactase deficiency, mucosal damage, delayed intestinal transit, or colonic flora in the small intestine.	Child must be NPO before the procedure. Expired air is collected before ingesting a carbohydrate drink and at 30-minute intervals for 3 hours afterward. Instruct family to bring child's usual bottle or cup from home to facilitate intake of drink and a favorite toy or activity to provide distraction during waiting time.

(Continued)

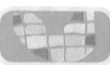   **TESTS AND PROCEDURES** for Evaluating Altered Gastrointestinal Status *(Continued)*

Diagnostic Test or Procedure	Purpose	Findings and Indications	Health Care Provider Considerations
Gastric pH	To assess pH of gastric secretions; gastric secretions are aspirated from an NG or gastrostomy tube. Secretions are placed on pH paper, and resulting color is compared with color chart.	Low pH may indicate gastritis. Usual goal in treating gastritis is a gastric pH level more than 4. For checking newly inserted NG tubes, gastric placement indicators are an aspirate of pH less than 5 along with aspirate characteristics. Aspirate characteristics that indicate gastritic origin: grassy green color; clear, colorless, or off-white to tan mucus with sediment; brown mucus. Aspirate characteristics that indicate inadvertent respiratory placement: watery, straw-colored fluid, possibly with streaks of bright-red blood; mucus-containing fluid that resembles secretions obtained with tracheal suction. Aspirate characteristics that indicate intestinal placement: light to dark golden yellow or brownish-green color (from bile staining). If pH is more than 6, suspect inadvertent respiratory placement, especially if aspirate characteristics support this possibility.	pH may be altered by medications such as proton pump inhibitors and histamine-2 (H2)–receptor antagonists.
Alanine amino-transferase (ALT), aspartate amino-transferase (AST)	To assess the degree of hepatocellular damage in liver disease and graft function in liver transplantation; also used to monitor liver function in children receiving hepatotoxic medications and parenteral nutrition (PN)	ALT is the enzyme that most specifically indicates hepatocellular injury. AST is the enzyme that is present in heart, muscle, and liver; levels increase with hepatocellular injury.	For all blood tests, explain the procedure and support child during specimen collection. Blood sample collection is sent to lab in correct container. Assessment for best choice of local topical anesthetic agent and administer prior to venipuncture for serum studies. Use standard precautions.

Diagnostic Test or Procedure	Purpose	Findings and Indications	Health Care Provider Considerations
Gamma glutamyl transferase (GGT), alkaline phosphatase (ALP)	To assess liver function	GGT elevation indicates cholestasis, obstructive liver disease. ALP indicates cholestasis disorders or extrahepatic obstruction. ALP may also be elevated in children with rickets secondary to impaired intake or absorption of calcium and phosphorus.	
Ammonia	To monitor patients with severe liver failure	Normal level indicates liver is functioning and is able to excrete ammonia. Elevated in patients with hepatic encephalopathy	
Bilirubin (total, direct [conjugated], indirect [unconjugated])	To evaluate liver function and determine cause of various forms of jaundice	Levels are elevated in many forms of liver disease. Unconjugated bilirubin reflects altered function outside the liver; conjugated bilirubin reflects altered function within the liver. Total bilirubin is the sum of the two values.	Normal neonatal hyperbilirubinemia has elevated unconjugated bilirubin.
Hepatitis antigens, antibodies	To detect causative agents of hepatitis infection	Specific antibodies and antigens help to determine whether infection is active, chronic, or resolved.	
Total protein, albumin	To monitor nutritional status and liver function	Levels may be elevated with dehydration. Levels are decreased in patients with malnutrition, liver disease, and protein-losing enteropathies. Albumin takes a long time to become depleted in the body, so a low level reflects a long-term, chronic problem.	Low levels may manifest by peripheral edema or ascites.
Vitamins A, D, E, and K	To identify deficiencies and evaluate response to replacement therapy	Absorption of fat-soluble vitamins A, D, E, and K may be impaired in children with malabsorption syndromes or liver disease.	Vitamin A is important in maintaining skin and mucous membranes; plays a role with night vision.

(Continued)

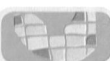

TESTS AND PROCEDURES for Evaluating Altered Gastrointestinal Status *(Continued)*

Diagnostic Test or Procedure	Purpose	Findings and Indications	Health Care Provider Considerations
			Vitamin D promotes intestinal absorption of calcium, phosphate; depleted in peripheral neuropathy, rickets, and osteoporosis. Vitamin E acts as an antioxidant; depleted in peripheral neuropathy. Vitamin K is synthesized by gut flora; necessary for blood clotting factors; depleted in coagulopathies; hemorrhagic manifestations such as bruising and bone mineralization.
Zinc	To determine zinc levels	Zinc is normally excreted through the GI tract. Children with excess losses through the GI tract from diarrhea or prolonged NG drainage may be at risk for deficiencies.	Zinc is an important element in protein synthesis and wound healing.

imaging techniques visualize both the structure and the function of GI organs. Endoscopic examination enables direct visualization of the inner lumen of the GI tract. Tissue samples from biopsies determine alterations in GI organs at the cellular level. State-of-the-art technology is providing newer methods to evaluate segments of the GI tract (see Tests and Procedures 18-1) that have been historically difficult to access—for example, the video capsule endoscopy can be used to visualize the small intestine between the ligament of Treitz and distal ileum.

The nurse must be familiar with both the purpose of and the procedures for the various diagnostic tests and studies used to evaluate alterations in GI status. This familiarity is important to ensure that both the patient and family are appropriately prepared and supported before, during, and after each diagnostic procedure. Preparing the child and family includes providing developmentally appropriate explanations of the test's purpose, steps, and duration as well as anticipatory guidance about sensations the child may experience during the test. Sedation is commonly used for many endoscopic procedures and requires vigilant monitoring of the child (see Chapter 10). Consult with a child life specialist, when available, to aid in preparing the child.

Obtain and handle diagnostic specimens carefully. Many agents that cause GI illness, such as viral and bacterial stool pathogens, are highly infectious. Maintain meticulous attention to standard precautions.

ANSWER: Although both ultrasound and CT scanning can provide images of the appendix, CT scanning with contrast will provide much more information. After the contrast has progressed through the bowel to the cecum, it will very quickly highlight images of the ruptured appendix. The contrast will then be absorbed and begin to collect in the bladder. If the child's kidneys are functioning normally, the CT scan will verify this as well.

TREATMENT MODALITIES

The disease and child's clinical condition determine the treatment needed. Treatment may include therapeutic endoscopy; surgical intervention; ostomy; or nutritional therapy with targeted infant formulas, modified oral diets, or enteral or parenteral nutritional support.

THERAPEUTIC ENDOSCOPY

Therapeutic endoscopy involves the use of endoscopic techniques to treat specific GI alterations. It may be used for dilation of strictures (most commonly in the esophagus), foreign body removal, sclerotherapy (use of an agent that leads to thrombosis and obliteration of the vein) to treat esophageal varices and dilated blood vessels, and excision of polyps. Gastrostomy tubes, such as a PEG tube, transpyloric tubes, or G-J tubes, used to deliver enteral nutrition, may be placed by endoscopy.

SURGICAL INTERVENTION

Surgical intervention is used to repair alterations in GI tract structures, remove diseased structures, or, in the case of liver transplantation, replace nonfunctional structures. Surgical intervention may also be used to place medical devices, such as gastrostomy tubes and central venous catheters, used for therapeutic interventions. Surgical interventions specific to the GI disorders described in this chapter, along with the associated nursing care issues, are discussed in the section covering that disorder. General care of the child undergoing surgery is discussed in Chapter 11.

Controlling pain and promoting deep breathing are particularly important for the child after abdominal surgery. Pain may prevent full diaphragmatic excursion and proper lung expansion, increasing the risk of atelectasis. Encourage the use of an incentive spirometer to promote lung excursion.

Peristalsis takes longer to return after abdominal surgery than after surgery in other systems. This delay depends in part on the extent of bowel manipulation during surgery. Monitor for the return of bowel sounds by auscultating the child's abdomen periodically (Tradition or Science 18-1). Assist with early ambulation to facilitate peristalsis and keep the child NPO until peristalsis returns.

Excess losses of fluid from the GI tract, such as with suction, vomiting, diarrhea, hypoproteinemia, and malnutrition, may cause fluid and electrolyte imbalance. Monitor the child's fluid and electrolyte status, and administer appropriate replacement therapy as ordered.

OSTOMY

An **ostomy**, or *stoma*, is a surgically created opening between the GI tract and the outside of the body (Fig. 18-3). Ostomies can be created at various sites in the GI and genitourinary (GU) tracts and may be temporary or permanent, depending on the child's clinical condition. An *esophagostomy* communicates between

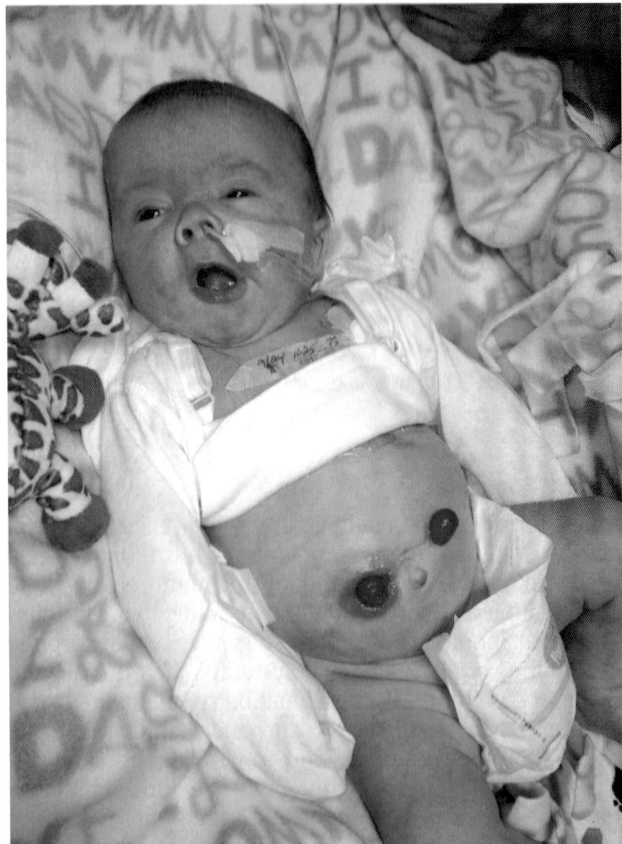

Figure 18-3 An ostomy with a healthy, pink, moist stoma.

the esophagus and an external site on the neck. A *gastrostomy* provides an opening between the stomach and the abdominal wall. Ostomies may be created at various sites in the small intestine (e.g., jejunostomy, ileostomy) or in the large intestine (e.g., colostomy).

A certified wound, ostomy, and continence nurse (CWOCN)—a registered nurse with specialized training and certification in the management of ostomies and skin care—is an essential resource and support person for the child with an ostomy and the child's family. The CWOCN collaborates with the surgeon in ostomy site selection, whenever possible, and provides information regarding product selection, pouching techniques, and patient and family education.

Interdisciplinary management of the child with an ostomy includes both interventions involving direct care and those that promote self-care or care by parents. Developmental issues are varied. The parents of an infant with an ostomy may need instructions about clothing options that protect the pouch system from the infant's exploring hands. School-aged children and their parents, along with school personnel, may need help in dealing with an ostomy in the school setting. The adolescent may have concerns regarding body image and sexuality that need to be discussed. Referral to community support groups may provide children and their families with additional resources to assist with adjustment issues.

More Inquiry Needed

TRADITION OR SCIENCE 18-1

Are bowel sounds adequate for assessing the return of GI motility after abdominal surgery?

Listening to bowel sounds has long been the traditional way to determine when GI motility resumes after abdominal surgery, but the usefulness of this practice has not been rigorously tested. Studies conducted on patients who had undergone abdominal surgery found that auscultation of bowel sounds was not a reliable postoperative clinical indicator of return of GI motility. The study findings indicate that the return of flatus and first postoperative bowel movement, abdominal distention, nausea, vomiting, and tolerance of diet are more appropriate for this purpose. More research is needed to provide evidence that these findings can be applied to pediatric postoperative ileus (Madsen et al., 2005; Massey, 2012).

NUTRITIONAL THERAPY

Modified infant formulas, specific oral diets, enteral nutrition and PN, and specialized feeding techniques are all used in treating the child with altered GI status. Nutritional therapy is an interdisciplinary effort and requires the participation of many health care team members. The nurse plays an important role not only in delivering the various nutritional therapies but also in assessing the child's response to therapy and in teaching the child and family about the therapeutic regimen.

 QUESTION: Will Cory require special nutritional therapy?

Infant Formulas

Infant formulas are available in a wide range of formulations designed to meet a variety of nutritional needs. *Breast milk* is the gold standard for infant feeding. The composition of breast milk is ideally suited to the term infant's nutritional needs and the digestive and absorptive capabilities of the infant's GI system. When breast milk is fed to a preterm infant, it must be supplemented with a *human milk fortifier*. This product supplements the caloric, protein, vitamin, and mineral (especially calcium and phosphorus) content of the breast milk to meet the increased requirements of the preterm infant.

Standard cow's milk infant formulas are designed to meet the nutrient needs of infants up to age 1 year. They are commonly available in powder, liquid concentrate, and ready-to-feed preparations. There is an increase in the number of infant formulas containing the long-chain polyunsaturated fatty acids docosahexaenoic acid (DHA) and arachidonic acid. These long-chain polyunsaturated fatty acids are components of lipids that make up cell and intracellular membranes. DHA is found in high amounts in the retina and brain, whereas arachidonic acid is essential for normal growth. For home use, the powdered form is usually the most economic. *Preterm infant formulas* contain increased concentrations of calories, protein, electrolytes, minerals, vitamins, and long-chain polyunsaturated fatty acids to meet the unique physiologic and nutritional needs of the premature infant's immature system. *Soy-based infant formulas* use a soy protein instead of cow's milk protein and are designed for infants with lactase deficiency, galactosemia, or allergy to cow's milk protein or those whose parents want to feed them a vegan diet.

A substantial number of infants with lactose intolerance or true cow's milk allergy also exhibit allergy to soy proteins. For these infants, as well as infants with various disorders of digestion and absorption, *protein casein hydrolysate formulas* may be indicated. These formulas are hypoallergenic; their protein component is broken down, and their fat and carbohydrate components are modified to facilitate digestion and absorption. Pregestimil and Alimentum have 55% and 33% fat, respectively, as medium-chain triglycerides, which do not require the normal fat digestive pathway. Pregestimil formula is most commonly used in the care of infants with short bowel syndrome and disorders that result in malabsorption of fat, such as biliary atresia or cystic fibrosis. Nutramigen, although it has casein hydrolysate, also has a regular fat source and is indicated only for milk and soy protein allergy. Pure amino acid–based formulas, Neocate and EleCare, are chemically defined formulas based on synthetic amino acids. These formulas are appropriate for infants who have cow's milk protein intolerance or multiple food protein allergies and cannot tolerate casein hydrolysate formulas (Venter et al., 2012).

Modular components can be added to the various infant formulas to increase the concentration of a specific component within the formulas. Individual fat (e.g., medium-chain triglyceride oil), carbohydrate (e.g., Moducal, Polycose), and protein (e.g., Casec) supplements are available that may be used to increase the caloric or nutrient density of the formula.

The caloric and nutrient density of infant formulas may also be altered by varying the amount of water used to mix the formula. Normal caloric density of infant formula is 20 cal/oz. An infant who has increased calorie and nutrient requirements but is fluid restricted or cannot tolerate a large volume of formula may need a concentrated formula. Formula is concentrated by mixing less than the standard amount of water to formula in the powder or liquid concentrate form. Formulas may be concentrated to as much as 30 cal/oz in this manner. Formulas may be diluted to various strengths by mixing them with more than the standard amount of water. This may be done when monitoring an infant for formula intolerance. In this case, an infant would be fed one-half strength formula, advanced to three-quarters strength, and then to full strength. Dilution is usually a short-term strategy.

Teaching parents and other caregivers about the proper use of infant formulas is an important nursing responsibility in both acute care and ambulatory settings. Topics to cover include appropriate formula selection, proper technique for mixing and storing formula, and assistance with formula procurement (see Chapter 4). Parents may try to save money by diluting formula or attempt to "give better nutrition" by feeding concentrated formula. Teach parents that altering caloric density by adding more or less water should be done only with the guidance of a health care provider. Also teach parents never to mix powdered infant formula with oral electrolyte or rehydrating solutions. Doing so can cause electrolyte imbalance.

Modified Oral Diets

Modified oral diets are another form of nutritional therapy used to treat children with GI disorders. The consistency of oral diets may be altered to facilitate ingestion of food for children with oropharyngeal, esophageal, or neuromuscular (e.g., cerebral palsy) impairments that make ingesting foods difficult. The nutrient composition of a child's diet may be altered to meet disease-specific requirements (Table 18-2).

Various oral supplements can be used to increase caloric and nutrient intake for a child unable to meet nutritional needs from usual dietary sources. Milk-based

TABLE 18-2 Modified Oral Diets		
Diet	**Description**	**Indications**
Puree, mechanical soft	"Blenderized," ground, or chopped whole foods	Dysphagia, esophageal stricture
High fiber	Dietary fiber increased in soluble and nonsoluble forms	Constipation, irritable bowel syndrome (IBS)
Lactose free	Milk, milk products, lactose-containing foods eliminated	Lactose intolerance, primary or secondary
High protein, high calorie	Added portions of food sources of protein, fat provided to increase calorie, protein content of diet	Weight less than ideal for age; increased calorie and protein needs for wound healing; cystic fibrosis
Fat controlled	Limiting of dietary fat	Pancreatitis, gall bladder disease
Protein restricted	Limiting protein intake to decrease nitrogenous waste products in bloodstream	Advanced liver disease, renal dysfunction
Salt restricted	Sodium intake restricted to varying degrees, depending on whether purpose is to reduce sodium, fluid retention, or both	Liver disease, children on corticosteroid therapy, renal dysfunction
Gluten free, gliadin free	Avoids gluten-containing foods; eliminates gliadin to reduce symptoms caused by sensitivity to gliadin from wheat, rye, oats, and barley	Celiac disease, celiac sprue (gluten intolerance)

oral supplements, such as Carnation Instant Breakfast or powdered milk, may be added to cow's milk to supplement calories and protein. Clear liquid oral supplements, such as Resource or Carnation Instant Breakfast Juice Drink, are supplemented with protein. Lactose-free oral supplements may be used as a supplement or as a sole source of nutrition. These formulas (e.g., PediaSure, Kindercal) have 1 cal/mL, are isotonic, and are formulated to meet the nutritional requirements of children 1 to 10 years of age when adequate volumes are tolerated. Adult lactose-free oral supplements may be used for older children and are available in a variety of preparations, including fiber-enriched, high-protein, and high-calorie formulas.

Although most oral supplements are available in a variety of flavors, many children may initially complain about their palatability. Collaboration with the child and parent, as well as creativity, is helpful in promoting acceptance of oral supplements.

KidKare To help promote acceptance of oral supplements, provide opportunities for the child to try different flavors. Altering the temperature and texture of the oral supplement to present it in a child-friendly form may also be helpful. Popsicles can be made by freezing the supplement, or a slushy drink can be made by blending the formula with ice. Some supplements offer flavor packets to avoid taste fatigue.

Formulas and nutritional supplements continue to be modified and expanded as a result of advances in nutrition. Prebiotics (nondigestible substances that stimulate the growth of normal flora) and probiotics (live bacteria that benefit the host) have gained increased attention. The purpose of these substances is to support the environment of the GI tract in restoring and maintaining a healthy immunologic state. Probiotics

have been shown to be effective in reducing the risk of antibiotic-associated diarrhea, decreasing the duration of acute diarrhea, and supporting growth of healthy infants during the first 6 months of life (Kligler et al., 2007) as well as preventing necrotizing enterocolitis and all-cause mortality in preterm infants (Deshpande et al., 2011). Studies have also examined their use to treat infant colic (Pärtty et al., 2012; Savino & Tarasco, 2010) and to establish the safety of administering probiotics to infants. However, more controlled studies are needed to provide evidence-based recommendations for use with children to identify specific products and doses to treat specific conditions.

Enteral Nutrition

Children with functional GI tracts who are unable to meet their fluid or nutrient requirements by oral feeding may require enteral nutrition (Chart 18-1). Enteral feeding allows fluids and nutrients to be delivered directly into the GI tract by means of an enteral feeding tube. Contraindications to enteral nutrition include complete intestinal obstruction, intractable vomiting, and severe enterocolitis.

Enteral Formulas

Various formulas are used for enteral feeding. Formula selection is dictated by the child's age, clinical condition, and nutrient requirements. Children younger than age 1 year may receive breast milk and standard or specialty infant formulas by enteral feeding tube. For older children, a number of enteral feeding formulas are available.

Standard tube feeding formulas are nutritionally complete and designed for use in children with normal digestion and absorption, such as the formulas used as a sole source of nutrition discussed earlier in the section "Modified Oral Diets" (e.g., PediaSure, Kindercal). *Elemental formulas* are designed for use in children who have impaired digestion and absorption. These

| CHART 18-1 | **Indications for Enteral Nutrition** |

Gastrointestinal Disorders

Esophageal atresia (EA), strictures

GERD

IBD

Liver disease

Malabsorption, chronic diarrhea

Motility disorders

Pancreatitis

Short bowel syndrome

Increased Metabolic Needs

Burns

Sepsis

Trauma

Congenital heart disease

Bronchopulmonary dysplasia

Cancer

Cystic fibrosis

Chronic Disease

AIDS

Renal disease

Neurologic Disorders

Head injury, coma

Cerebral palsy with oral–motor impairment

Dysphagia

Tumor

Prematurity

Psychiatric Disorders

Anorexia nervosa

formulas are partially predigested, with protein supplied as peptides or amino acids and a large proportion of fat supplied in the form of medium-chain triglycerides. Elemental formulas are available in both pediatric and adult formulations (e.g., Vivonex Pediatric, Peptamen Junior). Older children and adolescents may use formulas designed for adults, such as Ensure or TwoCal HN, depending on the underlying GI condition. Occasionally, an elemental formula may be used as an oral supplement. Flavor packets are available to increase the palatability of these formulas. Some tube feeding formulas are designed for use in specific disease states, such as renal failure or liver failure. Modular components may be added to elemental formulas to supplement their carbohydrate, fat, or protein concentrations.

Enteral Feeding Methods

Enteral feedings are delivered into the stomach or into the small intestine if the child is at risk for pulmonary aspiration. Feedings may be delivered on a continuous or an intermittent schedule. *Continuous enteral nutrition* feedings are administered slowly over 12 to 24 hours using an enteral pump. Continuous feedings are used when feedings are being delivered into the small intestine. They are also indicated whenever an enterally fed child is assessed to be at high risk for aspiration or has impaired digestion and absorption of nutrients. Nocturnal, continuous feedings may also be used to supplement the daily dietary intake in children with some chronic conditions who have increased nutritional needs (e.g., cystic fibrosis, IBD).

Intermittent enteral nutrition is administered by bolus or gravity drip method on an interval schedule. The frequency and volume of the feedings are determined by the patient's age, size, and nutritional goals. A small infant may receive intermittent feedings every 3 to 4 hours, whereas an adolescent may require feedings only every 6 to 8 hours. Intermittent feedings more closely approximate the normal physiologic hunger–satiety cycles.

Enteral Feeding Tubes

Various enteral feeding tubes may be used to deliver enteral nutrition. Tube selection depends on the child's age, clinical condition, nutrient requirements, desired feeding route, and the expected duration of therapy. The orogastric (OG) feeding tube is most commonly used for premature infants or infants younger than age 4 weeks who are obligate nose breathers and who might experience respiratory distress, airway obstruction, or both if a feeding tube is passed transnasally.

Nasoenteric feeding tubes (NG or nasojejunal tubes) are small-bore feeding tubes passed transnasally through the esophagus into the stomach or small intestine (see Nursing Interventions 11-6 and Evidence-Based Clinical Practice Guidelines 18-1; see also thePoint for Procedures). NG or nasojejunal tubes are used for short-term enteral nutrition when the length of therapy is expected to be less than 3 months. These tubes may stay in place continuously or may be inserted intermittently, as indicated by the child's feeding regimen (Fig. 18-4).

Nasoenteric tubes for short-term or intermittent use were previously made from polyvinyl chloride (contains di-[2-ethylhexyl] phthalate, a chemical compound that makes plastic products flexible, strong, and moldable). This substance was found to pose risks to the pediatric population. Today, nasoenteric tubes are made from polyurethane or silicone. These tubes are less irritating and may stay in place for up to 4 weeks. They come with a wire stylet, which may be inserted into the tube to stiffen it and facilitate placement. When the stylet is used, it is removed before using the tube for feeding. For feeding, select a tube of appropriate length with the smallest available exterior diameter. Polyurethane tubes are often preferred because their internal diameter is larger than that of comparably sized silicone tubes.

ALERT *If you encounter resistance during placement of a nasoenteric feeding tube, do not force the tube. Withdraw the tube and attempt placement again. Use of excessive force may cause perforation. Because of the potential for perforation, never reinsert a stylet while the tube is in the patient.*

EVIDENCE-BASED CLINICAL PRACTICE GUIDELINES 18-1
Insertion and Placement Verification of Nasogastric and Orogastric Tubes

Cirgin Ellett, M. L., Cohen, M. D., Perkins, S. M. et al. (2011). Predicting the insertion length for gastric tube placement in neonates. *Journal of Obstetric, Gynecologic, and Neonatal Nursing, 40*(4), 412–421.

Guidelines for determination of insertion length for NG and OG tubes.

Cirgin Ellett, M. L., Cohen, M. D., Perkins, S. M. et al. (2012). Comparing methods of determining insertion length for placing gastric tubes in children 1 month to 17 years of age. *Journal for Specialists in Pediatric Nursing, 17*(1), 19–32.

Guidelines for determination of insertion length for NG and OG tubes.

Freeman, D., Saxton, V., & Holberton, J. (2012). A weight-based formula for the estimation of gastric tube insertion length in newborns. *Advances in Neonatal Care, 12*(3), 179–182.

Guidelines for determination of insertion length for NG and OG tubes.

Cincinnati Children's Hospital Medical Center. (2011). *Best evidence statement (BESt). Confirmation of nasogastric/orogastric tube (NGT/OGT) placement.* Cincinnati, OH: Author. Retrieved from

http://www.cincinnatichildrens.org/service/j/anderson-center/evidence-based-care/recommendations/topic

Guidelines for verification of correct placement of NG and OG tubes.

ENA Emergency Nursing Resources Development Committee. (2010). *Gastric tube placement verification.* Des Plaines, IL: Author. Retrieved from

http://www.ena.org/IENR/CPG/Documents/GastricTubeCPG.pdf

Guidelines for verification of correct placement of NG and OG tubes.

Gastrostomy tubes and jejunostomy tubes (J-tube) are placed to support nutritional needs in a variety of conditions and routes (Fig. 18-5). Many types of tubes are available from a variety of manufacturers. Follow the manufacturer's instructions for use and ensure that you are familiar with the types used in your institution.

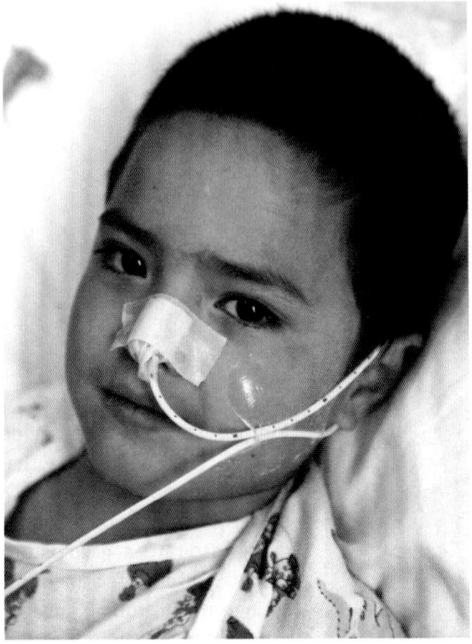

Figure 18-4 The child with an NG tube. Assess to ensure that the NG tube does not exert pressure on the nares to avoid skin breakdown. Commercially available securement methods or tape can be used to secure the tube.

Review and know the policies and procedures specific to each device (see thePoint for Procedures and Supplemental Information).

Interdisciplinary Interventions

Care of the child receiving enteral nutrition involves the following activities:

- Managing the enteral feeding tube and enteral nutrition delivery system to ensure accurate delivery of fluid and nutrients and prevent system-related complications
- Monitoring the child's response to enteral nutrition, including metabolic complications
- Supporting the child's and family's educational and developmental needs with regard to the therapy

Care of the child receiving enteral nutrition is an interdisciplinary effort, and interventions are enhanced through collaboration with other members of the health care team. The dietitian plays a key role in assessing nutritional status, calculating nutrient requirements, selecting formulas, monitoring response to therapy, and educating the patient and family. The occupational therapist may be involved in helping to promote oral feeding skills (see Chapter 17). Collaborate with the advanced practice nurse or CWOCN to teach complex care of the enteral tube site. The pharmacist is a valuable consultant for drug and nutrient interactions when medications must be administered by enteral feeding tubes.

Before administering a feeding, verify that the feeding tube is placed as is appropriate for the type of tube.

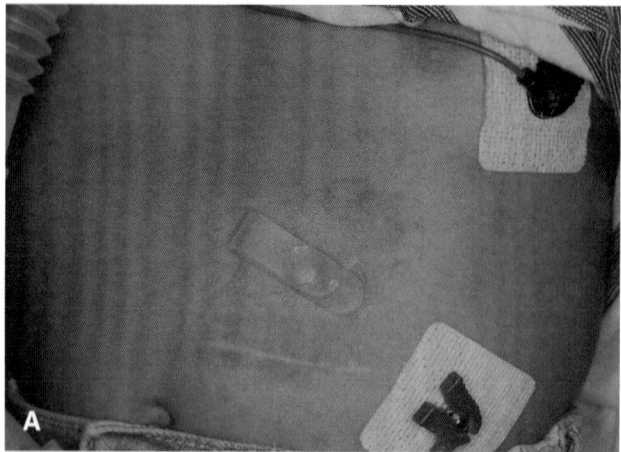
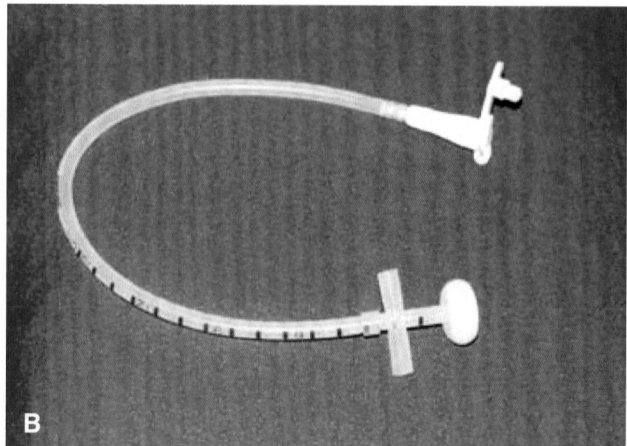

Figure 18-5 Gastrostomy tubes. (A) A skin-level gastrostomy access device has a low profile and therefore is not as bulky or obvious as other gastrostomy tubes. (B) A PEG tube has an internal tip that is dome shaped and anchors the tube in the body, which prevents the tube from falling out. The crossbar at skin level prevents internal tube migration.

To minimize the possibility of aspiration with enteral feedings, elevate the head of the bed to a minimum of 30 degrees, and preferably to 45 degrees, for all patients receiving enteral nutrition unless a medical contraindication exists (Bankhead et al., 2009). Administer feeding as ordered (Fig. 18-6). Although flushing enteral feeding tubes with cranberry juice or carbonated cola beverages is frequently cited as the most effective method for maintaining tube patency, research has indicated that prevention and water flushes are an effective flushing agent (Metheny et al., 1988) (see Tradition or Science 18-2 and thePoint for Procedures). Juices and cola may seem to initially unclog the tube, but the sugars line the tube and break down the proteins, causing more clogging. Commercially available devices with enzymes are now available for declogging tubes such as

the Intro-Reducer and Clog Zapper by Viasys (Dandeles & Lodolce, 2011; Forest-Lalande, 2012).

Research has suggested that the practice of providing nonnutritive sucking (NNS) experiences is beneficial to infants. NNS incorporates the use of a pacifier to stimulate oral–motor function when alternate feeding routes are indicated. Improved weight gain, decreased heart rate and energy expenditure, decreased restlessness, and increased alert states have all been documented with NNS, as have decreased length of stay and pain control (Pinelli & Symington, 2005). However, an extensive review of well-controlled studies in hospitalized preterm infants, in which NNS was examined as part of the plan of care, concluded that further research is needed to establish evidence that NNS provides a direct benefit in terms of behavioral outcomes, GI function,

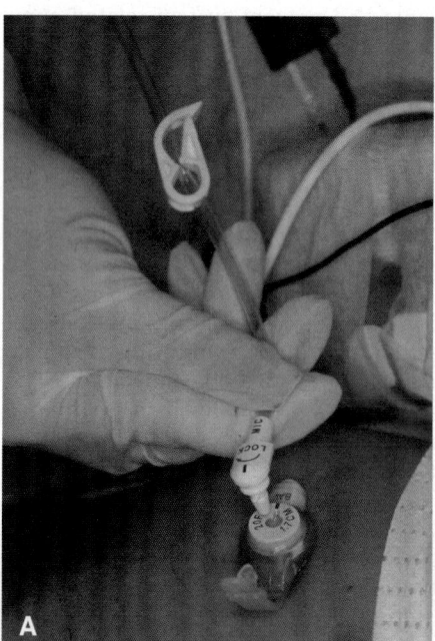
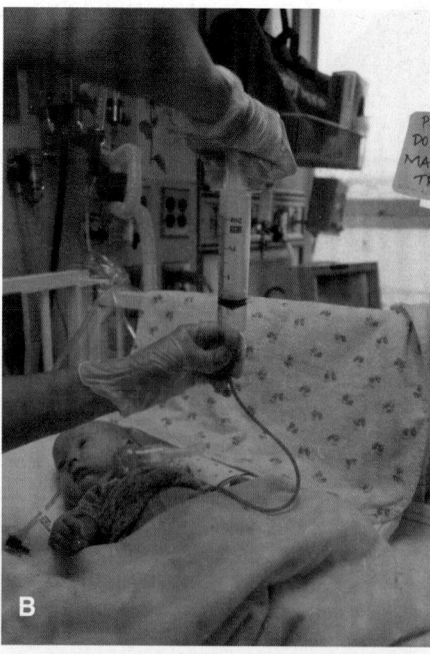

Figure 18-6 (A) Enteral devices such as the "button" require that a feeding tube be connected to the device to instill fluids. (B) Before beginning the feeding, gently aspirate a gastrostomy tube for gastric contents or attach the barrel of a syringe to the tubing and gently palpate the child's abdomen. Note the presence of gastric contents in the syringe. Avoid vigorous aspiration because it might pull gastric mucosa against the tube.

TRADITION OR SCIENCE 18-2

Evidence-Based Practice

Is the time-honored practice of auscultation after insufflation of air over the epigastric region adequate for verifying NG or OG feeding tube position?

Nursing research indicates that testing the pH of aspirates and evaluating the aspirated contents is a more reliable way of verifying enteral feeding tube placement than the commonly used practice of auscultating the abdomen while insufflating air through the feeding tube (Huffman et al., 2004; Metheny & Meert, 2004; Westhus, 2004). The Society of Pediatric Nurses recommends abdominal x-ray to verify placement if aspiration fails to confirm correct positioning (Longo, 2011).

or feeding (Bingham et al., 2010; Pinelli & Symington, 2005). No harmful effects of NNS were reported when a pacifier is used safely.

Assess GI, hydration, and nutritional status. Monitor the child for abdominal distention, nausea, or vomiting. Assess stool output and stooling patterns. When the child's nutritional status and enteral intake are being stabilized, monitor gastric residuals before each intermittent feeding and every 4 to 6 hours during continuous feedings. If residuals exceed ordered parameters, hold the feeding and notify the physician or advanced practice nurse. Gastric emptying is facilitated by a right-side-down or prone position. However, the child's position after feeding must be in accordance with the American Academy of Pediatrics' Back to Sleep recommendations for safety (American Academy of Pediatrics, Task Force on Sudden Infant Death Syndrome, 2011).

Obtain and document the child's weight daily. Check height and head circumference (in children younger than age 3 years) weekly. Compare current and previous values to evaluate the child's growth pattern. Also monitor for signs of dehydration or fluid overload; electrolyte imbalance; and vitamin, mineral, and trace element deficiencies.

Community Care

Most children with feeding tubes are sent home with the tube in place, making parent education and planning for home management a priority in the plan of care. Collaborate with discharge planning personnel to ensure that the child and family have appropriate formula, supplies, and home equipment. Teach the family (and child, as developmentally appropriate) how to care for the enteral feeding tube, to prepare and administer enteral feedings, to monitor for complications, and to attend to developmental and safety issues. Ensure that the outpatient follow-up plan is coordinated with the home health agency (Teaching Intervention Plan 18-1). Collaborate with the parents and school staff to facilitate transition back to school and the standard classroom (see Chapter 12).

ANSWER: Not necessarily. Cory will not receive any oral feeding immediately after surgery until his intestines are active and functioning. During this recovery period, he will receive fluid, glucose, and electrolytes via his peripheral IV. When he has evidence of return of bowel function, he will start with a soft diet and progress to a regular diet. However, as noted in Chapter 6, Cory's nutritional status was not optimal before this illness. He may benefit from nutritional supplements, particularly protein. Protein is necessary for wound and tissue healing, and Cory has poor protein stores and often refuses to eat foods that are high in protein.

NURSING PLAN OF CARE

 QUESTION: Which of the nursing diagnoses in Nursing Plan of Care 18-1 are applicable to Cory?

Analysis of assessment findings will identify nursing diagnoses pertinent to that child and family. Chapter 11 identifies nursing diagnoses commonly applicable to the psychosocial needs of the acutely ill child. Nursing diagnoses pertinent to the child with an alteration in GI status often reflect an alteration in nutrition or fluid and electrolyte status resulting from the GI condition. Nursing diagnoses generally applicable to a child with altered GI status are identified in Nursing Plan of Care 18-1. Nursing diagnoses more specific to each particular GI disorder are identified in the section covering that disorder.

ANSWER: Nursing diagnoses applicable to Cory may include the following:
- Deficient fluid volume related to inadequate intake
- Acute pain related to the effects of GI system dysfunction
- Imbalanced nutrition: Less than body requirements related to effects of alteration in GI tract function

ALTERATIONS IN GASTROINTESTINAL STATUS

Alterations in GI status can take many forms. The cause can be difficult to ascertain, as in failure to thrive (FTT) or, more obvious, as with physical malformations. GI status is also affected by inflammatory disorders; disorders that affect GI motility, function, and absorption; and hepatic disorders.

FAILURE TO THRIVE

FTT is often used as a diagnosis, yet it is actually a symptom. Continuing debate in the literature illustrates the lack of consensus in using FTT as a diagnosis as

TIP 18-1: A TEACHING INTERVENTION PLAN for the Child With a Gastrostomy Tube, J-Tube, or G-J Tube

Nursing Diagnoses and Family Outcomes

- Deficient knowledge: Care of enteral feeding tube; safety issues regarding enteral feeding
  Outcomes: Family and child, if developmentally appropriate, will demonstrate proper care of tube.
  Child will not develop complications associated with the presence of an enteral feeding tube (displacement, blockage, infection).
- Imbalanced nutrition: Less than body requirements related to effects of child's condition
  Outcomes: Child will demonstrate appropriate weight, height, and head circumference growth along own growth curve.
  Family and child will demonstrate appropriate feeding techniques.

Teach the Child/Family

Enteral Feeding Tube Care

Maintaining Placement
- Monitor integrity of system used to secure tube. Resecure as necessary.
- Monitor position of gastrostomy tube or G-J tube before each feeding and with site care by pulling back gently on the tube to ensure inner balloon or retention device is snug against abdominal wall (cannot be done with skin-level gastrostomy tubes). For tubes with an external segment, compare the graduated centimeter markings with the baseline measurement for tube position verification.
- If the tube becomes dislodged, cover site with clean gauze and tape and notify the health care provider.

Maintaining Patency
- Flush tube with water after each intermittent feeding or every 4–6 hours during continuous feedings, per protocol. Monitor total fluid volume of flushes to prevent fluid overload.
- Administer medications in liquid form. If medications must be crushed, consult with pharmacist regarding appropriate solution for dissolving medications. Never crush enteric-coated or time-release medications.
- Administer medications one at a time. Flush before, after, and in between multiple medications.
- Flush every 8 hours if tube is not being used.
- For G-J tubes, verify the port for medication administration (usually the feedings are given through the J-port; the G-port is used for gastric decompression). Maintain scheduled flushing; for example, flush J-tubes every 4–6 hours around the clock during the continuous delivery of feedings.

Preventing Infection
- Provide site care every 24 hours or whenever area around tube is moist or crusted with secretions.
- Use sterile saline or water to clean around newly placed tubes and to remove dried blood or crusted secretions at tube exit sites.
- Use of soap and water are recommended on well-healed tube sites.
- Dry site thoroughly after cleaning and apply external securing device as necessary for specific tubes.
- Avoid covering tube sites with ointments or occlusive dressings unless otherwise instructed. This practice may cause moisture retention at the tube site and may promote granuloma formation.
- Rotate the gastrostomy tube every 24 hours when performing skin care. Turn the tube 360 degrees, which helps to prevent the tube from embedding in the gastric mucosa. *Do not rotate J- or G-J tubes* because doing so may cause torque and retraction of the tube into the stomach or kinking of the tube.

Administration of Enteral Feedings

Preparing for Feeding
- Prepare formula, including type, concentration, and amount. Use premeasured volume of formula at room temperature.
- Check for gastric residual before starting feeding by gently aspirating from tube with a syringe or positioning the tube below the level of the stomach with only the barrel of the syringe attached.
- Position with head elevated 30–45 degrees, either upright in lap, lying on right side, or sitting and supported as indicated.

Administering Feeding
- By enteral pump, connect the tubing to the enteral feeding tube and adjust the rate.
- By syringe, connect the syringe barrel to the tube, pour the formula into the syringe, and let it free flow slowly by gravity. It should take about as long as it would if the child was sucking or drinking the formula.
- If formula does not flow freely, reposition the child slightly and give a brief but gentle push to start the flow with syringe plunger. Do not force, and do not use plunger to infuse entire feeding.

After Feeding
- Flush tube with a small amount of water unless contraindicated. Leave gastrostomy tube open for 5–10 minutes after feeding to allow for escape of air.

Preventing Infection
- Change enteral feeding pump bags every 24 hours.

- Limit formula in enteral feeding bags to no more than 4 hours worth or per policy.
- Refrigerate excess formula after opening and use within 24–48 hours.

Safety
- Never use parenteral infusion equipment for administration of enteral feedings. Inadvertent administration of enteral formulas through the parenteral route has been reported and has led to fatal complications.
- Keep the tube secured to the body to prevent dangling and accidental dislodgment.
- Elevate the child's head at least 30 degrees during feedings and for 30–60 minutes afterward to reduce the risk of aspiration.
- Avoid warming the formula using a microwave oven.

Developmental Considerations
- Provide infant with pacifier during enteral feedings.
- Provide all children with developmentally appropriate social interaction during enteral feedings.
- Use developmentally appropriate safety precautions to ensure integrity and safety of enteral feeding system. For example, cover site with a shirt so an infant cannot pull at tube. Use longer feeding tubing when child is learning to walk. If the child is on nighttime feedings, thread tubing through pajamas and out the bottom of the leg to avoid the child getting tangled up in tubing.
- Normalize the child's routine so that the feeding can be administered during mealtimes with family.

Contact Health Care Provider if
- Feedings will not infuse
- The tube looks shorter or the centimeter markings on the external tube segment have changed (the tube may have moved/migrated)
- Child has diarrhea or vomiting with no other signs of illness
- Child has signs of infection, such as increased amounts of yellow or green drainage from the skin exit site; tenderness, swelling, or increased redness around the skin exit site; fever
- Child has vomiting, diarrhea, constipation, increasing abdominal distention, general discomfort, or signs of dehydration (decreased urination, lack of tears, dry mucous membranes) or fluid overload (shortness of breath, edema)
- Child experiences pain with feeding
- The tube has leakage or redness around it
- The tube is accidentally dislodged

---

well as in defining it. Some experts propose abandoning the term *failure to thrive* altogether for one that is more accurate, such as *pediatric undernutrition, inadequate growth,* or *growth deficiency.*

Although consensus does not exist on the definition of FTT, a working definition for this text can be considered. FTT is the failure to grow at a rate consistent with expected standards most commonly diagnosed in children younger than 2 years of age but can occur in older children (Scholler & Nittur, 2012). FTT is thought to be a result of interaction between the environment and the child's health, development, and behavior.

Traditionally, discussion has included three types of FTT:

1. Organic FTT: associated with an underlying medical condition
2. Nonorganic FTT: most commonly diagnosed at age 5 years or younger; has no associated medical conditions affecting poor growth
3. A combination of both types

The etiology of organic-related FTT is linked to a vast number of diagnoses resulting in poor growth that may span all systems. Table 18-3 provides some selected examples in each system that may affect growth. More descriptive diagnoses for nonorganic (nonmedical) FTT are now identified as having developmental or psychological problems, such as sensorimotor disorder, disorder of infancy, family relationship problem, or oral–motor dyspraxia.

The precise incidence of FTT is not known. However, FTT is reported to occur in 5% to 10% of the pediatric population, and 1% to 5% of all hospital admissions of children younger than age 2 years are because of concerns about growth (Scholler & Nittur, 2012). Children younger than 2 years of age are at particular risk because this is a time of rapid brain growth, weight gain, linear growth, and psychomotor development.

Pathophysiology

Regardless of the etiology, FTT during the first year of life is a serious condition. The brain grows as much during the first year of life as it does throughout the rest of the child's life. Maximal postnatal brain growth occurs during the first 6 months of life.

The pathophysiology of organic FTT depends on the causative condition. Nonorganic FTT was recognized during the early 20th century. Historically, the mother's characteristics, such as depression, substance use, social isolation, and maltreatment during childhood, were attributed as the central cause of this condition. These characteristics rendered the mother unable to effectively nurture, parent, or feed her infant or child. "Maternal deprivation syndrome" or "maternal neglect" was a diagnosis given to infants and children whose FTT was thought to have a psychosocial origin. Certain infant behaviors also may contribute to growth failure. Some of these behaviors include being difficult to feed, apathetic, aversive to cuddling, passive, inactive, irritable, and not wanting to be touched. Despite these known

NURSING PLAN OF CARE 18-1:

The Child With Altered Gastrointestinal Status

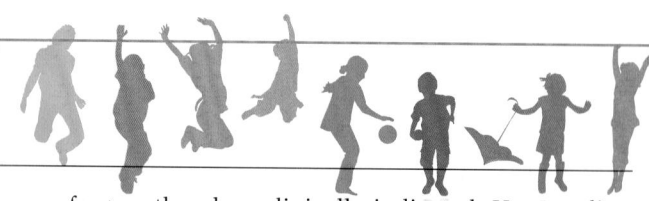

Nursing Diagnosis: Deficient fluid volume related to inadequate intake or excessive losses from GI tract

Interventions/Rationale

- Assess child's hydration status (moistness of mucous membranes, presence of tears when crying, skin turgor).

  Assessment provides baseline data to evaluate changes in child's status and facilitates early detection of changes.

- Monitor for factors that might cause deficient fluid volume (e.g., inadequate intake, diarrhea, vomiting, fever).

  Early identification of risk factors enables early intervention to minimize the fluid deficit.

- Weigh the child daily.

  Change in weight is a good estimate of fluid balance, especially in young children, who have a greater proportion of body water in the extracellular space.

- Record intake and output; weigh diapers.

  Measurements provide quantitative evidence that enables evaluation of fluid balance to detect imbalance.

- Monitor for signs of increasing dehydration (e.g., less elastic skin turgor, depressed fontanels, sunken eyes, weight loss, rapid pulse, dry mucous membranes, decreasing urine output) and report to physician or advanced practice nurse.

  Early identification of fluid deficit enables early intervention to replace lost fluid.

- Monitor laboratory reports (e.g., electrolytes, pH, hematocrit, serum albumin, urine specific gravity).

  Laboratory test results facilitate evaluation of child's status and response to therapy.

Expected Outcomes

- Child will achieve and maintain normal fluid and electrolyte balances.
- Child and parents will identify signs of fluid imbalance and implement interventions to treat it.

Nursing Diagnosis: Acute pain related to the effects of GI system dysfunction, procedures, and treatments

Interventions/Rationale

- Assess and document the onset, location, duration, character, intensity, and aggravating and relieving factors of pain during the initial evaluation. Assess pain with vital signs or more frequently when clinically indicated. Use a validated scale with which the child and staff are familiar.

  The bowel is sensitive to pressure; increased bowel transit time and a hyperosmotic load cause stretching and spasms in the intestines. When diarrhea or vomiting is present, abdominal cramping and distension are often accompanying symptoms. The initial assessment directs the pain management plan. The child's self-report is the most reliable evidence. To obtain accurate assessments, reliable and valid scales must be used correctly.

- Minimize crying; burp child as necessary.

  Crying may increase swallowing of air, which may lead to abdominal distention. Burping helps to expel swallowed air.

- Use biobehavioral methods to cope with pain. Position the child with knees flexed. If age appropriate, teach the child to use slow, controlled breathing.

  Positioning with knees flexed minimizes stretching of the peritoneum; relaxation may help reduce anxiety, which can intensify the pain experience and may provide distraction from the pain.

- Administer ordered medications when indicated (e.g., postoperative narcotics, topical anesthetic for IV insertion). If pharmacologic management is indicated but not ordered, contact the advanced practice nurse or physician to obtain orders.

  Appropriate medications may be necessary to ensure effective relief from pain.

- Prepare children and families for procedures and teach them pain relief interventions that they can use (e.g., deep breathing, relaxation, distraction).

  Anxiety may exacerbate pain. Knowing what to expect during medical encounters and how to manage discomfort through the procedure may help alleviate anxiety. Knowing how to manage pain may empower the child and family and also facilitates prompt implementation of comfort interventions. Collaborate with a child life specialist to incorporate multimodal interventions.

Expected Outcomes

- Child will verbalize complaints of discomfort.
- Child will state a decrease in pain level with appropriate interventions.
- Child will remain free of behavioral signs of discomfort.
- Child and family will describe interventions to be implemented if the child experiences pain.

Nursing Diagnosis: Imbalanced nutrition: Less than body requirements related to effects of alteration in GI tract function

Interventions/Rationale

- Assess and document growth parameters; activity; eating behaviors, patterns, and habits; dietary choices, including food likes, dislikes, and intolerances; and knowledge about development, diet, and nutrition using an interdisciplinary approach.

  An interdisciplinary approach with a nurse, physician, dietitian, occupational therapist, and child life specialist augments the assessment process to incorporate developmentally based nutritional goals for the plan of care.

- Include the parents and child in goal development and solicit input about their perceptions of and ability to meet the nutritional goals and plan of care.

  Parent and child "buy-in" is essential to the success of the plan of care.

- Encourage parents to bring in the child's favorite foods or those that are most culturally familiar within prescribed restrictions if appropriate if they cannot be provided within the organization.

  Favored or familiar foods are more likely to be accepted and consumed by the child.

- Consider placing the child on a reward system based on meeting nutritional goals, such as a sticker chart with incremental rewards. Computer or video game time may be effective in rewarding the older child.

  A reward system provides positive feedback and an incentive to the child to try to meet the goal or perform the desired behavior.

- Document intake and output and daily weights.

  Measurements provide objective data to evaluate the child's response to therapeutic nutritional goals.

- Determine and implement behavioral modifications as clinically indicated, including feeding and eating techniques, such as postural or oral control techniques; portion control; environment control, such as eating meals with family and others or creating a TV-free environment during mealtime; offering scheduled nutritional oral supplements and snacks; positioning to prevent aspiration; and avoiding odors that may stimulate nausea.

  Appropriate environmental controls may make it easier for the child to consume adequate nutrients.

- Explore the parents' and child's perception of body image and concerns of health status as it relates to nutrition. Solicit concerns and questions.

  Lack of knowledge or inaccurate perceptions may increase anxiety and result in activities that undermine the treatment plan. Knowing the child's and parents' perceptions enables teaching to address inaccurate beliefs or modification of the treatment plan to accommodate the concerns.

- Discuss and explore feelings about alternative feeding approaches if oral methods continue to place the child at nutritional risk. Emphasize that alternative feeding methods do not indicate failure on anyone's part but rather are needed to provide the recommended nutrition as a result of the underlying GI condition.

  Implementing an individualized plan of care with nutritional goals optimizes the likelihood of increasing nutritional intake and of implementing an ongoing plan to meet the needs of children at nutritional risk.

Expected Outcomes

- Child and family will identify ways to achieve appropriate nutritional intake.
- Child will demonstrate appropriate nutritional intake.
- Child will maintain growth velocity along own growth curve.

Nursing Diagnosis: Impaired skin integrity related to inadequate nutritional intake

See Nursing Plan of Care 25-1.

Nursing Diagnosis: Deficient knowledge: Child's GI condition and treatment

Interventions/Rationale

- Assess family's knowledge of child's condition and care needs.

  Baseline assessment assists in focusing teaching to family's needs.

- Use developmentally appropriate methods to teach child and family about the condition.

  Knowledge facilitates appropriate management of the condition and enhances the transition to successful home management.

- Instruct parents in the proper method of making, storing, and giving formula/meals.

  Inappropriately prepared or stored formula/ food may cause dehydration (concentrated, hyperosmolar solutions), inadequate weight gain and nutrition (overly diluted formulas do not provide sufficient calories), and disease (bacterial overgrowth may occur).

- Teach parents to manage child's condition (diet, treatments) and what symptoms to report to health care provider.

  Appropriate management facilitates optimal outcomes. Appropriate intake may reduce fluid and electrolyte imbalances and support weight gain.

(Continued)

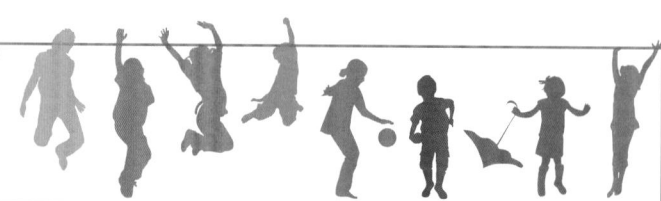

NURSING PLAN OF CARE 18-1:
The Child With Altered Gastrointestinal Status (*Continued*)

- Use facts and examples to teach good hand hygiene technique and sanitation habits; observe return demonstration.

  Hand hygiene reduces transmission of microorganisms.

Expected Outcomes
- Child and family will describe the illness and will identify important clinical manifestations and potential complications.
- Child and family will describe the treatment plan for the illness and will demonstrate the ability to administer the necessary medications and treatments.

Nursing Diagnosis: Delayed growth and development related to lack of opportunity or restrictions imposed by condition, parents, or self; inability to participate in developmentally appropriate activities

Interventions/Rationale
- Routinely compare weight and height measurements with previous measurements and age-appropriate norms.

  Comparisons can provide evaluation of the child's growth trajectory.
- Assist the family in evaluating the child's regressive response to illness or chronic health condition. Explain the effect of acute illness or a chronic condition on the child.

  Children typically regress when ill. A chronic condition may impose restrictions that limit the child's energy or ability to engage in age-appropriate activities. Parents who understand their child's responses are better able to support the child and assist him or her in achieving full potential.
- Provide developmentally appropriate activities, tailored to the child's needs and situation.

  Tailored activities facilitate the child's ability to participate and achieve milestones.

Expected Outcomes
- Child will perform developmentally appropriate tasks.
- Parents will identify normal developmental milestones for their child and ways to help their child achieve these milestones.

---

behavioral descriptions, the etiology of nonorganic FTT remains poorly understood.

Altered maternal–infant interaction is understood to play a major role, however. The transactional model is used to explain this relationship. The model examines the altered reciprocal interaction between the mother and infant, including environmental influences that affect the relationship over time. For example, the household is a disorganized and chaotic environment, the infant is apathetic and passive, and the mother misinterprets the infant cues and therefore does not meet the infant's needs. Over time, this ineffective interaction

System	Contributing Etiology
GI	GERD, celiac disease, malabsorption syndromes, structural anomalies that effect oral–motor function (e.g., cleft palate), tracheoesophageal fistula (TEF), pyloric stenosis, intractable diarrhea, Hirschsprung disease, IBD, chronic liver disease (e.g., biliary atresia, hepatitis)
Cardiopulmonary	Congenital heart disease, heart failure, chronic lung disease, asthma, cystic fibrosis
Renal	Chronic kidney diseases, renal tubular acidosis
Metabolic/genetic	Inborn errors of metabolism, congenital syndromes (e.g., Pierre Robin syndrome), chromosomal conditions (e.g., Cornelia de Lange syndrome)
Neuromuscular	Cerebral palsy, degenerative diseases (e.g., muscular dystrophy, spinal muscular atrophy), conditions that include dysphagia
Endocrine	Hypothyroid, hypoparathyroid, pituitary disorders (e.g., congenital hypopituitary, adrenal disorders, growth hormone deficiency), diabetes mellitus, diabetes insipidus
Infection	Intrauterine infections, HIV, tuberculosis, parasitic infections
Miscellaneous	Malignancy, lead poisoning

TABLE 18-3   Medical Conditions That Contribute to Organic Failure to Thrive

alters the mother–infant dyad. The poor fit between the infant and mother results in malnutrition. Many studies conducted on nonorganic FTT have described the characteristics of the mother, infant, and environment after the diagnosis. Greater understanding of how nonorganic FTT develops may be gained by prospectively assessing the mother–infant interaction to help sort out those characteristics of the mother–infant dyad that contribute to nonorganic FTT.

Assessment

A careful history is the cornerstone to direct the plan of care. This history includes the prenatal history with regard to maternal lifestyle, medication use, and illnesses; birth history; postnatal history; and the condition that triggered the current medical encounter. Verify the child's age to ensure that the child's growth parameters are plotted correctly on growth charts. After malnutrition or inadequate growth is established, a plan is developed to support the nutritional deficit while the workup for the etiology ensues.

Inadequate growth may result from inadequate caloric intake, inability to retain the calories (e.g., malabsorption), and/or increased caloric expenditure (e.g., chronic lung disease). Obtain a careful dietary history to assess whether intake is inadequate because the nourishment provided is inappropriate, or nourishment is appropriate but intake is inadequate. Ask about type of formula, volume consumed per 24 hours, and method of formula preparation. If the child is eating solid foods, a typical recall of the day's intake may be helpful, as will the frequency of meals and snacks. Inquire about the timing and type of food introduced in the diet. Elicit information about the characteristics and number of stools per day and wet diapers or voids. Also ask whether vomiting occurs, its characteristics, and amounts.

CROSS-CULTURAL CARE

Sensitivity to ethnic, cultural, and religious differences may help clarify information, lead to greater understanding of the use of home remedies, and help avoid misunderstandings about growth problems. For example, duration of breastfeeding and introduction of solid food may be culturally determined. Contemporary cultural norms regarding fear of obesity and the desire to maintain a "healthy" or "organic" diet may also play a role in some situations.

Diagnostic Tests

In general, when nonorganic FTT is suspected, no single study can verify this diagnosis. Studies are guided from positive findings from a careful history and physical examination. Basic screening tests may be performed to obtain baseline information. Screening for iron-deficiency anemia, tuberculosis, lead poisoning, and chronic urinary tract infection along with review of neonatal screening test results are recommended. Other tests include complete blood count (CBC); electrolytes,

including blood urea nitrogen; creatinine; and liver function tests, including total protein and albumin. Prealbumin, a hepatic protein also called *transthyretin*, may be obtained as a baseline nutritional marker because prealbumin levels are a good measure of visceral protein status. Prealbumin is more sensitive than albumin as an indicator of nutritional recovery because it has a half-life of 2 days, reflecting more recent changes in nutritional status than albumin's 21-day half-life (Loughrey & Duggan, 2005). Monitoring prealbumin trends and patterns provides information to help direct nutritional interventions. Findings from the history and physical examination determine indications for additional specific tests. For example, an infant with a history of frequent regurgitation may need a pH study to rule out GERD.

Nursing Diagnoses and Outcomes

Nursing Plan of Care 18-1 presents a variety of nursing diagnoses that can be applied to the child with altered GI status. Nursing diagnoses applicable to the child with organic FTT depend on the causative condition. The following nursing diagnoses and outcomes are specifically applicable to the child with nonorganic FTT:

Nursing Diagnosis: Impaired parenting related to parental low self-esteem, depression, or other psychosocial issues; negative perception of the child; poor fit between parent and child temperaments or interactional styles
Outcome: Parent will express acquisition of progress toward positive feelings and demonstrate adequacy in the parenting role.
Nursing Diagnosis: Ineffective health maintenance related to impaired family dynamics, lack of resources
Outcome: The family will identify existing medical and community services and accept assistance.

Interdisciplinary Interventions

When FTT is determined to be secondary to a medical diagnosis (i.e., organic), the ability to intervene with an effective plan of care is more direct than for FTT from a nonmedical and environmental/developmental/behavioral cause (i.e., nonorganic). Ongoing monitoring with supportive interdisciplinary interventions is necessary for all children. This discussion focuses primarily on nonorganic FTT.

An interdisciplinary team is most effective in this complex condition. The team consists of a physician, nurse, dietitian, medical social worker, occupational therapist, and child life specialist. Additional expertise, such as that of a psychologist or psychiatrist, may be indicated.

Providing adequate energy through calories for growth is the cornerstone of therapy. The physician and dietitian develop a plan of care to meet the nutritional goals based on assessment findings. Calorie-dense formulas for infants and high-calorie foods for older children are given, including oral nutritional supplements. Multivitamin supplements with minerals, including iron and zinc, are recommended.

The occupational therapist assesses oral–motor dysfunction; the medical social worker assesses the family system related to stressors, financial issues, support systems, and feelings the parents are experiencing. The nurse provides support, education, and accurate information about feeding and setting limits and feedback about interactions, reading behavioral cues, and developmentally based parenting skills. Careful measurement of weight, length, and, for children younger than 3 years of age, head circumference is done upon admission. Daily monitoring of weight is critical to assess the response to the plan of care and nutritional interventions. When possible, weigh the child before breakfast, at the same time of day, on the same scale, and without clothing, unless the child is older than 36 months of age.

Observing the primary caregiver and the child's response to him or her is a critical part of determining an individualized plan of care. Observing these interactions during feeding or mealtime can yield valuable information because caregiver–child relationships are demonstrated through these interactions. Insights into the nature of nonorganic FTT may be revealed. Note concerning behaviors on the part of the caregiver, such as making negative comments about the child, not paying attention to the child, lack of responsiveness or awareness of the child's feeding cues, inability to feel comfortable around the child, or rough handling of the child. Also note positive actions of the caregiver, such as talking to the child and positioning the child so that the child is comfortable for feeding and can make eye contact. Note concerning behaviors of the child, such as crying, agitation, or rigidity during feeding. Also note positive feeding behaviors of the child, such as appearing relaxed and interacting with caregiver.

Food refusal and aversion are types of feeding disorders seen in some children, especially those who were born prematurely, were small for gestational age, or who required tube feeding because they may be have been subject to intrusive feeding practices (Levine et al., 2011).

Community Care

After the child has demonstrated a successful weight-gaining pattern, a follow-up plan is determined. The interdisciplinary approach ensures that all aspects of community programs are accessed. If FTT is found to originate from a medical condition, then the follow-up plan and home care management are focused to meet the needs of the family and child with a new medical diagnosis and possibly a lifelong chronic condition. Subspecialist care and follow-up care are determined based on diagnosis.

Close follow-up with a monitoring plan for continuity of care when the infant shows developmental/behavioral problems related to FTT (e.g., occupational therapy) may be an option. When FTT is determined to be from neglect or maltreatment, referrals to Child Protective Services may be needed to determine the risk and safety factors if the child is returned home with the same caregiver. Family preservation and maintenance with close monitoring through home health visits and Child Protective Services to support the child's continued positive growth pattern may be the best option. Depending on the severity of their conditions, some children may be placed out of the home. The appropriate support systems, referrals, and education are directed to optimize transition to home and to normalize the family and child's function as much as possible. Referral to Women, Infants, and Children (WIC) to obtain formula and nutrient-rich foods is helpful when financial resources are stressed. Additional programs that provide coordinated interdisciplinary follow-up when the child or family meets criteria for these services are arranged; for example, they may qualify for Medicaid, Children's Medical Services, and parenting classes (see Chapter 2).

MALFORMATIONS OF THE UPPER GASTROINTESTINAL TRACT

Malformations of the upper GI tract that can affect GI function include cleft lip, cleft palate, EA, TEF, and pyloric stenosis.

CLEFT LIP AND PALATE

Cleft lip and cleft palate, which often occur together, are the most common congenital craniofacial anomalies. The overall incidence of cleft lip and palate (CLP) malformations varies by ethnic group—1 in 500 in Native Americans and Asians and 1 in 2,000 in those of African descent. The distribution of cleft types is approximately 46% for combined CLP, 21% for isolated cleft lip, and 33% for isolated cleft palate (Chigurupati, 2012).

Multiple causes have been identified for CLP. Familial patterns of inheritance have been established for CLP and, to a lesser extent, for cleft palate alone. Environmental factors have also been identified in the etiology of CLP, such as alcohol and tobacco use (resulting in fetal hypoxia). Drugs such as phenytoin and retinoids, dietary factors such as folic acid and vitamin deficiencies, and intrauterine irradiation have all been implicated. Folic acid is recommended as a supplement for women of childbearing age not only to prevent neural tube and abdominal wall defects but also to help prevent CLP (Molina-Solana et al., 2013). CLP is also associated with particular syndromes, and advances in genetics continue to add information to assist in differentiating etiologies.

The child with CLP may have long-term problems with impaired facial growth and dental anomalies. Speech disorders may also occur. Eustachian tube dysfunction is also associated with cleft palate and can increase risk for recurrent otitis media and associated hearing impairment. Mortality is related to the severity of associated syndromes.

Pathophysiology

Cleft lip results from incomplete or failed fusion of embryologic structures, the maxillary and medial nasal elevations, between the fifth and eighth weeks of gestation. The cleft may be unilateral or bilateral and may vary from a small indentation in the lip to a wide, deep fissure that extends to the nostril (Figs. 18-7 and 18-8).

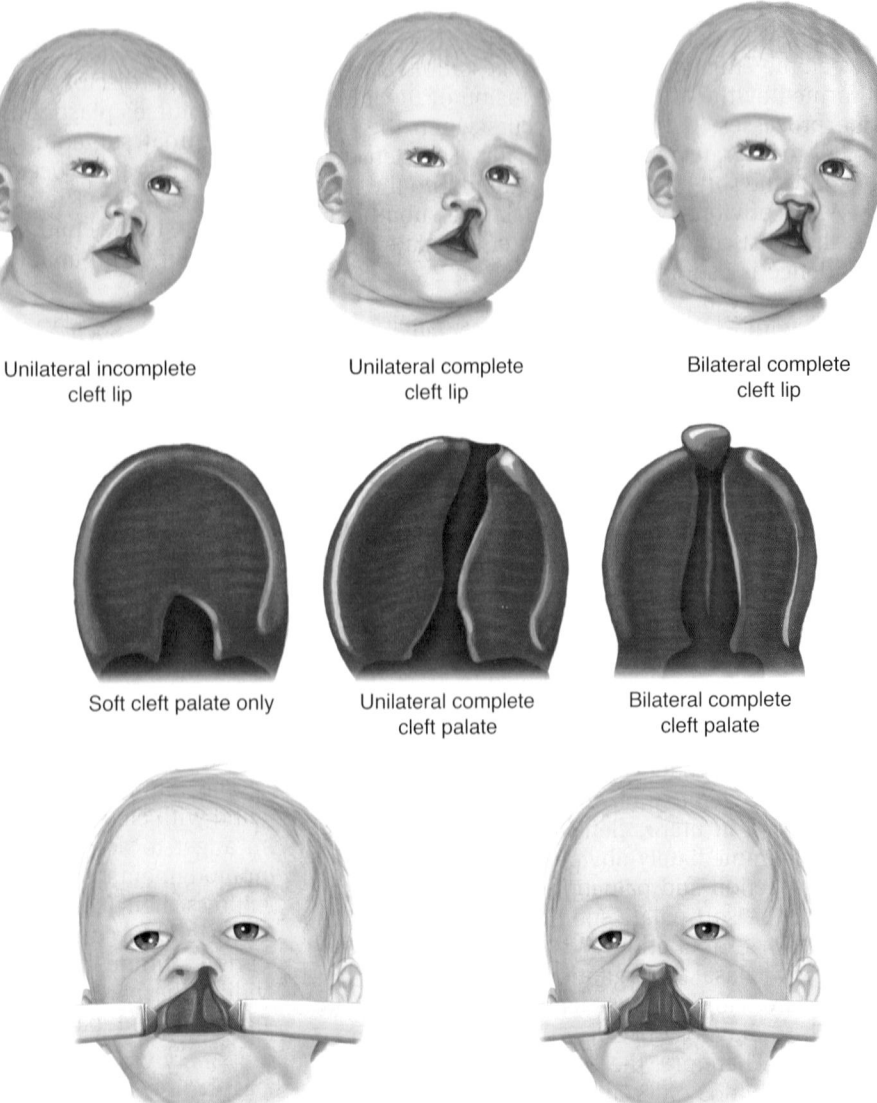

Unilateral incomplete
cleft lip

Unilateral complete
cleft lip

Bilateral complete
cleft lip

Soft cleft palate only

Unilateral complete
cleft palate

Bilateral complete
cleft palate

Figure 18-7 Variations of CLP.

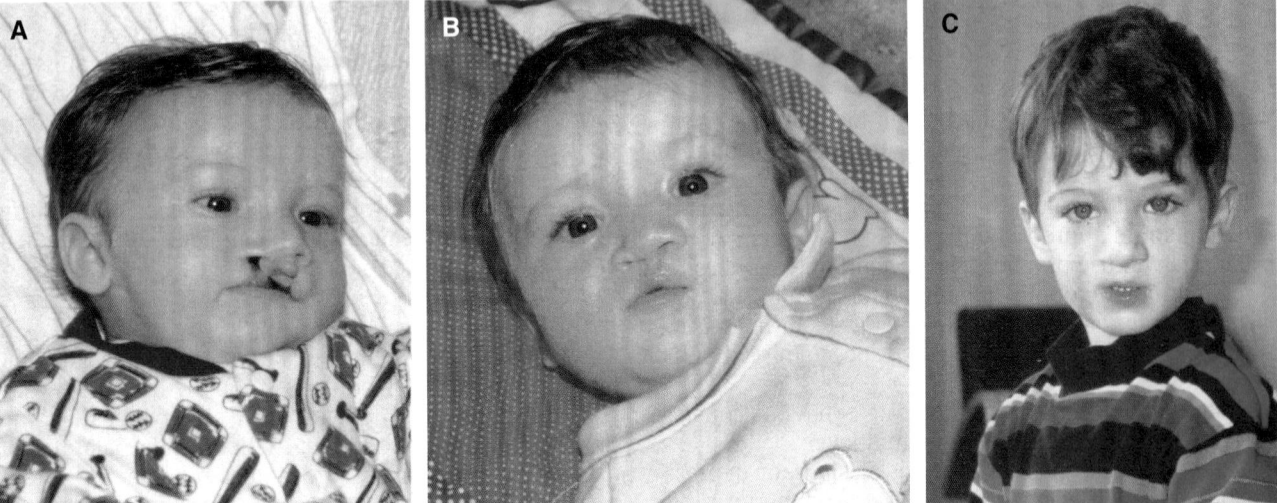

Figure 18-8 Child with CLP at birth (A), immediately after lip repair (B), and at 3 years of age (C).

Dental anomalies may also be present, with missing, malpositioned, or deformed teeth.

Between the 7th and 12th weeks of gestation, the palate is formed by the migration and fusion of the lateral palatine processes. Cleft palate occurs when the processes fail to migrate and fuse normally. The cleft may involve only the soft palate or may extend into the hard palate. A less obvious type of cleft palate, a submucous cleft, is the most common of the posterior palate clefts. The incidence is estimated to be between 2 and 8 per 10,000 (Sadove et al., 2004).

Children with CLP may have other associated anomalies. Although some may be relatively minor, others, such as cardiac malformations, may be life threatening. More than 300 different syndromes that include cleft defects, particularly cleft palate, have been reported. Cleft palate is most often part of a syndrome, whereas cleft lip is more often isolated (Harry et al., 2012). Trisomy 13, Pierre Robin syndrome, and Treacher Collins syndrome are associated with a cleft palate. Because of familial patterns of inheritance and the many associated syndromes, genetic counseling is recommended for families.

Assessment

If a diagnosis of CLP is made in utero by ultrasound early during the pregnancy, the family is referred to the interdisciplinary cleft team before the birth of the child. If not diagnosed in utero, cleft lip and, in most cases, cleft palate is immediately obvious at birth.

Visual inspection and palpation of the palate all the way back to the soft palate should be done as part of every newborn examination. When cleft palate is not noted at birth, nasal regurgitation of fluids may alert the health care team to its presence. Submucous clefts are difficult to diagnose because the entire palate may appear intact. Therefore, the defect may not be identified until the child is older and presents with hypernasal speech. A bifid uvula, a hard palate with a notched posterior, or a translucent area in the midline of the soft palate are anatomic clues leading to diagnosis.

Nursing Diagnoses and Outcomes

In addition to those listed in Nursing Plan of Care 18-1, the following nursing diagnoses and outcomes may apply to the child with CLP:

Nursing Diagnosis: Impaired parenting related to perception of an infant with a cleft lip, palate, or both
Outcomes:
- Parents will verbalize acceptance of the child and demonstrate appropriate nurturing behaviors.
- Parents will use psychosocial support and services to facilitate their coping and adjustment responses.

Nursing Diagnosis: Chronic low self-esteem related to perception of facial deformity and speech impediment
Outcomes:
- Child will demonstrate appropriate behaviors consistent with his or her developmental level.
- Child will demonstrate absence of signs of depression and will report sleeping well and performing well in school.

Interdisciplinary Interventions

Care of the child with cleft lip or palate involves a large interdisciplinary team, including the pediatrician; nurse; plastic surgeon; oral surgeon; ear, nose, and throat surgeon; audiologist; orthodontist; dentist; speech therapist; occupational therapist; social worker; and geneticist. The nurse's role involves providing direct care to the child, along with supporting the parents, educating them about their child's care, and coordinating services.

Psychological Support

When the diagnosis of cleft lip is made at birth, after the initial stabilization and assessment, the parents need information about their neonate's condition. Because of the obvious and disfiguring nature of the defect, its presence is often very distressing to the family. Provide information about the anomaly and anticipated care needs in simple, direct terms. Providing the same information during more than one encounter is helpful because parents may easily become overwhelmed trying to process new information while dealing with the crisis of the birth of a child with a visible defect. Early involvement of a member of the CLP team is recommended to provide the family with accurate information about the child's condition and treatment plan.

The family's emotional response to the birth of a child with cleft lip, palate, or both may range from grief to anger to denial (see Chapter 12). Convey an open, nonjudgmental attitude to encourage the parents to express their feelings. Support the family's adjustment to the child's condition by demonstrating an accepting, caring attitude toward the child and family and by providing the parents with opportunities and support for normal infant–parent interactions.

caREminder

Point out positive qualities in the infant, such as hair and eye color, turning toward the parents' voice, and alertness to surroundings.

A systematic review of psychosocial effects of CLP reported the overall majority of children and adults do not experience major psychosocial problems. Behavioral problems, satisfaction with facial appearance, and particular aspects of social functioning were some of the reported difficulties. Self-esteem was generally reported as good. More well-controlled studies are needed to clarify discrepancies in the literature (Hunt et al., 2005; Klassen et al., 2012).

Feeding

The infant with cleft lip or palate presents special challenges in terms of feeding. Although the infant with cleft lip alone may do well with either breastfeeding or bottlefeeding, the infant with a cleft palate may experience problems if the defect renders the infant unable to generate negative suction pressure in the oropharynx and milk is regurgitated into the nasal cavity.

Breastfeeding may be more successful because the compliant breast forms a seal on the lip, palate, or both. Consultation with a lactation specialist may be helpful. Bottlefeeding may require modification of the nipple.

❚ ALERT *Closely monitor an infant with CLP who is being breastfed for weight gain and hydration status.*

Many feeding methods have been described to facilitate feeding the infant with cleft palate, including use of various nipple designs, crosscut nipples, and palatal obturators. No single feeding technique is best; any method that enables the infant to complete feeding in a 20- to 30-minute period and supports adequate growth is acceptable.

Use feeding methods that promote sucking, whenever possible, because use of the orofacial muscles is necessary to develop those muscles and to develop feeding and speech skills. Rarely, feeding must be done using a large syringe with rubber tubing at the tip to instill formula in the side of the infant's mouth or by NG tube. If these feeding methods are necessary, involve an occupational therapist, a speech and language therapist, or both to assess, develop, and maintain oral–motor skills. The Pigeon Bottle may be recommended for an infant with bilateral or a wide unilateral cleft. A compressible-type squeeze bottle is helpful when the infant cannot feed within an appropriate time frame with a standard bottle. Other products used include the Haberman Feeder and Mead Johnson Cleft Palate Nurser (Fig. 18-9). Remind parents that patience is the key to the feeding process.

Surgical Interventions

Operative repair of a cleft lip usually takes place at age 2 to 3 months. The goals of the surgery are to close the defect and to achieve a balanced, symmetric appearance. The timing of cleft palate repair is controversial and varies from age 6 months to 2 years. It also depends on the nature of the defect, the presence of other anomalies, and surgeon preference. Earlier repairs are believed to support normal speech development, whereas later repair is thought to support palatal growth with less disruption of the midfacial hypoplasia. The lack of clear evidence favoring one approach over the other has led to a compromise: Most cleft palate repairs are done at age 12 to 24 months, and preferably prior to 18 months of age, before development of speech patterns. The insertion of bilateral ventilation tubes (in the ears) has become the standard of care. Tube insertion has been correlated with better outcomes by reducing hearing screening failures and by preventing otitis media.

Cleft lip repair usually involves only a 24-hour hospital stay or is done as an outpatient procedure, whereas cleft palate repair typically involves a 2-day hospital stay. Preoperative preparation of the family focuses on providing information regarding the surgical procedure and the child's postoperative care needs both in the hospital and at home (Teaching Intervention Plan 18-2).

Immediate postoperative care focuses on airway management, hemostasis, and pain control. The child is at risk for airway compromise because of laryngeal edema caused by intubation during surgery and incisional edema. After palate repair, the child must learn to breathe through smaller nasal passages. Blood clots may also fall off the incision and obstruct the airway. Use of a high-humidity oxygen tent may be ordered. Observe the child carefully for signs of respiratory distress, bleeding, and excess mucus in the mouth.

❚ ALERT *Use a bulb syringe for suctioning. A soft catheter or low suction should be used only in an emergency, avoiding the suture lines. Remember that the roof of the mouth is also the floor of the nose.*

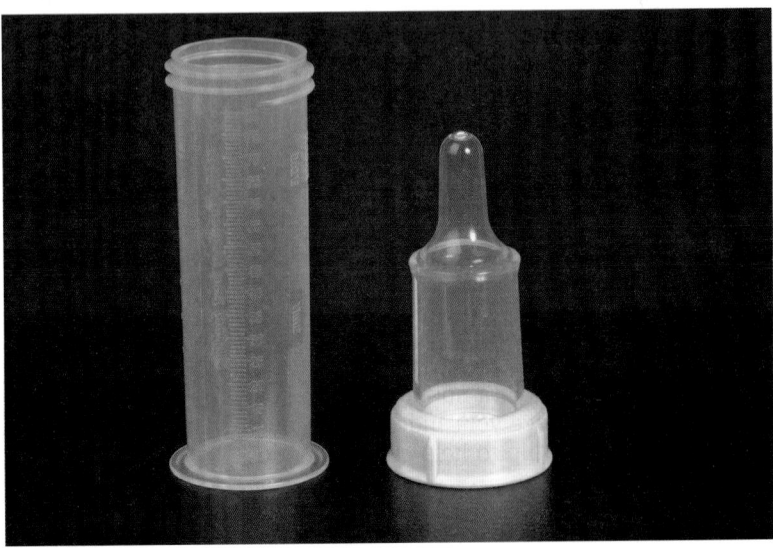

Figure 18-9 The Haberman Feeder is used for children with cleft palate and other orofacial problems that hamper the child's ability to nurse.

TIP 18-2: A TEACHING INTERVENTION PLAN for the Family of the Child With Cleft Lip/Palate

Nursing Diagnoses and Family Outcomes

- Imbalanced nutrition: Less than body requirements related to impaired ingestion of nutrients
  Outcomes: Infant will take in adequate nutrients for normal growth and development.
  Infant will show weight/length increases along growth curve.
  Parents will demonstrate the ability to feed the infant in a manner that facilitates optimal intake of nutrients.
- Risk for infection related to effects of dysfunctional eustachian tubes, aspiration, or surgery
  Outcomes: Child is free from ear, respiratory, and incisional infection postoperatively.
  Parents verbalize an understanding of the symptoms of infection and appropriate follow-up measures.
- Risk for injury related to potential trauma at operative site post cleft lip/palate repair
  Outcomes: Operative site will be protected from injury using developmentally appropriate measures.
  Family will demonstrate an understanding of how to prevent injury to the operative site.
- Deficient knowledge: Cleft lip/palate pathology and treatment, feeding and suctioning techniques, surgical site care
  Outcomes: Child is free from complications associated with cleft lip/palate.
  Family is able to describe the pathology of cleft lip/palate, short- and long-term potential complications, and treatment plan.
  Family verbalizes the need for corrective surgery and possible later revisions.
  Family demonstrates appropriate feeding, suctioning, and restraint techniques and surgical site care.

Teach the Family

Preoperative Care
Feeding
- Children with cleft palates in particular may have trouble generating enough pressure to feed.
- If breastfeeding, manually extend nipple and place it in child's mouth. Talk with a lactation consultant.
- If not breastfeeding, use squeezable bottles, which may be easier for the child to feed from.
- Place the nipple in the child's mouth; ensure that the nipple is in a normal feeding position, not the cleft. Place your index finger lengthwise over the cleft in lip to help create suction.

- Encourage sucking by stroking cheek or moving jaw.
- Compress the bottle with infant's sucking cues and allow rest time.
- Feed the child slowly in an upright position. Watch for cues that infant is getting too much or not enough formula (if formula flow is a consistent problem, the feeding system may need to be modified) or needs to rest. Burp frequently but not so often that it frustrates the infant, causing increased distress.
- Hold and feed the infant in a relaxed manner to avoid communicating anxiety to the infant.
- Position the infant in an infant seat or on right side after feeding.

Oral Hygiene
- Offer the infant water after every feeding to clean the mouth of formula.
- If the infant has a removable maxillary prosthesis, remove and clean it every day.

Preventing Infection
- Monitor for signs of infection, such as fever over 101° F (38.3° C), excessive mucus, coughing, rubbing ears, diarrhea, and irritability.
- Keep child away from persons with upper respiratory tract infections.
- Use good feeding techniques to prevent aspiration; suction oropharynx with bulb syringe as needed.
- Reposition the child every 2 hours.

Preparation for Surgery
- Practice feeding technique that will be used postoperatively. Check with surgeon to verify which technique will be used; some may allow breastfeeding or bottlefeeding with enlarged nipple, whereas others prefer a syringe with feeding tube at the end. It is helpful to teach the syringe-feeding technique, regardless, so the child will be familiar with it because pain may prevent the child from sucking postoperatively.
- Use rubber tubing or 8 French feeding tube cut to 1 in., attach to 30-mL syringe, and pull formula into syringe; fill enough syringes for the feeding to avoid having to stop feeding, possibly frustrating the infant.
- Hold infant upright as for normal feeding; direct tube to side of cheek away from surgical site.
- Drip formula into mouth by gently pushing on the plunger.
- Burp after every 15 mL.
- Practice this until comfortable; this may help avoid distress postoperatively.
- Apply elbow immobilizers for a few hours each day so the infant becomes used to wearing them.

- Secure immobilizers snugly enough so they do not slip but not so tight that they impair circulation; your index finger should be able to fit under the immobilizer. To make sure they are not too tight, check the child's hands to make sure they are warm and pink.
- Remove the immobilizers every hour, one at a time, so the child can exercise that arm; check the skin under the immobilizer at this time for signs of irritation.

Postoperative Care

Pain Management
- Administer analgesic, as prescribed, for pain; do not hesitate to medicate for pain because a comfortable child is less likely to cry and put stress on the suture line. Discomfort usually lasts 2–4 days after surgery.
- Use biobehavioral measures such as distraction, putting in swing, reading books, or playing music to comfort child.

Positioning
- Position the child upright in infant seat, on side or back; do not put the infant on his or her abdomen after lip repair to avoid rubbing the incision on the sheets and injuring it.

Incision Care
- Clean the lip incision three times a day with sterile water or ordered solution, and apply thin layer of antibiotic ointment (how often to clean, solution, and ointment will be prescribed by the surgeon).

Feeding
- Use the feeding method practiced preoperatively; avoid touching or putting stress on the suture line. Usually for lip repairs, breastfeeding or bottlefeeding is permitted; for palate repairs, use syringe with feeding tube at end.

- Avoid putting things into the child's mouth, such as pacifiers, feeding utensils, straws, or cups with a spout.
- Feed only liquids or pureed foods as ordered; do not give foods that need to be chewed or that have chunks in them.
- Offer infant water after every feeding to clean mouth of formula.

Immobilizers
- Keep the elbow immobilizers on at all times; to check fit, use the same technique as practiced preoperatively; monitor for adequate circulation and skin irritation.
- Remove immobilizers every hour, one at a time, and closely monitor the child so nothing goes near the mouth.
- Offer a variety of developmentally appropriate distractions to keep the child content: holding, cuddling, looking at books, touching different textured objects, picking up small objects and putting them in a container, puzzles, clay, or wagon rides.
- Use the immobilizers until the surgeon says to stop, usually 2–6 weeks.

Contact Health Care Provider if

Preoperatively
- Child has signs of infection fever over 101° F (38.3° C), excessive mucus, coughing, rubbing ears, diarrhea, and irritability

Postoperatively
- There is bright-red bleeding from mouth or nose
- Aforementioned signs of infection, swelling, increasing redness, or pus around the suture line is present
- Pain is not controlled with the prescribed medications and child cannot be comforted
- Child refuses to eat

Position the child with the head of the bed elevated 30 degrees to prevent secretions from pooling in the oropharynx. If only the palate has been repaired, position the child on his or her abdomen.

Bleeding may occur at the suture line. Apply gentle pressure or ice to the lip incision, as ordered. If the child is bleeding from the palate repair, intervene as needed for respiratory distress and notify the physician.

Pain is not unusual during the first 24 to 48 hours postoperatively. Assess the need for analgesics and evaluate their effectiveness after administration (see Chapter 10). Anticipate the child's needs and meet them *before* the child becomes distressed. Medicate for pain relief. Also minimize pain and discomfort from other sources (e.g., hunger, wet diaper, need for attention or repositioning) to prevent crying, which results in tension on the suture line.

The child must be prevented from putting his or her hands near the mouth to avoid disturbing the incision.

Therefore, elbow immobilizers are used for the first 10 to 14 days postoperatively. The child's hands are still free, but the elbow immobilizers prevent elbow flexion and touching or injuring the operative site. The elbow immobilizers must be secure enough so they do not slide off but loose enough so a finger can slide underneath. Perform and document neurovascular checks on a routine basis. Release the immobilizers every hour, one at a time, to allow motor activity that encompasses the child's entire range of motion.

After cleft lip repair, the child will have sutures on the exterior portion of the lip that remain in place for up to a week. Provide wound care by cleaning the suture line regularly with normal saline or sterile water to remove any crusted drainage. Apply an antibiotic ointment. Clear liquids are usually offered after the child recovers from the anesthesia. The infant's usual breastfeedings or bottlefeedings are commonly resumed within 6 to 24 hours of cleft lip repair. Resumption of oral feeding is usually delayed up to 48 hours after cleft palate repair. Use caution during the first 10 to 14 days postoperatively to avoid injury to the palatal suture line. During bottle-feeding, position the nipple so that it does not touch the palatal suture line. Avoid using straws or cups with spouts. Pureed or soft foods may be carefully fed to the child by spoon or cup. Offer water after feedings to cleanse the oral cavity.

Community Care

After surgical repair, the child with cleft lip or palate faces various ongoing health challenges. The child with cleft palate is at risk for hearing loss because eustachian tube dysfunction may cause recurrent otitis media. Speech impairments may be present because the repair may affect the function of the pharyngeal and palatal muscles, requiring long-term speech therapy. An increase in plaque, gingivitis, and dental caries and abnormal dental development and malocclusion require the ongoing involvement of pediatric dentists and orthodontists (Hazza'a et al., 2011). Maxillofacial surgery and rhinoplasty may be required later in life if midfacial growth is impaired and the nasal septum is deviated. Alterations in appearance and speech impairment may have a negative effect on the child's self-image. The involvement of social workers or other mental health practitioners is important in dealing with these concerns.

ESOPHAGEAL ATRESIA AND TRACHEOESOPHAGEAL FISTULA

EA is a congenital anomaly that results from failure of the esophagus to develop normally between the fourth and sixth weeks of fetal development. The proximal esophagus ends in a blind pouch instead of communicating normally with the stomach. In most cases, EA is associated with TEF, an abnormal communication between the esophagus and trachea. TEF results from failure of the trachea and esophagus to separate, an event that normally takes place between the sixth and seventh weeks of gestation.

EA, with or without TEF, occurs in 1 per 3,500 live births worldwide (the majority are EA with TEF; EA and TEF may also occur as isolated defects) (Harmon & Coran, 2012). The etiology is unknown. In 50% to 70% of cases, associated congenital anomalies, such as cardiac defects, or anorectal or renal abnormalities are seen (Harmon & Coran, 2012). Approximately half of cases are associated with a recognizable malformation syndrome such as a part of a chromosomal syndrome, VACTERL (Vertebral, Anal, Cardiac, Tracheal, Esophageal, Renal/Radial, Limb anomalies), CHARGE (Coloboma, central nervous system anomalies, Heart defects, Atresia of the choanae, Retardation of growth and/or development, Genital underdevelopment, Ear anomalies and sensorineural hearing loss), Goldenhar, Opitz G, and Fanconi anemia (Harmon & Coran, 2012).

Overall survival among children with EA and TEF approaches 95% as a result of improvements in neonatal care and surgical techniques (Pinheiro et al., 2012). Prematurity and low birth weight along with congenital anomalies, most commonly cardiac, increase the mortality risk. Children with EA and TEF may experience long-term problems with esophageal dysmotility and GERD. After surgical repair, esophageal stricture at the surgical anastomosis may occur, requiring recurrent esophageal dilation.

Pathophysiology

The esophagus and trachea normally begin to develop from a common foregut between the third and fourth weeks of gestation. During the sixth to eighth weeks of embryologic development, the mesodermal ridges form and separate the esophagus from the trachea. EA and TEF result when the trachea and esophagus fail to separate normally during this period. Epithelialization and recanalization of the esophagus also occur at this time. Failure of these normal recanalization processes has been hypothesized as a cause of EA.

EA and TEF present in various ways (Fig. 18-10). In 80% of cases, the esophagus ends in a blind pouch, with a fistula communicating between the distal esophagus and the trachea. EA without TEF is the next most common form, occurring in up to 8% of cases. TEF without EA occurs in approximately 4% of cases. This form is also known as the "H" type of TEF. Other configurations of EA and TEF have been classified.

Assessment

Clinical manifestations of EA and TEF may be noted prenatally. A maternal history of polyhydramnios is usually present in one third of cases of EA and in some cases of TEF. Inability to identify the fetal stomach with radiology strongly suggests EA.

At birth, the infant demonstrates excessive oral secretions accompanied by coughing, choking, and cyanosis, which become worse when feeding is attempted (Clinical Judgment 18-1).

caREminder

Excessive drooling of saliva may be the first symptom of TEF. When fed, the infant sucks well but then chokes and coughs as the feeding enters the lungs.

Be alert for potential problems in the newborn, particularly when a maternal history of polyhydramnios exists. During physical assessment, attend to signs that may indicate a more severe problem. Problems with initiating oral feeds and signs that the infant's response to feeding is ineffective are early signals that indicate a need for further critical assessment. Assess respiratory status and position the infant supine with the head elevated to decrease aspiration risk and to protect the airway. Respiratory distress may ensue from aspiration of pooled secretions in the proximal esophageal pouch or from secretions passing through a proximal fistula. In the presence of distal TEF, gastric juices can reflux into the respiratory tract, causing a chemical pneumonitis. Overt clinical manifestations of cardiac, musculoskeletal, or other GI anomalies may also be present.

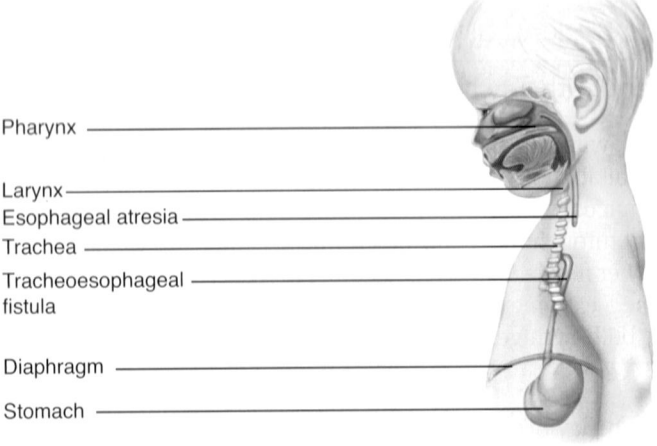

A   EA with distal TEF

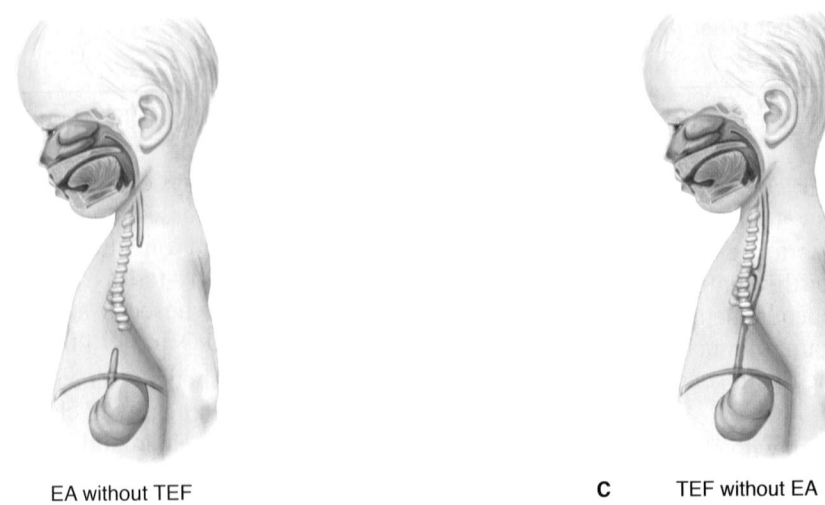

B   EA without TEF   C   TEF without EA

Figure 18-10 (A) The esophagus ends in a blind pouch with a fistula between the distal esophagus and trachea. (B) Esophageal atresia (EA) without fistula. (C) Tracheoesophageal fistula (TEF) without EA.

When TEF is present without EA, diagnosis may be difficult, and the defect may not be diagnosed for several months. The infant may choke during some feedings as the formula crosses the fistula and enters the lungs. Other feedings may proceed without symptoms.

Diagnostic Tests

When TEF is suspected, a feeding tube is passed into the esophagus. If EA is present, the tube will pass only a few centimeters before resistance is felt. The diagnosis is confirmed by radiographs, which will show the tube in an air-filled upper esophageal pouch and will also indicate the presence or absence of gas in the stomach. The presence of gas in a distended stomach indicates a distal TEF. The absence of gas in the stomach is associated with EA without TEF. Chest radiographs also screen for the presence of pneumonia, cardiac defects, or vertebral anomalies. Contrast studies, bronchoscopy, or endoscopy may also be used to establish the presence of TEF with or without EA. Contrast medium is used with caution because the risk of aspiration is high. An echocardiogram is done to evaluate cardiac anatomy and function.

Nursing Diagnoses and Outcomes

In addition to those listed in Nursing Plan of Care 18-1, the following nursing diagnoses and outcomes may be applicable to the child with TEF:

Nursing Diagnosis: Ineffective airway clearance related to inability to swallow secretions preoperatively
Outcome: Infant will demonstrate a clear, patent airway, without signs of airway compromise.
Nursing Diagnosis: Risk for aspiration related to secretions or fluids entering the respiratory tract secondary to structural defect
Outcomes:
• Infant will remain free of signs and symptoms of aspiration of secretions or fluids.
• Infant will remain free of infection secondary to aspiration.
Nursing Diagnosis: Risk for injury related to procedures disrupting integrity of postoperative suture line
Outcomes:
• Infant will exhibit an intact surgical site without signs of disruption of anastomosis.

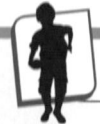

CLINICAL JUDGMENT 18-1

An Infant With Tracheoesophageal Fistula

Anh is a term newborn female, 2 hours old, with Apgar scores of 9 and 9 with no obvious congenital anomalies. The nurse noted a large amount of mucus, which she attributed to the infant's rapid descent through the birth canal. Anh's father is bottle-feeding her first feeding. Anh started sucking and then turned extremely blue. The nurse suctioned Anh with a bulb syringe, getting copious amounts of secretions, and gave free-flow oxygen. Anh responded immediately and regained a pink color. The nurse tried to feed Anh herself to determine whether the cyanotic episode would be repeated. Anh eagerly began sucking, then started coughing, and became extremely cyanotic. Again, Anh responded promptly to suction and oxygen.

Questions

1. Is Anh demonstrating normal newborn behavior?

2. What behaviors are of concern?

3. Are the symptoms that Anh presents classic signs of TEF? What other pathologic process might be considered?

4. What should the nurse do?

5. Anh is 36 hours postoperative TEF repair and has a chest tube in place. What should the nurse evaluate? What are signs of complications?

Answers

1. No.

2. Duskiness with feeding and excessive saliva during the first few hours after birth are not normal. Acrocyanosis is to be expected for the first few hours after birth; central cyanosis around the mouth and mucous membranes is not normal. A moderate amount of mucus is normal for the first 24 hours as the infant goes through the transition to extrauterine life.

3. Anh does present with classic TEF, particularly the immediate color change with feeding and swallowing of fluid. Cardiac or respiratory pathology manifests as cyanosis that does not respond as well to suctioning and oxygen administration. Such cyanosis is prolonged after feedings or continuous and can be exacerbated by other things such as stress.

4. Position Anh upright. Maintain a clear airway with intermittent or continuous suction as necessary. Notify the physician or advanced practice nurse. Continue to assess Anh's cardiorespiratory status and maintain a neutral thermal environment during diagnostic testing such as chest radiograph. Provide psychosocial support for Anh's parents. Maintain NPO and IV fluids as ordered.

5. The nurse should evaluate respiratory status, functioning and integrity of chest tube, efficacy of pain management, fluid and electrolyte balance including nutritional support, incision site for integrity and infection, and parental coping. Signs of complications resulting from anastomosis leak include respiratory distress with tachypnea, cyanosis, the presence of saliva in the chest tube tubing, and signs of sepsis caused by the leak (e.g., temperature instability, hypoglycemia, apnea, bradycardia).

- Infant will demonstrate secure positioning and appropriate placement of the NG tube.

Nursing Diagnosis: Impaired swallowing related to presence of esophageal stricture or impaired peristalsis secondary to surgery

Outcomes:

- Infant will remain free of signs of stricture development, and dilation will be performed as needed.
- Child will use methods to enhance effective swallowing, such as eating slowly, chewing foods well, and maintaining an upright position.

Interdisciplinary Interventions

Surgical repair of EA and TEF is delayed until the infant is medically stable. The goal of preoperative care is to prevent and treat any complications that may arise from aspiration or reflux of secretions into the respiratory tract.

caREminder

The surgeon writes specific orders for positioning the infant. Orders usually specify maintaining the infant with EA in an upright position preoperatively to reduce the risk of aspiration. However, some surgeons prefer to have the infant positioned prone to facilitate drainage of the blind pouch by gravity. Clarify the desired position if no specific orders are provided.

Ensure that emergency equipment is readily available at the bedside. A sump catheter can be maintained in the upper esophageal pouch to provide continuous suction of pooled secretions. Respiratory support and broad-spectrum antibiotics are given as needed to treat aspiration pneumonia. In many cases, a gastrostomy may be performed to provide gastric decompression and, eventually, enteral nutrition. Nutritional support with PN is initiated after the infant is stabilized.

The timing of definitive surgical repair of EA and TEF depends on the infant's condition. The infant who is close to term and is without other significant medical problems, such as aspiration pneumonia, may undergo repair within 24 to 72 hours of birth. If cardiac defects are present, they are corrected first. Premature infants with major respiratory distress or associated severe anomalies are maintained with proximal esophageal low suction, gastric decompression, and PN until medically stable enough to undergo definitive repair of EA and TEF.

Surgical repair may be done through a thoracotomy or thoracoscopically. Thoracoscopic repairs may have more successful outcomes and better cosmetics, along with a promise of fewer musculoskeletal complications, such as scoliosis, as the child's development progresses (van der Zee & Bax, 2007).

During surgery, the TEF is ligated, and then the proximal and distal segments of the esophagus are anastomosed. If primary anastomosis is not possible because the length of the esophageal segments is inadequate, then the esophagus may be replaced with portions of the stomach (gastric interposition). If the infant's condition does not permit esophageal replacement during the initial surgery, a cervical esophagostomy may be done, with subsequent esophageal replacement at age 6 months to 1 year by gastric or colonic interposition, during which a portion of the stomach or colon is used to replace the esophagus.

During the initial postoperative period, the infant will have a chest tube, gastric decompression, and continued respiratory support. Interventions such as fluid management, pain management, and hemodynamic support are used as clinically indicated. Special care to prevent aspiration is vital. A suction catheter with markings to indicate the distance from the infant's nose to the point just above the anastomosis may be kept at the bedside. This tool can be used to guide consistent depth of insertion for the suction catheter to avoid trauma at the anastomotic site. Effective pain control is important so the infant does not disrupt the anastomosis by crying and moving excessively in response to pain.

ALERT *Insert suction catheters less than the distance to the anastomosis. An approximate measurement can be done from the tip of the nose to the earlobe. Secure the NG tube well and use extreme caution to avoid displacement. If displacement occurs, do not reinsert the tube. Introducing catheters around the area of the suture line increases the risk of disrupting the suture line and causing leaks.*

Antibiotics are continued and nutritional support with PN is maintained until full enteral feedings are tolerated. Enteral nutrition through an NG or gastrostomy tube may be started as early as the fourth postoperative day. Small-volume drip feedings are usually instituted because bolus feedings may cause GER. Acid suppression therapy is instituted to reduce irritation at the anastomosis. A radiographic study with water-soluble contrast medium is done by postoperative days 5 to 7 to assess the integrity of the esophageal anastomosis. If no leak is seen, the chest tube is removed and oral feedings are begun.

Ongoing assessment for anastomotic leak or stricture is essential. Anastomotic leaks occur in about 12% of cases (Holcomb et al., 2005). The infant typically exhibits respiratory distress with tachypnea, cyanosis, and signs of sepsis. Continued NPO status and PN support are required, along with antibiotics and respiratory care, until the leak heals. Most leaks heal spontaneously within 1 to 3 weeks.

The infant with an esophageal stricture at the anastomotic site may demonstrate coughing, regurgitation, recurrent aspiration, and FTT. A stricture may not be evident in an infant until after solid foods are introduced. The older child may complain of **dysphagia** (inability to swallow or difficulty swallowing) or may exhibit difficulties swallowing solid foods. Strictures are managed with esophageal dilations.

Tracheomalacia (softening of the tracheal cartilage) occurs in 10% to 20% of children with TEF. These children exhibit bradycardia, cyanosis, and apnea, usually after feedings. They also have a characteristic harsh cough and are at risk for frequent respiratory infections during infancy and early childhood. The diagnosis is made by flexible bronchoscopy. The symptoms of a child with mild distress may improve spontaneously during the first 2 years of life.

GERD commonly occurs after a repair. Medical management may be initially successful, but many children need surgical intervention. All children should adhere to nursing interventions for GERD.

Lifelong esophageal dysmotility is present in a large number of these children. Infants with EA and TEF are at risk for oral feeding dysfunction related to prolonged NPO status, subsequent reliance on NG or gastrostomy feeds, and frequent problems with esophageal function. Early attention to oral–motor stimulation and involvement of an occupational therapist in the infant's plan of care may help address such dysfunction. As the child advances in age, teach parents to cut table foods into small pieces and avoid foods that are difficult to chew and swallow, such as hot dogs. Children must be supervised during mealtime and need reminders to chew well, take small bites, and wash down their food with fluids as needed to ease swallowing.

Community Care

Management of the infant with EA and TEF presents challenges across the continuum of care when preparing the child and family for the transition to home and coordinating care with multiple health care providers. The child with EA and TEF frequently has other associated medical conditions that can make discharge teaching very complex. The child with EA and TEF as a part of VACTERL association requires follow-up with numerous health care providers. The nurse plays a key role in case management of these children by promoting coordination of care and facilitating communication among the various health care providers as well as by providing ongoing parental support and education.

PYLORIC STENOSIS

Pyloric stenosis, also called *hypertrophic pyloric stenosis* (HPS), is the most common cause of gastric outlet obstruction in infants. It is more common in firstborn males and occurs in approximately 2 to 4 per 1,000 live births in western populations; it is less common in African and Asian populations (Pandya & Heiss, 2012; Schwartz, 2012). The exact cause is not known, but, because of regional differences in incidence, environmental factors are thought to play a role. Pyloric stenosis has a strong familial aggregation and an association with maternal smoking during pregnancy, preterm delivery, small weight for gestational age, cesarean section, and congenital malformations (Krogh et al., 2012). An association of HPS with orally administered erythromycin for *Bordetella pertussis* treatment or prophylaxis in infants younger than 1 month of age has been reported. For these infants, the risk of developing pertussis outweighs the possible risk of developing HPS. Educate caregivers when therapy is needed in this age group.

Surgical correction of pyloric stenosis is curative. With prompt diagnosis and treatment, the operative mortality for treatment of pyloric stenosis is less than 1%.

Pathophysiology

In pyloric stenosis, hypertrophy and hyperplasia of the circular smooth muscle of the pylorus of the stomach occurs (Fig. 18-11). The lumen of the pylorus narrows and lengthens, and the gastric outlet is progressively obstructed.

Assessment

Typically, manifestations of pyloric stenosis become apparent at age 3 to 5 weeks. The infant usually presents

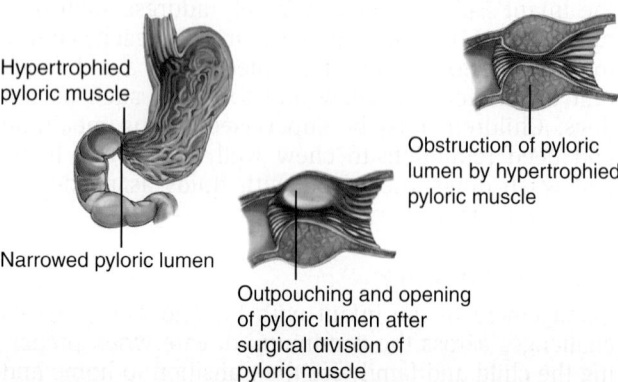

Figure 18-11 In pyloric stenosis, the pyloric muscle hypertrophies and obstructs the passage of stomach contents into the intestines. Surgically splitting the muscle relieves the obstruction.

with a history of regurgitation and nonbilious vomiting during or shortly after feeding. Within a week of onset of symptoms, the vomiting may become projectile. The vomitus usually consists of gastric contents but may become "coffee ground" in color if esophagogastritis causes bleeding. Parents may describe the infant as irritable and hungry all the time. Weight loss and FTT may be noted. Because of persistent vomiting, the infant with pyloric stenosis presents with varying degrees of dehydration. As dehydration caused by vomiting progresses, the parents may report lethargy, decreased urine output, and constipation.

On physical examination, the infant may appear fussy and fretful. With severe dehydration, the infant may seem apathetic and even moribund. The upper abdomen is typically distended, and visible peristaltic waves may be seen moving from left to right across the upper abdomen. When the abdomen is palpated, a mass may be felt in the epigastric region. The mass is hard, mobile, nontender, and usually is described as an "olive." Palpation of the olive may be difficult to appreciate in an irritable infant. It is best identified when the infant is calm.

Diagnostic Tests

Diagnosis of pyloric stenosis can usually be made based on health history and physical assessment findings. If the examiner is unable to palpate the olive-sized mass in the epigastrium, an ultrasound study may be used to establish the diagnosis. It is also used to measure the length and diameter of the pyloric muscle, which can determine whether stenosis is present. A barium study will demonstrate the "string sign," which indicates a narrowed pyloric channel and retained gastric contents.

Blood tests may be performed to determine the extent of dehydration and electrolyte disturbances. A hypochloremic metabolic alkalosis and hypokalemia result from depletion of sodium, potassium, and hydrochloric acid.

Interdisciplinary Interventions

After establishing the diagnosis of pyloric stenosis, the initial goal of therapy is to correct any fluid and electrolyte imbalances. IV fluid replacement is initiated to rehydrate the child and to correct electrolyte imbalances. The infant may be made NPO to prevent further fluid losses from vomiting. If excessive vomiting is present, an NG tube may be inserted to empty and decompress the stomach. Carefully monitor IV fluid intake, and quantify and document urine output and losses from emesis. Implement comfort measures for the infant as well as parent reassurance and support.

The definitive treatment of pyloric stenosis is surgical pyloromyotomy via an open, transumbilical, or laparoscopic approach. After fluid and electrolyte balance is reestablished (this may take hours to days, depending on severity), the infant is taken to surgery. A small abdominal incision is made, and the pyloric mass is incised longitudinally, splitting the underlying muscle. This procedure allows the gastric mucosa to bulge up between the split, relieving the obstruction.

CROSS-CULTURAL CARE

Medical management, primarily outside of North America, involving IV fluid administration, oral atropine, and fluid and electrolyte therapy has been reported. In one study, oral therapy was continued for several months, and the infants were closely monitored with favorable outcomes compared with those undergoing pyloromyotomy. It is thought that atropine decreases muscle spasms and peristalsis, which contribute to the fixed obstruction that leads to the hypertrophied and stenotic pylorus. Although this approach will not replace surgical correction, it may have a role in treating an infant with contraindications to anesthesia or infants who are a high surgical risk (Aspelund & Langer, 2007).

Postoperatively, the infant receives IV fluids until shortly after recovering from anesthesia, when oral feedings are usually started. A small amount of breast milk, formula, or an oral electrolyte solution, such as Pedialyte, may be offered for the initial feeding. Traditionally, if this solution is tolerated, the volume and concentration of feedings are quickly advanced until full feedings are achieved, usually within 24 hours postoperatively. Frequent burping is recommended.

Up to 50% of infants may have some vomiting postoperatively as a result of persistent edema of the pylorus and inefficient gastric emptying (see thePoint for Care Path: An Interdisciplinary Plan of Care for the Child With Pyloric Stenosis). Decrease in the swelling of the muscles takes place by 3 weeks, and at 6 weeks, normal muscle thickness is expected. Parent education about intermittent postoperative emesis is crucial to minimize parent anxiety.

Community Care

Infants with pyloric stenosis may be discharged at 24 to 48 hours, depending on the postoperative feeding approach and when normal feedings are reestablished. Parents require instruction regarding the infant's feeding schedule and any necessary wound care for the abdominal incision. Teach them about the signs of complications, such as recurrent vomiting, wound infection, fever, abdominal pain, and signs of dehydration. Reinforce with the parents that some emesis is expected but that persistent vomiting requires a call to the physician. Explain that the risk for wound infection may be higher if the infant experienced malnutrition preoperatively. Follow-up referral to a community pediatric caregiver is recommended to ensure that the infant is monitored for normal growth and weight gain after surgery.

MALFORMATIONS OF THE LOWER GASTROINTESTINAL TRACT

Malformations of the lower GI tract include intestinal atresia and stenosis, hernias and hydroceles, gastroschisis and omphalocele, congenital diaphragmatic hernia (CDH), Meckel diverticulum, malrotation and volvulus, intussusception, Hirschsprung disease, and anorectal malformations.

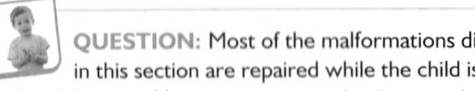

QUESTION: Most of the malformations discussed in this section are repaired while the child is an infant. How would you compare nursing interventions for infants and school-aged children, such as Cory, who is undergoing GI surgery?

INTESTINAL ATRESIA AND STENOSIS

Intestinal atresia is a congenital defect that results in complete obstruction of the bowel. *Duodenal atresia*, which accounts for approximately 50% of all atresias of the small intestine (Stellar & Widmer, 2013), is frequently associated with other congenital defects, including trisomy 21, intestinal malrotations, congenital heart defects, and VACTERL. Vertebral and renal problems are also common. *Jejunoileal atresia* results in the obstruction of one or multiple segments of the jejunum or ileum. It is not commonly associated with other congenital defects. *Stenosis* of the intestine results in a partial or incomplete obstruction.

The prognosis for duodenal atresia after surgical repair is excellent, with most patients experiencing no long-term sequelae. The prognosis for infants born with jejunoileal atresia is affected by the amount of bowel involved and the birth weight of the infant. Overall survival rates have improved greatly during the past decade, with survival as high as 95% for infants with isolated duodenal atresia (Applebaum & Sydorak, 2012).

Pathophysiology

Because of the congenital malformations with which duodenal atresia is commonly associated, it is believed to occur very early during embryologic development, resulting from a failure of the lumen of the intestine to recanalize during the 8th to 10th week of gestation. Jejunoileal atresia is believed to occur at a much later stage of gestation because of the observation that meconium is commonly present in the bowel distal to the atretic segment. A mesenteric vascular insult, resulting in ischemia of the affected portion of intestine, may be the causative factor in jejunoileal atresia.

Various forms of duodenal and jejunoileal atresia result in intestinal obstruction. Type I atresia occurs when a mucosal membrane or web occludes the inner lumen of the bowel. In type II atresia, the proximal intestine ends in a blind loop and is connected to the collapsed distal intestine by a fibrous cord. Type III atresia results in both the proximal and distal segments of intestine ending in blind loops with no connection. In cases of jejunoileal atresia, a type IV defect may also occur, resulting in multiple atretic segments of bowel, often described as having the appearance of a string of sausages.

Assessment

Polyhydramnios is observed in many cases of both duodenal and jejunoileal atresia. Most infants become symptomatic within the first 24 hours of life. Bilious vomiting and abdominal distention occur in most cases. Infants with duodenal atresia may present with upper abdominal distention but with a scaphoid abdomen because of the lack of distal intestinal air. Failure to pass meconium may be observed, although normal meconium may be present with more distal atresia. Conduct a careful physical assessment, noting abdominal contour, and palpate the abdomen for softness or distension. Monitor for passage of meconium; report progressive gastric distention and vomiting to the physician.

Diagnostic Tests

Intestinal atresia may be diagnosed by prenatal ultrasound. In cases of intestinal atresia, the ultrasound examination demonstrates polyhydramnios during the third trimester, along with fluid-filled cysts in the abdomen of the fetus.

When intestinal atresia is not diagnosed in utero, initial evaluation of a symptomatic infant includes a flat-plate abdominal radiograph. The infant with duodenal atresia customarily demonstrates a "double-bubble" sign on radiograph where both the stomach and proximal duodenum are dilated and filled with gas. The infant with jejunoileal atresia demonstrates distended loops of intestine with multiple air–fluid levels. In some cases of jejunoileal atresia, when obstruction is evident in the distal intestine, a water-soluble contrast enema is the test of choice. This reveals a microcolon because the colon has not filled with meconium and remains undilated with a smaller diameter colon (Stellar & Widmer, 2013).

Interdisciplinary Interventions

Prenatal diagnosis enables parents to plan for the infant to be delivered in a facility where further diagnostic workup and intervention can be done soon after birth. The nurse may provide anticipatory guidance to the parents so that they understand the infant's condition and know what to expect at the time of delivery.

At birth, or when clinical symptoms otherwise become evident, the infant requires initial stabilization with IV fluids to ensure that maintenance needs are met and that ongoing losses are replaced. An NG tube is placed to provide gastric decompression and to prevent aspiration of gastric contents. Serum electrolytes and blood cell counts are monitored and any abnormalities are corrected. The infant's blood glucose levels are closely monitored. Broad-spectrum IV antibiotics may be administered prophylactically. Respiratory support may be necessary because of the risk for aspiration, the stress that altered GI function places on the newborn, or other anomalies that compromise the infant's condition.

Surgical correction of duodenal atresia involves resection of the atretic segment of duodenum and duodenoduodenal or duodenojejunal anastomosis. Resection and primary anastomosis are also commonly done during surgical correction of jejunoileal atresia.

In cases involving extensive resection of bowel, massive dilation of proximal bowel, or colonic atresia, a two-stage procedure is done. A jejunostomy or ileostomy is created initially to drain the proximal bowel, with final anastomosis to the remaining distal intestine done some months later. In all cases, the surgical goal is to preserve as much intestine as possible. Massive resection of the small intestine may leave the infant with short bowel syndrome (described later in this chapter), leading to long-term problems with meeting fluid and nutrient requirements using the GI tract.

In infants with both duodenal and jejunoileal atresia, a gastrostomy tube may be placed at the time of surgery to facilitate gastric decompression during the initial postoperative period and to administer enteral nutrition support if poor tolerance to oral feedings is anticipated. If a large amount of bowel has been resected or a very proximal ostomy exists, a central venous catheter may be inserted to administer PN.

Postoperative care continues with many of the interventions begun during the preoperative period. Respiratory support may continue during the early postoperative period. Continue gastric decompression by NG/OG tube or gastrostomy until intestinal motility normalizes. Monitor progress by measuring and observing gastric aspirates, which should decrease in quantity and change from bilious to a clear, saliva color. Normalization may take from 5 days up to 3 weeks, depending on the location and the extent of the atresia. Monitor the surgical site and provide pain management.

Maintaining the patency of the gastric drainage system and close monitoring of output are essential. PN is initiated to meet the infant's nutritional needs. Administer IV fluids and replacement as indicated by losses. Carefully monitor the infant's fluid and electrolyte status. Expect to continue IV antibiotics for 5 to 7 days postoperatively.

Begin enteral or oral feedings when the intestinal motility normalizes. Formula choice varies depending on the extent of bowel resected. Infants with limited resection may be given breast milk or cow's milk infant formula; infants with massive intestinal resection or an ostomy placed high in the intestinal tract will require a protein hydrolysate or elemental formula. As formula intake increases, wean the infant from PN. Careful monitoring is important to ensure adequate growth and weight gain as well as GI tolerance.

Monitoring and supporting the infant's physiologic needs are important during the postoperative period. Assess fluid status carefully, including all losses from gastric drainage, stools, and an ostomy, if present. Monitoring GI function, including return of bowel sounds, gastric residuals, and feeding tolerance, is a key aspect of care. Support and educate the family. Hospitalization may be prolonged, and the parents may need support and guidance in establishing their parental role with their sick newborn. Social services can help the family deal with the crisis of the birth of an infant with health problems and the stress of the child's prolonged hospitalization.

Community Care

Incorporate family education regarding home care for their infant into the plan of care from the start. Address gastrostomy and ostomy care, administration of feedings, and signs of intestinal dysfunction. If PN will be required for a prolonged period, the family will need extensive preparation to manage administration of PN and a central venous catheter care at home (see Chapter 17).

HERNIAS AND HYDROCELES

A hernia is a protrusion of an organ, part of an organ, or another structure through the wall of the cavity in which it is contained. Inguinal and umbilical hernias are two of the most common types. Gastroschisis, omphalocele, and diaphragmatic hernias are types of hernias that require special considerations. They are discussed later in this chapter.

A hernia in the abdominal region is considered *reducible* when its contents are easily manipulated back into the peritoneal cavity. An *incarcerated* hernia occurs when the abdominal contents become trapped and difficult to reduce. A *strangulated* hernia occurs when the herniated intestines become twisted and edematous, compromising blood flow. Intestinal obstruction and ischemia may occur. This is a surgical emergency, and the child should be taken to the emergency department immediately.

A hydrocele results from peritoneal fluid communicating with the scrotal area through a patent processus vaginalis, collecting in the tunica vaginalis. Inguinal hernias and hydroceles are among the most common congenital anomalies in infants that require surgical repair.

Pathophysiology

The processus vaginalis is an outpouching of the peritoneum that develops during the third month of gestation. In males, it descends along the inguinal canal to the area of the scrotum. In females, it terminates in the area of the labia majora. During the seventh month of gestation, the testes descend through the processus vaginalis into the scrotum. The processus vaginalis typically remains patent until birth and closes at birth or during early infancy. Protrusion of abdominal contents through the patent processus vaginalis into the inguinal area causes the hernia.

Inguinal hernias (Fig. 18-12) are caused by abdominal contents exiting the peritoneal cavity and protruding into the processus vaginalis. In girls, it is not uncommon to palpate an ovary that is protruding. An umbilical hernia results from imperfect closure or weakness of the umbilical ring that allows portions of intestine or omentum to protrude. This type is more common in low-birth-weight, female, and African American infants. Umbilical hernias usually cause no problems and often regress spontaneously. Surgical repair is not indicated unless the hernia becomes strangulated or incarcerated, persists beyond age 3 years, or continues to enlarge after age 2 years.

Inguinal hernias occur in about 3% to 5% of term infants and 13% of infants born at less than 33 weeks' gestational age (Wang, 2012). Indirect inguinal hernias, which are developmental defects rather than a direct inguinal hernia caused by a weakened wall, are most common. Unilateral right-sided hernias are more common (60%) than left-sided ones, a difference thought to result from the fact that the right testis descends later than the left. Hernias may also occur in children with conditions characterized by increased intra-abdominal pressure, which forces the abdominal contents into the processus vaginalis, a peritoneal sac that normally closes early during infancy. These children include those with ventriculoperitoneal shunts, those with chronic cough secondary to cystic fibrosis, and those receiving peritoneal dialysis.

Hydroceles are caused by peritoneal fluid communicating with the scrotal area through a patent processus vaginalis. A hydrocele may be communicating (processus vaginalis remains patent and allows peritoneal fluid to cause intermittent scrotal swelling that waxes and wanes related to activity) or noncommunicating (processus vaginalis is completely obliterated, with fluid collecting in the scrotal area that does not increase in size). A noncommunicating hydrocele usually disappears by age 1 year (see Fig. 18-12).

Assessment

The diagnosis of hernia or hydrocele is most commonly made by history and physical examination. The parents of the child with an inguinal hernia typically report

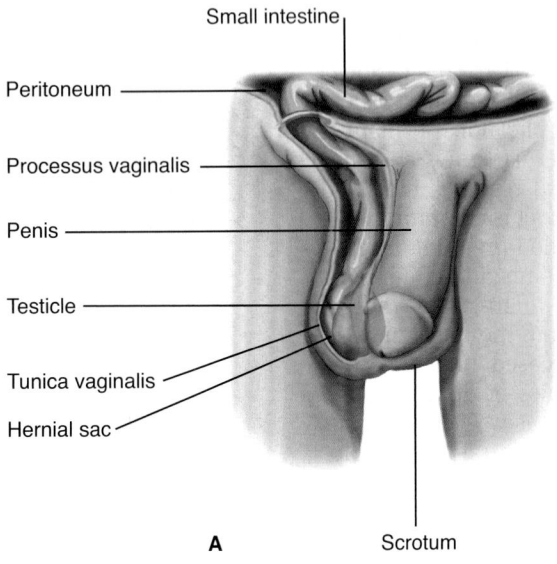
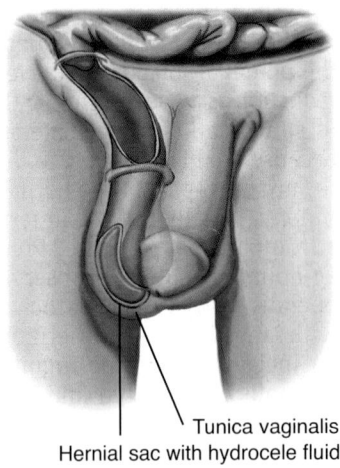

Figure 18-12 (A) In an inguinal hernia, the bowel protrudes into the patent processus vaginalis. (B) A noncommunicating hydrocele has no connection with the abdominal cavity, so the amount of scrotal swelling does not fluctuate with activity. In a communicating hydrocele, the processus vaginalis remains patent and the amount of scrotal swelling may vary with the child's activity.

seeing a bulge in the groin area that occurs only when the child cries, strains, or coughs. Pain is not typically reported unless the hernia becomes incarcerated or strangulated. In this case, the child may be irritable, with cramping abdominal pain and vomiting that may progress from nonbilious to feculent as obstruction of the trapped bowel progresses. The inguinal area may become swollen, hard, and purple.

The swelling associated with a hydrocele is not painful. The scrotal sac is translucent on transillumination (shining a light through the scrotum). For the child with a communicating hydrocele, observe for a scrotal bulge or swelling that increases with crying or straining and decreases when the child is at rest.

On physical examination, an inguinal hernia appears as a bulge in the inguinal or scrotal area; thickening of the structures of the inguinal canal may be felt with palpation. The examination may include attempts to palpate the hernial sac over the cord structures in the inguinal region. This sliding sensation of the sac and cord structures over the pubic bone is described as a positive "silk glove sign." It is not diagnostic of a hernia but is suggestive of one. An umbilical hernia is observed as an intermittent bulging of the umbilicus. It is typically not associated with pain.

CROSS-CULTURAL CARE

Teach parents that home remedies, such as using belly bands or taping a coin over the umbilicus, will not prevent or cure an umbilical hernia. If parents insist on using such remedies, encourage them to use a small coin and clean the umbilical area with soap and water if soiled and to leave the area open to dry whenever possible.

Interdisciplinary Interventions

Manual reduction of an incarcerated hernia of any type is attempted before surgical repair. The child is sedated, the lower torso is elevated, and the incarcerated contents of the hernia are gently manipulated back into the peritoneal cavity. If the reduction is successful, elective surgical repair is scheduled 24 to 48 hours later. Delaying the surgery allows time for resolution of any edema of the bowel resulting from the incarceration and substantially reduces the potential for postoperative complications. If manual reduction is unsuccessful or the hernia shows evidence of strangulation, immediate surgical repair is indicated because the blood supply to the bowel is compromised.

Surgical repair of the hernia, called *inguinal herniorrhaphy*, usually is done in term infants and children as an outpatient procedure. Preterm infants may require 24 hours of acute care observation in the hospital postoperatively because of their increased risk of apnea with anesthesia. The herniorrhaphy is done through an incision above the inguinal crease. The processus vaginalis is identified and ligated. Contralateral exploration and herniorrhaphy are done in children younger than age 1 year who are at high risk for occurrence of "second-side" hernia after repair of the initial hernia.

Surgical intervention for a hydrocele is similar to that for a hernia with a high ligation of the processus vaginalis. The distal portion of the excess sac may be carefully trimmed down to and around the testis.

Preoperatively, assess the hernia site and the child's vital signs. Be alert for signs of incarceration or strangulation. These signs include an increase in behaviors that indicate pain and the presence of a firm, tender mass in the inguinal region. Vomiting and abdominal distension may also be present.

caREminder

Carefully assess the skin condition in the inguinal area. Diaper rash or skin breakdown may lead to poor wound healing or wound infection and can necessitate delay of elective surgery.

Postoperatively, assess the surgical site for bleeding or drainage, recurrence of the hernia, and any vascular compromise to the gonads. Monitor for apnea and desaturation of oxygen for infants younger than 1 year of age with a history of prematurity. Educate parents regarding the surgical procedure, preoperative routines, postoperative care, signs and symptoms of recurrence or complications, and avoidance of constipation. Usual activities can be resumed after several days; contact sports are restricted for at least 2 weeks.

GASTROSCHISIS AND OMPHALOCELE

Abdominal wall defects include gastroschisis (a full-thickness defect of the abdominal wall, usually to the right of the umbilical cord, through which loops of bowel eviscerate) and omphalocele (herniation of intestines into the base of the umbilical cord covered with a large peritoneal sac; Fig. 18-13). These defects occur in 1 per 4,000 live births (Fountaine & Knight, 2013). Gastroschisis has been associated with young maternal age and maternal smoking; gender distribution is not a factor (Fountaine & Knight, 2013). Omphalocele occurs sporadically, with 40% being associated with

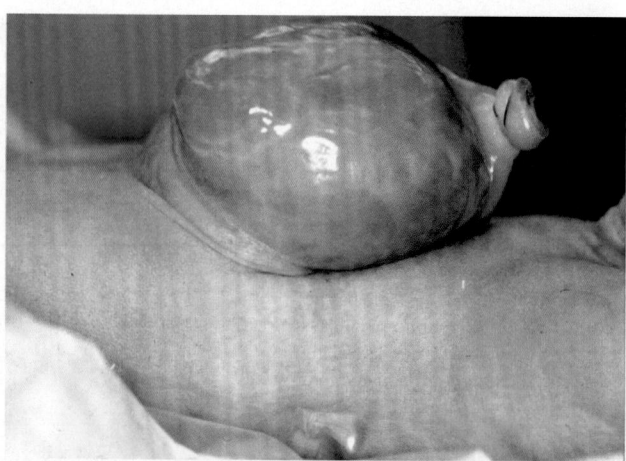

Figure 18-13 Omphalocele in a newborn. Note the large protruding sac.

chromosomal anomalies (Fountaine & Knight, 2013). The etiology of these abdominal wall defects is poorly understood. A mechanical or teratogenic event early during fetal development is hypothesized.

Infants born with gastroschisis have a survival rate of 90% to 95%. Outcome in those born with omphalocele is usually related to associated congenital anomalies and life-threatening complications (Ledbetter, 2012).

Pathophysiology

The defect associated with gastroschisis is believed to occur between the fourth and eighth weeks of fetal development. Although the exact mechanism is unclear, gastroschisis may be the result of an early tear in the umbilical cord before the umbilical ring closes. The bowel eviscerates into the amniotic cavity, where prolonged contact with amniotic fluid creates a fibrous peel over the exposed loops of bowel. The fibrous peel apparently contributes to the intestinal dysmotility often seen in infants with gastroschisis. Another hypothesis advances that a failure exists of one or more folds of the abdominal wall to fuse properly and completely, leading to a defect and herniation into the amniotic fluid. Associated anomalies are usually confined to the GI tract, with intestinal atresia occurring in 5% to 15% of all cases. Intestinal malrotation may also be seen.

The pathophysiology that leads to the development of omphalocele is poorly understood. An early defect in abdominal wall development may result in a disparity between the size of the abdominal cavity and the abdominal viscera, leaving inadequate space for the midgut to return to the abdominal cavity during the 10th week of gestation after its normal extracolonic phase of development. All infants with omphalocele have a malrotation because of the nature of the developmental defect. It is often associated with other congenital defects. In contrast to gastroschisis, omphalocele is associated with advanced maternal age and abnormal karyotypes. Associated malformations are present in up to 80% of these infants. Trisomies 13, 18, and 21 are the most common chromosomal anomalies (Islam, 2012). Cardiac anomalies are found in 30% to 50% of cases (Ledbetter, 2012). The size of the defect can be classified as small or as giant. There is no agreement in the definition of a giant omphalocele; however, some classify it as larger than 5 cm and as a large as 8 cm. It is also described by the integrity of the membranes as being intact or ruptured. The defect may contain small and large intestine, liver, and other abdominal structures.

Assessment

Both gastroschisis and omphalocele are evident immediately in the delivery room. With a planned delivery, interdisciplinary health team members, such as neonatologist and surgeon, are present in the delivery room. If the defect was undetected prenatally, the infant is stabilized and transported to a tertiary care nursery. The nurse assesses the color of the viscera and may approximate the degree of the defect related to the volume of externalized viscera.

Diagnostic Tests

Abdominal wall defects may be detected prenatally. Elevated maternal serum α-fetoprotein is detected through routine surveillance. The amount of α-fetoprotein secreted is directly proportional to the size of the defect. In addition, most abdominal wall defects are diagnosed with routine ultrasound. Differentiating the type of abdominal wall defect is important to direct other prenatal testing such as an echocardiogram. Prenatal diagnosis allows the family and medical team to plan for the delivery in a tertiary-level hospital, where a team of specialized health care providers can manage the infant postnatally.

Prenatal diagnosis also allows for family counseling and for a decision to terminate or proceed with the pregnancy after all the prenatal studies are completed. Studies have not been conclusive regarding the benefits between a vaginal or cesarean section delivery.

In some centers, the infant with gastroschisis may be delivered electively at 36 weeks' gestation to reduce the exposed bowel's contact with amniotic fluid, thereby minimizing formation of the fibrous peel. There is no evidence that elective early delivery changes the outcome.

Nursing Diagnoses and Outcomes

In addition to those listed in Nursing Plan of Care 18-1, the following nursing diagnoses and outcomes may apply to the child with an abdominal wall defect:

Nursing Diagnosis: Ineffective breathing pattern related to the effects of diaphragmatic elevation by bowel
Outcome: The child will demonstrate adequate lung expansion and blood oxygenation.
Nursing Diagnosis: Hypothermia related to effects of increased heat loss through exposed viscera
Outcomes:
- The child will exhibit signs and symptoms of minimal heat loss.
- The child's body temperature will remain within normal limits.
Nursing Diagnosis: Risk for infection related to presence of exposed viscera
Outcome: The child will remain free of signs and symptoms of infection.
Nursing Diagnosis: Risk for injury related to presence of exposed viscera and potential for torsion of bowel or supporting vessels
Outcome: The child will remain free of injury, including maintenance of bowel position and blood supply.

Interdisciplinary Interventions

At birth, handle the exposed bowel or peritoneal sac carefully to prevent twisting or torsion of the mesentery. Protect the bowel by wrapping the exposed viscera with warm saline-soaked gauze and cover and seal with a plastic wrap or place in a "bowel bag," which should contain the defect, torso, and legs to prevent heat and fluid loss from the exposed viscera. Monitor and maintain a normothermic environment. Obtain IV access. Give fluid resuscitation and correct any

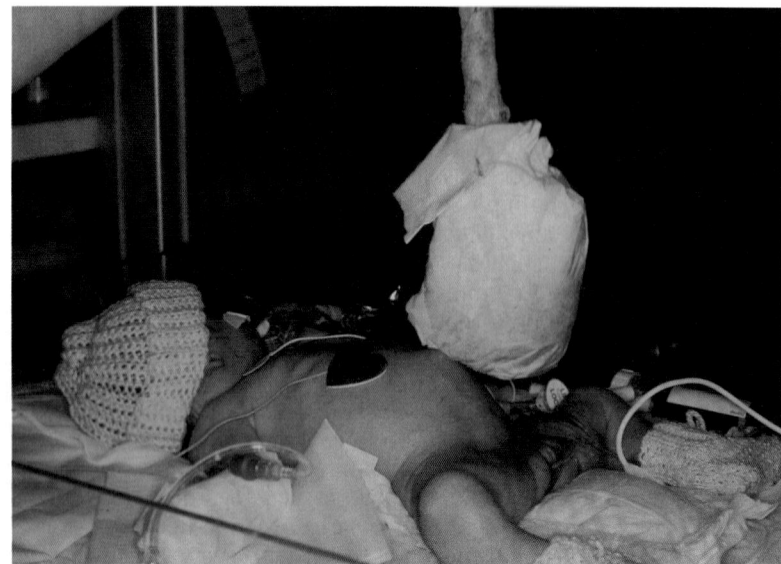

Figure 18-14 If an omphalocele or gastroschisis is too large to repair immediately, a Silastic silo is placed over the exposed viscera and the intestines are gradually reduced into the abdominal cavity over a period of days.

electrolyte abnormalities. Administer broad-spectrum antibiotics as ordered. Provide hemodynamic and respiratory support, including mechanical ventilation, as needed. Insert an OG or NG tube to prevent aspiration and decrease abdominal distention. Anticipate insertion of a urinary catheter to monitor urine output.

Surgical intervention is necessary to close the abdominal wall defect. Small defects may be treated with reduction of the eviscerated bowel into the abdominal cavity, followed by primary closure of the abdominal wall. Larger defects require a staged repair. A Silastic silo is placed around the exposed viscera (Fig. 18-14) and the protruding bowel is slowly reduced into the abdominal cavity every 12 to 24 hours until complete reduction is achieved. This technique enables the cavity to expand gradually to accommodate the bowel. After the bowel is fully reduced into the abdominal cavity, the abdominal wall is surgically closed.

If a silo has been placed, monitor for signs of hypothermia and for shock from fluid depletion caused by heat loss and insensible water loss through the exposed viscera. Position and move the infant with extreme caution to avoid tension on the site or torsion of the mesentery. Monitor the contents in the silo for color changes (symptoms of ischemia). Monitor for respiratory distress, which may be caused by elevation of the diaphragm from returning too much bowel to a small abdominal cavity. Also monitor for cyanosis of the lower extremities, which may indicate pressure on the descending aorta and its femoral branches. The infant is usually sedated before reduction to minimize movement.

Continue to protect the abdominal wall after surgical closure. Patient goals include monitoring respiratory and hemodynamic status, managing fluids, maintaining vascular access, facilitating gastric decompression, managing pain (see Chapter 10), and preventing infection. Providing parenteral support is a priority. Nutritional support with PN through a central venous catheter is usually initiated 1 or 2 days after surgery,

after fluids and electrolytes stabilize. Feedings are initiated when the child is medically stable and bowel function has returned. Bilious vomiting and occult blood in the stools and gastric residuals may indicate necrotizing enterocolitis or obstruction; report these findings to the surgeon.

The child with gastroschisis may have a prolonged postoperative ileus and may require parenteral support for several weeks before feedings can be initiated. In some cases, enteral drip feedings by NG or gastrostomy tube are necessary because of persistent intestinal dysmotility that causes intolerance to oral or bolus feedings. A semielemental formula typically is used when initiating enteral feedings. In cases in which intestinal atresias are associated with gastroschisis, short bowel syndrome results from bowel resection and requires prolonged dependence on PN.

Maintaining parent involvement in the care of the infant is central to the plan of care. Discharge planning and parent education must be coordinated for the home enteral feeding program, oral–motor stimulation, skin care, and home PN, including central venous catheter care (see Chapters 12 and 17).

Community Care

The infant discharged with these conditions has the same needs as all other infants for follow-up to ensure optimal growth and development. Ensuring family function is intact, with appropriate bonding for high-risk infants, must be considered in the discharge plan. Teach parents to report signs of complications early. Bilious vomiting, abdominal distention, poor appetite, constipation, diarrhea, or fever may be associated with bowel complications, such as intestinal obstruction. Continued support and care for the infant is directly related to the extent of bowel resected and the function of remaining bowel. Infants may require a discharge plan for a home enteral program, a home parenteral program, or a combined program. Extensive planning and education are needed for transition to home care when this intensive support is required. Evaluate ongoing therapy for developmental and oral–motor function and make appropriate referrals to optimize outcomes.

CONGENITAL DIAPHRAGMATIC HERNIA

CDH is the protrusion of abdominal contents into the chest cavity through a defect in the diaphragm. The incidence is approximately 1 per 2,200 births (Rollins, 2012). Associated anomalies such as cardiac defects, trisomy 18, EA, omphalocele, and disorders of the central nervous system have been reported. CDH may be an isolated anomaly or associated with multiple malformations. Delayed presentations have occasionally been reported.

The overall survival rate for live births varies with the severity of the defect but has reached as high as 85% in some reports as a result of advances in preoperative physiologic stabilization and medical and surgical advances and protocol-driven management; early term infants have the greatest survival rate (Rollins, 2012).

Pathophysiology

CDH results from the failure of the pleuroperitoneal canal (the opening between the chest and abdomen) to close completely during fetal development or from an early return of the intestines to the abdomen after the normal herniation into the umbilicus during fetal development.

The defect in the diaphragm may be large or small, allowing proportional amounts of abdominal contents to herniate. The herniation is most commonly on the left side, through the posterolateral foramen of Bochdalek. Bilateral hernias are rare and are typically fatal.

More threatening to the infant's survival are the associated effects on the pulmonary system. The ipsilateral lung is usually hypoplastic, with decreased numbers of airway generations, alveoli, and arterioles. The arterioles also show increased muscular mass. The contralateral lung has similar abnormalities, but to a lesser extent, from pressure from a shift to the mediastinum. Compression of the lungs by the herniated viscera during fetal development may contribute to the hypoplasia and persistent pulmonary hypertension. Abnormal development of the mesenchyme is another possible cause.

Assessment

Most infants with CDH experience respiratory distress at birth or within the first few hours of life. As the infant swallows air, the herniated segment distends and further compromises lung and diaphragmatic excursion. Assessment findings include decreased or absent breath sounds on the affected side, although bowel sounds may be heard. If the defect is on the left, which is most common, heart sounds are shifted to the right. Chest sounds are dull on percussion. Tachypnea and cyanosis are present. Assess the need to assist with or initiate resuscitation in the delivery room, which is often required. A high incidence of pneumothorax with left-sided defects is observed. Blood gas analysis reveals acidosis.

Physical examination reveals a barrel-like chest, particularly on the affected side. In contrast to the normal protruding abdomen, the abdomen of the infant with CDH looks scaphoid, or sunken, because of the absence of abdominal contents.

Diagnostic Tests

CDH is often diagnosed during pregnancy by fetal ultrasound. After birth, chest radiograph is usually diagnostic, showing gas-filled intestinal loops in the chest, displacement of the cardiac silhouette, and a gasless abdomen.

Nursing Diagnoses and Outcomes

In addition to the nursing diagnoses listed in Nursing Plan of Care 18-1, the following nursing diagnoses and outcomes may apply to the infant with CDH:

Nursing Diagnosis: Impaired gas exchange related to effects of lung hypoplasia and lung compression
Outcome: The infant will demonstrate oxygen saturation levels adequate to sustain life and prevent the sequelae of oxygen deprivation.
Nursing Diagnosis: Grieving (by the family) related to child's high risk of death
Outcomes:
- Family will verbalize feelings related to infant's high-risk condition.
- Family will spend as much time as possible with the infant.
- Family will demonstrate understanding of the infant's condition and prognosis.

ALERT *Ventilatory support is usually required. Support includes insertion of an endotracheal tube if the infant requires ventilatory assistance. Infants with CDH should not receive bag-and-mask ventilatory support because air insufflation causes further distention of the intestinal loops in the chest, causing further lung compression and thus decreasing the infant's ability to oxygenate.*

Interdisciplinary Interventions

CDH is a life-threatening emergency. Initially, the primary concern is to stabilize cardiopulmonary status.

Intubate and ventilate using a low peak pressure and gentle ventilation (<30 cm H_2O), if possible. The infant may be treated with paralytic agents to avoid further swallowing of air and further pulmonary compromise. An umbilical artery catheter or arterial line is usually placed to monitor blood gas values. A central venous catheter may be inserted to provide full hemodynamic and pulmonary support. A dual lumen (vented) OG tube is passed to decrease the amount of air in the hernia, decrease the lung compression, and allow for continuous suction. Keep the infant NPO and administer and monitor IV fluids and antibiotics.

Surgical Intervention

Traditionally, surgery was done on an emergency basis. Today, the current approach in most medical centers is with nonemergent surgery; however, there is no clear evidence to support nonemergent versus immediate surgical repairs (Harting & Lally, 2007). The parameters for surgical readiness are center dependent but generally include hemodynamic stability, acid–base balance within physiologic range, and ability to tolerate conventional ventilation with adequate oxygenation.

Preoperative treatment with extracorporeal membrane oxygenation (ECMO) is one management option when the infant fails conventional medical therapy. ECMO is similar to cardiopulmonary bypass, which allows the cardiopulmonary system to rest while allowing oxygen and carbon dioxide to be exchanged mechanically outside the body. The goal of initial stabilization is to address the cardiorespiratory compromise caused by pulmonary hypertension and hypoplasia before surgery is attempted. Pharmacologic treatment of the pulmonary hypertension has proved to be of limited value.

Surgery may be done open, thoracoscopically, or laparoscopically. With the open approach, the hernia is most commonly reduced using a subcostal incision on the ipsilateral side. The defect in the diaphragm is corrected using primary closure, if possible. If primary closure will cause excessive tension on the intestines, diaphragm, and large vessels and thereby compromise total thoracic compliance, then a synthetic patch or an abdominal muscle flap procedure is used (Szavay et al., 2012).

Postoperatively, an infant with CDH usually remains critically ill and a challenge to manage. The infant's respiratory status continues to be of primary concern. The goal is to prevent persistent pulmonary hypertension caused by vasoconstriction and acidosis and to preserve the "good lung" from barotrauma. Oxygen therapy is continued; infants are weaned carefully from mechanical ventilation. The infant remains at high risk for pneumothorax because of the pulmonary abnormalities. The use of tube thoracostomy to treat pneumothorax has fallen out of favor because it is postulated to cause iatrogenic pulmonary injury via a mediastinal shift after pleural suction. The lungs usually will gradually displace fluid and air as they enlarge.

Monitor and assess breath sounds and respiratory status for signs of pneumothorax. If such signs occur, notify the physician or advanced practice nurse promptly. Routine postoperative care includes pain management, careful monitoring for changes in the infant's status, and administering IV fluids and antibiotics. The OG tube remains in place for gastric decompression. A gastrostomy tube may be placed during surgery to facilitate postoperative GI decompression and feeding.

Provide developmentally supportive care (dim the lights, decrease noise, handle gently) to decrease stress on the infant. Involve social services or clergy as appropriate to help support the family.

Nutritional Interventions

Initiate feedings gradually, and wean the infant from PN as tolerance to feeding progression is demonstrated. Infants with CDH frequently have GERD. Monitor for signs of GERD and use appropriate positioning and feeding techniques. Problems with sucking and swallowing and aversion to oral stimulation may be observed, resulting from prolonged NPO status. Consult the occupational therapist to provide assessment and interventions for oral–motor dysfunction. Early involvement with the occupational therapist may help to reduce some of the oral–motor problems. Feedings should be small and frequent; avoid overfeeding. Feed the infant in a semiupright position and burp frequently. Enteral nutrition may be continued to support growth and development because FTT is a common complication. Other complications include chronic lung disease, chronic aspiration pneumonia, and GERD that requires surgical intervention.

ALERT   *The infant with CDH is prone to abdominal obstruction. Vomiting, abdominal distention, or a change in bowel elimination pattern should be reported immediately.*

Community Care

Involve the family in the infant's care to the greatest extent possible. Before discharge, ensure that family members can demonstrate appropriate feeding techniques. Also, teach the family how to recognize signs of respiratory distress, respiratory infection, and bowel obstruction and to notify their health care provider if such signs occur. Emphasize the need for long-term follow-up care to identify and intervene for any long-term sequelae.

MECKEL DIVERTICULUM

The most common congenital malformation of the GI tract, Meckel diverticulum, is asymptomatic in most cases, but it may cause disease in approximately 2% of those affected (Pepper et al., 2012). It is often referred to as the rule of twos: It occurs in 2% of population, has a 2:1 male-to-female ratio, is located within 2 ft of ileocecal valve on the antimesenteric border, is commonly 2 cm in diameter and 2 in. in length, can contain 2 types of ectopic tissue (pancreatic and gastric), and is more common before 2 years of age (Pepper et al., 2012). With early identification and surgical intervention, Meckel diverticulum is usually resolvable.

Pathophysiology

Meckel diverticulum arises from a vestigial segment of the embryonic yolk sac that fails to separate from the primitive intestine during the fifth and seventh week of gestation. Meckel diverticulum can occur anywhere in the abdomen but is most commonly found in the right lower quadrant. It is found on the antimesenteric border of the ileum, usually within 40 to 50 cm of the ileocecal valve. A range of distances from the ileocecal valve may occur as well as the size of the Meckel diverticula, depending on the age and size of the child at time of diagnosis. Ectopic tissue, most commonly gastric tissue, may be found in the distal tip of a Meckel diverticulum. Secretion of acid and pepsin from the ectopic gastric tissue causes peptic ulceration and, ultimately, bleeding in the lower GI tract.

Assessment

Most symptomatic children present younger than age 2 years. Intermittent, painless rectal bleeding is the most common clinical manifestation of Meckel diverticulum. The blood is most often bright red or maroon and may be passed independent of stool, resulting from ulceration at the junction of the ectopic tissue and the normal ileal mucosa. Emphasize to the family that they must save all output so a full assessment can be completed. Careful assessment and measurement of blood loss will determine further interventions. Bleeding may be so severe as to cause severe anemia or hemorrhagic shock.

Physical assessment findings may include pallor, lethargy, and hemodynamic instability. Intestinal obstruction (secondary to intussusception or volvulus) can occur and presents with bilious vomiting, abdominal pain, and distention. Perforation is a potential complication but is uncommon. Presentation of symptoms may also be similar to acute appendicitis with nausea, vomiting, and right-sided abdominal pain.

Diagnostic Tests

Depending on the degree of bleeding, a CBC may reveal severe anemia. Standard radiographic imaging and barium studies of the GI tract are of little value in identifying Meckel diverticulum. Definitive diagnosis is most commonly made with a Meckel scan (technetium-99m pertechnetate scan), which uses IV injection of a technetium isotope to visualize the ectopic gastric mucosa commonly found in bleeding Meckel diverticulum. If the Meckel scan is not diagnostic, a tagged red blood cell study may be done to localize the bleeding site.

Interdisciplinary Interventions

Because rectal bleeding is the most common manifestation of Meckel diverticulum, assessing and restoring circulating fluid volume is the most important initial step in patient management. Administer IV fluids and possibly a transfusion of packed red blood cells to restore circulating fluid volume. After the child is stabilized, further diagnostic workup can take place. Place the child on NPO status and give antibiotics if peritoneal signs present, as ordered.

A diverticulectomy is performed via an open approach or laparoscopically. Under most circumstances, intestinal resection is not required, recovery is complete, and complications are uncommon. Laparoscopic surgery is frequently used and is helpful in evaluating the child with unusual symptoms (Chan et al., 2008). Resection can be performed safely either open or laparoscopically; a laparoscopic approach is recommended for its benefits for postoperative recovery (Pepper et al., 2012).

Promoting the child's comfort during both the preoperative and postoperative periods is an important aspect of care. Provide information and support to the child and family regarding diagnostic procedures and therapeutic interventions to help allay anxiety during the course of the hospitalization. Postoperatively, monitor for the return of bowel function, encourage early ambulation, and monitor tolerance to progression of diet. The hospital stay is usually short, and the child will go home when there is no evidence of fever and when ambulation and a regular diet are tolerated.

Community Care

Instruct the family to report any signs of infection to their surgeon. The child's return to school and to full activities may vary depending on the surgeon.

MALROTATION AND VOLVULUS

Although the incidence of malrotation is reported to be approximately 1 in 6,000 live births, its true incidence is difficult to ascertain because many affected infants are asymptomatic. Volvulus occurs most commonly during the first month of life, but it can occur anytime during childhood (Juang & Snyder, 2012).

Malrotation is the result of incomplete or deviated rotation of the midgut during embryologic development between the 8th and 10th week of gestation, which causes incomplete fixation of the mesentery on the posterior abdominal wall at the duodenum and proximal colon. *Volvulus* is a life-threatening complication of malrotation in which the malrotated bowel twists in a clockwise direction on itself, causing vascular compromise and, ultimately, necrosis of the bowel. Because of the nature of their structural defects, omphalocele, gastroschisis, and CDH are all associated with volvulus. Other associated conditions include intestinal atresias, Hirschsprung disease, and Meckel diverticulum.

Infants who lose little or no intestine have an excellent prognosis. The infant or child will recover from surgery with minimal problems. The outcome for the child with associated medical complications such as infarcted bowel, complications with associated congenital anomalies, or who age younger than 1 month has increased risks for morbidity.

Pathophysiology

The midgut comprises the duodenum distal to the entry of the bile duct, jejunum, ileum, appendix, cecum, and colon up to the midtransverse segment. Between the 5th and 10th weeks of gestation, the midgut grows rapidly and, because of lack of space, is forced to rotate out of the abdominal cavity into the umbilical cord. Between the 10th and 11th weeks of gestation, the abdominal cavity enlarges to a point that allows the midgut to reenter the abdominal cavity. The midgut normally rotates 270 degrees counterclockwise as it returns to the abdominal cavity. If the midgut fails to complete this rotation, the mesentery usually cannot fix completely onto the posterior abdominal wall, and a foreshortened mesenteric base forms. This foreshortening results in a stalklike, "poorly fixed" structure, creating a risk for the bowel to twist on itself, kinking and knotting the intestinal loops and causing abdominal pain and intestinal obstruction. Congenital bands of adhesions, known as *Ladd bands*, are usually present. These bands extend from the right upper quadrant across the duodenum to the cecum and may cause duodenal obstruction.

Malrotation can present as a chronic problem, with intermittent abdominal pain and vomiting alternating with asymptomatic periods. Infants with malrotation and midgut volvulus present acutely with intense symptoms, and their condition can deteriorate rapidly (Saito, 2012).

Assessment

Assess the patient's general color, activity level, and the volume and characteristics of emesis, which is usually bilious and possibly more pronounced in young infants. Assess the abdomen for progressive distention accompanied by constant (vs. intermittent) pain. Presentation of symptoms may be less pronounced in older children. Signs of acute or intermittent intestinal obstruction, crampy abdominal pain, FTT, constipation, bloody diarrhea, and hematemesis may be observed in the older child with malrotation. In some cases of malrotation, the presentation of symptoms can be intermittent with few obvious physical findings.

ALERT *To avoid serious complications of malrotation with volvulus, any acute onset of bilious emesis in an otherwise healthy infant requires immediate workup that includes malrotation with volvulus in the differential. This symptom must be treated as an emergency situation.*

Infants with volvulus usually present through the emergency room with a history of a healthy infant experiencing sudden onset of vomiting, progressing to bilious vomiting. When substantial vascular compromise has occurred, the child may demonstrate abdominal distention and tenderness, signs of peritonitis, with rapid deterioration leading to hypovolemic shock. The presence of blood in the stool is a serious sign because it indicates vascular compromise of the intestine.

Diagnostic Tests

Diagnosis of malrotation is supported by radiographic evaluation. In 20% of cases, a plain radiograph of the abdomen may demonstrate either an air-filled stomach and duodenum with a proximal obstruction (commonly termed a *double-bubble sign*) or gas-filled intestinal loops with distal obstruction (Zerpa & Shapiro, 2013). Free air in the peritoneum may be seen if perforation has occurred. An upper GI barium swallow contrast study is the gold standard for diagnosing volvulus. The classic finding is the small intestine rotated to the right side of the abdomen, indicating the malrotation, with contrast narrowing at the obstruction site, causing a "corkscrew" appearance (Lampl et al., 2009). Ultrasound is also used as a diagnostic tool.

Interdisciplinary Interventions

Surgical correction of malrotation with signs of obstruction or volvulus is necessary in symptomatic infants. Preoperatively, an NG tube is inserted for gastric decompression and IV fluids are administered to aggressively correct any fluid volume deficits. IV antibiotics are also given. During surgery, the malrotation is identified and "untwisted." All adhesive bands are divided, and the cecum is placed in the left abdomen. This surgery is commonly referred to as *Ladd procedure*. Often, an appendectomy is done in conjunction with the Ladd procedure to prevent confusion later on if the patient develops appendicitis; the appendix will be in a different position because of the untwisting and relocation of the intestines.

If a volvulus is identified, emergency surgery is necessary to minimize intestinal necrosis, untwist the bowel, and reestablish the blood supply. Nonviable bowel is resected. If bowel necrosis is extensive, or viability of the bowel is questionable after the volvulus has been untwisted, "second-look" surgery may be done 24 to 48 hours after the initial surgery to achieve maximal salvage of bowel.

Postoperative management is affected by the amount of bowel that is resected. The child with volvulus and extensive bowel necrosis may be critically ill during the immediate postoperative period and may require prolonged hospitalization. Care is similar to that for other intestinal surgeries. Monitor vital signs and hydration status, and provide pain management. Provide scrupulous care of the NG tube, including assessment of the skin condition of the nares, to avoid complications related to skin breakdown. If the infant required a significant length of bowel resection resulting in short bowel syndrome, a gastrostomy tube and a central venous catheter may be placed at the time of surgery.

Volvulus needs to be considered as a catastrophic event for the child and family. Provide physiologic and educational interventions within a framework of emotional support that recognizes and responds to the family's reaction to this acute and extreme change in the child's health. A social worker or psychologist may be helpful to the child and family in dealing with the acute crisis of the child's illness and in making long-term adjustments. Child life specialists may provide developmentally appropriate play experiences to help the child cope with the effects of hospitalization and changes in health and bodily function.

Community Care

Education is essential. Teach the family to recognize signs of bowel obstruction resulting from the increased risk for adhesions. Educate the family in the care specific to their infant's needs. Some infants may require enteral feeding through a gastrostomy tube; education may be required for parenteral therapy and for central line management, depending on the extent of the resection and the amount of bowel remaining. Teach the family routine care and problem-solving skills that will help them to cope with nonroutine situations.

INTUSSUSCEPTION

Intussusception is a common cause of intestinal obstruction. More than 75% of cases occur in children younger than 24 months old, with peak incidence between 5 and 10 months and a male-to-female ratio of 2:1 (Pepper et al., 2012). It occurs when a proximal segment of bowel prolapses or telescopes into the lumen of an immediately distal segment of bowel. This prolapse results in vascular compromise, edema, and, eventually, mechanical obstruction. The ileocecal junction is a common site of intussusception (Fig. 18-15).

Intussusception can be classified as is idiopathic or pathologic. The idiopathic form, which occurs more than 90% of the time, is believed to be a result of a viral illness, during which hypertrophied lymphoid tissue develops (Peyer patches) in the bowel (an identified change in the intestinal mucosa). This lymphoid tissue becomes a lead point for the intussusception, accounting for the majority of infant presentations. Usually, in older children, a pathologic lead point can be identified, most commonly as a Meckel diverticulum, polyp, or hemangioma, to name a few from a lengthy list of potential triggers. An individual with cystic fibrosis may develop intussusception resulting from the thick, inspissated stool that may result from inconsistent ingestion of replacement pancreatic enzymes. The multiple lead points can be classified into anatomic, malignant, genetic, vascular, infectious, traumatic, and postsurgical. After age 3 years, common lead point pathologies include Meckel diverticulum, lymphoma, and polyps (Pepper et al., 2012).

The prognosis for the child with intussusception is good if detection and treatment are prompt. Recurrence occurs in 0.5% to 15% of cases after nonoperative reduction and is usually within the first 24 hours. Therefore, these children are admitted and observed. Long-term sequelae are uncommon.

Pathophysiology

Edema develops within the telescoped bowel wall secondary to vascular and lymphatic compression. Bleeding occurs, resulting in the passage of blood and mucus in the stool. As the bowel becomes more edematous, mechanical obstruction of the bowel occurs. If left untreated, this obstruction may lead to significant complications including necrosis, perforation, and death (Pepper et al., 2012).

Assessment

The child with intussusception classically presents as a usually healthy infant with severe abdominal pain that is crampy and intermittent, causing the knees to be drawn up to the chest. Vomiting is nonbilious at first but may become bilious as the disease progresses and complete intestinal obstruction occurs. Check the child's diaper or underpants. Dark-red blood and mucus are passed through the rectum; this discharge is commonly described as *currant jelly stools*. Although this type of stool is classically described in the literature, it is a late sign, and absence of bloody stools does not alter the workup.

During the early stages of intussusception, the physical findings from assessment may reveal no abnormalities other than episodic pain. The infant or child's level of consciousness may reveal increased irritability progressing to lethargy and listlessness as the disorder progresses. Monitoring the temperature may reveal a low-grade fever. Palpate the abdomen, which should be soft and nontender. A sausage-shaped mass is commonly palpable in the mid to upper right quadrant, with bowel signs absent in the right lower quadrant. With progressive obstruction, the abdomen may become more distended and tender, and the mass may become nonpalpable. Palpate the groin for incarcerated hernia or testicular torsion, which must be ruled out as a possible cause of intermittent acute pain.

Diagnostic Tests

A CBC and electrolyte panel may be part of the evaluation. The CBC may show a slight increase in white blood cells, reflecting inflammation, and the electrolyte panel may reflect some degree of dehydration if the child has had excessive fluid losses from vomiting. The urinalysis shows signs of dehydration with elevation of specific gravity.

Radiographic evaluation begins with a plain radiograph of the abdomen, which often reveals nonspecific findings but may demonstrate some density in the area of the intussusception or show presence of small bowel obstruction. A contrast enema, done with air alone or with barium, is used as both a diagnostic and therapeutic tool in treating intussusception. The air enema under fluoroscopy is now widely used because air is safer than contrast media, exposes the child to less radiation, and avoids further peritoneal complications if perforation occurs. The contrast enema is done after the child has received NG

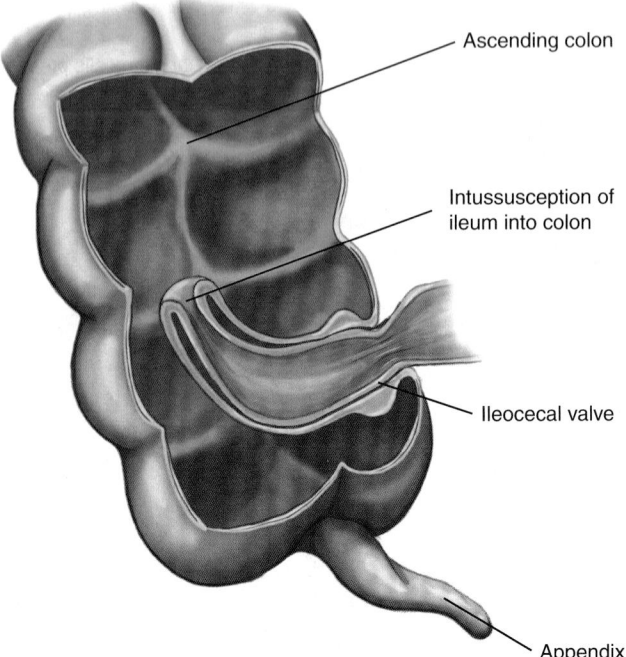

Figure 18-15 In intussusception, a portion of the bowel telescopes into itself, causing signs and symptoms of intestinal obstruction.

Ascending colon

Intussusception of ileum into colon

Ileocecal valve

Appendix

decompression, IV access with fluid resuscitation, and IV antibiotics. A surgeon is present in the event of bowel perforation during enema administration. The child is sedated before the procedure. The contrast material infused during the enema delineates the area of intussusception on radiograph, which appears like a coiled spring within the lumen of the bowel. The pressure of the contrast material is maintained for as long as 5 minutes; this causes reduction of the intussusception in more than 90% of cases (Pepper et al., 2012). The radiograph technician is able to visualize the reflux of air into the small bowel as the tissue mass is successfully reduced. The child is observed for 24 to 36 hours for signs of recurrence. Ultrasound may also be used for the diagnosis.

Interdisciplinary Interventions

Surgical reduction of intussusception is required in cases in which overt signs of peritonitis, bowel perforation, or septic shock are present or when radiographic interventional methods fail. Fluid resuscitation and IV broad-spectrum antibiotics are given preoperatively. A laparotomy is performed through a transverse right lower quadrant incision. Manual reduction of the intussusception is attempted after the bowel is mobilized. If this approach is not successful, the affected bowel is resected, with end-to-end anastomosis. If bowel perforation is detected during surgery, a temporary ostomy may be created.

A key intervention in the care of the child with intussusception is teaching the family about the signs and symptoms of recurrent intussusception. Recurrence may also develop months later in a small percentage of patients, even after a surgical reduction. Early recognition and treatment are important to avoid severe illness.

Community Care

Instruct the family to return to the medical facility if vomiting, abdominal pain, or bloody stools recur. If a surgical procedure was performed, provide instruction on signs of wound infection, such as fever, redness, swelling, or drainage from the incision.

HIRSCHSPRUNG DISEASE

Hirschsprung disease, or congenital megacolon, is a congenital absence of ganglion cells (ganglia) from variable lengths of the terminal bowel. Short-segment Hirschsprung disease accounts for as many as 80% of cases and affects the rectosigmoid colon; long-segment Hirschsprung disease (approximately 15% to 20% of cases) extends proximal to the sigmoid colon; in approximately 5% of cases, total colonic aganglionosis is present (Bergeron et al., 2013).

Hirschsprung disease occurs in 1 of 5,000 live births and has a 4:1 predominance in males; short-segment disease occurs five times more frequently in males than females (Bergeron et al., 2013). Both familial and sporadic cases have been identified through molecular genetics, and specific genes have been identified as the cause of Hirschsprung disease in some patients. The RET proto-oncogene on chromosome 10 accounts for 50% of familial cases and is most common in

long-segment disease (Bergeron et al., 2013). As many as 12% of children with Hirschsprung disease have associated chromosomal anomalies, most commonly trisomy 21, and 18% present as part of a syndrome with other congenital defects (Bergeron et al., 2013).

Long-term follow-up studies report that these children overcome postoperative problems and do well over time (Dasgupta & Langer, 2008). Social satisfaction, quality of life, and sexual function are reported to be relatively normal for most individuals living with Hirschsprung disease. Children with coexisting conditions are at greater risk for complications, but this risk decreases over time as well.

Pathophysiology

During the 5th to 12th weeks of gestation, neuroblasts (precursors of the intestinal ganglia) migrate to the GI tract. Neurons arise from the embryonic neural crest cells that normally populate the distal colon during this time. The portion of the enteric nervous system in the gut wall consists of two major plexuses of ganglia connected by bundles of axons: the myenteric intermuscular (Auerbach) and submucous (Meissner) plexuses, located between the circular and longitudinal muscle layers and the submucous layer. The absence of these plexuses leads to inadequate relaxation in the affected bowel. In response to stool in the rectum, the internal sphincter of the rectum contracts instead of relaxing. This abnormal response obstructs passage of the stool and results in dysmotility, bacterial overgrowth, and enterocolitis. In response to the obstruction, the proximal normal bowel distends, thus the term *megacolon* (Fig. 18-16). As the bowel distends, intraluminal pressure increases, putting pressure on the bowel wall. This pressure decreases blood flow, causing ischemia and deterioration of the mucosal barrier. Stasis also allows bacterial overgrowth, through which bacteria proliferate

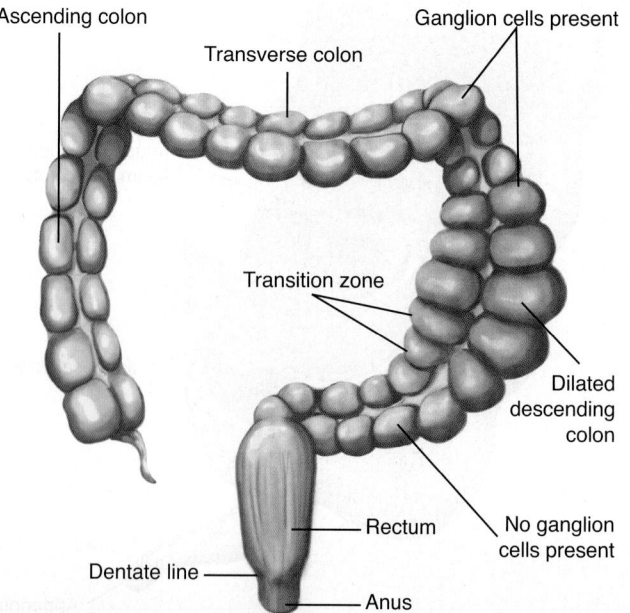

Figure 18-16 In Hirschsprung disease, dilation of the colon occurs proximal to the aganglionic section.

with translocation into the abdominal wall. Inflammation and infection of the bowel wall (enterocolitis) can result—a potentially life-threatening complication.

Assessment

Clinical manifestations of Hirschsprung disease vary depending on the extent of the bowel segment involved and the child's age at the time of diagnosis (Developmental Considerations 18-1). Suspect Hirschsprung disease when the newborn does not pass meconium during the first 24 hours after birth and has bilious vomiting or has abdominal distention, feeding intolerance, and with bilious aspirates and vomiting. For the older child, a history of severe constipation from birth, FTT, abdominal distention, and an empty rectal ampulla on digital rectal examination are clinical indicators for Hirschsprung disease.

Enterocolitis is the presenting symptom in approximately 6% of newborns with Hirschsprung disease.

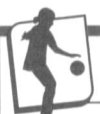

DEVELOPMENTAL CONSIDERATIONS 18-1

Presentation of Hirschsprung Disease

Newborn

Breastfed infants may present with less severe manifestations:
- Failure to pass meconium within 48 hours after birth
- Abdominal distention
- Bilious vomiting
- Liquid stool (from seepage around fecal impaction, must be differentiated from diarrhea of enterocolitis)
- Enterocolitis
  - Abdominal distention
  - Diarrhea
  - Fever
- Hematochezia

Older Infants and Children
- Chronic constipation
- Characteristic stools
  - Foul smelling
  - Consistency varies: small pellets, ribbonlike, or liquid (from seepage around fecal impaction, must be differentiated from diarrhea of enterocolitis)
- Abdominal distention
- Enterocolitis
  - Abdominal distention
  - Diarrhea
  - Fever
  - Hematochezia
- FTT

Risk factors for enterocolitis in this group include delay in diagnosis beyond age 1 week and Down syndrome (Austin, 2012).

Physical examination most often reveals a distended abdomen and the absence of stool in the rectum. During the rectal examination, upon withdrawal of the digit, there may be an explosive release of foul-smelling liquid stool and air as a result of decompression of the proximal normal bowel.

Diagnostic Tests

Abdominal radiographs can be helpful to determine the air patterns present in the colon. A water-soluble contrast enema is commonly the first step in establishing the diagnosis of Hirschsprung disease. In most cases, the study demonstrates a characteristic transition zone where the aganglionic segment of bowel and the dilated proximal segment meet (see Fig. 18-16). Contrast enemas are avoided when a patient presents with suspicion of enterocolitis. Rectal manometry may be used as a diagnostic tool, particularly in the older child. Definitive diagnosis is made by histologic evaluation with suction rectal biopsy from 1, 3, and 5 cm above the dentate line, demonstrating the absence of ganglion cells in the submucosa and myenteric plexus. If insufficient tissue is obtained, a full-thickness biopsy and exam under anesthesia (EUA) is done in the operating room.

Nursing Diagnoses and Outcomes

In addition to the nursing diagnoses listed in Nursing Plan of Care 18-1, the following nursing diagnoses and outcomes may apply to the infant with Hirschsprung disease:

Nursing Diagnosis: Constipation related to effects of aganglionic bowel
Outcome: The child and family will verbalize understanding of signs of altered elimination and implement appropriate interventions.
Nursing Diagnosis: Risk for infection related to potential complication of postoperative atelectasis and enterocolitis
Outcomes:
- The child will be free of infection.
- The child and family will recognize the signs of enterocolitis and contact the health care provider when such signs are present.

Interdisciplinary Interventions

Preparing and supporting the child during tests and procedures and providing parent education and support are important activities throughout the diagnostic workup. Surgery is the definitive treatment. The aganglionic segment of bowel is removed, and the normal bowel is anastomosed to the rectum. Historically, this surgery was done in two stages, an approach still used at some institutions. With two-stage surgery, the child undergoes a diverting colostomy just proximal to the transition zone. This procedure allows the normal bowel to decompress and return to normal size. At a later date, usually when the child is 6 to 12 months old or has reached a body weight of 5 to 10 kg and is medically stable, a second-stage pull-through procedure is done to reestablish bowel continuity. Surgical approaches have undergone numerous revisions, and debate continues over the best surgical approach. The most common approach is the Soave endorectal pull-through procedure. This surgery is a primary pull-through in which the aganglionic rectum is stripped of its mucosa and normal innervated colon is pulled through the muscular layer ("muscular cuff") of the rectum and anastomosed 1.0 to 1.5 cm above the dentate line. Colostomy is indicated in a subgroup of patients, such as a very sick child with enterocolitis, a child with massive megacolon, a neonate with pneumoperitoneum, a child with developmental delay, or a child with total colonic aganglionosis.

Surgical correction also may be done laparoscopically. A laparoscopic biopsy is initially done to identify the transition zone, and then the procedure is performed. Another more recent approach is the transanal (perineal) pull-through, first described in 1999. This technique consists of a transanal mucosectomy, followed by a full-thickness transanal resection of the aganglionic rectum and sigmoid colon and coloanal anastomosis.

Initial preoperative care of the child diagnosed with Hirschsprung disease includes the standard care for any child with suspected bowel obstruction. The child is kept NPO, and gastric decompression is instituted. IV fluids and electrolytes are administered to meet maintenance requirements and correct any deficits, along with IV antibiotics. If enterocolitis is suspected, additional interventions include rectal irrigations and possibly a colostomy. Bowel preparations are surgeon dependent; however, literature has shown that there is no significant difference in length of stay, anastomotic leakage, or complications when comparing bowel preparation to no bowel preparation (Güenaga et al., 2011; Leys et al., 2005). If the child must have an ostomy, the CWOCN will be involved during the preoperative period. The CWOCN will mark the site for the stoma and provide education and support to the child, family, and clinical nurse while preparing the family for surgery.

Provide routine postoperative care for the child after surgery. The CWOCN will collaborate with the bedside nurse to monitor the appearance and function of the colostomy and to select appropriate pouching appliances. After the pull-through, monitor the child closely for signs of intra-abdominal abscess, such as fever, irritability, and abdominal distention. Assessing skin condition is important with patients having a pull-through procedure because they will have frequent liquid stools postoperatively. Aggressive skin care using skin barrier creams to avoid maceration or skin breakdown is required. Early involvement of the CWOCN to assist with skin care recommendations and a skin care program is an essential part of the plan of care, both postoperative and home care. Rectal dilations are initiated at 2 to 3 weeks after surgery to reduce the risk

of stenosis. These are continued for about 6 months until the anastomotic scar tissue becomes supple. Many children are placed on a home bowel program to maintain full evacuation of the colon. Other therapies may include rectal washouts (similar to enemas) for 3 to 4 months to reduce the incidence of enterocolitis.

ALERT   *Do not administer anything per rectum for the first 2–3 weeks after a pull-through procedure, including suppositories, thermometers, or catheters. Place a sign on the patient's bed so that others will avoid these measures.*

Community Care

The child with Hirschsprung disease has special care needs at home after both primary and staged surgeries. Assess the family's understanding of Hirschsprung disease and the treatment plan. Prepare the family to meet the child's anticipated care needs at home. When two-stage surgery is performed, the family will need instruction in colostomy care. Include the child in all teaching, as developmentally appropriate. Provide instruction in skin care, pouch application and management, and signs of complications. The CWOCN will collaborate with the bedside nurse in the teaching process and in referring the family to community resources, such as a home health agency, for support and to reinforce family education. The family should receive needed ostomy care supplies at discharge and should be given information about where to obtain additional supplies.

After pull-through, the child and family will need to be taught about postoperative complications. Emphasize signs of anastomotic stricture, bowel obstruction, and enterocolitis. Provide them with the appropriate follow-up contacts. Teach the family to contact their physician for signs of enterocolitis (see Developmental Considerations 18-1). In addition, teach the parents and patient signs of bowel obstruction, which include abdominal distention, bloating, vomiting, or severe constipation and pain. These complications can occur at any time.

Long-term problems may include delays in toilet training, staining, fecal incontinence, constipation, and an overall negative effect of the disease on the quality of life. Although many children attain satisfactory bowel function, families need to be prepared for these problems, supported during toilet training of the child, and encouraged to have realistic expectations about the child's ability to achieve continence. Constipation and fecal soiling are late sequelae that deteriorate with increasing age; many adolescents and adults attain social continence but some may require a specific bowel management regime (Rintala & Pakarinen, 2012). Quality of life in children, adolescents, and adults with Hirschsprung disease has been reported to be comparable to the general population with little limitation in physical activities, social contacts, or occupation (Rintala & Pakarinen, 2012).

Children and families may benefit from peer support in dealing with Hirschsprung disease (see thePoint for Organizations). Community organizations such as the local ostomy association offer opportunities for children and families to interact with others who have been similarly affected.

ANORECTAL MALFORMATIONS

Anorectal malformations encompass disruptions in anal development that result from altered prenatal development of the GI and GU tracts during the 4th to 16th weeks of gestation. Anorectal agenesis (also referred to as *imperforate anus*), anal stenosis, and fistulas (rectovaginal fistula or fistulas in females and rectourethral fistula in males) are examples of anorectal malformations. Persistent cloaca is a complex congenital malformation in which the rectum, vagina, and urinary tract are fused together in a single common channel communicating externally through a single perineal orifice located at the normal urethral site. The posterior sagittal anorectoplasty (PSARP) is the most common surgical approach.

Anorectal malformations occur in 1 in 4,000 live births and are slightly more common in males than females. Although their precise etiology is not known, anorectal malformations are sometimes associated with the presence of other congenital anomalies, often as a part of VACTERL association.

Anorectal malformations are classified as high, when the infant has no perineal fistula, or low, when a perineal bowel opening is present. Specific malformations are generally common to each classification (Table 18-4). GU anomalies, other than fistulas, are associated with low lesions in 20% of cases and with high lesions in 50% of cases.

The prognosis for a child with an anorectal malformation depends on the type of malformation and the presence of other congenital anomalies. Morbidity usually results from associated defects and the complexity of the lesion.

Pathophysiology

During the fourth week of gestation, the cloaca (a transitory embryologic cavity) forms at the end of the primitive hindgut. The cloaca serves as the early common channel of the rectum and the urogenital structures. The urorectal septum develops at 4 to 6 weeks' gestation, descending in a cephalocaudal direction to unite with the cloacal membrane that divides the rectum from the urogenital structures. Rupture of the cloacal membranes at 8 weeks' gestation forms the urogenital and anal orifices. Further differentiation takes place during the next 8 weeks to form the bladder, the urethra, and seminal vesicles in males and the urethra and vagina in females. Failure of embryologic development at any point in this process can result in anorectal anomaly. The form of the anomaly is closely related to the timing of the disruption in embryologic development, with high anomalies occurring around the 4th week of gestation and low anomalies occurring between the 10th and 12th weeks.

Assessment

Anorectal malformations are usually immediately obvious at birth. On the initial physical examination, the anus is absent or displaced (Fig. 18-17). Affected females may have a variable number and configuration of openings noted in the perineal area. The presence of a fistula may be noted when gas or stool is expelled from the urethra or vagina. In males, fistulas may be seen anywhere along the tract between the usual location of the anus and the tip of the penis, appearing as epithelial pearls or spots of meconium. Meconium may be seen in the urine if a fistula is present between the bowel and urinary tract.

An anal malformation that is not immediately noted may present with signs of lower intestinal obstruction, such as abdominal distention and bilious vomiting within the first 18 to 24 hours after birth. The presence of a midline groove with well-formed buttocks and an obvious anal dimple indicates a good prognostic sign that the malformation is low in contrast to flattened buttocks (with no midline groove) and the absence of an anal dimple, which indicates a high malformation.

Diagnostic Tests

Male infants need a urinalysis to detect the presence of meconium in the urine. Radiographic evaluation is necessary to determine the extent of the malformation. A cross-table lateral radiograph with the infant positioned prone with the pelvis elevated can be used to differentiate a high lesion from a low lesion. It can also disclose the presence of gas in the bladder or urethra, which indicates the presence of a fistulous connection with the bowel. Ultrasound of the abdomen and pelvis determines whether the malformation includes the urinary tract. If the study is positive, a more detailed urologic evaluation is conducted.

CT or MRI may also be used to visualize the anorectal anatomy. Radiopaque dye studies of any obvious

TABLE 18-4	Classification of Anorectal Malformations	
Classification	**Male**	**Female**
High	Anorectal agenesis	Anorectal agenesis
	Anorectal agenesis with rectourethral fistula	Anorectal agenesis with rectovaginal fistula
	Rectal atresia	Rectal atresia
Intermediate	Rectobulbar urethral fistula	Rectovestibular fistula
	Anal agenesis	Rectovaginal fistula
		Anal agenesis
Low	Anocutaneous fistula	Anocutaneous fistula
	Anal stenosis	Anal stenosis
		Anovestibular fistula

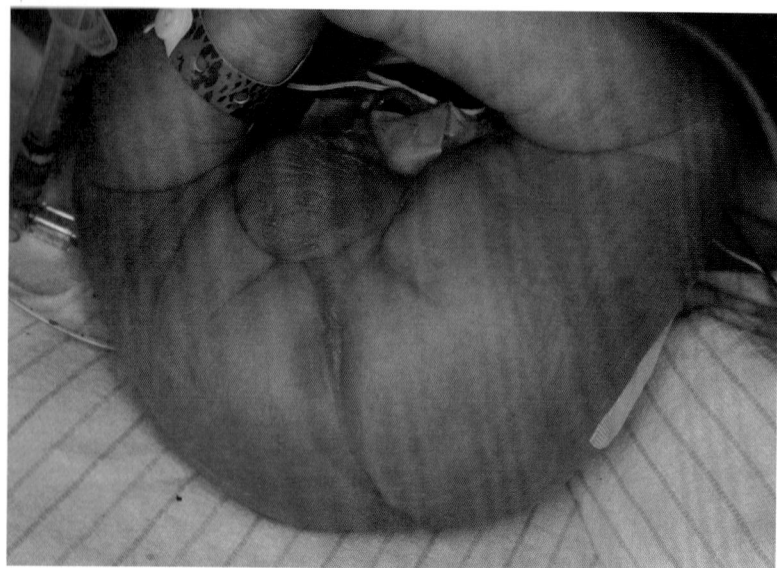

Figure 18-17 An anal dimple may be present in low types of anal agenesis but not in high types.

fistulous tracts may be done to determine the exact anatomy of the tract.

Interdisciplinary Interventions

The infant with anorectal malformation requires a careful physical examination to determine the presence of other anomalies that may be life threatening. The more complex and higher the defect, the greater the chance for an associated anomaly. In addition, a determination is made if the presenting defect requires a colostomy. Immediate stabilization focuses on relieving intestinal obstruction by NG decompression. The infant is put on NPO status, and IV fluids and antibiotics are administered. Strict monitoring of intake and output is recorded. Provide standard preoperative care.

Surgical intervention depends on the nature of the malformation. Children with low lesions require anoplasty (creation of an anal opening) in a single-stage procedure.

Perform routine postoperative care with special attention to prevention of perineal skin excoriation from passing small, frequent, liquid-type stools. Antibiotic ointment is applied to this area after each diaper change for 2 weeks and as indicated. The plan of care includes nothing per rectum. Signage may be posted on the crib to communicate this to the health care team. Two to 3 weeks after surgery, anal dilations are begun and continued for approximately 2 months to prevent stenosis of the operative site. Dilations may be continued on a tapering schedule.

Children with high lesions require a diverting colostomy within the first 24 to 48 hours of life. Definitive repair is done in two subsequent stages. The first stage is done after 1 month of age, although some surgeons may wait until an older age, when the rectovaginal or rectourethral fistula (if present) is repaired. The PSARP procedure is done to create an anal opening. A laparotomy is performed with a PSARP when the rectum is too high and cannot be

visualized from the posterior approach. Postoperative care is more complex after an open abdominal procedure with the PSARP. Dilations of the newly created anus begin 2 weeks after surgery and continue for approximately 6 to 8 weeks, at which time the desired size is achieved. The second stage of the surgery, final closure of the colostomy, is then planned. Dilations continue on a tapering schedule for a total of 6 months. In recent years, pediatric surgeons have attempted one-stage repairs to avoid a colostomy, future surgeries, and thus additional trauma to the patient. Decisions are individualized based on many factors, such as the complexity of the malformation and peripheral circumstances.

Besides the usual postoperative care, inspect the anoplasty site for mucosal prolapse, which may occur if an inadequate amount of sphincter has been preserved. The postoperative plan of care includes administering IV antibiotics and fluids and managing pain. A urinary catheter is placed if a cloacal repair was required to correct the malformation. This measure protects the suture line in the urethra; notify the surgeon if the catheter becomes dislodged.

Interventions for skin care generally are surgeon specific but may include applying antibiotic ointment to the perineum with each diaper change for at least 2 weeks (Guardino & Pieper, 2013). Stool-softening agents may be administered. The surgeon initially carries out anal dilations. Before the patient's discharge, the parents are instructed (either by the surgeon or by the surgical nurse at the follow-up visit) to continue anal dilations at home.

After closure of the colostomy, the child is not discharged until he or she has passed stools and demonstrated diet tolerance. Frequent, small, liquid stools resulting in perineal excoriation must be addressed. Many skin barriers are available. Consult with the CWOCN to determine the most effective skin barrier and skin care program.

Constipation is a long-term problem after PSARP and may also be experienced with low lesions. The spectrum of problems experienced directs bowel management interventions. Interventions may include diet, increased activity, oral agents, enemas, biofeedback, and bowel management programs. For the child on a bowel program with daily enemas that is effective in controlling soiling or constipation, an antegrade continence enema procedure may be considered as an option when he or she reaches school age so the child may be independent in performing the daily bowel management plan. This procedure involves creating a one-way conduit between the skin and the cecum using the appendix, sometimes referred to as the *Malone procedure*. An abdominal stoma is created to allow easier access for daily flushes/enemas with evacuation through the rectum to achieve more efficient bowel management and promote independence.

Community Care

Management for the infant with an anorectal malformation includes family education about colostomy care. Refer the family for home health nursing follow-up as needed. Concerns related to fecal incontinence have long-term implications in both the clinic and school settings. Provide anticipatory guidance for parents, including support with bowel management programs. The goal of bowel management is "social continence" for children who are unable to be fully continent. Follow-up care is essential for the coordination of individualized interventions and for the provision of long-term support needed to progress toward normalization of elimination patterns.

ANSWER: A primary difference of GI surgery among infants through school-aged children such as Cory is the parent–child relationship. For many infants with a malformation, surgery occurs before a parent–child relationship is well established. Nurses should spend additional time supporting the parent–infant relationship and encouraging the parent to master caregiver skills.

INFLAMMATORY DISORDERS

Inflammatory disorders of the GI tract include gastroenteritis, appendicitis, IBD, and pancreatitis.

GASTROENTERITIS

Gastroenteritis, an inflammation of the GI tract, may be caused by GI irritants such as bacteria, viruses, and toxins produced by fish and mushrooms (Table 18-5). Outbreaks of gastroenteritis routinely occur in daycare centers, schools, institutions for the handicapped, and other places where overcrowding is prevalent and hygiene is inadequate. Food-borne outbreaks occur fairly regularly. Hospital-acquired infections resulting in gastroenteritis involve two main organisms: rotavirus

TABLE 18-5   Causes of Gastroenteritis

Bacteria	Viruses	Parasites
Campylobacter	Adenovirus	Cryptosporidium
Clostridium difficile	Astrovirus	Entamoeba histolytica
Clostridium perfringens	Calicivirus	Giardia lamblia
Escherichia coli (four types)	Norwalk virus	Isospora
Salmonella	Rotavirus	
Shigella		
Staphylococcus aureus		
Vibrio cholera		
Yersinia		

Nonmicrobial Food-Borne Agents	
Agent	Food
Anatoxin	Poisonous mushrooms (Amanita phalloides)
Ciguatera fish neurotoxin	Barracuda, snapper, amberjack, grouper, oysters, mollusks
Histamine scombroid (fish)	Tuna, mackerel, bonito, mahimahi

and *Clostridium difficile*. Both organisms can linger in the environment for a long time and can be easily transmitted from child to child on the unwashed hands of health care workers. Acute diarrhea may also result from overfeeding with hyperosmolar fluids; use of antibiotics; and extraintestinal infections such as pneumonia, urinary tract infection, or otitis media, which are usually self-limited and mild in severity. Generally, acute gastroenteritis has about a 5-day duration. Life-threatening gastroenteritis seldom occurs in the United States.

Diarrheal diseases are a worldwide leading cause of illness and death among children younger than 5 years of age (Lozano et al., 2013). Infants are particularly vulnerable to gastroenteritis with subsequent dehydration. Treatment for these children includes breastfeeding, oral rehydration solution, and zinc supplementation. Studies have shown benefits of probiotics in preventing and treating GI diseases (Ritchie & Romanuk, 2012).

Pathophysiology

Microbes that cause gastroenteritis are transmitted by the fecal–oral route. Hands are contaminated with stool by not washing them after toileting or changing an infant's diapers. These contaminated hands are then placed directly into the mouth or on foods, and then the contaminated food is consumed. The bacteria or viruses either remain unchanged in the food or continue to grow and multiply, possibly producing toxins.

Assessment

Typical signs and symptoms include diarrhea, nausea, vomiting, and abdominal pain. However, specific findings vary with the causative organism. For example, some organisms produce watery diarrhea, whereas others produce bloody diarrhea. Fever, nausea, and vomiting may be present with some infections but missing with others. History regarding duration of symptoms, underlying or preexisting condition including an immunocompromised status, sick contacts, dietary changes, presence of blood in stool, recent travel, exposure to pets, recent use of antibiotics, and history of fever may assist in directing the workup. A physical examination is done to rule out other extraintestinal causes, such as a urinary tract infection or otitis media. The physical examination also allows the health care provider to assess for clinical evidence of dehydration. Signs such as capillary refill less than 2 seconds, dry mucous membrane, absence of tears, and ill general appearance are associated with a greater sensitivity to fluid volume deficit.

Diagnostic Tests

Examination of the stool both physically (noting color, consistency, odor, and volume) and microscopically (leukocytes, ova or parasites, culture) is essential. Fresh stool is sent to the laboratory for culture. However, in a healthy infant or child who presents without fever and no blood in the stools, stool cultures may not be ordered. The laboratory reports positive culture results for *Salmonella*, *Shigella*, *Campylobacter*, *Yersinia*, or hemorrhagic *Escherichia coli*. Other tests include enzyme immunoassay for *Clostridium difficile* toxins and rotavirus as well as neutralizing antibody for other viral agents. Many laboratories use DNA probes and polymerase chain reaction for certain organisms.

If the child is febrile, a urine culture may be considered to rule out urinary tract infection, and serum electrolytes may be obtained for evaluation of dehydration.

Interdisciplinary Interventions

Treatment consists of rehydration and correcting any electrolyte imbalances (see thePoint for Care Path: An Interdisciplinary Plan of Care for the Child With Gastroenteritis). Antibiotic therapy depends on the severity of the illness or whether a specific pathogen is isolated. Often, antibiotics do not alter the course of the illness significantly and contribute to the development of resistant strains and/or a carrier state of infection. However, antibiotics may be useful for life-threatening infections.

Assess and monitor the child for signs of fluid and electrolyte imbalance (see Chapter 17 for an in-depth discussion of assessment and treatment). Oral rehydration therapy is the method of choice for treatment of children with gastroenteritis who have mild to moderate depletion. Oral rehydration therapy does not necessitate hospitalization, so it is advantageous in maintaining family cohesion. Provide parents with detailed teaching about how to implement oral rehydration therapy—what fluid to use, how long to continue, how to advance the child's diet, signs of worsening status in the child, and when to notify the health care provider. If the child is severely dehydrated, or fails to improve on oral rehydration, hospitalization may be necessary for IV hydration. Observe contact precautions when handling stool or stool-contaminated items. When caring for patients with gastroenteritis, educate all caregivers to clean hands with soap and water until an organism is identified. Waterless alcohol-based products for hand hygiene do not kill the spores of *C. difficile*.

Probiotic use has been extensively studied for acute diarrhea. Recommendations to use probiotics are gaining much attention because of their safety and minimal side effects. Some practitioners recommend using probiotics in the treatment of rotavirus infection. Studies, in general, have limitations in the methodology; thus, more controlled studies are needed to validate this practice. Nonetheless, the use of probiotics may play a treatment role in some cases and has been shown to decrease the duration and severity of acute diarrhea (Ritchie & Romanuk, 2012). There is also some evidence that *Saccharomyces boulardii* may be helpful in preventing recurrent *C. difficile* infection (Kelesidis & Pothoulakis, 2012)

Diarrheal stools are irritating to the perianal area. Instruct the older child to wipe gently but thoroughly. If the area is excoriated, use moist, soft towelettes. If not toilet trained, change children's diapers as soon as possible after stooling. Wash with a moist, soft cloth and apply a thick layer of petroleum jelly, zinc oxide ointment, or other skin barrier product.

Community Care

Poultry is often positive for *Campylobacter* and *Salmonella*; therefore, teach family members to wash their hands and cooking implements thoroughly after handling poultry. Often, daycare centers are sources of outbreaks for *Campylobacter*, *Salmonella*, *Shigella*, and rotaviral gastroenteritis. Again, teach effective hand hygiene, especially after diapering an infant, and proper disposal of diapers in occlusive bags prior to disposing outside the home. Emphasize separating food preparation areas and diaper-changing areas. Serve as a liaison between the daycare center and the family by providing accurate information. Advise the family to keep infants not yet toilet trained out of the daycare center until diarrhea stops.

Report food-borne outbreaks of gastroenteritis to the local health department for tracing and prevention of further cases of food poisoning.

Currently, there are two rotavirus vaccines available (Rotarix and RotaTeq), administered as oral preparations with schedules set forth by the Centers for Disease Control and Prevention. There is much hope that these vaccines will reduce the burden of rotavirus disease in children in the United States. There is also great promise, as the details of availability to areas outside the United States are processed, for advancement of greater global health care issues to reduce the number of deaths from gastroenteritis.

APPENDICITIS

 QUESTION: How typical is Cory's experience with appendicitis?

Appendicitis is an obstruction of the vermiform appendiceal lumen at the end of the cecum. It is a common condition, with approximately four appendectomies per 1,000 children performed annually (Pepper et al., 2012). It is most common in children between age 6 and 14 years, with peak incidence at age 9 to 11 years. Appendicitis is rare in children younger than age 2 years. Diagnosis of acute appendicitis in children younger than age 7 years may be difficult because they may not have the typical presentation.

The prognosis for appendicitis is good with early recognition and surgical intervention. Perforation is most common in children. Perforation rates vary from 30% to 42%, influenced by access to surgical care (Lee et al., 2012). Perforation leads to potential complications such as wound infection, intra-abdominal abscess, and peritonitis, in addition to increased length of stay and costs. Mortality from appendicitis is rare.

Pathophysiology

Appendicitis begins with obstruction of the lumen of the appendix by a fecalith (a concrete mass of fecal material) or by lymphocytic hyperplasia. With obstruction, the flow of normal mucosal secretions is inhibited, resulting in increased intraluminal pressure and compromised venous drainage. Ischemic breakdown with simultaneous bacteria of the lumen wall occurs. These events lead to appendicitis, which may become complicated by gangrene and perforation.

Assessment

The health history and physical assessment provide valuable information in the diagnosis of appendicitis and often are the only diagnostic tools needed. Focus the history on determining the time of onset and location of the pain. The parent or child may describe the pain as initially being periumbilical and then migrating to the lower right quadrant. Younger children may describe the pain as more generalized, whereas older children are better able to localize the pain. The pain is initially crampy as the appendix distends against obstruction, but it becomes more constant as inflammation increases and the appendix distends further. Also elicit any recent history of nausea, anorexia, vomiting, and fever. In appendicitis, low-grade fever, nausea, anorexia, and vomiting typically occur after the onset of abdominal pain. Diarrhea may be present in very young children.

 ALERT   *With perforation of the appendix, abdominal pain is suddenly relieved; however, it returns (along with signs of a generalized acute abdomen) as peritonitis develops. Therefore, sudden cessation of appendicitis pain is an ominous sign.*

During the physical examination, observe whether the child guards the area of pain or winces with movement, such as walking or climbing onto the examination table or hospital bed. The abdomen appears flat with imperforated appendicitis; abdominal distention may be present after perforation occurs. The child with imperforated appendicitis may have only mild temperature elevation. After perforation, the temperature may rise to 101° to 104° F (38.3° to 40° C), and the child may appear dehydrated. Signs of shock may be present if peritonitis is advanced.

On auscultation, bowel sounds are normal to hyperactive early during the course of appendicitis but become hypoactive with perforation. Percussion reveals irritation and pain in the right lower quadrant. Rebound tenderness is present with palpation in the right lower quadrant, referred to as *McBurney's point* (point of tenderness, one third of the distance from the right anterior superior iliac spine along a line extending to the umbilicus).

caREminder

Palpate the right lower quadrant last during the physical assessment of the child with suspected appendicitis. Doing so enables you to assess the child's response more accurately in comparison with the response in quadrants that should be free of pain.

Diagnostic Tests

A CBC and urinalysis are obtained as a part of the workup of the child with suspected appendicitis. Although laboratory tests may not be helpful in establishing a definitive diagnosis of appendicitis, they are important tools in ruling out other potential causes of illness. White blood cell counts are elevated in 80% of patients with acute appendicitis. These counts may be normal early during the course of the disease but increase as inflammation progresses. Therefore, a second CBC is often done for comparison. Urinalysis may reveal a small number of white blood cells in the urine as a result of urethral irritation from the proximity of the urethra to the inflamed appendix.

Ultrasound is also used as a first-line imaging tool. Some reports state it is less sensitive and more operator dependent and is thus not as helpful as a diagnostic tool. Some institutions have adopted the practice to use ultrasound first to reduce the child's exposure to ionizing radiation and to determine whether additional imaging is necessary if a confident diagnosis cannot be made.

Radiographic evaluation is not a standard part of the workup of the child with suspected appendicitis but may be useful if the diagnosis is uncertain. When a plain radiograph of the abdomen is obtained, it is not diagnostic. Imaging studies assist the surgeon in making an accurate diagnosis when the clinical findings are inconsistent. CT scanning is often used because of its high sensitivity. It provides a complete assessment of the imaged region, defining a perforated appendix or, with a complicated appendectomy, identifies abscess formation. However, there is growing concern over the widespread use of CT scanning and the radiation risk it poses to children.

Interdisciplinary Interventions

Surgical appendectomy through a right lower quadrant transverse incision is the definitive treatment for appendicitis. In some centers, laparoscopic appendectomy may be a treatment option for the child with uncomplicated, imperforated appendicitis. For those children in whom the diagnosis is in doubt, such as adolescent females, or for obese children, a laparoscopic approach may be advantageous. This approach avoids a larger incision than may be needed with the traditional open approach. The laparoscopic approach enables intraperitoneal exploration and a wider visual field. All children with suspected appendicitis receive preoperative IV antibiotics. Postoperative administration of antibiotics after an uncomplicated appendectomy for appendicitis without perforation is thought to reduce the incidence of wound infection. The hospital stay may be 1 to 2 days.

Management includes comfort measures, pain control, and IV hydration until an oral diet is tolerated. Discharge criteria include a normalized white blood cell count, afebrile status, tolerance of oral diet, and adequate pain control with oral medicines (see thePoint for Care Path: An Interdisciplinary Plan of Care for the Child With Nonperforated Appendicitis). Traditionally, pain management for simple imperforated appendicitis included acetaminophen with codeine. About 10% of children are now known to lack the receptors for converting codeine into a bioavailable form (see Chapter 10). When poor relief is obtained from this medication, other analgesics are recommended.

In the event of complicated appendicitis by perforation, intraoperative debridement of necrotic material and lavage of the peritoneal cavity are performed. The optimal antibiotic treatment has not been determined. Narrow-spectrum antibiotics such as aminoglycoside-based triple-antibiotic therapy, which achieve adequate coverage for the most common organisms and reduce the incidence of antibiotic resistance, have traditionally been used. There is a growing trend, however, toward broad-spectrum monotherapy (piperacillin/tazobactam or cefoxitin), which has had at least equal efficacy to the traditional method and which may decrease the length of hospital stay and hospital costs (Lee et al., 2012).

Intestinal ileus may persist for 3 to 5 days after surgery, making it necessary for the child to remain NPO and receive NG decompression and IV fluids until oral intake can be resumed. In some cases, the child may be discharged early and may complete the IV antibiotics at home.

When children present with a perforated appendix that has become a localized abscess with right lower quadrant peritoneal irritation, an interval appendectomy may be considered in a select group of patients. These children are treated with IV antibiotics following CT-guided drainage of the abscess. The appendectomy is scheduled for several weeks after this treatment.

Complications of appendicitis occur more frequently after appendectomy for a perforated appendix. The most common complication is a wound infection and abscess. When this complication occurs, opening the wound to achieve healing by secondary intention is the treatment. Wound cultures and antibiotics may be ordered. A wound abscess may be drained under CT guidance.

Preoperative management of the child with appendicitis requires careful and ongoing assessment of the child's vital signs, pain, and hydration status. Promptly report changes in vital signs and any changes in the character of the child's pain that are consistent with the onset of perforation and peritonitis to the medical team. Traditionally, pain medication has been held until the diagnosis is firmly established to avoid masking symptoms.

More recently, studies have reported that administration of analgesics did not seem to interfere with identifying a diagnosis of appendicitis (Green et al., 2005; Manterola et al., 2011; Yuan et al., 2010). Other reports indicate that the physical examination may be altered with administration of analgesics but does not result in an increase of incorrect management decisions (Ranji et al., 2006). More randomized, controlled studies are needed to support a practice change and to address comfort in this population.

Allow the child to assume the position that permits greatest comfort; incorporate relaxation techniques. The child will be NPO and will have an IV for antibiotics and fluids. Teach the child about patient-controlled analgesia if it may be used postoperatively (see Chapter 10).

Both child and parents may be fearful and anxious about the child's pain, multiple procedures, examinations, and the impending surgery. Offering clear, developmentally appropriate explanations of all interventions and providing emotional support to the child and family may help alleviate their fear and anxiety (Fig. 18-18; see Chapter 11).

After surgery, the child requires routine postoperative care and comfort measures. Monitor the child who has been treated for a perforated appendix for signs of wound infection. Routinely assess for return of bowel function and respiratory complications such as atelectasis or pneumonia. Provide interventions to maintain the proper function of the NG tube, and administer and monitor IV fluids and antibiotics. A drain may be placed to promote excretion of infected peritoneal fluid.

Reinforce preoperative instruction with the child and parents on the use of patient-controlled analgesia and the incentive spirometer. Analgesia is administered

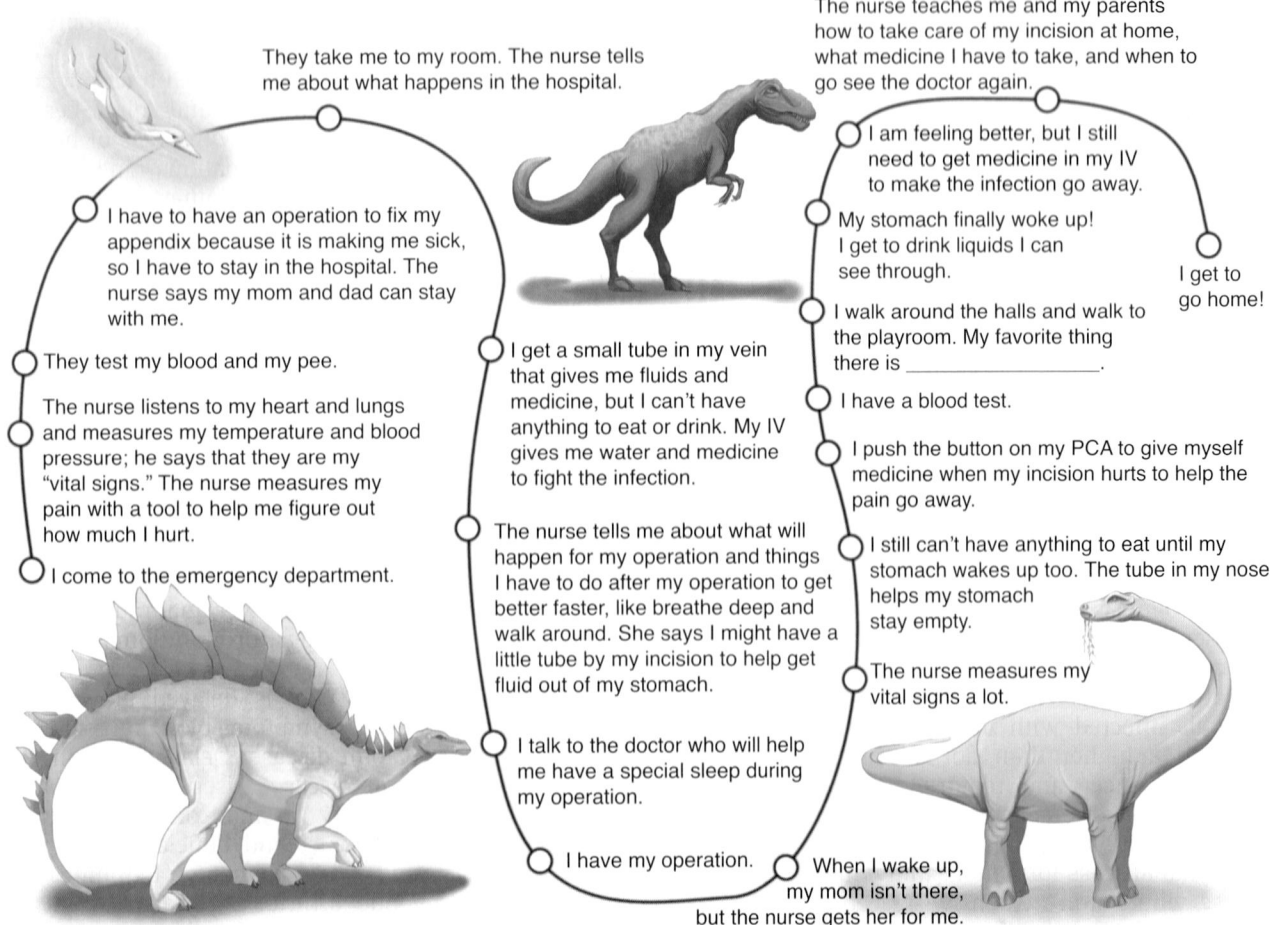

They take me to my room. The nurse tells me about what happens in the hospital.

I have to have an operation to fix my appendix because it is making me sick, so I have to stay in the hospital. The nurse says my mom and dad can stay with me.

They test my blood and my pee.

The nurse listens to my heart and lungs and measures my temperature and blood pressure; he says that they are my "vital signs." The nurse measures my pain with a tool to help me figure out how much I hurt.

I come to the emergency department.

I get a small tube in my vein that gives me fluids and medicine, but I can't have anything to eat or drink. My IV gives me water and medicine to fight the infection.

The nurse tells me about what will happen for my operation and things I have to do after my operation to get better faster, like breathe deep and walk around. She says I might have a little tube by my incision to help get fluid out of my stomach.

I talk to the doctor who will help me have a special sleep during my operation.

I have my operation.

When I wake up, my mom isn't there, but the nurse gets her for me.

The nurse teaches me and my parents how to take care of my incision at home, what medicine I have to take, and when to go see the doctor again.

I am feeling better, but I still need to get medicine in my IV to make the infection go away.

My stomach finally woke up! I get to drink liquids I can see through.

I get to go home!

I walk around the halls and walk to the playroom. My favorite thing there is _____.

I have a blood test.

I push the button on my PCA to give myself medicine when my incision hurts to help the pain go away.

I still can't have anything to eat until my stomach wakes up too. The tube in my nose helps my stomach stay empty.

The nurse measures my vital signs a lot.

Figure 18-18 A care path for a child with perforated appendix.

before use of the incentive spirometer or ambulation to progress the child toward recovery with maximum cooperation from the child.

Community Care

Families of a child who is eligible for early discharge require instructions regarding wound care, line care, and administration of IV antibiotics. Request a referral for home health nursing and home pharmacy services to support the family in the home transition. Instruct the parents to contact the surgeon if signs of infection, fever, anorexia, abdominal pain, vomiting, or diarrhea occur. Clarify the child's permitted activity level with the surgeon. Often, children can return to school in a week and resume normal activities, such as participating in physical education, within 4 weeks.

ANSWER: Much of Cory's experience with appendicitis is typical; however, Cory is younger than most children who have appendicitis. Remember, the peak ages are 9–11 years. Cory's inflammation also progressed until the appendix ruptured, which occurs in only 35% of cases.

INFLAMMATORY BOWEL DISEASE

IBD is actually a group of diseases characterized by inflammation of the GI tract. Crohn disease and ulcerative colitis are the most common forms of IBD and together account for more than 80% of all cases. Ulcerative colitis results in an inflammation of the mucosal layer of the large intestine and rectum. Inflammatory disease associated with Crohn disease can occur in any part of the GI tract, from the mouth to the anus, and is transmural. The classification of indeterminate colitis has been used to describe those children who have ambiguous characteristics and cannot be accurately designated as having Crohn disease or ulcerative colitis (Gramlich & Petras, 2007).

The incidence of IBD in the United States is estimated at 71 per 100,000 people, with 20% to 25% developing in children and adolescents with a median age of 15 years at diagnosis (Gray et al., 2011). The most important risk factor for developing IBD is a positive family history. Children with IBD more often have a family history of IBD than do adults with IBD (Day et al., 2012). Genetic, immunologic, and environmental factors have been cited in the etiology of IBD. Although the precise interaction between these factors is not well understood, individuals with IBD are thought to have a genetic predisposition to an immunologically mediated inflammatory response to certain environmental triggers.

Increased incidence and prevalence of IBD has been documented worldwide. One explanation is the "hygiene hypothesis," which advances a fundamental lifestyle change has resulted in a low microbial exposure from a formerly high microbial exposure. Exposure to fewer microbial antigens during early years leads to a less robust immune system. This ultimately results in the body's inability to mount a strong immunologic response to potential exogenous challenges to offending agents in later years and thus may consequently lead to chronic inflammation (Kugathasan & Fiocchi, 2007).

The prognosis for all forms of IBD depends on the type, severity, and extent of disease and the response to medical therapy. Surgery is ultimately curative for ulcerative colitis. Over the long term, however, individuals affected with ulcerative colitis have demonstrated a higher than normal risk of developing colorectal cancer and require ongoing monitoring. Crohn disease is a recurrent disease. Long-term complications may include stricture, fistula, and intra-abdominal abscess formation. Individuals with severe disease who require extensive resection of diseased bowel may be left with short bowel syndrome and long-term dependence on PN.

Pathophysiology

The exact pathophysiology of IBD is not known, but it is believed to involve defective regulation of the intestine's immune-mediated response to an environmental trigger, resulting in varying degrees of injury to the inner lumen of the GI tract. The patterns of injury vary by disease, both grossly and histopathologically (Table 18-6). The inflammation associated with ulcerative colitis is confined to the rectum and large intestine. The inflammatory lesions are continuous and involve only the mucosal layer. The inflammation associated with Crohn disease may occur in any part of the GI tract but commonly involves the terminal ileum and colon. Lesions are intermittent and transmural, with areas of healthy tissue between areas of inflammation. Linear ulcerations, aphthous ulcers, and granulomatous lesions are all associated with Crohn disease.

Assessment

Clinical manifestations of IBD can be seen not only in the GI tract but systemically as well. The characteristic GI manifestation of ulcerative colitis is bloody diarrhea accompanied by crampy, typically left-sided, lower abdominal pain. Disease severity is assessed based on stool frequency and the severity of abdominal pain, along with the degree of fever, weight loss, anemia, and hypoalbuminemia. The diarrhea associated with Crohn disease is often watery, as opposed to bloody. Abdominal pain is a common complaint and is usually located in the right lower quadrant. Perianal disease with fistula, skin tags, or granulomas may be present.

Systemic symptoms such as delayed growth and anorexia may precede GI symptoms by months to years in many cases of Crohn disease. Delayed growth and weight loss in Crohn disease arises from decreased nutrient intake secondary to anorexia; early satiety; malabsorption of nutrients; and deficiencies of vitamins, minerals, and trace elements. Extraintestinal manifestations include arthritis, arthralgias, oral ulcerations, dermatologic changes (erythema nodosum), ophthalmologic changes, and osteopenia.

Diagnostic Tests

Diagnostic evaluation of the child with suspected IBD is done to rule out other potential causes of disease and to classify the type of IBD the child has. Laboratory studies are used as an initial screening measure. The CBC of the child with IBD frequently demonstrates microcytic anemia. The erythrocyte sedimentation rate is elevated in active Crohn disease; this finding is

TABLE 18-6 Characteristics of Inflammatory Bowel Disease

Characteristic	Ulcerative Colitis	Crohn Disease
Gross Morphologic		
Areas of involvement	Rectum and variable length of colon	Any area of GI tract, terminal ileum, and colon are common sites
Distribution of lesions	Continuous, uniform	Intermittent, "skip" lesions with healthy tissue between areas of inflammation
Fistulas, strictures	Absent	May occur
Histologic		
Ulcerations	Shallow; limited to mucosal and submucosal layers	Transmural, penetrating all layers of GI tract
Granulomas	Absent	May be present

less common in ulcerative colitis. Low serum albumin and iron levels are common, as are other nutritional markers that indicate malabsorption and malnutrition from GI losses and inflammation, such as total protein, total albumin, and fat-soluble vitamin levels. Normal values do not exclude a diagnosis of IBD (Mack et al., 2007). Stool samples are obtained to look for gross or occult blood and to rule out the presence of enteric pathogens. Fecal markers such as calprotectin and lactoferrin (proteins released from activated neutrophils in the bowel mucosa) assess for inflammation. Baseline liver enzyme levels are obtained to monitor for potential side effects of pharmacologic management and to screen for associated liver disease (primary sclerosing cholangitis).

Other serologic tests may include an assay for C-reactive protein, which is an inflammatory marker. Commercially developed tests using perinuclear anti-neutrophil cytoplasmic antibodies, anti-*Saccharomyces cerevisiae* antibodies IgG and IgA, and other antibodies as well as genetic and inflammatory markers are available. Once IBD has been diagnosed, they can be helpful in differentiating between ulcerative colitis and Crohn disease and predicting the severity of disease. Because these tests are expensive and have a sensitivity of about 60%, it is preferable not to use them as a screening tool.

Endoscopy and intestinal biopsy, which are the gold standard, are done to establish and differentiate the diagnosis of IBD with histologic confirmation. Subsequent endoscopic evaluation may be done during the course of treatment to assess the child's response to therapy. Radiographic studies are done to visualize the pattern and extent of lesions and to screen for strictures or fistulas. A small bowel follow-through or MRI study may be obtained to evaluate the small intestine for disease involvement. Ultrasound and MRI may be used to document complications such as abscess formation, fistulae, and bowel wall thickening. Recently, concerns regarding the amount of radiation exposure that children with IBD may receive have surfaced (Fuchs et al., 2011), and because of the increased risk of cancer, the use of studies which use large amounts of radiation, such as computed axial tomography, should be minimized.

Nursing Diagnoses and Outcomes

In addition to those listed in the Nursing Plan of Care 18-1, the following nursing diagnoses and outcomes may apply to the child with IBD:

Nursing Diagnosis: Risk for impaired skin integrity related to effects of diarrhea
Outcomes:
- Child will be free from perineal erythema or excoriation.
- Child's skin will remain intact.
Nursing Diagnosis: Disturbed body image related to perceptions of disease and effects of therapy, restricted diet, effects of medications, retarded growth, and delayed sexual maturation

Outcome: Child will verbalize a positive self-image.
Nursing Diagnosis: Ineffective coping related to chronicity of the condition
Outcomes:
- Child will verbalize feelings and identify own strengths.
- Child will develop alternative, positive coping strategies.
- Child will identify and use external resources, such as peer support, group participation, one-on-one support, camp for teens with special needs or IBD, or counseling with a mental health practitioner.

Interdisciplinary Interventions

Interventions for managing IBD involve a variety of treatment methods, including medical, nutritional, and surgical therapies. IBD is a chronic condition with symptoms that are frequently distressing and may alter the child's usual activities of daily living. Ongoing psychosocial assessment and support as well as sensitivity to the stresses that the disease and its treatment place on the child and family are essential.

Medical therapy for IBD uses various agents. Treatment regimens are individualized depending on the type, location, and severity of the disease and the presence of extraintestinal or systemic manifestations. Patient and family education and monitoring for response to therapy and side effects are important nursing activities.

Pharmacologic Therapy

Corticosteroids were once the pharmacologic mainstay of medical therapy in treating both Crohn disease and acute moderate to severe ulcerative colitis. Today, their role is limited to acute exacerbations and as a bridge to maintenance therapy. Although their specific mechanism of action in IBD is not precisely understood, the manner in which they modulate cell-mediated immunity produces an anti-inflammatory effect that can induce remission of IBD symptoms. These medications are not optimal for long-term therapy because they fail to prevent relapse and they cause adverse side effects. Thus, other medications are used with corticosteroids, with the goal of weaning the patient off the corticosteroids as soon as possible. Corticosteroids are administered as oral prednisone or prednisolone or as IV methylprednisolone. In severe disease, in which malabsorption may be present, corticosteroids are initiated in the IV form and then transitioned to the oral form when enteric absorption becomes more reliable. These agents are administered at high doses initially, followed by a slow-tapered schedule until a maintenance dose is achieved. Continual tapering of steroids is a goal. These medications are adjusted according to the child's response to therapy. Children require ongoing monitoring for side effects while receiving corticosteroid therapy. Acute side effects during high-dose therapy include glucose instability, hypertension, fluid and sodium retention, and mood swings. Long-term side effects of special concern in children include growth impairment and bone demineralization. The cushingoid changes associated with corticosteroid use (moon facies, hirsutism, acne) may create body image concerns for the adolescent that can affect adherence to drug therapy.

KidKare Educating adolescents about the management of oral medications (e.g., steroids) and not to quit "cold turkey" or abruptly stop these medicines is vital for this developmental age, which is characterized by "omnipotence" as a central theme in psychosocial development.

First-line therapy in treating mild disease consists of sulfasalazine, and other aminosalicylate-containing medications are used to treat mild to moderate ulcerative colitis and colonic disease in Crohn disease. 5-Aminosalicylic acid (5-ASA) is the active agent in sulfasalazine and is primarily activated in the colon. 5-ASA inhibits prostaglandin synthesis in the colon, leading to a localized anti-inflammatory effect. 5-ASA–containing products are available in oral, enema, or suppository forms.

Metronidazole, an antibiotic with both antibacterial and antiprotozoal properties, has been used to treat IBD. Its primary benefit is in treating Crohn disease when perianal complications are present. Ciprofloxacin has also been used to reduce the microbial intestinal flora associated with inflammation.

Immunomodulating agents are used to treat moderate to severe IBD. These include azathioprine, 6-mercaptopurine (6MP), and methotrexate. Azathioprine and 6MP are commonly used for their steroid-sparing properties to reduce inflammation and maintain remission. A blood test for thiopurine methyltransferase (TPMT) should be obtained prior to the initiation of therapy. TPMT is the enzyme that metabolizes 6MP, and patients with low or absent activity are at increased risk for bone marrow suppression. Therapy must be administered for at least 3 months before efficacy can be established. Close monitoring for side effects, including suppressed bone marrow function, pancreatitis, and hepatitis, is necessary. There is a concern that in very rare cases, patients, especially young males, taking 6MP or azathioprine in combination with infliximab (Remicade), can develop hepatosplenic T-cell lymphoma (Mackey et al., 2009); for this reason, methotrexate is being used more frequently to treat IBD. Methotrexate can be administered weekly by intramuscular or subcutaneous injection in patients who have not responded to other first-line therapies. Side effects include nausea, stomatitis, diarrhea, and pulmonary interstitial pneumonitis, although this last effect is rare.

Biologic agents are genetically engineered antibodies to the inflammatory cytokine tumor necrosis factor alpha (TNFα), one of the proteins responsible for producing inflammation in IBD. Biologics reduce inflammation and help the tissue to heal, as evidenced by endoscopic and histologic evaluation. They thereby induce and maintain remission. The biologic drugs typically used to treat IBD are infliximab, adalimumab (Humira) and certolizumab (Cimzia). Infliximab is approved for use in Crohn disease and ulcerative colitis in pediatric patients. Adalimumab and certolizumab are approved for use in adults with Crohn disease. Infliximab is administered intravenously over 2 hours and repeated at scheduled intervals. Monitoring is required for acute infusion reactions, such as flushing, chills, chest pain, shortness of breath, and pruritus. Most infusion reactions are managed with antihistamines or corticosteroids and by slowing the infusion rate. Immunomodulatory and biologic therapies can make a patient more susceptible to infectious diseases. Counsel parents to inform their health care provider if their child has a fever or comes into contact with anyone with a contagious illness. Patients receiving these agents should not be given live virus vaccinations because they may develop the disease.

Nutritional Interventions

The goal of nutritional intervention is to provide adequate nutrient intake to optimize normal growth and development, including pubertal development (which is frequently delayed), and to prevent and correct nutrient deficiencies. Dietary management focuses on enhancing protein and calorie intake. Generally, a high-protein, high-calorie diet is recommended. During an exacerbation, the child may require dietary restrictions such as a lactose-free or low-fiber, low-residue diet to facilitate intestinal recovery. Many patients will self-restrict their diets as a result of nausea, abdominal pain, vomiting, and anorexia, creating more vulnerability to growth failure and poor nutrition.

Patients with IBD, especially those with Crohn disease, are at risk for fat-soluble vitamin deficiency from malabsorption caused by bile salt deficiency and inadequate intake. Iron-deficiency anemia is common from blood loss or impaired use of iron. Steroid use may increase urinary excretion of minerals. IBD affects bone metabolism, and the incidence of osteopenia and osteoporosis is high (Ghishan & Kiela, 2011). Monitor oral intake and assess for deficiencies. Routine supplementation includes a daily multivitamin and calcium. Vitamins D and B$_{12}$, plus folate, zinc, and iron, should be given, as necessary, along with fat-soluble vitamins in their water-soluble forms. The use and application of omega-3 fatty acids in the treatment of Crohn disease has been studied for its anti-inflammatory role. Results indicate that they are safe to administer, but the data do not support using omega-3 fatty acids to maintain remission in Crohn disease (Turner et al., 2009).

Studies have shown that enteral therapy is an effective induction therapy for children with newly diagnosed Crohn disease. It is given as the primary source of nutrition for 8 to 12 weeks, usually by NG tube (Critch et al., 2012). Elemental, semielemental, and polymeric formulas have similar efficacy. Efforts are underway to encourage enteral therapy use because of few adverse effects and the advantage to the child's overall growth and nutrition. For children with Crohn disease who require prolonged bowel rest for the treatment of fistulas or who have lost substantial amounts of intestine because of resection, long-term PN in the home may be necessary (see Chapter 17).

Surgical Interventions

Indications for surgical intervention in IBD vary depending on the type of disease present. For the child with ulcerative colitis, surgery is indicated in the presence of the following conditions: colonic perforation or hemorrhage, toxic megacolon, and growth failure from corticosteroids. Removing the diseased colon cures ulcerative colitis. In the past, colectomy with a standard ileostomy was the traditional operative approach. During the past 15 years, the ileal pouch anal anastomosis has become more common. With this approach, after colectomy, an internal pouch is constructed from the distal ileum and is anastomosed to the anus (Fig. 18-19). Complications of this procedure include pouch stenosis, which results in the obstruction of the outflow of stool from the pouch, and pouchitis, an inflammation of the pouch resulting from stool stasis. Various therapies are used for treatment, including antibiotics, probiotics, and topical agents. Although 90% of children achieve acceptable stool continence and frequency after the surgery, a small number may experience soiling or nighttime fecal staining.

Surgical intervention does not cure Crohn disease because Crohn disease is a recurrent disease. Surgical intervention, thus, is reserved to treat complications of Crohn disease. As with ulcerative colitis, emergency surgical intervention is necessary in the case of bowel perforation or hemorrhage. Intestinal obstruction from chronic inflammation and fibrosis may be treated with bowel resection and primary anastomosis. Stricture-plasty may be used in cases of partial obstruction. Surgical intervention may be indicated to treat a fistula or abscess that does not respond to medical therapy. If colectomy is required for intractable disease, a standard ileostomy is performed. The ileoanal pull-through is contraindicated for individuals with Crohn disease because of the risk of recurrent disease.

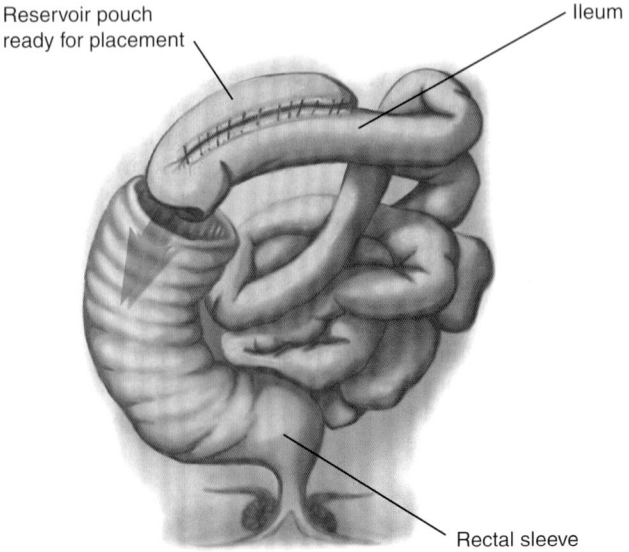

Figure 18-19 Ileoanal anastomosis with a pouch reservoir is commonly used for ulcerative colitis.

Community Care

The symptoms of IBD, as well as the side effects of therapy, may affect the daily life of the child and adolescent considerably. Shame and secrecy regarding GI symptoms, body image concerns, anxiety, and depression may all occur in the child with IBD. Supportive relationships with family, peers, and health care workers may be very therapeutic. Provide ongoing education, and encourage open discussion of concerns relating to symptoms, treatments, and side effects. Referral to community support organizations for target psychosocial interventions, such as specialized camps (Shepanski et al., 2005), has been shown to reduce overall psychosocial morbidity. Coordination with the school nurse for restroom privileges, as needed, and to use the school clinic bathroom for privacy and preservation of self-esteem is helpful.

PANCREATITIS

Pancreatitis in children is characterized by inflammation of the pancreas that causes clinical signs of abdominal pain and vomiting and is accompanied by elevated pancreatic enzymes. Pancreatitis may be acute or chronic. Acute pancreatitis is a reversible process; chronic pancreatitis results in permanent changes in the anatomy and function of the pancreas. Although the causes are numerous, the clinical pattern in all types is similar. The intensity of the disease and its complications may vary depending on the etiology.

The prevalence of acute pancreatitis is reportedly increasing, but the reason for this increase is unclear. In children, acute pancreatitis is caused by numerous factors. A review of past studies indicates that the main etiologies are biliary, medications (valproic acid, L-asparaginase, prednisone, and 6MP are most commonly implicated), idiopathic, systemic disease (sepsis, systemic lupus erythematosus), and abdominal trauma, followed by infectious, metabolic (diabetes), and hereditary causes (Bai et al., 2011). Biliary obstruction may prevent the ducts of the pancreas from draining. Disease of the biliary tract includes gallstones and gallbladder sludge as well as structural abnormalities, such as pancreatic divisum, and is seen in 10% to 30% of patients. Idiopathic, or acute pancreatitis of no identifiable cause, occurs in approximately 25% of cases (Kandula & Lowe, 2008). Pancreatitis caused by infection is seen in less than 10% of cases. Viral infections associated with pancreatitis include mumps, hepatitis A, rotavirus, varicella, adenovirus, and coxsackievirus B4. Most children with uncomplicated acute pancreatitis do well with supportive care. In rare cases, children can develop multisystem organ failure; the lungs and kidneys are most severely affected.

Chronic pancreatitis originates from similar causes as acute pancreatitis, and there are toxic/metabolic, idiopathic, hereditary, autoimmune, and obstructive forms. Several genes have been implicated in the hereditary form. Mutations have been identified in the cationic trypsinogen gene ($PRSS_1$), the pancreatic inhibitor gene ($SPINK_1$), the cystic fibrosis transmembrane conductance regulator gene (*CFTR*), chymotrypsin C (*CTRC*), and calcium-sensing receptor (*CASR*) (Whitcomb, 2012). Exacerbations of chronic pancreatitis and acute pancreatitis are similar and treated with the same approach, but children with chronic pancreatitis can go on to develop symptoms of chronic abdominal pain, obstructive jaundice, malabsorption, and diabetes mellitus.

Pathophysiology

The pathogenesis of pancreatitis is poorly understood, but inflammation results in edema of the pancreas and necrosis, apoptosis, and hemorrhage within the pancreatic tissue. Acute pancreatitis (most common) is usually self-limited. Recurrent acute pancreatitis can occur with normal pancreatic function in between cycles of inflammation. Recurrent acute pancreatitis is most commonly seen in children with underlying structural alterations and in those with familial or idiopathic pancreatitis. Pseudocysts or abscesses can develop, although these complications are infrequent.

Assessment

The child admitted with the suspicion of pancreatitis typically has a complaint of abdominal pain, either epigastric, upper left, or upper right quadrant pain (or some combination) that may radiate to the back. In the younger child, abdominal pain may not be as evident but rather may be manifested as irritability (Kandula & Lowe, 2008). Nausea and vomiting are common, particularly with ingestion of food. A history of anorexia is common. Fever, tachycardia, hypotension, and jaundice may be present. Abdominal signs such as abdominal distention, decreased bowel sounds, rebound tenderness, and guarding may also be noted.

Diagnostic Tests

Routine laboratory tests are done, including a CBC and blood chemistry panel. An elevated white blood cell count may be seen, and serum amylase and lipase levels are usually more than three times the normal value. Both amylase and lipase levels are monitored frequently for trending patterns throughout the course of the illness but do not correlate with the severity of illness (Kim et al., 2008). Total bilirubin, ALP, and blood glucose may also be elevated. CT and abdominal ultrasound are done to confirm diagnosis, determine severity, and identify complications. These studies assist in identifying a pancreas enlarged by inflammation, dilated pancreatic ducts, cysts in the common bile and intrahepatic bile ducts, or abscess formation. Endoscopic retrograde cholangiopancreatography and MRCP may also be done to evaluate the biliary and pancreatic ducts. Endoscopic retrograde cholangiopancreatography is used for both diagnosis and therapeutic interventions, such as a biliary sphincterotomy, dilation of a stricture, stone removal, stent placement, or drainage of pseudocysts. MRCP is useful for identifying structural abnormalities such as stenotic or dilated ducts or cholelithiasis. It offers the promise for even more frequent use in pediatrics because it is less invasive.

Nursing Diagnoses and Outcomes

Nursing diagnoses and outcomes for the child with a GI alteration are identified in Nursing Plan of Care 18-1. Pain management is a major issue for the child with pancreatitis because the inflamed pancreas causes severe pain. The following nursing diagnoses may also apply to the child with pancreatitis:

Nursing Diagnosis: Ineffective breathing pattern related to splinting (guarding) because of severe pain
Outcome: Child will demonstrate a breathing pattern that maintains oxygenation within the child's normal range.
Nursing Diagnosis: Dysfunctional GI motility related to irritation of the GI system leading to nausea
Outcomes:
- Child and family will discuss and use methods to decrease nausea.
- The child will report relief of nausea.

Interdisciplinary Interventions

The main interventions for pancreatitis are supportive, including administration of antibiotics, stress ulcer prophylaxis, pain relief by analgesic administration, fluid management, glycemic control, promotion of pancreatic rest during the acute phase until the child is stabilized (pancreatic enzyme levels are not increasing and pain is controlled), and monitoring for complications. Keep the child NPO to rest the pancreas. When severe emesis is present, an NG tube may be placed to decompress the stomach to prevent gastric distention. When the child is stabilized, nasojejunal feeding is started. This type of feeding is associated with improved immune function in adult studies (Marik, 2009) and, subsequently, is used in the treatment of children. PN via a central venous catheter (e.g., peripherally inserted central catheter) may be administered to support nutrition through recovery. Feedings are advanced slowly. A low-fat diet is used when nausea, abdominal pain, and decreased levels of amylase and lipase occur.

Patient positioning may play a role in nonpharmacologic comfort measures. Remind the patient to try a fetal position to minimize stretching or tension of the peritoneum. Pseudocysts and abscesses, if present, may require surgical drainage and antibiotic therapy.

Chronic pancreatitis treatment is also supportive but may evolve into a debilitating condition. Ongoing need for analgesics, loss of school attendance, and depression may be experienced as a result of the chronic nature of the condition.

Community Care

Educate the child and family about managing a low-fat diet and ways of incorporating the diet into the child's lifestyle when the child returns to school and in other social circumstances.

DISORDERS OF GASTROINTESTINAL MOTILITY AND FUNCTION

Disorders of GI motility and function involve a diverse group that includes functional abdominal pain and IBS (types of chronic abdominal pain), colic, GERD, and constipation.

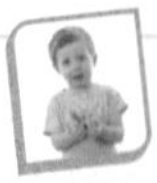

> QUESTION: Identify ways in which disorders of GI motility and function are different from the acute illness Cory experienced. What is the role of the nurse when children are cared for at home?

FUNCTIONAL ABDOMINAL PAIN AND IRRITABLE BOWEL SYNDROME

Numerous definitions exist in the literature that describe chronic abdominal pain, using terms such as *recurrent abdominal pain* and *chronic, functional, nonorganic,* and *psychogenic abdominal pain*. Efforts have focused not only on defining and clarifying terminology for the clinician but also on developing guidelines for evaluating and treating the spectrum of conditions based on extensive literature review, consensus of the expertise of the committee members, and evidence-based practice when available.

Chronic abdominal pain, formerly called recurrent abdominal pain, is one of the most common complaints of school-aged and adolescent children. In 1999, symptom-based criteria, known as the Rome II criteria, were developed to define functional bowel disorders associated with abdominal pain. Revisions were published again in 2006, known as Pediatric Rome III Criteria for Functional GI Disorders. These criteria address the following disorders:

1. Abdominal pain–related functional GI disorders, including IBS, functional dyspepsia, abdominal migraine, and functional abdominal pain
2. Cyclic vomiting syndrome, aerophagia, and rumination
3. Functional constipation and nonretentive fecal incontinence

The term *functional* is used to differentiate GI symptoms of a chronic or recurrent nature that cannot be explained by structural or biochemical studies (Rasquin et al., 2006).

This discussion is limited to functional abdominal pain and IBS. Functional abdominal pain is defined as weekly occurrences of intermittent or continuous abdominal pain for at least 8 weeks. Functional pain syndrome includes the previous definition with the addition of pain occurring 25% of the time and either some loss of daily function or additional somatic complaints such as headache, extremity pain, or sleep problems. IBS is defined as at least weekly abdominal discomfort or pain for 8 weeks, with at least two of the following three conditions present, at least 25% of the time:

1. Abdominal pain or discomfort improved with defecation
2. Abdominal pain or discomfort associated with a change in the frequency of stool
3. Abdominal pain or discomfort associated with a change in form (appearance) of stool

In addition, there is no indication of an inflammatory, metabolic, structural, or neoplastic condition that may explain the patient's symptoms.

Prevalence of functional abdominal pain is reported to range between 0.3% and 19% in children; IBS is reported to range from 6% to 14% in children and 22% to 35.5% in adolescents (Chio & Nurko, 2011). In adult studies, IBS is more prevalent in women, but no such pattern has been found in pediatric studies. Although the etiology is not as clearly defined as conditions having an organic etiology, remember that the pain is not imaginary. The child's experience of pain is *real*.

Pathophysiology

Complex factors influence GI function, including inflammation, positive family history of GI conditions, allergy, and psychoemotional states that can result in altered sensory experiences arising from these stimuli on the gut. The current understanding of pathophysiology in these disorders includes a disordered brain–gut communication between efferent and afferent pathways that signal messages between the central nervous system and the intestine. These disrupted signals may result from a postinfectious state disrupting the mucosal nerves, a genetically susceptible individual related to serotonin reuptake abnormalities, altered intestinal microflora, ineffective coping with perceived stressors, and associated psychiatric disorders that may influence the individual's experience but do not cause the symptoms. Visceral hypersensitivity, a child perceiving normal GI function as pain, was thought to be a factor in functional GI disorders, but newer studies have not been able to replicate the original findings. In IBS, altered motor function of the colon leading to increased or sluggish transit has been implicated (Camilleri & Di Lorenzo, 2012).

Assessment

Diagnosis of functional abdominal pain and IBS is based on typical health history data and normal physical assessment findings. Assess carefully to identify red flags that may indicate the need for a more extensive workup to rule out organic etiologies (Chart 18-2). Elicit specific information about the nature of the pain and associated factors. Obtain a thorough diet history to evaluate for food allergies or intolerances. Include the child in the interview, in a developmentally appropriate manner, to

CHART 18-2 **Some Indicators of Organic Causes of Abdominal Pain**

Unexplained fever
Weight loss
Deceleration of linear growth velocity
Evidence of GI blood loss
Severe vomiting
Chronic severe diarrhea
Persistent pain in right upper or lower quadrants
Family history of IBD

elicit his or her perceptions of the cause of pain as well as exacerbating and alleviating factors.

Functional abdominal pain typically manifests in children as episodic attacks of abdominal pain. Pain episodes may cluster in the morning or the evening. They may delay the onset of sleep at night but typically do not awaken the child from sleep. The episodes are not consistently associated with activities such as meals or bowel movements. Pain is usually localized in the periumbilical area without radiation and is nonspecific in character. A history of frequent school absences is common in functional abdominal pain. In some cases, it may be associated with physical, emotional, or sexual abuse.

IBS is characterized with pain and either diarrhea- or constipation-predominant symptoms. The pain is generally relieved by defecation. The individual experiences cycles of increased symptoms and symptom-free periods. Triggers that exacerbate the symptoms are identified, such as food, stress, and hormonal changes. Environmental stressors are frequently reported. Alterations in family dynamics may be present. For both conditions, physical assessment reveals no obvious abnormalities. Growth is not impaired, and weight loss is not seen.

Diagnostic Tests

A simple laboratory evaluation may be done to screen for organic disease. This evaluation includes a CBC, erythrocyte sedimentation rate, and urinalysis and culture because urinary tract infections can present as symptoms of abdominal pain. Stool specimens may be obtained to test for ova and parasites, *Giardia* (by enzyme-linked immunosorbent assay), and occult blood. A basic liver panel and albumin with amylase and lipase may be obtained. If lactose intolerance is suspected, a lactose hydrogen breath test may be done. If results are normal in the presence of a normal physical examination, further testing is likely not necessary to determine a diagnosis of functional abdominal pain or IBS.

Interdisciplinary Interventions

After a positive diagnosis of functional abdominal pain or IBS is determined, education and reassurance of the child and parents are the key elements in the treatment plan. As with many GI conditions, an interdisciplinary team approach is most beneficial for these complex problems. The physician, nurse, social worker, dietitian, and other health care professionals work with the family to outline the plan of care and goals. Reassure the child and family that the symptoms are not uncommon and explain the underlying mechanism of the abdominal pain. An analogy can be made to the treatment approach for a headache. A headache can be from a variety of causes, including diet, stress, fatigue, or tension. Most people recognize that many things cause headaches and that an individual's tolerance to headache discomfort also varies. Explain that the pain arises from a heightened excitability of the nerves that communicate to the brain, which is expressed by a feeling of stretching or spasm in the gut, to validate their pain experience. Assist the child and family to identify

triggers that exacerbate bowel symptoms and pain and ways to eliminate or modify them. Evaluate the child's and parents' specific perceptions and concerns about the pain, explore their coping skills, and help them develop methods to manage anxiety when pain is present (Clinical Judgment 18-2). One study reported that the intervention of distraction by their parents during pain episodes made the children feel better compared with the parents providing additional attention, reassurance, and sympathy (Walker et al., 2006).

Diet modification to avoid identified triggers has been suggested. Evidence that increased fiber in the diet provides a benefit is inconclusive. There is evidence that cognitive behavioral therapy may provide the skills to reframe, and thereby modify, the pain experience and reduce disability on a short-term basis (Di Lorenzo et al., 2005). Family therapy may be helpful to assist parents to reinforce adaptive and positive behaviors. There is also evidence that treatment with peppermint oil may benefit the child with IBS because of its properties to relax smooth muscles (Rahimi & Abdollahi, 2012). Tricyclic antidepressants have been used to reduce central pain perception. They are used in lower doses than for the treatment of depression. Selective serotonin reuptake inhibitors have also been used in the treatment of functional abdominal pain. With increased acknowledgment of the mind–body–spirit connection, multimodal therapies may become the strongest approach to long-term treatment; more studies are needed to tease out those interventions that are of most benefit (Camilleri & Di Lorenzo, 2012).

Community Care

If school absence has been an issue, help the child and family develop a plan for school reentry and for handling episodes of pain in the school setting. With parental permission, involve the school nurse and teacher in the plan to ensure a consistent approach. The nurse in the outpatient setting can serve as a valuable support and communication link for the family in treating these disorders.

Children with chronic abdominal pain may be at risk for later emotional symptoms and psychiatric disorders (Di Lorenzo et al., 2005). More research is needed to direct the care of children and families affected by these common problems.

COLIC

Colic, also known as the irritable infant, is a term used to describe a constellation of infant behaviors characterized primarily by prolonged periods of inconsolable crying in an otherwise healthy, thriving infant. The condition has been recognized for decades, yet complete understanding continues to elude the experts.

Colic is reported to occur in 10% to 30% of infants (Kheir, 2012). Differences in the incidence of colic by sex, cultural background, breastfeeding versus bottle-feeding, or birth weight have not been identified.

Colic is thought to be a multifactorial phenomenon. Its exact etiology remains unclear, although many theories,

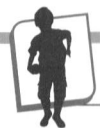

CLINICAL JUDGMENT 18-2

A Child With Functional Abdominal Pain

Rose is a 9-year-old girl brought in to the clinic by her mother and is complaining of abdominal pain. This pain has occurred before.

Questions

1. What other history would the nurse want to obtain?
2. What factors in the history are significant?
3. Does Rose have symptoms of organic disease?
4. What is the next step in the evaluation?
5. All laboratory results are normal. Rose and her mother are taught about functional abdominal pain, pain relief interventions (warm baths, distraction, talking about stressors), and Rose is referred for counseling to help her cope with her parents' divorce. What are symptoms of organic disease that warrant further follow-up?

Answers

1. *Past medical history*, including previous and current illnesses, immunizations, fever, allergies, food intolerances, normal weight, has Rose started puberty (occasional colds, otitis media, diarrhea, immunizations up to date, typical weight is 62 lb, she has not started puberty); *daily routines*, including patterns of elimination (describe number, amount, appearance), diet history, sleep patterns (voids four to six times per day; yellow urine; no dysuria; one stool every 1–2 days; brown, formed, no pain with evacuation; abdominal pain unrelated to stooling pattern; no change in sleep habits); *pain history*, including how long the pain has been occurring, how often, when does it occur (time of day, location such as school or home), where is it located, what is done when the pain occurs, does anything relieve or exacerbate it, has it been interfering with activities of daily living or school attendance or performance, Rose's and family's response to the pain, what does the family think is wrong (pain has been occurring one to two times per week for about 5 months, is crampy pain, located in the periumbilical region lasting 1–3 hours, usually in the evening, no medications are given, mother sits with Rose and distracts her with "talking about happy times" until the pain resolves, does not impact activities of daily living, Rose and her mother think Rose may have some disease); *family history*, including IBD, ulcer disease, recurrent or chronic pain, anxiety disorders (unremarkable except mother suffers from occasional migraines); and *psychosocial history*, including family functioning, school performance, peer relationships, previous stressors and typical coping style and response (parents are getting a divorce, Rose is doing her typical B and C work in school, has many friends, no major stressors previously, Rose usually reads or goes out to play when she is stressed).

2. History is predominately unremarkable except for recurrent abdominal pain, mother's history of migraines, and impending parental divorce.

3. No.

4. Explain to Rose and her mother that this type of pain may be caused by dysfunctional motility and things other than disease and that some laboratory tests will be done. A CBC, sedimentation rate, urinalysis, and possibly stool for Hematest will be done. Extensive testing may indicate to Rose and her mother that the health care team thinks something is seriously wrong and can increase their anxiety further.

5. Weight loss, fever, blood in emesis or stool, abdominal distention, or fatigue

---

both physiologic and psychological, have been proposed. Physiologic factors that apparently play a role in colic include the immaturity of the infant nervous system (which makes it difficult for the infant to screen out sensory stimuli). Another theory includes GI disorders ranging from such minor conditions as gas, cramps, and overeating to major disorders such as food allergy and GERD. Psychosocial factors that have been cited include parental anxiety and variations in infant temperament. Most cases of colic apparently result from some interaction between physiologic and psychosocial factors. Karp

(2004) has advanced the theory of the *fourth trimester*, suggesting that the infant essentially is born too soon, with all functions still immature. It proposes that the infant does not "wake up" and actively respond to the environment until the third month after birth.

Pathophysiology

Like the etiology of colic, the pathophysiology of colic also is unclear. In most cases, crying is a normal physiologic response on the part of the infant to distress or discomfort and serves to communicate the infant's needs to the parents. The normal 6-week-old infant may cry up to 3 hours a day, decreasing to 1 hour per day by age 3 months (Brazelton, 1962). In the case of colic, unexplained crying will generally begin at about 2 weeks of age, with a peak at 6 weeks to 2 months of age. The inconsolable crying lasts about 3 to 4 hours and can continue to 4 to 6 months of age. The episodes usually occur around the same time of day, often in the evening. No long-term negative physiologic sequelae are associated with colic. Although studies have supported all of the theories mentioned here as having a role in the pathophysiology of colic, none of them fully explain colic. Keefe et al. (2006) proposed an etiology as a delay or disturbance in the sleep–wake cycle of the infant's ability to self-regulate. The "fourth trimester" theory (Karp, 2004) is also compatible with previously described colic characteristics. Karp's research identified a "calming reflex" that occurs in utero that forms the foundation for his proposed interventions.

Assessment

A thorough history and physical examination rules out any organic sources of discomfort or distress. The infant with colic has prolonged episodes of crying but appears otherwise healthy and demonstrates appropriate weight gain. The crying episodes are often accompanied by abdominal distention and flatus. The infant may be noted drawing the knees in toward the chest. The colicky symptoms are consistent over time, unlike those of other GI conditions in infancy, which may present with abdominal pain but progress with other signs such as vomiting, diarrhea, abdominal distention, and fever. Parents may report that simple soothing measures are ineffective during the crying episodes. Note what methods have been used to calm the baby or to help the parents cope.

ALERT   *Assess the effect of the infant's behavior on the parents' feelings about parenting and on the family and marital relationship. The stress of caring for a colicky baby can result in shaken baby syndrome (see Chapter 29). Colic has been implicated as a trigger for infant maltreatment and parental dysfunction, such as neglect or inattentiveness (Keefe et al., 2006).*

Nursing Diagnoses and Outcomes

In addition to those listed in Nursing Plan of Care 18-1, the following nursing diagnosis and outcomes may apply to the family of an infant with colic:

Nursing Diagnosis: Risk for impaired parenting related to effects of prolonged, distressed crying
Outcomes:
• Parents will demonstrate an ability to read their infant's cues and respond quickly and appropriately.
• Infant will demonstrate a decrease in the amount of daily crying.
• Parents will identify sources of support for feelings of increased stress.

Interdisciplinary Interventions

Family education and counseling are the key interventions in managing infant colic. Teach the family to read the infant's cues to determine what infant need is being communicated. Teach them to determine what is normal infant crying and to understand the importance of meeting the infant's needs in a timely fashion. Make family members aware that by dealing with the crying episodes, they can also avoid escalation of crying to a point at which the infant cannot be consoled. Teaching soothing techniques and ways to handle the infant offers the family caregivers a sense of control (Nursing Interventions 18-1). Reassure the parents that too much holding will not spoil the infant.

Caring for the infant with colic can be very stressful and frustrating. Family members may feel a sense of failure because they cannot calm their infant. Acknowledge the parents' feelings and provide support. Assist the parents to identify family and community resources for respite. Emphasize the time-limited nature of colic, which usually diminishes by 3 to 4 months of age. This knowledge may help the family cope with their immediate frustrations.

CROSS-CULTURAL CARE

Many populations use star anise tea as a treatment for infant colic. Star anise tea has been documented to have neurologic and GI toxicities and should not be administered to infants because of its potential danger in this population.

GASTROESOPHAGEAL REFLUX DISEASE

GER is the passage of gastric contents into the esophagus. It is a normal physiologic process that occurs at all ages several times a day. It results in regurgitation in infants and young children because of the small size of their esophagus. GER is common in infancy and usually resolves by about 1 year of age.

GERD is present when complications arise (Sherman et al., 2009). Conditions that carry a high frequency of association for the development of GERD include EA, neurologic impairment, cystic fibrosis, motor dysfunction, increased intragastric pressure, delayed gastric emptying, and central nervous system disorders. Other high-risk groups of children include those who have a repaired omphalocele or a repaired CDH and chronic lung disease.

The prognosis for the child with GERD is related to the severity of symptoms and whether associated anomalies are present. By 1 year of age, most infants with mild to moderate reflux will become symptom free and able to discontinue medications. When medical therapy has failed or the symptoms are severe, surgery is indicated.

Pathophysiology

The body has a natural barrier system at the gastroesophageal junction to prevent the reflux of gastric contents into the esophagus that includes both anatomic

NURSING INTERVENTIONS 18-1

The Crying Infant

- Reduce sensory stimuli: minimize noise, light, extraneous movements; handle infant with firm, deliberate movements
- Contain the infant: keep extremities close to the body, swaddle tightly, use caution to avoid overheating
- Provide opportunities for sucking: nonnutritive or feeding
- Position on side or stomach for calming (not for sleeping), or hold infant with stomach pressed against your shoulder or in a football hold (infant's stomach against your forearm, infant's crotch at your antecubital fossa, and your hand supporting the head); the last two positions provide warmth and pressure against the infant's stomach, which may help calm
- Use low, calming, rhythmic voice; mimic (verbally or with commercially produced tapes) the "shhh" sounds infants hear in utero; play rhythmic 60-cycle music (e.g., Pachelbel's Canon in D)
- Use rhythmic movement: rocking, swaying, or swinging; use jiggly, rapid, small movements two to three times a second, interspersed with slow, broad swaying; teach parents never to shake an infant

and physiologic elements. Anatomically, the length of the esophagus, its orientation with the surrounding intra-abdominal ligaments, and the angle of His (made by the esophagus and axis of the stomach) play a role as a barrier to reflux. The LES is not an anatomic structure but a zone of specialized muscle that remains tonically contracted most of the time and aids in preventing reflux of gastric contents. Esophageal motility and gravity facilitate clearance of refluxed material as well as saliva. Effective gastric emptying is also a factor in preventing reflux. Under normal circumstances, the LES remains functional as a result of the combined anatomic and physiologic elements. The LES is controlled by the vagus nerve, and transient relaxations are triggered by gastric distension after a meal.

Conditions that cause a decrease in LES pressure lead to the development of GERD. Continuous LES hypotonia, incompetent LES, inappropriate LES relaxation, and anatomic disruption of the esophagogastric junction (e.g., hiatal hernia) are the most common mechanisms of decreased LES pressure. Esophageal motor dysfunction, increased intragastric pressure, and delayed gastric emptying are other contributing factors.

Both intrinsic and extrinsic factors can cause decreased LES. Children with central nervous system disorders have demonstrated an increased incidence of LES hypotonia. Medications such as theophylline and foods containing fat, chocolate, or caffeine, or those that are highly spiced, may cause transient decreases in LES pressure. Children who are fed enterally are at risk for reflux related either to gastric distention from bolus feedings or the presence of an NG tube.

When the esophagus is repeatedly exposed to gastric secretions, esophagitis results. The associated inflammation can cause pain (often called *heartburn* by older children), dysphagia, ulcerations, and chronic occult blood loss leading to anemia. Chronic esophagitis can result in stricture formation and altered esophageal motility. Barrett esophagus is a rare related condition that, even in children, can eventually lead to adenocarcinoma. Long-term studies on the sequelae experienced by adults when GERD is diagnosed in childhood are needed to provide a life span view of this condition.

Severe GERD can cause vomiting, which over time may lead to inadequate nutrient intake and FTT. Vomiting may also put the child at risk for pulmonary aspiration of gastric contents. Reflexive responses to the presence of refluxed material in the esophagus may trigger bronchospasm, laryngospasm, and, in some cases, apnea.

Assessment

Conduct a thorough history and physical examination when evaluating a child with suspected GERD to assess for causative factors and severity of symptoms and to rule out other pathologic conditions. A spectrum of symptoms is associated with GERD, and presentation may vary with age (Chart 18-3).

A careful feeding history and direct observation of feeding technique may be helpful in distinguishing GERD from more benign problems, such as overfeeding or inadequate burping technique. Additional history includes disruption of sleep pattern and behavioral changes.

Ascertain whether the child is experiencing regurgitation or vomiting. Parents may describe regurgitation and vomiting as the same entity. However, vomiting is forceful expulsion of gastric contents.

Diagnostic Tests

GERD is essentially a clinical diagnosis based on symptoms, but certain tests may be ordered to evaluate the severity of the disease as well as to look for any anatomic anomaly that may be contributing to the symptoms. Radiographic evaluation commonly includes an upper GI series to assess for anatomic or structural abnormalities, such as malrotation, hiatal hernia, or stricture. A gastric emptying study may be done to assess for delayed function. Upper GI endoscopy may

CHART 18-3 **Clinical Manifestations of Gastroesophageal Reflux Disease**

Gastrointestinal Manifestations

- Effortless regurgitation or vomiting after feeding in infants (this symptom is also seen with normal GER without any other symptoms present)
- Weight loss or FTT from decreased nutrient intake associated with vomiting
- Irritability
- Feeding refusal
- Older children may not experience vomiting but may report episodes of chest pain or heartburn associated with reflux
- Dysphagia and anemia associated with esophagitis
- Hematemesis

Pulmonary Manifestations

- Chronic cough, frequently noted at night when the child is supine
- Recurrent bronchopulmonary infections
- Bronchospasm, laryngospasm, apnea, and bradycardia can be associated with reflux episodes
- Reactive airway disease
- Chronic hoarseness

Other

- Sandifer syndrome: The child assumes a spasmodic posture, often after feeding, to facilitate esophageal clearance with neck extension and rotation of the head and neck to one side; typically, the back is arched with spine hyperextension

be done, with biopsies to assess for esophageal erosions and histologic changes from esophagitis.

Continuous intraesophageal pH monitoring (for 24 to 48 hours) is the gold standard diagnostic test. It is used to determine the frequency and duration of reflux episodes and their temporal relationship with the child's activity and symptoms. The parent or nurse must maintain a thorough record of all the child's activities and symptoms during the study, including the beginning and ending of feedings, sleep–wake periods, position changes, and any GI or respiratory symptoms. Carefully observe the child to ensure that the pH probe is not dislodged. The study may be done in the hospital or in the outpatient setting. In either setting, educate and support parents in their role in monitoring and recording their child's activity during the study period; parental monitoring and accurate record keeping contribute to meaningful test outcomes.

A more advanced technology for the pH study is available at some centers. This technology uses multichannel intraluminal impedance monitoring, which detects all reflux episodes, both acidic and nonacidic, as well as the direction of flow of the esophageal contents. It uses the principle of low voltage between placed electrodes on a multichannel intraesophageal catheter and measures differences in conductivity of refluxed

contents that are either gas, liquid, or mixed material between different esophageal segments. It can therefore identify a bolus in the esophagus and determine the height of the column of reflux in the esophagus. With this technology, it is also possible to assess whether symptoms, such as cough, apnea, or chest pain, are related to reflux (Mousa et al., 2011).

Interdisciplinary Interventions

Various treatment strategies are used to manage GERD. The choice of treatment depends on the severity of the child's symptoms and associated medical problems.

Conservative Management

Conservative management is a common approach taken for infants with mild GERD symptoms. Parental reassurance regarding a thriving, healthy infant is a critical intervention. Additionally, time-honored approaches involve modifications in positioning, diet, and feeding.

Evidence that infants have substantially fewer GERD symptoms in the prone position has been demonstrated with pH monitoring. This should not be recommended in children younger than 1 year of age because of the increased risk of sudden infant death syndrome (Vandenplas et al., 2009), but the infant can be held upright and prone on the parent's chest after feeding. For children who are older than 1 year of age, including adolescents, the guidelines state that there is a likely benefit to left-side positioning during sleep and elevation of the head of the bed. There is not sufficient evidence to support elevation of the head, although this is widely practiced, perhaps because many children with GERD also may be fed via an enteral tube. Positioning with the right side down promotes gastric emptying and can be used after feedings when the infant is well supported. Car seats hold an infant in a position that induces reflux. If a car seat is used, teach parents to ensure that the infant is not slouching, thus increasing intra-abdominal pressure.

The infant should be offered smaller, more frequent feedings. A meta-analysis demonstrated that thickened feedings are moderately effective in reducing GER in infants and is not associated with serious adverse effects (Horvath et al., 2008), thus they are often recommended. Teach parents to thicken feedings with rice cereal (1 tablespoon/oz with standard 20-cal/oz formula) and implement a feeding schedule with smaller feeding volumes at more frequent intervals. Formula thickened with rice cereal is commercially available. In some infants, GERD may be caused by cow's milk protein allergy or intolerance (Borrelli et al., 2012; Semeniuk & Kaczmarski, 2006). Studies have shown that changing these infants to an extensively hydrolyzed or amino acid formula significantly reduces symptoms. If the infant with GERD caused by cow's milk intolerance is breastfed, cow's milk should be eliminated from the mother's diet.

The effect of diet on GERD for older children and adolescents has not been widely studied, but it is agreed among pediatric gastroenterologists that caffeine, chocolate, alcohol, and spicy foods should be avoided if they aggravate symptoms (Vandenplas et al., 2009). Counsel patients not to eat for several hours before bedtime. Weight loss will decrease reflux, and smoking should be discouraged.

Neurologically impaired children and others with dysmotility often suffer from GERD, along with poor gastric emptying and constipation. They may have impaired swallowing and be unable to protect their airways from refluxed material. These patients will require enteral tube feeding, usually via gastrostomy tube. If reflux continues to be problematic, feeding via a gastrojejunal tube can be helpful. The gastric port can be used to decompress the stomach to prevent gastric juices refluxing into the esophagus while the patient is being fed into the small bowel. This approach can sometimes avoid or delay the need for surgery.

Pharmacologic Therapy

For moderate and severe cases of GERD, pharmacologic therapy is used in conjunction with conservative management strategies. Antacid preparations and H2 blocking agents (e.g., famotidine, ranitidine) are used to provide symptomatic relief of esophagitis and to reduce the damaging effects of refluxed gastric contents on the esophageal mucosa. Proton pump inhibitors (omeprazole, lansoprazole) are effective acid-suppressing agents and are superior in relieving symptoms. Prokinetic agents such as metoclopramide, low-dose erythromycin, and cisapride (available in the United States under extremely limited conditions because of the drug's potential for cardiotoxicity) are used to enhance gastric emptying.

Educating the parents about side effects of these medications is important. For example, metoclopramide can produce central nervous system side effects such as extrapyramidal reactions and dystonia. Accordingly, provide the parents with verbal and written instructions regarding medication administration, drug interactions, and ways to recognize untoward reactions promptly.

Surgical Interventions

Surgical intervention for GERD is indicated when symptoms do not respond to medical therapy, when severe complications exist, or when episodes are life threatening. The goal of surgical intervention is to create an anatomic barrier to reflux. The most common surgical antireflux procedure in children is the Nissen fundoplication. The fundoplication creates a one-way "valve" by wrapping the gastric fundus 360 degrees around the lower end of the esophagus. If fundoplication is performed as an open operative procedure, it requires a 5- to 7-day hospitalization. Laparoscopy is often used because this approach offers a more rapid recovery period, earlier discharge, earlier initiation of feedings, less postoperative pain, and is more cosmetically pleasing.

Immediately after the fundoplication, the junction between the stomach and esophagus (the "wrap") may be "tight" as a result of postoperative swelling, making belching and vomiting difficult. A temporary gastrostomy tube is often placed at the time of surgery to vent air from the stomach during the immediate postoperative period. The gastrostomy tube may be removed approximately 6 to 8 weeks after surgery, unless the child has a continued indication for enteral nutrition through the gastrostomy tube, which may be a common scenario.

Postoperative management includes assessing the effectiveness of gastric decompression by either NG or gastrostomy tube and assessing the surgical incision. Intake and output are monitored. Pain management is scheduled to optimize comfort and maximize progression of recovery. Effective pain management enables the child to perform activities to promote ambulation and to prevent pulmonary complications.

Feedings are initiated when bowel function returns. If a gastrostomy tube is in place, vent it before and after feedings and for retching and abdominal distention. Monitor and intervene early for constipation to avoid the child straining to stool. Collaboration with a pediatric registered dietitian and physical therapist may be beneficial when the child's condition is complicated by obesity.

Discharge planning and family education are important. Assess the parents' knowledge of postoperative care, management of the gastrostomy tube, and feeding schedule. Consider any underlying disease of the child when planning discharge and family education regarding treatment strategies. Instruct the family regarding dietary modifications, feeding techniques, positioning, and medication administration. Direct observation while the parents feed and position the child helps provide meaningful feedback. Provide education about medications, dosing schedules, and potential side effects verbally and in writing.

The child undergoing surgical intervention for GERD will need instruction regarding gastrostomy tube home management in addition to routine pre- and postoperative instructions. Teach the child, as developmentally appropriate, and family about gastrostomy tube site care, use of the gastrostomy tube for gastric venting, and feeding as indicated. Additional education includes problem solving for mechanical, feeding, and infectious complications as well as safety issues related to the child's developmental level. The family also needs education about gastrostomy tube replacement if accidental dislodgment occurs. Most surgeons and gastroenterologists identify a safe postplacement time frame during which this procedure may be done at home. Collaborating with hospital-based or health care insurance case managers is important to link the family to appropriate community resources for obtaining supplies and equipment necessary for home care.

Community Care

Home health follow-up is helpful to support the family during the initial postoperative period and to help the family transfer their knowledge successfully to the home setting. Ongoing monitoring of response to medical therapy is done in both the outpatient and home settings. Develop a plan for the child to return to daycare or school during the discharge process. When a child requires a gastrostomy tube, direct the family to contact the school and to complete required school forms to avoid delays in school attendance. Consider including child care and school personnel or other caregivers in the discharge plan. The school nurse is an important collaborator in this effort.

CONSTIPATION

Constipation is a delay or difficulty in defecation that has been present for longer than 2 weeks and causes considerable distress. In the past, there has been a lack of a generally accepted definition. A consensus of experts defined a spectrum of disorders of defecation in an attempt to provide uniform definitions to classify these problems for diagnosis and treatment and to collect information that directs outcomes based on consistent definitions (Rasquin et al., 2006). An elaboration of the previous simple definition from the Pediatric Rome III Criteria includes at least two of the following characteristics of constipation: hard or painful stools, defecations two or fewer times a week, at least one episode of incontinence per week, presence of a large fecal mass in the rectum, and a history of large-diameter stools that can obstruct the toilet (Rasquin et al., 2006). Further, the definition states that these characteristics must be present for 1 month in children up to 4 years of age and present at least once a week for at least 2 months in children older than 4 years and adolescents. Normal stool frequency varies developmentally, so the definition of constipation must be made relative to the expected developmental norm. *Encopresis* (fecal incontinence) is the involuntary loss of formed, semiformed, or liquid stool into the child's underwear after the child has achieved a developmental level of 4 years. Encopresis is usually a symptom of chronic constipation.

Constipation is a common pediatric problem, with a prevalence ranging from 0.7% to 29.6% (median 12%) (Mugie et al., 2011). Constipation prevalence reports vary by age and gender. One epidemiologic review reported an increased prevalence around the preschool age, which is a typical time for toilet training (van den Berg et al., 2006), yet overall prevalence gender rates are considered to be similar. Encopresis is more common in males (van den Berg et al., 2006).

Constipation may arise from a variety of disorders, both organic and nonorganic (Chart 18-4). Most commonly, it is the result of functional causes. After other underlying causes such as structural, metabolic, or endocrine have been ruled out, constipation may be called *functional constipation*. Encopresis most commonly arises from functional constipation in a child with no evidence of physical abnormality. It is manifested by the history of an expulsion of a normal bowel movement, usually involuntary, in an inappropriate place or inappropriate social context. Fecal incontinence, with or without constipation, arising from organic disease is less common. Children with special needs or chronic conditions are at higher risk than others for constipation and may experience constipation as a complication of their condition. This section covers only the topic of constipation.

CHART 18-4   Causes of Constipation in Children

Functional (Nonorganic)
Toilet training (starting too early, routine, or coercive)
Excessive parental intervention
School bathroom avoidance
Busy lifestyle
Very sedentary lifestyle
Immobility
Sexual abuse
Cognitive handicaps
Attention-deficit/hyperactivity disorder
Depression

Organic
Genetic predisposition
Dietary
- Excessive dairy intake
- Low-fiber diet
- Dehydration
- Malnutrition, underfeeding
Anal malformations
- Imperforate anus
- Anal stenosis
- Anterior anus
Intestinal motility disorder
- Intestinal pseudo-obstruction
Neurogenic
- Hirschsprung disease
- Spina bifida
- Tethered cord
- Hypotonia
- Myelomeningocele
- Cerebral palsy
Metabolic/endocrine disorders
- Hypothyroidism
- Hypercalcemia
- Diabetes mellitus
- Diabetes insipidus
- Lead poisoning
Medications
- Opiates
- Antacids
- Antihypertensives
- Anticholinergics
- Antidepressants
- Nonsteroidal anti-inflammatory drugs
- Diuretics
Situational
- Febrile or prolonged illness
- Surgery or bed rest
- Anal fissure or diaper dermatitis
- Change in child's diet or routine

Pathophysiology

The process of normal defecation depends on the interaction between numerous sensory and motor mechanisms. The rectum forms a right angle with the anal canal. The urge to defecate is initiated by distention of the rectum with stool. This event induces a reactive relaxation of the internal anal sphincter and contraction of the external anal sphincter. Squatting or sitting straightens out the angle between the rectum and the anal canal, enabling stool to pass easily. Increasing intra-abdominal pressure, as with the Valsalva maneuver, and voluntarily relaxing the contracted external anal sphincter permits feces to be expelled. It is important to have small children sit appropriately on the toilet with feet flat on the floor or a footstool so they may relax the muscles to help the defecation process.

Constipation is a symptom and, in children, is commonly the result of voluntary fecal withholding resulting from an experience of painful or frightening defecation. Another frequently cited time for constipation to emerge is during toilet training. Change in diet, illness, stress, beginning school, and not taking time from play to defecate have all been implicated as causes to functional constipation. Painful lesions, such as fissures of the anal or perianal region, or hardened stools may result in pain when feces are passed, causing the child to withhold stool to avoid pain. Psychosocial or behavioral factors also may contribute to constipation. Overly aggressive toilet training, childhood anxieties that cause the child to avoid school bathrooms, or intrusive parental interventions surrounding toileting habits may all result in stool withholding.

After a pattern of withholding is begun, a vicious cycle develops. As defecation is delayed, progressively larger amounts of stool are built up in the rectum for longer periods of time, resulting in more pain and more withholding. Fecal soiling results when a large stool mass stretches the walls of the colon and rectum, desensitizing the rectum, and involuntary leakage of semiformed or liquid stool occurs around the fecal mass.

Assessment

The goals of the initial history and physical examination of the child with functional constipation or encopresis are to assess causative factors and to rule out any potential organic causes. Note information regarding stool frequency, size, and stooling pattern; time first stool was passed after birth; and associated symptoms, such as fever, abdominal distention, anorexia, nausea or vomiting, weight loss, or failure to gain weight. Obtain a thorough diet and toilet training history, noting any pertinent psychosocial stressors.

Complaints of abdominal pain may be expressed. Assess the contour of the abdomen and note distention. Palpate for fecal masses, particularly in the left lower quadrant. Appetite may be poor. After passage of stool, parents may note that the child's mood and appetite improve. Question about urinary tract symptoms and incontinence, which can also be seen in the child with functional constipation and encopresis. Symptoms occur as a result of the dilated rectum placing pressure on the bladder, causing spasms. Recurrent urinary tract infections have been reported, particularly in females, usually related to ascending bacteria from fecal soiling.

Assess the sacral area for dimpling, which may indicate a spinal abnormality. Inspect the perianal area to note fissures, position of the anus, dermatitis, and rectal prolapse.

Diagnostic Tests

Barium enema or anorectal manometry may be done when problems persist or an organic etiology is suspected, such as Hirschsprung disease. Stools are tested for occult blood. A flat abdominal film allows the extent of the constipation to be evaluated and response to clean out, if performed.

Interdisciplinary Interventions

The treatment plan for the child with constipation is individualized depending on the severity of symptoms and on the child's developmental level. For simple constipation, incorporating more fiber, fruits and vegetables, and whole grain foods; discontinuing medications associated with constipation; and using laxatives may be effective. Increasing hydration, although commonly recommended, has not been shown to affect stool output or consistency (Rajindrajith & Devanarayana, 2011). Constipation in children with specialized chronic conditions requires additional evaluation and treatment that may be beyond the scope of primary care. For the child whose symptoms are more severe, the treatment plan is generally designed in three stages: (1) disimpaction (bowel cleanout) and patient education, (2) prevention of reimpaction/maintenance, and (3) establishment of regular bowel habits.

During the initial phase of education, the goal is to "demystify" the process of defecation and to help decrease feelings of guilt or blame. Describe the normal process of defecation and explain the pathophysiologic alterations associated with constipation. Using the abdominal radiograph to provide a visual image may reinforce the extent of the problem and understanding of the treatment plan with the parents and child. Explain the treatment or approach; provide options when able; and include the purpose of each therapeutic intervention, anticipated outcomes, and potential problems. Disimpaction is necessary to eliminate any fecal mass from the rectum that may be present. Disimpaction may be achieved with polyethylene glycol electrolyte-free solution (PEG 3350) at a dose of 1.5 g/kg/day until resolution or a maximum of 6 days (Savino et al., 2012) or, in severe cases, a colonic lavage solution. The colonic lavage may be administered through an NG tube by a continuous drip method. Some clinicians may routinely use enemas in severe cases, although this method may be traumatic for both child and family and can contribute to the cycle of aversive experiences the child associates with defecation. Enemas are also difficult for the parents to carry out at home. High doses of oral medications have been shown to be an effective cleanout method.

Children with special needs or chronic illness may require enemas in combination with oral agents. They may require admission to acute care for more aggressive interventions, such as administration of polyethylene glycol–electrolyte solution (GoLYTELY) via an NG tube plus use of an enema preparation. These children may be at increased risk for complications from administering enemas. When enemas are deemed necessary, the child should have small volumes with short retention times to reduce the risk for potential complications. Cardiopulmonary and intravascular volume status should be evaluated before administering hypertonic enemas.

The goal of phase 2 is to prevent reimpaction or maintenance. Treatment is designed to overcome the child's tendency to withhold stool. Various agents are used for this purpose—most commonly mineral oil and osmotic agents such as milk of magnesia, lactulose, or sorbitol. Polyethylene glycol, electrolyte free (Miralax), has been found to safely treat chronic constipation. This drug is not readily absorbed and is therefore an excellent bowel evacuating agent. It is better accepted than older agents because it is tasteless, odorless, colorless, and has no grit. It can be mixed with liquids such as Kool-Aid or Gatorade. Therefore, it is the agent of choice both for treating disimpaction and for maintaining stooling patterns (Benninga et al., 2005). If mineral oil is used, it should not be given to children at risk for pulmonary aspiration; it is also contraindicated in infants younger than 1 year of age. Oral agents are usually continued until 4 to 6 months after the last painful stool. The child must be weaned off the laxative slowly.

KidKare Give the child choices regarding how the Miralax or mineral oil is taken. Miralax can be mixed with beverages (water, juice, soda) and offered chilled. Serving mineral oil cold or mixing it with orange juice or carbonated beverages enhances its palatability. Emulsified mineral oil should be shaken before use and given with meals. It is more palatable than nonemulsified mineral oil.

The role of fiber is controversial; however, educating the child and parents about the importance of a balanced diet that includes whole grains, fruits, and vegetables promotes overall health. Increasing fluid intake will not correct the problem unless dehydration is present. A program to encourage regular toileting behaviors is also initiated at this time. Behavioral management is more helpful in conjunction with oral agents than oral agents alone. Children are asked to sit on the toilet for 5 to 10 minutes to 20 to 30 minutes after every meal and attempt to evacuate the rectum. This practice takes advantage of the natural gastrocolic reflex. A system of positive reinforcements/incentives, such as stickers, can be instituted to reward adherence to medications and toileting sessions. Proper alignment and positioning is important to flatten the anorectal angle and facilitate the passage of stool by supporting young children's dangling feet on a footrest. Encourage the parents to communicate the treatment plan to appropriate school and child care personnel to promote

consistency. Psychological and behavioral issues can present ongoing concerns for the child and family and may require intervention from a psychologist, social worker, or child development professional. Biofeedback may be beneficial for a select subgroup of children with persistent symptoms. The child is weaned off the medications as regular bowel habits become reestablished.

Community Care

The child with chronic constipation and fecal soiling can experience many negative psychological and social sequelae. Low self-esteem, poor school performance, and impaired peer relations have been reported. Family relationships can be affected negatively. Parents who do not understand the physiologic mechanisms that cause constipation with fecal soiling may become frustrated and angry with their child's recurrent soiling.

A collaborative effort between the child, family, and health care team is essential to successful outcomes during the treatment phase. The nurse, in the outpatient and school settings, plays an important role in the treatment plan. Child and family evaluation, education, and support, along with phone and clinic follow-up to monitor progress and make necessary modifications in the treatment plan, are key. Educate and support the family through the treatment phase, because a great deal of patience and time may be required to achieve successful outcomes. Follow-up is recommended for at least 1 year after initial successful treatment to reinforce success and provide treatment with laxatives if relapse occurs.

ANSWER: In many chronic conditions, parents assume the responsibilities of caregiving. In these instances, the role of the nurse centers on the family unit. The nurse provides education, reassurance, and support through telephone follow-up or outpatient visits.

DISORDERS OF MALABSORPTION

Disorders of malabsorption include chronic diarrhea, short bowel syndrome, celiac disease, and lactose intolerance.

CHRONIC DIARRHEA

Chronic diarrhea is defined as diarrhea that persists for more than 3 weeks. Because normal stool consistency and frequency varies developmentally, diarrhea is defined as an increase in stool frequency and alteration in stool consistency compared with the child's norm.

The incidence of chronic diarrhea varies depending on the etiology (Chart 18-5). In Munchausen syndrome by proxy, a rare form of child abuse (see Chapter 29), diarrhea may be induced by the administration of laxatives.

The prognosis of a child with chronic diarrhea depends on the underlying etiology. Some causes of chronic diarrhea are easily resolved, such as eliminating

CHART 18-5 Causes of Chronic Diarrhea

Infectious
Viral
Bacterial
Protozoal

Malabsorption
Congenital carbohydrate malabsorption
Lactase deficiency
Malabsorption secondary to mucosal damage
• Postinfectious enteropathy
• Cow's milk, soy protein intolerance
• Intractable diarrhea of infancy
• Celiac disease
Pancreatic insufficiency
• Cystic fibrosis
Short bowel syndrome
Malnutrition

Inflammatory Bowel Disease
Crohn disease
Ulcerative colitis

Immune Deficiency States
AIDS
Severe combined immune deficiency

Oncology
Hormone-secreting tumors
Radiation enteritis
Graft-versus-host disease

Drugs
Antibiotic-associated diarrhea
Sorbitol-containing drugs

Dietary
Overfeeding
Fruit juice
Excessive sweets, sorbitol

Anatomic
Partial obstruction
Malrotation
Blind loop syndrome

Other
Young child's diarrhea
Motility disorders
Encopresis
Bacterial overgrowth
Munchausen syndrome by proxy

the offending agent and treating an infectious process, whereas other causes, such as IBD or diarrhea related to pancreatic insufficiency, may have serious, lifelong consequences for the child.

Pathophysiology

The pathophysiology of chronic diarrhea depends on the cause of the diarrhea. Numerous physiologic mechanisms can result in diarrhea. Osmotic diarrhea results from malabsorption of an absorbable solute. This event creates a solute load in the intestine that results in increased fluid losses. Malabsorption of carbohydrates, whether because of mucosal injury or congenital defects of carbohydrate absorption, results in osmotic diarrhea. Overfeeding or excessive fruit juice consumption creates a high solute load in the intestine that also will result in osmotic diarrhea.

Certain intestinal infections, severe GI mucosal injury, or tumors may result in secretory diarrhea. The hallmark characteristic of secretory diarrhea is large volumes of watery diarrhea despite complete bowel rest. Other causes of diarrhea include mechanical obstruction and bowel resection. In the case of mechanical obstruction, formed stool cannot pass beyond the area of blockage, but liquid stool may leak around it. Massive resection of intestine reduces the absorptive surface area of the bowel and decreases bowel transit time, resulting in diarrhea.

Assessment

The child with chronic diarrhea requires a comprehensive diagnostic evaluation to establish the etiology of the illness.

When taking the history, ask questions to identify risk factors for infection. Carefully review the child's diet history and history of growth and weight gain. Assess for signs of dehydration, malnutrition, or other indicators of GI dysfunction during the focused physical assessment. Ask the child or family to save the stool so direct observation and quantification of the stool can be done.

Clinical manifestations of chronic diarrhea can vary depending on its etiology. Assess the appearance (consistency, size, and color), frequency, odor, and urgency of stool, which can provide clues regarding the underlying cause. Assess for blood in the stool, and ask about associated symptoms such as abdominal pain, fever, and vomiting. Assess and query about the stool pattern because stools may cycle between normal and abnormal daily or intermittently. The child with chronic diarrhea secondary to pancreatic insufficiency will have the large, bulky, foul-smelling stools characteristic of fat malabsorption. The child with diarrhea secondary to an inflammatory illness, such as ulcerative colitis, may have liquid stool with mucus and bright-red blood.

Physical assessment findings also vary. Although some children may appear quite well, others may appear acutely or chronically ill. The child's pattern of growth and weight gain will reflect the duration and severity of the diarrhea. Some children do not exhibit any alteration in growth and weight gain, whereas others demonstrate delayed growth, substantial weight loss, and FTT. Overt signs of nutrient deficiencies may be present in these cases. If the child has experienced severe fluid and electrolyte losses from the diarrhea, dehydration and metabolic imbalances may be evident on physical examination.

Diagnostic Tests

Laboratory evaluation of the stool can help differentiate between infectious, inflammatory, or malabsorptive causes. Stool culture for bacteria and for ova and parasites are obtained to assess for infection. Stool specimens for white blood cell counts, occult blood, and alpha 1-antitrypsin assess for inflammatory causes. Screening for malabsorptive disorders is done by measuring stool pH, reducing substances, fecal fat, and fecal pancreatic elastase-1. A sweat test is done to rule out cystic fibrosis. DNA analysis may also be done in conjunction with a sweat test to further evaluate for genetic mutations associated with cystic fibrosis.

Blood specimens are taken to evaluate for systemic disease, fluid and electrolyte imbalance, and nutritional status. A CBC with erythrocyte sedimentation rate or C-reactive protein, chemistry panel with electrolytes, liver and renal function tests, and serum protein level determination are done. Trace mineral and vitamin levels may be assessed. A hydrogen breath study may be done if malabsorption is suspected. Immunologic studies may be included in the workup, such as serum Ig with IgA and IgG subsets.

Radiographic studies are typically used only in situations in which the results of the history and physical examination suggest an anatomic defect, obstruction, or IBD. Endoscopic evaluation with intestinal biopsy, which includes small intestinal biopsy, is reserved for the child with suspected celiac or IBD, infection from a source not identified by stool culture, suspected mucosal injury of unidentified origin, or unexplained chronic diarrhea.

Interdisciplinary Interventions

Treatment of the child with chronic diarrhea involves treating the underlying organic source of the diarrhea, along with nutritional intervention to optimize digestion and absorption of nutrients and foster growth and weight gain. For the child with chronic diarrhea related to overfeeding or excessive juice consumption, treatment consists of nutritional counseling to normalize the child's diet. Modifying formula or diet may be necessary in malabsorptive disorders. Casein hydrolysate formulas, amino acid–based formulas, and modified protein–based formulas are commonly used in these cases. In cases of severe mucosal injury, enteral or PN may be necessary to support the child's fluid and nutritional requirements until mucosal healing takes place. The child with secretory diarrhea may require complete bowel rest and support with PN until the cause of the diarrhea resolves.

Management of the child with chronic diarrhea involves meticulous attention to fluid and electrolyte balance. Carefully assess and document all of the child's intake—whether oral, enteral, or by IV—and all output, including stool volume and characteristics. Ongoing assessment and management of any venous access device is essential to maintain delivery of parenteral therapies.

caREminder

Assess infant stool volumes by weighing diapers. If mixing of urine and stool makes accurate assessment difficult, separate stool and urine using an infant urine bag. To obtain a stool specimen, a disposable diaper can be applied inside out. The plastic barrier will not absorb the stool, which can then be removed and placed in the specimen container.

Replacement of fluid losses should be considered when stool volumes exceed 15 to 20 g/kg body weight per day. Carefully assess the child's hydration status and feeding tolerance. Skin integrity may be impaired secondary to frequent diarrheal stools. Prompt, frequent diaper changes and meticulous skin care are important. Collaboration with the CWOCN may be helpful to ensure that optimal skin barrier products are available for use. Educate the parents regarding medical and dietary management of the child's diarrhea. Also provide instruction in specialized nutrition support therapy techniques and home monitoring.

SHORT BOWEL SYNDROME

Short bowel syndrome is a condition in which extensive resection of small bowel results in malabsorption, fluid and electrolyte loss, and malnutrition. Short bowel syndrome in neonates is associated with congenital anomalies of the GI tract, such as jejunoileal atresia, gastroschisis, and omphalocele. Preterm infants with severe necrotizing enterocolitis may undergo intestinal resections that result in short bowel syndrome. Infants and older children who experience malrotation with midgut volvulus may sustain severe ischemic injury to the small intestine that requires massive intestinal resection. Children with Crohn disease who undergo repeated resections of diseased bowel may also be left with a short bowel.

Necrotizing enterocolitis, midgut volvulus, or congenital anomalies such as jejunal or ileal atresia and gastroschisis are the most common reasons for intestinal resection resulting in short bowel syndrome. Reported survival rates for the child with short bowel syndrome exceed 85% to 90%; 80% to 95% of children who require intestinal transplantation become independent of PN (Lopushinsky et al., 2007).

Pathophysiology

The small bowel is the primary site for digestion and absorption of nutrients. At 26 to 38 weeks' gestation, the small bowel undergoes extensive development, doubling in length. The full-term neonate is born with 200 to 300 cm of small bowel, which has an absorptive surface area of 950 cm. By adulthood, small bowel length grows to 600 to 900 cm with an absorptive surface area of 7,500 cm. These facts are important in understanding the infant's response to massive small bowel loss.

Short bowel syndrome occurs when extensive resection of small bowel reduces the absorptive surface area, causing malabsorption of nutrients, fluid, and electrolytes. During a process called *intestinal adaptation*, the remaining bowel develops the capability to do the work of digesting and absorbing adequate fluid and nutrients to support life. Although the very small infant does not initially tolerate resection of large segments of small bowel as well as an adult does, over the long term, the infant has greater potential for intestinal adaptation because of the greater capacity for growth of the small bowel.

A number of factors affect the small intestine's ability to adapt. The length of remaining bowel, the site of the resection, and whether the ileocecal valve is intact after the resection all play an important role in determining long-term outcomes. As a general rule, infants with as little as 15 cm of small bowel with an ileocecal valve or 40 cm of small bowel without an ileocecal valve at the time of their neonatal resections have a greater chance to become independent of PN (Harris, 2007). Prognosis with older children with this bowel length would be worse.

Resection of the jejunum is less well tolerated than resection of the ileum because the ileum has greater capacity for adaptation. The presence of the ileocecal valve is an important prognostic factor because this valve functions to slow the intestinal transit time and prevent reflux of bacteria from the large bowel into the small bowel. The quality and function of the child's residual bowel is also an important factor, with residual disease and surgical complications such as strictures, fistulas, and dysmotility having a negative influence.

Intestinal adaptation in short bowel syndrome occurs through various mechanisms. The presence of nutrients in the lumen of the small intestine leads to dilation of the residual bowel and mucosal hyperplasia, which results in increased villous height and crypt depth. This reconfiguration increases the absorptive surface area in the small bowel. The very young neonate's inherent capacity for intestinal growth may also contribute to the process of adaptation. The process of adaptation can take from months to years. Providing adequate nutritional support during this process is essential. Full or partial support with PN is required until intestinal adaptation to full enteral feedings takes place.

Assessment

Clinical manifestations of untreated short bowel syndrome include profuse, watery diarrhea; malabsorption; and FTT. Dehydration, electrolyte imbalances, and vitamin and mineral deficiencies may also occur. Skin breakdown may occur on the buttocks and perineum because of ongoing contact with diarrheal stools. Infants with short bowel syndrome are also at risk for oral feeding aversions because of prolonged nutritional support with parenteral and enteral feedings.

Children with short bowel syndrome are at risk for hepatobiliary complications. **Cholestasis** (stasis of bile flow) and cholelithiasis (gallstones) can result from malabsorption of bile salts and gallbladder stasis. Prolonged PN may put the child with short bowel syndrome at risk for cirrhosis, liver failure, and death. Liver disease in the parenterally fed child is believed to be multifactorial but is poorly understood. Prematurity, lack of enteral nutrition, and recurrent infection are all believed to play a role in the development of PN-associated liver disease. A contributing factor is thought to be related to fat emulsion. Currently, the fat emulsions comprise soy and safflower oil or soy oil alone, which are high in omega-6 fatty acids. This formulation is thought to contribute to the proinflammatory effect from the omega-6 fatty acids. Studies are currently being conducted to investigate the use of omega-3 fish oil to formulate fat emulsions (Tillman & Helms, 2011). Initial reports are promising.

Diarrhea and malabsorption in the child with short bowel syndrome may be exacerbated by bacterial overgrowth syndrome, a condition involving abnormal bacterial colonization of the small bowel. This condition can result from impaired motility secondary to adhesions or strictures and absence of the ileocecal valve.

Diagnostic Tests

At the time of surgery, the surgeon notes the length of remaining bowel and the presence or absence of the ileocecal valve. Other diagnostic studies may be needed to further define the functional status of the remaining bowel related to GI complications. These studies may include (but are not limited to) upper and lower endoscopy. Radiographic studies are used to determine growth of bowel length. Additional studies are done periodically to determine patient progress or to define ongoing problems.

Interdisciplinary Interventions

The basic principles of managing the child with short bowel syndrome are to initiate early and aggressive use of enteral nutrition to facilitate small bowel adaptation and to provide ongoing support with PN until adaptation takes place. Careful management of fluids, electrolytes, and nutrition along with prevention, early identification, and treatment of complications are also essential. Care of the child with short bowel syndrome is a collaborative effort across the continuum of care. In addition to nurses, the team includes the pediatrician, pediatric gastroenterologist, pediatric surgeon, dietitian, pharmacist, occupational therapist, and social worker.

The initial diagnosis of short bowel syndrome is established at the time of operative intervention for the underlying intestinal anomaly or disease state. During the initial postoperative period, the immediate goal is to stabilize fluid and electrolyte levels. Accurately measure and document all output, including urine, stool, NG or gastrostomy tube drainage, and ostomy output. Careful ongoing replacement of excess fluid loss is vital.

Gastric hypersecretion is typical during the early stages after intestinal resection and is treated by administering an H2 blocker (e.g., ranitidine) or a proton pump inhibitor (e.g., lansoprazole). Frequent laboratory evaluation of electrolyte balance is done. PN is initiated after the initial postoperative stabilization and is advanced gradually until the child's nutritional requirements are met (see Chapter 17). Meticulous care of the central venous access device, the child's lifeline, is essential to minimize the potential for catheter-related bloodstream infections. Baseline PN laboratory values, including liver and renal function tests, calcium, magnesium, phosphorus, total protein, and albumin, are done at the time PN is initiated and on a regular basis throughout the course of therapy.

When the child's GI function returns postoperatively, enteral feedings are started at low volumes by continuous drip through an NG tube, for the short term, or gastrostomy tube to promote nutritional tolerance. The primary goal of enteral nutrition during the immediate postoperative period is to stimulate the intestine's adaptive response. Elemental or casein hydrolysate formulas are frequently used, although in some cases, breast milk is given if available. Provide maternal support to establish and maintain a breast milk supply while the infant is NPO or unable to feed by mouth. Small-volume oral feedings and oral stimulation through a pacifier are established as early as possible to prevent oral feeding aversion.

Assess the infant's tolerance of PN and enteral feedings by careful, ongoing evaluation of weight gain, fluid and electrolyte balance, and stool output. Evaluate stools for malabsorption by testing for occult blood, pH, and reducing substances. Replace excess fluid losses with IV electrolyte solutions. Advance enteral feedings slowly and wean the child from PN proportionally as tolerance to enteral feeding progresses.

Bowel tapering and lengthening procedures for long-term functional improvement are considered when the remaining bowel segment is impaired. During intestinal adaptation, the remaining bowel may become dilated with subsequent dysmotility from attempts to increase the surface area. In the Bianchi procedure, the dilated bowel is resected longitudinally and anastomosed end to end from the divided bowel. The end result is a bowel segment that is half the former diameter and twice the length. A newer procedure—serial transverse enteroplasty—is performed by stapling the bowel segment in a "Z" or zigzag pattern, which effectively increases the absorptive surface area while also tapering the bowel. The benefit of this procedure reduces the risk of an anastomotic leak because the bowel lumen is not disrupted (Harris, 2007).

Community Care

Infants and children transitioned to home require coordinated services to provide optimal growth and development and to direct successful home care. Home health nurses play a pivotal role to assist families in applying principles of safety, appropriate to the infant's or child's developmental level, as individual milestones in growth and development occur. When the infant or child is medically stable, discharge to home on PN and enteral nutrition can be considered. Teach the family to become expert in PN administration and central venous access care.

Continually reinforce infection prevention techniques because catheter-related bloodstream infections are a common but preventable complication. Provide instruction on the home enteral program, gastrostomy tube care, skin care, and oral stimulation. An occupational therapist monitors and follows the progress of oral–motor skills.

The infant's complex medical needs must be balanced by opportunities for normal growth and development. Social services and home care nursing provide ongoing support. Evaluation of the family's and child's coping styles and functioning is ongoing and necessary because the duration of complex home therapy is often unpredictable.

CELIAC DISEASE

Celiac disease, also known as *celiac sprue* or *gluten enteropathy*, is an immune-mediated disorder that develops as a reaction to gluten, the protein component of wheat, in genetically susceptible individuals (Catassi et al., 2010). Celiac disease can develop at any age, and the incidence of celiac disease varies greatly geographically. In the United States, celiac disease was thought to be relatively rare when the presentation relied on the classic malabsorptive symptoms of diarrhea and growth failure. Recent reports have confirmed that it is more common than once believed, with an estimated prevalence in the United States of approximately 1 in 100 children (Tully, 2008). The prevalence of celiac disease is higher among children with type 1 diabetes mellitus, Down syndrome, Turner syndrome, Williams syndrome, and autoimmune disorders such as autoimmune thyroiditis and autoimmune hepatitis and among children with a first-degree relative diagnosed with celiac disease (Kneepkens & von Blomberg, 2012). The prognosis for the child with celiac disease is good with the institution of a lifelong gluten-free diet. Symptoms typically improve within the first week of starting the diet, and mucosal damage resolves within 6 months.

Pathophysiology

The child with celiac disease produces auto-antibodies which can be tested for in the blood. These include the antitissue transglutaminase IgA and the antiendomysial antibody IgA. Over time, villous atrophy of the proximal small intestine develops. The mucosal layer of the small intestine appears "flat" instead of having the normal fingerlike projections of healthy villi. Lack of functional villi results in impaired digestion and absorption of nutrients. The damage to the intestinal mucosa is believed to be mediated by immunologic mechanisms, with mucosal injury arising from an adverse immunologic reaction to gliadin, a polypeptide protein fraction of gluten. Injury to the mucosa of the small intestine and malabsorption is manifested after gluten from wheat, oats, barley, or rye is introduced into the diet. Symptoms resolve when the child is placed on a gluten-free diet.

Assessment

The workup of the child with suspected celiac disease includes an initial history and physical examination that contains a detailed nutritional assessment to evaluate the child's pattern of growth and diet history and to look for signs and symptoms of malabsorption and nutritional deficiencies. Diagnostic tests are also performed.

The clinical presentation of celiac disease may vary depending on the child's age and the degree of injury to the intestinal mucosa. Assess the child's general appearance and color, along with growth parameters. Classically, a young child, after demonstrating normal growth during the first months of life, presents with a history of FTT between 6 and 24 months of age after gluten products are introduced into the diet. Chronic diarrhea with foul-smelling, bulky, greasy stools is typical, although in some cases, constipation is present and is accompanied by dilation of the colon and rectal prolapse. Abdominal distention, pain, vomiting, muscle wasting, and hypotonia are common. Anorexia, irritability, and lassitude are also common. In severe cases, overt signs of nutritional deficiencies may be present on physical examination. In adolescence, celiac disease may present as growth retardation with delayed puberty or menses, or short stature. Anemia is frequently present.

Assessment beyond the GI system also provides indicators of celiac disease. Assess the skin, particularly the trunk and the interior aspects of the elbows and knees, for an intensely itchy, vesicular rash (dermatitis herpetiformis). Inspect the oral cavity for the presence of aphthous ulcers and for dental enamel irregularities. Question the child and family about these extraintestinal manifestations in the history, including neurologic complaints. Evaluation for osteomalacia and osteoporosis is recommended. Iron-deficiency anemia unresponsive to iron therapy is the most common non-GI manifestation.

Diagnostic Tests

Laboratory tests evaluate for malabsorption and nutritional deficiencies. Blood cell counts and serum iron, protein, mineral, and vitamin levels may all be decreased in chronic malabsorption, and total IgA levels are measured to rule out selective IgA deficiency (Tully, 2008). Serum levels of antiendomysial antibodies and antitissue transglutaminase antibody are recommended in the workup and are indicated for those at increased risk for celiac disease (Husby et al., 2012). However, if the selective total IgA level is deficient, then the antitissue transglutaminase antibody and antiendomysial levels are unreliable. Testing may also be done to assess lactose tolerance and to detect malabsorption of dietary fat.

If suspicion of celiac disease is high after initial screening and from the results of serologic tests, a referral to a pediatric gastroenterologist is indicated. An upper GI endoscopy with small bowel biopsy from multiple sites is recommended while the child is receiving a typical oral intake of gluten. To conclusively make the diagnosis of celiac disease, multiple biopsy specimens of the small intestine must demonstrate the characteristic histologic appearance of celiac disease, and the child must demonstrate a clinical response to a gluten-free diet. Reevaluation by small bowel biopsy within 4 to 6 months of initiating a gluten-free diet is no

longer recommended; however, this may be indicated for those individuals who have an unsatisfactory clinical response. Capsule endoscopy may become a tool to evaluate mucosal healing and to screen for intestinal complications (Shamir & Eliakim, 2008).

Testing is available for genetic markers to identify a high- or low-risk propensity for developing celiac disease. The presence of *HLA-DQ2* or *HLA-DQ8* markers indicates the potential for disease development. Not all individuals who have the markers will develop the disease (Tully, 2008).

Nursing Diagnoses and Outcomes

In addition to those presented in Nursing Plan of Care 18-1, the following nursing diagnosis and outcomes may apply to the family of a child with celiac disease:

Nursing Diagnosis: Ineffective family therapeutic regimen management related to lifelong maintenance of dietary restrictions
Outcomes:
• Child will demonstrate avoidance of products that contain gluten.
• Child will remain free of injury to the intestinal mucosa.
• Child and family will list palatable alternatives to gluten products.
• Child and family will confirm receipt of information and resources on how to identify gluten-containing products.
• Child and family will verify knowledge of how to connect with a support group to assist with effective coping and management.

Interdisciplinary Interventions

The goal of therapy is to resolve the symptoms and minimize the complications using the best known strategies. Initiating the gluten-free diet as early as possible and adhering to it for life are essential to symptom management. The main offending proteins are wheat, barley, and rye. In the past, oats were also identified as causing intestinal damage. More recently, pure oats have been determined to be safe, although concerns regarding wheat contamination during harvest and milling of oats render their safety questionable, and avoidance is still recommended. See and Murray (2006) summarize the management approach using CELIAC as an acronym:

Consultation with a skilled dietitian
Education about celiac disease
Lifelong adherence to a gluten-free diet
Identification and treatment of nutrition deficiencies
Access to a support group
Continuous long-term follow-up

Education regarding the diet is an essential part of the treatment plan and is a collaborative endeavor that includes the physician, dietitian, nurse, patient, family, and community members. An experienced dietitian who is knowledgeable about gluten-free diets is essential to the child's and parents' education and understanding. The teaching plan emphasizes information about the following aspects of care: the importance of adhering to the diet, sources of gluten (both food and nonfood), alternatives to gluten foods, places to obtain gluten-free products, label reading and shopping, managing eating away from home (whether at school, with friends, or in restaurants), support groups, and follow-up.

Gluten, in the form of malt, modified food starches, or dextrins, is used as a stabilizer or preservative in many processed foods and nonfood products. The Food Allergen Labeling and Consumer Protection Act of 2004 helped to identify ingredients in processed foods and make them safer for people on restricted diets. This law requires that peanuts, tree nuts, soy, fish, shellfish, milk, eggs, and wheat be listed on all food labels. The U.S. Food and Drug Administration has also defined and permitted the use of "GF" (gluten free) on labels (See & Murray, 2006).

Provide ongoing education to reinforce that damage may occur, despite a lack of overt symptoms, with nonadherence to the diet. Refer the family to community resources for gluten-free foods and to peer support organizations such as the Celiac Sprue Association (see thePoint for information on Organizations).

In addition to a gluten-free diet, the child is monitored for vitamin deficiencies such as calcium, iron, zinc, magnesium, and fat-soluble vitamins. Supplements are provided as indicated. It is important to ensure that all prescription and over-the-counter medications are gluten free.

Community Care

Ongoing monitoring is necessary to evaluate the child's response to therapy. Failure to respond to the gluten-free diet or exacerbation of symptoms may be the result of nonadherence. Developmental factors in younger children and social pressure on older children and adolescents may make adhering to the diet difficult (Community Care 18-1). Because adherence is so

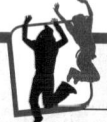

COMMUNITY CARE 18-1

Maintaining a Gluten-Free Diet

- All forms of wheat, rye, barley, and usually oats (some people can tolerate) should be omitted.
- Other foods are permitted as desired or as specified by the physician.
- *Caution:* Always read labels on commercially prepared foods. When in doubt, contact the producer.

Foods	Allowed	Not Allowed
Beverages	Milks Fruit juices Carbonated beverages Cocoa (read label to check that no wheat flour has been added) Coffee (ground; read label on instant) Tea	Malted milk Ovaltine Beer
Bread/cereal	Breads made from rice, corn, soybean, potato, tapioca, sago, or gluten-free wheat flour Dry cereals made only with rice or corn; cornmeal, hominy	Breads, rolls, crackers, cakes, cookies, cereals, noodles, spaghetti, and so forth; made from wheat, rye, wheat germ, barley, bran, oats
Fruit	As desired	
Meat/fish/fowl/eggs/cheese/nuts	As desired, plain Peanut butter	None with breading, cream sauce, thickened gravy Cold cuts (unless labeled "all meat")
Vegetables	As desired	None with cream sauce or breading
Fats	Butter, margarine, oil, pure mayonnaise Salad dressing thickened with allowed flours	Commercial salad dressings (read label)
Condiments/sweets	Salt, pure spices Sugar, honey, molasses, syrup, jam, jelly, candy (read label) Gelatin, homemade ice cream, rice pudding, pudding thickened with allowed flours	Some candies are dusted with flour to prevent sticking, or made with flour Ice cream, sauce, and gravy mixes may contain wheat flour without listing on label Soy sauce

difficult, finding developmentally sensitive ways to include children in all dietary counseling is important to increase their sense of involvement and responsibility in the treatment plan. The child and family must understand the importance of the lifelong diet and the ramifications of nonadherence.

 KidKare Remind children and parents that wheat free does not always equate with gluten free.

Follow-up is necessary to determine whether goals are achieved and to reinforce the plan of care. Encourage parents to work with school food service personnel to identify gluten-free foods that the child can enjoy with peers. Parents can also contact those adults who host "play dates" or serve food at school parties about the need for gluten-free foods and can send gluten-free snacks and treats with the child. Caution parents about well-intended people who may offer the child gluten-containing food because they do not understand the importance of medical diets. Encourage parents to reinforce education and empower the child by having him or her make appropriate choices at the market and at restaurants and by including the child in meal planning and preparation.

LACTOSE INTOLERANCE

Lactose intolerance, also known as *primary lactase deficiency*, is the most common cause of carbohydrate malabsorption. Symptoms may begin in early childhood, may be subtle, and may progress over many years. The incidence of primary lactase deficiency varies greatly by ethnic group. Up to 80% of African American and Ashkenazi Jewish adults and approximately 50% to 80% of Hispanics experience primary lactase deficiency. It approaches almost 100% in Asian and American Indian adults (Heyman, 2006), whereas only about 2% of northern Europeans experience this condition despite having a diet rich in dairy products.

CROSS-CULTURAL CARE

In parts of the world such as Asia and Africa, where primary lactase deficiency is very common, milk products are not a large part of the usual adult diet, so symptoms of lactose intolerance are relatively rare.

Pathophysiology

Lactose is the primary carbohydrate found solely in mammalian milk. Lactase, an enzyme located on the brush border near the tip of the intestinal villi, breaks down lactose so that its component parts can be absorbed. When lactase activity is inadequate, lactose is malabsorbed. An increased osmotic load to the gut is generated where fluids and electrolytes are drawn into the intestinal lumen, resulting in loose stools. The likelihood of developing symptoms depends on the amount of residual lactase activity, the amount of lactose

ingested, and the composition of the meal. Premature infants have substantially lower levels of lactase activity until at least 34 weeks' gestation. Caucasian children may not demonstrate symptoms of primary lactase intolerance until 4 to 5 years of age, whereas 20% of Hispanic, Asian, and African American children may show some relative signs of deficiency younger than 5 years of age (Heyman, 2006). GI disease can adversely affect lactase activity. Acute infectious gastroenteritis, such as that caused by rotavirus, can cause partial villous atrophy, resulting in a transient lactase deficiency. Individuals with disease characterized by inflammation of the GI tract, such as Crohn disease, ulcerative colitis, or celiac disease, may also experience secondary lactase deficiency. At-risk infants, younger than 3 months old, who develop gastroenteritis and suffer from subsequent lactase deficiency may experience a complicated recovery process.

Primary lactase deficiency results from the normal physiologic decline in lactase activity that usually begins during childhood at various ages and across different racial groups. Secondary lactase deficiency results from small bowel mucosal injury resulting from insults from infection (e.g., *Giardia*, chemotherapy, or bacterial overgrowth). The intestinal disease or inflammation can cause transient lactose intolerance. Developmental lactase deficiency is defined as relative lactase deficiency seen in infants younger than 34 weeks' gestation. True congenital lactase deficiency, in which symptoms are present shortly after birth, is extremely rare.

Assessment

A thorough history is the initial step in evaluating the child with suspected lactose intolerance to correlate the relationship of lactose ingestion to clinical symptoms. A detailed diet history may not offer accurate information because of the relative variance of lactose consumed and the degree of lactase deficiency. Primary lactose intolerance is manifested by one of the following symptoms: abdominal pain, bloating, diarrhea, nausea, and flatulence. In some cases, complaints of recurrent abdominal pain may be the only presenting symptom. Those with low lactase activity may be able to tolerate some lactose intake, particularly when it is part of a meal. The most reliable diagnostic tool in establishing the diagnosis of lactose intolerance is the hydrogen breath test. An increase in breath hydrogen levels after ingestion of a load of lactose indicates lactose malabsorption. When secondary lactase deficiency is suspected, additional studies are performed related to the differential diagnosis, such as stool specimens and serology, to rule out an infectious process and celiac disease, respectively.

Interdisciplinary Interventions

Lactose intolerance is treated by reducing or eliminating lactose-containing foods in the diet. The amount of lactose that can be tolerated is highly variable. Dietary counseling focuses on helping children and parents identify both obvious and hidden sources of lactose in processed foods. Milk products treated with a microbially derived lactase may be used. Lactase enzymes are also available in tablets or drops, which may be ingested with lactose-containing foods to improve tolerance. Many children can tolerate small amounts of lactose such as yogurt, hard cheeses, and ice cream without discomfort.

Dietary counseling also includes ensuring that daily calcium and vitamin D requirements are adequately met through other sources, particularly when a strict diet is recommended. The nurse, in collaboration with the dietitian, makes sure that counseling is developmentally and culturally sensitive to enhance adherence.

HEPATIC DISORDERS

Hepatic disorders that alter GI function include biliary atresia, cirrhosis, and end-stage liver disease.

BILIARY ATRESIA

Biliary atresia is characterized by obstruction of bile flow out of the liver caused by absence of, or progressive sclerosis of, the extrahepatic bile ducts. Biliary atresia is currently the most common indication for liver transplant in children. It occurs in 1 in 12,000 to 14,000 births in the United States (Hollen et al., 2012). The process begins during the prenatal period and is slightly more predominant in females than males.

If recognized and treated early, biliary atresia has a better outcome. Without surgical intervention, the child will succumb to end-stage liver disease by age 12 to 24 months. Advances in the surgical management of biliary atresia and liver transplantation have greatly improved the outlook for the child with biliary atresia.

Pathophysiology

Biliary atresia is postulated to stem from five possible causes: (1) a defect in the development of the biliary tract, (2) a defect in the prenatal circulation, (3) viral infection or toxin exposure, (4) genetic predisposition, or (5) inflammatory or immunologic dysregulation (Bezerra, 2006). A proposed working model provides insight into the disease mechanism and progression. The model divides the causes of biliary atresia into two types: those that are toxic or environmental and those that act directly on the host, including defects in fetal or prenatal circulation, immunologic dysregulation, and defects in morphogenesis. It proposes that biliary atresia is initiated by an insult that leads to an inflammatory response. In a normal host, the tissue is repaired, with resumption of physiologic homeostasis, and the host becomes disease free. In genetically susceptible hosts, progression of injury to the biliary tract results in biliary atresia. Approximately 10% to 20% of infants with biliary atresia have associated malformations (situs inversus, polysplenia, congenital heart defects, and absent inferior vena cava [splenic malformation syndrome]) (Kelly & Davenport, 2007) that suggest a defect during early embryologic development.

The child with biliary atresia experiences chronic obstruction of bile flow that results in progressive damage to the liver. Cholestasis leads to edema and inflammation of the portal tracts of the liver, destruction of the portal bile ducts by bile plugs, secondary proliferation of intralobular bile ducts, and inflammation of the parenchyma of the liver. Progressive fibrosis and, eventually, cirrhosis of the liver tissue result in end-stage liver disease (described later in this chapter).

Assessment

Infants with biliary atresia typically present with jaundice between 3 and 8 weeks of age. The jaundice is persistent and progressive. Stools are acholic (pale, clay colored), and the urine is usually dark. The abdomen is usually enlarged early during the course because of hepatomegaly. On physical examination, the liver feels large and firm. Splenomegaly may develop after the first 6 weeks. Infants with biliary atresia often thrive and appear well during the first month of life but then demonstrate progressive malnutrition and growth failure as the disease progresses. As liver function deteriorates, the child demonstrates the manifestations of end-stage liver disease, including **ascites** (accumulation of large amounts of serous fluid in the peritoneal cavity), splenomegaly, portal hypertension, and decrease in liver size as fibrosis progresses.

Diagnostic Tests

Laboratory evaluation is used to rule out causes of jaundice that are unrelated to the biliary tract and to establish the degree of liver damage sustained (Chart 18-6).

CHART 18-6　**Diagnostic Evaluation of the Child With Liver Dysfunction**

Laboratory Evaluation

ALT, AST

ALP

Gamma glutamyl transpeptidase

Bilirubin, total/direct

Hepatitis A, B, and C serologies

TORCH titers

HIV screen

Alpha 1-antitrypsin

Metabolic screen

CBC

Prothrombin time, partial thromboplastin time

Sweat chloride

Radiographic Studies

Abdominal ultrasound

HIDA scan

Cholangiogram (intraoperative)

MRCP

Liver Biopsy

Percutaneous or intraoperative

TORCH, toxoplasmosis, other infections, rubella, cytomegalovirus, herpes simplex.

Imaging studies are used to visualize the architecture and function of the biliary tract. Liver biopsy and cholangiography may be done percutaneously or intraoperatively as a means to definitively establish the diagnosis. A HIDA scan is an imaging study during which an IV-administered radioactive material is taken up by the liver and normally excreted by the biliary system into the intestine and eventually excreted in the stool. If bile flow is undetected, a 24-hour follow-up scan is done. When there is bile obstruction, as in the case of biliary atresia, excretion of bile is not detectable. Efforts are underway to determine a sensitive screening method for early detection (Kelly & Davenport, 2007).

Nursing Diagnoses and Outcomes

In addition to those presented in Nursing Plan of Care 18-1, the following nursing diagnoses and outcomes may apply to the child with biliary atresia:

Nursing Diagnosis: Risk for infection related to impaired liver function and poor nutritional status
Outcome: Child will remain free of acquired infection.
Nursing Diagnosis: Risk for impaired skin integrity related to pruritus secondary to liver dysfunction
Outcomes:
• Child will exhibit intact skin.
• Child will verbalize a reduction in complaints of pruritus.

Interdisciplinary Interventions

Because jaundice and liver failure have many possible causes (see the section on cirrhosis), a comprehensive evaluation is needed to establish the diagnosis. Care during the diagnostic period focuses on supporting the child's physiologic and psychosocial needs as well as on meeting the parent's information needs throughout the many diagnostic procedures.

Surgical Interventions

Hepatic portoenterostomy, also known as the *Kasai procedure*, is the first-line operative intervention. Historically, portoenterostomy has been done before 2 months of age for optimal results; however, surgery may be of benefit beyond the recognized 60-day parameter to "bridge" the infant until transplant is arranged. Infants diagnosed later are referred directly for liver transplant. Numerous modifications have been made to the Kasai procedure, but the principle remains the same: A conduit is made to bypass the fibrotic extrahepatic biliary tree and reestablish bile drainage. Anastomosis of a jejunal bowel segment to the transected surface of the porta hepatis creates a Roux-en-Y structure that provides a pathway for bile drainage. Postoperative goals include stimulating bile flow and providing nutritional therapy to promote growth and development and to prevent complications, such as ascending cholangitis.

Postoperative care is similar to other surgical conditions of the abdomen. Fluid management, IV antibiotics, abdominal decompression via NG tube, and pain management are central to the infant's recovery. Monitor the NG output and ensure that the system is effectively functioning. The NG tube may require irrigation to keep it patent. Management also includes administering agents such as phenobarbital or ursodeoxycholic acid to stimulate secretion of bile. Corticosteroids are administered in many centers for their well-recognized anti-inflammatory effects.

Nutritional Interventions

Aggressive nutritional support is critical to postoperative and long-term management. The infant is at high risk for FTT and malnutrition because of malabsorption of dietary fat and fat-soluble vitamins caused by decreased intraluminal concentrations of bile acids. Infant formulas are given that provide a high percentage of fats as medium-chain triglycerides and therefore are readily absorbed (e.g., Portagen, Pregestimil). NG feedings or IV fat emulsions may also be used to ensure adequate caloric intake. PN may be administered if the infant is not showing progress toward meeting nutritional goals. Supplements of fat-soluble vitamins A, D, E, and K are given in their water-soluble forms. Collaboration between the dietitian, nurse, physician, and family is essential in ongoing monitoring of nutrition, liver function, and other parameters.

Interventions to Prevent or Manage Complications

Bacterial ascending cholangitis is a frequent complication after hepatic portoenterostomy, with an incidence of 40% to 60%, most commonly during the first several years after surgery (Cowles, 2012). Bacterial organisms ascending from the intestinal tract are frequently implicated along with bile stasis. Prophylactic antibiotic therapy with trimethoprim–sulfamethoxazole is given as long-term therapy to minimize these episodes. Fever, increased jaundice, and acholic stools are the overt clinical signs of ascending cholangitis. If ascending cholangitis occurs, treatment is with broad-spectrum IV antibiotics. Teach parents to recognize the signs and symptoms of bacterial ascending cholangitis to ensure that their child receives prompt medical attention. Instruct parents to notify their physician if they observe fever, decreased appetite, or increased jaundice (evidenced by skin color, color of sclera, and return of pale, acholic stools). Another complication is portal hypertension from impaired blood flow. This complication progresses to hypersplenism, ascites, and bleeding from esophageal varices, which can be life threatening. Variceal bleeding is treated by sclerotherapy or, in older children, with variceal banding.

Pruritus is a bothersome result of cholestasis. Rifampin has been found to alter bile acid metabolism and reduce systemic and intrahepatic levels of bile acid levels, thus lending relief from cholestatic pruritus. This medication must be monitored carefully during long-term use because of the potential for side effects. Inform parents that this medication turns the urine orange. Ensure that the child's fingernails are clipped to avoid damaged skin integrity (see Chapter 25 for other appropriate nursing interventions). These children may also experience altered sleep patterns because the pruritus is intense.

Discuss methods that may help parents cope, such as alternating times (or nights) that they get up to tend to the child, sleeping when the child sleeps, or having family and friends sleep over to provide respite.

Community Care

The family of the child with biliary atresia faces multiple psychosocial stressors resulting from the chronic and often degenerative nature of the disease. Complicated medical care in the home, multiple acute hospitalizations, and, for many, the prospect of liver transplant may present a source of ongoing anxiety and may strain family and personal relationships, work performance, and finances. The family's coping can be enhanced by ongoing involvement with a social worker or other mental health professional and by referral to peer support organizations.

CIRRHOSIS AND END-STAGE LIVER DISEASE

Cirrhosis is defined by the World Health Organization as a diffuse liver process characterized by fibrosis and the conversion of normal liver tissue into structurally abnormal nodules. The end result of most forms of liver disease, cirrhosis, has many possible causes (Table 18-7). The precise incidence of cirrhosis in children is difficult to ascertain.

The national increase in childhood obesity has led to an increase in the condition of nonalcoholic fatty liver disease (NAFLD). It is defined as a chronic liver disease with excessive accumulation of hepatic fat, representing a spectrum of liver disease. The manifestations may range from steatosis (fat accumulation in the hepatocyte without inflammation) to steatohepatitis. Nonalcoholic

steatohepatitis (NASH) marks a more progressive disease that also manifests with fat accumulation along with inflammation and fibrosis. Cirrhosis can be a long-term complication. There is some controversy regarding whether the origin of NAFLD is the first step toward NASH or whether they exist as two separate conditions (Lerret & Skelton, 2008).

The long-term outlook for the child with cirrhosis varies depending on the nature and severity of the disease. Although the child with compensated cirrhosis may experience very little impairment, the child with active cirrhosis or fulminant hepatic failure will require liver transplant to achieve long-term survival.

Pathophysiology

Cirrhosis and end-stage liver disease are the end result of the liver's response to injury. The mechanisms of injury may vary, but the liver's response follows a typical pattern. Injury to the hepatocyte leads to cell necrosis. Cell necrosis releases factors that lead to fibrous regeneration of connective tissue. Normal liver structures are disrupted by fibrosis and nodule formation, leading to compression and distortion of intrahepatic vascular structures. This distortion and compression, in turn, causes further ischemic and hypoxemic injury to the hepatocytes.

In compensated cirrhosis, cirrhosis presents without biochemical or clinical evidence of impairment in liver function. In active cirrhosis, the signs and symptoms of cirrhosis are manifest and progressive. In fulminant hepatic failure, sudden impairment in liver function with acute massive necrosis leads to hepatic encephalopathy within 8 weeks of symptom onset.

Assessment

Clinical manifestations of cirrhosis and end-stage liver disease depend on the etiology of the injury to the liver and on how rapidly hepatic failure progresses. General manifestations of cirrhosis often mimic other systemic illnesses. FTT may be noted, along with anorexia and easy fatigability. Jaundice may be present but is not always evident. Nausea, vomiting, and abdominal pain and distention may occur. Children with compensated cirrhosis may have few findings on physical examination or laboratory evaluation. Children in fulminant hepatic failure demonstrate multiple alterations, both physically and biochemically.

On physical examination, with advanced disease, muscle wasting may be noted. The liver may be large and tender during the early stages of cirrhosis but progresses to becoming small and shrunken as it becomes increasingly nodular. Hepatomegaly may be difficult to appreciate when obesity coexists. Marked enlargement of the spleen and abdominal ascites are noted when portal hypertension is present. Ascites may also be noted when hypoalbuminemia is present. Cyanosis and digital clubbing occur in the presence of chronic hypoxemia from pulmonary systemic collateral shunting. Easy bruising or overt signs of bleeding may be seen, related to clotting factor deficiencies and low platelets.

TABLE 18-7	Diseases Leading to Cirrhosis
Etiology	**Disease**
Infectious	Viral hepatitis Herpesvirus
Metabolic disorders	Alpha 1-antitrypsin deficiency Cystic fibrosis Glycogen storage disease Hemochromatosis Wilson disease
Biliary malformations	Biliary atresia Alagille syndrome Choledochal cyst
Toxic exposure	Acetaminophen Isoniazid Natural toxins (mushrooms)
Vascular disease	Budd-Chiari syndrome Congestive heart failure Veno-occlusive liver disease
Other	Parenteral nutrition liver disease Neonatal hepatitis Primary sclerosing cholangitis

Diagnostic Tests

Laboratory evaluation is done to detect serologic evidence of causative factors. Evaluation of liver function tests, blood indices such as CBC with differential, clotting parameters, and visceral protein status helps to establish the degree to which liver function is impaired. These studies are abnormal with advanced disease. Radiographic and imaging studies detect any structural abnormalities within the liver and biliary duct system. Liver biopsy provides histologic evidence to confirm the diagnosis and the severity of the fibrosis or cirrhosis.

Interdisciplinary Interventions

The goal of the initial diagnostic evaluation of the child with suspected cirrhosis is to establish the underlying cause of liver disease and to determine the degree of injury to the liver. Similar to the management of the child undergoing evaluation for suspected biliary atresia, the goal during the diagnostic phase is to support the child's physiologic and psychosocial needs and to meet the parent's information needs throughout the many diagnostic procedures.

Care of the child with cirrhosis is geared toward preventing and treating the complications associated with cirrhosis and end-stage liver disease. Therapy to treat the underlying cause of the liver disease is undertaken, with the goal of eliminating or modifying whatever agent or mechanism is causing injury to the liver.

Supportive Interventions

Nutritional therapy is geared toward optimizing calorie and protein intake without exacerbating the underlying symptoms of cirrhosis. Ascites is managed with fluid and sodium restrictions; diuretics are commonly administered to enhance fluid excretion. However, diuretic therapy may cause fluid and electrolyte imbalances and can also impair renal function. Hypoalbuminemia can contribute to the accumulation of ascites and edema in the child with end-stage liver disease and may necessitate intermittent albumin transfusions. Portal hypertension can lead to the development of esophageal or gastric varices that are potential sites of upper GI bleeding. Coagulopathies related to abnormal prothrombin production and associated thrombocytopenia put the child at risk for GI bleeding, particularly when varices are present. Endoscopic sclerotherapy or a banding procedure may be used to treat such varices. Monitoring the child for changes in the level of consciousness is key to identifying the development of hepatic encephalopathy. Hepatic encephalopathy is treated by reducing and modifying protein intake and by administering neomycin or lactulose.

Surgical Interventions

Liver transplantation, offered at specific tertiary care centers, offers definitive treatment for the life-threatening complications of cirrhosis and end-stage liver disease. The liver transplant team manages the child through all phases of transplant, from evaluation to the ongoing follow-up care after surgery. The nurse coordinator on the team plays a vital role in coordinating the child's care and providing child and family education during the preoperative and postoperative periods.

See thePoint for a summary of Key Concepts.

REFERENCES

American Academy of Pediatrics, Task Force on Sudden Infant Death Syndrome. (2011). SIDS and other sleep-related infant deaths: Expansion of recommendations for a safe infant sleeping environment. *Pediatrics, 128*(5), 1030–1039.

Applebaum, I. H., & Sydorak, R. (2012). Duodenal atresia and stenosis—Annular pancreas. In A. G. Coran, N. S. Adzick, T. M. Krummel et al. (Eds.), *Pediatric surgery* (7th ed., pp. 1051–1057). Philadelphia, PA: Saunders Elsevier.

Aspelund, G., & Langer, J. C. (2007). Current management of hypertrophic pyloric stenosis. *Seminars in Pediatric Surgery, 16*(1), 27–33.

Austin, K. M. (2012). The pathogenesis of Hirschsprung's disease-associated enterocolitis. *Seminars in Pediatric Surgery, 21*(4), 319–327.

Bai, H., Lowe, M., & Husain, S. (2011). What have we learned about acute pancreatitis in children? *Journal of Pediatric Gastroenterology and Nutrition, 52*(3), 262–270.

Bankhead, R., Boullata, J., Brantley, S. et al. (2009). Enteral nutrition practice recommendations. *JPEN. Journal of Parenteral and Enteral Nutrition, 33*(2), 122–167.

Benninga, M. A., Candy, D. C., & Taminiau, J. A. (2005). New treatment options in childhood constipation? *Journal of Pediatric Gastroenterology and Nutrition, 41*(Suppl. 1), S56–S57.

Bergeron, K. F., Silversides, D., & Pilon, N. (2013). The developmental genetics of Hirschsprung's disease. *Clinical Genetics, 83*(1), 15–22.

Bezerra, J. A. (2006). The next challenge in pediatric cholestasis: Deciphering the pathogenesis of biliary atresia. *Journal of Pediatric Gastroenterology and Nutrition, 43*(1), S23–S29.

Bingham, P., Ashikaga, T., & Abbasi, S. (2010). Prospective study of non-nutritive sucking and feeding skills in premature infants. *Archives of Disease in Childhood. Fetal & Neonatal Edition, 95*(3), 194–200.

Borrelli, O., Mancini, V., Thapar, N. et al. (2012). Cow's milk challenge increases weakly acidic reflux in children with cow's milk allergy and gastroesophageal reflux disease. *Journal of Pediatrics, 151*(3), 476–481.

Brazelton, T. B. (1962). Crying in infancy. *Pediatrics, 29,* 579–588.

Camilleri, M., & Di Lorenzo, C. (2012). Brain-gut axis: From basic understanding to treatment of IBS and related disorders. *Journal of Pediatric Gastroenterology and Nutrition, 54*(4), 446–453.

Catassi C., Kryszak, D., Bhatti, B. et al. (2010). Natural history of celiac disease autoimmunity in a USA cohort followed since 1974. *Annals of Medicine, 42*(7), 530–538.

Chan, K. W., Lee, K. H., Mou, J. W. et al. (2008). Laparoscopic management of complicated Meckel's diverticulum in children: A 10-year review. *Surgical Endoscopy, 22*(6), 1509–1512.

Chigurupati, R. (2012). Cleft lip and palate: Timing and approach to reconstruction. In S. C. Bagheri, R. B. Bell, & H. A. Khan (Eds.), *Current therapy in oral and maxillofacial surgery* (pp. 726–750). St. Louis, MO: Elsevier.

Chiou, E., & Nurko, S. (2011). Functional abdominal pain in children and adolescents. *Therapy, 8*(3), 315–331.

Cowles, R. (2012). The jaundiced infant: Biliary atresia. In A. G. Coran, N. S. Adzick, T. M. Krummel et al. (Eds.), *Pediatric surgery* (7th ed., Vol. 2, pp. 1321–1330). Philadelphia, PA: Saunders Elsevier.

Critch, J., Day, A. S., Otley, A. et al. (2012). Use of enteral nutrition for the control of intestinal inflammation in pediatric Crohn disease. *Journal of Pediatric Gastroenterology and Nutrition, 54,* 298–305.

Dandeles, L. M., & Lodolce, A. E. (2011). Efficacy of agents to prevent and treat enteral feeding tube clogs. *Annals of Pharmacotherapy, 45*(5), 676–680.

Dasgupta, R., & Langer, J. C. (2008). Evaluation and management of persistent problems after surgery for Hirschsprung disease in a child. *Journal of Pediatric Gastroenterology and Nutrition, 46*(1), 13–19.

Day, A. S., Ledder, O., Leach, S. T. et al. (2012). Crohn's and colitis in children and adolescents. *World Journal of Gastroenterology, 18*(41), 5862–5869.

Deshpande, G., Rao, S., & Patole, S. (2011). Progress in the field of probiotics: Year 2011. *Current Opinion in Gastroenterology, 27*(1), 13–18.

Di Lorenzo, C., Colletti, R. B., Lehmann, H. P. et al. (2005). Chronic abdominal pain in children: A technical report of the American Academy of Pediatrics and the North American Society for Pediatric Gastroenterology, Hepatology, and Nutrition. *Journal of Pediatric Gastroenterology and Nutrition, 40*(3), 249–261.

Forest-Lalande, L. (2012). Needs for peds feeding gastrostomies: Prevention and management of tube-related complications. *World Council of Enterostomal Therapists Journal, 32*(3), 22–27.

Fountaine, E. A., & Knight, K. M. (2013). Ultrasound for abdominal wall defects. *Ultrasound Clinics, 8*(1), 55–67.

Fuchs, Y., Markowitz, J., Weinstein, T. et al. (2011). Pediatric inflammatory bowel disease and imaging-related radiation: Are we increasing the likelihood of malignancy? *Journal of Pediatric Gastroenterology and Nutrition, 52*(3), 280–285.

Gishan, F. K., & Kiela, P. R. (2011). Advances in the understanding of mineral bone metabolism in inflammatory bowel disease. American Journal of Physiology. *Gastrointestinal and Liver Physiology, 300*(2), G191–G201.

Gramlich, T., & Petras, R. E. (2007). Pathology of inflammatory bowel disease. *Seminars in Pediatric Surgery, 16*(3), 154–163.

Gray, W. N., Denson, L. A., Baldassano, R. N. et al. (2011). Disease activity, behavioral dysfunction, and health-related quality of life in adolescents with inflammatory bowel disease. *Inflammatory Bowel Diseases, 17*(7), 1581–1586.

Green, R., Bulloch, B., Kabani, A. et al. (2005). Early analgesia for children with acute abdominal pain. *Pediatrics, 116*(4), 978–983.

Guardino, K., & Pieper, P. (2013). Anorectal malformations in children. In N. Browne, L. Flanigan, C. McComiskey et al. (Eds.), *Nursing care of the pediatric surgical patient* (3rd ed., pp. 359–370). Burlington, MA: Jones and Bartlett Learning.

Güenaga, K. F., Matos, D., & Wille-Jørgensen, P. (2011). Mechanical bowel preparation for elective colorectal surgery. *Cochrane Database of Systematic Reviews, (9),* CD001544.

Harmon, C. M., & Coran, A. G. (2012). Congenital anomalies of the esophagus. In A. G. Coran, N. S. Adzick, T. M. Krummel et al. (Eds.), *Pediatric surgery* (7th ed., pp. 893–918). Philadelphia, PA: Saunders Elsevier.

Harris, J. B. (2007). Neonatal short bowel syndrome. *Newborn and Infant Nursing Reviews, 7*(3), 131–142.

Harry, B., TeBockhorst, S., & Deleyiannis, F. (2012). The impact of congenital cardiovascular malformations on the assessment and surgical management of infants with cleft lip and/or palate. *Cleft Palate-Craniofacial Journal.* Advance online publication.

Harting, M. T., & Lally, K. P. (2007). Surgical management of neonates with congenital diaphragmatic hernia. *Seminars in Pediatric Surgery, 16,* 109–114.

Hazza'a, A., Rawashdeh, M., Al-Nimri, K. et al. (2011). Dental and oral hygiene status in Jordanian children with cleft lip and palate: A comparison between unilateral and bilateral clefts. *International Journal of Dental Hygiene, 9*(1), 30–36.

Heyman, M. B. (2006). Lactose intolerance in infants, children, and adolescents. *Pediatrics, 118*(3), 1279–1286.

Holcomb, G. W., Rothenberg, S. S., Bax, K. M. A. et al. (2005). Thoracoscopic repair of esophageal atresia and tracheoesophageal fistula: A multi-institutional analysis. *Annals of Surgery, 242*(3), 422–430.

Hollen, J., Eide, M., & Gorman, G. (2012). Early diagnosis of extrahepatic biliary atresia in an open-access medical system. *PLoS One, 7*(11), e49643.

Horvath, A., Dziechciarz, P., & Szajewska, H. (2008). The effect of thickened-feed interventions on gastroesophageal reflux in infants: Systematic review and meta-analysis of randomized, controlled trials. *Pediatrics, 122*(6), e1268–e1277.

Huffman, S., Jarczyk, K. S., O'Brien, E. et al. (2004). Methods to confirm feeding tube placement: Application of research in practice. *Pediatric Nursing, 30*(1), 10–13, 21–22.

Hunt, O., Burden, D., Hepper, P. et al. (2005). The psychosocial effects of cleft lip and palate: A systematic review. *European Journal of Orthodontics, 27*(3), 274–285.

Husby, S., Koletzko, S., Korponay-Szabó, I. R. et al. (2012). European Society for Pediatric Gastroenterology, Hepatology, and Nutrition guidelines for the diagnosis of coeliac disease. *Journal of Pediatric Gastroenterology & Nutrition, 54*(1), 136–160.

Islam, S. (2012). Advances in surgery for abdominal wall defects: Gastroschisis and omphalocele. *Clinics in Perinatology, 39*(2), 375–386.

Juang, D., & Snyder, C. L. (2012). Neonatal bowel obstruction. *Surgical Clinics of North America, 92*(3), 685–711.

Kandula, L., & Lowe, M. E. (2008). Etiology and outcome of acute pancreatitis in infants and toddlers. *Journal of Pediatrics, 152*(1), 106–110.

Karp, H. (2004). The "fourth trimester": A framework and strategy for understanding and resolving colic. *Contemporary Pediatrics, 21*(2), 94–116.

Keefe, M. R., Kajrlsen, K. A., Lobo, M. L. et al. (2006). Reducing parenting stress in families with irritable infants. *Nursing Research, 55*(3), 198–205.

Kelesidis, T., & Pothoulakis, C. (2012). Efficacy and safety of the probiotic *Saccharomyces boulardii* for the prevention and therapy of gastrointestinal disorders. *Therapeutic Advances in Gastroenterology, 5*(2), 111–125.

Kelly, D., & Davenport, M. (2007). Current management of biliary atresia. *Archives of Disease in Childhood, 92*(12), 1132–1135.

Kheir, A. E. M. (2012). Infantile colic, facts and fiction. *Italian Journal of Pediatrics, 38.*

Kim, Y. S., Lee, B. S., Kim, S. H. et al. (2008). Is there correlation between pancreatic enzyme and radiological severity in acute pancreatitis? *World Journal of Gastroenterology, 14*(15), 2401–2405.

Klassen, A. F., Tsangaris, E., Forrest, C. R. et al. (2012). Quality of life of children treated for cleft lip and/or palate: A systematic review. *Journal of Plastic, Reconstructive & Aesthetic Surgery, 65*(5), 547–557.

Kligler, B., Hanaway, P., & Cohrssen, A. (2007). Probiotics in children. *Pediatric Clinics of North America, 54*(6), 949–967.

Kneepkens, C. M. F., & von Blomberg, M. E. (2012). Coeliac disease. *European Journal of Pediatrics, 171*(7), 1011–1021.

Krogh, C., Gørtz, S., Wohlfahrt, J. et al. (2012). Pre and perinatal risk factors for pyloric stenosis and their influence on the male predominance. *American Journal of Epidemiology, 176*(1), 24–31.

Kugathasan, S., & Fiocchi, C. (2007). Progress in basic inflammatory bowel disease research. *Seminars in Pediatric Surgery, 16*(3), 146–153.

Lampl, B., Levin, T. L., Berdon, W. E. et al. (2009). Malrotation and midgut volvulus: A historical review and current controversies in diagnosis and management. *Pediatric Radiology, 39*(4), 359–366.

Ledbetter, D. J. (2012). Congenital abdominal wall defects and reconstruction in pediatric surgery: Gastroschisis and omphalocele. *Surgical Clinical of North American 92*(3), 713–727.

Lee, S. L., Yaghoubian, A., Stark, R. et al. (2012). Are there differences in access to care, treatment, and outcomes for children with appendicitis treated at county versus private hospitals? *The Permanente Journal, 16*(1), 4–6.

Lerret, S., & Skelton, J. A. (2008). Pediatric nonalcoholic fatty liver disease. *Gastroenterology Nursing, 31*(2), 115–119.

Levine, A., Bachar, L., Tsangen, Z. et al. (2011). Screening criteria for diagnosis of infantile feeding disorders as a cause of poor feeding or food refusal. *Journal of Pediatric Gastroenterology and Nutrition, 52*(5), 563–568.

Leys, C. M., Austin, M. T., Pietsch, J. B. et al. (2005). Elective intestinal operations in infants and children without mechanical bowel preparation: A pilot study. *Journal of Pediatric Surgery, 40*(6), 978–981.

Longo, M. (2011). Best evidence: Nasogastric tube placement verification. *Journal of Pediatric Nursing, 26*, 373–376.

Lopushinsky, S. R., Fowler, R., Kulkami, G. S. et al. (2007). The optimal timing of intestinal transplantation for children with intestinal failure: A Markov analysis. *Annals of Surgery, 264*(6), 1092–1099.

Loughrey, C. M., & Duggan, C. (2005). Laboratory assessment of nutritional status. In K. M. Hendricks & C. Duggan (Eds.), *Manual of pediatric nutrition* (4th ed., pp. 70–82). Hamilton, Canada: B. C. Decker.

Lozano, R., Naghavi, M., Foreman, K. et al. (2013). Global and regional mortality from 235 causes of death for 20 age groups in 1990 and 2010: A systematic analysis for the Global Burden of Disease Study 2010. *Lancet, 380*(9859), 2095–2128.

Mack, D. R., Langton, C., Markowitz, J. et al. (2007). Laboratory values for children with newly diagnosed inflammatory bowel disease. *Pediatrics, 119*(6), 1113–1119.

Mackey, A. C., Green, L., Leptak, C. et al. (2009). Hepatosplenic T cell lymphoma associated with infliximab use in young patients treated for inflammatory bowel disease: Update. *Journal of Pediatric Gastroenterology and Nutrition, 48*(3), 386–388.

Madsen, D., Sebolt, T., Cullen, L. et al. (2005). Listening to bowel sounds: An evidence-based practice project. *American Journal of Nursing, 105*, 40–49.

Manterola, C., Vial, M., Moraga, J. et al. (2011). Analgesia in patients with acute abdominal pain. *Cochrane Database of Systematic Reviews*, (1), CD005660.

Marik, P. E. (2009). What is the best way to feed patients with pancreatitis? *Current Opinion in Critical Care, 15*(2), 131–138.

Massey, R. (2012). Return of bowel sounds indicating an end of postoperative ileus: Is it time to cease this long-standing nursing tradition? *Medsurg Nursing: Official Journal of the Academy of Medical-Surgical Nurses, 21*(3), 146–150.

Metheny, N., Eisenberg, P., & McSweeney, M. (1988). Effect of feeding tube properties and three irrigants on clogging rates. *Nursing Research, 37*(3), 165–169.

Metheny, N. A., & Meert, K. L. (2004). Monitoring feeding tube placement. *Nutrition in Clinical Practice, 19*, 487–495.

Molina-Solana, R., Yáñez-Vico, R. M., Iglesias-Linares, A. et al. (2013). Current concepts on the effect of environmental factors on cleft lip and palate. *International Journal of Oral and Maxillofacial Surgery, 42*(2), 177–184.

Mousa, H. M., Rosen, R., Woodley, F. W. et al. (2011). Esophageal impedance monitoring for gastroesophageal reflux. *Journal of Pediatric Gastroenterology and Nutrition, 52*(2), 129–139.

Mugie, S. M., Benninga, M. A., & Di Lorenzo, C. (2011). Epidemiology of constipation in children and adults: A systematic review. *Best Practice & Research. Clinical Gastroenterology, 25*(1), 3–18.

Pandya, S., & Heiss, K. (2012). Pyloric stenosis in pediatric surgery: An evidence-based review. *Surgical Clinics of North America, 92*(3), 527–539.

Pärtty, A., Kalliomäki, M., Endo, A. et al. (2012). Compositional development of Bifidobacterium and Lactobacillus microbiota is linked with crying and fussing in early infancy. *PLoS One, 7*(3), e32495.

Pepper, V., Stanfill, A., & Pearl, R. (2012). Diagnosis and management of pediatric appendicitis, intussusception, and Meckel diverticulum. *Surgical Clinics of North America, 92*(3), 505–526.

Pinelli, J., & Symington, A. (2005). Nonnutritive sucking for promoting physiologic stability and nutrition in preterm infants [Review]. *Cochrane Database of Systematic Reviews*, (4), CD001071.

Pinheiro, P. F. M., Simões e Silva, A. C., & Pereira, R. M. (2012). Current knowledge on esophageal atresia. *World Journal of Gastroenterology, 18*(29), 3662–3672.

Rahimi, R., & Abdollahi, M. (2012). Herbal medicines for the management of irritable bowel syndrome: A comprehensive review. *World Journal of Gastroenterology, 18*(7), 589–600.

Ranji, S. R., Goldman, L. E., Simel, D. L. et al. (2006). Do opiates affect the clinical evaluation of patients with acute abdominal pain? *Journal of the American Medical Association, 296*(14), 1764–1774.

Rajindrajith, S., & Devanarayana, N. M. (2011). Constipation in children: Novel insight into epidemiology, pathophysiology and management. *Journal of Neurogastroenterology and Motility, 17*(1), 35–47.

Rasquin, A., Di Lorenzo, C., Forbes, D. et al. (2006). Childhood functional gastrointestinal disorders: Child/adolescent. *Gastroenterology, 130*(5), 1527–1537.

Rintala, R. J., & Pakarinen, M. P. (2012). Long-term outcomes of Hirschsprung's disease. *Seminars in Pediatric Surgery, 21*(4), 336–343.

Ritchie, M. L., & Romanuk, T. N. (2012). A meta-analysis of probiotic efficacy for gastrointestinal diseases. *PLoS One, 7*(4), e34938.

Rollins, M. D. (2012). Recent advances in the management of congenital diaphragmatic hernia. *Current Opinion in Pediatrics, 24*(3), 379–385.

Sadove, M. A., van Aalst, J. A., & Culp, J. A. (2004). Cleft palate repair: Art and issues. *Clinics in Plastic Surgery, 31*(2), 231–241.

Saito, J. (2012). Beyond appendicitis: Evaluation and surgical treatment of pediatric acute abdominal pain. *Current Opinion in Pediatrics, 24*(3), 357–364.

Savino, F., & Tarasco, V. (2010). New treatments for infant colic. *Current Opinion in Pediatrics, 22*(6), 791–797.

Savino, F., Viola, S., Erasmo, M. et al. (2012). Efficacy and tolerability of peg-only laxative on faecal impaction and chronic constipation in children. A controlled double blind randomized study vs a standard peg-electrolyte laxative. *BMC Pediatrics, 12*, 178.

Scholler, I., & Nittur, S. (2012). Understanding failure to thrive. *Paediatrics and Child Health, 22*(10), 438–442.

Schwartz, M. Z. (2012). Hypertrophic pyloric stenosis. In A. G. Coran, N. S. Adzick, T. M. Krummel et al. (Eds.), *Pediatric surgery* (7th ed., pp. 1021–1028). Philadelphia, PA: Saunders Elsevier.

See, J., & Murray, J. A. (2006). Gluten-free diet: The medical and nutrition management of celiac disease. *Nutrition in Clinical Practice, 21*(1), 1–15.

Semeniuk, J., & Kaczmarski, M. (2006). Gastroesophageal reflux (GER) in children and adolescents with regard to food intolerance. *Advances in Medical Sciences, 51*, 321–326.

Shamir, R., & Eliakim, R. (2008). Capsule endoscopy in pediatric patients. *World Journal of Gastroenterology, 14*(26), 4152–4155.

Shepanski, M. A, Hurd, L. B., Culton, K. et al. (2005). Health-related quality of life improves in children and adolescents with inflammatory bowel disease after attending a camp sponsored by the Crohn's and Colitis Foundation of America. *Inflammatory Bowel Diseases, 11*(2), 164–170.

Sherman, P. M., Hassall, E., Fagundes-Neto, U. et al. (2009). A global, evidence-based consensus on the definition of gastroesophageal reflux disease in the pediatric population. *American Journal of Gastroenterology, 104*(5), 1278–1295.

Stellar, J., & Widmer, T. (2013). Intestinal atresias, duplications, and meconium ileus. In N. Browne, L. Flanigan, C. McComiskey et al. (Eds.), *Nursing care of the pediatric surgical patient* (3rd ed., pp. 313–329). Burlington, MA: Jones and Bartlett Learning.

Szavay, P., Obermayr, F., Maas, C. et al. (2012). Perioperative outcome of patients with congenital diaphragmatic hernia undergoing open versus minimally invasive surgery. *Journal of Laparoendoscopic & Advanced Surgical Techniques, 22*(3), 285–289.

Tillman, E. M., & Helms, R. A. (2011). Omega-3 long chain polyunsaturated fatty acids for treatment of parenteral nutrition–associated liver disease: A review of the literature. *Journal of Pediatric Pharmacology and Therapeutics, 16*(1), 31–38.

Tully, M. A. (2008). Pediatric celiac disease. *Gastroenterology Nursing, 31*(2), 132–140.

Turner, D., Zlotkin, S. H., Shah, P. S. et al. (2009). Omega 3 fatty acids (fish oil) for maintenance of remission in Crohn's disease. *Cochrane Database of Systematic Reviews*, (1), CD006320.

van den Berg, M. M., Benninga, M. A., & Di Lorenzo, C. (2006). Epidemiology of childhood constipation: A systematic review. *American Journal of Gastroenterology*, *101*(10), 2401–2409.

van der Zee, D. C., & Bax, K. M. A. (2007). Thoracoscopic treatment of esophageal atresia with distal fistula and of tracheomalacia. *Seminars in Pediatric Surgery*, *16*(4), 224–230.

Vandenplas, Y., Rudolph, C. D., Di Lorenzo, C. et al. (2009). Pediatric gastroesophageal reflux clinical practice guidelines. Joint recommendations of the North American Society for Pediatric Gastroenterology, Hepatology, and Nutrition (NASPGHAN) and the European Society for Pediatric Gastroenterology, Hepatology, and Nutrition (ESPGHAN). *Journal of Pediatric Gastroenterology and Nutrition*, *49*(4), 498–547.

Venter, C., Laitinen, K., & Vlieg-Boerstra, B. (2012). Nutritional aspects in diagnosis and management of food hypersensitivity—The dietitians role. *Journal of Allergy (Cairo)*, *2012*(269376).

Walker, L. S., Williams, S. E., Smith, C. A. et al. (2006). Parent attention versus distraction: Impact on symptom complaints by children with and without chronic functional abdominal pain. *Pain*, *122*(1–2), 43–52.

Wang, K. S. (2012). Assessment and management of inguinal hernia in infants. *Pediatrics*, *130*(4), 768–773.

Westhus, N. (2004). Methods to test feeding tube placement in children. *Maternal Child Nursing*, *29*(5), 282–287, 290–291.

Whitcomb, D. (2012). Framework for interpretation of genetic variations in pancreatitis patients. *Frontiers in Physiology*, *3*, 440.

Yuan, Y., Chen, J. Y., Guo, H. et al. (2010). Relief of abdominal pain by morphine without altering physical signs in acute appendicitis. *Chinese Medical Journal*, *123*(2), 142–145.

Zerpa, J., & Shapiro, T. (2013). Malrotation and volvulus. In N. Browne, L. Flanigan, C. McComiskey et al. (Eds.), *Nursing care of the pediatric surgical patient* (3rd ed., pp. 333–344). Burlington, MA: Jones and Bartlett Learning.

See thePoint for additional organizations.

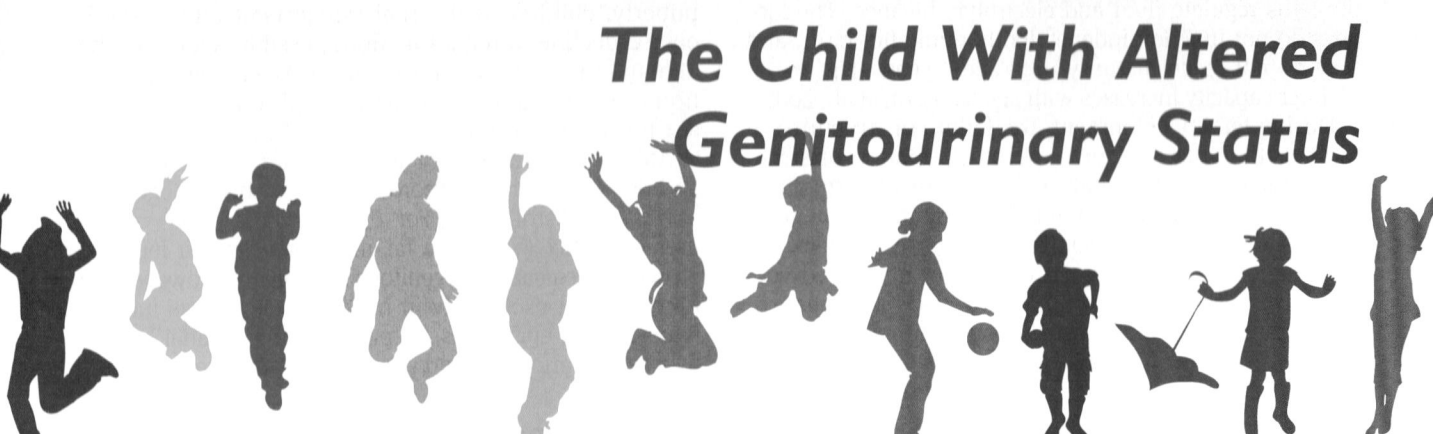

CHAPTER 19

The Child With Altered Genitourinary Status

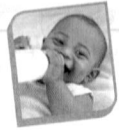

CASE HISTORY

B. J. and J. D. Johnson were first introduced in Chapter 5. They are African American fraternal twins with one older sister. When they were born, J. D. was noted to have a glanular hypospadias without chordee. B. J. was circumcised the day after the twins were born, but the health care provider recommended that J. D. not be circumcised until after his surgery to repair the hypospadias. The boys' father, James Johnson, has expressed concerns about the anomaly, the surgical repair of his son's penis, and the delay of circumcision. J. D. is now 9 months old and is scheduled to have hypospadias repair as an outpatient.

CHAPTER OBJECTIVES

1 Correlate the child's history, symptoms, and physical signs with manifestations of genitourinary abnormalities.

2 Identify various diagnostic procedures and their applications in genitourinary evaluation.

3 Identify evidence-based therapies available to children with alterations in genitourinary status.

4 Describe common alterations in health patterns related to the genitourinary system.

5 Identify the teaching needs of the child experiencing challenges related to urinary elimination.

6 Discuss the types of renal replacement therapies available for the child experiencing acute renal failure or chronic renal disease.

7 Choose evidence-based nursing interventions that support the interdisciplinary plan of care for the child with a genitourinary disorder.

See thePoint for a list of Key Terms.

Pediatric urology and nephrology are complementary, but distinct, practice disciplines. Urology studies the structure and function of all parts of the urinary tract. Nephrology studies kidney function: how the kidneys regulate serum chemistries, maintain fluid balance, and produce hormones.

Urologic and nephrologic disorders in children run the gamut, from problems such as hydrocele, proteinuria, and urinary tract infections (UTIs) to complex disorders including bladder exstrophy and renal failure. Recurrent UTIs, enuresis, and dysfunctional voiding are the most common genitourinary conditions affecting children. Urologic and nephrologic sequelae often result from neurologic disorders such as myelomeningocele, neuromuscular dysfunction, or accompanying abdominal or sacral tumors, such as rhabdomyosarcoma or sacral teratoma. Trauma to the genitourinary tract, or shock resulting from trauma, can cause renal or urologic problems. Malformations of the genitalia and urinary system structures can occur during fetal development. Although some of these malformations are life threatening, many can be surgically corrected when the child is young.

Medical advances have led to development of more types of diagnostic tools, improvement in surgical techniques, and refinements in the equipment used to treat genitourinary abnormalities. As a result, the lives of many children have been prolonged and improved by treatment of these disorders.

DEVELOPMENTAL AND BIOLOGIC VARIANCES

The genitourinary system begins to form during the first month of gestation with the rudimentary development of the kidneys. Between the 11th and 12th weeks of gestation, the fetal kidneys begin to produce urine. In utero, the placenta serves as a "pseudokidney," helping the fetus regulate fluid and electrolyte balance. The kidneys do not function independently until after birth, and they do not reach maturity until age 2 years (Fig. 19-1). Bladder capacity increases with age (Jansson et al., 2005).

During fetal development, the failure of structures to form or the abnormal or duplicate formation of structures result in congenital genitourinary abnormalities (see thePoint for Supplemental Information: Congenital Anomalies and Associated Genitourinary Defects). Obstruction of urine flow, as a result of misplaced vessels or abnormal innervation, can cause back-pressure of urine and damage to renal tissue before birth. This pressure may result in **hydronephrosis**, a condition in which urine backs up into the renal pelvis and calyces, which dilate and impair renal function.

In young children, renal blood flow is slow, the reabsorption of amino acids is limited, autoregulation is not fully developed, and concentration of urine is not as effective as in an adult. Thus, during periods of fluid loss (caused by diarrhea, fever, fluid restrictions, or reduced fluid intake), the child is at increased risk for dehydration.

Most children with genitourinary disorders are younger than 7 years old, because the most common disorders are usually congenital, with symptoms manifesting early in life. The most common noncongenital genitourinary condition is UTI. UTIs are more common in girls until they reach school age, with an incidence of about 8% compared to 2% in males, likely because of a short urethra and close proximity to fecal bacteria (Habib, 2012). UTIs increase in incidence in females after the commencement of sexual activity.

Diseases in children younger than 5 years of age that result in end-stage renal disease (ESRD) are generally congenital. Those leading to ESRD in older children are usually the result of other urologic abnormalities. At puberty, children with renal impairment often experience a decline in renal function, possibly related to the demand of increasing muscle mass exceeding the function of the remaining functional nephrons or related to sex hormones, or both.

Although genitourinary abnormalities occur in males and females, certain disorders have a distinct gender-associated distribution. For example, UTIs and vesicoureteral reflux (VUR) are far more prevalent in females. Structural defects of the genitourinary organs, however, are found almost exclusively in males. These defects include hypospadias, epispadias, cryptorchidism, inguinal hernia, hydrocele, varicocele, and posterior urethral web or valve.

ASSESSMENT

Signs and symptoms of genitourinary and renal conditions, such as mild abdominal pain, low-grade fever, slow weight gain, and edema, are often subtle. Determining when symptoms began may be difficult because clinical signs may have gone unnoted for some time before the child presents for evaluation.

FOCUSED HEALTH HISTORY

 QUESTION: Which aspects of J. D.'s focused health history are most important to obtain?

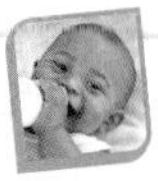

In the focused health history, collect data that may indicate a primary or secondary condition that affects genitourinary function (Focused Health History 19-1).

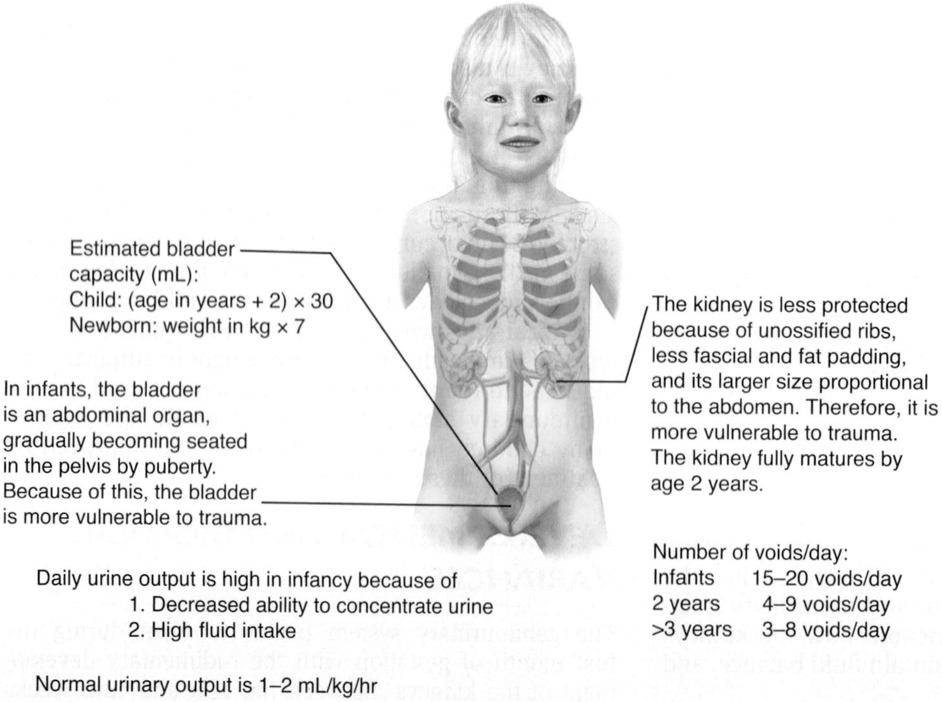

Estimated bladder capacity (mL):
Child: (age in years + 2) × 30
Newborn: weight in kg × 7

In infants, the bladder is an abdominal organ, gradually becoming seated in the pelvis by puberty. Because of this, the bladder is more vulnerable to trauma.

The kidney is less protected because of unossified ribs, less fascial and fat padding, and its larger size proportional to the abdomen. Therefore, it is more vulnerable to trauma. The kidney fully matures by age 2 years.

Daily urine output is high in infancy because of
1. Decreased ability to concentrate urine
2. High fluid intake

Normal urinary output is 1–2 mL/kg/hr

Number of voids/day:
Infants   15–20 voids/day
2 years   4–9 voids/day
>3 years   3–8 voids/day

Figure 19-1 Developmental and biologic variances: genitourinary system.

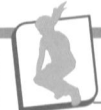

The Child With Altered Genitourinary Status

Current history	Poor growth
	Weight gain/edema, most recent weight
	Malaise, fatigue
	Intermittent fevers, chronic infections and treatment of seizures (may be a sign of electrolyte abnormalities)
	Changes in or abnormal voiding patterns
	  - Frequency of urination, urgency
	  - Presence of pain or burning during voiding
	  - Quality of urinary stream, dribbling
	  - Straining with voiding
	  - Pre- and postvoid leaking
	  - Holding maneuvers (in which the child sits on the heels in such a way to suppress the urge to void)
	  - Color and odor of the urine
	  - Presence of day or nighttime enuresis
	Discharge from urethra or genitals
	Hematuria, proteinuria, hypertension
	Changes in consistency and frequency of stools, chronic constipation or encopresis
	Enlargements, lumps, or masses in groin, abdomen, or scrotum
	Abdominal or flank pain (duration, intensity, precipitating factors, anything that improved or increased the symptoms)
	Current medications and recreational drugs (nonsteroidal anti-inflammatory drugs can be particularly nephrotoxic)
	Home remedies for current genitourinary/renal conditions and their success or failure
	Presence and treatment of any chronic genitourinary/renal disease or other conditions

Past medical history	**Prenatal/Neonatal History** *Maternal* Polyhydramnios or oligohydramnios Diabetes or hypertension Toxemia Alcohol ingestion or cocaine exposure Use of nephrotoxic drugs Abnormal antenatal ultrasounds (if present, what gestational age the alterations were noted) *Infant* Birth weight Gestational age Asphyxia Ear abnormalities Presence of a single umbilical artery (often associated with renal abnormalities) Abdominal mass Abnormal newborn screening test results Chromosome anomaly Malformations (spina bifida, cardiac, esophageal, rectal, pulmonary) *Previous Health Challenges* Bleeding disorders Streptococcal infections and treatment Varicella Hospitalizations or surgeries, circumcision at birth Status of current immunizations, especially varicella Latex sensitivity If prior genitourinary or renal problem: information about the condition, any ongoing treatments, medications, or special appliances that the child is using as a result of the condition

(Continued)

FOCUSED HEALTH HISTORY 19-1

The Child With Altered Genitourinary Status *(Continued)*

Nutritional assessment	Types and quantity of fluid and food intake Sodium intake Dietary preferences or difficulties; episodes of thirst, anorexia, nausea, vomiting, craving for salty foods
Family medical history	Familial renal disease or uropathology Familial type 1, or insulin-dependent, diabetes Hypertension Hematuria, proteinuria Systemic lupus erythematosus/lupus nephritis Dialysis or renal transplantation may signify inheritable renal disorder Deafness (Alport syndrome) Chronic UTIs Renal or urinary tract calculi Parental enuresis and age at resolution If any of these are present, presentation, evaluation, and treatment
Social and environmental history	Any recent life changes (e.g., in school, family, death, parental divorce or separation)
Growth and development	Normal growth trajectory, failure to thrive, short stature Age at which child achieved daytime and nighttime bowel and bladder control Delayed puberty, age of onset of menses Sleep habits (e.g., does child sleep deeply and not arouse to void) School performance, as age appropriate

Note: See Chapter 8 for a comprehensive health history.

Obtain a detailed history of the child's voiding pattern (Chart 19-1). A bowel history helps to evaluate constipation, which can be connected to incontinence and UTIs.

Note any recent colds or other respiratory or dermatologic infections. Streptococcal infections may lead to antigen–antibody reactions that can affect renal function as much as 2 to 3 weeks after the infection has resolved (see the sections in this chapter on "Hemolytic–Uremic Syndrome" and acute "Postinfectious Glomerulonephritis").

Gather a comprehensive family medical history; many genitourinary abnormalities in children are more likely to occur if other family members have had the same condition. For instance, functional incontinence, urinary tract anomalies, and renal calculi have familial distributions.

ANSWER: When obtaining J. D.'s health history, important aspects include information about any familial issues related to genitourinary function, including a family history of anomalies. Information related to the mother's pregnancy and labor, and J. D.'s birth, as well as information about any other anomalies, is also important.

FOCUSED PHYSICAL ASSESSMENT

Although direct examination of the kidneys and urinary tract is difficult, inspecting, auscultating, percussing, and palpating parts of the genitourinary system and other body systems may provide information about renal function (Focused Physical Assessment 19-1). Direct special attention toward the abdomen, spine, and external genitalia and to neuromuscular status of the lower extremities. Genitourinary conditions, renal disease, and renal failure have particularly far-reaching effects on different body systems because of the renal system's critical role in regulating fluid and electrolyte balance. Furthermore, abnormalities in other body systems are often associated with genitourinary disorders because gestational events that affect genitourinary development may also affect other developing systems. In addition, evaluate bowel habits because urinary dysfunction is sometimes brought on by bowel dysfunction.

While obtaining the health history, formulate a general impression of the child's renal health. Observe for poor skin color, fatigability or lethargy, bony configurations, and abnormal speech patterns,

CHART 19-1   A Voiding Profile

1. How often does your child urinate? During the day? _____ During the night? _____

2. Is the urine stream Strong, Weak, Dribbling, Small? (circle applicable answers)

3. Does your child have difficulty initiating the urine stream? Yes   No

4. Can your child tell when he or she needs to void during the day? Sometimes   Always   Never
   What does your child do when he or she needs to void? Ignore the sensation Go to the bathroom Squat or cross legs to avoid going to the bathroom

5. Does your child experience pain with urination? Yes   No
   How old was your child when he or she was toilet trained (dry during the day)? _____ years _____ months

6. Does your child have any daytime wetting accidents? Yes   No
   If yes, how many a day? _____
   How long has this been going on? _____ months _____ years

7. Does your child soak his or her underwear when he or she wets? Yes   No

8. Have you tried any treatment? Yes   No

9. Does your child leak urine (dribble) after going to the bathroom? Yes   No

10. Does your child have dribbling caused by activities such as coughing, sneezing, laughing, running, or playing sports? Yes   No

11. Does your child have damp underwear during the day? Yes   No

12. Does your child wear protective pads for any wetting accidents? Yes   No

13. Does your child wet the bed? Yes   No
    If yes, how many times a night does he or she wet the bed? _____

14. How long has your child wet the bed? _____

15. Has there ever been a time when your child was dry at night? Yes   No

16. Have you ever tried treatment? Yes   No
    If yes, what treatment? _____

17. Has your child ever had a UTI? Yes   No
    If yes, what were the symptoms _____

18. Has your child had unexplained fevers? Yes   No

19. Does your child have frequent stomachaches? Yes   No

20. How often does your child have a bowel movement? _____

21. What is the consistency of the bowel movements? Hard, round balls Soft and log shaped

22. How much fluid does your child drink during day? _____

23. What fluids does your child drink during the day? _____

24. How does your child bathe? Shower Bath

all of which can occur in urinary conditions or renal failure. In particular, assess for signs of fluid overload and electrolyte imbalance, including changes in vital signs and the presence of edema and ascites. Electrolyte imbalance can lead to skeletal and cardiac manifestations, such as fractures and murmurs. Chapter 17 presents more information on fluid and electrolyte imbalances and their effects on all body systems.

On physical examination, the child's abdomen should appear flat when the child is lying supine. On percussion, dullness or flatness should be heard along the left costal margin over the spleen and kidneys and 1 to 3 cm below the right costal margin over the liver. Dullness heard above the symphysis pubis indicates a full bladder. Tympany should normally be heard throughout the rest of the abdomen.

It is difficult to palpate most genitourinary organs. The kidneys are rarely palpable, except in neonates. A distended bladder may be palpated above the symphysis pubis. Palpation that elicits complaints of abdominal tenderness is common in UTI.

Examine genitalia for structural anomalies, such as labial fusion in a female and hypospadias or epispadias in a male. In an uncircumcised male older than age 3 years, the foreskin of the penis is usually retractable without difficulty; narrowing of the preputial opening of the foreskin that prevents it from being retracted over the glans penis is called **phimosis**. Palpate the testes to ensure that they have descended. Chapter 8 presents a more detailed description of abdominal and genital assessment.

DIAGNOSTIC CRITERIA

 QUESTION: Would J. D. have had to undergo any diagnostic tests or procedures to confirm his condition?

Various diagnostic procedures and laboratory tests are used to evaluate genitourinary function. Tests and Procedures 19-1 describes common diagnostic studies for evaluating the genitourinary system. Procedures can be invasive and frightening, particularly for the young child. Catheterization is especially feared because of the coinciding features of urologic function and sexual expression that shape the child's concept of the genital organs. Teachings of "good touch/bad touch" sexual abuse programs may further compound the child's apprehension.

KidKare Before the procedure, prepare the child and family by describing the internal structures that will be examined. Helpful steps include giving demonstrations using anatomically correct dolls; showing pictures of or touring the radiology department; and describing the visual, auditory, and somatic experiences the child will encounter during the study or procedure. Be honest with the child, and use age-appropriate information.

Teach the child coping skills (e.g., guided imagery, relaxation and deep breathing, use of music or distraction techniques) and reinforce use of these skills during the procedure.

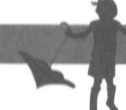

FOCUSED PHYSICAL ASSESSMENT 19-1
The Child With Altered Genitourinary Status

Assessment Parameter	Alterations/Clinical Significance
General appearance	Child may be listless because of electrolyte imbalance or anemia.
	Chronic kidney disease (CKD), UTI, or renal failure may cause poor growth.
	Poor skin turgor, dry mucosa, or recent weight loss may indicate dehydration.
	Sudden weight gain may indicate fluid excess.
	Child may have vague complaints or none because the decrease in renal function progresses slowly.
Integumentary system (skin, hair, nails)	Pallor suggests anemia resulting from decreased erythropoietin (EPO) levels.
	Dry, pruritic skin with petechiae can be caused by uremia.
	"Doughiness" can be caused by poor nutrition or fluid excess.
	Hypopigmented spots, seen in tuberous sclerosis, can be associated with polycystic kidney disease.
	Café-au-lait spots may indicate neurofibromatosis, which is associated with renal artery stenosis.
	Dysplasia of nails may be a sign of nail–patella syndrome, which is associated with nephrotic syndrome (NS).
	Malar rash, photosensitivity, and discoid rash are associated with systemic lupus erythematosus, which may include lupus nephritis.
	Purpura is seen in Henoch-Schönlein purpura.
Head and neck	Microcephaly is a syndromal feature that can be associated with obstructive uropathy or chronic renal failure in infants.
	Potter facies can occur with renal agenesis and oligohydramnios.
	Periorbital edema is caused by fluid retention from nephritic syndrome or renal failure.
	Low-set ears or high-arched palate may be indicators of multisystem syndrome with associated urologic abnormalities.
	Short neck and low hairline is associated with Klippel Feil syndrome, which may include renal adysplasia.
	Pale mucosa can indicate anemia.
	Circumoral cyanosis can indicate a heart defect with associated renal anomalies.
	Webbed neck occurs with Turner or Noonan syndromes, genetic conditions also associated with renal or gonadal malformations.
Eyes	Cataracts, Lisch nodules, and colobomata are associated with retinitis pigmentosa; renal disease may be associated.
	Splinter hemorrhages and cotton-wool patches are indicative of hypertension.
Ears	Structural abnormalities (e.g., preauricular pits) of the ears or deafness are associated with renal malformation.
Face, nose, and oral cavity	Caries and tooth discoloration are common in chronic renal disease.
Thorax and lungs	Rapid or deep breathing may be a sign of respiratory compensation for acidosis.
	Rales may indicate fluid excess.
	Widely spaced nipples are associated with Turner syndrome, which may include horseshoe kidneys.

Assessment Parameter	Alterations/Clinical Significance
Cardiovascular system	Rapid, irregular pulse may indicate fluid excess.
	Elevated blood pressure can occur with renal failure, fluid excess, or certain medications; alternately, improper cuff size may have been used to obtain measurement.
	Murmurs are associated with anemia as well as cardiac defects.
	A friction rub can indicate pericarditis caused by uremia, inadequate dialysis, or infected hemodialysis access (catheters, grafts, fistulas).
Abdomen	Fluid excess can lead to edema, ascites, and descent of the liver margin.
	A protuberant abdomen may suggest fluid retention, organomegaly, peritonitis, or ascites.
	Distended veins may indicate abdominal or vascular distention.
	Flank masses may be unilateral or bilateral and in children are usually of renal origin: multicystic kidney disease, hydronephrosis, autosomal recessive polycystic kidney disease (ARPKD), Wilms tumor.
	Slack abdominal muscles may indicate prune-belly syndrome.
	Fever and local swelling, redness, and discharge at exit sites for urinary drainage tubes and peritoneal dialysis (PD) catheters are signs of infection.
	Hydronephrotic kidneys or distended bladder may be palpable.
	Chronic constipation/encopresis correlates with UTI and voiding dysfunction.
Lymphatic system	Lymphedema may be related to Turner syndrome, which may include horseshoe kidneys.
External genitalia (includes anus) and breasts	Unusual genital appearance may result from birth defects and other anomalies.
	Masses, lesions, and inability to palpate testes on palpation of scrotal sac suggest testicular anomalies or undescended testicles.
	Tanner stage of puberty can be delayed in CKD.
	Amenorrhea, anovulation, impotence, and sterility are common in postpubertal young people with chronic renal disease.
Musculoskeletal system	"Renal rickets" (changes and pathologic fractures of ribs and long bones of arms and legs) occurs with renal osteodystrophy in children; bones are weakened by changes in calcium and phosphorus metabolism with renal failure.
	Short stature associated with numerous conditions that involve kidney abnormalities.
	Postaxial polydactyly, absent or small patella seen in nail–patella syndrome, which may include NS.
	Muscle wasting occurs in advanced chronic renal disease.
	Muscle weakness occurs in many renal conditions.
Neurologic system	Developmental delay may result from chronic condition and its treatment.
	Fatigability, muscle wasting, and lethargy can occur with renal failure.
	Level of consciousness may be decreased in renal failure.
	Temporary psychosis with hallucinations can result from very high levels of blood urea nitrogen (BUN).
	Gait can change as a result of fluid in abdomen for PD.
	Sacral abnormalities such as deformed gluteal cleft, tuft of hair, vascular markings, a dimple, or lipomeningocele are associated with myelodysplasia, the most common cause of neuropathic bladder dysfunction in children.
	Fine/gross motor development delay may be associated with enuresis.

TESTS AND PROCEDURES for Evaluating Genitourinary Status

Diagnostic Test or Procedure	Purpose	Findings and Indications	Health Care Provider Considerations
Blood Studies			
Complete blood count (CBC), white blood cell (WBC) count	Determines number of WBCs in blood	Normal Newborn: 9,000–30,000 cells/mm^3 0–2 years old: 6,000–17,000 cells/mm^3 >2 years old: 5,000–10,000 cells/mm^3 Elevated in presence of infection or inflammation Decreased in lupus/viral illnesses	Deliver specimen to laboratory within 4 hours of drawing blood.
Hemoglobin	Determines total concentration of hemoglobin in peripheral blood; tests for anemia	Normal Newborn: 14–24 g/dL Infant: 10–15 g/dL Child: 11–16 g/dL Lower in presence of renal parenchymal disease, obstructive uropathy, CKD	Shortened red blood cell life span and decreased erythropoiesis with renal disease
Hematocrit	Determines percentage of red blood cells to total volume of blood	Normal Newborn: 44%–64% Infant: 30%–40% Child: 31%–43% Lower in presence of renal parenchymal disease, obstructive uropathy, CKD	
Clotting studies: Prothrombin time (PT), partial thromboplastin time (PTT), international normalized ratio (INR)	Determines PT and PTT, thus evaluating the extrinsic coagulation system	Normal PT: Newborn: 12–17 seconds Child: 11–13 seconds Normal PTT: Newborn: 25–45 seconds Child: 30–45 seconds Normal thrombin time: Newborn: 12–16 seconds Child: 7–12 seconds Prolonged in children experiencing renal complications Thrombocytopenia	If insufficient blood is added to a citrate-containing tube, a falsely elevated PT may result. Do not obtain blood sample for test within 3 hours of a heparin dose.
Serum chemistries (BUN, creatinine, electrolytes, glucose)	Evaluates fluid and electrolyte status in presence of acute renal failure or chronic renal disease	Elevated levels indicative of renal disease	Sodium can be decreased with polyuria or urinary-concentrating defects.

Diagnostic Test or Procedure	Purpose	Findings and Indications	Health Care Provider Considerations
Cholesterol, triglycerides	Evaluates for hyperlipidemia	Elevated in children with acute renal failure or chronic renal disease and NS	Child should fast 12–14 hours before sample is drawn.
Erythrocyte sedimentation rate (ESR)	A nonspecific test to detect inflammatory or infectious disease	Normal Newborn: 0–2 mm/hr Child: 0–20 mm/hr Elevated levels suggest inflammatory state.	
C-reactive protein (CRP)	Nonspecific test to diagnose infection or inflammation	Normal, <0.8 mg/dL Elevated levels indicate presence of inflammatory process.	
Antinuclear antibody (ANA) C3	Evaluates abnormal levels in the complement system	High level of false-positive ANA levels Low C3 level indicative of postinfectious glomerulonephritis (PIGN) or systemic lupus erythematosus	

Urinalysis

Specific gravity	Measures the concentration of particles in the urine to evaluate the concentrating and excretory ability of the kidneys	Normal Newborn: 1.001–1.015 Child: 1.001–1.025 Low: diabetes insipidus, pyelonephritis, renal damage High: dehydration	To accurately determine specific gravity, use first morning void. If not analyzed immediately, refrigerate the urine.
pH	Indicates acid–base balance of patient	Normal, 4.6–8.0 (average, 6.0) Increased in presence of bacteriuria	Urine becomes alkaline upon standing. Foods may affect pH: citrus fruits, dairy products, and vegetables cause alkaline urine; meat and fruits (e.g., cranberry) cause acidic urine.
Blood	Determines presence of red blood cells in urine	Normal: 0–2 red blood cells per high-power field Elevated levels indicate possible UTI, calculus, trauma, urethral obstruction, renal parenchymal disease.	When obtaining urine sample from adolescent females, question about presence of menstruation.

(Continued)

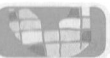

TESTS AND PROCEDURES for Evaluating Genitourinary Status *(Continued)*

Diagnostic Test or Procedure	Purpose	Findings and Indications	Health Care Provider Considerations
Protein	Indicates renal disease	Negative: <8 mg/dL Positive test indicates renal disease; the presence of protein is indicative of glomerulonephritis and requires immediate intervention.	False-positive result occurs after strenuous activity or stress. Obtain first morning void. A 24-hour specimen is more accurate than a spot urine and is usually paired with a similarly collected urine creatinine to standardize the results. Keep refrigerated
Glucose	Determines presence of sugar in urine	Presence of glucose may indicate diabetes mellitus, a potential cause for nocturnal enuresis. Also associated with renal tubular damage	
Leukocyte esterase (LE)	Detects LE, an enzyme that breaks down WBCs	Normal: negative Positive dipstick testing indicates probable UTI.	Obtain midstream clean-catch urine sample. Test may not be accurate for children. False-positive results are seen in urine mixed with vaginal secretions. False-negative results are seen in urine with high protein levels or increased ascorbic acid levels.
Nitrites	Indicates conversion of nitrate to nitrite by bacteria	Negative Positive test may indicate bacteriuria.	False-negative result occurs often with children. Obtain midstream clean-catch sample from adolescent females.
Urine Microscopic Studies			
WBCs	Detects WBCs in urine	Normal: 0–4 cells per high-power field More than 5 cells indicates pyuria.	Obtain midstream clean-catch urine from females.
Red blood cells	Detects red blood cells in urine	Normal: 0–3 cells per high-power field	
Casts	Detects "clumps" of cells; can be WBCs, red blood cells, hyaline casts	Hyaline casts: 0–3 cells per low-power field, normal; any other cast are abnormal Red blood cell casts need further investigation for acute glomerulonephritis.	

Diagnostic Test or Procedure	Purpose	Findings and Indications	Health Care Provider Considerations
Bacteria	Detects UTI	Normal: negative Positive: visible bacteria	Difficult to detect Obtain midstream clean-catch sample to avoid contamination.

Microbiologic Studies

Urine culture and sensitivity	Determines the presence of bacterial pathogens Determines the type of bacteria Determines how effectively various antibiotics will inhibit bacterial growth	Normal: no growth More than 100,000 colony-forming unit (CFU)/mL are indicative of UTI. Sensitivity reported by zone of inhibition or by degree of sensitivity/resistance per antibiotic	Obtain midstream clean-catch samples. Young or non–toilet-trained children may require suprapubic aspiration or catheterization. If unable to process urine within 30 minutes, refrigerate sample. Obtain sample before initiating antibiotic therapy.

24-Hour Urine Collection

Creatinine clearance	Assesses glomerular filtration rate (GFR) from timed urine collection *and* blood sampling	Creatinine clearance values should be close to GFR values. Increased levels indicate CKD.	Refrigerate urine collection as retrieved. Attach a sticker to the collection bottle indicating the date and times urine collection started and stopped and the child's height and weight.

Radiographic Studies

Kidney, ureter, and bladder (KUB, or flat plate) radiograph	Screening study to check for urinary calculi and to assess location, size, and shape of urinary organs	Normal organ placement and size, no calculi, normal gas pattern Abnormal findings require further testing.	Barium from other radiographic studies may interfere. Older children may be asked to hold their breath for a part of the picture.
Ultrasound (sonogram)	Use of reflected sound waves to evaluate kidney, bladder, ureters, and fetal urinary system	Useful initial study to evaluate urinary structures, abdominal masses, hydronephrosis, urinary calculi, cysts, and renal tumors Used during shock wave lithotripsy to focus on the urinary stone	No preparation No radiation No contrast material used
Intravenous pyelogram (IVP) or excretory urogram	Evaluates kidneys and internal drainage structures; renal function demonstrated by contrast material being filtered and excreted by kidney	Can diagnose multiple congenital anomalies, calculi, obstruction, tumors	Bowel preparation is required. Barium in bowel interferes with study. Contraindication is allergy to iodine or shellfish. Increase fluids after study.

(Continued)

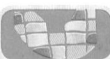 **TESTS AND PROCEDURES for Evaluating Genitourinary Status** *(Continued)*

Diagnostic Test or Procedure	Purpose	Findings and Indications	Health Care Provider Considerations
Voiding cystourethrogram (VCUG)	Visualizes bladder and urethra, evaluates urine flow during bladder emptying, grades the severity of reflux	Normal: complete emptying, no reflux, smooth bladder, no urethral anomalies VUR, lower urinary tract trauma, tumors, pelvic masses, urethral obstruction, posterior urethral valves and strictures	Not to be performed in the presence of a UTI Requires catheterization
Renal scan (scintigraphy) Dimercaptosuccinic acid (DMSA) Diethylenetriamine pentaacetic acid (DTPA, 99mC-DTPA) Mercaptoacetyltriglycine (MAG3, 99mTc-MAG3)	Injected radioisotope evaluates anatomy and function of renal parenchyma Defines the parenchymal tissue and outlines defects in the cortex, detects renal scarring Evaluates split renal function and renal blood flow; used to detect kidney obstruction when diuretic medication is included with the scan	Normal renal function, normal time to excrete dye Pyelonephritis, urinary obstruction, nonfunctioning kidney (which may not be visualized by an IVP), tumor, abscess, trauma	Do not schedule within 24 hours after IVP. Minimal radiation exposure Child should be well hydrated. Radioactive tracer is excreted within 24 hours. Requires intravenous (IV) injection.
Computed tomography (CT)	Visualizes horizontal or vertical cross-section of kidney to determine nature of tissue material Use of iodine contrast dye enhances the image	Renal trauma, tumor, cyst, hematoma, calculi, congenital anomalies	Patient must not move during procedure; child or infant is sedated. CT with contrast requires IV injection. Inquire about allergy to shellfish or iodine.
Computed tomographic angiography	Depicts renal vessels, often used in evaluation of hypertension	Renovascular disease	
Renal angiography	Evaluates the renal blood vessels	Renal vascular malformation, definitive or preoperative embolization of vascular tumors	Requires IV injection Patient must not move during procedure; child or infant is sedated. Inquire about allergy to shellfish or iodine.
Magnetic resonance imaging (MRI)	Characterizes and stages renal lesions	Acute pyelonephritis	Equipment may induce feelings of claustrophobia.

Diagnostic Test or Procedure	Purpose	Findings and Indications	Health Care Provider Considerations
Additional Tests			
Cystoscopy	Directly visualizes urethra and bladder, bladder trigone, ureteral orifices	Urethral strictures, urethral webs, posterior urethral valves, cystitis, ectopic or displaced ureteral orifice, calculi	Requires anesthesia Preoperative preparation Dysuria noted up to 24 hours, may be intense with initial void
Urodynamics	A series of tests evaluates bladder and urethral function and innervation. Cystometrogram measures bladder capacity and pressure during the filling phase. Urinary flow rate measures volume of urine voided in a specific time. Urethral pressure profile measures urethral and sphincter competency. Electromyography measures neurologic activity of sphincter. Postvoid residual	Detrusor sphincter, dyssynergia, urethral obstruction, hyperreflexia, hyporeflexia, uninhibited bladder contractions, neurogenic bladder, congenital sphincter anomaly (e.g., bladder exstrophy)	Requires externally placed perineal electrodes Requires catheterization Requires cooperation of child, who is asked to void on command and to lie still
Percutaneous renal biopsy	Determines type of kidney disease or cause of renal failure and likelihood of recovery or disease progression	Abnormal cellular structure, inflammation, scarring, immunofluorescent staining, or electron microscopy	Sedation required Observe for signs of bleeding for 18 hours after biopsy.

Several methods are used to obtain urine samples. The choice of method is based on the reason for testing the urine and on the child's ability to void (Nursing Interventions 19-1).

caREminder

Many children have difficulty voiding on command. When a urine sample will be needed during an examination, remind the family to offer fluids to the child on the trip to the office or clinic, or have the specimen collected at home using the appropriate collection technique.

In toilet-trained children, clean-catch midstream urine samples are the easiest samples to obtain and are satisfactory for most routine urinalysis and culture and sensitivity studies. Obtaining a urine sample from a non–toilet-trained child presents a major challenge. Methods to collect urine include using a urine collection bag, urethral catheterization, and suprapubic aspiration

(Tradition or Science 19-1; see also thePoint for Procedures/Interventions: Urine Collection: Routine Voided; Urine Collection: Urinary Catheterization: Insertion and Removal; Urine Specimen Collection Methods).

Bacterial count criteria used to establish the diagnosis of UTI are determined by the method used to collect the sample (Tradition or Science 19-2). Freshly voided samples are preferred for routine urine tests, and they are necessary for urine culture and sensitivity tests.

caREminder

If the sample cannot be sent to the laboratory within 30 minutes, refrigerate it to prevent false-positive results.

ANSWER: In most cases, hypospadias is diagnosed by physical examination. Further diagnostic testing would be warranted if J. D. was experiencing difficulty voiding or if additional anomalies of the genitourinary tract or other body systems were suspected.

NURSING INTERVENTIONS 19-1

General Considerations for Urine Specimen Collection

Consideration	Intervention
Language used by the nurse may be misunderstood by the child.	Use the child's words (e.g., "pee-pee") to make a request.
Adolescent may be reluctant to have test completed because of concerns over body image, body functions, privacy, or suspicion that specimen is requested for drug testing.	Inquire about concerns; try to elicit specific information. Explain why test is needed.
Child may have difficulty complying with request.	Provide potty chair or urine collector in toilet. Run water in sink to trigger urge to void. Offer child something to drink; most infants void shortly after feeding. Offer moderate amounts of fluid (too much fluid may dilute the specific gravity of the urine). Enlist the assistance of the family, which may increase the child's cooperation.
Disposable diapers with absorbent gel are difficult to aspirate from and yield inaccurate results.	See thePoint for Procedure: Urine Collection: Routine Voided

TREATMENT MODALITIES

Treatment to maintain or restore genitourinary function is aimed at compensating for alterations in gravity flow or muscular contraction that impede normal urine flow and reestablishing the free flow of liquid waste (urine) from the body. When renal failure occurs, multifaceted treatment must be initiated to rid the body of toxins and perform the work of the nonfunctioning kidneys.

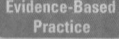 TRADITION OR SCIENCE 19-1

Should lidocaine gel be used routinely for urinary catheterization?

Two randomized controlled trials (RCTs) involving pediatric patients compared use of lubricant gel to lidocaine gel. Lidocaine gel was placed on genital mucosa and intraurethrally. Both studies showed decreased pain response and recommended use of lidocaine gel as part of a standard approach to urethral catheterization in the pediatric patient (Boots & Edmundson, 2010; Mularoni et al., 2009). Recent research recommends the use of lidocaine lubricant to decrease pain during urethral catheterization in children. This is recent research and may yet to be translated into clinical bedside care, which provides an opportunity for individuals to advocate nursing practice change.

URINARY DIVERSION

Urine normally flows unimpeded from the kidneys through the ureters and collects in the bladder. At a time that is physiologically and socially appropriate, the sphincter relaxes to allow micturition by a bladder contraction (by the smooth muscle component of the bladder). Anomalies or conditions that restrict urine flow, such as ureteral strictures or kinking, massive VUR, or spinal cord trauma, may require urologic management by urinary diversion. Diversion techniques either incorporate the use of tubes or are tubeless. Urinary diversion is most often a temporary measure, although some functional disabilities require permanent diversion.

Drainage Tubes

Various drainage tubes are used to divert urine flow. Foley catheters, ureteral stents, and nephrostomy or ureterostomy tubes provide an exit for urine from the body either proximal to an obstruction or through a section that may be occluded after surgical manipulation. In some cases, a stent or catheter is also used to create hemostasis within incised urinary mucosa or to act as a splint after ureteral reconstruction.

Advantages of externalized urinary drainage tubes are their uncomplicated design, multiple applications, and easy removal. However, because of their drawbacks, such as increased risk for infection, mucus plugs, and urolithiasis, plus the potential for accidental dislodgment, intubated urinary diversion is used for short-term management.

TRADITION OR SCIENCE 19-2

What is the best method of obtaining urine to evaluate for UTI?

In an extensive systematic review to determine the accuracy of tests to detect UTI in children younger than 5 years of age, Whiting et al. (2006) determined that, in toilet-trained children, clean, voided midstream urine (CVU) samples had similar accuracy to those obtained by suprapubic aspiration. Although urethral catheterization has been considered a reliable method to diagnose UTI, newer research indicates that samples obtained by catheterization should be interpreted similar to CVU (Lau et al., 2007). Agreement between CVU and catheterized specimens analyzed by the presence/absence of growth was good in boys but poor in girls; agreement was poor when samples were analyzed by colony counts, with CVU having higher counts than catheter (Lau et al., 2007). Catheterized specimens produced fewer false positives than CVU, but both rates were unacceptably high (Lau et al., 2007).

In non–toilet-trained children, suprapubic aspiration is reliable and has been considered the gold standard, but many parents and health care providers consider it unacceptably invasive, and it may not always be successful (Roberts et al., 2011; Etoubleau et al., 2009). American Academy of Pediatrics guidelines (Roberts et al., 2011) recommend urethral catheterization as a reliable method to diagnose UTI in children younger than age 2 years. Catheterization is also invasive, requires technical expertise, and risks introducing bacteria into the bladder. Noninvasive methods are preferable but typically yield less accurate results. If a sample collected by a urine collection bag is negative, one may feel confident about the results. If, however, the urine sample is positive, this result may be from contamination, especially if the urine collection bag was left in place for an extended time. Therefore, reliability of such results is questionable. Specimens obtained using urine collection bags yield unacceptably high false-positive results. When a urine collection bag is used, a negative result is considered accurate but a positive result requires confirmation with a catheterized specimen prior to the start of treatment (Roberts et al., 2011; Etoubleau et al., 2009; Karacan et al., 2010; Tosif et al., 2012).

Nursing care for the child with tubed urinary diversion focuses on preventing infection, maintaining tube patency, avoiding dislodgment of the apparatus, and providing comfort measures. For a child with urinary drainage tubes, teach all aspects of home care to the family (and child as appropriate), demonstrate, and observe their performance before the child is discharged. Review the signs and symptoms of complications, emergency procedures, and methods of telephone contact in case of emergency. Home care nursing visits, as needed, and telephone follow-up ensure consistent care and provide additional reassurance to the family.

Stents

An indwelling stent facilitates continuous flow of urine within the ureter, so one may be used after corrective ureteral procedures or as an adjunct to shock wave lithotripsy in treating large renal calculi. Children with internalized urinary diversion require no special care or activity restrictions, although a repeat cystoscopic procedure is necessary to remove the stent. When a double-J stent is used for short-term diversion (e.g., after removal of stones), a string is left protruding from the urethra (taped to the child) to allow the stent to be removed in the health care provider's office.

Stomal Diversion

Nonintubated diversion is accomplished by externalizing a urinary structure, allowing urine to drain through a stoma. This technique is the treatment of choice for long-term management of children with urologic malfunction secondary to neurologic compromise, trauma, or severe congenital outlet defects. Short-term, tubeless urinary diversion is useful to quickly drain the hydronephrotic kidney and to stabilize renal function before definitive corrective surgery. The stoma is located proximal to the diseased, obstructed, or atonic urinary structure, most commonly as a *ureterostomy* (detaches the ureter from the bladder and brings it to the surface of the abdomen), *pyelostomy* (creates an opening to the kidney pelvis), or *vesicostomy* (creates an opening to the bladder) (Fig. 19-2).

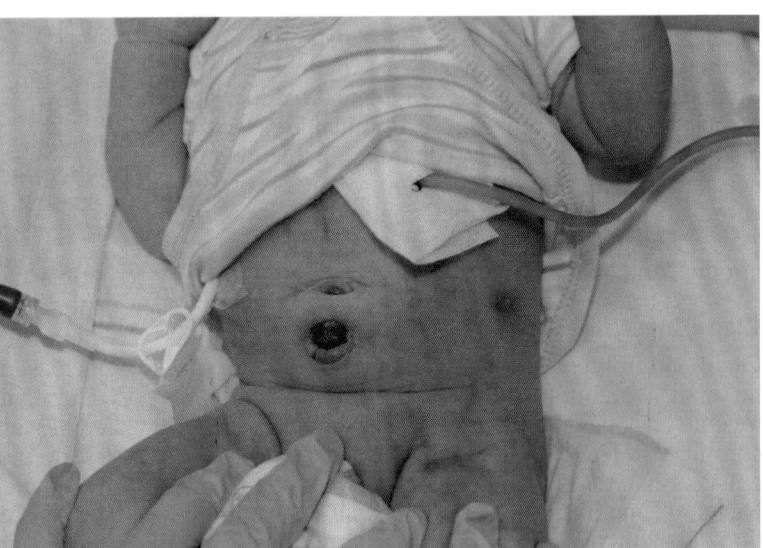

Figure 19-2 A vesicostomy creates an opening to the bladder to divert urine flow.

Once hailed as a life-saving procedure, permanent urinary diversion through a stoma led to such overwhelming negative consequences that the management of children who would previously have been treated with stomal diversion has shifted. (For more information, see thePoint for Supplemental Information: Urinary Diversion Through a Stoma.) The current trend is to combine surgical and pharmacologic approaches to restore function to the lower urinary structures while conserving the upper tracts. For most children, the potential to become continent is great. A key positive factor has been the introduction of clean intermittent catheterization to maintain regular and complete bladder emptying.

Urinary Reconstruction

Evaluating bladder capacity, contractility, and sphincteric competency is essential to determine a treatment plan. A small, inelastic bladder must be enlarged to provide an adequate reservoir. Bladder augmentation material is typically supplied by ileum, sigmoid, or (rarely) gastric tissue. If the bladder has normal capacity and good detrusor (bladder muscle) contractility, it is left alone. Urethral resistance is considered next in attempting to determine the capability for continence and complete bladder emptying. High sphincteric resistance, which blocks urine flow, is managed by clean intermittent catheterization. Insufficient resistance requires either a procedure to reconstruct the bladder neck or surgical implantation of an artificial sphincter to prevent dribbling. Clean intermittent catheterization may be instituted to ensure complete bladder emptying. Any impairment to catheterization, such as poor fine motor control or extreme skeletal deformity, may necessitate the creation of a continent catheterizable stoma (Mitrofanoff procedure). Pharmacologic agents that mediate detrusor function may be administered as adjuncts to achieve the goal of continence.

Benefits from reconstructing the urinary tract rather than creating an external stomal diversion include less disfigurement, no need for an external collection device, improved preservation of the upper tracts, and improved continence. Disadvantages are either procedure dependent or related to poor patient adherence to the postoperative regimen or lax patient follow-up. Complications related to the augmented bladder or the associated gastrointestinal resection include electrolyte disturbances, mucus plugs, calculi in the bladder, bladder cancer, reflux, and ascending pyelonephritis (from chronically neglected catheterization). Stomal problems include stomal stenosis, leakage, false passage, atrophy, and stomal breakdown.

Clean Intermittent Catheterization

Clean intermittent catheterization has revolutionized the management of voiding dysfunction related to neurogenic or congenital causes. By reversing the cycle of chronic bladder distention, which creates mucosal ischemia, urinary stasis, and an environment conducive to bacterial colonization, clean intermittent catheterization substantially lowers UTI rates. Additionally, clean intermittent catheterization alleviates the persistently elevated intravesical pressure, a precursor for VUR and upper tract damage. An added benefit of clean intermittent catheterization involves the therapeutic effects on detrusor function. A regularly emptied bladder, drained before distention occurs, maintains detrusor contractility and prevents overflow incontinence.

Technique

Clean intermittent catheterization can be performed on children of any age, using a 6- to 14-French-diameter catheter. A variety of catheters are available, including latex, latex-free, and hydrophilic catheters.

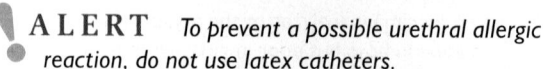

ALERT   *To prevent a possible urethral allergic reaction, do not use latex catheters.*

Clean technique is used by the family and child when catheterizing. Most people who catheterize routinely will have bacteria in the bladder, but this condition is not treated as a UTI unless the child also has symptoms such as fever, abdominal pain, or back pain.

Teach the family and child, as appropriate, how to perform clean intermittent catheterization (Teaching Intervention Plan 19-1). Before teaching the child or family how to perform clean intermittent catheterization, review the pelvic and perineal anatomy, clearly highlighting the urethral pathway. Depending on the child's gender, demonstrate how the normal male urethra is much straighter when held erect and perpendicular to the abdomen or that the female urethral tract is angled toward the umbilicus. Have the family perform the procedure on an anatomically correct doll until proficiency is achieved before attempting the procedure on the child. Boys have little difficulty locating the external meatus, but girls often need to use a mirror. When the child is able to easily locate and enter the urethra with a tube, the mirror can be removed.

The age to teach a child self-catheterization depends on developmental and emotional factors, such as attention span, fine motor and manipulative control, family support, emotional readiness, and ability to perform sequential behaviors. Individualized judgment and procedural adaptation are required for children who are physically, emotionally, or developmentally challenged. Full independence with the procedure occurs when the child acquires a concept of time and record keeping, typically around age 6 to 8 years (Clinical Judgment 19-1).

Adolescent Acceptance

Poor adherence to clean intermittent catheterization is often seen during adolescence and is associated with increased rates of epididymitis and recurrent UTIs (Holmdahl et al., 2007). The psychosocial chaos of adolescence may impinge on the teen's acceptance of clean intermittent catheterization and on the teen's willingness to commit to a long-term bladder-emptying routine. Driven to fit in with peers, teens who have never previously balked at the technique may refuse to

TIP 19-1: A TEACHING INTERVENTION PLAN for the Child Requiring Clean Intermittent Catheterization

Nursing Diagnosis and Family Outcomes

- Readiness for enhanced self-health management
  Outcomes: Child and family will perform clean intermittent catheterization proficiently.
  Child and family will catheterize in a timely manner to prevent urine leakage and skin breakdown.
  Child and family will identify signs and symptoms of stomal stenosis and infection.

Teach the Child/Family

To Catheterize via Urethra or a Continent Diversion (Stoma)

- Educate regarding the importance of regular bladder drainage and the consequences of negligence. Strategize with the family to devise a workable catheterization routine for the child. Timing of clean intermittent catheterization should be every 3–4 hours, although more frequent drainage may be needed initially for continence. Because the child with a neurogenic bladder lacks sensory pathways to detect a full bladder, an alarm can be set to provide the needed cue for bladder emptying. Ask the surgeon/primary provider if the child needs to awaken at night to catheterize. It may be sufficient to catheterize before bedtime and immediately upon waking. If it is necessary to awaken the child at night, have the child set an alarm and remind him or her that most people awaken at least once at night to urinate; this is more common in older children.
- Some children will need to use an indwelling Foley catheter during the night if hydronephrosis is a concern. If so, instruct them on Foley insertion and the use of a night drainage bag.
- Cleanse the perineum with mild soap and water once a day.* Menstruating females may wish to cleanse prior to each clean intermittent catheterization. Females should use three front-to-back swipes with clean wipes each time; males should use a circular motion around the meatus. If the child has a stoma, cleanse around the stoma using three strokes in a circular motion; avoid "scrubbing" back and forth. In uncircumcised males, pull back the foreskin to clean the head of the penis.
- Assemble all supplies as needed (e.g., catheter, lubricant, wipes, container to collect urine if not draining into toilet). Carry disposable towelettes and lubricant with the catheter for adequate meatal hygiene. For an infant, placing a protective pad under the child's bottom can help minimize mess.

- Perform hand hygiene using soap and water or alcohol-based hand gel.
- Position urine collection container if needed, or reposition self to sit on, stand, or sit in wheelchair facing the toilet using a catheter extension tube if needed (available through medical supply companies).
- Lubricate the catheter with a water-based gel. If a hydrophilic catheter is being used, the catheter may come prelubricated with water in its package or water may need to be added to the package. Exposing the hydrophilic catheter to water activates the special coating and the entire catheter is slippery. Gel is not necessary when using hydrophilic catheters.
- Insert the catheter gently into the urethra (stoma) until urine begins to flow. After urine is flowing, insert the tube a little farther and instruct the child to keep holding the catheter and watch for urine to stop. Urine flows more readily when the child raises intra-abdominal pressure using methods such as the Valsalva technique, laughing, or blowing (e.g., blowing bubbles or a pinwheel). Teach the child/family to use the Credé maneuver to massage the vesical dome only if the child has no VUR, per physician approval.
- When urine flow stops, slowly remove the catheter, stopping to wait if the urine begins to drain again. When finished draining the bladder, teach the child to pinch the tube so that as he or she removes it, urine will not drip on clothing.

Catheter Care

- Rinse the tube with soap and water after catheterization, and dry and place it in a breathable container such as a plastic zip-lock bag with holes in it, a toothbrush holder, or a paper bag. It may be helpful to use a syringe filled with water to flush the catheter.
- Once a week, either soak the tube in a 1:3 solution of vinegar and water, rinsing well before use, or boil in water for 5–10 minutes.
- Plastic tubes last for 2–4 weeks.

For Children Attending Daycare/School

- Upon family request/approval, teach designated staff clean intermittent catheterization techniques and/or how to support the child in self clean intermittent catheterization.
- Help staff/child to provide flexibility in the school day schedule and identify a private area to store supplies and perform clean intermittent catheterization.

(Continued)

TIP 19-1: A TEACHING INTERVENTION PLAN for the Child Requiring Clean Intermittent Catheterization (*Continued*)

To Monitor Urinary Function
- Evaluate amount of urine output; note consistent decrease in volume.
- Observe urine for mucus, odor, or discoloration.
- Check stoma for signs of irritation, bleeding, shrinkage, protrusion, or other change in appearance.

Contact Health Care Provider if
- Child has high temperature or persistent or unexplained fever more than 101° F (38.3° C).

- There is a foul odor, consistent discoloration, or excess mucus in the urine.
- Child has flank pain or aching, extreme fatigue, or loss of appetite.
- Child has abdominal pain or pain when catheterizing stoma.
- Child has difficulty passing the catheter or there is a large amount of blood when catheterizing.

*Some practitioners recommend cleansing before each clean intermittent catheterization, but there is limited evidence to support this practice (Bray & Sanders, 2007).

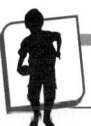

CLINICAL JUDGMENT 19-1

The Child With Spina Bifida Seen for a Self-Catheterization Program

Five-year-old Michelle was born with myelomeningocele at the L1 level. She is seen in the rehabilitation outpatient clinic for an instructional program in self clean intermittent catheterization. Until now, Michelle has been incontinent and has continued to wear diapers. This has not presented a problem in the past, but she is now preparing to enter a public school.

Questions

1. What information will you need regarding Michelle's elimination patterns?
2. What self-care techniques should be introduced to Michelle?
3. How would you determine that Michelle is ready to participate in this program?
4. What steps would be followed in introducing self clean intermittent catheterization to Michelle?
5. How would you determine that Michelle is ready for discharge?

Answers

1. How much fluid does Michelle usually drink per day, especially in the evening? How frequently does she wet diapers? When changed, is the diaper damp, wet, or fully saturated? Is she aware of voiding and does she seem bothered if wet?
2. Perineal care, recognition of relationship of volume of intake and types of fluids to output of urine
3. Michelle shows interest in "keeping dry" and wearing underwear, Michelle is able to understand that she will be able to "go to the bathroom" using the catheter and will not be wet in between times
4. A clean intermittent catheterization program should be initiated by the nurse, explaining the purpose and technique to Michelle step by step (a visual aid, handout, picture book, or video/DVD may be helpful). An anatomically correct doll can be used to introduce the topic and explain how the body works.

Michelle can also "try" the techniques on this doll. Michelle should assist in gathering supplies and in setting up for the procedure and watch the catheterization using a mirror. Michelle should initiate steps of the procedure (cleansing with soap and water, identifying urethral opening with mirror). Michelle should try to insert the catheter after she has been cleansed and prepared by the nurse. Michelle should try the procedure while sitting on the toilet.

5. Michelle is able to perform each step of the procedure independently with only occasional reminders or verbal cues. Michelle's parents demonstrate independence in performing the procedure. Michelle's parents support their daughter in completing each task and understand the steps that Michelle must practice to gain complete independence. The family can solve different scenarios and complications (management of limited supplies, UTIs, scheduling catheters around community social activities).

perform clean intermittent catheterization. Teens will often deny their need for assisted bladder emptying in a self-deceptive attempt to be like other teens. Offer the family anticipatory guidance about this problem as the child approaches puberty. The following suggestions can enhance the teen's cooperation:

- Acknowledge and validate the teen's conflicting feelings about his or her body.
- Maintain privacy and confidentiality.
- Avoid shaming the teen, especially around peers.
- Help the teen create a contract of responsibility.
- Offer either developmentally appropriate rewards or negative feedback to promote expected behavior.

PHARMACOLOGIC MANAGEMENT

Managing many genitourinary and renal conditions involves the use of pharmacologic agents. Medications may be curative, as in the administration of an antibiotic to treat UTI, or used as adjuncts to other treatment modalities, as in the management of voiding disorders. Thus, the nurse needs to be familiar with common genitourinary medications used in children and their urologic and renal applications (see thePoint for Medications: Medications Used to Manage Genitourinary Conditions). Steroid therapy is used to treat several renal conditions, as described in this chapter's section on "Nephrotic Syndrome." (See Chapters 22 and 25 for more information regarding steroid therapy.)

RENAL REPLACEMENT THERAPIES

Altered laboratory values or fluid imbalance from renal causes that cannot be controlled with conservative measures such as diet or medication require some form of renal replacement therapy. These therapies include PD, hemodialysis, and kidney transplantation.

Peritoneal Dialysis

PD may be used to provide renal replacement therapy in acute kidney injury (AKI) or chronic renal disease. Methods for children include intermittent PD, continuous ambulatory PD, and continuous cycling PD (also called automated PD).

All PD methods use the same physiologic principles of metabolic and fluid control and require similar nursing care. Diffusive and convective clearance (solute and fluid clearance) occur when the peritoneal membrane's rich blood supply comes into apposition with sterile dialysate instilled into the child's abdominal (peritoneal) cavity through the dialysis catheter. The dialysate stays in the peritoneal cavity for a predetermined period (dwell time) based on the child's metabolic control and acuity. The dwell time ranges from 2 to 12 hours, after which the dialysate is drained out. Fresh dialysate is instilled to complete the cycle. In PD, the dialyzing membrane for each child is exactly the right size compared with body surface area (BSA) because it is the child's own peritoneum.

The rate of solute clearance and the ultrafiltration rate in PD are determined by the amount of dialysate put into the child's abdomen. To maximize therapy, the amount of dialysate instilled into the peritoneum is calculated using the patient's BSA (Verrina et al., 2009). Very sick, catabolic children requiring acute PD and intensive care, extra volume, and nutritional supplementation may require hourly exchanges, whereas otherwise healthy children on chronic PD may require fewer exchanges each day.

Commercially prepared dialysate is available in three dextrose concentrations: 1.5%, 2.5%, and 4.25%. The dextrose concentration governs the rate of ultrafiltration: the higher the dextrose concentration, the more fluid is removed during an exchange. In the acute setting, custom dialysate solutions prepared by a pharmacy may be used to provide better metabolic control.

For all types of PD, access to the peritoneum is achieved with a Tenckhoff or other commercially available catheter. The catheter is placed in the peritoneum through a midline incision below the umbilicus. The distal portion is tunneled to a lateral exit site on the abdomen where it does not interfere with the child's clothing (Fig. 19-3).

Catheter function can be compromised by poor catheter position, fibrin or omentum clogging the holes, abdominal adhesions from past surgeries, or constipation. If dialysate flows in slowly, the rate can be increased by raising the level of the inflow bag or by squeezing the bag gently to increase the rate of flow. Outflow problems are more difficult to overcome. Lowering the outflow bag by raising the child's height (e.g., picking up the child or seating the child on a taller piece of furniture) or having the child change position (roll from side to side, sit up, stand up, or walk around) are the only methods that are easily done at home (Developmental Considerations 19-1). If outflow is still a problem, the physician may prescribe an oral medication, usually sorbitol, to induce diarrhea. The increased intestinal peristalsis may change the position of the catheter to one that allows more flow. If none of these are effective, the dialysis nurse may be asked to perform forceful flushes of the catheter with normal saline using sterile technique.

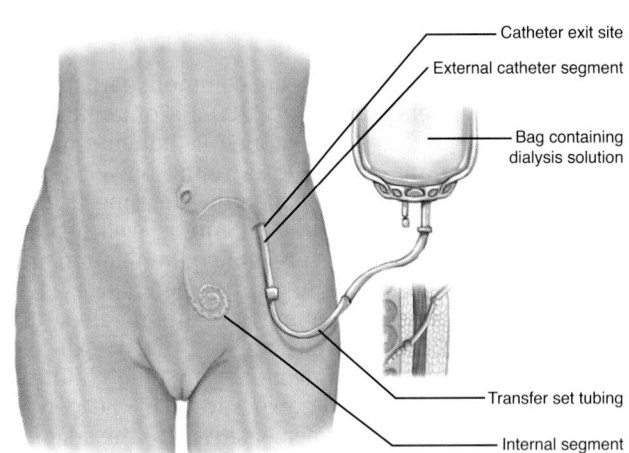

Figure 19-3 During PD, an implanted tube allows instillation of the dialysate fluid into the child's peritoneal cavity.

Catheter exit site
External catheter segment
Bag containing dialysis solution
Transfer set tubing
Internal segment

DEVELOPMENTAL CONSIDERATIONS 19-1

Participation in Peritoneal Dialysis at Home

Age	Age-Appropriate Activities
Infancy	Wears a mask during sterile procedures without distress and without removing it Tolerates catheter exit site care without undue distress Easily distracted by diversional activities during exchange procedure
Early childhood	Same as infancy Does not attempt to pull on catheter tubing
Middle childhood	Assists in gathering supplies or preparing the room where an exchange will be performed Fully cooperates during an exchange procedure
School-aged child	Assists in disposing of supplies after procedure Gathers supplies and prepares room where exchange will be performed Completes exchanges or sets up cyclers with family or other adult supervision Examines effluent for cloudiness Assists in disposing of supplies after procedure
Adolescence	Gathers supplies and prepares room where exchange will be performed Completes exchanges with minimal or no supervision Disposes of supplies after procedure Informs family when supplies are low and need to be reordered Recognizes early signs of peritonitis

If forceful flushes do not correct the outflow problem, radiopaque dye is instilled under sterile conditions and its flow is followed with fluoroscopy. If these studies show that a fibrin sheath has formed around the catheter, urokinase may be used to dissolve the fibrin. A volume sufficient to fill the catheter is instilled using sterile technique, allowed to dwell for 30 to 60 minutes, and then is aspirated out of the catheter. A dialysate exchange is done to check the catheter function. If outflow is still poor, surgical replacement of the catheter is the only option.

Exit site or tunnel infections are common, particularly in younger children (Aksu et al., 2007). Contamination of the exit site by feces can happen if the child is still wearing diapers and has a loose, runny bowel movement. Teach the family to change the dressing if fecal contamination occurs and the exit site is well healed. An occlusive dressing helps prevent contamination and decreases the need for frequent dressing changes. If a newly placed catheter dressing is contaminated, tell the family to call the dialysis nurse. Diligent exit site care can usually prevent infections. In some children, eosinophilia develops at the exit site or in the peritoneal cavity as a result of hypersensitivity to the silicone catheter. Teach the child and family to keep the catheter immobile to avoid pulling and exit site trauma, which may lead to infection (Teaching Intervention Plan 19-2).

The major causes of morbidity with PD are catheter-related infections and peritonitis (van Diepen et al., 2012; Warady et al., 2012) (Chart 19-2). Peritonitis can result from a break in sterile technique when changing the dialysate, from a break in the closed PD system, or from an exit site infection migrating along the tunnel and into the peritoneal cavity.

ALERT *Monitor for signs of peritonitis in a child receiving PD and immediately report them to the physician or Advanced Practice Registered Nurse. Signs of peritonitis include abdominal pain and tenderness upon examination, fever, nausea, vomiting, and/or cloudy dialysis fluid. Any time the dialysis fluid is cloudy or has visible flecks or clumps, a fluid sample should be sent for culture.*

Completing an exchange earlier than scheduled may be necessary to immediately evaluate the character of the dialysate. If the fluid is not cloudy and abdominal pain is not generalized, peritonitis may be ruled out by the health care provider. Some older children who have had peritonitis several times may be able to recognize the prodromal symptoms before the dialysate becomes cloudy (Clinical Judgment 19-2). Standardized treatment and

TIP 19-2: A TEACHING INTERVENTION PLAN for the Child With a Tenckhoff Catheter

Nursing Diagnoses and Family Outcomes

- Impaired skin integrity related to effects of presence of catheter
  Outcomes: Skin at catheter entrance site remains intact and free from breakdown.
  Family performs cleaning and catheter maintenance procedures.
- Risk for infection related to catheter and dialysate exchange process
  Outcomes: Child/family protect catheter exit site from trauma.
  Family identifies signs and symptoms of infection.
  Family verbalizes measures to prevent infection.

Teach Child/Family

Newly Placed Catheter (First 1–14 Days After Placement)

- Sterile exit site dressing changes will be done once per week by the dialysis nurse; schedule appointments for weekly dressing change.
- The nurse will remove the old dressing, inspect exit site/tunnel for drainage and redness (mild redness is normal), cleanse exit site, and apply a new dressing, making it occlusive around the catheter and securing it with netting/band.
- Child and family should reinforce dressing if needed, not change it. Ensure that the dressing is occlusive around the catheter; keep the catheter from dangling with netting/band at all times. Do not pull on the catheter.
- No showers.

Well-Healed Catheter Site (14 Days After Insertion)

- Dressing is optional.
- Daily exit site cleaning is still required.
- Child should shower daily and not bathe in a way that allows the exit site to soak in dirty water. If using dressing, leave dressing on until after cleaning body.

- Use regular soap on washcloth to wash rest of body.
- Remove dressing (if using) and clean around exit site with a new, clean washcloth with antibacterial soap (from a pump).
- Rinse under shower.
- Dry rest of body with bath towel, avoiding exit site. Allow exit site to air dry or use clean 4 × 4 gauze.
- Apply new dressing if desired.
- Secure solution transfer set with tape to abdomen to prevent pulling on exit site or secure with expandable gauze net.

Safety Concerns

- Examine Tenckhoff catheter and solution transfer set daily for signs of splits or cracks. Check that catheter adapter between Tenckhoff and solution transfer set is firmly seated and that solution transfer set is *tightly* screwed on to adapter.
- Child should avoid contact sports or games likely to affect exit site or pull on catheter or solution transfer set.
- Some dialysis centers allow children with Tenckhoff catheters to swim; others do not. If swimming is permitted, remind the child and family to swim only in well-chlorinated private pools or the ocean. Public pools, ponds, lakes, and rivers can have high bacteria counts, putting the child at risk for an exit site infection.

Contact Health Care Provider if

- Exit site or tunnel is hot, red, painful, or swollen
- Exit site is draining or smells bad
- Exit site is bleeding
- Any signs of splits or cracks in the Tenckhoff catheter are observed
- Child receives an injury to abdominal insertion site of catheter

---

training approaches to avoid peritonitis exist (Verrina et al., 2009; Bakkaloglu, 2009) and include prevention of PD catheter exit site infections, sterile considerations for connecting and disconnecting to dialysis, and hand hygiene.

Frequent episodes of peritonitis can lead to thickening of the peritoneal membranes and reduced ability to ultrafiltrate or remove solute. Inadequate peritoneal membrane function can mean that a child must be switched permanently from PD to hemodialysis.

Intermittent Peritoneal Dialysis

Intermittent PD is often used for acutely ill children who require a dialysis exchange every 1 to 2 hours. Their serum chemistries fluctuate and dictate frequent adjustments in the composition of their dialysate. The intermittent PD system is an open system, with air

---

CHART 19-2 Clinical Indicators of Peritonitis

Cloudy dialysate outflow (effluent)

Abdominal pain

Rebound abdominal tenderness

Acute discomfort during fill phase of dialysis

Fever

General malaise

Nausea

Vomiting

Increased WBC count of dialysate outflow

Positive bacterial culture of dialysate outflow

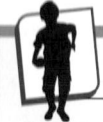

A Child With Chronic Renal Disease

Neal is a 6-year-old boy who has been on home PD for the past 6 weeks. His grandparents are the primary caregivers and have been responsible for managing all of his care at home. This past weekend, Neal complained of abdominal pain, especially during infusion of the dialysate. He vomited once this morning and has a temperature of 101.6° F (38.6° C). Neal and his grandfather come to the outpatient renal clinic for evaluation.

Questions

1. What other assessment data would be important to elicit?

2. When a child has peritonitis, what would you expect the dialysate to look like after an exchange?

3. Does Neal need to be hospitalized?

4. What measures should be instituted to reduce Neal's pain and discomfort?

5. Two days later, the home health nurse visits Neal. What data would indicate that his peritonitis is improving and that the grandparents are taking measures to prevent another infection?

Answers

1. When was an exchange last completed? What did the dialysate look like after drainage from the abdomen? When does Neal experience pain? Do any specific events produce abdominal pain? What does the catheter exit site look like? Have the grandparents describe their technique for catheter site care and for connecting and disconnecting the child to the dialyzer.

2. The dialysate looks cloudy. A specimen of the dialysate should be evaluated for culture and sensitivity study. Gram stain and cell count of the fluid should also be completed to determine the infecting organisms.

3. If Neal has not demonstrated severe weight loss or signs of dehydration, and if the grandparents feel they can manage his care at home with the assistance of home health care, then Neal need not be hospitalized.

4. Begin antibiotic therapy immediately. Acetaminophen can be given to reduce fever and promote comfort. The dialysate should be warmed before instillation. A slow introduction of the fluid during inflow may also help reduce abdominal discomfort.

5. Neal has no fever, complaints of abdominal pain are minimal, the dialysate fluid is clear after infusion, and the grandparents demonstrate the use of aseptic techniques to clean the catheter site and to connect and disconnect the child for an infusion.

---

vents and other openings in the tubing. This arrangement, along with recurrent breaks in the system caused by frequent dialysate bag changes, increases the likelihood of peritonitis. Changing to a closed PD system as soon as the child's condition stabilizes helps prevent such complications.

Continuous Ambulatory Peritoneal Dialysis

Continuous ambulatory PD involves three to four exchanges during the child's waking hours, timed to fit into the child's daily schedule. A usual schedule is to do the exchanges upon arising, after school, midevening, and before bed. On weekends, the schedule may be adjusted to coincide with meals.

Continuous Cycling Peritoneal Dialysis

Continuous cycling PD uses an automated, programmable machine that delivers dialysate to the peritoneum, measures the dwell period, and ensures that all the dialysate and ultrafiltrate is drained from the peritoneal cavity. Prescription and compliance data can be obtained from the machine to monitor for mechanical or adherence problems. Usually, continuous cycling PD is completed at night while the child sleeps, and most centers prescribe a last fill, which the child ambulates with through the day. When the abdominal cavity is filled with a large volume of dialysate, the liquid exerts less pressure on the abdominal wall and the inguinal canal if the child is in a recumbent position than it does in a standing position; thus, hernias are less likely to occur with continuous cycling PD than with continuous ambulatory PD. Many practitioners use continuous cycling PD exclusively for children, believing that it lessens the burden of family responsibility because the system is opened only twice daily: at bedtime and upon awakening. Because of the small dialysate volumes used, using continuous cycling PD machines for infants can be difficult; continuous ambulatory PD or hemodialysis may be required instead.

Hemodialysis

Hemodialysis removes waste products and corrects serum chemistry values of the child's blood by circulating it through an extracorporeal circuit. The artificial kidney, or dialyzer, contains a blood compartment and a dialysate compartment. Substances in the blood but not in the dialysate, such as BUN or creatinine, cross the semipermeable membrane of the dialyzer into the dialysate by osmosis and are carried away as waste.

During hemodialysis, children require vigilant assessment because they can be more unstable than adults (Fig. 19-4). Continuously monitor the child's weight (with a metabolic scale if the child's dry weight is less than 12 kg), check blood pressure frequently (every 1 to 15 minutes), and constantly observe the child for changes in hydration status or for early signs of complications. This monitoring has become much easier with the use of noninvasive monitoring devices (Patel et al., 2007). Monitor for complications such as fever, fluid overload or excessive removal, hyperkalemia, hypernatremia, hypocalcemia, and muscle cramps. Also assess for machine malfunctions, blood leaks, and allergic reactions, and address these emergencies as they arise.

Alarms and safety mechanisms in the hemodialysis machine are triggered by problems arising in the circuit. Blood or dialysate flow shuts off if safety parameters are exceeded; this event requires intervention by the nurse or technician. Blood lines must be selected carefully based on the volume of blood they hold.

caREminder

The total volume of the extracorporeal circuit (bloodlines plus dialyzer) should not exceed 10% of the child's circulating blood volume (Sebestyen & Warady, 2011). If it does, then blood priming becomes necessary.

Initial studies indicate that daily home hemodialysis leads to improved growth, metabolic and blood pressure control, fewer diet and fluid restrictions (Fischbach et al., 2011), and improves health-related quality-of-life (Culleton & Asola, 2011; Goldstein, 2007). Nocturnal home hemodialysis provides excellent biochemical and metabolic control; however, it requires more extensive training and technical expertise than PD.

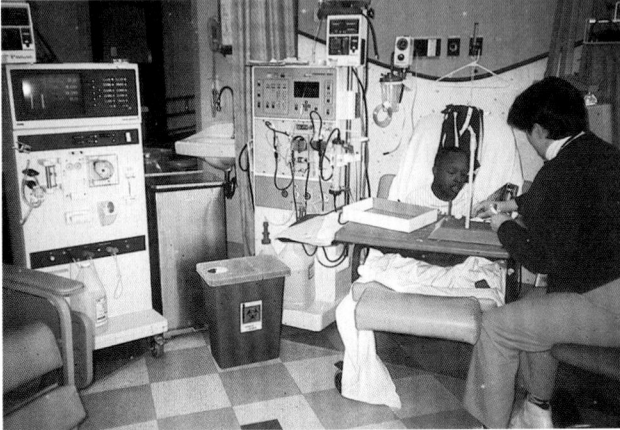

Figure 19-4 Hemodialysis must be performed at a specialized center where the child's status can be constantly monitored by the specialty nursing staff.

Access for hemodialysis is achieved by percutaneous catheter or by an arteriovenous fistula (AVF) or arteriovenous graft (AVG).

Percutaneous Catheter

The percutaneous catheter for acute hemodialysis can be placed in the subclavian, jugular, or femoral veins, depending on the size of the child and the size of the veins. The surgeon or nephrologist selects the site. These catheters are designed to be removed after a time, usually after a few days to a month. However, permanent catheters, most commonly placed in a subclavian vein or jugular vein, can last for many years. Maintain diligent attention to sterility when attaching the catheter to, or detaching it from, the hemodialysis circuit or when performing exit site care. Adequate functioning of the catheter is often highly related to the position of the child's body. Sometimes, children with subclavian catheters must hold unusual body positions to maintain adequate blood flow through the catheter.

As with any device passing through the skin, potential complications of hemodialysis are infection at the exit site and septicemia if proper sterile technique is not observed during attachment or detachment for a treatment. Catheter kinking and thrombosis may also occur. Assess for signs of infection and poor flow through the catheter. Teach children with subclavian catheters not to swim, take showers, or bump or pull on the catheter or the exit site and to keep a sterile occlusive dressing over the exit site at all times.

Arteriovenous Fistula or Graft

The preferred form of vascular access for most children on maintenance hemodialysis (when hemodialysis is expected for longer than 1 year) is by AVF or AVG (National Kidney Foundation, 2006).

An AVF or AVG requires time to heal and "mature" after placement surgery—typically, 3 to 6 months. A second surgery may be needed to raise the fistula closer to the skin surface before use. Thus, if interim dialysis is needed, a catheter is also placed. After the AVF/AVG is accessed and in use, the catheter will be removed. Teach the family to assess patency daily by feeling for a "thrill," the gentle vibration of blood flow through the AVF/AVG. Also assess by listening with a stethoscope for a "bruit," a blowing sound. If the thrill or bruit cannot be detected, notify the physician; intervention may be required.

Fewer complications occur with fistulas than with percutaneous catheters because they are indwelling. The infection risk is much lower. They also do not clot like catheters. The biggest complication is pain while accessing the fistula. Minimize this problem by using topical anesthetics before dialysis.

Continuous Renal Replacement Therapy

Renal replacement therapy uses the same basic principles as hemodialysis. Blood is removed from the child, pumped through a dialysis filter, and returned after removal of surplus water and wastes. The major difference is that intermittent hemodialysis removes large amounts of water and wastes in a short time, whereas continuous renal replacement therapies remove water and wastes at a slow and steady rate. Continuous renal replacement therapy is used to treat critically ill children with AKI and metabolic abnormalities.

Although hemodialysis and acute PD provide therapeutic options for critically ill children with AKI, neither may be appropriate under specific conditions (Goldstein, 2011). Hemodialysis can place the child at risk for potential dialysis disequilibrium and may be untenable because of hemodynamic instability. PD has been associated with respiratory compromise by mechanically restricting diaphragmatic movements and increasing the risk of hydrothorax. Additionally, PD may be less effective than continuous renal replacement therapy in treating inborn errors of metabolism and poisonings (Goldstein, 2011; Sebestyen & Warady, 2011). These issues may be compounded in treating very small infants, particularly those who weigh less than 3 kg.

Kidney Transplantation

A successful kidney transplant is the ultimate treatment goal for children with CKD. Most centers try to accomplish it as quickly as possible by performing preemptive transplants before dialysis is needed. This approach may not be possible with some underlying diseases that require a short period of dialysis before transplant or when a living donor is not available. Kidneys for transplant can come from a living related, living unrelated, or deceased donor.

In order to determine an appropriate donor, human lymphocyte antigen typing and serum crossmatch are completed. Human lymphocyte antigen typing is a process that examines the WBCs in serum for markers (antigens) that are involved in immune response; these markers help the immune system discriminate self from nonself. A crossmatch test determines whether the serum of the potential donor reacts with that of the potential recipient. These tests are performed for living and cadaver donation. The prospective donor must also have a compatible blood type. A well-matched kidney can reduce the likelihood of rejection. The best possible kidney donor is an identical twin; next best is a human lymphocyte antigen–identical sibling. For more information, see thePoint for Supplemental Information: Kidney Transplantation: Matching Recipients and Donors.

Transplanted kidneys last varying lengths of time. Hyperacute rejection causes the loss of the kidney in the operating room as the transplant is being performed. Acute rejection usually occurs within the first 7 to 14 days after transplantation. Rejection can occur at any time after transplantation, particularly if the child stops taking immunosuppressive medications. Even if medications are taken as prescribed, chronic rejection—a slow, insidious process—can result in the loss of the kidney. However, the longer the transplant remains in place without complications, the more likely it is that it will never be rejected. Survival 1 year after kidney transplant is 98.2% with organs from living donors and 97.1% with organs from deceased donors; 5-year survival rates are 95.6% for patients with living donors and 92.6% for patients with deceased donors (Smith et al., 2007).

Acute or chronic rejection can cause loss of transplant function. This complication is treated in the same manner as the initial loss of native kidney function: conservative management, followed by dialysis. Retransplantation at a future date is usually an option, except when hyperacute rejection occurs for an unknown cause, when the likelihood of the basic disease recurring in the transplant is too great, or with an elevated panel-reactive antibody.

Posttransplant Medication

Medications for immunosuppression are used to prevent the immune system from rejecting the allograft while maintaining sufficient immunity to prevent infection. Immunosuppressive medications are the only therapy available to prevent acute and chronic rejection and maintain adequate graft function. These agents can be grouped into those used for induction, maintenance, and antirejection immunosuppression.

Induction therapy starts pretransplant or immediately following transplantation. These drugs are given at high doses to prevent acute rejection and include antithymocyte globulin (Thymoglobulin), methylprednisolone, basiliximab (Simulect), and Daclizumab (Zenapax).

Maintenance therapy is given posttransplant to maintain the graft. Maintenance drugs include azathioprine (Imuran), mycophenolate mofetil (CellCept), prednisone, cyclosporine, sirolimus, and tacrolimus.

Antirejection medications, including methylprednisolone, Thymoglobulin, basiliximab, daclizumab, and muromonab (OKT3), are given to treat episodes of acute rejection. Some of the medications can be given by IV infusion during the immediate postoperative period. By the time the recipient is discharged home, the medication can be taken orally.

Teach the child and family that immunosuppressive medications to prevent rejection of the transplanted organ must be taken, in the exact amount prescribed, for as long as the transplanted kidney is functioning. In addition, transplant recipients receive medications to prevent infections and may require medications to treat hypertension. Before discharge, teach the child and family which medications to take, the amounts prescribed, and the effects and side effects of each medication. In addition to preventing rejection, these medications increase the recipient's susceptibility to infection and can cause other side effects including hypertension, weight gain, hirsutism, and impaired growth.

Community Care

Transplant patients are not "cured." These children never reach a point at which they no longer require medical attention or drug therapy. However, a well-stabilized transplant patient requires only daily or every-other-day medication. Clinic visits are usually twice a week initially, but as the child continues to do well, the visits are slowly decreased to every 3 to 4 months. Monthly checks of blood chemistries, CBCs, and medication levels are required to monitor kidney function and drug levels and to detect signs of rejection. Some centers recommend periodic biopsies of the transplanted kidney to detect rejection before it has caused enough damage to change laboratory values.

caREminder

Adolescents are particularly at risk for transplant medication nonadherence because the side effects of immunosuppressants, such as "chubby cheeks," acne, and hirsutism, may negatively affect their body image. Talk with the teen about such feelings, and reinforce the importance of the medications.

Lifelong immunosuppressive medication use puts these children at increased risk for community-acquired infections. During outbreaks of infectious illnesses, monitor these children closely and treat them aggressively because of their altered immune status. Teach the family that the child should receive a yearly influenza vaccine and be evaluated at the first sign of infectious illness.

Despite the short-term risks and the long-term side effects, successful transplantation still offers the child with renal failure the best chance at the most normal lifestyle possible (Community Care 19-1).

NURSING PLAN OF CARE

QUESTION: Which nursing diagnoses are most appropriate to include in the plan of care for J. D. and his family?

The nursing plan of care for a child with a genitourinary disorder should address the potentially dangerous alterations in fluid and electrolyte status that can result from these disorders (Nursing Plan of Care 19-1). Adequate urinary and renal function is central to efficiently excreting toxins from the body. Failure to remove waste products through urinary excretion can lead to dysfunction of other body systems, such as the cardiovascular and musculoskeletal systems.

Most children and their families find it difficult and embarrassing to discuss conditions that affect elimination patterns and competency of the genitalia. If the condition is congenital, the parents may feel guilty and question whether they could have prevented the anomaly. If the condition is acquired, family members may feel frustrated because of their inability to determine what is wrong with the child and to obtain effective treatment. The nurse plays a pivotal role in helping the child and family follow the treatment regimen that allows the child to live a full and normal life within any constraints imposed by the condition. Work with the family to help the child feel self-confident and comfortable with any changes in appearance resulting from the condition. Various support organizations can provide information and other help to the child with a genitourinary condition.

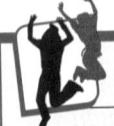

COMMUNITY CARE 19-1

Concerns of the Newly Transplanted Patient

Concern	Response
Can I go back to school soon and do all activities?	You will not be able to return to school for 6 weeks or until healing is complete. Driving is not allowed until healing has occurred, you are not taking pain medications, and are stable on your posttransplant medications (show no behavioral side effects). Do not lift anything heavier than 10 lb for 8 weeks. Do not participate in contact sports (e.g., tackle football, wrestling, or hockey) or sports that could severely jar the kidney (e.g., skydiving).
Can I be with my friends once I get out of the hospital?	For the first 6 weeks, you need to stay away from people to prevent infection. A few friends can come see you during this time as long as they do not have any signs of a cold or other illness.
Are there any restrictions on what I can eat?	You can have as much protein and fluid as you want, but concentrate on low-salt food to prevent high blood pressure. Remember, prednisone will increase your appetite, so be sure you eat healthy, low-calorie snacks and keep a close eye on your weight.
Do I have to take my medications every day?	All medications must be taken every day, on time, and at the correct dose to keep your new kidney healthy. Your family will help you to remember to take these medications. When you go back to school, you will have to help the nurse remember that you need to take your medication every day.

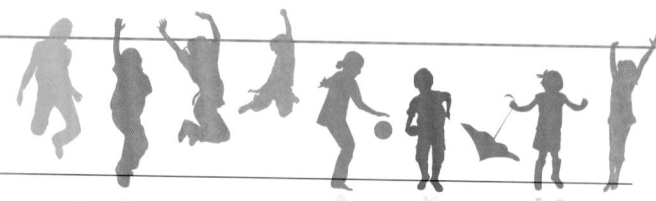

NURSING PLAN OF CARE 19-1:

The Child With Altered Genitourinary Status

Nursing Diagnosis: Excess fluid volume related to effects of accumulation and retention of fluids, electrolytes, and waste products

Interventions/Rationale

- Record strict and accurate intake and output. Include incidental fluids such as those taken with medications, ice chips, and ice pops.
  Accurate intake and output is necessary to determine renal functioning and fluid replacement needs.
- Weigh twice daily, always with the same scale, wearing same amount of clothing, at the same time every day.
  Monitors fluid status. In older children, a weight gain of greater than 0.5 kg can indicate fluid retention.
- Monitor vital signs, especially heart rate and blood pressure.
  Tachycardia and hypertension can occur because of excessive fluid.
- Auscultate lung and heart sounds.
  Excessive fluid or fluid overload can lead to pulmonary edema and heart failure. Listen for adventitious breath sounds and/or extra heart sounds.
- Assess level of consciousness.
  Fluid shifts can lead to accumulation of toxins, acidosis, and electrolyte imbalances.
- Monitor specific gravity.
  Indicates ability of kidneys to concentrate urine.
- Monitor laboratory values (e.g., BUN, creatinine, urine and serum sodium, serum potassium, hemoglobin, and hematocrit) and diagnostic studies (chest radiographs).
  Assess progression and management of renal failure or dysfunction.
- Administer medications (antihypertensives, diuretics, prostaglandins) as ordered.
  Side effects of medication may alter and affect renal function. See specific medication for physiology of effects of medication.
- Monitor and assess IV site carefully, giving solution at prescribed rate and prescribed solution.
  Avoids IV infiltration and helps maintain consistent infusion of fluids.

Expected Outcomes

- Child will exhibit decreased evidence of fluid retention.
- Child will maintain stable weight.
- Child will maintain blood pressure within prescribed parameters.
- Child will maintain normal electrolyte levels.

- Signs and symptoms of fluid volume excess will be recognized promptly and treatment will be initiated.

Nursing Diagnosis: Impaired urinary elimination related to effects of condition or disease process

Interventions/Rationale

- Monitor vital signs, peripheral pulses, skin turgor, capillary refill, and oral mucosa.
  Indicates fluid balance, level of hydration, and effectiveness of fluid replacement.
- Auscultate lungs, particularly noting adventitious breath sounds.
  Adventitious sounds may indicate fluid overload.
- Monitor respiratory rate and effort.
  May indicate developing complications such as diaphragmatic pressure.
- Monitor electrolytes, arterial blood gases, and calcium.
  Impaired renal function increases the risk of electrolyte and/or acid–base problems. Increased calcium may increase risk of crystal/stone formation.
- Monitor and document urine characteristics such as specific gravity, odor, and color.
  Assesses for urine infection; monitors fluid status. Provides a baseline for kidney function and presence of infection. Urine characteristics may provide information about alterations in renal function (e.g., decreased specific gravity may indicate problems concentrating urine or overhydration; hematuria may indicate bleeding).
- Visually inspect and palpate the lower abdomen for bladder fullness and suprapubic distension.
  The bladder lies in the suprapubic region of the abdomen. Retention of urine can cause tissue distention of bladder and kidneys and increases risk for infection.
- Observe for signs of urine retention or bladder infection (e.g., voiding small amounts, dysuria, frequency, fever).
  Helps detect and treat problems promptly.
- Keep accurate intake and output; weigh daily, at same time, same scale, in same clothes.
  Monitors fluid balance; helps estimate fluid-needs replacement. Fluid intake should approximate fluid losses (urine, nasogastric, wound drainage, and insensible losses).
- Assess for and follow up on reports of flank or abdominal pain.
  Pain may indicate pathology and may be a medical emergency itself. Complete obstruction can cause perforation into peritoneal cavity.

- Assess indwelling urinary catheter, when used, for patency; irrigate as necessary; report a decrease in urine output.

  Alerts nurse to inadequate output. Tubes can be occluded by stones or kinks. Failure to drain may cause urinary retention.

- Ensure adequate fluid intake.

  If fluid intake is not maintained, child may revert to oliguric phase.

- Facilitate access to the toilet and teach child to make scheduled trips to the bathroom.

  May need to train the child to empty the bladder at specified intervals.

- Educate the child and family on signs and symptoms of overdistended bladder, adequate intake, and signs and symptoms of UTI.

  Reduces the risk of infection.

Expected Outcomes

- Child will excrete 0.5–2 mL/kg urine per hour.
- Child will maintain fluid balance, with intake equaling output.
- Child will not experience urinary retention or bladder distention.
- Signs and symptoms of altered urinary output will be recognized early, and interventions will be initiated promptly.
- Child and family will participate in activities or adopt techniques to normalize the child's urinary elimination.
- Child and family will demonstrate skill in care and hygiene measures in response to altered urinary elimination.
- Child and family will demonstrate interventions to avoid urinary retention.

Nursing Diagnosis: Risk for infection related to effects of disease, chronic illness, medications, and invasive procedures or catheters, urinary retention

Interventions/Rationale

- Promote hand hygiene by child, family, and staff.

  Reduces risk of infection by cross-contamination.

- Assess for presence of, existence of, and history of risk factors such as incontinence, urine obstruction, indwelling catheters, lack of skin integrity, and types of medication.

  Risk factors may weaken body's line of defense for fighting infection.

- Monitor WBCs, increased frequency, burning on urination, bladder spasms, foul-smelling urine, and changes in output or intake.

  May indicate an infection.

- Document urine characteristics.

  Cloudy urine and odor may indicate infection.

- Assess nutritional intake and fluid intake, including weight and serum albumin, BUN, and creatinine levels.

  Patients with poor nutritional and fluid intake may be at risk for infection.

- Encourage intake of protein and fluid as appropriate for the child.

  Maintains optimal nutritional and fluid status to fight infection.

- Teach child to take medications as ordered.

  Maintains fluid and electrolyte balance and state of health.

- Demonstrate and allow return demonstrations of all high-risk procedures the child and family will perform after discharge.

  Helps ascertain safe performance of procedures and may decrease the risk of infection.

Expected Outcomes

- Child will not develop infection.
- Child's signs and symptoms of infection will be recognized early, and interventions will be initiated in a timely manner.
- Child and family will identify signs and symptoms of UTI.
- Child and family will express their understanding of the need for prompt medical intervention if an infection occurs.

Nursing Diagnosis: Ineffective family therapeutic regimen management related to complex health care needs and lack of understanding of importance of regimen

Interventions/Rationale

- Assess child and family's perceptions and knowledge of regime.

  Allows for correction of and opportunity for increased knowledge.

- Schedule a team conference with family and child, including teachers and friends as appropriate and approved by family, to provide information and explore feelings and attitudes. Encourage the child to take part in the selection of conference participants.

  Child becomes a comanager and assists in having mutual support and information.

- Provide verbal and written instructions regarding regime.

  Enhances and fosters adherence; provides reference for later referral.

- Stress importance of regular, frequent follow-up appointments to ensure proper health care needs.

  Enhances opportunities to alter regime as health care needs improve or deteriorate.

- Explain the side effects of the medical regime, including the medications.

  Nonadherence is frequently caused by not knowing what to do and by side effects of medications.

- Use a variety of teaching methods.

  Children and families learn in different ways.

- Allow the child and family to practice new skills, providing immediate feedback on performance.

  Allows for enhanced retention and for making corrections of necessary skills.

(Continued)

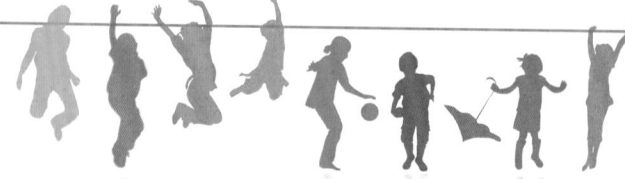

NURSING PLAN OF CARE 19-1:

The Child With Altered Genitourinary Status (*Continued*)

Expected Outcomes
- Child and family will show that they understand the child's health care needs and know how to manage current needs.
- Child and family will develop a plan to incorporate components of therapeutic regimen into their lifestyle (diet, medications, activities).
- Child and family will effectively manage the child's health care needs.

Nursing Diagnosis: Disturbed body image related to effects of illness

Interventions/Rationale
- Arrange for child and family to meet others who have had similar experiences and managed them successfully.
  Provides a support system.
- Provide openings to enable the child to express feelings by validating your observations and feelings (e.g., "You look down. How are things going?")
  Assists in identification of concerns and problems.
- Be a good listener and accept what the child verbalizes. Remember not to take anger or hostility personally.
  Provides the child an opportunity to discuss issues and misconceptions.
- Focus on the child's feelings and deal with the presenting behavior.
  Keeping focus on the child helps him or her feel that he or she is being heard.
- Determine what the body image change means to the child and what effect the child thinks it will have on life. Do not challenge perceptions you think are unrealistic, but continue to provide opportunities for the child to share these perceptions and feelings with you.
  Developmental changes normally occur as the child grows.
- Be accepting of child's body changes.
  If child is repulsed or ashamed of physical changes, he or she will be watching the faces of others for negative signs, which may reinforce the child's negative feelings.
- Assist the child to normalize the change; use developmental strategies.
  Child may perceive changes that are not present or real.

Expected Outcomes
- Child will verbalize positive self-concept.
- Child and family will be prepared for potential alterations in the child's appearance caused by the disease process and treatment interventions.
- Child's peers will be prepared for the child's altered appearance and provide support for the child.

Nursing Diagnosis: Deficient knowledge: Physiology and pathology of condition and care needed by child

Interventions/Rationale
- Assess family's knowledge of the child's condition and care needs.
  Assists in focusing teaching to family's needs.
- Explain condition and all treatments and procedures. Be present when other health team members give information. Reinforce and clarify information.
  Helps the child and family to understand condition and treatments and to make informed decisions.
- Identify signs and symptoms that require further evaluation.
  May assist in early detection and assist in prompt intervention of developing problems.
- Emphasize the need for ongoing medical care.
  Monitors disease process and provides opportunity for further teaching and discussions.
- Discuss potential complications related to specific therapeutic regime.
  Giving appropriate strategies to deal with side effects and complications may enhance adherence.
- Provide a list of medications, with dosage and schedule; list the side effects of each; explain the importance of adhering to prescribed dosages and where and how to obtain refills; and advise not to take over-the-counter drugs unless prescribed.
  Giving information and a tangible list may facilitate adherence to regime.
- Explain food and fluid restrictions and allow the child and family to plan daily menus and intake. Discuss the importance of maintaining an accurate intake and output as an indicator of fluid balance and renal functioning.
  Giving information may enhance adherence. Promotes healing and provides energy for tissue repair.
- Instruct in daily weights, frequent blood pressure check, and wearing of MedicAlert bracelet.
  Self-monitoring can provide early detection of complications.

- Initiate referrals, appointments with community support groups, mental health clinics, and so forth, as needed for continued psychosocial support.
  Provides for continued support.
- Encourage regular activity and exercise as tolerated.
  Immobility increases renal stasis and calcium shift out of bones.

Expected Outcomes

- Child and family will verbalize their understanding of the physiology and pathology of the condition, its effect on urinary tract function, and its medical and surgical management.
- Child and family will state rationale for care needed and will demonstrate care and hygiene measures needed to manage the child's care.

Nursing Diagnosis: Anxiety related to child's diagnosis and uncertainty of outcomes for the child

Interventions/Rationale

- Assess the level of fear in the child and the family. Observe for signs of denial and depression.
  Assists in determining the type of interventions needed.
- Acknowledge the feelings of the child and family; acknowledge normalcy of the situation.
  Acknowledgment of feelings can sometimes help the child and family gain control over their fears.
- Answer questions and concerns of the child and family, and provide opportunities for asking questions and voicing concerns.
  Creates feelings of cooperation; assists in identification of fears and concerns.
- Encourage the child and family to participate in the care of the child.
  Involvement promotes a feeling of control and feelings of usefulness.

Expected Outcomes

- Child and family will be able to manage their anxiety and perform activities of daily living.
- Child and family will verbalize their feelings of grief, loss, fear, powerlessness, or spiritual distress to an appropriate support source.

Nursing Diagnosis: Interrupted family processes related to presence of child with chronic or acute genitourinary disorder

Interventions/Rationale

- Assess family members' perceptions of problems.
  Each family member has perceptions that need to be understood.
- Evaluate strengths, coping skills, and support systems.
  Facilitates use of previous successful techniques.
- Consider cultural factors and incorporate into care practices as indicated and appropriate.
  May decrease serious conflict.
- Provide opportunities to express concerns, fears, expectations, or questions.
  Promotes communication and support.
- Assist family in setting realistic goals.
  Helps family gain control over the situation.
- Encourage family to obtain information and resources.
  May provide clarification.

Expected Outcomes

- Child and family will verbalize their feelings to each other and to the health care team.
- Child and family will demonstrate effective decision making and mutual support activities.
- Child and family will participate in treatment activities at developmentally appropriate levels.
- Child and family will implement effective coping mechanisms to work through problems associated with the illness.
- The family will verbalize their awareness of stressors that compromise their caregiving role.
- The family will express their feelings regarding their child's condition and its long-term management.
- The family will seek emotional, physical, and financial support from significant others, professionals, or other parents.
- The family will demonstrate parenting/caregiving behavior that is positive and appropriate for the age of their child.

ANSWER: For J. D. and his family, appropriate nursing diagnoses include deficient knowledge (condition, treatment, effect on functioning and appearance), anxiety related to the anomaly and impact on J. D.'s body image and functioning, interrupted family processes related to J. D.'s anomaly, and impact on the father's view of his son and concerns about the condition.

ALTERATIONS IN GENITOURINARY STATUS

Alterations in genitourinary status have many causes—from infection to developmental, structural, and neurologic problems. Trauma can also alter genitourinary status.

URINARY TRACT INFECTION

UTI is the inflammatory process that results from bacterial invasion into the sterile urinary tract. The epithelial cells that line the urinary tract respond quickly to bacterial infiltration, flooding the area with pathogen-destroying leukocytes. Voiding rids the body of the substances; however, endotoxins released during bacterial breakdown irritate mucosal nerve endings and cause localized inflammation. WBCs and bacteria in the urine (**pyuria** and **bacteriuria**, respectively) confirm the diagnosis of a UTI (see thePoint for Supplemental Information: Terminology Used to Describe Urinary Tract Infections).

UTI is the most common serious bacterial infection in childhood (Bitsori & Galanakis, 2012). In the United States, UTIs result in almost 50,000 hospitalizations per year in children younger than age 18 years (Spencer et al., 2010). UTI prevalence is about 5% in children 2 to 24 months of age with fever (Finnell et al., 2011). Circumcised boys have a threefold to fourfold decreased risk of UTI compared to uncircumcised boys (Shaikh et al., 2008). UTIs are more common in females than males after the neonatal period, and the incidence is high in sexually active adolescent females.

Escherichia coli, prevalent in the gastrointestinal tract, and *Klebsiella* are the organisms predominantly responsible for pediatric UTIs (Jerardi et al., 2012).

UTI can occur anywhere along the urinary tract but is most often confined to the bladder (cystitis). Urethritis in children can result from haphazard perineal hygiene or from contact with various products, such as bubble bath solutions or soaps, that irritate the child's urinary tract. Upper tract infections (pyelonephritis) are the most common serious infection of young children.

If cystitis is left untreated, it can progress to pyelonephritis with potential for kidney damage, hypertension, or renal insufficiency. Risk factors for UTI include anatomic and host factors. Anatomically, the female's short, straight urethra, situated in close proximity to the rectum, provides a convenient access route for invading bacteria. Female infants are especially vulnerable because of perineal colonization from fecal soiling. Urinary stasis is a prominent risk factor. VUR is the most commonly associated abnormality of children with UTI. Numerous studies have correlated UTI with bowel dysfunction (Alsaywid et al., 2010; Bower et al., 2006; Kasirga et al., 2006; Mattoo, 2007). This connection is believed to stem from pressure of the distended rectal segment and possibly from colonic seeding of bacteria by the hematogenous route.

Pathophysiology

Normally, the urinary tract is a sterile system, and the slightly acidic urine creates a hostile environment for most alkaline-favoring microorganisms. Bacteria that invade the urinary tract meet the first line of defense—expulsion by bladder flushing, or voiding. Anything that compromises total and frequent voiding, such as an anatomic defect, constipation, or neurologic dysfunction, increases the risk of mucosal infiltration of the bladder.

Bacterial growth triggers an immune response. Within hours, leukocytes flood the area. The affected tissue becomes inflamed and edematous. Bacteria-released endotoxins, alkaline in nature, promote disease progression. Sensitized nerve endings respond with uninhibited, painful bladder spasms in an attempt to flush out the pathogens. Localized mucosal infiltration produces hemorrhagic areas. Distorted by tissue inflammation, the ureterovesical junction may be temporarily incompetent.

If the infection is untreated, transient reflux permits it to ascend into the kidneys, resulting in pyelonephritis. Severe reflux is closely associated with permanent renal damage (M. Chen et al., 2013). Chronic or recurrent pyelonephritis resulting in renal damage and scarring may progress to chronic renal disease if it continues (Roberts et al., 2011). The cycle from initial bacterial influx to pyelonephritis can be rapid, reaching completion in 48 hours or less.

Pyelonephritis in children younger than age 2 years seems to be especially troublesome. Bladder trigone instability promotes ureterovesical junction shifting during infection, magnifying the likelihood of reflux and renal involvement. Scarring of the renal tissue and frequent UTI recurrence are more likely following initial infection. Children are at greatest risk for renal scarring during the first year of life. Early detection and treatment, coupled with long-term surveillance, are paramount to improve the prognosis for these children.

Pyelonephritis may progress to gram-negative septic shock, a response to circulating bacterial endotoxins. The child appears moribund and may experience seizures, hypotension, subnormal temperature, and loss of consciousness. Gram-negative septic shock is a medical emergency that requires life-saving treatment (see Chapter 31 for specific management).

Pyelonephritis traditionally requires hospitalization to administer IV fluids and parenteral antibiotics. This regimen provides rapid, high-dose drug therapy and fluid replacement to reduce or prevent renal parenchymal infiltration. It is appropriate for the child who is acutely ill or who is unable to maintain a high fluid intake.

Assessment

Determine the child's symptoms. Classic symptoms of UTI—urinary frequency, urgency and hesitancy, dysuria, hematuria, and stranguria (stopping and starting the urinary stream)—vary somewhat based on the child's age and cognitive level (Developmental Considerations 19-2). Constitutional symptoms, such as high temperature (>102° F [39° C]), flank pain, vomiting, lethargy, and generalized malaise, are more serious and point to pyelonephritis.

When the child's symptoms suggest a UTI, the nurse is often responsible for properly collecting and handling a urine sample. Accurate diagnosis depends on selecting a collection method with the least risk of contamination (see Tradition or Science 19-2).

Positive findings of blood and protein in the urine, using a urine Chemstrip, are suggestive of a UTI.

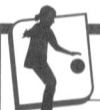

Signs and Symptoms of Urinary Tract Infection Based on Age

Neonate: Jaundice, fever, failure to thrive, poor feeding, vomiting

Infant: Irritability, poor feeding, fever, vomiting, diarrhea, strong odor of urine

Early childhood: Vomiting, diarrhea, abdominal or flank pain, fever, enuresis, urgency, frequency, new incontinence, strong odor of urine

Middle childhood: Fever, vomiting, flank or abdominal pain, frequency, urgency, dysuria, new incontinence, strong odor of urine

LE and nitrite readings, although accurate in adults, are problematic in children. LE is an enzyme that is released during WBC destruction. Positive findings are closely correlated to a UTI. However, negative findings can occur even when an infection is present because of frequent voiding and lower esterase levels in the child's blood. To obtain a positive nitrite reading, urine must be in the bladder for at least 4 hours in the presence of the bacteria containing reductase, so nitrate is reduced to nitrite. Infants typically void frequently, so a positive nitrite test is often not obtained in infants with infection.

Diagnostically, a UTI is identified by the presence of WBCs in the urine (pyuria) and by a urine culture that grows bacteria (bacteriuria) of a significant number. Cultures that grow mixed flora usually represent contamination. Obtain urine collection for culture prior to beginning antibiotic therapy and IV therapy for dehydration.

If a febrile infant appears severely ill or does not demonstrate improvement, a renal/bladder ultrasound (RBUS) evaluation of the urinary tract is recommended during the first 2 days of treatment (Roberts et al., 2011). If the infant demonstrates significant improvement, then the RBUS is recommended 1 to 2 weeks after the infection resolves (Roberts et al., 2011). VCUG is indicated only if the RBUS shows scarring, hydronephrosis, or findings indicative of high-grade VUR or obstructive uropathy (Roberts et al., 2011). VCUG is indicated after the second UTI (Roberts et al., 2011). The ultrasound may rule out obstructive uropathy but is a poor screening tool for VUR. A standard VCUG depicts urethral and bladder anatomy and VUR. Nuclear cystography uses less radiation than the standard VCUG and can help visualize the bladder and detect VUR. Grading of VUR is less precise, however, and associated bladder abnormalities cannot be detected with nuclear cystography. Therefore, a standard VCUG is preferred as the initial study, and nuclear cystography is used in

follow-up studies. A DMSA renal scan is the best tool for detecting tubular damage and renal scarring; unfortunately, the DMSA renal scan cannot detect VUR. Obtaining a VCUG too soon after a UTI may result in a false-positive study because of inflammation.

Elevated WBC counts, CRP, and ESRs are often present with pyelonephritis.

Interdisciplinary Interventions

The goal of treating UTIs is to eliminate the infection, prevent urosepsis, and reduce renal damage. Prompt intervention for UTI is necessary to provide symptomatic relief, halt the spread of infection, eliminate systemic infiltration of bacteria, and preserve the kidney. Short-term interventions combine antibiotic therapy, increased fluid intake, frequent voiding, and daily bowel movements. Long-term management involves further urinary evaluation and monitoring for recurrence.

Antibiotic Therapy

Antibiotics used to treat infection of the lower urinary tract include combined trimethoprim–sulfamethoxazole, nitrofurantoin, penicillins, and cephalosporins administered orally for 7 to 10 days. The antibiotic regimen may be altered when the bacterial sensitivity results are available, generally 48 hours after inoculation of the culture medium.

Increased Fluid Intake

A high daily fluid intake (as much as 1,000 mL for the older child) dilutes and washes out endotoxins and tissue debris. Water is the recommended fluid, along with juice, soup, milk, ice cream, gelatin, and frozen liquid desserts. Teach the child to avoid bladder irritants such as chocolate and caffeine-rich beverages. Although no studies have been replicated among children, encouraging the consumption of cranberry juice entails little risk (Tradition or Science 19-3). Maintaining a fluid record (Fig. 19-5) helps to encourage fluid intake. Children enjoy coloring the pictures and are proud to receive a reward sticker or star each day.

Another predisposing factor to bladder instability and recurrent UTI is constipation, which should be managed aggressively. Unstable bladder contractions and inability to relax the pelvic floor muscles, problems often associated with constipation, may result in incomplete bladder emptying. Adequate fluid intake can help prevent constipation.

Frequent Voiding

Most children with UTI experience uncontrolled frequency of urination resulting from detrusor hypersensitivity. However, the accompanying dysuria and bladder spasm may cause some children to withhold urine. Localized relief can be afforded by a tub or sitz bath or with a perineal rinse during voiding. A mild analgesic, such as acetaminophen, is recommended every 4 hours for comfort. Frequent voiding decreases urinary stasis and helps prevent UTIs. Because children spend a

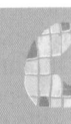

More Inquiry Needed

TRADITION OR SCIENCE 19-3

Are cranberry juice and cranberry products effective for preventing or managing UTIs in children?

Research demonstrates that cranberry affects the urinary tract by eliminating adhesion of microorganisms to epithelial cells that are in the urinary tract (Howell, 2007; Y. Liu et al., 2006).

Studies in adults demonstrate inconclusive evidence that cranberry may protect against UTIs. Although some small studies demonstrate a slight benefit, when including results of larger studies in a systematic review, no significant differences were found between cranberry juice and antibiotics for prevention of UTIs (Jepson et al., 2012). An RCT with 176 premenopausal women demonstrated no significant differences between cranberry juice and placebo juice (Stapleton et al., 2012). Another systematic review and meta-analysis, which tempered their results cautioning substantial heterogeneity across the included RCTs, found that cranberry-containing products did have a protective effect against UTIs but were more effective in certain subgroups, including women with recurrent UTIs, females, children, cranberry juice drinkers, and those who used cranberry-containing products more than twice a day (Wang et al., 2012). A systematic review found no evidence that cranberry effectively treats UTI once an infection is present (Jepson et al., 2010.).

Cranberry may be effective only in certain subpopulations. The evidence is inconclusive regarding whether it is effective in the elderly. McMurdo et al. (2005) examined the effectiveness of cranberry juice in hospitalized elderly patients with a mean age older than 81 years. Although they did find fewer UTIs caused by *Escherichia coli*, they caution against using the results without further study because the number of UTIs was a secondary outcome, and the study was underpowered (McMurdo et al., 2005). The evidence does not support its effectiveness in patients with a neurogenic bladder (B. B. Lee et al., 2007).

Although numerous studies have examined the effectiveness of cranberry products to prevent UTI/chronic cystitis in adults, particularly women, few studies have investigated the use of cranberry products in children. An RCT found that cranberry juice did not significantly reduce number of children with UTI recurrence but did reduce number of recurrences and associated antimicrobial use (Salo et al., 2012). An RCT comparing cranberry juice with high concentrations of proanthocyanidin to cranberry juice with no proanthocyanidin found a significant reduction in UTI risk in the high proanthocyanidin group (Afshar et al., 2011). Children accept cranberry juice well, but there is no change in bacterial flora in the nasopharynx or the bacterial fatty acid composition of stools and no effect on common infectious diseases or their symptoms (Kontiokari et al., 2005). Many parents give cranberry juice to their children with renal problems. One study examined the effects of cranberry juice on bacteriuria in children with neurogenic bladder who were receiving intermittent catheterization and found that cranberry concentrate had no effect on bacteriuria (Schlager et al., 1999).

Cranberry is not a substitute for antibiotics in the treatment of acute UTI. There is a strong scientific basis for recommending its use in adult women. More inquiry is needed to determine cranberry dosing, optimal preparation (e.g., concentrate, juice, capsules), and effectiveness in children.

---

substantial amount of time in school, work with school staff if possible to arrange schedules that allow voiding on a regular basis, every 2 to 3 hours.

Community Care

UTIs are managed at home, but when UTIs progress to pyelonephritis, hospitalization is usually required to manage fever and pain (see Chapter 11). When the diagnosis of UTI is confirmed, direct child and family teaching to include all aspects of disease progression and management. Discuss medication administration, risk factors that affect the child's potential for reinfection, and recommended prevention techniques. Give the family a home care instruction sheet to reinforce the information (Teaching Intervention Plan 19-3). Encourage the family to share this information with babysitters, teachers, or other adult caregivers. Emphasize the importance of long-term follow-up to identify and reduce the effects of long-term sequelae.

A urine culture is typically obtained 48 to 72 hours after completing the antibiotic therapy to ensure that the urine is sterile. Most uncomplicated UTIs respond to treatment, and cultures are negative after 2 days of antibiotics, which has led some to argue that repeat cultures to demonstrate cure cause unnecessary trauma and expense (Oreskovic & Sembrano, 2007). The child with a negative urine culture should undergo repeat cultures every 3 months during the ensuing year.

If a UTI recurs, the child may be given prophylactic therapy, using low-dose antibiotics. Nitrofurantoin or a combined trimethoprim–sulfamethoxazole preparation is the usual choice because of these agents' low serum and high urine concentrations.. Antibiotic prophylaxis to prevent UTI in children with low-grade VUR is no longer recommended, however. A systematic review concluded that the evidence of benefit is weak (Williams et al., 2006). Recent research indicates that antibiotic prophylaxis does not reduce incidence of UTI and increases the prevalence of resistant organisms (Conway et al., 2007; Garin et al., 2006), and that increased surveillance with prompt treatment of UTI may be indicated instead of prophylaxis (Roberts et al., 2011).

URETHRITIS

Young girls experiencing symptoms of burning, dysuria, frequency, or vaginal itching may possibly have a UTI; more commonly, the symptoms are caused by irritation of the skin at the opening of the urethra (urethritis) or around the vaginal area (vulvovaginitis). Before puberty, sensitive urethral tissue is easily irritated by chemicals or mechanical factors (see Teaching Intervention Plan 19-3). Vaginal discharge could suggest vaginal washout resulting from the child's position during urination or can signal a vaginal infection or sexual abuse.

Chronic urethral and introital irritation causes some young girls to develop labial adhesions (synechiae), beginning at the posterior fourchette and advancing anteriorly. In severe cases, the vagina may be completely occluded. Labial adhesions appear as a translucent line

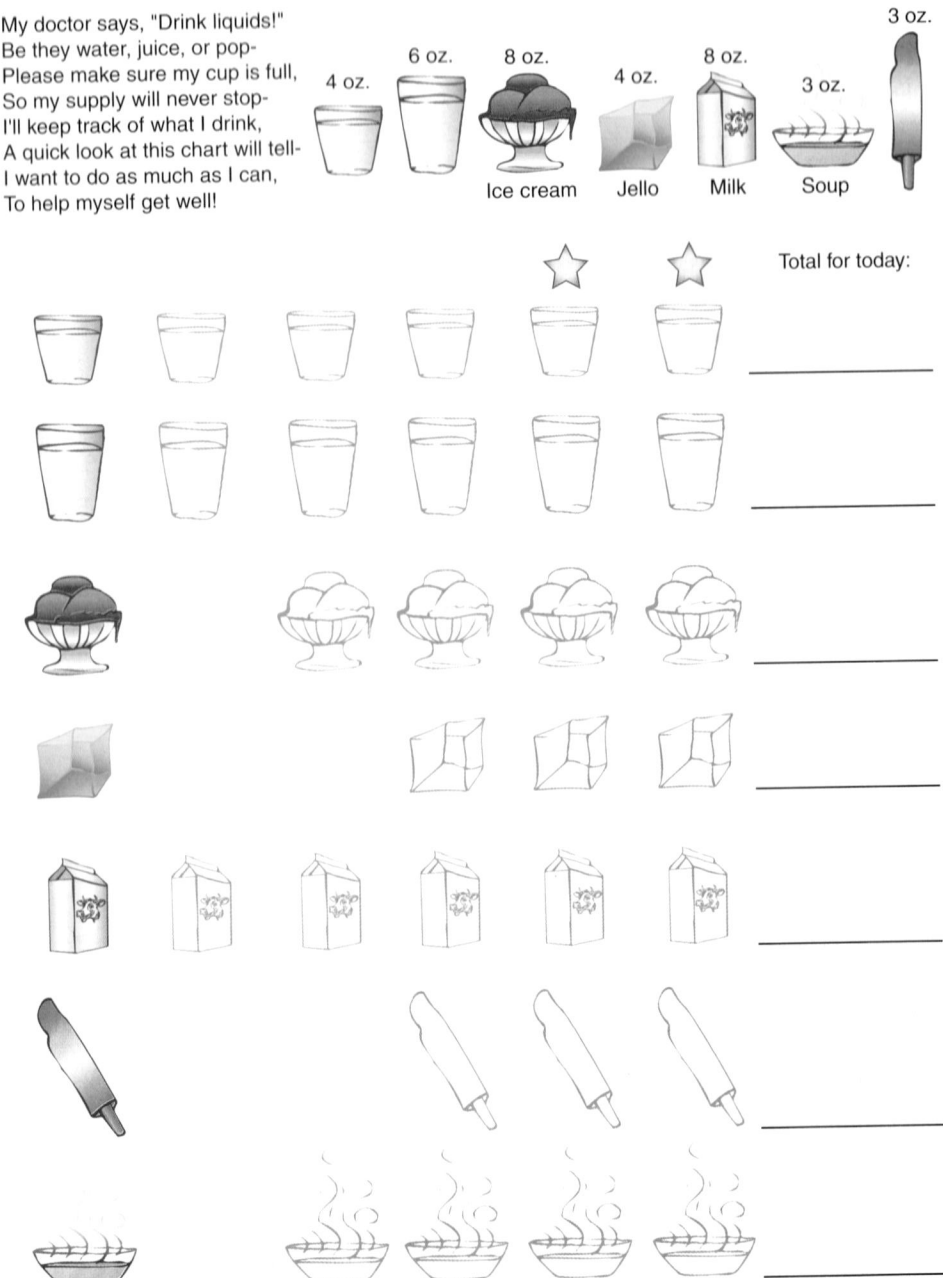

My doctor says, "Drink liquids!"
Be they water, juice, or pop-
Please make sure my cup is full,
So my supply will never stop-
I'll keep track of what I drink,
A quick look at this chart will tell-
I want to do as much as I can,
To help myself get well!

4 oz.   6 oz.   8 oz.   4 oz.   8 oz.   3 oz.   3 oz.

Ice cream   Jello   Milk   Soup

Total for today:

Figure 19-5 Having the child keep a fluid record may help motivate him or her to consume more fluids.

of central fusion and act as a hood that deflects urine into the vagina, producing dysuria. Severe cases may require treatment with a topical estrogen cream and gradual separation of the labia.

Although benign, urethritis is alarming because the symptoms may be similar to those of cystitis. Differentiating cystitis from a UTI is important to prevent misdiagnosis, unnecessary medication, and overaggressive urologic evaluation. The health care team obtains a meticulous history and a urine sample to confirm urethritis (Clinical Judgment 19-3).

The symptoms of urethritis can be distressing for the child and frightening to the family. Nursing care begins with reassuring the child and family of the benign nature of this condition and continues with guided questioning to find the precipitating cause (e.g., bubble bath, pinworms, inadequate hygiene). The goals of treatment for urethritis are to relieve symptoms and eradicate the underlying irritant. Home management is summarized in Teaching Intervention Plan 19-3.

VOIDING DISORDERS

The successful achievement of urinary bladder control is a highly anticipated childhood milestone. Delay or difficulty in achieving control after a socially acceptable age provokes a spectrum of negative responses from the child and family: anxiety, disgrace, frustration, anger,

TIP 19-3: A TEACHING INTERVENTION PLAN for the Child With a Urinary Tract Infection or Urethritis/Vulvovaginitis

Nursing Diagnoses and Family Outcomes

Urinary Tract Infection

- Impaired urinary elimination related to effects of infection
  Outcomes: Child returns to normal voiding pattern. Child and family will demonstrate skill in managing protocol to treat UTI.
  The family will verbalize signs and symptoms that indicate the child has a UTI.
- Acute pain with urination related to bladder spasms
  Outcomes: Family will implement relief measures that ease urination.
  Child will be free from pain.
- Health-seeking behaviors: Prevention of UTI
  Outcome: Child and family will identify methods that decrease risk of reinfection.

Urethritis/Vulvovaginitis

- Impaired skin integrity related to chemical or mechanical irritation of the genital area
  Outcomes: Child and family will identify irritants that precipitate or exacerbate the condition.
- Child's skin will remain free from secondary infection and will regain integrity.
- Child and family will pursue comfort measures that reduce urethral and vulvovaginal inflammation.

Teach the Child/Family

Cause of Urinary Tract Infections

- UTIs are infections of the bladder or kidneys caused by bacteria (germs) that travel up the urethra and start to grow in the bladder.
- UTIs are more common in girls, possibly because they have a short, straight urethra.
- Constipation is commonly associated with UTI.
- Causes of UTI include
  - Abnormalities of the urinary tract
  - Improper wiping after urination or bowel movement
  - Infrequent urination
  - Chemicals that irritate the urethra, including chlorine, bubble bath, soapy bath water

Cause of Urethritis/Vulvovaginitis

- Exposure to harsh soaps or chemicals causes inflammation of urethral meatus
- Bubble bath, chlorine, soapy bath water
- Use of cleansing towelettes to clean genital and rectal area
- Inadequately rinsed laundry items
- Poor genital hygiene
- Other causes
- Itching from rectal pinworms (worse at night)
- Wearing tight jeans or spandex pants
- Masturbation

- Presence of constant moisture in genital area if overweight
- Treatment delay may lead to infection of bladder

Signs and Symptoms of Urinary Tract Infection

- Bladder pressure/spasm before and after urinating
- Painful, frequent urination in small amounts
- Difficulty holding urine, wetting the bed or underwear
- Cloudy, dark, or foul-smelling urine
- Stomachache
- Temperature more than 100° F (37.8° C)
- Vomiting or weight loss, decreased appetite
- Diarrhea or constant diaper rash
- Crankiness or listlessness
- Poor color to skin

Signs and Symptoms of Urethritis/Vulvovaginitis

- Painful urination
- Mild frequency or avoidance of urination
- Genital rash or burning
- May experience wetting or leaking of urine during daytime
- Bed-wetting rare

Treatment of the Child With a Urinary Tract Infection
Antibiotics

- Take _____
- Dose _____ use proper measuring spoon.
- Give medicine _____ times a day for _____ days.
- Store per pharmacy instructions.
- The child should finish all medicine, even if feeling well; do not skip doses.
- Instruct daycare, school personnel, or babysitter to give medication.

Fluids

- Encourage drinking of six to eight glasses of fluid daily, especially water.
- Do not give carbonated sodas, tea, and coffee.

Pain and Fever Control

- Give acetaminophen at dose of _____ every 4 hours as needed.

Diet

- Increase child's fiber and bran intake.
- Increase child's daily intake of fresh fruits and vegetables.

Skin Care for Urethritis/Vulvovaginitis

- Soak two times a day in basin or bathtub for 10–15 minutes; use plain water. Baking soda or vinegar may be added. Make sure the area is dry before donning clothes.
- *Or*, apply to irritated area compresses of witch hazel three times a day.

- *Or*, apply boric acid compresses. Mix 1 teaspoon boric acid powder in 2 cups of water; apply with paper towel or cotton balls three times a day.
- *Or*, apply protective ointment (e.g., A&D ointment, zinc oxide), and low-potency hydrocortisone cream (if prescribed) twice daily; symptoms should be gone after 2–3 days.
- If pinworms are detected, further instructions will be given.

Preventive Care
- Drink enough fluids each day to keep urine light in color.
- Monitor pattern of bowel movements.
- Teach girls to wipe carefully from front to back after urinating or having a bowel movement.
- Encourage showers.
- If baths are given, limit bath time to 15 minutes. Do not use bubble baths or soapy bath water, and do not let bar of soap float in tub. Shampoo hair at end of bath with the child standing, and rinse genital area after the bath. Have child urinate after the bath.

- Rinse and dry genital area after swimming in a pool. Don dry clothes; do not allow child to stay in wet bathing suit.
- Encourage urination every 3 hours during the day.
- Because the child has a high-risk of another UTI, urine cultures must be checked every 3 months for 1 year.
- Child should wear cotton underpants and should not wear tight pants or nonbreathable materials, such as spandex and nylon.
- Wash new clothes before the child wears them.
- Discontinue use of irritating laundry additives (e.g., fragrances, dyes).
- Keep child's fingernails short and free from dirt buildup.

Contact Health Care Provider if
- Temperature of more than 100.4° F (38.0° C) develops
- Urine is pink or bloody
- Child looks sick, has a seizure, or has chills
- Child complains of back pain
- There is no improvement in child's condition after 2–3 days of antibiotic therapy

insecurity, and lowered self-esteem. The particular age depends on the culture of the family. Uncorrected, a childhood voiding disorder can affect the child's social and emotional development and may lead to acting-out behaviors, childhood depression, dysfunctional family interactions, and a marked risk for child abuse. Voiding disorders are classified as dysfunctional voiding, functional incontinence, or neurogenic and anatomic incontinence.

Dysfunctional Voiding

Dysfunctional voiding is a dysfunction of the lower urinary tract in which the actions of the bladder muscle and the external sphincter are not coordinated. This dysfunction can cause incontinence, incomplete bladder emptying, inability to voluntarily start or stop voiding, or high pressure in the bladder. When no neurologic or anatomic cause can be identified, the voiding patterns in children with dysfunctional voiding are believed to originate from behavioral issues. These behavioral issues may evolve from adverse situations that occur around toilet training and inhibit the maturation of normal urinary control.

Dysfunctional voiding may be associated with UTI, urinary retention, or VUR and can include abnormalities in voiding patterns such as staccato voiding (interruptions in the urine flow that prolong voiding time and leave postvoid residual urine, increasing the risk of UTI), fractionated voiding (incomplete and infrequent small-volume voids), postponement of voiding, and urge syndrome. In urge syndrome, the child has overactive detrusor contractions and a small bladder capacity, resulting in frequent voiding. The child has a strong desire to void and maneuvers into squatting positions

that externally compress the urethra to retain urine and avoid leakage. The associated incomplete bladder emptying leads to urinary stasis and infection, causing inflammatory changes in the bladder wall that stimulate overactivity of the detrusor. This voiding pattern can also be seen in children with cerebral palsy, spinal cord injury, sacral agenesis, and myelodysplasia. Conversely, a child with "lazy bladder" has a large-capacity bladder and a pattern of infrequent voiding. This child postpones responding to the urge to void with a weak or absent detrusor contraction and voids only once or twice a day, usually by abdominal straining; typically, the child feels no urge to void upon awakening in the morning. The volume voided usually exceeds the normal age-correlated capacity.

Vaginal voiding, another form of bladder dysfunction, is postvoid dribbling, which often causes external vaginal irritation or vaginal odor. It occurs in healthy girls after toilet training. These girls complain of leaking when they stand up after voiding, or damp underwear after voiding, from urine being deflected off the labia and into the vagina, where it is temporarily trapped during micturition. This deflection occurs when the child fails to void with the legs wide enough apart to allow urine to escape freely from the introitus. It can occur in any girl but is most common among those who are obese.

Of children with voiding dysfunction, 40% experience dysfunctional elimination syndrome, in which concomitant constipation or fecal soiling occurs (Feldman & Bauer, 2006). Dysfunctional elimination syndrome includes gastrointestinal disorders that contribute to dysfunction of the lower urinary tract, including unstable or overactive detrusor bladder muscle, infrequent voiding syndrome, or functional bowel disturbance.

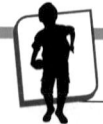

CLINICAL JUDGMENT 19-3

The Child With Painful Urination

Mrs. Sternberg received a call from her daughter's teacher at preschool, reporting that 4-year-old Sally was complaining of vomiting, abdominal pain, and pain with urination and had a temperature of 100° F (37.8° C). Mrs. Sternberg immediately picked up Sally from daycare and brought her to the community clinic where you work. Mrs. Sternberg thinks Sally must have a stomachache from all of the candy she ate at a party the day before.

Questions

1. What assessment data would be important to collect?
2. Which of the data in this vignette would suggest Sally has a stomachache?
3. Select a nursing diagnosis that reflects the family's need for information and home care regarding UTIs.

4. Laboratory analysis reveals bacteria present in the urine, and the diagnosis of UTI is confirmed. Based on your assessment and nursing diagnosis, what is your next plan of action?
5. How would you determine whether Mrs. Sternberg understood the plan of care?

Answers

1. Did Mrs. Sternberg notice any symptoms before today? Has Sally experienced any enuresis? Is anyone else sick at home? Assess weight and blood pressure. A clean-catch urine specimen or a urine specimen obtained by catheterization is needed.
2. Abdominal pain and vomiting. However, in light of the other symptoms, such as fever and pain on urination, the health care team should suspect that Sally has a UTI.
3. Deficient knowledge: Management and prevention of UTIs
4. Teach Mrs. Sternberg the following points:
   - Importance of administering oral antibiotics for the full course of therapy

   - Need for follow-up urine culture 48–72 hours after initiating treatment
   - Need to monitor urine cultures every 3 months for a 1-year period
   - Need for radiographic evaluation to rule out other genitourinary conditions
   - Need to increase Sally's fluid intake, especially of water
   - Need to maintain proper hygiene and avoid irritants such as bubble baths
5. Mrs. Sternberg brings Sally in for repeat urine cultures, as requested. She reports that Sally is drinking more fluids and that she is maintaining good perineal hygiene.

Functional Incontinence

Functional incontinence is a lack of urinary control beyond the developmental age when bladder control should be achieved, usually thought to be 5 years. It is secondary to a multitude of exogenous causes. Usually called *enuresis*, functional incontinence implies mild or episodic urine leakage. Enuresis can occur during the day (diurnal) or at night (nocturnal). Children with *primary enuresis* have never achieved complete continence. In *secondary enuresis*, the child achieves continence for at least 6 months but then resumes incontinence.

The incidence of functional incontinence is age dependent. An estimated 2% to 7% of school-aged children continue to experience functional incontinence. Over 10% of 6-year-olds and approximately 5% of 10-year-olds have nocturnal enuresis (Franco et al., 2013), which is more common in boys (Nevéus, 2011). Because most children experience spontaneous resolution of functional enuresis, it only becomes a problem when the child or the family becomes concerned about the interference that enuresis exerts on their lifestyle.

Heredity is a factor in the development of enuresis, although the mechanism is unclear. The risk for a child to develop enuresis is only 15%; that risk escalates to 44% if one parent experienced enuresis and 77% if both parents were affected (Ward-Smith & Barry, 2006).

Enuresis is thought to be precipitated or exacerbated by various interconnected factors based on the perspective that enuresis is a symptomatic response, not a disease entity. The prevailing thinking interprets enuresis as a neuromaturational/developmental lag with superimposed familial, social, environmental, psychological, or organic mediating components.

To appreciate the concept of *neuromaturational lag* requires understanding bladder physiology. In infants, voiding occurs as a spontaneous response to the activation of stretch receptors, following the sensation of bladder filling. In spinal arc fashion, the stretch stimulus is carried to the spinal cord and rerouted along motor neurons back to the bladder and sphincter, bypassing higher neurologic centers. Micturition results from the simultaneous involuntary action of a bladder detrusor contraction and sphincter relaxation. Between age 2 and 4 years, myelination of the lumbosacral neural circuits is gradually accomplished, completing the neuromaturation of the detrusor and sphincter. The theory of neuromaturational lag proposes that enuretic children possess bladders with small capacity and also experience delayed myelination of the lower spinal nerves. The result is that these children respond with premature detrusor contractions during the filling state and cannot effectively contract the sphincter. Rather, they rely on forced constriction of the bladder neck or sphincter to remain continent during the day, but they are unable to exert sphincter pressure at nighttime to prevent bed-wetting. Because most children with functional enuresis eventually acquire complete bladder control, even without treatment, the cause is believed to be a neuromaturational delay.

Other physiologic factors may contribute to enuresis. Bladder stretch receptors may be abnormal or dulled during early childhood. As the child acquires the ability to interpret bladder fullness, he or she acquires urinary control by contracting pelvic floor muscles or by waking to void. Episodes of involuntary sphincter relaxation may allow urinary seepage. Enuretic children do not rouse to the sensation of a full bladder. They are deep sleepers (Nevéus, 2011), but the depth of sleep does not relate to the severity of the enuresis (Ozden et al., 2007). Sleep patterns are similar for both enuretic and nonenuretic children, and enuretic episodes occur during all stages of sleep (Bader et al., 2002). Primary nocturnal enuresis has been shown to be associated with habitual snoring (Alexopoulos et al., 2006); treating the airway obstruction improves enuresis (Firoozi et al., 2006).

Organic factors are also known to predispose a child to enuresis. Antidiuretic hormone follows a circadian rhythm that increases at night, increasing renal tubular reabsorption of water, resulting in decreased urine output. Conditions that produce polyuria, such as diabetes mellitus, diabetes insipidus, or chronic renal disease, may be underlying causes of enuresis.

Food allergens have been periodically identified as precipitating factors in enuresis, but few studies back up this phenomenon. Some children have experienced improvement or eradication of enuresis or urgency, with reduced sensation of bladder irritability, when chemical additives or artificial sweeteners were eliminated from the diet. These additives may exert a diuretic effect that increases urine production.

UTI and constipation, which can increase bladder irritability and reduce functional bladder capacity, can be another factor in enuresis. Eradicating bladder infection may stop bed-wetting.

Psychosocial and developmental influences can also play a part in enuresis. For example, enuresis is more common among children from lower socioeconomic groups and deprived backgrounds (Van Hoecke et al., 2003), but this relation may stem from the disorganization that often is present in these children's daily life. Psychological factors that affect the child may affect the persistence of primary enuresis or incite secondary enuresis. Children with enuresis have decreased self-esteem and are more likely to be the target of bullying behavior and to have attention/activity problems, oppositional behavior, and conduct problems (Joinson, Heron, Emond et al., 2007). They tend to be less conscientious and more neurotic (Van Hoecke et al., 2006). As a result of enuresis, these children may not participate in age-appropriate activities, such as sleepovers or overnight camps. After successful treatment, these children report greater self-esteem and happiness, improved appearance, and reduced acting-out behaviors, suggesting that emotional disorders are expressions of distress related to the inability to control the voiding function (Ward-Smith & Barry, 2006). Enuresis has been found to be associated with relatively low IQ scores (Joinson, Heron, Butler et al., 2007).

Neurogenic and Anatomic Incontinence

Neurologic control of the lower urinary tract (bladder, urinary sphincter, pelvic floor muscles, and urethra) involves the coordinated efforts of cerebral structures and spinal pathways. The urologic end result of lesions in these segments of the nervous system is a neurogenic bladder. Neurologic defects with detrimental effects on urologic function are wide ranging and include congenital neuromuscular disorders such as myelomeningocele, spina bifida, sacral agenesis, spinal lipoma, sacral teratoma, or tethered spinal cord and acquired conditions such as spinal trauma, transverse myelitis, osteomyelitis, muscular dystrophy, degenerative disorders, or residual sequelae from rectal or genital surgical procedures. Generally, children with this type of incontinence experience moderate to complete loss of bladder function.

Some anatomic anomalies of the lower urinary tract may precipitate severe incontinence by distorting the sphincter mechanism. These defects include bladder exstrophy, epispadias, posterior urethral valves, ureterocele, and marked or multiple urethral strictures. Ureteral **ectopia**, in which the ureter terminates at a site within or distal to the sphincter, likewise causes constant dribbling.

There is no uniformity to the types of neurogenic bladder problems that children can manifest, even among those with similar neuromuscular deficits. Furthermore, the neurogenic effects may change in response to changes during growth and development. Therefore, children with a neurogenic bladder must be monitored closely to accurately assess their bladder function and response to treatment. Improper management of the child with a neurogenic bladder can have ominous consequences in the upper urinary tract. Renal damage or failure can develop from chronic ascending infection or reflux following bladder atony, which causes urinary retention.

Assessment

The evaluation of a child with a voiding disorder includes a complete health history, physical examination, and diagnostic testing.

A detailed history of voiding habits is necessary. Because family members are often unaware of "normal" voiding and age-appropriate bladder control, ask precise questions and obtain explicit details.

Assess urgency, frequency, age at onset of enuresis (primary vs. secondary), type of enuresis (nocturnal, diurnal, or combined), history of UTI, associated daytime control problems, and presence of other health problems that induce polyuria. Creating a multigenerational family tree may highlight a genetic predisposition for enuresis. The amount of urine voided during a typical enuretic episode can be estimated by evaluating the size of a wet spot or the extent to which bed linens are soaked. Discuss previous treatment measures, the child's diet, and any concomitant bowel problems, particularly chronic constipation. Encopresis may indicate that the voiding disorder has a neurologic component.

Explore psychosocial factors such as recent lifestyle changes, the effect of the voiding disorder on the child and family, and school performance. Assess family dynamics by observing family–child interactions for nonverbal clues. Ascertain the family's commitment to resolving the child's problem, situations that may influence timing or choice of treatment, and factors that may impede adherence to a treatment regimen. For example, if the child has several caregivers, it is imperative that they all cooperate in the management plan and do not send the child contradictory messages.

A thorough voiding history is the cornerstone in differentiating voiding disorders; it also directs the treatment regimen. The following tools are useful to ensure that you gather all salient data:

- Voiding profile: This questionnaire is used to glean important details about the child's voiding problem. Designed to be completed before the child's first visit, it also helps the family gain a clear perspective of the child's problem (see Chart 19-1).
- Voiding diary: This 3-day record of the child's drinking habits, voiding/stooling pattern, daytime activities, and emotional state should include weekend days as well as school days.
- Child interview: Using developmentally appropriate wording, inquire about urinary habits, daytime symptoms, emotional response, and motivation level. Sample questions might include the following: "Can you tell when you need to void during the day—usually, sometimes, or never? At night?" "When you feel the urge to void, what do you do? Ignore the sensation? Try to get to the bathroom? Assume a squatting position, cross your legs, or press your thighs together to stop the urge or hold the urine?" "Is your underwear damp very often?" "How worried are you about this problem?" "What bothers you the most?" "What would change if you become dry?" A lack of motivation on the child's part predisposes all initiatives to failure. If assessment shows poor motivation,

counsel the family to delay treatment for 6 months, then reassesses the child's readiness.

Perform a careful physical examination to detect signs of anatomic or neuromuscular abnormalities (see Focused Physical Assessment 19-1). Specifically note any genital abnormalities and palpate the abdomen for a distended bladder or for stool in the colon. Inspect the lumbosacral spine for dimpling or sacral malformation, a lipoma, a hairy patch, sinus tract, deviated or absent cephalad segment of the gluteal clef, or a flattened buttock. If any of these signs are present, perform a neurologic assessment of lower extremity function, rectal tone, perineal and anal sensation, and intactness of the bulbocavernosus reflex. Evaluate the child's gait and perform a developmental assessment, when applicable.

If possible, observe the child while he or she is voiding. Note a weak or intermittent stream, dribbling, or straining to initiate urination. These signs suggest organic involvement. Vaginal voiding can be detected if the girl leans backward or does not separate her legs during a void.

Diagnostic Tests

Collect a urine sample to check levels of glucose and presence of blood or protein. Measure urine concentration of the first morning void by specific gravity. Obtain a urine culture to test for bacterial infection.

At this point, all data are scrutinized and compiled to determine a diagnosis and to consider the need for further studies. If a neurologic deficit is suspected, a VCUG and renal ultrasound are performed, and serum creatinine and BUN levels are obtained to define the lower urinary tract and screen for renal dysfunction. Sacral deformities are highlighted by MRI of the lower spine. Urodynamic testing of the bladder is crucial to establish the specific type of bladder dysfunction; this test is usually reserved for children in whom conservative therapy has failed (Feldman & Bauer, 2006).

Most children with voiding disorders are diagnosed with functional incontinence. An overwhelming proportion of this group consists of children with uncomplicated nocturnal enuresis—meaning, they have no history of UTI and minimal daytime symptoms. No further diagnostic studies are recommended because the rate of organic anomaly mirrors that of the general pediatric population.

However, children with a history of UTI, significant diurnal symptoms, or encopresis are at risk for a superimposed uropathologic condition and constitute a group with complicated enuresis. They should be evaluated with VCUG, renal ultrasound, and spinal radiographs to screen for effects of lower tract dysfunction. Urodynamic or renal function studies are pursued if warranted.

Nursing Diagnoses and Outcomes

Nursing Plan of Care 19-1 presents nursing diagnoses generally applicable to the child with a genitourinary condition. The following diagnoses address some more specific care needs of the child with a voiding disorder:

Nursing Diagnosis: Impaired parenting related to child's inability to achieve continence
Outcomes:
- Parents will verbalize their acceptance of the child.
- Parents/family will identify the stressors related to the voiding disorder.
- Parents/family will use positive coping mechanisms in response to the child and the voiding disorder.
- Parents/family will refrain from blaming the child for the voiding disorder while encouraging the child to take responsibility in managing the consequences.

Nursing Diagnosis: Readiness for enhanced self-health management: Managing urinary incontinence
Outcomes:
- Child and family will participate in a management protocol.
- Child, family, or both will verbalize an understanding of the therapeutic goals of managing the voiding disorder.
- Child or family will demonstrate accurate and safe use of medications.
- Child, family, or both will express realistic expectations and an appropriate time frame for completing the management protocol.

Interdisciplinary Interventions

Management of the child with a voiding disorder requires an interdisciplinary effort using medical, nursing, nutritional, and psychosocial health care professionals, whose skills are combined to ameliorate the child's problem, guided by the child's acceptance of and response to treatment.

Management of dysfunctional voiding and enuresis is symptomatic and may include pharmacologic agents such as anticholinergics, behavior modification techniques to modify voiding patterns, bladder retraining, bowel management (see the discussion of constipation in Chapter 18), and diet management (Evidence-Based Clinical Practice Guideline 19-1). Management of neurogenic and anatomic voiding disorders may include surgery, pharmacologic agents, and clean intermittent catheterization.

Surgical Management

Congenital anomalies detected during the diagnostic evaluation are assessed by a pediatric urologist to determine the appropriateness of corrective or reconstructive surgery. Various procedures include reimplantation of the ureters for VUR or ureteral ectopia, bladder neck reconstruction for defects of the sphincteric mechanism, and endoscopic fulguration (destruction with electric current) of urethral webs or strictures. Implantation of an artificial sphincter has been used

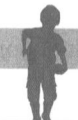

EVIDENCE-BASED CLINICAL PRACTICE GUIDELINES 19-1
Management of Enuresis

European Association of Urology and European Society for Paediatric Urology

Tekgül, S., Riedmiller, H. S., Dogan, P. et al. (2013). *Guidelines on paediatric urology*. Arnhem, The Netherlands: European Association of Urology & European Society for Paediatric Urology. Retrieved from

http://www.uroweb.org/gls/pdf/22%20Paediatric%20Urology_LR.pdf

Offers guidelines for diagnosis and management of enuresis.

American Academy of Pediatrics, European Society for Paediatric Urology, European Society for Paediatric Nephrology

Vande Walle, J., Rittig, S., Bauer, S. et al. (2012). Practical consensus guidelines for the management of enuresis. *European Journal of Pediatrics, 171*(6), 971–983. Retrieved from

http://link.springer.com/article/10.1007/s00431-012-1687-7/fulltext.html

Provides guidelines for evaluation and treatment of enuresis.

National Institute for Health and Clinical Excellence. (2010). *Nocturnal enuresis: The management of bedwetting in children and young people.* Retrieved from

http://www.nice.org.uk/nicemedia/live/13246/51367/51367.pdf

Provides best practice guidelines on care of children and young people with nocturnal enuresis.

The International Children's Continence Society

Neveus, T., Eggert, P., Evans, J. et al. (2010). Evaluation of and treatment for monosymptomatic enuresis: A standardization document from the International Children's Continence Society. *Journal of Urology, 183*(2), 441–447. Retrieved from

http://download.journals.elsevierhealth.com/pdfs/journals/0022-5347/PIIS0022534709026822.pdf

Recommends strategies for evaluating and treating enuresis in children with no other lower urinary tract symptoms.

to manage neurogenic bladder. Bladder atrophy or a noncompliant, rigid detrusor may require bladder augmentation to increase urine capacity. Urinary diversion may be a temporary or a permanent choice in cases of massive obstructive uropathy or when sphincteric reconstruction fails or to provide bladder access for intermittent catheterization. For the child with spinal agenesis or tethered spinal cord, neurosurgical intervention such as laminectomy is used to release neural compression. Bladder function may return fully or only partially (Guerra et al., 2006); ongoing urodynamic evaluation is necessary to monitor progress. Surgical intervention within a year of symptom onset results in the best symptom improvement (Hajnovic & Trnka, 2007).

Surgery, even when successful in correcting urologic anomalies, does not always eradicate incontinence completely. Supplemental techniques are implemented based on the residual symptoms.

Pharmacologic Management

Medications are used to treat UTI and to modify bladder activity that is detrimental to continence. Urinary antibacterials are administered when a UTI is documented; long-term suppressive therapy may be necessary for the child at risk for recurring infections. Medications that moderate neurotransmission to the lower urinary tract are used to treat urgency or to increase bladder capacity. The anticholinergic agent oxybutynin chloride (Ditropan) exerts an antispasmodic effect on the detrusor, counteracting uninhibited contractions. This drug is effective for an unstable or noncompliant bladder. Imipramine hydrochloride (Tofranil), an anticholinergic and antidepressant drug, has mild sympathetic action on the detrusor and a strong effect on sphincteric constriction. It may also lower the sleep arousal threshold, making the child more responsive to the nocturnal filling sensation. Desmopressin acetate (DDAVP), a derivative of antidiuretic hormone, reduces the volume of urine produced during sleep. DDAVP is not considered a cure for enuresis; rather, it serves as a treatment for the symptom. It is available in a nasal spray or in tablet form. Alpha-adrenergic antagonists such as doxazosin (Cardura) inhibit detrusor contractility, improve bladder compliance, and increase bladder capacity. They may be used in children with recalcitrant voiding dysfunction and hyperreflexic noncompliant neurogenic bladders (El-Hefnawy et al., 2012).

Numerous studies report initial high success rates for these pharmacologic agents, but relapse rates are high when the drugs are discontinued (Glazener et al., 2008; O'Flynn, 2011). Many families are reluctant to administer medications to their children on a long-term basis, fearing side effects or personality changes. Safety issues are a concern, particularly for imipramine, which has caused death in overdosed children. These medications appear to be most effective as adjuncts to other enuretic therapies, to enhance management of neurogenic or unstable bladder, or to offer short-term alleviation of enuresis before such experiences as camping or vacation.

Behavior Modification Techniques

Behavioral methods to treat enuresis and dysfunctional voiding include rewards for accomplishing predetermined goals or behaviors, such as dry nights, adherence to medication or diet changes, or appropriate responses to the moisture alarm; family modeling of healthy urinary habits; timed daytime voiding or waking the child to void; and encouraging the child to assume responsibility for behavior (e.g., by changing bed linens). For enuresis, simple behavioral methods may be used initially because they are less demanding than moisture alarms and have less risk of adverse effects than medications. In one study, almost half the patients with good adherence to timed voiding for daytime incontinence improved substantially within 4 months (Allen et al., 2007).

Moisture alarms work by applying moisture-sensing devices to the child's bed or underwear. An alarm awakens the child as wetting occurs. The child is gradually conditioned to associate the sensation of a full bladder with arousal and learns to inhibit micturition. The long-term success rate is best when combined with behavior interventions. The alarm and/or behavioral interventions require intensive effort on the part of the child and the family and may not be suitable for all families (Glazener et al., 2008, O'Flynn, 2011). This system is highly effective, with 66% to 79% (Cutting et al., 2007) of users achieving dryness. In one study, initial dryness was achieved in a median time of 10 weeks, and 64% of subjects remained dry at 24 months (Cutting et al., 2007).

Bladder Retraining

Biofeedback therapy is effective in treating children with dysfunctional voiding and enuresis (Kibar et al., 2007). It is used to retrain the pelvic muscles, promoting relaxation of the pelvic floor and improving bladder function.

Kegel exercises are pelvic floor contractions that simulate the stopping and starting of urine flow. They can be performed as the child experiences urgency during bladder filling. Kegel exercises can be taught to children as young as 5 years of age but require a great deal of practice and involved support. These maneuvers effectively suppress involuntary detrusor contractions and improve nocturnal enuresis (Schneider et al., 1994).

Children with hyperextended bladders develop a pattern of delayed daytime voiding, up to 4 hours or longer, followed by urgency, or wetting, resulting from the desensitization of the bladder during the fill stage. They require an opposite method of therapy. Encourage these children to void every 2 hours, even before they sense bladder fullness, as a means to restore detrusor sensitivity. Alarm watches are useful reminders to void on schedule; they come in both vibrating and audible forms.

Clean intermittent catheterization permits regular, complete bladder emptying of an atonic bladder (see "Treatment Modalities" section). In addition to preventing infection from urinary stasis, this procedure stops overflow incontinence. It also counteracts hydronephrosis, which results from a constantly filled bladder.

Dietary Manipulation

Along with the nutritional recommendations for improved bowel functioning, such as fiber, fruit, and extra fluids, eliminating foods with dyes, preservatives, and, especially, artificial sweeteners may be effective. Discourage caffeinated foods, such as cola, tea, and coffee, which exert a diuretic effect. Although many families restrict fluids before bedtime, this precaution does not seem to reduce enuresis. Butler et al. (2005) found that fluid restrictions were similar in children who did and did not wet the bed.

Psychotherapy

Although most children with voiding disorders do not manifest psychopathologic symptoms, concurrent distressing life circumstances, discipline problems, depression, and family conflicts warrant assistance from mental health professionals. Successfully managing these issues is important to prevent complicating the already tenuous emotional climate for the child. Unresolved issues drain the family's ability to formulate and adhere to a long-term, often complex, management program.

Nursing Management

Assist the child and family to manage and to cope with this condition through education about treatment options. The nurse's role in the interventions for a child with a voiding disorder is varied (Nursing Interventions Classification 19-1). All aspects of therapy require comprehension and acceptance by the child and family; therefore, child and family education is instrumental to the success of a chosen mode of therapy.

When surgical intervention is indicated, provide preoperative, postoperative, and follow-up teaching. Teach the child and family about medications, including dosage, expected results, side effects, and home safety measures. Skin care and hygiene measures, such as the use of protective emollients and enzyme washing solutions, prevent chafing or skin breakdown related to chronic exposure to urine. Changes in diet may require creative problem solving to ensure that the child accepts them.

Developmental, temperamental, and motivational assessments provide the child and family with predictions regarding the appropriateness of a subscribed therapeutic intervention. Be alert for expressions of intolerance directed by the family toward the child and the voiding problem; this evaluation assesses the risk for child abuse and the potential for the family's successful participation in a long-term management regimen. Offer parenting and coping techniques gleaned from feedback from other families or from personal experience. By taking the role of a consistent resource person, the nurse can monitor progress and offer encouragement. Remind the child and family that, in most cases, enuresis is self-limiting. The benefits derived from reducing enuresis and dysfunctional voiding can be generalized to include enhanced self-esteem, improved outlook on life, and a positive sense of self-control.

OBSTRUCTIVE UROPATHY

Obstructive uropathy is a term used to describe damage caused by a congenital or acquired condition that impedes urine excretion, often caused by VUR or ureteropelvic junction (UPJ) obstruction. Common obstructive lesions within the tubular structures (urethra or ureters) include redundant tissue leaflets (valves) or strictures at sites of segmental attachment. Insufficiently innervated ureteral segments halt the wavelike flow of muscular contractions from the renal pelvis to the bladder. Ureteral placement outside of the trigone affects compression of the ureteral orifice during voiding. Anomalous ureteral placement creates an ectopic orifice in the proximal urethra or in the vagina. Despite continuous dribbling, the ectopic ureteral opening is often too stenotic for complete urine drainage.

During early fetal development, the kidney originates in the pelvis. It gradually ascends to a retroperitoneal site, acquiring new vasculature while the outgrown blood vessels degenerate. An aberrant vessel remnant may constrict the ureter during the migratory process, causing obstruction. If the kidney fails to rise from the pelvis (the so-called pelvic kidney), ureteral growth may become redundant, and the ureter may kink. Likewise, kinking or twisting may occur as a result of either a sharply angled UPJ or following inadequate rotation of the renal unit shortly before birth.

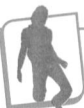 **NIC 19-1 NURSING INTERVENTIONS CLASSIFICATION:** Urinary Incontinence Care: Enuresis

Definition: Promotion of urinary continence in children

Activities:

Assist with diagnostic evaluation (e.g., physical examination, cystogram, cystoscopy, and lab tests to rule out physical causation)

Interview parent to obtain data about toilet-training history, voiding pattern, urinary tract infections, and food sensitivities

Determine frequency, duration, and circumstances of enuresis

Discuss effective and ineffective methods of prior treatment

Monitor family's and child's level of frustration and stress

Perform physical examination

Discuss techniques to use in reducing enuresis (e.g., night-light, restricted fluid intake, scheduling nocturnal bathroom trips, and use of alarm system)

Encourage child to verbalize feelings

Emphasize child's strengths

Encourage parents to demonstrate love and acceptance at home to counteract peer ridicule

Discuss psychosocial dynamics of enuresis with parents (e.g., familial patterns, family disruption, self-esteem issues, and self-limiting characteristic)

Administer medications as appropriate for short-term control

From Bulechek, G. M., Butcher, H. K., Dochterman, J. M. et al. (Eds.). (2013). *Nursing interventions classifications (NIC)* (6th ed.). St. Louis, MO: Mosby. Used with permission.

Pathophysiology

Forces that maintain urinary excretion originate in the renal pelvis because accumulated urine is propelled through the ureter. Low-pressure peristaltic contractions, initiated within the pelvic musculature, transmit urine in a wavelike fashion past the UPJ to the ureter. The distal ureteral segment burrows into the bladder wall and is tunneled within the inner bladder mucosa. The ureteral orifice emerges within the bladder interior at the trigone. Initially, a bolus of urine spurts into the empty bladder sac unimpeded; as bladder distention stretches and thins the submucosal tunnel, increasing bladder pressure eventually collapses the ureteral lumen to prevent urine regurgitation. During micturition, the sphincter relaxation is coordinated with high-pressure detrusor (bladder muscle) contractions to expel urine.

Urinary tract obstruction interferes with the normal urine drainage process, resulting in pathophysiologic changes ranging from mild to severe (Fig. 19-6). Partial urethral blockage is initially compensated for by hypertrophy of the bladder wall, which is necessary to generate the elevated pressure for bladder emptying. Failure of this protective effect produces retrograde ureteral dilation and progressive loss of tissue elasticity. The most serious insult from obstructive uropathy is the visceral destruction induced by hydronephrosis. Escalated pressures within the renal tubules and glomerular structures compromise the filtration process.

Vesicoureteral Reflux

VUR is abnormal backflow of urine from the bladder into the ureter and, sometimes, the kidneys during voiding through an incompetent ureterovesical junction. Although the incidence is estimated at 0.4% to 1.8% in children without urologic symptoms, 30% to 50% of children (depending on age) with a history of symptomatic UTI have VUR (Tekgül et al., 2012). Siblings of patients with known reflux have a 27.4% (range 3% to 51%) chance of reflux (Tekgül et al., 2012). For this reason, routine screening of siblings of children with reflux is recommended.

VUR seems to be related to the valve mechanism of the ureterovesical junction. Primary VUR, the most common variant of VUR, results from a congenital deficiency in the formation of the ureterovesical junction and is related to a short mucosal tunnel length that compromises the flap valve mechanism. Secondary VUR occurs from decompensation of a normally formed ureterovesical junction because of neurogenic bladder, anatomic abnormality, or outlet obstruction, which results in increased bladder pressure. Managing the underlying causes often resolves reflux.

The International Reflux Grading System classifies VUR into five grades (Lebowitz et al., 1985), depending on the degree of retrograde filling and dilation of the renal collecting system (Fig. 19-7). The degree of

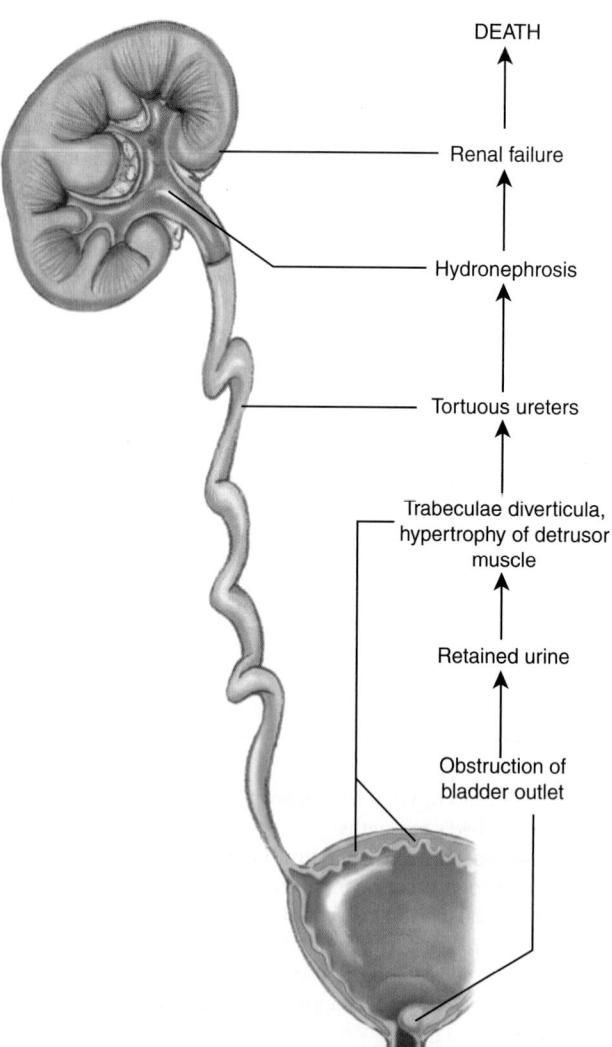

Figure 19-6 Urinary tract obstruction can occur anywhere in the upper or lower tract; some of the most common sites and the related effects are indicated.

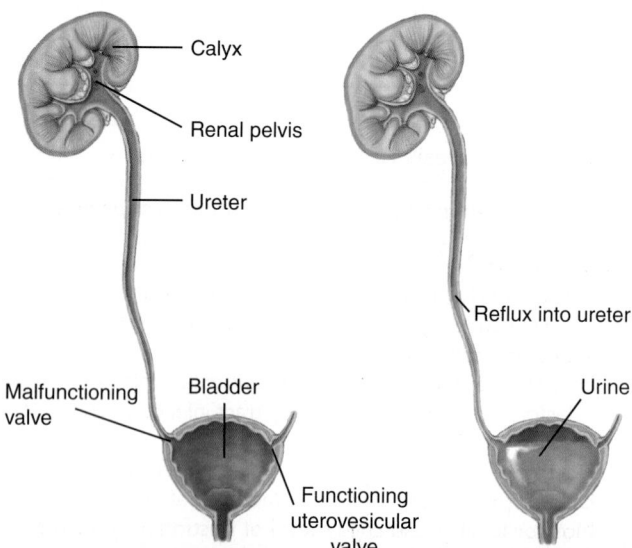

Figure 19-7 In VUR, a defect in the vesicoureteral junction allows urine to flow back into the ureter during voiding. After voiding, the urine returns to the bladder from the ureter, resulting in incomplete bladder emptying.

grading is important to the child's management and prognosis. The more severe the reflux, the lower the rate of spontaneous resolution and the higher the incidence of renal scarring.

Ureteropelvic Junction Obstruction

UPJ obstruction is the most common cause of antenatal hydronephrosis. With an incidence of 1 in 1,250 live births, it is more common in males than in females (2:1) (Groth & Mitchell, 2012). Routine ultrasound screening during the second trimester has resulted in more infants being diagnosed with antenatal hydronephrosis.

Successful passage of urine from the renal pelvis to the ureter requires a patent UPJ. Thus, in UPJ obstruction, the intrapelvic pressure created by hydronephrosis exerts a direct negative effect on glomerular filtration. As pressures within the nephron exceed glomerular capillary pressure, reverse fluid and solute transport occurs. Concentration of urine is hampered because of restricted renal blood flow and long-standing distal tubular damage. The acceleration of fluid buildup provides a nourishing broth for bacterial colonization, and altered hydrogen excretion creates metabolic acidosis.

In its most severe form, hydronephrosis leads to obliteration of the functional renal unit. However, factors such as degree and duration of obstruction, plus the presence or absence of calculi or infection, are mediating variables in the expression of renal involvement.

Assessment

The evaluation of a child with UPJ obstruction includes a complete health history, physical examination, and diagnostic testing.

The most common sign leading to a diagnosis of obstructive uropathy is UTI; the second most common sign is the presence of a voiding disorder. Ask about the presence of flank pain. Children with obstruction, particularly UPJ defects, experience flank pain either intermittently or after high fluid intake with infrequent voiding. Also, hematuria may occur after minimal trauma. Measure height and weight, because delayed growth and weight gain may occur in the child with VUR, even when reflux is low grade and without infection. Boys with mild to moderate obstruction from posterior urethral valves (see the**Point** for Supplemental Information: Obstructive Uropathy: Posterior Urethral Valves) typically void infrequently, emptying their bladders with a weak, intermittent stream or a thin, forceful one. Having experienced this abnormal voiding pattern since birth, these boys (and their families) wrongly assume this micturition to be normal. To help detect this anomaly, obtain a detailed voiding history and observe the child's urinary stream.

Diagnostic Tests

Antenatal diagnosis of obstructive uropathy has become commonplace since the addition of ultrasonography in routine prenatal care. Hydronephrosis, ureteral enlargement, and a "keyhole" hypertrophic bladder are signs of a major urologic anomaly. Reduced amniotic volume is pathognomonic for obstructive uropathy as well as

for other genitourinary and gastrointestinal disorders. Because oligohydramnios is not apparent until 18 weeks of gestational age, a screening sonogram should be delayed until after that time. Prenatal findings suggestive of an obstructive lesion may be transient or idiopathic; therefore, radiographic evaluation should be repeated during the neonatal period to confirm the diagnosis. The value of prenatal detection rests not with its ability to predict the degree of renal function but rather as a signal to facilitate early therapeutic intervention on a nonemergent basis.

Because VUR can delay growth and weight gain, urologic studies should be a part of the diagnostic evaluation of any child with failure to thrive. Urologic radiographic techniques are used to thoroughly investigate the nature of obstructive uropathy. The basic workup requires a VCUG and an RBUS. The ultrasound may not be sensitive to detect low grades of reflux; however, it is useful in detecting hydronephrosis and can be used as a baseline study to monitor kidney growth for follow-up. Nuclear cystogram may be used in follow-up evaluation in patients with established reflux. A DMSA renal scan can help to detect renal cortical scars. Some infants incur benign hydronephrosis, which is stable and causes no impairment to renal function. Differentiating physiologic hydronephrosis from pathologic UPJ obstruction can be difficult. A diuretic renogram, which uses furosemide augmentation to induce high-volume urine, helps identify which infants could benefit from surgical intervention.

Kidney function and other tests may be performed, including urinalysis, specific gravity, urine culture, serum BUN, creatinine, creatinine clearance, CBC with differential, urinary pH, and electrolytes. Unless renal function is substantially impaired, these values will be in a normal range.

Interdisciplinary Interventions

Optimal care for children with obstructive uropathy combines a mixture of medical and surgical approaches tailored to the degree of obstruction, the child's age, and the renal status. For example, the newborn with severe hydronephrosis is critically ill from metabolic acidosis, fluid overload, uremia, and possibly respiratory compromise and must be treated promptly to stabilize the child's condition before urologic reconstruction is begun.

Nursing Management

The child with obstructive uropathy will require support in the prenatal and hospital settings that continues in the home, school, and camp settings. The nurse working in these settings is uniquely positioned to support the child and family's decision making and adherence to treatment.

During the evaluation phase, expand the family's knowledge base, clarifying and supplementing information presented by other health care team members. Explain diagnostic studies and prepare the child and family for procedures (see Chapter 11). Families easily become overwhelmed by the shock that an apparently healthy child has a major organ anomaly that may undermine a vital body function. Siblings may likewise be affected. Basic facts of urologic anatomy and physiology require constant review.

After a diagnosis has been made, the family and the child need information and support to help them accept a management program. Educate the child and family about medications, including therapeutic effects, dosage, side effects, and safety precautions. If surgical intervention has been recommended, assist with preoperative preparation for the child and family, and monitor the postoperative course.

Medical and Surgical Management

The primary goal of medical management is to prevent infection and renal scarring by adhering to a long-term regimen of prophylactic antibiotics. Medications of choice include nitrofurantoin (Furadantin, Macrodantin), trimethoprim–sulfamethoxazole (Septra), nalidixic acid (NegGram), or methenamine mandelate (Mandelamine) augmented by ascorbic acid. Breakthrough infections while on suppression therapy, nonadherence to prophylactic medication, or persistence of reflux into puberty may direct a change from medical management toward surgical correction of the anomaly.

Acute relief of the urinary obstruction should be performed by placing a urinary catheter. When the infant is stable, a posterior urethral valve can be obliterated by endoscopic ablation. Temporary insertion of a catheter is used in rare cases to reduce postoperative bleeding. In most cases, the child is discharged after postsurgical recovery and an initial voiding.

When the child's condition is complicated by VUR, reimplantation of the submucosal ureteral segment can be undertaken at the same time, or the child can be reevaluated several months later to detect unresolved reflux and undergo the procedure at that time. After surgical correction, any residual negative effects on voiding or urinary continence need further attention. Medical or surgical interventions can be implemented based on the remaining symptoms (see "Voiding Disorders" section).

The infant with high-grade urethral valve disease and severely affected upper tracts demands immediate medical attention to correct metabolic acidosis and antibiotics to eradicate urosepsis. Surgical intervention for urinary tract decompression can be provided by bladder catheterization or temporary urinary diversion (see "Treatment Modalities" section). Procedures such as loop–cutaneous pyelostomy, ureterostomy, or vesicostomy carry minimal surgical risk and are safe for the unstable infant. Definitive procedures such as reimplantation, bladder diverticulectomy, and valve ablation can be delayed to allow for renal rejuvenation, reduction of ureteral tortuosity, and improved bladder compliance.

Management decisions are individualized based on the child's age, gender, grade of reflux, bowel and bladder dysfunction, and susceptibility to UTI and renal scarring (Fonseca et al., 2012). Antibiotic prophylaxis has not been shown to provide benefit against pyelonephritis and renal scarring for children with grade I or II VUR (Cooper, 2012); increased surveillance and prompt treatment of UTI may be indicated (Fonseca et al., 2012). Antibiotic prophylaxis does appear to benefit children with grade III or higher VUR (Cooper, 2012). High-grade reflux in a young child and any reflux in a child older than age 5 years will probably not be spontaneously outgrown. Episodes of breakthrough UTI compound the risk of renal parenchymal scarring and usually require surgical management. Severe reflux with massive hydronephrosis and aperistaltic megaureters may be initially treated with temporary urinary diversions (see "Treatment Modalities" section). When medical management fails, surgery may be performed to reimplant the ureter. Surgical correction of VUR involves separating the ureter from the bladder and creating a tunnel between the layers of bladder mucosa. The ureter is threaded within the tunnel so that its opening into the bladder is within the trigone. Surgical correction leads to a 57% reduction in febrile UTIs but does not decrease overall risk of new or progressive renal disease (Fonseca et al., 2012).

Endoscopic treatment of VUR by injecting a polymer is an alternative to open reimplantation and long-term antibiotic therapy. During the endoscopic procedure, the child is under general anesthesia. A cystoscope aids the surgeon in identifying the ureteral orifice; the substance is injected a few millimeters distal and medial to this orifice.

Hydronephrosis secondary to UPJ obstruction is most often treated with pyeloplasty or ureteroplasty. The focus of these procedures is to dissect the obstructive ureteral component and either anastomose the ureteral segments or suture the remaining ureter to the renal pelvis. Best results are obtained when the surgical correction is performed before the child's first birthday because renal function may improve markedly. When the initial renal scan demonstrates less than 10% of function, the diseased organ is excised to avoid the long-term manifestation of hypertension. For the infant with severe or bilateral UPJ obstruction, a temporary percutaneous pyeloplasty can be performed with the expectation that low-pressure urinary draining will improve function. Permanent surgical repair is done after the infant is 1 year old.

Postoperative Care

Managing pain, maintaining fluid balance, keeping tubes patent, and preventing infection are important components of postoperative care.

Assess for pain and intervene as indicated. Incisional pain is most prominent for the first 2 days after surgery. Relief can be afforded by parenteral administration of morphine sulfate or by extradural nerve blockage in the spinal canal. Patient-controlled analgesic devices can be especially useful for the older child with a flank incision after pyeloplasty or ureteroplasty. The child who has undergone reimplantation of the ureter needs medication to subdue bladder spasms until the urinary drainage tubing is removed and full bladder reexpansion occurs, approximately 1 to 2 days later.

After the urologic obstruction is corrected, the child may experience postobstructive diuresis. During the immediate postoperative period, carefully monitor urine output and specific gravity, keeping in mind that these children have reduced concentrating ability.

❗**ALERT** *Urine output that approaches the IV intake is an early indicator of diuresis; an increasing specific gravity approaching 1.020 and dwindling urine output are later signs of dehydration from excessive fluid loss.*

Measuring urine output for the infant with a temporary urinary diversion requires weighing stomal dressings and diapers. Maintain a bedside record showing dry and wet dressing weights to accurately assess output. Disposable diapers wrapped girdle fashion (see thePoint for Supplemental Information: Urinary Diversion Through a Stoma) around pyelostomy or ureterostomy sites are often used over sterile dressings; record their weight as well.

A bolus of IV fluids may be needed to compensate for the high urine output. Fluid balance stabilizes within 1 to 2 days; after removal of the IV fluids, encourage oral intake.

A ureteral stent, a urethral catheter, or a suprapubic tube may be used after uncomplicated reconstructive repairs of obstructive uropathy. If the child's surgical repair is extensive or involves ureteral tapering, stents are necessary to prevent obstruction from postoperative edema (Nursing Interventions 19-2).

❗**ALERT** *In the postoperative child with ureteral, suprapubic, or urethral drainage tubes, bladder spasms may indicate a mucus plug in the tube. Monitor patency of the system, checking for urine flow and milking the tubes every 2 hours or in accordance with the facility's policy.*

The use of urinary tubes places the child at high risk for nosocomial infection. Pay meticulous attention to incisional and urinary tube care. Observe the child's urine for cloudiness or foul odor, and note any changes in vital signs that indicate infection. Administer antibiotics as ordered to prevent gram-negative infection.

NURSING INTERVENTIONS 19-2

Postoperative Care of the Child With a Ureteral Stent

During reconstructive urologic surgery, stents are placed to divert urine from the surgical site. These devices prevent urinary extravasation through the incision and prevent urine flow obstruction caused by edema. Depending on the procedure and on surgeon preference, the stents may either exit the body through the incision and attach to external collection containers or drain into a diaper. Removal of the stent is readily accomplished shortly before the child's discharge from the hospital, and the ureteral exit site epithelializes quickly.

A ureteral double-J stent is placed at the anastomosis site of pyeloplasty. This stent passes from the renal pelvis to the bladder; it is an internal stent with no external site. The double-J stent is generally removed cystoscopically 4–6 weeks postoperatively.

Imaging studies are usually done 6–8 weeks after surgery to assess renal function and to help rule out residual obstruction. Additional imaging studies may be ordered 6 months to 1 year postoperatively to check for a silent obstruction or stricture at the anastomosis site.

To Ensure Tube Patency

Encourage high fluid intake.

Monitor output; ongoing output is a good indicator of patency.

Teach these techniques to the family, including older siblings, and incorporate their participation in the child's care.

For external drains, observe tubes for mucous shreds or debris, which may block tube; use gravity to help move these potential obstructions through the tube; check for tube kinking and straighten as needed.

To Prevent Infection With External Drains

Keep the collection device below the level of incision.

Observe urine for signs and symptoms of infection (e.g., foul odor, cloudiness).

Monitor the child's temperature.

Aspirate urine sample for culture.

Apply antibacterial ointment to tube site.

Maintain a closed urinary drainage system.

To Manage Bladder Spasms With External Drains

Ensure tube patency as noted earlier.

Tape tubes securely to the leg or body.

Medicate for spasms with oxybutynin or belladonna and opium suppositories as ordered.

Prevent bladder stimulation secondary to a full rectum by completing a preoperative bowel evacuation, encouraging a high fluid intake, promoting early ambulation postoperatively, and administering a stool softener or glycerin suppository postoperatively.

To promote wound healing, encourage the child to consume a diet high in protein and fluids. Nutritious snacks such as milkshakes or instant breakfast drinks are excellent ways to meet both dietary goals. Consult the dietitian for the child with special dietary needs, lactose intolerance, or poor appetite.

Reconstructive surgery of the genitourinary tract can be psychologically traumatic to children of all ages. Discuss with the child and family issues of body image, sexual identity, and modesty violation to alleviate negative responses to such emotionally charged concerns; collaborate with a child life specialist.

Community Care

Home care after surgical procedures to alleviate urologic obstructions is directed toward restricting activity, preventing infection, maintaining high fluid intake, and preventing potential long-term complications. Inform the child and family that any residual voiding discomfort dissipates more quickly if the child has a high fluid intake, which promotes bladder stretching. Mild analgesics are rarely needed after the child's first day or two at home. Teach the child and family that vigorous activity, especially jumping or bouncing, is prohibited for the first week or until the first postoperative visit. The child may return to school when he or she feels comfortable as long as activity is restricted. Baths and showers are permitted after wounds are healed. After ureteral reimplantation, antibiotics may be continued until a follow-up VCUG documents successful resolution of reflux.

Infants with ureterostomies or pyelostomies are generally comfortable at the time of discharge. Demonstrate girdle-style diapering to the family, placing another diaper in the usual fashion for bowel movements and the occasional urine that may dribble from the bladder. This dribbling, although not harmful, may cause bladder spasms; mild analgesics, such as acetaminophen, offer adequate pain relief.

Stomal sites usually require minimal skin care. Soap and water cleansing is generally adequate. If irritation occurs, emollients such as zinc oxide or vitamin A and D ointments usually suffice. Chronic irritation may signal a UTI; teach the family to bring such conditions to the health care provider's attention. Tub bathing is allowed after clearance by the surgeon.

Prepare the child and family for ongoing urologic radiographic studies, which assess for unresolved obstruction and monitor renal function. If one kidney is severely compromised, restriction from contact sports is wise and may be mandated by the child's school system. The nurse can help the physical education department create an adaptive sports program for the child. Families often require emotional support to alter their expectations for their child and to rechannel the child's energies into other, less physical outlets.

Potential long-term ramifications of hydronephrosis include the risk of hypertension, urinary calculi, pregnancy-related infections, renal compromise, and genetic transmission of congenital defects to offspring. The nurse's role is to present families with strategies to prevent these complications or enable early detection, such as encouraging a lifelong habit of high fluid intake and frequent voiding, daily bowel movements, and yearly blood pressure monitoring. Teach children to ensure that every health care provider is aware of their urologic history and that their offspring are evaluated for congenital urologic anomalies shortly after birth.

ANOMALIES OF THE BLADDER AND URETHRA

Anomalies of the bladder and urethra include exstrophy–epispadias complex, hypospadias, patent urachus, and prune-belly syndrome. This section covers exstrophy–epispadias complex and hypospadias. For information about patent urachus and prune-belly syndrome, see thePoint for Supplemental Information: Anomalies of the Bladder and Urethra.

EXSTROPHY–EPISPADIAS COMPLEX

The bladder exstrophy–epispadias complex is a serious congenital anomaly affecting multiple organs of the urologic and musculoskeletal systems. Interrupted abdominal development during early fetal life produces an exposed bladder and urethra, pubic bone separation, and associated anal and genital abnormalities. The three variations of this complex are cloacal exstrophy, classic exstrophy, and epispadias.

Bladder exstrophy–epispadias complex is rare, occurring in 4.63 per 100,000 singleton live births and affecting males twice as often as females (Jayachandran et al., 2011). The cause of this anomaly is unknown, but it appears to be unrelated to genetic or teratogenic exposure.

Pathophysiology

The three general variants of the exstrophy–epispadias complex share a common precipitating factor: persistence of the cloacal membrane beyond the point of expected resorption during embryologic development. During early gestational life, the embryo has an alimentary tract that terminates as an enlarged chamber—the *cloaca*. Its posterior border is the *cloacal membrane*, which runs from the umbilicus to the tail gut. A mound of tissue, the *urorectal septum*, protrudes into the upper cloacal chamber, migrating toward the cloacal membrane. The urorectal septum separates the cloaca into the anterior *urogenital sinus* and the posterior *anal canal*. Meanwhile, the cloacal membrane recedes as it is filled in with strong mesodermal tissue. In rare instances, the cloacal membrane becomes overly prominent and blocks the proliferation of mesodermal cells. Later, the membrane weakens and ruptures, leaving cloacal structures uncovered. The timing of cloacal membrane rupture determines which of the three exstrophy variations will occur.

Cloacal Exstrophy

If the cloacal membrane disintegrates before the completed cloacal division of its anterior and posterior compartments, the exposed surface is a combined bladder and rectal structure. Both ureters are lateral and have an incompetent bladder junction, and the internal sphincter and urethra are split. This condition results in bilateral reflux and total incontinence after initial bladder closure. This version of the defect is rare and occurs between the fourth and sixth weeks of gestational life.

Classic Exstrophy

In classic exstrophy, rupture of the cloacal membrane occurs after the anterior–posterior separation has been completed, exposing the urinary structures only. An everted bladder with lateral ureteral orifices is noted, along with a splayed internal sphincter and urethra (Fig. 19-8). Bilateral reflux and total incontinence occur postoperatively to bladder closure. The defect occurs during the first trimester.

Epispadias

The least involved presentation in the exstrophy–epispadias complex triad is epispadias, which results from cloacal membrane disintegration after the eighth fetal week. A urethral groove extends along the dorsal penile shaft (Fig. 19-9) or along the entire female urethra. If the internal sphincter is affected, total incontinence results.

Assessment

At birth, the infant with bladder exstrophy–epispadias complex is healthy and physiologically normal, except for the affected structures. Classic bladder exstrophy is apparent at birth, with the inner mucosal surface of the bladder exposed in the suprapubic area, appearing red, shiny, and rugated and constantly seeping urine. When cloacal exstrophy is present, the rectal segment protrudes within the bladder mucosa. In males, the penis is short, splayed, and exhibits dorsal curvature (chordee). Cryptorchidism is often present. In females, the urethra and the vagina are short. If primary reconstruction is delayed beyond infancy, the vagina may prolapse. Orthopedic manifestations are minimal after

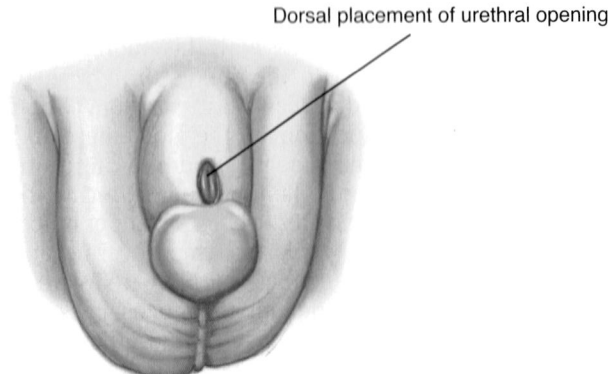

Epispadias

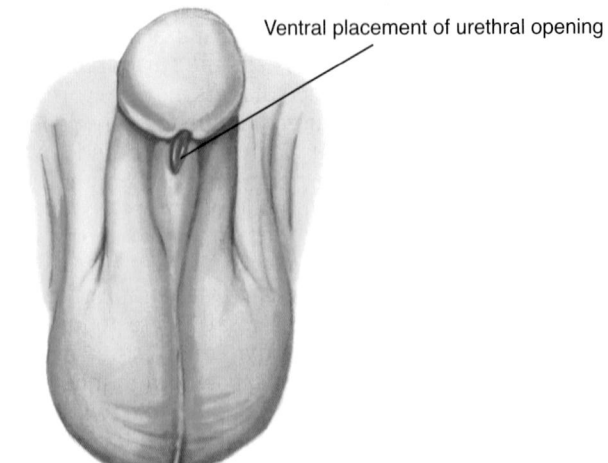

Hypospadias

Figure 19-9 Epispadias and hypospadias with chordee. Note the possible locations of the urethral opening.

early pelvic ring closure. When surgery is delayed, the child may ambulate with a waddle.

Renal structures are evaluated by a newborn ultrasound or renal scan. Beyond the neonatal period, an IVP may be substituted. A pubic computed tomographic scan highlights the severity of pubic separation.

Interdisciplinary Interventions

Management of these congenital anomalies centers on surgery to correct the defect.

Surgical advances have dramatically improved the management for children with bladder exstrophy–epispadias complex. Rather than resort to urinary diversion, the focus of care is on early surgical correction. Within days after birth, the bladder is covered with peripheral tissue and the pelvic ring is closed. Postoperatively, the infant is placed in Bryant traction until fibrous healing of the symphysis pubic occurs, generally after 3 to 4 weeks.

Because postoperative edema of the bladder is expected, ureteral stents and a suprapubic tube are temporarily inserted to prevent urinary obstruction. Successive surgical procedures to correct reflux, reconstruct a sphincter mechanism, close the urethra, and repair the phallus are individualized depending on the child's anatomy and response to previous surgery.

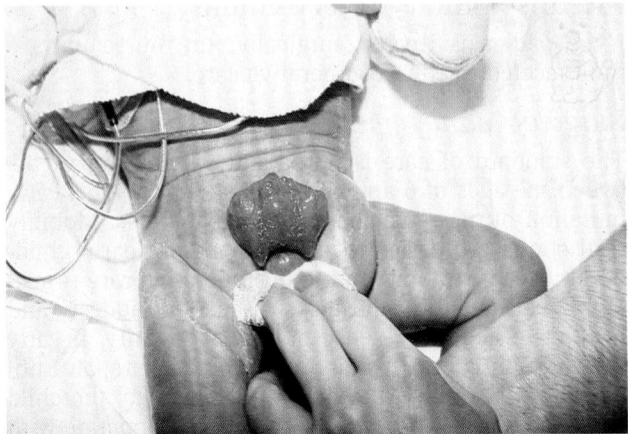

Figure 19-8 The bladder is open and exposed on the abdomen in classic exstrophy.

Because of the physical disfigurement of the genitalia and the family's unfamiliarity with this anomaly, family members often react to the child's birth with this disorder with horror, disbelief, and revulsion. Provide emotional support, education, and reinforcement of the proposed medical management. In addition to routine newborn care, educate the family about skin care, diapering, and hygiene measures. Delicate bladder mucosa should be protected by a plastic wrap covering at all times. Do not use gauze, either wet or coated with petroleum jelly, which may denude the mucosal tissue, or ointments or creams, which may occlude the ureteral orifices and impede urine flow. Soaps and powders may be abrasive and can promote bacterial growth. Therefore, all of these hygiene products are contraindicated. Clear water is best for cleansing, and a hair dryer set on a low setting effectively keeps the surrounding skin surface dry. Loosely fastened diapers may be worn. Tub bathing is avoided. Postoperative nursing care depends on the child's specific surgical procedure and on the preference of the attending surgeon. See Chapter 20 for management of the child in traction.

Community Care

Educate the family that regular evaluation studies to monitor reflux and to assess for UTI are required to conserve renal function. Urodynamic testing may be used to demonstrate bladder capacity and sphincteric activity. Urinary continence for the child with bladder exstrophy–epispadias complex may be an ongoing concern. Management of this problem often requires a multifaceted approach, incorporating pharmacologic agents, behavioral and motivational techniques, and skin care to provide optimal urine control. Pediatric-sized absorbent products and undergarments are available over the counter or in many specialty catalogues.

Negative emotional sequelae from repeated hospitalization, altered parenting response, or dysfunctional coping techniques may require psychological intervention. Assess for these problems, initiate discussions, and refer for more intensive intervention as indicated.

HYPOSPADIAS

QUESTION: Mr. Johnson has many questions and concerns about the hypospadias and why the repair has been postponed until now. He also voices concerns about his son's appearance and how it might affect J. D. in the future. How should the nurse respond to his questions and concerns?

Hypospadias is a congenital anomaly of the penis in which the urethral folds fail to fuse in the midline and the urethral meatus opens on the ventral surface of the penis. It can be classified according to the location of the urethral meatus along the ventral surface of the penis (glanular, coronal, midpenile, penoscrotal, perineal). Hypospadias is often associated with chordee, a condition in which a deficiency of the normal

structures on the ventral side of the penis cause curvature in the penis (see Fig. 19-9). This congenital curvature of the penis may result in infertility secondary to difficulty in semen delivery. Megameatus is a variant of hypospadias in which the urethral meatus is larger than expected and hidden beneath a full foreskin.

The cause of hypospadias is not clear. Hypospadias affects 1 in 200 to 300 live male births, with an incidence of 14% in male siblings and 6% to 8% in offspring (Stein, 2012).

Pathophysiology

Creation of the male urethra begins with the appearance of a urethral groove in the forming genital tubercle, at about the sixth fetal week. Fusion of the urogenital folds that border this groove is initiated during week 9, proceeding along the ventral line from the perineum toward the distal shaft. Simultaneously, a glanular dimple forms at the tip and carves a notch to the corona, splitting the glans. This groove then becomes contiguous with the penile urethra and undergoes ventral fusion. The prepuce develops during week 12, following completed urethral development; scrotal fusion also occurs at this time.

Assessment

A thorough neonatal examination of the male genitalia should reveal hypospadias. In rare instances, hypospadias can be diagnosed after a completed or aborted circumcision. Infants with severe hypospadias and cryptorchidism should be investigated for intersex disorders and undergo karyotyping with endocrinologic workup. Additional testing including renal, bladder, and abdominal ultrasound may be warranted in children who have additional organ system anomalies such as cardiac murmur, imperforate anus, or pyloric stenosis.

caREminder

If any degree of hypospadias is present, a circumcision should not be performed without a urologic evaluation because the prepuce is used for the reconstructive surgery.

Interdisciplinary Interventions

Hypospadias is treated surgically; the nurse plays a multifaceted role in postoperative care.

Surgical Management

The standard of care is outpatient surgical repair between the ages of 6 and 12 months (AAP, 1996); early initiation of the repair has many advantages. Mobility restrictions are easier to maintain before early childhood. Psychic trauma during postoperative care is negligible because the child lacks a sense of modesty and has yet to acquire a sense of gender identity. If early intervention is not feasible, postponing the repair until after age 2½ years is advisable. By this age, the child can be prepared for hospitalization, can cooperate with postoperative care and restrictions, and can verbalize his needs or concerns. Two-stage procedures are often begun at age 6 to 12 months, followed by a final urethral advancement 3 to 6 months later.

The goals of surgical repair are to provide symmetric appearance to the penis and prepuce, produce a sexually functional phallus by correcting chordee and straightening the penis, advance the glans along the meatus to enable physiologically and socially appropriate ejaculation and allow the child to stand while voiding, create urethral integrity unimpeded by residual stricture or stenosis, and make the penis cosmetically acceptable. Corrective surgery to create a new urethra is usually performed in one-stage outpatient surgery. A two-stage procedure may be necessary for proximal shaft, penoscrotal, and perineal defects. To improve surgical results in children with small glans, preoperative treatment with testosterone may be used: administered as testosterone enanthate 25 mg in three injections 4 weeks apart or testosterone cream applied directly to the penis.

Postoperative care for the child undergoing hypospadias repair focuses on urinary diversion, wound care, pain management, and activity restrictions (see thePoint for Care Paths: An Interdisciplinary Plan of Care for the Child With Surgical Correction of Hypospadias). Several bladder drainage systems may be used, including a Foley catheter, urethral stent drainage, or (rarely) a suprapubic cystotomy. (In some cases, depending on the degree of hypospadias, tissue adequacy, and the urologist's preference, the repair may be completely tubeless.) The drainage tube may be connected to a closed drainage unit or may remain as an open system, in which case a "double-diaper" technique shields the operative site from moisture, fungal infections, and breakdown in skin integrity. With this technique, the open drainage tube is sandwiched between two diapers. The bottom diaper, covering the penis, remains dry. Some urologists choose to insert a penile stent, a tube that is inserted within the penile urethra only. The stent diverts urine past the internal incision but spares the child from bladder catheterization and resultant bladder spasms. This type of stent, which extends only 2 to 3 mm past the meatus, is secured to the glans by sutures, which dissolve in 7 to 10 days. The child painlessly expels the tube during normal voiding.

Nursing Management

Assess the parents' emotional response to their son's anomaly. Parents mourn the loss of the "perfect" son and fear for his sexual ability and satisfaction, gender identity, and peer acceptance. The idea of delicate reconstructive surgery on a body part that is integral for urologic, sexual, and psychosocial response is abhorrent to many parents, especially fathers. Emphasize that the genitalia, although definitely male, is incompletely formed rather than defective or inadequate. Use illustrations of surgical procedures and before-and-after photographs to address parental anxieties and promote bonding.

Nursing care for the child undergoing hypospadias correction is guided by the specific surgical procedure and the child's age. Hospitalization can vary from less than 24 hours to 5 days. Indwelling stents are typically removed by cutting a stitch that secures the catheter

to the glans. Use developmentally appropriate interventions to prepare the child preoperatively and to facilitate psychological adjustment.

Nursing care for the closed drainage catheter or stent follows the principles described for postoperative care after reimplantation of the ureter. To ensure that the fragile urethral incision remains free from tension, the tube must be taped to angle for ventral penile exposure. Urinary retention, although uncommon, is possible if the stent malfunctions because it is blocked or kinked. Monitor urine output and assess for distention over the lower abdomen. An oral antibiotic may be administered prophylactically while the tube is in place to reduce the risk of infection. An antibiotic ointment is dabbed on the urethral meatus daily.

A compression bio-occlusive dressing is applied to the penis to reduce incisional edema and control ecchymosis. The dressing remains undisturbed until the glanular edema visibly decreases, usually for 3 to 5 days, and is then removed. Dressing removal can be facilitated by a 30-minute tub bath, which the child can undergo even if the urinary apparatus remains in place (Gormley et al., 2007).

Postoperative discomfort is surprisingly minimal after hypospadias repair. Penile block and caudal block, administered during the procedure, afford adequate analgesia for most children. Postoperative pain can usually be controlled with acetaminophen with codeine. Bladder spasms in response to the tube rubbing against the bladder mucosa and trigone are controlled with oxybutynin to reduce detrusor contractility. Bowel evacuation before surgery helps to lessen this problem. Tubeless repair eliminates bladder spasms, but the child may experience painful voiding postoperatively and refuse to urinate. In such cases, catheterization is required.

The preschool-aged child who remains hospitalized after hypospadias surgery has some degree of activity restriction. Because most boys feel alert and well postoperatively, provide diversional activities to dissipate stored energy constructively. Gross motor activities and games, such as wheelchair kickball or rhythm movements, are especially important.

Because the hospital stay typically is limited to less than 24 hours, provide discharge teaching expeditiously. Demonstrate how to care for urinary drainage systems, paying particular attention to tube anchoring and patency. Family members should perform a repeat demonstration of catheter irrigation to remove a mucus plug. Emphasize that the tubing should never be clamped or kinked, and explain the double-diaper process. Encourage the child to eat a nutritious diet high in protein and fiber, with extra fluids. Educate about prescribed medications. Instruct the family how to care for postoperative wound edema and explain how ecchymosis normally resolves. Explicitly describe activities that need to be curtailed until healing is complete (usually 2 to 3 weeks), such as rough play, swimming, and contact sports. Emphasize that the child must not play on any straddle-type toys for at least 2 to 3 weeks. Review bathing techniques based on the surgeon's instructions. Give the family these instructions in writing, along with instructions for scheduling post-discharge visits to the surgeon.

The most common postoperative complications include urethrocutaneous fistula (communication between the new urethra and penile skin, which allows urine to drain through two holes) or meatal stenosis (regression or scarring that narrows the meatal opening). Discuss the potential for these complications and remind the family to regularly observe the child's voiding pattern. Indicators of problems include a thin, forceful stream; infrequent voiding; a spray-type stream; dysuria; or ventral leaking during a void. Instruct families to report these symptoms to the surgeon. Teach older children to recognize the signs and symptoms that indicate complications and encourage them to assume self-care.

ANSWER: The nurse should first explain the anomaly and then the rationale for delaying the repair and circumcision, including the use of the prepuce for reconstructive surgery. The nurse should emphasize the advantages of repair at this age, such as easier restriction of mobility and negligible psychological trauma because J. D. still lacks a sense of modesty and has not yet acquired a sense of gender identity. In addition, the nurse needs to assess the parents' emotional response, in particular Mr. Johnson's response, to J. D.'s anomaly. His concerns may reveal worry about his son's sexual ability and satisfaction, gender identity, and peer acceptance. In addition, thoughts about surgery on a body part such as the penis can be overwhelming. The nurse needs to emphasize that the genitalia is definitely male and that it is incompletely formed rather than describing it as inadequate or defective. Using photographs of before-and-after repair may be helpful.

CONDITIONS AFFECTING THE MALE GENITALIA

Conditions that affect the male genitalia include cryptorchidism, testicular torsion, circumcision, and varicocele.

CRYPTORCHIDISM

In a normally developed male child, each testicle is secured within its sac in either side of the scrotum. Although the testicles are retractable by the cremasteric muscle when necessary for warmth or protection, each testicle should be palpable in its normal location outside the body of the child. Cryptorchidism, also called *cryptorchidia* or *hidden testicle*, is a condition in which a testicle has not descended normally.

An undescended testis is noted in approximately 3% of term male infants and in 25% to 30% of preterm male infants (Merriman et al., 2012). Spontaneous descent may occur during the first few months of life; therefore, a decreased incidence of 0.8% to 1.1% is reported from 3 to 12 months of age (Merriman et al., 2012). The risk of cryptorchidism among offspring whose father had the defect is double that of the average population, although how the inheritance mechanism affects the child is unclear. Risks for undescended testes are high in premature infants with low birth weight and in multiple births.

The cause is unknown, but several hypotheses have been presented. Possible hormonal causes include inadequate testosterone production or insufficient response to the androgenic hormone. Ineffective development of the inguinal canal, abnormal epididymal development, and reduced intra-abdominal pressure represent possible structural causes.

Cryptorchidism is a risk factor for testicular germ cell tumors (Trabert et al., 2013). Prepubertal orchiopexy decreases the risk of testicular cancer (Merriman et al., 2012).

Pathophysiology

Cryptorchidism has etiologic roots in early fetal development. The testicular germ cells first appear along the mesonephric duct. Between 6 and 9 weeks after conception, hormones secreted by the structure stimulate cellular growth and maturation into an organized testicle. The testicle remains in a perinephric position until a fibrous band exerts downward tension on the organ. By the end of the 12th week, the gonad has journeyed to the internal inguinal ring, where it rests until the 7th month.

During the third trimester of pregnancy, the inguinal canal opens and a hollow space is created in the scrotal sac. The testicle migrates into the scrotal sac, where it bonds to the scrotal lining. Closure of the internal ring of the inguinal canal concludes the process of testicular descent. In cryptorchidism, this process is not completed, and the testicle occupies an anomalous position.

Assessment

The diagnosis of cryptorchidism is made by physical examination. Begin assessment for testicular descent with the interview. Because the cremasteric reflex is weak during the neonatal period, ask about the family's observation of testicular descent during the first 3 months after birth. Inquire whether the family has noticed normal testicular descent when the child is relaxed, such as during a bath.

On visual inspection of the scrotum, a flaccid, nonpendulous scrotum suggests an absent testis. Observe the size, contour, and skin surfaces of the scrotum.

Scrotal palpation requires that the examiner have warm hands and that the child be relaxed. Relaxation can be encouraged by placing the young child in his parent's lap, assuming a frog-leg position. To counteract recoil of the testes, apply pressure at the external inguinal ring (see Fig. 8-12). After the testicle is isolated, use a milking action to coax it into the sac. Coating the finger with talc or soap may ease this process. Older boys may be examined as they sit cross-legged, leaning slightly forward to facilitate palpation.

A nonpalpable testis may be absent, atrophic, or located in a position where it cannot be palpated by physical examination. Palpable testes are classified into three categories: retractile, ectopic, or truly undescended. A *retractile* testis is most often found in the inguinal area but can be palpated at any point along the pathway of descent. These testes are normally descended but are found in the extrascrotal position because of an active cremasteric reflex, usually in response to fear, cold, pain, or touch. They can usually be manually repositioned into the scrotum. An *ectopic* testis is misdirected from the normal pathway of its descent. These testes may be located in the perineal or femoral area. A *truly undescended* testis may be palpable intermittently; it may be located in the intra-abdominal region, scrotal canal, or inguinal ring.

The retractable, but normally descended, testis is equal in size to its contralateral mate, whereas the cryptorchid testis is smaller and softer. If no testicle can be discerned, examine the lower abdomen, perineum, or femoral regions for an ectopic gonad.

Interdisciplinary Interventions

Cryptorchidism is managed surgically, with orchiopexy.

Surgical Management

Surgical manipulation of the undescended testis is the treatment of choice. Spontaneous descent after 9 months is unlikely, and orchiopexy is recommended at or soon after 9 months of age (P. A. Lee & Houk, 2013). Surgical placement accomplishes three goals: it preserves as much testicular function as possible, thereby potentially avoiding infertility; it offers the child a normal scrotal appearance and avoids trauma and torsion; and it facilitates regular testicular self-examinations, which could increase the likelihood of detecting cancer during young adulthood.

Management of the child with a nonpalpable testis includes a presurgical laparoscopic evaluation to ascertain the presence and viability of the intra-abdominal organ. Laparoscopy enables testicular tissue and spermatic vessels to be visualized with 90% to 100% accuracy. If the spermatic vessels are atretic (undeveloped), the gonad will be absent, and no surgery is required. A testicular prosthesis is surgically implanted when the child reaches puberty.

Intra-abdominal testes must be identified because of the risk of malignancy. Surgical options include gonadal excision or Fowler-Stephens orchiopexy in one or two stages. Fowler-Stephens orchiopexy involves division of the spermatic vessels before movement of the testis.

Some have advocated intervention with hormones such as human chorionic gonadotropin or gonadotropin-releasing hormone to encourage testicular descent or to facilitate surgical exploration by enlarging the gonad. This approach is not recommended for unilateral cryptorchidism because of poor efficacy, cost, and risk of side effects (Ludwikowski & González, 2013).

Nursing Management

Nursing care for the child with an undescended testis and his family begins when the defect is first suspected. Educate the family regarding the importance of timely surgical correction and the endocrinologic consequences of cryptorchidism. Include information regarding hospitalization, preoperative and postoperative procedures, and developmentally appropriate coping techniques.

After a management plan has been provided by the urologist or surgeon, the nursing focus is to reinforce teaching and clarify any misconceptions held by the child or his family. Use illustrations to explain the defect and the chosen treatment regimen.

Postoperative nursing care after orchiopexy is usually provided in an outpatient surgical suite. See Chapter 11 for a description of routine postoperative care.

Community Care

Discharge instructions encompass incision care and activity restriction. Most surgeons either cover the operative site with a transparent dressing or leave it open to air. No special care is necessary other than inspecting for signs of infection and promptly cleansing urine and stool off the operative site. The return to tub bathing depends on the surgeon's preference. Educate the child and family to avoid vigorous activity, straddle toys, and contact sports for 7 to 10 days.

Long-term follow-up care is imperative for the child with cryptorchidism. The parents should be referred for endocrinologic consultation if infertility or hormonal dysfunction is suspected. Counseling with a psychoendocrinologist and, in time, a reproductive endocrinologist may be necessary when the boy reaches adulthood, becomes sexually active, or considers paternity.

Because of the potential for endocrinopathy and malignancy, many urologists continue to see the child with cryptorchidism on a yearly basis.

caREminder

> *Monthly testicular self-examination is recommended for all males beginning in puberty, and it is essential for the male with cryptorchidism.*

As a part of discharge teaching, provide the family with an instructional brochure on testicular self-examination. Offer it to the child's father as an added reminder that he should also perform the procedure. Nurses who care for adolescents in any setting should be prepared to teach testicular self-examination as part of routine health maintenance. Also, nurses in clinic settings can display brochures on testicular self-examination in a prominent area with other health teaching publications.

TESTICULAR TORSION

Torsion, or rotation, of the testicle constitutes one of the few urologic emergencies. This condition occurs when the testicular suspensory apparatus, the spermatic cord, twists and obstructs circulation to the testis. In such a case, emergency medical attention is needed to prevent tissue necrosis.

The incidence of testicular torsion is estimated at 4.5 per 100,000 males younger than 25 years of age (DaJusta et al., 2012). The precipitating factor for testicular rotation is unknown, but a rising testosterone level with increased testis weight is a possible cause. The condition affects the left testicle more often that the right, possibly because it has a longer spermatic cord. No familial or racial tendencies toward the defect have been documented nor is it associated with other congenital anomalies.

Scrotal examination of the child with testicular torsion often discloses a "bell-clapper" defect. Normally, the testis resides partially encased within a scrotal sheath, and the exposed spermatic cord–epididymal layer is securely attached to the scrotal lining. This attachment stabilizes the testicle and places it in a vertical position. In some boys, the scrotal sheath completely encases the testicle, epididymis, and spermatic cord, blocking adherence of these structures to the scrotum. This arrangement results in a loosely suspended gonad, which lies horizontally within the sac: a bell-clapper deformity.

Although the anomalous testicular attachment is often bilateral, torsion is generally restricted to one testis. Because an undescended testis can also become twisted, acute abdominal pain in the child with cryptorchidism should raise suspicion of torsion.

A variation of testicular torsion involves the twisting of a testicular or epididymal appendix. Torsion of these congenital appendages usually occurs during preadolescence, but the condition may manifest at any age. Damage is confined to the appendix, sparing the testicle.

A second, rarer, form of testicular torsion occurs during testicular descent, either antenatally or within the neonatal period. Because the process is usually painless, the child undergoes treatment for cryptorchidism. At the time of surgical exploration, however, testicular atrophy is evident. The bell-clapper deformity is often seen in the remaining testis, which is then secured to the scrotum as a precaution.

Pathophysiology

Twisting of the spermatic cord occludes testicular circulation. The initial response is tissue congestion and testicular edema; unrelieved obstruction leads to vascular thrombosis and necrosis. If the occlusion is complete and unrelieved, tissue death occurs swiftly, possibly within 2 hours and certainly after 12 hours. Intermittent or self-resolving episodes are possible and may cause varying degrees of tissue damage. The prognosis for adequate hormonal function is consequently unpredictable.

Assessment

Acute scrotal pain, often associated with nausea and vomiting, is the hallmark sign of this disorder. Because testicular torsion can occur in association with scrotal trauma, always evaluate complaints of scrotal pain to rule out a diagnosis of torsion. During the history and the physical examination, be sure to address psychosexual issues. Reassure the child that the pain is not related to self-manipulation or to arousal from sexual fantasies.

ALERT *The boy who complains of scrotal pain may be experiencing a testicular torsion. He must receive immediate medical attention to prevent infarction of the gland.*

A history of previous inguinal or scrotal surgery does not discount the potential for torsion. Obtain historical data with the physical examination. Ask for details about the child's condition, such as onset and duration of pain, and any similar episodes of scrotal pain that resolved spontaneously. Question the adolescent male about sexual activity or urethral symptoms. Affirmative responses to these queries suggest epididymitis or orchitis. Persistent but mild scrotal discomfort is more suggestive of torsion of the testicular appendages.

Conduct the examination in privacy and assure the child that his responses are confidential. Explain that testicular torsion is a secondary effect from a congenital anomaly and that it is unrelated to sports or vigorous activity. Do not imply that the child or the family is to blame for any delay in seeking treatment. Teens typically ignore early signs of illness, and family members are frequently unaware that scrotal pain may have such serious consequences.

Begin the examination with the boy in a standing position to check for horizontal placement of the opposite testis. With the boy lying down, assess the abdomen for tenderness and pain or swelling in the inguinal area, especially if the boy has an undescended testis on the side corresponding to the pain.

Inspect the scrotum for edema. A blue dot suggesting torsion of the testicular appendix may be noted in light-skinned males. Stroke the inner thigh of the affected side to elicit a cremasteric sign. If it is present, testicular torsion is unlikely. On palpation, the twisted testicle is exquisitely tender throughout the organ. Torsion of the appendix, in contrast, creates localized discomfort, with a palpable upper pole nodule.

Diagnostic Tests

Microscopic urinalysis without evidence of pyuria and bacteriuria provides additional diagnostic confirmation. If the examination does not provide a clear diagnosis, high-resolution sonograms with color Doppler are used to assess testicular perfusion and intrascrotal contents. This noninvasive technique has a high degree of accuracy. A drawback to the color Doppler sonogram is that accuracy depends on the technique and expertise of the technician (DaJusta et al., 2012). Also, the sonogram may give a false negative if the torsion is intermittent. If the physical examination and diagnostic studies do not conclusively exclude testicular torsion, the boy must undergo surgery.

Interdisciplinary Interventions

Suspected testicular torsion is a surgical emergency. Testicular viability diminishes dramatically after 6 hours. Open exploration is performed through a midline scrotal incision, the testis is derotated and surgically fixed to the scrotal wall, and a contralateral orchiopexy is performed. If infarction has occurred, the necrotic gland is removed to prevent detrimental effects to the remaining testis. A pinched testicular appendage is excised for the same reason.

Nursing care after correction of a testicular torsion is directed toward enabling the child and his family to cope with the long-term effects of the condition. If the function of the affected testis has been severely impaired, or if the organ was unsalvageable, counsel the boy to avoid high-impact contact sports. Many municipalities prohibit children with only one of a paired organ set from participating in organized sports; for many adolescents, the forced redirection of their energy and skills may seem punitive and unfair. The nurse can facilitate a positive adjustment by candidly discussing the issue and providing referrals to counseling facilities if necessary.

Community Care

Nurses can exert the greatest effect on this disorder within the community health sphere. The best way to ensure an optimum outcome for boys with testicular torsion is by raising public awareness of the disorder and the need to seek immediate medical care. Numerous vehicles exist to educate the public about this condition, including boys' clubs, Boy Scout troops, parent groups, religious youth organizations, school health classes, and health publications in print and on the Internet.

CIRCUMCISION

QUESTION: Suppose J. D. was going to have a circumcision at this age. How would his circumcision compare to what his brother had the day after birth?

Circumcision, surgical removal of the prepuce (or foreskin) of the penis, is the most ancient and common operative procedure performed on males in the world for cultural, religious, or medical reasons. Although circumcision itself is not a pathologic condition, the nurse commonly encounters the procedure in the United States, and appropriate management is required.

CROSS-CULTURAL CARE

The practice of circumcision varies dramatically worldwide. Globally, approximately 30% of males are circumcised (World Health Organization & Joint United Nations Programme on HIV/AIDS, 2007). Male circumcision is common among Jews and Muslims (Pinto, 2012) and in the East Cape of Africa (Meissner & Buso, 2007). Circumcision rates are likely underestimated at approximately 56% to 59% of male neonates in the United States (AAP, Task Force on Circumcision, 2012b), 90% of Filipino men (R. B. Lee, 2006), and 87% of males in Nigeria (Okeke et al., 2006). Male infants from Central and South America, Europe, or Asia, however, are only rarely circumcised (Steadman & Ellsworth, 2006).

The AAP, Task Force on Circumcision (2012a) policy states that there are benefits to circumcision and the benefits outweigh the risks; however, it does not take the controversial stance of recommending circumcision as routine. Many pediatric organizations do not recommend routine circumcision of newborns (British Medical Association, 2004; Canadian Paediatric Society, Fetus and Newborn Committee, 1996; Royal Australasian College of Physicians, 2010). This stance has been challenged (Dickerman, 2007; Morris et al., 2006; Schoen, 2006), making routine circumcision one of the most controversial issues in modern pediatric health care (Tradition or Science 19-4).

TRADITION OR SCIENCE 19-4

Does circumcision reduce incidence of specific diseases?

Multiple studies have demonstrated that male circumcision reduces the incidence of UTI (Morris & Wiswell, 2013; Shaikh et al., 2008; Simforoosh et al., 2012); meta-analysis demonstrated a 90% reduction (Singh-Grewal et al., 2005). Debate arises about the magnitude of this benefit; some argue that the benefit applies only to those at high risk of UTI (Singh-Grewal et al., 2005); others argue that the benefit of preventing renal scarring after UTI might make this benefit cost-effective (Malone, 2005).

Circumcision may reduce the risk of a male acquiring a sexually transmitted infection (STI) by 48% (Fergusson et al., 2006). Circumcision reduced the incidence of acquiring syphilis, cancroid, and genital herpes (Weiss et al., 2006); risk of chlamydial infection in female partners by 82% (Castellsagué et al., 2005); and the incidence of human papillomavirus (Baldwin et al., 2004; Davis et al., 2013), the causative agent in cervical and penile cancer. Circumcision also reduces the risk of candidal infections (Aridogan et al., 2009; Richters et al., 2006).

Women are more likely to acquire cervical cancer from uncircumcised partners (Drain et al., 2006). The risk of penile cancer is greatly reduced in circumcised men (Daling et al., 2005; Provencio-Vasquez & Rodriguez, 2009).

Circumcision reduces transmission of HIV. Systematic reviews and meta-analysis of observational studies provide evidence of this association (Siegfried et al., 2005; Siegfried et al., 2003; Weiss et al., 2000). RCTs of male circumcision in Africa demonstrate that it provides a protective effect against HIV infection of more than 50% in these high-risk populations (Auvert et al., 2005; Bailey et al., 2007; Gray et al., 2007; C. M. Liu et al., 2013; Plank et al., 2009). Contrary to this strong evidence, Turner et al. (2007), after adjusting for other risk factors, reported no protective effect of circumcision associated with women's risk of acquiring HIV, although findings suggest that further investigation of the effect in high-risk women is warranted. Controlling viral load in HIV-positive men may reduce transmission to female partners (Wawer et al., 2005).

The complication rate after neonatal circumcision in developed nations is 0.2% (Wiswell, & Geschke, 1989) to 0.34% (Ben Chaim et al., 2005); a study of Nigerian infants reported a rate of 20% (Okeke et al., 2006). Complication rates reported after circumcision beyond the neonatal period was 1.2% in boys younger than 15 years old in England (Cathcart et al., 2006) and 1.8% in men in Africa between 18 and 24 years old (Krieger et al., 2007). Most complications are minor; they include bleeding, wound infection, redundant foreskin from inadequate removal, and penile–glandular tissue bridge. Major complications include urethral fistula, concealed penis (excision of shaft epithelium with adhesions), penile necrosis, hypospadias, and penile amputation. Research has not shown a difference in sexual satisfaction between those who are or who are not circumcised (Collins et al., 2002; Senkul et al., 2004).

Aside from religious or cultural beliefs, routine male circumcision has generated extensive debate. Evidence demonstrates that circumcision has a protective effect against some diseases. Because of the ethical and cost–benefit issues that the topic engenders, circumcision remains a choice that requires consideration of individual beliefs and risks.

Pathophysiology

Creation of the foreskin begins during the third fetal month. Originating at the base of the glans, the prepuce proceeds distally to envelop the penile tip, and the adjacent tissue layers become adherent. As fetal growth nears completion, clefts of cells resembling holes in a sponge develop within the preputial–glanular layer to begin the separation process. At birth, only 4% of males have a retractile prepuce, but by age 3 years, the foreskin is retractable in 90% of boys.

In children, smegma is a by-product of preputial separation. As the epithelial cells degenerate, they form white clumps, which are expelled normally during micturition. During puberty, sebaceous cell secretions mix with epithelial cells to lubricate the glans.

Two pathologic conditions are related to foreskin development: phimosis and paraphimosis. Phimosis is a nonretractile foreskin. Because most infants exhibit physiologic phimosis, the description among young males is confined to foreskin constriction that obstructs urine flow. A foreskin that balloons during urination indicates phimosis. Ulceration of the glans resulting from this phenomenon may lead to balanoposthitis, an infectious condition of the glans. Phimosis can be treated with topical steroids, and circumcision need only be used if steroid treatment fails.

Paraphimosis is a painful condition resulting from forced retraction of a tight or stenotic foreskin below the coronal ridge, usually during an overzealous attempt to clean the glans before separation is complete (Fig. 19-10). The resulting constriction creates pain, distal edema, and difficulty replacing the foreskin. Emergency medical intervention is needed to relieve the obstruction through manual compression of the edematous glans or, in severe cases, surgical release of the constricting foreskin with a dorsal slit.

Assessment

Detailed scrutiny of the genitalia is necessary before neonatal circumcision. Signs suggestive of a congenital anomaly include chordee, a hooded prepuce, or meatus dislocation. A newborn with bilateral undescended testes and severe hypospadias should be evaluated for an intersex condition. A male infant with an apparently small phallus should also be examined by a urologist before a decision regarding circumcision is made. Palpate the bladder for distention and assess voiding.

ALERT *Examine the infant for signs of a bleeding dyscrasia, such as unexpected ecchymotic spots or prolonged bleeding after newborn testing.*

Administer vitamin K, as ordered, before the procedure to offset potential bleeding complications. Also, question the family regarding a family history of coagulation disorders. If the history is positive, circumcision should be deferred until it is determined that the child does not have a bleeding disorder.

Interdisciplinary Interventions

With well-baby education condensed into shortened hospital stays after delivery, many parents have little opportunity to make a thoughtful decision about circumcision. Nurses have ample opportunity to provide anticipatory guidance during prenatal visits and childbirth education programs. If the parents choose not to have their son circumcised, provide instructions for proper genital care (Teaching Intervention Plan 19-4).

Circumcision is ideally performed within the first 48 hours after delivery, but it can be performed anytime through the first month of life without general anesthesia. The procedure begins with a thorough cleansing of the glans, then the inner preputial epithelium is separated from the glans. A dorsal slit is made through the foreskin, which allows a clamp mechanism to be applied over the glans. The prepuce covering the clamp is excised. Hemostasis is provided where needed, and a lubricated gauze pad is wrapped circumferentially over the raw edges. Circumcision for the older infant or child is similar, but sutures are needed to approximate the skin edges.

Pain management during and after circumcision is necessary because newborns likely experience even more pain than an adult would with the same stimulus. Therapeutic options include caudal block, dorsal penile block, and topical analgesics (e.g., EMLA, LMX4), all of which offer continued relief for 4 to 8 hours after the procedure. Also use sucrose and nonnutritive sucking (see Chapter 10). Discomfort after circumcision in infants may persist for 24 to 48 hours. Mild analgesics are generally adequate to extinguish pain (Garry et al., 2006).

After circumcision, observe the child's penis for bleeding or signs of infection. In many cases, the first sign of a blood dyscrasia is prolonged oozing after the procedure. Although most infants void within 6 hours after circumcision, an excessively tight dressing may induce urinary retention. Reapply the bandage to correct the problem.

Community Care

Discharge teaching includes providing families with information about wound care. Instruct them to reapply the dressing for 1 to 2 days; petroleum-coated gauze bandages can be used and applied to the tip of the penis.

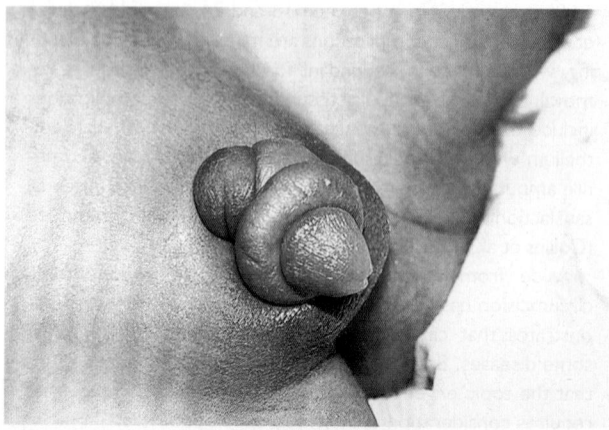
Figure 19-10 Paraphimosis. Note the swollen prepuce.

TIP 19-4: A TEACHING INTERVENTION PLAN for a Boy Who Is Uncircumcized

Nursing Diagnoses and Family Outcomes

- Deficient knowledge: Normal preputial separation
  Outcome: The family will express an understanding of appropriate hygiene measures, which vary by age of the child.
- Risk for infection related to inappropriate hygiene measures
  Outcomes: The family will adhere to recommended hygiene measures and teach them to the child.
  Child will gain independence in adopting a consistent hygiene regimen.

Teach the Child/Family

Hygiene Measures: Birth to 3 Years
- The foreskin and the glans (the end of the penis) are normally fused during these years.
- No specific care of the foreskin is recommended.
- Occasionally retract the foreskin to check for separation.
- The foreskin should *only* be retracted with gentle pressure until resistance is felt.

After Complete Foreskin Separation
- Retract the foreskin fully to expose the glans.
- Cleanse the glans with a mild soap and water and dry completely.
- Return the foreskin to its normal position.
- Perform this routine daily.

Adolescence
- White discharge, called *smegma*, needs to be removed daily.
- Retained smegma can be irritating and may be a source of infection.
- When sanitation facilities are inadequate (such as long hiking trips) or in hot, humid climates, disposable wash towelettes may be used.

Contact the Health Care Provider if
- The glans becomes sore or excoriated
- There is an unusual odor, rash, or discharge around or from the penis
- The foreskin cannot be retracted

This dressing helps prevent the circumcised area from rubbing against the diaper or sticking to the diaper as the healing process is occurring. Teach the family that the penis will appear edematous and ecchymotic during the process of wound healing. If the child is not an infant, caution the child and family to avoid straddle toys and vigorous play for 3 to 4 days. Tub baths may be instituted after the fifth day to help the sutures dissolve.

> ANSWER: Care for the older infant or child having a circumcision is similar to that for a newborn. However, sutures are needed to approximate the skin edges. Pain management as well as family teaching related to wound care and monitoring for signs and symptoms of bleeding and infection are key for a child at any age. Tub baths can be used after the fifth day to help dissolve the sutures in the older infant or child.

VARICOCELE

A varicocele is a scrotal mass resulting from engorgement of the spermatic vein and scrotal vasculature. Blood return from the scrotum into the renal vein is impeded, producing antegrade vascular dilation and stasis. The pooled blood raises the temperature around the testicle, with potentially adverse effects on the organ.

Varicoceles are seldom evident before the second decade of life, reaching their peak incidence by the midteens. The prevalence of scrotal varicoceles is 15% in postpubertal males aged 12 to 18 years old (Fine & Poppas, 2012). Varicoceles are clinically detectable on the left side in 90% of cases and are bilateral in 3% (Diamond et al., 2011). No genetic, racial, or congenital risk factors are associated with the phenomenon.

The etiologic basis for a varicocele rests with a discrepancy in the attachment angles of the right and left spermatic veins to their corresponding renal vein. The right spermatic renal junction is obliquely angled, allowing unobstructed circulation, whereas the left junction is a 90-degree angle, which reduces blood velocity. It is probable that anatomic changes in relative renal position and vascular configuration, secondary to the pubertal growth spurt, trigger the development of the varicosed venous network.

Pathophysiology

By the time the child reaches mid to late adolescence, the deleterious effects of a varicocele can be noted. Increased glandular volume, which normally occurs during puberty, is delayed in the affected testicle. Histologic evaluation of the affected gonad demonstrates delayed maturation and decreased spermatogenesis. These changes are progressive into adulthood, reducing the density and motility of spermatozoa. The presence of a varicocele is a common cause for male infertility, and its effects are cumulative.

The youth's response to surgical correction of the varicocele seems to depend on the severity and duration of the condition. Studies suggest that correction in older adolescents results in catch-up growth of the testis and markedly improved sperm concentration and motility (Choi & Kim, 2013). Although evidence that catch-up growth affects fertility is limited, varicocelectomy may improve fertility (Choi & Kim, 2013).

Assessment

The cardinal sign of a varicocele is a palpable scrotal mass of veins, typically described as a "bag of worms." The defect is noted when the boy is in an upright position, and it resolves when the adolescent is examined in a supine position. Occasionally, boys describe a heavy or dragging sensation to the scrotum, but most varicoceles are asymptomatic. They are usually detected as a scrotal fullness during a routine scrotal examination or when teaching the child to perform testicular self-examination.

When a varicocele is palpated, determine testicular volume, monitoring for a discrepancy between the affected gland and its mate. Measure testicular volume on a regular basis with an orchidometer or by ultrasound. A reduction in the volume of the affected testicle is an indicator of testicular damage.

Hormonal tests are not indicated unless the child has signs of hypogonadism. Follicle-stimulating hormone and testosterone levels vary as boys go through puberty. Gonadotropin-releasing hormone stimulation test may help identify early testicular dysfunction, but a normal test does not indicate absence of risk for future infertility, and an abnormal result does not indicate future infertility.

Interdisciplinary Interventions

Early detection of the varicocele and vigilant monitoring for testicular changes are necessary to avoid testicular damage.

caREminder

Institute thorough genital examinations when the boy enters puberty and repeat yearly, along with monthly testicular self-examination.

Surgical correction is recommended when signs of testicular impairment are present, such as abnormal semen analysis or change in testicular size (Diamond et al., 2011). The recommended procedure is ligation of the varicosity and removal of the spermatic vein as either an open or laparoscopic procedure.

Nursing care for the adolescent undergoing a varicocelectomy includes routine postoperative stabilization, pain relief, and wound assessment. The hospital stay is minimal, and home instructions focus on activity restrictions for 10 to 14 days.

Community Care

Important components of discharge teaching by the nurse are to review the possible postoperative complications with the child and his family and to stress to the boy himself the necessity of performing monthly testicular self-examination. Long-term problems, although infrequent, include the development of a hydrocele or the recurrence of a varicocele arising from varicosed collateral vessels. A postoperative hydrocele is asymptomatic and is typically left unrepaired. A recurring varicocele requires additional surgery to ensure that the affected testicle will catch up to its contralateral mate in volume size.

RENAL FAILURE

The kidneys are vital in regulating fluid and electrolyte balance in the body. Kidney failure may result from acute or chronic processes that cause kidney injury, congenital conditions, or acquired disease.

ACUTE KIDNEY INJURY

AKI, previously called acute renal failure, develops rapidly over days or weeks. It can be classified according to the site of injury to the kidney:

- Prerenal, resulting from impaired blood flow to or oxygenation of the kidneys
- Intrinsic renal (or parenchymal), resulting from glomerular, tubular, or interstitial injury
- Postrenal, resulting from obstruction of the urinary flow at some level between the kidney and the urinary meatus

Prerenal AKI may be abated with early supportive treatment and correction of the low flow state. Intrinsic renal AKI may require pharmacologic intervention. Postrenal AKI usually requires physical removal of the obstruction. All have the potential for requiring dialytic intervention if they are not amenable to supportive or corrective intervention. Long-standing pre- or postrenal AKI may lead to intrinsic AKI.

AKI most commonly results from prerenal causes secondary to systemic illness (Fortenberry et al., 2013). Infants are most vulnerable because of their immature kidneys and large BSA compared with body mass. The most common causes of prerenal AKI are related to excessive fluid losses from trauma and bleeding or losses from the gastrointestinal, genitourinary, or integumentary systems. In developing countries, prerenal AKI is primarily caused by infections such as gastroenteritis and malaria (Radhakrishnan & Kiryluk, 2006). In children, the causes of intrinsic renal AKI vary by age. In infancy, multiple factors can contribute to failure, including hypoxic insults, drug toxicities, renal artery and venous thrombosis, and congenital renal malformations. In school-aged children, glomerular diseases are the most common causes. Glomerular diseases can affect adolescents as rapidly progressive forms of glomerulonephritis, but trauma also contributes in this age group. Postrenal AKI in younger children is commonly caused by congenital defects. The incidence of AKI in critically ill children is estimated to be 10% (Basu et al., 2011).

Pathophysiology

Prerenal AKI results from the kidneys' protective responses to diminished renal blood flow in an effort to regain normal intravascular volume, blood pressure, and renal perfusion. In the first response (the myogenic reflex), the glomerular afferent arteriole dilates to maintain glomerular blood flow. With the second response (glomerulotubular feedback), constriction or dilation of the afferent arteriole is further regulated by sodium and chloride delivery to the macula densa area of each nephron. During the third response, decreased blood pressure in the kidneys causes release of renin, which leads to production of angiotensin, a potent vasoconstrictor, and increased aldosterone synthesis, which increases sodium resorption from the distal tubule. Also, vasopressin secretion is increased, which results in more water being resorbed from the distal tubule. These protective responses work for a limited time, but unless the initial insult is resolved, the compensatory mechanisms become overwhelmed. This eventuality results in decreased glomerular blood flow and decreased GFR, which may not be reversible.

In intrinsic renal AKI, the pathology is caused by parenchymal injury from ischemia, intravascular coagulation, and microvascular injury. Common causes of intrinsic renal disease include hemolytic–uremic syndrome (HUS), glomerulonephritis, nephrotoxic drugs, acute tubular necrosis, and interstitial nephritis (Gulati, 2012).

UPJ stricture, posterior urethral valves, calculi, tumors, or compression of the ureters or the urethra may cause postrenal AKI. However, deposition of substances such as uric acid crystals, xanthines, or casts in the tubular lumens can also cause postrenal AKI. Renal blood flow increases in early hours after an obstruction occurs, but it slowly declines with prolonged obstruction from renal vasoconstriction; therefore, rapid identification of the cause and repair are imperative.

The prognosis and recovery of the child with AKI depend on the underlying cause. Mortality is often related to comorbid conditions and not directly to the renal failure itself.

Assessment

The symptoms of AKI have a sudden onset and are related directly to the lack of kidney function. Assess for **oliguria**—production of less than 0.5 mL urine per kilogram body weight per hour in children and less than 1 mL/kg/hr in infants—which may be the first sign of AKI. Anuria, essentially no urine production, is a less common sign of AKI. Children can also have AKI and have normal urine output or nonoliguric renal failure. A stratification system has been proposed to evaluate AKI in children: pRIFLE (pediatric Risk, Injury, Failure, Loss, End-stage) (Akcan-Arikan et al., 2007). Severity of renal injury increases as estimated creatinine clearance and urine output decreases.

Assess for hypertension, edema, or shortness of breath, which may indicate volume overload resulting from retained fluid. Monitor also for gastrointestinal disturbances (anorexia, nausea, vomiting, diarrhea), cardiac arrhythmias, altered level of consciousness (lethargy, drowsiness, coma), or central nervous system disturbances (headache, seizures), which may be signs of acidosis or serum electrolyte imbalance.

Assess for the first sign of recovery from the oliguria of AKI, which is usually diuresis marked by polyuria. This phase is heralded by a slow increase in urine volume, often greatly exceeding normal volumes, followed by slow decline in serum creatinine and BUN.

ALERT   *Assess for electrolyte imbalances and dehydration during the polyuric phase of AKI. Massive urine output can quickly cause electrolyte or fluid imbalance.*

Diagnostic Tests

Renal failure can affect the results of various laboratory tests. Elevated serum BUN and creatinine are most diagnostic. With decreasing renal function, severe electrolyte imbalances can occur, most notably hyperkalemia and acidosis. Hypocalcemia and hypoalbuminemia can also be noted.

Interdisciplinary Interventions

The goals in treating AKI are to reduce symptoms and to provide supportive care until renal function returns. Treatment can range from conservative management to some form of dialysis, depending on the severity of the symptoms (see "Treatment Modalities" section at the start of this chapter). Medication, dietary restrictions, or dialysis may be needed to control fluid overload, acidosis, electrolyte imbalance, or central nervous system disturbances. Erythrocyte-stimulating agents (e.g., epoetin alfa [Epogen, Procrit], darbepoetin alfa [Aranesp]) should be administered to prevent the anemia of renal failure. Teach and model good hygiene practices, such as diligent hand hygiene and daily baths, to prevent infections.

CHRONIC KIDNEY DISEASE

CKD is a progressive loss of kidney function. In children, the more prevalent causes of CKD are uropathies (31%) and glomerular disease (27%) (Sebestyen & Warady, 2011; Wong et al., 2006). The National Kidney Foundation (2002) guidelines define CKD as (1) kidney damage (either pathologic abnormalities or markers of damage, including abnormalities in blood or urine tests or imaging studies) for longer than 3 months, with or without decreased GFR; or (2) GFR less than 60 mL/min/1.73 m^2 for longer than 3 months, with or without kidney damage.

A CKD staging system (Table 19-1) was developed to help the care provider understand the severity of renal dysfunction, address changes in medical management, and make referrals to appropriate medical teams to prevent or delay adverse outcomes of CKD. Children can remain at a specific level of GFR, or their overall function may progressively worsen.

Pathophysiology

CKD in children has many causes. It can be related to an inherited disorder, congenital abnormalities, injury during the neonatal period, glomerulonephritis, nephritic syndrome/NS, tubulointerstitial disease, or renal transplant. Although many different diseases can cause CKD, morphologic changes associated with the progression to ESRD are somewhat standard. Sclerotic glomeruli with proliferative matrix changes as well as interstitial fibrosis are common. Chronic interstitial inflammation and tubular atrophy are also seen. The few remaining functional glomeruli may develop hypertrophic tubules as the kidney attempts to compensate for lost function. As kidney function deteriorates, secondary complications arise because the kidneys are unable to meet the body's physiologic demands (see Table 19-1).

TABLE 19-1   Stages of Chronic Kidney Disease, Complications, and Interventions

Description	Secondary Complications	Interventions
Stage I		
Normal or increased GFR (≥90 mL/min/1.73 m²)	No complications caused by kidney dysfunction because kidney function does not decline; kidneys may even be hyperfiltering	Provide interventions to prevent progression of disease by managing proteinuria and hypertension. Provide teaching to reduce risks of cardiovascular disease, including regular aerobic exercise, healthy weight, and heart-healthy diet.
Stage II		
Mild decrease in GFR (60–89 mL/min/1.73 m²)	May occur when kidney is unable to keep up with the body's demands. Alterations in electrolyte balance from decreased kidney filtration of blood, typically acidosis and hyperkalemia. The kidney produces the hormone EPO, which is essential in the formation of red blood cells. Declining GFR reduces the kidney's ability to produce adequate amounts of EPO, causing renal anemia. As a result of the reduction in growth hormone secretion, alterations in growth patterns can begin.	Preventive measures as noted earlier. Monitor for electrolyte imbalances. Dietary intervention (low potassium). Medications for acidosis (sodium bicarbonate). Monitor for anemia. Medications to supplement iron and EPO. EPO requires subcutaneous injections. Monitor growth velocity. Rule out alternative causes for growth failure (acidosis, poor nutrition, endocrine abnormalities). Dietary restriction of phosphorous
Stage III		
Moderate decrease in GFR (30–59 mL/min/1.73 m²)	Further alterations in bone metabolism and growth can occur. The kidney excretes 70% of dietary phosphate intake; as function declines, hyperphosphatemia develops. A decrease in calcium absorption in the gut leads to hypocalcemia. Phosphorous–calcium imbalance affects the parathyroid gland. A decrease in the number of calcium receptors on the parathyroid gland in individuals with CKD occurs.	Monitor and manage as noted earlier, plus monitor for bone disease. Monitor growth velocity. Restrict phosphorous. Medicate to treat bone disease/growth failure. • Phosphorous binders • Vitamin D • Growth hormone (daily subcutaneous injection) Anticipatory teaching and planning for renal transplant
Stage IV		
Severe decrease in GFR (15–29 mL/min/1.73 m²)	The previous alterations become more pronounced and more difficult to control.	All of the interventions mentioned earlier, plus begin anticipatory teaching and planning for renal replacement therapy.
Stage V		
Kidney failure/ESRD (GFR <15 mL/min/1.73 m²)	Signs and symptoms of uremia typically present.	Requires renal replacement therapy • PD • Hemodialysis • Kidney transplant

Adapted from National Kidney Foundation. (2006). KDOQI clinical practice guidelines and clinical practice recommendations 2006 updates: Hemodialysis adequacy, peritoneal dialysis adequacy and vascular access. *American Journal of Kidney Diseases, 48*(Suppl. 1), S1–S322.

Assessment

Obtain a detailed prenatal and antenatal history. Antenatal findings may include polyhydramnios, oligohydramnios, and abnormal antenatal ultrasound.

Signs and symptoms of CKD in children are vague and differ by stage of disease. With the benefit of laboratory and radiographic studies, children are presenting earlier for long-term follow-up care. Overall signs and symptoms of chronic progressive kidney disease can include, but are not limited to, fatigue, exercise intolerance, delayed growth and sexual maturation, dry and itchy skin, hypertension, headaches, renal osteodystrophy or bony changes, muscle cramps or myopathy, and generalized malaise. Decreased renal function also increases susceptibility to infection. In young children, findings may include failure to thrive or short stature. Older children and adolescents may present with delayed puberty and poor school performance.

Assess the child and the family for their responses to CKD. As with any other chronic condition, the psychological effects of CKD on the child and family can be devastating. Both the diagnosis and the treatment cause stress for all family members. The family mourns the loss of their "normal, healthy" child and experiences anger, denial, and hopelessness. Even though they intellectually understand that CKD can progress and lead to ESRD, families still may repeatedly question the necessity of recommended treatments and ask for second opinions. Children, too, mourn the loss of their good health. If nephrectomy is necessary, they mourn the loss of this body part, even if no normal kidney function remained. Some children believe that being "bad" has brought on the illness and that only being "good" will result in a cure. Explain the condition, as age-appropriate, and provide frequent reassurance to decrease fright and increase the child's sense of well-being. Ask about the child's school performance. Multiple factors contribute to poor performance: anemia, uremia, absences, and depression; intervene as indicated.

If the cause is a hereditary disease, guilt is a common parental feeling. Families who believe that the disease may result in the child's death may become distant and less supportive of the child because they are experiencing anticipatory grief. See Chapter 12 for a discussion of the effects of chronic conditions on the child and family.

Diagnostic Tests

The gold standard measurement of GFR is creatinine clearance. This test requires a 24-hour urine collection and a serum creatinine level drawn during, or at the end of, the urine collection. This cumbersome task is not feasible in younger children who are not toilet trained. An *estimated* GFR is commonly calculated instead, using the Schwartz formula:

Height (in centimeters) $\times$ CF/serum creatinine = GFR (in milliliters per minute per 1.73 m^2)

where CF is the coefficient factor (0.45 in infants, 0.55 in children, and 0.7 in adolescent males).

Improved formulas to estimate GFR are under development (Furth et al., 2006).

caREminder

Creatinine is a measure of muscle breakdown, so results can be misleading in very thin or malnourished children.

Multiple lab values are monitored based on the child's stage of CKD. These include serum electrolytes, CBCs, iron stores, calcium, phosphorous, intact parathyroid hormone levels, cholesterol panels, and nutritional parameters such as albumin, total protein, and prealbumin levels. Intermittent measurements of serum creatinine can guide treatment but cannot predict the rate of decline or likelihood of renal failure.

Nursing Diagnoses and Outcomes

The slow onset of CKD and the anticipation of future dialysis and transplantation govern the selection of diagnoses, which reflect the child's psychosocial needs. Nursing diagnoses and outcomes typically applicable to the child with renal disease are presented in Nursing Plan of Care 19-1. The child and family require extensive teaching to prepare them for each different phase of the child's disease progression. Evaluate nursing diagnoses that can be applied to direct the child's psychosocial

care needs, including those related to activity intolerance and body image disturbance. In addition, the following nursing diagnoses may be applicable to reflect alterations in family and individual coping:

Nursing Diagnosis: Compromised family coping related to the effects of the presence of chronic condition and ongoing care requirements of child
Outcomes:
- Child and family will demonstrate effective decision making and mutual support activities.
- Child and family will share ongoing concerns with one another and with members of the health care team.
- Child and family will participate in treatment activities at developmentally appropriate levels.

Nursing Diagnosis: Grieving related to response to loss of kidney function and restricted lifestyle
Outcomes:
- Child and family will verbalize feelings of grief and accept these responses as appropriate to the situation.
- Child and family will seek support from appropriate resources to assist in dealing with grief.

Plan nursing care to address the child's current level of kidney function, to slow progression, and to treat secondary issues that arise out of decreased function.

Interdisciplinary Interventions

Treatment for CKD ranges from conservative medical and dietary management to dialysis or kidney transplantation. All treatment modalities for children require a major investment of family time and energy as well as commitment from an interdisciplinary care team. Each team member must address family members' knowledge deficits and support the other team members in caring for the child and family. Because work overlaps significantly, schedule regular team meetings to discuss care plans, ensuring consistent care and a unified approach to the child and family.

During the early stages of CKD, regular observation of the child's condition may be all that is required. However, when a child is first diagnosed with kidney disease requiring treatment, explain all the appropriate treatment modalities to the family and the child, as developmentally appropriate. Include extended family or significant others who support the family and assist in caring for the child. As the child progresses into stage IV, begin planning for transplantation and renal replacement therapy. Planning ahead reduces anxiety and decreases the need for emergent decision making if a rapid decline in function occurs.

Nursing care of the child with stage V CKD includes teaching the child and family about the long-term implications of each treatment option (Teaching Intervention Plan 19-5). Assess family coping mechanisms and intervene if indicated. Educate both the child and family of the consequences of not adhering to the prescribed treatment regimen; help the family to focus on promoting the most normal lifestyle possible. Close interaction with a social worker and renal dietitian are imperative at this stage of kidney disease. Children may need assistance in school scheduling to accommodate

TIP 19-5: A TEACHING INTERVENTION PLAN for the Child With Renal Disease

Nursing Diagnoses and Family Outcomes

- Excess fluid volume related to excess sodium intake or fluid retention
  Outcomes: Child maintains fluid intake within ordered parameters.
  Child maintains baseline weight.
  Child and family demonstrate skill in monitoring child's fluid intake and sodium intake.
- Risk for impaired skin integrity related to delayed healing, pruritus, edema, and/or Tenckhoff catheter insertion
  Outcomes: Child's skin remains intact.
  Child and family institute measures to monitor and maintain skin integrity.
- Delayed growth and development related to effects of disease and medications
  Outcome: Child demonstrates age-appropriate skills and behaviors to the extent possible.

Teach the Child/Family

Fluid Intake

- If fluids need to be encouraged, offer small amounts (30–60 mL) of the child's favorite fluid every hour while the child is awake.
- Keep a chart of the fluids consumed to assist in monitoring intake.
- If fluids are restricted, pour out the day's fluid allotment in a single container to be kept in the refrigerator. Set aside enough fluid to consume with medications.
- Any food substance that melts (e.g., ice cream, ice, gelatin dessert) counts as liquid intake.
- Ensure that all fluids have some calories in them to maximize the number of calories that the child receives. Do not offer low-calorie and diet drinks unless the child is significantly overweight.

Nutrition

- If the child is in renal failure, protein intake is restricted to recommended daily allowance for age group.
- If the child is receiving PD, protein intake may be up to 100 g/day.

- A potassium-restricted diet (2 g/day) is generally recommended. High-potassium foods include citrus fruits, dried fruits, bananas, potatoes, chocolate, nuts, and tomatoes.
- No-added-salt diet
  - No more than 4 g sodium/day
  - Do not use table salt at all
- Low-salt diet
  - No more than 2 g sodium/day
  - Do not use table salt at all
- Encourage intake of high-carbohydrate and/or high-fat foods, such as hard candy, bread, and butter, and add Polycose or vegetable oil to formulas.
- Calcium supplements should be given to prevent bowing of the long bones and joint swelling (renal rickets).

Skin Care

- Because healing times are prolonged, monitor skin integrity daily and provide routine skin care.
- Clean the Tenckhoff catheter, hemodialysis access catheter, or urinary diversion tube site daily.
- Itching is common in renal failure. Keep the child's nails trimmed to prevent scratching, and use a moisturizing cream (e.g., Eucerin) to help minimize itching.

Health Maintenance

- Practice proper hand hygiene to prevent infections in the child with immunosuppression.
- Ensure that immunizations (especially varicella vaccine) are current before kidney transplantation.
- Platelet function is decreased. Observe child for bleeding. If bleeding occurs, apply direct pressure to the site, elevate the affected area, and apply a dressing or ice to the site.
- Promote good dental hygiene to prevent cavity formation and the need for extensive dental work.

Developmental Considerations

- Encourage independence and activities appropriate to the child's developmental level.
- Encourage school attendance.
- Set behavioral limits and reward desired behaviors.
- Give the child choices, allowing some participation in decisions about his or her care.

dialysis and frequent medical appointments. Adherence to dietary management can be very difficult, especially in the teenage population; provide ongoing reeducation. Child life specialists help provide coping skills and diversion during dialysis.

Conservative Management

Conservative management is used for children with impaired renal function before dialysis is required. The main focus of conservative management is to treat the symptoms of CKD and prevent further damage.

Controlling blood pressure is a priority. Teach the family how to measure blood pressure, what their child's normal blood pressure is, and at what level to contact their health care provider about elevated or low measures. Facilitate obtaining automatic blood pressure devices as indicated (e.g., for infants, when it is difficult to obtain accurate readings).

Teach families how to give injections (see Chapter 9 and thePoint for Procedures/Interventions for Medication Administration: Subcutaneous). Children with CKD may require erythropoietic-stimulating agents to treat anemia. These injections are given from three times weekly to as infrequently as monthly with the new longer acting erythropoietic-stimulating agent formulations. Children may also require recombinant human growth hormone injections, which are given daily at bedtime. Frequently assess child and family coping and proper injection technique; inspect injection sites.

When caring for a child undergoing conservative management, frequently assess the child's nutritional status by appetite, weight and height measurements, and activity level. Nausea and vomiting are common symptoms of renal failure, particularly as the child gets closer to requiring dialysis. These symptoms are thought to result from the body compensating for protein load or may be related to an altered taste pattern. If medications are vomited, instruct the family to consult the health care provider to determine whether they should be readministered.

Although laboratory tests are a good method to monitor serum chemistries, laboratory tests should be kept to a minimum. Decrease the trauma associated with laboratory tests as much as possible. For instance, drawing blood from a child's heparin lock or implanted venous access device eliminates the need for multiple needle sticks. Use topical anesthetics for needle procedures (see Chapter 10).

ALERT   *Renal failure affects the body's ability to form blood clots. Children who have been in renal failure for a while are at risk for prolonged bleeding. Teach families to control excessive bleeding from laboratory tests or injuries by applying ice and direct pressure.*

Renal failure causes immunosuppression. Teach the child and family to avoid exposure to contagious diseases, avoid skin breakdown, and take antibiotics as ordered.

Dietary Management

The diet recommended for a child with renal failure is individualized and designed based on the child's level of CKD. In stages I to IV, the renal diet consists of restricted amounts of protein, low potassium and phosphorus, and low to moderate sodium. Permitted levels may be modified depending on the child's requirements. To achieve fluid balance, the child's underlying disease process is considered. For children in stages I through IV, fluids are not usually restricted; in fact, they often are told to "push" fluids.

The diet for a child in stage V CKD is essentially a balanced diet, and, in contrast to the diet in stages I through IV, a more liberal protein intake is allowed because of the catabolic nature of dialysis; fluids are restricted. Educate the family regarding dietary restrictions, and suggest ways to help the child adhere to the regimen. Grandparents or friends, if they are unaware of the scope of restrictions, may inadvertently sabotage the diet by handing the child a candy bar or a banana.

Encourage the child with CKD to live as normal a life as possible. Attending school, after-school activities, sports, scouting, and camp is important. Assist the child and family, as requested, to explain dietary limitations to school and camp personnel. Most institutions can adjust menus for children with dietary restrictions.

Support the family in developing practices to prevent the child with renal failure from feeling different or deprived because of dietary limitations. Having the whole family eat the renal failure diet at home helps the child to normalize the diet. In addition, the family's food preparer avoids the stress of preparing two different menus at each meal; salt, spices, or butter can be added to individual portions after they have been served.

The child on a limited-potassium diet must limit intake of citrus fruits, bananas, potatoes, chocolate, nuts, dairy products, and tomatoes, which are all high in potassium. Dried fruits of all kinds are also high in potassium because the dehydration process concentrates the substance.

ALERT   *Many salt substitutes use potassium as their main ingredient. These substances exacerbate hyperkalemia in children with CKD.*

Renal Replacement Therapies

If conservative measures fail to manage the child's condition, some form of renal replacement therapy is necessary. The child with severe hyperkalemia, hyponatremia, increased BUN levels, fluid retention, and metabolic acidosis is a candidate for dialysis (see "Treatment Modalities" section). Monitor for symptoms or complications of uremia such as anorexia, nausea and vomiting, poor growth, lethargy, and an inability to concentrate, which are also indications to begin dialysis. Specific serum creatinine and creatinine clearance values and other criteria have been established as indications for dialysis in adult patients. However, such specific criteria have not been adopted for children because serum creatinine levels depend on the child's muscle mass. Thus, because of the disparity in muscle mass, a serum creatinine level of 3 mg/dL in a newborn may demonstrate the same need for dialysis shown by a level of 8 mg/dL in an adolescent. Creatinine clearance may be more useful in determining the need for dialysis in smaller children. Symptoms of ESRD are sufficient reason to begin dialysis even if laboratory values do not indicate that it is needed. For children with AKI, the rapidity of onset, duration, severity of abnormalities, and symptoms govern the decision to begin dialysis (Table 19-2).

CONGENITAL RENAL DISEASE

Congenital renal disease results from improper embryonic development of urinary tract structures. It occurs in several forms. Agenesis is the complete absence of kidney tissue. If agenesis is unilateral, it may not be discovered until later in life. At birth, the contralateral kidney is stimulated to undergo compensatory hypertrophy to maintain normal renal function. As long as renal function in the sole kidney is normal, children can grow and function normally, with no adverse effects to the single kidney. Usually, the left kidney is absent, and

TABLE 19-2   Comparison of Dialysis Modalities

Modality	Advantages	Disadvantages
Peritoneal dialysis	Easy to start Easy for staff to learn Liberal diet Liberal fluids Consistent therapy Most normal lifestyle, can usually attend school uninterrupted No heparinization Can travel with/have equipment shipped to destination	Results are not rapid; this method produces slow, gentle fluid removal and solute correction Not appropriate after recent abdominal surgery Unrelenting, must be done 7 days per week Risk of peritonitis; tunnel and exit site infections More responsibility on family
Hemodialysis	Rapid fluid and solute chemistry correction Therapy three to four times a week Less work at home	Expensive equipment Trained and experienced staff required Blood vessel access required Heparinization required Diet and fluid restrictions Intermittent therapy/missed school time Travel time/expense to dialysis unit Extracorporeal circuit required
Continuous renal replacement therapy	Slow, gentle fluid removal and solute correction for the hemodynamically unstable patient	Blood vessel access required Requires high staff-to-patient ratio with highly trained and experienced staff Heparinization required Extracorporeal circuit required Continuous arteriovenous hemofiltration requires mean arterial pressure more than 60 mm Hg

the right kidney is normal. The condition predominates in males (Schwaderer et al., 2007).

A small kidney with fewer nephrons than normal is called a *hypoplastic kidney*. Like other congenital malformations, hypoplasia can be unilateral or bilateral. Bilateral hypoplastic kidneys is a leading cause of ESRD during the first decade of life.

Dysplastic kidneys and polycystic kidney disease, congenital conditions that cause renal disease, are discussed in this section.

DYSPLASTIC KIDNEYS

Aplastic and *dysplastic* are terms that are often used interchangeably to describe kidneys that have not developed normally. Aplastic or dysplastic kidneys can occur bilaterally or unilaterally. Dysplasia often occurs along with a functional obstruction of the collecting system, such as neuropathic bladder (González Celedón et al., 2007), posterior urethral valves, or prune-belly syndrome.

Pathophysiology

Dysplastic kidneys show abnormal differentiation of renal tissues, with primitive glomeruli and tubules, cysts, and nonrenal tissues, such as cartilage. Altered gene expression or obstruction in the renal system can contribute to development of renal dysplasia (Jain et al., 2007; Shibata & Nagata, 2003).

Assessment

The function of dysplastic kidneys varies as widely as the types of anomalies do. Presenting signs and symptoms can be apparent (flank mass, UTIs, hematuria,

proteinuria) or can be somewhat concealed by other conditions, such as failure to thrive.

Children with dysplastic kidneys can show the signs and symptoms of CKD. The degree of renal impairment often progresses as the child grows and is related to degree of proteinuria, number of febrile UTIs, presence of hypertension, GFR at onset of deterioration, and puberty (González Celedón et al., 2007). Bilateral dysplastic kidneys may have enough function to maintain a newborn but are not able to keep a larger child healthy. If a child has unilateral dysplasia, the contralateral side may develop well, hypertrophy, and provide normal renal function.

Dysplastic kidneys can be seen on ultrasound; their size can be measured, and any scarring can be noted. However, a kidney biopsy is needed to differentiate between dysplastic and hypoplastic tissue.

Interdisciplinary Interventions

As the child with dysplastic kidneys progresses through the stages of CKD, first, conservative management, then some form of renal replacement therapy will be required (see "Chronic Kidney Disease" section).

POLYCYSTIC KIDNEY DISEASE

Polycystic kidney disease is an inherited disease characterized by diffuse cystic lesions in both kidneys. Polycystic kidney disease has no ethnic or gender predilection. Two types of polycystic kidney disease exist: autosomal dominant and autosomal recessive. Autosomal dominant polycystic kidney disease (ADPKD) is the most common inherited human kidney disease; incidence is 1 in 500 to 1 in 1,000 live births (Boyer et al., 2007).

ARPKD predominantly presents in infancy, occurring in 1 in 20,000 live births (Torres & Harris, 2006).

Pathophysiology

In addition to the renal cysts in ADPKD, cysts are present in other organs, such as the liver, pancreas, seminal vessels, and arachnoid membranes. Other abnormalities can be present, such as intracranial aneurysms, aortic root dilation and aneurysms, mitral valve prolapse, and abdominal wall hernias (Torres et al., 2007). ADPKD is less aggressive than ARPKD, and progression to ESRD in childhood is rare; however, many progress to ESRD as adults (Torres et al., 2007). When renal insufficiency appears, the GFR typically decreases at a rate of 4.4 to 5.9 mL/min/year (Torres et al., 2007).

In ARPKD, in addition to the renal cysts, some degree of biliary dysgenesis and hepatic fibrosis is always present (Goilav et al., 2006). Regardless of the genetic etiology (ARPKD or ADPKD), kidney transplantation may be indicated in the presence of ESRD. Kidney and liver transplantation may be needed depending on the degree of liver impairment caused by biliary dysgenesis and hepatic fibrosis in ARPKD or if polycystic liver disease accompanies ADPKD. If a child with ADPKD dies, the cause is usually attributed to cirrhosis, portal hypertension, or ruptured esophageal varices resulting from liver disease.

Long-term prognosis is variable. The earlier the disease manifests, the greater the number of nephrons affected and the poorer the prognosis. About 30% of newborns die from lung hypoplasia with oligohydramnios sequence (Bisceglia et al., 2006). In ARPKD diagnosed in an infant, decreased GFR is usually evident early but can remain stable or even slightly improve during the first year of life. Most children require renal replacement therapy before adolescence (Goilav et al., 2006). Much of the morbidity associated with ARPKD is related to the hepatic disease rather than the renal disease. With advances in renal transplantation, renal survival rates are high.

Assessment

Manifestations of ADPKD may not appear until late childhood or even adolescence, but occasionally, they may affect neonates. An abdominal mass, flank pain, hematuria, hypertension, and (less frequently) renal insufficiency may be the presenting symptom (Boyer et al., 2007).

ARPKD typically presents during early infancy as bilateral flank masses that do not transilluminate. The presence of respiratory distress, infantile hypertension, and a history of oligohydramnios is highly suggestive of the disease.

ADPKD and ARPKD may be diagnosed by prenatal ultrasound that demonstrates renal cysts. Renal ultrasonography is often used for assessment and diagnosis; CT or MRI may also be used.

Interdisciplinary Interventions

Treatment of either type of polycystic kidney disease is symptomatic. In addition to treatment of hypertension, congestive heart failure, respiratory distress, or other symptoms of CKD, surgical removal of the polycystic kidneys is often necessary. Maintenance dialysis is then required until renal transplantation is successful (see "Treatment Modalities" section).

Because polycystic kidney disease is hereditary, older children with the disease and their parents should receive genetic counseling along with teaching about dialysis and transplantation. This preparation permits them to make informed decisions about reproductive choices.

GLOMERULAR DISORDERS

Injury to the glomerulus leads to impaired kidney filtration. As a result, blood components normally excluded (e.g., red blood cells, protein) can pass into the urine and be excreted. The type and severity of the defect determines the degree of functional impairment.

Various renal disorders are grouped under the larger diagnosis of glomerulonephritis. There is proliferation and inflammation of the glomeruli and evidence of both hematuria and proteinuria. Many of the glomerulopathies are believed to be a direct result of an immune mechanism. For more information, see the Point for Supplemental Information: Causes of Glomerulonephritis. A kidney biopsy is the only way to identify the type of glomerulonephritis. A specific diagnosis is essential in determining treatment for the underlying disease, in assessing the likelihood of retaining or regaining normal renal function, and for assessing the probability that disease will recur. Disorders discussed in this section include NS, proteinuria, HUS, PIGN, and Alport syndrome.

NEPHROTIC SYNDROME

NS is characterized by a sudden onset, with edema as its first presenting symptom, and a diagnostic triad of proteinuria, hypoalbuminemia, and hypercholesterolemia. NS may be congenital, caused by a genetic mutation or secondary to congenital infection. More commonly, NS is acquired and typically idiopathic, classified based on the response to corticosteroids as steroid sensitive or steroid resistant. NS can also be secondary to infection, medications, or neoplasia.

Annually, NS develops in 16 per 100,000 children (Gipson et al., 2013). Most cases develop in 2- to 6-year-old children. Boys are affected almost twice as often as girls (Krishnan, 2012). Minimal change NS is the most common cause (77%) of idiopathic NS in children. Minimal abnormalities are found on renal biopsy, and these children have the highest likelihood of complete disease resolution by their early teens. The incidence of focal segmental glomerulosclerosis appears to be increasing (Krishnan, 2012). This is clinically important because focal segmental glomerulosclerosis is the lesion most likely to be a precursor to CKD.

Pathophysiology

The primary pathophysiologic event in NS is increased permeability to albumin in the glomerular basement membrane. This permeability results in massive albumin loss into the urine and hypoalbuminemia, causing circulating fluid volume depletion and decreased intravascular oncotic pressure. Compensatory physiologic mechanisms result in sodium retention (renin–angiotensin–aldosterone) and free water retention. Hyperlipidemia in NS is thought to result from hypoalbuminemia stimulating hepatic protein synthesis, including lipoproteins, and loss of lipoprotein lipase into the urine. Nonalbumin proteins lost in the urine include immunoglobulins, clotting factors, and several important binding proteins in the plasma, including several hormonal binding proteins. As a result of the loss of immunoglobulins, a child with NS is prone to infection even before immunosuppressive therapy is initiated, and severe ascites may be complicated by spontaneous bacterial peritonitis. Thrombotic events have been reported in the portal vein, sagittal sinus, and various limb vessels (Schachter, 2004).

Categorizing NS by response to therapy helps to delineate prognosis and treatment plans. Steroid therapy is the first-line treatment, and response is categorized as steroid-resistant, steroid-responsive, or steroid-dependent. Steroid resistance is diagnosed after no response is obtained after 12 weeks of steroid treatment. These children require renal biopsy and second-line agents for treatment. In steroid-responsive children, the amount of protein in the urine decreases to negative or trace amounts within 10 to 15 days after initiation of steroid therapy. Steroid-dependent children relapse when alternate day therapy is begun or within 2 weeks after all steroid therapy has been discontinued. Most children are steroid responsive and respond to prednisone therapy within 2 weeks.

Assessment

Typically, the first sign of NS is periorbital edema; it is often originally thought to be an allergy. Periorbital edema is most noticeable upon arising but subsides as the child is upright during the day; however, it may shift to peripheral, scrotal, or vaginal edema. Weight gain usually occurs, but the family may mistake it as being caused by growth. Urine becomes diminished, foamy, or frothy. Ascites and pleural effusion may develop from the fluid shifts. Blood pressure is usually normal to slightly decreased.

The child is as edematous on the inside of the body as on the outside. Gastrointestinal edema can cause diarrhea, anorexia, and poor food absorption. If the protein loss is prolonged, signs of malnutrition, such as hair changes, pallor, or shiny skin with prominent veins, may ensue. The child may be irritable from the swelling, lethargic, fatigued, and increasingly susceptible to infection, especially pneumonia, peritonitis, cellulitis, and septicemia.

Interdisciplinary Interventions

Treatment aims to decrease urinary protein loss (thus controlling edema), balance nutrition, restore normal metabolic function, and prevent or treat any infection (see thePoint for Care Paths: An Interdisciplinary Plan of Care for the Child With Nephrotic Syndrome). Children with steroid-sensitive NS should be treated for at least 3 months with corticosteroids (Hodson et al., 2010). The child is usually hospitalized for the first episode of NS so that the diagnosis may be confirmed, therapy can be initiated, and the family can be taught about the disease and its management. Recurrences can usually be managed at home; however, severe edema causing respiratory distress, ascites, skin breakdown, or massive scrotal swelling requires hospitalization.

The child may ambulate as tolerated and is given a low-sodium, well-balanced diet with fluid restriction only if the edema is severe. Hydrotherapy is often helpful to assist in fluid shifting. Instruct the child to soak in a warm bath or swim in a pool to aid in mobilizing fluid back into the intravascular space. Elevate the lower extremities or scrotum if indicated to reduce fluid pooling. Monitor for skin breakdown, a particular risk with marked edema, and intervene as indicated. Peritonitis is the most common infection in actively nephrotic children. Because steroid therapy may suppress physical findings of infection such as fever, carefully assess the child. Severe abdominal pain that impedes activity should be evaluated emergently.

Community Care

Most children have had their childhood immunizations by the time NS first develops. After NS is diagnosed, consider the child's current use of steroids when making decisions to immunize. Educate the family that if the child is not receiving steroids, immunizations should occur at regular intervals, with the understanding that they may cause the child's NS to relapse. The risk of contracting a preventable disease likely far outweighs the risk of NS relapse. Immunizations administered to a child taking steroids may not evoke adequate response and therefore may not fully protect the child from illness.

Viral illnesses, especially upper respiratory infections, are an unavoidable part of childhood. If an NS relapse occurs because of viral illness, instruct families to seek medical care so that steroid treatment can be reinitiated.

Educate families on the importance of treating the child normally, particularly during periods of remission, and of having age-appropriate expectations of the child (e.g., discipline, chores).

PROTEINURIA

Many healthy children excrete protein in their urine, up to 100 mg/m² BSA daily (Hladunewich & Schaefer, 2011). The causes of proteinuria can be classified into three main categories. In *postural*, or *orthostatic*, proteinuria, a nonpathologic form, children excrete normal or slightly increased amounts of protein when they are recumbent. When they arise, however, protein excretion increases. *Nonpathologic transient* proteinuria can occur with a temperature of 101° F (38.3° C) or more, after vigorous exercise, with heart failure, with seizures, after exposure to cold, or with emotional stress. *Fixed* proteinurias are more likely to be pathologic. The abnormal proteinurias are caused by glomerular or tubular disorders, overload of protein in the blood, and alterations in intrarenal blood flow.

Pathophysiology

Glomerular proteinuria results from changes in the electrostatic charge or size of the pores of the glomerular capillary membranes, which increase membrane permeability, resulting in increased levels of plasma proteins in the filtrate. In tubular proteinuria, normal levels of smaller molecular weight proteins are filtered but are not reabsorbed from the proximal tubule as they should be.

Overload proteinuria occurs when excessive amounts of low-molecular-weight proteins, present because of a disease process, are present in glomerular filtrate. The levels exceed the resorptive capacity of the proximal tubules. The compensatory changes in a single functioning kidney give rise to altered blood flow within that kidney and can lead to proteinuria.

Assessment

Protein in urine can sometimes be detected by a foamy appearance, but this is an unreliable indicator. A dipstick test, a turbidimetric test with sulfosalicylic acid, or both types of tests are required for accurate detection. The accuracy of dipstick testing can be affected by the concentration of the urine. If proteinuria is detected first by dipstick, it must be verified by laboratory measures of actual protein excretion. Measurement of protein-to-creatinine ratio in a first-morning urine sample correlates to the 24-hour protein excretion value (Rashman et al., 2006).

Interdisciplinary Interventions

Children with pathologic proteinuria should have a physical examination, urinalysis with microscopic examination, a first-morning protein-to-creatinine ratio, urine culture, serum albumin, BUN, creatinine, and C3 levels. If hematuria, hypertension, or impaired renal function is found, a kidney biopsy is necessary.

If a child loses less than 1 g of protein in the urine every 24 hours, no treatment is required. The child should have a yearly well-child visit including a first-morning protein-to-creatinine ratio and blood pressure check.

A child who excretes more than 1 g of protein every 24 hours, in whom the cause is not orthostatic proteinuria, should have a kidney biopsy. Prolonged proteinuria can cause glomerular scarring and accelerate progression of CKD.

HEMOLYTIC–UREMIC SYNDROME

HUS is the most common cause of acute renal failure in children younger than age 5 years (Keir et al., 2012). The disease itself is characterized by hemolytic anemia with fragmented red blood cells and thrombocytopenia. The specific renal pathology is thrombotic microangiopathy, in which platelet–fibrin thrombi form in the kidneys. Typically, children present in renal failure as a result of the disease.

Assessment

Childhood HUS can be divided into two entities: according to clinical presentation and outcomes. About 90% of HUS cases in children have a prodromal illness involving diarrhea caused by Shiga toxin–producing *E. coli*—typically, O157 (Keir et al., 2012). Prognosis is generally good, although lethargy, oliguria, dehydration, and high WBC count ($>20 \times 100$ cells/L) and hematocrit levels ($>23\%$) upon presentation are associated with mortality (Oakes et al., 2006). Death occurs in up to 5% of cases, and 25% of survivors develop CKD, proteinuria, or hypertension (Keir et al., 2012). The second category, children with no diarrheal prodrome, encompasses a heterogeneous group of disorders, and prognosis is often

poor (Waters et al., 2007; Zimmerhackl et al., 2006). Some are caused by genetic mutations that predispose to HUS, such as mutations in complement regulatory proteins (Sellier-Leclerc et al., 2007). HUS may also be associated with infections caused by *Streptococcus pneumoniae* (Waters et al., 2007).

From 5 to 10 days after onset of the prodromal illness, HUS begins, with the child manifesting a sudden onset of pallor, bruising or purpura, irritability, and oliguria. The child usually has a slight fever, anorexia, abdominal pain, vomiting, watery and blood-stained diarrhea, and mild jaundice. Signs of circulatory overload also may occur. With central nervous system involvement, lethargy and seizures develop (Clinical Judgment 19-4). Between days 4 and 7, renal manifestations peak and can range from mild renal insufficiency to AKI that requires dialysis.

 A L E R T *Immediately refer a child with vomiting and watery, bloody diarrhea who develops purpura or pallor to the primary health care provider for workup for HUS.*

Interdisciplinary Interventions

Supportive therapy should begin early (see the Point for Care Paths: An Interdisciplinary Plan of Care for the Child With Acute Renal Failure Resulting From Hemolytic–Uremic Syndrome). Frequent dialysis and transfusions of packed red blood cells to maintain the hemoglobin level usually result in recovery. For survivors, screening for microalbuminuria may facilitate early recognition of renal sequelae and intervention. Children who develop CKD are managed accordingly.

Community Care

Educate families about the importance of cooking meat fully because HUS may be transmitted in undercooked ground beef containing *E. coli* bacteria. Also, reinforce good hand hygiene to reduce fecal–oral contamination and transmission of *E. coli* bacteria.

POSTINFECTIOUS GLOMERULONEPHRITIS

Acute PIGN, previously called acute poststreptococcal glomerulonephritis, is one of the most common acute renal syndromes. PIGN is most commonly caused by group A streptococci but can be caused by other organisms including other strains of streptococci (groups C and G), staphylococci, gram-negative bacilli, mycobacteria, parasites, fungi, and viruses The child has symptoms of varying severity after infection.

Pathophysiology

PIGN results from the immune response to antigens, with circulating immune complexes triggering complement and the inflammatory process (Welch, 2012). Biopsy specimens from children with PIGN show that pathologic findings vary with the severity of the disease. Mild cases show minimal to moderate proliferation of mesangial cells and matrix. In severe cases, mesangial

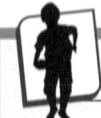

CLINICAL JUDGMENT 19-4

The Child With Hemolytic–Uremic Syndrome

Leo is a 3-year-old with HUS. He presented in the emergency department with a temperature of 100.4° F (38° C); lethargy; vomiting; abdominal pain; and watery, blood-stained diarrhea. His skin is pale, slightly jaundiced, and bruises easily. Within several hours after admission to the hospital, a decision is made to initiate PD. The physician explained the purpose of dialysis and the need for surgery to place a Tenckhoff catheter. As you enter the child's room, the mother is crying and asks, "Is my baby going to die?"

Questions

1. During your health assessment, what additional information would be beneficial to elicit to clarify the diagnosis?

2. Why does Leo's skin appear pale, with slight jaundice, and have evidence of bruising?

3. What should be the focus of your nursing plan of care at this time?

4. What actions would you take to implement your plan?

5. How would you determine that the parents understood the treatment plan?

Answers

1. Has Leo recently had a bacterial or viral illness? HUS is commonly associated with these conditions.

2. Leo is pale as a result of anemia, which results from damaged red blood cells. The jaundice and easy bruising are results of thrombocytopenia.

3. Providing comfort to the parents, addressing the parents' concerns by reemphasizing and clarifying the plan of care as explained by the physician, and determining what other concerns the parents may have

4. Show parents pictures of the Tenckhoff catheter and PD process. Discuss how they can help support their child and hold him during dialysis. Help parents select diversionary activities for their child. Review with parents the clinical indicators that the health care team will be evaluating to determine when kidney function is returning.

5. Parents verbalize that they understand the plan of care, they are able to discuss the plan of care with their child and other family members, and they select activities to keep the child calm and content during dialysis treatments.

---

cell, matrix, and endothelial cell proliferation as well as infiltration with polymorphonuclear cells and monocytes can be so extensive that the capillary lumens are occluded. In fact, severe disease is called *diffuse endocapillary exudative proliferative glomerulonephritis*.

The disease usually runs its course in about 1 month. Prognosis is excellent; more than 95% of children recover completely (Nast, 2012). Serum complement levels may remain low for 12 to 16 weeks. Mild proteinuria may last for several months, and microscopic hematuria may be present for up to a year. In some children with oliguria, rapidly progressive glomerulonephritis develops; in others, chronic glomerulonephritis develops more slowly. In general, children with prolonged proteinuria and an abnormal GFR have a poor prognosis.

Assessment

Severe clinical manifestations may include AKI with sudden onset of gross hematuria, edema, hypertension, and renal insufficiency. However, up to half the children are asymptomatic, with only microscopic hematuria. A typical case might show the sudden onset of mild proteinuria, hematuria, and periorbital edema. The urine is tea or cola colored from the presence of red blood cells. The child is usually irritable and complains of flank or midabdominal pain, general malaise, and fever. Hypertension can cause headache, vomiting, somnolence, and other central nervous system symptoms, including seizures. Fluid overload can cause cardiovascular symptoms such as dyspnea and tachypnea as well as an enlarged, tender liver.

Laboratory testing for serum creatinine, albumin, hemoglobin, hematocrit, and complement levels and urine testing for complete urinalysis and urine protein excretion help identify the presence of disease. Kidney biopsy is the only way to distinguish between the various types of glomerulonephritis. The biopsy specimen is examined by both light microscopy and electron microscopy, and it is stained for immunofluorescence.

Interdisciplinary Interventions

Treatment of acute PIGN is symptom specific. Dietary restrictions of fluid, sodium, and potassium are recommended. Bed rest, antihypertensives, and diuretics are also helpful in treating this condition. Early treatment of streptococcal infections with antibiotics does not always prevent development of the disease, but an evidence review noted some protection (Del Mar et al., 2006). The affected child and all other family members with positive cultures should undergo antibiotic treatment for 10 to 14 days. See "Chronic Kidney Disease" section for information on supportive care for renal sequelae.

HEREDITARY NEPHRITIS (ALPORT SYNDROME)

Of the several types of hereditary glomerulonephritis, Alport syndrome, or hereditary nephritis, is the most common, accounting for approximately 3% of cases of ESRD in children (Kashtan, 1999). Mutations in the genes for type IV collagen, the major constituent of basement membranes, cause this syndrome. About 80% of children have the X-linked form, 15% have an autosomal recessive form, and 5% have an autosomal dominant form (Kashtan et al., 2013).

Pathophysiology

In children younger than age 5 years with Alport syndrome, biopsies are normal except for a few fetal glomeruli. As the child grows older, microscopic changes occur in the glomeruli: mesangial cells and matrix proliferate, capillary walls thicken, and tubules atrophy or dilate. These changes usually start to occur during the teenage years, but presentation of the disease can vary widely. Progression to renal failure may occur.

Assessment

The presenting symptom of Alport syndrome may be a persistent asymptomatic microscopic hematuria or an episode of gross hematuria after an upper respiratory infection. Some children with Alport syndrome have progressive bilateral sensorineural hearing loss, which begins in the high frequencies and progresses to total deafness. Most also have eye disorders, such as whitish or yellowish flecks around the macula and anterior lenticonus.

Interdisciplinary Interventions

For children with hearing or vision loss associated with Alport syndrome, facilitate their obtaining hearing aids and glasses as needed. Genetic counseling helps both the parents and the child make informed reproductive choices in the face of this hereditary disease. If Alport syndrome progresses to ESRD, as it generally does in males, dialysis and transplantation are the usual treatments.

RENAL CALCULI

Renal calculi (urolithiasis) are relatively uncommon in children. They can be broadly classified into three categories, defined by the precipitating condition: infection-related calculi, calculi resulting from a metabolic imbalance, and pharmacologically induced calculi. For more information, see thePoint for Supplemental Information: Renal Calculi.

RENAL TRAUMA

Renal injury usually occurs in conjunction with abdominal trauma, although it can occur as an isolated event. Based on information from the National Electronic Injury Surveillance System, the annual incidence of GU injuries ranged from 25,399 to 33,163, resulting in about 28,000 emergency department visits annually (Tasian et al., 2013). The most common mechanism of injury is falls; injuries are most frequently associated with sporting and exercise equipment, furniture, and clothing items (Tasian et al., 2013). Renal trauma rarely causes death but may compound the effects of other life-threatening injuries. Certain characteristics of the child's renal structure increase its susceptibility to damage. The child's kidney fills proportionately more space in the abdomen compared with the adult organ. Its position is lower in the retroperitoneum, and it is less protected by fat and fascia. Supporting structures have greater elasticity, which allows for excessive renal motion after bodily force. Immature ossification of the encircling ribs further compromises protection to the kidney. Congenital anomalies or an aberrant renal location (e.g., hydronephrosis, fused kidneys, or a pelvic kidney) increase the potential for damage after even minimal force (El-Atat et al., 2011).

Pathophysiology

Blunt abdominal trauma can compress the renal unit against skeletal structures (i.e., ribs or vertebrae), rupturing its surrounding renal capsule or causing a subcapsular hematoma. In situations such as a bicycle–automobile accident, the child's increased kidney motility can create an acceleration–deceleration injury, which can shear or thrombose the vascular attachment site or disrupt the UPJ. Penetrating forces, such as a bullet, knife, or rib, can cause injury by puncturing or shattering a renal segment. Iatrogenic injuries can occur during invasive procedures such as biopsy, tube placement, or stone manipulation.

Most children who sustain renal trauma heal completely, with little or no residual negative sequelae. The child's long-term prognosis more closely depends on the severity of other wounds.

Assessment

Assess any child who sustains a compressing, penetrating, or blunt wound to the abdomen, chest, flank, or spine for renal trauma. Hematuria may be gross or microscopic but is not always diagnostic of renal trauma. Carefully evaluate the liver and spleen, additional potential sources of hematuria. Other indications of renal trauma include tenderness or pain to the flank or upper abdomen, ecchymosis of the trunk, palpable abdominal mass, nausea and vomiting, and hypotension. Elevated BUN and creatinine, oliguria, and anuria that accompany a history of trauma are also indications of severe renal injury.

Diagnosis of renal trauma is best determined by computed tomographic scan, which provides detailed views highlighting organ involvement (Y. J. Lee et al., 2007). Renal injury is classified based on extent of injury: grade I, contusion or subcapsular hematoma; grade II, shallow cortical laceration or confined perirenal hematoma; grade III, deep cortical injury without extension into the medulla; grade IV, laceration extending into the medulla and collection system or a vascular injury; and grade V, shattered kidney or avulsion of the renal hilum, which devascularizes the kidney (Moore et al., 1989). This classification system has useful predictive value for management, need for surgical intervention, and follow-up care.

Interdisciplinary Interventions

Emergency care and stabilization is the first priority for the child with multiorgan trauma. After this goal is accomplished, results of the renal computed tomographic scan direct management of this injury. Reattachment of renal vessels or the ureter, evacuation of blood clots, and closure of renal lacerations are surgical goals for major injuries that involve the collecting system or major blood vessels and branches with hemodynamic instability.

Conservative treatment, the management of choice, historically required bed rest; however, early ambulation as tolerated is being studied (Aguayo et al., 2010). The child is hospitalized, and fluids are increased by IV therapy or by mouth if tolerated. Monitor urine for volume and degree of hematuria and vital signs for indications of hemorrhage and shock. Fever can be treated with increased fluids and antipyretics. Control discomfort by implementing pain interventions such as medications, positioning the child to keep pressure off the affected site, and applying ice packs to the affected area. Diversional activities are extremely important during this phase because resolution of gross hematuria may require confinement of a week or longer. The healing progress is monitored by computed tomographic scans, and hospital discharge is considered when gross hematuria fades. Outpatient follow-up with activity restrictions continues until microscopic hematuria disappears.

When conservative treatment is chosen, monitor the child for the following complications: infection, persistent or recurring bleeding, perirenal bleeding or hematuria, urinary leakage or obstruction, or renal necrosis. Be alert for changes in vital signs, decreased urine output, increasing level of hematuria, or increased flank or abdominal pain, all of which are clues to potential problems.

Community Care

At discharge from the hospital, review with the family the need for long-term follow-up. Late complications include hydronephrosis, hypertension, renal atrophy, or AVF or aneurysm, conditions that generally develop slowly and silently. Blood pressure monitoring should occur periodically during the ensuing year to monitor for hypertension. For the child who underwent a nephrectomy or who has a severely compromised residual kidney, restriction from contact sports may be prudent as well as legally mandated, although review of the evidence demonstrates that cycling causes more than three times more kidney injuries than football and that such restriction may be unwarranted (Grinsell et al., 2006). Focus child and family counseling around acceptable low-impact sports and help plan the child's physical education program at school, in daycare, or in extracurricular sports settings.

See thePoint for a summary of Key Concepts

REFERENCES

Afshar, K., Stothers, L., Scott, H. et al. (2011). Cranberry juice for the prevention of pediatric urinary tract infection: A randomized controlled trial. *Journal of Urology*, *188*(4)(Suppl.), 1584–1587.

Aguayo, P., Fraser, J. D., Sharp, S. et al. (2010). Nonoperative management of blunt renal injury: A need for further study. *Journal of Pediatric Surgery*, *45*(6), 1311–1314.

Akcan-Arikan, A., Zappitelli, M., Loftis, L. L. et al. (2007). Modified RIFLE criteria in critically ill children with acute kidney injury. *Kidney International*, *71*(10), 1028–1035.

Aksu, N., Yavascan, O., Anil, M. et al. (2007). A ten-year single-centre experience in children on chronic peritoneal dialysis—Significance of percutaneous placement of peritoneal dialysis catheters. *Nephrology Dialysis Transplantation*, *22*(7), 2045–2051.

Alexopoulos, E. I., Kostadima, E., Pagonari, I. et al. (2006). Association between primary nocturnal enuresis and habitual snoring in children. *Urology*, *68*, 406–409.

Allen, H. A., Austin, J. C., Boyt, M. A. et al. (2007). Initial trial of timed voiding is warranted for all children with daytime incontinence. *Urology*, *69*, 962–965.

Alsaywid, B. S., Saleh, H., Deshpande, A. et al. (2010). High grade primary vesicoureteral reflux in boys: Long-term results of a prospective cohort study. *Journal of Urology*, *184*(Suppl. 4), 1598–1603.

American Academy of Pediatrics. (1996). Timing of elective surgery on the genitalia of male children with particular reference to the risks, benefits, and psychological effects of surgery and anesthesia. *Pediatrics*, *97*(4), 590–594.

American Academy of Pediatrics, Task Force on Circumcision. (2012a). Circumcision policy statement. *Pediatrics*, *130*(3), 585–586.

American Academy of Pediatrics, Task Force on Circumcision. (2012b). Male circumcision. *Pediatrics*, *130*(3), e756–e785.

Aridogan, I. A., Ilkit, M., Izol, V. et al. (2009). Glans penis and prepuce colonisation of yeast fungi in a paediatric population: Pre- and postcircumcision results. *Mycoses*, *52*(1), 49–52.

Auvert, B., Taljaard, D., Lagarde, E. et al. (2005). Randomized, controlled intervention trial of male circumcision for reduction of HIV infection risk: The ANRS 1265 trial. *PLoS Med*, *2*(11), e298.

Bader, G., Nevéus, T., Kruse, S. et al. (2002). Sleep of primary enuretic children and controls. *Sleep*, *25*, 579–583.

Bailey, R. C., Moses, S., Parker, C. B. et al. (2007). Male circumcision for HIV prevention in young men in Kisumu, Kenya: A randomised controlled trial. *Lancet*, *369*, 643–656.

Bakkaloglu, S. A. (2009). Prevention of peritonitis in children: Emerging concepts. *Peritoneal Dialysis International*, *29*(Suppl. 2), S186–S189.

Baldwin, S. B., Wallace, D. R., Papenfuss, M. R. et al. (2004). Condom use and other factors affecting penile human papillomavirus detection in men attending a sexually transmitted disease clinic. *Sexually Transmitted Diseases*, *31*, 601–607.

Basu, R., Devarajan. P., Wong, H. et al. (2011). An update and review of acute kidney injury in pediatrics. *Pediatric Critical Care Medicine*, *12*(3), 339–347.

Ben Chaim, J., Livne, P. M., Binyamini, J. et al. (2005). Complications of circumcision in Israel: A one year multicenter study. *Israel Medical Association Journal*, *7*, 368–370.

Bisceglia, M., Galliani, C., Senger, C. et al. (2006). Renal cystic diseases: A review. *Advances in Anatomic Pathology*, *13*, 26–56.

Bitsori, M., & Galanakis, E. (2012). Pediatric urinary tract infections: Diagnosis and treatment. *Expert Review of Anti-infective therapy*, *10*(10), 1153–1164.

Boots, B. K., & Edmundson, E. E. (2010). A controlled randomized trial comparing single to multiple application lidocaine analgesia in pediatric patients undergoing urethral catheterization procedures. *Journal of Clinical Nursing*, *19*(5–6), 744–748.

Bower, W. F., Sit, F. K., & Yeung, C. K. (2006). Nocturnal enuresis in adolescents and adults is associated with childhood elimination symptoms. *Journal of Urology*, *176*, 1771–1775.

Boyer, O., Gagnadoux, M. F., Guest, G. et al. (2007). Prognosis of autosomal dominant polycystic kidney disease diagnosed in utero or at birth. *Pediatric Nephrology*, *22*, 380–388.

Bray, L., & Sanders, C. (2007). Teaching children and young people intermittent self-catheterization. *Urologic Nursing*, *27*, 203–209.

British Medical Association. (2004). The law and ethics of male circumcision: Guidance for doctors. *Journal of Medical Ethics*, *30*(3), 259–263.

Butler, R. J., Golding, J., Heron, J. et al. (2005). Nocturnal enuresis: A survey of parental coping strategies at 71\2 years. *Child: Care, Health and Development*, 31(6), 659–667.

Canadian Paediatric Society, Fetus and Newborn Committee. (1996). Neonatal circumcision revisited. *Canadian Medical Association Journal*, 154(6), 769–780.

Castellsagué, X., Peeling, R. W., Franceschi, S. et al. (2005). *Chlamydia trachomatis* infection in female partners of circumcised and uncircumcised adult men. *American Journal of Epidemiology*, 162, 907–916.

Cathcart, P., Nuttall, M., van der Meulen, J. et al. (2006). Trends in paediatric circumcision and its complications in England between 1997 and 2003. *British Journal of Surgery*, 93, 885–890.

Chen, M., Cheng, H., & Chio, Y. (2013). Risk factors for renal scarring and deterioration of renal function in primary vesico-ureteral reflux children: A long-term follow-up retrospective cohort study. *PLoS One*, 8(2), e57954.

Choi, W. S., & Kim, S. W. (2013). Current issues in varicocele management: A review. *The World Journal of Men's Health*, 31(1), 12–20.

Collins, S., Upshaw, J., Rutchik, S. et al. (2002). Effects of circumcision on male sexual function: Debunking a myth? *Journal of Urology*, 167, 2111–2112.

Conway, P. H., Cnaan, A., Zaoutis, T. et al. (2007). Recurrent urinary tract infections in children: Risk factors and association with prophylactic antimicrobials. *Journal of the American Medical Association*, 298, 179–186.

Cooper, C. S. (2012). Individualizing management of vesicoureteral reflux. *Nephro-Urology Monthly*, 4(3), 530–534.

Culleton, B. F., & Asola, M. R. (2011). The impact of short daily and nocturnal hemodialysis on quality of life, cardiovascular risk and survival. *Journal of Nephrology*, 24(4), 405–415.

Cutting, D. A., Pallant, J. F., & Cutting, F. M. (2007). Nocturnal enuresis: Application of evidence-based medicine in community practice. *Journal of Paediatrics and Child Health*, 43, 167–172.

DaJusta, D. G., Granberg, C. F., Villanueva, C. et al. (2012). Contemporary review of testicular torsion: New concepts, emerging technologies and potential therapeutics. *Journal of Pediatric Urology*. Advance online publication.

Daling, J. R., Madeleine, M. M., Johnson, L. G. et al. (2005). Penile cancer: Importance of circumcision, human papillomavirus and smoking in in situ and invasive disease. *International Journal of Cancer*, 116, 606–616.

Davis, M. A., Gray, R. H., Grabowski, M. K. et al. (2013). Male circumcision decreases high-risk human papillomavirus viral load in female partners: A randomized trial in Rakai, Uganda. *International Journal of Cancer*. Advance online publication.

Del Mar, C. B., Glasziou, P. P., & Spinks, A. B. (2006). Antibiotics for sore throat. *Cochrane Database of Systematic Reviews*, (4), CD000023.

Diamond, D. A., Gargollo, P. C., & Caldamone, A. A. (2011). Current management principles for adolescent varicocele. *Fertility and Sterility*, 96(6), 1294–1298.

Dickerman, J. D. (2007). Circumcision in the time of HIV: When is there enough evidence to revise the American Academy of Pediatrics' policy on circumcision? *Pediatrics*, 119, 1006–1007.

Drain, P. K., Halperin, D. T., Hughes, J. P. et al. (2006). Male circumcision, religion, and infectious diseases: An ecologic analysis of 118 developing countries. *BMC Infectious Diseases*, 6, 172.

El-Atat, R., Derouiche, A., Slama, M. R. et al. (2011). Kidney trauma with underlying renal pathology: Is conservative management sufficient? *Saudi Journal of Kidney Diseases and Transplantation*, 22(6), 1175–1180.

El-Hefnawy, A. S., Helmy, T., El-Assmy, M. M. et al. (2012). Doxazosin versus tizanidine for treatment of dysfunctional voiding in children: A prospective randomized open-labeled trial. *Urology*, 79(2), 428–433.

Etoubleau, C., Reveret, M., Brouet, P. et al. (2009). Moving from bag to catheter for urine collection in non-toilet-trained children suspected of having urinary tract infection: A paired comparison of urine cultures. *Journal of Pediatrics*, 154(6), 803–806.

Feldman, A., & Bauer, S. (2006). Diagnosis and management of dysfunctional voiding. *Pediatrics*, 18, 139–147.

Fergusson, D. M., Boden, J. M., & Horwood, L. J. (2006). Circumcision status and risk of sexually transmitted infection in young adult males: An analysis of a longitudinal birth cohort. *Pediatrics*, 118, 1971–1977.

Fine, R. G., & Poppas, D. P. (2012). Varicocele: Standard and alternative indications for repair. *Current Opinion in Urology*, 22(6), 513–516.

Finnell, S. M. E., Carroll, A. E., Downs, S. M. et al. (2011). Diagnosis and management of an initial UTI in febrile infants and young children. *Pediatrics*, 128(3), e749–e770.

Firoozi, F., Batniji, R., Aslan, A. R. et al. (2006). Resolution of diurnal incontinence and nocturnal enuresis after adenotonsillectomy in children. *Journal of Urology*, 175, 1885–1888.

Fischbach, M., Fothergill, H., Zaloszyc, A. et al. (2011). Intensified daily dialysis: The best chronic dialysis option for children? *Seminars in Dialysis*, 24(6), 640–644.

O'Flynn, N. (2011). Nocturnal enuresis in children and young people: NICE clinical guideline. *British Journal of General Practice*, 61(586), 360–362.

Fonseca, F. F., Tanno, F. Y., & Nguyen, H. T. (2012). Current options in the management of primary vesicoureteral reflux in children. *Pediatric Clinics of North America*, 59(4), 819–834.

Fortenberry, J. D., Paden, M. L., & Goldstein, S. L. (2013). Acute kidney injury in children: An update on diagnosis and treatment. *Pediatric Clinics of North America*, 60(3), 669–688.

Franco, I., von Gontard, A., & De Gennaro, M. (2013). Evaluation and treatment of nonmonosymptomatic nocturnal enuresis: A standardization document from the International Children's Continence Society. *Journal of Pediatric Urology*, 9(2), 234–243.

Furth, S. L., Cole, S. R., Moxey-Mims, M. et al. (2006). Design and methods of the Chronic Kidney Disease in Children (CKiD) prospective cohort study. *Clinical Journal of the American Society of Nephrology*, 1, 1006–1015.

Garin, E. H., Olavarria, F., Nieto, V. G. et al. (2006). Clinical significance of primary vesicoureteral reflux and urinary antibiotic prophylaxis after acute pyelonephritis: A multicenter, randomized, controlled study. *Pediatrics*, 117, 626–632.

Garry, D. L., Swoboda, E., Elimian, A. et al. (2006). A video study of pain relief during newborn male circumcision. *Journal of Perinatology*, 26(2), 106–110.

Gipson, D. S., Messer, K. L., Tran, C. L. et al. (2013). Inpatient health care utilization in the United States among children, adolescents, and young adults with nephrotic syndrome. *American Journal of Kidney Diseases*, 61(6), 910–917.

Glazener, C. M. A., Evans, J. H. C., & Peto, R. E. (2008). Complex behavioural and educational interventions for nocturnal enuresis in children. *Cochrane Database of Systematic Reviews*, (1), CD004668.

Goilav, B., Norton, K. I., Satlin, L. M. et al. (2006). Predominant extrahepatic biliary disease in autosomal recessive polycystic kidney disease: A new association. *Pediatric Transplantation*, 10, 294–298.

Goldstein, S. L. (2007). Advances in renal replacement therapy as a bridge to renal transplantation. *Pediatric Transplantation*, 11(5), 463–470.

Goldstein, S. L. (2011). Advances in pediatric renal replacement therapy for acute kidney injury. *Seminars In Dialysis*, 24(2), 187–191.

González Celedón, C., Bitsori, M., & Tullus, K. (2007). Progression of chronic renal failure in children with dysplastic kidneys. *Pediatric Nephrology*, 22, 1014–1020.

Gormley, A., Fishwick, J., & Whinall, B. (2007). Home dressing removal following hypospadias repair. *Journal of Child Health Care*, 11, 158–166.

Gray, R. H., Kigozi, G., Serwadda, D. et al. (2007). Male circumcision for HIV prevention in men in Rakai, Uganda: A randomised trial. *Lancet*, 369, 657–678.

Grinsell, M. M., Showalter, S., Gordon, K. A. et al. (2006). Single kidney and sports participation: Perception versus reality. *Pediatrics*, 118(3), 1019–1127.

Groth, T. W., & Mitchell, M. E. (2012). Ureteropelvic junction obstruction. In A. G. Coran, N. S. Adzick, T. M. Krummel et al. (Eds.), *Pediatric surgery* (7th ed., pp. 1411–1425). Philadelphia, PA: Elsevier Saunders.

Guerra, L. A., Pike, J., Milks, J. et al. (2006). Outcome in patients who underwent tethered cord release for occult spinal dysraphism. *Journal of Urology, 176,* 1729–1732.

Gulati, S. (2012). Acute kidney injury in children. *Clinical Queries: Nephrology, 1*(1), 103–108.

Habib, S. (2012). Highlights for management of a child with a urinary tract infection. *International Journal of Pediatrics, 2012,* 943653.

Hajnovic, L., & Trnka, J. (2007). Tethered spinal cord syndrome: The importance of time for outcomes. *European Journal of Pediatric Surgery, 17,* 190–193.

Hladunewich, M. A., & Schaefer, F. (2011). Proteinuria in special populations: Pregnant women and children. *Advances in Chronic Kidney Disease, 18*(4), 276–272.

Hodson, E., Willis, N., & Craig, J. (2010). Corticosteroid therapy for nephrotic syndrome in children. *Cochrane Database of Systematic Reviews,* (4), CD001533.

Holmdahl, G., Sillén, U., Abrahamsson, K. et al. (2007). Self-catheterization during adolescence. *Scandinavian Journal of Urology and Nephrology, 41*(3), 214–217.

Howell, A. B. (2007). Bioactive compounds in cranberries and their role in prevention of urinary tract infections. *Molecular Nutrition & Food Research, 51,* 732–737.

Jain, S., Suarez, A. A., McGuire, J. et al. (2007). Expression profiles of congenital renal dysplasia reveal new insights into renal development and disease. *Pediatric Nephrology, 22,* 962–974.

Jansson, U. B., Hanson, M., Sillén, U. et al. (2005). Voiding pattern and acquisition of bladder control from birth to age 6 years: A longitudinal study. *Journal of Urology, 174,* 289–293.

Jayachandran, D., Bythell, M., Ward Platt, M. et al. (2011). Register based study of bladder exstrophy-epispadias complex: Prevalence, associated anomalies, prenatal diagnosis and survival. *Journal of Urology, 186*(5), 2056–2061.

Jepson, R. G., Mihaljevic, L., & Craig, J. C. (2010). Cranberries for treating urinary tract infections. *Cochrane Database of Systematic Reviews,* (4), CD001322.

Jepson, R. G., Williams, G., & Craig, J. C. (2012). Cranberries for preventing urinary tract infections. *Cochrane Database of Systematic Reviews,* (10), CD001321.

Jerardi, K. E., Auger, K. A., Shah, S. S. et al. (2012). Discordant antibiotic therapy and length of stay in children hospitalized for urinary tract infection. *Journal of Hospital Medicine, 7*(8), 622–627.

Joinson, C., Heron, J., Butler, R. et al. (2007). A United Kingdom population-based study of intellectual capacities in children with and without soiling, daytime wetting, and bed-wetting. *Pediatrics, 120,* e308–e316.

Joinson, C., Heron, J., Emond, A. et al. (2007). Psychological problems in children with bedwetting and combined (day and night) wetting: A UK population-based study. *Journal of Pediatric Psychology, 32,* 605–616.

Karacan, C., Erkek, N., Senel S. et al. (2010). Evaluation of urine collection methods for the diagnosis of urinary tract infection in children. *Medical Principles and Practice, 19*(3), 188–191.

Kashtan, C. E. (1999). Alport syndrome: An inherited disorder of renal, ocular, and cochlear basement membranes. *Medicine, 78,* 338–360.

Kashtan, C. E., Ding, J., Gregory, M. et al. (2013). Clinical practice recommendations for the treatment of Alport syndrome: A statement of the Alport Syndrome Research Collaborative. *Pediatric Nephrology, 28*(1), 5–11.

Kasirga, E., Akil, I., Yilmaz, O. et al. (2006). Evaluation of voiding dysfunctions in children with chronic functional constipation. *Turkish Journal of Pediatrics, 48,* 340–343.

Keir, L. S., Marks, S. D., & Kim, J. J. (2012). Shigatoxin-associated hemolytic uremic syndrome: Current molecular mechanisms and future therapies. *Drug Design, Development and Therapy, 6,* 195–208.

Kibar, Y., Ors, O., Demir, E. et al. (2007). Results of biofeedback treatment on reflux resolution rates in children with dysfunctional voiding and vesicoureteral reflux. *Urology, 70,* 563–566.

Kontiokari, T., Salo, J., Eerola, E. et al. (2005). Cranberry juice and bacterial colonization in children: A placebo-controlled randomized trial. *Clinical Nutrition, 24,* 1065–1072.

Krieger, J. N., Bailey, R. C., Opeya, J. C. et al. (2007). Adult male circumcision outcomes: Experience in a developing country setting. *Urology International, 78,* 235–240.

Krishnan, R. G. (2012). Nephrotic syndrome. *Paediatrics and Child Health, 22*(8), 337–340.

Lau, A. Y., Wong, S. N., Yip, K. T. et al. (2007). A comparative study on bacterial cultures of urine samples obtained by clean-void technique versus urethral catheterization. *Acta Paediatrica, 96*(3), 432–466.

Lebowitz, R. L., Olbing, H., Parkkulainen, K. V. et al. (1985). International system of radiographic grading of vesicoureteric reflux. *Pediatric Radiology, 15*(2), 105–109.

Lee, B. B., Haran, M. J., Hunt, L. M. et al. (2007). Spinal-injured neuropathic bladder antisepsis (SINBA) trial. *Spinal Cord, 45*(8), 542–550.

Lee, P. A., & Houk, C. P. (2013). Cryptorchidism. *Current Opinion in Endocrinology, Diabetes, & Obesity, 20*(3), 210–216.

Lee, R. B. (2006). Filipino experience of ritual male circumcision: Knowledge and insights for anti-circumcision advocacy. *Culture, Health & Sexuality, 8,* 225–234.

Lee, Y. J., Oh, S. N., Rha, S. E. et al. (2007). Renal trauma. *Radiologic Clinics of North America, 45,* 581–592.

Liu, C. M., Hungate, B. A., Tobian, A. A. R. et al. (2013). Male circumcision significantly reduces prevalence and load of genital anaerobic bacteria. *mBio, 4*(2), e00076-e13.

Liu, Y., Black, M. A., Caron, L. et al. (2006). Role of cranberry juice on molecular-scale surface characteristics and adhesion behavior of *Escherichia coli. Biotechnology and Bioengineering, 93,* 297–305.

Ludwikowski, B., & González, R. (2013). The controversy regarding the need for hormonal treatment in boys with unilateral cryptorchidism goes on: A review of the literature. *European Journal of Pediatrics, 172*(1), 5–8.

Malone, P. S. (2005). Circumcision for preventing urinary tract infection in boys: European view. *Archives of Disease in Childhood, 90,* 773–774.

Mattoo, T. K. (2007). Medical management of vesicoureteral reflux. *Pediatric Nephrology, 22,* 1113–1120.

McMurdo, M. E., Bissett, L. Y., Price, R. J. et al. (2005). Does ingestion of cranberry juice reduce symptomatic urinary tract infections in older people in hospital? A double-blind, placebo-controlled trial. *Age and Ageing, 34,* 256–261.

Meissner, O., & Buso, D. L. (2007). Traditional male circumcision in the Eastern Cape: Scourge or blessing? *South African Medical Journal, 97,* 371–373.

Merriman, L. S., Herrel, L., & Kirsch, A. J. (2012). Inguinal and genital anomalies. *Pediatric Clinics of North America, 59*(4), 769–781.

Moore, E. E., Shackford, S. R., Pachter, H. L. et al. (1989). Organ injury scaling: Spleen, liver, and kidney. *Journal of Trauma, 29,* 1664–1666.

Morris, B. J., Bailis, S. A., Castellsague, X. et al. (2006). RACP's policy statement on infant male circumcision is ill-conceived. *Australian and New Zealand Journal of Public Health, 30,* 16–22.

Morris, B. J., & Wiswell, T. E. (2013). Circumcision and lifetime risk of urinary tract infection: A systematic review and meta-analysis. *Journal of Urology, 189*(6), 2118–2124.

Mularoni, P. P., Cohen, L. L., DeGuzman, M. et al. (2009). A randomized control trial of lidocaine gel for reducing infant distress during urinary catheterization. *Pediatric Emergency Care, 25*(7), 439–443.

Nast, C. C. (2012). Infection related glomerulonephritis: Changing demographics and outcomes. *Advances in Chronic Kidney Disease, 19*(2), 68–75.

National Kidney Foundation. (2002). K/DOQI clinical practice guidelines for chronic kidney disease: Evaluation classification and stratification. *American Journal of Kidney Diseases*, *39*(Suppl. 1), S1–S266.

National Kidney Foundation. (2006). KDOQI clinical practice guidelines and clinical practice recommendations 2006 updates: Hemodialysis adequacy, peritoneal dialysis adequacy and vascular access. *American Journal of Kidney Diseases*, *48*(Suppl. 1), S1–S322.

Nevéus, T. (2011). Nocturnal enuresis—Theoretic background and practical guidelines. *Pediatric Nephrology*, *26*(8), 1207–1214.

Oakes, R. S., Siegler, R. L., McReynolds, M. A. et al. (2006). Predictors of fatality in postdiarrheal hemolytic uremic syndrome. *Pediatrics*, *117*, 1656–1662.

Okeke, L. I., Asinobi, A. A., & Ikuerowo, O. S. (2006). Epidemiology of complications of male circumcision in Ibadan, Nigeria. *BMC Urology*, *6*, 21.

Oreskovic, N. M., & Sembrano, E. U. (2007). Repeat urine cultures in children who are admitted with urinary tract infections. *Pediatrics*, *119*, e325–e329.

Ozden, C., Ozdal, O. L., Altinova, S. et al. (2007). Prevalence and associated factors of enuresis in Turkish children. *International Brazilian Journal of Urology*, *33*, 216–222.

Patel, H. P., Goldstein, S. L., Mahan, J. D. et al. (2007). A standard, noninvasive monitoring of hematocrit algorithm improves blood pressure control in pediatric hemodialysis patients. *Clinical Journal of the American Society of Nephrology*, *2*, 252–257.

Pinto, K. (2012). Circumcision controversies. *Pediatric Clinics of North America*, *59*(4), 977–986.

Plank, R. M., Makhema, J., Kebaabetswe, P. et al. (2009). Acceptability of infant male circumcision as part of HIV prevention and male reproductive health efforts in Gaborone, Botswana, and surrounding areas. *Aids Behavior*, *14*, 1198–1202.

Provencio-Vasquez, E., & Rodriguez, A. (2009). Circumcision revisited. *Journal of the Society of Pediatric Nephrology*, *14*(4), 295–300.

Radhakrishnan, J., & Kiryluk, K. (2006). Acute renal failure outcomes in children and adults. *Kidney International*, *69*, 17–19.

Rashman, M. M., Azad, K., Ahmed, N. et al. (2006). Spot morning urine protein creatinine ratio and 24 hour urinary total protein excretion rate. *Mymensingh Medical Journal*, *15*, 146–149.

Richters, J., Smith, A. M., de Visser, R. O. et al. (2006). Circumcision in Australia: Prevalence and effects on sexual health. *International Journal of STD & AIDS*, *17*, 547–554.

Roberts, K. B. & Subcommittee on Urinary Tract Infection, Steering Committee on Quality Improvement and Management. (2011). Urinary tract infection: Clinical practice guideline for the diagnosis and management of the initial UTI in febrile infants and children 2 to 24 months. *Pediatrics*, *128*(3), 595–610.

Royal Australasian College of Physicians. (2010). *Circumcision of infant males*. Sydney, Australia: Author.

Salo, J., Uhari, M., Helminen, M. et al. (2012). Cranberry juice for the prevention of recurrences of urinary tract infections in children: A randomized placebo-controlled trial. *Clinical Infectious Diseases*, *54*(3), 340–346.

Schachter, A. D. (2004). The pediatric nephrotic syndrome spectrum: Clinical homogeneity and molecular heterogeneity. *Pediatric Transplantation*, *8*, 344–348.

Schlager, T. A., Anderson, S., Trudell, J. et al. (1999). Effect of cranberry juice on bacteriuria in children with neurogenic bladder receiving intermittent catheterization. *Journal of Pediatrics*, *135*, 698–702.

Schneider, M. S., King, L. R., & Surwit, R. S. (1994). Kegel exercises and childhood incontinence: A new role for an old treatment. *Journal of Pediatrics*, *124*, 91–92.

Schoen, E. J. (2006). Ignoring evidence of circumcision benefits. *Pediatrics*, *118*, 385–387.

Schwaderer, A. L., Bates, C. M., McHugh, K. M. et al. (2007). Renal anomalies in family members of infants with bilateral renal agenesis/adysplasia. *Pediatric Nephrology*, *22*, 52–56.

Sebestyen, J. F., & Warady, B. A. (2011). Advances in pediatric renal replacement therapy. *Advances in Chronic Kidney Disease*, *18*(5), 376–383.

Sellier-Leclerc, A. L., Fremeaux-Bacchi, V., Dragon-Durey, M. A. et al. (2007). Differential impact of complement mutations on clinical characteristics in atypical hemolytic uremic syndrome. *Journal of the American Society of Nephrology*, *18*, 2392–2400.

Senkul, T., Iseri, C., Sen, B. et al. (2004). Circumcision in adults: Effect on sexual function. *Urology*, *63*, 155–158.

Shaikh, N., Morone, N. E., Bost, J. E. et al. (2008). Prevalence of urinary tract infection in childhood: A meta-analysis. *Pediatric Infectious Disease Journal*, *27*(4), 302–308.

Shibata, S., & Nagata, M. (2003). Pathogenesis of human renal dysplasia: An alternative scenario to the major theories. *Pediatrics International*, *45*, 605–609.

Siegfried, N., Muller, M., Deeks, J. et al. (2005). HIV and male circumcision: A systematic review with assessment of the quality of studies. *Lancet Infectious Diseases*, *5*, 165–173.

Siegfried, N., Muller, M., Volmink, J. et al. (2003). Male circumcision for prevention of heterosexual acquisition of HIV in men. *Cochrane Database of Systematic Reviews*, (3), CD003362.

Simforoosh, N., Tabibi, A., Khalili, S. A. et al. (2012). Neonatal circumcision reduces the incidence of asymptomatic urinary tract infection: A large prospective study with long-term follow up using Plastibell. *Journal of Pediatric urology*, *8*(3), 320–323.

Singh-Grewal, D., Macdessi, J., & Craig, J. (2005). Circumcision for the prevention of urinary tract infection in boys: A systematic review of randomised trials and observational studies. *Archives of Disease in Childhood*, *90*, 853–858.

Smith, J. M., Stablein, D. M., Munoz, R. et al. (2007). Contributions of the Transplant Registry: The 2006 Annual Report of the North American Pediatric Renal Trials and Collaborative Studies (NAPRTCS). *Pediatric Transplantation*, *11*, 366–373.

Spencer, J. D., Schwaderer, A., McHugh, K. et al. (2010). Pediatric urinary tract infections: An analysis of hospitalizations, charges, and costs in the USA. *Pediatric Nephrology*, *25*(12), 2469–2475.

Stapleton, A. E., Dziura, J., Hooton, T. M. et al. (2012). Recurrent urinary tract infection and urinary Escherichia coli in women ingesting cranberry juice daily: A randomized controlled trial. *Mayo Clinic Proceedings*, *87*(2), 143–150.

Steadman, B., & Ellsworth, P. (2006). To circ or not to circ: Indications, risks, and alternatives to circumcision in the pediatric population with phimosis. *Urologic Nursing*, *26*, 181–194.

Stein, R. (2012). Hypospadias. *European Urology Supplements*, *11*(2), 33–45.

Tasian, G. E., Bagga, H. S., Fisher, P. B. et al. (2013). Pediatric genitourinary injuries in the United States from 2002 to 2010. *Journal of Urology*, *189*(1), 288–293.

Tekgül, S., Riedmiller, H., Hoebeke, P. et al. (2012). EAU guidelines on vesicoureteral reflux in children. *European Urology*, *62*(3), 534–542.

Torres, V. E., & Harris, P. C. (2006). Mechanisms of disease: Autosomal dominant and recessive polycystic kidney disease. *Nature Clinical Practice Nephrology*, *2*, 40–55.

Torres, V. E., Harris, P. C., & Pirson, Y. (2007). Autosomal dominant polycystic kidney disease. *Lancet*, *369*, 1287–1301.

Tosif, S., Baker, A, Oakley, E. et al. (2012). Contamination rates of different collections methods for the diagnosis of urinary tract infections in young children: An observational cohort study. *Journal of Paediatrics and Child Health*, *48*(8), 659–664.

Trabert, B., Zugna, D., Richiardi, L. et al. (2013). Congenital malformations and testicular germ cell tumors. *International Journal of Cancer*. Advance online publication.

Turner, A. N., Morrison, C. S., Padian, N. S. et al. (2007). Men's circumcision status and women's risk of HIV acquisition in Zimbabwe and Uganda. *AIDS*, *21*, 1779–1789.

van Diepen, A. T., Tomlinson, G. A., & Jassal, S. V. (2012). The association between exit site infection and subsequent peritonitis among peritoneal dialysis patients. *Clinical Journal of the American Society of nephrology, 7*(8), 1266–1271.

Van Hoecke, E., Baeyens, D., Vande Walle, J. et al. (2003). Socioeconomic status as a common factor underlying the association between enuresis and psychopathology. *Journal of Developmental and Behavioral Pediatrics, 24,* 109–114.

Van Hoecke, E., De Fruyt, F., De Clercq, B. et al. (2006). Internalizing and externalizing problem behavior in children with nocturnal and diurnal enuresis: A five-factor model perspective. *Journal of Pediatric Psychology, 31,* 460–468.

Verrina, E., Cappelli, V., & Perfumo, F. (2009). Selection of modalities, prescription, and technical issues in children on peritoneal dialysis. *Pediatric Nephrology, 24*(8),1453–1464.

Wang, C. H., Fang, C. C., Chen, N. C. et al. (2012). Cranberry-containing products for prevention of urinary tract infections in susceptible populations: A systematic review and meta-analysis of randomized controlled trials. *Archives of Internal Medicine, 172*(13), 988–996.

Warady, B. A., Bakkaloglu, S., Newland, J. et al. (2012). Consensus guidelines for the prevention and treatment of catheter-related infections and peritonitis in pediatric patients receiving peritoneal dialysis: 2012 update. *Peritoneal Dialysis International, 32*(Suppl. 2), S32–S86.

Ward-Smith, P., & Barry, D. (2006). The challenge of treating enuresis. *Urology Nursing, 26,* 222–224.

Waters, A. M., Kerecuk, L., Luk, D. et al. (2007). Hemolytic uremic syndrome associated with invasive pneumococcal disease: The United Kingdom experience. *Journal of Pediatrics, 151,* 140–144.

Wawer, M. J., Gray, R. H., Sewankambo, N. K. et al. (2005). Rates of HIV-1 transmission per coital act, by stage of HIV-1 infection, in Rakai, Uganda. *Journal of Infectious Diseases, 191,* 1403–1409.

Weiss, H. A., Quigley, M. A., & Hayes, R. J. (2000). Male circumcision and risk of HIV infection in sub-Saharan Africa: A systematic review and meta-analysis. *AIDS, 14,* 2361–2370.

Weiss, H. A., Thomas, S. L., Munabi, S. K. et al. (2006). Male circumcision and risk of syphilis, chancroid, and genital herpes: A systematic review and meta-analysis. *Sexually Transmitted Infections, 82,* 101–110.

Welch, T. R. (2012). An approach to the child with acute glomerulonephritis. *International Journal of Pediatrics, 2012,* 426192.

Whiting, P., Westwood, M., Bojke, L. et al. (2006). Clinical effectiveness and cost-effectiveness of tests for the diagnosis and investigation of urinary tract infection in children: A systematic review and economic model. *Health Technology Assessment, 10*(36), 1–154.

Williams, G., Wei, L., Lee, A. et al. (2006). Long-term antibiotics for preventing recurrent urinary tract infection in children. *Cochrane Database of Systematic Reviews,* (3), CD001534.

Wiswell, T. E., & Geschke, D. W. (1989). Risks from circumcision during the first month of life compared with those of uncircumcised boys. *Pediatrics, 83,* 1011–1015.

Wong, H., Mylrea, K., Feber, J. et al. (2006). Prevalence of complications in children with chronic kidney disease according to KDOQI. *Kidney International, 70,* 585–590.

World Health Organization & Joint United Nations Programme on HIV/AIDS. (2007). *Male circumcision: Global trends and determinants of prevalence, safety, and acceptability.* Geneva, Switzerland: World Health Organization.

Zimmerhackl, L. B., Besbas, N., Jungraithmayr, T. et al. (2006). Austria epidemiology, clinical presentation, and pathophysiology of atypical and recurrent hemolytic uremic syndrome. *Seminars in Thrombosis and Hemostasis, 32,* 113–120.

See the**Point** for additional organizations.

The Child With Altered Musculoskeletal Status

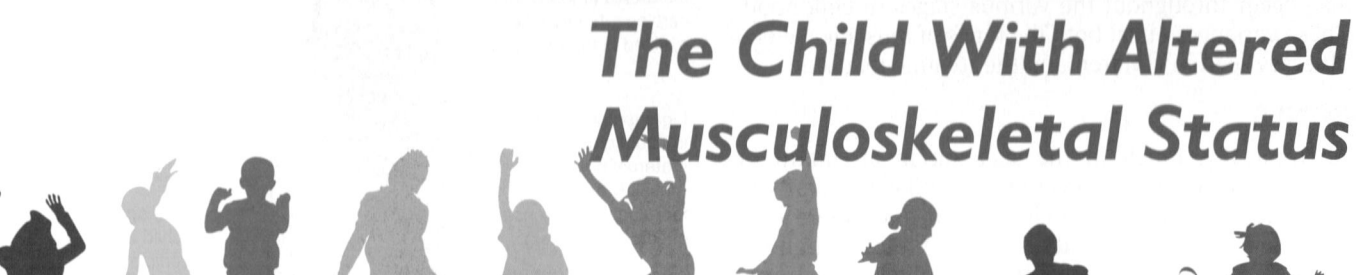

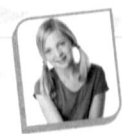

CASE HISTORY

Remember the Whitworth family and Cory, who we introduced in Chapter 6 and featured in Chapter 11? Cory has several siblings: Ken, Collin, Chris, Clarissa, and Cathy. Cory's scoliosis was diagnosed by radiograph obtained as a component of his presurgical assessment. Cory is now in kindergarten and is receiving no treatment for his scoliosis. He has a strong family history of scoliosis; his mother and his sister Cathy also have scoliosis. Cathy's scoliosis was diagnosed when she was 13 years old and in the seventh grade. At first, there were no interventions, and she saw the physician every 6 months. Then her back began to hurt anytime she had to sit for a length of time, such as in school or at a movie. Now she is in the eighth grade and growing rapidly. She has a brace, which was made for her and which she wears at home and at night, but she does not have to wear it to school. Cathy has had her brace for almost a

year and she hates it. It is uncomfortable, she has trouble falling asleep in it, and she sweats in it. It is embarrassing to wear to anyone's house if she is sleeping over with friends. Cathy often removes her brace in the middle of the night.

Cathy's older siblings enjoy teasing and tormenting her. Collin, a very athletic senior in high school, was taunting her when Cathy lost her temper and punched her brother. Collin turned so that the punch landed on his shoulder. Pain shot up through Cathy's arm. She could not clench and open her fist. When the pain would not subside and her hand began to swell, Cathy had to tell her mother that she might have broken a bone in her hand from hitting her brother. Her mother took her to the emergency department, where radiograph verified that she had broken the fifth metacarpal, often referred to as a *boxer's fracture*. A cast was placed on her right hand.

CHAPTER OBJECTIVES

1 Recognize clinical signs and symptoms that would indicate a musculoskeletal disorder or injury.

2 State the interdisciplinary interventions that are commonly used for each musculoskeletal disorder or injury.

3 Explain nursing care interventions to promote healing and prevent further injury and skin breakdown in the child receiving treatment for a musculoskeletal disorder or injury.

4 Provide family education regarding home care, activity, and dietary modifications for the child with a musculoskeletal disorder or injury.

5 Describe measures to protect children from musculoskeletal injury.

See thePoint for a list of Key Terms.

The musculoskeletal system provides the framework for the human body. The symmetry of muscle and bone propelling a body through space is apparent in elite athletes. Not as visible to the naked eye is the force it takes for a child to walk across a room for the first time. Bone is resilient and, particularly in children, has a remarkable ability to remodel itself.

This chapter focuses on various congenital and hereditary disorders that alter this balance. It also explores growth-related disorders, infectious and inflammatory disorders, and trauma specific to pediatrics.

DEVELOPMENTAL AND BIOLOGIC VARIANCES

Many anatomic and physiologic differences exist between the musculoskeletal systems of children and those of adults. Just as children should not be treated as "little adults," children's bones and muscles cannot be treated like adult bones and muscles (Fig. 20-1). Differences also occur throughout the various stages of childhood. These variances affect both the types of musculoskeletal illnesses seen in children and the treatments used.

BONES

Anatomically, much of the skeleton in an infant or young child consists of preosseous cartilage and growth plates called **physes**. The child's bones are more flexible, have a higher porosity, and have a lower mineral count. The osteogenic **periosteum** is thick and strong, producing **callus** more rapidly and in greater amounts than in adults. Because of these structural differences, a child's bone absorbs more energy before breaking and may even bow rather than break (fracture) when trauma occurs. When fractures do occur, the thick periosteum is likely to remain intact. Therefore, femoral fractures in nonambulating infants, particularly spiral fractures, are believed to be highly specific for inflicted injury.

> **ALERT**   *A child younger than age 1 year who presents with a fracture should be evaluated for possible physical abuse or an underlying musculoskeletal disorder that would cause spontaneous bone injury.*

The young bone can bend to a 45-degree angle and then straighten when the bending force is removed. This flexibility accounts, in part, for the high incidence of greenstick fractures seen in young children. As the child matures, the type of fracture reflects the porosity and strength of the affected bone.

Young children have an active growth area at each end of the long bones (humerus, radius–ulna, femur, and tibia–fibula) known as physeal or **epiphyseal plates**. Longitudinal growth of the long bones takes place through a process known as *endochondral ossification*. The epiphyses at the ends of each bone are cartilaginous in infants and become more ossified with time.

caREminder

> *The calcium deposits in bones make them appear white in radiographs. Cartilage, like many soft tissues, is not visible on radiographs. Therefore, because of the cartilaginous nature of their skeletal systems, it may be difficult to detect fractures in young children.*

The process of converting cartilage to bone continues until skeletal maturity is completed during adolescence. At that time, increasing levels of androgenic hormones produced during puberty cause the growth plates to gradually stop functioning. Alterations in the growth of a child's bones can occur as a result of trauma, nutritional deficits, metabolic disorders, and soft-tissue disorders. The epiphyseal plate is an area of vulnerability and structural weakness in the bone. The

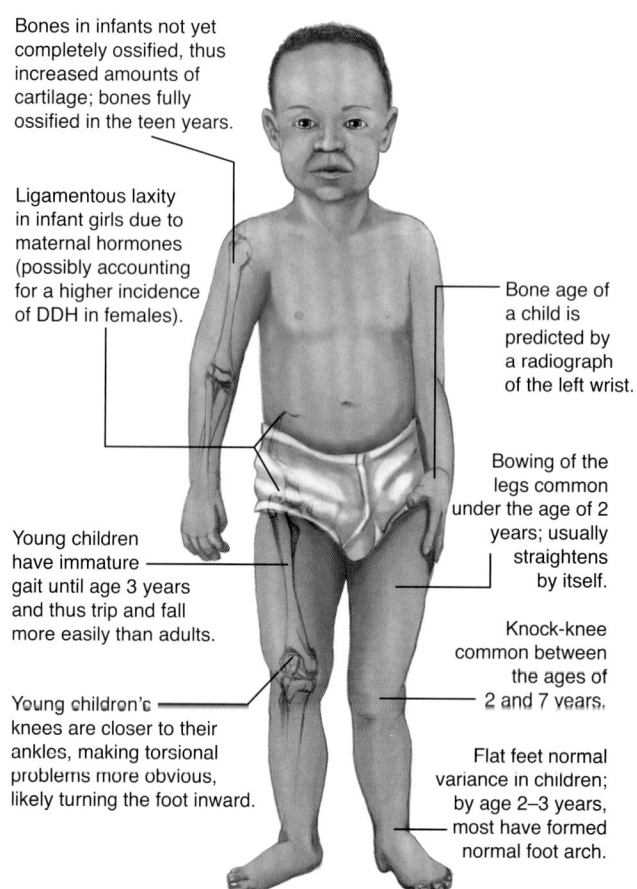

Bones in infants not yet completely ossified, thus increased amounts of cartilage; bones fully ossified in the teen years.

Ligamentous laxity in infant girls due to maternal hormones (possibly accounting for a higher incidence of DDH in females).

Bone age of a child is predicted by a radiograph of the left wrist.

Bowing of the legs common under the age of 2 years; usually straightens by itself.

Young children have immature gait until age 3 years and thus trip and fall more easily than adults.

Knock-knee common between the ages of 2 and 7 years.

Young children's knees are closer to their ankles, making torsional problems more obvious, likely turning the foot inward.

Flat feet normal variance in children; by age 2–3 years, most have formed normal foot arch.

Figure 20-1 Developmental and biologic variances in the musculoskeletal system. DDH, developmental dysplasia of the hip.

physes are not as strong as metaphyseal or diaphyseal bone (mature calcified bone). Ligaments frequently insert into the epiphyses. Thus, traumatic forces that are applied to an extremity may be transferred to the physes, causing injury. Trauma to the growth plate can result in complete or partial closure. Consequently, angular deformities or shortening of the bone can occur, depending on the physes involved and the amount of remaining growth.

When a child injures a bone, healing follows the same processes as in adult bone. In a child, however, the thick periosteum has an abundant blood and nutrient supply. The metabolically active periosteum, combined with the child's growth potential, creates a more rapid healing process in the child. During adolescence and with further skeletal maturity, the rate of healing slows to that of the adult.

Remodeling is the process by which correction of the fracture site occurs through a combination of periosteal reabsorption and new bone formation. Factors that affect remodeling include the child's age, proximity of the fracture to a joint, and relation of the angular deformity to the plane of the joint axis of motion. If the child is young, the fracture occurs adjacent to a physes, and the deformity is in the plane of motion; therefore, the remodeling potential is great. Thus, for certain pediatric fractures, **reduction**—restoring proper anatomic alignment—is not necessary.

Children often outgrow many of the abnormalities in structure seen in the young, immature skeleton. For instance, in utero positioning can cause physiologic alterations in the child's musculoskeletal status that may take up to 4 years to completely resolve. Normal newborns have 20- to 30-degree hip and knee contractures, which usually resolve by age 4 to 6 months. The infant frequently has inward rotation of the lower leg, creating a bowed appearance in which the feet may be turned slightly inward. This bowed appearance results from the legs and feet being tucked close to the body while the fetus is developing in the uterus. Metatarsus adductus (intoeing or pigeon-toed) is a common finding in infants and young children. For some children, medical management is used to correct the malformation if it does not spontaneously resolve as the child's bones and muscles grow.

At birth, the child's spine has a C-shaped appearance. Spinal curvature undergoes several changes as the child gains the ability first to hold the head erect, then to sit, and finally to stand and bear weight. The child's weak abdominal musculature contributes to a "potbellied" or hyperlordosis appearance that is common in young children.

MUSCLES

Voluntary muscle control changes as the child's overall development proceeds in a cephalocaudal fashion. The primary protective reflexes seen in the infant (e.g., rooting, palmar grasp, stepping) are replaced by the purposeful movements associated with an intact, growing nervous system and an increasing muscle mass. The infant's muscles account for only 25% of total body weight, whereas in adults, they account for 40% to 45%. Muscle mass increases with use and as innervation proceeds. In children with cerebral palsy, or other conditions in which connections between nerve fibers and muscle fibers are abnormal, muscle development is abnormal. Muscle atrophy and contractures are common.

During adolescence, muscle growth is influenced by hormonal changes, primarily the increased production of androgenic hormones. Higher levels of androgen and testosterone are partly responsible for more extensive muscle growth in males than in females. Androgen excess, as seen in young athletes taking anabolic steroids, can accelerate muscle development and skeletal maturation. This practice can result in short stature, interfere with normal testosterone levels, and impair spermatozoa production.

The incidence of sports injuries increases dramatically in adolescents. The young child has resilient soft tissue, so dislocations and sprains are unusual occurrences. However, an adolescent's increased participation in athletics increases the opportunity for fractures, dislocations, and ligamentous tears. In addition, rapid bone and muscle growth may contribute to the appearance of "clumsy" and awkward motions of the adolescent who is trying to adjust to new body dimensions. These factors, combined with the risk-taking attitude of many adolescents, can lead to a higher rate of personal injury.

ASSESSMENT

Assessment is based on a focused health history, beginning with the birth of the child to his or her presenting complaint and physical assessment aided by diagnostic imaging.

FOCUSED HEALTH HISTORY

> **QUESTION:** Referring to the case study, what are the aspects of the focused health history that reveal the most pertinent information related to Cathy's scoliosis and the most pertinent information for the metacarpal fracture?

Assessment of the musculoskeletal system begins with a history of the child's past health concerns from the prenatal period to the present (Focused Health History 20-1). Start with a history of the birth and delivery. The type of delivery (vaginal or cesarean) and the condition of the infant at birth, including Apgar score, will aid in identifying potential orthopedic disorders. Certain orthopedic problems are congenital (e.g., polydactyly and limb deformities), developing in utero as the fetus matures. Orthopedic injuries (e.g., a brachial plexus injury or a fractured clavicle) may occur during the birthing process. For example, breech delivery has been highly associated with the diagnosis of developmental dysplasia of the hip (DDH) (Imrie et al., 2010). Other orthopedic disorders may be noted only as the child grows or may be acquired as a complication of another primary illness such as polio, tetanus, or an infection in a bone.

Note whether the child has reached appropriate developmental milestones (see Chapters 4 to 7). Primitive reflexes that persist longer than 3 months of age may indicate a fixed motor–brain defect. In the older infant or child, missed milestones may be the first clue that a child has a musculoskeletal disorder, such as cerebral palsy, or some other degenerative disease.

Explore the family history for any hereditary disorders. The presence of scoliosis, clubfoot, hip or skeletal dysplasia, or neuromuscular disorders in family members may help in diagnosing genetically linked orthopedic disorders.

ALERT *Children who have had repeated exposures to latex during hospitalizations and surgery are at higher risk than others for latex allergies. Investigate the possibility of a latex allergy in all children with a suspected musculoskeletal disorder, especially in those who have had surgical procedures.*

Obtain a thorough history of the current problem, including the onset and duration of symptoms, extent of the disability, and any home remedies or medical treatments that have already been used. Common concerns include pain, swelling, deformity, clumsiness, weakness, stiffness, and limitation of movement (Tradition or Science 20-1).

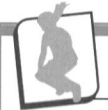

The Child With Altered Musculoskeletal Status

Current history	Reports of musculoskeletal or neuromuscular pain, including onset, what makes it better or worse, does it interfere with sleep Noticeable deformity Stiffness or swelling of a joint or extremity Gait changes (e.g., limping) Recent accident or injury, including description of event (e.g., speed of the car or bicycle) and any report of a snapping sensation felt or heard before or after the injury or fall
Past medical history	**Prenatal/Neonatal History** Maternal exposure to teratogens, infections, medications, or illegal drugs or alcohol Type of delivery (vaginal or cesarean) and complications Positioning of the child in utero, presentation (e.g., cephalic, breech) Neonatal history (e.g., Apgar scores, periods of anoxia) **Previous Health Challenges** Any chronic conditions or congenital anomalies History of surgery, hospitalizations, fractures, or bone and joint infections History of hyperactivity or attention deficit disorder **Childhood Illnesses** Polio Tuberculosis Conditions that can affect the spine **Immunizations** Status of current immunizations, especially polio and *Haemophilus influenzae* type b (Hib) Date of last tetanus shot **Allergies** Medications Latex, especially in children with myelomeningocele or with indwelling shunts **Current Medications** Medications that may affect bone density, wound healing, or bleeding time Use of medications for calcium deficiency or rickets
Nutritional assessment	Recent weight change or decreased appetite Use of vitamin supplements Intake of calcium-containing foods
Family medical history	History of developmental dislocated hip, clubfoot, or other skeletal or neurologic disorders
Social and environmental history	Any exposure to unsafe physical or structural settings Consistent, proper use of car seat Use of safety gear with activities (e.g., helmet with bicycling; wrist supports, knee pads, and elbow pads when skateboarding or roller blading) Child's interaction with friends; risk taker; history of thrill-seeking behavior Cultural practices influencing musculoskeletal development (e.g., use of papoose board)

Growth and development	Physical milestones
	First time for crawling, walking, running
	Previously achieved developmental milestones that the child no longer is able to accomplish
	Developmental milestones
	School grade for child
	Child's participation in age-appropriate activities
	Habits
	Activities when not in school
	Games child likes to play
	Usual bedtime; usual awakening time
	Involvement in sports; number of hours per week of practice or competition

Note: See Chapter 8 for a comprehensive health history.

ANSWER: The strong family history, with Cathy's mother and brother both having scoliosis, is pertinent information. So is the information that Cathy's back is uncomfortable when she sits for any length of time. Because she was involved in an acute incident, the description of the incident and the physical symptoms are most pertinent.

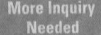

More Inquiry Needed

TRADITION OR SCIENCE 20-1

Do adolescents really experience "growing pains?"

Growing pains, first identified in 1823, are experienced by an estimated 4%–34% of young adolescents. Criteria for diagnosis include limb pain of at least 3 months' duration, intermittent pain with symptom-free intervals of days or months, pain occurring bilaterally not related to joints, pain severe enough to interfere with regular activities, and normal physical examination and laboratory findings (Evans, 2008; Uziel & Hashkes, 2007). The cause of growing pains remains unclear; however, psychosocial factors may be indicated. A pronated (or flat) foot posture is not correlated to growing pains (Evans, 2008). The pain usually appears late in the day or is nocturnal, often awakening the child (Uziel & Hashkes, 2007). Growing pains are physically benign, with resolution occurring within 1–2 years. The most important intervention is to explain the natural benign course of the growing pains, thus decreasing anxiety and fear (Uziel & Hashkes, 2007). Treatment interventions include massage, heat application, and use of nonsteroidal anti-inflammatory medications. It is possible that a diet enriched in calcium and vitamin D might affect bone status and pain episodes, but this theory has not been investigated (Uziel & Hashkes, 2007).

FOCUSED PHYSICAL ASSESSMENT

QUESTION: Describe the focused assessment related to Cathy's scoliosis. What would be included in the focused assessment related to the metacarpal break in her right hand?

Physical assessment of the musculoskeletal system includes inspection and palpation, range of motion (ROM) evaluation, and neurologic examination (Focused Physical Assessment 20-1, see Chapter 8). In the newborn, assess ROM of the head (to look for congenital torticollis, a condition in which the head is tilted to one side) and palpate the clavicles for tenderness or lumps, especially if the history shows that delivery was difficult. Assess the hips, with the diaper removed, for dislocation. Examine the limbs for any syndactyly or webbing.

Assess older children unclothed, except for undergarments, to ensure visualization of all aspects of the musculoskeletal system. Examine younger children while they sit on a parent's lap or move around the examination room. Observe movements such as gait, mobility, arm swing, hand preference, guarding, climbing, and playing. During inspection, note the degree of symmetry of size and configuration between limbs as well as the child's ability to move them. Unequal growth, paralysis, or spasticity in a limb may be subtle. Note any absence of parts, duplication of parts, or abnormal swelling. Assess ROM of all joints, either passively or actively. To analyze gait, ask the child to walk down a hall or to follow a parent who is walking and note any limp, tiptoeing, or foot drop.

Palpate the limbs to detect any areas of tenderness, swelling, masses, crepitus, or warmth. Begin the examination at the most distal joints (the toes) and work up to the hip joint or begin with the fingers

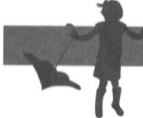

Musculoskeletal System

Assessment Parameter	Alterations/Clinical Significance
General appearance	Observe child undressed except for diapers or underclothes.
	Level of irritability, fever, and pain may indicate general state of well-being.
	Café-au-lait spots suggest neurofibromatosis.
	Maculopapular rash may indicate juvenile idiopathic arthritis (JIA)
Musculoskeletal system	Gait
	• Observe walking, sitting, and climbing up on the examination table.
	• Difficulty running, waddling gait, frequent falls, and using hand to walk up legs (Gowers sign) may suggest muscular dystrophies.
	• Limp: unequal leg lengths, pain, muscle or joint weakness or injury
	• Gait abnormalities in infancy and early childhood may indicate: septic arthritis, osteomyelitis, DDH, child abuse or neuromuscular disease
	• Gait abnormalities in middle childhood may indicate: septic arthritis, osteomyelitis, Legg-Calvé-Perthes disease (LCPD), JIA, cancer, sickle cell crisis, trauma, or neuromuscular disease
	• Gait abnormalities in adolescence may indicate: fractures, tumor, slipped capital femoral epiphysis (SCFE), osteomyelitis, Osgood-Schlatter, scoliosis, tarsal condition, JIA, trauma
	Neck
	• Observe for alignment and ROM.
	• Tilting of head to one side with chin pointing to opposite side in a newborn may indicate torticollis.
	Shoulders and upper extremities
	• Decreased movement or ROM, or guarding, may indicate clavicular fracture or nursemaid's elbow; pain or tenderness at the elbow or wrists may be caused by inflammation, infection, or fracture.
	• In the newborn or very young child: Pseudoparalysis of arm on affected side may indicate clavicular fracture or brachial plexus injury.
	• Infant or child does not voluntarily use arm: Look for radial head subluxation, nursemaid's elbow, or congenital dislocation.
	• In the older child with history of trauma secondary to fall with the arm outstretched or falling on the shoulder: Observe for pain, tenderness, bruising, and swelling at the fracture site (clavicle).
	Wrists and fingers
	• Decreased movement, decreased ROM, or guarding may indicate arthritis, sprain, strain, or infectious process.
	• Decreased sensation or impaired motor function may indicate ulnar, radial, or medial nerve injury or compromise, especially when cast or splint is applied.
	• Amount of swelling usually reflects severity of injury.
	• Tenderness or swelling in wrist or elbow may indicate joint disruption.
	• In the newborn, look for webbing of digits, lack of digits, or duplication of digits.
	• Joint swelling or effusion, limitation of joint motion and tenderness, pain with motion, and increased heat or warmth of joints may indicate JIA.

Assessment Parameter	Alterations/Clinical Significance
	Spine • Alignment: Spinal curvature, rib hump, asymmetric rib cage, or tenderness at spinal processes may indicate scoliosis, infection, arthritis, sprain, strain, or neoplasm. • Newborn: Observe for hairy patches in the sacral area or a dimple in the gluteal fold—may indicate spina bifida occulta. • School age, 8 years and older: scoliosis screening at each well-child visit and group screening in the schools • Tingling or decreased sensation in fingers may indicate spinal cord injury (such as that seen in cheerleaders, wrestlers, gymnasts, or those engaging in other sports in which whipping motions, flips, or cervical compression are common) **Hips** • ROM, extra skinfold in groin or buttock area, or decreased ROM with adduction may be indication of DDH, septic arthritis, or JIA. • Newborn or infant: Shortening of femur in flexion (Galeazzi sign), shortening of limb in extension, Ortolani sign, or Barlow sign may indicate DDH. • Middle childhood or adolescence: Pain in hip or groin area and limping may indicate SCFE. • Vague hip or knee pain with painless limp and decreased ROM of hip, abduction, or internal rotation may indicate LCPD. **Lower extremities** • Asymmetry of limbs or abnormal alignment may indicate metatarsus adductus or neuromuscular clubfoot. • Intoeing from age 3 years to maturity suggests internal femoral torsion. • Newborn with hypotonia or hypertonia may indicate neurologic deficit. • Muscle weakness and wasting may indicate muscular dystrophies. **Knees** • Infant and child: Angulation deformity may indicate genu varum or genu valgum, internal tibial torsion, or external tibial torsion. • Middle childhood or adolescence: Pain in knee or thigh may indicate SCFE. • Joint swelling or effusion, limitation of motion, tenderness, pain on motion, and increased warmth in knee may suggest JIA. • Pain in medial femoral condyle may indicate osteochondritis dissecans. • Dull, achy pain exacerbated by impact loading (running, jumping, stairs) may indicate Osgood-Schlatter disease. • Adolescent with history of knee giving way, with immediate pain or swelling, suggests an anterior cruciate ligament tear. **Ankles** • School-aged child and adolescent: Pain, tenderness, and warmth may suggest sprain or strain injuries **Feet** • Intoeing for ages 0–1 year may indicate metatarsus adductus; for 1- to 3-year-olds may indicated internal (medial) tibial torsion. • Heel pain may indicate Sever's disease or plantar fasciitis. • Foot drop suggests peritoneal nerve injury

NURSING INTERVENTIONS 20-1

Neurovascular Assessment

Assessing circulation to an extremity is done frequently for the first 24 hours after a cast has been applied, after surgery has been performed on an extremity, or when nerve injury is suspected. After that, time assessment every 4–8 hours is sufficient if there is no neurovascular compromise. The categories for assessment include the following:

- *Pain*—Ask the child if he or she has pain in an extremity. Pain is common at the injury site. If the pain is not relieved by narcotics, or pain becomes worse when the finger or toes are flexed, the child may have compartment syndrome and the physician should be notified immediately.
- *Sensation*—Determine if the child can feel touch on the extremity. Two-point discrimination is decreased when there is neurovascular compromise.

- *Motion*—Ask the child to move his or her fingers or toes; lack of movement may signal nerve damage.
- *Temperature*—Assess the extremity for temperature (warm vs. cool) compared to unaffected limb. A cool extremity may become warm if a blanket is placed over it and the extremity is elevated. If these actions do not warm the extremity, there is poor circulation.
- *Capillary refill*—Apply brief pressure to the nail beds and note how quickly pinkness returns. Sluggish capillary refill signals poor circulation.
- *Color*—Note the color of the extremity and compare to the unaffected extremity.
- *Pulse*—Check pulses distal to the injury or cast. This may not be possible if the cast covers the foot or hand. If the pulse is difficult to locate, check it with a Doppler machine and mark it with an "X."

and work up to the shoulders. Estimate the size of any bony or soft-tissue masses. Palpate the spine and examine it for any dimples or hairy patches; note the general contour of the spine. Look for hip or shoulder asymmetry.

caREminder

If injury has occurred, examine that area last and be gentle when palpating the injury site.

Perform a neurovascular assessment of the extremities (described in Nursing Interventions 20-1). Compare the affected extremity with the unaffected one for neurovascular status and strength. Extremities should be pink, warm, and have strong (+2) pulses. The child should be able to move the extremity and sense pinpoint discrimination. Frequent assessments for changes noted early will aid in identifying potential complications and guiding treatment.

Examine limb ROM to assess hip flexion, contractures or spasm of the extremities, and limitation of motion. Test muscle strength to assess for neuromuscular problems such as poliomyelitis and muscular dystrophy. To assess motor ability, ask the child to bend his or her arm and to push and pull against your hand; then, using his or her foot, ask the child to push down and pull up against your hand. Test superficial and deep tendon reflexes in each extremity.

Observe the child as he or she stands up from a sitting or lying position. If you note abnormal reflexes or muscle weakness, encourage the family to talk to the primary health care provider.

ANSWER: Inspection and palpation should be used to assess Cathy's spine. Ask Cathy to bend at the waist to determine whether the scapula and posterior iliac crests are symmetric. Palpate along the spine to assess the location of curvature. Inspection, limitations of movement, and gentle palpation should be incorporated into Cathy's assessment of the metacarpal break in her right hand. Inspect the degree of swelling, comparing right and left. Ask Cathy to open and shut her fist and observe the limitations. Gently palpate along the metacarpals for swelling.

DIAGNOSTIC CRITERIA

QUESTION: Which of the described diagnostic tests are most applicable for each of Cathy's musculoskeletal problems?

Blood, joint fluid, and bone analyses are diagnostic tests used to evaluate musculoskeletal alterations. In addition, diagnostic imaging techniques also are very useful (Tests and Procedures 20-1). The sensitivity and specificity of each test may vary with the disease process and the child's age. A regular radiograph (plain x-ray) is often acquired initially and guides the selection of additional imaging (Fig. 20-2).

ALERT   *If the child has a history of trauma, maintain cervical spine precautions during diagnostic testing until the physician rules out a cervical spine injury.*

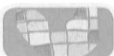 **TESTS AND PROCEDURES for Evaluating Musculoskeletal Conditions**

Diagnostic Test or Procedure	Purpose	Findings and Indications	Health Care Provider Considerations
Complete blood count	Blood sample analysis to evaluate several indicators (e.g., infection, anemia)	Normal range, 6,000–11,500/μL Elevated white blood cell (WBC) count found in presence of infection, septic arthritis, osteomyelitis.	Explain to child and family that this test helps to evaluate conditions that may alter normal ranges of components of the blood.
C-reactive protein (CRP)	Measures protein in the blood that is released when infection is present	Normal, <1.0 mg/dL Level >0.9 mg/dL may indicate infection, septic arthritis, inflammatory bowel disease, rheumatoid arthritis, or lupus	Explain that CRP level rises as an inflammatory process worsens and falls as healing occurs. Urge the child/family to avoid aspirin, acetaminophen, or ibuprofen before test because these drugs may lower CRP levels.
Calcium and phosphorus levels	Tests amount of these minerals in blood sample; assists in diagnosis of renal and skeletal diseases	Normal ranges: • Calcium, 8.5–11 mg • Phosphorus, 3.0–4.5 mg/dL Low levels may indicate rickets, malabsorption syndrome, and starvation Increased levels may indicate bone tumor, healing fracture, skeletal disease, high milk intake, bone metastasis of cancer	Explain that the test evaluates the balance of chemicals in the body, specifically calcium and phosphorus. Handle specimen gently to avoid hemolysis.
Rheumatoid factor (RF)	Measures the body's autoimmune response to an antigen	Negative, <60 International Unit/mL May indicate juvenile arthritis (JA), systemic lupus erythematosus (SLE)	Ensure that specimens are tested as soon as possible or within 72 hours of collection. Keep in mind that gold therapy decreases the Rh titer.
Erythrocyte sedimentation rate (ESR)	Evaluates presence of an inflammatory process; does not assist in revealing the site or cause of inflammatory process	Normal range, 0–10 mm/hr Indicates how much inflammation in the body	Keep specimen at room temperature. If the ESR is elevated, anticipate that other diagnostic studies will be completed. If the ESR is elevated and the child is already being treated for a known disease, expect a change or increase in medications or therapy.
Blood culture and sensitivity	Diagnoses bacteremia or septicemia; identifies pathogenic microorganisms present in blood and determines their sensitivity to antimicrobial agents	Causative organisms seen with bacteremia or septicemia; positive blood culture in 40% of children with septic arthritis	Use strict aseptic technique to gather specimen. If more than one culture is ordered, the specimens should be drawn separately, at no less than 30 minutes apart, to rule out the possibility of transient bacteremia. Be aware that antimicrobial therapy given prior to blood collection may result in false-negative findings. Allow a minimum of 24–72 hours for culture reports to identify pathogens. Some pathogens, such as fungi and mycobacteria, may take weeks to incubate and provide identifiable growth.

(Continued)

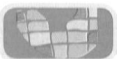

TESTS AND PROCEDURES for Evaluating Musculoskeletal Conditions (Continued)

Diagnostic Test or Procedure	Purpose	Findings and Indications	Health Care Provider Considerations
Bone biopsy	Allows microscopic examination of bone tissue; usually performed to diagnose a lesion found by radiograph examination	Normally, no abnormal cells or tissue Abnormalities possibly indicate infection, malignant tissue	Obtain informed consent. Anticipate administering intravenous antibiotics prebiopsy to prevent postoperative infection. Assist in providing conscious sedation and pain medication. Explain that discomfort at the site will persist for several days after the test.
Fluid aspiration from joints	Determines cause and type of joint disorder and effusion; allows for fluid drainage from a joint or to administer local pharmacologic therapy	Increased or abnormal levels possibly indicate noninflammatory abnormalities (e.g., traumatic arthritis), inflammatory abnormalities (e.g., rheumatoid arthritis, SLE), septic abnormalities (e.g., septic arthritis), or hemorrhagic abnormalities (e.g., trauma)	Obtain informed consent. Assist in providing local sedation and pain medication. Explain that discomfort may be felt when the needle enters through the synovial membrane into the joint capsule. Apply ice packs for 24–36 hours after test to decrease pain and swelling. Apply elastic bandage after test to maintain good joint stability. Observe site for erythema, tenderness, warmth, or exudate.
Arthrography	Uses fiberoptic endoscope to visualize selected joints for injuries or abnormalities; assists in monitoring degenerative processes or joints; aids in evaluating effects of medical or surgical interventions; may also be used to perform minor surgical repair	Abnormal findings possibly indicate tears, injury, dislocation, fracture, subluxation, or synovial abnormalities	Obtain informed consent. Check for allergies and monitor for reaction to contrast medium. Assist in providing local sedation and pain medication. Explain that discomfort may be felt when the needle enters through the joint cavity and from pressure of the tourniquet. Administer intravenous antibiotic if ordered to prevent infection of the bone after manipulation. Assess joint areas for rashes or signs of infection after procedure.
Bone scan	Detects early bone disease from cancer and metastasis of cancer to the bone (highly sensitive); measures the response of bone tissue to therapeutic interventions	No differentiation between benign and malignant processes; directs attention to areas of the skeleton that may need further study	Obtain informed consent. Explain that there is some radiation exposure to entire body. A large scanning camera is positioned over the child and moves slowly above and around the body, taking 1–3 hours for completion of the scanning. Determine whether child is claustrophobic or unable to remain still for long periods of time. Administer sedation, if ordered. Inform child and family that test takes about 4 hours to complete. Ensure intravenous access necessary to administer contrast agent. Inform child and family that contrast medium takes 2–3 hours to be absorbed in the bone tissue prior to test. Have child void prior to test; a distended bladder will decrease visibility of the pubic bone. Encourage fluids after test to facilitate renal clearance of contrast agent.

Diagnostic Test or Procedure	Purpose	Findings and Indications	Health Care Provider Considerations
Computed tomography	Evaluates and diagnoses a large number of clinical conditions of the musculoskeletal system, with radiographs taken at multiple angles to provide cross-sectional anatomic display	Abnormalities visualized include tumors, cancer, lesions, abscesses, fluid collection, and inflammation	Obtain informed consent. Assess for allergies to contrast agent, which may be used; observe for reaction to contrast media. Determine whether child is claustrophobic or unable to remain still. Administer sedation if ordered.
Magnetic resonance imaging (MRI)	Detects structural, circulatory, and metabolic abnormalities in the body; visualizes hard and soft tissue and bone marrow	Abnormal findings include tumors, edema, hemorrhage, abscesses, skeletal abnormalities, intervertebral disk abnormalities, spinal cord compression, and muscular disease	Obtain informed consent. Determine whether child is claustrophobic or unable to remain still. Administer sedation if ordered. Remove all metal objects from child's body. If family members are allowed to stay with child during procedure, ensure they remove all metal objects from their bodies. Explain to child that machine makes various noises as the radio waves are turned on and off. Provide child with earplugs if necessary.
Plain film radiograph	Examines bones to evaluate child's pain or discomfort and confirm suspected injury or disease; provides a two-dimensional view; visualizes most fractures well; does not visualize cartilage and other soft tissues well	Abnormalities may indicate fracture, osteomyelitis, growth plate abnormalities, injury, cancer, infection, nutritional alterations	Keep in mind that radiographs are an easily available and inexpensive testing method. Inform child and family that the child will need to be positioned properly.
Ultrasound	Aids in verifying other diagnostic tests to verify or confirm presence of musculoskeletal abnormality; provides good view of soft-tissue masses and cysts	Abnormalities may indicate a mass, inflammation, abscess, or tumor	Tell the child and family that no sedation is needed. Explain that the test is painless. Explain that an ultrasound lubricant will be applied to the area being viewed. Remove the lubricant after test is completed.

ANSWER: For both of Cathy's musculoskeletal problems, a radiograph will confirm the diagnosis. Both problems are related to the bone, not the surrounding soft tissue, and are readily visible on a radiograph.

TREATMENT MODALITIES

QUESTION: Of the following treatment modalities, which is traditionally used for scoliosis and which for fracture? Compare the nursing care associated with each treatment modality and select the treatment best employed for Cathy's fractured hand.

Various treatment modalities are used to manage musculoskeletal alterations. These may include heat and cold applications; brace and splint applications; serial manipulation; casting; traction; external fixation; and continuous passive motion (CPM), ambulatory devices, and prosthetic devices. The complications of immobilization, nutritional interventions, pain management, and diversional activities are discussed. To implement or support these health care interventions, be sure to understand their principles and mechanics. Also, allow the child to be involved in his or her own care as much as possible. For a child too young to manage self-care, encourage caregivers to manage or assist. By involving the family, the health care team can achieve better cooperation from the child and family and improve adherence to treatment (Developmental Considerations 20-1).

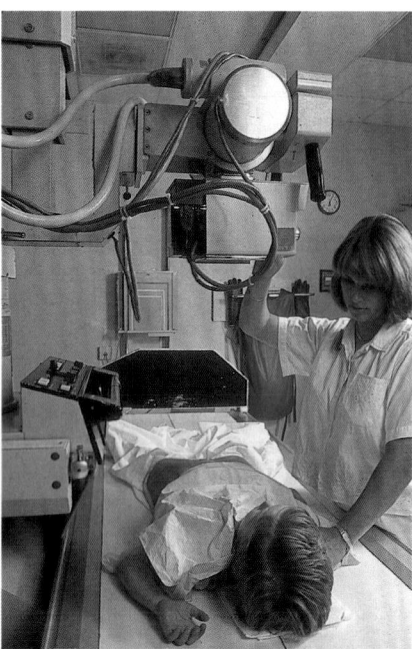

Figure 20-2 A radiograph is a noninvasive diagnostic procedure that most children will complete in a cooperative manner.

COLD AND HEAT APPLICATIONS

Simple application of cold and heat has long been used as therapy for soft-tissue injuries. In some cases, both may be used.

Cold Application

By decreasing tissue temperature, cold can cause vaso-constriction; diminish pain, metabolism, and muscle spasm; minimize the inflammatory process; and aid recovery after soft-tissue trauma. After injury, cold is primarily used to reduce metabolism, thereby mini-mizing the degree of tissue damage. During rehabilita-tion, it is used primarily to relieve pain. Ice is often used in combination with compression and elevation. Cold can be delivered by disposable ice bags, ice col-lars, cold packs, gels, moist compresses, immersion in cold water (55° F) via soak or sitz bath, or the use of a cooling blanket. Intermittent application of cold is rec-ommended for the first 24 to 48 hours after injury to re-duce edema. It is usually applied for 15 to 20 minutes followed by a 30-minute rest period. Cold compresses and sitz baths should only be used for approximately 10 minutes because moisture intensifies the cooling process (Metules, 2007).

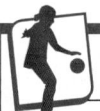

DEVELOPMENTAL CONSIDERATIONS 20-1

Age-Appropriate Self-Care Activities for the Child With a Musculoskeletal Condition

Infancy

Family or caregivers provide all self-care needs.

Diversionary activities may be needed to prevent infants from pulling at straps, pins, and wires.

Child indicates pain and discomfort in a manner recognizable to primary caregivers.

Early Childhood

Child wears or uses supportive devices without disturbing the integrity and safety of the device.

Child learns to be mobile with use of assistive devices as needed and as physically capable.

Child takes medications with assistance.

Child indicates pain and discomfort in manner recognizable to primary caregivers.

Middle Childhood

Child uses walker, crutches, or wheelchair to assist in mobility.

Child verbalizes feelings of pain and discomfort related to condition.

Child takes medications as instructed.

Child selects biobehavioral methods to manage pain and discomfort.

Child performs pin care.

Child selects foods to eat that provide a well-balanced diet.

Child wears clothes that are easy to put on and take off given the restrictions of his or her condition.

Adolescence

Child uses walker, crutches, or wheelchair to assist in mobility.

Child administers own medications.

Child verbalizes feelings of pain and discomfort re-lated to condition and independently implements or seeks assistance in implementing biobehavioral methods to manage pain and discomfort.

Child selects activities that enhance mobility and do not cause additional pain or discomfort.

Child performs pin care.

Child selects foods to eat that provide a well-balanced diet.

Child monitors diet to prevent weight gain.

Child selects clothes that enhance body image and self-esteem.

Cold therapy is not recommended for persons with hypersensitivity to cold or with impaired circulation. Assess the child's skin for changes in color, integrity, sensation, or any other signs of injury before and after cold application. Cold application is not placed on an open wound. Cold applications are not placed directly on the skin. Many cold applications have a protective cloth covering; if this is not the case, the cold pack can be wrapped in a thin towel or pillowcase before applying to the skin. After the treatment, dry the skin well.

KidKare Gel packs cool skin faster than an ice bag and should be applied for no more than 10 minutes. Ice can be applied for 20 minutes but should also be monitored carefully to prevent skin and tissue damage.

Heat Application

Heat is generally used for subacute or chronic conditions to warm muscle groups, cause vasodilation, relieve inflammation, and relieve pain from muscle stiffness or spasm. Application of heat allows the muscles to stretch further and increases the circulation of oxygenated blood to muscles and joints.

Heat therapy can be used in a dry or wet form. Dry heat is provided by means of infrared lamps, heating pads, electric heating blankets, and commercial hot packs. To prevent burning, heat sources applied to the skin should have a protective covering. Tub baths, immersion in a hot tub, compresses, and hot water bottles are sources of wet heat. Do not apply heat for more than 15 to 20 minutes at a time (Metules, 2007). After an hour of heat therapy, capillary vasoconstriction occurs as a secondary effect, making the therapy more destructive than beneficial. For this reason, do not reapply heat sooner than 1 hour after the initial application.

KidKare When using electrical sources of heat, the caregiver should not make a point of showing the child how plugging in the apparatus makes the light come on or the dial glow. A young child is likely to consider this a game and may want to play with the plug after the caregiver leaves the room.

During heat therapy, evaluate the skin for changes in color, integrity, and sensation. Monitor the child for profuse sweating or an increase in respirations or pulse rate, which indicate the need to immediately stop the therapy. Do not allow electric sources of heat to become wet or let the child go to bed with a heating pad in place. Heat lamps are not recommended for home use with children because of the risk of burns.

caREminder

The child should never be left unattended during a tub bath. A child who is feeling weak, ill, or lethargic may not be able to support himself or herself adequately in the tub.

BRACES AND SPLINTS

Braces and splints are devices made from a solid material, such as molded plastic. Straps (Velcro, or leather with buckles) hold the splint or brace in place. The device is either custom made for the child by a trained orthotist or therapist or is a standard-sized device that is adjusted to fit the child. The purpose of a splint or brace is to immobilize a body part to provide support for weak limbs or to prevent deformities by maintaining optimal functional position of the joints.

A brace or splint can be removed for bathing, sleeping, or exercise. The amount of time each day that the child must wear the brace or splint is dictated by the type of device and the medical reasons for the treatment. For instance, a child with scoliosis may need to use a Milwaukee or Boston brace. These plastic braces must be worn between 16 and 23 hours a day. For some children, the brace is removed only for bathing. The Pavlik harness is a cloth brace used in children with DDH. This brace must be worn at all times for 4 to 6 weeks. A wrist or knee splint may be applied to immobilize an area during the acute phase of an arthritic condition or after an athletic injury. In these cases, the child may select not to wear the splint during periods of inactivity.

Priorities for care of a child with a splint or brace include ensuring that the device is fitted and used correctly to achieve its maximal effects and maintain skin integrity. If the device does not fit properly, the skin can become irritated and can break down. Wearing cotton clothing underneath the brace or splint can minimize skin irritation. Daily baths or skin care, followed by thorough drying of the skin, helps to maintain cleanliness, stimulate the skin, and minimize skin irritation. Give the child and family verbal and written instructions regarding how and when to apply the device, how it should look on the child, what activities should be allowed and prohibited during the treatment, and how to care for and clean the device.

The child who wears a splint or brace may feel self-conscious about his or her physical appearance. This feeling may negatively affect adjustment and adherence to the treatment regimen. Encourage the child to participate in all care decisions surrounding brace or splint wear. Assisting the child to select appropriate and attractive clothes to wear over the brace is helpful. Encourage the child to verbalize feelings associated with brace or splint wear. Direct the child toward positive coping behaviors and remind him or her of the positive eventual outcomes of therapy.

SERIAL MANIPULATION

In serial manipulation, passive ROM exercises are used to manipulate a joint or muscle group. The purpose of serial manipulation is to restore joint alignment or to maintain functional mobility of a joint. The passive movements of the joint should not cause pain. An example is passive manipulation during diaper changes, used for the child with metatarsus adductus to attempt to straighten the child's forefoot. Serial manipulation may also be used in conjunction with other techniques such as casting. For example, the child with clubfoot may use serial manipulation techniques to stretch the foot by hand, and then use a cast to hold the position of the foot in place. The cast serves to help stretch the soft tissues of the foot. Every few weeks, the cast is removed, serial manipulation is again performed, and a new cast is placed on the foot.

Serial manipulation of a joint or muscle group is not recommended for all musculoskeletal disorders. The treatment is usually taught to the family by a physical therapist. The family should be aware that the treatment might not be successful and that other therapies, such as a brace or casting, might be required.

CASTING

Casts hold fractured extremities in alignment, prevent or reduce contractures, and provide postoperative immobilization. Casts, made from either plaster or synthetic materials, can be made to fit an extremity or the trunk. The location of the musculoskeletal problem and the degree of immobility needed to achieve healing or correction determine the type of cast to be applied (Fig. 20-3) (see thePoint for Procedures: Cast Care; a comprehensive step-by-step procedure for care and management of the child in a cast).

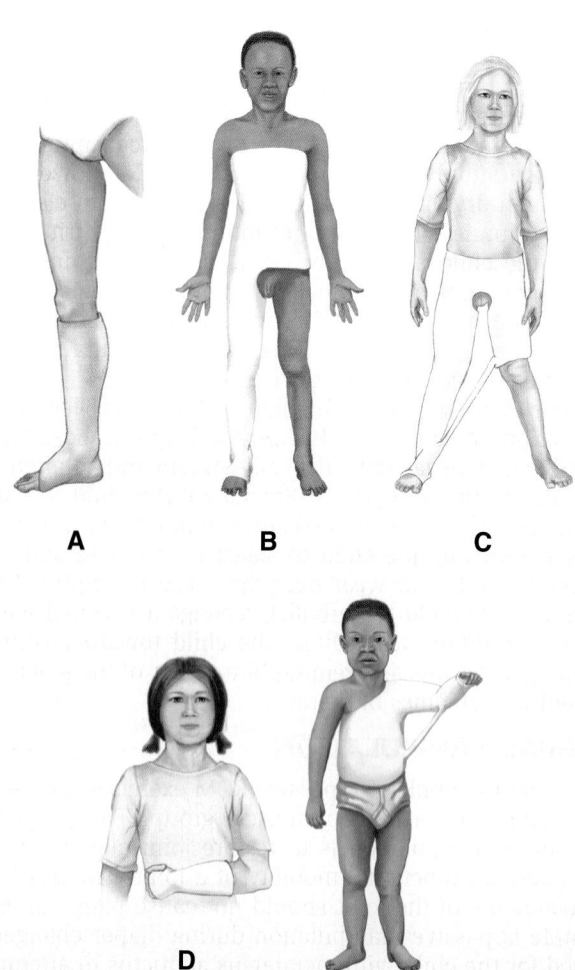

Figure 20-3 Types of casts. (A) Short leg cast. (B) Unilateral hip spica cast. (C) One and one-half hip spica cast. (D) Short arm cast. (E) Shoulder spica cast.

A   B   C

D

Casts are generally applied and removed in an acute care setting or specialized outpatient clinic by a trained physician or orthopedic technician. Unless the child has an illness or injury that requires extensive hospitalization, after cast application, the child promptly returns home, where cast care must be managed by the child and family (see thePoint for Supplemental Information: Teaching Information for the Child With a Cast).

KidKare Fiberglass casts are available in a variety of colors and designs, such as neon, stripes, and camouflage. Ask the child or parents what design they prefer before the cast is placed.

Neurovascular compromise, skin breakdown, and misalignment of a fracture can occur if the cast is not properly fitted. Careful assessment aids in prompt recognition and treatment of these complications. Teach family members neurovascular assessment and cast maintenance techniques. Other aspects of home care include maintaining good nutrition and modifying activities as needed to promote the healing process.

ANSWER: Braces are a common treatment modality for scoliosis, and casting is a treatment modality for fractures. Both of these treatments immobilize the child and have the potential to apply pressure to the skin and tissue. Critical nursing interventions for both treatment modalities include assessment of perfusion and skin integrity to identify areas of potential skin breakdown. With her fractured hand, Cathy would be evaluated by the health care team and placed in a cast to immobilize the extremity.

TRACTION

Traction is defined as the application of a pulling force to an injured or diseased part of the body or extremity; countertraction pulls in the opposite direction (see thePoint for Procedures: Traction Care). Traction is used for four primary purposes:

1. To reduce or prevent spasm or contracture of muscles and relieve pain
2. To immobilize a part of the body or a joint to promote rest and healing of bones and soft tissue
3. To reduce a subluxation, dislocation, or fracture and maintain alignment
4. To prevent, lessen, or correct deformities

Traction and suspension are required to override the natural muscle tension and to restore alignment. Several basic traction principles must be maintained to enable the traction to work effectively. First, *countertraction* is provided as sandbags, metal weights, or the child's body weight. Second, the prescribed *line of pull* is maintained. This principle requires a child to lie still in one position—a challenging task. Third, the traction is *continuously applied.* Fourth, there must be *prevention or reduction of friction* that interferes with the effectiveness of the traction.

Three types of traction are used: manual, skin, and skeletal. *Manual traction* uses force applied to the bones by a physician, nurse, or technician to keep them in alignment. Manual traction is used in cases of stable fractures or dislocations to reduce the bone or re-align joints before splinting or casting (see thePoint for Supplemental Information: Types of Skin Traction and Types of Skeletal Traction).

Skin traction is applied to the skin using skin adherents, Ace wraps, commercial traction tapes, or special foam boots to which the pull is applied (usually a 1- to 5-lb weight for children). Weights applied to skin traction should not exceed 3.5 kg or 8 lb. Intact skin integrity is essential because this type of traction cannot be applied over an open wound or when the skin is at high risk for impairment. Assessment of neurovascular and motor status is also essential prior to traction application so that changes from baseline can be noted. Assess neurovascular and motor status at least every 4 hours or more frequently for children at risk for neurovascular impairment. Skin traction may be intermittently removed by health care prescriber order.

Skeletal traction refers to any traction apparatus where the pull force is applied directly to the skeleton via pins, wires, screws, and/or tongs that are inserted into the appropriate area of bone. Weights applied can be 4.5 to 11.5 kg (10 to 25 lb). Skeletal traction is beneficial for unstable or fragmented fractures that are not amenable to surgical intervention. Skeletal traction would also be used if there were skin damage associated with the fracture. Skeletal traction carries a risk of pin tract infection and osteomyelitis. Frequent skin and neurovascular assessments are important components of care for a child in skeletal traction as well as pin site care (Tradition or Science 20-2).

Never remove or add traction weights without specific physician orders. Do not allow weights to touch the floor or drag on the bed parts; keep weights hanging free.

EXTERNAL FIXATION

External fixation uses a system of percutaneous pins, rods, and wires connected to a rigid frame placed on the outside of the body to hold fractured bones in place while they heal. It is used to treat complex, unstable fractures of both upper and lower extremities. An external fixator can hold the bone fragments much more rigidly than a cast. It is usually left in place for 6 weeks, and continued splinting is required for some time after removal.

An external fixator may also be used to lengthen bones or correct angular or rotational defects. In these cases, the wires, rings, and telescoping rods allow limb lengthening to occur by the process of distraction: two opposing bone ends are separated, and new bone regeneration occurs to fill in the gap.

Care of the child with an external fixator device involves maintaining skin integrity and preventing infection or injury. Skin and neurovascular assessments are needed. Skin care is similar to that for a child in skeletal traction. Pin care must be completed daily to prevent infection. To prevent dryness, lotions can be applied to skin away from the entry sites of pins and wires.

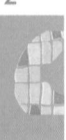

TRADITION OR SCIENCE 20-2

Should pin care be completed daily, and, if so, what cleansing solution should be used?

The National Association of Orthopaedic Nurses (Holmes & Brown, 2005) and the Royal College of Nursing Society of Orthopaedic and Trauma Nursing (Timms et al., 2011) have established evidence-based practice guidelines for skeletal pin site care. The guidelines make the following recommendations:

1. Pins located in areas with considerable soft tissue should be considered at greater risk for infection.
2. Pin sites should be covered with a dressing that applies light compression and keeps any excess exudate away from the wound.
3. At sites with mechanically stable bone–pin interfaces, pin site care should be done on a daily or weekly basis (after the first 48–72 hours). The frequency of a dressing change increases in the presence of infection or if the dressing becomes saturated.
4. Chlorhexidine 2 mg/mL may be the most effective cleansing solution for pin care.
5. Patients and their families should be taught pin site care before discharge from the hospital. They should be required to demonstrate whatever care must be done and should be provided with written instructions that include signs and symptoms of infection (Holmes & Brown, 2005; Timms & Pugh, 2012).

Activities in which the fixator might be hit or bumped are restricted during the treatment. In some cases, the child may be able to bear weight on the affected limb.

Teach the child not to pick at or manipulate any of the wires or pins. The child may wear baggy sweatpants or skirts over the device. Velcro can be sewn into the seams of pants to allow them to easily slip over the fixator device.

SURGICAL INTERVENTIONS

Pediatric musculoskeletal surgery is performed for two main reasons: (1) to correct a deformity or broken bone and (2) to prevent a deformity. The goal in either case is to enable the child to live a functional life. Surgical interventions aim to restore mechanical balance to the body through bone fusions, bone lengthening or shortenings, muscle realignments or releases, joint reconstruction, or even amputations. Internal fixation is a method to position and support a fractured bone until it is strong enough to bear weight. Materials such as stainless steel or, more recently, cobalt and titanium are used to support the body. These materials are compatible with tissue and rarely cause an allergic reaction. The most common types of internal fixation are wires, plates, rods, pins, nails, and screws.

Nursing care of the postoperative child is discussed in Chapter 11. ROM exercises or restrictions of movement may be necessary to protect the surgical area. For instance, logrolling is used to turn the child who has had a spinal fusion, whereas continuous passive ROM machines may be used on the adolescent who has had knee surgery. Postoperatively, the child is likely to experience significant pain. The assessment and management of pain in children is discussed in Chapter 10.

 Care of the Hospitalized Child: Pain Management

CONTINUOUS PASSIVE MOTION

CPM is a treatment method used to provide early controlled motion after surgery or injury of an upper or lower extremity. Joint motion is provided passively by a device to diffuse synovial fluid without compromising the integrity of the repaired tissue. The goals of CPM are to decrease edema and pain while maintaining ROM. CPM can be used for elbows, knees, hips, ankles, and fingers. Some are adaptable for use in children.

The physician specifies how many hours the patient must use the device, the ROM (both extension and flexion), and the speed of the cycle. Most devices have a small, handheld keypad that is programmed either by the nurse or physical therapist. The nurse or physical therapist places the patient in the machine with the joint properly aligned. The nurse also monitors patient adherence and skin integrity and adjusts the settings as ordered. When the CPM machine is used at home, teach the patient and family how to properly position the joint in the machine and how to adjust the ROM settings.

AMBULATORY DEVICES

The child may need assistance with ambulation after surgery, injury, or immobilization of a lower extremity. The ambulatory device transfers a portion of the body weight to the arms and provides additional support during walking. The device can also help the child get up from and down to a sitting position. The type of device selected is based on the child's age, overall functional ability, degree of strength in the arms and legs, balance, and ability to maintain an upright position. A physical therapist works with the child and family to choose the most appropriate device and teaches the child how to use the device correctly and how to best achieve an effective gait pattern.

The types of ambulatory devices that children can use include canes, crutches, and walkers. A *cane* is used to widen the base of support on the side of the affected limb. The cane is held on the same side as the affected leg and is moved in coordination with the affected leg. A regular cane has a single base; a quad cane has a four-pronged base of support. When a cane is used, the affected leg experiences partial weight bearing. Canes are more effective for school-aged and older children who have good gait and upper extremity coordination.

Crutches relieve weight bearing from the affected limb by transferring body weight and gait control to the arms and hands. The muscles of the arms, shoulders, back, and chest are all used during crutch walking. Exercises may be initiated before crutch use to strengthen these muscles. Instruction regarding the position and proper manipulation of the crutches is essential to prevent further injury to the child. To prevent nerve palsy, the top of the crutches should be between two and three finger widths below the axilla. The position of the crutches during periods of rest and movement is important to ensure that stability is maintained and gait is not compromised (Fig. 20-4). Gait is described in terms of the

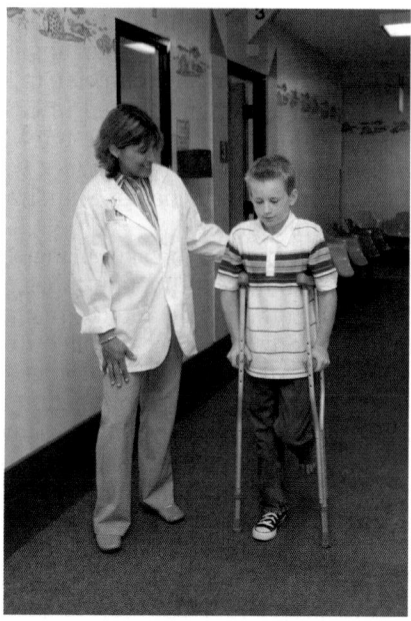

Figure 20-4 Crutches are placed under the child's arms. To avoid shoulder nerve injury, the child should not lean on the crutches. The crutches are placed approximately one ft in front of the child, and the child's legs should swing up to, but not beyond, the crutches.

number of points in contact with the floor. For instance, a three-point gait occurs when the two crutches and the unaffected limb are touching the floor.

Walkers are useful ambulatory devices for young children and those with limited functional abilities. A walker uses a four-legged base to provide support during ambulation. A parallel stationary walker requires the child to lift and advance the entire walker when ambulating, which may be difficult for the child with more severe musculoskeletal challenges. The rolling walker has two to four wheels attached to the base and merely requires the child to gently push the device to assist in ambulation. This type of walker is less stable, however, especially on wet or slippery surfaces.

PROSTHETIC DEVICES

Children with limb deformities and those who have experienced permanent loss of a body part may elect to use a prosthetic device to enhance mobility and body image. Prostheses are individually fitted to the contour of the remaining body part. The prosthetic device can be a completely formed body part such as a hand or foot, or it can be a device with myoelectric controls that enable the child to move and use the extremity.

Experience has indicated that children who have been fitted with prostheses earlier than 4 years of age function better than those fitted at a later age. Fitting an artificial limb within a year after birth or traumatic injury is optimal. Frequent adjustments will be needed for growth, evaluation may be needed every 3 to 4 months, and a new prosthesis may be needed as frequently as every 18 months. Each child's physical condition, aspirations, and life circumstances are reflected in the prosthetic prescription and treatment plan. Management is a team effort, with special attention to effects of growth and changes that characterize childhood.

Family education is extremely important in managing prosthetic training, applying the prosthesis, monitoring skin tolerance, and promoting good maintenance of the prosthetic device to prevent wear and tear.

PREVENTION OF COMPLICATIONS OF IMMOBILIZATION

Conditions that affect a child's muscles, bones, or connective tissues generally lead to immobility. A primary focus of the interdisciplinary team is to prevent formation of contractures, loss of muscle tone, or fixation of joints during immobilization. The immobilized area may be limited to a specific body part, or immobilization may affect every aspect of the child's activities and mobility. Immobility can also be hazardous to the child if the health care team and the family do not take measures to prevent systemic complications and disability. Nursing Interventions 20-2 summarizes the hazards of immobility and the interventions to prevent these hazards.

NURSING INTERVENTIONS 20-2

Promoting Healing and Preventing Complications of Immobility

Nursing Diagnosis	Clinical Manifestations	Nursing Interventions	Rationale
Ineffective breathing pattern	Slow, shallow respirations Pooling of secretions Decreased cough reflex	Evaluate respiratory status each shift. Encourage child to cough and breathe deeply. Initiate use of an incentive spirometer and chest physiotherapy as needed. Mobilize patient as soon as possible.	Immobilization leads to decreased lung expansion, decreased respiratory effort, decreased cough reflex, and pooling of secretions. Baseline assessment provides data for early interventions. Pulmonary status is evaluated to prevent atelectasis. Early interventions reduce respiratory complications.
Ineffective peripheral tissue perfusion	Absent pulses Altered skin color, elasticity, sensation, temperature, moisture Capilary refill >3 seconds Edema of extremities	Turn the patient and ensure clothing and bed lines are not restricting blood flow and movement of extremities. Encourage active and passive ROM activities. Apply elastic stockings to lower extremities. Mobilize the patient as soon as possible.	Vasodilation and impaired venous return may result from muscular inactivity and response to injury.
Risk for peripheral neurovascular dysfunction	Decreased capillary refill Pain, pallor, pulselessness, paresthesia, and/or paralysis of extremities Changes in extremities, including increased or decreased temperature, increased swelling, decreased sensation and movement	Assess the child's extremities for clinical manifestations of neurovascular dysfunction, comparing affected and unaffected extremities. Monitor motor function and ROM by having the child move fingers and toes.	The unaffected extremity can be used as a baseline for assessment. Starting the examination on the healthy limb may calm the child. Normal capillary refill is 1–3 seconds. Longer than 3 seconds indicates inadequate arterial supply. Swelling peaks within 24–48 hours unless tissue damage is extensive. Document responses indicating sensation as present, absent, or abnormal. If the child's nerves are intact, sensation should be felt at areas of innervation above and below the injury. Document motion distal to the fracture as normal ROM, painful, or minimal.

(Continued)

NURSING INTERVENTIONS 20-2

Promoting Healing and Preventing Complications of Immobility (*Continued*)

Nursing Diagnosis	Clinical Manifestations	Nursing Interventions	Rationale
Hyperthermia	Increase in body temperature Flushed skin Increased respiratory rate and heart rate Warm to touch	Monitor child's temperature for fever. Monitor laboratory values for elevated WBCs or elevated ESR.	Elevated temperatures may indicate infection. Fever of 101°F or higher should be reported. Elevated WBC count and elevated ESR are indications of infection and or inflammation.
Impaired physical mobility	Decreased muscle mass and strength Decreased bone mass and strength	Encourage active and passive ROM activities. Encourage isometric and isotonic exercises. Mobilize patient as soon as possible.	Imbalance between osteoblastic and osteoclastic activity leads to calcium and phosphorus loss, resulting in decreased muscle tone and decreased bone stress.
Imbalanced nutrition: Less than body requirements	Decreased efficiency in using nutrients Increased potassium and calcium excretion Decreased appetite	Give small, frequent meals. Give increased fiber, protein, vitamin C, and acidifying foods. Limit calcium intake. Mobilize the patient as soon as possible.	Inactivity will result in decreased basal metabolic rate and oxygen consumption. Nitrogen loss and negative nitrogen balance can occur because of protein loss from loss of muscle mass. Balanced nutrition is needed to promote healing.
Impaired skin integrity	Increased potential for skin breakdown	Inspect the child's skin for rashes, redness, irritation, or pressure sores. Avoid positions that put pressure on bony prominences. Turn the patient regularly. Keep the patient's skin clean and dry. Apply lotion to dry skin areas. Apply pressure-equalizing and pressure-reducing devices.	Skin assessment includes looking at the bony prominences and at any area that is in contact with the traction or suspension apparatus, cast, and bedding material. Continuous pressure on bony prominences can compromise skin integrity.
Constipation	Constipation Urinary retention Renal calculi Anorexia	Evaluate the individual's established elimination patterns for amount, consistency, and frequency of bowel movement and urination. Encourage fluid intake and roughage. Encourage small, frequent meals. Provide privacy for elimination. Administer stool softeners or suppositories as ordered. Monitor urine output and characteristics of urine every shift. Offer acidic juices such as apple or cranberry.	General muscle weakness and atrophy with inactivity slow peristalsis and cause urinary stasis in the renal pelvis. Promote intake of water and juices; limit milk intake to maintain bowel and bladder function because constipation and renal calculi are both related to immobility. Privacy is especially important to children who are school aged through adolescence. A stool softener or suppository helps facilitate bowel movements.

Nursing Diagnosis	Clinical Manifestations	Nursing Interventions	Rationale
Acute pain	Discomfort Observed evidence of pain Sleep disturbance Guarding behavior Changes in appetite and eating	Assess for cause of pain. Use pharmacologic and biobehavioral measures for pain management. Position for comfort.	Actual or potential tissue damage can cause pain. Pain may indicate compartment syndrome.
Deficient diversional activity	Boredom Irritability Regressive behaviors	Provide a stimulating environment with age-appropriate toys, posters, and music. Provide age-appropriate toys or activities for the child in traction. Encourage a family member to stay with the young child. Allow friends and classmates to visit. Have classmates telephone or write letters to the hospitalized child. Encourage movement by having the child perform appropriate self-care. Enlist child life specialist and physical therapist in providing activities that will encourage movement without disrupting traction. A hospital or school tutor can be contacted to continue the school-aged child's schooling. Encourage age-appropriate behavior. Allow for regressive behavior without punishment. Provide methods by which the child can express anger appropriately.	Imposed immobility associated with musculoskeletal conditions and traction can cause disruptions in patients' independence, body image, and self-esteem. Stress and changes in role can bring about anxiety and fear. Sensory deprivation can lead to boredom and a sense of being forgotten. Peer interactions are especially important to school-aged children and adolescents. Move the bed to the playroom daily to change the environment. An immobilized child may regress to an earlier developmental level.

NUTRITIONAL INTERVENTIONS

 QUESTION: Cathy is a rapidly growing 13-year-old girl with a broken hand and scoliosis. How can she meet her calcium and vitamin requirements?

Children with musculoskeletal disorders do not generally require any special dietary considerations unless the child is immobile or acutely injured. In most cases, a healthy, well-balanced, age-appropriate diet provides for the nutritional needs of the child (see Chapters 4 to 7). Foods high in calcium and phosphorus are of particular importance in promoting the development of strong bones and teeth (Table 20-1). Also, adequate calcium intake during childhood and adolescence is a key strategy in preventing osteoporosis and skeletal fractures later in life. Vitamins A and D are also needed to regulate absorption and deposition of calcium and phosphorus, thus aiding bone growth and contributing to bone strength.

When the child is immobile and has a low caloric expenditure, weight gain may become a concern. The child's diet can be modified to reduce the number of calories ingested while continuing to provide vitamins and minerals to promote growth.

Children who have experienced an acute injury to the bone, skin tissues, or muscle may require increased intakes of calcium, phosphorus, vitamins, and minerals. Calcium and phosphorus promote bone formation and growth to damaged areas. Vitamin A is needed for the creation of collagen, scar formation, and growth of new epithelial cells. Vitamin C is necessary for collagen synthesis, to improve resistance to infection, and to form capillaries to bring blood to the damaged musculoskeletal areas. Minerals such as zinc, copper, and iron also assist in the synthesis of collagen (Lanou et al., 2005).

TABLE 20-1	Important Nutrients to Promote Strong Bones	
Nutrient	**Food Sources**	**Results of Deficiency on Musculoskeletal System**
Calcium	Milk, cheese, yogurt, cottage cheese Clams, oysters Broccoli, cauliflower, cabbage Molasses	Improper bone growth (rickets, bowed legs, osteomalacia, osteoporosis) Porous bones Tetany and muscle spasm
Phosphorus	Milk, cheese, egg yolks Meat, fish Nuts Whole-grain cereals Legumes	Rickets, bowed legs Porous bones Stunted growth
Vitamin A	Liver and liver sausage Butter, cream, whole milk, egg yolks Green and yellow vegetables, yellow fruits Ripe tomatoes Fortified margarine Fish liver oils	Poor bone formation
Vitamin D	Vitamin D–fortified milk Butter, egg yolk, liver, and saltwater fish (small amounts) Fish liver oils	Soft bones Bowed legs Poor posture

ANSWER: Between the ages of 9 and 18 years, 1,200–1,500-mg calcium is recommended per day. Families need to be aware that given how food is labeled, this means 120%–150% of the recommended daily allowance. During this critical period of rapid growth, teenagers store calcium in their bones and establish the bone density for their adult years. Medical studies also show that there may be a relationship between inadequate calcium intake and broken bones. A variety of foods are needed for vitamin requirements, but four 8-oz glasses of milk will meet a teenager's calcium requirements. Some fruit juices are also calcium fortified, but read the nutritional labels carefully.

PAIN MANAGEMENT

Sources of pain and discomfort for the child with a musculoskeletal disorder include diagnostic and surgical procedures, muscle spasms, development of contractures, injury to the bone and tissues, joint inflammation, swelling, stiffness, and the processes of healing. Children want to move and explore their world. Even in the presence of pain, children are likely to find ways to adapt their movements and motion to remain as active as possible.

Providing pharmacologic and biobehavioral measures are essential to ensure the child's comfort, maintain the integrity of the child's musculoskeletal status, and promote continuing achievement of developmental milestones. Because motion is so crucial to the child, the child's mobility must not be negatively affected by pain. Chapter 10 provides a summary of pain management techniques that are effective in children.

DIVERSIONAL ACTIVITIES

The child's physical activities are based on the amount of motion allowed and the child's need for stimulation,

peer interaction, and opportunities to promote normal development (Fig. 20-5). When a child is immobilized, passive and active ROM exercises should be completed three or four times a day to maintain functional ability. In the acute care setting, the child life therapist can provide age-appropriate toys to place around the bed. Children should be provided with a playroom setting, when possible. Photographs of family members or the child's favorite movie or TV characters can be taped to the crib and traction bars to provide visual stimulation. If necessary, social services personnel can provide assistance for family members who stay with their child during the hospitalization, and they can assist with the family's anticipated needs on discharge.

Attendance at school, when possible, is strongly encouraged. The school nurse can work with the family to adapt the child's environment, schedule, and physical

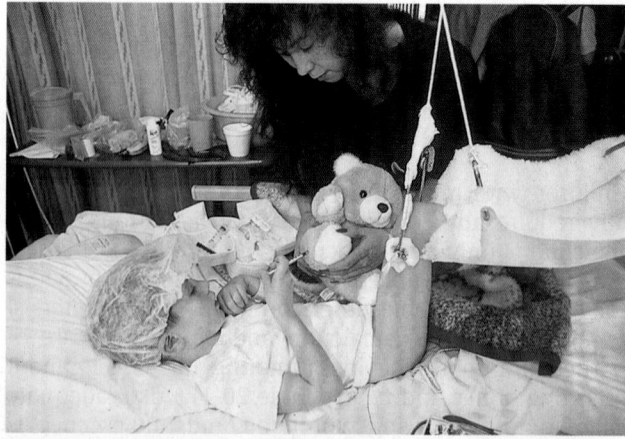

Figure 20-5 The immobilized child should be provided with age-appropriate toys and diversional activities.

activities as necessary. If the child is unable to attend school, diversionary activities in the home or in the acute care setting must be incorporated into the daily plan of care. The child can become easily bored and regress socially, personally, and academically. Providing age-appropriate activities and encouraging visits from friends can help the child adapt to the immobilized state.

NURSING PLAN OF CARE

QUESTION: Using Nursing Plan of Care 20-1, what is the nursing diagnosis most appropriate for Cathy? Select a nursing diagnosis that is applicable to Cathy but is not found in Nursing Plan of Care 20-1.

The child with a musculoskeletal disorder or injury faces challenges in mobility and movement. Such challenges may require long-term adaptation by the child and family to change the environment, their daily living activities, and their developmental expectations to complement the child's abilities. When temporary injury has occurred, alterations in the child's lifestyle usually require only short-term modifications. However, the active young child or the adolescent concerned with body image issues may have difficulty meeting the demands of the treatment regimen. The nursing plan of care addresses the impaired or altered mobility and movement that the child may experience. In addition, concerns regarding body image and achieving optimal levels of growth and development are likely to emerge. The nursing plan of care should reflect these concerns. Most musculoskeletal disorders or injuries are managed in the home. Formulate the plan of care to address the teaching, family support, and resources that will be required to manage the child's illness at home, in school, and as the child participates in community activities (Nursing Plan of Care 20-1). For some children, the musculoskeletal condition may be lifelong, with periods during which symptoms are exacerbated and the child may need hospitalization. The Nursing Plan of Care in Chapter 12 addresses the care needs of the child with a chronic condition and the child in need of rehabilitation or habilitation services. Nursing Plan of Care 11-1 provides the plan of care when the child's condition requires hospitalization for acute management.

ANSWER: The nursing diagnosis that is relevant for both the fractured metacarpal and Cathy's scoliosis is impaired skin integrity related to surgical incision, wounds, or application of treatment devices such as casts, braces, and external fixators. Another appropriate diagnosis is related to the fact that Cathy is not wearing her brace for the amount of time required to effect change in her spine. An appropriate diagnosis is ineffective self-health management: noncompliance with therapeutic regimen.

ALTERATIONS IN MUSCULOSKELETAL STATUS

Alterations in musculoskeletal status can result from congenital and hereditary disorders, growth-related disorders, infectious or inflammatory disorders, or traumatic injuries.

CONGENITAL AND HEREDITARY DISORDERS

Disorders that are caused by an inherited gene or that occur within the intrauterine environment are referred to as *congenital disorders*. The child is born with the disorder, although it may not be apparent at birth. For example, a clubfoot is visible at birth, whereas mild osteogenesis imperfecta (OI) may escape detection until the child becomes active and experiences numerous fractures.

METATARSUS ADDUCTUS

Metatarsus adductus or intoeing is a mild deformity in which the bones of the forefoot turn inward (Fig. 20-6). It is a common congenital problem that occurs in both males and females and presents bilaterally in 50% of the cases. It is defined as a transverse plane deformity in the tarsometatarsal joint in which the metatarsals are deviated medially. The cause of metatarsus adductus is unknown, although many affected children have a family history. Intrauterine positioning, especially with breech positioning, may also play a role because the feet are tucked medially in utero. Prone sleeping position of the baby may increase the tendency of the feet to turn inward. Absence of a medial cuneiform or abnormal growth of the medial cuneiform has been considered to affect development of metatarsus adductus. In addition, arrest of normal rotation of the foot during fetal development plays a role in the development of metatarsus adductus. Children with metatarsus adductus have an increased incidence of hip dysplasia.

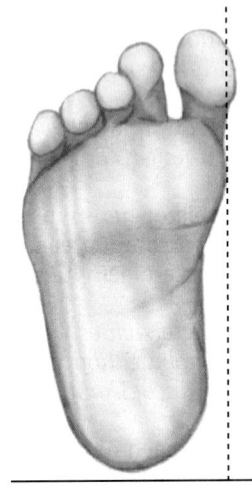
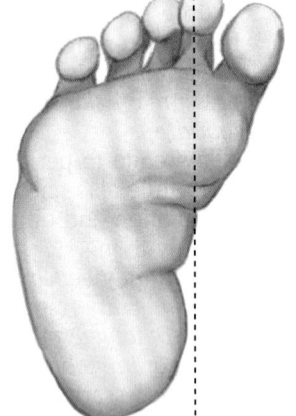

Normal   Metatarsus varus

Figure 20-6 Metatarsus adductus is graded according to the degree of inward toeing that passes beyond the medial border of the foot.

NURSING PLAN OF CARE 20-1:

The Child With Altered Musculoskeletal Status

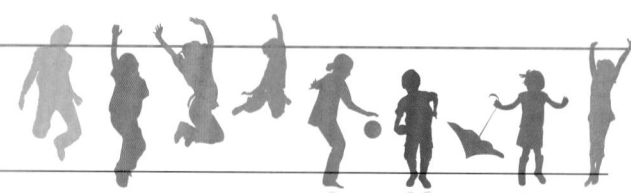

Nursing Diagnosis: Acute or chronic pain related to musculoskeletal condition or treatment regimen

- See Nursing Plan of Care 10-1 for a complete description of pain management interventions.

Nursing Diagnosis: Impaired physical mobility related to restriction of movement/activities, physical and cognitive impairments, traction, deformity, or brace

Interventions/Rationale

- Assess for muscle strength in all extremities.
  Rehabilitation and habilitation will be geared toward maximizing the strength of unaffected extremities and maintaining and potentially maximizing strength of affected extremities.
- Assess for complications of immobility (e.g., ineffective breathing pattern, constipation, imbalanced nutrition), and use interventions to prevent and treat complications.
  Even children on temporary bed rest or with restricted physical mobility can experience the complications associated with immobility. Ongoing assessments, preventive care, and prompt intervention when complications are apparent will minimize additional impairment.
- Assist the child or encourage the child to perform ROM exercises twice daily, or as prescribed; praise correct performance of exercises and positive attitude.
  ROM exercises promote venous return, prevent stiffness, and maintain muscle strength and endurance.
- Turn and position the child every 2 hours or as needed. Ensure limbs are maintained in functional alignment using pillows, wedges, and so forth. Support feet in dorsiflexed position. Use other antipressure devices as needed (e.g., specialty beds, sheepskin mattress).
  Optimizes circulation to all tissues and relieves pressure on skin and bony prominences. Prevents foot drop.
- Allow child to perform tasks at his or her own rate while also encouraging and facilitating early ambulation and other age-appropriate activities of daily living.
  Child may be fearful of initiating activities given mobility restrictions. Early mobilization will enhance long-term recovery and reduce debilitating effects of immobility.
- Place necessary items within easy reach of the child. Alter environment to ensure the child's belongings are accessible and easy to use and operate given the child's mobility restrictions. Keep side rails up and the bed in the low position.

Promoting a safe environment for child to perform self-care activities will prevent further injury and will support mobilization.

- Provide a list of restricted activities based on condition (e.g., for a child with scoliosis, no weight lifting, trampoline, or gymnastics).
  Restricted movement caused by a cast or brace and restriction of some activities might discourage or limit participation in beneficial physical activities.
- Review with the family, school officials, and other community personnel (as identified by the family) practical changes for school and home environment (e.g., modifications to enable participation in physical education class, access to classes without going up stairs).
  Ensures that the child's mobility limitations are communicated to the family, school, and other community agencies so that a safe environment can be provided for the child and ensures that the child's ongoing plan of care can be implemented and supported.

Expected Outcomes

- Child will maintain muscle strength, endurance, and joint flexibility in unaffected extremities.
- Child will remain free from the complications of immobility.
- Child will be as mobile as possible as soon as possible, using assistive devices if needed.
- Child will perform as many activities of daily living as possible.

Nursing Diagnosis: Risk for peripheral neurovascular dysfunction related to the effects of the musculoskeletal disorder

Interventions/Rationale

- Frequently monitor all extremities for pulses, sensation, movement, color, capillary refill, edema, ROM, and complaints of pain; compare findings bilaterally.
  Frequent monitoring provides baseline data to recognize early development of complications. Prolonged bed rest, restrictive devices such as casts and braces, reductions in muscle strength and function, and decreased mobility may all contribute to changes in neuromuscular and neurovascular status, including the development of compartment syndrome.
- Assess for developing thrombophlebitis (e.g., calf swelling, Homans sign, redness, localized swelling, and increased temperature).
  Prolonged bed rest or immobility can promote clot formation.
- Assist child or encourage child to perform ROM exercises twice daily, or as prescribed; praise correct performance of exercises and positive attitude.

ROM exercises promote venous return, prevent stiffness, and maintain muscle strength and endurance.

- Monitor fit of casts, braces, and appliances to ensure that devices are not causing constriction that would lead to neurovascular compromise.

   Ill-fitting braces and appliances may constrict blood flow and sensation to the extremities. Peripheral swelling and edema will alter fit of appliances. Normal physical growth of the child will alter fit of appliances over time.

Expected Outcome

- Child will exhibit signs and symptoms of adequate neurovascular function.

Nursing Diagnosis: Impaired skin integrity related to surgical incision, wounds, or application of treatment devices such as casts, braces, and external fixators

Interventions/Rationale

- Conduct a complete assessment of the skin, including evaluating for signs and symptoms of skin breakdown and infection. Assess skin for color, texture, moisture, general appearance, signs of redness, and appearance of wounds and incisions. Assess vital signs.

   Assessment provides baseline data about the skin to allow for early detection and prompt intervention should problems such as infection, as evidenced by increased temperature and heart rate, occur.

- If child is on bed rest, change position, logroll, or assist child to turn every 2 hours; check for correct position of feet and forehead when in prone position.

   Frequent position changes prevent pressure areas from developing and prevent tissue from breaking down.

- Keep skin clean, dry, and free from irritants.

   Skin breakdown may be caused by shear, friction, and irritation.

- Inspect pressure areas and bony prominences.

   Visual inspection helps identify areas at risk for breakdown as well as areas that are beginning to break down.

- Apply pressure relief device to bed as appropriate.

   Flotation devices, air mattresses, and so forth, assist in preventing the development of pressure areas.

- Teach the child how to assess for proper fit of brace or appliances.

   A poorly fitting cast or brace may rub against the skin, causing skin breakdown.

- Teach care of wound or incision site, including assessment of site for signs of infection (e.g., redness, odor, excessive drainage).

Surgical procedures and breaks in the skin (e.g., pin sites) provide potential sites for infection.

Expected Outcomes

- Child will remain free of any signs of skin breakdown or infection.
- Child will exhibit signs and symptoms of healing to regain skin integrity of wound or incision site.
- Child or family will demonstrate skill in care of wound, incision, or treatment devices to maintain or enhance skin integrity.

Nursing Diagnosis: Constipation related to decreased activity level and impairments in musculoskeletal status

Interventions/Rationale

- Assess the child's usual patterns of elimination and compare with current pattern, including frequency, color, and quality of stool. Assess dietary patterns. Evaluate current medication usage that may contribute to constipation.

   Baseline data provide information about deviation from normal stool patterns. Constipation may result from decreased metabolic need, changes in nutritional patterns, inactivity, and use of certain medications.

- Encourage a high-protein, high-fiber diet with small, frequent meals and increased fluid intake. Encourage the child to consume "natural" cathartics such as prunes, beans, or green leafy vegetables.

   Protein will enhance the healing process, and protein and fiber add bulk to stool to make defecation easier. Inadequate fluid intake may contribute to constipation.

- Manage environmental conditions to enhance regular elimination patterns (e.g., encourage a regular time for elimination, provide adequate privacy, assist child in bathroom or in using bedpan).

   Children will often avoid going to the bathroom (even when they feel the urge) if they think others may be able to see them while they eliminate, if the toileting equipment is not familiar to them, and if they feel it will "hurt" when they have to defecate.

- Give bulk fiber (e.g., Metamucil), stool softeners, laxatives (e.g., milk of magnesia, Citrucel, or mineral oil), and suppositories as ordered; record effectiveness.

   A variety of over-the-counter agents can be used to change the bulk of intestinal contents, soften stool, lubricate intestinal mucosa, and/or stimulate rectal mucosa.

Expected Outcomes

- Child will pass stool according to his or her usual elimination pattern.
- Child will demonstrate an increased fluid and fiber intake.
- Child will report easy and complete elimination of stool.

(Continued)

NURSING PLAN OF CARE 20-1:

The Child With Altered Musculoskeletal Status (*Continued*)

Nursing Diagnosis: Impaired urinary elimination related to effects of immobility

Interventions/Rationale

- Monitor bladder function daily. Observe for signs of urinary retention, incontinence, or infection (e.g., voiding small amounts, dysuria, frequency, fever).

  Urinary tract infections are hazards of immobility because a recumbent position may cause urinary stasis in the renal pelvis. Increased calcium excretion from inactivity causes alkaline urine, which promotes bacterial growth.

- Record intake and output. Ensure hourly urine output is 1 mL/kg/hr.

  Intake and output provide evidence of the adequacy of fluid balance. Urine output less than 1 mL/kg/hr indicates dehydration.

- Assess need for intermittent or Foley catheterization.

  The incontinent child or the child with decreasing urinary output may require catheterization to ensure accurate measurement of urinary output.

- Explain the necessity of high fluid intake. Collaborate with the child and family to encourage fluid consumption.

  Increasing fluids will reduce the likelihood of urinary tract infections.

Expected Outcomes

- Child will maintain normal urinary elimination patterns postoperatively and while mobility is restricted.
- The child will remain free of signs and symptoms of a urinary tract infection.

Nursing Diagnosis: Delayed growth and development related to lack of stimulation, immobility, physical limitations of musculoskeletal condition (e.g., joint stiffness, limitations in ROM)

Interventions/Rationale

- Perform complete developmental screening and compare with norms for age of child.

  Developmental screening provides baseline data to determine areas of fine motor, gross motor, language, and social skills that need enhancement.

- Collaborate with the family to determine factors that may impede the child's participation in age-appropriate activities and self-care activities.

  The child's health status, environmental conditions, overprotection by family members, and child's own fears may be issues that impede participation in activities. A comprehensive assessment of these factors will assist in determining which of these factors can be managed or changed to better support achievement of developmental milestones.

- Collaborate with child life services and school services to determine age-appropriate play activities for the child that enhance developmental skills. Share strategies with the child and family. Encourage the child to do as much for himself or herself as possible; assist in resuming as many normal activities as possible.

  Children on forced bed rest and forced immobility (braces, casts) have restricted activities, thereby limiting routine opportunities for growth and development.

- Work with the child and family to develop a plan for involving the child in self-care activities and self-management of the treatment regimen (e.g., learning to put on a brace, self-administering medications) as age appropriate. Refer to rehabilitation services as needed.

  Encourage the child to perform skills at a level appropriate to his or her assessed abilities. Over time, the child should become more independent in managing the chronic condition.

Expected Outcomes

- Child will demonstrate skills appropriate for developmental stage and age.
- Family members will demonstrate an understanding of child's special needs.
- As the child matures, the child will demonstrate increasing responsibility for maintaining the treatment regimen.

Nursing Diagnosis: Chronic or situational low self-esteem related to physical manifestations of condition, use of devices such as braces or splints, disturbed body image, feelings of powerlessness, and unrealistic self-expectations

Interventions/Rationale

- Provide openings to enable child or adolescent to express feelings. Be a good listener and accept what the child or adolescent verbalizes. Be accepting of the child's body image changes and limitations related to the child's condition.

  Allowing the child to talk provides an outlet to discuss his or her frustrations and concerns. Listening to the child provides an opportunity to validate his or her concerns and discuss ways to help build his or her self-esteem. Visual differences such as a body cast or brace may contribute to low self-esteem.

- Schedule a team conference with the family, child, teachers, school nurse, and health care team members to provide information and explore feelings and attitudes; encourage the child to take part in selecting conference participants.

  Team conferences facilitate open discussion among all family members. Active listening and open acceptance of the child's physical changes will model acceptance of the child and will assist family members, including the child, to accept changes.

- Give the child a sense of control by providing realistic decision-making opportunities.

   The child may feel powerless, further adding to feelings of low self-esteem.

- Assist the child or adolescent to develop strategies to enhance self-esteem (e.g., changing physical appearance, participating in enjoyable activities in which the child can excel, developing new friendships).

   Appropriate strategies help the child or adolescent to explore new methods for developing positive feelings about himself or herself.

- Arrange for the child and other family members to meet others who have a similar condition or experiences and who have managed these issues successfully.

   Meeting others provides an opportunity for the child or adolescent and family to identify with someone who is experiencing the same type of situation. It also provides an opportunity to learn new coping strategies and to have realistic perceptions of how others have managed their condition over time.

Expected Outcomes
- Child will verbalize positive statements about self.
- Child will discuss concerns related to feelings about self and body.
- Child will maintain age-appropriate interaction with peers.

Nursing Diagnosis: Deficient knowledge: Child's condition, treatment, exercises, and care of appliances and assistive devices

Interventions/Rationale
- Provide instruction regarding treatment plan (e.g., exercises, restriction of activities, proper application of braces or appliances, frequency of follow-up appointments, diet, and skin care).

   If deficient knowledge exists, the child and family cannot appropriately adhere to treatment, manage the appliance, or detect signs of complications.

- Allow time for questions, provide a written summary of what the health care team has said about the child's condition and recommended plan of treatment, and reinforce or repeat initial explanation as needed.

   Questioning provides opportunities to clarify misconceptions and ensures that the child and family are able to manage care when in the home environment.

- Observe the child and caregivers demonstrate home care skills.

   Return demonstration provides an opportunity to ensure the child and family can independently perform the skill in a safe and accurate manner.

- Make appropriate referrals to community service agencies (e.g., home health, physical therapy, education, mental health counseling) as needed.

   Many musculoskeletal conditions require ongoing, long-term management to assist the child in achieving maximum developmental abilities.

Expected Outcomes
- Child and family will describe the illness, identifying the child's specific manifestations and the planned treatment regimen.
- Child and family will demonstrate necessary skills for care.

The natural history for flexible metatarsus adductus is spontaneous correction with further growth. Although passive stretching is often suggested, no studies document its effectiveness. Inappropriate aggressive treatment could lead to valgus hindfoot deformity and skewfoot (The Pediatric Orthopaedic Society of North America [POSNA], 2012). The ultimate goal of therapy is to straighten the forefoot so that it is aligned with the heel, the soft-tissue vertical crease is present, and the deformity is structural and rigid or "nonflexible."

caREminder

To differentiate metatarsus adductus from clubfoot, hold the infant's heel in one hand and try to position the foot to midline with the other hand. If you are able to straighten the foot, the child has metatarsus adductus, not clubfoot.

Radiographs are not usually necessary. However, radiographs are acquired if passive correction indicates the metatarsus adductus is inflexible to determine whether other deformities exist.

Interdisciplinary Interventions

Treatment of flexible metatarsus adductus in the infant consists of gentle, passive manipulation, performed by the caregivers during diaper changes, and stretching exercises. The caregiver holds the child's heel still with one hand while attempting to straighten the forefoot with the other hand. The child may also benefit from slightly overcorrecting the position of the foot by wearing splints or reverse-last shoes. The splints or shoes are worn 22 hours a day, and the child's condition is reevaluated in 4 to 6 weeks (Hosalkar et al., 2007).

Flexible deformities that persist beyond 8 months or rigid deformities need serial casting. Serial casting, done as often as biweekly, gently molds the foot into proper position. After casting, a straight or reversed shoe may be worn to maintain the foot in the correct position. Surgical correction is rare but may be indicated in persistent rigid adductus. Persistent adductus deformity does not appear to cause disability or degenerative arthritis.

Teach the family passive manipulation, correct infant sleeping positions, and cast care, if indicated (see thePoint for Procedures: Cast Care). Reassure the family that the deformity need not interfere with the child's development and ability to participate in full activities.

CLUBFOOT

Clubfoot, or *talipes equinovarus*, is a congenital deformity that typically has four main components: inversion and adduction of the forefoot, inversion of the heel and hindfoot, equinus (limitation of extension) of the ankle and subtalar joint, and internal rotation of the leg. Clubfoot is a complex, multifactor deformity with genetic and intrauterine factors, although the etiology of idiopathic clubfoot remains unknown (Chung & Rooks, 2008). It is common (1 per 1,000 live births), occurs twice as often in males as in females, and has a higher incidence in persons of Hispanic and Asian heritage (Baindurashvili et al., 2012; Morcuende, 2006). Approximately 80% of all children born with clubfoot live in developing countries, and many of these children and their families lack the financial and medical resources to seek treatment.

Pathophysiology

The exact mechanisms that results in the anatomic abnormalities of clubfoot are unknown. Several hypotheses exist regarding mechanism of injury, including uterine constriction; abnormalities of the bones, joints, and/or connective tissues; distal limb vasculature; muscle migration; and presence of underlying developmental or neurologic abnormality or arrest. It has been demonstrated that severe clubfoot resembles an embryonic foot at the beginning of the second month of fetal development and, because the deformity is accompanied by underdevelopment of the bones and muscles, this implies that the abnormality may occur between 9 and 38 weeks of gestation (Morcuende, 2006).

The clubfoot malformation, which can be unilateral or bilateral, is usually obvious at birth. The main anatomic components of clubfoot are a flexed ankle, a turning in of the heel, and adduction of the forefoot (Fig. 20-7). Clubfoot can be classified into extrinsic (supple) type, which is essentially a severe positional soft-tissue deformity, and intrinsic (rigid) type, in which manual reduction is impossible. The type of clubfoot determines the specific treatment.

Assessment

On examination, the foot appears small, with a flexible, soft heel because the calcaneus is hypoplastic. The heel is usually small and internally rotated, making the soles of the feet face each other in the case of bilateral deformity. Evaluation of the foot includes

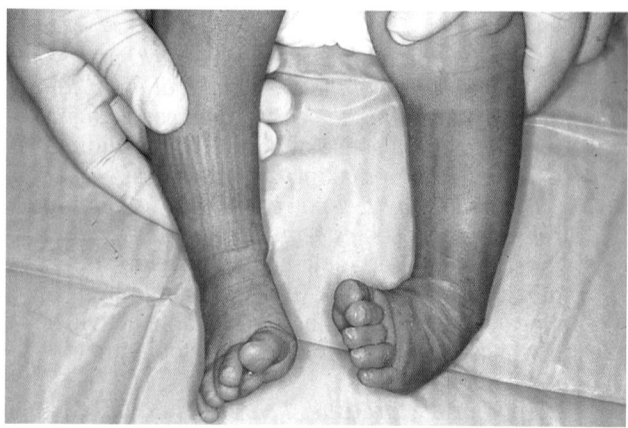

Figure 20-7 The child with clubfoot has a flexed ankle, a turned heel, and an adducted forefoot.

measuring foot size and shape, ROM of the joints, and radiographic evaluation. Radiographs reveal roughly parallel axes of the talus and calcaneus.

Interdisciplinary Interventions

In the case of supple or extrinsic clubfoot, the universally accepted treatment consists of a casting and manipulation technique known as the *Ponseti method*. In rigid (intrinsic) clubfoot, casting followed by surgery may be the treatment of choice. In either type, the treatment begins immediately after diagnosis.

With the Ponseti method, specific manipulation and casting is performed weekly in the physician's office for 6 to 8 weeks. When correction has been achieved, a foot abduction brace is used until the child is 6 months of age. Part-time use of the abduction brace is recommended during sleep until the child is 3 to 4 years of age. The Ponseti method may not be successful, and the condition may reoccur, thus requiring additional treatment (Hennessey, 2012; Ponseti et al., 2006).

The *French method* may also be used, either alone or in conjunction with the Ponseti method. The French method starts with a trained physical therapist for three sessions each week (30 to 60 minutes per session) with the infant, mobilizing and stretching the foot, taping it to maintain correction, and fitting it with a molded plastic splint. Parents are taught how to conduct the mobilization, stretching, and taping at home. Most improvement occurs in the first 3 months, but home therapy may continue for up to 2 years.

For a rigid clubfoot that does not respond to treatment, surgery is recommended. The goal of surgery is to obtain a straight, painless, plantigrade (child stands with the sole of the foot on the ground, not on his heels or the outside of his foot), and mobile foot with normal radiographic appearance (Ippolito et al., 2005). The two surgical procedures most widely performed are Achilles tenotomy and arthrodesis, which is performed for more severe cases with residual varus and forefoot adduction. The Achilles tenotomy is performed before the child is walking, and the second procedure is done if the tendon release does not allow the foot to be in a functional position. Surgery requires brief hospitalization. Nursing care includes postoperative pain management, neurovascular assessment of the involved foot, and cast care teaching for the caregivers. A below-the-knee cast is applied for up to 12 weeks, with a cast change every 4 weeks. After cast removal, follow-up is usually done at 6-month intervals.

Depending on the treatment protocol, teach caregivers cast care procedures and, as treatment progresses, care and application of foot braces (see "Treatment Modalities" section). Ensure the caregivers understand the importance of daily assessment of the child's skin to monitor for skin breakdown from cast or brace wear or infection from surgical incisions. Treatment of this condition extends over several months. Encourage caregivers to be diligent with regard to following the treatment protocol and to complete all follow-up appointments. A delay in attainment of gross motor skills at 9 and 12 months of age has been noted in children treated for clubfoot (Garcia et al., 2011). Reassure parents that these delays in the first year of the child's life will not extend and impact later development of gross motor skills. The ultimate goal of therapy is to restore the look and function of the foot, thus allowing the child to walk correctly, and to prevent any long-term disabilities.

DEVELOPMENTAL DYSPLASIA OF THE HIP

DDH is a condition in which the femoral head has an abnormal relationship with the acetabulum. The term includes **luxation** (frank dislocation: complete loss of contact of the femoral head with the acetabulum), **subluxation** (partial dislocation: femoral head able to move within or outside the confines of the acetabulum), instability, and a number of radiologic abnormalities that demonstrate inadequate formation of the acetabulum (Shipman et al., 2006). Hip dysplasia can occur in utero, perinatally, or during infancy or childhood. Because, in some cases, the condition may not be apparent at birth, the term *developmental dysplasia of the hip* has replaced the term *congenital dysplasia of the hip*. However, the earlier a dislocated hip is detected, the more simple and effective the treatment.

DDH is one of the most common defects in the newborn infant, with incidence influenced by genetic and racial factors. The incidence of DDH in developing countries ranges from 1 to 20 per 1,000 births. Among Native Americans, the prevalence of hip dysplasia is nearly 25 to 50 cases per 1,000. The prevalence is very low among southern Chinese and black populations. There is a tenfold increase in children whose parents had developmental hip dysplasia compared with those who have not. And the rate of DDH with breech positioning is approximately 20% (McCarthy, 2011). Eighty percent of persons with DDH are female. The greater incidence in females may reflect the fact that they are more susceptible to the maternal hormone relaxin, which may contribute to ligamentous laxity.

Pathophysiology

At birth, the femoral head and the acetabulum are primarily cartilaginous. The acetabulum continues to grow postnatally. The growth of the fibrocartilaginous rim (the labrum) that surrounds the bony acetabulum deepens the socket. This continued development of the femoral head and acetabulum is needed to form a normal adult hip joint.

In general, hip development is normal during the fetal period and then gradually becomes abnormal for a variety of reasons. These reasons may include fetal position in utero, presentation at birth (e.g., breech), and generalized ligamentous laxity of the hip joint (McCarthy, 2011).

Assessment

Current clinical guidelines include screening of all newborns' hips by physical examination. Thanks to aggressive screening, late presentation of DDH is becoming less common.

Obtain information about the type of delivery and any family history of DDH to aid in determining the newborn's risk. Examine the infant while the child is relaxed and lying on a firm surface. Look for apparent limb length discrepancy and restricted or diminished motion, especially with abduction of the affected side. With the infant supine and the pelvis stable, abduction to 75 degrees and adduction to 30 degrees should be possible. Limitations in abduction may indicate DDH. Also perform Ortolani and Barlow tests (see Nursing Interventions 8-2 for an illustration and explanation of these maneuvers). A newborn with a positive Ortolani or Barlow sign at the 2-week examination should be referred to an orthopedist. At 3 to 4 months of age, the capsule laxity decreases and muscle tightness increases, making the two maneuvers no longer reliable indicators of DDH.

In the 3-month-old infant, limited adduction of the affected hip is the predominant sign when the hip becomes fixed in the dislocated position. Asymmetric thigh folds and a positive Galeazzi sign (one femur shorter than the other when measured with the hips and knees flexed) are physical findings that may be an indication of acetabulum abnormalities. Examine the hips at every well-baby visit until the infant is walking. Document all findings. If the physical findings arouse suspicion of DDH or if strong family history or concern exists, refer the child to an orthopedist for age-appropriate imaging.

Additional physical examination findings for late dislocation include asymmetry of gluteal thigh and/or labral skinfolds, decreased abduction on the affected side, standing or walking with external rotation, and leg length inequality (McCarthy, 2011). In the older child, physical findings may include short leg with toe walking on the affected side, positive Trendelenburg sign, or waddling gate (McCarthy, 2011).

caREminder

If a child's hip is known to be dislocated, do not repeatedly assess it because repeated manipulation of the joint may increase risk of vascular compromise.

Diagnostic Tests

Accurate diagnosis of abnormalities in the acetabulum requires imaging. Ultrasound is a safe method to evaluate for infant DDH that assesses hip morphology and hip stability. Once DDH has been diagnosed, sonograph can be used to evaluate hip position and acetabular development during treatment (McCarthy, 2011; Torres & DiPietro, 2009).

Interdisciplinary Interventions

If DDH is diagnosed early, simple and effective non-invasive treatment options usually result in excellent long-term anatomic and functional outcomes. Early detection of DDH limits malformation of the joint, and early treatment allows the hip to remodel and form properly. Remodeling is facilitated by maintaining the hips in a position of flexion and abduction using a Pavlik harness. Delayed diagnosis increases the risk of complications from treatment. Infants diagnosed after 6 to 8 months of age may require surgery for a closed reduction, followed by spica casting. Closed or open reduction and casting may also be needed when the child's condition does not improve after Pavlik harness treatment. As a child grows, the dislocation produces secondary changes in the shape of the hip. These changes can be corrected only with a surgical procedure to recreate a socket that is similar to a normal hip joint.

Although rare, complications from DDH and its treatment do occur. One common complication is lack of concentric reduction, which necessitates further operative procedures. In its severe form, and even with surgical treatment, DDH results in shortening of the affected leg and early osteoarthritis (Rosendahl et al., 2010). The child will need to be monitored until age 17 years, when the adolescent growth spurt is complete.

Bracing

The Pavlik harness is the most common device used for newborns or infants younger than 6 months of age (Gelfer & Kennedy, 2008; U.S. Preventive Services Task Force, 2006). This harness promotes hip flexion and abduction by prohibiting hip extension or adduction while allowing some kicking and movement. It consists of a chest strap, held at the nipple line by two shoulder straps. The leg and foot are adjusted with anterior and posterior straps, which hold the hips in proper position. Hip flexion is set to 100 to 110 degrees, and abduction is set at 50 to 70 degrees. Treatment is continued until the hip joint stabilizes or ultrasound or radiographs are normal. The Pavlik harness has been found to be effective in about 90% of the infants treated during the first 6 months of life

The harness must be applied by a physician and adjusted throughout the course of treatment. A poorly adjusted harness may make the dislocation worse and is associated with other complications (Fig. 20-8). Skin breakdown can occur underneath the harness or in groin folds if skin is not kept clean and dry. Tightly or poorly fitting shoulder straps can compress the brachial plexus, and improperly positioned leg straps can lead to subluxation of the knee and hyperflexion of the hips. Abduction is not without risk, with avascular necrosis

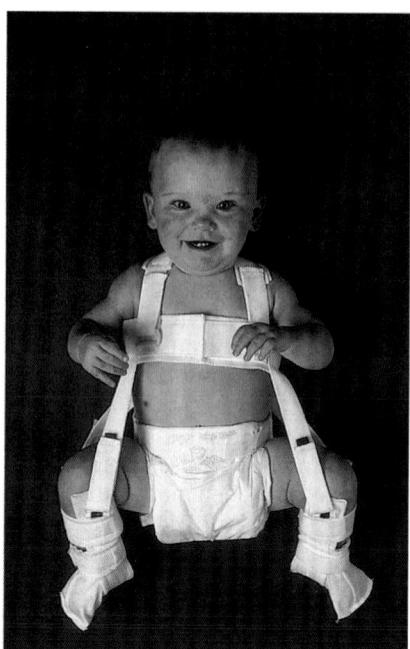

Figure 20-8 The Pavlik harness is used to maintain the hips in a position of flexion and abduction. Wheaton Pavlik Harness. Courtesy of Wheaton Brace Co. Reprinted with permission.

(AVN) being reported in approximately 2% of patients referred before 2 months of age (Rosendahl et al., 2010).

Traction

In cases in which DDH is not corrected by the harness, or when a late diagnosis is made, traction is used for about 2 weeks, followed by closed reduction and a body cast for 8 to 12 weeks. One type of traction, Bryant traction, aims to stretch the soft tissues around the hip and allows the femoral head to move back into the hip socket (see thePoint for Procedures: Traction Care). After 1 to 3 weeks in traction, the child is taken to the operating room, where the hip is reduced manually and a hip spica cast is applied. Often, an arthrogram is done at the same time to confirm that the hip has been reduced.

The spica cast is worn for 3 to 6 months. The position of the hip is checked periodically to make sure it remains satisfactory. Computed tomography may be used to get a three-dimensional (3-D) view.

caREminder

Unless the crossbar (as found in some spica casts) has been specifically reinforced so that it can be used for lifting or turning, do not use it for these purposes. Check with the physician or orthopedic technician if you are unsure about the safety of using the crossbar.

Surgical Interventions

If traction does not adequately stretch the muscles, surgical intervention may be indicated. In the child older than 2 years of age, if the hip has been dislocated for some time, the muscles around the hip shorten and become contracted. In such children, surgical intervention is recommended (Hart et al., 2006). A percutaneous adductor **tenotomy** consists of cutting an adductor tendon of the hip to decrease the risk of AVN (a potential complication of forced reduction and abduction) by taking pressure off the hip joint.

An open reduction of the hip consists of an **osteotomy** (incision or transaction of the bone) of the acetabulum or femur and removal of soft tissues. This operation cuts the bone and realigns it, allowing the hip to be concentrically placed so that it can continue to grow correctly as the child ages. After an open reduction, the child is placed in a hip spica cast for 6 to 8 weeks and then in an abduction splint for up to 3 more months.

This surgery is painful, and children generally are in the hospital for 2 to 3 days afterward. Intravenous narcotics are required for the first day after surgery, and oral narcotics are often needed for several days thereafter. Reassure the family that the incision will heal even though it is under the cast.

Community Care

Beginning in the outpatient setting, family education and support are key. The parents and other family members may experience a variety of reactions to the diagnosis, including shock, fear of the potential risks of surgery, feelings of loss and anger at the unexpected news, and uncertainty and anxiety about the future. Parents are often reluctant to hold the baby or change a diaper for fear of hurting the hip. Also, mothers tend to blame themselves for causing the dislocated hip. Seeing a small baby placed in a Pavlik harness for the first time can be upsetting. When the parents realize that the harness does not hurt the child and the baby can still move, some of their fears and anxieties may lessen (Clinical Judgment 20-1).

If the diagnosis of DDH is made when the child is older, family members may become angry with their health care provider for not finding the disorder earlier. The stress may be compounded by hospitalization of the child for traction or surgical procedures and by long-term follow-up.

After the plan of treatment is established, instruct the family on proper application of the Pavlik harness, skin care, and other activities of daily living such as diaper changing (Teaching Intervention Plan 20-1). Provide referrals to community resources, as necessary, to help the family cope with the child's care, such as frequent transportation between the home and clinic. Children do not need specialized transportation unless they cannot fit into a car.

Additional family education and modifications to the home environment may be necessary if the child is placed in a spica cast. Before surgery, prepare the family

---

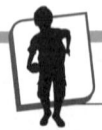

CLINICAL JUDGMENT 20-1

The Child With Developmental Dysplasia of the Hip

Lauren is a 2-month-old female who comes to the community health clinic with her mother for her immunizations. During her physical examination, you note that the fat folds in her thighs are not even.

When interviewing the mother for the birth history, she says that Lauren is her first child and that she was delivered via cesarean section because of her breech presentation.

Questions

1. During your assessment, what other information would help you to determine the problem?

2. What diagnostic studies would help you to determine the problem?

3. The mother is upset that the condition has not been noted sooner. What could you say to her at this time?

4. How can DDH be treated?

5. How would you determine that the harness is keeping the hip in the correct position?

Answers

1. Is there any family history of DDH or of joint laxity? Were Lauren's hips examined at birth or at any other time before this visit?

2. Ultrasound of the hip, possibly a plain radiograph. Ortolani and Barlow maneuvers would help to confirm the diagnosis.

3. Signs of DDH may not be present at birth or during the initial assessment of the child. Now that it has

been noted, corrective therapy can begin and the child should have a very good outcome.

4. Use the Pavlik harness for a few months. If this does not work, traction and casting, or possibly surgery, may be needed.

5. Ultrasound of the hip or a plain radiograph of the child while she is in the Pavlik harness

---

TIP 20-1: A TEACHING INTERVENTION PLAN for the Child With a Pavlik Harness

Nursing Diagnoses and Family Outcomes

- Deficient knowledge: Care of the child requiring a Pavlik harness
  Outcome: Caregivers will demonstrate measures to care for the child with a Pavlik harness.
- Risk for impaired skin integrity related to the use of a Pavlik harness
  Outcomes: Caregivers will demonstrate proper skin care techniques to maintain the child's skin integrity while a Pavlik harness is being used.
  Child will exhibit intact skin without redness, irritation, or breakdown.

Teach the Family

Positioning of the Harness

- Explain the purpose and function of the Pavlik harness.
- Ensure that the harness remains in place on the child at all times until the hip is stable (unless otherwise instructed by the physician). For this reason, only one harness is distributed and it is applied at the physician's office or clinic.
- Instruct the caregivers on how to correctly reattach the buckles or straps of the harness should they loosen or become detached.
- Use indelible ink to make black lines to show where the straps should pass through the buckles.
- Use letter coding to match the straps to their respective buckles.
- Fasten diaper tapes under the straps to prevent any pull on the straps.

Care of the Harness

- Sponge the harness clean with mild soap if it becomes soiled.

- If needed, place the harness in the washing machine for cleaning on cold water/gentle cycle and then line dry. (This necessitates that a second harness be obtained and placed on the child by a person trained to do so.)
- Do not remove the harness unless otherwise instructed by a health care provider.

Skin Care

- Give the child a daily sponge bath, paying close attention to the skin under the straps and stirrups.
- Check the skin under the harness daily for irritation, and gently massage the skin to stimulate circulation.
- Do not use powders or lotions that will cake and irritate the skin.
- Use padding beneath the shoulder straps to prevent discomfort at pressure points.
- Unfasten the shoulder straps to slip a shirt on the child. This should not affect hip position.
- Provide perineal care in the usual manner because the harness does not affect it and there are no straps covering that area.
- Do not pull the legs when changing the diaper because of the possibility of forced dislocation. Instead, lift the child from under the buttocks and slide the diaper under the bottom.
- Try using disposable diapers with elastic around the legs (recommended) to prevent the brace from becoming wet or soiled.

Contact the Health Care Provider if

- Harness becomes heavily soiled and needs to be replaced
- Skin underneath the harness becomes red or swollen or if areas of skin breakdown are noted
- Child appears to be in pain
- Harness comes off

---

for how the child's lower extremities are placed and how the cast is applied to ensure abduction of the hips. Other important areas for teaching include handling the child in a cast; petaling or waterproofing the cast; and feeding, dressing, and bathing the child in a cast (see thePoint for Procedures: Cast Care). Car seats and high chairs may be unusable or may require modification for a child with a spica cast. For infants, a bouncing seat can be used as a feeding chair, and car seats that have been adapted for children in hip spica casts can be purchased or rented. Strollers, wagons, or reclining wheelchairs also provide mobility for the child.

CONGENITAL LIMB DEFECTS

Congenital malformations of the limbs are typically classified into seven categories:

1. Failure of formation (absent parts)
2. Failure of differentiation (lack of part separation)
3. Duplication
4. Overgrowth
5. Undergrowth
6. Congenital constriction band syndrome
7. Generalized abnormalities

The most common congenital defects are absence of limb, duplication of fingers or toes, overgrowth or undergrowth of a limb, and amniotic band syndrome. Amniotic band syndrome is a set of congenital birth defects believed to be caused by entrapment of fetal parts (usually a limb or digits) in fibrous amniotic bands while in utero. Syndactyly, or webbing of two digits, is common, as is polydactyly (Fig. 20-9).

Pathophysiology

Chapter 3 describes the normal development of bone formation and the development of the extremities in utero. Altered growth and development patterns are likely to result in impairment of function and malformation of

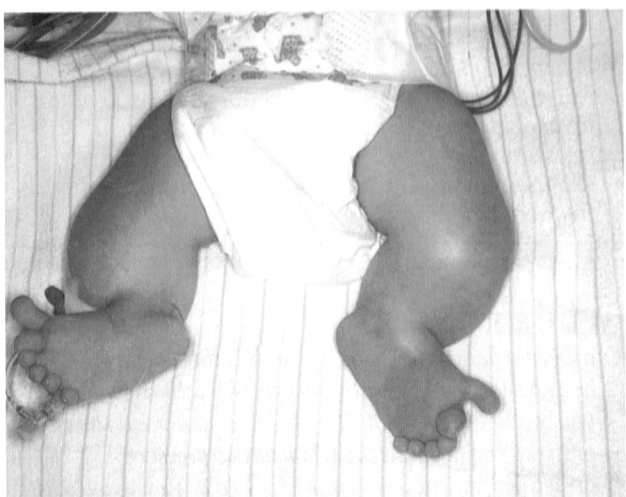

Figure 20-9 This infant with polydactyly has additional toes on each foot.

the anatomic structure of the limb. Abnormal in utero positioning may cause congenital deformities. Malformations may also be associated with genetic syndromes, such as trisomy 13, trisomy 18, trisomy 21, Carpenter syndrome, and orofaciodigital syndrome. Risk factors that may increase the likelihood of congenital limb defect include conditions that affect the developing fetus, such as maternal exposure to chemicals, viruses, or specific medications while pregnant.

Interdisciplinary Interventions

Early diagnosis and management of congenital anomalies is mandatory to prevent progression of certain deformities, to detect any limb-threatening conditions when there is neurovascular impairment, and to provide early psychological support to the child and the family. No standard interventions or treatments have been identified for congenital limb defects. If the child is functioning well, no treatment interventions may be instituted. Many children with limb deformities learn to adapt to their condition and do not consider themselves limited in performing any normal developmental skills and abilities. A limb deformity does not necessarily prohibit a child from participating in any age-appropriate activities. As the child matures, encourage caregivers to support the child's independence and self-care abilities.

Prosthetics may be selected to equalize limb lengths, correct malrotation, and improve body mechanics (Fig. 20-10). A prosthesis is expensive and requires maintenance. For the growing child, the prosthetic device must be replaced every year until age 5 years. Thereafter, annual assessment determines when the size of the prosthesis needs to be altered again. Some families choose not to obtain the prosthesis and to teach the child to function without it.

Surgical procedures are used to create a stump that is amenable to prosthetic fitting, to lengthen a deficient bone, or to improve limb function. In some cases, the defect can be repaired with a minor surgical procedure. Children with more severe defects may need several

corrective procedures over time. The ultimate goal of surgery is to provide the child with a limb that has good function and appearance. Function usually takes precedence; a hand that looks good but does not work correctly is of little help to the child. Rehabilitative services are used to optimize function of the limb after surgery.

Community Care

Child and family education and coordination of needed health care services are key components of community care. If the child has a prosthesis, the family must learn to assess the skin for redness and irritation. The child is most likely to experience these complications with a new brace or prosthesis. Teach the caregivers to report any signs and symptoms. For example, if the skin becomes irritated, the brace or prosthesis needs adjustment; in cases of severe skin breakdown, wear may need to be discontinued for a time. Care of the stump is also important. Rubbing alcohol can be applied to toughen the stump skin. However, lotions or oils are avoided. A cotton sock or other piece of clothing can be worn underneath the brace or prosthesis to absorb the moisture from perspiration.

Physical and occupational therapy can assist the child to become independent in activities of daily living and in the use of the prosthesis. Social services can provide the family with information regarding where to find assistive devices, alternative funding opportunities, and support groups. Children with limb deformities are fully capable of adapting to this condition such that it does not affect their ability to pursue competitive and noncompetitive physical activity. Support from the

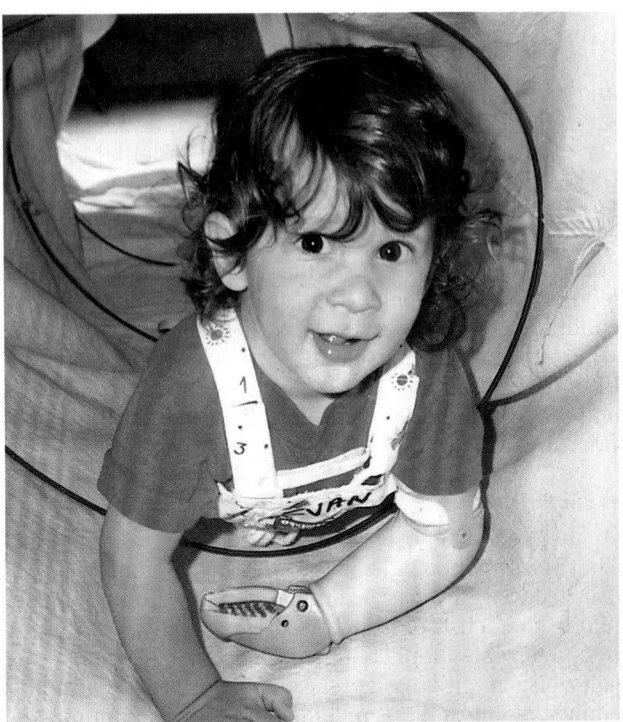

Figure 20-10 The child with a limb deformity and prosthesis should be encouraged to participate in age-appropriate activities to the limit of his or her abilities.

family, the health care team, and community groups will assist these children in achieving their desires to participate in activities with their peers.

OSTEOGENESIS IMPERFECTA

Often referred to as *brittle bone disease*, OI is an autosomal dominant inherited disorder (see Fig. 3-3) characterized by bone fragility and low bone mass. Occasionally, a child will develop OI through a spontaneous genetic mutation. OI occurs in all racial and ethnic groups and is equally prevalent in males and females. The incidence ranges from 1 in 10,000 to 1 in 20,000 live births (Monti et al., 2010).

Pathophysiology

This genetic condition stems from a variety of mutations of the genes COL1A1 and COL1A2, which encode the α1 and α2 chains that, when organized into a triple helix, constitute type I collagen (Monti et al., 2010). Collagen is the major protein of the body's connective tissue and is the framework on which bone and tissue are built. Children with OI produce less collagen, or a poorer quality of collagen, than healthy children do. Subsequently, this defect leads to bone fragility (the bones fracture easily), low bone mineral density, short stature, fractures, blue sclerae, dentinogenesis imperfecta (poor tooth development), joint laxity, and deafness later in life (Cheung & Glorieux, 2007; Krakow, 2008).

A classification system has been developed that identifies four main types of OI. *Type I mid nondeforming* is the most common and mildest form. Children with type I have bones that are predisposed to fractures. Other than spinal curvature, bone deformity is minimal. *Type II perinatal lethal* is the most severe type and is frequently lethal at or shortly after birth. *Type III severely deforming* and *type IV moderately deforming* are more serious than type I but not as lethal as type II. More recently, researchers have reported four additional types of OI: *type V moderate to severe disease* causing deformity and short stature, with normal teeth and sclerae; *type VI moderate disease with severe vertebral body involvement with compression*; *type VII*, a condition similar to type II with a smaller head and white or faintly blue sclerae; *type VIII*, similar to type III with a round face, normal sclerae, and barrel chest; and *type IX*, a milder condition than types VII and VIII (Monti et al., 2010).

Assessment

OI is often diagnosed through physical examination. The assessment starts with a review of family medical history. Physical examination commonly reveals major characteristics such as bone fragility leading to fractures, **osteopenia** (insufficient bone tissue), short stature, and progressive skeletal deformity. Additional clinical manifestations include blue sclerae, dentinogenesis imperfecta, joint laxity, and maturity-onset deafness. A unique feature of a fracture in a child with OI is lack of bruising or swelling at the fracture site. However, the child has tenderness at the site of the fracture.

ALERT *When taking blood pressures, guard against inflating the blood pressure cuff too tightly because this could lead to bruising or fractures in patients with severe OI. Do not use an automatic blood pressure cuff because the cuff inflation pressure is preset and cannot be controlled. Avoid obtaining a blood pressure in an extremity that has repeatedly fractured and/or has a bowing malformation because the bone in the limb may be especially predisposed to fracture (National Institutes of Health, 2005).*

Laboratory tests will confirm the diagnosis and rule out diagnoses such as rickets and hypophosphatasia. Biochemical tests can evaluate the collagen, and molecular testing can confirm the genetic pattern and type of OI. Radiographs reveal multiple normal callus formations at new fracture sites, generalized osteopenia, evidence of previous fractures, and skeletal deformities.

As children grow older, many become disabled by their severe deformities. Children with OI have normal intelligence, but social development may be delayed because of increased dependence on family members and decreased social interactions.

Interdisciplinary Interventions

OI cannot be cured. Management depends on the severity of the condition and on the age of the child. For example, the desired outcome for the child with the mild form (type I) is to lead as normal a life as possible, whereas in the lethal perinatal form (type II), survival at birth is the immediate goal. Treatment focuses on preventing injury and providing prompt and aggressive orthopedic management. Early treatment and correction of fractures or bowing and bending of the bones helps to maximize mobility and prevent deformities. Fractures are a part of life for these children, and hoping to completely eliminate fractures is not realistic.

When a fracture occurs, acute management consists of precise alignment to prevent deformity and application of a lightweight cast or splint for immobilization. Early return to weight-bearing activity is crucial to stimulate formation of new bone. Often, splints and braces are used on the lower extremities to assist with ambulation and to protect against fractures (see "Treatment Modalities" section earlier in this chapter).

Surgical Interventions

Children with OI often require surgery to reduce fractures, correct spinal deformities, and straighten long bones. A common procedure is intramedullary "rodding" with solid or telescoping rods. Solid rods are easier to insert, but they do not "grow" with the child and must be replaced every 2 to 4 years. Telescoping rods require more extensive surgery, but they can be adjusted as the child grows. Placement of the rods is not a perfect solution because the small diameter of the bone and the abnormal collagen can cause complications. However, intramedullary rodding can provide stability to a deformed bone and help prevent progressive deformities.

Postoperative care includes pain management, neurovascular checks, assessing for bleeding at the surgical site, and special attention to positioning as a result of the child's limited ROM and the potential for fractures and skin breakdown. Children with OI are prone to have slightly higher than normal body temperature, sensitivity to heat and cold, excessive sweating, and pseudomalignant hyperthermia after anesthesia (National Institutes of Health, 2005). The exact cause of these symptoms is unknown but is believed to be due to an increased metabolic rate. Therefore, intravenous fluid therapy initiated preoperatively is continued postoperatively. Ensure adequate hydration throughout hospitalization, with frequent weight checks and careful monitoring of intake and output. Avoid the use of warming blankets and heavy drapes (during surgery) and blankets (during recovery) to prevent hyperthermia. The length of the recovery period depends on the extent of the surgery, the child's age, and the child's previous activity level. After surgery, the limb is supported by a lightweight cast or splint for about 4 weeks. Bracing may be used after the cast is removed to provide additional support for standing and walking as the child continues to heal.

Physical Therapy

Physical therapy is a mainstay of treatment for children with OI and focuses on ROM and muscle-strengthening exercises. After a fracture or surgical intervention, the physical therapist helps the child to regain mobility. Swimming has been found to be one of the most beneficial forms of therapy. The presence of deformities may require the child to use ambulatory devices such as a walker or a wheelchair. The physical therapist ensures that the child can use the device safely.

Pharmacologic Interventions

During the last decade, bisphosphonates administered orally or parentally to children and adults have produced favorable results. Pamidronate has been shown to increase bone mass, decrease skeletal pain, and decrease fracture incidence in children (Krakow, 2008). The effect is most marked in the spine, where vertebral remodeling may improve vertebral height. Growth hormone treatment may also be considered to increase short stature (Monti et al., 2010).

Nutritional Interventions

Nutrition and diet are important to maintain a healthy weight and to support overall health. Although no food or vitamin supplement has been shown to reverse or prevent symptoms, calcium and vitamin D are essential to maintaining strong bones and helping to prevent osteoporosis. Daily calcium and/or vitamin D supplements may be prescribed if an analysis of the child's diet indicates they are not meeting dietary requirements of these substances.

Community Care

Most families are unaware of the different types of OI, the prognosis for the disorder, and the special care needs of a child with OI. Genetic counseling is aimed at primary prevention. Ensure that information given to the family is specific to the child's type of OI. Families are anxious about the possibility of causing a fracture in their child. Provide specific instructions on how to hold, change, and position the infant to reduce fractures and to help decrease anxiety. Families of children with OI must achieve a delicate balance between protecting the child and allowing the child to have normal life experiences (Community Care 20-1).

caREminder

Signs of a fracture, especially in an infant, are important to teach to caregivers. In an infant, these signs include general symptoms such as fever, irritability, and refusal to eat.

Older children with OI become aware that if they injure themselves, they need to be evaluated for a possible fracture. Symptoms of a fracture in an older child include pain, swelling, and, possibly, deformity at the site.

MUSCULAR DYSTROPHY

The muscular dystrophies are a group of genetic diseases characterized by progressive weakness and degeneration of the skeletal muscles that control movement. These disorders vary in age of onset, hereditary pattern, and area of weakness. Most dystrophies begin during childhood or adolescence, and all are progressive to some degree. The most common type of muscular dystrophy is Duchenne muscular dystrophy (DMD), also known as *pseudohypertrophic dystrophy*. Other types include limb–girdle (involving weakness of the pelvic and shoulder girdles) and facioscapulohumeral (involving the face and shoulder girdle).

DMD is the most common X-linked recessively inherited disease, occurring in approximately 1 in 3,600 to 6,000 newborns. An estimated one third of cases result from new mutations, with no family history (Bushby et al., 2010a). DMD is predominately a male disease; females are the carriers. In the rare instance that a female has the disease, it is usually a milder form with a slower progression. The advancement of molecular biology techniques have focused on the genetic code for dystrophin, a 427-kd skeletal muscle protein (Dp427). These defects result in the various clinical manifestations found in muscular dystrophy (Do, 2012). Genetic counseling should be considered for females in the family.

A steady and progressive increase in weakness and disability occurs with DMD. Muscle weakness tends to occur in a proximal-to-distal direction. Decreasing muscle

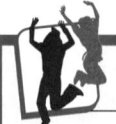

COMMUNITY CARE 20-1

Recommendations for Promoting Health and Safety for the Child With Osteogenesis Imperfecta

In the Home

Encourage active ROM exercises for children of all ages.

Avoid jerking or pulling when moving the child. The child should be allowed to move independently whenever possible.

Fractures can occur. Watch for signs of a fracture, which include pain, swelling, or deformity at the site.

Encourage the child to wear rubber-soled shoes to assist with traction while ambulating.

Remove throw rugs from the floors to help prevent falls.

Monitor toys placed on the floor to prevent the child from tripping on them.

If a wheelchair is needed, the home may need ramps installed to permit easy transportation.

Encourage the child to do as much self-care as possible.

The Osteogenesis Imperfecta Foundation has literature, support groups, social gatherings, and conferences for the children and their family members.

In the School

Encourage the child to attend regular school if possible.

Arrange for home tutors during periods of hospitalization and home recovery.

Discourage participation in contact sports.

Recommend activities such as swimming, arts, crafts, and computer activities.

Body image disturbances are common. Evaluate the child's acceptance of self and acceptance by others, and provide interventions to support positive peer interactions.

Evaluate hearing annually to ensure that no loss has occurred, which may affect school performance.

After an Injury

If the caregiver or child suspects a fracture, the child should see a health care provider immediately.

Before transportation of the child, immobilize the affected area.

Continue treatment measures instituted by the health care team (e.g., splinting, braces) until follow-up care reveals no further need for these interventions.

Consider ordering acetaminophen for pain after an injury.

Dietary Needs

Inactivity and short stature may lead to obesity. Recommend a low-fat, high-fiber diet, with a reduced number of calories.

Encourage fluid intake to prevent dehydration from increased diaphoresis.

Oral Care

Encourage yearly dental checkups. Teeth are frequently prematurely eroded or broken. Teeth may need to be capped.

Complete dental hygiene after every meal.

Skin Care

Because of the problems with diaphoresis, advise the child to wear lightweight clothes that allow ventilation.

Use a sheepskin or softly padded mattress on all bedding.

---

strength can affect the patient's ambulatory ability. With loss of ambulatory ability, children become wheelchair dependent by age 7 to 13 years. With loss of ambulation, there is usually a rapidly progressive course of muscle or tendon contractures and scoliosis. Death usually occurs in the third decade of life as a result of cardiopulmonary compromise (Do, 2012). Currently, DMD has no cure. Gene therapy techniques are being investigated as a way to prevent muscle degeneration and as a potential cure (Manzur et al., 2008). Glucocorticoid corticosteroids (prednisone and deflazacort) have been shown to benefit DMD patients by increasing muscle strength, pulmonary function, and functional abilities in these patients.

Pathophysiology

In DMD, the defect on the X chromosome results in a deficiency or absence of the protein dystrophin. This protein, which is thought to help strengthen the muscle cell membrane, is a part of the complex of interacting proteins in the dystrophin–glycoprotein complex. The dystrophin–glycoprotein complex may play a key role in the cascade of events that lead to muscle cell necrosis. Dystrophin can be found on the surface membrane of muscles and in the brain. Without dystrophin, the sarcolemma membrane is prone to tearing during muscle contraction, which allows muscle cells to break open and their contents to enter the bloodstream. An increase in creatinine kinase levels indicates that muscle damage is occurring. Creatinine kinase levels are high in DMD patients at birth; high levels persist throughout life.

Assessment

Neonates typically display no clinical symptoms. However, occasionally, an infant with DMD displays mild delay in attaining milestones as an early symptom.

In most cases, the diagnosis of DMD is made around age 5 years, although it may be suspected earlier if the child has delays in major milestones such as independent walking or language. The family may report initial symptoms of delayed walking, frequent tripping or falling, or difficulty running or climbing stairs (Bushby et al., 2010a). Note the child's gait; children with DMD appear clumsy. Initial and regular neuromuscular and skeletal assessments are completed by a neuromuscular specialist to evaluate the presence of the condition and the disease progression. Muscle strength, ROM, posture, and gait are evaluated. The classic finding for DMD is Gowers sign (Fig. 20-11). Because of the muscular weakness in the pelvis and legs, children must use one or both hands to brace the lower extremities and to raise themselves off the floor from a sitting or prone position. Tiptoe walking is also common.

Apparent hypertrophy of the calf muscles marks the progression of DMD and is the reason for the term *pseudohypertrophic muscular dystrophy*. Although the calf muscles look big and strong, fat and fibrous tissues have infiltrated the muscle, actually making it weaker. Deep tendon reflexes eventually diminish or disappear. However, the child with DMD does not lose sensation in the extremity.

Motor function of the child is categorized in three phases: making progress, plateau, and decline. The child who is making progress will be clinically identified as having DMD yet will still be gaining motor skills, albeit at a slower rate than one's peers. The plateau phase, occurring usually around ages 4 to 8 years, is noted when the child is no longer progressing in motor skills yet shows no decline of skills. This phase may last only a few months. It is during this phase that glucocorticoid therapy is initiated; it is more beneficial at this time than when the child is in the decline phase (Bushby et al., 2010a).

Diagnostic Tests

An elevated creatinine kinase level is the hallmark laboratory value in children with DMD. Severely elevated levels, as high as 15,000 to 20,000 units/L, reflect the primary damage at the sarcolemma membrane as creatinine kinase leaks out of the muscle fibers. Serum creatinine kinase elevation can be detected at birth, but the test is rarely done at that time because infants lack symptoms. Elevated alanine transaminase (ALT) and aspartate transaminase (AST) may also be present. Although primarily seen as an indicator of liver damage, these transaminases are also produced by muscle (Bushby et al., 2010a). Electromyography is sometimes used if creatinine kinase levels are not elevated. The most definite diagnosis is made on the basis of either muscle biopsy or DNA analysis, with blood sampling completed prior to biopsy. The characteristic muscle biopsy demonstrates scattered groups of regenerating and

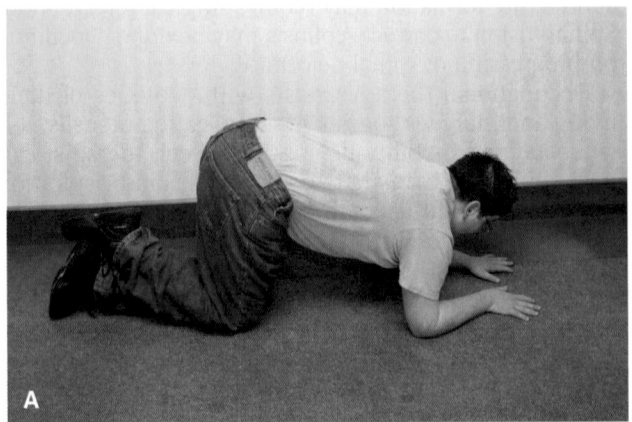 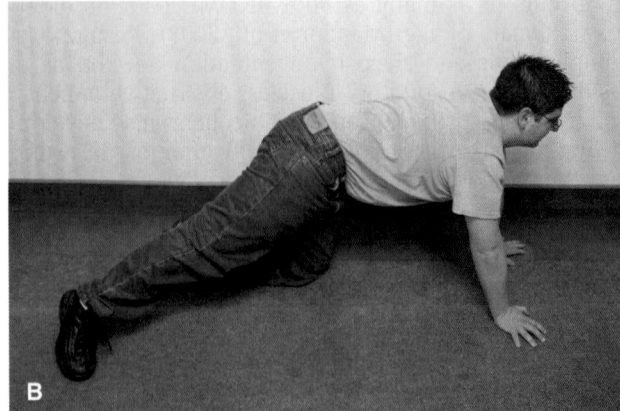 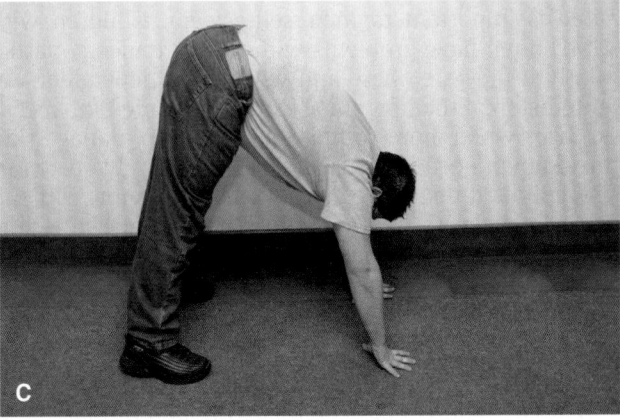 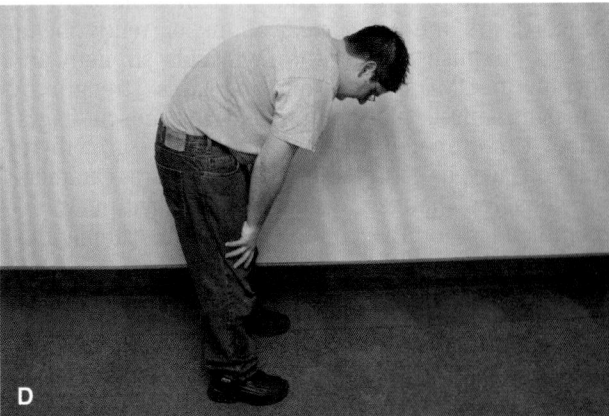

Figure 20-11 Gowers sign. (A–D) The older adolescent must use one or both hands to brace the legs and then raise himself off the floor to a standing position.

necrotic muscle fibers. DNA analysis reveals the defect on the X chromosome.

Interdisciplinary Interventions

Management of the child with DMD requires an interdisciplinary team consisting of a nurse, orthopedist, neurologist, pediatrician, geneticist, physical therapist, occupational therapist, orthotist, dietitian, social worker, and psychologist. When possible, follow-up should be done at a specialty clinic where the team approach is best facilitated. The goals of treatment are to maintain daily functioning for as long as possible and to prevent deformities, which can further disable the child. Good supportive care can increase comfort and the life expectancy of the child with DMD. Palliative care is implemented to relieve or prevent suffering and to help improve the quality of life for the child.

Progressive muscle deterioration and long term glucocorticoid therapy can lead to an increase in pain, lower limb contractions, risk of scoliosis, risk of vertebral fracture, decreased pulmonary function, cardiomyopathy, swallowing difficulties, and deterioration in speech intelligibility (Bushby et al., 2010b). Hospitalization is required when the child faces acute exacerbations related to their condition, such as pneumonia and severe weight loss requiring aggressive nutritional intervention. As the child ages, the teenage years may be marked by respiratory and cardiac complications and the progressive development of scoliosis. Cardiomyopathy occurs in as many as 90% of DMD patients older than 18 years of age (Manzur et al., 2008). Respiratory complications and sleep hypoventilation develop as a result of weak respiratory muscles, obstructive apneas, and hypoxemic dips during sleep. Scoliosis may develop during the pubertal period, especially after loss of walking. Progression of curvature of the spine affects respiratory function, feeding, sitting, and overall comfort. Surgical spinal fusion may be indicated. Each of these conditions requires referral to an appropriate medical specialist for treatment. Otherwise, the child's condition is managed by practitioners in their community medical home in collaboration with the family caregivers. The goals of treatment are to keep the child independent and at a high functioning level for as long as possible.

Glucocorticoid corticosteroids (prednisone and deflazacort) are the only medications currently being used to diminish the decline in muscle strength and function in DMD. Prednisone increases strength by increasing muscle mass and decreasing muscle degradation. Unfortunately, side effects include growth retardation, weight gain, moon face, hirsutism, cataracts, and behavior changes. Glucocorticoid therapy is not recommended for the child who is still gaining motor skills. Thus, children younger than 2 years of age are generally not started on this therapy, which often may not be initiated until the child is between 4 and 8 years of age, when a decline in muscle strength is visible (Bushby et al., 2010a). The major long-term benefit of glucocorticoid therapy is prolonged independence or braced ambulation and minimalization of respiratory, cardiac, and other orthopedic complications.

caREminder

Ensure the child is up to date on his or her immunizations and that varicella immunity has been established prior to the initiation of long-term glucocorticoid therapy.

Community Care

The impact of the diagnosis of DMD on a family cannot be underestimated. All members of the family will be affected by the care needs of the child. Encourage the family to seek support and health care assistance from the many local, state, and national resources available for children with muscular dystrophy. See Chapter 12 for more information on intervening for a family of a child with a chronic illness.

Physical therapy and occupational therapy are an important part of the life of a child with DMD. Physical therapy initially focuses on stretching tight muscles. Conservative treatment for DMD generally begins with resting night splints to slow ankle contractures, followed by long leg braces to delay progression to a wheelchair. Ankle contractures may be corrected with heel cord release, and muscle transfers (such as posterior tibialis muscle transfer) may be considered to preserve functional ability. As weakness progresses, physical therapy can provide appropriate equipment and assistive devices to maintain functional mobility. Progressive scoliosis and contracture formation may require surgical intervention. Spinal fusion to correct scoliosis may be done depending on progression of spinal deformity.

Occupational therapy assists with activities of daily living and includes special clothing, eating utensils, toilet seats, and mobility devices. A speech therapist can help with issues related to dysphagia and aspiration risks as the child gets weaker. A recreational therapist can help the family to connect with resources within the community, such as the parks and recreation department for activities, groups that provide adaptive physical education, and disabled student service organizations. The Muscular Dystrophy Association can be a great social and financial support to families (see thePoint for Organizations).

Letting children with DMD be as independent as possible is important to their self-esteem. Children with DMD often have problems with pressure ulcers, particularly if they are obese and wheelchair dependent. An enterostomal therapy nurse can be consulted for specific cases when more complex strategies to manage skin breakdown need to be used. Obesity not only decreases the child's functioning but also makes it more difficult for caregivers to lift the child. Nutritional counseling is important, both to ensure an adequate diet and to control constipation. Neurogenic bowel can be a complication of DMD.

caREminder

Obesity related to inactivity is common in the child with DMD.

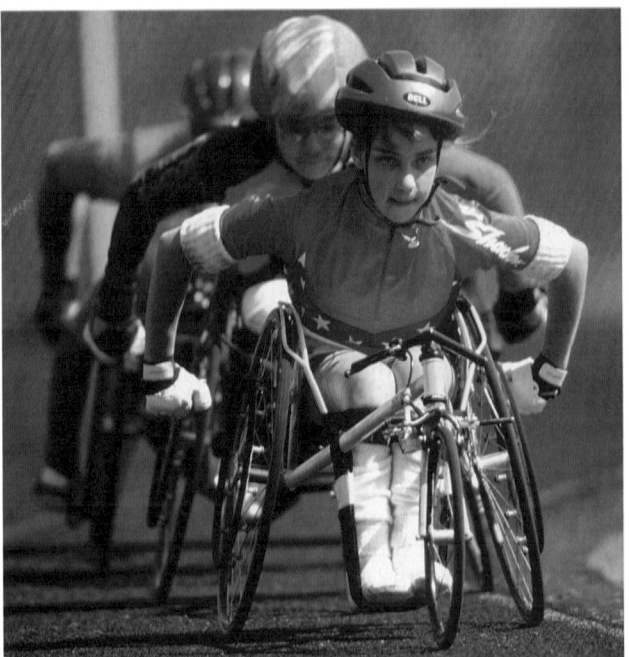

Figure 20-12 Wheelchair sports provide an opportunity for the child with muscular dystrophy to enjoy physical activity and interact with peers.

Appropriately selected activities can boost self-esteem, provide social interaction, and normalize life for the child with DMD. Children attend school until they are not able to sit up. When the child cannot attend school, a home tutor can be arranged. School personnel meet with the family and selected members of the health care team to develop an individual education program to meet the child's educational needs. (See Chapters 2 and 12 for more discussion about individualized education programs [IEPs]). Activities such as arts and crafts, board games, and computer games are favorites. Many children with DMD attend camps for children with disabilities and participate in wheelchair sports. Many options are available for the wheelchair athlete, including tennis, swimming, rowing, skiing, and track and field (Fig. 20-12). Teams are organized at the state level and through rehabilitation programs. Local tournaments and national championships provide opportunities for all levels of athletes to participate.

Anticipatory guidance is ongoing. As the child's status deteriorates, the family and child will most likely need counseling related to decision making for placement of a tracheostomy tube for positive-pressure ventilation and airway and secretion management. Early education on the progression of the disease can assist the patient and family with decision making and advance directives.

GROWTH-RELATED DISORDERS

Growth-related disorders become evident as the musculoskeletal system matures. Multiple diagnoses are related to delayed or accelerated growth. Many of these conditions are associated with endocrine or metabolic disorders (e.g., growth hormone deficiency, hypothyroidism, hypophosphatemia, rickets) (see Chapters 26 and 27). Growth disorders may also be secondary to other chronic conditions

such as cystic fibrosis, renal disease, and cardiac disease. Many growth-related disorders are self-limiting; as the child grows, the disorder resolves itself. In other cases, such as LCPD or scoliosis, a joint is destroyed or the child is left with a permanent disfigurement. In all these cases, the cause is either not known or not fully understood.

TORSIONAL DEFORMITY: FEMORAL ANTEVERSION

A torsional deformity is a musculoskeletal condition in which the bone is "twisted." Such twisting can occur in the femur or tibia. In femoral anteversion, also called *internal femoral torsion*, the femur is medially rotated (Fig. 20-13). It is often associated with metatarsus adductus, neuromuscular disorders (e.g., cerebral palsy, myelodysplasia), LCPD, and DDH. It is postulated that femoral anteversion increases the likelihood of development of osteoarthritis in adulthood. Torsional deformities affect females twice as often as males, and a familial tendency has been noted.

Pathophysiology

The rotational and angular alignments of the legs change during a child's growing years. Children begin life with the femurs anteverted. In most children, femoral anteversion will remodel (resolve spontaneously) by age 8 years (Gordon et al., 2005). In a child with a neuromuscular problem (e.g., cerebral palsy), resolution may not occur as a result of the underlying neurologic defect and/or the musculoskeletal sequelae of the disorder, and treatment is needed.

Assessment

Begin the assessment by asking family members if they have any concerns regarding their child's gait. The history of the problem, including onset, progression, and

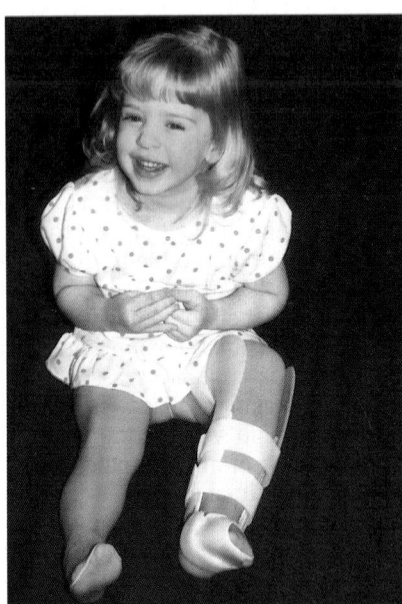

Figure 20-13 In femoral anteversion, the thighs rotate medially and the knees and patellae turn inward. Braces can be used to correct this problem. Courtesy of Wheaton Bracing System.

any previous management, plus information about the perinatal period and motor development are essential. Next, evaluate the child's gait by having the child walk the length of a hallway unclothed except for underclothing. Observing gait provides information on muscle strength, coordination, and foot angle. Assessment of femoral anteversion frequently includes a subjective complaint that the child is walking "pigeon toed" or seems to trip over his or her feet when running (running may accentuate dysfunction or rotation).

On physical examination, the child's thighs medially rotate, and the knees and patellae turn inward. The legs appear bowed when the feet are pointed straight ahead. Clinical measurements determine medial and lateral rotation of the hip. In children with femoral anteversion, measurement shows decreased lateral rotation of the femur and increased medial rotation. Radiologic examination may be done to rule out other pathology, such as acetabular dysplasia.

Interdisciplinary Interventions

Normally, no treatment is necessary because of spontaneous remodeling of the femoral anteversion. If femoral anteversion is severe (limiting participation in normal activities of daily living or sports) and does not resolve spontaneously or the child has a neuromuscular disorder, derotation femoral osteotomy may be done to correct alignment. An osteotomy involves a cut through the femur; the bone is then rotated to the desired position, and screws are used to hold it until the bone heals. A hip spica cast is then applied for approximately 6 weeks.

Assure the family and child that this problem often resolves on its own. When surgery is necessary, educate the family on caring for the hip spica cast and arrange for a wheelchair rental and a home tutor. In most cases, postoperative physical therapy is not needed.

TORSIONAL DEFORMITY: TIBIAL TORSION

The most common cause of intoeing in young children is internal tibial torsion, which is a medial twisting of the tibia along the axis of the tibia, and has been attributed to position in utero or in sleep. Pressure from the uterus or mattress on the legs as the fetus or child tucks the legs under the body is thought to twist the tibia. Medial torsion causes an intoeing gait; lateral torsion causes an out-toeing gait. Alignment problems of the lower extremities are related to alterations in normal limb development and rotation of the hip, femur, and tibia in utero.

Abnormal medial tibial torsion rarely occurs as a single deformity. It is commonly associated with femoral anteversion, congenital metatarsus varus (intoeing), or developmental genu varum (knock-knee). It occurs in approximately 5% of adult females and 3% of adult males. The degree of tibial torsion varies with the child's age. At birth, the tibia rotates medially, but with normal growth and development, it spontaneously derotates.

Assessment

The child with medial tibial torsion usually presents with a history of being pigeon toed. Often, a family history of medial tibial torsion is noted.

Lateral tibial torsion is seen as an out-toeing gait. Children usually do not have a positive family history for lateral tibial torsion. Unlike medial torsion, which may improve during late childhood, lateral torsion usually worsens. Worsening results from a contracture of the iliotibial band, the congenital deformity that has caused the torsion.

Diagnosis is made by physical examination. Two methods can be used to screen for tibial torsion. First, the child sits with the knees at a 90-degree angle, and the examiner palpates the malleoli. Normally, the medial malleolus lies farther forward than the lateral malleolus. Second, with the child lying prone, the examiner measures the thigh–foot angle (see Fig. 8-14). Family members will often report that the child has intoeing. Radiographs are not very useful in diagnosing tibial torsion in young children. Most cases spontaneously resolve with growth. Correction can be seen as early as 4 years of age and in some children by 8 to 10 years of age (Wells & Sehgal, 2012). Persistent tibial rotation in an older child requires referral to an orthopedic surgeon.

Interdisciplinary Interventions

Most often, treatment consists of observation and reassurance because most cases resolve spontaneously as the child grows. Thus, yearly observations are all that is needed in most cases. For children with persistent deformity and functional impairment, treatment with supramalleolar osteotomy is recommended (Wells & Sehgal, 2012). Generally, the surgery is not done until 8 to 10 years of age so that normal physiologic remodeling can occur.

LEGG-CALVÉ-PERTHES DISEASE

LCPD is a common pediatric hip disorder that causes pain and decreased hip motion, possibly leading to a femoral head deformity. It has an incidence of 1 per 850 children in northern Europe and the United States (Perry et al., 2012). LCPD occurs four times more often in males, and there is bilateral involvement in 8% to 24% of cases. The peak age is 4 to 8 years (Hailer et al., 2010).

Pathophysiology

LCPD is a form of AVN of the proximal capital femoral epiphysis (growth plate) in children. A limited study has suggested that abnormalities in vascular structure and function may be the mechanism by which the disease develops, but further research is need to support this theory (Perry et al., 2012). LCPD progresses through four distinctive phases:

1. Avascularity: interrupted blood supply to the femoral head; cessation of bone growth with no change in bone density and intact surface cartilage
2. Revascularization: restoration of blood supply to the femoral head with reabsorption of dead bone with laying down of immature new bone; possible remodeling of femoral head in a deformed position
3. Reossification: laying down of new bone with continued remodeling
4. Residual deformity: completion of healing; hip normal or deformed forever

Assessment

The first symptoms of LCPD typically include pain, limping, and decreased ROM in the affected hip. These symptoms usually have been plaguing the child for months, with no history of trauma, before the child complains. The child will report hip or groin pain, which may be referred to the knee or thigh. Pain increases with activity and decreases with rest.

On observation, the child may hold the leg in slight flexion, and a hip contracture may be present. Limited hip motion, especially internal rotation and abduction, is a classic sign of LCPD. The limited abduction is secondary to synovitis and muscular spasm. Most children with LCPD walk with a limp that becomes more pronounced during later stages of the disease. Additional findings include leg length discrepancy, thigh atrophy on the affected side, and a positive roll test. The roll test is done with the child lying supine. The examiner rolls the hips of the affected extremity into internal and external rotation. The maneuver will evoke guarding or muscle spasm on the affected side.

Diagnostic Tests

Radiographs are the standard technique for diagnosing LCPD and evaluating treatment. Based on the location and degree of involvement of the epiphysis, the disorder is classified using the two basic classification systems: the Catterall system, used retrospectively; and the Salter-Thompson classification system, which aims to predict outcome. Involvement of only the posterior epiphysis has a good prognosis. When the entire epiphysis is involved, the prognosis is poor because the growth plate is often severely damaged, further increasing the risk of residual deformity.

Bone scans are particularly useful in diagnosing the early stage of LCPD when changes may not be evident on radiographs. A bone scan shows decreased uptake of dye in an affected femoral head and more clearly demarcates the area of avascularity; MRI and arthrography also may be performed.

No laboratory studies are relevant for LCPD. However, a complete blood count and an ESR or CRP may be done to rule out infectious or inflammatory processes.

Interdisciplinary Interventions

The goals of treatment for LCPD are to achieve and maintain ROM, relieve weight bearing, and position the femoral epiphysis within the acetabulum with traction. The earlier that treatment begins, the less risk there is of residual deformity to the hip joint. Also, children whose LCPD is diagnosed at a young age tend to have fewer long-term problems. Approximately 80% of children have a good recovery, although they may have difficulty later in life with hip degeneration.

Pain Relief Interventions

The first step in treatment is to regain motion around the hip joint and relieve pain resulting from **synovitis** (inflammation of the synovial membrane) or muscle spasm around the hip. Nonsteroidal anti-inflammatory drugs (NSAIDs) help decrease inflammation and pain.

Some physicians place the child in Buck traction (see thePoint for Procedures: Traction Care) at home or in the hospital until ROM improves and pain diminishes (approximately 1 to 2 weeks). The child must be on strict bed rest, and even sitting in bed (except to eat meals) is discouraged. When the child is placed on home traction, a home care company provides the traction equipment, trains the family to set up traction, and sends nurses or physical therapists to the home periodically. Home traction requires an enormous time commitment from the family, and the child will need home tutoring. Also, staying in traction may be an issue for some children at home. Children who are younger or whose disease is detected early may require only observation and follow-up, with radiographs obtained every 2 to 4 months.

Containment Interventions

After the inflammation in the hip has decreased and ROM has improved, the next goal, containment, can be addressed. Containment involves holding the femoral head in abduction to prevent the edge of the acetabulum from denting the head. However, some movement of the hip is desirable to mold the soft head round.

Containment can be achieved in a variety of ways, and the treatment chosen depends on the stage of the disease and physician preference. Nonsurgical options for containment include braces and Petrie casts (thigh-to-ankle casts connected by a brace that holds the legs apart). The most commonly used brace is the Atlanta–Scottish Rite orthosis, which enables weight bearing. A child may be placed in Petrie casts for a few weeks and then braced, or the child may be put in a brace immediately. Both options have advantages and disadvantages, and both maintain the hips in abduction.

To be effective, bracing must be used for 6 to 18 months. The brace is worn constantly, except for bathing. Children can wear the brace over regular clothes and some can even participate in other activities, such as baseball, while wearing the brace. The child must be monitored routinely. Some physicians prefer to treat the child with physical therapy or no brace at all.

Surgical options for containment of the hip are reserved for children with severe deformity. Surgical options achieve containment via an osteotomy of the femur. A pelvic osteotomy can be used to increase abduction and correct the various existing deformities, alleviating the associated symptoms. The child is hospitalized for approximately 3 days and is discharged home in a hip spica cast for 6 to 8 weeks. When the cast is removed, no further treatment is needed. The advantages of this treatment method are that the child is restricted in a cast for only 2 months and that the hip containment is permanent. The disadvantages are those related to any surgery and the possibility of a leg length discrepancy as a result of the osteotomy. As an adult, the child may be at higher risk for degenerative joint disease.

Community Care

Community care begins with educating the family and child about the disease process and the use of corrective devices (i.e., traction, casting, or bracing). Despite the healthy appearance of the affected child, family members and other caregivers must come to understand the seriousness of this disease and the importance of adhering to the treatment regimen. The treatment for LCPD can span a few years, which can be a stressful time for families emotionally as well as financially. Social services can assist families to find the resources they need to manage long-term care.

If home traction is required, family members must learn the principles of traction and immobilization. Assist with arranging home health care services to monitor the child's progress and to evaluate the family's ability to manage the traction device. If parents work, the home health agency may be able to assist in locating a daytime caregiver for the child. Home tutoring arrangements should be made with the child's school so that the child does not fall behind in schoolwork.

If casting is used, be aware that these types of casts vary widely (see "Treatment Modalities" section at beginning of this chapter). Fitting through the door of a house or car may be impossible unless the child turns sideways. A reclining wheelchair allows some mobility, although it is limited. Special transportation services in a van or ambulance can be arranged by social services or the home care nurse, if required.

If the child is in a brace, he or she may attend school and participate in many of the activities with other children. Give the child specific instructions regarding how and when to wear the brace. If the brace becomes soiled, instruct caregivers to wash it with a damp cloth. If the brace breaks, urge the caregivers to contact the company that issued the brace promptly to provide an immediate replacement.

SLIPPED CAPITAL FEMORAL EPIPHYSIS

SCFE is defined as a posterior and inferior slippage of the proximal femoral epiphysis at the femoral neck, occurring through the physeal plate (Fig. 20-14).

SCFE is the most common hip disorder. The incidence is 1 case per 100,000 children. It occurs most frequently in adolescents, with a slightly greater incidence in males. SCFE most commonly occurs just after the onset of puberty. Often, the child is overweight. African American children have a slightly higher occurrence. The average age of occurrence is 12 years in girls and 13.5 years in boys (Peck, 2010). Other underlying risks include malnutrition, endocrine abnormalities, and prior developmental hip dysplasia. Slippage is unilateral in 20% to 37% and bilateral in 9% to 18% of cases (Adler, 2008). With prompt treatment, many children do well after a slip. Barring the complication of AVN, the prognosis is good. However, the child is at risk for degenerative hip arthritis later in life, a risk that increases with the severity of the slip.

Pathophysiology

The exact cause of SCFE is unknown. Numerous theories have been proposed, but none have been proved. A genetic component has been noted, and the most plausible theory is that SCFE is related to an endocrine abnormality. Idiopathic SCFE may be caused by many factors, including obesity, physeal orientation, abnormalities in physeal architecture, and hormonal changes during adolescence that affect physeal strength. Some researchers believe the incidence of SCFE is related to the child's geographic location and the time of the year (Tradition or Science 20-3). Obesity results in increased shear stress across the physeal plate, which is already orientated more vertically and posteriorly in children than in adults. Researchers are noting a rise in the incidence of SCFE that correlates with the rise in childhood obesity (Benson et al., 2008; Murray & Wilson, 2008).

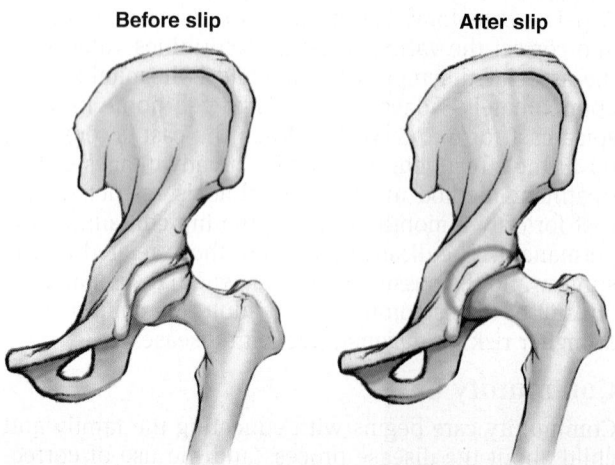

Figure 20-14 In SCFE, the femoral head moves upward and forward while the capital epiphysis becomes displaced backward and downward.

Evidence-Based Practice   **TRADITION OR SCIENCE 20-3**

Is seasonal variation evident in the onset of SCFE symptoms?

Several researchers have been interested in the relationship between the seasons and the onset of SCFE symptoms. Furthermore, seasonal variation has been examined as it relates to gender, ethnicity, and geographic location. Study data remain inconclusive. Lehmann et al. (2006) found that slips occurred significantly more often during the summer north of 40° latitude and during the winter south of 40° latitude in the United States. Brown (2004) found significantly more seasonal variation in the northern United States, in both boys and girls, than in the southern United States, but less seasonal variation occurred among blacks than among whites. Maffulli and Douglas (2002) completed their work in Scotland and determined that for male patients, seasonality was significant, with an autumnal peak that was highest in November. No significant seasonal variation was present among female patients, although there was a trend similar to that in male patients, again with the highest incidence in November.

Why this interest in seasonal variation of SCFE? Although the cause of seasonal variation in SCFE remains unknown, the effect is believed to differ by latitude and skin pigmentation, suggesting a possible link to impaired vitamin D synthesis. More research is needed to strengthen the associations indicated between seasonal changes and the physiologic rhythms that may affect the onset of SCFE.

TABLE 20-2   Classification of Slipped Capital Femoral Epiphysis

Stage	Severity
Preslip phase: The child complains of weakness in the leg and pain in the hip or knee when standing or walking for prolonged periods of time.	Grade I (preslip): The physis widens without actual displacement of the epiphysis.
Acute slip: A child falls and then reports hip pain.	Grade II (minimal slip): The femoral neck is displaced from the femoral head by up to one third.
Chronic slip: The femoral head gradually slips off the femoral neck and remodels.	Grade III (moderate slip): The femoral neck is displaced by more than one third but less than one half of the femoral head.
Acute on chronic slip: Slow, progressive slippage becomes more displaced when a child falls.	Grade IV (severe slip): The epiphysis is displaced by more than 50%.

Trauma also has a role in the development of a slip. If a heavy child's growth plate is already weak, and the child falls on the weakened hip, SCFE may result. Other conditions associated with SCFE include hypothyroidism, renal osteodystrophy, and postradiation therapy.

SCFE is classified by the stage and the severity of the disease, which in turn influence prognosis (Table 20-2). Complications that can occur as a result of SCFE are chondrolysis (acute necrosis of the cartilage of the hip) and AVN (loss of blood supply) of all or part of the femoral head.

Assessment

Typically, the child with SCFE has a history of intermittent limp and pain for several weeks or months in duration, which may be in the hip, groin, or knee. A vague history of trauma often exists. As the epiphysis continues to slip, the child loses hip motion, including internal rotation, flexion, and abduction. The gait is often **antalgic** (limping on the affected side). Although the knee examination and distal neurovascular examination are normal, the child often refuses to move the hip. The hip may be held in external rotation at rest, whereas the hip is typically held in a position of flexion, internal rotation, and abduction. In a moderate or severe slip, the affected leg also may be shorter, with an atrophied thigh muscle. Radiographs of the pelvis are the best tools for diagnosing SCFE.

ALERT *Do not attempt ROM evaluation in a child with a suspected acute slip because this evaluation could worsen displacement.*

Interdisciplinary Interventions

Distinguishing between stable and unstable SCFE is important in directing care. In stable SCFE, ambulation is possible, with or without crutches; in unstable SCFE, ambulation is not possible, with or without crutches. The patient with an unstable hip has a poorer prognosis because this condition carries an increased risk of AVN.

The goal of treatment for SCFE is to prevent further slippage and to achieve closure of the physeal plate. Delay in diagnosis is associated with increased slip severity and is associated with higher risk of AVN and

chondrolysis. Increased slippage is associated with poorer long-term outcomes including pain, limitation of motion, and degenerative joint disease. When SCFE is diagnosed, the child should stop all weight-bearing activities, be placed on crutches or use a wheelchair, and be referred to an orthopedic surgeon. The most widely accepted treatment for stable SCFE (90% of cases) is in situ, one-screw internal fixation—a surgical intervention that pins the hip together with a single central screw. Results of this type of surgery are excellent, and blood loss and complications are minimal. For the child with unstable SCFE without surgical dislocation, treatment is urgent reduction with decompression and internal fixation (Loder & Dietz, 2012; Sonnega et al., 2011).

After internal fixation, the child is discharged on bed rest, followed by partial weight bearing with crutches. A follow-up visit with the physician will determine when the child can fully bear weight on the affected leg. The pin is removed later. Children with SCFE are monitored by their physicians until they have reached skeletal maturity to ensure that they do not develop contralateral SCFE or experience residual deformity and pain of the femur.

Assist the child and family in adjusting to sudden hospitalization, no weight-bearing activity, and surgery. Manage postoperative pain with oral or intravenous narcotics. Monitor the neurovascular status of the affected extremity closely (see Nursing Interventions 20-1). The physical therapist instructs the child in crutch walking.

KidKare Instruct the child that safe crutch walking starts with wearing low-heeled, rubber-soled shoes (sneakers are ideal). The child should not try to move quickly on crutches because a fall may result.

Community Care

The child is ready for discharge from the hospital when he or she can ambulate safely with crutches and when the pain is well controlled with an oral narcotic, such as acetaminophen with codeine. Crutches will be needed for ambulation for 3 to 6 months postoperatively. The child may then gradually resume normal activities, including running and contact sports. The child is closely monitored for 6 to 12 months for hip, groin, or knee pain in the nonaffected leg as a result of the high incidence of bilaterality seen in SCFE.

OSGOOD-SCHLATTER DISEASE

Osgood-Schlatter disease is one of the most common causes of knee pain in the adolescent. The diagnosis requires consideration in a child who presents with pain, swelling, and tenderness at the anterior tibial tuberosity. It is often seen in adolescence after a rapid growth spurt. The typical patient is a 13- to 14-year-old boy or a 10- to 11-year-old girl. It can occur unilaterally and presents bilaterally in about 30% of cases (Chang, 2010).

The prognosis for Osgood-Schlatter disease is very good. Symptoms can be expected to resolve about the time that the child's skeletal growth ceases (in boys, around age 17 years; girls, age 15 years). This condition does not result in long-term complications; however, many patients with Osgood-Schlatter disease may have pain on kneeling as an adult.

Pathophysiology

The underlying cause is believed to be a partial traumatic avulsion of the proximal tibial tuberosity at the insertion of the patellar tendon. The patella is particularly susceptible to trauma during rapid growth spurts, when the tibial tuberosity is susceptible to strain as a result of repetitive, submaximal stress from the quadriceps muscles.

Assessment

The child will often give a history of participation in sports that requires repetitive quadriceps contractions, such as football, basketball, soccer, gymnastics, and ballet. Discomfort is exacerbated with running, jumping, kneeling, and going up and down stairs. The child will often report pain relief with rest. The diagnosis is made by physical examination. The major clinical manifestations include visible soft-tissue swelling and tenderness to direct pressure over the proximal tuberosity at the site of the site of the patellar tendon insertion. Upon palpation, a soft mass (or bump) can often be felt in the area. This bump is called the anterior tibial tubercle.

Osgood-Schlatter disease is rated as grades 1 through 3, according to severity. Grade 1 involves pain after activity that resolves within 24 hours, grade 2 involves pain during and after activity that does not limit activity and resolves within 24 hours, and grade 3 consists of constant pain that limits sport and daily activity. Grades 1 and 2 require conservative treatment for a short time. Grade 3 may require conservative treatment for 3 to 6 months.

 KidKare Asking the child to squat or extend his or her knee against resistance usually elicits pain and is a good indicator of Osgood-Schlatter disease.

Irregularity of the tibial tuberosity is often seen on radiographs; however, they are usually unnecessary for diagnosis.

Interdisciplinary Interventions

In most cases, Osgood-Schlatter disease is self-limiting and can be managed by the primary care physician. Conservative management is directed at limiting physical activities that require frequent knee bending, jumping, or repetitive motion of the knee. Analgesics are recommended

for pain, and anti-inflammatory agents are used to reduce inflammation. Ice may be applied during the acute phase. Exercises during the rehabilitation phase include quadriceps isometrics, straight-leg raising, and isotonic resistance exercises for the hamstring. Occasionally, a splint or protective padding is applied, especially when the child has difficulty restricting activities.

In the rare cases when a child develops a painful ossicle in the distal patellar tendon, surgical excision may be recommended. Displaced avulsion fracture, a very rare complication, typically requires surgical repair.

Treatment of Osgood-Schlatter disease requires up to 3 months before the child can resume full sports involvement. Support the child and family at this time. A note from the physician or nurse to the school is needed if the child participates in a physical education program. If a child participates in multiple sports activities, choosing one sport to remain involved in will enable the child to recover and feel that he or she has some control. Involvement of the team coach may be needed to increase adherence to rehabilitation. Treatment should continue until the child can enjoy activities without discomfort or noticeable pain afterward. Too rapid a return to sports will cause symptoms to recur. If symptoms are not controlled by conservative management, the child will need referral to an orthopedic surgeon.

SCOLIOSIS

> **QUESTION:** Cathy has idiopathic structural scoliosis. Cathy and her family want to know if she might need surgery for her scoliosis. How would you explain the rationale for surgical versus nonsurgical intervention for idiopathic scoliosis appropriate for Cathy?

Scoliosis is defined as 3-D torsional deformity of the spine and trunk (Negrini et al., 2012). The primary deformity is a lateral curvature in the frontal plane, an axial rotation in the horizontal one, and a disturbance of the sagittal plane normal curvatures.

Scoliosis can be idiopathic or functional. Causes of functional scoliosis include postural compensation for leg length discrepancy and irritation of the sciatic nerve. Approximately 20% of cases are functional; the remaining 80% of cases are idiopathic (Negrini et al., 2012). The prevalence of idiopathic scoliosis (>10 degree curve) is 2% to 3% of the U.S. population. Approximately 0.03% affected have a curve greater than 30 degrees. The incidence is roughly equal in girls and boys for small curves, but girls have 10 times the risk of developing a curvature of greater than 30 degrees (Spiegel & Dormans, 2011).

Negrini et al. (2012) describe idiopathic scoliosis as a torsional deformity of the spine, which combines a translation and rotation of a variable number of vertebrae, which changes the 3-D geometry of the spine. The Cobb angle measurement is used to assess and define the degree of curvature in the frontal (coronal) plane. Visualizing an anteroposterior upright radiograph of the child's spine, the location of an upper end vertebra and a lower end vertebra are used as reference points to measure the Cobb angle. The diagnosis of scoliosis is confirmed if the angle is 10 degrees or higher and axial rotation can be seen (Negrini et al., 2012).

Kyphosis and *lordosis* are two terms used to describe a spinal curvature in the sagittal plane. Kyphosis is commonly described as a "humpback" or excessive forward concavity of the spine. Lordosis is a "swayback" or excessive backward concavity of the spine. Both curves are present in the normal spine, but when they become excessive, families may seek treatment. Lordosis, usually of the lumbar spine, is not a major deformity in children. Kyphosis and lordosis are not as commonly seen as scoliosis. The following discussion focuses on scoliosis.

Pathophysiology

Current theories hold that scoliosis is multifactorial, involving both genetic and environmental components. Four major curve patterns occur in children with idiopathic scoliosis: thoracic, lumbar, thoracolumbar, and double major (Fig. 20-15).

The age at onset and the location of the curve affect the prognosis of scoliosis considerably. The younger the child at the time of diagnosis, the greater the degree of curvature because of the amount of growth remaining. Adolescents with a curvature of less than 30 degrees at the time of bone maturity are unlikely to experience further progression. Adolescents with a curve between 30 and 50 degrees are likely to progress an average of 10 to 15 degrees of curvature after bone maturity. Curves greater than 50 degrees will progress at about 1 degree per year.

Curvature tends to progress more severely in females than in males. Congenital curves are also more likely to progress and to cause respiratory compromise. Life-threatening effects on pulmonary function increase as the curve angle worsens.

Assessment

When obtaining the history, include questions about family history of scoliosis and presence of pain or neurologic changes, including bowel or bladder dysfunction. The presence of severe pain or neurologic symptoms would be atypical of scoliosis. Include the date that the curve was first noticed and the history of progression of the curve. A slowly progressing curve is less worrisome than a sudden increase in severity of a curve.

THORACIC

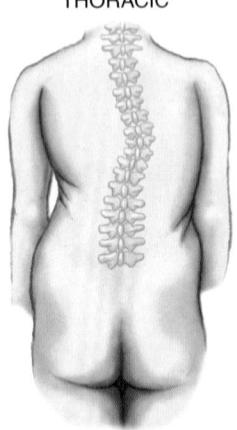

90% occur on the right side above T-11

LUMBAR

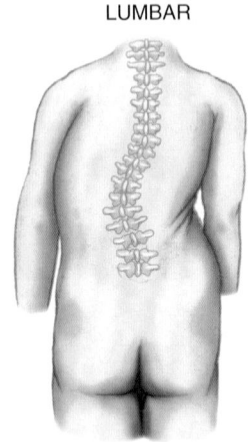

70% occur on the left side at L-1 or lower

THORACOLUMBAR

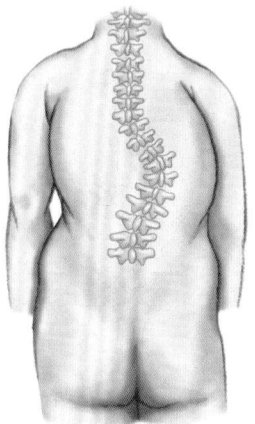

80% occur on the right side at T-11 – T-12

DOUBLE MAJOR

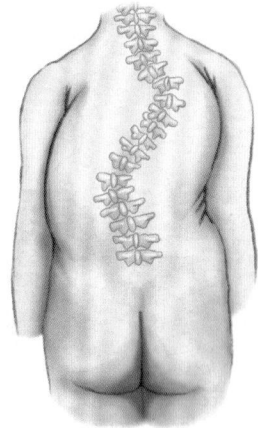

Usually involves right-sided and left-sided lumbar curves

Figure 20-15 The four major curve patterns in idiopathic scoliosis.

ALERT *If pain is reported as a symptom of the child's scoliosis, investigate immediately. Pain is not a normal finding for idiopathic scoliosis, and the presence of this particular symptom could signal an underlying condition, such as a tumor of the spinal cord.*

Physical examination should include an assessment of Tanner stage (see Figs. 3-23 and 3-24) and a complete neurologic examination. Peak curve progression occurs during Tanner stage 2 or 3. If neurologic signs such as a limp, weakness, or change in gait pattern are evident, pursue a full neurologic workup. Observe gait, measure leg length, and assess overall physical maturity.

Scoliosis screening is done routinely in schools and during well-child physicals by nurses. A scoliometer or "humpometer" can be used during screening to obtain a rough measurement of the curvature and to help identify scoliosis. The child bends forward at the waist while holding the palms together with arms extended (Fig. 20-16).

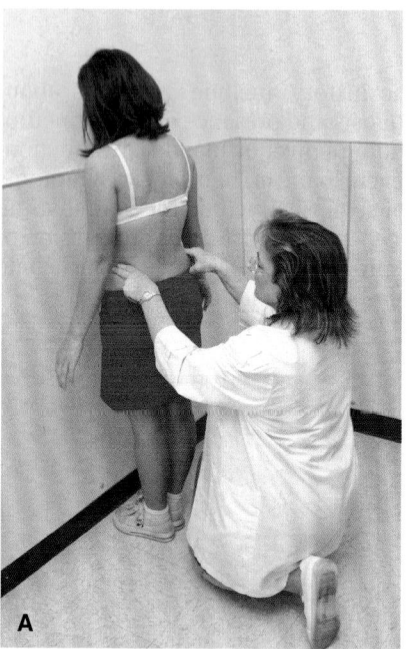
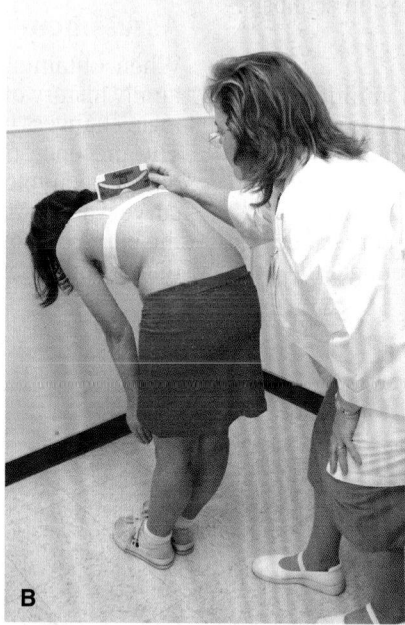
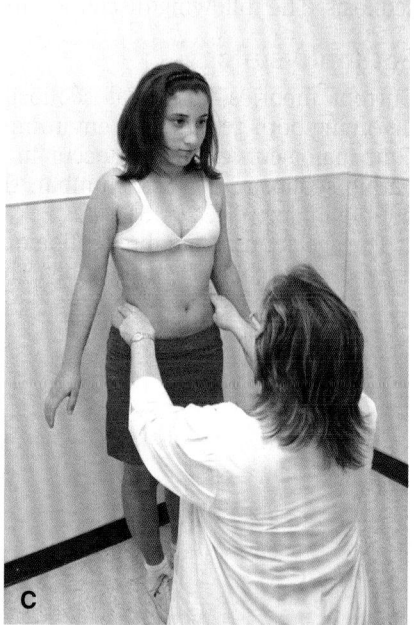
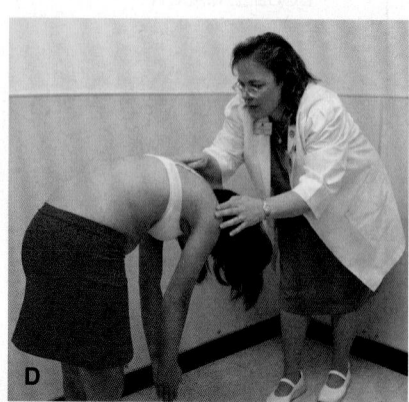
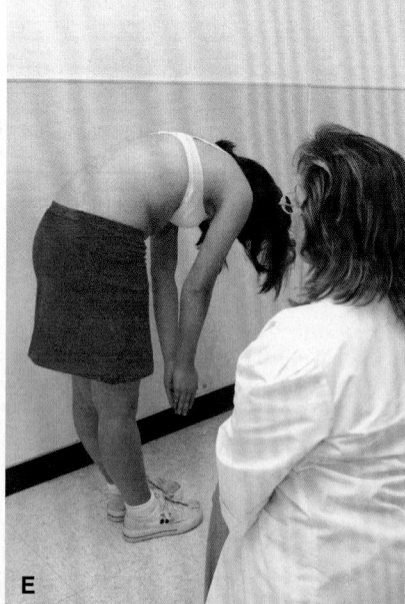

Figure 20-16 Scoliosis screening is performed by the school nurse. (A) The examiner begins by viewing the child from the back, looking for symmetry of the shoulders, scapulae, and waist creases. (B) Next, the child is asked to place her hands together and bend forward. The examiner uses a scoliometer to obtain a rough estimate of the degree of spinal curvature. (C) The examiner looks from the front for anterior chest deformity or asymmetry. (D) When the child bends forward toward the examiner, particular curves may become more visible. (E) Observing the child from the side allows the examiner to assess for kyphosis and lordosis.

The examiner looks along the horizontal plane of the spine from the back and side to detect an asymmetry in the contour of the back, known as the *rib hump* (the hallmark of scoliotic curves); those greater than 10 degrees require referral to a physician for radiography.

Diagnostic Tests

Abnormalities on physical examination require radiographic evaluation with a single standing, posteroanterior radiograph to enable measurement of the curve using the standardized Cobb or Risser grading scale. MRI is indicated for a left thoracic curve, pain, or positive neurologic examination.

Nursing Diagnoses and Outcomes

Many of the nursing diagnoses and outcomes for the child with a musculoskeletal disorder presented in Nursing Plan of Care 20-1 apply to the child with scoliosis. In addition, the following nursing diagnoses may apply to the newly diagnosed child and the child undergoing surgical intervention:

Nursing Diagnosis: Ineffective breathing pattern related to effect of curvature on ventilation and mobility

Outcome: Child will achieve maximal lung expansion with adequate ventilation.

Nursing Diagnosis: Acute pain related to surgical intervention to treat scoliosis

Outcomes:
- Child will experience minimal pain during the post-surgical recovery period.
- Child will identify measures effective in relieving pain.
- Caregivers will express awareness of the child's pain and perform measures to comfort the child.

Interdisciplinary Interventions

Education is an important component of the care for a child with scoliosis. At the time of diagnosis, many children and families are often upset and scared. Basic explanations and truthfulness are the best approach with teenagers. Progression of a curve is the basis for deciding whether the child will need treatment. The selected treatment regimen then is based on the child's age, the degree of curvature, and the child's willingness to adhere to the treatment program. Treatment options for scoliosis fall into two groups: nonsurgical and surgical interventions. The goals of treatment are to stop (or even reduce) curve progression at puberty, to prevent or treat respiratory dysfunction and spinal pain syndromes, and to improve aesthetics via postural correction (Negrini et al., 2012). See Evidence-Based Clinical Practice Guidelines 20-1.

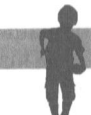

EVIDENCE-BASED CLINICAL PRACTICE GUIDELINES 20-1
Management of Scoliosis

American College of Radiology & The Society for Pediatric Radiology. (2009). *ACR–SPR practice guideline for the performance of radiography for scoliosis in children.* Retrieved from

http://www.acr.org/ ~ /media/FD620650A1B346579E89909FB3BFBB45.pdf

Guidelines for use of radiology to assess and monitor presence and progression of scoliosis in children.

Downs, J., Bergman, A., Carter, P. et al. (2009). Guidelines for management of scoliosis in Rett syndrome patients based on expert consensus and clinical evidence. *Spine, 34*(17), e607–e617. Retrieved from

http://www.rettsearch.org/Outcome/files/Guidelines_Management_Scoliosis_Spine_34_607.pdf

Scoliosis is a common condition seen in patients with Rett syndrome. These consensus guidelines were developed to help manage this frequently seen comorbidity

Negrini, S., Aulisa, A., Aulisa, L. et al. (2012). 2011 SOSORT guidelines: Orthopaedic and rehabilitation treatment of idiopathic scoliosis during growth. *Scoliosis, 7*(3), 1–35. Retrieved from

http://www.scoloiosisjournal.com/content/7/1/3

A review of the evidence on management of conservative treatment of idiopathic scoliosis (CTIS).

Richards, B. S., & Vitale, M. (2007). *AAOS-SRS-POSNA-AAP position statement: Screening for idiopathic scoliosis in adolescents.* Retrieved from

http://www.aaos.org/about/papers/position/1122.asp

Guidelines for screening adolescents for scoliosis.

van Bosse, H. J. P. (2010). *Guidelines on scoliosis monitoring and treatment for children with Prader-Willi syndrome.* Retrieved from

http://www.pwsausa.org/syndrome/Guidelines%20on%20Scoliosis%20Monitoring%20and%20Treatment%20MA-65.pdf

Children with Prader-Willi syndrome have an incidence of scoliosis between 40% and 90%. These guidelines provide specific guidance for these children.

U.S. Preventative Services Task Force. (2004). *Screening for idiopathic scoliosis in children.* Retrieved from

http://www.uspreventiveservicestaskforce.org/3rduspstf/scoliosis/scoliors.pdf

Evidence indicating that early screening of adolescents for scoliosis is no better than not screening in detecting the condition.

Nonsurgical Interventions

If the curve of the child's scoliosis is less than 20 degrees, most health care providers observe the child for any further progression of the curve. The child is assessed approximately every 6 months on an outpatient basis until the physician determines either that the curve is progressing or more aggressive treatment is needed.

Physiotherapeutic specific exercises (PSEs) consist of a variety of exercises completed in the outpatient setting by the caregiver and with the child's cooperation. Depending on the exercise, they may be conducted daily or several times a week. The schedule of exercises, which is directed by a physical therapist, serves to help prevent or limit progression of the scoliosis. PSEs are also employed in collaboration with bracing (Negrini et al., 2012).

When the scoliosis measures between 20 and 39 degrees of curvature, and evidence of progression exists, bracing is generally the next course of action. Bracing has proved effective to alter the natural curve progression of scoliosis if the brace is worn as prescribed. The effectiveness of other approaches, such as physical therapy, chiropractic care, biofeedback, and electrical stimulation, has not been proven.

During the past 50 years, a variety of braces, or orthoses, have been developed to treat scoliosis. The Milwaukee brace is the most familiar brace, although the Boston brace (the most common form of the thoracic–lumbar–sacral orthosis brace) has become more popular (Fig. 20-17). This is likely a result of its acceptance by teenagers because it is not visible when worn under clothing. However, the Boston brace is not effective for high thoracic curves. A brace also may be custom-designed specifically for a child.

 KidKare If the child expresses strong resistance and noncompliance with wearing a brace, a surgical approach to care may be required.

If the child must wear a brace, the brace should be worn full time or no less than 18 hours per day. The hours of bracing per day are prescribed in proportion with the severity of deformity; the age of the child; the stage, aim, and overall results of treatment; and the achievable compliance (Negrini et al., 2012). The brace is specifically constructed to treat the type of curvature that is unique to that child. During brace treatment, children are seen in the physician's office every 4 to 6 months. After the child reaches skeletal maturity, the amount of time wearing the brace is tapered. When braces work, they prevent progression of the curve by holding it in place until the child reaches skeletal maturity. Teaching Intervention Plan 20-2 summarizes a teaching intervention plan for the child with a brace. Despite adherence to a bracing regimen, however, the curve does progress in some children, necessitating surgical intervention.

Surgical Interventions

Most experts believe that if a spinal curve reaches 40 degrees or more, surgery should be considered because the possibility is great that the curve will worsen. With a curve measurement of more than 50 degrees, surgery is almost always needed. Each case is considered for neurologic status, bone age, diagnosis, curve size, physical and psychological effect of the deformity, and readiness for a major surgical intervention.

The goals of scoliosis surgery are to fuse the vertebrae so that the spine cannot bend and to correct the deformity. The most common surgical approach for idiopathic scoliosis is posterior spinal fusion (Table 20-3). This procedure consists of a long, straight, midline incision extending to two levels above and below the segments of the spine to be fused. Iliac crest bone graft is used to augment the fusion (see the Point for Care Path: An Interdisciplinary Plan of Care for the Child With Posterior Spinal Fusion).

Surgical intervention for the child with neuromuscular scoliosis is different because it often occurs at a younger age and the fused portion of the spine is longer. The surgical technique is anterior and posterior to enable increased stabilization of the spine and sacrum. To

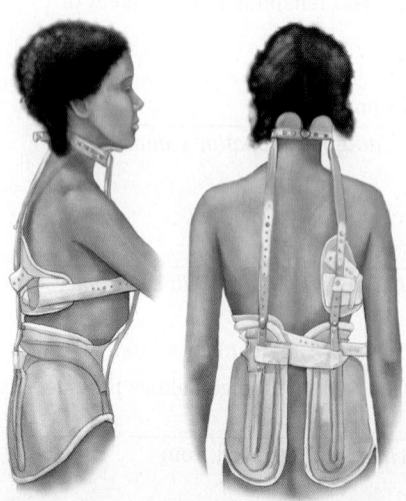

A. Milwaukee brace

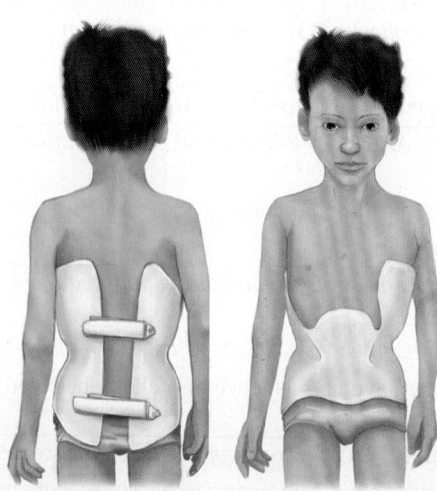

B. Boston brace

Figure 20-17 (A) Milwaukee brace (side and back views). (B) Boston brace (front and back views).

TIP 20-2: A TEACHING INTERVENTION PLAN for the Child Wearing a Brace for a Back Condition

Nursing Diagnoses and Family Outcomes

- Noncompliance related to discomfort and alteration in body image from brace
  Outcome: Child will wear brace for prescribed period of time.
- Risk for impaired skin integrity related to presence of brace
  Outcome: Child will exhibit intact skin without evidence of pressure areas or skin breakdown.
- Risk for injury related to presence of brace
  Outcome: Child will remain safe and free of injury.

Teach the Child/Family

Schedule for Brace Wear

- Inform about the amount of time the child is to wear the brace each day. The number of hours the brace must be worn depends on the severity of deformity; age of the child; the stage, aim, and overall results of treatment; and the achievable compliance
- Encourage wearing the brace during sleep to use up the most hours.

Skin Care and Comfort

- With a new brace, gradually increase wearing time so that the skin can develop tolerance for the pressure of the brace.
- Bathe or shower each day.
- Wear a 100% cotton T-shirt underneath the brace to absorb moisture.
- Do not use powders or lotions under the brace.
- Watch for areas of redness that do not disappear in 20 minutes, tingling, and numbness.
- Cover the chin pad (if present) with a smooth cloth to preserve skin integrity.
- Wear the brace as tightly as possible; if it is loose, it will rub the skin and cause skin breakdown.
- Consult the orthotist who made the brace if the brace does not seem to fit well. Fit and comfort are important factors.
- Loosen the brace during meals if necessary.

- Urge the child to avoid sitting in one position for long periods of time.

Appearance

- Select loose clothing that will camouflage the brace.

Brace Care

- Clean the brace each day by hand with mild soap and water and allow it to air dry completely. Once a week, wipe the brace down with rubbing alcohol.
- Examine the components of the brace regularly. Contact the physician and/or orthotist if there are any signs of "wear and tear" that may affect the function of the brace.

Activity and Safety

- Check the home for possible environmental hazards. Normal defense mechanisms and mobility are altered in a brace. Either remove hazards or find ways to avoid them.
- Urge the use of safety precautions and devices (e.g., handrail when using stairs).
- Allow bicycle riding while in the brace.
- Do not allow participation in swimming, gymnastics, skating, skiing, or contact sports while in the brace.
- Complete exercises as prescribed by the physical therapist. These exercises help adapt to the brace, encourage the active correction of the spinal deformity, and maintain the trunk musculature. Exercises focus on actively shifting laterally in the direction of the correction (away from the brace pad), extending the trunk while in the brace, and taking deep breaths.

Contact the Health Care Provider if

- Signs of redness, numbness, or tingling persist under or around the brace
- Brace seems to become uncomfortable despite having fit well in the past
- Parts of the brace become loose, cracked, or broken
- Child is not wearing the brace for the prescribed amount of time each day

---

obtain the desired outcomes, rods, sublaminar wires, or a combination are used. Postoperative care is more challenging because these children need pulmonary support, fluid status monitoring, and nutritional support in addition to routine postoperative monitoring.

As an adjunct to surgery, halo–gravity traction is used preoperatively and postoperatively in children with severe trunk decompensation, failed previous spinal fusion, or severe pulmonary compromise. This process can be long and costly and can be a drain on the family. The halo traction is in place for a few weeks before

surgery and for up to 6 weeks after surgery. Potential complications of loose pins and wound infections add risk during the perioperative and postoperative courses.

Preoperatively, the health care team reviews the surgical plan with the family. Education begins with explaining the degree of the curve, the surgical procedure, possible surgical complications, and duration of hospital stay. The teaching includes postoperative dressing change, bracing needs, pain management, activity level, and home care needs. See Chapter 11 for additional information on preoperative and postoperative care of the child.

TABLE 20-3	Types of Surgery for Posterior Spinal Fusion				
Type of Instrumentation and Description	**Indications**	**Area of Fixation**	**Early Postoperative Positioning**		**Brace Needed**
Harrington: single rod with two hooks	Scoliosis, not commonly used	Top and bottom of curve	Logroll and bed rest for 1 week until casted; do not logroll to convex side of thoracic curve		Yes; or cast
Texas Scottish Rite Hospital/ Cotrel-Dubousset (TSR/CD): double rod with multiple hooks and crossbars	Idiopathic scoliosis, lordosis	Segmental	Head of bed up 30–45 degrees Hip flexion over crease of bed Logroll until ambulating Bed flat when on side No overhead frame		No
Luque: double rod with wires	Neuromuscular disease (scoliosis, muscular dystrophy, cerebral palsy)	Segmental	Logroll Head of bed up 30 degrees		No

After surgery, children may go either to the intensive care unit for one night or to the pediatric unit. Care during the first 24 to 48 hours focuses on optimizing respiratory status, monitoring fluid volume shifts, and managing pain. Subtle changes in vital signs, such as decrease in blood pressure and increase in pulse rate, may be early indicators of hypovolemia. Occasionally, the child needs mechanical ventilation for a brief period to assist with breathing and to optimize respiratory status. Often, chest tubes are necessary after anterior spinal surgery. The tube is usually left in place until postoperative day 3, when it is removed by the surgeon.

Preventive pulmonary care is essential to avoid pneumonia. Such care may include oxygen by nasal cannula or mask and coughing and deep breathing along with the use of an incentive spirometer and chest physiotherapy. Pulse oximetry is useful for monitoring respiratory depression resulting from the surgery or analgesics. Respiratory therapy may be required to assist with mobilizing secretions.

After the child is transferred to the pediatric care unit, ongoing postoperative assessments for a child with a spinal fusion include evaluating fluid balance (intake and output), monitoring wound healing and drains, assessing neurovascular status of the extremities, and facilitating ambulation. Because of the amount of muscle exposed during this surgery, children tend to have more blood loss than with other orthopedic procedures. Monitor vital signs and hemoglobin and hematocrit levels to determine the need for blood transfusions after surgery.

Turn the child, using a logroll technique (Fig. 20-18), every 2 hours to decrease pooling of secretions in the lungs. Encourage coughing and deep breathing. The incentive spirometer and early ambulation are also important in preventing pulmonary complications. Assess bowel sounds and gradually progress fluid and diet intake as bowel motility is fully restored.

The wound from a spinal fusion is closed with dissolvable sutures on the inside and Steri-Strips or staples on the outside. It is then covered with gauze bandages and a pressure dressing. The incision is kept covered with a dressing for 2 to 3 days. Assess the area for bleeding and note any unusual drainage on the dressing. A Hemovac or similar surgical drain may be used to help evacuate excess blood from under the skin. Output from the Hemovac is generally greatest during the first 24 hours, gradually tapering off during the next few days. The drain usually is discontinued at about postoperative day 2 or 3. Monitor the amount of accumulated drainage, and assess the child for infection at the incision site.

The administration of prophylactic antibiotics for the first 72 hours postoperatively is a common practice to prevent infection. Stool softeners or a laxative may be needed to prevent constipation, which is a common side effect of pain medications.

Syndrome of inappropriate antidiuretic hormone secretion (SIADH) is common in spinal fusion patients after surgery because of a number of factors, including

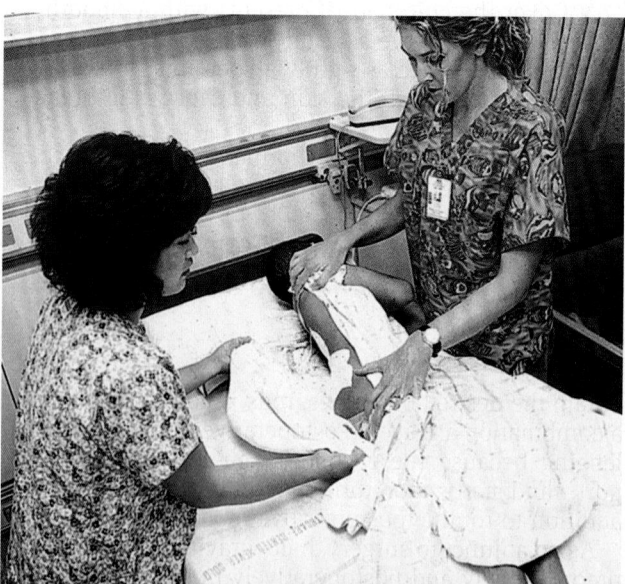

Figure 20-18 The logrolling technique is used after back surgery to prevent the child from flexing the back while being turned from side to side in bed.

change in blood volume, anesthetic medications, and the physical and emotional stress of the surgical procedure itself (see Chapter 26). The body responds by releasing antidiuretic hormone to retain fluids. The first sign of developing SIADH is usually a decrease in urine output, with an associated increase in urine specific gravity. Measure the serum level of sodium. Monitor blood pressure; if it decreases, administer additional fluids or blood transfusions as ordered. In mild hyponatremia with minimal symptoms, the treatment is to restrict fluid. SIADH usually resolves spontaneously in 2 to 3 days as the patient starts diuresis.

Pain after a spinal fusion cannot be eliminated, but it can and should be controlled (see Chapter 10). For some patients, especially nonverbal ones, a continuous intravenous infusion of opioids works well. Patient-controlled analgesia is very effective in managing pain and is a common method of pain treatment. Other children benefit from an epidural infusion of a local anesthetic or opioids, placed in the incision during surgery, to block transmission of pain impulses. After approximately postoperative day 3, the child can be switched to oral pain medications (Clinical Judgment 20-2).

Early mobilization helps to prevent pulmonary emboli, phlebitis, and skin breakdown. Assess the child's level of pain and provide pain relief, as needed, before turning or ambulation. Physical therapy after surgery assists the child in ambulation training, including teaching how to step and make transfers. Encourage family caregivers to accompany the child to therapy. Remind children to move their extremities while they are on bed rest; the physical therapist can also teach strengthening and isometric exercises to the child who is bedridden. Children who are wheelchair bound may need their wheelchair adjusted to conform to their new shape. If the child has a brace or cast after the surgery, review brace or cast care and general skin care before discharge. Ensure that family members can correctly demonstrate how to apply the brace. Make brace adjustments before the child goes home.

Community Care

Although special equipment is usually not needed after a spinal fusion, some children require an elevated toilet seat, hospital bed, or a shower chair in their home after discharge. These needs can be assessed in the hospital as the child's activity progresses. Plans must be

---

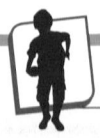

CLINICAL JUDGMENT 20-2

The Child After Spinal Fusion

Whitney is a 13-year-old black female who is admitted to the hospital for a posterior spinal fusion for idiopathic scoliosis. She is brought to your unit from the postanesthesia care unit (PACU) after her surgery. She has an intravenous line in her left hand, a nasogastric tube set to low intermittent suction, and a Foley catheter. Her orders state that she is NPO (nothing by mouth), on strict intake and output, and must logroll every 2 hours. Her vital signs are as follows: temperature, 99.5° F; pulse rate, 90 bpm; respiratory rate, 28 breaths/min; and blood pressure, 135/78 mm Hg. She is moaning.

Questions

1. During your assessment, what other data would be important to elicit from the PACU nurse who is giving you the report?

2. What are some of the important aspects of care you will want to evaluate in this postsurgical child?

3. Is Whitney in pain currently?

4. How can her pain be managed?

5. What factors would indicate that her pain is well controlled?

Answers

1. How much blood was lost in the operating room and how much blood did Whitney receive? How much fluid did she receive in the operating room? Assess the appearance of the wound and the amount of drainage in the Hemovac. Note the type of procedure that was done and any complications that occurred in the operating room. Also, check pain medication orders. When was the last pain medication given, and is the dose appropriate for her weight?

2. Fluid balance, pain management, and respiratory status

3. She is probably in pain, as evidenced by increased pulse, respirations, and blood pressure. Whitney should be asked to rate her pain to validate your assessment.

4. Intravenous or epidural infusion of opioids via patient-controlled analgesia pump or bolus

5. Whitney is able to logroll easily, she is sleeping, she verbalizes relief of pain, and her vital signs return to baseline

made regarding supervision of the child at home and to ensure that the child is able to continue with school studies during the recovery period at home. The child can usually return to school within 4 to 6 weeks.

During the home recovery period, children should avoid activities that require twisting, bending, or lifting heavy objects. The child should not participate in contact or high-impact sports for up to 2 years. Swimming and cycling are encouraged, however, and can be resumed within 3 to 4 months (Community Care 20-2).

Good nutrition is an important aspect of wound healing and general health. By the time of discharge, children are eating a regular diet. Some children need iron supplementation after surgery because of anemia caused by blood loss during surgery. Vitamin C and protein are important for healing; thus, the child should be encouraged to eat foods that contain those dietary elements. Extra calcium intake is not needed if the diet is well balanced. If the child has constipation caused by decreased activity and medication, encourage eating foods high in fiber and increasing fluid intake. A stool softener such as docusate sodium (Colace) may also be necessary.

The diagnosis of scoliosis often happens at an emotionally vulnerable time: the teenage years. Because body image is at the forefront of a teenager's mind, the hump on his or her back may be considered enormous. Anything that makes a teenager feel different from his or her peers is stressful. Contact with another teenager who is undergoing the same problems can be helpful. Family members also need to be supported with counseling because they can be frightened by the unfamiliar situation as well. Difficulties can arise when the parents and teenager disagree on the type of treatment to be undertaken. Most teenagers comprehend what is happening to their bodies and should be included in decision making from the start. (See Chapter 2 for more information on informed consent, autonomy, and self-determination issues.)

> **ANSWER:** An example of an explanation for surgical versus nonsurgical interventions appropriate for Cathy is, "If you are wearing your brace and it is slowing down the rate your spine is curving, then you might not need surgery. If the curvature in your back becomes more than 50 degrees or the rate of curvature increases quickly, then you will probably need to have surgery."

INFECTIOUS AND INFLAMMATORY DISORDERS

Musculoskeletal disorders classified as inflammatory or infectious affect the bones and joints. Infections are generally caused by bacteria that invade bones or joints.

COMMUNITY CARE 20-2

Activity Guidelines for Children After Back Surgery

Time Frame	Activities Encouraged	Activities Discouraged	Activities Restricted
Discharge from hospital to 4–6 weeks	Walking Quiet activities Study with home tutor; may start back to school in 3–4 weeks Riding in car, but not driving Swimming	Lifting more than 5 lb Running Diving in a pool Playing contact sports Riding dirt bikes, all-terrain vehicles, or mountain bikes	Gymnastics Parachuting Bungee jumping Motorcycle riding Trampoline jumping
6 weeks to 3 months	Same as above, but driving is allowed	Same as above	Same as above
3–6 months	Riding a bike Light jogging Lifting 5–10 lb	Running Diving in a pool Playing contact sports Riding dirt bikes, all-terrain vehicles, or mountain bikes	Same as above
6 months to 1 year	Return to most of the normal activities done before surgery Bowling, skiing, skating, aerobics, golfing, horseback riding, diving, racquet sports, lifting weights	Playing contact sports until 1 year from surgery Water park amusement rides or roller coasters until 1 year after surgery	Same as above unless approved by physician

Osteomyelitis and septic arthritis are the most common infectious disorders. The most common inflammatory disorders of children are JIA and SLE.

OSTEOMYELITIS

Osteomyelitis is an infection of the bone and the tissues around the bone. The two most common types in children are acute and subacute hematogenous osteomyelitis.

ALERT *All types of osteomyelitis require immediate treatment if suspected because they can cause massive bone destruction and life-threatening sepsis.*

Osteomyelitis occurs in 2 per 10,000 children. Approximately 50% of cases occur in preschool-aged children (Kocher et al., 2006). Except for the increase in incidence in patients with sickle cell disease, there is no predilection for osteomyelitis based on race (Kaplan, 2011).

Osteomyelitis most often involves the long bones of the lower limbs, although it can occur in any bone of the body. Numerous organisms cause osteomyelitis. The most common cause of acute hematogenous osteomyelitis is *Staphylococcus aureus*. Group A beta-hemolytic streptococci are the next most common causative organisms in the neonate, followed by *Streptococcus pneumoniae*, *Haemophilus influenzae* type b, and *Kingella kingae*. As a result of the widespread use since the late 1980s of conjugate vaccine against *H. influenzae*, acute hematogenous osteomyelitis caused by this organism has been virtually eliminated. With increased use of the 7-valent conjugate vaccine against *Streptococcus pneumoniae*, incidence of invasive infections caused by this organism is expected to decrease. However, *Candida lusitaniae* is emerging as an opportunistic causative pathogen in premature infants.

Early recognition of osteomyelitis in young patients before extensive infection develops and prompt institution of appropriate medical and surgical therapy minimizes permanent damage (Kaplan, 2011).

Pathophysiology

Organisms causing osteomyelitis can gain access through a variety of routes, including an open fracture, penetration of the skin by a contaminated object, spread from a septic joint or infected wound, or spread from a bacterial infection somewhere in the body, such as dental caries or ear infection. Blunt trauma also may precede osteomyelitis because the hematoma formed from the trauma acts as an entry port for microorganisms. Premature infants; infants with birth complications such as ventilator dependency, central line, and umbilical catheter placement (Kocher et al., 2006); children with sickle cell disease; and children with malignancies or JA who are taking immunosuppressive agents and are malnourished have the highest incidences of osteomyelitis.

Osteomyelitis results in inflammatory destruction of bone, bone necrosis, and new bone formation. In children older than 1 year of age, infection starts in the metaphyseal sinusoidal veins and is contained by the growth plate. The joint is spared unless the metaphysis is intracapsular. In infants younger than 1 year of age, some metaphyseal vessels may transverse the epiphyseal plate and permit spread of infection to the epiphysis and adjacent joint.

The infection spreads laterally and breaks through the cortex, lifting the periosteum to form a subperiosteal abscess. The presence of vascular connections between the metaphysis and the epiphysis makes infants particularly prone to infection in the adjacent joint. The cortical bone of neonates and infants is thin and loose, consisting predominately of woven bone, which permits pressure caused by infection to escape and promotes rapid spread of the infection into the subperitoneal region. Two common areas of osteomyelitis are the proximal tibia and the distal femur (Kaplan, 2011; Kocher et al., 2006).

Assessment

The earliest signs of osteomyelitis are often nonspecific. Older infants and children will most likely have fever, pain, and localized signs such as edema, erythema, and warmth. The infant may exhibit irritability, lethargy, and decreased motion of the limb. Note family reports of a recent infection, such as a cold or otitis media. Alternatively, the child may have a history of falling or trauma to an extremity.

Also investigate the duration of symptoms and any history of prior bone infection after surgery or trauma. The child with chronic osteomyelitis exhibits symptoms similar to those of acute osteomyelitis, but the history reveals symptoms persisting for longer than 3 weeks or prior bone infection weeks or months ago. Because of the increased awareness of the need for prompt, aggressive treatment for acute osteomyelitis, the incidence of chronic osteomyelitis in children is decreasing.

Physical examination of the affected area reveals localized tenderness, redness, warmth, and pain on palpation of the area. Occasionally, children have soft-tissue swelling around the area. With involvement of the lower extremities, limp or refusal to walk is seen in approximately half the patients (Kaplan, 2011).

Diagnostic Tests

Radiographs are often used for initial evaluation to rule out other causes, such as fracture or foreign body. MRI has emerged as the most sensitive and specific test for osteomyelitis. It is the best imaging technique for identifying abscesses and for differentiating between bone and soft-tissue infection (Kaplan, 2011). Radionuclide imaging can be valuable in suspected bone infection at multiple sites.

Laboratory studies that may aid in the diagnosis are a WBC count, CRP, and ESR. The WBC count is elevated in about half the patients, and CRP and ESR are almost always elevated. A blood culture should be done in all suspected cases. Aspiration or biopsy of bone provides the optimal specimen for culture to confirm the diagnosis.

Nursing Diagnoses and Outcomes

Nursing diagnoses, nursing interventions, and desired patient outcomes for the child with a musculoskeletal disorder are presented in Nursing Plan of Care 20-1.

Depending on the assessment data, the following nursing diagnoses may also apply to the child with osteomyelitis:

Nursing Diagnosis: Risk for injury related to effects of infectious process on bone mass
Outcomes:
- Child will maintain the affected extremity in proper alignment.
- Child will refrain from bearing weight on the affected extremity.
- Child will complete entire course of antibiotic therapy to promote full recovery.

Nursing Diagnosis: Risk for imbalanced body temperature related to the infectious process
Outcome: Child's body temperature will remain within normal range.

Interdisciplinary Interventions

Interdisciplinary interventions for both chronic and acute osteomyelitis are the same and focus on eradicating the infection via antibiotic therapy, ensuring the child's comfort, and promoting growth and development.

Antibiotic Therapy

The initial empirical antibiotic therapy is based on knowledge of likely bacterial pathogens at various ages and the result of gram stain of any aspirated material. In the neonate, nafcillin or oxacillin and a broad-spectrum cephalosporin such as cefotaxime are used. If methicillin-resistant *Staphylococcus aureus* (MRSA) is suspected, vancomycin is substituted for nafcillin (Kaplan 2011; Peltola et al., 2010). In the older infant or child, the choice of empiric antibiotic therapy is dependent on community MRSA rates. If MRSA accounts for greater than 10% *S. aureus* rates, then vancomycin or clindamycin would be the antibiotic of choice. Cefotaxime or ceftriaxone is recommended for positive pneumococcal cultures (Kaplan, 2011; Peltola et al., 2010). When blood culture or aspirate results are obtained, antibiotic therapy is tailored to the causative organism. After the patient demonstrates a response to antibiotic therapy (usually within 2 to 3 days) and final blood cultures obtained are negative, the parenteral medication is stopped and the patient is switched to oral antibiotics, usually for 4 to 8 weeks. However, children who do not respond well initially to intravenous antibiotics may remain on intravenous antibiotic therapy much longer. Monitoring ESR or CRP may be of value in assessing response to antibiotic therapy.

caREminder

The antibiotics used to treat osteomyelitis are caustic to veins. Be diligent about diluting the medication and infusing it slowly

Monitor the intravenous site closely for signs of infiltration. Usually, the child with osteomyelitis receives long-term antibiotic therapy. Duration of treatment is based on the type of infection, and no standard length of treatment has been determined. Four to 6 weeks of therapy is not atypical, although a longer period of time may be needed if infection persists. Whenever possible, advocate for the patient to have a long-term intravenous line inserted, such as a peripherally inserted central catheter (PICC). Because frequent laboratory tests can also be drawn from a PICC line, the child will receive fewer needle sticks. (See Chapter 17 for a more complete discussion of care of the PICC line.)

Comfort Interventions

Making the child comfortable and ensuring relief from pain are key for the child with suspected or known osteomyelitis. Splinting the involved extremity may be helpful during the first few days of treatment (see "Treatment Modalities" section earlier in this chapter). However, splinting should not be used indefinitely because it may discourage use of the affected extremity. If required, oral analgesics such as acetaminophen, ibuprofen, or narcotics can be given to relieve pain. After antibiotics have been administered for at least 24 hours, bone and tissue pain should start to subside.

Child Life Specialist Interventions

The hospitalized child can become easily bored and frustrated by the limitations imposed by lengthy intravenous therapy. The involvement of a child life specialist can be extremely helpful in providing age-appropriate diversions and activities that do not compromise the intravenous site or cause the child pain in the affected limb. These activities also can help to foster growth and development.

Community Care

Some children with osteomyelitis are discharged on a regimen of home intravenous antibiotic therapy. Discuss this option with the family at the start of treatment. Collaborate with home care nursing services to ensure the family has the education, supplies, and support personnel to manage home intravenous therapy. The nurse helps in assessing whether a family can maintain a child on home intravenous antibiotics and teaches the family intravenous therapy skills. If the antibiotics can be scheduled every 8 to 12 hours, adherence increases. Family members who are administering one or two antibiotics every 4 to 6 hours can easily become sleep deprived.

Some children may return to school while they are receiving intravenous antibiotics at home depending on the schedule for administration, such as administration every 12 hours. Other children use a home tutor until they have completed the medications. ESR or CRP is monitored by the physician to determine the response to antibiotic therapy. Instruct the family to notify the physician if the child becomes febrile or experiences pain in the affected area.

The child with chronic osteomyelitis may benefit from increased psychological support to help deal with depression associated with physical limitations and frequent hospitalizations. Treatment is prolonged, painful, and frustrating for the child and family.

SEPTIC ARTHRITIS

Septic arthritis, a bacterial invasion of a joint space, can occur in any joint in the body. Septic arthritis occurs in all age groups, although the most common age of occurrence is 1 to 2 years. The annual incidence of septic arthritis remains 4 to 10 cases per 100,000 patients per year. In persons with underlying joint disease or prosthetic joints, the incidence is increased to 30 to 60 cases per 100,000 population (Lynn & Matthews, 2012). The most common causative organisms are *S. aureus* and MRSA, followed by *K. kingae* (Faust et al., 2012). Before antibiotics became available, the mortality rate among children with septic arthritis was 50%. Septic arthritis is a medical and surgical emergency that must be treated as soon as possible.

Pathophysiology

The process of septic arthritis begins when bacteria enter the joint space. The organism can invade the joint through hematogenous seeding (transmitted by the bloodstream), by extension of an adjacent bone infection (osteomyelitis), by seeding from a distal site of infection (otitis or upper respiratory infection), or by a penetrating wound or foreign body in the joint. An inflammatory reaction occurs, resulting in fluid and WBCs entering the joint. The WBCs release an enzyme that breaks down the surface of the articular cartilage. Scar tissue replaces the articular cartilage, restricting joint motion. If not treated promptly and aggressively, septic arthritis results in permanent loss of function. Large joints are more commonly affected than small joints. Approximately 60% of cases affect the knee or hip (Mathews & Coakley, 2008). Other sites for septic arthritis, in decreasing order of incidence, are the ankles, elbows, wrists, shoulders, and pelvis.

Assessment

Typically, assessment of the child with septic arthritis reveals a 1- to 2-week history of pain in the affected extremity, with decreased activity tolerance and passive ROM. Warmth, tenderness, and swelling over the joint are common. The child usually complains of pain in an extremity and often has a limp that is associated with pain. If the hip joint is the affected area, the child may exhibit slight flexion, abduction, or external rotation of the affected extremity. An infant may present with or without fever, symptoms of irritability, failure to eat, and crying when handled.

The child may resist or guard the joint when asked to move it. If the hip or lower extremities are involved, the parent usually reports that the child will not walk or crawl. History may reveal reports of a recent ear infection, cold, or joint trauma. Any history of a bite or penetrating wound, such as with a needle or thorn, is also important to note when trying to ascertain the cause for the septic arthritis.

Diagnostic Tests

Laboratory tests used in diagnosing septic arthritis include a complete blood count with differential for WBCs, neutrophil count, band cell count, ESR or CRP, and blood cultures. The identification of pathogens in the synovial fluid remains the most definitive diagnosis of septic arthritis. The WBC count may be normal or elevated, with an increased neutrophil count. Blood cultures will reveal the causative organism. The ESR and CRP rate test are not reliable in diagnosis of septic joint disease because they only indicate inflammation or infection. Also, these levels may not be raised when the infection is confined to the synovial fluid in the joint.

Radiologic tests for septic arthritis include a plain radiograph, ultrasound, and bone scan. Radiographs may show a subtle increase in the joint space or soft-tissue changes (such as swelling) and can rule out any lesions. Ultrasound may be done, especially if the hip is affected, to observe for fluid in the joint. Although bone scans are ineffective in demonstrating septic arthritis, they may be helpful in ruling out osteomyelitis as the cause of the child's symptoms.

Definitive diagnosis requires joint aspiration using fluoroscopy to obtain fluid for cultures and determine WBC count. If fluid sample contains more than 50,000 WBC cells per cubic millimetere and 90% are polymophonucleocytes confirms the diagnosis.

Interdisciplinary Interventions

The goals of treatment of septic arthritis are to prevent destruction of the articular cartilage and to retain motion, strength, and function. Care of the child with septic arthritis also includes managing pain, reducing body temperature, and ensuring consistent medication administration.

Procedural Interventions

In septic arthritis, the inflammatory process, not the bacteria itself, causes damage to the joint. Thus, the inflammatory exudates that cause the damage to articular surfaces must be released. This may be accomplished with needle aspiration of the fluid. If the fluid continues to accumulate, then arthroscopy can be used to clean out the joint and obtain a synovial biopsy. In certain joints, such as the hip or shoulder, an arthrotomy, or surgical opening into the joint, is needed. The fluid and biopsy samples are sent for laboratory examination to ascertain the causative organism.

Perform wound management of an open arthrotomy site. Secure the dressing, note the color and amount of secretions, and change the dressing if necessary.

Infection Management

The administration of antibiotics for a 4- to 6-week period is an important aspect of the treatment plan. Broad-spectrum intravenous antibiotics are started after a culture has been obtained. After an organism has been identified, the antibiotic may be changed to one that is specific for the causative organism. If the causative agent is not identified, broad-spectrum intravenous antibiotics are continued for the entire course of therapy. If the causative agent is identified, and if the child has a good response to the treatment regimen (decreased pain and swelling, a downward trend in laboratory values, and fever resolution), the child may be switched to oral antibiotics for 3 to 6 weeks or the length of time it takes for the ESR or CRP to return to normal.

During the acute phase of the infection, monitor the child's temperature frequently. Administer antipyretics as ordered. Implement other cooling measures, such as a tepid sponge bath and removing blankets or clothing. To prevent dehydration secondary to fever, encourage fluids.

Pain Management

If the child is uncomfortable, administer oral pain medications and monitor their effectiveness. Give analgesics before beginning daily activities or treatments that may cause discomfort.

If necessary, initially splint the affected limb or joint for comfort. The splint can be removed after a few days. Observe the child to note the extent of joint mobility, voluntary movement, and weight-bearing capabilities. Encourage the child to participate in daily activities as he or she feels able. Provide assistive devices, such as crutches or a walker, as needed to support ambulation.

Community Care

Intravenous antibiotic therapy can be managed by home care when it is determined that the ESR or CRP level is decreasing and the antibiotics are effective. Before discharge, teach the family about administering the child's medication and collaborate with home care services, as needed, to ensure the child receives daily medication. Emphasize the importance of not missing scheduled doses and the need to continue administering the medication (whether intravenous or oral) even if the child feels better. Insufficient treatment can result in permanent damage to the articular cartilage or in chronic osteomyelitis. Follow-up care is needed to assess the effectiveness of the treatment.

Families require support during the acute and home management phases of the child's illness. With a diagnosis of septic arthritis, concern about loss of joint function is paramount. If treatment was delayed, family members may feel guilty about not seeking medical attention earlier. Encourage the family members to seek support from social services, clergy, and friends.

JUVENILE IDIOPATHIC ARTHRITIS

JIA, also referred to as *juvenile rheumatoid arthritis* (JRA) and *juvenile arthritis*, is the most common chronic inflammatory condition of children. The prevalence of JIA is 1 per 1,000 persons younger than 18 years of age. Depending on the arthritis subset, girls are affected more frequently than boys (Beukelman et al., 2011; Secor-Turner et al., 2011).

Pathophysiology

The cause of JIA and the mechanisms that lead to the chronic synovial inflammation are unknown. Heredity is thought to play some part, but researchers believe that something in the environment triggers the disease. JIA is considered to be an autoimmune disorder. It occurs when the body's immune system mistakenly identifies the body's own tissue as foreign and attacks the tissue, as if trying to rid the body of an invader. Although the clinical onset of JIA may follow an acute systemic infection or physical trauma to a joint, no research supports a direct cause-and-effect mechanism.

JIA starts with an inflamed synovial membrane and adjacent joint capsule. The inflammation of the synovial tissues produces increased amounts of fluid, which are secreted into the joint. The increased fluid volume causes the joint to become swollen and boggy, a condition termed *joint effusion*. The joint feels edematous and warm to the touch. The synovial membranes become infiltrated with lymphocytes and plasma cells, which cause the normally clear joint fluid to become cloudy. Prolonged synovitis can erode joint structures and narrow joint spaces. Eventually, bone deformity, subluxation, and **ankylosis** (immobility and consolidation) of joints occur. Growth disturbances adjacent to the affected joint can cause overgrowth or undergrowth of the affected part.

The joint pain and stiffness associated with JIA are initially caused by the pressure applied to sensory nerves in the area of the edematous membranes. As the disease progresses, pain and discomfort may also be a result of joint destruction or contractures, which lead to stiffness and immobility.

There are five subtypes of JIA defined by the International League of Associations for Rheumatology (ILAR) (Petty et al., 2004) according to the symptoms at disease onset:

- **Systemic** disease—involves one or more joints and characterized by fever of at least 2 weeks in duration and accompanied by one or more of the following: rash, generalized lymphadenopathy, and systemic involvement that may include organs as well as joints
- **Oligoarticular** arthritis—involves one to four joints during the first 6 months after disease onset and may extend to more joints after 6 months (extended oligoarticular arthritis)
- **Polyarticular** arthritis— involves five or more joints during the first 6 months after disease onset
- **Psoriatic** arthritis— identified if there is arthritis and psoriasis (rash)
- **Enthesitis-related** disease—identified if there is arthritis and/or enthesitis (inflammation of sites where tendon or ligaments attach to the bone)

Some familial tendencies have been demonstrated in early-onset oligoarticular JIA. Siblings appear to be at increased risk for development of JIA. Some genetic markers (e.g., human leukocyte antigen [HLA]-B27, -DR5, -DR8, and -DR4) can be linked to certain types of JIA. However, more research is needed in this area.

Assessment

Physical manifestations of JIA vary according to the type. Most commonly, family members state that the child has become cranky or irritable. The child may tire easily, have a poor appetite with scant weight gain, and demonstrate some growth delays. Ask questions about the child's daily activities and comfort. Children with JIA have a difficult time getting out of bed in the morning because of joint stiffness. They may not participate in play or sports activities that are painful to them. The child's gait may be altered to avoid putting pressure on a distal joint.

Children with systemic JIA often present with a history of spiking fevers with temperatures more than 103° F (39.5° C) daily for 2 weeks, in conjunction with a rash that comes and goes with the fever. They often have swollen lymph nodes and an enlarged liver and spleen; they may also have pleuritis or myocarditis. They will be listless and unwell during the fever and become more engaged when the temperature returns to normal. During the course of the fever spikes, the child may complain of weakness, lose weight, and suffer from anemia. The child may present with pain; warmth; and swelling of knees, ankles, wrists, or elbows. For some children, however, no signs of joint inflammation may be evident until months or even years later. During physical assessment, inspect and palpate each joint for redness, swelling, warmth, and tenderness; note any nodules on the joints that may be present in polyarticular-onset JIA. To assess for limping or guarding behavior, observe the child walking down a hall. Children with JIA tend to keep their joints flexed, which can cause contractures. Accurate measurement of height and weight is also essential because JIA can retard growth.

In addition to examining the musculoskeletal system, assess the child for other systemic changes resulting from the inflammatory process. Carditis, pleurisy, pneumonia, and organomegaly are typically manifestations of progressive illness. Inflammation of the iris and ciliary body, called *anterior uveitis*, *iritis*, or **iridocyclitis**, may occur. This complication is most typically seen with oligoarticular JIA. The inflammation can cause eye pain and diminished vision; in some cases, permanent blindness occurs. Remind family members to seek medical treatment if visual changes are noted that could indicate iridocyclitis, such as sensitivity to light, blurred vision, or redness of the eye. Encourage annual ophthalmologic examination including slit-lamp examination to promote early detection and treatment.

Diagnostic Tests

Diagnosis of JIA is often made on the basis of the child's constellation of symptoms. No laboratory test can diagnose JIA. Some nonspecific indicators of inflammation may be noted, including elevated WBC count, ESR, and CRP level. Additional laboratory analysis should include antinuclear antibody (ANA), RF, and anti-cyclic citrullinated peptide.

Radiographs do not show any changes until late during the disease course, but they are useful for comparing bone growth or damage from the time of diagnosis onward. Other radiologic tests, such as MRI, computed tomography, or bone scan, may be performed to rule out other diagnoses.

Nursing Diagnoses and Outcomes

Nursing diagnoses and outcomes for the child with a musculoskeletal disorder are presented in Nursing Plan of Care 20-1. The following nursing diagnoses should

also be considered for the child with JIA, especially for the child with a subtype of JIA in which fever is a frequent occurrence:

Nursing Diagnosis: Risk for imbalanced body temperature related to inflamed synovial tissues
Outcomes:
- Child will maintain normal body temperature.
- Child will remain free of joint swelling and pain.

Nursing Diagnosis: Deficient fluid volume related to fever
Outcome: Child will maintain normal fluid volume as evidenced by good skin turgor, moist mucous membranes, and adequate urine output.

Nursing Diagnosis: Imbalanced nutrition: Less than body requirements related to anorexia, dietary inadequacies, drug–nutrient interactions, limitations in physical activity, mechanical feeding difficulties, and susceptibility to food fads
Outcomes:
- Child will exhibit weight gain appropriate to his or her age, height, and physique.
- Child and family members will implement measures to ensure that the child consumes adequate amounts of nutritious food.

Interdisciplinary Interventions

The desired outcomes for children affected with JIA are to prevent deformities, minimize discomfort, promote mobility, and preserve the ability to perform activities of daily living. Drug therapy and physical therapy are mainstays of treatment for JIA. The health care team in the acute setting may encounter the child when he or she is experiencing a severe exacerbation of illness that requires intense physical therapy and nutritional support; when a change of medications is required; or when surgical intervention, such as muscle or tendon release, is needed to treat severe musculoskeletal complications. However, most children are cared for at home. The interdisciplinary team collaborates to ensure continuity of care regardless of the setting for treatment. Implement an interdisciplinary teaching plan to provide family members with the knowledge and skills needed to attend to the child's care needs at home (Teaching Intervention Plan 20-3). Review the plan with the child periodically so that, as the child grows and matures, he or she can continue to learn more about the condition and accept increasing responsibility for managing self-care.

Pharmacologic Interventions

Various drugs are used to treat JIA. These include NSAIDs, disease-modifying antirheumatic drugs (DMARDs), and glucocorticoids.

Treatment usually starts with NSAIDs, which include a variety of medications that affect the processes involved in inflammation. A reduction in pain, swelling, and stiffness help the child to participate in normal day-to-day activities. Some of the more commonly prescribed medications in this group include naproxen (Naprosyn), tolmetin sodium (Tolectin), indomethacin (Indocin), and ibuprofen (Advil or Motrin). Aspirin is not used in treatment of JA because of its side effects (Beukelman et al., 2011).

TIP 20-3: A TEACHING INTERVENTION PLAN for the Child With Juvenile Arthritis

Nursing Diagnoses and Family Outcomes

- Risk for impaired physical mobility related to joint inflammation, swelling, and pain
  Outcomes: Child will take medications as ordered.
  Child will follow daily exercise program.
  Child will moderate activity with adequate periods of rest and relaxation.
- Chronic pain related to joint inflammation and contracture
  Outcomes: Child and family members will describe interventions to reduce pain and discomfort associated with the child's condition.
  Child will experience no pain or acceptable levels of reduced pain as evidenced by play and participation in daily self-care activities.
- Delayed growth and development related to physical limitations, discomfort, and clinical progression of the child's condition
  Outcomes: Child will maintain a normal weight for age and height.
  Child and family will acknowledge the importance of well-balanced meals and rest periods.
  Child will participate in age-appropriate activities that are modified as needed based on the child's current status.

Teach the Child/Family

Medications

- Administer anti-inflammatory and analgesic medications per health care provider orders to maintain a therapeutic blood level and reduce the likelihood of joint pain and swelling.
- Reduce gastric irritation associated with medication administration by taking salicylates with food or milk.
- Review adverse side effects of prescribed medications, and report any adverse signs and symptoms to the health care provider.

Activity and Safety

- Encourage the child to participate in low-impact exercises, especially swimming.
- Avoid overexercising and stimulating swollen joints, which aggravate pain.
- Assist child to complete exercise program daily at home, at school, or at another community location.
- Incorporate exercise program into daily play activities such as throwing a ball, riding a bike, or molding clay.
- Encourage child to attend regular school.
- Schedule daily rest periods for the child.
- Encourage the child to participate in daily self-care activities and tasks around the home.
- Use splints, sandbags, or casts to maintain position of function and to prevent muscle contractions.

- Provide assistive devices, such as elevated commodes and handrails, to aid in body mechanics.
- Choose clothing that is easy for the child to put on and take off.
- Modify eating utensils, brushes, combs, and toothbrushes for easier grasp.
- Ensure the child is evaluated by an ophthalmologist for slit-lamp examination and routine eye care on a regular basis.

Pain Management

- Encourage the child to take a warm bath for 20 minutes upon awakening in the morning.
- Use an electric blanket, if a bath is not feasible, to warm and relax the muscles and joints.
- Use warm, moist packs and heating pads to relieve joint discomfort.
- Use paraffin baths to reduce joint pain.
- Use a firm mattress and lie flat in bed to reduce flexion deformity.

Nutrition

- Provide a well-balanced diet to avoid weight gain or weight loss.
- Select foods high in iron if anemia is a concern.
- Monitor weight on a weekly basis. If the child becomes overweight, an extra burden can be put on weight-bearing joints.
- Monitor the child's hematocrit level on a regular basis to assess for anemia, which can be associated with the inflammatory process.
- During febrile periods, monitor the child for adequate hydration and encourage intake of fluids.

Psychosocial

- Encourage the child to verbalize his or her feelings regarding the condition.
- Encourage the child to meet other children with JIA.
- Encourage independence. Do not do for the child what the child can do for himself or herself.
- Encourage the child to participate in therapy and treatment decisions to promote self-care, a sense of autonomy, and control over the situation.
- Encourage the child to engage in activities in which he or she can be successful and thus promote positive self-esteem.

Contact the Health Care Provider if

- Joint pain and inflammation worsen despite current medication regimen
- Child's temperature increases to more than 103.1° F (39.5° C) and is not reduced by such measures as medication, tepid baths, and cool clothes
- Child appears to be dehydrated (lips dry and cracked, no tearing present, urine output low)
- Child has signs of drug toxicity
- Child's vision appears to be impaired

ALERT *The use of aspirin has been strongly associated with Reye syndrome in children who have had chickenpox or flu. Because aspirin may be an ongoing part of the regimen of the arthritic child, warn caregivers of the relationship between viral illnesses, aspirin, and Reye syndrome; teach them to identify the symptoms of Reye syndrome.*

It may be necessary to try several NSAIDs to determine which one works best. The most common side effect of this class of drugs is stomach upset, which can frequently be avoided by taking the medication with food. Indomethacin is contraindicated in children younger than 12 years of age.

For children with prolonged arthritis in several joints that may lead to permanent damage, second-line drugs called *disease-modifying antirheumatic drugs* are often prescribed. This is a category of unrelated drugs defined by their ability to slow the progression of the disease. Drugs in this group include methotrexate, leflunomide, sulfasalazine, etanercept, gold salts, and antimalarials (e.g., penicillamine, hydroxychloroquine). DMARDS operate by different mechanisms yet are used alone or in combination to limit the disease progression and reduce the signs and symptoms of moderately to severely active rheumatoid arthritis in patients who have had an inadequate response to other disease-modifying agents. The DMARDs can take up to 6 months to take effect. Each drug has its own side effects that require careful monitoring by regular examination and laboratory tests. Tumor necrosis factor (TNF)-α inhibitors may also be used as a means to help inhibit the inflammatory response associated with JIA.

ALERT *Hepatitis B and C screening is recommended for children with risk factors for infection prior to initiation of methotrexate or TNF-α inhibitors (Beukelman et al., 2011).*

The use of glucocorticoids is not generally considered unless severe, systemic complications of JIA are present and are not responding to other drug therapies. These agents suppress the symptoms of JIA but do not induce remission or prevent joint damage. In addition, the side effects of steroid use may lead to even more physical complications for the child. If steroids such as prednisone are used, the dosage of the medication should be reduced and then gradually discontinued as soon as symptoms have been suppressed. With persistent arthritis, injections of steroids directly into the joint can be helpful.

Use of alternative therapies may include herbal medicines, acupuncture, and dietary management. Complementary therapies may include relaxation techniques such as massage, imaging, controlled breathing, yoga, and exercise (Arthritis Foundation, 2010).

Physical Therapy

Goals of physical therapy and rehabilitation include controlling pain, preventing limitation, restoring ROM in affected joints, maintaining and improving muscle strength, increasing and maintaining endurance for activities of daily living, minimizing effects of inflammation, and ensuring normal growth and development. Methods used include heat–cold application, massage, electrical stimulation, and ultrasound. These therapies are aimed at reducing pain and stiffness so the child will be able to participate in an exercise program to reduce contractures and develop specific muscle groups.

For children who develop permanent contractures in the joints, a stabilizer splint must be used as an orthosis (to stabilize flexion contractures by stretching). Gradual casting is also used for this purpose. Ideally, the cast is removed at 24- to 48-hour intervals to enable aggressive stretching before the next cast is reapplied (see thePoint for Procedures: Cast Care). During an illness flare-up, an inflamed joint can be continually maintained in a neutral position by using an immobilization device. When the flare-up is under control and inflammation has diminished, the splint or brace may be worn only at night.

Passive, active, and resistive exercises are carried out daily by the child to preserve ROM, muscle strength, and gross motor activity. Exercises can be completed at home, at school, in an acute care setting, or at a local health club. Age-appropriate activities are encouraged and modified as needed based on the severity of the child's symptoms.

Children with JIA can participate in normal school and family activities. Gymnastics and high-impact contact sports are to be avoided. However, swimming is an excellent exercise for children with JIA. Other therapeutic exercises include playing with clay, bicycling, playing the piano, and softball. Extreme stress and fatigue may trigger exacerbations of JIA. Encourage rest, relaxation, leisure activities, and relief from emotional distress to reduce the risk of exacerbations.

For children with progressive debilitation caused by their disorder, occupational therapy can be beneficial. Measures are taken to adapt the child's environment and to train the child to use assistive devices to continue to perform independent daily tasks and activities. Assistive devices may include comb handle extenders, thicker handles on eating utensils, and shoehorns to put on shoes. Clothes with easy Velcro openings can facilitate putting on and removing clothing.

Heat therapy to alleviate pain and stiffness is important for the child with JIA. Other treatments include warm baths; moist, warm packs; and paraffin (wax) baths for the small joints of the hands once a day (see "Treatment Modalities" section). A warm morning bath can help the child overcome early morning stiffness, but it may be impractical for busy families. An alternative is to have the child use a sleeping bag at night to stay warm. Another alternative is to have an electric blanket with a timer that turns on 1 hour before the child awakens. Use of a waterbed is another option for easing stiffness. Teach children and families about different measures to promote comfort and reduce generalized body stiffness.

Surgical Interventions

Surgery to treat JIA is rare. Arthroscopic synovectomy may be performed to decrease pain. Occasionally, some patients require or request a total joint replacement. This procedure should be performed only on older children because joint replacements wear out in about 20 years.

Nutritional Support

Children with JIA are at risk for nutritional problems. Stiffness decreases activity and increases the tendency to gain weight, thus exacerbating the problems associated with mobility. Arthritis of the temporomandibular joint can affect the child's ability to chew, causing pain and limited jaw movement. Undernutrition and wasting can contribute to poor linear growth and low lean body and muscle mass. Anorexia can lead to acute or chronic undernutrition as a result of an inadequate intake of both calories and protein. Many of the medications taken by the child with JIA have potential adverse effects on nutritional status, including anorexia, constipation, nausea, fatigue, diarrhea, and gastrointestinal distress. Additionally, family members of children with JIA may select unconventional dietary remedies to "treat" their child. These therapies can interfere with the child's medical therapy and may be a source of malnutrition.

Several measures can be instituted to enhance the child's growth and development by addressing dietary concerns (Nursing Interventions 20-3). Frequent assessment of the child's nutritional status should be an integral part of the contacts between the child and the health care team. Obtain height and weight measurements on a regular basis. Ask the child and family about side effects of any medications, appetite and appetite changes, frequency of meals and snacks, types of foods eaten on a day-to-day basis, and the presence of discomfort or any mechanical difficulties when chewing.

Promotion of Normal Development

Chronic illness has a great effect on a child's psychosocial well-being (see Chapter 12). Normal developmental milestones, such as starting school, socialization, and achieving independence in activities of daily living, may be delayed. The family may overprotect the child and restrict play activities for fear of injury. To promote growth and development, the child should be encouraged to interact with peers in school and social settings by participating in age-appropriate activities as much as the child's physical condition allows. Assist the family and child in modifying the child's environment and schedule to account for the child's physical limitations and to decrease the likelihood of fatigue.

The child may be at risk for self-esteem or body image disturbances because of the limitations imposed by illness and any physical manifestations. Encourage the child and family members to speak openly about the child's condition and to feel comfortable asking others for assistance when needed. Support organizations can provide educational materials, specialized services, and financial aid for qualified children and their families (see thePoint for organizations). Important measures that promote adaptation to the disease and enhance development include encouraging the child's natural skills and characteristics to develop. Provide opportunities for the child to reach his or her maximum potential while ensuring personal safety and management of their condition.

Community Care

The child with JIA can be managed primarily in the home. Clinic, home health, and school nurses are primarily responsible for collaborating with the health care team to monitor and manage the needs of the child with this condition. Issues of impaired physical mobility, altered nutrition, risk for impaired skin integrity, and chronic pain must be

---

NURSING INTERVENTIONS 20-3

Measures to Promote Adequate Dietary Intake for the Child With Juvenile Arthritis

- Encourage children with poor appetites to eat higher calorie, nutrient-dense, tasty foods such as nuts, peanut butter, sandwiches, milkshakes, and cheese.
- Encourage children with small appetites to eat small, frequent meals throughout the day.
- Make mealtime a pleasant event. Nagging and food battles only serve to decrease the child's appetite.
- Provide calcium and vitamin D supplementation under the guidance of a dietitian.
- Choose iron-fortified cereals and other products.
- Follow the standard of the *MyPlate* guide to plan meals with serving sizes appropriate to the child's age (see Chapter 5).

- If mechanical feeding difficulties are present, provide the child with a soft diet and teach him or her to take small bites. If eating difficulties persist, referral to an occupational therapist may be necessary.
- Assist the child to select activities that will keep him or her mobile and active without causing undue pain and joint problems.
- Assess and treat the side effects of drug–food interactions (e.g., constipation, diarrhea, nausea).
- Discourage children and family members from using unconventional remedies to treat their child's condition.
- Refer the child to a registered dietitian if dietary issues continue to be an ongoing threat to the child's growth and development.

managed on a daily basis. The child also faces challenges related to altered growth and development and the potential for body image disturbances caused by the debilitating nature and sometimes disfiguring outcomes of the child's arthritic condition (see Teaching Intervention Plan 20-3).

SYSTEMIC LUPUS ERYTHEMATOSUS

SLE is a systemic inflammatory disease that affects many organs in the body. *Lupus*, the Latin term for wolf, was combined with erythema to name this disease—lupus erythematosus—because one of the presenting symptoms is a facial rash that looks like the face of a wolf. Lupus is an autoimmune disorder that may involve any organ system but most commonly involves skin, joints, and kidneys. The onset may be sudden, affecting one or more major organ systems, or it may be insidious in nature, with nonspecific symptoms such as fever, fatigue, or joint and muscle pain. When the onset is insidious, diagnosis is often delayed for weeks or months.

The reported prevalence of SLE in children and adolescents is 1 to 6 per 100,000 people. The incidence is highest among African Americans, Hispanics, Native Americans, and Pacific Islanders. SLE predominantly affects females, with reported 5:1 ratio prior to puberty. SLE is rarely seen in children younger than 5 years of age and is usually diagnosed in adolescence. When males are affected, they manifest symptoms at an earlier age and have more severe form of the disease (Ardoin & Schanberg, 2011). The mortality rate has decreased with the evolution of newer treatment options. Infection is currently the leading cause of death.

Pathophysiology

The cause of SLE is unknown, but genetic, hormonal, environmental, and immunologic factors are believed to interact and lead to disease expression. Studies indicate there is a genetic predisposition to lupus. Genome studies have indicated a gene on chromosome 1 that is associated with lupus in certain families. In addition, genes on chromosome 6 called *immune-response genes* were also associated with the disease.

SLE is a multisystem autoimmune disease involving both the humoral and cellular aspects of the innate and acquired immune systems. The autoimmune reactions are directed against the cell nucleus, especially the DNA. Autoantibodies are produced against the nuclear antigens, cytoplasmic antigens, and blood cell surface antigens. When the autoantibodies bind to their specific antigens, complement activation occurs, and immune complexes accumulate within the blood vessel walls, causing ischemia. Ischemia within the blood vessels leads to thickening of the internal lining, fibrinoid degeneration, and thrombus formation. At this point, manifestations of SLE appear.

Assessment

The manifestations of SLE vary depending on the organs affected and degree of their involvement. The American College of Rheumatology has established criteria of 11 manifestations to distinguish SLE from other connective tissue diseases (Chart 20-1). Evidence of

---

CHART 20-1 American College of Rheumatology Classification Criteria for Systemic Lupus Erythematosus

The diagnosis of SLE requires the presence of 4 or more of the following 11 criteria, serially or simultaneously, during any period of observation.

1. Malar rash: fixed erythema, flat or raised, over the malar eminences, tending to spare the nasolabial folds
2. Discoid rash: erythematous, raised patches with adherent keratotic scaling and follicular plugging; possibly atrophic scarring in older lesions
3. Photosensitivity: skin rash as a result of unusual reaction to sunlight, as determined by patient history or physician observation
4. Oral ulcers: oral or nasopharyngeal ulceration, usually painless, observed by physician
5. Arthritis: nonerosive arthritis involving two or more peripheral joints, characterized by swelling, tenderness, or effusion
6. Serositis: pleuritis, by convincing history of pleuritic pain, rub heard by physician, or evidence of pleural effusion; pericarditis documented by electrocardiography, rub heard by physician, or evidence of pericardial effusion
7. Renal disorder: persistent proteinuria, >500 mg/24 hr (0.5 g/day) or >3+ if quantitation is not performed; or cellular casts (may be red blood cell, hemoglobin, granular, tubular, or mixed cellular casts)
8. Neurologic disorder: seizures or psychosis occurring in the absence of offending drugs or known metabolic derangement (e.g., uremia, ketoacidosis, electrolyte imbalance)
9. Hematologic disorder: hemolytic anemia with reticulocytosis; or leukopenia, <4,000/mm³ (4.0 × 10³/L) on two or more occasions; or lymphopenia, <1,500/mm³ (1.5 × 10³/L) on two or more occasions; or thrombocytopenia, <100 × 10³/mm³ (100 × 10³/L) in the absence of offending drugs
10. Immunologic disorder: antibody to double-stranded DNA antigen (anti-dsDNA) in abnormal titer; or presence of antibody to Sm nuclear antigen (anti-Sm); or positive finding of antiphospholipid antibody based on an abnormal serum level of immunoglobulin (Ig) G or IgM anticardiolipin antibodies, a positive test result for lupus anticoagulant using a standard method, of a false-positive serologic test for syphilis that is known to be positive for at least 6 months and is confirmed by negative *Treponema pallidum* immobilization or fluorescent treponemal antibody absorption test
11. ANAs: an abnormal ANA titer by immunofluorescence or equivalent assay at any time and in the absence of drugs known to be associated with drug-induced lupus

Adapted with permission from Tan, E. M., Cohen, A. S., Fries, J. F. et al. (1982). The 1982 revised criteria for the classification of systemic lupus erythematosus. *Arthritis and Rheumatism, 25,* 1274; Hochberg, M. C. (1997). Updating the American College of Rheumatology revised criteria for the classification of systemic lupus erythematosus [Letter]. *Arthritis and Rheumatism, 40,* 1725.

four manifestations in the absence of other definable disease entities is sufficient for the diagnosis of SLE. Generally, nonspecific findings that may be assessed at the time of disease onset include fever, malaise, weight loss, recurrent abdominal pain, anorexia, and fatigue. Headaches are present in more than 10% of children at the time of diagnosis. Conjunctivitis also is a common early manifestation.

Arthritis and arthralgia are the most common presenting symptoms of SLE. The child may complain of morning stiffness and joint pain or swelling. The arthritis of SLE is usually symmetric and affects both small and large joints. Commonly affected joints are hands, wrists, and knees. Joint deformities or erosions are rare. Rheumatoid nodules may appear during periods of disease exacerbations and may disappear as the disease activity diminishes.

Dermatologic findings are the second most common manifestations. These may include maculopapular and vasculitic rashes, livedo reticularis (reddish blue mottling of skin, exacerbated by exposure to cold), and periungual erythema or other nail bed changes. Many acutely affected individuals may have a butterfly rash across the bridge of the nose and on the cheeks that may spread to the scalp, neck, chest, and extremities. The rash may become bullous, possibly leading to a secondary infection. Photosensitivity is a classic dermatologic sign of SLE, especially if it occurs in the presence of arthritis.

Other skin eruptions may include vasculitic lesions with ulceration; purpuric lesions; and subcutaneous nodules on the palms, fingertips, soles, extremities, or trunk. Macular and painless ulcerative lesions in the mouth and nose may be present. Alopecia, resulting from inflammation around the hair follicles, may lead to patchy or generalized loss of hair. Hair may be coarse, dry, and brittle.

Polyserositis, inflammation of several mucous membranes, is another clinical manifestation of SLE. Pericarditis, peritonitis, or pleuritis may be present. Cardiovascular symptoms that may develop over time include pericarditis, substernal or precordial pain, murmurs, persistent tachycardia, transient dysrhythmias, and pleural and pericardial effusions. Raynaud phenomenon, in which vasoconstriction causes blanching, cyanosis, and erythema in the toes and fingers in response to cold or stress, may be noted.

Renal involvement is common in children. Nephrotic syndrome and acute glomerulonephritis may develop and are considered life-threatening occurrences. Renal insufficiency is manifested by weight gain, hypertension, edema, increased serum creatinine levels, and decreased creatinine clearance. Additionally, urinalysis reveals hematuria, proteinuria, and increased urinary sediment.

Almost all children with SLE have one or more hematologic abnormalities, including anemia, leukopenia, and thrombocytopenia. Lymphoid involvement may be noted in the form of generalized lymphadenopathy and hepatomegaly.

Central nervous system symptoms may arise as indications of the central nervous system vasculitis, as toxic symptoms resulting from the medication regimen, or

as behavioral outcomes of this chronic illness. Central nervous system vasculitis can lead to irritability, depression, headache, lethargy, dizziness, seizures, ataxia, and hallucinations. Ongoing use of corticosteroids lowers the threshold for seizure activity and may cause personality changes such as depression or euphoria. Depression can also occur as a result of learning that one has SLE or from coping with the issues associated with acute disease activity that limit the child's activities.

With SLE, exacerbations and remissions that vary in severity, depending on the particular organ system involved, occur. After the first 2 years, the disease only rarely involves previously unaffected organ systems. Distinguishing the symptoms of disease exacerbation from those of infectious complications may be difficult. Suspect infection if fever, coughing, shortness of breath, chest pain, and changes in behavior and visual acuity occur until proved otherwise.

Diagnostic Tests

Initial screening for SLE includes the following tests: a complete blood count with differential, ESR, CRP measurement, ANA count, and a test to detect RF. Additional laboratory values may be determined to rule out other disease processes. The ANA test identifies the presence of ANAs in the blood. The presence of ANAs is a marker of an autoimmune process and is most commonly seen in SLE.

Interdisciplinary Interventions

No one treatment for SLE exists; management depends on the manifestations and severity of the disease. Medical management is tailored to meet the individual child's needs based on organ system involvement and on the severity of inflammation at the time of evaluation. The goal of therapy is to control both the acute exacerbations of the illness and the ongoing chronic disease manifestations to enable optimal functioning, to prevent scarring in any organ system, and to prevent intolerable side effects of the therapy. Collaboration among health care professionals is necessary. Child life specialists in the hospital setting and a variety of allied health professionals in outpatient settings, including social workers and psychologists, may help the family and child to cope with issues (e.g., body image concerns related to disease and medications) in a positive manner.

Interventions for Joint Involvement

Joint involvement, specifically, arthralgias, are usually controlled with NSAIDs and antimalarial medications such as hydroxychloroquine. Aspirin is not recommended because the large doses needed may cause liver toxicity.

ALERT   *Ibuprofen has been associated with an aseptic meningitis syndrome in SLE; therefore, it should not be administered to children with SLE (Nguyen et al., 2004).*

Medications must be taken daily to maintain adequate blood levels. NSAID therapy requires careful monitoring of renal function because these agents decrease glomerular blood flow and can precipitate acute renal failure in children with SLE.

A physical therapy program can be implemented to help the child manage joint pain, enhance ROM, and prevent injury and contractures. Periods of rest should be incorporated into the child's daily routine, especially during periods of exacerbation.

Interventions for Skin Involvement

The rash of SLE is generally treated with an antimalarial drug, preferably hydroxychloroquine. Topical steroids may also be used if cutaneous involvement is limited. Because hydroxychloroquine carries a risk of retinal damage, an eye examination should be performed every 6 months in patients receiving this drug.

Rashes and lesions require careful monitoring for signs of infection. In addition, assess the toes and fingers for vascular compromise. Urge the child and caregivers to keep the extremities warm during cold weather by using socks, gloves, and layered clothes. Also instruct them to avoid tight clothing.

Photosensitivity can be well controlled by using sunscreens, avoiding sun exposure, and using steroid therapy. When the child must be exposed to the sun, emphasize the importance of using broad-spectrum sunscreens that block both ultraviolet A and B rays (sun protection factor [SPF] 15 or higher); avoiding long-term exposure; and wearing long-sleeved clothing, pants, large-brimmed hats, and sunglasses. Not only can sun exposure exacerbate the skin rash but it may also precipitate systemic exacerbations.

Interventions for Systemic Involvement

Major organ system involvement in SLE usually necessitates the use of corticosteroids. Symptoms such as fever, skin manifestations, pleuropericarditis, and lymphadenopathy usually can be effectively treated with low-dose prednisone or hydroxychloroquine. Alternate-day steroid therapy is currently being used to minimize the linear growth and sexual maturation problems associated with steroid use.

 KidKare A child with SLE should wear a MedicAlert bracelet to alert emergency personnel to his or her dependence on steroids.

High-dose oral prednisone for a period of 4 to 6 weeks may be indicated for the child with central nervous system and renal involvement. Long-term use of high-dose prednisone is avoided whenever possible because of the serious complications (e.g., cataracts, fractures, hypertension, and metabolic disturbances) that may occur. The aim of therapy is to control activity of the disease with the lowest possible dose of prednisone. To aid in this process, steroid-sparing agents such as azathioprine, methotrexate, and hydroxychloroquine may be used. When the child's condition has been stabilized, the high-dose steroids are tapered to prevent the negative effects of sudden medication withdrawal.

Instruct caregivers regarding the need for an ophthalmic evaluation for retinal damage within the first 30 to 60 days after initiating drug therapy and every 6 months thereafter. These evaluations aid in detecting and preventing macular inflammatory problems.

Periodic blood work for evaluating drug toxicity and disease activity must also be discussed with the child and family.

Sexually active adolescent females need counseling about birth control and pregnancy. Inform them that SLE can become more active with the use of certain oral contraceptives and during pregnancy. It is usually recommended that a diaphragm and spermicide be used for birth control because they do not have adverse side effects that affect the adolescent's SLE. However, low-dose oral contraceptives may be used if the patient is carefully monitored, especially if compliance with barrier contraception is poor. The fetus is at risk for injury both by the mother's disease and by the side effects of the drugs required to treat the mother's disease.

Nutritional Support

The child receiving steroid therapy needs to be monitored for weight gain and fluid retention. If renal involvement is a concern, a low-sodium, low-protein diet may be instituted. Adolescent females on steroid therapy should ingest increased amounts of calcium.

Interventions to Enhance Growth and Development

The child commonly needs help to deal with any problems that he or she may have related to self-image and self-esteem. The undesirable effects of medication therapy such as weight gain and "moon face," the restrictions related to photosensitivity, and the increased risk for depression are among the factors that can affect the child's self-concept. The child may refuse to follow preventive measures, thereby precipitating an acute episode of the condition (Developmental Considerations 20-2).

The health care team and family members should strive to help the child achieve as normal a lifestyle as possible within the constraints of the illness. Encourage independence in decision making while still monitoring for safety and wellness. Social workers or psychologists trained to deal with chronic illness in children may be helpful in assisting them to learn to cope with their frustrations. Support groups that enable children to meet others with SLE and to discuss common concerns are useful for some children. Several organizations offer written information about SLE and can direct families to local support groups and activities in their community (see thePoint for Organizations).

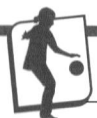

DEVELOPMENTAL CONSIDERATIONS 20-2

Management Issues for Children With Systemic Lupus Erythematosus

Concerns of the Child	Actions Demonstrated by Child	Health Care Provider and Family Interventions
"I don't want to be different than other children."	Refuses to take medications while at school	Arrange medication schedule to eliminate or minimize need to take medications during school and social activities.
"I don't like the effects of medications on how I look."	Avoids taking medication	Have caregiver unobtrusively monitor child taking medication.
"I want to participate in summer activities in the sun."	Refuses to avoid the sun	Help child select hats, clothing, lotions, and other protective gear that can be used to protect against overexposure to the sun.
"Applying sunscreen is messy and not cool."	Does not use sunscreen consistently each day when out in the sun	Review with the child the importance of using sunscreen. Have the child select a favorite type of sunscreen to use. Have the child apply sunscreen at home before meeting friends.
"Rashes make me look funny."	Does not want to socialize with others or go out in public	Encourage the child to use hypoallergenic cosmetics to cover rashes.
"I can't do anything. I can't be like my other friends."	Feels depressed or different	Assist family members to emphasize child's positive attributes and accomplishments. Encourage participation in counseling or support group.
"I look fat."	Feels depressed; cries	Help the child select clothes that camouflage weight gain.
"I am too tired to play with other kids."	Wants to be excused from school activities and extracurricular activities because of fatigue	Assist the child to pace activities and periods of rest to minimize fatigue. Assist the child to select activities that are not as physically demanding, such as playing piano, art, and computer activities.

MUSCULOSKELETAL TRAUMA

QUESTION: The radiograph in the emergency department shows that Cathy has an oblique fracture of the fifth metacarpal. It is a closed fracture and the bone is not out of alignment. She has a fiberglass cast applied to her right hand. What are the developmental principles of working with adolescents that you will use to develop an individual teaching plan for Cathy, who now has a cast?

Childhood trauma has been the leading cause of death among children for nearly 50 years, and it has been the second leading cause of morbidity. The most common childhood musculoskeletal trauma includes sprains, followed by lacerations, fractures (excluding the skull), intracranial injuries, and internal injuries. The most serious injuries tend to be fractures and intracranial injuries.

During the past 20 years, participation in organized athletics by children and adolescents between ages 6 and 21 years has grown considerably. In the United States, about 30 million children and teens participate in some form of organized sports, with about 3.5 million injuries each year. The most common injuries are sprains and strains (National Safe Kids Campaign, 2012). Approximately 25% to 30% of sports injuries occur during organized sports and another 40% occur during unorganized sports (Bautista & Flynn, 2006). More than 200,000 injuries per year are related to use of playground equipment, with 88% of these injuries occurring on monkey bars, jungle gyms, swings, and slides. The highest injury rate among high school athletes is in baseball, followed by soccer, basketball, and football. Gymnastics, tennis, track and field, and cross-country events have lower injury rates (Bautista & Flynn, 2006).

In recent years, injury rates have been dramatically reduced because of changes in safety requirements for children involved in sports. Preseason examinations, medical coverage at sports events, proper coaching, adequate hydration, proper officiating, proper equipment, and improved field and surface playing conditions have the potential to reduce sports injuries. Chapters 6 and 7 discuss safety concerns and sports activities in more detail. Table 7-1 discusses the ergogenic aids, such as steroids, that young athletes use, or consider using, in hopes of enhancing their athletic performance. Use of these aids may have severe health outcomes for the youth and may contribute to sports injuries.

This section describes the care of children with fractures, overuse injuries, sprains and strains, and dislocations.

FRACTURES

Fractures are common in the pediatric patient. The risk for sustaining a fracture in childhood is 42% to 64% in males and 27% to 40% in females (Valerio et al., 2010).

Fractures in children vary in several important ways from fractures in adults, and these variables affect care. First, a child's bone heals faster than an adult's bone. The younger the child, the faster the bone heals because younger children have a proportionately higher metabolic rate. Children's bones are also softer than an adult's bones, and their bones may bend or buckle rather than break. Another crucial difference between managing adult and pediatric fractures is that children's bones have an open growth plate (epiphysis). Any damage to the growth plate can result in limb length discrepancy, joint incongruity, and progressive angular deformity of the limb.

During the birthing process, fractures may occur in the newborn. However, fractures generally are rare during the first year of life because the child has limited mobility. Multiple, severe fractures in an infant may be an indication of a metabolic bone disease, such as OI. During the first 2 years of life, many fractures in children may be the result of physical abuse.

ALERT *In a nonambulatory child, the accidental occurrence of a spiral fracture is rare. Thus, spiral fractures in young children are most often the result of twisting of the extremity by an abusive adult.*

When the child starts to walk, the clavicle and radius are the most commonly fractured bones. Fractures can occur from trauma, such as sudden twisting of a limb or a force applied to the limb, such as a kick. Pathologic fractures occur when preexisting diseases weaken a bone, as happens with bone tumors.

In general, fractures in children heal without complications. Possible complications such as limping, decreased ROM, and nerve deficits rarely occur.

Pathophysiology

The amount of force required to fracture a bone depends on the strength of the bone, the size of the bone, and other extrinsic factors, such as the direction of the force. After the fracture occurs, inflammation develops at the site. Osteoblasts (bone-forming cells) activate within 24 hours to begin making new bone. During the ensuing few weeks, callus forms and knits together into compact bone. This process takes 4 to 12 weeks in children, depending on their skeletal age. Remodeling, a process that rounds off angles and fills in hollows, continues for up to 1 year after the fracture. Because the ability of bone to remodel is enhanced in children, the ends of the fracture do not have to be aligned perfectly, as they do in adults.

A fracture is either closed or open. A closed fracture involves no break in the skin. An open fracture occurs when a portion of the bone protrudes through the skin or when an external wound connects to the fracture site. Open fractures are classified as types I, II, or III, depending on the degree and severity of the soft-tissue damage or loss, the size of the wound, and the amount of wound contamination. For example, with a type I open fracture, the wound size is less than 1 cm and there is minimal contamination and soft-tissue damage. For a type II fracture, the wound size is larger than 1 cm and there is moderate contamination and tissue damage. For a type III fracture, the wound is large, with a high degree of contamination and extensive tissue damage. One fracture type is not more complicated than the other, but the potential for infection is greater with an open fracture.

Classification of fractures also involves identifying the location and describing the nature of the fracture. The location refers to where the fracture occurs along the shaft of the bone (Fig. 20-19). Fractures can also be described in terms of the type of injury that has occurred (Table 20-4).

The prognosis varies according to the type of fracture and its location. If the injury involves the growth plate in an immature bone, growth disturbance may follow. The growth plates of the lower extremities are primarily responsible for determining the height of the child. Disturbance of their function may result in slow growth, overgrowth, or cessation of growth. Table 20-5 illustrates the Salter-Harris classification system that describes the injury and the potential for growth disturbance.

Assessment

Assessment for fractures is part of the emergency trauma care of a patient after initial stabilization. Obtaining a history of the accident helps determine the nature and extent of the injuries. Motor vehicle accidents and falls have a high index of suspicion for fractures, especially if the child was unrestrained in the vehicle.

KidKare Ask the child to tell how the fracture occurred in his or her own words. If possible, ask this question without the family members present if abuse is suspected and an honest response is desired from the child.

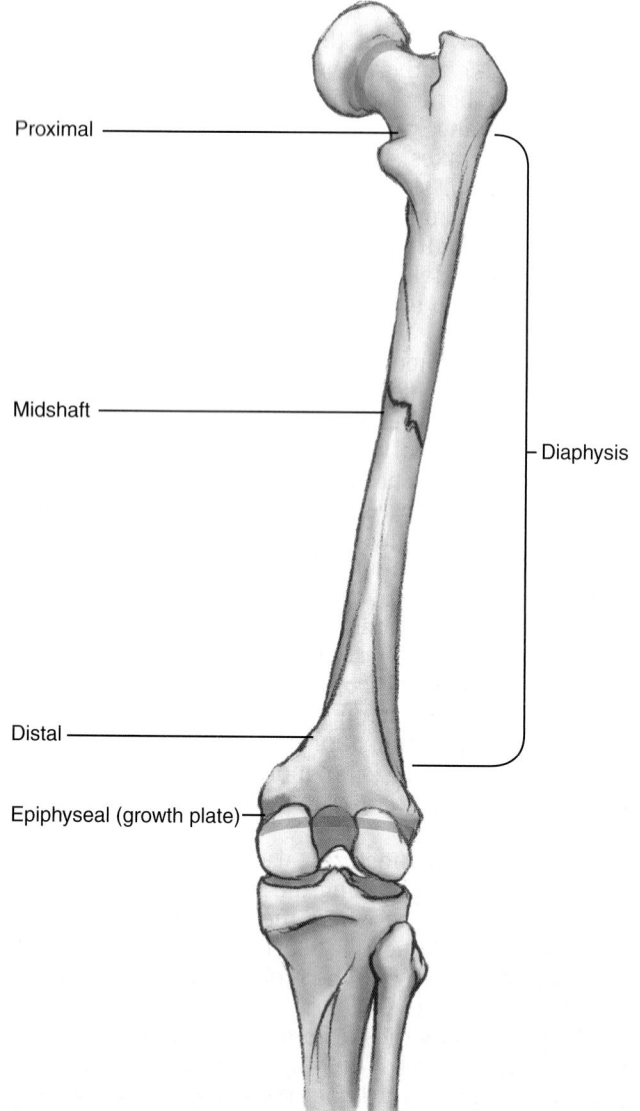

Proximal

Midshaft

Diaphysis

Distal

Epiphyseal (growth plate)

Figure 20-19 Classification of fracture by location.

The child may complain of pain, numbness, or tingling in an extremity. Remove all clothing to facilitate assessment. Open fractures may be obvious; a closed fracture can make the limb grossly distorted. However, some fractures, such as of the spine or pelvis, are not as evident. For all trauma patients, the cervical spine must be protected by a cervical collar until radiographs rule out a fracture.

Other abnormal physical findings with a fracture include shortening of the limb, swelling, muscle spasm, crepitus, and discoloration of the limb. The child may refuse to move the limb, or a change in neurovascular status may be apparent. A fracture always causes pain, although the intensity and severity of the pain varies among children. Ask the family about the child's normal response to pain or previous experience with pain to help define the pain associated with a possible fracture. In nonverbal children, facial grimacing, whimpering, or crying may

be elicited when the child is repositioned or when articles of clothing are removed.

Diagnostic Tests

Radiographs are the primary method used to evaluate fractures. Both anteroposterior and lateral views are recommended. The joints above and below the suspected fracture also must be included to evaluate potential associated injuries. If child abuse if suspected, radiographs are used to detect the presence of old fractures and to determine the extent of healing that has taken place at other fracture sites. In certain cases, other tests can be ordered to evaluate a suspected fracture. These tests include computed tomographic scans, MRI, fluoroscopy, and myelograms.

Interdisciplinary Interventions
Interventions to Reduce the Fracture

The choice of treatment for a fracture depends on the type, the location, and other associated injuries. For the bone to heal, the edges of the fracture must be close together or aligned and relatively immobile. A general treatment principle is to allow the child to mobilize as quickly as possible while the fracture is reduced and the bone is immobilized. Although bone healing is important, restoring the use and appearance of the extremity is also crucial. Fracture reduction involves one of two main methods: closed reduction or open reduction.

Closed reduction aligns the fracture fragments by manually manipulating the extremity or applying traction. Procedural sedation (see Chapter 10) or general anesthesia are used before attempting a closed reduction. Ideally, the fracture is reduced as soon as possible. However, certain situations, such as when a large amount of swelling is present at the site or when the child's life is in danger, make immediate reduction impossible. In those cases, the physician may have to delay reducing the fracture for a few days. If fractures are not displaced, they do not need to be reduced.

An orthopedist uses open reduction when a fracture cannot be reduced by closed methods or when torn muscles or ligaments must be repaired. Usually, some type of internal fixation stabilizes the fracture until it is healed. A variety of pins, screws, plates, and rods are available for fixation, depending on the type of fracture and the age of the child (see "Treatment Modalities" section earlier in this chapter). Internal fixation with screws, plates, or rods is standard treatment with older children. Intramedullary fixation places a rod in the shaft of the femur to provide stabilization. After the bone has healed, the rods are removed. Telescoping rods are ideal for children who have a chronic bone disease such as OI, but they are not indicated for the treatment of femur fractures in otherwise healthy children.

After reduction, the fracture is immobilized by one of a variety of different methods including splints, braces, casts, external fixators, or traction (see "Treatment Modalities" section). Immobilization is used to prevent rotation and shearing of the fracture site, to maintain the position of the fracture after reduction, and to permit active muscle contraction. Also, keeping the site in

TABLE 20-4   Classification of Fractures by Description of the Type of Break

Type	Illustration	Description
Transverse		Line crosses the shaft at a 90-degree angle
Spiral		A diagonal line coils around the bone; caused by a twisting force
Oblique		A diagonal line across the bone
Greenstick	 **Greenstick** A fracture in which one side of a bone is broken and the other side is bent	Bone is bent but not broken; more common in children than adults

(continued)

TABLE 20-4	Classification of Fractures by Description of the Type of Break	
Type	**Illustration**	**Description**
Comminuted	**Comminuted** A fracture in which bone has splintered into several fragments	Three or more fracture fragments
Compression	**Compression** A fracture in which bone has been compressed (seen in vertebral fractures)	Bone becomes wider and more flat; usually seen in the spine

good alignment relieves pain and allows more ease in movement of the adjacent, unaffected areas of the body.

Wound Care for Open Fractures

The treatment of open fractures differs from that of closed fractures. Either external or internal fixation can be used to treat open fractures. The potential for infection from wound contamination is great. Typically, the wound is irrigated and debrided and the fracture is stabilized. The size of the wound determines whether the wound is closed after the initial procedure (primary closure) or is left open for further irrigation and debridement. The child receives antibiotics before the procedure. If the child has a draining wound and the wound culture is positive, antibiotic therapy continues for a few weeks.

Pin site care (see Tradition or Science 20-2) for child in skeletal traction is essential. Anticipate administering analgesics about an hour before pin care if the child experiences discomfort with the treatment. Encourage older children to assist with pin care, even if they simply open the packages of cotton applicators. Participation gives them some feeling of control over a frightening situation.

Pain Management

Pain management for a fracture is essential. Intravenous opioids, such as morphine, provide relief for the first 24 hours. After the fracture is reduced and immobilized, administer oral narcotics, such as acetaminophen with codeine, to control discomfort. Muscle spasms, especially with a femur fracture, can be extremely painful. Diazepam, which relaxes the muscle, is highly effective. Muscle spasms generally subside after the first week.

Prevention of Complications

Early complications from a fracture can occur despite prompt treatment and careful observation. These complications can include shock, fat emboli, **compartment syndrome**, deep vein thrombosis, pulmonary embolism, and infection. Late complications—such as nonunion or delayed union, refracture, joint stiffness, posttraumatic arthritis, or pseudoarthritis—can often be prevented or their effects minimized by aggressive treatment and proper evaluation.

Compartment syndrome is one of the most feared complications associated with musculoskeletal surgery and trauma. This syndrome occurs when the nonelastic fascia that covers bone, muscle, nerves, blood vessels, and soft tissue cannot expand adequately to compensate for the bleeding or swelling from trauma or the pressure from splints or casts. As the pressure increases, circulation slows; if the pressure is unchecked, the tissues and nerves may die. The compartments of the lower leg and forearm are most commonly affected.

TABLE 20-5	Salter-Harris Classification of Epiphyseal Fractures	
Classification	**Illustration**	**Description**
Type I		Separation of the epiphysis May be mistaken for a sprain Does not usually affect growth
Type II		Fracture separation of the epiphysis Circulation remains intact; growth usually not affected
Type III		Fracture through the epiphysis into the joint Does not usually affect growth if reduced properly
Type IV		Fracture of the epiphysis extending into the joint and the metaphysis Open reduction and internal fixation usually necessary to prevent growth disturbance
Type V		Crush injury to the epiphyseal plate Results in premature closure of the epiphyseal plate and growth arrest (occurrence is rare)

ALERT *The color and pulses of a limb with compartment syndrome remain intact at first. The classic sign of compartment syndrome is unrelenting pain that is not relieved by narcotics. Notify the physician immediately.*

If the child in a cast develops compartment syndrome, initially the cast is split or bivalved on one side. If that measure does not relieve the symptoms, a fasciotomy, a surgical incision made through the fascia to release the pressure, is performed. The incision remains open but is wrapped with a sterile dressing for a few days. At that point, either the physician closes the fasciotomy site or allows it to heal by itself. The best treatment for this complication is to prevent excessive swelling and to detect neurovascular compromise as quickly as possible. Always assess neurovascular status frequently and notify the physician of any change. In addition, elevate the extremity above the level of the heart to decrease swelling, and apply cold packs to the injured site for the first 24 hours.

Nutritional Support

Typically, children with fractures do not have extra nutritional needs if they eat a well-balanced diet containing sufficient amounts of protein, calcium, and iron to promote the healing process. However, a child in a body cast should eat small, frequent meals to avoid abdominal distention. The diet should have increased amounts of fluid and fiber to prevent constipation. A laxative or stool softener is helpful for some children who are in traction or a body cast. Appetite may decrease because of the inactivity.

Supportive Interventions

The child who enters the acute care setting for treatment of a fracture probably has not had any preparation for the experience and has most likely undergone some sort of trauma. The family may also be in a state of shock. Crisis intervention for both the child and family is essential. If the family was part of a motor vehicle accident or community disaster, multiple family members or friends may be hospitalized. Siblings are encouraged to visit, especially if they witnessed the accident or causal event. A visit helps to reassure siblings that their brother or sister is alive. See Chapter 11 for a more complete discussion of care of the hospitalized child, including managing regressive behaviors, child life interventions, and social service support.

Community Care

Teaching is an important component of the care of a child with a fracture. Instructions on the treatment plan, basic principles of bone healing, neurovascular assessments, and cast care by the nurse can help family members feel more confident about caring for their child in the home (see thePoint for Procedures: Cast Care and Supplemental Information: Teaching Information for the Child With a Cast).

Depending on the type of fracture, the child's physical mobility may be limited after he or she returns home. Adaptations to the home environment may be needed to accommodate the child in a cast or in traction. Specialized devices such as a rolling wheelchair may be needed. Crutches and walkers are other aids used to restore mobility (see Fig. 20-4). Wagons for small children are fun and useful. A physical therapist can help the family to learn methods of transfer and use of assistive devices. Demonstrate good body mechanics and safety practices to the child to prevent further injury.

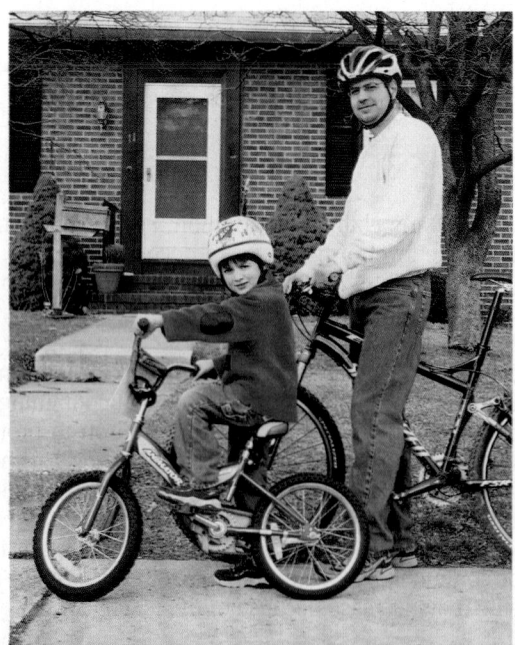

Figure 20-20 Children should be introduced at a young age to wearing protective gear to prevent physical injury. Parents and adult family members can be role models for their children by also wearing bike helmets.

A primary role of the health care team is to promote public awareness of measures that can prevent accidental injury and trauma to children. Safety fairs held at malls and other public places educate families and children about ways to prevent accidents, childproof the home, and develop a family escape plan for fires. Safety programs, often ones that involve the use of puppets or interactive displays, can be used by schools for education. These programs commonly focus on street safety, fire safety, and emergency routines as well as seat belt and helmet use. In recent years, legislation has been passed in many states that requires certain safety precautions for children, such as the mandatory use of helmets when bike riding (Fig. 20-20) and of car safety restraint devices. The National Safe Kids Campaign is one example of a nationwide program that has local coalitions in every state to focus on community education about accident prevention (see thePoint for Organizations).

> **ANSWER:** Cathy will prefer to care for the cast and her hand herself. Direct your teaching to Cathy, but have her mother listen to the care instructions as well:
>
> - The cast must be kept dry. To shower, place the casted hand in a plastic bag and secure it with a rubber band.
> - Keep the hand clean. You can use baby wipes or alcohol on paper towels to clean your hand.
> - Do not put anything in the cast. Do not scratch inside the cast.
> - Your fingers should stay pink, warm, and dry. Call your doctor if you have any severe pain, numbness, or tingling in your hand.

OVERUSE INJURIES

Overuse injuries occur from the repetitive application of stresses to otherwise healthy tissue. This type of injury is common in organized sports (Table 20-6). Most overuse injuries have a good prognosis.

Pathophysiology

The process starts when repetitive activity fatigues a specific structure, such as tendon or bone. Without adequate recovery, microtrauma develops and stimulates the body's inflammatory response, causing the release of vasoactive substances, inflammatory cells, and enzymes that damage local tissue. Cumulative microtrauma can cause degenerative changes, leading to weakness, loss of flexibility, and chronic pain. Children are particularly susceptible to overuse injuries in tissues associated with growth cartilage in the articular surfaces, physes, and apophyses.

- Articular injuries are associated with articular cartilages, secondary areas of ossification found where major tendons attach to bone. These growth centers are the weakest link in the musculoskeletal chain.
- Physeal injuries can be caused by repetitive loading of the physes (primary ossification centers located at the ends of the long bones). Ischemia to these areas can disrupt or even arrest growth.

TABLE 20-6   Common Overuse Injuries

Type	Cause	Physical Findings
Jumper's knee (patellar tendonitis)	Repetitive pulling action on the distal pole of the patellar tendon	Point tenderness at proximal aspect of tibia associated with tendonitis
Little leaguer's elbow	Repetitive valgus stress Common in adolescent pitchers	Osteochondral injuries Damage to proximal radial epiphysis and growth plate
Little leaguer's shoulder	Repetitive overhead throwing	Stress fracture of proximal humeral growth plate
Osgood-Schlatter disease	Irritation of tibial tubercle from excessive running or jumping exercises	Point tenderness to proximal tibia Inflammation Possible avulsion injury
Osteochondritis dissecans	Cause unknown May be familial or result of metabolic bone problem	Knee pain Inflammation Swelling Portion of articular cartilage separates
Sever disease	Activities that include vigorous running or jumping resulting in heel pain	Limp Apophysitis of the calcaneus Point tender heel pain Tight Achilles tendon
Shin splints	Excessive running Improper shoes Running on hard surfaces	Pain Inflammation in anterior aspect of the tibia
Sinding-Larsen-Johansson disease	Excessive extension action on the patellar tendon associated with jumping activities	Knee pain Diagnosed with radiographs Avulsion fracture of the lower pole of patella
Spondylolisthesis	Excessive flexion and extension activities; commonly seen in gymnasts, skaters, and football linemen	Back pain Diagnosed with radiographs Anterior displacement of L5 on S1
Spondylolysis	Excessive flexion and extension activities	Back pain Diagnosed with radiographs

- Shin splints are an inflammation of tendons and muscles of the shin. The shin bone (tibia) is covered by the periosteum, a band of soft tissue that has both nerve tissue and a blood supply. Just above the ankle and below the knee, tendons help attach muscles to the periosteum. When the shin is overstressed by impact forces of exercise, these structures can become inflamed.

Assessment

Overuse injuries are generally diagnosed based on history and physical examination. Focus the history on recent growth spurts, changes in training, and playing surfaces. Radiographs may be needed to rule out other diagnoses. With overuse injuries, the pain generally worsens with activity and improves with rest.

The child may complain of pain across the lower back and muscle spasm resulting in changes in posture and gait if a stress fracture (spondylolysis and spondylolisthesis) occurs. Radiographs will show the position of the vertebrae.

Interdisciplinary Interventions

Treatment aims to restore as much function as possible in the shortest time and to enable the athlete to return to preinjury performance. Children experience pressure from coaches, peers, and even parents when they are absent from a sport. Emphasis must be placed on the player's personal capabilities because serious injuries result when the child returns prematurely.

Conservative treatment methods for the child with an overuse injury include avoiding the causative activity for 6 to 8 weeks. Applying ice to the injured area will help to reduce the inflammation and irritation. NSAIDs (ibuprofen) are used for inflammation and pain control. The physical therapist institutes a stretching and strengthening program for the appropriate muscle groups.

The goals for a child's return to play are determined by the health care team. The physician and the nurse should discuss realistic expectations for the treatment plan with the patient and the family.

The physical therapist also plays an important role here. Vital facts regarding the athlete's rehabilitative progress and potential can determine outcome. Nurses can link the chain of communication in this interdisciplinary approach.

SPRAINS AND STRAINS

A *sprain* is a tear or a stretch in a ligament resulting from a pulling or twisting injury to a joint. A *strain* is a tear to the musculotendinous unit. Sprains and strains are uncommon in younger children and are usually seen in the adolescent age group. The growth plate (physis), which is an area of new bone formation, is weaker than the ligaments in younger children; as a result, it is prone to fracture. When children reach puberty, skeletal growth declines and the growth plates begin to close. Thus, the growth plate is less susceptible to injury, and the ligaments and tendons are more vulnerable to sprains and strains. Ankle and wrist sprains are most common.

Sprains are classified according to severity. *First-degree*, or mild, sprains result when the ligament is stretched and the affected joint is stable. *Second-degree*, or moderate, sprains occur when the ligament is partially torn and joint laxity is noted on examination. *Third-degree*, or severe, sprains are produced when the ligament is completely torn and the injured joint is unstable. The prognosis is favorable for first- and second-degree sprains. However, severe sprains carry an increased risk of recurrent injury, persistent instability, and traumatic arthritis, particularly if the athlete does not adhere to the rehabilitation regimen.

Pathophysiology

Ankle sprains and strains are usually the product of an inversion injury, in which the lateral aspect of the ankle joint is thrust outward and the foot is turned inward as if stepping on its side. This mechanism of injury causes insult to the anterior talofibular ligament and, in severe cases, involves the posterior talofibular ligament (Fig. 20-21).

Wrist sprains often occur as a result of repetitive motion injuries. Sprain occurs when the ligaments of the wrist are stretched beyond their normal limits or, in severe cases, completely torn, thus leading to instability of the joint. Wrist sprain may also lead to carpal tunnel syndrome.

Assessment

Obtain a history of the event that caused the injury to help determine the extent of the injury. Information about the mechanism of the injury is important. The

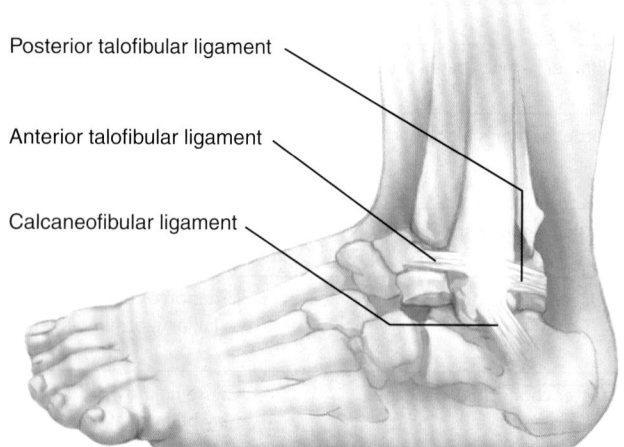

Figure 20-21 Ankle sprains occur when the foot is suddenly turned inward, causing tearing of the outside ligaments.

timing of swelling and local hemorrhage at the injury site indicates the amount of joint injury sustained. The presence of an audible sound at the time of injury may also indicate the severity of the problem.

Palpate the affected area and the surrounding structures to determine the site of injury and the ligaments injured. Palpate the most painful areas last. A first-degree sprain is characterized by minimal pain, swelling, and ecchymosis. Full ROM of the joint and weight bearing are possible. The joint is stable, with mild tenderness noted over the point of injury. The child with a second-degree sprain has moderate pain, swelling, and ecchymosis. Motion of the extremity is slightly limited and painful. Mild joint laxity is present, with tenderness noted over the joint. The child may be unable to bear weight or perform daily activities with the extremity. When a third-degree sprain has occurred, substantial swelling and severe ecchymosis occur rapidly, usually within the first 30 minutes after the injury. Severe pain over the joint may make it difficult to examine the injury and evaluate the extent of immobility. The child cannot bear weight on or otherwise use the extremity.

Diagnostic Tests

A radiograph of the injured extremity is done if there is evidence of an obvious fracture or misalignment or if physical examination reveals a third-degree sprain. Fractures may not be easy to identify because of the cartilaginous nature of the young child's bones. The child who does not show improvement within 4 days of therapy should be reevaluated for a potential fracture at the site.

Nursing Diagnoses and Outcomes

The nursing diagnoses for a child with a musculoskeletal condition are presented in Nursing Plan of Care 20-1. In addition, because a sprain or strain can severely limit

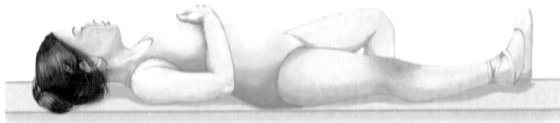

Rest

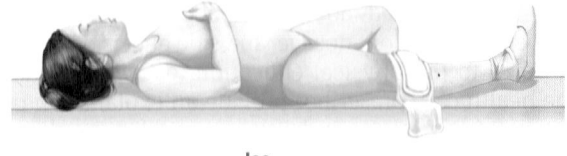

Ice

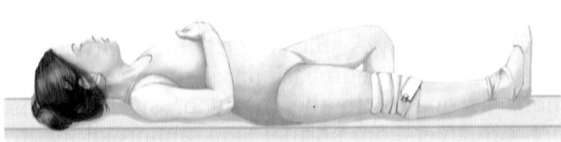

Compression

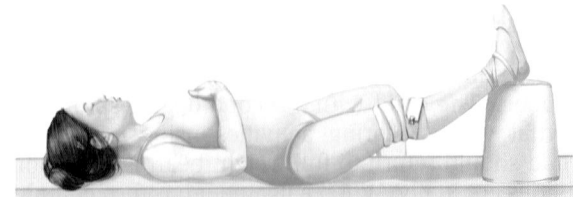

Elevation

Figure 20-22 The RICE protocol: rest, ice, compression, and elevation.

the mobility of an active youth, the following diagnosis may be applicable:

Nursing Diagnosis: Noncompliance related to degree of mobility restrictions over an extended period
Outcomes:
• Child will adhere to treatment regimen as demonstrated by use of elastic wraps, slings, braces, crutches, or other orthopedic supportive devices.
• Child will refrain from weight-bearing and sports activities as prescribed.

Interdisciplinary Interventions

Initially, all sprains and strains are treated with a period of rest, ice packs, compression, and elevation (RICE); early motion of the limb is also encouraged (Fig. 20-22). RICE can be done immediately at the location in which the child was injured. Do not apply heat during the acute phase because it may cause increased swelling and inflammation through hyperemia.

caREminder

In an injury to the foot or ankle, be sure to keep the child's shoe in place to help control swelling. The possibility of any fractures are ruled out using radiographs.

The severity and location of injury guide further management decisions. External support can be provided with an elastic bandage, brace, sling, or ankle lacer in mild sprains (Fig. 20-23). In grades I and II ankle sprains, rehabilitation can begin immediately. Prolonged immobilization is not recommended. In grade III sprains, in which a ligament is completely torn, the limb is usually immobilized in a cast or brace. Surgery may be needed to relieve pain and restore function.

Early motion after acute injury of the soft tissue will help the child make a more rapid recovery. A stretching and strengthening program is instrumental in returning the child to full function. Physical therapists instruct the patient in quadriceps and hamstring exercises for knee sprains and strains. For ankle and wrist injuries, an ROM program is implemented. The nurse or physical therapist can teach crutch walking. When crutch walking, the child should bear weight on the hands, not the underarms, to avoid nerve damage (see Fig. 20-4).

Community Care

Home care instructions vary based on the injury and on the treatment indicated. To decrease the potential for swelling, teach the patient and the family the proper technique for wrapping the injured extremity. The wrap should be started distal from the affected area. If the joint is located below the level of the heart, swelling is alleviated by elevating the limb. If anti-inflammatory

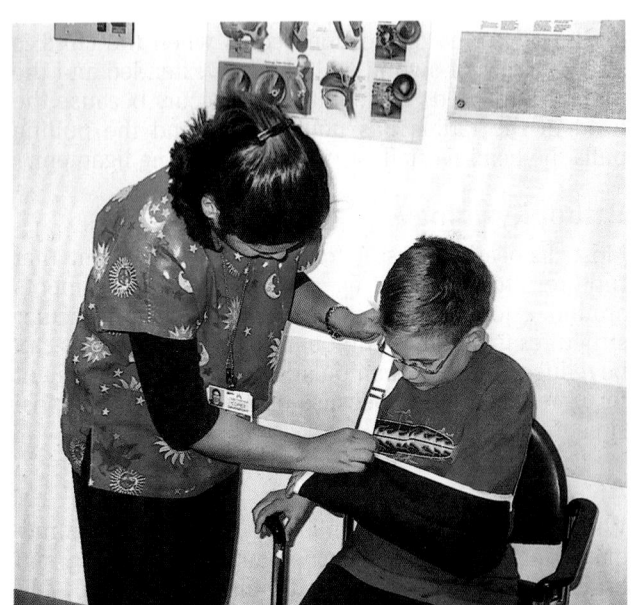

Figure 20-23 For the child with a sprain, the nurse is responsible for teaching the child how to put on and adjust the device.

medicines are used, advise the patient and family of the proper route, action, dosage, and side effects of the agent.

Notes to the physical education teacher or coach by the health care prescriber provide an explanation of the extent of the injury and list any restrictions the child may have. The note can also state what the child is permitted to do. For example, if the child sustained a knee strain and is walking with the assistance of crutches, upper body strengthening exercises can continue. The child with a first-degree injury can return to sport activities within 2 to 3 weeks if the affected joint has proper support. The child with a second-degree sprain can do partial weight-bearing activities using crutches. The child should return to full weight-bearing and sport activities gradually. When a ligament has torn completely, the return to sport activities should not occur for 4 to 8 weeks after the injury.

DISLOCATIONS

A dislocation occurs when extreme force is placed on a ligament, causing two bone ends to become partially or completely displaced or the head of a bone to be dislodged from its socket. The shoulder and proximal interphalangeal joint of the hand are the joints most often dislocated in sports. A dislocation of the knee or hip is rare but must be treated as an emergency. Massive force is needed to dislocate the knee, and with dislocation, the peroneal nerve and popliteal artery may be involved.

Dislocations can occur alone or can be accompanied by an avulsion or growth plate fracture. As in sprain and strain injuries, dislocations are not as common in younger children because the epiphysis is less susceptible to stress and more likely to fracture. However, dislocations are common in children with ligamentous laxity, as is seen in patients with trisomy 21, who are prone to subluxation (partial displacement) or dislocation of the hips. Nursemaid's elbow (subluxation of the proximal radial head) is commonly seen in 1- to 4-year-olds. This dislocation occurs when the child is lifted, jerked, or swung with the arm extended and the forearm pronated. The subluxation occurs because the head of the radius has not matured and the pulling pulls the head partially out of the encircling ligament.

Pathophysiology

Most dislocations result from one acute incident that ruptures the surrounding soft tissues and ligaments around a joint. Insult to vascular and neurovascular structures is possible. Although simple dislocations can be reduced quickly, manipulation may be more difficult for unreduced joints because of the swelling and possible interposed tissue.

Assessment

With a dislocation, the child experiences pain immediately after the injury, accompanied by swelling and bruising. Movement of the extremity is decreased, and obvious deformity may be seen. The opposite joint is assessed first so that a baseline comparison can be made with the affected joint. Radiographs are acquired to rule out any fractures.

Interdisciplinary Interventions

Dislocations are treated conservatively. The area of dislocation is reduced, usually with the child receiving procedural sedation and analgesia or general anesthesia. After reduction, acute dislocations are treated with RICE and immobilization. Slings, splints, or casts are used for 3 weeks after reduction for patient comfort and to allow healing of the capsular structures. Recurrent dislocations require possible surgical intervention.

Frequently assess neurovascular status to detect any variations secondary to the injury or swelling. Also instruct caregivers on normal and abnormal neurovascular findings. Review any medication information such as dosage, route, action, and side effects; provide cast care instructions as appropriate (see thePoint for Supplemental Information: Teaching Information for the Child With a Cast).

Community Care

Mobilization of the joint begins approximately 3 weeks after the injury has occurred to prevent joint stiffness. The physical therapist instructs the patient and family on a home exercise program to aid the patient in returning to full ROM with joint stability. As previously discussed, written notes to coaches and teachers should detail permitted and nonpermitted activities.

See thePoint for a summary of Key Concepts.

REFERENCES

Adler, B. (2008). *Imaging in slipped capital femoral epiphysis*. Retrieved from http://emedicine.medscape.com/article/413810

Ardoin, S., & Schanberg, L. (2011). Systemic lupus erythematosus. In R. M. Kliegman, B. F. Stanton, J. W. St. Geme et al. (Eds.), *Nelson textbook of pediatrics* (19th ed., pp. 2800–2811). Philadelphia, PA: Elsevier/Saunders.

Arthritis Foundation. (2010). *Alternatives and natural therapies*. Retrieved from http://www.arthritistoday.org/treatments/alternativetherapies/index.php

Baindurashvili, A., Kenis, V., & Stepanova, Y. (2012). Soft-tissue complications during treatment of children with congenital clubfoot. *European Wound Management Association Journal, 12*(3), 17–19.

Bautista, S., & Flynn, J. (2006). Trauma prevention in children. *Pediatric Annals, 35*(2), 83–91.

Benson, E., Miller, M., Bosch, P. et al. (2008). A new look at the incidence of slipped capital femoral epiphysis in New Mexico. *Journal of Pediatric Orthopedics, 28*(5), 529–533.

Beukelman, T., Patkar, N., Saag, K. et al. (2011). 2011 American College of Rheumatology recommendations for the treatment of juvenile idiopathic arthritis: Initiation and safety monitoring of therapeutic agents for the treatment of arthritis and systematic features. *Arthritis Care & Research, 63*(4), 465–482.

Brown, D. (2004). Seasonal variation of slipped capital femoral epiphysis in the United States. *Journal of Pediatric Orthopaedics, 24*(2), 139–143.

Bushby, K., Finkel, R., Birnkrant, D. et al. (2010a). Diagnosis and management of Duchenne muscular dystrophy, part 1: Diagnosis, and pharmacological and psychological management. *Lancet Neurology, 9*(1), 77–93.

Bushby, K., Finkel, R., Birnkrant, D. et al. (2010b). Diagnosis and management of Duchenne muscular dystrophy, part 2: Implementation of multidisciplinary care. *Lancet Neurology, 9*(2), 177–189.

Chang, A. (2010). *Osgood-Schlatter disease.* Retrieved from http://emedicine.medscape.com/article/827380-overview

Cheung, M., & Glorieux, F. (2007). Bisphosphonates in osteogenesis imperfecta. *Clinical Reviews in Bone & Mineral Metabolism, 5*(3), 159–164.

Chung, E., & Rooks, V. (2008). *Clubfoot imaging.* Retrieved from http:/emedicine.medscape.com/article/407294

Do, T. (2012). *Muscular dystrophy.* Retrieved from http://emedicine.medscape.com/article/1259041

Evans, A. (2008). Growing pains: Contemporary knowledge and recommended practice. *Journal of Foot and Ankle Research, 1,* 4. Retrieved from http://www.jfootankleres.com/content/1/1/4

Faust, S., Clark, J., Pallett, A. et al. (2012). Managing bone and joint infection in children. *Archives Disease in Children, 97*(6), 545–553.

Garcia, G., McMulkin, M., Tompkins, B. et al. (2011). Gross motor development in babies with treated idiopathic clubfoot. *Pediatric Physical Therapy, 23*(4), 347–352.

Gelfer, P., & Kennedy, K. (2008). Developmental dysplasia of the hip. *Journal of Pediatric Health Care, 22,* 318–322.

Gordon, E., Pappademos, P., Schoenecker, P. et al. (2005). Diaphyseal derotational osteotomy with intramedullary fixation for correction of excessive femoral anteversion in children. *Journal of Pediatric Orthopaedics, 25*(4), 548–553.

Hailer, Y., Montgomery, S., Ekbomm, A. et al. (2012). Leg-Calve-Perthes Disease and the risk of injuries requiring hospitalization: a registered study involving 2579 patients. *Acta Orthopaedics, 83*(6), 572–576.

Hart, E., Albright, M., Rebello, G. et al. (2006). Developmental dysplasia of the hip: Nursing implications and anticipatory guidance for parents. *Orthopaedic Nursing, 25,* 100–109.

Hennessey, T. (2012). Congenital clubfoot and the Ponseti method: A review of recent literature. *Current Orthopedic Practice, 23*(5), 442–447.

Holmes, S., & Brown, S. (2005). Skeletal pin site care. *Orthopaedic Nursing, 24*(2), 99–107.

Hosalkar, H., Spiegel, D., & Davidson, R. (2007). The foot and toes. In R. M. Kliegman, R. Behrman, H. Jenson et al. (Eds.), *Nelson textbook of pediatrics* (18th ed., pp. 2776–2777). Philadelphia, PA: W. B. Saunders.

Imrie, M., Scott, V., Stearns, P. et al. (2010). Is ultrasound screening for DDH in babies born breech sufficient? *Journal of Children's Orthopaedics, 4*(1), 3–8.

Ippolito, E., Farsetti, P., Caterine, R. et al. (2005). Long-term comparative results in patients with congenital clubfoot treated with two different protocols. *Journal of Bone and Joint Surgery, 85A*(7), 1287–1294.

Kaplan, S. (2011). Osteomyelitis. In R. M. Kliegman, B. F. Stanton, J. W. St. Geme et al. (Eds.), *Nelson textbook of pediatrics* (19th ed., pp. 2365–2376). Philadelphia, PA: Elsevier/Saunders.

Kocher, M., Lee, B., Dolan, M. et al. (2006). Pediatric orthopedic infections: Early detection and treatment. *Pediatric Annals, 35*(2), 112–122.

Krakow, D. (2008). Heritable diseases of connective tissue. In G. Firestein, R. Budd, E. Harris et al. (Eds.), *Kelle's textbook of rheumatology.* Philadelphia, PA: W. B. Saunders.

Lanou, A. J., Berkow, S. E., & Barnard, N. D. (2005). Calcium, dairy products, and bone health in children and young adults: A reevaluation of the evidence. *Pediatrics, 115*(3), 736–741.

Lehmann, C., Arons, R., Loder, R. et al. (2006). The epidemiology of slipped capital femoral epiphysis: An update. *Journal of Pediatric Orthopaedics, 26*(3), 286–290.

Loder, R., & Dietz, F. (2012). What is the best evidence for the treatment of slipped capital femoral epiphysis? *Journal of Pediatric Orthopedics, 32*(Suppl. 2), S158–S165.

Lynn, M., & Mathews, C. (2012). Advances in the management of bacterial septic arthritis. *International Journal Clinical Rheumatology, 7*(3), 335–342.

Maffulli, N., & Douglas, A. (2002). Seasonal variation of slipped capital femoral epiphysis. *Journal of Pediatric Orthopedics, 11*(1), 29–33.

Manzur, A., Kinali, M., & Muntoni, F. (2008). Update on the management of Duchenne muscular dystrophy. *Archives of Disease in Childhood, 93*(11), 986–990.

Mathews, C., & Coakley, G. (2008). Septic arthritis: Current diagnostic and therapeutic algorithm. *Current Opinion in Internal Medicine, 7*(5), 532–537.

McCarthy, J. (2011). *Developmental dysplasia of the hip.* Retrieved from http://emedicine.medscape.com/article/1248135-overview

Metules, T. (2007). Hands-on help. Practical tips for the bedside. Hot and cold packs. *Healthcare Traveler, 14*(9), 36–40.

Monti, E., Mottes, M., Fraschini, P. et al. (2010). Current and emerging treatments for the management of osteogenesis imperfecta. *Therapeutics and Clinical Risk Management, 6,* 367–381.

Morcuende, J. (2006). Congenital idiopathic clubfoot: Prevention of late deformity and disability by conservative treatment with the Ponseti treatment. *Pediatric Annals, 35*(2), 128–136.

Murray, A., & Wilson, N. (2008). Changing incidence of slipped capital femoral epiphysis: A relationship with obesity? *Journal of Bone and Joint Surgery, 90*(1), 92–94.

National Association of Orthopaedic Nurses (2008)

National Institutes of Health. (2005). *Osteogenesis imperfecta: A guide for nurses.* Bethesda, MD: Author. Retrieved from http://www.niams.nih.gov/Health_Info/Bone/Osteogenesis_Imperfecta/nurses_guide.pdf

National Safe Kids Campaign. (2012). Retrieved from http://www.safekids.org

Negrini, S., Aulisa, A., Aulisa, L. et al. (2012). 2011 SOSORT guidelines: Orthopaedic and Rehabilitation treatment of idiopathic scoliosis during growth. *Scoliosis, 7*(3), 1–35.

Nguyen, T. N., Gal, P., Ransom, J. L. et al. (2004). Recurrent ibuprofen-induced aseptic meningitis. *Annals of Pharmacotherapy, 37,* 229–233.

Peck, D. (2010). Slipped capital femoral epiphysis: Diagnosis and management. *American Family Physician, 82*(3), 258–262.

The Pediatric Orthopaedic Society of North America. (2012). *Metatarsus adductus.* Retrieved from http://www.posna.org/education/StudyGuide/MetatarsusAdductus.asp?css,media

Peltola, H., Pääkkönen, M., Kallio, P. et al. (2010). Short- versus long-term antimicrobial treatment for acute hematogenous osteomyelitis of childhood: Prospective, randomized trial on 131 culture-positive cases. *Pediatric Infectious Disease, 29*(12), 1123–1128.

Perry, D., Green, D., Bruce, C. et al. (2012). Abnormalities of vascular structure and function in children with Perthes Disease. *Pediatrics, 130*(1), e126–e131.

Petty, R. E., Southwood, T. R., Manners, P. et al. (2004). International League of Associations for Rheumatology classification of juvenile idiopathic arthritis: Second revision, Edmonton, 2001. *Journal of Rheumatology, 31,* 390–392.

Ponseti, I., Zhivkov, M., Davis, N. et al. (2006). Treatment of the complex idiopathic clubfoot. *Clinical Orthopaedics and Related Research, 451,* 171–176.

Rosendahl, K., Dezateux, C., Fosse, K. et al. (2010). Immediate versus sonographic surveillance for mild hip dysplasia in newborns. *Pediatrics, 125*(1), e9–e16.

Secor-Turner, M., Scal, P., Garwick, A. et al. (2011). Living with juvenile arthritis: Adolescents' challenges and experiences. *Journal of Pediatric Health Care, 24*(5), 302–307.

Shipman, S., Helfand, M., Moyer, V. et al. (2006). Screening for developmental dysplasia of the hip: A systematic literature review for the U.S. Preventive Services Task Force. *Pediatrics, 117,* e557–e576.

Sonnega, R., van der Sluijs, J., Wainwright, A. et al. (2011). Management of slipped capital femoral epiphysis: Results of a survey of the members of the European Paediatric Orthopaedic Society. *Journal of Child Orthopaedics, 5*(6), 433–438.

Spiegel, D., & Dormans, J. (2011). The spine. In R. M. Kliegman, B. F. Stanton, J. W. St. Geme et al. (Eds.), *Nelson textbook of pediatrics* (19th ed., pp. 2365–2376). Philadelphia, PA: Elsevier/Saunders.

Timms, A., & Pugh, H. (2012). Pin site care: Guidance and key recommendations. *Nursing Standard, 27*(1), 50–55.

Timms, A., Vincent, M. Santy-Tomlinson, J. et al. (2011). *Guidance on pin care, report and recommendations from the 2010 consensus project on pin care*. Royal College of nursing. Retrieved from http://rcn.org.uk/_data?assets?pfg_file/0009/413

Torres, M., & DiPietro, M. (2009). Developmental dysplasia of the hip. *Ultrasound Clinic, 4*(4), 445–455.

U.S. Preventive Services Task Force. (2006). Screening for developmental dysplasia of the hip: Recommendation statement. *Pediatrics, 117*, 898–902.

Uziel, Y., & Hashkes, P. (2007). Growing pains in children. *Pediatric Rheumatology, 5*(5). Retrieved from http://www.ped-rheum.com/content/5/1/5

Valerio, G., Gallé, F., Mancusi, C. et al. (2010). Patterns of fractures across pediatric age groups: Analysis of individual and lifestyle factors. *BMC Public Health, 10*, 656. Retrieved from http://www.medscape.com/viewarticle/735238

Wells, L., & Sehgal, K. (2011). Torsional and angular deformities. In R. M. Kliegman, B. F. Stanton, J. W. St. Geme et al. (Eds.), *Nelson textbook of pediatrics* (19th ed., pp. 2344–2351). Philadelphia, PA: Elsevier/Saunders.

World Health Organization. (2012). *Congenital anomalies*. Retrieved from http://www.who.int/surgery/challenges/esc_congenital_nomalies/en/

See thePoint for additional organizations.

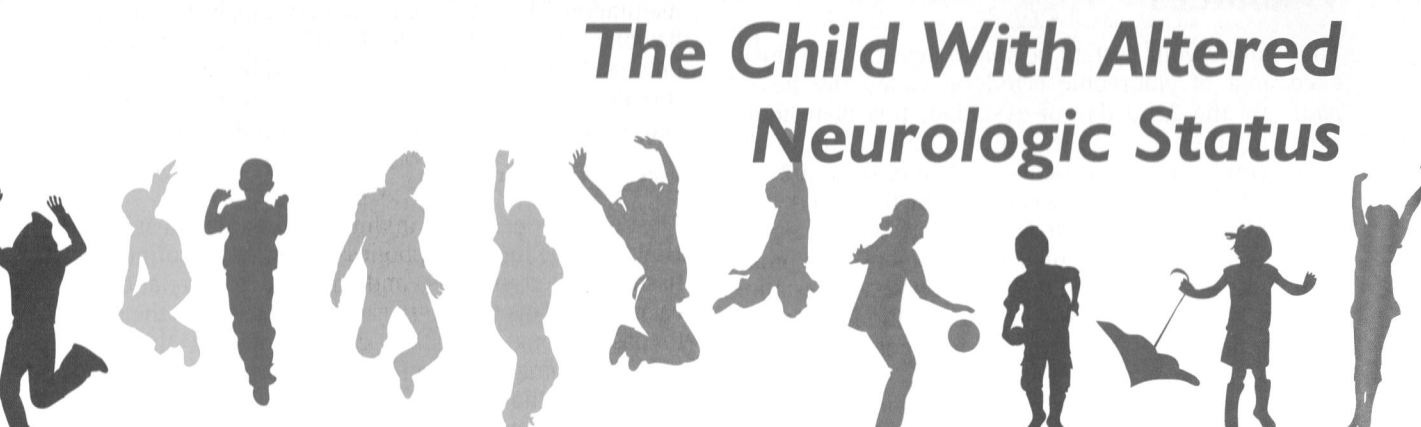

The Child With Altered Neurologic Status

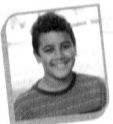

CASE HISTORY

Joey Curricio is 11 years old. He is the most athletic of the Curricio children and also the greatest risk taker. Since he was a young child, Joey has found the extreme in any activity; he climbs higher and jumps further. He loves most sports, especially soccer.

On a beautiful spring day, Joey's team has a soccer game against their most evenly matched rival. His parents and siblings are all there to watch. The ball is kicked high in the air, and Joey and a boy from the opposing team both jump to head the ball. With an audible thud, their heads collide, and both boys fall down. The referee reaches them first, then their coaches, and then the parents. Both boys are conscious, but Joey has a laceration at his hairline that is bleeding profusely.

Supported by his father, he walks to the sidelines. Joey sits next to his father, talking as his father applies pressure to the cut and his brother returns with a sandwich bag of crushed ice. Then Joey's speech slows, his eyes roll, and he loses consciousness.

Upon arrival at the hospital emergency department, Joey is still unconscious. The nurse's assessment determines his pupils are bilaterally sluggish; he does withdraw from painful stimuli and will open his eyes in response to painful stimuli as well. Within 30 minutes, Joey is opening his eyes to verbal command; he is mumbling incomprehensibly and will purposefully withdraw from painful stimuli. His parents estimate that he was unconscious at the soccer field and en route to the hospital for about 20 minutes.

CHAPTER OBJECTIVES

1 Identify components of the neurologic assessment.

2 Examine the effect of embryonic development on the child's neurologic functioning.

3 Explain the purposes of diagnostic tests used in the assessment of the child with altered neurologic status.

4 Discuss the treatment modalities that can be selected to therapeutically manage the needs of the child with altered neurologic status.

5 Identify common neurologic conditions that children may experience and their causes and defining characteristics.

See thePoint for a list of Key Terms.

The child with altered neurologic status presents a variety of complex health care concerns. This chapter highlights some common disorders and offers guidelines for developmentally appropriate interventions that address the child's physiologic, emotional, and social needs. Include the family as an integral component of care for the child.

Nurses are often in the best position to coordinate the interdisciplinary teams that manage children with neurologic problems. Depending on the facility, personnel available to the child and family may include physicians, advanced practice nurses, nurses, psychologists, social workers, child life specialists, physical therapists, occupational therapists, pastoral care staff, recreation specialists, nutritionists, and speech therapists. When these services are unavailable to a family whose child has a complex neurologic problem, referral to a regional medical center for evaluation is indicated. Support groups and national organizations can provide assistance, education, and networking for specifically affected populations. Virtual, online, and social media methods may also be recommended to the family for support and information. Always prescreen resources that are recommended to families.

DEVELOPMENTAL AND BIOLOGIC VARIANCES

The fetal nervous system begins to develop as a thickened area of embryonic ectoderm called the *neural plate*. By the 22nd day of gestation, this plate folds, becoming the neural tube, which ultimately forms the spinal cord and the ventricular system of the brain.

Neuronal proliferation is complete by birth, and most full-term infants are born with a full complement of neurons. However, neuronal development and proliferation during the second to fourth months of gestation can be influenced by exogenous (nutrition, infection, toxic exposure, ischemia) or endogenous (genetic) factors, leading to brain malformation.

After birth, the nervous system continues to mature through the processes of myelination and synaptogenesis. Myelination is the process of formation and deposition of myelin (a phospholipid protein) on nerve fibers, which insulates the fibers and enhances the efficiency of impulse conduction. Myelination begins at about 30 weeks' gestation and continues for several years after birth. Synaptogenesis is the process by which nerve cells develop connections with each other. Proliferation and overproduction of synaptic connections start prenatally and continue after birth. In a process that is highly dependent on experience and exposure, synaptic connections are gradually eliminated for some time after birth. Synapses that are used frequently are maintained, so early experiences are vital to developing and maintaining synapses and are therefore vital to brain development and maturation. The development of increasingly complex behavioral, sensory, and motor functioning depends on this process. Early life neglect characterized by decreased sensory input alters growth and organization of the brain and causes neurologic dysfunction (Taylor & Rogers, 2005).

SKULL BONES

Most of the bones of the infant skull are ossified at birth. However, the individual bones are joined by connective tissues, called **sutures**, and they move in relation to each other. This flexibility is essential to allow the head to pass through the birth canal. However, the pressures of vaginal birth can cause **molding**, an abnormal skull shape that may be evident for several days after prolonged labor or after deliveries requiring forceps or vacuum-assisted extraction. Molding may indicate a difficult delivery but does not indicate neurologic problems. In most cases, the head becomes normocephalic within 1 to 2 days. **Fontanels** (wider areas of unossified membranous tissue) occur at the intersections of sutures. Ossification of the bones of the skull is not fully complete until approximately 12 years of age.

BRAIN GROWTH

During the first year of life, the brain grows to 50% of its adult size (Fig. 21-1). The skull grows and takes shape in response to pressure from the growing brain

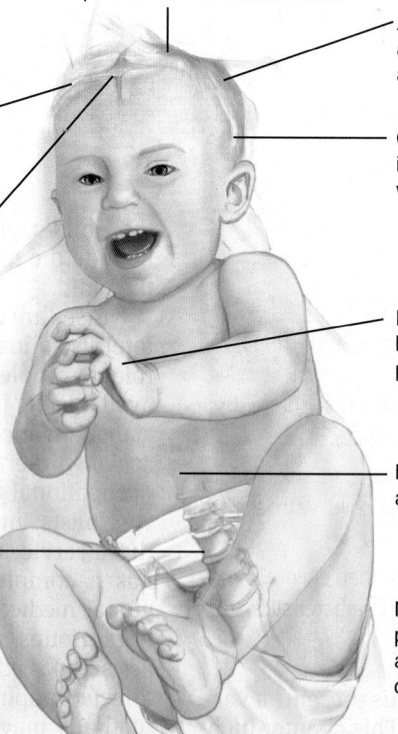

The child's brain is constantly undergoing organization of function and myelinization; thus, the full implications of a neurologic insult or injury may not be immediately apparent and may take up to several years to manifest.

A child may exhibit focal or generalized electrical discharges on an EEG that would be considered abnormal in an adult.

Increased intracranial pressure (ICP) may separate the sutures, especially the sagittal suture, until age 10–12 years.

A neonate's neurodevelopmental age is calculated to be the neonate's chronologic age minus the number of weeks born before term.

In the neonate, the spinal cord terminates at L3, compared with an adult, where it terminates at L1–L2. This affects the site of needle insertion for the lumbar puncture.

Accurate and complete neurologic assessment of infants and young children is limited by their developmental level.

Open sutures and fontanels in infancy and early childhood help compensate for increases in ICP.

At birth, the brain is about 25% of adult size; at age 1 year, 50% of adult size; and at age 5 years, 90% of adult size.

Cerebrospinal fluid volume is 50 mL in the neonate, compared with 150 mL in the adult.

Premature development of handedness before age 1 year is not usual and may point to a focal neurologic lesion.

Myelinization begins in the third fetal month and usually is complete by puberty.

Many developmental reflexes are present at birth and disappear by age 1 year. Persistence or asymmetry of the reflexes may indicate an abnormality.

Figure 21-1 Developmental and biologic variances: neurologic system.

and cerebrospinal fluid (CSF) spaces. The size and shape of a child's head should follow proportional dimensions and grow proportionately with the rest of the child's body. If intracranial pressure (ICP) is increased, as with hydrocephalus, head growth will occur out of proportion to height and weight. Conversely, in the presence of certain genetic conditions, malnourishment, or neglect, brain and head growth will be less than expected. Premature closure of one or more sutures causes craniosynostosis (abnormal head shape), which can occur as an isolated defect or as part of a syndrome.

Children have proportionately large and heavy heads, which make them prime candidates for cerebrospinal trauma secondary to inadequate head control. For example, young children learning to walk are clumsy and top heavy; when they fall, the head usually leads. Before the fontanels and sutures are completely fused, young children are at higher risk than older children and adults for serious consequences of head injury.

VENTRICULAR SYSTEM AND CEREBROSPINAL FLUID

The ventricular system plays an important part in the overall function of the central nervous system (CNS). The ventricles are interconnected cavities in the brain where 90% of the body's CSF is produced. CSF bathes the brain and acts as a liquid shock absorber, decreasing the force of impact to the head on the brain. It also carries away waste products from tissues in and around the brain. Normally, the rate of CSF production, approximately 0.35 mL/min, equals the rate of absorption. The circulating volume of CSF in children is approximately 65 to 140 mL; for adults, it is 90 to 150 mL (Aicardi, 1998).

CEREBRAL BLOOD FLOW

Cerebral blood flow (CBF) in various age groups is estimated and averaged. In adults, it is thought to be 50 mL/100 g brain tissue per minute. Age and gender differences exist, and CBF is highest during early childhood. The rate in newborns is similar to that in adults, with normal CBF estimated at 40 mL/100 g brain tissue per minute. At around 2 to 4 years of age, CBF peaks at 130 mL/100 g brain tissue per minute then stabilizes back to adult values at about 7 to 8 years of age (Wintermark et al., 2004). Cerebral blood flow velocity (CBFV) in newborns is about 24 cm/sec; it increases with age, peaking at 6 to 9 years when it is about 97 cm/sec. After age 10 years, CBFV decreases to adult values of about 50 cm/sec (Udomphorn et al., 2008).

ASSESSMENT

Assessing a child with altered neurologic status requires both a comprehensive health history and a physical assessment focused on the child's neurologic system and appropriate to the specific situation.

FOCUSED HEALTH HISTORY

QUESTION: To evaluate Joey's current neurologic status, what information is an important part of Joey's health history and establishes his baseline?

The most important factor in evaluating a child with altered neurologic status is the history. Gather the health history by interviewing the child and parents and reviewing medical records. The urgency of the child's problem, age of the child, and availability of reliable historians guide the health history (Focused Health History 21-1).

Obtain a description of the presenting problem. In emergency or critical care areas, this history may be given by emergency or transport personnel. Although the health interview should focus on the child's presenting neurologic signs, evaluating non-neurologic signs and symptoms can also provide useful information. For example, neurologic disorders may initially present as nonspecific viral illnesses, failure to thrive, or developmental delay or regression, or they may occur at the same time as other systemic diseases.

Consider aspects of the past medical history to place the current problem in perspective. For example, premature infants may have a history of intracranial bleeding, seizure activity, or episodes of apnea that can substantially affect current neurologic functioning. Likewise, the child with a history of bacterial meningitis is at increased risk for hydrocephalus and hearing impairment.

Nutritional status, both past and current, is an important aspect of the history. Poor nutritional intake can affect the child's attention span and ability to concentrate. A history of failure to thrive may indicate a metabolic disorder that affects neurologic functioning. Ingestion of nonfood substances (pica) can cause harmful toxicities that may affect neurologic function.

For a complete assessment, use developmental and biologic milestones to determine whether the child's patterns of development are normal, delayed, or demonstrate regression. Developmental milestones include activities such as when the infant or child first rolled over, sat unsupported, took steps, and rode a tricycle. The ages at which babbling and first words began are also important cognitive milestones to evaluate. History of school achievement and current school placement offer insight into current cognitive functioning.

ANSWER: It is important that the health care team knows that Joey is a healthy, athletic, 11-year-old boy with no neurologic deficits and no obvious risk factors.

FOCUSED PHYSICAL ASSESSMENT

Neurologic assessment of the infant and young child can be challenging. The child's emotional state and cognitive ability affect the examination. Document

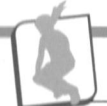

FOCUSED HEALTH HISTORY 21-1

The Child With Altered Neurologic Status

Current history	Duration, frequency, and character of presenting problem Precipitating or related factors Relief measures or home remedies Interference with daily activities, such as missed school days Static or progressive nature of condition Recent changes in ability to meet developmental milestones Weakness of any body part Asymmetry of movement or sensation Significant lethargy or irritability Trembling, shakiness, or abnormal movements Any loss of consciousness, vomiting, visual disturbances, or changes in breathing patterns
Past medical history	**Prenatal/Neonatal History** Gestational age at birth, birth weight Apgar scores Results of prenatal maternal α-fetoprotein, amniocentesis, or chorionic villi sampling Any significant pre-, peri-, or postnatal events causing asphyxia, trauma, jaundice, apnea Need for ventilator support during neonatal period **Previous Health Challenges** Previous hospitalizations, serious illness, injury, or surgeries History of child abuse Recent infection (e.g., upper respiratory, ear, and sinus) Metabolic disorder Past neurologic or developmental testing Psychological disorders Malignancies Chickenpox or any type of herpes infection
Nutritional assessment	History of pica or malnutrition
Family medical history	Seizures/epilepsy Headaches/migraines Cognitive challenge, learning problems Hypotonia Neurocutaneous lesions Problems similar to those for which the child is being evaluated Early deaths in the family
Social history	Perceived stressors for the child or among other family members Changes in lifestyle, activities, academic performance
Environmental history	Exposure to radiation Lead exposure
Growth and development	Sleep patterns Ability to meet developmental milestones

Note: See Chapter 8 for a comprehensive health history.

the presence of any factors, such as anxiety, pain, limited mobility, or the influence of medication, which may alter optimal responses. Also, consider development when interpreting the results of the examination. For example, the presence of a startle reflex is normal until about 4 months of age, but if this reflex persists past 4 months, it is evidence of neurologic dysfunction.

Much information can be obtained by observing the child carefully during the history taking. Continue observation as the child remains in a comfortable position, perhaps playing or sitting on the parent's lap. This approach gives the child an opportunity to become comfortable with the examiner and increases the chance that the child will cooperate with the examination. Observe how the child interacts with both his or her parents and the examiner. At about 8 or 9 months of age, the child should begin to demonstrate stranger anxiety; absence of this response may indicate neurologic dysfunction. As the child plays, note symmetry and smoothness of muscle movements as well as any abnormal postures (Focused Physical Assessment 21-1). Assess muscle strength by watching the child crawl, pull up to a standing position, squat and resume standing, and walk. Evaluate the child's intellectual and language skills while watching him or her play. Assess behavior; note impulsivity, distractibility, hyperactivity, or unusual patterns of social interaction. Observe how the parent deals with the child's behavior to gain insight into the quality of parent–child interactions.

caREminder

Follow a systematic approach while examining the level of consciousness, cranial nerves, motor skills, sensory responses, and cerebellar function. Perform the most intrusive or distressing portions of the examination last to keep the child calm and cooperative for as long as possible during the examination.

Incorporate developmentally appropriate toys or games as part of the assessment. Examples of familiar and inexpensive items that may be helpful in assessing the child include the following:

- Blocks, crayons and paper, and clay to assess dexterity, handedness, and grip strength
- Pencil and paper to have the child write his or her name or specific letters if able to do so; this assesses fine motor skill in addition to cognitive knowledge
- Pull toys, a jump rope, and a ball to assess cerebellar functions such as gait, balance, and functions dependent on cranial nerve (CN) VIII
- Brightly colored picture books and beanbag toss toys to assess visual acuity and eye movement served by CNs III, IV, and VI
- Salty snacks, lemon juice, sugar, and tonic water to assess CN I function and sensory portions of CNs VII and IX; this is typically only employed when the child is suspected to have a CN I dysfunction
- Books, magazines, and flash cards to assess language skills

Inspect the child's head for disproportionate growth and unusual shape. The best way to evaluate cranial growth patterns is to obtain serial head circumference measurements, plot them on a standardized growth chart for head circumference, and compare them with weight and length at each well-child visit (see Chapter 8).

Consider the child's status when performing the physical assessment. Typically, assessments of children's neurologic systems can be divided into three common types:

1. The brief screening examination
2. The acute neurologic check
3. The comprehensive neurologic assessment

Most often, portions of these examination types are combined, depending on the child's status and on the nature of the problem.

The Brief Screening Examination

Brief screening examinations are usually performed in emergency situations to triage neurologic deficits, to establish baseline data for later evaluation, and to develop an initial plan of care. When cardiac and respiratory status are deemed stable, perform a limited neurologic assessment, which includes

- Cerebral function, vital signs, level of consciousness, mental status, and verbal response
- Cranial nerves, usually CNs II, III, IV, and VI, for pupil reactivity, cardinal fields of gaze, and eye movement
- Motor system: strength, movement, and symmetry
- Sensory system: tactile and pain sensation in extremities
- Reflexes: deep tendon reflexes and superficial reflexes

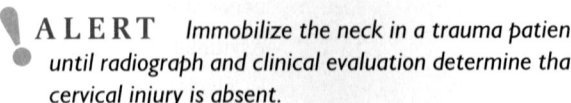 **ALERT**   *Immobilize the neck in a trauma patient until radiograph and clinical evaluation determine that cervical injury is absent.*

Immediately report **decorticate** and **decerebrate posturing**, which are characteristic body positions that indicate brain dysfunction (Fig. 21-2).

The Acute Neurologic Check

 QUESTION: What is Joey's initial score on the modified pediatric Glasgow Coma Scale (GCS)? What is his score after 30 minutes in the emergency department? What are the implications of these scores?

Acute neurologic checks are performed to monitor at-risk patients closely because subtle changes in neurologic function may precede rapid deterioration. Perform the acute examination repeatedly and frequently (Chart 21-1) and document each examination. Compare sequential assessments with the child's baseline state, note acute changes as well as trends to determine deterioration or improvement, and document.

FOCUSED PHYSICAL ASSESSMENT 21-1

The Child With Altered Neurologic Status

Assessment Parameter	Alterations/Clinical Significance
General appearance	Head nodding, lip tremors, eye blinking, and staring may be evidence of epilepsy or motor tics.
	Dysmorphic features may be present with certain genetic syndromes.
	Stuttering, dysarthria, nasal speech, or dysphonia may indicate cranial nerve or cerebral abnormalities.
Integumentary system	Café-au-lait spots, port-wine stain, or abnormal areas of pigmentation may be indicative of a neurocutaneous syndrome.
	Presence of a sacral dimple or tuft of hair may indicate spina bifida occulta.
Head and neck	Bulging fontanels may indicate increased ICP; sunken fontanels may indicate dehydration. Asymmetry of head shape may indicate plagiocephaly or craniosynostosis.
	Changes from child's growth trajectory may indicate hydrocephalus (if increasing) or malnutrition and decelerating brain growth (if decreasing).
	Head circumference less than the 5th percentile indicates microcephaly.
Eyes	Asymmetry of eye movements, ptosis, or inability to follow an object through the cardinal fields may indicate cranial nerve abnormality.
	Asymmetry of pupillary response may indicate increased ICP, an intracranial mass, or brain stem herniation.
	Vertical nystagmus indicates brain stem dysfunction.
Ears	Failure to respond to voice or sounds may indicate cranial nerve impairment or conductive hearing impairment but may also indicate inattention.
	Nausea, ataxia, and vertigo suggest vestibular pathology.
Face, nose, and oral cavity	Absent or asymmetric gag reflex, stridor, hoarseness, or dysphonia suggests cranial nerve abnormality.
	Asymmetry of facial expression suggests cranial nerve abnormality.
	Fasciculations of the tongue suggests neuromuscular disease.
Musculoskeletal	Spasticity with increased deep tendon reflexes suggests upper motor neuron disease.
	Flaccidity with decreased deep tendon reflexes suggests lower motor neuron disease, peripheral neuropathy, or myopathy.
	Hypertrophy of the calf muscles and positive Gowers sign suggest a muscular dystrophy.
	Generalized hypotonia with decreased deep tendon reflexes suggests neuromuscular disease.
Neurologic	*Consciousness:* Irritability, restlessness, and inability to be consoled by the parent are early signs of increased ICP. Lethargy and diminished or no response are late signs of increased ICP or may be the effect of drugs.
	Mentation: Impulsivity, short attention span, and distractibility may indicate attention-deficit/hyperactivity disorder or other behavior disorder. Impaired verbal and nonverbal communication, short- and long-term memory, and inability to perform age-appropriate activities of daily living may indicate cognitive impairment.
	Motor skills: Inability to perform rapid alternating hand movements or finger-to-nose movement, ataxia, or positive Romberg sign may indicate cerebellar dysfunction.
	Reflexes: Absence, asymmetry, or persistence of developmental reflexes may indicate cerebral abnormalities.

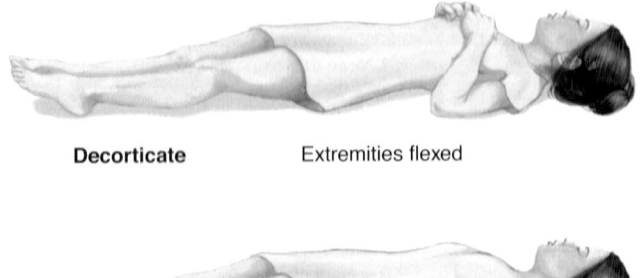

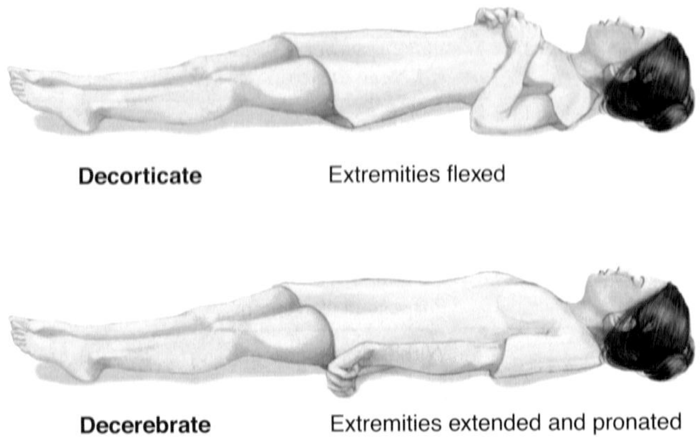

Decorticate   Extremities flexed

Decerebrate   Extremities extended and pronated

Figure 21-2 Decorticate and decerebrate posturing.

Vital signs, which are sensitive to changes in neurologic function, require prompt intervention to avoid potential life-threatening situations. For example, ICP initially slows heart rate and elevates blood pressure (Cushing triad). Base the frequency of assessments on the child's acuity level; the type of injury, illness, or surgery; and nursing judgment.

In addition to acute neurologic checks to evaluate the child with a depressed level of consciousness, a modified pediatric GCS can be used (Table 21-1). The GCS uses eye opening, motor response, and verbal response

to quantify level of consciousness, allowing objective comparisons over time.

> **ANSWER:** Using the modified pediatric coma scale, Joey's initial score is a 7 out of 15 possible points. He will open his eyes to painful stimuli (2 points), he withdraws from painful stimuli (4 points), and he is making no verbal responses (1 point). After 30 minutes, Joey's coma score has improved to 9 points. He is opening his eyes to verbal command (3 points), withdraws from painful stimuli (4 points), and is making sounds (2 points). The nurse will continue to assess Joey to determine whether there are changes in his assessment. If Joey's score decreases, the medical intervention will become more aggressive. If his score continues to improve, the response will be more conservative.

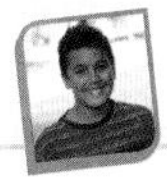

The Comprehensive Neurologic Assessment

The comprehensive neurologic assessment, used in nonacute situations or after the child's status has been stabilized, is described in Chapter 8. This examination includes a health history and evaluation of mental status, behavior, achievement of developmental milestones, motor and sensory functions, infant reflexes (see Table 8-9), cranial nerve function (see Table 8-10), and deep tendon reflexes (see Table 8-11).

CHART 21-1   Acute Neurologic Check: Assessment Parameters

Vital Signs
- Blood pressure
- Pulse
- Respiratory pattern

Level of Consciousness
- Stimulus needed to achieve a response (voice, light touch, deep pain?)
- Quality of response (arousal with ability to answer questions appropriately, arousal with momentary eye opening and no meaningful verbalizations, no response?)
- Duration of response (awake and conversant for 15–20 minutes after arousal, awake and able to maintain alertness for only 1–2 minutes?)

Verbal Responses
- Spontaneous?
- Appropriate?

Pupil Size and Reactivity
- Observe first via indirect light, then via bright-light stimulus; pupils should constrict promptly and briskly
- Record description of pupillary response: nonreactive, sluggish, absent, or unequal (anisocoria)

NOTE: Extremely small pupils may be a side effect of narcotic medications used during anesthesia or used postoperatively for pain control.

Eye Movements
- Assess eye movements as indicated in Table 8-10
- If child is comatose, assess the *oculocephalic reflex* (*doll's eye movement*) by moving the child's head left to right or up and down; when the reflex is present, the eyes look left when the head is moved right, and vice versa; absence indicates brain stem injury

Motor Function
- Note movement of all extremities and whether movement is
  - Symmetric
  - Spontaneous
  - Elicited only by stimulus (note type of stimuli required and the response elicited)
- Note abnormal motor responses to noxious (painful) stimulation: decorticate and decerebrate posturing
- Assess tone by feeling the resistance of the child's extremities to passive movement
- Assess strength by testing the child's ability to move against resistance
- Describe muscle tone and strength as
  - Flaccid (hypotonic)
  - Normal
  - Spastic (hypertonic)
  - Clonus: hypertonic response indicating motor pathway abnormalities; ankle clonus seen as repetitive movements elicited by quick flexion of the foot

TABLE 21-1   Pediatric Coma Scale*

Assessment Component	Score	>1 Year Old	<1 Year Old
Eyes opening	4	Spontaneously	Spontaneously
	3	To verbal command	To shout
	2	To pain	To pain
	1	No response	No response
Best motor response	6	Obeys	Purposeful movement
	5	Localizes pain	Withdraws from touch
	4	Withdraws from pain stimuli	Withdraws from pain stimuli
	3	Abnormal flexion (decorticate posturing) response to pain	Abnormal flexion (decorticate posturing) response to pain
	2	Extension (decerebrate posturing)	Extension (decerebrate posturing)
	1	No response	No response
		>5 Years Old	2–5 Years Old
Best verbal response	5	Oriented and converses	Appropriate word and phrases
	4	Disoriented and talks	Inappropriate words
	3	Inappropriate words	Cries and/or screams
	2	Incomprehensible sounds	Grunts
	1	No response	No response
Total	3–15		

*Modification of GCS.

DIAGNOSTIC CRITERIA

> **QUESTION:** Which of the following diagnostic criteria will be most effective for Joey? How can the nurses support Joey and his family during the diagnostic tests?

Numerous diagnostic studies are available to help health care practitioners diagnose neurologic dysfunction. Tests and Procedures 21-1 describes various procedures, invasive and noninvasive, for evaluating neurologic status, including specific preparations for each test. The nurse's role in helping children and their families who are undergoing these tests includes teaching and preprocedure preparation.

For children, any diagnostic procedure can be frightening. When preparing the child, consider the child's developmental level, cognitive ability, and physical status, including level of consciousness and pain threshold. In emergency situations, there may be little time to provide teaching; therefore, offer the child comfort measures during the study and support the family until the child is stabilized. Minimize painful interventions, which may require premedicating the child (if not contraindicated) to reduce anxiety.

Many nonpainful diagnostic procedures may be considered uncomfortable to the child because he or she must remain still or be awkwardly positioned. Use measures to help the child relax during procedures such as computed tomography (CT) or magnetic resonance imaging (MRI). Effective interventions include use of guided imagery, music therapy, and audiotapes to tell stories to the child during the procedure. Such methods help to minimize the use of sedatives to assist the child in remaining calm (Stouffer et al., 2007; Train et al., 2006).

caREminder

In some cases, hair ornaments (e.g., beads) or orthodontic metal (braces) may cause an artifact on a CT scan or MR image. Inform the family about the specific requirements of the radiology department for their child's diagnostic tests. Treat children with head lice or tinea capitis before they undergo electroencephalogram (EEG).

> **ANSWER:** CT is ordered to determine whether any subdural bleeding is present. The CT scan will produce an image that shows both bone and soft tissue. To obtain the best image possible, Joey must keep still for the procedure. It is not possible to predict when he will regain consciousness, and sedation would mask neurologic changes, so use of immobilizers is preferable. Supporting Joey's physical status includes positioning Joey so that his head is in alignment and, if possible, slightly elevated, which may prevent an increase in ICP during the procedure. Supporting Joey's family includes assuring them that Joey is not uncomfortable and keeping them informed throughout the procedure.

 **TESTS AND PROCEDURES for Evaluating Neurologic Status**

Diagnostic Test or Procedure	Purpose	Findings and Indications	Health Care Provider Considerations
Lumbar puncture	A hollow needle with a stylet is introduced into the lumbar subarachnoid space of spinal canal to withdraw CSF.	Diagnostic: Measures CSF pressure, collects CSF sample for laboratory tests for blood or microorganisms, contrast dye injected for radiographic studies, and evaluates CSF flow dynamics. Therapeutic: Injection site for spinal anesthesia or intrathecal medications. Presence of blood may be the result of trauma during needle insertion or may signal CNS hemorrhage.	Assist as necessary with positioning, securing, and calming child (see thePoint for Lumbar Puncture Procedure: Procedures/Interventions). Encourage fluids before and after lumbar puncture. Have child empty bladder before lumbar puncture because child must remain supine for 4–6 hours after procedure. Premedicate for pain, and monitor for signs and symptoms of headache related to decreased amount of CSF. Maintain strict asepsis. Be aware test is contraindicated in patients with substantially increased ICP because brain stem may herniate downward, causing tissue compression, which may lead to death.
Plain radiographs	Detects structural abnormalities. Common views are posteroanterior, lateral, Towne (semiaxial, half axial), and any portion of spinal column.	Identifies the presence of fractures, widened skull sutures, calcifications, bone erosion, or skeletal anomalies.	Remind child to be still during procedure. Ensure that support person wears protective apron.
Ultrasound (sometimes called an *echoencephalogram*)	Pulsed ultrasonic beam (Doppler) is used to locate midline brain structures. Probe is placed at a vertical angle, reflecting sound waves off structures. Images are created on a screen and produce measurable pictures.	Diagnoses intracranial abnormalities such as mass lesions and enlarged ventricles. Measures two tables of the skull and the third ventricle. May be used in prenatal testing for fetal anomalies such as spina bifida.	Be aware child must have open fontanel and remain still for the study. Teach child and family that ultrasound is a painless procedure and usually takes 15 minutes.
CT	Views the brain in three dimensions. Radiographic beam scans cranium in successive layers (cuts), and computer digitizes image. Differentiates density of bone (lighter) and air (darker). Test becomes invasive if radioisotope dye is injected to enhance views of blood vessels, vascular lesions, and localized changes in blood–brain barrier.	Used for effective visualization of tumors, ventricles, brain tissue, CSF, hematomas, and cysts.	Inform child that noncontrast study is painless. If CT is enhanced, prepare child for intravenous (IV) access. Anticipate sedation; motion destroys clarity of scan. Tell child test takes about 20–30 minutes. Because of the concern about the amount of radiation absorbed during CT scans, the use of CT is limited to specific circumstances. Children are at greater risk from radiation via CT because of their greater body surface area and a long potential lifetime to be exposed and to manifest long-term radiation effects such as cancer (Bulas et al., 2009). ALARA (as low as reasonably achievable) must always be considered by the radiologists and technicians performing the scan (Brody et al., 2007).

(Continued)

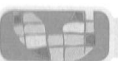 TESTS AND PROCEDURES for Evaluating Neurologic Status *(Continued)*

Diagnostic Test or Procedure	Purpose	Findings and Indications	Health Care Provider Considerations
MRI	Creates images without radiation using radiofrequency emissions that are converted to computer images. Child is supine and placed in a cylindrical opening that encases a strong magnet. MRI machines make loud humming and intermittent tapping noises. MRI produces images that differentiate between gray and white matter.	Provides sharp anatomic detail and information about the chemistry of living tissue. Useful in tumor identification. T1-weighted images may be done to determine hydrogen–tissue density. T2-weighted images detect changes in tissue biochemistry, indicating early disease.	Be aware that contrast MRI requires IV access. Inquire about allergy to MRI contrast material. Anticipate sedation if child is restless or dislikes confined spaces. Avoidance of motion is critical. Most children younger than 6 years of age require sedation. Remove all metal/magnetic items. Surgical implants such as pacemakers, bone pins, or cerebral clips are contraindications. Orthodontic braces may affect accuracy of MRI interpretation. Noncontrast study is painless. Suggest ear plugs or headphones to dampen noise. If age appropriate, allow child to see MRI machine before study. Depending on imager, tell child that study takes 45–60 minutes.
Positron emission tomography (PET) scan	Online cyclotron creates positron-emitting radionuclides. Patient is injected with or inhales radioactive tracer, which crosses the blood–brain barrier. The positron reacts to electrons, creating gamma rays. The biochemical and physiologic function of living tissue is studied as gamma rays are measured and coded by a computer.	PET scans can measure cellular processes, cerebral metabolism, CBF, membrane transport, synthesis, and receptor binding. They identify specific areas of the brain that are functioning or malfunctioning.	Obtain consent because of the nature of radioactive tracer substance. Anticipate sedation so child will remain still. Be aware that PET scans are clearer than conventional radionuclide scans.
Myelography	Images produced via radiograph, fluoroscopy, or CT. Water-based contrast media more commonly used than oil-based media. When in the CSF, the media enters nerve tissue by upward diffusion. This eliminates the need to reposition the patient. The rate of uptake is reduced by maintaining the child in a sitting position. If water-based media enters the cranial vault, seizures are likely to occur. There is no need to remove contrast fluid when the myelogram is completed because it is absorbed and excreted in the urine. Metrizamide can cause extreme diuresis.	Visualizes any or all of the spinal axis for diagnosis of tumor, congenital lesions, or bony changes. Significant risk factors include allergic reaction to iodine, headache, aseptic meningitis/infection, and seizures.	Obtain history of iodine allergy. Child must be NPO (nothing by mouth) 4 hours before myelogram. Obtain frequent neurologic assessment and vital signs. Maintain seizure precautions. Minimize activity. Strictly monitor intake and output. *Water-based medium:* Discontinue all neuroleptic drugs, monoamine oxidase inhibitors, and psychostimulants 48 hours before myelogram. After study: Avoid administration of phenothiazines, maintain a quiet environment, and keep child supine with head of bed elevated 30–45 degrees for 12–24 hours. *Oil-based medium:* Premedicate as ordered, such as with meperidine (Demerol) or atropine. After study: keep child flat in bed for 6–24 hours per physician's order.

Diagnostic Test or Procedure	Purpose	Findings and Indications	Health Care Provider Considerations
EEG and video EEG	Graphic recording of electrical activity of the brain via 17–21 electrodes glued to the scalp. Differences in electrical activity between electrodes create brain wave patterns, which are classified based on the number of cycles per second (cps). Four frequency bands are identified: (1) delta (1–4 cps), (2), theta (4–8 cps), (3) alpha (8–13 cps), and (4) beta (13–35 cps). Brain waves are usually recorded at rest, after hyperventilation, during photic (flashing light) stimulation, and during sleep. Video EEG involves recording the child's EEG and ECG, with continuous videotaping 24/7, except while toileting. The EEG electrodes are placed on the head and then the head is wrapped to keep them in place.	Detects and locates abnormal electrical discharges produced in the brain. It is used to detect seizure activity; monitor patients with head injury, stroke, metabolic coma, and some psychological illness; and assist with brain death determination. EEG may also be used during intracranial surgery for intractable seizures. EEG strips "map" electrical activity on the surface and guide the extent of cortical resection. Abnormal findings are epileptiform activity, slowing of normal waves, abnormal amplitude, or disorders of age-specific patterns. Can be used to diagnose and witness infrequent seizures that may be difficult to treat.	Withhold medications or foods known to alter brain wave activity per physician's order, such as stimulants, depressants, antiepileptics, tranquilizers, chocolate, colas, and tea. Ensure that child's hair is clean, without oils, sprays, or lotion. Alleviate common fears such as that the EEG will cause electrical shock or reads minds. Inform child that EEGs are painless procedures and usually take 45–60 minutes. After the EEG, clean hair of glue and gel, and resume medication. Requires hospital admission for 3–5 days and a family member at the bedside continuously to indicate when a seizure has occurred. Medication doses are lowered or stopped prior to admission to attempt to elicit seizure activity during the video EEG; therefore, the nurse may see more seizures and must be ready to respond appropriately. The child is not ill but is confined to the hospital room to stay within the video camera's recording ability. Preparation for this procedure is important, and involvement of child life or recreation therapy can be very helpful.
Evoked potential studies (EVPs)	Small electrodes attached to a wire and placed over the skull and a visual or auditory stimulus is given (visual auditory). Electrodes are placed on either arm or leg and stimulus is given (somatosensory).	*Visual EVP:* Determines that visual pathway is intact. In infants, light-emitting diode goggles are used. *Auditory EVP:* Determines that auditory pathway is intact. Earphones are used. *Somatosensory EVP:* Determines both spinal cord and critical appreciation of electrical stimulus. These can be obtained in the upper extremities by stimulation of midarm nerve and in lower extremities by stimulation of popliteal nerve.	Keep in mind that complete cooperation and immobility are required. In young or uncooperative children, maintain NPO status for 4 hours, and anticipate the need for sedation.

(Continued)

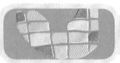

TESTS AND PROCEDURES for Evaluating Neurologic Status *(Continued)*

Diagnostic Test or Procedure	Purpose	Findings and Indications	Health Care Provider Considerations
Electromyography (EMG) and nerve conduction velocity (NCV)	Small Teflon-coated needles attached to a wire are inserted into muscle, and the brief electrical discharge is recorded. Patient contracts muscle, causing electrical activity, and motor unit action potential is studied. Electrodes are placed over a peripheral nerve in two locations: reclining and sending. An electrical impulse is sent from sending to receiving with the speed and amplitude of the response measured.	Analyzes electrical events associated with skeletal muscle fiber contraction. EMG and NCV are usually ordered together to diagnose and differentiate between peripheral nerve and muscle disorders.	Be aware that NCV can slow if child is hypothermic.

TREATMENT MODALITIES

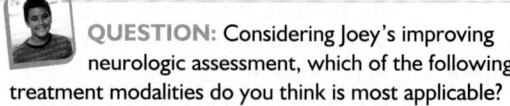

QUESTION: Considering Joey's improving neurologic assessment, which of the following treatment modalities do you think is most applicable?

Management of the child with a neurologic disorder varies based on the condition. General measures—medication, surgery, and supportive care—are discussed in this section; more tailored management is discussed in the section on specific conditions.

PHARMACOTHERAPY

Pharmacologic agents are used to treat a variety of neurologic conditions. Antibiotics or antivirals are used to treat infectious disease processes. Broad-spectrum antibiotic or antiviral therapy is typically initiated until CSF, blood, and wound cultures indicate that no infection exists or that the type of agent used must be changed because the child has a sensitivity to the current agent. Start antibiotic or antiviral therapy after CSF, blood, and wound samples are obtained. Acetaminophen is given concurrently to reduce fever associated with the infectious process.

Antiepileptics are used to treat and prevent seizures. Glucocorticoids and diuretics are used to reduce cerebral edema. Paralytic agents may be used if the child is receiving mechanical ventilation to control restlessness and agitation in the child at risk for increased ICP. Pain medications may be necessary, as may sedatives, to relieve anxiety and agitation. Sedatives should be administered in an intensive care setting where close monitoring of neurologic status is available.

CRANIAL SURGERY

Treating many neurosurgical injuries or problems requires direct access to the brain through the bony structures of the skull. The following discussion addresses the general care given to children having cranial surgery involving craniotomy and craniectomy.

A **craniotomy** refers to a "flap" opening of the skull in which the bone is removed and then replaced at the completion of surgery. If part of the cranium (skull) is excised and not replaced, the procedure is termed a **craniectomy**. When large portions of bone are not replaced, a **cranioplasty** may be done to repair the cranial defect and to protect the brain by placing a molded piece of synthetic material, usually Silastic, or autologous or donor bone over the opening.

Anatomically, the brain can be divided into two regions for surgical access. The tentorium cerebelli is a double fold of the dura mater that forms a separation between the **supratentorial** region (the upper brain structure, or the cerebrum) and the **infratentorial** region (the lower area of the cerebellum and brain stem, which includes the midbrain, pons, and medulla). Most surgical procedures in the supratentorial region of the brain are indicated for resection or biopsy of tumors or cysts, resection of epileptogenic cortex (seizure foci), placement of ventricular catheters to drain CSF, draining collected blood after head injury, or placement of ICP monitors. Surgical procedures in the infratentorial region are usually indicated for tumor or cyst resection. Care of the child with a tumor is discussed in Chapter 22.

Preoperative Care

Preparing children and families for intracranial surgery is not always possible. If the child is admitted following trauma or another emergency situation, little time is available for teaching. In these cases, the physician's priority is to obtain informed consent from the parents by discussing the purpose of the surgery, the possibility of alternative treatment or lack of treatment, the potential risks, and the expected outcomes. Ideally, the nurse should be present during the physician's discussion with the family to reinforce and clarify the information presented.

If the admission is planned, begin education before surgery. Assess the family's ability to comprehend the diagnosis and planned treatment. The family is often overwhelmed with fear and anxiety; therefore, incorporate the family's coping mechanisms into the teaching plan and review information as needed. Emotional support is essential from the first contact with the family and throughout the child's recovery period. Provide education and emotional support for the child according to the child's developmental stage and ability to understand. Specific topics important to discuss with the child and family prior to a neurosurgical procedure are outlined in Teaching Intervention Plan 21-1. Because neurosurgical procedures often involve the head and

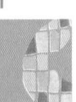

Evidence-Based Practice

TRADITION OR SCIENCE 21-1

Is hair removal necessary for cranial surgery?

Shaving the hair was thought to decrease the risk of postoperative wound infection. Studies demonstrate that cranial surgery without hair removal is safe and not associated with increased risk of wound infection (Adeleye & Olowookere, 2008; Broekman et al., 2011; Gil et al., 2003; Miller et al., 2001; Ratanalert et al., 1999; Sebastian, 2012; Tang et al., 2001). Not removing the hair also may prevent additional psychological stress for the child and family.

face, some of the child's and family's preoperative anxiety and fears may be related to shaving the hair and worrying about visible scars (Tradition or Science 21-1).

Neurologic surgery that involves the frontal or temporal bones often results in marked periorbital edema for several days after surgery. Prepare the family for

---

TIP 21-1: A TEACHING INTERVENTION PLAN for the Child Undergoing Cranial Surgery

Nursing Diagnoses and Family Outcomes

- Risk for infection related to presence of surgical incision
  Outcome: Child's incision site remains free from infection.
- Disturbed body image related to physical appearance after cranial surgery
  Outcomes: Child and family will discuss feelings about altered appearance.
  Child will express positive feelings about self.
  Child and family will implement positive coping skills to deal with altered appearance.
- Deficient knowledge: Child's condition, treatment plan, and home care requirements
  Outcomes: Child and family will express interest in learning about child's condition.
  Child and family will demonstrate health care behaviors needed to manage child's care at home.
  Child and family will express understanding of postoperative plan, routines, and expectations.

Teach the Child/Family

Postoperative Plan
- Expected length of surgery and recovery
- Intensive care unit routines and policies
- Necessity of assessments and their frequency
- Necessity for and types of monitors, access lines, catheters, and so forth
- Necessity for and types of tests and medications
- Progression of diet and activity orders
- Plan for pain management

- Expectations for family involvement in postoperative care

Postoperative Appearance
- Complete or partial head shave possible
- Location of incision and type of dressing
- Potential for facial edema
- Potential for postoperative motor/sensory deficits

Community Care Postoperatively
- Care of incision and dressings (staple or stitch removal)
- Signs and symptoms of potential short- and long-term complications
- Plan for medical/surgical follow-up: clinic appointments, diagnostic tests
- Medications
- Diet and feeding
- Plan for rehabilitation if needed (physical, occupational, speech therapies)
- Anticipatory guidance about potential neurologic deficits, safety measures, and adaptations
- Referrals to appropriate community agencies if indicated (home health care, social services, public health)
- Plan for resumption of usual activities, return to school

Contact Health Care Provider if
- Redness or drainage is noted from surgical incision site
- Child has a fever
- Child displays changes in neurologic status as demonstrated by changes in level of consciousness, lethargy, irritability, vomiting, and fontanel fullness

this postoperative event. Often, the child and the family understand the reasons for the postoperative effects of surgery, and they simply need the nurse's presence for support, reassurance, and as a sounding board to express their feelings or to begin an anticipatory grief process.

An accurate, well-documented, preoperative neurologic baseline assessment is essential in monitoring the child's postoperative functioning for potential complications. Carefully document problems with vision, hearing, communication, and any other preexisting neurologic deficits or developmental delays.

If the child has seizures preoperatively, document the description of the events in detail and implement seizure precautions, such as padding the side rails of the bed to prevent injuries. If the child has been taking antiepileptic medications, they are usually given before surgery so that serum levels remain constant. Medications can be given with a sip of water or in parenteral forms while the child is NPO.

Postoperative Care

The type and location of surgery will affect the postoperative nursing assessments. Surgery in the supratentorial area is most likely to be associated with postoperative seizures, focal motor deficits, or confusion. Infratentorial surgery may involve entry to the area from a midline incision at the back of the skull. This procedure carries a risk of respiratory compromise because midline entry into the cranial vault is close to the medulla oblongata, which contains the major respiratory center of the brain. The child may remain intubated for a longer time, especially if surgery was done to remove a tumor of the spinal cord, cerebellum, or brain stem.

CROSS-CULTURAL CARE

If hair is shaved, do not discard it during the surgery. Return it to the postoperative unit where the child is managed, in case the family requests it. In some cultures, loss of the hair is considered to be a serious loss to the child's spiritual well-being.

The nursing role after cranial surgery involves frequent acute neurologic monitoring and assessment of vital signs, intake and output, dressing, drainage, and pain to monitor the child for any potential complications. Nursing responsibilities may include caring for internal and/or external drains and shunts and ICP measurement. Complications may include increased ICP, seizure, hemorrhage, leakage of CSF, local tissue hypoxia, hyperthermia, hydrocephalus, hypovolemic shock, syndrome of inappropriate antidiuretic hormone secretion (SIADH), infection, and respiratory compromise resulting from edema in the respiratory center. In addition, the child is at risk for complications associated with immobility.

As soon as the child is in the postoperative setting, frequently assess vital signs and neurologic status to identify subtle changes and trends. Measure intake, output, and urine specific gravity to monitor for signs

that the child is developing SIADH (see Chapter 26). Identify any complications of postoperative immobility including pneumonia, deep vein thrombosis, constipation, and skin breakdown. Do not overlook these possibilities, even during the acute monitoring phase.

Note and report any substantial drainage on the dressing. It is a common practice to gently outline the border of the fluid with a surgical marker, indicating the time and change in amount of drainage. Follow strict infection control measures because the child with a healing surgical wound is very vulnerable to infection.

ALERT   *Closely monitor drainage from the dressing, incision, nose, or ears after neurosurgery for any similarity to CSF. If the dura mater tears during surgery, CSF can leak into the ear or nose.*

The possibility of CSF drainage is greater when the surgery is done after a traumatic injury in which a skull fracture may have occurred or after infratentorial surgery for a tumor. Collect suspected drainage in a sterile test tube for CSF glucose determination. To minimize sources of infection, do not pack, suction, or disturb these areas until the drainage is identified. Discourage the child from touching the drainage or the dressing and instruct the child not to blow his or her nose. Encourage the child to remain quiet.

Implement both pharmacologic and biobehavioral comfort measures to keep the child comfortable during the postoperative period. Carefully titrate analgesics to provide comfort for the child while enabling adequate neurologic assessment.

Nursing Interventions 21-1 summarizes the guidelines for immediate postoperative nursing management of the child after intracranial surgery. A drain may be used for the first 24 hours postoperatively. Sutures or staples are usually removed in 7 to 10 days.

SUPPORTIVE CARE

The child who experiences an alteration in neurologic status is at high risk for experiencing altered responsiveness during the course of his or her condition. **Responsiveness** is the child's ability to interact with the environment. It includes the ability to receive and prioritize sensory stimuli (input); process, analyze, and integrate the input (throughput); and produce a response (output). Responsiveness is expressed by thoughts, verbalizations, movement, behavior, and mood. Responsiveness is affected by developmental age and by the current level of maturity of the nervous system.

Altered responsiveness involves the impairment of input, throughput, or output. For example, input may be altered in a child with congenital blindness or deafness. Throughput may be altered in a child with a perceptual problem, such as a visual motor deficit, or a child who experiences delays in processing time after a severe head injury. Output is altered in a child who experiences paralysis, sensory motor deficits, or speech impairment.

NURSING INTERVENTIONS 21-1

Assessments and Interventions After Cranial Surgery

System	Assessment	Interdisciplinary Interventions
Neurologic	Level of consciousness Pupillary reaction Corneal reflex Ocular movement Gag reflex Motor function Sensory function Vital signs including ICP Reflexes Monitor for seizures	Monitor frequently. Test cranial nerve function. Note medications that may affect pupillary response. Maintain ICP less than 20 mm Hg. Note widening pulse pressure, bradycardia, and altered respirations (Cushing triad) and report immediately. Maintain neutral position of head and neck. Elevate head of bed 30 degrees. Palpate infant fontanel. Provide safe environment with side rails up. Minimize activity. Maintain internal and/or external shunt as indicated; maintain exact position as indicated, measure output color and amount. Consult neurology and ophthalmology as needed.
Respiratory	Breath sounds Oxygen saturation Cyanosis Respiratory rate Airway patency Blood gases	Turn child every 2 hours to promote postural drainage. Adjust ventilator settings per physician's order. Gently suction secretions. Provide humidified oxygen per physician's order. Encourage deep breathing exercises. Consult respiratory therapy.
Elimination	Urine output, 0.7 mL/kg/hr Indwelling urinary (Foley) catheter intact Constipation Monitor blood urea nitrogen, creatinine, specific gravity	Strictly monitor input and output. Provide catheter care to prevent infection. Give daily stool softener to reduce hard stools or straining (Valsalva maneuver), which increases ICP. Consult nutritionist.
Fluid and electrolytes	Mucous membranes and eyes for dryness	Restrict fluids per prescriber's orders. Provide hydration/medication. Use IV pump to avoid fluid bolus. Use artificial tears in eyes. Provide oral care.
Musculoskeletal	Pressure ulcers Flexibility of joints	Provide range-of-motion exercises daily. Provide skin care/sheepskin pad on bed. Consult physical therapy.
Psychosocial	Level of pain Level of fear or anxiety	Administer pain medication. Provide emotional support. Encourage parental participation in care. Explain all interventions before touching child. Anticipate and answer questions. Consult child life specialist.

Altered responsiveness may appear as an acute, self-limiting process (e.g., after cranial surgery) or may be a long-term condition (e.g., after a traumatic brain injury [TBI]). Additional hazards may result if the child is immobilized or at risk of physical injury resulting from sensory and perceptual deficits.

Managing Altered Responsiveness

Nursing care for the child with altered neurologic functioning varies according to the nature of altered responsiveness. In general, goals for nursing care are to continue assessment for alterations in health status, protect the child from additional injury, and assist the family in adapting to the child's needs.

Physical safety is a concern for the child with altered responsiveness. To prevent falls from the bed, keep the side rails up at all times. Use adaptive supports as necessary to prevent falls when the child is out of bed (e.g., when the child is positioned in a chair, use safety belts as necessary to maintain the child comfortably in an upright position and ensure support so the child will not slip from the chair to the floor or become entangled in the belt). The mobile child may be prone to falls because of altered spatial perception, altered motor ability, or altered mental processing, which can lead to impulsive behavior. Protective helmets can be used to protect the mobile child's head from further injury. However, restraints and protective equipment do not replace close monitoring and supervision. Preventing the hazards of immobility is also important.

> **ANSWER:** Supportive care and careful monitoring are critical for Joey. Be aware of the potential for rapid change. Should Joey's ICP increase, he could decompensate very quickly. By the same token, if he should regain consciousness, he may be disoriented, confused, and potentially angry and requires careful monitoring.

Minimizing Disuse Syndrome

Complications from altered responsiveness and immobility can include respiratory complications, musculoskeletal problems, gastrointestinal problems, urinary tract problems, and altered skin integrity. These complications place the child at risk for *disuse syndrome*, a state in which the child is at risk for deterioration of a body system as a result of musculoskeletal inactivity or immobility.

The immobile child also has decreased lung capacity because the inspiratory muscles are not aided by gravitational pull; chest expansion is limited by the weight of the body against one aspect of the chest; and, when the child is in a horizontal position, the abdominal contents push against the diaphragm. Furthermore, stimulus for fully expanding the lungs is minimal when little or no muscular activity occurs. Pooling of secretions within the lungs and exposure to microorganisms may lead to serious respiratory infection.

Although chest physiotherapy for the unresponsive child cannot include voluntary deep breathing and coughing, turning the child from side to side, at least

every 2 hours, helps to expand different areas of the lungs and reduces pooling of secretions in the lungs. Elevate the head of the child's bed periodically, if the child can tolerate it, and position the child in a sitting posture for short periods, if the physician's orders permit. Health care personnel in contact with the unresponsive child must wash their hands carefully and avoid persons with active respiratory infections.

Airway management also helps to prevent infection in the child. Gently suction nasal and oral secretions, and maintain good hygiene of oral and nasal mucous membranes, keeping them free of dried secretions; lubricate regularly to prevent breaks in membrane integrity. Oral health maintenance is often complicated by the bite reflex in children with neurologic damage.

caREminder

Never insert your fingers in the child's mouth, and do not insert anything in the child's mouth that could damage the teeth or gums in case the child's jaws close unexpectedly.

Muscles that are not used regularly lose strength, tone, and mass rapidly. Also, contractures may form at unused joints, permanently limiting the child's musculoskeletal functions. Exercise therapy, including passive range-of-motion exercises (unless contraindicated by volatile ICP) and attention to body alignment when positioning the child, can prevent these complications. The heavier the child, the more care is needed in positioning because the weight of the limbs may strain major joints, muscles, ligaments, and tendons. Place pillows under the arms and between the legs to minimize this stress. Shoulder supports can help to prevent dislocation. Washcloths, small gauze rolls, or hand splints can help keep the fingers in functional alignment. High-top athletic shoes or ankle–foot orthoses can help prevent foot drop.

When the child begins to recover, reinstitute weight bearing as soon as it can be tolerated. Physical therapy regimens include range-of-motion exercises and use of a tilt table, a standing frame, and parallel bars to help gradually restore weight bearing and active range of motion.

Altered oral–motor function, chalasia of the cardiac sphincter, and delayed gastric emptying put the child with altered consciousness at risk for regurgitation and aspiration of gastric contents. If the child requires enteral feeding, elevate the child's head during feeding to help prevent aspiration of food particles. Give infants who retain a sucking reflex a pacifier during enteral feedings to help prevent the development of oral–motor defensiveness and to help retain the suck reflex for future oral feeding.

caREminder

Do not attempt oral feedings until oral–motor function is evaluated and gag and swallow reflexes are known to be intact.

Nutritional monitoring, including careful calculation of caloric needs, is important to prevent muscle wasting. Because metabolism decreases with inactivity, also take care not to overfeed the child.

If possible, hold infants and small children for feedings to preserve the social contact and caring interactions they have previously associated with feeding. Holding, rocking, and other caring interactions with the family and the nursing staff are equally important for older children. If the child's condition contraindicates being held, techniques such as massage (tactile stimulus), singing to the child (auditory stimulus), and frequent contact that keeps the caregiver's face in the child's line of vision may be appropriate substitutions.

Assess bowel function by auscultating bowel sounds in all abdominal quadrants and by maintaining a record of the child's bowel movements. Diarrhea may accompany a change in the feeding regimen and may be a sign that the feeding is not being tolerated. Adjustments may be required to enteral volume, rate, or formulation.

Constipation may be a sign of inadequate fluid intake or sluggish peristalsis related to the child's immobility. Lack of bowel movements; passage of hard balls of stool; or abdominal palpation for firm, full intestines can help to confirm suspicions that bowel evacuation is inadequate. Assess and intervene promptly to manage constipation and avoid impaction. Stool softeners may be given to prevent constipation, because the Valsalva maneuver, which is used when moving bowels, may increase ICP.

Bladder tone and bladder emptying may also be affected by altered motor and sensory function. Neurogenic bladder is a common sequela of spinal cord injury (SCI) and myelodysplasia. With neurogenic bladder, clean intermittent catheterization may be required to provide urinary continence, to prevent overdistention of the bladder, and to protect the upper urinary tract from damage (see Chapter 19).

Immobility is a major assault to the integumentary system. Constant rubbing on bed linens, body pressure against wrinkled garments, pressure of body weight on delicate tissues, reduced blood flow in pressure areas, mechanical irritation from tubing, and chemical irritation from wet and soiled diapers all contribute to the risk for altered skin integrity. Use pressure-relieving mattresses, keep linen wrinkles to a minimum, and ensure that no small objects (e.g., plastic sheaths from disposable needles) are left in the child's bed. Protect opposing skin surfaces and pressure points with pillows and foam supports. Inspect the skin thoroughly during regular care for any areas of redness. Reposition non-red, bony prominences and massage them to increase circulation; do not further irritate reddened areas of the child's skin with massage.

Promoting Health Maintenance

For some children, altered neurologic functioning may be a lifelong condition. Involving the family members who will help care for the child at home as early as possible in discharge planning and teaching helps to ensure that they develop the skills needed to care for

the child. Include the child in planning, teaching, and self-care to the extent possible.

Explain how the illness or disorder affects the child, including the anatomy and physiology of the neurologic processes involved. Give the family written material on symptoms that indicate the need for medical intervention so they know when to call the health care provider. Teach care techniques by demonstrating and having the family members, and child as appropriate, perform the technique. Such techniques may involve feeding the child through a nasogastric tube, tracheostomy care, eye care, oral care, positioning, use of various equipment, passive range-of-motion exercises, skin care, and safety precautions (see Chapter 11). Provide information about medications, including purpose, administration, and side effects. Emphasize the need for medical follow-up, including laboratory studies to monitor therapeutic drug levels.

Family members need time to accept alterations in the child's level of responsiveness and may need help in modifying their expectations. Help them recognize the child's capabilities and strengths by pointing out those skills and abilities that have been preserved; point out events that indicate progress. Some families find it helpful to keep a journal or video log; looking back helps them see the progress that their child is making. At the same time, the family may need help accepting the child's new limitations. For example, the family may need help distinguishing reflex movements from voluntary movements so that movements such as posturing are not mistaken for purposeful responses.

CROSS-CULTURAL CARE

Cultural approaches to the care of a child with a neurologic deficit are varied. Some cultures promote the idea that such a child is a blessing sent from God which enhances the worthiness of the parents. Blacher and McIntyre (2006) found that religious interpretation is one probable reason why Latina mothers have reported higher positive impact from having a child with a disability than Anglo mothers.

The incidence of behavioral problems in children with developmental delay and cognitive disabilities is higher than in typically developing children (Fox et al., 2007). Provide information about techniques for behavior management and discipline and about community resources for ongoing support after hospital discharge. Some families may benefit from professional counseling.

The family also needs information about the availability of physical and financial support for the child's care after discharge. In most states, supplemental insurance plans are in place to assist in meeting the health care expenses related to caring for a child with a disability. Community agencies are available to assist families in identifying financial resources. Arrange for referral to a social worker. Barriers such as language often pose impediments to obtaining necessary services for children with neurologic deficits or disabilities.

Caring for a child with altered neurologic functioning has a tremendous effect on the entire family. Counsel the family about the physical and emotional hazards associated with full-time care of the child with a disability. Encourage them to take advantage of respite care offered by friends, relatives, and community resources. As the family adapts to the child's condition, roles and responsibilities may shift. Disability-free siblings likely play a large role in socialization and normalization of the child with a neurologic or developmental disability. Parents gain added responsibilities, which place increased demands and restrictions on the entire family. Even though parents may adapt to their child's disability, they may never fully accept it. Chronic sorrow often develops and periodically waxes and wanes. Times of transition, or life changes, are especially difficult (Coffey, 2006). Sensitivity, presence, availability, communication skills, and knowledge help the nurse provide support to the family.

Family members often have questions about the child's prognosis and whether to seek additional opinions from other health care professionals. Such discussions call for sensitivity on the part of the nurse. It takes time for the family to understand and to accept the reality of a neurologic deficit, whether temporary or permanent. The nurse can help the family obtain needed information and ensure that their questions are adequately addressed. In many cases, arranging a meeting for the family with the multidisciplinary team will address the family's concerns while all the care providers are present. Often, the presence of a social worker who has been involved with the family is very helpful.

NURSING PLAN OF CARE

QUESTION: Which of the nursing diagnoses, interventions, and outcomes in Nursing Plan of Care 21-1 is most pertinent to Joey?

Conditions affecting the child's neurologic status are of special concern to the health care team because such conditions create the potential for long-term sequelae that can affect the child's cognitive and motor functioning. In addition, the child's social and personal development may become impaired. Therefore, the goals of health care management are to intervene immediately to prevent progression of neurologic insult while, if possible, simultaneously treating the underlying condition. During these early critical stages of the child's care, monitor and maintain physiologic functioning of all body systems because the brain and its functions are vitally linked to other systemic body functions. Support the family as the child is stabilized, a diagnosis is reached, and treatment interventions are initiated. As the child responds to the interdisciplinary interventions, the goals of the health care team become directed toward optimizing the child's outcomes through rehabilitation activities. Nurses in the home, the school,

and the rehabilitation center help the family evaluate the child's capabilities and help the child reach his or her highest level of growth and development. Nursing Plan of Care 21-1 summarizes the nursing diagnoses that can be applied to children experiencing a neurologic disorder. These diagnoses reflect the broad scope of problems that confront the child and family as they deal with both the emergent and long-term issues surrounding the child's condition.

ANSWER: A potential nursing diagnosis for Joey would be ineffective tissue perfusion related to injury. Except for the intervention regarding assessing fontanels, all the interventions are appropriate and all the expected outcomes apply to Joey.

ALTERATIONS IN NEUROLOGIC STATUS

Neurologic events that can affect neurologic function include increased ICP, seizures, epilepsy, breath-holding spells, and headaches. Alterations in neurologic status may stem from adverse outcomes of neurologic conditions, congenital disorders, craniofacial abnormalities, infectious and parainfectious processes, neuromuscular disorders, neurocutaneous syndromes, or neurologic trauma.

QUESTION: What adverse outcomes could result from a head injury like Joey sustained?

INCREASED INTRACRANIAL PRESSURE

ICP is determined by the space occupied by the three intracranial components: brain, blood, and CSF. The incidence of increased ICP cannot be determined because its etiologies vary widely.

Pathophysiology

ICP is dictated by CBF and cerebral perfusion pressure (CPP). If initial compensatory mechanisms and autoregulation cannot maintain optimal ICP, brain tissue can herniate into other brain structures.

For ICP to remain constant, if the volume of one of the components increases, the volume of the other components must decrease. These components—brain, blood, and CSF—can alter their volume to maintain normal ICP, a mechanism known as **compensation**. When an increase in volume occurs, the brain begins a complex series of activities aimed at decreasing the overall ICP and maximizing perfusion of sensitive brain tissue. These compensatory mechanisms enable a normal volume–pressure relationship to be maintained for as long as possible. If these mechanisms become exhausted, an imbalance occurs, volume increases, and increased ICP results. This explanation of cerebral volume dynamics is known as the **Monro-Kellie doctrine**.

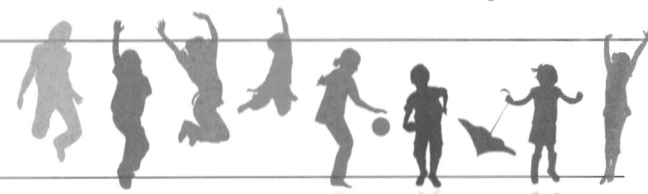

NURSING PLAN OF CARE 21-1:

Child With Altered Neurologic Status

Nursing Diagnosis: Ineffective breathing pattern related to effects of seizures, neurotrauma, and CNS damage

Interventions/Rationale

- Assess child's respiratory status.
  Provides baseline data from which to evaluate changes in the child's status.
- Maintain a patent airway; use airway adjuncts as needed.
  Promotes oxygenation and helps avoid increases in carbon dioxide (CO_2), which can cause vasodilation and increase intracranial blood volume. Anoxic events can increase brain size; both anoxic events and increased brain size can decrease cerebral perfusion.
- Monitor respiratory rate, rhythm, and depth; auscultate breath sounds.
  As ICP increases, vital centers located in the brain stem are affected, causing abnormal respiratory patterns. Monitoring status allows for early detection of problems and implementing interventions.
- Assess color, amount, and consistency of pulmonary secretions.
  A change in consciousness or responsiveness may impair the child's ability to clear pulmonary secretions. Accumulated secretions provide a good medium for bacterial growth and may result in increased partial pressure of carbon dioxide (PCO_2), which may cause increased ICP.
- Assess circulatory status (e.g., pulse, blood pressure, and skin color).
  Assists in detecting hypoxia.
- Monitor arterial blood gas values.
  Enables early detection of acid–base abnormalities and decreases in oxygen saturation, allowing for early intervention. Monitoring of CO_2 must also be addressed to avoid hypercapnia. Using hyperventilation to reduce CO_2 will assist in decreasing ICP.
- Administer oxygen as ordered; assess effectiveness.
  A change in consciousness or responsiveness may impair the child's ability to clear pulmonary secretions or aerate adequately, causing hypoxemia and acid–base disturbances.
- Encourage deep breathing and limit coughing.
  Deep breathing aids in aeration and preventing stasis. Coughing increases ICP.

Expected Outcomes

- Child's respiratory rate will remain within age-appropriate parameters.
- Child will exhibit arterial blood gases within normal range.
- Child will maintain respirations without ventilatory support.

Nursing Diagnosis: Risk for ineffective cerebral tissue perfusion related to effects of brain injury or seizure activity

Interventions/Rationale

- Assess neurological status and vital signs every 1–2 hours as needed.
  If deviations from normal are noted promptly, interventions can be implemented in a timely manner. An alteration in either arterial pressure or ICP alters cerebral perfusion.
- Assess fontanels in children younger than 2 years of age.
  In children younger than 2 years of age, a bulging fontanel may indicate increasing ICP.
- Elevate the head of the bed 30 degrees, and align the head and neck.
  Head elevation up to 30 degrees may reduce ICP without affecting CPP. Head alignment facilitates venous outflow from the brain, maintaining balance in intracranial volume (i.e., brain tissue, blood, and CSF).
- Describe and record behavior carefully.
  Changes in behavior may be some of the earliest signs of alteration in neurovascular status.
- Administer fluids within fluid restrictions to prevent cerebral edema.
  Overhydration expands intravascular volume, potentially increasing ICP.

Expected Outcomes

- Child will maintain or improve current level of consciousness.
- Child will exhibit ICP within normal range.
- Risk factors for altered cerebral perfusion and complications will be reduced as much as possible.
- Child will achieve adequate oxygenation and nutrition at the cellular level.

Nursing Diagnosis: Ineffective thermoregulation related to neurologic trauma or illness

Interventions/Rationale

- Assess child's vital signs and monitor routinely.
  Provides baseline data from which to evaluate changes in the child's status. Hypothalamic injury or disease can alter the child's ability to thermoregulate. Monitoring enables early detection of deviations from normal, allowing for early intervention.

(Continued)

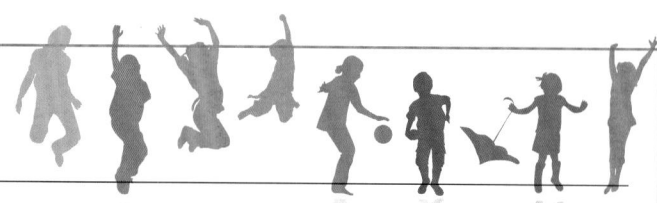

NURSING PLAN OF CARE 21-1:

Child With Altered Neurologic Status (*Continued*)

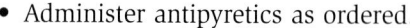

- Administer antipyretics as ordered.
  Hyperthermia increases metabolic rate, stressing homeostasis and increasing insensible water loss, disrupting fluid balance. Antipyretic therapy is a central cooling intervention.
- Implement cooling or warming measures, as indicated.
  Physical cooling or warming methods also help the child maintain normothermia in the presence of thermoregulatory dysfunction.

Expected Outcome
- Child's body temperature will be maintained within normal limits.

Nursing Diagnosis: Risk for acute confusion related to effects of neurologic injury or illness

Interventions/Rationale
- Assess child's thought processes and level of orientation and monitor routinely.
  Provides baseline data to evaluate changes in child's status and facilitates early detection of changes.
- Orient child to name, time, place, and surroundings at every contact. Teach family to reorient a conscious child periodically to surroundings.
  Neurologic injuries may result in an alteration in consciousness that may be short- or long-term. Including familiar persons may decrease confusion and anxiety for the child.
- Remain with the child who is not fully conscious and oriented until the child is stable.
  Impaired consciousness may place the child at risk for injury to self or others.

Expected Outcomes
- Child will receive treatment for physiologic causes, resulting in restoration of thought processes.
- Child will demonstrate improvement in sensorium via care activities that help to restore thought processes.
- Child will remain safe and free from injury.

Nursing Diagnosis: Risk for infection related to presence of surgical incision, head trauma, or bacteria infecting the neurologic system

Interventions/Rationale
- Assess for signs of infection (e.g., increase in temperature, erythema) and behavior indicating neurologic infection (e.g., irritability, decreased level of consciousness).
  Facilitates early detection of infection.

- Implement interventions such as wound care to reduce risk of infection. Maintain a closed drainage system for external venous drainage.
  Surgical intervention, the use of external drains, and head trauma result in a break in skin integrity. The use of shunts introduces a foreign object into the head that is a potential source for infection.
- Report any changes in vital signs or behavior (e.g., irritability, decreased level of consciousness) immediately.
  Prompt detection of deviations from normal allows timely intervention.
- Monitor operative sites, shunt sites, and sites of injury for signs of redness and swelling.
  Prompt detection of deviations from normal allows for timely intervention.

Expected Outcomes
- Child will remain free from infection.
- Child will receive prompt treatment for infectious process, if present.
- Child will demonstrate resolution of infectious process without complications to neurologic integrity.

Nursing Diagnosis: Risk for injury related to effects of sensory and motor deficits

Interventions/Rationale
- Assess the child's level of consciousness to determine changes and to determine ability to participate in self-care activities.
  Physical injury may occur during periods of altered consciousness and seizure activity.
- Monitor for seizure activity.
  Children with a history of epilepsy are at increased risk for additional seizures. Cerebral edema may alter neuronal functioning, leading to the development of seizures. Metabolic imbalances such as hypoxia, hypoglycemia, and electrolyte imbalances secondary to neurosurgery or neurologic insult can also contribute to the development of seizures.
- Protect from potential injury related to seizures (e.g., keep bed in low position, keep side rails up and padded).
  Changes in cognitive functioning and sensorimotor impairments place the child at risk for injury.

Expected Outcomes
- Child and family will identify factors that increase potential for injury.
- Family members will assist in identifying and implementing safety measures to prevent injury.

- Child will increase self-care activities within parameters posed by sensorimotor limitations.
- Child will remain safe in the environment.

Nursing Diagnosis: Delayed growth and development related to physical or neurologic impairment

Interventions/Rationale
- Assist parents to individualize growth and development expectations for child. Help develop methods to promote achievement of milestones.
  Parents may not have realistic expectations regarding growth and development of their child, especially if the neurologic condition was sudden in onset and the child lost previously achieved developmental milestones.

Expected Outcomes
- Child will demonstrate age-appropriate skills as able, given sensorimotor limitations.
- Parents will express understanding of their child's growth and developmental potential as defined by the child's condition.
- Child and parents will participate in activities to enhance child's achievement of developmental milestones.

Nursing Diagnosis: Disturbed body image related to altered physical capabilities, lifestyle changes, or physical appearance following neurologic injury or illness

Interventions/Rationale
- Assess child's perception of body image.
  Provides baseline data from which to evaluate changes in the child's perception of self.
- Encourage discussion concerning misconceptions, fears, the reality of public discrimination, and social stigma.
  Children with neurologic disorders and their families must cope with social stigma and rejection because of the public's misconceptions and prejudices about these conditions (e.g., epilepsy, meningomyelocele). The child may be embarrassed and may feel insecure and resentful about the condition and about his or her inability to participate in typical activities for age. Expressing and discussing feelings may help child to cope.
- Inform parents of the importance of treating their child as any other child.
  Helps the child to feel normal and may avoid behavioral problems from lack of limits.
- Assist the parents to plan age-appropriate developmental activities for the child based on the child's capabilities.
  Will help the child master skills to achieve developmental potential.

- Prepare the child to assume self-care responsibilities.
  Will help the child achieve developmental potential.

Expected Outcomes
- Child will discuss feelings about change in body image.
- Child will express positive feelings about self.
- Child will implement positive coping skills to deal with change in body image.

Nursing Diagnosis: Deficient knowledge: Child's condition, treatment plan, and home care requirements

Interventions/Rationale
- Assess family's knowledge of child's condition and care needs.
  Assists in focusing teaching to family's needs.
- Explain all treatments and procedures, and be present when information is given by other health care team members. Reinforce and clarify information.
  Helps the child and parents to understand condition and treatments and make informed decisions.
- Demonstrate required care. Provide opportunity for return demonstration.
  Helps the child and parents master care needs.
- Teach and counsel family regarding child's condition and need for adhering to current interdisciplinary regimen.
  Child and parents cannot manage treatment program if deficient knowledge exists. Misconceptions and poor care are fostered when the family lacks understanding or knowledge.
- Teach child and family to identify and report symptoms that indicate a change in the child's condition or a deleterious side effect of medications or other treatments.
  Enables prevention or early detection of problems and early intervention.

Expected Outcomes
- Child and family will express interest in learning about child's condition.
- Child and family will participate in teaching sessions to learn about child's condition.
- Child and family will demonstrate health care behaviors needed to manage child's care at home.
- Family will verbalize confidence in caring for child's ongoing health needs.
- Family will manage child's health care in the home.

Nursing Diagnosis: Disabled family coping related to response to severity of child's condition and potential or actual long-term disability

Interventions/Rationale
- Assess family's coping and identify needs regarding child's care related to condition.
  Allows identification of family strengths and areas where support is needed.

(Continued)

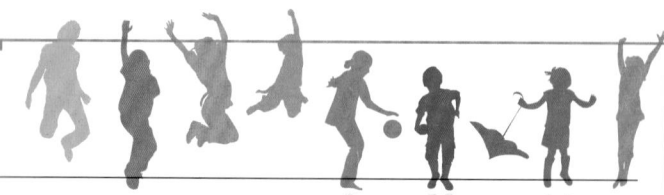

NURSING PLAN OF CARE 21-1:

Child With Altered Neurologic Status (*Continued*)

- Encourage family expression of fears and feelings of helplessness, guilt, anger, and despair outside the child's hearing range. Arrange for spiritual and counseling support as needed.

    Family may find it difficult to maintain open communication under stress. They often need validation that their feelings are normal.

- Enlist other personnel (e.g., child life specialist, social worker, clergy) to assist child and family in coping with child's condition.

    Recognition of individual perceptions and previously successful methods of coping can help families in coping with their child's condition.

- Provide a list of community resources and support for emotional and spiritual needs.

    Ongoing support can help with coping and meeting emotional needs.

Expected Outcomes
- Family will express their concerns about coping with child's illness.
- Family will be able to identify their needs.
- Family will seek resources and sources of emotional and spiritual support.
- Family will be able to meet their needs as well as the child's to their mutual satisfaction.
- Family will obtain financial and physical resources to manage child's care in the home.

Cerebral Blood Flow

CBF provides oxygen to the brain and transports metabolic components to and from its cells. CO_2 causes vasodilation in cerebral blood vessels, which increases blood volume and, therefore, increases ICP. Oxygen content can also affect ICP, although to a much lesser degree. Profound hypoxia (partial pressure of arterial oxygen [PaO_2] <50 mm Hg) can lead to cerebral vasodilation as the body tries to send more oxygen to the brain tissue. For these reasons, airway management for the child at risk for, or experiencing, increased ICP is paramount.

Cerebral Perfusion Pressure

CPP, a major factor affecting CBF, is the pressure gradient that determines blood flow and oxygenation to the brain tissue. It is calculated by subtracting the ICP value (determined by using an ICP monitor) from the mean arterial blood pressure. CPP is affected by changes in arterial blood pressure as well as by changes in ICP. A normal CPP is approximately 80 mm Hg, with values more than 60 mm Hg considered acceptable in children with acutely increased ICP secondary to trauma.

Mechanisms That Increase Intracranial Pressure

Several mechanisms are known to increase ICP, including increased brain mass, increased cerebral blood volume, increased CSF volume, and obstructed CSF flow. Increased brain mass can result from brain tissue edema secondary to cell anoxia after head injury, brain surgery, infections, and inflammatory diseases such as encephalitis. Lesions within the brain also increase brain mass.

Vasodilation, which occurs for numerous reasons, including oxygen deprivation and increased systemic blood pressure, increases cerebral blood volume. Cerebral blood volume is also increased by decreased venous outflow and increased intrathoracic pressure.

Increased CSF volume can result from increased production of CSF by the choroid plexus, obstructed flow of CSF through the ventricular system, or decreased absorption of CSF in the subarachnoid space. Increased CSF volume secondary to hydrocephalus or meningitis is common in children. The mechanisms of increased ICP are interrelated, and more than one process can occur at one time.

Compensatory Mechanisms

Several compensatory mechanisms serve to maintain ICP in response to increasing volume within the skull. These mechanisms include (1) a displacement of CSF from within the cranial cavity to the distensible subarachnoid space around the spinal cord, (2) an increase in the rate of CSF absorption into the venous system, and (3) a reduction in cerebral blood volume resulting from compression of the low pressure venous system.

Cerebral blood vessels alter their diameter to maintain a constant blood supply to brain tissue despite fluctuation in the arterial blood pressure via a mechanism termed *autoregulation*. When arterial pressure increases, vasoconstriction occurs; when arterial pressure decreases, vasodilation occurs. However, dramatic changes in arterial blood pressure (to <50 mm Hg or >150 mm Hg) impair cerebral autoregulation. When the systemic blood pressure declines to less than 50 mm Hg, cerebral ischemia occurs and cell function is impaired. When severe hypertension occurs, the blood–brain barrier breaks down, and cerebral edema results. When autoregulation is impaired, CBF and CPP become passively dependent on systemic arterial pressure.

Herniation of Brain Tissue

Herniation can be described as a physical displacement of a portion of the brain through and into other brain structures, usually because of an increase in the volume of brain, blood, or CSF. When pressure in one area is excessive, the brain may displace to an area of less resistance, causing serious and potentially life-threatening consequences. The best treatment is prevention of increased ICP through early management.

The most common type of supratentorial herniation is uncal herniation, which can be unilateral or bilateral. As the uncus of the temporal lobe pushes into midline structures, it puts pressure on the oculomotor nerve, causing pupil dilation and sluggish or absent response to light. Other signs and symptoms of uncal herniation include declining consciousness, decerebrate posturing, increased blood pressure, slow pulse, and respiratory irregularity.

Infratentorial herniation is less common and can involve herniation of the cerebellar tonsils up through the tentorium or down through the foramen magnum. The brain stem can also herniate down through the foramen magnum. Signs of infratentorial herniation include decerebrate or decorticate posturing, declining consciousness, impaired upward gaze, irregular respiration, pupillary constriction or dilation, and lower cranial nerve palsies. Medullary compression can result in death from cardiac or respiratory arrest.

ANSWER: Intracranial swelling or bleeding resulting from a head trauma such as Joey sustained could result in increased ICP, necessitating placement of an ICP monitor.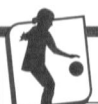

Assessment

Signs of increased ICP vary depending on the age of the child (Developmental Considerations 21-1). In infants and young children, open sutures allow the cranial bones to spread apart to accommodate increased cranial volume during the initial phases of increased ICP, especially when the buildup of pressure is slow or chronic. In instances of acute increased ICP, however, the skull may not change as readily to compensate for the added volume. Because of this phenomenon, the signs and symptoms of acute and chronic increased ICP in infants and young children vary. The skulls of older children are less accommodating.

Differences in the signs and symptoms are also related to whether the underlying process is acute or chronic and to the child's developmental level and ability to communicate subjective symptoms. A complete assessment of factors in the child's history, including changes in behavior, attainment of developmental milestones, or level of alertness or responsiveness, is vital.

Ask about headache, a common symptom of increased ICP at all ages. Headache is generalized and is worse in the morning on awakening or on rising to a standing position. The pain is usually constant but varies in intensity. Vomiting, especially on arising in the morning, is often present. Visual disturbances, including diplopia and strabismus, may also occur. Pertinent physical assessment findings include impairment

---

DEVELOPMENTAL CONSIDERATIONS 21-1

Clinical Manifestations of Increased Intracranial Pressure

Headache in the morning that decreases with vomiting or lessens throughout day
Cranial enlargement secondary to hydrocephalus
Vomiting
Diplopia
Papilledema
Lethargy and somnolence (late signs)
Headache present with Valsalva maneuver

Child Younger Than 3 Years Old
Marked irritability
Bulging fontanel
Disrupted sleep patterns
Resistance to being held or comforted
Decreased appetite
Developmental delays or loss of acquired milestones
Increased head circumference
Delayed closure of anterior fontanel (usually between 8 and 18 months of age)

---

of upward gaze and papilledema (passive swelling of the optic disk).

Palpate the anterior fontanel of a quiet infant to assess ICP. Bulging of the fontanel above the level of the bone edges and an inability to palpate the bone edge indicate increased ICP.

After establishing a baseline, monitor neurologic status and vital signs as necessary in accordance with the child's condition and the prescriber's orders. Monitoring may be required as frequently as every 15 minutes for a child whose condition is unstable and changing rapidly, or it may be several times daily for a more stable patient.

Diagnostic Tests

Diagnostic tests are obtained to identify the specific cause of increased ICP. These tests may include skull radiographs, CT scans and MR images, CBF studies, EEG, and evoked potentials.

Nursing Diagnoses and Outcomes

Nursing Plan of Care 21-1 presents a variety of nursing diagnoses that may be applicable to the child with a neurologic condition. The following diagnosis applies specifically to the child with increased ICP:

Nursing Diagnosis: Decreased intracranial adaptive capacity related to changes in intracranial components
Outcome: Child's ICP will remain in normal range.

Interdisciplinary Interventions

> **QUESTION:** Should Joey's parents be allowed to stay with him during his assessment in the emergency department?

The treatment of increased ICP is complex and specific to the causative factors. Prevention programs to prevent head and brain injury focus on the use of helmets, seat belts, and barriers to water access. Recent programs have also focused on preventing high-risk behaviors and violence.

Increased ICP may require medical and surgical methods of treatment. Generally, medical measures are instituted while the need for surgery is assessed. In many instances, surgical and medical management occur simultaneously.

Monitoring Intracranial Pressure

Continuous monitoring of ICP is used to assess the effects of treatment in maintaining adequate CPP. ICP is measured in millimeters of mercury or in centimeters of water. Monitoring devices range from a noninvasive transducer that may be placed over a fontanel to more commonly used invasive devices, such as an epidural transducer, a subarachnoid bolt or screw, and an intraventricular catheter transducer. An ICP monitor is placed by a neurosurgeon, either at the bedside or in the operating room. The nurse assists in gathering supplies, ensuring strict asepsis during the procedure, and supporting the family with information.

Normal ICP ranges from 0 to 15 mm Hg, although temporary elevations to as high as 100 mm Hg can occur with activities such as coughing and the Valsalva maneuver. Increased ICP may be moderate (20 to 40 mm Hg) or severe (>40 mm Hg). The placement of an ICP monitor enables calculation of CPP, which is a more accurate predictor of long-term outcome for children with increased ICP.

When the child's ICP is being monitored, the goal is to keep the ICP at less than 20 mm Hg and the CPP at more than 40 mm Hg (Rohlwink et al., 2012). To attain this goal, mean arterial blood pressure must be 70 mm Hg or more.

A sudden increase in ICP can occur as a result of a change in head and neck position, a partially obstructed airway, hyperthermia, and increased patient agitation caused by noxious external stimuli. Stroke, intracranial hemorrhage, and impending herniation are also potential causes of a change in ICP. If ICP suddenly increases, quickly assess the child to note any change in vital signs or in neurologic parameters (Nursing Interventions Classification 21-1).

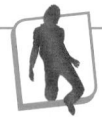

NIC 21-1 NURSING INTERVENTION CLASSIFICATION: Cerebral Edema Management

Definition: Limitation of secondary cerebral injury resulting from swelling of brain tissue

Activities:

Monitor for confusion, changes in mentation, complaints of dizziness, syncope

Monitor neurologic status closely and compare to baseline

Monitor vital signs

Monitor CSF drainage characteristics: color, clarity, consistency

Record CSF drainage

Monitor CVP, PAWP, and PAP, as appropriate

Monitor ICP and CPP

Analyze ICP waveform

Monitor respiratory status: rate, rhythm, depth of respirations; PaO_2, pCO_2, pH, bicarbonate

Allow ICP to return to baseline between nursing activities

Monitor patient's ICP and neurologic response to care activities

Decrease stimuli in patient's environment

Plan nursing care to provide rest periods

Give sedation, as needed

Note patient's change in response to stimuli

Screen conversation within patient's hearing

Administer anticonvulsants, as appropriate

Avoid neck flexion, or extreme hip/knee flexion

Avoid Valsalva maneuvers

Administer stool softeners

Position with head of bed up 30 degrees or greater

Avoid use of PEEP

Administer paralyzing agent, as appropriate

Encourage family/significant other to talk to patient

Restrict fluids

Avoid hypotonic IV fluids

Adjust ventilator settings to keep $PaCO_2$ at prescribed level

Limit suction passes to less than 15 seconds

Monitor lab values: serum and urine osmolality, sodium, potassium

Monitor volume pressure indices

Perform passive range-of-motion exercises

Monitor intake and output

Maintain normothermia

Administer loop-active or osmotic diuretics

Implement seizure precautions

Titrate barbiturate to achieve suppression or burst-suppression of EEG as ordered

Establish means of communication: ask yes-or-no questions; provide magic slate, paper and pencil, picture board, flash cards, VOCAID device

From Bulechek, G. M., Butcher, H. K., Dochterman, J. M. et al. (Eds.). (2013). *Nursing interventions classifications (NIC)* (6th ed.). St. Louis, MO: Mosby. Used with permission.

Assess for hypercapnia (elevated partial pressure of arterial carbon dioxide [$PaCO_2$]) and hypoxia (decreased PaO_2) by means of blood gas analysis and pulse oximetry. If suctioning is necessary to maintain the airway, do this in short intervals to prevent suction-induced hypoxia. When mechanical ventilation is necessary, maintain $PaCO_2$ between 35 and 38 mm Hg and PaO_2 more than 85 mm Hg (Orliaguet et al., 2008). In the presence of refractory increased ICP, $PaCO_2$ less than 35 mm Hg may be used (Orliaguet et al., 2008). When positive end-expiratory pressure is used for pulmonary hypoxia, avoid excessive intrathoracic pressure, which may also contribute to elevated ICP. Reducing the $PaCO_2$ by controlled hyperventilation causes vasoconstriction of cerebral blood vessels, which in turn decreases ICP. Because of this unique phenomenon, manual hyperventilation to decrease $PaCO_2$ may be used in the critical care setting.

Closed Ventricular Drainage/Ventriculostomy

In cases of increased ICP in which ventricular access is obtained to measure ICP, controlled drainage of CSF may be used during the acute phase of treatment. Sterile closed-drainage systems enable close monitoring of CSF drainage and easy access to inline ports for drawing CSF specimens to monitor infection and other parameters.

Ventriculostomy is the procedure that creates the opening into the ventricle to place the catheter. The term is also used in reference to the ventricular drainage system. The ventricular drainage catheter is usually inserted through a burr hole in the skull into the lateral ventricle. The catheter is tunneled under the subcutaneous tissue and exits the scalp some distance from the burr hole, an approach that decreases the risk of intraventricular infection. The catheter is connected to a drainage system, which works by gravity, so the amount of CSF drainage depends on the position of the drip chamber in relation to the lateral ventricle. The physician may order continual drainage or intermittent drainage when the ICP reaches a specific level.

Nursing care for the child with a ventricular drainage system includes carefully recording the color, amount, and rate of drainage. Ensure that the system is at the proper level with the correct settings. The key to accurate ICP measurement is to use the same landmark each time; for example, tragus of the ear or outer canthus of the eye. An institution should have a universally accepted location used consistently in order to avoid confusion and inaccurate measurements. Overdrainage of a ventricular drainage system can also cause an alteration in CSF and electrolytes, which must be monitored and treated accordingly (American Association of Neuroscience Nurses [AANN], 2011). Keep in mind the effects of positioning on ICP. Use strict aseptic technique and maintain a closed system. Monitor electrolytes closely and anticipate that fluid lost with CSF may have to be replaced with IV fluids.

Positioning

Neck flexion and head rotation appear to increase ICP. Keep the head and neck in a neutral position in relation to the shoulders and upper trunk, and elevate the head

15 to 30 degrees (Fan, 2004). Use pillows to prevent the child from sliding down in bed and to support the head in a neutral position when the child lies on his or her side. Support the child's head in a neutral position during turning and lifting. Increases in ICP have also been seen in response to lateral and prone positioning, which should be avoided. Overdrainage of CSF can result in CSF hypovolemia. Overdrainage of spinal fluid can result in lower pressure in the lumbar spine than in the brain. If CSF overdrainage occurs resulting in mental status changes, place the patient in a Trendelenburg position to reverse the pressure gradients and increase CSF volume (AANN, 2011).

Temperature Regulation

Fever causes vasodilation and increased CBF. Fever treatment can decrease the vasodilation and reduce systemic and cerebral metabolic requirements. Administering antipyretics and using tepid water sponge baths and cooling blankets are recommended to maintain body temperature at 97.7° to 100.4° F (36.5° to 38.0° C). Lower the body temperature slowly to prevent shivering, which increases ICP.

Pharmacologic Interventions

A common treatment for ICP is the use of the hyperosmolar therapy with agents such as mannitol or hypertonic saline. These agents increase the osmotic pressure in the cerebral blood vessels, thereby causing water to move from the brain tissue to the vascular space. Hyperosmolar therapy may be most effective during the first 48 hours of administration. Frequently monitor neurologic status, urinary output, and fluid and electrolyte balance. Assess for potential hypovolemia.

Sedation (e.g., midazolam) reduces the stress response and lowers ICP. Analgesics such as fentanyl provide pain relief and help depress airway reflexes in the intubated patient; antianxiety agents should never be used in place of appropriate analgesics. If initial medical management is not successful, a barbiturate coma may be induced.

Pancuronium (Pavulon), a paralyzing agent, may be used during the initial phases of management to decrease muscle responses to voluntary, central, and environmental stimuli. Although a child treated with pancuronium cannot move or respond to stimuli, sensory functions are not altered, so the child may still be able to hear and feel. Nursing care includes meticulous skin care, the application of artificial tears and eye lubricant, and frequent neurologic assessments. Sedatives should always be given in conjunction with paralytic agents.

Antiepileptics, such as phenobarbital, phenytoin, levetiracetam, or lamotrigine, may be ordered if the child has a history of seizures. Monitor drug levels frequently to avoid toxicity. Giving a patient with brain injury an antiepileptic on a prophylactic basis is controversial if a seizure has not occurred (Liu & Bhardwaj, 2007).

If an ICP monitor is in place, the child will receive prophylactic antibiotics. Monitor peak and trough drug levels to prevent toxicity and to optimize the drug's effect.

Steroids such as dexamethasone are used primarily to reduce edema surrounding mass lesions. Antacids must be given concurrently to minimize side effects, including gastritis and stress ulcer.

Surgical Interventions

Surgery to relieve rapidly increasing ICP may be acutely needed in cases of severe head injury resulting in large hemorrhages. A decompressive craniectomy is performed to relieve ICP in children with severe TBI, diffuse cerebral swelling, and intracranial hypertension (Bor-Seng-Shu et al., 2012). Chronic clinical conditions may also present as a surgical emergency, especially if they are undiagnosed for a long time. Examples include brain tumors and subdural hematomas secondary to nonaccidental trauma in shaken baby syndrome. In these latter cases in particular, medical management is necessary to lessen the substantial risk of morbidity or mortality during surgery on a highly pressurized brain. In some cases, this risk cannot be avoided. In most cases, an ICP monitor is inserted during surgery to assist in postoperative management of ICP.

Comfort and Support Interventions

In addition to assessing and monitoring, nursing care of the child with increased ICP focuses on reducing the child's pain, crying, and agitation with comfort measures, including the timely use of analgesics and sedatives as necessary. Also, enlist the family's help to provide comfort measures (see Chapter 10). Encourage the presence of family members at the child's bedside. In some cases, family presence will lead to more agitation and increased ICP, and the family will need frequent explanations and support through the acute phase of treatment. Suggest that the family bring security objects from home to comfort the child. Plan care activities so that the child has uninterrupted periods of rest and sleep, and reduce the number of care activities at any one time. Support for the family during this crisis is vital.

> **ANSWER:** Yes, an important component of family-centered care is to keep parents with their child. An important aspect of nursing management of a child with increased ICP is to prevent distress and agitation that can elevate ICP.

SEIZURES

Seizures can be categorized as epileptic or nonepileptic. An epileptic seizure is a transient clinical event that results from abnormal and excessive activity of cerebral neurons. The abnormal activity, which can be seen on an EEG, results in paroxysmal disorganization of one or more brain functions. The resulting effects may be excitatory (motor, sensory, or psychic), inhibitory (loss of awareness or muscle tone), or a combination of the two. Nonepileptic seizures, such as a psychogenic seizure or a brief convulsion as the result of a syncopal event, are not associated with an epileptic discharge in the brain. Seizure episodes may affect the child in any one or combination of the following ways: altered responsiveness; altered sensation, perception, or both; or altered movements, mobility, or muscle tone.

The clinical features of an epileptic seizure depend on the characteristics of the abnormal electrical discharge and the area of the brain involved. Children may have occasional seizures as the result of a specific event, such as a febrile illness, hypoglycemia, or CNS infection. Some children may have recurrent seizures without a specific provoking event. This pattern is considered epilepsy. Epilepsy may be idiopathic (without an identified cause) or symptomatic (resulting from an acquired cause). This section covers care of the child experiencing a seizure of any kind, regardless of circumstances, cause, and seizure type, and also reviews status epilepticus. Febrile seizures, mentioned briefly in this section, are described in detail in Chapter 31. Epilepsy is covered in the following section.

Pathophysiology

About 5% of children in the United States will have a seizure before age 20 years. About 25% of these children will develop epilepsy, a condition characterized by recurrent, unprovoked seizures (MacAllister & Schaffer, 2007).

Seizure susceptibility changes with age and developmental stage (Developmental Considerations 21-2).

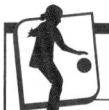

DEVELOPMENTAL CONSIDERATIONS 21-2

Common Causes of Seizures

Neonate
- Hypoxic–ischemic encephalopathy
- Intracranial hemorrhage
- Blood chemistry imbalance such as hypoglycemia, electrolyte imbalances
- Intracranial infection
- Cerebral malformations
- Genetic factors such as genetic syndromes, benign familial neonatal seizures (autosomal dominant inheritance), familial congenital cerebral malformation, inborn errors of metabolism, neurocutaneous syndromes
- Neonatal abstinence syndrome
- Head trauma

Beyond Neonatal Period
- Seizure onset after neonatal period may result from causes listed earlier
- Intracranial infection
- Head trauma
- Exposure to drugs of abuse or other toxins
- Tumor or malignancy
- Idiopathic
- Hypoxia
- Fever

Several factors may contribute to the immature brain's propensity to have seizures. Many of these factors relate to the normal developmental process of synapse formation in infants and children:

- Excitatory process developing before inhibitory process
- Differences in the ionic microenvironment
- Immaturity of circuits that modify expression of seizures
- Reduced threshold for activating seizures

In normal brain activity, certain groups of neurons are active during the processes of thinking, hearing, moving, or other activities. Other groups of neurons are less active, and still others are inactive at any given moment. During a seizure, groups of neurons all activate at the same time, causing a sudden burst of electrical activity in the brain and disrupting normal function. Two factors account for neuronal tissue's potential to produce an epileptic seizure. First, disruptions of cellular depolarization and repolarization mechanisms result in abnormal excitability, causing cells to fire randomly. Second, abnormal synchronization of a group of neurons may occur, which initiates the electrical burst of an epileptic seizure.

Many nonepileptic paroxysmal events occur in childhood that can be mistaken for seizure activity. These events can range from the benign (e.g., breath-holding spells, hyperventilation, night terrors, gastroesophageal reflux) to life threatening (e.g., cardiogenic syncope, hypoglycemia). Tourette syndrome and other related tic disorders are not seizures and require different medical management. In rare circumstances, it may be necessary to obtain an EEG to determine if a movement is a tic or a seizure. In the majority of cases, EEGs are not indicated nor should they be obtained.

Classification of Seizures

A system to classify epileptic seizures was developed by the Commission on Classification and Terminology of the International League Against Epilepsy (1989). Epileptic seizures are first classified as partial or generalized, based on the origin of the event, and are then further classified based on the clinical symptoms present. Seizures are termed *unclassified* if the available information is not enough to classify them as partial or generalized.

Partial Seizures

In partial seizures, the abnormal neuronal firing is initially localized to one or more groups of neurons or areas within the same hemisphere of the brain. The effect on brain function is limited, or focal. The abnormal activity may spread to involve the entire brain, an event called *secondary generalization*. Partial seizures are further classified as simple or complex, according to whether consciousness is lost during the event.

Simple partial seizures are usually brief events, often lasting less than 1 minute, during which consciousness is preserved. Simple partial seizures may consist of motor, sensory, autonomic, and/or psychic signs or symptoms. Motor involvement, the most

common, involves rhythmic movement, alternating contraction and relaxation (clonic) typically limited to one muscle group (such as the fingers) or to a contiguous group of muscles (as in an arm or a leg). Involvement may spread from this initial site to involve all the muscles on one side of the body. **Todd paralysis**, a transient paralysis of the involved muscle groups, may follow a simple partial seizure and may last as long as 24 hours.

Simple partial seizures beginning in the parietal lobe are associated with somatosensory symptoms, such as a "pins-and-needles" sensation or a feeling of numbness. Involvement of the occipital lobe may cause visual symptoms consisting of flashes of light or color or loss of vision in a specific area (scotoma or hemianopia). Autonomic symptoms may include vomiting, pallor, flushing, sweating, dizziness, erection of body hairs, pupillary dilation, tachycardia, incontinence, and other autonomic functions. Psychic symptoms may include cognitive symptoms, affective symptoms, illusions, or hallucinations.

Complex partial seizures, the most common type of seizures in children, often originate in the temporal lobe, an area concerned with memory and emotion. Symptoms may be variable and may include a wide range of behaviors.

Some children with complex partial seizures experience a *prodrome*—that is, they are aware of an impending seizure days or hours before it occurs. Others experience an *aura*. A prodrome differs from an aura in that the prodrome is not part of the actual **ictal** (seizure) event. An aura is an ictal phenomenon; it is part of the actual seizure activity. It is the portion of the seizure that occurs before consciousness is lost and for which memory is retained when consciousness is regained. Auras vary considerably among individuals; children may experience sensory (e.g., visual, auditory, olfactory, gustatory) symptoms, visceral sensations, or complex subjective experiences such as fear, embarrassment, or dizziness. Children may also state that they have an indescribable "funny feeling" before the onset of a seizure.

Following the loss of consciousness, various types of automatic behavior (automatisms) may occur, such as chewing, gagging, choking, lip smacking, spitting, waving, clapping, scratching, masturbating, walking, skipping, running, screaming, crying, or laughing. On regaining consciousness (the **postictal** period), the child often feels tired and falls asleep.

Generalized Seizures

In a generalized seizure, the abnormal electrical activity occurs throughout the brain, and cortical functions are disrupted. Generalized seizures can be primary—that is, both hemispheres are involved from the outset—or secondarily generalized from a partial seizure. Consciousness is impaired in a generalized seizure.

Generalized tonic–clonic seizures may be preceded by both a prodromal phase and an aura. An aura indicates that the seizure began focally (as a partial seizure) and then spread throughout the brain. Typically, generalized tonic–clonic seizures involve five recognizable phases: flexion, extension, tremor, clonic, and postictal. During the brief (5-second) flexion phase, consciousness is lost. Seizure activity usually begins in the face with the eyes rolling upward and the mouth opening with jaw muscles rigid. Flexion of the extremities follows. The extension (tonic) phase (which lasts 10 to 30 seconds) begins with extension of the back and the neck and includes extension of the legs. The jaws clamp together tightly, and tongue biting can occur. Apnea may begin during the tonic phase, with rigid extension of the thoracic and abdominal muscles, and may persist through the clonic phase. The tremor phase (5 to 10 seconds) marks the transition between the tonic and clonic phases. Fine tremors usually begin in the extremities and spread proximally. The clonic phase may last 30 to 50 seconds. A characteristic rhythmic jerking is produced by the rapid contraction and relaxation of opposing muscle groups. The jerking decreases in frequency as this phase nears completion. Apnea frequently lasts through the clonic phase, causing increasing cyanosis. Secretions pool in the mouth and throat, leading to noisy respirations. This stage can be difficult for observers because the child appears to be in great distress, yet nothing can interrupt the seizure. After the last clonic jerk, the bladder sphincter relaxes, and incontinence may occur. During the immediate postictal phase, the child is still unconscious, but relaxation of muscles results in a flaccid posture. Cyanosis resolves as breathing returns to normal, but pallor often lingers. The child may either gradually awaken or progress directly into a sleeping state.

Clonic seizures consist of episodes involving loss of awareness followed by rhythmic jerking movements of the arms and legs. The length of the seizure varies, and the jerking can be unilateral or bilateral. These seizures are relatively rare, but they can occur in all ages, including neonates.

Myoclonic seizures are characterized by sudden, brief jerks of muscle groups. Flexor muscles are often involved on both sides of the body, resulting in sudden falls for older children or spasms for infants. Loss of consciousness may be momentary and unobserved. Myoclonic seizures may occur several times in a row.

Tonic seizures consist of a brief, sudden onset of increased tone of the extensor muscle. If the child is standing, he or she typically falls to the floor. *Atonic seizures* involve a sudden loss of muscle tone and loss of consciousness. During a brief attack, the seizure may be confined to a particular group of muscles and, although the child's head may drop suddenly, the child may not fall. Seizures of larger muscle groups may initiate falls and are often referred to as *drop attacks*. More prolonged attacks may begin with a fall but then continue with the child lying limp and unresponsive for seconds or minutes. Longer attacks are usually followed by drowsiness.

Absence seizures consist of a sudden, brief (usually no longer than 30 seconds) arrest of the child's motor activity accompanied by a blank stare and loss of awareness. The child maintains posture. At the end of the seizure, the child returns to the activity that was in progress as though nothing has happened. Interruption of mental activity may be incomplete, allowing the child to continue simple or automatic behavior during the lapse of full mental function. The child retains no memory of the seizure but may be aware of a "time loss." Postictal confusion and sleepiness do not occur.

Febrile Seizures

Febrile seizures are defined as seizures that occur in association with a febrile illness in the absence of CNS infection, electrolyte imbalance, or previous afebrile seizure. It is not necessary for the child to have a fever at the time of the seizure for the seizure to be considered a febrile seizure. Higher fevers are associated with a greater risk of febrile seizure. These seizures most frequently occur in children from 6 months to 5 years of age (Hampers & Spina, 2011).

Simple febrile seizures are less than 15 minutes in length, are generalized, and occur as a single event during a single febrile illness. Complex febrile seizures are longer than 15 minutes, have a focal component, and occur repeatedly during the same illness.

The prognosis for febrile seizures is generally good, and children rarely have any short- or long-term deficits. Recurrent febrile seizures are associated with younger age of onset, family history, low peak temperature at time of first febrile seizure, and a complex first seizure. Less than 1% of children who have a simple febrile seizure will develop epilepsy (Hampers & Spina, 2011).

Diagnostic evaluation of a child who presents with a seizure associated with fever is aimed at determining whether the child had a febrile seizure or if a more serious underlying condition is present. The presence of CNS infection is determined by lumbar puncture, which is indicated in a child younger than 18 months and in older children if there are clinical signs of meningitis. Except for blood glucose documentation, additional diagnostic studies are not indicated unless signs and symptoms other than fever and seizures are present.

For the child who has a history of febrile seizures, using daily antiepileptic medication to prevent further seizure is not recommended because the medication causes substantial adverse effects (Lux, 2010). Rectal diazepam is often recommended for emergency treatment of febrile seizures and is indicated for children with a history of prolonged or multiple febrile seizures and for those who live long distances from medical care. Although the family must be trained in its use, the drug is easy to administer and provides the family with a sense of control. Counsel the family of a child with a febrile seizure that the seizure is not life threatening and does not cause permanent injury. Evidence-based recommendations for evaluating infants or young children after a simple febrile seizure direct clinicians to identify the cause of the child's fever. Evaluation for meningitis should take place quickly via lumbar puncture. Simple febrile seizures do not usually require further evaluation, specifically EEG, blood studies, or neuroimaging. If seizures occur in the absence of fever in an infant or young child, evaluation will include a more in-depth workup (American Academy of Pediatrics Subcommittee on Febrile Seizures, 2011).

Neonatal Seizures

Neonatal seizures do not resemble the seizures of infants or older children. Myelinization of the CNS is incomplete during the neonatal period, and epileptic discharges are not transmitted well in the neonate's brain. As a result, partial or fragmentary motor events or subtle behavioral changes such as apnea may be manifestations of seizures. Types of seizures that are recognizable in the infant include

- Focal clonic seizures: repeated, irregular jerking affecting one or both limbs on one side
- Multifocal clonic seizures: migratory jerking movements noted first on one limb then another, and on one side then the other; facial muscles may be involved
- Focal tonic seizures: rigid posturing of the extremities and trunk; fixed deviation of eyes may be present; may be associated with apnea
- Myoclonic seizures: brief, repeated extension and flexion movements of arms, legs, or all limbs
- Subtle seizures: chewing motions, excessive salivation, apnea, blinking nystagmus, bicycling or pedaling movements, and changes in skin color

Common causes of neonatal seizures are listed in Developmental Considerations 21-2. Pyridoxine dependency, a rare metabolic disorder, may also precipitate seizures in the neonate. Seizure activity in neonates may be difficult to distinguish from nonepileptic activity (Chart 21-2). Observation is crucial for appropriate diagnosis.

In neonatal seizures, interictal EEG patterns (activity in between seizures) are helpful in predicting outcome. Normal interictal patterns are associated with a good prognosis, with no seizures beyond the neonatal period, and normal developmental progress. Abnormal patterns are associated with a poor prognosis, generally continued seizures, and abnormal or delayed development.

Treatment of neonatal seizures is aimed at identifying and treating the cause. Care involves maintaining a patent airway and supporting cardiovascular function. A trial of pyridoxine is usually given to treat potentially pyridoxine-dependent seizures. Antiepileptic therapy

CHART 21-2	Distinguishing Neonatal Seizure Activity From Nonepileptic Movements
Seizure Activity	**Nonepileptic Movements**
Tachycardia and increased blood pressure	No changes in vital signs
Movement not suppressed by gentle restraint	Movement suppressed easily with gentle restraint
Seizure activity unchanged by sensory stimuli	Enhanced nonepileptic movements with sensory stimuli

includes lorazepam, phenobarbital, or phenytoin. Therapy is usually very short-term and may be discontinued after 2 weeks of complete seizure control.

Status Epilepticus

Status epilepticus occurs when seizures last longer than 30 minutes or recur without return of consciousness between seizures. It is a common neurologic emergency in children and can be life threatening. Children younger than 3 years of age are most likely to develop status epilepticus, and most who present with status epilepticus do not have a prior history of seizure. The most common cause of status epilepticus in children is febrile seizure (Ng & Maganti, 2012). For a child with a history of epilepsy, the most likely cause of status epilepticus is poor adherence to medication regime or acute antiepileptic drug withdrawal.

The clinical outcome of status epilepticus depends on the etiology and is worse for children with status epilepticus precipitated by serious intracranial insults. Death is usually the result of the underlying cause rather than the seizure itself. Sequelae include epilepsy and motor or cognitive deficits. Outcome is greatly improved by rapid intervention and cessation of the seizure activity.

Assessment

Some seizures are more easily recognized than others because the signs and symptoms are so variable among the different types of seizures. For example, generalized tonic–clonic seizures are easily recognized, whereas simple or complex partial seizures may be more difficult to recognize, possibly occurring repeatedly before being recognized. Absence of a preexisting history of seizures can also make recognition more difficult.

A seizure has three distinct parts: the ictal phase, the postictal phase, and the interictal phase, which describes the period between seizures and is considered the child's baseline. Clinical manifestations depend on the area of the brain that is involved. Observe the seizure or obtain an accurate description of the seizure from the family member or caregiver to assist in accurate diagnosis and treatment. Simultaneously, intervene as appropriate (Nursing Interventions 21-2).

In the event of a first-time seizure or status epilepticus, assess to determine causative factors. Conduct a thorough physical examination, and evaluate urine, blood, and CSF (e.g., serum glucose, electrolytes, and drug levels) as indicated for infectious, metabolic, or toxic cause of seizure. Urgent brain imaging with CT can determine whether there is a traumatic or neoplastic cause. EEG and MRI are conducted when the child is stable.

Interdisciplinary Interventions

Caring for a child with a seizure involves providing initial management, pharmacologic therapy, and simultaneous investigation of the cause (Evidence-Based Clinical Practice Guidelines 21-1). Also, institute safety measures to reduce the potential for injury to the child if another seizure occurs.

NURSING INTERVENTIONS 21-2

Seizure Assessment and Management

Assessment

Seizure Onset
- Note activities and potential precipitating factors prior to onset.
- Did the child indicate an aura or knowledge of impending seizure?
- Did the child alter activities? If so, how?
- Observe the sequence of events.

Level of Awareness
- Note level of responsiveness to self, others, and environment.
- Observe whether responses were rote or more complex and how much they were affected (e.g., partially, totally).
- Assess response to stimuli: tactile (e.g., touch lightly, gently shake or move arm or leg), auditory (e.g., state child's name, give a command), and visual (e.g., make sudden movement toward child, wave hands in front of child's face).
- Is the child performing inappropriate activities (verbalization: strange words, mumbling, cursing; combative, agitated; wandering, performing activities without awareness)?

Muscle Movement/Tone
- Note general postural change or specific muscle movements; observe location and specific activity. If bilateral, note whether it was symmetric.
- Observe for purposeful movements and automatisms (repetitive, purposeless movements).
- Assess muscle tone. Is it normal, increased (tonic, spastic, rigid), or decreased (limp, flaccid)?

Physiologic Responses
- Assess for autonomic symptoms (color change, perspiration, skin temperature change, drooling, increased heart rate, blood pressure, bladder and sphincter tone).
- Check pupil reactivity.
- Note apnea.

Postictal
- Assess for possible incontinence resulting from muscle relaxation.
- Describe child's behavior.
- Ask child what he or she remembers before, during, and after seizure.
- Note length of time until child resumes normal behavior and activities.

- If confusion or disorientation is present, describe and note duration.
- Note presence of any temporary deficits (memory loss, aphasia, paresis).

Interventions
- Remain with child; provide privacy as possible.
- Direct movements during seizure to prevent injury:
  - Do not restrain or restrict the child's movements.
  - Move any harmful objects away from the child.
  - If the child is walking and headed for a dangerous situation (e.g., open stairs), attempt to steer the child in a safe direction.
  - Assist or move child into a lying position on the floor, if necessary and possible.
- Monitor neurologic status, behavior, and vital signs.
- Administer medication, as ordered, and monitor for side effects.
- Reassure and provide psychosocial support to child and bystanders.
- When the event is finished
  - Turn the child to a side-lying position.
  - Position to maintain airway.
  - Turn head toward the side to prevent choking and aspiration.
  - If the child is lying on the floor, place something soft under the head.
  - Monitor until child returns to baseline status.

Documentation
- When and where the seizure began (date, time of day, preseizure activity of child)
- Whether the onset and entirety of seizure were observed
- Duration of seizure, preseizure activity.
- Any warning signs that the seizure was about to happen (aura)
- Clinical characteristics (specific description of movements and behaviors, including description of progression)
- Level of consciousness
- Signs and symptoms after the seizure stopped (postictal events)
- Child's memory of events

EVIDENCE-BASED CLINICAL PRACTICE GUIDELINES 21-1
Seizure Management

American Association of Neuroscience Nurses

American Association of Neuroscience Nurses. (2009). *Care of the patient with seizures* (2nd ed.). Glenview, IL: Author. Retrieved from

http://www.aann.org/pdf/cpg/aannseizures.pdf

Provides information about the classification, epidemiology, and pathophysiology of seizure disorders and neurologic assessment and management of the patient with seizures.

Neurocritical Care Society

Brophy, G. M., Bell, R., Claassen, J. et al. (2012). Guidelines for the evaluation and management of status epilepticus. *Neurocritical Care, 17*(1), 3–23. Retrieved from

http://www.springerlink.com/content/58p64531795312j1/fulltext.html

Recommendations for the evaluation and management of status epilepticus in critically ill patients.

American Academy of Neurology

Go, C. Y., Mackay, M. T., Weiss, S. K. et al. (2012). Evidence-based guideline update: Medical treatment of infantile spasms. Report of the Guideline Development Subcommittee of the American Academy of Neurology and the Practice Committee of the Child Neurology Society. *Neurology, 78*(24), 1974–1980. Retrieved from

http://www.neurology.org/content/78/24/1974.full.pdf + html

Recommendations regarding pharmacologic treatment of the child with infantile spasms.

American Academy of Neurology

Hirtz, D., Berg, A., Bettis, D. et al. (2003). Practice parameter: Treatment of the child with a first unprovoked seizure. Report of the Quality Standards Subcommittee of the American Academy of Neurology and the Practice Committee of the Child Neurology Society. *Neurology, 60*(2), 166–175. Retrieved from

http://www.neurology.org/content/60/2/166.full.pdf

Recommendations regarding the child with an unprovoked seizure; includes differential diagnosis and workup.

American Academy of Pediatrics

Steering Committee on Quality Improvement and Management, Subcommittee on Febrile Seizures. (2008). Febrile seizures: Clinical practice guideline for the long-term management of the child with simple febrile seizures. *Pediatrics, 121*(6), 1281–1286. Retrieved from

http://pediatrics.aappublications.org/content/121/6/1281.full.pdf + html?sid = aaec9a56-c1d9-42b6-a37a-8a4c620463b9

Reviews evidence for long-term management of the child with simple febrile seizures.

Initial Management

Initial management of the child with a seizure involves basic first aid and is similar regardless of the seizure type:

- Remain calm and stay with the child.
- Protect the child from any additional injury; use common sense.
- Provide time for the child to recover after the seizure stops.
- Reassure and provide support to the child and to others (see Nursing Interventions 21-2).

caREminder

Do not insert a tongue blade or similar object into the child's mouth because it may cause injuries. Do not give the child anything to eat or drink until he or she has clearly recovered from the seizure as evidenced by complete recovery from seizure activity, full alertness, and return of normal motor function.

Protecting the child from injury depends on what happens during the seizure. Individuals experiencing only staring or altered responsiveness may require no initial intervention other than someone standing by to make sure that the child does not fall or lose balance. Speak softly, if at all, to the child with altered responsiveness to avoid agitating or confusing the child.

If the child is having altered sensations or perceptions, acknowledge these states. Reassure the child that he or she is safe and that the experience will soon be over.

Recovery time after a seizure varies. Some children can immediately return to activities. Other children may be confused or may fall deeply asleep for several hours.

 KidKare After recovery, reassure the child in a manner similar to this: "You just had a seizure and it is over now; everything is OK."

The child's questions determine whether he or she needs more information to understand the experience. Young children witnessing a seizure may think that the child is dying, having a tantrum, choking, or misbehaving. Adults often think the same thing. Again, simple explanations are helpful. Statements, such as, "It's OK; he's having a seizure and it will be over soon," can be tremendously reassuring if delivered in a calm, confident manner by the nurse.

It may not be necessary to call for emergency help during a seizure because the event is self-limiting and, by itself, does not injure the child. However, seek emergency help if

- The child does not start breathing after the seizure, in which case initiate artificial ventilation
- The seizure activity continues for longer than 5 minutes
- The child has one seizure after another without regaining consciousness between the seizures
- The child has sustained serious injuries

If this is the child's first seizure, or if the child is experiencing status epilepticus, emergency care is warranted to treat, monitor, and stabilize the child's condition.

Treatment of the child with status epilepticus includes rapidly treating the seizure itself, treating the underlying cause, and providing supportive care. Almost simultaneously in an emergency setting, an airway is secured, cardiac status is evaluated, vital signs are measured, an IV line is established, blood is drawn, antiepileptic drugs are given, and diagnostic tests are completed. Blood is usually drawn to obtain glucose level, complete blood count, electrolytes, calcium, magnesium, phosphorus, and antiepileptic drug levels (if appropriate) and for blood culture. IV glucose is administered using a 2-mL/kg dose of 25% glucose in children and a 5-mL/kg dose of 10% glucose in infants younger than 6 months of age.

Pharmacologic Interventions

In treating status epilepticus, the most common mistake is failing to give a sufficient amount of drug early enough. In the acute care setting, first-line therapy is a benzodiazepine (lorazepam as first choice) given intravenously, followed by phenytoin or fosphenytoin, then phenobarbital, valproate, or levetiracetam. If IV access cannot be established, diazepam rectal gel may be used. In the prehospital phase, because establishing IV access in a child with seizures can be challenging and time consuming, intramuscular treatments are given more quickly and reliably with equal or better efficacy. Intramuscular midazolam is as safe and effective as IV lorazepam for seizure cessation (Silbergleit et al., 2012). If the seizures persist, an infusion of midazolam, pentobarbital, or propofol may be started (Brophy et al., 2012). Monitor electrocardiogram and blood pressure closely while administering medications. Immediately treat any identified abnormalities. After early, aggressive treatment has brought status epilepticus under control, maintenance therapy is initiated. Antiepileptic drugs are always tapered in dosage to the point of complete withdrawal; the drug should not be stopped suddenly. Further information on maintenance antiepileptic drug therapy can be found in the discussion of epilepsy.

The dosages of antiepileptic drugs used to treat status epilepticus cause decreased responsiveness, with the potential for ineffective breathing patterns and ineffective airway clearance. Less common, but more serious, reactions may include allergic and other idiosyncratic responses. Nursing care involves monitoring serum drug levels and seizure activity; laboratory testing; monitoring oxygenation, vital signs, and lung sounds; assessing the adequacy of breathing patterns; and airway clearance. To minimize aspiration and airway problems, position the child in a side-lying position, and turn every 2 hours.

Safety Measures

Protect a child undergoing a seizure from falls and injuries, aspiration pneumonia, hyperthermia, and drug side effects. Children with seizure-related falls and injuries may have fractures, dislocations, lacerations, or hematomas. Risk also exists for injury secondary to continued seizure activity. Nursing care includes continuous observation of the child. Institute seizure precautions as indicated, including padding the side rails, keeping the bed in the lowest position with raised side rails, removing harmful objects from the child's environment, and having bag–valve–mask ventilation and suction readily available. In addition, administer medications as ordered, monitoring the child for possible side effects and checking drug levels as ordered. Teaching the child and family about precipitating factors, medications, use of a MedicAlert identification, and basic seizure management is also important to maintain the child's safety (Community Care 21-1).

Aspiration pneumonia can occur from choking on food or other objects in the child's mouth or from aspiration of vomitus. Nursing care may include suctioning, positioning of the child in a semiprone or side-lying position, monitoring vital signs and lung sounds, inserting a nasogastric tube, and ensuring that the child is NPO until he or she has recovered from the seizure and from the depressant side effects of antiepileptic drugs and gag and swallow reflexes are adequate.

Hyperthermia may occur as a symptom of CNS infection, or it may occur as a result of continued status epilepticus, especially when motor symptoms are involved. Nursing care may include keeping the child in minimal, light clothing; giving tepid sponge baths; monitoring temperature; and using cooling devices.

Supportive Care

The level of self-care deficit depends on the type of seizure and how consciousness and responsiveness are affected. If the child is unconscious, nursing care includes providing adequate fluids and nutrition, starting with NPO status, IV fluids, and enteric feeding until the child recovers, then progressing to oral food and fluids as tolerated. Assess skin integrity; turn and position at least every 2 hours; and provide hygiene related to urine and bowel incontinence, eye care if the eyelids do not shut, and oral hygiene.

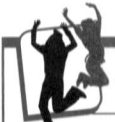

COMMUNITY CARE 21-1

Safety for the Child With Poorly Controlled Seizures

General
- Have the child wear a MedicAlert bracelet.
- Keep emergency treatment medication readily available, if prescribed.
- Teach care providers outside of family about child's condition and treatments.

Falls and Injury Prevention
Increase safety of child's environment:
- Remove potentially harmful objects from child's environment (sharp corners, objects).
- Use carpeting and padding.
- Place barriers at open stairways.
- Use chairs with arms.
- Have child wear a protective helmet.
- Have child avoid stairs or use with supervision.
- Allow child to participate in age-appropriate activities with appropriate safety equipment (e.g., bike helmets, elbow and knee pads); do not allow participation in antigravitational activities (e.g., wall/rope climbing, monkey bars).

Water Safety
- Have the child bathe with supervision, using minimal water levels, and pad the fixtures.
- Allow older children to shower, if preferred, when a responsible other can routinely check on their safety. Leave the door unlocked.
- Ensure that the child swims under lifeguard supervision with a buddy.

Sleep Safety
- Use low bed, away from furniture.
- Use thin pillow and minimal padding in sleep area (pillows, stuffed animals, comforters).
- Use infant monitor.

EPILEPSY

Epilepsy is a chronic condition characterized by recurrent seizures, but the terms *seizure* and *epilepsy* are not synonymous. Many types of seizures do not fall under the classification of epilepsy. Epilepsy has numerous causes and is not a single disease entity; rather, it is an indication of brain dysfunction.

Epilepsy may be the only evidence of an underlying brain abnormality, or it may be one of many symptoms. The younger the child at the onset of symptoms, the greater the likelihood that the cause of the disorder will be identified. A familial predisposition to epilepsy appears to exist. Evidence from sibling, offspring, and twin studies points to a genetic component, although it is poorly defined. In most cases, epilepsy is idiopathic (without an identifiable cause).

Epilepsy syndromes are defined as clusters of signs and symptoms that tend to occur together. They are classified as focal or generalized and as idiopathic or symptomatic (associated with a known disorder). Identifying a specific epilepsy syndrome is helpful in making treatment decisions and determining prognosis. Some epileptic syndromes include the following:

- Benign rolandic epilepsy: One of the most common syndromes; usually occurs between 4 and 11 years of age, typically in boys. Characterized by partial seizures at night (described as tingling sensations on the side of the face), inability to talk without loss of consciousness; possible secondary generalization; normal neurologic examination, typically with normal development and intelligence in child. There often is a positive family history. An EEG demonstrates a distinctive diagnostic pattern. Antiepileptic agents (carbamazepine) are given only if seizures are occurring frequently or during the day.
- Infantile spasms: Age-dependent epilepsy syndrome, usually between 3 and 12 months of age. Characterized by clusters of myoclonic seizures. Cause is known (symptomatic, such as neurocutaneous disorders, brain malformations, metabolic and degenerative diseases) or unknown (cryptogenic). Seizures consist of sudden flexor or extensor movements of the neck, trunk, and extremities and occur in clusters of up to 100 spasms. It is possibly difficult to differentiate from colic or a startle reflex. An EEG will demonstrate a distinctive pattern called *hypsarrhythmia*. Infantile spasms are associated with developmental delay, although early treatment may lead to improved development. Spasms are resistant to conventional antiepileptic medications, and treatment usually consists of daily intramuscular injection of adrenocorticotropic hormone with potential side effects (hypertension, hyperglycemia, and gastrointestinal bleeding). *West syndrome* is a subtype of infantile spasms with a triad of symptoms: infantile spasms, intellectual disability or developmental delay, and hypsarrhythmia on EEG.
- Lennox-Gastaut syndrome: Is characterized by multiple seizure types, including tonic, atonic, atypical absence, and episodes of tonic and nonconvulsive status epilepticus, with an onset usually between ages 1 and 7 years. Multiple causes are associated with this syndrome, but most children have a brain lesion. EEG demonstrates a typical pattern of slow spike and wave. Most children have cognitive deficits. Seizures are highly resistant to treatment and require multiple medications.

Assessment

A diagnosis of epilepsy is made on the basis of clinical data and historical information. A specific history obtained from someone who witnessed the seizure is extremely helpful in establishing the diagnosis. An EEG can provide supportive evidence and can aid in classification and treatment of the disorder. Indications for further workup may include failure of medications or specific findings on the neurologic examination that indicate an underlying brain abnormality.

Interdisciplinary Interventions

The child with epilepsy requires intervention from an interdisciplinary health team. From acute to chronic care, nurses are often the best resource for organizing, planning, and evaluating the complexities of epilepsy management. The manifestations of this condition are frightening, yet most pediatric epilepsies can be successfully controlled.

Management of the child with epilepsy includes managing seizures, educating the family and the child, and addressing associated emotional or learning disabilities (Clinical Judgment 21-1). Treatment with medications is the mainstay of epilepsy management. Alternative therapies, including surgery, ketogenic diet, or vagal nerve stimulation, may be options for the child with seizures that are unresponsive to drug therapy. Supportive care is discussed in the section on "Seizures."

Pharmacologic Interventions

The goal of drug therapy is optimal seizure control with minimal side effects (see thePoint for Medications and Administration: Antiepileptic Medications). Drug

---

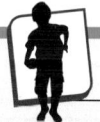

CLINICAL JUDGMENT 21-1

The Child Who Presents With Seizures

Four-year-old Dwayne is brought to the clinic by his mother because he had a seizure earlier in the morning. His mother describes the seizure as jerking movements of the arms and legs with drooling from the mouth. Dwayne was very tired after the seizure and fell asleep. Dwayne has had three similar episodes in the past, so his mother decided to wait until he awoke to come to the clinic. His previous seizures occurred when he was 1 year, 2½ years, and 3½ years old. All these seizures were associated with a fever and illness. Dwayne has had a cold for the past 4 days. His mother has not taken his temperature but has been giving him acetaminophen because he felt warm.

Questions

1. What other information would you collect from the mother at this time?

2. What type of seizure might Dwayne be exhibiting?

3. Dwayne has an EEG that reveals consistent findings for the diagnosis of epilepsy. He will be placed on an antiepileptic medication. What nursing diagnosis would you select to reflect the family's teaching needs at this time?

4. When Dwayne returns to the clinic 1 month later, what data should be reviewed with the family?

5. What information would help you determine that Dwayne and his family are responding well to his treatment plan?

Answers

1. More information regarding diagnostic tests and treatment measures that occurred when Dwayne had other seizures; family history of seizures; Dwayne's ability to meet age-appropriate developmental milestones; history of recent ear infections, other illnesses, or immunizations; medications he is taking. Ask mother to provide more details of when the seizure occurred, how long it lasted, the child's responsiveness during and after the seizure, and behaviors seen during the seizure.

2. Simple febrile seizure, complex febrile seizure, exposure to medications or toxins, or epilepsy

3. Deficient knowledge: Management of epilepsy, or health-seeking behaviors: Management of epilepsy

4. Review parent and child's perception and understanding of diagnosis, treatment plan, and future course of illness; discuss the importance of monitoring the child's development. Review medication schedule, dosage, and side effects. Review parental interventions if Dwayne has another seizure. Determine whether other child care providers are prepared to assist Dwayne if he has a seizure when in their care.

5. Family reports medications are given as scheduled with no difficulty encountered in refilling the prescription as needed, family attends all scheduled clinic visits, Dwayne has no seizure activity, drug levels are within therapeutic ranges, and Dwayne continues to progress well developmentally

treatment typically begins with one antiepileptic agent, and the dosage is increased gradually until seizures are controlled, clinically significant toxicity is experienced, or serum drug levels reach the high end of the therapeutic range without controlling the seizures. If the first drug is ineffective, a second is added, or another drug is tried. Pay careful attention to the potential for drug interactions when the child is being treated with more than one medication. During this process, ensure that the child and family are aware of the need to report changes in sensation, behavior, or clinical symptoms, such as poor balance, bleeding, or icteric sclera, that may signal a toxic reaction and that they understand the importance of close follow-up care. Some antiepileptic medications require periodic serum blood levels to assess drug metabolism and effectiveness. Many newer antiepileptic medications do not require blood testing; efficacy is determined by dose and seizure control as described by the child and family.

Antiepileptic therapy is usually continued until the child has been seizure-free for 18 to 24 months and the EEG is normal. Antiepileptic medications must be tapered and not stopped abruptly.

Surgical Interventions

Epilepsy surgery may be indicated for children with intractable or uncontrolled seizures who have not gained seizure control after therapeutic trials with the most appropriate antiepileptic drugs. In the absence of a tumor causing the epilepsy, the epileptic focus is removed. Such children should be referred to a medical center for a comprehensive epilepsy evaluation. Prolonged EEG monitoring with surgically implanted depth electrodes or an electrode grid may be required to more clearly define the epileptogenic focus. Potential candidates for lobectomy may also undergo an intracarotid amobarbital test (Wada) angiogram to localize the speech center. Neuropsychological testing as well as evaluations with psychologists and speech, physical, and occupational therapists are usually completed. Appropriate medical selection of the children who may benefit from this procedure is essential. Seizures must be focal, intractable to medical management, and must arise from an area of the brain that could be removed without significant neurologic deficit.

Alternative Therapies

Alternative therapies such as the ketogenic diet have been used to treat refractory epilepsy. This diet has been found to be especially effective for myoclonic epilepsies, but it is effective for other types of epilepsy as well. It is often tried for seizures associated with Lennox-Gastaut syndrome, with varying results. A multidisciplinary team is needed to manage the child on the ketogenic diet, including the nurse, dietitian, neurologist, primary care provider, and pharmacist. Because the ketogenic diet is high in fat and low in carbohydrates, monitor the child carefully for hypoglycemia and ketonuria. The diet requires commitment by the family because it is very restrictive. Use of less restrictive diets such as modified Atkins or low-glycemic index diets are also being used in managing epilepsy (Kossoff & Hartman, 2012).

Electrical Therapies

Vagus nerve stimulator therapy controls seizures by delivering an intermittent electrical impulse to the brain. A pacemaker-like device, implanted under the skin in the left chest, sends mild, intermittent electrical impulses through a lead to the left vagus nerve, which then sends signals to the brain.

Community Care

Family members must make a commitment to maintain close medical follow-up through outpatient clinic visits, consent to periodic diagnostic evaluations, and comply with recommended drug therapy. Education should be an ongoing, individually tailored process. Because of the chronic nature of epilepsy, the plan of care must allow for changes based on physical growth and emotional maturation. Siblings and extended family may provide valuable support if they are included in the overall treatment regimen.

Educating children and their family is crucial to seizure control. Children want to know as much as their parents and to have information presented at their level (McNelis et al., 2007). Parents want to know about all aspects of the conditions. In one study, parents felt that they were not given enough information about the condition, treatment plans, or medications and felt that information should be given over time (McNelis et al., 2007). Provide the family with information about the child's seizure type, events that can trigger seizures, seizure recognition, initial seizure management, medications, and the potential effect of seizures and medication on early development and behavior (Teaching Intervention Plan 21-2). Also include teaching about status epilepticus and the need for emergency care.

The Epilepsy Foundation of America (see thePoint for Organizations) offers a comprehensive teaching and support program and can provide information appropriate for children, families, and teachers in both English and Spanish.

Although most children with epilepsy have normal intelligence, comorbid conditions such as attention-deficit/hyperactivity disorder, depression, and anxiety may occur. These may result from the epilepsy itself, or they may be side effects from antiepileptic drugs. These conditions affect the child both at home and at school and can influence academic success considerably. Upon family request, facilitate a conference with school staff to identify the child's specific needs and treatment plan and to alert the school staff of any potential side effects of medications. The child may qualify for special education services under the Individuals with Disabilities Education Act. Adaptations may have to be made in the educational plan so that the child can succeed (see Chapters 2 and 12).

Encourage the family to provide a MedicAlert bracelet for the child to wear at all times. A helmet may be necessary for children with kinetic, or "drop," seizures or for those children with substantial delays in motor development. Encourage the family to focus attention on well siblings who may have unexpressed fears about

TIP 21-2: A TEACHING INTERVENTION PLAN for the Child With Epilepsy

Nursing Diagnoses and Family Outcomes

- Risk for injury related to hypoxia, aspiration, and loss of or impaired consciousness
  Outcome: Child will remain free from injury, aspiration, or respiratory distress during a seizure.
- Deficient knowledge: Medications, diet, and management of child during a seizure
  Outcomes: Family administers medications safely to the child.
  Family verbalizes side effects of medications.
  Family identifies when treatment plan is not controlling child's seizures.

Teach the Child/Family

Management of the Child During a Seizure
- Refer to Interventions section in Nursing Interventions 21-2.
- Remove sharp objects and hazards from area around the child.
- Loosen tight clothing.
- Do not put anything into the child's mouth.
- Remove the child's eyeglasses to prevent injury to face.
- Allow seizure to end without interference.
- After the seizure, position the child in side-lying position with head in a midline position. Do not hyperextend the neck. If child vomits, carefully turn the child to the right side to prevent aspiration.
- Observe and document details of the child's seizure, including activity before, during, and after; date, time, and length of episode; and child's physical status during seizure (e.g., incontinence, difficulty breathing, paralysis, loss of consciousness).
- Observe the child's respiratory status during seizure. If breathing becomes impaired, call for emergency medical assistance.

Preventing Seizures
- Give medications as ordered. Consistent drug therapy is critical.

- Avoid events, activities, or stimuli that trigger seizure activity.
- Inform teachers or daycare providers about child's condition and how to intervene if a seizure occurs.

Medications
- Ensure that family knows names of drugs, amount, time to be administered, why they must be given consistently, why antiepileptics cannot be stopped abruptly, and possible side effects.
- Monitor for side effects such as drowsiness, lethargy, ataxia, nystagmus, and gastrointestinal upset.
- Take the child to the health care provider for scheduled evaluations of therapeutic drug levels and blood counts if indicated.
- Ensure that family and child care providers/school know when and how to administer "rescue" seizure mediations such as rectal diazepam.

Nutrition
- Provide instructions regarding ketogenic diet if used for seizure control.
- Encourage adequate intake of vitamin D and folic acid if child is taking phenytoin or phenobarbital.

Activity
- Be aware of the need for possible activity restrictions depending on frequency of seizures and degree of seizure control that is maintained.
- Provide supervision during activities such as swimming or bicycle riding.
- Avoid having the child become overtired.

Contact Health Care Provider if
- Child experiences an increase in seizure activity
- Child is lethargic or listless
- Child has a high fever
- Child is experiencing depression or negative feelings about self because of seizure disorder
- Child experiences breathing difficulties during a seizure

---

the disease or may harbor guilt or anger toward the affected sibling.

BREATH-HOLDING SPELLS

Breath-holding spells are the voluntary cessation of breathing in response to a painful, noxious, or frustrating stimulus. This nonepileptic paroxysmal event may resemble seizures. Breath-holding spells, although dramatic, are considered to be benign. If prolonged, however, they can lead to unconsciousness or convulsion. These spells are most common in children 1 to 3 years of age. In the child older than 6 years of age, breath-holding spells are unusual and require further investigation.

Pathophysiology

Two types of breath-holding spells occur: pallid and cyanotic. Pallid breath-holding spells are vagally mediated events that follow a trivial, unpleasant stimulus such as a bump on the leg or a mild injury to the head. A sudden collapse, pallid color, diaphoresis, and rigid posture with a few extremity jerks are typical. After the precipitating event, the child may lose consciousness. The hypersensitive vagal response also results in bradycardia and, sometimes, asystole. Crying is usually not noted. Sleep may follow the episode.

Cyanotic breath-holding spells are more complex events, precipitated by anger or frustration. In the midst

TABLE 21-2 Differentiating Breath-Holding Spells From Seizures

Characteristic	Breath-Holding Spell	Seizure
Age at onset	6–18 months	Variable depending on cause
Precipitating event	Cyanotic spell: frustration, anger Pallid spell: minor injury, fear	Rarely noted
Crying at onset	Typically present	Not typically noted
Cyanosis	Typically present at onset	Rare at onset of seizure, may occur if seizure is prolonged
Convulsive activity	Occasionally seen	Typically noted
Incontinence	Never	Sometimes occurs
Level of consciousness	Unconscious	Unconscious
Postictal confusion	Uncommon	Common; lethargic, sleepy
Physical examination	Typically normal Bradycardia	Variable Tachycardia
EEG	Typically normal	Typically abnormal

of crying, the child stops breathing during expiration to the point of cyanosis. Cerebral oxygenation decreases, and loss of consciousness follows. There may be associated clonic movements of the extremities.

Pallid and cyanotic breath-holding spells are differentiated from seizures by the events that trigger the spell, time of occurrence (never during sleep), and the progression of events (Table 21-2). EEG is normal between attacks. During an episode, the EEG may show diffuse slowing with rhythmic slowing during the tonic–clonic activity. In both types, cardiac evaluation may be warranted because prolonged QT syndrome or other cardiac events may be the cause (Akalin et al., 2004). Iron-deficiency anemia and autonomic dysregulation may also contribute to breath-holding spells (Kolkiran et al., 2005). Breath-holding spells usually resolve spontaneously, without sequelae.

Interdisciplinary Interventions

Treatment for breath-holding spells is not usually necessary. The child may be treated with iron, which has been demonstrated to decrease the number of spells (Boon, 2002).

If unconsciousness occurs during either type of breath-holding spell, carefully place the child on the floor on his or her side to prevent aspiration. These events may be very frightening, and the family requires explanation and support. Focus family interventions on behavior modification and assisting the child to express anger and frustration in other ways. Advise family members of normal developmental parameters and suggest they not give undue attention to the child after the breath-holding event because attention may unintentionally reinforce continued demonstration of these behaviors.

HEADACHES

Headaches are a common neurologic symptom in childhood; about 20% to 89.5% of children studied have headaches at least once a week (Kernick et al., 2009;

Nyame et al., 2010). Children experience a variety of different headache types, including tension headache, migraine headache, and chronic daily headache.

In general, the term *headache* is used to describe pain or discomfort in the skull or facial structures because the brain has no pain receptors. The pain is referred from dura, blood vessels (traction), dilation of blood vessels, or sustained contraction of muscles.

Headaches are broadly classified as primarily neuronal (migraine or tension type) or secondary to another process (brain tumor, increased ICP, infection) (Table 21-3). Headaches are described as acute, resulting from an acute illness such as meningitis or subarachnoid hemorrhage; acute recurrent, caused by migraine; chronic progressive, caused by intracranial hypertension or tumor; and chronic nonprogressive, possibly caused by muscle contraction (tension). Acute and chronic progressive headaches are of the most concern as potential indicators of underlying neurologic problems. In children, documentation of a specific cause, such as tumor or stroke, is uncommon.

Assessment

Conduct a complete clinical history and examination. Characterizing a headache helps to define the cause (e.g., tumor, tension, migraine). Headaches associated with meningitis or subarachnoid hemorrhage are often described as bursting, with a rapid progression of pain that radiates down the neck and spine. The chronic progressive headache of intracranial hypertension usually presents as aching and throbbing, which is increased by coughing or straining and is present on arising in the morning. Both acute headaches and those associated with intracranial hypertension are associated with other neurologic symptoms, such as papilledema or alterations of consciousness. Muscle contraction (tension-type) headaches are described as bilateral, manifesting diffuse tightness or pressure in a bandlike distribution.

TABLE 21-3   Headaches in Children

| | Primary Headaches | | Secondary Headaches | | | |
	Migraine	Tension Type	Traumatic	Rebound	Infectious	Structural Disorder
Etiology	Primarily a neuronal process, trigeminal activation, hyper-excitable cerebral cortex Likely genetic basis Production of norepinephrine and serotonin resulting from stimulation of brain structures, leading to inflammation of pial and dural blood vessels, stimulation of the trigeminal nerve, and pain	Pathophysiology poorly understood Probably a combination of muscular and central emotional factors	Head or neck trauma; hemorrhage	Substance use/withdrawal (alcohol, drugs), carbon monoxide exposure Medication overuse (e.g., analgesics)	Intracranial infection; occasionally systemic infection	Increased ICP; neoplasm; arteritis; teeth, sinus, or vision disorders
Epidemiology	Occurs at any age, but frequency increases with age. Before puberty, boys more than girls; after puberty, more frequent in girls Atypical migraine variants more common in younger children	Older children	Any age	Older children	Younger children	Any age
Characteristics	Without aura more common in children; unilateral, pulsating, intense pain aggravated by routine physical activity; associated with anorexia, nausea, vomiting, photophobia, phonophobia, overall feeling of exhaustion; relieved by sleep Abdominal symptoms more frequent in children than adults	Bilateral, nonpulsatile, pressing/tight quality; intensity mild or moderate	May be present without obvious sign of trauma Neurologic signs: altered mental status, abnormal eye movement, optic disk distortion	No typical qualities	Diffuse continuous pain, aggravated by straining, nausea, or focal neurologic signs	Diffuse pain, with increased ICP, often worse in morning with associated vomiting (no nausea); symptom onset may be gradual Head circumference may increase if fontanels not fused
Management	Prophylaxis: regular schedule for sleep, meals, exercise Avoidance of caffeine and trigger foods Biobehavioral: biofeedback, relaxation, cognitive control of stress, acupuncture Acute treatment: analgesics, triptans, biobehavioral methods as noted earlier, sleep	Over-the-counter analgesics, sleep, biobehavioral interventions as under Migraine	Manage trauma	Eliminate exposure to toxin (or offending agent) Decrease frequency of analgesic use	Treat infection: antibiotics for bacterial	Manage structural disorder

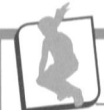

FOCUSED HEALTH HISTORY 21-2

The Child With Headaches

Acute History
- Recent illness
- Injury
- Change in sensory perception or mobility
- Diet or weight change
- New medication or oral contraceptive use
- Level of activity
- Onset of puberty or menses

Chronic History
Pertinent past history of
- Illness, infection, surgery
- Developmental abnormalities
- Dental problems
- Alcohol or drug use
- Allergies
- Visual disturbances or corrections
- Diet, include caffeine and sugar intake
- Sleep patterns
- Family history of migraine or other disorders

Psychosocial Factors
- Perceived stressors
- Scholastic ability
- Feelings of depression or sadness
- Changes in lifestyle
- Concept of self
- Affect
- Appearance
- Relationship with family and friends
- Social activities and hobbies
- Nonverbal cues

- Family history of headache and effect on patient
- Patient's perception of significance of headache (e.g., fear of cause, outcome, diagnosis)
- Past experience with hospitals or health care providers
- Identification of other person in the patient's confidence

Headache Data
- Location
- Duration
- Frequency
- Quality
- Time of occurrence
- Severity
- Accompanying symptoms
- Treatment attempts
- Outcome of treatment
- Documentation of headache pattern
- Presence or lack of prodromal warning (aura)

Pain Assessment
- Type of pain
- Pattern of progression or intensity
- Identification of factors that make pain worse or better
- Specific causes related to headache pain (e.g., bright lights, foods)
- Biobehavioral therapy and effectiveness
- Medication and effectiveness
- Patient's experience with other types of pain

Identification of Headache Triggers
- What factors seem to start headache? Activity, foods, medication, menses, specific stressors, change in environment or seasons, work or school atmosphere?

Note: See Chapter 8 for a comprehensive health history.

Assessment of the child begins with a detailed history of the child's condition (Focused Health History 21-2) to evaluate the characteristics of the headaches and to distinguish any findings that may indicate pathologic abnormality. Indicators such as a recent onset or recent increase in frequency or severity; an occipital or consistently localized headache; head trauma accompanying the headache; behavioral, personality, or gait changes accompanying the headache; complaints that the headache interrupts sleep, is exacerbated by changes in position, or occurs on arising and is accompanied by vomiting and then fades; or headache in a child younger than 3 years of age warrant immediate evaluation.

When examining the child with headaches, include a neurologic assessment, percussion of the sinuses, and notation of blood pressure. Evaluate visual acuity and listen for cranial bruits. The presence of a bruit warrants

further investigation. Children with tension or migraine headaches usually have a normal physical examination.

Diagnostic Tests

Extensive diagnostic investigation is required in acute and chronic progressive headaches to rule out brain tumors or meningitis. This investigation would include neuroimaging and possibly CSF examination.

Nursing Diagnoses and Outcomes

Nursing Plan of Care 21-1 presents a variety of nursing diagnoses that can be applied to the child with a neurologic condition. The following diagnosis also applies specifically to the child with headaches:

Nursing Diagnosis: Acute pain related to effects of pathology

Outcomes:
- Child will not experience pain from headaches.
- Child and family will use measures to reduce factors that precipitate onset of headaches.
- Child and family will implement pain control measures to reduce child's discomfort.

Interdisciplinary Interventions

The goal of therapy is to stop the headaches (see Table 21-3). Treatment for acute or chronic progressive headaches focuses on treating the underlying organic cause and most likely requires hospitalization to provide health care interventions such as surgery, ICP management, or IV antibiotic therapy. Management of chronic nonprogressive headaches usually includes administering mild analgesics and teaching stress management techniques. Treatment of migraines involves using medications and behavioral management as well as teaching patients to avoid headache triggers.

Pharmacologic Interventions

Symptomatic medications (analgesics) to manage pain are available in both over-the-counter and prescription forms. They are most effective if taken at the first sign of a headache. Exercise caution when giving acetaminophen or aspirin to children. Excessive doses of acetaminophen have been linked to hepatic toxicity. Salicylates, such as aspirin, contribute to Reye syndrome. Acetaminophen, ibuprofen, and aspirin are contained in many combination over-the-counter medications. Teach the family that they must read medication labels and not exceed the recommended dose. Acetaminophen and ibuprofen should not be taken more than two to three times a week because of the risk of rebound headache (see Table 21-3) and the development of chronic daily headache.

Pharmacologic therapy for migraine consists of three basic approaches: symptomatic (as noted earlier), abortive, and preventive. *Abortive* medications modify migrainous changes in blood vessels such as triptans. Triptans are serotonin agonists that are available in multiple types of preparations (nasal spray, disintegrating tablets, tablets, or injectable). As with many medications, the U.S. Food and Drug Administration has not approved triptans for use in children, but they are often used off label (see Chapter 9). As with symptomatic medications, it is important that abortive medications be taken as soon as the aura or the headache starts. If the medication is not taken until the headache is well established, it is less likely to relieve the pain.

Preventive therapy is instituted if the frequency of headache has a significant effect on the child's daily life. Preventive therapy includes use of daily doses of tricyclic antidepressants, calcium channel blockers, beta-blockers, alpha-agonists, or antiepileptics. Preventive medications gradually decrease the frequency and intensity of the headaches and may take 4 to 6 weeks to be fully effective. Ensure that the family understands that such medication must be taken every day, not just when the child is experiencing headache. Preventive medications are gradually discontinued several months after the headaches stop.

Biobehavior Management

Headache pain can be incapacitating and may cause children to lose valuable time in school and social activities. A wide variety of foods and other substances are known to be migraine triggers (see thePoint for Supplemental Information: Foods and Products Associated With the Onset of Migraine). Use a headache calendar or diary to assist the family in identifying which substances and activities may be acting as triggers. Avoiding these substances may prevent recurring headaches. If stress is a major factor in triggering headaches, suggest supportive counseling through hospital, school, community, or religious resources. School attendance should be mandatory. Encourage the family to arrange for medication to be available at school and, with parental permission, provide information for school personnel so they understand the importance of providing the medication as soon as the headache starts. Enlist the support and observation of school counselors. If the child needs to remain at home, encourage bed rest, with a return to school the same day if the headache recedes. Teach the family to give minimal attention to the headache to avoid creating a situation in which the child uses headaches to draw unnecessary attention or as a means to avoid school.

Other interventions include providing a dark, quiet environment. Therapeutic touch or massage therapy may help. The use of biofeedback mechanisms is also useful and may help avoid heavy use of pharmaceuticals.

Provide education to the child and family regarding types of headaches, preventive measures, and judicious use of medication. If the child requires acute pain management, pharmacologic interventions must precede implementation of the longer term strategies. Teach the child to maintain a regular schedule of sleep, intake (do not skip meals), and physical activity and to limit caffeine consumption and avoid smoke (both active and secondhand).

CENTRAL NERVOUS SYSTEM ANOMALIES

Most CNS anomalies present at birth result from abnormalities in the formation of the neural tube or disordered development of neurons in the fetal brain. Others result from abnormal formation of the bony covering of the nervous system. Many of these anomalies are genetic. The most serious defects involve large portions of the spinal column and brain. Smaller defects may be limited to specific areas. Severity of the anomaly is related to its location, size, and degree to which the nerve tissue is involved. Neural tube defects (NTDs), hydrocephalus, Chiari malformation, and craniofacial abnormalities are examples of congenital disorders discussed in this chapter.

NEURAL TUBE DEFECTS

Defects in the formation of the neural tube (neurulation defects) result in **dysraphic defects**: structural malformations of the brain and spinal cord arising from interplay among genetic and environmental factors. Anencephaly, encephalocele, and spina bifida are examples of dysraphic defects resulting from incomplete closure of the neural tube. Thus they are termed *neural tube defects* (Table 21-4).

TABLE 21-4   Common Neural Tube Defects

Type	Description	Outcomes
Anencephaly	Failure of anterior neural tube closure, resulting in only rudimentary development of the brain stem and basal ganglia with no bony covering of the dorsal skull area	Sustained extrauterine life is virtually impossible; most stillborn, remainder die during neonatal period.
Encephalocele	An external sac or mass that may occur at any point over the vertex or base of the skull May be covered with either scalp or a transparent membrane	Dependent on presence of hydrocephalus, infection, actual rupture of the encephalocele, and amount of neural tissue in sac.
Spina bifida cystica	Incomplete fusion of one or more vertebral laminae, resulting in an external protrusion of the spinal tissue; occurs most commonly in lumbosacral area Meningomyelocele: protruding saclike structure contains meninges, spinal fluid, and neural tissue Meningocele: protruding sac contains meninges and CSF	Spinal roots may terminate in sac, which significantly affects motor and sensory function below that point. Neurologic complications are less severe than in meningomyelocele.
Spina bifida occulta	Incomplete fusion of vertebra at one level that may be signaled only by an overlying dimple or tuft of hair	Usually, there is no evidence of dermatologic, neurologic, or musculoskeletal disorders. It may present some of these problems in late childhood.

Since the introduction of folic acid supplementation three decades ago, the overall prevalence of NTDs has decreased. In addition, antenatal testing procedures can be used to detect NTDs early, permitting termination of the pregnancy, if desired.

The cause of NTDs is multifactorial. NTDs may occur as a result of various chromosomal aberrations or after fetal exposure to teratogenic drugs, but exact reasons for abnormal closure of the neural tube remain unclear. Factors associated with NTDs include

- Poor nutrition: Folic acid deficiency; zinc and generalized vitamin deficiencies are also thought to be contributing factors, as is maternal obesity.
- Maternal age: Adolescents and women older than 35 years of age are at greater risk for newborns with NTDs.
- Pregnancy history: Women who miscarry during the pregnancy immediately preceding the current pregnancy are thought to be at higher risk.
- Birth order: Firstborn children are at highest risk.
- Socioeconomic status: The prevalence of NTDs is higher in groups with low socioeconomic status, possibly because of poor nutrition.

The increased incidence of NTDs in siblings underscores the importance of genetic counseling and proper periconceptual nutrition. Dietary sources of supplemental folic acid seem imperative, particularly in genetically vulnerable families.

Pathophysiology

Malformations of the neural tube usually involve malformations of the laminae and pedicles of the vertebral column. The formation of the bony vertebral column occurs simultaneously with the formation of the neural tube, except that the vertebral column originates from mesodermal, rather than ectodermal, cells. If the neural tube either fails to close properly on either end or becomes overdistended and ruptures after initial normal closure, then the NTD occurs.

Anencephaly is one of the most severe congenital neurologic anomalies. There is no treatment.

Spina bifida, or myelodysplasia, refers to incomplete closure of the primary neural tube. Of the defects collectively termed *spina bifida*, 95% are meningomyeloceles, the most severe form of spina bifida. The remaining 5% are meningoceles, and because they do not involve the spinal cord, they may be easier to repair and are often asymptomatic. The most common site of involvement in the spine is the lower thoracic, lumbar, or sacral area (Fig. 21-3).

Although the pathologic abnormalities observed at the site of the open spinal defect are the most obvious, other abnormalities are often found throughout the brain, spinal canal, and other body systems, such as the genitourinary and cardiovascular systems. The degree of functional impairment associated with the various types of spina bifida depends on the level and the extent of the associated defects. The neurologic findings usually correlate with the particular muscle groups (myotomes) that are innervated by affected spinal cord segments.

Assessment

An infant with anencephaly presents with portions of the forebrain and parts of the brain stem that appear to have little definable structure. The exposed neural tissue resembles a mass of hemorrhagic, fibrotic, degenerated neural tissue; the frontal, parietal, and parts of the occipital bone structure are usually absent. The physical appearance of the infant is grossly abnormal.

Immediately after delivery of a newborn with spina bifida, a team of specialists completes a comprehensive evaluation.

caREminder

In addition to the appropriate delivery room routines, take care to protect the newborn's spinal or cranial lesion from injury and infection.

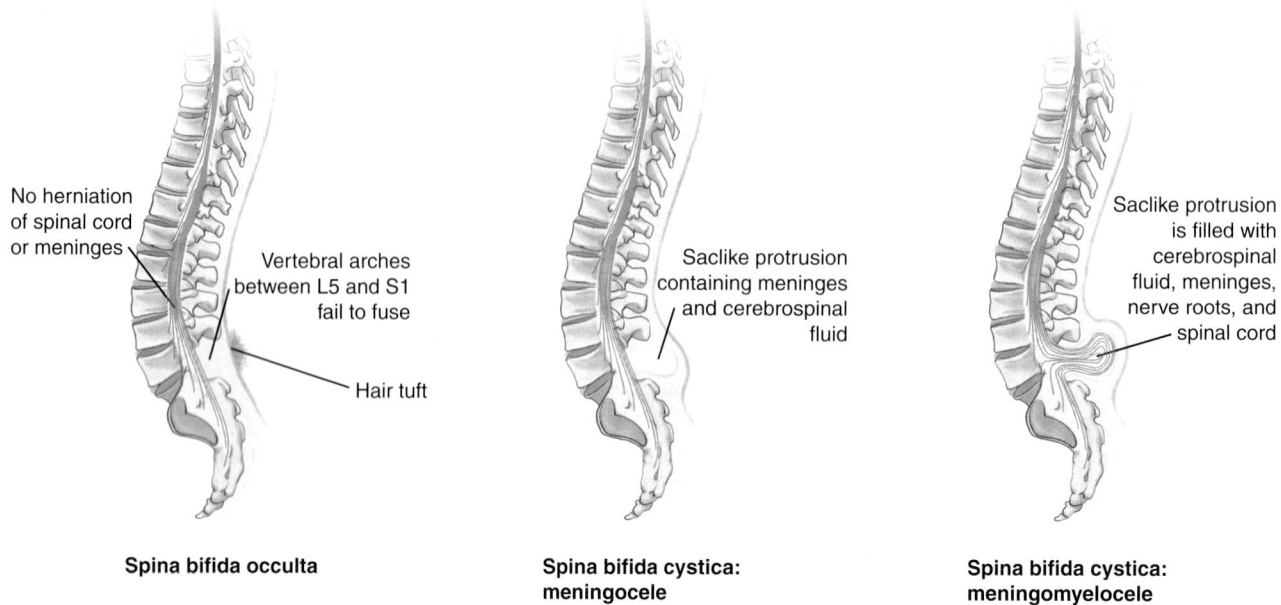

No herniation
of spinal cord
or meninges

Vertebral arches
between L5 and S1
fail to fuse

Hair tuft

Saclike protrusion
containing meninges
and cerebrospinal
fluid

Saclike protrusion
is filled with
cerebrospinal
fluid, meninges,
nerve roots, and
spinal cord

Spina bifida occulta

**Spina bifida cystica:
meningocele**

**Spina bifida cystica:
meningomyelocele**

Figure 21-3 Malformations of the spine.

As soon as possible, take the infant from the delivery room to the specialty care nursery for close monitoring and examination. A complete physical examination with attention to the NTD itself, the presence or absence of hydrocephalus, degree of nerve involvement, and motor and sensory functional capacities is needed. The possibility of associated cardiac, renal, or gastrointestinal conditions that might interfere with early surgery must also be ruled out. This evaluation is best accomplished in medical centers with spina bifida teams and may require transporting the infant to a tertiary care hospital.

The defect is examined in regard to size, level, and nature of tissue covering. Any leakage of CSF is noted. The cranial sutures and fontanels are palpated, and head circumference is measured. Development and movement of upper and lower extremities are assessed. An initial evaluation of bowel and bladder function is also carried out.

Assess the degree of neurologic dysfunction. The dysfunction secondary to spina bifida can range from complete paralysis to minimal involvement; most often, it is somewhere in between. A lesion at the middle thoracic level causes total paralysis of the lower extremities. The more common lumbosacral lesions generally leave children with some degree of hip, knee, or ankle flexion, enabling them to walk, either with braces and crutches or with minimal assistive devices, depending on the functional level of the lesion. Closed or nonvisible lesions (spina bifida occulta) often go undiagnosed until later in childhood and are frequently not associated with any impairment.

In most lumbosacral lesions, the muscles of the legs are affected, and the electrical responses of these muscles may vary. Sensory disturbances are usually symmetric but patchy. Determine sensory level with a dermatome chart, which is used to delineate areas of skin innervated by each sensory spinal nerve.

Clubfeet, scoliosis, contractures, and dislocated hips are common in children born with lesions of the lumbosacral area. Bowel and bladder dysfunction such as constipation, incontinence, or urinary tract infections are almost always apparent because the nerves that supply these organs are located in the sacral area. The clinical manifestations associated with all the lesions of spina bifida are only as clear as the diagnostic assessment of functional capacity.

Diagnostic Tests

With many NTDs, prenatal diagnosis is possible using assays of fetal amniotic fluid, ultrasonography, or maternal serum to determine elevated maternal serum α-fetoprotein concentrations. However, false-positive results may occur with maternal serum α-fetoprotein assays, resulting in unnecessary prenatal anxiety for parents.

Measurement of maternal serum α-fetoprotein between 16 and 18 weeks' gestation aids in determining NTDs. This level is typically elevated in open NTDs. Level II ultrasonography can determine specific structural defects and is typically performed after detection of high levels of maternal serum α-fetoprotein. Three- or four-dimensional ultrasound provides additional clarity. Ultrasonography is also useful in prenatal detection of closed NTDs, in which α-fetoprotein levels are not elevated. Amniotic α-fetoprotein, which detects a majority of all open NTDs, can be obtained; however, amniocentesis increases the risk of pregnancy loss.

CT or MRI will be performed to delineate the anatomy of the herniated mass. Ultrasound or CT studies of the head are done to determine the degree of hydrocephalus present. Diagnostic studies to monitor urinary tract and renal function may be obtained.

Nursing Diagnoses and Outcomes

Nursing Plan of Care 21-1 identifies a variety of nursing diagnoses that can be applied to the child with a neurologic condition. The following diagnoses also apply specifically to the child with spina bifida:

Nursing Diagnosis: Risk for infection related to inadequate primary defenses (broken skin), sequelae of invasive procedures (shunt placement)

Outcomes:
- Child's lesion or incision will remain protected to prevent infection (e.g., meningitis, urinary tract infection, decubitus).
- Child will be free from urinary stasis.
- Child will be free from breaks in skin integrity.

Nursing Diagnosis: Bowel incontinence related to effects of decreased innervation of lower intestinal tract

Outcomes:
- Child will not be constipated.
- Child will learn measures to control bowel function.
- When appropriate for age, child will participate in bowel-training program.

Nursing Diagnosis: Impaired urinary elimination related to urinary retention associated with decreased innervation of bladder and sphincter

Outcomes:
- Child will remain free from urinary tract infection.
- Child's bladder will be emptied at regular intervals.
- When appropriate for age, child will participate in bladder-training program.

Nursing Diagnosis: Risk for injury related to exposure to latex

Outcomes:
- Child and family will be able to identify and avoid substances containing latex.
- Child will remain free of exposure to latex and will take latex precautions during all health care encounters.

Interdisciplinary Interventions

In light of the physical defects, be particularly sensitive in handling the postpartum experience with involved family members. Supportive care is given to the infant with anencephaly until all body functions cease. Social work and pastoral care may provide the most beneficial interventions. Parents will likely require medical and nursing services to answer genetic and physiologic questions. Each family responds to the situation in different ways; assess their needs individually.

Surgical Interventions

Fetal surgery for NTDs, specifically for meningomyelocele, covers the defect with skin to protect it from further damage from contact with amniotic fluid, which may lessen the resulting neurologic deficit. Early results of this approach suggest a lower incidence of hydrocephalus and hindbrain herniation in infants who underwent prenatal closure of the NTD (Saadai & Farmer, 2012). However, further long-term study and development of fetal surgical techniques are needed before fetal surgery can be considered a treatment option for NTDs.

After birth, early neurosurgical treatment for the infant is aimed at preventing infection such as meningitis by surgical reduction and closure of the open lesion. The infant undergoes ultrasound or CT studies of the head to determine the degree of hydrocephalus present. In most cases, a ventriculoperitoneal shunt is placed to aid CSF drainage and to reduce ICP.

Surgical repair of symptomatic spina bifida occulta (see Table 21-4), regardless of the specific anomaly, is undertaken relatively soon after diagnosis, although it need not be an emergency procedure. The primary surgical aim in these cases is to free up the spinal cord, which may be tethered or tied by the defect, so that progressive deterioration of function is arrested.

In cases of encephalocele, the timing of surgical intervention may vary depending on the size, location, and extent of nervous tissue involvement. Early death is common in severe cases, usually related to complications of hydrocephalus, infection, or actual rupture of the encephalocele. In any of the aforementioned cases, meticulous postoperative care is essential to maintain wound integrity, prevent infection and CSF leaks, and promote timely healing of the repair.

Early operative care for spina bifida cystica (see Table 21-4) focuses on preserving all neural tissue, providing a normal anatomic barrier, and controlling early progressive hydrocephalus. Maintain a sterile, constantly moistened saline dressing on the sac until the surgery is performed so that it will not dry out. The surgical procedure involves dissecting the exposed sac and closing the dura mater and skin over the preserved neural tissue. Skin grafting may be performed over the lesion. If hydrocephalus is present at birth, a ventriculoperitoneal shunting device may be inserted at the time of initial closure. If the clinical features of hydrocephalus are not apparent initially, the child should be evaluated for this condition frequently because hydrocephalus eventually develops in over 90% of children with meningomyelocele (Saadai & Farmer, 2012).

General Postoperative Management

After surgery, ensure adequate cardiopulmonary function and nutrition, which are essential to wound healing. The infant must lie prone for several days postoperatively to avoid pressure on the wound and infection. When the infant is less restricted in positioning and is allowed to be supine, obtain orthopedic, rehabilitative, and urologic consultations to better understand the child's functional capacity. Hip and spine radiographs, renal ultrasound, electrical muscle testing, and auditory testing are commonly done before discharge from the hospital. Close follow-up of fontanel size and head circumference is also important. As for any child, perform normal well-child care routines and monitor infant development; do not let these measures be overshadowed by the special care requirements of these children.

Assist with determining the child's functional abilities, including motor performance and sensory deficits. Perform skin assessment, including observation of incisions from surgical closure or shunt placement and any pressure points or areas of breakdown. Also evaluate bowel and bladder function, monitoring for symptoms of urinary tract infection or bowel obstruction. Assess nutrition, mobility, and psychosocial adjustment of the child and the family to the defect and to its associated problems.

Assess shunt function and monitor for increased ICP. Monitoring for increased ICP includes obtaining serial daily head circumference measurements, checking for bulging fontanels, and noting changes in the child's level of consciousness.

Infection Prevention

During the neonatal period, care of the protruding sac is extremely important. For an encephalocele covered with skin, position the infant to avoid pressure on the lesion. If the encephalocele is in the occipital area, a foam "half donut" may be useful in positioning. The more common lumbosacral spinal meningomyelocele are usually protected only by a thin membrane. Apply a sterile, saline-soaked dressing after the sac is examined for gross tears or leakage. Rather than changing it frequently, keep the dressing moist with a sterile saline solution at regular intervals. The infant may be placed on a prophylactic broad-spectrum antibiotic if the defect appears to be infected. Take meticulous care to avoid any contamination of the sac by the child's stool and urine. Monitor for signs and symptoms of meningitis, which may include irritability, fever, feeding intolerance, and seizures. Alert the physician if any of these symptoms become apparent.

After surgery, treat the wound aseptically and maintain the infant in the prone position for several days to avoid both pressure on the incision and CSF leak. Use a protective barrier drape to prevent contamination by stool or urine, and change the drape when necessary. Frequently change the diaper if the infant has continuous urine and stool leakage. Notify the neurosurgeon of any potential wound contamination.

Urinary tract infections are prevented by a bladder program that includes intermittent catheterization or, in more severe cases, surgical diversion techniques to protect the kidneys from infection. Teach the child (when old enough) and family members how to perform intermittent catheterization and how to recognize urinary tract infections. Odorous or cloudy urine, pain on urination, increased irritability, and hematuria are common symptoms. Educate the family to alert the urologic specialist about changes in bladder function throughout the child's developing years.

Skin Care Measures

Prevent pressure ulcers by optimizing skin integrity and avoiding pressure on any at-risk area. Areas that require special attention include the spinal defect area, perianal area, sacrum, knees, elbows, ankles, and any area with diminished sensation. The use of a skin barrier (DuoDerm or Stomahesive wafer), cut and applied in two parallel strips or a windowpane fashion, prevents skin breakdown from continual tape removal when frequent dressing changes are needed after initial closure. After the dressing is changed, pull a barrier drape over the dressing to prevent contamination from stool below the closure. Often, the best nursing care for skin breakdown in the anal area is to leave the infant's buttocks exposed to air or to use a heat lamp safely to promote drying of the area. Ensure adequate nutrition for the child.

As children grow, teach them to inspect their skin routinely and to avoid skin contact with potentially abrasive or thermal sources to prevent unnoticed skin breakdown secondary to decreased sensation.

Prevention of Latex Allergy

Sensitivity to latex products, such as gloves and urinary catheters, poses a life-threatening health risk for patients with meningomyelocele. Although only 15% of patients with spina bifida demonstrate a clinical allergy, about 50% are latex sensitive and at high risk of anaphylaxis when exposed to latex (Rendeli et al., 2006).

caREminder

Carefully screen for latex and rubber allergies in the patient and family.

The incidence of allergic reactions increases with age because the older child is exposed repeatedly over time to latex products. Consider all children with NTDs as latex sensitive and place them on latex precautions.

The child with latex sensitivity should be premedicated with steroids or diphenhydramine before surgery or diagnostic testing. Have nonlatex products available in operating rooms, emergency departments, and all other settings where care is likely to be given to latex-sensitive children. Help the family understand this risk and supply them with educational materials and latex-free equipment. Chapter 11 discusses the management of latex allergies.

Prevention of Neurologic Injury

Rupture of the fluid-filled sac could lead to immediate death as a result of sudden decompression of CSF from the cranial cavity. Correctly position infants with spinal lesions in either the prone or side-lying positions, depending on the function of the child's lower extremities. A flat position is also favored. A cloth roll under the infant's hips in the prone position helps to enable proper alignment of the lower extremities and promotes downward flow of stool and urine away from the open lesion.

Most children with spina bifida manifest hydrocephalus. Many children require the insertion of a shunt during the time of the back closure, whereas others are followed with serial ultrasound examinations and then have a shunt placed, if needed, at a later date. Most children require shunting within the first few months of life.

Assess the appearance and nature of the fontanel, the sutures, and the infant's head circumference. Use cardiopulmonary monitoring for infants who do not have shunts in place to evaluate for signs of apnea and bradycardia secondary to increased ICP. Lethargy, feeding intolerance, and seizures are also evidence of increasing ICP and of the need for shunt placement.

Prevention of Orthopedic Injury

Neuromuscular and sensory deficits can lead to orthopedic problems, including scoliosis, kyphosis, hip dislocation, and ankle deformities. Joint stability may be affected by contractures, muscle control, and altered sensation. Teach the child and family which activities are safe and which are potentially risky. As a child with spina bifida becomes more mobile, teach the family to monitor the child's use of or function of his or her limbs. Hip dislocation and limb fractures may go unnoticed for long periods because of decreased sensation. Encourage routine orthopedic follow-up.

Promotion of Elimination

More than 90% of children with spina bifida have a neurogenic colon. Fecal incontinence and constipation, the two most common problems, are related to the loss of parasympathetic innervation of the colon and the pelvic floor, sensation in the rectum, and motor innervation of the external anal sphincter. Encourage the family to institute a bowel program in early childhood, incorporating the five elements of timing, diet, exercise, posture, and rectal stimulation. Teach the family and the child to plan bowel evacuation after a meal, and encourage the child to eat a well-balanced diet that is high in fiber and low in carbohydrates. Exercising the lower portion of the body after the meal and adopting a knee–chest position to put pressure on the abdomen can aid in bowel evacuation. Finally, encourage rectal stimulation with a suppository or by digital stimulation to initiate or sustain the defecation reflex.

Clean intermittent catheterization for bladder elimination has generally replaced the use of the Credé maneuver (manual pressure applied from the umbilicus toward the symphysis pubis to express urine). Drug therapy with anticholinergic drugs (ACDs) and surgical procedures, including bladder augmentation and placement of an artificial sphincter, are also common. Nursing care includes maintaining bladder programs, teaching family members signs of urinary tract infection, and addressing psychosocial issues related to bladder elimination.

Supportive Interventions

The initial crisis after the birth of the infant with an NTD must be effectively resolved if the family is to function well as a unit. This is a time of major crisis for families as they deal with an unexpected outcome of the pregnancy. Their expectations of a perfect baby are shattered by the reality of the birth defect, separation from the infant if the infant is transported, and the critical need for medical intervention. When assessment of the infant is completed, the child's long-term prognosis should be discussed with the family. Emphasize to the family that surgery does not restore normal neurologic function; it merely preserves existing function.

Allow the family to grieve by being with them and listening to them. An example of a phrase that might be helpful in eliciting some of their feelings is, "This isn't really what you expected, is it?" or "This whole event must be so overwhelming to you." Give the family honest information about the most immediate aspects of medical care.

As the infant heals from the surgery and discharge is planned, assess the family's coping skills and available resources to ensure a successful transition to home. It is normal for parents to continue grieving the birth of a child with a congenital malformation even as they feel relief that their child has recovered from surgery.

The nurse is often the one person who has the knowledge, skill, and time to clarify any misconceptions, repeat any information as necessary, and assess the family's values and perceptions about NTDs. Assess the family's support system and available resources as well, providing contacts and assistance as needed.

Community Care

Caring for the child with an NTD such as spina bifida is a lifelong commitment for families. The effect of medical costs, as well as social and emotional concerns, can be overwhelming. Direct care toward maximizing the child's abilities rather than focusing on disabilities (Developmental Considerations 21-3; Teaching Intervention Plan 21-3).

Although children with spina bifida tend to score in the low average range of intellectual function, they have problems in socialization, academic function, and vocational accomplishment and demonstrate impaired attention and executive function, which may contribute to their social difficulties (Rose & Holmbeck, 2007). Many children with spina bifida are able to attend regular schools and, with proper evaluation, are able to maintain attendance in age-appropriate classes.

Many factors affect the self-esteem of a child with spina bifida, including mobility, physical appearance and weight, family support, and experiences within the health care system. Obesity is a common problem, particularly in adolescents. Promote healthy eating habits at an early age in accordance with the child's activity level. Encourage involvement in wheelchair sports activities. Self-esteem may have a direct effect on the child's desire to maintain a normal weight. Involving the whole family in self-esteem–building activities is paramount.

Because children with spina bifida may have many surgical procedures throughout their lives, providing for a successful operative experience is essential. Provide preoperative preparation such as age-appropriate play activities and honest, but not scary, developmentally appropriate explanations about the procedure. Many of the orthopedic procedures required for these children involve long periods of rehabilitation to achieve the best results. Continual support and positive

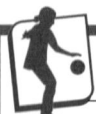

DEVELOPMENTAL CONSIDERATIONS 21-3

Teaching Needs of the Child With Spina Bifida

Infancy
Focus teaching toward parents, siblings, and relatives:
    Teach skin care.
    Teach bowel and bladder function.
    Discuss nutrition.
    Discuss signs of increased ICP.
    Discuss activity and mobility.
    Demonstrate methods to promote achievement of developmental milestones.
    Select methods to promote family coping.

Early Childhood
Continue teaching with family, begin including child:
    Continue bowel- and bladder-training program.
    Teach diet and weight management.
    Discuss child's concept of spina bifida.
    Discuss behavior management.
    Teach activities to promote independence and autonomy.
    Consult specialists to maximize mobility (braces, wheelchair).
    Obtain "Handicapped" tags for family cars.
    Discuss availability of preschool or daycare.
    Encourage socialization and age-appropriate activities.
    Encourage use of developmental toys and games.
    Teach skills to adapt home environment for child safety and mobility.
    Perform baseline intellectual function testing.

Middle Childhood
Teach more advanced concepts to child and parents:
    Discuss body image.
    Begin to use more medically correct terminology.

Encourage discussion of emotions and social supports.
Encourage peer interaction via summer camp and school groups.
Plan activities to promote sense of achievement.
Discuss accomplishments as well as failures.
Provide teaching and consults to school staff.
Begin teaching intermittent bladder catheterization.
Parental involvement:
    Outline self-care activities within the child's ability level.
    Assist parents with the child's psychosocial changes.
    Discuss parent's concept of child's progress and needs.

Adolescence
Focus teaching on the adolescent:
    Discuss issues of body image, sexuality, and social interactions.
    Teach self-care regarding bladder emptying, hygiene, and skin care.
    Encourage peer interaction to develop group identity.
    Refer to nutritionist for diet and weight management.
    Discuss theory of personal identity within family structure.
    Suggest patient begin a journal for questions and concerns.
Parental involvement:
    Stress importance of the child's need to be included in decisions.
    Discuss methods to promote independence at home and school.
    Begin transition to adult health care facility.

---

reinforcement from the nursing staff are important to the child's optimal recovery and function.

Teachers and other school personnel are an important part of the team caring for the child with spina bifida. Prolonged absences affect the child's success at school. Help the family make a plan for the child to continue his or her schoolwork while in the hospital or at home recovering from hospitalizations. Adaptations may be necessary to account for cognitive impairments. School also provides an important social outlet for the child, so make every effort to keep the child involved in a school program even if involvement is less than full time. School success has a positive effect on self-esteem and on future life success.

HYDROCEPHALUS

Hydrocephalus is defined as a dilation of the ventricles inside the brain caused by an imbalance in the rate at which CSF is produced and absorbed. The two primary

causes, whether congenital or acquired, are (1) blocked flow of CSF and (2) impaired venous absorption of CSF in the subarachnoid space. A third, but rare, cause is over-production of CSF caused by a tumor, called a *choroid plexus papilloma*. The clinical manifestations of hydrocephalus vary with its precise cause and duration, the age of the child, and the ability of the skull to expand.

Congenital hydrocephalus occurs in approximately 0.47 to 0.59 per 1,000 live and still births (Garne et al., 2010; Jeng et al., 2011) and may be diagnosed prenatally by ultrasound or may be overt at birth. Congenital etiologies include spina bifida, Chiari malformations, congenital arachnoid cysts, congenital stenosis of the aqueduct of Sylvius, Dandy-Walker cyst, and other intracranial masses, including congenital tumors.

Acquired hydrocephalus occurs secondary to mass lesions. Acquired lesions in infancy are most commonly a result of intracranial bleeding, meningitis, or both, resulting in fibrosis of the meninges, which prevents

TIP 21-3: A TEACHING INTERVENTION PLAN for the Child With a Repaired Neural Tube Defect

Nursing Diagnoses and Family Outcomes

- Risk for infection related to consequences of surgical incision, presence of shunt, urinary retention, and immobility
  Outcomes: Child's incision site remains free from infection.
  Child remains free from urinary tract infections.
  Child's skin remains intact.
- Urinary retention related to effects of lack of innervation of bladder and sphincter
  Outcomes: Child remains free from urinary tract infection.
  Child remains free from constipation.
  Child participates in bowel- and bladder-training program when age-appropriate.
- Risk for injury related to effects of neuromuscular and sensory deficits
  Outcome: Child remains free of contracture, alterations in skin integrity, and trauma to extremities with altered sensation.
- Delayed growth and development related to sensorimotor limitations
  Outcomes: Parents participate in activities to promote child's developmental outcomes.
  Child achieves developmental milestones to highest level of ability given the sensorimotor limitations.

Teach the Child/Family

Skin Care
- Examine skin daily for areas of redness or a break in the skin integrity.
- Provide wound care and dressing changes (if necessary).
- Reposition child every 2 hours.
- Use sheepskin or air mattresses on areas of bony prominence.
- When removing splints and braces, assess skin for reddened areas.

Bowel and Bladder Function
- Establish routine and regular bowel program with suppository and stimulations.
- Effect clean intermittent catheterization.
- Institute bowel- and bladder-training program when age appropriate.

Nutrition
- Maintain good fluid intake and high-fiber diet to prevent constipation.
- Encourage intake of fluids such as cranberry, grape, and prune juices or those high in vitamin C to prevent urinary tract infections.

- Monitor child's weight; a low-calorie diet may be necessary.

Activity and Mobility
- Observe the child's movements for signs of loss of sensation of lower extremities.
- Consult a specialist to maximize mobility as child grows (braces, wheelchair).
- Perform passive range-of-motion exercises.
- Use proper positioning with pillows, pads, and rolls, as needed.
- Have child ambulate or sit in wheelchair whenever possible.
- Periodically evaluate adaptive equipment for damage, loose screws, alignment, or similar faults.

Growth and Development
- Modify home environment as child grows to ensure child's safety.
- Encourage stimulation with age-appropriate activities.
- Encourage child to be as independent as possible.
- Teach alternative methods for personal hygiene and mobility.
- Praise child's independent behaviors.
- Allow child to ventilate feelings about self and interactions with peers.

Monitoring for Complications
- Monitor for signs of increased ICP (changed level of consciousness, changes in behavior, headache, vomiting, fever) that may be signs of shunt malfunction.

Health Maintenance
- Organize and maintain child's medical records.
- Access community resources and support groups.
- Seek financial assistance as needed.
- Discuss babysitting and child care options.

Contact Health Care Provider if
- Redness or discharge is noted from site of surgical incisions
- Areas of the child's skin become reddened or there is a break in the skin surface
- Urine becomes cloudy or foul smelling
- Child displays changes in neurologic status as demonstrated by changes in level of consciousness, lethargy, irritability, vomiting, and fontanel seeming to be full
- Child has fever

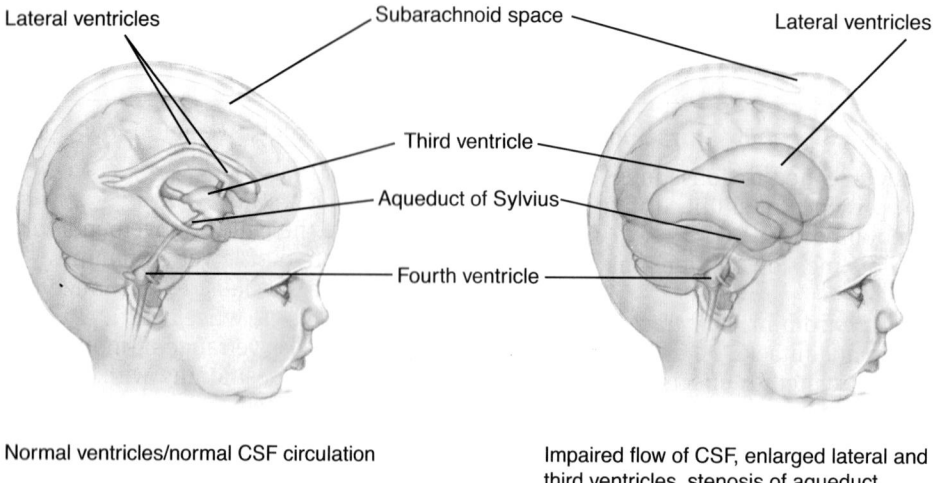

Figure 21-4 Normal CSF circulation and alterations caused by hydrocephalus.

reabsorption of CSF by the arachnoid villi. Infants born prematurely are at increased risk of intraventricular hemorrhage.

Pathophysiology

CSF is primarily manufactured in, and secreted by, the choroid plexus. This structure lines the base of the paired lateral ventricles and the roof of the third and fourth ventricles (Fig. 21-4). CSF is produced and then propelled, in a pulsatile fashion, from the choroid plexus through a small passageway called the *intraventricular foramina of Monro* to the third ventricle. From there, it travels through the aqueduct of Sylvius to the fourth ventricle. From the fourth ventricle, the CSF flows through the foramen of Magendie and the paired foramina of Luschka into the subarachnoid space, up over the surface of the brain, and downward around the spinal cord. The CSF is then reabsorbed by the arachnoid villi located in the dural sinuses, which are the large blood vessels that drain the venous blood from the head, and through the walls of capillaries of the CNS and pia mater. Small amounts of CSF are absorbed in the cells lining the ventricles and through the lymphatic system of the spinal cord.

The terminology used to describe hydrocephalus has been confusing because the terms used were coined before the era of modern diagnostic testing, when the site of the blockage may have been implied rather than precisely identified. The terms *communicating* and *noncommunicating* hydrocephalus are still used occasionally to describe the status of the ventricles in this disease. Communicating hydrocephalus describes a blockage "outside" the ventricular system (e.g., meninges). The implication is that the ventricles can still communicate, despite the blockage. Noncommunicating hydrocephalus implies a blockage somewhere in the ventricular system that prevents CSF from reaching the subarachnoid space for reabsorption. Another way to classify hydrocephalus is to categorize the disorder as either *congenital* or *acquired*, as described earlier. Most believe it best

to classify hydrocephalus by the site of the blockage, by the cause, and by the state of progression. Prognosis for the child with hydrocephalus depends on these and other factors.

Assessment

Ask about any history of trauma, CNS infection, familial megalencephaly, birth injury, or prematurity; note the onset and duration of symptoms. Measure head circumference. An abnormal increase above the established growth curve, a circumference above the 95th percentile at birth, or a rapidly increasing head circumference should raise suspicion of hydrocephalus. Note spilt sutures or a full or bulging fontanel, especially one that is nonpulsatile, indicating high pressure. Other clinical signs and symptoms become apparent as hydrocephalus progresses. Cranial nerve palsies result in the classic "sunset" appearance of the eyes, in which the sclera are visible above the iris and the infant is unable to look upward with the head facing forward. Collier sign (upper eyelid retraction) may also be present and may occur with third ventricle lesions. Scalp veins are prominent, and the infant may demonstrate lethargy, irritability, high-pitched cry, poor feeding habits, and projectile vomiting. Increased motor tone, spasticity, or opisthotonic posturing (arched back) may be present. Developmental delays are also common in children younger than 2 years of age.

In the older child with a fused cranium, signs and symptoms of hydrocephalus may develop either slowly or rapidly. Rapid development leads to acute neurologic deterioration. Symptoms of increased ICP in these children include frontal headache, nausea, and vomiting that may be projectile. If these symptoms occur on awakening, suspect increased ICP. CO_2 retained during sleep and decreased venous drainage while the child is lying flat may contribute to morning symptoms. Other signs and symptoms include poor school performance, restlessness, changes in personality or activity level, double vision, papilledema, spasticity, hyperreflexia, ataxia, and new onset or change in seizure pattern.

In later stages, bradycardia or altered respirations and seizures are life threatening if not treated.

Diagnostic Tests

Level II ultrasonography of the fetus can confirm a prenatal diagnosis of hydrocephalus. This condition is not always detected by a screening ultrasound. Trans-uterine placement of ventriculoamniotic shunts during late pregnancy is being developed, but the technique involves risk to the fetus and mother and remains controversial (Bruner et al., 2006).

In infants and children, evidence of hydrocephalus is most frequently obtained with a CT scan. In infants with an open fontanel, ultrasound may be used. When a complex lesion is suspected, MRI may be used initially. Skull radiographs may show widened or split sutures, and the skull may have a "beaten silver" appearance, characteristic of chronically increased ICP.

Interdisciplinary Interventions

After hydrocephalus is identified, treatment is directed toward resolving the cause of obstruction. Doing so may not be possible in congenital hydrocephalus. When acquired hydrocephalus occurs in an older child, the lesion causing the obstruction (most frequently neoplasm) can be removed to enable CSF flow to return to normal. In some cases, however, even complete resection of a tumor fails to reestablish normal CSF pathways.

Cerebrospinal Fluid Removal

Medical management of hydrocephalus is limited to withdrawal of CSF by lumbar puncture or by ventricular tap. This procedure is usually performed on a short-term basis in infants with inflammatory processes or intracranial hemorrhage. In some cases, acetazolamide (Diamox) is prescribed, which may decrease CSF production. However, electrolyte disorders and long-term administration are problematic (Tsitouras & Sgouros, 2011).

Surgical Interventions

Advances in neuroendoscopy have led to the development of smaller scopes and powerful light sources, allowing the neurosurgeon to gain access to the ventricular space in the brain through a small burr hole. Once there, the surgeon can visualize the ventricles, fenestrate cysts, and place indwelling catheters.

The most common treatment for hydrocephalus is to reduce the ICP by surgically shunting the CSF from the ventricles to another body cavity, such as the peritoneal cavity, where it is absorbed.

The three main components of mechanical shunting devices are (1) ventricular catheter, (2) reservoir and valve to regulate flow of CSF (and thus ICP), and (3) distal tubing. The CSF is drained by the ventricular catheter to the distal cavity, where the CSF is resorbed into the body's fluids. The soft shunt tubing is placed directly under the scalp on the skull bones and is palpable under the skin of the scalp; it then travels along the neck, after which it is placed into the distal site.

The *ventriculoperitoneal* location is chosen for most mechanical shunts (Fig. 21-5). After insertion of the ventricular tube through a cranial burr hole, the length of the shunt is tunneled subcutaneously to the upper quadrant of the abdomen. A small incision is made and the shunt is guided into the peritoneal cavity with plenty of extra tubing to enable the child to grow without having to undergo further surgery to lengthen the shunt. Specific risks of this procedure include bowel perforation and ascites if the CSF is poorly absorbed.

The *ventriculoatrial* shunt is placed only if a concurrent abdominal problem exists that precludes insertion of a ventriculoperitoneal shunt. This shunt can be inserted into the right atrium of the heart by passing it through the jugular vein, or, in more extensive cases, directly into the heart. Risks include catheter movement, dysrhythmias, operative risks associated with more extensive surgery, endocarditis, septicemia, and congestive heart failure.

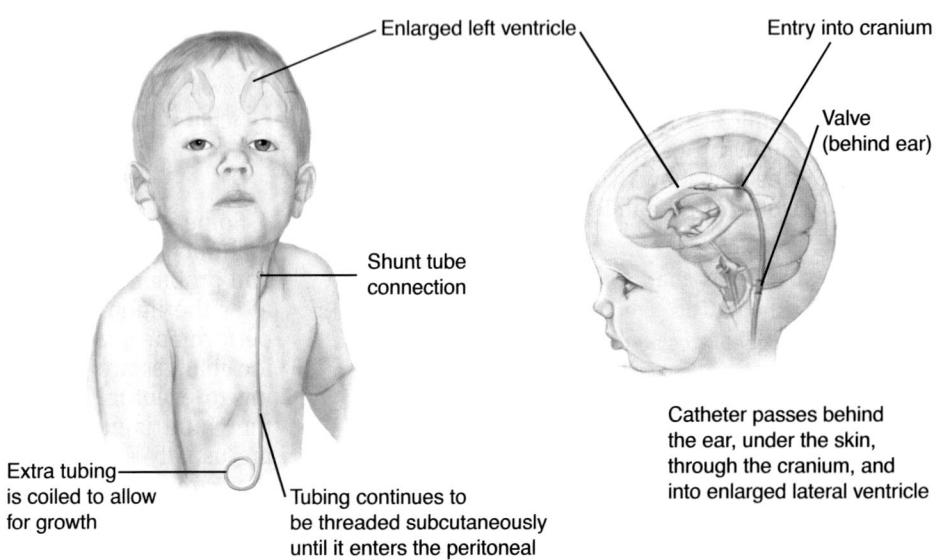

Enlarged left ventricle

Entry into cranium

Valve (behind ear)

Shunt tube connection

Extra tubing is coiled to allow for growth

Tubing continues to be threaded subcutaneously until it enters the peritoneal cavity

Catheter passes behind the ear, under the skin, through the cranium, and into enlarged lateral ventricle

Figure 21-5 Placement of ventriculoperitoneal shunt.

A third ventriculostomy is an endoscopic procedure to treat hydrocephalus without the need to place a shunt. Criteria for candidacy include large ventricles at baseline, no evidence of abnormal absorption of CSF in the subarachnoid space (i.e., communicating hydrocephalus), and absence of previous infection or bleeding into the brain. Older children with acquired obstructive hydrocephalus are often appropriate candidates. Through a small incision, the scope is placed into the lateral ventricles and moved into the third ventricle, where a small hole is punctured to allow CSF to flow into the subarachnoid space. The recovery time is 1 to 2 days. The size of the ventricles on postoperative CT does not change rapidly, as is sometimes the case with a shunt. This procedure fails in some children, for whom placement of a shunt is eventually required (Yadav et al., 2012).

In addition to preparing the child and family for surgery, a key preoperative intervention is monitoring for increased ICP and instituting measures to reduce the risk of increasing the pressure. Cardiorespiratory monitoring and frequent monitoring of pupil size, motor movements, and level of consciousness are essential. Immediately report changes in status and administer medications as ordered. Be ready to assist if a ventricular shunt tap is needed. Regularly assess fontanels and note bulging or flatness. If the child is vomiting, IV hydration may be necessary. Hydration should be administered at a rate of no more than 75% to 80% of *maintenance* fluid requirements to prevent fluid overload, which may increase ICP. Elevate the head of the bed 30 degrees, and decrease external stimuli. Have oxygen and suction ready at the bedside in case the child has a seizure. In some centers, a preoperative dose of IV antibiotics may be ordered as prophylaxis against infection. Follow individual surgeon preferences for laboratory work or skin shampoo preparation.

Begin teaching and preparation of the child and family as soon as the decision to place a shunt is made. Provide information about the procedure as well as what to expect after it. Assist families in understanding the terminology and the equipment used. Make written handouts, preprinted booklets, and a structured teaching session a part of the preoperative plan. Provide the child with age-appropriate information. Evaluate family understanding of the shunt, its function, and how to manage follow-up care. Photographs of normal CT scans and scans that show hydrocephalus offer compelling comparisons for the family.

KidKare Allow the older child to handle a demonstration shunt. This exercise can alleviate many fears and often generates additional questions.

In addition to basic postoperative care following cranial surgery (covered earlier in this chapter), perform postoperative care specific to the child with a shunt:

- Observe for signs of neurologic deterioration after an initial period of recovery or signs of slow and incomplete recovery. Report any of these trends to the physician so that appropriate radiographs can be ordered. Children who experience a rapid decrease in ventricular size after shunt placement are susceptible to developing subdural fluid collections.
- Avoid applying any cardiac lead patches, temperature probes, or unnecessary tape over the shunt site because of the fragility of the skin. Be particularly careful with the scalp because it is often stretched and is therefore more susceptible to breakdown. A newborn infant may be placed on a waterbed initially to prevent pressure on the skin around the shunt.
- Monitor for potential complications, especially infection, shunt malfunction, and excessive drainage of CSF.
- Pay close attention to the integrity of surgical incisions, and ensure that children keep their hands away from fresh incisions (use a stockinette cap if appropriate). Monitor the child's temperature, and administer antibiotics, if ordered. The organisms most commonly isolated from infected shunts are *Staphylococcus epidermidis* and *Staphylococcus aureus*. If the organism is difficult to eradicate, intraventricular instillation of antibiotics may be useful. In most cases of shunt infection, the distal end of the shunt is externalized to a CSF-collecting system until the bacteria are eradicated and a new shunt is placed. In nearly all cases, the shunt must be completely removed and replaced to achieve a cure.
- Monitor for shunt malfunction that *may* be hardware related or the result of obstruction (often resulting from infection or buildup of fibrin debris and protein substances). Assess for signs of increased ICP.
- Assist with preparing the child for diagnostic tests to evaluate shunt function, including radiographs, brain imaging, shunt tap, radionuclide shuntography, and ICP monitoring.

ALERT *Monitor for signs and symptoms of shunt infection or malfunction, which can be acute or chronic, depending on the cause and the child's abnormality and brain compliance. Acute presentation includes rapid onset of vomiting, severe headache, irritability, lethargy, fever, redness along the shunt tract, and fluid around the shunt valve.*

Some children with shunt failure from infection or malfunction present with more insidious symptoms, and problems may not be noted until weeks or months after the initial surgery. Occasional changes in school performance, intermittent headaches, and mild behavior changes are noted by those around the child, leading to eventual evaluation and the determination that the shunt is malfunctioning. Because family members are usually aware of their child's day-to-day behavior, they are sensitive to the changes that indicate shunt malfunction. Listen to a parent's intuition, even if a shunt has recently been placed, because shunts may require several revisions (Clinical Judgment 21-2).

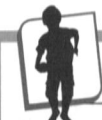

CLINICAL JUDGMENT 21-2

The Child With a Ventriculoperitoneal Shunt

Three-month-old Shila had a ventriculoperitoneal shunt placed 2 weeks ago following a diagnosis of congenital hydrocephalus. The family has returned to the clinic for a follow-up appointment.

Questions

1. How could the diagnosis of hydrocephalus be assessed in a child so young?
2. What concerns might parents have at this time?
3. Shila has a temperature of 101° F (38.3° C) and it is noted that the shunt incision site is reddened and not healing well. What nursing diagnosis would be appropriate for the child with a shunt infection?
4. What health care interventions are appropriate to treat Shila's ventriculitis?
5. Family teaching is given regarding management of Shila's shunt. What information should the family be able to relate back to the nurse to indicate that effective teaching has taken place?

Answers

1. During well-child visits at 1 and 2 months of age, an abnormal increase in head circumference may be noted. Other findings that are suspicious include a full or bulging fontanel, increased motor tone, developmental delays, irritability, high-pitched cry, poor feeding, projectile vomiting, and cranial nerve palsies resulting in the classic "sunset" appearance of the eyes.
2. Is the shunt working? How can they tell if it is working? Will their child be normal?
3. Risk for infection related to placement of ventriculoperitoneal shunt
4. First, the shunt is tapped to look for suspected bacteria. Antibiotics are given correctly and in a timely manner. Vancomycin in conjunction with gentamicin or a broad-spectrum cephalosporin is initially given. Antibiotics are readjusted based on the determination of the cultures and susceptibility outcomes. Acetaminophen is given for fever. Monitor for signs of improvement or worsening. Provide comfort measures.
5. Family can state signs and symptoms of increased ICP and shunt malfunction, demonstrate proper handling of child with new shunt and home safety measures, and identify indications for calling the health care provider if problems occur.

Shunt overdrainage is a complication of a functioning shunt. This complication may lead to **slit ventricle syndrome**, in which overdrainage causes the ventricles to become accustomed to a very small or slitlike configuration. When normally occurring variations in ICP arise, the ability of the ventricles to act as a buffer is limited, leading to symptoms consistent with intermittent catheter occlusion such as headache, dizziness, and nausea. Children with slit ventricle syndrome present challenging management problems and may require changes in valves to more finely regulate pressure and siphoning.

Community Care

Home care instructions for family include monitoring for signs and symptoms of shunt malfunction, proper handling of the child with a new shunt, home safety, and indications for calling the physician if problems occur. For example, instruct the family to place the child on the unoperated side to prevent pressure on the shunt valve (if directed by the physician) and to elevate the head of the bed to enhance gravity flow through the shunt. Educate them to observe the operative site for redness, puffiness, or oozing of fluid. Teach them the signs and symptoms of blockage or infection such as increasing drowsiness, vomiting, headache, irritability, restlessness, swelling around the pump, persistent bulging of fontanel, fever, poor feeding, and seizure activity and to notify the health care provider should any occur. In some cases, the shunt requires pumping. Teach the family, if ordered by the physician, to depress the valve area firmly and quickly with forefinger, leaving the finger on pump to feel it refilling. Advise them not to force the depression if it is difficult and to call the health care provider immediately.

It is imperative that the health care team and the family establish trust and good communication. Maintenance of a therapeutic relationship involves ongoing education, mutual decision making, and the creation of a supportive atmosphere for verbalizing questions and concerns. Nurses facilitate this process by teaching, initiating care conferences, and organizing resources to assist families.

Children should be closely monitored with developmental screening, either in the school setting or with routine medical checkups. Most families are concerned about the effect that hydrocephalus may have on their child's intelligence and development. The degree of disability depends on the severity of hydrocephalus; the presence of other brain anomalies; and the presence of conditions such as intraventricular hemorrhage, infection, and hypoxia. Generally, normal intelligence is enhanced if shunts are placed early, proper function is maintained, and infection is avoided.

CHIARI MALFORMATION

Chiari malformations are congenital anomalies of the structures at the junction of the brain and the spinal cord. This anatomic area is often referred to as the *cervicomedullary junction.*

Two other diagnoses associated with Chiari malformations are **syringomyelia**, or *syrinx*, and **hydromyelia**. Syringomyelia is a cavity lying outside the central canal area of the spinal cord that is not lined by ependymal cells, and hydromyelia is a cavity within the spinal cord that is partially or completely lined with ependyma. These two diagnoses are frequently discussed in conjunction with Chiari malformation because of their similar clinical presentations and their probable common pathophysiologic development. Chiari malformation is associated with several cranial and vertebral abnormalities as well as genetic syndromes and is thought to have a genetic basis.

Pathophysiology

Chiari malformation is characterized by abnormalities of anatomy and physiology (Fig. 21-6), which in turn produce mechanical deformities. Four variations of the Chiari malformation exist. Each type is defined by associated structural anomalies and by the symptoms they produce. Chiari type I presents most often in adolescents and adults. The condition is characterized by a displacement of the cerebellar tonsils into the cervical canal. The clinical features include malformation of the base of the skull and upper cervical spine. Hydromyelia, syringomyelia, and diastematomyelia (longitudinal splitting of the spinal cord) are frequently present. Because symptoms often progress slowly, Chiari type I malformation may go undetected for many years.

Chiari type II, which is uniquely associated with meningomyelocele, is found in infants and is the most common of these malformations. Chiari type II is characterized by downward displacement of the cerebellar tonsils and medulla through the foramen magnum. As the cerebellar tonsils at the base of the spine protrude downward into the foramen magnum of the cervical spine, normal CSF pathways are blocked, and the fourth ventricle becomes dilated with CSF. Signs and symptoms of hydrocephalus occur. Nearly every case of thoracolumbar, lumbar, and lumbosacral meningomyelocele is accompanied by the Chiari type II malformation. Hydrocephalus is also associated with the Chiari type II malformation in 90% of cases (Tubbs et al., 2012). In addition to the complications of the meningomyelocele lesion, other common problems include apnea, laryngeal stridor, and feeding disturbances such as reflux and aspiration. Functional compromise of lower cranial nerves may occur. Ataxia and nystagmus indicate cerebellar impairment, and there may be increased deep tendon reflexes, loss of vibration and position sense, and recurrent occipital and frontal headaches. About half of deaths that occur among infants with meningomyelocele can be attributed to hindbrain anomalies that affect vital physiologic processes. The age at which symptoms of Chiari type II appear has implications for prognosis: the earlier the symptoms appear, the more likely it is that brain stem nuclei are hypoplastic and the poorer the prognosis.

Type III Chiari malformation is essentially an occipital encephalocele, consisting of an opening of the skull and cervical area, through which the cerebellum protrudes. Type IV consists of a single abnormality, failure of the cerebellum to develop, and may be a variation of the Dandy-Walker syndrome (a congenital malformation of the cerebellum and fourth ventricle).

Assessment

The clinical examination focuses on the most common signs and symptoms of the Chiari type II malformation. These signs and symptoms include nystagmus, nuchal

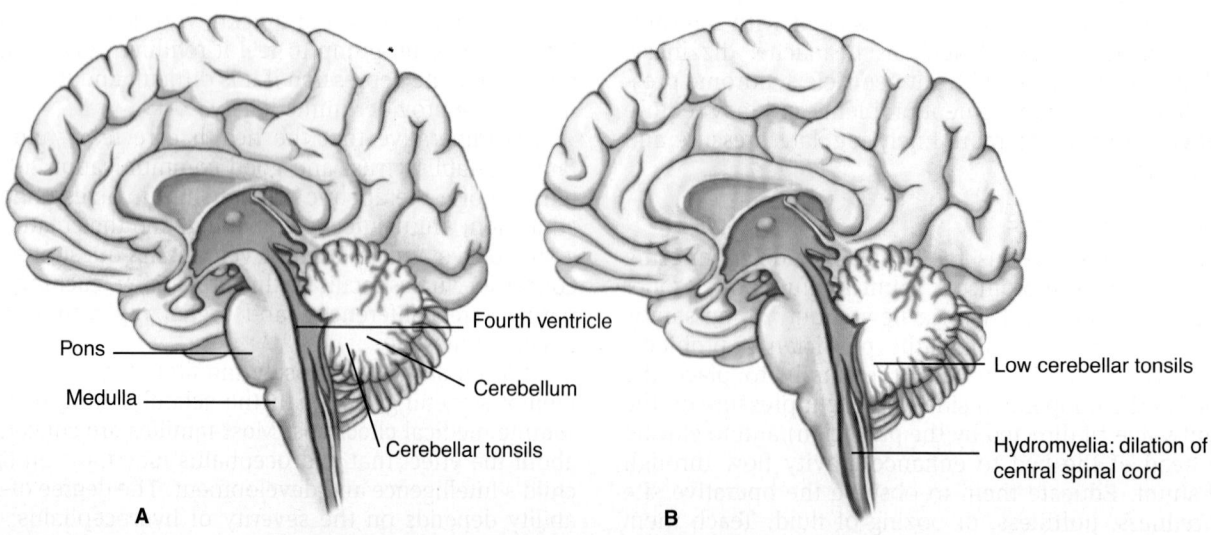

Figure 21-6 Normal posterior fossa (A) and Chiari malformation with hydromyelia (B).

rigidity, poor suck reflex, drooling, difficulty swallow-ing,' vomiting, weak or absent cry, and inspiratory stri-dor during agitation. In more severe cases, episodes of apnea may be reported. Be alert for these signs and symptoms in a child with meningomyelocele because they can progress very rapidly and may require imme-diate surgical intervention. In older children, decreased strength in upper extremities, with increased tone and exaggerated deep tendon reflexes, may also be present.

A type I malformation may not be detected for years, possibly until adolescence. The adolescent with Chiari type I malformation is likely to have a more chronic presentation, which includes occipital headaches, neck pain, urinary infrequency, progressive lower limb spas-ticity, and scoliosis.

Radiographic techniques are used to demonstrate the type and extent of the lesion, including the presence of hydromyelia or hydrocephalus. MRI is particularly useful in identifying the anatomy to provide accurate diagnosis.

Interdisciplinary Interventions

Children with a Chiari malformation require careful monitoring and MRI to determine the extent of neu-rologic involvement associated with the condition. If symptoms are not life threatening, a conservative approach is undertaken in the hope that the child will stabilize and outgrow the symptoms. Surgery may be recommended to decompress the suboccipital and cer-vical areas.

Surgical decompression involves removing the posteri-or aspect of the foramen magnum and excising the upper cervical vertebral arches. This decompression alleviates the pressure on the fourth ventricle and the affected cra-nial nerves, arresting symptom progression. Besides per-forming bony decompression of the area, many surgeons incise the dura and place a graft to allow further decom-pression of the anatomic structures. Postoperatively, some of these children who have received grafts develop symptoms of meningeal irritation, which require close monitoring to rule out infection. Some children show little objective improvement, and deficits that existed preoperatively may be permanent. The goal of the sur-gery is to prevent further symptoms rather than to relieve existing ones, although existing symptoms are usually relieved to some degree. Ventriculoperitoneal shunts are placed to treat hydrocephalus, and because they are usu-ally permanent, patients are monitored throughout life by a neurosurgery team.

Postoperative care is the same as that described for cranial surgery. Give special attention to avoiding respiratory distress and respiratory infection. Airway function and protection may be altered as a result of preexisting symptoms and respiratory compromise dur-ing surgery. Ensure that oxygen and suction are readily available at the child's bedside if needed. Feed children with poor gag and swallow reflexes slowly, and place them in an upright position after feeding to avoid aspi-ration and pneumonia.

Ensure adequate pain control. Neurologic assess-ments help to determine whether overmedication or postoperative complications have occurred. Teach the family to assess for changes in their child's neuro-logic status, recognize impending signs of respiratory problems, and report any signs of incisional redness or irritation. Before discharge, address any need for occupational therapy to adapt feeding or stimulation programs to meet the child's functional capacity if the child will later require a referral.

CEREBRAL PALSY

Cerebral palsy (CP), the most common cause of physi-cal disabilities in developed countries, is defined as a disorder of movement and posture. CP is best described as a constellation of symptoms with many causes and etiologies, which are usually not known. The extent of symptoms is variable, ranging from imperceptibly mild to debilitating severity. It is often associated with epi-lepsy and abnormalities of speech, vision, and intellect. As gestational age and birth weight decreases, the inci-dence of CP increases. The incidence of CP in preterm infants has increased as a result of neonatal intensive care and multiple births. The rates of CP in term infants have remained steady.

Pathophysiology

The precise pathophysiology of CP is not known. Typi-cally, CP results from a defect or lesion of the develop-ing brain. However, in some cases, no specific lesion or area of infarct can be found. Although the enceph-alopathy itself does not progress, it produces a perma-nent disorder of posture and movement that results in progressive musculoskeletal pathology in most affected children. The brain injury may occur before, during, or after birth, usually before age 5 years. Sometimes, CP can be the result of a traumatic accident, such as a near-drowning episode, whereby the brain is deprived of oxy-gen for some period of time. Risk factors associated with CP may include perinatal factors, such as exposure to teratogens, intrauterine infection, fetal/placental dys-function, maternal preeclampsia, complications of labor and birth, prematurity, asphyxia, and sepsis; and child-hood factors, such as TBI, carbon monoxide poisoning, respiratory distress syndrome, meningitis/encephalitis or brain abscess, near drowning or other asphyxiating in-jury, respiratory obstruction, hemorrhage, and embolus or thrombus. Increased use of brain imaging has dem-onstrated that perinatal influences may be stronger than previously thought.

The patterns of dysfunction seen in the child are relat-ed to whether damage is limited to one area of the brain, is scattered in multiple areas, or is unilateral or bilateral. Dysfunction is also related to the cause of the damage and the stage of brain development at the time of injury. In all cases, the lesion cannot be repaired. Although the lesion or injury does not worsen, symptoms can and do worsen unless close attention is paid to occupational and physical therapy to maintain range of motion.

The essential motor problem in CP is lack of muscle control. This lack of control usually stems from fail-ure to inhibit specific reflexes of the CNS. The reflexes

TABLE 21-5   Types of Cerebral Palsy

Type and Incidence	Characteristics
Spastic type (65%)	Increased muscle tone with clasp-knife character Increased deep tendon reflexes Pathologic reflexes Spastic weakness Difficulty with fine and gross motor skills Muscle contractures common Scoliosis
Hemiplegia (30%)	Primary unilateral involvement, often with the arm more involved than the leg
Quadriplegia (5%)	Four-limb involvement, with legs more involved than arms, although legs still show substantial involvement
Diplegia (30%)	Four-limb involvement, with legs more involved than arms; arms may have only minimal impairment and no functional handicaps
Athetoid type (20%)	Purposeless, involuntary, uncontrollable movements of face and extremities Fluctuating muscle tone Deep tendon reflexes and movements increase with stress and voluntary movements; deep tendon reflexes absent during sleep Symmetric four-limb involvement
Ataxic type (5%)	Disturbed coordination Unsteady gait Hypotonic muscles Slurred speech In general, good motor prognosis
Mixed type (10%)	Usually a mixture of spastic athetoid types

involving muscle movement are stretch, crossed extension, long spinal, symmetric tonic neck, asymmetric tonic neck, vestibular, and startle. Each of these reflexes is normally present in infancy. Normally, these reflexes fade or are inhibited as development progresses. Injury to the brain may cause these reflexes to persist, barring control of muscle movement. Without control of these movements, functional ability is lost or cannot be attained. As the child grows, motor and nonmotor manifestations, such as scoliosis and muscle contractures, may become more disabling. Scoliosis can cause lung compression, loss of ambulation, or inability to sit; muscle pull imbalances can cause a subluxated or dislocated hip, leading to pain and problems with sitting.

Children with CP are classified by the area (extremity) most affected and by the degree of involvement (Table 21-5). Children with CP often have other physical abnormalities such as seizures; vision, hearing, or speech deficits; difficulty with feeding; and learning difficulties (Chart 21-3). Intelligence may be average or below average. These associated deficits reflect the fact that motor areas of the brain work together; it is rare for a specific area to be affected in isolation.

Assessment

Developmental surveillance is a key part of assessing a child with CP. Abnormal patterns emerge as the damaged nervous system matures. Observe for suspicious signs such as excessive docility or irritability. Poor feeding during the neonatal period combined with irritability, poor sleep patterns, difficulty in cuddling, and poor visual attention merit additional screening or referral. Note evidence of early motor signs including poor head control, asymmetric fisting, and increased tone in limbs. Often, CP cannot be diagnosed until the child is 6 to 12 months old, a time when the child's inability to achieve a developmental milestone becomes more evident. An infant identified with any of the previous findings requires referral for further evaluation.

caREminder

Presentation of reflexes that persist beyond the expected age of disappearance (e.g., tonic neck reflex) or the absence of expected reflexes is highly suggestive of CP.

Neuroimaging tests can be performed on the child with CP to determine the site of the brain impairment and to provide clues regarding the potential cause. The results of these tests do not affect the child's treatment. Other diagnostic tests may be performed to rule out other potential causes of the child's current condition. These tests include cytogenic studies (genetic evaluation of the child and other family members) and metabolic studies.

Nursing Diagnoses and Outcomes

Nursing Plan of Care 21-1 and Nursing Plan of Care 20-1 outline the plan of care for the child with altered neurologic and musculoskeletal status, respectively. The physical disabilities and impaired neuromuscular status of the child with CP are addressed with nursing

CHART 21-3	Deficits Associated With Cerebral Palsy

Musculoskeletal and Reflexive Deficits

Hypotonia

Spastic hypertonia

Hypertonus: lead pipe rigidity that can be "shaken out" by rapid movements of the extremities

Persistent primitive reflexes

Contractures

Osteoporosis

Scoliosis

Neurologic Deficits

Intellectual disability (30%–77%)

Language disorder (approximately 40%)

Learning disability (approximately 40%)

Range of neurobehavioral disorders (up to 50%), attention-deficit/hyperactivity disorder, autism, hyperkinetic or distract-ible behavior

Visual disorders (50%–90%)

Hearing disorders (10%)

Somatosensation (up to 50% of hemiplegia)

Seizures (30%–40%)

Gastrointestinal and Nutritional Problems

Drooling

Malnutrition

Bowel and bladder incontinence

Constipation

Other Systemic Complications

Growth failure

Genitourinary complaints

Respiratory infections

Fatigue

diagnoses that focus on impaired physical mobility, skin integrity, and neurovascular function. In addition, the child with CP experiences difficulty in self-care activities as a result of physical and cognitive limitations. The nursing plan of care should reflect the stress on family members as they relate to a child with a life-long disability. In addition to these considerations, the following diagnoses could apply to the child with CP:

Nursing Diagnosis: Impaired verbal communication related to effects of condition
Outcomes:
• Child will communicate and express his or her needs as much as possible.
• Child will communicate needs and desires without undue frustration.
• Child will use alternative means of communicating, including the use of adaptive equipment, as needed and as able.

Nursing Diagnosis: Imbalanced nutrition: Less than body requirements related to inability to ingest food or retain food in the presence of gastroesophageal reflux
Outcomes:
• Child will receive optimal nutrition to maintain ideal body weight.
• Child will tolerate gastrostomy tube feedings, if needed, to maintain ideal body weight.

Interdisciplinary Interventions

CP is a disorder that cannot be corrected. Therefore, interventions focus on preventing or minimizing deformities and maximizing the child's functioning in the home, school, and community via an integrated health care plan using the expertise of a variety of professionals. The health care team works to maximize the child's potential, considering neurologic and other impairments. The child is encouraged to learn to function independently.

Children younger than 3 years old can benefit from early intervention services. Early intervention is a system of services to support infants and young children (see Chapter 30). For older children, special education and related services are available through the public school system to help each child achieve and learn.

Medical and Surgical Interventions

Management of the child with CP is challenging. The musculoskeletal pathology is much more complex than simple contractures. Torsion of the long bones, joint instability, and degenerative changes in the weight-bearing joints are common and debilitating. The primary management goal is to prevent development of fixed contractures.

Managing spasticity has been shown to delay the onset of orthopedic problems; treatments are classified as focal or generalized. One of the most commonly used agents is BTX-A, a potent neurotoxin produced by the bacterium *Clostridium botulinum* under anaerobic conditions. It binds to cholinergic nerve endings and inhibits release of the neurotransmitter acetylcholine. It decreases a spastic muscle's ability to generate forceful contraction, therefore decreasing the spastic response. BTX-A is injected by the health care provider into the affected muscles and can be used in combination with serial casting. Its safety has been established in a number of open-ended studies.

Conservative measures such as bracing may be used to provide support for ambulation and to discourage contractures. If contractures do develop, orthopedic surgery may be indicated. Various muscle releases and tendon transfers can be done to correct or to relieve contracture. For example, to correct a subluxated or dislocated hip, a hip osteotomy and release of soft tissues and tight tendons may be performed to hold the hip in place. Spinal stabilization with instrumentation can greatly improve or stop the progression of scoliosis.

Neurosurgical Interventions

Selective dorsal rhizotomy is a neurosurgical procedure performed to reduce muscle stiffness and spasticity in children with CP. For some children, the procedure reduces spasticity, resulting in improved walking; it enables others to sit more comfortably in a wheelchair. Selective dorsal rhizotomy may also improve respiratory function, improve arm and head control, and decrease leg spasticity. The procedure takes about 4 hours and involves making a 4- to 6-in. incision in the lower back to uncover and test small nerve rootlets that make up the sensory nerve fibers in the spinal cord. Using a surgical microscope, the surgeon locates, divides, and tests the rootlets of each nerve and cuts rootlets with abnormal responses. Ideal candidates for rhizotomy are children between the ages of 3 and 10 years.

This procedure is most beneficial for the child with spastic diplegia who has some form of forward movement and can take steps by himself or herself without falling. Here, the goals of surgery are better gait and improved leg function. It is also helpful for children with severe spastic quadriplegia or spasticity in all extremities with very limited movement. The goal of surgery is to increase the child's independence by enabling the child to sit for longer periods of time, use a potty seat, and power a wheelchair independently. Selective dorsal rhizotomy involves intensive follow-up, so the family's ability to cooperate is essential.

Pain Management

Pain management in children with CP is complex. Although opioids are useful for incisional pain after surgery, they do not ease muscle spasms. Because of positioning and immobilization in casts, children with CP have more problems with muscle spasms than other children. Muscle relaxants, such as diazepam or other benzodiazepines (e.g., clonazepam), can be administered along with narcotics to relieve discomfort. Muscle relaxants and seizure medications may be needed on a long-term basis, depending on symptoms.

caREminder

Undermedication of children with CP is common because of their communication difficulties. Assess nonverbal pain cues carefully (see Chapter 10). Epidural analgesia is a good option for pain management in children with CP who have had lower extremity surgery, particularly if they are nonverbal. Administering a constant infusion maintains a steady level of analgesia.

Community Care

Acute care of the child with CP is usually necessary only during initial evaluation to perform surgical procedures, to deal with mobility or nutritional issues, or to provide supportive care during serious illnesses such as pneumonia, dehydration, or systemic infection. To optimize the child's level of functioning and provide for the child's basic health care needs, orthopedic and neurosurgical services collaborate with a variety of other professionals in outpatient and community settings. These services continue throughout the child's life, with modifications in the treatment goals as the child grows and matures.

Physical and Occupational Therapies

The interventions provided by the physical and occupational therapist are essential in helping to reduce the risk of contractures and promote the optimal use of motor function. The child's ambulation is likely to be difficult or inefficient. Formal gait analysis and ongoing therapy can assist the child to ambulate. Abnormalities of tone and reflexes can interfere with the child's abilities to perform daily functions. The therapist can introduce techniques or adaptive equipment to help the child achieve activities of daily living that he or she is cognitively capable of completing. The therapist ensures continuity of the plan of care by providing teaching to both the nurse and family regarding the specific measures that will enhance the child's motor functions. Activities such as swimming or horseback riding can help strengthen weaker muscles and relax the tighter ones.

Nutritional Therapy

The nutritional status of children with CP must be addressed. Oral–motor dysfunction leads to limited food intake, which can lead to growth failure, especially in children with severe CP. Severe feeding dysfunction is associated with lower weight, height, and muscle mass. Food must be easy to swallow (chopped or mashed), and jaw support must be given to help the child chew. Gavage or gastrostomy feedings may be needed to meet the child's caloric requirements or if risk of aspiration is severe. A nutritionist can provide the family with suggestions to increase caloric intake, including high-calorie milkshakes and formulas. Reinforce the nutritional information provided to the family and ensure that menu selections reflect guidelines established by the dietitian. Evaluating and documenting the child's intake will provide further evidence of compliance with the dietary plan.

Speech and Language Therapies

Twenty percent of children with CP display hearing or language problems because CP affects the muscles used to produce speech, resulting in slow and slurred speech with a nasal quality. The child's facial features may also seem distorted when he or she is speaking. The child should be evaluated by a speech therapist to determine the best method to help the child communicate most effectively. For the child with good receptive language skills who has difficulty speaking, alternative forms of expressive communication (e.g., computer, "touch-talker," communication board, sign language, or facial gestures) can be used. Families are usually adept at interpreting their child's needs and can help decrease the child's frustration with his or her inability to communicate.

Vision Support

Up to 75% of children with CP have some sort of visual problem or impairment. They may have acuity loss, field loss, occulomotor problems, or processing problems. These conditions may impair eye–hand coordination. Referring these children to an eye care specialist for treatment such as glasses, eye patching, or surgery is important.

Hearing Support

Children with CP are prone to hearing loss, which is often not detected because of their communication difficulties. Failure to follow directions or be attentive to sounds can be wrongly associated with the child's level of cognitive ability. Thus, all children with CP should be referred to an audiologist to ensure accurate and sensitive assessment of their hearing. In most cases, an amplification device (hearing aid) is recommended (see Chapter 28 for more information on hearing loss and treatment). Treating hearing loss early can substantially improve the child's overall outcomes.

Psychosocial Support

The family of a child with CP may experience emotional, physical, and financial challenges because of the ongoing demands of the child's condition. Social services can help the family to find support groups, respite care, and other community resources for needed equipment (see Chapters 2 and 12 for more information on community care, chronic conditions, and rehabilitation). Ramps, vans, electric wheelchairs, computers, and mechanical feeders are just a few of the devices that can make the child more independent. The United Cerebral Palsy Association can help families dealing with the issues of children with CP (see thePoint for Organizations).

Special Education

Problems that may affect learning for some children with CP include learning disabilities, cognitive challenge, and seizures. The interdisciplinary health care team collaborates with the school to ensure that these issues are addressed by developing and implementing an individualized educational plan and providing the necessary adaptations, modifications, and services the child needs to succeed (refer to Chapters 2 and 12 for detailed information on developing an individualized educational plan). Depending on the child's mental capacity and physical disabilities, additional interventions such as physical therapy, occupational therapy, or speech therapy may be needed. In addition to therapy services and special equipment, children with CP may need assistive technology. Examples of assistive technology include communication devices, such as communication boards and voice synthesizers, and computer-based assistive technology. Computers range from electronic toys with special switches to sophisticated computer programs operated by simple switch pads or keyboard adaptations. The health team's goals are to integrate the child into normal school activities as much as possible and to provide a learning environment that is structured to meet the child's unique learning and developmental needs. Every effort should be made to allow the child the intellectual and social stimulation that school provides (see Chapter 12 for more detailed descriptions of the rehabilitative and home care measures that can be provided for the child with CP).

CRANIOFACIAL ABNORMALITIES

Craniofacial malformations may occur as a result of genetic influences, multifactorial prenatal influences, acute craniofacial trauma, and disfigurement associated with cranial or facial tumor resection. Advances in imaging techniques and three-dimensional reconstructive surgery techniques have resulted in improved methods to enhance the physical appearance of affected children. Developments in fetal surgery offer the potential of treating selected anomalies in utero. The most common craniofacial malformations seen in children that occur as a result of alterations in normal development are microcephaly and craniosynostosis (Fig. 21-7). Table 21-6 provides a summary of these abnormalities.

Meningitis

Infectious processes can affect the brain and spinal cord. *Meningitis* refers to inflammation of the membranes of the brain, spinal cord, or both. The three meningeal layers that can be affected include (1) the dura mater (pachymeningitis), (2) the subarachnoid mater, and (3) the pia mater (leptomeningitis). The etiologic agents involved in meningitis include bacterial, viral, and fungal organisms. Chemical toxins such as lead and arsenic, contrast media used in myelography, and metastatic malignant cells can also trigger an inflammatory process that, although not infectious, is similar in clinical appearance.

BACTERIAL MENINGITIS

Bacterial meningitis is a pyogenic (purulent) infection that involves the pia mater and arachnoid mater layers of the meninges and the subdural space, including the CSF. Over 75% of cases occur in children younger than 5 years of age (Agrawal & Nadel, 2011). Because of infant immunizations, the incidence of some types of bacterial meningitis has decreased (Table 21-7). Outbreaks of *Haemophilus influenzae* meningitis can occur, however, in unvaccinated populations and immunocompromised children.

Bacterial meningitis can be a devastating illness because of the systemic involvement and severity of its clinical course. Rapid diagnosis and early treatment contribute to the most favorable recovery.

Pathophysiology

The pathogens responsible for meningitis usually disseminate from a distant site of infection and then spread into the meninges. Bacterial colonization and infiltration of the meninges most commonly occur after an upper respiratory infection or bacteremia accompanying otitis media, sinusitis, or mastoiditis. Pathogens can also enter through penetrating wounds or through the skin in the presence of a structural defect, such as a myelomeningocele. In the neonate, additional risk factors include maternal infection, premature rupture of amniotic membranes, premature birth, low birth weight, prolonged labor, and the immaturity of the neonatal immune system. After the pathogen is implanted,

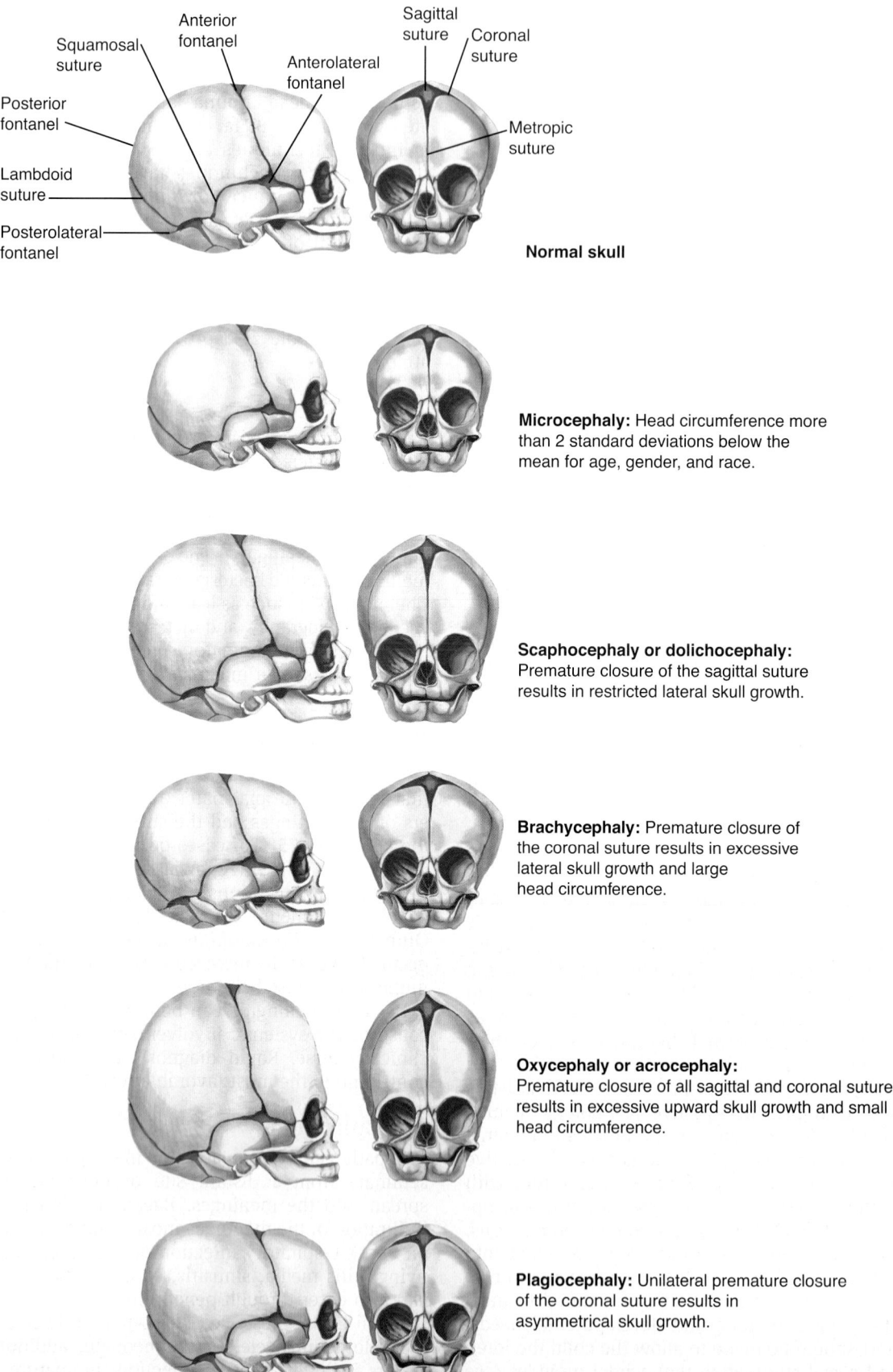

Squamosal suture

Anterior fontanel

Sagittal suture

Coronal suture

Anterolateral fontanel

Posterior fontanel

Metropic suture

Lambdoid suture

Posterolateral fontanel

Normal skull

Microcephaly: Head circumference more than 2 standard deviations below the mean for age, gender, and race.

Scaphocephaly or dolichocephaly: Premature closure of the sagittal suture results in restricted lateral skull growth.

Brachycephaly: Premature closure of the coronal suture results in excessive lateral skull growth and large head circumference.

Oxycephaly or acrocephaly: Premature closure of all sagittal and coronal sutures results in excessive upward skull growth and small head circumference.

Plagiocephaly: Unilateral premature closure of the coronal suture results in asymmetrical skull growth.

Figure 21-7 Normal skull and variations that result from premature closure of cranial sutures.

TABLE 21-6   Craniofacial Abnormalities

Description	Assessment	Interdisciplinary Interventions
Microcephaly		
HC that measures 2 *SD* below the mean for the child's age and gender. *Primary* (genetic) microcephaly caused by a genetic inheritance pattern or syndrome (e.g., trisomy 21, trisomy 18, cri du chat, Cornelia de Lange). *Secondary* (nongenetic) microcephaly can result from exposure to noxious agents in utero or during times of rapid brain growth (e.g., radiation, congenital infections, maternal ingestion of drugs or alcohol, meningitis or encephalitis, malnutrition, maternal diabetes, hyperthermia, or hypoxic ischemic encephalopathy).	Measurement of HC (at birth or over time) and visual inspection may reveal a very small head. Record HC of parents and siblings to evaluate for familial tendencies. Assessment for other physical and congenital abnormalities (e.g., abnormal facies, short stature, deformities of the hands, congenital heart disease). Karyotypes are obtained if chromosomal syndrome is suspected. CT or MRI used to assess structural abnormalities of the brain or intracerebral calcifications. Blood or urine analyses are done to determine specific causative agents (e.g., cytomegalovirus, rubella, or herpes simplex infection).	No treatment to alter or reverse the child's small HC. Treat causative agent (if known) to minimize involvement of further body systems. Work in collaboration with the family to optimize the child's development (see Chapter 30 for care of the child with a developmental disability). Most children with microcephaly experience some degree of cognitive deficit.
Craniosynostosis		
Absence of, or premature fusion of, one or more cranial sutures; the process of early suture closure. *Craniostenosis* (often used synonymously with *craniosynostosis*) describes the deformity that results from early fusion of sutures. *Primary, simple synostosis:* involvement of one suture; *primary, compound synostosis:* absence or early fusion of two or more sutures. Most cases present as an isolated problem not associated with other syndromes or anomalies. *Secondary* occurs as a result of a known disorder causing failure of brain growth and expansion or early fusion of sutures. *Syndromic* involves closure of multiple sutures and occurs in conjunction with other morphologic syndromes or developmental anomalies, (e.g., Crouzon and Apert syndromes; see thePoint for Supplemental Information: Genetic Disorders Associated With Craniosynostosis). In these cases, development of facial bones is also affected, and increased ICP can be a serious secondary complication. The number of sutures involved and the rate and degree of fusion determine cranial asymmetry. Growth is inhibited at right angles to the fused suture, whereas compensatory expansion occurs at the sutures that are functional. The earlier in fetal or infant life that synostosis occurs, the greater the effect in cranial growth and appearance.	Parents are often the first to notice abnormalities in the infant's head shape. Palpate the head for suture location and mobility; note bony ridges along suture lines and any facial or cranial asymmetry. Evaluate asymmetry by comparing the location of the external ear canals and the outer canthi of the eyes from right to left; best made with the examiner looking down on the infant or child from a superior position. Move the child's hair away from the forehead during examination, especially when synostosis of the metopic or either coronal suture is suspected. Plot serial measurements of HC on growth chart to provide an early indication of the development of craniosynostosis. Measure height, weight, and HC simultaneously to ensure that the child is not failing to grow on all parameters for other reasons. Perform a complete neurologic examination; evaluate sensory and motor function, cranial nerves, and for signs indicative of chronic increased ICP (progressive papilledema, impairment of vision, and changes in mental status such as increased irritability or lethargy), which may occur if the cranial bones are not able to expand with brain growth.	Assess the family's goals. It is hard for a parent of an otherwise healthy-appearing child to consent to surgery of this magnitude, even in the presence of obvious deformity. Elicit concerns and provide positive reinforcement. Surgical intervention to prevent increased ICP and correct cosmetic deformity is usually done between 3 and 12 months of age, when the child's bone is still pliable. Preoperatively, make parents aware of the potential for blood loss in the child; the family may wish to donate blood. Educate family members about skull anatomy and how surgery will change it. Show before-and-after photographs of children who have undergone similar corrective surgery. Prepare parents for the postsurgical appearance of their child with a turban-style head dressing, orbital edema that may cause the child's eyelids to swell shut, and irritability for the first few days. Postoperatively, monitor the child's neurologic status, including level of consciousness, pupillary responses (not done if eyes are swollen shut), and signs of increased ICP. Monitor vital signs for changes indicating infection or changes in ICP. Assess surgical dressings and drains and monitor fluid and electrolyte balances because children undergoing this surgery often have mild to moderate cerebral edema. Facial swelling and severe eye and periorbital swelling require skin surveillance to prevent further trauma, skin breakdown, or infection.

(Continued)

TABLE 21-6   Craniofacial Abnormalities (*Continued*)

Description	Assessment	Interdisciplinary Interventions
	Conduct a full developmental evaluation. Check the family history for indications of genetic findings in other family members, living or dead. Radiographic studies and a CT scan assist in detailing the bony structure and associated intracranial abnormalities.	Elevate the head of the head at least 20–30 degrees, per surgeon preference. Increased intrathoracic pressure, which results from elevating the torso, has been known to increase ICP. For this reason, children recovering from surgery are maintained on moderate fluid restrictions. Prophylactic antibiotics may be administered for a few days. Monitor the child for CSF leak. Prevent the child from touching the incision after removal of the head dressing; this may require use of elbow splints. Administer prophylactic eye drops or ointments as ordered if prolonged eye swelling increases risk of conjunctival infection or ulcer. Provide pharmacologic pain management, implement biobehavioral methods as adjuncts (see Chapter 10); considerable postoperative pain is typical. Be aware that easing the fear and anxiety of a young child who cannot see is a challenge, but sedatives are rarely ordered because they mask true neurologic status and make assessment difficult. Ask parents which biobehavioral measures help their child to cope. Maximize use of the senses of touch, taste, smell, and hearing to assure a child that his or her familiar and comforting world has not disappeared. Ensure adequate rest periods, even as the child appears to get back to normal activity.
Positional Plagiocephaly		
A nonsynostotic disorder resulting from molding caused by repeat positioning on the same side of the head	Assess as with craniosynostosis.	To prevent or minimize positional plagiocephaly, teach parents to alternate the sleep position of the child (e.g., put the child's feet at one end of the bed for a week, then at the other end the next week), alternate feeding positions, hang decorations or move crib to encourage child to look to both sides, and put the child prone daily while awake. *Dynamic orthotic cranioplasty* incorporates the use of special hard-shell helmets, designed by orthotic technicians or physical therapists, which have internal inserts that place gentle pressure on the skull aligned opposite to the affected area. The helmet is worn 24 hours a day, generally for 3–6 months. Controversy exists over whether the helmets are necessary because many children outgrow this deformity without them (de Ribaupierre et al., 2007). Teach the parents to assess the scalp daily for redness or abrasions and to provide good hygiene to the scalp. As the child adjusts to the helmet, acetaminophen may be needed to decrease irritability and to promote comfort. Teach the family the importance of follow-up evaluations for assessment of the child and to adjust the helmet based on the progression of the therapy.

HC, head circumference; *SD*, standard deviation.

TABLE 21-7   Bacterial Meningitis

Pathogen	Predisposing Factors	Considerations	Prevention
Pneumococcus (*Streptococcus pneumoniae*)	Otitis media, mastoiditis, basilar skull fracture, sickle cell disease, asplenia	Has a 25% mortality rate with treatment	Pneumococcal conjugate vaccine recommended for all children aged 2–23 months Pneumococcal polysaccharide vaccine recommended for high-risk children aged 2 years old or older
Meningococcus (*Neisseria meningitidis*)	Close contact with a previous case at daycare center, nursery school, or college dorm	Has a 5%–10% mortality rate with treatment	Rifampin, ceftriaxone, or ciprofloxacin for all close contacts Meningococcal polysaccharide diphtheria toxoid conjugate vaccine for high-risk children aged 11 years or older Meningococcal polysaccharide vaccine for high-risk children aged 2–10 years
Haemophilus influenzae	Otitis media, pharyngitis, sickle cell anemia, asplenia	Has a 5% mortality rate with treatment	Rifampin for all household contacts *H. influenzae* type B conjugated vaccine recommended for all children beginning at 2 months of age
Gram-negative enteric bacteria	Maternal vaginal or perineal colonization, congenital dural defects (myelomeningocele)	Has a 50%–75% mortality rate with treatment	No chemoprophylaxis or vaccine available.
Group B *Streptococcus*	Maternal vaginal or perineal colonization	In twin delivery, requires treatment of both twins even if only one is symptomatic.	No chemoprophylaxis or vaccination is required. Intrapartum administration of ampicillin by mother may prevent infection of newborn.
Listeria monocytogenes	Maternal vaginal or perineal colonization. Maternal infection from consuming contaminated dairy products, meats, and vegetables.	Pregnant women should avoid unpasteurized milk and soft cheeses, such as goat cheese.	No chemoprophylaxis or vaccine is available
Shunt-associated meningitis (coagulase-negative or coagulase-positive *Staphylococcus*, gram-negative rods, enterococci)	Ventriculoatrial or ventriculoperitoneal shunt	Requires scrupulous technique Requires adequate skin asepsis when accessing shunt	Based on causative pathogen

it proliferates and spreads into the CSF and through perivascular channels and meningeal folds to the brain parenchyma. Later, clumps of purulent exudate collect around the base of the brain, obstructing CSF and potentially causing hydrocephalus and cranial nerve palsies. Blood vessel walls and endothelium become involved, and cerebral perfusion may be compromised, leading to cerebral edema. Vasculitis associated with thrombosis can cause infarctions (strokes), seizures, and focal deficits. Continued necrosis of cells in the brain cortex and hydrocephalus can lead to permanent damage, increased ICP, and death.

Assessment

In neonates, the manifestations of infection and meningeal irritation may be minimal or absent. Consider bacterial meningitis in any newborn who fails to thrive and who exhibits irritability, apnea, seizures, a tendency for **opisthotonos** (a form of spasm in which the head and heels are bent backward and the body is bowed forward), poor feeding, emesis, hypothermia, hyperthermia, hypotonia, hypertonia, grayish skin, jaundice, or other evidence of sepsis. Bulging fontanels are present as ICP rises.

The infant may have few striking signs. The family may notice only that the infant is resistant to being cuddled or diapered, displays irritability, and has a mild fever. The infant may have a high-pitched cry, a transient vacant stare, and anorexia. A bulging, tense fontanel is a common signs and may indicate increased ICP. Older children may have nonspecific complaints, such as high fever, vomiting, and fatigue. Severe headache, altered consciousness, stiff neck (nuchal rigidity), and convulsions are often present and suggest neurologic involvement.

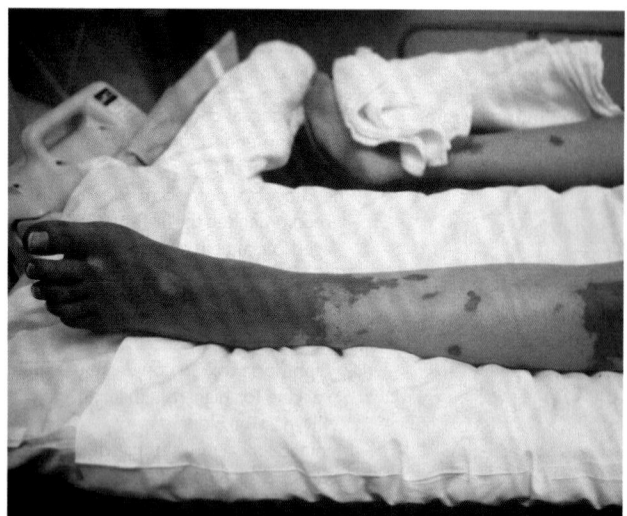

Figure 21-8 This child's legs exhibit the characteristic purpuric lesions of meningococcal disease.

Ask the child to try to touch the chin to the chest. If pain prevents the child from doing so, nuchal rigidity, caused by inflamed meninges, may be present.

The Kernig sign (inability to extend the legs fully when lying supine) and the Brudzinski sign (flexion of the hips when the neck is flexed from a supine position) are frequently present.

Document any rash. Both *H. influenzae* meningitis and meningococcal meningitis can cause a petechial rash. As the rash rapidly progresses, darker purpuric eruptions occur. These eruptions are associated with meningococcemia septic shock, known as Waterhouse-Friderichsen syndrome (Fig. 21-8).

ALERT *Advise any family inquiring about a "purple rash," especially one associated with other symptoms such as fatigue, fever, and vomiting, to have the child seen by a health care provider immediately.*

Meningococcemia, an overwhelming septic infection, may develop in patients with *Neisseria meningitidis* meningitis. Its high fevers, purpuric lesions, and circulatory collapse from adrenal insufficiency constitute a medical emergency. The accompanying inflammatory response is marked by disseminated intravascular coagulation, encephalitis, lung abscess, and organ hemorrhage leading to tissue necrosis. This collection of symptoms may result in death only hours after the onset of fever. Meningococcemia has a mortality rate of 5% to 20% (Pace & Pollard, 2012). Rapid diagnosis and antibiotic therapy can be lifesaving.

Diagnostic Tests

Bacterial meningitis can be diagnosed through signs and symptoms, plus a CSF culture. The fluid is examined for cloudiness, blood cell counts, white blood cell differential, and protein and glucose levels (Table 21-8).

caREminder

The glucose and protein content of the CSF provide clues to the etiology of meningitis. A low glucose level and high protein count in spinal fluid indicate bacterial meningitis. A normal to high glucose level and a normal to low protein count typically indicate viral meningitis.

Common microbiologic tests for bacterial meningitis also include a Gram stain and a blood culture. These tests are positive in 80% to 90% of infected patients for spinal fluid and 30% to 60% for blood specimens. Counterimmunoelectrophoresis and latex agglutination tests can detect bacterial antigen in spinal fluid, urine, or blood in less than 1 hour. These rapid tests are helpful when children have been pretreated with antibiotics before the lumbar puncture or blood culture. Although these rapid diagnostic tests are available, they cannot be used as the sole basis of diagnosis because false results can occur.

Other laboratory tests may include cultures of blood, urine, nasopharynx, and CSF leaks to identify the source of septicemia. Complete blood cell counts may show an increased total white blood cell level with elevated numbers of immature granulocytes. Serum C-reactive protein levels increase acutely with bacterial infection. CT or MRI may be used to monitor the course of the illness and to determine the need for specific interventions.

TABLE 21-8	Analysis of Cerebrospinal Fluid for Central Nervous System Infections				
	Pressure (mm H₂O)	**Appearance**	**Leukocytes (/mm³)**	**Protein (mg/dL)**	**Sugar (mg/dL)**
Normal CSF	60–200 (5–15 mm Hg)	Clear	0–5	10–30	40–80
Bacterial meningitis	Elevated	Turbid, cloudy	Elevated, 100–60,000; polymorphonuclear cells predominate	Elevated, 100–500	Decreased
Aseptic meningitis	Normal or slight elevation	Clear	10–1,000	Not greater than 100	Normal to low, <40
Tuberculosis meningitis	Elevated	Clear	25–100	100–200	<50
Brain abscess	Elevated	Clear	Elevated, 10–200	Elevated, 75–500	>50

Interdisciplinary Interventions

Treating bacterial meningitis requires prompt, intensive medical management and nursing care; it also frequently requires pain management.

Pharmacologic Interventions

Treatment for bacterial meningitis calls for aggressive intervention with appropriate IV antibiotics given for 7 to 14 days. Broad-spectrum antibiotic therapy is initiated before the results of CSF cultures are obtained. After organism sensitivities are known, antibiotic therapy is refined based on sensitivities identified by the culture, and dosages are adjusted to maintain therapeutic serum antibiotic levels, when appropriate. IV corticosteroids, such as dexamethasone, may be used as an adjunct to antibiotic therapy to decrease short-term neurologic sequelae and prevent hearing loss (Brouwer et al., 2010).

Infection Control Interventions

Droplet precautions are recommended until at least 24 hours of effective antibiotic therapy have elapsed. Generally, continuing isolation beyond 24 hours is not recommended for any of the forms of bacterial meningitis except those caused by *H. influenzae* and *N. meningitidis*.

Surgical Interventions

Surgical treatment may be necessary for infants or children with severe seizures, increased ICP, ventriculomegaly, hydrocephalus, subdural effusion, or empyema. Treatment may include ventriculostomy to drain infected or obstructed fluid. A shunt may be necessary. Some organisms may require careful intraventricular administration of antibiotics. Subdural effusions may be treated with subdural antibiotic irrigation and drainage performed by a physician or advanced practice nurse.

Supportive Interventions

Supportive interventions include managing fever and hydration, which entails monitoring response to treatment. Avoid overhydration to prevent the onset of SIADH that would further exacerbate cerebral edema and lead to life-threatening compromise of cerebral tissues. Fluids are often restricted to a combined oral and IV total of one half to two thirds of maintenance fluids (see thePoint for Care Path: The Child With Uncomplicated Bacterial Meningitis). Supportive care may also include recognition and treatment of increased ICP, seizures, cerebral edema, hydrocephalus, subdural effusion, and empyema.

If seizures have occurred, the child may receive a loading dose of phenobarbital, phenytoin (Dilantin), or fosphenytoin sodium (Cerebyx), followed by maintenance doses. If seizure activity persists beyond 4 days, risk of residual damage and chronic seizure disorders increases.

Additional interventions include acute neurologic monitoring, evaluating vital signs and head circumference, palpating the anterior fontanel, measuring daily weight, measuring intake and output, and assessing the IV site (Clinical Judgment 21-3). Assess the child for discomfort, irritability, behavioral problems, seizures, vomiting, appetite, thirst, and other potential complications. The child is at risk for seizure activity, so keep bedside rails up and ensure that someone stays with the child in the bathroom. If a seizure occurs, provide appropriate immediate care, observe and document seizures, and administer antiepileptic medications as ordered by the prescriber. Teach family members and the child about seizure observation, management, and medications.

Monitor the child for potential hearing loss caused by meningitis or ototoxic side effects of aminoglycoside antibiotics and diuretics by assessing the child's response to auditory stimuli and the ability to localize sounds. If hearing loss is suspected, notify the prescriber to ensure that the child is tested appropriately. An otologist can determine treatment and ongoing follow-up.

Assessment for potential arthritis and stress ulcer is also indicated in the child with meningitis.

Pain Management

The child with meningitis is likely to experience pain related to meningeal irritation. In addition, some diagnostic tests, such as lumbar punctures, blood draws, administration of IV fluids and antibiotics, and immobility associated with bed rest, may cause discomfort. Although completely relieving the child's pain and discomfort may not be possible, use pharmacologic and biobehavioral measures to maximize the success of pain relief interventions (see Chapter 10). Discuss pain with the child honestly, indicating how much a procedure will hurt, how long it will last, and what will help to lessen the pain. Ensure that the child understands that the pain is *not* a punishment.

Community Care

Community care begins with prevention measures for meningitis and control so that existing cases do not cause others. Ongoing home care is crucial.

Prevention and Control

Preventive measures against bacterial meningitis include prompt treatment for upper respiratory infections, otitis media, sinusitis, mastoiditis, and other infections, especially in younger infants and children. Immunization with *H. influenzae* type B, 7-valent pneumococcal conjugate vaccine, 23-valent pneumococcal polysaccharide vaccine, meningococcal (groups A, C, Y, and W-135) polysaccharide diphtheria toxoid conjugate vaccine, or meningococcal polysaccharide vaccine primes the child's immune system and facilitates effective response to subsequent exposure, thus preventing meningitis. See Chapter 8 for a discussion of immunizations.

For family members and exposed staff, chemoprophylaxis is only necessary in cases of exposure to meningococcus or *H. influenzae*. Family members who share the same household with the infected child should receive rifampin prophylaxis; adults can receive a single dose of ciprofloxacin. Any daycare or school contacts should also receive prophylaxis because the duration and extent of contact with the infected child may be difficult to determine. Generally, if close, intimate

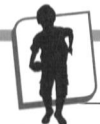

The Child With Meningitis

Kara is 9 years old and is brought to the emergency department by her guardian because of severe headaches and a stiff neck for the past 24 hours. Kara did not want to go to school today. Upon arrival in the emergency department, she vomited. She has had no history of a recent cold or other illness. Her temperature is 102° F (38.9° C).

Questions

1. To determine whether Kara has meningitis, what diagnostic tests and procedures should be completed?
2. What clinical finding is classically associated with meningococcal meningitis?
3. The CSF is cloudy with an increased white blood cell count, low glucose level, and elevated protein level. What nursing diagnosis could be selected to reflect Kara's potential for neurologic dysfunction?
4. Kara is transferred to the pediatric unit. What nursing measures should be taken to make Kara comfortable and minimize pain?
5. Twenty-four hours later, Kara demonstrates no improvement. She remains febrile, continues to vomit, and has become very irritable and lethargic. What action should the nurse take?

Answers

1. Lumbar puncture; cultures of blood, urine, and nasopharynx; CT or MRI of the head for child with symptoms of increased ICP
2. Rapidly spreading purpuric skin lesions
3. Risk for injury related to complications of meningitis including increased ICP, seizures, and hearing loss
4. Analgesics should be given as ordered. Head of bed should be elevated and the room should be kept quiet, with subdued lighting. Health care activities should be arranged to cause the least amount of disturbance to Kara. Comfort objects should be provided.
5. Report these findings immediately to the physician. The antibiotics may need to be changed. New lumbar puncture and blood cultures may be performed.

mouth-to-mouth contact has occurred, then prophylaxis is necessary. However, many families of children in the same classroom or school demand prophylaxis because meningitis is so devastating. Rifampin is relatively inexpensive and causes few side effects. Thus, most health departments give prophylaxis generously. Ciprofloxacin is an attractive alternative to rifampin for persons older than 18 years of age because it is given as a single dose.

caREminder

Unless a health care worker has unprotected, intimate contact with the patient, prophylaxis is not indicated. Intimate contact involves face-to-face encounters, such as intubating the child, assisting with a lumbar puncture, or giving mouth-to-mouth resuscitation without using a mask.

Many employee health and infection control programs offer prophylaxis to health care workers regardless of the extent of the exposure. However, the American Academy of Pediatrics and the Centers for Disease Control and Prevention (CDC) recommend prophylaxis for health care workers based on actual exposure rather than heightened concern (American Academy of Pediatrics, 2012).

Home Care and Rehabilitation Interventions

Home care and rehabilitation are based on the residual effects of the disease and vary for each child. The child may be discharged while still on IV antibiotic therapy if the child is stable, afebrile, has no complications, and the family is able to manage care at home. Make arrangements with the home health nurse before discharge to ensure a smooth transition of care from acute to home care settings. Instruct the family how to assess neurologic status and to evaluate changes in vital signs, and encourage collaboration with the health care team. Compare developmental findings with previously recorded assessments to evaluate developmental delays. In addition, the health care team works with the family to provide rehabilitation as needed to address problems with other systems that arise during the course of the illness. Before discharge, brain stem auditory-evoked potentials or audiometry for older children is usually done. If hearing loss occurs, early intervention is possible. Careful follow-up is advisable, with developmental testing and information about appropriate infant stimulation.

CHAPTER 21 · · · The Child With Altered Neurologic Status **1085**

TUBERCULOUS MENINGITIS

Tuberculous meningitis, a complication stemming from primary lung infection with tuberculosis (see Chapter 24), is seen infrequently in developed countries but is a common cause of bacterial meningitis in developing countries. The highest incidence is seen in children 1 to 3 years of age and is unusual in infants younger than 3 months old (Agrawal & Nadel, 2011; Donald & Schoeman, 2009); congenital cases are rare. Occasionally, tuberculous meningitis may occur many years after the primary infection, resulting from the rupture of one or more tubercles, which discharge bacilli into the subarachnoid space.

Outcomes are favorable with early diagnosis and treatment. However, if untreated, death is likely. Complications are related to the effectiveness of treatment and the stage of infection at which the child is diagnosed. Long-term sequelae can include hearing loss, communicating hydrocephalus, intellectual and emotional disturbances, seizures, and muscle spasticity.

Pathophysiology

Mycobacterium tuberculosis is the organism responsible for tuberculosis infections. In children younger than 20 years of age, the lungs are the predominant site for *primary* tuberculosis infections, followed by the lymph nodes, pleural space, and meningeal covers of the brain. *Secondary* infection occurs as *M. tuberculosis* bacteria enter the lungs and rapidly spread throughout the body via the lymphatic system and bloodstream. When organisms reach the highly vascular meningeal covering of the brain, the child becomes at risk for tuberculous meningitis; therefore, the infection may be classified as either primary or secondary.

Assessment

The onset of tuberculous meningitis may be rapid or gradual. Rapid onset is more common in infants and younger children, with acute hydrocephalus, seizures, and cerebral edema developing after only a few days of symptoms. More commonly, onset is gradual, with signs and symptoms developing over weeks. Initial manifestations are nonspecific and include fever, lethargy, headache, and malaise. Within 10 to 14 days, positive meningeal signs (nuchal rigidity, Kernig sign, severe headache) develop.

Diagnostic Tests

Analysis of CSF may show little abnormality because the fluid is obtained from a site proximal to the inflammation and obstruction. CT scans or MR images are usually normal during the early stages of the illness. Diagnosis is typically based on clinical suspicion because laboratory, radiographs, and clinical findings are often nonspecific.

Interdisciplinary Interventions

The child requires treatment for tuberculosis (see Chapter 24). In addition to long-term treatment with isoniazid, rifampin, and pyrazinamide, steroids have been shown to improve outcome (Marx & Chan, 2011).

If neurologic sequelae are present, other therapy (e.g., physical or occupational therapy) may be warranted.

Provide emotional support to the family; ongoing disease sequelae and long-term medication regimes are stressors. Teach and reinforce with children and their families the importance of adhering to the medication regime.

ASEPTIC MENINGITIS

Aseptic meningitis is one of the most common causes of infection of the meninges. It occurs at all ages but is more common in children. Meningitis with negative bacterial cultures from CSF is termed *aseptic*. It can be caused by many agents, such as fungi, rickettsiae, drugs, or postinfection, but enteroviruses are the most common cause (Riddel & Shuman, 2012). Common enteroviruses include echoviruses, coxsackievirus, and polio. Herpes simplex types I and II may cause aseptic meningitis in adolescents and life-threatening encephalitis in neonates and children.

Pathophysiology

Viruses gain access to the CNS through systemic circulation. They enter cells in the meninges, causing inflammation and edema. Incidence of infection by enteroviruses is highest during the summer months.

Assessment

The clinical manifestations are similar to those of bacterial meningitis; however, they do not progress as rapidly and are usually less severe. Assess the child for fever, headache, vomiting, and stiff neck. Seizures are seen less frequently in aseptic meningitis than in bacterial meningitis. Irritability, drowsiness, and lethargy may occur but are milder than in patients with encephalitis. The child's history usually reveals the presence of a recent or concurrent viral illness.

Document the presence of any rash or other physical signs. When aseptic meningitis occurs with or follows a discrete, red, maculopapular rash, enterovirus or coxsackievirus infection is likely. When coxsackievirus is the offending pathogen, symptoms may also include the appearance of vesicles and ulcers on the soft palate, paroxysmal pain in the intercostal muscles caused by irritation of pleural surfaces, and symptoms of pericarditis. If aseptic meningitis is caused by mumps virus, parotiditis may also occur.

Diagnostic Tests

Lumbar puncture is completed to obtain CSF for examination and potentially differentiate aseptic meningitis from bacterial meningitis (Fig. 21-9) (see thePoint for Procedures: Lumbar Puncture). The CSF in aseptic meningitis usually contains a greater amount of white blood cells than normal but fewer than in bacterial disease. CSF glucose may be normal, and protein may be only mildly elevated. Virus or virus antibodies may be isolated from CSF, blood, sputum, stool, or other specimens. The lumbar puncture may also help to alleviate symptoms of increased ICP.

Interdisciplinary Interventions

Health care interventions for aseptic meningitis are primarily supportive and are aimed at ameliorating symptoms. The child may be hospitalized to monitor and

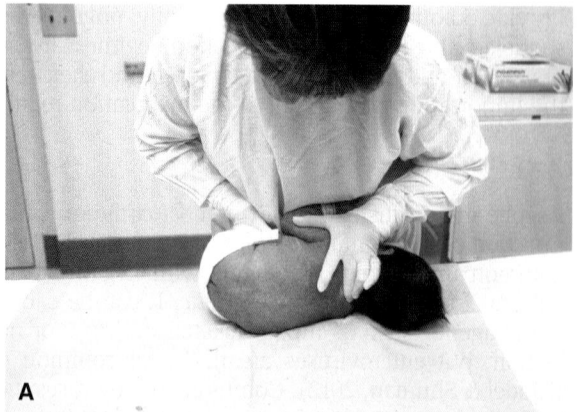

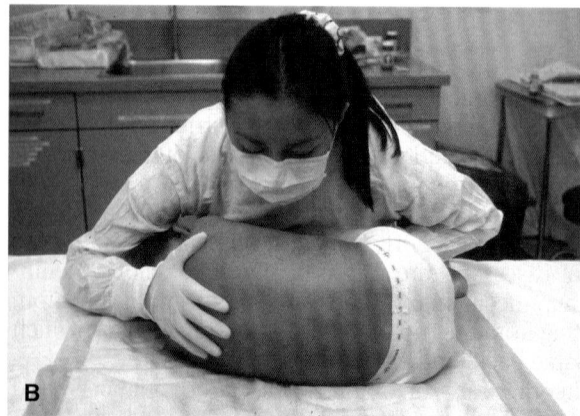

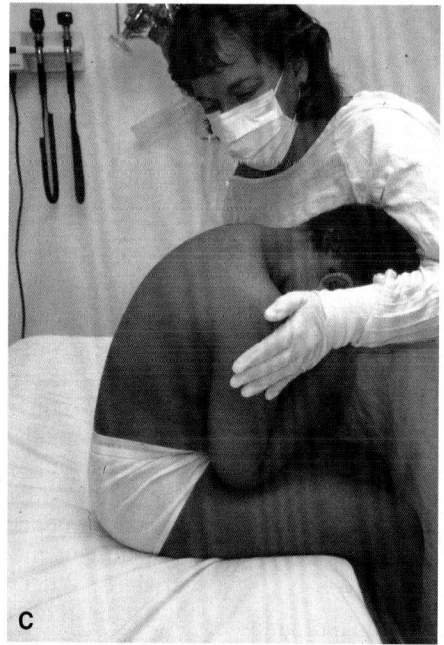

Figure 21-9 Positions for lumbar puncture. (A) Knee-chest position. (B) Recumbent position. (C) Sitting position.

manage neurologic status, monitor fluid and electrolyte balance, control hyperthermia, provide supportive care, control pain, maintain adequate nutrition, and treat seizures, if they occur.

Young infants are routinely hospitalized because of the risk of meningitis caused by bacterial infection. Because bacterial meningitis can be so devastating, young infants receive broad-spectrum antibiotics (ampicillin and cefotaxime) until CSF bacterial cultures are negative and thus bacterial meningitis is ruled out. Older and less severely affected children may be managed on an outpatient basis, with analgesics and antipyretics administered as needed.

ENCEPHALITIS

Encephalitis is defined as an inflammation of the brain. When the meninges are also involved, the term *meningoencephalitis* is used. If the spinal cord is involved, the term *myelitis* or *encephalomyelitis* is used. Although encephalitis closely resembles meningitis in origin and

presentation, the clinical course may be more severe because the infection affects actual brain tissue.

A wide variety of infectious agents may cause encephalitis. Viral encephalitis is most commonly seen in children. The viruses most frequently identified as causative agents are enteroviruses, arboviruses, and herpes simplex virus. Viral encephalitis is particularly common in children who are immunosuppressed. The advent and widespread use of measles, mumps, rubella, and chickenpox vaccines has substantially decreased the incidence of viral encephalitis.

Nonviral causes of encephalitis include bacteria, spirochetal infections, cat scratch disease, parasites, fungi, rickettsial infections, protozoa, and helminths. These organisms may be inadvertently introduced into the body during administration of certain chemotherapeutic agents, diagnostic imaging dyes, detergents, or alcohol into the CSF.

The prognosis of encephalitis depends on the degree and duration of cerebral and CNS involvement and the ability to successfully manage secondary complications.

Neurologic sequelae are present at discharge in 60% of children who recover from acute infection (Fowler et al., 2008).

Pathophysiology

CNS involvement is believed to be secondary to an infectious process occurring elsewhere in the body. The CNS may be severely affected, with associated dysfunctions as seen in Guillain-Barré syndrome (GBS) and Reye syndrome. As the brain tissue becomes inflamed, fever, headache, seizure, agitation, and altered states of awareness result from increasing cerebral or cerebellar dysfunction.

Assessment

The onset of symptoms may be acute or gradual, with complaints of general muscle pain, fever, gastrointestinal distress, and mild respiratory symptoms. Clinically, the neurologic presentation is similar to that in meningitis, including headache, changes in arousal and consciousness, and possible persistent seizures. Complete a thorough history to evaluate any recent viral illnesses or exposures that may identify the causative organism. Assess for signs of increased ICP and meningeal irritation, including headache, fever, and stiff neck.

Diagnostic Tests

Laboratory evaluation includes examination of CSF, blood, stool, and sputum to help establish the cause of the disease. In many cases, CSF values are unspecific. Lymphocyte count may be increased, glucose is usually normal, and protein levels are often mildly elevated. If localized CNS hemorrhage has occurred, red blood cells and hemoglobin may be present in the CSF. CSF should also be examined for acid-fast organisms, parasites, and bacteria. Fourteen to 21 days after the onset of encephalitis, the CSF should again be evaluated and tested.

CT and MRI may show cerebral edema, hydrocephalus, or lesions. An EEG may show abnormalities consistent with seizure activity.

Interdisciplinary Interventions

The care of the child with encephalitis is directed toward managing and preventing secondary complications such as seizures, increased ICP, and respiratory involvement. Severely affected children may receive mechanical ventilation, ICP monitoring, and ventriculostomy care as warranted (see the discussion on increased ICP earlier in this chapter).

If a causative organism is identified, appropriate antimicrobial medications are prescribed. Herpes simplex encephalitis should be treated with IV acyclovir for 10 days. Until cultures reveal a specific etiologic agent, children with fever and acute encephalic symptoms are generally given acyclovir and an antibacterial agent.

If seizures have occurred, treatment is initiated by administering IV diazepam or lorazepam. Characteristically, the seizures associated with encephalitis are difficult to control. If benzodiazepine is ineffective, IV phenytoin is administered. Further seizure activity may require the use of phenobarbital. Aggressive and prolonged use of antiepileptic medications creates the need for mechanical

ventilation to support the child's respiratory status and cardiac monitoring to assess for cardiac conduction defects. As always, monitor the child for side effects.

The child's precarious condition and the lack of a definitive treatment for the child's illness are likely to cause the family a great deal of stress and fear. Provide frequent communication to the family regarding the child's status. Arrange support services to help the family through this difficult time. Involve the family in care decisions and in direct care for the child.

BRAIN ABSCESS

A brain abscess is a localized infection that extends into the brain parenchyma. Brain abscess can be multiple or single and is most often located in the frontal and temporal lobes.

Brain abscesses are rare, yet serious. They are typically caused by streptococci, staphylococci, enteric bacteria, or mixed flora. Gram-negative enteric pathogens are most common in neonates (Chowdhry & Cohen, 2012). *S. aureus* is the primary cause of direct infection following head trauma or intracranial procedures. Blood-borne spread of organisms is likely to cause multiple abscess formation, whereas other mechanisms generally result in single lesions. Risk factors for brain abscess in children include sinusitis, otitis, pulmonary infection, cyanotic congenital heart disease, endocarditis, meningitis, bacteremia, and immunodeficiency.

The mortality rate associated with brain abscess has been reported at 3.7% (Shachor-Meyouhas et al., 2010) to 5.9% (Felsenstein et al., 2013). The likelihood of recovery without substantial neurologic deficit is increased by rapid diagnosis, antimicrobial medications, and diligent monitoring.

Pathophysiology

The origin of brain abscesses can usually be traced to one of three situations:

1. Extension of local infections of the middle ear, mastoid, or sinuses
2. Distal infections in the chest or lungs or spread through the bloodstream in an immunocompromised host (metastatic abscess)
3. Direct infection as a result of open head trauma, intracranial surgery, bacterial meningitis, or cranial traction

Within 2 weeks of initial microbial entry, the abscess becomes an encapsulated lesion filled with pus.

Assessment

Symptoms occur in two stages and vary according to the location of abscess. At the onset of infection, the child may complain of earache, fever, or vomiting. Assess for neurologic changes, such as drowsiness and sensory deficits, which may be present but unnoticed because they are mild. Organization and enlargement of the abscess lead to compression of brain tissue, causing signs of increased ICP. Severe headaches, changes in ocular function, seizures, and ataxia may occur, signaling the family to seek medical attention. Elicit any history of recent otitis media, mastoiditis, sinusitis, or dental abscess. If a child presents with these symptoms, alert and collaborate with a physician to complete diagnostic studies.

Diagnostic Tests

Diagnosis is confirmed by CT and MRI. In infants with an open fontanel, cranial ultrasonography may also be used for diagnostic purposes. Radiographs of the chest and skull help to locate the primary source of infection, such as an object aspirated into the lungs.

ALERT *Lumbar puncture is contraindicated in patients with brain abscess because increased ICP creates a risk of cerebral herniation.*

Blood analysis is usually inconclusive regarding the causative organism. The white blood cell count may be normal, but an elevated erythrocyte sedimentation rate is not consistently present.

Interdisciplinary Interventions

Managing brain abscess involves both IV antibiotic therapy and surgical draining of the lesion. The type of antibiotic used depends on the causative organism, the site of the abscess, and the child's state of health. Antibiotic therapy is adjusted after the abscess drainage is cultured and organism sensitivities are obtained. Antibiotic therapy continues for 4 to 8 weeks.

Surgical excision and drainage of the abscess remains the definitive treatment for brain abscess. The child and the family will require reassurance regarding surgery. Monitor children postoperatively for increased ICP and drainage or bleeding from the incision site.

Community Care

When fever is reduced and aspiration or excision of the abscess has reduced ICP, the family can be taught to administer IV antibiotics at home and to assess the child for changes in neurologic status. A central venous access is usually inserted before discharge to avoid repeat punctures of the child's skin. If the family feels uncomfortable administering the medications, a home care nurse can be employed to complete the task and to monitor the child's progress.

In some cases, if the child is medically stable, conservative treatment with antibiotics only, administered in the home or outpatient setting, may be scheduled. The child's progress is monitored by follow-up CT and by careful clinical examinations.

TETANUS

Tetanus is an acute infectious process caused by the exotoxin *Clostridium tetani*, a gram-positive anaerobic rod. The infectious process leads to a spastic, paralytic illness. The illness has been reported to occur after penetrating or crushing wounds, burn injury, pregnancy, and general surgery and in neonates with umbilical stump infections. The disease is preventable with proper health care and a series of vaccinations.

The paralysis of tetanus rapidly becomes severe during the first week of onset, stabilizes during the second week, and gradually recedes over an ensuing 1- to 4-week period. Long-term sequelae may include CP, hypoxic brain injury, diminished intellectual capabilities, and behavioral problems. Shorter onset periods and the presence of complications are associated with a poorer prognosis (Bankole et al., 2012).

Pathophysiology

C. tetani spores are found in soil, house dust, animal intestines, and human feces. The spores are harmless until they enter a susceptible host. Any inadequately immunized patient who has been exposed to high levels of bacterial contamination from an injury is at high risk for tetanus.

After injury, local production of exotoxins occurs in the wound, and these toxins are then carried centrally via neural pathways. The primary sites affected are the spinal cord and brain stem. Tetanus toxin blocks normal inhibition of antagonist muscles, causing affected muscles to sustain maximal contraction. The autonomic nervous system also becomes unstable as a result of the infectious process. Airway obstruction and asphyxiation can occur as a result of laryngeal and respiratory muscle spasms.

CROSS-CULTURAL CARE

Tetanus neonatorum is more common in developing countries where women are not immunized against tetanus, contaminated instruments are used to cut the umbilical cord, or native poultices such as cow dung or fermented milk are used for umbilical cord care.

Assessment

Ask about recent injuries. The incubation period from time of injury to onset of symptoms is usually between 7 and 14 days. Early signs of tetanus vary but may include low back pain, stiffness in the jaw and lower limbs, and dysphagia. As the disease progresses, the classic lockjaw or trismus is seen, which is the spasm of the masticatory (chewing) muscles. As the facial muscles become more rigid, the corners of the mouth are drawn up and outward, resulting in what appears to be a fixed smile, a condition referred to as *risus sardonicus*, which is caused by intractable spasm of facial and buccal muscles. Paralysis extending into the abdomen, lumbar spine, hip, and thigh muscles can cause the child to assume an arched posture (opisthotonos) in which only the back of the head and the heels touch the ground.

The seizures associated with tetanus appear suddenly and are characterized by tonic contractions of muscles with clenched fists, flexion and abduction of the arms, and hyperextension of the legs. Seizures last a few seconds to a few minutes, with intervening periods of rest. As the illness progresses, the seizures become sustained and exhausting. Seizure activity may be triggered by sight, sound, or touch.

Ask about output; dysuria and urinary retention occur from bladder sphincter spasm. Bowel incontinence may occur during seizures. Temperature as high as 104° F (40° C) is generally present as a result of the sustained metabolic energy generated by spastic muscles. Tachycardia, arrhythmias, labile hypertension, diaphoresis, and cutaneous vasoconstriction occur as the autonomic nervous system becomes involved. The child does not lose consciousness and experiences extreme pain.

Neonatal tetanus is characterized by poor sucking, irritability, and fever occurring 3 to 12 days after birth. As the infection progresses, the infant develops facial grimaces, muscle rigidity, and opisthotonos. If the child is untreated, death occurs secondary to asphyxia. Diagnosis of tetanus is based on the clinical presentation because wound cultures often fail to detect *C. tetani.*

Interdisciplinary Interventions

The most critical goals of interdisciplinary management of tetanus are to maintain a patent airway, control seizures, neutralize the circulating toxin, and eradicate the *C. tetani* organisms.

Airway Maintenance

Endotracheal intubation may be required to prevent aspiration and respiratory arrest resulting from laryngospasm. In many cases, oxygen therapy and suctioning to manage oral secretions are sufficient. Approach suctioning cautiously because manipulation of the airway can provoke muscle spasm and seizures. In severe cases, a tracheostomy may be performed.

Seizure Control

Diazepam is considered to be the most effective sedative for control of tetanic activity. The medication is given by continuous IV infusion and is titrated as needed to control spasms. The dosage is slowly reduced as the child's symptoms recede. Phenobarbital also may be used to control seizures. Apnea can occur as a result of high doses of these medications; thus, mechanical respiratory support may be needed.

Control of Infection

The bacteria must be killed to halt continuation of the infectious process, and the neurotoxin within the child's system must be neutralized. Penicillin G, given intravenously for 10 to 14 days, remains the antibiotic of choice. Erythromycin and tetracycline can be given if the child is allergic to penicillin.

To neutralize toxin that is diffusing from the wound, human tetanus immunoglobulin (TIG) is administered as a single intramuscular dose. If TIG is not available, human intravenous immunoglobulin (IVIG) or equine tetanus antitoxin can be administered. In addition, after the child is actively recovering from the disease,

immunization with DT (diphtheria–tetanus) or DTaP (diphtheria–tetanus–acellular pertussis) can be given if

- Five years have lapsed since the child's last tetanus shot
- The child is younger than 6 years of age
- The child has never been immunized for tetanus

Wound debridement is essential to the healing process. Meticulous care of the umbilical cord site or wound site is needed to ensure no further growth of spores.

Supportive Interventions

Provide care to minimize stimulation. A quiet, darkened setting is preferred. The child must be sedated to manage pain and prevent seizure activity. Monitor cardiorespiratory status and initiate suctioning as needed.

Monitor fluid and electrolyte status and bowel and bladder function. Seizure, sustained rigid paralysis of the muscles, and instability of the autonomic nervous system predispose the child to many complications. The child is likely to be hemodynamically unstable, and thermoregulation may be difficult to manage. When the child's condition becomes more stabilized, consult physical therapy personnel to begin rehabilitation of affected muscle groups.

Community Care

Tetanus is preventable through active immunization. Chapter 8 discusses pediatric immunization schedules; Appendix C provides links to these schedules. Immunizing pregnant women with tetanus toxoid can prevent neonatal tetanus.

Tetanus prophylaxis should be followed as a part of wound management. Tetanus toxoid should always be given after a dog or other animal bite. Treatment of all wounds, except those experienced by fully immunized patients, should include administration of human TIG. If the immunization status of the child is unclear or if the child receives a tetanus-prone wound (e.g., crush or projectile wound, contaminated wound), TIG should be administered intramuscularly. Immediately clean and debride the wound itself. A tetanus toxoid booster is given to all persons with a wound if

- Immunization status is unknown or incomplete
- The wound is clean but more than 10 years have passed since the last booster
- The wound is serious and more than 5 years have passed since the last booster (CDC, 2012)

Work to ensure that a child's immunization status is up to date. Providing education to high-risk communities with limited health care resources is a valuable activity. Encourage the family to keep organized immunization records that are easily accessed by family members if the child is injured.

REYE SYNDROME

Reye syndrome is an acute, noninflammatory encephalopathy with fatty degenerative changes in the liver, brain, and kidneys first described in 1963 by Reye et al.

The syndrome, which reached peak incidence in the 1980s, is now relatively rare. Although identification of potential causes enables avoidance of some agents, the potential for epidemic recurrence still remains (Johnsen & Bird, 2006).

Evidence supports the hypothesis that Reye syndrome is associated with aspirin (salicylate) use during the febrile prodrome of viral infections such as influenza A or B or varicella; some argue a causal linkage exists (Glasgow, 2006). Reye-like illness has been linked with agents such as valproic acid, aflatoxin, and chemical toxins, but research has not supported this association (Glasgow, 2006). Warning labels placed on containers of salicylate are believed to have reduced the incidence of this disease.

Early diagnosis and implementation of supportive care can prevent progression of the syndrome. Prompt intervention is crucial because the disease can have a rapid onset, leading to coma or death within hours. Full neurologic recovery is usually achieved if cerebral edema does not progress.

Pathophysiology

The pathophysiology of Reye syndrome is complex and appears to involve a defect in mitochondrial function. Chemical metabolic imbalances are a hallmark feature. Examples include hyperammonemia from decreased levels of the enzymes that convert ammonia to urea, hypoglycemia and lactic acidosis from prolonged vomiting, and increased amounts of short-chain fatty acids. Any combination of these metabolic dysfunctions can generate cerebral edema and increased ICP.

Assessment

Evaluate the child's history generally for recent mild respiratory or gastric illness. Clinical signs and symptoms include persistent vomiting and diarrhea during the recovery phase of a viral illness and altered levels of consciousness such as lethargy, agitation, combativeness, or seizures. Also question the family and child about the use of aspirin or aspirinlike products during the illness.

Diagnostic Tests

Abnormalities in hepatic function are demonstrated by elevated aspartate transaminase, activated clotting time, lactate dehydrogenase, and ammonia levels. A liver biopsy, completed only if the diagnosis is unclear, reveals microvascular fat and mitochondrial alterations. A staging system is used to describe the clinical course and the severity of the syndrome (Table 21-9).

Interdisciplinary Interventions

Children with Reye syndrome are cared for in an intensive care setting because of the high risk for increased ICP and liver dysfunction. No specific treatment exists. Supportive care is directed toward monitoring and managing cerebral edema (see earlier discussion on increased ICP). Interventions include nasotracheal intubation with ventilatory control to maintain low PCO_2 levels and to decrease CPP. Mannitol is administered to decrease elevated serum osmolarity. A barbiturate-induced coma may be used if cerebral edema cannot be controlled. Vitamin K may be administered to correct prolonged prothrombin time. Phenytoin may be given to control seizures.

Ensure frequent and open communications are maintained between the health care team and the family. Explain all equipment and treatment measures. Family members may desire social services or clerical support to help them to deal with this unexpected crisis.

To prevent Reye syndrome, teach children and adults not to administer salicylate products to children, especially if the child has respiratory or gastrointestinal symptoms. Salicylate can be found in a number of over-the-counter products.

GUILLAIN-BARRÉ SYNDROME

GBS is an acute, demyelinating polyneuropathy of primarily peripheral nerves, which occurs as a postinfectious process. This immune-mediated process is triggered by a viral or bacterial illness such as a respiratory or gastrointestinal illness. The rate per 100,000 person-years of GBS in children from birth to 9 years of age is 0.62 and in those 10 to 19 years of age is 0.75, increasing 20%

TABLE 21-9	Stages of Reye Syndrome
Stage	**Symptoms**
Stage I	Vomiting, lethargy, sleepiness, mild confusion, elevated serum liver enzymes, normal blood ammonia level, grade I EEG
Stage II	Disorientation, delirium, combativeness, hyperventilation, hyperreflexia, appropriate response to noxious stimuli, elevation in blood ammonia and serum liver enzymes, grade II or III EEG
Stage III	Coma, decorticate posturing, preservation of pupillary light reflexes, pupils dilated, persistent elevation in blood ammonia and serum liver enzymes, grade III or IV EEG
Stage IV	Deepening coma, decerebrate rigidity and posturing to painful stimuli, oculocephalic response, fixed pupils, hypoventilation, decreased blood ammonia and serum liver activity, grade III or IV EEG
Stage V	Coma, seizures, absent deep tendon reflexes, respiratory arrest, flaccidity, hypotension, decreased blood ammonia and serum liver enzyme activity, grade IV or electrocerebral silence on EEG

for each 10-year age increase (Sejvar, Baughman et al., 2011). GBS is a reversible disease with a good prognosis for most children.

Pathophysiology

During the viral illness that precedes GBS, the myelin sheath surrounding the peripheral nerves is altered. The altered myelin is perceived as a foreign protein, and sensitized lymphocytes attack it, leading to edema, destruction, and nerve root compression. Normal nerve conduction is interrupted, resulting in symmetric ascending weakness that progresses over about 2 weeks, in most cases (some up to 4 weeks), although rapidly progressive weakness reaching nadir in several hours may be seen. Clinical improvement is seen over weeks or months. Infants and children have a more rapid recovery than adults and tend to have a complete recovery (Sejvar, Kohl et al., 2011). GBS is thought to include several subtypes based on pathology. These include acute inflammatory demyelinating polyradiculoneuropathy (AIDP), seen most commonly in North America and Europe, and acute motor axonal neuropathy (AMAN), seen in other parts of the world. Acute motor and sensory axonal neuropathy (AMSAN) is less common. Fisher syndrome is another subtype consisting of ataxia, areflexia, and ophthalmoplegia seen more commonly in eastern Asia (Sejvar, Kohl et al., 2011).

Assessment

The clinical examination focuses on motor, sensory, cranial nerve, and autonomic functions. Assess for progressive, ascending motor weakness of more than one limb. Note any areflexia or complaints of excruciating pain in the upper legs and back. Rapid progression of symptoms makes prompt diagnosis imperative because respiratory failure, loss of swallow and gag reflexes, and need for ventilatory support can develop quickly. Respiratory failure may be preceded by progressive involvement of truncal musculature and cranial nerves as well as sensory impairment. Elicit history of recent viral infection and determine the child's immunization status to eliminate the possibility of poliomyelitis.

Blood and urine cultures are completed to search for a causative agent and underlying systemic or immune-mediated disorders. Analysis of CSF reveals few white blood cells, with elevation of protein. Peripheral nerve conduction time studies and electromyogram demonstrate decreased nerve velocities.

Interdisciplinary Interventions

The treatment of GBS is primarily supportive. Because of the potential for rapid deterioration and respiratory failure, the child must be admitted to a high-observation area with possible rapid transfer to intensive care. During the acute phase of the disease, frequently assess respiratory function, heart rate, and blood pressure so that rapid intervention can be implemented if deterioration occurs.

The immune basis for GBS suggests use of IVIG or plasma exchange (PE) to prevent demyelination. A Cochrane review demonstrated that IVIG started within 2 weeks of onset is as effective as PE, but completion of IVIG therapy is much more likely (Hughes et al., 2012). The goal is to prevent respiratory compromise and the need for ventilatory support, thereby promoting a shorter recovery course.

During the acute period, provide supportive measures to sustain life, prevent complications, and promote comfort. Preventing the complications of immobility is of paramount importance, so initiate interventions as early as possible during the acute phase. The child is at risk for mobility problems such as joint contractures, skin breakdown, and deep vein thromboses. Perform passive range-of-motion exercises, frequent repositioning, and meticulous skin care to minimize these complications. Parenteral nutrition is provided if the child is intubated. Solid foods are introduced after extubation, once the child's ability to swallow is established. If severe pain is present during the initial stages of the disease, administer comfort measures. Pain medications should not interfere with the child's respiratory function or ability to cough.

Children with severe respiratory insufficiency may be intubated and placed on a ventilator. The inability to verbalize needs and loss of bodily functions are frightening to the child and the family. Incorporate developmental assessments and psychosocial support measures throughout the acute course.

When urinary retention is present, an indwelling or intermittent catheter is indicated. Tachycardia and arrhythmias may occur, and cardiac monitoring should continue. Sleep disturbances are common and are caused by pain, lack of scheduled rest periods, noise, and treatment interventions. Ensure adequate pain management. Organize care and create a schedule to provide quiet time for the child.

During recovery, children slowly regain muscle strength and sensation, and they experience reduced pain. Comprehensive care is still vitally important in the five most commonly affected areas: respiration, mobility, nutrition, autonomic nervous system, and psychological response. The early phases of the recovery program must balance activities with adequate rest. Fatigue or exhaustion can cause symptoms to return, which may be devastating for the child. Provide support and encouragement as progress is made in each area.

Community Care

Encourage parents to accept relatives' and friends' offers of help and respite. Educate parents about exercise, diet, and measures to provide psychosocial support to their child. Ideally, discharge planning begins with the child's admission to the hospital. Provide the family with resources to ease the return to normal life. The family may require home health nursing services. Good communication between the acute care setting and outreach teams facilitates high-quality continuity of care. GBS is an illness that requires a highly skilled, interdisciplinary health care team to manage the many facets of patient care. To the team, the nurse contributes clinical skills and expertise as an educator, patient advocate, supportive listener, and coordinator of resources.

The illness creates an abrupt interruption of established routines. If mentally and physically able, some children are able to continue their education using home teaching sessions. Child life specialists may offer suggestions for developmentally appropriate activities to alleviate boredom. The stress of pain, isolation, and dependency may cause feelings of anger or depression. The child likely will regress to previous developmental stages to meet security needs. When family members are aware of these natural responses, they can provide better support.

SPINAL MUSCULAR ATROPHY

Spinal muscular atrophy (SMA) is a disorder characterized by degeneration of the anterior horn cells of the spinal cord and some cranial nerve nuclei, resulting in weakness and wasting of voluntary muscles. SMA is the most common autosomal recessive neuromuscular disorder and, after cystic fibrosis, the most common recessive condition leading to death in children (D'Amico et al., 2011). SMA is linked to an abnormality on chromosome 5 that is consistent across all forms of the disorder. Although the disorder is inherited, a high rate of spontaneous mutation has also been noted.

Pathophysiology

In SMA, anterior horn cells in the spinal cord and motor nuclei of the brain stem are progressively lost. Loss of function in one motor neuron results in abnormalities and loss of function in the muscles supplied by that motor neuron. As deterioration or loss of motor neuron function increases, muscle fiber and function are also lost. There is no cardiac involvement. Intelligence is normal.

Historically, three forms of SMA have been described. Common to all forms is the presence of more proximal, lower extremity weakness. SMA I, also known as Werdnig-Hoffmann disease, is the most severe form and begins in utero or early infancy. These infants can perform few spontaneous movements, are unable to lift the head, have difficulty with sucking and swallowing, and deep tendon reflexes are lost. Initial examination may also document **fasciculations** (continuous, involuntary "wormlike" movements that are best observed in the tongue). They may also be present in the child's deltoid, biceps, and quadriceps muscles. Intercostal muscles are also weakened, resulting in respiratory failure.

SMA II, the late infantile form, has a later onset (6 to 24 months of age) than SMA I and causes less initial weakness. These infants may achieve sitting and, with orthotic support, may achieve ambulation. On clinical examination, deep tendon reflexes are absent, and fasciculations may be present.

SMA III, also called Kugelberg-Welander disease, is the juvenile form of SMA, with onset occurring between 3 and 17 years of age. Early symptoms are nonspecific and include delayed developmental milestones and motor clumsiness. Atrophy of proximal muscles may be present.

Assessment

When taking the history, note early infant deaths within the family, family members with similar problems, and any maternal observations of decreased fetal movements, all of which suggest SMA I. Focus the clinical evaluation on assessment of the motor system and cranial nerves. Document any findings of hypotonia, generalized weakness, thin muscle mass, the presence of fasciculations, and altered tendon stretch reflexes. Inability to meet motor developmental milestones is one of the first diagnostic clues of concern to family members.

Diagnostic Tests

When the diagnosis is suspected, a specific gene deletion study by blood sample should be performed. Documentation of the defect in chromosome 5 eliminates the need for muscle biopsy. However, weakness and hypotonia in infants have many potential causes. Therefore, an EMG is usually performed to document specific muscle responses. The EMG results vary by type of SMA in the quantity and character of fibrillations and fasciculations.

When the blood deletion study is negative, but the EMG suggests SMA, a muscle biopsy is performed. The histologic specimens differentiate SMA from other intrinsic muscle diseases. Specifically, large group muscle atrophy is seen in SMA.

Interdisciplinary Interventions

Treatment of SMA is supportive and involves monitoring respiratory and nutritional status. In SMA I, the most common cause of death is loss of respiratory function because muscle weakness leads to ineffective airway clearance and diminished vital capacity. Involvement of cranial nerve nuclei and swallowing problems lead to inadequate nutrition. Alternative feeding methods may be required.

In SMA types II and III, loss of respiratory function may also occur but is usually not as rapid as that seen in type I. Monitor respiratory status, growth, and development. As the child grows and continues to have weakness, contractures and scoliosis may occur because of immobility. Orthopedic care is instituted to provide support and maintain strength of functional muscles. Monitor and treat skin as immobility increases.

For the family, the rapid deterioration characteristic of SMA I requires many decisions regarding the extent of medical intervention that should be instituted. Measures taken may prolong the child's life without improving its quality. Encourage the child with SMA type II or III to participate in age-appropriate activities to the extent that he or she is able. Monitor nutritional intake, and ensure that immobility of a muscle group does not lead to further musculoskeletal alterations. Ensure that the family's psychosocial, emotional, cognitive, and interpersonal needs are being addressed (see Chapter 12 regarding care of the child with a chronic condition).

MYASTHENIA GRAVIS

Myasthenia gravis (MG) is a neuromuscular disease caused by immunologic neuromuscular blockade. The disease is characterized by progressive weakness of certain voluntary muscles. The disease most commonly affects the oculomotor, facial, laryngeal, pharyngeal, and respiratory muscles.

Pathophysiology

MG is related to an antibody-mediated autoimmune attack directed against acetylcholine receptors in the postsynaptic membrane. In affected children, antibodies destroy acetylcholine receptor sites, resulting in diminished muscle response and weakness. The condition may be acquired or congenital. Acquired MG includes *transient neonatal MG* and *juvenile MG*. The genetic forms of MG are rare.

Transient neonatal MG occurs in approximately 10% of infants born to mothers with MG (Masters & Bagshaw, 2011). Infants acquire maternal acetylcholine receptor antibodies transplacentally, and symptoms occur shortly after birth. Symptoms of transient neonatal MG disappear without residual neurologic or developmental complications within 2 to 4 weeks of birth. These infants are not at risk for developing MG later in life.

Juvenile MG accounts for 10% to 15% of MG cases in North America and Europe, whereas up to 50% of MG cases in Asian countries present by 15 years of age (Trouth et al., 2012). The pathophysiology for juvenile MG involves antibody depletion of acetylcholine receptors. With juvenile MG, patients who experience muscle weakness only in the extraocular and facial muscles generally have a milder course. Permanent, spontaneous remission of symptoms is inversely proportional to the severity of the symptoms. With treatment, prognosis is good, and the child has a normal life expectancy.

Congenital (genetic) MG is a familial abnormality of neuromuscular transmission with a little understood pathophysiology. It differs from the transient form in that

- It is not immunologically mediated
- Mothers do not have MG
- Symptoms first appear from birth to age 12 months
- Extraocular muscles are more severely affected
- Response to medication or surgery (thymectomy) is limited
- Symptoms are present throughout life

Treatment and supportive care for congenital MG improve the outcome overall (Khan et al., 2011).

Assessment

Low Apgar scores for respiratory effort, muscle tone, and reflex irritability should alert to the possibility of transient neonatal MG. The baby may appear cyanotic, "floppy," expressionless, and too weak to cry. Attempts to feed are marked by poor sucking and rapid fatigue.

Initial symptoms of juvenile MG include unilateral or bilateral ptosis or diplopia in a diurnal pattern (symptoms worsen as the day progresses). For more severely affected children, dysarthria, dysphagia, skeletal muscle weakness, and respiratory problems can occur. The onset of these symptoms may develop over years or as quickly as within 24 hours.

Diagnostic Tests

Diagnosis of MG is confirmed by the edrophonium chloride (Tensilon) test. An injection of Tensilon is given at an age-determined dosage. Initial administration of 20% of the dose is followed by a full dose, after no adverse effects have been noted. The injection should result in immediate, but brief, improvement in muscle tone.

Electrodiagnostic evaluation of muscle response identifies the defect at the myoneural junction, indicating MG. Repeated stimulation of the nerve results in sequential reduction of muscle response (decremental response). A positive decremental response is seen in 80% of children with MG.

Interdisciplinary Interventions

Treatment is based on the type of MG, the child's age, and the severity of symptoms. In all cases of MG, provide supportive care to ensure airway protection and adequate oxygenation.

Supportive Interventions

For the newborn with transient MG, intubation, mechanical ventilation, and enteral feedings may be necessary until the condition resolves naturally. Promote bonding by encouraging parents to hold their infant and assist with daily care activities. If the mother wishes to nurse her infant, and the infant shows no signs of respiratory distress, she can attempt short periods of breastfeeding. She may also express milk and freeze it for later use. Supplemental nutrition should be administered by feeding tube to conserve the infant's energy.

Monitor the infant's respiratory function by assessing breath sounds, rate, and oxygen saturation (especially during feedings). Ensure that suction equipment is available at the bedside if the airway becomes blocked with secretions. Continuous pulse oximetry is a useful tool in ongoing evaluation of the infant's oxygenation status.

Pharmacologic Interventions

Controversy still exists regarding the most effective management of MG. Anticholinesterase drugs, usually pyridostigmine (Mestinon), are the first line of treatment to control symptoms. Short-term use of anticholinesterase drugs is effective in transient neonatal MG. The dosage of medication is closely monitored to detect toxicity.

If symptoms are disabling, steroid therapy (prednisone) is used. When long-term steroid therapy is initiated, potassium supplements, antacids, or histamine-$_2$ (H_2)-blocking agents; vitamin D; and calcium supplements may be required to promote healthy bone development and healing.

Surgical Interventions

Thymectomy remains a controversial therapy in the pediatric population. The entire thymus and mediastinal fat are removed during the procedure. If removal of the thymus gland is indicated, provide pre- and postoperative care.

Emergency Interventions

Emergency situations (cholinergic crisis) may also arise with elevated levels of acetylcholinesterase drugs and may require intubation and ventilatory support. The Tensilon test is used to differentiate between myasthenic and cholinergic crises (Table 21-10).

As with MG diagnosis, if the injection of edrophonium improves muscle strength, the likely diagnosis is myasthenic crisis. More medication is then needed for treatment. If the Tensilon test does not improve symptoms, or they worsen, they are most likely being caused by cholinergic crisis. Anticholinergic medications should be temporarily withheld.

Educational Interventions

Because of the chronic nature of persistent and juvenile MG, teaching is a lifelong part of the treatment plan. Teach the family to reduce factors that may exacerbate the disease to the point of myasthenic crisis, including stress, infection, or prolonged physical activity. Be knowledgeable about drug therapy, side effects, and disease course to develop a teaching plan for the child and family.

❗ALERT *Certain medications can exacerbate weakness in the child with MG. These drugs include aminoglycosides, procainamide, quinidine, curare, succinylcholine, and possibly calcium channel blockers and beta-blockers. Teach the child and family to avoid sedatives, antibiotics, and cold remedies that contain these products by ensuring that health care providers are aware of the MG diagnosis and the medications that may exacerbate symptoms.*

As the child grows older, help the family to adjust roles so the child assumes appropriate responsibility for managing his or her disease to foster independence through self-care.

NEUROCUTANEOUS SYNDROMES

The most frequently occurring neurocutaneous syndromes are collectively called *phakomatoses*. These diseases are characterized by their tendency toward tumor formation in the CNS, skin, and visceral linings of various organ systems and by their recognizable cutaneous manifestations. Because of the rarity of these diseases, this chapter covers only the three most common phakomatoses: tuberous sclerosis, neurofibromatosis (NF), and Sturge-Weber syndrome (Table 21-11).

TABLE 21-10 Myasthenic Versus Cholinergic Crisis	
Myasthenic Crisis	**Cholinergic Crisis**
Etiology	
Severe weakness with bulbar and respiratory compromise occurring during natural course of disease May be preceded by an infection Symptoms may lead to an overdose of anticholinesterase drugs	ACD toxicity
Symptoms	
Anoxia Cyanosis Bowel and bladder incontinence Decreased urinary output Absence of swallow reflex and cough	Hypotension Nausea Vomiting Diarrhea Abdominal cramps Pallor Blurred vision Facial muscle twitching
Tensilon Test	
Produces temporary improvement	Produces no improvement or worsening of symptoms
Treatment	
Early detection Managing respiratory function Medical support of other body functions Plasmapheresis Increase anticholinesterase medications	Discontinue ACDs and gradually reinstate medications as symptoms improve Manage respiratory function

TABLE 21-11	Neurocutaneous Syndromes
Condition/Inheritance	**Characteristics**
Tuberous sclerosis complex, autosomal dominant	Cognitive deficits, autism, epilepsy, adenoma sebaceum (red, highly vascular papules on the face) Lesions called *tubers* may invade the brain and the retina; other types of tumors may invade the heart and the kidneys; skin, lungs, and skeleton may be affected
NF previously referred to as *von Recklinghausen disease*, autosomal dominant	Areas of increased skin pigmentation (café-au-lait spots), central and peripheral nervous system tumors (neurofibromas), and other skeletal, endocrine, and vascular findings Initial symptoms are usually cutaneous changes, neurologic symptoms often occur, language disorders and learning disabilities common Difficulty with tasks that require planning, attention, and organization common, leading to higher incidence of attention-deficit/hyperactivity disorder NF1: Peripheral nerve tumors and a higher incidence of brain tumors; neurofibromas usually develop at 10–15 years of age NF2: Much rarer; multiple tumors of the brain, spinal cord, auditory nerves; hearing loss may become evident in adolescence; the vestibular nerve may also be affected, resulting in poor balance
Sturge-Weber syndrome (encephalo-facial angiomatosis), only phako-matosis without a recognizable hereditary pattern	Port-wine stain (facial nevus) usually apparent at birth, often associated with congenital glaucoma; focal or generalized seizures, usually begin before 1 year of age and are difficult to treat; intracranial calcification, hemiparesis, and often cognitive deficits and behavioral problems Abnormalities of the dura mater over the occipital lobe, calcification and necrosis of underlying brain tissue common

Assessment

The diagnosis of neurocutaneous diseases is often made by the characteristic findings of each disease. A thorough genetic history is helpful. Focus assessment on developmental, behavioral, and psychosocial issues. Obtain neurologic baseline assessment, and examine systems that are known to be affected by tumors, tubers, or other findings associated with these disorders.

Diagnosis is based on clinical features. Specific genes for tuberous sclerosis complex and NF have been identified, and genetic testing may confirm these diagnoses. Because the manifestations of these diseases vary widely, some possible tests include EEG, CT, MRI, PET, skin biopsy, ophthalmologic examinations, and various other tests, depending on the organ systems involved.

Interdisciplinary Interventions

No cure exists. Care for children with these disorders is individualized and depends on the specific disease, with the focus of care aimed at alleviating symptoms. When seizures are present, antiepileptic regimens may be tried until control is achieved. Brain lesions such as tumors, tubers, or neurofibromas may be surgically excised, especially if they cause increased ICP or seizures. In some cases of Sturge-Weber syndrome, the lobes of the brain causing the seizures are surgically removed.

When these children are hospitalized, seizure precautions may be necessary. The child may also display some degree of cognitive disability or behavior that is difficult to control. Guard the child's safety at all times, modifying the plan of care to adapt to the child's behavioral needs.

Help the family to cope with the diagnosis, and assist with genetic counseling to assess the probability of abnormalities occurring in future children. Allow the family to express the initial denial and guilt that may manifest shortly after diagnosis.

Families facing these diseases require ongoing support, particularly when the family is faced with many hospitalizations. In some instances, encourage the family to explore long-term resources. A nurse may interact with the same child many times during a number of separate hospitalizations. Continuity of nursing care can promote trust and a more positive view of the health care system for the child.

HEAD INJURIES

Head injury is the general term for several different types of injury. This section covers scalp injuries; skull fractures; concussions, contusions and lacerations; vascular injuries and hematomas; and cranial nerve and TBI, where the brain itself is injured.

 QUESTION: Which elements of Joey's experience are typical for a head injury?

TBI in the pediatric population is a major cause of death and disability (Alexiou et al., 2011; Asemota et al., 2013). The spectrum of injury with TBI ranges from minor concussion that requires a few hours of observation to major trauma with dismal long-term consequences for the child. Rates are highest among children aged 0 to 4 years, followed by adolescents aged 15 to 19 years (Coronado et al., 2011).

The most common causes of head trauma in infants and children are falls, child abuse, and motor vehicle accidents. Infants may experience head trauma during a difficult delivery with forceps or a prolonged, traumatic labor and delivery. Infants or young children may sustain a head injury because of a fall from a caregiver's arms, out of windows, or down stairs. These children are also at the age when they may be victims of child abuse, particularly shaking injuries. During early and middle childhood, children are susceptible to being injured while playing or climbing. Falls are the leading cause of TBI in adolescents 10 to 13 years of age (Asemota et al., 2013). Motor vehicle occupant accidents are the most common causes of TBI in adolescents 14 to 19 years of age (Asemota et al., 2013). Athletic injuries also contribute to head injuries in this age group. Other factors that may predispose a child to head injury are seizure disorders, gait instability, alcohol or drug ingestion, and cognitive delays, including poor judgment.

ANSWER: Joey is a male and was injured while participating in an athletic activity—both are common elements of preadolescent head injuries.
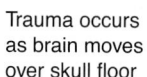

Pathophysiology

The pathophysiology of head injuries is complex in that the extent of the visible injury may not indicate the extent of actual brain injury. A head injury may involve any or all of the cranial and skull layers, including scalp, skull, dura, brain, and blood vessels as well as neurons and supportive glial cells. Injuries can be classified as *primary*, meaning they result from the actual traumatic event, or as *secondary*, indicating that the damage is caused by pathologic processes that occurred as a result of the initial injury. Secondary injury may be related to how quickly treatment is initiated after the injury has occurred.

Injury in pediatric head trauma occurs though several mechanisms. Blunt or nonpenetrating injury can distort brain tissue and shear neurons, even without outward evidence of injury or trauma. Penetrating or open injuries can produce either focal or diffuse damage, depending on the velocity and the type of penetration.

Compression injuries are the result of the skull being compressed between two forces, crushing the brain and compromising its integrity. Other commonly used terms are **coup** (pronounced "coo") and **contrecoup** injuries. These terms are used to describe an injury to brain tissue that results when a blow to the head causes the brain to hit the skull at the location of impact (*coup*), and then rebound to the opposite side of the skull, where injury can also occur (*contrecoup*) (Fig. 21-10).

Scalp Injuries

The scalp is composed of five layers, including connective tissue and vascular structures. Together, these layers offer tremendous protection to the skull. Scalp injuries include abrasions and lacerations.

Skull Fractures

 QUESTION: Could Joey have a skull fracture? If so, which type is most likely?

The human skull is composed of two layers, the inner and outer tables, separated by a spongy tissue called the *diploic space*. In a head injury, a fracture may occur at the site of impact or in areas of the skull with less tensile strength. There are five types of skull fractures: linear, depressed, comminuted, diastatic, and basilar.

Nearly 70% of skull fractures are *linear* and involve the cranial vault. Fracture lines may be simple or complex and follow no predictable pattern. Children with uncomplicated linear fractures are usually admitted to the hospital for a short period of observation and are likely to resume normal activities within a few days. The bone heals on its own, and the fracture is not likely to be evident on skull radiographs 6 months to 1 year after the injury.

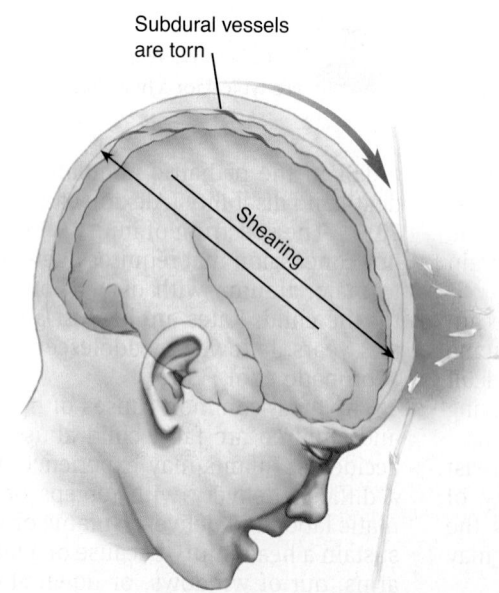

Subdural vessels are torn

Counter or deceleration injury (contrecoup)

Shearing

Trauma occurs as brain moves over skull floor

Acceleration injury from initial impact (coup)

Figure 21-10 Mechanisms of coup–contrecoup injury.

There are two concerns with linear fractures. First, an unrecognized tear may occur in a layer of meninges that permits CSF to escape. If the tear is unrepaired, a "growing fracture of childhood" may occur as the CSF collects and begins pulsating outward. The fracture widens, and a small lump develops over the area of the fracture. The second concern is the presence of a linear fracture over the middle meningeal artery in the temporal region. Because the artery adheres closely to bone in this area, a linear fracture can tear the artery, resulting in an epidural hematoma.

Depressed skull fractures are often associated with scalp lacerations. The exception is "ping-pong" fractures or other fractures of the infant skull. A fracture is considered depressed when the inner table is displaced by more than the thickness of the skull. Compound depressed skull fractures (those with lacerations) should be debrided and elevated as soon as possible after the injury. Surgical elevation of the fragments is considered in closed injuries in which fragments are depressed more than 0.5 to 1 cm. Depressed fractures with many fragments are referred to as *comminuted*.

Diastatic skull fractures occur along the suture line. The separation is usually visible on skull radiograph. These fractures often do not occur at the site of impact; they are seen most frequently in newborn babies and infants.

The most serious type of skull fracture is a *basilar skull fracture*. These fractures involve a break in the basal portions of the frontal, ethmoid, sphenoid, temporal, or occipital bones. Two signs of this type of skull fracture are the Battle sign (bruising or ecchymosis behind the ear, caused by blood leaking into the mastoid sinus) and raccoon eyes (blood leaking into the frontal sinuses, causing an edematous and bruised periorbital area). Children with these fractures may also have CSF leakage from the nose (rhinorrhea) or ears (otorrhea) because of tears in the meninges. CSF leaks are rare but can be serious, especially if they do not stop spontaneously. Basilar skull fractures are associated with cranial nerve injuries. Optic, extraocular, and acoustic nerve injuries are the most common.

> **ANSWER:** Although Joey does have a scalp laceration and edema surrounding the laceration, there is no external evidence of a compression fracture. Furthermore, he does not display the Battle sign or raccoon eyes, and he does not have any CSF leaking from his ears or nose, so it is unlikely he has a basilar skull fracture. The most likely type of fracture is a linear fracture, and the CT scan will determine this.

Concussions, Contusions, and Lacerations

The most common injury from blunt trauma is a concussion. In minor, reversible head trauma, a concussion may occur. Concussions tend to occur from impact when the head is in motion rather than in a fixed position. This injury is a transient and reversible neuronal dysfunction that produces instantaneous loss of awareness and responsiveness on the part of the child that may last minutes or hours. The child has amnesia of events immediately surrounding the head trauma. Most concussions are mild and do not require either hospital observation or admission.

Contusions are "bruises" to the brain. They occur either at the site of impact or at a point directly opposite the impact (coup–contrecoup injury). The injury may cause focal edema or generalized cerebral edema or bleeding at either location; increased ICP may occur. Symptoms may not peak until 48 to 72 hours after the injury, and complications from the edema last for days.

Lacerations are discontinuity of brain tissue caused by penetrating craniocerebral trauma such as gunshot wounds. Lacerations are considered to be serious because of the substantial intracerebral bleeding that can be caused by this type of injury.

Vascular Injuries and Hematomas

> **QUESTION:** Could Joey have a "bleed?" If so, which type would be most typical, and why is this worrisome?

Hematomas occur when the shearing force created by impact tears bridging vessels that supply blood to the various layers of the dura mater. Epidural hematomas are likely to be acute and usually result from a tear in an artery, although 25% have a venous origin. An epidural hematoma occurs between the bone and the dura (Fig. 21-11). The child usually has a short period of unconsciousness followed by a period of lucidity in which he or she is believed to have recovered; within 4 to 8 hours, the child begins to experience a rapid decline in neurologic function that causes severe cerebral shift and even death if left untreated. Common locations for epidural hematomas are the temporal fossa, subfrontal, and occipital areas. Surgical treatment is emergent and arrests the serious symptoms if done rapidly.

Acute subdural hematomas are usually of venous origin and are often associated with an underlying contusion. These hematomas occur under the dura mater. Subdural hemorrhage has also been shown to occur from shaking injury. This type of hematoma occurs more frequently in infants and is usually bilateral, whereas epidural hematomas are unilateral. Common symptoms are increased ICP and seizures.

Chronic subdural hematomas are usually related to trauma, but they may not be identified until long after the injury, usually after skull growth has accelerated beyond the normal level. The characteristic signs are irritability; full, nonpulsatile fontanel; failure to thrive; and low hematocrit levels.

> **ANSWER:** Joey might possibly have a bleed. A CT scan is ordered primarily to determine whether there is any intracranial bleeding. An epidural bleed would be most likely, given his age and injury. This is problematic because he might seem to recover but could then quickly decompensate and even die.

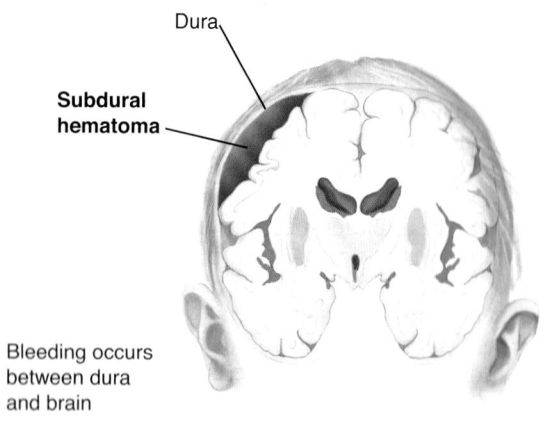
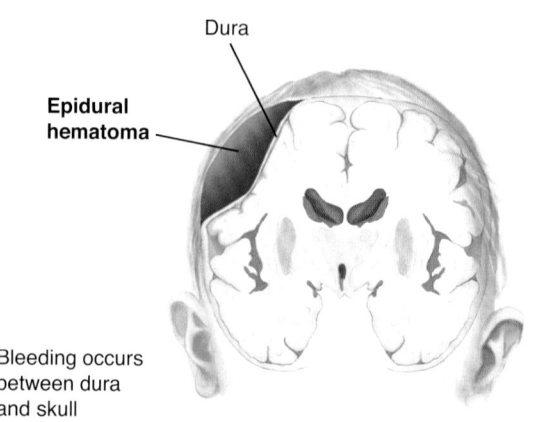

Figure 21-11 Subdural hematoma and epidural hematoma.

Cranial Nerve and Traumatic Brain Injury

Although basilar skull fractures are the most common cause of cranial nerve injury, nerve damage can also be caused by compression, stretching, or severe laceration, most commonly involving CNs I (loss of smell), VII (facial paralysis), V and VI (eye movements), II (optic fields), and VIII.

Damage to neurons is called *diffuse axonal injury* (also known as *shearing*), one of the most common TBIs. When the head is subjected to impact, the gray matter on the cortical surface is displaced more than the deep white matter. As a result, the axons degenerate, and their ability to transmit impulses effectively diminishes. The course and outcome for the child depend on the extent of the injury.

Assessment

 QUESTION: In addition to his GCS score, what parameters would a nurse assess on Joey?

The primary components of the assessment are a thorough history and physical examination and appropriate imaging studies.

Note the actual mechanism of injury or state of consciousness after the injury, or both, which can be a useful tool in diagnosing the type of trauma. Another major aspect of history taking is to determine whether there has been posttraumatic amnesia, as in concussion injuries, or a seizure at the time of injury, predisposing the child to injury. Also note a family history of bleeding disorders. If retinal hemorrhages are present in an infant with signs and symptoms of hematoma, be alert for the possibility of shaken baby syndrome (see Chapter 31).

After the family history and the history of the event have been gathered, carry out a complete neurologic assessment. Assess cognitive and mental functions and cranial nerves. Evaluate for signs of increased ICP. If the injured child arrives at the health care facility in a state of rapid neurologic decompensation, assessment and interventions are often done simultaneously. If any evidence exists of a pressure buildup great enough to threaten herniation of the cerebral lobes, immediate action must be taken to alleviate the pressure.

Determine and document level of consciousness, ability to follow commands, presence of confusion or irritability, pupil responsiveness, extraocular eye movements, and generalized strength and tone of extremities. In severe cases of neurologic trauma, posturing may be present. Begin each assessment by providing the same degree of stimuli to the child so that a comparison of responses can be made over time. Observe whether any CSF is leaking from the ear canals or nares and whether changes have occurred in external findings (increased swelling or tenderness over scalp abrasions or wounds). Record any abnormal motor movements or potentially seizure-related activity. Finally, monitor cardiorespiratory and vital sign parameters closely, and immediately report evidence of increasing ICP.

ANSWER: The nurse would assess Joey's vital signs, quality of respirations, pupils, and physical signs such as the presence of leaking CSF from the ears or nose.

Diagnostic Tests

Radiographic studies for head injury generally include skull and cervical spine films and a CT scan. If the injury is minor and the child appears to be neurologically intact, a CT scan may not be necessary, although plain skull films are usually obtained to rule out a skull fracture. MR images are being used more frequently, particularly in children with more severe injuries, as a way to follow white and gray matter changes over time.

If seizure activity occurs after the injury, an EEG is necessary. Injuries involving the cranial nerves may be followed with brain stem auditory-evoked responses or with visual-evoked responses, or both. A child with long-term cognitive deficits may require neuropsychological evaluation to assess functional, learning, and, eventually, vocational abilities.

Interdisciplinary Interventions

Care of the child with head trauma varies according to the mechanism of injury, the location, and any association with multisystem injuries (e.g., fracture of ribs, femur, laceration of liver). For scalp injuries, gentle cleaning followed by hemostasis, conservative debridement of dead tissue, and suturing without tension is the recommended approach to management.

Conservative Interventions

The treatment for mild head injury is generally a conservative observational approach that may involve monitoring the clinical manifestations for several hours before discharging the child. Most nondepressed skull fractures heal over time. A moderate head injury may involve a prolonged hospital stay and the use of methods to decrease ICP. Keeping some children hospitalized may be necessary to follow cranial nerve functions and to ascertain that there is no worsening disease process.

Surgical Interventions

Surgical management of head injury may be necessary, most commonly to elevate a depressed skull fracture or remove an acute epidural or subdural hematoma. Chronic subdural hematomas may require mechanical shunting to the peritoneal space. Severe injuries necessitate a critical care environment with close monitoring of vital functions. The insertion of an ICP measuring device by the neurosurgeon may be necessary to monitor changes in ICP and to initiate medical therapy based on these changes.

Supportive Interventions

The child with head injury is at high risk for altered cerebral perfusion. Carefully monitor oxygen saturation with pulse oximetry and administer oxygen as necessary. When a child's oxygenation status is questionable, administering oxygen is prudent even before a pulse oximetry reading is obtained. Monitor the child's hemoglobin and hematocrit levels closely to ensure adequate oxygen-carrying capacity within the blood. To promote optimal cerebral tissue perfusion, closely monitor systemic perfusion parameters, such as blood pressure and other vital signs. Monitor fluid and electrolyte status to avoid fluid overload and resultant cerebral edema. Administer antiepileptics as ordered, implement seizure precautions, and document any seizure activity.

Slightly elevating the head of the child's bed is important in managing increases in ICP, and it is useful in optimizing airway position. Slight hyperextension of the neck can be achieved by placing a towel roll underneath the child's shoulders. Never attempt this measure, however, until cervical spine injury has been ruled out. Oral or deep suction may be necessary every 2 to 4 hours to clear secretions and to stimulate a cough. Have an appropriate-sized bag and mask available at the bedside to ventilate the child in an emergency, as needed.

Ongoing Interventions

 QUESTION: Joey has now been in the emergency department for 30 minutes. How frequently is the nurse obtaining vital signs and neurologic checks on Joey?

Perform ongoing assessment of the child's neurologic function, including level of awareness or responsiveness and the presence of confusion, every 1 to 2 hours after injury. Document any changes in the child's condition and assess the child more frequently if warranted. Changes in level of consciousness are often the first indication of changes in ICP and cerebral perfusion.

ANSWER: Joey is still unstable and could change rapidly. Assessments should be done at least every 15 minutes, and the nurse or an adult should remain with him at all times.

Investigate the possibility of a CSF leak from the nose or ears, or from scalp lacerations, and report to the physician as soon as possible. Suspect a CSF leak if copious, clear fluid is draining from the nose, ears, or scalp lesion. Differentiating CSF from other fluids may be difficult. One method is to measure the glucose of the suspected fluid. If the fluid is CSF, the glucose level will be equivalent to that in CSF obtained by lumbar puncture. Antibiotics will likely be administered prophylactically when the scalp has been lacerated or when an open injury is present. Cleanse wounds as indicated, perform frequent oral care, and monitor for signs of skin and systemic infection.

Community Care

Ongoing involvement after the child leaves the hospital centers on helping the family to cope with the effects of the injury and preventing further injury to the child. After a minor head injury, educate the family to observe the child closely for 24 hours for signs as previously discussed; check the child every few hours when sleeping. If abnormal signs occur, notify the health care provider.

If the child is severely brain injured, the biggest task facing the family is the grief of losing the child they once had. Frequently, the personality changes in the child are dramatic and disturbing. The entire structure of the family is likely to change. Initially, when progress seems to occur daily, families have strong hope that their child will recover completely. As the family realizes their loss, depression and related stress can set in. Offer the family realistic expectations and support throughout their grief work. Refer the family for further counseling if needed. Encourage the family to take part in their child's care, and encourage them to take breaks for themselves.

Provide the child and family with assistance in making sound judgments in daily activities. Comprehensive rehabilitation programs that involve a component of behavior modification, such as increased helmet use, are usually effective in helping children become aware of their own safety.

For children with long-term sensory deficits (vision, hearing, smell), address the need for adaptations to prevent further injury. Educate family members about seizure precautions, if they are needed. Also discuss toxic side effects of antiepileptics with children and families, as appropriate.

The sequelae from a head injury in childhood can become a lifetime burden. Seizure activity becomes posttraumatic epilepsy. Postconcussion syndrome can be apparent for a year or more after the injury. Hydrocephalus can occur as the result of an infectious process. The most difficult aspects of long-term outcome are the ensuing personality and behavioral changes that can prevent the child from achieving a completely independent lifestyle. Persistent physical difficulties may affect independence. Nevertheless, most pediatric head injuries are minor occurrences that require no hospitalization and engender no long-term damage.

ACUTE SPINAL CORD INJURY

Although SCI is an infrequent occurrence in the general pediatric population, the incidence of these injuries increases substantially after age 15 years. Boys are much more likely to sustain an SCI than girls (Parent et al., 2011). Motor vehicle accidents are the most common cause (Basu, 2012) and account for 40% of pediatric SCI in the United States, with improper seatbelt restraint increasing the risk of injury (Achildi et al., 2007). Other causes of SCI are falls and firearm and athletic injuries. Birth injuries can affect the cervical spine.

caREminder

> Treat all injured children as if an SCI has occurred until the potential for this problem has been eliminated. This approach includes immediately immobilizing the head and spine on a spine board before transfer from the scene of the injury.

Most spinal fractures result in no neurologic deficit. However, SCI with no evidence of radiographic abnormality is well documented in children.

Pathophysiology

SCIs are often described in relation to the mechanism and anatomic location of injury. Flexion–dislocation, hyperextension, vertical compression, and rotation are the major mechanisms of injury. Flexion–dislocation injuries are common in motor vehicle accidents, whereas vertical compression injuries are associated with diving or trampoline injuries. The location and classification of an SCI is usually referred to as the level of injury below which sensory and motor function are impaired (Chart 21-4).

Several factors influence the severity of the actual injury to the spinal cord. The mechanism for cellular damage and functional impairment is usually compression

---

CHART 21-4   ASIA Impairment Scale (AIS)

A = Complete: No sensory or motor function is preserved in the sacral segments S4-S5.

B = Sensory Incomplete: Sensory but not motor function is preserved below the neurological level and includes the sacral segments S4-S5 (light touch, pin prick at S4-S5: or deep anal pressure (DAP)), AND no motor function is preserved more than three levels below the motor level on either side of the body.

C = Motor Incomplete: Motor function is preserved below the neurological level**, and more than half of key muscle functions below the single neurological level of injury (NLI) have a muscle grade less than 3 (Grades 0-2).

D = Motor Incomplete: Motor function is preserved below the neurological level**, and at least half (half or more) of key muscle functions below the NLI have a muscle grade ≥ 3.

E = Normal: If sensation and motor function as tested with the ISNCSCI are graded as normal in all segments, and the patient had prior deficits, then the AIS grade is E. Someone without an initial SCI does not receive as AIS grade.

** For an individual to receive a grade of C or D, i.e. motor incomplete status, they must have either (1) voluntary anal sphincter contraction or (2) sacral sensory sparing <u>with</u> sparing of motor function more than three levels below the motor level for that side of the body. The Standards at this time allows even non-key muscle function more than 3 levels below the motor level to be used in determining motor incomplete status (AIS B versus C).

NOTE: When assessing the extent of motor sparing below the level for distinguishing between AIS B and C, the **motor level** on each side is used; whereas to differentiate between AIS C and D (based on proportion of key muscle functions with strength grade 3 or greater) the **single neurological level** is used.

From American Spinal Injury Association. (2011). *International standards for neurological classification of spinal cord injury.* Atlanta, GA: Author. Reprinted with permission.

---

and contusion rather than actual transection. During the first hours after injury, decreased blood flow and ischemia result in extensive tissue destruction. Compression injuries may result from spinal epidural or subdural hematomas that can be surgically alleviated.

The immediate response to SCI is called *spinal shock*. In this phenomenon, the reflexes controlled by nerves below the level of the injury are temporarily suppressed. Spinal shock can last from a few hours to many months. The appearance of perianal reflexes signifies the end of spinal shock and the beginning of recovery. During the recovery period from the acute phase, hyperreflexia and spasticity may appear.

A common physiologic consequence of SCI is a phenomenon referred to as *central cord necrosis*. As further edema and ischemia develop, vascular stasis and thrombosis occur, propagating the vicious cycle; the eventual outcome is necrosis of gray matter.

Assessment

Immediate signs and symptoms of SCI vary depending on whether the injury is complete or partial. Because complete SCI is rare, this section focuses on partial injury.

A symmetric flaccid paralysis and loss of reflexes below the portion of damaged cord occur. Pain, temperature, and proprioception below the level of the injury may be preserved somewhat. Moderate vasomotor instability and lowering of the blood pressure usually occur.

Cervical cord injury is characterized by respiratory insufficiency caused by disruption of innervation to the diaphragm. Another condition that occurs immediately after injury is called *neurogenic shock*. This condition is characterized by hypotension, caused by vasodilation of the vascular bed below the level of injury; bradycardia; and loss of the ability to sweat below the level of injury.

Quadriplegia results from injuries at the cervical level and implies complete loss of leg function and limited, if any, use of the arms. Paraplegia results from thoracic or high lumbar injury and is characterized by a loss of leg function alone. Most SCIs are incomplete and result in variable degrees of motor and sensory loss below the level of the lesion. Neurologically complete lesions are rare.

Clinical manifestations in chronic SCI are related to the degree of recovery and functional return after the initial injury. Complications, such as autonomic dysreflexia and bladder dysfunction, occur during the post-acute phase.

Any child who has sustained an injury is presumed to have SCI until proved otherwise. The child with cervical spine injury frequently requires intubation to maintain the airway. Assess and maintain the airway while maintaining the neck in a neutral position. Immobilize the neck and spine before moving the child. Perform frequent assessments of vital signs and neurologic status to monitor for signs of shock or other injuries. Assess sensory and motor functions systematically to determine the level of injury. Obtain a history of the injury, if possible, for clues to the type of injury the child may have suffered.

Diagnostic Tests

After the clinical examination has been carried out, a thorough radiographic examination is completed. Anteroposterior, lateral, and oblique views of the spine, down to the suspected level of injury, are obtained. Routine films of the spine and pelvis below the level of the injury are necessary to rule out any other hidden fractures. Spinal CT scans and MR images may each be useful, depending on the type of injury and information desired.

Nursing Diagnoses and Outcomes

Nursing Plan of Care 21-1 presents a variety of nursing diagnoses that may be applicable to the child with a neurologic condition. The following diagnosis applies specifically to the child with SCI:

Nursing Diagnosis: Impaired skin integrity related to limitation of voluntary movement
Outcome: Child's skin will remain intact.

Interdisciplinary Interventions

Treatment of acute SCI begins immediately. Initial management at the scene of the trauma includes stabilizing the spine and establishing an adequate airway. Other appropriate measures during the acute phase include administering IV dexamethasone to reduce swelling around the spinal cord and initiating aggressive pulmonary hygiene measures to prevent pneumonia. Stress ulcer is common and is often prevented by administering antacids or histamine blockers. Frequent repositioning is ordered. The child may be placed in a special frame or bed for turning. Urinary catheterization is also necessary until bladder function can be determined.

Throughout the acute care phase, institute rehabilitative measures to ensure the best possible outcome for the child. Safe and early mobilization is attempted by using a variety of stabilizing devices.

Monitor the child for cardiovascular complications, which may include *orthostatic hypotension* and *autonomic hyperreflexia* (also called *dysreflexia*). Orthostatic hypotension associated with changes in position is caused by interruption of the reflex arc in the upright position, which produces vasoconstriction and pooling of blood in the abdomen and lower extremities. Some patients with quadriplegia may not be able to tolerate even a slight elevation of the head, which makes mobilization difficult. Closely observe vital signs before and after position changes. Compression stockings and abdominal binders can be used to improve venous return and to reduce the incidence of orthostatic hypotension.

Autonomic hyperreflexia occurs when an uncontrolled increase in sympathetic activity occurs that cannot be inhibited because of the SCI. The syndrome is characterized by acute pounding headache, paroxysmal hypertension, profuse diaphoresis, nausea, nasal congestion, and bradycardia. The sudden increase in blood pressure may rupture cerebral blood vessels. Autonomic hyperreflexia can be caused by a variety of avoidable triggers, including overdistended bladder; distension of visceral organs, such as the bowel by constipation; or stimulation of the skin. If symptoms are observed, immediately place the child in a sitting position to lower the blood pressure. Quickly assess the child to identify and relieve the triggering stimuli. If these measures do not alleviate hypertension, administration of a ganglionic blocking agent may be necessary.

After acute SCI, children are at risk for thromboembolism and respiratory compromise. Many children with cervical lesions require a tracheostomy. Bowel and bladder care to prevent urinary tract infection need to be adapted as mobility increases. Prevention of skin breakdown is a task assumed by all personnel who provide care for the child with SCI. Physical, occupational, and speech therapies, as well as an assessment of learning and nutritional and psychosocial needs, are essential. The complex and emotional medical care of these children is best managed in an interdisciplinary rehabilitative center. Reintegrating the disabled child into the family requires a group of individuals committed to the ultimate goal of providing the child with the best possible quality of life. Chapter 12 provides more information regarding the rehabilitation needs of these children.

SCI has a profound effect on both the child and family. The family experiences shock, denial, and anger as they grieve the loss of their healthy child. Many families require professional counseling to come to terms with their child's injury. In addition, the family must learn complex medical procedures to care for their child. The amount of time that must be spent meeting basic needs changes the structure of daily family life. Financial burdens may be overwhelming as well. Besides the medical costs, the family home may need structural changes to accommodate the change in the child's mobility. Early recognition of family coping strategies, anticipatory guidance, and referral to appropriate community agencies will help the family deal with the effects of their child's injury.

To help prevent injuries, nurses can participate in vehicle safety, substance use education, and violence prevention programs and give anticipatory guidance to deal with conflict and avoid violence.

See thePoint for a summary of Key Concepts.

REFERENCES

Achildi, O., Betz, R. R., & Grewal, H. (2007). Lapbelt injuries and the seatbelt syndrome in pediatric spinal cord injury. *Journal of Spinal Cord Medicine, 30*(Suppl. 1), S21–S24.

Adeleye, A. O., & Olowookere, K. G. (2008). Nonshaved cranial surgery in black Africans: A short-term prospective preliminary study. *Surgical Neurology, 69*(1), 69–72.

Agrawal, S., & Nadel, S. (2011). Acute bacterial meningitis in infants and children: Epidemiology and management. *Paediatric Drugs, 13*(6), 385–400.

Aicardi, J. (1998). *Diseases of the nervous system in childhood* (2nd ed.). London, United Kingdom: MacKeith Press.

Akalin, F., Turan, S., Guran, T. et al. (2004). Increased QT dispersion in breath-holding spells. *Acta Paediatrica, 93*(6), 770–774.

Alexious, G. A., Sfakianos, G., & Prodromou, N. (2011). Pediatric head trauma. *Journal of Emergencies, Trauma, and Shock, 4*(3), 403–408.

American Academy of Pediatrics. (2012). Summaries of infectious diseases: Meningococcal infections. In L. K. Pickering (Ed.), *Red book: 2012 report of the Committee on Infectious Diseases* (29th ed., pp. 500–509). Elk Grove Village, IL: American Academy of Pediatrics.

American Academy of Pediatrics Subcommittee on Febrile Seizures. (2011). Neurodiagnostic evaluation of the child with a simple febrile seizure. *Pediatrics, 127*(2), 389–394.

American Association of Neuroscience Nurses. (2011). *Care of the patient undergoing intracranial pressure monitoring/external ventricular drainage or lumbar drainage: Clinical practice guideline series*. Glenview, IL: Author.

Asemota, A. O., George, B. P., Bowman, S. M. et al. (2013). Causes and trends in traumatic brain injury for United States adolescents. *Journal of Neurotrauma, 30*(2), 67–75.

Bankole, I. A., Danesi, M. A., Ojo, O. O. et al. (2012). Characteristics and outcome of tetanus in adolescent and adult patients admitted to the Lagos University Teaching Hospital between 2000 and 2009. *Journal of the Neurological Sciences, 323*(1–2), 201–204.

Basu, S. (2012). Spinal injuries in children. *Frontiers in Neurology, 3*, 96.

Blacher, J., & McIntyre, L. L. (2006). Syndrome specificity and behavioural disorders in young adults with intellectual disability: Cultural differences in family impact. *Journal of Intellectual Disability Research, 50*(Pt. 3), 184–198.

Boon, R. (2002). Does iron have a place in the management of breath holding spells? *Archives of Disease in Childhood, 87*, 77–78.

Bor-Seng-Shu, E., Figueiredo, E. G., Amorim, R. G. et al. (2012). Decompressive craniectomy: A meta-analysis of influences on intracranial pressure and cerebral perfusion pressure in the

treatment of traumatic brain injury. *Journal of Neurosurgery, 117*(3), 589–596.

Brody, A. S., Frush, D. P., Huda, W. et al. (2007). Radiation risk to children from computed tomography. *Pediatrics, 120*(3), 677–682.

Broekman, M. L. D., van Beijnum, J., Peul, W. C. et al. (2011). Neurosurgery and shaving: What's the evidence? *Journal of Neurosurgery, 115*(4), 670–678.

Brophy, G. M., Bell, R., Claassen, J. et al. (2012). Guidelines for the evaluation and management of status epilepticus. *Neurocritical Care, 17*(1), 3–23.

Brouwer, M. C., McIntyre, P., de Gans, J. et al. (2010). Corticosteroids for acute bacterial meningitis. *Cochrane Database of Systematic Reviews*, (9), CD004405.

Bruner, J. P., Davis, G., & Tulipan, N. (2006). Intrauterine shunt for obstructive hydrocephalus: Still not ready. *Fetal Diagnosis and Therapy, 21*(6), 532–539.

Bulas, D. J., Goske, M. J., Applegate, K. E. et al. (2009). Image gently: Why we should talk to parents about CT in children. *American Journal of Roentgenology, 192*, 1176–1178.

Centers for Disease Control and Prevention. (2012). Tetanus. In *Epidemiology and prevention of vaccine-preventable diseases* (The Pink Book) (12th ed.). Atlanta, GA: Author.

Chowdhry, S. A., & Cohen, A. R. (2012). *Citrobacter* brain abscesses in neonates: Early surgical intervention and review of the literature. *Child's Nervous System, 28*(10), 1715–1722.

Coffey, J. S. (2006). Parenting a child with chronic illness: A metasynthesis. *Pediatric Nursing, 32*(1), 51–59.

Commission on Classification and Terminology of the International League Against Epilepsy. (1989). Proposal for revised classification of epilepsies and epileptic syndromes. *Epilepsia, 30*, 389–399.

Coronado, V. G., Xu, L., Basavaraju, S. V. et al. (2011). Surveillance for traumatic brain injury–related deaths—United States, 1997–2007. *Morbidity and Mortality Weekly Report, 60*(SS05), 1–32.

D'Amico, A., Mercuri, E., Tiziano, F. D. et al. (2011). Spinal muscular atrophy. *Orphanet Journal of Rare Diseases, 6*, 71.

de Ribaupierre, S., Vernet, O., Rilliet, B. et al. (2007). Posterior positional plagiocephaly treated with cranial remodeling orthosis. *Swiss Medical Weekly, 137*(25–26), 368–372.

Donald, P. R., & Schoeman, J. F. (2009). Central nervous system tuberculosis in children. In H. S. Schaaf & A. Zumla (Eds.), *Tuberculosis: A comprehensive clinical reference* (pp. 413–423). London: Saunders Elsevier.

Fan, J. (2004). The effect of backrest position on intracranial pressure and cerebral perfusion pressure in individuals with brain injury: A systematic review. *Journal of Neuroscience Nursing, 36*, 278–288.

Felsenstein, S., Williams, B., Shingadia, D. et al. (2013). Clinical and microbiologic features guiding treatment recommendations for brain abscesses in children. *Pediatric Infectious Disease Journal, 32*(2), 129–135.

Fowler, A., Stodberg, T., Eriksson, M. et al. (2008). Childhood encephalitis in Sweden: Etiology, clinical presentation and outcome. *European Journal of Paediatric Neurology, 12*(6), 484–490.

Fox, R. A., Keller, K. M., Grede, P. L. et al. (2007). A mental health clinic for toddlers with developmental delays and behavior problems. *Research in Developmental Disabilities, 28*(2), 119–129.

Garne, E., Loane, M., Addor, M. C. et al. (2010). Congenital hydrocephalus–prevalence, prenatal diagnosis and outcome of pregnancy in four European regions. *European Journal of Paediatric Neurology, 14*(2), 150–155.

Gil, Z., Cohen, J. T., Spektor, S. et al. (2003). The role of hair shaving in skull base surgery. *Otolaryngology, Head and Neck Surgery, 128*(1), 43–47.

Glasgow, J. F. T. (2006). Reye's syndrome: The case for a causal link with aspirin. *Drug Safety, 29*, 1111–1121.

Hampers, L. C., & Spina, L. A. (2011). Evaluation and management of pediatric febrile seizures in the emergency department. *Emergency Medicine Clinics of North America, 29*(1), 83–93.

Hughes, R. A. C., Swan, A. V., van Doorn, P. A. et al. (2012). Intravenous immunoglobulin for Guillain-Barré syndrome. *Cochrane Database of Systematic Reviews*, (7), CD002063.

Jeng, S., Gupta, N., Wrensch, M. et al. (2011). Prevalence of congenital hydrocephalus in California, 1991-2000. *Pediatric Neurology*, *45*(2), 67–71.

Johnsen, S. D., & Bird, C. R. (2006). The thalamus and midbrain in Reye syndrome. *Pediatric Neurology*, *5*, 405–407.

Kernick, D., Reinhold, D., & Campbell, J. L. (2009). Impact of headache on young people in a school population. *British Journal of General Practice*, *59*(566), 678–681.

Khan, A., Hussain, N., & Gosalakkal, J. A. (2011). Bulbar dysfunction: An early presentation of congenital myasthenic syndrome in three infants. *Journal of Pediatric Neurosciences*, *6*(2), 124–126.

Kolkiran, A., Tutar, E., Atalay, S. et al. (2005). Autonomic nervous system functions in children with breath-holding spells and effects of iron deficiency. *Acta Paediatrica*, *94*(9), 1227–1231.

Kossoff, E. H., & Hartman, A. L. (2012). Ketogenic diets: New advances for metabolism-based therapies. *Current Opinion in Neurology*, *25*(2), 173–178.

Liu, K. C., & Bhardwaj, A. (2007). Use of prophylactic anticonvulsants in neurologic critical care: A critical appraisal. *Neurocritical Care*, *7*(2), 175–184.

Lux, A. L. (2010). Treatment of febrile seizures: Historical perspective, current opinions, and potential future directions. *Brain & Development*, *32*(1), 42–50.

MacAllister, W. S., & Schaffer, S. G. (2007). Neuropsychological deficits in childhood epilepsy syndromes. *Neuropsychology Review*, *17*(4), 427–44.

Marx, G. E., & Chan, E. D. (2011). Tuberculous meningitis: Diagnosis and treatment overview. *Tuberculosis Research and Treatment*, *2011*, 798764.

Masters, O. W., & Bagshaw, O. N. (2011). Anaesthetic considerations in paediatric myasthenia gravis. *Autoimmune Diseases*, *2011*, 250561.

McNelis, A., Buelow, J., Myers, J. et al. (2007). Concerns and needs of children with epilepsy and their parents. *Clinical Nurse Specialist*, *21*(4), 195–202.

Miller, J. J., Weber, P. C., Patel, S. et al. (2001). Intracranial surgery: To shave or not to shave? *Otology & Neurotology*, *22*(6), 908–911.

Ng, Y. T., & Maganti, R. (2012). Status epilepticus in childhood. *Journal of Paediatrics and Child Health*. Advance online publication.

Nyame, Y. A., Ambrosy, A. P., Saps, M. et al. (2010). Recurrent headaches in children: An epidemiological survey of two middle schools in inner city Chicago. *Pain Practice*, *10*(3), 214–221.

Orliaguet, G. A., Meyer, P. G., & Baugnon, T. (2008). Management of critically ill children with traumatic brain injury. *Paediatric Anaesthesia*, *18*(6), 455–461.

Pace, D., & Pollard, A. J. (2012). Meningococcal disease: Clinical presentation and sequelae. *Vaccine*, *30*(Suppl. 2), B3–B9.

Parent, S., Mac-Thiong, J.-M., Roy-Beaudry, M. et al. (2011). Spinal cord injury in the pediatric population: A systematic review of the literature. *Journal of Neurotrauma*, *28*(8), 1515–1524.

Ratanalert, S., Saehaeng, S., Sripairojkul, B. et al. (1999). Non-shaved cranial neurosurgery. *Surgical Neurology*, *51*, 458–463.

Rendeli, C., Nucera, E., Ausili, E. et al. (2006). Latex sensitisation and allergy in children with myelomeningocele. *Child's Nervous System*, *22*(1), 28–32.

Reye, R. D., Morgan, G. & Baral, J. (1963). Encephalopathy and fatty degeneration of the viscera, a disease entity in childhood. *Lancet*, *2*(7311), 749–752.

Riddell, J., & Shuman, E. K. (2012). Epidemiology of central nervous system infection. *Neuroimaging Clinics of North America*, *22*(4), 543–556.

Rohlwink, U. K., Zwane, E., Fieggen, A. G. et al. (2012). The relationship between intracranial pressure and brain oxygenation in children with severe traumatic brain injury. *Neurosurgery*, *70*(5), 1220–1231.

Rose, B. M., & Holmbeck, G. N. (2007). Attention and executive functions in adolescent with spina bifida. *Journal of Pediatric Psychology*, *32*(8), 983–994.

Saadai, P., & Farmer, D. L. (2012). Fetal surgery for myelomeningocele. *Clinics in Perinatology*, *39*(2), 279–288.

Sebastian, S. (2012). Does preoperative scalp shaving result in fewer postoperative wound infections when compared with no scalp shaving? A systematic review. *Journal of Neuroscience Nursing*, *44*(3), 149–156.

Sejvar, J. J., Baughman, A. L., Wise, M. et al. (2011). Population incidence of Guillain-Barré syndrome: A systematic review and meta-analysis. *Neuroepidemiology*, *36*, 123–133.

Sejvar, J. J., Kohl, K. S., Gidudu, J. et al. (2011). Guillain–Barré syndrome and Fisher syndrome: Case definitions and guidelines for collection, analysis, and presentation of immunization safety data. *Vaccine*, *29*(3), 599–612.

Shachor-Meyouhas, Y., Bar-Joseph, G., Guilburd, J. N. et al. (2010). Brain abscess in children - epidemiology, predisposing factors and management in the modern medicine era. *Acta Paediatrica*, *99*(8), 1163–1167.

Silbergleit, R., Durkalski, V., Lowenstein, D. et al. (2012). Intramuscular versus intravenous therapy for prehospital status epilepticus. *New England Journal of Medicine*, *366*(7), 591–600.

Stouffer, J. W., Shirk, B. J., & Polomano, R. C. (2007). Practice guidelines for music interventions with hospitalized pediatric patients. *Journal of Pediatric Nursing*, *22*(6), 448–456.

Tang, K., Yeh, J. S., & Sgouros, S. (2001). The influence of hair shave on the infection rate in neurosurgery: A prospective study. *Pediatric Neurosurgery*, *35*(1), 13–17.

Taylor, E., & Rogers, J. W. (2005). Practitioner review: Early adversity and developmental disorders. *Journal of Child Psychology and Psychiatry*, *46*(5), 451–467.

Train, H., Colville, G., Allan, R. et al. (2006). Paediatric 99mTc-DMSA imaging: Reducing distress and rate of sedation using a psychological approach. *Clinical Radiology*, *61*(10), 868–874.

Trouth, A. J., Dabi, A., Solieman, N. et al. (2012). Myasthenia gravis: A review. *Autoimmune Diseases*, *2012*, 874680.

Tsitouras, V., & Sgouros, S. (2011). Infantile posthemorrhagic hydrocephalus. *Child's Nervous System*, *27*(10), 1595–1608.

Tubbs, R. S., Hankinson, T. C., & Wellons, J. C. (2012). The Chiari malformations and syringohydromyelia. In R. G. Ellenbogen, S. I. Abdulrauf, & L. N. Sekhar (Eds.), *Principles of neurological surgery* (3rd ed., pp.157–168). Philadelphia, PA: Elsevier.

Udomphorn, Y., Armstead, W. M., & Vavilala, M. S. (2008). Cerebral blood flow and autoregulation after pediatric traumatic brain injury. *Pediatric Neurology*, *38*(4), 225–234.

Wintermark, M., Lepori, D., Cotting, J. et al. (2004). Brain perfusion in children: Evolution with age assessed by quantitative perfusion computed tomography. *Pediatrics*, *113*(6), 1642–1652.

Yadav, Y. R., Parihar, V., Pande, S. et al. (2012). Endoscopic third ventriculostomy. *Journal of Neurosciences in Rural Practice*, *3*(2), 163–173.

See thePoint for additional organizations.

CHAPTER 22

The Child With a Malignancy

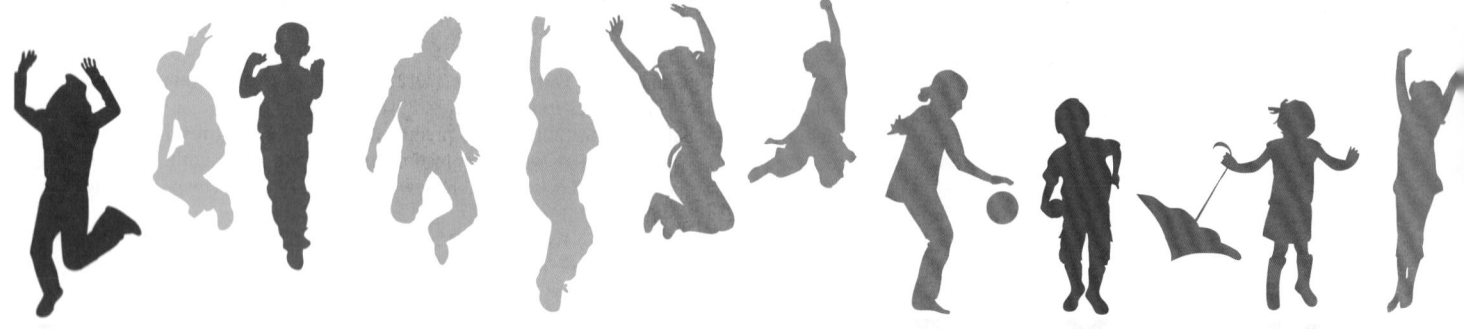

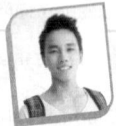

CASE HISTORY

George Tran is Ashley Tran's younger brother. They were introduced in Chapters 1 and 13. George is 14 years old and an eighth grader. As Ashley often laments, George is an excellent student. He is not involved in any sports but spends most of his leisure time on the computer.

George has always been small for his age. This summer, he started a growth spurt and is now more than 5 ft tall. He started having pain in his right leg, in his "shin bone," several months ago. George's parents, Tung and Loan, told him it was "a growing pain" and it would go away on its own. He has been keeping off his leg as much as possible, keeping it elevated while he is on the computer, and taking over-the-counter analgesics for the pain. The pain, however, has not gone away. His leg hurts when he walks and is swollen and tender when compared with the left leg. George's parents take him to the health care provider. An x-ray of his leg shows a lesion in the tibia. The doctor tells George and his parents that it could be cancer, such as an osteogenic sarcoma. He refers them to the oncologist at a tertiary medical center.

George's diagnostic procedures include a radiograph, magnetic resonance imaging (MRI), and computed tomography

(CT). The physician's report on the radiograph of the right leg documented "an area of radiolucency in the proximal right tibia measuring approximately 12 cm with a pattern of permeative destruction: poorly defined borders, cortical destruction, periosteal elevation, and extraosseous extension into soft tissue." In other words, there is a cancerous tumor of the bone. The MR image of the extremity confirmed these findings and also indicated a pathologic fracture through the lesion. A CT scan was then performed to determine the extent of metastasis. The chest CT showed 10 nodules consistent with metastatic lung disease.

George has been a healthy child with no serious illnesses or hospitalizations. There is a family history of cancer, including osteogenic sarcoma. His family genogram (as shown in Chapter 8, Fig. 8-1) shows his maternal grandmother died of breast cancer and his mother's older brother died as a teenager in Vietnam from a "leg bone cancer." Loan, George's mother, remembers only a little about her brother's disease because she is 11 years younger than her brother and both of her parents are dead.

CHAPTER OBJECTIVES

1 Identify abnormal findings in the physical assessment of a child with a malignancy.

2 Describe the nursing care for children undergoing diagnostic tests to detect and diagnose pediatric malignancies.

3 Select the treatment modalities that are most effective for specific pediatric malignancies.

4 Describe the interdisciplinary interventions to minimize the treatment-related side effects associated with each type of malignancy.

5 Identify the psychosocial needs of children with malignancies and their families.

6 Discuss the types of malignancies commonly found in the pediatric population.

See thePoint for a list of Key Terms.

Cancer is the second leading cause of death in children, exceeded only by accidents. In the United States, approximately 12,500 new cases of cancer in children and adolescents (younger than age 20 years) are reported each year, with cancer being accountable for an estimated 2,500 deaths (National Cancer Institute, Surveillance, Epidemiology, and End Results [SEER] Program, 2009). The likelihood that a child will be diagnosed with cancer by age 20 years is approximately 1 in 300 for males and 1 in 333 for females (Heath & Ross, 2010).

Caring for children with cancer presents the health care provider with unique challenges and opportunities. The challenge of pediatric oncology is to provide the aggressive therapy needed to eradicate the disease or slow its progress while at the same time minimizing toxicities and improving long-term quality of life by decreasing late effects. The opportunities arise from working in a field that has demonstrated dramatic advances in treating and curing childhood cancer during the past few decades. The mortality rate among children with cancer has decreased by 42% since the 1960s. The 5-year survival rate for all childhood cancers combined has increased from 58% (1975 to 1977) to 81% (2002 to 2008) (National Cancer Institute, SEER Program, 2009). The increasing survival rate is the result of aggressive multimodal therapy and improved supportive care. **Multimodal therapy** is accomplished by providing various combinations of therapies, such as multiagent chemotherapy, radiation, surgery, hematopoietic stem cell transplantation (HSCT), and biologic response modifiers (BRMs). The combination used depends on the type of malignancy and extent of disease at the time of diagnosis or relapse.

The field of pediatric oncology can be as emotionally draining as it is challenging and exhilarating. Various health care personnel (physicians, nurses, advanced practice nurses) are involved in the short- and long-term care of the child with cancer. The interdisciplinary team involved in the care of the child with cancer may also include social workers, psychologists, child life specialists, teachers, pharmacists, dietitians, religious advisors, and a rehabilitation team. The interdisciplinary team must work in harmony, collaborating and communicating effectively to develop a trusting therapeutic relationship with the child and family and to demonstrate support and confidence in the plan of care that is selected for each child.

DEVELOPMENTAL AND BIOLOGIC VARIANCES

Cancers in children differ substantially from cancers in adults (Developmental Considerations 22-1). Cancers can arise from all three germ cell layers: endoderm (inner), mesoderm (middle), and ectoderm (outer). Most childhood cancers arise from the embryonic mesodermal germ layer, which becomes connective tissue, muscle, bone, cartilage, kidneys, sex organs, blood, blood and lymph vessels, and lymphoid organs. As a result, 92% of childhood cancers (leukemias, lymphomas, and sarcomas)

develop from primitive embryonal tissue. The remaining 8% of childhood cancers arise from neuroectodermal tissue and give rise to central nervous system (CNS) tumors (Ruccione, 2011). In contrast, most adult cancers involve the epithelial tissue and are called *carcinomas*. Epithelial cancers are quite rare in children younger than 15 years of age.

Tumors derived from mesodermal and neuroectodermal tissue are more deeply seated than epithelial tumors (i.e., endodermal tissue) and thus are not easily detected until they are quite large. In almost 80% of pediatric oncology cases, distant **metastasis** (spread) is present at the time of diagnosis (Ruccione, 2011).

Certain pediatric malignancies clearly occur at times of peak physical growth and cellular maturation (Fig. 22-1). This coincidence suggests that cellular growth and development are central to the mechanism of cancer in children. In contrast, adult cancers are more commonly associated with environmental exposures (e.g., radiation exposure, pesticides). Data gathered by the SEER Program from 1975 to 2009 have clearly demonstrated that cancer incidence rates for persons younger than 20 years of age are related to age, sex, race, and body site. Environmental exposures (e.g., electromagnetic fields, cellular devices) at geographic sites have not been conclusively proved as epidemiologic causes of cancer in children (National Cancer Institute, SEER Program, 2009). Peak incidence classically occurs in the 0- to 4-year age group for many childhood cancers (e.g., leukemias, hepatoblastoma, neuroblastoma, Wilms tumor, and retinoblastoma), and incidence increases with age in others (e.g., Hodgkin lymphoma, non-Hodgkin lymphoma [NHL], and CNS and bone tumors,). Age is also an important factor because prognosis for some histologically identical cancers differs based on the age at onset. For example, acute lymphoblastic leukemia (ALL) has a favorable prognosis in children aged 1 to 9 years but a very poor prognosis for infants younger than 1 year and children 10 years and older. For all sites combined, cancer incidences are generally higher for males than females. For example, males younger than 15 years of age have almost double the incidence rate of NHL. In 2000 to 2004, black children had significantly lower cancer incidence rates than white children overall for many specific sites (National Cancer Institute, SEER Program, 2009).

ASSESSMENT

Childhood cancers may be detected early during the course of the illness or may be diagnosed after symptoms have been present for several weeks or months. Delayed diagnosis may be attributable to the vagueness and nonspecificity of symptoms or to a health care provider's lack of experience and knowledge of childhood cancers. In some cases, a child may have been under the recent care of a health care provider and no malignancy was suspected. Yet, within a few weeks, a fast-growing cancer can completely alter the child's previous healthy status. In other cases, the child may have already undergone treatment for vague symptoms that mimic many common childhood illnesses such as the

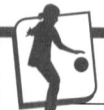

DEVELOPMENTAL CONSIDERATIONS 22-1

Comparison of Childhood and Adult Cancers

Factor	Childhood Cancers	Adult Cancers
Incidence	Rare; 2% of all cancer cases in United States	Common; more than 98% of all cancer cases in United States
Sites	Involve tissue (e.g., reticuloendothelial system, CNS, muscle, bone)	Involve organs (e.g., lung, breast, colon, prostate)
Histology	Most common type: nonepithelial leukemia, lymphoma, sarcomas, embryonal	Most common type: epithelial carcinomas
Time period from initiation to diagnosis	Relatively short period; weeks to months; years rarely	Long period; months to years; may be more than 20 years
Influence of environmental factors in causation	Some environmental factors; few lifestyle factors; overall, no strong influence shown; more likely interaction of genetic alterations and environmental factors (i.e., ecogenetics)	Strong relationship to environmental exposures and lifestyle factors (e.g., sun, ionizing radiation, smoking, alcohol)
Prevention	Minimal strategies known	80% estimated to be preventable
Early detection	Generally accidental; small percentage known as genetically at high risk can be followed more closely	Possible with adherence to early detection screening tests and examination recommendations
Stage at diagnosis	Metastatic disease present in 80%	Local or regional disease in 20%
Response to treatment	Very responsive to chemotherapy; higher doses tolerated	Less responsive to chemotherapy
Treatment of side effects	Less difficulty with acute toxicity but more substantial long-term consequences	More difficulty with acute toxicity but fewer long-term consequences
Prognosis	Leading cause of death from disease in United States; survival rate approximately 80%	Second leading cause of death from disease in United States; less than 60% survival rate

Data from Baggott, C., Fochtman, D., Foley, G. et al. (Eds.). (2011). *Nursing care of children and adolescents with cancer and blood disorders* (4th ed.). Glenview, IL: Association of Pediatric Hematology/Oncology Nurses; Smith, M. A., Seibel, N. L., Altekruse, S. F. et al. (2010). Outcomes for children and adolescents with cancer: Challenges for the 21st century. *Journal of Clinical Oncology, 20*, 2625–2634.

flu, gastroenteritis, or headaches. In most instances, the child's health history and physical examination are limited to the chief complaint. For example, a child complaining of headaches and blurred vision may appear to have eye strain requiring glasses and is referred to an optometrist for follow-up prior to being referred to an oncologist for a suspected brain tumor.

Cancer is usually not suspected until the primary health care provider has ruled out a variety of different diagnoses based on clinical presentation. Diagnostic tests may reveal an abnormal complete blood count (CBC), or a mass detected on plain radiographic films may cause the health care provider to suspect cancer. At this point, the child is usually referred to an oncologist for a diagnostic workup.

The signs and symptoms of childhood cancer are different from those associated with cancer in adults. Adult cancers are generally detected as a result of

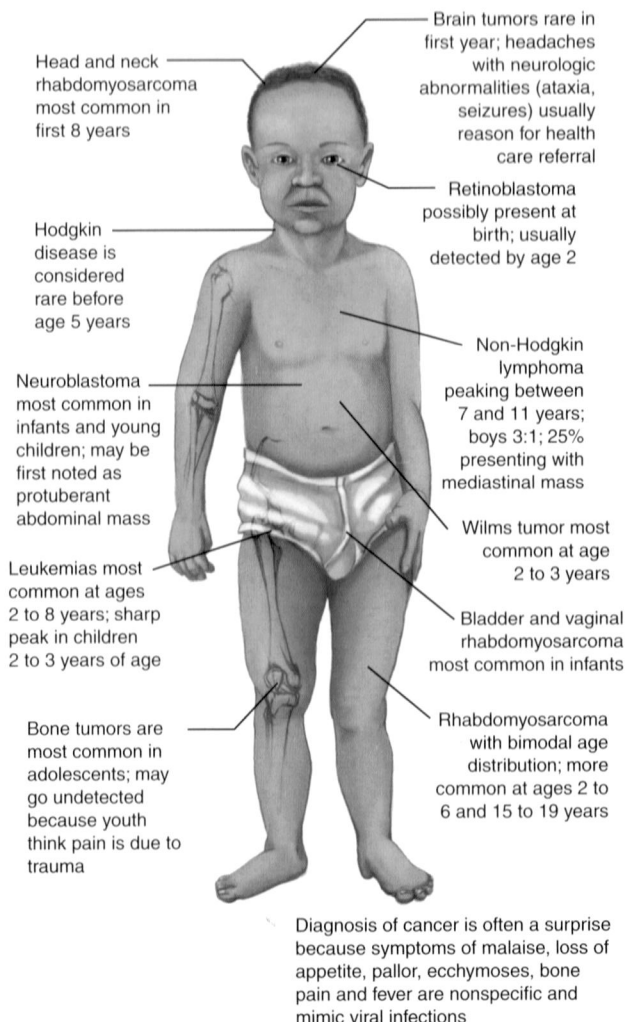

Head and neck rhabdomyosarcoma most common in first 8 years

Brain tumors rare in first year; headaches with neurologic abnormalities (ataxia, seizures) usually reason for health care referral

Retinoblastoma possibly present at birth; usually detected by age 2

Hodgkin disease is considered rare before age 5 years

Non-Hodgkin lymphoma peaking between 7 and 11 years; boys 3:1; 25% presenting with mediastinal mass

Neuroblastoma most common in infants and young children; may be first noted as protuberant abdominal mass

Wilms tumor most common at age 2 to 3 years

Leukemias most common at ages 2 to 8 years; sharp peak in children 2 to 3 years of age

Bladder and vaginal rhabdomyosarcoma most common in infants

Rhabdomyosarcoma with bimodal age distribution; more common at ages 2 to 6 and 15 to 19 years

Bone tumors are most common in adolescents; may go undetected because youth think pain is due to trauma

Diagnosis of cancer is often a surprise because symptoms of malaise, loss of appetite, pallor, ecchymoses, bone pain and fever are nonspecific and mimic viral infections

Figure 22-1 Developmental and biologic variances: pediatric malignancies.

changes in bowel or bladder habits, rectal bleeding, an unusual lump, a chronic cough, a nonhealing wound, a nosebleed, or complaints of pain when certain body areas are palpated. In contrast, the signs and symptoms of cancer in children are primarily the result of one or more of the following factors:

- Compression, infiltration, or obstruction caused by the tumor (e.g., bone pain, abdominal pain, mediastinal mass)
- Changes in blood cell production such as decreased hemoglobin, hematocrit, white blood cell (WBC) count, or platelets (e.g., the child is pale, tired, bruises easily, and has petechiae)
- Metabolic, electrolyte, hormonal, or immunologic alterations caused by tumor metabolism or cell death (e.g., increased frequency of infections, hypercalcemia)

A limited health history and physical assessment can lead to delays in the detection and diagnosis of cancer in children. Conversely, a systematic health history and complete physical examination can assist in the early detection and diagnosis of a suspected malignancy.

FOCUSED HEALTH HISTORY

QUESTION: What is George's presenting symptom? Knowing that George is Vietnamese American, what is an important topic to assess during the during the health history interview?

A systematic approach to obtaining a focused health history is necessary to elicit the most relevant data for detecting a possible malignancy in a child (Focused Health History 22-1). The presenting signs and symptoms and the chief complaint, as stated by the child or family, provide the most important clues regarding the type of cancer that should be suspected. Elicit specific information about the sequence of events related to the current illness, such as the date the symptoms appeared (onset), the sequence and duration of symptoms, and any diagnosis that was made or treatment that was prescribed by another health care provider. Determine whether culturally based remedies (e.g., vitamins, organic compounds, holy water, or herbs) were tried before conventional medical treatment was sought.

Ask pertinent questions about each body system to elicit additional symptoms that the family may not have recognized or considered as important. Check the child's past medical history to assist in identifying clinically important symptoms that the family or other health care providers may not have associated with the current diagnostic evaluation. Often, family members downplay or self-diagnose certain symptoms and attribute them to normal childhood findings (e.g., "growing pains," "frequent colds," "finicky eater"). Information regarding past medical history should include the child's prenatal and neonatal history, allergies, immunizations, childhood illnesses, and previous hospitalizations.

If the child has a history of a previous malignancy, obtaining information regarding the malignancy and all treatments used is especially important. This information is crucial in assessing the potential for a secondary malignancy. Chemotherapy and radiotherapy are known to be powerful carcinogens. In children who survive 5 years after the diagnosis of cancer, another cancer is 10 to 20 times more likely to develop than for children without a history of cancer (National Cancer Institute, 2008a). Certain childhood cancers are associated with an increased incidence of a secondary cancer site. Children with Hodgkin lymphoma, leukemia, ovarian cancer, retinoblastoma, or the genetic form of Wilms tumor, and children who received radiation or alkylating agents (type of chemotherapy), are among those at particularly high risk (National Cancer Institute, 2008a). Hodgkin lymphoma is the most common tumor that precedes both hematologic and nonhematologic secondary tumors. A secondary malignancy may also be associated with the treatment of the primary tumor, or there may be a genetic association between the primary and secondary cancer (e.g., children with retinoblastoma are at risk for secondary osteosarcoma).

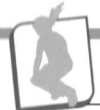

FOCUSED HEALTH HISTORY 22-1

Pediatric Malignancies

Current history	Recurrent fever, nausea, vomiting, diarrhea, constipation Fatigue, pallor, bleeding of mucous membranes Cough or dyspnea unrelated to infectious illness Bruising, unexplained injuries, tissue pain unrelated to an injury Recent traumatic injury associated with current complaint of pain in bone or tissue Masses, swollen or tender lymph nodes Morning headache with vomiting Unsteady gait, limping Visual disturbances Chronic drainage from ear Immunizations up to date Allergies Current medications, including prescription, over-the-counter, and home remedies
Past medical history	**Prenatal/Neonatal History** Maternal drug or substance use Maternal history of miscarriage, fetal death Parental exposure to chemicals, radiation, alkylating agents Newborn infection; mass noted at birth **Previous Health Challenges** History of persistently occurring infections, nontraumatic bone fractures, unusual bleeding (nose, mouth, rectum), unusual bruising, failure to thrive, anemia **Childhood Illnesses** History of childhood illness (e.g., chickenpox) Recent contagious exposure
Nutritional assessment	Weight loss, decreased appetite, nausea, vomiting, constipation, diarrhea
Family medical history	Family history of cancer, especially childhood malignancies, immune disorders Family history of genetic abnormalities (e.g., Down syndrome, neurofibromatosis)
Social and environmental history	Primary cultural group of the family Family support systems Past experiences with stressors and coping mechanisms Recent out-of-country travel Exposure to environmental hazards: • Drugs containing radioisotopes or immunosuppressive agents, in utero or during childhood • Toxic chemicals, fumes, aerosols, smoke, radiation • Household members' smoking behaviors • Power lines, chemical treatment plants, waste dumps
Growth and development	Significant variation from or delay in achieving normal patterns of growth and development The child's habits, including toileting, sleeping, speech patterns, and daily activities Previous exposures to and coping mechanisms for stress and illness

Note: See Chapter 8 for a comprehensive health history.

The family medical history is a very important aspect of history taking when cancer is suspected. Familial and genetic diseases such as autoimmune diseases, immune deficiencies, Down syndrome, and neurofibromatosis have been linked to various types of cancer in children.

CROSS-CULTURAL CARE

The incidences of certain cancers differ notably among ethnic groups from different geographic locations. For instance, ALL is the most common cancer among white children in the Western countries, but its incidence is low among black children in the United States and in Africa and among Arab and Indian children. In tropical Africa, Burkitt lymphoma accounts for more than half of all cases of childhood cancer. In Ankara, Turkey, acute myelomonocytic leukemia accounts for more than half the childhood cases of cancer (National Cancer Institute, 2008a).

A family genogram completed by the health care provider is helpful in plotting health problems of parents, grandparents, aunts, uncles, siblings, and first cousins. The information collected should include ages, a list of serious illnesses, and, if deceased, the cause of death. Give special attention to a family history of malignancies.

A history of environmental exposures may be important whenever a malignancy is suspected. Environmental factors have long been implicated in the increased risk of certain cancers, most commonly *ionizing radiation* (such as radiographs or radiation given off by radioactive materials), electromagnetic fields, radon, drugs, viruses, and alkylating agents or topoisomerase II inhibitors. Information collected should include exposures to these and other hazardous materials, pollutants, insecticides, and environments where the child may have been in contact with hazardous substances. Exposures to these elements by parents before conception, by the mother during fetal development, or by the child after birth have all been associated with cancer development. Some cancers are associated with certain genetic syndromes, such as Li-Fraumeni syndrome, neurofibromatosis, and Down syndrome.

Collect a social history, which provides important information about family functioning and support systems. Include psychosocial and cultural aspects such as parents' race, marital status, age, socioeconomic status, names and ages of all children and their familial relationship to the ill child, and cultural beliefs. In addition, assess the strengths and weaknesses of each family member to determine the effect of the diagnosis, previous experience with stressors, and ability to cope with the stress. Assess the group dynamics within the family and determine whether there are other stressors present (e.g., financial difficulty, divorce). Cancer is a chronic illness that affects the entire family. Over time, family relationships and dynamics change as the family adjusts to the varying demands of the child's illness.

An early understanding of family roles, strengths, and coping mechanisms assists the health care team in helping the family deal with the emotional impact of the illness.

Document baseline physical and developmental milestones as well as the child's eating, sleeping, and toileting habits. Also note any recent regressions in behavior that may be related to the current illness. For example, a 14-month-old child who has been walking and drinking from a cup may regress to crawling and have difficulty sitting unsupported or holding a bottle. These regressions are common in young children with brain tumors.

ANSWER: The presenting symptom is pain in the tibia. The pain was first noticed about 3 months prior to seeking medical assistance, but it did not interfere with George's normal activities. It is important to ask what cultural remedies George's family may have tried at home. When the nurse asked, George's mother described several traditional Vietnamese methods of healing that have been performed on George. His mother placed a silver coin inside a hardboiled egg and rolled it over the affected area of his shin. They also placed suction cups over the painful area of his leg. This was not painful for George, but it did leave little pink circles on his shin.

FOCUSED PHYSICAL ASSESSMENT

QUESTION: What do you anticipate a focused physical assessment of George will reveal?

When cancer is suspected in a child, perform a head-to-toe assessment, with special attention to areas related to symptoms. Focused Physical Assessment 22-1 provides a detailed review of findings by body region that should be evaluated during the physical assessment when a malignancy is suspected.

Begin the assessment by observing the child's overall appearance. Note skin color, presence of ecchymoses or petechiae, nutritional status, asymmetry of facial features or extremities, lymph nodes, and level of activity. A child with cancer often appears pale and thin, with symptoms of lethargy and generalized malaise. Children may have experienced recent weight loss and appear malnourished if they have experienced prolonged nausea, vomiting, or loss of appetite. The presence of pallor, ecchymoses, and petechiae may indicate that the cancer has invaded the bone marrow and is interrupting the normal production of red blood cells and platelets, as in leukemia. Asymmetry of facial features may indicate a retinoblastoma or nasopharyngeal rhabdomyosarcoma (RMS). Asymmetry of an extremity may indicate a bone tumor or soft-tissue sarcoma. Enlarged lymph nodes that are firm and painful on palpation and that are associated with weight loss, fever, and an abnormal chest radiograph may indicate a lymphoma, such as Hodgkin lymphoma or NHL.

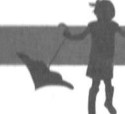

Pediatric Malignancies

Assessment Parameter	Alterations/Clinical Significance
General appearance	Unexplained weight loss, fever, and night sweats may indicate cancer.
	Weight loss may be secondary to decreased appetite, nausea, vomiting, or diarrhea.
	Fever may be secondary to infection or disease process.
	Night sweats may be present in Hodgkin lymphoma.
Integumentary system	Pallor, bruising, petechiae, or mucous membrane bleeding may indicate leukemia or other cancer involving the bone marrow.
Head and neck region	Masses on the cranium may indicate a soft-tissue or bony mass.
	Drainage from ear, asymmetry of face, jaw pain, or swelling may indicate an infection or the presence of a soft-tissue mass.
	Bruising or swelling around eyes (proptosis) may indicate soft-tissue mass.
	Bleeding gums may indicate thrombocytopenia; pallor of the gums may indicate anemia.
	Enlarged or tender cervical lymph nodes may indicate lymphadenopathy caused by cancer cells in the lymph nodes.
	Presence of white reflection in pupil of the eye (cat's eye reflex) may indicate retinoblastoma.
Thoracic and axillary region	Asymmetry may indicate the presence of a soft-tissue mass.
	Difficulty breathing or respiratory distress may indicate mediastinal mass (may be seen on a radiograph).
	Enlarged or tender axillary lymph nodes may indicate lymphadenopathy caused by cancer cells in the lymph nodes.
Gastrointestinal (GI) system	Asymmetry, a palpable mass, rectal bleeding, or vaginal discharge may indicate the presence of an abdominal tumor.
	Hepatomegaly or splenomegaly (enlargement of the liver or spleen) may be caused by an infection or tumor in the liver or abdomen.
Musculoskeletal system	Asymmetry, bone pain or tenderness, limited range of motion, or palpable bony or soft-tissue mass may indicate a bone tumor such as osteosarcoma or Ewing sarcoma.
Neurologic system	Cranial nerve abnormalities, ataxia, gait disturbances, alterations in level of consciousness, or diminished reflexes may indicate the presence of a brain tumor.

The presence of pain, limping, or decreased range of motion requires further investigation. Obtain a thorough history of the location, onset, duration, frequency, and intensity of the pain as well as precipitating and alleviating factors. Headaches, especially when associated with vomiting, must be further evaluated to rule out a possible brain tumor.

ANSWER: George's physical assessment is unremarkable except for his complaint of pain with activity and a firm soft-tissue mass fixed to the underlying bone with slight tenderness.

DIAGNOSTIC CRITERIA

QUESTION: Identify measures you could implement to support George and his family during his diagnostic procedures. Each diagnostic test has given the family bad news. What kind of strategy would help to communicate the results of the tests?

Diagnostic and staging procedures are used to detect the presence of a malignancy, identify the type of malignancy, identify the location of the malignancy, and determine the extent of disease. When cancer is suspected, these procedures are usually carried out quickly so that the appropriate treatment plan can be initiated quickly. The cancer evaluation process includes clinical assessment, laboratory and radiologic tests, and, most important, a biopsy of tissue or fluid for pathologic confirmation. Recent advances in radiologic techniques have dramatically improved the ability to diagnose cancer. Noninvasive imaging studies such as CT, ultrasonography, positron emission tomography (PET), and MRI enable earlier detection of a malignant growth (Tests and Procedures 22-1). However, a definitive diagnosis of cancer cannot be made without pathologic confirmation. In addition, the use of radiolabeled isotopes and monoclonal antibodies is making scanning procedures more thorough and cancer specific. These techniques enable the oncologist to follow treatment response or disease progression.

The nurse caring for children suspected of having cancer is in a unique position to offer support and guidance to the child and the family as they undergo the numerous diagnostic and staging procedures. The nurse must possess a thorough understanding of these procedures and the usual sequence in which they are completed. In most instances, the child's nurse plays a key role in preparing the child and family for tests and procedures and for ensuring the child's safety.

KidKare Establishing an open, honest nurse–child relationship is important. One of the easiest ways to do this is to give simple, honest answers when children ask questions. If the procedure is going to hurt, the child should be told so and be prepared for it. Let the child know that it is OK to be afraid and to cry. Do not tell the child to "act like a big boy" or "big girl."

Provide children who are undergoing tests with an age-appropriate explanation of the procedure and why it is necessary. Children are more apt to cooperate if they understand what is being done and why the test or procedure is necessary. During diagnostic tests, avoid restraining the child if possible. Avoid asking the parent or family member to restrain the child. They should be present for emotional support and comfort. If children have some freedom of movement, they feel they have some control over the situation.

Evaluation and treatment for cancer frequently requires painful procedures, such as venipunctures, lumbar punctures, bone marrow aspirations, and biopsies. The nurse caring for children with cancer must intervene to prevent or minimize pain from such procedures or from the cancer itself. Pharmacologic and biobehavioral interventions can be implemented to maximize the child's comfort. Pharmacologic interventions include sedation and analgesia or general anesthesia for invasive procedures (e.g., lumbar punctures and bone marrow aspirations or biopsies), topical anesthetic for injections and venipunctures, and nonsteroidal anti-inflammatory drugs to decrease cancer pain. Biobehavioral interventions such as age-appropriate preparation, reassurance, diversion, relaxation, breathing exercises,

music therapy, and imagery have been cited as effective measures to reduce the pain of a child or adolescent during invasive procedures. The nurse can easily teach these interventions to the family and the child or adolescent, thereby increasing their sense of control. (See Chapter 10 for a comprehensive discussion of pain management techniques.)

ANSWER: During this diagnostic period, the Tran family will meet many new health care providers. Nurses, however, are the ones who remain with the Tran family throughout George's illness. The nurse should provide preprocedure explanations and prepare George and his family for the diagnostic tests. Unlike the difficulties with younger children, George is able to cooperate even in a lengthy test and is fascinated by the different technology involved in imaging. The nurse should also help the family understand the results of the diagnostic procedures. One strategy to both facilitate communication and allow the presence of the tumor to become real is to allow the adolescent and his family to see all the images. The challenge is to relay the results in a manner that is well understood despite language barriers. The nurse should provide emotional support when the family receives the diagnostic results showing a lesion and again when the results show metastases.

TREATMENT MODALITIES

The therapeutic plan for the child with a malignancy includes initial and ongoing treatment plus supportive care, all using an interdisciplinary approach. Supportive care includes managing the numerous side effects and adverse outcomes associated with the therapies used to eradicate the cancer. This section will discuss the interdisciplinary interventions that may be selected to treat the child with cancer. In collaboration with the child and family, decisions about the course of treatment are based on the type of cancer, the location of the cancer, and the extent of the disease. The primary goal of treatment is to *cure* the child without causing substantial harm or impairment. Advances have been made during the past decade in understanding cancer biology, and technologic advances have enabled development of multimodal therapy (the combination of two or more therapeutic modalities—radiation, chemotherapy, and/or surgery—to treat cancer), which is considered the gold standard (the best possible treatment).

An individualized therapeutic plan is developed for each child based on the child's unique presentation using multimodal therapy to offer the best chance of survival. The modes of therapy currently include surgery, chemotherapy, radiation therapy, biotherapy, and HSCT. Gene therapy for treating childhood cancers is in the early phases of clinical application. The therapeutic plan is individualized and includes supportive care to treat the adverse outcomes that may present as a result of multimodal therapy. Supportive care measures include, but are not limited to, managing pain, nausea, and vomiting; infection prevention; providing

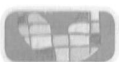 **TESTS AND PROCEDURES** for Evaluating Pediatric Malignancies

Diagnostic Test or Procedure	Purpose	Findings and Indications	Health Care Provider Considerations
CBC with differential	Determines abnormal loss or destruction of cells that may indicate cancer or bone marrow suppression. Changes in values may indicate complications such as anemia, neutropenia, and thrombocytopenia.	Increased WBC count with the presence of lymphoblasts can indicate leukemia. Malignancies with bone marrow involvement may cause hemoglobin, hematocrit, and platelet levels to be low. Decreased red blood cells and hemoglobin, seen in anemia. Decreased neutrophil count indicates neutropenia, which is often a presenting sign of malignancy, or a relapse in cancer treatment or immunosuppression secondary to chemotherapy and/or radiation treatment. Platelet count less than 150,000/mm³ indicates thrombocytopenia.	Be aware that children who require numerous venipunctures may become fearful and uncooperative. Provide good explanations, use topical anesthetic before initiating a venipuncture; consider using an intermittent infusion device for obtaining venous blood samples.
Absolute neutrophil count (ANC)	Measures the number of neutrophil granulocytes (type of WBC that fights infection) present in the blood.	The normal range for the ANC is 1.5–8.0 (1,500–8,000/mm³). An ANC less than 1,000 in infants 2 weeks to 1 year of age or less than 1,500 in children older than 1 year of age indicates neutropenia.	ANC is not measured directly; it is calculated by multiplying the WBC count by the percentage of neutrophils (segmented [fully mature] and bands [almost mature]) in the differential WBC count. Use good infection control measures during lab draw to protect child from exposure to infection. Advise family of neutropenic precautions if ANC is low.
Serum chemistries	Indicates metabolic state as well as renal and liver function. Helps to evaluate the body's response to the cancer treatment.	Elevations in potassium, phosphorus, uric acid, and lactate dehydrogenase (LDH) levels and decrease in calcium may be seen at the start of chemotherapy and indicate tumor lysis syndrome. High uric acid, blood urea nitrogen (BUN), and creatinine levels are associated with renal failure. Changes in levels are important as prognostic indicators and evidence to manage disease and evaluate treatment response.	Ensure that proper tubes are used and that volume of blood is adequate for lab analysis.
Urinalysis	Provides general information about renal function.	May indicate urinary tract infection secondary to child's immunosuppressed state. May indicate altered renal function secondary to chemotherapy and/or radiation treatments.	When obtaining urine sample from adolescent females, question about presence of menstruation. Obtain midstream, clean-catch sample to avoid contamination.

Diagnostic Test or Procedure	Purpose	Findings and Indications	Health Care Provider Considerations
Urine catechol-amines vanil-lylmandelic acid (VMA), homovanillic acid (HVA) (catecholamine metabolites)	Identifies specific tumor markers used to differenti-ate neuroblastoma from other tumors.	VMA and HVA levels are elevated in 90%–95% of chil-dren with neuroblastoma.	Obtain sample before CT scan because the contrast medium affects the results.
Tumor markers	A characteristic or substance that indicates the presence of a specific tumor.	α-Fetoprotein (AFP) levels are commonly elevated more than 20 mg/mL in children with hepatoblastoma, hepatocellular cancer, or germ cell tumors. Beta human chorionic gonado-tropin (β-HCG) is elevated in children with hepatoblastoma and germ cell tumors.	Prepare child for venipuncture to obtain blood sample. Ensure that proper tubes are used and that volume of blood is adequate for lab analysis.
Immunopheno-typing of monoclonal antibodies and cytogenetic studies	Used to identify, clas-sify, and describe specific types of cells in a sample of blood, marrow, or lymph node cells. Determines whether a chromosomal abnormality exists within a tumor. This procedure can be important in helping to decide on the best treat-ment for a child.	Findings include distinguishing myelogenous leukemic cells from lymphoblastic leukemic cells. Normal lymphocytes can be distinguished from leukemic lymphocytes, and B-cell lymphocytes can be distinguished from T-cell lymphocytes. Also provides information about whether the patient's cells are monoclonal (derived from a single malignant cell).	Prepare child for specific lab test (venipuncture, bone marrow aspi-ration, or lymph node biopsy) to obtain cell sample for analysis.
Lumbar puncture	Introduces a hollow needle with stylet into the lumbar subarachnoid space of spinal canal to withdraw CSF. Used to introduce chemotherapeutic agents into the spinal canal and circulating CSF.	Provides diagnostic or staging workup in children with leukemia, lymphoma, parameningeal RMS, and medulloblastoma.	Nurse may need to assist with posi-tioning, securing, and calming child (see thePoint Procedure: Lumbar Puncture). Encourage fluids before and after lum-bar puncture. Empty bladder before lumbar puncture because child must remain supine for 4–6 hours after the procedure. Premedicate for pain and monitor for signs and symptoms of headache related to decreased amount of CSF. Maintain strict asepsis. Contraindicated in children with sub-stantially increased ICP because brain stem may herniate downward, causing tissue compression, which may lead to death.

(Continued)

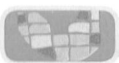 **TESTS AND PROCEDURES** for Evaluating Pediatric Malignancies *(Continued)*

Diagnostic Test or Procedure	Purpose	Findings and Indications	Health Care Provider Considerations
Bone marrow aspiration and biopsy	Aspirated bone marrow is used for microscopic examination of cell type and morphology. Test performed to determine when leukemia is present, if the tumor has spread to the bone marrow, or when a CBC suggests malfunctioning bone marrow.	When leukemia is present, bone marrow aspiration can reveal more than 25% blasts (immature and undifferentiated cells). In tumor metastasis, carcinogenic cells may be present in bone marrow.	Procedure is done using aseptic technique. Topical anesthetic is used to anesthetize the skin; an injectable anesthetic is used to anesthetize the bone. Prepare the child for the procedure; explain where the sample will be obtained. Position the child properly based on the site of aspiration; place pillows or folded blanket under the child's abdomen to elevate the hips (for iliac crest site). Allow a family member to stay in the room during the procedure. Position the family member at the head of the table, allowing the adult to provide verbal and physical support. The family member should not help to restrain the child. Provide procedural sedation monitoring for children receiving sedatives and analgesics in a treatment room; the procedure can also be done while the child is in the operating room for biopsy, resection, or line placement. Apply pressure dressing to site after aspiration. Remove dressing and inspect site after 24 hours.
Radiographs	Uses radiation to examine soft tissue and bony structures of the body. Aids in detecting tumors and metastasis to bones and vital organs.	Abnormal masses in the chest wall, lungs, and mediastinum may indicate tumors in this area. Lesions on the bone may indicate tumors (e.g., Ewing sarcoma, osteosarcoma) or metastasis of tumors and warrant further investigation by bone scan, CT, or MRI.	Determine whether adolescent female patients may be pregnant. Advise the child to hold absolutely still. Provide age-appropriate explanations (such as the radiograph machine being a "camera" that takes pictures of "your insides") to assist in gaining the child's cooperation. Provide reassurance that family members are nearby. Anticipate the need for assistance in positioning and maintenance of the positioning for infants and young children.

Diagnostic Test or Procedure	Purpose	Findings and Indications	Health Care Provider Considerations
Computed Tomography (CT)	Uses serial scans of each plane in the area studied to provide a three-dimensional view and represents a cross-sectional view of body structures. Uses a contrast medium (intravenous [IV] for brain CT; oral for abdominal or pelvic CT) to enhance visualization. Visualizes known or suspected solid tumors. Detects masses, locates lesions, and evaluates response to treatment.	CT of chest may reveal presence and extent of pulmonary lesions. Abnormal body masses, lesions, or enlarged organs provide further evidence of presence of tumors or metastasis.	Inform the child that he or she must remain very still for 30–90 minutes. Anticipate the need for immobilization or sedation in young children. IV or oral contrast dye may be ordered. If oral contrast medium is used, mix in a clear fluid and ensure that the medium is cold and that the child drinks the entire volume within 45–60 minutes. The oral contrast dye is usually given the night before the tests and again 2 hours before the test. The child may then have nothing else to eat or drink until the test is completed. If the child is unable to tolerate the contrast by mouth, expect to administer the oral contrast medium via nasogastric tube. Ensure IV access, especially if IV contrast medium is to be used. Educate child and family about the scan, especially if the scan is done on an outpatient basis.
Magnetic Resonance Imaging (MRI)	Uses radio waves and magnets to produce a highly defined, computerized image of the body. Provides extremely precise visualization and information (as much as direct visualization). Helps to determine exact location and size.	Abnormal body masses, lesions, or enlarged organs provide further evidence of presence of tumors or metastasis.	MRI is the image of choice for brain stem and bone tumors. Keep in mind that the strong magnetic field precludes MRI study of persons who have any implanted metallic objects in their body. Inform the child and family that the test lasts about 60 minutes and that the child must lie very still. Anticipate sedation for children who cannot lie still, who may become frightened by the loud noise made by the machine, or who become claustrophobic because of the close quarters. Provide continuous monitoring of pulse oximetry and heart rate during and after the scan for children who are sedated. Ensure that jewelry and other metallic objects are removed.
Bone scan	A nuclear scanning test to rule out cancer involving the bones. Determines the extent of bone involvement.	Abnormal body masses, lesions, or enlarged organs provide further evidence of presence of tumors or metastasis. Areas of disease will have an increased uptake of the radioactive dye. Highly sensitive method of detecting bony lesions but does not distinguish between cancer and inflammatory processes.	Inform the child and family that the scan lasts 30–60 minutes. Two to 4 hours before the scan, a radioisotope dye is injected intravenously into the child. Encourage the child to lie still during the test; instruct in measures to facilitate lying still. Sedation may be required to keep the child still.

(Continued)

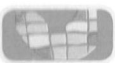

TESTS AND PROCEDURES for Evaluating Pediatric Malignancies *(Continued)*

Diagnostic Test or Procedure	Purpose	Findings and Indications	Health Care Provider Considerations
Positron Emission Tomagraphy (PET) scan	Combines conventional nuclear medicine techniques with transaxial tomography to study blood flow and volume and protein metabolism of specific regions or organs. Uses isotopes to detect physiologic and metabolic activity. Aids in differentiating viable tumors from necrotic or scar tissue.	Abnormal body masses, lesions, or enlarged organs provide further evidence of presence of tumors or metastasis. Most effective for diagnosis and evaluation of neuroblastoma, Hodgkin lymphoma, NHL, bone tumors, lung and colon cancers, and brain tumors.	Inform child to avoid intake of caffeine, nicotine, and alcohol for 24 hours before scan. Child must fast at least 4 hours prior to the scan. IVs with dextrose should be avoided 6 hours before the scan to prevent a false-positive result. Ensure adequate IV access, which is required for isotope injection. Child may need sedation to remain still. PET scans are clearer than conventional radionuclide scans.
Metaiodobenzylguanidine (MIBG) scan	Uses a radioactive substance to detect certain types of nervous tissue. MIBG is taken up and stored in adrenergic tissues.	Increased uptake indicates the presence of neuroblastoma, a tumor of the sympathetic nervous system.	A special medicine (potassium iodide [SSKI]) is given to protect the thyroid gland from the radioactive substance in the tracer.
Ultrasound	Uses sound waves to create images that visualize body structures and locate masses.	Unusual mass or enlarged lymph nodes or organs may indicate a tumor.	Be aware that ultrasound is the initial screening test for the child with a palpable mass. Inform child and family that this test is noninvasive, but that it may take as long as 30 minutes to complete. Allow an adult family member to stay with child during the procedure, if appropriate. Inform the child that the transducer may "tickle" and that a gel is used that may feel cold. Provide infants with a juice bottle during the procedure to alleviate crying. Check to determine if a full bladder is needed for the test; some ultrasounds require this to differentiate organs.
Tissue specimen biopsy	Analyzes tissue such as lymph node or unidentifiable mass to determine pathology of tissue cells. Identifies specific type of tumor cells for initiating optimal treatment.	Tissue specimen reveals abnormal cells.	Ensure proper labeling and handling. Local anesthetic is used. After the procedure, the area may be tender or sore for a few days.

psychosocial support; and promoting growth and development. A discussion of these and other interventions is included in this section.

In order to remain consistent across the care continuum, treatment is guided according to standards and protocols created by the Children's Oncology Group (COG) and the Association of Pediatric Hematology/Oncology Nurses (APHON). COG is a large group of multidisciplinary health care professionals who collaborate with one another and other national and international treatment groups. Their focus is to conduct clinical trials aimed at increasing the long-term survival rates and minimizing late effects associated with aggressive cancer treatment. APHON is the professional nursing organization for the nursing care of children, adolescents, and young adults with blood and cancer disorders and their families. Their core purpose is to support and advance nurses in optimizing outcomes for this patient population and their families.

SURGERY

QUESTION: Surgery is an important treatment for George. A limb salvage or limb-sparing procedure may be the best option. This surgery allows the surgeon to remove the tumor while saving the limb. How can the nurse support George after he is told that he will have a limb salvage procedure on his right leg?

The primary goal of surgery in pediatric oncology is to remove all visible disease while maintaining or restoring normal body function. The best prognosis is related to early detection and removal of disease. Thus, surgery is considered a definitive treatment in more than half of all cancer patients. Surgery may also be used for diagnosis. In this case, a biopsy is performed in which a tissue sample is taken and examined for evidence of cancer. Surgery is also likely for insertion of central venous catheters (CVCs) or implantable venous access devices that will be used to obtain blood specimens and to administer chemotherapy, antibiotics, and total parenteral nutrition (Wallace, 2009).

Recent advances in surgical oncology have provided major improvements in the surgical management of children with cancer. These improvements have allowed a better quality of life for the child, both physically and psychosocially. Surgery is most frequently combined with chemotherapy, radiation therapy, or biotherapy. Surgery and adjuvant therapy can increase disease-free and long-term survival for children with cancer.

Nursing care of the child with cancer following surgical treatment is similar to the care given to any child who undergoes surgery. (See Chapter 11 for more discussion of presurgical and postsurgical care.) Monitor the child for complications from the surgery and for pain control using an age-appropriate pain rating scale (see Chapter 11). Assess the surgical site for any bleeding or signs of infection. Offer support to families anxiously awaiting biopsy results or news of the effectiveness of the surgical intervention.

ANSWER: The nurse will give George his preoperative and postoperative information, just as he or she would for any surgery. George requires additional assessment and interventions that include focusing on what he will still be able to do and enjoy after the surgery is complete and he begins to heal. In addition, the nurse needs to address George's psychosocial needs, especially related to how the surgery may affect his body image.

CHEMOTHERAPY

QUESTION: Chemotherapy is also an important component of George's treatment. He will receive two courses of chemotherapy before the surgical resection of the tumor. He will receive additional courses after surgery. The consultants have recommended a combination of three drugs, including doxorubicin. What is the nurse's role related to George's chemotherapy treatment?

Chemotherapy is a systemic mode of cancer treatment. This approach has been extremely effective in the treatment of childhood cancers, especially leukemia and lymphoma. The development of new drugs and combinations of drugs, along with new administration techniques, has resulted in advanced treatment regimens and increasing survival rates. Children with cancer undergo chemotherapy regimens for periods ranging from a few months to years. Side effects range from minimal to severe. The nurse plays a key role in providing children and their families with the appropriate information and support throughout treatment. The side effects of chemotherapy include neutropenia, thrombocytopenia, anemia, nausea, vomiting, and mucositis. Nursing management of these side effects is discussed later in the "Treatment Modalities" section.

Chemotherapy affects the **cell cycle**. Cells go through four phases to complete cell growth cycle: G1 (the first "gap"), S (synthesis phase), G2 (the second gap), and M (mitosis). Cells move into G0 (the resting phase) after mitosis; during the G0 phase, cells are not actively dividing. The G1 phase varies the most in duration (8 to 48 hours) and is the phase in which DNA synthesis is beginning and active RNA and protein synthesis occurs. Cells then enter the S phase, during which most DNA synthesis occurs. This phase takes from 10 to 30 hours, during which time the DNA content of the cell doubles. After the S phase, cells move into G2. During this phase, the RNA and protein necessary for mitosis are synthesized. This process takes 1 to 12 hours. During the last phase of the cell cycle, the M phase, mitosis (cell division) occurs, which takes approximately 1 hour. Mitosis is a four-step process (prophase, metaphase, anaphase, and telophase) that results in two identical daughter cells.

Cancer cells are difficult to treat in the G0 phase because the cell is not dividing. Malignant cells are believed to have a shorter cell cycle time and grow at a faster rate because of their uncontrolled, erratic growth patterns.

Chemotherapeutic Agents

Generally, chemotherapeutic agents fall into one of two classifications: *cell cycle–specific* or *cell cycle–nonspecific agents*. Cell cycle–specific agents exert their maximal effect during a specific phase of the cell cycle. Cell cycle–nonspecific agents act on cells regardless of their phase. The maximal amount of cell destruction is directly proportional to the dose and combination of drugs given. Combining drugs that act at different phases of the cell cycle produces optimal cell cycle disruption and cell destruction. Combining drugs also helps to prevent drug resistance, which occurs when a cancer cell builds up a tolerance to a single agent, thus rendering therapy with that agent ineffective. Finally, combination therapy allows multiple drugs to be given at safe dosages, an approach that minimizes toxic side effects while maximizing cancer cell destruction.

Chemotherapeutic agents are pharmacologically classified into seven categories. Table 22-1 summarizes the

TABLE 22-1	Types of Chemotherapy Agents	
Type	**Action**	**Examples**
Alkylating agents	Cell cycle–nonspecific, destroying both resting and dividing cells. During alkylation, the hydrogen atoms of some molecules within the cell are replaced by an alkyl group. This group interferes with DNA replication and RNA transcription.	Busulfan Carboplatin Carmustine Cisplatin Cytoxan Dacarbazine Ifosfamide Lomustine Mechlorethamine hydrochloride Melphalan Procarbazine Temozolomide Thiotepa
Antimetabolites	Cell cycle–specific, most active during the S phase and acts similar to normal cellular metabolites that are necessary for cell function and replication. These drugs damage cells by acting as a substitute for a natural metabolite in an important molecule, thereby altering the function of the molecule.	5-Fluorouracil Clofarabine Cytarabine Fludarabine Gemcitabine Hydroxyurea Mercaptopurine Methotrexate Thioguanine
Antitumor antibiotics	Cell cycle–nonspecific agents, synthesized naturally by various bacterial and fungal species. They interfere with cellular metabolism, thereby blocking DNA transcription, RNA transcription, or both.	Bleomycin sulfate Dactinomycin Daunomycin Doxorubicin Idarubicin Mitoxantrone
Plant products	Cell cycle–specific because they crystallize microtubular proteins and arrest mitosis. Agents are derived from the periwinkle plant (*Vinca rosea*) and are sometimes called vinca alkaloids.	Etoposide Paclitaxel Teniposide Vinblastine Vincristine
Hormones (corticosteroids)	Not chemotherapeutic drugs per se but are effective in treating cancers that arise in tissues that depend on hormones for cellular proliferation. The hormonal environment of the cancer cell is altered, thereby affecting cancer cell division. Hormones and corticosteroids can interfere with protein synthesis and modify the DNA transcription process.	Dexamethasone Hydrocortisone Prednisone
Miscellaneous agents	Medications with a mechanism of action that is not fully understood or not like any of the other categories described. This group includes enzyme inhibitors, platinum agents, and nonclassic alkylating agents.	Asparaginase Carboplatin Cisplatin Hycamtin Hydroxyurea Procarbazine Retinoic acid Trisenox

Information from Kline, N. E. (Ed.) (2009). *Essentials of pediatric hematology/oncology nursing: A core curriculum* (3rd ed.). Glenview, IL: Association of Pediatric Hematology/Oncology Nurses.

action of these agents and lists examples. Some agents cause more severe side effects than others. Chemotherapy agents do not distinguish between cancer cells and other rapidly dividing normal cells and therefore cause predictable side effects. The hematopoietic system, GI tract, and integumentary system are composed of rapidly dividing cells and thus are highly susceptible to toxic effects. Nursing care of these side effects is discussed later in the "Treatment Modalities" section. Myelosuppression (suppression of bone marrow function), nausea, vomiting, diarrhea, hair loss, and skin problems are common side effects in children receiving chemotherapy.

Chemotherapeutic Regimens

A chemotherapy regimen is composed of several phases. During *induction*, the initial phase, intensive therapy is given to kill enough cancerous cells to induce a remission. **Remission** occurs when a temporary or permanent response to therapy causes a decrease in, or absence of, the primary malignancy. During the next phase, the *consolidation phase*, intensive therapy is given to destroy the remaining cancer cells. The *maintenance phase* is a designated period during which less intensive treatment is continued to destroy any residual cancer cells. This phase can continue for a few years. During the *observation phase*, therapy has ended and the child is monitored for recurrent disease or late effects of treatment. The observation phase can be a stressful period for the family. Although they are thankful to have completed chemotherapy and frequent monitoring, they may experience increased anxiety related to the possibility of a relapse. During any of these phases, the child may relapse. In these cases, the treatment protocol is changed and the child goes through each of the phases again, beginning with induction. A child is considered to be a cancer survivor when he or she has been disease free for 5 years from time of diagnosis.

Chemotherapy Administration

Chemotherapy doses for children are most often calculated according to the child's body surface area or are based on the child's weight in kilograms (for infants younger than 1 year of age) to minimize toxic effects to tissues and organs (see nomogram in Fig. 9-1, for calculating body surface area). Chemotherapeutic agents are administered intrathecally via lumbar puncture; into the veins either peripherally or via CVCs; into the lateral ventricle using the Ommaya reservoir; or into intraperitoneal, intracavitary, or intra-arterial sites using implantable pumps. Portable infusion pumps deliver continuous therapy to children in ambulatory settings.

Chemotherapy administration necessitates safety precautions for both the child and the nurse or caregiver administering the medication (Nursing Interventions 22-1). The National Institute for Occupational Safety and Health (NIOSH, 2004) has developed guidelines to protect health care workers from unwarranted exposure to cytotoxic agents caused by accidental absorption, inhalation, or ingestion.

ANSWER: George's physician or nurse practitioner is primarily responsible for discussing the need for chemotherapy and the delivery system that will be used to administer the chemotherapy (e.g., infusion devices). George's nurse should follow up with the family and further explain the procedure of receiving chemotherapy as well as the expected side effects in order for George and his family to know what to expect. The nurse will assess for side effects and use interventions to reduce those side effects as needed.

In response to metabolizing, detoxifying, and excreting many chemotherapy agents, certain organs may experience toxic side effects. Every child must be evaluated for baseline organ function before chemotherapy administration. Liver and renal function blood tests (i.e., BUN, creatinine clearance tests, bilirubin levels) are conducted and evaluated for normal function. An electrocardiogram or echocardiogram may be indicated to evaluate heart function. Pulmonary function tests are used to evaluate lung capacity. Neurologic examinations indicate any loss of deep tendon reflexes or sensory function. Increased creatinine levels, the presence of proteins, or hematuria in urine indicate drug toxicity. Changes in organ function or laboratory values require appropriate drug modifications, dose deletions, or modified timing of drug delivery. The decision to modify therapy is complex because the goal of eradicating the cancer must always be maintained while supporting the child through the toxic side effects.

RADIATION THERAPY

Radiation therapy is used frequently in conjunction with chemotherapy, surgery, or HSCT to treat cancer in children. It can be used as curative treatment for radio-sensitive tumors or as a palliative measure to relieve symptoms. New advances in the delivery of radiation have led to less acute and long-term side effects and to better targeted sites of delivery. For example, intensity-modulated radiation therapy (IMRT), gamma-knife radiosurgery, and proton beam radiation allow for the precise delivery of high radiation doses to the tumor site while minimizing damage to surrounding tissue.

Radiation is cytotoxic by damaging the synthesis of nucleic acids, causing breaks in the DNA or RNA molecule, or causing double-stranded breaks in the molecules. Radiated cells cannot divide or they lose their function and die during division. Thus, normal and malignant cells that divide rapidly are most susceptible to the effects of radiation.

Many of the acute side effects of radiation are the result of damage to normal cells that divide rapidly, including the cells of the mucous membranes, hair follicles, and bone marrow. Acute side effects are usually anticipated 7 to 10 days after treatment has been initiated and may last for several weeks or even several months after therapy is completed.

Nursing responsibilities for the child receiving radiation treatments include providing concrete explanations

NURSING INTERVENTIONS 22-1

Safety Guidelines for Chemotherapy Administration

Event	Guidelines
Preparation	Use a CVC for administration whenever possible to minimize the risk of extravasation.
	A health care provider who is competent in peripheral IV access selects the peripheral vascular access site and places the catheter.
	Pharmacists mix and prepare chemotherapy agents in a biologic safety cabinet, wearing protective gear (i.e., latex gloves, gown, face shield) and using sterile techniques.
	Nurses wear protective gear, ensure IV connections have a Luer-Lok and are secured, and use a plastic-backed absorbent pad under the site of administration to catch any leakage when administering chemotherapy.
Disposal	Consider equipment that has contained chemotherapy drugs, body excretions after chemotherapy administration, and linens and clothing contaminated with chemotherapeutic agents or excretions as hazardous waste.
	Chemotherapeutic agents may be excreted in the urine for up to 48 hours after administration. Dispose of these materials in designated, properly labeled hazardous waste containers.
Extravasation	Notify a physician immediately if suspected or definite extravasation is identified.
	Immediately perform procedures (i.e., elevate extremity, apply ice, apply topical or injectable antidotes) according to institutional guidelines for extravasation.
Spills	Cleanup of accidental spills of chemotherapy drugs should occur immediately by specially trained registered nurses (RNs) and environmental services.
	Confine spills and restrict the area until appropriate cleaning procedures have been completed.
Family teaching	Teach family members safety procedures for home chemotherapy administration and disposal. These procedures should be used for a minimum of 48 hours after administration.

From Kline, N. E. (Ed.) (2009). *Essentials of pediatric hematology/oncology nursing: A core curriculum* (3rd ed.). Glenview, IL: Association of Pediatric Hematology/Oncology Nurses.

to the child and family regarding the radiation procedure and its side effects (Nursing Interventions 22-2). Before therapy is started, the area on the child's body to define the radiation field is marked (Fig. 22-2). During the procedure, the child must lie still and not change position. Plastic casts and molds may be used to immobilize the child during the treatments. Shielding devices made of lead are used to protect surrounding healthy tissues and organs against unnecessary radiation exposure. These shields may feel heavy to the child. The machinery involved in the treatment can create a variety of noises that may frighten the child. The child is alone in the treatment room, although he or she can communicate verbally with the staff. All of these sensations can make the child feel uncomfortable, claustrophobic, anxious, or bored. Young children may need sedation or general anesthesia. Older children can be taught distraction techniques. Family members, who

are located outside the room, can talk or read to the child to focus attention away from the procedure. After radiation treatment, nursing and family interventions focus on managing the side effects of the therapy and preventing further complications.

BIOTHERAPY

For many years, researchers have studied the complex functions of the immune system as it relates to cancer. Through research and technologic advances, *biotherapy*, the use of *biologics and targeted therapy*, has emerged as a mode of cancer treatment. Researchers have known that certain substances in the body can influence the immune system, thereby helping to fight cancer or the side effects of cancer treatment. Targeted therapy drugs are known to enhance the destruction of cancer cells by binding to their surface and inducing cell death (Bernstein, 2011). These substances include a host of naturally occurring or

NURSING INTERVENTIONS 22-2

Management of the Side Effects of Radiation Therapy

Site	Response	Nursing Interventions
General	Fatigue	Address possible causes such as anemia, poor nutrition, pain, and medications. Encourage light or moderate activity with frequent rest breaks.
Skin	Loss of epidermal layer Erythema, dryness Wet desquamation	Keep skin clean with daily baths. Avoid applying creams, perfumes, or lotions during radiation treatments. After treatments, moisturize skin with vitamin E, aloe vera, or lanolin. Help child to avoid sun exposure and to use sunscreen with minimum sun protection factor (SPF) of 30. Do not remove radiation markings. Contact skin care specialist for severe skin toxicities. Avoid applying tape adhesives when radiation is to be delivered. May need to remove CVC occlusive dressing during radiation treatments. Cover CVC site with gauze dressing/paper tape.
GI tract	Mucositis Pain Dysphagia Ulceration Swelling of esophagus, stomach, or intestines Nausea, vomiting Diarrhea	Provide daily oral and dental care. Recommend dental visit prior to initiation of radiation. Treat mucositis per health care provider orders. Give antiemetics before and during radiation treatments. Encourage oral fluid intake. Encourage small, frequent meals. Advise avoidance of spicy, fried, or high-fiber foods. Assess for dehydration. Give analgesics as needed.
Salivary glands and parotid glands	Decreased formation of saliva Dryness of mucous membranes Taste disorder Parotiditis	Encourage daily oral hygiene. Give analgesics as needed. Encourage oral fluid intake.
Kidney or bladder	Cystitis Ulceration	Encourage fluid intake. Assess for blood in urine.
Bone marrow	Myelosuppression Anemia Thrombocytopenia	Exercise infection precautions. Observe for temperature more than 38° C and notify physician. Observe for signs of bleeding. Teach child to avoid crowds. Observe for any signs of inflammation or infection.
Hair follicle	Alopecia	Recommend wigs or accessories (e.g., scarves, caps). Help with skin hygiene.
Lungs	Decreased levels of surfactant in lungs Shortness of breath Less tolerance for physical activity Pneumonitis Pulmonary fibrosis	Assess respiratory status. Provide oxygen as ordered. Encourage frequent rest periods.

(Continued)

NURSING INTERVENTIONS 22-2

Management of the Side Effects of Radiation Therapy (*Continued*)

Site	Response	Nursing Interventions
Heart	Myocarditis or pericarditis	Assess cardiac status. Note palpitations and complaints of chest pain that are relieved by sitting up and leaning forward.
Brain or spinal cord	Edema	Assess neurologic status. Assess for memory loss. Assess achievement of cognitive milestones (see Chapter 3).
Ovary/pelvic area	Permanent sterility possible. Scarring in pelvic area. Thinning and inflammation of vaginal lining	Inform patient and family about potential sterility. Provide sexually active adolescents with guidelines for intercourse during radiation. Encourage use of water-soluble lubricant during intercourse.
Testes/pelvic area	Produces temporary low sperm count. Azoospermia (complete absence of sperm in the ejaculate) may persist for several years	Provide sperm banking option when appropriate for the older adolescent.

synthetic agents that elicit clinically important responses in cancer patients (Nursing Interventions 22-3).

The exact mechanism of action of biologic or targeted therapy varies. They may

- Modify the immune response to the cancer
- Act directly against the tumor by suppressing tumor growth or killing the tumor cell

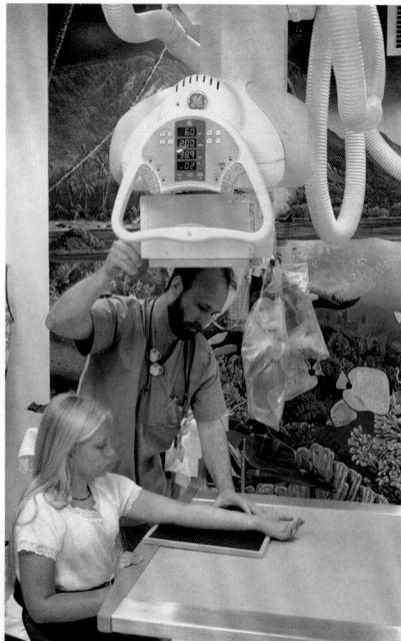

Figure 22-2 Prior to initiating radiation, the child radiologist will carefully evaluate the child and the areas to be radiated.

- Act directly against the tumor by attaching to the surface and killing the cell
- Alter other biologic factors that can directly or indirectly influence the viability of the tumor (McCune, 2009)

Management of children receiving biotherapy is a challenge because each individual is biologically different, so reactions or side effects from receiving these agents may differ. Some side effects associated with administration include general flulike symptoms, fluid retention, low-grade fevers, bone pain, chills, rash, and neuropathic pain.

Obtain baseline assessments of the child's vital signs prior to biotherapy administration, and continue to monitor these vital signs during infusion per protocol. Medications (e.g., acetaminophen, diphenhydramine, hydrocortisone) may need to be administered prior to infusion to decrease the flulike symptoms and other unwanted side effects.

ALERT   *Report adverse reactions (e.g., temperature >103.3° F [39.6° C], shortness of breath) to the primary health care provider and be prepared to discontinue administration. Emergency supplies should be readily available should the child experience a hypersensitivity reaction.*

Use interventions to minimize the discomfort associated with side effects and complications of biotherapy.

NURSING INTERVENTIONS 22-3

Biotherapy Agents

Type of Agent	Potential Side Effects
Hematopoietic growth factors (erythropoietin, granulocyte–macrophage colony-stimulating factor [GM-CSF], granulocyte colony-stimulating factor [G-CSF]): A family of glycoproteins responsible for stimulating and regulating hematopoiesis. Includes CSFs, which encourage the growth of bone marrow stem cells.	Erythropoietin (Epogen): hypertension, headaches, fever, myalgia, rashes, flulike symptoms GM-CSF: flulike symptoms (e.g., fever, bone pain, headache) and "first-dose phenomena" (flushing, hypoxia, tachycardia, oxygen desaturation) G-CSF: bone pain, joint pain, fever, rashes, pain at injection site
Interleukins: Cytokines that relay information between leukocytes to modulate their activities. Interleukin is a recombinant growth factor that activates the body's immune system.	Flulike symptoms, vascular leak syndrome, skin and mucosal changes, nausea, vomiting, CNS changes, altered laboratory values
Monoclonal antibodies: A cancer-specific antibody produced in a laboratory for a target antigen. Used to detect the presence of tumors and linked with chemotherapy as a treatment measure.	Allergic reactions, fever, chills, rigors, malaise, nausea, vomiting, hypotension
Interferons: Members of the cytokine network, capable of inhibiting viral replication, modulating immune responses, and altering cellular proliferation	Flulike symptoms, fatigue, malaise, anorexia, diarrhea, changes in mental status, abnormal liver function tests, neutropenia, thrombocytopenia, skin irritation, bone pain
Protein tyrosine kinase inhibitors: Enzymes that are involved in many cellular processes such as cell proliferation, metabolism, survival, and apoptosis. Several protein tyrosine kinases are known to be activated in cancer cells and to drive tumor growth and progression. Protein tyrosine kinases inhibitors are used to block the interactions of these enzymes and thus stop cancer growth.	Diarrhea, cardiac dysfunction, skin rash, pruritus, folliculitis, hair changes, paronychial inflammation of nails, hand–foot syndrome, skin discoloration, hypertension
Vaccines: Therapy being developed to initiate an immune response to foreign antigens. In this case, vaccines are investigational in pediatrics. Some vaccines have been developed to prevent cancer development and reoccurrence (e.g., hepatitis B vaccine and Gardasil [for cervical cancer caused by human papillomavirus]).	Soreness at infection site

Nursing Interventions

- Assess child and family knowledge of the drug administration, including purpose, side effects, dosing instructions, and food–drug interactions. Provide additional education when needed.
- Ensure emergency supplies are on hand during drug administration should the child have an adverse reaction to the substance.
- Obtain baseline vital signs and mental status. Monitor changes in these baseline parameters during administration.
- Administer premedications (acetaminophen, diphenhydramine, hydrocortisone) when needed.
- Monitor for signs and symptoms of side effects.
- Ensure measures to maintain skin integrity are followed by all caregivers.
- Administer supportive medical therapies for capillary leak syndrome (e.g., IV fluids, blood product administration, vasopressors).
- Monitor intake and output. Monitor child's weight.

Information from McCune, R. (2009). Biologic response modifiers. In N. E. Kline (Ed.), *Essentials of pediatric hematology/oncology nursing: A core curriculum* (3rd ed., pp. 108–112). Glenview, IL: Association of Pediatric Hematology/Oncology Nurses.

HEMATOPOIETIC STEM CELL TRANSPLANTATION

Current advances and technologic progress in HSCT have benefited many children with cancer. The phrase *hematopoietic progenitor cell transplant* has also been used when referring to this type of treatment modality. All the body's blood and immune cells originate as stem cells in the bone marrow in a process called *hematopoiesis*. Stem cells for HSCT are obtained from bone marrow or from peripheral or cord blood. HSCT is used to treat solid tumors and diseases that affect the hematopoietic (blood-forming) system, the immune system, and metabolism.

Types of Hematopoietic Stem Cell Transplantation

Two types of stem cell transplantation are performed: **autologous** (auto HSCT), which uses the child's own stem cells; and **allogeneic** (allo HSCT), which uses a matched donor's stem cells (Fig. 22-3). An allo HSCT donation most often comes from a sibling, rarely from a twin (syngeneic HSCT). However, it can also come from a parent or an unrelated donor. Healthy stem cells for reinfusion can also be donated from cord blood from the child's newborn sibling or from an unrelated donor from a cord blood bank. The goal is to provide the child with the most genetically compatible bone marrow donor achieved by matching the histocompatibility (the degree of compatibility of tissues: the degree of similarity between some antigens that determines the degree of success of a tissue graft or stem cell transplant) types of patient and donor.

Human leukocyte antigen (HLA) and DNA blood analyses are used to determine histocompatibility. HLAs, protein antigens on the cell surfaces of all nucleated cells, recognize foreign tissues and activate the immune system to fight them. The HLA types of donor and recipient must match to prevent the recipient from rejecting the donor marrow or having an increased potential for developing graft-versus-host disease.

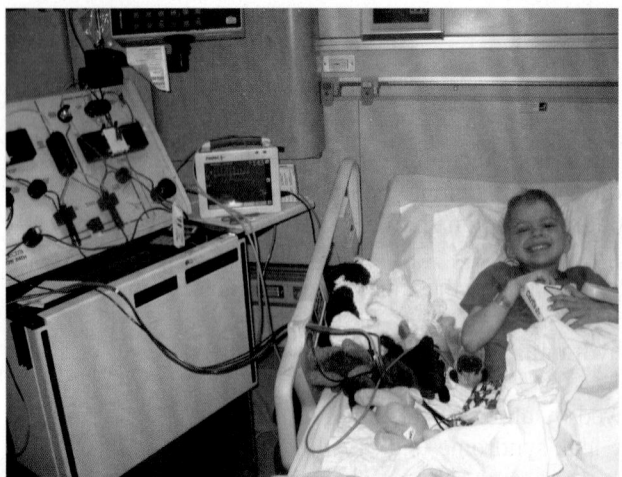

Figure 22-3 In preparation for an autologous stem cell transplant, the child's peripheral blood stem cells are harvested, frozen until needed, then given back (transplanted) after the child has received high doses of chemotherapy, radiation therapy, or both to destroy the cancer cells.

Phases of Hematopoietic Stem Cell Transplant

Before undergoing HSCT, the child undergoes extensive physical and psychosocial evaluation to confirm that he or she is eligible. The child is hospitalized, isolated, and monitored, sometimes for several weeks or months. During *conditioning*, the initial 7 to 10 day phase of HSCT, the child receives very high (lethal) doses of chemotherapy or total body radiation depending on the child's diagnosis and type of bone marrow he or she is to receive. Conditioning, which ablates (destroys) bone marrow, is an attempt to eliminate any remaining disease and to prepare the child's body to accept the new, healthy bone marrow. During this time, the bone marrow is unable to make neutrophils. The child develops **neutropenia**, an unusually low blood concentration of these immune cells, and is therefore at high risk for infection. Protective measures must be instituted. For children receiving allogeneic stem cell transplants, such measures include use of high efficiency particulate air (HEPA) filtration and positive pressure to reduce pathogens in the child's room and strict handwashing technique. Many institutions do not require such strict isolation precautions, and children receiving autologous stem cell transplants may be managed on the oncology unit simply with careful handwashing and standard precautions. IV gamma globulins and prophylactic antiviral, antifungal, and antibiotic medications may also be administered to prevent infection. If infection occurs, antibiotics are used as needed.

After conditioning, there is 1 day of rest (day −1). On the following day, day 0, the child's or donor's hematopoietic stem cells are infused into the child using a process similar to a blood transfusion. These healthy stem cells migrate into the empty spaces in the child's bone marrow, where they take root, grow, and ideally repopulate into healthy, new bone marrow.

During the *post-HSCT phase*, the child is at high risk for complications, including susceptibility to infection, until new blood cells and immune cells are present and optimally functioning. **Engraftment** is the process by which the hematopoietic stem cells begin making new blood cells; it is considered successful when the ANC reaches 500/mm^3 for 2 consecutive days. An effective transplant produces new, cancer-free hematopoietic and immune systems in the recipient.

Throughout the phases of HSCT, complications can occur; these are weighed against the benefits of curing the child's disease (Nursing Interventions 22-4; Fig. 22-4). The acute toxicities can be life threatening; thus, the nurse must assess the child daily for any organ toxicities, infections, bleeding complications, fluid and electrolyte imbalances, or skin and mucous membrane toxicities. Management of these side effects is addressed later in the "Treatment Modalities" section.

Late effects also can occur. These may include cataracts, growth hormone deficiency, thyroid dysfunction, delayed puberty, pulmonary fibrosis, cardiomyopathy, renal toxicity and renal failure, amenorrhea, and sterility. Interventions vary depending on the exact effect (Fig. 22-5). For all complications, provide supportive care.

NURSING INTERVENTIONS 22-4

Complications of Hematopoietic Stem Cell Transplantation (HSCT)

Complication	Manifestation	Nursing Interventions
Nutritional alterations	Nausea Vomiting Mouth ulcerations	Administer total parenteral nutrition as indicated. Provide meticulous oral care. Provide diet to maximize caloric intake. Administer antiemetics.
Infection risk	Neutropenia	Implement neutropenic precautions. Administer prophylactic antimicrobials as ordered to prevent herpes, cytomegalovirus, and fungal and bacterial infections. Use radiated and leukocyte-depleted blood products. Obtain cultures when clinically indicated. Provide routine personal hygiene. Ensure good skin integrity. Avoid rectal medications or temperature measurements.
Thrombocytopenia and anemia	Platelet count less than 50,000/mm³ Hemoglobin less than 8 g/dL Fatigue Tachycardia Shortness of breath Pallor Dizziness Bruising, petechiae, epistaxis, oozing from the gums or CVC Blood in urine, emesis, or feces	Administer platelet and red blood cell transfusions as needed (all blood products should be radiated and leukocyte depleted). Initiate bleeding precautions and safety precautions to avoid injury. Administer oxygen to prevent tissue hypoxia.
Mucositis	Deterioration of mucosa and GI tract Excessive secretions Difficulty swallowing and breathing Anorexia Difficulty eating Abdominal cramping Watery diarrhea	Provide meticulous oral care, including use of oral rinses. Anticipate intubation to facilitate breathing. Provide measures to control pain, such as viscous lidocaine, diphenhydramine, and sucralfate. Treat diarrhea with antidiarrheal medications (e.g., loperamide, octreotide).
Veno-occlusive disease (VOD)/ sinusoidal obstruction syndrome (SOS)	Congestion of venules of the liver Sudden, unexpected weight gain Thrombocytopenia refractory to platelet infusions Jaundice Hepatomegaly Right upper quadrant pain Ascites Encephalopathy	Observe oral and IV fluid restrictions. Obtain daily weights and abdominal girth measurements. Elevate head of bed. Monitor hepatic function. Assess mental status.
Interstitial pneumonia	Nonproductive, dry cough Fever Tachypnea Nasal flaring Dyspnea Hypoxia	Assess respiratory and ventilation status, including use of pulse oximetry and blood gases. Provide respiratory treatments as needed. Administer supplemental oxygen or ventilation as needed. Raise head of bed. Promote rest.

(Continued)

1126 UNIT 3 · · · Managing Health Challenges

NURSING INTERVENTIONS 22-4

Complications of Hematopoietic Stem Cell Transplantation (HSCT) (Continued)

Complication	Manifestation	Nursing Interventions
Renal complications	Dehydration Third spacing Hemorrhage Hypovolemia Septic shock Hypoproteinemia	Assess fluid and electrolyte status. Maintain adequate intravascular volume and renal perfusion (e.g., administer renal dose of dopamine to promote renal transfusion). Adjust dose and frequency of medications that are toxic to renal function. Correct fluid and electrolyte imbalances. Minimize use of nephrotoxic agents. Implement dialysis if renal failure is severe.
Graft-versus-host disease, acute: occurring within the first 100 days after HSCT Graft-versus-host disease, chronic: occurring 100 days or more after HSCT	Maculopapular rash on the palmar and plantar surfaces of the hand and feet evolving into erythematous rash over most of body (ranging from slight redness of the skin to complete skin desquamation [see Fig. 22-4]) Diarrhea (positive occult blood) Fever Jaundice Hepatomegaly Hypertension Infection (especially fungal and viral for children with chronic graft-versus-host disease)	Ensure daily evaluation of blood counts. Provide platelet infusion. Provide packed red blood cell transfusion. Administer immunosuppressive/antigraft-versus-host disease medications.
Graft rejection or failure	Fever Infection Decrease in blood counts	Reinfuse blood stem cells into child. Check CBC with differential on a daily basis. Provide supportive measures to prevent infection.

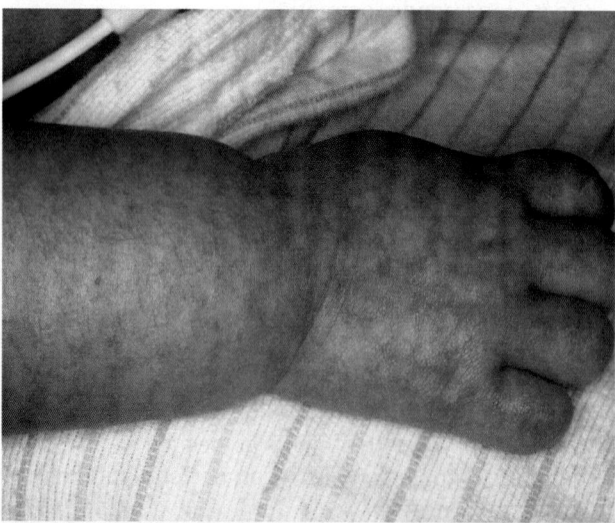

Figure 22-4 Graft-versus-host disease typically presents as a maculopapular rash that starts on the palms and soles and evolves to an erythematous rash over most of the body.

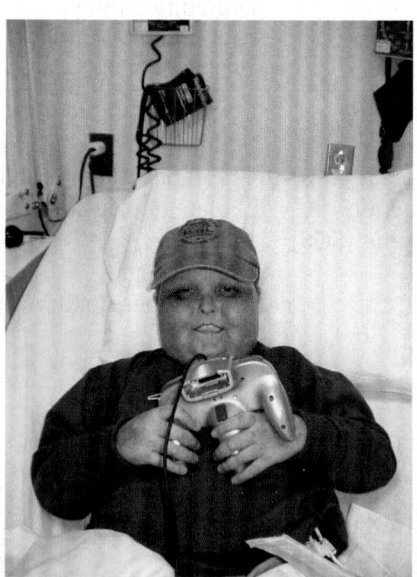

Figure 22-5 High-dose corticosteroid therapy for this child after HSCT has produced a characteristic "moon face" appearance.

PAIN MANAGEMENT INTERVENTIONS

> QUESTION: While George was in the hospital after his surgery, the nurse noted that he was reluctant to admit his pain. Identify issues related to George's age and stoicism and effective management of his pain. What plan would you develop to assess and manage George's pain?

Children with cancer may experience pain for a variety of reasons. Initially, children may experience pain caused by the disease itself—for example, bone pain in leukemia, headaches in brain tumors, abdominal pain with abdominal tumors. More commonly, children with cancer experience treatment-related pain that results from the numerous procedures and tests that are done at the time of diagnosis and throughout the treatment course and from side effects of treatment, such as postoperative pain, oral mucositis, skin irritation and breakdown, and esophageal and abdominal pain from GI irritation or ulcerations. Interest in pediatric cancer pain research is strong, and the literature is growing. Initially, most literature focused on the pain and discomfort associated with certain diagnostic procedures, such as bone marrow aspiration and lumbar puncture, although, even in this area, pain management techniques vary considerably among practitioners. Topics of ongoing research include describing the trajectory of a child's pain over the course of the illness, the late effects of pain, the reported incidence of pain after the disease has been eradicated, and evaluating traditional and nontraditional pain management approaches that can be effective before, during, and after procedures and treatments.

Both pharmacologic and biobehavioral interventions are important in managing pediatric pain. Mild analgesics, topical anesthetics, and opioids can be used to treat pain. Sedatives such as midazolam (Versed) or anesthetic medications such as ketamine or propofol may be used to assist children undergoing painful procedures that are required routinely during their cancer treatment.

Chronic or terminal pain may be managed in the home with continuous administration of opioids, orally or intravenously, as a bolus injection or infusion (see Chapter 10). Managing pain in the home setting requires a collaborative effort among the child and family, home health nurse, home care pharmacist, and oncologist.

Several biobehavioral pain management strategies have been successful in dealing with the pain associated with procedures. These interventions include complementary and alternative medicine (CAM) therapies such as music therapy, hand holding, imagery, hypnosis, relaxation, diversion, rest and sleep, massage, heat, breathing exercises, and biofeedback. Chapter 10 discusses these pain management techniques in detail. A variety of techniques can be taught to the child and the child's family to provide a repertoire of coping skills and an effective alternative or adjunct to pain medications.

> ANSWER: George is old enough to report and describe his pain accurately, so the issues of pain assessment for a younger child do not apply in his case. However, George's vital signs and physical symptoms indicate he is reluctant to admit his pain. Rather than have him receive pain medications on an as-needed basis, the hospital nurses established a round-the-clock schedule of pain relief to help maintain a constant blood level of pain medication, a schedule that continues at home. The home care nurse developed the idea of establishing a database in George's computer for him to enter his pain rating and any descriptions of his symptoms at regular intervals throughout the day. George prefers the privacy of documenting his symptoms on the computer, which provides the physician and nurse with more data to develop George's pharmacologic pain management interventions.

INTERVENTIONS RELATED TO VENOUS ACCESS

A **central venous catheter (CVC)**, also called a *central line*, is a device inserted for many children undergoing cancer treatment to enable easy administration of chemotherapy, blood products, nutrition, IV fluids, and IV medications. It also provides a means for obtaining blood samples without the need for repeated venipunctures. The types of devices include peripherally inserted catheters (PICCs), externally tunneled Silastic catheters, and implanted ports. The child, if age-appropriate, and the primary caregivers are thoroughly instructed on how to manage these devices at home. Use and maintenance of PICCs and external CVCs at home include dressing changes, cap changes, heparin flushes, blood draws, medication administration, and emergency care guidelines. In addition to nursing instruction, aids such as booklets, videos, and hands-on demonstration with a doll should be used to support teaching interventions (Fig. 22-6). A thorough discussion of these devices is presented in Chapter 17, including information regarding home management of the child with a CVC and

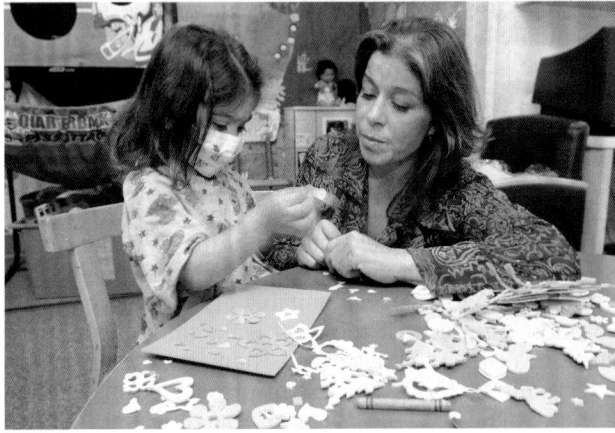

Figure 22-6 The child life specialist encourages the child with cancer to participate in playroom activities.

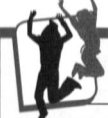

COMMUNITY CARE 22-1

School Reentry

The child with a malignancy may experience problems that can affect school attendance and performance. These problems include periods of absenteeism, increased school anxiety, negative attitudes by school officials, taunting by peers, social isolation, and learning difficulties induced by illness or treatment. Reentering the classroom can be emotionally, physically, and mentally difficult for the child, the teacher, and the other students.

To facilitate the child's successful reentry into the classroom

- Contact the school nurse and the child's teacher to discuss the child's reentry, providing teachers and school officials with adequate information regarding the child's condition.
- Use federally mandated education planning for students with special needs (individualized education plan) to establish educational goals for the child and to identify mechanisms to achieve these goals.
- Provide teachers with books and other resources about cancer.
- Provide teachers with a toll-free number so they can contact a health care provider regarding any questions or concerns they may have about having a child with cancer in their classrooms.

- If the child, the family, and school officials agree, have a nurse, child life specialist, or social worker attend the child's classroom before the child reenters the class to discuss with classmates the causes of cancer and the physical changes caused by treatment. Classmates should be allowed to ask questions, but respect the child's privacy at all times.
- Use skits or puppet shows to educate the child's peers and gain their support.
- Film the child with cancer in the hospital setting. Include a tour of the hospital, views of the child's room and places where procedures are done, and footage of the child. Take the movie to the child's class for viewing before the child's reentry. Use the video as a means to discuss the child's cancer.
- Provide instruction at home until the child is able to return to school.
- During home instruction, encourage the child to remain in contact with peers and teachers through pictures, letters, e-mail, and visits.
- Refer family to counseling if school phobia or truancy is a problem.
- Monitor for any problems related to school performance or relationships with teachers or peers at school.

---

developmental considerations when securing the CVC. If a child with a CVC returns to school, school officials must be informed of CVC instructions and emergency care (see Community Care 22-1).

Children with CVCs are at risk to develop infections in the blood or at the exit site, a primary portal for entry of microorganisms. Children may tamper with the dressing covering the site; the solutions, tape, and dressings used to clean the site may cause irritation, potentially leading to infection. Therefore, careful local skin care is imperative to reduce the incidence of infection and sepsis. Institutions vary in their approach to CVC site maintenance. It is highly recommended that an antiseptic solution be used to clean the site, which is then covered by a sterile occlusive dressing. The length of time between dressing changes also varies with institutional policy and the condition of the CVC site.

When chemotherapy is administered peripherally or through a CVC or an implantable access device, extravasation can occur if the drug leaks into surrounding areas, causing cellular tissue damage (see Nursing Interventions 22-1). The extent of damage may range from a small, reddened area to a large lesion that becomes necrotic and requires plastic surgery. Most extravasations can be prevented by maintaining good

assessment techniques before, during, and after chemotherapy administration. Note the vein size and device location and patency. If areas of redness or ulceration occur at the administration site during the infusion, stop the chemotherapy immediately and assess patency. The child may also complain of burning or loss of sensation or movement. If extravasation does occur, prompt intervention using an antidote to the particular chemotherapeutic agent is indicated.

NUTRITIONAL INTERVENTIONS

Many factors contribute to appetite suppression and decreased food intake in the child undergoing cancer treatment. Anorexia and weight loss may result from anorexia-inducing substances secreted by the tumor cells, pain, nausea, vomiting, stomatitis, metabolic disturbances, and alterations in taste. A child may experience increased appetite, fluid retention, and weight gain with the use of steroids. Nutritional problems may also be psychosocially related. The child may feel apathetic, depressed, or fearful and not wish to eat. The child may also use eating or drinking as a way to manipulate parental behavior and responses or as a way to feel some control over the events that are occurring.

Maintaining the child's nutritional status is important because it allows the body to better tolerate the cancer treatment. Nutritional assessment should include daily weights; intake and output; calorie counts; and laboratory test results of elements such as sodium, potassium, albumin, calcium, magnesium, glucose, and protein. Also assess the child for factors that may be contributing to the anorexia, such as pain, nausea, diarrhea, or stomatitis. Side effects associated with the treatment regimen must be prevented, alleviated, or minimized before the child's nutritional status can be improved.

KidKare Supplemental nutrition can be achieved orally by providing small, frequent meals; high-protein shakes; and nutritional supplements such as Ensure or Sustacal and by allowing the child to eat whatever he or she desires and can tolerate.

The oral route is always preferable for supplemental nutrition. If increasing oral intake is not possible, the enteral route (tube feedings) is the second choice in children whose GI tract is intact and can tolerate it. Nasogastric or nasojejunal tubes are used on a short-term basis; gastrostomy tubes are considered if prolonged support is required. Parenteral nutrition is indicated if the child cannot tolerate the oral or enteral route (Rock et al., 2012).

The dietitian can be an excellent resource in designing a diet plan to address the child's health problems. If rapid weight loss is a problem, foods high in protein and carbohydrates are recommended. For the child experiencing weight gain related to steroid therapy, for example, the plan must meet the child's nutritional needs while minimizing fluid retention. Low-sodium foods without added salt are recommended. The child may be experiencing an increase in appetite; thus, meals and snacks should be satisfying but not overly high in calories.

ORAL HYGIENE INTERVENTIONS

The oral cavity is a common site of stomatitis, mucositis, infections, or bleeding. The terms *stomatitis* and *mucositis* are often used interchangeably. Some clinicians distinguish between the two by clarifying that **stomatitis** can be any oral mucosal reaction to local factors (e.g., infection, injury, poor oral care). **Mucositis** is the mucosal reaction that can occur throughout the GI system as a side effect of systemic administration of chemotherapeutic agents (Chen et al., 2004).

The rapidly dividing mucosal epithelial cells lining the oral cavity and the GI tract are easily damaged by chemotherapeutic agents, with mucosal changes appearing within 2 to 3 days after chemotherapy administration. Changes in the oral mucosa can also be a result of anorexia, radiation to the oral cavity, and poor oral care. Radiation to the oral cavity decreases saliva production. Saliva is needed to provide a natural defense against tooth decay. Poor nutritional status and dental care can indirectly affect the oral cavity and the integrity of the mucous membranes (Fig. 22-7). In addition, children

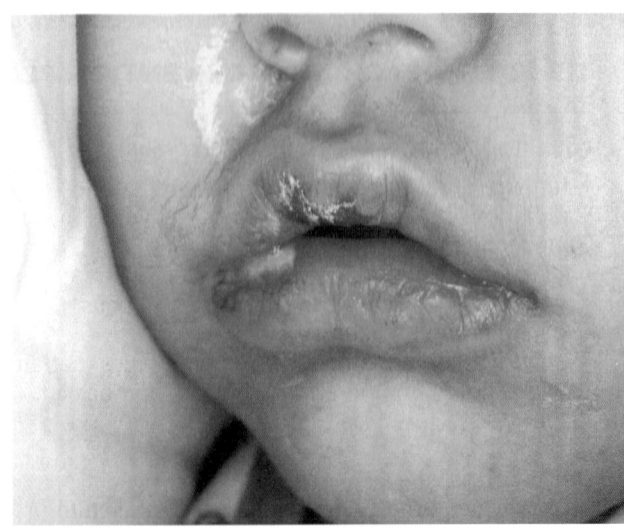

Figure 22-7 Oral inflammation (stomatitis) and ulceration around the lips and in the mouth (mucositis) causes great discomfort and makes it difficult for the child to open the mouth, eat, and swallow.

who are neutropenic are more at risk for oral infections such as with *Candida*, herpes simplex, herpes zoster, gram-negative organisms (*Pseudomonas*), and gram-positive organisms (*Streptococcus*).

Obtain a baseline assessment of the child's oral cavity, including evaluation of the integrity and color of the lips, tongue, gingivae, and mucous membranes. Note if child has any orthodontic hardware. Determine the child's ability to produce saliva, swallow, and eat. Baseline dental examinations should be performed before beginning therapy and on a routine basis to assess and treat any dental problems. Perform oral assessments daily during chemotherapy treatments, when radiation to the head or neck regions is being given, or when the child has undergone HSCT.

caREminder

An ulcerated or inflamed oral area can cause emotional distress to the infant and young child who use sucking on a thumb or pacifier as a form of coping. Diligent assessment of the oral cavity to prevent stomatitis is important.

The goals of oral care are to preserve the integrity of the oral cavity, promote oral comfort, and promptly treat any oral problems that occur. Teach the child and family how to perform meticulous oral care, which is essential in the home, school, and hospital settings (Teaching Intervention Plan 22-1). Measures to treat the discomfort caused by tender gums or oral lesions can be used to ensure that the child can speak, eat, and swallow.

A variety of interventions have been developed to reduce the severity of mucositis; however, available evidence does not recommend any particular treatment as optimal for all children. The type of disease and the chemotherapeutic agents the specific child is receiving affect

TIP 22-1: A TEACHING INTERVENTION PLAN for Oral Hygiene for the Child With Cancer

Nursing Diagnosis and Family Outcomes

- Impaired oral mucous membranes related to radiation therapy, chemotherapy, dehydration, or ineffective oral hygiene

  Outcomes: Child and family will demonstrate measures to prevent or minimize mucous membrane breakdown.

  Child will demonstrate mucous membranes that are intact, free from infection, soothed, and healed.

Teach the Child/Family

Daily Care

- Oral hygiene should be completed by the child or primary caregiver three to four times a day and as needed whether the child is hospitalized, at home, or participating in activities away from home.
- To promote healthy oral mucosa, the child needs to do the following:
  - Brush with soft toothbrush (that is changed on a regular basis) to prevent bleeding of the gums. Floss when oral mucosa is healthy and platelet counts are at acceptable levels.
  - Rinse and spit with 0.1% chlorhexidine mouthwash (Peridex), saline, or sodium bicarbonate after meals, at bedtime, and as needed to clean the oral mucosa. These solutions should not be swallowed because they kill the normal flora of the GI tract.
  - Avoid hard foods that can cause abrasions to the gum line.
  - Avoid acidic foods that can irritate tender or sore areas in the mouth.
  - Avoid chewing gum and candy.
  - Maintain good fluid intake to keep mucous membranes moist.
  - Keep the lips lubricated with Vaseline or some type of lip balm to prevent cracking.
  - Participate in regular dental checkups.

Stomatitis or Mucositis Management

- To promote comfort in the presence of stomatitis or mucositis, the child may use oral analgesic agents that contain an antacid, diphenhydramine (Benadryl), and a topical anesthetic (Dyclone or viscous lidocaine) for mild discomfort. These agents can be applied directly to sore areas of the mouth or swished and spit.
  - Avoid spicy, salty, and bitter foods.
  - Avoid hot foods; choose tepid or cold liquids.

- Choose foods that require little chewing (e.g., pudding, cottage cheese, soft cheeses, bananas, applesauce, milkshakes, smoothies, popsicles).
- Use a straw to ingest liquids.
- Cut food into small pieces prior to ingestion.
- Use topical analgesics before eating.
- When moderate to severe stomatitis or mucositis is present
  - Continue meticulous oral hygiene. Oral rinses can be used to clean the teeth, with a toothette used to remove debris loosened by the rinse.
  - Do not use chlorhexidine to treat established oral mucositis.
  - Use nutritional supplements (e.g., Boost, Ensure) or supplemental IV fluids and nutrition as appropriate, depending on the child's ability to eat and swallow.
  - If the pain from mucositis is moderate to severe, IV analgesics (opioids, such as morphine or fentanyl) may be needed.
  - When severe mucositis is present, premedicate to manage pain before completing oral care.

ALERT *The side effects of viscous lidocaine include a decreased gag reflex, tingling, and seizures. Teach the child never to swallow a solution containing this agent.*

Management of Infection

- For fungal infections, swish and swallow with nystatin or other antifungal agents as ordered. Oral intake should be restricted for 30 minutes afterward to promote absorption of the medication into the mucosa.
- Per physician's orders, administer medications for treatment of systemic candidiasis or herpetic lesions.

Contact Health Care Provider if

- Stomatitis or mucositis does not show signs of healing with improved tissue integrity
- Child develops new lesions that appear different in color, shape, and location than previous/current mucositis lesions
- Child refuses to eat or drink
- Child develops a fever
- Child complains of oral pain

Information from Keefe, D. M., Schubert, M. M., Elting, L. S. et al. (2007). Updated clinical practice guidelines for the prevention and treatment of mucositis. *Cancer, 109*(5), 820–831. Retrieved from http://www.mascc.org/content/125.html; Landers, R., & O'Hanlon-Curry, J. (2009). Gastrointestinal complications. In N. E. Kline (Ed.), *Essentials of pediatric hematology/oncology nursing: A core curriculum* (3rd ed., pp. 134–140). Glenview, IL: Association of Pediatric Hematology/Oncology Nurses.

decisions about oral care. If oral infections occur, appropriate medications specific to the suspected organism are prescribed. Children with severe mucositis may be hospitalized because the effects are likely to involve other parts of the GI tract such as the esophagus, stomach, or intestines. Severe mucositis with excessive secretions may cause localized swelling or tissue sloughing, which can place the child at risk for airway occlusion and aspiration.

INTERVENTIONS FOR NAUSEA AND VOMITING

Nausea and vomiting may be mild to severe, depending on the chemotherapeutic drug being administered and the tolerance of the child receiving the drugs. The key to optimal prevention and control of chemotherapy-induced nausea and vomiting is the timing of the antiemetic that is given (Nursing Interventions 22-5).

caREminder

It is vital that antiemetic therapy be given orally or intravenously before the start of chemotherapy and that it be continued on a regularly scheduled basis. This treatment plan provides the maximal effect to minimize nausea and vomiting.

Ondansetron (Zofran) is an antiemetic drug that is commonly administered to children receiving chemotherapy. Other agents used include metoclopramide (Reglan), diphenhydramine (Benadryl), lorazepam (Ativan), promethazine (Phenergan), dexamethasone (Decadron), granisetron (Kytril), dolasetron (Anzemet), palonosetron (Aloxi), and aprepitant (Emend). A combination of drugs and modifications of timing are useful in individualizing a child's antiemetic regimen (Tipton et al., 2007).

Biobehavioral measures may help to control nausea and vomiting. For example, salty, dry foods such as soda crackers and toast can be offered. Carbonated beverages that are consumed through a straw to ensure slow fluid uptake may be acceptable to the child.

The child may have specific food preferences as he or she begins to feel less nauseous. Every effort should be made to provide food and fluid that is palatable to the child and that provides optimal nutrition.

Maintain accurate records of the child's intake and output; measure emesis and test it for blood using guaiac measures. A guaiac-positive result can indicate irritation of the GI tract from vomiting. These results should be discussed with the physician because a more effective antiemetic regimen may be needed.

The child and family should be prepared to handle posttreatment nausea and vomiting that may occur at home. Teaching Intervention Plan 22-2 summarizes the content to cover in discussions with the family about home management of nausea and vomiting.

BOWEL ELIMINATION INTERVENTIONS

 QUESTION: What are some strategies that George can undertake to prevent constipation from the narcotics that he takes?

Constipation or diarrhea can occur in the child being treated for cancer. Certain chemotherapeutic agents, particularly vincristine, and many opioids cause constipation. In addition, tumor growth, decreased mobility, and altered fluid and nutritional intake may also play a role in constipation that could then lead to the development of hemorrhoids and aggravation of rectal fissures or perineal abscesses. Diarrhea may occur as a side effect of surgery, radiation therapy, or chemotherapy. The use of antibiotics and nutritional supplements, tumor growth, infections, and stress can also cause diarrhea. If prolonged, diarrhea can lead to fluid and electrolyte imbalances, dehydration, and perineal discomfort.

Question the child or parent about the child's usual pattern of bowel elimination. In the acute care setting, maintain accurate intake and output records, noting the number, amount, color, and consistency of the stool.

NURSING INTERVENTIONS 22-5

Interventions to Minimize and Manage Nausea and Vomiting

- Formulate an individualized plan of care for the child based on previous responses and mechanisms that are successful in assisting the child to cope with nausea and vomiting.
- Encourage fluids and small, frequent meals as tolerated. The child should avoid spicy or strongly odorous food.
  - Assist the child in using relaxation techniques, such as guided imagery and distraction (videos, video games, other games, reading), to focus thoughts away from physical discomforts.

- Monitor environmental triggers such as sights, smells, and sounds that may heighten feelings of nausea and vomiting. Administer oral dose of lorazepam (if ordered) the night before and the morning of the chemotherapy administration.
- Administer antiemetic agents, as ordered, 30 minutes before initiating chemotherapy and on a regularly scheduled basis for up to 24 hours after the chemotherapy ends.
- Keep accurate records of intake and output.
- Test all emesis for blood.
- Give IV fluids as ordered to maintain hydration.

TIP 22-2: A TEACHING INTERVENTION PLAN for Gastrointestinal Complications

Nursing Diagnoses and Family Outcomes

- Deficient fluid volume related to nausea, vomiting, mucositis, or diarrhea
  Outcome: Child is able or assisted to maintain adequate fluid intake by mouth or by naso-gastric or IV access.
- Imbalanced nutrition: Less than body requirements related to disease process and medication-induced vomiting, anorexia, changed taste sensations, depression, or changes in intestinal epithelium
  Outcomes: Child is able to eat frequent, small nutritious meals.
  Child's caloric intake is adequate for age.
  Child is able to maintain weight that is normal for age.
- Constipation related to effects of chemothera-peutic agents
  Outcome: Child and family use measures to prevent or minimize constipation.
- Diarrhea related to effects of chemotherapeutic agents
  Outcome: Child and family use measures to prevent or minimize diarrhea.

Teach the Child/Family

Management of Nausea and Vomiting
- Implement diet measures such as eating small, frequent bland meals; avoiding noxious smells; eating foods high in protein; and drinking plenty of fluids.
- Administer antiemetic as ordered.

- Recognize side effects of antiemetic.
- Recognize signs and symptoms of dehydration.
- Stress importance of oral hygiene.

Management of Mucositis (also see Teaching Intervention Plan 22-1)
- Recognize signs and symptoms of dehydration.
- Recognize signs and symptoms of fungal infection.
- Eat small, frequent meals to prevent feelings of bloating, indigestion, and heartburn

Management of Constipation
- Recognize signs and symptoms of fecal impaction.
- Maintain toileting routines.
- Increase fiber and fluids in diet.
- Avoid rectal manipulation and medications.
- Promote physical activity.

Management of Diarrhea
- Recognize signs and symptoms of diarrhea.
- Maintain accurate records of stool patterns.
- Institute bland, low-residue diet or a lactose-free diet.
- Institute meticulous perianal hygiene and strict handwashing.

Contact Health Care Provider if
- Child experiences uncontrolled vomiting
- Child is unable to eat or drink
- Child is experiencing weight loss
- There is a change in the frequency of the child's stool
- Child is experiencing hard or loose stools

If changes have been noted in the child's elimination patterns in the home, instruct families to keep a record of the child's elimination pattern (see Teaching Intervention Plan 22-2). The stool can be tested for occult blood as an indication of bowel integrity.

Also monitor the child's weight, noting any significant losses. If diarrhea is the problem, assess for signs of dehydration, including dry mucous membranes and sunken fontanel and poor skin turgor. Check laboratory test results for fluid and electrolyte imbalances. Obtain stool cultures, if ordered, to determine the presence of infectious agents.

Measure abdominal girth daily in the presence of constipation. Palpate the abdomen, noting areas of tenderness, swelling, or rigidity. Inspect the perineal and perianal area for redness, skin breakdown, hemorrhoids, fissures, or abscesses.

caREminder

The use of enemas, suppositories, digital manipulation, or rectal thermometers should be avoided to help prevent trauma to the rectal mucosa.

For the constipated child, a stool softener such as docusate sodium (Colace) can be administered. A sitz bath or perineal irrigations can be used to treat abscesses or fissures in the perineal and rectal area. A high-fiber diet, an active lifestyle, and good perineal and rectal hygiene can prevent such complications. Reducing distractions and allowing ample private, quiet time for bowel elimination are important.

 KidKare High-fiber foods that may entice the older child include granola bars, cookies with raisins, popcorn, and apple slices.

In the presence of severe dehydration or electrolyte imbalances resulting from diarrhea, administer IV fluids as ordered. Anticipate the need for medications to thicken the child's stool, decrease peristalsis, or treat infection. A bland, low-residue diet or a lactose-free diet may be instituted to curb further problems with diarrhea (see Teaching Intervention Plan 22-2).

ANSWER: For a 14-year-old boy, bowel movements are a topic that he may not want to discuss with either his parents or the nurse. Strategies that provide George with lots of information and options would increase his sense of control and his privacy. Specific guidelines for when to alert the health care team would help prevent George from becoming impacted. George would be instructed to monitor his bowel movements and increase his water intake and given advice on how to add natural fiber and fiber supplements to prevent constipation. Promoting activity and exercise would be helpful as well.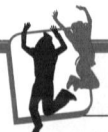

INFECTION PREVENTION AND CONTROL INTERVENTIONS

QUESTION: A review of George's immunizations shows that he is current on vaccines. The state where George lives requires the hepatitis A vaccines and the series of hepatitis B prior to seventh grade. He had chickenpox when he was 6 years old. What interventions are appropriate for George and his family to implement to prevent George from developing an infection?

Children receiving cancer treatment are **immunosuppressed**—their immune systems are suppressed—and thus are at increased risk for infection, particularly 7 to 10 days after receiving chemotherapy. This period is called the **nadir** because the immune cell count is lowest at this point. Preventing infection is essential for these children because any infection can become serious and could lead to death. Community Care 22-2 highlights key aspects of infection prevention in the home.

Children receiving chemotherapy may also receive prophylactic medications to help prevent certain opportunistic infections. For example, trimethoprim–sulfamethoxazole (Bactrim) is administered to prevent severe respiratory infections, such as *Pneumocystis jiroveci* pneumonia; acyclovir may be administered to prevent herpesvirus infections; and fluconazole or ketoconazole may be administered to prevent fungal infections. Another preventive medication, G-CSF, is administered by subcutaneous injection or IV route for up to 14 days after chemotherapy. This agent stimulates the bone marrow to repopulate granulocytes more quickly and efficiently, decreasing the duration of neutropenia and thereby reducing the risk of infection.

A L E R T   *Varicella zoster infection (chickenpox) can be life threatening to the immunosuppressed child. The child with cancer who is exposed to chickenpox should receive varicella zoster immune globulin within 5 days of exposure if the child has not had this communicable disease. The varicella vaccine has not yet been approved for use in children with cancer.*

With regard to vaccine administration, children who have decreased immunity (e.g., those receiving chemotherapy) have compromised immune systems and are thus not able to fight infection effectively. Live-bacteria and live-virus vaccinations are contraindicated for all immunosuppressed children. Inactivated vaccines may be administered. These include diphtheria–tetanus–pertussis (Tri-Immunol), hepatitis B (Engerix-B), inactivated poliovirus (Poliovax), pneumococcal (Pneumovax), and influenza virus (Fluogen) vaccines.

COMMUNITY CARE 22-2

Infection Prevention at Home

- Practice good handwashing habits.
- Do not share eating utensils, drinking glasses, baby bottles, pacifiers, etc.
- Eat a well-balanced diet.
- Include high-fiber foods and maintain good fluid intake to prevent constipation; notify the physician if constipation occurs.
- Avoid unpeeled raw vegetables and fruits, salad bars, raw eggs, natural cheeses, and raw meats or fish because they might carry bacteria.
- Avoid exposure to molds (e.g., digging in soil).
- Practice good oral care (brush teeth after each meal and before bedtime using a soft toothbrush).
- Practice good personal hygiene, with particular attention to keeping the perineum and other skin-fold areas clean.

- Avoid crowds and decrease the child's exposure to others when the child's ANC is less than $500/mm^3$.
- Keep the child away from individuals known to have an infection.
- To prevent perianal fissures and infection, do not insert anything into the rectum (e.g., no rectal thermometers, suppositories, or enemas).
- Do not use tampons.
- Avoid fresh flowers and plants because of the spores or organisms in the soil and leaves.
- Postpone immunizations until infections or anemia resolve.
- Contact a health care provider if the child has a temperature more than 101° F (38.3° C) or has any signs of infection.

TIP 22-3: A TEACHING INTERVENTION PLAN for the Child at Risk for Infection

Nursing Diagnosis and Family Outcome

- Risk for infection related to neutropenia, immunosuppressive therapy, and presence of CVC
  Outcome: Child and family will recognize and report signs of infection to their health care provider.

Teach the Family

Interventions

- If the child appears to be sick
  - Observe the child's skin for pallor or bruising.
  - Observe CVC site for signs of infection or leaking.
  - Check the child's temperature (under the arm or by mouth) any time that he or she feels warm to the touch or is uncomfortable; do not check the temperature rectally.
  - Do not give the child medication for fever unless instructed by health care provider; if prescribed, administer acetaminophen; *never* give aspirin.
  - Encourage intake of fluids and small, frequent offerings of nutritious food.

- Observe whether the child's urine or stool appears bloody.

Contact Health Care Provider if

- Child has a temperature of 101.5° F (38.6° C) or higher or a temperature of 100.5° F (38.1° C) or higher lasting more than 1 hour
- Child appears seriously ill without a fever
- Child has shaking chills, fever, or both after flushing the vascular access device
- Child is confused, has slurred speech, or is difficult to arouse
- Child is extremely weak or pale
- Child has bruising or bleeding
- Child has repeated excessive vomiting or diarrhea
- Child has decreased urinary output or blood in urine
- Child exhibits redness, swelling, or leakage at the central venous access site, or if the device has cracks, is pulled out, or does not flush

---

ANSWER: The obvious interventions include reviewing hand hygiene techniques with George and his family and limiting contact with visitors for 2 weeks.

Unfortunately, even with these prevention measures, the child may develop sepsis, a common complication of chemotherapy treatment. Fever can be the first indication of sepsis; however, symptoms can be subtle in the immunosuppressed child. Thus, the family and the nurse must assess the child for fever and must recognize and prevent its progression to septic shock (Teaching Intervention Plan 22-3).

ALERT   *If a child's temperature spikes to 101.5° F (38.6° C) or remains at 100.5° F (38.1° C) or higher for 4 hours or longer, the child must be evaluated by a provider immediately.*

Blood and other specimen cultures (e.g., urine, wound drainage) are obtained from all possible sources, including the CVC if indicated. In the presence of fever, broad-spectrum antibiotics are administered immediately, and the child is closely monitored until the origin of the fever is established. If no source of fever is identified, the child continues to receive broad-spectrum antibiotics for approximately 48 to 72 hours and then is reevaluated for continuing treatment (Tradition or Science 22-1 and

Evidence-Based Practice   TRADITION OR SCIENCE 22-1

Can children with febrile neutropenia be treated on an outpatient basis?

Outpatient strategies to manage the child with fever and neutropenia focus on two methods: no hospitalization, with symptoms managed entirely with oral antibiotics administered at home; or early hospital discharge with conversion to oral antibiotics administered at home. Holdsworth et al. (2003) reviewed available clinical trials and determined that although these two practices are common in the literature, such interventions should only be used in low-risk populations (children with negative blood cultures, evidence of hematopoietic recovery, and no comorbid condition). Teuffel et al. (2011) reviewed 1,448 articles on clinical trials for the outpatient management of febrile neutropenia. The authors summarized that outpatient management and treatment for febrile neutropenia is a safe and effective alternative to inpatient, although age of patient and administration route of antibiotic may influence outpatient treatment plan. The costs of inpatient versus outpatient care of neutropenic patients must also be considered in the evaluation of the efficacy of outpatient services (De Lalla, 2003). Guidelines to safely manage children with neutropenia and fever at home should be provided to all families, and comparative studies should continue to be employed to assess differences between inpatient and outpatient services of febrile neutropenia in relation to factors such as costs, time to clinical response, interventions employed, and survival rates.

thePoint Care Path: An Interdisciplinary Plan of Care for the Child With Neutropenia and Fever). If an organism is isolated, more specific antimicrobial agents are given. IV fluids are given to prevent dehydration and further complications, such as septic shock. In severe cases of septic shock, the child is at risk for disseminated intravascular coagulation and liver failure.

BLOOD COMPONENT THERAPY

Anemia, neutropenia, and **thrombocytopenia** (an abnormally low concentration of platelets in the blood) are common results of bone marrow suppression after chemotherapy. Blood counts are monitored closely, a minimum of once a week or more frequently if clinically indicated.

❗ A L E R T *Spontaneous bleeding may occur at platelet counts of less than 10,000–20,000/mm³.*

Red blood cell and platelet transfusions are often given to maintain a hemoglobin concentration of at least 7.0 to 8.0 g/dL and a platelet count of 10,000 to 20,000/mm³ or higher as clinically indicated. For example, a hemoglobin of ≥10 g/dL should be maintained for children undergoing radiation therapy. Oxygen containing hemoglobin is considered a radiosensitizer, which makes cancer cells more sensitive to the effects of radiation. Some oncologists advocate that children with brain tumors should maintain platelet counts of more than 50,000/mm³ to minimize the risk of intracranial bleeding. Other precautions for the child with thrombocytopenia include

- Avoiding aspirin and aspirin-containing products
- Using a soft toothbrush or sponge for mouth care
- Avoiding contact sports, rough play, and amusement park rides using increased centrifugal force
- Postponing elective procedures such as dental work
- Avoiding intramuscular injections, rectal temperatures, and enemas
- Increasing intake of roughage and fluids to prevent constipation and straining
- Using stool softeners to prevent constipation or hard stools, which can lead to mucosal damage and bleeding

Certain chemotherapy drugs may alter blood coagulation studies, and children may need to receive thawed plasma, cryoprecipitate, or factor VIII to correct coagulopathy. For example, the drug L-asparaginase, which is used to treat acute leukemia, may decrease the fibrinogen level, which then necessitates checking of weekly fibrinogen levels and administration of cryoprecipitate as ordered.

INTERVENTIONS FOR ONCOLOGIC EMERGENCIES

At the time of diagnosis and during cancer treatment, certain emergencies may arise that must be swiftly recognized and treated by the health care team

(Table 22-2). These emergencies can arise from secondary effects of the cancer or from toxicities of chemotherapy administration. Critical ongoing nursing assessment and immediate expert medical attention are required to treat and minimize deleterious outcomes of these emergencies.

INTERVENTIONS FOR LATE EFFECTS

QUESTION: What long-term sequela is important to discuss with George and his family?

Most children with cancer become long-term survivors, defined as being disease free for at least 5 years from diagnosis. In the United States, 1 in 900 people between the ages of 15 and 45 years is a survivor of childhood cancer. Almost 80% of childhood cancer survivors will be alive 5 years after the diagnosis, and almost 75% will be alive after 10 years (National Cancer Institute, SEER Program, 2009). Survival rates have increased dramatically during the past three decades because of advances in medicine and technology related to surgery, radiation therapy, chemotherapy, biotherapy, and supportive care. As a result of increased long-term survival, considerably more *late effects* of treatment are being observed. Late effects may be treatment related (e.g., chemotherapy, biotherapy, radiation therapy) or by tissue injury, scar tissue formation, or impaired cell growth resulting from treatment. All cells and organs of the body can experience some late effects. Some of the systems and organs that more commonly experience late effects are discussed in Nursing Interventions 22-6.

To help the child and family identify and monitor long-term complications, pediatric oncology nurses need to be knowledgeable about the possible late effects of cancer treatment (Evidence-Based Clinical Practice Guidelines 22-1). Pediatric nurses have a great responsibility and opportunity to provide this family education and to reinforce the importance of short- and long-term follow-up care. They must also provide guidance to children and adolescents regarding health care decisions and risk-taking behaviors (e.g., smoking, drug use). The child's treatment history, organ damage, and potential for late effects place the child at higher risk for injury from these behaviors.

Long-term psychosocial issues may also arise for childhood survivors. Interruptions in the child's developmental milestones; alterations in family dynamics; and concerns regarding return of the malignancy, defining a new identity, and coping with long-term physical complications are issues that must be addressed to ease psychosocial rehabilitation. The nurse plays a pivotal role in providing anticipatory guidance for the child and the family to assist them in coping with uncertainty, living with compromised health and possible disabilities, and fear of discrimination.

TABLE 22-2   Interventions to Manage Oncologic Emergencies

Oncologic Emergency	Description	Clinical Presentation	Health Care Interventions
Hyperleukocytosis	Peripheral WBC count is >100,000/mm³, causing increased blood viscosity, blast cell aggregates, and thrombi in the microcirculation.	Shortness of breath Tachypnea Cyanosis Blurred vision Papilledema Agitation Ataxia Confusion, delirium, stupor	Infuse IV fluids (approximately 3,000 mL/m²/day), sodium bicarbonate, and allopurinol or rasburicase. Exchange transfusion or apheresis may be necessary to substantially decrease the number of circulating WBCs.
Tumor lysis syndrome	Rapid release of large quantities of electrolytes and metabolites from the cancer cells during induction of chemotherapy resulting from rapid lysis (breakdown) of tumor cells agents.	Hyperuricemia Hyperkalemia Hyperphosphatemia Hypocalcemia Flank pain Hematuria Decreased urine output Lethargy Muscle cramps and twitching Seizures Respiratory distress Diarrhea Renal failure Cardiac dysfunction	Provide IV hydration to flush cell by-products through the kidneys. Administer diuretics. Administer antihyperuricemics (allopurinol [Zyloprim] or rasburicase [Elitek]) to reduce uric acid production. Monitor serum chemistry levels. Manage hyperkalemia, hyperuricemia, hyperphosphatemia, and hypocalcemia using oral and IV solutions specific to electrolyte needs. Monitor intake and output. Provide early renal and critical care consultation
Septic shock	Presence of infection and the subsequent systemic inflammatory response to that infection, which results in physiologic alterations occurring at the capillary endothelial level. This can lead to decreased tissue perfusion, cellular hypoxia, and death.	Fever or hypothermia Tachycardia Tachypnea Peripheral vasodilation Leukocytosis Leukopenia Reduced mental alertness Organ failure	Initiate volume resuscitation with isotonic or crystalloid boluses. Administer broad-spectrum antibiotics. Provide supportive care and symptom management to maintain organ function.
Disseminated intravascular coagulation	Pathologic activation of coagulation factors and mechanisms that happens in response to the child's disease. Alterations in blood-clotting mechanisms are manifested by decreased platelets, increased prothrombin, and decreased fibrinogen.	Uncontrolled bleeding Petechiae, ecchymosis, purpuric rash Prolonged prothrombin time and partial thromboplastin time Platelet count, 100,000/mm³ Increased D-dimer assay Decreased antithrombin III levels Below-normal fibrinogen levels Increased fibrin degradation products	Manage symptoms. Provide blood product transfusions (fresh-frozen plasma, cryoprecipitate, platelets, red blood cells). Apply pressure to bleeding sites. Monitor urine, stool, emesis, and needle puncture sites for presence of blood.
Typhlitis	Bacterial infection of the cecum. May lead to necrotizing colitis.	Neutropenia Fever Severe abdominal pain in right lower quadrant Distended abdomen Diminished or absent bowel sounds Diarrhea Nausea Vomiting	Administer broad-spectrum antibiotics intravenously. Provide supportive care to manage symptoms. Anticipate surgical intervention to remove area of inflammation or infarct may be necessary.
Spinal cord compression	Compression of the spinal cord caused by tumor mass on or near the spinal cord. This can be a result of primary tumor of the spine or from spinal metastases.	Motor weakness Difficulty bearing weight Paresthesia Shooting back pain Changes in bowel and bladder function	Arrange a neurosurgical consult to determine extent of neurologic impairment. Use MRI or myelography to assess location and extent of cord compression. If indicated, perform emergency surgery to relieve compression.

TABLE 22-2   Interventions to Manage Oncologic Emergencies (*Continued*)

Oncologic Emergency	Description	Clinical Presentation	Health Care Interventions
Syndrome of inappropriate antidiuretic hormone secretion (SIADH)	Inappropriate release of antidiuretic hormone resulting in fluid retention. Vincristine and cyclophosphamide administration can precipitate SIADH.	Hyponatremia Low serum osmolarity High urine specific gravity and osmolarity Decreased urinary output	Restrict fluids to below maintenance levels. Monitor intake and output. Monitor specific gravity of each voiding. Monitor serum sodium levels. Administer diuretics. Monitor for seizure activity.
Superior vena cava syndrome	Mediastinal compression of the superior vena cava caused by size and location of tumor mass, usually a lymphoma	Airway obstruction Respiratory distress Edema Changes in mental status	Arrange emergency radiation consult. Initiate emergency radiation or steroids to reduce tumor mass from vena cava.
Anaphylaxis	Acute and severe allergic reaction	Individual responses vary, including eruption of skin and mucous membranes, lesions, and itching; respiratory symptoms (coughing, sneezing, stridor, dyspnea); cardiac complications (tachycardia, hypotension, decreased peripheral perfusion); and GI symptoms (diarrhea, nausea, vomiting).	Test doses of medications that are at high risk for causing an anaphylactic reaction should be given prior to medication administration. Pretreat child with diphenhydramine (Benadryl) or hydrocortisone (Solu-Cortef) prior to medications likely to cause anaphylaxis. Administer epinephrine and oxygen if reaction occurs. Intubate as indicated by child's respiratory effort.

Information from Secola, R., & Reid, D. (2009). Oncologic emergencies. In N. E. Kline (Ed.), *Essentials of pediatric hematology/oncology nursing: A core curriculum* (3rd ed., pp. 153–158). Glenview, IL: Association of Pediatric Hematology/Oncology Nurses.

ANSWER: A potential late effect for George, who received chemotherapy, can be sterility. Adolescents should be given the information about their future ability to become parents. Boys have the option of banking sperm before chemotherapy treatments. Newer technology also provides girls with options for fertility preservation. Nurses need to assess the physical and psychosocial maturity of the boy to determine whether this is an appropriate topic for a family. The religious and cultural values of the family should also be discussed and considered in this decision-making process.

EDUCATIONAL INTERVENTIONS

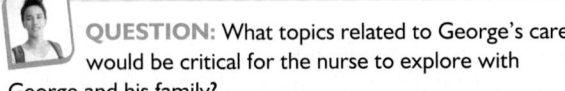

QUESTION: What topics related to George's care would be critical for the nurse to explore with George and his family?

Education for children and families dealing with childhood cancer begins at the time of diagnosis and continues through each phase of the child's treatment. This necessary education process is sustained to assist the child in the years following his or her cancer treatment or to assist the family after the death of the child. From the moment that cancer is suspected, the family is thrown into a new world in which they must learn new medical terminology, procedures, tests, and methods to care for the needs of their child. Through education,

most families acquire a sophisticated level of knowledge of pediatric oncology. All members of the health care team play a critical role in providing information to help the child and family cope and make informed decisions during the trajectory of their child's cancer illness.

Topics to address during the long-term educational process with the child and family include

- Pathophysiology, prognosis, and signs and symptoms of the malignancy
- Diagnostic testing methods and procedures, including interpretation of laboratory test results
- Disease-specific treatment options and outcomes, treatment-induced side effects
- Tumor and treatment-related pain management techniques
- Infection prevention measures
- Management of treatment side effects, such as nausea, vomiting, stomatitis, alopecia, diarrhea, constipation, dehydration
- Nutritional needs and measures
- Care of devices such as CVCs
- Promotion of growth and development, including at home and at school
- Home management of medications, medical equipment, and assistive devices
- Needs of child and family members
- Coping techniques
- Management of long-term sequelae related to the child's tumor and specific therapy regimen

NURSING INTERVENTIONS 22-6

Interventions to Manage the Late Effects of Cancer Therapy

System/Organ	Long-Term Effect	Nursing Interventions
Endocrine: ovaries/testes	Infertility Sterility	Refer the child to endocrinologist. Refer the family for counseling, sperm banking or egg harvesting before treatment, and replacement hormones.
Endocrine: thyroid, hypothalamus	Hypothyroidism Thyroiditis Graves disease Benign or malignant tumor of the thyroid	Refer the child to endocrinologist and for replacement hormones for hypothyroidism or persistent thyroiditis. Prepare child for possible surgical removal of part or all of thyroid if Graves disease or tumor present.
Cardiovascular	Cardiomyopathy Pericarditis Valvular damage Coronary artery disease	Monitor cumulative lifetime anthracycline dosages. Refer the child to cardiologist. Anticipate need for medications such as digoxin and diuretics. Prepare for possible sodium restriction and low-fat foods. Prepare child for surgical replacement of damaged valves or cardiac transplantation (in extreme cases of cardiomyopathy).
Musculoskeletal	Scoliosis Kyphosis Spinal shortening Osteoporosis Osteopenia Avascular necrosis Delayed or arrested tooth development	Refer the child for rehabilitation services. Encourage nutritional balance and maintenance. Prepare the child and family for shortened growth of bones. Refer the child to orthopedic surgeon. Advise the child to avoid rough sports. Calcium supplementation and bisphosphonates may be needed for osteopenia and osteoporosis. Encourage frequent dental evaluations.
Vision	Cataracts	Refer the child to ophthalmologist. Prepare the child for surgical removal.
Hearing	Hearing loss	Refer the child to audiologist; hearing aid may be needed. Refer the child for speech therapy consult, especially when hearing loss occurs at a younger age.
Respiratory	Pulmonary fibrosis	Encourage smoking prevention/cessation. Provide immediate care for respiratory infections. Encourage yearly flu vaccines. Avoid activities that may increase lung pressure (e.g., scuba diving)
GI	Chronic enteritis Cirrhosis or fibrosis of the liver	Refer the child for nutrition consults. Assist the child and family in dietary modifications if necessary.
Genitourinary	Chronic nephritis Chronic hemorrhagic cystitis Nephrectomy	Refer the child to nephrologist; dialysis may be needed. Ensure adequate hydration. Plan for possible bladder irrigations and antibiotics if needed and ordered.
Hematopoietic	Prolonged immunosuppression	Teach infection control precautions. Administer adequate antibiotic therapy and prophylactic antibiotics, as ordered. Monitor blood count.

EVIDENCE-BASED CLINICAL PRACTICE GUIDELINES 22-1

Late Effects of Childhood Cancer

Children's Oncology Group. (2008). *Establishing and enhancing services for childhood cancer survivors: Long-term follow-up program resource guide.* Retrieved from

http://www.survivorshipguidelines.org/pdf/LTFUResourceGuide.pdf

A guide to establishing and enhancing long-term follow-up programs for childhood cancer survivors.

National Cancer Institute. (2012). *Late effects of treatment for childhood cancer (PDQ).* Retrieved from

http://www.cancer.gov/cancertopics/pdq/treatment/lateeffects/HealthProfessional/page1

Comprehensive, peer review summary of late effects of 11 types of childhood cancer.

These topics are not discussed at a single visit; rather, they are introduced and reviewed as the need arises. As the child grows and develops new levels of cognitive understanding, topics should be revisited to ensure that the child's understanding is age-appropriate.

CROSS-CULTURAL CARE

In some cultures, children's autonomy is not encouraged. Family members and children are not likely to discuss difficult issues. Information about the child's illness may be filtered or not discussed at all among family members. The health care team should share their beliefs about the importance of fully disclosing information to the child. The family may agree to have the health care provider discuss the illness and treatment with the child, but they may choose not to participate in these discussions.

ANSWER: Initially, the educational focus will be to help George and his family understand the implications of George's diagnosis and treatment modalities. During his chemotherapy treatments, infection prevention will be an important topic of education. Throughout George's care, pain management will also be a subject of education.

PSYCHOSOCIAL INTERVENTIONS

QUESTION: The diagnosis and treatment of a child with a malignancy is inherently stressful for families. Nurses should identify stressors that can be changed. How might you help the Tran family get through this stressful time?

Children with cancer and their families are placed in stressful situations throughout the course of the child's illness. Stressors include the diagnosis itself, chemotherapy or radiation treatments, unplanned hospitalizations, added financial demands, unexpected complications, involvement of other family members (or lack of involvement), relapse or progression of the disease, completion

of therapy, awareness of other children's deaths, and possibly the impending death and actual death of the child. Peer support groups (Fig. 22-8) and assistance from other interdisciplinary team members, such as child life specialists, social workers, and psychologists, can assist with stress management and coping strategies.

Establishing open communication and trust with the child and family is key to providing optimal psychosocial support. At the time of diagnosis, family members are often in a state of shock or denial and are unable to accept or comprehend the vast amount of information that is given to them. After the initial family conference, at which time the diagnosis and treatment plan are discussed with the family, review and clarify the information. When the child is hospitalized, daily contact with a consistent oncology team member allows for ongoing guidance, education, and support. It also provides an opportunity for the family to ask questions and verbalize concerns and enables them to participate in daily decision making about their child's treatment plan.

The nurse is the health care provider who has the most direct contact with the child and thus plays a key role in providing psychosocial support. Useful strategies include establishing a trusting relationship with the child by communicating honestly and answering questions

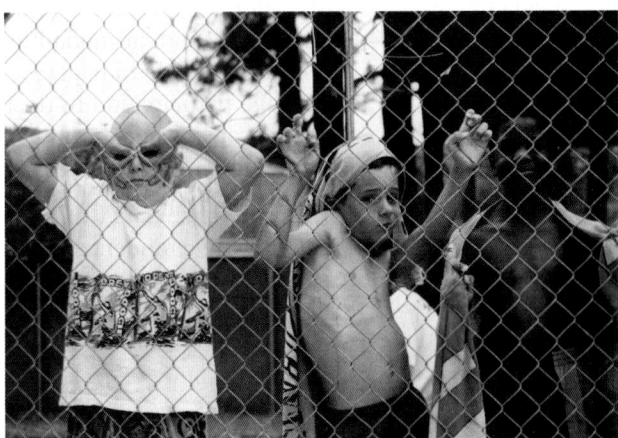

Figure 22-8 Summer camps and other planned social activities provide opportunities to build relationships with other children who have cancer. These friendships provide sources of support, understanding, and encouragement. Courtesy of Camp Ronald McDonald for Good Times.

directly. In addition to providing age-appropriate explanations for daily routines and procedures, encourage the child to verbalize fears and concerns regarding his or her disease and treatment. Many pediatric oncology patients will be asked to participate in clinical drug trials or other research studies to test the efficacy of new treatment regimens. In such cases, it is the investigator's responsibility to discuss the specifics of the research with the family. Nurse participation in these discussions is essential to ensure that required protocols are followed and to serve as an additional source of information and support to the family as needed. See Chapter 2 for further discussion of the role of nurses in pediatric research and the rights of children and their families.

KidKare Children aged 7 years and older have a right to decide whether to participate in clinical research studies. The nurse caring for these children should assess the child's basic understanding of the clinical research study and provide adequate time for the child to ask questions regarding his or her treatment. Equally important is the nurse's role as the child's advocate if the child refuses to participate.

Give special attention to adolescents (aged 11 to 21 years) because they have unique needs and sometimes experience greater difficulties adhering to their treatment regimens and grappling with the consequences of their disease (Developmental Considerations 22-2).

DEVELOPMENTAL CONSIDERATIONS 22-2

Concerns of the Adolescent With Cancer

Concern	Family and Health Care Provider Interventions
Peer acceptance	Use school reentry program to educate peers about child's condition.
Changes in friendships	Assist adolescent to find new supportive relationships. Encourage relationships with other adolescents who have cancer. Encourage participation in activities such as summer camps and rap sessions with other adolescents with cancer. Be a friend. Provide computer access for social media networking. Assign to room with another adolescent during hospitalization. Stress importance of spending time visiting with friends in a "teen lounge" environment during hospitalization.
Physical changes	Help adolescent to maintain normal appearance by using wigs and wearing loose clothing. Emphasize the temporary nature of many of the side effects of therapy. Investigate with the adolescent his or her fertility and sexual concerns.
Desire to be "normal"	Encourage adolescent to engage in usual activities. Control the amount of information given out about the adolescent's condition.
Desire to be independent and have sense of control	Respect adolescent's privacy during physical care. Assist adolescent to learn measures to control anxiety and pain related to procedures or treatment modalities (e.g., biofeedback, self-hypnosis, progressive muscle relaxation, guided imagery). Encourage participation in decision making regarding care. Do not encourage adolescent to be overly dependent on nurses and family for physical care. Discuss interactive websites designed to educate and assist with his or her disease and treatment.
Poor self-esteem	Communicate confidence in adolescent's ability to succeed. Assist adolescent to participate in activities in which he or she will be successful. Plan for adolescent to return to school as soon as possible after an illness or hospitalization. Assist adolescent to develop effective mechanisms to cope with stress. Ensure that family expectations for the adolescent and how the adolescent sees such expectations are congruent and realistic.
Future life expectations	Encourage adolescent to make plans for the future. Openly discuss the long-term sequelae of cancer. Provide education on health insurance and employment strategies.

The social isolation from their peers as a result of hospitalization or homebound illness adds to feelings of loneliness and depression. Nonadherence, excessive anxiety, moodiness, depression, and fear of changes in body image are common reactions expressed by adolescents who delay, modify, or stop their treatment.

Strategies used by health care personnel to help children and adolescents to cope with their chronic condition include therapeutic play, art therapy, music therapy, pet therapy, storytelling, keeping a journal or scrapbook of drawings, using CAM therapy (i.e., guided imagery, relaxation, biofeedback, massage, acupressure, and traditional Chinese medicine), and social interaction with other children (see Chapters 10 and 11). Encourage the child and family to participate in programs designed to support and strengthen children and families coping with a serious illness. For example, in the Beads of Courage program, children are able to tell their cancer story using colorful beads that symbolize their courage and milestones that they have achieved during their unique treatment journey.

When cancer is diagnosed in a child, families experience overwhelming stress as a result of coping with their own feelings and needs and with the physical and emotional needs of the ill child and other family members, especially those of the siblings. Stressors include the following:

- The shock of the diagnosis of cancer
- Role changes necessary to meet the demands of caring for a chronically ill child
- The financial burden caused by medical costs and a possible loss of income (if it becomes necessary for a family member to stay home with the child)
- Fear of losing the child
- Marital discord
- Feelings of guilt related to spending less time with the siblings and with one's spouse
- The need to learn technical and medical information to better understand the child's disease and its treatment

Many of these stressors continue throughout the course of the child's illness and posttreatment period. Although families know that the child's illness will include periods of exacerbations and remissions, additional stress comes from constantly being on the alert for the situation to get worse. Chapter 12 provides an in-depth discussion of the effects of a child's chronic condition on the family and gives practical interventions to assist family members as they cope with these stressors. The nurse is often the health care team member who initially provides psychosocial support for the family and facilitates consultations with other health care team members.

Siblings must also adjust to the diagnosis of cancer, although this may not be acknowledged by the parents (Tradition or Science 22-2). The major stressors experienced by siblings include short- or long-term separation from one or both parents, decreased attention from the parents even in the presence of the ill child, the need to assume additional household responsibilities, fear of losing their brother or sister, and guilt that their thoughts or wishes may be responsible in some way

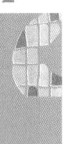

TRADITION OR SCIENCE 22-2

More Inquiry Needed

Do parents recognize that the brothers and sisters of children with cancer may have emotional difficulties as a result of the changes brought by the diagnosis?

Nurses have long been concerned about the effect of childhood cancer on well siblings. Recognition of this need has prompted development of sibling classes, educational materials for siblings, and sibling support groups. But are siblings using these interventions, and are parents assisting and encouraging siblings to use them? Ballard (2004) obtained views from parents in 86 families about siblings' needs and support being offered. About one half of all parents of children with cancer did not expect their well children to have any problems as a result of the experience. They were not willing to have the siblings participate in interventions aimed at providing for the needs of the well child. This finding indicates that families may not see their well children as being at risk for problems. This research was consistent with that of Murray (2002), who found that siblings and parents did not agree on the types of support most helpful for the siblings, and that siblings are not being provided with the type of support they believe would be most helpful. This research is both a call and a challenge to nurses to critically evaluate participation in sibling programs to determine whether these programs are useful and helpful to the sibling population. Gursky (2007) provided educational interventions to well siblings of hospitalized children. Her pre- and posttest design demonstrated that the children who participated in the educational interventions had significantly lower anxiety levels after interventions than did siblings who did not participate in the interventions. It is clear that measures are still needed to better inform parents about the needs of well siblings and to provide easier access to professional support for siblings in the form of literature, media materials, support groups, and individual counseling as needed.

for causing the cancer (Fig. 22-9). These stressors may become evident through changes in the sibling's behavior both at home and in school. (See Chapters 12 and 13 for more information about supporting siblings of the ill child.)

The child and the family members also experience grieving. Grieving and disappointments may occur along various points of the child's treatment regimen. The loss of hair or a limb; inability to achieve remission using a certain combination of chemotherapeutic agents; and missing school dances, plays, and family vacations because of unexpected hospitalizations are examples of situations that can intensify the child's or family's sense of grief. Grieving also may be a result of the actual death of the child. Members of the health care team must be cognizant of and sensitive to the issues that may cause great disappointment to a particular child or member of the child's family. Chapter 13 summarizes interventions to help the family deal with grief and loss.

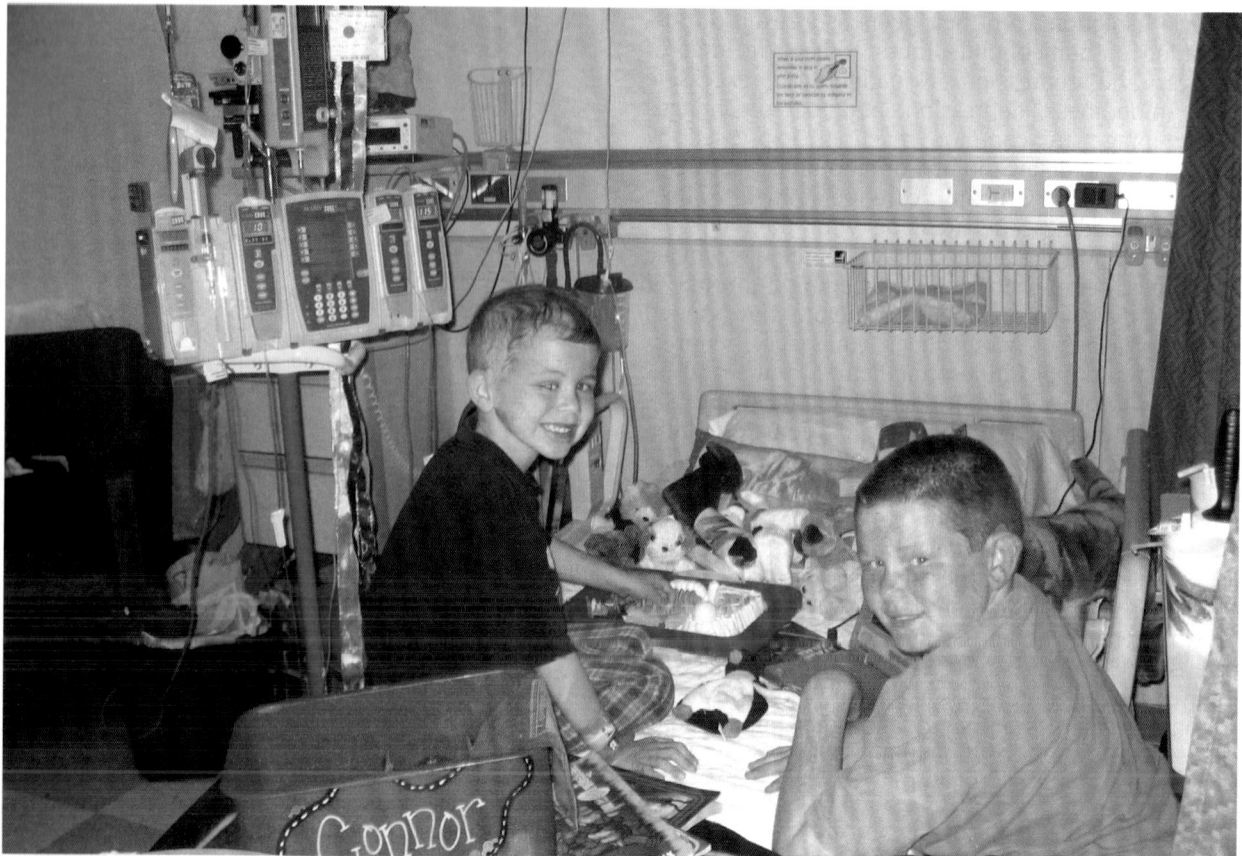

Figure 22-9 Brothers share time together in the hospital.

ANSWER: The discovery of George's illness was quickly followed by a surgery on the affected limb. George is the only son in his family, and his parents have ambitions and dreams of his career and success. One stressor the nurse can help alleviate is the language barrier. George's mother's English is not very fluent and she does not understand the medical explanations. She is relying on Tung or George to translate for her. Obtaining a medical translator is more appropriate than using the patient to translate.

The hospital nurses and a nurse case manager can provide information and some support. However, a more critical role of the nurse is to assist the family to mobilize its own social and emotional support systems. Ask the family about their religious affiliations such as church or a community group. Question them about whom they would want to know about George's illness. The Health Insurance Portability and Accountability Act (HIPAA) regulations prevent the release of information, so it must be given by family.

Loan and Tung look first to their family for support and then to the Vietnamese community and their church. Loan is very close to her sisters, and they have offered to help in any way they can. As members of the community hear about George's condition, they begin dropping by the Tran home to give food and offer prayers and support. George's family is his primary support. His friends are initially frightened to come see him, but Ashley returns to live at home and spends her afternoons with her brother. She feels that she cannot add any further stress to her family.

INTERVENTIONS TO PROMOTE GROWTH AND DEVELOPMENT

 QUESTION: How can you assess and promote growth and development for George?

Children with cancer face challenges to their physical, social, emotional, and intellectual growth. The treatment regimen and its side effects may inhibit normal physical development. For instance, chemotherapy and steroids can cause delays in pubertal development. *Radiation* can impair bone growth and growth hormone production. Chronic malnutrition, anorexia, and lethargy can affect weight gain and development of muscles.

The child's social, emotional, and intellectual development may be impaired because of frequent hospitalizations and chronic health problems that restrict the child's activities to the home. Absence from school and social activities can impair the child's ability to sustain meaningful relationships with peers. Overprotection by well-meaning family members can prevent the child from learning self-care and decision-making skills.

Many measures can be used to promote age-appropriate development for the child with cancer. Allow children of all ages to maintain a sense of control by providing them choices in their daily care whenever possible. Establish a schedule of daily activities with the child. The schedule should incorporate necessary health care interventions with the child's usual activity schedule (such as attending school). If the child is hospitalized, ensure that the schedule provides opportunities for visits from school friends and activities with other hospitalized children. If the child requires isolation, ensure that visitors and items are screened so that activities and schoolwork can be brought to the child's room to maintain the child's social and intellectual development.

caREminder

The Centers for Disease Control and Prevention (CDC) does not recommend allowing flowers and plants in the rooms of patients who are immunocompromised.

School reentry may be difficult for the child who is returning after a prolonged absence or with notable changes in his or her appearance. These children may fear that other children will make fun of them, try to pull off their wig, or gossip about them. Classmates may be afraid that they will "catch" cancer, or they may wonder whether the child is going to die. Community Care 22 1 summarizes interventions that can be used to help children rejoin their classmates. These interventions focus on easing the transition to the classroom through peer programs and by providing medical information to key school officials.

Children returning to the classroom should be encouraged to participate in sports and in musical and artistic activities that they enjoy and in which they find a sense of accomplishment. Activities need only be limited by the child's imagination and his or her physical ability to perform, especially during periods of disease exacerbation.

ANSWER: Consider all aspects of George's development: emotional, intellectual, and social. Discuss with George and his family his specific needs as a 14-year-old with cancer. George has always been an excellent student. Determine how he will continue his intellectual development. Will he be able or willing to return to a large public high school? Discuss alternative opportunities for him to keep up on his academics. Discuss what can be done to continue his school friendships if he does not return to school.

HOME CARE INTERVENTIONS

QUESTION: As an adolescent, George wants to feel in control of his life. The osteogenic sarcoma has a series of repercussions that cause George to feel out of control. He has experienced surgery on his leg, which causes a change in body image. George does not want to return to school. The prognosis for George is not yet known. What aspects of George's care do you think can be managed at home? What will be some of the challenges of providing home care?

Given the current demands of managed care, as well as the technologic advances related to medical and nursing care, home care and palliative care services for children with cancer have become considerably more common. Professional home care services may be requested by a family when a child becomes terminally ill. Hospice care provides psychosocial support and interdisciplinary health care for dying children and their families. Home care and hospice services allow such children to remain with their families in familiar surroundings while continuing to receive interventions that make them comfortable and that minimize visits to the hospital.

The scope of home care in pediatric oncology ranges from single interventions, such as antibiotic administration, to complex plans of care requiring multiple services. Infusion therapy is a common regimen that can be used to provide total parenteral nutrition, pain medications, chemotherapeutic agents, antimicrobials, and blood products in the home. Other routine home care that can be provided by the family with little or no assistance from a home care nurse include caring for and maintaining the CVC, supporting daily oral hygiene, providing daily skin care, administering oral or subcutaneous medications, and staying vigilant for signs and symptoms of infection.

The home care nurse conducts ongoing assessments of the family's ability to care for the ill child in the home, assists in the procurement of medical equipment and supplies, provides needed health care interventions, and coordinates the delivery of home care services by other members of the team. Collaboration with the home care pharmacist, primary oncologist, physical and occupational therapist, nutritionist, speech therapist, and respiratory therapist is essential to ensure that all aspects of the child's development are supported. (See Chapter 12 for more detailed information regarding the nurse's role in home care.)

When cancer treatment is completed, home care management is not finished. Research indicates that many children and families experience difficulty reintegrating the child into family, school, and community settings and transitioning to less intensive medical oversight of the child's health status (Labay et al., 2004). Obstacles to successful reintegration include the lack of ongoing community and extended family support structures, lack of reimbursement for medical and psychological interventions to assist the family in the reintegration process, and the child's state of physical and psychological well-being. More research is needed to better assess the needs of the reintegration process. In addition, nursing care to provide ongoing assessment and intervention of the family must be extended to promote optimum family adjustment.

ANSWER: Most of George's care will take place at home. After the surgery, George spent several days in the hospital but was then discharged home. A home care nurse visits to continue to monitor and change the dressing on his surgical site. One of the challenges is Loan's lack of English fluency. The home care agency is trying to find a nurse who speaks Vietnamese to be the case manager for the Tran family. Loan does not work outside the home and is very willing to provide the care her son needs. The challenge is communicating accurately.

PALLIATIVE INTERVENTIONS

Palliative care is designed to prevent or diminish the emotional and physical suffering from life-threatening illnesses. The goal of the health care team is to promote quality of life for the child and the family as the child transitions from curative care to end-of-life care (Crozier & Hancock, 2012). Interventions focus on managing symptoms (e.g., pain, nausea, anorexia) and providing emotional and spiritual support to the child and family. Research has indicated deficiencies in meeting parental needs during this time of their child's life. These deficiencies include a lack of communication and information from the health care team, a perception of being disrespected and avoided, a need for more emotional support, and a need for more continuity of care (Aschenbrenner et al., 2012). Nurses play an important role in helping families transition to end-of-life care. Care for the family extends beyond the child's death to provide support as family members grieve the loss of the child and adapt to a world without their beloved child's presence. Chapter 13 covers pediatric palliative care in depth, including interventions to support the dying child, the family, and the professionals caring for the child.

NURSING PLAN OF CARE

QUESTION: Applying the information related to supportive care, what are the nursing diagnoses that may be relevant to George's care at this time?

The nursing plan of care for a child with cancer and the child's family reflects the complex nature of the disease and the need to implement creative care strategies (Nursing Plan of Care 22-1). Whenever possible, the child's treatment should be guided by an interdisciplinary team at a specialized facility with the technology to quickly diagnose and treat the child's disease. The interdisciplinary treatment plan is focused on eradicating the cancer and minimizing and treating the effects of the multimodal treatment regimen (see thePoint Care Path: An Interdisciplinary Plan of Care for the Child With Neutropenia and Fever). In addition, the Nursing Plans of Care in Chapter 10 (Pain Management), Chapter 12 (Chronic Conditions as a Challenge to Health Maintenance), Chapter 13 (Palliative Care), and Chapter 23 (The Child With Altered Hematologic Status) also describe nursing diagnoses and interventions useful in managing care of a child with cancer.

The nurse plays an instrumental role in humanizing the cancer experience to enhance the dignity, strengths, and uniqueness of each child and his or her family. Providing education to the family is an ongoing part of the plan of care. Concerns about the child's ability to achieve developmental goals and about the family's ability to maintain effective levels of coping must be addressed during all phases of the child's treatment program.

ANSWER: Examples of appropriate nursing diagnoses include

Deficient knowledge: Diagnosis, treatment plan

Anxiety related to the uncertainty of the future

Acute pain related to operative procedure

Risk for constipation related to opioid use

Risk for infection related to neutropenia

PEDIATRIC MALIGNANCIES

Pediatric malignancies can arise in almost any tissue, including blood, organs, bone, and nervous tissues, and therefore affect many body systems. Prognosis varies with the type of cancer and the extent of disease at diagnosis.

CHILDHOOD LEUKEMIAS

Leukemia is a cancer of the blood or bone marrow characterized by an abnormal proliferation of blood cells, usually WBCs (leukocytes). Leukemia is the most common childhood cancer and accounts for approximately one third of all cancer cases diagnosed in children younger than 15 years of age. The French–American–British (FAB) cooperative group has established a classification system for acute leukemia based on the form, structure, and chemistry (morphology) of the blast cells. The World Health Organization (WHO) has developed a more comprehensive system to categorize leukemia based on morphology, immunophenotyping, and cytogenic and clinical features. There are four major types of leukemia based on whether it had an acute or chronic onset and whether the involved cancer cell is a lymphoid or myeloid stem cell lineage:

1. ALL, also known as *acute lymphocytic leukemia*. This is the most common type of leukemia in young children and the most common type of cancer in children, although it also affects adults, primarily those aged 65 years and older (Carroll & Finlay, 2010).
2. Acute myeloid leukemia (AML), also referred to as *acute myeloblastic leukemia*. Approximately 15% to 20% of children with leukemia have AML.
3. Chronic myeloid leukemia (CML), also referred to as *chronic myelogenous leukemia*. This occurs predominantly in adolescents and adults. Approximately 5% of children with leukemia have this form of the disease.
4. Chronic lymphocytic leukemia (CLL), which most often affects adults older than the age 55 years. It sometimes occurs in younger adults, but it almost never affects children and therefore is not covered in this chapter.

Some chromosomal abnormalities are associated with childhood leukemia. For example, leukemia is 15 times more likely to develop in children with trisomy 21 (Down syndrome) than in other children and has also been associated with other autosomal recessive disorders (e.g., Fanconi anemia). Other less

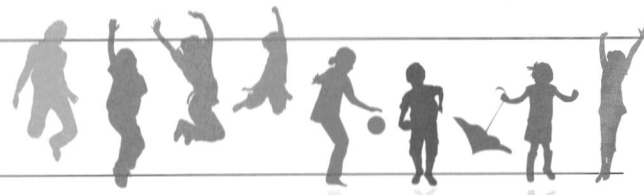

NURSING PLAN OF CARE 22-1:

The Child With a Malignancy

Nursing Diagnosis: Deficient knowledge: Diagnosis, treatment plan, and health care needs of the child

Interventions/Rationale

- Assess current knowledge level. Educate the child and family about the treatment plan and health needs.
- Encourage family members to ask questions or write them down as they think of them. Answer questions in a nonthreatening, brief, and honest manner; provide information at child's level of understanding.

    The diagnosis of cancer will evoke anxiety in the child and family because treatment is complex and, in some cases, prognosis for the child may be poor. The family will need information to be given many times to help them better understand the complex and unfamiliar changes in their life that will occur as a result of their child's diagnosis.

- Enlist assistance of interdisciplinary team to provide education to the child and family. Give the child and family written instructions to enhance verbal instruction and to enable them to review information at their own pace. Provide opportunities to demonstrate care skills on mannequins and on the child before discharge.

    If knowledge deficit exists, families cannot appropriately maintain the child's level of functioning or prevent complications.

- Give instructions at a developmentally appropriate level in terms of what the child will see, hear, feel, taste, and smell. Encourage the child to participate (as age-appropriate) in discussions about the treatment plan, and provide the child with as many opportunities as possible to make decisions about daily care (e.g., when to take a bath, complete a dressing change).

    Respect for a child's developing capacity for autonomy and emerging self-determination requires that the child's wishes be considered. Doing so involves the concept of assent, which is the child's agreement with the decision. To involve the child in the decision-making process and to decrease anxiety, provide information in a manner that the child understands.

- Refer child and family to community support/home health care services as appropriate to help reinforce, review, and reeducate.

    Family may need assistance, reinforcement, and reeducation at home to manage the child's care and to adapt to lifestyle changes. This support is especially important immediately after the diagnosis and first discharge home from the hospital.

Expected Outcomes

- Child and family will verbalize understanding of diagnosis, treatment, and child's health care needs.
- Child and family will participate in the informed consent process and care of the child based on their understanding of the child's illness and treatment options.

Nursing Diagnosis: Acute (or chronic) pain related to effects of disease process, diagnostic procedures, and/or treatment modalities

Interventions/Rationale

- Assess pain using a reliable and valid method that is developmentally appropriate and appropriate for the situation. Elicit the family's assessment of child's pain.

    The subjective rating of pain is most reliable, but it may not be an option in a nonverbal child (infant, intubated, comatose). Validated tools provide the most accurate assessment. The absence of behaviors that indicate pain does not necessarily mean that the child is not experiencing pain. Parents and other family members know their child best and are familiar with typical behaviors.

- Implement pharmacologic and biobehavioral interventions to alleviate pain, including anticipated procedural pain (see Nursing Plan of Care 10-1). Use a preventive approach to keep pain at or below an acceptable level. Involve the family in pain management. Instruct them in using oral anesthetics as ordered for mouth pain.

    Unrelieved pain has deleterious physiologic effects, such as tachycardia, suppressed immune function, and atelectasis, as well as negative psychological effects. Opioid analgesics are indicated for moderate to severe pain. Pain is better managed if it is not allowed to escalate. Having the family provide pain relief measures may be more comforting to the child than having them provided by a nurse. Pain from oral mucositis may prevent the child from eating, drinking, and taking his or her oral medications.

- Assess for the probable cause of the pain to direct the choice of pain relief measures. Monitor for changes in the child's condition that may identify a need to change pain relief methods.

    For the child with a malignancy, pain may come from the tumor site, as rapidly growing cancer cells invade bone and tissue; and from the administration and side effects of chemotherapy, radiation, and surgery (e.g., mucositis, skin blistering, and incision site pain). Techniques of pain relief may have to be added or changed to relieve the pain.

(Continued)

NURSING PLAN OF CARE 22-1:

The Child With a Malignancy (*Continued*)

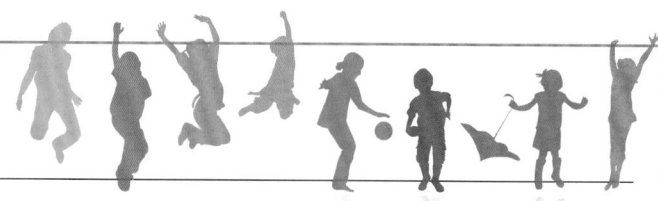

- Assess response to pain and coping strategies, including medications and distraction. Assess cultural, environmental, personal, and psychic factors that may contribute to pain, expression of pain, and relief or pain.

  Assessment of responses identifies strategies that may have worked previously. Identification of factors enables evaluation of child's unique response to pain and helps to individualize management strategies.

- Provide periods of rest and sleep.

  Fatigue can contribute to the perception of pain.

- For the child with chronic pain, encourage the child to keep a diary to help identify aggravating stressors and relieving factors.

  Maintaining a diary may help the child and family identify factors contributing to pain, strategies to modify lifestyle, and help alter the plan of care to relieve or prevent pain.

Expected Outcomes

- Child will experience minimal discomfort during and after procedures.
- Child will state that adequate pain relief has been obtained.
- Child and family will demonstrate use of effective pain relief measures.

Nursing Diagnosis: Risk for infection related to neutropenia, immunosuppressive therapy, or presence of CVC

Interventions/Rationale

- Monitor WBC counts, differential, and ANC for decreases that indicate the child is at greater risk for infection.

  The large numbers of immature WBCs that proliferate in the body during the malignancy process do not provide a defense against infection and at the same time drastically reduce normal composition of the blood. Treatment regimens of chemotherapy and/or radiation further reduce the bone marrow's ability to produce necessary blood components.

- Isolate the child from any persons with infectious diseases, especially chickenpox. Use neutropenic precautions (prevention measures for infection) when ANC is less than 500/mm^3.

  Neutropenia means that the neutrophil count is too low to adequately fight infection. Precautions must be used to keep the child from exposure to infectious agents. Immunocompromised children are at higher risk for chickenpox. In addition, children who have had varicella in the past are at risk for viral

reactivation of herpes zoster when in state of immune compromise.

- Maintain good hygienic practices and ensure that child and family follow these practices; ensure that all children wash hands after toileting. Stress the importance of good hand hygiene for the child, family, and staff.

  Hygienic practices prevent transmission of microorganisms.

- Monitor the child for signs of infection (e.g., increased temperature, pulse, and respirations). Examine child's skin and mucous membranes daily for lesions or breaks; provide oral care several times a day (see Teaching Intervention Plan 22-1). Monitor IV sites and incision sites for signs of infection.

  Early identification leads to prompt treatment.

- Obtain cultures as appropriate.

  Cultures provide data about microorganisms causing infection and about antibiotic drug sensitivity.

- Administer antibacterial, antifungal, and antiviral medications as prescribed.

  Use of appropriate medications is essential in treating infections and preventing progression to sepsis.

- Teach family to recognize the signs and symptoms of infection early (e.g., fever, chills, productive cough, and malaise) and to use neutropenic precautions in the home (see Community Care 22-2).

  The child and family can learn to avoid situations that will increase the likelihood of infection and can implement wellness behaviors that will enable the child to remain healthy.

Expected Outcomes

- Child will remain free from infection.
- Child and family will recognize and report signs and symptoms of infection to their health care providers.
- Child and family will describe measures to reduce risk of infection.
- Child and family will demonstrate measures to reduce the likelihood of infection from the CVC.

Nursing Diagnosis: Impaired urinary elimination related to chemotherapy or disease process

Interventions/Rationale

- Determine whether child is at risk for urinary retention.

  Tumors involving the abdomen (Wilms tumor, neuroblastoma) can alter normal bowel and bladder function; these changes can be reversed by tumor removal or shrinkage. Treatment measures (chemotherapy, radiation, surgery) may cause urinary retention.

- Assess pretumor bladder patterns and current bladder patterns.

  Assessment provides baseline of child's habits.
- Monitor intake and output. Observe for signs of urinary retention or infection (e.g., voiding small amounts, dysuria, frequency, fever).

  Close monitoring provides evidence of fluid balance and prompt identification of problems to ensure adequate intake and fluid replacement. Urinary retention may indicate urinary tract infection.
- Assist with bladder function until the tumor effects are diminished (e.g., Credé method, diapering, catheterization).

  Assisting with bladder function facilitates emptying of the bladder, thereby reducing the risk for an infection.

Expected Outcome

- Child will demonstrate adequate voiding patterns with evidence of adequate renal function during course of therapy.

Nursing Diagnosis: Diarrhea and/or constipation related to effects of chemotherapeutic agents, radiation, or disease process

Interventions/Rationale

- Determine whether the child is at risk for bowel dysfunction.

  Tumors involving the abdomen (Wilms tumor, neuroblastoma), graft-versus-host disease, and bacterial endotoxins can alter normal bowel and bladder function. Treatment measures (chemotherapy, radiation, surgery) may cause constipation or diarrhea.
- Assess pretumor bowel patterns and current bowel patterns. Assess quantity, consistency, color, odor, and frequency of stools. Maintain accurate intake and output. Auscultate bowel sounds every 4 hours.

  Assessment provides baseline of child's habits, hydration status, and bowel activity. Hyperactive bowel sounds are present with diarrhea; hypoactive sounds, with constipation.
- Monitor general condition, vital signs, skin turgor, and mucous membranes every shift and as necessary. Monitor child's weight daily.

  Diarrhea can quickly lead to dehydration and electrolyte imbalances in the pediatric population. Severe dehydration will cause dry mucous membranes, absence of tearing, and weight loss.
- Check stools for reducing substances (Clinitest) and for occult blood (guaiac) every shift. Obtain stool cultures as ordered.

  Evaluation of stool identifies reducing substances (unabsorbed sugars), blood, and bacteria in stool and assists with differential diagnosis of cause of diarrhea.
- Change diapers with each stool. Clean and dry perineal area, wear gloves, and practice scrupulous handwashing when in contact with stool. Provide sitz baths or tub baths for comfort and cleaning.

  Perianal skin care prevents skin breakdown in perineal area. Sitz or tub baths provide comfort measures for tender skin and mucosal areas.
- Assess ongoing nutritional status; provide roughage and fluids for constipation. Offer low-residue, low-lactose foods for diarrhea. Administer adequate hydration and high-fiber diet for constipation.

  Low-residue and low-lactose foods do not irritate the GI mucosa. Fiber, when it reaches the colon, absorbs water and adds bulk to stool, thus making defecation easier.
- Assist with bowel function (e.g., with stool softeners, laxatives) until the tumor effects or effects of chemotherapy and radiation are diminished. Instruct the child and family to place nothing in the rectum.

  Use of stool softeners or laxatives helps prevent constipation. Tearing of the rectal mucosa in the neutropenic child can occur with rectal insertion.
- Administer antispasmodic medication as prescribed. Administer laxatives, stool softeners, or emulsifiers as ordered. Monitor effectiveness.

  Antispasmodic agents help to decrease or prevent diarrhea. Laxatives, stool softeners, or emulsifiers help to relieve and prevent constipation.
- Give the child privacy for toileting. Assist the child to establish a regular bowel pattern.

  The child may experience difficulty having a bowel movement using a bedpan or bedside commode. Setting aside time for elimination encourages establishment of a regular pattern.
- For constipation, encourage ambulation and other activity as tolerated.

  Prolonged bed rest, lack of exercise, and inactivity contribute to constipation.

Expected Outcomes

- Child and family will use measures to prevent or minimize diarrhea and constipation.
- Child will maintain normal pattern of bowel elimination.

Nursing Diagnosis: Risk for injury related to defect in hemostasis (e.g., factor deficiency, low platelet count)
See Chapter 23, Nursing Plan of Care 23-1.

Nursing Diagnosis: Risk for impaired skin/tissue related to radiation therapy, chemotherapy, presence of a CVC, graft-versus-host disease, and immobility

Interventions/Rationale

- Inspect the child's skin and mucous membranes for signs of radiation effects (erythema and darkening, desquamation, thin epidermis, blistering).

(Continued)

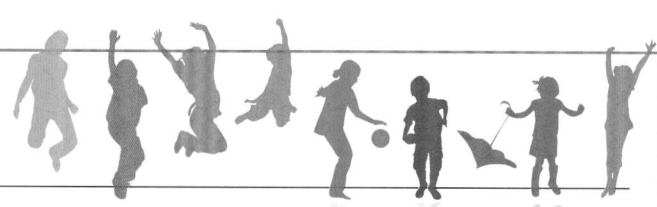

NURSING PLAN OF CARE 22-1:

The Child With a Malignancy (*Continued*)

Melanocytes in the skin are stimulated during radiation treatment, making skin darker in color. Basal cells of the epidermis are affected during radiation. Epithelial cells of the GI tract proliferate rapidly. Because chemotherapy affects fast-growing cells, it causes stomatitis and mucositis.

- Change the child's position every 2 hours.
  Frequent position changes relieve trauma and pressure over bony prominences and may prevent skin breakdown.

- Provide meticulous hygiene practices, keeping skin dry and clean and keeping mucous membranes moist and intact:
  - Assist with daily bath; avoid rubbing the skin. Use mild, nonperfumed soap and tepid water.
  - Complete CVC dressing changes per institutional policy.
  - Complete perineal care after each voiding or defecation.
  - Apply lubricating lotions or creams.
  Keeping skin and mucous membranes intact reduces potential sites of entry for organisms and the development of opportunistic infections.

- Use topical and systemic antibiotic or antifungal medications as ordered.
  Medications may be ordered to prevent infection or for treatment for specific causative organism of skin infection.

Expected Outcomes
- Child and family will demonstrate measures to prevent or minimize skin and mucous membrane breakdown.
- Child's skin and mucous membranes will remain intact, free from infection, soothed, and healed.

Nursing Diagnosis: Impaired oral mucous membrane integrity related to radiation therapy, chemotherapy, dehydration, or ineffective oral hygiene

Interventions/Rationale
- Assess oral health and oral pain using a valid and reliable oral assessment tool. Assessment should include inspection of oral mucosa for
  - Bleeding; sores; ulcerations involving intraoral soft tissue, palate, tongue, gums, and lips in and around mucous membranes
  - Evidence of infection (e.g., candidiasis, herpes simplex, bacterial infections)
- Assess for impairments in speech, swallowing, and drooling.
  Chemotherapy affects fast-growing cells, thus causing stomatitis and mucositis. Cottage cheese–like white or pale patches on the tongue, buccal mucosa, and palate may indicate candidiasis.

Painful itching vesicles (especially on the upper lip) may indicate herpes simplex. Yellowish brown plaque (gram-positive bacteria) and creamy white patches (gram-negative bacteria) located on the buccal mucosa indicate presence of oral infection. Speech and swallowing difficulties may result from ulcerated, bleeding, and painful oral mucosa.

- Assess child's nutrition status, including child's ability to eat and drink. Weigh child daily.
  Dehydration may lead to dry mucous membranes and subsequent open lesions on the lips. Inability to chew and swallow may occur secondary to painful and inflamed oral mucous membranes. Weight loss may indicate inadequate nutritional consumption.

- Provide meticulous hygiene practices, keeping mucous membranes moist and intact:
  - Implement oral hygiene protocol (see Teaching Intervention Plan 22-1), including brushing teeth with soft toothbrush that is replaced on a regular basis and rinsing mouth with chlorhexidine or other recommended oral solution.
  - Apply lubricating ointment to the lips.
  Keeping mucous membranes intact reduces potential sites of entry for organisms and the development of opportunistic infections. Oral rinsing using sterile water or solutions such as chlorhexidine will decrease the incidence of developing mucositis.

- Use topical and systemic antibiotic or antifungal medications as ordered.
  Medications may be ordered to prevent infection or for treatment for specific causative organisms of oral mucous membrane infection. Topical anesthetics may be necessary to decrease oral pain. Thinning of oral mucous membrane linings increases sensitivity to oral pain.

- Use measures to promote adequate dietary intake (see Teaching Intervention Plan 22-2), including referral to a dietitian.
  Dietary modifications may be necessary to ensure the child remains hydrated and receives adequate caloric intake to promote healing and tissue integrity.

Expected Outcomes
- Child and family will demonstrate measures to prevent or minimize mucous membrane breakdown.
- Child's mucous membranes will remain intact, free from infection, soothed, and healed.

Nursing Diagnosis: Imbalanced nutrition: Less than body requirements related to nausea, vomiting, or oral mucositis

Interventions/Rationale
- Obtain nutritional history to include food likes and dislikes, daily consumption, patterns of nausea and vomiting, and effective strategies for increasing nutrient intake and managing nausea and vomiting.

  The child's nutritional patterns and responses to nutritional interventions are individual. Plan of care should build on successful strategies used at home or during previous hospitalizations.
- Document intake and output, daily weights, enteral or parenteral intake, and episodes and amounts of vomiting and diarrhea.

  Assessment provides baseline information and evidence of change in dietary patterns.
- Monitor for signs of increasing dehydration (e.g., tachycardia, less elastic skin turgor, depressed fontanels, sunken eyes, weight loss, rapid pulse, dry mucous membranes, decreasing urine output, changes in urine specific gravity).

  Early recognition may decrease or prevent dehydration.
- Monitor laboratory tests indicative of nutritional status (e.g., hemoglobin, red blood cell indices, and total protein).

  Evaluation of laboratory test results provides information about whether intake of nutrients is adequate.
- Adjust diet based on child's specific needs and challenges (e.g., nausea, mucositis). Institute and teach measures to reduce or prevent nausea and vomiting (see Nursing Interventions 22-5).

  Behavioral and dietary interventions can be effective to enhance dietary intake and manage nausea and vomiting.
- Use creative and developmentally appropriate approaches to enhancing nutritional intake (e.g., offer attractive, colorful foods in small, frequent servings; encourage family and friends to bring in favorite foods; allow child to select foods; reward intake with stickers, stars, special privileges), allow child to use feeding skills already mastered (e.g., sit young child in high chair, if able, and encourage self-feeding), and experiment with food textures and temperatures to find foods most palatable to the child.

  Participation in care may encourage the child to ingest fluids and nutrition.
- Administer supplemental vitamins and minerals as prescribed. Provide between-meal protein supplements.

  Supplements replace missing nutrients and assist with tissue repair.
- Administer IV fluid (including total parenteral nutrition and hyperlipids) as ordered (see Nursing Plan of Care 17-1).

  IV fluid replacement may be necessary to maintain hydration.
- Administer antiemetics as ordered.

  Medications can be effective in controlling nausea and vomiting. Regimen must be tailored to child's specific needs.
- Brush teeth with soft toothbrush or sponge, provide oral care every 2–4 hours, and rinse mouth with water after feedings.

  Oral care provides a clean, fresh mouth; may decrease or prevent infection; and may enhance nutritional intake.
- Coordinate nutritional approaches with nutritionist; request that special foods be available or stocked on the unit around the clock.

  Coordinating with nutritionist assists in providing the child with necessary nutrients. Inadequate nutrition further compromises the child's immune system.
- Coordinate with health care prescriber about initiating feedings or total parenteral nutrition if child is unable to maintain adequate oral intake.

  Feedings or total parenteral nutrition may be necessary to ensure that the child receives adequate nutrition.

Expected Outcomes
- Child will be able or assisted to maintain adequate fluid intake by oral, nasogastric, or IV access.
- Child's caloric intake will be adequate for age.
- Child will maintain weight that is normal for age.

Nursing Diagnosis: Anxiety related to uncertain prognosis, actual or perceived loss of body integrity, threat to self-concept
See Nursing Plan of Care 12-2

Nursing Diagnosis: Disturbed body image related to being different than peers, perceiving self as sick, loss of body part
See Nursing Plan of Care 12-2.

Nursing Diagnosis: Spiritual distress related to crisis of the illness, suffering, or death of a child
See Nursing Plan of Care 13-1.

common chromosomal abnormalities and familial tendencies (in identical twins and siblings) have also been associated with an elevated risk for childhood leukemia.

In addition to genetics, environmental factors (e.g., exposure to radiation, toxic chemicals, and chemotherapy), viral infections (e.g., Epstein-Barr virus [EBV] or HIV), and immunodeficiencies or abnormalities of the immune system have been linked with leukemia (National Cancer Institute, SEER Program, 2009). The reason that leukemia develops in any particular child is rarely known, but tendencies or similarities that have been documented remain of interest to health care providers.

ACUTE LYMPHOBLASTIC LEUKEMIA

ALL accounts for approximately 78% of childhood leukemia in the United States. Annually, ALL occurs at a rate of approximately 35 cases per million. Approximately 2,900 children and adolescents younger than 20 years of age are diagnosed with ALL each year in the United States. The incidence of ALL is highest in Hispanic children (43 cases per million) and also substantially higher for white children than for black children, with a nearly three-fold higher incidence at 2 to 3 years for white children when compared with black children (National Cancer Institute, 2008a). Genetic factors are presumed to play an important role in the origin of ALL.

The initial WBC count is perhaps the most important prognostic factor. Children with WBC counts greater than 50,000/mm³ tend to have a poorer prognosis, and those with WBC counts greater than 100,000/mm³ have a particularly poor prognosis. Age at diagnosis also influences the prognosis, with children younger than age 2 years and older than age 10 years at diagnosis having a relatively poor prognosis. Children younger than 1 year of age have the least favorable prognosis. In most reports, girls have a better prognosis than boys. Current statistics indicate that slightly over 85% of children with ALL survive at least 5 years past diagnosis (National Cancer Institute, SEER Program, 2009).

Pathophysiology

ALL causes extreme proliferation of immature lymphocytes referred to as **blast cells**. This disease originates in B or T lymphoid cells (with B-lymphoblastic leukemia more prevalent [>80% of cases] than T-lymphoblastic leukemia [National Cancer Institute, 2006]). The leukemic cells proliferate (multiply) rapidly and pack the bone marrow. They compete for space and interfere with normal blood cell development (hematopoiesis), possibly spreading to other lymph tissues and organs. Therefore, a child with ALL often presents with signs and symptoms related to failure of normal hematopoiesis (anemia, neutropenia, and thrombocytopenia).

Immunobiologic study of ALL determines which lymphocytes have been transformed into leukemic cells and identifies the stage of cellular development in which the leukemia occurred. Abnormalities in chromosomal numbers and structures are also examined to assist in predicting response to treatment and long-term prognosis.

A common feature of ALL is **extramedullary** disease (systemic disease outside the blood and bone marrow). The most common sites of extramedullary spread are the CNS, testes, liver, kidneys, and spleen. Extramedullary disease can be present at time of diagnosis or at the time of recurrence.

Assessment

Most children diagnosed with leukemia usually have been symptomatic for several weeks, with symptoms being assumed by the family and/or primary care provider to be the flu or other common childhood illnesses. Signs and symptoms of leukemia are directly related to

---

CHART 22-1 **Clinical and Diagnostic Features of Leukemia**

Fatigue, weakness

Pallor

Fever

Bruising

Bleeding (e.g., petechiae or purpura)

Weight loss, anorexia

Swollen gums

Sore throat, recurrent infections, flulike symptoms

Abdominal pain, nausea, vomiting

Bone pain

Lymphadenopathy

Splenomegaly or hepatomegaly

Elevated leukocyte count

Decreased hemoglobin

Decreased platelet count

---

the degree of bone marrow infiltration and the spread of disease (Chart 22-1). A CBC followed by a lumbar puncture, bone marrow aspiration, and biopsy are the first diagnostic procedures completed to confirm the diagnosis of leukemia.

Interdisciplinary Interventions

Treatment for children with ALL is determined by the child's WBC count, age, chromosomal abnormalities, and extent of disease. When all factors have been evaluated, a risk category is determined and combination therapy is initiated. The first goal is to induce a remission with combination chemotherapy. Children with ALL achieve remission 98% of the time with induction therapy. After remission is attained, children receive further intensive chemotherapy and then maintenance chemotherapy over a 2- to 3-year period. Males traditionally are treated for a longer time than females because of the concern with testes as a "sanctuary site" (place where leukemia cells hide). Chemotherapy and possibly radiation therapy to the CNS may also be used to kill leukemia cells that are present in the cerebrospinal fluid (CSF) because the CSF is also considered a sanctuary site for leukemia. Supportive care is ongoing throughout treatment to prevent acute bleeding or infectious complications.

ALERT *Acute bleeding can be a potentially life-threatening emergency for children with leukemia. The platelet count should be more than 10,000–20,000/mm³ at all times, and the child with evidence of bleeding or extreme bruising should receive a platelet transfusion.*

Thorough handwashing or using antibacterial gel, limiting visitors and exposure to germs, and prophylactic antibiotics are key components for the care of the child with leukemia.

Children with extremely high-risk prognostic factors at diagnosis, children in whom initial therapy fails to achieve remission (i.e., refractory), and children who relapse receive more intensive combination chemotherapy and possibly HSCT. This aggressive approach has helped to increase disease-free long-term survival rates. Supportive care and observation are more prolonged and intense for this group of children.

Community Care

Children with all types of leukemia are primarily managed in the home. Hospitalizations are required for infusion of certain chemotherapeutic agents and when the child's health status is severely compromised (e.g., fever, child is dehydrated). Many tertiary care centers are able to provide chemotherapy infusions on an outpatient basis in an infusion center specifically designed for providing these types of treatments. Managing the child's care needs in the home depends on the side effects of treatment the child is experiencing. The "Treatment Modalities" section of this chapter discusses these therapeutic interventions in detail. The goal of home care is to promote the child's personal growth and development while managing the complex physical and psychosocial challenges the diagnosis of cancer brings to the child and his or her family. The child is encouraged to participate in school and community activities while always being mindful of his or her current health status and limiting activities as needed to prevent injury, protect from ill contacts, and ensure the child is comfortable.

ACUTE MYELOID LEUKEMIA

AML represents approximately 15% to 20% of all childhood leukemia cases. AML is equally distributed among races and sexes. Most research indicates that children with a high WBC count at diagnosis have a poorer outcome (Creutzig et al., 2004). Although much progress has been made during the past decade in treating this disease, the 5-year survival rate for children younger than age 15 years is 60% (National Cancer Institute, SEER Program, 2009).

The exact cause of AML is unknown; however, certain risk factors are associated with the development of this disease, including radiation exposure in utero, previous treatment with alkylating agents, maternal cigarette or marijuana use during pregnancy, history of a previous malignancy, trisomy 21, Fanconi anemia, and environmental exposure to chemicals (especially benzene) and pesticides (National Cancer Institute, SEER Program, 2009).

Pathophysiology

Most cases of AML are believed to result from a malignant transformation of a single blood stem cell in the bone marrow. Most often, this transformation occurs in a myeloid cell line. The malignant clone causes a proliferation of immature, relatively undifferentiated cells that replace healthy bone marrow elements. The

immature cells accumulate in the bone marrow and in extramedullary sites, interfering with bone marrow function.

The term *acute myeloid leukemia* refers to a heterogeneous group of malignancies that have been classified into subtypes according to the pathology and biology of the malignant cells. The FAB system is the former classification system used to describe the eight subtypes of AML based on morphology, which range from M0 and M1 for AML without differentiation, through M7, which indicates acute megakaryoblastic leukemia. The WHO classification system has replaced the FAB classification system for AML because it uses relevant morphologic, cytogenetic, immunophenotypic, and clinical information.

Assessment

Children with AML may present with a few seemingly benign, flulike symptoms or they may have severe, life-threatening symptoms (see Chart 22-1). Bleeding or severe hemorrhaging, as well as extremely high WBC counts ($>100,000/mm^3$), is often seen in these children. Extramedullary spread of disease, particularly in the CNS at diagnosis, may occur. Initially, the same diagnostic procedures and nursing assessments are done as for the child with ALL, including bone marrow aspiration biopsy and a lumbar puncture.

Interdisciplinary Interventions

Initial treatment of AML is targeted at preventing life-threatening complications and achieving remission. Immediate blood component therapy, infection prevention, and initiation of combination chemotherapy drugs to reduce leukemia burden are crucial treatments.

After remission is achieved and complications are no longer life threatening, treatment of the CNS with more intensive chemotherapy is recommended. Allogeneic HSCT is used for high-risk patients with an appropriately matched donor (siblings preferred) and for low-risk patients who relapse. Biotherapy, or targeted therapy, has also been incorporated into the treatment plan for some children with AML. Children are often hospitalized for extended periods to undergo aggressive treatment and for treatment of subsequent infections that require vigilant supportive care and protective isolation (Clinical Judgment 22-1).

CHRONIC MYELOID LEUKEMIA

CML is a proliferation of mature myelocytic cells in which mutation can begin years before the onset of symptoms. This disease presents, is diagnosed, or may progress through three different phases: chronic phase, accelerated phase, and blast crisis phase. A hallmark chromosomal abnormality is the translocation of chromosomes 9 and 22 t(9;22), identified as the *Philadelphia chromosome*. CML presents as an increased proliferation of myeloid cells, up to 100 times the normal amount. The elevation of the WBC count and the degree of organ and lymph node involvement affect the prognosis. The phase of the disease at the time of clinical presentation also determines the outcome.

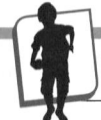

CLINICAL JUDGMENT 22-1

The Immunosuppressed Child With Fever

Jasmine is a 4-year-old girl with leukemia. She completed her most recent course of chemotherapy 7 days ago. She is now being admitted to the hospital with a fever of 101.8° F (38.8° C), chills, a WBC count with an ANC of 475/mm^3, a platelet count of 59,000/mm^3, and hemoglobin level of 8.8 g/dL.

Questions

1. What additional assessment data should be obtained at this time by members of the health care team?
2. The father states that Jasmine has not been around any sick people. He is confused as to how she could have gotten ill. What should the nurse tell him?
3. The physician orders include blood cultures, a chest radiograph, urine and throat cultures, IV fluids, and antibiotics. Which of these orders should be completed first?
4. What precautions should be taken given the child's vital signs and blood analysis findings?
5. Jasmine's 6-year-old brother is standing outside the room crying. He says, "It's all my fault she's sick. I spit on her." What should he be told about his sister's current situation?

Answers

1. Vital signs, type of chemotherapy last received, presence of mouth sores, redness or irritation at the venous access device site, intake and output history, ANC, and oxygen saturation measured using a pulse oximeter.
2. Most infections are from commonly occurring bacteria in the child's system; these bacteria are harmful to Jasmine only because of her depressed immune system.
3. Cultures of the blood, urine, and throat should be taken before starting antibiotics. As soon as these tests are completed, IV fluids should be started and antibiotics given immediately.

Vital signs should be monitored carefully. Chest radiographs can be obtained after antibiotic therapy has been initiated.

4. Jasmine is neutropenic, thrombocytopenic, and anemic. Neutropenic precautions (see Community Care 22-2) as well as precautions to prevent and reduce the risk of bleeding should be used.
5. Reassure the boy that his spitting did not cause his sister to be sick. Encourage him to go in the room and be with his sister. Instruct him on good handwashing techniques to help protect his sister from getting sicker and explain how he can do this at home to help her avoid getting an infection.

Pathophysiology

Little is known about the cause of CML. It is a rare disease in children, accounting for 1% to 3% of all cases of childhood leukemia (National Cancer Institute, 2008a). There are no significant differences in incidence among race or sexes. Ionizing radiation exposure may be the only environmental risk factor associated with this disease.

Most patients are diagnosed during the chronic phase of the disease. During this phase, CML symptoms are less intense and the WBCs can still fight infection. During the accelerated phase, the child may develop anemia, the number of WBCs may increase or decrease, or the number of platelets may decrease. During this phase, the number of blast cells increases. The spleen may swell, and the child may truly feel ill. During the blast crisis phase, the number of blast cells increases in the bone marrow and blood. Red blood cells and platelets decrease, and the child is prone to infection. The child may also be lethargic and have shortness of breath, stomach pain, bone pain, and/or bleeding during this phase.

Assessment

As mentioned, children with CML may present during the chronic, accelerated, or the blast phase of the disease. In many cases, the onset of the disease is chronic: slow and not easily detected. The diagnosis may be made when a blood count is performed for another reason. During this chronic phase, children may present with nonspecific symptoms of pallor, low-grade fever, weight loss, anorexia, and night sweats. The chronic phase can last up to 3 to 4 years before progressing to a myeloid or lymphoid **blast crisis**, in which only immature leukemia cells are produced. In this case, the blast phase symptoms appear more like those of acute leukemia, with the presence of splenomegaly, bone marrow dysfunction, and lymphadenopathy.

Interdisciplinary Interventions

The initial goal of therapy is to achieve remission with chemotherapy and biotherapy. Children in the chronic phase of CML respond very well to tyrosine–kinase inhibitors such as oral imatinib (Gleevec), dasatinib (Sprycel), or nilotinib (Tasigna). The treatment usually returns the level of blood cells to normal and shrinks the spleen to normal size. Most children will not experience bleeding or unusual infections at this time. Some may need chemotherapy initially to decrease their WBC count. Most children being treated for chronic phase CML can participate in their day-to-day activities. With drug treatment, most children are in remission and symptom free for long periods of time. However, drug treatment does not cure these children of CML. Regular checkups, including blood and bone marrow analyses, are needed to assess for any signs that a relapse has occurred and the CML has returned. CML is likely to return if drug treatment is stopped. Children who do not respond to these oral agents, who develop resistance to the drugs, or who progress to the accelerated or blast phase may undergo an allogeneic HSCT for curative treatment.

CENTRAL NERVOUS SYSTEM TUMORS

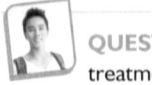 QUESTION: What is the incidence, prognosis, and treatment of brain tumors compared to bone tumors like George has?

Tumors of the CNS are the second most common malignancy in childhood. In the United States, approximately 2,500 to 3,500 (National Cancer Institute, 2012a) children younger than 20 years of age are newly diagnosed each year (National Cancer Institute, SEER Program, 2009). Brain tumors, although rare during the first year of life, tend to occur most frequently in children younger than age 10 years. Incidence is roughly equal in males and females. Approximately 74% of all children with CNS tumors demonstrate a 5-year survival rate (National Cancer Institute, 2008a).

There are important differences between the types and locations of tumors in children when compared with adults. Astrocytomas account for 50% of all childhood brain tumors; however, some can be benign. Medulloblastomas account for 20% of all childhood brain tumors and are the most common malignant CNS tumor. Both are infratentorial tumors (Watral, 2009). In children, 50% to 60% of brain tumors are *infratentorial* (located in the cerebellum, fourth ventricle, or brain stem), whereas in adults, they are primarily *supratentorial* (located in the cerebrum). Also, 75% or more of brain tumors in children occur in the midline (third and fourth ventricles, optic chiasm, and brain stem) (Kuttesh et al., 2011).

The cause of CNS tumors remains unknown. Direct correlations exist between certain hereditary and familial syndromes (e.g., neurofibromatosis [50-fold increased risk], tuberous sclerosis, Li-Fraumeni syndrome, retinoblastoma) and CNS tumors (National Cancer Institute, 2008a). Environmental factors are also related to the incidence of CNS tumors and include industrial and chemical toxins, ionizing radiation, and exogenous immunosuppression, as seen in transplant recipients. Studies have investigated prenatal and perinatal exposures to these risk factors that may correlate with the increased incidence of brain tumors in children. Brain tumors have been associated with certain parental occupations, particularly those in which parents were exposed to electromagnetic fields or ionizing radiation (National Cancer Institute, 2008a).

Various types of ionizing radiation exposures in children also have been associated with CNS tumors. These events include therapeutic doses of ionizing radiation to the head (i.e., treatment of tinea capitis, exposure to radiographs, radioisotopic contrast media, ultraviolet radiation, and nuclear bomb fallout). Several reports document the development of a primary brain tumor after cranial radiation received for a prior malignancy such as ALL (National Cancer Institute, 2008a).

Pathophysiology

Brain tumor is a general term for many histologic categories. Each type has distinctly different clinical manifestations, modes of treatment, and outcomes. Of all pediatric CNS tumors, astrocytomas located at cerebellar, cerebral, and brain stem sites are the most common (approximately 50% of cases), followed by medulloblastoma (22%), other gliomas (15%), ependymomas (10%), and others (3%) (Blaney et al., 2010). Table 22-3 summarizes the major types of pediatric CNS tumors.

CNS tumors are categorized by their histologic characteristics and degree of malignancy. This is termed **tumor grading**. CNS tumors are frequently described as low-grade or high-grade. Low-grade tumors are slow growing, contain a few mitotic cells, and show no evidence of necrosis or vascular proliferation. Although they are less malignant than high-grade tumors, their progress may go undetected for some time, causing major damage to adjacent tissue. High-grade tumors are rapid growing, contain multiple mitotic cells, and show evidence of necrosis and endothelial and vascular proliferation.

Assessment

Children with a suspected CNS tumor require a thorough physical and neurologic examination. The clinical presentation of a child with a CNS tumor depends on the size and location of the tumor and the child's age and developmental stage. Most brain tumors in children arise in the posterior fossa and result in initial symptoms associated with increased intracranial pressure (ICP) and hydrocephalus caused by compression of the fourth ventricle. The most common complaint in children older than 2 years of age associated with increased ICP is headache (see Chapter 21). Activities such as straining with a bowel movement, coughing, or, in severe cases, changing the position of the head cause the headache to worsen. However, the occurrence of a headache does not always fit the classic picture of headache associated with increased ICP. The head pain may be more vague and nonspecific.

ALERT   *Any headache associated with vomiting or lethargy should be evaluated immediately by a physician to rule out increased ICP.*

TABLE 22-3   Types of Central Nervous System Tumors

Type	Description	Assessment	Interdisciplinary Interventions
Cerebellar astrocytoma	Accounts for 15%–25% of all types of astrocytomas Occurs most often during the first decade of life, with a peak incidence at age 5–8 years Two types: classic or pilocytic	Insidious onset, slow progression, most symptomatic for 2–7 months (some possibly several years) before diagnosis Majority presenting with symptoms of increased ICP Focal neurologic signs such as ataxia, nystagmus, and head tilt Decreased muscle tone, abnormal reflexes, and speech characterized by pauses between syllables (scanning speech)	Surgical resection Radiation therapy only if residual tumor exists Chemotherapy not useful; typically reserved for recurrent or progressive tumor growth or as adjunct therapy for children with high-grade astrocytomas
Cerebral astrocytoma	Grading as high (highly malignant) or low Accounts for approximately 25% of all types of astrocytomas Located in cerebrum; infiltrative Prognosis favorable with complete surgical resection, minimal neurologic deficits postoperatively, low-grade tumor, and slower onset of symptoms; poorer prognosis than cerebellar astrocytomas	Initial symptoms variable with tumor location within cerebrum; symptoms progressive and increasing Nonspecific and nonlocalizing signs of increased ICP (in 75% of children, regardless of tumor location) Papilledema (edema of the optic nerve) common at diagnosis Grand mal–type seizures (in 25% of children)	Complete resection difficult (location of tumor dictating extent of surgical resection possible) Preoperative anticonvulsant therapy Adjunctive radiation or chemotherapy (under investigation in national clinical trials) Radiation delayed until evidence of recurrence appears
Medulloblastoma	Cerebellar tumor composed of medulloblasts (undifferentiated neural tube cells) Usually located in the midline of the cerebellum; possibly occurring in cerebellar hemispheres Most common primary posterior fossa tumor (approximately one in five cases of childhood brain tumors [National Cancer Institute, 2006]) Peak incidence at age 5–7 years Have highest rate of extraneural (outside CNS) spread, with bone and bone marrow accounting for 80% of metastatic sites; also possible spread to lungs, liver, and lymph nodes Children younger than age 3 years frequently with poorer prognosis; children older than age 3 years who undergo surgery and total neuraxis (brain and spine) radiation with better chance of long-term survival than those younger than age 3 years and in whom the entire tumor was not removed and the disease has spread to other areas of the body (National Cancer Institute, 2006)	Symptomatic for less than 2 months before diagnosis resulting from rapidly growing tumor and location in the posterior fossa Initial symptoms associated with increased ICP: • Headaches, decreased alertness, visual disturbances, irritability, seizures, and motor impairment • Progressive lower extremity ataxia as tumor enlarges and displaces surrounding brain tissue • Diplopia and multiple cranial nerve deficits with pressure and tumor infiltration at the brain stem	Complete surgical resection CT or MRI at 72 hours postoperatively to evaluate tumor resection Radiation therapy (tumor very radiosensitive) routinely to entire brain and spine Chemotherapy in high-risk cases, such as when child has recurrent disease, and in very young children (younger than age 2–3 years) to delay the use of radiation to the brain

TABLE 22-3	Types of Central Nervous System Tumors *(Continued)*		
Type	**Description**	**Assessment**	**Interdisciplinary Interventions**
Brain stem glioma	Accounts for 10% of all CNS tumors Median age of occurrence is 5–9 years Pons the most common site of occurrence, although tumors can also arise in the medulla or midbrain (Rosenblum, 2005) Poor overall prognosis; survival rate less than 10%, with a median survival time of 2 years (Rosenblum, 2005)	Insidious onset of symptoms, with a duration of approximately 3–5 months Characteristic triad of signs and symptoms arising from early interference with the functioning of the cranial nerve nuclei, pyramidal tracts, and cerebellar pathways Paresis of conjugate gaze (eye movement not in unison); most important sign for localizing the lesion; occurring in more than half of these children Pyramidal tract involvement (present in 80%–90%); possibly masked by the more obvious ataxia or may present chiefly as subtle changes in gait, handedness, or posture of an extremity; hemiparesis and bilateral reflex changes Cerebellar pathway signs: horizontal nystagmus (in almost one third of cases) and truncal and extremity ataxia, indicating involvement of corticopontocerebellar fibers running through the brain stem	Most nonresectable because of location Radiation (main treatment modality) Adjuvant chemotherapy not used because of unproved efficacy; possible use for palliation Biotherapy used
Ependymoma	Third most common infratentorial tumor Accounts for 5%–10% of posterior fossa tumors; highest incidence among children during first 7 years of life (Blaney et al., 2006) Arise from ependymal cells Histologically two types: low-grade (highly cellular, with a characteristic pattern of rosettes around blood vessels) and high-grade (anaplastic ependymomas with rosette formation and necrosis, mitoses, and increased cellularity) Survival variable from several months to 10 years or longer; children with complete resection have best prognosis (Blaney et al., 2006)	Average duration of symptoms: 2–3 months. Symptoms variable based on tumor location If tumor in posterior fossa, increased ICP with papilledema most common If tumor supratentorial, local motor weakness, visual disturbances, and seizures	Complete resection followed by radiation Total and near-total resections more easily achieved in supratentorial tumors; such resections less common in the posterior fossa as a result of common infiltration of brain stem and higher operative morbidity

Information from Watral, M. (2009). Central nervous system tumors. In N. E. Kline (Ed.), *Essentials of pediatric hematology/oncology nursing: A core curriculum* (3rd ed., pp. 28–32). Glenview, IL: Association of Pediatric Hematology/Oncology Nurses.

An array of symptoms specific to certain tumor locations assists the health care team in localizing the particular tumor region in the brain (Chart 22-2).

Diagnostic Tests

Initial evaluation for a child with a suspected brain tumor can be achieved by either CT or MRI. A CT scan is more appropriate for children in whom sedatives are contraindicated—for example, children with increased ICP, a history of seizures, or changes in neurologic status. When performed with and without contrast, CT can detect 95% of CNS tumors. MRI is the image of choice for a medically stable and cooperative child because of its safety and its ability to collect detailed information. Because of its ability to image in three planes, MRI is particularly useful in diagnosing infiltrative tumors of the brain stem. The presence of calcification, hemorrhage, or cysts may assist in identifying certain types of tumors. Sedation and analgesia or general anesthesia may be used to keep the infant or younger child quiet and calm during the

CHART 22-2 Signs and Symptoms of Brain Tumors

Infratentorial Tumors (Brain Stem and Cerebellar)

Increased ICP

Ataxia (gait, truncal)

Nystagmus

Head tilt

Diplopia

Cranial nerve deficits

Hypotonia

Abnormal reflexes

Changes in speech

Hemiparesis

Positive Babinski sign

Supratentorial Tumors (Tempoparietal, Temporal Lobe, Frontal Lobe, Occipital, Midline)

Headaches

Seizures

Hemiparesis

Hyperreflexia

Sensory losses

Visual disturbances

Aphasia

Personality changes

Growth failure

Endocrine changes

procedure. PET, where available, is also used to image the tumor and assess its level of activity.

A lumbar puncture is usually performed to obtain CSF for analysis when no signs of obstructive hydrocephalus or increased ICP are present (see Fig. 21-9). The fluid is tested for the presence of tumor cells as well as for decreased sugar, increased protein, and increased enzymes.

Nursing Diagnoses and Outcomes

General nursing diagnoses and outcomes are presented in Nursing Plan of Care 22-1. In addition, the following diagnosis may apply to the child with a brain tumor:

Nursing Diagnosis: Risk for injury related to seizure activity

Outcome: Child will remain free of injury during a seizure.

Interdisciplinary Interventions

Complete surgical resection, when possible, is the treatment of choice for children with brain tumors. The location of the brain tumor is the factor that determines the surgical approach and resectability of the mass and surrounding brain tissue. In some instances, a resection is too risky, and a biopsy is done for histologic confirmation.

The child usually requires monitoring in a pediatric intensive care unit for 48 to 72 hours postoperatively

(Clinical Judgment 22-2). Frequent assessment of vital signs, neurologic status, and mental status is crucial to identify early signs of increased ICP secondary to cerebral edema. IV steroids are used intraoperatively to minimize edema of the brain tissue. Anticonvulsants may also be ordered prophylactically to prevent seizures. Children who have hypothalamic, pituitary, or other suprasellar tumors are at high risk for SIADH or diabetes insipidus (DI) and should be managed in collaboration with an endocrinologist. In these cases, special attention must be paid to abnormal urine output and serum sodium levels.

Radiation therapy may be used alone or in combination with surgery. The success of radiation therapy depends on the location and radiosensitivity of the tumor and on the expertise of the radiation oncologist. Young children are at high risk for severe sequelae associated with radiation of immature brains (learning disorders, varying degrees of cognitive challenge). Thus, radiotherapy is not recommended in children younger than age 3 years.

The nurse plays a key role in educating the child and family and in managing side effects related to radiation therapy, such as nausea, hair loss, and anorexia (Fig. 22-10). It is extremely important that the child lie still during the entire radiotherapy session. Precision is required to maximize the dose of radiation delivered to the tumor and to minimize the effects in surrounding tissue. Very young children require sedation or general anesthesia for each therapy session. Special devices such as soft blocks, Styrofoam molds, tape, and Velcro straps may also be used to immobilize the head and neck. The nurse is responsible for preparing the child for sedation and for monitoring the child's status during sedation and throughout the recovery period. (See Chapter 10 for an in-depth discussion of sedatives and nursing responsibilities associated with sedation and analgesia.)

The efficacy of chemotherapy in treating brain tumors requires further investigation. Many studies have

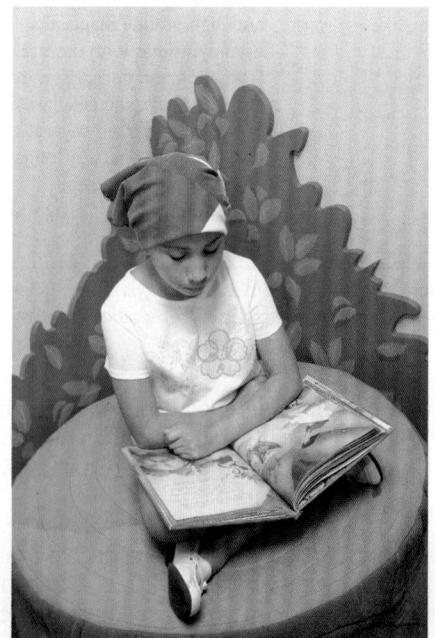

Figure 22-10 A young girl wears a bandanna to conceal her lack of hair.

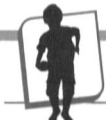

CLINICAL JUDGMENT 22-2

Postoperative Care of a Child With a CNS Tumor

Remus, a 4-year-old boy, was brought to his health care provider with complaints of irritability, headaches, morning vomiting, and clumsiness. Examination of the child revealed papilledema, photophobia, and ataxia. A CT scan was performed that revealed a large mass in the fourth ventricle with significant hydrocephalus. The child was started on steroids overnight and had a craniotomy the next day. The pathologic diagnosis was medulloblastoma. You are caring for Remus 3 days after surgery on the pediatric hematology/oncology unit.

Questions

1. What aspects of the physical assessment are of particular importance?
2. Which information might reveal the presence of neurologic compromise?
3. The grandparents come to visit Remus and are overheard telling his mother that no therapy will do any good and that she should just take him home to die. Using your knowledge of medulloblastoma treatment and outcomes, how would you intervene?
4. In anticipation of the child's future needs for chemotherapy and ongoing IV therapy, placement of a CVC was completed at the same time as the craniotomy. What are the nursing interventions associated with care of Remus's CVC?
5. Based on the treatment plan of chemotherapy and radiation therapy, what teaching elements will be necessary for the family before discharge?

Answers

1. Vital signs, neurologic assessment, signs of infection, drainage from surgical or external ventriculostomy site, intake and output.
2. Decrease in level of consciousness, vomiting, ataxia, major variations between intake and output.
3. Reassure the grandparents that successful treatments are available for children with brain tumors. If approved by the child's parents, invite the grandparents to the family conference during which the plan for determining the spread of disease and the accompanying treatment plan will be discussed.
4. Assess the CVC for patency and the CVC site for signs of infection; ensure that the dressing is dry and intact. Make sure the CVC is properly secured. Participate in educational interventions with the family to ensure they know all aspects of CVC care and medication administration.
5. A comprehensive teaching plan with the child and family will include assessment of and managing for side effects/toxicities of the treatment regimen (chemotherapy and radiation); medication administration; managing nutritional needs; home care of the CVC, managing pain, and providing comfort measures; mouth care instruction; and information about neutropenia, anemia, thrombocytopenia, signs and symptoms of infection, and fever precautions.

demonstrated either regression of symptoms or tumor regression with the use of several chemotherapeutic agents that are capable of penetrating the blood–brain barrier. Care of children undergoing treatment for a brain tumor with either one or a combination of the modes discussed requires collaboration among many disciplines and clear and effective communication with the family.

ANSWER: CNS tumors usually affect children younger than 10 years of age and osteogenic sarcoma usually occurs during midadolescence. The CNS tumors and bone tumors have about the same statistical rate of survival—around 65%. For both, the first treatment of choice is surgery, and for both, there is an indication of genetic predisposition.

Community Care

As with most pediatric malignancies, after the diagnostic phase and initial treatment phase (e.g., surgery) are complete and the child is clinically stable, the child is discharged home. Ongoing care for a CNS tumor will include both inpatient admissions and outpatient visits for chemotherapy and radiation treatments (see "Treatment Modalities" section earlier in this chapter for a comprehensive review of interventions to manage complications of therapy, growth and development concerns, and late effects of therapy).

Children with CNS tumors may need additional support such as physical therapy, speech therapy, and other rehabilitative services, depending on the degree and extent of neurologic loss as a result of the tumor and/or treatment sequelae. Recovery may take weeks or months, depending on the severity of symptoms the child is experiencing. Some children may never fully regain certain physical and cognitive functions.

LYMPHOMAS

Malignant lymphomas represent the third most common type of childhood cancer. These neoplasms occur in the lymphoid and reticuloendothelial systems, which are widely distributed throughout the body. Hodgkin lymphoma and NHL are the two major types of lymphomas. Hodgkin lymphoma is generally fairly localized and can be treated as a solid tumor. NHLs are often disseminated and must be treated as systemic disease.

HODGKIN LYMPHOMA

Hodgkin lymphoma is a lymphoid malignancy that arises from a single lymph node or lymph node region. It accounts for 6% of pediatric malignancies diagnosed in the United States. The annual incidence in the United States is 7.3 per million white children and 5.2 per million black children younger than age 15 years. The exact cause is unknown, but epidemiologic studies suggest an infectious agent. Studies have reported an increased risk of Hodgkin lymphoma in close relatives, particularly same-sex siblings and twins. Children who have had EBV are also known to have higher risk for Hodgkin lymphoma (Metzger et al., 2010). This higher risk may be linked to genetic or environmental factors associated with immunocompetence.

Pathophysiology

The lymphoma spreads by extending to contiguous (connected) lymph node areas. In advanced disease, it disseminates and may involve any organ in the body but particularly involves the spleen, liver, bones, lungs, and bone marrow. Histologic diagnosis of Hodgkin lymphoma is determined by the presence of Reed-Sternberg cells. The presence of these cells alone is not diagnostic, however, because similar cells can be seen in infectious mononucleosis, other reactive lymphoid hyperplasias, and other neoplasms. Hodgkin lymphoma is classified by the predominating cells. The most common classification system used for Hodgkin lymphoma is the WHO classification. This classification describes two broad classes of Hodgkin lymphoma: nodular lymphocyte predominant and classical Hodgkin lymphoma. Classical Hodgkin lymphoma is divided into four subtypes: (1) nodular sclerosis (40% children, 70% adolescents); (2) mixed cellularity (30%; more in children); (3) lymphocyte-rich (5%); and (4) lymphocyte-depleted (rare in children). They are listed in relative prognostic order, from best to worst (Baggott et al., 2011).

Staging is a method of defining the anatomic extent of detectable disease at the time of diagnosis. The standardized staging system for Hodgkin lymphoma provides prognostic information and serves as the primary rationale for treatment decisions. Children with stage I and stage II lymphoma have 10-year survival rates of more than 90% and relapse-free survival rates of 70% to 90%. Children with stage III lymphoma have 5-year survival rates of 95%. The prognosis for children with stage IV lymphoma continues to improve, with a 5-year survival rate of 80% (National Cancer Institute, SEER Program, 2009).

Assessment

Characteristically, the first sign of Hodgkin lymphoma is painless, progressive lymph node enlargement, with two thirds of the cases involving a site above the diaphragm and one third of the cases involving a site below the diaphragm. Other signs and symptoms vary according to the sites of the enlarged nodes, resulting in local tissue compression. For example, mediastinal lymphadenopathy may produce a persistent nonproductive cough. Signs and symptoms of Hodgkin lymphoma include

- Cervical or supraclavicular lymphadenopathy (60% to 90% of cases)
- Painless, firm nodes that are movable in surrounding tissue
- Hepatomegaly, splenomegaly, or both in generalized disease
- Anorexia
- Weight loss of 10% or more within previous 6 months
- Malaise
- Lethargy
- Drenching night sweats
- Fever of 38° C (100.4° F) or higher occurring for at least 3 consecutive days

Certain systemic symptoms are considered prognostically important. Children with unexplained weight loss of more than 10% during the past 6 months, unexplained fever with temperatures of more than 100.4° F (38° C), or drenching night sweats are classified "B" in the staging procedure. The absence of these symptoms places the child in the "A" classification. The percentage of children with B classification increases in advanced disease.

Diagnostic Tests

Diagnostic evaluation of the child with suspected Hodgkin lymphoma involves many tests and studies including a CBC; erythrocyte sedimentation rate (ESR); serum copper, liver, and renal function tests; alkaline phosphatase assay; baseline thyroid stimulating hormone; and free thyroxine (T_4) measurement. Bilateral bone aspiration and biopsy are completed to assess for the presence of leukemia. Posteroanterior and lateral chest radiographs, chest CT scan, gallium scan or PET scan (now considered the gold standard in evaluating Hodgkin lymphoma), bone scan (for bony involvement), abdominal and pelvic CT scan, and MRI are used to determine location and extent of lymph node and organ involvement. Surgical biopsy of the involved site is necessary to analyze tissue for histologic, morphologic, cytogenic, immunophenotypic, molecular, and enzymatic properties.

Interdisciplinary Interventions

The goal of treatment is to cure the child of the disease while minimizing treatment-related toxicities. Children with localized lymphoma may be treated with radiation therapy alone. However, most children are treated with both radiation and chemotherapy (Yahalom, 2006). Radiation treatment may be involved field for localized lymphoma (radiation limited to areas of confirmed lymph node involvement) or extended field for advanced disease (treatment of adjacent uninvolved lymph node regions). In unfavorable or advanced disease, the child may receive total nodal radiation. When possible, radiation therapy is delayed until the child is 8 years old to prevent retardation of bone growth and soft-tissue development. Chemotherapy is the primary treatment in advanced disease.

Community Care

Care of the child at home focuses on managing side effects of therapy (e.g., nausea, vomiting, risk for infection) and supporting the child's desire and ability to maintain normal developmental activities. The "Treatment Modalities" section discusses such issues as reentry into school and coping with the psychosocial effects of the diagnosis of cancer on the child and family. Most relapses of Hodgkin lymphoma occur within 3 years of diagnosis (Androkites, 2009). Thus, the need to ensure the child completes all chemotherapy and radiation treatments is paramount, as is the need to be evaluated on a regular basis to ensure no relapse has occurred and the child and family are coping adequately with the diagnosis, treatment, and long-term outcomes.

NON-HODGKIN LYMPHOMA

NHL is a malignant disorder of the lymphocytes that affects the cells and organs of the immune system. Generally, there is rapid onset, with widespread disease noted at the time of diagnosis. Peak incidence occurs at ages 7 to 11 years. Incidence in boys is three to four times greater compared to girls. The highest incidence rates of NHL exist in the United States and Canada (National Cancer Institute, SEER Program, 2009). A higher incidence of NHL has been noted in several population groups, specifically individuals infected with HIV or EBV and those with congenital immunodeficiency syndromes such as Wiskott-Aldrich syndrome, Bloom syndrome, and severe combined immunodeficiency syndrome. In addition, patients whose immune systems have been suppressed with medications for other illnesses have a higher risk for this cancer (Metzger et al., 2010; National Cancer Institute, 2008a).

Tumor burden (the number and size of tumors present determined by laboratory analysis of LDH, uric acid, and lactic acid) at the time of presentation is generally considered the most important prognostic factor. Current staging systems do not accurately reflect tumor burden. Whether disease is localized or advanced is also important. For instance, CNS involvement is thought to be a poor prognostic indicator. The 5-year survival rate in children is 83.8% (National Cancer Institute, SEER Program, 2009).

Pathophysiology

In NHL, the malignant cells appear undifferentiated, and the pattern of infiltration is diffuse. The disease has a rapid onset and presents with widespread involvement. NHL is believed to result from genetic aberrations that influence cell proliferation, differentiation, and cell death (Androkites, 2009). The WHO, along with European and American scientists, developed the Revised European-American Classification of Lymphoid Neoplasms (the REAL system), which is now the most widely accepted classification for pediatric NHL (Baggott et al., 2011). The REAL system classifies NHL by histology into four types: (1) lymphoblastic lymphoma; (2) Burkitt or Burkitt-like lymphoma; (3) diffuse large B-cell lymphoma; and (4) anaplastic large-cell lymphoma. A staging system is also used to identify the extent of the disease and thereby dictate the extent and duration of therapy. The most common and widely used staging system for pediatric NHL is the St. Jude Staging System (Chart 22-3).

Assessment

Because most lymphomas are generalized at the time of diagnosis, most children are diagnosed with stage III or IV disease. The most common sites of nodal involvement are intra-abdominal, mediastinal, peripheral nodal, and nasopharyngeal. The course of symptoms is generally brief, ranging from a few days to a few weeks. Signs and symptoms vary based on the cell type or histologic appearance and the specific organs

---

CHART 22-3 | **Staging for Non-Hodgkin Lymphoma (St. Jude Staging System)**

Stage I
- A single tumor (extranodal) or single anatomic area (nodal) with the exclusion of mediastinum or abdomen

Stage II
- A single tumor (extranodal) with regional node enlargement
- Two or more nodal areas on the same side of the diaphragm
- Two single (extranodal) tumors with or without regional node on the same side of the diaphragm
- A primary GI tumor with or without mesenteric node involvement, grossly resected

Stage III
- Two single extranodal tumors on opposite sides of the diaphragm
- Two or more nodal areas above or below the diaphragm
- All of the primary chest tumors
- All extensive primary abdominal tumors
- All paraspinal or epidural tumors

Stage IV
- Any of the above plus central nervous system (CNS) and/or bone marrow involvement at diagnosis

TABLE 22-4   Clinical Presentation of Non-Hodgkin Lymphoma

Type	Common Clinical Presentation
Lymphoblastic lymphoma (30% of all cases)	Mediastinal mass, pain, cough, wheezing, dysphagia, dyspnea, tracheal compression, tachypnea, pleural effusion, supradiaphragmatic lymphadenopathy; superior vena cava syndrome (swelling in the back, neck, and upper extremities); respiratory distress; propensity for rapid spread to bone marrow, CNS, and gonads
Burkitt or Burkitt-like lymphoma (40% of all cases)	Abdominal primary; tumor lysis syndrome (increased uric acid and LDH); jaw tumor (African); propensity for spread to bone marrow and CNS; tumor burden may be massive May mimic appendicitis; intussusception; ovarian, pelvic, or retroperitoneal masses; ascites, pain, or swelling; nausea, vomiting, GI bleeding; lymphadenopathy of the inguinal or iliac regions
Diffuse large B-cell lymphoma (20% of all cases)	Two thirds of cases present with advanced disease, most commonly in the abdomen Lymph node involvement Bone marrow, mediastinal, and CNS disease are not common
Anaplastic large-cell lymphoma (10% of all cases)	Hepatosplenomegaly, fever, weight loss Involvement of peripheral, intrathoracic, or intra-abdominal lymph nodes Bone involvement common

involved (Table 22-4). For example, lymphomas in the abdomen would produce symptoms such as abdominal pain, nausea, vomiting, changes in bowel patterns, and abdominal distention.

ALERT *Intussusception (telescoping of the bowel) may be caused by lymphoma. As a rule, symptoms of intussusception in children older than age 5 years are highly suspicious for NHL.*

Lymphomas in the mediastinum would lead to symptoms of wheezing, stridor, dysphagia, and superior vena cava syndrome; bone marrow involvement would cause pallor, anemia, or thrombocytopenia.

Diagnostic Tests

Diagnostic studies include CBC; renal and liver function studies; serum electrolytes, calcium, phosphorus, magnesium, LDH, and uric acid determinations; EBV titers; urinalysis; chest radiograph; bone marrow aspirate; CSF cytologic study; and diagnostic images of the involved tumor sites—in particular, CT studies of the head and neck, chest, or abdomen. The stage of disease has important implications for both prognosis and selecting optimal therapy.

Accurate staging of lymphomas is extremely important in determining the extent of disease and ensuring that the appropriate treatment regimen is followed. The staging system in childhood NHL generally reflects the tumor burden.

In stage I childhood NHL, cancer is found in a single area or lymph node outside the abdomen or chest. In stage II childhood NHL, cancer is found in only one area and in the lymph nodes around it, in two or more areas or lymph nodes on one side of the diaphragm, or in the stomach or intestines and has been completely removed by surgery. The lymph nodes in the area may or may not have cancer.

In stage III childhood NHL, cancer is found in areas or lymph nodes on both sides of the diaphragm, beginning in the chest, in more than one place in the abdomen, or in the area around the spine. In stage IV childhood NHL, cancer is found in the bone marrow, brain, or spinal cord. Cancer may also be found in other parts of the body (Gorlick et al., 2010).

Stages I, II, and III have relatively clear-cut definitions, whereas stage IV has substages based on the extent of bone marrow involvement. Much controversy surrounds these designations because more than 25% blasts in the bone marrow usually is classified as ALL rather than as lymphoma. Stage IV NHL is commonly defined as "bulky disease," as evidenced by large amounts of tumor and less than 25% blasts in the bone marrow.

Nursing Diagnoses and Outcomes

Nursing diagnoses applicable to the child with cancer are presented in Nursing Plan of Care 22-1. In addition, the following diagnosis may apply to the child with NHL:

Nursing Diagnosis: Impaired urinary elimination related to the effects of tumor lysis syndrome
Outcome: Child will be free from complications of fluid and electrolyte imbalance and renal failure related to tumor lysis syndrome.

Interdisciplinary Interventions

The intensity and duration of therapy are directly related to the extent of disease. Children in stages I and II with a relatively low tumor burden generally require briefer and less intense therapy. Children in stages III and IV with a higher tumor burden require more aggressive and longer term therapy.

ALERT *As tumor burden increases, as in advanced disease, so does the likelihood of spontaneous or therapy-induced tumor lysis syndrome.*

Tumor lysis syndrome may present before the initiation of therapy and often worsens after chemotherapy is begun (see Nursing Interventions 22-6 for a summary of the management of tumor lysis syndrome).

NEUROBLASTOMA

Neuroblastoma is a tumor that primarily occurs in infants and young children. Composed of cells that are very similar to those of the sympathetic nervous system, the tumor can be found anywhere that sympathetic nervous tissue is present. Neuroblastomas most commonly occur on the adrenal gland.

Neuroblastoma is the fourth most common childhood cancer, accounting for 8% to 10% of all childhood tumors (D'Andrea, 2009). It is the most common tumor found in children younger than 1 year of age. Neuroblastoma occurs slightly more in males than females and most frequently in white children (National Cancer Institute, 2008b). The overall 5-year survival rate for children diagnosed between 2002 and 2008 for all stages combined was 75.4%. Two well-known factors predict a favorable prognosis for children with neuroblastoma. Children younger than 1 year of age who are in stage I, II, or IVS (see discussion on staging) have a favorable prognosis. Children with these stages characteristically demonstrate disease-free survival rates ranging from 75% to 100% (National Cancer Institute, SEER Program, 2009).

The cause of neuroblastoma remains relatively unknown. Epidemiologic studies do not have sufficient statistical power to provide evidence of any certain etiologic risk factors.

Pathophysiology

Neuroblastoma is a solid, commonly encapsulated tumor that is usually composed of small, round cells (rosettes) surrounding a region of neural or ganglion cells. Neuroblastoma may occur at a primary site only, or it may metastasize to other sites, including the bone marrow. Neuroblastomas often secrete two catecholamine metabolites: HVA and VMA. These metabolites can be found in the child's urine. Screening infants by analyzing urine samples can detect neuroblastoma before the presentation of any other clinical signs in some children (Sawada, 1992). However, current data do not support neuroblastoma screening because such screening results in overdiagnosis. This leads to unnecessary diagnostic and therapeutic procedures with consequent physical and psychological morbidity, including death from treatment complications. There is no evidence from controlled studies or randomized trials of decreases in mortality associated with catecholamine metabolite screening (National Cancer Institute, 2008b).

The International Neuroblastoma Staging System is the commonly used staging system. Stage I reflects localized minimal disease. Stage II involves incomplete gross total resection and ipsilateral lymph node involvement. Stage III is used when the tumor crosses the midline and includes contralateral lymph node involvement. Stage IV refers to disseminated disease to the bone, lymph nodes, bone marrow, liver, and perhaps organs. Stage IVS is a type of neuroblastoma in neonates that is disseminated to all areas except the bone, which occurs briefly and subsequently spontaneously regresses.

Assessment

The signs and symptoms of neuroblastoma depend primarily on the site of the primary tumor and the extent to which it has metastasized to other sites (i.e., bone marrow involvement). The most common site is the abdomen. Less common sites include the thorax, neck, and pelvis. Metastases are found in approximately 60% of newly diagnosed children, accounting for the poor prognosis rates associated with this disease (D'Andrea, 2009; Mazur, 2010). Bone pain, spinal cord compression, neurologic deficits, and abdominal pain may all be present, depending on tumor size and location. Sphenoid bone and retro-orbital involvement can cause ecchymosis of the eyelids and **proptosis** (protruding eyeballs). The child has a "raccoon-eyed" presentation and may appear to be abused (Fig. 22-11). Manifestations of other bone involvement may cause limping or refusal to walk.

Analysis of the urine for excessive amounts of the catecholamine metabolites VMA and HVA is useful in the diagnosis of neuroblastoma.

Interdisciplinary Interventions

To provide an optimal chance of cure, multimodal treatment is based on the stage and important prognostic indicators at diagnosis. Surgery plays a major role in treatment. When the tumor is localized, complete surgical resection may be feasible and is often curative. Children with disseminated disease are poor candidates

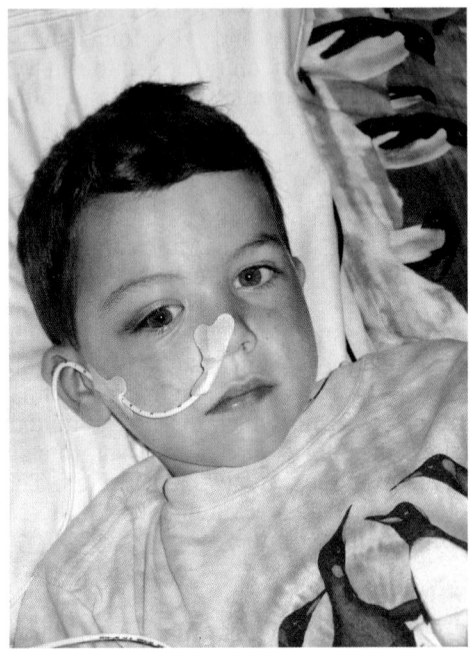

Figure 22-11 Metastasis of neuroblastoma to the periorbital area can cause a child to have a "raccoon-eyed" or bruise-like presentation around the orbital area.

for surgery. In these cases, chemotherapy is the primary treatment method. Chemotherapy may render a large tumor resectable, allowing for the possibility of a delayed or second-look surgery to remove the remaining tumor. Radiation may be used for local control of the tumor or for local palliation of metastatic disease. Children with more advanced neuroblastoma (unresectable or metastatic disease) undergo aggressive chemotherapy and radiation as well as autologous HSCT and biotherapy.

The child with neuroblastoma requires general oncology supportive care, similar to that previously discussed. Such care includes psychosocial support; teaching; and physical preparation for procedures, surgery, side effects of chemotherapy, and radiation therapy in standard doses or in the higher doses associated with HSCT. Because of this tumor's commonly poor prognosis, every treatment option is offered to the child and the family.

WILMS TUMOR

A primary tumor of the kidney, Wilms tumor accounts for 7% of cancers in children younger than age 15 years (National Cancer Institute, SEER Program, 2009). The majority of cases are diagnosed before the age of 5 years. The average age at diagnosis is 2 to 3 years. Wilms tumors are rare after the age of 10 years. Approximately 500 new cases of Wilms tumor occur each year, with a slightly higher than average incidence in black children and females. Five-year survival rate is 90% of all children with the disease (National Cancer Institute, SEER Program, 2009). Recurrence of disease is possible and most often occurs in the lungs.

Most cases of Wilms tumor occur without any genetic predisposition. However, there are a number of congenital anomalies and genetic conditions that are associated with an increased risk of developing a Wilms tumor, such as Beckwith-Wiedemann syndrome (macroglossia, omphalocele, and visceromegaly), WAGR syndrome (Wilms tumor, aniridia, genitourinary abnormalities, and mental retardation), and sporadic hemihypertrophy.

Pathophysiology

Wilms tumor is usually a large, rapidly growing tumor, often very soft and vascular. After surgical resection, the composition of the tumor cells is examined microscopically and determined to be either a favorable or an unfavorable tissue type. The tumor may be present in one or both kidneys, which is a very important prognostic factor. The pathologic staging for Wilms tumor ranges from stage I, in which disease is limited to the kidney and allows for complete removal, to stage V, in which bilateral kidney involvement occurs. This staging system is currently recommended by the National Wilms Tumor Study Group.

Assessment

A firm, nontender abdominal mass is the most common sign in the otherwise asymptomatic child at the time of diagnosis. Some children may experience abdominal pain, hematuria, or hypertension. The tumor is confined to one side, not crossing the midline as neuroblastoma does. The presence of distended abdominal veins may indicate that the mass is occluding the inferior vena cava.

ALERT *If Wilms tumor is suspected, the abdomen should not be palpated. Palpating the abdomen may cause the tumor capsule to rupture, resulting in tumor spillage. Tumor spillage can change the tumor from stage I to stage II or III, depending on the amount of spillage that occurs.*

Interdisciplinary Interventions

Multimodal therapy is recommended for the child with Wilms tumor. Immediate surgical removal of the affected kidney is imperative even if pulmonary metastasis is present. The goals of surgery are to remove the tumor without producing hematogenous spread, prevent rupture of the tumor capsule and subsequent spillage of tumor cells, and provide a tissue sample for pathologic evaluation to determine spread and staging. Members of the health care team have an opportunity to provide preoperative education for the child and the family while they await surgical intervention. Preoperative teaching should include a discussion of other treatment modes that may be used, such as radiation and chemotherapy.

Postoperative care involves pain management and ongoing abdominal assessment to observe for intestinal obstruction and signs of infection, bleeding, or fluid and electrolyte imbalance. This care also involves frequently monitoring the child's blood pressure because manipulation of or pressure on the kidney or the removal of a kidney may alter renin production and cause hypertension. Postoperatively, the tumor site is highly sensitive to radiation therapy, and adjuvant chemotherapy improves overall survival rates. The intensity and duration of chemotherapy is determined by the completeness of the surgical resection and the extent or staging of the tumor. Most children can be cured of this tumor, and ongoing investigations continue to improve outcomes for children with unfavorable or metastatic Wilms tumor.

Home care includes ensuring the child attends all health care visits and completes the chemotherapy and radiation treatment plan. The "Treatment Modalities" section discusses management of treatment side effects.

RHABDOMYOSARCOMA

RMS is the most common soft-tissue tumor in children, accounting for approximately 5.3% of the cases of cancer among children from birth to 14 years of age and 3.2% of the cases among adolescents 15 to 19 years of age (National Cancer Institute, SEER Program, 2009). Approximately 350 cases are diagnosed each year in the United States. Almost two thirds of RMS cases are diagnosed by 6 years of age. This tumor is slightly more common in males than females.

The cause of RMS is unknown. However, RMS has been associated with familial cancer syndromes, such as Li-Fraumeni, and with neurofibromatosis. Epidemiologic studies of RMS have demonstrated that maternal use of marijuana and cocaine in the year before the child's birth was associated with increased incidence of RMS in the child; similarly, marijuana, cocaine, and other recreational drug use by the father has also been associated with an increased risk of RMS in the child (Wexler et al., 2010).

The most important factors associated with prognosis appear to be the location and the extent of disease at the time of diagnosis. Children with no detectable metastases at diagnosis (group I) have much better outcomes than those with widespread disease (group IV). Children with tumors of the head and neck have a better prognosis than those with genitourinary tumors. In most children with localized disease, it is a curable disease when multimodal therapy is initiated. More than 70% of children survive 5 years after diagnosis. Relapses are uncommon after 5 years of disease-free survival (National Cancer Institute, SEER Program, 2009).

Pathophysiology

All sarcomas originate in primitive mesenchymal cells. Mesoderm cells form tissue known as mesenchyme. The mesenchyme cells give rise to fibrous and adipose connective tissue, blood vessels, lymphatic structures, and smooth and striated muscles. Thus, sarcomas can arise in many sites throughout the body. Sarcomas differ histologically and are identified by the mature cell type that they most closely resemble. RMSs arise from tissue that resembles striated muscle and are named for primitive muscle cells called *rhabdomyoblasts*, which are located throughout the body. The tumors occur in four anatomic sites: the head and neck, the genitourinary tract, the extremities, and the trunk.

The International Classification of Rhabdomyosarcoma has identified five broad histologic subtypes of RSM:

1. The *embryonal* type is the most common subtype and has an intermediate prognosis.
2. The *spindle cell* type is a less common variant of embryonal RSM, and it generally has a superior prognosis. The spindle cell variant arises disproportionately in the paratesticular region but may also be seen in the head and neck, extremities, and orbit.
3. The *botryoid* type has a particularly favorable prognosis and tends to arise almost exclusively from the bladder and vagina in infants and young children or from the nasopharynx in older children.
4. The *alveolar* type most commonly involves the muscles of the extremities and trunk and is associated with the poorest prognosis.
5. The *undifferentiated sarcoma* is the least common subtype, usually arising in the muscles of the extremities. It also has a poor prognosis.

The histologic diagnosis of RMS is based on the overall cellular pattern and the presence of rhabdomyoblasts with or without characteristic cytoplasmic cross-striations.

CHART 22-4   Intergroup Rhabdomyosarcoma (IRS) Study Group Clinical Grouping and Staging System

IRS Clinical Group

Group I: A localized tumor that is completely removed with pathologically clear margins and no regional lymph node involvement

Group II: A localized tumor that is grossly removed with (A) microscopic disease at the margin; (B) involved, grossly removed regional lymph nodes: *or* (C) both A and B.

Group III: A localized tumor with gross residual disease after incomplete removal or biopsy only.

Group IV: Distant metastatic disease is present at diagnosis.

IRS Stage

Stage I: Localized tumor involving the orbit (the area near the eye), head, and neck area except for parameningeal sites (next to the membranes covering the brain) or genitourinary tract tumors except bladder and prostate.

Stage II: Localized small tumors of any site not in stage I. The tumor must be less than 5 cm (about 2 in.), with no regional lymph node spread.

Stage III: Localized tumor at any site not included in stage I. The tumor is greater than 5 cm (2 in.) in diameter and/or has spread to regional lymph nodes.

Stage IV: Distant metastatic tumor is present at diagnosis.

From National Cancer Institute. (2009). *Childhood rhabdomyosarcoma treatment (PDQ)*. Retrieved from http://www.cancer.gov/cancertopics/pdq/treatment/childrhabdomyosarcoma/HealthProfessional/page4

The most commonly used staging system (Chart 22-4) for RMS in the United States was developed in 1972 by the Intergroup Rhabdomyosarcoma Study Group. This staging system is based on disease extent and resectability, defining groups I through IV by local disease status, the involvement of regional lymph nodes, and the extent of residual tumor after primary surgery.

Assessment

Signs and symptoms of RMS vary according the location of the primary site and the presence and extent of metastasis. Presenting symptoms can be caused by the primary tumor, metastases, or both. The signs and symptoms are usually attributed to the mass lesion or to obstructive phenomena.

RMS in the head and neck occurs predominantly in the orbit; nasopharynx; maxillary antrum; middle ear; and soft tissues of the scalp, face, and neck. Tumors in the orbit grow rapidly and are usually detected early because of the obvious changes they produce. Evaluation of the eyes may reveal symptoms such as ptosis (with or without lid swelling), exophthalmos, orbital cellulitis, or cranial nerve deficits.

Approximately one half of head and neck RMSs and undifferentiated sarcomas arise in nonorbital parameningeal sites (paranasal sinuses, nasopharynx, and middle ear). Tumors originating in the paranasal sinuses can cause nasal obstruction, chronic sinusitis, epistaxis, swelling, or local pain. Signs of nasopharyngeal tumors include hypernasal speech, nasal obstruction, discharge, visible polypoid masses in the nasopharyngeal cavity, and serous otitis. Middle ear RMS can present as chronic otitis media. Signs may include mucopurulent or sanguinous drainage from the affected ear, facial nerve palsy, conduction types of hearing loss, or a polypoid mass seen in the external ear canal.

Parameningeal tumors have a high probability of direct extension into the meninges. Multiple cranial nerve palsies occur as the tumor invades the neurovascular sheath. As the tumor extends, it may cross multiple foramina and fissures and invade the epidural space. Intracranial spread can produce symptoms associated with increased ICP, such as headache with vomiting or diplopia. Overall survival rates are drastically reduced when intracranial extension is present.

Within the genitourinary tract, RMS in younger children presents in the urinary bladder, prostate, and vagina. In adolescent males, the tumor occurs in the paratesticular soft tissue or spermatic cord. Tumors of the retroperitoneal area are usually asymptomatic until their growth is quite extensive. At the time of diagnosis, the child may complain of vague abdominal pain or genitourinary or bowel obstruction. A palpable mass may be present. Local lymph nodes are commonly affected. A tumor arising in the bladder may cause urinary retention, straining to void, hematuria, or passage of tissue in urine. Paratesticular tumors usually present as asymptomatic, nontender masses in the scrotum, lying above and separate from the testes. They may be associated with abdominal or pelvic masses resulting from metastasis. Half of all vaginal RMSs are associated with abnormal vaginal bleeding, and the other half are associated with a protruding polypoid mass.

Tumors originating in the extremities are usually deep-seated, palpable masses with soft to firm consistency that may be mistaken for a traumatic hematoma, especially in middle childhood. Tumors are relatively fixed to the underlying musculature and occasionally involve the skin. Sarcomas of the extremity are recognized by swelling in the affected limb. Pain, tenderness, and redness may be present.

Tumors of the trunk are similar to those of the extremities in exhibiting all histologic types and in their tendency for local recurrence and for distant spread despite wide local excision. Tumors of the trunk are of relatively large diameter compared with head and neck and bladder tumors.

RMS that involves the bone can produce pain, swelling, and limited function of the affected body part. Bone marrow metastasis can result in symptoms of pancytopenia such as anemia, bleeding, or infection. Most children with bone marrow involvement have extremity or truncal RMS and have concomitant metastases to bone, lung, or lymph nodes. Primary lesions of the prostate and maxillary sinus are also frequently associated with bone marrow metastasis.

Diagnostic Tests

Before biopsy of a suspected tumor mass, imaging studies of the mass and baseline laboratory studies are obtained to further delineate the location of the mass and any signs of metastasis. After the diagnosis of RMS has been made, an extensive evaluation to determine the extent of the disease is completed prior to initiating therapy. This evaluation should include a chest radiograph, CT scan of the chest, bilateral bone marrow aspirates and biopsies, bone scan, lumbar puncture, MRI of the base of the skull and brain (for parameningeal primary tumors only), and CT scan of the abdomen and pelvis (for lower extremity or genitourinary primary tumors).

Interdisciplinary Interventions

Multimodal treatment of RMS has greatly improved long-term survival rates. Surgical resection of the primary tumor usually offers the best prospect for local tumor control in limited disease cases. The addition of radiotherapy and multiagent chemotherapy has decreased indications for radical surgery, allowing more limited surgical intervention or potentially eliminating the need for surgery.

The goal of surgical intervention is complete tumor resection whenever possible. It is always desirable to preserve the child's vital or functionally useful structures or organs. In many cases, however, the location of the tumor, the degree of metastasis, and the infiltration of adjacent organs prohibit complete tumor excision. In combined-method treatment, surgery includes the initial incisional biopsy and evaluation of disease extent. Gross total resection is the most rapid way to eradicate the disease and should always be used if subsequent function or cosmetic appearance will not be greatly impaired.

Community Care

After surgical resection and discharge from the acute care facility, radiation and chemotherapy will continue to be administered to the child. Both overnight and outpatient visits are to be expected to ensure the child receives the optimal combination of therapies. As with other pediatric malignancies, it is important to educate the family regarding neutropenia, anemia, thrombocytopenia, signs and symptoms of infection, and fever precautions (see "Treatment Modalities" section earlier in this chapter).

BONE TUMORS

Malignant bone tumors account for approximately 5% of all childhood malignancies. Most of these tumors occur during adolescence. The two most common bone tumors are osteogenic sarcoma and Ewing sarcoma. The cause of most bone cancers is unknown.

OSTEOGENIC SARCOMA

 QUESTION: How typical is George's experience with osteogenic sarcoma?

Osteogenic sarcoma (OS), also called *osteosarcoma*, is a malignant tumor of the bone derived from osteoid tissue. The most common sites are in the long bones such as the distal femur, proximal tibia, and proximal humerus. Osteogenic sarcoma accounts for approximately 56% of all primary sarcomas of the bone. Peak incidence occurs between age 10 and 20 years, coinciding with the time of rapid bone growth (Baggott et al., 2011).

A genetic predisposition for osteogenic sarcoma has been suggested, with some cases developing in multiple members of the same family. Children with a history of hereditary retinoblastoma have an increased risk for osteogenic sarcoma. The p53 oncogene has been associated with this tumor (Gorlick et al., 2010).

The prognosis for osteogenic sarcoma continues to improve. The most important prognostic factor for osteogenic sarcoma is the extent of the disease. Children with overt metastatic disease have an unfavorable outcome. Other factors that affect prognosis include age (children younger than age 10 years fare worst; those older than age 20 years have good outcomes), tumor size (the smaller the size, the better the outcome), and sex (females fare better than males) (Gorlick et al., 2010).

Pathophysiology

Osteogenic sarcoma is characterized by the production and proliferation of malignant osteoid tissue and immature bone. The malignant bone growth of osteogenic sarcoma is detected at the time that bone-forming tissue is growing rapidly during the adolescent years. Five distinct tissue types of osteogenic sarcoma have been described: conventional (most common), periosteal, telangiectatic, multifocal, and miscellaneous. Some of these types are more common and some are more aggressive—factors that assist the health care professional in determining the chances for the child's long-term survival.

Assessment

Most children present with pain in the affected limb that increases with activity or weight bearing. Refusal to walk and limited range of motion are common findings. Tenderness and the presence of local edema or redness may also be noted. The older child should be able to specify the location of the pain. In the younger child, irritability, crying, and decreased movement or locomotion may be the only indicators of a problem. Many times, the diagnosis is made after a traumatic injury in which radiographs reveal the presence of a previously unknown tumor site.

Interdisciplinary Interventions

After diagnosis has been confirmed, surgical intervention is a vital treatment for children with osteogenic sarcoma. Tumor removal, limb salvage procedures, and amputation are all viable surgical options. Limb salvage procedures provide tumor removal while preventing the physical and psychosocial complications that occur with amputation (Fig. 22-12). Amputation is used if no other surgical options will provide the child the best chance of disease-free survival.

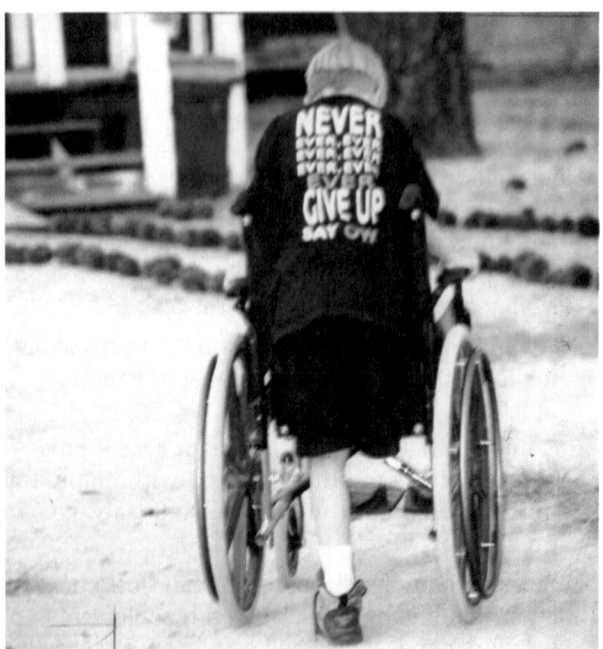

Figure 22-12 One child's strategy to deal with amputation for osteogenic sarcoma: "Never ever give up, say ow." Courtesy of Camp Ronald McDonald for Good Times.

Historically, surgery alone was used as the primary treatment, but 5-year survival rates were less than 20% (Gorlick et al., 2010). Chemotherapy is currently used for all patients, and it plays a substantial role in improving survival rates to 65% to 75% (Baggott et al., 2011). Preoperative and postoperative multiagent chemotherapy is used to prevent metastasis. Additional limb salvage procedures are more successful if performed after tumor viability and extent are modified by chemotherapy (Betcher et al., 2011). Osteogenic sarcoma is highly resistant to radiation. If radiation is considered as a treatment option, it must be delivered in high doses. Radiation is more often used for pain control and palliation. Most children with osteogenic sarcoma require intensive physical and psychosocial management postoperatively and during their intense therapy.

Thorough pain assessment and effective management are vital components of nursing care for children with osteogenic sarcoma (see Chapter 10 for further discussion of pain management). Children may experience specific bone pain and tenderness before or during treatment as well as "phantom" limb pain after amputation. Providing pain management without hesitation is important to promote physical and psychosocial well-being for these children (Nursing Interventions 22-7).

Community Care

An intensive and structured rehabilitation program is highly recommended. After the surgeon has cleared the child postoperatively, physical therapy and occupational therapy are instituted as soon as possible to maintain and improve the child's motor function and

NURSING INTERVENTIONS 22-7

Support for the Child Diagnosed With Osteosarcoma

Help child to make informed decisions about treatment options, understand the surgery planned, and know what to expect from postoperative routines and treatments. Prepare the child for the possibility of amputation or limb salvage.

Allow the child to verbalize fears or concerns about the loss of a limb or changes in appearance or function.

Encourage the child to examine an actual prosthesis and to see other children with amputated limbs or who have undergone limb salvage procedures.

Discuss the options for managing hair loss caused by chemotherapy, especially with adolescents, for whom appearance and self-image are crucial. These options include wearing wigs, hats, bows, scarves, and other items of apparel.

Prepare the child for the possibility of phantom limb pain. Explain that the child might feel itching, tingling, or pain sensation even though the limb is no longer there.

Discuss the drugs, such as antidepressants, that are used to treat these symptoms.

Provide discharge teaching about follow-up rehabilitation programs. Provide help and support to address the child's emotional readiness to face peers and family members.

Encourage the child to wear loose clothing to distract attention from the deformity or the prosthesis.

Give information on peer support groups, camps, and education and organization resource websites.

Review the risks and complications associated with chemotherapy and radiation that accompany surgical intervention for the osteosarcoma.

---

quality of life. Reconstructive surgery may be needed at some point to reshape or rebuild a limb or body part that may have been altered during initial therapies to remove the tumor. Rehabilitative services are essential if the child has lost a limb. These services can assist the child to gain new skills, learn to manage adaptive devices, and improve motor function (see Chapter 12). Because most of these patients are adolescents, body image is a major issue. Social and psychosocial intervention from peers and health care workers is a vital component of the child's plan of care (Fig. 22-13).

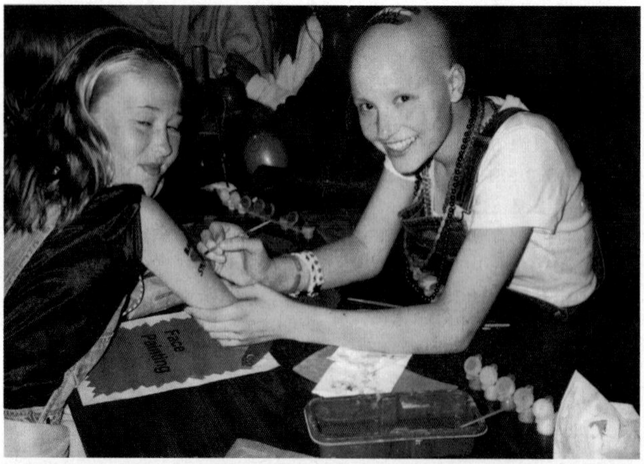

Figure 22-13 The adolescent undergoing treatment for osteogenic sarcoma can grow to accept changes in her appearance and continue to develop a positive self-image. Courtesy of Camp Ronald McDonald for Good Times.

ANSWER: For the most part, George's presentation and treatment are typical of other children with osteogenic sarcoma. Note the possibility of familial predisposition. George's mother is certain that her older brother also had osteogenic sarcoma. The most atypical aspect is that George represents the minority of patients (10%–20%) who present with metastasis to the lungs.

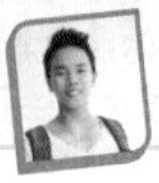

EWING SARCOMA

Ewing sarcoma is a highly malignant tumor, primarily of the bone, but it also can arise in soft tissue. These tumors may arise in any bone but are most often located in flat bones (pelvis, chest wall, and vertebrae) and the diaphyseal region of the long bones. It is often seen in the extremities with soft-tissue involvement. Ewing sarcoma is rare in children younger than age 5 years. The incidence is slightly higher in males. It is most commonly seen in whites and rarely seen in blacks. There is no known hereditary factor (Hawkins et al., 2010). The extent of the disease at the time of diagnosis is most important in determining outcome. Children with metastatic disease to the bone, bone marrow, or lungs have a poor prognosis.

Pathophysiology

Ewing sarcoma is characterized by densely packed, small round cells. Even when the tumor detected is very small, there may be microscopic spread to other areas. Ewing sarcoma commonly occurs in the pelvis, tibia, fibula, and femur. It is not known what causes Ewing sarcoma or what cells give rise to it. Approximately

10% to 30% of children have metastases at diagnosis (Betcher et al., 2011).

Assessment

Pain and a soft-tissue mass around the affected bone are the common clinical presentations of Ewing sarcoma. These signs may be misdiagnosed for some time as an injury related to sports or other physical activities. Children who have metastatic disease may present with anorexia, malaise, fever, fatigue, and weight loss. Other clinical signs depend on the location of the sarcoma.

Diagnostic Tests

In addition to a complete medical history and physical examination, the child with suspected Ewing sarcoma will have diagnostic evaluation that includes blood tests such as a CBC and LDH levels. Tissue breakdown elevates LDH, and this finding is associated with Ewing sarcoma and other cancers. ESR may also be elevated.

Radiograph and imaging tests will include bone scans to detect bone disease and evaluate the causes of bone pain or inflammation, MRI and CT imaging of primary tumor to secure accurate images of the tumor as well as chest radiographs, and CT of chest and bilateral bone marrow aspirates and biopsies to determine tumor spread in the body. A biopsy is also completed to distinguish Ewing sarcoma from any other type of cancer that may be present and to help examine the morphology of the cancer cells to determine treatment. The biopsy may be done under general anesthesia, and if the tumor is small and in an accessible location, the entire tumor may be removed at this time. If the tumor is too large or cannot be removed without risk to adjacent tissue, then only a portion of the tumor may be removed during the biopsy.

Interdisciplinary Interventions

Surgery, radiation, and chemotherapy are used for primary lesions. Surgery is used to resect the primary tumor while maintaining an intact limb. Amputation is rarely indicated. Local radiation is given to primary and metastatic sites. The use of multiagent chemotherapy improves survival rates and has become the mainstay of therapy. Treatment advances for bone tumors result in more long-term survivors but also more late effects. Skeletal impairments and the risks of secondary malignancies reinforce the necessity for long-term patient follow-up.

The psychosocial adjustments related to Ewing sarcoma are usually less traumatic than those seen with osteosarcoma because, in most cases, the affected limb is preserved. A thorough explanation of the side effects of chemotherapy and radiation therapy is still a vital component of the child and family's plan of care. A physical therapy program is often needed to strengthen the affected limb or to assist in the recovery from orthopedic reconstructive surgery that may be required following tumor removal.

RETINOBLASTOMA

Retinoblastoma, the most common intraocular childhood tumor, is a malignant tumor composed of embryonal retinal cells. The incidence is 1 in 16,000 live births in the United States, constituting 11% of cancers in the first year of life but only 3% of all childhood cancers (National Cancer Institute, 2008a). Although the tumor may be present at birth, most tumors (63%) are detected before age 2 years. The average age at diagnosis is 11 months for children with bilateral tumors and 22 months for those with unilateral tumors. Incidence does not vary significantly with sex or race (National Cancer Institute, 2008a).

The prognosis in retinoblastoma depends on the location and size of the tumor, and the presence and degree of ocular or extraocular involvement. If the tumor is unilateral and small, and the eye is treated promptly, the long-term survival rate is more than 90% (National Cancer Institute, 2008a). After the tumor has extended into the optic nerve, the cure rate decreases to 50%. Children with extraocular extension fare poorly, with a 25% survival rate. Numerous studies have indicated that survivors of retinoblastoma are at increased risk for secondary malignant tumors. These tumors are not associated with the ocular disease but are primary tumors of other organs.

Pathophysiology

Retinoblastoma usually develops in the posterior portion of the retina. The malignancy may appear as a single tumor in the retina, appearing in a rosette formation. The tumor can also have multiple foci that extend locally to adjacent structures or spread distantly. Local extension usually occurs within the intraocular space before invading the structures surrounding the globe. Distant spread, or metastasis, occurs when tumor cells grow along the optic nerve, enter the subarachnoid space, and spread to the CNS. Intracranial extension is the most common cause of death (National Cancer Institute, 2012d).

The tumor has a tendency to outgrow its blood supply, resulting in necrosis. Calcification appears in necrotic areas, especially in large tumors. The intraocular calcium is readily detected on radiographs and is an important diagnostic sign.

Retinoblastoma occurs in two types: hereditary and nonhereditary. The nonhereditary and unilateral type accounts for 60% of cases, 15% are hereditary and unilateral, and the bilateral hereditary type accounts for 25% of cases (National Cancer Institute, 2008a). The nonhereditary type of tumor arises by spontaneous mutation in somatic cells such as retinoblasts. Children with nonhereditary retinoblastoma have unilateral disease and no family history or increased risk of other malignancies. Hereditary retinoblastoma is suspected when a positive family history exists or, in the case of sporadic disease, when the child is affected bilaterally. This is caused by the mutation of the RB1 gene (National Cancer Institute, 2012d).

caREminder

Because of the strong hereditary influence of retinoblastoma and its ability to be cured during early stages, children with a positive family history should be monitored very closely. The child should receive a complete eye examination a few days after birth, at age 6 weeks, every 2–3 months until age 2 years, and then every 4 months until age 3 years.

CHART 22-5   Reese-Ellsworth Staging Classification of Retinoblastoma

Group I: Very Favorable Prognosis

- Solitary tumor, smaller than 4 disk diameters* at or behind the equator
- Multiple tumors, none larger than 4 disk diameters, all at or behind the equator

Group II: Favorable Prognosis

- Solitary tumor, 4–10 disk diameters, at or behind the equator
- Multiple tumors, 4–10 disk diameters, behind the equator

Group III: Doubtful Prognosis

- Any lesion anterior to the equator
- Solitary tumors, larger than 10 disk diameters, behind the equator

Group IV: Unfavorable Prognosis

- Multiple tumors, some larger than 10 disk diameters
- Any lesion extending anteriorly to the ora serrata

Group V: Very Unfavorable Prognosis

- Tumors involving more than half the retina
- Vitreous seeding

*1 disk diameter = 1.5 mm.

Hereditary retinoblastoma arises in one of three ways: inheritance from an affected parent by autosomal dominant transmission, inheritance from an unaffected gene carrier parent, or acquired as a new germinal mutation from a parent who did not inherit the gene. Children with the hereditary type of retinoblastoma are at increased risk for other malignancies.

The Reese-Ellsworth staging classification is the standard system for prognostic evaluation of retinoblastoma for the extent of intraocular disease (Chart 22-5). The staging system predicts the likelihood of tumor control and preservation of vision, but it does not predict survival. It classifies children with retinoblastoma according to tumor size, number, and location of tumors and presence of vitreous seeding. No standard staging system exists for disease that has extended beyond the orbit of the eye.

Assessment

The signs and symptoms of retinoblastoma vary according to the stage at the time of diagnosis. When the tumor is small, the child may initially present with strabismus secondary to impaired vision. As the tumor enlarges, a creamy white pupillary reflex, known as *leukocoria*, or *cat's eye*, develops, and the tumor may be visualized easily. Children with red, painful eyes demonstrate late symptoms, resulting from inflammation, uveitis, or vitreous hemorrhage.

Diagnostic Tests

Early detection and diagnosis is extremely important because early intervention is effective and may preserve the child's vision. Without pathologic confirmation, the diagnosis must be made by the ophthalmoscopic, ultrasonographic, and radiographic appearance. A definitive diagnosis of retinoblastoma can usually be made during a complete funduscopic examination. Pupillary dilation and examination under sedation or general anesthesia are necessary to evaluate the retina fully. The tumors appear as creamy pink or white masses, but they may be obscured by retinal detachment, hemorrhage, or cloudy fluid in the anterior chamber.

Ultrasonography is a particularly valuable diagnostic tool in demonstrating the presence of a mass in the posterior segment of the eye if the fundus is obscured by retinal detachment or hemorrhage. Radiographic identification of intraocular calcium strongly suggests retinoblastoma because it is extremely rare for any other ocular disorder of childhood to produce such a finding. CT of the orbit is more sensitive than plain radiographic film in detecting the presence of calcium. MRI is usually not necessary but may be helpful in confirming the diagnosis in the absence of calcium.

Nursing Diagnoses and Outcomes

Nursing diagnoses applicable to the child with cancer are presented in Nursing Plan of Care 22-1. In addition, the following nursing diagnosis may be applicable to the child with retinoblastoma:

Nursing Diagnosis: Disturbed sensory perception: Visual, related to effects of vision loss resulting from tumor location and/or compression
Outcome: Child will adapt to receiving visual input from one eye or to blindness if severe bilateral involvement has occurred.

Interdisciplinary Interventions

The treatment plan for a child with retinoblastoma is individually tailored and based on the extent of disease. The following are considered when planning treatment: unilateral or bilateral involvement; evidence of vision or any potential for vision; extent of disease (confined to the globe or extension to the optic nerve); and occurrence of orbital, CNS, or distant metastases. Treatment options include surgery, radiotherapy, phototherapy, and cryotherapy.

The surgical intervention in the treatment of retinoblastoma is enucleation, or removal of the eye. Enucleation must be considered in children with severe retinal disruption with no possibility that sight can be restored, extension of the tumor into the anterior chamber, painful glaucoma with permanent loss of vision, or unresponsiveness to other forms of treatment. A cosmetic disadvantage for children younger than age 3 years is that the orbit ceases to grow normally after an eye is removed. As the face continues to grow, the orbit appears increasingly sunken.

Preparation of the family for the child's appearance after surgery or radiation is essential. Initially, the child has an eye patch in place that is changed regularly by the ophthalmologist. The orbit and the face are edematous during the postoperative period, making it difficult to fit a prosthesis until the edema subsides. Fitting for a prosthesis usually takes place 3 weeks after surgery, unless complications occur.

Radiotherapy is used to control local disease while attempting to preserve vision. Retinoblastoma is known to be highly radiosensitive. Radiotherapy can be administered via external beam or via radioactive applicators. External beam radiation produces the same appearance as surgery because it interferes with bone growth. Radioactive surface applicators (plaques) are indicated if recurring small tumors remain after external beam therapy or as initial therapy for small solitary tumors. A surgical procedure is performed to suture the radioactive applicators to the sclera. The device is left in place for 7 days and then removed. The child is placed under general anesthesia for the application and removal of the radioactive devices.

caREminder

The child with radioactive devices is placed alone in a single room to prevent radiation exposure to other children and staff. Staff members follow radiation precautions and wear radiation-sensitive badges to ensure that their exposure is minimal and within the guidelines determined by the National Council on Radiation Protection and Measurements.

Photocoagulation therapy destroys the blood vessels supplying the tumor. It is generally used in conjunction with external beam radiation in tumors in the posterior part of the eye that fail to respond after 4 to 6 weeks of radiation or that recur after radiation therapy. Photocoagulation must be performed under direct visualization and is appropriate for tumors located posterior to the equator. It may also be used for small tumors that are located away from the optic nerve and macula. Photocoagulation is performed with the child under general anesthesia.

Cryotherapy destroys the tumor cells by forming intracellular ice crystals that interfere with the microcirculation of the tumor, ultimately resulting in cell death. Cryotherapy may also be used in conjunction with external beam radiation. The treatment is indicated for small primary or recurrent tumors in the anterior part of the retina or for small recurrences of the disease after radiotherapy has been administered. Cryotherapy does not require direct visualization of the tumor. Cryotherapy is performed with the child under general anesthesia.

Chemotherapy may be used in cases of metastatic disease. It is administered intravenously or intrathecally. Despite chemotherapeutic treatment, prognosis is poor in the presence of metastatic involvement.

Community Care

After enucleation, the child and family need support and guidance, including postoperative care of the socket, discharge teaching, and information about the prosthesis. The child's family also may need additional support and counseling if the retinoblastoma is hereditary. They may feel guilty for transmitting the defect to their child. The child and family need preparation for the prospect of the child losing vision in the affected eye as well as loss of the affected eyeball. Emphasize that the vision in the affected eye is probably already lost and that the child can still have a normal life with one functioning eye. It is also helpful to show the child pictures of a child with a prosthetic eye. Doing so helps the child and family to picture how the prosthetic eye will look.

Care of the socket includes maintaining a clean, dry dressing or eye pad. The eye pad should be changed daily until the socket is healed. The family may need additional discharge instructions on cleaning the socket or applying an antibiotic ointment if one is prescribed.

Initial instructions for care of the prosthesis are given by the ocularist who fits and manufactures the device. The prosthetic eyeball is removed only when cleaning is necessary. It is cleaned by placing it in water that is slightly warmer than room temperature and soaking for several minutes. Families are instructed by the ocularist in removing and replacing the prosthesis.

GERM CELL TUMORS

Germ cell tumors emerge from embryonal cells, known as germ cells, which originate in the embryonic yolk sac during gestation (Olson et al., 2010). Germ cell tumors are extremely rare, occurring at a rate of 20.6 per 1 million children younger than 20 years of age, with prevalence slightly higher in males than in females. Incidence approximately doubles in adolescents aged 15 to 19 years. The overall 5-year survival rate in children diagnosed between the years 2002 and 2008 was 91.2%; rates for intracranial and intraspinal germ cell tumors were slightly lower, at 86.7% (National Cancer Institute, SEER Program, 2009). Little is known about the cause of germ cell tumor. There is an association with sex chromosome abnormalities. For example, 50% of patients with mediastinal germ cell tumors have Klinefelter syndrome (XXY phenotype). Heredity may also be a mild contributor in adolescent cases (Olson et al., 2010).

Pathophysiology

Germ cell tumors are most commonly found in the gonads and usually discovered during puberty. However, these tumors can also occur in other areas along the path in which the germ cells migrate and can be malignant or benign. These other areas include the cervical neck, upper jaw, nasopharynx, intracranium, retroperitoneum, and mediastinum (Olson et al., 2010). Germ cell tumors are histologically classified into mature teratomas, immature teratomas, malignant germ cell tumors, and CNS germ cell tumors. It is not uncommon for one tumor to include different cell types; this is classified as a mixed germ cell tumor (National Cancer Institute, 2012c).

Both classes of teratomas contain different types of tissues, such as hair, bone, and muscle. Mature teratomas are benign, although they can create complications for patients because they have the potential to secrete enzymes and hormones, such as insulin, growth hormone, and vasopressin. Immature teratomas are most often found in the gonads and are graded based on the amount of immature neural tissue found upon biopsy. Malignant germ cell tumors consist of frank malignant cells and are further classified by location. CNS germ cell tumors generally emerge from the pineal and suprasellar region of the brain. Pineal tumors are more common; however, 5% to 10% of patients have involvement in both regions. Patients with CNS germ cell tumors can experience hypopituitarism and often present with DI (National Cancer Institute, 2012b).

Assessment

Testicular germ cell tumors will present as a painless, irregular palpable mass, often with inguinal hernias or hydroceles. Clinical manifestations of ovarian tumors may include a palpable mass, pain, swelling, nausea, vomiting, constipation, and genitourinary complications. Extragonadal malignant germ cell tumors will generally present with palpable masses and pain at the site. Children with CNS germ cell tumors may present with visual loss, growth hormone deficiency, increased urine output, anorexia, and psychosocial complications (National Cancer Institute, 2012b).

Diagnostic Tests

Blood samples are obtained to evaluate the child's serum chemistry levels. Furthermore, germ cell tumors secrete tumor markers, which include elevated levels of AFP, β-HCG, and LDH. For those with CNS germ cell tumors, serum sodium must be closely monitored because of the common presentation of DI. Imaging tests will include ultrasound, CT scan, and MRI to evaluate for disease at the site and detect any metastases to other areas. A biopsy is also completed to confirm diagnosis.

Interdisciplinary Interventions

Combination chemotherapy is currently the most effective treatment strategy because germ cell tumors generally have favorable response rate. Initial surgical intervention is most appropriate when there is little risk of damaging surrounding structures. However, resection is often avoided in cases involving a vital structure because of the efficacy of chemotherapy protocols. In cases where surgery cannot be avoided, males with testicular tumors will undergo an orchiectomy, whereas females with ovarian tumors will receive an oophorectomy. In cases of CNS germ cell tumors, the child will receive a combination of surgery, chemotherapy, and autologous stem cell rescue. Germ cell tumors are most commonly found in adolescents and young adults, and the nurse should remain astute to the psychosocial needs of these children, who may experience struggles with body image. The nurse should remember to include the child and family in teaching about all procedures, surgical interventions, and chemotherapy as well as keep them involved in planning their care.

See thePoint for a list of Key Concepts.

REFERENCES

Androkites, A. (2009). Hodgkin's lymphoma. In N. E. Kline (Ed.), *Essentials of pediatric hematology/oncology nursing: A core curriculum* (3rd ed., pp. 25–28). Glenview, IL: Association of Pediatric Hematology/Oncology Nurses.

Aschenbrenner, A., Winters, J., & Belknap, R. (2012). Integrative review: Parent perspective on care of their child at the end of life. *Journal of Pediatric Nursing, 27*(5), 514–522.

Baggott, C., Fochtman, D., Foley, G. et al. (Eds.). (2011). *Nursing care of children and adolescents with cancer and blood disorders* (4th ed.). Glenview, IL: Association of Pediatric Hematology/Oncology Nurses.

Ballard, K. (2004). Meeting the needs of siblings of children with cancer. *Pediatric Nursing, 30*(5), 394–401.

Bernstein, M. L. (2011). Targeted therapy in pediatric oncology. *Cancer, 117*, 2268–2274.

Betcher, D. L., Simon, P. J., & McHard, K. M. (2011). Bone tumors. In C. Baggott, D. Fochtman, G. Foley et al. (Eds.), *Nursing care of children and adolescents with cancer and blood disorders* (4th ed., pp. 1084–1105). Glenview, IL: Association of Pediatric Hematology/Oncology Nurses.

Blaney, S. M., Haas-Kogan, D., Poussaint, T. Y. et al. (2010). Gliomas, ependymomas, and other nonembryonal tumors. In Pizzo, P. A. & Poplack, D. G. (Eds.), *Principles and practice of pediatric oncology* (pp. 717–771). Philadelphia, PA: Lippincott Williams & Wilkins.

Carroll, W. L., & Finlay, J. L. (Eds.). (2010). *Cancer in children and adolescents*. Boston, MA: Jones and Bartlett

Chen, C., Wang, R., Cheng, S. et al. (2004). Assessment of chemotherapy-induced oral complications in children with cancer. *Journal of Pediatric Oncology Nursing, 21*(1), 33–39.

Creutzig, U., Zimmermann, M., Reinhardt, D. et al. (2004). Early deaths and treatment-related mortality in children undergoing therapy for acute myeloid leukemia: Analysis of the multicenter clinical trials AML-BFM 93 and AML-BFM 98. *Journal of Clinical Oncology, 22*(21), 4384–4393.

Crozier, F., & Hancock, L. (2012). Pediatric palliative care: Beyond the end of life. *Pediatric Nursing, 38*(4), 198–203, 227.

D'Andrea, L. (2009). Neuroblastoma. In N. E. Kline (Ed.), *Essentials of pediatric hematology/oncology nursing: A core curriculum* (3rd ed., pp. 32–36). Glenview, IL: Association of Pediatric Hematology/Oncology Nurses.

De Lalla, F. (2003). Outpatient therapy for febrile neutropenia: Clinical and economic implications. *Pharmacoeconomics, 21*(6), 397–413.

Gorlick, R., Bielack, S., Teot, L. et al. (2010). Osteosarcoma: Biology, diagnosis, treatment, and remaining challenges. In P. A. Pizzo & D. G. Poplack (Eds.), *Principles and practice of pediatric oncology* (5th ed., pp. 1015–1044). Philadelphia, PA: Lippincott Williams & Wilkins.

Gursky, B. (2007). The effect of educational interventions with siblings of hospitalized children. *Journal of Developmental and Behavioral Pediatrics, 28*(5), 392–398.

Hawkins, D. S, Bolling, T., Dubois, S. et al. (2010). Ewing sarcoma. In Pizzo, P. A. & Poplack, D. G. (Eds.), *Principles and practice of pediatric oncology* (pp. 987–1014). Philadelphia, PA: Lippincott Williams & Wilkins.

Heath, J. A., & Ross, J. A. (2010). Epidemiology of cancer in children. In W. L. Carroll & J. L. Finlay (Eds.), *Cancer in children and adolescents* (pp. 3–14). Boston, MA: Jones and Bartlett.

Holdsworth, M., Hanrahan, J., Albanese, B. et al. (2003). Outpatient management of febrile neutropenia in children with cancer. *Pediatric Drugs, 5*(7), 443–455.

Keefe, D. M., Schubert, M. M., Elting, L. S. et al. (2007). Updated clinical practice guidelines for the prevention and treatment of mucositis. *Cancer, 109*(5), 820–831.

Kuttesh, J., Rush, S., & Ater, J. (2011). Brain tumors in childhood. In R. M. Kliegman, B. F. Stanton, J. W. St. Geme et al. (Eds.), *Nelson textbook of pediatrics* (19th ed., pp. 1746–1752). Philadelphia, PA: Elsevier/Saunders.

Labay, L., Mayans, S., & Harris, M. (2004). Integrating the child into the home and community following completion of cancer treatment. *Journal of Pediatric Nursing, 21*(3), 165–169.

Mazur, K. A. (2010). Neuroblastoma: What the nurse practitioner should know. *Journal of the American Academy of Nurse Practitioners, 22*, 236–245.

Metzger, M., Krasin, M. J., Hudson, M. M. et al. (2010). Hodgkin lymphoma. In Pizzo, P. A. & Poplack, D. G. (Eds.), *Principles and practice of pediatric oncology* (pp. 638–662). Philadelphia, PA: Lippincott Williams & Wilkins.

McCune, R. (2009). Biologic response modifiers. In N. E. Kline (Ed.), *Essentials of pediatric hematology/oncology nursing: A core curriculum* (3rd ed., pp. 108–112). Glenview, IL: Association of Pediatric Hematology/Oncology Nurses.

Murray, J. S. (2002). A qualitative exploration of psychosocial support for siblings of children with cancer. *Journal of Pediatric Nursing, 17*(5), 327–337.

National Cancer Institute. (2006). *Childhood cancers.* Retrieved from http://www.cancer.gov/cancertopics/types/childhoodcancers

National Cancer Institute. (2008a). *National Cancer Institute research on childhood cancers, cancer facts.* Retrieved from http://www.cancer.gov/cancertopics/factsheet/Sites-Types/childhood

National Cancer Institute. (2008b). *Neuroblastoma screening(PDQ).* Retrieved from http://www.cancer.gov/cancertopics/pdq/screening/neuroblastoma/HealthProfessional/page1

National Cancer Institute. (2012a). *Childhood brain and spinal cord tumors treatment overview (PDQ).* Retrieved from http://cancer.gov/cancertopics/pdq/treatment/childbrain/healthprofessional

National Cancer Institute. (2012b). *Childhood central nervous system germ cell tumors treatment (PDQ).* Retrieved from http://cancer.gov/cancertopics/pdq/treatment/childCNS-germ-cell/healthprofessional

National Cancer Institute. (2012c). *Childhood extracranial germ cell tumors treatment (PDQ).* Retrieved from http://cancer.gov/cancertopics/pdq/treatment/extracranial-germ-cell/healthprofessional

National Cancer Institute. (2012d). *Retinoblastoma treatment (PDQ).* Retrieved from http://cancer.gov/cancertopics/pdq/treatment/retinoblastoma/healthprofessional

National Cancer Institute, Surveillance, Epidemiology, and End Results Program. (2009). *SEER cancer statistics review, 1975–2006.* Retrieved from http://seer.cancer.gov/csr/1975_2006/index.html

National Institute for Occupational Safety and Health. (2004). *Preventing occupational exposure to antineoplastic and other hazardous drugs in health care settings* (NIOSH Publication No. 2004-165). Cincinnati, OH: Author. Retrieved from http://www.cdc.gov/niosh/docs/2004-165/2004-165d.html

Olson, T., Schneider, D., & Perlman, E. (2010). Germ cell tumors. In P. A. Pizzo & D. G. Poplack (Eds.), *Principles and practice of pediatric oncology* (5th ed., pp. 1045–1067). Philadelphia, PA: Lippincott Williams & Wilkins.

Rock, C. L., Doyle, C., Denmark-Wahnefried, W. et al. (2012). Nutrition and physical activity guidelines for cancer survivors. *CA: A Cancer Journal for Clinicians, 62*(4), 242–274.

Rosenblum, R. (2005). Brain stem glioma: Two case studies. *Journal of Pediatric Oncology Nursing, 22*(2), 114–118.

Ruccione, K. (2011). The biological basis of cancer. In C. Baggott, D. Fochtman, G. Foley et al. (Eds.), *Nursing care of children and adolescents with cancer and blood disorders* (4th ed., pp. 36–113). Association of Pediatric Hematology/Oncology Nurses.

Sawada, T. (1992). Past and future of neuroblastoma screening in Japan. *American Journal of Pediatric Hematology and Oncology, 14*(4), 320–326.

Teuffel, O., Eithier, M. C., Alibahi, S. et al. (2011). Outpatient management of cancer patients with febrile neutropenia: A systematic review and meta-analysis. *Annals of Oncology, 22*(11), 2358–2365.

Tipton, J. M., McDaniel, R. W., Barbour, L. et al. (2007). Putting evidence into practice: Evidence-based interventions to prevent, manage, and treat chemotherapy-induced nausea and vomiting. *Clinical Journal of Oncology Nursing, 11*(1), 69–78.

Wallace, J. (2009). Central venous access devices. In N. E. Kline (Ed.), *Essentials of pediatric hematology/oncology nursing: A core curriculum* (3rd ed., pp. 165–168). Glenview, IL: Association of Pediatric Hematology/Oncology Nurses.

Watral, M. (2009). Central nervous system tumors. In N. E. Kline (Ed.), *Essentials of pediatric hematology/oncology nursing: A core curriculum* (3rd ed., pp. 28– 32). Glenview, IL: Association of Pediatric Hematology/Oncology Nurses.

Wexler, L. H., Meyer, W., & Helman, L. J. (2010). Rhabdomyosarcoma. In P. A. Pizzo & D. G. Poplack (Eds.), *Principles and practice of pediatric oncology* (5th ed., pp. 923–953). Philadelphia, PA: Lippincott Williams & Wilkins.

Yahalom, J. (2006). Don't throw out the baby with the bathwater: On optimizing cure and reducing toxicity in Hodgkin's lymphoma. *Journal of Clinical Oncology, 24*(4), 544–548.

See the**Point** for additional organizations.

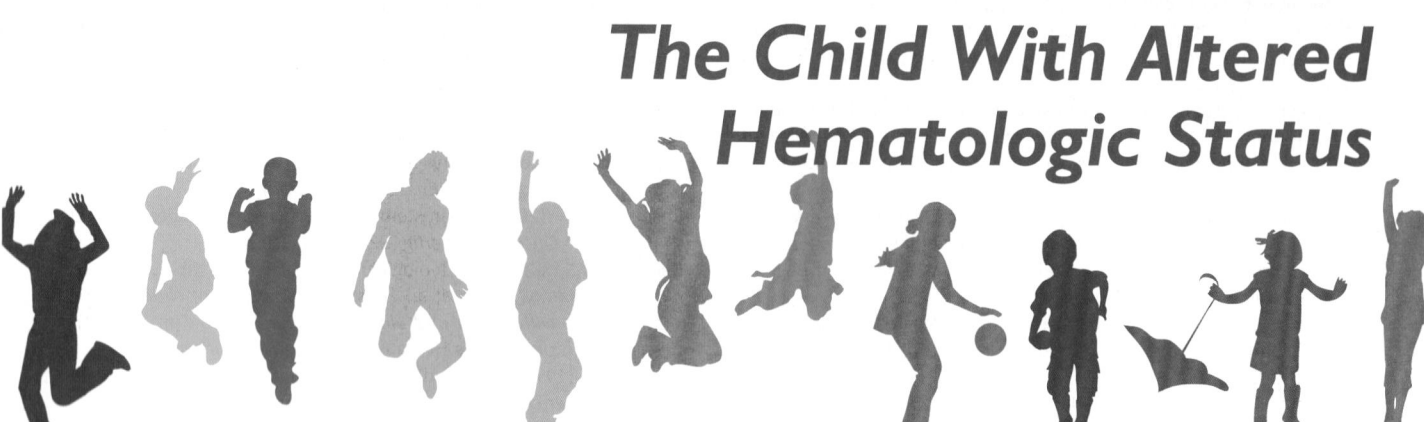

CHAPTER 23

The Child With Altered Hematologic Status

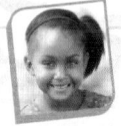

CASE HISTORY

The Johnson family, an African American family with twins J. D. and B. J., were first introduced in Chapter 5; J. D. was also featured in Chapter 19. The boys have an older sister, Shawanda, who is 6 years old and has sickle cell disease. The parents, James and Lanese Johnson, divorced about a year ago. James knew that he had sickle cell disease in his family; his aunt also has the condition. Lanese was surprised to discover that she, too, is a carrier of the trait.

Shawanda was diagnosed as a newborn following the state's neonatal screening. She had mild anemia but very few problems until she turned 2 years of age. One evening, shortly after her second birthday, she began crying and saying, "Owie," and holding her chest. Lanese gave her acetaminophen

(Tylenol) and encouraged her to drink juice. When Shawanda could not stop crying, they went to the emergency department and Shawanda was admitted to the hospital. The admitting nurse on the pediatric floor documented the following: temperature of 102.9° F (39.4° C), pallor, irritability, mild nasal flaring, tachypnea, and decreased breath sounds. Her oxygen saturation on room air was 89%, and her chest radiograph showed bilateral pulmonary infiltrates. Admitting laboratory studies included hemoglobin, 5.7 g/dL; reticulocytes, 24%; and white blood cell count, 35,000/mm³. Arterial blood gases revealed pH, 7.44; partial pressure of arterial oxygen (PaO_2), 78 mm Hg; and partial pressure of arterial carbon dioxide ($PaCO_2$), 35 mm Hg

CHAPTER OBJECTIVES

1 Describe how assessment data are used to identify and manage bleeding disorders, anemias, and hemoglobinopathies in children.

2 Discuss the role of the health care team in preparing children and families for various diagnostic studies that help to identify and manage hematologic disorders.

3 Summarize the interventions by the health care team during transfusion therapy.

4 Discuss the rationale for the interdisciplinary interventions used in managing pediatric hematologic alterations.

5 Describe the nursing care of children with bleeding disorders, anemias, and hemoglobinopathies.

See thePoint for a list of Key Terms.

A healthy hematologic system is essential to overall well-being. Composed of blood-forming organs, plasma, blood cells, and blood vessels, the hematologic system is responsible for transporting essential elements to, and waste products from, cells throughout the body. The hematologic system plays a crucial role in **hemostasis** (blood clotting), immunity, and heat regulation. Alterations in hematologic status can result in serious illness and death.

The hematologic system in children and adolescents can deviate from normal in a number of ways. This chapter describes the more important of these hematologic alterations. In addition, this chapter provides information to enhance the nurse's role in collaborating with the interdisciplinary health care team as they work together to correct or minimize the effects of pediatric hematologic disorders on children and families.

DEVELOPMENTAL AND BIOLOGIC VARIANCES

QUESTION: Shawanda has sickle cell disease. What blood cells are affected by her condition?

The hematologic system forms early during fetal development. Blood formation can be detected by the 14th day of gestation. By the 3rd to 4th week of gestation, blood islands are evident in the yolk sac. The peripheral cells of the blood islands become blood vessel walls in the developing embryo; the central cells of the blood islands become the embryo's primitive blood cells. By the 4th week of gestation, circulation is evident.

The liver shows evidence of **hematopoiesis**, the formation and development of blood cells, by the sixth week of gestation and becomes the major site of blood cell production during the prenatal period. The spleen, thymus, and lymph nodes are also engaged in hematopoiesis in the developing fetus.

At about the 20th week of gestation, the bone marrow, primarily the bone marrow of the long bones, pelvis, sternum, ribs, and vertebrae, becomes involved in blood cell production. It is the primary site of hematopoiesis during the childhood and adult years (Fig. 23-1).

STEM CELLS

The *stem cell* is the earliest stage in the development of all blood cells. Hematopoiesis depends on the stem cell for two major reasons: (1) the stem cell can differentiate to form progenitor (precursor) cells for red blood cells, white blood cells, and platelets; and (2) the stem cell is capable of self-renewal, providing a continuous supply of the cells required for hematopoiesis. Fetal blood and umbilical cord blood are rich sources of stem cells.

RED BLOOD CELLS

The *erythrocyte* (red blood cell) undergoes several developmental changes as it progresses through the prenatal period to infancy and childhood. These changes include shifts in production rate, life span, appearance, and type of *hemoglobin* (the erythrocyte's oxygen-carrying molecule).

The rate of red blood cell production is relatively high as gestation draws to a close. It decreases after birth, reaching its low point during the neonatal period. Red blood cell production increases somewhat during infancy, again during early childhood, and, for males, during the adolescent years. Those living in high-altitude environments generally produce a greater number of red blood cells and develop physiologic **polycythemia** (an excess of red blood cells).

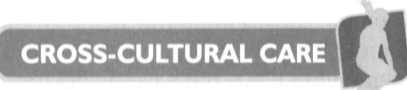

CROSS-CULTURAL CARE

Ethnic variations exist in red blood cell indices. In particular, black children tend to have lower hemoglobin values than white or East Asian children.

The life span of red blood cells gradually increases with gestational age. Red blood cell survival duration at birth for a full-term newborn is 60 to 70 days. For a premature infant, the red blood cell survival time is briefer, and the amount of decrease is positively correlated with the degree of the infant's immaturity. By the end of the neonatal period, it reaches the normal life span of 100 to 120 days.

Newborns' red blood cells vary in size and shape. These cells are larger and are more likely to be irregularly shaped than the red blood cells of older children and adults.

Hemoglobin is the major component of red blood cells. Normally, it consists of two pairs of globin

---

Infants and adolescents are especially susceptible to iron-deficiency anemia as a result of high growth requirements and dietary deficiencies.

Hematopoiesis beginning in the liver by the sixth week of gestation; this is the primary site of prenatal blood cell production.

The yolk sac is the earliest site of blood cell production in the embryo.

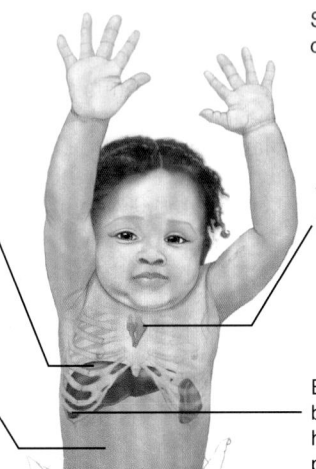

Sickle cell anemia is more common in black children.

The thymus is a site of perinatal hematopoiesis.

By the 20th week of gestation, the bone marrow becomes involved in hematopoiesis. The long bones, pelvic bones, sternum, ribs, and vertebrae are significant sites of blood cell production for children and adolescents.

In most states, newborn screening using a blood sample taken from a heel stick is used to determine the presence of sickle cell anemia.

Figure 23-1 Developmental and biologic variances: hematologic system.

polypeptide chains. Various types of globin chains exist, differing in their amino acid composition. Hemoglobin F, hemoglobin A, and hemoglobin A₂ are the most common types.

Hemoglobin F, composed of alpha and gamma globin chains, is the predominant hemoglobin during the fetal stage of development and at birth. During the first 6 months after birth, it gradually declines, but it continues to be present in trace amounts throughout life. An excess of hemoglobin F may be associated with hemoglobinopathies, such as sickle cell disease and certain other disorders.

Hemoglobin A, composed of alpha and beta globin chains, is predominant after early infancy, constituting more than 95% of hemoglobin. A deficiency of hemoglobin A is associated with certain forms of sickle cell disease and thalassemia.

Hemoglobin A₂, composed of alpha and delta globin chains, is a minor hemoglobin, constituting only approximately 2.5% of hemoglobin. An increase or decrease in its concentration may, however, contribute important diagnostic information in hematologic disorders such as thalassemia.

Red blood cells experience several phases during their maturation process. Initially, erythropoietin (a hormone) stimulates certain stem cells to commit to the red blood cell lineage. The committed stem cells then sequentially develop into erythroblasts, normoblasts, reticulocytes, and, finally, red blood cells. Reticulocytes and red blood cells, present in the peripheral circulation, are nonnucleated cells, unlike red blood cells during earlier stages of development.

As previously mentioned, red blood cells have a life span of about 120 days. When the cells die, the iron from the hemoglobin is recycled to make more red blood cells. Sufficient iron is needed to form hemoglobin and thus ensure the red blood cells have enough hemoglobin to carry oxygen to the entire body. As a result of growth requirements, it is essential that children and adolescents have a diet that contains iron-rich foods to ensure adequate intake of iron for hemoglobin production.

> **ANSWER:** Sickle cell disease involves a problem with hemoglobin, which is carried by the red blood cells.

WHITE BLOOD CELLS

White blood cell production begins in the liver at approximately week 5 of fetal development. Additional production occurs in the thymus (8 to 9 weeks), the spleen (11 weeks), and the lymph nodes (12 weeks). At birth, the number of circulating white blood cells is equal to that found in adults. As with red blood cell development, specific stem cells commit to the various white blood cell lineages: myeloid, monocytic, and lymphoid.

Myeloid Lineage

Stem cells that commit to the myeloid lineage sequentially progress in their development to myeloblasts, then neutrophil/eosinophil/basophil granulocytes or

monoblasts, then monocytes, then macrophages. *Bands* or *stabs*, juvenile forms of neutrophils, may increase during times of hematopoietic stress, such as infection. Circulating granulocytes have a short life span of approximately 12 to 14 hours.

After a decline during infancy, the white blood cell differential shows a steadily increasing percentage of neutrophils (also known as *polys* or *segs*). The peak level is achieved during adolescence and continues into the adult years. The percentage of eosinophils and basophils in the differential remains fairly constant throughout the life span (see Appendix D for a summary of all normal laboratory values).

Monocytic Lineage

Stem cells that commit to the monocytic lineage sequentially proceed in their development to monoblasts, promonocytes, and monocytes. Mature monocytes appear in the peripheral circulation for about 12 hours and then enter body tissues. Monocytes phagocytose pathogens, present antigens, and secrete cytokines. Apart from minor changes during infancy, the percentage of monocytes in the white blood cell differential remains quite steady throughout the life span.

Lymphoid Lineage

Stem cells that commit to the lymphoid lineage sequentially progress in their development from lymphoblasts to prolymphocytes to mature T or B lymphocytes. T cells, or thymus-derived lymphocytes, are involved in cell-mediated immunity. B cells, or bone marrow–derived lymphocytes, are involved in humoral immunity. The life span of lymphocytes is variable, ranging from a few days to months or years. After an increase during infancy, the white blood cell differential shows the percentage of lymphocytes gradually decreasing throughout childhood. A plateau occurs during adolescence and remains through the adult years.

PLATELETS

Platelets (also called *thrombocytes*) develop from stem cells that commit to the platelet lineage. These committed stem cells sequentially develop into megakaryoblasts, promegakaryocytes, and then mature megakaryocytes or platelets. The number of circulating platelets is relatively constant throughout the life span and ranges from 150,000 to 450,000/mm³ (see Appendix D).

ASSESSMENT

Alterations in hematologic status can affect the function of multiple body systems besides the hematologic system. Thus, when acquiring data during the health history and physical assessment, consider not only the hematologic abnormalities but also how these abnormalities can alter other physiologic processes. Keep normal hematologic developmental and biologic variances in mind when assessing children and adolescents because what is normal at one age may be abnormal at another age. For instance, the newborn has a higher hemoglobin level than an adolescent (see Appendix D for all laboratory values).

FOCUSED HEALTH HISTORY

QUESTION: What additional information would be important for the nurse to obtain when assessing Shawanda's current illness?

A focused health history contributes important information for determining a particular hematologic disorder. Components of this health history are identified in Focused Health History 23-1.

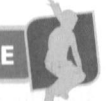

CROSS-CULTURAL CARE

The child's demographic data are important because some hematologic diagnoses are more commonly associated with a certain age group, sex, race, or geographic location. Examples include iron-deficiency anemia (IDA) during late infancy and adolescence, hemophilia in males, sickle cell disease among blacks, and thalassemia among those of Mediterranean ancestry. The child's religious background is important because some religious groups may not consent to health care or they may refuse specific interventions. Jehovah's Witnesses, for example, may not consent to the use of blood or blood products, even in life-threatening situations. If the child is a minor and parental or guardian consent cannot be obtained, a court order is required to give transfusions.

Because hematologic alterations can affect multiple body sites, ask the family for information that may identify abnormalities involving all body systems. Begin with the birth history and proceed to the child's current age. Ask about bleeding, anemia, and infection. For each occurrence, identify the child's age, prescribed treatment, and subsequent course of events. Note instances of abnormal bleeding and delayed wound healing associated with accidental and surgical wounds, such as scalp lacerations, circumcision, extraction of teeth, tonsillectomy, and adenoidectomy.

When reviewing childhood illnesses, make particular note of infections, which are frequently responsible for hematologic alterations in children. Note any allergies, which also can cause hematologic alterations, particularly eosinophilia.

The child's nutritional status and dietary habits provide helpful data for assessing and managing hematologic disorders that are associated with nutritional deficiencies, such as IDA and megaloblastic anemia. The child's environmental history also may be important. For example, exposure to certain chemicals may precede the onset of aplastic anemia, pica may be a sign of IDA and can also be associated with increased lead levels because of heavy metal consumption, and low humidity in the home may lead to **epistaxis**, bleeding from the nose. A child who has lived in or visited other countries may have been exposed to infectious agents not common in the United States. The dengue virus, for example, found in Southeast Asia, Central America, and South America, can interfere with normal hematopoiesis (Kroeger et al., 2004).

The family medical history and the social history provide data that may be important in diagnosing a hereditary hematologic disorder such as hemophilia, von Willebrand disease, sickle cell disease, thalassemia, or hereditary spherocytosis. Inquire about hematologic abnormalities in parents, siblings, aunts, uncles, cousins, and relatives from preceding generations. Note the name or description of the hematologic disorder and the relationship of the affected family member to the child.

When a chronic hematologic disorder such as hemophilia or sickle cell disease has been diagnosed, note the development and management of long-term sequelae as well as the incidence and course of events associated with acute health problems.

ANSWER: It would be important to seek additional information about Shawanda's symptoms and the time of their onset. Ask for further details about what was done at home, particularly the amount of fluid she had and the dose and frequency of the analgesic medication (acetaminophen) given. Also, inquire about any changes in her activities that may provide clues to possible factors contributing to Shawanda's current status, such as inadequate fluid intake, exposure to heat and/or humidity or cold, excessive physical activity, travel to high altitude, or exposure to infectious organisms. Keep in mind that, often, a precipitating factor cannot be identified.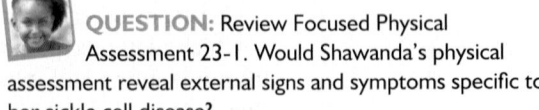

FOCUSED PHYSICAL ASSESSMENT

QUESTION: Review Focused Physical Assessment 23-1. Would Shawanda's physical assessment reveal external signs and symptoms specific to her sickle cell disease?

Although a specific hematologic disorder is usually identified or confirmed by laboratory studies, the physical assessment contributes important information for determining which laboratory studies are needed and provides data that aid in management of the hematologic disorder.

Pediatric hematologic alterations usually are characterized by

- Atypical hemostasis (bleeding longer than normal)
- **Anemia** (decreased oxygen-carrying capacity of the blood caused by abnormally low red blood cell mass, hemoglobin levels, or blood volume)
- **Neutropenia** (abnormally low percentage of neutrophils compared with total white blood cells; decreases a child's ability to fight pathologic bacteria)

These abnormalities may occur separately or together, and because they can affect multiple body systems, physical assessment must address each system. Particular physical alterations may be associated with bleeding disorders, anemia, and neutropenia (Focused Physical Assessment 23-1).

The skin provides valuable information about the hematologic system. Often, it is the first site to provide

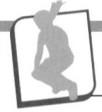

FOCUSED HEALTH HISTORY 23-1

The Child With Altered Hematologic Status

Current history	Prescribed medications, over-the-counter medications, or home remedies child is taking for a known hematologic condition; note the use of aspirin, aspirin-containing medications, nonsteroidal anti-inflammatory drugs, anticoagulants, or other medications that may alter hematologic status. Time and date of last use of all medications and factor replacement therapy used to treat current condition (e.g., steroids, chelators, factor-stimulating products, antifibrinolytic agents, antibiotics)
Past medical history	**Prenatal/Neonatal History** Prenatal history of mother (for all children); note infections, anemia, nutritional deficiencies, medications, and postpartum hemorrhage History of prolonged bleeding at umbilical cord, circumcision, and injection sites Bleeding from telangiectatic lesions or hemorrhagic bullae Infection, jaundice, anemia during neonatal period **Previous Health Challenges** Epistaxis or other bleeding episodes and their precipitating events; any other indications of unusual response to injury Surgical procedures (including dental extractions) and traumatic injuries; child's hematologic and immunologic response to those events History of soft-tissue abscesses, cellulitis, wound infections Presence of known HIV infection or other immunologic disorder, leukemia, or malignant tumor Recipient of blood or blood products; note any adverse reactions and if premedication was used prior to administration Childhood illnesses contracted, including influenza, chickenpox, hepatitis, mononucleosis, or other infectious diseases; note exposure to parvovirus (fifth disease), which may precipitate aplastic crisis in children with sickle cell disease Immunizations and whether they are up-to-date Presence of allergies to medicines, foods, latex, plants, animals, pollen, and so on
Nutritional assessment	Inadequate weight gain or unexplained weight loss Decreased appetite Dietary habits indicative of anemia; particularly note intake of milk, meat, and vegetables; vitamin and mineral dietary supplements; particularly note ascorbic acid intake
Family medical history	Family history of unexplained bruising, bleeding, anemia, thrombosis, neutropenia, immune disorder Family history of specific hematologic disorders such as hemophilia, von Willebrand disease, or sickle cell disease
Social history	Exposure to chemicals, such as home treatment to exterminate insects Observed ingestion of lead, lead-based paint; previous lead level evaluation Dehumidifier or low humidity in the home Ethnicity and geographic origin of ancestors Family history of consanguineous marriages or partnerships Beliefs about health care; especially beliefs related to the use of blood and blood products
Growth and development	Child's activities for a typical day and any recent changes in these activities (e.g., reduction in activity level or cessation of specific activities) Failure to achieve developmental milestones

Note: See Chapter 8 for a comprehensive health history.

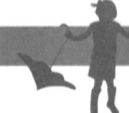

FOCUSED PHYSICAL ASSESSMENT 23-1

Hematologic System

Assessment Parameter	Alterations/Clinical Significance
General appearance	Fever may be present with infections related to neutropenia.
	Pallor, inadequate weight gain, and unexplained weight loss are common signs of anemia. Family may reported child is easily fatigued.
	Bleeding, bruising, and petechiae are signs of thrombocytopenias, idiopathic thrombocytopenic purpura (ITP), and bleeding disorders.
	Jaundiced sclera may be present with hemolytic anemia, sickle cell disease, and thalassemia.
	Joint and muscle swelling is a sign of hemophilia.
	Dactylitis, especially in an infant, is a common sign of sickle cell crisis.
Integumentary system (skin, hair, nails)	Easy bruising; petechiae; ecchymoses; purpura; bleeding from wounds, line sites, or invasive procedure sites; telangiectatic lesions; and hemorrhagic bullae may indicate thrombocytopenia, ITP, or bleeding disorders.
	Pallor, jaundice, bronzed skin, waxy skin, spooned nails, and lower extremity ulcers may be indications of an anemia.
	Skin lesions; skin breakdown at skinfolds or perianal area; cutaneous cellulitis; abscesses; and wound infections at line sites, procedure sites, surgical sites, or trauma sites may indicate neutropenia.
	Vascular changes are associated with telangiectasia and hemangiomas.
Head and neck	Frontal bossing is common with thalassemia.
Eyes	Icterus can be present with hemolytic anemias, sickle cell disease, and thalassemia.
Face, nose, and oral cavity	Pale mucous membranes are present with anemia.
	Epistaxis (common) and hemoptysis (rare) are associated with bleeding disorders.
	Angular stomatitis is a sign of anemia.
	Thrush and sores in oropharynx may indicate neutropenia.
Thorax and lungs	Tachypnea may be present with anemia or infection.
	Sinusitis, pharyngitis, bronchitis, and pneumonia may be signs of neutropenia.
	Fungal respiratory infections should present a high index of suspicion of neutropenia.
Cardiovascular system	Tachycardia and hypotension are associated with loss of blood in bleeding disorders, decreased hemoglobin level in anemias, and fever and infection in neutropenia.
	Palpitations, arrhythmias, and murmurs may be associated with anemia.
	Sepsis or septic shock may be a complication of neutropenia.
	Enlarged heart and heart failure are associated with anemia.
Vasculature	Swelling proximal to central line sites, presence of collateral blood vessels, or both may indicate thrombosis.
Gastrointestinal system	Enlarged spleen is often present in sickle cell disease and hemolytic anemias.
Lymphatic system	Persistently swollen lymph nodes may indicate neutropenia.
External genitalia and breasts	Delayed development of secondary sex characteristics is common in sickle cell disease and other anemias.

(Continued)

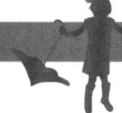

FOCUSED PHYSICAL ASSESSMENT 23-1

Hematologic System (Continued)

Assessment Parameter	Alterations/Clinical Significance
Musculoskeletal system	Short stature and absent or triphalangeal thumbs are associated with Fanconi and Diamond-Blackfan anemias.
	Avascular necrosis is often a cause of hip pain in children with sickle cell disease.
	Joint or muscle swelling, especially after trauma, is associated with hemophilia.
Neurologic system	Headache, scleral or conjunctival bleeding, retinal hemorrhage, intracranial hemorrhage, focal neurologic changes, seizures, and altered level of consciousness may all be associated with bleeding disorders.
	Headache, dizziness, decreased ability to concentrate, and irritability may occur with anemia.
	Dizziness, decreased ability to concentrate, altered level of consciousness, listlessness, and confusion may be associated with infection resulting from neutropenia.

clinical evidence of a hematologic alteration. For example, petechiae and purpuric bleeding that show initially on extremities or mucosa are typical of platelet disorders (Fig. 23-2). Raised **ecchymoses** (blotchy areas of hemorrhage in the skin) are more typical of vascular disorders. Severe bruising to specific areas, such as the head or buttocks, although indicating the need to evaluate the child for possible abuse, may also be signs of bleeding disorders. For example, children with hemophilia often have bruises in areas such as the chest or buttocks.

The complete documentation of physical findings provides information that may point to, or rule out, specific hematologic disorders. Follow-up physical assessment provides information for evaluating the response to treatment and contributes data for planning for ongoing health care needs.

For the child with a chronic hematologic disorder, be alert for changes that may occur with disease or long-term treatment. Examples are the onset and development of cardiac abnormalities in the child with chronic anemia secondary to disease and iron overload caused by blood transfusion therapy.

ANSWER: No, although Shawanda may be smaller for her age and appear pale, she does not have physical signs indicating the presence of sickle cell disease. Her presentation is that of respiratory distress, pain, and fever. It is the laboratory test results and history of sickle cell disease that lead to a diagnosis.

DIAGNOSTIC CRITERIA

Laboratory studies provide important data for assessing the physical status of the child with a hematologic disorder. Three common hematologic laboratory studies are

1. Coagulation profile (partial thromboplastin time, prothrombin time, platelet count, fibrinogen, and platelet function analysis [or PFA 100]) to determine clotting status
2. Blood cell profile (complete blood count or [CBC] with differential) to evaluate cellular components
3. Bone marrow examination (aspiration and biopsy) to evaluate blood cell development

ALERT   *Monitor children with a known or suspected hematologic disorder for prolonged bleeding after a blood specimen collection, bone marrow aspiration, or other invasive procedure.*

A number of other laboratory studies provide information related to the hematologic system (Tests and Procedures 23-1). The nurse may be responsible for obtaining blood samples. For more specialized procedures such as bone marrow aspiration, the registered nurse provides ongoing monitoring of the child, particularly during sedation, and assists the physician, advanced practice nurse, and clinical laboratory personnel to obtain the specimen and monitor the child's response to the procedure.

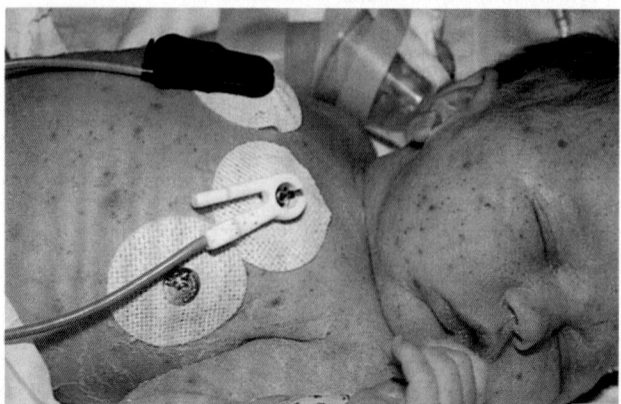

Figure 23-2 Petechiae are 1- to 2-mm red or purple spots under the surface of the skin caused by blood leaking from capillary vessels.

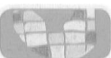

TESTS AND PROCEDURES for Evaluating Hematologic Status

Diagnostic Test or Procedure	Purpose	Findings and Indications	Health Care Provider Responsibilities
CBC with differential	Determines abnormal loss or destruction of cells that may indicate blood disorders. Changes in values may indicate complications such as anemia, neutropenia, and thrombocytopenia.	Decreases in red blood cell number, size, and hemoglobin content identify anemias. Reduced platelet numbers identify thrombocytopenia. Increased white blood cell number and distribution identify infection; decreased granulocytes and white blood cells suggest neutropenia.	Obtain specimens when child is calm; specimens obtained when child is upset may show increased white blood cell count. Mix blood sample with anticoagulant in tube gently to prevent clotting.
Absolute neutrophil count (ANC)	Measures the number of neutrophil granulocytes (type of white blood cell that fights infection) present in the blood. ANC is not measured directly but is calculated by multiplying the white blood cell count by the percent of neutrophils (segmented [fully mature] + bands [almost mature]) in the differential white blood cell count.	The normal range for ANC is 1.5–8.0 (1,500–8,000/mm^3). ANC less than 1,000/mm^3 in infants 2 weeks to 1 year or less than 1,500/mm^3 in children older than 1 year indicates neutropenia.	Use good infection control measures during lab draw to protect child from exposure to infection. Advise family of neutropenic precautions if ANC is low (see Chapter 22).
Antithrombin III	Assesses level of antithrombin III.	Normal levels vary with age. Antithrombin III deficiency indicates hypercoagulability, as in genetic antithrombin III deficiency or DIC.	Fill tube to line with blood; mix gently with anticoagulant in tube to prevent clotting. Transport specimen to laboratory quickly.
Bilirubin fractions	Measures direct (conjugated) and indirect (unconjugated) bilirubin levels.	Elevated levels of unconjugated bilirubin may be associated with hemolytic conditions.	Protect sample from light.
Bleeding time	Screens for platelet function and von Willebrand factor.	When test is done correctly, prolonged time shows that platelets have decreased ability to adhere to blood vessel wall and form a platelet plug.	No longer used routinely in pediatrics because accuracy depends on technician's skill and on child remaining still for more than 5 minutes. As an alternative, use platelet function analysis.
Coagulation Tests			
Activated partial thromboplastin time	Measures intrinsic clotting system, which needs factors VII, VIII, IX, X, XI, XII, fibrinogen, and prothrombin.	Values may be prolonged during heparin administration, in hemophilia, von Willebrand disease, and DIC and in the presence of circulating inhibitors.	Must be drawn swiftly with a clean venipuncture (no hematoma). May be performed on the same collection tube as prothrombin time and fibrinogen. Apply cotton or a bandage to the puncture site if there is any continued bleeding.

(Continued)

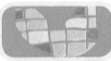 **TESTS AND PROCEDURES for Evaluating Hematologic Status** *(Continued)*

Diagnostic Test or Procedure	Purpose	Findings and Indications	Health Care Provider Responsibilities
Prothrombin time	Measures extrinsic clotting system, which needs fibrinogen, prothrombin, and factors V, VII, and X.	Values may be prolonged in vitamin K–associated factor deficiencies, DIC, during warfarin administration, or in the presence of circulating inhibitors; also in malabsorption and liver disease.	Apply cotton or a bandage to the puncture site if there is any continued bleeding.
Platelet function analysis	Screens for platelet function and von Willebrand disease.	Positive results indicate need for hematology workup.	Be aware that adequate hemoglobin level is needed for test. Send with CBC or hemoglobin and hematocrit.
Coombs test direct (antiglobulin test)	Detects antibodies attached to red blood cells.	Antibody presence helps detect hemolytic disease of newborn.	Handle specimen gently to prevent hemolysis. Transport to laboratory immediately.
Disseminated intravascular coagulation (DIC) profile	Provides data for various indicators of DIC.	Test includes prothrombin time, activated partial thromboplastin time, fibrinogen, platelet counts, thrombin, and D-dimer assay for fibrin derivatives. Prolonged or altered values will indicate presence of DIC.	Anticipate need for additional testing; no standard exists.
Factor assays	Detects specific factor deficiencies.	Low level of factor VIII may indicate von Willebrand disease or hemophilia A. Low level of factor IX may indicate hemophilia B. Levels of factors V, VII, X, XI, XII, and XIII and fibrinogen may also be ordered but are rare.	If sending out for processing, ensure that laboratory knows that samples must be spun and frozen until processed. Apply pressure to venipuncture site for 10 minutes; apply cold pack. Factor assays do not routinely need to be repeated for children who have been diagnosed with a factor deficiency.
Folate, red blood cells	Evaluates for folate deficiency.	Low levels present in megaloblastic anemia.	Protect sample from light.
Hemoglobin electrophoresis	Quantifies hemoglobins.	Identifies hemoglobinopathies such as sickle cell disease (+Hgb S). Used to confirm positive results from newborn screening for specific hemoglobinopathy.	May be inaccurate if drawn within 4 months of blood transfusion.
Osmotic fragility	Determines presence of spherical red blood cells.	Positive results are diagnostic for spherocytosis.	Check CBC or hemoglobin and hematocrit with test. Low hemoglobin level may give false-positive test results.
Peripheral blood smear	Identifies morphologic alterations in blood cells.	Shape abnormalities help to detect sickle cells, spherocytes, abnormal platelets, etc.	Gently mix blood sample with anticoagulant in specimen tubes to prevent clotting.

Diagnostic Test or Procedure	Purpose	Findings and Indications	Health Care Provider Responsibilities
Plasminogen activity	Determines plasminogen levels.	Low levels are associated with DIC and thrombosis.	Place collected specimen on ice. Note use of medications that may interfere with normal coagulation. Draw blood for coagulation studies last when more than one blood sample is being obtained.
Protoporphyrins (free erythrocyte protoporphyrins)	Determines levels of iron stores.	Low iron stores identify IDA, lead poisoning.	Note current hematocrit; send with CBC or hemoglobin and hematocrit. Send to lab on ice.
Reticulocyte count	Determines red blood cell production by the bone marrow.	Low production may be caused by a lack of vitamin B_{12}, folic acid, or iron in the diet or by illnesses affecting the bone marrow such as cancer. The reticulocyte count increases when the bone marrow produces more red blood cells in response to blood loss or treatment of anemia.	Apply cotton or a bandage to the puncture site if there is any continued bleeding. Request CBC to be completed at the same time because the reticulocyte count is dependent on red blood cells.
Ristocetin cofactor	Measures the ability of the plasma to agglutinate platelets in the presence of the antibiotic Ristocetin.	Low levels are associated with von Willebrand disease.	Anticipate repeat testing necessary to confirm von Willebrand disease diagnosis. Be aware that stress elevates levels. Send blood type sample along with testing because levels vary by blood type.
Schilling test	Determines whether a vitamin B_{12} deficiency exists. Detects pernicious anemia and intestinal malabsorption syndrome.	Low level of vitamin B_{12} in urine suggests impaired absorption caused by lack of intrinsic factor. Intestinal malabsorption results in less vitamin B_{12} being excreted in urine.	Administer capsule of radioactive 57-cobalt-tagged liquid vitamin B_{12}, followed 1–2 hours later by administration of an intramuscular injection of vitamin B_{12}. Collect urine to determine whether vitamin B_{12} is being absorbed normally. If not, less is excreted in the urine. Prepare child in advance for this procedure, including withholding foods and fluids for 4 hours before starting the test. After the test is started, allow the child to eat normally.
Serum ferritin (SF)	Identifies levels of iron stores.	Low levels are associated with iron deficiency (ID); high levels are associated with iron overload.	Transport specimen on ice.

(Continued)

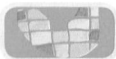

TESTS AND PROCEDURES for Evaluating Hematologic Status (Continued)

Diagnostic Test or Procedure	Purpose	Findings and Indications	Health Care Provider Responsibilities
Total iron-binding capacity and transferrin	Total iron-binding capacity evaluates iron-binding capacity and levels. Transferrin evaluates levels of circulating iron. The tests are typically drawn and measured at the same time.	Increased levels are associated with IDA and polycythemia vera. Low levels are associated with anemia of chronic disease, hemolytic anemia, and sickle cell disease.	Ensure that the child is fasting in the morning (circadian rhythm affects iron) prior to lab draw. Have sample drawn before child is given therapeutic iron or blood transfusion. Iron determinations in children who have had blood transfusions should be delayed for at least 4 days.
Type and crossmatch	Identifies blood type and presence or absence of Rh factor.	Results aid in matching donor cells with host cells for compatibility.	Review institutional policies for blood typing and cross-matching procedures.
von Willebrand factor antigen	Determines amount of von Willebrand factor present.	Low levels are associated with von Willebrand disease.	Anticipate repeat testing to confirm diagnosis of von Willebrand disease. Stress causes elevated levels. Send blood type sample along with specimen; levels vary by blood type.
von Willebrand factor multimer analysis	Quantifies amounts of multi-mers present.	Reduced amount of large multimers assists in determining subtype of von Willebrand disease.	Call laboratory for sample requirements; usually must be sent out to specialty lab.
Vitamin B_{12}	Assesses levels of serum B_{12}.	Low levels identify B_{12} deficiency and megaloblastic anemia.	Protect sample from light.
Bone marrow aspiration and biopsy	Aspirated bone marrow is used for microscopic examination of cell type and morphology. Identifies and evaluates specific hematologic disorders.	Abnormalities of cells in fluid or tissue can differentiate between malignant and nonmalignant hematologic conditions.	Procedure is done using aseptic technique. Topical anesthetic is used to anesthetize the skin; an injectable anesthetic is used to anesthetize the bone. Position the child properly based on the site of aspiration; place pillows or folded blanket under the child's abdomen to elevate the hips (for iliac crest site). Allow a family member to stay in the room to provide verbal and physical comfort Provide procedural sedation monitoring for children receiving sedatives and analgesics in a treatment room The procedure can also be done while the child is in the operating room for biopsy, resection, or line placement. Apply pressure dressing to site after aspiration. Remove dressing and inspect site after 24 hours.

caREminder

Assessment of the hematologic system depends on scrupulous techniques for obtaining, transporting, and testing blood or bone marrow specimens. Pay careful attention to ensure that sufficient quantities of specimen are transported in the appropriate container under appropriate conditions. Invalid or misleading levels can result if specimens are not handled properly. Ensure that the correct technique is used to obtain the specimen, including the use of standard precautions. Validate that the correct sample amount is secured. The specimen should be appropriately smeared on a slide or placed in the correct specimen receptacle (e.g., blood tube, Microtainer). Last, be sure that the sample is correctly labeled with the child's name and a second identifier prior to leaving the room.

Transporting blood samples requires properly preserving the specimens so that accurate test results can be secured. Handle specimens gently to prevent **hemolysis** (destruction of the red blood cells). Place the specimen on ice, if appropriate, and transport all samples to the laboratory as soon as possible to avoid specimen deterioration.

Laboratory testing of blood samples is conducted by specific criteria to provide reliable test results. However, normal values for some hematologic tests, such as coagulation studies, may vary from laboratory to laboratory depending on the specific test methodology and the reagents used. To evaluate test results, use the normal values from the laboratory that performed the test. When feasible, use the same laboratory for all testing for consistent test results.

Whenever blood or bone marrow sampling is required, the nurse has an important role in preparing the child and family. Accurate information about the test's purpose and procedure and appropriate responses to questions such as "Will it hurt?" help the child and family know what to expect before, during, and after the procedure. Offer topical anesthesia such as LMX or EMLA cream (see Chapter 10). In addition, involve family members in comfort holding, distraction techniques, and developmentally appropriate play to help the child prepare for and cope with the test.

TREATMENT MODALITIES

Primary interventions for the child with a hematologic disorder begin with environmental measures that prevent complications associated with the disorder, such as padding the pant knees for the crawling child to prevent bruising, using good handwashing technique and avoiding crowds for the neutropenic child to prevent infection, and providing dietary modifications for the child with anemia to enhance iron stores. Treatment for children with hematologic abnormalities may involve intravenous (IV) transfusion and chelation therapies. In certain circumstances, splenectomy may be required.

BLEEDING PRECAUTIONS

Nursing interventions for the child with a potential for excessive bleeding begins with teaching the child and family measures to prevent bleeding (Nursing Interventions 23-1). Instruct families to not only provide a safe environment for children with bleeding disorders but also to normalize the environment as much as possible. Review with the family the child's developmental milestones, and anticipate sources of injury based on each new developmental stage. Although infancy is rarely a period of stress or bleeding problems, the early childhood stages may expose the child to new sources of trauma and thus, in some cases, reveal the presence of a bleeding disorder. In general, the safety precautions used for all children (Chapters 4 to 7) also apply to the child with a bleeding disorder. Reassure the families of children with the potential for bleeding that age-appropriate toys are generally safe. Encourage children to participate in age-appropriate physical activities and sports to enhance muscle strength and coordination and to develop a sense of well-being. Advise caregivers and children to implement precautions when the child engages in contact sports and any activities that carry risk for injury and trauma (e.g., ice hockey, football). Developmental Considerations 23-1 addresses sports guidelines for the child with a bleeding disorder.

Instruct family members, older children, and adolescents to notify health care providers of a bleeding disorder before any invasive procedures to enable use of specific measures to prevent bleeding. Such prophylactic measures include applying pressure for at least 3–5 minutes after a procedure such as a venipuncture, the use of antifibrinolytics for dental work, and the use of factor replacement therapy for surgical procedures. Good dental hygiene is important to reduce bleeding caused by gingival disease. Children with bleeding disorders are encouraged to wear medical IDs that describe their conditions and treatment.

Fever and pain in children with bleeding disorders are often managed with acetaminophen or acetaminophen with codeine.

caREminder

Aspirin, ibuprofen, and ibuprofen-containing medications—such as Excedrin, Midol, Pepto-Bismol, and Percodan—are contraindicated in children with bleeding disorders because they interfere with normal platelet function.

CONTROL OF HEMORRHAGE

When bleeding occurs, health care interventions focus on managing the bleeding promptly. Oral cavity bleeding can result from injury, tooth extraction, or surgery such as a tonsillectomy. Other areas of bleeding are revealed by ecchymoses, epistaxis (nosebleeds), **hematuria** (blood in the urine), **hematemesis** (vomiting blood), and **hematochezia** (bloody stool, also called *melena*).

First aid for someone with a bleeding disorder is the same as it would be for other children. RICE measures (rest, ice, compression, and elevation; see Fig. 20-22)

NURSING INTERVENTIONS 23-1

Preventing Bleeding and Controlling Hemorrhage

Signs and Symptoms of Bleeding
- Bruising
- Bleeding from a cut or other wound
- Reddish, pinpoint rash on skin or in mouth
- Bleeding from nose or mouth
- Blood in sputum, vomitus, stool, urine
- Increase in bleeding with menstrual period
- Intracranial bleeding as evidenced by headache, vomiting, irritability, confusion, seizure, sleeping more than usual, difficulty arousing the child
- Pallor
- Rapid pulse
- Clammy skin
- Shortness of breath
- Dizziness
- Abdominal pain if internal abdominal bleeding
- Decreased blood pressure (late sign in pediatric patient)

Interventions to Prevent Bleeding
- Avoid intravascular, intramuscular, and subcutaneous injections and lab specimen collection.
- Administer intramuscular injections (e.g., immunizations) using Z-track technique; apply pressure and cold for 10 minutes after injection.
- Instruct child to use soft toothbrushes or toothettes for oral care. Rinse and brush teeth after each meal.
- Discourage nose picking, vigorous wiping of the nose, or vigorous nose blowing.
- Avoid rectal procedures (temperatures, suppositories, enemas).

- Promote diet and adjunct therapies to help child avoid constipation.
- Administer oral antifibrinolytic agents before invasive procedures (e.g., dental work).
- Avoid contact sports, heavy lifting, and strenuous activity.
- Shave with an electric razor, not a razor blade.
- Use an emery board for trimming nails; avoid use of nail clippers and/or scissors.
- Teach child and family to avoid activities that can cause trauma.
- Teach child and family signs of bleeding and appropriate actions to take if bleeding occurs.

Interventions to Manage Hemorrhage
- RICE (rest, ice, compression, and elevation)
  - Maintain bed rest when child is actively bleeding.
  - Place ice pack over area of bruising.
  - Apply manual pressure over the bleeding area.
  - Elevate the bleeding extremity.
- Apply pressure dressings to a potential bleeding area.
- Assess vital signs.
- Monitor the child's hemoglobin and hematocrit levels before and after blood loss.
- Monitor for signs of persistent bleeding (e.g., blood in secretions).
- Administer factor replacement, DDAVP, or blood products as appropriate (e.g., fresh-frozen plasma, platelets).

should be used to treat minor bumps and bruises. Children with a bleeding disorder often bleed for a longer time; therefore, the volume lost is greater than children who do not have a bleeding disorder.

Teach the child, family, and school or sports activity personnel how to manage epistaxis: apply constant pressure for 10 minutes to the soft mid nose, with the head tilted forward, and repeat for an additional 10 minutes if necessary. Instruct the child not to blow his or her nose if it is bleeding. Bleeding that persists after this treatment may require treatment with factor replacement, antifibrinolytic therapy, or both. More severe trauma may require use of a synthetic hormone, desmopressin acetate (DDAVP; see discussion later in this chapter). Teach children and their families the skills necessary to administer DDAVP and factor replacement therapy in the home. Many children with more severe bleeding disorders have central venous access; their families are taught to use these devices to infuse factor doses at home.

NUTRITIONAL THERAPY

QUESTION: How could nutritional therapy potentially improve Shawanda's well-being?

Several nutrients play important roles in blood cell formation. Production and maturation of red blood cells is affected by nutritional intake of iron, vitamin B$_{12}$, and folic acid.

Iron is essential to the formation of hemoglobin. Iron is also a component of myoglobin, a protein located in muscle tissue, and is present in enzymes that permit the oxidation of glucose to produce energy for the body. About 80% of iron in the body is available to carry oxygen. The remainder is stored in the body as a protein iron compound called *ferritin* (Lutz & Przytulski, 2010). Vitamin B$_{12}$ is a coenzyme used in the synthesis of

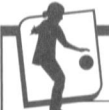

DEVELOPMENTAL CONSIDERATIONS 23-1

Sports Guidelines for Children With a Bleeding Disorder

Usually Safe	Riskier and May Be Discouraged; However, Physical and Psychosocial Benefits Likely Outweigh Risks	Risks Outweigh Benefits; Not Recommended
Archery	Baseball	Boxing
Badminton	Basketball	Diving
Fishing	Bicycling	Football
Golf	Bowling	Hockey
Hiking	Cross-country skiing	Motorcycling
Ping-pong	Frisbee play	Racquetball
Swimming	Gymnastics	Rugby
Walking	Horseback riding	Skateboarding
	Ice skating	Skiing
	Jogging	Snowboarding
	Roller skating/blading	Wrestling
	Running	
	Soccer	
	Tennis	
	Volleyball	
	Water-skiing	
	Weight lifting	

DNA, RNA, and myelin and is necessary for red blood cell formation. Folic acid is involved in the maturation of red blood cells and is closely involved with the functions of vitamin B$_{12}$. Without vitamin B$_{12}$, folic acid is unable to assist in the manufacturing of red blood cells.

Intake of iron, vitamin B$_{12}$, and folic acid is enhanced by ensuring a balanced, healthy diet that includes foods high in these substances (Chart 23-1). The health care provider may also recommend over-the-counter vitamin supplements as an integral part of the child's home therapy. Acute episodes of sickle cell disease, bleeding associated with hemophilia, and IDA may require increased dosages of these vitamins and minerals; in some cases (e.g., use of interferon with severe IDA), IV administration may be required to replenish depleted stores. Collaborate with the nutritionist to provide family education about dietary sources of these vitamins and minerals, and ensure that family members know the signs and symptoms of deficiencies.

ANSWER: Shawanda would most likely benefit from a diet high in iron, vitamin B$_{12}$, and folic acid. Iron is essential to the formation of hemoglobin. Vitamin B$_{12}$ is important in red blood cell formation. Folic acid is involved in the maturation of red blood cells.

TRANSFUSION THERAPY

Transfusion therapy involves the administration of blood or a blood component from a healthy donor to a recipient whose blood has a specific quantitative or qualitative

deficiency. Transfusing specific components of blood is routine in pediatrics. It decreases the risk of circulatory overload and allows the donor blood to benefit more than one person in need. The most frequently transfused blood components are packed red blood cells (PRBCs), platelets, and fresh-frozen plasma (Table 23-1).

The primary concern associated with transfusion therapy is safety. Meticulous care is required when obtaining, processing, typing, and crossmatching blood to ensure compatibility between donor and recipient and to prevent the transmission of disease-causing microbes such as HIV and hepatitis viruses.

Before administration, blood products may be radiated. Radiation interferes with lymphocyte proliferation and prevents transfusion-associated graft-versus-host disease in the recipient who is immunodeficient. Also, blood products are often purposely leukocyte depleted, by means of special microaggregate filters, to minimize the probability of febrile reactions and to decrease the incidence of alloimmunization. PRBCs are occasionally washed to remove residual leukocytes.

It is essential to ensure that consent is obtained and that the right child is the recipient of any transfused blood product by checking two patient identifiers. Adhere carefully to specific institutional policies and procedures when administering blood products to ensure patient safety. When preparing to give blood products, educate the child and family regarding the purpose and procedure of the transfusion.

Be alert for signs and symptoms of a transfusion reaction during and after a transfusion of blood products

CHART 23-1   Dietary Sources of Iron, Vitamin B₁₂, and Folate

Iron

Liver, other red meats

Clams, oysters

Lima and navy beans

Dark-green leafy vegetables

Dried fruit

Vitamin B₁₂

Poultry

Fish

Meat

Eggs

Milk products (e.g., cow's milk, cheese, yogurt)

Fortified breakfast cereals

Folate

Leafy, green vegetables (e.g., romaine lettuce, cooked spinach, broccoli, brussel sprouts)

Whole-grain cereals and fortified breakfast cereals

Wheat germ

Legumes

Oranges

Beets

Cooked asparagus

Beef liver

(Table 23-2). Most transfusion reactions occur during the first 15 minutes of transfusion, so begin the transfusion slowly at first and monitor the child closely. If no transfusion reactions are apparent, increase the infusion rate as appropriate. Continue regular monitoring throughout the transfusion. If a transfusion reaction occurs, stop the transfusion immediately, keep the IV line patent with normal saline, monitor the child closely, and notify the physician. Additional interventions depend on the nature and severity of the reaction.

Experiencing transfusion reactions, especially severe ones, is likely to be stressful for the child and family. Be sure to provide emotional support and ongoing progress reports about the child's status.

Exchange Transfusion

Exchange transfusion involves substituting donor red blood cells for recipient red blood cells. During exchange transfusion, small quantities of the recipient's blood are alternately removed and replaced with donor blood until the desired volume of blood has been exchanged.

Clinical situations in which exchange transfusions might be prescribed include the following:

- When the increased blood volume from a simple transfusion might not be tolerated. Examples include the newborn, who is at risk for fluid overload, and the child with severe anemia, who is at risk for heart failure.
- To decrease the quantity of an abnormal element in the blood or to remove an excessive amount of a normal component. Examples include the child with a severe sickle cell crisis (caused by a large number of sickled red blood cells) and the child with polycythemia.

Exchange transfusion is described in more detail in Chapter 14.

Chronic Transfusion Therapy

Chronic transfusion therapy is an ongoing program in which blood transfusions are given at regular intervals (usually about every 3 weeks). Chronic transfusion therapy is used when the benefit—avoiding potentially serious medical complications—justifies the risks of alloimmunization, infection, and iron overload. By regularly providing normal red blood cells, chronic transfusion suppresses production of abnormal erythrocytes. Beta-thalassemia major (Cooley anemia) and certain severe vaso-occlusive crises associated with sickle

TABLE 23-1	Commonly Transfused Blood Components	
Product	**Indications for Use**	**Administration**
PRBCs	Symptomatic anemia Replacement therapy (e.g., during surgery)	Children usually receive 10–15 mL/kg, generally transfused over 2–3 hours, with 4 hours being the maximum infusion time. Severely anemic children are at risk for heart failure if PRBCs are given too rapidly. Anemic state must be gradually corrected with separate transfusions.
Platelets	Bleeding associated with thrombocytopenia or platelet dysfunction Preoperatively when thrombocytopenia present High risk for bleeding related to severe thrombocytopenia	Given as quickly as the child can tolerate, usually over 20–30 minutes.
Fresh-frozen plasma	Replacement of noncellular coagulation factors	Given as quickly as the child can tolerate, usually over 20–30 minutes.

TABLE 23-2   Transfusion Reactions

	Hemolytic Reaction	**Febrile Reaction**	**Allergic Reaction**
Description	Red blood cell destruction that occurs when the blood product is not compatible with the recipient's blood type or when the donor blood contains minor blood group antigens to which the recipient has been previously sensitized (alloimmunized). Reactions can be immediate or delayed.	Not associated with hemolysis. Generally occurs when the recipient has developed antibodies to leukocyte, platelet, or plasma protein antigens in the donor blood. These reactions are more likely in children who have previously received blood products.	Nonhemolytic reactions that occur when the donor blood contains plasma proteins or other antigens to which the recipient is hypersensitive.
Signs and symptoms	Fever Chills Urticaria Restlessness Headache Chest pain, tachycardia, hypotension Abdominal/lower back pain Oliguria Shock	Fever Chills Diaphoresis	Rash, pruritus Urticaria Swelling Severe reactions: respiratory distress, bronchospasm, hypotension, and shock Anaphylaxis
Treatment	Fluids, corticosteroids, vasopressors, and mannitol may be required to maintain circulation and urinary output.	Usually treated with acetaminophen and corticosteroids.	Rash and pruritus usually respond to the antihistamine diphenhydramine. Severe reactions require treatment with epinephrine, IV fluids, airway protection, oxygen, vasopressors, and other interventions as needed.
Preventive measures	Sensitization is most likely in children who have previously received multiple transfusions and have been exposed to allogeneic antigens. Type and crossmatch accurately. Use leukocyte-depleted blood products to help prevent alloimmunization.	Pretreat with antipyretic and corticosteroid. Use leukocyte-depleted blood products.	Pretreat with antihistamine and corticosteroid. Wash red blood cells before transfusing.

cell disease are clinical situations in which a chronic transfusion program may be prescribed.

Goals of a chronic transfusion therapy program for children with severe chronic anemia include

- Maintaining a hemoglobin S level between 30% and 50% in children with sickle cell disease
- Providing primary stroke prevention or preventing stroke recurrence
- Treating chronic debilitating pain, pulmonary hypertension, and anemia associated with chronic renal failure
- Increasing the quality-of-life for children with chronic heart failure
- Delaying the onset of splenomegaly with hypersplenism and the accompanying need for splenectomy

Children receiving chronic therapy are at increased risk for infection from blood-borne viruses; therefore, they should receive immunization against hepatitis B.

The major complication of an ongoing transfusion therapy program is the development of toxic iron overload, which leads to pathologic changes in body

systems, including the hepatic, endocrine, and cardiac systems. Hepatic changes are among the earliest to occur and include fibrosis and cirrhosis. Endocrine changes include pancreatic destruction, which causes insulin-dependent diabetes mellitus, and hormone deficiencies that impair growth and delay the appearance of secondary sex characteristics. Cardiac changes include arrhythmias and heart failure. If iron chelation therapy is not started during early childhood, the cardiac alterations become severe and often lead to death during the teenage years.

Iron chelation therapy, usually started by age 3 or 4 years, is accomplished with the use of deferoxamine. The drug acts by binding free iron in the bloodstream and excreting it via urine from the kidneys. Deferoxamine is contraindicated for children with severe renal disease. Chelation therapy is prolonged and painful, which makes adherence difficult for many children and adolescents. Deferasirox (Exjade), an effective oral chelating agent, can be given once daily and has demonstrated efficacy in children (Tunc et al., 2012).

KidKare To improve compliance with parenterally administered chelation therapy, combine behaviorally oriented programs with education, and include family members.

SPLENECTOMY

Removal of the spleen is sometimes necessary for children with severe hematologic abnormalities or those refractory to transfusion, nutritional measures, and pharmacologic treatment. Although splenectomy is the most effective treatment available for some conditions such as sickle cell disease, hereditary spherocytosis, and chronic ITP, it leaves children immunologically impaired and therefore is not first-line therapy for most diseases of the hematologic system. Children should receive *Haemophilus influenzae* type b and polyvalent pneumococcal vaccines before splenectomy to stimulate antibody production for future protection against sepsis. A splenectomy may be done via a laparotomy. However, laparoscopic splenectomy provides a less invasive technique for children who need this treatment.

SUPPORTIVE CARE

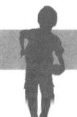

QUESTION: When caring for Shawanda and her family, what supportive care will be necessary?

Management of the child with a hematologic disorder requires attention to the psychosocial needs of the child and all members of the family.

Support of the Child

Helping children with any hematologic disorder requires accurate knowledge about the disorder, its management, and its complications to promote the child's physical and psychological well-being. Although children with hematologic conditions score well on quality-of-life measures (Bullinger & von Mackensen, 2003; Yalcin et al., 2007), they need to develop effective coping skills. They may fear bleeding, pain, or infection. They may wonder what will happen to them when they do experience a bleeding episode or vaso-occlusive crisis. Knowing the signs and symptoms that require attention, how to respond when they occur, and what to expect others to do helps children cope. Instruct children to notify their family, teachers, or other caregivers when they experience any concerns or symptoms so that interventions can be implemented promptly. For children with hemophilia, for example, these measures usually include factor replacement. Older children and adolescents have probably learned how to prepare and administer their own factor, whereas family members or home health nurses usually perform this procedure for younger children. School visits by a nurse or social worker knowledgeable in the child's specific care can provide support for school personnel (Evidence-Based Clinical Practice Guidelines 23-1).

Children may be concerned about pain associated with IV insertion and laboratory testing. The use of topical anesthetic creams and family involvement with comfort holding techniques and distraction can help children cope (see Chapter 10).

EVIDENCE-BASED CLINICAL PRACTICE GUIDELINES 23-1
Children With a Bleeding Disorder in School and Daycare Settings

National Hemophilia Foundation. (2006). *Back to school with a bleeding disorder*. Retrieved from

http://www.hemaware.org/story/back-school-bleeding-disorder

Article aimed at helping parents to better understand how to prepare child with a bleeding disorder to be safe in the school setting.

National Hemophilia Foundation. (2001). *The child with a bleeding disorder: First aid for school personnel*. Retrieved from

http://www.hemophilia.org/NHFWeb/MainPgs/MainNHF.aspx?menuid=204&contentid=27

Publication for school nurses and teachers who have a student with a bleeding disorder. Describes typical injuries associated with a bleeding disorder and the steps that need to be followed to treat the condition in the school setting.

National Hemophilia Foundation. (2011). *Guidelines for growing: An action plan for parents of children with bleeding disorders*. Retrieved from

http://www.cdc.gov/ncbddd/hemophilia/documents/8PG_G4G_5-8.pdf

Brochure to provide guidance for parents of children 5–8 years old with a bleeding disorder. Guidelines are also available for other age groups.

National Hemophilia Foundation. (2012). *The student with a bleeding disorder*. Retrieved from

http://www.hemophilia.org/NHFWeb/Resource/StaticPages/menu0/menu5/menu58/menu98/Studentwithableedingdisorder.pdf

School nurses' guide to bleeding disorders.

Children with hematologic conditions must establish their identities as individuals with a particular chronic disorder. Help them to identify their positive qualities, realize what they can do, develop healthy self-images, and formulate realistic goals for their futures (see Nursing Plan of Care 12-1).

Support of the Family

Families of a child with a hematologic condition are likely to have psychosocial concerns. Provide informational and emotional support to meet family needs. Informational support means providing families with timely information regarding the disorder and its effect on their child. Develop an ongoing teaching plan that includes the information that family caregivers commonly require (see Teaching Intervention Plans 23-1 and 23-2 later in this chapter). Families also need counseling about specific aspects of the disease—for example, the genetic nature of sickle cell disease and what it means for their other children, both now and in the future.

Although the desired outcomes of providing information include improved family coping and the ability to parent a child with a hematologic condition effectively, the information family members receive is likely to be emotionally disturbing at first. As the family begins to learn about the child's condition, families may worry that they will not recognize a bleeding episode or will not respond appropriately. They may also fear that the child will easily become anemic or neutropenic. The diagnosis of a bleeding disorder, the early bleeding episodes thereafter, and any painful or serious bleeding episodes are all sources of emotional stress for most families. Also, parents (especially the mother) may feel guilty if the child's condition was transmitted genetically.

Health care expenses may generate stress, especially if the child has a severe condition and frequently requires costly factor replacement therapy or medications. Factor products are very expensive, and children can surpass insurance lifetime maximums quickly. A social worker or financial counselor can advise families about available benefits and offer other resources for support.

Emotional support for family members includes listening, identifying previously effective coping skills, providing positive reinforcement, and offering practical information. Support groups provide an opportunity for caregivers to share, learn from others, and encourage one another.

As in other chronic or genetic disorders, the well siblings of children with a hematologic condition need attention. Sometimes they feel left out, or they may feel guilty because they are well. Siblings need a sense of belonging within the family. They need to feel that their parents have time for them and value them just as much as they value the child with the chronic condition. Also, siblings need accurate knowledge about the child's condition, its etiology, its management, and its complications; information about how they can help during bleeding episodes or other complications; and their own need for genetic testing for the condition if necessary.

ANSWER: Supportive care needs to be focused on all members of the family. Supportive care for Shawanda involves teaching her about her disease at an age-appropriate level and assisting her to develop age-appropriate coping skills and a positive self-image. Pain relief measures also are important. Supportive care for the family includes providing emotional support to all family caregivers and siblings and providing them with information about the disorder and effective coping strategies. Shawanda's brothers need attention, too. They need to feel that their parents have time for them. In addition, they need teaching to assist them in understanding what is happening with their sister so that they can help, as appropriate.

NURSING PLAN OF CARE

The primary foci of health care interventions for pediatric hematologic alterations are to prevent injury to the child and to provide the child and family with a strong knowledge base about the disorder, crisis prevention, and supportive measures. Nursing Plan of Care 23-1 summarizes the nursing diagnoses and outcomes that might apply to the child experiencing a disorder of hemostasis or a form of anemia. In addition, the nursing plan of care in Chapter 12 is applicable to the child with a chronic hematologic condition.

ALTERATIONS IN HEMATOLOGIC STATUS

Alterations in hematologic status can be broadly categorized as disorders of hemostasis, anemias, and hemoglobinopathies.

DISORDERS OF HEMOSTASIS

Hemostasis is a complex process designed to prevent hemorrhage. Effective hemostasis requires ongoing interaction among the vascular walls, platelets, and certain plasma factors. Hemostasis comprises four major events that occur in a set order following the loss of vascular integrity:

1. Injury to a blood vessel evokes a vasoconstrictive response that slows blood loss from the damaged vessel.
2. Platelets become activated by thrombin and aggregate, leading to the formation of a platelet plug at the site of injury. The protein *fibrinogen* is primarily responsible for stimulating platelet clumping. Platelets clump by binding to collagen that becomes exposed after rupture of the endothelial lining of vessels. Upon activation, platelets release adenosine diphosphate and thromboxane A_2 (which activate additional platelets), serotonin, phospholipids, lipoproteins, and other proteins important for the coagulation cascade. In addition, activated platelets change their shape to accommodate formation of the plug.
3. A fibrin mesh (called a *clot*) forms and entraps the plug, ensuring the stability of the initially loose

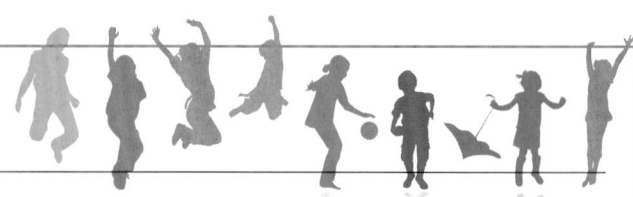

NURSING PLAN OF CARE 23-1:

For the Child With Altered Hematologic Status

Nursing Diagnosis: Risk for injury related to effects of hematologic disorder (e.g., factor deficiency, low platelet count)

Interventions/Rationale

- Assess child's vital signs and hydration status. Assess for any increase in active bleeding, bruising, or petechiae. Assess for frank bleeding from nose, mouth, or urinary and gastrointestinal tract. Monitor stools and urine for occult blood.

    Promotes early assessment to facilitate prompt treatment.

- Assess child's tissue perfusion including skin color, warmth, pulses, capillary refill, complaints of numbness or tingling of extremities, vital signs, and oral mucosa.

    Indicates fluid balance, level of hydration, and effectiveness of fluid replacement.

- Monitor laboratory values (hemoglobin, hematocrit, red blood cells, platelets, white blood cells).

    Evaluates for reduced oxygen-carrying capacity of blood, potential infection, and ability to stop bleeding.

- Encourage consolidation of laboratory blood sampling.

    Reduces the number of venipunctures and risk of blood volume depletion.

- Institute supplemental oxygen as needed.

    Increases oxygen-carrying capacity of the blood.

- Institute measures to prevent bleeding or control hemorrhage, as indicated (see Nursing Interventions 23-1). Monitor for effectiveness of interventions, including any adverse reactions such as transfusion reactions (see Nursing Interventions 23-2).

    Ensures effective and prompt administration of interventions such as administering factor replacement to reduce the incidence and severity of bleeding episodes and resultant complications.

- Review with the family the child's treatment plan, including medications and common side effects, injury prevention, and hemorrhage control measures. As requested by the family, provide information to school/daycare about child's condition (see Community Care 23-1).

    Enables correction of misunderstandings and increases knowledge.

Expected Outcomes

- Child will remain free of injury, experiencing minimal to no bleeding as a result of injuries such as falls, punctures, cuts, or other environmental hazards.
- Child will maintain laboratory values consistent with normal hemostasis.
- Child will exhibit signs and symptoms of adequate tissue perfusion.
- Child and family will identify common types of bleeding associated with the child's particular bleeding disorder.
- Child and family will identify signs and symptoms associated with overt and covert bleeding and will use interventions to prevent or immediately treat bleeding.

Nursing Diagnosis: Acute pain related to vaso-occlusive crisis, hemarthrosis associated with trauma to a limb, bleeding in joints, and/or traumatic injury to muscles

Also see Nursing Plan of Care 10-1.

Interventions/Rationale

- Assess pain using a reliable and valid method that is developmentally appropriate and appropriate for the situation. Elicit assessment of child's pain from the perspective of the family caregivers.

    The subjective rating of pain is most reliable, but it may not be an option in a nonverbal child (infant, intubated, comatose). Validated tools provide the most accurate assessment. The absence of behaviors indicative of pain does not necessarily mean that the child is not experiencing pain. Families know their child best and are familiar with their typical behaviors.

- Assess location and character of pain. Assess for ability to move affected limbs. Assess for paresthesia.

    Frequent episodes of bleeding or vaso-occlusive crises can result in joint inflammation, impaired mobility, and resulting nerve compression. Pain may be occurring in other sites related to soft-tissue hemorrhage.

- Use comfort measures. Position child comfortably, using pillows, lightweight blankets, and other measures to decrease pressure on tissues. Use splints for joint discomfort. Use foam overlay mattresses. Use ice packs or moist heat as indicated. Offer use of whirlpool bath.

    Excessive bleeding in the joints and from traumatic injury can cause joint pain, swelling of the joints, and tenderness to affected sites. Positioning devices and use of splints can increase the child's comfort. Ice may decrease swelling. Moist heat may increase circulation to the area.

- Implement pharmacologic and biobehavioral interventions to alleviate the pain (see Chapter 10 for a detailed discussion). Use a preventive approach to keep pain at or below an acceptable level. Involve the family in pain management.

Unrelieved pain has deleterious physiologic effects, such as tachycardia, suppressed immune function, and atelectasis as well as negative psychological effects. Opioid analgesics are indicated for moderate to severe pain. Pain is better managed if it is not allowed to escalate. The family can provide measures that may be more comforting to the child than those provided by a nurse.

- Administer treatments (e.g., factor VIII, cold treatment, oxygen therapy) to control bleeding and/or underlying cause of pain such as a vaso-occlusive crisis.

  Treating the primary hematologic cause will help control current pain and prevent future pain.

- Reassess pain level and evaluate effectiveness of interventions frequently.

  Frequent reassessments are required to ensure effective control and to prevent exacerbation of the pain. Children respond differently to interventions; what is effective for one may not work for another.

- Provide rest periods. Encourage child to progress from passive range of motion to active exercise as tolerated. Provide assistive devices as needed to help child be mobile.

  These measures assist child in maintaining optimum physical mobility while remaining pain free.

Expected Outcomes

- Child will state that adequate pain relief has been obtained.
- Child will demonstrate pain relief by absence of crying, restlessness, agitation, irritability, facial grimacing, splinting, or rigid body posture.
- Child will perform activities of daily living and developmentally appropriate activities with minimal interference from pain and medication side effects.

Nursing Diagnosis: Anxiety related to perceptions about receiving a transfusion

Interventions/Rationale

- Allow family to express fears, concerns, and anger. Acknowledge concerns; reassure that others have expressed similar concerns.

  With public awareness of AIDS and other blood-borne pathogens, the family is likely to express some concerns about receiving blood/ blood products. Likewise, the family may have concerns about their ability to complete other aspects of the treatment plan. Listening to their concerns provides the opportunity to identify their fears and problems. Fears may immobilize the family and interfere with adequate care. These fears must be addressed to facilitate patient care.

- Assess family ethnic, cultural, and religious background.

  Information about family background provides clues about potential resistance or concern of family members about having the child receive blood, be sedated, or undergo other procedures or therapies.

- Reinforce health care provider explanations about the proposed treatment plan. Offer a brief explanation of precautionary measures used by the blood bank to ensure safety of blood product administration.

  Transfusions and many other procedures and treatments require informed consent for treatment. Sufficient information prior to administration is required for informed consent.

- Explain the usual protocol for administering blood products (e.g., taking vital signs before, during, and after administration; having two nurses validate that the correct product is being administered).

  Knowledge of the protocol helps to alleviate family and child concerns when these measures are enacted.

Expected Outcomes

- Child and family will express concerns regarding blood/blood product transfusion.
- Child and family will describe protocol for administering transfusion.

Nursing Diagnosis: Risk for injury related to effects of transfused blood/blood product

Interventions/Rationale

- Allow child and the family to express feelings, fears, and concerns (see previous diagnoses).

  Provides opportunities to clear up misconceptions and to provide accurate and factual information.

- Follow hospital policy and procedure manuals for blood transfusions.

  Administration protocols follow evidence-based practice guidelines to ensure patient safety.

- Use measures to prevent transfusion reactions:
  - Identify child and verify blood (type, Rh factor, donor number, expiration date) with another nurse or physician.
  - Prime infusion line with normal saline to decrease risk of hemolysis of red blood cells.
  - Monitor prescribed flow rate of infusion, use an infusion pump to regulate flow, administer slowly during the first 15 minutes of infusion for all children, and continue slow rate for children at risk for fluid overload.
  - Remain with the child during the first 15–30 minutes of transfusion.
  - Note and report changes in skin color (pallor, duskiness) and mentation (restlessness,

(Continued)

NURSING PLAN OF CARE 23-1:

For the Child With Altered Hematologic Status (*Continued*)

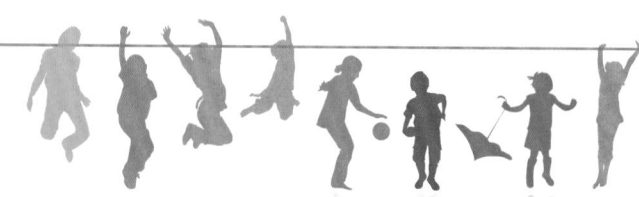

confusion, agitation) when taking vital signs. Note facial flushing, bounding pulses, and complaints of headache and flank or chest pain.

- Auscultate lungs for the presence of rales, rhonchi, or muffled breath sounds prior to initiating transfusion and when changes in vital signs, skin color, or mentation occur.
- Identify possible transfusion reactions promptly (see Nursing Interventions 23-2).
- Inform child and family of key symptoms of adverse reactions before leaving child and show them how to notify nurse should such reactions occur.

    Early identification of transfusion reaction allows for prompt treatment. Most reactions will occur during the first 30 minutes of administration. Administration of blood/blood products increases circulating blood volume. If the child is unable to compensate for this additional fluid volume, pulmonary congestion may develop, altering the ventilation–perfusion ratio and impairing gaseous exchange. Family members can assist in identifying problems.

- Initiate immediate measures to correct transfusion reactions (see Nursing Interventions 23-2).

    When a hemolytic reaction occurs, an antibody–antigen response causes blood cells to agglutinate, resulting in obstruction of blood flow to vital organs, including the lungs. Emergency treatment may be necessary for respiratory distress, hypotension, shock, or fluid overload.

- Continue to monitor vital signs; report significant changes.

    The child requires ongoing assessment to evaluate effectiveness of treatment and resolution of reaction.

- Obtain blood sample, and forward specimen and remaining blood product with attached tubing to laboratory.

    Follow-up specimen collection enables repeat typing and crossmatch of blood to determine compatibility.

Expected Outcomes

- Child will remain free of complications of blood/blood product administration.
- Child will maintain adequate ventilation and perfusion of all body tissues.

Nursing Diagnosis: Deficient knowledge: Hematologic disorder, treatment, care, and potential complications

Interventions/Rationale

- Assess child and family members' perceptions and knowledge of child's condition, treatment regimen, and preventive care.

    Teaching requires a solid base from which to start. It helps enable correction of misconceptions and provides opportunity for additional teaching as indicated.

- Provide genetic counseling as indicated.

    Many hematologic conditions have an underlying genetic basis.

- Schedule a team conference with key family caregivers, child, friends (as appropriate), and teachers to provide information and explore feelings and attitudes. Encourage child to take part in selecting conference participants.

    Child becomes a comanager; assists in having mutual support and information.

- Stress importance of regular, frequent follow-up appointments to ensure that health care needs are met properly. Initiate referrals, appointments with community support groups, mental health clinics, etc., as needed for continued psychosocial support.

    Health care needs are constantly changing. Frequent follow-up enhances opportunities to alter regimen as health care needs improve or deteriorate and provides for continued support after discharge.

- Teach child and parents how to administer medications, factor replacement, and dietary therapy/modifications in the home and school.

    Effective home management of the child's condition can reduce subsequent complications of the child's condition.

- Instruct family regarding safety procedures to use to prevent a hematologic crisis (e.g., avoid contact sports for child with hemophilia; avoid high altitudes for child with sickle cell disease).

    Preventive measures are essential to reduce injury and the need for hospitalization.

Expected Outcomes

- Child and family will verbalize understanding of child's condition, its treatment, and ongoing home care.
- Child and family will demonstrate interventions to provide emergency care for child if child sustains a hematologic injury or insult at home or school.

- Child and family will use measures to create a home environment that protects the child from injury.

Nursing Diagnosis: Ineffective protection related to neutropenia, thrombocytopenia, bleeding, and/or loss of macrophage activity after splenectomy
Also see Nursing Plan of Care 22-1.

Interventions/Rationale
- Monitor laboratory values that indicate hematologic deficiencies (e.g., white blood cell count, partial thromboplastin time, platelet count).
  Reduced values indicate need to implement strategies to protect the child from infection and bleeding.
- Assess for bleeding (frank blood from nose, gums, wounds, etc., and blood in urine and stools). Assess for infection (elevated temperature, increased heart rate, diaphoresis).
  Risk of bleeding is increased as platelet counts decrease. Risk of infection occurs in the presence of neutropenia.
- Institute bleeding precautions, including minimizing number of venipunctures for laboratory tests; avoiding rectal procedures (temperatures, enemas, suppositories); using a soft toothbrush for oral care; not using ibuprofen or aspirin; avoiding contact sports, heavy lifting, or strenuous activity; and using bed rails, pads, or blankets on and around furniture to protect child from injury (see Nursing Interventions 23-1).
  Venipuncture sites will ooze and bleed more in the presence of low platelet counts. Anything placed in the rectum may cause tearing and bleeding of the anal mucosa. Ibuprofen decreases the ability of the blood to clot. Aspirin can increase bleeding, especially when platelets are low. A soft toothbrush is gentler on the gums and thus helps prevent bleeding. Vigorous and rigorous activity can cause bruising and injury to soft tissue. Younger children are prone to falls, and the environment can be altered to protect them from hurting themselves against furniture and beds.
- Administer factor replacement, DDAVP, or blood products as ordered.
  Transfusion therapy may be warranted to ensure restoration of lost or depleted platelets.
- Teach family to recognize early the signs and symptoms of infection (e.g., fever, chills, productive cough, malaise) and to use neutropenic precautions in the home (see Community Care 22-4).

The child and family can learn to avoid situations that will increase the incidence of infection and to implement wellness behaviors that will enable the child to remain healthy.
- Stress importance of handwashing by child and family caregivers.
  Handwashing reduces transmission of microorganisms and the risk for infection.
- Instruct family regarding administration of prophylactic antibiotics. Monitor child's adherence in taking medication.
  Prophylactic antibiotics counteract opportunistic infections.
- Instruct family to ensure that child completes routine immunizations.
  Immunization ensures child remains protected from certain childhood diseases.
- Instruct child to avoid contact with persons who have colds or infections.
  Avoiding sick people protects child from contracting bacterial and viral infections from others.
- Reinforce importance of need for daily hygiene, mouth care, and perineal care.
  Proper hygiene protects against bacterial invasion.
- If child is hospitalized, provide a private room for protective isolation.
  Isolation may be necessary if the ANC is less than 500/mm³. These children are at high risk for infection.

Expected Outcomes
- Child will remain free from infection; any infection will be detected and treated early.
- Child and family will institute measures to prevent infection and injury (e.g., careful hygiene, immunizations up to date).
- Child will have reduced risk of bleeding as indicated by adequate platelet levels and absence of bruising and petechiae.

Nursing Diagnosis: Anxiety related to prognosis, actual or perceived loss of body integrity, threat to self-concept
See Nursing Plan of Care 12-2.

Nursing Diagnosis: Disturbed body image related to being different than peers, perceiving self as sick, loss of body part
See Nursing Plan of Care 12-2.

Nursing Diagnosis: Spiritual distress related to response to crisis of the illness, suffering, or death of a child
See Nursing Plan of Care 13-1.

platelet plug. Platelet plugs are usually adequate to seal off tiny ruptures in blood vessels, but clot formation is necessary to close larger vascular injuries. If the plug contains only platelets, it is called a *white thrombus*; if red blood cells are present, it is called a *red thrombus*.

4. When bleeding is controlled, plasmin degrades and dissolves the clot and releases fibrin degradation products. This final step enables normal blood flow to resume after tissue repair.

Two biochemical pathways lead to the formation of a fibrin clot: the intrinsic pathway and the extrinsic pathway. Although these pathways are initiated by distinct mechanisms, the two converge on a common pathway that leads to clot formation. The **intrinsic pathway** leads to formation of a red thrombus or clot in response to an abnormality in the vessel wall in the absence of tissue injury. The **extrinsic pathway** leads to formation of a fibrin clot in response to tissue injury. Both pathways are complex and involve numerous different proteins called *clotting factors* (Table 23-3).

A disorder in hemostasis is called a **coagulopathy**. These disorders are caused by deficiencies or imbalances of clotting factors. The most common deficiencies seen in children involve factor VIII (hemophilia A), factor IX (hemophilia B), and von Willebrand factor (von Willebrand disease). These disorders can cause rapid, excessive blood loss, which can quickly place a child in a life-threatening situation. Prompt interventions are necessary to prevent and control hemorrhage (see Nursing Interventions 23-1). DIC and ITP are also disorders in hemostasis that are seen in the pediatric population and are discussed later in this section.

TABLE 23-3	Clotting Factors
Clotting Factor	**Name**
Factor I	Fibrinogen
Factor II	Prothrombin
Factor III	Tissue thromboplastin
Factor IV	Calcium
Factor V (no factor VI)	Proaccelerin
Factor VII	Proconvertin
Factor VIII	Antihemophilic factor
Factor IX	Plasma thromboplastin component; Christmas factor
Factor X	Stuart factor
Factor XI	Plasma thromboplastin antecedent
Factor XII	Hageman factor
Factor XIII	Fibrin-stabilizing factor Prekallikrein; Fletcher factor High-molecular-weight kininogen; Fitzgerald factor Platelets

HEMOPHILIA

Hemophilia is a serious bleeding disorder, affecting an estimated 20,000 males in the United States. About 400 children are born with this disorder each year (Centers for Disease Control and Prevention, 2011). The most prevalent forms, hemophilia A (classic hemophilia) and hemophilia B (Christmas disease), are usually inherited in a recessive manner through a genetic defect on the X chromosome (see Fig. 3-3). Among the offspring of a carrier female and a normal male, half the daughters are carriers of hemophilia and half are disease free. Half the sons have hemophilia and half are disease free. Among the offspring of a normal female and a male with hemophilia, all the daughters are carriers of hemophilia and all the sons are disease free. Some females who are carriers have an increased tendency to bleed, similar to a male with mild hemophilia, and require treatment. In some rare genetic circumstances, females can have moderate to severe hemophilia.

Hemophilia also can result from a spontaneous genetic mutation, with approximately one-third of children with hemophilia having no family history of this disorder. Among people who have hemophilia, 9 out of 10 have hemophilia A, and 70% of those individuals have the severe form of the disease (National Heart, Lung, and Blood Institute, 2011). Hemophilia affects all ethnic groups.

The prognosis for children with hemophilia has improved considerably during recent years. The development of comprehensive treatment centers, the availability of virally inactivated and recombinant factors for replacement therapy, and the advent of home infusion therapy have improved treatment success.

Pathophysiology

Hemophilia A and hemophilia B are distinguished by the particular procoagulant factor that is decreased, absent, or dysfunctional. In hemophilia A, it is factor VIII; in hemophilia B, it is factor IX. A disorder in either factor inhibits the formation of thrombin, which is essential to normal coagulation.

Hemophilia A and hemophilia B are subclassified as mild, moderate, or severe on the basis of the level of factor VIII and factor IX, respectively (Srivastava et al., 2013):

- *Mild hemophilia* is characterized by a factor level of 5% to 40% of normal (0.05 to 0.40 International Units/mL). People with mild hemophilia experience prolonged bleeding only when injured. Thus, their condition may not be diagnosed unless they have trauma or surgery.
- *Moderate hemophilia* is distinguished by a factor level of 1% to 5% of normal (0.01 to 0.05 International Units/mL). People with moderate hemophilia usually have prolonged bleeding with trauma, surgery, or muscle overuse, but they may experience occasions of spontaneous bleeding as well.
- *Severe hemophilia* is characterized by a factor level less than 1% of normal (<0.01 International Units/mL). People with severe hemophilia have prolonged

bleeding with trauma or surgery. They also may have frequent episodes of spontaneous bleeding (bleeding that occurs in the absence of injury).

Regardless of the type, if bleeding is not treated effectively, target joints are particularly at risk for deterioration and the development of chronic, disabling hemophilic arthropathy (joint disease). Other common types of bleeding in children with hemophilia are intramuscular **hematomas** (localized masses of extravasated blood) and oral cavity bleeding. Any extensive internal or external blood loss, particularly episodes involving the head or central nervous system, neck, or abdomen (e.g., iliopsoas intramuscular hemorrhage), is potentially life threatening.

Assessment

The clinical hallmark of hemophilia A or hemophilia B is **hemarthrosis** (deep bleeding into joints, muscles, and soft tissue). Frequently, the person with hemophilia develops a "target" joint that is repeatedly the site of bleeding episodes. Assess the child for hemarthrosis, which most often affects the knee, elbow, and ankle joints. Monitor for tingling, tenderness, pain, warmth, swelling, and decreased mobility at the affected site. Gently assess range of motion of all extremities. Repeated bleeding into a joint causes cartilage erosion and joint space narrowing, decreased range of motion, and proximal muscle weakening; disabling arthropathy may follow.

Intramuscular hematomas cause swelling, heat, and tenderness and can restrict movement. If deep, they can be difficult to palpate and the child may complain of only a vague sense of discomfort or pain, even when serious hemorrhage has occurred. Hematomas that block the airway, compress vital organs, or result in extensive internal bleeding and shock can be life threatening. Some hematomas compress nerves and cause paralysis.

Bleeding episodes can also be related to the child's stage of development. For example, neonates may have a marked cephalhematoma, bleeding with circumcision, or bleeding from the umbilical cord or site. Infants may experience oral bleeding with eruption of a tooth. Young children are prone to falls and injuries. In middle childhood, children are more likely to experience bleeding episodes when they dare to engage in high-risk physical activities or during loss of deciduous teeth. Adolescents are at risk for bleeding episodes when they yield to peer pressure and participate in high-risk physical activities.

Diagnostic Tests

Laboratory data identify hemophilia A or hemophilia B. In both disorders, fibrinogen levels, platelet count, and prothrombin time are normal; partial thromboplastin time is prolonged. Factor VIII is decreased in hemophilia A; factor IX is decreased in hemophilia B. If substantial blood loss occurs, the blood cell profile (CBC) may also point to anemia.

Interdisciplinary Interventions

Hemophilia treatment centers employ professionals from various disciplines, such as physical therapy, social work, hematology, orthopedics, gynecology, nutrition, and genetics, who provide complete, comprehensive health care for children with hemophilia. Teaching is a critical aspect of the child's care. The primary treatment for hemophilia includes the use of factor replacement therapy to replace clotting factors and the use of adjunct medications to increase clotting factors prior to undergoing certain medical or dental procedures.

Factor Replacement Therapy

The most important aspect of management is prompt and appropriate factor replacement to raise the factor level as quickly as possible, thereby shortening the bleeding episode and decreasing the probability of long-term complications. Prompt therapy is so essential that treatment usually precedes diagnostic testing to assess fully the current injury or bleeding episode.

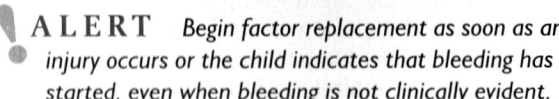 **ALERT**   *Begin factor replacement as soon as an injury occurs or the child indicates that bleeding has started, even when bleeding is not clinically evident.*

Factor replacement therapy is the IV infusion of *factors VIII and IX concentrates* to prevent or control bleeding. *Factor VIII concentrates* are used for hemophilia A. *Factor IX concentrates* are used to manage acute hemorrhage or to decrease the risk of bleeding associated with surgery in children with hemophilia B. These concentrates are derived from either human plasma or a genetically engineered cell line made by DNA technology called *recombinant*. For both types, the factor VIII or IX protein is nearly identical to the protein that is lacking in the blood of hemophiliacs. After the infusion is complete, the recipient has all the proteins needed for clotting to occur. This replacement of missing clotting factors is not permanent. Half the infused clotting factor activity is removed by the body every 12 to 24 hours. Thus, within 2 or 3 days, almost all the infused factor VIII or IX concentrate is gone from the bloodstream and the child may not be able to form clots again. However, by this time, the factors will have been effective in assisting clot formation at the site where the bleeding occurred, which initiated the need for factor replacement.

The level of factor correction required to achieve hemostasis depends on the nature of the injury or specific bleeding episode. Mild to moderate hemorrhage requires factor correction to 30% to 50% of the normal factor level. This goal is often achieved with a one-time infusion of factor, but an additional one or two doses may be needed. Severe or life-threatening hemorrhage necessitates immediate factor correction to 100%, followed by a 50% to 100% factor level, maintained for a number of days. Similar factor correction and maintenance are prescribed when surgical procedures are required. Maintenance levels are achieved by intermittent or continuous infusion.

Factor replacement therapy is not curative. However, the genes for factor VIII and factor IX have been cloned, and gene transfer methods are currently being developed that are likely to have future clinical application.

The goal of gene transfer therapy is to facilitate endogenous production of factor VIII and factor IX in quantities that cure hemophilia or at least decrease its severity (Branchford et al., 2013).

caREminder

Use of 23- or 25-gauge needles is recommended for IV access to protect the veins and prevent bleeding at the IV site. When venipuncture is necessary, apply pressure after the venipuncture for 3–5 minutes (Srivastava et al., 2013).

Management of Complications

The child with hemophilia will require management for complications caused by replacement therapy. Two major concerns include the development of inhibitors (antibodies) and transmission of viral diseases.

Approximately 46% of patients with factor VIII deficiency develop an inhibitor, 15% to 20% of them at high titers. Five percent of patients with factor IX deficiency develop an inhibitor, and many of them also develop anaphylactic reactions to factor IX infusions. The presence of an inhibitor is suspected when a child does not achieve the expected factor level or clinical response after replacement therapy (Branchford et al., 2013).

Most children with inhibitors receive the same factor replacement as children without inhibitors. However, they may need a larger dose to attain the desired factor level. Some children with inhibitors require individualized alternative therapy with procoagulant factor bypassing agents, such as factor VIII inhibitor bypassing agent or activated factor VII (NovoSeven).

The transmission of viral diseases, particularly hepatitis and HIV infection, was a major concern among those who received factor VIII or factor IX concentrates before the mid-1980s. Since 1985, factor replacement concentrates have been treated with heat or chemicals to inactivate HIV and substantially reduce the risk of hepatitis and other viral diseases. Recombinant factor products greatly reduce viral exposure risk; thus, concerns families may have about HIV transmission from products administered to their child are not substantiated.

Medications

Certain medications can be used in conjunction with factor replacement therapy or can be used independently in situations when there are concerns that the child may experience bleeding (dental procedures, surgery).

DDAVP, a synthetic analogue of a natural antidiuretic hormone, can be used to increase the level of factor VIII by causing its release from endogenous storage sites. DDAVP is used only for children with mild, and possibly moderate, hemophilia A who demonstrate a satisfactory response to a trial of DDAVP therapy (Srivastava et al., 2013). For these children, DDAVP is the treatment of choice for mild to moderate hemorrhage. DDAVP is not prescribed for children with hemophilia B. DDAVP is usually given diluted in normal saline for a 30-minute IV infusion or by nasal spray once daily. Two forms of DDAVP nasal spray are available. One type is used for enuresis and is not effective for hemostasis. Stimate is the only DDAVP nasal spray that can be used to control bleeding. Side effects of DDAVP (as an antidiuretic hormone) include headache, hypertension, and flushing. DDAVP should not be used for more than 3 consecutive days (Curry, 2004).

Two *antifibrinolytic agents* useful in treating both hemophilia A and B and von Willebrand disease are tranexamic acid (Cyklokapron) and aminocaproic acid (Amicar). These drugs do not help to form a clot; rather, they act by stopping the activity of the enzyme plasmin, which dissolves blood clots in the mucous membranes of the mouth, nose, and urinary tract. The medications are used alone or in conjunction with clotting factor replacement for treating nosebleeds (epistaxis) and to prevent bleeding in the mouth prior to dental surgery. Amicar is contraindicated for children with DIC and renal bleeding. It should be used cautiously in those with cardiovascular, renal, or hepatic disease and in those receiving estrogen therapy.

KidKare During antifibrinolytic therapy, do not allow children to use drinking straws, baby bottles, or pacifiers; prevent them from sucking on hard candy, eating chips, or placing any hard objects in their mouths. These measures help to avoid clot dislodgment.

Fibrin glue is a product made of solutions of fibrogen and thrombin. When these substances are mixed together, they mimic the last stages of the clotting cascade to form a fibrin clot. The pasty substance can be applied topically on a wound and is most often used to stop bleeding after dental procedures or to stop bleeding from other types of wounds. *Thrombin powder* is a dry powder that can be applied directly to the top of a wound to stop minor bleeding. These products are used for individuals with hemophilia or von Willebrand disease to help control bleeding.

Preservation of Joint Mobility

Complications associated with bleeding most often involve joints and muscles. Adjunct measures include RICE (see Nursing Interventions 23-1). In addition, corticosteroids such as prednisone may be used to reduce inflammation in the joint.

Hemarthroses in target joints frequently lead to weakness and dysfunction in adjoining musculature. Thus, muscle-strengthening exercises that do not cause tissue damage or bleeding are likely to be incorporated into a rehabilitation program for those with hemophilia. A physical therapy program designed to maintain normal range of motion may also be instituted.

Community Care

Health care for the child with hemophilia is a coordinated effort between family, school nurses, and the child's outpatient health care team. Major points of focus include ensuring smooth transitions from inpatient to outpatient care, providing education about the disorder, and preventing bleeding episodes. In addition, ongoing psychological support of the family is essential. Home therapy can be used to manage mild and moderate bleeding episodes (Srivastava et al., 2013).

Outpatient visits for ongoing assessment and management generally occur at a comprehensive treatment center at least once per year. Desired outcomes for these visits are related to the child's physical and psychosocial needs on the basis of an updated history and current physical assessment.

Discharge planning for outpatient visits can include referral or follow-up information for a local physician, a home care company, and a community health agency. It may entail contact with community groups, such as the child's daycare center or school (Community Care 23-1). It might involve assisting a family with travel plans by informing them of sources of health care for the child while away from home and by identifying an appropriate storage place for the child's particular type of factor replacement.

KidKare Summer camps specific for children with bleeding disorders provide them opportunities to learn more about their conditions and to be with other children who have hemophilia in a supportive and mentored environment.

An important component of the teaching process is to assess the family's understanding of the child's home care needs and the family's ability to care for the child at home. Be alert for the developing child's readiness to learn more about hemophilia and for the need to correct misconceptions the child and family may have. Also, as the child and family reach new developmental milestones, be alert for the need to discuss the child's activities and specific concerns associated with each developmental phase.

Teaching may encompass a variety of topics, depending on the specific nature of the child's visit to the health care provider. For example, when a child with hemophilia has orthopedic surgery on a lower extremity, teaching is likely to include cast care, crutch walking, pain management, signs and symptoms of bleeding at the surgical site, administration of factor replacement therapy at home, and a schedule for outpatient follow-up appointments. It will emphasize the need to call the physician if bleeding, fever, increased pain, or other complications occur (Clinical Judgment 23-1).

 ALERT *All children with hemophilia should have some form of identification with them at all times (bracelet, necklace, something in the wallet) that indicates their condition, the severity of the disorder, the type of treatment product used, and emergency contact information.*

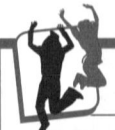

COMMUNITY CARE 23-1

The Child With Hemophilia in School

Children with hemophilia usually attend school on a regular basis when they are not having active bleeding. It is important that their teachers know they have a bleeding disorder. Also, the teaching staff should know the guidelines that have been established to prevent and manage an individual child's bleeding episodes and to promote the child's normal growth and development.

The school nurse collaborates with the comprehensive health care team and joins the child and family in providing information to the teaching staff. Outcome objectives for teachers and teaching assistants include the following:

- State the type and severity of the child's hemophilia, and correlate an increased severity with an increased risk of bleeding, including spontaneous bleeding.
- Identify body joints and muscle tissue as the hallmark sites of bleeding for the child with hemophilia.
- Describe signs and symptoms associated with covert bleeding, such as tingling, tenderness, pain, warmth, and altered motor function of the affected body site (e.g., refusal to walk or to participate in usual physical activities).

- Discuss the need for prompt factor replacement for bleeding episodes to prevent joint injury, tissue damage, and possible life-threatening hemorrhage.
- State the rationale for not giving aspirin to the child with a bleeding disorder.
- Discuss the importance of the child's participation in physical activities except for activities that are identified as high-risk and inappropriate for the child. School personnel should be informed of the activities in which the child is not to participate.
- Explain the importance of telephoning the designated family member whenever the child is injured or says he is bleeding, *even when there are no signs and symptoms of bleeding*. The family may advise school personnel that it is not necessary to telephone them regarding small, superficial cuts and scrapes because factor replacement is usually not required in such situations.
- Describe the significance of treating the child as the classmates are treated. Although there is a need to be aware of the bleeding disorder, the teaching staff should not focus on it or single the child out for special attention or privileges.

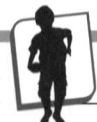

CLINICAL JUDGMENT 23-1

A Child With Hemophilia A

Jason is a 7-year-old boy with severe hemophilia A. He is admitted to the hospital this morning for a scheduled tonsillectomy later today. The health history reveals that hemophilia was diagnosed during infancy shortly after prolonged bleeding occurred with circumcision. Recently, he experienced a tonsillar bleeding episode in conjunction with pharyngitis. Today's physical examination findings are within normal limits. There is no evidence of bleeding or pharyngitis. Admission laboratory studies are within normal limits except for a prolonged partial thromboplastin time of 74.2 seconds and a factor VIII level of less than 1%.

Questions

1. What additional information would you elicit to assess Jason's readiness for surgery?
2. Is Jason's hemophilia classified as mild, moderate, or severe? Why?
3. Why is Jason a candidate for a tonsillectomy?
4. How can Jason's bleeding be controlled after surgery?
5. Identify two significant clinical findings associated with posttonsillectomy bleeding.

Answers

1. Inquire about what Jason has been told regarding his surgery and what to expect after surgery. Ask whether he has attended a preoperative class for children and, if so, ask about his response to it. Ask what Jason knows about the precautions that will be taken to control bleeding during and after surgery—that is, continuous infusion of factor VIII and close monitoring by nursing staff for signs and symptoms of bleeding.
2. Jason has severe hemophilia because his uncorrected factor VIII level is less than 1%.
3. A history of a tonsillar bleeding episode together with severe hemophilia places Jason at increased risk for another tonsillar bleeding episode, particularly if there is recurrent pharyngitis.
4. Jason's bleeding can be controlled after surgery by factor VIII infusion, antifibrinolytic medication, avoidance of hard or sharp foods and objects in the mouth, and a soft diet with no hot or spicy foods and beverages.
5. Two significant clinical findings associated with posttonsillectomy bleeding are bleeding at the surgical site and rapid pulse rate.

Thoroughly teach the child and family about measures to prevent and control bleeding (see Nursing Interventions 23-1). The potential for serious, life-threatening bleeding underscores the need for prudence in selecting daily activities. This may prove to be somewhat difficult as the child grows and begins to participate in activities, including sports. All children need regular exercise to help them develop a strong musculature that supports their joints and decreases the risk of bleeding. Decisions regarding sports participation can be especially challenging (see Developmental Considerations 23-1). The family should consult with the comprehensive health care team and must consider the child's developmental level and physical ability as well as the severity of the hemophilia.

VON WILLEBRAND DISEASE

von Willebrand disease is the most common hereditary bleeding disorder. It results from a quantitative, structural, or functional abnormality of von Willebrand factor.

In general, von Willebrand disease is inherited in an autosomal dominant fashion through a genetic defect on chromosome 12. The exact incidence of von Willebrand disease is not known because, in its mild form, it may not be diagnosed until an episode of prolonged bleeding occurs at a time of surgery or trauma. The estimated incidence is close to 1.3% of the population (Bowman, 2010). Males and females and the various racial groups are affected in equal numbers. In general, the prognosis for children with von Willebrand disease is good, particularly because most of them have a mild form of the disease.

von Willebrand disease may also be acquired with certain clinical disorders such as hypothyroidism, collagen vascular disease, and Wilms tumor. Acquired von Willebrand disease usually resolves when the accompanying clinical disorder has been treated.

Pathophysiology

von Willebrand factor consists of groups of glycoproteins or multimers of varied molecular weight. von Willebrand factor has two primary functions in hemostasis. First, it acts as an adhesive bridge between platelets and injured vascular subendothelium. After vessel injury, plasma von Willebrand factor high-molecular-weight multimers bind to the endothelium and support platelet adherence. The adhered platelets recruit more platelets and promote fibrin clot formation.

Second, von Willebrand factor low-molecular-weight multimers serve as a carrier protein for the procoagulant factor VIII. Without von Willebrand factor, factor

VIII has a markedly decreased survival time, which may decrease the level of factor VIII.

There are three major categories of von Willebrand disease: type I, type II, and type III (Table 23-4). Types I and III are characterized primarily by a quantitative deficiency in von Willebrand factor. Type II is characterized primarily by structural and functional abnormalities of the factor.

Assessment

The primary clinical manifestations of von Willebrand disease are bruising and mucous membrane bleeding from the nose, mouth, and gastrointestinal tract. Determine whether the child has had recent dental work or accidental injury. Prolonged bleeding after trauma or surgery, including tooth extraction, may be the first evidence of abnormal hemostasis in those with mild von Willebrand disease. For females, obtain a detailed menstrual history, including length of menstrual flow and quantity of bleeding. Menorrhagia and profuse postpartum bleeding may occur. Bleeding associated with von Willebrand disease may be severe and may lead to anemia and shock, but deep bleeding into joints and muscles, like that seen in hemophilia, is rare except with type III von Willebrand disease.

Diagnostic Tests

The level of von Willebrand factor may vary in conjunction with certain physiologic factors. High estrogen levels during pregnancy are associated with increased von Willebrand factor levels, which decrease the probability of prolonged bleeding during the prenatal period. Inflammation, exercise, and stress also are correlated with increased levels of von Willebrand factor. If blood samples are drawn at these times, or if children experience particular stress from the venipuncture procedure itself, the presence of von Willebrand disease may be masked.

Fluctuating levels of von Willebrand factor may make von Willebrand disease difficult to diagnose, especially in its milder form. Initial screening studies may or may not document a prolonged activated partial thromboplastin time or abnormal platelet function analysis. Factor VIII levels may be decreased or within normal limits. The von Willebrand factor antigen level is usually decreased or absent but can be borderline in mild von Willebrand disease. The *ristocetin cofactor level*, an indirect laboratory measure of von Willebrand disease factor activity (see Tests and Procedures 23-1), generally reflects decreased von Willebrand factor activity, but this level, too, may be borderline in mild von

TABLE 23-4 Major Types of von Willebrand Disease				
	Type I	**Type II**		**Type III**
Percentage affected among those with von Willebrand disease	70%–90%	15%–20%		1%–10%
		Type IIA	**Type IIB**	
Severity of bleeding	Mild to moderate	Mild to moderate	Moderate to severe	Severe
Distinctive characteristics	Decreased quantities of all sizes of von Willebrand factor multimers Decreased activity of von Willebrand factor	Absence of intermediate-sized and large von Willebrand factor multimers Increased levels of small von Willebrand factor multimers Decreased activity of von Willebrand factor; possibly disproportionate with quantity of von Willebrand factor	Abnormal attraction of von Willebrand factor to platelets Only small- and intermediate-sized von Willebrand factor multimers because of large multimers binding to platelet surfaces Increased platelet agglutination Possible thrombocytopenia	Absence (or near absence) of all sizes of von Willebrand factor multimers Absent or minimal activity of von Willebrand factor Low factor VIII level
Interventions	Usually, single dose of DDAVP; may repeat infusions every 12–24 hours for major surgery until healing is complete	DDAVP for minor bleeding Plasma-based von Willebrand–containing factor VIII replacement therapy for moderate bleeding	Replacement therapy for bleeding episodes and surgery DDAVP contraindicated (facilitates release of additional, abnormal von Willebrand factor, enhancing platelet agglutination and thrombocytopenia) Platelets and von Willebrand factor for severe thrombocytopenia	Replacement therapy with factor VIII concentrates that contain von Willebrand factor Children with this type of von Willebrand disease may have spontaneous bleeding, including deep joint and muscle bleeding.

Willebrand disease. A von Willebrand factor multimeric analysis test is helpful in distinguishing among the various types of von Willebrand disease.

A diagnosis of von Willebrand disease cannot be established or ruled out by one set of laboratory values alone. A definitive diagnosis of von Willebrand disease requires documentation of two sets of abnormal von Willebrand factor studies. When the child's history indicates the possibility of von Willebrand disease, laboratory studies should be repeated periodically and can be more definitive when procured at times of active bleeding episodes.

Interdisciplinary Interventions

Management of the child with von Willebrand disease depends on the classification of the disease (see Table 23-4). The most common treatment is DDAVP, which acts to temporarily increase von Willebrand levels, although it may be ineffective in type IIA or type IIB. It is given intravenously or intranasally (see discussion regarding hemophilia treatment). Monitor von Willebrand factor levels before and after the administration of DDAVP because repeated dosing can cause tachyphylaxis and lessened response (Ben-Ami & Revel-Vilk, 2013).

When DDAVP is ineffective or tachyphylaxis develops, von Willebrand factor replacement therapy is needed. Such therapy is provided with a plasma-based factor VIII concentrate, such as Humate-P, Koate DVI, or Alphanate, which contain von Willebrand factor as well as factor VIII (see Table 23-4). These medications are given intravenously and may be used for children with type I von Willebrand disease in certain situations such as major trauma or major surgery.

Community Care

Steps to prevent bleeding and measures to provide for the psychosocial needs of children with von Willebrand disease and their families are similar to those described in the section on hemophilia and in the "Treatment Modalities" section at the beginning of the chapter.

DISSEMINATED INTRAVASCULAR COAGULATION

DIC is an acquired coagulopathy that, paradoxically, is characterized by both thrombosis and hemorrhage. Its acuity level ranges from low-grade compensated DIC to fulminant, multisystem, life-threatening DIC.

DIC is not a primary disorder but occurs as a result of a variety of alterations in health status, such as burns, traumatic injuries, hypoxia, severe shock, hemolytic transfusion reactions, cardiovascular disorders, acute myelogenous leukemia, metastatic malignancies, infection or sepsis, liver disease, and hypo- or hyperthermia. Conditions that precipitate DIC may, in turn, be complicated by DIC. The etiology of DIC is not well understood. The prognosis for DIC varies according to the prognosis for the underlying disorder and the severity of DIC. Fulminant DIC can be life threatening.

Pathophysiology

Although DIC can be precipitated by different disorders, its basic pathophysiology is the same, leading to the development of both thrombosis and hemorrhage. Extensive microvascular damage, accompanied by vasodilation and loosening of endothelial junctions, leads to capillary leaking and shock. Unregulated activation of the coagulation pathways promotes excess thrombin generation, widespread microthrombi, and ischemic damage to multiple organs. Coagulation factors are consumed and platelets are exhausted, leading to disseminated bleeding.

Thrombosis in DIC occurs when the coagulation system is overstimulated by a primary triggering disorder. Overstimulation leads to an excessive amount of circulating thrombin, which in turn leads to increased fibrin clot formation. Microvascular and, at times, macrovascular thrombosis occurs, hindering normal blood flow, and may result in ischemia and organ damage.

Also, red blood cells become fragmented as they circulate among the numerous fibrin deposits in the vasculature. Subsequently, a hemolytic anemia may develop.

Hemorrhage associated with DIC may occur as a consequence of various pathophysiologic events. First, the intravascular thrombi, which form as a result of excessive thrombin in the circulation, trap platelets, resulting in hemorrhage secondary to **thrombocytopenia** (an abnormally low concentration of circulating platelets). Second, excessive amounts of circulating plasmin are produced, leading to excessive fibrinolysis and an abnormally high amount of circulating fibrin degradation (split) products (FDPs or FSPs). FDPs function as anticoagulants, thereby contributing to hemorrhage. Also, FDPs cover platelet membranes, making the platelets dysfunctional and leading to hemorrhage. Third, levels of clotting factors involved in normal coagulation are substantially decreased or absent in DIC, resulting in hemorrhage.

Assessment

The most obvious clinical feature of DIC is bleeding. However, be alert for clinical manifestations of the other major pathophysiologic event in DIC: thrombosis. Bleeding and thrombosis may occur in multiple, unrelated anatomic locations. All anatomic sites affected by DIC are at risk for ischemia, tissue damage, organ failure, and necrosis. The most common sites affected by DIC involve the kidneys, lungs, skin, gastrointestinal tract, and central nervous system (Chart 23-2).

Also, monitor for the systemic manifestations of DIC, such as fever, hypotension, acidosis, and hypoxia.

Diagnostic Tests

Although no test is specifically diagnostic for DIC, certain alterations in hematologic laboratory data can contribute to its identification (Table 23-5). Such laboratory data must be assessed, however, within the context of the child's history, underlying disorder, and general clinical state. Also, the absence of laboratory findings commonly associated with DIC does not necessarily exclude its presence.

CHART 23-2 **Common Complications of Disseminated Intravascular Coagulation by Body System**

- Renal involvement: hematuria, oliguria, and anuria
- Pulmonary involvement: hemoptysis, tachypnea, dyspnea, and chest pain
- Cutaneous involvement: petechiae, ecchymoses, hemorrhagic bullae, pallor, jaundice, acrocyanosis, and gangrene; also possible bleeding from surgical or traumatic wounds and from invasive procedure sites
- Gastrointestinal involvement: hematemesis, hematochezia, and absent or hypo- or hyperactive bowel sounds
- Central nervous system involvement: possible headaches, increased intracranial pressure, sensory deficits, seizures, altered mental status, and decreased level of consciousness

Nursing Diagnoses and Outcomes

Nursing diagnoses and outcomes for the child with a bleeding disorder are presented in Nursing Plan of Care 23-1. The following nursing diagnosis and outcome also applies to the child with DIC:

Nursing Diagnosis: Ineffective tissue perfusion related to intravascular thrombosis and hemorrhage
Outcome: Child will exhibit adequate tissue perfusion of all body systems affected by DIC and regain adequate laboratory values for hemostasis.

Interdisciplinary Interventions

Management of the child with DIC is individualized based on the underlying disorder and the degree of DIC. Thus, specific treatment may vary from no treatment, in the absence of clinical manifestations, to intensive treatment in the presence of fulminant DIC.

TABLE 23-5 Laboratory Data Commonly Associated With Disseminated Intravascular Coagulation

Laboratory Test	Result
Antithrombin III	Decreased
D-dimer assay	Increased
Fibrinogen	Decreased
Fibrinogen/fibrin degradation (split) products	Increased
Fibrinopeptide A level	Increased
Partial thromboplastin time	Prolonged
Plasminogen	Decreased
Platelet count	Decreased
Prothrombin time	Prolonged
Schistocytes	Present

When clinical manifestations are present, primary interventions are directed toward (1) effective treatment of the disorder that precipitated DIC and (2) supportive care to correct physiologic alterations resulting from DIC.

Treatment of the precipitating disorder may include, for example, surgery to remove diseased body tissue; antibiotic therapy to treat infectious disease; chemotherapy to destroy malignancies; and measures to correct shock, hypoxia, and acid–base imbalance.

Supportive care includes the administration of platelet concentrates, cryoprecipitate, factor concentrates, and fresh-frozen plasma to replace depleted platelets and coagulation factors.

Collaborate with the health care team to plan and provide the therapeutic and supportive measures needed. A key aspect of the nurse's role is to assess the child for signs and symptoms of impaired tissue perfusion in the various body systems that may be affected by DIC. Important outcomes for the child and related nursing interventions are delineated in Nursing Interventions 23-2.

Concerns about bleeding, clotting, and organ failure with serious DIC are likely to produce considerable emotional stress in both the child and family. The health care team must be sensitive to this stress. Education about DIC, ongoing progress reports, and emotional support for the child and family are important components of the interdisciplinary management of DIC.

Community Care

Posthospitalization care is related to managing the underlying condition that precipitated DIC (e.g., metastatic malignancy, liver disease, cardiovascular disorder). In addition, ongoing care will be needed based on the degree of organ impairment and limb involvement related to impaired tissue perfusion during the DIC crisis. Rehabilitation services may be required for any loss of extremities (see Chapter 12).

IDIOPATHIC THROMBOCYTOPENIC PURPURA

ITP is an acquired, self-limiting disorder of hemostasis characterized by destruction and decreased numbers of circulating platelets. ITP is primarily an autoimmune disease; the immune system attacks and destroys the body's own platelets for an unknown reason. Because "idiopathic" means "of unknown cause," the condition is also referred to as *immune thrombocytopenic purpura* or *autoimmune thrombocytopenic purpura*. ITP is the most common thrombocytopenic disorder among children.

ITP is frequently preceded by a viral illness within 1 month of onset, most often an upper respiratory infection but sometimes another infection such as varicella or infectious mononucleosis. ITP has also occurred after vaccination for smallpox and measles. Infection or vaccination may somehow trigger the immune reaction that leads to ITP in these children. In adults, ITP does not seem to be linked to infections.

NURSING INTERVENTIONS 23-2

Objectives and Interventions for the Child With Disseminated Intravascular Coagulation

Outcome Objectives	Nursing Interventions
Maintain adequate renal function	Measure intake and output accurately Report the following: • Intake greater than output • Hematuria • Oliguria, anuria
Maintain adequate pulmonary function	Assess breath sounds in all lobes of the lungs Report the following: • Abnormal breath sounds • Tachypnea • Dyspnea • Chest pain • Hemoptysis • Abnormal pulse oximetry readings
Maintain cutaneous integrity	Inspect the skin Report the following: • Overt bleeding • Pallor, jaundice • Petechiae, ecchymoses • Hemorrhagic bullae • Acrocyanosis • Poor healing at sites of injury or invasive procedures
Maintain adequate gastrointestinal function	Assess bowel sounds in all quadrants Report the following: • Absent or hypo- or hyperactive bowel sounds • Blood in emesis or stool
Maintain adequate neurologic function	Assess neurologic status Report the following: • Unstable or abnormal blood pressure, temperature, pulse, and respiratory rate • Unequal size of pupils • Absent or unequal pupillary responses to light • Headaches • Seizures • Changes in sensory perception, such as altered vision or hearing; numbness • Changes in motor function, such as altered speech or mobility • Irritability • Changes in behavior • Decreased level of consciousness • Rigid posturing

ITP can be acute or chronic. Acute ITP, the predominant form among children, is characterized by thrombocytopenia of sudden onset, which resolves spontaneously within 6 months. Typically, acute ITP in children occurs between 1 and 6 years of age; it affects males and females in equal numbers. The prognosis for ITP is good, especially for children who have had a preceding viral illness, with at least two thirds recovering spontaneously (Provan et al., 2010). Chronic ITP is characterized by continuous or recurrent thrombocytopenia of more than 6 months' duration. It is more likely to affect children older than 10 years of age, females, and have an insidious onset (Blanchette & Bolton-Maggs, 2010). Children with chronic ITP may experience spontaneous remission, with one study indicating 30% of children experienced remission within 5 years of diagnosis (Bansal et al., 2010).

Pathophysiology

The pathophysiologic mechanisms of ITP have traditionally been attributed to platelet autoantibody production and the resulting accelerated destruction of circulating platelets. Recent evidence indicates that complex multifactorial processes are present which lead to ITP. Impaired platelet production, T-cell–mediated effects, and failure of the bone marrow to increase production of platelets contribute to a process in which the disorder perpetuates itself (Gernsheimer, 2009; Provan et al., 2010). The cause or precipitating event triggering ITP can be attributed to a myriad of conditions including infection (60% of pediatric cases), post measles–mumps–rubella vaccination, bleeding after surgery, and exposure to environmental toxins or a certain drug (Provan et al., 2010).

Assessment

A thorough assessment of the skin reveals the hallmark of ITP: random purpura in the presence of an otherwise normal physical examination. In addition to the cutaneous petechiae and ecchymoses, look for petechiae and hemorrhagic bullae of the mouth and pharynx. The extent of purpura is usually related to the degree of thrombocytopenia. When the platelet count is less than 20,000/mm³, spontaneous bleeding is more likely and may occur. Determine whether the child has a history of epistaxis, hematuria, hematemesis, hematochezia, or menorrhagia.

Intracranial hemorrhage, although rare, is a life-threatening form of spontaneous bleeding associated with ITP. Assess for headaches, vomiting, retinal hemorrhage, irritability, seizures, lethargy, and coma as clinical indicators of intracranial bleeding.

ALERT *The child with evidence of intracranial hemorrhage requires immediate medical attention. Notify the physician of the child's condition, prepare the child and family for emergent computed tomography of the child's head, monitor closely, and be prepared to provide oxygenation and other supportive care.*

Diagnostic Tests

Thrombocytopenia, with a platelet count less than 100×10^9/L, is the only laboratory abnormality expected with ITP (Neunert et al., 2011). However, if major blood loss has occurred, a CBC can show evidence of anemia or iron deficiency (ID).

Bone marrow examination, although previously recommended as a diagnostic tool, is no longer necessary in children who present with typical ITP findings (Neunert et al., 2011).

Interdisciplinary Interventions

Management of the child with ITP is directed toward preventing serious, life-threatening bleeding and involves supportive care; possible pharmaceutical intervention; and, occasionally, splenectomy (Tradition or Science 23-1). Giving platelet transfusions is not customary because of the destructive process that affects platelets in ITP. However, at times of surgery or life-threatening bleeding, platelets may be used. Children with no bleeding or mild bleeding (petechiae and bruising) are managed by observation alone regardless of platelet count (Neunert et al., 2011).

Pharmacologic Interventions

Pharmacologic interventions include corticosteroids or immune globulin (as indicated) for extensive bleeding or if the child is at risk for life-threatening bleeding related to severe thrombocytopenia (platelet count <20,000 mm3).

Corticosteroid therapy (prednisone), as a single-dose treatment or a short-course therapy, can be given to enhance vascular stability, decrease production of antiplatelet antibodies, and decrease clearance of phagocytic-susceptible platelets, thereby improving platelet survival, increasing the platelet count, and decreasing bleeding. However, prolonged use of corticosteroids is not considered beneficial and may actually suppress platelet production. If severe thrombocytopenia or major bleeding recurs, alternative therapy is recommended.

Evidence-Based Practice   TRADITION OR SCIENCE 23-1

Should children with ITP and a platelet count of 20,000 cells/mm³ or less be treated?

Data suggest that two thirds of the cases of children with ITP and a platelet count of 20,000 cells/mm³ or less recover their platelet counts within 6 months of diagnosis. Of the remaining children, approximately 76% will achieve spontaneous remission sometime after this initial period (Blanchette & Bolton-Maggs, 2010). Watchful waiting, with no treatment unless clinical symptoms occur in addition to cutaneous signs, is considered valid therapy and should be offered to families in addition to the options of treatment with intravenous immunoglobulin (IVIG), corticosteroids, or anti-D immunoglobulin (Neunert et al., 2011; Provan et al., 2010; Sevier & Houston, 2005; Tarantino & Bolton-Maggs, 2007).

IVIG therapy is given daily for 2 to 5 days and usually brings about a quick increase in the platelet count. IVIG is thought to act by interfering with the attachment of antibody-coated platelets to Fc receptors on the macrophage cells of the reticuloendothelial system. IVIG is expensive, but if it decreases hospitalization time and the likelihood of splenectomy, it can be a cost-effective intervention for ITP (Blanchette & Bolton-Maggs, 2010).

Anti-D-RhO (WinRho) immunoglobulin increases the platelet count in most Rh-positive patients with ITP. Response with anti-D immunoglobulin is slower than with IVIG, but it is easier to administer and costs less (Blanchette & Bolton-Maggs, 2010).

❗ A L E R T *Monitor hemoglobin of children receiving anti-D immunoglobulin. Because anti-D antibody binds to Rh-positive erythrocytes, most children experience some hemolysis, some severe enough to warrant transfusion.*

Rituximab, high-dose methylprednisolone, and dexamethasone have demonstrated efficacy in managing children with persistent or chronic ITP who continue to have bleeding despite treatment with IVIG, anti-D immunoglobulin, or conventional doses of corticosteroids (Neunert et al., 2011; Provan et al., 2010).

Ensure that children and the family know that neither corticosteroids nor IVIG shortens the duration of ITP. The primary purpose of these agents is to increase the number of circulating platelets and thereby reduce the risk of life-threatening bleeding. If severe thrombocytopenia recurs, intermittent pharmacologic intervention using IVIG, anti-D immunoglobulin, corticosteroids, or some combination may be used to prevent the platelet count from dropping dangerously low until the ITP spontaneously resolves (Blanchette & Bolton-Maggs, 2010).

Surgical Interventions

Splenectomy is reserved for children with life-threatening bleeding; those with chronic ITP who are at risk for serious bleeding; those with a lack of responsiveness or intolerance to therapies such as corticosteroids, IVIG, and anti-D immunoglobulin; and children who have a need for improved quality-of-life (Neunert et al., 2011). The purpose of splenectomy is twofold: (1) to remove the primary site of antiplatelet antibody production and (2) to remove the major site for the destruction of antibody-coated platelets. In the presence of chronic ITP, when possible, splenectomy is delayed for at least 12 months to ensure the procedure is necessary and because children are at greater risk for developing life-threatening postsplenectomy sepsis. When splenectomy is planned, specific vaccines are given to help decrease the risk of postoperative sepsis. The polyvalent pneumococcal vaccine is given at least 2 weeks before surgery to allow time for an effective antibody response. The vaccine for *H. influenzae* may be given

as well. Prophylactic antibiotics are also initiated. After a splenectomy, the long-term complications include risk for infection and postsplenectomy sepsis.

Community Care

Bleeding and the fear of bleeding are stressful for children with ITP and their families. Health care providers must be sensitive to this stress. Educating about ITP and providing ongoing assessment and emotional support are important parts of the interdisciplinary management of ITP. Steps to prevent bleeding and measures to provide for the psychosocial needs of children with ITP and their families are similar to those described in the section on "Treatment Modalities" at the beginning of the chapter and in Nursing Interventions 23-1.

ANEMIAS

 QUESTION: Based on the laboratory test results at the time of Shawanda's hospital admission, is her anemia moderate or severe?

Although the anemias of childhood have distinguishing features, they share a common characteristic: the hemoglobin concentration or the red blood cell count is less than normal. Anemias are usually detected or confirmed by CBC analysis. Both moderate and severe anemias (hemoglobin <8 g/dL) lead to decreased oxygenation of body tissues. When symptomatic and life-threatening anemia is present, red blood cell transfusions increase hemoglobin levels and improve oxygenation.

Anemias are classified by morphologic features and by physiologic characteristics. Morphologically, red blood cell size categorizes anemias as microcytic (small cell size), normocytic (normal cell size), and macrocytic (large cell size). Physiologic characteristics categorize anemias as disorders of red blood cell production and red blood cell destruction. IDA, megaloblastic anemia, lead poisoning, and aplastic anemia are examples of disorders that interfere with normal red blood cell production. Abnormalities involving the red blood cell membrane, such as hereditary spherocytosis, together with the various hemolytic anemias, are examples of disorders involving red blood cell destruction. In addition to productive and destructive physiologic disorders, anemia may result from major internal and external bleeding.

ANSWER: Shawanda's laboratory test results reveal a hemoglobin level of 5.7 g/dL. Thus, her anemia would be considered severe (<8 g/dL).

IRON-DEFICIENCY ANEMIA

IDA is the most common nutritional anemia of childhood. It is a microcytic (red blood cells are smaller than normal), hypochromic (red blood cells are paler than normal) anemia that occurs when the body's iron stores are depleted. ID occurs when there is insufficient iron to maintain physiologic functions that require iron absorption (American Academy of Pediatrics, 2010). IDA is present when the hemoglobin concentration is more than two standard deviations below the mean. IDA may be diagnosed if the hemoglobin is less than 11.0 to 13.3 g/dL (depending on age) and increases after a course of therapeutic iron supplementation (U.S. Preventive Services Task Force, 2006). For male and female children aged 12 through 35 months, anemia is defined as a hemoglobin less than 11.0 g/dL (American Academy of Pediatrics, 2010).

CROSS-CULTURAL CARE

In developing countries of the world, the World Health Organization (2011) estimates that ID affects 2 billion children and adults. This deficiency is the result of poor diets, lack of iron fortification, infections such as malaria, and parasitic infestations such as hookworm. IDA in developing countries is frequently associated with deficiencies in other nutrients such as folic acid, vitamin C, and vitamin A. Thus, when children with nutritional anemia come to the United States, health care providers need to consider that lack of iron may not be the only nutrient deficiency.

The increased availability and use of iron-fortified food products and infant formulas and an increase in breastfeeding have contributed to a substantial decrease in the incidence of IDA in the United States. ID is present in 6.6% to 15.2% of children in the United States aged 12 to 35 months, and IDA is present in 0.9% to 4.4% of children in this age range (Baker et al., 2010). Risk factors associated with IDA in infants and young children include low socioeconomic status; a history of prematurity or low birth weight; exposure to lead; breastfeeding beyond 4 months of age without supplemental iron; and weaning to whole milk, formulas, and cereals that are not iron-fortified (Baker et al., 2010). In older children and adolescents, ID is more prevalent in females, recent immigrants, obese children, and fad dieters (U.S. Preventive Services Task Force, 2006). IDA is easily treated; thus, the prognosis is good if IDA is managed early and effectively (Tradition or Science 23-2).

Pathophysiology

IDA is most likely to occur when children experience ID because of rapid physical growth, inadequate iron intake, inadequate iron absorption, or loss of blood. IDA develops most commonly during infancy and adolescence, when physical growth is rapid and iron intake is frequently insufficient.

ID is described in three stages:

1. Stage 1 is characterized by depletion of ferritin; hemosiderin; and other iron storage compounds in the liver, spleen, and bone marrow. Anemia is not present during this stage.

Evidence-Based Practice   **TRADITION OR SCIENCE 23-2**

Do infants with IDA have long-term developmental delays?

IDA appears to have long-lasting effects on motor development, mental development, and auditory and visual system functioning. Iron is required for normal myelination, which affects both motor and sensory development. Studies have substantiated that infants who had IDA demonstrated motor development delays (Antunes et al., 1997; Carter, 2010), lower mental test scores (Carter, 2010; Grantham-McGregor & Ani, 2001; Lozoff et al., 1996), longer auditory brain stem and visual evoked potential responses (Algarin et al., 2003; Congdon et al., 2012), alterations in normal development of sleep patterns (Peirano et al., 2007), and adverse social and emotional behavior (Carter, 2010; Lozoff et al., 2008) during early childhood. These deficits can occur even with moderate anemia, and they may remain despite correction of the IDA (Eden, 2005). Evidence continues to build that the presence of IDA during infancy demands immediate intervention to prevent adverse motor and cognitive sequelae that affect these children as they continue to grow and mature (Baker et al., 2010; Carter, 2010; Lozoff et al., 2000).

2. Stage 2 is characterized by a lack of transport iron. Iron saturation of transferrin decreases and, although anemia is generally not yet present, the hemoglobin concentration trends toward low normal.

3. Stage 3 is characterized by a marked deficit in transport iron that inhibits normal production of hemoglobin. Erythrocyte protoporphyrin increases because there is inadequate iron with which it may combine to form heme. Transferrin receptors, located on cell surface membranes in various body tissues, become more numerous in response to the iron-poor environment. A microcytic, hypochromic anemia develops during this stage of ID.

In addition to inadequate dietary intake, impaired iron absorption may lead to IDA. The intestinal mucosal cells are particularly important because they act as a holding zone and gatekeeper for iron. When the body does not need iron, it is lost with desquamation of intestinal mucosal cells; however, when the body needs iron, it enters the circulation via the intestinal mucosa. Impairment of the intestinal mucosa may inhibit adequate iron absorption. Iron malabsorption may also occur with inflammatory and infectious disorders.

Assessment

The American Academy of Pediatrics recommends universal screening for all anemias at 12 months of age. IDA may not be readily apparent when the anemia is mild, thus routine screening for at-risk children (low socioeconomic status, poor dietary intake) is important. Starting in adolescence and throughout their childbearing years, females should be routinely screened for anemia (Baker et al., 2010).

As anemia progresses, signs and symptoms may become apparent. Note any family concerns that the child is easily fatigued, experiences shortness of breath, is irritable, and has decreased tolerance for physical work and exercise. Physical assessment may reveal pallor, fissures at corners of the mouth, inflammation of the tongue, and spoon-shaped nails. Heart murmurs and heart failure are noted with severe anemia. Skeletal abnormalities also may be noted.

Dietary assessment is important. Children whose diet consists almost exclusively of cow's milk may have occult blood loss and suppression of appetite along with severe anemia. Pica, the appetite or craving for nonnutritional substances (e.g., soil, chalk, foam), persisting for more than 1 month is associated with both IDA and celiac disease (Borgna-Pignatti & Marsella, 2008).

Children with ID absorb greater amounts of lead and thus are at greater risk of developing lead poisoning. In addition, ID may impair cognitive and psychomotor development (see Tradition or Science 23-2). During the assessment process, complete developmental screening to assess for any lags in achieving age-appropriate milestones (see Chapter 3).

Diagnostic Tests

Generally, a hemoglobin test is used when children are initially screened for IDA. As the child progresses through the three stages of ID, laboratory evidence of this deficiency increases. During the first stage, the depletion of iron stores is most commonly identified by a decrease in SF. A normal SF result does not rule out IDA, however, especially during inflammation or infection; thus, a simultaneous measure of C-reactive protein (CRP) is completed to rule out inflammation (Baker et al., 2010). Reticulocyte hemoglobin content (CHr) testing is available and provides a measure of the iron available to cells recently released form the bone marrow. A low CHr concentration has been shown to be the strongest predictor of ID in children (Baker et al., 2010).

During the second stage of ID, the lack of transport iron is identified primarily by a decrease in transferrin saturation (TSAT). A decrease in serum iron and an increase in total iron-binding capacity are likely to be evident as well. However, these tests individually are not as reliable as TSAT. In addition, during this stage, early red blood cell changes may be noted, with the hemoglobin decreasing to low normal.

Laboratory manifestations of the third stage of ID include changes in red blood cell indices. These changes include an increase in erythrocyte protoporphyrin and transferrin receptors and a decrease in hemoglobin, hematocrit, mean corpuscular volume (MCV), mean corpuscular hemoglobin (MCH), and mean corpuscular hemoglobin concentration (MCHC).

Interdisciplinary Interventions

In most cases, the child with IDA is managed on an outpatient basis (see discussion in "Community Care" section that follows). However, severe IDA and iron malabsorption may require treatment with parenteral forms of iron supplementation, which include iron dextran (Imferon), sodium ferric gluconate, and iron sucrose. In such cases, hospitalization is required, with careful monitoring of the child during IV or intramuscular administration of iron. Adverse effects of administration include skin staining at site of intramuscular injection, severe pain at the injection site, fever, and anaphylaxis. Use the Z-track injection technique when administering the iron intramuscularly.

Children with severe anemia may also require supportive therapy such as supplemental oxygen, IV fluids, bed rest, and consultation with a nutritionist. In some cases, the child may require PRBC transfusion (see discussion earlier in the chapter in "Treatment Modalities" section). Provide ongoing monitoring of the child's progress as he or she receives these therapies, and provide education to family members.

Community Care

Outpatient management of the child with mild or moderate IDA is aimed at correcting the anemia, replenishing the depleted iron stores, and preventing further ID. As with inpatient interventions, these goals are achieved primarily with iron supplementation, nutritional counseling, and ongoing family education.

Iron Supplementation

Iron supplementation is generally the first line of treatment when there is suspected, but unconfirmed, IDA in a child who is otherwise healthy. Anemia in children is most often caused by ID; thus, a trial period of administering iron supplementation is often given prior to the completion of costly, elaborate laboratory tests. The trial period is usually 1 month. If the hemoglobin concentration increases substantially during this period, the presumed diagnosis of IDA is supported. Iron supplementation continues for up to 4 additional months to complete correcting the anemia and to replenish the iron stores. To avoid iron overload, do not continue therapeutic iron supplementation thereafter.

Iron supplements are generally given orally as elemental iron in the form of ferrous sulfate, a well-absorbed and inexpensive iron preparation. Supplemental iron should be stored out of the reach of children to guard against accidental poisoning.

caREminder

Iron is absorbed better on an empty stomach, and it is most often given to infants as a single dose before breakfast. For older children, the daily amount of iron supplementation is usually divided into two or three doses and is given between meals. Children receiving oral iron supplements have dark stools and may experience gastrointestinal side effects such as nausea and constipation. Also, teeth may be temporarily stained by liquid iron preparations. To avoid staining the teeth, give liquid iron using a straw or a syringe to place the medication toward the back of the child's mouth.

During infancy, ID is especially common after the iron stores that are present at birth are depleted. Thus, special care must be taken to ensure that infants have an adequate supply of iron. Prophylactic iron supplementation is given whenever an infant's dietary intake is inadequate. Full-term infants require an iron intake of 1 mg/kg/day starting at 4 months of age until iron-rich foods are introduced into the child's diet. Formula-fed infants should receive iron-fortified formula; breastfed babies should receive iron-fortified infant cereal two times per day. Whole milk should not be given to children younger than 12 months of age.

Preterm infants require an iron intake of 2 mg/kg/day until 12 months of age. As with the full-term infant, iron-fortified formula can be given. Infants receiving human milk require iron supplementation of 2 mg/kg/day by 1 month of age until they are old enough to receive iron-fortified infant cereal (Baker et al., 2010).

Children between infancy and adolescence with sufficient food intake usually do not require iron supplements. However, supplements may be needed during adolescence, especially among teenagers who are experiencing rapid physical growth and are prone to fad diets and poor nutrition. Also, teenage girls who are pregnant, lactating, or heavily menstruating require iron supplements because their total iron need is not met by diet alone.

Nutritional Counseling

Nutritional counseling is an important intervention in treating and preventing IDA. Certain dietary habits enhance iron intake and increase the bioavailability of iron.

For infants, iron intake is better with iron-fortified infant formula than with fresh cow's milk. In addition to being poor in iron content, fresh cow's milk is associated with intestinal blood loss, which contributes to ID, especially during the first 6 months of infancy. The distribution of iron-fortified infant formula in the federal Special Supplemental Nutrition Program for Women, Infants, and Children is a major factor in the decreased incidence of IDA in the United States. In addition, the increased use of iron-fortified products and better iron availability in some food products may contribute to the continuing decline in the incidence of IDA (Baker et al., 2010; Eden, 2005).

Iron intake is enhanced with the use of iron-fortified infant cereal. Including meat in infants' diets, along with foods and juices fortified with ascorbic acid, promotes the absorption of iron from a meal. Also, avoiding solid foods at or near the time of breastfeeding enhances the bioavailability of the limited amount of iron in human milk.

Although many foods for children and adolescents contain iron, this iron may be in different forms. Heme iron, found primarily in foods from animal sources (meat, poultry, and fish), is readily absorbed by the intestinal mucosa and thus is the best source of iron for the body. In contrast, nonheme iron is found mainly in foods derived from nonanimal sources, such as vegetables, fruits, cereals, and breads. It must be changed from the ferric to the ferrous form to facilitate absorption. Factors that will increase the iron absorption from nonheme foods include eating a heme and nonheme food together (e.g., tuna with beans), eating nonheme foods with foods that are sources of vitamin C (ascorbic acid; e.g., strawberries, oranges, broccoli), and cooking nonheme foods in an iron pot such as a cast iron pan.

Just as the absorption of nonheme iron can be facilitated by certain foods such as soy, it can also be hindered by other dietary components. Inhibitors of nonheme iron absorption include bran foods, milk, and tannin-containing beverages such as tea and coffee. Certain antacids and antibiotics also may impede the absorption of nonheme iron.

Vegetarians consume mainly nonheme iron. When planning meals, they need to be aware of the role of ascorbic acid in facilitating the absorption of nonheme iron and to avoid those foods and beverages that decrease the bioavailability of their iron intake.

Education

The nurse has an important role in providing education about treating and preventing IDA (Teaching Intervention Plan 23-1). In addition to providing education to children and families in the health care setting, the nurse also provides community education. By arranging for educational programs at schools, daycare centers, health fairs, and so forth, the nurse can make an important contribution to preventing IDA. Children and families who develop dietary habits that facilitate iron intake and absorption and who receive prophylactic iron supplements during times of increased iron need are less likely to experience IDA (Clinical Judgment 23-2).

MEGALOBLASTIC ANEMIA

Megaloblastic anemia is a nutritional anemia that most often results from a deficiency of either vitamin B_{12} or folate (folic acid) resulting from inadequate intake, malabsorption, or a metabolic disorder. Vitamin B_{12} deficiency is more likely to occur among people who are strictly vegetarian than among those who eat meat and other animal products. The newborn may have inadequate vitamin B_{12} as a result of maternal vitamin B_{12} deficiency. Malabsorption is associated with pernicious anemia, in which intrinsic factor, which is required for absorption of vitamin B_{12}, is either absent or dysfunctional. Malabsorption of vitamin B_{12} may also stem from gastric and intestinal disorders, such as necrotizing enterocolitis, and from HIV infection. In addition, vitamin B_{12} deficiency may be caused by an inborn error of vitamin B_{12} metabolism.

Folate deficiency can occur at any age but is more likely to occur among infants, especially among premature infants who are experiencing rapid physical growth and have increased folate needs. Pregnancy, lactation, alcoholism, sickle cell disease, and infections such as hepatitis and HIV also increase demand for folate. Malabsorption of folate can occur with intestinal disorders such as chronic diarrhea. Folate deficiency can also stem from altered folate metabolism, which has been reported with ongoing use of anticonvulsant

---

TIP 23-1: A TEACHING INTERVENTION PLAN for the Child With Iron-Deficiency Anemia

Nursing Diagnoses and Family Outcomes

- Deficient knowledge: Iron-deficiency anemia, sources of dietary iron, and management
  Outcomes: Child and family describe IDA and the need for adequate dietary iron to prevent this anemia.
  Child and family identify sources of dietary iron.
- Risk for injury related to effects of anemia
  Outcomes: Child and family identify short-term and long-term effects of impaired tissue oxygenation caused by IDA.
  Child and family identify child's need for iron supplements to correct anemia and replenish iron stores.

Teach Child/Family

Managing the Child's Condition

- Instruct about IDA: inadequate iron, decreased hemoglobin in red blood cells, decreased oxygenation of body tissues.
- Inform about causes of IDA: inadequate iron intake, especially during times of rapid physical growth (infancy, adolescence); malabsorption of iron; iron loss related to excessive bleeding.
- Educate concerning dietary sources of iron.
- Heme iron (easy to absorb): meat, poultry, fish
- Nonheme iron (harder to absorb): vegetables, fruits, cereals, breads
- Discuss dietary habits to facilitate absorption of nonheme iron:
  - *Include* meat, poultry, fish, and foods or beverages with vitamin C in the same meal.
  - *Exclude* bran foods, milk, tea, and coffee in the same meal.
    Note: Milk is not a dietary source of iron.
- Teach regarding dietary sources of iron for infants: iron-fortified formula and cereal.
- Advise breastfeeding mothers to avoid giving the child solid foods near breastfeeding time to enhance bioavailability of the limited amount of iron in human milk.

Note: Breastfed babies need iron supplements or iron-fortified infant foods because the amount of iron in breast milk is insufficient.

- Suggest meals providing adequate iron intake within the context of family's ethnic group and budget limitations.
- Provide instructions regarding signs and symptoms of IDA in children:
  - Less active, less playful
  - Poor appetite
  - Sleeping more
  - Pale in color
  - Short of breath
  - Irritable
  - Increase in infections
  - Abnormal growth and development
- Inform that children often adapt to a gradual decline in hemoglobin. Thus, signs and symptoms of anemia may not be readily apparent at first.
- Teach concerning iron supplements, when prescribed:
  - For best absorption, give iron with water or juice between meals; do not give with antacids, milk, bran foods, tea, or coffee.
  - If liquid iron prescribed, give with a straw or use syringe to place toward back of child's mouth to prevent teeth staining.
  - Give full dose of iron, but do not give extra amounts or extra doses.
  - Expect color of child's stools to become dark while iron is supplemented.
  - Store iron medicine where children cannot reach it.

Contact the Health Care Provider if

- Child continues to show signs and symptoms of IDA despite dietary changes and supplement administration
- Child experiences side effects of iron supplementation such as constipation, nausea, or vomiting
- Child takes too much iron (immediately call physician or poison control center for your community)

---

medication (e.g., phenytoin). In general, vitamin B_{12} and folate deficiencies are readily treated. Thus, the prognosis for megaloblastic anemia is good.

Pathophysiology

Although megaloblastic anemia can develop with either vitamin B_{12} deficiency or folate deficiency, anemia takes longer to occur with vitamin B_{12} deficiency because the body's stores of vitamin B_{12} are greater than its stores of folate. The liver is the primary site for storage of vitamin B_{12} and folate.

A deficit of vitamin B_{12} or folate interferes with normal DNA synthesis within the red blood cells. The deficient

cells fail to synthesize enough DNA for normal **erythropoiesis** (formation of erythrocytes). The result is scant, immature red blood cells in the bone marrow and peripheral blood that appear nucleated and macrocytic and fail to reproduce normally.

The prolonged reproductive process does not interfere with RNA formation, but the cells acquire more RNA than normal. This alteration appears to increase the amount of hemoglobin and other cellular components, which in turn results in the cellular enlargement commonly associated with megaloblastic anemia.

Megaloblasts evidence immaturity, showing the presence of nuclei and the absence of the biconcave disks

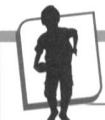

CLINICAL JUDGMENT 23-2

A Young Child With Iron-Deficiency Anemia

Cody is a 15-month-old boy who comes to the clinic. His mother reports that he was doing well until about 1 week ago. Since then, he has been less playful and sleeping more than usual. His past history is negative for hematologic disorders and other abnormalities. There is no history of recent illness, injury, or foreign travel; his mother has not noted any blood loss. Apart from skin pallor and decreased activity, Cody's physical examination is unremarkable. His laboratory results include the following: hemoglobin, 7.7 g/dL; MCV, 54 fL; and MCH, 17 pg.

Questions

1. What additional information would you elicit concerning Cody?
2. Assuming that Cody's diagnosis is IDA, at what stage is it?
3. Why is ID the most probable reason for Cody's anemia?
4. How is IDA managed?
5. What data would indicate that an IDA is resolving?

Answers

1. Obtain a diet history for Cody. Particularly, elicit information to help assess Cody's intake of dietary iron. For example, does Cody drink formula or cow's milk? If formula, is it iron fortified? If cow's milk, is Cody taking iron supplements? How many ounces of milk or formula does Cody drink on a typical day? (Too much may interfere with Cody's appetite for solid foods.) Does Cody eat solid foods? If yes, are they a source of iron?

2. The IDA would be stage III because Cody is anemic (hemoglobin, 7.7 g/dL), and his red blood cells are small in size and decreased in hemoglobin content (MCV, 54 fL; MCH, 17 pg). These changes are not characteristic of the first two stages of IDA.

3. IDA is the most frequent reason for microcytic, hypochromic anemia in infants and young children. Generally, it is the result of an inadequate intake of dietary iron coupled with depletion of the iron stores that are present at birth.

4. When IDA appears to be the result of a dietary deficiency, it is managed with the following:
   - Iron supplementation to correct anemia and replenish iron stores
   - Nutritional counseling to promote an adequate dietary intake of iron and to prevent further iron deficiency

   If these measures are not effective, further studies are needed to assess for malabsorption of iron or loss of iron through bleeding.

5. Data that indicate that IDA is resolving include a decrease in the signs and symptoms that are present at diagnosis and a return to normal hematologic laboratory values. With Cody, look for increased activity and playfulness and the return of normal skin color and normal sleep pattern. Also, note the return of normal-for-age hematologic values. For a 15-month-old, these are as follows: hemoglobin, 9.6–15.6 g/dL; MCV, 76–92 fL; MCH, 23–31 pg.

---

that characterize mature red blood cells. They are also fragile, with a life span that is one-half to one-third that of normal red blood cells. Despite these alterations, circulating megaloblastic cells are capable of transporting oxygen normally.

Assessment

Megaloblastic anemia is not an early manifestation of vitamin B_{12} deficiency or folate deficiency; it appears after these deficiencies have been present for some time.

Assess children for pallor, weakness, unsteady gait, irritability, poor feeding, failure to thrive, and developmental delay. They may experience abnormal sensations and, with severe anemia, there may be evidence of heart failure and inflammation of the tongue.

With vitamin B_{12} deficiency, in particular, neurologic and gastrointestinal disturbances can occur in the absence of or before the onset of megaloblastic anemia.

Diagnostic Tests

Laboratory evidence of megaloblastic anemia can be categorized as follows: (1) evidence that shows the presence of megaloblastic anemia, (2) evidence that identifies or rules out vitamin B_{12} or folate deficiency, and (3) evidence that points to the etiology of vitamin B_{12} or folate deficiency.

Megaloblastic anemia is characterized by typical changes in the bone marrow and blood cell profile. Bone marrow shows the presence of megaloblasts. Blood cell profile changes include decreased hemoglobin and hematocrit and increased MCV and MCH. In addition to oval, macrocytic red blood cells, hypersegmented neutrophils are present. With severe anemia, neutropenia and thrombocytopenia also may be noted.

Vitamin B_{12} deficiency may be identified by a low vitamin B_{12} level in serum, tissue, or both. In megaloblastic anemia, the serum level is usually low before megaloblasts become evident. Tissue vitamin B_{12} deficiency is indicated by elevated levels of urinary methylmalonic acid, serum methylmalonic acid, and total homocysteine. Tissue deficiency may be evident in children with neurologic and gastrointestinal disturbances in the absence of megaloblastic anemia. When vitamin B_{12} deficiency is identified or suspected, the Schilling test (see Tests and Procedures 23-1) is helpful in determining a malabsorptive etiology such as pernicious anemia. However, neither a normal vitamin B_{12} level nor a normal Schilling test rules out vitamin B_{12} deficiency.

Folate deficiency is likely to be recognized by a low serum or red blood cell folate level. Decreased serum folate usually becomes apparent before evidence is seen of a reduced level of red blood cell folate or the onset of megaloblastic anemia.

caREminder

Folate deficiency may be masked by a normal serum folate level when the folate deficiency exists simultaneously with a vitamin B_{12} deficiency. Along with serum folate level, expect to check the serum or tissue level for B_{12} or perform a Schilling test.

Interdisciplinary Interventions

The child with megaloblastic anemia can be managed on an outpatient basis by the interdisciplinary team. Management of the child with megaloblastic anemia has four goals: identifying the cause of the anemia, correcting the anemia, replenishing vitamin B_{12} and folate stores, and preventing further deficiency and anemia.

The cause of megaloblastic anemia is identified by carefully evaluating the child's history, clinical presentation, and the results of diagnostic laboratory tests. A deficit of both vitamin B_{12} and folate may be present rather than deficiency of just a single nutrient. The anemia is corrected, vitamin B_{12} and folate stores are replenished, and further deficiency and anemia are prevented by supplementation and nutritional counseling. Follow-up care includes physical assessment and laboratory studies to ascertain that the anemia is corrected and that the stores of vitamin B_{12} and folate are replenished.

Vitamin B_{12} caused by inadequate intake is replenished by oral supplementation. When the deficiency is secondary to malabsorption, parenteral injections of vitamin B_{12} are likely to be prescribed, although oral and intranasal routes are being investigated. Children with congenital alterations in vitamin B_{12} metabolism may receive injections or large doses of oral vitamin B_{12}.

Folate supplementation is given orally. Even when folate deficiency is caused by malabsorption, some folate is absorbed when it is given orally in large doses. However, children who are receiving oral vitamin B_{12} therapy for vitamin B_{12} deficiency should avoid large doses of folate, because if vitamin B_{12} supplements do not correct the vitamin B_{12} deficiency, the folate may protect against megaloblastic anemia but fail to prevent the neurologic impairment associated with vitamin B_{12} deficiency.

Preventing further deficiency and anemia entails nutritional counseling, particularly when megaloblastic anemia is caused by inadequate intake of vitamin B_{12} or folate. The nurse has a key role in ensuring that the child and family receive information concerning dietary sources of these nutrients (see Chart 23-1). In addition, the nurse can instruct staff in daycare centers, schools, and other community groups about the importance of including foods with vitamin B_{12} and folate in the diets of children and adolescents.

APLASTIC ANEMIA

Aplastic anemia is a disorder in which the normal production of blood cells in the bone marrow is absent or decreased. This defect leads to altered peripheral blood counts that reflect **pancytopenia** (abnormally low numbers of all types of blood cells) and not merely the presence of anemia. Aplastic anemia can be acquired, occurring at any age, inherited, or congenital, which may not become evident until some years after birth. Fanconi anemia is the most common inherited form of aplastic anemia seen in children.

Acquired aplastic anemia (AAA) is characterized by a lack of precursor cells for the platelets, red blood cells, and white blood cells that are normally present in the peripheral circulation. As a result, the blood cell profile typically shows thrombocytopenia, anemia, and neutropenia. The cause of AAA is often unknown, particularly in children. However, in a number of cases, it is associated with a history of exposure to drugs (e.g., chloramphenicol), chemicals (e.g., benzene), toxins (e.g., ionizing radiation), or infection (e.g., hepatitis). Occasionally, AAA has been diagnosed during pregnancy, and increased estrogen levels might contribute to the onset of this disorder during the antepartum period. In addition, genetic factors may play a role in susceptibility to AAA. In general, the disorder affects all racial groups, and its incidence among females and males is similar. The prognosis for AAA is related to the severity of the disorder. Generally, mild to moderate disease can be easily managed and has a good prognosis. However, children with severe disease require more aggressive treatment and, even then, approximately one in five does not survive to adulthood.

Fanconi anemia is a rare, inherited form of aplastic anemia that is associated with an autosomal recessive inheritance pattern. The hematologic abnormalities associated with this disorder may occur with other physical alterations. Generally, Fanconi anemia is diagnosed during childhood or adolescence. Although current treatment of bone marrow failure associated with Fanconi anemia has improved the prognosis for children with this disorder, most do not live beyond the third decade of life. Allogeneic stem cell transplantation has been curative for some children with Fanconi anemia (Xing et al., 2013).

Pathophysiology

Much remains unknown about the pathophysiology of AAA and Fanconi anemia. However, it appears that the stem cells of the bone marrow are affected and that these cells incur both qualitative and quantitative deficits. These deficits lead to pancytopenia in the peripheral blood, placing the child at increased risk for bleeding, secondary to thrombocytopenia; tissue hypoxia, secondary to anemia; and infection, secondary to neutropenia. In addition, Fanconi anemia is associated with an increased number of chromosomal breaks.

Assessment

The primary clinical manifestations of aplastic anemia are related to bone marrow failure and pancytopenia. Assess for abnormal findings related to bleeding, tissue hypoxia, and infection (see Focused Physical Assessment 23-1). In addition, for the child with Fanconi anemia, observe for possible multiple physical anomalies that most commonly include

- Café-au-lait spots and other areas of hyper- or hypopigmentation
- Short stature, frequently because of a short trunk
- Anomalies of the hands and forearms, such as absent thumb
- Renal anomalies
- Hypogonadism, particularly in males
- Microcephaly
- Characteristic facial appearance, including a broad nasal base, epicanthal folds, small eyes, microdontia, and a small jaw

Diagnostic Tests

Thrombocytopenia, anemia, and neutropenia are revealed by respective abnormalities in the blood cell profile. Severe aplastic anemia is evidenced by an ANC of less than 500/mm³, a hemoglobin level less than 7 g/dL, a platelet count less than 20,000/mm³, and a reticulocyte count less than 1%. The anemia associated with AAA is most often normocytic, but at times, the red blood cells appear macrocytic. Bone marrow aspirations and biopsies reveal hypocellular and fatty marrow. These tests are particularly important not only in diagnosing AAA but also in ruling out other possible reasons for pancytopenia, such as leukemia.

To distinguish between AAA and Fanconi anemia, chromosome breakage analysis after exposure of cultured cells to DNA cross-linking is performed on peripheral blood lymphocytes. With Fanconi anemia, an increased number of chromosome breaks are noted. Other physical alterations associated with Fanconi anemia may be identified or ruled out with additional diagnostic studies such as a skeletal survey or renal ultrasonography.

Nursing Diagnoses and Outcomes

Nursing diagnoses and outcomes for children with bleeding and anemia are given in Nursing Plan of Care 23-1. In addition, the following nursing diagnosis and outcomes apply when the child has aplastic anemia:

Nursing Diagnosis: Fear related to possibility of child's death resulting from severe aplastic anemia
Outcomes:
- Child and family will verbalize fears concerning potential for premature death of child.
- Child and family identify information and acknowledge the need for emotional support to manage anticipatory grief.

Interdisciplinary Interventions

In addition to necessary supportive care, management of the child with aplastic anemia centers on restoring normal hematopoiesis. Children with mild or moderate aplastic anemia may require only supportive care, provided on either an inpatient or outpatient basis, depending on the severity of current symptoms. However, for those with severe aplastic anemia, bone marrow transplantation is the treatment of choice when a suitable donor is available.

Pharmacologic Interventions

Immunosuppressive therapy is used for children with severe AAA who are not candidates for bone marrow transplantation. Antithymocyte globulin is often the first line of such treatment. Although this cytotoxic agent is effective in about one-third of those who receive it, its mode of action in AAA is unclear. Generally, antithymocyte globulin is administered intravenously, once a day, for about 4 days. Before the first dose, a test dose is recommended to identify hypersensitivity. Observe children receiving antithymocyte globulin for adverse reactions such as fever, chills, rash, urticaria, pruritus, dyspnea, chest pain, nausea, vomiting, leukopenia, and thrombocytopenia. Other less frequent side effects that may occur and can be life threatening include hypotension, pulmonary edema, laryngospasm, and anaphylaxis. Serum sickness may also occur. In addition to antithymocyte globulin, corticosteroids and cyclosporine may be incorporated into the treatment plan for severe AAA.

Generally, children who respond to immunosuppressive therapy do so within 3 months. However, they may continue to have some degree of abnormal hematopoiesis rather than the complete restoration of bone marrow function that usually follows successful bone marrow transplantation.

Androgen therapy may be used alone or in combination with corticosteroids to stimulate hematopoiesis in a child with Fanconi anemia. The therapy must be administered continuously to be effective. However, the beneficial effects may not be evident in laboratory tests for several weeks.

Bone Marrow Transplantation

Bone marrow transplantation is the treatment of choice for a child with severe AAA. It is also a possible option for a child with Fanconi anemia when androgen therapy is no longer effective. Bone marrow transplantation is a complex process, requiring numerous tests and procedures. In addition to the usual tests to identify a suitable marrow donor, the potential donor for a child with Fanconi anemia must be evaluated for covert Fanconi anemia. When bone marrow transplantation is successful, it offers the hope of a cure for aplastic anemia associated with Fanconi anemia.

Children receiving such transplants are hospitalized in an environmentally controlled, intensive care setting to prepare for, receive, and await marrow engraftment of donor stem cells. These children require intensive prophylactic and supportive therapy, particularly while they await the restoration of hematopoiesis and the resolution of pancytopenia. Care is provided by specially prepared physicians, nurses, social workers, dietitians, pharmacists, and others. Chapter 22 provides more information about bone marrow transplants and the care of child undergoing this intervention.

Supportive Care

Supportive care for children with aplastic anemia involves close monitoring of blood counts for evidence of thrombocytopenia, anemia, and neutropenia as well as close observation for indicators of bleeding, tissue hypoxia, and infection. Although blood product support is sometimes necessary, every effort is made to refrain from such transfusions. Transfusions place the child at risk for becoming sensitized to the surface antigens on donor blood cells (alloimmunization). Alloimmunization decreases the probability that the bone marrow, when transplanted, will successfully engraft and increases the probability of graft-versus-host disease among bone marrow transplant recipients. When a suitable marrow donor is available, it is likely to be a family member. Thus, to decrease the risk of alloimmunization when pretransplantation blood products are necessary, it is important that the blood products not be from family members. Blood products are usually radiated and then filtered during administration, a procedure that decreases the number of white blood cells and, in turn, reduces the risk of alloimmunization.

If thrombocytopenia is present, therapeutic platelet support is given when there is evidence of bleeding. In addition, antifibrinolytic agents and topical agents are used to control bleeding. Prophylactic platelet support may be considered for children whose platelet count falls to less than 5,000/mm³, primarily to decrease the risk of intracranial hemorrhage. During thrombocytopenia, instruct the child and family to observe certain precautions.

caREminder

For children with thrombocytopenia, apply firm pressure to venipuncture and intramuscular injection sites for 3–5 minutes immediately after each procedure, and apply a pressure dressing to the site.

PRBCs are given when transfusion support is required for symptomatic anemia and dangerously low hemoglobin levels. However, children often adapt to chronic anemia, and when they can tolerate hemoglobin levels as low as 6 g/dL, they should be allowed to do so. If red blood cell transfusion therapy is required for a long time, monitor the child for iron overload.

Neutropenia increases risk for infection, especially when the ANC is less than 500/mm³. Fever in the child with neutropenia is a serious sign and is presumed to indicate sepsis until proved otherwise. Common inflammatory responses associated with infection are likely to be absent in children with neutropenia. Instruct the child and family on the increased risk of rapidly progressing, life-threatening sepsis during neutropenia and the importance of notifying the physician immediately when fever of 101° F (38.3° C) or higher occurs.

ALERT *The child with fever and neutropenia requires immediate evaluation for sepsis, even if the child looks well. When sepsis is suspected, follow hospital protocol to obtain bacterial (both anaerobic and aerobic) and viral blood cultures as well as cultures from any obvious source (e.g., throat, if child complains of sore throat). Initiate broad-spectrum parenteral antibiotics as ordered, preferably within 1 hour of presentation.*

Ensure that the child with fever and neutropenia receives a septic workup, including physical examination, blood cultures, and blood counts, and begins IV antibiotics. Antibiotics are continued at least until the child is afebrile, blood cultures are negative, and any sepsis has been treated. However, long-term oral prophylactic antibiotics are not given to the child with neutropenia associated with aplastic anemia. Neither are granulocyte transfusions used, except in the presence of life-threatening sepsis that is not responding well to IV broad-spectrum antibiotic therapy.

Community Care

Preventing infection in the child with neutropenia, especially sepsis caused by endogenous microorganisms, is not always possible. However, ensure that the child and family are taught infection prevention measures for people with neutropenia (see Community Care 22-2).

Instruct the child and family to identify activities that are tolerated by children with anemia. Typically, these activities are less strenuous, help the child conserve energy, and provide adequate oxygenation to support the child's vital body functions and activities of daily living. Remind them to be alert for and report signs that indicate that the child is not tolerating the anemic state, such as dyspnea, irritability, listlessness, and marked fatigue.

Experiencing a life-threatening disorder is usually stressful for children and their families. Health care providers must be sensitive to this stress. Education about aplastic anemia; its treatment; and the ongoing need to provide laboratory data, physical assessment data, and emotional support are important components of the interdisciplinary management of aplastic anemia. The Aplastic Anemia & MDS International Foundation is a source of support (see thePoint for Organizations). In addition to managing the aplastic anemia, the interdisciplinary team is involved in identifying and treating nonhematologic health problems that may be present in the child with Fanconi anemia. Referrals for ongoing informational and emotional support and genetic counseling after discharge are important interventions for the child and family experiencing Fanconi anemia.

HEREDITARY SPHEROCYTOSIS

Hereditary spherocytosis is characterized by loss of surface area on the red blood cell membrane. Spherocytic erythrocytes are prone to premature destruction, placing the child at risk for hemolytic anemia, especially with severe hereditary spherocytosis.

Most often, hereditary spherocytosis becomes evident during childhood, but it can be discovered during any phase of life. Hereditary spherocytosis is common; it affects an estimated 1 in 5,000 people. The actual incidence is probably higher because asymptomatic or mild hereditary spherocytosis may not be diagnosed. Although hereditary spherocytosis can occur in various racial and ethnic groups, its highest incidence is among those of northern European heritage.

For 75% of those with hereditary spherocytosis, the disorder follows an autosomal dominant inheritance pattern; for the remaining 25%, it follows an autosomal recessive inheritance pattern. Hereditary spherocytosis can also occur as a result of a spontaneous genetic mutation in individuals who have no family history of this abnormality. In general, the prognosis for hereditary spherocytosis is good. However, life-threatening complications, such as severe hemolytic anemia and aplastic crises, are possible, especially among children with severe hereditary spherocytosis.

Pathophysiology

The normal red blood cell membrane has a large surface area relative to the cell's volume, which permits red blood cells to adapt their shape to their environment and safely navigate through the vascular system, even through narrow capillaries. Spherocytic erythrocytes have a diminished membrane surface area with a reduced surface-to-volume ratio, which decreases their ability to adapt their shape to their environment. Also, spherocytes are osmotically fragile, leading to premature rupture and a considerably shorter life span than that of normal red blood cells.

The spleen poses the greatest challenge for erythrocytes. Although normal erythrocytes can contort themselves to pass through spaces that are more narrow than they are, spherocytic red blood cells are more likely to be trapped in the splenic cords or to rupture as they journey through the venous sinus walls.

Assessment

Although the clinical presentation can be quite varied, with some children even being asymptomatic, the primary manifestations of hereditary spherocytosis are anemia, splenomegaly, and jaundice.

The degree of anemia tends to parallel the severity of spherocytosis. Assess the child with severe hereditary spherocytosis for pallor, fatigue, weakness, and other manifestations of anemia such as delayed growth and development.

Palpate the spleen. Splenomegaly is a common physical finding in children with hereditary spherocytosis and may be associated with abdominal distention, tenderness, and pain. Although the degree of splenomegaly may range from minimal to marked, the size of the spleen does not necessarily correlate with the severity of the spherocytosis.

Most children with hereditary spherocytosis intermittently manifest acholuric jaundice (jaundice without bilirubin in the urine). Jaundice in the neonate with undiagnosed hereditary spherocytosis can pose a particular challenge because neonatal jaundice may occur in conjunction with a variety of other disorders, such as sepsis and hemolytic disease of the newborn.

Anemia, splenomegaly, and jaundice are often accelerated during infection. Children who are otherwise asymptomatic are likely to show these manifestations when viral illnesses and other infections occur.

In addition, children with hereditary spherocytosis may experience indigestion and biliary colic secondary to gallstone formation. This cholelithiasis is more likely to occur in older children and adolescents than in younger children. Complete a nutritional assessment, noting the child's dietary and elimination patterns. Determine whether the child experiences a stomachache after eating and whether any association exists between abdominal pain and the type of foods eaten.

Diagnostic Tests

The primary laboratory evidence for hereditary spherocytosis consists of (1) a positive osmotic fragility test, (2) an elevated reticulocyte count (usually >6%), and (3) the presence of spherocytes on the peripheral blood smear. In addition, the bilirubin level is usually elevated, and the red blood cell indices are likely to exhibit low normal or abnormal hemoglobin and hematocrit levels, with an increased MCHC. MCV and MCH are generally within normal limits.

Interdisciplinary Interventions

Treatment for hereditary spherocytosis includes surgical management (splenectomy) and nutritional interventions.

Splenectomy is the most effective intervention for symptomatic hereditary spherocytosis. Although spherocytic erythrocytes are still present in the blood after removal of the spleen, their life span generally improves to about 80% of normal as hemolysis decreases. Anemia and jaundice usually disappear soon after splenectomy. In addition, removal of the spleen is associated with a reduction in symptomatic gallbladder disease among children and adolescents with hereditary spherocytosis.

Make sure the child has been immunized with the *H. influenzae* type b vaccine and a multivalent pneumococcal vaccine before splenectomy and receives prophylactic penicillin after splenectomy.

The benefits of splenectomy must be balanced with the potential complications. The risk of life-threatening sepsis is a particular concern for asplenic individuals, especially young children. Thus, every effort is made to delay splenectomy until the child is at least 5 years of age. When young children with hereditary spherocytosis experience marked hemolytic anemia, they are generally supported with red blood cell transfusions until they reach the age at which the postsplenectomy course is safer.

Children with hereditary spherocytosis are likely to have an increased need for folic acid. Folic acid supplements may be required to maintain adequate folate stores and to prevent the megaloblastic crises that can complicate hereditary spherocytosis.

Community Care

Instruct children with hereditary spherocytosis and their families to notify their health care provider or nurse practitioner when signs and symptoms of anemia, splenomegaly, or infection develop. Fatigue, pallor, weakness (anemia), and jaundice may be signs of an aplastic crisis, especially if preceded by a viral or other infection with chills, fever, lethargy, vomiting, diarrhea, and a "slapped cheek" maculopapular rash (parvovirus infection).

Even with mild hereditary spherocytosis, severe hemolysis and splenomegaly can occur with infections. Red blood cell transfusions may be required at such times even though, generally, the child is not transfusion dependent.

Also, instruct children with hereditary spherocytosis and their families about appropriate physical activities. Contact sports and strenuous physical activities should be avoided because, even with mild hereditary spherocytosis, these activities may increase red blood cell hemolysis and lead to anemia.

HEMOGLOBINOPATHIES

Hemoglobinopathies are anemias that result from a structural or quantitative abnormality involving hemoglobin. These alterations range in severity from clinically insignificant to profound and life-threatening disease.

Sickling disorders are hemoglobinopathies in which a structural alteration in the hemoglobin molecule causes red blood cells to assume a sickle shape under certain circumstances. Hemoglobin S is an example of a structurally abnormal hemoglobin. Its presence, instead of the normal hemoglobin A, is associated with the most common sickling disorder, hemoglobin SS disease.

Thalassemia disorders are hemoglobinopathies in which one or more of the globin chains necessary for the synthesis of hemoglobin is deficient or absent. The normal hemoglobin A molecule is composed of paired alpha and beta globin chains. A deficiency in the alpha chain results in alpha-thalassemia, a deficiency in the beta chain is associated with beta-thalassemia.

SICKLE CELL DISEASE

 QUESTION: If neither of Shawanda's parents have sickle cell disease, what is the probability that any of Shawanda's future siblings will have sickle cell disease?

Sickle cell disease is a hereditary disorder characterized by any one of a number of structural abnormalities in the beta globin chains of the hemoglobin molecule. These abnormalities may be clinically unimportant or may result in serious overt disease.

Sickle cell disease affects approximately 0.1% of the African American population in the United States. In Africa, it is estimated to affect 4% of black Africans (National Institutes of Health [NIH], 2009). About 30% of children with sickle cell anemia also have beta-thalassemia (Steinberg, 2005). The widespread distribution of sickle cell disease has led to neonatal screening programs to identify children with this disorder.

CROSS-CULTURAL CARE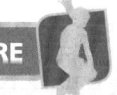

Sickle cell disease has a widespread geographic and ethnic distribution. It is most common among those of African descent. Sickle cell disease also affects a large number of children whose ancestral roots are in the Mediterranean, Caribbean, Central American, and South American parts of the world. White children can also have sickle cell disease, although it is rare in this population.

Sickle cell disease follows an autosomal recessive inheritance pattern, with the genetic defect present on chromosome number 11 (see Fig. 3-3). When both parents are heterozygous for the hemoglobin S gene, there is a 25% probability that each child will have hemoglobin SS disease and a 50% probability that each child will have the sickle cell trait. In addition, there is a 25% probability that each child will have normal hemoglobin. When one parent is heterozygous and the other parent is homozygous for the hemoglobin S gene, there is a 50% probability that each child will have hemoglobin SS disease; children who do not have hemoglobin SS disease will have the sickle cell trait. Persons with the trait need counseling about the genetics of the disorder because of the potential consequences for their children. Most children with sickle cell disease are homozygous, having inherited the same abnormal beta globin gene from each parent. The long-term prognosis for sickle cell disease varies depending on its type and clinical severity. In general, the median survival is 42 years for males and 48 years for females (Quinn et al., 2010).

ANSWER: Shawanda's parents each have the sickle cell trait but not the disease, which means that they are heterozygous for the condition. Therefore, each of her future siblings have a 25% chance of the disease, a 50% chance of having the trait, and a 25% chance of having normal hemoglobin.

Pathophysiology

QUESTION: Shawanda's younger brothers develop a parvovirus infection. How might their infection affect Shawanda and her condition?

The red blood cells of children with hemoglobin SS disease are prone to become sickle shaped and fail to function in a normal manner. Circumstances such as increased body temperature, high hemoglobin concentration, decreased blood pH, dehydration, and decreased blood oxygen level enhance the sickling process. Erythrocytes may be reversibly or irreversibly sickled. The former lose their sickle shape with reoxygenation, whereas the latter remain sickled despite their return to an oxygenated environment.

Sickle cells are characterized by rigidity, which limits their ability to adapt their shape to their surroundings, particularly in the microvasculature (Fig. 23-3). Sickle cells undergo premature hemolysis, accounting for the chronic anemia seen with this disease. In addition, sickle cells enhance blood viscosity, increasing adherence of sickle cells to the vascular endothelium, which is an important factor in the vaso-occlusion commonly associated with sickle cell disease.

The clinical hallmark of sickle cell disease is the vaso-occlusive (acute pain) crisis caused by sickle cells obstructing the circulation. This leads to painful ischemia and infarction. The bones, lungs, liver, spleen, brain, and penis are common sites of crisis events (Fig. 23-4). Other important sickle cell crises include the following:

- *Acute splenic sequestration:* Sickled red blood cells are trapped and a large amount of blood accumulates within the spleen. It occurs among children whose spleen is still functional. With hemoglobin SS disease, the spleen generally ceases to function during early childhood. Thus, the incidence of acute splenic sequestration decreases when children with hemoglobin SS disease reach middle childhood.

❗ **ALERT**   *Acute splenic sequestration can rapidly progress to cardiovascular collapse and death. Prepare the child for emergent transfusion with PRBCs.*

- *Aplastic crises:* Transient episodes of bone marrow suppression in which red blood cell production is markedly decreased. Normally, children with sickle cell disease have increased bone marrow activity and produce an above-average number of red blood cells to compensate for the shortened survival time of their atypical erythrocytes. In hemoglobin SS disease, red blood cells live for approximately 10 to 20 days, in contrast to the 120-day average in the general population. These crises also may occur in conjunction with bacterial and viral infections, including parvovirus B19, which can interfere with normal erythropoiesis (development of mature red blood cells), triggering erythroid aplasia.
- *Infections:* Occur frequently and tend to be severe, even life threatening, among children with sickle cell disease because their immune status is altered. A primary factor is the development of a nonfunctional spleen. Generally, this event occurs early in life among children with hemoglobin SS disease and places them at high-risk for sepsis, meningitis, pneumonia, and other infections.

❗ **ALERT**   *Even in the absence of other clinical manifestations of infection, febrile children with sickle cell disease require emergency health care. A child with sickle cell disease and a temperature more than 101° F (38.3° C) should be treated with parenteral antibiotics before obtaining radiographs or laboratory results. A child with a temperature of more than 104° F should be admitted promptly.*

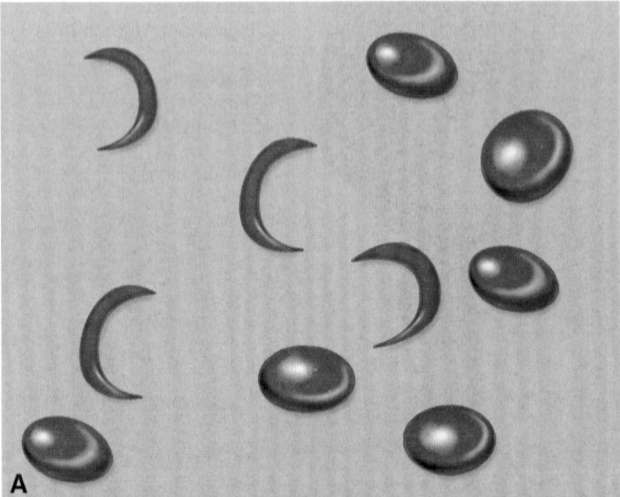

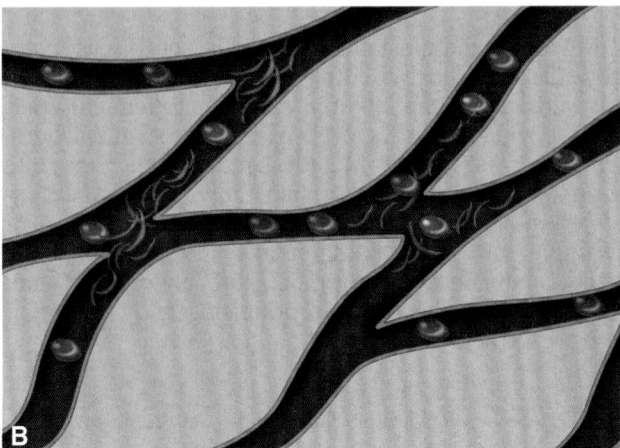

Figure 23-3 (A) Sickle cells contain abnormal hemoglobin that causes the cells to have a sickle shape. (B) The cells are rigid and tend to form clumps that block the blood vessels. Blocked blood vessels can cause pain, serious infections, and organ damage (vaso-occlusive crisis).

In addition to acute complications, the chronic complications of hemoglobin SS disease may be multiple.

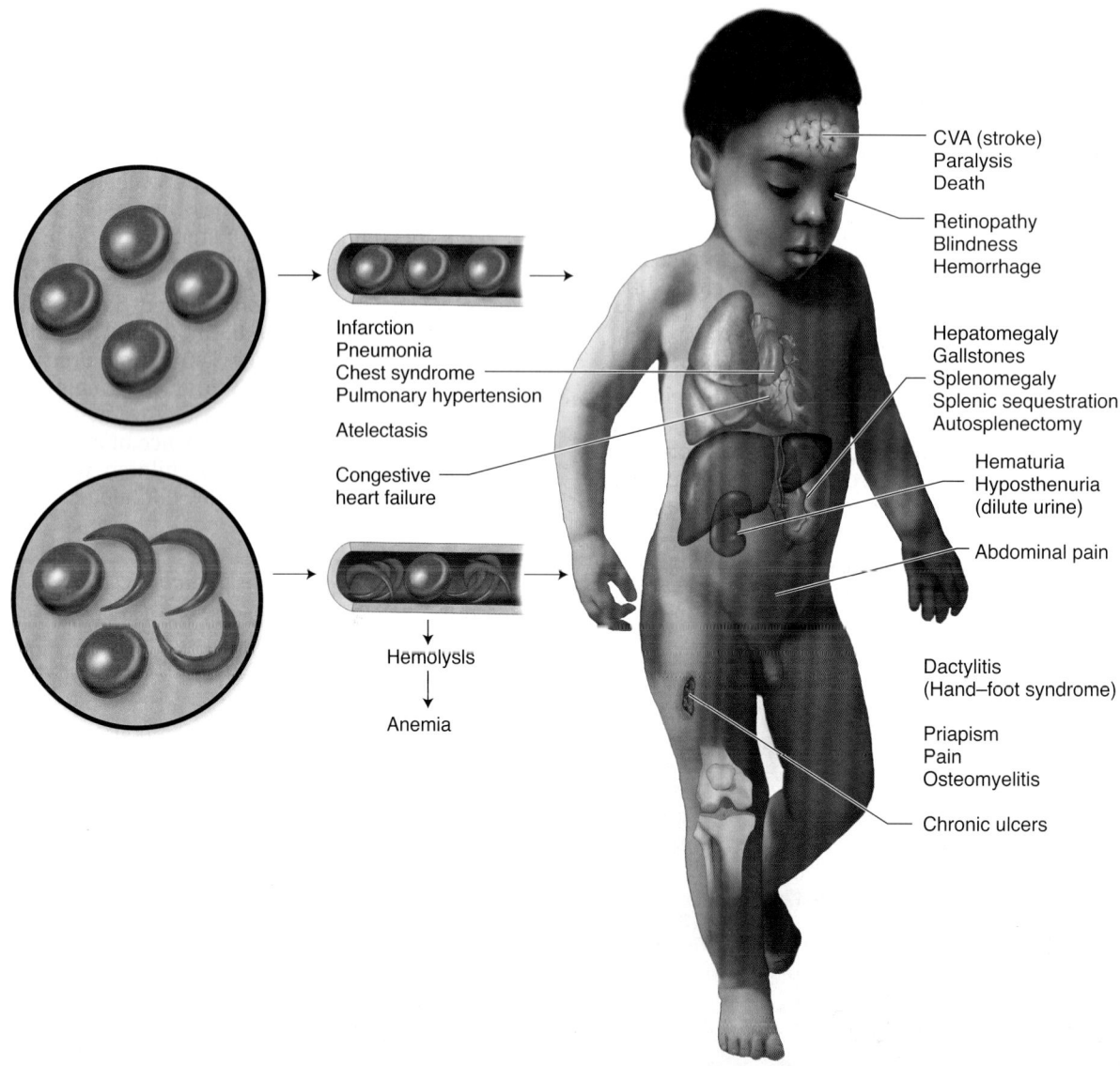

Infarction
Pneumonia
Chest syndrome
Pulmonary hypertension

Atelectasis

Congestive
heart failure

Hemolysis
↓
Anemia

CVA (stroke)
Paralysis
Death

Retinopathy
Blindness
Hemorrhage

Hepatomegaly
Gallstones
Splenomegaly
Splenic sequestration
Autosplenectomy

Hematuria
Hyposthenuria
(dilute urine)

Abdominal pain

Dactylitis
(Hand–foot syndrome)

Priapism
Pain
Osteomyelitis

Chronic ulcers

Figure 23-4 Effects of sickle cell anemia on various parts of the body.

They can involve the eyes, ears, heart, lungs kidneys, liver, and bones (Chart 23-3). General growth and development are often delayed.

ANSWER: Exposure to parvovirus (fifth disease) may precipitate an aplastic crisis for Shawanda. This virus can interfere with normal erythropoiesis (development of mature red blood cells), triggering erythroid aplasia. In addition, any infection can be severe and possibly life threatening because Shawanda's immune system is altered.

Assessment

QUESTION: Based on Shawanda's manifestations, what would the nurse most likely suspect as her current problem?

The clinical manifestations of sickle cell disease vary considerably. Most children experience occasional crises, although some children experience frequent crisis events, whereas others rarely experience such episodes. Ongoing assessment includes monitoring the child with sickle cell disease for signs and symptoms of crisis events and chronic complications (Table 23-6). For example, vaso-occlusive crisis may present with bone pain, acute chest syndrome, acute abdominal pain, cerebrovascular accident, or priapism.

! A L E R T   *Respiratory failure may occur rapidly with acute chest syndrome. Provide supplementary oxygen, promptly administer medications ordered for pain, provide incentive spirometry, and prepare the child for transfusion of PRBCs.*

CHART 23-3	Chronic Complications of Sickle Cell Anemia
Organ/System	**Complications**
Skin	Skin ulcerations, with ankles and lower legs as the primary sites
Eyes	Vascular changes in the eyes, most of which are not harmful
	Proliferative retinopathy, which can lead to blindness
Ears	Sensorineural hearing loss resulting from hair cell destruction in the inner ear
Cardiovascular	Increased cardiac output, cardiomegaly
	Cardiac murmurs
Lungs	Chronic lung disease related to repeated pulmonary infarctions and pneumonia
Kidneys	Some degree of renal impairment
	Hyposthenuria (inability to produce urine with high specific gravity); excretion of large amounts of dilute urine leading to nocturia and enuresis
Liver and biliary system	Hyperbilirubinemia and high liver enzyme levels resulting from intrahepatic sickling; hepatomegaly
	Gallstones
Sexual development	Delayed development of secondary sexual characteristics
	Possible decreased fertility among males
Skeletal	Skeletal changes, usually resulting from expansion of the bone marrow cavity and bone infarction (e.g., frontal bossing, maxillary overgrowth, and flattened vertebrae)
	Avascular necrosis of the femoral head after repeated bone infarctions (more likely to occur among adolescents than children)

Also assess the child with sickle cell disease for chronic complications. Children with sickle cell disease are normal in size at birth, but subsequent growth and development are altered. Increases in standing and sitting height occur more slowly than usual. Weight gain and development of secondary sexual characteristics are delayed. Although full height is generally achieved by the completion of adolescence, weight gain frequently continues to be less than normal. This delay in weight gain is thought to stem from the body's increased need for calories to support increased bone marrow activity and cardiovascular compensation.

ANSWER: Children with sickle cell disease who present with respiratory symptoms, chest pain, and fever, like Shawanda, are generally diagnosed with acute chest syndrome. Its etiology is usually difficult to identify with certainty, and it is assumed that both sickling and infection are present. Manifestations include fever, hypoxia, and tachypnea; decreased hemoglobin concentration; increased reticulocyte count; and leukocytosis. Shawanda's chest radiograph shows pulmonary infiltrates, also indicative of acute chest syndrome.

Diagnostic Tests

Newborn screening for sickle cell is mandated in the United States. For the initial testing, most states use either thin-layer isoelectric focusing or high-performance liquid chromatography using blood samples collected by heel stick. These testing materials have high sensitivity and specificity for sickle cell anemia. Regardless of the birth setting, all infants should undergo screening between 24 and 72 hours of age. Verification of the results is made by the health care provider during the infant's first office visit. If repeat testing is needed, this should be completed no later than 2 months of age (U.S. Preventive Services Task Force, 2007).

caREminder

Specimens must be drawn prior to the administration of any blood transfusions because of the potential for a false-negative result. Also, premature infants may have false-negative results when adult hemoglobin is undetectable (U.S. Preventive Services Task Force, 2007).

Screening is not done widely in older children; if sickle cell disease is suspected in an older child, hemoglobin electrophoresis is used to confirm the diagnosis. Alterations in laboratory studies can differ among the various forms of sickle cell disease.

With sickle cell disease, anemia is generally evident by 4 months of age. Reticulocytosis is present, and baseline hemoglobin levels usually range between 6.0 and 10.0 g/dL. By the time the child reaches early childhood, a peripheral blood smear typically shows the presence of abnormal red blood cells, such as sickle cells (crescent or sickle shaped) and target cells (which have a "doughnut" appearance). When the spleen is nonfunctional or absent, red blood cells also may contain inclusions such as *Howell-Jolly bodies* (nuclear fragments of condensed DNA) and *Heinz bodies* (caused by oxidative injury to and precipitation of hemoglobin).

Note current laboratory data for hematologic status, liver function, and renal function. Review the results of special studies such as arterial blood gas studies, pulmonary function tests, electrocardiography, and radiography.

Nursing Diagnoses and Outcomes

 QUESTION: What outcomes would be appropriate for Shawanda?

In addition to those presented in Nursing Plan of Care 23-1, general nursing diagnoses and outcomes for the child with sickle cell disease are presented in Teaching Intervention Plan 23-2 (see also thePoint for Care Path: An Interdisciplinary Plan of Care for the Child With Sickle Cell Disease and Acute Chest Syndrome). Additional nursing diagnoses applicable to the child with sickle cell disease may be found in Chapters 10 and 12.

TABLE 23-6   Sickle Cell Crises and Associated Assessment Findings

Type of Crisis		Assessment Findings
Vaso-occlusive crisis		Presentation variable depending on location of vaso-occlusion
	Bone pain	Most commonly in lumbosacral spine, knee, shoulder, elbow, and femur
		Small bones of the hands and feet (dactylitis) in infants and young children
		Avoidance of activities involving use of affected extremities
		Leukocytosis, fever, ill appearance
		Radiographic evidence of bone changes within 2 weeks of the onset of dactylitis (usually reversible over several months)
	Acute chest syndrome	Chest pain and pulmonary infiltrates
		Pneumonia (more extensive and slower to resolve)
		Abnormal chest findings not immediately evident on radiographic studies
		Cough, fever, hypoxia, and tachypnea
		Decreased hemoglobin concentration, increased reticulocyte count
		Leukocytosis
	Acute abdominal pain	Distended abdomen with enlarged liver, spleen, or other organs
		Guarding, tenderness, including rebound tenderness
		Elevation of white blood cell count (less than what would be associated with a "surgical abdomen")
		Stabilization/improvement of pain with hydration and mild sedation
	Cerebrovascular accident	Hemiparesis, hemiplegia, impaired speech, impaired comprehension, visual disturbances, severe headache, seizures, and coma
		Computed tomography, magnetic resonance imaging, or magnetic resonance angiography identifying sites of sickling and vaso-occlusion
		Possible resulting chronic impaired motor function and decreased IQ
		Abnormal results of screening Doppler ultrasonography (initiation of transfusion program if abnormal)
	Priapism	Painful, nonsexual erection of the penis occurring for an extended time, more than 24 hours, or as a short episode; repeated brief episodes ("stuttering" priapism)
		Urine retention with prolonged episodes
Acute splenic sequestration		Sudden and quickly progressing splenic enlargement, abdominal distention, pallor, weakness, dyspnea, tachycardia, and hypotension
		Left upper quadrant abdominal pain and vomiting
		Decreased hemoglobin, hematocrit (number and size of red blood cells), and platelet count
		Increased reticulocyte count
		Presence of nucleated red blood cells
Aplastic crisis		Absence of reticulocytes
		Decreased hemoglobin and hematocrit
		Decreased red blood cell precursors in the bone marrow

ANSWER: Desired outcomes for Shawanda most likely would include afebrile status, evidence of adequate gas exchange, and effective breathing pattern with normal respiratory rate and rhythm with no signs of respiratory distress, ability to tolerate oral fluids, pain relief, and return to previous level of age-appropriate functioning (being more talkative and playful) with continued growth and development.

Interdisciplinary Interventions

Whenever possible, management of the child with sickle cell disease is directed by an interdisciplinary professional team that is affiliated with a center for comprehensive treatment of pediatric hematologic disorders. This team collaborates with health care providers in the child's home community to ensure complete health care for the child. The interdisciplinary team bases care practices on clinical practice guidelines such as those provided by the NIH (2002). These guidelines include recommendations for neonatal screening, health maintenance measures, family education, and assessment and treatment of the child who presents for emergency care.

Health supervision guidelines have also been recommended by the American Academy of Pediatrics (Hagan et al., 2008). These guidelines emphasize the importance of an ongoing health maintenance program to manage sickle cell disease effectively. Such a program begins with an accurate diagnosis of the specific type of sickle cell disease. Thereafter, it includes regular visits to the health care center to update the health history and physical assessment data and to provide needed interventions. Baseline data obtained during routine clinic visits are especially helpful in managing future crises such as an impending aplastic crisis. For example, a hemoglobin level of 6.5 g/dL is more likely to indicate an impending crisis in a child whose

TIP 23-2: A TEACHING INTERVENTION PLAN for the Child With Sickle Cell Disease

Nursing Diagnoses and Family Outcomes

- Deficient knowledge: Diagnosis of sickle cell disease
  Outcome: Child and family describe sickle cell disease in general and the child's hemoglobinopathy in particular.
- Risk for injury related to sickle cell crises
  Outcomes: Child and family identify signs and symptoms of the following types of crisis events:
  - Vaso-occlusion
  - Infection
  - Acute splenic sequestration
  - Bone marrow aplasia
  Child and family seek emergency health care for fever and signs and symptoms of life-threatening or severely painful crisis events.
- Acute or chronic pain related to blocking or stacking action of sickled cells in the lungs, bone, and muscles
  Outcomes: Child exhibits adequate hydration status.
  Child reports relief from pain.
  Child and family identify pain relief measures that may be used at home.
- Risk for injury related to chronic complications of sickle cell disease
  Outcomes: Child and family identify common chronic disorders that may develop with sickle cell disease.
  Child receives ongoing health care to identify and manage chronic complications associated with sickle cell disease and, when possible, to prevent such complications.
- Disturbed body image related to perceptions of physical alterations associated with sickle cell disease
  Outcomes: Child and family verbalize concerns regarding physical alterations and receive informational and emotional support.
- Risk for impaired parenting related to child's chronic physical disorder
  Outcomes: Parents identify normal developmental milestones and their role in helping their child achieve these milestones.
  Parents identify positive attributes about their child and ways in which they can promote the child's self-esteem.
  Parents engage in appropriate interactions with their child.

Teach Child/Family

Information About the Child's Condition
- Characteristics of sickle cell disease: abnormal hemoglobin, sickling of red blood cells, abnormal function of sickled cells

- Child's type of sickle cell disease and its usual clinical course
- Etiology of sickle cell disease and the risk of future children having sickle cell disease or sickle cell trait
- Factors that may precipitate sickling of red blood cells:
  - Fever
  - Infection
  - Dehydration
  - Hot and/or humid environment
  - Cold air and/or water temperature
  - High altitude
  - Excessive physical activity

General Signs and Symptoms of Sickle Cell Crises
- Fever
- Pain
- Hand–foot syndrome (painful swelling of hands and feet)
- Respiratory distress
- Abdominal distention
- Pallor, weakness
- Penile erection
- Neurologic deficits such as impaired vision or speech, impaired motor function or paralysis, seizures

Types of Crisis, Associated Signs and Symptoms, and Chronic Complications
- Vaso-occlusion: bone pain, acute chest syndrome, acute abdominal pain, cerebrovascular accidents, priapism
- Infection
- Acute splenic sequestration
- Aplastic crises
- Complications: cardiac, renal, hepatic, skeletal, pulmonary, visual, auditory, and dermatologic complications; delayed growth and development

Managing the Child's Condition
- Need for emergency health care for fever, severe pain, and other signs and symptoms of crisis events
- Measures to relieve pain associated with sickle cell crises: rest, increased fluid intake, analgesics
- Need for ongoing health care to identify and manage chronic complications
- Opportunities to express concerns regarding altered body image related to sickle cell disease; follow up with emotional support and additional information, as needed

Promoting Growth and Development
- Measures to promote normal growth and development:
  - Safety
  - Nutrition and extra fluid intake

(Continued)

TIP 23-2: A TEACHING INTERVENTION PLAN for the Child With Sickle Cell Disease *(Continued)*

- Exercise
- Dental care
- Stress management
- Avoidance of tobacco, alcohol, and unpre-scribed drugs
- Immunizations, including hepatitis B, *Haemophilus influenzae* B, and pneumococcal vaccines
- Guidelines for activities that are appropriate for the child's physical state and developmental level
- Nonphysical disciplinary measures, balancing overly protective and overly permissive parental behaviors
- Communication with siblings and affected child about sickle cell disease
- Communication with school and child care personnel about child's needs

Contact the Health Care Provider if
- Child has temperature of 101° F (38° C) or higher
- Child has pain that is not relieved by oral medication
- Child experiences
  - Chest pain
  - Shortness of breath or trouble breathing
  - Severe headaches or dizziness
  - Severe stomach pain or swelling
  - Jaundice or extreme paleness
  - Painful erection in males
  - Sudden change in vision
  - Seizures
  - Weakness or inability to move any part of the body
  - Loss of consciousness

---

baseline hemoglobin is 8.8 g/dL than it is in a child whose baseline hemoglobin is 6.8 g/dL.

Vaso-occlusive pain crises that are mild to moderate frequently can be managed at home with increased fluid intake, analgesics, and biobehavioral measures such as relaxation, warmth, and bed rest. Crises with persistent and severe pain require hospitalization to administer IV fluids, IV analgesics, and other interventions appropriate to the particular crisis event (Clinical Judgment 23-3). Supplemental oxygen is usually reserved for children who demonstrate hypoxia (Fig. 23-5). Exchange, partial exchange, or simple blood transfusions may be indicated for children with continuing hypoxia or cerebral hyperemia.

Repeated, severe vaso-occlusive crises or a history of cerebrovascular accident may require an ongoing transfusion program to suppress production of sickled cells. However, such programs carry the typical risks of blood transfusions. In addition, a long-term transfusion program eventually results in iron overload that requires ongoing iron chelation therapy.

An alternative intervention for severe vaso-occlusive disease is bone marrow transplantation (Yesilipek, 2007). It offers the hope of a cure and may be recommended when a suitable bone marrow donor is available (see Chapter 22). In the future, children with sickle cell disease may be cured with gene transfer therapy.

Acute splenic sequestration requires emergency intervention to restore normal blood volume and tissue oxygenation. Most often, restoration is achieved with blood transfusions. As normal cardiovascular status is restored, blood trapped in the spleen is again mobilized, and the sequestration episode resolves.

Aplastic crises are generally transient. Although the resulting anemia may become severe, necessitating blood transfusion and other supportive interventions, aplastic crises usually resolve spontaneously.

Pain Management

Pain associated with sickle cell crises can be excruciating, and adequate analgesia is necessary to provide relief. Managing severe pain generally includes the use of strong narcotic analgesics such as morphine sulfate, nalbuphine, and hydromorphone. These medications may be given at higher doses than usual, and they are most effective when given as a continuous infusion with patient-controlled analgesia. As the child improves, patient-controlled analgesia alone, weaker opioids alone, or weaker opioids in combination with nonnarcotic analgesics (e.g., acetaminophen with codeine) are substituted, and the child is subsequently weaned as the painful crisis resolves.

caREminder

Meperidine is contraindicated for ongoing pain management because it increases the risk of seizures.

Assess the child for verbal and nonverbal indicators of pain (e.g., withdrawal, crying, grimacing) and use a developmentally appropriate pain assessment tool. Collaborate with the interdisciplinary health care team to ensure interventions that provide pain relief for children with sickle cell crises (see Chapter 10).

Fluid Therapy

Fluid therapy is initiated during a crisis event to restore circulating blood volume and to decrease the vaso-occlusive effects of the sickled cells circulating in the blood. Provide IV fluids and monitor the child's state of hydration. IV fluids can be combined with oral fluids to ensure the child receives 1.5 times the maintenance fluid requirements for the child based on his or her age and weight.

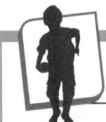

CLINICAL JUDGMENT 23-3

A Young Child With Sickle Cell Disease

Tyrone is a 2-year-old boy with hemoglobin SS disease. Last evening, he was admitted to the hospital via the emergency department after an acute onset of chest pain. The pain was not relieved at home by increased fluid intake and acetaminophen with codeine. Pertinent findings from the admitting physical examination include fever with a temperature of 104° F (40.0° C), irritability, mild nasal flaring, tachypnea, and decreased breath sounds. Tyrone's oxygen saturation on room air is 87%. His chest radiograph shows bilateral pulmonary infiltrates. Admitting laboratory studies include hemoglobin, 4.7 g/dL; reticulocytes, 24%, white blood cell count, 30,000/mm³; and platelet count 90,000/mm³.

Questions

1. What additional information would you elicit to assess Tyrone's current illness?
2. What data from Tyrone's medical record will help you interpret his admitting laboratory test results?
3. What is most likely to be Tyrone's current health problem?
4. How can Tyrone's pain be managed?
5. What assessment data would indicate that Tyrone's physical condition has improved?

Answers

1. Seek additional information about Tyrone's symptoms and the time of their onset. Ask for further details about home interventions, particularly the amount of fluid intake and the dose and frequency of analgesic medication. Inquire about conditions that may have precipitated sickling in Tyrone, such as inadequate fluid intake, exposure to heat and/or humidity or cold, excessive physical activity, travel to high altitude, and exposure to infectious organisms. *Note:* There are many times when the precipitating factor cannot be identified.
2. Tyrone's baseline laboratory values help to interpret his current laboratory values. With certain crisis events, it is not unusual to note a decrease in hemoglobin and an increase in reticulocyte count. Also, the white blood cell count is elevated above its baseline value.
3. Children with sickle cell disease who present with respiratory symptoms, chest pain, and fever are generally diagnosed with acute chest syndrome and infection. The etiology is usually difficult to identify with certainty, and it is assumed that both sickling and infection are related to the current symptoms he is experiencing.
4. Because Tyrone's pain was not relieved by oral fluids and oral analgesics at home, he should receive IV fluids and an IV narcotic, such as morphine sulfate, on a regular schedule around the clock. As his condition improves, oral fluids and a weaker analgesic will be substituted. The analgesic will be discontinued when the painful crisis resolves.
5. The following assessment data would indicate that Tyrone's physical condition has improved: afebrile, normal respiratory rate and rhythm with no signs of respiratory distress, tolerating oral fluids, normal sleep pattern, and more talkative and playful.

Managing Infections

Infections among children with sickle cell disease can be caused by various microorganisms, including pneumococcus and *H. influenzae*. The potentially severe nature of these infections requires that fever be regarded seriously and that prophylactic antibiotic therapy be initiated. Broad-spectrum antibiotics are used to manage acute chest syndrome and vaso-occlusive crises caused by infection. Instruct the child and family about the increased risk of rapidly progressing, life-threatening sepsis in sickle cell disease, and stress the importance of immediately calling their health care provider in the event of fever.

They should anticipate a septic workup, including physical examination, blood counts, blood culture, urine culture, and chest radiograph as well as parenteral antibiotic therapy.

The availability of ceftriaxone, a broad-spectrum, long-acting antibiotic, permits selected children with a febrile illness to be cared for at home after a few hours of observation in the clinic or emergency department. Outpatient care is a safe, convenient, and less costly option for children who are relatively well and free of complications and whose caregivers are reliable in providing the prescribed follow-up health care. Febrile children who are quite young, especially infants, and

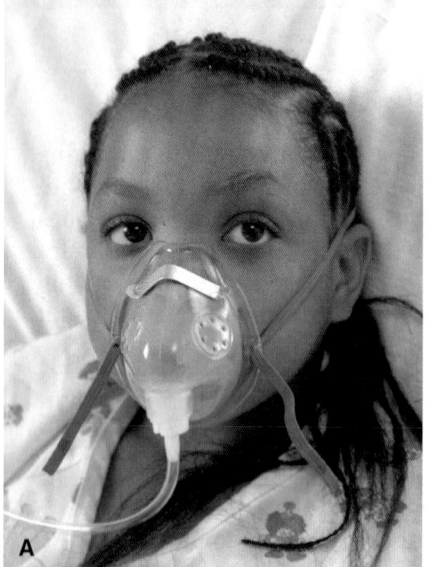 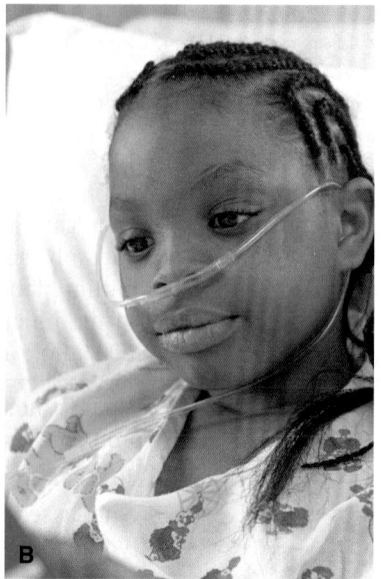 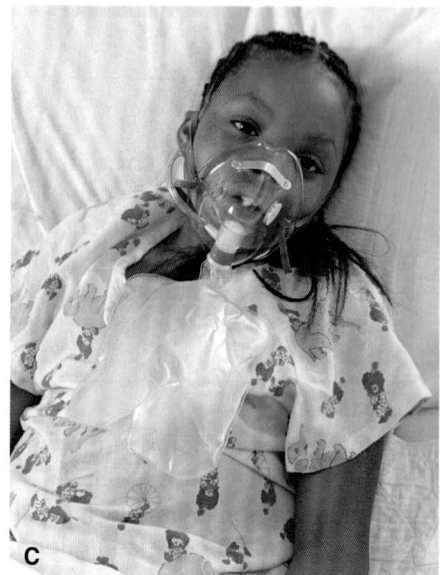

Figure 23-5 (A–C) Oxygen may be needed during a sickle cell crisis or an episode of acute chest syndrome to help relieve symptoms.

children with severe illness and complications are generally hospitalized.

Therapeutic antibiotics are continued at least until cultures are negative and any infection has been treated. Thereafter, antibiotic prophylaxis is resumed. Other measures to prevent serious infection in children with sickle cell disease include immunization with polyvalent pneumococcal and *H. influenzae* vaccines.

Stimulation of Hemoglobin Production

Hydroxyurea may be used to improve hematologic values by stimulating hemoglobin F production, thereby decreasing vaso-occlusive complications. Benefits have included decreasing painful episodes, hospitalizations, number of blood transfusions, and acute chest syndrome (NIH, 2008). Complications from therapy can range from nausea to moderate bone marrow suppression to malignancy. Hydroxyurea does not adversely affect growth. Although strong evidence exists for the therapeutic use of hydroxyurea in adults and adolescents, efficacy of this medication has not been firmly established in infants and preadolescents. Clinical trials of this medication in the pediatric population are ongoing.

Nutritional Interventions

Adequate folic acid intake is especially important during recovery from an aplastic crisis. Normally, the diet supplies a sufficient amount of folic acid. However, to ensure adequate intake in hemoglobin SS disease, folic acid supplements may be prescribed.

Surgical Management

Children who have experienced splenic sequestration crises may subsequently have an elective splenectomy. However, this surgical procedure is not indicated during times of acute splenic sequestration.

Surgical procedures for children with sickle cell disease require perioperative measures to prevent sickling. Preoperative transfusion corrects anemia and provides an increased number of hemoglobin A erythrocytes. Transfusion also decreases the body's need to engage in erythropoiesis, thereby reducing the number of hemoglobin S erythrocytes entering the circulation. Other common measures that help prevent sickling during the perioperative period are adequate fluid support, oxygenation, environmental warmth, and preventing acidosis.

Community Care

For children with sickle cell disease, view discharge planning from two perspectives. One involves planning related to specific events such as vaso-occlusive crises, infections, and surgical procedures. The second relates to planning associated with outpatient appointments for ongoing assessment and management of sickle cell disease. In both situations, identify desired outcomes and plan appropriate interventions to attain these outcomes by the end of a hospital stay or an outpatient visit.

Discharge planning for episodic events must consider the needs related to the particular event as well as the needs associated with sickle cell disease. When special supplies and services are required, referral to a home care company may be necessary.

Education is a major part of discharge planning (see Teaching Intervention Plan 23-2). Start teaching as early as possible and plan time for review. Teaching may encompass a variety of topics, depending on the specific situation. For example, when a young child with sickle cell disease has an elective splenectomy after two earlier episodes of splenic sequestration, education is likely to include measures to promote good hydration; signs of abnormal wound healing; signs of wound infection; ways to identify nonverbal indicators of pain; pain management techniques; schedule for outpatient follow-up appointments; and the need to call the physician for bleeding, fever, increased pain, or other complications.

An important component of the teaching process is to assess the family's understanding of the child's home care needs and their ability to provide them. Management of sickle cell disease also requires attention to the psychosocial needs of the child and the family (see "Treatment Modalities" section earlier in this chapter).

Outpatient visits for ongoing assessment and management of sickle cell disease generally occur at least two times per year. These visits occur more frequently with children who are newly diagnosed or quite young or whose health needs require close monitoring. Desired outcomes for these visits address physical and psychosocial needs indicated by the updated history and current physical assessment.

Be alert for the developing child's readiness to learn more about sickle cell disease as well as the need to correct misconceptions that the child and family may have about the disorder, its effect, its complications, and its management. Also, as the child and family reach new developmental milestones, be alert for the need to discuss the child's activities and specific concerns during each developmental phase. As children develop, teaching must be an ongoing process that assesses their previous knowledge and expands upon it. Knowing the beneficial effects of keeping well hydrated and warm, as well as the negative effects of cold, dehydration, and other physical stressors, can assist children in managing their disorder.

Children with sickle cell disease need to develop effective coping skills for dealing with both physical and psychosocial concerns. They may fear painful crisis events. They may wonder what will happen when they experience a crisis event. Knowing the signs and symptoms of crises, knowing what to do, and knowing what to expect others to do helps children cope with crisis events. Instruct children to notify family members when they experience pain or other indicators of sickle cell crises and that measures should be taken promptly to abate crisis events.

Like their peers, children with sickle cell disease are involved in establishing their identities. Help them to identify their positive qualities; recognize what they can do; and develop realistic, healthy self-concepts. This process is particularly important for adolescents with sickle cell disease whose peers achieve physical growth and develop secondary sex characteristics sooner than they do.

Discharge planning for outpatient visits may include follow-up information or referral to a local health care provider, a home care company, and a community health agency. It may involve contact with community groups such as the child's school or daycare center (Community Care 23-2). It may entail helping a family with planning for camp or vacation by providing a letter detailing the child's need for emergency health care if a crisis event occurs. It may incorporate a referral to the Sickle Cell Disease Association of America, Inc. for literature and information about the services and local chapters of this and related organizations (see thePoint for Organizations).

BETA-THALASSEMIA

Thalassemia comprises a variety of microcytic hemolytic anemias that are characterized by a decrease or absence of one or more of the normal globin chains in the hemoglobin molecule and by ineffective erythropoiesis. Thalassemias are classified according to the defective globin chain and the clinical severity. Alpha-thalassemia, seen primarily in Southeast Asia, is less common than beta-thalassemia. In beta-thalassemia, children homozygous or doubly heterozygous for beta (0) thalassemic genes cannot make normal beta chains and are, therefore, unable to make any hemoglobin; thus, there is an absence of absence of production of beta globin (Benz, 2013). In beta (+) thalassemias, children are able to make some hemoglobin A and are generally less severely affected than those homozygous for beta (0) thalassemic genes. Beta-thalassemia is classified in terms of its clinical intensity (Chart 23-4).

Beta-thalassemia is a hereditary disorder. It follows an autosomal recessive inheritance pattern, with the genetic defect present on chromosome number 11. The disorder affects equal numbers of females and males. Children who are heterozygous for the defective gene usually do not show clinically significant disease; those who are homozygous tend to have serious disease, especially if the disorder is not diagnosed and appropriate interventions are not implemented.

In addition, some children inherit a gene for hemoglobin S from one parent and a gene for beta-thalassemia from the other parent. This inheritance results in sickle beta-thalassemia. The severity of this disorder depends on the extent to which the beta-thalassemia gene contributes to production of hemoglobin A. When no hemoglobin A is present in the red blood cells, the disorder tends to be severe. When some hemoglobin A is present in the red blood cells, the disorder is usually milder.

CROSS-CULTURAL CARE

Beta-thalassemia is most common among people of Mediterranean descent. Also, it affects a substantial number of those whose ancestral roots are in the Middle East, India and Southeast Asia, and Africa. Screening programs are common in Europe and Asia, where the incidence of thalassemia is greater. In the United States, hemoglobin electrophoresis is recommended for at-risk populations to identify those with thalassemia and thalassemia trait.

The prognosis for beta-thalassemia depends on its severity. If untreated, children with thalassemia major die during the first year of life. Children with thalassemia minor generally experience no disease-related health problems; those with thalassemia intermedia experience moderately severe anemia, bone deformities, and splenomegaly.

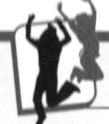

COMMUNITY CARE 23-2

The Child With Sickle Cell Disease in School or Daycare

Children with sickle cell disease will participate in school and daycare in both public and private settings. It is important for the child's teachers and caregivers to know that the child has sickle cell disease. Also, staff should know the guidelines that have been established to prevent and manage crisis events and to promote normal growth and development in children with sickle cell disease.

The nurse may assist the child's family in providing information to the staff. Outcome objectives for the child's caregivers include the following:

- Describe sickle cell disease, in general, and how it affects the child who will be cared for at the daycare center, in particular.
- State factors that may precipitate crisis events in the child with sickle cell disease, such as humidity, heat, cold, and excessive physical activity.
- Describe common types of crisis events associated with sickle cell disease:
  - Vaso-occlusive crises
  - Infections
  - Acute splenic sequestration
  - Aplastic crises
- Discuss common signs and symptoms associated with crisis events:
  - Pain
  - Fever

  - Pale color
  - Difficulty breathing
  - Enlarged abdomen
  - Vomiting, diarrhea
  - Refusal to eat or drink
  - Irritability
  - Increased somnolence
  - Weakness or numbness of arms or legs
  - Swelling of hands or feet
- Discuss the need for prompt medical care for crisis events associated with sickle cell disease.
- Discuss the importance of the child receiving extra fluids and pausing for rest periods during times of physical activity. Daycare center personnel should be informed of any activities in which the child is not to participate, such as swimming in cold water.
- Relate the child's more frequent use of restroom facilities to the effect of sickle cell disease on kidney function.
- Describe the significance of treating the child as other children are treated. Although there is a need to be aware of sickle cell disease and what to do if a crisis event occurs, the school or daycare center staff should not focus on it or single the child out for special attention or privileges.

CHART 23-4 **Classification of Beta-Thalassemia**

Thalassemia minima: referred to as "silent" because it causes no clinically important hematologic abnormalities.

Thalassemia minor: the term applied to heterozygotes who have inherited a single gene leading to reduced beta globin production. Associated with some abnormal hematologic findings; most are asymptomatic on physical examination.

Thalassemia intermedia: becomes apparent during early childhood with hematologic abnormalities in conjunction with classic findings of hyperbilirubinemia, splenomegaly, hepatomegaly, delayed growth and sexual maturation, and abnormal facial appearance. These children have later onset and a milder degree of anemia, which may or may not require transfusional support.

Thalassemia major (*Cooley anemia*): the most severe form, with symptoms of pallor, fatigue, and weakness and poor feeding, failure to thrive, and delayed growth and development generally appearing during the first year of life. These children have either no effective production (as in homozygous beta [0] thalassemia) or severely limited production of beta globin.

Adapted from Benz, E. (2013). *Treatment of beta thalassemia*. Retrieved from http://www.uptodate.com/contents/treatment-of-beta-thalassemia

Pathophysiology

Beta-thalassemia stems from a defect in the beta globin gene. The result is inadequate production of the beta globin chains, necessary for hemoglobin A synthesis.

People who are heterozygous for beta-thalassemia generate about half the normal quantity of beta globin chains. Those who are homozygous for beta-thalassemia are subclassified as having beta+ thalassemia and beta0 thalassemia. Those in the beta+ group synthesize up to one-third the normal quantity of beta globin chains; those in the beta0 group produce no beta globin chains.

Alpha globin chains, which are also required for the synthesis of hemoglobin A, continue to be produced in their normal quantity. However, the lack of beta globin chains with which they can be paired creates an excess of free alpha globin chains. These free alpha globin chains precipitate and appear as inclusion bodies within developing red blood cells. The inclusion bodies have a destructive effect, leading to the demise of most red blood cells while they are still maturing in the bone marrow.

The red blood cells that enter the peripheral circulation in decreased number are characterized by microcytosis (small size), hypochromia (less color as a result of poor staining properties because of decreased hemoglobin), poikilocytosis (abnormal shape), and the presence of inclusion bodies. Their life span is usually limited to a few hours or days, with damaged cells being removed from circulation by the spleen and liver. Red blood cells that contain a substantial amount of hemoglobin F survive longer. People with thalassemia may produce an increased amount of hemoglobin F to compensate for the deficiency of hemoglobin A.

When severe anemia occurs, the bone marrow greatly expands and produces an increased number of erythroid precursor cells. However, these cells meet an early demise, just like their predecessors, and increased erythropoiesis is negated by hemolysis.

Assessment

The clinical manifestations of beta-thalassemia vary considerably depending on its severity. Typically, the child with thalassemia minima and minor will be asymptomatic. However, for the child with thalassemia intermedia and major, observe for facial changes that begin during infancy, including frontal *bossing* (prominence of the frontal bone), prominent cheekbones, depression of the nasal bridge, maxillary overbite, and mandibular prominence. This classic "thalassemic" facies is caused by the expanding bone marrow (Fig. 23-6). In addition, urine may appear dark and tea-colored as a result of red blood cell hemolysis. Extramedullary areas of hematopoiesis occur as compensation for ineffective erythropoiesis. Features of the ineffective erythropoiesis include enlargement of involved anatomic sites, such as the liver, spleen, and lymph nodes. Although the clinical manifestations of beta-thalassemia can be severe, they are seen less frequently today because of the use of transfusion therapy.

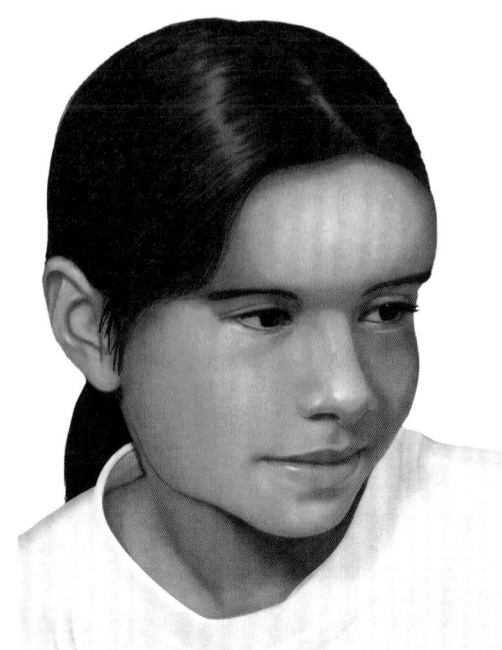

Figure 23-6 Iron overload related to thalassemia leads to bony changes such as frontal bossing and maxillary prominence.

Diagnostic Tests

Diagnosis of beta-thalassemia is generally made after the third month of life, when the normal switch from predominantly hemoglobin F to predominantly hemoglobin A fails to occur, and the child becomes anemic (see Tests and Procedures 23-1). The infant with thalassemia is born with only hemoglobin F or, in some cases, hemoglobin F and hemoglobin E. Children with beta-thalassemia have severe anemia with few reticulocytes (<8%), numerous red blood cells, and microcytosis. Unconjugated serum bilirubin levels are usually elevated. Other blood chemistry values will appear normal during the early stages of the condition. Elevated SF levels and Hemoglobin A_2 are present. Radiography is used to assess for bone marrow hyperplasia.

In addition, serum bilirubin levels may be increased as a result of red blood cell hemolysis. Leukocytosis also may be present. A normal white blood cell differential distinguishes this leukocytosis from that associated with infection.

Radiography may detect bone changes, such as a thinning of long bone cortices, which makes these bones fragile and prone to pathologic fractures (Salama et al., 2006). It also may detect sites of extramedullary areas of hematopoiesis that develop as the body attempts to compensate for ineffective erythropoiesis in the bone marrow. These sites may appear as masses in the chest, for example.

Nursing Diagnoses and Outcomes

Nursing diagnoses and outcomes for the child with a hematologic condition are described in Nursing Plan of Care 23-1. In addition, the following nursing diagnosis and outcomes apply to the child with beta-thalassemia:

Nursing Diagnosis: Risk for injury related to effects of iron overload
Outcomes:
• Child and family will demonstrate understanding of the etiology of iron overload.
• Child and family will identify the physical changes associated with iron overload, including their life-threatening potential.
• Child and family will demonstrate acceptance of the importance of iron chelation therapy in preventing severe iron overload.

Interdisciplinary Interventions

Management of beta-thalassemia varies depending on its severity. Most children with thalassemia minima or minor do not require blood transfusion therapy because they do not tend to have anemia. An exception occurs during pregnancy, when transfusion support may be necessary. Treatment for children with thalassemia intermedia and major includes transfusion therapy, iron chelation therapy, and bone marrow transplantation. Current investigations for new treatment modalities include the use of medications to stimulate increased synthesis of hemoglobin F as well as the development of curative gene transfer therapy.

Transfusions and Iron Chelation Therapy

The primary intervention for beta-thalassemia is a chronic transfusion program of PRBCs with iron chelation. Such a program facilitates adequate oxygenation of body tissues and practically eliminates all symptoms of thalassemia.

CROSS-CULTURAL CARE

In some countries, limited blood supply and the risk of transfusion-transmitted viral infections may make it difficult to effectively provide beta-thalassemia children with the PRBCs they need for treatment. In such cases, newer treatments are being investigated, such as hydroxyurea, which is an oral agent widely used in the treatment of myeloproliferative disorders. Hydroxyurea has been shown to help reduce the transfusion requirements of these children and thereby lengthen the time intervals between when transfusions are necessary (Anasari et al., 2007).

Transfusions of PRBCs are generally required every 2 to 4 weeks. Management of the condition by numerous transfusions results in excess iron in the body (transfusional hemosiderosis). Removal of the excess iron is necessary to prevent damage to major organs. Iron chelation therapy is used to remove the excessive iron. Deferoxamine is most commonly used to chelate the iron, allowing excretion in the urine and stool. Side effects include nausea, joint pain, stomachache, and low white blood cell counts (Roberts et al., 2007).

Children with minima or minor types of beta-thalassemia, who do not require ongoing transfusion, may need supportive transfusions during times of infection and other events that trigger hemolytic or aplastic crises. Oral folic acid supplements may be prescribed to maintain adequate folate stores.

Bone Marrow Transplantation

A newer mode of treatment for beta-thalassemia intermedia and major is allogenic bone marrow transplantation (see Chapter 22). This procedure has been shown to be most effective in children younger than 15 years old without excessive iron stores and hepatomegaly (DeBaun et al., 2011). When successful, it offers the hope of a cure. Although it is not an option for every child with severe beta-thalassemia, bone marrow transplantation may be recommended when a suitable donor (preferably a human leukocyte antigen–matched sibling) or stem cells are available.

Community Care

Interdisciplinary management of beta-thalassemia requires ongoing physical assessment and laboratory studies to monitor for anemia and its sequelae. Although children in a transfusion program often lead nearly normal lives, they need regular follow-up assessment for iron overload and its associated physical alterations. The psychosocial interventions for children with beta-thalassemia and their families are similar to those described in the section on "Sickle Cell Disease."

The nurse and other members of the health care team play a major role in beta-thalassemia. In addition to family-centered care and education, they provide community education about the disorder and its management and genetic counseling about the probability of having a child with heterozygous or homozygous beta-thalassemia. The Cooley's Anemia Foundation is an additional source of information (see thePoint for Organizations).

See thePoint for a summary of Key Concepts.

REFERENCES

Algarin, C., Peirano, P., Garrido, M. et al. (2003). Iron deficiency anemia in infancy: Long-lasting effects on auditory and visual system functioning. *Pediatric Research*, 53(2), 217–223.

Ansari, S., Shamsi, T., Siddiqui, F. et al. (2007). Efficacy of hydroxyurea (HU) in reduction of pack red cell (PRC) transfusion requirement among children having beta-thalassemia major: Karachi HU trial (KHUT). *Journal of Pediatric Hematology Oncology*, 29(11), 743 746.

Antunes, H., Goncalves, S., Dinis-Ribeiro, M. et al. (1997). Iron deficiency anemia: Effects of iron therapy on infants' development test performance. *Journal of Pediatric Gastroenterology and Nutrition*, 24(4), 492.

Baker, R., Creer, F., & The Committee on Nutrition. (2010). Diagnosis and prevention of iron deficiency and iron-deficiency anemia in infants and young children (0–3 years of age). *Pediatrics*, 126(5), 1040–1050.

Bansal, D., Bhamare, T. A., Trehan, A. et al. (2010). Outcome of chronic idiopathic thrombocytopenic purpura in children. *Pediatric Blood & Cancer*, 54(3), 403–407.

Ben-Ami, T., & Revel-Vilk, S. (2013). The use of DDAVP in children with bleeding disorders. *Pediatric Blood & Cancer*, 60(Suppl. 1), S41–S43.

Benz, E. (2013). *Treatment of beta thalassemia*. Retrieved from http://www.uptodate.com/contents/treatment-of-beta-thalassemia

Blanchette, V., & Bolton-Maggs, P. (2010). Childhood immune thrombocytopenic purpura: Diagnosis and management. *Hematology/Oncology Clinics of North America*, 24(1), 249–273.

Borgna-Pignatti, C., & Marsella, M. (2008). Iron deficiency anemia in infancy and childhood. *Pediatric Annals*, 37, 329–337.

Bowman, M. (2010). A prospective evaluation of the prevalence of symptomatic von Willebrand disease (VWD) in a pediatric primary care population. *Pediatric Blood & Cancer*, 55(1), 171–173.

Branchford, B. R., Monahan, P. E., & Di Paola, J. (2013). New developments in the treatment of pediatric hemophilia and bleeding disorders. *Current Opinions in Pediatrics*, 25(1), 25–30.

Bullinger, M., & von Mackensen, S. (2003). Quality of life in children and families with bleeding disorders. *Journal of Pediatric Hematology/Oncology*, 25(Suppl. 1), S64–S67.

Carter, C. (2010). Iron deficiency anemia and cognitive function in infancy. *Pediatrics*, 126(2), e427–e434.

Centers for Disease Control and Prevention. (2011). *Hemophilia: Facts*. Retrieved from http://www.cdc.gov/ncbddd/hemophilia/facts.html

Congdon, E., Westerlund, A., Algarin, C. et al. (2012). Iron deficiency in infancy is associated with altered neural correlates of recognition memory at 10 years. *The Journal of Pediatrics*, 160(6), 1027–1033.

Curry, H. (2004). Bleeding disorder basics. *Pediatric Nursing*, 30(5), 402–405, 428–429.

DeBaun, M., Frei-Jones, M., & Vichinsky, E. (2011). Thalassemia syndromes. In R. M. Kliegman, B. F. Stanton, J. W. St. Geme et al. (Eds.), *Nelson textbook of pediatrics* (19th ed., pp. 1674–1676). Philadelphia, PA: Elsevier/Saunders.

Eden, A. (2005). Iron deficiency and impaired cognition in toddlers: An underestimated and undertreated problem. *Paediatric Drugs, 7*, 347–352.

Gernsheimer, T. (2009). Chronic idiopathic thrombocytopenic purpura: Mechanisms of pathogenesis. *The Oncologist, 14*, 12–21.

Grantham-McGregor, S., & Ani, C. (2001). A review of articles on the effect of iron deficiency on cognitive development in children. *Journal of Nutrition, 131*, 649S–668S.

Hagan, J. F., Shaw, J. S., & Duncan, P. M. (Eds.). (2008). *Bright futures: Guidelines for health supervision of infants, children, and adolescents* (3rd ed.). Elk Grove Village, IL: American Academy of Pediatrics.

Kroeger, A., Nathan, M., & Hombach, J. (2004). Dengue. *Nature Reviews. Microbiology, 2*(5), 360–361.

Lozoff, B., Clark, K., Jing, Y. et al. (2008). Dose–response relationships between iron deficiency with or without anemia and infant social–emotional behavior. *Journal of Pediatrics, 152*, 696–702.

Lozoff, B., Jimenez, E., Hagan, J. et al. (2000). Poorer behavioral and developmental outcomes more than 10 years after treatment for iron deficiency in infancy. *Pediatrics, 105*, ES1.

Lozoff, B., Wolf, A., & Jimenez, E. (1996). Iron-deficiency anemia and infant development: Effects of extended oral iron therapy. *Journal of Pediatrics, 129*(3), 382–389.

Lutz, C., & Przytulski, K. (2010). *Nutrition and diet therapy: Evidence-based applications*. Philadelphia, PA: F. A. Davis.

National Heart, Lung, and Blood Institute. (2011). *What is hemophilia?* Retrieved from http://www.nhlbi.nih.gov/health/dci/Diseases/hemophilia/hemophilia_all.html

National Institutes of Health. (2002). *The management of sickle cell disease* (NIH Publication No. 02-2117). Washington, DC: U.S. Government Printing Office.

National Institutes of Health. (2008). NIH consensus development conference statement on hydroxyurea treatment for sickle cell disease. *NIH Consensus and State-of-the-Science Statement, 25*, 1–30.

National Institutes of Health. (2009). *Sickle cell disease*. Retrieved from http://science.education.nih.gov/supplements/nih1/genetic/activities/activity2_database.htm#incidence-africa

Neunert, C., Lim., C., Crowther, M. et al. (2011). The American Society of Hematology 2011 evidence-based practice guideline for immune thrombocytopenia. *Blood, 117*(16), 4190–4207.

Peirano, P., Algarin, C., Garrido, M. et al. (2007). Iron deficiency anemia in infancy is associated with altered temporal organization of sleep states in childhood. *Pediatric Research, 62*(6), 715–719.

Provan, D., Stasi, R., Newland, A. et al. (2010). International consensus report on the investigation and management of primary immune thrombocytopenia. *Blood, 115*(2), 168–186.

Quinn, C. T., Rogers, Z. R., McCavit, T. L. et al. (2010). Improved survival of children and adolescents with sickle cell disease. *Blood, 115*(17), 3447–3452.

Roberts, D., Brunskill, S., Doree, C. et al. (2007). Oral deferiprone for iron chelation in people with thalassaemia. *Cochrane Database of Systematic Reviews*, (3), CD004839.

Salama, O. S., Al-Tonbary, Y. A., Shahin, R. A. et al. (2006). Unbalanced bone turnover in children with beta-thalassemia. *Hematology, 11*(3), 197–202.

Sevier, N., & Houston, M. (2005). Chronic refractory ITP in children: Beyond splenectomy. *Journal of Pediatric Oncology Nursing, 22*(3), 145–151.

Steinberg, M. (2005). Predicting clinical severity in sickle cell anaemia. *British Journal of Haematology, 129*(4), 465–481.

Srivastava, A., Berwer, A. K., Mauser-Bunschoten, E. P. et al. (2013). Guidelines for management of hemophilia. *Haemophilia, 19*(1), e1–e47.

Tarantino, M., & Bolton-Maggs, P. (2007). Update on the management of immune thrombocytopenic purpura in children. *Current Opinion in Hematology, 14*(5), 527–534.

Tunc, B., Tavil, B., Karakurt, N. et al. (2012). Deferasirox therapy in children with Fanconi aplastic anemia. *Journal of Pediatric Hematology/Oncology, 34*(4), 247–251.

U.S. Preventive Services Task Force. (2006). *Screening for iron deficiency anemia including supplementation for children and pregnant women: Recommendation statement*. Publication no. AHRQ 06-0589. Rockville, MD: Agency for Healthcare Research and Quality. Retrieved from www.ahrq.gov/clinic/uspst06/ironsc/ironrs.htm

U.S. Preventive Services Task Force. (2007). *Screening for sickle cell disease in newborns: U.S. Preventive Services Task Force recommendation statement*. Rockville, MD: Agency for Healthcare Research and Quality.

World Health Organization. (2011). *Worldwide prevalence of anaemia 1993-2005: WHO global database on anaemia*. Retrieved from http://www.who.int/nutrition/publications/micronutrients/anaemia_iron_deficiency/9789241596657/en/index.html

Xing, W., Xu, M., & Yang, F. (2013). Bone marrow microenvironment defects in fanconi anemia. In M. Puiu (Ed.), *Genetic disorders*. Rijeka, Croatia: InTech. Retrieved from http://www.intechopen.com/books/genetic-disorders/bone-marrow-microenvironment-defects-in-fanconi-anemiabone-marrow-microenvironment-defects-in-fancon

Yalcin, S., Durmusoglu-Sendogdu, M., Gumruk, F. et al. (2007). Evaluation of the children with beta-thalassemia in terms of their self-concept, behavioral, and parental attitudes. *Journal of Pediatric Hematology Oncology, 29*(8), 523–528.

Yesilipek, M. A. (2007). Stem cell transplantation in hemoglobinopathies. *Hemoglobin, 31*(2), 251–256.

See the**Point** for additional organizations.

CHAPTER 24

The Child With an Infectious Disease

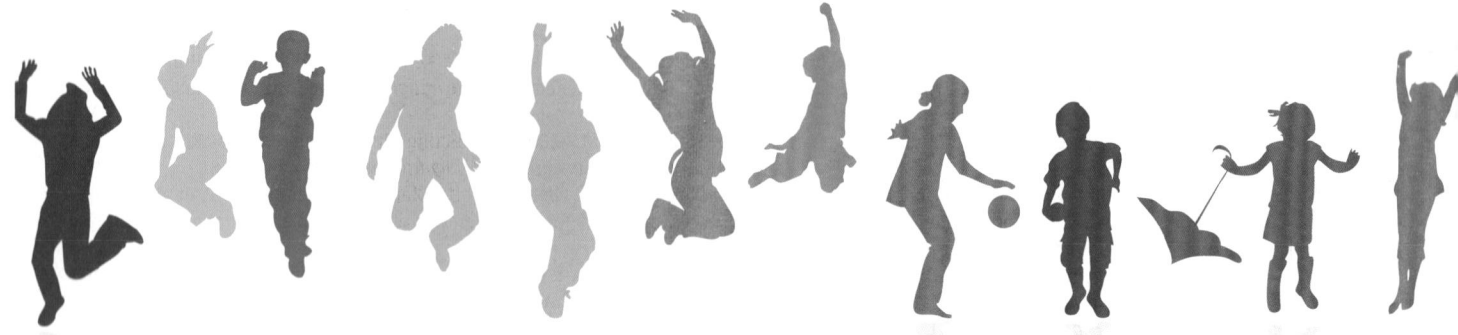

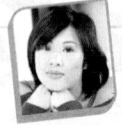

CASE HISTORY

Remember Ashley Tran from Chapter 7? Ashley is occasionally having unplanned and unprotected intercourse with her boyfriend. Ashley is experiencing frequent urination and a burning sensation when she urinates. She has also noticed an increase in vaginal discharge with an unusual odor. She is worried that she may have a sexually transmitted infection (STI). She decides to go talk to the school nurse.

CHAPTER OBJECTIVES

1 Identify assessment findings specific to pediatric infections and the diagnostic criteria used to confirm diagnoses.

2 Discuss nursing interventions to prevent the transmission of disease-causing organisms

3 Describe the nursing care for congenitally and perinatally infected infants.

4 Compare the different herpesviruses and discuss the nursing care for each.

5 Describe at least one evidence-based intervention to decrease the risk of transmission of HIV from a pregnant female to her fetus.

6 Identify the symptoms of at least three tick-borne infections and teaching needed to reduce transmission of tick-borne infections.

7 Name two sexually transmitted infections and interventions to prevent transmission.

8 Identify two infectious diseases that should be reported to the local health department for follow-up contact tracing.

See thePoint for a list of Key Terms.

Microorganisms are as ancient as life itself. They are essential to life. Yet, they can also be a great nemesis worthy of annihilation. Although some organisms live quietly in a symbiotic relationship with the body, benefiting the organism and the human host, others cause devastating disease and acute illness. Disease-producing microorganisms, such as bacteria, viruses, fungi, and parasites, are often called **infectious agents** (see thePoint for Supplemental Information: Summary of Infectious Agents and Disease-Producing Characteristics). This chapter explores these infectious agents and the diseases they produce, and the epidemiology (e.g., incubation, mode of transmission), assessment, and related nursing interventions for such diseases.

DEVELOPMENTAL AND BIOLOGIC VARIANCES

Every healthy child is born with an innate (natural) immune system. This system enables the body to recognize when it is being invaded by foreign microorganisms and to quickly respond to the invasion before healthy body tissue cells are destroyed. It also includes the first line of defense for preventing diseases from entering the body: the skin and mucous membranes.

Children also receive passive immunity from their mothers, transplacentally and through the breast milk. This immunity varies based on the diseases to which the mother has been exposed and the antibodies she has developed. The antibodies passed from the mother to the infant offer only temporary protection, typically for the first year of life.

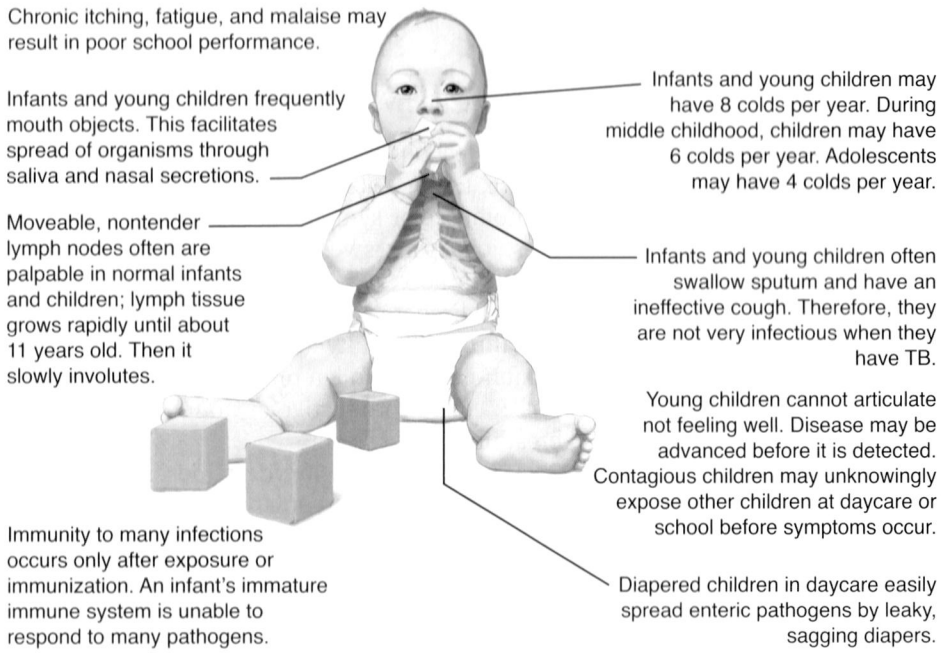

Chronic itching, fatigue, and malaise may result in poor school performance.

Infants and young children frequently mouth objects. This facilitates spread of organisms through saliva and nasal secretions.

Moveable, nontender lymph nodes often are palpable in normal infants and children; lymph tissue grows rapidly until about 11 years old. Then it slowly involutes.

Immunity to many infections occurs only after exposure or immunization. An infant's immature immune system is unable to respond to many pathogens.

Infants and young children may have 8 colds per year. During middle childhood, children may have 6 colds per year. Adolescents may have 4 colds per year.

Infants and young children often swallow sputum and have an ineffective cough. Therefore, they are not very infectious when they have TB.

Young children cannot articulate not feeling well. Disease may be advanced before it is detected. Contagious children may unknowingly expose other children at daycare or school before symptoms occur.

Diapered children in daycare easily spread enteric pathogens by leaky, sagging diapers.

Figure 24-1 Developmental and biologic variances: infection in children.

The adaptive, or active, immune system develops throughout the life span in response to the diseases to which we are exposed or against which we are immunized with vaccines. Children, especially infants and young children, experience higher incidences of infections than adults because of physiologic and immunologic immaturity (Fig. 24-1). It is not unusual for a child, especially one who attends daycare, to have six to nine infections a year during the first 2 years of life.

Some infections are particularly prevalent in specific age groups:

- Infancy: upper respiratory infections, enteric infections, vaccine-preventable diseases such as pertussis (because of incomplete immunity), gastroenteritis, and other diseases transmitted by the oral–fecal route
- Early childhood: upper respiratory infections, enteric infections (in those not toilet trained), communicable diseases transmitted by adults and other caregivers, soil-borne diseases (parasites), food-borne illnesses
- Middle childhood: ectoparasites (lice), food-borne illnesses, upper respiratory illnesses, pharyngitis
- Adolescence: sexually transmitted infections, mononucleosis

Infections acquired in utero or in the immediate postnatal period also place the fetus and newborn at risk. Known as congenital and perinatal infections, these include both bacteria and viruses. The TORCH constellation (*toxoplasmosis, other infections, rubella, cytomegalovirus* [CMV], *herpes simplex virus* [HSV]) was once used as an acronym for a panel of serologic diagnostic testing. Now, many additional organisms must be considered (e.g., enteroviruses, hepatitis B and C, group B *Streptococcus* [GBS], *Escherichia coli*, etc.). A diverse range of diagnostic tests is available for confirming neonatal infection, so diagnostic testing should be based on history and clinical presentation.

QUESTION: Ashley goes to see the school nurse. What aspects of her situation would be most important for the school nurse to address during the health history and physical assessment?

ASSESSMENT

It is difficult to focus on one system when discussing infectious diseases. The infection may be localized to one system or it may be systemic. Infections may have a rapid onset or occur long after exposure to the infectious agent. Infections may also mimic other diseases. Thus, the nurse needs astute questioning and assessment skills (see thePoint Supplemental Information: Features of Immunodeficiency).

History of response to previous infections and of the current illness, as well as meticulous documentation of physical findings, is essential for the health care team to diagnose the child accurately and decide on effective therapy. Depending on the causative organism and resulting disease, infectious illness may manifest in different ways. The first sign may be a deviation from normal behavior, such as altered sleep pattern, irritability, or increasing lethargy. Inflammation, fever, rash, or some combination may also be seen as general signs. More system-specific signs of infection include rhinitis, cough, diarrhea, and jaundice.

FOCUSED HEALTH HISTORY

Infectious disease processes cover such a wide range of health concerns that the nurse must start with a broad systems approach when obtaining a health history. Use responses to general questions to focus the assessment (Focused Health History 24-1).

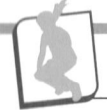

The Child With an Infectious Disease

Current history	Known infectious contacts; their symptoms (and diagnosis, if known) Presence, timing, site of onset, and home management of • Neuromuscular symptoms: headache, stiff neck, ataxia, muscle pain or weakness, joint pain, swelling, or erythema (describe) • Eyes, ear, nose, throat, neck: change in vision, drainage, conjunctivitis, ear pain or discharge, otitis media, rhinitis (describe), mouth sores or lesions, sore throat, difficulty swallowing • Lymph nodes: swollen or painful lymph nodes • Chest: cough (productive or nonproductive), shortness of breath or difficulty breathing, new murmur • Skin: rash (describe), pruritus (describe), pain • Gastrointestinal symptoms: vomiting, diarrhea (frequency, appearance), abdominal pain • Genitourinary symptoms: discharge (describe), flank pain or pain on urination, rash or lesions (describe), generalized edema or recent weight change • Fever: describe fever extremes and pattern, diaphoresis, chills, rigor • Change in level of consciousness or behavior (e.g., lethargy, irritability, weakness), headaches, seizures • Medications: current and recent including nonprescription. Recent use may affect ability to interpret negative culture results.
Past medical history	**Prenatal/Neonatal History** Birth history: maternal infectious disease history, delivery method, prematurity, neonatal illnesses, skin lesions noted at birth, postnatal exposures, method of infant feeding **Previous Health Challenges** Recurrent or chronic illness, prior hospitalizations, transfusion, surgery, evidence of complete resolution of infection between episodes Childhood illnesses: previous communicable diseases, recent exposure to disease Immunizations: immunizations received, dates, any rashes, unusual responses to live vaccines Allergies: allergic reactions to drugs, antibiotics, food, plants, or products (describe reaction)
Nutritional assessment	Recent changes in food or fluids consumed; recent weight change; formula preparation (describe); ingestion of honey, raw or undercooked meats, seafood, or restaurant food
Family medical history	Family history of early infant mortality, immunodeficiency, autoimmune disease, or malignancy History of child's presenting illness in other family members or close contacts (describe)
Social and environmental history	Recent changes in family lifestyle, daycare or school attendance (name and location), living arrangements (home, apartment, homeless, number of family and extended family living there), living location (rural, urban, suburban), drinking water source, family pets (list), exposure to farm or exotic animals, travel history (domestic and foreign), exposure to foreign-born individuals General hygiene, hand hygiene routines of child and caregivers, bathing History of pica; animal or insect bites or scratches; living or playing near or recent visit in wooded area, pond, lake, or farm

Growth and development	Child's growth plotted along own height and weight growth curves, head circumference in children younger than 3 years of age Body mass index Achievement of age-appropriate developmental milestones

Note: See Chapter 8 for a comprehensive health history.

Start with general questions regarding the presenting symptoms of illness, such as fever, rash, enlarged lymph nodes, and cough. Obtain information regarding the child's recent illness exposures, daycare or school exposures, environmental exposures, exposures to animals, and any travel history. Document immunization status and any history of past infections. This information often provides valuable clues that can lead to the diagnosis of the child's illness.

CROSS-CULTURAL CARE

Different infectious agents are prevalent in different parts of the world. To uncover clues about the causative agent, ask about recent immigration, travel within the country or abroad, and exposure to people who have traveled or immigrated recently.

Augment the focused health history with specific questions about the presenting illness. For example, if the child presents with failure to thrive and esophageal thrush, focus the health history on maternal and birth history to determine the risks of serious illness such as HIV infection. Similarly, a child presenting with severe bloody diarrhea and cramping would need a detailed nutritional assessment focusing on the names and locations of restaurants or social gatherings where the child has eaten or the name of the child's infant formula and the methods used to prepare formula in the home.

Use the history to try to determine whether the child has features suggestive of impaired host defense. The practitioner should determine whether the child has infections that are too frequent, too severe, or rare in the child's demographic group. For example, five to six upper respiratory infections each year can be expected during the early and middle childhood years. However, more than one episode of pneumonia during a 5-year period would be unusual in children without asthma, cystic fibrosis, or another underlying pulmonary pathology. Also, the time required to clear infections may be prolonged in children with compromised immune function.

A history of infection with an unusual pathogen (e.g., *Aspergillus*, *Serratia*, or *Pneumocystis* species) suggests a defect in immune surveillance. The site of infection may also imply specific immune deficits. For example, children with neutropenia may experience frequent dermatologic infections, and children with antibody deficiency syndromes usually experience recurrent

upper and lower respiratory infections. Equally important, ascertain whether infections resolve completely between episodes.

FOCUSED PHYSICAL ASSESSMENT

After a thorough history, examine the child, carefully reviewing each major system. Assess growth parameters. Children with severe immunodeficiency often have growth failure, which can be an important indicator of disease severity. Weight is typically impaired first, so low weight for height may be an early indicator of failure to thrive.

In children with competent immune systems, the infectious process may be localized to one system but often has systemic effects (Focused Physical Assessment 24-1).

caREminder

If one child in the family has symptoms of an infection, assess the siblings for infection as well.

In contrast to the typical appearance of some diseases in adults, such as tuberculosis (TB) or hepatitis, clinical findings in children may be few. Most children cannot produce sputum or mucus when they cough, and what little is produced is usually swallowed. Therefore, children with TB rarely present with a coughing illness. Jaundice is rare in childhood hepatitis. In many cases of hepatitis, the child does not even look ill.

ANSWER: Key aspects of the health history would include identification of the onset of Ashley's symptoms as well as any other overall complaints, her sexual history and current sexual activity, and information to determine whether her boyfriend is experiencing any symptoms. Physical assessment would focus on identifying any fever, evaluation of her urinary complaints and appearance of urine to rule out possible urinary tract infection, and evaluation of the appearance of her vaginal discharge, such as color, amount, characteristics, and odor.

DIAGNOSTIC CRITERIA

Numerous methods can be used to analyze immune system function and to identify causative organisms of infectious diseases (Tests and Procedures 24-1). Prudent use of laboratory tests requires that they be selected on the basis of history and physical examination findings. Rapid and accurate identification of causative

Infectious Disease

Assessment Parameter	Alterations/Clinical Significance
General appearance and vital signs	Deviation from normal behavior, lethargy, irritability, disinterest in environment, or assuming specific position may indicate infectious process. Abnormal vital signs; for example, fever can indicate possible systematic infection, tachypnea is common in pneumonia, and low blood pressure is seen in septic shock.
Integumentary system (skin, hair, nails)	Color: erythema (on cheeks: fifth disease, scarlet fever), jaundice (hepatitis), pallor (generalized in some chronic infections, such as intestinal parasites; circumoral: scarlet fever)
	Rash: appearance—macular (rubella, rubeola), papular, vesicular, pustular (varicella), crusts (impetigo), hives, blanches with light pressure (roseola), petechial (meningococcemia)
	Location and distribution on trunk, extremities, or face (e.g., varicella starts on trunk and spreads to face and extremities); eczema may be present in immunodeficiency syndrome; lymphadenopathy often present during infection
	Nails: clubbing, embolic lesions (endocarditis); thickened, discolored (fungal infection)
	Hair: hair loss (tinea), thinning (chronic infection)
Head and neck	Head: normocephalic (microcephaly could indicate neonatal infection)
	Neck: stiff neck, painful or swollen lymph nodes (many infections)
Eyes	Eyes: conjunctivitis (rubella, rubeola, adenovirus), jaundice (hepatitis)
Ears	Ears and neck: earache, parotid swelling and tenderness (mumps)
Face, nose, and oral cavity	Face: facial tenderness or headache (sinusitis, cellulitis)
	Nose: congestion, rhinorrhea, excoriation (cold, sinusitis)
	Throat and mouth: swollen tonsils, if present (tonsillitis); oral ulcers; adherent white patches on tongue, palate, inner cheeks (candidiasis); membrane in pharynx, adherent, gray white (diphtheria, scarlet fever); Koplik spots on buccal mucosa opposite molars (rubeola); vesicles (HSV), white strawberry tongue (white coat on tongue with red, edematous papillae projecting through) or later red strawberry tongue (white coat desquamates leaving red, edematous papillae projecting [scarlet fever])
Thorax and lungs	Cough (rubeola, TB, pertussis); note whether cough is productive, associated with cyanosis, vomiting (pertussis)
	Oxygen saturation less than 97% (respiratory infection)
	Presence of rales or rhonchi, use of accessory muscles to breathe (respiratory infection)
Neuromuscular	Change in level of consciousness, sluggish pupillary response (meningitis, encephalitis), Brudzinski or Kernig sign (meningitis)
	Limited range of motion: arthritis, arthralgia (rheumatic fever, fifth disease, Lyme disease)
	Muscle pain or weakness (influenza)
Cardiovascular system	Tachycardia above expected for fever (especially with diphtheria, scarlet fever, rheumatic fever)
	New-onset murmur (endocarditis)
Vasculature	Swollen or painful vessels associated with intravenous (IV) lines (infection, phlebitis)
Abdomen	Appearance: distention (intestinal parasites), pain with palpation, hepatomegaly (hepatitis, visceral larva migrans, mononucleosis, congestive heart failure resulting from rheumatic heart disease), splenomegaly (mononucleosis)
Lymphatic system	Multiple, scattered, swollen, and tender lymph nodes (Epstein-Barr virus [EBV])
External genitalia and breasts (includes anus)	Vaginal or urethral discharge (sexually transmitted infections)
Musculoskeletal system	Painful, swollen, or tender joints or refusal to walk (*Staphylococcus* infection, malaria)
Neurologic system	Peripheral weakness or ataxic gait, hyper- or hyporeflexia, sluggish or asymmetric pupillary response, disorientation (meningitis, encephalitis)

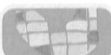 **TESTS AND PROCEDURES for Evaluating the Child With an Infection**

Diagnostic Test or Procedure	Purpose	Findings and Indications	Health Care Provider Considerations
Complete blood count (CBC) with differential	To compare the status of specific blood elements. Detailed evaluation of the white blood cell count and morphology may help to detect infection.	Values outside age-appropriate laboratory reference ranges indicate how the body is responding to the infection and adequacy of response. Infection usually causes leukocytosis. Neutropenia in a neonate often indicates sepsis. Neutrophilia after the neonatal period indicates an infectious process. An increase in bands (immature neutrophils) may indicate bacterial infection. Immunocompromised patients may not be able to mount a response that is reflected in an increased white blood cell count or change in the differential.	Provide psychosocial support. Obtain specimen, label appropriately, and send to laboratory.
Serum C-reactive protein (CRP)	To detect elevated levels of CRP, a non-specific measure of inflammation in the body. CRP is normally present in trace amounts; production is increased after tissue injury or destruction.	Levels of 10–19 mg/L suggest viral infection or noninvasive bacterial infection. Levels more than 20 mg/L suggest invasive bacterial infection or fungal septicemia. In neonates, levels more than 10 mg/L suggest sepsis or meningitis.	Provide psychosocial support. Obtain specimen, label appropriately, and send to laboratory.
Erythrocyte sedimentation rate (ESR)	A screening procedure to identify children who may have an infectious or inflammatory process	An elevated ESR is generally indicative of the presence of infection or an inflammatory process; it is nonspecific (not diagnostic for any particular pathology).	Provide psychosocial support. Obtain specimen, label appropriately, and send to laboratory.
Urine culture	To diagnose a urinary tract infection. To monitor microbial colonization after urinary catheter insertion	Cultures are reported as "no growth" if urine is sterile (no infection). Bacterial count of more than 100,000 organisms/mL of a single species is indicative of infection. Bacterial count of 10,000–100,000 organisms/mL of a single species from a catheterized specimen may indicate infection. Counts less than 10,000 organisms/mL or multiple organisms indicate contamination.	Use gloves when handling all specimens. Obtain a sterile catheterized specimen (preferred) or a clean-catch specimen from continent children and adolescents. Collect at least 3 mL urine and send to the laboratory immediately or store in a specimen refrigerator until transport to the laboratory.

(Continued)

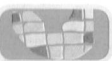

TESTS AND PROCEDURES for Evaluating the Child With an Infection (Continued)

Diagnostic Test or Procedure	Purpose	Findings and Indications	Health Care Provider Considerations
Stool culture	To identify pathogenic bacteria	Normal fecal flora consists of gram-negative aerobic and anaerobic bacteria. Pathogenic bacteria include *Salmonella, Shigella, Campylobacter, Escherichia coli* O157:H7, *Clostridium difficile, Clostridium botulinum, Yersinia,* and *Vibrio*.	Send a fresh specimen collected from a bedpan or diaper. Use a tongue blade to transfer it to a sterile container. If a rectal swab is used, insert the swab into the anus just past the anal sphincter. Rotate the swab gently. Withdraw it and place it in a transport tube.
Sputum culture	To identify the cause of pulmonary infection	Expectorated sputum has normal flora (alpha streptococci and *Neisseria*) and is Gram stained before processing to determine the quality of the specimen. The presence of the following organisms usually indicates infection: *Mycobacterium tuberculosis, Haemophilus influenzae, Klebsiella* spp., *Staphylococcus aureus, Pseudomonas* spp.	Send early morning specimen (before eating breakfast) for TB. Have the child rinse or gargle with water and then cough deeply into a sterile container. Transport specimen to laboratory within 2 hours. Small children may not be able to produce sputum. Consider using gastric lavage as an alternative.
Blood culture	To confirm sepsis To identify the microorganism in bacteremia and sepsis	The presence of any organism usually indicates infection. Common skin contaminants (coagulase-negative *Staphylococcus, Bacillus, Corynebacterium*) isolated from a single bottle frequently represent contamination.	Disinfect blood culture bottles (two in a set) with appropriate disinfectant. Clean venipuncture site with appropriate disinfectant. Allow to dry. For endocarditis, send two specimen sets taken from two sites at least 2 hours apart.
Gastric lavage	To identify TB in a child when bronchoscopy cannot be performed Often gives better results than bronchoscopy in children	The presence of TB in the specimen by acid-fast staining and culture techniques indicates infection.	In the early morning, before eating, introduce a nasogastric tube. Withdraw a sample and place in a sterile container. Lavage 20–30 mL sterile water if unable to spontaneously withdraw gastric fluid. Transport to the laboratory within 15 minutes at room temperature.
Enzyme-linked immunosorbent assay (ELISA)	Direct detection of viral antigens in body fluids	Specific viral antigens are tested and are either positive or negative.	Obtain a blood specimen for most tests. Obtain a nasal wash for respiratory syncytial virus or influenza testing. Stool or urine can also be tested.
Nucleic acid probes	Diagnostic and screening test that can detect specific viral or bacterial DNA or RNA	If sample is positive for the presence of specific organisms (e.g., *Neisseria gonorrhoeae, Chlamydia,* various strains of *Mycobacterium*), infection with the organism is indicated.	Send throat, urogenital, or rectal swabs to the laboratory. Other specimen sources include blood, CSF, urine, and bone marrow.

Diagnostic Test or Procedure	Purpose	Findings and Indications	Health Care Provider Considerations
Direct fluorescent antibody (DFA)	Detects specific enzyme-labeled antibodies Usually used for respiratory viruses, herpes, rabies, some respiratory bacteria (pertussis)	If positive, results are virus and bacteria specific.	Send sputum samples or throat swabs to the laboratory on transport medium. Lesion scrapings should be sent on DFA slides.
Western blot	Lysate of concentrated virions is placed on specialized gel. Viral proteins separate by molecular weight. Used as a confirmatory test with ELISA for HIV but can be specific for other viruses	Positive results are reported as bands. The specimen has bands in specific molecular weight ranges for the virus being tested. For example, HIV has p24, gp120, and so on.	Send a blood specimen. If a patient has a positive ELISA for HIV, perform a confirmatory Western blot test before explaining the results to the patient.
Rapid antigen extraction	To test rapidly for the presence of group A streptococci (GAS) (antigen) or influenza A and B viruses	Result is positive if GAS or influenza A or B viruses are present. For GAS, negative tests require a 24-hour incubation for conventional growth on agar.	Send a throat swab to the laboratory. Swab both tonsillar pillars. Have the child take a deep breath to reduce gagging.
Delayed hypersensitivity skin testing	To test for certain diseases (e.g., coccidioidomycosis, TB) To serve as a positive control when conducting these tests; one or more antigens (e.g., *Trichophyton*, tetanus, *Candida*, mumps) are injected intradermally at the same time; if the child responds to any of them, it demonstrates effective T-cell function and results of the others can be considered valid Sometimes used to test T-cell–mediated immunity, although it has limited value in the HIV era	A positive reaction (induration at site) to the antigens indicates the body has mounted a T-cell–mediated immune response. Findings depend on antigens injected. All children older than 1 year of age should demonstrate a reaction to *Candida*, which is ubiquitous, as well as tetanus, mumps, and diphtheria, to which they have been exposed via routine immunizations. A positive reaction to purified protein derivative indicates a history of infection with TB. Immunocompromised or chronically ill children or those with severe nutritional deficiencies may not demonstrate a response (anergy).	Review the child's history for hypersensitivity to the test antigens. Observe the child for signs of anaphylaxis. Each antigen is injected intradermally to the forearm using a separate needle for each antigen; a control antigen must be used in chronically ill children. Use a pen to circle each site and label appropriately. Teach the child and family that the test involves injecting small doses of antigens under the skin; that the area needs to be monitored at 24, 48, and 72 hours after the test; and that the circles should not be washed off until the test has been completed. A negative reaction may require placement of additional or stronger antigens. When reading the test, record erythema and induration in millimeters.

organisms facilitates initiation of appropriate therapy and improves outcomes.

TREATMENT MODALITIES

The key to controlling infectious diseases is prevention (Evidence-Based Clinical Practice Guidelines 24-1). Childhood immunization is the primary intervention to prevent disease. Immunizations not only prevent disease in the child but they also protect unvaccinated individuals who come into contact with the child. Immunizations are responsible for preventing and controlling many of the once common and often fatal childhood diseases. See Chapter 8 for more about immunization. Breastfeeding also can reduce the incidence of infection (Tradition or Science 24-1).

Regardless of the agent causing the infection, use standard precautions (see Siegel et al. [2007] for guidelines). Care for all children as if they may have a communicable infection to prevent the spread of infection throughout the hospital or community.

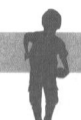

EVIDENCE-BASED CLINICAL PRACTICE GUIDELINES 24-1
Infection Prevention and Control

Siegel, J. D., Rhinehart, E., Jackson, M. et al. (2007). *2007 guideline for isolation precautions: Preventing transmission of infectious agents in healthcare settings.* Retrieved from

http://www.cdc.gov/hicpac/pdf/isolation/isolation2007.pdf

Provides recommendations to prevent health care–associated infections across the spectrum of health care delivery settings.

Centers for Disease Control and Prevention. (2002). Guideline for hand hygiene in health-care settings: Recommendations of the Healthcare Infection Control Practices Advisory Committee and the HICPAC/SHEA/APIC/IDSA Hand Hygiene Task Force. *Morbidity and Mortality Weekly Report, 51*(RR-16), 1–44. Retrieved from

http://www.cdc.gov/mmwr/PDF/rr/rr5116.pdf

Presents guidelines for hand hygiene to prevent nosocomial infections in patients and health care personnel.

World Health Organization. (2009). *WHO guidelines on hand hygiene in health care.* Retrieved from

http://whqlibdoc.who.int/publications/2009/9789241597906_eng.pdf

Reviews the evidence on hand hygiene in health care and presents recommendations for practices that reduce transmission of pathogens to patients and health care workers.

Centers for Disease Control and Prevention. (2011). *Guidelines for the prevention of intravascular catheter-related infections.* Retrieved from

http://www.cdc.gov/hicpac/pdf/guidelines/bsi-guidelines-2011.pdf

Presents guidelines to reduce the incidence of infections associated with intravascular therapy.

National Institute for Health and Clinical Excellence. (2013). *Infection: Prevention and control of healthcare-associated infections in primary and community care.* Retrieved from

http://guidance.nice.org.uk/CG139

Provides evidence-based guidelines to prevent and control health care–associated infections in community and primary care settings.

Pickering, L. K., Baker, C. J., Freed, G. L. et al. (2009). Immunization programs for infants, children, adolescents, and adults: Clinical practice guidelines by the Infectious Diseases Society of America. *Clinical Infectious Diseases, 49*(6), 817–840. Retrieved from

http://www.guideline.gov/summary/summary.aspx?view_id = 1&doc_id = 15442

Presents guidelines for immunization of different populations for optimal disease prevention through vaccination while maintaining safety.

Centers for Disease Control and Prevention. (2009). Guidelines for prevention and treatment of opportunistic infections among HIV-exposed and HIV-infected children. *Morbidity and Mortality Weekly Report, 58*(RR-11), 1–166. Retrieved from

http://www.cdc.gov/mmwr/preview/mmwrhtml/rr58e0826a1.htm

Guidelines present how to prevent opportunistic infections in HIV-exposed and HIV-infected children that occur in the United States and those that can be acquired during international travel. The guidelines also describe epidemiology, clinical presentation, and diagnosis and treatment of opportunistic infections.

Centers for Disease Control and Prevention. (2010). Sexually transmitted diseases treatment guidelines, 2010. *Morbidity and Mortality Weekly Report, 59*(RR-12), 1–110. Retrieved from

http://www.cdc.gov/std/treatment/2010/STD-Treatment-2010-RR5912.pdf

Guidelines on approaches to sexually transmitted disease prevention. Also gives guidelines for treatment of those who have, or are at risk for, sexually transmitted diseases.

TRADITION OR SCIENCE 24-1

Does breastfeeding during early infancy decrease the risk of infection during infancy?

Multiple studies have demonstrated that human milk feeding decreases gastrointestinal (Arifeen et al., 2001; Dewey et al., 1995; Howie et al., 1990; Lopez-Alarcon et al., 1997; Quigley et al., 2007) and respiratory infections (Arifeen et al., 2001; Bachrach et al., 2003; Blaymore Bier et al., 2002; Gdalevich et al., 2001; Quigley et al., 2007). Delaying complementary feeding until after 3 months of age was associated with reduced risk for respiratory infection and improved growth (Kalanda et al., 2006). Compared with exclusive breastfeeding for only 4–6 months, exclusive breastfeeding for 6 months or longer decreased morbidity from respiratory infections and otitis media (Chantry et al., 2006) and did not negatively affect growth (Khadivzadeh & Parsai, 2004; Kramer & Kakuma, 2002; Onayade et al., 2004). Many health professionals, including the American Academy of Pediatrics (AAP) (Eidelman & Schanler, 2012) and the World Health Organization (2010b), recommend breastfeeding exclusively for the first 6 months of life.

There are also significant beneficial effects of feeding human milk to preterm infants. Although a number of early studies noting the infection-reducing properties of human milk feedings for premature infants (Blaymore Bier et al., 2002; el-Mohandes et al., 1997; Hylander et al., 1998; Narayanan et al., 1984) had flawed study designs (de Silva et al., 2004), more recent studies found lower rates of sepsis and necrotizing enterocolitis (NEC), indicating that human milk contributes to the development of the preterm infant's immature host defense (Eidelman & Schanler, 2012; Sullivan et al., 2010).

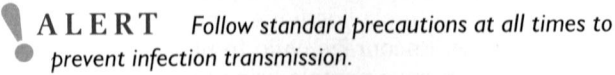

ALERT *Follow standard precautions at all times to prevent infection transmission.*

Most communicable diseases must be reported to the local health department. Check local regulations; they vary in terms of which communicable diseases are reported.

Individual treatment of the child depends on the disease process. Prophylactic antibiotics are often used in children with immunodeficiencies to prevent serious infections. A variety of other treatments may be used, depending on the specific immunodeficiency. These modalities include IV gamma globulin, enzyme replacement, gene therapy, interleukin-2 infusions, and bone marrow transplantation. Refer to Chapter 31 for more about managing fever.

NURSING PLAN OF CARE

QUESTION: Which nursing diagnosis from Nursing Plan of Care 24-1 would be most appropriate for Ashley?

The history and physical assessment should identify health issues that need to be addressed. Applicable nursing diagnoses depend on specific assessment findings. Chapter 11 identifies nursing diagnoses commonly applicable to the psychosocial needs of the acutely ill child. Nursing diagnoses and care generally applicable to a child with an infection are identified in Nursing Plan of Care 24-1. More specific diagnoses depend on the specific pathology and its effect on the child's health.

ANSWER: Appropriate nursing diagnoses may include deficient knowledge about the infection, transmission, and ways to reduce the risk of transmission; and noncompliance towards the drug regimen related to Ashley's current stage of development (being an adolescent).

PEDIATRIC INFECTIONS

Infectious diseases are generally classified into five major categories on the basis of causative agents: bacteria, viruses, fungi, parasites, and rickettsiae. Sepsis results when the body is overwhelmed by infection and may be caused by various infectious agents. Infections may occur when the immune system does not function properly; thus, persistent infection despite treatment, or infection with an unusual pathogen, may signal an underlying immunodeficiency (see thePoint Supplemental Information: Summary of Infectious Agents).

SEPSIS

Sepsis is microbial invasion of the bloodstream from bacteria, viruses, fungi, and parasites or their toxic products, resulting in a spectrum of disease from mild systematic symptoms and circulatory compromise to massive circulatory collapse and multiorgan failure (Bateman & Seed, 2010). Systemic inflammatory response is diagnosed in the presence of at least two of the following features (one of which must be abnormal temperature or leukocyte count) (Goldstein et al., 2005):

- Core temperature (measured via rectal, oral, bladder, or central catheter) more than 101° F (38.5° C) or less than 96° F (36° C)
- Tachycardia (mean heart rate greater than two standard deviations above normal for age not caused by external stimuli) *or*, in children younger than 1 year of age, bradycardia (mean heart rate less than 10th percentile for age not caused by external agents or congenital heart disease)
- Mean respiratory rate more than two standard deviations above normal for age
- Leukocyte count depressed or elevated for age or more than 10% immature neutrophils

Sepsis is the major cause of mortality in children worldwide, causing almost 70% of deaths in children younger than the age of 5 years (Riley & Wheeler, 2012) and causing 60% to 80% of deaths per year in childhood (Kissoon et al., 2011). Overall mortality is 10%

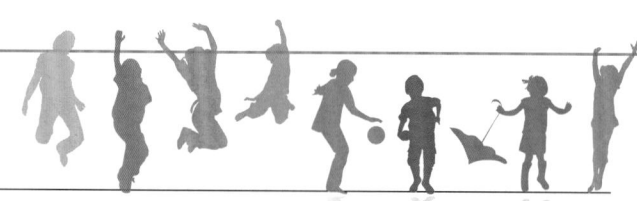

NURSING PLAN OF CARE 24-1:

The Child With an Infectious Disease

Nursing Diagnosis: Hyperthermia related to effects of pathogen

Interventions/Rationale
- Institute cooling measures as indicated (see thePoint Procedures: Cooling Measures).
- Monitor temperature trends.
    Fever is a result of endotoxin effects on the hypothalamus. Monitoring helps detect changes early.
- Assess for the presence of contributing factors such as dehydration, environmental warmth, and exercise.
    May identify the source of contributing risk factors.

Expected Outcome
- Child will report or evidence minimal discomfort related to fever.

Nursing Diagnosis: Imbalanced nutrition: Less than body requirements related to effects of decreased intake and increased metabolic demands

Interventions/Rationale
- Weigh daily.
    Assesses adequacy of nutritional absorption and use.
- Auscultate bowel sounds.
    Decreased gastric motility can interfere with absorption.
- Palpate peripheral pulses.
    Weak pulses are indicative of hypovolemia.
- Observe for increased fatigue, abdominal pain, and nausea.
    May indicate fluid and electrolyte deficits.
- Monitor CBC (i.e., white blood cells, red blood cells, hematocrit, hemoglobin) and electrolytes (i.e., potassium, sodium, calcium, blood urea nitrogen, creatinine).
    Assesses level of hydration and cellular breakdown and reflects fluid shifts, indicating fluid losses and dehydration.
- Monitor intake and output and evaluate fluid balance. Monitor urine specific gravity.
    Helps identify risk of dehydration and balance of fluids. Decreasing urine output may indicate hypovolemia. Increased intake with decreased output may indicate third spacing and tissue edema.
- Establish hourly intake schedule; instruct child to drink and eat slowly.
    Reduces risk of dehydration and may increase ability to tolerate intake.

- Discuss/identify food preferences; encourage choosing meals from available menus.
    May enhance intake and promote sense of participation and control.
- Refer child to dietitian.
    May assist in planning a diet that meets nutritional needs.
- Administer vitamin supplements and IV fluids as ordered.
    Supplements may be needed to ensure adequate intake and assist in healing and fighting infection.

Expected Outcome
- Child will maintain adequate calorie and nutrient intake (oral, enteral, or IV) to meet maintenance and growth needs.

Nursing Diagnosis: Deficient diversional activity related to effects of isolation, fatigue

Interventions/Rationale
- Encourage family members and support system to mobilize around child.
    Family knows the child best and can provide social interaction targeted to the child's needs and temperament.
- Encourage one-on-one social interaction with the child.
    Allows child to concentrate on social interaction without excessive disruption.
- Provide periods of rest.
    Fatigue can discourage social interaction.
- Determine favorite play activities and hobbies prior to illness. Encourage child to play at developmental level; have parents bring in toys or favored objects (e.g., doll, blanket) from home.
    Play helps children process and cope with events in their world; familiar objects and routines provide security, comfort, and a sense of control.
- Encourage participation in a variety of activities (e.g., music, crafts, games, social interactions), as developmentally appropriate.
    Varying activities provides different mechanisms with which to cope and helps the child to master different skills.
- Refer to occupational therapist or play therapist.
    Can introduce and design new programs for stimulation.
- Increase activity levels as tolerated.
    Promotes gradual return to normal activity level and improves stamina. Increases self-esteem and sense of control.

Expected Outcomes
- Child will engage in situationally and developmentally appropriate activities.
- Child, if fatigued, will engage in sedentary activities such as painting, reading, or watching television.
- If pruritic rash is present, caregivers will distract child from scratching.

Nursing Diagnosis: Deficient knowledge: Disease process

Interventions/Rationale
- Assess child's and family's understanding of the disease process.
  Provides baseline of family knowledge. Allows for clarification of misinformation.
- Encourage expression and acknowledge feelings.
  Provides an open line of communication and safe environment for children to express themselves.
- Reinforce accurate knowledge and provide accurate information at current level of understanding.
  May reduce misconceptions and fears.
- Educate the child and family on the child's needs; provide written instruction.
  Provides reinforcement and a source of reference.
- Identify, review, and reinforce current therapeutic regimen.
  Provides a continuous progression of recovery and prevents complications.
- Identify signs and symptoms of individual risks, side effects, and self-care needs.
  Recognizing problems provides opportunities for prompt and ongoing evaluation and intervention.
- Identify individual roles of child and family members.
  Identifies responsibilities and roles to assist family with coping.
- Encourage family members to participate in care of the child.
  Facilitates communication and provides a sense of control for family.
- Identify community resources, social worker, and support groups for family.
  Provides additional assistance to family as the need arises.

Expected Outcome
- Child and family will demonstrate an accurate understanding of the infection and describe its signs and symptoms, transmission, isolation, treatment, and complications.

Nursing Diagnosis: Risk for infection related to potential for exposure

Interventions/Rationale
- Maintain standard precautions. Perform hand hygiene after each care activity.
  Reduces the risk of cross-contamination.
- Place the child in a private room or, as appropriate, cohort with others who have the same condition. Encourage parents to keep sick children home from school and activities.
  Reduces risk of transmitting infection.
- Limit visitors as indicated; screen visitors for infection.
  Reduces risk of exposure for compromised host.
- Assess signs and symptoms of infection (e.g., fever, chills, pain, productive cough), history of exposure to infectious diseases, presence of wounds, and nutritional deficiency.
  Intervention can be implemented to control related factors; early identification leads to prompt intervention. Chills frequently precede temperature spikes in presence of generalized infection.
- Obtain specimens (e.g., urine, blood, sputum, wound, invasive lines) as indicated for culture and sensitivity.
  May reflect inappropriate or inadequate antibiotic therapy or an overgrowth of resistant or opportunistic organisms.
- Monitor laboratory studies (e.g., white blood cells, neutrophils, bands).
  Reflects success of the body's attempts to respond to infection.
- Monitor for changes in physiologic functions (e.g., headaches/confusion, flushed skin, fatigue, loss of appetite).
  Changes may indicate worsening of child's condition.
- Educate child and family regarding methods of transmission of infection.
  Provides a baseline of knowledge.
- Evaluate child's hygiene habits. Educate on appropriate hygiene habits and demonstrate hand hygiene techniques.
  Hygiene, especially hand hygiene, is key in preventing nosocomial infection.
- Encourage changes in position and deep breathing.
  May provide good pulmonary toilet and reduce respiratory compromise.
- Discuss the influence of nutrition in preventing infection; encourage and maintain adequate nutrition (caloric and protein intake).
  Adequate intake of calories and protein can boost the immune system and provide necessary elements for tissue repair.
- Assess for adequate immunizations against childhood diseases. Educate parents regarding the benefits of immunization.
  May reduce susceptibility to infection.
- Educate child and family on signs and symptoms of infection.
  Provides a baseline of knowledge.

(Continued)

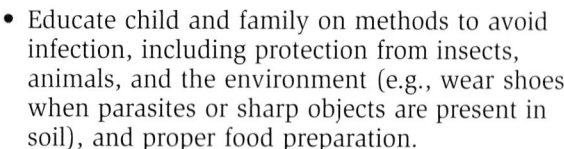

NURSING PLAN OF CARE 24-1:

The Child With an Infectious Disease (Continued)

- Educate child and family on methods to avoid infection, including protection from insects, animals, and the environment (e.g., wear shoes when parasites or sharp objects are present in soil), and proper food preparation.
    Provides knowledge base to initiate preventive measures.
- Collaborate with local health department when disease outbreaks are noted.
    Helps identify and prevent infection; helps identify the mode of transmission.

Expected Outcomes
- Child and siblings will have age-appropriate immunizations.
- Family will be educated regarding the importance of immunizations.
- Child will not expose others to the disease and will not contract another infection.

Nursing Diagnosis: Noncompliance (drug regimen)

Interventions/Rationale
- Create a trusting environment by listening to concerns and being available to child and family.
    Respect and rapport must be established before child will take part in the learning process.
- Use a variety of teaching strategies.
    Promotes retention of material.
- Explore child's and family's feelings regarding drug regimen.
    May improve communication; may clear up misconceptions. Includes child in the decision-making process.
- Discuss essential information needed for the plan of treatment.
    Provides a knowledge base for the child to make informed decisions.

- Discuss side effects and preventive measures.
    Promotes adherence and strategies to deal with side effects.
- Discuss dietary plan to increase adherence and limit nausea, vomiting, and side effects from medications.
    Dietary planning improves nutrition, which may improve adherence to medication regimen.
- Discuss importance of follow-up care and appointments and explore potential barriers to accomplishing these goals.
    Helps to continue follow-up of disease process. Discussing potential barriers may aid in meeting treatment needs.
- Have child self-monitor (e.g., on a calendar, chart) drug regimen on a daily basis.
    Places a sense of responsibility on the child for making sure the plan is followed.
- Review signs and symptoms that require medical evaluation, intervention, or both.
    May promote prompt intervention to prevent serious complications or nonadherence.
- Discuss stress management strategies (e.g., relaxation, deep breathing, visualization).
    Promotes relaxation and stress control.
- Discuss ways in which the child can participate in self-care.
    Increases self-control and self-confidence.
- Discuss potential conflicts between parents and child.
    May decrease issues of control and improve adherence.
- Refer to social services and support groups.
    Provides additional resources for child and family.

Expected Outcome
- Child (and family, if applicable) will complete prescribed course of medication and will verbalize the importance of continuing to take medications even after symptoms disappear.

(Dellinger et al., 2008). Neonates and young infants have immature immune systems and can rapidly become critically ill with infection, resulting in overwhelming sepsis. These infants are commonly admitted to the hospital with an acute febrile illness in which the source of the fever is unknown, even after a careful history and physical examination. The management of acute febrile illness in young infants is challenging because the risk of serious overwhelming bacterial illness in this age group is high. During the initial assessment, distinguishing bacterial or fungal infections from other, often less serious, viral infections is nearly impossible.

Children with skin defects, such as aplasia cutis, epidermolysis bullosa, or ichthyosis, often have breaks in the skin that provide an opening for bacteria to invade, causing a secondary bloodstream infection. Defects in skin closure, as with gastroschisis or exstrophy of the bladder, expose underlying tissues and organs to outside microbial contamination and invasion, resulting in sepsis. Children who are immunocompromised (e.g., because of chemotherapy, steroid therapy, asplenia, or immune cell dysfunction) or who have invasive devices such as indwelling lines are also at increased risk for sepsis.

Low-birth-weight infants and infants with respiratory distress syndrome, longer duration of parenteral nutrition, genetic factors, and maternal perinatal risk factors, such as maternal infection or prolonged rupture of membranes, are at particular risk for sepsis (Bizzarro et al., 2011; Polin & Committee on Fetus and Newborn, 2012). Neonatal sepsis can be caused by viruses such as herpes simplex or enteroviruses and by protozoa (e.g., *Toxoplasma gondii*). However, bacteria are typically the culprits. Infants are infected during the birthing process or by transplacental transmission. Events such as prolonged rupture of the membranes (longer than 18 hours) and amnionitis contribute to contamination at birth or ascending infections. Hospitalized neonates, especially premature infants, run an extremely high risk for sepsis because of invasive devices, endotracheal tubes, and central venous catheters. Fungi also play a role in sepsis, particularly in the hospitalized neonate. Multiple antibiotics may be used in the hospitalized infant, altering the infant's normal flora and leaving the infant susceptible to opportunistic organisms such as fungi. Common skin fungi, such as *Candida* spp., are often causes of sepsis.

Assessment

Evaluate the child's temperature, heart and respiratory rates, and laboratory values in light of the definition of systemic inflammatory response and sepsis. Look for risk factors and maintain a high index of suspicion for sepsis in any infant who is ill during the first 90 days of life. Infants with sepsis may present with nonspecific symptoms (Chart 24-1). Measure temperature rectally and remember that the magnitude of the fever may not reflect the seriousness of the illness (Henker & Carlson, 2007).

Children with suspected sepsis should have a CBC with differential, blood culture, and urine culture. A lumbar puncture should be performed in infants and should be considered in older children with neurologic symptoms. Those with respiratory symptoms should also have a chest radiograph.

Nursing Diagnoses and Outcomes

Common nursing diagnoses and outcomes for the child with an infection are identified in Nursing Plan of Care 24-1 (see also thePoint Care Paths: An Interdisciplinary Plan of Care for the Child With AIDS Pneumonia).

Interdisciplinary Interventions

Because of the high morbidity and mortality associated with severe sepsis, aggressive treatment must begin immediately. Institute interventions to support and maintain circulation and tissue oxygenation (see Nursing Plan of Care 31-1). Identify the source of infection and initiate antibiotic therapy within the first hour after sepsis is recognized (Kissoon et al., 2010). Empiric treatment typically consists of ampicillin plus an aminoglycoside or cefotaxime, depending on the neonate's risk factors. Vancomycin or ceftazidime may be added to reduce risk of nosocomial infection or provide coverage for infection by methicillin-resistant *Staphylococcus aureus* (MRSA) or *Pseudomonas*. Amphotericin should be added if fungal infection is suspected. Acyclovir should be added if herpes infection is suspected. Antimicrobial

CHART 24-1 Signs and Symptoms of Neonatal Sepsis

General
Temperature instability
Hypothermia (more common) or fever
Decreased activity levels
Irritability, lethargy, or coma
Decreased urine output
Floppiness (hypotonia)
Poor feeding, vomiting, diarrhea
Hypoglycemia
Seizures

Cardiac
Bradycardia or tachycardia
Mottling or pallor
Poor capillary refill
Hypotension
Cyanosis

Pulmonary
Apnea or tachypnea
Sternal retractions
Grunting
Nasal flaring
Irregular respirations

therapy can be tailored after a causative organism has been identified (see thePoint Medications: Summary of Antimicrobial Therapy for Sepsis).

Maintain aseptic technique and good nutrition and decrease stress for the child, which may help promote immunocompetence, thus bolstering the ability to resist infection. Closely observe the child for subtle changes in vital signs, behavior, feeding tolerance, and physical assessment to promptly detect signs of sepsis (Clinical Judgment 24-1). When sepsis is suspected, IV antibiotic therapy is necessary (see thePoint Care Path: An Interdisciplinary Plan of Care for the Child With AIDS Pneumonia).

Community Care

Maternal screening for GBS and prophylactic intrapartum antibiotics can greatly reduce the risk of neonatal GBS sepsis.

Educate parents regarding signs of disease in their infant and advise them when to rapidly seek care for any behaviors that are not typical for their child. This education could be the key to preventing overwhelming sepsis in the young infant. Also, educate parents that timely immunization of the child can provide some immunity to serious infectious diseases such as hepatitis and pertussis.

BACTERIAL INFECTIONS

Although vaccination programs have virtually eliminated many of the serious bacterial diseases in developed countries, no vaccines are yet available for most bacterial

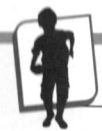

CLINICAL JUDGMENT 24-1

An Infant With Sepsis

Melissa is a 4-day-old infant who was admitted to the pediatric intensive care unit after an episode of cyanosis and difficulty breathing. Her mother states that she has not been "doing well." The mother describes Melissa as fussy, irritable, and not nursing well. Admitting vital signs showed tachycardia and tachypnea with grunting and sternal retractions. She was intubated, given mechanical ventilation, and was placed on a cardiac monitor. Baseline laboratory tests included blood cultures, CBC with differential, arterial blood gas, and spinal fluid for cultures and cell counts.

Questions

1. During your assessment, what other information would it be important to have concerning Melissa's current illness?
2. What is the current problem?
3. What is the best way to support the family during this crisis?
4. Why was Melissa having difficulty feeding?
5. What nursing consultations might be considered?

Answers

1. The birth history is always important, along with information concerning other sick family members or siblings. If she was born at your facility, request that the old medical record be sent to the nursing unit.
2. Respiratory distress, behavioral changes, and poor feeding, which are signs of sepsis. Melissa is admitted with a diagnosis of suspected sepsis. The culture results reveal GBS as the causative organism.
3. Keep the family informed. Explain all tests and procedures. Provide paper and pencils so that the parents can write down questions for the nurses or the physicians. Offer to call the hospital-based clergy for support.
4. Melissa has a respiratory infection resulting in blocked nares and tachypnea. Neonates are obligate nose breathers, and feeding is difficult when they cannot breathe through their noses. To suckle, an infant must coordinate breathing with sucking and swallowing, which is difficult when the infant is tachypneic.
5. Consult a lactation specialist to help the mother express milk during the current crisis and assist with any problems when the infant begins to breastfeed again.

infections. Therefore, prompt identification and treatment are key in preventing overwhelming bacterial infection.

Mycobacterial Infections

Mycobacteria cause both non-TB and TB disease. Non-TB mycobacterial infections are not spread person to person, whereas TB is.

NONTUBERCULOUS MYCOBACTERIAL INFECTIONS

Nontuberculous mycobacteria (NTM) species are found everywhere in nature: soil, food, water, and animals. A few of these species cause infection in children, especially immunocompromised children such as those with HIV or cystic fibrosis. Reliable estimates of the incidence of infection are limited. NTM may also be known as atypical mycobacterial infections or *Mycobacterium avium* complex.

Assessment

Although NTM may cause disseminated disease in the immunocompromised child, the most common presentation in children is cervical lymphadenitis that does not respond to typical antibiotic therapy (American Academy of Pediatrics [AAP], 2012o). An otherwise healthy child typically presents with cervical lymph nodes that are usually firm, mobile, and nontender. The history shows that the lymph node has continued to enlarge over time, and the overlying skin has turned a bluish purple color.

A tuberculosis skin test (TST; or Mantoux test) may be ordered to assist in the diagnosis of NTM. NTM and TB share many of the same antigens, which may cause the TST to react (AAP, 2012o), but in NTM, the induration (reaction) is usually less than 10 mm. If the TST is reactive, a chest radiograph should be obtained to rule out TB. Definitive diagnosis of NTM disease requires isolation of the organism. NTM can be cultured in the laboratory and can be easily grown from excised lymph tissue. Polymerase chain reaction (PCR) testing is available in some reference laboratories.

Interdisciplinary Interventions

Excision of affected lymph nodes is considered a curative treatment for NTM cervical lymphadenitis (Scott et al., 2012). Antimicrobial therapy is very complex and typically is not successful. Because antibiotic resistance is common, drug therapy involves the use of two or three drugs over a 6- to 12-month period.

Children with HIV should receive antibiotic prophylaxis for NTM.

TUBERCULOSIS

TB is caused by an infection with *Mycobacterium tuberculosis*. TB is spread person to person in respiratory droplets. In children and adolescents, most TB infections are asymptomatic. This type of infection is called *latent tuberculosis infection* (LTBI). LTBI is defined as infection in an asymptomatic person with a positive TST, no clinical findings of disease, and a normal chest radiograph (AAP, 2012z).

TB rates are highest in urban, low-income areas and in non-white racial and ethnic groups. Foreign-born children account for 25% of all diagnosed cases in children younger than the age of 14 years. The homeless, residents of correctional facilities, people with immune suppression, immigrants, international adoptees, refugees, and travelers to and from endemic regions (e.g., Asia, Africa, Latin America, and the former Soviet Union) are at high risk for LTBI and active TB (AAP, 2012z). The risk of disease progression and dissemination is higher among children than adults, with risk being highest in infants younger than 12 months of age (Wiseman et al., 2012).

During the early 1990s, outbreaks of a strain of TB that was resistant to many familiar antitubercular drugs were documented (Centers for Disease Control and Prevention [CDC], 2006a). These resistant strains of TB, called *multidrug-resistant TB*, are resistant to the main first-line TB drugs, isoniazid and rifampin. Multidrug-resistant TB continues to be an increasing problem because of nonadherence to completing TB drug regimens as ordered and decreased funding for public health clinics used for TB control, which includes distributing TB drugs, monitoring TB patients, and tracking exposures.

In 2006, a new highly resistant TB strain was identified that, to date, has been virtually untreatable. This strain, known as extremely drug-resistant TB, is resistant to the first-line TB drugs and to many of the second-line TB drugs as well. Although both multidrug-resistant TB and extremely drug-resistant TB may initially result from treatment mismanagement that selects for multiresistant strains, once acquired, they can spread from person to person, posing a potential global health threat.

Assessment

In children, TB presents a great diagnostic challenge. Unlike adults, children, especially young ones, are usually asymptomatic, even when the TST is positive. History of exposure is often the most vital piece of information obtained. Chest radiographs are seldom positive. When TB infection progresses to disease, clinical findings usually occur within the first 6 months of exposure to *M. tuberculosis*; however, many years may elapse before infection progresses to disease.

Up to 50% of children with TB are asymptomatic. Notable exceptions include children with HIV infection and infants. Children also may manifest TB in forms other than the traditional pulmonary symptoms. Assess for nonspecific symptoms such as fever, growth delay or weight loss, persistent cough, fatigue, and night sweats (rare). Radiographic findings range from normal to pulmonary and extrapulmonary abnormalities. Non-remitting cough of more than 2 weeks' duration, documented weight loss during the preceding 3 months, and fatigue provide good diagnostic accuracy in HIV-free children 3 years of age or older (Marais et al., 2006).

The first obvious signs and symptoms of TB after an asymptomatic pulmonary infection may be extrapulmonary (TB that occurs outside the lungs), most commonly cervical lymphadenitis, meningitis, bone infection, and miliary TB. In infants and some children, the lymph nodes continue to enlarge to the point that bronchial obstruction results. Miliary TB, a form of extrapulmonary TB, is also more common in childhood TB. In miliary TB, massive numbers of tubercle bacilli are released into the bloodstream and then disseminate to other organs. Central nervous system (CNS) involvement—TB meningitis—is a serious and often fatal complication seen almost exclusively in children younger than age 4 years (see Chapter 21). TB meningitis usually develops gradually, 3 to 6 months after the primary infection. Older children complain of headache, irritability, and insomnia. Infants and younger children lose developmental milestones.

ALERT   *In children exposed to TB, assess neurologic signs frequently and notify the health care provider of changes. An abrupt onset of lethargy, convulsions, and nuchal rigidity precedes the development of hydrocephalus and increasing intracranial pressure. Coma and irregular pulse and respiration may follow, culminating in death.*

Diagnostic Tests

The TST (or Mantoux test) is the primary method used for determining TB exposure. Intradermal administration of purified protein derivative is the most accurate and reliable test method. Creating a 6- to 10-mm wheal is crucial for accurate testing (AAP, 2012z). The skin test must be read in 48 to 72 hours by measuring the size of the reaction (induration). Control tests may be performed at the same time as the purified protein derivative test in patients who are immunocompromised. The control skin tests are usually *Candida* or tetanus. One or two controls are chosen and administered on the opposite forearm. Because most children have been exposed to *Candida* in the environment and to tetanus through immunization, the control test should be positive. A nonreactive control test indicates that the child is anergic. **Anergy** is a condition in which the immune system is so deficient that it cannot mount a reaction to the skin tests. Thus, TB cannot be ruled out in a child with a negative TST and nonreactive control tests. Interferon-gamma release assay (IGRA) is recommended in asymptomatic children older than 4 years of age who have been immunized against BCG (AAP, 2012c).

Chest radiographs may be of little diagnostic value because they usually appear normal. Children also have great difficulty in producing sufficient sputum and coughing productively. They often swallow their secretions. Obtaining a sputum specimen for an acid-fast bacteriologic culture and smear from a young child may be difficult; therefore, gastric washings are recommended rather than sputum samples. The tubercle bacilli pass through the digestive system completely intact and unharmed by stomach acid and other digestive processes. Hence, sputum smears may be negative for TB, but gastric washings may be positive.

The standard for diagnosis is still a positive culture for *M. tuberculosis*. Acid-fast smears are helpful but cannot be specific for *M. tuberculosis*.

Interdisciplinary Interventions

Because *M. tuberculosis* takes up to 6 weeks to grow in the laboratory, therapy is started on the basis of a positive smear or strong clinical evidence of pulmonary, meningeal, or extrapulmonary infection. Standard drug

therapy consists of isoniazid, rifampin, and pyrazinamide given for 2 months, followed by isoniazid and rifampin for 4 months. However, specific drug therapy is based on the organism's drug sensitivity.

Preventive therapy is given to children with positive skin tests (purified protein derivative) and no clinical evidence of disease (i.e., LTBI). Treatment consists of isoniazid for 9 months. For children with HIV infection, preventive therapy may be extended to 12 months. Rifampin is given as preventive therapy in cases of known exposure to multidrug-resistant TB.

Nursing care of children with known or suspected pulmonary TB must be individualized (Fig. 24-2). Because young children are often asymptomatic, their relative infectiousness varies. If hospitalized, most children do not need airborne precautions in a **negative-pressure isolation** room (room in which air flows into the room from the hallway and is removed by a separate, filtered exhaust to the outside); only those with significant pulmonary infection should be in this isolation. Infants and small children with pulmonary TB rarely cough up sputum. What little sputum they do manage to cough up contains few tubercle bacilli because their cavitary lung lesions have few bacilli. Therefore, as these cavitary lesions break open, few or no bacilli escape into the bronchi to be coughed up.

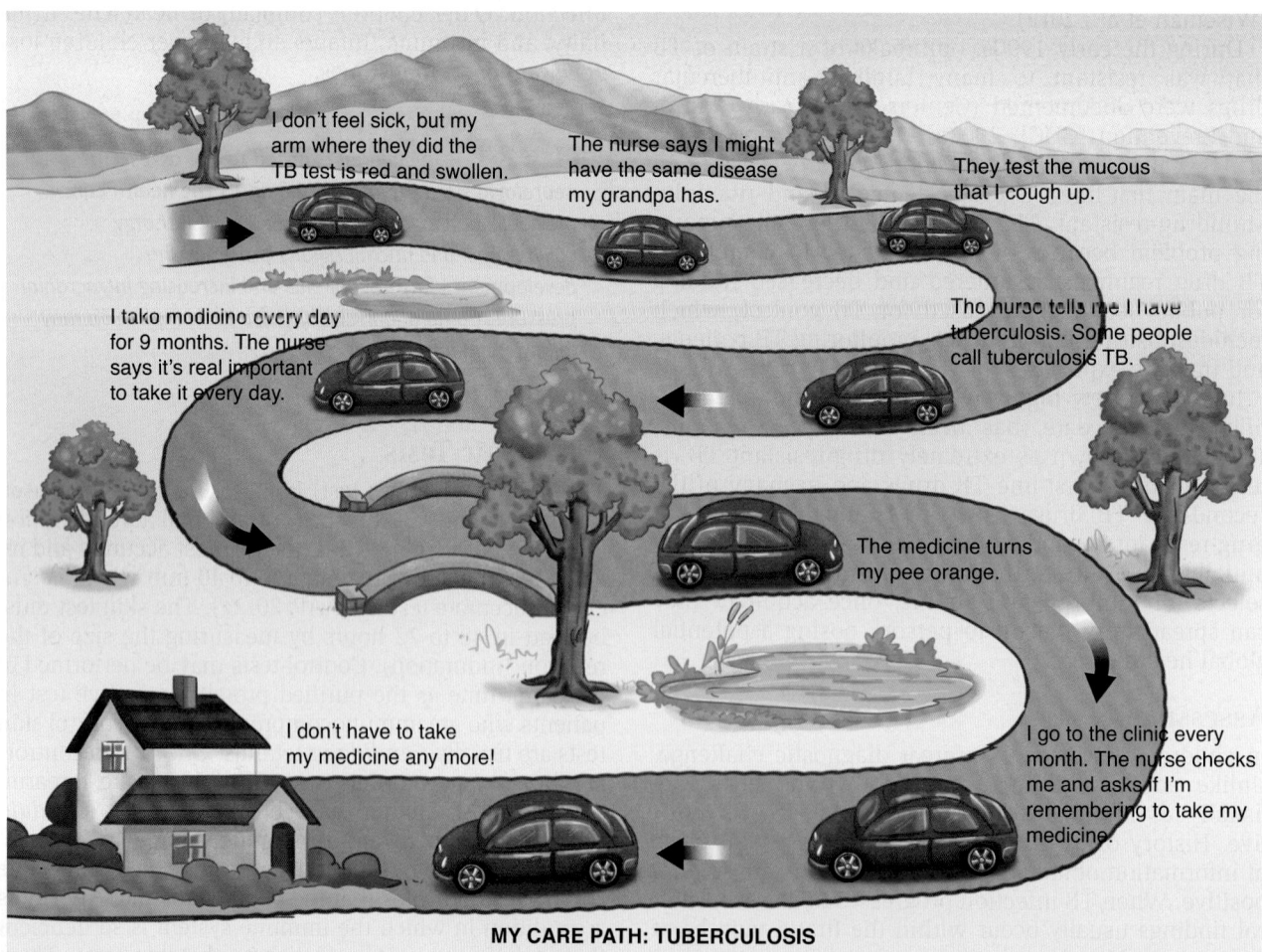

Figure 24-2 A care path for a child with TB.

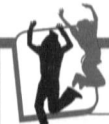

COMMUNITY CARE 24-1

Tuberculosis Follow-up

The health care provider, diagnosing laboratory, and treating institution (clinic, hospital, or private physician's office) are legally responsible for informing the local health department of all cases of TB. The local health department then initiates contact investigations. Contacts are persons exposed to the child with pulmonary TB and could be in many locations, such as church, school, or daycare center. The health department

- Determines who in the community has been exposed to the child
- Performs screening tests (skin tests) on exposed individuals, such as family members, neighbors, and schoolmates
- Provides preventive drug therapy (isoniazid)
- Provides drug treatment, follow-up laboratory work, and radiographic evaluation
- Provides for directly observed therapy to families who may be nonadherent because of homelessness, parental drug abuse, or other reason
- Assists with arranging temporary placement in halfway housing or other state-run facilities

As children mature, the ability to cough and infect others increases, especially during adolescence. Place adolescents and children with positive sputum smears in a negative-pressure room. Wear an N95 respirator or a high-efficiency particulate air respirator in the room.

Frequently, the TB source for the child is a parent or close relative. Thus, the child in isolation may not pose an infection risk, but the parents or visitors may. Refer relatives and close family contacts to the local health department (Community Care 24-1) for testing and treatment. Children need their parents, especially when they are ill and in the strange surroundings of a hospital. Parents or close relatives with pulmonary TB can wear a mask to and from the isolation room when visiting. Other accommodations can also be arranged, including having food trays for the parents delivered to the child's room.

Community Care

Long-term follow-up of the child with TB is particularly important because of the potential for nonadherence in completing the typically lengthy treatment regimen. Strains of TB that are resistant to common antitubercular drugs arise as a result of partial treatment. Monitor the child for the presence of drug side effects (Nursing Interventions 24-1) and adherence to therapy. If nonadherence is an issue, directly observed therapy may be implemented. In this approach, the medication is taken in the presence of the nurse.

Assess nutritional status and provide diet counseling, if needed, to prevent poor healing stemming from inadequate nutrition, which affects immune function. Refer the child to social services if poor intake is related to inadequate finances.

PERTUSSIS

Pertussis, also known as *whooping cough*, begins as an upper respiratory illness and progresses to a persistent cough characterized by an inspiratory whoop. Pertussis is endemic worldwide. Even in countries with high rates of vaccination coverage, a resurgence of pertussis has been noted (Bechini et al., 2012).

An estimated 50 million cases of pertussis occur globally each year, most in developing countries, causing 400,000 deaths, primarily in infants (Guiso et al., 2011; Forsyth, 2007). Vaccine-induced immunity to pertussis wanes after 5 to 10 years, leaving adolescents and adults susceptible and an important reservoir for infection. Adolescents and adults play a critical role in the spread of pertussis.

Pertussis is caused by the bacterium *Bordetella pertussis* and is transmitted by respiratory droplets that are coughed or sneezed by the child in the **catarrhal** (characterized by inflamed mucous membranes) and early **paroxysmal** (occurring with a sudden onset) stages of the illness. This infectious period can last for 6 weeks or longer (AAP, 2012q). Common comorbidities associated with pertussis include pneumonia, seizures, and encephalopathy.

Assessment

The incubation period for pertussis is 7 to 10 days, during which the child is most contagious. The *catarrhal phase* occurs during this initial incubation period, producing coldlike symptoms (runny nose, scratchy throat, and mild cough). This stage is followed by the *paroxysmal phase*, characterized by periods of paroxysmal coughing, during which the child coughs violently, vomits, has apneic spells, and becomes cyanotic. At the end of the coughing attack, the patient gasps (whoops) for air. Infants younger than 6 months may not exhibit classic whooping. These intense spells of coughing often interfere with feeding and sleep. The paroxysmal phase lasts 2 to 6 weeks and is followed by a *convalescent stage* characterized by a persistent (but not paroxysmal) cough.

Nasopharyngeal swab samples, obtained using Dacron or calcium alginate swabs, are sent to the laboratory for pertussis culture. These samples are plated on special media and must incubate for 7 days. The laboratory must be informed of the potential diagnosis so that the swab is handled appropriately. A positive culture is diagnostic for pertussis, but the organism is not likely to grow if obtained 2 weeks or longer after the onset of coughing or if antibiotics have already been started.

DNA amplification (PCR) testing is increasingly being used in preference to culture because of its increased sensitivity and shorter turnaround time. The use of PCR testing and single-serum serology is recommended to

NURSING INTERVENTIONS 24-1

For the Child Receiving Antitubercular Drugs

Drug/Route	Nursing Interventions
Isoniazid (INH) PO	Potential liver toxicity. Monitor liver function tests and assess for jaundice.
Rifampin (Rif) PO	Orange discoloration of secretions or urine. Could stain contact lenses. Teach family about discoloration.
Pyrazinamide (PZA) PO	Potential liver toxicity. Monitor liver function tests.
Streptomycin IM	Usually given only in meningitis because of ototoxicity. Conduct hearing screens at initiation of therapy, midway, and at the end of therapy. Observe for skin rashes. Rotate injection site, use pain reduction techniques, and provide psychosocial support.
Ethambutol (EMB) PO	Use for older children only. Can cause reversible optic neuritis. Assess visual acuity, visual fields, and red/green color discrimination daily.

IM, intramuscular; PO, per os (oral).

confirm the diagnosis of cases that meet the clinical definition of pertussis (Cherry et al., 2005).

Nursing Diagnoses and Outcomes

Common nursing diagnoses and outcomes for the child with an infection are identified in Nursing Plan of Care 24-1. Additional nursing diagnoses and outcomes for infants with pertussis may include the following:

Nursing Diagnosis: Ineffective breathing pattern related to effects of prolonged coughing attacks
Outcome: Child will maintain adequate oxygenation, evidenced by an oxygen saturation of 97% to 99%, and no alteration in level of consciousness.
Nursing Diagnosis: Disturbed sleep pattern related to effects of coughing spells interrupting rest
Outcome: Child will obtain adequate sleep and resume previous sleep patterns.

Interdisciplinary Interventions

Infants younger than 6 months of age may require hospitalization for supportive care to manage apnea, hypoxia, or feeding difficulties. The macrolides (erythromycin, azithromycin, and clarithromycin) are the drugs of choice for pertussis in children 6 months of age or older. Azithromycin and clarithromycin are not U.S. Food and Drug Administration (FDA) approved for use in infants younger than 6 months of age; however, infants younger than 1 month of age should be treated with azithromycin because erythromycin is associated with increased risk of infantile hypertrophic pyloric stenosis. Trimethoprim-sulfamethoxazole is an alternative antibiotic for children who cannot tolerate erythromycin. Antibiotics given during the catarrhal phase of the illness may halt disease progression. Unfortunately, pertussis is often not

suspected until the more characteristic symptoms (especially paroxysmal coughing) develop. Antibiotics given at the paroxysmal stage or later usually have little or no effect on the outcome of the illness but are used to limit the spread of pertussis to others.

Use droplet precautions until 5 days after antibiotic therapy has been started or until 3 weeks after the onset of paroxysmal coughing. Offer macrolide chemoprophylaxis for a 5-day course to all close contacts of the child.

caREminder

In the ambulatory setting, place a child suspected of having pertussis in a private examination room as soon as he or she enters the clinic or office. Advise personnel who enter the room to observe standard precautions and wear a mask.

During the paroxysmal phase, the child can have up to 20 coughing attacks a day and may vomit after the attacks. Avoid stimulating the child, which may precipitate a coughing paroxysm. Maintain a calm manner while supporting the child and parents during coughing paroxysms, which are quite frightening. Such coughing also disturbs sleep and nutrition. Focus nursing care on keeping the child adequately hydrated and nourished and alleviating coughing episodes with antitussives. Gentle suctioning after coughing may be needed to maintain a patent airway. The nursing and respiratory care staff must make it a priority to maintain ventilatory support (see Chapter 16).

To prevent pertussis, universal immunization with pertussis vaccine is recommended for all children younger than 7 years old. Pertussis immunity wanes 4 to 12 years after completion of childhood vaccination. As such, adolescents and adults serve as a reservoir of disease and are the most common source of pertussis infection in infants. Booster doses of pertussis vaccine are recommended to protect infants from the disease.

PNEUMOCOCCAL DISEASE

Pneumococcal infections are common in the extremes of life—the very young and the very old. Before routine use of the childhood pneumococcal conjugate vaccine, *Streptococcus pneumoniae* was the most common bacterial cause of otitis media, pneumonia, and sepsis in young children (AAP, 2012s). Pneumococcus is also a common cause of meningitis.

Many children and adults are colonized with pneumococcus in the upper respiratory tract. Transmission is person to person by respiratory droplets. The progression from pneumococcal colonization to invasive disease is multifactorial. Preceding viral infections lower resistance to disease and may contribute to invasive disease. Agents and diseases that decrease the normal self-cleaning functions of the respiratory system, such as bronchial obstruction, irritants, or allergens that decrease ciliary function, can also push colonization toward invasive disease. Errors in immune response in such conditions as HIV, splenectomy, agammaglobulinemia, leukemia, and sickle cell disease inhibit the body's natural defenses and lead to invasive disease (Table 24-1). Epidemics of pneumococcal pneumonia occur most frequently in the winter in overcrowded situations. Infants, with their immature immune systems, are particularly prone to develop invasive disease.

Pneumococcal disease occurs in many forms, including meningitis, sinusitis, otitis media, occult bacteremia, and pneumonia. Because pneumococci commonly colonize the upper respiratory tract, pneumonia, otitis media, sinusitis, and mastoiditis are a direct result of this colonization.

Pneumococcal meningitis usually results from the bacteria crossing the blood–brain barrier into the CNS and seeding the meninges. Invasion may happen as the result of a pneumococcal infection of the bloodstream or by direct extension from a pneumococcal infection in the mastoid or paranasal sinuses to the meninges.

Children younger than 2 years old and those with congenital immunodeficiencies, asplenia, sickle cell disease, and HIV infection are at increased risk for pneumococcal disease, as are Native Americans, Native Alaskans, and African Americans.

Assessment

Pneumococcal pneumonia often occurs abruptly, with the child exhibiting a temperature of 102° to 103° F (38.9° to 39.4° C), chills, productive cough, and otitis media. Listen for rales on auscultation of the lungs and dullness to percussion. Assess the sinuses by pressing the fingers along the sinus tracts of the face; the child may complain of pressure or pain. Children with bacteremia or meningitis may exhibit fever and irritability. In cases of meningitis, nuchal rigidity (neck stiffness) may occur.

caREminder

Ask the child to try to touch their chin to their chest. If pain prevents the child from doing this, it may be from nuchal rigidity caused by inflamed meninges.

In pneumococcal pneumonia, chest radiographs reveal subsegmental lobar consolidation. Bacteriologic cultures of blood, spinal fluid, and other body fluids are commonly collected and Gram stained to reveal pneumococci. Elevated white blood cell counts are helpful in diagnosis but are not conclusive. Rapid antigen tests can detect pneumococcal capsular antigen in urine, spinal fluid, pleural fluid, and blood. These tests are of limited value, however, because they lack sensitivity and specificity.

Nursing Diagnoses and Outcomes

Common nursing diagnoses and outcomes for the child experiencing an infection are identified in Nursing Plan of Care 24-1. The following nursing diagnosis and

TABLE 24-1	Risk for Pneumococcal Disease Associated With Altered Immune Function	
Immune Defect	**Reason for Increased Risk**	**Interventions**
Immature immune system (premature infant or term neonate) response	Decreased phagocytic activity Varied levels of protective maternal antibodies (immunoglobulin G [IgG]) Decreased response to polysaccharide antigen	Antibiotic therapy Proper nutrition to increase infant's response to infection Hand hygiene in hospitals, clinics, daycare centers, and other child care settings
Asplenic infants, children, and adolescents	Diminished or absent neutrophil function	Pneumococcal vaccine for all children Daily prophylaxis with oral penicillin until adulthood
Acquired or congenital immunodeficiency (such as in HIV infection or agammaglobulinemia)	Dysfunctional immune system Increased respiratory infections	Antibiotic therapy Pneumococcal vaccine for all children
Sickle cell disease	Decreased immune function related to functional asplenia	Daily prophylaxis with oral penicillin starting at age 4 months Pneumococcal vaccine

outcome may also apply to a child with pneumococcal disease:

Nursing Diagnosis: Ineffective airway clearance related to effects of excessive mucus production
Outcome: Child's airway will remain patent.

Interdisciplinary Interventions

Penicillin and cephalosporins are the drugs of choice for treating *S. pneumoniae* infection. Because resistant pneumococcal strains are increasingly common, vancomycin plus ceftriaxone or cefotaxime may be used as an alternative to treat serious infections, such as meningitis or bacteremia. High-dose amoxicillin or amoxicillin clavulanate is effective treatment for mild-to-moderate infections, such as otitis media. Extended-spectrum cephalosporins, such as cefdinir, cefuroxime, and ceftriaxone, are also useful, especially in cases of penicillin allergy. As with any antibiotic, teach the family to complete the full course exactly as prescribed.

Community Care

Standard precautions are recommended for children with pneumococcal infections, including those caused by penicillin-resistant strains. The primary goal is to prevent invasive pneumococcal disease. Teach parents the importance of immunization. Two pneumococcal vaccines are available against pneumococcal disease (see Chapter 8). Children at high risk of developing invasive pneumococcal disease should also be offered prophylactic low-dose antibiotics for preventive therapy. Refer to the specific disease forms caused by pneumococcus for other nursing care (e.g., otitis media).

STAPHYLOCOCCAL INFECTIONS

Staphylococcus aureus and *Staphylococcus epidermidis* are normal flora of the skin. Infection results when staphylococci enter normally sterile body fluids or sites. *S. aureus* produces localized and invasive infections as well as three toxin-mediated illnesses: toxic shock syndrome (hypotension, skin desquamation, fever, and multisystem involvement), scaled skin syndrome (blistering and peeling), and food poisoning.

Staphylococci are the cause of 40% of all skin and wound infections, 23% of all lower respiratory tract infections, 22% of all bloodstream infections, and 15% of all other infections (urinary tract, brain, abdominal) in infants and children (Mandell et al., 2005). *S. aureus* is the leading cause of nosocomial infections and is responsible for 50% to 70% of community-acquired osteomyelitis. Furuncles, cellulitis, lymphatitis, impetigo, and wound infections are common childhood staphylococcal infections (see also Chapter 25).

Toxic shock syndrome gained national attention during the late 1980s, when women who used superabsorbent tampons became quite ill with fever, vomiting, a desquamating rash, and hypotension. Later, a toxic shock–like syndrome was observed in nonmenstruating women and children who had one thing in common: positive cultures for *S. aureus*.

Pathophysiology

Staphylococci can infect the blood, the pulmonary system (pneumonia), bones, joints, skin and soft tissue, and surgical wounds; meningitis is rare. A major complication of a staphylococcal blood infection is endocarditis. Although staphylococcal endocarditis is most common in IV drug abusers, children with congenital heart disease or those with artificial heart valves, grafts, and patches can also develop this infection. The lesions formed by a *Staphylococcus* infection may break off to form septic emboli in other locations, such as the brain or lungs.

MRSA is common in large hospitals and is responsible for 50% of health care–associated infections (AAP, 2012u). MRSA is also increasingly responsible for community-associated infections. The major reservoir for MRSA is the lower part of the nose (anterior nares). Hands become contaminated by touching or rubbing the nose. Then health care workers, colonized with MRSA in their nose, spread the organism unwittingly from patient to patient on their hands. Children can easily become colonized with MRSA if they frequently encounter health care workers or spend time in community settings such as daycare or schools. Children can also develop MRSA as a result of antibiotic therapy for persistent infections, such as chronic otitis media or lung infections.

Coagulase-negative staphylococci, common flora of the skin and mucous membranes, are frequently seen in hospital-associated infections, infections of medical devices, and urinary tract infections.

Assessment

Species of staphylococci that produce exfoliating toxins can cause scalded skin syndrome. In this syndrome, assess for skin bullae that evolve into generalized desquamation. The child's skin can be painful to the touch, and even the slightest touch can lead to skin peeling.

Bone and joint infections resulting in septic arthritis or osteomyelitis often begin as a bloodstream infection. These infections often begin in the metaphyseal portions of the long bones. Assess for refusal to move the limb, painful joints, crepitus, and heat. Soft-tissue swelling is evident either on physical examination or radiograph.

Surgical wound infections and device-related infections produce yellow, foul-smelling pus at the operative site or device insertion site. The wound becomes red, inflamed, and hot to touch. Pus oozes from the suture line or can be expressed by applying gentle pressure along the sides of the suture line. Areas of fluctuance are often palpable.

Diagnosis is confirmed by Gram stain of the infected body fluids. Cultures determine whether the gram-positive cocci in clusters are coagulase-positive or coagulase-negative staphylococci. Microbiologic evaluation of the cultures further identifies the organism and its susceptibility pattern.

Nursing Diagnoses and Outcomes

Nursing diagnoses and outcomes for the child with an infection are identified in Nursing Plan of Care 24-1. Additional nursing diagnoses and outcomes most commonly associated with staphylococcal infections include the following:

Nursing Diagnosis: Activity intolerance related to effects of joint pain in septic arthritis

Outcome: Child will report or evidence adequate pain control and will participate in age-appropriate activities.

Nursing Diagnosis: Impaired skin integrity related to effects of *Staphylococcus* causing desquamation

Outcomes:
- Child will not develop secondary infection.
- Child's skin integrity will be restored.

Interdisciplinary Interventions

Many staphylococci are resistant to penicillin. Vancomycin is the drug of choice for serious infections involving multidrug-resistant strains. However, sensitive strains respond to most antibiotics, including oxacillin, nafcillin, methicillin, most cephalosporins, erythromycin, and clindamycin. Most community-acquired MRSA infections can be treated on an outpatient basis with trimethoprim–sulfamethoxazole or clindamycin.

Maintain scrupulous hand hygiene when caring for patients with staphylococcal infections. *Staphylococcus* is present in the normal flora on the child's and nurse's skin. Provide wound care wearing gloves. Wear a gown if there is any risk that your clothing may become soiled.

Implement contact precautions for children with MRSA infections or those who are colonized with MRSA. Continue contact precautions until antibiotic therapy is discontinued and repeated cultures are negative.

During outbreaks of MRSA infection, cultures may be taken of health care workers' anterior nares, axilla, and groin as part of an epidemiologic workup. The infection control practitioner can use the results to determine a common source of the outbreak. Individuals found to be positive may undergo CDC-recommended decolonization by taking daily showers with chlorhexidine gluconate, applying mupirocin ointment to the anterior nares, or taking a prolonged course of oral trimethoprim–sulfamethoxazole.

Community Care

Educate daycare and school staff regarding hand hygiene for all staff and students to reduce the spread of community-acquired MRSA. Because emergence of community-acquired MRSA has been documented among sports and athletic teams during the past several years, educating team leaders and members is particularly important (Stanforth et al., 2010; Turbeville et al., 2006). To prevent the spread of MRSA among family members, teach the family to keep fingernails short, not to share washcloths and towels, and to change sleepwear and underwear daily (Newby et al., 2011).

Streptococcal Infections

Two types of streptococci cause disease: group A and group B.

GROUP A STREPTOCOCCAL INFECTIONS

GAS disease is one of the most common diseases of childhood, causing a variety of cutaneous and systemic infections and complications with variable severity and prognosis (Table 24-2). Invasive GAS disease has received media attention as "flesh-eating" bacteria. Because GAS disease is so common and not reportable to the health department, estimating the true incidence of the disease is impossible. Globally, over 660,000 new cases of invasive GAS disease occur each year, with an estimated 163,000 deaths, although these figures

TABLE 24-2 Types of Group A Streptococcal Infections		
Infection	**Clinical Manifestations**	**Complications**
Streptococcal pharyngitis	Sore throat, malaise, fever, enlarged tonsils studded with gray-white exudate, enlarged lymph nodes	Peritonsillar abscess Scarlet fever Rheumatic fever Damage to mitral valve may necessitate replacement in midlife
Erysipelas	Red, edematous, warm, raised lesions with sharply demarcated margins Edema that advances rapidly	Bullae can leave open weeping lesions that may develop secondary infection
Streptococcal impetigo	Fragile vesicles that evolve into pustules Pustules that enlarge and erode	Secondary bacterial infection Streptococcal toxic shock Glomerulonephritis
Streptococcal cellulitis	Warm, erythematous, painful, edematous lesion with ill-defined margins that rapidly spreads History of trauma, varicella lesions, burns, or surgery	Invasion of lymph nodes and bloodstream Streptococcal toxic shock
Necrotizing fasciitis (invasive GAS disease)	Within 24 hours of trauma, site swelling and cellulitis that spreads to surrounding tissue Deep infection of subcutaneous tissue that destroys fascia and fat Frank gangrene that develops by 4–5 days	Life-threatening infection Need for surgical drainage or amputation

underestimate disease burden because of lack of quality data from developing countries (Steer et al., 2012). Mortality from GAS toxic shock syndrome is 34% in children (Rodríguez-Nuñez et al., 2011). The severity of GAS disease is determined, in part, by the susceptibility of the host and the serotype of the GAS.

Pathophysiology

Streptococci inhabit the upper respiratory tract in 15% to 50% of asymptomatic children. Pharyngitis is spread primarily through droplets as the infected child coughs or sneezes. In daycare centers and nursery schools, hand-to-hand-to-mouth transmission may occur, especially among young children. Food can be a mode of transmission if handled by an infected or colonized individual. The incubation period is 2 to 5 days for streptococcal pharyngitis and 7 to 10 days for impetigo (AAP, 2012v).

Before the antibiotic era, scarlet fever, rheumatic fever, and glomerulonephritis were common complications of GAS disease. The incidence of all three complications has decreased since World War II. They are now relatively preventable with appropriate antibiotic therapy. Rheumatic fever typically occurs a week after the onset of pharyngitis, with the development of fever, polyarthritis, and carditis. Nephritis is more common after streptococcal skin infections than after pharyngitis, but long-term renal sequelae are seldom seen in children.

Assessment

GAS pharyngitis typically presents as fever, malaise, and a sore throat. Lymph nodes in the neck are palpable. Examine the tongue, which at first appears white, then within 2 days becomes red (strawberry tongue). If GAS pharyngitis progresses to scarlet fever, the rash appears about 12 hours after onset of the disease. The rash follows an ordered progression and has been compared to a "sunburn with goose pimples" (Figs. 24-3 and 24-4).

Invasive GAS disease begins as a mild infection such as strep throat and rapidly progresses to a severe illness. Be alert for signs of bacteremia (blood infection), a toxic shock–like syndrome, multisystem organ failure, a rapid decrease in blood pressure, and necrotizing fasciitis, which destroys muscle, fat, and underlying tissue.

A positive throat culture for GAS disease makes the definitive diagnosis for streptococcal pharyngitis. However, rapid antigen tests have proved useful in diagnosing patients quickly to begin antibiotic therapy. Because these tests are not as sensitive as a throat culture, a negative test must be confirmed by a culture.

Common serologic tests used for diagnosis include antistreptolysin O and a latex agglutination test (Streptozyme). These serologic tests are frequently used to diagnose rheumatic fever. Expect a positive result if GAS are present.

Skin infections are usually diagnosed by skin or wound cultures. Invasive GAS infections are diagnosed by positive cultures of cerebrospinal fluid (CSF) or

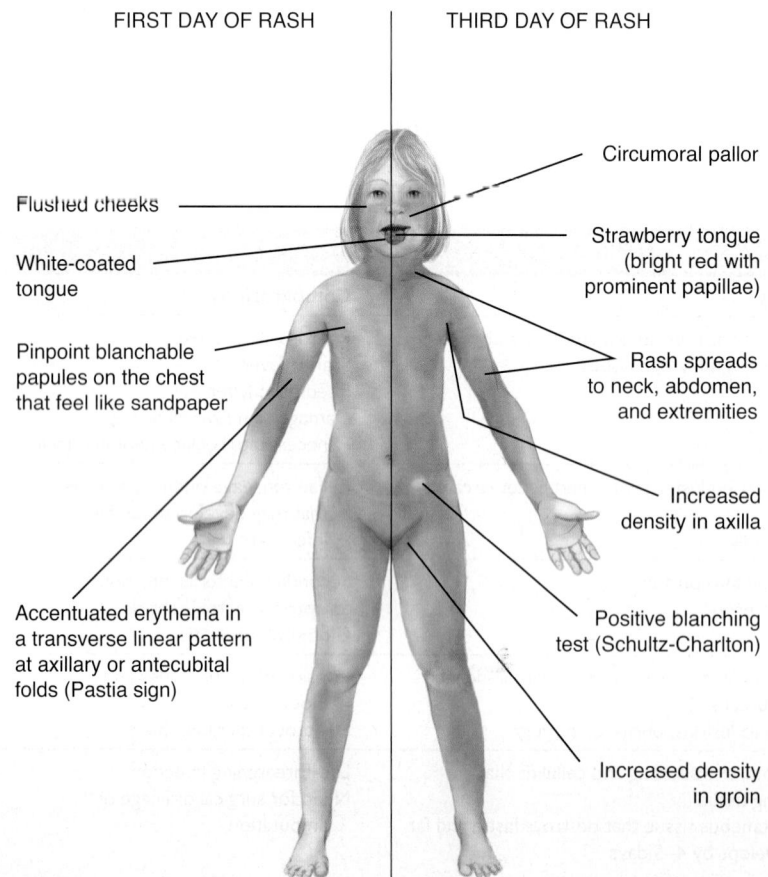

FIRST DAY OF RASH | THIRD DAY OF RASH

Flushed cheeks

White-coated tongue

Pinpoint blanchable papules on the chest that feel like sandpaper

Accentuated erythema in a transverse linear pattern at axillary or antecubital folds (Pastia sign)

Circumoral pallor

Strawberry tongue (bright red with prominent papillae)

Rash spreads to neck, abdomen, and extremities

Increased density in axilla

Positive blanching test (Schultz-Charlton)

Increased density in groin

Figure 24-3 Progression of rash in scarlet fever.

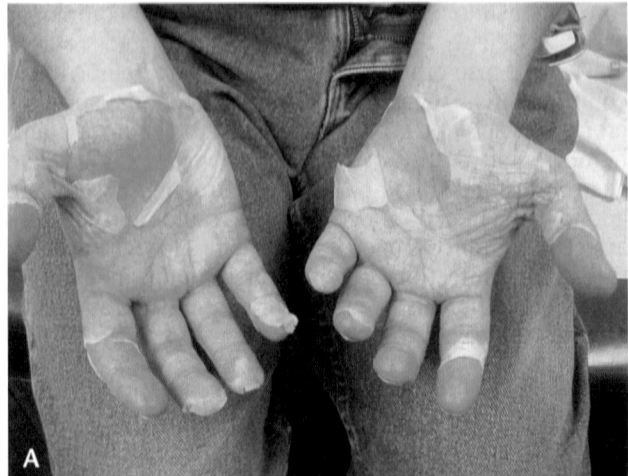

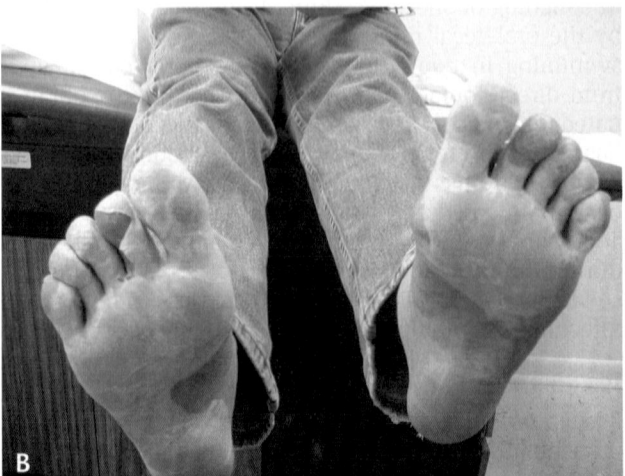

Figure 24-4 (A and B) During the convalescent phase of scarlet fever, the skin of the palms and soles frequently peels.

synovial, peritoneal, or pleural fluid. Tissue biopsies may be performed in cases of suspected gangrene.

Nursing Diagnoses and Outcomes

In addition to those identified in Nursing Plan of Care 24-1, the following nursing diagnosis and outcomes may apply to the child with GAS pharyngitis:

Nursing Diagnosis: Impaired swallowing related to painful sore throat
Outcomes:
* Child will experience minimal throat pain.
* Child will maintain adequate fluid and nutritional intake.

The following nursing diagnosis and outcomes may apply to the child with invasive GAS disease:

Nursing Diagnosis: Impaired tissue integrity related to effects of pathogen
Outcomes:
* Child will experience minimal tissue damage.
* Child will not develop secondary infection related to effects of cellulitis or necrotizing fasciitis.

Interdisciplinary Interventions

The agent of choice is penicillin, which is the most effective therapy available for treating streptococcal infections (Chiappini et al., 2011). Cephalosporins, the macrolides, and clindamycin are also effective but should be reserved for children with penicillin allergy. In necrotizing fasciitis, drainage and debridement are often necessary. In severe cases of gangrene, fasciotomy or amputation may be necessary.

For hospitalized children with GAS pharyngitis or pneumonia, maintain droplet precautions until antibiotic therapy has been given for 24 hours (AAP, 2012v). Unfortunately, this regimen excludes the child from the playroom or other group activities. Provide psychosocial support as indicated to help the child adjust to body image changes and to activity limitations.

Community Care

Nurses should advise parents of nonhospitalized children with group A pharyngitis to exclude the child from daycare or school until after 24 hours of effective therapy.

caREminder

Instruct parents of the child with group A pharyngitis to discard the child's toothbrush. The organism can survive on the toothbrush and reinfect the child after antibiotic therapy is completed.

Observe strict hand hygiene between patients and adhere to aseptic techniques to prevent nosocomial spread of infection. In outbreaks, group the patients with GAS infection into a cohort and have the same nurse or nurses care exclusively for these infected patients.

GROUP B STREPTOCOCCAL INFECTIONS

GBS is a leading cause of neonatal sepsis and death. Group B streptococci are gram-positive, aerobic diplococci that are divided into nine serotypes. Serotype III is the primary cause of GBS meningitis and most late-onset GBS disease (Edmond et al., 2012).

Pathophysiology

Colonization of the lower genitourinary tract occurs in approximately 15% to 40% of pregnant women (AAP, 2012v). Group B streptococci may ascend the birth canal to infect infants, or infants may acquire the bacteria as they descend through the birth canal. The implementation of maternal GBS screening and the initiation of intrapartum antibiotic prophylaxis has substantially decreased the incidence of early-onset GBS disease but not late-onset disease (Edmond et al., 2012).

Assessment

Early-onset GBS disease often begins as an overwhelming systemic infection within the first few days of life. Early-onset GBS is characterized by respiratory distress, apnea, shock, pneumonia, and (less often) meningitis. Watch for signs and symptoms of sepsis. Late-onset GBS disease typically occurs at 1 to 3 months of age and often presents with meningitis, osteomyelitis, septic arthritis, or cellulitis.

A positive culture from the infant with gram-positive cocci in chains can provide a presumptive diagnosis of GBS infection. Positive maternal cultures and the signs and symptoms of sepsis in the neonate are also evidence of infection. Cultures of GBS from any sterile body site, such as blood, spinal, or pleural fluid, or from an area of focal infection are diagnostic. Rapid antigen tests, which test for the presence of GBS in CSF, blood, or urine, are available but are not recommended because of their poor specificity.

Nursing Diagnoses and Outcomes

Common nursing diagnoses and outcomes for the child with an infection are identified in Nursing Plan of Care 24-1.

Interdisciplinary Interventions

Treatment for GBS disease requires penicillin or ampicillin plus an aminoglycoside. This combination of antibiotics is often used to treat suspected bacterial infections empirically when the organism has not yet been identified.

The length of hospitalization for an infant admitted with GBS sepsis can vary from 3 to 5 days to 1 to 3 weeks. The length of treatment for GBS ranges from 10 days for sepsis to 2 to 3 weeks for meningitis. GBS osteomyelitis or endocarditis may require 4 to 6 weeks of IV antibiotic therapy. The infant may be sent home with IV antibiotics. Instruct the parents how to give IV antibiotics and care for the IV access line and emphasize the importance of finishing all the medication (see earlier discussion of sepsis). Also, teach parents the signs of infection and which ones should trigger a call to their health care provider.

Isolation is not necessary for GBS disease but may be needed for outbreaks of GBS in nurseries. Frequent updates to the family of a sick infant are appreciated and critical in communicating information that may be difficult for laypeople to understand.

VIRAL INFECTIONS

Disease-causing viruses include such viruses as adenovirus, various enteroviruses, herpesviruses, HIV, measles, mumps, parvovirus, rubella, and hepatitis. See Chapter 16 for information on respiratory syncytial virus infection and influenza. Vaccines have been developed for many common and easily transmissible viral infections. Many new antiviral agents are also available to treat specific viral infections.

ADENOVIRUS INFECTION

Adenovirus commonly infects the upper respiratory tract in infants and young children during the late winter, spring, and early summer months. Adenovirus typically presents with symptoms of the common cold, sore throat, tonsillitis, and otitis media. It is also commonly associated with fever and conjunctivitis. Adenovirus may also cause other disorders, including hemorrhagic conjunctivitis; severe respiratory infections such as croup, bronchiolitis, or a pertussis-like syndrome; and hemorrhagic cystitis. A few adenoviruses infect the gastrointestinal tract and cause gastroenteritis. Enteric adenovirus infection occurs year-round and usually affects children younger than 4 years old. Serious life-threatening infections such as pneumonia, meningitis, or encephalitis can occur in infants and immunosuppressed children (AAP, 2012a).

Pathophysiology

Adenovirus infection is common in all pediatric age groups. Respiratory infections are transmitted by direct contact through exposure to respiratory secretions (as in coughing or sneezing). Enteric strains are transmitted by the oral–fecal route. Eye infections may result from swimming in pools that are not properly chlorinated, from direct contact with the conjunctiva with contaminated fingers, or from ophthalmologic equipment that has not been properly disinfected. Nosocomial infection can result from contact with infected health care workers or contaminated equipment. The incubation period for adenovirus is 2 to 14 days. Children are most contagious during the first few days of illness but may continue to shed adenovirus for up to several months. Asymptomatic infection is common, and reinfection may occur.

Assessment

Respiratory tract infections can present as pharyngitis, bronchiolitis, croup, or severe pneumonia (see Chapter 16 for specific signs and symptoms of these respiratory disorders). The pharyngitis is typically exudative and is often confused with streptococcal pharyngitis. The nurse can differentiate adenoviral pharyngitis from GAS pharyngitis if conjunctivitis is present because conjunctivitis suggests a viral etiology. Adenoviral upper respiratory tract infections often mimic pertussis, with prolonged episodes of paroxysmal coughing.

Suspect adenoviral eye infection (epidemic keratoconjunctivitis) when the conjunctiva appear red and granular, with clear drainage, and the child has frequent tearing and photophobia. Eye irritation and redness can last for 1 to 2 weeks. Superficial erosion of the cornea and subepithelial corneal infiltrates can be seen by ophthalmologic examination.

caREminder

Adenovirus is not inactivated by ethanol, commonly used in eye clinics to disinfect equipment. After cleaning the contaminated instrument, immerse it in 1% sodium hypochlorite for 10 minutes or steam autoclave.

Gastroenteritis infections caused by enteric strains of adenovirus are second only to rotavirus in frequency. Symptoms include diarrhea that lasts for 6 to 9 days, accompanied by vomiting.

Hemorrhagic cystitis caused by adenovirus occurs more often in males than in females. The child excretes grossly bloody urine for 1 to 2 weeks.

Diagnostic Tests

Viral cultures of samples from pharyngeal swabs or rectal swabs, urine, or eye drainage all yield adenovirus. Serologic tests by complement fixation can detect adenovirus if acute and convalescent sera are used. PCR testing is available to rapidly detect adenovirus.

Nursing Diagnoses and Outcomes

In addition to those identified in Nursing Plan of Care 24-1, the following nursing diagnosis and outcome may apply to the child with epidemic keratoconjunctivitis:

Nursing Diagnosis: Acute pain related to effects of conjunctivitis
Outcome: Child will report or evidence only minimal discomfort.

The following nursing diagnoses and outcomes may apply to the child with adenovirus gastroenteritis:

Nursing Diagnosis: Impaired skin integrity related to effects of diarrheal stool in contact with perianal skin
Outcome: Child's perianal skin integrity will be restored.
Nursing Diagnosis: Deficient fluid volume related to excessive diarrheal output and decreased intake
Outcome: Child will maintain adequate fluid volume and tissue perfusion evidenced by urine output of 1 mL/kg and capillary refill less than 2 seconds.

Interdisciplinary Interventions

No effective antiviral therapy exists for adenovirus. Treatment is supportive care.

If soothing saline eye drops are used for conjunctivitis, instruct the parents to wash their own hands after instilling the drops to avoid infecting themselves. Thorough hand hygiene after diapering an infant with diarrhea is essential to prevent further spread in the family.

Children with croup seem to benefit from cool-mist humidifiers. During acute exacerbations, it is often helpful for the child to breathe the water vapor created by running hot water in the shower or the cool night air (see Chapter 16).

Health care workers with adenoviral infection should avoid direct patient care for 14 days after onset of illness.

Community Care

Children in daycare centers are at increased risk for respiratory and enteric infections with adenovirus. Encourage parents to exclude their child from daycare if the child has diarrhea, conjunctivitis, or respiratory infection symptoms or if children at the center exhibit these symptoms.

ENTEROVIRUS (NONPOLIOVIRUS) INFECTIONS

Enteroviruses—classified as group A and B coxsackieviruses, echoviruses, and enteroviruses—are frequently responsible for asymptomatic, mild, and widespread illnesses in infants and children. Children with enteroviruses may present with the following signs and symptoms:

- Respiratory: coldlike symptoms, sore throat, herpangina, stomatitis, pneumonia
- Skin: rashes
- Neurologic: aseptic (viral) meningitis, encephalitis
- Gastrointestinal: nausea, vomiting, diarrhea, abdominal pain
- Eye: conjunctivitis
- Heart: myopericarditis

Children with immunodeficiencies may have persistent infection lasting for months (AAP, 2012f).

Pathophysiology

Enteroviruses are spread by respiratory droplets, by the fecal–oral route, and from mother to infant during the peripartum period. They also live for long periods on surfaces, allowing transmission by fomites. Infections occur most commonly in the summer and fall, except in tropical climates, where infections occur year-round. Respiratory viral shedding typically lasts 1 week; however, fecal viral shedding may last for several weeks. The incubation period is usually 3 to 6 days.

Assessment

Enterovirus infection most commonly presents as a nonspecific febrile illness. Because they cause a variety of illnesses, enterovirus infections may manifest in diverse ways; assess for the signs noted here.

Group B coxsackieviruses and echoviruses can cause serious disseminated disease in the newborn, which can be fatal. These infections may be transmitted either transplacentally or from mother to infant during the newborn period.

Enteroviruses commonly cause febrile illnesses in infants and young children. Many of the enteroviruses also cause rashes, particularly the coxsackieviruses and echoviruses. Hand, foot, and mouth disease is a common enterovirus illness characterized by fever, a vesicular rash on the buccal mucosa and tongue, and a maculopapular rash on the hands and feet, which may also become vesicular.

The enteroviruses commonly cause viral meningitis (Mohseni & Wilde, 2012); assess for characteristic signs and symptoms of fever, headache, malaise, and signs of meningeal irritation. This illness is self-limited, and most children have minimal morbidity (Mohseni & Wilde, 2012). Children with immunodeficiencies who develop enterovirus CNS infections may have an infection that persists for years. These children may have frequent recurrent symptoms of meningitis, encephalitis, or progressive deterioration of the CNS.

Enterovirus type 70 and coxsackievirus A24 cause subconjunctival hemorrhage with swelling, redness, congestion, tearing, and pain. Patients usually recover fully in 1 week.

Herpangina is usually caused by group A coxsackieviruses and is characterized by tiny vesicles on the tonsils, uvula, posterior pharynx, and soft palate. The illness is also accompanied by high fever, sore throat, loss of appetite, and difficulty swallowing. Some children may also experience vomiting. Herpangina typically occurs in the summer and fall and may occur in epidemics.

Group B coxsackieviruses and echoviruses cause myocarditis or pericarditis in older children. Illness ranges from a mild, self-limited pericarditis to severe chronic or even fatal myocardial disease. The enteroviruses have also been implicated as the cause of some viral cardiomyopathies.

Diagnostic Tests

The enteroviruses can be cultured from stool, rectal swab, throat specimens, urine, blood, and CSF; however, many group A coxsackieviruses do not grow well in culture. PCR is available to rapidly detect enterovirus RNA, but it cannot characterize the type of enterovirus.

Interdisciplinary Interventions

No specific therapy is available for enterovirus. IV immunoglobulin (Ig) has been used in immunodeficient patients with CNS infection, in infants with life-threatening disseminated infection, and for viral myocarditis. Provide supportive care as indicated.

Community Care

Use contact precautions for infants and young children during their illness. Educate caregivers to pay particular attention to hand hygiene when changing diapers. Also, educate caregivers, particularly child care providers, to clean contaminated surfaces with soap and water and then disinfect them with a chlorine bleach solution (¼ cup bleach to 1 gallon water), which inactivates the virus.

Herpesvirus Infections

Seven herpesviruses produce clinically important infection in humans:

1. CMV
2. EBV
3. Herpes simplex virus type 1 (HSV1)
4. Herpes simplex virus type 2 (HSV2)
5. Human herpesvirus type 6
6. Human herpesvirus type 7
7. Varicella zoster virus (VZV)

All herpesviruses can remain dormant in the body after the primary infection has subsided, producing periodic, recurrent, or latent infections. Recurrent infections are usually not as severe as the primary infection but may be life threatening in the immunocompromised host.

CYTOMEGALOVIRUS INFECTIONS

Like all herpesviruses, CMV can be reactivated after primary infection. Almost everyone encounters CMV eventually. However, the infection is usually asymptomatic and of little consequence. An infectious mononucleosis-like syndrome may occur in adolescents and adults. CMV can cause pneumonia, colitis, and retinitis in immunosuppressed individuals, such as those undergoing organ transplantation, receiving chemotherapy, or infected with HIV.

CMV congenital infection also occurs and is typically asymptomatic. Approximately 10% of infants with congenital CMV infection present with serious illness, however, such as growth retardation, jaundice, purpura, microcephaly, intracranial calcifications, or retinitis. Between 10% and 20% of congenitally infected infants are diagnosed with intellectual disability or sensorineural deafness in childhood (AAP, 2012d).

Transmission of CMV is by direct contact with virus-containing secretions, such as urine or saliva. This contact can occur in daycare centers or nurseries when drooling, teething babies share toys that they bite or gum. Adolescents may acquire CMV through sexual intercourse and kissing (saliva). Transmission from an infected mother to her infant may occur by transplacental passage of the virus in utero, passage of the neonate through an infected birth canal, or ingestion of infected breast milk. Other modes of transmission include blood transfusions and solid organ transplants.

Reactivation of CMV after transplantation could contribute to organ rejection. It is believed that CMV is in itself immunosuppressive, suppressing the activity of natural killer cells and contributing to immunosuppression in children with HIV infection and other infections.

Assessment

Most CMV infections are asymptomatic. A few individuals may exhibit a vague mononucleosis-like illness with fatigue, fever, and mild hepatitis. Immunocompromised children may experience pneumonia, gastritis, colitis, arthralgia, arthritis, encephalopathy, retinitis, fever, and lymphadenopathy. AIDS patients with reactivated CMV, if untreated, may develop vision loss caused by CMV retinitis.

Most infants with congenital CMV infection are asymptomatic, but about 12.7% manifest fetal damage at birth (Kadambari et al., 2011), as summarized in Chart 24-2. Long-term sequelae such as hearing loss or cognitive or neurologic impairment occur more often and are more severe in symptomatic infants than in asymptomatic infants (40% to 58% vs. 13.5%) (Dollard et al., 2007).

Despite the physical signs with which a symptomatic newborn typically presents, and even if cerebral

---

CHART 24-2   Effects of Congenital Cytomegalovirus Infection

- Intrauterine growth retardation
- Jaundice, hepatitis, hepatosplenomegaly
- Anemia, thrombocytopenia
- "Blueberry muffin" rash (deep, bluish, purpuric lesions)
- Celery stalking (radiographic lines in the long bones)
- Chorioretinitis
- Cerebral calcifications, intellectual disability, microcephaly, seizures, hearing loss

calcifications are evidenced on radiographs, viral culture or serologic testing is still needed to confirm the diagnosis. Viral culture specimens can be obtained from urine or from pharyngeal or cervical secretions. CMV can also be isolated from human milk, semen, and leukocytes. In addition, the presence of Ig CMV antibodies in cord blood can identify congenitally infected infants. The shell vial assay is the standard rapid culture method for detecting CMV infections. Newer methods for CMV detection include a CMV antigenemia assay, which detects a viral protein in the infant's white blood cells, and PCR, which detects CMV DNA.

Nursing Diagnoses and Outcomes

In addition to those listed in Nursing Plan of Care 24-1, the following nursing diagnosis and outcomes may apply to the infant affected with congenital CMV:

Nursing Diagnosis: Interrupted family processes related to reaction to extremely ill infant
Outcomes:
• Parents will express concerns regarding the infant's treatments and prognosis.
• Family will visit the newborn frequently, maintain mutual support, and seek external resources as needed.
• Parents will be involved in the infant's care.

Interdisciplinary Interventions

Treatment for CMV, especially retinitis, is with ganciclovir or foscarnet. Antiviral drugs are given by induction therapy (doses that gradually increase over 3 weeks to the therapeutic dosage). Limited studies show that ganciclovir is beneficial in children (Kadambari et al., 2011). However, more studies are needed to verify its safety and effectiveness in children (AAP, 2012d). After therapeutic levels are reached, some HIV-infected children and bone marrow transplant recipients are given 6 to 12 weeks of maintenance therapy with reduced dosages. Even with reduced dosages, ganciclovir and foscarnet are highly toxic. Ganciclovir may induce bone marrow toxicity, and foscarnet can trigger renal tubular dysfunction.

Focus nursing care of infants or children who may have congenital CMV syndrome or who may be shedding CMV on supportive care and good hand hygiene. The risk of acquiring CMV infection during pregnancy can provoke anxiety among health care workers who are pregnant or planning to become pregnant because of the risk of congenital CMV syndrome.

However, the common notion that nurses and other health care workers are at increased risk for acquiring CMV from pediatric or neonatal patients is a misconception. Many studies of CMV transmission in health care settings have concluded that health care workers acquire CMV at the same rate as the general population (Balcarek et al., 1990; Morgan et al., 2003). Standard precautions are important, however, because any patient could reactivate CMV at any time because of stress and could shed the virus in the urine, saliva, and other body fluids. Neonates can also shed CMV. Therefore, infants and children who have not been identified as infected may pose a greater risk to others, especially if standard precautions are not followed.

caREminder

The CDC does not recommend isolating infants with congenital CMV infection (Siegel et al., 2007). Instead, the CDC recommends using standard precautions and educating health care workers (especially pregnant ones) about hand hygiene.

EPSTEIN-BARR VIRUS INFECTION

EBV, the causative agent in mononucleosis, infects up to 90% of the population (Odumade et al., 2011). Mononucleosis is transmitted primarily by oral–salivary spread in young children and close intimate contact (kissing) in adolescents and young adults. Illnesses with EBV range from asymptomatic to fulminant lymphoproliferative disease (AAP, 2012e). EBV is also associated with malignancies such as Burkitt lymphoma, nasopharyngeal cancer, Hodgkin disease, and some autoimmune disorders, such as Sjögren syndrome.

EBV is a member of the herpes family of viruses and, like all herpesviruses, can be reactivated after primary infection.

Assessment

Symptoms of mononucleosis present as a triad: sore throat (exudative pharyngitis), fever, and lymphadenopathy. Ask about other common signs and symptoms, which include fatigue, headache, and an enlarged liver or spleen. Jaundice is uncommon, occurring in only 5% to 10% of cases (Odumade et al., 2011). Although a rash is not typical, a central rash may occur during the first few days of the illness.

The disease can begin insidiously over 30 to 50 days after the 4- to 6-week incubation period, or it may begin abruptly after the incubation period. In general, symptoms are more pronounced in adolescents than in children who may be asymptomatic. Coinfection with group A strep pharyngitis is common and could mask the symptoms of EBV, leading the health care practitioner to overlook the diagnosis of mononucleosis during the early stages of illness (Fig. 24-5).

Diagnostic Tests

The total number of atypical lymphocytes in the blood characteristically increases, along with a high titer of heterophil antibody. Monocytes constitute 50% of the total white blood cell count. The overall leukocytosis that is present early in the disease can be so elevated that leukemia is suspected.

Diagnosis is based on a blood count showing lymphocytosis and at least 10% atypical lymphocyte formation, symptoms, and testing for heterophil antibody. In young children, the heterophil antibody test is usually negative.

Viral cultures can be obtained from saliva, blood, or lymph tissue but can take up to 8 weeks to cultivate.

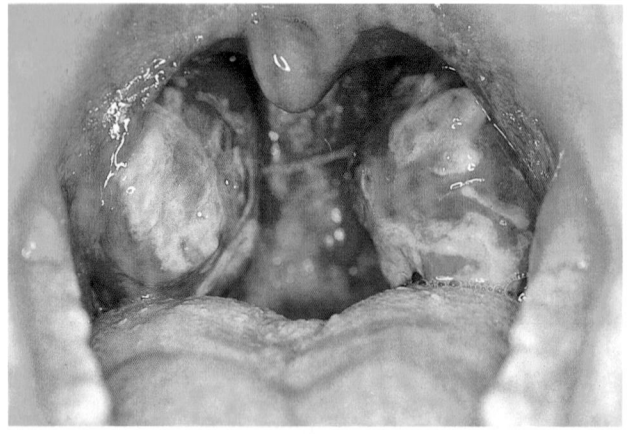

Figure 24-5 Appearance of tonsils in a child with infectious mononucleosis. Note the degree of erythema, enlargement, and purulent covering. Copyright Dr. P. Marazzi/SPL/Science Source/Photo researchers. Reprinted with permission.

EBV-specific antibody tests are most commonly used to diagnose EBV. During the course of mononucleosis, EBV produces an initial antiviral capsid antigen immunoglobulin M (anti-VCA IgM). This VCA IgM declines to barely detectable levels over time. As VCA IgM starts to decline, there is a detectable increase in anti-VCA IgG. Antibodies to EBV nuclear antigen appear during the recovery phase of infection. EBV VCA IgG and EBV nuclear antigen persist for life.

PCR testing is also useful in determining the presence of EBV DNA. A positive test is indicative of infection but must be quantitated to differentiate acute infection from past infection.

Nursing Diagnoses and Outcomes

In addition to those listed in Nursing Plan of Care 24-1, the following nursing diagnosis and outcome may apply to the child with EBV:

Nursing Diagnosis: Fatigue related to effects of disease process
Outcome: Child will obtain adequate rest and perform age-appropriate quiet activities as tolerated.

Interdisciplinary Interventions

In general, no therapy is currently recommended for EBV. Steroids should be used only to control life-threatening complications such as enlarged tonsils blocking the airway, fulminant hepatitis, or hemolytic anemia. Ganciclovir is used to treat EBV infection in the immunosuppressed population.

caREminder

> *Avoid ampicillin if concomitant streptococcal pharyngitis is present. Use of ampicillin causes a rash in most individuals with mononucleosis.*

No isolation precautions are recommended for the hospitalized patient. Most otherwise healthy children and adolescents recover with no sequelae. Provide supportive nursing care and educate the family regarding comfort techniques such as antipyretics for fever reduction and pain relief (e.g., medications; dark, quiet room).

Suggest a soft or liquid diet for children with throat pain. Encourage enough liquids to prevent dehydration. Because of their chronic fatigue, children and adolescents usually self-limit their activity; thus, forced bed rest is not necessary. Recommend home teachers for children with prolonged fatigue who cannot attend school. Teach children and parents to notify the health care provider if abdominal pain, especially in the left upper quadrant, or left shoulder pain occurs (may indicate splenic rupture).

KidKare Advise children with an enlarged spleen to limit activity until they are cleared by their health care providers. The risk of splenic rupture is highest in the first 3 weeks of illness, but cases have been reported 7 weeks after symptom onset. There is no consensus on when contact activity can be resumed. Resolution of any complications and clinical judgment determine when activity can be resumed. If an athlete is asymptomatic, afebrile, and well hydrated, he or she may resume activity to his or her level of physical fitness 3 (Putukian et al., 2008) to 4 weeks (O'Connor et al., 2011) after diagnosis.

HERPES SIMPLEX VIRUS INFECTIONS

HSV1 and HSV2 produce similar clinical syndromes. Generally, HSV1 is associated with oral lesions (above the waist) and HSV2 is associated with genital lesions (below the waist). However, HSV1 infections can occur in the genital area, and HSV2 infections can occur orally. The appearance of HSV1 and HSV2 lesions is identical: vesicular lesions on an erythematous base.

Transmission and acquisition of HSV infection is most often asymptomatic, which has contributed to a worldwide epidemic. In the United States, it is estimated that more than 50% of young adults are infected with HSV1, and 20% to 30% are infected with HSV2 (AAP, 2012j).

HSV infection can also be passed to the fetus or neonate by maternal genital HSV infection. Because most genital HSV infections are asymptomatic, the mother is often unaware of her infection or the risk to the infant. Maternal transmission to the fetus occurs during passage through an infected birth canal or as an ascending infection with prolonged (longer than 6 hours) rupture of amniotic membranes (Straface et al., 2012). Occasionally, during a primary maternal infection, the virus crosses the placenta during the maternal viremic phase, when a high volume of virus is circulating in the maternal blood.

The incidence of neonatal HSV infection ranges from 1 in 3,000 live births to 1 in 20,000 live births. The greatest risk of infection is in infants born to mothers with primary infection (33% to 50%). The risk is much lower in infants of mothers with recurrent infection (<5%). The presence of maternal HSV antibodies from past recurrent infection can serve to protect the infant during pregnancy. Neonatal HSV infection is caused by HSV2 at least 75% of the time (AAP, 2012j).

Children with dermatitis are at increased risk of developing eczema herpeticum, a disseminated HSV infection of the skin. Teach the family to use caution to avoid exposing the skin of children with dermatitis to cold sores whenever possible.

Untreated infants with disseminated disease soon develop respiratory and circulatory collapse, with death following. Even with antiviral treatment, the mortality rate among neonates with disseminated disease is 25%. Surviving infants often face the lifelong sequelae of neurologic impairment, blindness, and recurrent skin lesions. Although most infants with isolated CNS involvement survive, almost all sustain considerable neurologic sequelae. The best outcome is in infants with disease limited to the skin, eyes, and mouth (Wolfert et al., 2011).

 QUESTION: Based on Ashley's complaints, would the school nurse suspect a genital herpes infection?

Assessment

Primary genital infections often involve painful labial and cervical lesions in females or penile lesions in males; assess for such lesions. Inguinal lymphadenopathy may be present. Systemic illness including fever, muscle aches, and malaise lasting about a week may also occur with primary infection. Recurrent infections are generally less severe and, in females, may be limited to the cervix, which has few nerve endings for pain. Thus, many recurrent infections are asymptomatic. For these reasons, monitor pregnant females for signs of primary genital herpes infection. HSV2 infections typically are acquired from sexual activity; evaluate for sexual molestation when the infection is present in nonneonates.

Neonatal herpes presents in three distinct groups: disseminated disease; isolated CNS involvement; and localized infection of the skin, eyes, and mucous membranes. However, infants with CNS involvement can also have localized disease as well. Neonatal HSV infection manifests within the first 3 weeks of life, typically 7 to 10 days after birth (Chart 24-3).

Oral HSV infections range from mild "cold sores" to gingivostomatitis. Shedding of herpesvirus occurs in

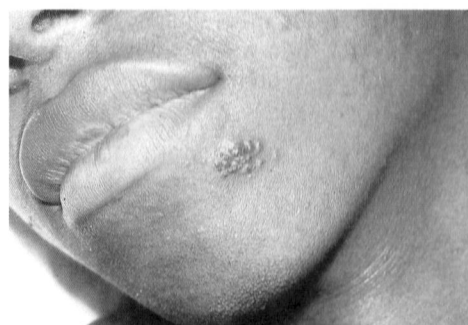
Figure 24-6 Lesions in herpes simplex.

the saliva. Monitor for dehydration because the mouth becomes intolerably sore with severe gingivostomatitis, resulting in decreased intake. Illness usually begins with a fever, sore mouth, and anorexia. Lesions can extend to the entire mouth area, tongue, gums, and inside of the cheek (buccal mucosa). Infants or children who suck their thumbs or fingers can develop herpetic whitlow (herpetic lesions appearing on the fingers or thumb).

Primary infections begin with an "aura" or tingling sensation; note this when obtaining a history. Then, 24 to 48 hours later, painful vesicular lesions with an erythematous base erupt. The lesions typically last 10 to 14 days (Fig. 24-6).

HSV1 infection has been transmitted during athletic competitions that involve close physical contact and frequent skin abrasions (AAP, 2012j). Wrestling and rugby are the sports most commonly associated with the transmission of HSV1. Transmission may occur through active lesions or asymptomatic viral shedding. Teach coaches and athletes to clean mats and sports equipment with a bleach solution between matches to limit or prevent the spread of HSV.

Diagnostic Tests

HSV is easily cultured from skin lesions; 1 to 3 days are required for viral detection. Rapid diagnosis is made with detection of HSV antigens in lesion swabs using commercially available ELISA kits. Commercially available ELISA antibody blood test kits can be used to identify recent (IgM) or past (IgG) HSV infection. A Western blot for HSV can distinguish between HSV1 and HSV2. PCR testing rapidly detects HSV DNA in CSF and blood.

ANSWER: The school nurse might suspect a genital herpes infection because it is an STI. However, genital herpes infection would involve painful labial and cervical lesions. Ashley has complained of burning on urination and increased vaginal discharge but no pain in the genital area.

Nursing Diagnoses and Outcomes

The common nursing diagnoses and outcomes discussed in Nursing Plan of Care 24-1 apply to the infant with congenital herpes simplex infection. Depending on the

---

CHART 24-3 Effects of Congenital Herpes Simplex Virus Infection

- Nonspecific symptoms: irritability, fever, poor feeding, lethargy
- Intrauterine growth retardation
- Jaundice, hepatitis, hepatosplenomegaly
- Anemia, thrombocytopenia (characterized as blueberry muffin purpura), disseminated intravascular coagulopathy
- Vesicular lesions on the infant's skin, eyes, or mucous membranes
- Chorioretinitis
- Meningoencephalitis, cerebral calcifications, intellectual disability, microcephaly, seizures
- Pneumonitis

disease manifestations, other diagnoses may also be appropriate. For the child with acquired herpes simplex disease, the following nursing diagnosis and outcomes may apply:

Nursing Diagnosis: Impaired oral mucous membrane related to effects of herpesvirus
***Outcomes*:**
- Child will ingest sufficient fluid to prevent dehydration.
- Child and family will implement interventions to minimize discomfort and speed healing.

Interdisciplinary Interventions

Treatment for congenital infection is with IV acyclovir. Disseminated and CNS disease should be treated for a minimum of 21 days; localized (skin, eyes, or mucous membrane) disease should be treated for 14 days. Topical treatment for eye involvement is usually with trifluridine, idoxuridine, or vidarabine. The pregnant mother or the adolescent with genital HSV infection can be treated with oral acyclovir, valacyclovir, or famciclovir to decrease viral shedding and encourage faster resolution of the lesions. Suppressive therapy may be offered to patients with more than six outbreaks a year. Because the lesions of varicella and herpes simplex resemble each other, varicella infection is considered in the differential diagnosis for an infant who may have a congenital herpes infection.

Educate postpartum women with active herpes lesions on the value of hand hygiene. Transmission of HSV to the infant can occur if the mother touches the baby with contaminated hands. HSV transmitted to the mother's hands after postpartum pericare can be washed off with soap and water. Mothers, fathers, grandparents, or any visitor who has active oral HSV lesions should not kiss the infant because they can transmit their virus to the infant.

Use contact precautions with the infant with congenital herpes simplex infection. Advise parents to exclude their child with HSV mouth sores from daycare only if the child *cannot* control oral secretions (drooling). Ensure that health care workers with active oral lesions wear surgical masks to cover the lesions, avoid touching the lesions, and pay scrupulous attention to hand hygiene.

HUMAN HERPESVIRUS INFECTIONS

Infection with human herpesvirus type 6 or type 7, also known as *roseola*, is a common childhood rash disease. Roseola is typically characterized by a high fever that is followed by a rash and may lead to febrile convulsions. The virus is thought to be transmitted primarily through the respiratory secretions of infected children. Infection seldom occurs before the age of 6 months, and nearly all children are infected by 2 to 3 years of age. Viral shedding continues after the rash and fever subside. The incubation period is approximately 9 days (Dyer, 2007).

Assessment

Suspect roseola in a child who does not appear ill despite 3 to 5 days of high fever (103° to 104° F [39.4° to 40° C]); typically, the child is quite playful. A rash appears briefly after the fever subsides. The rash begins centrally (on the trunk) and then spreads to the neck, arms, and legs. The rash is rose colored and blanches under pressure. It can disappear within hours of its initial appearance.

The diagnosis of roseola is based on the clinical presentation. PCR testing is available, but standardized interpretation has not been established. Some research virology laboratories may be able to isolate the virus from blood.

Nursing Diagnoses and Outcomes

In addition to those listed in Nursing Plan of Care 24-1, the following nursing diagnosis and outcomes may apply to the child with roseola:

Nursing Diagnosis: Risk for injury related to the effects of the fever (febrile seizures)
***Outcomes*:**
- Child will experience no sequelae of the fever.
- Parents will implement fever management interventions.

Interdisciplinary Interventions

Isolating the infant is not necessary if the infant is hospitalized. Nursing care consists of standard precautions and supportive care. Acetaminophen or ibuprofen is given to reduce fever. Implement seizure precautions and anticonvulsants, such as phenobarbital, as ordered for children with a history of febrile convulsions (AAP, 2012k). Tepid baths can be given to augment the effects of antipyretic agents (see thePoint Procedures: Cooling Measures).

VARICELLA ZOSTER VIRUS INFECTION

Primary VZV infection is commonly known as *chickenpox*; the recurrent form is known as *shingles*. Varicella is a common, relatively benign childhood illness; however, complications of varicella are increasingly common. They include secondary bacterial infections of the skin, pneumonia, and encephalitis. Varicella tends to be more severe in adolescents and adults, and the immunocompromised are at risk for more serious complications, including disseminated disease or even death.

Varicella is transmitted by direct contact with the vesicles and by the airborne route (AAP, 2012aa). As the child talks, coughs, and sneezes, viral particles can become airborne. Although 95% of all adults are immune to varicella because of a history of the disease, maternal varicella can occur, leading to fetal infection. Fetal infection during the first or second trimester can cause limb atrophy, scarring of the arms and legs, eye and CNS disorders, or fetal death.

Once a person is infected with varicella, the virus remains in the body, hidden among the dorsal root and trigeminal nerve ganglia. Reactivation of varicella causes shingles, which can occur years to decades later and can produce painful lesions along the ganglia (nerve pathways). Reactivation is triggered by exposure to a stressor, such as excessive sunlight, extreme cold, labor, the loss of a loved one, job loss, chemotherapy, or other forms of immune suppression.

Assessment

After an incubation period of 10 to 21 days, the illness begins with a low-grade fever and malaise. Assess for the vesicular lesions that characterize the disease, which usually begin as superficial vesicular lesions that resemble dewdrops on the skin. A red base develops, followed by pustules. The rash is extremely pruritic. The lesions appear in successive crops over several days and affect the trunk, scalp, face, and extremities. Lesions can appear on the mucous membranes of the eyes, vagina, rectum, mouth, and throat. Sunburned skin and diapered areas have significantly more lesions, but they are often smaller than in other areas. Between 5 and 7 days after onset, the lesions begin to crust (Fig. 24-7).

The VZV PCR test is the method of choice for quickly diagnosing VZV. ELISA is the most common antibody test used to determine immunity. Paired sera for acute and convalescent antibodies can be used to determine acute infection. Collecting the virus using skin scrapings and then staining with immunofluorescent monoclonal antibodies can rule out herpes simplex. Because the tests are specific for VZV, test results are positive for an infected child.

Interdisciplinary Interventions

As with all vaccine-preventable illnesses, prevention is the best management (see Chapter 8 for discussion of the varicella vaccine). Varicella zoster immune globulin (VZIG) is given to immunosuppressed children immediately after exposure to someone with varicella. VZIG is given in the hope of preventing varicella, because varicella infection in an immunosuppressed child can be life threatening. VZIG decreases the infection's effects on the already weakened immune system. For hospitalized children who receive VZIG prophylactically, use airborne isolation precautions from day 10 to day 28 after the exposure occurs.

Treatment for immunocompromised patients and pregnant patients with severe complications involves administration of IV acyclovir.

Children with active varicella are rarely hospitalized. If a child with varicella is hospitalized, maintain isolation precautions. Place the child in a private room, preferably a negative-pressure room. If the child must leave the room for tests or procedures, ensure that the child wears a mask. Examine the child's skin for new lesions daily. When lesions have begun to crust and no new lesions appear, isolation precautions can be discontinued after 5 more days. To relieve the child's boredom of being confined in an isolation room, ask the child life specialist to bring washable toys, videotapes, DVDs, or games into the room.

The most common complication of varicella is secondary bacterial infection caused by the child scratching the lesions. Teach the child and parents interventions that promote comfort and prevent infection or scarring caused by scratching the lesions (Teaching Intervention Plan 24-1).

Parents may sometimes need to bring a child with active varicella to the health care provider's office. Teach parents to alert the office staff about the child's potential diagnosis. Many physicians' offices have an alternative entrance for contagious children.

Community Care

Varicella has a large effect on families in which both parents work and the child attends daycare. Because the child is highly contagious, a parent must often stay home with the sick child. Nurses can encourage parents to explore alternative babysitting arrangements with agencies that accommodate sick children.

HIV AND AIDS

HIV is a retrovirus that attacks the immune system by destroying T lymphocytes (cells that are critical to fighting infection and developing immunity). Untreated, HIV infection renders the immune system useless, and the child is unable to fight even the most benign infection. HIV infection leads to AIDS. There are two types of HIV: HIV type 1 and HIV type 2 (most commonly found in Africa).

Globally, approximately 2.5 million children younger than 15 years of age were living with HIV in 2009 (Joint United Nations Programme on HIV/AIDS [UNAIDS], 2010). An estimated 390,000 children younger than 15 years of age became infected in 2010, a 30% decrease from 2002 to 2003 (WHO, 2011). In 2010, an estimated 250,000 children younger than 15 years of age worldwide died from AIDS-related causes; 20% fewer than in 2005 (WHO, 2011). Worldwide, AIDS accounts for 3% of deaths in children younger than 5 years of age (WHO, 2011).

Three chief modes of transmission exist for HIV (Chart 24-4). Blood transfusions and administration of clotting factors are rarely modes of transmission, because donated blood is tested and clotting factors are heat treated. Mother-to-child transmission (MTCT) accounts for almost all new HIV infections in the preadolescent population (AAP, 2012l). In developed countries, the total number of children with AIDS has dropped dramatically during the past decade, thanks to routine use of antiretroviral therapy in HIV-infected women. MTCT rates are less than 2% in developed countries but 25% to 40% in developing countries (Prendergast et al., 2007). One

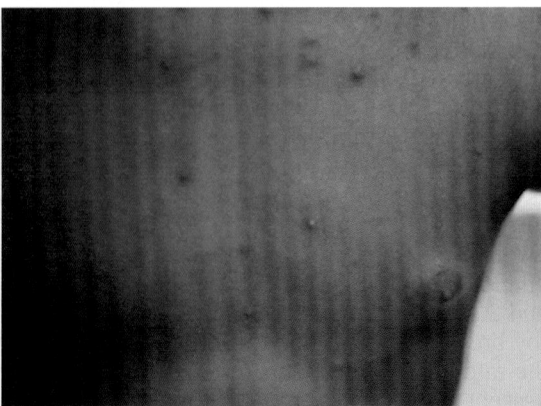

Figure 24-7 Varicella lesions.

TIP 24-1: A TEACHING INTERVENTION PLAN for the Child With Varicella

Nursing Diagnoses and Family Outcomes

- Risk for impaired skin integrity related to effects of pruritic skin lesions
- Risk for infection related to effects of scratching
  Outcomes: Child will not develop secondary infection.
  Child will experience minimal discomfort from pruritus.

Teach Child/Family

Managing Discomfort and Rash

- The best treatment for skin discomfort is a cool bath with soothing colloidal oatmeal (e.g., Aveeno) every 3–4 hours for the first few days. Calamine lotion may help decrease itching. If the itching becomes severe or interferes with sleep, give the child a nonprescription antihistamine (diphenhydramine hydrochloride [Benadryl]).
- Keep fingernails short. Wash child's hands frequently with antibacterial soap to reduce bacterial colonization.
- Remind child not to scratch lesions. If the young child scratches at lesions, consider applying mittens or cotton socks over hands.

- If urination becomes painful, apply some 2.5% lidocaine (Xylocaine) or 1% dibucaine (Nupercainal) ointment (nonprescription) to the genital lesions every 2–3 hours to relieve pain.
- Administer acetaminophen for fever. Aspirin should be avoided in children and adolescents with varicella because of the link with Reye syndrome.
- If child is uncomfortable because of oral lesions, offer cool fluids; ice pops; or soft, bland food. Avoid citrus, spicy, or salty foods. If mouth ulcers become troublesome, have the child gargle or swallow 1 tsp to 1 tbsp of an antacid solution four times a day after meals.

Contact Health Care Provider if

- Red, tender areas are noted on skin or a speckled, fine rash develops
- Child seems very sick or develops the following: difficulty awakening, stiff neck, trouble walking, difficulty breathing or rapid breathing, or vomiting more than three times
- Scabs become soft and drain pus
- Fever lasts more than 4 days

CHART 24-4 Transmission of HIV

Modes of Transmission

- Sexual contact (both heterosexual and men having sex with men [MSM] or women having sex with women [WSW])
- Percutaneous or mucous membrane exposure to needles or other sharp instruments contaminated with blood or bloody body fluids
- Mother-to-infant transmission before or around the time of birth

Timing of Transmission

- Intrauterine: HIV can be detected in aborted fetal tissue as early as 8 weeks.
- Intrapartum: In twin pregnancies, the incidence of infection is higher among the first twin born.
- Postpartum: HIV-positive mother breastfeeds the infant, and the infant acquires HIV infection from the breast milk.

Maternal Factors That Determine Transmission of HIV

- Low maternal CD4+ lymphocyte counts (<100): advanced HIV disease
- High maternal viral load
- Presence of sexually transmitted infections, such as syphilis, which tax the immune system and cause placental inflammation, compromising the placental barrier
- Zidovudine therapy during pregnancy: reduces transmission of HIV to the baby by 67%

of the United Nation's Millennium Development Goals is to eliminate MTCT of HIV (WHO, 2010a). Coverage with antiretroviral regimens to prevent MTCT in low- and middle-income countries was 48% in 2010 (WHO, 2011).

Several maternal factors determine the likelihood of HIV transmission to the infant (see Chart 24-4). The main goal in prenatal care of the pregnant woman with AIDS is to decrease her viral load by giving her highly active antiretroviral therapy (HAART) during the pregnancy. Prolonged rupture of the membranes in a mother with a detectable viral load increases the risk of transmission of HIV to her infant. In these cases, cesarean section may lessen the risk of HIV transmission. Diagnosing and promptly treating occult STIs is necessary.

Babies born to HIV-positive women may test positive for HIV antibody. This result is actually a measure of maternal antibody and not indicative of true infection. Usually, 13% to 39% (one in four) of babies born to untreated HIV-positive mothers are actually infected (AAP, 2012l). Infants may remain HIV antibody positive for as long as 18 months because of the slow rate of decay of maternal HIV antibody. Therefore, true infections in infants must be confirmed by detecting HIV in culture or by PCR testing for HIV DNA or RNA.

HIV can be transmitted postnatally through breastfeeding. Although this risk of transmission is low in the United States, worldwide HIV is thought to be transmitted by breastfeeding in one third to one half of cases.

The rate of HIV infection continues to increase in the adolescent population, primarily through sexual exposure. Adolescents account for approximately 50% of new

HIV cases each year (AAP, 2012l). Most HIV-infected adolescents are asymptomatic.

caREminder

Routinely offer HIV testing to all pregnant adolescents. If test results are positive, administration of HAART significantly decreases (from 25% to 8%) the likelihood of perinatal transmission.

Pathophysiology

The sole purpose of HIV is to replicate or make copies of itself. It enters a cell, basically takes over the DNA, and commandeers the cell to make copies of HIV. Although HIV selects T4 lymphocytes as the preferred cells, it invades many other cells as well. However, T4 cell invasion is important because T4 lymphocytes defend the body against invading pathogens. HIV either renders T4 cells dysfunctional or creates "holes" in the membranes of T4 cells, resulting in osmotic pressure differences between the outside and the inside of the cell that cause the cells to literally destroy themselves. Thus, T4 cells are depleted in number and cannot signal B cells to form protective antibodies to fight off the invading virus. In short, HIV targets the immune system to leave the body defenseless.

The prognosis for an HIV-infected child who has the first AIDS-defining illness (Chart 24-5) during the first year of life is usually grim, especially if the first illness is *Pneumocystis jiroveci* pneumonia (PCP). Children who can fend off the first AIDS-defining illness have the best prognosis. The use of early HAART and adjunctive therapies, including PCP prophylaxis, has substantially improved survival rates among children with HIV infection (Nesheim et al., 2007).

Assessment

Most children infected with HIV develop symptoms within the first year of life. The remainder become symptomatic sometime before age 5 years. HIV-infected children typically present with generalized lymphadenopathy, enlarged liver and spleen, failure to thrive, thrush, diarrhea, growth and developmental delays, and frequent recurrent infections.

Examine the history carefully. Untreated children, with their immature immune systems, may have recurrent opportunistic infections (see Chart 24-5). PCP is one of the most common AIDS-defining diseases in children. Along with PCP, children may experience at least two serious bacterial infections in 2 years. These infections are typically sepsis, otitis media, chronic sinusitis, meningitis, gastroenteritis, and pneumonia (see also thePoint Care Path: An Interdisciplinary Plan of Care for the Child With AIDS Pneumonia). The causative organism varies, although *S. pneumoniae* is a common cause.

Differential diagnosis in children with HIV is often difficult. Many conditions mimic HIV and the failure to thrive that it causes (Chart 24-6). For example, children born with congenital heart defects often fail to thrive because of the severity of their lesions. Inborn errors of metabolism and genetic causes of immunodeficiency must also be ruled out. Typical TORCH infections could be opportunistic infections in the HIV-infected child.

CHART 24-5   AIDS-Defining Illnesses in Children With HIV Infection

- Candidiasis: esophagus, trachea, bronchi, or lungs
- Coccidioidomycosis: disseminated or extrapulmonary
- Cryptococcoses: extrapulmonary
- Cryptosporidiosis: chronic intestinal
- CMV disease: (other than liver, spleen, lymph nodes) in children older than 1 month of age
- CMV retinitis: loss of vision
- Chronic herpes simplex: ulcer (longer than 1 month), pneumonitis, esophagitis in children older than 1 month of age
- Histoplasmosis: disseminated or extrapulmonary
- HIV encephalopathy
- Isosporosis: chronic (longer than 1 month)
- Kaposi sarcoma: rare in young children
- Lymphoid interstitial pneumonitis
- Lymphoma, primary brain
- Lymphoma (Burkitt or immunoblastic sarcoma)
- *Mycobacterium avium* complex or *Mycobacterium kansasii* (disseminated or extrapulmonary)
- *Mycobacterium tuberculosis:* disseminated or extrapulmonary
- *Pneumocystis jiroveci* pneumonia
- Progressive multifocal leukoencephalopathy
- Toxoplasmosis of brain: onset in child older than 1 month of age
- Wasting syndrome caused by HIV

CHART 24-6   Conditions That Mimic Pediatric AIDS

Condition: Description

- Cardiac syndrome: poor contractility, myocarditis, heart failure
- Chronic pneumonitis: lymphoid interstitial pneumonitis, pulmonary lymphoid hyperplasia
- Encephalopathy or myelopathy: progressive encephalopathy, subcortical dementia, impaired brain growth, neoplasm, stroke
- Hematologic syndrome: idiopathic thrombocytopenic purpura, lymphadenopathy
- Hepatitis syndrome: hepatosplenomegaly, hyperbilirubinemia
- Malignancies: lymphoreticular tumors, Burkitt lymphoma, leiomyosarcomas
- Opportunistic infections: *Pneumocystis jiroveci* pneumonia
- Renal syndrome: progressive glomerulopathy
- Wasting syndrome: failure to thrive, wasting

Diagnostic Tests

During infancy, diagnosis of HIV requires detection of HIV by culture or of HIV DNA or RNA by PCR, because ELISA and Western blot tests for HIV antibody may be positive from the presence of maternal antibody. A presumptive diagnosis of HIV can be made on the basis of a single positive HIV culture or PCR; however, two negative tests are required to rule out HIV infection. Routine ELISA and Western blot tests for HIV antibody may be used to diagnose HIV in children after the age of 12 to 18 months.

Interdisciplinary Interventions

Maternal treatment consists of oral zidovudine during the pregnancy and intravenously during delivery. Zidovudine reduces the likelihood of transmission without harming the fetus. The newborn also receives zidovudine for 6 weeks after birth (AAP, 2012l).

The goal of treatment is to keep the child as healthy as possible for as long as possible. Zidovudine effectively interferes with HIV replication but can cause bone marrow suppression and nausea. If it fails, or the child cannot tolerate it, the health care provider may select another antiretroviral drug.

PCP prophylaxis with trimethoprim–sulfamethoxazole (Septra or Bactrim) should begin at 4 to 6 weeks of age and continue through the first year of life. After 1 year of age, PCP prophylaxis should be started when CD4 cell counts start to decrease. Age-appropriate immunizations are given on schedule as long as CD4 counts are normal. Live-virus vaccines should be held if CD4 counts are low or the child is severely immunocompromised.

Antiretroviral therapy is indicated for most children and adolescents with HIV; however, in asymptomatic patients with normal CD4 counts, antiretroviral therapy may not be started right away. Combination antiretroviral therapy (HAART) is more effective than monotherapy, preferably with three drugs when possible (Panel on Antiretroviral Therapy and Medical Management of HIV-Infected Children, 2011). The nurse plays an important role in supporting adherence to medication regime. Caregiver report, pharmacy refill report, and maintenance of appointments together are predictive of adherence (Burrack et al., 2010).

Nursing care of HIV-positive infants and children involves using standard precautions. Because these children have many needs and the mothers of HIV-positive infants may not have health insurance because of homelessness, IV drug abuse, or unemployment, involve social services as soon as possible. Refer mothers and infants to the dietitian for counseling to prevent the general decline in nutritional status of HIV-positive children. In developed countries, teach mothers with HIV not to breastfeed. In developing countries, the risk of infant mortality from nutritional deficiency and other infectious diseases outweighs the risk of HIV transmission. Explain all current medications, especially antiviral drugs and PCP prophylaxis, to the primary caregiver. HIV disease is a chronic condition. Encourage children to practice healthy lifestyles and lead well-rounded lives. Discuss discipline and family standards with parents

(see Chapter 12). Collaboration between adolescent and adult care providers and adequate preparation for transitioning the youth to adult care can maintain continuity of care and improve adherence (Maturo et al., 2011).

Community Care

Many educators and government officials believe that education and prevention are the best ways to manage HIV disease. Recommend safer sex practices. Although the only 100% safe sex practice is abstinence, safer sex can be achieved through using latex condoms; having a monogamous relationship; and avoiding substances, such as drugs and alcohol, that cloud judgment.

Children cope with the diagnosis of AIDS in different ways at different ages (Developmental Considerations 24-1). Assist the family by listening to their concerns and making appropriate referrals to the various agencies and organizations that can offer both social and financial support.

MEASLES

Measles is a serious disease that is highly communicable. It is an acute viral illness characterized by fever, cough, **coryza** (acute rhinitis), conjunctivitis, rash, and Koplik spots. Measles complications include otitis media, pneumonia, and encephalitis. Acute encephalitis resulting in permanent brain damage occurs in approximately 1 out of every 1,000 cases in the United States (AAP, 2012m). Measles can be fatal in children younger than 5 years of age, immunocompromised children, and children with severe malnutrition.

The routine use of the measles vaccine has dramatically decreased the incidence of measles (see Chapter 8 for a discussion of vaccines). In 2000, measles was declared eliminated from the United States, but cases of measles continue to occur when the virus is imported from other countries. There was a median of 60 cases and four outbreaks per year from 2001 to 2010 (CDC, 2011a).

CROSS-CULTURAL CARE

Underimmunized populations, especially in large urban areas, are at risk for measles. Immigrants, members of religious groups that prohibit vaccination, and homeless or impoverished people are frequently unvaccinated. Some have limited access to health care; others lack adequate knowledge of the health care system.

Pathophysiology

Measles is a seasonal disease. Outbreaks peak during the winter and spring. It is highly contagious and is transmitted by the airborne route. It can be spread directly by coughing or sneezing or indirectly by airborne-suspended droplets. The child harbors the virus in nasopharyngeal secretions during the acute stage of the illness. The typical incubation period is 8 to 12 days. Children are contagious from 1 to 2 days before the rash appears until 4 days after the onset of

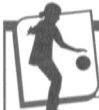

DEVELOPMENTAL CONSIDERATIONS 24-1

Psychosocial Issues Related to Pediatric HIV Infection

Children	Families
Infancy Unable to grasp concept of illness and death Infants and young children have immediate concern about physical trauma and parent separation. **Early Childhood** Begin to conceptualize death process involving physical harm Concerns center around medical tests and procedures. **Middle Childhood** Children begin to understand "something is wrong." By age 10 or 11 years, understand death is permanent and universal Fear of ostracism and rejection Guilt regarding origin of illness **Adolescence** Diagnosis often produces denial, fear, withdrawal, and fear of being rejected by peers. There is a disruption in forming relationships outside the family. Anxieties may lead to poor school performance, depression, isolation, and acting-out behavior.	Trauma of diagnosis falls on the caregiver. Biologic mother may have found out her status upon diagnosis of child. Guilt: Regardless of mode of acquisition, all parents experience some degree of guilt. Anger: Against medical system if contracted through a transfusion, against themselves if prenatal Families tend to move past this phase when reassured of ongoing comprehensive family care. Task overload, whether from scarce resources, lack of support, or burden of secrecy Caring for a child with HIV infection is overwhelming. Isolation: Most parents are unwilling to share child's diagnosis. Therefore, the traditional supports available to families of a child with a life-threatening illness are not available from friends, community, and clergy. Medical home may be the only source of support for these families. Depression: Reactive depression may result from facing HIV infection in the family, and parents may also have chronic depressive state that is a result of the coexistence of multiple problems. Fears of multiple losses: Parents begin to mourn alienation from other family members and loss of lifestyle, trust of friends, and self-esteem.

the rash. The cycle of illness typically lasts 10 days; therefore, this illness is often called the *10-day measles*.

Occasional complications include otitis media, mastoiditis, pneumonia, encephalomyelitis, and (rarely) subacute sclerosing panencephalitis. Subacute sclerosing panencephalitis is a degenerative CNS process associated with progressive behavioral and intellectual deterioration followed by convulsions, coma, and death. Measles vaccination programs have reduced the incidence of subacute sclerosing panencephalitis to nearly zero.

Assessment

The hallmark of measles is the appearance of Koplik spots. Look for them first appearing as red spots along the inside of the cheek (Fig. 24-8). They evolve over time to form pinpoint white papules on a rose-red base. Two days after the appearance of Koplik spots, a red maculopapular rash appears with fever. The rash first

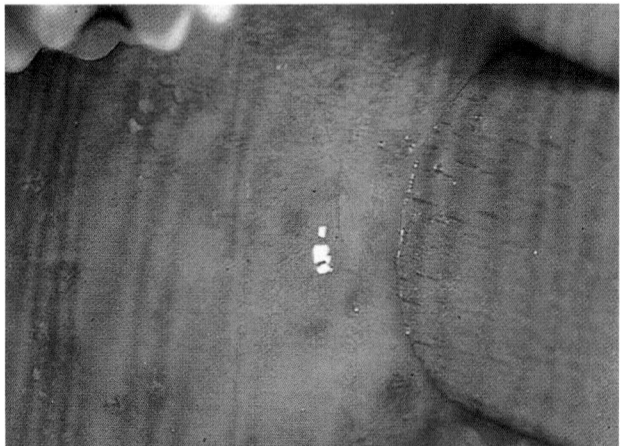

Figure 24-8 The rashes of measles. Koplik spots appear as red spots along the inside of the cheek. From SPL/Custom Medical Stock Photo. Reprinted with permission.

appears on the face and neck and then progresses down the body.

Other typical symptoms include fever, conjunctivitis, coryza, and a cough. Symptoms peak between the second and third days. The rash generally begins to fade by the third day. By the fourth day, symptoms begin to resolve, with the fever decreasing and conjunctiva clearing.

Diagnosis is typically made by the presenting clinical features. The measles virus can be isolated in tissue culture from nasopharyngeal secretions, blood, urine, and conjunctival fluid. Viral cultures are generally not used, however, because most laboratories are not equipped to cultivate the viruses.

The most useful antibody test is a paired sera test comparing the difference in titers between an acute specimen and a convalescent specimen taken 2 to 4 weeks later. Measles IgM antibodies can be detected in a single specimen if it is collected after the second day of the rash and before 30 days after the onset of illness.

Nursing Diagnoses and Outcomes

In addition to those identified in Nursing Plan of Care 24-1, the following nursing diagnoses and outcomes may apply to the child with measles:

Nursing Diagnosis: Risk for injury related to effects of measles photophobia
Outcome: Child will undergo interventions to decrease the discomfort associated with photophobia.
Nursing Diagnosis: Hyperthermia related to effects of measles
Outcome: Child will experience minimal discomfort and no injury associated with fever.

Interdisciplinary Interventions

No specific antiviral treatment is available. Uncomplicated measles is self-limiting and usually requires only supportive care.

If the child is hospitalized with measles, use airborne precautions for the duration of the illness. Provide care that includes supportive therapy and fluids. Coughs are sometimes difficult to control, and common cough suppressants seem inadequate. Therefore, encourage fluid intake to lubricate the mucous membranes. Do not treat associated conjunctivitis with antibacterial drops or ointments. The virus is unaffected by the antibacterial medication. If photophobia is present, dim the lights. However, avoid completely darkening the room because it may be depressing to a child whose activity is already curtailed. Provide quiet, diversionary activities.

ALERT   *As with all viral illnesses, avoid aspirin products because of the increased risk of Reye syndrome.*

Community Care

Susceptible persons exposed to measles may be given the measles vaccine to prevent disease. Prevention after exposure is possible because the body's immune response to the measles vaccine is elicited in 7 days, whereas the incubation period of natural measles is 8 to 12 days. Vaccination is certainly the method of choice in outbreaks in schools or daycare centers. For outbreaks in daycare centers, the vaccination age may be lowered to 6 months. These children can then resume the normal vaccination schedule, with the first immunization at 15 months and the next before school entry or at age 11 or 12 years, depending on local school requirements. Pregnancy is a contraindication for the measles vaccine (measles, mumps, rubella vaccine [MMRV]) because it is a live-virus vaccine. However, measles is not known to cause congenital birth defects. Administration of MMRV is not harmful if it is given to a person who is already immune to one or more of the viruses.

MUMPS

Before a vaccine was developed, mumps was a common childhood disease. Mumps is a vaccine-preventable disease that occasionally occurs in outbreaks in undervaccinated populations (see Chapter 8 for a discussion of vaccines). Known as *infectious parotitis*, it is a systemic disease characterized by acute inflammation of the salivary glands, particularly the parotid glands. It is seasonal in its occurrence, with most cases arising during late winter and spring.

The incidence of mumps in developed countries has been low during the postvaccine era (e.g., 200 to 300 cases per year in the United States from 2001 to 2005 [CDC, 2008]). However, outbreaks involving mainly older youths and young adults (aged 11 to 26 years) have occurred in developed countries such as the United States (Atkinson et al., 2012), the United Kingdom (CDC, 2006b), Canada (Watson-Creed et al., 2006), and Korea (Park et al., 2007). These outbreaks highlight the importance of immunizations. Globally, more than 718,000 cases of mumps occurred in 2011 (WHO, 2012b).

Pathophysiology

Complications of mumps are rare. Occasionally, adolescent or adult males experience orchitis (inflammation of the testis), but sterility rarely occurs. Mumps during pregnancy is not known to result in birth defects. However, pregnancy is a contraindication for the mumps vaccine or MMRV because of the theoretic risks (AAP, 2012n).

Assessment

Swelling of the salivary glands is the hallmark of mumps (Fig. 24-9). In the classic illness, the child complains of an earache made worse by chewing. Fever, headache, and generalized malaise are often accompanying symptoms. The health care team will rule out other causes of parotid swelling. Such causes include stones that block Stensen ducts; CMV; coxsackievirus; parainfluenza virus infections; and various tumors, hemangiomas, and lymphangiomas of the parotid gland.

Mumps can be diagnosed by isolating the mumps virus from throat swabs, urine, and spinal fluid. Mumps-specific IgM antibody or mumps virus by PCR can be detected in serum. Specific mumps serologic

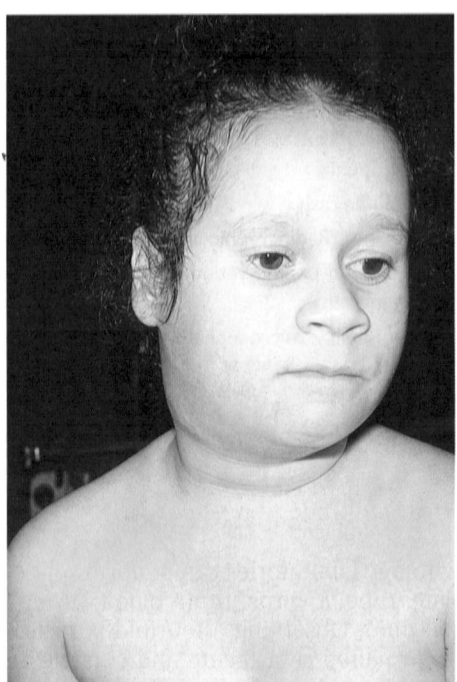

Figure 24-9 In mumps, the parotid glands swell and obscure the angle of the jaw. Copyright Morris Huberland/Science Source/Photo Researchers. Reprinted with permission.

tests include mumps hemagglutination inhibition test, complement fixation, and enzyme immunoassay.

Nursing Diagnoses and Outcomes

See Nursing Plan of Care 24-1 for pertinent nursing diagnoses and outcomes. The diagnosis of "Imbalanced nutrition: Less than body requirements" may be especially applicable for a child with mumps because of pain associated with chewing.

Interdisciplinary Interventions

No antiviral therapies are available to treat mumps, so supportive care is indicated. Children with mumps are seldom hospitalized. Mumps vaccine may be helpful in controlling outbreaks.

When a child with mumps is hospitalized, place the child in a private room with droplet precautions until 9 days after the onset of swelling. In an outbreak, when two or more children with mumps are admitted, they may share a room.

Community Care

In the home, educate the family to keep the child with mumps out of school or daycare until 9 days after the onset of swelling. Assist the family to arrange for home teachers for school-aged children.

Nursing care of children with mumps is supportive. Swollen parotid glands may cause discomfort while eating. Because the child often complains of increased pain upon chewing, recommend a soft diet. Educate the child to avoid citrus foods and some sour candies or foods that may elicit pain and increased salivation.

PARVOVIRUS B19 INFECTION

Parvovirus B19 infection is also known as *erythema infectiosum* or *fifth disease*. It is called *fifth disease* because it was the fifth childhood disease recognized to cause a rashlike illness in children. The other four diseases are measles, rubella, varicella, and scarlet fever. The mode of transmission is through respiratory secretions. It is contagious upon close contact with the infected individual. Outbreaks among elementary and middle school classmates are often demonstrated; secondary transmission among family members accounts for 50% of new cases (AAP, 2012p). The incubation period is 4 to 14 days. Complications are rare in children.

Assessment

In children with the well-known "slapped cheek" facial appearance, look for a lacelike rash on the abdomen and extremities (Fig. 24-10). The lacelike rash increases in color with heat, such as after a warm bath, and may last for several weeks.

The unique rash and facial appearance in children with parvovirus B19 are diagnostic. However, acute infection can be confirmed with the serologic test that measures parvovirus B19–specific IgM antibody. The presence of

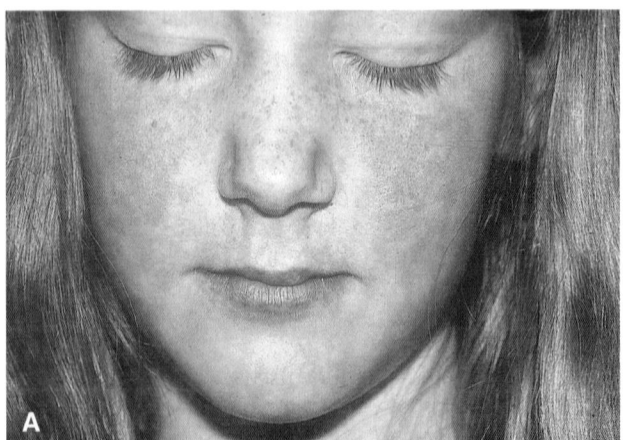
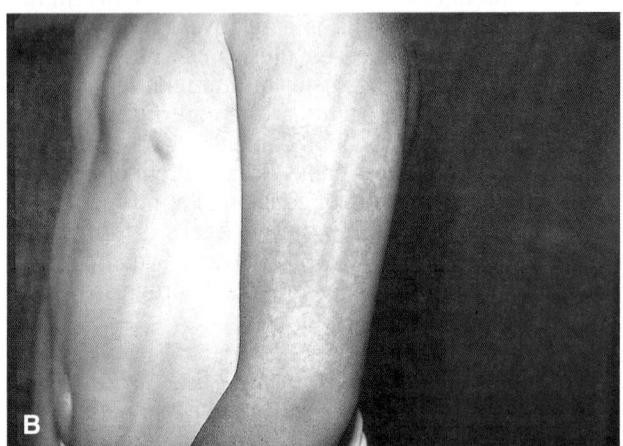

Figure 24-10 Rashes of parvovirus B19. (A) The hallmark sign is the "slapped cheek" appearance of the face. (B) The lacelike rash (from CDC). Reprinted with permission.

parvovirus B19 IgG antibody indicates past infection and immunity. Parvovirus B19 antigens can be detected by radioimmunoassay or by enzyme assay. Viral detection by PCR is also available, but the parvovirus DNA must be quantitated to distinguish acute infection from past infection.

Interdisciplinary Interventions

Treatment for parvovirus B19 infection is generally supportive. Because parvovirus B19 infections can trigger an aplastic crisis in patients with hemolytic anemias such as sickle cell disease, provide supportive care, such as oxygen and transfusion with red blood cells, for these patients as indicated. IV Ig is helpful for the immunocompromised patient.

By the time the rash appears, most children are no longer infectious, so isolation is unnecessary. However, in the immunodeficient child and those with sickle cell disease or other chronic hemolytic conditions, parvovirus B19 infection may cause aplastic crisis, rendering them infectious during the entire course of the illness. For these individuals, implement droplet precautions. Because only about half the population has had parvovirus B19, health care personnel could be susceptible. Fetal infection can result in fatal nonimmune hydrops. Therefore, pregnant employees and visitors must observe droplet precautions. For children managed with droplet precautions, arrange for play therapy, video games, and other diversions, because trips to the playroom are not possible.

RUBELLA

Rubella, also known as *German measles*, is a vaccine-preventable rash disease. It is also called *3-day measles* because it produces a rash that lasts approximately 3 days. Rubella has an incubation period of 14 to 21 days.

Pathophysiology

Rubella is a relatively mild disease in children but is significant in nonimmune pregnant females. If maternal infection occurs during the first trimester, transplacental infection can have disastrous effects on the fetus. In the pregnant woman, rubella is a relatively mild disease. In 25% to 50% of the cases, the woman has no symptoms at all. The rash occurs as an immune response to viral invasion, which occurs at the end of the incubation period. Much of the fetal damage occurs during the viremic stage, when the viable virus is circulating in the maternal blood. The risk of congenital abnormalities is 90% if rubella is acquired during weeks 2 through 10 of pregnancy (Duszak, 2009). The risk of fetal damage from rubella declines as the pregnancy progresses.

Assessment

In children with acquired rubella, a fine rash appears. A slight fever and generalized lymphadenopathy, particularly in the suboccipital, postauricular, and cervical areas, may be found. In infants with congenital rubella, skin lesions, such as a blueberry muffin rash, and major organ system defects (Chart 24-7) are the hallmarks.

CHART 24-7   Effects of Congenital Rubella

- Intrauterine growth retardation
- Hepatosplenomegaly
- Thrombocytopenia
- Blueberry muffin rash
- "Celery stalking" (Radiographic lines through long bones)
- Cataracts, salt-and-pepper retinopathy, glaucoma, microphthalmia
- Intellectual disability, microcephaly, encephalitis, seizures, hearing loss
- Pneumonitis
- Ventricular septal defect, valvular stenosis, myocardial stenosis

---

Most virology laboratories can perform serologic tests that isolate rubella virus from blood, urine, throat, and spinal fluid. Observing a fourfold increase in antibody titer in paired sera (acute and convalescent) is a common test for distinguishing between immunity and acute infection. Detection of rubella-specific IgM and IgG antibodies is especially useful for confirming congenital infection.

Nursing Diagnoses and Outcomes

In addition to those identified in Nursing Plan of Care 24-1, the following nursing diagnosis and outcome may apply to the child with congenital rubella:

Nursing Diagnosis: Risk for delayed development related to visual and auditory effects of rubella

Outcome: Child's sensory deficits will be recognized early, and interventions will be implemented to minimize their deleterious effects on growth and development.

Interdisciplinary Interventions

Rubella immune globulin is available for postexposure prophylaxis for pregnant women in whom pregnancy termination is not an option. It may prevent or limit the disease in these women.

Nursing care of children with rubella is largely supportive. Maintain contact precautions for 7 days after the onset of the rash or, for a child with congenital infection, for the duration of the hospital stay. Teach parents to maintain these precautions. Provide specific care related to the number and type of defects the child exhibits. Discharge planning along with parent teaching eases the transition from the hospital to the home.

All health care personnel should be vaccinated with rubella vaccine (MMRV) or demonstrate immunity by titer. Most individuals born before 1957 have had rubella, ensuring immunity. Those born after 1957 need a second MMRV to guard against waning immunity.

Community Care

Infants with congenital rubella can shed rubella virus in urine and nasopharyngeal secretions for a year or longer. Educate parents that congenitally infected infants must be excluded for this period from large groups, such as daycare and church nurseries. Passive maternal antibodies wane after 4 to 6 months. Because the MMRV is usually given at ages 12 to 15 months, all infants between the ages of 6 and 12 months are susceptible.

VIRAL HEPATITIS

The hepatitis group of viruses (hepatitis A, hepatitis B, hepatitis C, hepatitis D or delta, and hepatitis E) are related in name but are different. For example, although hepatitis A virus (HAV) is an RNA virus and hepatitis B virus (HBV) is a DNA virus, they do share a common pathology: infection of the liver. Hepatitis can cause liver inflammation, jaundice, an increase in liver enzymes, and liver failure. Hepatitis A and B are the most common hepatitis infections in infants and children and are covered in this section.

HAV infection (also known as *infectious hepatitis*) is commonly transmitted from person to person by fecal–oral contamination. Infected children shed HAV in the stool. Transmission can occur between children and caregivers in the home and in daycare centers. For example, a daycare worker could change the diaper of an infant who is shedding HAV, and then the worker might prepare food without proper hand hygiene. Although prolonged or relapsing hepatitis A infection can occur, chronic infection does not (AAP, 2012i).

In recent years, HAV has affected more adolescents and young adults than in the past, when most infections occurred among young children. This shift is likely the result of the introduction of routine hepatitis A immunization.

HBV is transmitted by exposure to blood and body fluids. People with chronic HBV infection are the primary reservoirs for infection. Transmission commonly occurs through sharing unclean needles, needle sticks, sexual contact, and perinatal exposure to an infected mother. However, young children can be at great risk for HBV infection from household child-to-child transmission or transmission from inanimate objects, such as washcloths and toothbrushes. Children in institutions or those who are immunosuppressed or on dialysis are also at high risk for HBV infection. Sexually active adolescents are at high risk for HBV infection as well as for other STIs. Chronic infection can occur, resulting (rarely) in fulminant hepatitis. This highly fatal complication of HBV infection may lead to hepatic coma and death unless a liver transplantation occurs. The implementation of routine childhood immunization for hepatitis B has dramatically reduced the number of infections in infants and children.

Assessment

Hepatitis A typically presents with fever, malaise, and nausea. Younger children are often asymptomatic and without jaundice, whereas older children are typically symptomatic, with infection lasting several weeks and accompanied by jaundice 70% of the time.

Hepatitis B may present in a variety of ways. Signs and symptoms range from nonspecific illness such as anorexia, nausea, or malaise to hepatitis with jaundice or, rarely, fulminant liver failure. Generally, children have mild symptoms without jaundice or are asymptomatic. Symptoms in children without jaundice include headache, malaise, anorexia, nausea, vomiting, and abdominal pain. Symptoms in children with jaundice include dark urine, clay-colored (light) stools, and jaundiced skin and sclera.

Diagnostic Tests

Serologic testing for hepatitis A IgM and IgG is available. HAV IgM is present at the onset of illness and typically disappears by 4 to 6 months. HAV IgG may be detected shortly after the appearance of IgM and persists after IgM disappears, indicating past infection and immunity.

A variety of serologic tests are available to detect hepatitis B; PCR testing can detect HBV DNA. Serologic tests for specific hepatitis viruses and their corresponding IgM and IgG antibodies confirm the diagnosis. In acute hepatitis, hepatitis IgM antibodies are present. Later in the infection, hepatitis IgG antibodies are present. The presence of IgG antibodies alone suggests that hepatitis occurred sometime in the past and that the patient is no longer infectious.

Serologic tests for hepatitis B can help confirm the diagnosis. Generally, the presence of any hepatitis B *antigen* always indicates that circulating virus is present and that the child's blood and body fluids are infectious. The presence of hepatitis B *antibody* means that the body is responding to the infection and that immunity is beginning. Those with chronic infection have circulating hepatitis B antigen and core antibody.

In hepatitis, liver enzymes are elevated, including lactate dehydrogenase, serum glutamic-oxaloacetic transaminase, and serum glutamic-pyruvic transaminase.

Nursing Diagnoses and Outcomes

In addition to those identified in Nursing Plan of Care 24-1, the following nursing diagnosis and outcome may apply to the older child with hepatitis:

Nursing Diagnosis: Activity intolerance related to fatigue
Outcome: Child will be increasingly able to tolerate activity and maintain school requirements.

Interdisciplinary Interventions

No treatment or cure exists for acute hepatitis infection. Vaccines have been developed for some of the hepatitis viruses, and routine childhood immunization for hepatitis A and B is recommended (see Chapter 8).

Antiviral therapy is available for chronic HBV infection, including interferon alfa, lamivudine, adefovir, or entecavir therapy.

caREminder

Liver transplantation has been used as a treatment for end-stage liver disease resulting from hepatitis B infection. However, because other body tissues still harbor HBV, the new liver may also become infected.

Focus nursing care for children with hepatitis A infection on teaching preventive measures, good sanitation, and careful hand hygiene. Through family hygiene instruction, nurses can help prevent outbreaks in families. Educate that standard hand hygiene after toileting or diaper changing is essential specifically in preventing HAV infection. Teach family members about proper food handling. Counsel that HAV-infected infants or food handlers should be excluded from daycare or work for 1 week after the onset of illness.

Educate adolescents about sexual activity during the acute phase of HBV infection, when transmission may be likely. Health care workers should advise abstinence or the use of condoms.

Focus nursing care of an infant born to a hepatitis B antigen–positive mother on standard precautions such as wearing gloves when handling the infant after delivery and until all amniotic fluid is wiped off. Because hepatitis B has a long incubation period (up to 6 months), the infant of a chronic carrier or a woman with active HBV infection should receive hepatitis B immune globulin (HBIG). Active immunization with hepatitis B vaccine is also initiated. Giving hepatitis B vaccine to the child along with HBIG can prevent disease in 95% of infants (AAP, 2012i).

Community Care

Routine testing of *all* pregnant women for hepatitis B surface antigen (HBsAg) is recommended (U.S. Preventive Services Task Force, 2009). Without intervention, approximately 90% of infants born to women who are HBsAg positive will develop chronic hepatitis B infection (Smith et al., 2012). Hepatitis B infection is 85% to 95% preventable in infants of HBsAg mothers with the administration of HBIG and hepatitis B vaccine (Smith et al., 2012).

caREminder

Pregnant women should ideally be tested for hepatitis B early during pregnancy and before delivery (in patients at high risk) to identify infants who need immediate prophylaxis at birth.

Routine immunization for hepatitis A and B is recommended for all infants and children. In general, methods for preventing and controlling viral hepatitis transmission include hand hygiene after toileting or diapering infants, giving immunoprophylaxis after exposure (immune globulin), and active immunization. Limiting environmental contamination and sanitizing water can decrease the potential for exposure to hepatitis A. The inability to identify children who are infected, because they lack symptoms, emphasizes the importance of routine infection control procedures such as hand hygiene, sterilization of medical equipment, and standard precautions.

SEXUALLY TRANSMITTED INFECTIONS

STIs typically affect adults or sexually active teenagers. An STI in a child (other than a newborn) suggests sexual abuse, which the health care team must report to the appropriate authorities. In STIs, females usually exhibit vaginitis; males, urethritis. In infants and young children, some forms of vulvovaginitis result from chemical irritation rather than infection. For example, vulvar irritation can be induced by ammonia (from wet diapers), and allergic or chemical irritation of the vulva can result from the use of harsh soaps or bubble baths.

STIs include syphilis, gonorrhea, chlamydia, human papillomavirus, genital herpes, hepatitis B and C, and HIV infection. Herpes, hepatitis B, and HIV infection have been discussed previously in this chapter. Venereal warts are caused by human papillomavirus. Syphilis, gonorrhea, and chlamydia are discussed in this section.

The sexual activity leading to infection includes genital–genital, oral–genital, oral–anal, and genital–anal contact during heterosexual sex, MSM, or WSW. Approximately 19 million new cases of STIs are reported in the United States each year, with more than 50% of these infections occurring in the adolescent or young adult population (CDC, 2010).

SYPHILIS

Acquired syphilis is an STI that occurs in three stages: primary, secondary, and tertiary. Syphilis is a disease caused by a motile spirochete, *Treponema pallidum*. Congenital syphilis occurs when transplacental transmission of *T. pallidum* occurs any time during pregnancy or at birth. Transmission from an infected, untreated mother occurs 70% to 100% of the time in primary syphilis; the risk decreases with progression of maternal disease (Chakraborty & Luck, 2007). The incidence of acquired syphilis has declined in developed nations since the 1990s; however, rates remain high in large urban areas, the southern United States, among MSM, and in HIV infection (AAP, 2012w). Some European countries have seen a resurgence of congenital syphilis, and it remains an important issue globally; annually, an estimated 2.1 million pregnant women have active syphilis worldwide (Hawkes et al., 2011).

Pathophysiology

The incubation period of syphilis is typically 3 weeks but ranges from 10 to 90 days after exposure. *T. pallidum* is a sexually transmitted organism acquired by direct contact with the highly infectious ulcerative skin lesions or mucous membranes or through transplacental transmission from an infected mother to her fetus. An infected person who does not get treatment may infect others during the first two stages of the disease. Untreated syphilis in the tertiary stage, although not contagious, can cause serious heart abnormalities, mental disorders, blindness, other neurologic problems, and death.

Syphilis is a treatable disease, even in pregnancy. In untreated active maternal infection, adverse outcomes occur in up to 69% of infected women, including stillbirth (25%), prematurity or low birth weight (13%), neonatal death (11%), and neonatal infection (20%) (Hawkes et al., 2011). Lack of treatment or late treatment during pregnancy often results in hydrops fetalis or preterm birth. Infants born with congenital syphilis may have many body systems affected.

Assessment

Infants with congenital infection may present with illness at birth, or symptoms may develop within the first 4 to 8 weeks of life (Chart 24-8). If untreated, infants may go on to develop late disease, which typically involves the CNS, bones and joints, teeth, eyes, and skin.

The spirochete can be visualized using darkfield microscopy or with DFA tests of lesion fluid, the placenta, or the umbilical cord. Serologic tests include nontreponemal and treponemal tests. The nontreponemal test is the Venereal Disease Research Laboratory (VDRL) slide test and the rapid plasma reagin (RPR) test. Treponemal tests include the fluorescent treponemal antibody absorption test and the *T. pallidum* particle agglutination test. All women seeking prenatal care are screened for syphilis with a VDRL or rapid plasma reagin test early during pregnancy and again at delivery. The fluorescent treponemal antibody absorption or the *T. pallidum* particle agglutination test is used as a confirmatory test and remains positive for life.

Diagnosis in the newborn is confirmed by persistent or increasing VDRL titers or a titer that is fourfold greater than the maternal titer. Radiographs of long bones in the legs and arms may show metaphysitis (inflammation of the growing end of the bone). Spinal fluid of the newborn is also sent for a VDRL test. A positive result is indicative of infection (see thePoint Diagnostic Tests: Stages of Syphilis for review of the clinical characteristics of the three stages of acquired syphilis).

CHART 24-8 **Effects of Congenital Syphilis**

Early

- Intrauterine growth retardation
- Snuffles (persistent, sometimes bloody rhinitis containing *Treponema pallidum*), associated with hoarse cry
- Hepatosplenomegaly, jaundice, lymphadenopathy, thrombocytopenia, anemia
- Macropapular rash on palms and soles followed by desquamation
- Osteochondritis, periostitis

Late (Appearing After Age 2 Years)

- Saber shins (long bones at lower leg are broad at the knee and narrow at the ankle, resembling a saber)
- Perforated hard palate, saddle nose (cartilage in the nose is deformed so that it has a saddlelike appearance)
- Mulberry molars (molars are deformed and take on the appearance of a cluster of mulberries) Hutchinson teeth (teeth are malformed and small, resembling shoe-peg corn)
- Interstitial keratitis, iridocyclitis, and chorioretinitis
- Neurosyphilis: hearing loss
- Localized rash, nodules, and gummas (granulomatous-like lesions)

Interdisciplinary Interventions

Maternal treatment consists of intramuscular or IV penicillin G, even in individuals who are allergic to it. Women with penicillin allergy are desensitized to penicillin and then receive penicillin therapy. Desensitization is accomplished while the woman is hospitalized to ensure adequate emergency care is available should a severe reaction occur. Alternatives to penicillin are less effective. IV crystalline penicillin G is the treatment of choice for the infant.

Community Care

Nursing care for the infant with congenital syphilis consists of hand hygiene and careful handling of all secretions, particularly nasal secretions. Observe contact precautions for at least 24 hours after antimicrobial therapy has started.

Report syphilis and congenital syphilis to the local health department. For pregnant women with syphilis, offer testing for HIV and other STIs.

For infants with congenital syphilis, recheck the VDRL or rapid plasma reagin test at 2 to 4, 6, and 12 months after treatment or until the test is negative. Educate parents on the need for intensive follow-up health care visits for their infant during the first year of life.

Congenital syphilis is preventable. Consistent prenatal care and education are essential.

GONORRHEA

Gonorrhea is one of the oldest STIs described. Gonorrhea is caused by a gram-negative diplococcus, *Neisseria gonorrhoeae*. Like its cousin, *Neisseria meningitidis*, *N. gonorrhoeae* is a fragile organism with strict growth requirements. It rapidly dies on inanimate objects, such as toilets. Transmission occurs during vaginal, anal, or oral intercourse. Transmission to the neonate (neonatal eye infection) occurs when the infant descends through an infected birth canal. The incubation period is usually 2 to 7 days. The incidence of infection in the United States is highest in females aged 15 to 19 years, and more than 300,000 cases of infection are reported annually (CDC, 2011b).

Assessment

Gonorrhea infections occur in three distinct age groups: neonates, adolescents, and adults (AAP, 2012h). Neonates typically develop an eye infection (ophthalmia neonatorum), which formerly was a leading cause of neonatal blindness. Young girls may exhibit vulvovaginitis as a result of sexual abuse by an infected individual.

Sexually active adolescent girls tend to exhibit vaginitis, which may progress to pelvic inflammatory disease. Some infected persons, such as those with rectal or pharyngeal infections, remain asymptomatic. Assess for hallmark symptoms of gonorrhea, which include a thick yellow or white vaginal or urethral discharge, painful or burning urination, and, in females, abdominal cramping or pain. Infection could extend beyond vulvovaginitis to include abscesses of Bartholin glands, salpingitis, and perihepatitis.

In males, the infection is often limited to urethritis. A thick yellow or white penile discharge or painful urination may be present. However, some males exhibit acute epididymitis and prostatitis. In all cases, the organism could gain access to the circulatory system, causing sepsis, arthritis, endocarditis, and meningitis.

Diagnostic Tests

The standard for diagnosis is a culture of eye drainage, cervical secretions, urethral discharge, or a rectal or throat swab sample that is positive for *N. gonorrhoeae*. Smears with Gram stains of these fluids that are positive for gram-negative diplococci can also be helpful in making the diagnosis. Nucleic acid amplification testing is available for urethral or endocervical swabs and urine. These tests are highly sensitive and specific.

caREminder

Notify the laboratory of the possible diagnosis of gonorrhea pharyngitis when throat swabs are submitted. A throat swab in most laboratories is evaluated for GAS only; additional methods are needed to isolate gonorrhea.

The laboratory should differentiate the gonococci from other *Neisseria* species, especially meningococci. Both appear as gram-negative diplococci. Individuals with disseminated gonorrhea often appear clinically as if they have infection with *N. meningitidis*.

Nursing Diagnoses and Outcomes

Refer to Nursing Plan of Care 24-1 for general nursing diagnoses and outcomes for the child with an infection. Nursing diagnoses and outcomes for the child with gonorrhea depend on how the child or adolescent acquired the infection and clinical manifestations. If rape was involved, the following nursing diagnosis and outcome may apply:

Nursing Diagnosis: Rape trauma syndrome related to forced sexual activity
Outcome: Child will verbalize feelings, and interventions will be implemented to assist the child with coping.

If pelvic inflammatory disease is present, the following nursing diagnoses and outcomes may apply:

Nursing Diagnosis: Acute pain related to effects of disease
Outcome: Child will experience minimal discomfort.
Nursing Diagnosis: Deficient knowledge: STI prevention
Outcome: Adolescent will state and implement methods for preventing STIs (e.g., abstinence, condoms).

Interdisciplinary Interventions

Gonorrhea is often treated in the emergency room or ambulatory setting. Single-dose therapy with an extended-spectrum cephalosporin is recommended and generally effective. Implement pain management (e.g., topical analgesia, distraction) for intramuscular injections. On occasion, the infection spreads to the cervix and fallopian tubes. Pelvic inflammatory disease ensues, requiring

parenteral antibiotic therapy that includes an extended cephalosporin and doxycycline regimen, followed by oral doxycycline. Conditions such as appendicitis, cystitis, and pyelonephritis must be ruled out in the differential diagnosis. Disseminated infection should be treated with 7 to 14 days of IV cefotaxime. Gonorrhea continues to develop drug resistance over time; therefore, consult CDC STI guidelines before starting treatment (CDC, 2010).

The current practice of applying prophylactic eye drops (silver nitrate, tetracycline, or erythromycin) at birth decreases the incidence of ophthalmia neonatorum drastically. Ceftriaxone is the drug therapy of choice for gonococcal ophthalmia neonatorum. Patients should be empirically treated simultaneously for chlamydia because these two infections frequently occur together.

Community Care

Educate adolescents that abstinence or the use of condoms effectively prevents transmission of gonorrhea and most other STIs. Report gonorrhea to the local health department to initiate contact tracing and treatment. Report gonorrhea in children older than 1 month of age to the local department of health and human services because of suspicion of sexual abuse.

 QUESTION: Ashley is diagnosed with a chlamydia infection. For what other STI would the school nurse need to assess?

CHLAMYDIA

Chlamydia has become a serious public health issue. *Chlamydia trachomatis* infection is caused by an intracellular bacterial agent that has multiple serotypes. Trachoma is usually caused by serotypes A through C, whereas genital and perinatal infections are caused by B and D through K. *C. trachomatis* infection is one of the most common STIs worldwide, with high rates among sexually active adolescents and young adults (Machado et al., 2012). The CDC recorded over 1.3 million cases of chlamydia in the United States in 2010—the largest number of cases reported for any condition (CDC, 2011b).

Pathophysiology

Genital infection is transmitted sexually. *C. trachomatis* infection and gonorrhea are often coinfections, so treatment for both is recommended if either is confirmed. Neonatal infection is acquired as the infant passes through an infected birth canal. Infection occurs in 50% of infants born to untreated mothers (AAP, 2012c). Conjunctivitis and pneumonia are of the greatest risk to these infants. The incubation period varies but is at least 1 week.

ANSWER: Because Ashley has chlamydia, the nurse also needs to assess for gonorrhea because these two infections often occur together.

Assessment

Be alert for signs of chlamydia. This STI can be asymptomatic or can produce urethritis in both sexes, vaginitis in girls, cervicitis in adolescent girls, and epididymitis in boys. In girls, the infection may ascend the vaginal tract and progress to pelvic inflammatory disease that may ultimately lead to infertility or increase the risk for ectopic pregnancy. Signs in girls may be abnormal vaginal discharge or bleeding, painful urination, abdominal pain, fever, or nausea. Signs and symptoms in boys may be watery, white, or yellow penile discharge or painful urination.

Infants may acquire neonatal chlamydial conjunctivitis or pneumonia. The conjunctivitis appears as a keratoconjunctivitis with purulent discharge. The risk of chlamydial conjunctivitis in the exposed neonate is 25% to 50%. The infant may also have an asymptomatic infection of the pharynx, rectum, or vagina that can persist for 2 years (AAP, 2012c). The risk of pneumonia in the neonate is 20%. The signs and symptoms of pneumonia include a staccato cough without fever and hyperinflation of the chest as seen on radiographic evaluation.

C. trachomatis, the causative agent, can be grown in tissue culture cells. Rapid antigen detection includes DFA, enzyme immunoassay, and genetic probe testing. The DNA probe methods can rapidly and accurately test for the presence of both gonorrhea and chlamydia.

Nursing Diagnoses and Outcomes

Nursing diagnoses and outcomes for adolescents with sexually transmitted chlamydial infections are similar to those for gonorrhea. For the infant or child with chlamydial pneumonia, the following nursing diagnoses and outcomes may apply:

Nursing Diagnosis: Ineffective breathing pattern related to effects of disease
Outcome: The child will be assisted to maintain an effective breathing pattern and tissue oxygenation.
Nursing Diagnosis: Sleep deprivation related to coughing
Outcome: The child's cough will be controlled to obtain adequate sleep.

> **QUESTION:** Ashley has a trusting relationship with the school nurse. What interventions would be the priority for Ashley, and how might the school nurse promote Ashley's compliance with the treatment regimen?

Interdisciplinary Interventions

Treatment of chlamydial infection in adolescents usually involves doxycycline for 7 days or a one-time dose of azithromycin. Sexual partners should also be treated. Conjunctivitis in the newborn is treated with oral erythromycin to ensure that asymptomatic carriage is eradicated; topical application of erythromycin eye drops is ineffective. Pneumonia can be treated with oral azithromycin or erythromycin.

Oral erythromycin in infants younger than 6 weeks of age has been associated with infantile hypertrophic pyloric stenosis; however, it continues to be the drug of choice for chlamydia.

Nurses who work with adolescents may have the opportunity to discuss STI prevention with adolescents who have already been infected or are sexually active. If so, explain abstinence and the use of latex condoms as ways to prevent transmission. Teaching must include instructions on finishing the prescribed dose of medication completely and returning for follow-up care as needed.

> **ANSWER:** Priorities for Ashley would include antibiotic treatment for her and her boyfriend and an emphasis on the need to adhere to the medication therapy regimen to ensure that the infection completely resolves. As an adolescent, it might be more helpful for her and her boyfriend to receive the one-time dose of azithromycin rather than a 7-day regimen of doxycycline for chlamydia treatment. Both also would need simultaneous treatment for gonorrhea (a single-dose, broad-spectrum cephalosporin). In addition, both would need instruction on safe sex practices, including the use of condoms to prevent transmission. The nurse also needs to emphasize that the infection does not always cause symptoms, so adhering to safe sex practices reduces the risk of transmission and recurrence of the infection, which could ultimately lead to problems in the future.

FUNGAL INFECTIONS

Fungal infections often occur when the child's immune system has been suppressed because of chemotherapy, radiation, illness, or transplantation. Fungi are opportunists that take advantage of a vacated ecologic niche. When antibiotics are used to kill pathogenic strains of bacteria, they often kill useful bacteria (normal flora) as well. These useful bacteria normally keep fungi in check, and when they are gone, fungi can take over and cause serious infections. (See thePoint Supplemental Information: Fungal Infections for a discussion of aspergillosis, coccidioidomycosis, histoplasmosis, and *Malassezia furfur* infections.)

PARASITE AND VECTOR-BORNE INFECTIONS

Parasites have infested humans worldwide throughout the centuries. Parasites can range in size from the microscopic *Plasmodium* spp., which cause malaria, to the guinea worm, which can measure up to 3 m. Parasites have one aspect in common: they are free-living organisms. In many instances, humans are merely incidental hosts. In other cases, humans are a vital part of an elaborate life cycle that could include other animals or insects. Of all the infectious and parasitic diseases, few cause more distress to nursing staff than lice and scabies. These parasites are discussed in detail in Chapter 25. This chapter will discuss giardiasis, pinworm infestation, roundworm infestation, toxocariasis, toxoplasmosis, and arboviral infections.

Many bacteria or viruses must rely on vectors such as mosquitoes, ticks, or other arthropods to transmit diseases to humans and other mammals. These diseases are known as *vector-borne infections* (see thePoint Supplemental Information: Malaria).

GIARDIASIS

Giardia lamblia (also called *Giardia intestinalis*) is a protozoal organism that lives in freshwater streams. It infects both humans and wildlife. *G. lamblia* is the most common disease-causing parasite in the United States (AAP, 2012g). It exists as a trophozoite and as a cyst. The cyst form is infectious. Transmission is through ingestion of cyst-contaminated water or direct hand-to-mouth inoculation from cyst-contaminated hands; transmission by infected food is rare. Infection with this organism causes giardiasis. Infections range from asymptomatic to severe, life-threatening diarrhea.

Assessment

Suspect giardiasis in a child who has acute watery, foul-smelling diarrhea with abdominal pain, particularly if he or she has recently been camping or hiking. Watery stools are often accompanied by flatulence and abdominal distention. Anorexia is often seen, leading to weight loss and failure to thrive. Infections may last from a few days to years.

Identification of trophozoites or cysts in a direct stool smear is diagnostic. These smears can be observed directly (wet mount) or after being stained with iodine. Enzyme immunoassay tests for *Giardia* are commercially available.

Interdisciplinary Interventions

The treatment of choice is a 5- to 7-day course of metronidazole or a 3-day course of nitazoxanide. Therapy may be repeated if relapse occurs. Treatment of asymptomatic carriers is not recommended.

Community Care

Because outbreaks of giardiasis have occurred in daycare centers, instruct the parents to withdraw their infected child from daycare until the diarrhea resolves. If more than one child is involved, notify local health department officials. Instruct family members and caregivers to wash their hands carefully after diapering infants and toileting to avoid infection.

Advise families who camp and hike that the pristine appearance of cool mountain water may be deceiving. Beavers and other wildlife can harbor *Giardia* cysts and contaminate streams. Therefore, advise families who enjoy camping to boil all water and avoid drinking from streams.

PINWORM INFESTATION

Because it is caused by worms, pinworm infestation is often troubling to families. The causative agent of pinworm infestation (enterobiasis) is *Enterobius vermicularis*. Pinworm infestation occurs frequently in early and middle childhood, children who attend daycare centers, and primary caregivers of infested children.

Up to 50% of these populations in the United States may be infested with pinworm (AAP, 2012r). Clusters of infestation are also known to occur in families.

Pathophysiology

The mode of transmission is oral–fecal. The gravid female pinworm lays eggs at the child's perianal region at night. It usually dies after depositing the eggs. Rectal itching leads to scratching. Autoinoculation results if the child scratches the rectal area and then puts the hand in his or her mouth (e.g., thumb-sucking). Eggs can remain viable and infective on inanimate objects for 2 to 3 weeks. Eggs are swallowed and then hatched in the duodenum. The larvae live and grow, then slowly make their way toward the colon. Molting twice, adults mature in 1 to 1½ months. Then gravid females once again migrate to the anus to lay eggs.

Assessment

Suspect pinworm infestation in a child with perianal itching and localized irritation. Children heavily infested have been reported to exhibit sleeplessness, hyperactivity, weight loss, tooth grinding, abdominal pain, and vomiting, although a causal relationship has not been documented.

Aberrant migration of gravid female worms to the vagina may cause vaginitis. Subsequent aberrant migration from the perineum can contribute to salpingitis and pelvic peritonitis in female children (AAP, 2012r).

Diagnosis is confirmed by direct visualization of worms by the parents or by microscopy. Tell parents to view the child's anus with a flashlight 2 to 3 hours after the child is asleep. The worm is white, thin, about a half-inch long, and it moves. A simple technique, the cellophane tape slide method, is used to capture worms and eggs. Transparent adhesive tape is lightly touched to the anus and then applied to a slide. The tape is examined under low power for worms and eggs. The best specimens are obtained as the child awakens, before toileting or bathing.

Nursing Diagnoses and Outcomes

In addition to those identified in Nursing Plan of Care 24-1, the following nursing diagnosis and outcomes may apply to the child with pinworm infestation:

Nursing Diagnosis: Impaired skin integrity related to scratching perianal region from pruritus caused by pinworm
Outcomes:
• Child will receive treatment to eradicate pinworm and, thus, pruritus.
• Child's skin integrity will be restored.

Interdisciplinary Interventions

Treatment is with a single dose of albendazole or pyrantel pamoate (neither drug is approved by the FDA), with a second dose repeated 2 weeks later. Retreatment is often necessary. Entire families or daycare groups may need to be treated simultaneously.

Children infested with pinworms are rarely hospitalized. Nursing care centers on teaching parents and children appropriate eradication techniques. Linens and bedclothes can harbor eggs that remain infective. Therefore, emphasize rigorous hand hygiene after contact with the child, linens, or clothes. Teach parents to wash all linens and contaminated clothing using the hot cycle of the washing machine. Personal hygiene measures, such as good hand hygiene and avoiding scratching of the perianal region, may prevent transmission.

Community Care

Educating family members, schools, and daycare centers that recurrence is common can reduce some anxiety. Controlling infestations in schools and daycare centers can be difficult. Keeping fingernails clipped short and emphasizing handwashing seem to help.

ROUNDWORM INFESTATION

Ascaris lumbricoides, a helminth, is the most common cause of human roundworm infestations (ascariasis). Roundworm infestations most frequently affect young children, particularly those from developing nations who are living in poverty (Bethony et al., 2006). Infestation occurs after ingestion of soil contaminated by infective eggs. Larvae hatch in the small intestine and are transported first to the liver and then to the lungs, from which they ascend to the pharynx and are swallowed back into the intestine, where they mature. The adult worm lives in the lumen of the intestine, and the female can produce 200,000 eggs a day, which are excreted in the stool. Adult worms can live for 12 to 18 months if untreated (AAP, 2012b).

Roundworm infestations are more common in warm climates, in areas of poor sanitation, or where human feces are used as fertilizer. Globally, an estimated 807 million people are infested with roundworms (Bethony et al., 2006). The incubation period (from ingestion of egg to adult worm) is 8 weeks. Person-to-person transmission does not occur.

Assessment

Most infestations are asymptomatic; however, nonspecific gastrointestinal symptoms may occur. During the larval migration phase, the child may present with fever, cough, congestion, and shortness of breath. The eosinophil count is often high, and allergic symptoms such as itching and wheezing may occur with recurrent infestations. Children may complain of vague abdominal pain with nausea, vomiting, and anorexia. Partial obstruction of the intestine may occur. Worms may occasionally emerge through the nose or mouth, so ask parents if they have observed this. The child's history may reflect impaired growth, poor fitness, and poor cognitive and school performance (Brooker, 2010).

Ova can be detected by direct microscopic examination of the stool. Adult worms cans be identified if they are passed from the rectum, nose, or mouth.

Interdisciplinary Interventions

Deworming campaigns using antihelminthic drugs have helped to reduce worm burden in endemic countries (WHO, 2012a). Albendazole or ivermectin in a single dose or mebendazole for 3 days is the recommended treatment for roundworm infestation.

Community Care

Educate parents that roundworm infestation can be prevented by sanitary disposal of human feces away from children's play areas and vegetable gardens. Household bleach is ineffective in killing roundworms.

TOXOCARIASIS

Toxocariasis (infestation with *Toxocara*, a group of roundworms) causes two conditions in children: visceral larva migrans and ocular larva migrans. Toxocariasis is caused by second-stage larval migration of roundworms to the liver, lungs, CNS, and eyes of humans, usually children. The adult worms are commonly found in dogs (*Toxocara canis*) and cats (*Toxocara cati*). Young children become accidental hosts when they ingest soil contaminated by infective eggs, which can exist in the soil for years, or play with infested puppies. Many puppies younger than 10 weeks of age are congenitally infested with *T. canis* and excrete eggs in their feces.

Pathophysiology

A child ingests the eggs. The incubation period in humans is unknown. The eggs hatch in the intestine, and the larvae penetrate the intestinal wall. Using the intestinal capillary system, the larvae gain access to the bloodstream and migrate to the liver. Most of the larvae remain in the liver, but some pass on to the lungs, CNS, and eyes. Eventually, the larvae gravitate to a single location (either the liver or the eyes).

Assessment

A history of exposure to puppies or a history of **pica** (eating nonfood items such as dirt) is useful in establishing the diagnosis. The degree of symptoms depends on the number of eggs ingested. Most infestations are asymptomatic. Fever, increased white blood cell count, persistent eosinophilia, hypergammaglobulinemia, and hepatomegaly are typical. Malaise, anemia, and cough are sometimes present. Rare manifestations include myocarditis, encephalitis, and pneumonia.

Ocular manifestations occur as a visual decrease or even total vision loss in one eye. The retinal damage may go unnoticed until adolescence and may be noted only when the child applies for a driver's license and fails the eye examination.

Diagnostic Tests

Eosinophilia and hypergammaglobulinemia, along with high titers of isohemagglutinin to the A and B blood groups, are suggestive of *Toxocara* infection. Antibody titers for *Toxocara* are positive in infected children.

Liver biopsies and retinal examinations can reveal larvae, either by histologic preparation and staining of biopsy specimens or by direct visualization of the larvae in the eye. Other eye damage, such as retinal detachment, can also be directly observed.

Nursing Diagnoses and Outcomes

In addition to those identified in Nursing Plan of Care 24-1, the following nursing diagnosis and outcome may apply to the child with ocular larva migrans:

Nursing Diagnosis: Risk for delayed development related to effects of eye infestation on vision
Outcome: Child will obtain corrective visual aids as applicable.

Interdisciplinary Interventions

Treatment is with corticosteroids to reduce the allergic, inflammatory reaction and with antihelminthic drugs, such as albendazole or mebendazole, to destroy the parasite. Antihelmintic drugs may not successfully treat ocular larva migrans, and steroids may be indicated (AAP, 2012x).

Community Care

Toxocariasis infestation is preventable. Instruct parents to cover sandboxes when not in use to keep cats from using them as litter boxes. Instruct them also to keep children's play areas free of dog and cat feces and to have puppies dewormed at ages 2, 4, 6, and 8 weeks.

Parents may need to administer eye drops to a child with ocular larva migrans. Because some types of drops are administered hourly, the parents of a school-aged child may need to discuss eye drop administration with the school nurse. Parents may need to arrange for a home teacher if their child's school does not have a school nurse.

TOXOPLASMOSIS

T. gondii is one of the world's most common parasites. Toxoplasmosis is caused by *T. gondii*, a protozoan that lives in the intestinal tract of many animals, including domestic cats. The parasite occurs in three forms. tachyzoites (an amoebalike form), bradyzoites (a cast form), and highly infectious oocysts. Transmission occurs by eating foods contaminated with *T. gondii* cysts or inhaling dust that contains oocysts from cat feces. Eating fruits or vegetables harvested in countries that use fecal fertilizer sprays, drinking unpasteurized milk, and eating unfrozen or undercooked lamb, pork, or beef are the principal ways in which transmission occurs. The immunosuppressed and those with HIV are at increased risk for toxoplasmosis. A pregnant woman who empties cat litter boxes can inhale oocysts from the litter dust, develop toxoplasmosis, and transmit the parasite to her fetus. The incidence of fetal infection is 1 in 1,000 live births (AAP, 2012y).

Congenital toxoplasmosis occurs when a woman contracts toxoplasmosis for the first time during pregnancy. The organism can cross the placenta and infect the fetus. The risk of transmission to the fetus increases from 6% at 13 weeks to 72% at 36 weeks' gestation (Dunn et al., 1999). Damage to the fetus depends on the trimester in which the infection occurs. Maternal infection during the first trimester causes the most fetal damage; infection during the last trimester may cause little apparent damage.

> **CHART 24-9   Effects of Congenital Toxoplasmosis**
>
> - Intrauterine growth retardation
> - Jaundice, hepatitis, hepatosplenomegaly
> - Anemia, thrombocytopenia, disseminated intravascular coagulopathy
> - Blueberry muffin rash
> - Chorioretinitis, microphthalmia, optic atrophy, blindness
> - Intracranial calcifications, seizures, hydrocephalus, microcephaly, intellectual impairment, developmental delay

Assessment

Acquired toxoplasmosis in otherwise healthy children is usually asymptomatic. The signs and symptoms of congenital toxoplasmosis are summarized in Chart 24-9. Maternal symptoms are vague, usually consisting of fatigue. Most neonates are asymptomatic, but without treatment, congenital toxoplasmosis has adverse neurologic, intellectual, visual, and audiologic outcomes (Kaye, 2011).

Ocular *Toxoplasma* infection can result from congenital or acquired infection. It can cause tissue necrosis in the retina, vitreitis, iridocyclitis, and cataracts. Undetected and, therefore, untreated congenital infections usually manifest during adolescence as ocular disease (chorioretinitis).

Diagnostic Tests

A positive result for maternal IgM antibody to *T. gondii* is diagnostic. Fetal blood samples can be tested for the presence of IgM-specific antibodies. A PCR specific for *T. gondii* is becoming available to more laboratories; it can be performed on blood from the fetus, infant, or mother.

Fetal ultrasonography can show the presence of cerebral calcifications. After birth, ophthalmologic and neurologic examinations of the infant can be performed to look for chorioretinitis, hydrocephalus, microcephaly, and meningoencephalitis. Computed tomography or magnetic resonance imaging of the infant's head can show calcified brain lesions indicative of congenital toxoplasmosis.

Nursing Diagnoses and Outcomes

In addition to those identified in Nursing Plan of Care 24-1, the following nursing diagnosis and outcome is applicable to a severely affected infant who may be in the neonatal intensive care unit and requires mechanical ventilation:

Nursing Diagnosis: Ineffective breathing pattern related to effects of disease process
Outcome: Infant will maintain adequate tissue oxygenation, as evidenced by an oxygenation saturation of 97% to 99%.

Interdisciplinary Interventions

Treatment for maternal infection and for infected children is with pyrimethamine and sulfadiazine. These two agents act together (synergistically) and, along with leucovorin (folinic acid), serve as standard therapy. Pyrimethamine may cause severe depression of bone marrow function; leucovorin is given to counteract the suppression. Infants with congenital disease are treated for 12 months.

Because the infection cannot be transmitted from human to human, no special isolation precautions are observed. Explain the necessary ophthalmologic examinations and diagnostic laboratory tests and provide emotional support to the parents to help them cope with this adverse outcome of pregnancy.

Preconception and prenatal teaching includes washing all fruits and vegetables and freezing all meats, then cooking them thoroughly before consuming them. Avoid steak tartar and other raw meat pâtés. Encourage cat owners to have someone other than the pregnant woman empty the cat litter box daily. It takes 1 to 5 days before the oocyst can turn into the highly infectious spore form; thus, daily attention to the litter box is a must. Teach families to use disposable plastic litter box liners or disinfect the box with boiling water for 5 minutes.

Arboviral Infections

Arboviruses are spread by mosquitos, ticks, sandflies, and other biting arthropods and can cause CNS disease, fever with rash and headache, joint pain, and, occasionally, hemorrhagic fever with hepatitis. Illnesses range from a self-limited febrile illness with headache to aseptic meningitis or acute encephalitis resulting in seizures, coma, or even death. Arboviral infections commonly seen in the United States include West Nile virus (WNV), La Crosse encephalitis, eastern equine encephalitis, western equine encephalitis, Powassan encephalitis, and St. Louis encephalitis. They also include tick-borne infections such as Rocky Mountain spotted fever (RMSF), human monocytotropic ehrlichiosis (HME), and Lyme disease.

Birds and small mammals are the primary reservoir for most arboviruses. Humans and domestic animals are infected incidentally when an arthropod bites an infected animal, picks up the virus, and then bites a person or pet. Person-to-person transmission does not occur except through blood transfusions, intrauterine transmission, and possibly through human breast milk.

Definitive diagnosis is made by viral isolation from serum or CSF. Virus-specific antibody tests for IgG and IgM are also available. The presence of antibody in the serum or CSF of a patient with CNS symptoms is evidence of recent infection. A fourfold increase in antibodies 2 to 4 weeks apart confirms the diagnosis. PCR testing is available in reference laboratories. No specific treatment or immunizations are available. Treatment is supportive. The primary intervention is to prevent infection by such measures as using insect repellents containing diethyltoluamide (DEET), wearing protective clothing, and implementing mosquito control programs.

WEST NILE VIRUS

WNV is transmitted to humans primarily through the bite of infected mosquitoes. The *Culex* mosquito, which feeds at dawn and dusk and breeds in standing water, is the primary vector of WNV. The mosquito acquires the virus by feeding on infected birds and then transmits the virus to humans and other mammals.

WNV can also be transmitted through blood transfusions and organ transplantation. Intrauterine transmission and transmission in human milk have been described, but such cases are rare, and transmission in human milk has not been confirmed (Truemper & Romero, 2007). Some concern exists that aerosolized transmission can also occur. In the United States, WNV occurs during the late spring, summer, and early fall.

About 80% of WNV infections are asymptomatic, 20% of all infected patients develop West Nile fever, and fewer than 1% develop WNV neuroinvasive disease (Truemper & Romero, 2007). Children younger than 18 years old have a reduced incidence of morbidity and mortality associated with WNV and WNV neuroinvasive disease (LaBeaud et al., 2006), which occurs primarily in the elderly or immunocompromised (Truemper & Romero, 2007).

Assessment

Children with West Nile fever typically present with a sudden onset of fever, headache, muscle aches, and weakness. They may also often have abdominal pain with nausea, vomiting, or diarrhea. Some patients also have a rash. This phase of the illness lasts several days; however, the fatigue and weakness may linger for weeks.

Those with CNS disease present with typical signs of meningitis or encephalitis. Flaccid paralysis can also be part of this syndrome or can occur in isolation, without fever or other signs.

Although most women known to have had WNV infection during pregnancy have delivered infants without signs of infection or clinical abnormalities, evaluate these infants for signs of infection (Truemper & Romero, 2007).

Consider WNV in any child with a febrile illness or CNS disease who has had recent exposure to mosquitoes. Virus-specific antibody tests for WNV IgG and IgM are available for serum and CSF. The presence of antibody in the serum or CSF of a patient with CNS symptoms is evidence of recent infection. A fourfold increase in antibodies 2 to 4 weeks apart confirms the diagnosis. PCR testing is available in reference laboratories.

Interdisciplinary Interventions

Treatment for WNV infection is supportive, and standard precautions are recommended. Prevention is key. Educate families to take steps to avoid being bitten by infected mosquitoes. Teach them to stay indoors during dawn and dusk, when mosquitoes are active; to wear long-sleeved shirts, pants, and socks; and to apply insect repellents. See Teaching Intervention Plan 24-2 for a discussion of DEET and permethrin; picaridin, lemon eucalyptus oil, or clove oil may be alternatives to DEET (Kendrick, 2006; Shapiro, 2012).

TICK-BORNE INFECTIONS

Many organisms produce tick-borne infections in humans. Most organisms belong to the Rickettsiaceae family of bacteria. Because RMSF, HME, and Lyme disease are the most

TIP 24-2: A TEACHING INTERVENTION PLAN to Avoid Tick-Borne Disease

Nursing Diagnoses and Family Outcomes

- Risk for injury related to environmental conditions (tick-infested areas)

  Outcome: Child and family will describe and implement preventive measures to avoid tick attachment. Child will not become infected with rickettsial disease.

Teach Child/Family

Preventive Measures to Avoid Tick Attachment

- Spray clothing with permethrin and exposed skin with tick repellent containing DEET; follow label directions for use. For young children, use products containing DEET sparingly; do not use on children younger than 2 months of age. Do not use products with more than 30% DEET. Do not put DEET on eyes or mouth and use sparingly around ears; do not apply to a young child's hands (to prevent getting the product in the mouth or eyes). Do not apply to skin with wounds, sunburn, or irritated skin (where it is absorbed more readily). Length of protection from DEET products is concentration dependent (e.g., 6.5% lasts about 2 hours, 24% lasts about 5 hours). Wash repellent off skin with soap and water after child comes indoors. Do not use combination insect repellent and sunscreen products because sunscreen products must be applied more frequently, thus risking overuse of DEET. Apply regular sunscreen first, then insect repellent.
- Wear light colors and long sleeves, long pants, socks, and shoes. Tuck shirt or blouse into pants and pants into socks.
- Check skin and scalp for ticks every 2–3 hours, when leaving infested areas, after playing with outdoor pets, and when coming indoors. Ticks can be as small as a pinhead.
- Inspect pets daily for ticks.

Tick Removal Techniques

- Inspect and detect promptly; ticks are easier to pull off when not firmly attached.
- Grasp the tick as close to the head and as close to the skin as possible with fine-tipped tweezers.
- Apply steady upward pull. Do not twist or exert enough pressure to crush the tick.
- If the head remains in the skin, leave it and wash the site with soap; attempts to remove it may cause tissue damage, and leaving it does not increase the risk of disease.
- Wash the site and your hands with soap and water.

Contact Health Care Provider if

- Tick cannot be removed
- Child develops redness, swelling, a rash, or fever the week after the bite

---

common tick-borne infections, they are described in this section. In the United States, the incidence of tick-borne disease follows the seasonal pattern of tick exposures; the incidence is generally highest in the spring and summer. Most cases of tick-borne infections occur in children between ages 2 and 15 years because children play outdoors in tick-infested areas. Most ticks live in grasses and plants, especially in heavily wooded areas. As a child brushes past the grass or plant, the tick crawls onto the child and attaches. Unattached ticks on a family pet may climb onto a child who is playing with or grooming the animal. As the tick ingests blood, the warmth of that blood activates the bacteria. After the tick feeds for 6 to 10 hours, the organisms are released from the tick's salivary glands.

Not every tick is infected. The total number of organisms in infected ticks varies, and the severity of the resulting disease is dose related.

Treated early, prognosis of tick-borne disease is generally good; delaying treatment increases morbidity and mortality (Graham et al., 2011). Complications of untreated RMSF and HME can lead to death. Mortality from RMSF is 2% to 3% and lowest in children younger than 9 years of age; if antibiotic administration is delayed beyond 5 days, the fatality rate increases to 22.9% (Graham et al., 2011). Mortality associated with HME is 3%; disease severity is greater in immunocompromised patients (St. Clair & Decker, 2012). Mortality is rare with Lyme disease, typically involving cardiac disease if it occurs (Rim & Eppes, 2007).

Assessment

Obtain a thorough history and physical examination. Thoroughness is important because symptoms may be vague in all three of these tick-borne diseases (Table 24-3). Ask whether the child or parents have found a tick or remember an insect bite.

The rickettsiae in the spotted fever group of diseases cause a vasculitis that involves the skin (as a rash; Fig. 24-11) and major organ systems. Untreated cases with high numbers of organisms can present as overwhelming meningitis, multisystem organ failure, and disseminated intravascular coagulopathy.

HME symptomatically resembles RMSF. Some patients with Lyme disease are completely asymptomatic. During the early, localized stage, which occurs 3 to 30 days after the tick bite, a distinctive rash known as *erythema migrans* appears (Fig. 24-12). Early treatment of erythema migrans should prevent other manifestations, including later stages of the disease.

Diagnosis is based primarily on a history of a tick bite (especially one with an attached tick) and specific serologic tests for each of the three organisms. Acute and

TABLE 24-3   Clinical Features of Selected Tick-Borne Diseases

Disease	Bacterial Agent and Vector	Clinical Manifestations
Rocky Mountain spotted fever (RMSF)	*Rickettsia rickettsii* Dog tick Lone star tick Wood tick	Fever, headache, malaise, myalgia, nausea, and vomiting Rash: occurs before sixth day of illness, begins on wrists and ankles, and spreads centrally and to palms and soles; 10%–15% of cases have no rash (spotless fever) Severe cases: disseminated intravascular coagulopathy, organ failure, and death
Ehrlichiosis	*Ehrlichia chaffeensis* Deer tick	Fever, headache, chills, and malaise; rarely rash, which may help differentiate from RMSF Severe cases: renal failure, meningitis, encephalopathy, and respiratory failure
Lyme disease	*Borrelia burgdorferi* Deer tick	Early localized stage: erythema migrans (erythematous macule or papule with central clearing) at site of tick bite, fever, arthralgia, and myalgia Early disseminated stage: headache, fever, chills, malaise, multiple erythema migrans smaller than the original lesion, hepatosplenomegaly, sore throat with a nonproductive cough, conjunctivitis, lymphadenopathy, meningitis, and carditis Late disseminated stage: seizures, ataxia, chronic fatigue, numerous ocular lesions (panuveitis, retinal vasculitis), and chronic arthritis

convalescent antibody titers for RMSF, ehrlichiosis, and Lyme disease show a fourfold increase in the indirect fluorescent antibody test. These titers are usually accurate 7 to 10 days after the onset of the illness and are diagnostic at 1:64 (AAP, 2012t). IgM and IgG antibodies for each of the specific organisms can be measured by enzyme immunoassay.

Interdisciplinary Interventions

Treatment usually begins empirically while waiting for the test results. For a child who requires hospitalization, the treatment of choice for RMSF is doxycycline.

Fluoroquinolones are alternative treatments. Doxycycline may be given orally during convalescence or in less severe cases. The course of therapy is 7 to 10 days.

❗ ALERT   *Administration of tetracyclines to children younger than 9 years of age is typically avoided because of the risk of permanently staining developing teeth. However, some experts consider doxycycline to be the drug of choice at any age in acute life-threatening cases of rickettsial infection (AAP, 2012t).*

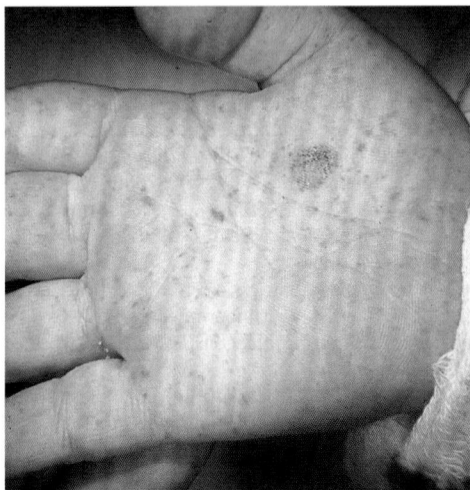

Figure 24-11 The rash of RMSF begins on the wrists and ankles and then spreads to become more generalized. Courtesy of Stuart Starr, MD, The Children's Hospital of Philadelphia. Reprinted with permission.

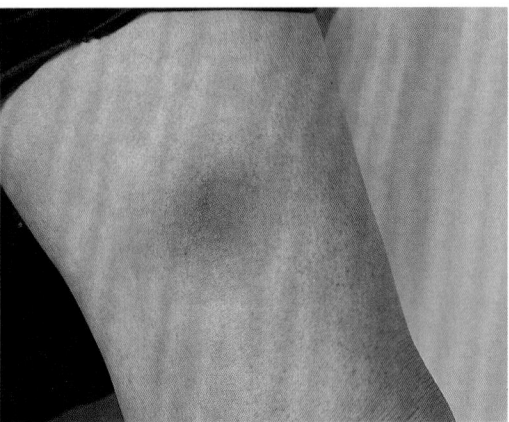

Figure 24-12 The erythema migrans of Lyme disease begins as a small, circular, reddened area and then expands with a central zone of clearing. Copyright Larry Mulvehill/Science Source/Photo Researchers. Reprinted with permission.

For ehrlichiosis, doxycycline is also the drug of choice. The treatment for Lyme erythema migrans and early disease is oral doxycycline. This drug should be given to children older than 8 years of age; children younger than 8 years of age should receive amoxicillin (Graham et al., 2011). Cefuroxime is the alternative for children younger than 9 years of age who are allergic to penicillin. Early Lyme disease is treated for 14 to 21 days. For early disseminated or late Lyme disease, IV penicillin or ceftriaxone is used for 14 to 28 days.

Community Care

Children with tick-borne illnesses are not contagious and therefore do not need isolation. Prevention is paramount; teach the family how to avoid tick attachment and remove ticks safely (see Teaching Intervention Plan 24-2). Agents other than DEET (e.g., picaridin, lemon eucalyptus oil, clove oil, IR3535) have been suggested as effective insect repellents (Cilek et al., 2004; Kendrick, 2006; Shapiro, 2012), but their effectiveness against ticks has not been determined.

Report all tick-borne infections to the state and local health departments. Although the child is not contagious, suggest to parents that they notify the school nurse when the child is being treated to dispel unwarranted fear among classmates.

See thePoint for a Summary of Key Concepts.

REFERENCES

American Academy of Pediatrics. (2012a). Adenovirus. In L. K. Pickering, C. J. Baker, D. W. Kimberlin et al. (Eds.), *Red book: 2012 report of the Committee on Infectious Diseases* (29th ed., pp. 220–222). Elk Grove Village, IL: Author.

American Academy of Pediatrics. (2012b). Ascaris. In L. K. Pickering, C. J. Baker, D. W. Kimberlin et al. (Eds.), *Red book: 2012 report of the Committee on Infectious Diseases* (29th ed., pp. 239–240). Elk Grove Village, IL: Author.

American Academy of Pediatrics. (2012c). Chlamydia. In L. K. Pickering, C. J. Baker, D. W. Kimberlin et al. (Eds.), *Red book: 2012 report of the Committee on Infectious Diseases* (29th ed., pp. 276–281). Elk Grove Village, IL: Author.

American Academy of Pediatrics. (2012d). Cytomegalovirus. In L. K. Pickering, C. J. Baker, D. W. Kimberlin et al. (Eds.), *Red book: 2012 report of the Committee on Infectious Diseases* (29th ed., pp. 300–305). Elk Grove Village, IL: Author.

American Academy of Pediatrics. (2012e). Enterovirus. In L. K. Pickering, C. J. Baker, D. W. Kimberlin et al. (Eds.), *Red book: 2012 report of the Committee on Infectious Diseases* (29th ed., pp. 315–318). Elk Grove Village, IL: Author.

American Academy of Pediatrics. (2012f). Epstein–Barr virus. In L. K. Pickering, C. J. Baker, D. W. Kimberlin et al. (Eds.), *Red book: 2012 report of the Committee on Infectious Diseases* (29th ed., pp. 318–321). Elk Grove Village, IL: Author.

American Academy of Pediatrics. (2012g). Giardia. In L. K. Pickering, C. J. Baker, D. W. Kimberlin et al. (Eds.), *Red book: 2012 report of the Committee on Infectious Diseases* (29th ed., pp. 333–335). Elk Grove Village, IL: Author.

American Academy of Pediatrics. (2012h). Gonococcal infections. In L. K. Pickering, C. J. Baker, D. W. Kimberlin et al. (Eds.), *Red book: 2012 report of the Committee on Infectious Diseases* (29th ed., pp. 336–343). Elk Grove Village, IL: Author.

American Academy of Pediatrics. (2012i). Hepatitis. In L. K. Pickering, C. J. Baker, D. W. Kimberlin et al. (Eds.), *Red book: 2012 report of the Committee on Infectious Diseases* (29th ed., pp. 361–397). Elk Grove Village, IL: Author.

American Academy of Pediatrics. (2012j). Herpes simplex virus. In L. K. Pickering, C. J. Baker, D. W. Kimberlin et al. (Eds.), *Red book: 2012 report of the Committee on Infectious Diseases* (29th ed., pp. 398–408). Elk Grove Village, IL: Author.

American Academy of Pediatrics. (2012k). HHV6. In L. K. Pickering, C. J. Baker, D. W. Kimberlin et al. (Eds.), *Red book: 2012 report of the Committee on Infectious Diseases* (29th ed., pp. 441–417). Elk Grove Village, IL: Author.

American Academy of Pediatrics. (2012l). HIV. In L. K. Pickering, C. J. Baker, D. W. Kimberlin et al. (Eds.), *Red book: 2012 report of the Committee on Infectious Diseases* (29th ed., pp. 418–438). Elk Grove Village, IL: Author.

American Academy of Pediatrics. (2012m). Measles. In L. K. Pickering, C. J. Baker, D. W. Kimberlin et al. (Eds.), *Red book: 2012 report of the Committee on Infectious Diseases* (29th ed., pp. 489–499). Elk Grove Village, IL: Author.

American Academy of Pediatrics. (2012n). Mumps. In L. K. Pickering, C. J. Baker, D. W. Kimberlin et al. (Eds.), *Red book: 2012 report of the Committee on Infectious Diseases* (29th ed., pp. 514–517). Elk Grove Village, IL: Author.

American Academy of Pediatrics. (2012o). Nontubercular mycobacterial (NTM) infections. In L. K. Pickering, C. J. Baker, D. W. Kimberlin et al. (Eds.), *Red book: 2012 report of the Committee on Infectious Diseases* (29th ed., pp. 759–767). Elk Grove Village, IL: Author.

American Academy of Pediatrics. (2012p). Parvovirus B19. In L. K. Pickering, C. J. Baker, D. W. Kimberlin et al. (Eds.), *Red book: 2012 report of the Committee on Infectious Diseases* (29th ed., pp. 539–541). Elk Grove Village, IL: Author.

American Academy of Pediatrics. (2012q). Pertussis. In L. K. Pickering, C. J. Baker, D. W. Kimberlin et al. (Eds.), *Red book: 2012 report of the Committee on Infectious Diseases* (29th ed., pp. 553–565). Elk Grove Village, IL: Author.

American Academy of Pediatrics. (2012r). Pinworms. In L. K. Pickering, C. J. Baker, D. W. Kimberlin et al. (Eds.), *Red book: 2012 report of the Committee on Infectious Diseases* (29th ed., pp. 566–567). Elk Grove Village, IL: Author.

American Academy of Pediatrics. (2012s). Pneumococcal infections. In L. K. Pickering, C. J. Baker, D. W. Kimberlin et al. (Eds.), *Red book: 2012 report of the Committee on Infectious Diseases* (29th ed., pp. 571–581). Elk Grove Village, IL: Author.

American Academy of Pediatrics. (2012t). Rickettsial diseases. In L. K. Pickering, C. J. Baker, D. W. Kimberlin et al. (Eds.), *Red book: 2012 report of the Committee on Infectious Diseases* (29th ed., pp. 620–621). Elk Grove Village, IL: Author.

American Academy of Pediatrics. (2012u). Staphylococcal infections. In L. K. Pickering, C. J. Baker, D. W. Kimberlin et al. (Eds.), *Red book: 2012 report of the Committee on Infectious Diseases* (29th ed., pp. 563–667). Elk Grove Village, IL: Author.

American Academy of Pediatrics. (2012v). Streptococcal infections. In L. K. Pickering, C. J. Baker, D. W. Kimberlin et al. (Eds.), *Red book: 2012 report of the Committee on Infectious Diseases* (29th ed., pp. 668–685). Elk Grove Village, IL: Author.

American Academy of Pediatrics. (2012w). Syphilis. In L. K. Pickering, C. J. Baker, D. W. Kimberlin et al. (Eds.), *Red book: 2012 report of the Committee on Infectious Diseases* (29th ed., pp. 690–702). Elk Grove Village, IL: Author.

American Academy of Pediatrics. (2012x). Toxocariasis. In L. K. Pickering, C. J. Baker, D. W. Kimberlin et al. (Eds.), *Red book: 2012 report of the Committee on Infectious Diseases* (29th ed., pp. 719). Elk Grove Village, IL: Author.

American Academy of Pediatrics. (2012y). Toxoplasmosis. In L. K. Pickering, C. J. Baker, D. W. Kimberlin et al. (Eds.), *Red book: 2012 report of the Committee on Infectious Diseases* (29th ed., pp. 720–727). Elk Grove Village, IL: Author.

American Academy of Pediatrics. (2012z). Tuberculosis. In L. K. Pickering, C. J. Baker, D. W. Kimberlin et al. (Eds.), *Red book: 2012 report of the Committee on Infectious Diseases* (29th ed., pp. 736–758). Elk Grove Village, IL: Author.

American Academy of Pediatrics. (2012aa). Varicella zoster virus. In L. K. Pickering, C. J. Baker, D. W. Kimberlin et al. (Eds.), *Red book: 2012 report of the Committee on Infectious Diseases* (29th ed., pp. 774–788). Elk Grove Village, IL: Author.

Arifeen, S., Black, R. E., Antelman, G. et al. (2001). Exclusive breast-feeding reduces acute respiratory infection and diarrhea deaths among infants in Dhaka slums. *Pediatrics, 108*(4), e67. Retrieved from http://pediatrics.aappublications.org/cgi/content/full/108/4/e67

Atkinson, W., Wolfe, C., & Hamborsky, J. (2012). *Epidemiology and prevention of vaccine-preventable diseases* (12th ed., second printing). Washington, DC: Public Health Foundation. Retrieved from http://www.cdc.gov/vaccines/pubs/pinkbook/table-of-contents.html

Bachrach, V. R., Schwarz, E., & Bachrach, L. R. (2003). Breast-feeding and the risk of hospitalization for respiratory disease in infancy: A meta-analysis. *Archives of Pediatrics & Adolescent Medicine, 157*, 237–243.

Balcarek, K. B., Bagley, R., Cloud, G. A. et al. (1990). Cytomegalovirus infection among employees of a children's hospital: No evidence for increased risk associated with patient care. *Journal of the American Medical Association, 263*(6), 840–844.

Bateman, S. L., & Seed, P. C. (2010). Procession to pediatric bacteremia and sepsis: Covert operations and failure of diplomacy. *Pediatrics, 126*(1), 137–150.

Bechini, A., Tiscione, E., Boccalini, S. et al. (2012). Acellular pertussis vaccine use in risk groups (adolescents, pregnant women, newborns and health care workers): A review of evidences and recommendations. *Vaccine, 30*(35), 5179–5190.

Bethony, J., Brooker, S., Albonico, M. et al. (2006). Soil-transmitted helminth infections: Ascariasis, trichuriasis, and hookworm. *Lancet, 367*(9521), 1521–1532.

Bizzarro, M. J., Jiang, Y., Hussain, N. et al. (2011). The impact of environmental and genetic factors on neonatal late-onset sepsis. *Journal of Pediatrics, 158*(2), 234–238.

Blaymore Bier, J., Oliver, T., Ferguson, A. et al. (2002). Human milk reduces outpatient upper respiratory symptoms in premature infants during their first year of life. *Journal of Perinatology, 22*, 354–359.

Brooker, S. (2010). Estimating the global distribution and disease burden of intestinal nematode infections: Adding up the numbers—A review. *International Journal for Parasitology, 40*(10), 1137–1144.

Burrack, G., Gaur, S., Marone, R. et al. (2010). Adherence to antiretroviral therapy in pediatric patients with human immunodeficiency virus (HIV-1). *Journal of Pediatric Nursing, 25*(6), 500–504.

Centers for Disease Control and Prevention. (2006a). Emergence of *Mycobacterium tuberculosis* with extensive resistance to second-line drugs: Worldwide, 2000–2004. *Morbidity and Mortality Weekly Report, 55*(11), 301–305.

Centers for Disease Control and Prevention. (2006b). Mumps epidemic: United Kingdom, 2004–2005. *Morbidity and Mortality Weekly Report, 55*(07), 173–175.

Centers for Disease Control and Prevention. (2008). Notifiable diseases/deaths in selected cities: Weekly information. *Morbidity and Mortality Weekly Report, 57*(41), 1131–1142.

Centers for Disease Control and Prevention. (2010). Sexually transmitted diseases treatment guidelines, 2010. *Morbidity and Mortality Weekly Report, 59*(RR12), 1–116.

Centers for Disease Control and Prevention. (2011a). Measles—United States, 2011. *Morbidity and Mortality Weekly Report, 61*(15), 253–257.

Centers for Disease Control and Prevention. (2011b). *Sexually transmitted disease surveillance 2010.* Atlanta, GA: Author. Retrieved from http://www.cdc.gov/std/stats10/surv2010.pdf

Chakraborty, R., & Luck, S. (2007). Managing congenital syphilis again? The more things change. *Current Opinion in Infectious Diseases, 20*, 247–252.

Chantry, C. J., Howard, C. R., & Auinger, P. (2006). Full breast-feeding duration and associated decrease in respiratory tract infection in US children. *Pediatrics, 117*, 425–432.

Cherry, J., Grimprel, E., Guiso, N. et al. (2005). Defining pertussis epidemiology: Clinical, microbiologic and serologic perspectives. [1. Epidemiology of pertussis]. *The Pediatric Infectious Disease Journal, 24*(5), S25–S34.

Chiappini, E., Regoli, M., Bonsignori, F. et al. (2011). Guidelines for the management of acute pharyngitis in adults and children. *Clinical Therapeutics, 33*(1), 48–58.

Cilek, J. E., Petersen, J. L., & Hallmon, C. E. (2004). Comparative efficacy of IR3535 and DEET as repellents against adult *Aedes aegypti* and *Culex quinquefasciatus. Journal of the American Mosquito Control Association, 20*, 299–304.

Coutsoudis, A., Pillay, K., Spooner, E. et al. (1999). Influence of infant-feeding patterns on early mother-to-child transmission of HIV-1 in Durban, South Africa: A prospective cohort study. *Lancet, 354*(9177), 471–476.

Dellinger, R. P., Levy, M. M., Carlet, J. M. et al. (2008). Surviving Sepsis Campaign: International guidelines for management of severe sepsis and septic shock: 2008. *Critical Care Medicine, 36*(1), 296–327.

de Silva, A., Jones, P. W., & Spencer, S. A. (2004). Does human milk reduce infection rates in preterm infants? A systematic review. *Archives of Disease in Childhood Fetal and Neonatal Edition, 89*, F509–F513.

Dewey, K. G., Heinig, M. J., & Nommsen-Rivers, L. A. (1995). Differences in morbidity between breast-fed and formula-fed infants. *Journal of Pediatrics, 126*, 696–702.

Dollard, S. C., Grosse, S. D., & Ross, D. S. (2007). New estimates of the prevalence of neurological and sensory sequelae and mortality associated with congenital cytomegalovirus infection. *Reviews in Medical Virology, 17*(5), 355–363.

Dunn, D., Wallon, M., Peyron, F. et al. (1999). Mother-to-child transmission of toxoplasmosis: Risk estimates for clinical counselling. *Lancet, 353*(9167), 1829–1833.

Duszak, R. S. (2009). Congenital rubella syndrome—Major review. *Optometry, 80*, 36–43.

Dyer, J. A. (2007). Childhood viral exanthems. *Pediatric Annals, 36*(1), 21–29.

Edmond, K. M., Kortsalioudaki, C., Scott, S. et al. (2012). Group B streptococcal disease in infants aged younger than 3 months: Systematic review and meta-analysis. *Lancet, 379*(9815), 547–556.

Eidelman, A. I., & Schanler, R. J. (2012). Breastfeeding and the use of human milk. *Pediatrics, 129*(3), e827–e841.

el-Mohandes, A. E., Picard, M. B., Simmens, S. J. et al. (1997). Use of human milk in the intensive care nursery decreases the incidence of nosocomial sepsis. *Journal of Perinatology, 17*, 130–134.

Forsyth, K. (2007). Pertussis, still a formidable foe. *Clinical Infectious Diseases, 45*(11), 1487–1491.

Gdalevich, M., Mimouni, D., & Mimouni, M. (2001). Breast-feeding and the risk of bronchial asthma in childhood: A systematic review with meta-analysis of prospective studies. *Journal of Pediatrics, 139*, 261–266.

Goldstein, B., Giroir, B., Randolph, A. et al. (2005). International pediatric sepsis consensus conference: Definitions for sepsis and organ dysfunction in pediatrics. *Pediatric Critical Care Medicine, 6*(1), 2–8.

Graham, J., Stockley, K., & Goldman, R. D. (2011). Tick-borne illnesses: A CME update. *Pediatric Emergency Care, 27*(2), 141–147.

Guiso, N., Liese, J., & Plotkin, S. (2011). The Global Pertussis Initiative: Meeting report from the fourth regional roundtable meeting, France, April 14–15, 2010. *Human Vaccine, 7*(4), 481–488.

Hawkes, A., Matin, N., Broutet, N. et al. (2011). Effectiveness of interventions to improve screening for syphilis in pregnancy: A systematic review and meta-analysis. *Lancet Infectious Diseases, 11*(9), 684–691.

Henker, R., & Carlson, K. K. (2007). Fever: Applying research to bedside practice. *Advanced Critical Care, 18*, 76–87.

Howie, P. W., Forsyth, J. S., Ogston, S. A. et al. (1990). Protective effect of breast feeding against infection. *British Medical Journal, 300*(6716), 11–16.

Hylander, M. A., Strobino, D. M., & Dhanireddy, R. (1998). Human milk feedings and infection among very low birth weight infants. *Pediatrics, 102*, e38. Retrieved from http://pediatrics.aappublications.org/cgi/content/full/102/3/e38

Joint United Nations Programme on HIV/AIDS. (2010). *UNAIDS report on the global AIDS epidemic 2010.* Geneva, Switzerland: Author. Retrieved from http://www.unaids.org/globalreport/Global_report.htm

Kadambari, S., Williams, E. J., Luck, S. et al. (2011). Evidence based management guidelines for the detection and treatment of congenital CMV. *Early Human Development, 87*(11), 723–728.

Kalanda, B. F., Verhoeff, F. J., & Brabin, B. J. (2006). Breast and complementary feeding practices in relation to morbidity and growth in Malawian infants. *European Journal of Clinical Nutrition, 60*, 401–407.

Kaye, A. (2011). Toxoplasmosis: Diagnosis, treatment, and prevention in congenitally exposed infants. *Journal of Pediatric Health Care, 25*(6), 355–364.

Kendrick, D. B. (2006). Mosquito repellents and superwarfarin rodenticides: Are they really toxic in children? *Current Opinion in Pediatrics, 18*, 180–183.

Khadivzadeh, T., & Parsai, S. (2004). Effect of exclusive breast-feeding and complementary feeding on infant growth and morbidity. *Eastern Mediterranean Health Journal, 10*, 289–294.

Kissoon, N., Carcillo, J. A., Espinosa, V. et al. (2011). World Federation of Pediatric Intensive Care and Critical Care Societies: Global Sepsis Initiative. *Pediatric Critical Care Medicine, 12*(5), 494–503.

Kissoon, N., Orr, R. A., & Carcillo, J. A. (2010). Updated American College of Critical Care Medicine—Pediatric advanced life support guidelines for management of pediatric and neonatal septic shock: Relevance to the emergency care clinician. *Pediatric Emergency Care, 26*(11), 867–869.

Kramer, M. S., & Kakuma, R. (2002). Optimal duration of exclusive breast-feeding. *The Cochrane Database of Systematic Reviews,* (1), CD003517.

LaBeaud, A. D., Lisgaris, M. V., King, C. H. et al. (2006). Pediatric West Nile virus infection: Neurologic disease presentations during the 2002 epidemic in Cuyahoga County, Ohio. *Pediatric Infectious Disease Journal, 25*(8), 751–753.

Lopez-Alarcon, M., Villalpando, S., & Fajardo, A. (1997). Breast-feeding lowers the frequency and duration of acute respiratory infection and diarrhea in infants under six months of age. *Journal of Nutrition, 127*, 436–443.

Machado, M. S. C., Costa e Silva, B. F. B., Gomes, I. L. C. et al. (2012). Prevalence of cervical Chlamydia trachomatis infection in sexually active adolescents from Salvador, Brazil. *Brazilian Journal of Infectious Diseases, 16*(2), 188–191.

Mandell, G. L., Bennett, J. E., & Dolin, R. (2005). *Principles and practice of infectious diseases* (6th ed.). London, United Kingdom: Churchill Livingstone.

Marais, B. J., Gie, R. P., Hesseling, A. C. et al. (2006). A refined symptom-based approach to diagnose pulmonary tuberculosis in children. *Pediatrics, 118*(5), e1350–e1359.

Maturo, D., Powell, A., Major-Wilson, H. et al. (2011). Development of a protocol for transitioning adolescents with HIV infection to adult care. *Journal of Pediatric Health Care, 25*(1), 16–23.

Morgan, M. A., el-Ghany, S. M., Khalifa, N. A. et al. (2003). Prevalence of cytomegalovirus (CMV) infection among neonatal intensive care unit (NICU) and healthcare workers. *Egypt Journal of Immunology, 10*(2), 1–8.

Mohseni, M. M., & Wilde, J. A. (2012). Viral meningitis: Which patients can be discharged from the emergency department? *Journal of Emergency Medicine, 43*(6), 1181–1187.

Narayanan, I., Prakash, K., Murthy, N. S. et al. (1984). Randomised controlled trial of effect of raw and holder pasteurised human milk and of formula supplements on incidence of neonatal infection. *Lancet, 2*, 1111–1113.

Nesheim, S. R., Kapogiannis, B. G., Soe, M. M. et al. (2007). Trends in opportunistic infections in the pre- and post-highly active antiretroviral therapy eras among HIV-infected children in the Perinatal AIDS Collaborative Transmission Study, 1986–2004. *Pediatrics, 120*(1), 100–109.

Newby, J. M., Gorwitz, R., Lesher, L. et al. (2011). Risk factors for household transmission of community-associated methicillin-resistant staphylococcus aureus. *Pediatric Infectious Disease Journal, 30*(11), 927–932.

O'Connor, T. E., Skinner, L. J., Kiely, P. et al. (2011). Return to contact sports following infectious mononucleosis: The role of serial ultrasonography. *Ear, Nose & Throat Journal, 90*(8), E21–E24.

Odumade, O. A., Hogquist, K. A., & Balfour, H. H. (2011). Progress and problems in understanding and managing primary Epstein-Barr virus infections. *Clinical Microbiology Reviews, 24*(1), 193-209.

Onayade, A. A., Abiona, T. C., Abayomi, I. O. et al. (2004). The first six month growth and illness of exclusively and non-exclusively breast-fed infants in Nigeria. *East African Medical Journal, 81*, 146–153.

Panel on Antiretroviral Therapy and Medical Management of HIV-Infected Children. (2011). *Guidelines for the use of antiretroviral agents in pediatric HIV infection.* Retrieved from http://aidsinfo.nih.gov/contentfiles/lvguidelines/pediatricguidelines.pdf

Park, D. W., Nam, M. H., Kim, J. Y. et al. (2007). Mumps outbreak in a highly vaccinated school population: Assessment of secondary vaccine failure using IgG avidity measurements. *Vaccine, 25*, 4665–4670.

Polin, R.A. & Committee on Fetus and Newborn. (2012). Management of neonates with suspected or proven early-onset bacterial sepsis. *Pediatrics, 129*(5), 1006–1015.

Prendergast, A., Tudor-Williams, G., Jeena, P. et al. (2007). International perspectives, progress, and future challenges of paediatric HIV infection. *Lancet, 370*(9581), 68–80.

Putukian, M., O'Connor, F. G., Stricker, P. R. et al. (2008). Mononucleosis and athletic participation: An evidence-based subject review. *Clinical Journal of Sports Medicine, 18*(4), 309–315.

Quigley, M. A., Kelly, Y. J., & Sacker, A. (2007). Breast-feeding and hospitalization for diarrheal and respiratory infection in the United Kingdom Millennium Cohort Study. *Pediatrics, 119*(4), e837–e842. Retrieved from http://pediatrics.aappublications.org/cgi/content/full/119/4/e837

Riley, C., & Wheeler, D. S. (2012). Prevention of sepsis in children: A new paradigm for public policy. *Critical Care Research and Practice, 2012*, 437139.

Rim, J. Y., & Eppes, S. (2007). Tick-borne diseases. *Pediatric Annals, 36*, 390–403.

Rodríguez-Nuñez, A., Dosil-Gallardo, S., Jordan I. et al. (2011). Clinical characteristics of children with group A streptococcal toxic shock syndrome admitted to pediatric intensive care units. *European Journal of Pediatrics, 170*(5), 639–644.

Scott, C. A., Atkinson, S. H., Sodha, A. et al. (2012). Management of lymphadenitis due to non-tuberculous mycobacterial infection in children. *Pediatric Surgery International, 28*(5), 461–466.

Shapiro, R. (2012). Prevention of vector transmitted diseases with clove oil insect repellent. *Journal of Pediatric Nursing, 27*(4), 346–349.

Siegel, J. D., Rhinehart, E., Jackson, M. et al. (2007). *2007 guideline for isolation precautions: Preventing transmission of infectious agents in healthcare settings.* Retrieved from http://www.cdc.gov/hicpac/2007ip/2007isolationprecautions.html

Smith, E. A., Jacques-Carroll, L., Walker, T. Y. et al. (2012). The National Perinatal Hepatitis B Prevention Program, 1994–2008. *Pediatrics, 129*(4), 609–616.

Stanforth, B., Krause, A., Starkey, C. et al. (2010). Prevalence of community-associated methicillin-resistant Staphylococcus aureus in high school wrestling environments. *Journal of Environmental Health, 72*(6), 12–16.

St. Clair, K., & Decker, C.F. (2012). Ehrlichioses: Anaplasmosis and human ehrlichiosis. *Disease-a-month, 58*(6), 346–354.

Steer, A. C., Lamagni, T., Curtis, N. et al. (2012). Invasive group A streptococcal disease: Epidemiology, pathogenesis and management. *Drugs, 72*(9), 1213–1227.

Straface, G., Selmin, A., Zanardo, V. et al. (2012). Herpes simplex virus infection in pregnancy. *Infectious Diseases in Obstetrics and Gynecology, 2012*, 385697.

Sullivan, S., Schanler, R. J., Kim, J. H. et al. (2010). An exclusively human milk-based diet is associated with lower rate of necrotizing enterocolitis than a diet of human milk and bovine milk-based products. *Journal of Pediatrics, 156*(4), 562–567.

Truemper, E. J., & Romero, J. R. (2007). West Nile virus. *Pediatric Annals, 36*, 414–422.

Turbeville, S. D., Cowan, L. D., & Greenfield, R. A. (2006). Infectious disease outbreaks in competitive sports: A review of the literature. *American Journal of Sports Medicine, 34*(11), 1860–1865.

U.S. Preventive Services Task Force. (2009). Screening for hepatitis B virus infection in pregnancy: U.S. Preventive Services Task Force reaffirmation recommendation statement. *Annals of Internal Medicine, 150*(12), 869–873.

Watson-Creed, G., Saunders, A., Scott, J. et al. (2006). Two successive outbreaks of mumps in Nova Scotia among vaccinated adolescents and young adults. *Canadian Medical Association Journal, 175*, 483–488.

Wiseman, C. A., Gie, R. P., Starker, J. R. et al. (2012). A proposed comprehensive classification of tuberculosis disease severity in children. *Pediatric Infectious Disease Journal, 31*(4), 347–352.

Wolfert, S. I. M., de Jong, E. P., Vossen, A. C. T. M. et al. (2011). Diagnostic and therapeutic management for suspected herpes simplex virus infection. *Journal of Clinical Virology, 51*(1), 8–11.

World Health Organization. (2003). *Global strategy for infant and young child feeding.* Geneva, Switzerland: Author.

World Health Organization. (2010a). *Antiretroviral drugs for treating pregnant women and preventing HIV infection in infants.* Geneva, Switzerland: Author. Retrieved from http://whqlibdoc.who.int/publications/2010/9789241599818_eng.pdf

World Health Organization. (2010b). *Guidelines on HIV and infants feeding 2010.* Geneva, Switzerland: Author. Retrieved from http://whqlibdoc.who.int/publications/2010/9789241599535_eng.pdf

World Health Organization. (2011). *Progress report 2011: Global HIV/ AIDS response: Epidemic update and health sector progress towards universal access.* Geneva, Switzerland. Retrieved from http://www.who.int/hiv/pub/progress_report2011/en/index.html

World Health Organization. (2012a). *Soil-transmitted helminthiases: Eliminating soil-transmitted helminthiases as a public health problem in children: Progress report 2001–2010 and strategic plan 2011–2020.* Geneva, Switzerland: Author. Retrieved from http://whqlibdoc.who.int/publications/2012/9789241503129_eng.pdf

World Health Organization. (2012b). *WHO vaccine-preventable diseases: Monitoring system 2012 global summary.* Geneva, Switzerland: Author. Retrieved from http://apps.who.int/immunization_monitoring/en/globalsummary/timeseries/tsincidencemum.htm

See thePoint for additional organizations.

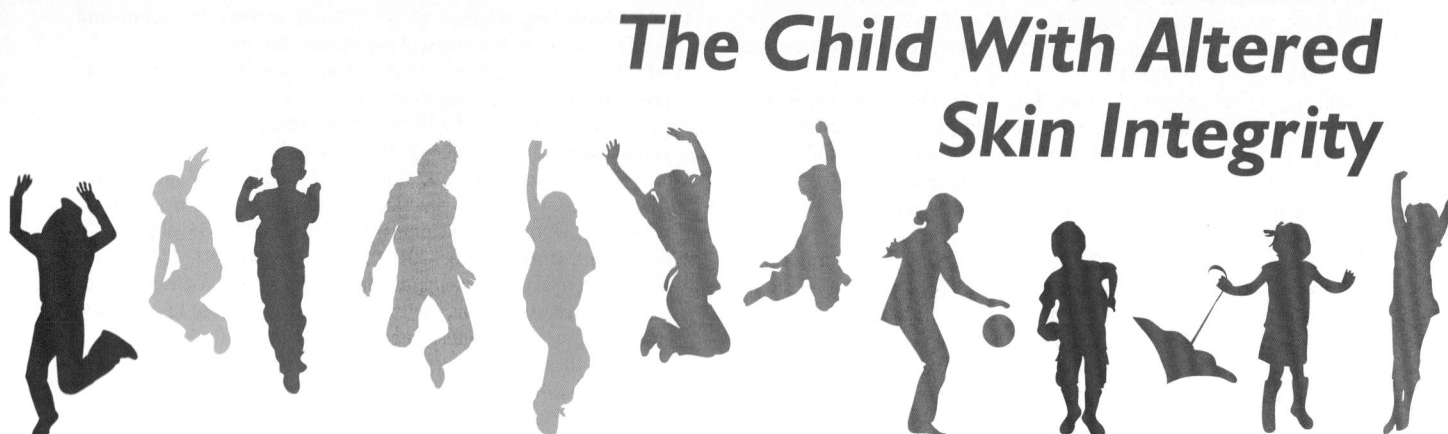

CHAPTER 25

The Child With Altered Skin Integrity

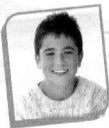

CASE HISTORY

In Chapter 21, you were introduced to Joey Curricio. Nick Curricio, Joey's 13-year-old brother, is a soccer player and Boy Scout. He is attending Boy Scout camp this summer between seventh and eighth grade. Unfortunately, he has returned home early from camp with an extensive rash. Nick has an olive complexion, he tans easily, and he is not prone to skin-related problems. He has seasonal allergies, ragweed in particular.

On Wednesday, pink patches began to appear on Nick's arms and neck. On Friday, the rash was continuing to spread, and Nick was sent home from camp. When his mother picked him up, his rash appeared as raised, pink blisters in patches across both forearms, on the inner aspect of the upper arms, on his torso where his arms came in contact with his torso, and on his neck up to the jaw line. Some of the blisters are still intact; many are ruptured and leaking fluid. Approximately one third of his skin above the waist is affected by the rash. Nick complains that he itches all the time, and he can't sleep.

His mother takes him to their family physician, who diagnoses this rash as a bad case of poison ivy. Nick has only had

a rash from poison ivy once, and it consisted of a spot about the size of a half dollar on the back of his hand. He asks the office nurse why it is so different this time. The nurse explains that like many other allergic reactions, the reaction is greater with subsequent exposure. It is the oils of the plant that cause the reaction. Because Nick did not realize he had come into contact with the plant, the oils on his shirt and arms continued to touch new areas of skin. He also did not shower that day or night.

The physician sends them home with a methylprednisolone dose pack, the recommendation to take an antihistamine at night, and instructions for topical care of the rash. Topical care includes using hydrocortisone cream or calamine lotion to help control itching. Cool compresses and tub soaks with colloidal oatmeal or baking soda may also help relieve itching. In addition, his mother should wash all the clothes that Nick brought home, including anything thrown in the duffle bag with the dirty clothes Nick wore in the woods.

CHAPTER OBJECTIVES

1 Identify characteristics of the child's skin that make the child especially susceptible to injury.

2 Perform a health history and physical examination that include a complete evaluation of the skin, hair, and nails.

3 Select nursing diagnoses that articulate the needs of the child, family, and community for the child who has a skin condition.

4 Describe the presenting signs and symptoms of skin conditions frequently seen in the pediatric population.

5 Use strategies to prevent further spread of a skin condition or further damage to tissue that has altered skin integrity.

6 Discuss therapies that are effective in treating conditions of the skin.

7 Identify the best evidence supporting treatment of conditions of the skin.

See thePoint for a list Key Terms.

The skin is an undervalued organ. Despite constant exposure to a changing environment, it provides an effective defense against disease and promotes homeostasis. To perform these functions, however, the skin must remain intact. Skin disorders are extremely common in infants, children, and adolescents and in many pediatric health care practices constitute the most frequent significant complaint for an office visit. Skin disorders can affect the daily life of the child by excluding him or her from school or daycare (Mancini, 2005; Popovich & McAlhany, 2007). Skin conditions are, by their nature, visible. Children with altered skin integrity have the same needs as all other children but must also cope with the ways their condition affects their lives and the perceptions of others. Health care providers must understand the basic principles of skin and wound diseases and appropriate interventions. This chapter explores various disorders that breach the skin's defense system, including infections, noninfectious conditions, and trauma.

DEVELOPMENTAL AND BIOLOGIC VARIANCES

The integumentary system begins to develop by the eighth week of gestation and continues to undergo many metamorphic events throughout the course of the individual's life. Skin, hair, and nail cells are constantly moving through stages of growth, replication, and maturation. The infant's fragile skin transforms during the first 3 years of life into a barrier of protection against a young child's many falls. During adolescence, hormonal changes trigger changes in skin appearance, contour, and smell. In addition, biologic variances such as color are more pronounced in the integumentary system than in most other body systems.

NEONATES AND INFANTS

The skin of the newborn serves a pivotal role in the transition from the "wet" (aqueous) intrauterine environment to the "dry" extrauterine environment. The skin, hair, and nails develop early in gestation. At less than 8 weeks of fetal life, the epidermis begins to form. Between the 14th and 16th weeks of gestation, nail and hair formation is established. A unique skin characteristic of the fetus is that the embryo and the early-gestation fetus (during the second and third trimesters) have the ability to heal a potentially scarring injury without scar formation. Although the exact processes of fetal wound healing are not fully understood, it is known that epithelial and mesenchymal tissues are regenerated to restore the tissues (Valencia et al., 2001).

Lanugo (fine, soft, lightly pigmented hair) covers most of the fetal skin. During the early neonatal period, vellus hair (also fine, short, soft, and lightly pigmented) replaces lanugo. Over time, terminal hair growth replaces vellus hair on the scalp, arms, and legs. Many other body areas continue to be covered with vellus hair until puberty (Fig. 25-1). Immediately after birth, vernix caseosa (a white, cheeselike substance produced in utero by the sebaceous glands) clings to the neonate's skin, especially on the neck, groin, and genital regions. This substance, which begins to form after the 20th week of gestation, protects the delicate fetal skin from abrasions, chapping, and hardening as a result of continuous exposure to amniotic fluid.

After birth, environmental and behavioral factors (e.g., ambient temperature, surface moisture, intermittent friction from clothing and blankets, and even being held) can affect skin structure and functions. Pigmentation is not well developed; the neonate's nail beds, ears, and scrotal areas are generally darker than the rest of the skin. **Milia** (white papules) caused by blocked sebaceous ducts appear over the nose, cheeks, and chin but disappear within a few weeks after birth. Because the vasomotor control of the skin in neonates is immature, a mottled appearance (cutis marmorata) may be observed in response to cooling, and the hands and feet may show acrocyanosis transiently. Prolonged cyanosis must be investigated.

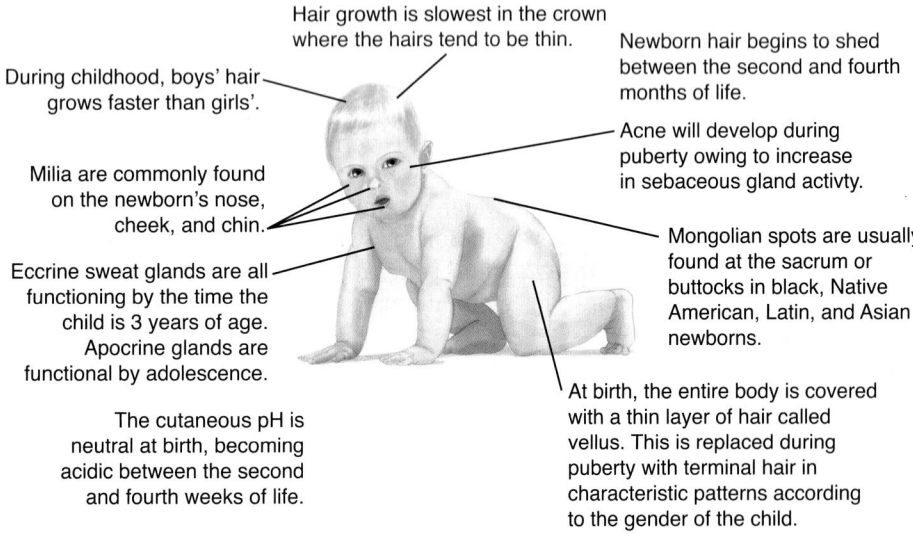

Hair growth is slowest in the crown where the hairs tend to be thin.

During childhood, boys' hair grows faster than girls'.

Milia are commonly found on the newborn's nose, cheek, and chin.

Eccrine sweat glands are all functioning by the time the child is 3 years of age. Apocrine glands are functional by adolescence.

The cutaneous pH is neutral at birth, becoming acidic between the second and fourth weeks of life.

Newborn hair begins to shed between the second and fourth months of life.

Acne will develop during puberty owing to increase in sebaceous gland activty.

Mongolian spots are usually found at the sacrum or buttocks in black, Native American, Latin, and Asian newborns.

At birth, the entire body is covered with a thin layer of hair called vellus. This is replaced during puberty with terminal hair in characteristic patterns according to the gender of the child.

The viscoelastic property of the dermis becomes completely functional at about 2 years of age.

The neonate's dermis is thin and very hydrated; thus, it is at greater risk for fluid loss and serves as an ineffective barrier.

Figure 25-1 Developmental and biologic variances: the skin and hair.

The structure of the term newborn's skin is similar to that of an older child and about 40% to 60% thinner than that of an adult (Eichenfield et al., 2008). The neonate's vascular and integument structures are immature, and melanin production and eccrine gland function are reduced; therefore, the skin has yet to develop all of its protective, metabolic, and interactive functions. Skin pH is more alkaline during the first few weeks of life, making it a better host for harboring microorganisms. As the pH becomes more acidic, the skin's capacity to fight infection improves.

The premature infant's skin reveals many unique features based on the degree of prematurity. The epidermis is very thin, transparent, permeable, and friable and is not equipped to handle the demands of thermoregulation, homeostasis, and protection (Developmental Considerations 25-1). In comparison, the skin of postmature and small neonates is thicker, appears dry and cracked, and may be meconium stained.

Skin functions in premature infants are primarily protective, one of the foremost being the regulation of water loss and intake. Permeability barrier immaturity in these infants has many consequences, primarily increased evaporative loss of free water from the skin surface, which could lead to energy loss through loss of heat by evaporation. This process can result in transepidermal water loss (evaporation of water from the skin). Numerous interventions are available to reduce the potential for fluid loss in premature newborns (see Chapter 14 for a complete discussion of these interventions).

The skin of term infants exhibits excellent barrier properties; in fact, its barrier function, as measured by transepidermal water loss, is superior to that of adult skin. The full-term neonate has well-developed brown fat stores—some internal (e.g., on the neck, behind the sternum) and some found over the scapular area in the connective tissue. The skin of the newborn has a greater ratio of body surface area to body weight than

---

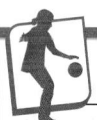

DEVELOPMENTAL CONSIDERATIONS 25-1

Characteristics of the Premature Infant's Skin

Thin, transparent, permeable, and poorly keratinized epidermis

The stratum corneum is not fully mature until about 34 weeks' gestation

Epidermal layer consisting of only a few layers of stratum corneum during first 3 weeks of life

Diminished cohesion between less cohesive epidermal and dermal layers

Dearth of sebaceous lubrication after first few weeks of life

Immature acid mantle

Enhanced permeability of the skin

Little subcutaneous fat

Wrinkled, gelatinous skin hanging loosely over limbs

Lanugo covering the body and increased vernix caseosa at birth

Increased loss of transepidermal water, leading to difficulty in fluid balance evaporation of water from the skin (called *transepidermal water loss*), which leads to difficulty in maintaining fluid balance

Nonfunctional apocrine sweat glands

Implications for Care

Neonate is prone to hypothermia. Keep the baby warm using an incubator.

Minimize the number of times health care providers enter the isolette, which changes the ambient temperature.

During bathing or procedures in which the neonate is out of the isolette, use heat lamps to keep the newborn warm.

Neonate is prone to skin breakdown, tearing, and blistering. Turn the neonate frequently to prevent skin breakdown.

Minimize use of adhesive-based products on the skin.

Use pectin-based barrier products to protect the skin.

Remove adhesives with water and diluted soap.

Do not bathe the neonate on a frequent basis.

Prevent intravenous (IV) catheter infiltration.

Neonate is at risk for fluid and electrolyte losses. Monitor fluid and electrolyte status diligently.

Provide fluid and electrolytes as needed via IV administration.

Neonate is at risk for potentially lethal topical absorption of chemicals (percutaneous toxicity). Minimize use of pharmacologic and cleansing compounds to the skin, such as neomycin, soap compounds, and lotions.

Information from Allwood, M. (2011). Skin care guidelines for infants aged 23–30 weeks' gestation: A review of the literature. *Neonatal, Paediatric and Child Health Nursing*, 14(1), 20–27; Larson, A., & Dinulos, J. (2005). Cutaneous bacterial infections in the newborn. *Current Opinion in Pediatrics*, 17, 481–486; Lund, C. (1999). Prevention and management of infant skin breakdown. *Nursing Clinics of North America*, 34(4), 907–920; Lund, C. H., Osborne, J. W., Kuller, J. et al. (2001). Neonatal skin care: Clinical outcomes of the AWHONN/NANN evidence-based clinical practice guideline. *Journal of Obstetric, Gynecologic, and Neonatal Nursing*, 30(1), 41–51.

that of the older child or adult. As a result, chemicals placed on newborn skin can be absorbed systemically at higher doses than might be desired.

caREminder

Maintaining and replacing fluid, and preventing fluid loss through evaporation, are vitally important, priority care issues in managing preterm and term infants.

CHILDHOOD AND ADOLESCENCE

As the child grows, both physical and developmental changes are manifested in the skin, hair, and nails. The skin thickens, hair grows at a faster rate, and sebaceous glands provide sebum, which lubricates the skin. Pigmentation darkens. The skin of the well-nourished child is elastic. The skin of young children and infants who eat an abundance of yellow vegetables, such as carrots and squash, may take on a yellowish cast (carotenemia) and is generally considered harmless.

As the child matures, substantial skin changes occur in both boys and girls. Most of these changes represent the onset of puberty. The apocrine and sebaceous glands increase in activity, causing more pronounced body odor and oily skin.

Secondary sex characteristics appear in response to hormonal release, which also stimulates integumentary alterations. For example, in the male, the pubic, axillary, and facial hair start to grow and darken. In the female, the areola of the breast darkens and enlarges, and pubic and axillary hair appears. Hair on the trunk and limbs increases during and after puberty, most noticeably in males. These changes occur as vellus hair converts to terminal hair in specific body regions. Concurrently, in the occipital and bifrontal areas of the male's scalp, some terminal hair converts back to vellus hair, resulting in a receding hair line. These changes in body function can generate problems with self-image in adolescents.

RACIAL VARIATIONS

Differences in the hair and skin pigmentation of children can be seen in persons of different races. For example, considerable variation exists in the hair of African Americans, which ranges from sparse and straight to dense and curly. Asians and Native Americans generally have straight, silky hair, but not in all cases.

Skin eruptions are not generally associated with specific racial differences. The most commonly cited biologic difference is in the appearance of mongolian spots in African American, Native American, Latin, and Asian newborns. Identifying skin lesions and assessing the degree of redness, jaundice, cyanosis, or pallor may be more challenging in children with darker skin tones. In these cases, observing for color changes in the mucous membranes, earlobes, conjunctivae, nails, and palms, or the abdomen and trunk (two areas less exposed to sunlight), may provide the best indicator of systemic problems.

ASSESSMENT

The health history and physical assessment serve as the clinician's tools to evaluate threats to the function, integrity, and cosmetic appearance of the skin, hair, and nails. Numerous environmental risks to the skin are inherent during childhood. Chemically and biologically contaminated air, water, soil, and foods present special risks to children's health. These environmental factors, which have a profound effect on adult health, affect children differently and perhaps more intensely. Children have "windows of vulnerability" while they are developing, during which their target organs and immune system may be more susceptible to environmental risks than an adult's. In addition, children spend their time in different physical locations than adults. For example, infants and young children spend lots of time on the floor; children, because of their height, inhale in a different breathing zone than adults. All these factors must be considered when managing wounds and other skin alterations in children.

FOCUSED HEALTH HISTORY

QUESTION: What information provided in the case study is pertinent in obtaining a focused health history on Nick?

The purpose of the health history is to collect data about the skin changes reported by the child or family and to successfully elicit information that indicates the primary source of the skin eruption. This assessment should provide clues to the diagnosis, management, and nursing care of the underlying issue. Careful observation and meticulous descriptions should cover the following areas: (1) history of the patient's skin condition, (2) physical assessment of the entire child as well as the specific skin condition, and (3) assessment of the child's and care providers' knowledge about the condition. Clinical findings from skin rashes, lesions, and infestations often lack specificity, and the etiologic agents may be elusive. Skin problems can be a source of acute embarrassment, yet assessment requires complete openness from the family. To ensure that all potentially affected individuals are identified and notified to limit further spread of the disorder, the nurse must approach such situations with sensitivity.

Focused Health History 25-1 details the dimensions of the health history specific to identifying skin disorders. Because the skin yields rich information about the child's general health, hygiene practices, and nutritional status, incorporating components of the skin assessment into all health interviews is essential. The skin also reveals many complex systemic pathologic processes. In these situations, the skin history may serve as the preliminary screen pointing to the need for a more in-depth review of a particular system.

The child's age and ethnicity are important data. For instance, distinguishing a bruise from a birthmark, such as a mongolian spot, is easier if the patient is a 7-day-old,

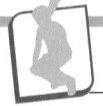

The Child With Altered Skin, Hair, or Nails

Current history	Time of onset
	Evolution of skin lesion
	Site of onset
	Normal appearance of the skin
	Presence of
	  • Itching
	  • Areas of wetness or dryness
	  • Cuts
	  • Rash: flat or raised
	  • Changes in color, shape, contour of nails
	  • Change in skin color: localized or generalized
	  • Areas of skin thinning or thickening
	  • Bruises
	  • Hair loss or excessive growth; change in texture
	Related systemic problems:
	  • Pyrexia
	  • Sore limbs
	  • Recent contact with other persons who have skin disorders
	Child's perception of the disorder

Past medical history	**Birth History**
	  Skin lesions noted at birth
	  Skin color changes after birth
	  Breastfeeding
	Childhood Illnesses
	  Previous communicable diseases
	  Recent exposure to a communicable illness
	Immunizations
	  Any immunizations recently given?
	  Previous postimmunization rashes/responses
	Allergies
	  Allergic reactions to latex, plants, medications, or food
	  Recent changes in food, diaper products, laundry detergents, soap, or other
	    skin products
	Current Treatment
	  Any medications child is taking: topical and systemic, prescribed and over
	    the counter
	  Length of time on medication
	  Recent changes in dosage
	  Home remedies to treat current condition

Nutritional assessment	Recent changes in food or fluids Recent weight loss Weight within normal limits
Family medical history	Family history of acne, psoriasis, impetigo, eczema, allergic reactions

Social and environmental history	Cultural or religious practices that may have caused the condition
	Any recent changes in family lifestyle?
	School attendance (note the name of the child's school or daycare center because communication with a teacher may be necessary)
	Any recent travel abroad
	Exposures to any household chemicals
	Amount of exposure to sun on routine basis
	Presence of insects/animals that may have bitten or scratched the child
Growth and development	**Health Promotion Activities**
	Concerns of child in relation to his or her skin
	Products used to care for child's hair, nails, and skin
	Frequency of bathing and hair washing
	Use of sunscreens, hats, and clothing to protect exposed skin

Note: See Chapter 8 for a comprehensive health history.

dark-skinned child compared to a 7-year-old child with very dark skin. Interview questions should also elicit descriptions of attempts at self-remedy to assess typical health promotion practices in the home.

Take the history from an individual who can describe the evolution of the eruption, potentially related factors, and measures taken to relieve the condition. Older children can provide their own histories, although they may be unable to provide information regarding immunization status, childhood illnesses, and family medical history.

Focus on the course, characteristics, and related systemic problems of the current skin condition. Ask the child or family caregivers to describe the lesions and to identify contacts with other children.

caREminder

With the family's permission, note the name of the child's school or daycare center because communication with the teacher may be necessary if the child's diagnosis proves to be contagious.

The medical history elicits information about events occurring during the prenatal, natal, and neonatal periods. In all children, changes in medication, diet, environment, and lifestyle can be causative factors. Brief encounters with animals, insects, plants, and other children can be key elements in explaining the source of the skin condition.

ANSWER: It is pertinent that Nick developed a rash in a new and different environment. It is relevant that rashes are unusual for Nick and that he does suffer from allergies.

FOCUSED PHYSICAL ASSESSMENT

QUESTION: What are the characteristics of Nick's rash that you would observe and document?

As the child develops, the skin, hair, and nails will change in appearance as a result of exposure to environmental elements and natural changes associated with human development.

Skin

Physical assessment of the skin involves two basic techniques: inspection and palpation. Focused Physical Assessment 25-1 summarizes the key data to assess during the examination. The ideal environment for the physical assessment is a well-lit room with white walls. Bright white fluorescent ceiling lighting is optimal because it does not cast a yellow hue on the skin.

caREminder

*Gloves are not necessarily required for skin assessment. However, if you suspect a contagious disorder, if body fluids are present on the skin, or if lesions are moist, then you must wear gloves. Use vinyl gloves if any possibility exists that the child may have a latex allergy. Touching the skin of an allergic child with latex may precipitate **urticaria** and airway edema.*

The examination room should be warm, and the child should wear an examination gown to provide easy access to all areas of the skin. The infant's diaper should be removed to inspect and palpate the genital area. Allow the child and the adolescent to wear underclothes

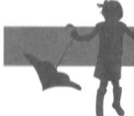

FOCUSED PHYSICAL ASSESSMENT 25-1

Skin, Hair, and Nails

Assessment Parameter	Alterations/Clinical Significance
General appearance of the skin and mucous membranes	Generalized color and condition of the skin versus local changes in skin color: pallor, cyanosis, jaundice, erythema • Yellow or jaundiced: liver disease, hemolytic disease, renal failure, myxedema, anorexia nervosa • Red or red-blue: alcoholism, local inflammatory process, fever, venous stasis • Blue: heart conditions, lung disease, disorder of hemoglobin, disorder of circulation • Pallor or loss of color: syncope, albinism, vitiligo, tinea versicolor, anemia, nephrosis, arterial insufficiency, anxiety states • Hyperpigmentation: mongolian spot, café-au-lait spots, port-wine stain Complexion: over- or underexposure to sun; pallor may indicate presence of illness, shock; blue-tinged complexion indicates cardiac or respiratory problems Turgor and mobility: dehydration, edema, swelling, presence of underlying mass Moisture: dryness found in dermatitis conditions; excessive moisture may indicate fever or hyperhidrosis (excessive sweating) Temperature: hypothermia, hyperthermia Odor; dry skin; presence of dirt may indicate poor hygienic practices Texture: previous scarring, sites of dermatitis outbreaks Vascular changes: telangiectasia, hemangiomas Evidence of scratching, such as erythema, scaling, or excoriated areas: atopic dermatitis (AD), scabies, lice, rash associated with infectious conditions Rash: environmental exposure, allergic reaction, infectious condition Plaques: AD Scaling: seborrheic dermatitis Macules, papules, vesicles: burns; Stevens-Johnson syndrome (SJS); erythema toxicum neonatorum (ETN); impetigo; AD; acne; milia; candidiasis; allergic contact dermatitis (ACD); cat scratch disease (CSD); hand, foot, and mouth disease; seborrhea; poison ivy, oak, sumac; sunburn
General appearance of the hair	Healthy scalp hair is shiny, silky, and strong; may be straight, curly, or kinky Normal distribution: light hair on all other body surfaces except palms, soles, inner labial surfaces (girls), and prepuce and glans penis (boys) Hair distribution appropriate to gender and Tanner staging of child: inappropriate distribution may indicate metabolic problems Quantity and areas of hair loss (alopecia) or balding that may be related to medical treatments (chemotherapy) or chronic hair pulling/tugging Texture: dry, brittle, or depigmented hair as seen in metabolic disorders Scalp condition and hygiene: lesions or scaling may indicate seborrheic dermatitis Presence of white eggs (nits) on hair shaft indicative of lice

Assessment Parameter	Alterations/Clinical Significance
General appearance of the nails	Healthy nail surface is slightly curved or flat (spoon shaped in newborn up to 3 years of age); may appear translucent in infants; edges are smooth, rounded, and clean; nails are clipped and clean, suggesting good hygiene practices
	Signs of nail biting may indicate stress
	Clubbing present with cardiac and chronic conditions; thickening may indicate fungal infection
	Color: discoloration of the nail or nail bed, such as cyanosis, suggests insufficient oxygenation; yellowing suggests fungal infection
	Slow capillary refill indicates problems with circulation
	Presence of hangnail
	Tender nail beds, swollen cutaneous area, pus or blood underneath the nail indicates infection, nail biting
Other systems	Evaluate as indicated by types of lesions, for example, burns will have systemic involvement secondary to fluid and electrolyte loss and damage to underlying tissue; periorbital cellulitis will affect vision and sinuses

during most of the examination to prevent any undue embarrassment and protect the child's emerging sense of modesty.

Begin the assessment with a general inspection of the total skin surface and then proceed to a focused assessment of the specific lesions noted during the health history. This method enables you to assess the general fitness of the skin. These observations can guide the health promotion and disease prevention discussions that conclude the health visit.

The child's pigmentation should be consistent with genetic background and age. Among the members of any population, a significant range of skin colors and hair types exists. Health care professionals must be able to recognize anomalies in children with deeply pigmented skin. For example, lesions that appear red or brown in children with white skin may appear black or purple in pigmented skin. Newborns may present with a bluish color in the nail beds, on hands and feet, and sometimes circumoral (around the mouth) for up to 10 days after birth. Discoloration is especially prominent during episodes of intense crying, breath holding, or exposure to colder environments. This condition, referred to as **acrocyanosis**, results from vascular insufficiency and resolves as the newborn adapts to extrauterine life; it is considered normal. In general, the white infant is usually pink to red, the Hispanic newborn may have an olive tint or slightly yellow hue, black infants may appear pinkish or even yellowish brown, and Asian newborns may be a rosy or yellowish tan. Freckles and moles appear in young children as a function of aging. Many birthmarks, such as mongolian spots, fade as melanocytes in the dermis mature. Inborn variations in skin color must be differentiated from transient changes (associated with crying,

acne, or sunburn) and from reflections of pathologic processes (see Focused Physical Assessment 25-1).

During inspection, use your sense of smell to detect skin odors. Sweat odors can be caused by hormonal changes and, depending on the child's age, may be a sign of poor hygiene. Intense odors can also signify infection. Throughout the assessment process, integrate the child's verbal and nonverbal cues into the examination findings. These can add important data to your assessment. For example, consistent scratching, persistent pulling at clothes, and attempts to discreetly cover certain body areas can indicate a skin condition. Allowing the child to verbalize freely during the physical examination can yield pertinent information.

Inspection and palpation yield information regarding skin moisture, color, thickness, temperature, and texture. Touching the child's skin provides valuable clinical information about skin texture, turgor, and temperature. Note the shape, color, size, consistency, character (e.g., redness, scaling, or excoriation), and distribution of any lesions or birthmarks. Many skin disorders have characteristic patterns of distribution. For example, candidiasis is usually found in the moist, dark intertriginous folds of the groin, axillae, and neck; warts and herpes lesions are most often located on mucous membranes. Eruptions that appear on previously healthy skin as a response to disease or trauma are called **primary lesions** (Table 25-1). **Secondary lesions** result from changes over time in the primary lesion, usually related to the progression of the disease process, scratching, or secondary infection (Table 25-2). Skin lesions can have characteristic shapes that clearly differentiate the diagnosis (see thePoint Supplemental Information: Common Configurations of Skin Lesions). For example, the skin lesions of ringworm (tinea corporis)

TABLE 25-1   Primary Skin Lesions

Type	Description	Example
Macule	Circumscribed change in skin color without elevation or depression; less than 1 cm	Freckle Petechia Flat nevi Measles Scarlet fever
Papule	Solid, elevated, circumscribed area; less than 1 cm	Mole Wart Lichen planus
Nodule	Solid, elevated, hard or soft lesion in the dermal or subcutaneous tissue; larger than 1 cm	Fibroma Intradermal nevi
Tumor	Solid, raised mass; firm or soft; benign or malignant; larger than 1–2 cm	Hemangioma Osteosarcoma
Wheal	Superficial raised area of localized skin edema, irregular, transient, and erythematous	Insect bite Allergic reaction Hive
Vesicle	Circumscribed elevated lesion containing serous fluid; less than 1 cm	Herpes simplex Early varicella (chicken pox) Contact dermatitis
Bulla	Circumscribed elevated lesion containing serous fluid; greater than 1 cm	Partial-thickness (second-degree) burn Blister Contact dermatitis

TABLE 25-1	Primary Skin Lesions *(Continued)*	
Type	**Description**	**Example**
Pustule	Vesicle containing pus	Impetigo Acne
Cyst	Encapsulated, fluid-filled cavity of dermis or subcutaneous layer	Sebaceous cyst Epidermal cyst

From Bickley, L. (2008). *Bates' pocket guide to physical examination and history taking.* Philadelphia, PA: Lippincott Williams & Wilkins. Used with permission.

are annular (circular); contact dermatitis usually forms in cluster shapes; and chicken pox appears as distinct, individual lesions.

Risk assessment is an important factor in preventing pressure sores; therefore, when a child is admitted to the hospital, document baseline skin integrity. Pressure ulcer (PU) development is an important issue with children as well as with adults. Although the majority of recommendations for skin assessment and care of children have been modified from adult practice guidelines, evidence-based guidelines specific to children and neonates are being developed (Tradition or Science 25-1).

ANSWER: It is important to note the distribution of the rash, the shape of the lesions (patches), and their color and character. The character of Nick's rash is that it comprises vesicles, small blisters, and bulla (larger blisters). It is also important to note that some of the blisters are intact and many others are not, thus increasing the risk of an infection.

Hair and Nails

Focused Physical Assessment 25-1 summarizes normal and abnormal findings of hair and nail examination. Hair that is matted and dirty or nail beds that contain dirt may signify poor hygienic practices. Further inspection of the hair and scalp may detect the presence of lice or other parasites. Dry, brittle, or depigmented hair and brittle nails can signal nutritional deficits. Children coping with a great deal of stress may exhibit chronic nail biting or pulling of the hair (trichotillomania). Diseases of the scalp and nails are not common in children, except in cases of infestations (e.g., lice and scabies), which spread easily in home, school, and daycare environments.

DIAGNOSTIC CRITERIA

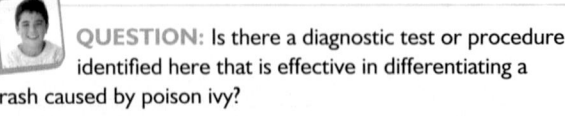 **QUESTION:** Is there a diagnostic test or procedure identified here that is effective in differentiating a rash caused by poison ivy?

A limited number of methods are available to confirm a diagnosis generated by a skin health history and physical examination. These include laboratory analysis by scrutiny of skin scrapings and culture, skin lesion biopsy, skin testing, and the use of special equipment, such as in **Wood lamp** examination (Fig. 25-2; Tests and Procedures 25-1).

Laboratory analysis of skin scrapings and cultures can provide excellent diagnostic assistance. For example, scabies, tinea, dermatophytes (ringworm), and candidal infection can be diagnosed with the use of superficial shavings or scrapings from the epidermis, and the **nits** or eggs from lice can be seen under the microscope. Cultures of the skin lesion or wound may identify bacteria and fungi. Skin biopsies can establish whether lesions are malignant or benign. Some minor biopsies can be completed in outpatient settings. Biopsy of the skin by excision is rarely required for diagnosis in children.

Skin testing is helpful in detecting the cause of an ACD. It is performed in one of three ways: intracutaneous, scratch, or patch testing.

ANSWER: No diagnostic criteria are effective in differentiating a rash caused by poison ivy. Poison ivy must be diagnosed by the history and the physical appearance of the rash.

TABLE 25-2   Secondary Skin Lesions

Type	Description	Example
Crust	Thickened, dried-out area formed when serum, blood, or purulent exudate dries on the skin	Impetigo Scab formed after abrasion
Scale	Thin, dry, or greasy flakes of skin; silvery or white in color	Psoriasis Drug reaction Seborrheic dermatitis Eczema Dry skin
Excoriation	Superficial, self-inflicted abrasion or scratch from intense itching	Insect bite Poison ivy Scabies Varicella
Fissure	Linear crack with abrupt edges, extends into the dermis	Tinea pedis
Erosion	Moist, circumscribed, depressed lesion that does not extend into dermis	Ruptured varicella lesion
Ulcer	Deep depression that extends into the dermis, irregular shape, may bleed	Pressure sore Chancre

TABLE 25-2 Secondary Skin Lesions (Continued)

Type	Description	Example
Scar	Fibrotic change resulting from the wound-healing process, normal tissue replaced with connective tissue (collagen)	Healed incision site or injury site Acne
Atrophic scar	Thinning of the epidermis, which results in skin-level depression	Striae associated with pregnancy or weight gain
Lichenification	Thickened skin area resulting from prolonged, intense scratching	Eczema
Keloid	Hypertrophic scar area that has built up tissue far greater than the size of the original injury	Site of multiple injuries or incisions
Petechia	Small, flat, nonblanchable vascular lesion caused by capillary hemorrhage	Rash evident with meningococcal meningitis Soft tissue injury
Ecchymosis	Large area of hemorrhage that change in color over time	Bruise caused by a fall or abuse

From Bickley, L. (2008). *Bates' pocket guide to physical examination and history taking*. Philadelphia, PA: Lippincott Williams & Wilkins. Used with permission.

TREATMENT MODALITIES

 QUESTION: Which of the following treatment modalities would be helpful to Nick? What is your rationale?

Skin and wound care has numerous objectives, principally, to preserve the integrity of normal skin. Care should incorporate these underlying concepts: first, the skin is a barrier that must be maintained; second, any insult that removes water, lipids, or protein from the epidermis alters the integrity of this barrier and compromises its function; and third, the normal epidermal barrier can be restored with the use of mild products, soaps, and appropriate emollient creams and lotions.

The nurse is responsible for completing skin surveillance measures to monitor skin conditions and to implement actions that maintain skin integrity. These measures include completing a thorough assessment of the skin (see Focused Physical Assessment 25-1), identifying children at risk for skin breakdown, and instituting measures to prevent further deterioration

TRADITION OR SCIENCE 25-1

Are valid scales available to assess skin integrity in the pediatric population?

Several valid and reliable skin assessment scales exist to assess adult patients. However, it is recognized that the factors that contribute to skin breakdown in children and premature infants differ from those for adult populations, making development of a pediatric risk assessment tool critical to determining the quality of pediatric skin care (Suddaby et al., 2005). Currently, there are more than 10 published scales for assessing the risk of skin breakdown in children. Reliability and validity testing of these instruments is ongoing, thus they have yet to establish the same level of credibility as tools used in the adult population. The pediatric scales have been primarily tested in the pediatric or neonatal intensive care settings and lack testing on general pediatric hospital populations and nonhospital populations (Baharestani & Ratliff, 2007). The most widely used scale is the Braden Q Scale, based on the Braden scale for adults. This scale is for PU risk identification in children aged 21 days to 8 years (Curley et al., 2002; Loman, 2000; Noonan et al., 2011; Quigley & Curley, 1996). The Neonatal Skin Risk Assessment Scale, modeled after the Braden scale, measures skin issues in the neonate population and is based on gestational age (Gray, 2004; Huffiness & Lodgson, 1997). The Starkid Skin Scale shows promise as a measure of risk of skin breakdown in the pediatric population (Suddaby et al., 2005). This one-page tool is based on the Braden Q Scale and is self-explanatory and easy to use. The Glamorgan scale, developed recently, has high sensitivity and evidence of interrater reliability (Parnham, 2012). Further research is needed to determine which assessment tools should be used for specific pediatric populations and to better identify what are the cutoff scores for identifying risk. In addition, research can help determine when risk assessments should be performed and when reassessments should be completed (Baharestani & Ratliff, 2007).

(e.g., overlay mattresses, frequent repositioning). In addition, the nurse is responsible for teaching children and their family hygienic practices that promote healthy skin and hair and help prevent the spread of a contagion (Community Care 25-1; Tradition or Science 25-2).

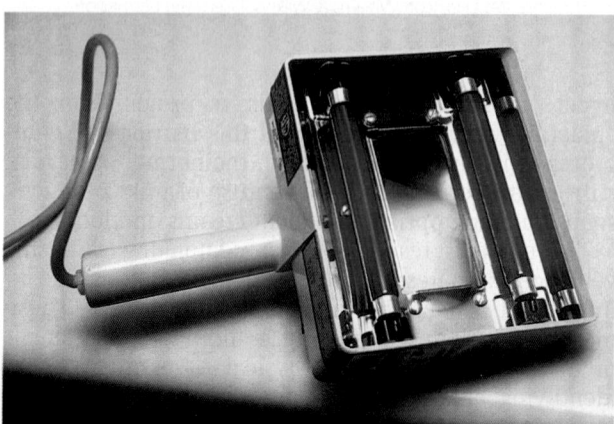

Figure 25-2 A Wood lamp uses UV light to fluoresce specific skin lesions.

Remember that the child with a skin condition may be in pain. Managing the pain, whether transient, chronic, or acute, is a nursing intervention that can be as simple as wiping away some tears or as complex as implementing patient-controlled analgesia (see Chapter 10).

Providing optimal skin care is an interdisciplinary effort. Many institutions have enterostomal therapists and wound, ostomy, and incontinence specialists. These expanded practice nurses are a valuable resource. Collaboration with the dietitian is also extremely vital to proper healing of the child's skin.

The physical therapist plays a role in skin care if physical mobility has become restricted and may provide alternative forms of treatment to enhance wound healing and facilitate elasticity of the affected area. Depending on the cause of the child's skin condition, a social worker consult and visits by a home care nurse may ensure continuity of care in the home setting and provide social support and educational resources for family members.

Amid the many interventions of the health care team, the psychological and cognitive needs of the child must be met. Approaches to skin care should account for the child's developmental stage and associated perception of the events surrounding the encounter with the health care team (Developmental Considerations 25-2).

MEASURES TO PROMOTE SKIN HYDRATION

Bathing and environmental considerations affect general skin hydration; moisturizers and lubricants can help to maintain or improve hydration.

Bathing

Bathing is often recommended to enhance hydration of the skin in dry climates or if the child has a condition in which the skin is very dry. Bathing in lukewarm (not hot) water can promote comfort and reduce itching (see Teaching Intervention Plan 24-1). The bath should not last long enough for the skin to become supersaturated. Soaps and oils may be used during the bath to cleanse and moisturize the skin. Mild soaps that can be used on the child's skin include Dove, Aveeno, and Neutrogena. Bath oils include Alpha Keri and Domol. Aveeno is an acceptable colloidal oatmeal bath. The child with a skin condition should avoid bubble baths because they can further irritate the skin. After the bath, the child should be gently dried. Children with skin conditions such as AD should immediately apply an emollient to the skin to maintain the skin's hydration.

Environmental Considerations

Environmental humidity affects skin hydration. Excessive humidity (>90%) or deficient humidity (<10%) can lead to alterations in skin integrity. Children with dry skin are especially susceptible to discomfort when the humidity is low. Use of a vaporizer, humidifier, and humidified heating during the winter months may help relieve itching. In warmer weather, air conditioning may help alleviate discomfort and itching.

Skin hydration is also affected by the child's fluid intake. To promote good skin hydration, the child should be encouraged to drink fluids frequently throughout the

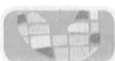 TESTS AND PROCEDURES for Evaluating Alterations of the Skin, Hair, and Nails

Diagnostic Test or Procedure	Purpose	Health Care Provider Considerations
Cultures • Skin • Wound • Nails • Hair	Samples of exudate, scales, and crusts are cultured to identify the bacterial, viral, or fungal causes of redness, irritation, or visible lesions.	Skin • Use polyester-tipped swabs to collect all skin and wound cultures. Cotton-tipped swabs are unsatisfactory because they may be treated with bacteriostatic solutions. • Wash affected site with 70% isopropanol or sterile water, allow to dry, and culture several lesion sites, swabbing the edges of the lesion. Wound • All superficial debris adjacent to the lesion and the wound itself must be gently wiped with a 70% isopropanol solution before culture is obtained. • Specimens collected from the wound edge are not very accurate. • Specimens should be delivered to the laboratory immediately so that testing can begin within 60 minutes of collection. Hair • Obtain hair and hair stubs or scrapings from areas of hair loss or infection sites without cleansing the scalp. • Both shaft and infected root or suspicious hairs are clipped or plucked with sterile forceps and sent to the laboratory in a Petri dish.
Scrapings for microscopic analysis	Samples of skin scrapings, nail clippings, or plucked hairs are stained and evaluated under the microscope to identify the bacterial, viral, or fungal causes of redness, scaling, irritation, or visible lesions.	Same considerations as for cultures.
Potassium hydroxide stain	Identifies fungi or yeast from skin, hair, and nails	Same considerations as for cultures.
Tzanck preparation • Giemsa method • Wright stain	Examines cells from the base of vesicles or bulla Smears are useful in diagnosing some viral infections (herpes simplex, varicella, herpes zoster, and eczema herpeticum) and in examining the white cell morphology of pustular disorders (ETN, candidiasis).	Wipe lesion with alcohol and allow to dry for 1 minute. Using a no. 15 blade, either remove crust or unroot the vesicle or pustule, then scrape the base of lesion with edge of blade. Transfer material to a glass slide, where stain is then applied.
Gram stain for bacteria	Identifies bacterial growth from a skin lesion	Same considerations as for cultures.
Scabies preparation	Identifies presence of scabies	Scrape intact vesicles, papules, or burrows with a no. 15 blade coated with immersion mineral oil. Sample as many primary lesions as possible to have a greater chance of having a positive scabies preparation.
Skin biopsy • Punch biopsy • Shave biopsy	Determines the histopathologic diagnosis of any skin tumor, palpable purpura, or persistent dermatitis as well as removal of small lesions	A local anesthetic using 1%–2% plain lidocaine should be given prior to biopsy. After the punch biopsy, bleeding may occur at the site. Firm pressure should be applied until bleeding stops. Suturing is optional.

(Continued)

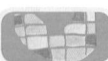

TESTS AND PROCEDURES for Evaluating Alterations of the Skin, Hair, and Nails *(Continued)*

Diagnostic Test or Procedure	Purpose	Health Care Provider Considerations
Skin testing • Intracutaneous • Scratch • Patch	Identifies the offending allergen, which may be the cause of allergic dermatitis responses.	Conduct the test after the allergic dermatitis has subsided and when the child is NOT taking antihistamines. Testing should be performed by a health care provider experienced in the interpretation and potential hazards of the procedures. Allergenic substance is injected under the skin (intracutaneous). The skin surface is irritated with a suspected allergic agent (scratch). The suspected trigger agent (antigen) is applied to the skin and occluded by hypoallergenic tape (patch). Patches should not be allowed to become wet while taped on the skin. The site is evaluated for a reaction 48–72 hours later, using standardized results for interpretation. Tell children to avoid bathing and strenuous activity while the patches are in place.
Wood lamp	Ultraviolet (UV) light is useful in the diagnosis of certain superficial pigmentary or infectious skin lesions.	Test must be performed in a darkened room. Procedure is noninvasive. No pain is associated with testing. Infected hair follicles have a grayish appearance in normal light but exhibit a yellow-green fluorescent appearance under Wood light.

day such as with meals, during snack time, and after play and exercise.

Moisturizers and Lubricants

Many moisturizers and lubricants are composed of petrolatum or a mixture of petrolatum and lanolin. These agents, which assist the child's skin to retain water, are most effective when applied to wet skin. They are used for children, such as those with AD, whose skin appears very dry or is unable to maintain hydration.

caREminder

Do not apply moisturizers and lubricants to the infant's or young child's diaper area. These products are likely to promote skin breakdown. They overhydrate the skin and act as a friction agent between the diaper and the baby's skin. Using appropriate ointments (e.g., petrolatum, Desitin, Balmex), and educating caregivers about their use, is paramount. Avoid products that contain fragrances.

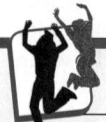

COMMUNITY CARE 25-1

Measures to Promote Skin Care and Hygiene

Personal Care
Ensure the child is bathed and the hair is washed on a regular basis.
Keep the child's nails trimmed.
Brush the child's teeth and tongue at least twice daily.
Use protective agents such as sunscreen and diaper rash ointments to protect the child's skin from injury.
Clean cuts and scrapes immediately and cover with an appropriate type of dressing.

Home, Daycare, and School
Introduce new foods gradually and monitor the skin for allergic reactions.

Note the presence of an unusual rash and report this information to a health care provider.
Ensure that clothing and other personal items such as hats, toothbrushes, and drinking cups are not shared.
Separate children with an unusual rash from other children until the causative agent can be determined.
Ensure that costumes used in play activities are washed frequently in hot water.
Instruct care providers and teachers to wash their hands frequently to prevent spread of infectious agents from one child to another.
Teach care providers to wear gloves when changing diapers, applying topical ointments, or treating wounds.

TRADITION OR SCIENCE 25-2

Is scientific evidence available regarding management strategies for the neonate's skin?

An important evidence-based standard for neonate and infant skin care was developed by the Association of Women's Health, Obstetric and Neonatal Nurses, and the National Association of Neonatal Nurses (Lund et al., 1999; Lund, Kuller et al., 2001; Lund, Osborne et al., 2001). The guidelines were based on a multicenter (51 hospitals) study completed to test the effectiveness of evidence-based clinical practice guidelines for neonatal skin care on selected clinical outcomes for newborns in neonatal intensive care units, special care units, and well-baby nurseries. Skin condition was assessed using the Neonatal Skin Condition Score based on dryness, erythema, and skin breakdown. Through implementation of these guidelines, neonatal skin improvement was noted as less visible dryness, redness, and breakdown. Furthermore, the study yielded recommendations for using emollients, decreasing frequency of bathing for this population, using pH-neutral cleaners, and using adhesives sparingly. All these recommendations were incorporated into the standard of care.

The guidelines have been updated based on an extensive review and evaluation of skin care–related research published between 2000 and 2007. The revised guidelines include discussions on newborn skin assessment, bathing, cord and circumcision care, disinfectants, diaper dermatitis, adhesives, emollients, transepidermal water loss, skin breakdown, and IV infiltration (Lund et al., 2007).

Supporting research concludes that daily prophylactic application of a topical ointment improves skin condition and decreases evaporative water loss, yet can also increase risk for infection, particularly with *Staphylococcus aureus*, in preterm infants (Conner et al., 2004). Current recommendations include not using topical ointments routinely on the skin of premature infants. In a recent review of newborn skin care practices, the evidence supports bathing the infant immersed in water is superior to washing; and bathing or washing with synthetic detergents or mild liquid baby cleansers was comparable or superior to water alone (Blume-Peytavi et al., 2012). These findings support the current guidelines.

Petrolatum-based agents include Vaseline pure petrolatum jelly and Moisturel. Petrolatum, lanolin, or mineral oil combination agents include Aquaphor ointment, Eucerin cream and lotion, Lubriderm, Keri Crème, Nivea Moisturizing, and UltraDerm. Popular zinc oxide–based products include Desitin, Balmex, generic zinc oxide, and Calmoseptine (also with calamine lotion).

TOPICAL MEDICATIONS

Topical medications can be used to treat skin conditions or prevent alterations in skin integrity. A topical medication consists of an "active" agent contained in a vehicle, or base. The topical application may also contain an "accelerant," which increases skin permeability, thus enhancing the mechanisms for medication absorption. Topical agents are widely used because of their ability to deliver an optimal concentration of a medication to the exact site where it is needed (Nursing Interventions 25-1). Topical therapies are beneficial to children who have cutaneous infections because they minimize the risk of systemic drug exposure that can occur with oral or IV medications. In addition, caregivers often find it easier to use a topical agent rather than convince a child to take an oral medication.

ALERT *Topical use does not guarantee safety. Systemic absorption and toxicity, local irritation, chemical burns, contact dermatitis, and poisoning from accidental ingestion can occur if safe administration techniques are not followed.*

The nurse applying a skin care agent to the child is responsible for monitoring the skin for effectiveness of the therapy. The child may have a sensitization to the agent that aggravates rather than relieves the symptoms or that creates new skin problems. Apply the agents following the frequency and dosage requirements recommended by the manufacturer or a pharmacist. Teach the family where and how to apply the agent. Suggest that reapplication of topical agents might be necessary if the child's skin becomes wet. Advise caregivers to wash their hands after applying the agent to remove it from their own skin.

SYSTEMIC DRUG THERAPY

Many of the skin conditions that occur in the pediatric population are a result of infection or immune responses within the body. In these cases, the primary cause of the skin condition must be treated using some type of systemic therapy. Medications are also given to relieve pain and reduce inflammation (see thePoint Medications and Administration: Systemic Drug Therapy).

If systemic therapy is indicated, assess the family's understanding of the need for this treatment and their ability to continue the course of therapy for the entire treatment. This includes financial ability as it relates to the family's health care plan. Some of the products are expensive, and reimbursement may not be adequately covered under the family's health care plan. Inform the family of the side effects of the medications. If IV administration is required, hospitalization may be necessary.

DRESSINGS

Wound healing may occur by primary, secondary, or tertiary intention. Primary intention refers to surgical closure, and these wounds generally heal very quickly. In secondary intention, the wounds are left open and allowed to heal by producing connective tissue; many products are available to use with these wounds, and

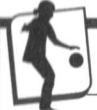

DEVELOPMENTAL CONSIDERATIONS 25-2

Skin Care

Stage Age	Developmental Principles	Nursing Strategies
Infancy	Exploration of the body is occurring. Infants are acutely aware of attitudes portrayed by caregivers. There is high need for comfort by a person who is familiar to the infant. Pain response may be difficult to interpret.	Involve the primary caregiver in the skin care. Distract the infant with toys during the procedure. Ensure that the infant is free from pain during procedures. Decrease the pain caused by frequent dressing changes by using Montgomery straps or protecting the skin with a skin barrier.
Early childhood	Child's thinking is egocentric, magical, and concrete. Child believes that two events contiguous in time are usually related. Child may perceive injury or hospitalization is a result of misbehavior. Limited experiences make it difficult to understand complicated explanations of events. Child learns about self and environment through play. Child is able to perform simple self-care tasks.	Use diversional play such as clay, crayons, or a favorite video during the procedure. Convey an attitude to the child that skin care is a process performed *with* them, not *to* them. Elicit cooperation and assistance when possible from the child; give choices. Provide careful, simple, present-oriented explanations. Use therapeutic play to foster expression of feelings and child's knowledge of the skin care activities. Allow child to perform skin care on a doll.
Middle childhood	Child follows rules or directions given by those in authority. Child is able to apply logical reasoning skills to familiar situations. Child comprehends cause-and-effect relationships. Memory is improved. One of the major fears is loss of control.	Allow child to help with skin care. The child may want to place the bandage on or assist in putting on the tape. Explain that the dressing should not be touched, picked at, pulled off, or gotten wet by the child. Use of rules and limits is important. Explain all aspects of the procedure, including the concept of sterile technique and germ transmission. Give specific guidelines regarding the degree of participation by the child and family in skin care. When medicating the child for pain, avoid drugs or doses that may make the child feel a loss of control.
Adolescence	Abstract thought processes develop. Body image is paramount. Privacy is important. Child is developing independence from family.	Teach the adolescent to manage skin care independently as appropriate. Family members should be included in care for support and as wanted by the adolescent. Address issues about body image in a positive, thorough, and honest manner. Consider the adolescent's body image concerns to be as important if not more important than the actual skin care.

NURSING INTERVENTIONS 25-1

Administering Topical Agents

Agent	Purpose	Key Points
Emollients	Lubricate and hydrate skin for dry, scaly skin conditions A bath additive to dry skin A soap substitute to cleanse the skin in treatment of all the inflammatory dermatoses	Apply with clean hands to avoid contaminating the contents of the container. Each family member should have a separate supply to avoid cross-contamination.
Barrier creams	Protect against irritation or repeated hydration Serve as water-repellent substance	In the diaper area, barrier creams should not be wiped away completely after each wet or dirty diaper. Such actions can cause further skin breakdown. Only clearly dirty or stained areas of cream should be removed. Additional cream may need to be applied with each diaper change.
Antiseptics and astringents	Cleanse skin and wounds	Povidone-iodine and hexachlorophene should not be used in neonates or those with badly burned or excoriated skin because of the risk of toxicity from absorption.
Keratolytics	Remove thickening of the surface of the skin (hyperkeratosis) in conditions with dry, scaling skin, such as ichthyosis, psoriasis, and eczema For acne, to relieve follicular obstruction by promoting peeling of the skin and inhibition of bacteria	The agent may leave a greasy feeling on skin. Generally, the agent needs to be used only every 12 hours.
Corticosteroids	Treat inflammatory conditions of the skin, particularly eczematous disorders	The more potent the steroid, the higher the incidence of side effects, including adrenal suppression and cushingoid effects. Also need to watch for thinning/weakening of the epidermis and regressive changes in the dermal connective tissue. In children, the risk is increased • By prolonged application • Under occluded areas, such as those covered by disposable diapers • On areas of thin skin Local side effects include skin atrophy, telangiectasia, purpura, and striae. Topical steroids may mask signs of infection.
Steroid/antibiotic mixtures	Treat inflammatory conditions of the skin, particularly eczematous disorders that have developed a secondary infection	Most steroid-responsive skin diseases do not require a topical antibiotic.
Coal tar	Treats psoriasis, although the mechanism for its therapeutic effect is unknown	Coal tar can be used alone, in ointment, or paste base. Scalp preparations and shampoos are also available.

(Continued)

NURSING INTERVENTIONS 25-1

Administering Topical Agents (Continued)

Agent	Purpose	Key Points
Antibacterials, antifungals, and antivirals	Treat localized infections Infection prophylaxis in traumatic and surgical wounds	Prolonged use may promote bacterial resistance and sensitization reactions. This treatment should be aimed at minor skin problems for 5–7 days only.
Antiparasitic preparations	Treat lice and scabies infestations	Give written instructions to the family to increase the likelihood of observing correct application procedure.
Sunscreens and sunblocks	Protect skin from effects of UV light	The higher the skin protection factor, the more efficient the preparation is in preventing burning. There is no internationally agreed-on standard of photoprotection.

the choice of product is guided by clinical factors. Most of the wounds described in this chapter, and most seen clinically, close by secondary intention. Tertiary intention closure occurs when there is a delay between the actual injury and closure; an example is a wound purposely left open for drainage, which is later closed.

Various wet, dry, and occlusive dressings may be used to treat a skin condition or wound (see thePoint Supplemental Information: Dressings for Wound Care). Today's dressings, which may be "dynamic" and "interactive" (e.g., hydrocolloids, calcium alginates, wound gels) or "static" (gauze), serve several functions:

- Reducing pain
- Providing a barrier to infection
- Helping clean the wound or lesion by debridement
- Promoting a moist environment conducive to healing
- Absorbing drainage from the wound or lesion
- Providing an aesthetic barrier while maintaining easy access to view the wound or lesion site

Wet Dressings

Wet dressings help moisturize the skin, decrease itching, and remove crusts. The dressing should be wet with lukewarm water and applied for 10 to 20 minutes, four to six times per day, for up to 1 week. During the treatment, the dressing should not be allowed to dry but should be rewetted or replaced with a new wet dressing as needed. Creams or ointments are usually applied after the wet dressing therapy to promote hydration. In some cases, after the application of a cream or ointment, another wet dressing followed by a dry dressing may be applied. For instance, in the treatment regimen for a child with psoriasis, a wet dressing is applied for 20 minutes, followed by application of a moisturizing agent. The body is then covered with a wet sleeper pajama or long johns, which is covered by a dry sleeper or long johns. The dressing and clothing are changed every 6 hours for a 24- to 72-hour period, or they may be used overnight for 5 to 10 hours.

caREminder

Avoid chilling the child by making sure the room is warm, but not hot. Also make sure a damp dressing remains damp and does not dry out. Change a dry dressing as needed to ensure that it remains dry and to help prevent chilling.

Dry Dressings

Dry dressings are most commonly used to cover a surgical wound or other break in the surface of the skin. A dry dressing may be as simple as a Band-Aid placed over a scraped knee.

Many children do not like bandages placed on their "owwies." To gain the child's cooperation, allow the child to place the bandage on himself or herself. The use of bandages with cartoon characters on them may make wearing the bandage more acceptable to the child.

Before placing a dressing, cleanse the wound gently with normal saline or other nontoxic wound cleanser. Treat surrounding normal skin in the same gentle fashion as the affected site to protect the healthy area from deterioration. Remove an old dressing carefully; never pull it off forcefully. Wetting the dressing and tape may be necessary to ease removal.

ALERT   *The neonate's skin has weak intracellular attachments. Rapid removal of tape can separate skin layers (epidermal stripping) and form blisters.*

Occlusive Dressings

Occlusive dressings enhance hydration of the skin, promote the absorption of topical medications, and prevent exposure of the area to microorganisms. Occlusive dressings are also effective in preventing epidermal stripping in preterm infants, by eliminating the need for tape, and skin irritation, by functioning as an artificial barrier (Lund, Kuller et al., 2001; Lund, Osborne et al., 2001; Lund et al., 2007). The effectiveness of polyure-thane dressings as a barrier to prevent microorganism growth on the excoriated skin of the preterm infant has been questioned. Data remain inconclusive, with some research indicating that high concentrations of bacterial growth under the dressings place the neonate at risk for infection (Strickland, 1997). A trend has also been noted toward increased risk of bacterial infection when occlusive topical ointments are used prophylactically on preterm infants (Conner et al., 2004).

Occlusive dressings are used in various ways. For instance, plastic wraps may be placed on the skin after hydrating the skin and applying a moisturizing agent. This type of occlusive dressing is left on for no lon-ger than 8 hours. Occlusive dressings are also used to protect the entry site of a vascular access device, to promote absorption of a topical agent such as EMLA cream, and to protect an open area of the skin from fecal contamination (e.g., in the child with myelome-ningocele).

WOUND CARE

The nurse is responsible for assessment of a wound and the surrounding tissue. These observations are impor-tant as baseline data from which the clinician can make judgments about progression of healing and course of treatment (see thePoint Supplemental Information: Wound Assessment).

❗ A L E R T *Signs of infection at the wound site may include a red streak running from the wound, a wound that progressively becomes more tender, dehiscing of the wound site, or a suture that comes out too early.*

The physician or nurse practitioner can choose to treat the wound either surgically or medically. Surgical interventions may consist of debridement and closure of an open, noninfected wound with sutures or staples (called a *flap*); medical interventions entail the use of medications and special dressings. Research during the late 1950s and early 1960s demonstrated that moisture provides the best microenvironment for wound regen-eration and repair. **Moist wound-healing** methods must be matched to the patient, wound, and setting and use dynamic products (see thePoint Nursing In-terventions: Dressings for Wound Care) as opposed to the traditional static gauze dressings. If antiseptics are applied topically to cleanse the wound area, use them only briefly, in low concentrations, and irrigate with normal saline, with the appropriate dressings applied. Normal saline is still considered the best solution to "wash out" wounds because of its relative isotonicity and minimal effect on tissue regeneration.

Chronic wounds may be managed using sterile, clean, or aseptic techniques. Research evidence does not dem-onstrate the superiority of one method over another in the management of chronic wounds nor does it support the use of one technique over another in specific patient care settings (Wooten & Hakins, 2005).

> *ANSWER:* Treatments that decrease itching include bathing in colloid oatmeal, such as Aveeno; keeping cool in air conditioning; and using cool compresses. Topical agents that decrease itching and help dry open blisters include calamine lotion and hydrocortisone ointment. Systemic drugs that are recommended for Nick include antihistamines and glucocorticosteroids. Dressings are not necessary for Nick's poison ivy rash.

MISCELLANEOUS TREATMENTS

Various physical and surgical interventions can be used to remove skin lesions or alter the appearance of the skin. For instance, makeup may be used to cover disfiguring birthmarks and scars. UV light therapy is used to treat psoriasis and acne. Repeated laser therapy treatments can remove vascular malformations such as a port-wine stain. Liquid nitrogen is used to remove warts. Disfiguring or irritating lumps or bumps can be removed from the skin surgically. All these therapies require the health care team to ensure that the child and family are well acquainted with the treatment op-tions. The treatment options may be painful and may themselves cause some disfigurement between the time of treatment and the complete healing of the skin. Al-ternative wound strategies include

- Surgical interventions: skin grafts, skin flaps, muscle flaps
- Negative pressure: vacuum-assisted closure
- Biologic agents: human skin equivalents (Dermagraft, Apligraf), growth factors (Regranex)
- Hyperbaric oxygen therapy, topical oxygen therapy
- Electrical stimulation
- Ultrasound therapy
- Free radical scavengers

NUTRITIONAL MANAGEMENT

When managing skin conditions, the importance of nutrition cannot be overlooked. Slow or insufficient wound healing, or the presence of certain skin disor-ders (e.g., dermatitis or hair loss), are manifestations of nutritional deficiencies. Protein deficiencies retard the formation of collagen. Vitamins and minerals are necessary for various metabolic processes and for epi-thelial tissue and collagen formation (Table 25-3). As a result of certain developmentally appropriate behav-iors (e.g., food jags), children can challenge the clini-cian's ability to provide sufficient nutrition. Metabolic and congenital disorders can also make the challenge of meeting energy requirements difficult. In a severely debilitated child, wound healing is often compromised because the nutrients crucial to the healing process are not available for metabolic purposes. For example, if albumin levels are below normal, protein depletion and edema impair wound healing. Parenteral protein and nutrients may be needed if the child is unable to ingest and digest foods taken orally.

TABLE 25-3   Nutrients and Wound Healing

Nutrient	Effect on Wound Healing
Carbohydrates	
Glucose	Provides energy for leukocytes and fibroblasts
Proteins	
Amino acids	Necessary for neovascularization and fibroblast production, lymphocyte formation, synthesis of collagen, phagocytosis, and wound remodeling
Albumin	Necessary to prevent edema by controlling oncotic pressure
Fats	
Essential fatty acids	Metabolized in prostaglandins and form cell membranes; primary energy source for infants
Vitamins	
Ascorbic acid	Necessary for collagen synthesis; improves immune response to infection
B complex	Cofactor of enzyme system and needed for energy; no direct link to wound healing
A	Promotes epithelialization and collagen synthesis
D	Necessary for calcium metabolism; no direct link to wound healing
E	May protect vitamin A oxidation during digestion; antioxidant; supports immune functions
K	Necessary for synthesis of prothrombin and other clotting factors; "hemostasis"
Minerals	
Zinc	Stabilizes cell membrane; promotes cell mitosis; helps with epithelialization
Iron	Necessary for collagen synthesis; enhances bactericidal action of leukocytes
Copper	Promotes formation of a stable collagen tissue
Magnesium	Important for protein synthesis

Nutritional management may also be of concern for the child who has to avoid certain foods that cause a localized or systemic skin reaction. In these cases, consultation with a nutritional specialist is imperative. The specialist can assist the family in identifying all the foods that may contain the allergic substance. In addition, a dietary plan must be established that ensures that, even though certain foods are avoided, a well-balanced diet is maintained (see Chapters 3 to 7 for information on the nutritional needs of healthy children).

NURSING PLAN OF CARE

 QUESTION: What is an appropriate nursing diagnosis and outcome for Nick and his family?

The data from the focused health history and physical assessment yield information about the child's skin, hair, and nails. Nursing diagnoses are formulated to direct the interdisciplinary team in a plan that addresses altered skin integrity (Nursing Plan of Care 25-1). Immediate goals for the child include treating the skin condition and relieving pain or itching. If the condition is contagious, measures must also be taken to prevent the illness from spreading to children and adults who have had contact with the affected child. When the condition limits physical mobility or alters body image, the interdisciplinary team must identify these concerns and provide measures to support the child and his or her family. Certain skin lesions are secondary symptoms of primary conditions that affect other organs. In these cases, health care must encompass a plan to treat the primary condition. Finally, nursing diagnoses must articulate the need for family education to prevent exacerbations of the skin condition and to manage the child's health needs in the home and at school. Nursing Plan of Care 12-2 provides additional information to assist in planning care for a child with a chronic condition.

ANSWER: Several nursing diagnoses are appropriate, including discomfort, risk for infection, and deficient knowledge regarding identification of poison ivy. However, "impaired skin integrity related to exposure to an environmental hazard" is the most comprehensive diagnosis. Appropriate outcomes include, "Child shows improvement in skin integrity."

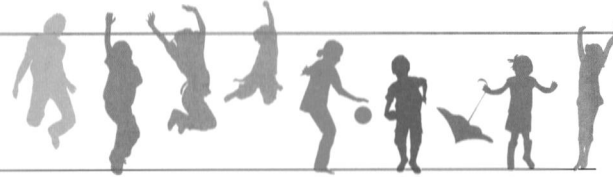

NURSING PLAN OF CARE 25-1:

The Child With Altered Skin Integrity

Nursing Diagnosis: Impaired tissue integrity related to primary break in the skin's surface, or exposure to physical, chemical, or environmental hazards

Interventions/Rationale
- Obtain baseline and ongoing assessments of skin and mucous membranes for alterations in integrity (see Focused Physical Assessment 25-1).
  Baseline assessments provide an index on which to compare changes. Ongoing assessment enables prompt detection of changes and interventions to address the alteration.
- Assess ongoing nutritional status, including intake and output, weights, calorie count, composition of diet, and serum albumin levels, as indicated by child's condition.
  Increased caloric intake may be needed to maintain nutritional intake and promote wound healing. Analyzing composition of the diet ensures that substances are ingested that will enhance wound healing (e.g., calcium, vitamin D). Weight loss or gain may indicate need for alterations in diet. Decreased serum albumin levels (<2.5 g/dL) indicate severe protein depletion and place the child at risk for skin breakdown.
- Assess environmental factors that may compromise skin integrity (e.g., wound drainage; humidity; friction; shear; pressure to bony prominences; immobility; presence of exacerbating agents such as pets, grass, exposure to sun).
  Identifying causative environmental agents can assist in prevention and early recognition and treatment of skin conditions.
- Implement measures to treat alterations in tissue integrity or to prevent potential alterations. Evaluate effectiveness of interventions.
  Use of topical agents, systemic drug therapy, protective dressings, skin hydration techniques, use of specialty beds, and nutritional support provide mechanisms to treat symptoms and pathology.
- Support caregiver competence in assessing the child's needs and in caring for the child.
  Reinforces new behaviors and bolsters the families' feelings of competence.

Expected Outcomes
- Child's areas of impaired tissue integrity will heal.
- Child's circulation and nutrients delivered to the wound site or lesion will remain adequate.
- Child and family will follow advised course of therapy to manage the child's skin condition.

Nursing Diagnosis: Acute pain related to skin disorder, healing process, diagnostic and treatment measures

Interventions/Rationale
- Assess pain using a reliable and valid method that is appropriate developmentally and for the situation. Elicit family members' assessment of child's pain.
  The subjective rating of pain is most reliable but may not be an option in a nonverbal child, (infant, intubated, comatose). Validated tools provide the most accurate assessment. The absence of behaviors indicative of pain does not necessarily mean that the child is not experiencing pain. Families know the child best and are familiar with typical behaviors.
- Implement pharmacologic and biobehavioral interventions to alleviate the pain (see Chapter 10). Use a preventive approach to keep pain at or below an acceptable level. Involve the family in pain management.
  Unrelieved pain has deleterious physiologic effects such as tachycardia, suppressed immune function, and atelectasis as well as negative psychological effects. Pain is better managed if it is not allowed to escalate. If the family can provide measures, that approach may be more comforting to the child than if measures are provided by nursing staff.
- Reassess pain level and evaluate effectiveness of interventions frequently.
  Frequent assessments are required to control the pain; children respond differently to interventions, so what is effective for one may not be for another.

Expected Outcomes
- Child will express a feeling of improved comfort or demonstrate pain relief through playful, smiling, responsive behaviors.
- Child and family will perform measures to relieve pain and comfort child.

Nursing Diagnosis: Risk for infection related to wound or open lesion

Interventions/Rationale
- Observe for signs and symptoms of infection (e.g., malodorous wound drainage, elevated leukocyte count, elevated temperature) and signs and symptoms of septicemia (e.g., positive blood cultures, hemodynamic changes).
  Loss of the first line of defense (skin) and formation of eschar provides an excellent culture medium for growth of infectious bacteria.

(Continued)

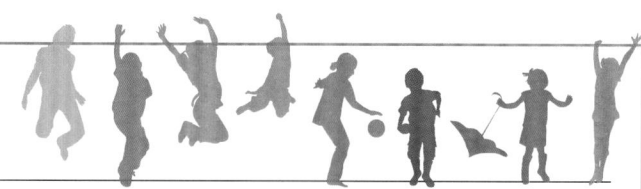

NURSING PLAN OF CARE 25-1:

The Child With Altered Skin Integrity (Continued)

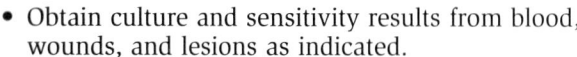

- Obtain culture and sensitivity results from blood, wounds, and lesions as indicated.

    Determines the presence of bacteria, fungal, or viral agents that may colonize and cause infection or septicemia. Determines sensitivity of causative agent to indicate most appropriate type of medication to treat the condition.

- Use aseptic techniques when managing external lines and tubes and when providing skin and wound care. Ensure that staff and visitors use universal precautions.

    Multiple exogenous factors contribute to the risk of infection (e.g., Foley catheter, IV, central venous catheters) as well as nonadherence to aseptic practices by staff and visitors. Universal precautions will help prevent transmission of child's infection to others.

- Administer antibiotics, topical antimicrobials, and bacteriostatic agents as ordered; evaluate and document effectiveness.

    Provides mechanism to treat causative agent and underlying pathology.

Expected Outcomes

- Child's vital signs, temperature, and laboratory values will remain within normal parameters.
- Child's wound or lesion site will remain free of signs and symptoms of infection.

Nursing Diagnosis: Disturbed body image related to real or perceived disfigurement caused by a skin condition

Interventions/Rationale

- Convey positive attitude about child; reinforce positive aspects of child's appearance and abilities.

    Child may be very self-conscious because of altered appearance related to skin condition. Positive feedback may enhance self-esteem.

- Help child to express feelings about current status and fears for the future; listen actively. Incorporate other health care personnel as appropriate.

    Fears and concerns may be real or unfounded, but in any case, the child will benefit from opportunities to discuss feelings and to develop a repertoire of coping strategies.

- Assist child to find methods to enhance physical appearance, personal comfort, and daily management of skin condition.

    Promotes active adaptation to condition, with variety of coping strategies to enhance self-esteem and to promote normalization in daily life.

Expected Outcomes

- Child will verbalize concerns regarding changes in body appearance or function.

- Child will express positive feelings about self.
- Family members will acknowledge variations or changes in child's appearance and verbalize acceptance of child.
- Child and family will institute measures to positively affect child's appearance (makeup, selection of clothing).

Nursing Diagnosis: Readiness for enhanced self-care related to demands of health care associated with chronic or acute skin condition

Interventions/Rationale

- Encourage participation and cooperation in care; reward all efforts; give choice and control over situation as appropriate.

    Minimizes perception of powerlessness. Maximizes personal responsibility of child for daily care.

- Provide predictability for the child and scheduling of self-care (e.g., do procedures/skin care at consistent time and place).

    Diminishes fears of unknown. Routine establishes structure and demonstrates how skin care can be incorporated into daily cares of child's life.

- Provide child and family education regarding skin care needs of child. Ensure that opportunities for redemonstration are provided and encourage family involvement in care prior to discharge.

    Ensures that child and family are comfortable with providing skin care measures and are capable of managing child when away from the health care setting. Validates that family will comply with treatments.

- Develop a plan with the family to prevent or minimize exacerbations of child's skin condition, prevent occurrence of infections, and/or prevent communicable transmission of skin condition.

    Identifies modifications in the home and child's social environments that may be required to protect child from recurrence or exacerbation of conditions. Provides concrete measures to protect other children and adults from causative agents.

Expected Outcomes

- Child and family will recognize need for family to assume ongoing management of skin condition.
- Child and family will implement measures to prevent spread of skin condition to other children and adults.
- Child and family will institute measures to alter environmental factors that may exacerbate the child's skin condition.

ALTERATIONS IN SKIN INTEGRITY

Alterations in skin integrity can result from a variety of sources and have implications for the overall health of the child.

NEONATAL SKIN LESIONS

Skin lesions unique to neonates may be congenital or acquired. Congenital abnormalities, which include vascular malformations, and disorders of pigmentation may pose specific problems because of their location on the body, their relation to other associated developmental defects, and their disfiguring appearance.

Acquired skin disorders include transient skin rashes, infestations, and infections. Acquired lesions usually have a short, benign course, although some neonates may be critically ill if involvement of other body systems is extensive. Examples include, but are not limited to, drooling rash, ETN, and dermatitis.

This section reviews some of the congenital lesions and common transient rashes found in the newborn population. Infestations and infections such as scabies, candidiasis, herpes simplex, and impetigo are discussed in subsequent paragraphs and are not unique to newborns.

VASCULAR BIRTHMARKS

Vascular malformations are caused by errors in vessel morphogenesis during embryogenesis, are virtually always visible from birth, and modify only slowly, over years or decades (Blei, 2005). Affecting vascular or epidermal tissue, birthmarks can vary in the degree to which they cause more serious physical problems. Vascular lesions in infants and children are broadly classified as hemangiomas and vascular malformations (Table 25-4). Hemangiomas are benign, vascular proliferations that rapidly enlarge during the first year of life, with slowing of growth during the next 5 years (Fig. 25-3). Involution, or natural degeneration of the tissue, occurs by 10 to 15 years of age (Herzog, 2011). Vascular malformations are developmental anomalies of blood or lymphatic vessel formation (Figs. 25-4 and 25-5).

Vascular birthmarks may range from relatively minor conditions, causing little if any disfigurement and pathologic consequences, to severe and potentially life-threatening conditions with visible skin alterations. The child's self-concept and development of body image may be negatively affected based on how the family and others respond to the child's condition and how the child perceives he or she is valued by others. Many of the conditions may regress spontaneously over time. Several treatment measures are available to help remove the lesion and cope with associated complications such as visual impairment and pulmonary obstruction. Nursing interventions include managing pain associated with surgery or laser therapy and assessing for complications of treatments (e.g., scarring, infection, hyperpigmentation). Response to therapy is slow. Assist the child and family to learn how to deal with the uncomplimentary comments made by others and with strategies to build the child's self-esteem.

Pigment Abnormalities

The amount and distribution of melanin in the epidermis accounts for the color of a person's skin. An alteration in melanin production, and the resulting hyper- or hypopigmentation, generally cannot be treated. Other manifestations of the underlying condition may be treated if their sequelae are threatening to the well-being of the child.

HYPERPIGMENTATION

Hyperpigmentation lesions are common at birth and may present during the first few weeks of life. Hyperpigmented lesions include mongolian spots, café-au-lait spots, and freckles (Fig. 25-6). Mongolian spots are blue-black macules or patches commonly located on the lumbosacral area. They are most common in Asian, black, and Hispanic infants. The sacrococcygeal area is most commonly affected, but lesions may occur on the buttocks, dorsal trunk, or extremities. Mongolian spots generally fade by age 2 to 3 years, although some traces of the lesions may persist into adulthood.

Café-au-lait spots are well-circumscribed, light-brown oval macules that may appear anywhere on the body. On black skin, the color of the spots may appear more dark brown. Black infants are more likely to have café-au-lait spots than white infants. The spots persist through childhood and may increase in number. Café-au-lait spots are a feature of several systemic disorders such as polyostotic fibrous dysplasia (large, usually solitary spot) and neurofibromatosis (more than five spots). The significance of café-au-lait spots, therefore, may be as a diagnostic tool for other disorders because treatment for this actual abnormality is generally unnecessary.

HYPOPIGMENTATION

Hypopigmentation occurs in newborns with phenylketonuria. These newborns have blond hair, blue eyes, and light-colored skin. The hypopigmentation is caused by the tight binding of the amino acid phenylalanine to the receptor sites of tyrosinase, which then does not allow the enzyme to oxidize phenylalanine to melanin (Weston et al., 2007).

Pigment loss is also a significant feature of *albinism*, a group of 14 syndromes characterized by congenital pigment loss in the skin, hair, iris, and retina. Nystagmus, strabismus, photophobia, decreased visual acuity, and astigmatism are common ocular findings. Blindness and skin cancer may occur in severe forms of albinism.

NEONATAL ACNE

Acne that is similar in distribution and appearance to adolescent acne may occur at birth and usually disappears within the first several weeks of life. However, this acne—small red bumps on the face, trunk, and extremities—can last as long as 6 months.

TABLE 25-4   Characteristics of Hemangiomas and Vascular Malformations

Characteristic	Hemangiomas	Vascular Malformations
Types	Classified as • Superficial (capillary or strawberry hemangioma) • Mixed (capillary–cavernous) • Deep (cavernous) New classification system • Localized • Segmented • Indeterminate • Multifocal	Telangiectatic (salmon patch) Hypertrophic capillary (angiokeratoma) Venous Arteriovenous Lymphatic Cutis marmorata telangiectatica Mixed
Etiology	Tumor of endothelial cells	Developmental anomaly
Growth	Rapid growth phase lasts several months up to age 1 year, followed by spontaneous regression by ages 10–15 years. Lesions usually do not more than double in size.	Slow, stable growth as child grows Does not fade or disappear over time
Incidence	Female predominance ranges 3:1 to 5:1	Ratio of male to female, 1:1
Presence at birth	Only 20% of lesions are seen at birth as blanched or erythematous macules; most appear at about 1 month of age.	Always present at birth, but may not be entirely evident
Clinical presentation	Lesion has a well-demarcated, hypopigmented flat area. Small telangiectatic vessels may course across the lesion. Color may be erythematous or white. During involution, lesion becomes pale centrally with lacy gray regions within the lesion.	Flat, cutaneous vascular lesion, possibly with a subcutaneous component
Associated complications and syndromes	Obstruction of vision Obstruction of respiration Thrombocytopenia Disseminated intravascular coagulation Infection Congestive heart failure Kasabach-Merritt syndrome Diffuse neonatal hemangiomatosis Maffucci syndrome Gorham syndrome Blue rubber bleb nevus syndrome Bannayan-Riley-Ruvalcaba syndrome	Glaucoma Sturge-Weber syndrome Beckwith-Wiedemann syndrome Klippel-Trenaunay syndrome Parkes-Weber syndrome Cobb syndrome
Treatment	Observation (most regress spontaneously) Corticosteroids (for visual or respiratory obstruction) Interferon alfa Surgical resection Embolization (for arteriovenous complications) Vascular-specific pulsed dye laser therapy	Observation Cosmetics as camouflage Tattooing (with flesh-colored insoluble pigments) Vascular-specific pulsed dye laser therapy

Information from Herzog, C. (2011). Benign vascular tumors. In R. M. Kliegman, B. F. Stanton, J. W. St. Geme et al. (Eds.), *Nelson textbook of pediatrics* (19th ed., p. 1772). Philadelphia, PA: Elsevier/Saunders; Miller, T., & Frieden I. (2005). Hemangiomas: New insights and classification. *Pediatric Annals, 34*, 179–187.

ALERT   *If blisters or pimples appear on the infant's skin, examine them immediately; the cause may be herpes simplex.*

No treatment is usually required because the condition is self-limiting. Antiacne medications are not recommended; however, topical benzoyl peroxide (BPO) creams, gels, or washes are generally safe and effective. Caregivers are cautioned not to apply baby oil or other ointments to the skin as a curative measure. The relationship (if any) between severe neonatal acne and severe adolescent acne later in the child's life is unknown.

MILIA

Milia are multiple, white or yellow, 1- to 2-mm papules appearing on the infant's cheeks, nose, chin, forehead, and occasionally the upper trunk and limbs. They can also appear on the midline of the palate where they are called *Epstein pearls*. These superficial epidermal cysts are caused by the blockage of the pilosebaceous glands by keratin and sebaceous materials. Although milia that appear on the face and limbs look like pimples, they are not infected.

Milia usually spontaneously disappear at age 1 to 2 months. Advise families not to apply cream or lotion to the lesion sites and not to squeeze or pick the lesions with a sharp instrument.

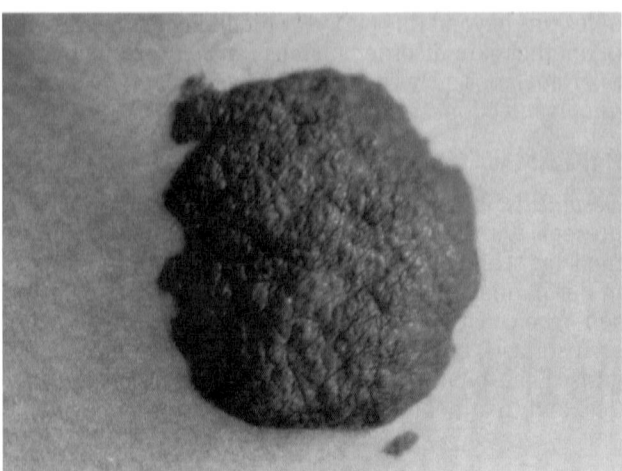

Figure 25-3 Strawberry hemangioma.

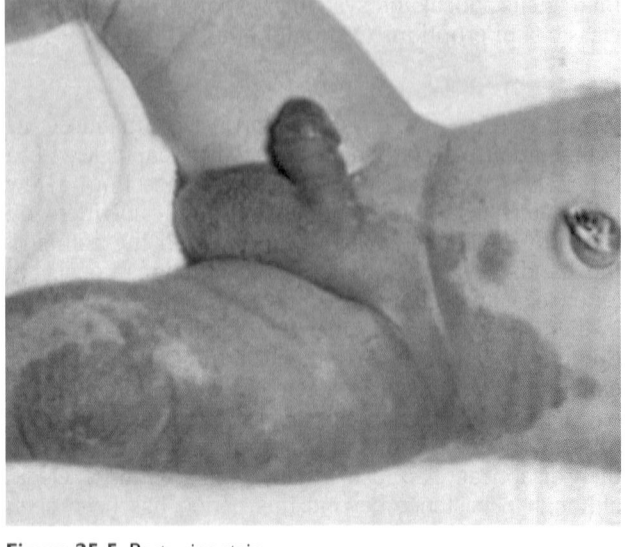

Figure 25-5 Port-wine stain.

DROOLING RASH

Transient rashes commonly develop on the chin or cheeks of an infant. Such rashes are similar to those seen in other cases of contact dermatitis, with erythema, edema, and vesicles likely. Two factors may cause the dermatologic changes. The first may be contact of the child's delicate skin with his or her own vomitus. The young infant is prone to wet burps, in which the food and the acid from the stomach contents may erupt and drool down the chin or, during sleep, may be absorbed into bed linen, resting against the cheeks. Some of this contact between the fluid and the skin may be averted by placing an absorbent diaper under the infant's face during naps and by rinsing the infant's face after feedings.

A drooling rash can also be caused by contact between the infant's cheek and the mother's breast during nursing. Changing the infant's position frequently and placing a cool washcloth on the infant's cheek will help to decrease the incidence of this rash.

ERYTHEMA TOXICUM NEONATORUM

ETN, or neonatal erythema, is one of the more well-known benign, self-limiting skin eruptions seen during the newborn period. Incidence estimates range from 50% to 70% of all healthy newborns (Marchini et al., 2005). It is virtually never seen in premature infants or those weighing less than 2,500 g. ETN occurs worldwide with no apparent gender, ethnic, racial, or seasonal predisposition (Eichenfield et al., 2008).

Most cases of ETN occur within 24 to 72 hours after birth, although lesions can erupt any time during the first 2 weeks of life. These lesions may wax and wane, usually lasting no longer than a week. The cause of ETN is unknown. Medications and the mode of feeding and skin care do not correlate with the emergence of the condition. It has been postulated that the skin appendages, especially the hair follicles, might act as an entry for microbes. The presence of these microbes

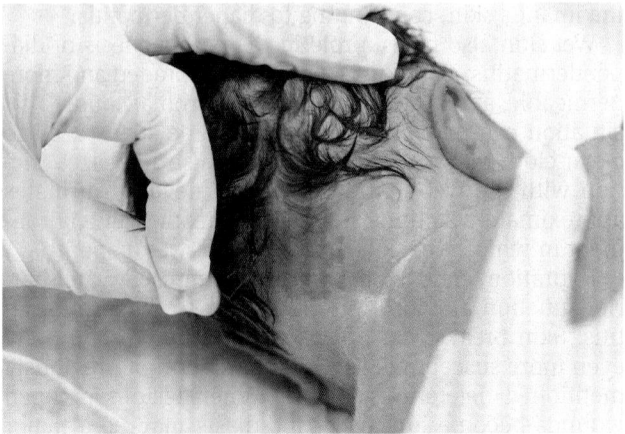

Figure 25-4 Salmon patch. When located on the nape of the neck (as shown here), this lesion is also referred to as a *stork bite*.

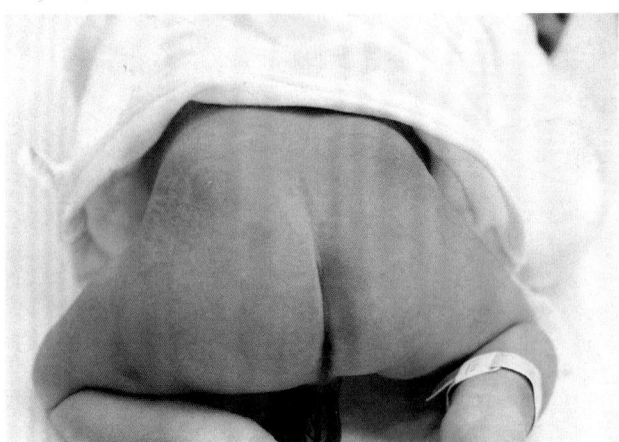

Figure 25-6 Mongolian spots are blue-black macules located on the lumbosacral area.

then elicits a local and systemic response, leading to the classic skin eruptions (Marchini et al., 2005).

Assessment

Within the first few days after birth, ETN manifests as combinations of erythematous macules, papules with a central vesicle, or pustules, ranging in size from a few millimeters to several centimeters, found anywhere on the body except the soles of the feet and the palms of the hands (Fig. 25-7). The classic eruptions consist of barely elevated yellowish papules or pustules (1 to 3 mm in diameter) with a macular flare similar to a flea bite. Common locations include the face, trunk, buttocks, and extremities. Lesions are discrete but can become confluent. Lesions that begin as macules often turn into pustules. Individual lesions may appear for a few days and then disappear. The rash usually remits within 1 week, although persistence beyond this period has been seen in some cases. In some cases, however, recurrences may occur within 5 to 11 days after the initial eruption. The secondary eruption is not as extensive as the original rash.

Diagnosis of ETN depends on microscopic examination of the lesions. In the diagnostic test of choice, scrapings of pustules are stained with Wright solution. If ETN is present, large numbers of eosinophils are detected. Also, microscopic examination of macules shows an accumulation of eosinophils in the dermis. However, neutrophils are rarely present. Cultures of lesions are sterile. A crucial factor differentiating ETN from other skin disorders is that, aside from eruption of the lesions, the neonate displays no other systemic involvement such as fever, lethargy, or poor feeding.

Interdisciplinary Interventions

Treating ETN is usually unnecessary, and lesions usually fade within 1 week. Monitor the affected neonate to ensure that the rash fades within 1 week. The persistence

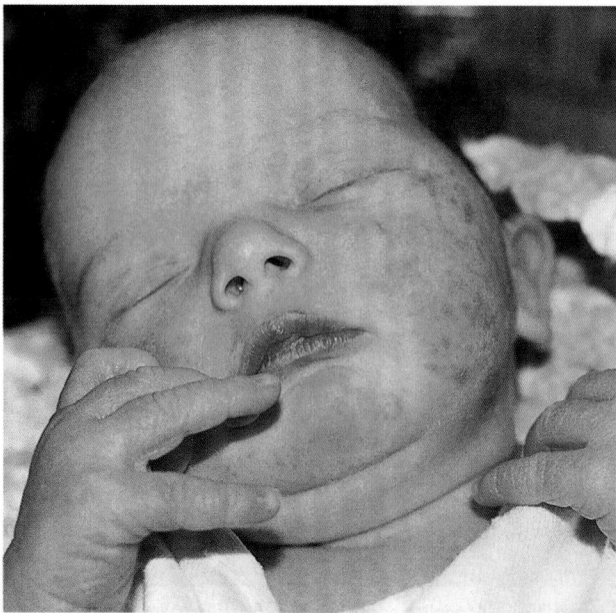

Figure 25-7 Erythema toxicum neonatorum.

of lesions beyond this period could indicate the presence of another skin disorder such as transient neonatal pustular melanosis, herpes simplex virus, *Staphylococcus aureus* infections, or candidiasis.

INFLAMMATORY SKIN DISORDERS

Dermatitis is a general term for skin conditions that present with erythema or with erythema accompanied by scaling, vesicles, or crusting. Common types of dermatitis are discussed: diaper, contact, atopic, and seborrheic. Other conditions included in this section are psoriasis, epidermolysis bullosa (EB), and acne vulgaris. Each type involves different causes, characteristics, and treatment plans.

DIAPER DERMATITIS

Diaper dermatitis, or *diaper rash*, is one of the most common skin rashes occurring during infancy. Diaper dermatitis is a type of irritant contact dermatitis (ICD). Because of its prevalence and specificity of interventions, the condition is discussed separately from contact dermatitis.

The exact incidence of diaper dermatitis is difficult to specify because less than 10% of episodes are referred for treatment to a health care provider (Bell, 2006). Most children have at least one episode of diaper rash during infancy, especially during a bout of gastroenteritis. Diaper dermatitis is most likely to occur within the first 2 years of life, peaking at age 6 to 9 months because of the change in dietary intake (Ravanfar et al., 2012).

Pathophysiology

Prolonged contact with an irritant, most commonly feces, urine, soaps, detergents, alcohol wipes, ointments, or friction, is a major contributing factor in diaper dermatitis (Adalat et al., 2007). However, an irritant alone does not cause diaper dermatitis; rather, the problem results from a combination of factors generated by the presence of the diaper. Urinary ammonia was once believed to be the primary etiologic factor for diaper dermatitis, but recent research has indicated that urine itself is not detrimental. It was found that urine and fecal enzymes interact to liberate ammonia and increase pH. Excessive alkalinity makes fecal protease and lipase even more irritating to the infant's skin, contributing to diaper dermatitis.

Wet skin also plays a role in the pathogenesis of diaper dermatitis. Wet skin is more easily abraded and more permeable, and it has an increased microbial count. This situation can be exacerbated by alkaline soaps used to clean cloth diapers. The wet diaper also increases friction with the wet skin. The average newborn urinates approximately 20 times in one day, creating an environment in which wet skin rubs against a wet diaper.

Hydration, elevated pH, and compromised water barrier function are contributing factors to diaper dermatitis. Skin breaks that breach the stratum corneum are even more susceptible to the combination of previously mentioned deleterious factors. When lesions or open wounds become infected, candidiasis may be a major culprit. *Candida albicans* can be cultured or recovered from the skin of 40% to 75% of infants with diaper dermatitis. It is rarely found in infants with healthy, unbroken skin (Ravanfar et al., 2012).

Assessment

The affected skin over the diaper area can take various configurations. In general, it is bright red, swollen, and sharply marginated; however, it may also have a glazed and wrinkled appearance (Fig. 25-8). There may be papular, vesicular, or bullous lesions, fissures, and erosions. If candidiasis develops, the rash consists of erythematous papular eruptions with satellite lesions. Diaper dermatitis rarely occurs in groin creases.

An infant with diaper dermatitis acts fussy and exhibits trouble sleeping and, in severe cases, even has difficulty with eating. Diaper changes can be extremely painful, especially if commercial diaper wipes are used for cleansing the genital area. Commercial wipes may contain alcohol and allergenic substances that may further irritate the child's skin.

Interdisciplinary Interventions

Essential to prevention is maintaining dry, protected skin (Ravanfar et al., 2012). Frequent diaper changes reduce skin exposure to urine and feces. For severe cases, further assessment and intervention to improve diapering practices and to identify causative agents may be necessary. Treatment strategies involve differentiating irritant dermatitis from candidiasis or staphylococcal infections. For mild irritant dermatitis, bathing daily in lukewarm water and using mild, irritant-free and fragrance-free soap is recommended. Cleansing the soiled diaper area with a mild cleanser and protecting the skin with a **barrier cream** (e.g., petrolatum, zinc oxide, dimethicone) is sufficient (Teaching Intervention Plan 25-1). Current practice recommends not using baby powder or talcum powder for many reasons, including possible inhalation into the infant's lungs, which could precipitate aspiration pneumonia. If a powder is used, one with cornstarch is recommended,

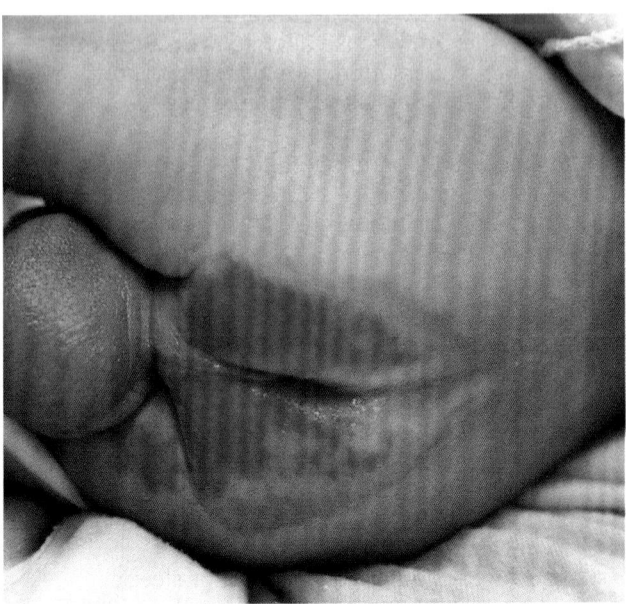

Figure 25-8 Diaper dermatitis.

and the powder should be placed in the caregiver's hand and then applied to the skin (Tradition or Science 25-3). A short course of hydrocortisone 0.1% cream, used twice daily, may be necessary.

caREminder

If the skin underlying the cream is clean, the cream does not have to be completely removed with each diaper change; rather, lightly wiping the area with a washcloth and mild cleanser is sufficient. The ointment prevents maceration and protects the skin from urine and feces. Ensure that the ointment is rubbed well into the skin so it serves as a true barrier.

Medical therapy is not usually required for diaper dermatitis, unless secondary infections develop.

ALERT *If steroid creams are ordered, they should be of a low potency (0.5%–1%), nonfluorinated type. High-potency steroids are rapidly absorbed through the infant's thin skin and can cause systemic toxicity. Take special care to avoid using combination products (e.g., antifungals and steroids) without verifying that the steroid is of the low-dose type.*

CONTACT DERMATITIS

 QUESTION: Is Nick's rash an ICD or an allergic dermatitis?

Contact dermatitis is an inflammatory skin condition involving a cutaneous response occurring when human skin is exposed to certain external natural or synthetic substances. Contact dermatitis is classified as either ICD or ACD.

In older children and adults, ICD most commonly results from exposure to irritants such as manufacturing processes, insecticides, or hobby supplies. In infants and young children, ICD is most commonly associated with saliva that causes a drooling rash or contact with abrasive soap and irritating detergents (Chart 25-1).

ACD results from a T-cell–mediated hypersensitivity reaction. The allergic reaction is commonly caused by exposure to plants (e.g., poison ivy, sumac, oak), nickel (in jewelry, dental appliances, metal fasteners), latex, animal fur, feathers, vegetables oils, synthetic fabrics, cosmetics, and perfumes or scented soaps that contain the offending allergen. ACD can occur in neonates because sensitization to an allergen and dermatitis can occur in as few as 10 days. The incidence of ACD is greatly increased after age 8 years. Children at high-risk for ACD reactions include those with a personal or family history of hay fever, AD (eczema), or asthma. Other risk factors include preexisting skin diseases, poor personal hygiene, and very dry–hot or dry–cold environmental conditions.

TIP 25-1: A TEACHING INTERVENTION PLAN for the Child With Diaper Dermatitis

Nursing Diagnoses and Family Outcomes

- Impaired skin integrity related to irritation of the diaper area
  Outcomes: Child regains skin integrity.
  Child exhibits no further evidence of skin breakdown.
- Deficient knowledge: Prevention and treatment of rash
  Outcomes: Family demonstrates skin care techniques to promote healing and to prevent further skin breakdown.
  Family caregivers verbalize measures to prevent diaper dermatitis.

Teach Child/Family

Medications

- If candidal infection is present, topical anticandidal agent (Nystatin, Lotrimin, Micatin, Nizoral) is applied to diaper area. Clotrimazole was superior to nystatin with respect to reduced symptom score. Cure rate was 100% for both clotrimazole and nystatin (Hoeger et al., 2010).
- If severe inflammation is present, apply a topical low-potency, nonfluorinated 1% hydrocortisone cream to rash site for 7–10 days.
- Children with recurrent diarrhea may be prescribed an oral anticandidal agent (nystatin) to sterilize the gastrointestinal tract and to prevent systemic infection.

Diaper Changes

- Change diaper frequently.
- Check diaper every 1–2 hours for wetness or soiling, and change wet or soiled diaper immediately.
- Use superabsorbent diapers if affordable. If using cloth diapers, consider placing a stay-dry liner in the diaper.
- With each wet or soiled diaper change, wipe the skin gently with plain water or a diaper wipe (nonallergenic, unscented).
- Wash the skin with water and a gentle, pH-neutral soap; rinse well.
- Pay particular attention to cleaning areas of skinfolds.
- Pat the baby's bottom dry; do not rub or use a hair dryer to dry.
- Avoid airtight occlusive diapers or diaper covers.
- Do not use plastic pants.
- Fasten the disposable diaper loosely.
- Brand-name disposable diapers can be altered to breathe better by snipping the elastic bands around the legs in a few places and cutting a few slits in the plastic diaper cover.
- Leave the baby's bottom exposed to air as much as possible.
- Put a towel or diaper open under the baby during nap time.
- Let the young child be "diaper free" for periods of time.

Creams and Ointments

- Do not use creams and lotions on most babies.
- Apply a layer of protective ointment or barrier cream (such as zinc oxide, petrolatum, or dimethicone base) to the noninfected diaper rash.
- Do not remove the barrier cream with every diaper change as long as a layer of paste remains on the skin and the skin underneath is clean.
- If the barrier cream must be removed, use a minimal amount of mineral oil to remove it.
- Do not use talcum powder. Cornstarch may be applied to areas where friction might occur. When wet, however, the cornstarch can clump and retain moisture on the skin. (There is some controversy regarding cornstarch. Some sources recommend not using it because microorganisms metabolize the cornstarch and aggravate yeast infections.)

Nutrition

- If the child has diarrhea, the child should be evaluated for dehydration. Dietary restrictions and hydration measures may be needed to stop the diarrhea and to prevent dehydration.

Nighttime Care

- Apply creams liberally to diaper area before bedtime, making sure to rub the product in completely, then apply a thin layer or coating.
- Avoid plastic pants at night.
- Until rash improves, awaken the child at least once a night to change the diaper.

Cloth Diapers

- Cloth diapers should always be washed in hot water with a combination of mild soap and distilled white vinegar and then double-rinsed. Wash, rinse, let the diaper soak in a water and ammonia mixture for 30 minutes, then rinse again.
- Do not use fabric softener or antistatic products because they may cause allergic rash. Be aware that some fabric softeners make fabrics non-absorbent and thus should not be used.

Prevention

- After the child's bath, let child be diaper free for a period of time.
- Change diapers frequently. Never leave a child in a soiled diaper.
- Wash cloth diapers appropriately (see above).
- Use appropriate barrier creams and ointments.

Contact Health Care Provider if

- Big blisters (more than one inch across) develop, as may open sores, or boils
- Rash does not look better in 3 days
- Rash becomes solid and bright red
- Rash becomes raw and bleeds
- The child is male and circumcised, and a sore or scab develops at the end of the penis
- Rash causes enough pain to disrupt sleep
- Child develops a temperature more than 100° F (37.8° C)

TRADITION OR SCIENCE 25-3

Should baby powder be used during diaper changes?

The use of baby powders containing talc (known as talcum powder) can cause accidental aspiration, pneumonia, and death (Brouillette & Weber, 1978; Moss, 1969). Aspiration is predominantly caused when the baby receives a "puff of smoke" when the powder is shaken from the container directly onto the baby's skin. In addition, the use of talcum powder is abrasive and is considered to contribute to the pathogenesis of diaper dermatitis (Atherton, 2004). All talcum powder containers should be closed and stored in a safe place, away from curious infants and young children. The parent should not self-administer talcum powder in an infant's or young child's presence.

Infants generally do not need any powder products on their diaper area. If the family wants to use a powder, cornstarch is an acceptable alternative to reduce friction in the diaper area. When wet, however, the cornstarch can clump and retain moisture on the skin. There is some controversy regarding cornstarch. Some sources recommend not using it because microorganisms metabolize the cornstarch and aggravate yeast infections (Janniger et al., 2005).

CHART 25-1 Common Causes of Contact Dermatitis

Irritant Contact Dermatitis

Saliva

Citrus juices

Bubble bath

Soaps, detergents, and body lotions with fragrances

Abrasive materials

Strong soaps

Occlusive shoes

Hobby supplies

Insecticides

Manufacturing agents

Allergic Contact Dermatitis

Poison ivy, poison oak, and poison sumac

Nickel (jewelry, buckles, clothing snaps)

Pierced earrings

Potassium dichromate (shoes, tanning agent)

Neomycin

Thimerosal, formaldehyde, and quaternium-15 (preservatives and topical agents)

Balsam of Peru (fragrance)

Wood alcohol (lanolin)

Colophony (rosin from wood)

Latex

Products containing formaldehyde (e.g., specific baby wipes, styling gel, shampoos)

ALERT   *The increased popularity in body piercing has led to an increase in allergic reactions related to nickel. Sensitization to nickel appears to increase with the number of piercings. For those with a suspected or diagnosed nickel allergy, test kits are available to identify the presence of nickel in a product (Copeland et al., 2007).*

Pathophysiology

In ICD, the irritating substance causes a nonspecific inflammatory reaction in the skin. Individual skin strength, concentration (dose) of the offending substance, and length of contact all contribute to the severity of reaction. Prolonged or repeated exposure to an irritating substance results in erythema and the potential for skin breakdown and lesions. A detailed health history, evaluation of the involved sites, and the child's age all can provide clues regarding the nature of the irritating substance.

ACD is caused by an allergen that penetrates the epidermis from the skin surface. An interaction between the T-lymphocyte component of the cellular immune system is mediated by antigen-presenting epidermal cells (Langerhans cells). When the antigen penetrates the skin, it is conjugated with a cutaneous protein and transported to the regional lymph nodes by the Langerhans cells. A primary immunologic response occurs locally in the nodes as the sensitized T cells circulate throughout the body. This process is called the *sensitization phase*. The duration of this phase depends on the potency of the allergen. For example, the oil urushiol, the offending agent in poison ivy, penetrates the epidermis, bonds with the dermis, and initiates the immune response usually after only one exposure. (Poison ivy, oak, and sumac are discussed in more detail in subsequent paragraphs of this chapter.) After sensitization occurs, children who are exposed to repeated contact by the same antigen experience an inflammatory reaction (ACD) within 8 to 24 hours. Children can remain sensitized to a certain allergen for many years.

The prognosis for contact dermatitis is very good if the offending substance is identified and exposure to the substance is prohibited. If the offending agent is removed, the skin's recuperative powers produce healing without treatment within 1 to 2 weeks. In more severe cases of ACD, the untreated dermatitis persists for 3 to 4 weeks. Any time a child has a break in the skin, risk for secondary infection is present. Therefore, prompt attention to the dermatitis and measures to stop exposure to offending agents should be instituted to prevent further alterations in skin integrity.

ANSWER: Nick's rash is an ACD caused by the body's allergic response to the oil or resin of the plant (urushiol). Poison ivy is unusual in that approximately 85% of the population will have an allergic response (American Academy of Dermatology, 2013).

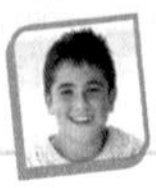

Assessment

Nurses are often the first to identify contact dermatitis during the history-taking process or physical examination. Contact dermatitis usually occurs in exposed skin areas: the face, neck, hands, forearms, legs, and feet. A characteristic inflamed response varies from erythema to large bullae on a reddened base and edema. The lesions may be well demarcated, exactly resembling the shape and size of the offending substance (e.g., red marks on the abdomen the size and shape of pajama snaps). Itching is intense and constant.

Diagnosis of contact dermatitis depends on a thorough history. Patch testing may be indicated if the etiology is not apparent (see Tests and Procedures 25-1). In addition to testing for the suspected allergen, the child undergoes testing with a standardized tested group of allergens that have been recognized by several medical associations as the most frequent causes of ACD. The classic positive patch test consists of erythema, edema, and small vesicles that do not extend beyond the border of the patch. Results must be examined within the context of the history and of the physical examination. A positive test does not necessarily mean that the identified allergen is responsible for the child's current dermatitis, although it does indicate that the child has sensitivity to a particular allergen. Skin cultures and biopsy may be used to rule out herpes simplex virus and staphylococcal infections.

Interdisciplinary Interventions

Untreated ACD slowly resolves over a 3- to 4-week period if contact with the allergen is avoided. Treatment for the itching and edema may include the use of Aveeno baths, calamine lotion, or Burow solution compresses. Mild- to medium-potency topical corticosteroid may be ordered by the health care prescriber to relieve inflammation and hasten the healing process. Oral corticosteroids may be prescribed for more severe reactions. Antihistamines may be ordered to decrease itching. If infected lesions are present, antibiotic therapy is usually initiated.

Community Care

QUESTION: What is the role of the nurse in educating the community about poison ivy?

Teach children and families ways to prevent contact dermatitis. First, they should remove the irritating and allergy-triggering substance from the home and school environment. Second, the child should wear protective clothing to minimize exposure to irritants, especially with plant allergies and caustic materials. After a contact allergen is confirmed by patch testing, the child must avoid all products or substances containing that allergen. Lists of products that contain the offending agents are usually available from a dermatologist. Teach the family how to read product labels to ensure that the allergen is not present.

Teach children and families proper skin hygiene, and emphasize that using mild antibacterial soaps and moisturizers can help to prevent painful scaling and cracking of the skin that can lead to a secondary infection, such as impetigo. The presence of a skin allergy may necessitate some restrictions of the child's activities to prevent contact with the offending agent. Young children may not understand or tolerate the limitations on their activities. Families can assist by providing enjoyable play alternatives for the child and by reinforcing the cause-and-effect relationship between the child's exposure to the irritant and the eruption of the skin rash.

ANSWER: Prevention is the most effective approach with poison ivy. Nurses can be instrumental in providing information to individuals, families, and organizations (e.g., Boy Scouts) concerning plant identification, properties of urushiol, strategies to use if one does come in contact with the plant, and products that are available to reduce the impact of contact. For example, when urushiol is transferred to an inanimate object, such as a ball, garden tools, and camping equipment, it can remain potent for months.

ATOPIC DERMATITIS

AD is a chronic, relapsing inflammation of the dermis and epidermis characterized by itching, edema, papules, erythema, excoriation, serous discharge, and crusting; it is a noncontagious condition that generally begins during infancy or early childhood. The term *atopic* refers to the fact that patients exhibit a heightened reaction to a variety of allergens. To the lay public, the condition is commonly known as *eczema*. The term *eczema* describes the combination of erythema, scaling vesicles, and crusts. Eczema-like lesions occur in several skin diseases; hence, the term *atopic dermatitis* is used in this book. AD is categorized into three stages according to the child's age (Developmental Considerations 25-3).

AD is a fairly common health problem. Research has indicated that about 50% of infants who develop AD will do so within the first year of life and that the prevalence has increased such that 20% to 25% of all 5- to 10-year-old children are affected (Nicol, 2011). Males and females are equally affected, and AD is more common in industrialized cities and in white and Chinese populations. Allergies have been thought to cause AD; however, research has not borne out a definitive association between AD and food allergies (Nicol, 2011).

A number of factors exacerbate AD, including sudden changes and extremes of temperature, irritating fabrics such as wool, excessive exercise that induces sweating, and direct contact with irritants such as detergents and perfumes. AD is also commonly associated with the ingestion of certain foods, such as dairy foods (Nicol, 2011).

The exact etiology of AD is unknown and may vary from child to child; however, it is part of the atopy syndrome that includes asthma, hay fever, and rhinitis/allergic rhinitis. Theories that have been proposed to describe the origin of AD include the inborn error of

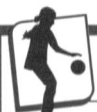

DEVELOPMENTAL CONSIDERATIONS 25-3

Stages of Atopic Dermatitis

Infantile Stage

Age 2–6 months, resolving in half of children between ages 2 and 3 years

Characteristics

Pruritus

Erythema

Exudate and crusts

Common sites: cheeks, forehead, scalp, extensor surfaces of arms and legs

Diaper area not usually involved

Childhood Stage

Age 4–10 years or following on continuously from infancy stage

Characteristics

Less exudate than the previous stage

Dry, itchy patches of skin

Common sites: wrists, ankles, antecubital and popliteal spaces

Adolescent and Adult Stage

Age 11 years (or puberty) and older

Characteristics

Exudation caused by external irritation or secondary infection

Dry, itchy patches of skin

Common sites: flexor folds, face, neck, back, upper arms, and dorsal aspects of the hands, feet, fingers, and toes

---

metabolism theory, the psychosomatic theory, and the immunologic theory. The first theory postulates that AD patients have a metabolic skin defect that causes excessive itching. The psychosomatic model holds that AD is caused by underlying stress and psychological dysfunctioning in the life of the child. The immunologic theory postulates that interactions between genes and environment contribute to the development of atopy (Guttman-Yassky et al., 2011a).

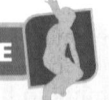
CROSS-CULTURAL CARE

The worldwide increase in the incidence of AD, which has paralleled an increase in asthma prevalence, is of great concern to clinicians. An increase in prevalence of both conditions is thought to be attributable to influences of the Western lifestyle, urbanization, and development. Industrialized Western countries have seen an increasing prevalence of AD during the past 30 years. This prevalence is higher in Western countries than in others, higher in industrialized countries with a market economy than in underdeveloped countries, higher in urban areas than in rural areas, and higher among privileged socioeconomic groups and smaller families. Epidemiologists believe that lifestyle changes prevalent in Western countries combined with increased environmental exposure to pollutants have influenced the "allergy pandemic" (Guttman-Yassky et al., 2011a; Nicol, 2011).

Pathophysiology

In AD, the stratum corneum, or outermost epidermal skin layer, is susceptible to damage from the environment with allergen penetration (Guttman-Yassky et al., 2011a; Nicol, 2011). There is impaired hydration with transepidermal water loss increase in lesional skin. Genetic studies focus

on the chromosome 1q21 containing genes known as the epidermal differentiation complex. Strong predisposing factors identified in AD are mutations of the filaggrin gene located in the epidermal differentiation complex. Mutations cause loss or reduction of the filaggrin protein, which is essential for formation and hydration of the skin barrier (Nicol, 2011).

Skin in patients with AD, deficient in antimicrobial peptides, has increased susceptibility to infections. Patients with AD are frequently colonized with *S. aureus*. Many of those patients colonized develop immunoglobulin E (IgE) molecules against the toxins produced by *S. aureus*. Toxins produced by *S. aureus* dysregulate normal immune response and result in the induction of corticosteroid insensitivity (Nicol, 2011). Biomarkers sE-selectin, interleukin-16 (IL-16), and thymus and activation-regulated chemokine (TARC) are proposed to be involved in pathogenesis (van Velsen et al., 2010). Serum TARC levels are elevated in patients with AD, when compared to healthy controls, and correlate with disease activity.

The condition may resolve spontaneously, especially in those children with milder cases who are able to effectively avoid environmental triggers. In general, the exacerbations become less frequent after adolescence, and most of these children can enjoy long periods in which they experience no symptoms. Up to 80% of children with AD will eventually develop allergic rhinitis or asthma later in childhood (Guttman-Yassky et al., 2011a).

Assessment

Diagnosis of AD depends on three clinical features: pruritus, dermatitis that fits into a typical age distribution, and a chronic or relapsing course. Most children have a family history of allergy (e.g., asthma, allergic rhinitis, food). The infantile form has lesions that are generalized on the trunk, scalp, cheeks, and extremities. The disorder spares the perioral and nasal areas. During childhood, the lesions occur in body creases such as the wrists, ankles, feet, and antecubital, flexural surfaces, and popliteal fossae. In the adolescent form, the face, feet, hands, flexural surfaces, and neck are affected.

The types of AD lesions also vary according to age. In the infantile form of the disorder, they include scaling, crusting, weeping, erythema, vesicles, papules, and oozing. In the childhood form, symmetric distribution of small erythematous papules or patches occurs along with lichenification (hardening of the skin) and hyperpigmentation. In adolescents, the pattern is similar to the childhood form, except that dry, thick plaques are more common.

Other accompanying symptoms that produce the most distressing components of AD include intense itching, drying of the unaffected skin areas, restlessness, irritability, lymphadenopathy, and other signs of allergic response (such as a bluish discoloration under the eyes). Many authorities believe that the intense itching and the resultant scratching (the "itch–scratch" cycle) are the main conditions that generate the lesions. If scratching is controlled, the lesions heal. No laboratory tests are diagnostic for AD, although increased eosinophil counts and serum IgE are common findings, and TARC levels correlated with AD disease activity (van Velsen et al., 2010). Patch testing with appropriate antigens is the gold standard for confirming AD.

caREminder

Differentiate between itch and scratch when determining nursing interventions. Itch is the underlying physiologic symptom that results in scratching, which, in AD, can lead to pain, excoriations, and skin breakdown. Scratching is a reflex action that is controlled at the spinal cord level and is, therefore, difficult to prevent in the presence of itch.

Interdisciplinary Interventions

The major goals of therapy are to prevent, alleviate, or control itching; reduce inflammation; hydrate the skin; avoid recurrence; and prevent secondary infection (Teaching Intervention Plan 25-2). Medical interventions do not cure this condition, but effective palliation can be achieved. Ensure that both child and the family understand that AD is both chronic and recurring. This knowledge can avoid concerns that therapy was withdrawn too soon and may diminish some anxiety when flare-ups occur.

The American Academy of Dermatology has an algorithm for AD treatment (Evidence-Based Clinical Practice Guidelines 25-1). By carefully controlling or reducing the exacerbations, and by diligently managing inflammation and **pruritus** (itching), the child or adolescent can have a normal lifestyle.

Frequently rehydrating the skin is a key element of the treatment regimen. To maintain healthy skin in the child with AD, hydration practices should be implemented to replace moisture in the stratum corneum and to prevent transdermal water losses. The numerous types of emollient therapies continue to be the cornerstone to successfully managing AD and are continued even in the absence of overt disease. To reduce inflammation, *topical corticosteroids* are administered to the affected area (Nursing Interventions 25-2). Topical corticosteroids are classified into groups, from class I (most potent) to class VII (least potent), based on cutaneous vasoconstriction tests. Topical ointments, which are the most occlusive than are creams, gels, lotions, or foams, also have a higher degree of systemic absorption. Skin penetration of the drug is highest in thin skin areas such as eyelids and genitals. Therefore, less potent preparations of corticosteroids should be used in those areas. Relapse and rebound of the skin disease may occur when treatment is discontinued. Low-potency corticosteroids are the medication of choice. However, treatment decisions should be based on extent and severity of disease. Additionally, the potent anti-inflammatory actions of these medications increase susceptibility to bacterial and fungal infections (Guttman-Yassky et al., 2011a, 2011b; Nicol, 2011). Systemic corticosteroids are rarely used; consequences include hypopigmentation, acne, secondary infection, and stretch marks.

Newer medications, and those considered as treating the underlying cause, are the topical nonsteroidal creams called *topical calcineurin inhibitors* (e.g., tacrolimus, pimecrolimus) (Yang & Curran, 2009). These compounds inhibit inflammatory cytokines within the immune system, which in turn decreases T-cell activation (Yang & Curran, 2009). *Tar preparations* can also be applied to the skin. These agents have a slower anti-inflammatory action than corticosteroid therapy and have fewer side effects. The use of *antihistamines*, both first (e.g., Benadryl) and second (e.g., Zyrtec, Allegra, Claritin) generation, may be considered for their antihistamine effect and their ability to help control itching. *Oral anti-infective therapy* may be indicated, because *S. aureus* colonization of the skin is common among children with AD. *Topical and oral antibiotics* are used for secondary infections. Keep the child's skin clean with tepid baths of nonirritating hydrophilic cleaners. Skinfolds and diaper areas need frequent cleaning with plain water.

Phototherapy has demonstrated effectiveness as an adjunctive intervention to control severe, generalized AD. UVA radiation is believed to trigger an immunologic response, mediated through Langerhans cells and eosinophils. UVB radiation is thought to work by immunosuppression, by inhibiting Langerhans cells and altering keratinocyte production (Guttman-Yassky et al., 2011b). However the lack of long-term, randomized controlled data limits clinical use of phototherapy (Guttman-Yassky et al., 2011b; Nicol, 2011). Other experimental therapies include methotrexate, mycophenolate mofetil, azathioprine, IV immunoglobulin, and cyclosporine A (Nicol, 2011).

Food allergy and other environmental triggers have been linked to AD. Hen's eggs, cow's milk, soy, fish, nuts, and wheat account for most of the food allergy triggers seen in children (Guttman-Yassky et al., 2011b).

TIP 25-2: A TEACHING INTERVENTION PLAN for the Child With Atopic Dermatitis

Nursing Diagnoses and Family Outcomes

- Impaired skin integrity related to chronic occurrence of dry skin, intense itching, erythema, and excoriation
  Outcomes: Child exhibits improved skin integrity. Child and family demonstrate skin care regimen.
- Risk for infection related to presence of lesions, higher concentration of flora on atopic skin, and decreased integrity of skin barrier
  Outcomes: Child and family demonstrate measures to prevent infection.
  Child and family identify signs and symptoms of skin infection.
  Child and family verbalize the actions to take if an infection is suspected or confirmed.
- Interrupted family processes related to child's discomfort and increased health care requirements
  Outcomes: Child reports increased comfort.
  Child and family correlate precipitating factors with appropriate skin care regimen.
  Child and family verbalize confidence in their ability to manage the child's care.

Teach Child/Family

Skin Care and General Hygiene
- Use a room humidifier or vaporizer to help provide moisture to the skin.
- Cool compresses and colloid baths can help control itching.
- Bathe child nightly for 15–20 minutes.
- Provide creative toys for water play or encourage the older child to read a book while soaking.
- Do not use bath additives such as oatmeal or baking soda, bubble bath, soaps, or bath oils.
- For adolescents with mild symptoms, a daily shower may be sufficient.
- Pat, rather than rub, the skin dry.
- Follow bath with immediate application of occlusive emollient such as Eucerin, Aveeno, or Lubriderm.
- Choose preparations with no artificial fragrance and chemical stabilizer additives that may cause further skin irritation.
- Wet wraps can be used on severely affected skin. Apply after soaking and after applying topical medications.
- For total body wrap, use wet pajamas, long underwear, or tube socks (for hands and feet). Layer dry clothing on top.
- Wet wraps of gauze or Kerlix with stockinette or surginet can be applied to smaller areas.
- Do not allow the wrap to dry.
- Chilling may occur if outer layer becomes wet.
- Use antibacterial soaps for handwashing.
- Keep child's nails clean and cut short. Gloves and cotton stockings may need to be placed on hands and feet to prevent itching.

Medications

Topical Steroids
- Medicine is used to control acute exacerbations.
- The potency of the medication is determined by the body area that it is applied to and the severity of the child's condition. In general, as low a level of potency as possible is used to achieve good effects.
- Side effects include thinning of the skin, hypopigmentation, acne, secondary infection, and stretch marks.

Topical Nonsteroidals (Topical Calcineurin Inhibitors)
- Medicine is used to control acute flare-ups and is believed to control the underlying cause.
- May be used in children as young as 6 months of age (pimecrolimus).
- Indicated for mild/moderate (pimecrolimus) as well as moderate/severe (tacrolimus) eczema.
- Side effects include occasional burning or itching upon application.

Tar Preparations
- Preparations are used to control acute exacerbation; they have a slower inflammatory action than topical steroids.
- Tar preparations should only be used when symptoms are mild.
- Tar preparations may cause burning and irritation if applied to skin areas with severe symptoms.
- Tar preparations have a bad smell, so many children dislike this treatment.

Antihistamines
- Medicine is used to reduce itching, primarily by causing drowsiness.
- Medicine may be taken at night to aid in comfort while sleeping.

Oral Antibiotics
- Medicine may be ordered if there is widespread skin breakdown or infection.

Phototherapy
- Once-weekly treatments, in conjunction with moisturizers and low-potency corticosteroids, can help control skin condition.
- Long-term use not studied and not feasible because of adverse effects of radiation exposure.

Nutrition
- Identify foods that exacerbate rash, and avoid these foods; use the standard elimination diet.
- Identify "hidden" ingredients in foods (e.g., eggs in baked goods) that might exacerbate the child's condition, and avoid these foods.
- Avoid cow's milk–based formulas; use soy-based or other special formulas such as partial whey.

Safety and Activity
- Outdoor activities are encouraged.
- Child should avoid getting sunburned.

(Continued)

TIP 25-2: A TEACHING INTERVENTION PLAN for the Child With Atopic Dermatitis *(Continued)*

- Swimming is permitted if followed by a shower to remove chlorine from skin, and then occlusive emollient is applied to skin.

Comfort and Support Measures

- Use first-generation antihistamines at night if scratching or rubbing of affected areas inhibits sleep; use second-generation antihistamines as preventive measures.
- Use mittens to prevent scratching during sleep.
- Remove clothing and bedding that increase itching.
- Maintain good skin care at all times to maintain optimal skin integrity and decrease pain.
- Maintain regular sleep/wake schedules despite disruptions in sleep patterns resulting from discomfort and itching.

Special Considerations

- Avoid known or suspected sensitivities to contact allergens, pets, or other environmental factors.
- Explain the "itch/scratch" cycle.

If infection occurs

- Use antibiotic creams as ordered.
- Use systemic antibiotics as ordered.
- Continue daily skin care.

Contact Health Care Provider if

- Child is in such discomfort that sleep and the ability to concentrate are affected
- Child spikes a temperature of 101.5° F (38.6° C) or more
- An area of the child's skin has a colored discharge, is warm to the touch, or has a foul smell

---

Breastfed infants may develop AD as a result of sensitization to foods or beverages ingested by the mother. Food-induced eczema should be diagnosed only after a thorough diagnostic evaluation that includes the child's history, the degree of sensitization, and the clinical relevance of the sensitization. If a food substance is an identified allergen, then it is removed from the diet as in the standard elimination diet, which usually consists of chicken, lamb, rice, banana, apple, and a vegetable from the cruciferous family. This diet is maintained for 2 to 4 weeks; if the child's symptoms are food-related, they will usually disappear within the first 2 weeks. However, the dietitian must reassure the family that a hypoallergenic diet does not always give immediate relief.

The child's condition may reach a point of remission, in which case using emollients and avoiding triggers will effectively manage the child's AD. When a flare-up occurs, acute control of pruritus and inflammation and managing secondary conditions (e.g., infection) are the prime focus of therapy.

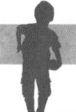

EVIDENCE-BASED CLINICAL PRACTICE GUIDELINES 25-1
Atopic Dermatitis

Hanifin, J. M., Cooper, K. D., Ho, V. C. et al. (2004). Guidelines of care for atopic dermatitis. *Journal of the American Academy of Dermatology, 50,* 391–404.

Care guidelines developed by the American Academy of Dermatology.

Leung, D. Y., Nicklas, R. A., Li, J. T. et al. (2004). Disease management of atopic dermatitis: An updated practice parameter. *Annals of Allergy, Asthma & Immunology, 93,* S1–S21.

Guidelines developed by the American Academy of Allergy, Asthma, and Immunology and the Joint Council of Allergy, Asthma and Immunology.

National Institute for Health and Clinical Excellence. (2007). *Atopic eczema in children: Management of atopic eczema in children from birth up to the age of 12 years.* Retrieved from

http://publications.nice.org.uk/atopic-eczema-in-children-cg57

Management of atopic eczema in children from birth up to the age of 12 years and guidance on diagnosis and assessment, management, and providing information and education for children and their caregivers.

Ring, J., Alomar, A., Bieber, T. et al. (2012). Guidelines for treatment of atopic eczema (atopic dermatitis) part I. *Journal of the European Academy of Dermatology and Venereology, 26(8),* 1045–1060.

Consensus document regarding management of AD.

Scottish Intercollegiate Guidelines Network. (2011). *Management of atopic eczema in primary care. A national clinical guideline.* Edinburgh, Scotland: Author. Retrieved from

http://guideline.gov/content.aspx?id=34951

Guidelines for care and management of patients with eczema.

NURSING INTERVENTIONS 25-2

Application of Topical Corticosteroids

Action
- Topical corticosteroids are effective anti-inflammatory agents that reduce inflammation of the skin by promoting vasoconstriction of the blood vessels in the skin and by preventing the shedding of inflammatory cells from the bloodstream to tissue sites. These medications reduce redness (erythema) and itching (pruritus) associated with inflammatory and hyperproliferation skin diseases.

Potency
- Potency is determined by the amount of skin blanching (vasoconstriction that correlates with the anti-inflammatory effects of the agent).
- Steroids are also categorized as **nonfluorinated**, having less potent and fewer side effects, and **fluorinated**, which are rarely used in pediatric practice.
- Potency may be increased by the vehicle (agent) with which the steroid is combined to create a gel or cream form of the medication.

Administration
- Corticosteroids are available in several forms: creams, gels, ointments, lotions, powders, aerosols, and tapes.
- At home, family caregivers should apply corticosteroids for their children.
- A thin layer is applied over the affected area; creams, lotions, and gels are rubbed in until no longer visible.
- Avoid unaffected areas.
- The agent may be applied with bare hands; wash hands thoroughly after application.
- A tongue depressor can be used to scoop the ointment out of a large container.

- On the face and scrotum, only low-potency glucocorticosteroids should be used. The epidermis is thin in these areas and side effects may be severe.
- Occlusive dressings or coverings (e.g., plastic pants covering a cloth diaper) should not be placed over an area in which a corticosteroid has been applied because this increases the absorption of the steroid and may lead to toxic side effects.
- The agents should not be used with conditions such as acne, rosacea, and some fungal infections or on severely eroded skin.
- Treatment is usually begun using a low-potency steroid. If lesions do not respond to therapy, the potency may be increased.
- Steroid therapy should be used for as short a time period as possible to achieve the desired effects.

Side Effects
- Striae
- Persistent erythema and telangiectasis
- Increased skin fragility
- Hypopigmentation
- Secondary infection
- Acneform eruption (steroid rosacea)
- Folliculitis, miliaria
- ACD
- Steroid addiction syndrome

Systemic Effects
- Cataracts
- Glaucoma
- Glycosuria
- Cushing syndrome
- Stunted growth in children (rare)

Community Care

AD causes much physical suffering, disability, and anguish for the child and the family. Prolonged discomfort and cosmetic disfigurement disrupt the activities of daily living. The child and the family need intense emotional support and assurance that lesions do not produce scarring unless secondarily infected. Families need to be taught that feeling overwhelmed by the disorder is a common experience. Poor adherence and maintenance to treatments as well as anxiety about using many of the medications mentioned are common features seen in families. Nurses can assist family members by allowing them to discuss their frustrations. Family members can alternately feel angry and then guilty about the demands of the child's care. Families need to be given emotional support and to be made aware of community sources of help. Older children and teenagers can be badly affected by AD because they are often rejected by peers who are offended by their skin condition.

The personal financial costs of managing this condition can be excessive for the family. In these cases, social workers can provide assistance by interviewing the child and family, assessing needs, and identifying available community resources. The social worker can help to improve the home environment and lifestyle, especially for impoverished children. If psychotherapy is necessary because of poor self-concept and associated behaviors, social services may be able to generate financial support for the family to receive this therapy.

School performance can be adversely affected by severe AD. Children may be unable to concentrate because of the itching. School nurses can act as a liaison with health care personnel to notify the family if they observe that the child's condition is worsening and affecting school performance. The school nurse's office can also be used by children with AD as a place where they can undress to apply moisturizing solutions to the skin. Assist the child with treatments if needed, assess the status of the condition, and help support a good self-concept. Educate school staff about the nature of the disease and the environmental conditions that need to be considered. For example, physical education (which generates sweating) and art class (exposure to paint and thinning agents) may have to be eliminated if they cause the dermatitis to worsen. Adolescents seeking employment should be guided to find work conditions that do not aggravate or activate their skin condition.

SEBORRHEIC DERMATITIS

Seborrheic dermatitis is a common, chronic, noncontagious dermatitis most likely caused by overproduction of sebum because it is common in areas with large numbers of sebaceous glands. Characterized by scaling and redness, seborrheic dermatitis lesions usually develop on the face, eyelids, scalp, body folds, external ears, and diaper area. This condition is frequently called *cradle cap* in infants or *dandruff* in older children.

The incidence of seborrheic dermatitis in the general population is 2% to 5%. Seborrheic dermatitis has been presented as a condition that occurs between the first 2 and 6 weeks of life, with recurrence seen during or after puberty. Most recently, classic seborrheic dermatitis in 2- to 10-year-olds has been noted to be fairly common (Williams et al., 2005). Seasonal fluctuation of the condition occurs, with most cases being reported during the spring and summer when sebaceous gland activity is increased by sweating. However, the child with an existing condition also has more symptoms in colder weather because of the low indoor humidity and lack of sunlight. A seborrhealike dermatitis is also common in children and adolescents infected with HIV.

In contrast to AD, seborrheic dermatitis is not genetically predisposed. The etiologic agents involved in seborrheic dermatitis include the presence of sebum, excessive perspiration, lipase activity, immune function, atmospheric humidity, the *Pityrosporum ovale* yeast organism that grows in hair follicles, poor hygiene, and stress (Williams et al., 2005). Occlusion of a skin area (e.g., diaper area), maceration, and moisture may also play a distinct exacerbating role.

Pathophysiology

Seborrhea is similar to psoriasis in that white blood cells migrate into the skin plaque. A hyperkeratosing process generates plaque formation (scaling). It may be difficult to distinguish psoriasis from seborrheic dermatitis.

Most cases of infantile seborrheic dermatitis clear up within 1 month, even without therapy. In the adolescent form, long-term prognosis is good if the treatment plan is adhered to faithfully.

Assessment

Seborrheic dermatitis has different manifestations in various age groups. In infants, yellow, waxy, adherent scales occur over the frontal and vertex areas of the scalp (cradle cap) and diaper area. Children aged 2 to 10 years have been found to exhibit both the "cradle cap" type of scalp scaling and the nonspecific fine, nongreasy scale commonly termed *dandruff* (Williams et al., 2005). In pubertal and postpubertal children, seborrheic dermatitis manifests as erythematous, oily plaques and patches of vesicles and papules occurring on the forehead, eyebrows, and symmetrically on the nasolabial folds.

Seborrhea may also cause scaling and erythema on the eyelids (blepharitis), on the external ears (otitis externa), and retroauricular areas. Blepharitis is often accompanied by styes. In severe cases, other affected areas include the intertriginous folds of the trunk, under the breasts in women, and the gluteal cleft.

Mild cases may involve no more than dealing with the nuisance of dandruff. However, severe cases can be extremely deleterious to body image and self-concept. The child can be assured that seborrheic dermatitis does not cause hair loss. Stress can activate an exacerbation in some children. No laboratory test or consistent pattern of laboratory abnormalities is associated with seborrheic dermatitis.

Interdisciplinary Interventions

Infantile seborrheic dermatitis usually responds well to cleansing the scalp with a mild shampoo. The thick, scaling lesions on the child's scalp can be treated by applying baby oil, salicylic acid in mineral oil, or a corticosteroid gel on the scalp for 10 to 15 minutes. The area is gently massaged with a soft toothbrush; then the scales can be rinsed away. A fine-toothed comb helps rid the hair of scale debris.

In the older child and adolescent, an antiseborrheic shampoo should be used daily to control scaling. Common names for these shampoos include Sebulex, Selsun Blue, and Head & Shoulders. When severe inflammation is present, a low-potency corticosteroid medication (0.5% to 1% hydrocortisone) may be administered two to four times a day, or ketoconazole 1% or 2% shampoo (e.g., Nizoral) may be used. Scaling may be so severe that a tar gel preparation (e.g., DHS Tar, Sebutone, Zetar) is prescribed that is left on the scalp all night. However, children are usually reluctant to have this medication applied because it is difficult to remove and has an offensive smell.

Teach family members and older children how to prevent seborrheic dermatitis of the scalp. Good scalp hygiene with a mild shampoo and gentle rubbing prevents the situation. If crusts are present, teach caregivers how to remove the crusts. Generally, topical ointments are not required; but, if they are prescribed, teach the family how to apply the ointments appropriately. Also teach them to avoid using greasy ointments or creams on the affected child.

PSORIASIS

Psoriasis is a chronic proliferative epidermal disease that usually manifests during the third decade of life, but it may develop at any time from birth onward. Characterized by flare-ups and remissions, psoriasis can, therefore, occur at any age.

Incidence of psoriasis peaks during adolescence and young adulthood and again during older adulthood. Psoriasis affects 1% to 3% of the population, with 25% to 45% of cases appearing before 10 to 16 years of age (Burns et al., 2013; Guttman-Yassky et al., 2011a). Psoriasis is much more common in white children and is seen twice as often in females.

Although the cause of psoriasis is unknown, a familial predisposition is present in 35% of cases, probably through polygenic inheritance patterns. Several hereditary and environmental mechanisms have been suggested. These include genetic inheritance, problems in cell division, and alterations in immune response. Other suggested causes are streptococcal and viral infections, hormones, contact with animal skins, increased weight, seasonal change (especially cold), drugs (lithium, indomethacin, and some beta-blockers), stress, and inflammatory bowel disease (Burns et al., 2013; Guttman-Yassky et al., 2011a).

Pathophysiology

The pathogenesis of psoriasis is not fully understood. In psoriasis lesions, basal cell layers reproduce cells too quickly, and these cells move upward in the skin in 3 to 5 days instead of 2 to 4 weeks. Normally, skin cells die as they move upward; in psoriasis, the quickly migrating cells do not. The partially living skin builds on the skin surface instead of being desquamated. As the heaped-up skin dries, it becomes brittle and cracks. Underlying this hyperactive epidermis is a swollen dermis congested with blood vessels and leukocytes; these conditions form minute abscesses that become pustules.

The course of management for psoriasis is prolonged and unpredictable. Spontaneous clearing is quite rare, but unexplained exacerbation, remission, or improvement is common (Guttman-Yassky et al., 2011a). If psoriasis persists to adolescence, it becomes a lifelong disease. Arthritis can be a noncutaneous complication. Patient outcomes focus on normalizing skin physiology as much as possible and promoting normal activities of daily living.

Assessment

The physical signs of psoriasis are varied. In some children, psoriasis is annoying; in others, it is a debilitating, devastating experience. Sharply demarcated red plaques covered in a silvery white, thick, adherent scale occur at the elbows, knees, scalp, back, genitals, and sacrum.

caREminder

Psoriasis closely resembles AD. Ask the child if the lesions are greasy. Psoriasis scales are erythematous and are not oily.

Facial psoriasis is rare, although facial lesions are more common in children than in adults. Affected skin thickens over the palms of the hands and the soles of the feet. Nail changes include pits, ridges, and brittleness. When the scales are peeled off, pinhead-sized bleeding can be seen (Auspitz sign). As the plaques clear, the skin beneath may show either increased or decreased pigmentation. Another characteristic sign is worsening of the eruptions during the winter.

Interdisciplinary Interventions

Treatment options for children with psoriasis are varied and are generally based on severity, size of areas involved, type of psoriasis, and the child's response to the initial therapy (Guttman-Yassky et al., 2011b). The goals of therapy include rehydrating the skin, removing scales, preventing infection, inhibiting the pathologic process and suppressing the immune response, and promoting acceptance of the child's condition (Nursing Interventions 25-3).

Community Care

The care of a child with psoriasis is demanding and emotional. Educate the family that psoriasis is not contagious and that the child should be encouraged to pursue normal activities. Neither overprotecting the child nor ignoring the problem is beneficial. Organizations such as the National Psoriasis Foundation are excellent resources for families (see thePoint for Organizations). Children and their families may experience a great deal of stress because of the meticulous measures that must be followed, the restrictions on the child's activities, and the unsightly appearance of the lesions. Help the family understand the long-term nature of psoriasis treatment. Lifestyle changes will help minimize recurrence. In addition, the family needs information regarding the side effects of the medications, how to monitor for fluid and electrolyte imbalances and for infection, and how to monitor the status of the skin.

EPIDERMOLYSIS BULLOSA

Although many skin disorders and infections can generate vesicles and bullae, the phrase "bullous skin disease" is usually reserved for the condition called *epidermolysis bullosa*. EB describes a family of inherited disorders characterized by exceptional skin fragility and the formation of bullae at the site of mechanical trauma. The disorders range in severity from mild (subtle small lesions) to severe (large, mutilating lesions with internal organ involvement). EB affects all races and both genders equally.

Pathophysiology

EB is classified into three major types, depending on the layer of skin in which blistering occurs. *EB simplex* is the most superficial type, in which mechanical trauma causes splitting of the epidermis within the basal layer. The most common forms of EB simplex are autosomal dominant. Although the lesions can be widespread, they occur predominantly on the extremities and heal

NURSING INTERVENTIONS 25-3

Psoriasis Therapy

Goal	Action
Rehydrate epidermis • Risk for impaired skin integrity • Deficient fluid volume	Apply moisturizers several times a day, after bathing and before bedtime. Apply topical emollients. Use soap substitutes. Protect from overexposure to sun. Prevent exposure to psoriasis triggers (e.g., cold stress, extreme heat, skin trauma) Maintain good fluid intake.
Remove scales • Impaired skin integrity	Apply keratolytic preparations.
Prevent infection • Risk for infection	Protect against injury. Maintain hydrated skin. Use aseptic hand-cleaning techniques. Monitor for infection. Administer systemic and topical antibiotics. Maintain protein-rich diet.
Reduce epidermal cell division and suppress immune response • Impaired skin integrity • Ineffective peripheral tissue perfusion	Administer PUVA, a combination of psoralen medication and UV light (has serious drawbacks; rarely used for children). Administer retinoid, a vitamin derivative, which can dramatically decrease scaling (has serious side effects). Administer methotrexate, an antimetabolite (serious side effects; rarely used for children). Avoid triggers: cold, stress, trauma to skin, infections of skin.
Promote acceptance of the child's condition • Impaired parenting • Ineffective family coping • Disturbed body image • Delayed growth and development	Allow family and child to verbalize concerns. Encourage activities that promote child's self-esteem and achievement of normal growth and developmental milestones. Refer child or family to support services and agencies.

without scarring. Fingernails may detach, but they grow back. The mucous membranes are not involved. By adolescence, blistering tends to lessen, and the child has the potential for a normal life span.

Junctional epidermolysis bullosa is predominantly an autosomal dominant inherited disease (see Fig. 3-3). The condition is characterized by bullae and erosions occurring on mucosal surfaces as a result of splitting within the lamina lucida, which is at the junction of the epidermis and dermis. This is considered a life-threatening condition because the erosions can lead to infection, sepsis, anemia, dehydration, and malnutrition. The mucous membranes of the respiratory, gastrointestinal, and genitourinary systems may all be involved.

Dystrophic epidermolysis bullosa has both autosomal dominant and recessive types, which are characterized by blistering in the dermis below the lamina densa. At birth, the child has large, dense bullae that heal slowly, leaving scars, fusion of scarred digits, and residual mucosal trauma. Blistering of the oral mucosa and larynx affects the child's nutritional intake. In addition to oral mucosal blistering, protein loss for the child may also occur through the skin, with anemia and chronic constipation. Dystrophic and dermatolytic EB have the poorest prognosis, the greatest degree of scarring, and the most contracture development.

Assessment

Diagnosis of EB is made by evaluating the family history and the child's clinical course and by completing a skin biopsy. EB usually manifests in neonates when blisters caused by delivery trauma appear. Lesions are clearly related to areas of handling or occur at sites of pressure or motion. The number and amount of blisters, scarring, and affected sites depend on the type of EB. Specific areas of the body commonly affected include the hands, feet, extremities, nails, and mouth. If the oral mucosa and larynx are involved, as in junctional EB, the child may have a hoarse cry. Involvement of other mucosal surfaces of the respiratory, gastrointestinal, and genitourinary tracts can lead to respiratory distress, severe dehydration, anemia, and chronic constipation. Musculoskeletal and eye involvement may result from scar formation.

A special maneuver called the Nikolsky technique is used to aid diagnosis. This procedure involves rubbing or rotating a portion of the child's skin with the examiner's fingers. Bullae that develop after this procedure are then sampled for standard light microscopy, transmission electron microscopy, and immunofluorescence mapping. Skin cultures may be assessed to rule out the presence of herpes simplex. Fetoscopy, a technique in which fetal skin samples are obtained between 18 and 21 weeks' gestation, can be used to elicit a prenatal diagnosis.

Interdisciplinary Interventions

Therapy is supportive and is aimed at optimizing nutrition, growth, and development. To prevent and treat infections, antibacterial baths and soaks, topical antibiotics, and, occasionally, systemic antibiotics may be ordered. Open wounds are treated with nontraumatizing dressings such as hydrogels (e.g., Vigilon), transparent dressings (e.g., OpSite), and petrolatum gauze.

Nursing care minimizes trauma to external skin and internal mucous membrane surfaces. Handle the child very carefully and take measures to avoid rubbing or chafing the skin. A hospital armband may cause enough irritation for blistering to develop. The child should wear loose, soft clothing. Pressure reduction devices such as overlays and special mattresses can be used to reduce skin friction. Wash the skin by soaking rather than by rubbing it with a washcloth.

To provide adequate nutrition, the health care team must counter both poor intake and losses caused by leaking of protein and body fluids from the blistering lesions. Breastfeeding is encouraged. If bottle-fed, the infant should have only cool formula with a soft nipple that does not irritate the oral mucosa. If severe nutritional problems exist, gastrostomy tubes can be used to administer feedings. Nasogastric intubation should be avoided to prevent possible irritation of the mucous membranes.

ACNE VULGARIS

Acne vulgaris is a chronic, inflammatory process of the pilosebaceous follicles. It is a skin condition affecting as many as 80% of all adolescents (Ramanathan & Hebert, 2011). Although girls often develop acne at a younger age than boys, severe disease affects boys 10 times more frequently (Ramanathan & Hebert, 2011). Ethnic variations also exist. Acne is more prevalent in white Americans than in either African or Asian Americans.

Acne may develop in children on corticosteroid therapy, anticonvulsant drugs, or antituberculosis drugs. External agents such as suntan oils, heavy makeup bases, or grooming agents can also cause acnelike eruptions. Acne seen in infants is rare and requires no treatment. Other factors that precipitate appearance of the lesions include stress, lack of sleep, and premenstrual hormone activity. Acne tends to be improved in the summer months. In general, food seems to play no specific roles (Ramanathan & Hebert, 2011). Genetic factors also seem to play an important role in the pathogenesis of acne.

Pathophysiology

Acne usually begins 1 to 2 years before the onset of puberty as a result of androgenic stimulation of the sebaceous glands. Increasing androgen levels trigger a hypertrophy of the sebaceous glands, resulting in increased sebum production. In addition, aberrant follicular keratinization of the pilosebaceous unit and excessive growth of microbial flora occur (Cotellessa et al., 2004). Inflammation is also added to this process. Overgrowth of certain bacteria on the skin, such as *Propionibacterium acnes* or *Staphylococcus epidermidis*, is thought to produce peptides or enzymes that exacerbate the inflammatory process.

When the normal flow of sebum of the skin is obstructed by the keratinization process, two types of comedones are formed. The open comedone (blackhead) is a firm, noninflammatory lesion filled with keratin and lipid, which block the mouth of the follicle. It has a blackened tip that is the result of oxidized melanin. Blackheads are easily managed except when traumatized or manipulated by the child. Inflammation rarely occurs with blackheads because the contents of the comedone easily escape to the skin surface.

The closed comedone (whitehead) is a semisoft, noninflammatory lesion caused by blockage at the neck of the follicle. It has a microscopic opening that does not allow easy escape of keratin and lipid. Therefore, as these substances build up, they rupture the follicular wall and expel sebum into surrounding dermis tissue. This event begins the inflammatory process that results in the presence of inflammatory papules, pustules, or nodules depending on the location and the extent of the inflammatory reaction.

Prognosis is individual in that no two children with acne react to treatment identically. Treatment takes time and good self-care. The ultimate goal for all children is the avoidance of the associated scarring.

Assessment

Acne lesions include comedones (blackheads, whiteheads), papules, pustules, nodules, cysts, and scars (Fig. 25-9). Lesions usually occur on the face, back, chest, and shoulders. As the condition resolves, the lesion site may appear red and hyperpigmented. Scar formation can occur. Atrophic scars appear as shallow, broad-based depressions or deep, steep-sided pits with irregular outlines (ice-pick scars). Hypertrophic or **keloid** scars most often appear on the back or chest as elevated, thick fibrotic plaques. Black adolescents have a greater propensity for this type of scarring. Facial lesions may extend into the scalp, with scarring alopecia (loss of hair) occurring as a result.

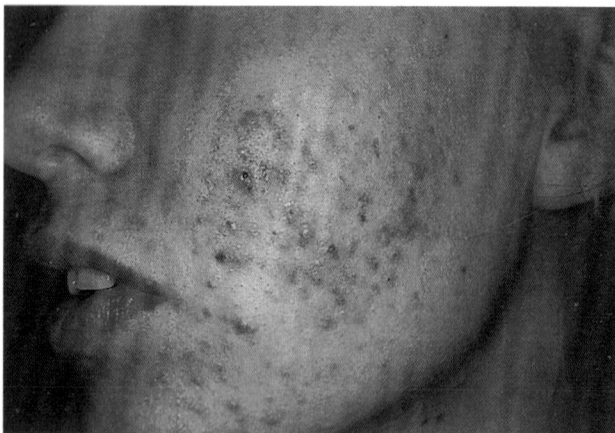

Figure 25-9 An adolescent with acne vulgaris.

Nursing assessment includes an evaluation of the factors that may exacerbate the onset of acne. Chart 25-2 provides a suggested grading of acne. Routine microbiologic testing is not necessary in the evaluation or management of acne (Ramanathan & Hebert, 2011; Strauss et al., 2007).

caREminder

Very young children with acne and other signs of pubertal maturity should be evaluated for precocious puberty.

Question the adolescent regarding his or her use of medications, makeup, and grooming products. In addition, information regarding contact with oils, greases, and waxes should be noted. Affected adolescents may work at gas stations, garages, or restaurants that serve greasy foods.

Adolescents may seek help for acne only after trying many home remedies. Question the adolescent about previous treatments, hygiene habits, stress, and diet.

CHART 25-2	Grading Scale for Acne Severity

Score	Definition
0	None, skin is clear
1	Few comedones
2	Mild comedones, few papules, minimal erythema
3	Comedones, papules, pustules, erythema
4	Moderate comedones; greater number of papules; pustules extending over wider area of face, chest, shoulders, back; increasing erythema
5	Comedones; increasing number of papules, pustules, nodules with erythema
6	Comedones, papules, pustules, nodules, cysts; scarring may or may not be present with hyperpigmentation

Interdisciplinary Interventions

The child or adolescent with acne may have serious concerns about his or her appearance, which are the usual triggering events for the first health care visit. Although the condition is not life threatening, the effect of acne on the adolescent can be great. Taunting by peers can be cruel in severe cases, and sometimes, professional psychological help is necessary. Early intervention does not prevent acne, but it does help control scarring.

Pharmacologic Interventions

Treatment usually revolves around medications, both topical and systemic, which are often combined because no single agent has proved effective against acne. Topical therapy, the preferred method of treatment, has a more rapid effect and few systemic side effects, although it can cause local irritation of the skin (Ramanathan & Hebert, 2011; Strauss et al., 2007). Instruct the adolescent to clean the skin with a mild soap before applying the topical agent. Abrasive soaps and astringents should not be used because these products only serve to cause drying and peeling of the skin and fail to prevent the lesions from appearing. These over-the-counter products may also interfere with the proper use of known, effective topical agents.

Topical therapy essentially consists of two categories: retinoids and antimicrobials (BPO and antibiotics—topical erythromycin) (see thePoint Medications and Administration: Use of Acne Medications) (Ramanathan & Hebert, 2011; Strauss et al., 2007; Zaenglein & Thiboutot, 2006). BPO and combinations of erythromycin or clindamycin have been found to be effective treatments for acne. *Retinoids* are the most potent agents available and have also been shown to reduce sebum production. Topical retinoids have now become a first-line treatment either alone or in combination with an antimicrobial agent (topical or oral). *Salicylic acid, an over-the-counter therapy, is moderately effective but* is deemed less effective than topical retinoids and is also less irritating. This anti-inflammatory agent is used in patients unable to tolerate retinoids and in the treatment of comedones found on the trunk. *Azelaic acid* is another keratolytic and anti-inflammatory agent used with patients having mild to moderate acne or in patients unable to tolerate retinoids (Ramanathan & Hebert, 2011). The principal effects of *topical antimicrobials* such as erythromycin or clindamycin are to reduce the follicular microbial colonization and decrease the inflammatory response. Monotherapy should not be used routinely because *P. acnes* may become resistant. Antibiotic resistant *Staphylococcus epidermidis* and *S. aureus* could also develop in monotherapy. When an antibiotic is combined with BPO, resistance may be avoided (Ramanathan & Hebert, 2011).

ALERT   *The use of topical antibiotics alone can be associated with the development of bacterial resistance (Ramanathan & Hebert, 2011; Strauss et al., 2007).*

Oral antibiotics are the most common systemic therapy prescribed and should be used in combination therapy with topical retinoid or BPO. Doxycycline and minocycline are considered more effective than tetracycline (Strauss et al., 2007). However, minocycline has an uncommon but significant adverse effect profile. The medications must be used for a minimum of 3 to 4 weeks to produce significant results. The systemic agents may produce side effects (see thePoint Medications and Administration: Use of Acne Medications). The patient should be instructed to stop taking the antibiotic and call the health care provider immediately if side effects occur.

Use of *oral contraceptives* may help to treat acne in some girls. Increased oil production can be caused by the body's androgen (male hormone) levels, which can be highest just before menstruation starts. Contraceptives work by decreasing endogenous androgen production.

Maintenance therapy in the form of topical retinoid may be continued to decrease microcomedone formation. Antibiotics (topical and oral) are discontinued after lesions are under control. If needed, antibiotics are used in combination with BPO and a topical retinoid (Ramanathan & Hebert, 2011).

Nutritional Interventions

Dietary restrictions, although no longer considered crucial to the progress and prognosis of acne care, convey the necessity of a well-balanced diet. Specific food restrictions have not been shown to be beneficial in the treatment of acne (Strauss et al., 2007).

Supportive Interventions

The dermatologist may perform comedone extraction or incision and drainage of cystic lesions. Therapy is targeted at controlling the inflammatory process by altering bacterial flora around the sebaceous glands with antibiotics and topically reducing the obstruction of sebaceous skin glands.

Advise the adolescent not to "pop" pimples because doing so can cause further inflammation at the site and scarring at sites of larger lesions. If teenagers are compelled to do it anyway, advise them to never open the pimple before it has come to a head. The hands and face should be washed first, and a sterile needle should be used to nick the surface of the yellow pimple. The pimple should not be squeezed, rather the pus should be allowed to run out and then be washed away with soap and water.

Community Care

Nurses often serve as the initial contact for adolescents who are affected by acne and can be instrumental to a teen by helping to decrease the fears of treatment and by offering hope about positive outcomes. Provide

---

CHART 25-3	Myths About Acne

Myth	Reality
Any acne medication works immediately.	It can take at least 8 weeks of a prescribed treatment regimen for the patient to see any improvement. Acne may even get worse before it gets better
Acne is the result of poor hygiene.	Because of this myth, people tend to overwash their skin, often scrubbing hard with abrasive cleansers. Acne is not caused by dirt or surface oil. Cleaning too often may, in fact, aggravate acne and cause flare-ups. The face should be washed twice per day with a mild soap and lukewarm water, then patted dry, followed by use of appropriate acne treatment.
Washing with abrasive soaps, cleansing granules, astringents, vigorous scrubbing, or a buff puff will clear up acne on the face.	Using fingertips or a soft washcloth is best.
Picking acne will make it go away.	This practice may cause scarring. Acne lesions should never be picked.
Once acne has cleared up, it will be gone forever.	There is no cure for acne. If acne medications are discontinued, acne will most likely flare up.
Stress causes acne.	Stress alone does not cause acne but may exacerbate psychological reaction to the acne. Acne is caused by overactive oil glands stimulated by androgens mixing with dead cells, which is one reason that this condition is seen during the teenage years, when androgen production is at its highest.
Eating chocolate, sugar, or greasy foods or drinking lots of soda will cause acne.	No evidence supports this belief. Certain foods may make some teenagers' acne worse, but no specific food has been proved to actually worsen acne. Also, although a balanced diet is important, no particular diet has been shown to be beneficial.
Teenagers are the only ones affected by acne.	Acne, although it predominates during the teenage years, can also affect adults, especially postmenstrual females. Neonates (acne neonatorum) and infants (infantile acne) can also experience acne.

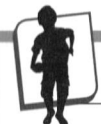

CLINICAL JUDGMENT 25-1

The Adolescent With Acne

Maggie is a 14-year-old who was admitted to the hospital with status asthmaticus. She is being discharged today. As you enter her room, you find her standing near a mirror, squeezing the pimples on her face. When she sees you, she says, "I just hate all of these zits. My face looks like frog skin. It is *so* embarrassing. My friend Kim has this neat medicine called 'Acu-something,' and when I am at home, I use some of that to clear up my face."

Questions

1. What questions should you ask Maggie regarding the comments she has just made?
2. What data in this scenario illustrate some poor health practices by Maggie?
3. What would be an appropriate nursing diagnosis based on the data you have collected?
4. What should be your plan of action regarding Maggie's concern about her acne?
5. As you discuss medication therapy with Maggie, what outcomes could you tell her can happen if she continues to squeeze her pimples and take her friend's medication?

Answers

1. Tell me more about this medicine you have been using (how often, how much, how long have you been using this). Have you been having any dry skin and lips; nosebleeds, muscle pain or stiffness, eye irritation; feel that your skin burns easily? Who knows that you are using this medicine?
2. Squeezing her pimples and taking someone else's medication. Further data would be needed to determine whether current hospital admission was related to poor home management of asthmatic condition.
3. Body image disturbance related to presence of skin lesions; deficient knowledge: skin care and management of acne; risk for injury related to use of friend's medication
4. Discuss the importance of not squeezing the acne lesions. Discuss some of the treatment options for acne. Discuss the extreme hazards of taking someone else's medication and the hazards associated with use of Accutane. Tell Maggie you would like to share her concerns with her parents and the doctor so that arrangements might be made for her to see a dermatologist. Tell Maggie's primary health care provider about her use of Accutane. Unmonitored use of this medication places her at risk for injury, especially in light of her asthmatic condition.
5. She may have further inflammation of the facial lesions. Scarring is more likely to occur if she continues to manipulate the lesions. Accutane is a prescription medication, and the person given the medication must be carefully monitored by a physician or nurse practitioner when it is being used. It has several hazardous side effects that could be harmful to Maggie's general health.

counseling related to the many myths (Chart 25-3) about appropriate treatment. Convey to the child that there is no true cure for acne; if untreated, however, it could last for many years, with numerous secondary complications. Teach about general lifestyle, hygiene, appropriate medication use, and realistic expectations of therapy (Clinical Judgment 25-1). The degree of patient adherence to the intervention plan will determine the effectiveness of therapy as well as long-term outcomes. Reinforce with teenagers that despite the severity of their acne, it is a temporary condition, and with present-day therapies, it can usually be very well controlled.

PARASITIC INFESTATIONS

Skin infestations in children are a common and growing concern to families, daycare providers, school officials, and health care providers. In the United States, the most common infestations affecting children are pediculosis (lice) and scabies (mites). Often misdiagnosed because of their appearance on healthy, "clean" children, these pesky insects are highly contagious and can be a source of embarrassment to the infected child and family. Eradication is possible when families closely follow prescribed instructions for treating the lice and mites, clean the home environment, and monitor those who have been in close contact with the infected child.

PEDICULOSIS

Pediculosis (lice) infestations have been identified for thousands of years. At one point, lice infestation was thought to be a sign of poor hygiene, with the only known cure being a complete head shave.

Lice have been known to transmit certain diseases, including typhus, trench fever, and relapsing fever. Fortunately, none of these diseases has been transmitted by lice in the United States for decades. Improved hygiene, better ability to wash and change clothes, immunizations, and the development of pediculicides and antibiotics have all played roles in decreasing the threat of disease transference. Lice infestation, however, remains a major community health problem throughout the world.

Humans can be infested by two subspecies of lice, each with its own unique set of characteristics and occupying a specific segment of the body: the head and body louse (*Pediculus humanus: capitis* or *corporis*), and the pubic or crab louse (*Phthirus pubis*). Head lice are the most common type seen in children, although adolescent sexual activity contributes to the incidence of pubic lice in this age population.

A familiar malady in schools and child care centers, head lice infestation occurs in all regions of the United States. Estimates range from 10 to 12 million cases per year (Centers for Disease Control and Prevention [CDC], 2010a; Gray, 2004). Although all socioeconomic groups are affected, lice are most common in school-aged white females, with the peak season occurring from August to November. Head lice are less common in blacks because lice do not attach easily to tight, curly hair. Head lice can infest both adults and children, but the incidence is greatest in children between ages 5 and 12 years.

Transmission of head lice occurs by direct contact with an infested person or indirect contact with personal articles. Carpeting, pillows, bed linens, hats, brushes, and ribbons from infested children are all possible sources of transmission.

Pubic lice have a more rounded body and prominent pincers than head lice. These lice generally infest the pubic region and sometimes the eyebrows, facial hair, and axillary hair. Pubic lice are most commonly transmitted through intimate bodily contact, although they may also be transferred by **fomites** (contaminated objects such as combs, brushes, and clothing). Infestation occurs most commonly in adolescents or adults; infestation in a younger child should raise the suspicion of sexual activity or abuse.

The least common form of pediculosis in the United States is body lice. These lice attach to infested clothing and bedding, living in the seams of these materials. The lice attach to the skin only long enough to feed.

Pathophysiology

Lice are parasitic insects that infest humans and can have an effect on the host. Their bites are relatively painless and may be felt as a slight tickling sensation. The signs and symptoms of pediculosis infestation are caused by the reactions of the host to the saliva or anticoagulants injected by the lice into the dermis. Intense itching may occur on the affected body part or in the scalp. Generally, the severity of symptoms is proportional to the degree of infestation. The adult louse lives only about 48 hours if not in contact with a human host, and the life span of the female is roughly 1 month. Eggs are laid at night, at the junction of a hair shaft and close to the skin; these nits will hatch within 7 to 10 days.

With treatment, these parasites can be eradicated successfully. Most often, resurgence of lice occurs because families fail to meticulously follow the treatment plan and eradicate the nits in all of the environments in which the child has contact with other carriers or fomites. In addition, no pediculicide is 100% effective or ovicidal, and improper application of the pediculicide and poor nit removal combing techniques can influence the reinfestation rate (CDC, 2010a).

Assessment

Families often confuse pediculosis with scabies (mites). Both infestations are caused by organisms that primarily choose the scalp as their feeding ground. Lice and scabies may occur in some of the same areas such as the axillary, cubital, popliteal, and inguinal areas. Both lice and mites cause pruritus, although mite infestation is characterized by nocturnal itching as opposed to the continuous pruritus associated with lice. Examination of the affected area and microscopic examination of the lice or nits are the classic discerning methods of analysis. Nits fluoresce white under Wood light. Mites are not visible using this technique; rather, scrapings from infected skin must be examined under a microscope to discern their presence.

ca**RE**minder

The hallmark of pediculosis is intense itching at all times of the day or night. Any body area, including the scalp, may show signs of the child's intense scratching, such as erythema, scaling, and excoriation of the skin.

Head lice infestation is commonly first suspected when children are observed scratching their heads vigorously. Listlessness or poor school performance may also be clues, indicating the child's high level of distraction. On inspection, the examiner observes whitish to sandy colored eggs (nits) on the hair shafts. Adult lice may be visualized under a microscope or a magnifying glass. They range in color from light beige to black and have six clawlike appendages.

Brown or cream-colored pubic lice nits attach themselves firmly to hair shafts, making removal difficult. As discussed earlier, pubic lice are often seen in the presence of other sexually transmitted infections, and affected children must be examined for signs of other such diseases, particularly gonorrhea and syphilis.

Interdisciplinary Interventions

Nurses play a crucial role in assessing children for lice and in obtaining a detailed health history. Families need to be taught the signs of lice infestation. An infested child typically scratches the infested area, most commonly the scalp, ears, and neck. Caregivers should examine the child's head in natural light near a window. The most readily identifiable sign is the presence of nits. Nits can easily be mistaken for dandruff, but the critical difference is that nits must be picked off to be removed.

When lice are detected, coordinate care to ensure that treatment of the child and affected family members begins immediately. Treatment for lice involves applying a pediculicidal agent, removing nits, and thoroughly cleaning (delousing) the environment (Teaching Intervention Plan 25-3). All three steps are crucial to

TIP 25-3: A TEACHING INTERVENTION PLAN for the Child With Pediculosis or Scabies

Nursing Diagnoses and Family Outcomes

- Impaired skin integrity related to infestation
  Outcomes: Child verbalizes a decrease in itching. Child maintains minimal integrity.
- Health-seeking behaviors regarding prevention of further infestations
  Outcomes: Family completes home treatment regimen to rid the child of the lice or mites and to treat itching.
  Family cleans the house to rid the home of all lice and mites.
  Family notifies others in close contact with the child of the contagious nature of the infestation.
- Risk for infection related to itching and potential breakdown of the skin
  Outcomes: Child will remain free from infection.
  Family notifies health care provider promptly if lesions appear infected or if a fever develops.

Teach Child/Family

Managing the Child's Condition

Pediculosis (Lice)
- Antilice shampoo
  - Strictly follow manufacturer's directions for application.
  - Pour about 2 oz of the antilice shampoo onto the hair, adding warm water to lather. Scrub the hair and scalp for 10 minutes. Rinse the hair thoroughly and dry.
  - Repeat application in 7–10 days if live lice are present.
- Removal of nits
  - Divide the child's towel-dried hair (not sopping wet) into four parts and insert the comb at the top of the head first. If nits fall into the lower hair, they will be removed with combing of the inferior areas. Use a fine-toothed comb. This is a time-consuming procedure that may be uncomfortable for the child.
  - Special attention should be given to the area around the ears and the nape of the neck, which are heavy infestation areas.

Scabies
- Have the child bathe or shower.
- Apply scabies cream or lotion.
  - Apply the cream or lotion to every inch of the child's body from the head down. Pay special

attention to the navel, between the toes, and body folds or creases. Leave some under the fingernails. Eight to 14 hours later, give the child a bath and remove the cream or lotion.
- Unless new lesions develop within 10 days, retreatment is unnecessary.

Cleaning the House
- Hot water wash all of the child's sheets, blankets, pillowcases, pajamas, underwear, and recently worn clothes. Dry in hot dryer for at least 20 minutes.
- Items that cannot be washed should be set aside in plastic bags for 3 days (for mites) or 23 weeks (for lice/nits) before being used again.
- Vacuum all floors, rugs, play and sleep areas, and furniture of home, school, and daycare facilities.
- *For lice,* combs and brushes should be soaked for 1 hour in a solution made from antilice shampoo or 1½ tablespoon Lysol and 1 qt water, followed by a hot-water rinse.
- It is not necessary to have the house sprayed or fumigated because this can be toxic to humans and pets.

Contagiousness
- *For pediculosis,* check the heads of everyone else in the home and treat any scalp rashes, sores, or itching with the antilice shampoo.
- Sexual partners should be notified of the diagnosis.
- *For scabies,* everyone living in the house should be treated preventively with one application of the scabies medicine. Close contacts of the infected child (friends, babysitter, daycare provider) should also be treated.
- Encourage children not to share hats, coats, combs, and similar personal items.
- The child's school or daycare facility should be notified of the diagnosis, and close contacts should be examined and treated prophylactically.
- Promote good general personal hygiene measures.

Contact Health Care Provider if
- Itching interferes with sleep; teach families that the rash or the itch may continue for 2–3 weeks after treatment
- Rash is not cleared within 1 week after treatment
- Rash clears, then returns
- Rash or sores begin to look reddened, warm to the touch, or oozing secretions
- Fever develops
- New nits or burrows appear

preventing recurrence. All potentially exposed persons should be examined and treated if infested.

Pediculicidal agents include permethrin (preferred agent) and pyrethrins; common brand names include Nix, Rid, and Pronto. Lindane use is not recommended by the American Academy of Pediatrics (CDC, 2010a,

2010b). None of the currently available pediculicides is 100% ovicidal, and resistance among lice to these more common and popular products has been increasing. Malathion (Ovide) has been shown to kill both nonresistant and resistant lice and is available by prescription (Bowden, 2012).

ALERT *Malathion has a foul odor, is flammable, and may cause respiratory depression if ingested. The agent should not be used on neonates and infants, and its safety in nursing mothers and children younger than 6 years of age is uncertain. Malathion should be considered for use only when other agents have failed.*

Toxic side effects, most often seen with lindane, may include nausea, vomiting, aplastic anemia, hypoplastic bone marrow, convulsions, and death. These serious side effects usually occur after repeated applications. When teaching families about pediculicide treatment, emphasize that more is not better. Directions for application must be strictly followed. Overuse and misuse may lead to absorption into the bloodstream and the possibility of adverse effects. The child's eyes must be carefully protected, and the caregiver should wear rubber gloves. Pediculicides cannot be used on eyebrows or eyelashes because they are irritating. Rather, lice infestation in these areas is treated by applying petrolatum to the lashes and brows three to four times a day for 2 weeks. The petrolatum seems to suffocate the insects. The nits can then be removed with a fine-toothed comb or tweezers.

Systemic agents have shown effectiveness in killing nymphs and lice, but not eggs. An oral dose of ivermectin (Stromectol) has been used to kill newly hatched nymphs. A second dose is administered 7 to 10 days after the first dose. No serious adverse reactions have been reported; however, the medication is not approved for use in children weighing less than 15 kg (33 lb). Infestation in infants should never be treated with pediculicidal products. Rather, the lice and nits should be manually removed or hand-combed. Pregnant women and persons allergic to pediculicidal agents should never use these agents. Families should be warned to avoid treating lice infestation with home remedies. Dog shampoo, vinegar, and kerosene have not been clinically proved to be effective against lice.

Community Care

Instruct families to follow the prescribed intervention plan carefully (see Teaching Intervention Plan 25-3). They also must be taught how to remove nits properly. The environment must be thoroughly cleaned. Pets are not a host for lice. Transmission occurs from direct contact (body to body, hair to hair) or indirect contact (clothing, brushes, hair apparel). Lice cannot live more than 72 hours off the human body. Therefore, the house should be vacuumed thoroughly, combs and brushes should be soaked in antilice shampoo, and all clothing and sheets should be washed in hot water.

School nurses play an important role in preventing and managing head lice epidemics. A social worker or visiting nurse may need to be called to investigate home conditions if lice infestation becomes recurrent or chronic. The school nurse educates teachers, officials, and the family to

- Have carpeted areas frequently vacuumed
- Discourage body contact and sharing of personal items between children

- Know how to examine for and identify lice
- Notify the nurse if a case is found
- Store naptime supplies in a clean area and send them home for frequent cleaning
- Have student clothes/storage areas (lockers) separated adequately by space and not be shared

Assist schools and daycare facilities to notify the family about prevention, detection, and treatment policies. The National Association of School Nurses' position statement on pediculosis management is that management should not disrupt the educational process. Children with live head lice should remain in class and be discouraged from close contact with other children (Pontius & Teskey, 2011). Screening programs for lice have not been shown to be cost-effective nor have they reduced the incidence of lice. Education programs may be helpful in reducing community head lice infestations. The National Pediculosis Association has free guidelines available for controlling head lice in child care environments and schools (see thePoint for Organizations).

SCABIES

A contagious skin condition caused by the human skin mite *Sarcoptes scabiei*, scabies affects children regardless of gender, age, or socioeconomic strata. Scabies occurs worldwide and increasingly in North America, with outbreaks occurring in association with crowded conditions, poor hygiene, and malnutrition. It is transmitted by close personal contact or shared clothing or linen. The scabies mite cannot survive for more than 3 days away from human skin. Therefore, it is not carried by fomites (combs, brushes, toys) as often as pediculosis, although some cases have been documented.

Pathophysiology

S. scabiei present on an infested person is attracted to the warmth and odor of an uninfested host. Once transmitted to the new host, the mite secretes a fluid that allows it to burrow into the stratum corneum, rarely penetrating through the epidermis. The mite sucks human tissue fluids for nourishment. The female mite lays one to three eggs per day for 15 to 30 days. The larvae mature and hatch in 10 days, emerging on the surface of the skin as eight-legged mites. After mating, the males die and the females begin to burrow under the skin to continue the reproduction cycle. The host's body begins to respond to the secretions of the mite or its feces, which are highly antigenic. This sensitivity response (itching, scratching) usually begins within 3 weeks of infestation, and incubation occurs 1 to 2 months after contact.

The prognosis for eradicating scabies is excellent. The currently available agents are strong scabicides with minimal toxic side effects. Treatment failure, which does occur, may be attributable to inadequate education and improperly applied treatment of the child and the environment. Underlying serious immune suppression (as in AIDS) can delay eradication of the mite infestation.

Assessment

The most common presenting symptom of scabies is pruritus, which is especially profound at night and at naptime. Younger children and infants who cannot scratch effectively respond to the constant itching by crankiness, fitful sleeping, rubbing their feet and hands together, and even refusing to eat. Severe cases can cause significant interference with the mood of the child and with the activities of daily living.

The primary lesion of scabies is the burrow, although vesicles, papules, nodules, and wheals also may appear. The linear, grayish burrows are present in 90% to 95% of all patients with scabies and are easy to find. Difficulty detecting the burrows may occur in the presence of excoriation and secondary infections such as impetigo. Infestation sites differ by age group. In infants and young children, the lesions may be generalized, with distribution on the palms, soles, scalp, face, and axillae being most common. The head and neck may also be affected. In older children, lesions are more often localized, being seen in finger webs, the axillae, body creases, the belt line, genitalia, and nipples.

Scabies is diagnosed by skin scrapings (see Tests and Procedures 25-1). Potassium hydroxide is not used because it will dissolve the mites, eggs, and feces; rather, a few drops of mineral oil are applied to a burrow, vesicle, or papule, and a dull edge of a scalpel is used to scrape the lesion. Scrapings are best obtained from interdigital areas or from flexor surfaces of the wrist. The burrow ink test, during which a drop of ink or rubbing a washable felt-tipped pen across the suspected burrow, may be done. It may be possible to detect a mite moving in the oil; the ova or feces of the mites may also be visible. Sometimes, finding either ova or feces is not possible, leaving the clinician the responsibility of treating the infestation based on the clinical history alone.

Interdisciplinary Interventions

As with pediculosis, treatment of scabies involves not only the affected infant or child but also the family and caregivers. Scabicidal agents available include permethrin (Elimite), ivermectin (Stromectol), lindane, and crotamiton (Eurax). Permethrin 5% cream is the drug of choice because of its high efficacy and low toxicity (Burns et al., 2013; CDC, 2010a, 2010b). It may be used in children as young as 2 months of age. It is applied once for 8 to 14 hours and removed, then reapplied 1 week later. Lindane lotion 1%, although U.S. Food and Drug Administration (FDA)–approved for treatment of scabies, is not now recommended as first-line treatment. Crotamiton is not FDA-approved for use in children. Ivermectin, an oral antiparasitic agent, is FDA-approved for treatment of worm infestations, not scabies. Oral ivermectin is reported effective in treating crusted scabies when topical lotions have failed or treatment is not tolerated. A total of two or more doses, 7 days apart, have been used. Safety in children weighing less than 15 kg has not been established (CDC, 2010a, 2010b).

Topical steroids and antihistamines, such as diphenhydramine (Benadryl), may be administered to help reduce pruritus in older children.

Community Care

Educate the family to apply the scabicidal agent, strictly following the manufacturer's directions. Most deleterious side effects result from overzealous application of these agents. Teach family caregivers to apply the agent to the whole body in infants and children (including the scalp and face), with special attention given to the ears, gluteal clefts, and toe and finger webs. Before application, the child should be given a tepid bath and be dried with a towel. Then, the agent should be applied evenly but thinly over the body. In older children, the scabicidal agent is applied from the neck down. The caregiver should wear rubber gloves during application.

Not all lesions clear immediately. Pruritus may persist after treatment, and postscabietic nodules may persist for months, even after the mites are eradicated. The child should not be bathed too aggressively because the subsequent skin dryness can result in excoriation of the skin. The child with excoriated skin is at risk for secondary infection caused by impetigo.

Teach families that, because a latent period of 1 month occurs after infestation, there may be other asymptomatic carriers present in the home or child's school. Instructing the family in good personal hygiene practices, cleaning the environment, and regular bath time checks can help prevent reinfestation (see Teaching Intervention Plan 25-3).

BACTERIAL SKIN DISORDERS

Infections of the skin are so common that few individuals escape without having had at least one bacterial skin infection during the childhood years. Most of these skin problems are easily handled and are benign in course. However, some can evolve into major illnesses if not promptly diagnosed and treated. Cutaneous bacterial infections are among the most frequent inflammatory skin disorders.

STAPHYLOCOCCAL SCALDED SKIN SYNDROME

Staphylococcal scalded skin syndrome (SSSS) is a disorder that is seen in infants and children but is rare in adults. In SSSS, infection by a particular strain of *S. aureus* causes blistering of the upper layer of skin. Severity can vary from localized blisters to generalized exfoliation affecting the entire body.

Pathophysiology

S. aureus, the causative agent of SSSS, produces an exfoliative toxin. The mechanism by which the bacteria cause this exfoliation remains elusive, although clinical studies are ongoing.

SSSS tends to occur only once and, if treated with antibiotics, usually resolves within a few days. Childhood mortality is approximately 4%. Mortality is associated with extensive skin involvement, overwhelming sepsis, and subsequent fluid and electrolyte imbalances.

Assessment

The child usually presents with a prodrome of sore throat or conjunctivitis. A culture of the eye drainage is frequently positive for *S. aureus*. Within 48 hours, the child develops fever, malaise, and extremely tender erythematous patches on the face, neck, axilla, and perineum. Flaccid bullae develop within the erythematous areas. Bullae enlarge and rupture to reveal a moist erythematous base; this process gives rise to the classic scalded appearance (Berk & Bayliss, 2010).

Surrounding skin appears normal, and no systemic symptoms are noted. Mucous membranes are not affected. A positive Nikolsky sign is typically elicited by gently rubbing uninvolved or healed skin to produce dislodgment of the superficial epidermis.

Lesion and drainage cultures are essential in identifying the causative organism, especially when infection is present. Blood cultures help to identify the source of the epidermic toxins. Skin biopsies may also assist in diagnosis.

Interdisciplinary Interventions

Health care interventions focus on eradicating the causative organism, preventing secondary infection, maintaining systemic support (nutritional, fluid, and electrolyte balances), and ensuring comfort. Prompt initiation of parenteral antistaphylococcal antibiotics (e.g., flucloxacillin, first- or second-generation cephalosporin, and clindamycin) is essential. Fluid and electrolyte loss during the illness is considerable, requiring oral or parenteral replacement. The eroded skin is at risk for secondary infections. Placement in the intensive care unit may occur, and additional antibiotics may be administered, as indicated by the child's condition (Berk & Bayliss, 2010).

Thermal dysregulation can occur as a result of the underlying infection, the severity of the illness, and peripheral vasodilation (Berk & Bayliss, 2010). Room temperature should be monitored and adjusted to compensate for changes in the child's core temperature.

In addition to monitoring fluid and electrolyte status, vital signs, and ongoing skin assessment, the nurse should attend to the child's pain. Adequate analgesic agents are administered to ensure that the child is comfortable. Opioids may be necessary to manage severe pain.

Blisters are left intact. Ongoing skin care includes covering eroded skin areas with petrolatum-soaked gauze, which helps to further reduce trauma to the skin. Pressure-relieving mattresses are used to reduce development of pressure sores. Diligent skin assessment and collaborative management ensures effective healing and reduces infection. The illness is usually brief, with no residual scarring of the skin.

IMPETIGO

A common superficial skin infection that most often occurs on the face, the arms, and the legs, impetigo usually affects children between the ages of 2 and 5 years. Impetigo contagiosa (nonbullous impetigo) and bullous impetigo (staphylococcal impetigo) are the two most common types of impetigo recognized (Table 25-5). Impetigo neonatorum is a form similar to bullous impetigo found specifically in the newborn. Common or secondary impetigo refers to the form that occurs as a complication of a systemic condition or secondary to another dermatologic problem. A child may have the characteristics of more than one type of impetigo at the same time.

Past studies established that the principal etiologic agent responsible for impetigo was group A beta-hemolytic *Streptococcus* (GABHS); if *Staphylococcus aureus* was cultured, it was considered a secondary invader. However, there exists sufficient and compelling evidence to suggest that *Staphylococcus aureus* is the primary agent in nonbullous and crusted impetigo and is almost always the exclusive agent in bullous types (McEvoy, 2000). The cause of impetigo and its characteristic appearance is related to the particular type of impetigo present. Impetigo contagiosa is primarily caused by GABHS and *Staphylococcus aureus* organisms.

Pathophysiology

The causative bacteria are carried in the nasal area and may pass on to the skin. The bacteria invade the superficial skin, most aggressively at areas of broken skin, causing a characteristic vesicular and pustular response and crusting. The infection may be disseminated after scratching an infected site. The infection can also be acquired through contact with other infected children or through contact with fomites such as combs or toys that come into contact with areas of the skin that have been compromised. Impetigo is more easily spread through crowded conditions, poor hygiene, and play situations in which children have skin-to-skin contact (e.g., contact sports). *S. aureus* is more prevalent in warm, humid climes, whereas GABHS is more prevalent in temperate zones. This disorder is also highly communicable among athletes and from contaminated equipment used by athletes (Feaster & Singer, 2010).

The prognosis for uncomplicated impetigo is usually excellent because the lesions are shallow and usually heal without scarring (Fig. 25-10). Transient pigmentation changes can occur in children with dark complexions. Lesions usually remain superficial, but organisms may invade deeper areas, causing cellulitis, lymphangitis, and more serious systemic infections including bacterial endocarditis. Acute poststreptococcal glomerulonephritis is a rare complication of impetigo, and early intervention with antimicrobial therapy does not seem to alter the risk.

Assessment

Children with impetigo do not generally appear ill or feverish. Nonbullous impetigo lesions are rarely painful. Thus, the family may delay seeking medical attention. Secondary symptoms, such as regional lymphadenitis, usually bring the child to the health care provider's attention. During this time, the infection may have been spread to other members of the household or the child's peers (Clinical Judgment 25-2). Refer to Table 25-5 for descriptions of the lesions.

TABLE 25-5   Types of Impetigo

Type and Common Sites	Cause	Characteristics of Lesions	Other Symptoms
Impetigo contagiosa (nonbullous impetigo) Sites: Skin surfaces exposed to environmental trauma Periorbital area Nares Face Extremities	GABHS *Staphylococcus aureus*	Lesions start with a single 2- to 4-mm erythematous macule that rapidly evolves to a vesicle or pustule. Vesicles are fragile and rupture easily, leaving a typical honey-colored, crusted exudate over the superficial erosion. Lesions spread rapidly to adjacent skin. There is often linear distribution, showing how patients scratched themselves.	Mild, localized lymphadenopathy
Bullous impetigo (staphylococcal impetigo) Sites: Buttocks Trunk Perineum Extremities Neck folds	*Staphylococcus aureus*	Flaccid and transparent bullae are usually less than 3 cm in diameter on previously untraumatized skin. When the blisters rupture, they leave a varnishlike superficial erosion with scant crusting.	Weakness Fever Diarrhea
Impetigo neonatorum Sites: Lesions may be few or many, favoring moist surfaces such as the groin, axilla, neck, and umbilicus.	Acquired during delivery, from fomites, or from human contact *Staphylococcus aureus* and *Streptococcus* most common	Lesions can range from bullous impetigo to the scalded skin syndrome. Bullae are tense; rupture easily; and leave red, glazed, oozing areas. Classic honey-colored crusting may be present. Lesions spread peripherally and clear centrally. Scale and satellite lesions are present.	Fever Adenopathy
Common or secondary impetigo Site: Location of primary lesions	Complication of systemic diseases such as diabetes mellitus, AIDS Dermatologic conditions that cause a break in the skin may lead to secondary impetigo (e.g., scabies, pediculosis, herpes simplex, insect bites).	Similar to impetigo contagiosa	Mild lymphadenopathy Symptoms of primary condition

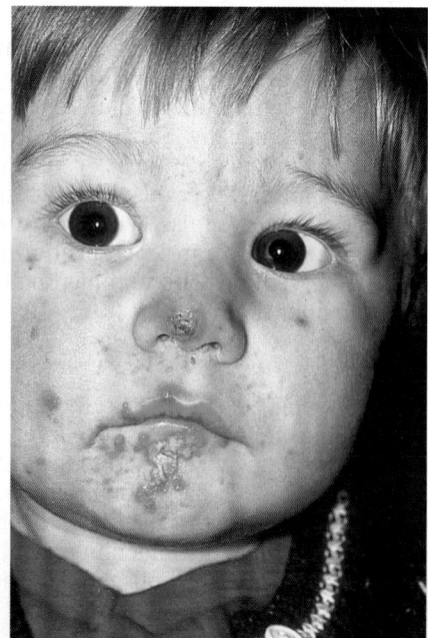

Figure 25-10 A child with impetigo.

Laboratory studies often reveal a slight increase in leukocytes in the bloodstream. Gram stains of scrapings from the lesions show gram-positive cocci in clusters, with neutrophils. Cultures and sensitivities are completed to guide therapy because the number of methicillin- and erythromycin-resistant strains of *S. aureus* is increasing.

! ALERT   *Some children are chronic carriers of S. aureus. Children with recurrent impetigo should be cultured for the organism in nares, perineum, and axillae.*

Interdisciplinary Interventions

Impetigo usually remains clinically stable for weeks, and many lesions heal spontaneously. In other cases, however, prompt therapy is crucial so that the impetigo does not spread to other children. Treating the child with impetigo involves performing daily hygiene to the affected areas, administering antibiotic therapy, and instituting measures to prevent further spread. Topical therapies may be used if the impetigo is superficial, nonbullous, or localized to

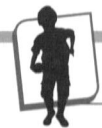

CLINICAL JUDGMENT 25-2

The Child With Impetigo

When Mrs. Sanchez picked up her daughter Ally from preschool, the teacher told her that Ally had a skin rash on her face that looked like impetigo. Mrs. Sanchez was informed that Ally could not come back to preschool until she had been seen by her health care provider, with treatment initiated if needed.

Questions

1. If Ally has impetigo, how would you expect the lesions to look?
2. What other characteristics of the lesions and history of this situation could help you confirm the presence of impetigo?
3. The nurse practitioner agrees with the evaluation of the lesions and tells Mrs. Sanchez that Ally has impetigo. What are the primary goals of care at this time?
4. What interventions should be implemented to treat the lesions?
5. What information should Mrs. Sanchez repeat to you to demonstrate her understanding of how to prevent spread of this skin condition?

Answers

1. Nonbullous lesions are vesicles that rupture, leaving moist, honey-colored, crusty lesions on erythematous, eroded skin. Bullous lesions are pustular blisters that rupture, leaving a varnishlike coating.
2. The most common site is the face, as seen in Ally's situation. Satellite lesions may occur near the primary site and on other body parts, especially the extremities or perineum. Impetigo is most often seen in children younger than 6 years of age. A history of pruritus and an earlier skin disruption at the site also confirm the current physical findings. Determine whether any other children at school have impetigo.
3. Treat the bacterial infection and prevent spread of the disease.
4. Gently clean and remove the crusts on the skin. Use topical antibiotics (mupirocin) three times a day for 5–14 days. If there is no improvement in 3 days, the child should be seen again by a health care provider, and oral antibiotics would be started and administered for a 10-day period.
5. Ally should be discouraged from touching or picking at the lesions. She should wash her hands frequently throughout the day. If she or anyone else touches the lesions, they should wash their hands immediately with antibacterial soap and water. Ally's fingernails should be cut short. Other members of the family should not use Ally's towel or washcloth. Ally can return to school after she has used the topical antibiotics for 48 hours.

one or two lesions. Some of the products available include mupirocin (Bactroban), retapamulin (Altabax), fusidic acid (Fucidin), bacitracin, neomycin, polymyxin B, triple antibiotic (bacitracin, neomycin, and polymyxin B;), and Gentamicin applied three to four times daily. Topical antibiotics are effective if hygiene and general health are good and the lesions are not widespread. Although many physicians treat impetigo only topically, others prefer to use systemic therapy for neonates and young children at risk for widespread disease and in whom no improvement is seen within 3 days of initiating topical therapy. Nursing responsibilities focus on educating the family about the treatment plan and helping the family to recognize the infection in case it recurs (Teaching Intervention Plan 25-4).

CELLULITIS

Cellulitis refers to a fairly common, full-thickness, nonsuppurative skin infection involving dermis and underlying connective tissue, often accompanied by lymphangitis and adenopathy. It affects slightly more males than females and occurs in all age groups. Any part of the body can be affected, but the most prevalent location is the legs.

Pathophysiology

Most cases of cellulitis develop in skin that has been compromised in some way, including debilitating disease, trauma (e.g., puncture wounds), human or animal bites, lymphatic damage, PUs, immune compromise, and tinea infections. In some hospitalized children, complex nosocomial cellulitis develops at IV infusion sites, surgery wound sites, and joint replacement sites. Periorbital cellulitis is often precipitated by infecting organisms from wounds, bites, and sinusitis. In children younger than age 3 years, facial cellulitis is commonly associated with otitis media. *Haemophilus influenzae* facial cellulitis has a violaceous hue that is commonly associated with otitis media.

The most common causative agents of cellulitis are GABHS and *Staphylococcus aureus*, acting alone or in combination. Other implicated microbes include *Escherichia coli*, *Proteus mirabilis*, group B streptococci, and anaerobes. *H. influenzae* and *Streptococcus pneumoniae* also can cause cellulitis, especially in children. The infecting agents, especially the streptococci, create a large amount of enzymatic spreading factors called *hyaluronidase*. These substances break down the fibrin

---

TIP 25-4: A TEACHING INTERVENTION PLAN for the Child With Impetigo

Nursing Diagnoses and Family Outcomes

- Impaired skin integrity related to presence of vesicles, erosions, and exudates
  Outcome: Child's skin shows evidence of healing within 42–78 hours of initiation of therapy.
- Risk for infection related to transfer of skin lesions from child to others during close personal contact with family and peers
  Outcomes: Child remains free from systemic infection.
  Family members and peers do not contract the skin infection.
- Deficient knowledge: Treatment and prevention of impetigo
  Outcomes: Family demonstrates measures to treat the child's skin condition.
  Family members participate in measures to prevent spread of the infection.

Teach Child/Family

Treatment of Lesions

- Apply warm water compresses to areas of lesions to remove crust and exudate several times daily.
- Clean lesions gently with mild soap to prevent secondary infection.
- Apply topical antibiotics or give oral antibiotics as ordered.

- Observe for treatment effectiveness such as decreased erythema and drainage.
- Follow-up appointment should be scheduled in 48–72 hours if there is no improvement and in 10–14 days.

Preventing Spread of Infection in Affected Child and to Others

- Observe skin carefully for signs of new infection (erythema, vesicles, erosions, exudate).
- Wash hands before and after caring for lesions using antimicrobial soap.
- Trim the child's nails and keep them clean.
- Keep the child out of school or daycare activities until after 24 hours of treatment with oral antibiotics or 48 hours with topical ointments.
- Keep infected athletes who compete in close-contact sports from competition until contagious period has passed. Sterilize athletic mats and equipment.
- Keep child's personal care items (towel, washcloth) separate from other family items until the lesions disappear.

Contact Health Care Provider if

- Presence of lesions does not diminish within 48–72 hours of initiating treatment
- Fever develops
- Lesions begin to appear infected
- Other members of the household exhibit the presence of similar lesions

---

network and other subcutaneous barriers that normally localize an infection. In addition, the hyaluronidase can also travel through the lymphatic system. As a result, severe cellulitis can rapidly progress to a life-threatening situation in a child if interventions are not prompt.

When sinusitis is the primary cause, the infection usually spreads from the ethmoid sinuses across the lamina papyracea and into the orbital area, causing periorbital cellulitis. Infection can also spread through the floor of the frontal sinus or the roof of the maxillary antrum. In all cases, the orbital septum is the only barrier protecting the infection from spreading from the eyelids to the orbit.

Prognosis for cellulitis depends on the promptness and efficacy of the interventions as well as on the child's general health status. If not eradicated, persistent cellulitis can lead to necrotizing fasciitis, bacteremia, or osteomyelitis.

Assessment

Characteristic health history and physical examination findings suggest the clinical diagnosis of cellulitis. Other signs include increased white blood cell count, positive blood culture (especially in facial cellulitis), and culturing of an organism from lesion aspirate.

Cellulitis is characterized by reddened or lilac-colored, swollen skin that pits when pressed by the fingertips (Fig. 25-11). The skin texture may resemble an orange peel, and the borders are usually indistinct and not palpable. Superficial blistering of the area is a common finding. The child may also have fever, chills, malaise, tachycardia, hypotension, and headache.

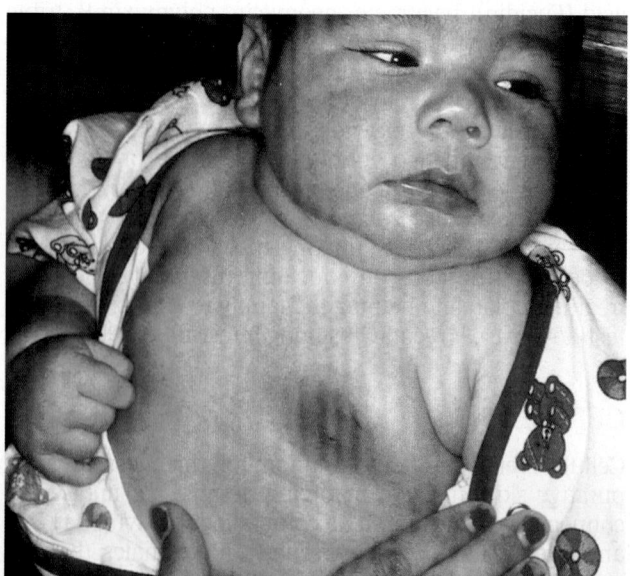

Figure 25-11 Cellulitis.

Regional lymphadenopathy and lymphangitis may occur. The child may appear prostrate and listless and may complain of severe pain over the affected area.

Interdisciplinary Interventions

Hospitalization is required for children with large areas of cellulitis or cellulitis of the face, systemic toxicity, high fever, or hypotension (see thePoint Care Path: An Interdisciplinary Plan of Care for the Child With Periorbital Cellulitis). If the skin ruptures or tears, the physician may order treatment with a nonocclusive dressing with saline-dampened gauze. Moisture-retaining dressings, such as the occlusive films (e.g., Tegaderm Opsite) and hydrocolloids (e.g., Duoderm, Tegasorb) are contraindicated in active cellulitis because they may contribute to the development of secondary infections.

Treating cellulitis typically involves administrating antibiotic therapy. The medication used depends on the infecting organism, the child's condition, and the site of infection. After the infection subsides, the antibiotic is typically changed to an oral anti-infective agent. Keep families informed of the medication regimen to prepare for continuing care of the child in the home after discharge from the acute care facility.

Members of the interdisciplinary team can monitor and facilitate the healing process. If the child is debilitated or unable to take foods orally, consultation with a dietitian may be necessary to plan ways to ensure adequate nutritional intake to support tissue healing. In a severely ill child, parenteral nutrition may be warranted.

During hospitalization, a child life specialist can assist in providing diversionary activities for the child. In addition, the child life specialist can provide play experiences that encourage expression of the child's feelings about hospitalization and pain. Chapter 11 discusses this aspect of the child's care in more detail.

Community Care

Family teaching before discharge should include the expected outcomes, the prescribed treatment regimen, and the coordination of home care and return clinic visits. The child and family members may need to learn aspects of dressing care and sterile technique. Instruct families to schedule outpatient visits so that the health care team can monitor the healing process and to call the health care provider promptly if signs of progressing infection develop, such as increased body temperature or increased swelling or pain near the lesion site.

CAT SCRATCH DISEASE

Transmitted by asymptomatic young cats, CSD is caused by a small gram-negative bacillus, *Bartonella henselae*. The condition is characterized by a benign subacute, chronic course of lymphadenopathy that usually resolves spontaneously in 2 to 3 months. Occasionally, CSD causes severe systemic sequelae; this development is seen more often in immunosuppressed children. CSD affects primarily children and adolescents, with the vast majority of cases in those younger than 20 years of age (Burns et al., 2013; Klotz et al., 2011).

Pathophysiology

In 87% to 99% of cases, a cat (usually a kitten) is involved, although other sources include dog scratches, monkey contact, and wood splinters (Klotz et al., 2011). The organism is believed to be spread from kitten to kitten. As the kittens age, they retain antibodies for *B. henselae* and the bacteremia subsides, which is why adult cats are less likely to be the culprits in transmission of this disease. The inoculation site may be a scratch, puncture, or abrasion and is usually nonpruritic and nonscarring.

Assessment

Symptoms of CSD manifest in a classic sequence. Usually 3 to 10 days after cat contact, maculopapular lesions appear on the skin in the inoculation area and progress to vesicles and pustules. The lymph nodes draining the site of the cat scratch become swollen 14 to 50 days after the contact. The nodes are tender, warm, reddened, and indurated, and they remain enlarged for up to a year.

Mild systemic signs and symptoms include malaise, anorexia, headache, body aches, sore throat, conjunctivitis, nausea, vomiting, abdominal pain, rashes, and arthralgia. Fever occurs in only about 25% of affected children, usually indicating systemic disease. More severe symptoms, such as central nervous system involvement, rarely occur. These symptoms can be severe and include seizures, myelitis, blindness, radiculitis, encephalitis, encephalopathy, paraplegia, cerebral arteritis, and coma.

Diagnosis is based on a history of contact with a young kitten, the presence of lymphadenopathy, positive skin test for *B. henselae*, and identified *B. henselae* organisms cultured from lymph nodes. The *B. henselae* immunofluorescent assay test is highly sensitive and specific for the detection of infection caused by this bacterium. A complete blood count may show leukocytosis and increased eosinophils; the erythrocyte sedimentation rate may be elevated early during the disease. Lymph node biopsy may also be performed.

Interdisciplinary Interventions

In most children, CSD resolves spontaneously in 2 to 4 months. Nursing care is supportive and children are rarely hospitalized. If desired, antimicrobial therapy may be ordered. Oral azithromycin (Zithromax) for 5 days is found to be effective in mild to moderate infections. Bed rest and analgesics may also be ordered if fever is present. Treatment of local lesions includes warm, moist soaks.

VIRAL SKIN DISORDERS

Any skin eruption associated with an acute viral syndrome is called a *viral exanthem*. If the mucosa is involved, it is called a *viral enanthem*, which tend to be nondescript, diffuse, and symmetric maculopapular rashes, often indistinguishable from a medication reaction. Viral exanthems include measles, rubella, enteroviral and adenoviral exanthems, roseola, the mononucleosis syndromes, herpes simplex, and herpes zoster. These conditions are discussed in Chapter 24. The discussion in this chapter is limited to warts, which are caused by the human papillomavirus (HPV); and hand, foot, and mouth disease, which is caused primarily by the coxsackievirus.

WARTS

Warts are common, harmless skin growths (small epidermal tumors of the skin) caused by a virus. They do not have "roots" or seeds as many believe; the dark specks sometimes seen in warts are actually the ends of capillaries. Verrucae, or warts, are one of the most common skin problems seen in children and are usually self-limiting (Dasher et al., 2009). The warts affecting children include the common wart (verruca vulgaris), flat warts (verruca plana), plantar warts, and, in adolescents, genital warts.

Pathophysiology

More than 200 types of HPV exist that can produce a broad spectrum of conditions ranging from asymptomatic warts to squamous cell carcinoma of the skin (Dasher et al., 2009). The clinical manifestations of HPV depend on the type of HPV and the immunologic status of the host.

HPV is transmitted through direct contact. Incubation periods range from 1 to 12 months, with an average of 2 to 3 months (Dasher et al., 2009). The virus invades the skin or the mucous membranes, and then skin changes occur. Children who are immunocompromised are at greater risk for development of the disease because HPV is known to be a latent asymptomatic infection. That is, once infected, the virus may remain latent in the basal layers of the epidermis, demonstrating manifestations when the child has a weakened immune system.

Most warts resolve spontaneously within several months to years. Some may require extensive treatment to remove if they are considered unsightly or occur in an area in which they are irritated by friction against clothing. The therapy should eradicate the problem without causing scarring.

Assessment

Slightly raised above the skin surface, *common warts* are growths that can be very small, or they can be large and clustering. Warts usually occur on the hands, but they can also be seen on the face, knees, and elbows. They are usually elevated, flesh-colored single papules with scaly, irregular surfaces. This type is usually asymptomatic and multiple in number. *Plantar warts* occur on the soles of the feet. They are often surrounded by a collar of hardened skin, and they can cause pain with walking. Warts that are not raised or rough are called *flat warts* and are often seen on the face, neck, and extremities.

Genital "moist" warts (*condylomata acuminata*) are single or multiple soft masses that usually appear around the anus, the vagina, or the penis. Occasionally, they can obstruct the urethral meatus or vaginal introitus. The incubation period for genital warts ranges between 6 weeks and 6 months, although much longer periods are possible. The virus is transmitted predominantly through sexual contact. These warts are usually asymptomatic, but they can itch, burn, or cause local pain. When untreated, venereal warts resemble cauliflowerlike masses.

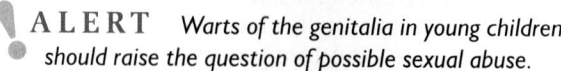

❱ **ALERT**   *Warts of the genitalia in young children should raise the question of possible sexual abuse.*

Interdisciplinary Interventions

Numerous health care modalities may be necessary, and the recurrence rate for warts is very high. Treatment usually involves either freezing the wart or chemically killing the skin that contains the wart virus. The decision to treat should be based on location, number, and size of the lesions; discomfort; and whether the warts are cosmetically objectionable. Active nonintervention is a viable option, given that many warts will resolve spontaneously (Dasher et al., 2009).

To freeze the warts, liquid nitrogen (cryotherapy) is applied to the site for 2 to 10 seconds, which may or may not be followed by electrosurgery to remove the wart. A blister or blood blister may develop at the site within 1 to 2 days. The blistered skin is soaked in warm, soapy water and then the blister can be gently opened, applying a thin layer of antimicrobial ointment to the area. Exposing warts to heat has been shown to clear the skin lesion. This treatment is completed by immersing the area in hot water, by applying exothermic patches, or by multiple 30- to 60-second exposures to heat at 122° F (50° C) (Dasher et al., 2009).

Over-the-counter chemical agents (e.g., maximum-strength wart remover, Mediplast, Compound W, Wart-Away) can be applied to eliminate the wart. These work by causing topical peeling and an inflammatory response and tend to turn the skin white. One study demonstrated that application of calcipotriol cream (a vitamin D_3 derivative) shows promise in treating warts (Labandeira et al., 2005).

Warts that are cut off are likely to spread. Plantar warts may respond with intermittent flattening of the lesion with a pumice stone or callus file.

❱ **ALERT**   *Concentrated drug store preparations of salicylic acid should never be used on venereal warts.*

Other destructive interventions that eliminate the wart by causing necrosis and blister formation include surgical excision, carbon dioxide laser therapy, photodynamic therapy, antimitotic agents (such as cantharidin), topical immunotherapy with contact sensitizers, immunotherapy modalities that stimulate an immune response to HPV, and intralesional injection of antigens (Dasher et al., 2009). Many of these surgical techniques are not preferred because, although they may remove the lesion, the resulting scar often becomes a more difficult problem than the wart itself (Tradition or Science 25-4).

TRADITION OR SCIENCE 25-4

Can duct tape be used to eliminate warts?

Occluding warts with duct tape or waterproof medical tape, either alone or in combination with a topical agent, has been shown in some studies to be effective as a standard treatment for warts. However, the mechanism for its use is unclear. Implementation involves leaving the tape in place for several days at a time, then simply changing the tape, for 1–2 months. One study demonstrated complete resolution of warts in 85% of adult patients treated with duct tape for 2 months, compared with 60% of those treated with cryotherapy (Focht et al., 2002). Complete resolution was reported in 6 weeks for 16% of those in the treatment group (*n* = 51) of the total 103 children ages 4–12 years in another study (de Haen et al., 2006). In another study, 21% of children and adults in the treatment group showed complete resolution after 2 months (Wenner et al., 2007). Duct tape has been shown to be more cost-effective than cryotherapy (Keogh-Brown et al., 2007) and could be considered first as a cost-effective noninvasive treatment. More vigorous trials are warranted using a pediatric population and larger samples.

Other treatments for multiple warts have included cimetidine and contact sensitizers. Cimetidine, an H_2-receptor antagonist used to suppress gastric acid secretion, at high doses has been found to augment delayed-type hypersensitivity and inhibit T-cell function. It has been used to treat multiple warts successfully in children. It has low side effects and easy administration. Treatment is a 2- to 4-month course at 20 to 40 mg/kg/day in two to three divided doses. Further controlled studies are needed. Contact sensitizers are believed to elicit a localized cell-mediation immune response triggering lysis of virus-infected cells. Three agents have been studied: dinitrochlorobenzene (DNCB), diphenylcyclopropenone (DPC), and squaric acid dibutyl ester (SADBE). However, none are FDA-approved and are used in only selected cases of when multiple warts are refractory to other treatments (Dasher et al., 2009).

Children and families need education about the cause and recurrence of warts. Families need to know that warts can disappear spontaneously but, even when treated, can be unpredictable. Teach that the spread of warts to other body parts is possible and that repeated irritation of the wart usually causes enlargement. Also educate adolescents about the transmission of genital warts and the cancer risk associated with condylomata. Genital warts can be cosmetically disfiguring, and the affected adolescent has the responsibility of protecting his or her sexual partner from infection.

HAND, FOOT, AND MOUTH DISEASE

Hand, foot, and mouth disease is a highly contagious viral syndrome seen most frequently in children during the summer and fall months. It is transferred from person to person by the fecal–oral route and possibly by the oral–oral route. Children younger than age 5 years are most commonly affected. The incidence among close contacts in the same household is also higher. Hand, foot, and mouth disease is usually caused by enterovirus 71 (EV71) or the coxsackievirus type A16. However, several other serotypes of enteroviruses such as A5, A7, A9, A10, B2, and B5 have been linked to outbreaks of the disease (Ooi et al., 2010).

Pathophysiology

The virus implants on the mucosa of the throat and ileum, followed by spread of the virus to the lymph nodes within 24 hours. By day 3, lesions on the oral mucosa appear, followed by extension of the disease to other secondary infection sites. Antibodies appear by day 7, with few newer lesions erupting at this time. The incubation period is from 3 to 6 days. Most cases completely resolve within 10 days.

Hand, foot, and mouth disease generally causes only mild difficulties for the child and is self-limiting. However, central nervous system involvement (paralysis, encephalitis, and meningitis) has been noted to occur as a result of the disease. The condition may be dangerous to the newborn and has been associated with spontaneous abortions. The lesions of the coxsackievirus A16 may be chronic, reappearing at later dates.

Assessment

Hand, foot, and mouth disease is generally a mild, self-limited disease that manifests with mild, nonspecific symptoms such as low-grade fever, malaise, anorexia, and sore mouth as well as symptoms of a cold. Mild abdominal pain and mild diarrhea may also be present.

Oral lesions are 3 to 6 mm in diameter, irregularly distributed on the buccal mucosa, tongue, gums, palate, and pharynx. Eruptions of lesions on other body surface areas generally occur within 48 hours after the appearance of the oral lesions. Painless, maculopapular eruptions, which may progress to vesicles 3 to 7 mm in diameter, are most frequently seen on the palms, soles, fingers, and toes. Lesions on the buttocks, extremities, and face are more likely to be evident in young children.

Diagnosis is made based on the clinical presentation and distribution of the lesions. The virus can be cultured from the cutaneous vesicles or the oral lesions.

Interdisciplinary Interventions

Symptomatic treatment is all that is usually required. IV immunoglobulin has been used in Asia and a benefit is suggested if given early in those children with severe CNS disease. Milrinone, a cyclic nucleotide phosphodiesterase inhibitor, used in a small sample of children with EV71-induced pulmonary edema had reduced tachycardia and lower mortality. Young children may need to be monitored for dehydration and fluid and electrolyte imbalance if the lesions interfere with their ability to eat and drink. Fluid management should be guided in the very sick child by central venous pressure. A soft, nonirritating diet for a few days and plenty of cool, clear fluids help prevent dehydration and food refusal. After meals, the child should rinse the mouth with warm water to prevent secondary infection of the oral lesions. Fever and discomfort can be managed with acetaminophen. Liquid Benadryl may be prescribed for the secondary lesion sites on the body if the child is particularly uncomfortable.

Community Care

Because hand, foot, and mouth disease is highly contagious, evaluate other family members who have had close contact with the affected child for signs of the condition. Spread of the disease is extremely difficult to prevent; therefore, infected but afebrile children may return to their daycare or school after their fever has subsided. If the child becomes confused or delirious, has a fever that persists for more than 3 days, refuses to eat, or shows signs of dehydration, then the child should be seen immediately by a health care provider.

Prevention is possible by teaching families, daycare providers, and teachers to use good hygiene practices. In child care settings in which caregivers are changing diapers, gloves should be worn during the diaper change, and hands should be washed with antibacterial soap after disposal of the diaper. Children should be taught to wash their hands with antibacterial soap before ingesting any food. For children with pacifiers or who are bottle-feeding, nipples that drop to the ground or are touched by other children should be cleansed thoroughly before being used again by the child.

FUNGAL SKIN DISORDERS

Infections caused by fungi are common throughout the world, especially in areas where general hygiene measures are poor. Nearly everyone is colonized with some form of fungi. Fungal infections account for a large portion of pediatric outpatient visits. During childhood, infections of the scalp, hair, and body surfaces are common; fungal infections of the hands, feet, and nails are rare before adolescence.

> ◣ A L E R T   *Fungal skin infections can be life threatening when the child is nutritionally depleted or is immunocompromised.*

DERMATOPHYTOSES

Formally called *dermatophytoses*, fungal skin infections are caused by the filamentous dermatophytes belonging to the classes *Trichophyton*, *Microsporum*, and *Epidermophyton*. These infections are commonly called either *ringworm* or by their Latin term, *tinea*. Dermatophytoses, or tinea infections, are seen in several forms, depending on their body location (Nursing Interventions 25-4) (Andrews et al., 2009; Parker, 2009; Theos, 2007). At least 40 dermatophyte species exist, but in the United States, most human infection is caused by a relatively small number of species (Theos, 2007).

Pathophysiology

Dermatophytes infect the keratin—that is, the stratum corneum layer of the skin, hair, or nails. Because keratin is shed constantly, fungi must multiply rapidly to keep pace with keratin production. As a result, tinea infections spread rapidly. These superficial fungi form an enzyme that enables them to digest keratin, causing scaling skin, crumbling nails, and breaking hairs. Inflammation associated with tinea infections is the result of an allergic response to fungal antigens that diffuse through the keratin to underlying living skin cells.

Tinea infections are usually transmitted from one infected person to another. This organism is acquired from three sources: organisms that live in the soil, animal fungi, or, most common, pathogens that will infect only humans and cannot survive elsewhere. Tinea infections can also be transmitted by asymptomatic carriers (e.g., school children) who harbor the organism but lack clinical symptoms (Andrews et al., 2009; Parker, 2009). Poor nutrition and hygiene, a tropical climate, debilitating diseases, atopy, and contact with infected animals, persons, or fomites all increase the likelihood of fungal infection.

caREminder

Dermatophytes do not depend solely on humans for growth. Transmission can also occur from infected pets and practically any items that touch the scalp, such as combs, towels, hats, and pillows.

Prognosis for tinea infections is excellent because current medical therapy usually eradicates the problem. Some forms, however, are resistant to therapy (tinea unguium). Underlying immune suppression can make treatment more difficult.

Assessment

The first sign of tinea in a child is scaling and hair loss on the scalp. Because treatment for any of the misdiagnoses differs substantially from that for tinea, patients may be treated incorrectly at first. Tinea lesions of the skin, nails, and hair are circular or annular (hence the name *ringworm*), with an active border that exhibits erythema and scaling. Nursing Interventions 25-4 summarizes the characteristics and health care interventions for the more common forms of tinea.

Diagnosis of a tinea infection can be confirmed by potassium hydroxide preparation treatment of lesion scrapings and microscopic examination to confirm the presence of fungi. In some cases, cultures of the lesions or a skin biopsy may be necessary to confirm the diagnosis. Examination of infected areas under Wood light was formerly routine in the diagnosis of tinea capitis; however, because the epidemiology is changing such that nonfluorescent *tinea tonsurans* is now the most common cause in the United States, Wood light is helpful only under some circumstances (Parker, 2009).

NURSING INTERVENTIONS 25-4

Management of Tinea Infections

Name	Appearance of Lesions	Common Location	Nursing Considerations
Tinea capitis	Round patches of hair loss that increase in size Broken hair shafts at surface, leaving a black-dot, stubbled appearance Scaling of scalp Mild itching Usually affects children ages 2–10 years, with males more often affected than females	Hair and scalp	Administer oral antifungal medication for 6–8 weeks. Use antifungal cream twice a week for 8 weeks; use antifungal shampoos. There is no need to shave or cut hair to prevent spread; hair regrowth is slow. Lesions are mildly contagious. The child can return to school after medications and antifungal shampoos have been started. Affected children should not share combs, brushes, or head wear.
Tinea corporis	Round, pruritic, expanding red lesions with well-circumscribed borders and central clearing Scaling on lesion borders Single or multiple lesions Annular lesions Uncommon after puberty	Entire body, especially face and extremities	Apply topical antifungal cream twice daily for 2–4 weeks, continuing for several days after clinical cleaning. Continue application of cream for 2 weeks after the lesions have disappeared. Lesions are mildly contagious. The child can return to school after treatment with topical medication has been started. To control spread, direct contact with infected children and animals should be avoided.
Tinea faciei	Erythematous, scaly lesions that commonly have a "butterfly" distribution	Face	Apply topical antifungal cream twice daily for 2–4 weeks, continuing for several days after clinical cleaning.
Tinea cruris (jock itch)	Erythematous, scaly eruption Not usually seen before adolescence Often seen in athletes	Inner thighs and inguinal creases	Apply topical antifungal cream twice daily for 2–4 weeks. Keep area dry. Wear loose-fitting cotton shorts. Cleanse area daily with water and carefully dry. Lesions are mildly contagious and will not affect dry, normal skin.
Tinea pedis (athlete's foot)	Vesicles and erosions on the instep of one or both feet Fissuring between the toes, with scaling and erythema Itchy and burning rash Unpleasant foot odor Most forms found exclusively in the postpubertal adolescent	Feet	For acute episodes, apply Burow solution compresses. Apply topical antifungal cream twice daily for 2–4 weeks to clean feet. Keep feet dry by wearing sandals, thongs, or no shoes. Wear cotton socks only and change them twice daily. Thoroughly dry feet after bath or shower. Lesions are not contagious.

(Continued)

NURSING INTERVENTIONS 25-4

Management of Tinea Infections *(Continued)*

Name	Appearance of Lesions	Common Location	Nursing Considerations
Tinea versicolor	Multiple annular to oval macules or patches with a fine scale On well-tanned or darkly pigmented children, lesions are hypopigmented	Neck, upper back, shoulders, upper arms	Wash affected areas with prescribed medicated shampoo of 1% selenium sulfide or (2.5%) selenium blue over-the-counter shampoo (Selsun Blue) daily for 2–3 weeks. Apply topical imidazole antifungal agent twice daily for a week then tapering may be ordered. Not contagious. Recurrence is likely. For chronic recurrence involvement, systemic antifungals may be indicated. Monthly treatment with the shampoo can prevent recurrence. Normal skin color does not return for 6–12 months.
Tinea unguium (onychomycosis)	Distal thickening and yellowing of the nail plate caused by separation of nail plate from bed and entrapment of air between the two structures Usually found in adolescents	Fingernails, toenails	Topical agents have not proved effective as a cure. Oral antifungal agents may be used.

Interdisciplinary Interventions

Care focuses on educating children and their families on how to follow the prescribed health care plan. The lesion sites should be cleansed thoroughly with water before applying any medications. Mild fungal infections of the skin may be managed with topical therapy with either imidazole preparations (miconazole and clotrimazole) or the allylamine terbinafine. Most patients require 2-week treatment courses. When several sites are involved, or topical treatments have failed, or if the hair and nails are affected, oral antifungals are used. Oral antifungal medications must be taken appropriately, and any side effects must be reported to the health care provider. Oral terbinafine is now considered superior to griseofulvin (Andrews et al., 2009). If terbinafine therapy is continued beyond 2 weeks, it is important to monitor full blood count and liver function tests. To prevent recurrence, teach child and family that all medications must be taken for the entire prescribed period, even if the lesions have faded.

Nurses in school settings assist in periodic screening of sports participants for tinea corporis to decrease the incidence of spread of the condition. Students participating in athletics should be encouraged to change their socks and shoes immediately after a sports activity and to expose their feet to warm, dry air by wearing sandals or thongs.

Children with tinea infections should refrain from applying oils or petroleum jelly to their skin or scalp because these agents act as an occlusive medium and can promote more fungal growth. All affected children should be advised not to share personal articles to prevent transfer of the fungi (Clinical Judgment 25-3).

CANDIDIASIS

Caused by the yeast *C. albicans*, candidiasis (candidosis or moniliasis) is an infection that occurs in the mouth, eyes, and anywhere on the skin. When the yeast is present in the oral cavity, it is commonly called *thrush*. Candida is a normal flora of which 20 species exist, but overgrowth can occur on the skin and mucous membranes. Most susceptible are newborns infected during the birthing process, chronically ill children, those receiving antibiotic therapy, and immunocompromised children.

Children with an immunologic deficit are at risk for development of chronic mucocutaneous candidiasis, a

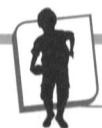

CLINICAL JUDGMENT 25-3

The Adolescent With Tinea Cruris

Mrs. Law brings her 16-year-old son, Kevin, to the clinic because he is complaining that he has a pink rash on his inner thigh and groin areas. Kevin is embarrassed about being at the clinic for this problem.

When his mother leaves the room during the examination, he asks you whether he got the rash from going skinny-dipping in a neighbor's lake with some of his buddies.

Questions

1. As you complete a physical examination, what characteristics of the lesions would indicate that Kevin has tinea cruris (jock itch)?

2. Is Kevin's age a significant factor in confirming this condition?

3. Is the fact that Kevin was skinny-dipping significant to the history of this skin condition?

4. What interventions should Kevin take to clear up the rash?

5. What is your response when Kevin asks, "What do I do if this stuff doesn't go away?"

Answers

1. The lesions should be symmetric, scaly with raised borders, erythematous, and slightly brown or pink. The penis and scrotum should have no lesions on them.

2. Tinea cruris is most common during adolescence.

3. No. Tinea cruris is most associated with hot, humid weather and wearing tight clothing. It is not associated with being in the water.

4. Keep the groin area dry. Wear loose-fitting cotton shorts. Wash clothes, towels, and athletic supporter daily. Using plain water, wash and then carefully dry the rash site daily. Apply topical antifungal cream to the site as ordered.

5. If the rash does not begin to improve within 1 week, or if it is not completely cured within 1 month, return to the clinic to be reevaluated. To prevent a reinfection, be sure to use the topical ointment for 1–2 weeks after the rash has vanished.

progressive infection characterized by large polycystic plaques resembling ringworm or psoriasis but with thick hyperkeratotic crusts. A defective cell-mediated immunity is a feature of this syndrome. After immunity is restored to normal, the cutaneous lesions resolve.

Pathophysiology

Congenital candidiasis is acquired in utero, affecting 1% of newborns. The infection is present at birth, characterized by pustular and vesiculopustular lesions that progress to a drying exfoliative stage. The lesions often clear within a few weeks. Lesions can be found anywhere, including the nails, oral mucosa (thrush), palms, and soles.

Neonatal candidiasis is acquired by the child during the birthing process by delivery through an infected birth canal. The mother usually has a history of a past or present vaginal yeast infection. Fungal infections are common during the newborn period, especially among premature neonates, and are responsible for considerable morbidity and mortality (Antaya & Robinson, 2010). A classic sign of the condition is the presence of a beefy, red, glazed, weeping dermatitis in the genital area. The lesions are well demarcated with raised borders and have slight scaling. Erythematous papules or vesiculopustular satellite lesions surround the periphery of the primary rash.

In infants and young children, candidal infections can develop as either an acute or chronic skin infection and may be either generalized or localized. In young children, candidal infection of the diaper area often transfers to other areas of the body, most commonly the oral mucosa (thrush). In the oral cavity, the lesions appear as white plaques that adhere to the oral surfaces tightly and that bleed when scraped. The outer lips appear chapped and cracked. The breastfeeding infant can transfer this infection to the mother's nipples if good hygiene is not promoted.

Candidiasis is often an opportunistic infection made possible by the weakened defense system of the child who is immunocompromised. Other contributing factors include trauma, malnutrition, and administration of broad-spectrum antibiotics. Eruption of the lesions has also been associated with excess perspiration or metabolic dysfunction. Local predisposing factors are moisture, macerated folds of skin, and warmth. Diapers make children particularly vulnerable to this infection. The prognosis is excellent, given the efficacy of antifungal agents. Systemic involvement must be considered if any of the following conditions are present: immunodeficient states (HIV or cancer), prematurity with low birth weight, pneumonia or sepsis, or previous treatment with a broad-spectrum antibiotic.

Assessment

Candidiasis presents as a deep, livid, red area of macerated skin with small satellite papules and pustules along the margin. Warm, moist body folds such as the axilla or the genital areas are the most common site of the rash (Fig. 25-12). Diagnosis of candidiasis is confirmed by

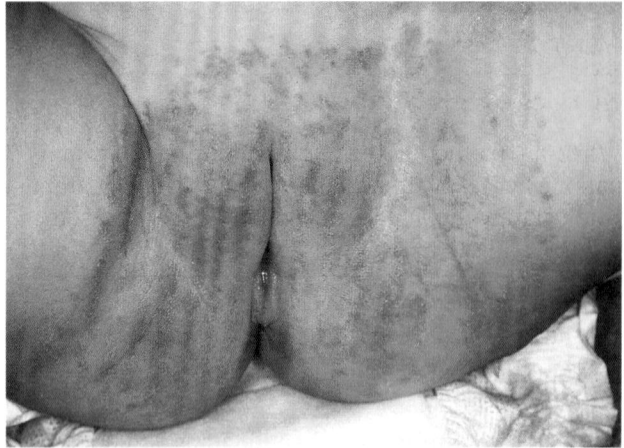

Figure 25-12 An infant with candidiasis.

potassium hydroxide slide examination showing budding yeasts and pseudohyphae. A positive fungus culture demonstrates white mucoid growth within 48 to 72 hours.

Older children with candidiasis may complain of discomfort and itching. Infants and young children may display fretful behavior and may have trouble sleeping.

Interdisciplinary Interventions

Management involves three primary interventions: (1) removal of any predisposing cause, (2) application of topical or oral antifungal agents, and (3) keeping the affected area dry. Commonly used medications include topical anticandidal agents such as nystatin, miconazole, and clotrimazole. Improvement should be noted within 3 to 5 days. Most patients require a 2-week course. Application of a low-potency corticosteroid cream, followed by a preventive petroleum, zinc oxide, or dimethicone water-repellent ointment to prevent the causative agent from continually reinfecting the area, may be required if inflammation is severe.

Oral infections are commonly treated with nystatin oral solution for 1 to 2 weeks. The solutions should be swabbed onto the mucous membranes using a cotton-tipped applicator (Teaching Intervention Plan 25-5). Older children may be treated with oral antifungals such as clotrimazole troches, itraconazole, or fluconazole. Systemic infections are treated with medications such as IV amphotericin B, itraconazole, fluconazole, and a new class of antifungals that includes caspofungin and micafungin (Parker, 2009).

Keep the affected area dry. The nurse and the family can assist the healing process with frequent diaper

---

TIP 25-5: A TEACHING INTERVENTION PLAN for the Child With Oral Thrush at Home

Nursing Diagnoses and Family Outcomes

- Impaired oral mucous membrane related to presence of candidiasis lesions
  Outcomes: Child's oral mucosa remains intact with no further breakdown.
  Child will experience effective swallowing.
- Risk for infection related to transfer of candidiasis from child to others during close personal contact with family and peers
  Outcomes: Child remains free from systemic infection.
  Family uses hygienic practices to prevent spread of infection.

Teach Child/Family
Medication Administration
- The prescribed solution is applied to the oral mucous membranes.
- A calibrated measuring device should be used to measure the amount of oral solution to be applied. One half of the dose is placed in each side of the mouth.
- A cotton-tipped applicator can be used to apply the solution to the oral mucosa of the young infant.
- Older children should be instructed to hold the suspension in their mouth or swish it throughout their mouth for several minutes.
- The solution is applied after feeding and cleaning of the mouth.

- The child should not drink immediately after application of the solution.
- The infant may swallow some of the solution. This is expected and does not harm the infant.
- If a dose is missed, the medication should be taken as soon as it is remembered but not if it is almost time for the next dose. Doses should never be doubled.

Medication Storage
- Oral solutions must be kept refrigerated.
- The solutions should be kept away from small children to prevent accidental ingestion.

Preventive Measures
- If the infant is bottle-fed, all nipples and pacifiers should be sterilized after each use.
- If breastfeeding, the mother should apply the solution or antifungal cream, as ordered, to her nipples to eliminate reinfection.
- The child's toothbrush should be cleansed thoroughly in hot water after each use.
- The infected child should not share drinking cups or eating utensils with others.

Contact the Health Care Provider if
- Irritation of the mucous membrane increases
- Child refuses to eat or drink
- Child shows signs of dehydration (poor urine output, lethargy, sunken eyes, sunken fontanel, poor skin turgor)
- Child shows other signs of illness (e.g., lethargy, fever, cold symptoms)

changes or by leaving the child's diaper off at times, thereby exposing candidal lesions of the groin area to the air, which helps them to dry. If topical antifungal agents are ordered, they should be applied after each washing or each diaper change and then covered with a protective cream as indicated earlier. Teach family members to recognize a candidal infection, especially if the child is receiving antibiotic therapy or is immunocompromised.

REACTIONS TO ENVIRONMENTAL FORCES AND SUBSTANCES

Environmental forces and substances pose different risks and hazards for children than for adults. PUs, formerly called *decubiti ulcers*, are a common reaction to environmental forces among long-term immobile patients. Poison ivy, oak, and sumac are plants that can cause cutaneous reactions ranging from mild to severe. Ambulatory and active children often come in contact with these environmental substances. In addition, reactions to medication can cause substantial alterations in skin integrity.

PRESSURE ULCERS

Pressure areas are localized areas of tissue destruction that occur when the tissue is compressed between a bony prominence and an external surface for an extended period. PUs occur in children and adolescents whose mobility, activity, or sensory perception is severely restricted because of prolonged immobilization or conditions that may impede movement (e.g., a child with myelomeningocele).

Pathophysiology

A PU arises secondary to tissue hypoxia caused by the prolonged pressure over a certain area. A critical relationship exists between time and pressure: a lower pressure over a longer time can generate an area of skin breakdown as easily as an area of high pressure for a short time. Preterm infants and children who are immobilized are two groups at high-risk for PUs.

The high-risk areas for ulcer formation are the bony prominences all over the body, such as the sacrum, heel, and elbow, because subcutaneous fat and superficial fascia are thinner and greater pressures are generated. PU locations differ in children according to age. In infants, the occiput is the most likely spot; in older children, sacral pressure is greatest. Other factors, including shear, friction, and nutritional deficiencies, all contribute to PU formation; however, pressure is the primary causative factor. Severity of the ulcer usually depends on the intensity and duration of the pressure and the tolerance of the affected tissue. Shear, the interplay between gravity and friction, results when gravity pushes down on the body while resistance (friction) occurs between the patient and a surface. Friction alone can cause minor or severe skin damage. Over time, however, friction and gravity may work synergistically to cause shear. Malnutrition, especially protein deficiency, should also be considered when assessing and managing PUs.

Assessment

The primary focus of the nursing assessment is to prevent alterations in skin integrity. Quigley and Curley (1996) developed a skin care algorithm to establish daily practices for assessment and prevention (see thePoint Evidence-Based Clinical Practice Guidelines). This tool identifies intrinsic and extrinsic factors such as immobility, incontinence, and health conditions that can precipitate a skin alteration. Upon recognition of altered integrity, immediate action should be taken to protect the skin.

If an ulcer has developed, the lesion must be continuously assessed for color, exudate, odor, and dimensions. PUs are organized into stages based on their severity (Wound, Ostomy and Continence Nurses Society, 2009):

- *Stage I*: Intact skin with nonblanchable redness of localized area usually over a bony prominence. In darker skin tones, the color may differ from surrounding skin.
- *Stage II*: Partial-thickness skin loss involving dermis. The PU is present with red pink wound bed and no slough. May be an intact or open/ruptured serum-filled blister.
- *Stage III*: Full-thickness skin loss. Tendon or muscle not exposed. Slough, undermining, and tunneling may be present. Depth of PU varies by site (e.g., bridge of nose, ears do not have subcutaneous tissue so stage III PU can be shallow).
- *Stage IV*: Full-thickness skin loss with extensive destruction, tissue necrosis, or damage to muscle, bone, or supporting structures (e.g., tendon or joint capsule). Undermining and sinus tracts may also be associated with stage IV PUs.
- *Unstageable*: Full-thickness tissue loss with PU base coverage by slough and/or eschar.
- *Suspected* deep tissue injury: Purple or maroon localized area of discolored intact skin or blood-filled blister due to damage of soft tissues underneath from pressure and/or shear.

Assessment factors include location of the wound, staging (I to IV, unstageable, and suspected deep tissue injury), size in centimeters (length, width, and depth), type of tissue at the wound base, presence of exudate or odor, presence and location of undermining or tracts, character of wound margins, condition of periwound skin, and dressing type.

Be cognizant of the child's nutritional status and relay all abnormal laboratory indices (especially decreased levels of albumin, low total protein, and altered serum electrolytes) to the health care provider.

Interdisciplinary Interventions

Recognizing the factors that predispose a child to PU formation and providing pressure relief to children at risk is crucial.

The best nursing care related to PUs is to prevent their occurrence. Hospitalized or immobilized children are prone to PU development because of the small amount of subcutaneous tissue and because these children are often debilitated by multisystem problems. A repositioning schedule should be developed for those children identified as at risk. Regular skin assessments then are able to evaluate the intervention's effectiveness. Pressure relief over bony prominences is an important part of a PU intervention program through repositioning or the use of foam mattresses or other pediatric specialty mattress systems (Parnham, 2012).

To standardize prevention and management, practice guidelines for treating PUs have been reviewed and synthesized (National Guideline Clearinghouse, n.d.; Wound, Ostomy and Continence Nurses Society [2010]). Nursing Interventions 25-5 summarizes many of the research-based PU guidelines for neonates and children. For more in-depth information, see thePoint Evidence-Based Practice Guidelines.

NURSING INTERVENTIONS 25-5

Prevention and Management of Pressure Ulcers in Neonates and Children

Assessments
- Upon admission, perform a comprehensive skin assessment and risk assessment for PUs on all neonates and children.
- Perform a head-to-toe skin assessment daily.
- Perform comprehensive nutritional assessment.
- Assess for pain.

Pressure Redistribution
- Evaluate skin under blood pressure cuffs, nasal prongs, arm boards, plaster casts, traction boots, nasogastric tubes, etc.
- As child grows, adjust orthotics, wheelchairs, and wheelchair cushions to changes in child's size.
- Ensure tubing, leads, toys, and syringe caps are not under or on top of child's skin when child is in bed, crib, or isolette.
- Tape invasive tubes without tension to the skin.
- Use age-appropriate low-air loss beds or overlays.
- In neonates younger than 32 weeks of age, use water, air, and gel mattresses and sheepskin and gel pads at the joints, behind the ears, and behind the occiput.
- Reposition the neonate every 4 hours and the older child every 2 hours.
- Use convoluted foam and gel pillows to reduce occipital and sacral pressure.
- Use draw sheet for lifting to minimize shearing.

Topical Treatments
- Select only those products that have been recommended for use in the neonate and pediatric population.

Wound Cleansing
- Use sterile water and normal saline for wound cleansing, with sterile water preferred for neonates.
- Warm cleansing solution to body temperature for use in neonates.

- Use a 20-mL syringe with a blunt needle or a polytetrafluorethylene catheter to flush wound exudate.
- Avoid use of antiseptics because of potential for tissue damage and absorption.

Debridement
- Fine mesh gauze with saline dampening can be used on the ulcer in a "wet-to-damp" method. When removed, the dressing removes necrotic tissue.
- Use whirlpool therapy to debride.

Managing Bacterial Colonization and Infection
- If extensive colonization is suspected, use antibiotic ointments.
- If infection is suspected, obtain cultures and Gram stains.
- Avoid use of silver sulfadiazine cream in neonates because of its potential for toxicity.

Dressings
- Use hydrogels, hydrocolloids, and film dressings for noninfected ulcers.
- Avoid products not recommended for neonate or pediatric populations.
- Use pectin-based skin barriers or hydrocolloid adhesive barriers where adhesive tape will be repeatedly removed and reapplied.
- For neonates, use cotton balls soaked with warm water to assist in the removal of adhesives.
- Avoid use of solvent adhesive removers and bonding agents in this population.
- Avoid products containing dyes, perfumes, and preservatives.

Pain Management
- If necessary, premedicate the child with pain relievers prior to management of the ulcer site.
- Use pain relief measures as needed.

Information from Ayello, E., & Sibbald, R. (2008). Preventing pressure ulcers and skin tears. In E. Capezuti, D. Zwicker, M. Mezey et al. (Eds.), *Evidence-based geriatric nursing protocols for best practice* (pp. 403–429). 3rd ed. New York, NY: Springer Publishing Company; Noonan, C., Quigley, S., & Curley, M. (2006). Skin integrity in hospitalized infants and children: A prevalence study. *Journal of Pediatric Nursing, 21,* 445–453; Parnham, A. (2012). Pressure ulcer risk assessment and prevention in children. *Nursing Children and Young People, 24*(2), 24–29.

POISON IVY, OAK, AND SUMAC

QUESTION: Would Nick also react to poison oak and poison sumac?

ANSWER: Because Nick has been sensitized to poison ivy, he will most likely also react to poison oak and poison sumac, even if it is his first exposure.

The significance and need to assess environmental risks during childhood has already been discussed. An important reason children's exposures are different from those of adults is because of their level of behavioral development. Most children actively explore their environments as well as exhibit frequent hand-to-mouth and object-to-mouth behaviors. This may bring them into contact with poison ivy, poison oak, and poison sumac, which are three potent antigens that characteristically produce an intense dermatologic inflammatory reaction upon contact with the skin. The source of the allergen is *urushiol*, a saplike oil, which is present on live or dead leaves. Sensitization to one plant produces cross-reactions with other plants containing urushiol.

The skin eruption is a form of contact dermatitis known as *rhus dermatitis*. One or 2 days after the encounter, the affected skin displays erythema, edema, and erythematous papular lesions in a streak or patch-like shape, representing the path in which the plant brushed across the skin. The lesions are itchy. Within 2 to 3 days, vesicular lesions develop and quickly rupture, leaking fluid that forms a crust over the lesion site. Fluid from the ruptured vesicles is not antigenic and does not spread the eruption. However, the rash can spread more during the first 2 weeks as a result of the allergenic response of the host. In addition, antigen retained under fingernails and on clothing initiates new eruptions if not removed by washing with soap and water. The offending antigen may also be carried on animal fur that comes into contact with the plants. The sap left on fur, clothing, and objects is contagious if not cleansed properly. Urushiol can remain potent for years, especially in dry environments, and becomes airborne when plants are cut with mowers. Lesions from the plant exposure usually resolve within 3 to 4 weeks. Complications from poison ivy, oak, and sumac exposure are low, although secondary skin infections can occur and hyperpigmentation and/or lichenification of skin lesions may occur in darkly pigmented children.

Learning to recognize the plants and to avoid contact with them is an important aspect of education for families. Community Care 25-2 describes the plants and summarizes the care that should be initiated if the child or other family member comes into contact with urushiol. The only preventative product approved thus far by the FDA to protect the skin from potential exposure is Ivy Block, a 5% quaternium-18 bentonite lotion that leaves a visible film on the skin. The lotion interferes with absorption of urushiol by physically blocking contact of the oil with the skin. Washing thoroughly with soap and water immediately after skin contact is also essential because if even 10 minutes have elapsed with the oil on the skin, only 50% will be removed.

ADVERSE DRUG REACTIONS

Adverse drug reactions (ADRs) are undesired effects arising from the appropriate use of medications. The actual incidence of ADRs is not known. The sudden eruption of skin lesions is the most common clinical feature of an ADR (Fig. 25-13).

Several factors have been associated with a high risk for ADRs in children. These include age younger than 12 months; the presence of serious, concomitant disease; the use of multiple drugs; and an increase in dose (Developmental Considerations 25-4). In many cases, ADRs are preventable by more carefully monitoring the administration of harmful drug–drug and drug–food combinations.

Pathophysiology

Mechanisms that cause ADRs include dose-related reactions, drug interaction reactions, idiosyncratic reactions, and allergic or immune-mediated reactions. *Dose-related reactions* are those experienced by a child because the dose ingested was either below or above the therapeutic level desired. A child may also have a dose-related toxic effect of a drug that is being given at a therapeutic level (e.g., hair loss with Accutane therapy). *Drug interaction reactions* are those caused by drug combinations that produce toxicity or lethal side effects. For instance, morphine and diazepam used together place a child at higher risk for apnea than if the drugs were used alone. *Idiosyncratic reactions* are attributed to an unusual characteristic specific to a certain child that causes him or her to have an adverse response to a certain medication. *Allergic or immune-mediated reactions* are created by immunologic mechanisms that produce a wide variety of systemic responses to the drug.

Assessment

Skin eruptions caused by a drug reaction are diverse in nature, and it may be difficult to identify the exact cause. For example, in the seriously ill child, the appearance of an unusual rash may be an allergic response to a drug or may be the result of a newly acquired viral infection. Ask the child and the family if the child is receiving any over-the-counter medications. Determine whether the child has had any changes in medications. Has the child had any allergic reactions in the past? Are there any other agents or processes that could be causing the skin lesions?

Morbilliform (measleslike) rashes are the most common type of skin manifestation seen in children in response to an ADR. However, drug reaction rashes can also assume several other forms (Table 25-6). The lesions may be accompanied by itching, malaise, fever, nausea, vomiting, and liver or kidney damage. Severe anaphylactic reactions can lead to respiratory compromise and shock. Anaphylaxis is discussed in more detail in Chapter 31. Any acutely occurring rash should be evaluated for a drug reaction.

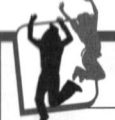

COMMUNITY CARE 25-2

Protecting Children Against Poison Ivy, Poison Oak, and Poison Sumac

Recognize the Plant

Poison Ivy

Small plant, vine, or low shrub with shiny green leaflets that grow in groups of three. The leaf stems have waxy, yellow-green flowers and, later, greenish berries. In the autumn months, the leaves turn red. Poison ivy grows all over the United States, except California and parts of adjacent states.

Poison Oak

Shrubs or vines with oak-shaped leaves that have a hairy, light-green underside and darker green surface. The leaves grow in groups of three. Some shrubs or vines have clusters of greenish or creamy white berries. The plant grows on the west coast of the United States and from Mexico to Colombia.

Poison Sumac

Colorful woody shrubs that grow from 5 to 25 ft tall, most commonly found in the eastern United States in swampy areas. A branch of the shrub contains 7–13 long, smooth, paired leaves, topped with a single velvety leaf. The plant is bright orange in the spring months, turns to a glossy dark green with a pale underside, and then to a reddish orange color in the fall. Poison sumac has drooping clusters of green berries. The nonpoisonous variety has upright red berries.

Protect the Child From Exposure

- Children should wear long pants and enclosed shoes with socks when walking in the woods or swampy areas.
- Rubber gloves and rubber boots are not considered protective because the catechols in urushiol are soluble in rubber.
- Apply Ivy Rest to the skin prior to the child's outing.
- Oil residue on clothes, pets, toys, and garden and sports equipment should be removed with liberal soap-and-water washing.

If the Child Is Exposed

- Immediately wash and rewash the affected area with yellow or brown laundry soap or nonperfumed

bath soap and cold water. Do not use a brush on the skin to avoid scratching the skin surface.
- Wash and rewash any clothes that came into contact with the plants.
- Wash any pets that came into contact with the plants. Wear gloves and do not touch the animal's fur with bare hands. Dispose of the gloves afterward.

To Help With Itching and Treatment of the Lesions

- Keep lesions clean by washing daily with mild soap and water.
- Do not use occlusive dressings. Allow vesicles to be open to drain.
- Apply tap water or Burow or Domeboro solution with a dressing to blistered or oozing lesions for 20 minutes, twice a day.
- Apply over-the-counter preparations to reduce itching and dry lesions (e.g., calamine lotion, Ivy Rest).
- Place the child in tepid baths with colloidal oatmeal (Aveeno). Hot water baths or showers will increase pruritus.
- Apply topical steroid creams as ordered by the health care provider.
- Administer antihistamines as ordered by the health care provider. Medications are usually given three to four times a day unless sedation interferes with the child's school work and other activities.
- Administer corticosteroids if ordered by the health care provider.
- Administer antibiotics if ordered by the health care provider to treat secondary bacterial infections.

Call Health Care Provider if

- Face, eyes, or lips become involved
- Signs of infection appear, such as redness, oozing, or pus at lesion sites
- Rash begins to blister
- Itching interferes with child's sleep

Common drug offenders include penicillins, cephalosporins, sulfa drugs, phenytoin, barbiturates, diazepam, isoniazid, and carbamazepine.

Interdisciplinary Interventions

The most immediate measure to take when an ADR occurs is to stop using the suspected drug. Treatment is individualized and may vary from simply monitoring

the child with no special interventions provided to treating the severe manifestations of anaphylaxis. If itching and rash formation are severe, oral antihistamines, oral steroids, or both may be ordered. If blistering occurs, the child's fluid and electrolyte as well as infection status should be monitored.

Review signs of an ADR with the family to assist in the early identification of problems that may recur in the

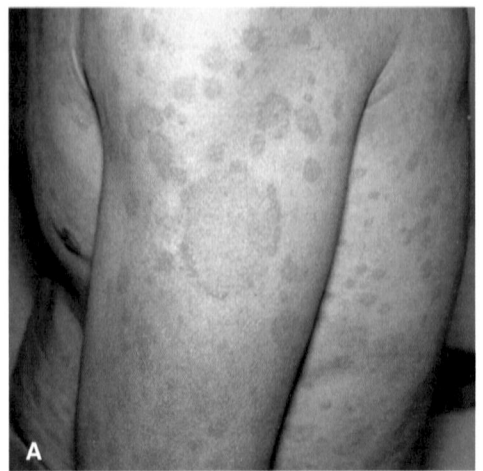

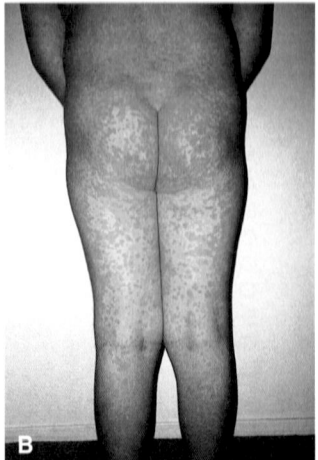

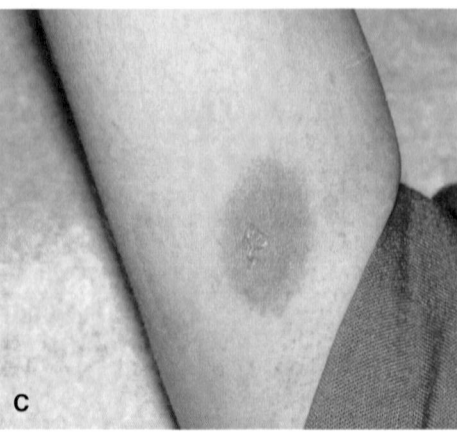

Figure 25-13 ADRs can manifest in various skin eruptions. For example, (A) a systemic eruption of itchy wheals or (B) measleslike lesions might occur, or (C) a fixed eruption might occur as a single oval lesion at the identical site where it had occurred previously.

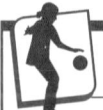

DEVELOPMENTAL CONSIDERATIONS 25-4

Why Children Are at Greater Risk for Adverse Drug Reactions

- The child's neurologic system is responsive and susceptible to impairment because it is still developing after birth (e.g., first-generation antihistamines are sedating in adults but are associated with paradoxic excitation in some children).
- Drugs given to mothers during pregnancy, delivery, and lactation can lead to adverse reactions for the child as a result of their teratogenic, pharmacologic, and toxic processes.
- Topical absorption of medications is enhanced in neonates and young children because of the increased permeability of their skin.
- The sick neonate and children with chronic conditions (e.g., cancer, asthma) are exposed to a large number of medications, thereby increasing their risk of an ADR.
- Symptoms of an adverse reaction may go undetected because the child's condition masks the side effects or are similar to those of an ADR.
- Premature infants and full-term neonates have a lesser capacity for renal elimination of drugs because of decreased glomerular filtration and tubular secretion.
- Many liquid medications for children contain excipients designed to improve the stability and tested acceptability of the medication. These additives can cause adverse side effects.

TABLE 25-6   Clinical Features of Drug Reactions

Type of Drug Eruptions	Drugs Associated With the Reaction	Clinical Signs	Interdisciplinary Interventions
Morbilliform	Allopurinol Amoxicillin Ampicillin Barbiturates Carbamazepine Cephalosporins Chloramphenicol Erythromycin Gentamicin sulfate Gold Isoniazid Nonsteroidal anti-inflammatory drugs (NSAIDs) Penicillins Phenytoin Sulfonamides Trimethoprim	Measleslike (morbilliform) or exanthematous lesions that start on the trunk and move to extremities Areas of normal skin may surround areas of eruption. Initial lesions become papular and then form plaques from joining of several individual lesions. Fever Malaise Arthralgia	Remove offending drug. Rash may fade with time, requiring no treatment. Give antihistamine therapy.
Urticarial	Acetylsalicylic acid (ASA) Amoxicillin Ampicillin Cephalosporins Horse serum Penicillins Sulfonamides	Edematous, flat, erythematous wheals that last less than 24 hours As lesions resolve, may leave a macular, brown, bruised appearance Angioedema of mucous membranes	Remove offending drug. Give antihistamine therapy. If needed in severe cases, give systemic steroids to maintain airway and diminish swelling associated with angioedema.
Serum sickness–like reaction	Cephalosporins Hydantoins Penicillins Sulfonamides Streptomycin Thiouracils	Fever Malaise Large urticarial plaques that resolve, leaving the skin areas with a dusky or bruised appearance Lesions may be accompanied by angioedema. Arthralgia Lymphadenopathy Edema Albuminuria	Remove offending drug. Take fever reduction measures. Apply symptomatic treatment using combination of analgesics, corticosteroids, and antihistamines.
Fixed	Barbiturates Carbamazepine Phenazone derivatives Phenolphthalein Sulfonamides Tetracycline Trimethoprim	Solitary or multiple sharply demarcated erythematous lesions that may look like urticaria or become bullous As lesions fade, skin remains hyperpigmented with residual, sharply demarcated outlines of the lesions.	Remove offending drug. Give antihistamine therapy.
Vasculitis	Allopurinol Barbiturates Gold Penicillins Sulfonamides Thiazide derivatives	Soft, small erythematous papules or urticarial wheals that blanch when pressure is applied Over several hours to several days, lesions become firm and dark red or purple.	Remove offending drug. Give antihistamine therapy.
Exfoliative dermatitis (Lyell syndrome, toxic epidermal necrolysis syndrome)	Allopurinol Barbiturates Hydantoin derivatives Penicillins Phenazone derivatives Sulfonamides Sulindac	Diffuse erythema followed by bullae and loss of large portions of epidermal tissue	Remove offending drug. Give cyclosporine therapy. Give intensive, specialized care similar to that given to a child with severe burns.

Data from Weston, W., Lane, A., & Morelli, J. (2007). *Color textbook of pediatric dermatology*. St. Louis, MO: Mosby.

future. Medication derivatives from the same family as the agent that caused the adverse reaction should be avoided. Recommend that the child wear a MedicAlert bracelet to notify others that the child has a medication allergy.

GENETIC AND IMMUNE-RELATED DISORDERS WITH DERMATOLOGIC MANIFESTATIONS

Several skin conditions appear linked to genetic susceptibility or to a systemic immunologic response. The conditions discussed in this chapter include urticaria and angioedema and SJS. Neurofibromatosis and dermatomyositis are rare disorders that may be encountered in the pediatric population but are not discussed in this chapter (see thePoint Supplemental Information: Neurofibromatosis and Dermatomyositis). Neurofibromatosis is a common autosomal dominant disorder in which affected children develop benign and malignant tumors. Childhood dermatomyositis is a multisystem inflammatory disease of uncertain origin that affects primarily skin and muscles.

In many cases, the exact mechanisms that trigger the dermatologic clinical features are unknown. The underlying insult that causes skin injury is likely to produce other clinical manifestations that can be severe. The child is cared for by an interdisciplinary team that includes support from dermatology, rheumatology, physical therapy, and nutrition specialists. Treatment is aimed at controlling skin lesions, preventing or reversing other systemic manifestations, and supporting the child and family through long-term therapy if required.

URTICARIA AND ANGIOEDEMA

Urticaria, a hypersensitivity reaction commonly called *hives*, is manifested by well-demarcated, raised erythematous lesions that blanch with pressure. The lesions are usually pruritic and involve the superficial layer of the dermis. Urticaria is a symptom that might be triggered by several disease states as well as medications, foods, animal stings, pollen, infections, heredity, and physical environment (cold). Urticaria and angioedema may occur at any age, although incidence is higher in young adults. Although in many cases the exact causative source may not be known, approximately 15% to 25% of the population has a history of one or more episodes of urticaria, most cases of which are acute and self-limiting and do not extend beyond a 6-week period. Acute or transient urticaria is more common in children and young adults. In some cases, the urticaria extends beyond the 6 weeks and may display periods of exacerbation for years.

When the urticaria extends deep into the dermis (subcutaneous or submucosal layers), it is known as **angioedema**. Angioedema is usually characterized by a tingling, burning sensation in normal-appearing skin with overlying swelling. Although urticaria is relatively common in children, angioedema is much less so.

Pathophysiology

Generally speaking, urticaria is caused by a complex interplay of immunologic-mediated antigen–antibody responses to the release of histamine from mast cells

CHART 25-4 · Mechanisms That Cause Urticaria

IgE-Mediated Urticaria

Allergic reactions (drugs, food, insect venom)

Physical urticaria (cold, heat, pressure, vibration, solar exposure, exercise)

Atopic diathesis

Complement-Mediated Urticaria

Collagen vascular diseases

Transfusion-related reactions

Hereditary angioedema

Acquired angioedema

Serum sickness (type III)

Necrotizing vasculitis

Non–IgE-Mediated Urticaria

Direct mast cell–releasing agents (opiates, muscle relaxants, radiocontrast media)

Histamine-releasing agents

Intolerance reactions (aspirin, nonsteroidal anti-inflammatory medications)

as a result of the trigger agent or toxin. The histamine release causes vasodilation and edema of the skin and mucous membranes, with vasodilation and increased vascular permeability causing the erythema and characteristic wheal (Bailey & Shaker, 2008). Urticaria may be the result of an immune-mediated reaction (IgE), a complement-mediated reaction, or a nonimmunologic-mediated mechanism (Chart 25-4). In the physical urticarias (those caused by cold, heat, etc.), histamine levels appear normal. The chemical mediator of physical urticarias appears to occur through cholinergic fibers of the autonomic nervous system.

Assessment

Begin evaluation of the child with a thorough family history of hives, angioedema, arthritis, atopy, and itching. Elicit information that specifically identifies when the lesions occur, how long the lesions last, and the events that might precipitate a flare-up. Note any association between some type of food or medication (such as aspirin) and occurrence of the lesions.

Acute urticaria and angioedema are defined by the sudden appearance of lesions or attacks of sensation (tingling). The location of the lesions may assist in determining the cause. The lesions are pruritic with erythematous raised wheals, 2 to 15 mm in diameter, scattered over the body. The center of the lesion is pale in color and has tense edema.

The wheals usually persist for 20 minutes to 3 hours, disappear, and then reappear at another location. An episode generally lasts 24 to 48 hours, although it may extend up to 6 weeks. When lesions appear for longer than 6 weeks, the urticaria is considered to be chronic. The subcutaneous extensions of the lesions, or angioedema, appear as large swellings around the eyelids, lips, face, trunk, genitalia, and extremities.

The physical urticarias are characterized by large (10 to 20 mm) blotchy erythematous areas surrounded by small (1 to 3 mm) central wheals. Heat, exposure to cold, ingestion of hot or spicy foods, a febrile illness, hot baths, and exercise sufficient to raise the body temperature by 0.5° C induce an attack. Delayed-pressure urticaria can initiate angioedema 4 to 6 hours after the pressure; the angioedema can last up to 24 hours. This condition is most commonly seen in adolescents who wear backpacks to carry their schoolbooks. If these lesions are fixed longer than 48 hours, it is most likely not urticaria. Angioedema has thick, edematous plaques usually involving the face. These are not associated with pruritus but rather with pain, burning, or both. This edema may last up to 72 hours, with gastrointestinal or laryngeal symptoms present (Bailey & Shaker, 2008).

The physical examination for urticaria involves light stroking of the skin with a blunt object, which may cause an intense wheal and flare reaction known as *dermatographism*. Applying a warm or cold stimulus that causes the appearance of wheals and intense itching can help to diagnose cold- or heat-induced urticaria. An exercise challenge may be used to help elicit exercise-induced urticaria.

Interdisciplinary Interventions

An acute attack of angioedema can be treated with oral antihistamines for 3 to 4 weeks until the antigen is eliminated. Hydroxyzine hydrochloride or diphenhydramine hydrochloride are most commonly used. Severe acute cases may require the use of subcutaneous or intramuscular epinephrine; in a few cases, systemic corticosteroids may also be needed.

If airway involvement results from angioedema, close monitoring in an acute care facility is indicated until the attack has been resolved. Opioids may be required for relief of abdominal pain, and nasogastric suction may be needed if the child has emesis. H_2-receptor antagonists may be useful in some children in controlling airway or bowel reactions.

Pharmacotherapy may include H_1 antihistamines. A prolonged course (3 months or longer) using second-generation drugs (e.g., cetirizine [Zyrtec], fexofenadine [Allegra], loratadine [Claritin]) may be needed to induce a remission. Failure to induce a remission may require dosage recalculation or change to a different antihistamine. Medication withdrawal must be gradual to prevent a rebound effect. If the urticaria recurs, the medication must be restarted at full strength.

Community Care

Because all triggers cannot be avoided, an anaphylactic emergency kit must be available to the child. Long-term care for the child should include avoidance of certain foods from the diet and avoidance of medications that contain aspirin or related compounds. A daily diet and symptom record can be initiated to help identify precipitating events. If a clear precipitating factor is not found, an elimination diet of lamb, chicken, rice, and

water for 2 to 4 weeks may be tried. If the child's symptoms do not improve, the urticaria was probably not caused by a food substance. A dietitian may provide suggestions for how nutritional requirements may be met through the diet phase and whether certain foods should be avoided for a long-term period.

Physical triggers should also be avoided. For example, thermal protection is important for children with cold-induced urticaria, and the generous use of sunscreen is helpful for the child with solar urticaria. The child with exercise-induced symptoms should be encouraged to decrease or stop the activity at the first sign of symptoms. Exercise-induced urticaria has been reported to be more pronounced in individuals who exercise after ingestion of certain foods such as shellfish, celery, peaches, grapes, and wheat. Therefore, some children must avoid exercise for 4 to 6 hours after ingesting a known offending food or medication.

No major complications arise from urticaria that is confined to the skin. Urticaria with respiratory manifestations, or involving vital structures by angioedema, is a more serious condition.

STEVENS-JOHNSON SYNDROME

SJS (also called *erythema multiforme major*) is the severe bullous form of erythema multiforme characterized by lesions of the skin and mucous membranes, fever, sore throat, headache, and systemic toxic effects. The lesions begin as macules and can develop into papules, vesicles, bullae, or urticarial plaques. The most extreme cases are called *toxic epidermal necrolysis syndrome* or *Lyell syndrome*; in these cases, the entire skin surface is affected.

SJS occurs in children and young adults and affects males more frequently than females. Acute and sudden onset often follows an upper respiratory infection, whereas the actual syndrome is generally triggered by medications. The drugs most commonly associated with SJS include sulfonamides, anticonvulsants, penicillin, antimalarial sulfadoxine–pyrimethamine, and barbiturates. Increasing evidence indicates that SJS may be the result of genetic susceptibility, although neither the etiology nor the exact mechanism is known (Papay et al., 2012; Vanfleteren et al., 2003). Finally, the association of SJS with patchy pneumonia, increased titers or cold agglutinins, and the isolation of *Mycoplasma pneumoniae* have suggested a relation to *Mycoplasma* infection.

The mortality rate of SJS may be as high as 10% during the acute phase, particularly in children with pulmonary involvement. Subsequently, the disease is self-limiting; skin lesions gradually subside without scarring in 1 to 4 weeks, although mucous membrane lesions may persist for months. Recurrences are rare (Papay et al., 2012; Vanfleteren et al., 2003).

Assessment

Most children with SJS have a prodrome of fever, headache, sore throat, and malaise; nonspecific respiratory infection; and possibly petechial rash. The hallmark of the syndrome is an erythematous papular skin lesion that enlarges by peripheral expansion and usually develops a central vesicle. This eruption may involve cutaneous surfaces, including the palms and soles. Lesions may be scattered or confluent, and new lesions appear for 2 to 4 weeks after onset. Cutaneous lesions tend to rupture, leaving the child at risk for fluid loss, anemia, bacterial superinfection, and sepsis. Vesiculobullous lesions also occur on mucous membranes of the conjunctivae, nares, mouth, anorectal junction, vulvovaginal region, and urethral meatus. Lesions have been described in the larynx, trachea, bronchi, bladder, and gastrointestinal tract. Esophageal stricture or visual impairment from corneal scarring may produce long-term sequelae such as eating difficulties and impaired vision. The diagnosis of SJS is made by history, presence of vascular lesions on at least two mucous membranes, fever, presence of systemic toxic effects, and appearance of classic cutaneous iris or target lesions.

Laboratory tests are not helpful in diagnosing SJS, so diagnosis is made clinically. However, complete blood count with differential; blood urea nitrogen; creatinine; electrolytes; urinalysis; and culture of lesions, blood, and urine are useful in supportive evaluation.

Interdisciplinary Interventions

The goals of therapy are to provide supportive care while the epidermis regenerates and minimize the potential for subsequent morbidity. An interdisciplinary specialty team of health care providers is required to adequately assess and manage SJS, including critical care intensivists and ophthalmologists. Nursing care is aimed at supportive measures and includes meticulous skin care, early detection and treatment of infection, careful attention to fluid balance, nutritional support, and alleviation of symptoms.

Pharmacologic Interventions

Antimicrobial silver sulfadiazine cream is generally not used because of the risk that the sulfa will trigger further eruptions. Use age-appropriate pain assessment tools for pain management. Viscous lidocaine may be used for pain relief on oral mucosa and in the perineal area.

ALERT   *When applying viscous lidocaine to the oral cavity with a cotton-tipped swab, do so sparingly. Swallowing viscous lidocaine interferes with the child's gag reflex and ability to swallow.*

Antibiotic therapy is indicated only when sepsis is diagnosed or strongly suggested. Neutropenia has been shown to indicate a poor prognosis and has been suggested as a criterion for prophylactic antibiotic therapy. Systemic steroid use is not indicated and may increase the risk of complications such as sepsis and gastrointestinal hemorrhage. Antimicrobials used may include macrolides, amoxicillin–clavulanic acid, and even acyclovir (Papay et al., 2012; Vanfleteren et al., 2003).

Nutritional Interventions

Nutritional management is based on severity of symptoms and ranges from a soft or liquid diet, in mild cases, to IV fluid management, in severe cases. The child may require parenteral nutrition during acute phases of the illness.

Surgical Management

Surgical consultation is required for children with severe skin lesions; treatment is similar to that for a child with burns, and the child may be managed in a burn unit or a pediatric intensive care unit. For severe damage, operative wound debridement and xenografts may be required.

Supportive Interventions

Children with SJS are usually admitted to a pediatric intensive care unit where supportive care for children who are potentially unstable, and particularly those with hypovolemia, can be cared for appropriately. Therapy includes daily bathing with saline, antibiotic ointments applied to eroded areas, and antibiotic mesh gauze applied to denuded areas.

Skin care includes use of sheepskin or air-fluid beds to reduce pressure on blistering or eroding skin. Lesions should be bathed daily with normal saline or Burow solution compresses and dressed with antibiotic or mesh gauze, depending on the extent of lesions. The child should be repositioned frequently. Children with extensive lesions should be placed in reverse isolation. Mucous membranes should also be cleansed with normal saline, followed by application of petroleum jelly ointment. Saline compresses can be used on eyes to reduce crusting of eyelid margins. Be alert to early symptoms of infection, such as elevated temperature, positive blood culture, change in vital signs, or increased irritability.

As for a burn patient, careful monitoring of fluid balance is required. Fluid resuscitation with colloids or crystalloids may be required for hypovolemia or sepsis-induced hypotension. Urine output should equal 1 to 2 mL/kg/hr. A Foley catheter may be required for children with difficulty voiding or with urethritis.

The ophthalmologist should examine the child's eyes daily, mechanically separating the lids and the palpebral from the bulbar conjunctiva, if necessary, and removing pseudomembranes obstructing vision. Children may need systemic as well as topical analgesia for this procedure. Topical antibiotics are prescribed for children with positive eye cultures. A follow-up appointment should be made with the ophthalmologist after discharge to ensure that no permanent visual impairment has occurred.

Community Care

If the onset of SJS is thought to be linked with a particular drug, the child and family should be taught to avoid that agent in the future. Long-term follow-up is necessary for children with mucosal or skin-scarring complications. Ophthalmologic consultation and follow-up visits are an important aspect of the overall plan of care.

THERMAL INJURIES

Thermal injuries are caused by hot or cold environmental forces and range from redness of the dermis to loss of circulation and cellular functioning in an extremity or other part of the body. Severe burns are among the most debilitating and disfiguring of all skin alterations. The third most common accidental injury in children, all but the most minor burns can have a traumatic effect on the child and the family. Even sunburn, although it is a type of minor burn and is substantially less ominous than major burns, may have long-term carcinogenic effects. Cold injury can also cause disfigurement and long-term discomfort to the child if exposure to cold–wet or cold–dry conditions is prolonged.

The most important interdisciplinary management strategy for thermal injuries is to teach prevention. Wearing proper attire, using protective skin creams and lotions, and regulating the time exposed to very hot or very cold weather conditions are important interventions to prevent thermal injury.

FIRE AND BURN INJURIES

Burn injury to children may be accidental or nonaccidental. Nonaccidental injury involves child abuse by burning or from neglect. For children younger than the age of 5 years, burns are likely to occur as a result of scalds or contact burns. Natural curiosity and increasing mobility in the child at this age contribute to the risk. Male children have a slightly higher risk for fire-related deaths, as do children living in rural areas. Black children are more than three times as likely as other races to die in a fire (Safe Kids Worldwide, 2011a, 2011b). The percentage of body surface area burned remains one of the most important factors associated with predisposing morbidity and mortality.

CROSS-CULTURAL CARE

Skin lesions and irregular markings on the child's body may be a result of folk practices used by the family to treat a specific illness. For instance, in the Chinese culture, the practices of cupping, skin scraping, and moxibustion can injure the child's skin. Cupping is a process that creates a vacuum in a cup by placing a heated material in the cup. The cup is then placed on the child's skin until easily removed. The treatment leaves a burn mark. Skin scraping is the process of applying oil to an area of the skin, then scraping the area with a coin repeatedly, leaving linear bruising on the skin. In the folk practice of moxibustion, the ignited moxa plant is applied to specific areas of the body to treat diseases that are caused from an excess of yin. This causes burn marks on the child. The nurse should emphasize to the family that, although these practices are meaningful, they can further injure the child. In addition, the burns and lesions on the skin caused by these folk practices can become infected.

Thermal injuries are the second most common cause of death in children in the United States, second only to motor vehicle accidents. An average of 496 children die every year in fires or from other burn injuries. The most common burn injury in a child younger than 5 years of age is from scalding by either spilling of hot liquids or from bath water.

> **ALERT** At 140° F (60° C), it takes 5 seconds for hot water to cause full-thickness burns. A temperature of 104° F (40° C) is the recommended maximum bathing temperature for children.

Burn injuries in children are preventable. More than one half of all pediatric burn injuries (59.5%) treated in emergency departments resulted from thermal burns. The most frequently injured body parts were the hand/finger (36%), followed by the head/face (21%) (D'Souza et al., 2009; Safe Kids Worldwide, 2011a, 2011b). Almost all of the burn injuries (92%) treated in emergency departments occurred at home (see thePoint Supplemental Information: Types of Burn Injuries).

Pathophysiology

Burn injury causes a multisystem cascade of effects. Many of its manifestations and outcomes are unique in the pediatric population because of physiologic differences between adults and children (Developmental Considerations 25-5). In addition to skin injury, the lungs, cardiovascular system, fluid and electrolyte balances, and metabolism may be damaged or altered; the potential for infection and sepsis also increases as the percentage of burned body surface area increases. Immediately after the injury, blood flow increases in the area around the injury. The burned tissue releases vasoactive substances, which increase capillary permeability. This increased permeability creates a fluid shift to the interstitial space (i.e., third spacing) with edema. This phase precedes the diuretic phase, which generally occurs 48 to 72 hours after burn injury, when the patient becomes more stable (Herndon, 2012). Managing fluids and electrolytes thus becomes vitally important.

Respiratory Compromise

Many noxious substances may be inhaled. The consequences of inhalation usually depend on the types of chemicals being released by the burning substance, the duration of contact, and whether the person was in a confined space. Obvious signs of inhalation injury include burns of the mouth, lips, nose, and face as well as sooty material deposited in those areas. Other signs include a hoarse voice, cough, wheezing, and dyspnea—all signs of respiratory distress.

Three types of respiratory system injury can occur with a burn: upper respiratory tract injury, pulmonary injury, and carbon monoxide inhalation and hypoxia injury (Table 25-7). As with all trauma patients, the first priority in managing the pediatric burn patient is to assess airway and breathing. Pulmonary complications of burn injuries account for a large percentage of patient deaths.

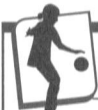

DEVELOPMENTAL CONSIDERATIONS 25-5

Pediatric Differences in the Effects of Burn Injury

- Very young children who have been severely burned have a higher mortality rate than older children and adults with comparable burns.
- Because a child's skin is thinner than an adult's, lower burn temperatures and shorter exposure to heat or chemicals can cause a deeper burn.
- A larger body surface area compared with adults places severely burned children at increased risk for fluid and heat loss. Children are also at increased risk for dehydration and metabolic acidosis secondary to diarrhea, evaporative water loss, and increased fluid requirements.
- The highest proportion of body fluid to mass in children increases the risk of cardiovascular problems because of their less effective cardiovascular response to changing intravascular volume.

- Burns involving more than 10% of TBSA require some form of fluid resuscitation.
- Infants and children are at increased risk for protein and calorie deficiency because they have smaller muscle mass and lower body fat reserves than adults. If they are not eating and their metabolism is increased, their protein and calorie needs will not be met.
- Hypertrophic scarring is more severe and scar maturation is prolonged.
- An immature immune system means an increased risk of infection for infants and young children.
- A delay in growth may follow extensive burns.
- In children, Curling ulcer occurs during the third or fourth week postburn, which is later than in adults.

Upper respiratory injury leads to swelling of the tissues in the throat and the upper airway, resulting in mechanical obstruction of the airway. Swelling starts within a few minutes of the injury, and the airway may occlude within a few minutes to a few hours. The edema remains in the tissues until it is slowly reabsorbed over a period of 2 to 5 days. Respiratory distress may be exhibited by abdominal breathing, head bobbing with respiratory efforts, nasal flaring, coughing, stridor, or wheezing. The young child may exhibit paradoxic inspiratory efforts, which draw the chest wall inward while thrusting out the abdomen. The small size of the pediatric airway may become occluded by tissue edema or mucus plugs, which increases the chance for a respiratory infection.

TABLE 25-7	Types of Respiratory Injury		
Type of Injury	**Cause**	**At Risk For**	**Interdisciplinary Interventions**
Upper airway obstruction	Edema of upper airway secondary to direct burn injury from inhaling superheated air, swallowing extremely hot liquids, or as a consequence of massive tissue swelling associated with extensive burns and burn shock therapy	Mechanical obstruction of upper airway	Intubation of airway; administration of warm, moist mist with oxygen as needed
Inhalation injury	Inhalation of toxic products of combustion (smoke), resulting in chemical irritation and trauma to lung tissue	Impaired gas exchange related to acute pulmonary failure 24–48 hours after burn injury	Early diagnosis of inhalation injury by bronchoscopy, or xenon-133 ventilation–perfusion scan, followed by intubation of airway and ventilatory support using a mechanical ventilator and oxygen as needed
Carbon monoxide	Carbon monoxide released as a by-product of combustion (especially common in structure fires) Carbon monoxide replaces oxygen on the hemoglobin molecule, leading to cellular hypoxia.	Systemic hypoxia, brain damage, death	Administration of 100% oxygen by mask if the child is awake, alert, and able to protect the airway until carboxyhemoglobin level returns to normal range; otherwise, intubation and ventilatory support as required Continued monitoring of blood oxygen levels and oxygen administration until hypoxia resolves

Burn Shock

Burn shock is a type of hypovolemic shock that begins to develop shortly after a burn injury of more than 15% to 20% total body surface area (TBSA) in children. In burns of up to 30% TBSA, the fluid leakage is around the injured area; when more than 30% is involved, the leakage becomes generalized (Herndon, 2012). Mechanisms of burn shock are not well understood, but the sequence of major burn injury followed by massive capillary leakage of circulating fluid into the surrounding tissues is well recognized.

ALERT *Untreated burn shock leads to death from hypovolemia. The larger the total body surface burned, the greater and more rapid the fluid loss.*

Within minutes of a major burn injury, all the capillaries in the circulatory system—not just those in the area of the burn—lose their capillary seal, resulting in leakage of intravascular body fluid into the interstitial spaces; this process is called *third spacing*. This leakage, which peaks during the first 18 to 24 hours after a severe burn, creates a tourniquet effect and results in compartment syndrome. Should this syndrome occur, surgical incisions of the burned tissue (escharotomy) or muscle sheaths (fasciotomy) will most likely be performed. Erythrocytes and leukocytes remain in the circulation and produce an elevated hematocrit and leukocyte count. Burn shock gradually decreases after 48 to 72 hours, at which time the capillary seal is generally restored, and more fluid stays in the circulating system, with increasing diuresis.

As with any other trauma patient in hypovolemic shock, concurrent systemic changes also occur after the burn injury, including the following events:

- Ileus, which persists for about 48 hours after the burn
- Decreased blood flow to the stomach and intestines, resulting in bacterial translocation into the peritoneum
- Curling ulcer, or true duodenal ulceration, which usually develops 10 to 14 days after burn injury
- Increased heart rate to increase cardiac preload
- Increased respiratory rate to meet the increased metabolic needs of the stressed body
- Decreased urinary output and increased specific gravity
- Increased blood urea nitrogen and creatinine
- Decreased hemoglobin and hematocrit

Fluid and Electrolyte Deficits

In addition to the large amount of intravascular fluid volume lost during burn shock, a child has a larger body mass-to-surface area ratio than an adult, thus increasing the extent of heat and evaporative water loss (Herndon, 2012). After the initial 24 hours—even though the capillary seal is restored and circulating volume is maintained—major fluid and electrolyte losses continue to occur through the burn wound until wound closure is achieved. Fluid loss through the skin after burn injury peaks after the fourth day but continues to be a concern until the area heals. Fluid and electrolyte imbalances can occur rapidly. Whenever hypotension develops in burn patients, the body's ability to fight infection at the tissue level is compromised by inadequate tissue perfusion to the skin. Infection usually develops quickly, and infected wounds lead to more tissue destruction. Overwhelming infection rapidly leads to sepsis.

Both renal blood flow and urinary output are curtailed after a severe burn. Conditions such as acute tubular necrosis may follow inadequate fluid replacement, glycosuria occurs in patients who are metabolically stressed, and urinary output is severely curtailed, which alters blood urea nitrogen and creatinine levels. This oliguric phase commonly persists for the first 24 to 36 hours after burn injury, followed by a diuretic phase. During these times, monitoring serum electrolytes, especially sodium and potassium, is essential.

Metabolic Alterations

The major metabolic responses to burn injury include

- Hypermetabolism
- Elevated catecholamine levels
- Hyperglycemia
- Increased nutritional needs
- Growth delay

Hypermetabolism characterizes the metabolic response to burn injury and occurs in proportion to the extent of the burn. Energy expenditures may increase from 40% to 100% above basal levels in children with burns of more than 30% TBSA. Core body temperature for a child with a major burn injury will reset at about 99.5° to 100.4° F (37.5° to 38° C) and will remain at that level or higher until skin coverage is achieved. When exposed to cooler temperatures, the child begins to shiver, increasing the oxygen and energy demands of the body tremendously. A warm environment minimizes the hemodynamic and metabolic stresses associated with major burn injury.

Elevated catecholamine levels result from the child's increased core temperature and metabolic rate. In addition, the stress associated with treatments, including the surface water evaporation that occurs with exposure of the child to room temperature air, increases catecholamine release, metabolic stress, and energy demands.

Hyperglycemia is common after burn injury because glucose metabolism is also altered. The elevation of fasting blood glucose levels above normal is related to the severity of the injury or to the presence of systemic infection. Young children may quickly deplete their glucose stores and may become hypoglycemic unless they receive adequate nutritional support.

Increased nutritional needs are associated with the hypermetabolic state required to heal a major wound. Major injury and infections can lead to weight loss and severe alterations in body composition, even when calories and protein are supplied in substantial amounts. Nitrogen imbalance is associated with failure to meet increased nutritional needs. Wound healing cannot occur when the child is in negative nitrogen balance; thus, the provision of adequate nutrition is essential to recovery. However, overfeeding results in increased carbon dioxide production that requires increasing respiratory rates to clear and, in addition, can cause fatty liver and other hepatic dysfunction. Thus, one goal of nursing care is to provide sufficient nutritional support.

Growth delay follows depression of growth hormone levels after major burn injury. The child will not increase in height for many months after the injury, while the body focuses on restoring and healing damaged tissue. A growth spurt is usually noted about a year after the recovery phase.

Infection and Sepsis

The warm, moist environment of a major burn wound is an ideal location for bacterial growth. Wound infection is a great risk because a burn injury presents a source of organisms capable of producing disease, a mode of transmission, and a susceptible host. The most common bacteria are found in the burn wound patient's own body, especially those bacteria normally present on the skin and in the gastrointestinal tract. Other bacteria can easily be spread to the patient by staff members who do not wash their hands after caring for other patients (nosocomial infection). Topical burn creams are used because the local blood supply to the area of burn injury is destroyed with the burn and systemic antibiotics are, therefore, not delivered to the burn wound.

Infection in partial-thickness burn wounds converts the area to a full-thickness injury, which then requires skin grafting. Hypovolemia for any reason, especially in children, greatly increases the incidence of wound conversion.

Systemic infection can result from aspiration of gastrointestinal fluid into the lungs, which may lead to pneumonia. Alternately, anaerobic bacteria may develop at the interface between the burn wound and the healthy tissue. If bacterial levels increase to the extent that invasion into the underlying tissue occurs, infection results. Bacteria then gain entrance into the systemic circulation and spread into other organs, causing sepsis.

The child's immune system is impaired after major burn injury and cannot protect the child from infection and sepsis caused by previously benign bacteria (Herndon, 2012). Monocyte and macrophage components of the immune system are not functioning well nor are white blood cells, such as neutrophils, granulocytes, and basophils. Phagocytosis, the normal mechanism for removing debris from a wound, does not occur.

Scarring and Disability

Although scarring is part of the healing process, burn scars can create substantial problems. Hypertrophic scarring results in an elevated, raised, reddened, and painful area that is very susceptible to traumatic injury from routine daily activities. Keloid scars form in the area of the burn and then expand onto unburned

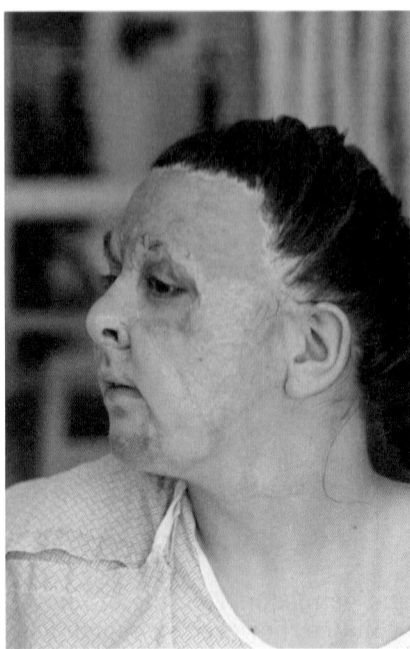

Figure 25-14 Child with burn scarring. Courtesy of Shriners Hospital for Children. Reprinted with permission.

tissue (Fig. 25-14). Burned areas become stiff and, without therapy, range of motion can become severely limited. Muscles tend to shorten, and skin contracts in burn areas involving the joints. Extension muscles are not as strong as flexor muscles, and injured areas over joints (especially the elbows, axillae, and knees) tend to become permanently fixed in the flexed position.

Assessment

The type and extent of burn injury will guide the assessment process. For instance, when child abuse is suspected, additional assessment factors to evaluate include descriptions of how the burn occurred (from the family and child), location (palms, soles, flexor surface of thighs or perineum), and patterns.

If the burn injury is severe, the physical assessment should begin with a primary assessment of the airways (the airway, breathing, and circulation [ABCs]). The most common cause of death during the first hour after an acute burn injury is respiratory impairment. Next, consider fluid and electrolyte parameters, appropriate fluid treatment, and pain issues. Finally, evaluate the extent of skin injury. This evaluation is based on many criteria. Burns can be described as superficial (first degree), partial (second degree; Fig. 25-15), or full-thickness (third degree), depending on the depth to which the skin has been destroyed (Table 25-8). The percentage of the TBSA must also be considered and can be calculated using the rule of nines. This method divides the surface area of the body into areas of 9% or multiples of 9% equal to 18%. When all body areas of 9% are summed, 1% remains, which is assigned to the

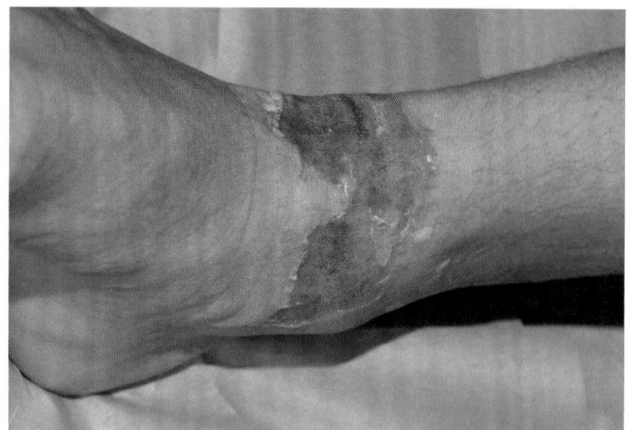

Figure 25-15 Child with partial-thickness (second-degree) burn. Courtesy of Shriners Hospital for Children. Reprinted with permission.

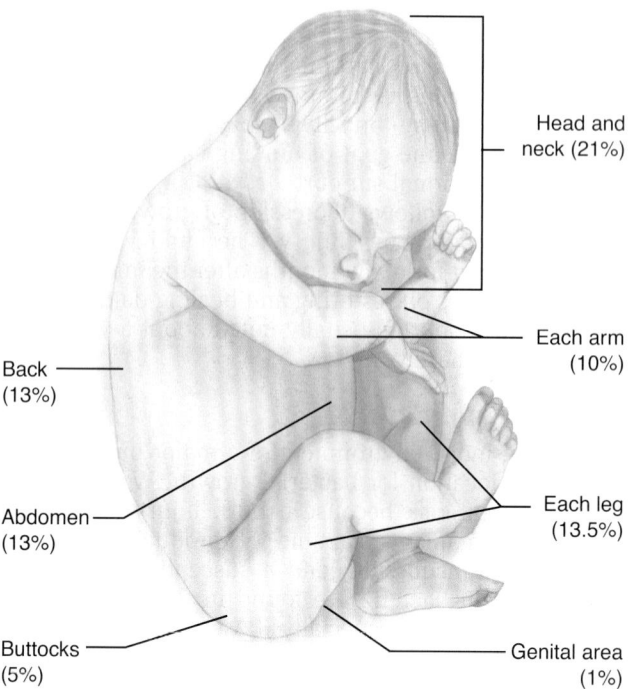

Head and neck (21%)

Each arm (10%)

Back (13%)

Abdomen (13%)

Each leg (13.5%)

Buttocks (5%)

Genital area (1%)

Figure 25-16 Rule of nines for babies and young children.

genitalia and perineum. The rule of nines is less accurate for children, however, so a modified version is presented in Figure 25-16.

For patients younger than 15 years of age, a second, more precise method of estimating burn size is used; burn estimation tables subdivide body areas into segments and assign a proportionate percentage of body surface to each area based on age (Fig. 25-17). The head of a newborn baby, for example, is proportionately much larger than any other area of the body. As a child grows, the lower extremities assume more body surface area; the head becomes relatively smaller compared with the rest of the body. Also, rather than being viewed as a whole, the lower extremity is divided into foot, leg, and thigh areas.

A third method of estimating burn injury extent uses the size of the patient's hand, assuming the palmar surface of the hand is roughly 1% of the total body surface. Visualizing the patient's hand covering the burn wound approximates the amount of body surface involved, especially if the burn areas are scattered.

Diagnostic Tests

A complete blood count should be obtained to establish baseline levels; many blood levels will be altered during the first 24 to 48 hours as a result of tremendous fluid shifts. For example, hematocrit will often be elevated secondary to fluid loss. White blood cell counts may also be elevated as an acute-phase reaction; increased counts later in the healing process could indicate infection. Assessing actual or potential pulmonary injury in children with flame injury involves measuring arterial blood gas and carbon monoxide levels. In addition, basic renal function tests, baseline clotting studies, type and crossmatch, chest radiographs, and pulse oximetry should be included (Herndon, 2012).

TABLE 25-8	Severity of Burns			
Depth of Burn	**Thickness**	**Appearance of Burn**	**Sensation**	**Example of Cause**
First degree	Superficial epithelium	Erythema	Painful	Sunburn
Second degree	Partial thickness Destruction into, but not through, epidermis	Blisters Peeling epidermis Swelling White or red mottling Weeping, wet	Painful Hypersensitive to air, touch	Very deep sunburn Scalds
Third degree	Full-thickness destruction of skin into hypodermis Death to all skin appendages and subcutaneous tissue	Translucent Mottled white or tan Waxy Leathery Basically dry	Painless (initially)	Fire Prolonged exposure to hot liquid Electricity
Fourth degree	Full thickness through all layers of skin down into the muscle and bone	Looks like third-degree burn	No sensation because of nerve damage	Prolonged flame contact High-voltage electrical injury

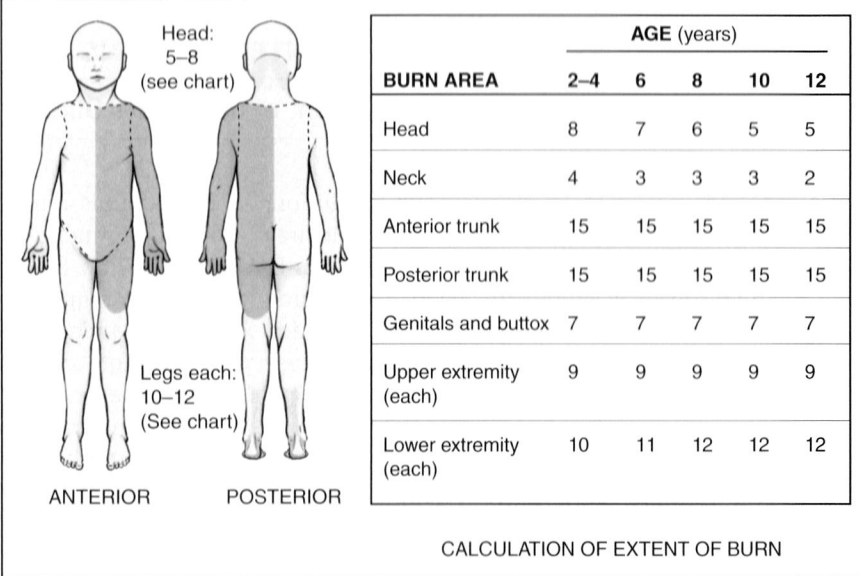

	AGE (years)				
BURN AREA	**2–4**	**6**	**8**	**10**	**12**
Head	8	7	6	5	5
Neck	4	3	3	3	2
Anterior trunk	15	15	15	15	15
Posterior trunk	15	15	15	15	15
Genitals and buttox	7	7	7	7	7
Upper extremity (each)	9	9	9	9	9
Lower extremity (each)	10	11	12	12	12

Head: 5–8 (see chart)

Legs each: 10–12 (See chart)

ANTERIOR   POSTERIOR

CALCULATION OF EXTENT OF BURN

Figure 25-17 Child burn size estimation table. Data from Boniol, M., Verriest, J., Pedeux, R. et al. (2007). Proportion of skin surface area of children and young adults from 2 to 18 years old. *Journal of Investigative Dermatology, 128*, 461–464.

Nursing Diagnoses and Outcomes

In addition to the nursing diagnoses presented in Nursing Plan of Care 25-1, the following diagnoses are appropriate for the child with a burn injury.

Nursing Diagnosis: Impaired skin integrity related to effects of burn

Outcome: Child's skin will heal without infection, as evidenced by restoration of the epithelial layer in partial-thickness injury or adherence of skin graft to area of full-thickness injury.

Nursing Diagnosis: Acute pain related to response to thermal injury and related procedures

Outcome: Child will experience pain relief, as evidenced by age-appropriate behaviors, adequate nutritional intake, and appropriate sleep patterns.

Nursing Diagnosis: Ineffective airway clearance/impaired gas exchange related to upper airway edema, smoke inhalation injury, or carbon monoxide/hypoxia

Outcomes: Child will maintain normal oxygen saturation, will have unlabored respirations at a rate appropriate for age, will have clear bilateral breath sounds, and carboxyhemoglobin is or will be normal.

Nursing Diagnosis: Ineffective peripheral tissue perfusion related to burn shock

Outcome: Child will maintain a urine output of 1 to 2 mL/kg/hr for the first 24 hours after the burn and will remain alert and oriented.

Nursing Diagnosis: Risk for deficient fluid volume related to loss of skin integrity in the area of the burn and systemic shifting of plasma and plasma components from the circulatory system into interstitial and intracellular spaces secondary to impaired capillary integrity

Outcome: Child will maintain normal fluid and electrolyte balance, as evidenced by intake and output measurements and serum electrolyte values that are within normal limits.

Nursing Diagnosis: Risk for infection related to burn wound contamination or to pulmonary complications

Outcome: Child will achieve wound closure without developing infection, systemic sepsis, or pneumonia.

Nursing Diagnosis: Imbalanced nutrition: Less than body requirements related to hypermetabolism and the increased energy requirements of wound healing

Outcomes:
- Child will maintain muscle mass and protein stores appropriate for age.
- Child's nitrogen balance and energy expenditure studies will consistently yield balanced results.

Nursing Diagnosis: Disturbed body image related to perception of appearance

Outcomes:
- Child will reenter previous social settings and will express a feeling of comfort in these areas.
- Family will provide emotional support for the child.
- Child will discuss feelings related to reactions of others to the child's change in appearance.

Interdisciplinary Interventions

Minor burn injuries (superficial or first-degree burns) are generally treated on an outpatient basis. Hospitalization is indicated for burn injuries greater than 10% TBSA in children; greater than 5% full thickness (third degree); any burns to eyes, ears, face, hands, feet, or genitalia; inhalation injuries; electrical burns; burns complicated by other comorbidities; or any burns with concomitant trauma (Herndon, 2012). Therapy for all burn injuries is designed to promote wound healing, prevent infection, and provide pain relief (Nursing Interventions 25-6). The goals of burn wound

NURSING INTERVENTIONS 25-6

Management of the Child's Burns

Eyes/Eyelids

Upon admission, irrigate the eyes with sterile solution. Eyelids will swell shut for 3–5 days. Cleanse the area gently; do not attempt to force the eyes open. After the edema resolves, wash the area every 8 hours and apply ointment and eye drops per physician's order. Inform the child that vision may be blurred because of the application of medications.

Ears

Upon admission, perform a gentle cleansing and use a cotton-tipped applicator to remove debris/eschar and blisters and secure hair away from the burned area. Position the child without using a pillow to prevent further trauma to the ears because wounds tend to adhere to pillows or bed linens. Apply Sulfamylon ointment as ordered by the physician.

Face

Upon admission, remove blisters and shave face (if age appropriate), except for eyebrows, as indicated. Apply bacitracin or other ointment per physician's order. Cleanse the area every 8 hours and reapply topical ointment. The area will heal quickly (7–10 days) if it is a superficial burn because of an abundant blood supply. Deeper burns are skin grafted early to decrease scarring. Pillows are not used with anterior neck burns to minimize scarring from chin to neck.

Hands

Upon admission, remove rings or other jewelry. Remove blisters and apply a topical antibiotic ointment (silver sulfadiazine), wrapping each finger individually and wrapping the entire hand in a manner that permits full range of motion. Cleanse the area every 8 hours, and reapply ointment and dressings. Encourage full range of motion and use of the hand. Elevate the child's hand above the level of the heart to promote edema reabsorption. Administer pain medication to facilitate use of the hand. The area will heal quickly (7–10 days) if it is a superficial burn because of abundant blood supply. Deeper burns should be skin grafted early to decrease scarring.

Feet

Upon admission, remove blisters. Apply topical antibiotic ointment (silver sulfadiazine) per physician's order. Wrap the toes individually; wrap the foot so that full range of motion is possible; and apply an elastic bandage, distal to proximal, over the dressing to promote comfort and reduce dependent edema. The patient should ambulate at least every 4 hours during the day unless contraindicated; pain medication should be administered to be effective at ambulation times. Elevate the patient's lower extremities when at rest.

Joints

Upon admission, remove blisters and shave areas with hair. Apply topical ointment per physician's order. Wrap the area to permit full range of motion. Cleanse the area every 8 hours, and reapply ointment and dressings. Shave areas of hair growth every 3–4 days. Encourage full range of motion. When at rest, joints should be kept in extension to prevent contracture formation.

Perineum

Upon admission, perform thorough cleansing and rinsing of the area, remove blisters, and shave the area. Insert a bladder catheter before edema accumulates. Apply silver sulfadiazine, per physician's order, directly to the perineum or onto diapers before application. Maintain the bladder catheter until the edema subsides. Cleanse the area after each stool/voiding, and reapply silver sulfadiazine. Scrotal edema can accumulate and may impair walking until resolved.

Circumferential Burns

Upon admission, identify areas of full-thickness circumferential burn. Cleanse the area, remove blisters, and shave as needed. Monitor distal pulses every 15 minutes using a Doppler monitor. If distal pulses diminish or disappear, notify the physician immediately and prepare for escharotomy or fasciotomy. After the procedure, check for pulses every 15 minutes for 24 hours postburn. If pulses diminish or disappear again, notify the physician. Apply topical ointment and dressings to the area per physician's order.

---

management are to close the wound and prevent infection. Wound closure is determined by depth and extent and is accomplished either by supporting spontaneous healing or by initiating surgical repair.

Many of the normal functions of the skin are altered by burn injuries (see thePoint Supplemental Information: Functions of Skin Altered by Burn Injury). Treatment of major burn injuries must correct respiratory compromise, burn shock, fluid and electrolyte deficits, and metabolic alterations; prevent infection and sepsis; and minimize scarring and disability.

Pharmacologic Interventions

For any burn, check the child's tetanus immunization status upon admission and ensure that tetanus toxoid is given if the child's immunizations are not up to date because anaerobic and aerobic bacteria can grow at the interface between burned and healthy tissue.

For minor burns, the burned area is covered with an antimicrobial ointment (usually bacitracin or silver sulfadiazine [Silvadene]) and a nonadherent dressing and light gauze (see thePoint Medications and Administration: Administering Topical Agents Commonly Used for Burns). Dressings are usually changed twice daily, with the patient premedicated for pain. Medications such as ibuprofen or acetaminophen are usually effective as an analgesic for minor burn injury, but the actual wound care will be very painful until healing is well established.

For major burn wounds, topical antibacterial agents are used to penetrate the **eschar** (necrotic skin and subcutaneous tissue) and to reduce bacterial growth in and around the wound. Silver sulfadiazine (Silvadene), the topical agent most commonly used, is not typically used on the face or for electrical burns. Facial burns are covered with a light layer of antimicrobial ointment. For burns to the ear or for electrical burns, mafenide (Sulfamylon) is the topical agent of choice because of its deep penetration into the eschar; do not apply it to the face. In a few burn units, protocol requires ointments to be placed on the wounds without a protective dressing. However, in most units, dressings are applied over the wound to keep the area moist and the topical agents in place. Systemic antibiotics are not used to control burn wound bacteria because there is no blood supply to the wound to deliver the drug. If systemic sepsis is diagnosed, systemic antibiotics are administered to eliminate the source of the sepsis, if possible.

caREminder

If systemic sepsis occurs, children exhibit all the signs of hypovolemic shock, but the actual timing of the symptoms depends on the volume status of the child at the time of onset of sepsis.

Pain and itching are both active components of recovery from a burn injury. With partial-thickness burns and in areas used for skin graft donor sites, nerve endings are exposed, and the areas are highly sensitive to pressure pain. Also, the joints underneath develop an arthritic type of pain that is activated with movement. Burn patients awaken each day with chronic pain, stiffness, and aching in the burned areas for many months after the burn is healed.

Itching occurs in all healing areas and causes great distress unless it is relieved with medication. Itching persists for several months after burns heal as new nerve endings and dermal elements reestablish themselves. Alterations in sweat glands after burn injury result in excessive sweat production, which leads to dry skin and itching, adding to the problem.

The perception of pain in the burned child varies widely, but it is usually related to procedural pain from dressing changes or physical therapy or from attempts to remain still to avoid the pain of movement. Chronically abused children learn not to verbalize pain and often withdraw into a trancelike state during painful procedures. Other children protest against each painful procedure with every bit of volume and energy available to them. The amount of protest a child manifests in response to painful procedures should not be the criterion for pain management. Procedural pain can be minimized by administering adequate analgesia 20 to 30 minutes before the procedure (to achieve maximal effect by the time the procedure is started), additional analgesia during the procedure, and analgesia at the completion of the procedure to allow the child to rest and recover. One effective method of pain control is the patient-controlled analgesia pump, which can be used by children as young as 6 years of age. For especially painful procedures, short-acting, memory-altering medications may be used so that the child does not recall the procedure.

caREminder

Administer pain medication before painful procedures so that maximal effectiveness coincides with the procedure. When the child undergoes a procedure, such as skin grafting, that is known to produce prolonged pain, administer pain medication on a scheduled basis rather than as needed after pain is reported.

Morphine is the analgesic of choice. It should be administered by IV. Ketamine is a widely used medication for conscious sedation during hydrotherapy and dressing changes. Oral medications such as acetaminophen with codeine may be used to diminish pain between dressing changes.

In older children, anxiety and anticipatory stress may respond to antianxiety medications. Ensuring adequate sleep and uninterrupted quiet time is essential to allow the child to restore inner resources. Visiting should be unrestricted and individualized to the child's needs and those of the family.

Itching of healing skin can be controlled by medications, such as diphenhydramine hydrochloride (Benadryl) or loratadine (Claritin), and by applying soothing lotions such as Nivea or Eucerin.

Nutritional Interventions

The child with a minor burn should increase fluid intake to replenish loss. The caloric requirements in the child with major burn injury are two to three times the normal basal requirements and necessitate aggressive nutritional support. In addition, healing cannot occur in the presence of negative nitrogen balance. Therefore, establishing and maintaining adequate nutritional intake is essential to survival. Several formulas have been proposed for estimating caloric requirements (see thePoint Supplemental Information: Estimating Calorie Requirements in Burned Patients Using the Galveston Formula).

Correct estimates are important because too little nutritional intake causes weight loss and protein mobilization from muscle, whereas administering excess calories can cause hyperglycemia, liver abnormalities, and increased carbon dioxide production. Weight, calorie and protein counts, and nitrogen balance are monitored daily; when possible, indirect calorimetric measurements of resting energy expenditure are obtained.

caREminder

Burn wounds cannot heal if the child is in negative nitrogen balance. Nutritional support is essential.

Most children with burns exceeding 25% of the TBSA are unable to consume an oral diet sufficient to meet their nutritional requirements. The child may refuse to eat because of the unfamiliarity of hospital food, because of pain, or in an effort to gain control over the environment. Many children require enteral tube feeding with supplemental liquid nutrition with vitamins (A, B, B_6, C, and E) and trace elements (iron, zinc, copper, and magnesium) to promote wound healing. If enteral feeding does not meet all of the child's nutritional needs, parenteral hyperalimentation can be administered. This route is used only as a last resort because of the risk of catheter-related infection and the desire to maintain intestinal integrity.

Surgical Management

Early burn wound excision is indicated for minor burns in which the wound would be slow (taking longer than 2 to 3 weeks) to heal. Only superficial burns with bright-pink wounds that indicate dermal circulation are suitable for conservative treatment (Herndon, 2012). Early surgery provides further benefits, which include removing potentially harmful bacteria, reducing the degree of scarring, and accelerating healing.

caREminder

Meticulous and regular performance of appropriate debridement and use of antimicrobial topicals and cover dressings are the cornerstones of successful burn wound management.

Major burn injury produces eschar, which releases chemical mediators that stimulate leukocytes to digest debris, but this digestion also damages capillaries and skin elements. Necrotic tissue within a wound prolongs inflammation and slows healing and epidermal coverage (Herndon, 2012). Biosurgical agents, such as maggots, are effective at debriding necrotic tissues in regions of deep burn where there is potential damage to tendons.

Debriding a wound removes the necrotic tissue. Initial debridement can be performed in the emergency department or on the unit in the **hydrotherapy** treatment room. Every 12 hours, burns are cleaned, old creams and ointments are removed, and loose tissue is trimmed from around the wound.

Full-thickness burn injuries and most deep partial-thickness burn injuries are managed surgically. Burn tissue is removed by excision. Wound coverage is achieved over healthy, unburned tissue. The skin used to cover the burn wound is harvested from an unburned area (donor site) of the child's own skin in a procedure called an **autograft**. The skin that is used is a paper-thin section of the upper layers of the skin (split-thickness skin graft). To cover a greater area, autograft skin is usually prepared with a skin mesher, which cuts small slits into the graft, enabling it to be stretched to cover an area 1½ to 9 times larger than the original graft. The slit pattern disappears as the graft heals (Fig. 25-18). If blood collects between the excised area and the skin graft, the skin graft will not adhere. Infection can also cause loss of skin grafts.

If the child does not have sufficient unburned skin for autografting, temporary coverage can be achieved by using a **homograft** (cadaveric skin) or **xenograft** (pig skin) that has been specially prepared for that use. A xenograft is applied when extensive early debridement is required; it is replaced every 2 to 3 days. These biologic skin coverings markedly reduce pain and facilitate movement of joints until suitable donor sites become available. Cultured epithelium, cell culture grafts, and synthetic skin substitutes such as Biobrane, Apligraf, and bio-occlusive also are available.

In some burn units, the burn eschar is removed in a two-stage excision and grafting procedure. On the first day, the burn is surgically excised, and the area is covered with antibiotic-soaked dressings. On the second day, the child is returned to surgery, where the autograft is obtained and applied to the previously excised burn areas. In other burn units, excision and skin grafting are accomplished in one procedure, with control of blood

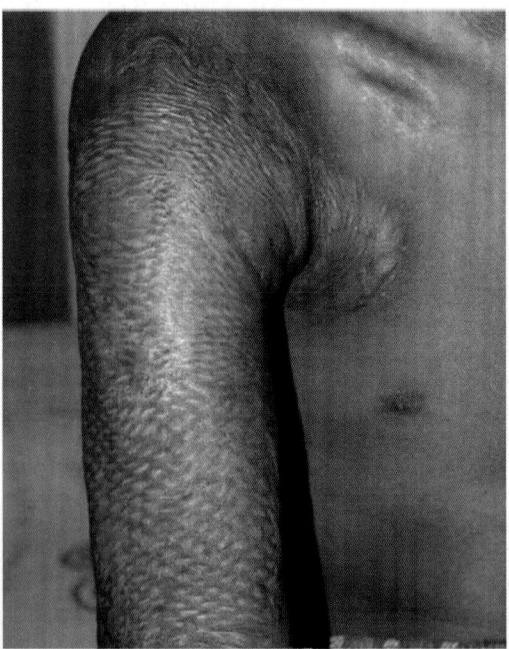

Figure 25-18 Child with healed mesh graft. Courtesy of Shriners Hospital for Children. Reprinted with permission.

loss occurring simultaneously. Blood loss with excision of large burns is massive and may require replacement of as much as one half of the child's circulating blood volume. Burn patients receive many blood transfusions during their hospital course.

Supportive Interventions

For minor burns, first ensure airway patency and evaluate hydration status. Then, remove any restrictive clothing or jewelry; keep the patient warm. If the burn is chemical, remove contaminated shoes and clothing, and flush the area with water. Clean the wound with mild soap and tepid water and debride the area of loose debris and necrotic tissue.

For severely burned children, initial treatment consists of establishing an airway and administering higher concentrations of oxygen to treat respiratory compromise until an assessment and treatment plan are completed.

Upper airway edema is managed by airway intubation and administration of humidified oxygen until the edema subsides, usually about 2 to 5 days later. When initial assessment indicates that airway edema is accumulating and will lead to airway compromise or occlusion, early, planned intubation is preferred over emergency intubation. Inhalation injury is managed by airway intubation and ventilation support at settings appropriate to the child's lung size. A full-thickness burn encircling the chest may limit full expansion of the lungs. In such cases, an escharotomy of the chest may be necessary to enable chest wall expansion.

ALERT   *Children who are severely burned and who do not have other injuries are awake, alert, and oriented. Loss of consciousness in a child with burn injuries is the result of factors other than the burn itself. The most common cause of unconsciousness in flame injury is hypoxia associated with smoke inhalation. If the child is unconscious, implement the ABCs, notify appropriate personnel, and prepare for possible intubation.*

Carbon monoxide inhalation and hypoxia are treated by administering high concentrations of oxygen by mask until the condition is resolved. Using a Venturi mask–type of oxygen delivery device will enable high-flow, high-concentration oxygen. When the inspired concentration of oxygen is increased, the half-life of carbon monoxide decreases.

ALERT   *Beware of extra cooling interventions, such as wet dressing or ice applications, which promote vasoconstriction and impair circulation.*

Therapy for burn shock is aimed at supporting the child through the period of hypovolemic shock until capillary integrity is restored. To maintain adequate circulating volume, fluids are administered intravenously at a rate greater than the rate of fluid loss. Many formulas

can be used to calculate the rate of fluid administration, the most common of which is the Parkland formula of fluid resuscitation (see thePoint Supplemental Information: Parkland Formula of Fluid Resuscitation for Burn Shock). Because urine output reflects end-organ tissue perfusion, IV fluids are administered at a rate sufficient to keep the child's urine output at 1 mL/kg body weight per hour—a rate that reflects adequate tissue perfusion. A Foley catheter is used to measure hourly bladder output. Ringer's lactate (crystalloid) most closely approximates the composition of the extracellular fluid being lost. Children younger than 5 years of age handle free water poorly, making them susceptible to pulmonary and cerebral edema. In infants younger than 1 year of age, a dextrose and saline solution may be used to prevent hypoglycemia.

caREminder

Major burns with large amounts of denuded skin should not be cooled. Additional heat loss will further decrease the core temperature and potentiate circulatory collapse.

If a child's urine output during burn shock is inadequate, the reason is insufficient administration of resuscitative fluids. Renal failure is not a component of burn shock if adequate fluids are administered. Burn shock fluid resuscitation formulas are only guidelines; individual children may require more than 4 mL/kg per percentage of TBSA burned during the first 24 hours.

Sensorium is an important guide to the adequacy of fluid resuscitation. The burn injury itself does not affect the sensorium, so any changes in mentation should be investigated. When burn shock fluid resuscitation is delayed, cerebral hypoperfusion and hypoxia may occur, predisposing the child to cerebral edema when massive fluid infusion is initiated.

caREminder

Elevating the head of the child's bed 10–15 degrees to decrease cerebral edema, along with monitoring for clinical signs of increased intracranial pressure, is essential to diminish the amount of cerebral edema during shock resuscitation.

Placing the head of the bed on wheel blocks to elevate the entire bed on a slant is preferable to elevating only the head of the mattress which results in edema accumulating in the groin and legs.

In certain cases, children may require fluid in excess of the calculated amount. Some of these exceptions include burn size that has been underestimated, pulmonary injury that sequesters fluid in the lungs, electrical injury with more tissue destruction than is visible, extremely deep injury, and delayed fluid resuscitation.

After burn shock has resolved, the child is given a colloid-containing solution to replace plasma lost from the circulating volume. When burn shock resuscitation is completed, a maintenance fluid plan is formulated using normal basal fluid requirements plus calculated evaporative water loss from the burn wound. The fluid infused is changed from Ringer's lactate to an electrolyte-free solution of 5% dextrose, with or without saline, depending on the patient's electrolyte status. The child's intake, output, and serum electrolyte balance are monitored closely. Fluids are administered in amounts equally divided throughout each 24-hour period. The child must continue to maintain adequate fluid intake until wound closure is achieved.

At times, fluid losses may increase, especially when the child's core body temperature exceeds 102.2° F (39° C), when tracheal intubation is required, when a paralytic ileus necessitates prolonged nasogastric suction, when perioperative procedures are accompanied by massive blood loss, and when diarrhea occurs.

ALERT *Fluid and electrolyte imbalance lasting for only a few hours can lead to sepsis, seizures, and death in burned children. It is imperative that ongoing nursing assessments and appropriate interventions be implemented to prevent unnoted fluid and electrolyte imbalances.*

Major burn wounds receive daily care until closure is achieved. Wounds are cleaned using mild soap before being covered with topical antimicrobial agents. Dressings are changed one to two times daily, depending on the agents used and on specific protocols. Dressings can be changed in hydrotherapy tanks, bathtubs, showers, or, if the child is too ill to be moved, at the bedside. Hydrotherapy (placing the burned area in water) makes cleaning easier and softens the eschar, thereby promoting range-of-motion. After debridement, the wounds are redressed.

Aseptic technique is used during dressing changes. In addition to pain control, measures to maintain the child's core body temperature, minimize shivering, and conserve energy must be part of wound care. To the degree possible, the child should engage in self-care. After dressings are applied, isolation is not necessary, and the child need not be restricted to an area of the hospital.

Hydrotherapy is used to clean the wound and the child and to engage in active range-of-motion exercises. Some facilities use disposable plastic hydrotherapy liners to prevent cross-contamination between patients. To prevent electrolyte loss through the skin into the water, hydrotherapy should last no longer than 20 minutes. The room should be very warm, and the child should be dried immediately after hydrotherapy.

Burn scars form in healed areas, including those that received skin grafts. Scarring starts when healing starts and continues for about 8 to 12 months. Preventing hypertrophic scarring is essential for optimal cosmetic and functional recovery.

After a wound is closed, scarring is minimized by applying pressure to the area using specially made anti-scarring compression garments. Garments such as gloves, shirts, pants, or face masks are individually measured and fitted to the burn area. They are worn 24 hours a day, except during bathing, for about 10 to 12 months after the burn. The time that children wear the special garments varies, depending on the rate at which the scar matures. For many years, these garments were available only in tan, but several manufacturers are now creating them in bright, interesting colors with attractive appliquéd figures and designs. Because donning and wearing these garments can be a difficult and painful process, adherence is often an issue, and the child's level of cooperation depends almost entirely on the attitude of the adult supervisor. Facial burns can be treated with rigid masks to restore a normal contour to the central face and chin.

Active range-of-motion therapy is continued for several months until the scars mature. Frequent exercise is required to prevent flexion contractures, which severely limit mobility and may require surgical correction. If the child is able and willing to cooperate, active range-of-motion and use of the burned areas promote optimal functional recovery. If the child is unable or unwilling to cooperate, passive range-of-motion, performed by staff, will help maintain function. The family and the child will be taught the physical therapy exercises before the child is discharged from the hospital because therapy must continue for about 12 to 18 months after the burn, until scar formation has peaked.

Immediate psychosocial stresses for the burned child include separation from family members and from home as well as all of the known psychological traumas associated with hospitalization. Children who are intubated cannot speak or cry out, and, often, their arms and legs are restrained to prevent pulling on IV lines and tubes. Physical restraint is terrifying to a young child. Older children, who may better understand the rationale for restraint, may experience anger and a lack of trust.

Children must be allowed "safe time" during the day when no medical procedure, painful or not, is performed. Identify the period as "safe" through a statement, such as, "I am going to sit and read to you for the next 15 minutes and nothing else will happen during that time." Daily periods of uninterrupted sleep must be planned so that the child has time to rest and regain mental and physical strength.

Infants manage stress by sucking. If the child cannot take liquids by mouth, provide a pacifier. Children who have recently given up bottles or pacifiers tend to regress during hospitalization; make these items available to them if desired. The feelings of safety and comfort afforded by their use far exceed any problems associated with weaning after discharge from the hospital.

Recently mastered toileting skills will be lost with the stress of a major burn injury, so children should be placed in diapers until they are once again able to invest effort in independent toileting. Reassure the child that this behavior is acceptable during burn treatment, that punishment will not occur, and that diapering is not intended as a punishment. After discharge, at a time that the child and the family feel is appropriate, toilet learning can begin again at home.

After the acute crisis of major burn injury is over and the child is nearing the time of discharge, short trips can be taken to nearby parks or shops to help the child and the family adjust to public reactions to the burn injury. The child may never look unburned, but the location of the burn and whether it can easily be covered with clothing during daily activities will affect the child's and family's adjustment. Some severely burned children lose all facial features, including ears, and going out in public becomes an ordeal that they and their family avoid. Other children lead well-adjusted lives despite major disfigurement. The inner strengths of the family and the value they ascribe to the child both before and after the burn appear to be deciding factors in the level of adjustment. More specifically, children appear to respond to the burn and to give it a meaning in a manner similar to the mother's reaction. Nevertheless, disfiguring burn scars have a tremendous long-term effect on the child and the family. Occasionally, family members will not be able to accept the child and will request foster placement.

Community Care

Involving the family in the care of the child facilitates acceptance and eases the transition to the provision of care in the community. For children with minor burns, teach the caregivers or the child to wash the burned area with mild soap and tepid water, to apply the prescribed ointment and a light dressing, and to promote use of the affected area. Instruct the family to soak the dressing in tepid water before removing it to loosen the dressing and to decrease the child's discomfort. Completing the wound care as quickly as possible reduces the pain because the contact of air and water on the exposed wound causes much of the pain. Burns of the face are usually left exposed, and antimicrobial ointment is applied twice daily. Inform the family of the importance of returning for follow-up visits.

Also provide instructions for meeting the child's nutritional needs and increasing caloric and protein intake. If the child is still receiving tube feedings, instruct the family on the procedures of tube feedings, on checking residuals, and on recognizing and reporting any complications. Provide the family with access to support groups for burn victims and their families. Be sure that the family members clearly understand the instructions for administering prescribed medications. Also instruct the family on the signs and symptoms that should be reported to the physician, the home health care nurse, or the clinic. To promote the child's normal growth and development, assess the family's understanding of the normal parameters for their child's age. If the family is not able to provide needed care, indicate community and hospital resources.

The long-term effects of burn injury are related to physical changes resulting from the healing and scarring process, developmental issues specific to burns in young children, or psychosocial alterations in the relationship between the child and family members (see Developmental Considerations 25-5). As soon as possible after discharge, the child and the family should resume normal daily activities. Most burn units have a formal program designed to facilitate the child's return

to school. A staff member may accompany the child on the first day back to school to explain what has happened to him or her and to describe the purpose of pressure garments or other therapeutic interventions. Age-related issues of intimacy and sexuality will eventually arise, as will self-esteem issues. Social workers and psychologists monitor the child's and family's adjustment during return clinic visits the first year after burn injury.

In the case of nonaccidental burn injuries, the child's placement after hospital discharge is determined by the legal system. Be prepared for the fact that the child may be returned to the home environment if it is believed that the child's safety can be ensured. The goal of protective services is always to restore and maintain the family unit if the child's safety can be ensured by close supervision by the agency.

Many burn prevention programs are taught in schools and youth groups, and both nurses and nursing students can implement these programs by contacting their local fire department or burn center (Karem et al., 2009; Lehna et al., 2010). Nurses' perceived knowledge and ability to teach about burn prevention was examined in 313 registered nurses (Lehna & Myers, 2010). It was found that all nurses, regardless of specialty area, had poor burn prevention knowledge. It was believed registered nurses, as a part of primary prevention education, could be at the forefront in teaching about burn prevention. In an instrument development study, an instrument was developed to measure nurses' burn prevention knowledge and the psychometric properties examined (Lehna & Myers, 2011). Nurses in a variety of settings (e.g., emergency departments, pediatric, and outpatient) were pre- and post-tested after completing a Web-based burn prevention education program (Lehna et al., 2011). Nurses showed significant gain and retention of burn prevention knowledge over time.

Public education emphasizing the importance of smoke detectors can also significantly decrease the incidence of burns. Children can be taught to evacuate the house in the event of a fire using fire drills that identify two or more exits from each room and a location for the family to meet outside the house. Other measures, such as the "stop, drop, and roll" program, can greatly decrease the severity of a burn injury.

Public campaigns to educate adults to turn water heater thermostats down to 120° F and to check the temperature of the water before placing a child in the bath can also reduce the number of accidental scald burns. Further educational tips should include the following:

- Caution children about touching fire place doors, heated radiators, space heaters, and floor furnace grates.
- Never leave a child unattended near a campfire or wood stove.
- Store all matches and lighters securely so they are inaccessible to children.
- Keep all chemicals in their original container and inaccessible to children.
- Ensure that all electrical outlets are inaccessible to young children.

ELECTRICAL INJURY

Electrical injury is a major injury that not only burns tissue but also often results in instant death because the electrical current disrupts the electrical rhythm of the child's heart, causing lethal arrhythmias. A common cause is household current, whereby the child inserts a conductive object into an electrical outlet. Other causes include defective electrical equipment, direct contact with either high- or low-voltage current, and lightning strikes.

The child who does not die instantly from contact with the electrical current is at risk for four major complications during the acute phase: cardiac arrest or arrhythmia, tissue damage caused by interrupted blood flow, myoglobinuria (urinary loss of globulin from muscles), and metabolic acidosis.

Pathophysiology

Entering through the skin, an electrical current follows a path of least resistance through the body, damaging skin layers, bone, nerves, tendons, and blood vessels. The heat of the current coagulates blood vessels and leaves the affected area without a blood supply. Gangrene develops in necrotic tissue unless it is removed, often requiring amputation.

The location of the damage depends on the child's position and exposure. Electricity may enter one hand and exit from the other, for example; or it may travel through the body and exit from one or both legs. The greatest damage occurs at the entrance and exit sites.

Myoglobinuria develops when products that are found in normal muscle are released into the blood after electrical injury. Myoglobin is a large molecule that mechanically obstructs the renal tubules and leads to acute tubular necrosis unless large amounts of IV fluid are administered to flush the myoglobin out of the kidney.

Metabolic acidosis follows electrical injury because of the associated cellular destruction and hypovolemic shock.

Cardiac arrest, tissue damage, myoglobinuria, or metabolic acidosis usually resolve within 24 hours after the injury. Other complications that follow electrical injury include loss of short-term memory and altered emotional states. The child can usually remember events up to the time of injury, including the names of family members and his or her address, telephone number, and personal information, but is unable to recall more recent events. This loss of memory can be distressing to the child and frustrating to the family. For example, the child may be unable to remember visits by the family and may feel abandoned by them. The child may also be unable to follow instructions because he or she is unable to retain them, and this inability may lead to difficulty with planning care. Altered emotional states may include an absence of affect and blank stares or may include the opposite type of emotional response, such as hyperactivity and feelings of paranoia. Emotional responses usually become normal after about a week, but they may persist longer in some children. The electrical injury need not be to the head for these altered states to occur.

Interdisciplinary Interventions

The immediate risk to the child is cardiac arrest or arrhythmia. If cardiac arrest occurs, standard cardiac life support measures are initiated.

Osmotic diuretics may be administered to promote increased urine volume. IV fluid is administered at a rate that maintains urine output at 2 mL/kg/hr until the myoglobinuria resolves.

Ringer's lactate contains sufficient bicarbonate to manage the acidosis that accompanies burn shock but not enough to correct the acidosis associated with shock after electrical injury (i.e., pathophysiologic hypovolemic shock, not a "shock" from the electrical current). Thus, sodium bicarbonate is added to the IV infusion to maintain pH balance.

Community Care

Long-term sequelae to electrical injury include development of ocular cataracts and gait-pattern instability resulting from neurologic deficits and alterations in spatial orientation. Ocular cataracts may occur in one or both eyes at varying times from within 3 months to 18 months after the injury. The very young child may not notice changes in visual acuity; therefore, eye examinations should be scheduled every 3 months for the first year after the injury.

SUNBURN

Sunburn, one of the most common skin injuries, results from excessive exposure to UV radiation in the sun's rays. Human skin has several defenses against UV radiation, including the stratum corneum, which absorbs some UV rays, and melanin, which increases pigmentation in the skin and protects against UV damage. Generally, children with darker skin pigmentation do not burn as quickly as fair-skinned children. Nonetheless, any child can be sunburned with sufficient sun exposure. The greatest risk of exposure is between 10 AM and 2 PM. Of increasing concern is the use of indoor tanning beds; dermatologists have expressed concern with the lack of regulation of this industry because these products emit up to 26 times more damaging UV light than an equivalent amount of sunlight (Herndon, 2012).

Most people receive 80% of their lifetime exposure to sun by the time they are 21 years of age.

Pathophysiology

The cutaneous photosensitivity in sunburn is a result of overexposure to UV radiation, particularly to the radiation of the UVB wavelength. The UVA wavelength can also cause burns but does so only after much longer exposure. The epidermis reflects 10% of the UVB rays, and 20% will penetrate to the dermis. UVA penetrates deeper, markedly accentuating UVB damage (Herndon, 2012). The exact cause of UV radiation damage is unknown. It is thought to result from a combination of direct effects, generation of toxic oxygen species, and the production of inflammatory mediators. Most children respond to UV radiation with increased skin pigmentation (tanning). Thus, tanning is one sign of cumulative UV injury to the skin. Cutaneous cells may demonstrate these cumulative effects many years later with fine and deep wrinkling of the skin, scaly red patches, and the potential for skin cancer formation.

Acute UV radiation exposure induces erythema secondary to vasodilation and increased blood volume in the dermis. Metabolic changes within the epidermis cause the cells to change shape and morphologic makeup. Peak reactions to sunburn occur 24 hours after the initial symptoms and may last up to 72 hours.

CROSS-CULTURAL CARE

Approximately 15% of white children have skin that never tans. These fair-skinned children should be taught to wear sunscreen throughout the summer and to avoid direct sun exposure whenever possible.

The prognosis for sunburn is good as long as the child is removed from sun exposure and receives prompt treatment. The more serious issue related to chronic sunburn is the increased risk of skin cancer. UV radiation is the primary cause of skin cancer. UV radiation also damages the connective tissue of the dermis, causing premature skin sagging and wrinkling later in life. Furthermore, chronic UV-induced damage actually causes changes in the skin's immune function. Although acute sunburn may be treated adequately, family members and older children must be taught about the aging and carcinogenic effects of chronic sun damage and overuse of tanning beds. It has been estimated that if sun protective clothing and sunscreens were used from early childhood on, then the incidence of nonmelanoma skin cancer in adulthood would decrease by 75% to 80% (Brown, 2007).

Assessment

Sunburned skin appears tender, reddened, and possibly slightly swollen. Severe sunburn may produce tense edema, vesicles, and bullae. On the head, the most prominent areas affected include the nose, cheeks, forehead, and ear lobes. On the extremities and trunk, skin areas unprotected by clothing are most affected.

Children with sunburn may have difficulty sleeping because of their discomfort. Sunburn over large areas of the body may result in systemic symptoms such as vomiting, headache, fever, chills, and malaise. In severe cases, extensive sunburn reduces the child's ability to sweat and may contribute to collapse from heat stroke.

Nursing Diagnoses and Outcomes

In addition to the nursing diagnoses presented in Nursing Plan of Care 25-1, the following diagnoses may apply. Additional information regarding care management for the child with an acute condition can be found in Chapter 11-1.

Nursing Diagnosis: Impaired tissue integrity related to reddened, tender, and swollen epidermis in response to overexposure to the sun
Outcome: Child will experience comfort and healing to areas that have been sunburned.

Nursing Diagnosis: Health-seeking behaviors regarding sun exposure protection and prevention
Outcome: The family and child will initiate preventive measures to protect the child's skin from excessive exposure to the sun.

Interdisciplinary Interventions

There is a lack of evidence to support the use of corticosteroids and NSAIDs in the treatment of sunburn (Land & Small, 2008). Symptomatic treatment of sunburn includes cool water or saline compresses, ice packs, local anesthetic sprays or creams, skin emollients, and extra fluids to compensate for any dehydration (Burns et al., 2013). When skin peeling occurs, a moisturizing cream or aloe vera gel may be applied. Jojoba oil and vitamin E are also sometimes helpful. Petroleum, butter, and other occlusive ointments may intensify the burn and should be avoided. The child also must be given plenty of cold water or flavored sports drinks, both during physical activity in the sun and afterwards. Acetaminophen or ibuprofen will soothe the discomfort. Severe blistering requires professional care.

Community Care

The best management for sunburn is to prevent it by limiting sun exposure and using an effective sun-screening agent on exposed skin (Fig. 25-19). Skin types dictate protection needs, though a SPF of at least 15 is recommended for all children (Burns et al., 2013):

- Skin type 1: Always burns, never tans; requires sun protection factor (SPF) of 15 or greater
- Skin type 2: Usually burns easily, tans minimally (fair skinned); requires SPF 15
- Skin type 3: Burns moderately, tans gradually (lightly pigmented, dark white); requires SPF 8 to 10
- Skin type 4: Burns minimally, tans readily (pigmented; for example, Mediterranean, Asian, Hispanic); requires SPF 4
- Skin type 5: Rarely burns, tans profusely (moderately pigmented; for example, American Indian, Hispanic, Middle Eastern); requires SPF 4
- Skin type 6: Never burns (darkly pigmented, black; for example, African American); no or low SPF needed

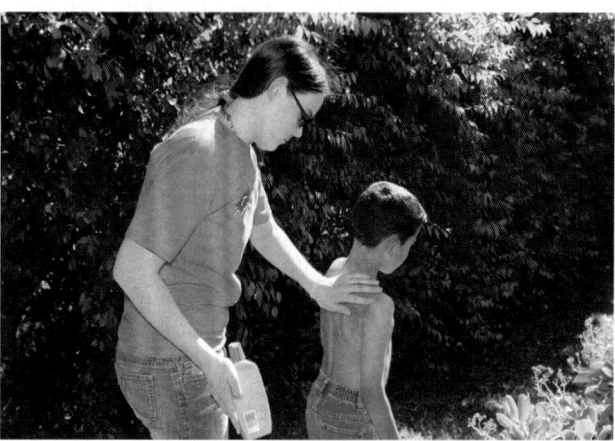

Figure 25-19 Sunscreens can be used to protect the skin through absorption, reflection, and scattering of UV radiation.

The American Academy of Pediatrics recommends that children younger than 6 months of age should not be exposed to direct sunlight because their sensitive skin and decreased sweating rate places them more at risk for heat stroke. If avoiding direct sunlight is not possible, dress infants in lightweight long pants, long-sleeved shirts, and brimmed hats (American Academy of Pediatrics, 2013).

Most sunscreens contain some combination of para-aminobenzoic acid, cinnamate, salicylates, and anthralin. A broad-spectrum sunscreen that protects against both UVA and UVB radiation should be used. Products with titanium dioxide or zinc oxide tend to provide the broadest protection. Sunscreens protect the skin by absorbing, reflecting, and scattering UV radiation. The quantifiable effectiveness of the sunscreen is expressed as the "sun protection factor." SPF is based on the UV-absorbing properties of the active chemical ingredient in the sunscreen. SPF reflects both duration and level of protection against UVB. For example, if a child normally burns within 15 minutes of exposure to the sun without sunscreen, use of a sunscreen with SPF 15 enables the child to stay in the sun 15 times 15 minutes or 225 minutes (3 hours 45 minutes) before achieving the same degree of erythema or burn. Reapplying the sunscreen does not prolong this time. SPF 15 sunscreen protects the child for only 225 minutes, no matter how many times it is applied during that period. Sunscreen agents that are waterproof with SPF 15 or more are recommended for children. Few data exist to show that any protection over SPF 30 renders any additional benefits. All sunscreens should be applied 30 minutes before sun exposure, and then reapplied every 2 hours or sooner, depending on the child's activity.

caREminder

Perhaps the most important consideration for using sunscreens effectively is not product characteristics but proper application and use. Applying an insufficient amount can decrease a product's SPF rating by 50%.

Instruct the family on management and prevention of sunburn (Community Care 25-3). Research suggests that although most people are fairly knowledgeable about the relation between sun exposure and skin cancer, many do not have a solid understanding of practical preventive strategies, such as how to choose the best sunscreen. Many adults use poor sun protection practices themselves, and their own habits have been found to reflect the degree of protection practiced for their children. Thus, the nurse needs to teach adult family members to protect themselves and serve as an example to their children. Point out that sunscreens do not protect the child's skin from all UV radiation; even with sunscreens, tanning or burning will occur if exposure is of sufficient duration.

Cold Injury

In cold–dry and cold–wet weather, children who play outdoors are at risk for cold injury and hypothermia (Community Care 25-4). In addition, one must be aware

---

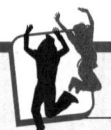

COMMUNITY CARE 25-3

Fun-in-the-Sun Safety: A Checklist

1. Choose a sunscreen that blocks both UVA and UVB radiation.
2. Choose a product that includes an SPF rating of 15 or greater.
3. Do not use sunscreens on children younger than 6 months of age. Instead, use hats or bonnets and light-colored clothes to protect the skin, and keep the infant away from direct exposure to the sun.
4. For children older than age 2 years, choose a sunscreen product based on the child's previous history of response to sun exposure. Sun-sensitive children should not remain outdoors for a long period of time, and an SPF product of at least 30 should be used to protect them.
5. Apply the sunscreen indoors before exposure to sun (some product labels recommend at least 30 minutes, others recommend up to 2 hours).
6. Reapply sunscreen after bathing, swimming, or perspiring if exposure to the sun is resumed. However, reapplication does not prolong the time frame of initial protection, which is provided by the selected SPF.
7. Some sunscreen products are labeled to denote that they offer protection in special circumstances:
   Sweat resistant: Protects for up to 30 minutes of continuous, heavy perspiration, then must be reapplied
   Water resistant: Protects for up to 40 minutes of continuous water exposure, then must be reapplied
   Waterproof: Protects for up to 80 minutes of continuous water exposure, then must be reapplied
8. Minimize exposure to the sun near the hour of noon.
9. Know whether any medication the child is taking causes photosensitivity.
10. Encourage children to wear lightweight, long-sleeved shirts and broad-brimmed hats during prolonged sun exposure.
11. If the child's skin feels warm, it is.
12. Take one or more of the following actions to protect the child's skin:
    Cover the skin.
    Apply sunscreen.
    Remove the child from sun exposure.

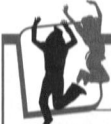

COMMUNITY CARE 25-4

Preventing Cold Injury

Families, especially those living in cold climates, must be educated about the hazards of cold injury. *The best health care management for cold injury is prevention.*

- Children should wear several layers of clothing under appropriate outerwear garments (including two pairs of socks, mittens, and a hat that covers the ears) to ensure warmth when playing outdoors.
- Outer garments should be waterproof, insulated, and offer protection against the wind.
- Children should wear well-fitted, insulated, waterproof, nonconstricting footwear in cold weather. Clothing that contains products such as polypropylene or Gore-Tex, wool, treated polyesters, or blends of synthetic wool fibers are best.
- If the child's hands, feet, or other body parts become wet while outdoors, a change to dry clothing or footwear should be made immediately.

- Children should rub their hands together or scrunch up their face when they are feeling cold to help warm up their bodies.
- Ample food and fluid should be provided during the time of outdoor activities.
- The child's exposure to extremely cold temperatures should be monitored and supervised by an adult with timely and appropriate rewarming opportunities.
- An adult who is feeling cold can be certain that children are also feeling cold and should bring them indoors.
- Children who participate in outdoor sports activities should be alert to the presence of numbing of body parts, particularly the nose, ears, fingers, and toes.

of the effects of windchill, which can significantly lower core body temperature.

Frostnip is a superficial cold injury that causes no damage to the skin tissue. *Frostbite* may be superficial or deep and can cause significant tissue damage or even tissue death. Exposed areas of the face are at greatest risk. *Immersion foot* (*trench foot*) occurs in cold weather when the feet are exposed to damp or wet, poorly ventilated shoes, causing tissue maceration and infection. *Hypothermia*, defined as a core body temperature of less than 95° F (35° C), is discussed in more detail in Chapter 31.

Extreme cold is an external force that freezes the cells of the skin. Ice crystals may form between or within cells, interfering with the activities of the normal sodium pump. This event leads to rupture of the cell membranes. Red cells or platelets may clump at the damaged site, causing microemboli or thrombosis. Blood may be shunted from the injured area, eventually causing cell death if not treated. The offending agent is not only the cold temperature but also the rapid motion of the surrounding wind or the presence of damp, cold conditions (Arford, 2008).

! ALERT   *Butane and propane propellants that are widely used in spray aerosols (e.g., hair spray, air fresheners) can cause moderately severe frostbite when sprayed directly on the skin at close range. Spray aerosols are a source of a variety of injuries and should be kept safely out of reach of children. Community and family education can help prevent occurrences.*

Susceptibility to cold injury may be increased by dehydration, fatigue, hunger, anemia, ingestion of alcohol or illicit substances, and the presence of other

illnesses. Therapy for any type of cold injury should begin as soon the injury is noticed.

FROSTNIP

Frostnip lesions are usually manifested as firm, white patches on the face, ears, and extremities that are numb. As the body is warmed, erythema develops with no immediate blistering. Over the ensuing 24 to 72 hours, blistering and peeling may occur. The affected area may have a residual hypersensitivity to cold that lasts for several days to weeks.

Care for the child with mild frostnip primarily involves providing first aid and teaching prevention measures. The child should be removed to a warm area quickly and examined for the possibility of more serious damage.

As the affected area rewarms, it can cause a stinging sensation, which may frighten the child. Explain by comparing the situation to that of a hand or foot "falling asleep." As the foot "wakes up," it tingles, almost to the point of hurting, but the feeling soon goes away.

FROSTBITE

Frostbite is the acute freezing of tissues when exposed to temperatures below the freezing point of intact skin. The severity of injury is related both to the temperature at the skin surface and to the duration of exposure. In frostbite, there are two mechanisms responsible for tissue injury. At the cellular level, the mechanism is freezing of the tissue and subsequent ice crystal formation in extracellular and intracellular tissues. In the second mechanism, the body during rewarming responds by alternating cycles of vasoconstriction and vasodilation (e.g., "*hunting reaction*") (Arford, 2008). A two-tiered classification is used: *superficial* no or minimal anticipated tissue loss, corresponding to first- and second-degree injury; and deeper injury and anticipated tissue loss, corresponding to third- and fourth-degree injury.

Interdisciplinary Interventions

The treatment of frostbite usually begins in the setting in which the child is found and to a body part that is noted to be extremely cold or frozen. The body part should be immediately protected from further damage. Elevate the extremity above level of heart to prevent dependent edema, whenever possible. Remove wet clothing; cover the child with blankets or other forms of insulation. When conditions are such that refreezing could occur, it is safer to keep the body part frozen. Most frostbite will thaw spontaneously and should be allowed to do so (McIntosh et al., 2011). In a supervised clinical setting, use warm water bath immersion for active external warming. Adding povidone-iodine or chlorhexidine to rewarming water reduces bacteria on the skin and is unlikely to be harmful. Water should be heated to 98.6° to 102.2° F. A risk of this process is core temperature afterdrop. When the extremities and trunk are warmed simultaneously, cold acidemic blood, which has pooled in the vasoconstricted extremities, returns to the core and causes temperature and pH to decrease. At the same time, removal from the cold environment results in peripheral vasodilation, potentially contributing to hypotension, inadequate coronary perfusion, and even ventricular fibrillation. For children suffering from this degree of hypothermia, the trunk should be warmed initially, and then the extremities. Also be aware of the potential for surface burns. Hypothermia frequently accompanies frostbite, and mild hypothermia may be treated concurrently. Moderate to severe hypothermia should be treated prior to treating frostbite.

Vascular stasis may result from frostbite. It is believed hydration and avoiding hypovolemia are important treatment strategies. Oral fluids are given to the alert child with no gastrointestinal symptoms (e.g., nauseous, vomiting) or who does not have altered mental status. Otherwise, IV normal saline should be given. Fluids should be warmed and given in small boluses. IV low-molecular-weight dextran (LMWD) decreases blood viscosity and prevents red blood cell aggregation and microthrombi formation.

NSAIDs are used when a child has frostbite to block the arachidonic pathway, potentially decreasing vasoconstriction, dermal damage, and further tissue destruction. Aspirin (ASA) has been proposed to be used as an alternative to NSAIDs therapy. No studies are available comparing the two types of therapy: NSAIDs versus ASA. Routine use of antibiotics is not supported by evidence. Antibiotics are administered to patients with significant trauma, potential sources of infection, or cellulitis or sepsis. Tetanus prophylaxis is administered according to guidelines.

No evidence supports use of dressings to a frostbitten part. Dressings used are placed between frozen digits and loose enough to allow for swelling.

Treatment with aloe vera ointment has been shown to improve outcomes by reducing prostaglandin and thromboxane formation. It is only beneficial for superficial injuries; topical ointments do not penetrate deep into tissues. Debridement of blisters may be done in the hospital setting. Common practice is to selectively needle aspirate clear blisters while leaving hemorrhagic blisters intact.

caREminder

Assess for core temperature afterdrop, a condition that occurs as peripheral vasoconstriction is reversed and blood is circulated through cold extremities, returning cold blood to the core.

Preventing long-term sequelae may include use of daily hydrotherapy to increase circulation, sympathectomy within 24 hours of frostbite to reduce tissue loss, and fasciotomy to prevent compartment syndrome. After frostbite occurs, it may take 1 to 3 months before the extent of tissue loss is known for amputation.

IMMERSION FOOT

When the feet, covered by poorly ventilated shoes, become damp or wet in cold weather, the extremity can become cold and numb. The foot becomes pale, edematous, and clammy. Tissue maceration and infection can occur, as can long-term hypersensitivity to temperature changes. As soon as the child's feet (or shoes) are known to be wet, the child's footwear should be changed. Treatment includes drying the skin, keeping the area well ventilated, and preventing or treating infection.

DISORDERS OF THE HAIR AND NAILS

Disorders of the hair and nails may result from such diverse causes as growth pattern disturbances, hereditary variances, disease, nutritional deficits, or trauma. A hair or nail problem is rarely the primary reason for a child to seek health care; rather, the problem is usually discovered by an astute nurse during routine or focused assessment.

HAIR DISORDERS

Inspect the hair for distribution, color, texture, amount, and quality. Hair color changes in response to certain dietary changes, ingested substances, or disease processes. For instance, kwashiorkor and zinc deficiencies can cause depigmented hair. Ingesting copper can turn the hair green, and ingesting cobalt can turn the hair blue. Discoloration can also be caused by the dithranol therapy for treatment of psoriasis. Premature graying (before age 20 years) can be an early sign of pernicious anemia or thrombosis.

Delayed or absent hair growth may indicate an ectodermal dysplasia. Alopecia (loss of hair) may occur for various reasons, including hair pulling, tinea capitis, and the use of chemotherapeutic agents. Hair disorders, including alopecia and structural anomalies of the hair shafts, are briefly described in Table 25-9. In most cases, disorders of the hair can be corrected by addressing or treating the underlying cause.

TABLE 25-9   Disorders of the Hair

Disorder	Definition
Hypertrichosis	Excessive hair growth in inappropriate locations
Hirsutism	Male-type secondary sexual hair growth in the female
Hypotrichosis	Deficient hair growth
Alopecia	Partial or complete hair loss, which may be hereditary or acquired, diffuse or patchy, scarring or nonscarring
Occipital alopecia of the newborn	Hair loss on the occipital area of the scalp resulting from friction between the child's head and, for example, a mattress or sheets
Telogen effluvium	Loss of scalp hair resulting from the premature conversion of hair loss in • The newborn during the first few years of life • Postpartum women • Patients after an acute febrile illness • Females after discontinuation of oral contraceptives
Congenital circumscribed alopecia	Localized areas of hair loss present at birth, usually overlying a birthmark or a sebaceous or epidermal nevus
Friction alopecia	Patchy hair loss caused by a variety of hairstyles: ponytails, curlers, rollers, tight braids
Toxic alopecia	Hair loss as a side effect of radiation therapy and certain drugs, such as chemotherapeutic agents
Trichotillomania	Hair loss with broken hairs resulting from the habit of pulling or twisting the hair
Alopecia areata	Rapid and complete loss of hair in round or oval patches on the scalp; cause unknown; 20% of patients have family history of the illness; increased incidence in patients with Down syndrome
Trichorrhexis nodosa	Structural defect that appears as a node or swelling on the hair shaft; defect caused by a fracture of the hair shaft with derangement of the cells in the cortex
Monilethrix	Autosomal dominant hair shaft defect in which the hair appears dry, lusterless, and brittle and fractures spontaneously or with mild trauma; affects eyebrows, lashes, body, and sexual hair; spontaneous improvement may occur at puberty
Trichorrhexis invaginata (bamboo hair)	Feature of Netherton syndrome; hair is dry, fragile with no apparent growth; thought to result from a transient defect in keratinization; hair growth may improve significantly at puberty
Trichoschisis	Hair shaft defect in which affected children have brittle hair; hair shaft is actually fractured
Pili torti	Autosomal dominant condition in which a structural defect of the hair shaft causes it to be twisted on its own axis; hair is normal at birth but is replaced by abnormal hair that becomes evident between ages 2 and 3 years; affected hairs have a spangled appearance, are fragile, and are often ash blonde in color
Pili annulati	Ringed hair that is characterized by hair shafts banded with bright rings when viewed in reflected light, not fragile; can be a familial or a sporadic defect
Wooly hair disease	Tightly curled, abnormal hair seen at birth; may occur as autosomal dominant condition in which most other hair is normal, as an autosomal recessive condition in which all hair is affected and appears short and pale, or in sporadic form (wooly hair nevus) in which localized areas of the scalp are affected
Menkes kinky hair syndrome	X-linked recessive disorder in which twisting of the hair is a result of a copper deficiency
Pityriasis amiantacea	Thick mat of scale on the scalp; reaction pattern of the scalp to inflammation, infection, or trauma
Tinea capitis	Fungal infection of the scalp caused by *Microsporum canis* or *Trichophyton tonsurans*; thick, white, scaling, broken hairs and areas of alopecia

TABLE 25-10   Nail Abnormalities

Name	Definition
Anonychia	Absence of the nail plate
Koilonychia	Flattening and concavity of the nail plate with loss of normal contour
Macronychia	Abnormally large nail
Micronychia	Unusually small nail
Leukonychia	White opacity of the nail plate, which may involve the entire nail plate, may be punctuated, or may be striated; can be the result of trauma, infection, dermatosis, malnutrition, anemia, heavy metal poisoning, or a benign hereditary defect
Onychogryposis	Acquired nail defect in which the nail plate is thick, overgrown, and distorted
Onycholysis	Separation of the nail plate from the nail bed resulting from trauma, psoriasis, fungal infection, contact dermatitis, porphyria, drugs, or drug-induced phototoxicity
Beau lines	Transverse grooves in the nail plate that represent an inability of the nail matrix to produce a nail plate of normal thickness as a result of periodic trauma or secondary to systemic disease
Yellow nail syndrome	Yellow nail, slow to grow; associated with congenital abnormalities of the lymphatic vessels and chylothorax
Pachyonychia congenita	Autosomal dominant disorder characterized by gross nail thickening
Pigmented nevi of the nail	Longitudinal band of pigment in the nail plate that is common in dark-skinned individuals
Lichen planus	Common longitudinal ridging of the nail plate; nail thinning and pterygium formation may occur
Twenty-nail dystrophy	Characterized by longitudinal ridging, fragility, distal notching, and opalescent discoloration of all the nails; tends to be self-limiting and reversible; eventually affects all 20 nails
Paronychia	Acute infection of the nail fold, which can be very painful, and is seen commonly in thumb or finger suckers; usually caused by staphylococcal, streptococcal, or pseudomonal infections; usually requires removal of the nail bed
Herpetic whitlow	Primary infection of the nail fold with herpes simplex
Ingrown toenail	Caused by incorrect cutting of toenail or ill-fitting footwear; produces pain, bacterial paronychia, and overgrowth of granulation tissue around the soft, pliable nail plate

NAIL DISORDERS

Disorders of the nails can cause changes in normal nail color, shape, texture, and size. Inspect the nails for these changes and for the presence of nail biting, skin picking, and infection. Nails can become discolored from antimalarial agents and certain other drugs; bacterial or fungal infections; and skin disorders such as alopecia areata, lichen planus, and psoriasis. Nail discoloration can also occur secondary to a systemic problem such as jaundice or cyanosis. Clubbing of nails may indicate chronic respiratory or cardiac disease. The curve of the nail in a convex or concave fashion may simply be hereditary or indicate injury, iron deficiency, or infection. Nail abnormalities in children that may reflect generalized skin diseases, systemic disease, bacterial or fungal infections, or trauma are reviewed in Table 25-10.

See thePoint for a summary of Key Concepts.

REFERENCES

Adalat, S., Wall, D., & Goodyear, H. (2007). Diaper dermatitis: Frequency and contributory factors in hospital attending children. *Pediatric Dermatology, 24,* 483–488.

American Academy of Dermatology. (2013). *Poison ivy, oak, and sumac.* Retrieved from http://www.aad.org/skin-conditions/dermatology-a-to-z/poison-ivy#.UWTbGJM3v2w

Andrews, R., McCarthy, J., Carapetis, J. et al. (2009). Skin disorders, including pyoderma, scabies, and tinea infections. *Pediatric Clinics of North America, 56,* 1421–1440.

American Academy of Pediatrics. (2013). *Summer safety tips.* Retrieved from http://www.healthychildren.org/English/news/Pages/Summer-Safety-Tips-Sun-and-Water-Safety.aspx?nfstatus=401&nftoken=00000000-0000-0000-0000-000000000000&nfstatusdescription=E

Antaya, R., & Robinson, D. (2010). Blisters and pustules in the newborn. *Pediatric Annals, 39*(10), 635–645.

Arford, S. (2008). Treatment of frostbite: A cold-induced injury. *Journal of Wound, Ostomy and Continence Nursing, 35*(6), 625–630.

Arndt, K. A., & Hsu, J. H. S. (2006). *Manual of dermatologic therapeutics: With essentials of diagnosis.* Philadelphia, PA: Lippincott Williams & Wilkins.

Atherton, D. (2004). A review of the pathophysiology: Prevention and treatment of irritant diaper dermatitis. *Current Medical Research Opinions, 20,* 645–649.

Ayello, E., & Sibbald, R. (2008). Preventing pressure ulcers and skin tears. In E. Capezuti, D. Zwicker, M. Mezey et al. (Eds.), *Evidence-based geriatric nursing protocols for best practice* (3rd ed., pp. 403–429). New York, NY: Springer Publishing Company.

Ayello, E., & Sibbald, G. (2009). *Preventing pressure ulcers and skin tears.* National Guideline Clearinghouse. Retrieved from http://www.guideline.gov/content.aspx?id=12262#Section420

Baharestani, M., & Ratliff, C. (2007). Pressure ulcers in neonates and children: An NPUAP white paper. *Advances in Skin & Wound Care, 20,* 208–220.

Bailey, E., & Shaker, M. (2008). An update on childhood urticarial and angioedema. *Current Opinion in Pediatrics*, 20, 425–430.

Bell, E. (2006). Much to consider when treating diaper dermatitis. *Infectious Diseases in Children*, 19(9), 12–13.

Berk, D., & Bayliss, S. (2010). MRSA, Staphylococcal scalded skin syndrome, and other cutaneous bacterial emergencies. *Pediatric Annals*, 39(10), 627–633.

Blei, F. (2005). Basic science and clinical aspects of vascular anomalies. *Current Opinion in Pediatrics*, 17, 501–509.

Blume-Peytavi, U., Hauser, M., Stamatas, G. et al. (2012). Skin care practices for newborns and infants: Review of the clinical evidence for best practices. *Pediatric Dermatology*, 29(1), 1–14.

Bowden, V. (2012). Losing the louse: How to manage this common infestation in children. *Pediatric Nursing*, 38(5), 253–254, 277.

Brouillette, F., & Weber, M. (1978). Massive aspiration of talcum powder by an infant. *Canadian Medical Association Journal*, 119, 354–355.

Brown, K. (2007). Dermatoses of summer. *Contemporary Pediatrics*, 24, 13–18.

Burns, C. E., Dunn, A. M., Brady, M. A. et al. (Eds.). (2013). *Pediatric primary care: A handbook for nurse practitioners* (5th ed.). Philadelphia, PA: W. B. Saunders.

Centers for Disease Control and Prevention. (2010a). *Head lice*. Retrieved from http://www.cdc.gov/parasites/lice/head/index.html

Centers for Disease Control and Prevention. (2010b). *Scabies*. Retrieved from http://www.cdc.gov/parasites/scabies.html

Conner, J. M., Soll, R. F., & Edwards, W. H. (2004). Topical ointment for preventing infection in preterm infants. *Cochrane Database of Systemic Reviews*, (3), CD003373.

Copeland, S., deBey, S., & Hutchison, D. (2007). Nickel allergies: Implications for practice. *Dermatology Nursing*, 19, 267–268, 288.

Cotellessa, C., Manunta, T., Ghersetich I. et al. (2004). The use of pyruvic acid in the treatment of acne. *European Academy of Dermatology and Venereology*, 18, 275–278.

Curley, M., Razmus, I., Roberts, K. et al. (2002). Predicting pressure ulcer risk in pediatric patients: The Braden Q scale. *Nursing Research*, 52, 22–33.

Dasher, D., Burkhart, C., & Morrell, D. (2009). Immunotherapy for childhood warts. *Pediatric Annals*, 38(7), 373–395.

De Haen, M., Spigt, M., van Uden, C. et al. (2006). Efficacy of duct tape versus placebo in the treatment of verruca vulgaris (warts) in primary school children. *Archives of Pediatric Adolescent Medicine*, 169, 1121–1125.

D'Souza, A., Nelson, N., & McKenzie, L. (2009). Pediatric burn injuries treated in US emergency departments between 1990-2006. *Pediatrics*, 124(5), 1424–1430.

Eichenfield, L., Frieden, I., & Esterly, N. (2008). *Textbook of neonatal dermatology*. Philadelphia, PA: W. B. Saunders.

Feaster, T., & Singer, J. (2010). Topical therapies for impetigo. *Pediatric Emergency Care*, 26(3), 222–230.

Focht, D., Spicer, C., & Fairchok, M. (2002). The efficacy of duct tape vs cryotherapy in the treatment of verruca vulgaris. *Archives of Pediatrics & Adolescent Medicine*, 156(10), 971–974.

Gray, M. (2004). Which pressure ulcer risk scales are valid and reliable in a pediatric population? *Journal of Wound, Ostomy and Continence Nursing*, 31, 157–160.

Guttman-Yassky, E., Nograles, K., & Krueger, J. (2011a). Contrasting pathogenesis of atopic dermatitis and psoriasis–Part I: Clinical pathologic concepts. *Journal of Allergy & Clinical Immunology*, 127(5),1110–1118.

Guttman-Yassky, E., Nograles, K., & Krueger, J. (2011b). Contrasting pathogenesis of atopic dermatitis and psoriasis–Part II: Immune cell subsets and therapeutic concepts. *Journal of Allergy & Clinical Immunology*, 127(6), 1420–1432.

Herndon, D. (2012). *Total burn care*. Philadelphia, PA: Saunders.

Herzog, C. (2011). Benign vascular tumors. In R. M. Kliegman, B. F. Stanton, J. W. St. Geme et al. (Eds.), *Nelson textbook of pediatrics* (19th ed., p. 1772). Philadelphia, PA: Elsevier/Saunders.

Hoeger, P., Stark, S., & Jost, G. (2010). Efficacy and safety of two different antifungal pastes in infants with diaper dermatitis: A randomized controlled study. *Journal of European Academy of Dermatology and Venereology*, 24, 1094–1098.

Huffiness, B., & Lodgson, M. (1997). The neonatal skin risk assessment scale for predicting skin breakdown in neonates. *Issues in Comprehensive Pediatric Nursing*, 20, 103–114.

Janniger, C., Schwartz, R., Szepietowski, J. et al. (2005). Intertrigo and common secondary skin infections. *American Family Physician*, 73, 15–17.

Karem, H., Probus, A. C., & Lehna, C. (2009). Local nursing students ignite the flame on fire prevention. *Kentucky Nurse*, 57, 8.

Keogh-Brown, M., Fordham, R., Thomas, K. et al. (2007). To freeze or not to freeze: A cost-effectiveness analysis of wart treatment. *British Journal of Dermatology*, 156, 687–692.

Klotz, S., Ianas, V., & Elliott, S. (2011). Cat-scratch disease. *American Family Physician*, 83(2), 152–155.

Labandeira, J., Vázquez-Blanco, M., Paredes, C. et al. (2005). Efficacy of topical calcipotriol in the treatment of a giant viral wart. *Pediatric Dermatology*, 22(4), 375–376.

Land, V., & Small, L. (2008). The evidence on how to best treat sunburn in children: A common treatment dilemma. *Pediatric Nursing*, 34(4), 343–348.

Lehna, C., Love, P., Holt, S. et al. (2010). Nursing students apply evidence based research principles in primary burn prevention projects. *Journal of Pediatric Nursing*, 25(6), 477–481.

Lehna, C., & Myers, J. (2010). Does nurses' perceived burn prevention knowledge, and ability to teach burn prevention correlate with their actual burn prevention knowledge? *Journal of Burn Care and Research*, 31(1), 111–120.

Lehna, C., & Myers, J. (2011). Development of an instrument that assesses individual's burn prevention knowledge. *Journal of Burn Care & Research*, 32, 26–30.

Lehna, C., Ramos, P., Myers, J. et al. (2011). A web-based educational module increases burn prevention knowledge over time. *Burns*, 37(7), 1255–1258.

Loman, D. (2000). Assessment of skin breakdown in children. *Journal of Child and Family Nursing*, 3, 234–238.

Lund, C., Kuller, J., Lane, A. et al. (1999). Neonatal skin care: The scientific basis for practice. *Journal of Obstetric, Gynecologic, and Neonatal Nursing*, 28(3), 241–254.

Lund, C. H., Kuller, J., Lane, A. et al. (2001). Neonatal skin care: Evaluation of the AWHONN/NANN research-based practice project on knowledge and skin care practices. *Journal of Obstetric, Gynecologic, and Neonatal Nursing*, 30(1), 30–40.

Lund, C. H., Kuller, J., Raines, D. et al. (2007). *Neonatal skin care* (2nd ed.). Washington, DC: Association of Women's Health, Obstetric and Neonatal Nurses.

Lund, C. H., Osborne, J. W., Kuller, J. et al. (2001). Neonatal skin care: Clinical outcomes of the AWHONN/NANN evidence-based clinical practice guideline. *Journal of Obstetric, Gynecologic, and Neonatal Nursing*, 30(1), 41–51.

Mancini, A. (2005). Pediatric dermatology. *Pediatric Annals*, 34(3), 161–162.

Marchini, G., Nelson, A., Edner, J. et al. (2005). Erythema toxicum neonatorum is an innate immune response to commensal microbes penetrated into the skin of the newborn infant. *Pediatric Research*, 58(3), 613–616.

McEvoy, M. (2000). Pediatric impetigo. *Advance for Nurse Practitioners*, 8(2), 69–71.

McIntosh, S., Hamonko, M., Freer, L. et al. (2011). Wilderness medical society practice guidelines for the prevention and treatment of frostbite. *Wilderness & Environmental Medicine*, 22, 156–160.

Moss, M. (1969). Dangers from talcum powder. *Pediatrics*, 43, 1058.

Nicol, N. (2011). Efficacy and safety considerations in topical treatments for atopic dermatitis. *Pediatric Nursing*, 37(6), 295–301.

Noonan, C., Quigley, S., Curley, M. (2011). Using the Braden Q scale to predict pressure ulcer risk in pediatric patients. *Journal of Pediatric Nursing, 26*, 566–575.

Ooi, M., Wong, S., Lewthwaite, P. et al. (2010). Clinical features, diagnosis, and management of enterovirus 71. *Lancet Neurology, 9*, 1097–1115.

Papay, J., Yuen, N., Powell, G. et al. (2012). Spontaneous adverse event reports of Stevens-Johnson syndrome/toxic epidermal necrolysis: Detecting associations with medications. *Pharmacoepidemiology and Drug Safety, 21*, 289–296.

Parker, J. (2009). Management of common fungal infections in primary care. *Nursing Standard, 23*(43), 42–46.

Parnham, A. (2012). Pressure ulcer risk assessment and prevention in children. *Nursing Children and Young People, 24*(2), 24–29.

Pontius, D., & Teskey, C. (2011). *Pediculosis management in school setting: Position statement.* Retrieved from http://www.nasn.org/PolicyAdvocacy/PositionPapersandReports/NASNPositionStatementsFullView/tabid/462/smid/824/ArticleID/40/Default.aspx

Popovich, D., & McAlhany, A. (2007). Accurately diagnosing commonly misdiagnosed circular rashes. *Pediatric Nursing, 33*, 315–321.

Quigley, S., & Curley, M. (1996). Skin integrity in the pediatric population: Preventing and managing pressure ulcers. *Journal of the Society of Pediatric Nurses, 1*(1), 7–18.

Ramanathan, S., & Hebert, A. (2011). Management of acne vulgaris. *Journal of Pediatric Health Care, 25*(5), 330–337.

Ravanfar, P., Wallace, J., & Pace, N. (2012). Diaper dermatitis: A review and update. *Current Opinion in Pediatrics, 24*(4), 472–479.

Safe Kids Worldwide. (2011a). *Fires, burns and scalds prevention.* Retrieved from http://www.safekids.org/fires-burns-and-scalds-prevention

Safe Kids Worldwide. (2011b). *Start safe: Fire resources for parents.* Retrieved from http://www.safekids.org/start-safe-fire-resources-parents

Strauss, J., Krowchuk, D., Leyden, J. et al. (2007). Guidelines of care for acne vulgaris management. *Journal of the American Academy of Dermatology, 56*, 651–663.

Strickland, M. (1997). Evaluation of bacterial growth with occlusive dressing use on excoriated skin in the premature infant. *Neonatal Network, 16*(2), 29–35.

Suddaby, E., Barnett, S., & Facteau, L. (2005). Skin breakdown in acute care pediatrics. *Pediatric Nursing, 31*(2), 132–138, 148.

Theos, A. (2007). Diagnosis and management of superficial cutaneous fungal infections in children. *Pediatric Annals, 36*, 47–54.

Valencia, I., Falabella, A., & Schachner, L. (2001). New developments in wound care for infants and children. *Pediatric Annals, 30*(4), 211–218.

Van Velsen, S., Knol, M., Haech, I. et al. (2010). The self-administered eczema area and severity index in children with moderate to severe atopic dermatitis: Better estimation of AD body surface area than severity. *Pediatric Dermatology, 27*(5), 470–475.

Vanfleteren, I., Van Gysel, D., De Brandt, C. et al. (2003). Stevens-Johnson syndrome: A diagnostic challenge in the absence of skin lesions. *Pediatric Dermatology, 20*(1), 52–56.

Wenner, R., Askari, S., Cham, P. et al. (2007). Duct tape for the treatment of common warts in adults: A double-blind randomized controlled trial. *Archives in Dermatology, 143*, 309–313.

Weston, W., Lane, A., & Morelli, J. (2007). *Color textbook of pediatric dermatology.* St. Louis, MO: Mosby.

Williams, J., Eichenfield, L., Burke, B. et al. (2005). Prevalence of scalp scaling in prepubertal children. *Pediatrics, 115*(1), e1–e6.

Wooten, M., & Hawkins, H. (2005). *WOCN position statement: Clean versus sterile: Management of chronic wounds.* Retrieved from http://c.ymcdn.com/sites/wocn.site-ym.com/resource/resmgr/advocacy_policy_white_papers/white_papers.pdf

Wound, Ostomy and Continence Nurses Society. (2009). *Position statement: Pressure ulcer staging.* Mount Laurel, NJ: Author.

Wound, Ostomy and Continence Nurses Society. (2010). *Guideline for prevention and management of pressure ulcers.* Mount Laurel, NJ: Author.

Yang, L., & Curran, M. (2009). Topical pimecrolimus. *Pediatric Drugs, 11*(6), 407–426.

Zaenglein, A., & Thiboutot, D. (2006). Expert committee recommendations for acne management. *Pediatrics, 118*, 1188–1199.

See **thePoint** for Organizations.

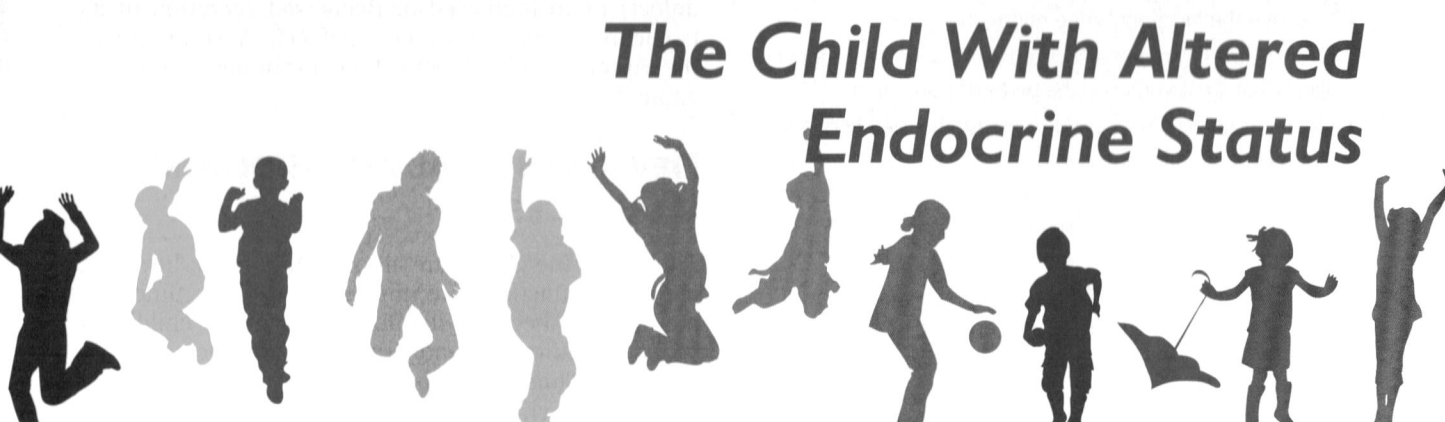

CHAPTER 26

The Child With Altered Endocrine Status

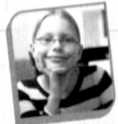

CASE HISTORY

Lindsay Jenkins was first diagnosed with type 1 diabetes mellitus (T1DM) when she was 6 years old (see Chapter 12). Right before Thanksgiving, her parents noticed that she seemed very thirsty and often would leave the dinner table to use the bathroom, but she did not seem sick. She had the energy of a normal 6-year-old. On Thanksgiving day, Lindsay romped with her cousins, although she was still very thirsty and her aunts commented on how thin Lindsay looked. The next day, Lindsay vomited and her parents decided to take her to the health care provider. Their health care provider tested her urine for glucose and ketones, and within 5 minutes, Lindsay received the diagnosis of T1DM. The health care provider told the Jenkins they would need to go to the hospital. Lindsay's initial blood sugar was more than 500 mg/dL. Lindsay and her family were in the hospital for 3 days to regulate Lindsay's glucose level and teach Lindsay's parents the basic skills of diabetes care.

Lindsay was discharged home on two insulin injections each day. Initially, Lindsay's parents drew up her insulin and gave her injections. Lindsay gave herself her first injection with a syringe when she was at diabetes camp at age 7 years; she had learned to draw up her own insulin by age 8 years. Her parents supervise her during this process. She checks her blood sugar before breakfast, before lunch, before dinner, and at bedtime. Her dad checks her at midnight, and her mom checks her at 3 AM if Lindsay has had a really active day. If the blood sugar is elevated at lunch, Lindsay uses an insulin pen of rapid-acting insulin at school, which greatly reduces the risk of an incorrect dosage.

Lindsay is now 8 years old and has reached an important milestone. She had been on a split-mixed dose of insulin since diagnosis but was recently switched to a multiple dose injection (MDI) regimen, which involves taking short-acting insulin for meals and snacks and a long-acting insulin every 24 hours. This has introduced flexibility to her life. Lindsay no longer needs to eat on a schedule, and meals and snacks can fluctuate in carbohydrate amount as she wishes. For the past 3 months, she has been proving to her pediatric endocrinologist that she is ready for an insulin pump. Lindsay has been counting her carbohydrates, testing her blood sugar, and giving herself multiple shots a day of rapid-acting insulin to cover meals and snacks and to mimic the manner in which the insulin pump will work. Lindsay has been wearing the pump with just a saline solution in it this week to prepare herself for wearing the pump permanently. The night before she begins the insulin pump, Lindsay will give herself the long-acting insulin to prepare for the pump start in the morning. The next day, Lindsay checks her blood sugar, injects her morning rapid-acting insulin, eats breakfast, and heads off to the endocrinologist's office with her parents. The pump is started that morning right after breakfast. The basal rate will temporarily be off until the time her long-acting insulin would have been due. Then the basal rate will begin and she will no longer require long-acting insulin. Lindsay's parents will write down all of her blood sugars, carbohydrates eaten, unusual activity levels, and pump settings and fax them daily to the diabetes nurse educator for a couple of weeks. Their goal is to keep Lindsay's blood sugars within a targeted range of 70–140 mg/dL. The nurse who works for the manufacturer of her insulin pump is coming to Lindsay's school to talk to the health technician and the school nurse about her new insulin pump. Lindsay's case study is also discussed in Chapter 2.

CHAPTER OBJECTIVES

1 Describe the functions of the endocrine system.

2 Describe the symptoms associated with disorders of endocrine glands that are common in the pediatric population.

3 Identify diagnostic tests used to assess the disorders associated with the endocrine glands.

4 Describe the interdisciplinary interventions unique to selected endocrine disorders, including the role of the nurse in managing the child's care.

5 Describe the educational plan for a child with a newly diagnosed endocrine disorder that encompasses both acute health care needs and long-term home management needs.

See thePoint for a list of Key Terms.

The endocrine system is a network of glands that work in parallel with the nervous system to regulate growth, development, and homeostasis. The parts of the endocrine system include the pituitary gland, thyroid gland, parathyroid glands, adrenal glands, and ovaries or testes. Endocrine glands secrete **hormones** directly into the bloodstream. Hormones are chemical messengers that exert physiologic effects on target cells in other endocrine glands, organs, or tissues. Thus, hormones transfer information and instructions from one set of cells to another set of cells that are genetically programmed to receive the message. Increased or decreased hormone levels are influenced by factors such as stress, infection, and changes in the balance of fluid and minerals in blood.

Endocrine function is regulated largely by negative feedback. One endocrine gland produces a hormone (tropic hormone) that affects functioning of either another endocrine gland or body tissue (the target gland or organ). In response, the target gland produces a hormone that inhibits the release of the tropic hormone. The target organ responds to the hormone acting on it but is not directly active in the feedback loop. The reverse is seen when the stimulating endocrine gland detects low levels of target gland hormone. In that case, tropic hormone secretion increases, which causes increased secretion of the target gland hormone. For example, the pituitary gland (hypophysis or master gland) controls the release of at least seven different hormones, including thyroid-stimulating hormone (TSH). This pituitary tropic hormone stimulates the thyroid gland (target gland) to release thyroxine (T_4) and triiodothyronine (T_3) (target gland hormones). Elevated levels of these hormones then, in turn, inhibit secretion of TSH, the tropic hormone.

Endocrine disorders are mainly of two types: hypofunction and hyperfunction. **Hypofunction** causes deficient target hormone secretion, and **hyperfunction** causes excessive target hormone secretion. Normal levels of hormones vary widely, and this range may overlap deficient and excessive hormonal blood levels. Analysis of hormones at various times may be necessary to establish glandular hypofunction or hyperfunction. Endocrine gland dysfunction may be attributable to disease of the gland itself (primary defect) or to increased or decreased secretion of its tropic hormone (secondary defect). A summary of the endocrine glands and their hormones is given in Table 26-1.

DEVELOPMENTAL AND BIOLOGIC VARIANCES

The endocrine glands are all present at birth; however, endocrine functions are immature. As these functions mature and become stabilized during the childhood years, alterations in endocrine function become more apparent. Thus, endocrine disorders may arise at any time during childhood development (Fig. 26-1). The endocrine disorders most prevalent in infancy are those that are congenital: hypopituitarism, congenital hypothyroidism (CH), congenital adrenal hyperplasia (CAH), aplasia of the parathyroid glands, and nesidioblastosis. Although disorders of the pancreas are less common in infancy, hyperinsulinism and insulin-dependent diabetes occur. Poor feeding, irritability, and poor growth (weight, length) may all be indicators that an infant has an endocrine disorder.

Growth disorders may begin in early childhood. Children who are walking are now compared with their peers in height, and discrepancies become evident. In middle childhood, the youth may present with a growth disorder or with signs of early puberty. During routine school health assessments, they may be measured in the school health setting or in the health care provider's office during routine visits. School-based health settings should refer children with perceived growth issues back to their primary care providers for evaluation.

Many endocrine disorders are detected during adolescence because of early pubertal onset or a delay in pubertal onset (see Chapter 3). Normal female adolescents begin pubertal development with development of breasts, growth of pubic and axillary hair, and **menarche** (the start of menstruation). In males, enlargement of the testes and penis and growth of pubic and axillary hair begin (see Figs. 3-23 and 3-24 for a review of pubertal staging). Girls with irregular menses may present to the primary care provider, gynecologist, or endocrinologist. A variety of autoimmune endocrine disorders may appear during this stage in development, including Hashimoto thyroiditis, Graves disease, autoimmune hypoparathyroidism, Addison disease, and T1DM. With the exception of T1DM, autoimmune disorders rarely occur before adolescence.

ASSESSMENT

Because the endocrine system varies greatly in its structures and functions, each gland requires its own specific assessment. The embryology, physiology, assessment, and disorders of each gland are discussed specifically and separately in this chapter.

TABLE 26-1 Hormones and Their Actions

Gland and Hormone	Major Target Tissue, Gland or Organ	Effect
Pituitary, Anterior		
Growth hormone (GH)	Bones, muscles, organs	Promotes growth of bone and soft tissue Mobilizes free fatty acids from adipose tissue Increases lean muscle mass Decreases fat mass Causes insulin resistance May induce hyperglycemia
TSH	Thyroid	Increases iodine uptake and iodide clearance from plasma Promotes growth of the thyroid Stimulates release of thyroid hormone from thyroid gland
Prolactin	Breasts	Initiates and maintains lactation Stimulates the formation and function of the corpus luteum
Adrenocorticotropic hormone (ACTH)	Adrenal cortex	Stimulates release of cortisol from the adrenal glands
Melanocyte-stimulating hormone (MSH)	Skin	Promotes skin pigmentation
Follicle-stimulating hormone (FSH)	Ovary (female) Testis (male)	Stimulates ovarian follicle growth and oogenesis Stimulates the activity of the seminiferous epithelium Controls spermatogenesis
Luteinizing hormone (LH)	Ovary and corpus luteum (female) Testis (male)	Aids in maturation of ovarian follicles Causes ovulation in the mature ovum Causes formation of the corpus luteum Stimulates progesterone secretion by the corpus luteum Stimulates the ovary to produce estrogen Stimulates Leydig cells of the testes to produce testosterone
Pituitary, Posterior		
Antidiuretic hormone (ADH)	Renal tubules	Increases kidney tubule permeability, thus increasing water reabsorption
Oxytocin	Uterus, mammary glands	Stimulates contraction of smooth muscles of the uterus Causes compression of the alveoli of the mammary glands (milk letdown reflex)
Thyroid		
T_4 and T_3	All tissues	Accelerates cell metabolism Works with GH to stimulate growth (very essential to development of nervous tissue) Increases glucose uptake by cells Increases rate of cholesterol removal by liver
Calcitonin	Bone and renal tubules	Lowers serum levels of calcium and phosphorus; decreases kidney excretion of calcium and phosphorus Increases calcium and phosphorus deposition in bone
Parathyroid		
Parathyroid hormone (PTH)	Gastrointestinal tract, bone, renal proximal tubules	Increases absorption of calcium, phosphorus, and magnesium from the intestine Promotes reabsorption of bony tissue and release of calcium into the bloodstream
Adrenal Cortex		
Aldosterone	Primarily renal distal tubules	Increases the reabsorption of sodium from distal tubule of the kidney Promotes water retention and potassium loss
Cortisol	All tissues	Increases protein catabolism, gluconeogenesis, and glycogenesis Is antagonistic to insulin and androgens Aids in erythrocyte formation and in maintenance of normal brain activity

(Continued)

TABLE 26-1	Hormones and Their Actions *(Continued)*	
Gland and Hormone	**Major Target Tissue, Gland or Organ**	**Effect**
Androgens	Many tissues, especially gonads and muscles	Increases retention of nitrogen, potassium, phosphorus, and sulfur Promotes growth and the development of male secondary sex characteristics Promotes axillary and pubic hair development in females
Adrenal Medulla		
Norepinephrine	Adrenergic receptors	Increases rate and strength of heart activity Dilates coronary vessels; constricts vessels in other organs (increases blood pressure) Stimulates alertness Mobilizes fatty acids from storage areas
Epinephrine	Heart, liver, lungs, brain, kidneys, and arteries	Dilates vessels to skeletal muscle Stimulates glycogenesis
Pancreas		
Insulin	Liver, muscle, adipose tissue	Increases glucose uptake by cells Stimulates the conversion of glucose to glycogen Promotes fatty acids and amino acid transport into cells Promotes lipogenesis and protein synthesis
Glucagon	Liver	Increases glycogenesis in the liver, thereby increasing blood glucose
Somatostatin	Alpha and beta cells in pancreas	Inhibits insulin and glucagon release
Ovaries		
Estrogen	Uterus, breasts, and bone	Causes initial stages of uterine regrowth during menstrual cycles Increases mammary duct growth Stimulates contraction of the uterus and uterine tubes Promotes development of breast tissue Accelerates epiphyseal closure Increases fat deposition in subcutaneous tissues Causes salt and water retention Improves bone mineral density
Progesterone	Uterus	Prepares the uterus for implantation of fertilized ovum Develops the secretory potential of the mammary gland Increases basal body temperature Promotes retention of salt and water
Relaxin	Pelvis	Softens pelvic ligaments before labor Creates sleepiness during pregnancy
Testes		
Testosterone	Spermatogenic tubules, penis, bone, and many other tissues	Ensures development of the male reproductive organs Promotes development of secondary sex characteristics Increases protein anabolism and calcium retention Increases rate of bone growth

FOCUSED HEALTH HISTORY

QUESTION: Review Focused Health History 26-1. What are the aspects of the case study that contain pertinent information for Lindsay's focused health history?

Endocrine disorders are not generally suspected as a primary clinical condition when a child presents with complaints of gastrointestinal, neurologic, or musculoskeletal problems in an outpatient setting. The serious nature of endocrine conditions means that most children are likely to present in the emergency department with severe metabolic distress. However, because endocrine dysfunction can affect all aspects of the child's growth, development, and physiologic functions, the health care provider must always keep a high index of suspicion for the possibility of endocrine dysfunction, especially in cases in which no other acute condition appears to be present.

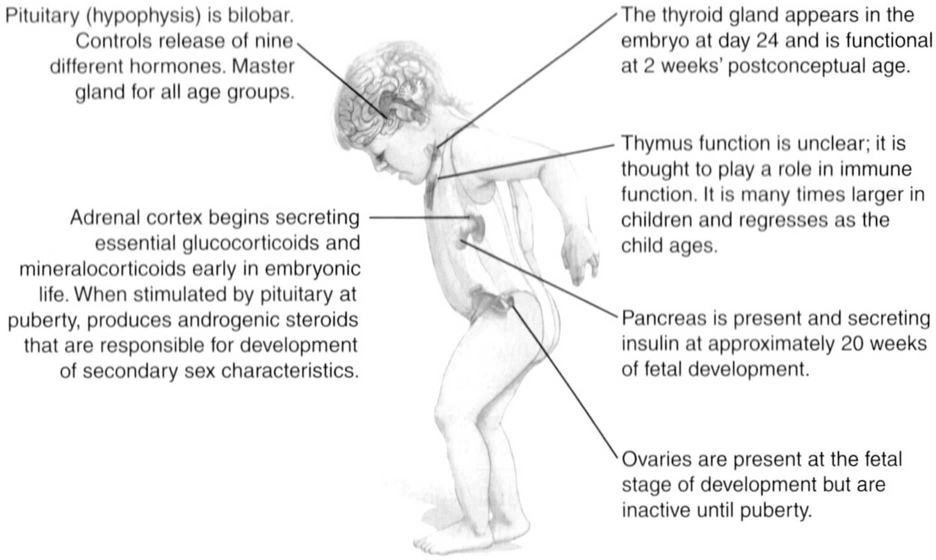

Pituitary (hypophysis) is bilobar. Controls release of nine different hormones. Master gland for all age groups.

The thyroid gland appears in the embryo at day 24 and is functional at 2 weeks' postconceptual age.

Thymus function is unclear; it is thought to play a role in immune function. It is many times larger in children and regresses as the child ages.

Adrenal cortex begins secreting essential glucocorticoids and mineralocorticoids early in embryonic life. When stimulated by pituitary at puberty, produces androgenic steroids that are responsible for development of secondary sex characteristics.

Pancreas is present and secreting insulin at approximately 20 weeks of fetal development.

Ovaries are present at the fetal stage of development but are inactive until puberty.

Figure 26-1 Developmental and biologic variances: endocrine system.

Endocrine disorders often cause changes in normal growth and activity patterns. Good records of general health assessment, including serial recording of growth parameters using Centers for Disease Control and Prevention (CDC) growth charts (see Appendix A), are especially helpful in making a diagnosis of endocrine dysfunction (Focused Health History 26-1).

Most general health assessment records in primary care settings include the child's height and weight, plotting growth parameters against norms. Correct measuring techniques must be used to complete these linear measurements (Tradition or Science 26-1). Reflective reports and memories shared by family members may be foggy and incomplete, but careful and thorough questioning by clinicians and family photographs of the child at various developmental ages can help pinpoint the origin and timing of problems with presenting symptoms. In addition, symptoms can be localized to individual glandular dysfunction more easily. Neonatal growth parameters, including weight, length, head and chest circumferences, and appearance at birth, are also useful to know when reconstructing a health history focused on possible endocrine dysfunction. When an endocrine dysfunction is suspected, primary care providers should seek the assistance of pediatric endocrinologists for diagnosis and further recommendations for treatment. Endocrinologists can also work as a team with the primary care provider to provide guidance for health surveillance throughout the child's growth and developmental cycle.

ANSWER: Critical information in Lindsay's case study includes sudden onset of symptoms, increased thirst, increased voiding, slight and gradual weight loss, and one incidence of vomiting.

FOCUSED PHYSICAL ASSESSMENT

QUESTION: If you were to conduct a head-to-toe physical assessment of Lindsay at age 8 years after she obtained her pump, what physical signs do you anticipate finding?

Dysfunctions of the endocrine system can result in a variety of physical changes because of the influence that circulating hormones have on growth and development, fluid and electrolyte balance, use of nutrients, and regulation of sex hormone levels. To pinpoint the exact systems affected by the dysfunction, and thereby more accurately determine the actual endocrine disorder, perform a systematic physical assessment (see Chapter 8). Inspection, palpation, and auscultation reveal specific findings that indicate certain conditions (Focused Physical Assessment 26-1).

Inspect the child's general appearance for abnormalities of facial structures and features; alterations in the appearance of the skin and hair; and the presence of abnormal, premature, or late secondary sex characteristics. Evaluate the child's size for his or her age.

Further evaluation of the child's respiratory, cardiac, gastrointestinal, and urinary functions is likely to reveal dysfunctions consistent with specific endocrine disorders.

ANSWER: There are very few physical signs of diabetes. The presence of the insulin pump is the most obvious. On her abdomen or hips, you can see small punctures at the previous insulin pump insertion sites. The insertion sites take a long time to fade and there may be as many as 10 old sites visible at any time. Her fingertips are calloused on both sides from multiple finger sticks; otherwise, her physical assessment reveals no clues to her diabetes.

FOCUSED HEALTH HISTORY 26-1

The Child With Altered Endocrine Status

Current history	Gradual versus sudden onset of symptoms
	Changes in child's lifestyle because of symptoms
	Changes in the child's physical appearance or general affect
	Recent changes in growth velocity or weight gain or loss
	Changes in sleep patterns
	Changes in appetite or thirst, food preferences
	Changes in vision
	Changes in voiding or stool patterns
	All medications the child is currently taking (prescribed, over the counter, herbal or home remedies)
Past medical history	**Prenatal/Neonatal History**
	Birth history
	Results of neonatal screening tests
	Feeding difficulties noted at birth and during infancy
	Child's size at birth
	Maternal factors that may have affected weight and height of growing fetus (e.g., tobacco or alcohol use)
	Previous Health Challenges
	Treatment in the past for the current problems or symptoms
	Recent minor illness such as gastroenteritis or a viral syndrome
	Current immunization status
	Any allergies to medications, food products, milk, or formula products
	Exposure to exogenous steroids, testosterone, or estrogen
	Exposure to endocrine disruptors such as tea tree oil, lavender, and bisphenol A (BPA)
Nutritional assessment	Recent change in diet, food intake
	Unusual hunger or thirst
	Recent weight loss or gain
	Current intake, usual intake
Family medical history	Family history of any endocrine disorders (e.g., thyroid disorders, diabetes mellitus)
	Family members who have had growth or development difficulties (e.g., very short or very tall, early or late puberty)
Social and environmental history	Normal daily activities
	Activity level (note fatigue vs. hyperactivity)
	Family resources to maintain a healthy diet, purchase needed medications, continue with consistent health care follow-up
Growth and development	Growth and development plotted on height and weight growth curves
	Achievement of age-appropriate developmental tasks
	Presence of learning disabilities or cognitive delays

Note: See Chapter 8 for a comprehensive health history.

DIAGNOSTIC CRITERIA

As with a focused physical assessment, no specific diagnostic criteria exist for general health challenges to the endocrine system. Serial serum hormone assays are performed for most endocrine conditions, and blood levels of these hormones often pinpoint the problems. Tests and Procedures 26-1 summarizes the hormones of the endocrine system and the diagnostic tests used to determine whether the presenting symptoms are endocrine related or of some other clinical origin.

TRADITION OR SCIENCE 26-1

Can nurses use strategies to ensure better accuracy of linear measurements?

Accurate measurements are essential for early detection of growth disorders in children, yet measuring linear growth is a technically difficult task (see Chapter 8 for measurement methods). Errors associated with linear measurement are generally attributed to error by the examiner and child in the measuring technique rather than error because of the measurement equipment (Himes, 2009). One multisite study used a didactic education program to teach appropriate linear measurement techniques to nursing staff. In 3- and 6-month follow-up evaluations, the treatment group (those who received education) showed significant improvement in accurately completing linear measures compared with the control group (no educational intervention). The educational background of the measurer was also found to be associated with accurate measurement, with registered nurses 1.8 times more likely than licensed practical nurses or nurses' aides to measure children using correct technique. The investigators demonstrated that correct technique and accurate measurement equipment are essential to ensure that a child's growth is monitored correctly (Hench et al., 2005; Lipman et al., 2004).

TREATMENT MODALITIES

 QUESTION: Briefly, what are the treatment modalities for TIDM?

Pharmacologic treatment modalities either replace insufficient hormone levels or block overproduction of hormones. These treatments are calculated based on the child's own serum blood levels of the hormones in question and on the child's physical appearance (e.g., short stature or premature development of secondary sex characteristics). Treatment options may involve surgical removal of a gland or portion of a gland that is oversecreting a hormone. If a tumor is causing endocrine dysfunction, surgical removal of the tumor is required. Many endocrine conditions require dietary modifications to manage the child's condition. Nursing Interventions 26-1 provides examples of endocrine conditions and their associated dietary management.

Treating most pediatric endocrine conditions requires the expertise of a team that is well versed in handling numerous cases; the child's ability to reach optimal growth and development hangs in the balance. With input from the endocrinology team, maximal growth potential can be realized. Normal well-child health care and appropriate surveillance of the endocrinologic issue may be administered by a primary care clinician, with oversight by the pediatric endocrine team.

ANSWER: The treatment for TIDM is to replace the insulin, which enables glucose uptake to the cells and maintains a desired range of serum glucose.

NURSING PLAN OF CARE

QUESTION: Which of the general nursing diagnoses found in Nursing Plan of Care 26-1 are most applicable to a family, like the Jenkins, whose child has TIDM?

Fortunately, with modern science and pharmacotherapy, most endocrine dysfunctions can be treated. Although the child with an endocrine condition and his or her family may have to manage the problem on a long-term basis, the outcomes of management are generally successful when treatment regimens are carefully followed. General nursing diagnoses for a child experiencing health challenges with the endocrine system are presented in Nursing Plan of Care 26-1. In addition, Nursing Plan of Care 12-2 provides additional diagnoses addressing family issues and home management concerns for the child with a chronic condition.

ANSWER: Nursing Diagnosis: Risk for ineffective family therapeutic regimen management is applicable for every family with a child with TIDM.

ALTERATIONS IN ENDOCRINE STATUS

Alterations in endocrine status can be categorized as disorders of the pituitary gland, thyroid gland, parathyroid glands, adrenal glands, and gonadal disorders.

DISORDERS OF THE PITUITARY GLAND

Disorders of the pituitary gland depend on the location of the physiologic abnormality. The posterior lobe is called the *neurohypophysis* because it is formed of neural tissue. It secretes ADH (vasopressin) and oxytocin. The anterior pituitary, or adenohypophysis, is made up of endocrine glandular tissue and secretes GH, ACTH, TSH, FSH, LH, MSH, and prolactin. Usually, several target organs are affected when there is a disorder of the pituitary gland, especially the adenohypophysis. Specific disorders are discussed with respect to their anatomic locations of origin and the effects of hyper- and hypofunction on target organs and the child as a whole.

Endocrine System

Assessment Parameter	Alterations/Possible Clinical Significance
General appearance	Abnormal growth velocity (i.e., too short or tall/large): hypopituitarism, pituitary disorders, thyroid and adrenal disorders
	Weight loss: pancreatic, thyroid, and adrenal disorders
	Weight gain or obesity: thyroid disorders, syndrome of inappropriate antidiuretic hormone secretion (SIADH), adrenal disorders
Integumentary system (skin, hair, nails)	Cold intolerance or cold extremities: hypothyroidism
	Change in color or texture: pituitary, adrenal and thyroid disorders, Cushing syndrome (CS)
	Easy bruising and striae: CS
	Sweating: thyroid disorders
Head and neck	Enlargement in anterior neck: goiter, thyroid disorders
	Brittle hair: hypothyroidism
	Hirsutism (excessive growth of hair): cortisol or androgen excesses
Eyes	Changes in vision: pituitary tumor, pancreatic disorders, precocious puberty
Face, nose, and oral cavity	Rounded face: CS
	Deformities or abnormal features: hypoparathyroidism, hypothyroidism, hypopituitarism
	Delay in dentition: hypocalcemia, hypopituitarism
Thorax and lungs	Fruity odor to breath: ketoacidosis/diabetes mellitus
	Kussmaul respirations: ketoacidosis/diabetes mellitus
Cardiovascular system	Palpitations: thyroid disorders
	Tachycardia: hyperthyroidism
	Hypertension: CS, hyperthyroidism, other adrenal disorders
Gastrointestinal system	Nausea: parathyroid disorders, diabetes mellitus, adrenal disorders
	Vomiting: parathyroid disorders, diabetes insipidus (DI), diabetes mellitus
	Changes in bowel habits (constipation or diarrhea): thyroid and parathyroid disorders, diabetes mellitus
	Polydipsia: DI, diabetes mellitus
	Dehydration: SIADH, diabetes mellitus, DI
Musculoskeletal system	Muscle weakness or lethargy: SIADH, hypothyroidism, hyperthyroidism, parathyroid disorders, hyperinsulinism, CAH, adrenal disorders
	Hyperactivity: hyperthyroidism
	Pathologic bone fractures: adrenal disorders
	Gait disturbances: hyperparathyroidism
	Diminished deep tendon reflexes: hypercalcemia, hyperparathyroidism
	Hyperreflexia/twitching: hypocalcemia, hypoparathyroidism
Neurologic system	Confusion: parathyroid disorders, diabetes mellitus
	Increased irritability/behavioral changes: DI, SIADH, precocious puberty
	Headaches: diabetes mellitus, adrenal insufficiency, CS, thyroid and pituitary disorders
	Changes in sleep patterns: pituitary disorders
Genitourinary system	Polyuria: diabetes mellitus, DI, parathyroid disorders
	Hematuria: parathyroid disorders
Genitalia	Onset, timing, deviation of menses: gonadal and thyroid disorders
	Testicular mass or pain: gonadal disorders
	Small genitalia: hypopituitarism, Prader-Willi syndrome or Klinefelter syndrome
	Ambiguous genitalia: CAH, disorders of sexual development (DSD)
	Presence of early pubertal changes or abnormal pubertal changes: precocious puberty, premature thelarche, gynecomastia
	Delayed pubertal changes: hypopituitarism, hypothyroidism, adrenal insufficiency

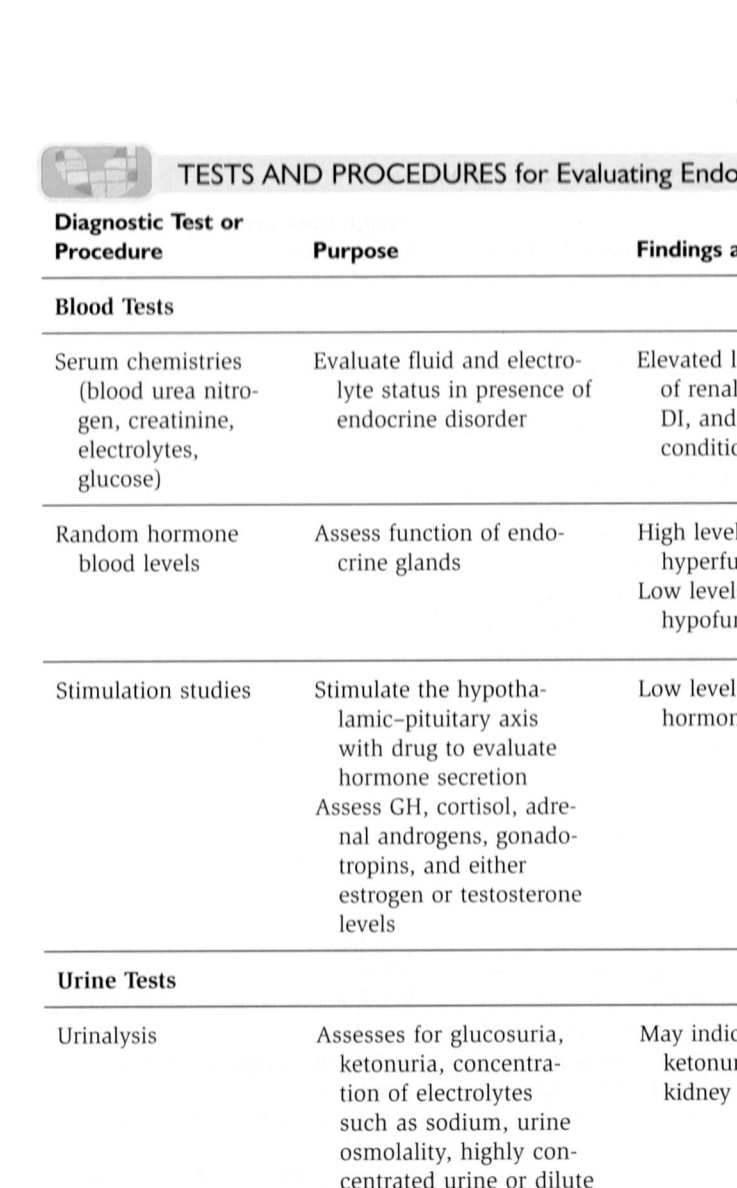

TESTS AND PROCEDURES for Evaluating Endocrine Status

Diagnostic Test or Procedure	Purpose	Findings and Indications	Health Care Provider Considerations
Blood Tests			
Serum chemistries (blood urea nitrogen, creatinine, electrolytes, glucose)	Evaluate fluid and electrolyte status in presence of endocrine disorder	Elevated levels indicative of renal involvement, DI, and other endocrine conditions.	Sodium can be decreased or increased with polyuria or urinary-concentrating defects.
Random hormone blood levels	Assess function of endocrine glands	High levels indicate hyperfunction. Low levels indicate hypofunction.	Draw labs at the same time as other serum chemistries to help decrease number of times child has to experience a needle stick.
Stimulation studies	Stimulate the hypothalamic–pituitary axis with drug to evaluate hormone secretion. Assess GH, cortisol, adrenal androgens, gonadotropins, and either estrogen or testosterone levels	Low levels indicate hormone deficiency.	Advise parents to keep child NPO (nothing by mouth) if assessing GH production. Explain procedure to child. Establish venous access. Obtain blood samples at precise times.
Urine Tests			
Urinalysis	Assesses for glucosuria, ketonuria, concentration of electrolytes such as sodium, urine osmolality, highly concentrated urine or dilute urine, and mineral loss such as calcium and phosphorus	May indicate diabetes, ketonuria, SIADH, DI, or kidney loss of minerals.	Attach urine bag to a child who is not toilet trained.
Fluid deprivation study	Evaluates the effect of fluid restriction on urine concentration, specific gravity, and urine volume. Monitors serum sodium and osmolality	Osmolality of urine more than 600 mOsm/kg with serum osmolality <300 mOsm/kg is a normal response. Osmolality of urine less than 600 mOsm/kg with serum osmolality >300 mOsm/kg and signs of dehydration are an abnormal response indicating DI.	Do not perform this test in children as an overnight study because severe dehydration may occur, leading to central nervous system (CNS) damage. Monitor input and output carefully. Assess vital signs every hour (blood pressure and pulse). Measure urine specific gravity and osmolality with each void. Obtain serum specimens for sodium, ADH, hematocrit, and osmolality. Monitor the child's weight closely (twice daily in some). Terminate the test and give desmopressin (DDAVP) if the child loses more than 3% of the baseline body weight or if tachycardia and substantial hypotension occur.

(Continued)

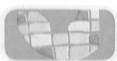 **TESTS AND PROCEDURES for Evaluating Endocrine Status** *(Continued)*

Diagnostic Test or Procedure	Purpose	Findings and Indications	Health Care Provider Considerations
Other Tests			
Radiography	Compares radiographs of the left hand and wrist against standards for age to determine bone age. Evaluates skeletal maturation	Delayed maturation indicates growth will continue for a longer time than normal. Accelerated maturation indicates growth will continue for a shorter time than normal. Skeletal age is more advanced than chronologic age in precocious puberty.	Radiography is easily available and an inexpensive testing method.
Computed tomography	Evaluates and diagnoses a large number of clinical conditions, with radiographs taken at multiple angles of the body to provide cross-sectional anatomic display	Abnormalities visualized include tumors, cancer, lesions, abscesses, fluid collection, and inflammation.	Assess for allergies to contrast agent, which may be used; observe for reaction to contrast media. Determine whether child is claustrophobic or unable to remain still. Administer sedation if ordered.
Magnetic resonance imaging (MRI)	Evaluates pituitary size and location as well as potential masses	May detect a brain lesion or mass to explain the cause of precocious puberty, DI, or GH production problems	Determine whether child is claustrophobic or unable to remain still. Administer sedation if ordered. Remove all metal objects from child's body. If parents are allowed to stay with child during procedure, ensure that they remove all metal objects from their bodies. Explain to child that machine makes various noises as the radio waves are turned on and off. Provide child with earplugs if necessary. Assess for allergies to contrast agent, which may be used; observe for reaction to contrast media.
Thyroid scan and radioactive iodine uptake test (RAIU)	Scan is used to determine the size, shape, and position of the thyroid gland. The RAIU is performed to evaluate the function of the gland by measuring how much radioactive iodine is taken up by the thyroid gland in a given time period.	Enlarged gland may indicate goiter. Small thyroid may indicate a congenital defect. Increased uptake of iodine would indicate hyperthyroidism; decreased uptake would indicate hypothyroidism. A nodule that doesn't uptake iodine (cold nodule) is more likely to be cancer.	Performed by giving a radionucleotide intravenously 2 hours before the scan. Ensure child has good intravenous (IV) access. 99m-Technetium is the preferred radionucleotide in children because it has the advantage of low radiation exposure. Used in the neonate to assess CH. I^{131} is the radionucleotide used in almost all other instances.

TESTS AND PROCEDURES for Evaluating Endocrine Status *(Continued)*

Diagnostic Test or Procedure	Purpose	Findings and Indications	Health Care Provider Considerations
Ultrasonography	Assesses thyroid Assesses uterus, ovaries or testes Assesses kidneys	Could indicate ectopic, enlarged, absent, or nodular thyroid Could indicate ectopic, enlarged, or absent gonads Could indicate horseshoe-shaped kidneys, as seen in Turner syndrome	Tell the child and parents that no sedation is needed and the test is painless. Explain that an ultrasound lubricant will be applied to the area being viewed. Remove the lubricant after test is completed.

DIABETES INSIPIDUS

 QUESTION: Compare DI with diabetes mellitus. Why do they share part of the same name? What do they have in common?

Central DI, also called *neurogenic, vasopressin-sensitive,* or *hypothalamic DI,* is a disorder of the posterior pituitary that results from deficient secretion of ADH. Nephrogenic DI is a result of the inability of the kidney to respond to ADH. Distinguishing between central DI and nephrogenic DI is important because treatment will be different. Central DI may result from

NURSING INTERVENTIONS 26-1

Nutritional Management of Selected Endocrine Disorders

Endocrine Disorder	Dietary Management	Rationale
Addison disease	High-protein, low-carbohydrate, high-sodium diet Small, frequent meals	Because of inadequate production of hepatic glucagons, the recommended diet prevents fatigue, hypoglycemia, and hyponatremia.
Cushing Syndrome	Low calorie, carbohydrate, and sodium diet Ample protein and potassium Reduced fluid intake	Helps control development of hyperglycemia, edema, and hypokalemia.
T1DM	Adherence to American Heart Association guidelines in addition to meeting guidelines for growth and development in child's age group	Helps prevent long-term effects of diabetes, including cardiovascular, neurologic, and renal effects.
Type 2 diabetes mellitus (T2DM)	Individualized meal plan with adherence to American Heart Association guidelines	Meal plan is aimed at improving eating habits, restricting caloric intake, achieving moderate weight loss, maintaining consistent carbohydrate intake, and decreasing fat intake.
Hypothyroidism	Low-calorie, low-cholesterol, low-saturated fat diet	Because of decreased metabolic rate, child requires fewer calories to support metabolic activity. Individuals with hypothyroidism tend to have high cholesterol levels.

NURSING PLAN OF CARE 26-1:

The Child With Altered Endocrine Status

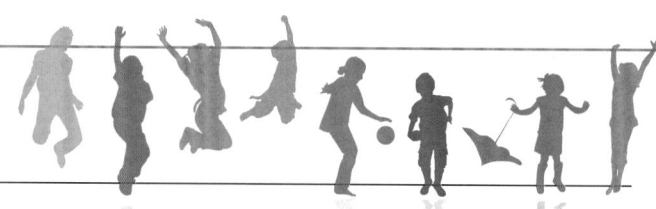

Nursing Diagnosis: Risk for excess or deficient fluid volume related to altered endocrine function

Interventions/Rationale

- Monitor and record vital signs.
  Retention or loss of sodium and water can cause dramatic shifts in fluid volume. Hypertension and edema can occur from expanded fluid volume with sodium and water retention. Hypovolemic shock (e.g., tachycardia, tachypnea, and hypotension) and dehydration can occur because of disturbances in water metabolism.
- Weigh child daily.
  Assists in detecting excessive fluid loss or gain.
- Monitor intake and output.
  With many endocrine conditions, urine volume is independent of fluid intake.
- Complete blood and urine analysis as ordered.
  Indicates electrolyte imbalances related to fluid volume excess or deficit. Indicates ability of kidneys to concentrate urine.
- Monitor fluid intake and provide access to fluids as warranted by the child's condition.
  Conditions such as CS may require restricted fluid intake, whereas the child with diabetes should have an easily accessible fluid source.
- Administer medication as prescribed.
  The goal of medication therapy is to return the child to normal hormone levels and/or maintain normal electrolyte levels.
- Instruct child and family in administering medications and managing fluids and nutrition. Include expected effects, dosage, and side effects when child does not adhere to regimen and monitor fluids and nutrition.
  Knowledge of the disease process and of the regimen for medication, fluids, and nutrition will promote adherence.

Expected Outcomes

- Child will remain well hydrated.
- Child will have normal serum hormone or electrolyte levels.
- Child and family will understand the need for replacement hormone or other medical therapy and long-term follow-up.
- Child and family will administer the hormone therapy as prescribed.
- Child and family will seek intervention when fluid volume excess or deficit occurs.

Nursing Diagnosis: Imbalanced nutrition: More or less than body requirements related to intake insufficient or in excess of activity expenditure and/or inability of body to utilize nutrients available

Interventions/Rationale

- Monitor trends in weight.
  Provides documentation of weight loss or gain that may indicate a need to change therapeutic regimen.
- Assess child's nutritional status, including appetite; presence of nausea, vomiting, or diarrhea; food intake; and food preferences.
  Endocrine dysfunction can impair gastrointestinal function, causing nausea, vomiting, and diarrhea. Appetite may increase when food preferences are determined and incorporated into regular meals and snacks.
- Provide diet specific to complement the metabolic hormonal excess or deficiency and thereby the nutritional needs of the child.
  The regimen to manage specific endocrine disorders may include specific dietary requirements. For instance, the child with Addison disease needs a high-protein, low-carbohydrate, high-sodium diet. The child with CS needs a diet low in calories, carbohydrates, and sodium, with ample protein and potassium (see Nursing Interventions 26-1).
- Provide child and family education regarding child's nutritional needs and the complications that may arise when dietary plan is not followed.
  Lack of knowledge or nonadherence to dietary guidelines can lead to severe complications of the child's condition.

Expected Outcomes

- Child and family will understand the need for specific nutritional therapy and long-term follow-up.
- Child will maintain weight within parameters for age and gender.
- Child will adhere to prescribed meal plan.

Nursing Diagnosis: Disturbed body image related to perception of changes in physical appearance resulting from hormonal imbalances

Interventions/Rationale

- Assess for changes in personal appearance caused by endocrine imbalance (e.g., obesity, increased body and facial hair, acne).
  Evaluation of physical changes may assist in the diagnosis of the condition.

- Assess child's feelings about changed appearance and evaluate coping mechanisms.
  Provides information about specific areas of concern for the child to help develop plan of action to help bolster child's self-esteem.
- Promote coping mechanisms that deal with changes in child's appearance (e.g., selecting flattering clothes, improving personal grooming and hygiene).
  Learning methods to compensate for changes in appearance can help improve child's self-esteem.
- Provide atmosphere of acceptance, including environment in which child feels supported.
  Child should feel that family, friends, and health care providers are providing care in an accepting manner. Child can be referred to a support group to learn additional coping strategies and to gain support from interacting with others who have a similar condition.

Expected Outcomes
- Child will express positive feelings about self.
- Child will use appropriate coping mechanisms to manage changes in physical appearance.
- Child will have access to support groups as needed.

Nursing Diagnosis: Risk for ineffective family therapeutic regimen management related to presence of chronic condition

Interventions/Rationale
- Evaluate child and family learning needs, self-management skills, and abilities.

Determines the amount and type of education and demonstration needed.
- Determine child and family members' ability (including developmental readiness) and willingness to learn.
  Assists in presenting educational information that is tailored to specific characteristics of the child and family members.
- Ensure that child and family have knowledge about causes of symptoms, treatment, and management regimen (e.g., dietary, medication). Instruct child to wear MedicAlert bracelet at all times.
  Allows others to identify the child as having an endocrine condition and provide appropriate care in an emergency.

Expected Outcomes
- Child and family will report ability to cope and adjust adequately.
- Child and family will show ability to accept and adapt to new health status and integrate learning.
- Child and family will identify factors that influence inability to adhere to plan.
- Child will demonstrate a level of adherence that promotes physiologic safety.

Nursing Diagnosis: Anxiety related to response to prognosis; actual or perceived loss of body integrity; threat to self-concept

See Nursing Plan of Care 12-2.

---

many different causes, including accidental or surgical trauma to vasopressin neurons; congenital anatomic hypothalamic or pituitary defects; neoplasms; infiltrative, autoimmune, or infectious diseases; increased metabolism of vasopressin; and genetic causes. Nephrogenic DI may have a genetic cause or can be acquired or caused from such conditions as polycystic kidney disease, an electrolyte imbalance, or a kidney defect. This section focuses on central DI, which is more commonly seen. The prognosis of children with central DI depends on the cause. Most children with proper treatment and follow-up can live fairly normal lives.

Pathophysiology

The hypothalamus produces ADH. After synthesis, the hormone is transported to the posterior lobe of the pituitary gland where it is stored for later release. The purpose of ADH is to concentrate the urine from the kidneys and to conserve water. ADH works directly on the renal collecting ducts and distal tubules to increase membrane permeability for water and urea. A deficiency in ADH causes the kidney to fail to reabsorb

water, which instead diffuses into the urine. Subsequently, a decrease in ADH secretion allows massive water loss, resulting in elevated sodium levels in the serum.

Assessment

The most common symptoms of central DI are **polyuria** (excessive urination) and **polydipsia** (excessive thirst). Children with central DI typically excrete 4 to 15 L urine/day despite fluid intake. The onset of these symptoms is usually sudden and abrupt. Ask about repeated trips to the bathroom, nocturia, and enuresis. Other manifestations may include dehydration, fever, weight loss, increased irritability, vomiting, constipation, and, potentially, hypovolemic shock.

caREminder

The first symptoms of central DI seen in children, especially in infants, are irritability and incessant crying that can only be alleviated with feedings of water. Formula or breast milk does not quench the child's thirst.

The child with diabetes mellitus also has polydipsia and polyuria but is satisfied with any type of fluid. With central DI, the child's urine is extremely dilute and often colorless, with a specific gravity usually not more than 1.005. Central DI may often be confused with diabetes mellitus because of the symptoms; however, in DI, no glucosuria occurs.

Diagnostic Tests

Diagnosis of central DI is usually confirmed by low urine specific gravity, serum osmolality greater than 300 mOsm/kg with urine osmolality less than 300 mOsm/kg, excessive urination despite fluid restriction, and elevated serum sodium levels when fluid is withheld. A water deprivation test may be ordered if the serum osmolality is less than 300 mOsm/kg, yet intake and output records in the home cannot be attributed to primary polydipsia. The water deprivation study can help to establish the diagnosis of central DI and differentiate between central and nephrogenic causes (see Tests and Procedures 26-1). MRI may be completed to help determine the underlying disease that is affecting pituitary function.

Nursing Diagnoses and Outcomes

In addition to the nursing diagnoses presented in Nursing Plan of Care 26-1, the following nursing diagnosis may apply to a child with central DI:

Nursing Diagnosis: Activity intolerance related to dehydration, excessive thirst, and frequent need to urinate
Outcome: Child will regain strength and desire to have increased level of activity.

Interdisciplinary Interventions

Treatment for central DI involves careful monitoring and management of the child to prevent fluid and electrolyte imbalances, providing nutritional support, and administering desmopressin (DDAVP), a synthetic analogue of ADH.

Monitoring

Monitor the child with central DI continually for signs and symptoms of dehydration (poor skin turgor, dry mucous membranes, sunken fontanels, weight loss, absence of tears, tachycardia, and decreased urine specific gravity) and hypernatremia (tachycardia, poor skin turgor, weak pulses, low blood pressure, cool skin, increased body temperature, dry mucous membranes, and changes in mental status). Administer sufficient fluids to maintain balanced intake and output over 24 hours. Record strict intake, output, and specific gravity measurements while the child is hospitalized. If urine output is more than 100 mL/hr for two consecutive voids, notify the health care provider. Weigh the child on the same scale at the same time every day.

Nutritional Interventions

Encourage high-calorie beverages, such as milk and juice, for children with central DI who are underweight because of inadequate calorie consumption. Instruct parents to note drinking patterns at home and to report changes to the health care provider. Parents need to understand the symptoms of water intoxication and dehydration to prevent acute episodes of decompensation that could require hospitalization (see Chapter 17 for a discussion of fluid and electrolyte status). In addition, remind parents and school nurses that adequate replacement fluid is needed during increased physical activity or extremely hot weather.

Pharmacologic Interventions

If postoperative or acute central DI cannot be controlled with fluid management alone, pharmacologic treatment is instituted. DDAVP may be administered intravenously, subcutaneously, intranasally, or by mouth. Long-term home therapy usually entails administration twice daily by the oral or intranasal route. The health care provider initially orders small doses, titrating the dose as needed. DDAVP acts immediately and lasts between 8 and 24 hours. Headaches, nasal congestion, and abdominal discomfort are rare side effects. Vasopressin (Pitressin) is usually administered parenterally in the acute treatment of central DI because of its shorter half-life.

Community Care

Provide education before discharge regarding home administration of DDAVP and fluid management (Teaching Intervention Plan 26-1). Ensure that the child's school nurse knows that the child is receiving treatment for central DI. It is unlikely that DDAVP will be administered in the school setting, but if the parents struggle with adherence to medication administration, the school nurse may be asked to assist. Any fluid intake guidelines should be clearly stated in a school health care plan that is on file with the school health office. Advise parents to inform teachers and coaches that their child needs liberal bathroom privileges and extra fluids to prevent embarrassing accidents or dehydration. Children should be encouraged to wear a MedicAlert bracelet indicating that they have DI.

caREminder

Parents must educate teachers thoroughly on the manifestations of dehydration and hypernatremia so they do not mistake these signs as bad or unruly behavior. A teaching session with the school nurse can prevent this misconception.

ANSWER: The word *diabetes* is derived from the Greek word for "passing through." It is used medically to describe diseases characterized by excessive urination. Both diabetes mellitus and central DI are a result of deficient secretion of a hormone by a gland; both, when untreated, result in excessive urination. The excessive urination in DI is from inadequate ADH to stimulate the absorption of water and thereby concentrate urine; excessive urination in diabetes mellitus is from excess glucose causing a hyperosmotic situation in both the bloodstream and the urine, which results in increased urination.

TIP 26-1: A TEACHING INTERVENTION PLAN for Administering Desmopressin (DDAVP)

Nursing Diagnosis and Family Outcomes

- Deficient knowledge: DDAVP administration
  Outcomes: The parents and child will understand the need for replacement hormone therapy and long-term follow-up.
  Parents and child will demonstrate how to give DDAVP.
  Parents and child will demonstrate strategies to monitor child's fluid balance.

Teach the Child/Family

Medication Administration
- Keep DDAVP refrigerated at all times.
- Clear the nostrils before giving medication.
- Insert measured tubing into the bottle of DDAVP.
- Fill the tube to the proper dosage.
- Hold the top of the tube closed.
- Insert the medication-filled end into the nostril.
- Blow the liquid out of the tubing and into the nostril.

Precautions
- Consult the health care provider initially to learn how to administer DDAVP.

- Do not repeat doses that have been swallowed or poorly absorbed.
- The medication is poorly absorbed if the child has nasal congestion.
- The dose may need to be repeated if the child sneezes immediately after the administration of the medication.
- Have an extra bottle of medication in case of breakage.
- Have child wear a MedicAlert bracelet, listing DI and the medications the child is using.

Monitoring the Child
- Closely monitor fluid balance, including daily weights (same time of day with same amount of clothing), fluid intake and output, and measurement of urine specific gravity.
- Look for signs of overdose, such as weight gain, concentrated urine, and decreased urine output.
- Look for signs of underdosage, such as polyuria, intense thirst, and dilute urine.

Contact the Health Care Provider if
- Child has signs of DI, including increased thirst, sudden weight loss, polyuria, urine specific gravity less than 1.005, or altered mental status

SYNDROME OF INAPPROPRIATE ANTIDIURETIC HORMONE SECRETION

SIADH results from hypersecretion of ADH. In SIADH, the negative feedback mechanism fails to regulate ADH release and inhibition. SIADH may occur with brain tumors, CNS disease (meningitis), head trauma, or after certain surgical procedures on the brain. It may also stem from the use of certain medications, such as chlorpropamide, imipramine, vincristine, and phenothiazines. SIADH may also be caused by excessive administration of vasopressin, which can be used for treating central DI, bleeding disorders, or enuresis.

Without immediate and effective interventions, CNS damage from SIADH can impair the child permanently. When the underlying disorder is corrected, the child should no longer be at risk, and the symptoms usually dissipate.

Pathophysiology

Normally, ADH is not secreted when excess fluid is in circulation because the fluid must be excreted. When ADH is hypersecreted, it shuts down the normal kidney function of water filtration and loss. Decreased sodium levels cause water to move into the cells, which causes brain cell swelling and increased intracranial pressure. Water remains in circulation, diluting all blood components. Metabolic toxins accumulate in the blood instead of being excreted. Hypokalemia and hypocalcemia

develop from the dilutional effects of SIADH. Weakness, lethargy, anorexia, nausea, vomiting, and behavioral changes develop as the fluid and electrolyte balance deteriorates and serum sodium levels decrease. CNS changes associated with hyponatremia include confusion, convulsions, and coma. Death may occur if treatment is not immediate and aggressive.

 A L E R T   *SIADH is a transient, but life-threatening, emergency that is usually treated in the intensive care setting.*

Assessment

Monitor weight, input, and output. The child with SIADH gains weight and has decreased urine output because fluids are retained. Assess the child's level of consciousness with vital signs assessment. Symptoms in SIADH resulting from dilutional hyponatremia may initially include headache, lethargy, slowness, poor concentration, lack of attention, nausea, restlessness, depressed mood, gait instability, muscle cramps, and tremors. As the condition progresses, the child develops confusion, disorientation, vomiting, hallucinations, acute psychosis, limb weakness, and dysarthria. In its most severe form, seizures, hemiplegia, respiratory insufficiency, coma, and death may occur (Gross, 2012).

Diagnostic Tests

Specific laboratory diagnostic criteria that define SIADH include the following:

- Serum osmolality <275 mOsm/kg
- Urine osmolality >100 mOsm/kg
- Serum sodium levels <135 mEq/L
- Urine sodium concentrations >40 mEq/L
- Normal adrenal and thyroid function(Gross, 2012; Kappy et al., 2009)

In addition, diagnostic tests reveal decreased levels of serum urea, creatinine, uric acid, and albumin. Renal, adrenal, and thyroid function tests are generally normal.

Nursing Diagnoses and Outcomes

In addition to the nursing diagnoses presented in Nursing Plan of Care 26-1, the following nursing diagnosis may apply to a child with SIADH:

Nursing Diagnosis: Disturbed thought processes related to effects of brain cell swelling and increased intracranial pressure as evidenced by confusion, disorientation, memory loss, seizures, and coma
Outcomes:
- Child's level of consciousness and orientation will remain normal or without further impairment.
- Child will remain free from injury during periods of altered level of consciousness.

Interdisciplinary Interventions

Emergency management and long-term interventions for SIADH are tied directly to the cause of the hormone imbalance. Indirect and direct interventions are aimed at maintaining fluid and electrolyte balance and regulating serum sodium and osmolality. Monitor intake, output, and weight records carefully. Place an indwelling urinary catheter to monitor hourly urine volume and specific gravity. Note any exposure to precipitating factors in the history.

The severity of the SIADH will guide supportive treatment options. For instance, in mild cases, treatment consists of fluid restrictions. Acute treatment is guided by the extent and duration of hyponatremia and the presence of any cerebral dysfunction. Maintaining airway, breathing, and cardiovascular stability is a primary concern and may require the child to be on ventilatory support. As serum sodium levels decrease, treatment consists of reducing the fluid overload and raising the serum sodium level and osmolality. Restricted IV fluids are ordered. Hypertonic saline solution (3% sodium chloride) may be administered as a sodium replacement. Diuretic agents such as Lasix are prescribed in conjunction with hypertonic or isotonic saline to diurese excess water. Rapid and complete recovery from SIADH is possible in most cases.

GROWTH HORMONE DEFICIENCY

Classic GH deficiency is the failure of the pituitary to produce sufficient GH to sustain normal growth in childhood or to produce minimally measurable GH after stimulation with two pharmacologic agents. In some cases, the causes of central GH deficiency are idiopathic. Males are twice as likely as females to be referred for idiopathic GH deficiency. Males are referred more often because of the societal expectation for males to be taller. Girls may have as high an incidence of GH deficiency but may not be referred because short stature is culturally more acceptable in females.

Beyond idiopathic GH deficiency, other frequently seen causes of GH deficiency include tumors (craniopharyngioma, optic glioma, adenoma, astrocytoma, and germinoma), septo–optic dysplasia (optic nerve hypoplasia, absence of septum pellucidum, and pituitary hormone deficiencies), long-term sequelae from cranial radiation, head trauma, congenital abnormalities and midline facial defects, or histiocytosis X.

Pathophysiology

GH stimulates the growth of all organs and tissues in the body, particularly the long bones. The synthesis of insulinlike growth factor 1 (IGF-1) in many tissues, especially the liver, is stimulated by GH. IGF-1, also known as *somatomedin C*, stimulates somatic growth. The child's nutritional state as well as several hormones influence the production of somatomedin C and resulting overall growth. Once growth is complete, some children may need to be evaluated to see whether or not they can produce adequate amounts of GH to meet their needs as adults. Adults who are GH deficient have increased cardiovascular morbidity and mortality, visceral fat, total cholesterol, and LDL cholesterol, leading to an increased coronary risk. In addition, they exhibit reduced bone mass and increased prevalence of fracture rates. Many report diminished quality of life, as evidenced by reductions in physical and mental energy, dissatisfaction with body image, and poor memory (American Association of Clinical Endocrinologists [AACE], 2009).

Assessment

The child with GH deficiency may present to the health care team at any time from birth to adolescence, depending on the causative factor. Conduct a complete evaluation, including family history, the child's birth history including gestational age at delivery, previous and current growth patterns, physical examination, bone age films, and specific endocrine studies.

Determine whether the child has had radiation treatments or a history of head trauma. Note information about short stature in the family history as well as the specific heights and weights of both parents and siblings. Obtain these measurements at the time of the initial visit. In the birth history, include any history of maternal illness, infections, tobacco or alcohol use, or malnutrition that could have affected the weight and height of the growing fetus. Plot birth length, weight, and head circumference for gestational age. Obtain growth charts, because deviation from the normal growth curve is always a cause for concern.

The physical examination is extremely valuable and informative when diagnosing the child with GH deficiency. Physical findings vary somewhat depending on the age of the child. The neonate with idiopathic GH deficiency usually presents with seizures secondary to severe hypoglycemia and may also be cortisol deficient. Prolonged hyperbilirubinemia may also be present. Males can have small testes and micropenis when a gonadotropin deficiency is also present. Infants usually have a cherubic facial appearance, frontal bossing (prominence of the forehead) is common, and the eyes appear prominent. The nasal bridge is not fully developed, the nose is small, and the infant may have micrognathia (abnormal smallness of the jaw). Truncal adiposity (excessive fat over the trunk area of the body) is common, along with small hands and feet. Dentition is often delayed, hair is sparse and thin, and the voice may be high pitched. Growth velocity is decreased, which eventually leads to short stature.

Children who develop GH deficiency beyond the neonatal and infancy period generally experience short stature and growth retardation. Developmental skills are normal because cognitive development is unaffected. The adolescent with GH deficiency may have a substantial delay of puberty in addition to short stature (Clinical Judgment 26-1).

Emotional difficulties related to small stature can occur. The short child is often treated as if younger by teachers and coaches, is teased by peers, and may become shy and withdrawn toward others. Body image is altered, and the child may dress as a younger child.

Diagnostic Tests

The child with GH deficiency usually has normal results of renal and liver function tests as well as thyroid function tests. The sedimentation rate is normal, indicating the absence of a chronic illness causing the short stature. IGF-1 and insulinlike growth factor–binding protein 3 (IGFBP-3) levels are usually below normal. Bone age, determined by radiograph, is usually interpreted as two or more standard deviations below the mean for age. Computed tomography or MRI of the head will generally reveal no abnormalities but may reveal a small pituitary gland or "empty sella" (the sella is the bony "cup" that holds the pituitary gland). Overnight sleep studies evaluating GH secretion reveal less than three peaks of GH more than 10 ng/mL. Provocative testing using at least two GH stimulants, such as arginine, clonidine, insulin, glucagon, or levodopa, will reveal GH levels less than 10 ng/mL.

Interdisciplinary Interventions

Pharmacologic therapy with GH is the treatment of choice for the child with GH deficiency. Educate the parent and child on the proper way to store, reconstitute,

---

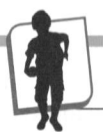

CLINICAL JUDGMENT 26-1

The Child With Growth Hormone Deficiency

Ten-year-old Wallace has been diagnosed with GH deficiency. As the nurse at his school, you have been working with Wallace and his family to help them adjust to the diagnosis and follow the treatment plan.

Questions

1. If left untreated, how would this condition manifest itself?
2. What therapy would you anticipate is being provided for Wallace by his pediatric endocrinology provider?
3. Based on Wallace's age and diagnosis, what are some important aspects of nursing care for him?

4. You have noted that other kids at school are teasing Wallace and have nicknamed him "Fly" because he is so little. How should you intervene?
5. How would you evaluate whether Wallace's parents and teachers are responding appropriately to his condition?

Answers

1. Child would continue to appear shorter than others of same chronologic age, with delayed onset of puberty.
2. Subcutaneous injections of GH usually given nightly. Treatment is carried out until growth is complete (a bone age of 15 years for girls and 17 years for boys).
3. Recognizing that Wallace may be experiencing threats to his self-esteem and body image and assisting Wallace to cope with these feelings.

4. Discuss the situation with Wallace's teachers, and ask them to intervene to stop and redirect the kids who are teasing Wallace. If Wallace feels comfortable with the idea, you could give a presentation about GH deficiency to his classmates.
5. Assess if the parents and teachers are interacting with Wallace according to his age rather than to his size.

and administer the GH. The parent or the child administers GH by subcutaneous injection usually 6 to 7 days per week (usually daily). It is generally given at bedtime to attempt to mimic the body's natural production and release during sleep. Discuss the possible side effects of GH with the child and family. These include an increase in blood glucose level, an increased incidence of slipped capital femoral epiphysis, scoliosis, local infection at the injection site, and pseudotumor cerebri.

Growth is greatest during the first year or two of therapy; however, after the initial catch-up growth, growth velocity is expected to be at or above normal for age. Currently, GH injections are given until the bones fuse or until the child ceases to respond to treatment with continued growth. Some endocrinologists believe that adults with GH deficiency diagnosed during childhood may need continued treatment (AACE, 2009).

Children with GH deficiency usually attain an acceptable height when given a supportive treatment plan to which they and their family can adhere.

Community Care

For maximal beneficial effects of treatment, emphasize the importance of regular follow-up care and adherence to prescribed medication dose and frequency of administration.

KidKare The child who has needle phobia may need extra attention. The child can help by selecting the injection sites, using an injector pen, and by participating in preparing the equipment. Psychological counseling may be necessary for children who are needle phobic; however, there are also some needle-less injector devices that can be used.

Precise heights and weights are obtained every 3 to 4 months at follow-up visits and are precisely plotted on the growth chart. The child may have a bone age study performed annually after therapy has been initiated to monitor advancing bone age.

PRECOCIOUS PUBERTY

Precocious puberty is development of sexual characteristics before the usual age of puberty. In developed countries, precocious sexual maturation is considered when characteristics such as breast development occur before age 8 years in girls or onset of menses occurs before age 9½ years. In boys, testicular enlargement occurring before 9½ years of age is considered precocious puberty. Girls are 10 times more commonly affected by precocious puberty than boys (Carel & Le'ger, 2008). However, boys are more likely to have a pathologic process, whereas girls usually have idiopathic precocious puberty.

The prognosis for a child with precocious puberty depends on the age at diagnosis and the immediacy of treatment. Appropriate treatment can halt sexual development and prevent severe short adult stature. The treatment prevents production of estrogen and testosterone. It is well known that estrogen causes closure of the epiphyses, which, if produced too early, will lead to severe adult short stature. Boys convert testosterone into estrogen, causing epiphyseal closure. Treatment for precocious puberty allows the child to achieve his or her maximum growth potential.

Pathophysiology

There are two primary categories of precocious puberty. *Peripheral precocious*, or *gonadotropin-independent, puberty* is less common and refers to conditions in which increased production of sex steroids is gonadotropin independent. Gonadotropin-independent precocious puberty does not involve hypothalamic–pituitary–gonadal activation. Rather, it is the result of the production of sex hormones by the adrenal gland or gonads and may be secondary to CAH; tumors that secrete human chorionic gonadotropin; tumors or cysts of the adrenal gland, ovary, or testis; exposure to exogenous sex steroid; or McCune-Albright syndrome (a genetic disease that affects the bones and skin and causes hormonal imbalances also called polyostotic fibrous dysplasia) (Carel & Le'ger, 2008).

Central precocious, or *gonadotropin-dependent, puberty* (CPP), the more commonly seen type of precocious puberty, is addressed in this section. CPP is initiated by hypothalamic–pituitary–gonadal activation and is similar to the mechanism seen in normal puberty. Gonadotropin-releasing hormone (GnRH) is secreted by the hypothalamus in periodic bursts that stimulate the pituitary to release the gonadotropins LH and FSH. These gonadotropins stimulate the gonads to produce sex hormones, causing sexual maturation. CNS abnormalities associated with CPP include tumors; hypothalamic hamartomas; acquired CNS injury caused by inflammation, surgery, trauma, radiation therapy, or abscess; or congenital anomalies such as hydrocephalus, arachnoid cysts, or suprasellar cysts.

Mental development in children with precocious puberty is normal, and developmental milestones are not affected; however, the child's behavior may change to that of a typical adolescent. Girls may have episodes of moodiness and irritability, whereas boys may become more aggressive.

Assessment

A comprehensive history, physical examination, and laboratory tests are essential in the diagnosis of precocious puberty.

Obtain and properly graph on the growth charts the current and previous height and weight measurements. Note growth spurts. In the history, include the chronologic timing of pubertal events, such as breast budding, phallic and testicular enlargement, body hair, acne, body odor, and deepening of the voice. Ask parents about changes in behavior such as increased moodiness, irritability, or aggressiveness. Elicit an extensive family history, including parental and sibling pubertal history, incidence of precocious puberty, CAH, neurofibromatosis, thyroid disease, and hypothyroidism. Note exposure to exogenous steroids; testosterone or estrogen; gonadotropins; or endocrine disruptors such as tea tree oil, lavender, or BPA and any perinatal abnormalities or previous head trauma. Also note signs or symptoms of neurologic involvement, such as headaches, visual disturbances, or motor incoordination.

Note the stage of sexual development according to Tanner classification (see Figs. 3-23 and 3-24). Note testicular and phallic size in boys, and check for gynecomastia. In girls, note breast development and examine the external genitalia for signs of labial fusion, estrogen production, or enlarged clitoris and labia. In both, examine the skin for café-au-lait spots, which can indicate neurofibromatosis or McCune-Albright syndrome, and for the presence of neurofibromas. Neurologic evaluation is essential, with special attention paid to visual fields, optic disks, and signs of increased intracranial pressure.

Diagnostic Tests

Laboratory testing may include different blood tests depending on the gender of the child. In boys, the health care provider may order a serum human chorionic gonadotropin test, which, if elevated, could indicate a human chorionic gonadotropin–secreting tumor. Suppressed serum LH levels indicate testotoxicosis, in which serum testosterone concentration is high. In both boys and girls, elevated adrenal androgens such as 17-hydroxyprogesterone (17OHP), androstenedione, dehydroepiandrosterone (DHEA), and testosterone indicate CAH. Nonclassical CAH presents with signs of premature adrenarche, specifically pubic hair and possibly body odor, as well as the elevated androgens listed above.

Additional laboratory testing may be done to evaluate the function of the adrenal glands and to rule out an adrenal virilizing tumor or hormone deficiencies. Pelvic or testicular ultrasounds are used to assess for the presence of cysts or tumors. An MRI of the brain is used to determine if the child has a hypothalamic lesion.

The child will need a bone age determination. A normal bone age is most consistent with benign premature **adrenarche** (growth of sexual hair), premature **thelarche** (breast development), or ingestion of exogenous sex steroids. An accelerated bone age is more suggestive of CPP, an adrenal or ovarian disorder, McCune-Albright syndrome, or familial male precocious puberty.

Interdisciplinary Interventions

Interventions and treatments vary depending on the cause of the precocious puberty. When a CNS tumor is detected, surgery, radiation, chemotherapy, or a combination of these treatment modalities is recommended.

Pharmacologic Interventions

In the absence of a CNS lesion, several treatment options may be considered. For CPP, long-acting GnRH agonists provide negative feedback and result in decreased levels of LH and FSH 2 to 4 weeks after initiating treatment. The agonists inhibit the release of LH and FSH, reduce gonadotropins and sex steroids to prepubertal levels, retard sexual maturation, and slow the linear growth velocity and skeletal maturation (see thePoint Medications and Administration: Pharmacologic Agents Used to Treat Precocious Puberty). The ultimate goal of therapy is to restore normal growth potential while allowing puberty to occur at the normal age with subsequent normal reproductive potential. Medications are administered subcutaneously on a daily basis or intramuscularly every 4 weeks or 3 months. One GnRH agonist (histrelin) is available in an implantable form that is placed in the inner aspect of the upper arm and provides continuous medication release for 12 months (Carel & Le'ger, 2008). At the onset of treatment with any of these medications, it is not unusual for a girl to have a menstrual bleed, but this rarely occurs twice. Pharmacologic interventions are usually discontinued when the child reaches the normal age for puberty (approximately age 11 years for girls and age 12 years for boys).

After treatment is initiated, GnRH testing is performed every 6 months to assess the effectiveness of the treatment. Normalization of accelerated growth, softening or no increase in size of breasts, and suppression of gonadotropin levels as well as normalization of estrogen or testosterone levels indicate effectiveness of the pharmacologic interventions.

Supportive Interventions

In addition to the medical treatment that may be needed, the child with precocious puberty needs psychosocial support. School-aged children with precocious puberty may become very self-conscious about their bodies around their peers and families. The child with precocious puberty may also have adverse psychological effects. The most difficult aspect for the child to endure may be teasing from other children about advanced sexual development. The child may feel isolated and rejected socially. Behavioral changes seen in boys and girls may cause problems in socializing with children in their own age group. Teachers, relatives, and neighbors often expect the child to behave older than his or her chronologic age based on physical appearance; this causes frustration for the child, who cannot live up to the expectations. Parents need clear and concise explanations concerning the causes of precocious puberty, treatment options, and counseling regarding the emotional and social implications of this condition on their child and the family. Provide the child with explanations in age-appropriate terms about what is happening to his or her body and strategies to cope with the physical changes he or she is experiencing.

Community Care

Encourage parents, teachers, and friends to interact with the child in an age-appropriate manner and promote realistic expectations. Encourage the child to participate in activities with same-age children. Clothing should also be age-appropriate, and parents may need assistance concerning how to minimize the appearance of breast development. Remind parents that intellectual, emotional, and social maturation does not keep pace with physical and hormonal changes. The child must be treated according to chronologic age and guarded against sexual abuse from older children or adults. Sexual curiosity is not usually advanced beyond the child's chronologic age. Educate parents and their precocious pubertal girls about the potential onset of menarche, if it has not yet occurred. Menstrual hygiene becomes an important concern for the child in elementary school and should be addressed with the teachers and nurses in the school. Most children who have precocious puberty adjust well, with some assistance; however, some may encounter serious problems adapting to their premature development. Provide counseling for children who experience any signs of substantial psychological effects, such as depression, withdrawal, or aggressive behavior.

DELAYED PUBERTY

Delayed puberty is the failure to develop sexually at an appropriate age or during the normal 3- to 5-year period at normal age of puberty onset. In girls who have not developed breasts by 13 years of age, or if more than 4½ years have passed between the initiation of breast development and menarche, delayed puberty is considered. Boys are considered to have delayed puberty if secondary sexual development has not started by 14 years of age.

Delayed puberty is more common in boys than girls and occurs in 2% to 3% of all adolescents. Constitutional growth delay is the most common cause. The serum gonadotropins are typically prepubertal, and the bone age, determined by radiograph, is delayed. The child may have a history of small stature during infancy and childhood. The two other major categories of delayed puberty are hypogonadotropic hypogonadism and hypergonadotropic hypogonadism. In hypogonadotropic hypogonadism, delayed puberty is associated with low serum gonadotropin levels secondary to abnormalities of the hypothalamus or the pituitary. These abnormalities include craniopharyngiomas, Kallmann syndrome, idiopathic hypopituitarism, autoimmune disease, isolated FSH deficiency, and hyperprolactinemia. In hypergonadotropic hypogonadism, delayed puberty is associated with elevated serum gonadotropin levels and low levels of testosterone or estradiol. This may be caused by ovarian or testicular failure secondary to chemotherapy with Cytoxan, abdominal or pelvic radiation, or autoimmune attack on the gonads.

Prognosis depends on the specific diagnosis (e.g., Turner syndrome or constitutionally delayed puberty). The aim of treatment is to assure continued advancement of secondary sexual characteristics and maturation of the uterus to allow for future pregnancy. In addition, estradiol and testosterone are critical in maintaining bone health and preventing early osteoporosis. There are also positive cardiovascular benefits.

Pathophysiology

In girls, the most common abnormality is Turner syndrome. Girls with Turner syndrome have delayed puberty, short stature, webbed neck, and cubitus valgus (deformity of the arm in which the forearm deviates laterally). The karyotype in girls with Turner syndrome is usually 45XO, although mosaicism will lead to a variety of karyotypes. In boys, abnormalities include Klinefelter syndrome; bilateral gonadal failure secondary to trauma, autoimmune destruction, infection, chemotherapy, or radiation; and congenital anorchia.

Assessment

Assessing the child with delayed puberty requires a detailed family history as well as the child's history, physical examination, and laboratory studies.

In the family history, include the onset of puberty; the patterns of growth and sexual development of the mother, father, and siblings; a history of consanguinity; and any history of infertility. Obtain growth charts documenting previous heights and weights. Note the child's history of chronic illness, nutritional disorders, birth trauma, and head trauma that may be indicative of causative factors.

During physical examination of the child with delayed puberty, include an accurate height and weight. Document any signs of puberty, noting breast development and presence of axillary hair and/or pubic hair. Measure testicular size and penile length carefully. Assess for the loss of a sense of smell, which would be present in Kallmann syndrome, one cause of delayed puberty.

Diagnostic Tests

Many laboratory studies are needed. Gonadotropin concentrations (LH and FSH) can be substantially higher than normal or in prepubertal ranges at an age when puberty would be expected. Electrolytes should be normal. Thyroid levels may indicate hypothyroidism, prolactin levels may be elevated (indicating a pituitary adenoma), and estradiol levels and testosterone levels decreased. A bone age determination, which is usually delayed, is performed along with MRI or computed tomography to rule out a hypothalamic or pituitary lesion.

A GnRH stimulation test can also be performed to distinguish between constitutional delay of puberty and hypogonadotropic hypogonadism. A human chorionic gonadotropin stimulation test can give information on testicular function. Often, the diagnosis can be made from baseline gonadotropin levels and the physical exam alone; however, imaging studies are required to rule out a brain tumor.

Interdisciplinary Interventions

Treatment for the child with delayed puberty depends on the specific cause of the problem and whether the delay in development will be temporary or permanent. When the diagnosis is constitutional delay of growth and puberty, the health care team should reassure the child and family that there is no serious problem and that pubertal development will occur with time.

Medical intervention has been used in the boy who has pubertal delay and whose emotional well-being is adversely affected, as evidenced by a decrease in school performance and a withdrawal from his social circle. A 3- to 6-month course of low-dose testosterone (50 mg testosterone enanthate or cypionate) given intramuscularly every 3 weeks for four doses is recommended, followed by reevaluation for possibility of continued treatment. Larger doses of testosterone were found to cause premature closure of the epiphyses and decrease the final height. Spontaneous growth velocity and sexual maturation usually follows this short course of treatment of low-dose testosterone, and therapy is no longer needed. Reassurance, close observation, and assistance with clothes selection are usually sufficient for girls with delayed puberty. However, a short course of estrogen can be used to begin the pubertal process.

The child with hypogonadotropic hypogonadism or hypergonadotropic hypogonadism requires replacement therapy with sex steroids. In boys, testosterone needs to be replaced; in girls, estrogen and progesterone need to be replaced. Testosterone enanthate or cypionate is also given intramuscularly every 4 weeks and is started when puberty normally begins in boys. Oral therapy or synthetic androgens do not stimulate complete pubertal development and are not an adequate therapy in boys. Oral ethinyl estradiol or transdermal patch is the replacement therapy of choice for girls. Estrogen is delivered by patch or orally in slowly increasing amounts. Once vaginal spotting occurs, progesterone is added to regulate the menstrual cycle.

Community Care

The child with delayed puberty has some of the same concerns and issues as the child with precocious puberty. Body image concerns may trigger withdrawal from age-appropriate activities and have led to decreased academic performance and altered self-concept. Teasing from peers about short stature and lack of physical maturation may be especially distressing to the child. Lindfors et al. (2007) examined the relationship between pubertal development and ego development in late-maturing boys. Researchers found that boys with delayed puberty were psychologically more immature than their nonaffected peers and that they experienced negative feelings about sexuality. It is believed that lower ego development may be related to the fact that boys with delayed puberty are treated more according to their stature than to their chronologic age, and the child develops in response to how he is treated by others. The adolescent brain undergoes a profound reorganization during puberty; thus, psychological immaturity in boys with delayed puberty may also be associated with the lack of brain maturation that would normally occur during puberty. Parental support and professional counseling can assist the youth to develop a healthy sense of self and to focus on personal strengths.

OTHER PITUITARY DISORDERS

Panhypopituitarism is the lack of all anterior pituitary function, resulting in the deficiency of TSH, GH, ACTH, LH, and FSH. The posterior pituitary may also be affected, and ADH may be deficient. The incidence of panhypopituitarism is 1 in 100,000 live births. Causes include tumors, radiation therapy, encephalitis, or head trauma (Marcus & Collins, 2004).

Pituitary gigantism (acromegaly) is an extremely rare disorder resulting from the hypersecretion of GH by the pituitary gland. Few cases of gigantism have been confirmed by appropriate hormonal testing and/or pathologic data. Hypersecretion of GH usually occurs as a result of a pituitary adenoma. Tumors of the hypothalamus may also produce an overabundance of GH. About 20% of the cases of gigantism have been associated with the McCune-Albright syndrome, which has other features, including café-au-lait pigmentation of the skin

and polyostotic fibrous dysplasia. Gigantism has also been associated with acanthosis, hyperinsulinism, obesity, and hyperandrogenism without elevated GH levels.

DISORDERS OF THE THYROID GLAND

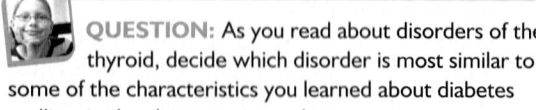

QUESTION: As you read about disorders of the thyroid, decide which disorder is most similar to some of the characteristics you learned about diabetes mellitus in the chapter case study.

The thyroid gland is responsible for the rate of all metabolic and chemical processes in the body, thereby affecting every cell, tissue, organ, and organ system. The thyroid gland is essential for life, growth, and development. Thyroid hormones affect body temperature and circulation; appetite; energy levels; growth; skeletal development; muscle tone and agility; cardiac rate (force and output); fluid balance; blood sugar levels; CNS function; bowel function; blood fat (cholesterol) levels; and the regulation of fat, carbohydrate, and protein metabolism in all cells.

The thyroid problems are among some of the most common medical conditions, yet because the symptoms appear gradually, the thyroid condition may go undiagnosed for some period of time. Thyroid conditions in children may be congenital, acquired, or secondary. Various congenital defects of the thyroid are caused by developmental malformations. This occurrence is called *thyroid dysgenesis*. The failure of the thyroid to descend to its proper position is manifested by the thyroid developing at the base of the tongue (a lingual thyroid) or in the upper part of the neck (a sublingual thyroid). Disorders may also be acquired, as in the case of Hashimoto thyroiditis, an autoimmune disease in which the child's own immune system attacks the thyroid gland and interferes with the production of thyroid hormones. Secondary thyroid disorders such as hypothyroidism may result when the pituitary gland fails to secrete enough TSH, which is necessary for normal stimulation of the thyroid gland.

HYPOTHYROIDISM

Hypothyroidism results from deficient production of thyroid hormone or a defect in thyroid hormonal receptor activity. Hypothyroidism in children may be congenital, acquired, or secondary. Acquired hypothyroidism usually refers to thyroid deficiency that becomes evident after a period of apparently normal thyroid function. Acquired hypothyroidism may result from a variety of causes. It may be caused by a congenitally defective thyroid gland that furnishes sufficient amounts of hormone early in life but is inadequate later in childhood. A thyroid gland that is ectopically located at the base of the tongue or upper neck (lingual thyroid or sublingual thyroid) can also cause acquired hypothyroidism in children. The most common cause of acquired hypothyroidism in iodine-sufficient regions of the world is lymphocytic thyroiditis (also called *Hashimoto thyroiditis* or *autoimmune thyroiditis*).

Lymphocytic thyroiditis is an autoimmune disorder, and antithyroid antibodies are present. It is often associated with other endocrine disorders, such as diabetes mellitus, and with certain chromosomal disorders, such as Down and Turner syndromes. With prompt diagnosis and treatment, children with acquired hypothyroidism will develop completely normally.

CH has a prevalence of 1 in 2,000 to 4,000 newborns (Rastogi & LaFranchi, 2010). CH is most commonly caused by defective thyroid gland development (dysgenesis) or a disorder of thyroid hormone biosynthesis (dyshormonogenesis). The thyroid gland may be ectopic (present in a site higher than the normal position in the neck), aplastic, or hypoplastic. Such defective glands often produce insufficient hormone to meet physiologic requirements. CH may also be caused by maternal ingestion of goitrogens (substances that produce a goiter) such as excessive amounts of iodide or antithyroid drugs. CH is further classified as either permanent or transient CH. Permanent CH is a persistent deficiency of thyroid hormone that requires lifelong treatment. Transient CH is a temporary deficiency of thyroid hormone, discovered at birth, but then the child recovers to normal thyroid hormone production typically within the first few months or years of life (Rastogi & LaFranchi, 2010).

Complications of CH are severe when treatment is delayed. Without treatment, children may die of respiratory obstruction because of macroglossia. Other severe effects of lack of treatment include dwarfism and severe cognitive challenge; these occurrences are rare in developed countries today.

Pathophysiology

The pathophysiology of hypothyroidism varies depending on the type of deficiency. Normally, the thyroid gland synthesizes sufficient T_4 and T_3. These hormones regulate metabolism, increase oxygen consumption, stimulate protein synthesis, affect carbohydrate and lipid metabolism, and promote growth and development. The thyroid also contains parafollicular cells, or C cells. These cells secrete calcitonin, which helps to maintain blood calcium levels. This hormone inhibits skeletal demineralization and promotes calcium deposition in the bone.

Thyroid hormone synthesis is regulated by TSH, which is secreted by the anterior pituitary. The secretion of TSH is under the control of thyrotropin-releasing hormone, which is synthesized in the hypothalamus. When thyroid hormone production decreases, as in primary hypothyroidism, there is a compensatory increase in levels of TSH. Therefore, thyroid hypofunction or hyperfunction may be caused by a defect in the thyroid gland (primary defect) or by a defect in the pituitary or hypothalamus (secondary/tertiary defect).

Assessment

Assessment of the child with a thyroid disorder includes a comprehensive history, physical examination, laboratory studies, and possibly a scan of the thyroid.

When taking the history, include questions about other family members with thyroid disease, growth and development, level of activity, the integumentary system (temperature and moistness of skin, texture of hair), gastrointestinal problems (diarrhea or constipation), calorigenesis, feeding problems, and weight gain or loss. Determine the child's gestational age at birth; 20% of cases have a gestational age greater than 42 weeks (Rastogi & LaFranchi, 2010). During the physical examination, include accurate measurements of height and weight, heart rate, and blood pressure; assessment of skin temperature and moisture; palpation of the neck to assess the size and location of the gland; neurologic evaluation (presence of tremors or hypoactive or hyperactive reflexes); and a developmental assessment. CH is nearly universally diagnosed within the first few days of life as a result of national newborn screening. Screening has allowed early diagnosis and initiation of treatment before symptoms of hypothyroidism occur.

Rarely, the diagnosis is missed or delayed and symptoms occur. Symptoms of CH appear in the bottle-fed infant before they appear in the breastfed baby as a result of the small amounts of thyroid hormone contained in breast milk. Affected infants have a history of feeding difficulties, inactivity, and constipation. They cry little and are often characterized as "good" babies who are quiet and passive. Developmental milestones are not acquired at age-appropriate times.

On physical examination, untreated children may have a characteristic facies that includes a dull appearance, pallor, a flat nasal bridge, puffy eyelids, a thick protuberant tongue, and low hairline (Fig. 26-2). Macrosomia is present at birth, and a large anterior or posterior fontanel may be palpated as well as an umbilical hernia.

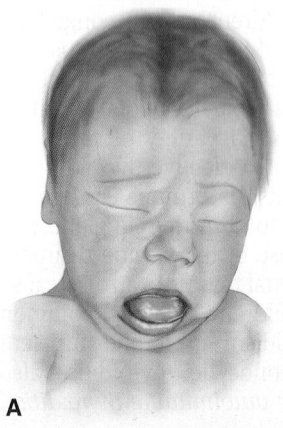

A

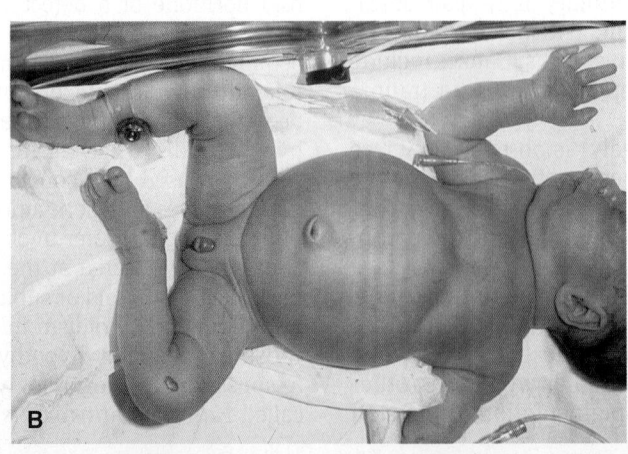

B

Figure 26-2 (A) CH in an infant produces facial puffiness, large tongue, and a dull expression. (B) A newborn with CH. Note the short, thick neck and enlarged abdomen.

Prolonged jaundice is common. The skin is cool, dry, and mottled; the infant may be hypothermic and have a hoarse cry. Cardiovascular manifestations consist of bradycardia and decreased pulse pressure. The muscles are hypotonic, and deep tendon reflexes are abnormal because of delayed relaxation after the reflex response. Umbilical hernias and congenital malformations (e.g., cleft lip, genitourinary malformations) may be present.

CH has been associated with speech delay, sensori-neural hearing loss, cognitive abnormalities, and poor growth if treatment is delayed.

The physical manifestations of acquired hypothyroidism depend on the age of the child. Mental development may be impaired in the very young child, as it is in CH. Deceleration of growth rate is often the first sign of acquired hypothyroidism in children. The child may or may not have an enlarged thyroid (goiter). Children may also present with cold intolerance, constipation, weight gain, and lethargy.

A deficiency of thyroid hormone causes decreased oxygen consumption, metabolic rate, and protein synthesis. A child with CH that goes untreated is at grave risk for cognitive challenge. Other children with juvenile or acquired hypothyroidism that is diagnosed later in life may perform well academically but will express cold intolerance, constipation, and decreased level of energy. Physically, children may demonstrate bradycardia, facial puffiness, and delayed reflexes.

caREminder

Early diagnosis and prompt treatment of CH is essential for normal growth and brain development. The greater the delay treating CH, the greater the degree of cognitive challenge that results. With early diagnosis and treatment, children with CH can develop normally.

Diagnostic Tests

Definitive laboratory findings for congenital or acquired hypothyroidism are low levels of T_3 and T_4 and high levels of TSH. However, in very mild (compensated) hypothyroidism, T_3 and T_4 levels may be normal, whereas TSH levels are elevated.

Neonatal screening for CH is mandatory; the assay usually consists of radioimmunoassay for T_4 on a drop of blood on filter paper. Blood specimens for neonatal screening are obtained by heel stick at the time screening for phenylketonuria and metabolic defects is performed.

Thyroid scans may be done to identify thyroid location, size, and function. Positive antithyroid antibodies are diagnostic of autoimmune thyroid disease.

Nursing Diagnoses and Outcomes

In addition to the nursing diagnoses presented in Nursing Plan of Care 26-1, the following diagnoses may apply to the child with hypothyroidism:

Nursing Diagnosis: Constipation related to decreased motility of the gastrointestinal tract
Outcome: Child's bowel habits will normalize with thyroid hormone treatment.

Nursing Diagnosis: Hypothermia related to decreased metabolic rate
Outcome: Child will remain normothermic.
Nursing Diagnosis: Activity intolerance related to fatigue and decreased strength and endurance
Outcomes:
• Child's excessive fatigue will resolve with thyroid hormone treatment.
• Child will regain physical strength and endurance.

Interdisciplinary Interventions

Treatment of hypothyroidism is pharmacologic and consists of replacement with L-thyroxine sodium (Synthroid, Levoxyl, Levothyroxine). Absorption of L-thyroxine is known to be adversely affected by soy protein formulas, concentrated iron, calcium, aluminum hydroxide, cholestyramine and other resins, fiber supplements, and sucralfate. In addition, the child's care providers should be warned that prolonged heat exposure may reduce the efficacy of L-thyroxine tablets (Rastogi & LaFranchi, 2010).

Serum levels of thyroid hormones and TSH are monitored by the health care provider to ensure that the proper dose is administered and that adherence is adequate. After therapy is instituted, growth rate and developmental levels are continually monitored.

Because of the importance of thyroid hormone for normal growth and development, identifying signs of hypothyroidism promptly is essential (Clinical Judgment 26-2). After hypothyroidism is diagnosed, instruct families on the importance of administering thyroid hormone as ordered (Community Care 26-1).

caREminder

Because children and adolescents do not "feel different" if they miss a dose or two of thyroid hormone, they may forget to take the medication. If one dose is missed, it can be taken the next day along with the usual daily dose.

Community Care

Since the advent of thyroid screening, hypothyroidism that occurs early in life remains undiagnosed in very few children, and fewer suffer irreversible developmental delay. If the child demonstrates developmental delays, refer the child to early intervention programs to help him or her achieve maximum potential. In the case of the child with acquired hypothyroidism, the quality of schoolwork may have declined before hypothyroidism was diagnosed and treated. Discuss the diagnosis with the child's teachers to teach them about the effect of hypothyroidism on learning ability and how treatment with thyroid hormone should return the child to his or her previous level of ability in school.

ANSWER: Autoimmune hypothyroidism is similar in onset to T1DM in that the gland has been functioning normally and then excretes an insufficient amount of hormone because of an autoimmune attack on the organ.

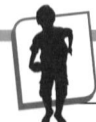

CLINICAL JUDGMENT 26-2

The Child With Hypothyroidism

Denise is a newborn diagnosed with hypothyroidism. Her parents, Mr. and Mrs. Brown, are very concerned about her disorder and about managing her care at home.

Questions

1. What diagnostic tests are used to assess for hypothyroidism in the newborn?
2. What clinical characteristics would be indicative of hypothyroidism?
3. What would be a major complication if Denise's condition had not been recognized and treated?
4. What steps should be included in the teaching plan for this family?
5. After your teaching is complete, what information should Mr. and Mrs. Brown be able to share with you to validate that they understand Denise's home care needs?

Answers

1. A simple blood test, done via heel stick, to diagnose hypothyroidism is required as part of the newborn screening tests.
2. Feeding difficulties, prolonged physiologic jaundice, lethargy, constipation
3. Intellectual disability
4. Teach family how to administer medications. Teach family the importance of lifelong therapy and the need for continual developmental surveillance. Provide family with ongoing education about normal growth and developmental milestones for the child.
5. Importance of administration of L-thyroxine sodium for life, importance of regular health care visits, and developmental surveillance to ensure child is meeting developmental norms

HYPERTHYROIDISM

Hyperthyroidism occurs less often in children than hypothyroidism. *Graves disease*, the most common cause of hyperthyroidism in children, is more frequently seen in females than males and is more likely to occur in adolescents than in young children (Vanderpump, 2011). The incidence of hyperthyroidism is increased in children with Down syndrome, diabetes mellitus, Addison disease, and with a family history of Graves disease. Less common causes include functional adenoma (Plummer disease), polyostotic fibrous dysplasia (McCune-Albright syndrome), acute suppurative thyroiditis, or pituitary tumor, which secretes excessive TSH.

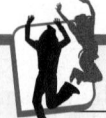

COMMUNITY CARE 26-1

Administration of Thyroid Hormone at Home to the Young Child

- No liquid preparation of thyroid hormone exists.
- Thyroid pills must be crushed for infants and very young children. Crush them in a small spoon. Add a few drops of water, breast milk, or formula to the spoon and mix. Put directly into the mouth; if residue remains, the parent can scoop it off with the finger and let the infant suck it off. The child can also lick the spoon. The goal is to minimize possible loss of medication by the use of multiple mixing/delivery implements. The medicine may be chewed and swallowed once developmentally able.
- Do not administer by mixing the medication with large amounts of milk or formula.
- Give approximately 30 minutes before a feeding.
- Give the medicine at the same time each day (easier to remember).
- Parents must supervise to ensure that thyroid hormone is taken as ordered.

 ALERT   *Soy products, calcium, and iron supplements prevent absorption of the medication and should not be given within 4 hours of the thyroid medication administration.*

Pathophysiology

Graves disease is characterized by the triad of hyper-secretion of thyroid hormone, presence of a goiter, and **exophthalmos** (bulging of the eyeballs). Exophthal-mos is less pronounced in children or not usually seen, except in long-standing disease. In this autoimmune disorder, thyroid-stimulating immunoglobulins (TSIs) affect the thyroid gland in much the same fashion as TSH. There is evidence for genetic and immunologic components to Graves disease.

Assessment

The signs and symptoms of hyperthyroidism are mani-fested in a variety of body systems. The onset is often insidious, with symptoms developing gradually. The most common early symptoms are related to emotional disturbances and increased motor activity. Ask about symptoms such as mood swings, poor attention span, and insomnia, which can be signs of hyperthyroidism.

caREminder

Hyperthyroid children are emotionally labile and cry easily. They are nervous, have short attention spans, and cannot sit still. Therefore, problems with schoolwork are common.

These children are usually considered to be hyperac-tive and to have behavior problems. Sleep disturbance is not uncommon. Weight loss, despite **polyphagia** (excessive hunger), is frequent. In addition, increased motility of the gastrointestinal tract may cause diar-rhea. Cardiac manifestations include tachycardia with palpitations, increased systolic blood pressure yielding an increased pulse pressure, cardiomegaly, and systolic murmurs. The skin may be flushed, warm, sweaty, and very smooth. Heat intolerance can be mild or severe.

The thyroid gland is usually enlarged by two to four times, making it visible and easily palpable. The gland is most commonly symmetric, and smooth and systolic bruits may be auscultated over it. The most common oc-ular manifestations are lid retraction with the appearance of staring. Growth rate may be accelerated, and hyperthy-roid children are frequently tall, with slightly advanced osseous development. Exophthalmos occurs in only one third of children, although ophthalmic abnormalities are found in most children at diagnosis (Fig. 26-3).

Complications of hyperthyroidism include atrial fi-brillation and **thyrotoxicosis** (thyroid "storm," or crisis). Thyroid crisis is rare in children, but it can be fatal. It is precipitated by stress, such as infection, trau-ma, and surgical emergencies, or by discontinuation of antithyroid therapy.

ALERT *The onset of thyroid storm is abrupt, and the symptoms are severe tachycardia, vomiting, diarrhea, hyperpyrexia, and confusion. If thyroid storm is not treated promptly, death may ensue.*

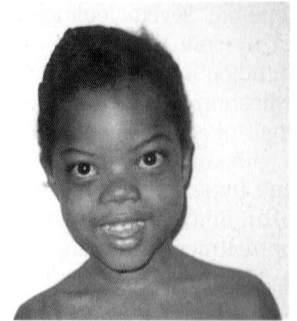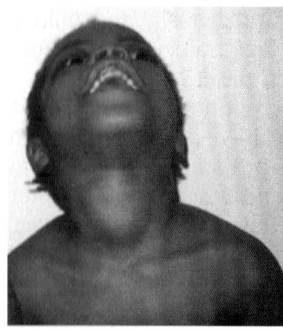

Figure 26-3 Children with hyperthyroidism exhibit hypermetabo-lism and accelerated linear growth. Facial characteristics shown here include "staring eyes" and enlarged thyroid gland (goiter).

Diagnostic Tests

A complete blood count should be done as a baseline because pharmacologic therapy used to treat hyperthy-roidism may cause neutropenia. Blood analysis will dem-onstrate levels of TSH that are very low because the high levels of thyroid hormone suppress the pituitary. Chil-dren with Graves disease have elevated levels of T_4 and T_3, suppressed levels of TSH, and elevated levels of TSI. If a thyroid ultrasound shows the presence of a nodule, a thyroid scan should be performed to differentiate be-tween a malignant nodule, a functional thyroid adenoma, and a benign thyroid nodule. A malignant nodule is usu-ally a "cold" nodule (a lesion with decreased concen-tration of radioisotope). A thyroid-secreting adenoma is usually "hot" (increased concentration of radioisotope).

Nursing Diagnoses and Outcomes

In addition to the nursing diagnoses presented in Nurs-ing Plan of Care 26-1, the following diagnoses may apply to the child with hyperthyroidism.

Nursing Diagnosis: Diarrhea related to effects of increased metabolic activity
Outcomes:
• Child's bowel habits will normalize.
• Child will not experience diarrhea.
Nursing Diagnosis: Disturbed sleep pattern related to increased metabolic energy production
Outcome: Child's insomnia and restlessness will resolve.
Nursing Diagnosis: Risk for decreased cardiac output related to atrial fibrillations
Outcomes:
• Child will maintain normal cardiac output.
• Child will receive prompt treatment for thyroid storm.

Interdisciplinary Interventions

Medical treatment for children with hyperthyroidism includes antithyroid drugs to block T_4 synthesis, I^{131} (ra-dioiodine) therapy, or near-total or total thyroidectomy (AACE, 2011b).

Methimazole (MMI) is the medication of choice for children with Graves disease. Improvement is usually no-ticed in 2 weeks, and the child becomes **euthyroid** (state of a having normal thyroid function tests). Most side effects of antithyroid medications are mild and include pruritus, rash, and mild leukopenia. Severe leukopenia or agranulocytosis—manifested by sore throat and sudden onset of high fever—or jaundice is an indication to discontinue the antithyroid medication and seek immediate medical care. Beta-adrenergic blocking agents, such as propranolol, may be used with antithyroid drugs to control tachycardia, tremors, and hyperactivity in the severely toxic patient (AACE, 2011b). Some children go into remission, with continuation of treatment extending over 1 to 2 years at a lower dosage. The majority of pediatric patients will eventually require I[131] therapy or surgery.

The outcome of treatment with I[131] therapy is related to the size of the thyroid gland at diagnosis. Children with a relatively small gland have a more successful treatment course. Some health care providers will recommend surgery if the gland is large or the child fails medical treatment and refuses radioiodine therapy or is younger than 5 years of age (AACE, 2011b). Radioiodine therapy carries less mortality and morbidity risk than surgery, but the risk of repeat hyperthyroidism and the subsequent expected hypothyroidism must be considered.

If the child is euthyroid after 2 to 3 years of therapy, therapy should be discontinued. The likelihood of permanent remission is good. However, if the thyroid is enlarged two times or greater, it is unlikely that remission will occur. Therapy may be continued, or ablation of the gland with radioactive iodine or total thyroidectomy may be performed.

In children in whom drug therapy is not possible, or in whom medical management has been unsuccessful, near-total or total thyroidectomy is indicated (AACE, 2011b). The child must be euthyroid before surgery and is therefore treated with methimazole. Complications of thyroid surgery are uncommon but include hemorrhage, vocal cord paralysis, and hypoparathyroidism.

Community Care

Although the appropriate dose of MMI will resolve symptoms, a time lag of a few weeks may occur between the start of therapy and the end of symptoms. During the transition from the start of therapy until the disappearance of symptoms, parents must be educated about the child's need for small, frequent, nutritious meals while polyphagic; lightweight clothing and good ventilation because of increased calorigenesis; and a low-pressure, nonstressful environment. Exophthalmos and a large goiter may cause alterations in body image.

 KidKare For children and adolescents, suggest the use of high-necked clothing to mask the goiter. Girls can use scarves to hide the goiter.

Educate teachers that excess thyroid hormone causes hyperactivity and poor attention span. Schoolwork should be structured accordingly until the child reaches a euthyroid state.

DISORDERS IN PARATHYROID FUNCTION

Located on the posterior surface of the thyroid gland, the four parathyroid glands secrete PTH, which maintains calcium homeostasis. PTH increases bone resorption,

thereby increasing the level of calcium in the serum. In the kidneys, PTH decreases urinary excretion of calcium and increases urinary excretion of phosphate. PTH also increases calcium absorption from the intestine. Parathyroid disorder occurs if the PTH level is too low (hypoparathyroidism) or too high (hyperparathyroidism).

HYPOPARATHYROIDISM

Hypoparathyroidism can be transient, congenital, or acquired. Transient hypoparathyroidism in children is most often seen in the first few days of life of preterm infants, infants of mothers with diabetes mellitus, infants of mothers with hypercalcemia, and infants with a prolonged delay in parathyroid gland responsiveness. Familial congenital hypoparathyroidism, transmitted by an X-linked recessive gene, has been reported only a few times. Sporadic occurrence of aplasia or hypoplasia of the parathyroid glands is a more frequent cause of congenital hypoparathyroidism, yet it is still extremely rare. Absence of the parathyroid glands is usually coupled with absence of the thymus gland. The absence of these glands is frequently associated with congenital heart defects, especially anomalies of the aortic arch. This constellation of defects, known as the DiGeorge syndrome, is associated with a deletion of the short arm of chromosome 22.

Pathophysiology

The release of PTH depends on the negative feedback relationship between the level of calcium in the serum and the level of PTH. A decreased level of serum calcium stimulates increased secretion of PTH. An elevated serum level of calcium causes decreased secretion of PTH. Low production of PTH in hypoparathyroidism results in hypocalcemia and hyperphosphatemia. Low serum calcium levels cause twitching, cramps, and tingling and, when severe, can induce tetany and seizures.

Acquired hypoparathyroidism may be caused by autoimmune destruction of the glands or inadvertent removal of the parathyroid glands during surgical thyroidectomy. Autoimmune hypoparathyroidism may be associated with Addison disease, mucocutaneous candidiasis, and alopecia.

Assessment

Assessment of the child with hypoparathyroid glands includes a health history, physical examination, and laboratory studies.

Physical signs of hypoparathyroidism are primarily a result of too little calcium in the blood. These symptoms include muscle spasm or cramping; tingling, numbness, or burning (especially around the mouth and fingers); headaches; hair loss; dry skin; malformed nails; and a history of yeast infections (candidiasis). Severe hypocalcemia can induce tetany, which is a state of hyperexcitability of the central and peripheral nervous systems. Tetany is manifested by carpopedal spasms, laryngospasms, paresthesias, convulsions, or some combination of these signs. In hypoparathyroidism, teeth may erupt late and be soft. Examination for dentition, skeletal growth, and any skeletal deformities is important. The child may also have intellectual deficiencies and a history of seizures. Diagnosis is based on a positive history of these signs and symptoms and on the physical examination. Assess for the presence of positive Chvostek or Trousseau signs, both of which indicate hypocalcemia.

caREminder

To test for the Chvostek sign, tap sharply over the facial nerve below the temple and anteriorly to the ear. The sign is positive when the mouth twitches (contraction of the lateral facial muscles). To check for the Trousseau sign, apply a blood pressure cuff to the child's upper arm. Inflate the cuff until the blood supply is occluded. If doing so causes carpal spasm (the fingers contract and the child is unable to open the hand), the Trousseau sign is positive.

Diagnostic Tests

Laboratory studies reveal low serum levels of calcium and PTH and an elevated serum level of phosphorus. Patients with long-standing hypocalcemia may exhibit calcifications in the basal ganglia, which may be apparent in radiographs of the skull. An electrocardiogram will show a prolonged QT interval, and electroencephalographic tracings usually show widespread, slow activity. Infants with tetany should have radiographs of the chest. DiGeorge syndrome must be part of the differential diagnosis in these infants; visualization of the thymus using chest radiographs will rule out this syndrome.

Diagnostic studies include measuring serum levels of calcium, phosphorus, alkaline phosphatase, magnesium, intact PTH, and, in some instances, vitamin D. Renal function studies may be necessary to rule out renal insufficiency. Radiographs of the bones, skull, and/or abdomen; an electrocardiogram; and an electroencephalogram may be helpful.

Nursing Diagnoses and Outcomes

In addition to the nursing diagnoses presented in Nursing Plan of Care 26-1, the following diagnoses are applicable for the child with hypocalcemia:

Nursing Diagnosis: Risk for injury related to seizures secondary to hypocalcemia
Outcome: Child will be seizure free when treated with calcium supplementation.
Nursing Diagnosis: Ineffective airway clearance related to laryngospasm secondary to hypocalcemia
Outcome: Child will have no breathing impairment when treated with calcium supplementation.
Nursing Diagnosis: Impaired skin integrity related to infiltration of calcium infusion
Outcome: Child's skin will not slough during or after calcium infusion.
Nursing Diagnosis: Ineffective perfusion (cardiopulmonary) related to rapid infusion of calcium
Outcome: Child's heart rate and rhythm will remain normal while the calcium infusion is given.

Interdisciplinary Interventions

The prognosis of hypoparathyroidism depends on the severity of the disorder. Children with mild hypoparathyroidism usually do very well with calcium and vitamin D therapy. However, during periods of illness (e.g., colds, vomiting), the child's calcium requirements may increase and the child may require increased doses of medication. Children with severe hypoparathyroidism require higher doses of medication, and their condition is more precarious. If doses of medication are missed, severe hypocalcemia may ensue.

Pharmacologic treatment is aimed at correcting hypocalcemia and maintaining a normal serum calcium level (9 to 11 mg/dL). Hypercalcemia must be avoided. Treatment of hypocalcemia consists of calcium and vitamin D. Calcium replacement therapy in the form of oral calcium carbonate or calcium glubionate are most commonly used. Oral calcitriol is the activated form of vitamin D (1,25 dihydroxyvitamin D). This medication improves absorption and use of calcium supplements. Calcium glubionate is most commonly used as a calcium supplement in neonates and younger children who require small amounts of supplementation. Other oral forms such as calcium carbonate, citrate, lactate, or gluconate may also be prescribed. For the child with tetany or seizures, give the calcium intravenously, slowly, as calcium gluconate. It can be administered orally later. Vitamin D is also necessary to maintain normocalcemia and serves as a suitable alternative for PTH. Monitor serum levels of calcium and phosphorus frequently, particularly during the early stages of treatment.

ALERT *Early identification of the child with hypoparathyroidism is crucial in preventing severe hypocalcemia, which can cause tetany and consequent laryngospasm and death.*

Children with severe hypocalcemia may require treatment with IV calcium gluconate, which the nurse must administer slowly intravenously over 1 hour while monitoring the heart rate because of the risk that this medication will cause bradycardia and circulatory collapse. Because calcium gluconate is caustic to tissue and infiltration causes sloughing, administer this drug with extreme caution, making sure that the IV line does not become infiltrated. Other forms of IV calcium, such as calcium chloride, are given safely only through a central line.

Community Care

The child should be attended by both a pediatric endocrinologist and the primary care provider to monitor growth, development, and electrolyte balances that could indicate a need for medication adjustment or nonadherence to medication schedule. No special diet is needed, although ensure the child's diet does contain adequate calcium and vitamin D intake.

HYPERPARATHYROIDISM

Hyperparathyroidism (PTH hypersecretion by one or more of the parathyroid glands) may be primary or secondary. Primary hyperparathyroidism may be caused by a defect of the parathyroid gland such as an adenoma or idiopathic hyperplasia of the parathyroid glands. Primary hyperparathyroidism is generally a disease of adults and is rare in children. Mild primary disease is usually identified in an older child or adolescent and is classified as familial hypocalciuric hypercalcemia (FHH). The majority of FHH is caused by autosomal dominant loss-of-function mutations in the plasma membrane G protein–coupled receptor known as CASR (calcium sensing receptor) gene. Secondary hyperparathyroidism is a compensatory increase in PTH in response to hypocalcemia that may be caused by a variety of disorders. Some causes of hypocalcemia that induce compensatory hyperparathyroidism include maternal hypoparathyroidism, vitamin D deficiency, and certain forms of rickets. The most common cause of secondary hyperparathyroidism is chronic renal failure and a complication of children receiving hemodialysis (Greenbaum et al., 2007). The prognosis of hyperparathyroidism and the resultant hypercalcemia depends on the disorder's etiology and severity.

Assessment

Physical manifestations of primary hyperparathyroidism are largely attributable to hypercalcemia. The systems affected in primary hyperparathyroidism are gastrointestinal, CNS, neuromuscular, skeletal, and renal. Ask about gastrointestinal symptoms, including anorexia, nausea, vomiting, and constipation. Document any CNS disturbances, such as confusion, impaired memory, and an altered level of consciousness. Look for neuromuscular manifestations such as weakness, muscle atrophy, paresthesias of the extremities, bradycardia, and cardiac irregularities. Note any bone pain, fractures, gait disturbance, or compression of the vertebrae. Renal changes related to increased urinary calcium loss are polyuria and polydipsia; in addition, renal calculi, hypertension, and renal colic have been described in children. Calcification in the cornea of the eye (band keratopathy) is an additional sign of hypercalcemia.

Signs and symptoms of secondary hyperparathyroidism depend on the disorder that induces the parathyroid gland(s) to hypersecrete PTH. Children with secondary hyperparathyroidism usually have some degree of hypocalcemia. Signs and symptoms related to the direct action of excess PTH are bone demineralization (bone pain, fractures), renal damage (hypertension, renal calculi), and pancreatitis.

The major complication of hyperparathyroidism is hypercalcemic crisis, which can adversely affect the cardiac, neurologic, and gastrointestinal systems.

ALERT   *Signs of hypercalcemic crisis include lethargy, muscle weakness, coma, and oliguria. Their early detection and treatment can help prevent sequelae and possible death.*

Diagnostic Tests

In children with primary hyperparathyroidism, the level of calcium in the serum is elevated (>10.8 mg/dL), the phosphorus level is decreased, and the magnesium level is low. PTH levels are elevated. Radiographs show demineralization of bone, subperiosteal resorption in the phalanges, and granular appearance of the skull. Abdominal films may show renal calculi. In secondary hyperparathyroidism, the serum level of calcium is decreased, whereas serum levels of phosphorus and PTH are elevated. Additional tests (e.g., renal function studies) must be done to determine the cause of secondary hyperparathyroidism.

Because FHH is primarily associated with mutations in a single gene (*CASR*), genetic testing can assist in the diagnosis of FHH.

Interdisciplinary Interventions

Treatment of hyperparathyroidism depends on whether the disorder is primary or secondary. Treating primary hyperparathyroidism consists of either surgical removal of the parathyroid adenoma or subtotal or total parathyroidectomy, depending on where the glands are hyperplastic. Treatment for FHH may not be required at the time of diagnosis, unless it occurs in a neonate with severe, life-threatening hypercalcemia. Otherwise, there is no treatment for FHH, and a parathyroidectomy is unnecessary and ineffective.

In secondary hyperparathyroidism, the underlying cause must be treated. In children with renal disease, treatment of secondary hyperparathyroidism includes oral administration of vitamin D (e.g., paricalcitol, a synthetic vitamin D_2), phosphate binders, and calcium (Greenbaum et al., 2007; Robinson & Scott, 2005). In addition, a low-phosphorus diet is prescribed. If secondary hyperparathyroidism is severe, parathyroidectomy may be necessary.

caREminder

Hypercalcemia can affect cardiac muscle contractility. Therefore, assess children with hyperparathyroidism for signs of bradycardia or cardiac arrhythmia.

When caring for a child after a parathyroidectomy, watch carefully for signs of postoperative complications, particularly hypoparathyroidism (see the earlier section on "Hypoparathyroidism"). Teach parents how to administer vitamin D, phosphate binders, and calcium. Intervention by a nutritionist is required to instruct the family on a low-phosphate diet to decrease hyperphosphatemia. In addition, if hypercalcemia persists, teach parents the importance of giving large amounts of fluids, particularly acidic fluids such as cranberry juice, to help prevent renal calculi.

Community Care

Instruct parents on safety precautions to be taken in the home and at school to prevent bone injury. If the child with hyperparathyroidism has skeletal deformities, the child may have an altered body image. Nurses and school counselors can be very helpful in assisting these children to identify positive, achievable goals for vocation and avocation.

DISORDERS OF THE PANCREAS

Disorders of the pancreas may develop at any age, including the fetal and neonatal periods. Common endocrine disorders of the pancreas in the pediatric population include diabetes mellitus (type 1 and type 2), hypoglycemia, and hyperinsulinemia.

Diabetes Mellitus

Diabetes mellitus is a group of metabolic diseases that are characterized by **hyperglycemia** resulting from defects in insulin action, insulin secretion, or a combination of the two (American Diabetes Association [ADA], 2013). Two major types of diabetes mellitus are recognized in children: T1DM, also called *immune-mediated diabetes*, results from beta-cell destruction and usually leads to insulin deficiency; and T2DM, previously referred to as *non–insulin-dependent diabetes*, which results from a progressive insulin secretory defect on the background of insulin resistance. T2DM may still be referred to as *adult-onset diabetes* despite the increasing incidence in children. A variety of clinical practice guidelines have been published to provide evidence-based standards for diagnosis and management of diabetes mellitus (Evidence-Based Clinical Practice Guideline 26-1).

TYPE 1 DIABETES MELLITUS

T1DM occurs when the pancreas is no longer able to produce insulin. The onset of symptoms of this disorder may be abrupt in children with T1DM or occur over months to years in children with T2DM. T1DM occurs as a result of an autoimmune process that results in destruction of pancreatic beta cells.

 QUESTION: In the case of Lindsay, what is an appropriate summary statement to explain how she "got" diabetes.

The annual incidence of T1DM in the United States is 13.8 to 16.9 per 100,000 white children and 3.3 to 11.8 per 100,000 black children. Approximately 176,000 children younger than 20 years of age have T1DM (ADA, 2013). The incidence of T1DM in children increases with age throughout childhood and reaches its peak at puberty.

T1DM has no single cause, although certain common characteristics can precede diagnosis, including seasonal variations (midwinter and spring) and a history of illness, emotional stress, or infection immediately preceding diagnosis. Many people with T1DM (40% to 60%) have no prior affected family member. Recent incidence of T1DM has been cited as 24.3 per 100,000 persons in the birth-to-19-year-old age group across all races (Dabelea et al., 2007). **Autoimmunity** (a condition in which the immune system attacks the body's cells), genetics, and environmental factors are all thought to contribute to the destruction of beta cells. Approximately 85% to 90% of newly diagnosed patients with T1DM have autoantibodies (ADA, 2013), and autoantibodies to islet cells, insulin, and certain key enzymes can also be found in relatives of people with T1DM. The presence of autoantibodies signifies an autoimmune response: the child's immune system is attacking the body and destroying beta cells. However, the mode of inheritance is not fully understood. The major hypothetical environmental factor in the development of T1DM is a virus that triggers the autoimmune process. Several viruses have been identified as possible triggers, including coxsackievirus B4; retrovirus; cytomegalovirus; and the viruses that cause mumps, hepatitis, and congenital rubella (Kelly et al., 2003).

T1DM can be controlled with proper medical attention, and acute complications are minimized if blood glucose control is maintained within a recommended target range for age. However, long-term complications such as disorders of the eye (diabetic retinopathy), kidney (diabetic nephropathy), circulatory system (heart disease, stroke), and nerve fibers (peripheral neuropathy) are common secondary conditions associated with poorly controlled diabetes. If left untreated, T1DM can result in death.

ANSWER: An example of a statement appropriate for Lindsay at age 6 years follows. "You have a gland called a pancreas and its job is to make insulin. Insulin makes it so that your body can use the glucose in the blood. Your pancreas stopped making enough insulin and so there is too much sugar in the blood. You did not do anything to make the pancreas stop making enough insulin. We don't know why, but in some kids, the pancreas stops working the way it should. So, for your body to use glucose, you will need to get extra insulin."

Pathophysiology

Insulin deficiency and resistance cause physiologic and metabolic changes throughout the body. Because of the insulin deficiency, glucose derived from dietary sources cannot be used by the cells (specifically muscle and fat cells) and begins to increase in the bloodstream (hyperglycemia). When serum glucose levels approach 180 mg/dL, the renal tubules have difficulty reabsorbing all the glucose, and glucose is spilled into the urine (**glucosuria**). Large amounts of electrolytes (sodium, potassium, calcium, phosphate, and magnesium) are also excreted by the kidneys as hyperglycemia increases, resulting in increased urination (polyuria) and dehydration. Excessive thirst (polydipsia) ensues in an attempt to relieve the dehydration. Polyphagia also results from the body's attempt to compensate for the calories lost during polyuria. The three "polys" are present in both T1DM and T2DM, but these signs are more dramatic in children with T1DM. Parents will usually report polyuria and polydipsia; in many cases, though, parents have not noticed polyphagia.

Insulin deficiency (and insulin resistance, to a degree) causes increased catabolism of protein, resulting in increased production of amino acids. At the same time, the liver converts triglycerides (lipolysis) to fatty acids,

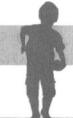

Care of the Patient With Diabetes Mellitus

American Association of Clinical Endocrinologists. (2011). American Association of Clinical Endocrinologists medical guidelines for clinical practice for developing a diabetes mellitus comprehensive care plan. *Endocrine Practice*, *17*(Suppl. 2), 1–53. Retrieved from

http://guideline.gov/content.aspx?id = 34038&search = Dietary + education + for + type + I + diabetes + mellitus +

Comprehensive guidelines for management of diabetes mellitus in adults and children.

American Diabetes Association. (2013). Standards of medical care in diabetes. *Diabetes Care*, *36*(Suppl. 1), S11–S66. Retrieved from

http://care.diabetesjournals.org/content/36/Supplement_1/S11.full

Official standards on care of the person with diabetes mellitus.

American Diabetes Association. (2013). Diabetes management at camps for children with diabetes. *Diabetes Care*, *35*(Suppl. 1), S72–S75. Retrieved from

http://care.diabetesjournals.org/content/35/Supplement_1/S72

Guidelines for clinicians and those who provide oversight of outdoor camps for children with diabetes.

American Diabetes Association. (2009). Nutrition recommendations and interventions for diabetes: A position statement of the American Diabetes Association, *Diabetes Care*, *31*(Suppl. 1), S61–S78. Retrieved from

http://care.diabetesjournals.org/content/31/Supplement_1/S61

Standards for nutritional management of diabetes mellitus.

Centers for Disease Control and Prevention. (2012). *National diabetes education program.* Retrieved from

http://wwwn.cdc.gov/pubs/ndep.aspx

Comprehensive materials to provide patient education about diabetes mellitus.

Inzucchi, S., Bergenstal, R., Buse, J. et al. (2013). Management of hyperglycemia in type 2 diabetes: A patient-centered approach. Position statement of the American Diabetes Association (ADA) and the European Association for the Study of Diabetes (EASD). *Diabetes Care*, *35*, 1364–1379. Retrieved from

http://care.diabetesjournals.org/content/35/6/1364

International guidelines for the treatment of hyperglycemia.

Copeland, K. C., Silverstein, J., Moore, K. R. et al. (2013). Management of newly diagnosed type 2 diabetes mellitus (t2dm) in children and adolescents. *Pediatrics*, *131*(2), 364–382. Retrieved from

http://pediatrics.aappublications.org/content/early/2013/01/23/peds.2012-3494.full.pdf

Practice guidelines for clinicians caring for children with T2DM developed by the American Academy of Pediatrics.

International Society for Pediatric and Adolescent Diabetes. (2011). *IDF/ISPAD global guideline for diabetes in childhood and adolescence.* Retrieved from

http://www.ispad.org/resource-type/idfispad-2011-global-guideline-diabetes-childhood-and-adolescence

Guidelines for optimal management of T1DM.

McIntosh, A., Peters, J., Young, R. et al. (2003). *Prevention and management of foot problems in type 2 diabetes: Clinical guidelines and evidence.* Sheffield, United Kingdom: University of Sheffield. Retrieved from

http://www.nice.org.uk/nicemedia/live/10934/29242/29242.pdf

Guidelines for managing long-term care of diabetic patients who may have foot problems.

Peters, A., & Laffel, L. (2011). Diabetes care for emerging adults: Recommendations for transition from pediatric to adult diabetes care systems. *Diabetes Care*, *34*, 2477–2485. Retrieved from

http://care.diabetesjournals.org/content/34/11/2477

Standards to minimize gaps that can occur when transitioning pediatric diabetic patients to adult care services.

which in turn change to **ketone bodies**. Ketone bodies, organic acids that are used for energy by the peripheral tissues, are not well used in insulin-deficient states. Excessive ketone bodies accumulate and are excreted by the kidneys (**ketonuria**). Ketone bodies can produce excessive amounts of free hydrogen ions, resulting in metabolic acidosis. Serum pH is lowered because the body cannot compensate. In severe acidosis, the depth and rate of respirations increases and becomes persistent as the body attempts to compensate by excreting excess carbon dioxide; this respiratory pattern mimics a deep panting pattern (Kussmaul respirations).

Insulin deficiency, in association with increased levels of counterregulatory hormones (glucagon, GH, cortisol, catecholamines) and dehydration, is the primary cause of **diabetic ketoacidosis** (DKA), a life-threatening form of metabolic acidosis that is a frequent complication of uncontrolled diabetes. Counterregulatory hormones, which have an anti-insulin effect, increase during times of stress and worsen insulin deficiency. Peripheral glucose use decreases, and hepatic gluconeogenesis increases (increased glucose production by the liver). Severe insulin deficiency causing DKA is a medical emergency and is characterized by hyperglycemia (serum glucose >300 mg/dL), hyperketonemia, ketonuria, glucosuria, metabolic acidosis (arterial pH, <7.30; bicarbonate, <15 mEq/L), and severe alterations in electrolyte and fluid balance. The degree of hyperglycemia does not predict the severity of DKA.

Assessment

> **QUESTION:** How typical was Lindsay's presentation of symptoms?

The child with diabetes usually presents with the classic symptoms of polyuria and polydipsia. Enuresis is seen frequently in the young child who was previously toilet trained, and nocturia is seen in all children. Polyphagia is seen early in diabetes, although anorexia is also commonly seen later in the disease when the child feels extremely ill. Compare current and previous weights. Weight loss, which can be as much as 10% to 30% of the original weight, may be substantial before parents even become aware of it, particularly in the older child. Parents may describe a viral illness preceding the symptoms of polyuria, polydipsia, and polyphagia. Ask about recent illnesses because fatigue, headache, and malaise often seen at the presentation of diabetes, may be attributed to other illnesses or events, such as influenza, recent viral illness, urinary tract infection, or summer heat.

ALERT   *The diagnosis of T1DM is often delayed in the infant because evaluation by parents of diaper quantity or volume is insufficient; therefore, they do not notice polyuria. Not until diapers are literally "flooded" do parents notice the large amount of urine output.*

Consider diabetes as part of the differential diagnosis in the infant presenting with vomiting, diarrhea, or dehydration. Other common, but less characteristic, symptoms that are more evident in middle childhood or adolescence include personality changes, lethargy, vision changes, altered school performance, headaches, anxiety attacks, intermittent breathlessness, chest pain, nausea, and either diarrhea or constipation.

If insulin deficiency persists and ketone bodies continue to be excreted, the child begins to experience stomach pains, vomiting, and continued weight loss. Dehydration quickly develops as DKA progresses. The degree of dehydration is assessed while the child is weighed and examined. Assessment includes examining the mucous membranes for moistness, the eyeballs for degree of depression, the skin for turgor, and the anterior fontanel (if present) for depression. The child may also show signs of impending shock: tachypnea, decreased output, decreased level of consciousness, slowed capillary refill, and tachycardia. A late sign of shock in children is hypotension.

DKA is most commonly present in new-onset T1DM or during crises in children with known T1DM, but it may also be found in newly diagnosed T2DM in the adolescent age group. Kussmaul respirations and changes in mental status may ensue. The breath develops a fruity odor in all children with DKA. If the child becomes somnolent and advances into a coma, these are ominous signs of cerebral edema. The child must be treated promptly with medications to reduce the edema in the brain and then be transferred to a pediatric critical care setting.

Identifying DKA is critical to facilitate treatment and the child's return to good health (Nursing Interventions 26-2). Presenting signs and symptoms of DKA may include altered level of consciousness, dehydration, electrolyte disturbances, dysrhythmias, shock, and complete vascular collapse. Children with DKA are seriously ill and require immediate treatment (ADA, 2013). The condition is best handled by a pediatric critical care team or by skilled pediatric endocrinologists.

> **ANSWER:** For her age, Lindsay had a typical sudden-onset presentation. Her parents noted two of the three polys, polydipsia and polyuria; there was a gradual weight loss; and, immediately prior to diagnosis as her blood sugar continued to climb, Lindsay had episodes of vomiting.

Diagnostic Tests

Blood glucose levels in T1DM are usually more than 200 mg/dL, and a urine sample reveals glucosuria and ketonuria, depending on the degree of acidosis (Chart 26-1). Glucose in the urine alone can be indicative of a low renal threshold for glucose (Silverstein et al., 2005). A glucose tolerance test is not recommended for diagnosing T1DM in children because it may delay diagnosis. Blood glucose and urine test results, along with history and physical examination, confirm the diagnosis. The child may appear very healthy or acutely ill, depending on the degree of acidosis. When performing an oral glucose tolerance test (OGTT) in children, the glucose load should be 1.75 g/kg up to a maximum of 75 g.

NURSING INTERVENTIONS 26-2

Diabetic Ketoacidosis

Nursing Assessment	Signs and Symptoms	Laboratory Test	Nursing Interventions	Medical Management
Assess for dehydration.	Skin turgor Dry mucous membranes Sunken eyeballs Depressed fontanel Signs of shock: tachypnea, decreased output, hypotension, weak pulse	Hemoglobin, hematocrit Blood urea nitrogen, creatinine	Monitor vital signs every hour. Administer 0.9% sodium chloride (NaCl) at rate ordered. Maintain accurate input and output records.	Administer 0.9% NaCl intravenously at a rate of maintenance plus one half of deficit in first 8 hours. Appropriate amount of fluid should be administered to replace losses and treat any evidence of shock. Fluids should not exceed 4 L/m^2/day.
Assess for potassium depletion.	Muscle weakness Flattened T wave on ECG	Potassium elevated (or normal if early); may drop as acidosis is corrected	Before administering potassium, ensure • Urine flow has been established • Laboratory value has ruled out hyperkalemia Administer potassium as ordered.	Measure electrolytes. Add potassium chloride to IV fluid per prescriber's orders.
Assess for phosphate depletion.	Anorexia Muscle wasting Paresthesia Tremors	Phosphorus elevated (or normal if early)	Monitor blood phosphate levels.	In severe acidosis, IV potassium phosphate may be ordered.
Assess for hyperglycemia.	Polyuria Polydipsia Polyphagia Weight loss	Blood glucose >180 mg/dL Urine glucose positive	Monitor blood glucose every hour. Monitor urine glucose and ketones every void. Prepare IV insulin drip (100 units regular insulin/100 0.9% NaCl) and administer as ordered.	Obtain blood glucose every 1–2 hours. Give IV insulin (regular) as ordered: 0.05–0.1 units/kg/hr IV drip. IV push insulin is not effective because of its short half-life. Acidosis will continue due to insulin deficiency outside of the use of a continuous insulin drip. Prime IV tubing with insulin-containing solution to ensure accurate delivery.

Nursing Assessment	Signs and Symptoms	Laboratory Test	Nursing Interventions	Medical Management
Assess for hypoglycemia.	Diaphoresis Tremors Tachycardia Irritability	Blood glucose <60 mg/dL	Suspend insulin drip. Notify health care provider. Have fast-acting carbohydrate and IV dextrose available.	If child can take oral fluids, offer 2–4 oz juice or soda (non-diet). If child cannot take fluids orally, administer 0.5–1 g/kg of 50% dextrose (diluted to D25 prior to administration) via IV slow push. Recheck blood glucose in 15–20 minutes. Generally, IV fluids will be changed to glucose containing (D5, D10, D12.5) to avoid hypoglycemia while on an insulin drip instead of stopping the drip.
Assess for degree of acidosis.	Kussmaul respirations Acetone odor on breath Change in level of consciousness	Altered pH Altered carbon dioxide Serum bicarbonate Serum ketones	Monitor vital signs every hour. Measure urine ketones every void. For severely acidotic child, perform neurologic checks every hour and administer bicarbonate as ordered.	Measure serum pH and carbon dioxide every 2 hours. Insulin administration and fluid correction as ordered should correct acidosis except in those children who are most severely acidotic (pH <7.30).
Assess for factors precipitating DKA.	Signs of infection: fever, otitis media, dysuria, etc. Report of missed or insufficient insulin dose Report of emotional stress	Change in white blood cell count Positive urine culture Positive throat culture	Report signs of infection to physician. Administer antibiotic as ordered. Teach child and family about consequences of insulin errors and sick-day management. Evaluate diabetes plan to determine whether it can be altered to better fit lifestyle. Refer to social service, psychologist, school nurse, or visiting nurse as necessary.	Order indicated studies. If infection is bacterial, treat with an antibiotic.

Criteria for the Diagnosis of Diabetes

$A_{1C} \geq 6.5\%$. The test should be performed in a laboratory using a method that is NGSP certified and standardized to the DCCT assay.

OR

FPG >126 mg/dL (7.0 mmol/L). Fasting is defined as no caloric intake for at least 8 hours.

OR

Two-hour plasma glucose ≥200 mg/dL (11.1 mmol/L) during an OGTT. The test should be performed as described by the WHO using a glucose load of 75-g anhydrous glucose dissolved in water.

OR

In a child with classic symptoms of hyperglycemia or hyperglycemic crisis, a random plasma glucose ≥200 mg/dL (11.1 mmol/L).

DCCT, Diabetes Control and Complications Trial; FPG, fasting plasma glucose; NGSP, National Glycohemoglobin Standardization Program; WHO, World Health Organization.
From American Association of Clinical Endocrinologists. (2011a). American Association of Clinical Endocrinologists medical guidelines for clinical practice for developing a diabetes mellitus comprehensive care plan. *Endocrine Practice, 17*(Suppl. 2), 1–53; American Diabetes Association. (2013). Standards of medical care in diabetes. *Diabetes Care, 36*(Suppl. 1), S11–S66.

Nursing Diagnoses and Outcomes

The nursing diagnoses presented in Nursing Plan of Care 26-1 apply to the child with ongoing management of T1DM. Also see thePoint Care Paths: An Interdisciplinary Plan of Care for the Child With Diabetic Ketoacidosis.

Interdisciplinary Interventions

Diabetes treatment involves medical therapy with insulin and supportive measures to enhance glycemic control. Monitoring and testing of metabolic control is ongoing. Involving a dietitian experienced in caring for children with diabetes is essential for meal planning and adjustments and for providing information about exercise and interactions between foods and medications, whether insulin or oral medications. A diabetes educator can also assist the family in fitting diabetes management into the child's lifestyle, as opposed to the older method of fitting the child's lifestyle into diabetes management. Assure the child and family from the outset that diabetes should not prevent the child from participating in anything.

Pharmacologic Interventions

 QUESTION: What are the various modes of insulin administration that Lindsay has mastered between the time of her diagnosis at age 6 years to her newest milestone at age 8 years?

Insulin therapy is required for a child with T1DM. Without insulin, the child will die. A combination of fast- or rapid-acting insulin, intermediate-acting insulin, or long-acting insulin is used (Teaching Intervention Plan 26-2). Some children who are newly diagnosed may need insulin twice daily, before breakfast and before dinner. There are a number of different insulin regimens available, including

• Split-mixed dosing using short- and intermediate-acting insulin at breakfast and short- and long-acting insulin at dinner

---

TIP 26-2: A TEACHING INTERVENTION PLAN for Administering Insulin

Nursing Diagnosis and Family Outcomes
• Deficient knowledge: Mixing and administering insulin
  Outcomes: Child and family will administer the correct kind and doses of insulin to the child. Child will demonstrate the highest levels of skill of which he or she is developmentally capable when administering insulin.

Teach the Child/Family
Insulin Administration
• Remove insulin from the refrigerator. Insulin can also be stored at room temperature for 1 month before being discarded.
• The person preparing and administering insulin should wash his or her hands.
• Wipe the tops of insulin bottles with alcohol.
• Gently roll bottle of intermediate- or long-acting insulin to ensure uniform mixture of insulin and to avoid introducing air bubbles.

• Draw up short-acting insulin, removing all air bubbles.
• Draw up intermediate acting insulin. Long-acting insulins cannot be mixed in a syringe with any other insulin. (Follow the manufacturer's recommendations.)
• Pinch the skin being used for injection to separate subcutaneous tissue from muscle.
• Give insulin in the subcutaneous tissue at either a 45- or 90-degree angle, depending on the length of the needle.
• Withdraw needle immediately after injection is given. Dispose of the needle in an appropriate needle storage container.

ALERT *Instruct families to call their local pharmacy or city waste disposal office for container disposal sites.*

- MDIs using long-acting insulin daily and short-acting insulin at each carbohydrate-containing meal
- Insulin pump therapy using short-acting insulin delivered continuously (basal rate) with additional insulin for carbohydrate intake or to correct high blood glucose levels (bolus)

The child, family, and health care provider together will make the decision on which regimen is best for them (see thePoint Medications and Administration: Insulin Types and Actions). These combinations are used to ensure that the peak action of the insulin coincides with the child's postprandial blood glucose peaks. The MDI pattern mimics the basal–bolus pattern an insulin pump could provide. The long-acting insulins have little if any peak; they serve as the basal, or "background" insulin. The rapid-acting insulins are administered to cover meals and snacks, acting as the "bolus" insulin. Insulin pump therapy is rarely initiated at diagnosis, but it can be started soon thereafter. Pump therapy is also widely used in pediatrics and should be considered if the child and family are mature, capable, and interested (Fig. 26-4). Insulin pumps are ideal for children with T1DM or absolute insulin-deficient T2DM who need four or more insulin injections a day and must assess their blood glucose four or more times a day (AACE, 2011a). When determining if the child is a candidate for an insulin pump, the health care team must determine if the child and key family members can master carbohydrate counting, insulin correction and adjustment formulas, and troubleshoot problems that may arise with pump operation and plasma glucose levels (AACE, 2011a).

The insulin dose is initially calculated using the child's body weight, pubertal status, and age. Time of day for administration can be selected by the parents and child according to their home and school schedules when using either the MDI or pump therapy regimen. Otherwise, the split-mixed dosing schedule is used and requires injections before breakfast and dinner. When using the insulin pump, the rapid (fast-acting, or bolus) insulin, given before meals and snacks, is dosed according to how much carbohydrate the child will consume and what the current blood glucose result is. The parents or child also adjust the dose for any exercise that might be planned. The subcutaneous injections of insulin should be started at mealtimes in the hospital to mimic the home schedule. The earlier during the course of hospitalization the parents or caregivers start giving injections, the easier it becomes to administer them and the sooner the child is able to leave the hospital.

Insulin strength is measured in units: 1 mL insulin is equal to 100 units (U-100). In the very small child, changing the amount of insulin by 1 or 2 units can represent a 50% or even a 100% increase or decrease, considering that the doses are usually very small. Insulin syringes and insulin pens that measure in half units are now available and may be helpful in the child's care. For the very young child or one who is very sensitive to it, the insulin can be diluted to U-75, U-50, or less to improve dosing accuracy. Show the child and the family the best sites on the child's body for injection (Fig. 26-5).

Lipohypertrophy (thickening) of the local tissue can occur when insulin is injected into the same location repeatedly. Insulin is not well absorbed into hypertrophied tissue, and its action is unpredictable, making glycemic control more difficult. Therefore, the child and parents should select at least two or three sites (arms, legs, stomach, or buttocks) for injection. Encourage the child and parents to try all the sites while the child is

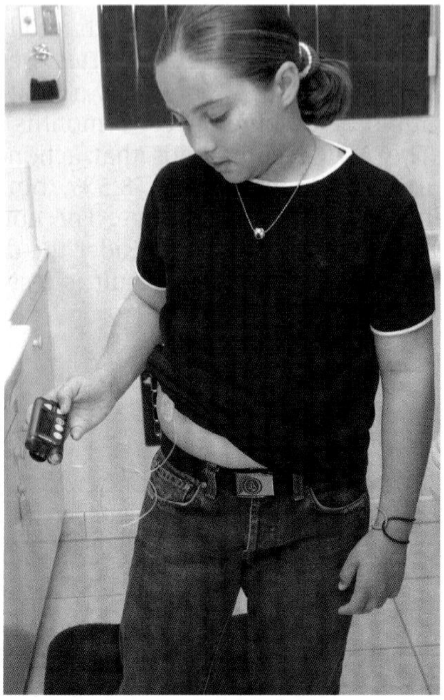

Figure 26-4 The patch for the insulin pump can be discreetly placed on the abdomen with the pump placed in the child's pocket.

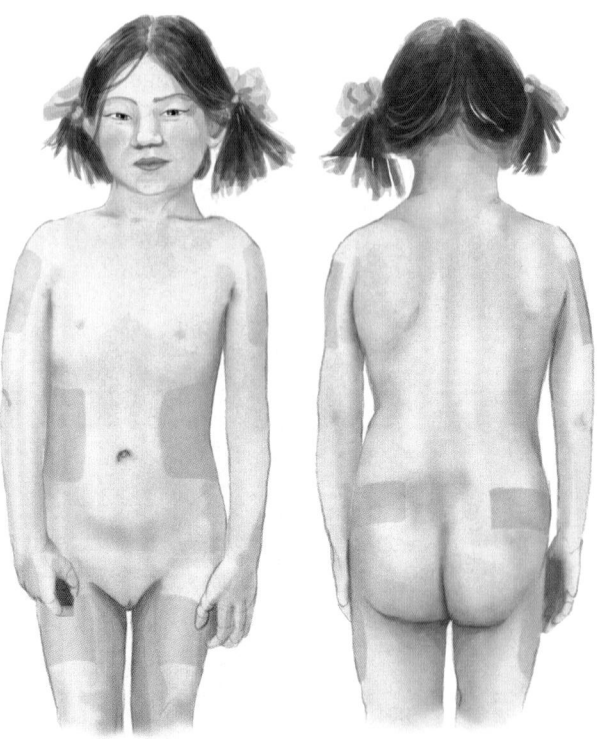

Figure 26-5 Sites for insulin injection should be rotated among the areas shown.

still hospitalized. Children can choose sites and then chart them so they remember not to overuse sites.

> **ANSWER:** By age 8 years, Lindsay has mastered three modes of insulin administration. Lindsay gave herself her first insulin injection with a syringe while at diabetes camp when she was 7 years old, she has used the insulin pen at school, and now she is managing the insulin pump.

Monitoring Metabolic Control

To ensure that treatment is working, blood glucose and urine ketones must be monitored.

Capillary blood glucose monitoring is usually done four to eight times a day for T1DM and two to three times a day for T2DM. This test can be performed by the child or a family member. The supplies are easily transportable, and many blood glucose meters are available to fit any child's lifestyle. Hypoglycemia, normoglycemia, and hyperglycemia are accurately assessed by capillary testing, and the results are immediate and specific. The disadvantages of blood glucose monitoring are the invasive nature of the procedure and the sometimes excessive cost of the equipment. The child with T1DM tests blood glucose four to eight times each day: before meals or snacks, before bed, occasionally overnight, and with any signs or symptoms of hypoglycemia or illness (see the section on "Hypoglycemia" in this chapter for more information on managing hypoglycemia). When the child's insulin dose has stabilized, the overnight test can be dropped and only done occasionally, for example with a new sports season, when metabolic demands might change.

Capillary blood glucose monitoring is accomplished by puncturing a finger (or toe in an infant or young child) with a lancet and placing a drop of blood on a blood test strip (Fig. 26-6). The finger should be cleaned with soap and water before testing. The test strip is inserted into a blood glucose meter, and results are usually received in less than 5 seconds. The accuracy of the reading depends on proper use of the test system. Quality checks should be completed using the control solution supplied with the blood glucose meter at purchase three to four times per year. The hotline number for the meter manufacturer can be found on the back of the meter, so children and families with questions or concerns can access help 24 hours a day.

Test results should be documented and used to regulate the insulin dose. Records should be brought to follow-up appointments and each subsequent health care visit. Many meters can download results into a computer program to provide ongoing documentation of the child's status.

> **QUESTION:** Lindsay's A_{1C} has always been less than 8% until she started a growth spurt. Her last A_{1C} was 8.1%. Is this an acceptable measurement, or will changes be made in her regimen?

Long-term metabolic control can be evaluated by measuring the glycosylated hemoglobin or hemoglobin A_{1C} (simplified now to the term A_{1C}). Glycosylation is the process by which glucose attaches to hemoglobin nonenzymatically—a slow, mostly irreversible process. The red blood cell, which contains the hemoglobin molecule, lasts in the bloodstream for 90 to 120 days. Increased levels of blood glucose increase the percentage of hemoglobin that is glycosylated and therefore reflect the average glucose concentration for the preceding 3 to 4 months (ADA, 2013). The A_{1C} level can be helpful in correlating the daily blood glucose results obtained by finger stick with the longer term picture (Table 26-2). The daily results really provide only a snapshot of diabetes control, 4 to 8 seconds out of the day, whereas the A_{1C} provides a long-term picture and should be obtained every 3 months at follow-up visits. The ADA recommends that action be taken when A_{1C} results are more than 8.5%, but this will vary depending on the child's age. For nonpregnant adults, ADA recommendations consider the diabetes to be under control when the A_{1C} result is less than 7% (ADA, 2013).

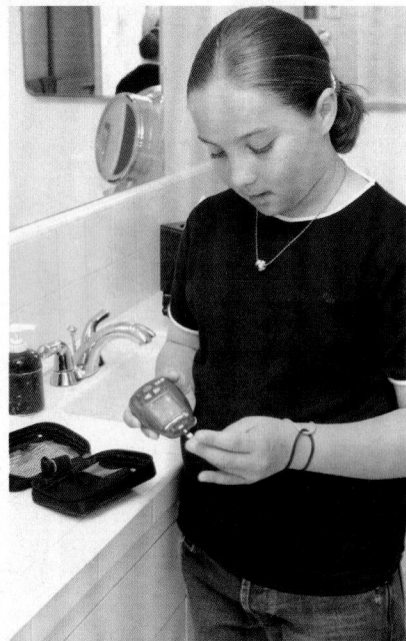

Figure 26-6 Many children perform blood glucose monitoring at home.

		Bedtime/	
Age	Before Meals	Overnight	HgbA$_{1C}$
0–6 years	100–180	110–200	<8.5%
6–12 years	90–180	100–180	<8%
13–19 years	90–130	90–150	<7.5%

TABLE 26-2   Plasma Glucose and A$_{1C}$ Goals for Type 1 Diabetes Mellitus by Age Group

From American Diabetes Association. (2013). Standards of medical care in diabetes. *Diabetes Care, 36*(Suppl. 1), S11–S66.

ANSWER: An A$_{1C}$ result of 8.1% is not within the target range for Lindsay's age. The recommendation is for action to be taken. Lindsay's endocrinologist made many changes, including the amount of insulin given per carbohydrate eaten.

Testing the urine for ketones is an easy and noninvasive monitoring method. However, the test is not considered useful as an effective way to monitor daily insulin doses. Urine ketones indicate fatty acid breakdown and may be present if an illness, insulin deficiency, starvation, or severe hypoglycemic reaction occurs. Teach the child and parents to test the urine for ketones whenever the blood glucose is 240 mg/dL or more or when the child is ill. The child should increase fluid intake if ketones are present in the urine and should notify the health care provider immediately if ketone levels are moderate to high. The family should have a sick-day management chart or handout to guide them in these instances. Extra insulin is essential to "clear" ketones. Initially, the diabetes care provider is needed to determine how much extra insulin the child with T1DM should administer.

ALERT *Urine ketones in association with vomiting may indicate ketoacidosis and should be handled as an emergency. The health care provider should be notified immediately after the first emesis, and the child may need to go to the emergency department.*

Nutritional Management

QUESTION: Which foods would you tell Lindsay that she cannot eat?

The goals of nutritional therapy for treating diabetes in children (ADA, 2013) are as follows:

- Maintaining target blood glucose by balancing food intake with insulin and activity
- Achieving blood glucose goals for age group without excessive hypoglycemia
- Achieving lipid and blood pressure goals
- Providing appropriate calories for normal growth and development in children and adolescents
- Preventing and treating acute complications and preventing long-term complications of T1DM

For children with T1DM, integrate insulin injections into usual eating and physical activity habits. Meal plans are based on the child's age, developmental level, preferences, culture, and ethnicity. The dietitian meets with the child and parents during the hospital stay or early in the outpatient setting. The ADA meal plan is virtually identical to the American Heart Association meal plan: both focus on healthy eating (Community Care 26-2). Children with diabetes should be told that any food they want can be worked into their meal plans. Portion sizes, selection and type of food, and activity are all considered to strike the healthy balance needed.

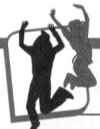

COMMUNITY CARE 26-2

Nutritional Guidelines for Individuals With Diabetes Mellitus

Protein
- Fifteen percent to 20% of daily caloric intake
- Derived from animal or vegetable source

Fat
- Thirty percent or less of the calories from total fat
- Less than 7% of calories from saturated fat
- Up to 10% of calories from polyunsaturated fat
- Minimize intake of trans unsaturated fatty acids

Carbohydrates and Sweeteners
- Carbohydrates and monounsaturated fats: 60%–70% of energy intake
- Sucrose and sucrose-containing foods: can substitute for other carbohydrates, but consider nutritional content
- Fructose: may be used as a sweetening agent; however, large amounts (>40% of calories) have adverse effects on serum cholesterol and low-density lipoprotein cholesterol

- Sorbitol, mannitol, and xylitol: produce a lower glycemic response than sucrose and other carbohydrates; however, excessive amounts have a laxative effect
- Saccharin, aspartame, and acesulfame K: U.S. Food and Drug Administration approved as nonnutritive sweeteners; can be used by people with diabetes

Fiber
- Twenty to 35 g dietary fiber, from varied sources

Alcohol
- Two alcoholic beverages per day for an adult male, one per day for an adult female (one alcoholic beverage = 12 oz beer, 5 oz wine, or 12 oz distilled spirits) can be ingested with, and in addition to, the usual meal plan. Children and adolescents should refrain from alcohol use. Alcohol diminishes gluconeogenesis by the liver and leads to hypoglycemia.

Adapted from American Diabetes Association. (2013). Standards of medical care in diabetes. *Diabetes Care*, *36*(Suppl. 1), S11–S66.

ANSWER: There is no food that Lindsay is not allowed to eat. Certainly, there are choices that are better than others. But as long as she keeps track of what she eats and programs her insulin pump correctly, there are no forbidden foods.

Community Care

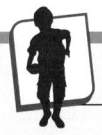

QUESTION: Lindsay plays on a basketball team. On the days she has a 1-hour basketball practice, her blood sugar will be affected for the next 24 hours. A midnight blood sugar of 150 mg/dL may become a 3 AM blood sugar of 50 mg/dL. What strategies can you develop to help stabilize Lindsay's blood glucose on the days when she has basketball practice?

Many children with new-onset T1DM are never hospitalized, even at diagnosis. Children can receive an initial injection of insulin in the emergency department and then return the next day to begin learning about their condition. Teaching is usually accomplished at large medical centers or communities that have active pediatric diabetes education programs. In smaller, outlying communities, hospitalization may still be routinely required for teaching purposes. The degree of acidosis and dehydration and the family social and support situation may also drive the need for hospitalization.

T1DM, when not managed carefully, can become a life-threatening acute illness. Management requires attention and caring from parents or another supportive person on an ongoing basis despite the child's perceived ability to manage the physical tasks of care, such as giving insulin injections. Often, children who do not do well, and thus come to the attention of the acute care system, either have an acute infection that exacerbates the chronic condition or lack parental and social supports, and may be indirectly asking for more adult attention by avoiding proper care of their chronic illness.

Caregivers, teachers, and physical education instructors need to have accurate information concerning the child and need to know how to identify and treat hypoglycemia (discussed later in this chapter). Inform teachers when a student is diagnosed with diabetes mellitus. When the child returns to school, encourage parents to give teachers, school nurses, and coaches instructions for their child, particularly instruction on recognizing and treating hypoglycemia in T1DM and those on insulin with T2DM (Clinical Judgment 26-3).

CLINICAL JUDGMENT 26-3

A Child With Type 1 Diabetes Mellitus

Pierre, age 10 years, has T1DM. He is admitted to the hospital at the time of diagnosis for initial management. In the pediatrician's office, Pierre's blood glucose level is 930 mg/dL.

Questions

1. During your admission assessment, what data would you collect to assist you to teach Pierre about his diagnosis and his management plan?

2. What factors would indicate good metabolic control for the child with T1DM?

3. On Pierre's fourth morning in the hospital, you note that he is pale and sweaty. Based on his symptoms, what is his problem at this time?

4. When teaching Pierre and his family about insulin administration, what strategies should be used?

5. When the home care nurse visits Pierre 1 week after discharge, what age-appropriate activities should she expect Pierre to be doing in regard to managing his diabetes?

Answers

1. Previous history of any serious or chronic illness, previous hospitalizations, Pierre's exposure to other family members who may have diabetes or another chronic condition

2. Hemoglobin A_{1c} values less than 7.5%, normal growth and development, and few episodes of hypoglycemia or hyperglycemia

3. Pierre is hypoglycemic. Rapid treatment would involve giving him 15-g glucose-containing solid, semisolid, or liquid such as orange juice.

4. Plan demonstration, supervision, and practice time with Pierre and his parents to learn injection and site rotation techniques, methods to draw up insulin, and the proper way to store medication and equipment.

5. Pierre is actively involved in testing his blood glucose levels. He gathers all the equipment for insulin administration. With parental assistance, he can draw up the correct dose of insulin. He can administer the injection himself, although sometimes he chooses to have a parent administer the injection, especially in hard-to-reach places. Pierre can discuss appropriate diet choices and restrictions. Pierre can recognize and treat hypoglycemia.

Children, particularly adolescents, may at times record results in their glucose logbooks that are not factual because high numbers may cause arguments between child and parent that the child wants to avoid. The child may be making up numbers rather than actually testing for them. The A_{1C} can help to determine whether this is the case because the A_{1C} and daily log should correlate. If they do not, an explanation for the differences should be sought. High and low results could be occurring at times the child is not testing, or the lack of correlation could be attributable to factitious numbers.

Exercise is a vital component in managing both T1DM and T2DM in children and offers many benefits. It assists in the use of dietary intake and may decrease the amount of insulin or oral agents that a child requires. Exercise enhances insulin absorption and facilitates weight loss or maintenance. Exercise is also important for the child's normal growth and development. The child should eat a snack before exercising to prevent hypoglycemia. Exercise lasting less than 1 hour usually requires a small snack consisting of a complex carbohydrate or a protein. More intense exercise or exercise lasting longer than 1 hour may require more frequent snacks throughout the activity and a combination of complex carbohydrates and protein before the activity. An insulin adjustment may also be needed if hypoglycemia occurs frequently with an activity. The family is instructed to check the child's blood glucose level before, during, and after activity and also before bedtime and overnight to prevent nighttime hypoglycemic events because exercise can cause delayed hypoglycemia (Community Care 26-3). Health care team members, parents, and school support personnel can teach adolescents effective coping skills that may help them deal with day-to-day management of their illness. Long-term care should include annual eye examinations and dental cleanings every 6 months. A fasting lipid panel should also be evaluated in the child within a year after diagnosis. Recommendations for lipid goals and management will vary according to the age of the child. Ongoing monitoring for other autoimmune illnesses, such as autoimmune thyroiditis and celiac disease, should be done annually as well.

 KidKare Hyperglycemia can be exacerbated if the child exercises when the blood glucose level is 240 mg/dL or more and ketones are present in the urine. Therefore, the child should generally avoid exercise if ketones are detected during this time. Guidance from the diabetes team should be sought if ketones are present. Exercise can be reinitiated when the urine is free from ketones.

ANSWER: If Lindsay's midnight blood sugar is less than 150 mg/dL, an effective strategy is to adjust the bedtime snack to include more protein or fat. This should ensure Lindsay's 3 AM blood sugar will not to be too low.

TYPE 2 DIABETES MELLITUS

QUESTION: What are the ways in which the onset of T2DM is different from that of T1DM?

T2DM is a condition characterized by insulin resistance. It has a slow and gradual onset and is most often related to obesity. T2DM is not considered an autoimmune disease.

Based on 2005 to 2009 data, about 215,000 people younger than 20 years of age in the United States have diabetes (either type 1 or type 2), with approximately 3,600 new cases of T2DM diagnosed annually (CDC, 2011). Native Americans, Hispanics, Asian/Pacific Islanders, and blacks have a higher incidence than other populations of T2DM in youth. Obesity (body mass index exceeding the 95th percentile) and **prediabetes** (individuals with blood glucose or A_{1C} levels higher than normal but not high enough to be classified as diabetes) among American children has increased, thereby impacting the numbers of children at risk for diabetes (CDC, 2011).

A strong family history of T2DM is often present, as is a familial tendency toward obesity and a sedentary lifestyle. A child whose mother had gestational diabetes is particularly at risk for T2DM (CDC, 2011). Although ethnic background and mother's gestational history are not a modifiable risk factor, weight and lifestyle certainly are. The challenge with T2DM in children is that often, the entire family's lifestyle, not just the child's, requires modification.

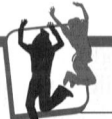

COMMUNITY CARE 26-3

Living With Newly Diagnosed Type 1 Diabetes Mellitus

Liberal bathroom privileges, because hyperglycemia creates polyuria

Snacks as needed to avoid hypoglycemia

Blood glucose checks as needed, to be performed by younger children in the presence of the school nurse; older children should be allowed to carry meter with them for testing

Fast-acting glucose in case of hypoglycemia available from teachers, coaches, or school nurses; glucagon available at school

In emergency, parents notified after 911 call

Peer support group recommended for middle childhood and adolescent patients

MedicAlert bracelet or necklace should be worn at all times.

T2DM is one of the leading causes of adult morbidity and mortality in the United States because of its role in the development of optic, renal, neuropathic, and cardiovascular disease. Children are at risk because T2DM can go unrecognized and untreated for many years while the hyperglycemic changes damage vital organs. Advocating for healthy lifestyles in children identified with T2DM can prevent many of the complications and the long-term economic burden on the individual of managing these complications in adult life.

Pathophysiology

T2DM is most often associated with obesity, hypertension, and elevated cholesterol (combined hyperlipidemia). The condition may also be associated with metabolic syndrome. It is also associated with acromegaly, CS, and a number of other endocrinologic disorders, including polycystic ovarian syndrome.

T2DM is characterized by peripheral insulin resistance with a defect of insulin secretion (hyperinsulinemia) that varies in severity with the individual. For T2DM to develop, both defects must be present. Many overweight individuals have insulin resistance, but only those with an inability to increase beta-cell production of insulin develop T2DM. During the progression from normal glucose tolerance to abnormal glucose tolerance, insulin resistance worsens. Hepatic glucose output increases with increased glycogen production and gluconeogenesis. The failure of the beta cells to hypersecrete insulin underlies the transition from insulin resistance to clinical diabetes, as demonstrated by overt fasting hyperglycemia and increased hepatic glucose function (ADA, 2013). Puberty is believed to play a role in the development of T2DM. During puberty, resistance to the action of insulin is increased, resulting in hyperinsulinemia. When pancreatic beta-cell functioning is normal, puberty-related insulin resistance is compensated by increased secretion of insulin. Increased GH secretion is believed most likely responsible for the increased insulin resistance. Not surprisingly, T2DM is extremely rare among children younger than 10 years of age (CDC, 2011).

Assessment

Look for signs and symptoms similar to those of T1DM, but much less severe. Determine if there is a family history of T2DM. Physical examination may reveal **acanthosis nigricans** (discoloration and skin thickening, most commonly found in the axillae, neck folds, and knuckles), which is a clinical sign of insulin resistance. Children with T2DM are usually older at diagnosis than those with T1DM, so a history may be easier to elicit. Children are usually older than 12 years of age and obese, but cases certainly do occur in early childhood and the diagnosis should be considered, regardless of age, if the child presents with risk factors. Children and parents may report urinary frequency, increased thirst, and, sometimes, difficulties in school. Weight loss is rarely a symptom; weight gain is usually the norm. Most children have no physical symptoms, and the diagnosis is discovered by routine urine screening during a school physical or acute visit. Female patients who are suspected of having T2DM should also be evaluated for signs of polycystic ovarian syndrome.

Diagnostic Tests

The child with T2DM usually has glucose in the urine ($\geq$200 mg/dL) and high fasting blood glucose ($\geq$126 mg/dL) or 2-hour plasma glucose value ($\geq$200 mg/dL) during an OGTT. Fasting insulin and fasting C-peptide levels are elevated. A diabetes autoimmune profile will be negative because T2DM is not an autoimmune-mediated illness. Acidosis can be present but is usually not as severe as in T1DM. The child can have ketones in the urine but does not appear acutely ill.

Children older than 10 years of age (or younger if pubertal onset is earlier) should be screened every 2 years for T2DM if they have certain risk factors: high-risk ethnicity (i.e., Native American, Hispanic, black), family history of T2DM, signs of insulin resistance (acanthosis nigricans, high blood pressure, polycystic ovarian syndrome, dyslipidemia), and overweight (body mass index >85th percentile for age and gender, weight for height >85th percentile, or weight >120% of ideal for height). A fasting plasma glucose is the preferred test. Random glucose testing can be done if concern exists that the family and child will not return for a fasting study (ADA, 2013).

Interdisciplinary Interventions

Management of the child with T2DM focuses on the following four objectives as outlined by the American Academy of Pediatrics (Copeland et al., 2013):

- Eliminating symptoms of hyperglycemia
- Assisting the child in maintaining a reasonable body weight (weight stabilization)
- Decreasing cardiovascular risk factors: hypertension, hyperlipidemia, hyperglycemia, microalbuminuria, sedentary lifestyle, and use of tobacco products
- Achieving overall improvement in the child's physical and emotional well-being

Eliminating Symptoms of Hyperglycemia

Children with T2DM usually complete blood glucose testing two to three times per day, generally before breakfast and 2 hours after the main meal. Motivating the child to test and understand the importance of testing is as important with T2DM as it is with T1DM. These issues may be more accentuated with T2DM because hypoglycemia is less common in these children; thus, they can become more complacent in their motivation to complete testing.

The American Academy of Pediatrics (Copeland et al., 2013) recommends that the primary health care provider monitor A_{1C} concentrations every 3 months and more frequently if the treatment goals for fingerstick blood glucose testing and A_{1C} concentrations are not being met.

The child with T2DM is usually not instructed to have urine ketone strips at home, unless he or she routinely receives insulin as part of care.

KidKare Encouraging the child to self-test can be a challenge. Help the parents to devise different motivating strategies. These strategies must be tailored to the age of the child. For example, parents may have a rule in their house that before a teenager is permitted to take the car keys or get in the driver's seat, a blood glucose test must be performed, regardless of whether the child has T1DM or T2DM. Testing before driving is required of anyone taking insulin.

Treating hyperglycemia in children with T2DM may require insulin at the outset if the child has random venous or plasma blood glucose concentrations $\geq$250 mg/dL or an A_{1c} >9% (Copeland et al., 2013). More commonly, the child can be managed initially with oral agents, meal planning, and increased activity. Metformin is the only oral agent approved for treatment of T2DM in children aged 10 years and older (Copeland et al., 2013). Metformin reduces the amount of sugar released by the liver into the bloodstream between meals. Side effects include nausea, upset stomach, diarrhea, and headache. The medication is better tolerated when taken with food. Angiotensin-converting enzyme (ACE) inhibitors (e.g., enalapril) are commonly used in children when microalbuminuria is evident because they have a protective effect on the kidneys. Lipid-lowering agents and blood pressure medications may be ordered to provide cardioprotection. Current medication references that focus on dosing and using medication in children should be consulted prior to prescribing.

Maintaining a Healthy Body Weight

The nutritional therapy goals for the child with T2DM include maintaining glycemic control and a healthy body weight. A weight-loss program can be implemented to accommodate the child's lifestyle and cultural preferences. Carbohydrate counting has been found to be an effective method to maintain glycemic control. In addition, a consistent low-carbohydrate meal plan can be effective in reducing caloric intake. The diet should include high-fiber foods. Fiber aids in improving postprandial hyperglycemia, weight loss, and satiety. To ensure dietary success, the entire family is encouraged to participate in the child's dietary and lifestyle choices.

Improving Overall Well-Being

Regular physical activity helps to treat T2DM and prevents cardiovascular complications and other complications from a sedentary lifestyle. Chapter 7 provides an in-depth discussion of physical activity guidelines for adolescents. These guidelines include encouraging adolescents to be physically active daily, engage in three or more sessions per week of physical activity that last 60 minutes or longer, and limit nonacademic screen time to less than 2 hours per day (Copeland et al., 2013). Following these guidelines will assist the youth to achieve improvement in his or her physical and emotional well-being.

Community Care

A primary goal of community care is tertiary prevention that targets youth at risk for developing T2DM. Youth programs are aimed at promoting appropriate nutritional intake and exercise patterns consistent with the child's age and developmental abilities. In addition, education must also focus on encouraging behavioral changes among family members. Parents typically purchase most of the groceries and make most of the decisions about the child's eating patterns at home. Parents should role-model making healthy, nutritional choices and participating in physical activities that promote cardiovascular health. The teaching plan to be used with children and their families includes discussing home care issues such as nutrition, exercise, and medication administration (Teaching Intervention Plan 26-3).

ANSWER: Whereas T1DM usually has a sudden onset, T2DM may have a very slow progression of symptoms and may remain undetected for a long time. Children who develop T2DM are usually obese; those with T1DM are not. In T1DM and T2DM, there often is a family history of diabetes; however, in T2DM, there is a greater chance that the mother experienced gestational diabetes during her pregnancy.

HYPOGLYCEMIA

Hypoglycemia (usually defined as blood glucose level <70 mg/dL) is a common complication for children with T1DM (ADA, 2013). It often occurs if a meal is missed or late, if the insulin dose is too high or drawn up incorrectly, or as a result of strenuous physical activity without an added snack. Alcohol ingestion, gastroenteritis, or extra insulin administration can also precipitate hypoglycemia. Alcohol intensifies insulin action and may inhibit gluconeogenesis, causing delayed hypoglycemia.

Children with no previous diagnosis of hypoglycemia should have a variety of tests completed to determine the differential diagnoses. These tests include glucose and electrolyte levels, OGTT, CBC, urinalysis to check for urinary ketones, serum insulin, cortisol levels, thyroid hormone levels, GH levels, C-peptide levels, serum amino acids and urinary organic acids.

KidKare The child and parents need to know that hypoglycemia can occur not only during or immediately after a strenuous activity but also several hours after the activity, when the child is resting quietly.

Assessment

Signs of hypoglycemia include diaphoresis, tremulousness, tachycardia, hunger, weakness, pallor, and dizziness. CNS symptoms include headache, irritability, poor coordination, combativeness, double vision, and confusion. Signs of severe CNS depression from hypoglycemia include unconsciousness and seizures.

TIP 26-3: A TEACHING INTERVENTION PLAN for the Child With Type 2 Diabetes Mellitus

Nursing Diagnoses and Family Outcomes

- Imbalanced nutrition: More than body require-ments related to intake in excess of activity and metabolic expenditure, lack of knowledge, and/or ineffective coping
  Outcomes: Child will maintain adequate caloric intake, as evidenced by achieving desired weight parameters.
  Child will maintain blood glucose and lipid levels within target parameters.
  Child will be able to make daily meal and snack choices that incorporate desired weight man-agement goals and physical activity schedule.
- Risk for noncompliance related to challenges required in changing one's lifestyle and maintain-ing these changes as child grows and develops
  Outcomes: Child and family will understand the management plan and be able to incorpo-rate dietary, physical activity, and medication administration changes into family lifestyle.
  Child or adolescent will make personal choices that are consistent with daily management plan for diabetes.

Teach the Child/Family

Managing the Child's Condition

Prevention
- Evaluate family lifestyle modifications that can be made to reduce risk of diabetes.

Stay at a Healthy Weight
- Establish goals for weight loss, blood glucose, and lipid values.
- Restrict carbohydrate intake to 45 g at each of the three main meals of the day.
- Eat smaller portions.
- Take your time eating. A good rule of thumb is to take 45 minutes to eat each meal.

Eat Healthy Foods
- Identify eating patterns that need changing.
- Read food labels to learn about the food and how much you should eat.
- Refer to registered dietitian for individualized diet plan.

- Eat meals and snacks about the same time each day; try not to skip any meals.
- If you eat too many carbohydrates at one time, your blood glucose may go too high. Choose high-fiber carbohydrates and foods low in saturated fats and high in monounsaturated fats.
- Drink water instead of juice and soda.

Be Active
- Determine frequency of exercise and type of moderate-intensity physical activity to be completed.
- Be physically active for at least 60 minutes every day.
- Discuss methods to maintain hydration and avoid hypoglycemia during exercise activities.

Medication Administration

Oral Agents
- Take oral medications for diabetes (i.e., metformin) as directed if needed to assist in control of diabetes.
- Side effects include nausea, cramping, diarrhea, and lactic acidosis. Take with a meal to minimize side effects.

Insulin
- May need to be used depending on severity of acidosis and hyperglycemia.
- Side effects include hypoglycemia and possible weight gain.

Monitoring
- Height and weight.
- Signs of DKA.
- Signs of hypoglycemia.

Contact the Health Care Provider if
- Child has manifestations of hyperglycemia (poly-phagia, polyuria, or polydipsia) or manifestations of hypoglycemia (hunger, nervousness and shaki-ness, perspiration, dizziness or light-headedness, sleepiness, confusion, difficulty speaking, feeling anxious or weak).
- Child experiences fatigue, malaise, or vomiting and the child is taking metformin. Stop the medication and notify health care provider imme-diately because these symptoms may indicate life-threatening lactic acidosis.

KidKare Infants cannot describe their symptoms and usually do not demonstrate many of the symptoms of hypoglycemia. Teach parents to rely on blood glucose monitoring and to administer glucose in the form of juice or tubes of decorative cake gel (not the larger tubes of icing) squirted inside the cheek pouch. In the case of an emer-gency, the parent administers glucagon either intramuscu-larly or subcutaneously.

Interdisciplinary Interventions

Hypoglycemia is treated based on the severity of the symptoms. In the case of mild or moderate hypoglyce-mia, simple carbohydrates are the treatment of choice; 15 to 20 g of carbohydrates is the recommended dosage for an older child. Recheck the glucose in 15 minutes. If still low, repeat the 15 g of carbohydrate. Once the glucose is above 70 mg/dL, a snack containing protein should be given if a meal will not be eaten in the next 1 to 2 hours. If a meal is due, give the protein-containing meal instead of the snack. Instruct the older child to ingest 4 to 6 oz of juice or regular soda, two to three glucose tablets, commercially available glucose gel, or a small tube of commercially available decorative cake gel. Children in the infant and early childhood age groups can be treated with 2 oz of juice, or two thirds of a tube of decorative cake gel, to equal 10 g fast-acting carbohydrate. Many parents of these young children find that milk flavored with a small amount of syrup that contains sugar enables the child to consume a fast-acting carbohydrate and a protein together and is easier for the child to consume (Silverstein et al., 2005). However, protein will slow absorption of the carbohydrate and delay euglycemia. The amount of carbohydrate should be adjusted according to the severity of the hypoglycemia and the blood glucose result. Mild to moderate hypoglycemia can occur in children with both T1DM and T2DM. It is common in children with T1DM from the action of insulin. It is less common in children with T2DM and depends on whether their treatment plan includes insulin or oral agents that carry hypoglycemia as a side effect.

Severe hypoglycemia results in loss of consciousness or seizures and must be treated with glucagon. Glucagon is a counterregulatory hormone that stimulates the liver to produce enough glucose to increase the blood glucose level by about 80 mg/dL. Instruct the parents how to administer glucagon properly. The child may be combative and thrashing, so administration can be difficult. Children 6 years of age and younger receive 0.5 mL (0.5 mg) glucagon subcutaneously or intramuscularly, and children aged 7 years and older receive 1 mL (1 mg) subcutaneously or intramuscularly. The child should respond within 10 to 15 minutes after the injection. The injection may be given right through clothing because trying to undress the child to give the injection wastes time and may be impossible with a thrashing child. Teach parents to obtain a blood glucose level before giving the glucagon or immediately after the injection has been given to document hypoglycemia. When glucagon is administered, the child is very likely to vomit while in a semiconscious state. Prepare the parents for this possibility, and instruct them to keep the child on his or her side after glucagon administration. The parent should take the child to the nearest emergency department or notify the rescue squad if the child does not respond within 15 minutes. If the child recovers at home, instruct the parents to call their primary care provider or endocrinologist to report the severe hypoglycemic episode and discuss any insulin adjustment that may be required within the next 24 hours. Severe hypoglycemia would be a very rare event for a child with T2DM, but any parent with a child with T1DM should be prepared with glucagon on hand at all times.

Community Care

Teach the parents and children the causes, symptoms, and treatment of hypoglycemia. Advise the child to wear an identification tag or MedicAlert bracelet, especially when away from home. Many types of emergency alert tags are available through mail-order houses, Internet sites, and jewelry stores. A bracelet or tag that the child finds appealing greatly increases the possibility that the child will wear it routinely. Adolescents, in particular, need to be educated concerning the effects of drugs and alcohol on diabetes. Judgment-altering substances or appetite suppressants affect the daily routine and create an imbalance among food, insulin, and exercise. Alcohol intensifies the glucose-lowering effects of insulin and also causes hypoglycemia (Silverstein et al., 2005). Diabetics who drive should check their glucose just before getting into the car and have glucose tablets, cake gel, Smarties, or some other substance to treat hypoglycemia stored in the car.

Explore the topic of alcohol ingestion routinely with children during follow-up visits for diabetes. As the children enter middle childhood and adolescence, ask parents to step out of the room for some topics, such as alcohol and drug use and sexual activity. Girls with poorly controlled diabetes may have difficulty conceiving, leading them to a false belief that they cannot become pregnant. Sexual activity must be discussed with these patients.

The risk-taking behaviors common among adolescents predispose this age group to frequent episodes of DKA. Groups that teach coping skills assist adolescents to prepare for situations (such as peer pressure to drink alcohol or use illicit drugs) and are an effective way to prevent health- and life-threatening behaviors (Silverstein et al., 2005). For medical and nursing management of DKA, see Nursing Interventions 26-2 and thePoint Care Paths: An Interdisciplinary Plan of Care for the Child With Diabetic Ketoacidosis.

HYPERINSULINEMIA

Hyperinsulinemia is an overabundance of insulin, which results in rapid depletion of exogenous and endogenous glucose and causes hypoglycemia. Hyperinsulinemia may present as a transient disease during the neonatal period, occurring almost exclusively among infants of mothers with diabetes. The most common cause of persistent hyperinsulinemia after the neonatal period is a combination of four genetic mutations on chromosome 11, a condition called *persistent hyperinsulinemic hypoglycemia of infancy* (PHHI). Hyperinsulinism seen in the older child is usually associated with a pancreatic adenoma, although this association is rare in the pediatric population.

Hyperinsulinism may cause hypoglycemic brain damage. Injury to brain tissue can cause cognitive challenge, cerebral palsy, seizure disorder, microcephaly, spasticity, and ataxia (Steinkrauss et al., 2005). When infants with hypoglycemia caused by hyperinsulinemia are identified early and oral feedings are initiated promptly, the prognosis is quite good. The neonatal form is transient and will dissipate as the infant adjusts to exogenous sources of glucose and develops an appropriate beta-cell response. Because the hypoglycemia of PHHI is more long-lasting than hypoglycemia in infants of diabetic mothers, infants with PHHI are at greater risk for the neurologic sequelae of repeated hypoglycemic events. PHHI must be identified and appropriately treated over the long term for the best prognosis; otherwise, neurologic damage may occur.

Pathophysiology

In infants of diabetic mothers in whom excellent blood glucose control (euglycemia) has not been achieved during pregnancy, second and third trimester hyperglycemia may result in metabolic complications. When blood glucose levels are elevated in the pregnant mother, the fetus then receives larger than required amounts of glucose, amino acids, and fatty fuels during growth and development. This supply far exceeds the growing fetus's demands and requires an increased supply of insulin from both mother and fetus. The immature beta cells in the fetal pancreas respond by proliferating more than is normally needed, producing excess insulin. After the infant is delivered, the pancreas continues to produce excessive amounts of insulin, which may result in neonatal hypoglycemia. Peak incidence of neonatal hyperinsulinemia and subsequent hypoglycemia is 6 to 12 hours after birth, but in severe cases, it can persist for several days after birth. In PHHI, the normal relationship of insulin release in response to glucose levels is disrupted; the pancreas and beta cells secrete excessive amounts of insulin in response to glucose levels.

Assessment

The infant with hyperinsulinemia is often macrosomic, or large for gestational age, at birth. Blood glucose levels in the term neonate may be less than 35 mg/dL. The infant may be lethargic, irritable, tachypneic, tremulous, diaphoretic, hypothermic, display episodic cyanosis, and have a high-pitched cry. Criteria for diagnosing hyperinsulinism include

- Plasma insulin concentrations >5 to 10 microunits/mL at time of documented hypoglycemia
- Insulin-to-glucose ratio is 0.4 or higher
- Low plasma ketones
- Low free fatty acid levels
- Rapid development of fasting hypoglycemia
- High exogenous glucose infusion rates needed to maintain euglycemia
- Absence of ketonemia or ketonuria
- Elevated C-peptide
- Increased plasma glucose after glucagon administration at time of hypoglycemia

Serum glucose and insulin levels are obtained every 2 hours. Every void should be checked for ketone bodies, although ketone levels are usually low or absent.

Interdisciplinary Interventions

Whether the underlying etiology is transient neonatal hyperinsulinemia or PHHI, the child with hyperinsulinemia may initially be given infusions of glucose and glucagon administered by the nurse. If the hypoglycemia does not resolve during the neonatal period, care at home will include providing frequent feedings throughout the day, awakening the infant for nighttime feedings, and initiating oral diazoxide.

Oral diazoxide suppresses the secretion of insulin by the beta cells without lowering the blood pressure (Steinkrauss et al., 2005). The initial dose is usually 5 to 20 mg/kg/day divided into three doses. A common acute side effect of diazoxide is the retention of salt and water. Water retention can be reduced by administering hydrochlorothiazide, which may also further decrease insulin secretion. Life-threatening complications, such as nonketotic hyperosmolar coma, congestive heart failure, and ketoacidosis, can be avoided by diligently monitoring fluid balance, electrolytes, and urine ketone levels.

Surgery for subtotal pancreatectomy or removal of focal lesions is indicated in infants who are unable to maintain euglycemia with pharmacologic treatment or who cannot be removed from IV therapy. A 95% to 99% subtotal pancreatectomy is performed by a pediatric surgeon. The spleen is left in place. Results of surgery can vary. Many children require insulin administration for weeks or months to control hyperglycemia while their bodies adapt, whereas other children have recurrent hypoglycemia shortly after surgery. In these cases, reexploration with a near-total pancreatectomy may be indicated. Any child who requires surgical intervention is considered at much greater risk to develop diabetes later in life.

Community Care

Provide parents clear and concise explanations for the cause of the hyperinsulinemia once it has been established and the specific therapy recommended. Teach parents the techniques to monitor blood glucose at home and to recognize the signs and symptoms of hypoglycemia. Instruct parents on the medical therapy and its possible side effects. Frequent feedings are required for nearly all these infants. If the infant must receive nighttime nasogastric feedings at home, teach the parents how to place a nasogastric feeding tube properly, and refer them to a home care company to obtain supplies, feeding pump, or formulas.

Preoperative preparation and psychological support are essential if surgery is recommended. Infants with hyperinsulinemia, whether transient neonatal or PHHI, usually improve rapidly with medical or surgical therapy.

DISORDERS OF THE ADRENAL GLANDS

The adrenal glands have two distinct portions: the adrenal medulla and the adrenal cortex. The two tissues have different embryonic origins, secrete different hormones, and have different regulatory mechanisms. The adrenal medulla secretes the catecholamines epinephrine (adrenaline) and norepinephrine (noradrenaline). Because these hormones are also produced by the sympathetic nervous system, the absence of a medullary adrenal supply is not life threatening. The adrenal cortex secretes steroid hormones that are essential to life (see Table 26-1). The three major groups of steroids are the mineralocorticoids, the glucocorticoids, and the sex steroids. The adrenal gland depends on pituitary secretion of ACTH. Therefore, a lack of adrenal steroids may be caused by inadequate ACTH production from the pituitary to stimulate the adrenal gland or a defect in the adrenal gland itself.

The conditions discussed in this section include adrenocortical insufficiency, CAH, CS, and premature adrenarche (see also thePoint Supplemental Information for a discussion of pheochromocytoma).

ADRENOCORTICAL INSUFFICIENCY

Acquired or chronic adrenocortical insufficiency results when the adrenal gland is absent or damaged. *Acquired adrenocortical insufficiency* is a relatively rare phenomenon in childhood. Common causes include traumatic, hemorrhagic, and neoplastic insults to the hypothalamic–pituitary axis. Trauma and hemorrhage may occur during the neonatal period as a consequence of prolonged labor. Treatment for illnesses such as neoplasms, nephrotic syndrome, severe respiratory distress, or rheumatoid arthritis with glucocorticoids can lead to suppression of the hypothalamic–pituitary function and secondary, usually temporary, loss of adrenocortical activity.

Abrupt withdrawal of corticosteroids in children who have been given large doses for a long time, or failure to give increased doses of corticosteroids during stressful situations such as surgery or severe infections, may precipitate acute *adrenal crisis*. This type of acquired adrenocortical insufficiency may be characterized by hypoglycemia without an associated illness (such as diabetes), failure of linear growth, lethargy, abdominal pain, vomiting, hypotension, or unexplained weight loss. Acute infections, such as meningococcemia, can lead to adrenal hemorrhage and shock (Waterhouse-Friderichsen syndrome). Other causes of adrenocortical insufficiency include metastatic cancer, familial glucocorticoid deficiency, defects of steroid biosynthesis (adrenal hyperplasia, discussed later in this chapter), isolated aldosterone deficiency, adrenalectomy for CS, hypopituitarism, and certain drugs.

Chronic adrenocortical insufficiency (Addison disease) is commonly caused by autoimmune destruction of the adrenal cortex, which results in dysfunction of steroidogenesis. The condition usually occurs during early adolescence. Children with T1DM are at increased risk for Addison disease (Babiker et al., 2011). It has been hypothesized that an environmental trigger initiates the autoimmune process that ultimately results in progressive dysfunction of the adrenal gland and the subsequent adrenal insufficiency of Addison disease, but no such trigger has yet been defined. Risk for adrenal autoimmunity is considered genetic. Many relatives of individuals with Addison disease have other autoimmune diseases such as T1DM or autoimmune thyroid disease (Barker et al., 2005).

If acute adrenocortical insufficiency is recognized and treated promptly, prognosis is good. Similarly, as long as the child with chronic adrenal insufficiency maintains appropriate daily hormone replacement therapy and increases doses during stress, the prognosis is good. Insufficient replacement therapy places the child at risk for adrenal shock and death during times of illness or stress.

Pathophysiology

Aldosterone is the most potent mineralocorticoid, and its principal action is in maintaining electrolyte balance and blood pressure. Aldosterone secretion is regulated by activation of the renin–angiotensin system, so adequate levels can be maintained even in the absence of ACTH. The predominant glucocorticoid is cortisol. It also maintains homeostasis of electrolytes, blood pressure, and blood glucose by its influence on the metabolism of most tissues. Without prompt treatment, acquired deficiency in the production of cortisol, and to a lesser degree aldosterone, may lead to life-threatening electrolyte and fluid imbalance. These imbalances must be treated, and the deficient steroid (cortisol and/or aldosterone) must also be replaced. After the acute manifestations of adrenal insufficiency are under control, its underlying causes must be investigated.

In chronic deficiency, the slow and progressive nature of the condition means that substantial damage occurs in the adrenal cortex before symptoms become evident. When there is enough damage to the adrenal cortex, insufficient amounts of cortisol (glucocorticoid) and aldosterone (mineralocorticoid) are released.

Assessment

The age at onset and the clinical manifestations depend on the underlying cause of acquired adrenal insufficiency. For example, those symptoms that are usually seen after birth, such as in adrenal hyperplasia, are characteristic of salt loss and include lethargy, nausea and vomiting, dehydration, fever, irritability, and pallor.

The onset of symptoms of chronic insufficiency is gradual, except in those children with undiagnosed deficiency who show signs of acquired adrenal insufficiency after a minor illness or trauma. Chronic symptoms include weakness, headache, irritability, anorexia, weight loss, nausea and vomiting, diarrhea, and signs of dehydration. Diminishing amounts of aldosterone from the adrenal cortex causes fluid and electrolyte imbalances and a subsequent decrease in blood pressure. Children with Addison disease who have T1DM will have symptoms of recurrent hypoglycemia with falling insulin requirements and will crave salty foods (because of their sodium deficit) (Babiker et al., 2011). Another characteristic finding is in the pigment of the skin. Children with Addison disease usually appear suntanned, but without suntan lines, because of excessive secretion of corticotropin and MSH. Hyperpigmentation is most noticeable on the face, hands, elbows, and knees as well as the groin, genitalia, areolae, and gums. Pubertal females may show less pubic hair because of diminished androgen production.

Diagnostic Tests

Laboratory data for both types of insufficiency reveal hyponatremia, hypoglycemia, and hyperkalemia. Serum cortisol, ACTH, electrolytes, and renin and aldosterone levels should be measured during the early waking hours, around 8 AM. The most definitive test for adrenal insufficiency is to measure plasma cortisol levels before and after administering exogenous ACTH, but this test is usually not necessary. Basal levels can establish the diagnosis without additional testing. In adrenal insufficiency, the baseline cortisol level is low, and no increase occurs after ACTH administration.

In chronic insufficiency with an autoimmune cause, high antibody titers to the adrenal gland are seen. Ultrasound images, computed tomographic scans, and abdominal radiographs are useful in visualizing the integrity of the adrenal glands. Because some of the conditions resulting in adrenocortical insufficiency have a genetic basis, the siblings of the child should also be evaluated.

Interdisciplinary Interventions

The child with adrenal insufficiency may or may not require hospitalization depending on the severity of the symptoms. Those children with severe electrolyte imbalance require immediate intervention. IV solutions are administered to restore electrolyte balance and intravascular volume. At the same time, parenteral cortisol is administered at 100 mg/m² as a loading dose and then 25 mg/m² every 6 hours. Dosing is based on measurement of body surface area in square meters that is calculated by the child's height and weight. If IV access is not immediately available, the hydrocortisone should be given intramuscularly. After 24 hours, these higher doses may be reduced, and oral doses of corticosteroids may be given.

Teach the child and family how to administer the replacement steroids cortisol (hydrocortisone) and aldosterone (fludrocortisone). Some children can be treated with hydrocortisone only if they maintain a liberal intake of salt in their diet. Hydrocortisone is usually given three times a day, and fludrocortisone can be given as a single daily dose. Fludrocortisone does not need to be increased during times of stress. The parents need to demonstrate proper mixing and intramuscular administration of hydrocortisone in the event of an emergency or excessive vomiting. Administration three times daily can be a barrier for some families, so twice-daily dosing can be attempted with close monitoring of clinical effects and laboratory studies such as ACTH or steroid levels. Give parents written guidelines regarding when and how much to increase maintenance doses during times of illness, trauma, or other periods of physical or emotional stress. If surgery is needed, the anesthesiologist must be told of the child's cortisol dependency. The family should feel comfortable contacting their pediatric endocrinology team whenever there is a question about adjusting medication.

KidKare All children with adrenal insufficiency should wear some form of medical identification alerting medical personnel that the child has adrenal insufficiency and is steroid dependent.

Parents need to be aware of potential side effects of the medications. Ensure that the family understands that the dosage of steroids used to treat adrenal insufficiency is meant to replace the deficit created by the condition. Much of the negative publicity about steroids is about glucocorticoids and androgens taken in excessive doses; side effects of this type of steroid use include poor growth, weight gain, poor wound healing, increased susceptibility to infection, and excessive bruising. A possible side effect with replacement doses of cortisol is gastric irritation, which can be minimized by taking cortisol with food or with an antacid. Manifestations of excessive fludrocortisone ingestion include generalized edema from water retention, hypertension, headaches, and signs of hypokalemia.

ALERT   *Families must maintain an adequate stock of medication and never allow the prescription to run out; acute withdrawal of cortisol can lead to adrenal crisis. Families should be reminded to check the expiration date on the injectable hydrocortisone and make sure it is current. An extra kit should be kept at school for emergency use.*

Community Care

Parents may need help finding a balance between protecting their child from potential life-threatening situations and the need to participate in age-appropriate activities necessary for physical, social, and emotional growth. Children's school and play activities should not be restricted. School and daycare personnel should be made aware of the need to notify the parents promptly if their child becomes ill or injured and to preplan cooperation with medication administration if a dose needs to be given during school hours.

CONGENITAL ADRENAL HYPERPLASIA

CAH is an autosomal recessive condition caused by an inborn deficiency of one of the enzymes needed to synthesize cortisol. Ninety percent to 95% of children born with CAH have a deficiency of 21-hydroxylase. The incidence of CAH is 1 in 15,000 births (Trakakis et al., 2009). Because the 21-hydroxylase enzyme is involved in cortisol and aldosterone synthesis, most children (75%) present with the more severe, salt-losing form of CAH.

Prognosis depends on the type and severity of CAH the child has inherited. If left untreated, the child with classic 21-hydroxylase deficiency, the salt-losing form, could die from severe hyponatremia. Children with partial deficiency have enough aldosterone to maintain sodium levels. If appropriately treated, children born with CAH enjoy a normal life expectancy. Cognitive and perceptual abilities in children with CAH are no different than among those without CAH.

For children with only the virilizing form of CAH, lack of treatment results in precocious puberty and adult short stature (Consortium on the Management of Disorders of Sex Development, 2006). In females born with CAH, the internal sex organs (uterus, ovaries, and fallopian tubes) are normal. With appropriate treatment, fertility should not be impaired. Menses should occur at the appropriate age if the girl's CAH is well controlled (Speiser & White, 2003).

Pathophysiology

Hormone synthesis by the adrenal cortex is controlled by the hypothalamic–pituitary–adrenal feedback system. Any condition that alters circulating blood levels of any adrenal hormone results in an imbalance in hormone production or inhibition. In CAH, blood levels of cortisol are inadequate. As a result, secretion of ACTH by the pituitary is increased in an effort to improve cortisol production. This prolonged hypersecretion results in adrenal gland hyperplasia and sex steroid overproduction. In females, this condition causes masculinization or virilization of the clitoris. In males, it may cause precocious puberty (Trakakis et al., 2009). Children with CAH who cannot maintain a sodium balance (salt-losing form of CAH) are at increased risk for severe hyponatremic dehydration, seizures, shock, and death from this electrolyte imbalance if they are not diagnosed and treated promptly.

Assessment

In the United States, newborn screening for CAH is required. Thus, most infants are generally diagnosed at, or shortly after, birth. However the newborn screening only identifies the most common form of CAH—21-hydroxylase deficiency. Female newborns with CAH almost always present with ambiguous genitalia (Fig. 26-7). Steroid synthesis occurs early during fetal life, so a lack of cortisol response within the pituitary–adrenal pathway results in excess ACTH production and, in turn, hypersecretion of the adrenal androgens and virilization. The external genitalia of females reveal an enlarged clitoris that resembles a penis. Urethral displacement onto the ventral shaft of the clitoris can be mistaken for hypospadias. The labia are fused and can take on the appearance

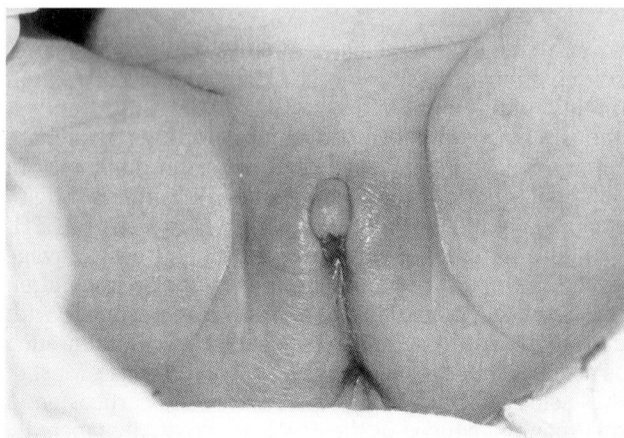

Figure 26-7 Genitalia of a female newborn with CAH. CAH may cause clitoral enlargement.

of a scrotal-like sac without testes. This condition may be misdiagnosed as cryptorchidism. The vaginal orifice may be incomplete. In general, more extreme virilization reflects greater severity of the enzyme defect.

Male newborns with CAH do not necessarily show abnormalities of the internal or external genitalia. The penis may be enlarged, and pigmentation of the scrotum may be darker than normal. Because CAH may have no obvious physical findings, male newborns not identified on newborn screening generally are not diagnosed until they present with signs of adrenal insufficiency. In both sexes, recurrent vomiting and irritability may be mistaken for reflux, pyloric stenosis, or colic. The symptoms progress and include lethargy, pallor, and dehydration. The child may be diagnosed with hypoglycemia, hyponatremia, and hyperkalemia.

Children with partial enzyme deficiency may not be diagnosed until childhood, when signs of premature adrenarche or menstrual irregularities appear.

Diagnostic Tests

Early prenatal diagnosis is possible through chorionic villus sampling, molecular techniques of DNA analysis, and amniocentesis.

Laboratory studies to confirm the diagnosis of CAH of the infant include serum levels of 17-hydroxyprogesterone, a cortisol precursor. Markedly elevated levels indicate CAH. ACTH, testosterone, DHEA, and androstenedione levels may also be obtained. Children with salt-losing CAH have low serum levels of sodium and chloride and elevated potassium and plasma renin activity. Chromosomal testing needs urgent attention to determine appropriate sex identification. Radiographic studies include pelvic ultrasonography to determine the presence of internal reproductive organs as well as the integrity of the adrenal glands (Trakakis et al., 2009).

Nursing Diagnoses and Outcomes

In addition to the nursing diagnoses and outcomes presented in Nursing Plan of Care 26-1, the following diagnoses and outcomes apply to the child with CAH:

Nursing Diagnosis: Risk for impaired parent/infant/child attachment related to reaction to sexual ambiguity of child
Outcomes:
• Parents will express concerns about sexuality issues to the health care team.
• Parents will initiate and maintain positive interactions with the infant.
Nursing Diagnosis: Risk for sexual dysfunction in females related to virilization of the genitalia
Outcome: Child will receive appropriate information regarding treatment for virilization.

Interdisciplinary Interventions

The care for children born with CAH varies; however, the goal for all children includes providing lifelong replacement doses of deficient steroids, preventing excessive androgen production, and maintaining adequate growth. Dietary salt supplements may also be required for the salt-wasting form of the disease. Treatment may include surgical interventions to normalize genital appearance and ensure proper genital function.

Pharmacologic Interventions

Neonates or children presenting in adrenal crisis require immediate intervention. This medical emergency includes providing appropriate IV solutions to correct fluid and electrolyte imbalances and hypoglycemia. Also, a parenteral form of hydrocortisone must be administered intravenously at double or triple the maintenance dose; it can also be given intramuscularly if IV access is not immediately available.

For children diagnosed in the absence of adrenal crisis, administering glucocorticoids inhibits the excessive production of androgens. Hydrocortisone (cortisol) is the treatment of choice for children and is considered a long-term therapy.

Children who are classified as having the salt-wasting form of the disease and also display diminished aldosterone production require a replacement mineralocorticoid called *fludrocortisone* and sodium chloride supplements. Doses for both replacement steroids are individualized throughout life by measuring renin and 17-hydroxyprogesterone levels (Speiser & White, 2003).

KidKare Fludrocortisone (Florinef) is not available in liquid form. The pill can be finely crushed and added to a small amount of formula or breast milk. Infants also require added salt in their formula or food. Children will naturally seek salty foods as needed and don't require additional salt supplementation.

caREminder

> Be sure to teach children with CAH and their families about the need for increased doses of cortisol (not fludrocortisone) during times of increased physical stress and illness. Without increased doses, inadequate corticosteroid supply could lead to adrenal crisis, which is life threatening.

Surgical Management

Female infants with ambiguous genitalia may require reconstructive surgery to ensure a normal function and appearance of the genitalia and adequate sexual functioning. If the female infant has an internalized vagina, it may be a source of pooling of urine, causing infection. In such cases, immediate surgery is necessary (Consortium on the Management of Disorders of Sex Development, 2006). With surgical intervention to correct appearance, the clitoris is not removed but is reduced in size and repositioned below the pubis, preserving the glans and all its blood and nerve components so that complete sexual gratification, including orgasm, can be achieved. The labia must also be separated (labioplasty) and a vaginal orifice (vaginoplasty) must be created. The timing of surgery depends on what surgery is to be done but generally starts in the younger aged child because repair is easier to accomplish when the distance to repair is smaller. Vaginal dilation may be required when the girl reaches puberty or becomes sexually active.

Genetic Counseling

Given the genetic nature of CAH, the parents will benefit from genetic counseling. A family history or genogram can identify previous infant deaths or sudden, unexplained deaths possibly caused by adrenal crises in infants, children, and adults with undiagnosed CAH. Parents need to understand that CAH is an autosomal recessive disorder, which means that both parents are carriers. Therefore, there is a 25% chance of having a child with CAH with *each* pregnancy. Prenatal testing for the 21-hydroxylase deficiency is available for parents who already have an affected child. For subsequent pregnancies, these mothers can be given high doses of cortisol, in the form of dexamethasone, during the first trimester to inhibit ACTH overproduction and to prevent or minimize virilization in the developing fetus. To be effective, this must be started as soon as pregnancy is confirmed and no later than the ninth week after the last menstrual period. Sexual differentiation begins in the ninth week of gestation. This is only necessary if the fetus is female.

Community Care

Teach parents about cortisol and aldosterone replacement and the need to increase cortisol doses, including those of intramuscular hydrocortisone, when the child is faced with stress, illness, and trauma (including extensive dental work). Review the potential side effects of the medications, and discuss the family's concerns about having a child on steroid therapy. Remind the family that the child is only taking a replacement dose of the steroid that his or her body cannot produce. School and daycare personnel must promptly notify parents in the event of illness or injury, and parenteral hydrocortisone should be available for administration in case of an emergency.

KidKare Children with CAH need to wear some form of medical identification at all times. The parent or older child should carry an emergency hydrocortisone injection kit with him or her.

CUSHING SYNDROME

CS is a characteristic cluster of signs and symptoms resulting from excessive levels of circulating cortisol. In infants and young children, CS is often caused endogenously by an adrenocortical tumor, usually a malignant carcinoma, and occasionally by a benign adenoma. In older children, the cause is more likely of pituitary origin, such as a pituitary tumor that produces excessive ACTH. This rare condition is known as Cushing disease (Savage et al., 2010). The more common cause of CS in children is side effects of prolonged or excessive treatment with exogenous corticosteroids for a medical condition such as asthma, lupus, or inflammatory bowel disease. Most of these side effects can be reversed after the corticosteroid treatment is reduced or the doses are gradually tapered.

Prognosis for children with CS depends on the underlying etiology. For children with the endogenous form of

CS caused by a neoplasm, symptoms usually disappear within 1 year of pituitary surgery. Primary adrenal tumors carry a poorer prognosis because the primary cancer often metastasizes to the lymph system, lung, liver, or bone before being diagnosed. Children experiencing symptoms of CS from an exogenous cause, such as increased doses or length of therapy with glucocorticoids, will do quite well if the medications can be tapered enough to eliminate the physiologic sequelae. However, in some diseases, such as severe forms of lupus, dose reduction may be difficult because high doses of glucocorticoids are needed to treat the primary condition.

Pathophysiology

Excess cortisol produces diverse side effects seen throughout the body. The most noticeable side effect is obesity or rapid weight gain with arrest in linear growth. Hypercortisolism retards linear growth by suppressing the release of GH. Alterations in the normal processes of carbohydrate, protein, and fat metabolism lead to increased protein catabolism, loss of muscle mass, and altered fat distribution. Fat distribution tends to be centrally located, with the child showing a characteristic rounded or moon face with flushed cheeks, a supraclavicular fat pad (known as a buffalo hump), and truncal obesity with red abdominal striae (Fig. 26-8).

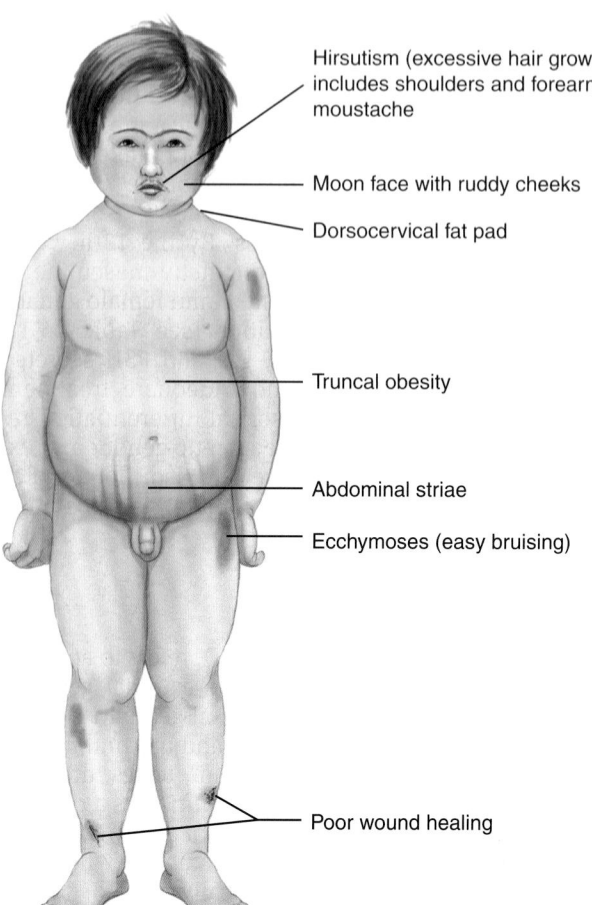

Hirsutism (excessive hair growth) includes shoulders and forearms; moustache

Moon face with ruddy cheeks

Dorsocervical fat pad

Truncal obesity

Abdominal striae

Ecchymoses (easy bruising)

Poor wound healing

Figure 26-8 Typical clinical manifestations of Cushing syndrome.

The thinned muscles of the extremities resulting from muscle wasting may be masked by generalized obesity.

Other physiologic consequences of excessive cortisol include poor wound healing, increased susceptibility to infections, and decreased inflammatory response. Excessive bruising, thin skin, and osteoporosis are also seen; hypertension, headaches, and mood disorders are less common. Production of androgens usually is excessive, which can cause virilization, characterized by increased body hair (hypertrichosis) on the face and trunk, pubic hair, acne, and deepening of the voice.

Assessment

Assessment focuses on evaluating the child for the characteristic physical signs of CS, such as a full, round face; truncal obesity; purple-red striae; and ecchymoses. Hypertension, hirsutism, acne, virilization, or menstrual irregularities are also commonly found, although these symptoms are prevalent in varying degrees in the general population. A very careful family history may reveal others with CS or endocrine neoplasias.

Diagnostic Tests

Diagnostic evaluation of CS is a challenge because the performance characteristics of the tests depend on the degree of severity of CS. In severe, overt CS, all diagnostic tests demonstrate high sensitivity and specificity to confirm the diagnosis. However, in subclinical or mild CS, test results may overlap with normal ranges defined for children without CS (Liu & Crapo, 2005). Laboratory studies include a complete blood cell count and blood and chemistry studies. Plasma cortisol levels are elevated, and the levels do not fluctuate throughout the day as they typically do. Urinary excretion of cortisol as measured by 24-hour collection is elevated. Computed tomography and MRI may locate pituitary or adrenal lesions. A low-dose (1 mg or 0.3 mg/m²) dexamethasone suppression test can be performed as an outpatient procedure. Parents administer dexamethasone orally during the evening and then bring the child in to measure the cortisol level the following morning. False-positive results may occur but are more common in adults. This test can also be performed with a high dose of dexamethasone (8 mg or 120 μg/kg); some clinicians believe that this test is more specific than the low dose. Tests such as salivary cortisol and combination corticotrophin-releasing hormone–dexamethasone testing have also been used to assist diagnosis (Liu & Crapo, 2005).

Nursing Diagnoses and Outcomes

In addition to the nursing diagnoses presented in Nursing Plan of Care 26-1, the following diagnosis applies to the child with CS:

Nursing Diagnosis: Risk for injury related to delayed wound healing, decreased inflammatory response, osteoporosis, and muscle weakness
Outcomes:
• Child will be protected from potential infections by practicing good health habits and avoiding exposure to pathogens.
• Child will remain free from injury.

Interdisciplinary Interventions

Treatment for CS depends on the specific reason for excess cortisol and may include surgery, radiation, chemotherapy, or the use of cortisol-inhibiting drugs. Surgery is the primary intervention for CS caused by adrenal or pituitary tumors. Microsurgery to excise only the tumor avoids the consequences of panhypopituitarism, and prognosis is quite good if metastasis has not occurred. In the event of adrenalectomy, appropriate stress and replacement doses of glucocorticoids are planned preoperatively to avoid adrenal crisis. Radiation and/or chemotherapy may also be used if the cause of the CS is ectopic ACTH syndrome. Cancerous tissue can be eliminated using surgery, radiation, and chemotherapy, thus curing the overproduction of cortisol caused by ectopic ACTH syndrome.

CS caused by exogenous steroid preparations requires a fine balance between continuing to use steroids to treat the underlying condition and avoiding their unpleasant side effects. If possible, the medication should be given early during the day to mimic the normal diurnal pattern of cortisol secretion. Alternate-day scheduling could also lessen stress on the hypothalamic–pituitary–adrenal pathway.

Various drugs have been used to manage CS, many with only limited effectiveness, depending on the underlying etiology of the hypercortisolism. Medications with potential efficacy at the hypothalamic–pituitary level (e.g., thiazolidinedione compounds and retinoic acid) are under investigation. A pharmacologic approach to the syndrome cannot be standardized because the pathophysiology of the syndrome varies from person to person (Sonino et al., 2005).

Community Care

Health care personnel treating children with long-term corticosteroid use should advise the child and family of the potential side effects before initiating treatment. Provide anticipatory guidance about diet, involvement in contact sports, injury prevention, and methods of avoiding exposure to infections.

PREMATURE ADRENARCHE

Adrenarche is the development of pubic hair, axillary hair, acne, and adult body odor that occurs when adrenal androgen secretion in the adrenal cortex matures. Premature adrenarche is the development of pubic hair that may be accompanied by axillary hair before age 8 years in girls and age 9 years in boys. This condition occurs more often in girls. In most cases, it is considered a normal variant in sexual development, especially if no other signs of pubertal development have occurred. However, premature adrenarche is gaining more attention from health care providers because it has been noted that girls with premature adrenarche are prone to have hyperinsulinemia, dyslipidemia, and hypertension, which may lead to atherosclerosis and metabolic syndrome later in life (Utrainen et al., 2008). In addition, premature adrenarche can be seen in exogenous exposure to androgens such as father's use of topical testosterone found in gels and patches.

An investigation may be required to determine whether premature adrenarche is of central (hypothalamic–pituitary) origin (see earlier section on "Precocious Puberty") if other signs of advancing puberty are evident such as clitoral enlargement or advanced bone age. These signs are also seen in primary adrenal dysfunction as well. Baseline 17-hydroxyprogesterone, androstenedione, dehydroepiandrosterone, and testosterone levels may be obtained. Cortrosyn stimulation testing may be necessary to diagnose nonclassical CAH or CAH in these children, even if the baseline studies are normal.

Treatment consists of reassuring the child and family of the benign nature of this condition. The child may develop a body image disturbance related to premature adrenarche. Attempt to help the child and family verbalize concerns about body image. Current literature reflects a concern that females with a history of premature adrenarche, intrauterine growth retardation, family history of T2DM, hypertension, and ovarian hyperandrogenism may represent a group at high risk for cardiovascular disease and T2DM. Given the association between premature adrenarche, hyperinsulinemia, dyslipidemia, and cardiovascular disease, long-term monitoring should be considered in such cases. Screening for T2DM with fasting plasma glucose and for cardiovascular risk with lipid panels may be warranted.

GONADAL DISORDERS

The genetic gender of an embryo is determined at the time of fertilization by the X- or Y-bearing sperm that penetrates the ovum; however, sex differentiation does not occur until the 7th week of gestation. At that time, the future ovaries or testes begin to take on their specific characteristics. The presence of the Y chromosome influences testicular development; its absence results in the creation of ovaries. By the 12th week, the external genitalia become distinctly masculine or feminine. The male gonads (testes) and female gonads (ovaries) have different functions (see Table 26-1). Both gonads are controlled by LH and FSH secreted by the anterior pituitary gland. Adequate treatment of children with disorders of sexual differentiation requires considering not only the genetic gender and external genitalia and appearance but also the complex effect of androgens during the prenatal and postnatal periods of life.

AMBIGUOUS GENITALIA

The term *ambiguous genitalia*, a DSD, refers to any condition in which the male or female external genitalia appear abnormal (Fig. 26-9). External genitalia include the clitoris, vaginal opening, labia, and urethral meatus of the female and the penis, scrotum, testes, and urethral meatus of the male. *Hermaphroditism* is a discrepancy between the gonads (ovaries or testes) and the external genitalia. In true hermaphroditism, which is a rare condition, the child is genetically male or female but has both testicular and ovarian tissue; most frequently, an ovotestis is found. Pseudohermaphroditism

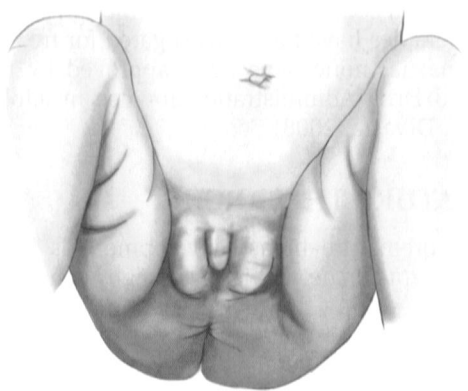

Figure 26-9 Male with ambiguous genitalia.

in the female reveals normal XX genotype and normal gonads, but the external genitalia are virilized. The male pseudohermaphrodite has normal XY genotype and testes, but the external genitalia are ambiguous or incompletely virilized.

With the exception of CAH, none of the conditions resulting in ambiguous genitalia is life threatening. Children with ambiguous genitalia may not be biologically capable of conceiving children depending on the extent of their hormone deficiency and the alteration of internal and external reproductive organs. Males with a micropenis can engage in sexual activities and father children through testosterone treatment to increase penile size.

Pathophysiology

Any interruption or abnormality in fetal sexual determination or differentiation results in ambiguous genitalia. Ambiguous genitalia may be caused by hormone imbalance or chromosomal aberrations. The most common cause of female pseudohermaphroditism is CAH. In CAH, androgen exposure on the developing female fetus creates virilization (see the discussion of pathophysiology in the section on "Congenital Adrenal Hyperplasia"). Male pseudohermaphroditism could be caused by defects in testicular differentiation, such as in gonadal dysgenesis, or in defective testicular or androgen hormone synthesis or action. Some males are insensitive to the effect of androgens and are classified as having a partial androgen insensitivity syndrome, which also results in genitalia (micropenis) that are not as developed as those of a male who is sensitive to the effects of androgens. In males with complete androgen insensitivity syndrome, the external genitalia are completely female in appearance.

Assessment

Ambiguous genitalia in genetic females (two X chromosomes) usually have some or all of the following clinical features:

- An enlarged clitoris that resembles a small penis
- A urethral opening (where urine comes out) anywhere along, above, or below the surface of the clitoris

- Fused labia that resemble a scrotum. Sometimes a lump of tissue is felt within the fused labia, further making them look like a scrotum with testicles

An infant with these features may be thought to be a male with undescended testicles.

Ambiguous genitalia in genetic males (one X and one Y chromosome) typically include some or all of the following features:

- A small penis (less than 2 to 3 cm or 0.8 to 1.2 in.) that resembles an enlarged clitoris
- A urethral opening anywhere along, above, or below the penis; it can be placed as low as on the peritoneum, further making the infant appear to be female
- A small scrotum with any degree of separation, resembling labia
- Undescended testicles, which commonly accompany ambiguous genitalia

For any child with delayed puberty or suspicious genitalia, hormone levels must be assessed to determine the integrity of the hypothalamus, anterior pituitary, and gonads (see earlier sections on "Precocious Puberty" and "Delayed Puberty"). Genetic testing is also completed to determine whether the child is a genetic male or female. Endoscopy, abdominal radiograph, and abdominal or pelvic ultrasound may be needed to determine the presence or absence of internal genital structures (such as undescended testes). In some cases, laparoscopy, exploratory laparotomy, or biopsy of the gonads may be necessary to confirm disorders associated with ambiguous genitalia.

Interdisciplinary Interventions

Ambiguous genitalia in the newborn creates anxiety for many. The parents have many questions and need assistance regarding what to tell inquisitive family members about the gender of the newborn. If there is any question about the external genitalia, a swift investigation must be undertaken to determine genetic sexual identification. Until the sex assignment has been determined, the health care team should refer to the newborn as "the baby" rather than "he" or "she." The name card placed in the newborn's bassinet should be white instead of pink or blue. Discourage the parents from giving the child an ambiguous name because it could serve as a reminder of the events surrounding the sexual ambiguity at birth. In addition, it would be wise to postpone sending birth announcements until the sex assignment is completed.

The first goal in treating ambiguous genitalia is to determine gender through chromosomal analysis. Unfortunately, this test can be time-consuming, and gender assignment is delayed. Health care providers must be honest and forthright with parents when gender identification is unclear because erroneous sex assignment can cause major lifelong social and emotional problems for the child and family.

If CAH is suspected, appropriate steroid replacement therapy is initiated. Genetic counseling is indicated, given the autosomal recessive nature of CAH (see the section on "Congenital Adrenal Hyperplasia" for details).

In some children, ambiguous genitalia are not obvious at birth. They are diagnosed at the time of adolescence or young adulthood when stunted growth, delayed puberty, or infertility raises the question of a broader chromosomal or hormonal abnormality. With this diagnosis also comes the developing awareness of possible permanent infertility or sexual dysfunction and a sense of loss.

With any genetic condition, a genetic counselor can give accurate information and prognoses. Issues for the child include differences from their peers in relation to sexual development, body image, and reproductive capabilities. Options are presented for alternative forms of raising a family (e.g., through adoption) as well as awareness that childless individuals and couples can also lead a very fulfilling life. Future advances in reproductive science may include the possibility of reproduction through donor gametes and hormonal support. Education and support groups for most syndromes are available to parents and families through local and national chapters for specific disorders. In addition, discuss how to support families on issues such as gender assignment, psychosocial support, timing of surgeries, hormonal therapy, and developing sexual well-being for the child (Consortium on the Management of Disorders of Sex Development, 2006).

GYNECOMASTIA

Gynecomastia is a condition in boys, usually occurring during early or midpuberty, that involves unilateral or bilateral breast enlargement. This common, transient occurrence usually lasts a few months to a year (Nordt & DiVasta, 2008). Gynecomastia is usually secondary to the normal hormonal imbalances between testosterone and estrogen that commonly occur during puberty. Hormone levels for FSH, LH, prolactin, testosterone, and estradiol are normal, but the ratio of testosterone to estradiol may be decreased. In younger children with gynecomastia who also show increased pigmentation of the nipple and areola, suspect exogenous estrogens in the form of creams, pills, or inhaled medications. The antifungal drug ketoconazole can also cause gynecomastia. Drugs of abuse such as alcohol, amphetamines, and marijuana can also cause gynecomastia in adolescent and adult males. Use of anabolic steroids and GH may also stimulate breast development, but adolescents abusing these medications tend to be athletes, so the gynecomastia may not be clinically evident because of increased muscle mass. Cases of gynecomastia have been linked to exposure to endocrine disruptors such as tea tree oil and lavender (Kalyan, 2007). Breast enlargement may also be a sign of other conditions, such as Klinefelter syndrome or other rare endocrine disorders.

The boy may develop body image disturbance related to gynecomastia. Therefore, encourage him and his family to verbalize concerns about body image. Treatment usually consists of reassurance to the boy and his family of the benign and transient nature of this condition. Surgical intervention is rarely indicated and should be considered only if the gynecomastia persists after the child completes puberty. Although several hormone therapies have been investigated for treatment of gynecomastia, none have been approved by the U.S. Food and Drug Administration for use in adolescents (Nordt & DiVasta, 2008).

PREMATURE THELARCHE

In girls, premature breast development is known as *premature thelarche*. It is a benign condition that may appear during the first 2 years of life. Breast development may be unilateral or bilateral, and regression usually occurs after a few years. These girls do not show maturation of the genitalia or presence of pubic hair, and menarche occurs at the expected age. Growth usually occurs at the normal rate and rarely is accelerated. This condition is thought to occur from an imbalance in the LH–FSH ratio within the hypothalamic–pituitary–gonadal pathway.

A girl with early breast development should be screened for true precocious puberty, especially if the age at onset is older than 2 years. Obtain plasma levels of LH, FSH, and estradiol. This condition may be caused by exogenous exposure to estrogens or endocrine disruptors. As with gynecomastia in boys, treatment includes reassuring the girl and family that this condition is benign and transient and that the other aspects of female pubertal progression should occur in normal sequence.

See thePoint for a summary of Key Concepts.

REFERENCES

American Association of Clinical Endocrinologists. (2009). Medical guidelines for clinical practice for growth hormone use in growth hormone deficient adults and transition patients: 2009 update. *Endocrine Practice, 15*(2), 1–29.

American Association of Clinical Endocrinologists. (2011a). American Association of Clinical Endocrinologists medical guidelines for clinical practice for developing a diabetes mellitus comprehensive care plan. *Endocrine Practice, 17*(Suppl. 2), 1–53.

American Association of Clinical Endocrinologists. (2011b). Hyperthyroidism management guidelines. *Endocrine Practice, 17*(3), 479–485.

American Diabetes Association. (2013). Standards of medical care in diabetes. *Diabetes Care, 36*(Suppl. 1), S11–S66.

Babiker, A., Leach, E., & Datta, V. (2011). Should we screen children with type 1 diabetes for Addison's disease? *Archives of Disease in Childhood, 96,* 700–701.

Barker, J., Fain, P., & Eisenbarth, G. (2005). Addison's disease and type 1 diabetes. *Current Opinion in Endocrinology & Diabetes, 12,* 280–284.

Carel, J. C., & Le'ger, J. (2008). Precocious puberty. *New England Journal of Medicine, 358*(22), 2366–2377.

Centers for Disease Control and Prevention. (2011). *National diabetes fact sheet, 2011.* Retrieved from http://www.cdc.gov/diabetes/pubs/factsheet11.htm

Consortium on the Management of Disorders of Sex Development. (2006). *Clinical guidelines for the management of disorders of sex development in childhood.* Retrieved from http://www.accordalliance.org/dsdguidelines/clinical.pdf

Copeland, K., Silverstein, J., Moore, K. R. et al. (2013). Management of newly diagnosed type 2 diabetes mellitus (t2dm) in children and adolescents. *Pediatrics, 131*(2), 364–382.

Greenbaum, L., Benador, M. N., Goldstein, S. et al. (2007). Intravenous paricalcitol for treatment of secondary hyperparathyroidism in children on hemodialysis. *American Journal of Kidney Diseases*, *49*(6), 814–823.

Gross, P. (2012). Clinical management of SIADH. *Therapeutic Advances in Endocrinology and Metabolism*, *3*(2), 61–73.

Hench, K., Shults, J., Benyi, T. et al. (2005). Effect of educational preparation on the accuracy of linear growth measurement in pediatric primary care practices: Results of a multicenter nursing study. *Journal of Pediatric Nursing*, *20*(2), 64–74.

Himes, J. (2009). Challenges of accurately measuring and using BMI and other indicators of obesity in children. *Pediatrics*, *124*(Suppl. 1), S3–S22.

Kalyan, S. (2007). Prepubertal gynecomastia linked to lavender and tea tree oils. *New England Journal of Medicine*, *356*(24), 2542.

Kappy, M., Allen, D., & Geffner, M. (2009). *Pediatric practice endocrinology*. New York, NY: McGraw Hill Professional.

Kelly, M. A., Rayner, M. L., Mijovic, C. H. et al. (2003). Molecular aspects of type 1 diabetes. *Molecular Pathology*, *56*(1), 1–10.

Lindfors, K., Elovainio, M., Wickman, S. et al. (2007). Brief report: The role of ego development in psychosocial adjustment among boys with delayed puberty. *Journal of Research on Adolescence*, *17*, 601–612.

Lipman, T., Hench, K., Benyi, T. et al. (2004). A multicenter randomized controlled trial of an intervention to improve the accuracy of linear growth measurement. *Archives of Disease in Childhood*, *89*, 342–346.

Liu, H., & Crapo, L. (2005). Update on the diagnosis of Cushing syndrome. *The Endocrinologist*, *15*(3), 165–179.

Marcus, B., & Collins, K. (2004). Childhood panhypopituitarism presenting as child abuse. *The American Journal of Forensic Medicine and Pathology*, *25*(30), 265–269.

Nordt, C., & DiVasta, A. (2008). Gynecomastia in adolescents. *Current Opinion in Pediatrics*, *20*, 375–382.

Rastogi, M., & LaFranchi, S. (2010). Congenital hypothyroidism. *Orphanet Journal of Rare Diseases*, *5*, 1–22.

Robinson, D., & Scott, L. (2005). Paricalcitol: A review of its use in the management of secondary hyperparathyroidism. *Drugs*, *65*(4), 559–576.

Savage, M., Dias, R., Chan, L. et al. (2010). Diagnosis and treatment of Cushing's disease in children. *Endocrine Development*, *17*, 134–145.

Dabelea, D., Bell, R. A., D'Agostino, R. B., Jr. et al. (2007). Incidence of diabetes in youth in the United States. *Journal of the American Medical Association*, *297*(24), 2716–2724.

Silverstein, J., Klingensmith, G., Copeland, K. et al. (2005). Care of children and adolescents with type 1 diabetes. *Diabetes Care*, *28*(1), 186–212.

Sonino, N., Boscaro, M., & Fallo, F. (2005). Pharmacologic management of Cushing syndrome. *Treatments in Endocrinology*, *4*(2), 87–94.

Speiser, P. W., & White, P. C. (2003). Congenital adrenal hyperplasia. *New England Journal of Medicine*, *349*(8), 776–788.

Steinkrauss, L., Lipman, T., Hendell, C. et al. (2005). Effects of hypoglycemia on developmental outcome in children with congenital hyperinsulinism. *Journal of Pediatric Nursing*, *20*(2), 109–118.

Trakakis, E., Loghis C., & Kassanos, D. (2009). Congenital adrenal hyperplasia because of 21-hydroxylase deficiency: A genetic disorder of interest to obstetricians and gynecologists. *Obstetrical & Gynecological Survey*, *64*, 177–189.

Utrainen, P., Jaaskelainen, J., Romppanen, J. et al. (2008). Childhood metabolic syndrome and its components in premature adrenarche. *Obstetrical & Gynecological Survey*, *63*, 312–313.

Vanderpump, M. (2011). The epidemiology of thyroid disease. *British Medical Bulletin*, *99*(1), 39–51.

See the**Point** for additional organizations.

CHAPTER 27

The Child With an Inborn Error of Metabolism

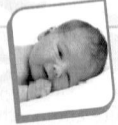

CASE HISTORY

The Rollins family was introduced in Chapter 3. Joellen and her husband, Chris, were expecting their third child. Their two other children are Selena, aged 5 years, and James, aged 2½ years. Joellen went into labor at 38 weeks' gestation and gave birth vaginally to their son, Sean, who weighed 6 lb 10 oz (3.01 kg) and was 20 in. (50.8 cm) in length. Joellen progressed through labor without complications and received epidural anesthesia during labor for pain management. Joellen has chosen to breastfeed her son.

Sean's 1-minute and 5-minute Apgar scores were 7 and 9, respectively. His initial physical examination revealed slight molding of the head with firm, flat fontanels. Head circumference was 34.5 cm and chest circumference was 32.5 cm. Skin was reddish pink with acrocyanosis. Vital signs were as follows: temperature, 99° F (37.2° C); apical pulse, 140 bpm; and respirations, 56 breaths/min. Some mucus was noted in his nose and mouth and was removed with a bulb syringe. Newborn reflexes were intact. Sean continued to adapt well to extrauterine life and was discharged from the hospital after 24 hours.

Joellen brings Sean to the clinic for a checkup. He is now 4 months old. Joellen mentions that she's noticed that Sean seems to be vomiting more often during the past 2–3 weeks. "It's not the usual baby spit-up either. It seems more forceful, and it's much larger amounts." Assessment reveals some hyperactivity with fine hand tremors. Sean's skin appears dry with some scaly patches noted. His cheeks are reddened with two dime-sized crusted areas bilaterally. Several areas on Sean's upper extremities appear erythematous with oozing vesicles. His wet diaper has a musty odor. Developmental assessment reveals that Sean is somewhat behind in achieving his milestones. Joellen reports she missed the follow-up appointment for testing after Sean's discharge from the hospital because she developed mastitis.

CHAPTER OBJECTIVES

1 Differentiate between inborn errors of metabolism that manifest at birth or in the immediate neonatal period (e.g., maple syrup urine disease) and those with later childhood onset (e.g., Wilson disease).

2 Describe key assessment factors that can assist in early identification of metabolic disorders in children.

3 Describe interventions performed by the health care team that are related to early identification of selected inborn errors of metabolism.

4 State the dietary management specific to each metabolic disorder that can prevent disease symptoms or decrease their severity.

5 Identify nursing interventions that assist the family and community to provide optimal care to the child with an inborn error of metabolism.

See thePoint for a list of Key Terms.

The body builds and maintains itself by *metabolizing* the food and fluid it ingests. The metabolic pathways used during this process may have inborn errors that cause an untoward reaction or lead to the creation of toxic substances. The mutation of single genes either results in a structurally altered enzyme that is not capable of normal catalytic activity or causes an inhibition of enzyme synthesis. Reduced enzymatic function produces a block in the metabolic pathway at a specific point. This block leads to an abnormal accumulation of substrate, or building block in the metabolic pathway, causing a block or "log jam" in the pathway. The accumulated substrate appears in the blood, urine, and tissues and can affect the body in many ways. The presenting symptoms are correlated with the potential effects of inborn errors during the intrauterine period of growth. For example, inborn errors of metabolism can cause defective development of the brain in utero. After birth, the infant's developing neurotransmitter system continues to be especially vulnerable to the abnormal biosynthesis of enzymes. Most inborn errors of metabolism are transmitted through autosomal recessive or X-linked inheritance. Type 1 diabetes mellitus, described in Chapter 26, is one of the most common errors of metabolism in children.

DEVELOPMENTAL AND BIOLOGIC VARIANCES

Inborn errors of metabolism can produce genetic changes that may vary from child to child depending on the degree of alteration and the system affected (Fig. 27-1).

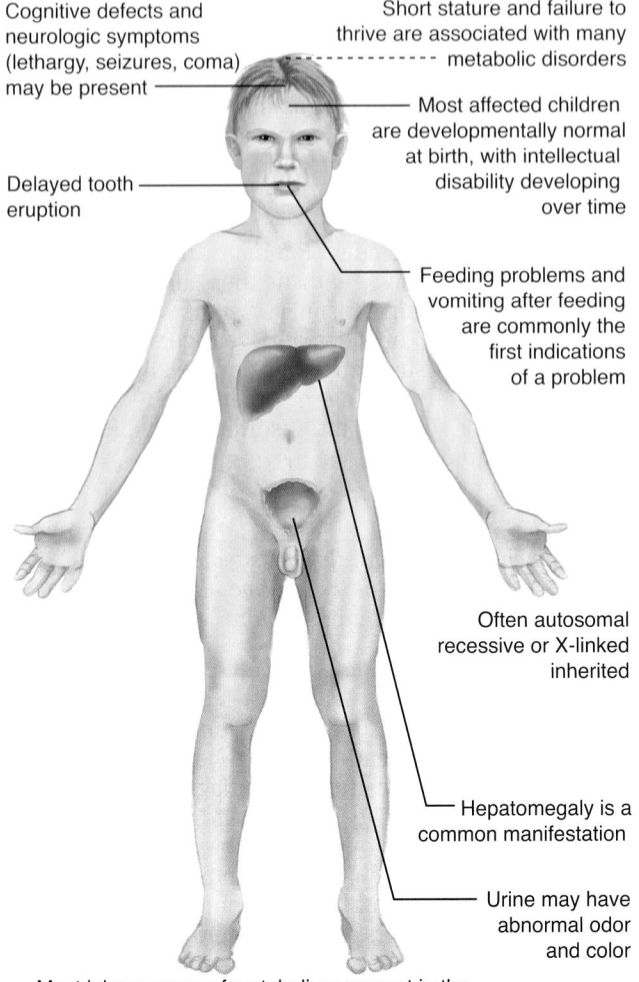

Cognitive defects and neurologic symptoms (lethargy, seizures, coma) may be present

Short stature and failure to thrive are associated with many metabolic disorders

Most affected children are developmentally normal at birth, with intellectual disability developing over time

Delayed tooth eruption

Feeding problems and vomiting after feeding are commonly the first indications of a problem

Often autosomal recessive or X-linked inherited

Hepatomegaly is a common manifestation

Urine may have abnormal odor and color

Most inborn errors of metabolism present in the childhood years and, if untreated, result in early death

Figure 27-1 Developmental and biologic variances: inborn errors of metabolism.

For some children, the clinical manifestations of these changes are inconsequential and are merely noted as some of the characteristics that make one person different from another. Other metabolic conditions produce symptoms that become apparent only under specific conditions that the child may or may not encounter during life. Still, other conditions produce disease states that vary from mild to fatal. Most inborn errors of metabolism become clinically evident during the neonatal period, although some may not manifest themselves until later (Developmental Considerations 27-1). Presentation in the adult years is not common, except with mitochondrial disorders, and is more likely to represent a metabolic disorder that has been activated or triggered by the presence of another disease state.

Certain ethnic and geographic origins confer risk for metabolic disorders. When these variances are known, carrier testing, genetic counseling, prenatal diagnosis, and newborn screening are initiated to help decrease the incidence of the disease and to enhance early identification of affected infants.

CROSS-CULTURAL CARE

Certain metabolic disorders are known to be more prevalent in specific ethnic groups and in people from specific geographic locations. For instance, the tyrosine defect tyrosinemia type I has a higher prevalence in patients with a French–Canadian ancestry. In the French–Canadian population of Quebec, the incidence of this condition is 1 in 1,846 newborn infants. The classic form of maple syrup urine disease (MSUD) is more common among members of Mennonite and Amish sects. Hyperglycinemia is more common in Finland than in other parts of the world. PKU is most common among Jews of Yemenite origin and in the populations of northern Europe, particularly Ireland, Scotland, Belgium, and Germany. Tay-Sachs disease, Gaucher disease, and Niemann-Pick disease occur more frequently among individuals of Ashkenazi Jewish descent. Although Tay-Sachs disease occurs 1 in 3,500 to 4,000 births, the carrier rate among Ashkenazi Jews is 1 in 30 (Kliegman et al., 2011).

ASSESSMENT

QUESTION: What might be the impact of Sean not having had diagnostic testing as scheduled after his discharge from the hospital?

Although the incidence of most inborn errors of metabolism is low, these biochemical disorders must be recognized and treated immediately because, for many children, early intervention can alter long-term outcomes. Without interventions, many disorders result in progressive loss of neurologic function, developmental disabilities, psychomotor retardation, growth abnormalities, seizures, and other severe symptoms that profoundly affect quality of life for the child and the family.

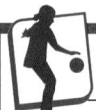

DEVELOPMENTAL CONSIDERATIONS 27-1

Developmental Age and Appearance of Selected Inborn Errors of Metabolism

Neonatal
Galactosemia
Hyperammonemia
Hyperglycinemia
Isovaleric acidemia
MSUD
Menkes disease
Phenylketonuria (PKU)
Sulfite oxidase deficiency
Tyrosinemia type I (acute form)

Infancy
Fructosuria
Hurler syndrome

Long-chain 3-hydroxyacyl-coenzyme A (CoA)
    dehydrogenase deficiency
Medium-chain acyl-CoA dehydrogenase
    deficiency
X-linked hypophosphatemic rickets

Early Childhood
Homocystinuria
Hunter syndrome
Hurler syndrome
Hyperammonemia
Tyrosinemia type I (chronic form)

Middle Childhood and Adolescence
Wilson disease

Early recognition is, therefore, the primary goal in diagnostic evaluation for inborn errors of metabolism. The sooner a metabolic disorder is detected, the sooner treatment can be initiated in an attempt to avert the negative consequences of the disease process.

> *ANSWER:* The lack of diagnostic testing as scheduled after birth may have significant effects on Sean's health, should he be diagnosed with an inborn error of metabolism. Early recognition is essential so that treatment can be initiated as soon as possible to prevent possible complications associated with this type of disease.

FOCUSED HEALTH HISTORY

Information obtained from a genetic history is important because genetic counseling provides guidance for families as they make decisions about childbearing. Genetic counseling may occur prior to conception, during the pregnancy, or after the child's birth based on when genetic issues come to the attention of the family and the health care provider. In utero diagnosis, which can occur early during pregnancy, is possible for many of the inherited metabolic disorders. **Newborn screening** programs provide early diagnosis for many of the more common metabolic disorders (see "Treatment Modalities" section for more information on newborn screening). Diagnosis enables timely intervention to prevent symptoms or to decrease their severity.

A detailed history of the child's health status and ffdevelopmental progress can provide many clues to the existence of a metabolic disorder. Common to most metabolic problems is a history of poor feeding, including rejection or dislike of protein foods, vomiting,

listlessness, failure to thrive, delayed development, and increasing weakness (Focused Health History 27-1). As the child grows, delays in reaching psychomotor developmental milestones or a regression in developmental achievements is noted. The child may have a history of an apparent life-threatening event (e.g., near-miss sudden infant death).

The pattern of heredity for many of the metabolic conditions is recessive, with neither parent presenting with clinically abnormal signs or symptoms. However, the health history of older and younger siblings may reveal symptoms similar to those of the child being assessed. Alternately, siblings or other close relatives may have a variant form of the disorder, with different or sporadic symptoms.

caREminder

> *If one child in the family has suspicious symptoms, counsel the family to have all other siblings evaluated, even if their symptoms are not exactly the same.*

The family history may reveal unexplained deaths (e.g., sudden infant death syndrome) during the infancy period, possibly indicating an undiagnosed, untreated metabolic disorder. The ill child and family members with suspicious symptoms should be questioned about the correlation between their symptoms and the presence of other common illnesses. Some variant forms of the metabolic disorders appear symptomatic only when exacerbated by a cold, vomiting, diarrhea, or other concurrent illnesses.

Ask parents whether newborn screening was completed and, if so, whether they were informed about the results.

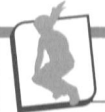

FOCUSED HEALTH HISTORY 27-1

Inborn Errors of Metabolism

Current history	Clinical deterioration in a previously normal neonate, infant, or child Neurologic abnormalities such as lethargy, hypotonia or hypertonia, seizures, migrainelike headaches, coma not responsive to intravenous glucose or calcium Apparent sepsis Respiratory insufficiency manifested by apneic episodes or tachypnea Cardiac failure, myopathy, pericardial effusion, arrhythmias Metabolic instability manifested as acidosis, ketosis, hyperammonemia, or hypoglycemia Gastrointestinal problems such as abdominal pain, poor feeding, vomiting, diarrhea, constipation, weight loss, hepatomegaly
Past medical history	**Birth History** Was newborn screening completed? What were the results? Any episodes of temperature instability Feeding difficulties Any history of apparent life-threatening event or prolonged apnea spells, inconsolable irritability, involuntary movements, or seizures during neonatal period Presence of dysmorphic features **Previous Health Challenges** Unexplained cognitive deficits, developmental delay, motor deficits, or seizures Unusual odor of urine or sweat, particularly during acute illnesses Intermittent episodes of unexplained vomiting, acidosis History of renal stones Cataracts, corneal clouding, or other ophthalmologic abnormalities Hematologic abnormalities (e.g., thrombocytopenia, neutropenia, anemia) in the presence of normal bone marrow findings Exaggerated response to minor stress or infection resulting in neurologic signs, acidosis, hypoglycemia
Nutritional assessment	Poor feeding, persistent vomiting Food likes and dislikes (e.g., salt craving, protein avoidance, lactose intolerance) Family eating patterns and health beliefs related to food
Family medical history	Any family history of miscarriages, stillbirths, or unexplained deaths during neonatal period or infancy Family history of consanguinity (birth as the result of a sexual relationship between blood relatives) Any parents, siblings, or cousins with symptoms similar to those presented by the patient Any family members with developmental delays, low intellectual functioning, or cognitive challenges
Growth and development	Growth (head circumference, weight, length) plotted on growth chart, recent weight loss or gain, failure to thrive Inability to meet growth and developmental norms, delay in the onset of puberty Failure to thrive Loss of previously acquired developmental milestones Decreased level of activity

Note: See Chapter 8 for a comprehensive health history.

CROSS-CULTURAL CARE

In the United States, the disorders that newborn screening programs test for vary from state to state. Tests for PKU and galactosemia are mandated by state law. Children born in other countries may not have been screened as neonates for metabolic disorders because other countries, especially the developing nations, do not have rigorous enforcement of or control over screening programs. Investigate the newborn screening requirements for the child's state or country of origin; determine whether the child underwent screening and what these clinical assessments showed.

Responses to the questions asked during a health history can possibly indicate a metabolic problem but must be considered in the context of the physical examination and laboratory findings before a diagnosis can be reached.

FOCUSED PHYSICAL ASSESSMENT

 QUESTION: Which assessment findings would lead you to suspect that Sean may have a metabolic disorder?

Hundreds of metabolic diseases have been described in the medical literature to date. Most of these disorders are clinically recognized during the newborn period or the first year of life. Unfortunately, many of the early signs of metabolic problems in children are vague. Presenting symptoms vary with age (see Focused Health History 27-1). The astute nurse recognizes that these symptoms are indices of many serious problems, including metabolic disorders, and motivates the interdisciplinary team to look more closely for underlying causes.

A crisis can develop rapidly in the presence of metabolic disturbance and cause irreversible symptoms or death. Identifying the cause of symptoms accurately and quickly is essential. A thorough physical assessment should be completed by the health care provider. Any member of the health care team may note some of the changes, particularly in urine and body odors, which are specific to certain metabolic disorders (Table 27-1).

The nervous system is most consistently affected. The physical examination should focus on evaluating neurodevelopmental functions. Abnormalities commonly revealed include impaired states of alertness and arousal, tremors, posturing, clonic jerking, tonic spasms, or seizures. Signs such as **opisthotonos** (extreme spasmic extension of the body resulting in arching of the back at severe angle) and disturbances of ocular movements may be noted. Limb movements are diminished or absent as neuromuscular function declines. Other neurologic responses that are affected include thermoregulation, causing hypothermia or

TABLE 27-1	Unusual Odors Associated With Metabolic Disorders	
Urine and Body Odors	**Disorder**
Maple syrup or burnt sugar	MSUD
Musty, mousey	PKU or tyrosinemia type I
Boiled cabbage, rancid butter, or rotting fish	Hypermethioninemia or tyrosinemia type I
Cat urine	Multiple carboxylase deficiency
Sweaty feet	Glutaric aciduria (type II) or isovaleric acidemia
Swimming pool	Hawkinsinuria
Rotting fish	Trimethylaminuria

poikilothermia (inability to maintain a consistent core body temperature), and cardiac and respiratory function. Irregular respirations, bradycardia, circulatory difficulties, and poor color may all be present (Focused Physical Assessment 27-1).

Nearly all metabolic disorders negatively affect growth and development. Therefore, assessment of the child's growth should be accurate and ongoing, and developmental status should be monitored with developmental screening tools (see Chapter 3 for a discussion of developmental screening tools). During infancy and early childhood, loss of previously attained milestones often occurs as the disease progress. Metabolic diseases that first manifest during late childhood and adolescence are usually less severe and progress less rapidly; however, they may still affect behavior, thinking, and emotions. Children with metabolic disease who are diagnosed and treated at a young age require continuing assessment to evaluate the effectiveness of therapy. If dietary or pharmacologic management regimens are failing, effects on the child's physical and cognitive functions can be noted.

ANSWER: Several assessment findings may suggest Sean has a metabolic disorder. Important findings would include evidence of tremors, reports of forceful vomiting, and appearance of skin lesions. Additionally, if Sean is lagging behind on achievement of developmental milestones, this would be a crucial indicator that would provide further evidence of a problem.

DIAGNOSTIC CRITERIA

Newborn screening programs have made early diagnosis of more than 30 inborn metabolic errors possible. Every state screens for PKU, galactosemia, and MSUD; however, there are numerous other conditions that vary from state to state in regard to if they require mandated testing (Tradition or Science 27-1).

Newborn screening refers to the public health programs that are available and employed after a child's

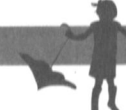

FOCUSED PHYSICAL ASSESSMENT 27-1
Metabolic System

Assessment Parameter	Alterations/Clinical Significance
General appearance	General appearance of clinical deterioration in previously normal child may indicate metabolic disorder.
	Failure to thrive
	Impaired states of alertness and arousal
	Poor temperature control
Integumentary system (skin, hair, nails)	Coarse, sparse, or brittle hair seen in Menkes disease
	Unexplained jaundice from hepatic involvement
	Hypothermia or poikilothermia (inability to maintain a constant core temperature)
	Sagging skin related to weight loss
	Tooth eruption delayed, abnormal shape, presence of many tooth abscesses seen in X-linked hypophosphatemic rickets
Head and neck	Dysmorphic features such as microcephaly, abnormal facial features (e.g., gargoylelike facial features seen in Hurler syndrome)
Eyes	Dislocated lenses, cataracts (galactosemia, Menkes disease, and Wilson disease)
	Disturbances of ocular movement, deterioration in vision including blindness (MSUD, mitochondrial disorders)
	Abnormal corneal pigmentation, Kayser-Fleischer rings seen in Wilson disease
Ears	Deafness (Hurler syndrome, Hunter disease)
Thorax and lungs	Irregular respirations, tachypnea, apnea related to metabolic acidosis (associated with many metabolic disorders)
	Pectus excavatum seen in Menkes disease
Cardiovascular system	Bradycardia, arrhythmias, circulatory difficulties related to hypoglycemia
	Advanced cardiac involvement such as hypertrophic or dilated cardiomyopathy, pericardial effusion
Gastrointestinal system	Hepatomegaly, splenomegaly associated with Wilson disease and hepatic dysfunction
	Jaundice from hepatic involvement (tyrosinemia type I, Wilson disease, galactosemia)
	Intermittent, unexplained recurrent episodes of vomiting related to protein imbalance, metabolic acidosis, or hyperammonemia
Genitourinary system	Unusual urine and body odors, particularly during acute illnesses, related to ketones and other metabolic substrates in urine
	Presence of renal stones (hyperparathyroidism)
Musculoskeletal system	Skeletal deformities (e.g., abnormal bone growth and formation) seen in Wilson disease, Hurler syndrome, and lysosomal storage diseases
	Involuntary, diminished, or absent limb or motor function (e.g., waddling gait, hypotonia, hypertonia) seen in Menkes disease, galactosemia, Tay-Sachs disease
Neurologic system	Neurologic deterioration, ataxia, tremors, clonic jerking, tonic spasms, and seizures; coma, encephalopathy related to effects of accumulating metabolites on the central nervous system (CNS)

TRADITION OR SCIENCE 27-1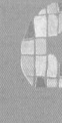

Do infants in all parts of the United States have equal access to newborn screening and its potential to prevent morbidity and mortality?

Variations exist among state newborn screening systems, and a national model for the structure and function of newborn screening systems has not yet been embraced. In addition, no uniform guidelines exist to direct periodic assessment for the conditions for which screening is performed. The American College of Medical Genetics recommended that all neonates in all states be screened for 29 treatable congenital conditions as well as 25 additional conditions detectable by screening which the American Academy of Pediatrics (AAP) endorsed in 2005 (AAP, Newborn Screening Authoring Committee, 2008). The American College of Obstetricians and Gynecologists (2011) endorses these recommendations and further encourages all care providers to make resources about newborn screening available to women and their families during prenatal visits. National standards continue to be developed to make newborn screening programs more comparable from state to state and service provider to service provider to address inequities in the provision of health care services. When completing a health assessment, note the state in which the child was born and determine whether further screening is needed because some tests may not have been completed during the newborn screening process in the state where the child was born.

birth to evaluate the infant for an array of treatable conditions that may not be visibly evident at birth. Among the screening tests are those for a variety of inborn errors of metabolism, hemoglobinopathies (e.g., sickle cell disease, beta-thalassemia), and miscellaneous multisystem diseases (e.g., cystic fibrosis) as well as an evaluation of hearing (see Chapter 28 for more about hearing screening). Evidence-Based Clinical Practice Guidelines 27-1 provides a number of resources related to newborn screening.

Although screening is available for numerous metabolic disorders, the cost-to-benefit ratio of such screening, in both economic and ethical terms, must be considered for each disorder. For the rarer metabolic disorders, the expense associated with testing all newborns may be perceived as unjustified. Therefore, specific criteria must be met before a metabolic disorder is included in a newborn screening program. Generally, disorders included in screening programs are those with

- Relatively high prevalence
- Clinical symptoms that are not present until irreversible damage occurs
- Clinical manifestations severe enough to affect society

- Known treatments and facilities available to provide treatment
- Diagnostic evaluation possible through a simple method of collection
- Follow-up available if test results are abnormal (including retesting; all screening tests can have false-positive and false-negative results)

If results of newborn screening are positive, or if the child presents with clinical manifestations consistent with a metabolic disorder, laboratory studies can differentiate the cause of the child's illness. High-pressure gas–liquid chromatography, ion-exchange chromatography, mass spectroscopy, and electron microscopy are used to analyze blood, plasma, urine, or cerebrospinal fluid to detect metabolic disorders (Tests and Procedures 27-1). The enzymatic defect that is interrupting the metabolic pathway results in either a deficiency of an essential substrate or the accumulation of a harmful metabolite. These deficiencies or elevations in the substrates can be detected in the body fluids. In some cases, when the presence of an inborn error of metabolism has been determined, further diagnostic testing may be done to determine the extent of organ involvement.

TREATMENT MODALITIES

 QUESTION: Why are newborn screening tests so important for newborns, such as Sean?

Advances in diagnosing and treating inborn errors of metabolism have greatly improved the prognosis for many children. Many of the treatable errors of metabolism require lifelong management, usually in the form of dietary restriction. Other metabolic diseases are fatal or result in severe intellectual disability, and no successful intervention has yet been developed. The management of children and families affected by inborn errors of metabolism includes a focus on prevention, early diagnosis, nutritional management, pharmacologic management, and other therapies specific to certain conditions. These treatment modalities are discussed in the following sections.

PREVENTION

Prevention, when it is possible, is the first intervention. For some diseases, such as Tay-Sachs disease, mild hyperphenylalaninemia, and Gaucher disease, **carrier testing** (heterozygote screening) is possible. Carrier testing is warranted for people who may have an elevated risk because of their ethnic or national origin. The nurse has an important role in providing genetic counseling to families who are suspected or known carriers of a metabolic disorder. This preventive intervention can serve as a way to provide full disclosure to couples regarding their risk of the disease, the burden of the disease, and their reproductive options before they make decisions regarding childbearing.

EVIDENCE-BASED CLINICAL PRACTICE GUIDELINES 27-1
Newborn Screening

American Academy of Pediatrics, Newborn Screening Authoring Committee. (2008). Newborn screening expands: Recommendations for pediatricians and medical homes—Implications for the system. *Pediatrics, 121*(1), 192–217. Retrieved from

http://pediatrics.aappublications.org/content/121/1/192.full

Policy for newborn screening programs.

American College of Medical Genetics. (2001). *Newborn screening ACT sheets and confirmatory algorithms.* Retrieved from

http://www.ncbi.nlm.nih.gov/books/NBK55827/

Patient information sheets on each newborn screening condition and the algorithm for screening and treatment.

American College of Obstetricians and Gynecologists. (2011). *Newborn screening.* Retrieved from

http://www.acog.org/Resources%20And%20Publications/Committee%20Opinions/Committee%20on%20Genetics /Newborn%20Screening.aspx

Policy statement on newborn screening with Web resources on the conditions that can be evaluated during newborn screening tests.

Centers for Disease Control and Prevention. (2012). *Newborn screening.* Retrieved from

http://www.cdc.gov/newbornscreening/

Information about newborn screening programs.

March of Dimes Foundation Genetics & Your Practice (2012)

http://www.marchofdimes.com/gyponline/index.bm2

Resources for health care professionals to help integrate genetics into their practice.

National Newborn Screening & Global Resource Center (2013)

http://genes-r-us.uthscsa.edu/%3Cfront%3E

U.S. national resource center on newborn screening. Includes guidelines for newborn screening internationally.

Secretary's Advisory Committee on Heritable Disorders in Newborns and Children. (2013). *Recommended uniform screening panel.* Retrieved from

http://www.hrsa.gov/advisorycommittees/mchbadvisory/heritabledisorders/recommendedpanel/index.html

Recommended tests to be included in newborn screening.

EARLY DIAGNOSIS

Early diagnosis is a critical intervention of the health care team and has the potential to avert the negative sequelae that are potential outcomes of a metabolic condition. In many cases, a diagnosis can be made in utero. Amniocentesis and chorionic villus sampling can detect many of the metabolic disorders. If a diagnosis is confirmed, a member of the health care team with genetic counseling experience and preparation can provide the family with information regarding the severity of the illness, the child's long-term prognosis, and the range of options available for maintaining or terminating the pregnancy. The family may experience turmoil and grief as they come to terms with the diagnosis for their unborn child. Providing emotional support to the family is an important aspect of care at this time. Chapter 13 provides an in-depth description of the interventions that can be implemented to support the family during the grieving process.

Newborn screening is also an aspect of early diagnosis (Nursing Interventions 27-1). When the neonate has been tested, results may be sent back to the health care provider in as few as 2 weeks. Positive results may be the first and only indicator of disease in an otherwise asymptomatic newborn. Further blood and urine testing is then initiated to confirm the diagnosis.

Another later aspect of early diagnosis is early recognition of symptoms during the neonatal period. Because children with inborn errors of metabolism may present with one or more of a large variety of symptoms (see Focused Physical Assessment 27-1), differentiating the condition from other childhood disorders may be difficult. Infants may present with lethargy, poor feeding, tachypnea or apnea, and recurrent vomiting. Because the clinical symptoms are usually nonspecific and may appear similar to those present with any number of generalized infections that can affect infants (G. Rezvani & Rezvani, 2011), opportunities to diagnose inborn errors may be missed. Thus, a primary intervention of the health care team is to consider and suspect a metabolic disorder when a neonate becomes severely ill, when developmental milestones are not met, or when developmental regression begins to appear in the previously healthy child.

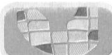 TESTS AND PROCEDURES for Evaluating Inborn Errors of Metabolism

Diagnostic Test or Procedure	Purpose	Findings and Indications	Health Care Provider Responsibilities
Blood Tests			
Newborn screening	Early diagnosis of inborn errors of metabolism; specific diseases assessed vary based on state regulations	Identifies presence of disorders such as PKU, galactosemia, hypothyroidism, and MSUD	Screening must be completed before discharge from the acute care facility (see Nursing Interventions 27-1).
Complete blood cell count, glucose, electrolytes, arterial blood gas, anion gap, plasma ammonium level	Used to rule out or confirm metabolic disorder	Alterations in glucose, ketones, blood pH and bicarbonate, and blood lactate all indicate metabolic disorder.	Note child's diet before the test because the ingestion of food or formula may impact lab results if a metabolic disorder is present.
Plasma amino acids, plasma carnitine	Detects changes in amino acid patterns, thus detecting abnormalities of amino acid transport or metabolism.	Defects related to metabolism of amino acids result in increased levels in the blood.	Note time of collection in relation to feeding. Fasting usually required prior to test. Verify length of fasting period needed with laboratory.
Blood urea nitrogen (BUN), creatinine	Evaluates renal function.	Elevations indicate renal involvement as seen in conditions such as Wilson disease.	Sample may be obtained at same time as completing other blood specimens.
Ammonia, lactic acid	Evaluates metabolism; ammonia is an end product of protein metabolism and lactate is an end product of carbohydrate metabolism	Lactate is elevated in disorders of carbohydrate and energy metabolism. Ammonia is markedly elevated in urea cycle defects. Obtain if child has altered level of consciousness, recurrent vomiting, or metabolic acidosis with increased anion gap is present.	Ammonia and lactate must be drawn without the use of a tourniquet. Blood should be free-flowing or result can be falsely elevated. Arterial sample is preferred for this reason. Blood sample is placed on ice and should be analyzed immediately.
Liver function panel or hepatic panel (should include bilirubin, transaminase, partial thromboplastin time, prothrombin time)	Evaluation of hepatic function	Hepatic involvement seen in conditions such as Menkes disease and Wilson disease	Sample may be obtained at same time as completing other blood specimens.
Urine Tests			
Ketones	Helpful in differentiating causes and types of metabolic disorders	Ketones are elevated in many metabolic disorders and low in others.	Urine kept at room temperature for 1 hour or more before testing may produce a false-negative result.

Diagnostic Test or Procedure	Purpose	Findings and Indications	Health Care Provider Responsibilities
Urine analysis, urine-reducing substances, assessment of urine odor	Deviation from normal ranges helpful in determining presence of metabolic disorder or in determining whether another causative factor exists for child's clinical presentation.	Accumulated substrates from faulty metabolic pathways will be present in the urine. Certain metabolic disorders have distinctive odors (e.g., maple syrup urine smells like burned sugar or maple syrup).	Note type of formula or food intake before the test. If 24-hour urine collection is needed, ensure that all urine is collected. Assist family to help young children who may be forgetful. For infants, drain the 24-hour collection bag frequently to help maintain stability of bag adhering to the child. Penicillin administration may cause a false positive for reducing substances.
Urine amino acids and organic acids	Detects changes in amino acid patterns, thus detecting abnormalities of amino acid transport or metabolism	Defects related to metabolism of amino acids result in increased levels in the urine.	No food or fluid restriction before test. Collect a clean random urine specimen. A 24-hour urine specimen may be requested.
Other Tests			
Mitochondrial DNA analysis	Determines presence of abnormal genes involved in inborn errors of metabolism	May identify primary genetic abnormality	Parental consent is required. Genetic counseling should be provided. Samples are obtained from a variety of body fluids and tissues. Test results may take weeks or months.
Liver biopsy	Determines extent of hepatic involvement	Hepatic involvement seen in Menkes disease and Wilson disease	Parental consent must be obtained. Monitor biopsy site, noting any bleeding and intervening if it occurs.
Skin biopsy, muscle biopsy	Evaluates skin and muscle fibroblasts and evaluates for presence of mitochondrial disease; skin biopsy may also determine enzyme assays	Mitochondrial disease will show alterations in muscle tissue.	Because these tests are more invasive, they would usually be performed only when index of suspicion for metabolic disease is high. Blood and urine tests should have been obtained prior to biopsies.

NURSING INTERVENTIONS 27-1

Guidelines for Completing Newborn Screening

- All newborns complete newborn screening before discharge from the newborn nursery, preferably between 24 and 72 hours of age and in no case later than 7 days of life.
- Screening of premature or sick infants is completed as close as possible to the time of discharge from the nursery or at or near the seventh day of age regardless of feeding status.

- If the initial specimen for newborn screening is collected before 12 hours of age, a second specimen should be collected at 1–2 weeks of age.
- Complete screening before transfusion or dialysis, if the child's condition permits. If the infant requires a blood transfusion or dialysis before the specimen is collected, complete newborn screening 24 hours after the blood transfusion/dialysis is completed.

NUTRITIONAL MANAGEMENT

The goal of dietary restriction, the primary treatment modality for inborn errors of metabolism, is to control the substrate accumulation by reducing or eliminating carbohydrates, proteins, or both. Special dietary restrictions and synthetic **medical foods** (formulas as well as foods) are the two most successful methods of controlling the enzyme deficiencies. Medical foods are prescribed by a health care provider to manage a disease or health condition in a child with special nutrient needs; use of these foods requires ongoing evaluation by the health care team. The label on the product must clearly state that the product is intended to be used to manage a specific medical disorder or condition. Provide nutritional counseling for children on special diets and their families (see Nursing Plan of Care 27-1). Strategies to assist the family include

- Assisting the family to obtain specialized infant formulas or medical foods
- Assisting the child and/or family to incorporate individual and ethnic food preferences into the diet of the older child
- Instructing the family and/or child on how to read labels and select appropriate food
- Observing the child and/or family's selection of foods appropriate to the prescribed diet
- Assisting the family in substituting ingredients to conform favorite recipes to the diet
- Providing written meal plans
- Teaching the child and/or family how to keep a food diary and use it as a method for evaluating the child's compliance with the dietary restrictions
- Providing the child and/or family with scenarios to preplan food selection at events such as parties, restaurants, and meals at other people's homes
- Providing written instructions for daycare, preschool, and school officials regarding dietary restrictions

Dietary management changes as the child grows, moving from a formula-based diet to solid foods. These medical foods are required throughout the life span. The pediatric health care provider, the nurse, and the nutritionist can work together to provide the family with a nutritional plan. The diet must incorporate the restrictions mandated by the particular metabolic disorder while considering the child's personal tastes and ethnic preferences. Ensuring that dietary restrictions are maintained outside the child's home environment is often difficult. Providing dietary instructions to daycare and school personnel is a key intervention. When the child attends a social event at which food is served, the family should either inquire beforehand whether appropriate foods will be served or take food items with them that are on the child's diet.

PHARMACOLOGIC MANAGEMENT

Pharmacologic dosages of vitamins and medications may be given in some instances. These products are used to supplement any deficient products or to assist in removing accumulated substrates. Work with the child and family to be certain they understand the importance of continuing pharmacologic therapy for an extended period. In most cases, the treatment is lifelong. The agreeable young child who easily adheres to the treatment regimen may become an independent adolescent who rejects being told what to do. Assisting the maturing child to be actively involved in his or her care and providing the child with a solid understanding of the importance of the pharmacologic and dietary regimen are aspects of the nurse's work with the family.

OTHER THERAPIES

Enzyme therapy is another treatment modality currently being used for some conditions (e.g., Cerezyme, currently in use for Gaucher disease) and researched for others. Enzyme activity can be delivered to such organs as the liver and spleen to treat non-CNS manifestations such as anemia, bone disease, and hepatosplenomegaly.

Liver and bone marrow transplantations have demonstrated some success in halting or slowing the progression of peripheral complications in conditions such as Hurler syndrome and Gaucher disease.

Advances in *gene therapy* bring new hope that metabolic disorders can be managed and, perhaps, cured. In gene therapy, normal genetic information is introduced into defective cells to compensate for genetic defects and correct disease phenotypes. Replacing the defective gene itself (*somatic gene therapy*) is currently being evaluated as a treatment alternative. Ethical issues concerning the harvesting of genetic material and the ability to construct or alter human tissue have kept gene therapy primarily in the research laboratory. However, as these ethical issues are resolved and the technical and medical problems of gene therapy are mastered, this management option is an increasingly attainable goal.

Advances in biochemistry continue to reveal previously unknown metabolic diseases and clarify the basic pathophysiology of known disorders, giving rise to hope for new treatments and improved outcomes for these children and their families. Provide counseling to the child and the family to ensure that they understand the risks, uncertain outcomes, and hardships that are associated with the initiation of therapies that have not yet proved their long-term effectiveness.

> *ANSWER:* Newborn screening tests are important for all newborns, including Sean, because they allow for early diagnosis of inborn metabolic errors. Additionally, these tests provide a baseline for helping to differentiate the wide variety of signs and symptoms of an inborn error disorder from other childhood disorders. Advances in diagnosing and treating these disorders have greatly improved the prognosis for many children. Moreover, positive results of screening tests may be the first and only indicator of a metabolic disorder in an otherwise asymptomatic newborn.

NURSING PLAN OF CARE

Although inborn errors of metabolism can be attributed to a variety of changes occurring in the metabolic pathway, the diseases present many common health care needs for the child and the family. Nursing diagnoses that can be applied to the child with a metabolic disorder reflect the need for long-term management and a focus on supportive care for the family of a child with a chronic, potentially fatal condition. The nursing plan of care focuses on prevention, early diagnosis, and prompt treatment (Nursing Plan of Care 27-1). Several other chapters in this text contain care plans that also apply to children with metabolic disorders. Children with metabolic conditions have chronic conditions that will affect their diets and activities for the rest of their lives, and changes in family roles and lifestyles may be necessary to adapt to these children's needs. Chapter 12 presents the plan of care for the child with a chronic condition and specifically addresses the nursing care concerns related to the family's adaptation to managing the child's chronic condition. Some metabolic disorders cannot be managed effectively, and these children have poor prognoses for survival. Families experience anticipatory grief and loss. Chapter 13 covers palliative care and provides a nursing plan of care for the grieving family. Last, many metabolic conditions are diagnosed during the neonatal period; therefore, the

nursing plan of care in Chapter 14 will be applicable to managing neonates with an altered health state.

ALTERATIONS IN METABOLIC STATUS

Alterations in metabolic status encompass disorders of amino acid, mineral, carbohydrate, and mucopolysaccharide metabolism as well as disorders of mitochondrial function and fatty acid oxidation.

AMINO ACID DISORDERS

Amino acids are the primary building blocks of proteins, which are key factors in many metabolic cycles and may function as neurotransmitters. Even in utero, amino acids are essential to life. Inherited errors of amino acid metabolism occur primarily in catabolic pathways. Most of the associated disorders can result in severe CNS dysfunction. However, early diagnosis, removal of toxic metabolites, promotion of anabolism, and adherence to dietary restrictions can prevent catastrophic outcomes. This section covers two of the most common amino acid disorders: PKU and MSUD. Table 27-2 provides a summary of important features of additional amino acid disorders.

PHENYLKETONURIA

Phenylketonuria, more commonly known as PKU, is the most frequently occurring aminoaciduria. PKU was first recognized in 1934 and is associated with an excess of phenylalanine in the blood.

> QUESTION: You suspect that Sean has PKU. You explain to Joellen that this is an inherited metabolic problem. She asks you, "Then why don't my other two children have the problem?" How would you respond?

The incidence of PKU in North America is approximately 1 in 14,000 to 1 in 20,000 live births (I. Rezvani, 2011). The highest incidence is found in Ireland and Turkey at a rate of 1 in 4,500 births. Ethnic variability occurs: The incidence is highest among whites and Native Americans and lower among blacks, Hispanics, and Asians (I. Rezvani, 2011).

PKU is an autosomal recessive genetic defect in which an enzyme deficiency renders the body unable to metabolize phenylalanine efficiently (see Fig. 3-3). Phenylalanine and its metabolites accumulate in the blood and urine and exert deleterious effects on brain development, especially during the periods of active myelination. A very small subset of patients with PKU does not develop cognitive deficits, however, even without treatment. This fact strongly suggests that modifier genes are responsible for this clinical variation, but none have yet been identified.

The recessive gene that transmits PKU is found on chromosome 12. The defect in the gene for phenylalanine hydroxylase is responsible for more than 400 mutations that allow for more than 10,000 genotype combinations

TABLE 27-2 Selected Amino Acid Disorders

Disorder and Inheritance	Pathophysiology	Significant Clinical Features	Key Diagnostic Findings	Management	Prognosis
Homocystinuria Autosomal recessive (chromosome 21)	Deficient cystathionine beta-synthase Prevents interaction of an intermediate product of the amino acid methionine with serine to form cystathionine	Dislocation of the lens (ectopia lentis) Intellectual disability Convulsions Osteoporosis Arterial and venous vascular thrombosis Limb overgrowth Fair hair and skin Connective tissue deficit, leading to scoliosis	Plasma homocystine 0.02–0.025 μmol/L Plasma methionine up to 2 μmol/L Plasma cystine low Increased homocystine in urine	High doses of pyridoxine (vitamin B_6), 100–500 mg per 24 hours Low-methionine, high-cystine diet Use of low-methionine formulas	Progress of the disease may not be stemmed.
Isovaleric acidemia Autosomal recessive (chromosome 15)	Deficient isovaleryl-CoA dehydrogenase	Intellectual disability Acidosis Vomiting Lethargy Coma Body has distinctive odor of sweaty feet during acute illness	Isovaleric acid in blood and urine	Low-protein, specific low-leucine diet	Near-normal intelligence if compliant with diet
Methylmalonic acidemia Autosomal recessive (chromosome 6)	Possible defect in the B_{12} coenzyme	Low blood pH Lethargy Vomiting Seizures Failure to thrive Intellectual disability	Methylmalonic acid in blood and urine	B_{12} unresponsive: low-protein diet B_{12} responsive: B_{12} in large doses	B_{12} unresponsive: death usually in infancy B_{12} responsive: normal growth and development
Tyrosinemia type I Autosomal recessive	Defect in which an enzyme is missing to break down the amino acid tyrosine	Poor appetite and failure to grow normally Vomiting Diarrhea, bloody stools A cabbagelike odor Jaundice (yellow skin and whites of eyes) Liver dysfunction leading to cirrhosis Irritability Lethargy (overwhelming tiredness) Kidney problems	Succinylacetone present in urine Abnormal liver function tests	Restriction of the amount of tyrosine and another amino acid, phenylalanine, in the baby's food Administration of nitisinone (Orfadin) to reduce toxic effects of tyrosine in the body Liver transplantation may be needed.	May cause death from liver failure

(Gambol, 2007). To have PKU, the child must receive the defective gene from both parents. Thus, the chance of a PKU birth when both parents are carriers is one in four. An estimated 1 person out of 50 is an asymptomatic heterozygous carrier of the PKU gene.

> ANSWER: You would need to explain to Joellen that PKU is an autosomal recessive genetic defect. For Sean to have the disorder, both parents must carry the recessive gene. However, even in this case, when both parents each carry the defective gene, the chance of a child having PKU is one in four.

If untreated, PKU almost always leads to severe, irreparable damage to the CNS. With adequate dietary treatment, however, the prognosis is good. The success of childhood treatment for PKU has led to increasing prevalence of maternal PKU. Childbearing women who have PKU are at risk for having infants with psychomotor retardation (92%), intrauterine growth retardation (40%), microcephaly (73%), or congenital heart defects (10%) (AAP, Committee on Genetics, 2008). High maternal phenylalanine levels have a teratogenic effect on the fetus, and defects are directly associated with the degree to which maternal phenylalanine levels are elevated. Dietary management throughout pregnancy must be extremely rigid for optimal neonatal outcomes to occur. Infants may or may not be born with PKU themselves, although the incidence of hyperphenylalaninemia is higher among infants born to PKU mothers. Approximately 1 in 120 infants born to a mother with PKU will inherit an abnormal gene from both parents and be affected by PKU (AAP, Committee on Genetics, 2008).

Pathophysiology

The exact pathogenic mechanisms of PKU have not been determined. Phenylalanine is an essential amino acid found in all protein foods. During a child's early growth period, approximately 50% of the phenylalanine in the normal daily intake is used for protein synthesis. As growth slows, the amount of phenylalanine needed by the body diminishes. Normally, excess phenylalanine is converted in the liver, pancreas, and kidneys to tyrosine (I. Rezvani, 2011). In the most severe (classic) form of PKU, the hepatic enzyme phenylalanine hydroxylase is completely inactive. This lack of enzymatic activity results in a buildup of phenylalanine and its metabolites, which affects numerous areas of metabolism, including the conversion of phenylalanine to tyrosine. Tyrosine plays an important role in the development of the CNS. It is the precursor of dopamine and norepinephrine. Tyrosine is also a substrate in the synthesis of thyroxine and melanin, which affect growth and pigmentation of the skin, hair, and eyes.

Assessment

 QUESTION: Sean was scheduled for testing after his discharge from the hospital. Why wasn't the testing done in the hospital before discharge?

Infants with PKU appear normal for about the first 3 to 6 months of life. Vomiting, sometimes mimicking the presentation seen in pyloric stenosis, may be severe and may lead to misdiagnosis. Be alert to this potential for misdiagnosis. After the first 6 months of life, an untreated child begins to excrete phenylacetic acid in the urine and perspiration and to manifest signs and symptoms of the tyrosine deficiency. These include severe psychomotor retardation, microcephaly, seizures, and hyperactivity. The child may develop a clumsy gait, fine tremors of the hands, poor coordination, odd posturing, or repetitious digital mannerisms. The inability to produce melanin causes hypopigmentation of the hair, eyes, and skin; untreated children with PKU are very blond and fair-skinned compared with their parents. Eczema occurs in 25% of untreated children. A musty or mousey odor from the child's urine and sweat is a classic sign of PKU but may not be noticed by the family because they are around the child daily. The nurse may note this odor during a routine physical examination or during the initial assessment of a child being evaluated for developmental delay. Clinical manifestations of PKU are rarely seen in countries where newborn screening programs are mandated and followed (I. Rezvani, 2011).

Diagnostic Tests

Plasma phenylalanine levels of >20 mg/dL are indicative of PKU. At birth, an infant with PKU has normal phenylalanine levels because of the rapid placental exchange of amino acids occurring in utero. However, these levels increase sharply after the baby has been fed because most formulas and breast milk contain

phenylalanine. Screening for PKU is mandated in all 50 states in the United States. Three screening methods are available: the Guthrie Bacterial Inhibition Assay, automated fluorometric assay, and tandem mass spectrometry (U.S. Preventive Services Task Force, 2008). The Guthrie Bacterial Inhibition Assay remains the most commonly used test to detect phenylalanine in blood. In this test, a drop of blood is obtained with a heel stick and is collected on special filter paper (Fig. 27-2). This test is performed routinely by nurses in the nursery, home setting, or health care provider's office. The screening is performed after 24 hours of life but before the infant is 7 days old. Infants tested within the first 24 hours after birth should receive a repeat screening test within 2 weeks. Premature infants and those with illnesses are tested at or near 7 days of age (U.S. Preventive Services Task Force, 2008).

caREminder

When obtaining blood for the Guthrie Bacterial Inhibition Assay, ensure that the first drop of blood is large enough to fill the imprinted space on the filter paper. Squeezing out more blood onto the paper creates a layering effect that can produce a false-positive test result.

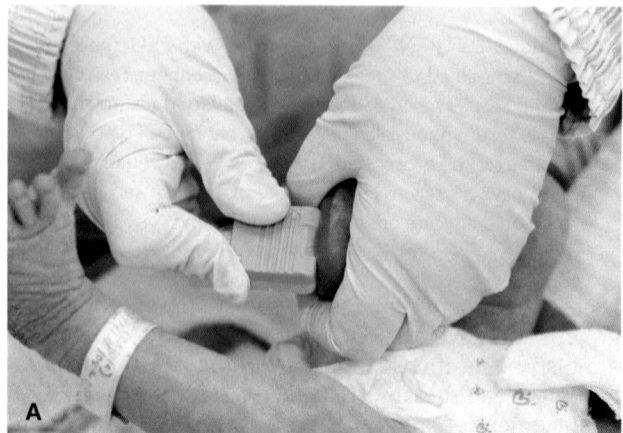
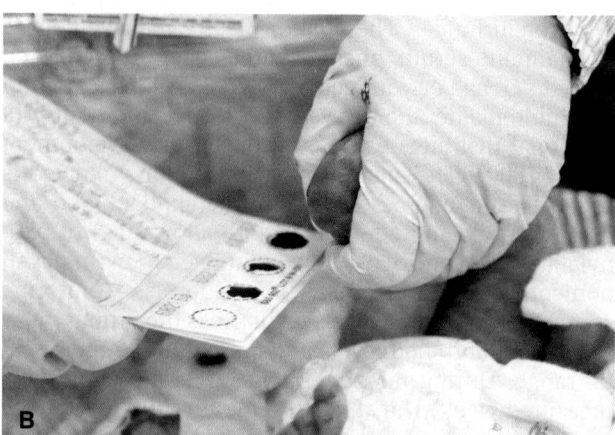

Figure 27-2 Screening for PKU. (A) Performing a heel stick. (B) Applying blood specimen to the card for screening.

Other diagnostic laboratory findings include a normal plasma tyrosine level and elevated urine metabolites such as phenylpyruvic acid, phenylacetic acid, and phenylacetylglutamine.

ANSWER: At birth, an infant with PKU has normal phenylalanine levels because of the rapid placental exchange of amino acids occurring in utero. However, these levels increase sharply after the baby has been fed because most formulas and breast milk contain phenylalanine. To ensure the accuracy of the testing results, testing should occur 48–72 hours after birth to make sure that the infant has had an adequate intake of breast milk or formula. Sean was discharged when he was 24 hours old. Therefore, testing was scheduled to occur after he was discharged.

Nursing Diagnoses and Outcomes

Management of the child with PKU focuses on early detection and intervention to avert the deleterious effects of the disease process. See Nursing Plan of Care 27-1 and thePoint Care Path: An Interdisciplinary Plan of Care for the Infant With PKU for examples of the nursing diagnoses and interdisciplinary care that can be instituted for the newly diagnosed child and his or her family.

Interdisciplinary Interventions

QUESTION: Sean is diagnosed with PKU. Joellen is scheduled to speak to a nutritionist about Sean's diet, and Sean is scheduled for follow-up blood testing to evaluate serum phenylalanine levels. What type of diet would you expect to be prescribed, how often would you expect Sean to have his serum levels checked, and what serum levels would indicate effectiveness of therapy?

Dietary treatment remains the safest option for optimal growth and development. Newer cell-directed therapies are also being investigated, including cell transplantation and gene therapy (Belanger-Quintana et al., 2011). Management of children with PKU focuses on preventing excessive accumulation of phenylalanine by restricting protein intake. The goal of dietary management is to maintain serum phenylalanine levels for children 12 years of age or younger between 2 and 6 mg/dL and for children older than 12 years between 2 and 10 mg/dL (National Institutes of Health Consensus Development Panel, 2000). The amount of phenylalanine allowed is based on ongoing assessment of the child's blood and urine phenylalanine levels. Dietary allowances of phenylalanine change depending on hunger, growth, development, and serum phenylalanine levels. Monitoring serum phenylalanine levels regularly is the primary way to ensure that blood levels remain within the therapeutic range. During infancy, blood levels are commonly measured weekly for the first 6 months and then every other week until 1 year of age. At 1 year and thereafter, monitoring usually occurs at the time of routine health surveillance visits (see Chapter 8).

Nutritional Management During Infancy

Begin dietary intervention within the first weeks of life. Typically, the infant and family are instructed by a nutritionist experienced with dietary restrictions for children with metabolic disorders. At each contact throughout the child's life, reinforce this teaching and assess adherence to dietary restrictions. Either the nutritionist or the nurse will assist the family in obtaining the formula for home use. A referral to social services is appropriate and will be a long-term need for the family to ensure that they have a reimbursement mechanism to purchase formula.

Infants diagnosed with PKU may continue to breastfeed. When a diagnosis has been made, the child's phenylalanine level needs to be reduced as quickly as possible. This is achieved through the use of a PKU medical food product. However, a small amount of natural protein is needed in the infant's diet and can be provided through breast milk. The phenylalanine content of breast milk varies from mother to mother. It is highest in the colostrum and declines with the duration of lactation. The phenylalanine content of the breast milk is counted toward the child's needs. Generally, the number of breastfeedings to be allowed in a 24-hour period is specified (two to four feedings), with phenylalanine-free formula given at the other times. Infants who are not breastfed are given a different medical food that contains some phenylalanine necessary for growth and development. Work with the mother to develop a system to keep track of the number of times she is breastfeeding each day.

Medical foods, sold in powder form, are a chief source of nutrition for infants and children with PKU. These foods are low in phenylalanine and contain vitamins, minerals, and, in some cases, carbohydrates and fats (e.g., Lofenalac, Phenyl-Free 2). Medical foods are reconstituted as formulas for infants and as milk substitutes for older children. The proteins in the medical foods have a characteristic flavor and, in some cases, aroma that are different from those of regular formula.

KidKare When the medical food is introduced within the first few months of life, infants usually grow accustomed to the flavor and readily accept the formula. If PKU is diagnosed late, the older infant or child is likely to find the taste of the medical food unacceptable. If the family encounters this problem, recommend that they try preflavored medical foods, which may be better accepted. Older children can use flavored powdered drink mixes to make the medical food more appealing.

The particular type and brand of medical food used are based on the child's age, dietary likes and dislikes, variations in dietary needs, and the cost and availability to the family. The cost of all formulas and many foods are covered by insurance or public health programs, but not all families and states have the same level of coverage.

If the family is having difficulty adhering to the nutritional recommendations, financial hardship might be the reason. If the family is not already in contact with social services, ensure that they are referred.

Nutritional Management Beyond Infancy

As solid foods are added to the diet, high-protein foods such as meat, fish, poultry, cheese, eggs, milk, nuts, beans, peas, and flour require the most severe limitations. Legumes, grains, and potatoes also have a relatively high phenylalanine content. The PKU diet is based on a food exchange list. Ingestion of a phenylalanine-free formula continues to be a key element of the child's diet throughout childhood, providing a significant portion of the child's protein calories, vitamins, and minerals. In addition, the food exchange lists include vegetables, fruits, breads, cereals, fats, miscellaneous, and "free" foods that are allowed on the diet.

ALERT *Advise families not to use products sweetened with aspartame, including those marked with the brand name NutraSweet and Equal, because they contain phenylalanine. Products sweetened with sucralose, marketed as Splenda, are allowable in the diet of a child with PKU.*

Assist the family and the older child to become adept at reading labels on packaged foods and beverages. Even in many foods not considered protein sources, phenylalanine may appear in the form of NutraSweet or Equal (Fig. 27-3).

Current recommendations are that all affected adults and children should be kept on a phenylalanine-restricted diet for life. Discontinuing dietary restrictions can cause deterioration of IQ and cognitive performance (I. Rezvani, 2011). Dietary counseling and monitoring of phenylalanine levels are recommended for all girls and women of childbearing age (AAP, Committee on Genetics, 2008).

ALERT *Elevated maternal phenylalanine concentrations during pregnancy can lead to adverse fetal outcomes such as microcephaly, intellectual disability, and fetal anomalies. Provide genetic and nutritional counseling to pregnant girls and women with PKU before (if possible) and after conception.*

Protein catabolism occurs during infection and may cause serum phenylalanine levels to become elevated. Illnesses that involve decreased appetite or vomiting may also affect the child's phenylalanine levels. In these cases, serum levels should be monitored, the medical food should be continued, and fluid intake must be increased. Tea, gelatin, and carbonated beverages are appropriate to offer.

ALERT *Overtreatment for PKU can cause a phenylalanine deficiency. The child with PKU does not synthesize phenylalanine. Teach families the signs and symptoms of phenylalanine deficiency: loss of appetite, vomiting, lethargy, failure to thrive, and malaise. The family can readily reverse these manifestations by feeding the child small volumes of milk.*

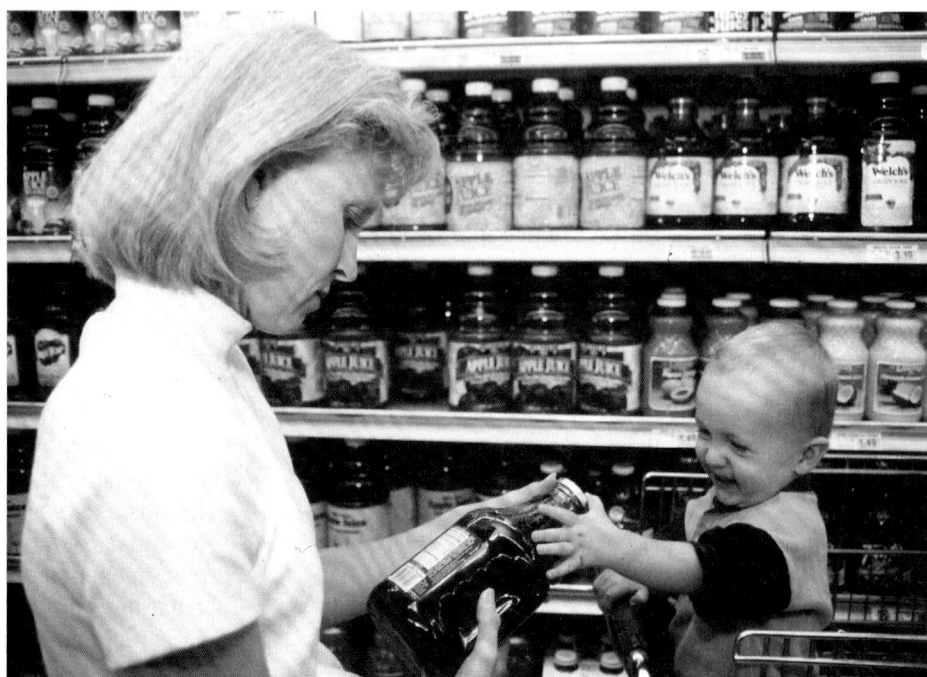

Figure 27-3 When buying food for the child with PKU, parents must examine product labels to check for aspartame (e.g., NutraSweet and Equal), which must be avoided. Products containing sucralose, marketed as Splenda, are acceptable.

ANSWER: Typically, a child with PKU receives a protein-restricted diet. For Sean, who is an infant, breast milk or medical food, sold in powder form, is the chief source of nutrition. Medical foods are reconstituted as formulas for infants and then as milk substitutes for older children. It is important to remember that phenylalanine is an essential amino acid necessary for growth and development. During infancy, the child obtains phenylalanine as a part of the medical formula or through breast milk. Diet is based on the child's blood and urine phenylalanine levels in conjunction with the child's hunger and growth and development. Follow-up testing of serum levels would be scheduled weekly for the first 6 months and then every other week until 1 year of age. Then it is checked during routine health visits, unless more frequent monitoring is warranted. Therapy is considered effective when Sean's serum phenylalanine levels are maintained between 2 and 6 mg/dL through the age of 12 years.

Community Care

The nurse's ongoing role in managing the care of the child with PKU centers on educating the family, the child, other caregivers, and school personnel. Teaching that reinforces the dietary regimen is critical to managing PKU successfully. Growth and developmental changes necessitate adaptation of the dietary plan. As the child matures, he or she must learn to manage the diet and take more responsibility for dietary choices. The family may seek advice and intervention to cope with the child who challenges the treatment plan (Developmental Considerations 27-2). Studies have shown that family cohesion and adherence to the restricted diet correlate positively with higher IQ levels. Thus, assessing family dynamics and implementing interventions to support the family under stress are important nursing interventions to enhance the long-term outcomes of these children and their families. Family counseling and participation in support groups

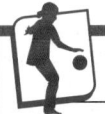

DEVELOPMENTAL CONSIDERATIONS 27-2

When the Child Does Not Want to Follow the Phenylketonuria Treatment Plan

Age	Reasons	Interventions
Infancy	Dislike taste of medical formula Dislike smell of formula when switching from bottle to the cup	Purchase formulas that can be easily served in a bottle to hide the smell. When foods are being introduced, begin with a paste of the medical food and water.
Early childhood	Assertion of autonomy Dislike taste Desire to explore tastes of "forbidden" foods	Encourage the introduction of the cup and self-feeding skills. Use flavorings to alter the taste of the medical food. Encourage the family not to be overly protective.
Middle childhood	Embarrassment or being self-conscious at school because they are eating something "different" from others Desire to have more control Eating lunch away from home, which makes it easy to disregard the diet	Be sure the child understands the condition. Give the child responsibility for the diet. Let the child choose and prepare his or her own medical food. Let the child select at what times the medical food is eaten. Let the child answer others' questions about the diet.
Adolescence	Rejection of authority Desire to have more control Poor eating habits of adolescence associated with busy schedule Development of physical and sexual identity	Allow the intake of free foods such as soda and candy, while still assisting the adolescent to maintain his or her weight. Have the adolescent explain the diet to friends as a vegetarian diet with a special formula. Provide genetic counseling and information regarding the risks and requirements of a PKU pregnancy.

can improve the family's coping abilities and strengthen the child's ability to manage the diet independently as the child becomes older.

Assist the family by providing information to all family caregivers, daycare providers, and school officials regarding the child's dietary restrictions. After the child enters the school setting, most school lunches can be adapted to fit the child's prescribed diet. These community care providers also need information regarding symptoms that indicate that appropriate phenylalanine levels are not being maintained.

Routine analysis of serum phenylalanine is a part of the continuing care of the child with PKU. Family members can be taught how to do routine blood collection but, at times, may need assistance in collecting the samples, especially if the child becomes combative and resistant to sampling.

MAPLE SYRUP URINE DISEASE

MSUD is an inherited autosomal recessive disorder of branched-chain amino acid catabolism—specifically, a deficiency of branched-chain 2-oxoacid dehydrogenase (see Fig. 3-3). The name comes from the sweet odor of maple syrup found in body fluids, particularly the cerumen (ear wax) and urine of infants with this condition.

Worldwide, the incidence of MSUD is 1 in 185,000 live births (Packman et al., 2012). The incidence is as high as approximately 1 in 380 live births in selected Mennonite settlements in Pennsylvania, Kentucky, New York, Indiana, Wisconsin, Michigan, Iowa, and Missouri (Strauss et al., 2009).

Untreated, the child with MSUD will die as early as 7 days of life. Early diagnosis and management substantially influence the prognosis for children with MSUD. Generally, the more severely the metabolic pathway is disturbed and the longer the resulting high levels of leucine remain, the poorer the child's prognosis. Injury to the child's brain from encephalopathy is the most common cause of developmental delays. Relatively normal intellectual outcomes are possible with early intervention, appropriate sick-day management under the guidance of a health care provider, and consistent dietary management.

Pathophysiology

 QUESTION: You know that Sean has been diagnosed with PKU. How are Sean's signs and symptoms similar to and different from those associated with MSUD?

In MSUD, the inborn error of metabolism results in deficient oxidative decarboxylation of the alpha-keto acids of the branched-chain amino acids: leucine, isoleucine, and valine. Accumulation of these amino acids, particularly leucine, causes severe neurologic symptoms. Variant forms of the disease, in which some residual activity of branched-chain oxoacid dehydrogenase occurs, have a more insidious onset and less severe course. The three variant forms are intermittent MSUD,

mild or intermediate MSUD, and thiamine-responsive MSUD. This chapter covers only the more prevalent, classic form of MSUD. The classic form produces severe intellectual disability unless intervention begins immediately after birth.

Infants appear normal at birth; but within the first week of life, acid–base, gastrointestinal, and neurologic problems appear. Initial signs of MSUD, usually occurring within 48 hours of delivery, include poor feeding, a maple syrup odor in cerumen, ketonuria, and vomiting. Subsequent to the first 2 days of life, infants develop deepening encephalopathy characterized by intermittent hypertonicity, lethargy, opisthotonos, and respiratory irregularities. Hypoglycemia is common, but infants do not clinically improve when glucose is administered intravenously as might be anticipated. Without intervention, symptoms progress to dehydration, convulsions, severe ketoacidosis, acute pancreatitis, coma, and death within 7 to 10 days. The three common causes of injury to the brain in MSUD are hyponatremia and cerebral edema, acute and chronic essential amino acid deficiencies, and inadequate follow-up care during recurrent and acute illnesses.

ANSWER: With PKU and MSUD, both inborn errors of metabolism, infants appear normal at birth. Vomiting also occurs; however, with MSUD, the vomiting occurs within 48 hours of birth. Sean did not experience vomiting until a couple of weeks ago. Additionally, neurologic symptoms are usually severe and symptoms progress rapidly with MSUD, such that death may occur. Sean's symptoms seem to have progressed slowly and the only neurologic-type findings noted were lagging developmental milestones, hyperactivity, and fine hand tremors.

Assessment

The key goal in assessment is early diagnosis. Newborn screening assists in early diagnosis. The nurse may be the first to recognize MSUD, typically by noting the characteristic maple syrup smell of the neonate's urine when changing his or her diapers; but this observation may not occur until 3 to 7 days after birth. Report any odd odor of the urine (often characterized as smelling like maple syrup or burned sugar) immediately to the health care provider. The maple syrup odor in cerumen (ear wax) is evident within 24 hours of birth and should be assessed if any suspicion or risk factors for MSUD exist (Strauss et al., 2009).

Diagnostic Tests

All states require newborn screening for MSUD. Tandem mass spectroscopy is the most reliable method of testing. If a suspicion of MSUD exists, testing routinely done includes plasma amino acids and urine organic acids. Ketonuria, as detected by use of standard urine strip tests, is present in MSUD. Additional laboratory findings that indicate MSUD are increased levels of leucine, isoleucine, valine, keto acids, and alloisoleucine in both plasma and urine.

As an autosomal recessive condition, when both parents carry the abnormal gene, the child has a 50% chance of being a carrier, 25% chance of being affected, and 25% chance of being normal. Molecular genetic testing of healthy children and prenatal testing is available if the condition has been detected in a family member.

Nursing Diagnoses and Outcomes

A nursing plan of care for the child with a metabolic disease is presented in Nursing Plan of Care 27-1. The Nursing Plan of Care in Chapter 14 is an additional resource for care planning for the neonate with altered health status. In addition, the following nursing diagnoses and outcomes apply to the child with MSUD during the neonatal period:

Nursing Diagnosis: Ineffective infant feeding pattern related to neurologic deterioration
Outcome: The family will demonstrate appropriate feeding techniques to ensure that the infant is receiving adequate nutrition.
Nursing Diagnosis: Risk for deficient fluid volume related to initiation of therapies to remove toxic metabolites (peritoneal dialysis, hemodialysis, hemofiltration)
Outcome: Infant will not experience vascular, cellular, or intracellular dehydration as a result of therapies to remove the toxic metabolites.

Interdisciplinary Interventions

The management goals for MSUD are to establish an early diagnosis, remove the toxic metabolites, and prevent tissue catabolism. Long-term treatment includes dietary leucine restriction; high-calorie, branched-chain amino acid–free formulas; and frequent monitoring. Liver transplantation is a reasonable treatment option for classic MSUD (Mazariegos et al., 2012).

Medical Management

Management of the neonate with suspected or confirmed MSUD in an intensive care setting is required. The complications from encephalopathy and metabolic decompensation necessitate frequent health care monitoring and interventions. Careful monitoring of the neonate's hydration and electrolyte status and treatment to adjust amino acid and electrolyte levels have been found to be effective for even the most extreme elevations of plasma leucine (Strauss et al., 2009). In MSUD, nutritional management alone does not decrease leucine levels quickly enough to reduce the risk of brain damage. Therefore, for the neonate, the initial treatment includes frequent adjustments in intravenous fluids and formulas with additives to control cerebral edema, minimize water retention, prevent catabolism, and maintain clinical stability while allowing weight gain and growth.

Debate exists about whether peritoneal dialysis, hemodialysis, or hemofiltration are required to remove the high levels of the branched-chain amino acids and their metabolites. These procedures involve a risk of infection and increased catabolism.

The family may feel intimidated and frightened by the sudden changes in their neonate's condition and the need to have the neonate in the intensive care unit. Work with the social worker and child life specialist to provide support and teaching to assist the family through the crisis associated with the initial diagnosis and rigorous treatment methods.

Nutritional Management

After the toxic metabolites have been removed, or their levels decreased, dietary management is the primary component of ongoing treatment of MSUD. The required diet is high in calories but restricted in leucine, isoleucine, and valine. The diet should be started immediately after diagnosis and at least by the fifth day of life. Breastfeeding can be continued to provide some nutrition and as a method of promoting bonding and nurturing between mother and child. However, all infants diagnosed with MSUD must be provided formula that meets their special dietary needs. Several proprietary formulas free of branched-chain amino acids are available. If the neonate demonstrates feeding difficulties, nasogastric feedings may be needed to ensure that nutritional health is maintained. As the infant gains strength and neurologic symptoms resolve, feeding problems may resolve and the infant can be bottle-fed once again.

Plasma levels are monitored at least every week during the rapid growth phase of infancy and frequently throughout the child's life. Plasma leucine concentration should range from 150 to 300 μmol/L with an age-appropriate intake.

Ongoing management with restricted intake of the branched-chain amino acids leucine, isoleucine, and valine must be adjusted according to plasma levels. Dietary management for the asymptomatic infant or young child also includes glutamine; alanine; Omega-3 polyunsaturated fatty acids as alpha linolenic acid; and age-appropriate intake for vitamins, minerals, and micronutrients (Strauss et al., 2009).

caREminder

Attention to the potential presence of catabolic states, even during minor illnesses, must continue throughout life. Instruct the family to contact the metabolic health care team to provide guidance during acute illnesses that may cause a catabolic state.

Community Care

When the child is ill, protein intake should be reduced and caloric intake should be increased by encouraging consumption of carbohydrate- and fat-containing foods (Strauss et al., 2009). Teach the family how to perform tests for urinary ketones, keto acids, or both at home if they note any changes in their child's behavior, if the child has an illness that could cause a metabolic imbalance, or if the child is having difficulty adhering to prescribed dietary restrictions. Early treatment of dehydration and acidosis may prevent death. When the affected child has surgery for any reason, postoperative management must focus on the accelerated breakdown of body proteins that occurs postoperatively, which results in high metabolite levels.

Family education goals should focus on reinforcing the need for the prescribed dietary regimen, the importance of follow-up appointments, and sick-day management. As the child grows, the frequency and severity of crisis events decrease, although lifelong dietary management is required. Genetic counseling should be provided to family members because identification of carriers of this metabolic condition is possible.

MINERAL DISORDERS

Mineral disorders are inherited defects characterized by alterations in metabolic pathways for the essential body metals: iron, copper, zinc, magnesium, molybdenum, and manganese. The defects can affect absorption, transport, cellular use, storage, or excretion of a mineral needed to perform certain body functions and thereby produce a variety of sequelae. Three of these disorders—Menkes disease, X-linked hypophosphatemic rickets, and Wilson disease—are covered in this chapter. Table 27-3 highlights other selected mineral disorders.

MENKES DISEASE

Menkes disease is also called *Menkes syndrome* or *trichopoliodystrophy*. An X-linked recessive gene causes Menkes disease. This rare disorder, most typically affecting males, is sometimes called kinky hair or steely hair syndrome because it causes a unique kinky conformation of the hair strands. Its hallmark is an extreme copper deficiency.

Infants with Menkes disease have a life expectancy of 4 months to 17 years. Certain mutations of the syndrome are receptive to treatment, but children with other mutations derive no benefit and progress to death by 3 years of age despite early treatment. Death is usually attributable to intracranial hemorrhages, uncontrolled convulsions, severe failure to thrive, infection, or some combination of these factors. In some variants of the disease with milder expression of the phenotype, survival into early adult years is possible with early treatment.

Pathophysiology

The primary defect in Menkes disease is caused by mutations of *ATP7A*, an X-chromosomal gene that leads to an abnormal cellular copper transport and reduced activities of numerous copper-dependent enzymes (Kodama et al., 2012). The available amount of the copper proenzymes dopamine hydroxylase and cytochrome-*c* oxidase are reduced, and levels of **ceruloplasmin** (a glycoprotein to which most of the copper in the blood is attached) are low. As a result, the brain's content of unsaturated fatty acids is decreased. Tissues such as the brain, liver, and muscle are subject to increased lipofuscin and degenerative changes. Malformation of connective tissue results in vascular, skeletal, dermal, and urogenital defects. Because copper does not cross the placenta, copper may be reduced in the liver and brain of affected individuals at birth.

Assessment

The mutated gene causing Menkes disease has been identified, making carrier testing possible. A detailed family history and genetic assessment can determine females at risk for producing affected offspring. Antenatal diagnosis in at-risk pregnancies can be made by measuring the uptake and retention of copper in vitro using cultured amniotic fibroblasts. Genetic testing may also identify family members with variants of the disease.

Most children with Menkes disease begin to exhibit symptoms by the age of 2 to 3 months. Some initial, nonspecific signs include poor feeding, failure to thrive, hypotonia, and hypothermia. Psychomotor developmental arrest, loss of developmental milestones, and general myoclonic seizures may occur if the disease continues undetected. Some affected children present later in childhood and show slowed growth, intellectual impairment, and neurologic deficits.

These signs should alert the nurse to perform a thorough physical assessment. Children with Menkes disease have several characteristic features. Scalp hair is classically short, twisted, coarse, sparse, and very brittle or kinky; the same hair is often noted on the eyebrows. The infant's face is "jowly," with sagging skin at the cheeks, and the ears appear large for the face. The palate tends to be high arched, and tooth eruption is often delayed. Pectus excavatum (a midline narrowing of the thoracic cavity, also described as *funnel chest*) is a common thoracic finding. Cognitive difficulties can also be noted. These children often have dysphagia, hypotonia, apnea, and spasticity with hyperreflexia. Ophthalmologic findings such as retinal degeneration, aberrant lashes with a texture similar to that of the rest of the hair, optic atrophy, cataracts, iris hypoplasia, and peripheral iris transillumination are usually present.

Diagnostic Tests

When the health care team's suspicions are aroused by the physical examination, laboratory values and genetic testing can confirm the diagnosis. Laboratory findings indicative of Menkes disease include hypocupremia (serum copper <11 μmol/L or <70 μg/dL), hypoceruloplasminemia (ceruloplasmin <200 mg/L), and low hepatic copper concentrations (<50 μg/g dry weight). The radiographic findings show abnormalities of bone formation in the skull (particularly of the wormian bones), metaphyseal spurring (primarily of the femur or other long bones), and anterior flaring or multiple fractures of the ribs. Magnetic resonance imaging often reveals tortuosity and elongation of cerebral and systemic arteries, with occlusion of some vessels, diffuse atrophy with ventriculomegaly, and white matter abnormalities that reflect impaired myelination.

Interdisciplinary Interventions

Therapy for Menkes disease is both palliative and supportive. Current treatment for classic Menkes disease consists of administering copper histidine (copper

TABLE 27-3	Selected Mineral Disorders				
Disorder and Inheritance	**Pathophysiology**	**Significant Clinical Features**	**Key Diagnostic Findings**	**Management**	**Prognosis**
Primary hypomagnesemia Autosomal recessive (chromosome unknown)	Intestinal malabsorption of magnesium	Small for gestational age Sleeping and feeding difficulties during infancy Progressive neurologic dysfunction (hyperactivity, tetany, convulsions) Renal tubular acidosis	Hypomagnesemia, <0.7 μmol/L Hypocalcemia Hypokalemia	Parenteral or intramuscular magnesium for acute symptoms, followed by oral supplements Calcium supplements	Well controlled if management maintained
Acrodermatitis enteropathica Autosomal recessive (chromosome unknown)	Systemic zinc deficiency	Irritability Dermatitis Alopecia Diarrhea Failure to thrive	Plasma zinc concentrations <50 mcg/dL	Zinc supplements of 1–3 mg/kg/day	Progressive deterioration without treatment In less severe cases, only growth retardation and delayed development are evident.
Hereditary hemochromatosis Autosomal recessive (chromosome 6); signs and symptoms rarely manifested in childhood	Excessive accumulation of iron causing extensive tissue damage	Joint pain Fatigue Weakness Various signs of major organ involvement (i.e., diabetes mellitus, hepatosplenomegaly)	Serum iron >25 μmol/L Serum transferrin saturation >45%	Phlebotomy to reduce iron	Organ damage can be prevented with treatment.

salts). Copper histidine is a copper replacement that is injected directly into the body to avoid absorption by the gastrointestinal system. Parenteral administration of copper histidine can correct the serum and hepatic copper deficiencies, deliver copper to brain cells, and make copper available for use by enzymes. In some variants of the disease, early treatment may be effective. However, copper histidine treatments will not reverse any of the child's presenting neurologic symptoms. A small subgroup of children benefit from these treatments if begun within days after birth. Pharmacologic management of seizures and infection should be initiated as these sequelae occur throughout the child's life span.

Beyond daily copper medications, other treatments are primarily symptomatic and supportive. Radiant heat using an infant warmer may be required to correct hypothermia, especially during the neonatal period. Vigilant monitoring of the child for early signs of infection (e.g., elevated temperature, vomiting, fussiness) enables specific workup and management. Observing for focal or generalized seizures permits early anticonvulsant therapy. Gentle handling of the child and padding of the crib sides help to minimize the risk of fracture and should also be carried out at home. Provide a high-calorie diet with careful monitoring of the child's weight gain. If vomiting caused by gastroesophageal reflux occurs, positioning and possibly nasogastric feedings may be necessary.

Assist the infant or child thrive to his or her greatest potential while supporting the family in the care techniques to achieve this goal. The families of children with Menkes disease are most likely to display grief as they cope with their child's terminal prognosis (see Chapter 13). Further stress is added because of the implications for future pregnancies. Groups of parents whose children have the same or similar problem are frequently helpful, as are groups focusing on palliative care support. Provide the family with contact information for these groups. The possibility of frequent hospitalizations for complications may require financial counseling. The coordination of acute care, home care agencies, and possibly a hospice service should be established by either social services or a nurse case manager as needs arise.

X-LINKED HYPOPHOSPHATEMIC RICKETS

X-linked hypophosphatemic rickets is a hereditary, X-linked dominant, renal phosphate wasting disorder (see Fig. 3-3). Spontaneous genetic mutations are also thought to occur because both autosomal recessive and autosomal dominant variants have been described. Prevalence in the United States is not known.

Pathophysiology

The defects associated with X-linked hypophosphatemic rickets are caused by mutations in the phosphate-regulating endopeptidase (*PHEX*) gene (Rajah et al., 2011). The condition is characterized by defective renal tubular reabsorption of phosphate, leading to phosphaturia (excess of phosphates in the urine) and

hypophosphatemia (deficiency of phosphates in the blood). Poor reabsorption of phosphate leads to abnormalities in bone and dental formation.

Early, adequate management of phosphorus and calcium levels usually results in normal bone development. In some patients, the phosphorus deficiency resolves spontaneously. Lack of or inadequate treatment may result in the need for corrective orthopedic surgery for leg lengthening and straightening procedures.

Assessment

Full-term infants appear normal at birth. The disease becomes clinically detectable about the first year of life, when a mild to moderate linear growth deficiency can be noted. Frontal bossing develops during early childhood. As the child begins to walk, the femur and tibia bow (genu varum, or bowlegs) as a result of weight bearing (Fig. 27-4). This malformation, combined with a developing tibial torsion (see Chapter 20), gives the child an unstable, waddling gait. Fractures, signs of swelling, and pain, especially in the extremities, indicate a need for further assessment in any infant or young child. Muscle weakness and decreased energy levels may also be noted. Teeth may erupt late but will be normal in appearance. A tendency toward dental decay and dental abscesses may be noted during the second decade of life. Thus, include a dental history and documentation of preventive dental activities in the assessment information gathered.

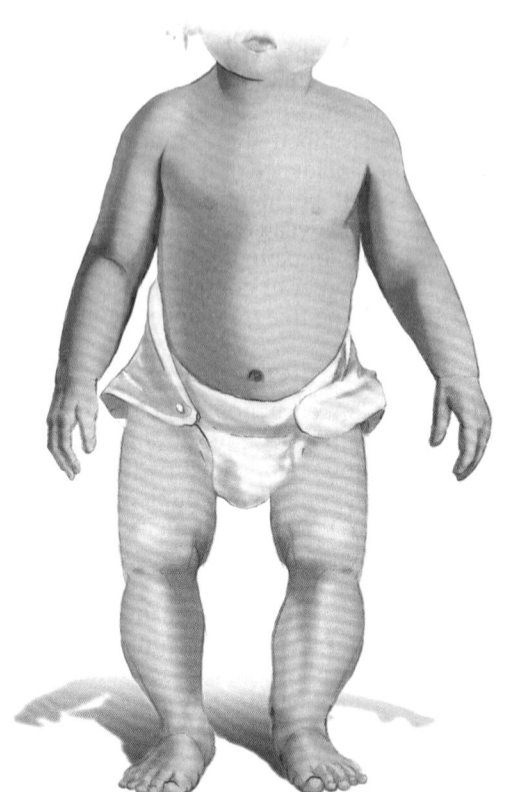

Figure 27-4 X-linked hypophosphatemic rickets affects skeletal development of the femur and tibia causing genu varum.

Diagnostic Tests

Significant laboratory findings include serum phosphorus less than 4 mg (although this constituent may remain normal up to age 9 months despite disease), alkaline phosphatase more than 200 International Units/L (in preterm infants, >300 to 400 International Units/L), and reduced transfer maximum for phosphate per unit volume of glomerular filtration rate in the presence of normal renal tubular function. Radiographic findings are most apparent in the lower body and include fractures of the long bones and ribs (which may be noted in the premature infant by 10 weeks of age); fraying, widening, and cupping of the metaphyses (especially of the tibia, femur, ulna, and radius); thickened cortices of long bone shafts with dense trabecular bone (first seen during late childhood); and calcification of tendons, ligament insertions, and joint capsules (seen in adolescence and later).

Nursing Diagnoses and Outcomes

The deficiency of phosphorus in children with X-linked hypophosphatemic rickets places the children at risk for orthopedic and dental problems. Therefore, in addition to the nursing plan of care presented in Nursing Plan of Care 27-1, the following nursing diagnoses and outcomes may apply to this patient population:

Nursing Diagnosis: Risk for activity intolerance related to potential for fractures, bone pain, and skeletal deformities
Outcomes:
• Child will participate in activities appropriate to his or her ability level that do not pose a threat of injury.
• Schoolteachers and the family will assist the child in pursuing activities that are safe and will build the child's self-confidence.
Nursing Diagnosis: Impaired oral mucous membranes related to higher incidence of dental abscesses
Outcome: Child will be identified early and treated promptly for dental decay and abscesses.
Nursing Diagnosis: Impaired verbal communication related to high number of dental extractions
Outcome: Child will be free from speech impairments.

Interdisciplinary Interventions

Management of X-linked hypophosphatemic rickets is designed to promote normal bone strength and growth. Interdisciplinary interventions begin with the prescription of a phosphate supplement, coupled with Calcitriol or another vitamin D analogue. Calcitriol is classified as a vitamin D analogue and a fat-soluble vitamin. Calcitriol's mechanism of action is to promote absorption of calcium in the kidneys and gastrointestinal tract to increase the serum levels of calcium. Calcitriol also decreases the serum phosphatase level and decreases bone reabsorption, enabling healthy bone to grow. Treatment is geared toward stabilizing the phosphorous level in the blood. Weight, calcium, parathyroid hormone, urinary calcium excretion, and alkaline phosphatase levels determine dosage levels. Frequent adjustment in dosages of the phosphate supplement and vitamin D

analogue helps to prevent hyperparathyroidism or hypercalcuria. Observe children for manifestations of hypercalcemia. These include weakness, fatigue, lassitude, headache, nausea, vomiting, and diarrhea. Serum and urine calcium levels should be monitored at least quarterly after the condition is stabilized, and the kidneys should be annually evaluated by ultrasonography.

As children reach adulthood, continued treatment with Calcitriol alone may be sufficient for those who remain asymptomatic. Treatment with growth hormone for **rachitic** children (those affected by rickets) who do not achieve normal linear growth may be initiated. Research on ways of correcting the basic metabolic error through genetic therapy is in progress. Treatment with thiazides may also be instituted to assist in counteracting the tendency for bone calcium loss.

caREminder

Consider the family's ability to adhere to medication dosing schedules when determining dosing for Calcitriol and phosphate supplementation. Multiple daily doses may not be the best frequency.

Special nutritional considerations are needed for the premature infant. Preterm breast milk contains adequate quantities of all the essential nutrients *except* calcium and phosphorus. Commercial preterm formula contains the necessary additional calcium and phosphorus, but premature infants must receive total parenteral nutrition until they are able to take and tolerate adequate amounts of formula. Counsel the family to avoid soy formulas, which have a phytase-binding quality that inhibits the intestinal absorption of phosphorus.

Community Care

Oral medications are required for years. Teach the family to give both medications together at set times of the day, which will help them remember to give medication regularly. This practice also establishes a routine pattern for children to use as they become more independent in taking responsibility for their medications.

Dental problems are a continuing challenge for the child with rickets because of the tendency to abscess. Primary teeth are usually extracted if abscessed. Depending on the site and number of extractions, speech could be adversely affected, and the child may need speech therapy. Root canals or other endodontic procedures are usually necessary for abscesses of the secondary teeth. Work with the child and the family to communicate the importance of good dental hygiene and regular visits to the dentist. Children should be encouraged to brush after every meal. The school nurse can support these actions by offering a place for children to store their cleaning materials and by encouraging them to brush their teeth.

Gentle handling of premature infants and any child with rickets is critical to prevent fractures. Family members need to be taught the importance of this concept as well. The nurse or social worker can discuss nonphysical forms of discipline with the family. In addition, the family, daycare providers, and school officials require guidance in selecting safe, soft toys for the child and in providing activities that safeguard against physical harm. For instance, contact sports and gymnastics are not recommended. The child's musical, science, or computer interests should be encouraged because these are safe activities that can enhance self-esteem and minimize physical injury. Self-image and esteem are important concepts to build. If growth has been slowed, the child may be sensitive about being shorter than his or her peers. Depending on the child's clinical status, the risk of fractures will probably limit the child's involvement in physical education, sports, and rough games. This, too, sets the child apart from others, and the child may become the focus of teasing. Family counseling and support groups can help prepare the child to cope with teasing and identify areas where he or she can excel to gain peer recognition.

The family may need financial support to manage the child's care properly. The cost of years of medications, laboratory tests, and follow-up visits, with the possible additional expenses of orthopedic surgery and extensive dental care, is considerable (see Chapter 2 for a discussion of financial support options for the family).

WILSON DISEASE

Wilson disease is an autosomal recessive disorder of copper metabolism characterized by cirrhosis of the liver and degenerative changes in the brain. Occurring in 1 in 30,000 children worldwide, Wilson disease results from mutations in a gene, ATP7B (Kodama et al., 2012). Although the symptoms are primarily hepatic, multisystem toxicity does occur. The disease is fatal unless recognized and treated early.

Pathophysiology

The metabolic defect in Wilson disease impairs normal hepatic excretion of dietary copper. As a result, soon after birth, copper begins to accumulate in the liver, causing progressive hepatic damage. Copper then escapes the liver and begins to accumulate in other major organs, such as the brain and the kidneys, and in the corneas. Fatty changes, inflammation, necrosis, and hepatic injury that can be virtually indistinguishable from chronic hepatitis become evident, and the brain and spinal column can be severely damaged.

Assessment

The diagnosis of Wilson disease should be considered in anyone between the ages of 5 and 30 years with liver abnormalities of uncertain cause (Roberts & Schilsky, 2008). The diagnosis can easily be missed because of the natural tendency to interpret the severe liver or neurologic manifestations as conditions of other disorders.

Note whether a sibling or first cousin has been previously diagnosed with the disease or has demonstrated symptoms similar to those of the child currently being evaluated. In addition, all patients with hemolysis or recurrent jaundice should be investigated for Wilson disease.

The physical manifestations of Wilson disease appear in multiple body systems. All affected children have hepatic involvement. However, only about 40% of children have hepatic disorders such as chronic or active hepatitis, cirrhosis, or hepatic insufficiency. Neurologic manifestations include encephalopathy, ataxia, fine tremors, dysarthria, dysphagia, dystonia, and epilepsy. Hematologic effects include acute hemolysis and coagulopathies. Ophthalmic signs include the characteristic **Kayser-Fleischer rings** (corneal copper deposits that appear as a rust-brown ring around the iris) visible on slit lamp ophthalmologic examination. Cataracts, strabismus, and impaired visual acuity may also be noted. Renal involvement is characterized by renal tubular acidosis, aminoaciduria, acute renal failure, and hematuria. Skeletal involvement includes osteoporosis and osteoarthritis. Amenorrhea and an increased incidence of spontaneous abortions are noted in affected adolescents. Other manifestations include abdominal pain, bacterial peritonitis, and blue lunules of the fingernails. About one third of affected patients exhibit neuropsychiatric disorders such as sudden onset of socially inappropriate behavior; depression; deterioration in school performance; or obsessive, bipolar, or schizophrenic behaviors (European Association for the Study of the Liver [EASL], 2012).

Diagnostic Tests

Diagnostic tests of the blood reveal low serum ceruloplasmin levels (<20 mg/dL). Basal 24-hour urinary excretion of copper is obtained and is significant if more than 40 µg. A penicillamine challenge study may be performed to further confirm diagnosis. During this test, 500 mg D-penicillamine is administered, and urine is collected and tested at 12 hours and 24 hours after administration. The agent acts as a chelating agent to help with the excretion of copper. Thus, a child with Wilson disease will have more copper excretes in their urine after taking this agent (Roberts, & Schilsky, 2008).

Interdisciplinary Interventions

Although Wilson disease is invariably fatal if not treated, administration of chelating agents or liver transplantation when the disease is identified may lead to a positive prognosis. Lifelong treatment with chelating agents and a low-copper diet is usually sufficient to reach a clinical remission in most cases. Management is aimed at minimizing liver and neurologic damage and controlling the effects of copper toxicity on other body systems.

Medical Management

D-penicillamine (the medication of choice) and trientine may be given to promote urinary excretion of copper and to detoxify excess copper remaining in the liver. These medications are given orally in two to four divided doses, 30 minutes before or 2 hours after meals. Because D-penicillamine causes antipyridoxine activity, a daily pyridoxine supplement is added to the patient's diet. Oral zinc gluconate and other zinc salts may also be prescribed. The zinc products have proved effective in arresting liver damage, although they cannot reverse existing hepatic cirrhosis, portal hypertension, or neurologic symptoms.

Emphasize to the child and family that the medications must be taken at all times and continued throughout the child's life. During the first month of treatment with D-penicillamine, the family needs to be alert for the development of fever and rash, sometimes accompanied by enlarged lymph nodes, which indicate hypersensitivity to the medication. Leukopenia or thrombocytopenia may also develop. If these adverse effects occur, the medication is discontinued until they subside, then is gradually reintroduced. If the adverse effects persist, D-penicillamine may be discontinued and trientine given instead. Proteinuria, a possible late adverse reaction, requires changing the chelating agent from D-penicillamine to trientine.

Nutritional Management

Treatment for Wilson disease commonly involves a low-copper diet in conjunction with chelation therapy (see "Treatment Modalities" section). Chart 27-1 lists foods with high and low copper content. The nutritionist can serve as an expert consultant to the health care team and the family. Working with the family, the nutritionist evaluates the child's urinary copper level and adjusts the child's diet accordingly. Foods rich in copper can be eaten in moderation as long as medication treatment is maintained. Drinking water should be analyzed to ensure it does not contain more than 100 µg copper/L. Bottled demineralized water may be used, and should contain only 1 µg copper/L. Alcohol should be avoided because it may harm the liver, which is already compromised as a result of Wilson disease. Use of copper cooking utensils is avoided.

Surgical Management

A child with fulminant hepatitis or hepatic failure related to Wilson disease may be a candidate for liver transplantation. The transplant cures the genetic defect and restores normal copper balance. Further neurologic deterioration is halted; however, no clear evidence exists that neurologic symptoms can be reversed. The family of a liver transplantation candidate needs assistance in becoming part of the organ transplant network. Social services can serve as liaisons between the family and the transplant agencies. During the evaluation and waiting period before transplantation surgery, the family needs intensive emotional support. The social worker and nurse can help the family to prepare for the transplantation and to get in touch with families of children who have already undergone the procedure.

CHART 27-1   Dietary Considerations for Wilson Disease

Foods Low in Copper (<0.1 mg/portion)	Foods High in Copper
Meat	**Meat**
• Beef, eggs, turkey, chicken (white meat only), cold cuts that do not contain pork, organ meats, or dark meat	• Lamb, pork, duck, goose, squid, salmon, organ meats, shellfish, soy protein meat substitutes, tofu, nuts, and seeds
Vegetables	**Vegetables**
• Most vegetables	• Vegetable juice cocktail, mushrooms
Fruits	**Fruits**
• Most fruits	• Nectarines, commercially dried fruits (e.g., raisins, dates, prunes), avocados
Starches/Breads/Grains	**Starches/Breads/Grains**
• Breads and pastas from refined flour, oatmeal	• Dried beans (e.g., lima, pinto, garbanzo, soy), lentils, millet, barley, wheat germ, bran breads and cereals, soy flour, soy grits, fresh sweet potatoes
Fats/Oils	**Fats/Oils**
• Butter, cream, mayonnaise, nondairy creamer, sour cream, oils, salad dressing	• No restrictions
Milk/Milk Products	**Milk/Milk Products**
• Most milk products	• Chocolate milk, soy milk, cocoa
Sweets/Desserts	**Sweets/Desserts**
• Jams, jellies, candies with allowable ingredients, flavoring extracts	• Candy with nuts, chocolate, or cocoa; desserts with ingredients rich in copper
Beverages/Miscellaneous	**Beverages/Miscellaneous**
• Coffee, tea, fruit juices, lemonade, fruit-flavored drinks, soups with allowable ingredients	• Instant breakfast drinks, mineral water, soy-based beverages, brewer's yeast, multivitamins with copper

Community Care

Through the phases of Wilson disease, including diagnosis, ongoing management, monitoring of its effects, and the liver transplantation process, numerous invasive procedures are required. Play therapy with child life specialists helps to alleviate the fear of these procedures. Children may experience symptoms that keep them from attending school. If this occurs, homeschooling should be arranged early.

The nurse plays an important role in the ongoing monitoring and management of the child with Wilson disease. Responses to medication and dietary regimens are evaluated at frequent intervals during the first year of therapy and on a routine basis thereafter. Blood and urine analyses are the primary modes of evaluation, so ensure that patient and family education stresses the importance of blood and urine collection.

KidKare Twenty-four-hour urine specimens are difficult to collect from children, who may forget to save their urine. Instruct the family to ensure that the child is at home during the entire collection process. They should encourage the child to void in only one bathroom, ensure that a collection device is always in place, and offer a reward for each successful collection of urine.

Also, help the family to determine whether the child's symptoms are improving or worsening once treatment has begun. Because overt signs of the disease may vary among children, review with the family the particular signs that their child has demonstrated, and explain which of these signs are expected to diminish with treatment. Diminished cerebral and hepatic signs and symptoms and fading Kayser-Fleischer rings are the best indicators of successful therapy.

As the child matures, work with the nutritionist, child, and family to expand the child's diet and personal responsibility for making dietary selections. Siblings should be screened for presymptomatic Wilson disease; if the metabolic defect is found, expression of the disease can be prevented by initiating the chelating agents promptly. In addition, genetic screening should be provided to all family members to detect asymptomatic homozygote carriers. Discuss with the family the results of the screening examinations and the implications for future family planning.

CARBOHYDRATE DISORDERS

Carbohydrates include starch, sucrose, and lactose. Various disorders related to interruptions in the pathway of carbohydrate metabolism result from specific genetic defects. Their classifications include galactose disorders, glycogen storage disorders, and fructose disorders. Galactosemia is discussed in this chapter. Table 27-4 highlights other selected carbohydrate disorders.

GALACTOSEMIA

Galactosemia is a rare, inherited metabolic disorder in which the body is unable to metabolize galactose, which reaches high levels in the body, damaging the liver, CNS, and various other body systems. Estimates of the incidence of classic galactosemia occurs about 1 in every 47,000 live births (Mayatepek et al., 2010). As an inherited autosomal recessive trait, galactosemia occurs in different forms, depending on the degree to which the metabolic pathway is blocked. Genotyping is required

TABLE 27-4	Selected Carbohydrate Disorders				
Disorder and Inheritance	Pathophysiology	Significant Clinical Features	Key Diagnostic Findings	Management	Prognosis
Fructose 1-phosphate aldolase (aldolase B) deficiency Autosomal recessive	Defect in fructose 1-phosphate aldolase B enzyme; fructose not converted to glucose	Asymptomatic until fructose introduced in diet Infants: anorexia, vomiting, failure to thrive, hypoglycemic convulsions, liver and kidney dysfunction Older children: spontaneous hypoglycemia and vomiting after ingestion of fructose	Increased serum and urine fructose	Diet free of fructose and sucrose	Good if diet followed
Pyruvate dehydrogenase deficiency X-linked or autosomal recessive	Defect in the multi-enzyme complex responsible for the generation of acetyl CoA from pyruvate for the Krebs cycle	Lactic acidosis (may be life threatening) Hypotonia Developmental delay Seizures CNS malformations and other postnatal changes (e.g., cystic lesions of the cerebral cortex, brain stem, and basal ganglia; ataxia; and psychomotor retardation)	Elevation of pyruvate and thus elevation of lactic acid levels	No clearly effective treatment Low-carbohydrate or ketogenic diet and dietary thiamine, carnitine, lipoic acid supplementation may be beneficial for some	CNS deterioration over time

to determine the specific classification. Affected tissues include the lens, liver, brain, kidney, and ovaries.

Severe, untreated cases of galactosemia are invariably fatal. Patients affected less severely have retarded psychomotor development, visual impairment, and residual cirrhosis. If chronic errors in metabolism persist, other complications appear despite treatment. Such complications may include speech abnormalities, ovarian failure, cognitive deficits, poor growth, and impaired motor function and balance. Among families who have a child affected by galactosemia, each pregnancy carries a one-in-four chance of producing a child with galactosemia (see Fig. 3-3). Prenatal testing by amniocentesis or chorionic villus sampling is available and should be offered for subsequent pregnancies.

Pathophysiology

The classic and most common form of galactosemia involves a defect in the enzyme galactose-1-phosphate uridyltransferase (GALT). This defect disrupts the conversion of galactose-1-phosphate to galactose uridine diphosphate. Consequently, galactose, a monosaccharide, is not converted to glucose. The accumulation of galactose-1-phosphate results in injury to the kidneys, liver, and brain.

Assessment

Infants with galactosemia appear normal at birth. Manifestation of symptoms can be noted within the first days of life after the infant has begun ingesting breast milk or formula that contains lactose because galactose is formed as a by-product of digestion. The infant may exhibit anorexia, vomiting, diarrhea, hypotonia, jaundice, liver dysfunction or hepatomegaly, and cataracts (sometimes during the first week of life) if dietary management is not instituted. Neonates may become septic; the mortality rate from sepsis caused by *Escherichia coli* in particular is very high among infants with galactosemia (Ohlsson et al., 2012). Other common signs in untreated infants include drowsiness, inattention, decreased vigor of neonatal reflexes, bulging fontanels, and bleeding from coagulopathies. An accumulation of galactitol in the lens leads to cataract development, which sometimes is evident during the first few days of life. Physical and cognitive challenges become evident over time.

Diagnostic Tests

Early identification of galactosemia is possible through the blood assay completed for state-mandated newborn screening. The Beutler method, which measures GALT in dried blood on filter paper, is used. Some states use total galactose quantization testing. Other laboratory findings indicative of galactosemia include elevated blood galactose level; low glucose level; galactosuria (urinary total reducing substances should be tested with a Clinitest tablet rather than a routine urine dipstick for glucose; test results usually yield a positive result, which is abnormal); positive Benedict test of urine; deficiency of galactose-1-phospate in red and white blood cells and liver cells; and elevated serum alanine aminotransferase (ALT), serum aspartate aminotransferase (AST), and bilirubin. Genetic testing may be conducted to determine if there is a mutation of the GALT-gene (Mayatepek et al., 2010). In acute illness, hypocalcemia and aminoaciduria are also present.

Nursing Diagnoses and Outcomes

The nursing plan of care to support the dietary management of galactosemia is consistent with the diagnoses associated with other metabolic conditions (see Nursing Plan of Care 27-1). The child with galactosemia is at risk for dehydration, speech problems, and the development of cataracts. Thus, the following nursing diagnoses and outcomes may apply:

Nursing Diagnosis: Deficient fluid volume related to vomiting and diarrhea related to ingestion of lactose
Outcomes:
- Child's vomiting and diarrhea will be corrected through a galactose-restricted diet.
- Child will maintain a balanced fluid and electrolyte status.

Nursing Diagnosis: Risk for injury related to visual impairment
Outcomes:
- Child will be evaluated on a regular basis for the presence of cataracts.
- Child's visual acuity will be optimized by maintaining a galactose-free diet.
- Child will remain free from injury related to visual impairments.

Nursing Diagnosis: Impaired verbal communication related to speech disorder and delayed development
Outcomes:
- Child's communication will be correctly interpreted.
- Child will receive from others communication that is directed at the child's appropriate developmental level.

Interdisciplinary Interventions

Dietary management is the primary intervention for galactosemia, with appropriate pharmacologic intervention as needed for infection, dehydration, and ovarian dysfunction.

The primary nutritional goal is to provide dietary intervention that will prevent manifestations of the condition. A galactose-restricted diet rapidly resolves and prevents most acute symptoms. Galactose is derived from the hydrolysis of lactose into glucose and galactose. The diet is therefore milk free, with *all* sources of lactose restricted (Chart 27-2). Breastfeeding is contraindicated. A soy protein isolate formula with added methionine and carnitine can provide all necessary nutrients for the infant. As processed foods are added to the child's diet, instruct the family to check labels for milk or milk products such as dry milk solids, lactose, curds, and whey. Casein (sodium caseinate, calcium caseinate), a milk protein sometimes called *hydrolyzed protein*, must also be avoided. The family should be advised that Kosher foods are usually lactose-free. These products can be a source of dietary options for the child. Reinforce the importance of this

CHART 27-2   The Galactose-Free Diet

Restricted Foods	Foods Allowed
Bread	Soy-based formula
Cheese, all types	(Nutramigen or
Medication preparations that contain lactose as a filler	Alimentum), soy milk, and soy cheese
Dried beans and peas	Unfermented soy sauce
Ice cream, sherbet	Cereals
Margarine	Vegetables
Milk (nonfat milk, nonfat dry milk, milk solids and derivatives, milk chocolate, buttermilk, butter)	Fruit
	Meats
	Kosher foods
Monosodium glutamates (MSGs) that contain lactose extenders	
Organ meats (brains, liver, kidney, heart, sweetbreads)	
Prepared foods containing galactose, lactose, whey, tragacanth gum, calcium caseinate (e.g., baked goods, confections, and frozen foods)	
Pudding	
Yogurt, sour cream	

prescribed diet with every family contact. Collaborate with the nutritionist to ensure that the child is receiving adequate calories, protein, vitamins, and minerals such as calcium. Calcium supplementation may be necessary given the numerous restrictions on dairy items in the child's diet. Recipes that use galactose-free milk substitutes can be provided to the family (Clinical Judgment 27-1). The restricted diet is generally recommended for life. The family must understand that the child does not develop an increased tolerance for milk products as he or she grows older.

In addition to dietary restrictions, the family must be aware of the many medications, particularly antibiotics, that use lactose as fillers. Examples include cephalosporins, erythromycin, lactulose syrup, and Neo-Calglucon. Be sure that the pharmacy from which the family obtains any prescriptions is aware of the child's diagnosis of galactosemia.

Infections, most commonly with gram-negative organisms, are treated with the appropriate antibiotic. If jaundice related to the galactosemia is present in the newborn, treatment may be required. Other supportive therapies include resolving any dehydration and electrolyte imbalances that have occurred as a result of the vomiting, anorexia, and diarrhea. Females who manifest symptoms of ovarian dysfunction later in life, including irregular menses and decreased fertility, may require hormonal therapy.

Community Care

Children with galactosemia, even those whose condition is controlled, may experience learning difficulties. Speech therapy is necessary to optimize outcomes from apraxia (Mayatepek et al., 2010). Many children also have cognitive impairments causing them to have lower educational achievement (Jumbo-Lucioni et al., 2012; Mayatepek et al., 2010). Family conferences with schoolteachers or daycare workers help school personnel understand the need for specialized classes and teaching techniques that enhance the child's developmental abilities. In addition, work with school officials to emphasize the need to monitor the child's diet when away from home and find ways to offer dietary alternatives when special class functions include food.

Evaluate all children diagnosed with galactosemia for cataracts. In many cases, introducing the galactose-free diet leads to spontaneous resolution of cataracts. Yearly evaluation of the child by an ophthalmologist is highly recommended. Children who do not adhere well to the diet are at risk for developing cataracts, as are those who were not diagnosed and treated for the metabolic condition at an early age.

MUCOPOLYSACCHARIDE DISORDERS

This group of lysosomal storage disorders involves abnormal storage of lipids in the neurons and polysaccharides in the connective tissues. This abnormal storage results in multiple neurologic and skeletal abnormalities. Specific mucopolysaccharide disorders include Hurler syndrome, Hunter syndrome, Tay-Sachs disease, Niemann-Pick disease, Gaucher disease, Fabry disease, Sanfilippo disease, Morquio syndrome, Shefe disease, and Maroteaux-Lamy disease. Most are autosomal recessive defects, although a few, such as Hunter syndrome, are X-linked. This section covers Hurler syndrome; an overview of the important factors of other selected lysosomal storage disorders is provided in Table 27-5.

HURLER SYNDROME

Hurler syndrome, or mucopolysaccharidosis I (MPS I), is the classic and most severe form of mucopolysaccharidosis. Hurler syndrome occurs in approximately 1 in 100,000 births and is inherited as an autosomal recessive trait (Muenzer et al., 2009). The disease is sometimes known as *gargoylism* because infants have distinctive gargoylelike facial features. Recent recommendations include dividing MPS I into two broader groups: severe MPS I and attenuated MPS I (Hurler-Scheie and Scheie syndromes) (Muenzer et al., 2009). In the past, children with Hurler syndrome deteriorated progressively, and death usually occurred by age 10 years from respiratory or cardiac failure resulting from organ damage.

Pathophysiology

A defect in the lysosomal enzyme, α-L-iduronidase, prevents the degradation of acid mucopolysaccharides, also known as *glucosaminoglycans*. As a result,

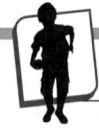

Nutritional Counseling

Nikki was born 2 months ago, normal for gestational age and without any postnatal complications. The results of Nikki's newborn screening test were positive for galactosemia. The parents, Melissa and Tom, both 17 years old, were called, and Nikki was brought back to the clinic for a repeated blood test.

The diagnosis is confirmed. You have been asked to provide teaching regarding the child's diet and home management. As you enter the room, Nikki's mother is clutching her baby and crying. Nikki's father has stepped out of the room to smoke a cigarette.

Questions

1. Before your teaching, what assessment data would it be helpful to collect about the family?

2. Although the infant is not eating solid foods, why do you want to know more about the family's diet?

3. What factors about the family would influence your teaching?

4. What topics should your nutritional counseling cover?

5. How could you evaluate the effectiveness of your teaching?

Answers

1. Family dietary patterns and dietary preferences related to ethnic or religious influences; whether health care insurance will cover the cost of medical food; primary caregiver of infant including daycare providers

2. Nikki may not be given breast milk. She needs a lactose-free diet. Milk products are found in a variety of products. Family members need to start learning which of those products they should not introduce to the child after feeding has begun.

3. Family's level of understanding of the metabolic condition itself; family's ability to accept the diagnosis realistically and take responsibility for the child's care

4. Name of diet, why the diet will help the child and why breastfeeding is contraindicated, formula that Nikki may drink, how to obtain formula, signs and symptoms of worsening condition, management of the child during childhood illnesses, how the diet will change as the child grows

5. Use scenarios to have family select appropriate formula. The family should relate the signs and symptoms of formula intolerance. Call the family in 1 week and again in 2 weeks for follow-up.

---

dermatan sulfate and heparan sulfates (polyglycosaminoglycans) accumulate in the tissues, producing the symptoms of Hurler syndrome. Because this metabolic pathway is part of cellular metabolism in many body organs, the defect results in damage to the brain, spinal cord, heart, viscera, bone, and connective tissue.

Assessment

Although Hurler syndrome produces distinctive clinical manifestations, diagnosis is not often reached during the neonatal period. Manifestations develop over time. Initial reasons to screen a patient for Hurler syndrome include rather common symptoms such as a swollen abdomen or a hernia. The growth of these children is usually within the normal range for the first year but falls below the third percentile thereafter. Physical examination will reveal hepatosplenomegaly, kyphosis, persistent nasal discharge, and noisy breathing. Neurologic development appears normal at first, but the child typically has delays in sitting, walking, and toilet training.

The skeletal deformities of Hurler syndrome are easily visible during a nursing assessment and include "gargoyle" facies (prominent supraorbital ridges with bushy brows, thickened lips, low nasal bridge, mild hypertelorism); large head with synostosis of the longitudinal suture; dwarfism; bone dysplasia, kyphosis, and gibbus, which produce a "catlike" posturing; broad hands with short, stubby fingers and clawlike deformities; flexion contractures of knees and elbows; and bilateral hip dislocation.

Neurologic manifestations include cystic areas in the white matter of the brain, severe intellectual disability, communicating hydrocephalus with possible increased intracranial pressure, and corticospinal signs. Other prominent manifestations include hepatosplenomegaly, protuberant abdomen, inguinal and umbilical hernias, conductive hearing loss, valvular heart disease, chronic rhinitis and respiratory infections related to a narrow pharynx and enlarged tongue, corneal opacities, and hirsutism.

As with other metabolic disorders, diagnosis relies heavily on blood, urine, and other radiographic tests. The nurse's role remains one of developmental surveillance. Changes in development or an inability of the child to meet developmental milestones should serve

TABLE 27-5   Selected Lysosomal Storage Disorders

Disorder and Inheritance	Pathophysiology	Significant Clinical Features	Key Diagnostic Findings	Management	Prognosis
Tay-Sachs disease Autosomal recessive	Deficient hexosaminidase A	Onset, 4–6 months of age Cherry-red macula Optic atrophy Loss of developmental milestones Hypotonia Seizures, late onset Dementia, early onset Almost all of Jewish ethnicity	Decreased hexosaminidase enzyme activity (serum, fibroblasts or leukocytes)	No treatment	Death by age 4 years
Niemann-Pick disease (types A, B, C, and D; type A most severe) Autosomal recessive	Deficient sphingomyelinase	Loss of developmental milestones Hepatosplenomegaly Enlarged lymph nodes Onset younger than age 6 months Cherry-red macula Optic atrophy 50% Jewish ethnicity (type A) Spastic paresis Dementia, early onset	Elevated serum lipids Aspartate amino-transferase Vacuolated lymphocytes Foam cells in bone marrow	No treatment	Death by age 3 years (type A)
Gaucher disease (type 1 mainly in Ashkenazi Jews; type 2 is severe and in infancy; type 3 in childhood) Autosomal recessive	Deficient glucocerebrosidase	Onset younger than 6 months of age Seizures Intellectual disability Hepatosplenomegaly Dementia Strabismus Bulbar palsy Spastic paralysis	Elevated acid phosphatase Elevated alkaline phosphatase Lipid-laden Gaucher cells found in bone marrow	Enzyme replacement therapy (types 1 and 3) Splenectomy (rarely used)	Death by age 2 years (type 2)

(Continued)

TABLE 27-5   Selected Lysosomal Storage Disorders (*Continued*)

Disorder and Inheritance	Pathophysiology	Significant Clinical Features	Key Diagnostic Findings	Management	Prognosis
Fabry disease Sex-linked recessive	Deficit of alpha-galactosidase A	Episodic, incapacitating pain, initially of fingers and toes Mild intellectual disability Seizures Peripheral red or purple macules or papules Renal disease Diabetes insipidus	Abnormal renal function	Management of pain crises Renal transplantation for renal failure	Death related to renal complications or stroke Renal treatment reverses symptoms
Hunter disease (mucopolysaccharidosis II) Sex-linked recessive	Deficient iduronate-2-sulfatase	Plethoric facies (coarseness) Hepatosplenomegaly Hydrocephalus Kyphosis without gibbus Claw-hand deformity Hypertrichosis Dwarfism Deafness Cardiomyopathy Obstructive airway disease Progressive neurologic decline	Excessive dermatan sulfate and heparan sulfate	Idursulfase (Elaprase—enzyme replacement) Success of bone marrow transplantation being evaluated	Late onset: live to age 40–70 years Some with average intelligence Juvenile type: death during adolescence
Sanfilippo disease (mucopolysaccharidosis III) Autosomal recessive	Deficit of heparan N-sulfatase (type A, most severe form); N-acetyl-alpha-D-glucosaminidase (NAG) (type B); acetyl CoA: alpha-glucosaminide (type C); or N-acetylglucosamine G-sulfate sulfatase (type D)	Severe retardation Mild shortness of stature Mild coarsening of facial features Hepatosplenomegaly Mild hirsutism Behavioral problems Progressive immobility	Heparan sulfate in urine	Bone marrow transplantation being evaluated	Severe retardation May live 40–50 years

as triggers to warrant referral to the primary health care provider for further investigation of the underlying cause of abnormalities in the physical and developmental assessments performed by the nurse.

Diagnostic Tests

The diagnosis is suggested by clinical examination and radiographic findings. Laboratory findings indicative of Hurler syndrome include dermatan and heparan sulfates in the urine. Definitive diagnosis requires detection of α-L-iduronidase deficiency in cultured skin fibroblasts, serum, or white blood cells.

Nursing Diagnoses and Outcomes

A plan of care for the child with Hurler syndrome can be implemented using diagnoses and interventions from Nursing Plan of Care 27-1. In addition, the skeletal deformities and oral–facial deformities characteristic in children with Hurler syndrome may prompt the following nursing diagnosis:

Nursing Diagnosis: Ineffective infant feeding pattern related to oral–facial deformities
Outcome: The family will demonstrate appropriate feeding techniques to prevent aspiration and ensure that the child is receiving adequate nutrition.

Interdisciplinary Interventions

Early diagnosis and supportive care (e.g., medications, respiratory treatments) focused on the respiratory and cardiac complications are the most common goals of management. Clinical progression can occur rapidly after the third year of life because of buildup of the storage material (mucopolysaccharides). Early diagnosis provides opportunities to get the missing enzyme into the body. Enzyme replacement therapy using laronidase has been shown to be effective in improving range of mobility. Some children treated before puberty also had increased growth. There may be some improvement in sleep apnea and also a decrease in hepatomegaly. Enzyme replacement has no effect on the progressive intellectual disability (Muenzer et al., 2009).

Bone marrow or cord blood transplantation has increased the life span of a child with Hurler syndrome by arresting its progress and reversing some of the most severe sequelae; however, it is associated with high morbidity and mortality. Transplantation can also greatly decrease the degree of cognitive damage associated with Hurler syndrome. Better health outcomes occur when the transplant occurs before age 2 years and in children with a developmental quotient of >70 (Muenzer et al., 2009).

Community Care

Families of children with a lysosomal storage disease require a great deal of emotional and social support. They are caring for a child whose physical and mental health deteriorates over a period of years, often resulting in severe neurologic impairment and death. Nursing personnel play a pivotal role in managing home care needs. Arrangements for medical equipment in the home, such as a wheelchair, are necessary. Depending on the family's situation, home health care assistance, respite care, or long-term care placement may be necessary. Coordination with transplant centers is indicated for the advanced practice nurse if the child is a candidate for bone marrow or cord blood stem cell transplantation.

Teach families that their child may not progress in motor activities, including walking and toilet training. Assistive devices to allow the child to sit comfortably, move about, and attain some use of the hands can be obtained by nursing personnel through occupational therapy and physical therapy consultations. The child may also experience behavioral problems such as emotional outbursts, excessive crying, and sleep disturbances in response to the neurologic deterioration. In these cases, sedatives may be administered to help manage the child.

The infant's large, protuberant tongue and narrowed nasopharynx cause difficulty sucking and feeding. Teach the family feeding techniques that prevent aspiration and assist the child to swallow (Nursing Interventions 27-2). Breastfeeding can certainly be tried but may not be successful. Bottles with a small-holed, soft nipple allow formula to flow slowly and may prevent choking. Nasal or deep suctioning may be required if aspiration does occur, so the family should be taught these techniques for home care.

As the disease progresses, the family has some difficult decisions to make regarding the child's care and the extent of medical interventions to be used to continue

---

NURSING INTERVENTIONS 27-2

Feeding the Child With an Enlarged Tongue

- Hold the child in an upright position with the head slightly tilted back to encourage the tongue to fall back.
- If bottle-feeding, initiate sucking by putting pressure on the tongue with the nipple and placing the nipple in a downward and posterior direction.

- When bottle-feeding, give cheek support so that the tongue curls around the nipple.
- If feeding with a spoon, place downward pressure on the tongue with the spoon to encourage swallowing and to displace the tongue.

to support the child's physical health. Provide the family with anticipatory guidance regarding measures to prolong the child's life. The family may elect not to subject their child to certain interventions. Serve as an advocate for the child and the family, ensuring that all members of the health care team respect the family's wishes.

MITOCHONDRIAL DISORDERS

Mitochondrial disease is considered to be a predominantly inherited disorder, but in some cases, a random mutation or an environmental toxin is thought to have contributed. All mitochondria are inherited from the mother, so the mutation in the DNA of the mitochondria will be passed on to all the children. However, only daughters will be able to pass that mutation onto their progeny. Because mitochondria serve as an energy center, converting the food we eat into sources of energy, the effects of mitochondrial disease can be broad reaching, and its effects on the individual child vary considerably. Mitochondrial disease affects every organ in the body, presents with many disease manifestations, and becomes evident at any age, from infancy through late adulthood. In a child affected by mitochondrial disease, always think: any organ, any disease, anytime—that is how far reaching the effects of this disease can be on children throughout their lives.

Mitochondrial disorders in adults are often related defects of mitochondrial functioning related to aging (e.g., Parkinson disease, stroke, Alzheimer disease). Most children with mitochondrial disorders appear normal at birth. Children most often present with developmental delays, failure to thrive, or neurologic disorders—some mild and some so severe at presentation that they require an intensive care admission. Some mitochondrial disorders, such as Leigh syndrome, have a rapid downhill course and are fatal within 1 year, whereas others appear milder. Prognosis, therefore, is extremely difficult to estimate; it depends on which organ systems are affected and how severely. Generally, the more systems affected, the poorer the prognosis.

Pathophysiology

The mitochondria serve as the energy powerhouse of the human body. Within the mitochondria, the chemical energy from food is harvested. This process results in the production of adenosine triphosphate (ATP). ATP is the predominant power source for all processes within the body. In addition to energy production, mitochondria carry out several other vital functions. These powerhouses are also involved in producing steroid hormones, manufacturing building blocks of DNA, and eliminating ammonia from the liver. Thus, the effects of a mitochondrial disorder on the overall functioning of the human body can be devastating. The more common mitochondrial disorders include mitochondrial myopathy, encephalopathy, lactic acidosis, and stroke-like episodes (MELAS); Leigh syndrome; Wolfram syndrome; mitochondrial respiratory chain disorders; and many other inborn errors of metabolism, such as fatty acid oxidation disorders and carbohydrate sensitivities.

Mitochondrial disorders can also be acquired through some pharmacologic treatment regimens, such as the use of ifosfamide in cancer treatment or zidovudine (AZT) in the treatment of HIV infection. Whether these medications unmask a previously, genetically determined mitochondrial disorder or actually cause the damage to the mitochondria themselves is not fully understood.

Assessment

A precise family history is essential when beginning any assessment of a child suspected of having an inborn error of metabolism. Mitochondrial disorders have a wide variety of symptoms that vary from person to person. Developmental and neurologic manifestations include poor growth, developmental delays, learning disabilities, intellectual disability, neurologic problems, confusion, memory loss, seizures, and dementia. Sensory impairments may include hearing loss, eye muscle paralysis, and progressive loss of vision. Loss of muscle coordination, muscle weakness, muscle cramping, muscle pain, and exercise intolerance affect motor development and skills. Organ involvement may include thyroid dysfunction and heart, liver, or kidney disease. Gastrointestinal disorders, severe constipation, respiratory disorders, diabetes mellitus, and pancreatic failure may also occur in children with a mitochondrial disorder.

Two people with the exact same defect in their mitochondrial DNA may not show the same symptoms. For this reason, family members who have all inherited a mitochondrial defect from their mother will not necessarily show the same symptoms or show them to the same degree. Some disorders are not evident until adulthood, and some never cause symptoms. Some cause the child to fall increasingly further behind in development. The symptoms of the specific mitochondrial disorder determine the treatment.

Diagnostic Tests

Many of the laboratory tests recommended for mitochondrial disease diagnosis are either extremely invasive or available at only a few centers. Muscle biopsies, for example, require an invasive procedure that the family may be hesitant to have their child undergo unless they are assured that a firm answer will result. Often, the results of biopsy are inconclusive, however, and the family should be aware of this fact before their consent is obtained. Other laboratory testing, such as testing on skin fibroblasts, can be extremely expensive because the samples must be packed and shipped to distant centers that can perform the tests. This expense is added to the expense required to complete the testing in the referral laboratory. Insurance companies may hesitate to pay for such testing or may require such exhaustive supporting data from the physicians and families that testing may not be done.

Laboratory studies should include mitochondrial DNA analysis; complete blood analysis including assessment of serum amino acids, lactic acid, carnitine, and ammonia; and urine analysis including assessment of carnitine and organic acids. Depending on the child's history and symptoms, other testing may be ordered, including brain magnetic resonance imaging, muscle or skin biopsy, electroencephalogram, electromyogram, and electrocardiogram. These lists are by no means exhaustive. Clearly, diagnosis of this disease can entail great expense, and the family may have to seek the expertise of many clinical specialists.

Nursing Diagnoses and Outcomes

Nursing diagnoses and outcomes for the child with metabolic disease are presented in Nursing Plan of Care 27-1. In addition, the following nursing diagnoses apply to the child with mitochondrial disease:

Nursing Diagnosis: Risk for injury related to seizure activity
Outcomes:
• Child and family will manage the environment to protect the child from injury if seizures occur.
• Child's medication regimen will be monitored and maintained so as to prevent seizures, accounting for changing demands related to illness and growth.
Nursing Diagnosis: Ineffective infant feeding pattern related to neurologic deterioration
Outcome: The family will demonstrate appropriate feeding techniques to ensure that the child is receiving adequate nutrition.

Interdisciplinary Interventions

After a mitochondrial disorder has been identified, management is primarily nutritional and supportive. The initial management goal of mitochondrial disease is to confirm the diagnosis. Definitive diagnosis will assist in planning treatment and, more importantly, in counseling the family about what to expect if the disease progresses. Nursing personnel assist in the diagnostic process by ensuring that ordered tests and procedures are completed. Providing information to the family on an ongoing basis will help reduce anxiety during this period of uncertainty about the diagnosis.

To date, there are no evidence-based treatment guidelines for mitochondrial disorders. Children may receive various vitamin "cocktails," antioxidants, amino acid supplements, and/or various medications considered useful in some specific mitochondrial disorders; dietary manipulation and exercise may also be used for various disorders (Goldstein & Wolfe, 2013; Sharma et al., 2012). A recent review of clinical trials conducted for patients with mitochondrial disorders found little benefit but stressed the need for continued pharmaceutical clinical trials (Kerr, 2013).

Investigational studies into other treatments such as bone marrow transplant and pharmacologic interventions continue, but many medications have carried far too many side effects for patients to tolerate. Bone marrow transplantation has shown promise for improving clinical manifestations of the disease and improving long-term survival. For many children with mitochondrial disorders, the best treatments are aimed not at the mitochondrial disorder itself but at the diseases that the mitochondrial disorder causes in the organs of the body. For example, many children require antiepileptic

medications for seizures, thyroid medication for thyroid disorders, or insulin for diabetes mellitus.

Supportive therapies such as physical therapy, occupational therapy, speech therapy, and adjustments to the educational plan in the school setting are essential. Act as coordinator and advocate for the child and family. Families require ongoing emotional support and respite care because the child's needs can become more intense and demanding as time goes on. A recent systematic review found significantly higher levels of stress, anxiety, and depression in families with a child with a mitochondrial disorder when compared to families with a child with other metabolic diseases; families have poorer quality of life (Sofou, 2013).

The goal of nutritional therapy is to promote optimal growth and development by meeting the child's nutritional needs for energy, protein, fluids, calories, vitamins, and minerals. Maintaining adequate nutrition will also assist in promoting as healthy an immune response as possible. Refer the family to a nutritionist experienced with metabolic disease to discuss ways to maximize the child's caloric intake, especially when muscle weakness and ataxia may make it difficult for children to feed or to simply have the energy to take in adequate calories.

Dietary interventions differ according to the suspected underlying etiology of the mitochondrial disorder. Dietary restrictions or additions will be different for a child with a fatty acid oxidation disorder than for a child with a carbohydrate sensitivity. The nutritionist will also collaborate with the health care provider to determine whether any nutrients such as thiamin, riboflavin, coenzyme Q10, or ascorbic acid should be added at pharmacologic doses rather than the over-the-counter strengths normally available.

Community Care

Refer families to a support organization such as the United Mitochondrial Disease Foundation (see thePoint Organizations). Many families have sought a diagnosis for years and are greatly relieved to learn that an international association, with education and support, is available. Informing the school nurse, who likely will not have had experience with a child with a mitochondrial disorder, is crucial. Often, adjusting the child's school day to incorporate frequent rest periods and snacks enables him or her to participate more fully in academics and activities. Encourage families to use spiritual support if doing so has been helpful to them in the past.

Families with children with mitochondrial disease are often much more knowledgeable about their child's disease than many of the health care professionals they encounter. This knowledge imbalance can lead to frustration on the family's part. Ask them to share information. Acknowledging what we, as health care providers, do not know is an important step in establishing a supportive relationship with the child and family. The family also needs assistance from their health care team to obtain insurance coverage for many medications, needed therapies, and home care assistance.

FATTY ACID OXIDATION DISORDERS

Fatty acid oxidation disorders are inherited mitochondrial conditions that affect the way the body can break down particular fats (fatty acids). Medium-chain-acyl-CoA dehydrogenase (MCAD) deficiency is the most common of the fatty acid oxidation disorders, with an incidence of 1 in 8,000 to 1 in 15,000 live births (Yusupov et al., 2010). All states assess for this disorder during newborn screening.

Prognosis for children with fatty acid oxidation disorders is good if the diagnosis is made prior to acute clinical presentation and metabolic decompensation. However, if the diagnosis is made after acute decompensation, and substantial organic failure has occurred, the prognosis can be very poor. Prior to being added to the expanded newborn screening in the United States, approximately 15% to 20% of children with MCAD deficiency died during their first acute presentation (Yusupov et al., 2010).

Pathophysiology

A child affected by a fatty acid oxidation disorder cannot break down stored fat for energy. The fatty acid oxidation process is complex and is composed of many processes for the oxidation of unsaturated fatty acids. Inherited enzymatic defects in the pathways for fatty acid oxidation create an accumulation of fatty acids that result in a variety of clinical manifestations. After the ingestion of food, the child will begin to experience problems such as hypoglycemia, vomiting, acidemia, lethargy, and difficulty breathing. For MCAD deficiency, the most common presentation is an acute life-threatening episode of hypoketotic hypoglycemia (a state in which plasma glucose and urine ketone concentrations are inappropriately low), often preceded by a prolonged fast or illness. Because of the absence of ketones, little or no acidemia occurs. Liver function tests are abnormal. Cardiomyopathy may be another manifestation at presentation.

Assessment

Infants appear normal at birth and continue to develop normally until they reach a stage when they no longer need to feed overnight and begin normal prolonged overnight fasting or they experience an intercurrent illness accompanied by vomiting and diarrhea that requires the body to mobilize energy sources from adipose tissue.

The family may describe going in to wake the child from a nap and being unable to awaken them. Other children are brought in to the emergency room with seizurelike activity or coma, unexplained lethargy, vomiting, or other signs of encephalopathy. Attacks of this illness may be misdiagnosed as Reye syndrome, severe dehydration, sudden infant death, or a seizure disorder. The clinical history of a child with no previous problems who has a sudden onset of severe clinical decompensation accompanied by any aspect of this clinical picture should have fatty acid oxidation disorder considered in the differential diagnosis.

Diagnostic Tests

Tandem mass spectrometry testing can be used to test for MCAD deficiency during newborn screening. This is the same heel stick blood sampling test used for screening phenylalanine. For the child not diagnosed during the newborn period, the following laboratory studies should be considered: basic metabolic panel that includes blood glucose, complete blood count with differential, blood gas, plasma ammonia, urine for reducing substances, urine ketones, quantitative plasma and urine amino acids, urine organic acids, and plasma lactate.

 ALERT   *Draw the lactate sample when the child is as calm as possible and without using a tourniquet. Using a tourniquet, or drawing blood from a struggling child, will yield falsely elevated serum lactate levels.*

Interdisciplinary Interventions

The immediate management goal for a child with acute metabolic decompensation is to suppress lipolysis as quickly as possible. Suppression is accomplished by administering 10% dextrose intravenously. Supplying an energy source is essential because the child is not able to access stored energy sources and acidosis will continue to worsen and possibly kill the child. After the initial crisis is past, management is primarily nutritional.

The infant or child with a fatty acid oxidation disorder needs to have frequent feedings. The diet must incorporate sustained-release carbohydrate and should minimize lipids. The primary goal of nutritional management is to prevent long-term fasting. Any fast longer than 10 hours can present an enormous stress to the child with any of these disorders. Children with MCAD deficiency usually increase in fasting tolerance as they age and experience less decompensation with acute illnesses. Children may incorporate a sustained-release carbohydrate, such as uncooked cornstarch mixed into pudding, into their diet with a bedtime snack to prevent negative effects of prolonged fasts during sleep hours.

Community Care

Providing family education regarding the interaction between diet, fasting, and symptom onset is an important nursing intervention. Teach the family the importance of monitoring blood sugar and urine ketones during acute illnesses (e.g., colds, gastrointestinal problems, chickenpox). Collaborate with the health care team to help the family develop a "rescue protocol" that will direct emergency care personnel on the immediate needs of the child if ill, such as the need for a high-concentrate glucose infusion and any necessary laboratory studies that should be monitored during a crisis. For infants and young children in daycare, the importance of adhering to the meal and snack schedule the family has set up with the health care provider must be strictly reinforced. Educate the family in meal and snack planning, and advise them that even apparently unaffected siblings may have the disorder. Testing siblings and parents will help to determine whether the disease is present.

See thePoint for a summary of Key Concepts.

REFERENCES

American Academy of Pediatrics, Committee on Genetics. (2008). Maternal phenylketonuria. *Pediatrics, 122,* 445–449.

American Academy of Pediatrics, Newborn Screening Authoring Committee. (2008). Newborn screening expands: Recommendations for pediatricians and medical homes—Implications for the system. *Pediatrics, 121*(1), 192–217.

American College of Obstetricians and Gynecologists. (2011). *Newborn screening.* Retrieved from http://www.acog.org/Resources%20And%20Publications/Committee%20Opinions/Committee%20on%20Genetics/Newborn%20Screening.aspx

Belanger-Quintana, A., Burlina, A., Harding, C. O. et al. (2011). Up to date knowledge on different treatment strategies for phenylketonuria. *Molecular Genetics and Metabolism, 104,* s19–s25.

European Association for the Study of the Liver. (2012). EASL clinical practice guidelines: Wilson's disease. *Journal of Hepatology, 56,* 671–685.

Gambol, P. (2007). Maternal phenylketonuria syndrome and case management implications. *Journal of Pediatric Nursing, 22,* 129–138.

Goldstein, A., & Wolfe, L. A. (2013). The elusive magic pill: Finding effective therapies for mitochondrial disorders. *Neurotherapeutics, 10,* 320–328.

Jumbo-Lucioni, P. P., Garber, K., Kiel, J. et al. (2012). Diversity of approaches to classic galactosemia around the world: A comparison of diagnosis, intervention, and outcomes. *Journal of Inherited and Metabolic Diseases, 35*(6), 1037–1049.

Kerr, D. S. (2013). Review of clinical trials for mitochondrial disorders: 1997–2012. *Neurotherapeutics, 10,* 307–319.

Kliegman, R. M., Stanton, B. F., St. Geme, J. W. et al. (Eds.). (2011). *Nelson textbook of pediatrics* (19th ed.). Philadelphia, PA: Elsevier/Saunders.

Kodama, H., Fujisawa, C., & Bhadhprasit, W. (2012). Inherited copper transport disorders: Biochemical mechanisms, diagnosis, and treatment. *Current Drug Metabolism, 13,* 237–250.

Mayatepek, E., Hoffmann, B., & Meissner, T. (2010). Inborn errors of carbohydrate metabolism. *Best Practice & Research Clinical Gastroenterology, 24,* 607–618.

Mazariegos, G. V., Morton, D. H., Sindhi, R. et al. (2012). Liver transplantation for classical maple syrup urine disease: Long-term follow-up in 37 patients and comparative United Network for Organ Sharing experience. *Journal of Pediatrics, 160,* 116–121.

Muenzer, J., Wraith, J. E., & Clarke, L. A. (2009). Mucopolysaccharidosis I: Management and treatment guidelines. *Pediatrics, 123,* 19–29.

National Institutes of Health Consensus Development Panel. (2000). Phenylketonuria: Screening and management. *NIH Consensus Statement Online, 17*(3), 1–27.

Ohlsson, A., Guthenberg, C., & von Döbeln, U. (2012). Galactosemia screening with low false-positive recall rate: The Swedish experience. *Journal of Inherited Metabolic Disease, 2,* 113–117.

Packman, W., Mehta, I., Rafie, S. et al. (2012). Young adults with MSUD and their transition to adulthood: Psychosocial issues. *Journal of Genetic Counseling, 21,* 692–703.

Rezvani, G., & Rezvani, I. (2011). An approach to inborn errors of metabolism. In R. M. Kliegman, B. F. Stanton, J. W. St. Geme et al. (Eds.), *Nelson textbook of pediatrics* (19th ed., pp. 416–418). Philadelphia, PA: Elsevier/Saunders.

Rezvani, I. (2011). Defects in metabolism of amino acids. In R. M. Kliegman, B. F. Stanton, J. W. St. Geme et al. (Eds.), *Nelson textbook of pediatrics* (19th ed., pp. 418–456). Philadelphia, PA: Elsevier/Saunders.

Rajah, J., Thandraye, K., & Pettifor, J. M. (2011). Clinical practice: Diagnostic approach to the rachitic child. *European Journal of Pediatrics, 170,* 1089–1096.

Roberts, E., & Schilsky, M. (2008). Diagnosis and treatment of Wilson disease: An update. *Hepatology, 47,* 2089–2111.

Sharma, M., Gulati, S., & Choudhary, A. (2012). Treatment of mitochondrial disorders. *Journal of Pediatric Neurology, 10,* 235–245.

Sofou, K. (2013). Mitochondrial disease: A challenge for the caregiver, the family, and society. *Journal of Child Neurology, 28*(5), 663–667.

Strauss, K., Puffenberger, E., & Morton, D. (2009). Maple syrup urine disease. In R. A. Pagon, M. P. Adam, T. D. Bird et al. (Eds.), *GeneReviews.* Retrieved from http://www.ncbi.nlm.nih.gov/books/NBK1319

U.S. Preventive Services Task Force. (2008). *Screening for phenylketonuria (PKU): U.S. Preventive Services Task Force reaffirmation recommendation statement.* Rockville, MD: Agency for Healthcare Research and Quality. Retrieved from http://www.annfammed.org/content/suppl/2008/03/07/6.2.166.DC1

Yusupov, R., Finegold, D. N., Naylor, E. W. et al. (2010). Sudden death in medium chain acyl-coenzyme a dehydrogenase deficiency (MCADD) despite newborn screening. *Molecular Genetics and Metabolism, 101,* 33–39.

See thePoint for Organizations.

CHAPTER 28

The Child With Altered Sensory Status

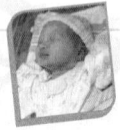

CASE HISTORY

Gabriella, introduced in Chapter 14, is now 1 month old or 32 weeks' gestation. Today, the ophthalmologist is coming to the neonatal intensive care unit to examine Gabriella's eyes. The nurse swaddles Gabriella and gives her a pacifier coated with sucrose in an attempt to provide comfort and address any pain that Gabriella may experience from the examination. The nurse also assists during the examination by holding Gabriella still while the ophthalmologist uses light and a special lens to see the retinal vasculature of the eye. The ophthalmologist determines that Gabriella does have an overgrowth of vasculature in her eye, or retinopathy of prematurity (ROP) stage II. At this time, there is no specific treatment and Gabriella's condition will be followed, but Abby and Ben Goldman, her parents, have lots of questions.

During a team conference, Abby and Ben are also told that before discharge, Gabriella will be tested by an audiologist for hearing loss because premature infants are at risk for sensorineural hearing loss. Gabriella has several specific risk factors that increase her risk for hearing loss: her increased serum bilirubin level, the use of furosemide (Lasix) to treat pulmonary edema, the use of indomethacin to close her patent ductus arteriosus, and the use of aminoglycosides to treat infection. Again, there is no precise answer—only the knowledge that there is the possibility of sensorineural hearing loss.

The week of Gabriella's discharge from the hospital arrives, and Gabriella has her auditory brain stem response (ABR) hearing screening test. She fails.

CHAPTER OBJECTIVES

1 Identify deviations from normal developmental patterns that indicate a visual, hearing, or communication disorder.

2 Describe assessment techniques commonly used to identify vision, hearing, and communication disorders in infants and children.

3 Identify the nursing interventions necessary to prepare children and their families for tests of sensory function.

4 Describe the etiology of common vision, hearing, and communication disorders of infants and children.

5 Discuss the pathophysiology related to common disorders of vision, hearing, and communication in infancy and childhood.

6 Identify the roles of the interdisciplinary team members in identifying and managing sensory disorders in children.

7 Develop a plan of care for an infant or child with an alteration in vision, hearing, or communication.

8 Summarize family and child education to prevent injuries and illness resulting in alterations in sensory function.

See thePoint for a list of Key Terms.

Infants and children depend on sensory input from the external world to assist them in their cognitive, social, and emotional growth. Sensory input comes in the form of visual and auditory stimulation and through the senses of touch, smell, and taste. To benefit fully from sensory stimulation to grow and develop, children must possess intact peripheral nerve pathways to receive the stimuli (sensory reception), and they must have brain development capable of recognizing and attaching meaning to the sensations received (sensory perception).

Communication is the child's ability to interact with the outside world in response to the sensations received.

This exchange of ideas, messages, and information involves both receptive and expressive abilities. The child who has intact sensory systems receives sensory input to which he or she cognitively and emotionally attaches significance. A child reacts to the environment by expressing behavioral and vocal responses. These responses complete the process of communication. Alterations in receiving or sending that make the child unable to share needs, desires, or ideas with others deeply affect the child's developmental process.

Children with altered sensory status, whether congenital or acquired, permanent or temporary, need interventions from other persons in the environment to facilitate their development. Nurses are uniquely positioned within the health care team to help prevent, screen for, and identify deviations from normal and intervene to assist the family in seeking a solution or adaption to the alteration in order to promote optimal development. The nurse's role in this process includes (1) promoting early identification and treatment of sensory alterations, (2) assisting and teaching families and children how to prevent or minimize trauma that could affect sensory abilities (Evidence-Based Clinical Practice Guidelines 28-1), (3) developing and implementing a care plan for the child with altered sensory function, and (4) helping family members to find ways to promote the development of the permanently impaired child. To this end, the nurse collaborates with a variety of specialists in sensory and communication disorders, such as ophthalmologists and optometrists for visual problems; audiologists, otolaryngologists, and otologists for hearing disorders; and speech–language pathologists and speech therapists for communication difficulties.

DEVELOPMENTAL AND BIOLOGIC VARIANCES

Development of sensory abilities is incomplete at birth. As the infant grows and develops, maturation of visual, auditory, and communication capabilities will occur, providing greater opportunities for children to engage with their environment and to grow emotionally, socially, and intellectually.

VISION

Early development of vision begins between the 2nd and 4th weeks of fetal life, along with development of the fetal brain. By the 16th week of fetal development, the eye has acquired its human appearance, and rudimentary internal structures are forming (Graven, 2004).

At birth, the optic nerve (cranial nerve II) is functional, and peripheral vision is fully developed (Fig. 28-1). However, development of visual acuity at birth is incomplete and is estimated to be 20/400. The *macula*, the portion of the retina that contains the color-sensitive rods, has yet to develop; and the *fovea*, the central portion of the macula, is unable to transmit an image to the brain. **Central vision**, which occurs as the fovea and macula mature, develops during the first few weeks and months of extrauterine life, when ocular structures are stimulated by normal sights of the infant's world. Within these first few months of life, physical changes to the eyes such as an increased distance between the cornea and retina, an increase in pupil dimensions, and strengthening of the rods and cones of the macula work together to improve the child's vision. If a defect or injury prevents images from reaching the retina,

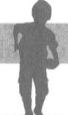

EVIDENCE-BASED CLINICAL PRACTICE GUIDELINES 28-1
Preventing Injury to Vision or Hearing

American Academy of Ophthalmology. (2003). *Protective eyewear for young athletes*. Retrieved from
http://www.aao.org/about/policy/upload/Protective-Eyewear-for-Young-Athletes.pdf

Policy statement about the types of protective eyewear children should use during sports activities.

Prevent Blindness America. (2011). *Preventing eye injuries from fireworks*. Retrieved from
http://www.preventblindness.org/prevent-eye-injuries-fireworks

Advice to prevent eye injury during events in which fireworks will be used.

Rodriguez, J., Lavina, A., & Agarwal, A. (2003). Prevention and treatment of common eye injuries in sports. *American Family Physician, 67*(7), 1481–1488. Retrieved from
http://www.aafp.org/afp/2003/0401/p1481.html

Review of common eye injuries from sports activities and the treatment for those injuries.

Centers for Disease Control and Prevention. (2013). *Hearing loss in children*. Retrieved from
http://www.cdc.gov/ncbddd/hearingloss/index.html

Guidelines and resources to help families prevent hearing loss in children.

Harvard Medical School. (2010). *Cleaning your ears*. Retrieved from
http://www.intelihealth.com/IH/ihtPrint/WSIHW000/35263/35268/337297.html?d = dmtContent&hide = t&k = basePrint

Instructions on how to prevent injury to the ear while completing ear care.

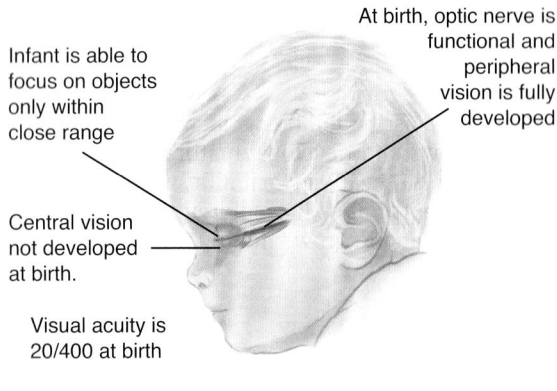

Infant is able to focus on objects only within close range

At birth, optic nerve is functional and peripheral vision is fully developed

Central vision not developed at birth.

Visual acuity is 20/400 at birth

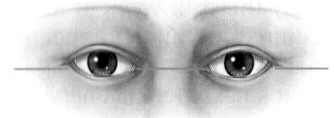

(A) Normal palpebral slant

Eye development complete by age seven

The normally white conjunctiva may have different color based on child's skin tone

In children of some ethnic groups, the outer canthus is normally slightly above the level of the inner canthus

Visual acuity is 20/20 by school age

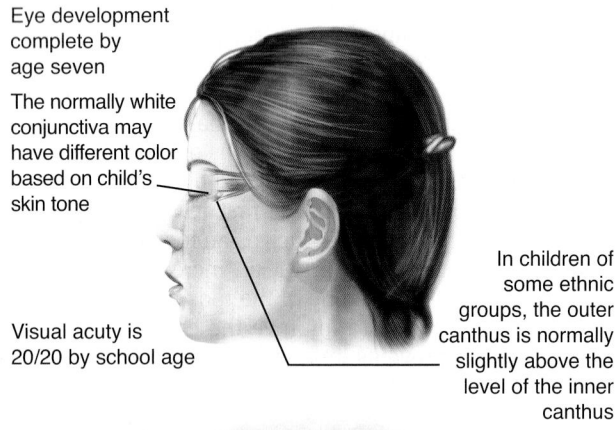

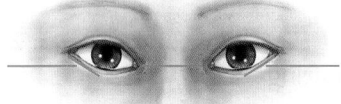

(B) Upward palpebral slant

Figure 28-1 Developmental and biologic variances: vision.

the macula and fovea are deprived of stimulation and do not develop the ability to transmit images. For example, congenital cataracts and ptosis of the eyelids are conditions that prevent visual development (Tuli et al., 2012). If not treated early, the eye loses its ability to continue to develop, and **amblyopia** (loss of functional vision in an otherwise normal eye) develops.

As visual acuity is developing, **accommodation**—the eye's ability to focus clearly—also improves. At birth, the infant can fix visually on near objects, depending primarily on sounds to recognize the approaching parent. The newborn's eyes are able to focus clearly only on objects within 8 to 10 in. During the next 4 months, the infant's eyes develop the ability to change shape (accommodate), allowing close and distant images to be focused on the retina. By ages 5 to 7 years, eye development is complete (Rozhkova et al., 2005). Developmental Considerations 3-1 presents the pattern of visual development in children.

Biologic variations are seen in different cultural groups and in children with different amounts of melanin in their skin. In children of Asian descent, the outer canthus of each eye may be located slightly above the imaginary line drawn from the inner canthus to the top of the ear. This slight upward slant is a normal biologic variation (see Fig. 28-1). Children with dark skin may have flecks of brown in the conjunctiva and have an orange-brown hue to the retina rather than the bright yellow-orange present in children with less melanin in the skin. Children of Hispanic descent may have brown flecks even if their skin color is light.

HEARING

Hearing is fully developed at birth; however, the neural pathways that enable the child to assign meaning to sounds in the environment are still being developed. Newborn infants quiet more quickly to a parent's voice than to the voice of a stranger. Music that the mother listened to during pregnancy has been shown to quiet the infant much more readily than unfamiliar music. These findings seem to indicate not only that the infant's hearing is fully developed at birth but also that it is fully developed well before birth. Developmental Considerations 3-2 presents the progression of hearing from birth to 15 months of age.

COMMUNICATION

Children's speech and language development begins at birth, with the differentiated cries that infants make to indicate discomfort, hunger, or loneliness. As the infant develops, syllables are differentiated, vowel sounds are articulated, and, finally, syllables are joined to make words and sentences. As the infant's cognitive skills grow, application of words to concrete objects progresses to the use of word symbols for abstract applications. Developmental Considerations 3-3 presents the progression of language acquisition in children.

Delays or deficits in speech or language are rarely attributable to biologic variations. Boys tend to begin to speak later than girls, and girls develop greater fluency at an earlier age, but the established "normal" ranges have been developed to include both sexes. Teaching prelingual infants to use sign language to communicate common needs has been found to be quite effective. As soon as infants can control their fingers, they can be taught to sign (Briant, 2009; Retnaba et al., 2011).

Developmental variations occur in the presence of hearing impairment or lack of stimulation. Infants and small children in bilingual families may take slightly longer than other children to develop full language skills because they are learning two language vocabularies and two language structures at the same time. The bilingual child's comprehension of abstract concepts is not delayed, however. Lack of stimulation is sometimes the reason children with visual impairment take longer to comprehend abstract concepts, but with assistance, they can also learn these concepts.

ASSESSMENT

Vision is assessed at birth and regularly throughout infancy and childhood. During early childhood, screening is imperative because uncorrected poor eyesight may impact a child's ability to learn and his or her subsequent educational performance once the child begins formal schooling (American Academy of Ophthalmology [AAO], 2007; American Academy of Pediatrics [AAP], 2007a; Berg & Wheeler, 2009). Even though an infant's eyes seem normal, the growth process can cause subtle changes in the shape and function of the eye. Abnormalities must be identified as soon as possible to enable normal development.

Vision screening begins at birth with ocular assessment by the health care provider and, if necessary, the ophthalmologist. Screening continues throughout childhood in the health care provider's office both during preschool examinations and during annual physical exams (Hered, 2011; Kemper & Clark, 2006). Vision screening should be performed at least once between the ages of 3 and 5 years and every 1 to 2 years for children older than the age of 5 years (AAP, 2012; U.S. Preventive Services Task Force, 2011). Schools often initiate screening programs to ensure that all children have their vision screened whether or not they go to the health care provider's office for an annual physical exam. As children grow and develop, they and their family may not be aware that they are experiencing subtle changes in their visual acuity, such as diminishing vision in one eye.

Hearing also must be assessed at birth and frequently thereafter during the first 36 months of life, particularly if the child is at risk for hearing impairment. The AAP endorses universal hearing screening for all newborns and infants as well as periodic screening for every child through adolescence. Children aged older than 5 years should be screened every 1 to 2 years (AAP, 2007b).

Not all hearing impairments manifest themselves at birth. Both late-onset genetic factors and factors within the child's medical history can contribute to the development of hearing impairment at any time during childhood. A child's behavior and responsiveness to parents and sounds in the environment will indicate to adults that the child may be unable to hear. Family concerns must always be followed up with appropriate professional assessment.

Hearing and language development are intertwined and so, too, is assessment. The ability of a young child with hearing impairment to learn language and speech is closely related to the time when remediation is begun; therefore, early identification and intervention are key to enhancing the child's opportunity for normal development.

Assessment of vision, hearing, and communication in infants and children begins with a focused health history followed by a physical examination. As children grow older and increasingly able to cooperate, the physical examination becomes more comprehensive (see Chapter 8). Depending on his or her expertise, the nurse may perform some or all of this examination. Nurse practitioners may perform the entire examination. Screening tests of visual acuity are often done in the school setting and may be completed by the school nurse and assistants.

Remind families that sensory screening is a valuable part of health assessment and that it should be done at regular intervals during childhood when the child visits their primary health care provider or during routine school-based assessments. A child's inability to cooperate, perhaps because the child does not speak the dominant language or is developmentally delayed, must not prevent accurate sensory screening. Children with special needs may need to be tested differently, but they should not be allowed to skip routine screening.

FOCUSED HEALTH HISTORY

Health history data concerning vision, hearing, and communication elicited from family members or the child, if old enough, enables the nurse to make inferences about possible deviations from normal sensory abilities. Suggested topics useful for eliciting this information are provided in Focused Health History 28-1. Additional data collected depend largely on the age of the child.

caREminder

Always pay attention to family members' observations. They are usually the first to detect abnormal signs or symptoms.

 QUESTION: Using Focused Health History 28-1, what are some risk factors that apply to Gabriella?

Visual History

Begin the visual history by questioning the family about any concerns they might have related to the child's vision. Also question the child about any complaints. Be aware that a young child may have difficulty answering questions about the quality of sight. Assess the child's visual acuity indirectly by asking whether the child enjoys looking at picture books and "reading." A child who seems to be frustrated by books or dislikes fine motor tasks that require close vision may truly have difficulty seeing the book or object (Fig. 28-2). For the child in school, ask whether the child can see the whiteboard easily without squinting or closing one eye. At this age, the child could also report blurring or double vision.

Hearing History

An infant's ability to attend to environmental sounds and parental voice is critical. Family members' observations concerning the child's responsiveness to their voices and of the child's general behavior are important. Family members are often the ones who first notice a problem with the child's ability to hear.

Carefully assess vocalization and language development as measures of hearing ability; also use them as measures of language, cognitive, and expressive development. The child who cannot hear sounds cannot imitate them and is less likely to make the developmentally appropriate vocalizations during infancy and early childhood. All infants are likely to babble in early infancy, but an infant of 9 to 12 months of age who is not attempting to repeat syllables (ma-ma-ma or da-da-da) should be referred for hearing assessment.

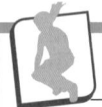

FOCUSED HEALTH HISTORY 28-1

The Child With Sensory Alterations

Current history	**General Information** • Family concerns related to vision, hearing, or communication • Completion of any vision, hearing, or communication testing **Eye-Related Concerns** • Poor school performance; child complains of difficulty seeing writing on blackboard at school or reading book and street signs • Squinting of one or both eyes • Headaches or complaints of pain in the eyes • Unexplained crying • Rubbing the eyes, tearing, redness, discharge, eyelid swelling • Rocking head side to side, abnormal head position • Complaints of blurred vision while reading, holding things close • Current medications related to treatment of eye disorder or medications or solutions used for contact lens wear **Ear-Related Concerns** • Complaints of ears "popping," feeling plugged or full, or difficulty hearing • Inattention to environmental sounds or human voice • Pulling and tugging at ears **Communication-Related Concerns** • Languages spoken and languages understood • Family members' perception of child's communication abilities
Past medical history	**General** • Congenital anomalies • Trauma to eyes, ears, or head • Eye or ear infections, seizures, meningitis • Previous referral for vision or hearing testing • Immunization status • Syndromes associated with vision or hearing loss **Prenatal/Neonatal History** • Problems during delivery or perinatal period • Prematurity or low birth weight • Mechanical ventilation • Hyperbilirubinemia; use of phototherapy • Perinatal or congenital infections (rubella, chlamydia, gonorrhea, cytomegalovirus, syphilis) **Health Challenges, Illness, or Injury Related to the Eye** • Glaucoma, cataracts • Discharge from eyes • Periorbital cellulitis • Unexplained crying, blurred vision, double vision • Strabismus • Amblyopia • Allergies, including those that may cause orbital redness or eye irritation **Health Challenges, Illness, or Injury Related to the Ear** • Bacterial meningitis, encephalitis • Infectious diseases associated with hearing loss (mumps, measles, Epstein-Barr virus) • Ototoxic drugs or radiation therapy • Neurodegenerative disorder known to be associated with hearing loss • History of otitis media (OM)

Health Challenges, Illness, or Injury Related to Communication
- Tonsillitis or enlarged adenoids
- Cleft lip or cleft palate
- Chronic OM
- Difficulty in chewing or swallowing
- Intellectual disability, cerebral palsy
- Trauma or strictures of trachea

Family medical history	**Vision Related** • Visual disorders, such as glaucoma, cataracts • Blindness • Metabolic or genetic disorders affecting vision (e.g., Marfan syndrome, Down syndrome) **Hearing Related** • Congenital or childhood-onset hearing loss **Communication Related** • Family members with speech or language disorders
Social and environ- mental history	Age-appropriate interactions with others Decline in academic grades or generally doing poorly in school **Vision Related** • Child's response to visual cues, ability to track objects, ability to see objects in the environment clearly (TV, pages in a book, puzzles) • Exposure to irritant environmental agents (e.g., smog, prolonged exposure to bright sunlight, frequent swimming) **Hearing Related** • Exposure to loud noises (music, lawnmowers, fireworks) • Family members' complaints that child "doesn't listen" or is "uncooperative" **Communication Related** • Bilingual family setting
Growth and development	Dates and results of previous vision and hearing testing Age-appropriate gross and fine motor skill development; delays Distance (near or far) child sits to watch television **Speech or Language Acquisition** • Age words first spoken • Progress of language acquisition; current level of language acquisition • Age-appropriate demonstration of expected knowledge (e.g., knows colors, body parts, points to named objects) • Use of visual communication (e.g., waves bye-bye, points, finger counts) • Methods used for expression of wants and needs **Speech** • Percentage of speech intelligible to family caregivers? To others? • Response of others to child's speech patterns • Child's perception of his or her speech patterns • Presence of stuttering

Note: See Chapter 8 for a comprehensive health history.

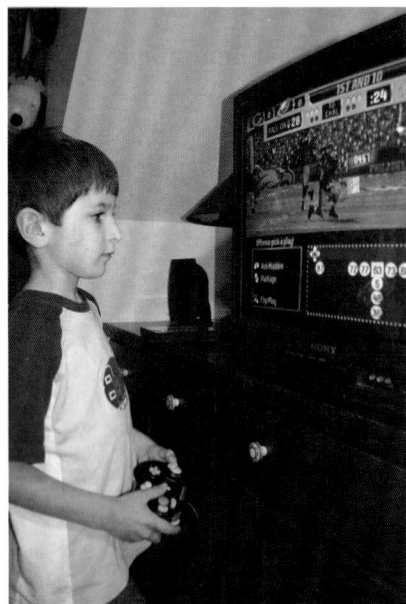

Figure 28-2 A child who stands close to the TV might do so because he or she has difficulty seeing.

caREminder

A child who does not hear directions, parental requests, or environmental sounds may not be able to respond appropriately. Although this behavior may be interpreted as uncooperative or unusual, it should be noted as potentially indicating hearing impairment. Ensure that the child's hearing is assessed.

Pay attention to other behavioral observations made by the family members that may be helpful in identifying a hearing deficit. For instance, suspect a hearing deficit in children who turn the television or radio volume up loud or who consistently turn their heads as if to catch the sound of the spoken word more easily. Also, suspect a hearing deficit in middle childhood if the child suddenly (1) begins to do less well in school, (2) misinterprets directions, or (3) fails to answer questions correctly. Children may be doing their best and may be unaware that they are not hearing all the information provided in class. The inability to hear directions may cause them to do poorly in school, which in turn can negatively affect the child's psychosocial development, especially if the child is punished or admonished to work harder because of failure to achieve in school.

ALERT *Infants and children who develop OM are particularly prone to development of either temporary or permanent hearing impairment.*

The child may use behavior in an attempt to cover up the problem. Silliness, using excuses, or joking may be conscious or unconscious attempts to distract peers, teachers, and family members from the fact that the child

did not clearly hear directions. Indeed, the youngster may not know that he or she did not hear all the directions. The child only knows that he or she did not perform as desired by the parent or teacher or as expected by peers.

Prenatal, environmental, and disease-related factors may affect development of the auditory systems and/or the ability to hear. Refer to Focused Health History 28-1 for examples of variables that can lead to hearing losses.

ALERT *Medications such as gentamicin or dihydrostreptomycin may be ototoxic (damaging to the cochlear mechanism of the inner ear) when given in high doses or under certain conditions. Space doses equally around the clock and measure peak/trough levels to avoid serum levels in the toxic range. Monitor renal function and hydration to ensure that they are within normal limits.*

ANSWER: Prematurity, hyperbilirubinemia, mechanical ventilation, and exposure to ototoxic medications are risk factors for impaired hearing, and all are present in Gabriella's health history.

Communication and Language Development History

The critical period for learning language is the first 36 months of life. Children who are unable to hear during that time are unable to learn the language necessary for normal verbal communication unless hearing intervention is provided. This deficit can affect learning, social development, and eventual vocational and economic potential. Learning the vocabulary and skills needed for communication is much harder after those first critical months have passed. Hearing deficit that begins after 36 months of age also diminishes the ability to profit from spoken words and sounds, but not to the same extent as a hearing deficit that begins prelingually.

Begin the health history with an assessment of articulation and language usage appropriate to the age of the child (see Focused Health History 28-1 and Developmental Considerations 3-3). If deviations from normal are found in the family's report, describe the characteristics of the child's speech and language ability with respect to articulation, fluency, voice quality, and word usage both by family report and by observation. Note psychosocial stressors or issues that could affect communication, such as bilingual environment.

FOCUSED PHYSICAL ASSESSMENT

Physical assessment of the sensory organs and affirmation that sensory function is intact begin immediately after birth and continue throughout our lives. Although many parts of the assessment requires the skills of a trained medical specialist, the nurse can complete an assessment that serves as the first level of screening to identify concerns that may require referral to a clinician who has more specialization in the area of concern. Focused Physical Assessment 28-1 provides an overview of the

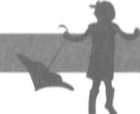

FOCUSED PHYSICAL ASSESSMENT 28-1
The Child With Sensory Alterations

Assessment Parameter	Alterations/Clinical Significance
General appearance	*Eyes* • Asymmetric placement and wide or close-set spacing of eyes may indicate congenital malformation. • Ptosis (drooping eye lids) and sunset eyes (appearance of upper portion of the sclera) may indicate neurologic conditions. • Slanted palpebral fissures are seen in children of Asian descent and in children with chromosomal abnormalities. • Swelling, tenderness, or lesions of the eyelid and surrounding tissue seen with blocked sebaceous gland or periorbital cellulitis. • Excessive tearing or discharge can indicate blocked tear duct, infection, or trauma. *Ears* • Presence of lop ears, skin tags, dimples, sinus tracts, and developmental anomalies (e.g., cleft lip or palate, abnormality of the pinna) may be associated with congenital disorders locally or in other organs (e.g., kidney). • Low-set or asymmetric placement may indicate congenital malformation or other congenital condition (e.g., chromosomal disorders, genitourinary disorders). • Excessive cerumen or discharge (yellow or greenish) from ear canal may indicate infection or presence of foreign body. • Structural abnormalities of head and neck may indicate congenital defect. • Presence of piercings and any signs of infection at piercing sites. *Oral Cavity* • Symmetry and facial expression may indicate cranial nerve defect or congenital defects. • Structural abnormalities such as cleft lip or palate or mandibular hypoplasia indicate congenital malformation. • Presence or absence of teeth may affect speech (e.g., young child who has recently lost front teeth). • Lesions, excoriations, or infections of the mouth or teeth may make speaking painful.
Structures	*Eyes* • Color changes of the sclera (yellow tint may be the result of jaundice; bluish tint, osteogenesis imperfecta) • Pupils unequal in size, shape, movement, or reaction to light may indicate trauma, accommodation disorders, strabismus, or nystagmus. • Black-and-white spots on the iris (Brushfield spots) are noted both in children with Down syndrome and in normal children. *Ears* • Inflammation of ear canal or tympanic membrane may indicate infection. • Pain with movement of the tragus may indicate otitis externa (OE). • Inability to visualize landmarks of middle ear, a pearly gray tympanic membrane, or other changes in the tympanic membrane (e.g., bulging, red, lack of mobility) may indicate inflammation, presence of a foreign body, or perforation. • Presence of fluid or bubbles behind tympanic membrane indicates OM or middle ear effusion (MEE). • Tympanic membrane that is scarred or an ashen gray color indicates previous perforations. *Oral Cavity* • Presence of a short or tight frenulum, as indicated by the child's inability to touch the tongue to the roof of the mouth, may impact speech and eating behaviors. • Lack of gag reflex may indicate damage to the glossopharyngeal nerve or vagus nerve. • Enlarged tonsils or increased redness or tonsillar exudate may indicate infection.

many aspects of the physical exam that are essential for the nurse to complete. Chapter 8 provides an in-depth description of the physical assessment of the eyes.

> **QUESTION:** The Goldman's first questions are, "How will you check her vision?" and "When will you know if her vision is impaired?" What explanation would you give to Abby and Ben?

Examination of the Eyes

Physical assessment of vision begins in infancy when the eye and sight are undergoing great change in a short period of time. Abnormalities identified and treated at this early age can prevent permanent loss of vision. Infants and young children are less able to understand directions and cooperate with the examiner, making assessment a challenge. However, children who are younger than 5 years of age should not forgo assessment because of development challenges; rather, they should be screened for vision problems such as amblyopia, strabismus, and near- and farsightedness (Agency for Healthcare Research and Quality, 2011; AAO, 2007; Schmucker et al., 2009). As children grow older, their cooperation makes physical assessment much easier and more accurate.

Children older than the age of 5 years should have their vision assessed every 1 to 2 years. Concerns raised by family members or teachers should prompt appropriate eye examinations, particularly because eye changes occur as physical growth progresses. The adolescent's ability to succeed and to reach his or her maximum potential in school and on the job could be jeopardized by the inability to see clearly.

> **ANSWER:** An example of the explanation the nurse might give to Abby and Ben is, "Right now, the ophthalmologists will examine the blood vessels of her retina weekly. It is possible that the blood vessels will stop spreading and growing, and no intervention will be needed. If the proliferation of retinal blood vessels increases dramatically, there are procedures that can be done to stop them, such as laser surgery or cryotherapy. There are also rare complications of ROP, such as a detached retina, that would immediately indicate her vision would be significantly impaired. Most of the time, we just don't know exactly how well she can see until she is older."

Examination of the Ears

Assessment continues with evaluation of the anatomic structures associated with hearing. Chapter 8 provides an in-depth description of the physical assessment of the head, neck, and ears. Inspecting the child's head and neck for structural anomalies or congenital defects is particularly important. Some facial structures arise from the same fetal tissue or are subject to the same genetic influences that affect the ears; thus, an abnormality in one should alert the health care provider to the possibility of other defects. Assessment of the ear includes evaluation of external structures, the ear canal,

and otoscopic examination of the internal structures of the middle ear (Vanderpool, 2009) (see Focused Physical Assessment 28-1). Several assessment techniques can be used to further assess hearing. These include techniques for hearing acuity and the Weber and Rinne tests.

When the assessment, performed by the nurse or other health care provider, indicates that a hearing deficit could or does exist, the child is referred to an audiologist. Criteria for referral include the following:

- Evidence of one or more risk factors
- Reported observations by family members or teachers of concern
- Questionable results with Rinne, Weber, or other screening test
- Decline in child's school performance
- Child complaints of inability to hear as well as before

>
> **QUESTION:** Abby and Ben ask, "How will Gabriella's hearing be tested? When will we know for sure if she does have a hearing loss?" How will you answer them?

Hearing Acuity

Behavioral assessment of hearing acuity is ideally done in a quiet room without external noise—a difficult task in the typical office or clinic. The whisper test, which is part of the basic physical assessment protocol used in many offices and clinics, requires the examiner to whisper a selected word while out of the line of vision of the child. The child's ability to hear the word is recorded as normal if the infant turns toward the examiner or exhibits pupillary response or blink reflex or if the older child is able to repeat the word. In the case of preverbal children, a change in behavior is considered an indication of hearing. Because of the variability in infant behavior, lack of consistency between examiners, and inability to control for either volume of the whisper or external noise, the whisper test is, at best, a gross measure of hearing acuity that should not be depended on to indicate normal hearing, particularly in high-risk infants and children.

Hearing in infants and young children may also be assessed in the home or office by making noise using a bell, a noisemaker toy, or a jangling set of keys out of the child's line of vision. A behavioral change, quieting behavior, or searching behavior is expected if the child hears the sound. The examiner may choose to look for the "startle response" by suddenly clapping the hands or otherwise making a loud noise out of the infant's line of vision. The hearing child would be expected to cry and act startled whereas the nonhearing infant would make no response. These tests also are, at best, rough estimates of the child's hearing ability and should not be depended on if other indicators of hearing deficit, such as delayed speech, occur.

Rinne and Weber tests

The Rinne and Weber tests can be used to assess hearing when the child reaches middle childhood. However, these tests may not yield accurate results until the child is 8 or 9 years of age because of behavioral factors and the child's desire to give the examiner the "correct" answer. A child who is at risk for or suspected of having a hearing deficit should be examined with tests that have been shown to be more accurate for the younger age groups. The Rinne and Weber tests are described here in case they are selected for use with older children.

The Rinne test evaluates for conductive and sensorineural hearing loss. The examiner strikes a tuning fork against his or her hand and then holds the base against the child's mastoid bone; the child hears the tuning fork through bone conduction. The child is asked to indicate when the sound is no longer heard. At that time, the tuning fork is held near the ear. The child with normal hearing hears the sound of the tuning fork again, this time through air conduction. Normal finding is air conduction (AC) greater than bone conduction (BC), and is recorded as AC > BC. If the child does not hear the sound through air conduction, the child should be referred to audiology for further testing. MEE or a middle ear anomaly may be present.

For the Weber test, the examiner again strikes the tuning fork on his or her hand, causing it to vibrate, and places the base in the midline on the child's forehead. The child is asked to indicate whether the sound is heard better on one side than on the other. Normally, the sound is heard equally on both sides. If the sound is heard better on one side than the other, a hearing impairment exists. The sound will lateralize to the ear with conductive hearing loss, as sometimes occurs in OM with effusion.

Evaluation of Communication

All children are assessed for developmental delays in communication on a regular basis during well-child examinations. Any tool used should rely on both family report and observations of the evaluator. Assessment will help to distinguish between variations in normal developmental patterns and true delay. With knowledge of normal speech acquisition patterns, the nurse may have opportunity to reassure family members (see Developmental Considerations 3-3). Children 18 to 24 months of age understand far more words than they will use. They will use an average of only 10 to 20 words, with less than 50% understandable by outsiders. By 24 months of age, the child's vocabulary averages 50 words, with 50% understandable. Various factors contribute to less-than-average vocabulary: (1) learning two languages at the same time, (2) having siblings who speak for the child, or (3) family members who meet the child's needs/wants without requiring use of words. When none of these is found to be applicable, the possibility of hearing deficit must be considered; refer the child for a full evaluation by a speech–language pathologist and audiologist.

Alterations in hearing often affect speech and language development; therefore, including speech and language during the evaluation of hearing is essential. Assessing the infant's vocalization, early syllable formation, and eventual verbalization and comparing the assessment with developmental norms provides additional clues to hearing impairment. An infant who fails to vocalize within the expected age range or who fails to form syllables may be unable to hear the vocalizations of other people. The nonhearing infant makes normal infant sounds; however, these sounds do not progress to syllabic babbling. Any infant or child with delayed speech should receive a full hearing assessment from an audiologist as soon as possible. Any child who fails to repeat new words in their entirety requires further assessment. A child who omits initial sounds or final sounds may not be hearing the sounds in a particular decibel range. For example, the final "ing" or "p" or "b" may simply be lost to the hearing of the child with residual fluid in the middle ear.

DIAGNOSTIC CRITERIA

In addition to the previously described elements of the physical examination, other technologic methods using sophisticated equipment are used to determine normal and abnormal sensory function and to monitor progress as a child undergoes treatment (Tests and Procedures 28-1). Family members need to be kept fully informed concerning the purpose of each test and how it is done. None of the tests are invasive or painful.

Vision

The use of automated vision screening technology (instrument-based vision screening) has been endorsed by the AAP (2012). Instrument-based screening is performed and interpreted by trained personnel and yields information about the presence and magnitude of optical and physical abnormalities of the eye (AAP, 2012). Photoscreening and autorefraction are examples of instrument-based screening. Photoscreening uses optical images of the eye's red reflex to estimate factors that place the child at risk for amblyopia, such as refractive error, media opacity, and ocular alignment. Autorefraction uses automated skiascopy or wavefront technology to objectively measure the eye's refraction error. Children who have difficulty holding still or undergoing examination with the ophthalmoscope or other equipment may be able to look at a particular object long enough for a photograph to obtain images of the pupillary reflexes (inflections) and the red reflex (Bruckner test). The ophthalmologist can review the screened images and the computer analysis to detect any positive findings. This graphic record also enables comparison with future photographs as a child with a detected disorder progresses in his or her therapy. Children who do not pass the assessment should receive a more complete eye examination.

Visual acuity in children older than 5 years of age who are verbal and cooperative can be assessed using a variety of wall charts. Several wall charts show pictures or shapes easily identified in any language: a boat, cup, circle, box, or heart. The Tumbling E chart requires the person to show which direction the arms on the E letters are pointing (E with arms pointing to the right, with arms pointing upward, to the left, or downward). For children who are literate, a chart with alphabet may be used. Various computer programs use a combination of boxes, letters, numbers, and pictures (Saunders, 2010).

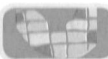 **TESTS AND PROCEDURES for Evaluating Sensory Alterations**

Diagnostic Test or Procedure	Purpose	Findings and Indications	Health Care Provider Considerations
Vision			
Visual acuity: Snellen E Kindergarten Test Chart Tumbling E chart Handheld Tumbling E or picture chart HOTV system (visual chart of letters H–O–T–V in various sizes) LEA Symbols Titmus Vision Screening	Test visual acuity	Acuity should be normal for age in each eye. To achieve credit for a line on the Snellen chart, the child must identify four out of six symbols on the line. For tests with larger letters/symbols where there are fewer per line, child must identify one more than half the letters/symbols on the line to pass. *Abnormal* scores: For ages 5 and younger, anything worse than 20/40 or a two-line difference between eyes needs referring. For ages 6 through adult, anything worse than 20/30 or a two-line difference between eyes needs referring,	Cover one eye at a time; test the uncovered eye. Child should avoid putting pressure on the eyeball that is covered. Any child who refuses to complete the test on one eye or the other is presumed to be unable to see well using that eye. If age 3 years, retest in 6 months; if age 4 years or older, retest in 1 month. If child refuses again, refer to the ophthalmologist. Children with deviations from normal should see the eye care specialist. Remind the family that visual acuity changes as the child grows in height and in maturity.
Blackbird Vision Screening System	Screens for visual acuity in young children who have short attention spans, are preverbal, and are preliterate	Normal acuity is indicated when the child is able to accurately tell position and direction of the bird in the story.	Child puts on a pair of cardboard "glasses" that allows first one, then the other eye to be occluded as the child listens to the story and watches the bird in the examiner's book fly to different positions and shows the examiner which way the bird is flying. The glasses, which the child takes home, contain a message to the family indicating that the child has participated in vision screening on that day.
Red reflex assessment	Screens for abnormalities of the back of the eye (posterior segment) and opacities in the visual axis, such as a cataract or corneal opacity	Both red reflexes should be of similar pink color of same hue with no opacities or white spots. Presence of white reflex or any white or dark spots is considered abnormal.	Ophthalmoscope is held close to the examiner's eye at 12–18 in. from the child's eyes. If color differs, or one is white and the other pink, report this to the health care provider for referral to the eye care professional.
Funduscopic examination	Identifies characteristics of internal ocular structures using an ophthalmoscope	Any abnormal findings in structure or appearance may indicate injury or compromises in vision.	Abnormal findings should be evaluated by the eye care specialist.

Diagnostic Test or Procedure	Purpose	Findings and Indications	Health Care Provider Considerations
Photoscreening	Uses optical images of the eye's red reflex to determine such factors as estimated refractive error, media opacity, and ocular alignment	Abnormal appearance of cornea and lens may indicate amblyopia and strabismus.	Handheld devices are particularly useful with infants, young children, and older children who are unwilling or unable to cooperate with visual acuity tests. The test takes less than 1 minute to perform. Stationary devices require the child to rest his or her chin on the machine's chin rest and look at a spot in the center of the camera. Tests can be completed by trained personnel. Photos can be taken at school or in any location and evaluated later by an eye care professional. Abnormal appearance requires further ophthalmologic testing using other technologies.
Vision field tests	Determine vision loss in any area of the visual field Screen for eye diseases, such as macular degeneration and glaucoma, which cause gaps in the visual field Completed as part of a neurologic examination after a stroke, head injury, or other condition that causes reduced blood flow to the brain	The complete visual field is seen by both eyes at the same time, and it includes the central visual field—which detects the highest degree of detail—and the side (peripheral) visual fields. Abnormal findings: visual cues in all visual fields are not accurately identified by the patient. May indicate presence of eye disease or nervous system disorder (e.g., tumor).	Difficult for young children to follow instructions and to complete this examination in an accurate fashion. Noninvasive tests
Color vision tests (e.g., Ishihara color plates)	Assess ability to distinguish color Used to screen for color blindness in people with suspected retinal or optic nerve disease or who have a family history of color blindness	People who have normal color vision are able to distinguish the colored numbers, symbols, or paths from the background of colored dots. Color vision tests merely detect a problem; further testing is needed to identify what is causing the problem.	Tests can be completed in a few minutes and are noninvasive. Refer for further testing if indicated. Color vision is usually tested only once, usually around age 5 years as children are entering their school years.

(Continued)

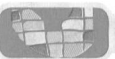 **TESTS AND PROCEDURES for Evaluating Sensory Alterations** *(Continued)*

Diagnostic Test or Procedure	Purpose	Findings and Indications	Health Care Provider Considerations
Autorefraction tests	Evaluate the refractive error of each eye	Identify presence of amblyogenic refractive error. Determine the correct prescription for eyeglasses or contact lenses.	Handheld devices are particularly useful with infants, young children, and older children who are unwilling or unable to cooperate. Test takes less than 1 minute to perform. Stationary device is used by an optometrist or ophthalmologist to evaluate the eyes with different lenses until the lens that corrects vision the best (sometimes better than 20/20 or 6/6) is found. Refraction is done as a routine part of an eye examination for people who already wear glasses or contact lenses. Child may have difficulty describing the effects of looking at an eye chart through various corrective lenses.
Hearing			
Auditory Brainstem Response (ABR)	Detects brain activity and quantifies the characteristics of the response when sounds are presented; may be used as part of newborn screening program. Earphones are placed on the child for introduction of clicking sounds. Electrodes are placed on the child's head to detect brain activity when sounds are heard. A computer averages these responses and displays waveforms.	There are characteristic waveforms for normal hearing in portions of the speech range. If brain activity is identified, test result is a "Pass." A normal ABR can predict fairly well that a child's hearing is normal in that part of the range. Characteristics of the response are measured and quantified by the audiologist. An abnormal ABR may be the result of hearing loss, but it may also be the result of some medical problems or measurement difficulties.	Discuss purpose of the test with the family. If not yet done, discuss family history for possible identification of risk factors for the infant. Ask the family to feed the infant immediately before the test is scheduled so the infant is quiet and calm. The child must remain quiet throughout the 15-minute test. If the child is at a very young age, the test may be performed under natural sleep; otherwise, the test is performed when the child is sedated. Provide the family with the results (pass/fail) and further information about follow-up if necessary.
Otoacoustic emissions (OAEs) Include transient-evoked otoacoustic emission (TEOAE) and distortion product otoacoustic emission (DPOAE)	Screen for middle and inner ear abnormalities contributing to diminished hearing Measure acoustic emissions generated in the cochlea in response to sounds; these emissions are picked up by sensitive microphones placed in the outer ear canal; these tests identify cochlear activity in each ear separately	Probes are placed in each ear canal, signals are delivered, and otoacoustic response (presence, absence, intensity) is recorded. The test does not measure transmission of sounds to the brain. Residual vernix in the ear or mild MEE can interfere with the recording of the OAEs, creating a false-positive result.	Test is performed by technicians trained in the use of the measurement device. Infant should be quiet during the test.

Diagnostic Test or Procedure	Purpose	Findings and Indications	Health Care Provider Considerations
Tympanometry	Assesses the status of the middle ear conduction system—that is, the tympanic membrane and the mobility of the bones of the middle ear A tone is introduced into the ear canal and the amount of sound reflected back from the tympanic membrane is measured as the pressure changes during the test.	The resulting graph should show a clear peak in the center as the mobile tympanic membrane moves in response to the sound. An ear with effusion (fluid behind the membrane) will show little, if any, mobility of the tympanic membrane.	Administered to children of all ages, although special equipment is needed to test infants younger than 4 months of age because of the small size of the external auditory canal. If abnormality is found, show the family the graph indicating that effusion is present and the child is probably not hearing well at this time.
Play audiometry	Evaluates hearing in each ear separately and evaluates behavioral responses to the sounds; after training and practice, earphones are placed on the child and sounds of specific frequencies and decibels are introduced; child's behavior in response to sounds is recorded	No response to sounds or inconsistent response to sounds indicates hearing loss.	Used with children who cooperate sufficiently to put a peg in a board or drop a block in a box in response to sounds Test is usually conducted in a specialized quiet location by a trained technician. Teach the child to perform an activity each time a sound is heard (e.g., putting a block in a box, placing pegs in a hole). Teach the child to wait, listen, and respond. Ideally, earphones are placed on the child's head so that independent information can be obtained for each ear. If the child refuses earphone placement or earphone placement is otherwise not possible, sounds are presented through speakers inside a sound booth. However, sound field screening does not give ear-specific information, thus hearing loss in only one ear may be missed.
Pure tone audiometry	Allows office screening for hearing loss for children aged 4 years and older In a quiet room, child is asked to indicate when a sound is heard. Various tones are presented by the instrument.	Success of the test depends on the child's cooperation and ability to focus on the sounds being presented. If hearing loss is identified, the primary care provider assesses the child's physical status and may refer the child to the audiologist if indicated.	Any health care provider may learn to use the equipment and to administer the screening test. The test is best done in a quiet room. Gain the child's cooperation and practice using midrange, louder sounds. Administer the test and record findings on the test report provided.

Hearing

Audiometry is used to evaluate two characteristics of sounds: intensity and pitch. The *intensity* of sounds that are heard by the human ear is measured in **decibels (dB)**. Extremely soft sounds that the hearing ear can hear are between 0 dB and 20 dB in intensity. Examples are whispers or rustling leaves. The sound of a train traveling rapidly on a nearby track measures approximately 90 dB. A normal conversation is about 60 dB. Chain saws, hammer drills, and bulldozers ring in at more than 100 dB. The *pitch* of a sound is its tonal quality, the speed at which the sound waves vibrate. High tones are caused by rapid vibration of sound waves, whereas the vibrations of low tones are slower. An example of high-pitched sounds is birds chirping; an example of low-pitched sounds includes motors and men's voices. Both intensity and pitch are important to the ability to hear and comprehend verbal communication. Audiometric testing assesses the infant's or child's ability to hear sounds of various intensities as well as various pitches.

The accuracy of hearing screening has improved with use of OAE tests and automated ABR testing (see Tests and Procedures 28-1). OAEs can be recorded from the ears of normal-hearing people but not from the ears of those with more than mild hearing losses (Holte, 2003). OAE tests are quick, noninvasive, and inexpensive, thus many states have adopted them to evaluate the hearing of all newborns prior to discharge. The ABR is an electrophysiologic measurement of activity in the auditory nerve and brain stem pathways (American Speech-Language-Hearing Association [ASHA], 2004).

Legislation in many states requires that all newborns undergo objective screening using the ABR. The Joint Committee on Infant Hearing (2007) recommends that infants admitted to the neonatal intensive care unit for more than 5 days should have ABR testing completed to screen for neural hearing loss. Infants who do not pass this screening are referred to an audiologist for rescreening and more comprehensive testing as indicated. It is also recommended that infants readmitted to the hospital in the first month of life should have a repeat hearing screening before discharge when the child has conditions associated with potential hearing loss (e.g., hyperbilirubinemia requiring exchange transfusion or culture-positive sepsis).

ANSWER: Gabriella will be tested at discharge for hearing loss with the ABR. The test uses click stimuli to evaluate the cochlear and brain stem response of the infant. The ABR does not specifically test what frequencies Gabriella can hear. It is possible for her to fail the ABR, have some hearing loss, but still be able to hear and understand conversation. Or, as happens rarely, she may pass the ABR and later be diagnosed with hearing loss in specific frequencies. Tone burst ABR and other newer sophisticated tests conducted by audiologists can be used to test specific frequencies. These tests can tell more about specific acoustic capacity of the child than earlier tests.

TREATMENT MODALITIES

The treatments for sensory alterations include measures to fully correct or reverse the underlying condition as well as measures to optimize vision, hearing, and communication to the greatest extent possible given the child's condition.

QUESTION: Ben and Abby also ask, "If Gabriella does have retinopathy of prematurity, how will it be treated?"

TREATMENTS FOR VISUAL PROBLEMS

Treatments for altered vision include corrective lenses, occlusion therapy, medication, and surgical intervention.

Corrective Lenses

Corrective lenses can be prescribed for children of any age to correct refractive errors (e.g., myopia, hyperopia, anisometropia), to protect a nonamblyopic eye, or to correct myopia in children with ROP. If a child has an unrecoverable loss of vision in one eye, polycarbonate protective lenses are highly recommended to protect the normal eye. Contact lenses may be substituted for eyeglasses when children are old enough to take responsibility for their care, insertion, removal, and cleaning (Tradition or Science 28-1).

Contact lenses are now being used for more than vision correction. Research is under way using the contact lens as a drug delivery system for treatment of glaucoma, as a way of measuring blood glucose, and as a way of measuring intraocular pressure. Research is also underway on restoring vision caused by corneal damage by infusing the contact lens with the patient's own stem cells and allowing them to repair the corneal damage (Benoit, 2012; Ciolino et al., 2009; Kading & Shen, 2012; Singh et al., 2011).

Evidence-Based Practice   **TRADITION OR SCIENCE 28-1**

At what age can children start wearing contact lenses?

For older children who really do not want to wear glasses, contact lenses are a good option. However, younger children aren't thought to be responsible enough to put lenses in, take them out, or clean and disinfect them without parental help. Walline et al. (2004) conducted a study to determine whether 8- to 11-year-old myopic children were able to wear and successfully manage the use of daily disposable contact lenses. The study demonstrated that these children were able to independently care for daily disposable lenses and wear them successfully. The disposable lenses eliminated the need for cleaning and disinfecting, which improved adherence to procedures required to avoid eye infections and eye injury. The researchers concluded that these lenses should be strongly considered as an option for younger children. Children in other studies reported significantly improved quality of life when allowed to wear contact lenses (Newman, 2011).

The rate of visual development is rapid during infancy and early childhood; thus, a young child who has corrective lenses prescribed should wear them all the time. All adults who work with the child should be encouraged to find ways to assist the child to keep the glasses on. The young child needs to see the ophthalmologist at regular, short intervals to monitor for possible changes in the prescription.

The majority of glasses for children are quite sturdy and have unbreakable lenses that are capable of withstanding much, but not all, of the wear and tear given to them by children. Breakage of glasses, as well as physical injury to the face and eyes, can occur because of falls.

 KidKare Protect active children from losing or breaking eyeglasses by using sports elastic during games such as basketball and soccer. Encourage children not to remove the eyeglasses during extracurricular activities.

Occlusion Therapy

Occlusion therapy is used to treat eye muscle weakness (see the section on "Strabismus"). The stronger eye is covered (e.g., with an eye patch), enabling the weaker eye to work alone for all or part of every day and thus become stronger. This can be accomplished with an eye patch or by clouding or covering one lens of the child's eyeglasses. Covering one lens of the eyeglasses loses its therapeutic value, however, if the child learns to peek around the covered or fogged lens. In that case, the eye patch is the treatment of choice (Fig. 28-3) (Gold et al., 2009).

During occlusion therapy, the ophthalmologist examines the child at frequent intervals to evaluate the progress made by the weaker eye and to detect any possible loss of vision in the patched good eye. The duration of treatment is determined by the ophthalmologist. Nursing responsibilities include working with the family to find ways to help the child accept the patching routine and thus strengthen the weaker eye. Gaining and keeping the child's cooperation is often a major challenge (Olitsky et al., 2009; Roefs et al., 2012). Note that family members who do not fully comprehend the importance of consistency in patching and frequent follow-up exams with the ophthalmologist tend to allow noncompliance

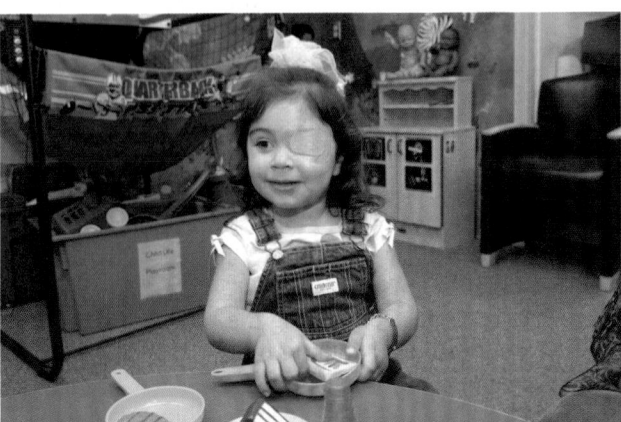

Figure 28-3 In occlusion therapy, the child keeps one eye patched to strengthen the other eye.

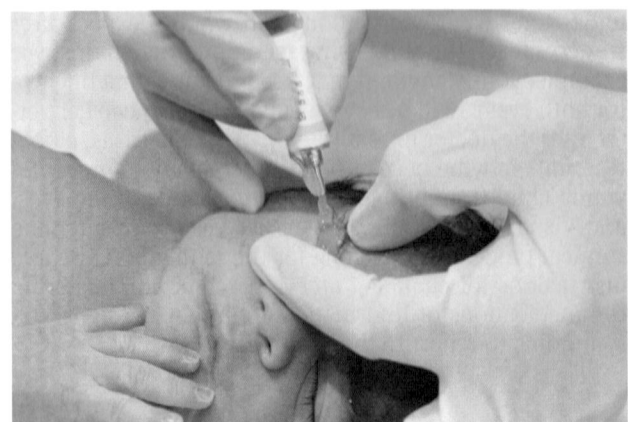

Figure 28-4 The nurse administers antibiotic eye ointment.

and thus jeopardize the child's vision. Therapy must continue over an extended period of time to be effective.

Pharmacologic Management

Antibiotics are used to treat bacterial infections of the eye and are administered topically, as drops or ointment (Fig. 28-4), or given orally. Decongestants, antihistamines, or a combination may be used topically or systemically to treat various ophthalmologic conditions such as allergic conjunctivitis. These medications may be prescribed to reduce ocular congestion, irritation, and itching (Burns et al., 2013).

In all cases, emphasize to the family the importance of using the medication according to directions, administering all doses each day, and finishing the prescription even if symptoms improve (see the**Point** Procedures/Interventions: Medication Administration: Ophthalmic). Warn older children and teenagers who may be self-administering the medication about the effects of using the medication more frequently than ordered. Additional information about administering ophthalmic medications is presented in Chapter 9.

Surgical Intervention

Surgical intervention may be necessary when the condition cannot be effectively treated with medical methods alone. Surgical alignment of the eyes may be considered for strabismus. Congenital cataracts are removed surgically, and laser surgery may be the treatment of choice for ROP, described later in this chapter.

Laser surgery, such as photorefractive keratometry and laser in situ keratomileusis, has been used in adults to correct refractory errors, but these procedures are considered experimental and are not approved by the U.S. Food and Drug Administration for children and adolescents younger than the age of 18 years. The procedures are difficult to perform in children because the child must remain still and cooperative during the procedures. In addition, children's eyes are still developing, and the refractive error remains in a state of change. The long-term effects of these procedures on a young child's eyes are unknown, so this mode of treatment is not generally recommended.

Preoperative and postoperative teaching is essential for the child and family. Ensure that the child and family understand what will be done and what to expect after surgery. Teach the child using age-appropriate terms. For example, young children may need to know that one eye (or both eyes) "will be covered up so it [they] can get better after the doctor fixes it [them]." In some cases, elbow restraints may be necessary postoperatively to prevent a young child from bringing his or her hands to the eyes, and visual therapy may be started very soon after the surgical procedure. Teaching for the family may include instructions for changing an eye patch or administering eye medications or information about danger signs and symptoms to report to the health care provider.

ANSWER: In response to Abby and Ben's question regarding treatment, you might provide the following explanation: "In most cases of ROP, the child's vision can be improved by wearing glasses. In situations when the growth of vessels warrants aggressive intervention, laser surgery might be performed."

TREATMENTS FOR HEARING PROBLEMS

QUESTION: If Gabriella is found to have a sensori-neural hearing loss, is there treatment for this problem?

The most important "treatment" for hearing loss is prevention. With the increased use of MP3 players, iPods, and other audio technology, children and adolescents are at increased risk for noise-induced hearing loss. Health care providers and families can partner to teach children to curtail hearing loss.

When children are born with or incur hearing impairment, treatment focuses on securing care and therapy for the child to maximize use of the residual hearing. The health care team works with the family to facilitate the child's developing independence and self-sufficiency and enhance communication through use of therapies such as hearing aids and cochlear implants.

Other treatment measures for disorders that may alter hearing include medication administration and surgery. Surgery may be indicated for reconstruction or cosmetic alteration of anatomic or structural defects. Surgical interventions may also be indicated to treat severe infections, and surgery is necessary when implanting certain types of hearing devices.

Prevention of Hearing Loss

A primary intervention of the health care team is to teach the family ways of preventing or minimizing injury to the ear and hearing loss. Routine health visits provide an excellent opportunity to discuss ear care with children and the family (Nursing Interventions 28-1).

NURSING INTERVENTIONS 28-1

Ear Care

Monitoring
- Monitor for drainage from ears, as appropriate.
- Monitor for episodes of dizziness associated with ear problems, as appropriate.
- Determine if cerumen in the ear canal is causing hearing loss.
- Monitor frequency of ear infections.

Preventative and Supportive Care
- Administer eardrops, as appropriate.
- Instill sweet oil in the ear to soften impacted cerumen before irrigation.
- Irrigate the ear canal with a Water-Pik on a low setting (or similar device) using warm water (80°–90° F), as appropriate.

Preventing Injury
- Avoid placing sharp objects in the ear.

Family Teaching
- Instruct family members how to clean infant's and child's ears.
- Instruct family members how to observe for ear infections in the infant and young child.

- Instruct family members about importance of completing antibiotic regimen when ordered for ear infections.
- Instruct family members to hold infant upright when bottle-feeding to avoid reflux into eustachian tubes.
- Demonstrate proper technique for ear irrigation to family/caregiver, as appropriate.
- Instruct about tubes as a medical treatment, as appropriate.
- Instruct to avoid immersing child's ears in water with tubes present.
- Instruct how to administer eardrops, as appropriate.
- Instruct about the importance of routine hearing testing.
- Instruct children not to put foreign objects in ears.
- Instruct how to monitor and regulate high-volume noise exposure.
- Instruct child to wear hearing protection for exposure to high-intensity noise.
- Instruct teenager concerning the potential danger of exposure to high-volume music, especially with headphones or ear buds.
- Instruct children with pierced ears how to avoid infection at the insertion site.

Review how to best clean the ear without causing damage to the sensitive tissues of the external canal. Urge parents and older children to never insert anything into the external canal. Advise them to clean the outer portion with a moist washcloth, leaving the cerumen in the external auditory canal to help maintain skin integrity inside the canal. Older children and adolescents may learn how to avoid infection at insertion sites on pierced ears by cleansing with soap and water if needed (see Chapter 7 for more information about care of piercings). For the child who has excessive cerumen buildup, use of an over-the-counter (OTC) product may be recommended. This treatment may include drops followed by gentle washing with warm water and a bulb syringe.

In a survey conducted by ASHA (2006), more than half of the surveyed adolescents reported at least one symptom of hearing loss. Teach the child and family about risk factors associated with hearing loss and how to minimize them, including preventing prolonged exposure to sound levels greater than 85 dB. Inner ear cells are sensitive to vibrations; excessive exposure to loud noise can damage the hairs in the cochlea (inner ear) and lead to hearing loss. Repeated exposure to loud noise can cause permanent damage and hearing loss, a condition known as *noise-induced hearing loss*. If the ears are damaged, sometimes the child with hearing loss will hear ringing or buzzing, even when there is no sound. Ringing in the ears, hissing, clicking, or buzzing sounds are all types of *tinnitus*, a common side effect of noise-induced hearing loss. An online survey completed by 9,363 adolescents and young adults indicated, by Likert scale, that hearing loss was considered a "very big problem" by only 8% of the respondents. However, most respondents had experienced tinnitus or hearing impairment after attending concerts (61%) and clubs (43%). Only 14% of survey participants had used earplugs at concerts and clubs to diminish the impact of loud music at these venues. A large number (66%) indicated they could be motivated to wear ear protection if they were aware of the potential for permanent hearing loss (Chung et al., 2005). Nurses are in a unique position to provide this information to vulnerable adolescents and young adults.

Repeated middle ear infections can also contribute to hearing loss. Reducing the incidence of respiratory tract infections in children, implementing breastfeeding for at least the first 6 months of life, avoiding supine bottle-feeding, and eliminating passive exposure to tobacco smoke have all been identified as effective in reducing the incidence of acute OM (Lieberthal et al., 2013).

Medication

Anti-infective drugs may be used topically in otic solution administered as eardrops when infections are present in the external auditory canal. Antibiotics may be given orally in liquid, chewable, or tablet form when the infection is located in the middle ear. Teach the family that prescriptions must be given for the length of time prescribed or the child runs the risk of recurrence or complications resulting from incomplete eradication of the organism. Chapter 9 describes the technique for administering otic medications (see thePoint Procedures/Interventions for procedure on Medication Administration: Otic).

Antipyretics and analgesics are useful in treating fever and pain associated with ear infections. Cerumenolytics are medications used to soften cerumen impacted in the external auditory canal for removal. Acidic eardrops help to prevent growth of bacteria or fungi in the external ear, particularly in children who swim frequently. To prevent swimmer's ear, the family may choose to use an OTC product, placed in the child's external auditory canal after swimming; alternatively, a solution of equal parts rubbing alcohol and white vinegar may be used.

Hearing Aids

Hearing aids are devices used to amplify and/or modify sounds to assist a person with a hearing loss. They are distinguished by where they are worn: behind the ear (BTE), in the ear (ITE), completely in the canal (CIC), and in the canal (ITC) (Chart 28-1). Hearing aids provide amplification in the pitch range where the individual child has a deficiency. Although the hearing aid can treat sound

CHART 28-1 Types of Hearing Aids

BTE (Behind the Ear)
- Suitable for all types of hearing losses, from mild to profound
- Electronics housed in a case that fits behind the ear; tubing and a custom-made ear mold direct the sound to the ear canal
- Type most often recommended for children, exceptionally sturdy; not limited by the size of the child's ear
- Made in several colors to match hair and skin tones

ITE (In the Ear)
- Used for a wide range of hearing losses
- Custom-made to fit the individual user's ear
- Worn inside the ear; usually recommended for mild to moderate, or sometimes even severe, hearing loss
- Available in several sizes; not usually recommended for young children (outer ears and ear canals are too small; still growing)
- Typically worn by children aged 8–10 years and older

CIC (Completely in the Canal)
- Smallest hearing aid style available, almost invisible in the ear
- All components housed in a small case that fits deep into the ear canal
- Suitable for mild to moderate hearing loss; not suitable for severe hearing loss
- Most children's ear canals not large enough to use CIC devices; possibly appropriate for older adolescents

ITC (In the Canal)
- A little bigger than the CIC; also fits deep into the ear canal
- Uses a slightly larger battery than CIC devices
- Used for mild to moderate hearing losses
- Not suitable for young children because their ear canals are too small and are growing rapidly; possibly appropriate for older adolescents

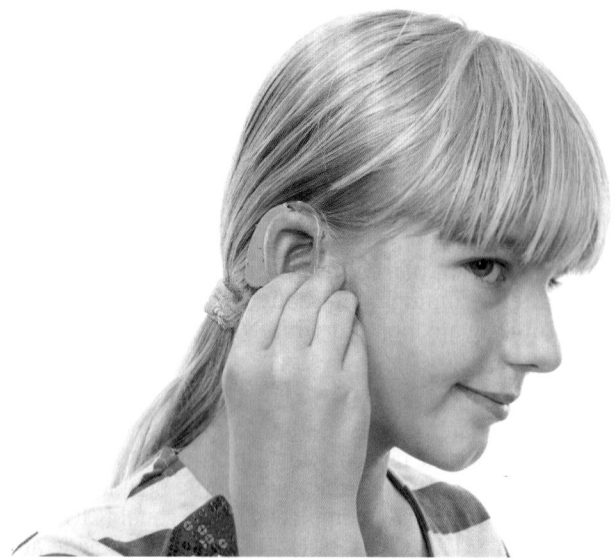

Figure 28-5 The child with a hearing aid.

electronically, it cannot completely differentiate between speech and background noises. The child using the hearing aid learns to recognize sounds as they are received, which may be quite different from the sounds received by children without hearing impairment (Fig. 28-5). The child may need to use speechreading in addition to the amplification device. Teaching Intervention Plan 28-1 summarizes the instructions for a family with a child using a hearing aid. When speaking with a child who uses a hearing aid, first get his or her attention, then be sure he or she can see your face as you speak. Enunciate words clearly, but do not speak more loudly than usual.

Cochlear Implant

Cochlear implant is recommended for children who are born with profound hearing loss or who sustain damage or injury that causes auditory nerve damage. Children with bilateral severe to significant sensorineural hearing loss and who do not benefit from conventional hearing aids are often candidates for cochlear implants.

Cochlear implants convert speech and environmental sounds into electrical signals and send these signals to the hearing nerve. The implant consists of a small electronic device, which is surgically implanted under the skin behind the ear, and an external speech processor. A microphone is worn outside the body as a headpiece behind the ear to capture incoming sound. Currently available devices have a magnet that holds the external system in place next to the implanted internal system. The external system may be worn entirely behind the ear and the speech processor may be worn in a pocket, belt pouch, or harness (Fig. 28-6). The speech processor translates the sound into distinctive electrical signals.

TIP 28-1: A TEACHING INTERVENTION PLAN for Care of the Child With a Hearing Aid

Nursing Diagnosis and Family Outcomes

- Deficient knowledge: Care and management of hearing aid
  Outcomes: Child will learn to care for own hearing aid.
  Child will adapt to use of hearing aid to enhance communication ability.

Teach Child/Family

General Information About Hearing Aids
- Information concerning children's hearing aid (amplification devices) styles and selection (see Chart 28-1)
- Characteristics of children's hearing aid such as
  - Are not easily broken
  - Do not require resizing as the child grows
  - Has sufficient power to meet the needs of the individual child

Adjusting to a Hearing Aid
- Both family and child need a period of time to adjust to the use and care of the hearing aid.
- At first, the amplification device may frighten the infant or confuse the older child.
- Some children may have physiologic responses, such as dizziness, when the amplification device is first used.

- An infant or child may require 1–3 months to adjust to wearing the hearing aid and attending to sounds.
- During and after the adjustment period, the infant or child must learn to assign meaning to sounds. Family members can help by making specific sounds to accompany pleasurable experiences.

Keeping the Hearing Aid Working Properly
- Examine the hearing aid daily, clean the ear mold, and test the battery.

Care of the Hearing Aid as the Child Matures
- By the age of 5 years, the child should be able to take on responsibilities for the care and maintenance of the hearing aid, which include:
  - Inserting and removing the ear mold and hearing aid
  - Notifying the family or teacher when a battery change is needed or the unit is malfunctioning
- When manual dexterity is present, taking on full responsibility for cleaning and testing the unit and for changing batteries

Contact Health Care Provider if
- Unit is not providing amplification as expected
- Ear mold is causing pain in the ear
- Child refuses to wear the hearing aid for any reason
- Ear mold or battery pack is broken

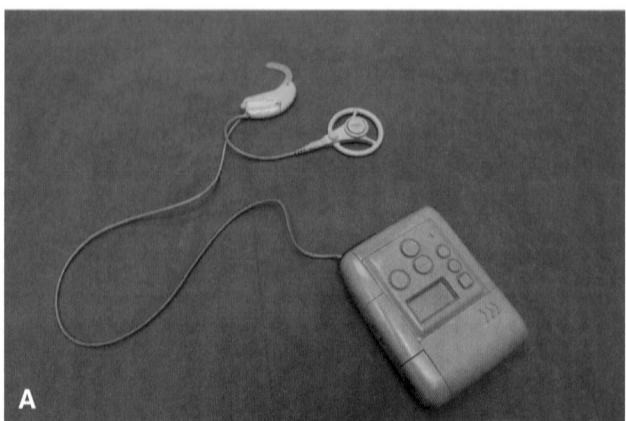
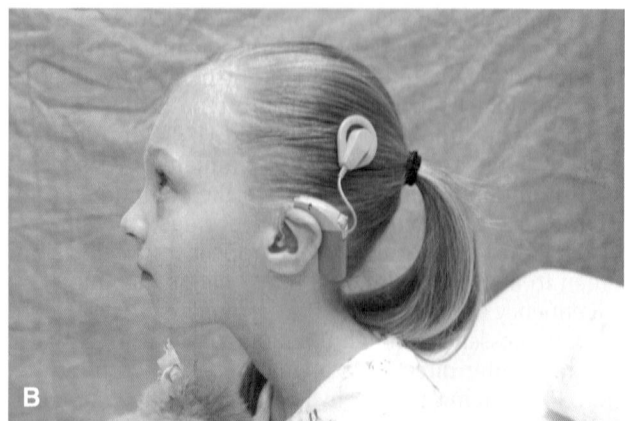

Figure 28-6 Cochlear implant device. (A) The external components of this cochlear implant device consist of an earpiece microphone, an external magnet to be placed near the internal device, and a speech processor. (B) The external components of a cochlear implant device are held in place by magnets placed in both the headpiece and the implant.

These signals or "codes" travel up a thin cable to the headpiece and are transmitted across the skin by radio waves to the electrodes implanted in the cochlea. The electrodes' signals stimulate the auditory nerve fibers to send information to the brain, where it is interpreted as meaningful sound. The brain learns to recognize this signal and the person experiences this as "hearing."

The implant is placed in a 2- to 3-hour outpatient procedure under general anesthesia. An incision is made to implant the device, thus the child will have a dressing on his or her head postoperatively and will require information about care of the dressing and assessment of the incision site for infection. Approximately 2 to 4 weeks after the implant is placed, the child returns to the implant center to have the external components of the device programmed and activated. The audiologist determines the child's threshold levels—that is, the minimum electrical current required to produce a response.

! ALERT *When the implant is turned off or not in use (e.g., while swimming, bathing, sleeping), the child cannot hear and is profoundly deaf.*

After the initial activation, the child will have several appointments with the audiologist within the first year to ensure maintenance and optimal performance of the device. Thereafter, annual appointments are scheduled to monitor the device. Speech and language therapy are initiated immediately after the device is activated and continue as long as needed to meet the individual needs of the child.

Cochlear implants are being used in children who have lost their hearing before the development of speech. Although these preverbal children cannot immediately tell us what they are hearing, observation by family members and subsequent testing demonstrate that these children communicate at least as well as those in whom cochlear implants were placed at a later age (Gifford et al., 2011; Rubinstein, 2002). The cochlear implant does not restore hearing to a normal range for deaf children; rather, it enables profoundly deaf children to detect sounds in the mild to moderate range of hearing loss. Thus, although the cochlear implant may dramatically affect speech and language development, the device alone does not guarantee the acquisition of spoken communication. Family involvement and ability to follow through with prescribed strategies to help the young child with hearing loss are critical to the child's ability to acquire language skills (DesJardin et al., 2006). Young children with cochlear implants have the potential to achieve language acquisition skills at the same level as their hearing peers (Caselli et al., 2012).

CROSS-CULTURAL CARE

Cochlear implants support communication within the home using spoken language. Studies have shown that exposure to a second language at home does not impair language acquisition in young children with cochlear implants. Children with cochlear implants can learn multiple spoken languages, and families need not fear introducing multiple languages to the child (Thomas et al., 2008).

Hearing Assistive Technology Systems

Several factors in the school and home setting can make hearing and communication a challenge for the hearing impaired child even if the child is using a hearing aid. These challenges include the distance between the child and the sound source (teacher, parent), competing noise in the classroom or home, poor room acoustics, reflections or echoes of sound (reverberations), and inability to attend to warning sounds (e.g., alarms) (ASHA, 2013).

Hearing assistive technology systems (HATS) are devices that maximize hearing and listening for people with a hearing loss. These devices can be used with or without hearing aids or cochlear implants. The primary goal of HATS is to provide the hearing impaired child with a safe environment where academic achievement, social skills, and speech and language development can be enhanced. A variety of HATS are available and can be selected, evaluated, fitted, and dispensed by a certified audiologist. Depending on the type of device, the purpose is to amplify sound. Some HATS are devices that use lights and vibrations to stimulate other senses used by the individual to enhance the communication experience (e.g., when the phone rings, the device makes lights flash or a message appear on a television screen to alert the individual that a call is incoming).

Frequency modulation (FM) sound systems send auditory messages through FM radio waves using a wireless transmitter directed to a small receiver worn by the child. FM systems are effective both indoors and outdoors and can be portable or permanently installed. An FM system allows the child to hear the teacher's voice at a constant intensity level and allows the teacher's voice to be heard more predominantly over other background noises.

Infrared systems are often used in the home to make television watching a pleasant experience for the hearing impaired. Sound is transmitted using infrared light waves to a transmitter that can be worn by the child. The TV sound can be set to a level all family members can be comfortable with because the child is able to amplify the sound to a degree that assists him or her to also hear the sounds at a distinguishable level.

Other HATS devices can help children use their visual or tactile senses to alert them to what others would hear in their environment (e.g., door bells, telephone calls, alarm clocks). For example, devices can light up when a doorbell rings, vibrate when an alarm goes off, or show text when a phone call is received.

Surgical Intervention

Surgical intervention may be indicated to correct a hearing impairment or enhance auditory functioning. Ear surgery is also performed to treat diseases, injuries, or deformities of the ear's auditory canal, middle ear, inner ear, and auditory and vestibular systems. Ear surgery is commonly performed to treat conductive hearing impairment, persistent ear infections, unhealed perforated eardrums, congenital ear defects, and tumors.

Surgery may be the primary mode of treatment, or it may be used when more conservative medical treatments have failed. Common types of ear surgery include stapedectomy, tympanoplasty, myringotomy, removal of tumors, and insertion of cochlear implants.

Ear surgery may also be performed for cosmetic purposes to set disproportionately large or prominent ears closer to the head. This corrective surgery, called *otoplasty*, can be considered for ears that protrude more than four-fifths of an inch (2 cm) from the back of the head. It can be performed at any age but is most commonly performed at 5 or 6 years of age, after the ears have reached full size. Having the surgery at a young age has two benefits: the cartilage is more pliable, making it easier to reshape, and the child's self-image may benefit from the cosmetic improvement.

Most ear surgery is performed with an operating microscope (microsurgery) to enable the surgeon to view the very small structures of the ear. The popularity of minimally invasive laser surgery for middle ear procedures is growing because it reduces the amount of trauma caused by vibration, enhances coagulation, and enables surgeons to access hard-to-reach places in the middle ear. Laser surgery can be safely performed in an outpatient operating suite.

ANSWER: There is not a single treatment for sensorineural hearing loss. Amplification devices may be of some assistance. The primary focus of the intervention is to prevent the hearing loss from altering communication and the child's development of clear language.

TREATMENTS FOR COMMUNICATION PROBLEMS

Treatment modalities designed to assist the child to overcome a communication disorder must necessarily involve a number of persons with whom the child comes into contact. This could include—in addition to the family—the health care provider, nurse, audiologist, speech-language pathologist, speech therapist, daycare teacher or schoolteacher, school nurse, and social worker.

The primary roles of the nurse and the physician include identifying problems, providing encouragement and support to the child and family, and maintaining the child's general health. In the primary care setting in the office, clinic, or school, the nurse may participate in case finding as a part of well-child examinations or screening programs, may make independent observations, or may be responding to concerns by family members. Guidelines for referral when a child is found to have communication impairment are found in Community Care 28-1.

The nurse may also be responsible for encouraging follow-up visits or encouraging the family and child to adhere to the recommendations of the speech-language pathologist or audiologist. Family involvement is essential to promote application of language skills learned in therapy sessions.

In cases of a communication disorder, the audiologist acts as a consultant to rule out or manage a hearing disorder. The audiologist can identify hearing disability and recommend the use of an amplification device (hearing aid) as needed.

The speech–language pathologist may provide a detailed description of the child's disability and plan a program of therapy to improve the child's communication ability. The speech–language pathologist may also provide the therapy or may delegate the daily or weekly therapy to a speech therapist.

Speech therapy may be provided in a private practice setting or in the school. Children assessed and identified with communication disorders and in need of speech therapy may be provided services free of charge through their public school system. An individualized education program (IEP) may be used to specify the child's learning needs and accommodations needed to enhance the child's classroom abilities. The school

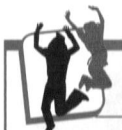

COMMUNITY CARE 28-1

Guidelines for Referral if Communication Impairment Is Suspected

Infancy
- Responsiveness to environmental sounds limited or absent
- Responsiveness to parental voice limited or absent
- Infant quieted by touch but not by voice
- Responsive vocalization limited or absent

Early Childhood
- Limited responsiveness to environmental sounds
- Does not seem to hear parental requests for the child's attention
- Does not use syllables or words
- Speech difficult to understand by 3 years of age
- Responds to visual cues but fails to respond to verbal cues
- Fails to follow directions when given verbally
- Inappropriate word usage for the age (e.g., vocabulary does not seem to grow with the child)

- Fails to use correct word endings (e.g., omits "ed," "ing," "s")
- Fails to form sentences correctly
- Stuttering or tonal dysfluency

Middle Childhood
- Any of the previous concerns identified in early childhood
- Consistent failure to follow directions presented verbally
- Failure to use appropriate voice quality or tone of voice (e.g., too loud, too soft, abnormally high or low pitch)
- Inability to construct complete and accurate sentences
- Consistent errors in pronunciation of specific sounds
- Inability to respond with verbally appropriate terms in social and play situations

speech therapist will meet with the child during school hours, working with the child outside of the classroom. The child's teacher and the school nurse are integral parts of the therapeutic team and should be kept fully informed of the program in progress. Chapters 2 and 12 provide further discussion about IEP.

NURSING PLAN OF CARE

QUESTION: Review Nursing Plan of Care 28-1. Which of the nursing diagnoses is most appropriate for Gabriella and her family at this time?

The nursing plan of care for a child with sensory alterations reflects the three-pronged scope of care in this area. First, the health care team should perform developmental surveillance to monitor the normal and healthy development of a child's vision, hearing, and communication. Second, they should provide education to prevent illness and injury that could impair sensory function. Third, they should select a plan of care that reflects the individual needs of the child with a diagnosed vision, hearing, or communication disorder (Nursing Plan of Care 28-1).

Family adaptation to alterations in the child's sensory status will vary based on the extent of the impairment and the health care resources available to the family. For instance, corrective lenses may appear to be a small and easy adjustment for the child and family to make to improve a child's vision. However, if that child is homeless, or the family lacks the resources to acquire corrective lenses and maintain annual visits to manage changes in vision, care management for the child can become more complex. The nursing plan must also always address the related physiologic, psychosocial, and educational factors. The attitudes of child and family toward the child's condition (i.e., psychosocial and emotional factors) greatly influence the child's ability to make the greatest use of his or her skills and abilities. Nursing Plan of Care 12-1 provides additional information to guide interventions when the child's sensory condition is identified as a lifelong chronic condition.

ANSWER: The most appropriate nursing diagnosis for Gabriella is compromised individual/family coping related to multiple adjustments secondary to child's diagnosis of vision, hearing, or communication impairments. At this time, family members are the focus of intervention to enhance understanding, coping, and strategies to ameliorate the consequences of hearing loss.

ALTERATIONS IN SENSORY STATUS

This section describes the various alterations in vision, hearing, and communication that are most common in the pediatric population. Various treatment plans are reviewed, although a more complete description of treatment modalities has been provided in the chapter. Prevention is always the first intervention of the nurse, and such measures may avert, in some cases, alterations in vision, hearing, and communication from occurring.

NURSING PLAN OF CARE 28-1:

The Child With Sensory Alterations

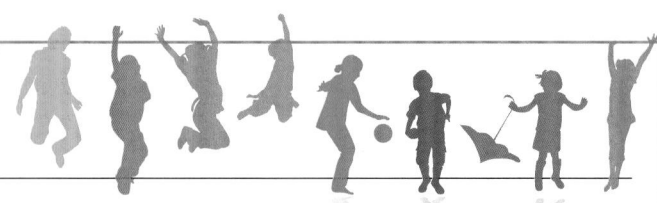

Nursing Diagnosis: Impaired comfort related to effects of altered sensory reception, transmission, or integration from visual or hearing impairment or loss of vision or hearing

Interventions/Rationale
- Introduce self to child and family, acknowledging child's sensory impairment.
  Orients child and helps reduce fears of being in unfamiliar environment.
- Assess vision/hearing/communication to determine child's functional capability. In-depth evaluation must be conducted by an optometrist, ophthalmologist, or otolaryngologist.
  Vision and hearing loss may occur gradually or abruptly (e.g., an accident) and may not affect both eyes and ears to the same extent. Evaluation provides baseline data regarding the extent of the child's visual or auditory loss.
- Review with the child and family the extent of the child's sensory impairment and management strategies the family has implemented to optimize the child's sensory perception.
  Ensures that home interventions to enhance the child's sensory perception are maintained during hospital or clinic visits. Communicate this information on the plan of care to ensure that adaptive measures are implemented, even when family members are not present with the child.
- Ensure that adaptive devices (e.g., glasses, contact lenses, magnifying glass, large-type books, and hearing aids) are accessible to the child and being used to optimize the child's vision or hearing and related activities.
  Use of adaptive devices may be essential for the child's optimal visual and auditory functioning. Ensuring that these devices are available and used provides optimum sensory perception for the child. Use play activities to engage the child's interest.
- When implementing new adaptive devices, demonstrate proper use and allow for return demonstration by child and family members.
  Ensures child and family will be able to use assistive devices at home and school.

Expected Outcomes
- Child will maintain sensory functioning at his or her highest level possible.
- Child will maintain optimal functioning within parameters of visual or hearing impairment, as evidenced by ability to care for self; navigate the environment safely; and participate in school, play, and family activities.
- Child will compensate for visual or hearing loss by using adaptive devices.
- Child and family will identify and use alternative methods to facilitate communication.

Nursing Diagnosis: Risk for delayed development related to lack of stimulation secondary to visual, auditory, or communication impairment

Interventions/Rationale
- Perform baseline assessment of child's achievement of developmental milestones. Reassess on routine basis following developmental surveillance guidelines (e.g., *Bright Futures* Guidelines).
  Baseline assessments provide an index on which to determine whether child meets age-appropriate developmental norms. Reassessment provides ongoing information about child's ongoing development and improvements when interventions have been used.
- Modify approach to child based on sensory deficits (e.g., approach from unaffected side of visual impairment, use touch, and talk to child).
  Interactions and interventions should be individualized to child according to abilities and not age.
- Increase/decrease stimuli and activities as appropriate to correct sensory deprivation/overload.
  Sensory deprivation and overload may both be detrimental. Sensory deprivation does not allow the child to have experiences that may be critical for stimulating new learning and behaviors; sensory overload may cause the child to "shut down" to protect self and maintain control.
- Collaborate with the interdisciplinary team (social worker, health care provider, school nurse, etc.) to develop a plan for the child to participate in family, school, play, and social activities to maximum capability.
  Provides additional support system for the family to ensure child's successful adaptation at home and school.

Expected Outcomes
- Child will attain age-appropriate developmental milestones within limits of functional abilities.
- Child will participate in family, school, and social activities using strategies that maximize child's sensory capabilities.
- Child's social development will progress according to developmental level.

Nursing Diagnosis: Risk for injury related to diminished sensory capabilities (visual, auditory, communication)

Interventions/Rationale
- Assess the environment to determine factors that may place child at risk for injury. Elicit parental feedback regarding ways to ensure a safe environment for the child.
  Modifying the environment may enhance the child's sensory perception and maintain the

child's safety. Examples of such modifications include increasing room lighting, ensuring that the bed is located in a low position with unobstructed access to the bathroom, ensuring that the floor is free of debris, and increasing the ring tone volume on a nearby phone.
- Assess for dizziness or disequilibrium.
  Disorders of the ear may be accompanied by dizziness because of the relationship between the inner ear and maintenance of equilibrium.
- Remove environmental barriers that may impede safe movement of child.
  Child's ability to see environmental obstacles may be impaired because of sensory deficit.
- Modify approach to and interventions for child according to deficits and specific sensory deficit.
  The child's ability to interpret the environment may be impaired by sensory deficits. Adaptations by family members (describing actions, writing in large print, speaking slowly) ensure that the child is not frightened by people and movement in the environment and can manage and interact appropriately with his or her environment.

Expected Outcomes
- Child's safety will be maintained.
- Child will be able to participate in activities while maintaining freedom from injury.

Nursing Diagnosis: Risk for impaired verbal communication related to diminished visual cues, auditory cues, or communication disorder (e.g., language delays, articulation or fluency disorder)

Interventions/Rationale
- Assess child's primary and preferred method of communication (e.g., sign language, written); ability to understand spoken word, written word, pictures, and gestures; and ability to convey information. Assess conditions or situations (e.g., tracheostomy, intubation) that may impair verbal communication.
  Communication may be impaired for a variety of reasons. Baseline assessment assists to determine the interventions that will have to be used to enhance communication with the child.
- Assess family's understanding of speech development and age-appropriate verbal milestones.
  Lack of understanding of age-appropriate norms for verbal communication may create unrealistically high expectations for the child's communication patterns or an inability to recognize that a speech problem exists and intervention is necessary.
- Use measures to enhance child's ability to understand communications from others:
  - Verbalize what you are doing.
  - Pause and wait for child to respond.
  - Provide stimuli to optimize functioning of other senses (e.g., tactile, auditory, kinesthetic).
  - Face child in good light, keeping hands away from your mouth.

- Speak close to child.
- Speak slowly and distinctly.
- Reduce environmental noise.
- Speak at normal volume unless requested to speak louder.
- Use short sentences and ask one question at a time.
- Avoid finishing sentences for the child.
  Taking time to communicate with child will assist child to feel valued and less fearful of the health care provider and health care setting.
- Refer child and family to community services to provide corrective therapy for speech disorders.
  Speech evaluation and therapy is available for all children aged 3 years and older from their local public school districts. Speech therapists provide in-depth evaluation of a speech impediment and use techniques to promote age-appropriate development of speech.

Expected Outcomes
- Child's ability to communicate will develop according to expectations for age.
- Child will produce understandable speech and communicate needs.
- Family members will demonstrate an understanding of verbal development in children and of alternative communication techniques.

Nursing Diagnosis: Ineffective coping or compromised family coping related to multiple adjustments secondary to child's diagnosis of vision, hearing, or communication impairments

Interventions/Rationale
- Assess child's and family's understanding of child's condition and anticipated short- and long-term outcomes.
  Establishes family knowledge base and expectations of outcomes. Provides data on which to engage family in teaching (as needed) and goal setting.
- Determine child's and family's psychological response to visual, hearing, or communication disorder.
  Responses may vary from acceptance to anger, withdrawal, and depression. Self-esteem may be negatively affected, especially if child is teased by peers about eyewear and visual limitations, wearing a hearing aid, or "talking funny."
- Explain tests and procedures, frequent assessments, and treatments in simple, concrete terms; repeat as necessary.
  Knowing what to expect may help reduce anxiety, distress, and feelings of uncertainty.
- Keep family informed about child's progress.
  Family is an integral part of child's care team. Regular updates on child's status assist the family in decision-making process.
- Use other health care personnel (e.g., child life specialist, clinical nurse specialist, social service

(Continued)

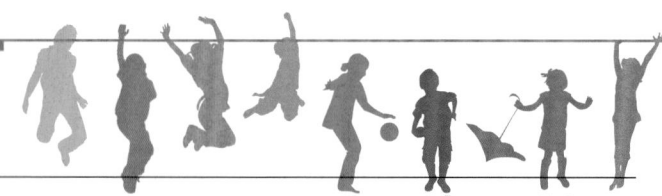

NURSING PLAN OF CARE 28-1:

The Child With Sensory Alterations *(Continued)*

worker) to assist child and family to cope with child's condition.

Child and family may need additional support services to effectively cope with the child's condition and to learn to manage home care.

Expected Outcomes
- Child will demonstrate appropriate use of coping mechanisms.
- Child will request help as needed and function independently when possible.

- Child and the family will effectively adapt to actual or potential altered abilities.
- Family will modify communication patterns to include new measures to communicate with the child.
- Family will use available support systems and coping mechanisms to adjust to their child's diagnosis.
- Child will demonstrate ability to communicate needs.
- Child will express decrease in frustration with regard to communicating with others.

ALTERATIONS IN VISION

Vision is one of the most important senses a child uses as he or she develops. Sight enables infants to bond with family members, explore their surroundings, move about, read, and interact with the world. Without the sense of sight, a child requires different approaches to and assistance in accomplishing developmental milestones. Children experience alterations in vision as a result of many conditions, including refractive errors, eye muscle disorders, conjunctivitis, injury, ROP, cataracts, and glaucoma. Refractive errors, conjunctivitis, and traumatic injury to the eyes are among the most common problems.

REFRACTIVE ERRORS

Visual images pass as light rays through the lens of the eye, bending so that the image focuses on the retina. The ability of the eye to focus an image clearly on the retina involves both accommodation and convergence. *Accommodation* is the eye's ability to change the shape of the lens so that the image, whether near or distant, is clearly focused on the retina. The ciliary muscles in the eye contract or relax to change the bending (refractive) angle of the lens. *Convergence* is the movement of the eyes toward the midline and occurs as objects are brought closer. Convergence occurs simultaneously with accommodation to enable the visual images in the two eyes to be focused at the same position on the retina of each eye, allowing **binocular vision** (fusion of the images from the two eyes) to occur.

During childhood, the child's eyes grow physically. As the child grows and the globe or lens changes shape, the eye muscles may be unable to compensate for the change in shape. As a result, the visual image focuses improperly in the retina, causing a refractive error that results in blurred near vision, blurred distant vision, or both. The four types of refractive errors include *myopia, hyperopia, astigmatism,* and *anisometropia* (Table 28-1). Regardless of the type of refractive error, treatment is with corrective lenses.

STRABISMUS

Each eye is controlled by six small muscles that move it into the six cardinal fields of gaze. These muscles must move with coordination and balanced strength so that both eyes can focus on the same location or object (binocular vision). Cranial nerves III, IV, and VI innervate these muscles.

ALERT   *Eye muscle disorders should not be ignored; ensure the child is assessed and treated as soon as concerns are identified, preferably before visual maturity at age 7 years.*

Disorders of eye movement may be a result of damage to one of the innervating cranial nerves or to one of the eye muscles. If any of the muscles that control eye movement are stronger or weaker than the opposing muscle in the same eye, that eye deviates from the line of vision, and the child develops strabismus. Strabismus, also called *lazy eye,* is a common eye problem in children (Fig. 28-7). If the eye turns inward toward the nose, the child has **esotropia**; if the eye turns outward, **exotropia**. Mild or transient strabismus is frequently found in infants younger than 3 months old and resolves spontaneously as the child develops and the eye strengthens.

Pathophysiology

At birth, the development of the infant eye is incomplete. During the first 4 months of life, binocularity (both eyes working together) is not consistent, thus intermittent esotropia or exotropia may normally occur. Beginning at about age 4 months, as the eyes work together more consistently, divergence decreases and binocularity increases. Eventually, the child sees a single, clear image. If the infant is unable to achieve central fusion of the visual image or if an eye muscle weakness or imbalance occurs (strabismus), possibly as a result of a congenital defect, systemic infection early in life, or intracranial

TABLE 28-1	Comparing Refractive Errors	
Refractive Error	**Description/Pathophysiology**	**Common Assessment Findings**
Myopia	Nearsightedness Light rays focused in front of retina Development especially during preteen and early teenage years	No difficulty reading Inability to see distant objects clearly (such as blackboard) If severe, child holding printed page very close to eyes
Hyperopia	Farsightedness Short axial length (shorter than normal distance from lens to retina) or decreased lens curvature Image focused behind the retina Possible overcoming of hyperopia if child's eye able to change shape via accommodation	Ability to see clearly at a distance Eyestrain with close work such as reading, headache Fatigue when reading or lack of interest in reading Squinting, rubbing eyes, tightly opening and closing eyes periodically Red, swollen eyelids
Astigmatism	Asymmetric shape and curvature of cornea	Eyestrain, headache Blurring or distortion of images
Anisometropia	Refractive errors in both eyes that are considerably different; the two eyes unable to work together	Possible development of amblyopia if severe Headache

injury, the eyes are unable to work together. The infant sees two images that cannot be merged (diplopia). The developing brain suppresses one image, and the infant develops amblyopia—functional blindness—in that eye. In many cases, however, appropriate therapy for strabismus can prevent this type of amblyopia.

Assessment

The assessment and diagnosis of strabismus is done during the routine eye examination (see Chapter 8 and Focused Physical Assessment 28-1). Suspect strabismus if

* The corneal light reflex is not symmetric
* Eye muscle movement is not smooth and consistent
* The cover–uncover tests demonstrate abnormal eye movement

CROSS-CULTURAL CARE

Among certain ethnic groups, the bridge of the nose in infants and young children is broad. Some children may have asymmetric epicanthal tissue that may give the appearance of convergence (deviation toward the midline) of one eye. These children have an "extra" fold of tissue at the inner canthus of one eye. If they do not have a symmetric fold on the other side, one eye appears to be closer to the bridge of the nose. This variation may cause the examiner to suspect an eye muscle imbalance; however, if the corneal light reflex is symmetric, the eyes are properly aligned, and the condition, called *pseudoesotropia* or *pseudostrabismus*, requires no treatment.

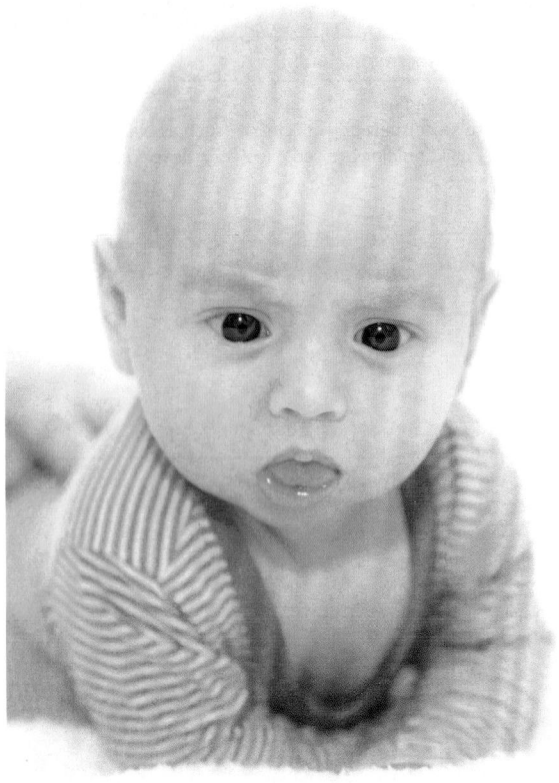

Figure 28-7 Strabismus in an infant

All deviations in eye muscle movement must be reassessed at each visit. If any deviations are accompanied by other symptoms that are new, such as ptosis of the eyelid or evidence of neurologic involvement, the child should be referred *immediately* to an ophthalmologist.

Nursing Diagnoses and Outcomes

Nursing diagnoses that are useful in planning the care of children with strabismus focus on supporting the family in their decision to seek medical attention for the child and in their efforts to adhere to any treatment protocol prescribed by the ophthalmologist. Assisting the family to adhere to treatment protocols may involve teaching them how to gain the child's cooperation by using principles of normal development.

 KidKare Make adherence into a game, in which the child gains rewards for wearing the patch or cooperating with the treatment protocol.

In addition to those listed in Nursing Plan of Care 28-1, the following nursing diagnosis and outcomes may apply:

Nursing Diagnosis: Noncompliance related to inconvenience of care and age of the child
Outcomes:
• Child and family will adhere to treatment protocol as recommended by the ophthalmologist.
• Child will experience no permanent visual impairment resulting from nonadherence to treatment protocol.

Interdisciplinary Interventions

Some cases of strabismus are obvious; others are detected by primary health care providers during routine examination. All should be referred immediately to an ophthalmologist for treatment. The earlier that treatment is initiated, the greater the likelihood of a good visual outcome.

Occlusion Therapy

The most common treatment for strabismus is occlusion therapy (see "Treatment Modalities" section). Vision in the stronger eye is occluded, continuously or intermittently, to strengthen the muscles of the weaker eye (see Fig. 28-3). Adherence depends on achieving an acceptable balance between occlusion and nonocclusion time, which may have to be explained carefully to and negotiated with the child.

Surgery

Surgical correction of strabismus may be necessary, depending on the child's condition and the success of occlusion therapy. It involves an eye muscle procedure designed to realign the eyes and enable binocularity to develop. Forbes and Khazaeni (2003) suggest that surgery is most successful if done between 4 and 24 months of age. See Chapter 11 regarding preoperative and postoperative care of the child.

An eye patch may be needed during the first day or few days after surgery to remind the child not to rub or put pressure on the eye. If the child is young, elbow restraints may need to be provided to prevent the child's hands from contacting the eye. Pain is seldom a problem; however, acetaminophen or ibuprofen may be given as needed.

Botulinum Toxin Injections

An alternative treatment being tested with some types of strabismus is injection with botulinum toxin to temporarily weaken the stronger muscle, allowing the weaker muscle to strengthen (Hauviller et al., 2007). With this treatment, some children achieve **orthotropia** (alignment of the eyes) in 2 to 4 weeks. The effects of the treatment persist for 5 to 8 weeks; treatment may have to be repeated before orthotropia is permanently achieved (Forbes & Khazaeni, 2003).

The injections are performed under local or general anesthesia, with general anesthesia preferable for children. Complications can occur if, when injected, the solution diffuses into the orbit, affecting other extraocular muscles, leading to ptosis or secondary vertical strabismus. To minimize side effects, the child should be positioned vertically during and after injections (Chatzistefanou & Mills, 2000). An expected side effect is soreness in the area that was injected. Ask the family to notify the health care provider if they notice any adverse side effects after the injections.

Community Care

When a child who is undergoing occlusion therapy is in daycare or in school, patching is monitored by teachers, volunteers, and the school nurse. Each of these adults needs to be knowledgeable about the purpose for eye patching and informed of the plan for the individual child. The school administrators need to be fully informed and have a written copy of the treatment plan in the school file.

The purpose of patching is to stimulate visual development in the nonoccluded eye, not to treat some malady of the patched eye, as some would believe. The child should be able to maintain consistent progress in school during treatment. If, however, wearing the eye patch during school hours prevents the progress of the child's education, the treatment plan should be reevaluated by the ophthalmologist.

The teacher and daycare providers may need to discourage teasing and educate the other children concerning the reason that the child wears the eye patch. Other children can learn to be a help rather than a hindrance in the treatment program and in the continued social development of the individual child.

The teacher or school nurse may need to replace the patch during the school day. A conference between the teacher, school nurse, and family can ensure that supplies (which the family can provide) are available and that school protocols are in place for the child to have the patch changed. The patch is put on loosely, but not so loosely that the child can peek around it. It is secured with nonirritating tape and may be decorated with drawings, stickers, or sequins. Channels of communication must be clarified with the school so that changes in the treatment plan can be implemented promptly and accurately and so that nonadherence is reported to the family without delay. Nonadherence could result in reevaluation of the treatment protocol, or it may simply be discussed with the child to establish the reason for it. Children may need rewards for adherence. If wearing the patch is a game, or if the patch can be decorated or treated as a fashion accessory, adherence will be much easier.

AMBLYOPIA

Amblyopia is diminished effective vision in one or both eyes, even with use of proper optical correction. Amblyopia results from altered or abnormal visual development despite apparently normal retinal and optic nerve anatomy (Granet & Khayali, 2011). The incidence of amblyopia may be higher than usual among some groups of children, such as those born prematurely, children of drug-dependent mothers, and children with other neurologic impairments.

Amblyopia is often preventable, yet many children with the condition are not identified until permanent damage has already occurred. Amblyopia is difficult to identify in infants; it is much more easily identified when children are old enough to follow directions and make simple choices. However, waiting for the child to grow old enough to cooperate can jeopardize vision in the affected eye.

Because amblyopia is usually asymptomatic, a complete ophthalmologic examination is necessary to confirm the diagnosis. Examination reveals reduced visual acuity but fails to identify any organic abnormality.

caREminder

If vision is obstructed for an extended time (e.g., because of cataracts), amblyopia and loss of vision can develop in any infant or child younger than age 7 years. For this reason, obstructions to vision should be resolved as soon as possible.

Pathophysiology

The critical period for visual center development in the brain is birth to ages 6 or 7 years. During the first 6 months of life, the neurologic pathways between the eyes and the visual centers of the brain mature, and binocular vision is achieved; the brain merges the images from the two eyes, allowing a single image to be perceived. Normally, these images are focused on the macular portion of the developing retina. If images are not focused on similar locations on the retina of each eye, the brain perceives a blurred image and reacts by suppressing vision in one eye. As a result, the portion of the brain associated with that eye is not stimulated and does not develop, leading to functional blindness in that eye. Similarly, if a congenital cataract prevents the image being transmitted to the brain from one eye, amblyopia can result. The longer visual suppression is present, the less reversible it becomes.

Amblyopia does not develop after the critical period for visual development is over, so it does not develop in an older child or adult who sustains an injury that causes eye muscle imbalance. Amblyopia can be subdivided according to its primary cause: deprivation, strabismic, or refractive. In each case, the visual image from the weaker eye is ignored by the visual center of the brain.

Assessment

Early identification of amblyopia is essential. Assessment of vision should begin with the first contact between health professional and family and should continue regularly throughout childhood (Developmental Considerations 28-1). Photoscreening has been suggested as a technique for screening children with risk factors associated with amblyopia who are difficult to assess because of their age and inability to cooperate with visual testing (e.g., infants, young children, and children with developmental delays) (AAP, 2008, 2012; Chou et al., 2011).

When amblyopia is present, testing of visual acuity assesses the effectiveness of treatment. As the amblyopia improves, visual acuity improves in the affected eye.

Interdisciplinary Interventions

The goal of treatment for amblyopia is to stimulate normal visual development. The earlier the condition is identified and treatment is begun, the greater the likelihood of a positive outcome. Treatment of the child with amblyopia should address its underlying cause and includes occlusion therapy (see "Treatment Modalities" section) and surgical correction of any related problem, such as strabismus, ptosis, cataract, or other anomaly. Occlusion therapy is usually the treatment of choice.

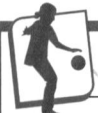

DEVELOPMENTAL CONSIDERATIONS 28-1

Screening for Amblyopia

Birth to Age 4 Months

History: Pay close attention to family's concerns about the infant's vision.

Inspection: Face and eyes should appear structurally normal:
- Eyes symmetric
- Lids open and close completely
- Color of pupil is variable
- Sclera white (without blue tinge)
- No drainage; no excessive blinking or tearing

With ophthalmoscope or penlight
- Identify red reflex
- Infant should "fix" vision on light source and briefly follow the light as it is moved

Age 4–12 Months

History: Continue to seek family reports or observations, which may indicate abnormal vision.

Inspect eyes for symmetry and normal appearance, including color of sclera and absence of drainage or excessive tearing.

Observe for symmetric corneal light reflection.

Identify red reflex again.

Do funduscopic examination if possible.

Between 1 and 4 Years

Continue all previous assessments.

Observe behavior during cover–uncover testing. Greater agitation when one eye is covered could indicate that the child does not see equally well with both eyes.

Attempt to get the child to fix vision on an object with each eye separately and to follow its movement.

By Age 4 Years

The child will probably be able to cooperate with the examiner who performs standard measures of ocular movement and visual acuity.

Testing should include measures of visual acuity in each eye separately as well as in both eyes together.

Middle Childhood

Vision should be checked annually. As physical growth and development occur, ocular changes may occur as well. Visual acuity significantly affects school performance and social adjustment.

School-aged children are anxious to please the examiner. Be particularly alert for "peeking" around the occluder card or other means of "cheating," such as memorizing the chart in use by watching other children taking the test.

Because development at young ages is more rapid, improvement may occur more quickly if the child is quite young when treatment begins. Although the best time to treat children with amblyopia is when they are younger than 7 years of age, Mohan et al. (2004) found significant improvement in visual acuity among children 11 to 15 years of age who had amblyopia caused by strabismus, anisometropia, or both and who adhered to full-time occlusion (De Weger et al., 2010). This type of research provides hope for children who are well beyond the age at which it was thought that no further improvement could occur (Astle et al., 2011; Holmes et al., 2011).

Community Care

Intervention for the child with amblyopia must always be a cooperative effort among all persons who come into daily contact with the child. This group may include family members and health care professionals—such as the pediatrician, family physician, ophthalmologist, optician, and nurse or nurse practitioner in the office, clinic, or school—as well as schoolteachers or daycare providers, all of whom need to know the treatment protocol being used and their responsibility in assisting the child and family to comply with it.

CONJUNCTIVITIS

QUESTION: Gabriella received a ribbon of erythromycin ointment in each eye at birth. Newborn eye prophylaxis is often a state requirement. What organisms cause conjunctivitis and why do all babies receive treatment instead of just the infected ones?

Conjunctivitis is an inflammation in and around the eye. It may be of bacterial, viral, allergic, or irritative origin. It occurs in children of all ages. The younger the child, the greater the likelihood of severe damage resulting from an eye infection. Conjunctivitis is usually less severe in older infants and children than it is in neonates. Table 28-2 summarizes the major types of conjunctivitis.

Neonatal conjunctivitis, also called *ophthalmia neonatorum*, is a broad term applied to the ocular reaction of newborn infants in response to either a viral (such as herpesvirus, cytomegalovirus) or bacterial invasion (most commonly *Chlamydia trachomatis* or *Neisseria gonorrhoeae*) or to the chemical substance instilled at birth to prevent the bacterial invasion. The chemical substances currently in use worldwide to prevent bacterial invasion include silver nitrate 1% drops,

TABLE 28-2   Types of Conjunctivitis

Type	Description/Etiology	Assessment	Interventions
Neonatal conjunctivitis (ophthalmia neonatorum)	Ocular reaction of newborn infants in response to viral or bacterial invasion or to the chemical substance instilled at birth to prevent bacterial invasion *Chemical:* silver nitrate 1%, erythromycin 0.5%, or tetracycline 1% *Bacterial: Chlamydia trachomatis* (most common), *Neisseria gonorrhoeae* *Viral:* herpesvirus, cytomegalovirus, other viruses	Variable symptoms ranging from mild to severe Maternal history related to prenatal care and exposure to sexually transmitted infections and treatment Generalized response: elevated or subnormal temperature, lack of interest in feeding, increased irritability *Chemical:* usually within 24 hours after eye prophylaxis; redness, irritation, negative cultures of drainage *Gonorrhea:* conjunctival inflammation and purulent discharge within 3–5 days of birth; fussiness, crying, especially when cleaning or examining eyes; possible progression to corneal ulcerations and destruction of ocular structures leading to scarring and blindness if left untreated *Chlamydia:* mild to moderate erythematous conjunctiva; moderate to large amounts of discharge within 5–14 days of birth; positive cultures (as early as 1–3 days after birth); fast spreading to other body organs such as lungs and gastrointestinal tract, leading to OM, pneumonia, rhinitis; possible isolation of organism in newborn's feces *Herpesvirus:* discharge, inflammation usually appearing during second and third weeks of life; mouth or skin lesions	Frequent cleansing of eye with normal saline Administration of topical agent (drops or ointment) Referral to ophthalmologist Infection control measures to prevent transmission If large amount of drainage present, hospitalization, intravenous or intramuscular aqueous penicillin or other antibiotic; hourly eye irrigation with normal saline until drainage subsides Ceftriaxone to newborn and mother if culture positive for *N. gonorrhoeae* Parental education about medication administration, eye cleaning, and follow-up appointments Parental education about severity of the condition & possible poor visual outcome if child does not receive the prescribed cleansing and medications and the recommended follow-up
Infectious conjunctivitis	*Bacterial:* usually accompanying a respiratory infection, most often resulting from *H. influenzae* or *S. Pneumoniae;* gonococcal possible in adolescents with genital infections or children exposed to it at home *Viral:* most commonly resulting from adenovirus	History to determine exposure to bacterial or viral contaminants Bilateral or unilateral *Bacterial:* itching, burning, yellow discharge with crusting, eyelid edema, conjunctival erythema; positive eye drainage culture for organism (see Clinical Judgment 28-1) *Viral:* redness of sclera and inner eyelids; clear, watery discharge; no purulent drainage or matting of eyelids; red conjunctiva; follicular hyperplasia (in older children); other signs of viral illness or gastrointestinal symptoms	Ruling out of other conditions such as glaucoma (because of tearing and photophobia), periorbital cellulitis (which involves the conjunctiva at the outset), foreign body or trauma (which causes redness, irritation, and tearing) Parental teaching about measures to prevent transmission (handwashing, care of child's clothing and care items [pillows, towels], keeping child's hands away from eyes and no rubbing, cleaning infected eye), administration of eye drops or ointment, comfort measures *Bacterial:* broad-spectrum topical agent until organism identified; possible oral antibiotic; parenteral antibiotics if other routes unsuccessful or treatment adherence is questionable; aqueous penicillin given parenterally as drug of choice for gonococcal conjunctivitis Child considered contagious until treated for 24 hours; usually kept out of school until cleared *Viral:* usually self-limiting; possible topical antibiotic to prevent superinfection; cool, moist compresses for comfort
Allergic conjunctivitis	Seasonal, induced by airborne antigens such as ragweed or pollen; year-round resulting from animal dander, dust mites, or other ever-present allergen Sole manifestation of child's allergy or possibly accompanied by respiratory or dermatologic responses. Irritation from contact lenses or use of makeup that causes an allergic reaction	History of allergy to foods, medicines, environmental triggers, rhinitis Bilateral Eyelid swelling Watery or clear, stringy, mucous discharge Inflamed conjunctiva Itching Rhinitis and related nose and throat symptoms Culture of drainage positive for eosinophils	Medications to treat symptoms and prophylaxis: topical, systemic, or both Vasoconstrictor eye drops (used sparingly and no longer than 3 days) Antihistamine and mast cell stabilizer eye drops; oral antihistamines Artificial tears to soothe and cool the eye Education related to elimination or avoidance of pollen-related allergies; measures to reduce exposure to triggers such as cleaning procedures for removal of dust mites or animal dander, restriction of pets Removal of contacts until redness and irritation has ceased

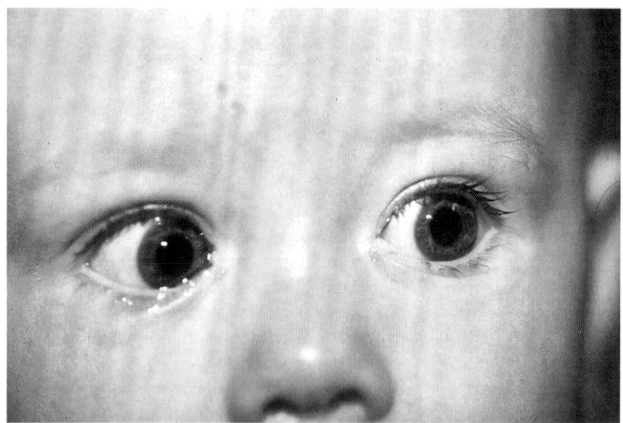

Figure 28-8 Neonatal conjunctivitis. A purulent, yellow discharge is noted draining from the conjunctiva.

erythromycin 0.5% drops or ointment, and tetracycline 1% drops or ointment (Simon, 2003; Teoh & Reynolds, 2003). Erythromycin and tetracycline drops or ointment may also cause a mild reaction, although such reactions are rare. Povidone-iodine 2.5% drops have been used in developing countries because they are inexpensive and easy to store. They turn the conjunctiva

brown for a short time but cause less ocular reaction than other prophylactic agents (Isenberg et al., 2002). Although effective against most bacterial conjunctivitis, povidone-iodine 2.5% drops seem to increase the risk of acquiring chlamydial conjunctivitis. Thus, additional measures would need to be used to prevent mother-to-fetus transmission of chlamydial infection (Ramirez-Ortiz et al., 2007). Ophthalmia neonatorum presents as an inflammation of the conjunctiva with redness, swelling, and purulent discharge (Fig. 28-8). Symptoms vary from mild to severe. The severity of the symptoms is not an indication of the causative organism. With better availability of erythromycin 0.5% ointment, it is now the medication of choice for ophthalmia neonatorum.

❗ ALERT   *Gonorrheal conjunctivitis is a medical emergency. Any newborn with eye drainage should be referred immediately to a pediatric ophthalmologist.*

Conjunctivitis in older infants and children is usually either infectious (bacterial or viral) or allergic in origin. Eye drainage cultures and sensitivity studies are used to identify the organism (Clinical Judgment 28-1). Allergic

---

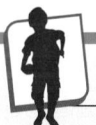

CLINICAL JUDGMENT 28-1

The Child With Eye Drainage

Cindy is a nurse practitioner who provides health care services to a number of daycare facilities. She receives a call from a daycare director regarding Daniel, age 4 years, who awoke from his nap and was unable to open his eyes because of the presence of crusty exudate. After Daniel's eyes were cleansed with a wet, warm cloth, Cindy was called. Cindy goes to the daycare center to see Daniel.

Questions

1. What other questions regarding Daniel's status should Cindy ask the daycare director at this time?

2. What actions should Cindy recommend be taken with Daniel?

3. What is Daniel's diagnosis?

4. What treatment measures should be instituted at this time for Daniel and the other children at the daycare center?

5. How would Cindy determine that Daniel's condition has improved?

Answers

1. Does he have a fever? Does he have any known allergies? Has any drainage been observed before this event? What color is the eye drainage? Has Daniel been rubbing his eyes frequently? Is he receiving treatment at home for this condition or for any other health problem? Do any family members or other children or workers at the daycare center have an infection?

2. Cindy should complete a physical assessment of the eye, noting signs of redness and the amount, color, and consistency of eye drainage. Recommend to the family that a culture of the eye drainage be completed.

3. Conjunctivitis of unknown etiology until culture results is returned. Yellow, purulent eye drainage indicates a likely bacterial cause. A watery discharge would indicate a viral conjunctivitis.

4. Antibiotic therapy should be ordered for a bacterial infection. The child should not return to daycare until he has been treated for 2 days. Towels, clothing, and pillows that have contacted the child's eyes should be washed. Viral conjunctivitis is usually self-limiting. A warm compress may also help decrease pain and discomfort.

5. Absence of eye drainage and fever.

conjunctivitis may be a reaction to allergens carried to the eyes by air currents or soiled hands or a reaction to substances placed in the eye for other purposes.

Conjunctivitis in infants and children must be identified and treated without delay. Consider any eye drainage that is yellow and sticky as contagious because this could indicate an infection. Instruct parents to wash their hands carefully with soap and water before and after wiping the baby's eyes. To clean the eye, wipe away the drainage with a clean tissue, working from the nose toward the temple. Use a clean spot on the tissue for each motion across the eye. Use a new tissue to wipe the other eye.

For most conjunctival conditions, a topical agent (drops or ointment) is prescribed. Ointments are preferred for bacterial conjunctivitis because treatment requires fewer doses over a shorter period. In addition, prescription ointments do not sting or burn and are not absorbed systematically to the extent that drops are. If the conjunctivitis is related to an allergic response, artificial tears can be used to soothe and cool the eye and possibly decrease the amount of allergen in the eye (Gold, 2011).

caREminder

The family must learn how to instill the eye ointment so that a maximum amount is spread across the conjunctiva. Teach them to keep the tube at room temperature and to help the child to hold the eye open while a thin line of ointment is spread along the lower conjunctival sac. The child should be encouraged to blink several times to spread the ointment then to hold the eyes lightly closed for a short time. Emphasize that it is critical that good handwashing techniques are used with this procedure before and after instilling the medication.

Teach parents to prevent other children from coming into contact with the infected child or eye drainage until an infection has been ruled out or an antibiotic has been given for 24 hours.

ANSWER: Several sexually transmitted infections cause conjunctivitis and may cause subsequent blindness, including gonorrhea and chlamydia. The presence of these organisms is not always known at the time of delivery. Most states have therefore legislated the mandatory but fairly benign treatment of all babies to protect a few from blindness.

EYE INJURIES

Eye injuries include those caused by accident, abuse, sports participation, fire, chemicals, or ordinary everyday play. In addition, chemical ingestion (e.g., antifreeze) or disease processes (e.g., hydrocephalus with shunt failure) may cause injury to structures of vision. Health care providers and adults need to be alert to the

potential for ocular and visual damage in each of these situations and do everything possible to prevent visual loss by preventing accidents and injury.

According to the AAP (2011), of the 42,000 sports- and recreation-related eye injuries during the year 2000, 43% occurred in persons younger than 15 years of age. A U.S. emergency department treats eye injuries because of sports every 13 minutes. Although most of these sports-related injuries occur to those aged 25 years and younger, only 15% of children wear protective eyewear during sports activities (Prevent Blindness America, 2012).

The incidence of various types of eye injuries varies with the age and sex of the child. Ocular injuries occur more frequently to boys than to girls (Forbes, 2001; Tomazzoli et al., 2003), presumably because of the more active nature of their play. In early childhood, children are prone to falls and sustain traumatic injuries from toys, scissors, or furniture more often than children in middle childhood and adolescence. They are also more likely to ingest toxic products such as antifreeze (methyl alcohol) and may spill chemicals on themselves, causing injury.

During early and middle childhood, children are inquisitive and very active. Eye injuries are most often caused by participation in a sports activity or other extracurricular activity without the necessary protection. School-aged children and teenagers may use sports equipment, guns, common tools, or toys to inflict injury on their peers. Children may also sustain blunt force injuries inflicted by another child's hand or foot. Glue injuries of the cornea and eyelashes are increasingly common in middle childhood.

An increasing source of ocular injuries among children in recent years is from youth participating in the sport of paintball. In a national study, the rate of ocular injuries from paintball more than doubled between 1998 and 2000. More than 40% of these injuries (1,200) were to children, most of whom were playing in unsupervised settings and with no eye protection. The AAP and others have recommended the development of rules and regulations for the sale and use of paintballs to prevent injuries and protect children's vision (AAP, 2011; Listman, 2004).

 KidKare Participants in paintball "war games" should always wear approved face shields with eye protection and be supervised by adults.

Eye injuries may also be caused by fire burns, fireworks, or other explosives such as chemical mixtures that children or teens experiment with or encounter. Fireworks can cause burn injuries in and around the eyes, contusions and lacerations of the eye, and penetrating injuries from exploding debris. Of all persons with burn injuries, 30% sustain burns to the head and neck. When tissues surrounding the eyes are burned, edema may cause the eyelids to swell shut. This condition is not only frightening to the child but also makes assessing the eye difficult.

Abuse must be ruled out in any injury sustained by a child. Calzada (2003) found that ocular injury (traumatic hyphema) can be the result of corporal punishment with a belt that accidentally strikes the child in the face. Shaken baby syndrome has different, but distinctive, effects on the retina and often results in blindness caused by bilateral retinal hemorrhages and bleeding into the vitreous humor.

Pathophysiology

Eye injuries are classified according to the anatomic parts involved: extraocular, anterior globe, or posterior globe injuries. *Extraocular injuries* include eyelid lacerations, soft tissue injuries with bruising, or fractures of the orbit. *Anterior globe injuries* are subdivided according to whether they are perforating or nonperforating injuries. *Nonperforating injuries* include corneal abrasions, foreign bodies on the conjunctiva, subconjunctival hemorrhage, and hyphema (Olitsky et al., 2011). *Perforating anterior globe injuries* include ruptured globe, perforated cornea, and conjunctival laceration. *Posterior globe injuries* include retinal edema, vitreous hemorrhage, and retinal detachment. Injury to the posterior globe is often accompanied by injury to the anterior globe or extraocular structures.

Blunt force injury, which causes hemorrhage in and around the eye, is a common injury in childhood. Eye injuries caused by repeated reciprocal movements of the head, as occurs when an infant or child is shaken, result in retinal tearing or intracranial bleeding involving the visual center located in the occipital region of the brain. These are injuries to the posterior globe, optic nerve, and brain parenchyma (Levine, 2004). When bleeding occurs around the eye (extraocular), it causes discoloration, commonly known as a *black eye* (Fig. 28-9). When small blood vessels of the conjunctiva are torn by an injury, subconjunctival hemorrhage may be seen as redness across a portion of the conjunctiva.

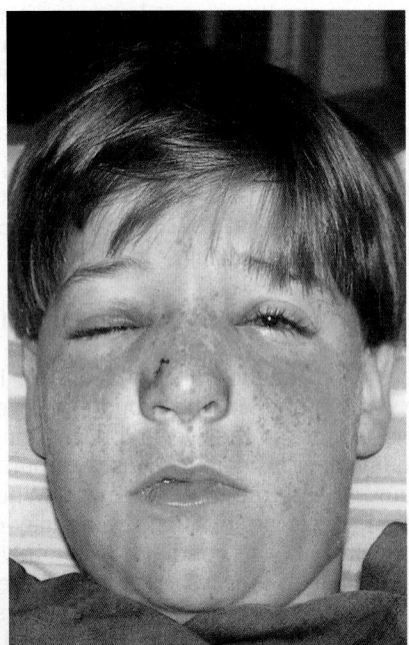

Figure 28-9 Eye injuries can cause temporary loss of vision as a result of swelling and bruising of the orbital area.

> **ALERT** *A large amount of bleeding into the globe of the eye, called hyphema, could result in increased intraocular pressure. Ensure that this injury is examined by an ophthalmologist as soon as possible. Increased intraocular pressure could damage the optic nerve.*

Facial burns from a chemical or fire may affect the eyes; however, eyes are usually well protected by the eyelids, which can close in 1/30th of a second, thus protecting the cornea. Most eye burns are caused by chemicals seeping into the eye or by sudden explosions involving steam or debris.

Paintball injuries are often severe because the size of the paintball (14 mm) enables it to slip past the bony orbit and hit the globe with much of the force with which it was propelled out of the gun, even though the eyelid closes spontaneously. Paintball injuries include hyphema (77%), retinal detachment/tear (27.5%), cataract development (28%), vitreous hemorrhage (33%), and ruptured globe (4.7%) (Listman, 2004). These are serious injuries, with poor visual outcomes. Visual acuity after treatment reached only 20/200 or worse in 43.1% of patients in one study, and only 44% had a satisfactory visual outcome (20/40 or better) (Listman, 2004).

Assessment

Assessing an eye injury begins with a detailed history of the events leading to the injury to identify the possible injuries the child may have sustained and the possible elements involved. Identification of the location and extent of the injury is made by the health care provider with appropriate diagnostic testing.

Diagnostic testing may include facial radiographs to identify possible orbital fracture and retinal examination to identify internal eye injury, damage, or bleeding into the eye. Computed tomography is helpful in identifying injury-related conditions that are not visible on x-rays.

Assessment for injury by chemicals and debris must be made very early during the treatment process to prevent corneal abrasion and burning. Chemicals should be washed away with copious amounts of water, and the debris should be removed immediately because edema of damaged tissues quickly makes both washing and examination difficult.

caREminder

> *Trauma victims who are unconscious when admitted to the health care facility should have their eyes cleaned as soon as possible if injury to the eyes is suspected.*

Interdisciplinary Interventions

The provider of first aid must follow appropriate protocols for removing small foreign bodies from the eye by everting the lid and using a cotton-tipped applicator to lift the foreign body from the surface of the conjunctiva.

If the damage is more extensive, the person providing first aid should encourage the child to close and cover the eye, keeping the eye and lid as still as possible. For chemical injuries, the first-aid provider begins the washing process prior to arrival of trained emergency technicians. Wash the eye with copious amounts of flowing water. In the case of injury with a blunt object, the first-aid provider will cover the eye and transport the child to a care facility. Most eye injuries require a follow-up visit to an ophthalmologist. Because of the intricacy of eye structure, even small injuries in a growing child can result in larger problems at a later date.

Community Care

In most cases, eye injuries are preventable. Children need to be encouraged to use safety equipment designed for specific sports or activities and to avoid misusing sports equipment, tools, and common objects such as pencils, black- or whiteboard erasers, sticks, stones, rubber bands, balls, paper wads, and toys (Fig. 28-10). Nurses, teachers, family members, and primary health care providers play key roles in stopping dangerous activities and educating children about avoiding behaviors that endanger their eyesight or that of other children and adopting behaviors that can help prevent eye injuries (Community Care 28-2). Providing information to the child concerning potential danger can help the child in his or her own decision-making process. Safety can become an internal motivator rather than a condition externally imposed by the family or other caregivers.

Sports are classified as high risk, moderate risk, or eye safe based on the risk of eye injury to the unprotected player. The AAO (2003) and the AAP (2011) recommend protective eyewear use, including polycarbonate face shields, in any sport in which risk of eye injury exists

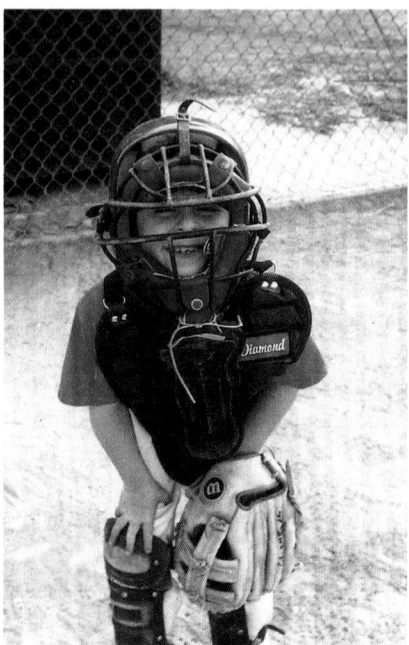

Figure 28-10 Safety equipment helps protect the child's eyes during sports activities.

(see thePoint Evidence-Based Practice Guidelines). The incidence of all types of injuries from high-impact sports (e.g., skateboarding, roller blading) is lower when participants wear safety equipment (Levine, 2004).

KidKare Wearing a helmet while riding a bike is the law in many states. Encourage children to always wear their helmet while participating in activities such as biking, skateboarding, and roller blading; it may help protect their head as well as other parts of their face from injury.

Protective eyewear should be mandatory for any sports participant who is either "functionally one eyed" or who has had eye surgery or trauma and whose ophthalmologist recommends eye protection. Functionally one eyed is defined as anyone who has visual acuity of 20/40 or worse in the eye with the poorest vision (AAP, 2011).

RETINOPATHY OF PREMATURITY

QUESTION: As Gabriella's nurse, you know that she has ROP and you know her parents are worried about how well she will be able to see. What are some of the roles that you can fill to meet the needs of Gabriella and her parents?

Retinopathy of prematurity is the term currently used to designate the aberrant and abnormal vascularization of the retina that occurs in some low-birth-weight preterm infants, causing impaired vision or blindness (AAP et al., 2013). The condition was first identified in 1942 and was called *retrolental fibroplasia*. The name was changed in 1984 after an international team of ophthalmologists met to identify a generally agreed upon classification system to describe the stages and severity of the disease process. ROP is described by location (zones) and severity (stages) as identified by the International Classification of Retinopathy of Prematurity (International Committee for the Classification of Retinopathy of Prematurity, 2005).

During the late 1940s and early 1950s, ROP occurred in epidemic numbers among premature infants because of the standard use of high concentrations of oxygen to treat respiratory complications in sick neonates. After the use of high concentrations of oxygen was curtailed in the mid-1950s, the incidence of ROP declined to almost zero. As technologic advances have enabled greater numbers of preterm infants to survive, the incidence of ROP is again increasing, with approximately 14,000 to 16,000 infants affected annually in the United States (Harrell & Brandon, 2007). White infants are more likely than African American infants to develop ROP. There are no differences in incidence between the genders. Oxygen therapy is a risk factor in the development of ROP, yet such therapy is a necessary element in the care of premature newborns. The use of blood products has shown no relationship to the development of ROP. The more severely ill the child at birth, the more likely he or she will develop ROP (Harrell & Brandon, 2007).

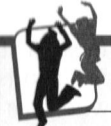

COMMUNITY CARE 28-2

Preventing Accidental Eye Injuries

At Home

- Always set a good example by using safety equipment and following safety rules.
- Begin childproofing the home as the infant becomes more mobile. Pad the corners of low tables (or temporarily remove the low table).
- Prevent access to toxic chemicals and cleaning supplies. Store them in a locked cupboard, well out of reach or outside the house where child has no access.
- Prevent access to automobile or lawn and garden chemicals, which the child may decide to taste.
  - Antifreeze smells and tastes good; however, ingestion can be lethal.
  - Garden chemicals often feel like coarse sand and come with colored pellets; however, they contain toxic substances.
- Prevent access to lawn and garden equipment that could cause injury.
  - Do not let young child ride on the riding mower.
  - Avoid letting the child play in the lawn while it is being mowed because flying debris can hit the child. When debris is thrown into the eye with the force of a mower, damage can occur.
- Buckle children securely into automobile safety seats and buckle the seat into the vehicle according to manufacturer's instructions. Teach older children to use seat belts correctly.
- Provide the child with age-appropriate, safe toys and play equipment.
  - Avoid toys with sharp points, sharp edges, shafts, spikes, or rods.
  - Avoid giving BB guns, pellet guns, bows and arrows, or darts to children as toys.
  - Keep toys meant for older children away from younger children.
- Teach children safety with toys and play equipment.
  - Avoid throwing toys.
  - Do not use toys as weapons.
  - Never pretend to point a gun at another person.
  - Avoid swinging on the swing when another child is too close.
  - Do not run while carrying any sharp or pointed objects—for example, scissors or sticks.

- Teach older children the proper use of safety equipment designed to prevent eye injuries.
  - Wear protective glasses when using a string trimmer or other lawn and garden tools and equipment.
  - Wear protective glasses when preparing and dispensing household or other lawn and garden chemicals.
  - Follow the directions when preparing and using any equipment or chemicals.
- Teach older children proper use of safety equipment designed to prevent eye injuries.
  - Wear helmets for inline skating and bike riding. Be sure that the helmet fits well enough to allow the child to see where he or she is going.

At School

- Set a good example for safety.
- Teach proper use of playground sports equipment—for example, swing sets with soft material (fabric or leather) seats, proper use of sliding boards.
- Consistently require appropriate use of classroom equipment—for example, scissors with rounded ends for young children.
- Set protective rules and require compliance.
  - Do not throw sand, toys, or other missiles.
  - Never hit another person in the face (or anywhere else).
  - Use school supplies (e.g., pens, pencils, rulers) for their intended purpose.
  - No throwing of any supplies or equipment.

During Sports Activities

- Consistently require the appropriate use of sports safety equipment.
- Teach proper use of equipment for organized sports activities and backyard or street sports.
- Use protective gear supplied.
  - Use batting helmets with polycarbonate face protector in youth baseball.
  - Use helmets with face protectors or face guards for ice and street hockey, football.
- Abide by the rules.
- Assign penalties for violation of the rules.
  - Hockey sticks are to be kept low, not used as weapons.
  - Bike helmets are to be worn whenever riding a bike or scooter.

Pathophysiology

In the normal newborn, retinal blood vessels are immature and the macula has yet to complete its development. The retinal blood vessels begin their development near the disk and grow toward the periphery of the retina between 16 and 44 weeks' gestation. Great variability exists with respect to the time of completion of this process; thus, when an infant is born prematurely, the status of eye development is not predictable.

ROP involves injury to the developing blood vessels and tissues of the retina, leading to regrowth or overgrowth of retinal vessels. Two factors are involved in the development of ROP. Vascular endothelial growth factor (VEGF) is the growth factor that is normally stimulated by hypoxia (low partial pressure of arterial oxygen [PaO_2]) in utero and stimulates vessel growth. Insulinlike growth factor 1 (IGF-1) is provided to the fetus in utero from the placenta and amniotic fluid. IGF-1 also contributes to the development of vascularization, and IGF-1 levels decrease immediately after delivery. Thus, a premature infant will experience immediate cessation of vascularization.

ROP is divided into two phases. During phase 1, the infant has termination of normal vessel growth and regression of some existing vessels. Levels of IGF-1 will slowly reestablish through endogenous production. Administration of supplemental oxygen after birth inhibits VEGF and causes death to the vascular endothelial cells. Subsequently, the lack of blood vessels in the retina initiates anaerobic metabolism and enhances the existing hypoxic situation. The retina becomes oxygen-deprived and its metabolic needs are not met. This hypoxic condition stimulates VEGF, which begins phase 2 of ROP (Harrell & Brandon, 2007).

During phase 2, IGF-1 levels return to normal (as a result of endogenous production) and act on the VEGF to cause vessel growth. However, this vessel growth is now considered pathologic and the resulting vessels are abnormal. As stated by Harrell and Brandon (2007) "ROP is caused by too little or too much oxygen at specific times during retinal vascularization, as well as by the suppression or stimulation of growth factors such as IGF-1 and VEGF at inappropriate times" (p. 372). In many infants with ROP, this overgrowth ceases or regresses spontaneously. In some, the overgrowth continues, making the development of useful vision unlikely because of the fibrotic changes of the retina or because of retinal detachment.

Assessment

All infants exposed to oxygen, weighing less than 1,500 g at birth, or with a gestational age of 32 weeks or less require assessment and screening for ROP by an ophthalmologist (AAP et al., 2013). The United Kingdom guidelines recommend screening all infants with a gestational age up to 30⁶/₇ weeks or with birth weights of less than 1,251 g (Jefferies, 2010). In addition, selected infants with a birth weight between 1,500 and 2,000 g or a gestational age greater than 30 weeks who have had an unstable clinical course or who have required cardiorespiratory support may be identified as at risk for ROP and therefore need to be assessed (AAP et al., 2013). Timing of the first eye examination is based on the child's gestational age at birth. The youngest infants at birth take the longest time to develop serious cases of ROP (AAP et al., 2013). Thus, timing for the examination varies between 31 and 36 weeks' postmenstrual age of the infant. For example, an infant who is born at 22 weeks' gestation will have an initial examination at 31 weeks' postmenstrual gestation (or 9 chronologic weeks after delivery); an infant who is born at 32 weeks' gestation will have an initial examination at 36 weeks' postmenstrual gestation (or 4 chronologic weeks after delivery) (see thePoint Evidence-Based Practice Guidelines). The schedule for follow-up examinations to monitor the progress of retinal vascularization is based on the findings from the initial examination and varies from 1 week or less in more severe cases to 2 to 3 weeks in less severe cases. ROP is not likely to develop in infants of 42 weeks' gestational age or older. The extensiveness of the acute form of ROP is described as stages 1 to 3 based on the amount of overgrowth of the retinal blood vessels.

Assess the family's adjustment to the condition. Also, assess family knowledge and understanding of the condition and the growth and development of the premature infant with a potentially disabling condition.

Provide assistance to the ophthalmologist during screening procedures. The child's pupils are dilated with mydriatic eye drops given 30 minutes before the examination. A binocular ophthalmoscope is used to examine the eyes. The procedure is uncomfortable and may increase stress responses in the vulnerable and compromised infant.

KidKare A topical anesthetic may be applied to the eyes prior to the examination to decrease the infant's discomfort. Swaddle the infant during the examination and provide oral sucrose and/or pacifiers.

Monitor vital signs during the examination because the mydriatic drops coupled with the ocular pressure may cause bradycardia, apnea, and hypertension. Applying nasolacrimal pressure and wiping away excess fluid can help prevent systemic absorption of the ophthalmic medications used during the examination.

Interdisciplinary Interventions

Interventions focus on preventing ROP. Prevention of premature birth is by far the best way to decrease the number of infants born before their eyes are fully developed. Any effort to decrease premature births would also decrease the incidence of ROP. It is well known that prenatal care decreases the incidence of premature birth; nurses play a key role in encouraging prenatal care, which helps in preventing premature births and, subsequently, in preventing the disabling effects of ROP.

Monitor and limit the amount of oxygen the premature infant is receiving. Ideally, major swings between periods of hypoxia and hyperoxia should be avoided. Research studies have recommended strict management guidelines that include maintaining oxygen saturation levels between 85% and 93%. These studies have indicated a decrease in the incidence of ROP when an infant's normal oxygen saturation range is maintained in this range (Chow et al., 2003; Vanderveen et al., 2006).

When ROP occurs, treatment focuses on arresting the growth of new and aberrant blood vessels in the retina to prevent complications such as detached retina and to enable continued normal development of vision. During the premature infant's hospital stay, the ophthalmologist monitors the progression of the condition with weekly eye examinations.

Surgical intervention to arrest the growth of retinal vasculature may be necessary. The choice and timing of treatments with cryotherapy or laser photocoagulation surgery (preferred treatment) is based on the progression of the disease and is determined by the ophthalmologist. Cryotherapy uses an extremely cold probe that is applied repeatedly to the eye to cauterize the hypoxic areas of the retina. An incision into the conjunctiva is required for this surgery. Complications include retinal scarring, cell destruction, and detachment of the retina. Laser photocoagulation involves use of argon or a diode laser to condensate the protein material in the eye, halting vessel growth. This procedure is less harmful to the eye than cryotherapy. Complications of the procedure include scarring; hemorrhage; burns of the cornea, iris, or lens; and development of cataracts (Harrell & Brandon, 2007; Jefferies, 2010).

The prognosis for infants with ROP is variable, and parents often require considerable support to be able to accept the long periods during which they will not know the degree of damage that their child has sustained. A referral to social services or clergy may be necessary to assist parents in adjusting to the possibility that their infant may have permanent eye damage.

Community Care

When the infant is discharged or transferred from one facility to another, follow-up by both the primary health care provider and ophthalmologist is essential. Results of the ROP screening must be shared with personnel at the receiving unit and with any new primary caregivers (Jefferies, 2010). All persons involved need to be aware of the increased risk for retinal detachment that exists in infants with ROP. If the infant has a poor visual outcome, parents may need guidance on how to best assist the infant to continue development in as near a normal pattern as is possible. Referral to a support group or to national organizations that provide assistive materials may be in order (see thePoint Organizations).

ANSWER: To meet Gabriella's needs, one role the nurse assumes is that of educator. The nurse spends more time with the parents than some other members of the health care team. The nurse should clarify and verify the parents' understanding of the diagnostic testing, the medical problem, and the potential treatments. Another key role of the nurse involves facilitating parent–infant bonding. Bonding occurs best when a family can spend time together, having eye-to-eye contact and lots of touching. All the senses are involved and stimulated in parent–infant bonding. Nurses who care for hospitalized infants, especially those with potential sensory impairments like Gabriella, must facilitate and encourage family–infant bonding.

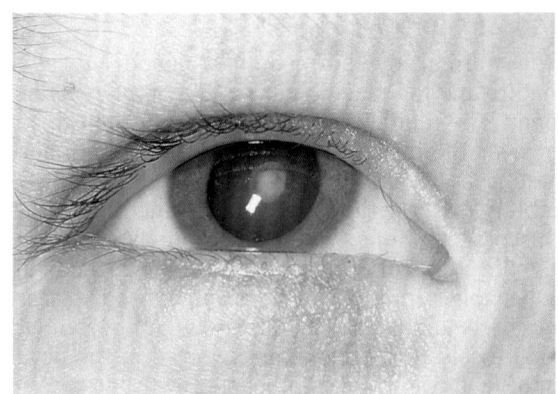

Figure 28-11 Cataracts may develop in infants or children of any age.

CATARACTS

Cataract refers to any opacity of the lens. Cataracts may be congenital or acquired after birth. Congenital cataracts may be observed at birth or may not be seen until later in infancy (Fig. 28-11). Congenital cataracts may result from exposure to infectious agents, such as rubella, toxoplasmosis, cytomegalovirus, herpes simplex, syphilis, and possibly varicella. Prematurity and genetic factors also contribute to the development of congenital cataracts. Cataracts are common in children with Down syndrome, although they are not always severe enough to be removed.

Cataracts may also be acquired during childhood as a result of trauma; toxic agents; or metabolic, endocrine, or other disorders. Trauma to the eye, such as from penetration injuries or contusions, may lead to scarring and thus lead to development of cataracts during childhood.

Pathophysiology

During the fourth and fifth weeks of fetal development, the lens capsule forms as a clear membrane. If the forming lens is attacked by an organism, it becomes milky white and cloudy and may fail to continue to develop. This opacification is called a *cataract* (Mickler et al., 2011).

The optic nerve and internal ocular structures continue to develop normally during fetal life unless the etiologic agent attacks these as well. Ocular development and visual development continue after birth. After birth, the infant's eyes also develop the ability to transfer images to the visual cortex of the brain. If a cataract is present, the visual image cannot reach the brain, and the visual cortex fails to continue to develop. If the cataract is removed before the infant is 2 months old, the visual center of the brain is able to resume development.

Assessment

Some cataracts may be detected easily during physical examination of the eye, whereas others may not be externally visible and may not be detected until visual acuity testing is done prior to school entrance. The absence of the red reflex and a white, opaque appearance of the lens are characteristic. Impaired visual acuity that accompanies a cataract may result in nystagmus (rapid oscillating movement of the eye) or strabismus (wandering eye) in the affected eye. Thus, carefully assess a child with any other ocular disorder or diminished acuity such as strabismus, amblyopia, or nystagmus because of the risk for an associated internal or superficial cataract.

Be alert for any history of poisoning with a toxic substance or history of severe infection, particularly with varicella or other viral condition, and for facial scars from burns, abuse, or other trauma.

Interdisciplinary Interventions

The primary goal is the preservation or development of useful vision for the child. The achievement of this outcome depends on the nature of the condition, the child's age when the cataract is identified and removed, and the diligence of the child and family in maintaining the visual therapy program.

Congenital cataracts must be surgically removed before the infant is age 6 weeks to prevent amblyopia and loss of useful vision (Mickler et al., 2011). Cataract removal is done by an ophthalmologist on an outpatient basis. Three types of surgical interventions can be performed. A **lensectomy** is typically carried out on children 18 months and younger. During this procedure, the whole lens and some of the vitreous "jelly" behind it are removed. For older children, and some younger children, an **aspiration** procedure is used, during which part of the lens is removed and some of the outer capsule of the lens remains. It is often possible to place an intraocular lens into the remaining capsule, either at the time of the procedure or at a later date. Last, an **intraocular lens implant** may be performed. In this case, the lens is removed and replaced by a permanent plastic lens. Intraocular lenses are not used with infants because of the rapid growth that occurs over a short time in the infant eye.

Postoperatively, although infections are rare, antibiotic drops may be prescribed prophylactically. If a child needs surgery in both eyes, the operations are usually completed within a week of each other to ensure one eye does not see before the other and thus become the stronger eye.

Corrective lenses are often recommended by the ophthalmologist after removal of the cataracts to replace the function of the natural lens for those children who did not receive an intraocular lens implant. Contact lenses that can be adjusted in power as the eye changes yield better results for young children. Use of contact lenses in infants and young children with cataracts is currently being studied, particularly with respect to difficulties faced by family caregivers with insertion and removal of the lenses in very young children. Ma (2003) found that in children younger than 8 years of age, contact lenses were well tolerated and were not found to be major stressors for the children or their families (see Tradition or Science 28-1).

Community Care

Teach family members how to administer eye ointment or drops correctly to avoid pressure on the globe of the eye. A patch and an eye protector made of hard plastic or metal is left in place (except for medication administration) until the follow-up visit with the ophthalmic surgeon. Instruct the caregivers to look at the eye as they instill medications and to look for any unusual redness, swelling, or drainage and to report this immediately to the ophthalmologist.

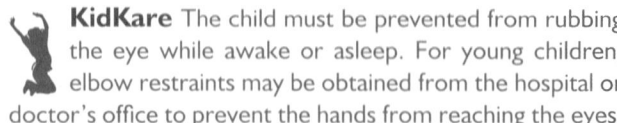 **KidKare** The child must be prevented from rubbing the eye while awake or asleep. For young children, elbow restraints may be obtained from the hospital or doctor's office to prevent the hands from reaching the eyes.

The infant who has undergone cataract surgery also requires aggressive treatment of amblyopia to achieve useful vision (see discussion earlier in this chapter). The success of treatment largely depends on the infant's age at diagnosis and removal and the cooperation of the infant and family with the occlusive patching regimen designed to stimulate the development of the weaker eye. Wilson et al. (2003) found that infants who had cataract removal by 6 weeks of age and whose parents were consistent with the patching regimen had visual acuity outcomes of 20/45 on average. For these parents, the age between 18 and 30 months was a difficult time to gain the child's cooperation with the patching routine. Parents were instructed to do their best during that time and to resume regular patching at 2½ years of age, when the child is more cooperative. The outcome was highly successful. The outcome was much less successful for children whose families abandoned the patching routine when the child objected to wearing the patch.

Adherence to follow-up, including evaluation of intraocular pressure, is important in minimizing the risk of **glaucoma** (increased intraocular pressure; discussed in the next section) resulting from cataract surgery (Lim et al., 2012).

When the child returns to the primary health care provider for well-child care, provide follow-up assessment of vision and monitor adherence to the therapeutic regimen developed by the ophthalmologist. As the child grows older, further assessment of visual status, using the assistance of developmental specialists, educators, and family support groups, may be necessary, depending on the amount of useful vision that develops. Support the family in their role as advocates for the child as they learn to access the services needed to facilitate the health care and education of their child.

GLAUCOMA

Glaucoma is a rare but potentially devastating condition when it occurs in infants and young children. *Glaucoma* is a general term used to indicate elevated pressure within the eye that leads to damage to the optic nerve with visual field loss. Glaucoma in children is classified as primary, or developmental, and secondary, or acquired (Chart 28-2). Primary glaucoma is characterized by abnormal circulation and drainage of aqueous humor from the intraocular space (Yadava, 2010). As the aqueous humor collects in the eye, intraocular pressure increases. Secondary glaucoma is associated with other ocular or systemic abnormalities.

CHART 28-2 **Classification of Childhood Glaucoma**

Primary (Developmental) Glaucoma

- Primary congenital glaucoma
  - Newborn congenital glaucoma
  - Infantile congenital glaucoma
  - Juvenile congenital glaucoma
- Juvenile open-angle glaucoma
- Developmental glaucoma associated with systemic diseases (e.g., Sturge-Weber syndrome, neurofibromatosis, trisomy 13)

Secondary (Acquired) Glaucoma

- Examples: traumatic glaucoma, glaucoma with intraocular neoplasms, glaucoma related to corticosteroids, glaucoma associated with increased venous pressure

The most common type of glaucoma is congenital/infantile glaucoma. The incidence of this glaucoma in infants and young children has been estimated at 1 in 15,000 infants in Western countries. It occurs more frequently in males and is usually bilateral. Among infants who have had surgery for congenital cataract removal, 6% to 45% will develop glaucoma (Kirwan & O'Keefe, 2006; Swamy et al., 2007). About 50% of primary glaucoma in children is related to other congenital conditions such as Marfan syndrome, neurofibromatosis, homocystinuria, Lowe syndrome, or congenital rubella. A few isolated cases of familial genetic transmission have been identified.

Pathophysiology

Congenital/infantile glaucoma results from a defect in the trabecular meshwork of the eye that prevents drainage of the aqueous humor out of the eye. The backup and accumulation of fluids causes increased pressure in the eye. The prognosis is good, although lifelong follow-up is required. *Juvenile glaucoma* is a disease with onset after age 3 years, usually secondary to some other disease process. Both infantile and juvenile glaucoma may occur secondary to a coexisting pathologic process. For example, in Marfan syndrome (an autosomal dominant congenital disorder affecting connective tissue, osseous development, and heart and eye structures), abnormal connective tissue of the trabecular meshwork is thought to prevent normal circulation of the aqueous humor out of the intraocular space, thus increasing intraocular pressure. Infantile and juvenile glaucoma may also be an acquired condition, resulting from an injury that causes scar tissue formation. If left untreated, infantile glaucoma progresses steadily and results in blindness.

Conditions such as trauma, ocular inflammatory disease, ocular tumors, and intraocular hemorrhage are also causes of glaucoma in the pediatric population. Such conditions may create elevated and sustained pressure within the eye that may lead to permanent nerve damage.

Assessment

Infants and children with glaucoma may experience a sudden or gradual onset of symptoms that includes epiphora (tearing), photophobia (sensitivity to light), and blepharospasm (eyelid squeezing). Signs and symptoms may be noted within a few days of birth or may develop insidiously. Family members' descriptions of the child's behavior are particularly important. Infants and young children may demonstrate unexplained behavior changes, such as irritability and episodes of unexplained crying, which alert the family that something is wrong. Families may not associate these behaviors with disease and may hesitate to mention behavior changes unless the health care provider specifically asks.

 ALERT   *Infants who have episodes of unexplained irritability and crying or unexplained behavior changes should be examined for eye pain and glaucoma, particularly if they have had cataracts removed.*

Ask the family about rubbing the eyes. Infants who are at least several months old and who have the dexterity to rub their eyes with their hands will do so if their eyes hurt. Family caregivers may consider this behavior another minor occurrence, without recognizing its potential importance to the diagnosis.

Assess the child for the comparative size of the eyes, corneal clouding (hazy, white area over the lens; Fig. 28-12), blue-tinged sclera, tearing or excess watering of the eyes without evidence of infection (*epiphora*), photophobia (sensitivity to light) even under low-light conditions, and blepharospasm (involuntary closure of eyelids). Inspect the eyes for buphthalmos (enlargement of one or both eyes), particularly if the condition is bilateral and if they consider large eyes a desirable trait. A difference in pupillary size of even 1 mm is considered abnormal, but deciding whether the smaller eye or the larger eye is abnormal may be difficult. Diagnosis at an early age is difficult because of lack of symptoms and difficulty in evaluating vision in infants and young children.

Assessment of the older child includes testing of visual acuity, pupil dilation, and visual field. Assessment of

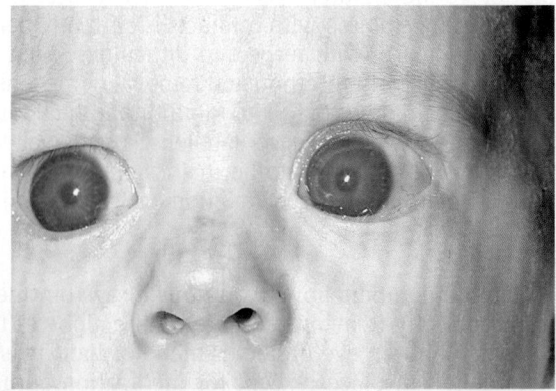

Figure 28-12 Corneal clouding in an infant with glaucoma.

intraocular pressure, using a procedure called tonometry, must be done by the specialist and often under anesthesia for infants, young children, and those who are unable to cooperate during the test. The "puff" test for intraocular pressure measurement may be used by the eye care specialist while testing children as young as age 4 to 4½ years; however, prior to this age, obtaining an accurate pressure measurement without anesthesia is difficult.

KidKare Before the puff test, the child needs to be fully prepared, usually by a family member, so that he or she will cooperate fully. The young child is much better able to cooperate if the test is approached as a game and the child is given the responsibility to hold his or her eyes "open wide" until the puff comes, then "you can close them tight." The eye care specialist performs the test first on one eye and then on the other.

All infants should be screened in the newborn nursery and at each well-child visit. Any suspicion of glaucoma must be treated urgently, with an immediate referral to an ophthalmologist. Prognosis improves with early diagnosis and treatment. Screening is recommended for those 20 years of age and older as part of a comprehensive eye examination (U.S. Preventive Services Task Force, 2005).

Interdisciplinary Interventions

The ophthalmologist may first administer medication to temporarily decrease ocular edema, clear the cornea, and improve visualization of both the surgical site and the iridocorneal angle. Oral acetazolamide, a carbonic anhydrase inhibitor, is the most effective initial therapy. Dorzolamide, a topical (ophthalmic) carbonic anhydrase inhibitor, may also be used. Topical beta-blockers suppress aqueous formation and may be used in conjunction with topical or systemic carbonic anhydrase inhibitor.

Surgery to either increase the outflow of fluid from the eye or to decrease the production of fluid within the eye may also be used to reduce the intraocular pressure. The goal is to have a level of equilibrium at which the eye will produce enough fluid to maintain its integrity yet allow enough fluid to exit to provide a normal intraocular pressure (Aponte, et al., 2011). The type of surgical technique is based on the pathophysiology of the child's condition. Goniosurgery, also known as *goniotomy* and *trabeculotomy*, are the surgeries of choice for congenital glaucoma. During these procedures, a surgical opening is made into the drainage area of the eye (the trabecular meshwork drainage system), establishing a more normal anterior chamber angle that allows the fluid to drain more freely. Children with more severe defects of the filtration channels often do not respond to goniosurgery, and filtration procedures may be required to bypass the malfunctioning system, creating a new egress passage for the aqueous humor. If filtration surgery is not effective, implants may be used to drain the aqueous fluid from the eye by way of a silicone tube to an episcleral reservoir (Walton, 2007).

Postoperative care may be provided initially by the nurse and later by the family. Eye patches or a protective eye shield may be used for a short time after the surgery to protect the child's eyes. Elbow restraints may be used to prevent the child from rubbing his or her eyes.

Community Care

The infant with glaucoma needs regular follow-up with the ophthalmologist throughout life. Both the nurse and the primary health care provider should encourage and facilitate such visits. Children do not outgrow glaucoma. Glaucoma is controlled so that further damage to the eye is avoided. Constant vigilance is necessary to ensure that pressure does not increase and damage delicate structures of the eye (Franzco & Franzco, 2011).

When the child enters school, urge the family to inform the school nurse of the child's past history of health problems. During the school years, the school nurse may be able to assist or encourage the family to obtain the health care follow-up that the child needs to prevent deterioration of vision. The school nurse also functions as a liaison among health care professionals, educators, and the family to help such children achieve their maximum potential.

Special attention should be given to the developmental and educational progress of children who have had a poor visual outcome. They may need alternative learning tools to make best use of limited visual acuity.

VISUAL IMPAIRMENT

Blindness is defined by educational and governmental agencies as having vision no better than 20/200 in the better eye or a visual field no better than 20 degrees at its widest diameter regardless of visual acuity. Persons with these limitations are said to be *legally blind*. However, they may still have considerable useful vision and may be able to use print as a major means of learning.

Partially sighted is the term used to describe the visual ability of those with visual acuity of more than 20/200 but worse than 20/70 in their better eye with correction (Education for All Handicapped Children Act, 1975). Both legally blind and partially sighted children are classified as *visually impaired*. They have certain rights in the community and in the educational system, which are addressed by the Americans with Disabilities Act.

CROSS-CULTURAL CARE

Visual impairment affects millions of people worldwide. Two thirds of all cases of blindness in the world are either preventable or curable, particularly those caused by infections or poor nutrition. Infections (with *C. trachomatis* and *N. gonorrhoeae*), parasites (onchocerciasis), and cataracts account for a large portion of blindness in adults and children in developing countries with poor nutrition (vitamin A deficiency) and limited access to soap and clean water (Patel et al., 2011). Visual impairment in more developed countries may be caused by genetic inheritance or by a local or systemic disease process that is acquired either pre- or postnatally.

CHART 28-3 Causes of Visual Impairment

Congenital defect: chromosomal abnormality

Systemic disease

Injury
- Head injury, occipital
- Penetrating injury to the ocular globe
- Blunt force injury to the head or globe
- Injury to the anterior globe with scarring

Infection (local or systemic)
- Maternal rubella
- Maternal infection with *Chlamydia trachomatis*
- Maternal gonorrhea
- Maternal varicella
- Infantile varicella
- Neonatal conjunctivitis caused by infection

Neisseria gonorrhoeae

C. trachomatis
- Meningitis
- Encephalitis

Other
- ROP
- Poisoning (e.g., methyl alcohol ingestion)

Any condition that causes damage to, or prevents development of, ocular structures may diminish the child's visual capacity (Chart 28-3).

Pathophysiology

The pathophysiology of visual impairment depends on the causative factors. The pathophysiology seen in shaken baby syndrome is that of bilateral retinal hemorrhages usually greater than compatible with injury described by the family. The shaken baby may also have other indicators of new or old injuries (see Chapter 29).

Ocular structures do not regenerate; thus, damage to the eye is permanent and may result in blindness. Blindness is the result of either optic nerve damage or damage to other parts of the eye that normally would help to focus the image on the retina. Blindness may also result from damage to the visual centers of the brain (cortical blindness). Visual impairment caused by injury or disease is usually not progressive; however, some genetic conditions are progressive over time and with physiologic development.

Assessment

Visual impairment is assessed grossly using eye screening and standard eye and vision assessments. The child with visual impairment requires follow-up by an ophthalmologist. Because of the difficulty of examining the ocular fundus in an infant, any infant who is suspected of having retinal damage caused by abuse should be examined by a specialist as soon as possible. If the assessment of the ocular fundus indicates abuse, and this

assessment is supported by other test results, immediate action is taken to protect the child and involve the local authorities. Other tests and radiographs may be completed to assist in the diagnosis.

caREminder

Be particularly aware that complications can develop rapidly in eye conditions; thus, any time an eye disorder is suspected, ensure that the child is referred and seen immediately. The "wait-and-see" approach has no place in a child's care when vision is at risk.

Interdisciplinary Interventions

Sudden onset of blindness or visual impairment requires immediate evaluation to determine the cause of visual loss and the extent of damage. When possible, interventions can be taken to correct the underlying problem (e.g., cataract surgery). Return of full sight may not be possible. When a child experiences any loss of vision, the goal is to assist the blind/visually impaired child to grow up and become a productive, fully functioning, independent adult.

There is no one "right" way to interact with blind or partially sighted infants and children. However, several interventions can facilitate care and increase the comfort of the visually impaired child and his or her family. Always keep in mind the child's developmental level. For example, a blind child who has not sustained brain damage usually has the capacity to reach the same developmental level and the same conceptual understanding of the world as his or her sighted peers, but the child may not have done so because of lack of experience. For this reason, the blind child may not understand the health care provider's descriptions at a level expected of a sighted child of the same age. Persons who work with blind or partially sighted children must provide the necessary information to help the child to understand the concepts being presented. Blindness does not affect the child's cognitive capacity, but it does affect how the content is presented.

Immediate interventions to ensure the child's safety are required when a child's visual impairment is suspected to be the result of abuse. The child should not be released from the office or emergency department without first having been fully assessed and a plan made for safe care, possibly including admission to the hospital for observation or to examine for further signs of injury. Infants with retinal hemorrhages or detachment, common in shaken baby syndrome, will have a substantial loss of vision and need immediate assessment by the ophthalmologist.

Community Care

Family members, teachers, and health care specialists need to assist the child in developing compensatory physical and communication skills to deal with the environment (James & Stojanovik, 2007). A child with limited or no visual ability must develop auditory and tactile senses earlier and to a greater skill level than their sighted peers (Ihsen et al., 2010; Withagen et al., 2010). Family members can begin the process at home using games similar to those played with sighted children for identification of objects, sizes, shapes, sounds, and textures. Children who have limited vision can benefit from having their attention drawn to specific objects or qualities to enhance their understanding of them. For example, sighted young children are very active, learning how to safely move about their space and conquer its challenges. Nonsighted children need to learn to feed themselves, bathe and dress themselves, and begin school as any child would do. Nonsighted children need the same degree of activity and the same physical challenges. They need to run, play, climb, jump, and manipulate their environment. Obviously, adults will structure playtimes for safety, always mindful of the activity needs of the age. These children need to have responsibilities at home and at school and to learn to make new friends wherever they find themselves.

Visually impaired children may be taught to read Braille very early in life. They can learn to use devices that transfer the printed page to a tactile format. They may be taught to type very early to prepare them for computer use. Using the computer, a vast array of materials can be converted to Braille directly from the printed page (see thePoint Organizations).

Creative play is frequently slower to develop in children with visual impairment; thus, these children benefit greatly by participation in a nursery school setting, where individual attention is possible and a wide variety of toys and activities are available. Children may need to be taught how to reach out to learn about their world and to experience things other children see and reach for (Ihsen et al., 2010).

Social interaction needs to be encouraged very early in life and sometimes taught to compensate for the child's inability to see facial expressions and nonverbal social responses of others. D'Allura (2002) found that when given a structured environment in which each child had something specific to contribute to a project, nonsighted preschoolers interacted with their peers at the same rate as their sighted peers. Prior to this research, nonsighted children had interacted far less than their sighted classmates. Galati et al. (2003) studied facial expressions used by sighted and nonsighted children aged 8 to 11 years and concluded that nonsighted children may need to be taught to purposefully use facial expressions more frequently to improve interpersonal communication.

Physical fitness skills are equally as important for the visually impaired child as for the sighted child. These children need help in developing skills of jumping, hopping, running, and other gross motor activities. Activities in which the visually impaired child can actively participate include swimming, gymnastics, and other individual sports rather than team sports such as basketball. The Special Olympics provides a wide variety of opportunities for persons with visual impairment to participate in sports activities.

Nurses are assuming greater responsibility in monitoring the well-child health care needs in the community and are frequently available to families of children with chronic disabilities. Nurses must be knowledgeable about the effect of visual impairment on child and family development, educational options, community resources, and general health care needs.

ALTERATIONS IN HEARING

Hearing and listening form the foundation for spoken communication. Infants and young children spend much of their day engaged in passive and active listening as a means of gathering information about their world; thus, hearing impairment during infancy and early childhood can have devastating effects on a child's development. Hearing deficit prevents the developmental stimulation provided by the auditory route and also prevents the child from learning speech by imitation, hindering the child's ability to verbally communicate needs, desires, and thoughts.

Approximately 1 to 2 newborns per 1,000 live births have moderate, severe, or profound bilateral sensorineural hearing loss. An additional 1 to 2 newborns per 1,000 live births have milder or unilateral impairments. Hearing loss can occur at any time during childhood; for children up to age 19 years, the prevalence of hearing loss is approximately 15% of the pediatric population (Centers for Disease Control and Prevention [CDC], 2012).

CROSS-CULTURAL CARE

In developing countries, the incidence of congenital bilateral hearing loss is 2 to 4 per 1,000 live births. Two thirds of people with hearing impairments worldwide live in developing countries. Although the cause of hearing loss is unknown in as many as 40% of all cases, known factors of hearing loss include congenital cytomegalovirus, rubella, and toxoplasmosis and the deleterious outcomes of measles, meningitis, mumps, and OM acquired by children who have not been vaccinated against such diseases (Olussanya & Newton, 2007).

In infants, hearing loss is most often associated with maternal infections (cytomegalovirus), complications after birth that result in intensive therapy in a neonatal intensive care unit, birth trauma, and congenital malformations. Early identification of these conditions will assist the child and family to make the necessary adaptations to ensure that the child meets appropriate developmental milestones. In young children and adolescents, alterations in hearing are most commonly caused by infections, blockages, or injuries that impair transmission of sound through the ear canal and inner ear structures. In these cases, prompt intervention is necessary to prevent permanent damage to the anatomic components of the auditory system.

Always keep in mind that *any* infant or child being examined or cared for could be one of a large number of children with an undiagnosed hearing deficit. Early identification of even partial hearing loss is essential to the development of communication skills and the lifelong learning process. Nurses are frequently in strategic positions in primary care settings, schools, hospitals, or home care to identify children at risk or who are suspected of having hearing deficit.

OTITIS MEDIA

OM is an inflammation of the middle ear and may be further defined as

- *Acute otitis media* (AOM) – rapid onset of signs and symptoms of inflammation of the middle ear
- *Uncomplicated AOM* – AOM without discharge from the ear (**otorrhea**)
- *Severe AOM* – AOM with the presence of moderate to severe **otalgia** (ear pain) or fever equal to or greater than 39° C (102.2° F)
- *Nonsevere AOM* – AOM with mild otalgia and a temperature below 39° C (102.2° F)
- *Recurrent AOM* – three or more well-documented and separate AOM episodes in the preceding 6 months, or four or more episodes in the preceding 12 months with at least one episode in the past 6 months
- *Otitis media with effusion* (OME) – inflammation of the middle ear with the presence of fluid in the normally air-filled space behind the tympanic membrane. This fluid exerts pressure on the tympanic membrane, causing pain as it bulges outward.
- *Middle ear effusion* (MEE) – fluid in the middle ear without reference to etiology, pathogenesis, pathology, or duration (Lieberthal et al., 2013).

AOM is one of the most common diseases of childhood. Eighty percent of children have had at least one episode of AOM by 3 years of age, although the greatest incidence is between 6 and 18 months of age. The incidence increases during winter and spring, paralleling the increased incidence of upper respiratory infection and sinus infections. AOM may give rise to MEE, which in turn causes temporary hearing loss. In 25% of cases, MEE persists for more than 3 months (Benge & Williamson, 2011).

Factors that contribute to AOM and OME include young age, allergies, HIV infection, genetic predisposition, craniofacial abnormalities, Down syndrome, and presence of other siblings. Breastfed infants often have a lower incidence of OM, possibly because of the composition of the breast milk itself and the immune factors provided from the mother. Infants who use a bottle or sippy cup for milk or juice at bedtime have a higher risk of developing OM than those who do not. Infants who use pacifiers are at higher risk for OM (Lieberthal et al., 2013; Marter & Agruss, 2007).

Children who attend daycare have a higher incidence of both AOM and nonsevere OM and a higher incidence of OME than those who do not attend daycare. These children also have more upper respiratory infections. Exposure to passive smoke increases the incidence of OM. Passive smoke damages the mucosa of the nasopharynx and eustachian tubes, thus increasing the susceptibility of the child to bacterial and viral invasion.

Pathophysiology

Organisms, most commonly pneumococci, *Haemophilus influenzae*, and *Moraxella catarrhalis*, gain entrance to the middle ear through the eustachian tube, which forms a normal connection between the pharynx and the middle ear. The infant's eustachian tube is shorter, wider, and more horizontal than those of older children and adults. Additionally, the infant's eustachian tube is made of cartilage and muscle with a flutter valve opening in the oropharynx. Its purpose is to equalize pressure between the ear and the environment and to drain normal fluid from the middle ear. This anatomic difference is thought to increase the infant's susceptibility to infection of the middle ear. Usually, the ear infection appears a few days after the onset of an upper respiratory infection. It is theorized that the flutter valve fails to prevent organisms from the oropharynx from entering the eustachian tube and subsequently the middle ear.

Inflammation and suppuration that result from the bacterial invasion prevent normal aeration and fluid drainage from the middle ear. When the middle ear fills with fluid, sound conduction is diminished because the vibration of the incus, stapes, and malleus is hindered by fluid. During this time, the infant does not hear as well as would be expected if the inflammatory process were not present. If the infectious process is long-lasting, the infant may miss developmental milestones in speech and language development.

Fluid that remains in the middle ear after the acute infection has abated may take 6 weeks to 3 months to clear. This fluid does not clear any faster with medication (antihistamines) and does not indicate an ongoing infectious process. It does, however, diminish hearing during this time.

The degree of hearing impairment in OM depends not on the severity of the infection but on the degree to which sounds are prevented from reaching the inner ear. Children with few OM infections catch up quickly when the effusion clears and hearing returns; however, the degree of hearing impairment is a critical factor in the progress of normal cognitive and language learning processes for the young child.

Assessment

Clinical manifestations of OM vary widely in infants and children. There may be evidence of ear pain (otalgia), as manifested by irritability, tugging or holding of the ear, changes in sleep or eating patterns, or complaints by the child that the ear hurts. Fever may be present, along with signs and symptoms of an upper respiratory infection and/or sinusitis. Purulent, bloody drainage from the ear may be present if the tympanic membrane has ruptured. The older child may complain of a sense of fullness or pressure in the ear, hearing loss, balance difficulties, or disequilibrium.

The primary health care provider examines the tympanic membrane using the otoscope to view the auditory canal and the tympanic membrane. For young children, the pinna must be pulled up and back for clear visualization. For older children and adults, the pinna is pulled either straight back or down and back to see the tympanic membrane fully. If the tympanic membrane is obscured by cerumen, the cerumen is removed prior to progressing with an otoscopic examination. The tympanic membrane is observed for contour, color, translucence, structural changes, and mobility. Otoscopic examination typically reveals a pearly gray, translucent tympanic membrane that is slightly concave in its contour. The tympanic membrane should be free of structural changes (scars, perforations) and be mobile. Pneumatic otoscopy is used to assess motility. When the ear is insufflated with a puff of air, the tympanic membrane usually moves. If the tympanic membrane does not move with applications of gentle positive or negative pressure, MEE is presumed to be present (Lieberthal et al., 2013).

The child is diagnosed with AOM if he or she presents with a moderate to severe bulging of the tympanic membrane or recent (less than 48 hours) onset of otorrhea not caused by OE (inflammation of the outer ear canal) or intense erythema of the TM (Lieberthal et al., 2013). Erythema of the TM may be a sign of inflammation or infection. AOM should not be diagnosed in children who do not have MEE as identified by pneumatic otoscopy and/or tympanometry.

caREminder

Crying may cause the tympanic membrane of the infant or young child to appear red.

Tympanometry, a test to indirectly assess the compliance (mobility) and impedance of the middle ear, can be done in the office to confirm the diagnosis of MEE. The test demonstrates an abnormal curve on the tympanometry graph if fluid is present in the middle ear. Tympanometry is usually not valid when done in infants younger than age 7 to 8 months because achieving a good fit between the instrument and the infant's ear is difficult.

Laboratory work that may be helpful in assessing the child with AOM includes a culture of the throat and any ear drainage that may be present. In addition, a complete blood count provides information about the white blood cell count (elevated in bacterial infections) and the hemoglobin level. Low hemoglobin is associated with increased susceptibility to infection. Follow-up assessment is essential after treatment for OM to determine whether the OM has cleared. Follow-up assessment of the child with MEE after AOM has cleared should be done monthly to assess developmental progress and to look for clearing of the effusion.

Nursing Diagnoses and Outcomes

In addition to those in Nursing Plan of Care 28-1, the following nursing diagnoses are appropriate for the child with OM. Additional information regarding care management for the child with an acute condition can be found in Nursing Plan of Care 11-1.

Nursing Diagnosis: Risk for infection related to middle ear inflammation, anatomy of eustachian tubes (in children younger than 3 years of age), and pooling of fluid and secretions in the pharyngeal cavity

Outcomes:
- Child will be free of infection.
- Child will not experience hearing loss as a result of OM.

Nursing Diagnosis: Risk for imbalanced fluid volume related to increased insensible fluid loss, fever, and decreased fluid intake

Outcome: Child will demonstrate signs and symptoms of adequate hydration.

Nursing Diagnosis: Pain (otalgia) related to inflammatory process.

Outcome: Child will be pain free and able to rest comfortably

Interdisciplinary Interventions

According to the guidelines for management of AOM developed by the AAP, a definitive diagnosis of AOM is made when the child has (1) history of acute onset of signs and symptoms, (2) presence of MEE, and (3) signs and symptoms of middle ear inflammation (Lieberthal et al., 2013). These children require antibiotic therapy. A child who does not display all three criteria is said to have nonsevere AOM or OME and may not be prescribed antibiotics as discussed in the following section.

Medications

Interventions for children with acute or chronic OM, with or without effusion, always include pain management with analgesics (acetaminophen or ibuprofen) and may include medication to treat the infection, when appropriate (Clinical Judgment 28-2). Pain assessment is completed on all children with OM, and regardless of findings from visualizing the tympanic membrane, if the child has pain, it should be managed using analgesics. Steroid therapy is not recommended for the treatment of OM (Tradition or Science 28-2).

National guidelines provide evidence-based recommendations for the use of antibiotics in the treatment of OM. Antibiotics must be used judiciously. Antibiotics change the flora of the respiratory and intestinal tracts, thus increasing the chance of allergy or undesirable side effects (diarrhea), decreasing the child's likelihood of developing immunity to the invading organism, and increasing the chance of the organism developing resistance to the antibiotic (Shaikh & Hoberman, 2010; Thornton et al., 2011).

Current guidelines recommend prescribing antibiotics under the following conditions:

- Diagnosis of AOM (bilateral or unilateral) in children aged 6 months and older with moderate or severe otalgia, or otalgia for at least 48 hours, or temperature equal to or greater than 39° C (102.2° F)
- Diagnosis of AOM (bilateral) in children younger than 24 months of age without severe signs or symptoms (mild otalgia for less than 48 hours and temperature less than 39° C [102.2° F]) (Lieberthal et al., 2013)

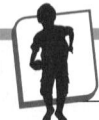

CLINICAL JUDGMENT 28-2

A Visit to Urgent Care

Brothers Christian, age 4 years, and Matthew, age 7 months, are brought to an urgent care facility on a Saturday night. Christian told his mom earlier in the evening, "I have a sword in my ear." Matthew has been pulling and scratching at his right ear since the previous night. Mom states the boys feel "hot."

Otoscopic examination of Christian's ears reveals red, bulging tympanic membranes with no visible landmarks. His temperature is 39° C (102.2° F). He is crying and wiggling during the examination.

Matthew's right ear also has a red tympanic membrane and no visible landmarks. The cone of light was difficult to assess because of the excessive wax in his ear. His temperature is 38.5° C (101.3° F). He is crying, and mom states he has been irritable and unwilling to drink from the bottle.

Questions

1. What questions would you ask the mother about the boys' current condition?

2. What can cause the tympanic membrane of the ear to be red?

3. What do you suspect is Christian's diagnosis? Matthew's diagnosis?

4. How does examination with the otoscope help differentiate a normal ear from an ear with OM?

5. Antibiotic therapy is ordered for the boys. The appropriate dose of amoxicillin is 80 mg/kg/day to be given twice a day. Christian weighs 15.9 kg; Matthew weighs 9 kg. Calculate the dosage of medication for each child.

Answers

1. Any presence of fever, complaints of hearing loss, pain in or around the ear, dizziness, impaired balance, or vomiting? How long has the child been pulling or tugging at the ear? Have the children been diagnosed with OM in the past? When?

2. Crying, AOM, infection

3. AOM with effusion for both boys

4. The normal ear has a pearl-gray tympanic membrane, with a visible cone of light and mobility of tympanic membrane observed with the pneumatic otoscope. The child with OM exhibits a swollen, opaque, and discolored (red or yellow) eardrum with no visible landmarks and little or no mobility. An air–fluid level may be seen.

5. Christian should receive 1,272 mg/day, or 636 mg per dose. Matthew should receive 720 mg/day, or 360 mg per dose. In addition, acetaminophen may be ordered for management of pain (otalgia).

Observation of the child first, with administration of antibiotics if the child worsens or fails to improve within 48 to 72 hours, is recommended for children (aged 6 to 23 months) with nonsevere unilateral AOM and for older children with nonsevere AOM (unilateral or bilateral) (Lieberthal et al., 2013). Amoxicillin is the medication of choice if the child has not received amoxicillin in the past 30 days or does not have a concurrent purulent conjunctivitis and the child is not allergic to penicillin. If the child does not meet these criteria for amoxicillin, an antibiotic with additional β-lactamase coverage for AOM can be prescribed. If the child fails to respond to the initial antibiotic treatment or the condition worsens, a change in therapy may be needed. Antibiotics are not prescribed prophylactically to reduce the occurrence of AOM (Lieberthal et al., 2013).

Surgical Management

Surgery for OM is indicated when episodes of AOM occur frequently (three episodes in 6 months or four episodes in 1 year, with one episode in the preceding 6 months); MEE persists too long and is accompanied by difficulty hearing; complications manifest such as mastoiditis, labyrinthitis, and facial paralysis; or symptomatic eustachian tube dysfunction exists (DeRosa & Grundfast, 2002; Lieberthal et al., 2013). The primary surgical option for treating OM is the placement of tympanostomy tubes. Under anesthesia, the surgeon inserts very small tubes into the eardrum to improve middle ear ventilation after

Evidence-Based Practice

TRADITION OR SCIENCE 28-2

Should steroids be used to treat otitis media?

Steroids given orally have been suggested by some practitioners as treatment for persistent MEE; however, the current guidelines do not recommend the use of steroids because of the limited scientific evidence of their benefit and the known adverse effects of steroid use. Steroids given in the ear canal are still used to decrease local inflammation. Antihistamines and decongestants are also not recommended as treatment measures because research has proved them to be ineffective in the management of ear infections (Grassia, 2004; Lieberthal et al., 2013).

fluid removal and to allow pressure equalization and normal drainage of middle ear. Tubes usually fall out by themselves in 6 to 18 months

Community Care

Nurses play a key role in teaching families how to reduce possible risk factors for OM. In particular, support the health care provider's plan of care and teach families that antibiotics are not always the best treatment. If a particular child's condition makes him or her a candidate for the observation approach, urge the family to bring the child back in 2 to 3 days for a reevaluation. If the condition has worsened, appropriate medication will be prescribed. If the condition has improved, the child is spared the necessity of taking antibiotics for a number of days and enduring any side effects that may develop.

The nurse is also responsible for teaching the child and family about tympanoplasty, including ear care after surgery. Instruct the family in measures to keep the ears dry, usually with insertion of a molded earplug or small cotton plugs whenever the child is around water. Tympanostomy tubes are tiny, possibly bordered on one end by a round, plasticlike plate. The tubes come in various styles, shapes, and sizes. Inform the family about the appearance and size of their child's tubes so that they can recognize them if and when they fall out.

To assist in the prevention of OM, the AAP recommends all children receive the pneumococcal conjugate vaccine and annual influenza vaccines. In addition, the AAP encourages exclusive breastfeeding for at least 6 months because this has been demonstrated to reduce the risk of early AOM (Lieberthal et al., 2013).

If the child has a chronic condition, spends time with adults who smoke, or has other risk factors, the OM may not clear, even with an initial round of antibiotics. Stress to the family the necessity of a follow-up ear examination, even if the child is feeling and acting well. To prevent development of chronic OM, the condition must be eradicated completely, and a second round of antibiotics may be prescribed for up to another 3 weeks. If treatment is not effective in eliminating the infection, the possibility of complications remains. Complications include generalized sepsis, meningitis, or mastoiditis.

When the child is exposed to cigarette smoke, the risk for OM increases. The nurse can use this opportunity to encourage adults to stop smoking or at least avoid smoking around the infant or young child. Adults who smoke and have infants in their home should smoke outside, cover their clothing, and leave the jacket or covering outside when returning to care for the infant. Handwashing prior to caring for the infant is essential as well.

OM may result in diminished hearing; thus, it is both a medical problem and an educational problem. Children whose hearing ability fluctuates from day to day cannot maximally benefit from any learning situation that involves voice or sound. They miss not only direct learning opportunities but also incidental learning opportunities that help a child fit into his or her social group.

If OME persists without resolution for 3 months, the child should have a hearing test. If the child's hearing is found to be deficient in the tonal range occupied by the spoken voice, a referral to the ear, nose, and throat specialist is made. Tympanostomy tubes could allow drainage of the fluid and restoration of hearing.

OTITIS EXTERNA

OE, also called *swimmer's ear*, is an inflammation of the tissue of the external auditory canal. Although it seldom threatens hearing, it can be very painful. Children who spend long hours in the swimming pool are prone to develop OE as a result of chronic irritation and maceration from excessive moisture in the ear canal. Inflammation of the ear canal may also be the result of herpesvirus, varicella zoster, various skin exanthems, and eczema.

Pathophysiology

Healthy skin of the external otic canal has an acidic pH (Eng & El-Hawrani, 2011). The cerumen found in the external auditory canal protects the thin layer of skin from the effects of moisture. If cerumen is removed with cotton-tipped applicators or is washed out by frequent introduction of water, as occurs when children swim for long periods, the pH changes and the skin becomes more vulnerable to organisms in the environment. The warm, moist atmosphere of the ear canal provides an ideal place for growth of bacterial or fungal organisms. The most common organism is *Pseudomonas aeruginosa*, although *Staphylococcus aureus*, *Enterobacter aerogenes*, *Proteus mirabilis*, *Klebsiella pneumoniae*, streptococci, staphylococci, and fungi have also been known to cause OE (Narayan & Swift, 2011). Inflammation causes the tissues to swell, which in turn causes pain. The swelling may extend from the external auditory canal to surrounding tissues of the face.

Assessment

The history presented by the child with OE may reflect extended periods in or around the water or a child with skin infections that affect the face (eczema). The child who washes his or her hair at night and goes to bed with wet hair is also prone to develop OE. The onset is usually sudden and without history of fever or upper respiratory symptoms. The classic sign of acute OE is pain on movement of the pinna or pain on pressure over the tragus. Edema; erythema; and thick, clumpy otorrhea (drainage) of the ear canal are present. Lymph nodes in the periauricular area may be palpable and tender. Otoscopic examination of the affected ear may not be possible because inserting the speculum causes extreme pain. When otoscopic examination is possible, it often shows that the tympanic membrane is not affected.

Interdisciplinary Intervention

Eardrops that provide antibacterial and antifungal medication to the external auditory canal are usually sufficient to eradicate the infection within 7 days, although the discomfort is gone in 2 to 3 days. Oral antibiotics are usually not necessary. Ear pain may be managed with Auralgan or other otic analgesic drops applied directly to the ear canal or with acetaminophen or ibuprofen taken orally. The child should avoid getting the ears wet either by swimming or shampooing until the OE has cleared, usually about 7 days. Ear drops placed in the external otic canal after swimming can maintain the acidic pH of the ear canal and prevent external OE.

Community Care

Prevention of OE includes

- Avoiding the use of cotton-tipped applicators in the ears
- Drying the ears well after shampooing or swimming (blow dry)
- Instilling dilute alcohol or 2% acetic acid eardrops after swimming or bathing

These eardrops may be purchased OTC or made at home by mixing equal parts rubbing alcohol and white vinegar. Vinegar changes the pH of the ear canal to discourage growth of organisms, and the alcohol encourages drying of the tissue.

caREminder

Caution caregivers not to use cotton-tipped applicators to remove cerumen because of the danger of either pushing the cerumen against the tympanic membrane or directly damaging the tympanic membrane with the cotton-tipped applicator stick.

HEARING IMPAIRMENT

QUESTION: Is the Goldman family in a unique situation regarding Gabriella's potential hearing loss? How similar might the experience be for other families of premature infants?

Hearing deficit is classified as minimal, mild, moderate, severe, or profound depending on the decibel threshold of sound required before the child can hear it. Normal speech has an intensity of 40 to 50 dB; thus, a child who requires a sound to be 50 dB before it is heard is unable to hear most speech with the unaided ear. Amplification (use of a hearing aid) may improve functional hearing. Hearing impairment is also classified according to the location of the defective hearing pathway (Table 28-3).

Each type of hearing deficit is managed differently; therefore, it is essential to obtain an accurate diagnosis as early as possible. The assistance of the audiologist in making the diagnosis is essential. A deficit may be temporary, as in transient OM, or permanent, as occurs when nerve damage is present.

When the diagnosis of hearing impairment is made, special attention must be given to teaching family members how to share abstract concepts with their child. Emotions are often displayed by tone of voice as well as body language and words. Children who cannot hear tonal variations need to learn to recognize behavioral indicators of emotion.

ANSWER: Prematurity alone is a risk factor for hearing loss, and the smaller and sicker the infant, the greater the risk for hearing loss. Most families of premature infants will have a similar experience to the Goldmans'. This experience includes the understanding that their child may have a hearing loss, the search for more information or a period of denial, and, as the child gets older, more diagnostic measures needed to determine the extent of hearing loss and appropriate interventions.

The origin of hearing deficit in infants and children is varied. Some types of hearing deficits are congenital, whereas others are acquired and related to identifiable events. Congenital hearing deficits may be familial, genetic, or associated with maternal infection (such as maternal rubella during the first trimester) or known congenital syndromes, such as Down syndrome or Turner syndrome.

TABLE 28-3   Types of Hearing Impairment

Type and Definition	Possible Causes
Conductive hearing impairment: inability of the outer and middle ear to transmit sound to the inner ear	Blockage by cerumen or foreign object Congenital malformation of external or middle ear OME (fluid in the middle ear) Scarring of the tympanic membrane
Sensorineural hearing impairment: inability of the inner ear to transmit sound impulses to the brain	Congenital malformation of the inner ear Genetic deterioration of the inner ear Damage to inner ear by disease or injury, child abuse, meningitis, encephalitis
Central hearing impairment: inability of the hearing centers of the brain to receive or process sound impulses	Congenital malformation or disorder of auditory center Brain damage by disease or injury Damage to cranial nerve VIII by disease or injury such as child abuse, meningitis, encephalitis, poisoning
Mixed hearing impairment: any combination of conductive and sensorineural factors	Blockages, malformations, damage to the ear by disease or injury

Risk factors for acquired hearing deficit include prematurity (possibly because of the fragile nature of the nerve endings in the inner ear), environmental noises (especially in older children and teenagers), infections such as meningitis or encephalitis during infancy or early childhood, and chronic OM, which can lead to scarring of the ossicles or tympanic membrane.

Pathophysiology

Hearing loss can be a result of malformation, damage, or disease process involving any of the four portions of the hearing mechanism: outer ear, which directs the sound waves to the eardrum; middle ear, which transmits the sound by means of vibrations of the malleus, the incus, and the stapes; inner ear, in which the cochlea transmits sound to the auditory nerve; and auditory center in the brain. Each requires different interventions with respect to medical or surgical management, sound amplification, and communication style.

Conductive Hearing Impairment

Conductive hearing impairment exists when malformation, inflammation, obstruction (such as cerumen or foreign object occluding the ear canal or fluid collection in the middle ear), or damage involves the outer or middle ear (such as perforation of the tympanic membrane), thus preventing sound from reaching the auditory nerve. Scarring of the tympanic membrane may also result in conductive hearing impairment. The most common cause of conductive hearing impairment, however, is OM (Kochlar et al., 2007).

Cerumen production is a normal process; however, excess production of earwax can cause cerumen impaction and hearing impairment. Approximately 10% of children either produce more than normal amounts or have difficulty with cerumen removal that results in hearing impairment. Cerumen is typically gold-colored when it is fresh and very dark when it is old. Normally, cerumen is moved to the external canal opening by constant movement of hair cells in the ear canal. In the outer ear area, the cerumen dries and flakes off. Cerumen impaction may develop in a child who wears hearing aids because the daily use of the ear mold prevents the cerumen from leaving the ear canal. All children who wear hearing aids should be monitored for the possibility of cerumen impaction.

Other conditions that can cause conductive hearing loss include congenital anomalies such as external auditory canal atresia or stenosis, abnormalities of the tympanic membrane, and ossicular malformation or fixation. Acquired abnormalities, such as tympanic membrane perforations and ossicular erosion resulting from middle ear infection or cholesteatoma, can also cause conductive hearing loss.

Sensorineural Hearing Impairment

QUESTION: If Gabriella does have sensorineural hearing loss, what does this really mean for her and her family? What does she hear?

Sensorineural hearing impairment exists when the cochlea does not relay sound pattern information to the brain. The usual cause is absence, malformation, or damage of some or all of the tiny structures in the inner ear (the hair cells, organ of Corti, membranes that form the cochlear partitions, or nerve fibers that link the hair cells to auditory nerves). This type of hearing impairment can be a result of many different factors affecting both the inner ear and the brain pathways. Risk factors include heredity; infections in the brain; exposure to intrauterine infections such as rubella, cytomegalovirus, and herpes simplex viruses; damage from loud sounds; exposure to ototoxic medications; and prematurity. Infants who are premature and of low birth weight are more prone to development of hearing deficit after intraventricular hemorrhage, anoxic periods, Rh incompatibility, or bilirubin encephalopathy. These tiny babies are more prone to nerve damage and hearing center brain damage than full-term infants. They are also, therefore, at higher risk for delays in comprehension and production of spoken language (Rinaldi & Caselli, 2009).

When nerve damage occurs, the volume and pitch of hearing is affected. The sounds heard are distorted, with certain sounds being lost altogether. For example, the "f," "s," and "d" sounds are frequently not heard, affecting the child's ability to understand speech. Persons with sensorineural hearing impairment often do not benefit greatly from amplification of sound by hearing aids because sounds are still distorted and verbal communication remains fragmented.

ANSWER: If Gabriella does have sensorineural hearing loss, she most likely will have hearing frequency loss. This means she does hear, but certain frequencies are distorted or lost. A positive aspect of Gabriella's situation is that assessment and intervention will begin very early. Gabriella should be enrolled in early intervention to clarify the articulation of her speech sounds.

Mixed Hearing Impairment

Mixed hearing impairment is caused by a combination of conductive and sensorineural factors that contribute to the hearing deficit. For example, OM may develop in a child with a mild sensorineural hearing loss, thus diminishing further his or her ability to hear and understand the sounds in the environment.

Central Hearing Impairment

Central hearing impairment is caused by damage or malformation within the brain itself or in the nerves that carry auditory information to the auditory portion of the brain. It results from direct damage to this portion of the brain or is secondary to sensory and experiential deprivation. Usually, the child with central hearing loss has difficulty paying attention to sounds and with recognizing, remembering, associating, and comprehending the significance of specific sounds.

This type of impairment is sometimes called *neural impairment* and is considered part of sensorineural hearing impairment, but, because the symptoms and the management are somewhat different, it is considered separately in this chapter. The conductive system and the auditory nerve pathways are intact through the inner ear, but the brain is unable to receive and process or assign meaning to the sounds. This inability prevents the child from understanding the sounds in the environment, including language. It may be a result of trauma, neurovascular changes such as may occur with perinatal asphyxia or intracranial hemorrhage, or a disease process. Usually, the child has difficulty in paying attention to sounds and in recognizing, remembering, and associating sounds with specific events. Only in rare cases do infections such as meningitis cause central deafness.

Assessment

Presenting signs and symptoms obvious to the outsider are usually the same in all types of hearing deficit; however, with testing, the audiologist can identify the type and degree of loss, which facilitates long-range plans for therapy, assistive devices, family teaching, and the child's educational needs. Physical assessment of a child with possible hearing impairment follows the pattern described previously. Frequently, however, deciding whom to assess is a larger question than deciding how to assess hearing.

In 1993, the National Institutes of Health Consensus Development Conference recommended that all infants be screened for hearing loss before being discharged from the hospital. Screening tests often yielded false-positive results, thus causing undue stress for many families. For this reason, the AAP (2007b) set guidelines and standards for the implementation of hearing screening programs. Technology has improved so that testing can be done rapidly and more accurately. At least two tests are in common use for newborn testing: the OAE test and the ABR (Kochlar et al., 2007) (see Tests and Procedures 28-1).

All infants who are at high risk for hearing deficit should be screened regularly at each well-child visit and at least annually by an audiologist. Any infant who has had repeated episodes of ear infection should also be screened annually. During school years, children should be screened at least every 2 years, with children who have had repeated or extended episodes of OM or effusion being screened annually. Children who are old enough to cooperate with the examiner may be given the standard hearing test that measures the child's ability to hear different tones at different volumes (Fig. 28-13).

> **❗ ALERT**   *Screening devices used in schools and clinics provide only a rough estimate of the child's ability to hear. Even after screening, if the family, physician, nurse, or child suggests that a problem exists, referral to an audiologist for testing with more sophisticated equipment is appropriate.*

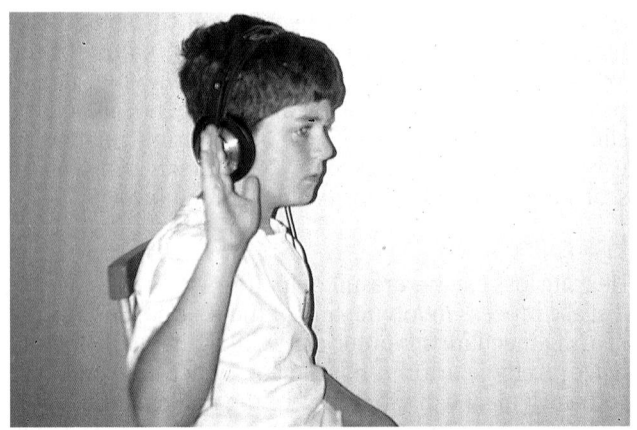

Figure 28-13 Children's hearing should be tested regularly.

When deciding whether to refer the child for more precise assessment, health care providers must consider the implications of not referring the child. For example, a child who frequently misbehaves in the classroom, fails to follow directions at home or at school, or suddenly does less well in school than usual is at risk for psychosocial and emotional effects as well as achievement delays in school. Early identification of hearing deficit can facilitate its treatment and avoid potential psychosocial, emotional, academic, and vocational problems. Waiting until development is lagging behind normal in early childhood or until behavioral effects of hearing deficit have developed in middle childhood is waiting too long.

Assessment should include history, particularly focusing on ear infections and on the previously mentioned behavioral factors as well as ear, nose, and throat examination. Fluid accumulating in the middle ear can substantially decrease hearing in the affected ear. Use of tympanometry in the office or clinic may be helpful in identifying an unrecognized MEE. Also, be alert for psychosocial manifestations of hearing impairment including communication difficulties, academic performance difficulties, and difficulty in social adjustment.

Interdisciplinary Interventions

> **QUESTION:** What is the role of the nurse in caring for Gabriella and her family and families like hers who may be dealing with children with a hearing impairment?

Interventions that are useful in managing hearing loss focus first on accurate diagnosis and second on identification of methods to facilitate normal development through life. Interventions must always involve the family as well as the child. A team approach is essential if the child is to benefit most from the available technology and therapy.

The primary care provider is often the interdisciplinary team leader, treating existing problems and referring the child as necessary for diagnosis or management of problems requiring a specialist. The nurse has a clear supportive role in assisting the family through the diagnostic process. The nurse may also have a role in assisting the family to accept the problem and participate in the treatment program. The audiologist identifies the nature and severity of the problem and makes recommendations to the family concerning its management. If necessary, the audiologist refers the child to a speech–language pathologist who works with the family and the child to provide speech readiness exercises or speech therapy for the child and training for the family. The audiologist makes recommendations to the family for the use of amplification devices. The speech–language pathologist teaches the child and family how to make best use of the amplification devices and monitors the child's progress. When the child is old enough to attend school, the school nurse, speech therapist, and teachers become involved as they provide an educational program for the child. Each person needs to have full information concerning the child's educational and speech therapy program.

Amplification devices (hearing aids) are more useful as assistive devices for children with conductive or mixed hearing deficit than they are for children with sensorineural hearing impairment. For these children, the device helps them to hear sounds in the environment and to learn to respond appropriately. The family and the child need to learn to manage and care for the hearing aid (see Teaching Intervention Plan 28-1).

Children with sensorineural hearing impairment may benefit somewhat from amplification devices; however, nerve damage may prevent amplification from improving the ability to understand the spoken language. They may need to learn to communicate through signing, speechreading, or both.

Cochlear implants are recommended for children with significant hearing loss. These devices are discussed in depth in the "Treatment Modalities" section earlier in the chapter.

caREminder

Children's hearing aids must be kept clear of cerumen. The audiologist will show the child and family how to clean the individual unit the child receives. Remind the child and family to clean it regularly, to avoid dropping it by always working over a folded towel, and to never get the aid wet.

Community Care

Three approaches to communication are taken by educators and families of children with a hearing deficit. Some subscribe to the oral approach, others to the signing approach, and a third encourage the use of both oral and signing methods. Children raised solely with the oral approach do not learn signing but depend on speechreading and amplification to communicate. Persons who subscribe to this approach believe that learning to sign distracts the child from attending to speech and alienates him or her from the hearing world. When communicating with the child who uses the oral approach, face the child when speaking, speak in a normal tone, and enunciate clearly. Keep environmental noise, such as air conditioners or other equipment sounds, to a minimum (Community Care 28-3).

Communication through sign language is a second approach (Fig. 28-14). In the United States, the sign language used most by persons who are deaf is called American Sign Language, a complete language in itself. The syntax is different from English, and persons using it do not voice the words as they communicate. Sign language used by hearing persons to communicate with persons who are deaf is usually a system of converting English into a manual code. Voicing words usually accompanies signs. Finger spelling may also be used. Baby sign language can be used to communicate with preverbal infants and young children and with children in this same age group who have hearing deficits. (Fig. 28-15). Hand gestures can be used to help the child communicate their needs. Working with children who sign is usually facilitated by the children themselves and their families who have developed a variety of coping skills for communicating with the hearing world. If the child is old enough to write, a pencil and paper may facilitate communication. If the child does not yet write, ask the family for information concerning some of the more common signs the child uses to indicate his or her needs and desires. A series of pictures from a magazine can be put together to use as a dictionary and can be very helpful in understanding what the child needs when nursing personnel are not familiar with sign language.

Many families like to ensure their children learn both oral and signing methods of communication. As the child matures, having a grasp of both methodologies provides greater opportunity to be able to communicate with others in a variety of settings and situations and to communicate with those who may not be well versed in one particular method.

caREminder

There is no single best method for communicating with the deaf child. Health care providers must have patience, be willing to learn, and be prepared to attempt any form of communication used by the child and family.

Children with profound hearing loss may have other comorbid chronic conditions or may experience developmental delays in social, gross, and fine motor areas related to their inability to hear. Care of the child with a hearing loss involves assessing all aspects of the child's life and providing medical care and habilitation as needed to ensure the child has the opportunity to meet all developmental norms for his or her age (Hyde et al., 2011).

Deaf children born into hearing families require adaptation of the family. The family must learn to be an advocate for the child until he or she can advocate for himself or herself. The family needs to adopt a philosophy with respect to communication and teach other family members to use that approach.

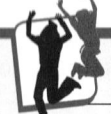

COMMUNITY CARE 28-3

Needs of the Child With Hearing Impairment

Hearing Disability	Sounds First Audible At	What Is Heard Without Amplification	Home and Educational Needs
Normal hearing	0–15 dB	All speech sounds	Prevent auditory damage through trauma, infection, or prolonged exposure to loud sounds.
Slight hearing impairment	16–25 dB	Voiced vowel sounds are heard clearly; may miss unvoiced consonant sounds like "p," "th," and "s." The child may display mild dysfunction. Possible demonstration of fatigue in trying to hear normal speech. Possible failure to hear and understand directions. Possible demonstration of effects of feeling left out (social isolation). Environmental sounds possibly preventing hearing voiced words clearly.	Be sure the child is paying attention. Ask the child to look at the speaker. Speak distinctly. Enunciate clearly. Encourage auditory training. Encourage speech therapy. Provide preferential seating in classroom. Evaluate need for hearing aid. Encourage social inclusion. Turn off environmental noise when possible (e.g., radio, television, air conditioner, and dishwasher). Use language frequently and consistently. Ask the child for input into conversations and discussions.
Mild hearing impairment	26–40 dB	Only louder voiced sounds audible. Seldom hearing enough of social interactions to benefit from social learning. Even with amplification, possibly missing full context of classroom interactions and directions	Anticipate the need for possible sound amplification through use of hearing aid. Use same techniques as noted earlier. Encourage the child to request clarification if words are unclear. Encourage social inclusion. Teach social skills. Teach peers how to interact and include this child. Provide directions in writing and provide summary of classroom interaction to assist in understanding its full content.
Moderate hearing impairment	41–65 dB	Failure to hear most speech sounds in normal conversational tones	Use amplification. If hearing impairment occurred prelingually, anticipate need for speech therapy or use of sign language.
Severe hearing impairment	66–95 dB	No speech sounds heard at normal conversational levels.	Use amplification. Anticipate use of sign language for maximal communication. Child may be a candidate for cochlear implant.
Profound hearing impairment	96+ dB	No speech or other sounds heard, but possible ability to feel vibrations from some sounds	Anticipate possible amplification (child may benefit somewhat). Use sign language for maximal communication. Child may be a candidate for cochlear implant.

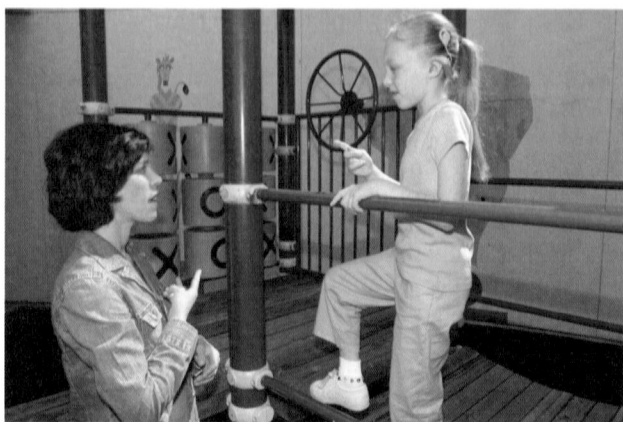

Figure 28-14 Sign language can be used by the child with a hearing impairment or by the child who has difficulty in communicating verbally as a result of his or her physical condition.

 ANSWER: The nurse focuses on Gabriella and her family's response to each aspect of her condition: the diagnostic process, the treatment or interventions, and the long-term consequences on growth and development.

ALTERATIONS IN COMMUNICATION

 QUESTION: Is Gabriella at risk for a communication disorder? Why or why not?

The processes of receiving, sending, and processing information are associated with different physiologic and cognitive abilities. The ability to receive verbal information is usually associated with the ability to see and hear. The ability to comprehend verbal information or information in symbols may be associated with the function of the central auditory centers or processing

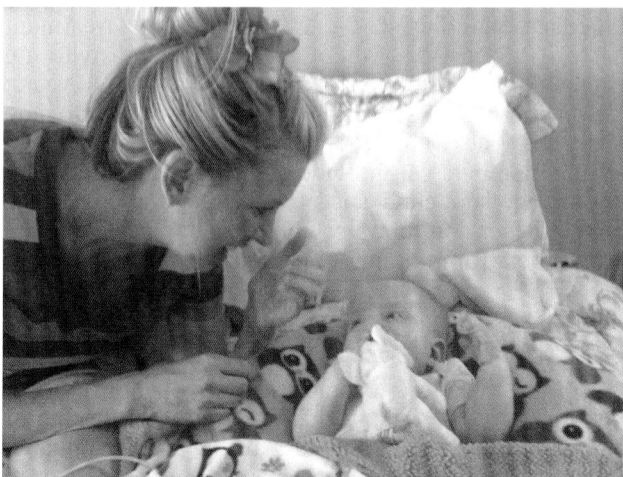

Figure 28-15 Sign language can be taught to infants with hearing loss to enhance communication with family members.

centers of the brain. The ability to send verbal or symbol messages (as in the case of sign language or gestures) is associated with cognitive abilities needed to formulate the message as well as coordination of speech centers and neuromuscular control centers needed to form the words so that others can hear and understand.

Children are said to have a communication disorder when their ability to receive, send, or process concepts or verbal, nonverbal, or graphic symbol systems is impaired. Thus, a child with a communication disorder may have a language, speech, or hearing disorder or some combination of these. Hearing disorders were discussed previously. A **speech disorder** includes impairment in articulation of speech sounds (forming words), fluency (saying words and sentences), or voice (tonal quality), whereas a language disorder includes impairment in comprehension (**receptive language**) or use of language in verbal, written, or symbol form (**expressive language**). A child with a speech disorder may have difficulty saying certain sounds after the time when he or she should have learned those sounds developmentally or may stutter after the time when brief repetitions or pauses are normal. The child with a **language disorder** (abnormality in formulating the content of speech) may be unable to understand what is being said to him or her or may have difficulty responding appropriately—for example, putting words together to express an idea intelligibly. A language disorder is frequently the first indication that a child has autism (Charman, 2004; Charman & Baird, 2003). The autistic child has altered ability in receptive and in expressive language. Children with any of the types of communication disorders must be assessed by the appropriate professional. Therapy is directed toward the specific communication disorder.

Remember that the child's ability to develop socially, both within and outside the family unit, depends largely on his or her ability to communicate. For this reason, early diagnosis is needed to make best use of the critical period for development of language—the first 36 months of life. Also, remember that although it does not always indicate that developmental delay is present, delayed development of speech and language ability is one of the most common indicators of developmental delay in children. Speech disorders, including various dysfluencies as well as delay, are more common and more readily observed than language disorders. Both speech disorders and language disorders occur more often in boys than in girls. Children who are learning two languages at the same time will do so more slowly but will catch up later.

LANGUAGE DISORDERS

Delay in a child's ability to use language as a means of communication may be a normal response to an environment that does not require verbal communication; it may indicate a language disorder; or it may be secondary to some other factor such as hearing impairment, autism, or brain damage. Language delay can also result when the child is developmentally occupied with learning other things such as concepts, motor skills, or some other aspect of life.

Children with a limited need to communicate may include twins who develop a personal communication system between themselves, a younger sibling born into a family with several older children who speak for the younger sibling, or possibly a child whose family members do not encourage independent speech. A child with limited comprehension of word symbols will be delayed in the use of words. Additionally, children with hearing impairments are likely to have language delays.

DISORDERS OF ARTICULATION

Articulation disorders may include atypical production of speech sounds that can interfere with intelligibility of speech. Children may substitute "th" for "s," may be unable to say certain sounds, or may add or omit other speech sounds from words.

Disorders of articulation often accompany structural anomalies such as cleft lip and palate, neuromotor disorders such as cerebral palsy, or hearing impairment. When a structural anomaly is corrected, the child's ability to form speech clearly is improved. For this reason, correction of structural defects is done as early as possible so that the child can learn to speak at normal times. If the structural abnormality cannot be corrected, the speech and language pathologist or the speech therapist may be able to assist the child to learn to form words in a way that improves intelligibility (ASHA, 2008).

For the child with neuromotor disorders, speech problems may be affected by a variety of issues such as poor respiratory control (resulting from weak muscles, laryngeal and soft palate dysfunction), an inability to articulate words (dysarthria; resulting from imprecise oral–facial structures, paralysis, spasticity of the muscles used in speaking), or emotional stress.

Developmental assessment is an essential component of the intervention process (see Chapter 3 for a discussion of developmental assessment tools that can be used by nurses and other health care professionals). In cases when the child has confounding or comorbid conditions that affect speech development, speech and language therapists and habilitation specialists (see Chapter 12) are involved to assist with feeding, drinking, and swallowing problems as well as muscular disabilities that may affect speech and language production. Speech–language therapists will work with the family and teachers to develop a program that focuses on the child's individual difficulties, including those that may affect development of social and motor skills. Speech–language therapists will also seek to provide communication devices to help the child with major communication difficulties.

DISORDERS OF FLUENCY

The most common fluency disorder is stuttering. Stuttering is the repetition of syllables or sounds, with frequent blockages in speech that can manifest as uncomfortable pauses accompanied by unusual mannerisms. It affects 5% of children at some point in their lives (Ashurst & Wasson, 2011).

Stuttering must be differentiated from normal dysfluency that occurs in young children between 2 and 4 years of age. At this age, children are learning the complexities of language structure as well as developing physical control of the oral movements needed to produce speech. Repetition of syllables or sounds at this age is usually part of normal development and does not require intervention. Children who stutter and are grade school aged are often recipients of teasing and bullying, which can have serious effects on their self-confidence and adjustment in the classroom. Teachers need to take appropriate action to prevent teasing and bullying (Nippold, 2011; Nippold & Packman, 2012).

Differentiating the normal dysfluency from the mild stutterer is often difficult. Baker and Blackwell (2004) suggested that children with normal dysfluency stutter using only one to two repetitions of the syllable and in fewer sentences (less than 1 in 10 sentences). Stutterers have more dysfluencies (i.e., more than 1 in every 10 sentences), and individual dysfluencies contain a greater number of repetitions of grammatic units. For example, the child with normal dysfluency may say "li-li-like," whereas the child with early stuttering would include three or more repetitions of the syllable before the word is completed, and the dysfluency would occur every two to three sentences during the conversation.

The causes of true stuttering are largely unknown; however, 15% of stutterers have a first-degree relative who currently stutters or did so in the past. Research has also shown that muscle coordination of the oral structures actually changes during stuttering and that stress, anxiety, and rate of speech also affect the dysfluency (Ashurst & Wasson, 2011).

Persistent dysfluency causes an increase in tension for the child who may then develop secondary characteristics that accompany the dysfluency. The child may blink the eyes, squint, and move the lips and face in particular ways in response to the dysfluency. These secondary characteristics increase the psychological effect of dysfluency and increase the tension the child feels.

The true stutterer needs to be referred to the speech–language pathologist for evaluation and treatment as early as possible. About 74% of children who are true stutterers experience remission within 4 years; however, 26% of stuttering persists beyond that time (Baker & Blackwell, 2004). Health care providers and family members can provide support to the child who stutters by modeling speech patterns that assist the child to feel comfortable while engaging in dialogue with others (Community Care 28-4).

DISORDERS OF THE VOICE

Voice disorders are characterized by sounds, pitch, volume, or voice quality that are abnormal for age or sex. A normal voice should have a pleasing quality and should not distract the listener. A wide variety of etiologies may contribute to voice disorders: voice misuse or abuse; vocal cord nodules, polyps, or paralysis; or

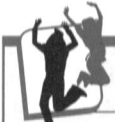

COMMUNITY CARE 28-4

Supporting the Child Who Stutters

- Model slow and relaxed speech (not so slow that it sounds abnormal, but unhurried speech with many pauses). Modeling relaxed speech is better than telling the child to slow down.
- Set aside a few minutes every day to do nothing but listen. Let the child talk about whatever is on his or her mind.
- When the child talks, pause a moment before answering. Doing so helps make talking less hurried and more relaxed.
- Try not to be upset or annoyed when the child stutters. He or she is learning many new skills, thoughts, ideas, concepts, and words all at the same time.

- If the child is frustrated or upset when stuttering happens, reassure him or her. Tell the child, "I know it's hard to talk sometimes, but that's OK. Lots of people get stuck on words sometimes."
- Reduce the number of questions you ask the child. Instead, comment on what the child has said.
- Let the child know you are listening to the content of what they have said rather than how he or she is talking.
- Be aware of how you are interacting with the child. Try to decrease criticism of the child's speech, and decrease your own rapid speech patterns, interruptions, and questions.
- Help family members to learn to take turns talking. Avoid interruptions while the child is talking.

---

gastroesophageal reflux disease (GERD). Both GERD and voice abuse can cause the development of nodules. Children with GERD are likely to present with hoarseness, sensation of a lump in the throat, pain on swallowing, frequent throat clearing, and dry cough. Hoarseness is a common symptom in voice disorders and may be caused by frequent upper respiratory infection or by overuse, such as seen when children scream loudly at sporting events or concerts or perhaps overuse their vocal cords in activities such as singing or acting. Children found to have nodules on the vocal cords should also be evaluated for GERD (Baker & Blackwell, 2004).

Children with voice disorders should be referred to the otolaryngologist or speech–language pathologist if hoarseness persists longer than 2 weeks, tonal quality is distracting (too loud, too soft, too high, or too low), frequent coughing or throat clearing occurs, or noisy breathing occurs at any time of day or night with normal activity or with exercise.

ANSWER: The potential for a visual disorder compounded by the possibility of sensorineural hearing loss does make Gabriella at risk for a communication disorder. She is at risk for a speech disorder, specifically, impairment in articulation of speech sounds. It is unknown whether she may have a language disorder, but learning disabilities, or information-processing disorders, are more prevalent in premature infants than the general population.

THE CHILD WITH MULTIPLE CHALLENGES IN SENSORY FUNCTION

The infant or child who has multiple deficits in sensory function and communication presents the greatest challenge to the family. Before widespread use of the rubella vaccine, congenital rubella was a major contributor to multiple sensory deficits. Since that time, prenatal or postnatal injury and illness have become the major etiologic agents for multiple sensory deficits. These deficits are sometimes accompanied by developmental delay and cognitive impairment.

MULTIPLE DEFICITS

The loss of both hearing and sight may be a result of congenital defect, acquired illness or injury, or a combination of these. In many cases, the combination of hearing and vision losses can affect language acquisition. Additionally, vision and hearing deficits are seldom complete; thus, the child's residual abilities must be identified and used to provide maximal benefit for the child. The desired outcome when working with a child with multiple sensory function challenges is for the child to have the opportunity to develop to his or her maximal potential. This requires the effort of the family and the entire health care team.

Assessment

QUESTION: How is the assessment of an infant born prematurely with potential vision impairment (ROP stage II) and potential sensorineural hearing loss, like Gabriella, different from a child without risk factors?

Assessment of a child with multiple sensory deficits, such as compromised vision and hearing, must include an assessment of the family strengths available to assist them in their care and teaching of the child. Initially, the family must deal with their sense of loss of the normal child they expected or once had. They must then implement coping strategies to facilitate family life and participation in the child's treatment program. Assessment of the child, therefore, must include assessment of parental adaptation to the needs of this infant or child.

Assess the child's impairments early and periodically as the child grows. Also include assessment of residual vision and hearing and of the child's ability to use these senses meaningfully. In addition, assess the child's other senses of touch, taste, and smell.

Cognitive and behavioral assessment provides information concerning the child's ability to explore the environment and learn from other senses. This is an area in which family members can contribute greatly in providing stimulation for the child. Anticipate performing these assessments regularly throughout infancy and childhood to foster optimal developmental progress. For the child in school, school systems commonly are responsible for cognitive and behavioral assessments. However, encourage the family to take an active part in securing these services and in providing information and follow-up.

Reinforce with the families of children with multiple sensory deficits that their observations of the child's abilities and responses are very important in the assessment process. For example, a child who has limited cognitive ability may demonstrate discomfort or pleasure in ways not common to other children. The family's knowledge of how the child demonstrates discomfort may be critical to the assessment of pain and care of this child during hospitalization for illness or while undergoing therapy. Family members' observations should be recorded for the benefit of all health care providers as they care for the child.

ANSWER: Sensory impairment and learning impairment are known problems (morbidities) for premature infants. Gabriella's parents are aware of the possibility of sensory impairment before her discharge from the hospital. The health care team and her parents will make certain that there is early detection and intervention for any problems that do appear. In addition, Gabriella will be monitored and regularly evaluated by a health care team with whom the family has already established a positive and trusting relationship.

Interdisciplinary Interventions

QUESTION: Consider the spectrum that exists for children with multiple disabilities. Gabriella may need to wear glasses to see clearly, and she may have difficulties hearing certain sounds. The other end of the spectrum is total blindness and deafness. How can nurses facilitate and support healthy relationships and healthy growth and development for children with known disabilities?

A child with multiple sensory challenges and his or her family can benefit greatly from the efforts of an interdisciplinary team of specialists. The pediatrician

and developmental pediatrician can monitor the child's growth, development, and general health. The nurse also assists in monitoring growth and development, and in providing support and teaching for the family. Other team members may include any person whose specialty and services the child may need, such as an ophthalmologist, speech-language pathologist, audiologist, social worker, or child life specialist. In addition, particularly when the etiology of the child's condition is unknown, referral to specialists in metabolic disorders and specialists in assessment of genetic disorders may be helpful. The family has a right to know whether the identified deficiencies are part of a genetic or metabolic syndrome that could recur in the family or whether the child's condition is a sporadic event. A young family thinking of having another child certainly needs to know the likelihood of having another child with multiple disabilities.

The nurse often works with the physician and assists in recommending referrals to other team members when consultation or therapy is needed. The nurse may function in a supportive role or as educator for a family with questions about the general care, developmental stimulation, or health of an infant or child. The nurse needs to know when to consult the physician and when to refer the family to the physician or other health care professional.

In the role of educator, the nurse helps the family plan ways to stimulate the child's remaining senses of touch, taste, and smell, and to encourage the child to learn the same things that normal children of the same age are learning. This is done by bringing experiences to the child rather than waiting for the child to reach out and learn. Early in life, an infant learns to differentiate among people. For instance, the visually and hearing impaired child makes differentiations by touch or smell. Encourage the family to reserve a specific and different action to identify each person. Offer suggestions about how to introduce the small child to different textures, and associate the texture with an activity.

Suggest stimulating residual vision, even if only for light and darkness, by placing the child in different light intensities for different activities. Propose stimulating residual hearing by using different types of sounds, such as music or sounds made by automobiles, trains, or drums. Taste and touch can be similarly stimulated and made part of the infant's learning environment.

A social worker may be needed to help the family access assistance from agencies that can help the child develop to his or her maximal potential. The child needs experiences outside the home, and the family members need time to do things without the child. A daycare experience for a portion of each week is an excellent opportunity for the child. The family may require funding assistance from an outside source to make these activities possible.

Daycare play opportunities during early childhood can also assist greatly in school readiness. Play opportunities become learning opportunities in a special class where the teacher is knowledgeable in teaching children with deficits. A child with cognitive deficiency needs much stimulation and one-on-one assistance to learn. The child with vision and hearing impairment needs early development of the sense of touch in preparation for finger spelling. Persons working with disabled children should not expect them to reach out to learn when they can neither see nor hear what is happening around them; rather, bring the learning experience to the child. Other children may need to be encouraged to participate in the teaching and stimulation process. Teach the child's peers and siblings about the challenges and how they can help the child to learn, regardless of whether the child is developmentally delayed or has normal cognitive ability. Chapter 12 provides additional information regarding care and home management of the child with a chronic condition and those requiring habilitation services.

ANSWER: Nurses will be present as a part of the health care team from birth when impairments may first be suspected through the development of IEPs in the school setting. Children are amazingly resilient and adaptive, and experienced nurses have wonderful success stories to share with parents. Nurses help the child and the family to see the character traits and the senses that compensate for impairment. Nurses provide resources, not only organizations but also specific individuals who will have a positive effect on a family. Nurses support families though long-term, caring relationships and by empowering families to advocate for their child.

See thePoint for a summary of Key Concepts.

REFERENCES

Agency for Healthcare Research and Quality. (2011). *Screening for visual impairment in children ages 1 to 5 years.* Retrieved from http://www.uspreventiveservicestaskforce.org/uspstf/uspsvsch.htm

American Academy of Ophthalmology. (2003). *Protective eyewear for young athletes.* Retrieved from http://www.aao.org/about/policy/upload/Protective-Eyewear-for-Young-Athletes.pdf

American Academy of Ophthalmology. (2007). *Vision screening for infants and children.* Available from http://one.aao.org/CE/PracticeGuidelines/ClinicalStatements_Content.aspx?cid = 0ad11e02-6a8b-437e-8d01-f45eb18bc0b6

American Academy of Pediatrics. (2003, reaffirmed 2007a). Policy statement: Eye examination in infants, children, and young adults by pediatricians. *Pediatrics, 111*(4), 902–907.

American Academy of Pediatrics. (2007b). Principles and guidelines for early hearing detection and intervention programs. *Pediatrics, 120*, 898–921.

American Academy of Pediatrics. (2008). Policy statement: Red reflex examination in neonates, infants, and children. *Pediatrics, 122*(6), 1401–1404.

American Academy of Pediatrics. (2004, reaffirmed 2011). Policy statement: Protective eyewear for young athletes. *Pediatrics, 113*(3), 619–622.

American Academy of Pediatrics. (2012). Instrument-based pediatric vision screening policy statement. *Pediatrics, 130*(5), 983–986.

American Academy of Pediatrics Section on Ophthalmology, American Academy of Ophthalmology, American Association for Pediatric Ophthalmology and Strabismus, & American Association of Certified Orthoptists. (2013). Screening examination of premature infants for retinopathy of prematurity. *Pediatrics, 131*(1), 189–195.

American Speech-Language-Hearing Association. (2004). *Guidelines for the audiologic assessment of children from birth to 5 years of age.* Retrieved from http://www.asha.org/policy/GL2004-00002.htm

American Speech-Language-Hearing Association. (2006). *Listen to your buds: Parents.* Retrieved from http://www.listentoyourbuds.org/parents.php

American Speech-Language Hearing Association. (2008). *Roles and responsibilities of speech-language pathologists in early intervention: Guidelines.* Retrieved from http://asha.org/policy/GL2008-00293.htm

American Speech-Language Hearing Association. (2013). *Hearing assistive technology.* Retrieved from http://www.asha.org/public/hearing/treatment/assist_tech.htm

Aponte, E. P., Diehl, N., & Mohney, B. G. (2011). Medical and surgical outcomes in childhood glaucoma: A population based study. *Journal of the American Association for Pediatric Ophthalmology and Strabismus, 15*(3), 263–267.

Ashurst, J. V., & Wasson, M. N. (2011). Developmental and persistent developmental stuttering: An overview for primary care physicians. *The Journal of the American Osteopathic Association, 111*(10), 576–580.

Astle, A. T., McGraw, P. V., & Webb, B. S. (2011). Can human amblyopia be treated in adulthood? *Strabismus, 19*(3), 99–109.

Baker, B. M., & Blackwell, P. B. (2004). Identification and remediation of pediatric fluency and voice disorders. *Journal of Pediatric Health Care, 18*, 87–94.

Benge, S., & Williamson, I. (2011). Hearing impairments part 1: An overview of glue ear. *British Journal of School Nursing, 6*(2), 69–72.

Benoit, D. P. (2012). Inflammation and contact lens wear. *Review of Optometry, 149*(4), 54–59.

Berg, P. H., & Wheeler, D. T. (2009). A review of primary care vision screening. *American Orthoptic Journal, 59*, 98–102.

Briant, M. (2009). *Baby sign language basics: Early communication for hearing babies and toddlers.* San Diego, CA: Hay House.

Burns, C. E., Dunn, A. M., Brady, M. A. et al. (Eds.). (2013). *Pediatric primary care: A handbook for nurse practitioners* (5th ed.). Philadelphia, PA: W. B. Saunders.

Calzada, J. (2003). Traumatic hyphema in children secondary to corporal punishment with a belt. *American Journal of Ophthalmology, 135*(5), 719–720.

Caselli, M. C., Rinaldi, P. Varuzza, C. et al. (2012). Cochlear implant in the second year of life: Lexical and grammatical outcomes. *Journal of Speech, Language, and Hearing Research, 55*(2), 382–394.

Centers for Disease Control and Prevention. (2012). *Hearing loss in children. Data and statistics.* Retrieved from http://www.cdc.gov/ncbddd/hearingloss/data.html

Charman, T. (2004). Matching preschool children with autism spectrum disorders and comparison children for language ability: Methodological challenges. *Journal of Autism and Developmental Disorders, 34*(1), 59–64.

Charman, T., & Baird, G. (2003). Practitioner review: Diagnosis of autism spectrum disorders in 2- and 3-year old children. *Journal of Child Psychology and Psychiatry, 43*, 289–305.

Chatzistefanou, K., & Mills, M. (2000). The role of drug treatment in children with strabismus and amblyopia. *Paediatric Drugs, 2*(2), 91–100.

Chou, R., Dana, T., & Bougatsos, C. (2011). Screening for visual impairment in children 1-5 years: Update for the USPSTF. *Pediatrics, 127*(2), e442–e479.

Chow, L., Wright, K., & Sola, A. (2003). Can changes in clinical practice decrease the incidence of severe retinopathy of prematurity in very low birth weight infants? *Pediatrics, 111*, 339–345.

Chung, J., Des Roches, C., Meunier, J. et al. (2005). Evaluation of noise-induced hearing loss in young people using a Web-based survey technique. *Pediatrics, 115*(4), 861–867.

Ciolino, J. B., Dohlman, C. H., & Kohane, D. S. (2009). Contact lenses for drug delivery. *Seminars in Ophthalmology, 24*(3), 156–160.

D'Allura, T. (2002). Enhancing the social interaction skills of pre-schoolers with visual impairments. *Journal of Visual Impairment & Blindness, 96*(8), 576–584.

De Weger, C., Van Den Brom, H. J. B., & Lindeboom, R. (2010). Termination of amblyopia treatment: When to stop follow-up visits and risk factors for recurrence. *Journal of Ophthalmology & Strabismus, 47*(6), 338–346.

DeRosa, J., & Grundfast, K. (2002). Surgical management of otitis media. *Pediatric Annals, 31*(12), 814–820.

DesJardin, J., Eisenberg, L., & Hodapp, R. (2006). Sound beginnings: Supporting families of young deaf children with cochlear implants. *Infants & Children, 19*, 179–189.

Education for All Handicapped Children Act, Pub. L. No. 94-142, 89 Stat. 773 (1975).

Eng, C. Y., & El-Hawrani, A. S. (2011). The pH of commonly used topical ear drops in the treatment of otitis externa. *Ear, Nose, & Throat Journal, 90*(4), 160–162.

Forbes, B. J. (2001). Management of corneal abrasions and ocular trauma in children. *Pediatric Annals, 30*(8), 465–472.

Forbes, B. J., & Khazaeni, L. M. (2003). Evaluation and management of an infantile esotropia. *Pediatric Case Reviews, 3*(4), 211–214.

Franzco N. S., & Franzco, S. C. (2011). Paediatric glaucoma: Baby steps to improved control. *Clinical & Experimental Ophthalmology, 39*(3), 191–192.

Galati, D., Sini, B., Schmidt, S. et al. (2003). Spontaneous facial expressions in congenitally blind and sighted children aged 8–11. *Journal of Visual Impairment & Blindness, 97*(7), 418–428.

Gifford, R. H., Olund, A. P., & DeJong, M. (2011). Improving speech perception in noise for children with cochlear implants. *Journal of the American Academy of Audiology, 22*(9), 623–632.

Gold, R. S. (2011). Treatment of bacterial conjunctivitis in children. *Pediatric Annals, 40*(2), 95–105.

Gold, R. S., Cheng, K. P., Olitsky, S. E. et al. (2009). Round table: Glasses vs patching in anisometropic amblyopia. *Ocular Surgery News, 27*(18), 44–46.

Grassia, T. (2004). Updated OME guideline helps clear up management misconceptions. *Infectious Diseases in Children, 17*(12), 29, 35.

Granet, D. B., & Khayali, S. (2011). Amblyopia and strabismus. *Pediatric Annals, 40*(2), 89–93.

Craven, S. (2004). Early neurosensory visual development of the fetus and newborn. *Clinics in Perinatology, 31*(2), 199–216.

Harrell, S., & Brandon, D. (2007). Retinopathy of prematurity: The disease process, classifications, screening, treatment, and outcomes. *Neonatal Network, 26*, 371–378.

Hauviller, V., Gamio, S., & Sors, M. V. (2007). Essential esotropia in neurologically impaired pediatric patients: Is botulinum toxin better primary treatment than surgery? *Binocular Vision and Strabismus, 22*(4), 221–226.

Hered, R. W. (2011). Effective vision screening of young children in the pediatric office. *Pediatric Annals, 40*(2), 76–82.

Holmes, J. M., Lazar, E. L, Melia, B. M. et al. (2011). Effect of age on amblyopia treatment in children. *Archives of Ophthalmology, 129*(11), 1451–1457.

Holte, L. (2003). Early childhood hearing loss: A frequently over-looked cause of speech and language delay. *Pediatric Annals, 32*(7), 461–465.

Hyde, M., Punch, R., & Grimbeek, P. (2011). Factors predicting functional outcomes of cochlear implants in children. *Cochlear Implants International: An Interdisciplinary Journal, 12*(2), 94–104.

Ihsen, E., Troester, H., & Brambring, M. (2010). The role of sound in encouraging infants with congenital blindness to reach for objects. *Journal of Visual Impairment & Blindness, 104*(8), 478–488.

International Committee for the Classification of Retinopathy of Prematurity. (2005). The International Classification of Retinopathy of Prematurity revisited. *Archives of Ophthalmology, 123*(7), 991–999.

Isenberg, S. J., Apt, L., & Campeas, D. (2002). Ocular applications of povidone–iodine. *Dermatology, 204*(Suppl. 1), 92–95.

James, D. M., & Stojanovik, V. (2007). Communication skills in blind children: A preliminary investigation. *Child: Care, Health and Development, 33*(1), 4–10.

Jefferies, A. (2010). Retinopathy of prematurity: Recommendations for screening. *Paediatric Child Health, 15*(10), 667–671.

Joint Committee on Infant Hearing. (2007). *Year 2007 position statement: Principles and guidelines for early hearing detection and intervention programs.* Retrieved from http://www.asha.org/docs/pdf/PS2007-00281.pdf

Kading, D. L., & Shen, K. (2012). Seeing the future with contact lenses. *Review of Optometry, 149*(1), 26–31.

Kemper, A. R., & Clark, S. J. (2006). Preschool vision screening in pediatric practices. *Clinical Pediatrics, 45*(3), 263–264.

Kirwan, C., & O'Keefe, M. (2006). Paediatric aphakic glaucoma. *Acta Ophthalmologica Scandinavica, 84*(6), 734–739.

Kochlar, A., Hildebrand, M., & Smith, R. (2007). Clinical aspects of hereditary hearing loss. *Genetics in Medicine, 9*, 393–408.

Levine, L. M. (2004). Pediatric ocular trauma and shaken infant syndrome. *Pediatric Clinics of North America, 50*(1), 137–148.

Lieberthal, A., Carroll, A., Chonmaitree, T. et al. (2013). The diagnosis and management of acute otitis media. *Pediatrics, 131*, e964–e999.

Lim, Z., Rubab, S., Chan, Y. H. et al. (2012). Management and outcomes of cataract in children: The Toronto experience. *Journal of the American Association for Pediatric Ophthalmology and Strabismus, 16*(3), 249–254.

Listman, D. (2004). Paintball injuries in children: More than meets the eye. *Pediatrics, 113*(1), 15–18.

Ma, J. J. (2003). Contact lenses for the treatment of pediatric cataracts. *Ophthalmology, 110*(2), 299–305.

Marter, A., & Agruss, J. (2007). Pacifiers: An update on use and misuse. *Journal for Specialists in Pediatric Nursing, 12*, 278–285.

Mickler, C., Bode, J., Trivedi, R. H. et al. (2011). Pediatric cataract. *Pediatric Annals, 40*(2), 83–87.

Mohan, K., Saroha, V., & Sharma, A. (2004). Successful occlusion therapy in 11- to 15-year-old children. *Journal of Pediatric Ophthalmology and Strabismus, 41*(2), 89–95.

Narayan, S. & Swift, A. (2011). Otitis externa: A clinical review. *British Journal of Hospital medicine, 72*(10), 554–558.

Newman, C. (2011). Literature review: Children and contact lenses. *Journal of Behavioral Optometry, 22*(4), 112–116.

Nippold, M. A. (2011). Stuttering in school age children: A call for treatment research. *Language, Speech, and Hearing in Schools, 42*, 99–101.

Nippold, M. A., & Packman, A. (2012). Managing stuttering beyond the preschool years. *Language, Speech, and Hearing Services in Schools, 43*, 338–343.

Olitsky, S. E., Hug, D., Plummer, L. et al. (2011). Disorders of the eye. In R. M. Kliegman, B. F. Stanton, J. W. St. Geme et al. (Eds.), *Nelson textbook of pediatrics* (19th ed., pp. 2148–2187). Philadelphia, PA: Elsevier/Saunders.

Olitsky, S. E., Schnall, B. Gunton, K. et al. (2009). Management issues in amblyopia treatment. *Journal of Pediatric Ophthalmology and Strabismus, 46*(1), 5–9.

Olussanya, B., & Newton, V. (2007). Global burden of childhood hearing impairment and disease control priorities for developing countries. *Lancet, 369*, 1314–1317.

Patel, D. K., Tajunisah, I., Gilbert, C. et al. (2011). Childhood blindness and severe visual impairment in Malaysia: A nationwide study. *Eye, 25*, 436–442.

Prevent Blindness America. (2012). *Leading cause of blindness in school-age children is sports-related.* Retrieved from http://www.prweb.com/releases/2012/8/prweb9817755.htm

Ramirez-Ortiz, M., Rodriguez-Almaraz, M., Ochoa-DiazLopez, H. et al. (2007). Randomised equivalency trial comparing 2.5% povidone–iodine eye drops and ophthalmic chloramphenicol for preventing neonatal conjunctivitis in a trachoma endemic area in southern Mexico. *British Journal of Ophthalmology, 91*, 1430–1434.

Retnaba, L., Parker, B., Lau, M. et al. (2011). *Baby sign language*. Retrieved from http://www.BabySignLanguage.com

Rinaldi, P., & Caselli, M. C. (2009). Lexical and grammatical abilities in deaf Italian pre-schoolers: The role of duration of formal language experience. *Journal of Deaf Studies & Deaf Education, 14*, 63–75.

Roefs, A. M., Tjiam, A. M., Looman, C. W. et al. (2012). Comfort of wear and material properties of eye patches for amblyopia treatment and the influence on compliance. *Strabismus, 20*(1), 3–10.

Rozhkova, G., Podugolnikova, T., & Vasiljeva, N. (2005). Visual acuity in 5–7 year old children: Individual variability and dependence on observation distance. *Ophthalmic and Physiological Optics, 25*, 66–80.

Rubinstein, J. T. (2002). Paediatric cochlear implantation: Prosthetic hearing and language development. *Lancet, 360*(9331), 483–485.

Saunders, K. (2010). Testing visual acuity of young children: An evidence-based guide for optometrists. *Optometry in Practice, 111*(4), 161–168.

Schmucker, C., Grosselfinger, R., Riemsma, R. et al. (2009). Effectiveness of screening preschool children for amblyopia: A systematic review. *BMC Ophthalmology, 9*(3), 1–12.

Shaikh, N., & Hoberman, A. (2010). Update: Acute otitis media. *Pediatric Annals, 39*(1), 28–33.

Simon, J. W. (2003). Povidone iodine prophylaxis of ophthalmia neonatorum. *British Journal of Ophthalmology, 87*(12), 1437.

Singh, K., Nair, A. B., Kumar, A. et al. (2011). Novel approaches in formulation and drug delivery using contact lenses. *Journal of Basic and Clinical Pharmacy, 22*, 87–101.

Swamy, B., Billson, F., Martin, F. et al. (2007). Secondary glaucoma after paediatric cataract surgery. *British Journal of Ophthalmology, 91*, 1627–1630.

Teoh, D. L., & Reynolds, S. (2003). Diagnosis and management of pediatric conjunctivitis. *Pediatric Emergency Care, 19*(1), 48–55.

Thomas, E., El-Kashlan, H., & Zwolan, T. (2008). Children with cochlear implants who live in monolingual and bilingual homes. *Otology & Neurotology, 29*, 230–234.

Thornton, K., Parrish, F., & Swords, C. (2011). Topical vs systemic treatments for acute otitis media. *Pediatric Nursing, 37*(5), 263–267.

Tomazzoli, L., Renzi, G., & Mansoldo, C. (2003). Eye injuries in childhood: A retrospective investigation of 88 cases from 1988 to 2000. *Journal of Ophthalmology, 13*(8), 710–713.

Tuli, S. Y., Kelly, M., Giordano, B. et al. (2012). Blepharoptosis: Assessment and management. *Journal of Pediatric Health Care, 26*, 149–154.

U.S. Preventive Services Task Force. (2005). Screening for glaucoma. *Annals of Family Medicine, 3*, 171–172.

U.S. Preventive Services Task Force. (2011). Screening for visual impairment in children ages 1 to 5. *Pediatrics, 127*, 340–346.

Vanderpool, P. (2009). Pediatric assessment: Guidelines for general practice nurses. *American Nurse Today, 4*(9), 10–12.

Vanderveen, D., Mansfield, T., & Eichenwald, E. (2006). Lower oxygen saturation alarm limits decrease the severity of retinopathy of prematurity. *Journal of American Association for Pediatric Ophthalmology and Strabismus, 10*, 445–448.

Walline, J., Long, S., & Zadnik, K. (2004). Daily disposable contact lens wear in myopic children. *Optometry and Vision Science, 81*(4), 255–259.

Walton, D. (2007). *Treatment of primary congenital glaucoma*. Retrieved from http://www.childrensglaucoma.com/_structure.php?content = treatment

Wilson, M., Jr., Trivedi, R., Hoxie, J. et al. (2003). Treatment outcomes of congenital monocular cataracts: The effects of surgical timing and patching compliance. *Journal of Pediatric Ophthalmology and Strabismus, 40*(6), 323–329.

Withagen, A., Vervloed, M., Janssen, N. et al. (2010). Tactile functioning in children who are blind: A clinical perspective. *Journal of Visual Impairment & Blindness, 104*(1), 43–54.

Yadava, U. (2010). Primary congenital glaucoma. *Journal of Current Glaucoma Practice, 4*(2), 57–71.

See thePoint for Organizations.

CHAPTER 29

The Child With Mental Health Challenges

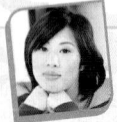

CASE HISTORY

Remember Ashley Tran from Chapters 7 and 24? Ashley has several stressors occurring simultaneously, and she feels as if she just can't deal with it all. A continuing source of conflict is school. Ashley's parents tell her she must bring her grades up. They are watching her do her homework each evening. She still does not understand her precalculus problems. She feels she cannot meet her parents' expectations and she has no control over her inability to get an A.

Another ongoing issue is social freedom. According to her parents, Ashley is not allowed to "date" until she is 18 years old. Her parents discourage her from just hanging out or going out with her friends. She is supposed to focus on her studies and not be distracted by dating. Ashley resents the restrictions her parents have imposed and feels they are unfair compared with the freedoms some of her friends from school have. "It is so hard going back and forth from the Vietnamese world in my parents' home to the American culture of school and work. I feel like the cultures are polar opposites and it is pulling me apart."

The most recent issue for Ashley is that her brother has been diagnosed with osteogenic sarcoma. He had to have surgery and treatments; he may even die. She feels guilty she is not the one with cancer. She is the one who causes the most family conflict. Her brother always does exactly as her parents wish.

At school, she is talking to her history teacher about her brother's diagnosis. Her teacher asks, "How about you, Ashley? How are you doing?" At first she says she is okay, she just hasn't been sleeping much. Then she begins to cry. The words start out slowly. Ashley starts to cry harder and the words spill out. "My brother has cancer in his bone and he may die. I can't do anything right. I never make my parents happy. I am just useless. I wish I would die instead of my brother." Ashley's teacher has been worried about Ashley because of her change in mood, but now she is frightened for Ashley and walks with her to the school nurse.

CHAPTER OBJECTIVES

1 Describe the mental status examination and the techniques used to assess alterations in children's mental health.

2 Explain the purpose and the use of the interdisciplinary categories (from the *Diagnostic and Statistical Manual of Mental Disorders*) used to diagnose, communicate, and treat alterations in children and adolescents' mental health.

3 Identify the criteria that indicate a need to refer children and adolescents to mental health professionals.

4 Describe interventions used to treat altered mental health in children and adolescents.

5 Describe the relation between cultural variables and alterations in mental health.

6 Discuss the influence of growth and development in relation to altered mental health.

7 Describe the behavioral, emotional, physical, and cognitive effects of abuse and neglect.

See thePoint for a list of Key Terms.

It is estimated that 20% of children and adolescents (e.g., ages 10 to 19 years) worldwide struggle with some form of disabling mental illness (Kessler et al., 2011). Most problems these children experience will go unnoticed, and those which are identified will go without treatment for an average of 7 years. More than 12% of adolescents experience depression and are at very high risk for suicide. An increasing number of younger children also have depression. An estimated 28.9% of children experience anxiety symptoms and disorders (Substance Abuse and Mental Health Services Administration, 2010).

The primary care provider is usually the person who first assesses the child or adolescent and discovers emotional or behavioral issues. Because these illnesses have lifelong effects on overall growth and development, family and peer relationships, academic achievement, and future employment and economic potential, identifying and treating them as early as possible is crucial. Regard every contact with a child or adolescent, no matter the reason for the contact, as an opportunity to screen for emotional, behavioral, and mental illness.

This chapter is written from a recovery model viewpoint. As such, language, examples, and so forth, are presented and designed from an optimistic empowerment client-/family-centered collaborative tone. **Recovery model** posits persons experiencing symptoms associated with a mental illness are capable individuals who respond well to treatment when they are empowered and involved in the planning of their care (Warner, 2010). Recovery model suggests a mental health diagnosis is no longer considered a lifelong disability. Empowerment and involvement includes discussions related to disease etiology, medication dosages, education, developing guidelines for care, and working in the field as a peer for others with similar symptoms and challenges. Goals are focused and developed based on the belief clients are capable of every life experience another person without a mental illness would expect to accomplish in life. Treatment goals are also steeped in client-/family-focused empowerment.

Based on recovery model, a diagnosis of mental illness no longer automatically means a person has a permanent disability. Rather, with proper treatment, anyone diagnosed with a mental illness has the potential for recovery. Most persons challenged by mental illnesses such as depression, bipolar disorder, and anxiety disorder work and live within their communities without anyone realizing they have a mental health challenge.

DEVELOPMENTAL AND BIOLOGIC VARIANCES

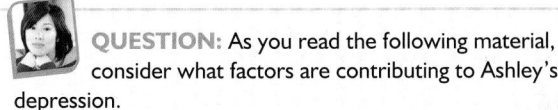

QUESTION: As you read the following material, consider what factors are contributing to Ashley's depression.

Mental health disorders in children and adolescents can originate from a variety of sources. For instance, the normal processes of growth and development may be sources of stress and emotional dysfunction for some children. How the child views the world, the meaning attached to events, and objects in the youngster's world provide important clues to the evolution of thought and behavioral disorders. Certain experiences during childhood, such as family disruption and child maltreatment, are strongly correlated with alterations in mental health.

The neurobiologic functioning of the brain is the foundation of all emotional or behavioral responses, disorders, and mental illness in children. Stress, genetics, environmental factors, or situational factors can affect the chemistry of the brain; an injury, genetic influences, or illness may cause structural changes. The brain controls thoughts, feelings, and behaviors; organizes and integrates incoming stimuli; and determines responses to stimuli, which are carried out through motor potential in other parts of the body. Dysfunction can be caused by a structural or chemical disorder. Brain function may be inherently impaired, as in autism and schizophrenia, or functional patterns may become distorted or impaired as a result of inappropriate stimuli, such as abuse, illness, injury, or as a result of genetic expression or psychosocial disruptions during the developmental processes.

Genetic expression is implicated in mental and behavioral alterations that affect children and adolescents. Studies of twins (monozygotic and fraternal) and family studies suggest that vulnerability for disorders such as schizophrenia, anxiety disorders, and mood disorders is transmitted genetically.

Research studies among adults point to a correlation between physical illness and alterations in mental health. For example, long-term chronic illness can alter mood, leading to depression. Additionally, endocrine function is increasingly believed to be a precipitating factor in mental illness. People with endocrine dysfunction, such as Cushing syndrome and Addison disease (disorders of adrenal function), tend to have a high incidence of depressive disorders (Kessing et al., 2011). Anxiety and depression are highly correlated with hyperthyroidism and hypo- or hyperparathyroidism. Levels of melatonin (a hormone produced in the pineal gland) are strongly correlated with the incidence of seasonal affective disorder; serotonin, norepinephrine, and dopamine also play a role (Levitan, 2007).

Symptoms of altered mental status can be relatively difficult to identify in children and adolescents (Fig. 29-1). Children will often outgrow symptoms associated with altered mental health because of the differences in their rate of emotional and physical growth. Children also tend to regress more readily than adults. Regressive symptoms, such as situational bed-wetting while on vacation or before starting a new school, are not always considered important in diagnosing altered mental status because they represent normal developmental reactions rather than true pathologic findings. If these behaviors persist, however, concern may be warranted.

The nurse must also take the cultural context of the child and the family into account. Based on culture, the family's social and behavioral expectations for the child, discipline, and definitions of abusive behavior may vary. For instance, in some cultures, families encourage a quiet and peaceful nature, so do not automatically

Some theorists believe maladaptive behavior is learned and reinforced by nonresponse toward the behavior by adults in the child's environment.

Children with endocrine dysfunction have a higher incidence of depressive disorders.

Suicide is the third leading cause of death among those aged 15–24 years.

Research studies have suggested that some mental disorders may have been transmitted genetically.

Use of substances interferes with development of problem-solving skills and use of effective coping devices.

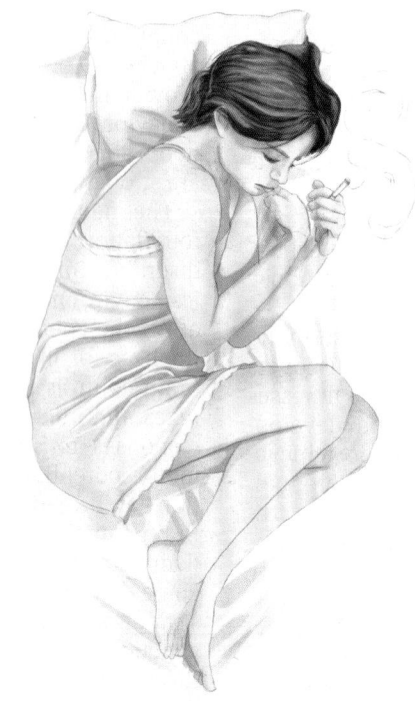

Severe childhood stress is believed to first occur at times when neural pathways are easily affected by experience.

Children regress more quickly than adults. These regressive symptoms may be the result of developmental stresses rather than represent true pathology.

Some theorists believe the child's mental health is influenced by interpersonal life experiences.

Acting-out behaviors may mask depression in children and adolescents.

Assessing family norms and culture is a critical element in evaluating the presence of mental health concerns in children in the family.

The physical manifestations of maturation (i.e., muscular tension, overwhelming fatigue, increased heart rate) can be interpreted by the adolescent as signs of physical illness and lead to undue stress and anxiety.

Figure 29-1 Developmental and biologic variances: mental health.

assess a child who is very quiet and passive in school as having school phobia or a learning disorder. Some culturally based practices can be physically harmful, however, and are inappropriate in the care of children. In these cases, the nurse is challenged to objectively assess as well as openly discuss cultural norms and differences. Too often, harmful practices are attributed to culture, when in reality, the behaviors are not the norm within the group's own culture. Some legal standards of behavior cross cultural lines, especially when distinguishing abusive from nonabusive behavior. In mental health nursing, as in other aspects of child health care, acknowledge the family's culturally based views, resources, and practices and show respect for them. Use culturally acceptable treatment approaches when possible, always clarifying with the individual and family what cultural norms they espouse, and work with the family to develop a shared definition of improvement in the child's behavior and level of functioning. Keep in mind, too, that having a particular cultural heritage does not automatically mean the family or individual will follow all or any of the cultural traditions associated with their group.

ASSESSMENT

View the child holistically, recognizing that many factors influence development and mental well being. Many alterations in mental health have a biologic basis, but also consider the child's interaction with the environment, his or her nutrition, temperament, genetic influences, physical health, and developmental status. Economic factors, living environment, peer interactions, resources available to the family, and the spiritual and cultural perspective of the family and community are important influences on children's mental health.

Thoroughly investigate any concern about emotional or behavioral changes. Early identification of possible mental health issues can assist with prompt diagnosis and treatment (Substance Abuse and Mental Health Services Administration, 2010). Assessment of mental health in a child or adolescent is complex. The nurse must assess a variety of systems and work with the child and the family to identify the behaviors that are acceptable, unacceptable, and most problematic.

FOCUSED HEALTH HISTORY

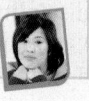 **QUESTION:** Cultural perspectives on mental health vary considerably. Ashley's parents see her depression as a shameful situation and do not wish to be involved in her care. Who would be involved in Ashley's assessment?

ANSWER: Ashley's depression has multiple sources: developmental challenges, cultural and intrafamily conflicts, and perhaps biologic vulnerability.

To assess a child or adolescent, gather information not only from the child or adolescent but also from the people who have meaningful relationships with the patient. Ideally, compile information from the child's teacher, family (including siblings), case worker, and other health care providers. Tools are available to make assessment easier. *Bright Futures in Practice* (Jellinek et al., 2002a), developed by the U.S. Department of Health & Human Services in partnership with the National Center for Education in Maternal and Child Health at Georgetown University, is a tool kit designed to help primary care providers promote mental health in children and adolescents and their families. It includes narrative guidelines, assessment tools, tool descriptions, and interviewing guides. The National Association of Pediatric Nurse Practitioners has developed the KySS (Keep your children/yourself Safe and Secure) Program (Melnyk et al., 2003), a survey for care providers and parents to assess mental health and psychosocial problems.

Information From the Child and Family

Elicit the child or adolescent's perspective on the problem for which he or she is being referred. By listening, the nurse is better able to establish a therapeutic alliance with the child, one of the nurse's primary objectives. Interview the parents separately, then the bring child and parents together to share information. Include the child's siblings, if possible, in the family session. During this session, observe patterns of family functioning and interactions, and interview all family members about their perceptions of the family's strengths, problems, and reasons for referral.

Focus interviews with children or adolescents on their strengths and weaknesses, including the reason for referral and the level of functioning within the school, family, and peer group. Ask questions based on the child's developmental level. Throughout the interview, assess the child's level of comprehension by asking the child to "Tell me in your own words what I mean by the question I just asked you." Never assume the child understands, even when questions are based on developmental level. Changes in mental status can also be accompanied by altered concentration, emotional delays, and a variety of stressors that impact communication (Chart 29-1).

caREminder

A child or adolescent's developmental level and chronologic age can vary widely. Many disorders and injuries in psychiatric patients lead to developmental delays. For example, a 9-year-old with a conduct disorder may need to be assessed at a 4-year-old level developmentally.

Assess the child or adolescent's ability to attend and participate in an interview. Some children and adolescents may be too hyperactive, anxious, depressed, or angry to participate fully in an intake interview. However, give such children the opportunity to do so.

The nurse must quickly assess the child's condition, prioritize family concerns, and gather the most important information.

When interacting with children and adolescents who may be angry and anxious about a referral, ask open-ended questions in a nonjudgmental manner. To decrease the child's anxiety, begin the interview by gathering nonthreatening information.

An important part of the mental health assessment is the mental status examination. When assessing older adolescents and adults, it typically includes questions such as "What year is it?" "Who is the president?" "What city are we in?" However, when assessing the mental status of a child, developmentally appropriate questions such as, "What color crayon is this?" "Do you have a dog?" and if so, "What is your dog's name?" or "Are you in school?" and if so, "What is your teacher's name?" can be used to evaluate cognition. Additionally, mental status examinations focus on behavioral observations made of the child or adolescent's appearance and behavior during 2 to 3 hours of interview. With children and adolescents, the mental status examination also includes information from family members, including siblings, and teachers about how the child interacts with peers.

A mental status examination conducted with a child or adolescent follows guidelines similar to those for the initial interview. Play can be used, especially for children younger than 7 years old. While observing play, a skilled clinician can assess most components of the mental status examination. Components of the mental status examination that cannot be observed can be obtained through nonthreatening verbal questioning. Conduct the mental status examination in a manner that decreases the child or adolescent's anxiety. An ability to establish a rapport with children and adolescents is essential in gathering necessary information without making the child overly anxious.

The nurse will gain most necessary information from older children and adolescents during a relaxed discussion, in an office, while observing their play, or while playing a game with them to engage them in conversation.

Typically, when a child or adolescent is referred for assessment, the entire family is in crisis. Families may feel stressed, embarrassed, exhausted, out of control, and scared. They may also fear the referral will culminate in the child being taken away from them. Often, one or more major events precipitate the referral. Gather information about the child's physical, emotional, behavioral, and cognitive states from birth to present (Focused Health History 29-1).

Discussions can become emotionally charged when professionals question families about their child-rearing practices. Therefore, when seeking information about family dynamics that might be perceived as judgmental, frame the question with, "In order to better understand your child, could you describe . . . " Families, particularly those from diverse cultural groups, tend to feel more comfortable when they are allowed to share their "story" rather than being bombarded with a series of questions. Remember, contact with health care

CHART 29-1   Child and Family Interviews

Child Interview

1. What name do you like to be called?
2. How old are you?
3. What grade are you in at school?
4. What is your favorite subject at school?
5. What subject do you not like?
6. What grades do you usually get in school?
7. Tell me about your teacher.
8. Tell me about why you are here today.
9. How do you get along with the kids in your neighborhood?
10. How do you get along with the kids in your class?
11. What do you usually do when you get mad?
12. What kinds of problems do you have in your family?
13. What things are you good at?
14. If you had three wishes, what would they be?
15. What are your favorite toys?
16. What kinds of things do your parents do that make you mad?
17. What do your parents do to let you know they love you?
18. What are three things that scare you?
19. How are you feeling right now?
20. Have you ever thought of hurting yourself? When? How?
21. Have you ever tried to kill yourself? When? How?
22 Has anyone ever touched you or tried to touch you in your private parts?
23. What is the worst thing that has ever happened to you?
24. Who do you miss the most?
25. What is the best thing that has ever happened to you?
26. Have you ever tried any drugs, alcohol, or cigarettes?
27. How often do you use them?
28. Are you sexually active? (as appropriate) (obtain specific information, e.g., oral sex, intercourse)

Parent/Legal Guardian Interview

1. Tell me about your main reasons for bringing your child here today.
2. What problems did you have during pregnancy?
3. How old was your child when he/she walked and was potty trained?
4. Have you ever wondered if your child was delayed in any area of development? Describe.
5. Describe your child's temperament.
6. What health problems has your child had since birth?
7. What medications does your child take?
8. Who lives in the household with your child?
9. How many hours per week has your child been in daycare?
10. Who cares for your child when you are gone?
11. How does your child get along with other family members?
12. How many friends does your child have?
13. Who does your child seem to get angry at? Why?
14. How old are your child's friends?
15. Does your child play mostly with boys, girls, or both?
16. How does your child get along with other children in school or the neighborhood?
17. In what areas does your child do well in school?
18. In what areas does your child have problems in school?

19. How does your child get along with his or her teachers?
20. Has your child ever been expelled from school?
21. What grades does your child usually get in school?
22. Is your child in a special program at school?
23. Who are your child's teachers and counselor?
24. What major stressors has your child been through?
25. How many homes has your child lived in?
26. Have you ever suspected that your child has been sexually molested?
27. Does your child use sexual language or have inappropriate sexual knowledge?
28. Does your child act or play sexually?
29. Have you ever noticed any trauma, bleeding, discharge, or redness on your child's genitalia?
30. Does your child play with matches or set fires?
31. Does your child ever urinate or defecate in his or her clothing?
32. Does your child ever do so when he or she is angry?
33. Have you ever noticed your child vomiting after meals?
34. Do you think your child has an eating problem? Describe.
35. What does your child do when he or she is angry?
36. How often does your child
    - Hit
    - Kick
    - Bite
    - Spit
    - Pinch
    - Butt head
    - Use profanity
    - Tear up property
    - Hurt animals
    - Throw tantrums
    - Lie
    - Steal
37. Do you suspect your child has used drugs, alcohol, or tobacco products?
38. How much drug and alcohol use is there by other family members in the home?
39. Do you think your child has ever intentionally tried to hurt himself or herself?
40. Has your child ever talked about or attempted suicide?
41. Do you think your child is sexually active?
42. Describe your child's self-esteem.
43. What losses has your child been through?
44. How do you discipline your child?
45. Have you ever noticed your child responding to things that aren't there?
46. Does your child ever say or do things that make no sense to you?
47. What do you enjoy about your child?
48. Which of the issues we have talked about is most problematic to you?
49. What treatment has your child received for these problems and where?
50. Is there anything else we need to know about your child that we have not covered?

FOCUSED HEALTH HISTORY 29-1

The Child With Altered Mental Health

Current history	Presence of delusions, loose associations, hallucinations, illusions, depression, mania, anxiety, phobias, obsessions, compulsions, impulsiveness, suicidal thoughts or behaviors, aggression (physical or sexual) Chronic sore throat or difficulty swallowing (forced oral sex, sexually transmitted infection [STI])
Past medical history	**Prenatal/Neonatal History** Maternal drug or substance use Birth trauma or injury **Previous Health Challenges** History of mental health disorder, suicidal thoughts or attempts, aggressive behaviors, homicidal thoughts, substance use Results of any neuropsychological testing Reports of sexual abuse or other forms of abuse Any allergies that cause child to appear highly distracted and unable to concentrate
Nutritional assessment	Recent weight loss or weight gain, decreased appetite, nausea, vomiting Child's perception of his or her weight Child's eating patterns/habits
Family medical history	Genetic and family history of mental health disorders, including depression, suicide attempts, substance/alcohol use
Social and environmental history	Presence of stressful events at home or school Child's peer group and its usual activities School performance Results of academic achievement tests Nature of relationship with parents/siblings/family Child's perception of how others view him or her
Growth and development	Child's plans for the future Child's perception of himself or herself (self-esteem) Previous exposures to stressful events Coping mechanisms used when encountering stressful events Any variations from achieving significant normal growth and developmental milestones

Note: See Chapter 8 for a comprehensive health history.

providers often occurs when families are under threat or stress from their child's illness. The family may perceive such questions as a challenge or a loss of control and may respond with increased anxiety and by becoming more controlling within the family. Families may become defensive, resentful, and angry. Families are an important resource for learning about the child's history and current behavior and need to be included in assessment, goal setting, planning, and evaluation.

Remember, also, that having a child diagnosed with a mental illness or emotional challenge carries a great deal of stigma. Although mental disorders, just as any illness, have biologic bases, society often finds fault with the individual or family if a child is diagnosed

with a mental disorder. Fear of what others will think or of how the child will be judged often causes families to delay seeking treatment for their children.

Information From Other Sources

Professional communication with involved teachers, counselors, advanced practice registered nurses (APRNs) in psychiatric nursing, social workers, probation officers, psychiatrists, psychologists, psychometrists, and physicians provides a more comprehensive picture of a child or adolescent's history and current level of functioning. Occasionally, the perceptions of family and professionals are vastly different. Typically, written referral summaries from involved psychiatric professionals provide the nurse with most necessary information. Further contact with psychiatric professionals requires parental/legal guardian consent. Communication with psychiatric professionals who are currently involved in the patient's care can provide vital information about family history, previous treatment, any placements outside of the home, and any legal entanglements in which a child may have been involved.

School personnel are knowledgeable about the children and families they serve. Before contacting school personnel, obtain a consent form signed by the child's legal guardian permitting the agency staff and the school to exchange information.

ANSWER: Unlike younger children, Ashley can be the primary historian. Her parents are not currently involved in her assessment and at this time are unwilling to be involved. Ashley is receiving her initial assessment from the school nurse. Ashley's history teacher also met with the school nurse to share her concerns.

FOCUSED PHYSICAL ASSESSMENT

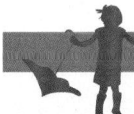 QUESTION: Do you anticipate Ashley's physical assessment will reveal any unusual findings?

Any child or adolescent referred for treatment should receive a thorough physical examination. While conducting the physical assessment of a child with emotional, behavioral, or mental illness problems, pay special attention to several areas of the examination that may indicate that the child's overall physical health is at risk or that there are signs of physical or sexual abuse (Focused Physical Assessment 29-1).

A common dilemma is whether to routinely conduct pelvic examinations on all girls suspected of having a psychiatric disorder. A child or adolescent may not have time to build up enough trust with the nurse to disclose sexual abuse, so a pelvic examination can provide useful information. On the other hand, pelvic examinations conducted on young girls, regardless of whether they have been sexually abused, can be traumatic for them. Chapter 8 provides a detailed summary of the pediatric physical assessment. Note any signs that indicate nutritional deficit (e.g., coarse, thin hair; gum and dental problems; delayed healing) and injury to the body that may have been inflicted by the child or others.

ANSWER: A physical assessment of Ashley by the school nurse reveals no unusual findings. Ashley confides that she is sexually active and the school nurse refers her to the local clinic for a pelvic examination.

DIAGNOSTIC CRITERIA

Evaluation of the child should be performed by a mental health professional. Tools such as lab or blood work and imaging studies are important first steps to detect and rule out potential physical explanations for presenting symptoms. Results from these tests, along with interview data, are beneficial in conjunction with the

---

FOCUSED PHYSICAL ASSESSMENT 29 1
The Child With Altered Mental Health

Assessment Parameter	Alterations/Clinical Significance
General appearance	Flat, sad, or irritable (especially in younger children) affect; depressed, unresponsive, lethargic, hyperactive related to specific mental health alteration; tremors, rigid movements, confusion, sedation may be side effects of medications
Integumentary	Presence of cuts, burns, abrasions, contusions, bruising, or other unusual marks on skin possible indication of self-inflicted mutilation or physical abuse
	Split fingernails; soft, sparse body hair related to malnutrition
	Unusual hair loss patterns may be caused by trichotillomania (an anxiety disorder in which the individual pulls out body hair to decrease anxiety).
Mouth, throat	Eroded dental enamel and reddened and inflamed gums may be caused by frequent, chronic vomiting (bulimia).
	Red, inflamed throat possibly resulting from trauma from self-induced vomiting, STI, forced oral sex
Vision, hearing	Deficits may be caused by physical abuse; may be misdiagnosed as oppositional behavior related to violent children repeatedly destroying their glasses or hearing aids
Genitalia	Bleeding discharge from genitalia, or complaints of burning or itching may result from sexual abuse or STI.

Diagnostic and Statistical Manual of Mental Disorders (*DSM*). The *DSM* provides the mental health professional with research-based criteria based on clinical symptom presentation for diagnosis of mental illness, even in children.

Brain Imaging Techniques

Recent advances in radiography, sound wave, and computer techniques have made imaging of the brain possible. Each technique produces different information, although positron emission tomography (PET) and single photon emission computed tomography produce similar images (Tests and Procedures 29-1). These techniques can be beneficial when used to diagnose some disorders.

Diagnostic and Statistical Manual of Mental Disorders Criteria

The American Psychiatric Association (APA), World Health Organization (WHO), Veterans Administration, and other professional organizations have developed and refined a classification system for mental disorders that is clinically focused. This system is described in the *DSM-5* (APA, 2013), which has become the

TESTS AND PROCEDURES for Evaluating Alterations in Mental Status

Diagnostic Test or Procedure	Purpose	Findings and Indications	Health Care Provider Considerations
Regional cerebral blood flow	Identifies cerebral perfusion abnormalities; the child sniffs radioactive gas; several radiographs delivered as a beam pass through the tissues; radiographs are layered through computer technology	An image of the brain is computed. Different sections of brain can be visualized to demonstrate blood flow through the brain tissue. Hypoperfusion or abnormal cerebral blood flow is seen in many brain disorders (e.g., depression, attention deficit disorder, schizophrenia).	Assess child for any allergic reactions to radioactive gas. Assure the family that the dose of radioactive substance is no greater than that used for diagnostic radiographs.
Magnetic resonance imaging (MRI)	Uses magnetic fields to visualize brain structure; several pulses of energy (sound waves) are used to stimulate atoms within tissue; an image of the brain is computed	Images show structure of the brain, anatomic deviations, and tissue damage.	Ensure that hairpins, eye makeup (with a metallic base), watches, and jewelry are removed and that child's gown does not have a metal snap. Prepare child for sounds of the machine. Child may need a sedative prescribed beforehand to assist him or her in lying quietly during the lengthy procedure.
Positron emission tomography (PET)	Involves very small amount of radioactive water injected into the arm, accumulating rapidly in the brain; positrons are emitted and multiple images are obtained and input into a computer; produces images of the brain and corresponding physiology	PET scans can measure cellular processes, cerebral metabolism, cerebral blood flow, membrane transport synthesis, and receptor binding. They identify specific areas of the brain that are functioning or malfunctioning.	Assist children to lie still during procedure. They may need a sedative administered beforehand to assist them in keeping still. Assure the family that, although procedure is lengthy, the actual radiation exposure is less than during regular radiographs.
Single positron emission computed tomography	The child is given a radioactive substance and multiple radiographs are obtained and input into a computer.	Images of normal and abnormal brain function are produced; these are similar to PET images but are less costly.	Same as for PET

internationally accepted standard for diagnosing mental disorders.

The purpose of the *DSM-5* is to provide clear descriptions of diagnostic categories. Common categories enable clinicians and researchers to diagnose, communicate about, study, and treat mental disorders systematically and consistently. The common language system also facilitates reimbursement. The use of the *DSM* diagnostic system demonstrates a commitment in the field to use research-based data to understand alterations in mental health (APA, 2013).

The *DSM-5* is used by a variety of mental health professionals, including advanced practice psychiatric nurses. However, it is inappropriate for use among professionals without the necessary knowledge base to assign a *DSM-5* diagnosis. Use of the *DSM-5* requires considerable training and experience in mental health. In addition to experience and training, most funding agencies and insurance boards require that mental health professionals who make diagnoses have a master's or doctoral degree.

TREATMENT MODALITIES

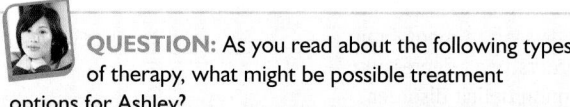

QUESTION: As you read about the following types of therapy, what might be possible treatment options for Ashley?

The needs of the child and the particular mental health alteration determine the treatment plan. Several disciplines are represented on mental health teams including the nurse generalist, APRN, psychiatrist, psychologist, social worker, occupational therapist, recreational therapist, special educator, family, and patient. Role boundaries tend to be blurred; each of the disciplines contributes to planning care and performs some part of the overall therapeutic plan. In many settings, all the disciplines are involved in the daily routine. In other settings, the team may not include all the potential members. Available resources, economic issues, and need play a major role in the number and kinds of members assigned.

COGNITIVE BEHAVIORAL THERAPY

Cognitive behavioral therapy (CBT) is one of the few evidence-based treatment methods, other than medication, available to treat mental health disorders. It requires a health care provider with specialized training, such as an APRN. CBT is based on the assumptions that thoughts mediate behavior, that causes assigned to behavior are related to how one perceives and assigns meaning to an event, and that changing one's patterns of dysfunctional thoughts (cognitions) and responses helps one cope with the event (Hofmann et al., 2010).

Thus, CBT focuses on cognitions, emotional responses, and the resulting behaviors and views them

as inextricably intertwined. Cognitions include the individual's perception of his or her world and the events and objects within it, including the self. Cognitions also include values, beliefs, attitudes, and causal attributions. Understanding the patient's cognitive system is the beginning step in CBT.

The therapeutic process helps the individual reframe perceptions, change ideas about a situation, or view a situation from a different perspective. Next, the patient is helped to see the relations among his or her thoughts and beliefs and his or her emotional responses. Finally, the patient is encouraged to use problem solving to identify alternative solutions or ways of behaving.

A variety of techniques based on CBT have been developed, such as coping skills therapy, assertiveness therapy, problem solving, and self-control therapy. In all CBTs, patients are taught specific skills such as thought stopping, reframing, relaxation skills, and assertive communication skills. Self-rights and the rights of others are emphasized. CBT is recommended for patients with many disorders, including depression, anxiety disorders, behavioral disorders such as conduct and oppositional defiant disorder (ODD), and obsessive–compulsive disorder (OCD).

INDIVIDUAL THERAPY

Individual therapy is an interpersonal process in which the patient and care provider together discover, explore, and resolve the patient's perceived and/or actual stressors, conflicts, behavioral responses, doubts, and anxieties. Individual therapy also requires specialized training. The broad goals of individual therapy include resolving conflicts, restoring developmentally appropriate functioning, improving self-understanding, and reducing symptoms. Individual therapy may be provided in outpatient clinics, community mental health centers, schools, inpatient hospital units, residential settings, or the patient's home. APRNs providing therapy in homes or residential settings often carry a variety of toys, games, craft materials, or books to use in their sessions.

The nature of the therapeutic sessions is determined by the patient's age, developmental status, and preference for interacting with the therapist. Play therapy is often used for young children. Activity therapy (structured activities such as clay modeling, sandtray therapy, drawing, and a variety of games) along with discussion works well with many school-aged children. Talk therapy is preferable for adolescents.

PLAY THERAPY

Play therapy is one form of individual therapy developed to address the needs of children through play. However, it also may be used in the family or group context. It allows children the freedom to experience their concerns and fears in a nonthreatening environment with an accepting and attentive adult. Play therapy is based on the assumption that play is therapeutic.

During therapy, play becomes the medium by which the child explores life problems, developmental issues, and interpersonal conflicts. The child is free to test new assumptions, feelings, and different kinds of behavior. The therapist provides and ensures safety and encourages the child to develop a more positive self-concept and realistic perception of the world. Behaviors that help the child to manage daily stressors are encouraged.

Play therapy is especially useful with children who have limited verbal abilities, those who have experienced trauma, and those who have experienced family separations or disruptions in early life.

GROUP THERAPY

Group therapy is used to prevent and treat childhood and adolescent mental health alterations. Group therapy is conducted in many settings, including schools, residential placements, hospitals, clinics, neighborhood centers, and community mental health centers. An advanced practice psychiatric nurse may be the therapist; alternately, a staff nurse may lead the group.

Group therapy is directed at improving socialization, promoting communication, and facilitating behavioral change. Various group models are used with children and adolescents. Children of preschool age benefit from play groups. Elementary school–aged children relate best in groups that are focused and use some structured activities and discussion. Adolescents often respond well to a variety of group interventions, such as recreational, occupational, communication, and self-esteem building.

Therapeutic effects of group therapy include expressing and sharing feelings, gaining a sense of community, inspiring hope, obtaining information and support, and role modeling. The peer group provides opportunities for youths to meet as equals within their own age group, communicate, understand others' perspectives, get along with others, compare themselves with others, define their social role, and perfect their social skills.

FAMILY THERAPY

Many models of *family therapy* exist, with diverse applications. All models focus on family dynamics. Interventions may be designed to develop family-based coping strategies, such as problem solving or stress management. In some families, the needs may include strengthening parental roles, improving communication, or improving interpersonal relationships.

In families with young children, play therapy is often incorporated to relax expectations and rules that might prevent children from expressing their feelings and needs. In families with adolescents, the focus may be on relaxing or strengthening rules and expectations to allow adolescents the appropriate amount of freedom to achieve their developmental tasks.

One form of nursing intervention that is especially helpful to families with a severely and persistently mentally ill member is family education. Family education, often provided by a staff nurse, provides information to help families understand the neurologic basis of the illness and the factors that may exacerbate or reduce symptoms of illness. Other goals of family education are to validate feelings associated with loss of the mentally healthy child or adolescent, improve problem solving, promote stress management, and access resources. The needs of families may go even further: Individualize care based on these needs.

MILIEU THERAPY

Milieu therapy, environmental structuring and management, is conducted in dynamic, specially structured settings designed to assist in the overall therapeutic process. Milieu therapy usually occurs in inpatient units but may be used in school settings, residential treatment settings, and the home. During milieu therapy, the environment is arranged to promote therapeutic goals, such as diminishing aggressive behavior and developing adaptive and social skills.

The therapeutic environment includes the people, activities, programs, and physical factors involved (Nursing Interventions 29-1). Children placed in therapeutic environments have usually experienced many failures and disruptions in their lives, such as not progressing in school, not meeting normal developmental tasks, or not having playmates. The milieu provides a safe and supportive environment for children and adolescents who are acutely ill, highly aggressive, and at high risk for abuse or self-harm.

Therapeutic milieus incorporate a variety of therapy strategies, such as family therapy, recreational and educational therapy, group therapy, social skills training, and behavioral management, used in conjunction with individual therapy. Active involvement of each child or adolescent is expected and facilitated. Successful milieus require excellent interdisciplinary collaboration.

BEHAVIORAL MANAGEMENT

Using *behavioral management*, the nurse collaborates with team members to develop appropriate goals, expectations, consequences (for failure to meet expectations), and rewards (for positive achievements). A problem-solving approach to behavior management, in which the team works with the child and family to identify needs and strengths, is optimal to help children change behavior and integrate new thoughts about themselves and their world. For change to occur, children need to experience their world and the people in it as caring and not just punitive, an experience that simulates the socialization process that most healthy children have experienced.

Behavioral management is built on a triad of components: empathy (understanding and respecting the child), communication (ask questions, listen, clarify, and give feedback), and discipline, which includes positive rewards (attention, celebration of positive behaviors) and negative consequences (inattention, reprimands, natural consequences, logical consequences, and penalties).

NURSING INTERVENTIONS 29-1

Maintaining a Therapeutic Environment for Inpatient Child/Adolescent Psychiatric Unit

Goal: Maintain Safety of Patients, Families, and Staff.

Interventions

- Ensure environment is safe and risk free.
- Make patient safety rounds every 15 minutes (or more often if needed) to ensure safety of patient.
- Provide structure for unit and maintain unit routine, making adjustments when needed.
- Closely monitor behavior of all patients; anticipate escalation of aggression, anxious behavior, or any threat to safety of patient, staff, or peers.
- Deescalate aggressive or anxious behavior, and take action to maintain safe and secure milieu.
- Role-model appropriate interaction with patients, family members, and other staff members.
- Provide adequate staffing.
- Encourage family involvement and facilitate appropriate interactions.
- Provide structured activities such as training in social skills, communication techniques, coping skills, and stress management.
- Post rules and be sure all patients, family members, and staff know them.
- Provide family and patient with a copy of unit rules and behavioral guidelines.

- Educate and train all staff in strategies to deescalate out-of-control behavior.
- Review with staff any situations that lead to disruptions on the unit.
- Implement strategies to closely monitor any suicidal or at-risk patients.
- Maintain restraint-free environment.
- Provide opportunity for patient and family feedback.

Goal: Implement Evidence-Based Plan for Each Patient.

Interventions

- Develop individual plan for each child with interdisciplinary team, including family and child; assess family and child understanding of treatment plan.
- Implement plan, including social skills training, communication techniques, stress management, coping skills, and symptom management.
- Assess overall health and effects of medication and therapeutic interventions; educate patient and family regarding importance of medication adherence.
- Document outcomes and celebrate successes with child and family.
- Review plan frequently with team, family, and child, and make changes as needed.

COMMUNITY-BASED WRAP-AROUND SERVICES

An effective treatment for children with severe emotional or behavioral disorders is *community-based wrap-around services* (Furman & Jackson, 2002). This treatment keeps the child in his or her home and school by providing the family and school with the professional support needed. This support may be an aide in school, individual and family therapy, medications, occasional respite care for the family, or any combination of supports that give the child, family, and school the assistance they need to avoid hospitalizing the child.

Wrap-around services are less costly than traditional hospitalization and build on the strengths and resources of the family and community. Nurses can help to keep the child in the home environment by connecting the child and family to community resources and providing education to, and serving as an information resource for, teachers. Advanced practice psychiatric nurses may conduct therapy in the school.

PSYCHOPHARMACOLOGY

A variety of medications are currently used to treat childhood and adolescent mental and behavioral disorders (Table 29-1), often **off label** (in a manner not recommended on the product labeling; for example, antipsychotics may be given to calm a child with attention-deficit/hyperactivity disorder [ADHD] who is taking Ritalin).

Medications are typically started at low dosages and titrated up to an effective level. A combination of medications may be more effective than one individual medication. Effectiveness of medications also changes over time, possibly because of the physical growth of the child and chemical changes in the body. Frequent changes in dosages and medications therefore may be needed to optimize therapeutic effect. Medications are usually used in combination with other forms of therapy.

The nurse's role in administering medications and observing and reporting responses, including therapeutic and adverse effects, is critical. Nurses often serve a

TABLE 29-1   Common Psychotropic Medications Used in Child and Adolescent Psychiatry

Classification and Examples	Disorder	Side Effects
Stimulants		
Methylphenidate (Ritalin), dextroamphetamine (Dexedrine), pemoline, amphetamine (Adderall)	ADHD, possibly depression	Insomnia, decreased appetite, weight loss, headache, tics
*Antidepressants**		
Tricyclics: imipramine, nortriptyline	ADHD, depression, tic and anxiety disorders	Anticholinergic effects (dry mouth, constipation, blurred vision), weight loss
Monoamine oxidase inhibitors (MAOIs): amitriptyline (Elavil), dibenzepin (Noveril)	As above	Dietary restrictions required, weight gain, drowsiness, insomnia, hypotension
Selective serotonin reuptake inhibitors (SSRIs): fluoxetine (Prozac), sertraline (Zoloft), paroxetine (Paxil), citalopram (Celexa), mirtazapine (Remeron), trazodone (Desyrel)	Depression, OCD, anxiety	Irritability, insomnia, gastrointestinal distress, headaches, nausea, increased blood pressure
Antimanic Agents		
Lithium	Bipolar disorder, depression, hyperaggression	Polyuria, polydipsia, tremor, nausea, diarrhea, weight gain, drowsiness; lithium requires close monitoring
Anticonvulsant Medications		
Carbamazepine (Tegretol), valproic acid (Depacon, Depakene, Divalproex , and Depakote [divalproex]), lamotrigine	Seizure, bipolar disorder, occasionally refractory depression, conduct disorder	Bone marrow suppression, dizziness, drowsiness, sedation, nausea
Antianxiety Agents		
Buspirone	Anxiety disorder, rage disorder; adjunct in mania, psychosis, depression, Tourette syndrome	Drowsiness, disinhibition, agitation, confusion, depression
Noradrenergic Agents		
Clonidine	Tourette syndrome, ADHD, aggression/self-abuse, agitation; alternative to stimulants	Sedation, hypotension, dry mouth, confusion, depression, constipation, urinary retention, rebound hypertension
Antipsychotic Agents		
Phenothiazines: thioridazine (Mellaril), chlorpromazine (Thorazine), haloperidol (Haldol)	Psychosis, mania, aggression; self-injurious, explosive, and violent and destructive behavior	Anticholinergic effects, extrapyramidal effects (dyskinesia, dystonia), drowsiness
Atypical Antipsychotics		
Risperidone, clozapine, olanzapine (Zyprexa), quetiapine (Seroquel)	Schizophrenia, pervasive developmental disorder, bipolar disorder	Granulocytopenia, seizures, agitation, headache, nausea, sedation, weight gain, dyslipidemia, parkinsonism, dizziness, dry mouth, constipation

*The U.S. Food and Drug Administration requires warning labels about the increased risk of suicide with antidepressant agents.

vital role in helping families to understand the need for the medication, the goals and expected outcomes, and how and when to administer medication. When medication does not appear to produce the desired results, nurses can help uncover patient and family factors that may be preventing success.

Families and children have a right to information about the medication, and their consent and cooperation must be elicited. Nurses serve an important function in school settings in monitoring medication administration and possible side effects. Nurses also teach teachers, helping them understand the use, potential benefit, and side effects of prescribed medications. The nurse may act as liaison between school personnel, family, and treatment team members.

ANSWER: The school nurse refers Ashley to an APRN who determines that CBT is an appropriate intervention and that a support group for adolescents may also benefit Ashley. Family therapy may also be beneficial, but Ashley's parents are not willing to come to counseling with her at this time. Medication may be an appropriate intervention in conjunction with another form of therapy for Ashley. The APRN prescribes paroxetine (Paxil), an SSRI. Education regarding medication is critical. The importance of taking the medication daily is stressed. It may take several days or even weeks for Ashley to feel any different. It is also very important that she not discontinue the medication abruptly. Teenage suicides have occurred when adolescents receiving SSRIs stop taking the medication. Although these suicides have received a great deal of publicity, they have not changed the value of pharmacotherapy but rather have emphasized the need for education, monitoring, and interpersonal therapy.

NURSING PLAN OF CARE

The nurse, as educator for both families and children, plays a critical role in helping the family make informed decisions in the best interest of the child. Refer children who are identified with a severe emotional or behavioral problem or mental illness to a mental health care provider. The APRN has an important role in assessing and treating children and adolescents with mental health problems and their families. He or she can perform mental and physical examinations; prescribe medications; and conduct individual, group, and family therapy.

 QUESTION: What nursing diagnosis would you develop for Ashley?

A variety of nursing diagnoses may be selected to address the needs of the child with an alteration in mental health status (Nursing Plan of Care 29-1). Altered thought patterns and behavior affect the child's self-esteem, ability to cope, and ability to interact appropriately with others. Another aspect to consider is the effect of mental status on the child's developmental and physical status. Stress reduction activities may help the child to cope adaptively with issues and challenges in his or her life (Nursing Interventions 29-2).

Changes and stressors within the family may contribute to the child's mental health condition or may be an outcome of the child's altered thought processes and inappropriate behaviors. Therefore, when developing a plan for the child's care, include the family as an integral part of both the discussion and planning the strategies to assist the child in meeting emotional, cognitive, and physical needs.

ANSWER: There are many diagnoses that would be applicable. One example is risk for situational low self-esteem related to actual or perceived problematic relationships and stress with family members or peers.

ALTERATIONS IN CHILDREN'S MENTAL HEALTH

Alterations in children's mental health vary widely in scope and severity, from separation anxiety and sleep disturbances to altered thoughts and perceptions, which could led to a diagnosis of schizophrenia later in life (note: Although signs and symptoms of schizophrenia may be present in childhood, the formal diagnosis is typically delayed until later to make sure symptoms are not associated with other issues such as developmental lags or social immaturity and to avoid early labeling and stigma in childhood).

ANXIETY DISORDERS

Anxiety is a common phenomenon of childhood and later life. Anxiety is often also a common occurrence in most mental health disorders. Children in particular experience multiple fears as they develop and as they encounter new experiences (see Chapters 4 to 7 for a discussion of typical fears in children). All individuals experience anxiety in response to a variety of life situations. Many are provoked to high anxiety at various times throughout childhood and later life. However, anxiety disorders are much more than stressful life experiences.

Approximately 20% of children aged 8 to 17 years have scores above the clinical cutoff on brief anxiety screening (Keeley & Storch, 2009). Anxiety is manifested in disorders such as generalized anxiety disorder, panic disorder, separation anxiety disorder, selective mutism, social phobia, and acute stress disorder.

Various factors are associated with, and may cause, anxiety disorders. Insufficient coping strategies, resources, or social support may contribute; some persons may be at higher risk because of genetic phenomena, disease states, neurotransmitter deregulation, or structural deficits in the brain. The amygdala is implicated in anxiety disorders, as are dysfunction of norepinephrine, dopamine, serotonin, and gamma-aminobutyric acid systems and abnormal chemoreceptor reactivity (Keeley & Storch, 2009). As the system becomes overwhelmed, patterns of deregulation may become established in the brain, resulting in continued manifestation of disabling anxiety.

Anxiety in children often manifests in somatic complaints such as feeling unsteady and dizzy, stomachaches, nausea, diarrhea, and sleeping difficulties (Keeley & Storch, 2009). Frequent somatic complaints should arouse some suspicion of an anxiety disorder or other mental health issue. Anxiety disorders have common characteristics as well as specific symptoms, so differential diagnoses can be challenging. Most of the disorders are treated similarly with CBT. Some respond to medications; others do not. Educating the child and family about the disorder, the implications for growth and development, and the importance of the treatment plan is always a part of the nursing role.

PANIC DISORDER

When a child is observed having a panic attack in a school or health care setting, implement immediate interventions (Nursing Interventions 29-3), then refer

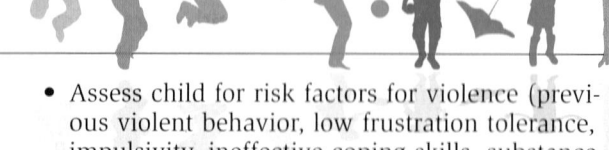

NURSING PLAN OF CARE 29-1:

The Child With Altered Mental Health

Nursing Diagnosis: Acute confusion* related to effects of mental health alteration

Interventions/Rationale
- Obtain medical history.
  Helps identify conditions that may be causative factors for mental status changes.
- Obtain baseline assessment of mental status.
  Provides baseline data to evaluate changes in child's status and facilitates early detection of changes.
- Adapt communication style to the child's needs and level. Speak slowly and calmly, avoid sudden movements, use short phrases, and allow child time to process information. Use pictures or props (e.g., a doll, puppet). Ask for clarification of child's statements if indicated.
  Simplifying communication may help the child process information and helps reduce stimulation. Clarification may help link seemingly incongruent statements to logical events.
- Interview child in familiar environment and reduce environmental stimuli (e.g., reduce noise, avoid too-bright lights, and limit number of persons in area).
  Excessive stimuli may overload the child and promote disorganization.
- Orient the child (e.g., call by name; introduce yourself with each contact; mention date, time, and place). Maintain routine and consistent staff if possible.
  Reinforces reality. Predictable routines promote security.

Expected Outcomes
- Child will remain oriented to person, place, and time.
- Child will communicate in a lucid manner.
- Child and family will identify internal and external factors that trigger or contribute to delusional episodes.
- Child will identify and perform activities that decrease delusions.
- Child will adhere to medication regimen to help modify psychological causes.

Nursing Diagnosis: Risk for self- or other-directed violence related to antisocial and aggressive character, excitement, or self-destructive behaviors

Interventions/Rationale
- Inform child and family of expectations for behavior and consequences for failure to meet the expectations.
  Provides structure for the child and makes child responsible for own actions.

- Assess child for risk factors for violence (previous violent behavior, low frustration tolerance, impulsivity, ineffective coping skills, substance abuse, bipolar disorder, conduct disorder).
  Knowing risk factors may enable structuring of the environment to avoid inappropriate behavior.
- Monitor the environment for situations that could precipitate violence; intervene to deescalate the situation.
  Early intervention may prevent violent behavior or reduce its intensity.
- Observe the child for feelings of anger (verbalization; facial expression of anger such as clenched jaw, eyebrows drawn together, increased restlessness, rigid posture) and acknowledge these feelings.
  Early recognition of potential escalation enables early intervention. The child may be unable to identify angry feelings; identifying these feelings may help the child to implement calming measures.
- Intervene to deescalate. Keep calm; speak in a low, even voice; minimize external stimuli; help the child implement self-calming and coping measures; assist the child to redirect energy into physical activity.
  Early intervention may prevent violent behavior or reduce its intensity. Physical activity may deplete excess energy.
- Remove others from the vicinity of a violent child.
  Minimizes risk to others.

Expected Outcomes
- Child will not harm self or others.
- Child will, depending on age, discuss feelings or use play to work through feelings and precipitating factors that led to destructive and/or violent acts.
- Child will learn new behavioral responses to curtail outbursts of rage, self-destructive behavior, or violence.
- Child will use positive coping strategies when he or she feels oncoming frustrations.
- Child and family will identify resources for crisis prevention and management.

Nursing Diagnosis: Impaired verbal communication related to altered mental status or neurologic impairment

Interventions/Rationale
- Keep statements simple; use short sentences and concrete terms. Convey that you have time to listen to the child and allow time for the child to respond. Use communication aids if indicated (letter/picture board, erasable slate).
  By maintaining simplified speech patterns, verbalizations are easier to understand, and communication patterns will be more effective.

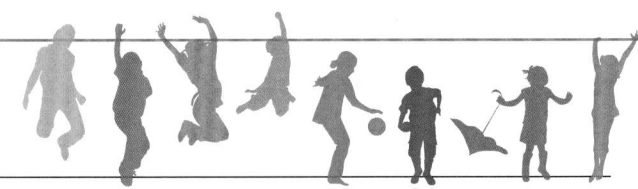

NURSING PLAN OF CARE 29-1:

The Child With Altered Mental Health *(Continued)*

Allowing the child time may reduce anxiety and encourage communication.

- Encourage the family to provide child with familiar objects (toys, pictures, books, and clothing) that evoke a positive response from child.

  Objects that are considered "friendly" will enable staff to attempt to engage child in a conversation that is nonthreatening and will enhance trust building.

- Do not prod the child to engage in dialogue. After several attempts, gently disengage and offer to return at a later time.

  If the child is not ready to communicate verbally, all attempts to force him or her to do so will lead to further alienation.

Expected Outcome

- Child will begin to demonstrate an ability to communicate feelings and needs, as evidenced by clear, understandable, and socially appropriate verbal and nonverbal behaviors.

Nursing Diagnosis: Ineffective coping related to sensory overload, lack of previously learned positive coping skills

Interventions/Rationale

- Discuss past and present coping mechanisms. Assist child to identify effective and ineffective coping mechanisms.

  Identification of coping mechanisms as effective or ineffective can provide guidance for selection of appropriate methods.

- Instruct the child in use of relaxation techniques (e.g., deep breathing, meditation, journaling). Role-play adaptive coping skills; support and reinforce use of these skills.

  Practicing the methods may help the child to use them when faced with a stressful situation.

Expected Outcomes

- Child will understand the relationship between emotional state and behavior.
- Child will accept responsibility for his or her behavior.
- Child will identify effective and ineffective coping techniques.
- Child will use available support system (friends, family, and therapist) to develop and maintain effective coping skills.

Nursing Diagnosis: Risk for situational low self-esteem related to actual or perceived problematic relationships with family members or peers

Interventions/Rationale

- Note manner of dress and state of hygiene and grooming (e.g., disheveled, unkempt appearance).

  Appearance may reflect self-perception.

- Actively listen while engaging child in dialogue or play regarding feelings about self and personal appearance (e.g., likes/dislikes, strengths/weaknesses).

  May reveal self-perceptions and allow discussion of reality versus perception. A child with altered mental status may have a distorted view of self in relation to the physical/social/emotional environment. Comparing self with a distorted environment can alter sense of self and subsequently decrease self-esteem. Dialogue enables discussion of methods to address perceived weaknesses and to focus on strengths; provides opportunity to educate the child regarding hormonal implications during puberty.

- Explore child's feelings about changes in body with onset of puberty.

  Pubertal changes can be stressful and require changes in self-perception.

- Encourage and reinforce positive self-statements; discuss ways to highlight good feelings about self (e.g., improving grooming, hygiene). Reinforce any attempts toward improvement in hygiene/grooming. Support socialization and conflict resolution skills. Introduce concept of accepting differences to promote individuality.

  Reducing negative thoughts can help increase self-esteem. Socialization skills may increase social support, and ability to resolve conflicts may increase sense of belonging, both of which may provide positive validation.

Expected Outcomes

- Child and family will describe areas of conflict.
- Child will openly express feelings toward family members and peers.
- Child and family will select measures to reinforce the child's positive qualities.
- Child will be able to describe his or her own positive qualities.

Nursing Diagnosis: Impaired social interaction related to effects of child's mental status or aberrant, antisocial behaviors

Interventions/Rationale

- Convey that you have time to spend with the child. Actively listen and observe verbal and nonverbal communication; verify communication.

  Can convey caring and increase child's trust and comfort with you.

- Model and role-play appropriate social interactions.

  Observing appropriate responses and productive interactions may help the child to develop a repertoire of positive responses.

Expected Outcomes
- Child and family will identify causes of problems in social interactions.
- Child will exhibit interactions and communication skills that enhance social interactions.
- Child will demonstrate behaviors that are socially acceptable.
- Child will report feeling less isolated as social interactions improve.

Nursing Diagnosis: Disturbed sleep pattern related to anxiety, mental status, or effects of medications

Interventions/Rationale
- Encourage consistent routines for sleep preparation.
  When routines are expected, child may find it easier to relax.
- Allow the child time for quiet transition by playing music or reading soothing materials.
  By decreasing stimuli, sleep will be induced naturally.
- Offer the child a massage.
  Decreasing muscle activity through therapeutic touch modalities often induces relaxation and sleep.

Expected Outcomes
- Child's sleep patterns will be adequate for rest.
- Family's sleep patterns will be adequate for rest.

Nursing Diagnosis: Interrupted family processes related to changes in family relationships, roles, and responsibilities

Interventions/Rationale
- Assess family's interaction patterns, family roles, stress levels, and coping mechanisms.
  Provides baseline data to develop plan of care, building on family strengths.

- Actively listen to family's perception of family functioning and concerns; acknowledge feelings.
  Feeling of "being heard" may help decrease anxiety and initiate problem-solving and coping behaviors.
- Assist the family to identify strengths and methods to develop effective interactions, improve ability to meet family members' needs, and facilitate individual growth. Videotape family interactions (preferably in the home), assist family to identify positive and negative interactions, and role-play to build on positive interaction patterns.
  Building on strengths helps the family feel hope that they can achieve their goals. Role-playing helps develop adaptive functioning patterns.

Expected Outcomes
- Family members will discuss changes in family dynamics and identify methods to deal with change in a therapeutic manner.
- Family members will seek appropriate resource services as needed to optimize family processes.
- Family members will understand the cause of the child's condition and available treatment modalities.
- Family members will support the child, discipline the child in a therapeutic manner, and remain involved in the child's treatment.

---

*Agitation is more commonly seen in children, confusion is more evident in adults

---

the child to his or her mental health care provider or primary health care provider.

caREminder
The most immediate goal of the nurse in panic and phobic disorders is to reduce anxiety to a manageable level and to reduce the child's physical discomfort.

In addition, encourage the child to master relaxation techniques and to avoid catastrophic thinking. Continued attacks suggest a need for antianxiety medication or behavior or cognitive therapy with a skilled mental health professional.

SEPARATION ANXIETY

The prevalence of separation anxiety disorder is cited as 7.6% in children aged 13 to 18 years (Merikangas et al., 2010), but more children have subclinical disturbances that are not diagnosed. Separation anxiety disorder is characterized by excessive anxiety when the child is separated from the home or the parents (primary attachment figure). School refusal or phobia (as it is commonly known) is a prime example of separation anxiety disorder.

Assessment

Factors that place children at risk for separation anxiety disorder are death of a parent or sibling, divorce, relocation, and chronic illness. Thus, a family history and assessment of current functioning are important.

NURSING INTERVENTIONS 29-2

Stress Reduction Activities

Stress is a generalized, nonspecific response of the body to any demand, change, or perceived threat and is unavoidable. Stressors are the circumstances or events that elicit this response and may be real or anticipated, positive or negative. Distress is damaging or unpleasant stress. Stress reduction techniques are usually most effective for children older than 6 years of age.

Techniques	Nursing Interventions
Develop effective coping mechanisms.	Role-play various ways of dealing with stressors. Discuss which methods would be the easiest and most useful for child and families.
Begin daily exercise program.	Suggest methods to reduce stress through exercise (e.g., walking, running, dancing, swimming, participating in sports, body movement exercises, yoga). Assist child in developing a plan of regular activity. Evaluate extracurricular school activities that would help the child deal with stressors. Refer to school and community gyms, health clubs, Young Men's Christian Association (YMCA), boys' and girls' clubs. Advise family to consult with child's primary care provider about contraindications to exercise program.
Develop alternate ways to relax.	Identify activities that the child enjoys (e.g., drawing, pottery, carpentry, writing, music, photography, and reading); assess for relaxing activities (e.g., watching the sunset, taking a bubble bath).
Practice relaxation techniques.	Guide child through a relaxation exercise to experience its usefulness. Begin relaxation with deep breathing. Use guided imagery to induce relaxation (e.g., "Take another deep breath and let all the tension release. With each breath you become more relaxed. Now imagine yourself in a peaceful, quiet setting [garden, beach, and so forth] . . . "). Refer child to audio media, books, and classes on learning and practicing relaxation techniques.
Practice diaphragmatic breathing and periodic deep breathing.	Steps for using diaphragmatic breathing with child: • Sit or recline in a comfortable position with legs uncrossed. • Place one hand on chest and other hand on diaphragm, approximately 2 in. below bottom center of breastbone. • Inhale so diaphragm expands and hand covering diaphragm moves out while other hand remains almost still. • As you exhale, diaphragm relaxes, and hand covering it moves inward.
Make positive affirmations.	Teach child to • Write out affirmation statements and place them in a visible area (e.g., mirror, steering wheel, refrigerator, desk) • Repeat the statements several times daily • Be specific, positive, and brief (e.g., "I am relaxed," not "I am not tense") • Use the present tense—"I am," not "I will" (e.g., "I am learning to express my feelings." "I am expressing anger in a positive way." "I am lovable.")
Improve self-care.	Discuss personal habits that contribute to distress: • Poor nutrition • Neglecting early warning signs of tension • Nonassertiveness • Drinking, smoking, substance abuse • Sexual activity (promiscuity resulting from peer pressure, lack of birth control)

Techniques	Nursing Interventions
Demonstrate positive ways to express and become more aware of feelings.	Discuss importance of setting priorities, taking one thing at a time.
Increase organizational skills.	Use strategies such as pocket folders or color-coded labels on shelves or boxes. Use calendar or list of things to do. Use reward system with stickers or small incentives.
Balance school and recreation.	Teach importance of • Regular study schedule so as not to become overwhelmed with all the work at one time and to be able to see progress • Learning to take relaxation breaks

Conduct a physical examination as well to determine any contributing physical problems.

Alcoholism, depression, agoraphobia, and panic disorder are relatively common among parents of children with separation anxiety disorder. Other family stressors (loss of home, emergency hospitalization, community violence, death in the family) should also be assessed. Observe the parent–child interaction; assess parental discipline, nurturance, dependence on the child, and encouragement of age-appropriate independence.

Findings often include problems associated with school. If the child has an academic deficit, is shy, or is awkward, the child may be teased by his or her peers. Family disruptions, chaos, or marital discord may compound the anxiety aroused by any problems experienced in school. In addition, extended absence from school may cause a child to fear embarrassment and ridicule by peers or punishment from teachers or school officials.

Nursing Diagnoses and Outcomes

In addition to the nursing diagnoses listed in Nursing Plan of Care 29-1 applicable to the child with separation anxiety or school phobia, the following diagnosis could be used to guide care:

Nursing Diagnosis: Anxiety related to separation from family or caregiver

Outcomes:
• Child will attend school, experiencing no anxiety related to separation or expectations at school.
• Child will stay overnight at a peer's house, experiencing minimal anxiety.

Interdisciplinary Interventions

Children with school refusal are best served when referred to a mental health professional skilled in treating anxiety disorders. The best approach is to involve the child and the family. The therapist (psychiatric APRN, psychiatrist, psychologist, or social worker) must act as a liaison between the school and family.

Cognitive–behavioral approaches produce the best results (Keeley & Storch, 2009). The therapist develops a trusting therapeutic relationship with the child, who is encouraged to think of anxiety as a manageable life situation that can be overcome in time by building a toolkit of skills during each therapy session. Additional step in the therapy process includes desensitization of the feared object (school or leaving home). Pictures of thermometers are often given to the child to indicate the amount of fear experienced and to evaluate progress.

Children may be hospitalized to help move them along and support a family when challenges prevent

---

NURSING INTERVENTIONS 29-3

Child Experiencing a Panic Attack

• Stay with the child or adolescent.
• Remain calm.
• Speak slowly, firmly, and reassuringly.
• Ask other persons to move away or move the child to a quiet, comfortable area.

• Encourage relaxation, focusing on a specific object or soothing thought.
• Administer medication if ordered.

success. Families are referred and encouraged to participate in community mental health programs as needed when they experience their own personal challenges such as marital discord, dependence on their child, depression, or substance abuse. By including all members of the family in an intervention, the likelihood of a successful outcome is greater.

Community Care

Nurses working in schools may be the first to recognize the problem of school refusal. Children are usually sent to the school nurse for somatic complaints. Frequent visits for minor complaints, especially if the child insists on going home, should alert the nurse to the possibility of a child and family in need and an opportunity to follow up and avoid the potential for school refusal.

The school or community health nurse may also be responsible for visiting children who have been absent for several days, and when illness is not verified, school refusal should be suspected (Clinical Judgment 29-1).

Nurses working in schools can intervene early by recognizing the warning signs and helping to prevent the anxious child from developing school refusal. Careful early assessment and identification of the child's challenges and fears can result in academic success or appropriate referral when warranted. The nurse may provide stress management techniques and support to the child and family returning to school.

Stress caused by a variety of family dynamics such as chaotic family structure/communication, parenting styles, or altered family relationships may be discovered. The nurse may also inform the family of the child's anxiety and refer them to a mental health clinic,

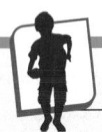

CLINICAL JUDGMENT 29-1

The Child With School Refusal

Nine-year-old Billy was brought to the community mental health center by his mother after a visit from the district truancy officer. Mrs. Johnson reported that Billy had refused to attend school for the past 3 weeks and had several absences since the school term began (3 months before).

Recent history acquired by the psychiatric nurse included the remarriage of Billy's mother 2 weeks before the beginning of school. Mrs. Johnson reported that Billy had always been a clingy child; when Billy was 4 years of age and she returned to work and placed him in a daycare center, he would cry for more than an hour after she left. The crying behavior continued every day for several months, although for shorter periods of time. This episode of school refusal actually began after Billy had been home for 3 days with a sore throat. During his 3-day

illness, his stepfather returned home early on the first 2 days and became involved in very loud arguments with Billy's mother. On the second day of arguing, Mr. Johnson hit his wife and then left the house, only to return several hours later, drunk but contrite and begging forgiveness. Billy had beseeched his mother to take him and their cat and leave the house, but his mother refused. After reluctantly being back in school for 3 days, Billy began refusing to go to school or to play with peers. Mrs. Johnson reported getting Billy to school on 2 days, but soon after she arrived at work, the school nurse called to request that Mrs. Johnson take Billy home because he was vomiting. Each morning since, Billy complained of feeling ill and remained in bed. Mrs. Johnson reported that there had been no more instances of Mr. Johnson's abusive behavior.

Questions

1. What additional information would you gather about Billy?
2. What elements of the history indicate Billy is at risk for alterations in mental health status?

3. What nursing diagnosis would be applicable to Billy at this time?
4. What steps can be taken to alleviate the school refusal and return Billy to school?
5. What other referrals should be made to assist this family?

Answers

1. Developmental and health history, family health history, academic achievements or challenges, peer relationships
2. Remarriage of Billy's mother, history of difficulty of separating from mother, witness to arguing and physical abuse between his stepfather and mother

3. Ineffective coping related to changes in family life and anxiety related to school attendance
4. Refer for play therapy or individual therapy to decrease anxiety regarding attending school and to determine other sources of stress for the child
5. Refer mother and stepfather to family counseling, and further assess home situation for spousal abuse and possible child abuse

although in managed care plans, the primary health care prescriber might have to make the referral. Individual and family therapy will be completed by an APRN or someone with advanced training in managing psychological issues (see thePoint Care Path: An Interdisciplinary Plan of Care for the Child With School Refusal).

POSTTRAUMATIC STRESS DISORDER

Posttraumatic stress disorder (PTSD) is a reactionary anxiety disorder occurring after a life-threatening event (or one perceived as life threatening or dangerous to physical integrity). PTSD may follow a single traumatic event or long-standing and repeated traumatic events, such as child maltreatment (especially sexual abuse). War, shootings, catastrophic environmental events (hurricanes, floods, earthquakes), and accidental disasters (automobile or airplane crashes) may evoke PTSD in the vulnerable child or adolescent.

An event triggering PTSD would usually be perceived as traumatizing by almost anyone experiencing it. The prevalence of PTSD in children and adolescents varies based on type of trauma and measurement tool. In a community sample of 1,420 children, 68% had experienced at least one potentially traumatic event and 37.0% had been exposed to more than one (Scheeringa et al., 2010).

DSM-5 (APA, 2013) criteria for acute stress disorder includes exposure to an extreme event accompanied by intense fear, horror, or helplessness; at least three dissociative symptoms; recurrence of the trauma; and extreme anxiety. The symptoms occur within 1 month after exposure and cause marked impairment.

Assessment

PTSD is characterized by repetitive uncontrolled memories (visual, auditory, physical sensations, and intrusive cognitions), repetitive behavior representative of the trauma and often observed in the child's play, trauma-specific fears, hyperalertness, and changed attitudes. Children with PTSD as a result of single-event trauma often exhibit denial, **dissociation** (a defense mechanism in which a group of mental processes are segregated from the rest of a person's mental processes to avoid emotional distress), psychic numbing, depersonalization, and rage. Regression, separation anxiety, and fearfulness may also be exhibited.

When assessing the child or adolescent suspected of having PTSD, a careful psychosocial and developmental history is imperative. Document the exposure to the trauma, including the type of trauma and length of exposure. Clear examples of behavior such as numbing (inability to feel psychic pain), sadness, avoiding activities, inappropriate responses to seemingly innocuous events, and increased physiologic arousal are clues to the disorder. Teachers and family members may describe behavior changes and identify the time when changes began. Anxiety scales for children may be helpful in assessing the degree of anxiety experienced.

A developmental history with a description of the previous coping style may provide information about the child's vulnerability. A neurologic examination should be conducted to eliminate the possibility of misdiagnosis.

A few scales may be useful in assessing stress symptoms in children. The Clinician-Administered PTSD Scale for Children and Adolescents (CAPS-CA) 8 to 18 years old, which rates the frequency and intensity of symptoms, includes pictorial scales for use with young children and offers items to assess overall severity, validity of ratings, associated symptoms, and coping strategies (Nader et al., 1996). The Children's PTSD Inventory (CPTSDI) has shown good reliability and validity with children between 7 and 18 years of age (Saigh et al., 2000). The Child Stress Disorders Checklist (CSDC), an observer–report instrument that measures acute stress and posttraumatic symptoms in children, has demonstrated good reliability and validity (Saxe & Bosquet, 2004; Saxe et al., 2003).

PTSD must be differentiated from phobic anxiety and conduct disorder. Phobic anxiety is related to a specific feared object, whereas PTSD is characterized by intrusive images that may be evoked by unrelated stimuli. Because of the potential for reactionary aggressive behavior in PTSD, it may be confused with conduct disorder. Unlike PTSD, conduct disorder is characterized by a continual and pervasive disregard for the rights of others.

Nursing Diagnoses and Outcomes

In addition to those presented in Nursing Plan of Care 29-1, the following nursing diagnosis and outcomes are applicable for the child with PTSD:

Nursing Diagnosis: Posttrauma syndrome related to response to accidental injury, assault, or other unexpected life event
Outcomes:
- Child will describe feelings and fears related to the traumatic event.
- Child will express feelings of safety.
- Child will use effective coping mechanisms to reduce fear.

Interdisciplinary Interventions

CBT is most effective for treating PTSD and related emotional and behavioral problems in children (Ollendick et al., 2008). Implement crisis intervention and family support measures immediately after the traumatic event. Help children to develop or improve their coping skills to help them manage anxiety, and educate families to equip them with the skills that will facilitate their child's recovery (Evidence-Based Clinical Practice Guidelines 29-1).

Although well-designed, randomized, controlled trials of medication efficacy in children with PTSD are lacking, medications are helpful in treating debilitating symptoms or comorbid conditions associated with PTSD (U.S. Department of Health & Human Services [DHHS], Administration on Children, Youth and Families, 2011). SSRIs target anxiety, mood, and reexperienced symptoms. Adrenergic agents, such as clonidine, may be used when symptoms of hyperarousal and impulsivity are problematic. In children with severe symptoms, mood stabilizers may be used (U.S. DHHS, Administration on Children, Youth and Families, 2011).

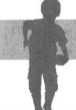

EVIDENCE-BASED CLINICAL PRACTICE GUIDELINES 29-1

Posttraumatic Stress Disorder

American Academy of Child & Adolescent Psychiatry

Cohen, J. A., Bukstein, O., Walter, H. et al. (2010). Practice parameter for the assessment and treatment of children and adolescents with posttraumatic stress disorder. *Journal of the American Academy of Child & Adolescent Psychiatry*, 49(4), 414–430. Retrieved from

http://www.cfbhn.org/Trauma informed care/practice parameter for the assessment and treatment of children and adolescents with posttraumatic stress disorder.pdf

Highlights the importance of early identification of PTSD, the importance of gathering information from parents and children, and the assessment and treatment of comorbid disorders.

International Society For Traumatic Stress Studies

Foa, E. B., Keanem T, M, Friedman, M. J. et al. (Eds.). (2009). *Effective treatments for PTSD: Practice guidelines from the International Society For Traumatic Stress Studies*. New York, NY: Guildford Press. Retrieved from

http://www.istss.org/TreatmentGuidelines.htm

Provides multiple guidelines for treatment of PTSD in children, adolescents, and adults.

National Institute for Health and Clinical Excellence, National Collaborating Centre for Mental Health, United Kingdom

National Collaborating Centre for Mental Health. (2005, reviewed 2011). *Post-traumatic stress disorder (PTSD): The management of PTSD in adults and children in primary and secondary care* (NICE Clinical Guideline 26). Retrieved from

http://www.nice.org.uk/nicemedia/live/10966/29769/29769.pdf

Provides guidelines for assessment and treatment of PTSD in children and adults as well as support for families and caregivers of individuals with PTSD.

OBSESSIVE–COMPULSIVE DISORDER

OCD is a chronic disorder closely associated with anxiety and is most often first identified in youth (1 of every 200 children and adolescents) or young adulthood (American Academy of Child & Adolescent Psychiatry, 2011). Diagnosis of OCD is based on the presence of a variety of obsessive and compulsive symptoms that so invade a child's thoughts and actions the child or adolescent is unable to complete normal functions and activities of daily living. The child or adolescent feels driven by his or her obsessions and/or compulsions to the point of ignoring his or her responsibilities such as work, school, and relationships. *Obsessions* are unwanted, unrealistic, irrational, recurring or persistent thoughts, impulses, or images beyond excessive worry. *Compulsions* are repetitive behaviors, rituals, or mental acts (American Academy of Child & Adolescent Psychiatry, 2011; APA, 2013) (Chart 29-2). Examples of compulsions are extreme handwashing, often to the point of broken skin and/or bleeding, and orderliness or counting that result in an inability to sleep, go to work or school, or maintain normal relationships.

As with other mental health disorders, the cause of OCD is not totally understood. However, evidence points to abnormalities in serotonin neurotransmission and, more recently, dopamine transmission within the brain. This evidence is supported by the effective treatment of OCD with SSRIs. Additionally, MRI and PET of a person experiencing obsessive and compulsive symptoms has shown increased blood flow and metabolic activity in the orbitofrontal cortex, limbic structures, caudate, and thalamus, with a trend toward

right-sided predominance (Greenberg et al., 2009; Simpson et al., 2011).

OCD is also considered a familial brain disorder and has also been noted to develop or worsen following a streptococcal infection. Although the disorder has been

CHART 29-2 Common Obsessions and Compulsions in Children

Obsessions
- Contamination
- Safety
- Doubting one's memory or perception
- Scrupulosity (need to do the right thing, fear of committing a transgression, often religious)
- Need for order or symmetry
- Unwanted, intrusive sexual/aggressive thought

Compulsions
- Cleaning/washing
- Checking (checking locks, stove, iron, safety of others)
- Counting/repeating actions a certain number of times or until it "feels right"
- Arranging objects
- Touching/tapping objects
- Hoarding
- Confessing/seeking reassurance
- List making

described as familial, a parent and/or grandparent's diagnosis of OCD does not necessarily lead to the child or adolescent developing symptoms.

Assessment

Children and adolescents can experience a variety of obsessions and compulsions. However, according to the *DSM-5*, when unwanted, irrational thoughts or behaviors associated with obsessions or compulsions produce severe physical and/or emotional discomfort and prevent normal activities of daily living, an assessment must be conducted to identify whether a diagnosis of OCD is warranted. Therefore, all unwanted, unrealistic, or irrational thoughts, impulses, images, behaviors, rituals, or mental acts reported or observed are to be evaluated for their impact on the child's ability to function and effectively conduct activities of daily living. As with any disorders identified in children or adolescents, early identification and treatment are imperative to enhance positive outcomes over time.

Ask the child or adolescent, "Is there anything you do over and over again and cannot resist doing, such as repeatedly washing your hands, counting up to a certain number, or checking something several times to make sure you had done it right?" It is also important to assess for the presence of any comorbid disorders.

A child or adolescent can experience either obsessions or compulsions or may describe a combination of both obsessions and compulsions. The foci of the obsessions and compulsions can often be connected. For example, an adolescent may have the obsessive, persistent thought that there are "bugs" crawling all over his or her hands and arms, resulting in the compulsion to wash his or her hands all day, thus preventing the youth from attending any of his or her assigned classes.

Children and adolescents tend to be self-conscious and/or ashamed of their obsessions and compulsions and often hide the fact they are struggling with various obsessions or compulsions. The child or adolescent may wake up during the night in order to perform his or her compulsive acts at a time when the child knows the family is asleep and will not become aware of these compulsions.

Interdisciplinary Interventions

Children and adolescents experiencing obsessive and/or compulsive symptoms often go to great lengths to hide their struggles from parents and other family members. Because of this, diagnosis and treatment is often delayed. Outcomes for children and adolescents challenged by symptoms associated with OCD are very good when diagnosed early.

Treatment generally involves a combination of medication (e.g., SSRIs), therapy (e.g., CBT), education, and support from family and school personnel. SSRIs have been effective in treating obsessive and compulsive symptoms. An average of 3 to 10 CBT sessions, combined with appropriate pharmaceutical management and family and teacher education about OCD, will typically place most youths with OCD on the path toward remission of symptoms.

ADJUSTMENT DISORDERS

A number of adjustment challenges may occur in children who experience loss or other traumatic life situations such as natural or man-made disasters, wars, abuse (especially sexual abuse), neglect, or exposure to violence. Continual unabated stress of poverty, homelessness, or family conflict or disintegration may have devastating effects on children or adolescents. They may be genetically vulnerable or physiologically vulnerable (e.g., chronically ill), or they may not have sufficient coping strategies or support to manage the psychological assaults. Many disorders occur as a result of life disruptions; this section addresses only those not discussed separately.

There tends to be frequent symptom overlap among adjustment disorders and mood disorders. For example, a child may have an adjustment disorder with depressed mood or disturbance in conduct. The distinction is the cause of the problem. **Adjustment disorder**, defined as a disturbance in behavior that develops as a result of adverse life circumstances and personal inability to cope with the resulting stress, is a common reason children are referred for mental health services.

The essential feature of adjustment disorder is clinically important emotional or behavioral symptoms within 3 months of an identifiable stressor found to overtax the individual's coping abilities. Bereavement is not considered to be an adjustment disorder, unless it incapacitates the individual beyond 3 to 6 months, depending on symptom severity. Stressors may be relocation (new school, new home), family changes (new sibling, parental separation or divorce), or accomplishment of a developmental milestone (starting school, going to camp). Bullying by another child is receiving increased attention as a possible cause of adjustment problems (Gibb et al., 2011).

An adjustment disorder of even a short duration (6 months or less) is of clinical importance because risk for suicide increases and potential for academic difficulties is high. With timely and appropriate intervention (support, understanding, and restabilization of family life), most children recover rapidly. In most children, a more severe disruptive disorder does not develop, and the conflict resolves, or the child adjusts to the change.

Assessment

Young children often manifest an adjustment disorder by whining and clinging behavior or by increased aggressive behavior or isolation. Children in the elementary school years and in adolescence often manifest adjustment disorders through somatic symptoms (stomach pains, nausea, headaches, fatigue), academic difficulties, or problems in social relationships. An adjustment disorder may be accompanied by anxiety or mood disturbance.

Whenever children are seen with the foregoing complaints, and when no physical reason is found for the behavior change, the nurse should investigate any changes in the child's life. Nursing assessment must include information about the precipitating stressor, its timing and severity, history of any previous alterations in mental health and behavior, and coping strategies. A suicide assessment is essential.

Interdisciplinary Interventions

Useful interventions are education (helping the youth and his or her family to understand the child's feelings and behaviors) and advocating for reduced stress and resources for the child. Providing family support, facilitating communication about the stressor, and assisting the child in the development of effective coping strategies are important interventions for preventing further deterioration.

Advocating for classroom changes by helping teachers to understand the reason for the child's behavior can help to relieve additional stress caused by educational pressures. If the child does not recover with brief problem-oriented therapeutic strategies, refer the child to a mental health clinic.

SLEEP DISORDERS

Sleep disruptions are common in children ages 3 to 7 years of age and may include nightmares, sleep terrors, or sleepwalking (Chart 29-3). With reassurance, appropriate bedtime activities (reading, quiet discussions), and comforting strategies by family members, most episodes last only a short while (see Chapters 4 to 7 for a summary of normal sleeping patterns of children of all ages).

Sleep disturbances usually erupt after times of high stress in the family or the child's daily routine, a frightening situation, or when self-expectations or family expectations for the child have increased. From ages 3 to 7 years, children learn new skills rapidly. Although the child can take pride in new accomplishments, expectations are increased as well; thus, they have the "stress" of success. Children of this age do not always have the language to express their feelings and worries, and families may not always find the time for quiet, nurturing activities (e.g., reading, singing, talking, holding, or cuddling) before bedtime. For these reasons, feelings and thoughts may spill over during sleep in the form of various sleep disturbances.

CHART 29-3   Types of Sleep Disorders

- Sleep disruptions: Unusual nighttime awakenings occur frequently, with no immediately known or observable cause (nightmares, sleep terrors, sleepwalking, confusion, and arousal).
- Nightmares: Child wakes during deep sleep, is frightened but alert, is able to report on what was frightening, and usually has difficulty returning to sleep. Nightmares occur in approximately 10% of children 3–6 years of age.
- Sleep terrors: Episodes occur usually after 1–2 hours of sleep; the child or adolescent looks terrified and very agitated. The child does not remember the sleep disruption. Sleep terrors are a developmental variable and not caused by anxiety or undue stress.
- Sleepwalking: The individual walks about while asleep. Sleepwalking usually occurs during the first part of the sleep cycle. Sleepwalking may be calm or agitated.

A family history is common in arousal disorders, which include confusional arousals (occur primarily in infants and young children during which moaning progresses to agitated, confused behavior with crying), sleepwalking, and sleep terrors (also called *night terrors*; the child looks terrified, has staring eyes, increased heart rate and sweating, and cries) (Stores, 2009).

Assessment

When assessing child or adolescent complaints about sleep disturbances, consider their overall health and developmental status. Document daily activities, bedtime routines, sleep pattern history, and a description of the sleep environment. It is important to elicit the family's perception of the child's sleep disturbance and the effect it has on family life.

Obtain a thorough description of the sleep disturbance, including any precipitating events, the length of time the disturbance has been occurring, the frequency of occurrence, any interventions used, and their success. The diagnosis of a sleep disorder is made when the precipitating event has passed and usual interventions to promote sleep have been tried for at least 1 month but have failed to bring about a change. Note any other physical or mental health conditions.

Interdisciplinary Interventions

Educate the families and the child to promote an understanding of the disorder and its management. Safety factors in the home of the sleepwalker should be identified and modified if warranted. For instance, the home should be secured so the child cannot easily leave the house. Items the child could run into or easily break should be relocated.

Discussing frightening or distressing events and the feelings aroused by them may help decrease the occurrence of nightmares and sleep terrors. Spending time with the child at bedtime (singing, reading, quietly talking) may help the child relax and sleep more restfully. The child needs reassurance that parents are available during the night to provide support, give reassurance, and help the child relax.

If the child is experiencing anger, frustration, or anxiety as a result of other underlying problems such as difficulty in school, family disruptions or parental conflict, recent or current trauma (e.g., such as sexual abuse), or anticipated trauma (e.g., anticipated loss of parent, punishment for wrongdoing, or recurrence of some tragedy), the underlying problem must be sorted out and addressed.

Families often allow children with sleep problems to sleep with them. It is best to discourage this intervention. It reinforces the child's belief that he or she is unable to master the problem. It may also give the message to the child that the parent is "frightened," unable to solve the problem, and perhaps needs to rely on the child. See Nursing Interventions 29-4 for other helpful techniques to prevent and treat sleeping disorders.

If the problem persists and the dreams do not abate, seek consultation with an APRN, psychiatrist, or other mental health professional. Persistent nightmares, sleep terrors, and sleepwalking may point to other issues that require further psychiatric evaluation.

NURSING INTERVENTIONS 29-4

Family Teaching to Prevent and Manage Sleeping Disorders

- Leave a night-light on.
- Leave the child's bedroom door open.
- Provide the child with a comforting blanket or stuffed animal.

- Avoid excessive anger and abusive discipline.
- Set and maintain realistic limits during the day.
- Reward the child for success.
- Keep expectations reasonable.

ATTENTION-DEFICIT/HYPERACTIVITY DISORDER

The *DSM-5* identifies three subtypes of ADHD based on symptoms (APA, 2013):

1. Predominantly inattentive, characterized by inability to attend to tasks and activities, tends to make careless mistakes, poor listener despite having normal hearing, often loses possessions
2. Predominantly hyperactive–impulsive, includes excessive motor activity, inability to sit or stay in one place, excessive fidgeting, excessive talking, impulsive behavior
3. Combined inattentive and hyperactive–impulsive

Prevalence of ADHD is 9.0% in children 8 to 15 years of age; it occurs twice as often in boys (12.3%) as in girls (5.5%) (Akinbami et al., 2011). Prevalence, at 10.3% and 10.6%, is greater for children with a family income, respectively, of less than 100% of the poverty level and between 100% and 199% of the poverty level (Akinbami et al., 2011). ADHD is serious and chronic, affects several areas of a child's life and functioning, and is highly comorbid with other disorders. The rate of comorbidity with externalizing disorders (e.g., ODD, conduct disorder) is about 50%; it is about 25% with anxiety and depression (Ollendick et al., 2008). Increasingly, these disorders are being viewed as potentially lifelong disorders.

ADHD is strongly linked to genetic and biologic factors, but psychosocial factors appear to interact in complex ways with such factors. In biologic parents of children with ADHD, 25% to 33% have ADHD (Cormier, 2008). Dopamine transmitter and receptor genes have been linked to ADHD, and abnormalities of brain structure and function have been noted (Cormier, 2008).

Assessment

The diagnosis of ADHD is most often made during the early school years. Symptoms of the disorder must be present for at least 6 months. The criteria fall into three areas of functioning: concentration, impulse control, and goal-directed behavior. The symptoms may not be demonstrated in early and short-term one-on-one situations, but after the child is comfortable in a situation, the behaviors begin to emerge.

Major problems for these children include interpersonal problems with age-matched peers, teachers, and, often, parents. Because of their impulsivity and poor problem-solving skills, children with ADHD are vulnerable to developing behavioral problems and a comorbid diagnosis of ODD or conduct disorder. These children are also susceptible to low self-esteem, anxiety, and depression. Behaviors associated with ADHD make them vulnerable to failure and negative feedback, which may contribute to these comorbid conditions.

ADHD should be assessed and diagnosed by an interdisciplinary team because several areas of functioning may be impaired. Psychometric testing helps to define the individual's cognitive and learning deficits. Children at various developmental levels function differently; thus, the evaluator must be familiar with age-appropriate norms. Obtaining information from teachers and family members is helpful because each is able to provide feedback about behavior in a different setting. Data obtained about the child's strengths can be used to enhance the program of interventions.

Interdisciplinary Interventions

Interdisciplinary interventions may include psychological assessment and assessment of the child's specific learning problems and intellectual ability (Evidence-Based Clinical Practice Guidelines 29-2). Psychology and special education experts are usually called upon for these assessments and to make recommendations for the individual educational program (see Chapter 12).

Children are hospitalized for ADHD if there is an exacerbation of symptoms/behaviors infringing on activities of daily life or there is an exacerbation or worsening of a comorbid condition such as depression or conduct disorder with very aggressive behavior.

A mental health provider (e.g., APRN, psychotherapist, or psychiatrist) is considered an invaluable part of the intervention when a child experiences challenges such as impaired self-esteem, depression, or conduct disorders. Psychiatric expertise is also included in an assessment when comorbidity is present such as when a child is diagnosed with depression or ADHD and conduct disorder or ODD.

Management of children with ADHD can include medication to control behaviors associated with this disorder (see Table 29-1). Stimulant medications are generally more effective than nonstimulants (Molina et al., 2009). Methylphenidate (Ritalin, Concerta), dextroamphetamine (Dexedrine), and dextroamphetamine and

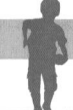

EVIDENCE-BASED CLINICAL PRACTICE GUIDELINES 29-2

Attention-Deficit/Hyperactivity Disorder

American Academy of Pediatrics

American Academy of Pediatrics. (2012). ADHD: Clinical practice guideline for the diagnosis, evaluation, and treatment of attention-deficit/hyperactivity disorder in children and adolescents. *Pediatrics, 128*(5), 1–18. Retrieved from

http://pediatrics.aappublications.org/content/early/2011/10/14/peds.2011-2654.full.pdf+html

Guideline presents assessment and treatment of ADHD in children and adolescents.

American Academy of Child & Adolescent Psychiatry

Pliszka, S. (2007). Practice parameter for the assessment and treatment of children and adolescents with attention-deficit/hyperactivity disorder. *Journal of the American Academy of Child & Adolescent Psychiatry, 46*(7), 894–921. Retrieved from

http://www.jaacap.com/content/pracparam

Guideline discusses assessment and treatment of ADHD in children and adolescents.

Scottish Intercollegiate Guidelines Network

Scottish Intercollegiate Guidelines Network. (2009). *Management of attention deficit and hyperkinetic disorders in children and young people. A national clinical guideline* (SIGN Publication No. 112). Edinburgh, Scotland: Author. Retrieved from

http://www.sign.ac.uk/pdf/sign112.pdf

Guideline discusses assessment of attention-deficit and hyperkinetic (hyperactivity) disorder in children and adolescents. Includes psychological interventions and pharmacologic and nutrition therapies in various age groups.

amphetamine (Adderall) are commonly prescribed and demonstrate a decrease in symptoms of ADHD (Gilchrist & Arnold, 2008). When stimulant medication fails or causes adverse effects, alternative forms of treatment are tried. A treatment algorithm, applied in the order presented, is recommended: atomoxetine (Strattera), bupropion or tricyclic antidepressants, other antidepressants, and alpha-agonists (Blader et al., 2010).

Health promotion and maintenance of general health are important considerations. Routine medical care should include all normal wellness care, such as immunizations, physical examinations, and dental and eye examinations and care. Assessment of nutritional status and physical growth and development are important because high activity levels and side effects of medication may decrease appetite and slow the rate of growth.

Additionally, there is an increasing risk of weight gain noted with some of the newer medications being used to treat mental health conditions. Monitor to determine whether medications are having the desired effects on the child's behavior and whether side effects are occurring. Ensure other members of the health care team know how treatment is going. Teach the child and family members how to assess the child's symptoms and behavior, look for side effects, and therapeutic responses to treatment.

Community Care

Nurses at school and in home care are responsible for family education (Teaching Intervention Plan 29-1). Positive reinforcement is effective for children with ADHD; educate family members and teachers to respond to (reward) positive behavior and to use consequences for or ignore negative behavior (Vierhile et al., 2009). Teach them to use "time-outs," having the child sit on a chair for a short period of time, when behavior persists. Behavior management is fairly effective in managing overactivity but is less effective in curtailing problems of inattention.

MOOD DISORDERS

 QUESTION: Why is it important for nurses to screen adolescents, such as Ashley, for a mood disorder such as depression?

The major mood disorders in children include major depressive disorder, dysthymia (depressed or irritable mood, less intense than major depression but more persistent), and bipolar disorder.

Mood disorders such as depression are characterized by a disturbance in mood (irritability, sadness, oppositionalism, negativity) that lasts for most of every day for a period of at least 2 weeks. Mood disorders in children and adolescents are common and serious for a number of reasons. Risk for suicide is common in youth with mood disorders (Kinnally & Mann, 2012). Mood disorders can also cause family, social, and peer relationships to deteriorate severely; school failure and poor academic achievement are common.

TIP 29-1: A TEACHING INTERVENTION PLAN for the Child With Attention-Deficit/ Hyperactivity Disorder

Nursing Diagnoses and Family Outcomes

- Impaired social interaction related to inability to control actions and behaviors
  Outcomes: Child gradually learns self-control and the ability to share peer acceptance and enjoyment in peer relations.
  Child completes self-care tasks and cooperates in school setting.
  Child follows instructions and is successful in academic activities.
- Chronic low self-esteem related to negative response from others regarding behavior
  Outcomes: Child identifies own strengths.
  Self-esteem is enhanced as evidenced by child's comments about self and about personal accomplishments.
- Risk for injury related to child's activity level and impulsiveness
  Outcome: Child's safety is ensured to the best extent possible.
- Readiness for enhanced knowledge: Medication side effects
  Outcomes: Child maintains adequate nutritional status.
  Child maintains adequate sleep pattern.
  Families express confidence in their ability to manage the medication regimen.

Teach Child/Family

Managing Child's Activity

- Encourage family members and teachers to decrease stimuli when concentration is important.
- Monitor adherence to medication regimen and reaction to medication.
- Decrease choices that child must make (limit to two for young child, three to four for older children).
- Practice problem-solving strategies with child.
- Give positive feedback for success (tokens, rewards), consequences for undesirable behavior.
- Tutoring may be necessary. Subdivide learning tasks so child is not overwhelmed and can maintain concentration.
- Give frequent positive feedback. Directions for each task should be clear, short, and broken into segments. For example:
  - Take your book out of your desk.
  - Open the book to page 10.
  - Read the second paragraph to yourself.
  - Answer the first question below the paragraph.
  - Now, answer the second question.
- Provide information about the characteristics and problems associated with ADHD.
- Assist parents with problem-solving ways of managing child's behavior and needs (e.g., a token reward and behavior management program).

- Assist in identifying community resources.
- Encourage assertive behavior with school system to obtain needed resources for the child's learning experience.
- Provide written resources and list of references that parents may use to increase understanding of the child's disorder and effective ways to manage child's behavior.

Safety

- Encourage parents to establish clear limits on where child may play or ride a bike and when higher risk activities may be undertaken. Monitor child's activities frequently.
- Reinforce positive behavior with feedback and intermittent rewards.

Improving Social Interactions and Self-esteem

- Provide supervision of peer play activities for the young child. Hold and soothe child when unable to provide self-control. Use time-outs (5 minutes for children in early childhood, 7–10 minutes for children in middle childhood). Young children benefit from structured preschool programs.
- Middle childhood: Consider social skills training in small groups to encourage
  - Turn-taking
  - Making appropriate requests
  - Communicating feelings and empathy
  - Problem solving in conflictual situations
  - Saying no to inappropriate behaviors
  - Expressing anger in appropriate (socially acceptable) ways
- Identify child's strengths and provide feedback to enhance positive self-thoughts.
- Reward positive behavior, provide limit setting as needed, and avoid negative comments that the child is "bad." Remove attention or special privileges for negative behavior. Help child to develop skills, with individual lessons to learn a special skill or with group activity that assists child to learn something of interest (a hobby, sport, or area of knowledge).

Medication Administration

- Teach families to administer medication after meals, decreasing amount in afternoons if it interferes with sleep; provide quiet activities before bedtime; and decrease stimulation at mealtimes.
- Explain what the medication is and how it works, its benefits, and its potential side effects.
- Discuss modifications for side effects.
- Assist in establishing a routine to prevent forgetfulness in giving the medication.

Contact Health Care Provider if

- Child appears very drowsy
- Child is unable to concentrate
- Child physically harms self or others
- No improvement is seen in school performance

Studies of mood disorders in children demonstrate a wide variety of factors are associated with alterations in mood and emotional states. Social factors such as family conflicts; bereavement; and physical, psychological, and sexual abuse have been implicated (Beardslee et al., 2011). Familial vulnerability (genetic), psychological factors (cognitive processing, cognitive distortions, temperament, and lack of adequate coping strategies), social and environmental factors (poverty, abuse, neglect), and biologic factors are all implicated or associated with mood disorders in preschool, elementary, and adolescent years.

Disorders that often occur with mood disorders include ADHD, PTSD, anxiety disorders, impulse control disorders, and learning disabilities. Mood disorders may result from excessive stress or an inherent error in the neurotransmitter system, especially the system associated with serotonin. Physical alterations caused by some endocrine, autoimmune, metabolic, and neurologic disorders also are associated with mood disorders.

MAJOR DEPRESSIVE DISORDER

Major depressive disorder has a prevalence rate of 2.8% in children and up to 8.3% in adolescents (Muñoz et al., 2010). Depression is being diagnosed more frequently in middle childhood as criteria for childhood disorders are clarified and differentiated. Gender disparity has been found to emerge after puberty, with a strong female preponderance (Thapar et al., 2012).

 ANSWER: Symptoms associated with mood disorders such as depression can produce suicidal feelings and increased risk for self-harm in adolescence; Ashley is at high risk for self-harm.

Assessment

 QUESTION: If you were the nurse assessing Ashley, what questions would you ask her?

Assess for severity (number of symptoms) and duration of symptoms. The interview with the child provides information about subjective symptoms of fatigue, suicidal ideation, and feelings of worthlessness. Families and teachers are best at providing information about the sequence of events and observable behaviors.

The school nurse may be able to provide information about somatic complaints, their frequency, and the response to nursing intervention. Teachers can provide important information about the child's progress or decline in academic performance, mood states, and coping and adaptation in the classroom. They also have information about peer relationships.

Families may report on changes occurring in appetite, weight gain or loss, and change in attitude and behaviors at home, such as increasing isolation,

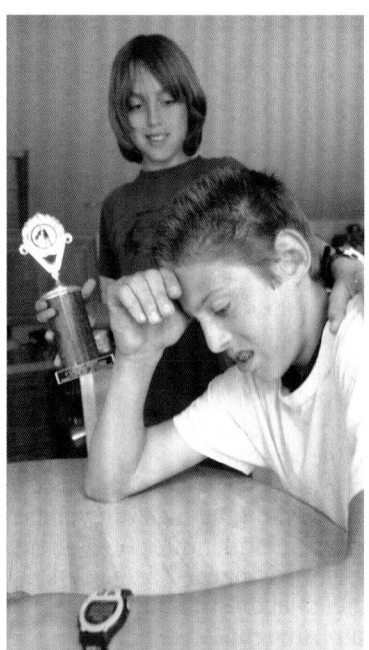

Figure 29-2 Adolescents are at risk for depression as they deal with the physical, emotional, and social changes that characterize this developmental stage.

anxiety, loss of pleasure in usual activities, and oppositional and aggressive behavior (Fig. 29-2). The child is most likely able to provide subjective information about how he or she feels, about sleep disturbance, and about worries.

caREminder

Children frequently exhibit depression in physical symptoms, irritability, and school failure. Adolescents may sleep excessively, appear sad, exhibit poor concentration and isolation, and complain of headaches. School performance often deteriorates. Assessing for suicidal thoughts or behaviors is essential.

Conduct a physical examination to rule out or identify illnesses or physical concerns that might contribute to a diagnosis of depression. The mental status assessment is usually best done through a semistructured interview to allow flexibility and to enable you to explore challenging areas or topics. For instance, if a child indicates he or she has thoughts of suicide, obtain additional information regarding any established plan and its lethality. Determine what resources are needed to ensure the safety of the suicidal youth.

Self-report measures may be used to help verify the diagnosis by trained mental health professionals. Some useful tools include the Center for Epidemiological Studies Depression Scale for Children (CES-DC), available through *Bright Futures in Practice: Mental Health—Volume II, Tool Kit* (Jellinek et al., 2002b); the Children's Depression Inventory (CDI) (Timbremont et al., 2004); and the Beck Depression Inventory (Krefetz et al., 2002).

ANSWER: Because of Ashley's current symptoms, the following questions could be used to determine if a referral is the next step:

- "Tell me about your sleep? What do you do before going to sleep? Do you have a routine, a pattern? Please describe it for me. When do you usually go to sleep and when do you wake? On the weekends, when you don't have school, how do you sleep?"
- "Tell me about sad feelings or thoughts. Are there times when you feel okay? Share a few examples of those times. When is the hardest or saddest time of day? What do you do to feel better? Do you drink alcohol or take any drugs to help you feel better?"
- "What worries you?"
- "Have you ever thought about hurting yourself?" (If the answer is yes, determine exactly how the adolescent is envisioning this self-harm and take measures to prevent an attempted suicide.)

Interdisciplinary Interventions

Interventions for selected mood disorders in children, including depressive disorder, are listed in Nursing Interventions 29-5. Interventions should also fit the specific situation (Tradition or Science 29-1). For instance, if the child has experienced a major loss, the intervention should be directed toward assisting the child through the grief process.

Bereavement therapy or a grief recovery program would be recommended to allow the child to work naturally through the normal grief process. However, if grief is not easily resolved and is prolonged because of a mood disorder, then medication such as a tricyclic antidepressant or SSRI would be recommended, usually in conjunction with CBT.

More Inquiry Needed

TRADITION OR SCIENCE 29-1

Is there an increased risk of suicide when antidepressants are used in children?

Studies have shown a trend toward suicidal thinking or behavior in children and adolescents who are taking antidepressants (Busch et al., 2010). Ghaemi and Vohringer (2013) demonstrated that the risks of SSRIs outweighed the benefits when unpublished data were included in a meta-analysis; others have demonstrated no effect on the likelihood of suicide attempt. The debate continues because data also demonstrate the benefits of antidepressants being greater than risk from suicidal ideation (Dudley et al., 2010). Possibly influencing the issue is the fact that medication improves mood and lifts the cloud of depression while also increasing energy. This can provide an opportunity for someone who is struggling to live because he or she finally has the energy it often takes to end one's life. Something else to consider is that in the past, suicides, especially those by children, were often classified as accidents. More inquiry is needed to determine whether there is a true association between use of antidepressant medications and suicide in children; in the interim, risks and benefits of use must be evaluated, and children must be closely monitored.

School-based behavioral programs and interventions can be effective in decreasing depressive symptoms and improving coping skills (Muñoz et al., 2010). These programs include psychoeducational interventions. The school nurse or school-based therapist can provide information about self-concept, relationships, communication, and coping and can promote acquisition of these skills by engaging adolescents in experiential

NURSING INTERVENTIONS 29-5

Mood Disorders

- Teach family and child about illness, associated symptoms, and behaviors. Explain therapeutic regimens: medications, psychotherapy, or behavior therapy; photo (light) therapy for seasonal affective disorder.
- Monitor child's response to medication, report lack of improvement or untoward side effects, and report changes from depression to mania and vice versa.
  - For depressive disorders, tricyclic antidepressants or serotonin reuptake inhibitors will likely be prescribed. Monitor for cardiotoxic effects of medication and for suicidal risk.

- For bipolar disorder, lithium, carbamazepine, or valproate will likely be prescribed. Monitor blood levels of medications as ordered.
- For seasonal affective disorder, light therapy or antidepressant medication will likely be ordered.
- Teach family and child about the medications: purpose, signs of improvement, side effects, when to report side effects, and withdrawal or termination of medication.
- Educate family to monitor adherence and changes (or lack of) in school behavior, attitude, and performance in collaboration with teachers and school nurse.
- Caution: All antidepressant medications take 10–21 days to begin showing an effect.

learning such as role-playing with other adolescents to identify the issues they are dealing with and engage them in problem solving to deal with them effectively.

BIPOLAR DISORDER

We now recognize children and adolescents experience bipolar disorder. *Bipolar disorder* is an altered mental status manifested as extreme changes in mood, activity, and behavior. Children often cycle through the mood swings very quickly, swinging several times an hour.

Because of the rapid mood swings, the **mania** (a phase of bipolar disorder characterized by expansiveness, elation, agitation, hyperexcitability, hyperactivity, and increased speed of thought or speech) or depression may be missed by care providers. These children often present as depressed children with aggressive acting out or with ADHD. Medications prescribed for depression frequently worsen the acting-out symptoms. Making a definitive diagnosis in young children is sometimes difficult.

Bipolar disorder affects an estimated 1% of adolescents, similar to adult prevalence rates; prevalence is much lower in preadolescents, about 0.1% (Lack & Green, 2009). A strong genetic link to the disorder seems to exist. First-degree relatives of individuals with bipolar disorder have elevated rates of bipolar disorder and major depressive disorder (Offord, 2012).

When one parent has bipolar disorder, the risk of each child also having the disorder is 15% to 30%. When both parents have the disorder, the risk of each child having the disorder increases dramatically to 50% to 75%. For example, if parents diagnosed with bipolar disorder have twins, both children have a 70% chance of also being diagnosed with bipolar disorder. When a mood disorder is present among first-degree relatives, individuals are prone to early onset of the disease.

Assessment

Bipolar disorder is manifested differently in children than in adults. Children often appear to have continuous mood disturbance, a mixture of mania and depression (Chart 29-4). Parents of these children often report that as infants, they had sleeping problems, demonstrated labile mood, and were hard to soothe (Leibenluft, 2011).

Because of rapid cycling behaviors and varying symptoms, it is helpful for families to keep a log of their child's daily behavior. The mental health care providers can use the log to monitor behavior and responses to treatment.

Children diagnosed with other disorders, such as depression, conduct disorder, and ODD, may actually have bipolar disorder or may develop bipolar disorder as a comorbid condition. Close monitoring and exploration for other conditions should continue.

Interdisciplinary Interventions

Treatment for children with bipolar disorder is complex and involves a great deal of trial and error because few child research studies currently exist and the most effective treatment for these children is based on

---

CHART 29-4   Symptoms of Bipolar Disorder*

- Irritable mood, depression
- Extreme changes in mood lasting a few hours to a few days
- Explosive rages
- Separation anxiety
- Defiance of authority
- Hyperactivity, agitation, and distractibility
- Sleep disturbances
- Enuresis
- Cravings for sweets or carbohydrates
- Impulsivity and or racing thoughts
- Daredevil behavior or grandiose beliefs of own abilities
- Inappropriate or precocious sexual behavior
- Delusions or hallucinations

*May include several.

---

anecdotal information and observations. CBT in conjunction with medication will help the child learn coping skills, self-soothing and self-regulating behaviors, socialization with peers, and a beginning understanding of how he or she can live a full life despite the diagnosis of bipolar disorder. Antipsychotic (e.g., olanzapine) and mood-stabilizing (e.g., lithium) medications are the mainstay of treatment (McDougall, 2009). Lithium blood levels must be monitored closely because too low a dose is not effective, but a high blood level can be toxic. Anticonvulsants such as carbamazepine (Tegretol), valproic acid (Depakene, Depakote [divalproex]), and oxcarbazepine (Trileptal) are effective for some children. Closely monitor children on these medications for side effects.

Diets rich in omega-3 fatty acids have been found to be helpful for children with bipolar disorder and are increasingly recommended. Light therapy, used for seasonal affective disorder, has helped some children with bipolar disorder as well.

Individual and family therapy is critical for these children and their families. These children struggle with many emotions, such as depression, anxiety, and guilt. These children often struggle to understand their confusing and varying emotions. These confusing feelings often lead to destructive and violent outbursts, after which they must deal with feelings of remorse and guilt. Caring for these children can take a large toll on parents, siblings, and extended family. Family therapy and support groups are helpful ways to share problems and solutions. Families may need help in developing structure and limits for their child; behavior management programs can also be useful.

School programs must also provide structure and support. Nurses should work with families to advocate for a classroom aide if needed as well as tutors and in-school counseling. Families and health care providers should work with the school system to develop individual educational programs for these children to provide the educational assistance needed.

Interventions include identifying a designated "safe place" where the child can refocus in a quiet and calm environment, arranging the child's seat to avoid distractions (being cognizant not to isolate the child), allowing transition time between activities, and performing routine multidisciplinary reviews of student status (performance, effectiveness of interventions, medication effectiveness and side effects) (Kutash et al., 2011). Use a calm and reassuring manner when interacting with the child, and work to identify mild behavioral changes that may lead to outburst early to circumvent the need for public interventions.

SUICIDE

Suicidal events, which include acts of self-destruction, life-taking acts, and threats of self-harm, are common among teenagers. Persons attempting or thinking about suicide experience hopelessness and despair and can think of no satisfactory way to solve their problems or to find satisfaction in daily living.

For young people 10 to 24 years old in the United States, suicide is the fourth leading cause of death; 7.8% had attempted suicide and 15.8% had seriously considered attempting suicide (Eaton et al., 2012). Male adolescents are much more likely to commit suicide than females (Cash & Bridge, 2009); the risk for suicide is the greatest among white males, but the rates are rapidly increasing for black males. Experts warn actual suicides could be even more common than data on suicide reports. As a result of increased public awareness campaigns improving recognition and understanding of suicidal behavior, many deaths attributed to incidents such as accidents, gang shootings, or police-involved shootings in the past are now being more carefully assessed, with many of those deaths now being attributed to suicide.

CROSS-CULTURAL CARE

Suicide is a major public health problem worldwide. Ethnic and cultural factors appear to play a role in the incidence of suicide (Twenge, 2011). Cultural and religious belief systems may mask the incidence of suicide in children and adolescents throughout the world.

Thoughts of suicide are frequently communicated to someone but are often discounted. Many myths still pervade societal thinking about suicide. Thus, many children contemplating self-harm are not taken seriously, are reassured inappropriately, or are inappropriately told "You will be okay" (Chart 29-5). Many risk factors are associated with suicide, including altered mental health status (e.g., depression, anxiety disorders) in combination with relational stress with families, friends, or significant others; abuse; academic failure; bullying; low self-esteem; relocation of family or friends; availability of firearms; and having a friend or peer who committed suicide.

CHART 29-5 Truths About Suicide (To Counter Common Myths)

- People contemplating suicide usually tell someone about it.
- Suicidal threats are real and must be taken seriously.
- Children and adolescents from good, intact homes do think about or commit suicide.
- Anyone who thinks about or commits suicide is or was not crazy; he or she cannot or could not see other alternatives.
- One should ask about thoughts or plans for suicide; this does not plant the idea but imparts the message that it is something that can be talked about.
- If a person talks about suicide, he or she has been thinking about it and may implement his or her plan.
- Accidents, gunshot wounds, and substance abuse are problems that can be associated with self-destructive and suicidal behaviors.
- Someone who is thinking about or who actually commits suicide is not always depressed.
- Suicidal persons can be helped to perceive other options and not to act on their thoughts.

Assessment

Most children give clues when they are thinking about suicide.

caREminder

When youngsters appeal for help or ask to talk about "a friend" who is upset and talking about suicide, the health care provider or teacher should be alerted to the potential risk for suicide. The child may be indirectly talking about, or asking questions about, his or her own concerns.

A common way for youths to communicate about suicidal thoughts is through a friend. They may pass a note to a classmate or ask the friend if they have ever thought about suicide, for advice about doing "it," or they may make threats in anger.

Conduct an assessment for suicidal thinking for adolescents and children who present with high-risk behaviors and high-risk factors in their life (Nursing Interventions 29-6). Ask all children and adolescents with depressive disorders, bipolar disorder, and substance abuse or who are despairing, feeling hopeless, and indicating despondency and powerlessness about suicidal thoughts, ideation, and plans. *Ideation* refers to thoughts and feelings that suicide is the only way to end the problem or misery that one is experiencing.

During assessment for suicide risk, children and adolescents may initially indicate suicidal thoughts or ideation but later deny them. This denial should not deter the caregiver from providing for the safety of the child.

Risk for suicide (at levels from low to high) is based on the hopelessness and despondency of the child, the

NURSING INTERVENTIONS 29-6

Guidelines for Assessing Suicidal Intent

- Establish rapport (show interest; actively listen; initiate talking in a friendly, respectful way).
- Use direct, simple questions (avoiding open-ended questions).
- Use language that the child can understand.
- Allow the child to tell his or her own story.
- Ask questions matter-of-factly, without judgment.

- Convey empathy and allow expression of feelings.
- Determine the intent, whether a plan has been formulated, and the degree of lethality.
- Ask about the child's support system and available resources.
- Discuss the need for protection and measures for prevention.

---

degree of lethality of a plan (if one exists), the intensity and frequency of thoughts about suicide, the quality and availability of resources and social supports for the child, and the child's ability to negotiate other ways of managing problems and feelings.

Commonly used highly lethal methods of suicide include using a gun (and having one available), jumping from a height, hanging, crashing in an automobile, carbon monoxide poisoning, and taking prescription sleeping pills. Children and adolescents often plan to run in front of a bus, truck, or train. Methods low in lethality include cutting wrists and taking nonprescription drugs (including aspirin and acetaminophen) or low-potency tranquilizers. All children who may be at risk should be evaluated.

Nursing Diagnoses and Outcomes

In addition to the nursing diagnoses presented in Nursing Plan of Care 29-1, the most important nursing diagnosis is related to the degree of risk for self-directed harm. Nursing diagnoses specific to the child with suicidal ideation include the following:

Nursing Diagnosis: Risk for self-harm related to hopelessness and/or powerlessness
Outcomes:
- Child or adolescent will not be exposed to or ingest dangerous substances.
- Child or adolescent will understand and accept the need for self-protection.

Nursing Diagnosis: Chronic low or situational low self-esteem related to feelings of inadequacy or perceptions of other's negative feedback
Outcomes:
- Child or adolescent will voice feelings related to self-esteem.
- Child or adolescent will engage in interventions and interactions with others that promote positive self-esteem.
- Child or adolescent will identify options other than suicide to stop emotional pain.
- Child or adolescent will use problem-solving skills to identify ways to cope with feelings.
- Child or adolescent will use adult support and resources when feeling helpless and despondent.

Nursing Diagnosis: Risk for suicide related to emotional distress and feelings of low self-worth

Outcomes:
- Child or adolescent will not harm self.
- Child or adolescent will report suicidal thoughts to others.

Interdisciplinary Interventions

The primary short-term goal is to ensure the child's safety and prevent self-harm. Nursing intervention must include referral to the appropriate resources. First and foremost, notify the child's family (parents, guardian). Referral for emergency care, such as psychiatric assessment and crisis intervention, may also be warranted. In some cases, the child may need to be hospitalized.

Community Care

School nurses should participate in educational programs for the community, families, school personnel, and children and implement strategies for suicide prevention (Chart 29-6). Suicide prevention contracts are a good idea after a relationship is established and the assessment is completed and before terminating the assessment session. The contract is best written by the child. The nurse may suggest sentences, words, and resources. The contract must be dated and signed by the child and the nurse. School-based prevention programs have proved effective, even with high-risk groups (Stein et al., 2010).

CHART 29-6   Strategies for Preventing Youth Suicide

- Train school and community leaders to identify young persons at highest risk for suicidal thoughts, threats, and attempts
- Educate young persons about suicide, risk factors, and interventions
- Implement screening and referral programs
- Develop peer support programs
- Establish and operate suicide crisis centers and hotlines
- Restrict access to highly lethal methods of suicide
- Intervene after a suicide to prevent other young persons from attempting or completing suicide

Suicide often raises fear in a community because of its contagion effect. Suicide contagion occurs when one suicide initiates a cluster of subsequent suicidal behaviors among the contacts of that person. Contagion effect can be seen in schools, communities, or inpatient settings. To prevent contagion effects, experts recommend friends, siblings, and classmates of the person who commits suicide receive immediate crisis intervention by mental health experts.

Few school systems have enough professional mental health personnel to successfully manage this type of crisis. It is, therefore, imperative that school systems make formal links with mental health agencies to handle school crises. In addition to these links, each school system should have a well-developed holistic plan to handle the dynamics of such a family and community crises.

The strategic plan used to respond to suicide (attempt or completion) in schools should include family contact; family support; interventions with siblings, peers, and classmates; and a list of local referral sources already linked to the system. Additional considerations include an organized method for early identification and referral of at-risk individuals, community and mental health partners/consultants, media campaigns, staff support and training, and an internal communication action plan.

IMPULSE CONTROL DISORDERS

Impulse control disorders are characterized by impaired inhibition to resist an impulse to perform an act that is harmful to self or others. Impulse control disorders include conduct disorder and ODD.

CONDUCT DISORDER

Conduct disorder is defined as persistent and repetitive patterns of behavior in which the rights of others are ignored and social norms and rules are violated. Anxiety and feelings are externalized and result in harmful behavior toward others. The behavior may be observed in a variety of settings (home, school, community) and interactions. For example, the child may act aggressively with the interviewer while denying his or her aggressive behavior. These children tend to use others as a scapegoat, initiate fights, and often use dangerous objects (sticks, hard objects, broken glass, knives, or guns). Their behavior may involve stealing, setting fires or otherwise destroying property, rape, assault, and, in the disorder's severest form, homicide. Lying, deceitfulness, and a lack of accountability for their behavior are characteristic of children with conduct disorder. Conduct disorder is a common reason that children are referred for mental health care.

Actual etiologic factors are unknown, but one of the most frequently cited characteristics of children with conduct disorder is temperament (the habitual style of reaction to situations). Other risk factors include parental factors (mental illness, criminal behavior, or conduct disorder behavior), abusive and coercive behavior toward the child by the family, learning disability or ADHD, substance abuse, intrauterine insults, neurologic impairment or injury, and frequent observance of crime or domestic violence, especially abuse of the mother.

The incidence of conduct disorder varies by gender and age. The range for males was 0.5% to 2.8% in childhood and 3.2% to 5.4% in 13- to 15-year-olds; for girls, the rate is under 1% in childhood and ranged from 1.4% to 3.3% in 13- to 15-year-olds (Keenan et al., 2010). Conduct disorder was found to be significantly more common in boys than girls and increased in prevalence with age (Fairchild et al., 2011). Two developmental pathways appear to exist: one beginning during childhood and one during adolescence. Most children with adolescent onset have a good chance of becoming responsible and productive adults (Leve et al., 2012).

Assessment

Assessment of the youth with conduct disorder is complex. A physical examination, including a neurologic examination, is recommended. Include the data outlined in Focused Health History 29-1. In addition, ask about possible involvement in gangs, cults, or unlawful behavior and previous involvement with law and justice systems. Ask directly if there has been any involvement in sexual behavior (coercive or noncoercive), childhood sexual abuse perpetrated by another, and/or foster care placements.

The types of acts committed and the situational context of the behavior (e.g., being involved with a gang or older group involved in crime, response to abusive behavior) should be clearly defined. Children with conduct disorders may have a previous or current diagnosis of learning disability, ADHD, or ODD. Assess the child for depression, suicidal or high-risk (self-harm) behaviors, and the intent or thought of bringing harm to others.

Conduct disorder must be differentiated from aggressive episodes caused by psychomotor seizures, brain injury, and PTSD. The aggressive outbursts occurring in these disorders are random and spontaneous, whereas the aggression of a child with a conduct disorder is more consistent and predictable. Conduct disorder is also not "delinquency." Delinquency implies committing criminal or illegal acts; it is a legal term. *Conduct disorder* is a diagnostic term. The behavior of the individual being assessed may indeed include acts that are illegal. The acts committed may include aggression toward people and animals, destruction of property, deceitfulness or theft, or serious violation of rules established in the home or by the school system.

Interdisciplinary Interventions

Interventions for children with conduct disorder include individual therapy, milieu therapy, recreational therapy, group therapy, family therapy, and social skills therapy. In some severe cases, the child may be placed in a special classroom where behavior can be more easily contained. A primary goal is to ensure that such children no longer harm others or seek to harm themselves. Remove all potentially harmful objects from the child's environment.

▌**A L E R T**   *Youths with conduct disorder who have comorbid depression are at very high risk for suicide. Implement suicide precautions.*

In the inpatient setting, place the child in a secure environment to prevent the child from running away. Develop a behavioral management contract with the child that includes safety expectations and sanctions for violations of these expectations. Pharmacologic interventions, dispensed and monitored by the nurse, may be used to control excessive violence or to treat underlying depression.

To help children reduce feelings of anger and rage, therapy focuses on teaching new problem-solving and stress management techniques. Children must learn to reinterpret the behaviors of others and ask questions to clarify the intent of others' behaviors to reduce their own feelings of threat or harm. Feelings of inadequacy potentiate the aggressive behavior. Therefore, children must learn to interact with others in nondefensive ways. In addition, children are encouraged to have a realistic view of self and to accept responsibility for their own behaviors. Group therapy can be used to focus on the communication skills of listening, reflecting, giving and receiving feedback, sharing feelings, expressing needs, and expressing desires in an assertive manner (Clinical Judgment 29-2).

OPPOSITIONAL DEFIANT DISORDER

ODD is a pattern of negative, resistant, and hostile behavior occurring in 1% to 16% of youths 7 to 21 years of age (Loeber et al., 2000; Steiner & Remsing, 2007). It is usually manifested after early childhood and before

---

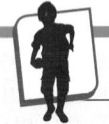

CLINICAL JUDGMENT 29-2

The Child With Conduct Disorder

Nancy is 13 years old and has a history of sexual abuse starting at 7 years of age. The perpetrator was 14 years old at the time, and the sexual abuse occurred over several months. Nancy is the older of two siblings. Her mother and father are divorced and she lives with her mother. Her father was injured in a hunting accident 3 years ago and has been a paraplegic since the accident. He wants to return home to live with his ex-wife and children. Nancy was referred by the school counselor to the community mental health center when she was 9 years old. She was seen three times and was then enrolled in an after-school learning improvement program by her mother. Since age 9 years, Nancy has had five inpatient psychiatric hospitalizations for behavioral problems. Nancy was recently admitted to the state hospital youth unit. She was expelled from school because of repeated assaults on younger children, persistently destroying books and papers of other students (which she denied), and, finally, because of physically assaulting one of her teachers. Nancy's mother reported that, during the past year, Nancy had killed her younger brother's two rabbits, deliberately broken several objects at home when enraged, and repeatedly stolen money from her mother and brother. Most recently, her mother found a stash of sharp knives, a baseball bat, and bullets (no gun) under Nancy's bed. Nancy's mother said that she was totally unable to control Nancy and said, "I hope you find a place for her where everyone will be safe from her." Nancy's mother has been treated for depression for the past 6 years. She compared Nancy with Nancy's father, saying, "She just doesn't care who or what she hurts, just like her father."

Questions

1. Is Nancy's family at risk for violence at this time?
2. Which of Nancy's behaviors indicate a conduct disorder?
3. What goal must take first priority at this time?
4. What nursing interventions will assist Nancy and her family in meeting this goal?
5. During therapy, what should be the outcomes for the behaviors displayed by Nancy?

Answers

1. The family is at risk. Nancy has the potential to harm a family member.
2. She often bullies, threatens, or intimidates others; she often initiates physical fights; she has been physically cruel to animals; she has deliberately destroyed others' property; she has stolen items of nontrivial value without confronting a victim.
3. Ensure the safety of others.
4. Teach Nancy conflict resolution skills, help Nancy practice appropriate expression of anger, routinely assess and remove potential weapons from Nancy and her environment, and work with Nancy to improve her self-esteem.
5. Positive rewards should be given for positive behavior; developmentally appropriate consequences should be given for negative behavior.

puberty. However, some of the behaviors are seen during the early childhood years. During the prepubertal years, the disorder is more common in boys, but equal gender prevalence is seen in adolescence. ODD often develops gradually, with increasing expressions of defiance, negativism, argumentativeness, loss of temper, and hostility.

DSM-5 criteria preclude a diagnosis of ODD in children who meet the criteria for conduct disorder; therefore, these incidence figures greatly underestimate the occurrence of clinically important oppositional behaviors in this population (Fahim et al., 2012). A child with ODD, particularly one who engages in physical aggression, has an extremely high likelihood of later being diagnosed with conduct disorder.

Causative factors, or factors with a strong correlation to ODD, are irritable temperament, history of abusive treatment, and ineffective coping strategies (e.g., projection, denial of own feelings, pain, hurt, or sadness). ODD is also commonly comorbid with mood disorders, anxiety disorders, and ADHD (Aebi et al., 2010).

Potential outcomes for children with ODD vary. In many cases, without early and effective treatment, conduct disorder and even criminal behavior ensue, resulting in incarceration. Other, less severe problems include academic difficulties or failure and continuous peer conflict, which may result in injury. These children often create enough family stress that treatment is sought; conflicts related to this stress may also precipitate parental separation and divorce.

Families often react to ODD with rigidly controlling and authoritarian behavior, which becomes increasingly detrimental as the child's opposition increases.

Assessment

To be diagnosed with ODD, the child must exhibit certain behaviors for 6 months or longer (Chart 29-7). When analyzing and synthesizing the assessment data, consider the developmental status of the child: Are any of the behaviors and concerns considered normal for the child's age or as a result of parenting style?

Evaluate children with ODD for depression. The underlying problem may be continuous, unmanageable life stresses and multiple losses. Dysthymia or

depressive traits may mimic ODD. ODD is also strongly associated with anxiety disorders. Mismanagement and lack of recognition of these underlying problems may lead to ODD.

Interdisciplinary Interventions

Counseling or problem-solving therapy with a mental health therapist is recommended. Nursing care includes working with the child and family to improve communication, problem-solving, and negotiation skills. Group therapy designed to develop listening, open communication, problem-solving, and perspective-taking skills is beneficial in helping these children to express themselves in more appropriate ways.

Therapeutic communication and behavior management techniques are helpful in decreasing resistance and stubborn refusal to engage in or complete expected activities. Teach family members behavior management strategies for communicating and negotiating with their child with ODD. School interventions include providing teachers with information about the disorder and teaching behavior management techniques.

Interdisciplinary intervention for ODD may also include medication. Many children show some improvement in mood and behavior when given an SSRI (see Table 29-1). After several attempts and minimal responsiveness to the interventions described, placement in a therapeutic foster home or residential facility may be necessary to relieve family stress and break the cycle of control and opposition.

SUBSTANCE ABUSE

Substance abuse is defined as a pattern of continued and inappropriate use of substances that causes substantial emotional, psychological, and physiologic effects. Marijuana is the illicit drug most widely used by children and adolescents (Behrendt et al., 2009). Use of inhalants such as butane, glue, aerosols, paint, and computer cleaner is increasing, however, and is being seen in younger children. Substance use often begins as early as age 12 years (grade 7) (Leatherdale & Burkhalter, 2012) (Chart 29-8).

Most adolescents are poorly informed about the effects of substance abuse. Adolescents and children who are using substances in a continuous and inappropriate way may experience repeated failure in school, difficulty in sports and social relationships, and conflict with the legal system. Youths who abuse substances are at increased risk for displays of aggression, being the recipient of aggressive acts, serious accidents, and homicide and suicide.

Assessment

The assessment goals for children and adolescents suspected of substance use and/or abuse include identifying the level of involvement, identifying motivating factors for beginning treatment, and matching their needs to the appropriate level and method of treatment (see Chart 29-9 for signs of substance use/abuse). As substance use progresses, signs become increasingly obvious and interpersonal problems heighten.

CHART 29-7 Diagnostic Criteria for Oppositional Defiant Disorder

Must exhibit at least four of the behaviors for at least 6 months.

Often loses temper

Often argues with adults

Often actively defies or refuses to comply with adults' requests or rules

Often deliberately annoys people

Often blames others for his or her mistakes or misbehavior

Is often touchy or easily annoyed by others

Is often angry and resentful

Is often spiteful or vindictive

CHART 29-8   Risk Factors for Substance Abuse

- Early age at first use
- Poor school performance
- High value for independence
- External locus of control
- Poor self-esteem
- Favorable attitude toward use of psychoactive substances
- High risk-taking behavior pattern
- Poor social skills
- Sexual and physical abuse
- Aggressive or impulsive behavior patterns
- Peer group influence
- Family influence (approval, exposure, abuse)
- Presence of psychiatric disorder, especially depression

Gather information from school, family, and peers about the child's activities and behaviors to note any recent changes in behaviors or issues that may influence the current abuse activities. Alcohol use (beer, wine) and cigarette smoking are early indicators of potential substance abuse; alcohol and tobacco are considered "gateway" substances.

When interviewing the child and family, ask direct, specific questions (Chart 29-10). If the adolescent resists talking or sharing information, asking for information about peers and being nonjudgmental about their behavior may assist in gathering information about the adolescent's own abuse. Question the family in the presence of the child to convey support of open, honest communication; both the family and child often deny the scope of the problem.

CHART 29-9   Signs and Symptoms of Substance Use/Abuse*

- Reddened eyes
- Dilated/pinpoint pupils
- Runny or stuffy nose (constant)
- Gastrointestinal upset (diarrhea)
- Weight loss or gain, change in eating habits
- Signs of needle tracks
- Slurred speech
- Unusual sleep patterns
- Restlessness or drowsiness, hallucinations or disorientation
- Awkward or clumsy physical movement, tremors
- Frequent minor illnesses (flu, colds)
- Change in friends; withdrawal from friends, activities, and family
- History of bizarre behavior
- Diminished academic performance

*Depending on the substance being abused; symptoms can be manifested in many different levels of intoxication and withdrawal.

CHART 29-10   Information to Obtain When Interviewing the Child/Adolescent About Substance Abuse

- Personal strengths of the child
- Coping strategies previously used successfully
- Dietary habits
- Use of over-the-counter medications
- Use of prescribed medications
- Use of other substances
  - Smoking cigarettes
  - Use of beer, wine, and other alcoholic drinks
  - Smoking marijuana
  - Use of other substances (e.g., inhalants, cocaine)

If substance use is revealed

- When used/surrounding what other activities (especially if participating in activities that require mental concentration such as driving, school, work)
- Where used
- With whom

Diagnostic Tests

Urine screening detects marijuana for up to 3 to 4 weeks after use. Other substances are present in urine for only 1 to 2 days after use. Adolescents who are using or abusing substances will strongly resist providing urine for a drug screen; they may question the examiner's trust in them or feign embarrassment.

Nursing Diagnoses and Outcomes

In addition to the nursing diagnoses and outcomes presented in Nursing Plan of Care 29-1, the following diagnoses can be applied to the child using substances:

Nursing Diagnosis: Decisional conflict: Substance use related to support system deficit, peer pressure, poor coping skills, and unclear personal values
Outcomes:
- Child or adolescent will express feelings about substance use.
- Child or adolescent will describe family, school, and peer issues and their potential effect on his or her substance use.
- Child or adolescent will make choices that are consistent with his or her personal values and are legally sanctioned.

Nursing Diagnosis: Risk for overdose related to substance abuse
Outcomes:
- Child or adolescent will express understanding of the harmful and potentially lethal effects of alcohol, tobacco products, and drugs.

- Child or adolescent will identify stressors or triggers that are likely to precipitate an episode of substance use.
- Child or adolescent will not ingest alcohol, tobacco products, or illegal drugs.

Interdisciplinary Interventions

A variety of methods are used to treat substance use and abuse in youths, and a variety of disciplines may be involved. The services actually provided depend on a number of factors, including the child's socioeconomic status, the length and severity of the problem, who may be harmed by the abuse, and what symptoms are exhibited by the individual child.

Education should be provided by persons with an understanding of the brain–body connection and the effects of alcohol or other abused substances on the body, its organs, neurotransmitters, brain cells, and observable behavior. Cognitive therapy with a strong confrontational component is used in individual and group therapy. Motivational therapy is a harm-reducing/problem-solving approach that helps the adolescent identify problems that the use of alcohol or drugs causes for him or her as well as reduce alcohol or drug use (Ramchand et al., 2011).

Family therapy is essential. The family must come to grips with any communication and nurturing deficits. A very structured and supportive environment is needed to assist the individual to remain drug free.

A three-pronged approach including education about substances, adult supervision when not in school, and the development of skills to resist peers and family members who may urge drug use has proved useful to prevent substance use by children and adolescents (Winters et al., 2011). Most children and adolescents are exposed to substance use by peers or by family members, such as older siblings and parents.

The nurse can educate and promote skills to resist drug use. These skills can include helping children and adolescents identify situations in which they are at high risk to use substances as well as assist them in finding ways to avoid or modify such situations. Additionally, the nurse can assist with developing a repertoire of cognitive and behavioral skills for modifying routine responses to high-risk situations, thus reducing the risk for substance use. Adaptive actions might be to talk with friends, attend a support group, or do something physical, such as play basketball.

CHILD ABUSE, NEGLECT, AND EMOTIONAL MALTREATMENT

Child abuse is a global problem, deeply rooted in cultural, social, and economic practices. The abuse of children and adolescents is so widespread no one knows its full cost. The effects of child maltreatment are profound: It is linked to most mental illnesses and addictions and causes human suffering; family disruption; increased violence; participation in gangs; absenteeism from work; lifelong unemployment; financial costs from acute and chronic hospitalization; welfare dependency; addictions; deaths from suicide, murder, and drunk driving; and perpetuation of the abuse on future generations.

Child abuse includes physical abuse, sexual abuse, neglect, and emotional or psychological abuse (Table 29-2). Children may be subjected to more than one type of maltreatment, and emotional abuse is usually a component of the other forms of abuse. Physical abuse suffered during childhood has been found to contribute substantially to psychological and physical problems in adulthood (Lansford et al., 2010). Child sexual abuse is covered in a separate section. This section will focus on physical abuse, neglect, and emotional maltreatment.

Each country and each state in the United States has its own legal definitions of physical abuse, neglect, and sexual abuse. Some definitions are more specific than others. For example, some states limit prosecution only to parents, excluding other perpetrators such as neighbors or other family members. Many definitions of abuse and neglect, which use phrases such as *resulting in bodily injury*, *deviant sexual conduct*, and *compelled by force or imminent threat of force* are vague and open to interpretation.

If health care professionals and individual states cannot reach consensus on definitions of abuse, it is difficult for professionals to exercise any authority in removing children to safer environments or in treating the victims and abusers. These unclear definitions, and the difficulty they create in substantiating abuse, create a system in which the abused child is often left in danger and untreated.

From 1992 to 2011, the rates of physical abuse declined 56%; sexual abuse, 63%; and neglect, 11% (Finkelhor et al., 2013). However, the number of deaths from

TABLE 29-2	Types of Child Abuse
Category	**Description**
Physical abuse	An injury intentionally inflicted on a child by a caregiver, paramour of a parent, or anyone residing in the child's home
Sexual abuse	The use of a child for sexual gratification or financial gain, by an adult or older child, whether by physical force, coercion, or persuasion; includes activities such as exhibitionism, pornography, genital fondling, attempted or actual anal, vaginal, or oral intercourse
Neglect	Acts or omissions by the perpetrator that fail to meet the child's needs for basic living, including food, hygiene, medical care, clothing, and a safe environment
Emotional or psychological abuse	Pattern of damaging interactions between parents and child (belittling, shaming, threatening or committing violence against the child or child's loved ones or objects, making the child feel unsafe, encouraging developmentally inappropriate behaviors, unreasonably limiting activities or social interactions, rejecting the child) that result in impaired growth, negative self-image, or disturbed child behavior

maltreatment did not change. Because many child deaths are not investigated, it is difficult to know the true extent of the problem. The highest rates of fatal child abuse are found among children aged birth to 4 years, with the most common cause of death being head injury, followed by abdominal injuries and intentional suffocation (Finkelhor et al., 2013). Millions of children are victims of nonfatal abuse and neglect. Rates of abuse and neglect vary by country, with 25% to 50% of children reporting physical abuse worldwide and 20% of women and 5% to 10% of men reporting sexual abuse when a child (WHO, 2010).

In the United States in 2011, an estimated 681,000 children were victims of maltreatment, a slight decrease from 2007 (723,000 victims) (U.S. DHHS, Administration on Children, Youth and Families, 2011). Neglect is the most common form of maltreatment. In 2011, 78% of victims were neglected, 17.6% were physically abused, and 9.1% were sexually abused (U.S. DHHS, Administration on Children, Youth and Families, 2011). In 2011, there were an estimated 1,570 child fatalities resulting from abuse and neglect, a slight decrease from 2007 (1,608 child fatalities) and 2009 (1,685 child fatalities) (U.S. DHHS, Administration on Children, Youth and Families). Children younger than 4 years old were the most vulnerable to fatalities. Various cultural norms, lack or fear of reporting, no other children in the home, and a number of other factors are believed to severely underestimate child adolescent maltreatment.

Vulnerability to child abuse depends, in part, on the child's age and sex (Chart 29-11). Young children between birth and 2 years of age are most at risk of physical abuse, and girls are at greater risk of sexual abuse than boys (U.S. DHHS, Administration on Children, Youth and Families, 2011). Perpetrators of abuse are often a mother acting alone (36.8%), a father acting alone (19%), both parents (18.9%), or a nonparent (12.8%) (U.S. DHHS, Administration on Children, Youth and Families, 2011).

Assessment

The effects of physical abuse, emotional abuse, and neglect are enormous and manifest in multiple ways. Emotional abuse may be inflicted without physical injury to the child, but it is what most seriously affects children. Children may also be physically or sexually abused, but the psychological impact of the abuse remains with the child after the bruises, burns, and broken bones have healed, often leading to a variety of psychological responses.

Many abused children respond in a manner that goes unnoticed by most adults, such as extreme efforts to please, withdrawal, and generalized anxiety. During assessment, in addition to physical signs, note the child's behavior. Behaviors that should raise suspicion of abuse include being wary of adults, cringing with sudden movements, apathy, excessive daydreaming, any signs of anxiety or depression, not turning to the parent for support, attentive to other children crying, poor hygiene (e.g., dirty, severe diaper rash, skin rash), and unusual dress (Is it appropriate for the weather? Long sleeves and pants may be worn to cover injuries even

CHART 29-11 Risk Factors for Child Maltreatment

Child
- Prematurity
- Difficult temperament
- Chronic illness
- Multiple birth
- Developmental or physical disabilities

Parent
- Poor impulse control and problem-solving skills
- Low self-esteem
- Mental health conditions
- Developmental delay
- Unrealistic/rigid expectations about child's needs and development
- Negative perception of child and child's actions
- History of childhood abuse

Family
- Social isolation
- Homelessness
- Disorganized, lack of cohesion
- Intimate partner violence
- Negative parent–child interactions
- Socioeconomic disadvantage: poverty, unemployment
- Stress
- Substance abuse
- Unrelated male adult living in the home

Community
- Violence
- Lack of support (child care, crisis intervention services)
- Socioeconomically disadvantaged

in warm weather; dirty clothing or inadequate attire for the weather may signal neglect).

Additional effects of abuse and neglect on school performance include a lack of motivation to achieve, fear of failure, an inability to establish positive relationships with unfamiliar adults, poor performance on standardized tests, lower grades, higher dependence on teachers, more trips out of the classroom as a result of behavioral problems, more suspensions, and lower social competence.

Assessment guidelines for signs of physical abuse are listed in Nursing Interventions Classification 29-1. Assess injuries in the context of medical, social, and developmental history; the explanation given; and the patterns of injury. Specific areas of the body are associated with accidental injury; other areas, with nonaccidental injury (Fig. 29-3). Bruises in nonmobile infants, over soft-tissue areas, and those that resemble an implement (e.g., loop marks of a hanger or doubled-over belt, linear petechiae resembling fingers on a cheek) suggest abuse.

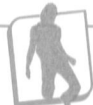

NIC 29-1 NURSING INTERVENTIONS CLASSIFICATION: Abuse Protection Support: Child

Definition: Identification of high-risk, dependent child relationships and actions to prevent possible or further infliction of physical, sexual, or emotional harm or neglect of basic necessities of life

Activities:

Identify mothers who have a history of no or late (4 months or later) prenatal care

Identify parents who have had another child removed from the home or have placed previous children with relatives for extended periods

Identify parents who have a history of substance abuse, depression, or major psychiatric illness

Identify parents who demonstrate an increased need for parent education (e.g., parents with learning problems, parents who verbalize feelings of inadequacy, parents of a first child, teen parents)

Identify parents with a history of domestic violence or a mother who has a history of numerous "accidental" injuries

Identify parents with a history of unhappy childhoods associated with abuse, rejection, excessive criticism, or feelings of being worthless and unloved

Identify crisis situations that may trigger abuse (e.g., poverty, unemployment, divorce, homelessness, and domestic violence)

Determine whether the family has an intact social support network to assist with family problems, respite child care, and crisis child care

Identify infants and children with high-care needs (e.g., prematurity, low birth weight, colic, feeding intolerances, major health problems in the first year of life, developmental disabilities, hyperactivity, and attention deficit disorders)

Identify caregiver explanations of child's injuries that are improbable or inconsistent, allege self-injury, blame other children, or demonstrate a delay in seeking treatment

Determine whether a child demonstrates signs of physical abuse (e.g. numerous injuries, unexplained bruises and welts, burns, fractures, unexplained facial lacerations and abrasions, human bite marks, whiplash, shaken baby syndrome)

Determine whether the child demonstrates signs of neglect (e.g. failure to thrive, wasting of subcutaneous tissue, consistent hunger, poor hygiene, constant fatigue and listlessness, skin afflictions, apathy, unyielding body posture, inappropriate dress for weather conditions)

Determine whether the child demonstrates signs of sexual abuse (e.g., difficulty walking or sitting, torn or bloody underclothing, reddened or traumatized genitals, vaginal or anal lacerations, recurrent urinary tract infections, poor sphincter tone, acquired sexually transmitted infections, pregnancy, promiscuous behavior, history of running away)

Determine whether the child demonstrates signs of emotional abuse (e.g. lags in physical development, habit disorders, conduct learning disorders, neurotic traits or psychoneurotic reactions, behavioral extremes, cognitive developmental lags, attempted suicide)

Encourage admission of child for further observation and investigation, as appropriate

Record times and durations of visits during hospitalizations

Monitor parent–child interactions and record observations

Determine whether acute symptoms in child abate when child is separated from family

Determine whether parents have unrealistic expectations for child's behavior or negative attributions for their child's behavior

Monitor child for extreme compliance, such as passive submission to invasive procedures

Monitor child for role reversal, such as comforting the parent, or overactive or aggressive behavior

Listen to pregnant woman's feelings about pregnancy and expectations about the unborn child

Monitor new parents' reactions to their infant, observing for feelings of disgust, fear, or disappointment in gender

Monitor for a parent who holds newborn at arm's length, handles newborn awkwardly, asks for excessive assistance, and verbalizes or demonstrates discomfort in caring for the child

Monitor for repeated visits to clinics, emergency rooms, or physicians' offices for minor problems

Establish a system to flag the records of children who are suspected victims of child abuse or neglect

Monitor for a progressive deterioration in the physical and emotional state of the infant or child

Determine parent's knowledge of basic care needs and provide appropriate child care information, as indicated

Instruct parents on problem solving, decision making, and child-rearing and parenting skills, or refer parents to programs where these skills can be learned

Help families identify coping strategies for stressful situations

Provide parents with information on how to cope with protracted infant crying, emphasizing that they should never shake the baby

Provide the parents with noncorporal punishment methods for disciplining children

Provide pregnant women and their families with information on the effects of smoking, poor nutrition, and substance abuse on the baby's health and their own

Engage parents and child in attachment-building exercises

Provide parents and their adolescents with information on decision-making and communication skills, and refer to youth services counseling, as appropriate

Provide older children with concrete information on how to provide for the basic care needs of their younger siblings

Provide children with positive affirmations of their worth, nurturing care, therapeutic communication, and developmental stimulation

Provide children who have been sexually abused with reassurance that the abuse was not their fault, and allow them to express their concerns through play therapy appropriate for age

Refer at-risk pregnant women and parents of newborns to nurse home visitation services

Provide at-risk families with a Public Health Nurse referral to ensure that the home environment is monitored, that

(Continued)

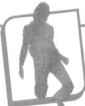

NIC 29-1 NURSING INTERVENTIONS CLASSIFICATION: Abuse Protection Support: Child *(Continued)*

siblings are assessed, and that families receive continued assistance

Refer families to human services and counseling professionals, as needed

Provide parents with community resource information (e.g., addresses and phone numbers of agencies that provide respite care, emergency child care, housing assistance, substance abuse treatment, sliding-fee counseling services, food pantries, clothing distribution centers, domestic abuse shelters)

Inform physician of observations indicative of abuse or neglect

Report suspected abuse or neglect to proper authorities

Refer a parent who is being battered and at-risk children to a domestic violence shelter

Refer parents to Parents Anonymous for group support, as appropriate

From Bulechek, G. M., Butcher, H. K., Dochterman, J. M. et al. (Eds.). (2013). *Nursing interventions classifications (NIC)* (6th ed.). St. Louis, MO: Mosby. Used with permission.

CROSS-CULTURAL CARE

Healing practices common in some cultures can resemble child abuse (see Cross-Cultural Care, Chinese Folk Practices, in Chapter 25), and injuries caused by these practices may warrant further investigation. Such practices can often be distinguished from abuse based on history and physical examination. Ask the family what was done to treat the child.

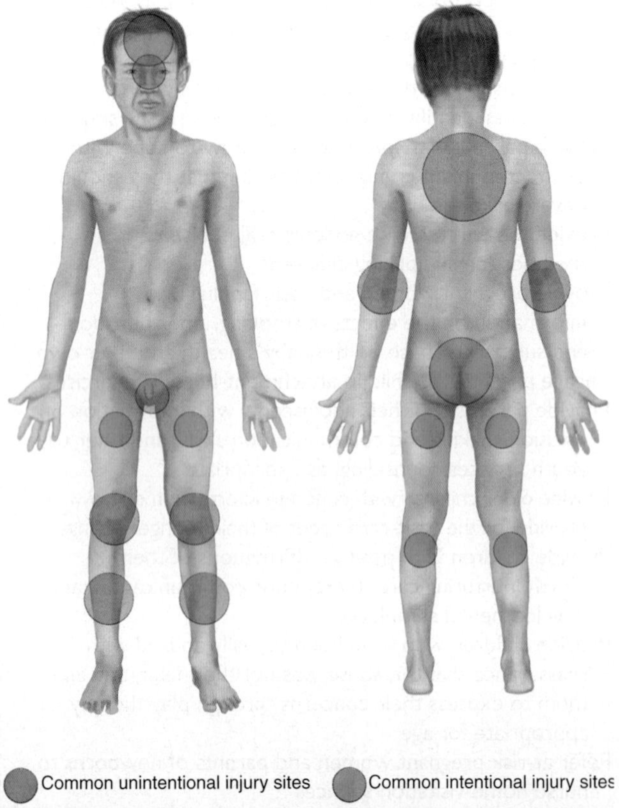

Some medical conditions may mimic a clinical picture (e.g., bruises with leukemia or idiopathic thrombocytopenic purpura) or skeletal findings that are associated with abuse (e.g., osteogenesis imperfecta, congenital syphilis, scurvy, rickets, and copper deficiency). Be cognizant of these conditions, and include health history questions and explore laboratory and diagnostic studies as indicated.

Diagnostic Tests

Diagnostic evaluation of child abuse depends on the symptoms and history. A primary screening tool in suspected abuse is a radiographic survey, including skull series, extremities (including hands and feet), and ribs. A bone scan is recommended when the skeletal survey is negative but a strong clinical suggestion of injury exists. Computed tomography and MRI may be ordered, depending on the symptoms. Ultrasonography may be done if visceral injury is suspected.

If abdominal trauma is suspected, urine and stool should be screened for blood. Blood studies should include bleeding studies to rule out a bleeding diathesis; serum calcium, phosphorus, and alkaline phosphatase if bone disease is a possibility; and liver and pancreatic enzymes if damage to these organs is suspected.

ALERT *Children who have been sexually abused must be evaluated for STIs. Conversely, if an STI is found in a prepubescent child or a sexually inactive adolescent, one must strongly consider sexual abuse.*

Identification of abuse of a child does not automatically lead to a psychiatric diagnosis for that child. Only if and when a child has demonstrated behavioral manifestations meeting *DSM* criteria can a diagnosis be made. Even when a diagnosis is thought to be related to unresolved factors precipitated by abuse, diagnoses are made solely based on the behavioral manifestations. Common diagnoses for abused children include conduct disorder, major depressive disorder, borderline personality disorder, and ODD.

● Common unintentional injury sites ● Common intentional injury sites

Figure 29-3 Unintentional injuries are typically seen in specific sites (purple areas). The nurse should suspect physical abuse in children with injuries in intentional injury sites (red areas).

Interdisciplinary Interventions

The nurse is obligated to report *suspicion* of abuse or neglect to the proper authorities; this does not require the nurse to *prove* the abuse or neglect has occurred. Often, reporting involves a judgment call on the part of the nurse. The purpose of reporting is to protect the child and others who may be at risk and to help the family. Mandated reporters are provided immunity from civil or criminal liability as a result of making a required report of known or suspected child abuse, unless reporting is done with malicious intent.

Mandated reporters who fail to report suspicious findings may be subject to criminal prosecution and sanctions imposed by licensing boards. Each state has a form for reporting suspected abuse or neglect (check with the state's attorney general's office); this form may also be used for reporting suspected medical neglect.

Treatment includes managing the acute condition. According to existing literature, nurses can perform several interventions thought to be successful in helping the child cope with the abuse (Nursing Interventions 29-7).

NURSING INTERVENTIONS 29-7

Abused and Neglected Children and Adolescents

Teach child anxiety-reducing techniques:
- Gradual relaxation (blowing bubbles helps with young children)
- Relaxation to music
- Visual imagery
- Exercise
- Talking with safe, appropriate people about feelings
- Choosing, building, and maintaining positive support systems
- Ensuring personal safety
- Setting boundaries
- Establishing a safe, supportive relationship
- Clarifying expectations and rules
- Self-soothing techniques

Assist child in managing his or her feelings; teach child to
- Identify feelings
- Express feelings appropriately
- Modulate and control feelings
- Identify events that elicit strong positive and negative feelings
- Express feelings verbally instead of physically
- Normalize feelings resulting from abuse
- Share feelings appropriately with peer group
- Find commonality and support within group for feelings resulting from abuse

Teach child assertiveness skills; teach child to
- Identify differences between assertiveness, passivity, and aggression
- Practice assertiveness skills
- Identify boundaries
- Understand when someone violates boundaries
- Practice responses when someone violates boundaries

Assist child in developing problem-solving skills:
- Provide simple problem-solving model.
- Increase awareness of child's control and decision making.
- Teach child to generate a list of possible solutions to problem situations.
- Help child look at consequences of each solution.
- Help child make best choice.
- Help child give self-positive and gentle negative feedback.
- Coach problem solving with actual situations as much as possible.
- Teach good touch/bad touch.
- Teach refusal skills.

Teach age-appropriate sexual expression.
Teach effects of substance abuse.
Assist child in value building and clarification:
- Define values.
- Identify role of values.
- Assist child in identifying and verbalizing values.
- Help link child's values to child's actions.
- Assist child in development of values.
- Help child practice value-based decision making.

Assist child in enhancing his or her coping mechanisms:
- Teach child to practice positive self-talk.
- Help child set realistic expectations for self.
- Assist child in learning to nurture self.
- Teach child to practice relaxation.
- Teach child to practice assertiveness and appropriate expression of feelings.
- Assist child in learning to accept defeat and failure.
- Help child identify and build skills and hobbies.
- Encourage child to identify and focus on strengths.
- Help child set and accomplish goals.
- Assist child in developing organizational skills.

Without accusing the family, tell them child protective services are being notified (e.g., "The symptoms are . . ., indicating they may not be accidental"). Encouraging the family to ask questions about the report may help the family to understand the process and anticipate social work visits and calls at home. Emphasize that the priority is to ensure the child's safety and well-being.

Provide emotional and social support for the family. Refer the family to support groups, self-help groups, or parenting classes, as needed. Remember the goal is to facilitate change so the family can live together as a functional, healthy unit.

CHILD SEXUAL ABUSE

In most cases of sexual abuse, the child knows the perpetrator. Common offenders are parents, step-parents, other adult relatives, trusted family friends, neighbors, or babysitters. Occasionally, more than one family member is involved in sexually abusing the child.

Adult substance abuse and child maltreatment are strongly related. Substance abuse tends to heighten sexual arousal while simultaneously decreasing inhibitions. This combination results in adults being far more aggressive and sexually violent. One in four families is reported to have problems with substance abuse (Hien et al., 2010).

Include a sexual assault assessment in every history of a child or adolescent. Keep in mind that victims often do not easily disclose the abuse and must be supported. Collect evidence within 72 hours of the event to document the occurrence of sexual abuse or assault. To do so, use an evidence kit, available in most emergency departments, that contains the necessary swabs, cultures, tubes, and envelopes to seal the specimens. Send any clothing worn during the abuse or assault with the medical specimens for investigation. For an adolescent who is not pregnant at the time of evaluation and not using birth control, offer postcoital contraception. This treatment is effective only up to 72 hours after the rape.

caREminder

If an abused or assaulted child is referred from your facility to another facility for specimen collection, instruct the child and family not to bathe the child or change his or her clothing until instructed to do so, to ensure evidence from the assault is not destroyed.

One of the most profound and tragic results of sexual abuse occurs when a parent is the abuser and the abuse affects the relationship between the victim and the nonoffending parent (Chart 29-12). Often, the nonoffending parent (in this discussion, the mother) has no knowledge of the sexual abuse until the child discloses it yet is treated with contempt and blame by family, friends, and professionals for "allowing" the abuse to continue. Occasionally, nonoffending parents have some knowledge or suspicion sexual abuse is occurring yet choose to continue to subject their children to

CHART 29-12   Factors That Prevent Children From Disclosing Sexual Abuse

- Child's young age
- Child's developmental level
- Dependency on adults for meeting basic needs
- Shame
- No witnesses to validate the abuse
- No observable physical injuries
- No outward manifestations of the sexual violation
- Disbelief and rejection by adults upon disclosure
- Threats (such as the perpetrator threatening to kill the victim's mother if the victim discloses the abuse)
- Force and aggression used by the perpetrator
- Fear of family breaking up
- Fear of abandonment
- Fear of loss of home
- Fear of foster placement
- Negative effect on the child's relationship with the nonoffending parent
- Parental disbelief and being labeled a "troublemaker"
- Loss of privacy and shame resulting from investigation and court proceedings
- Fear of reprisals, such as worsened physical and sexual abuse
- Fear that child will not be believed

abuse rather than give up their relationship with the perpetrator.

Victims may expect that their mother will always protect them from harm. When she does not, the victims may direct their rage at the mother. Often, the intensely conflicting feelings of love and hate for the actual perpetrator, who has a tremendous amount of power in the child's mind, are too threatening for the child to deal with. It is easier, therefore, for a child to direct the rage at a less threatening person, such as the mother or a younger sibling. Although the child's behavior becomes understandable after the abuse is disclosed, it is extremely difficult to live with on a daily basis.

The nonoffending parent is also thrown into crisis by the events. Often, the mother must terminate an important relationship, perhaps even end a marriage; deal with the stigma of incest; cope with the blame; and deal with the trauma to the child. She is often left to deal with this crisis alone, while simultaneously receiving the brunt of the child's anger.

When abuse is disclosed, the perpetrator is removed from the home. The nonoffending parent then must struggle alone to meet family needs, while attempting to provide the necessary mental health care with less time, money, and resources. It is imperative that the nurse takes a supportive stance rather than blame the nonoffending parent.

SHAKEN BABY SYNDROME

Abusive head injuries among infants result in mortality rates of 13% to 35% and substantial neurologic impairments in at least half of the survivors (Parks et al., 2012). *Shaken baby syndrome* involves intracranial trauma (e.g., subarachnoid or subdural hemorrhage or diffuse cerebral edema) and retinal hemorrhages, usually in the absence of skull fracture or external signs of traumatic injury, caused by vigorously shaking an infant. Shaking causes sudden deceleration of the infant's head, tearing the bridging vessels between the skull and the brain causing hemorrhage.

Other injuries such as fractures of the long bones or ribs may be present but not be readily apparent. The ribs are compliant in young children; therefore, in the absence of a history of accidental trauma bone fragility condition, rib fractures were considered to be pathognomonic of inflicted injury (Reyes et al., 2011). With recent changes in cardiopulmonary resuscitation (CPR) techniques, an increase in CPR-associated rib fractures in infants has been noted (Reyes et al., 2011). Posterior rib fractures are more common in child abuse, caused by the mechanical stress at the costovertebral junction when the child is grasped and shaken.

The child with shaken baby syndrome is typically younger than 2 years of age and commonly presents with complaints of lethargy, seizures, hyperirritability, poor feeding, bulging fontanel, breathing problems, or, in severe instances, coma or cardiopulmonary arrest. Hypothermia is a common finding in these children and is secondary to the occult central nervous system trauma. Consider abuse when presented with a child with encephalopathy without an obvious source.

The child who has been shaken is treated symptomatically. If trauma is suspected, immobilize the cervical spine. Assess airway, breathing, and circulation; support and stabilize; and frequently reassess. Continually monitor the child's neurologic status for signs of increasing intracranial pressure. Because shaking results in traumatic head injury, it is treated in the same way that trauma is managed (see Chapter 31).

MUNCHAUSEN SYNDROME BY PROXY

Munchausen syndrome by proxy, also known as pediatric condition falsification, is a form of medical abuse in which the child is subjected to an "illness" induced or fabricated by a parent or caregiver. The affected parent or caregiver seeks medical care for the child's fictitious illness and provides a fictitious history to support the illness. The fabricated or induced illness often results in the child being subjected to numerous unnecessary, invasive laboratory studies; hospitalizations; or surgeries. The syndrome can result in disability or death of the child.

The child's reported symptoms typically occur only when the parent is present and stop when the parent is not. Most cases present with some sort of neurologic disturbance, such as seizures or apnea. Less common presentations include hematuria, gastrointestinal bleeding, hypernatremia, or hyponatremia. The perpetrator may suffocate the child to produce apnea or seizures or may add his or her own blood to the child's urine or stool sample to fabricate bleeding.

In nearly all cases of Munchausen syndrome by proxy, the mother is the perpetrator and often has a health care background or is well versed in medical terminology (Kucuker et al., 2010; Squires & Squires, 2010). The mother is typically quite attentive to the child and is involved in the child's care but often lacks parental concern. For example, she may appear calm, not cry, and carry on with normal activities despite providing this dramatic, worrisome history. Assessment and interventions are summarized in Nursing Interventions 29-8.

The long-term outcome for these children has not been well researched. Mortality rates are estimated at about 10% (Squires & Squires, 2010); actual incidence is difficult to estimate because of the difficulty in identifying the diagnosis. When poisoning or suffocation is involved, mortality rates are as high as 33% (Squires & Squires, 2010). Many children develop a self-image as an ill or disabled person, which seriously harms the child's emotional and social development, causing emotional disorders, school-related problems, and poor concentration and school attendance. The victimized children are at risk of later developing the syndrome themselves and often have behavioral problems.

EATING DISORDERS

Eating disorders comprise a complex group of disorders, including anorexia nervosa (AN), bulimia nervosa, and binge-eating disorder. Anorexia is a disorder characterized by a distorted body image and the refusal to eat sufficient food to maintain normal weight. Those affected by AN often exercise compulsively and suffer from severe malnutrition. *Bulimia nervosa* involves binge eating of large amounts of food, followed by forced vomiting, excessive use of laxatives, enemas, or diuretics (Fig. 29-4). Children and adolescents affected with bulimia may also exercise compulsively. Binge-eating disorder is present when the child or adolescent frequently binge eats but does not purge the body (as with bulimia nervosa discussed later in this session).

Eating disorders are common among children and adolescents. Disordered eating behaviors and attitudes are reported in about 33% of girls and 15% of boys aged 11 to 17 years; this is particularly prevalent in those who are overweight (Herpetz-Dahlmann et al., 2008). Eating disorders are often comorbid with other disorders such as depression, OCD, personality disorders, and substance abuse. Adolescents with eating disorders also are more likely to have a history of abuse or trauma.

Risk factors associated with eating disorders include poor communication with parents, dissatisfaction with appearance or weight, lack of regular meals, use of tobacco, altered family dynamics (entangled relationships), and negative family food-related experiences (Hautala et al., 2008; Kluck, 2008; Waller et al., 2011). Other factors include sexual abuse, participation in activities that

NURSING INTERVENTIONS 29-8

Munchausen Syndrome by Proxy

Assessment

Social History
- Family history of previous, unexplained infant deaths/sibling illness
- Family dysfunction
- Marital discord, emotionally distant spouse

Child History
- Description of a prolonged, unexplainable illness that, despite medical attention and therapies, has not been resolved
- Discrepancy between clinical findings and history
- Symptoms that do not occur when others are present

Parental Behavior
- Seeming lack of concern for the child's condition and interest in performing many tests and procedures
- Remains calm when child is very ill (e.g., in cardiac arrest)
- Exemplary caregiver to child when health care members are present; ignores child when others are not present

Interventions
- Separate suspected perpetrator and child and see if symptoms persist.
- Try to talk with verbal children alone, away from the suspected perpetrator.
- Attempt to involve the other parent, if absent.
- Ask parents/family members separately how they are coping; suggest appropriate referrals.
- Objectively document: use nonaccusatory, fact-specific, detailed observations of behavior and interactions with the child, staff, and spouse (e.g., 12:01: mother standing on left side of bed where IV tubing is; 12:04: child became lethargic—blood glucose tested 40 mg/dL, IV tubing leaking, appears to be small puncture hole in tubing).
- Document relevant negatives (e.g., symptoms do not occur when the mother is absent).
- Covert video surveillance may be needed; follow institution protocol.
- Notify child protective services, institutional risk management, and local police.
- A multidisciplinary team will confront the perpetrator; the child may need to be protected at the same time as the perpetrator is confronted (e.g., a court order in place so the perpetrator cannot remove the child from the facility).
- Evaluate child's and family member's responses to interventions; they likely will require long-term follow-up and psychiatric referrals.

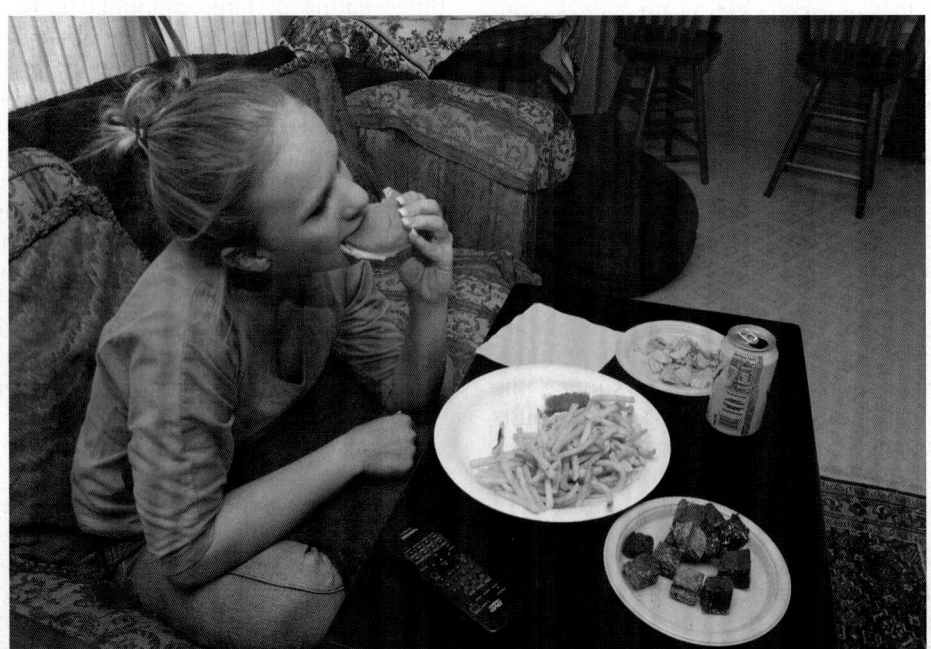

Figure 29-4 The adolescent with bulimia eats a large meal and then forces herself to vomit what she ate.

require attention to weight (e.g., ballet, gymnastics, wrestling, horse racing, modeling), and being adolescent and female (see Chapter 7 for further discussion).

Genetic vulnerability is suspected as one potential cause. Psychological factors contributing to risk include low self-esteem, perfectionist personality, distorted body image (perception of being fat), peer pressure, and media images (Cain et al., 2008; Courtney et al., 2008). Individuals diagnosed with anorexia display isolative tendencies, whereas individuals diagnosed with bulimia tend to have an extroverted personality type. Children with bulimia are often diagnosed late in their disease course because they are able to hide their behavior and maintain a more normal weight. Children with anorexia are often diagnosed earlier because their failure to eat and their extreme weight loss are more noticeable. However, the anorexic child may become quite skillful at hiding the weight loss under baggy, oversized clothes.

Assessment

Eating disorders contribute to profound metabolic disturbances, in addition to weight loss. Potential physical disturbances may include growth failure and cognitive deficits. Signs of AN in females include being underweight, delayed puberty, short stature, bradycardia, cardiomyopathy, osteoporosis, hair loss or lanugo (fine hair growth), and death if the disorder is not abated. Males often have similar signs, but, perhaps because they present to medical care later in their disease course, they are more likely to exhibit tachycardia and experience heart failure (Thomson et al., 2012). With bulimia, individuals display substantial alterations in health status, including sore throat, abdominal pain, constipation, and destruction of dental enamel (Devlin et al., 2012).

Note the child's current weight and elicit a history of the child's weight gain and loss patterns. Ask children about foods they eat, eating patterns, and what methods they have used to control their weight, if any. Also ask about the child's perception of his or her body image and the child's motivation to achieve a weight that is less than what their body requires to sustain life. The assessment in cases of bulimia should include the history of eating (how much, how often) and the compensatory behaviors used to maintain weight. The feelings associated with the behavior are important in making the diagnosis; they involve craving, an inability to control eating, and purging (forced vomiting).

Conduct a complete history and physical examination, emphasizing menstrual history; skin turgor; condition of the hair, teeth, and mucous membranes; and Tanner staging (see Chapter 3).

Physical examination may reveal gingivitis, parotid gland enlargement, and callused and irritated knuckles from using the finger to induce vomiting (with bulimia). Although amenorrhea is often used as diagnostic criterion for AN, it more accurately reflects weight loss and nutritional status less than what is needed to sustain life (Racine et al., 2011).

All children diagnosed with eating disorders require a referral to a mental health provider for a psychiatric assessment to include an assessment for any maltreatment. Additionally, the family will be assessed to determine personal, interpersonal, and social factors possibly contributing to the individual's current diagnosis. Assessment of the family's parenting style (e.g., values, discipline, nurturance, communication, and the family's perception of the problem) provides important data for treatment planning.

Many other factors may be contributing to the need for weight loss. If the desire for "thinness" and irrational body image of being "fat," characteristic of AN, are not present, other possible causes must be explored. These possibilities include depression and physical disorders such as Addison disease, Crohn disease, or brain tumors. Laboratory investigations are indicated to rule out such possibilities.

Nursing Diagnoses and Outcomes

In addition to the nursing diagnoses presented in Nursing Plan of Care 29-1, the following nursing diagnoses may be used to guide care interventions for the child or adolescent with an eating disorder:

Nursing Diagnosis: Disturbed body image related to inaccurate messages (self and others)
Outcomes:
- Child or adolescent will acknowledge health condition, express an understanding of the connection between food and the altered dynamics in their family relationships, and concede that exercise and weight loss have been excessive.
- Child or adolescent will participate in an eating disorder intervention program.
- Child or adolescent will express positive feelings about self.

Nursing Diagnosis: Impaired oral mucous membranes related to poor nutritional status and practices
Outcomes:
- Child's oral mucous membranes will remain intact.
- Child or adolescent will demonstrate good oral hygiene practices.

Interdisciplinary Interventions

Treatment of eating disorders involves multimodal therapy to attend to the child's physical, social, and interpersonal needs being affected by the eating disorder. A primary goal is to restore weight and reverse physical signs and symptoms of fluid, electrolyte, and nutritional imbalances. Treatment may involve hospitalization, ideally before the child exhibits medical instability such as vital sign changes (orthostatic hypotension with a heart rate increase of 20 bpm, a 20-mm Hg decrease in standing blood pressure, a heart rate of less than 40 bpm or more than 110 bpm, or inability to sustain body temperature [Mitchell & Crow, 2010]), cardiac dysrhythmias, or electrolyte disturbances.

A weight gain of 2 to 3 lb/week while hospitalized, and 0.5 to 1 lb/week in outpatient programs, is targeted (Mitchell & Crow, 2010). Caloric intake is increased gradually to avoid refeeding syndrome (fluid and other electrolyte disorders, particularly hypophosphatemia, and cardiac and neurologic dysfunction), which has significant risk, including coma and death; monitor serum electrolytes and vital signs.

The health care team works with the child and family to develop appropriate weight maintenance strategies and to improve the child's eating behaviors. Nursing interventions do not merely focus on the child's weight but include a holistic approach that encompasses dietary management, provides support to address the child's fear of excessive weight gain, monitors weight and adherence to the activity schedule, uses behavioral contracting, and provides behavior management to prevent purging behavior, excessive exercising, and to maintain the plan of care.

Psychiatric referral is strongly recommended to address cognitive distortions related to food and body image and to improve the child's social functioning skills. Directive and active individual therapy, family therapy, behavior therapy, and group therapy are all recommended as interventions.

CBT is superior to other psychological and drug treatments for treating bulimia nervosa (Schmidt et al., 2009). Young people with severe and protracted cases of anorexia or bulimia are hospitalized on inpatient psychiatric units to more closely attend to their medical and psychological needs (Clinical Judgment 29-3).

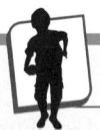

CLINICAL JUDGMENT 29-3

The Adolescent With an Eating Disorder

Emily, a 14-year-old female, was admitted to the inpatient adolescent unit of the children's hospital after collapsing at school. She was 5 ft 2 in. tall and weighed 79 lb. During the 5 months preceding admission, she had lost 26 lb. After losing 15 lb, she had been taken to the family's managed care facility. The physician prescribed an antidepressant and told her mother to restrict activities and monitor Emily's diet. Emily continued to lose weight. Emily had been an A student, but her grades had begun to deteriorate to Cs and Ds. She complained of fatigue and difficulty concentrating. She said whenever she got sleepy when studying, she would "relax" by exercising. Emily said she believed she was "too fat." Emily's history indicated eating had been a conflictual issue between her and her parents since she was a baby. Emily's mother said that when Emily was little, they were concerned she would be too fat. Her mother said, "But losing this much weight is just ridiculous! I think sometimes she is trying to kill herself." Emily's dad said, "Last year she looked really great! The boys were ogling her all the time. I couldn't stand it, but this weight loss has just gone too far!" Further investigation into family dynamics revealed that Emily's father was flirtatious with Emily and was outspoken about "keeping the boys away." His flirtations with Emily and constant reminder to his wife that Emily was his "little doll" caused considerable conflict between her parents. During the assessment, Emily revealed that she believed she was the cause of her parents' fights, and she was worried about how her father would handle her dating boys. She said that she avoided all boys because they were only interested in her body.

Questions

1. What data are significant in determining the presence of an eating disorder?

2. Why might Emily have developed an eating disorder?

3. What are the priority nursing diagnoses you could use to begin a care path for an adolescent with an eating disorder?

4. List one outcome goal for each of your diagnoses.

5. How would you determine whether Emily is in control of her eating disorder?

Answers

1. Current weight compared with height norms; history of weight loss; exercise patterns; and complaints of fatigue, sleepiness, and difficulty concentrating

2. Family conflict about her eating from an early age, adolescent rebellion against parents' control of social life, fear of growing up and becoming attractive, fear of losing father's attention

3. Imbalanced nutrition, less than body requirements; compromised family coping; disturbed body image

4. Emily develops a plan to eat a balanced diet (including sufficient calories) on or before day of discharge, family members sign a contract to participate in family therapy sessions for at least 8 hours, and Emily and parents state the importance of achieving Emily's target weight.

5. Emily maintains adequate weight for age, eats balanced meals that meet her caloric needs, and relates a positive self-identity.

SCHIZOPHRENIA

Schizophrenia is a severe brain disorder involving dysregulation of thought and perception and deterioration in adaptive abilities as its primary feature. (The term "thought and perception disorder" is increasingly used instead of "schizophrenia.") It has an insidious onset and results in severe and lifelong cognitive deficits and disordered behavior. Features of the disease must be present for at least 6 months before a diagnosis can be made (APA, 2013).

Although schizophrenia is rare in children, in many cases, altered thoughts, perceptions, and developmental difficulties noted during childhood are hints at possible very-early- or early-onset schizophrenia. The diagnosis of schizophrenia is often made during late adolescence or young adulthood. Schizophrenia onset is quite rare at age younger than 10 years or older than age 40 years. Schizophrenia diagnosed in children younger than age 13 years is defined as very-early-onset schizophrenia, with prevalence estimated at 1 in 10,000; early-onset diagnosis of schizophrenia occurs between ages 13 and 17 years, with prevalence estimated at 0.5% (Masi & Liboni, 2011).

Assessment

Making a diagnosis of schizophrenia in childhood can be difficult because the essential features may manifest differently with developmental level. Children manifest disorganized speech and behavior, which are seen in several other disorders. Adolescents and young adults diagnosed with schizophrenia are at especially high risk for suicide (APA, 2013), so give special attention to assessing this risk.

During the prodromal period (before complete manifestation), these children often exhibit deficits in several areas: peer relations, school performance, speech, motor milestones, unusual behaviors (hand flapping; twirling; rocking; unusual fascinations with light, smells, or textures). Other symptoms are unusual fears, unstable moods, inappropriate response in emotions or to social situations, perseveration (difficulty in moving from one activity to another), and ritualistic behavior. These same behaviors also are common among children with autism or developmental delays.

Assessment of childhood schizophrenia should include a complete physical examination, including a neurologic examination. Neurophysical findings demonstrate slow reaction times and abnormalities in eye tracking (ability to follow an object passed slowly from one side of the head to the other or up and down). Afflicted children are often awkward. They may show neurologic "soft signs," such as perseveration, right–left confusion (older children and adolescents), poor coordination, or mirroring (doing exactly the same behavior as the examiner). If you observe such signs, consider referring the child to a specialist.

Interdisciplinary Interventions

Initial studies have demonstrated the efficacy of neuroleptic agents with children and adolescents, but more research in children is needed (Masi & Liboni, 2011).

Neuroleptic agents used to treat schizophrenia are believed to block a specific dopamine receptor (D_2).

Although most neuroleptic agents are effective in treating the so-called positive symptoms (psychotic symptoms) of schizophrenia, they do not improve the negative symptoms. Negative symptoms include flat **affect** (the external expression of emotion attached to the ideas or representation of objects), lack of motivation, and poverty of speech. One problem with neuroleptic agents is sedation. This problem can be modified with lower (than adult) doses of the medication. Therapeutic effects usually occur in 7 to 14 days, and the drugs should be given a 4- to 6-week trial before a different medication is tried. Children and adolescents are susceptible to side effects of the medication (sedation and movement disorders such as dystonia, akathisia, tardive dyskinesia, and parkinsonian syndrome) even on low doses.

Additional interventions include clarifying the meaning of events and situations to counter cognitive distortions, **alteration of perception** (sensory impressions, such as sights, sounds, tastes, or smells that have no basis in external stimulation), and **alteration of thought** (false beliefs that are firmly maintained despite proof to the contrary and despite the fact that others do not share the belief). Help orient the individual to situations and provide needed protection (e.g., from peers or self-harm).

Interventions promoting independence and self-care are needed, including information concerning medication. Structured play activities, including social skills training, are recommended. Group therapy that is structured, skills oriented (e.g., communication and social skills), and presented in sessions of short length may be helpful.

Family interventions are also an important part of treatment. Families need help understanding the disorder and the medications (their purpose, side effects, and actions). They often need information on managing the behavior and promoting normal growth and development. Childhood schizophrenia is an extremely difficult experience for families. They must cope with the stress of losing the "healthy" child and manage the problems associated with the illness every day, while promoting the child's maximal development.

Accurate diagnosis of the disorder may take several years. Stigma is associated with any mental illness, but especially with a disorder such as schizophrenia. Families may experience blame, guilt, and isolation. It is essential that nurses offer support and convey the message that parents are not the cause of the disorder. Mutual support groups are helpful for many families.

Interventions also include consultation with a variety of personnel at the child's school (e.g., teacher, counselors) and involved community agencies. The nurse is frequently involved in accessing services for children with altered thought processes such as schizophrenia. Educating teachers about manifestations of these disorders is important. Teachers need to understand effects and side effects of medication. They need to understand that children tend to act out their hallucinations and delusions, whereas adolescents are more verbal.

Various treatment options are used to promote independence, social relationships, and health maintenance. These interventions include supportive therapy, social skills training, job coaching, symptom management, teaching activities of daily living (such as self-care, shopping for food and clothes, and using transportation), money management, housekeeping, and therapeutic ways to use leisure time.

PERSONALITY DISORDERS

A *personality disorder* is a long-term pattern of behavior deviating substantially from social norms (Cicchetti & Crick, 2009). Many believe this pattern of behavior affects functioning because of unmet needs originating in childhood. Personality disorders have historically included borderline personality disorder, dissociative disorder, antisocial personality, and obsessive–compulsive personality disorder where there is an overly rigid personality (unlike OCD where there are various compulsions acted upon and/or obsessions such as thoughts). However, APA (2013) has redefined personality disorders according to severity and dimension rather than categorical criteria. New domains include negative emotionality, introversion, antagonism, disinhibition, compulsivity, and schizotypy.

Personality disorders are most often diagnosed in the adolescent or young adult years. The prevalence of personality disorders range is 12.7% to 14.6%, increasing with age to an estimated lifetime prevalence of 28.2% at age 33 years (Johnson et al., 2008).

Self-injurious behaviors, such as cutting and scraping skin, and high-risk behaviors, such as substance abuse and sexual acting out, are symptoms often experienced by those diagnosed with a personality disorder. These high-risk behaviors can make a child or adolescent more susceptible to victimization.

Assessment

The features of personality disorders are difficult to identify in children. Symptoms are often identified and treated, but the diagnosis is avoided until later adolescence to allow for possible decrease in symptoms because of growth and maturity. In general, observe for combinations of the following behaviors: rapid mood changes, seeming inattention, rapid shifts in details when recounting events, situational amnesia, self-harm behaviors such as cutting, multiple piercings and tattoos, abuse, substance use, or other high-risk behaviors.

A diagnosis of personality disorder is avoided as long as possible in individuals before the age of 18 years. Rather, conduct disorder is often the diagnosis of choice until a long-term pattern is established. Additionally, the characteristics of a personality disorder must be present for at least 1 year before a diagnosis can be made. Children at varying stages of development manifest behaviors characteristic of normal growth and development that also are features of a personality disorder. Only when the behaviors persist and interfere with the developmental process and social well-being are they then applied to a diagnosis.

Interdisciplinary Interventions

If abuse is a causative factor, report it immediately. Reporting is both a legal obligation and helps ensure the future safety of the child. The second most important intervention is to develop a trusting relationship with the patient to provide appropriate feedback and interventions. Components of the treatment program used with personality disorders are a therapeutic behavior management program, group therapy, social skills training, recreational therapy, and participation in special education until discharged.

Nurses need to develop an accepting, open approach to the youth with personality disorder. Safety precautions are imperative because these children will use almost anything for self-harm when they are in a state of upset or feeling empty or "dead." Examples of potential weapons include pencils; erasers; sharp pieces of plastic, metal, or glass; and objects that may cause burns, such as matches or curling irons. The dead feeling is related to numbing of painful feelings and intrusive memories or images.

Clearly explain rules, and firmly yet empathetically adhere to them. Respond to unreasonable demands and expectations truthfully and realistically. These children often use abusive language and manipulation when realistic limits are set and reinforced. Remain calm but firm in insisting on appropriate behavior and adhering to rules established for the unit and the individual patient.

See thePoint for a summary of Key Concepts.

REFERENCES

Aebi, M., Müller, U. C., Asherson, P. et al. (2010). Predictability of oppositional defiant disorder and symptom dimensions in children and adolescents with ADHD combined type. *Psychological Medicine*, 40(12), 2089–2100.

Akinbami, L. J., Liu, X., Pastor, P. N. et al. (2011). *Attention deficit hyperactivity disorder among children aged 5–17 years in the United States, 1998–2009* (NCHS Data Brief No. 70). Hyattsville, MD: National Center for Health Statistics.

American Academy of Child & Adolescent Psychiatry. (2011). *Obsessive-compulsive disorder in children and adolescents.* Retrieved from http://www.aacap.org/page.ww?section=Facts for Families&name=Obsessive-Compulsive Disorder In Children And Adolescents

American Psychiatric Association. (2013). *Diagnostic and statistical manual of mental disorders* (5th ed.). Washington, DC: Author.

Beardslee, W. R., Gladstone, T. R. G., & O'Connor, E. E. (2011). Transmission and prevention of mood disorders among children of affectively ill parents: A review. *Journal of the American Academy of Child & Adolescent Psychiatry*, 50(11), 1098–1109.

Behrendt, S., Wittchen, H. U., Höfler, M. et al. (2009). Transitions from first substance use to substance use disorders in adolescence: Is early onset associated with a rapid escalation? *Drug and Alcohol Dependence*, 99(1–3), 68–78.

Blader, J. C., Pliszka, S. R., Jensen, P. S. et al. (2010). Stimulant-responsive and stimulant-refractory aggressive behavior among children with ADHD. *Pediatrics*, 126(4), 796–806.

Busch, S. H., Frank, R. G., Leslie, D. et al. (2010). Antidepressants and suicide risk: How did specific information in FDA safety warnings affect treatment patterns? *Psychiatric Services*, 61(1), 11–16.

Cain, A. S., Bardone-Cone, A. M., Abramson, L. Y. et al. (2008). Refining the relationships of perfectionism, self-efficacy, and stress to dieting and binge eating: Examining the appearance, interpersonal, and academic domains. *International Journal of Eating Disorders*, 41(8), 713–721.

Cash, S. J., & Bridge, J. A. (2009). Epidemiology of youth suicide and suicidal behavior. *Current Opinion in Pediatrics*, 21(5), 613–619.

Cicchetti, D., & Crick, N. R. (2009). Precursors and diverse pathways to personality disorder in children and adolescents. *Development and Psychopathology*, 21(3), 683–685.

Cormier, E. (2008). Attention deficit/hyperactivity disorder: A review and update. *Journal of Pediatric Nursing*, 23(5), 345–357.

Courtney, E. A., Gambox, J., & Johnson, J. G. (2008). Problematic eating behaviors in adolescents with low self-esteem and elevated depressive symptoms. *Eating Behaviors*, 9(4), 408–414.

Devlin, M. J., Kissileff, H. R., Zimmerli, E. J. et al. (2012). Gastric emptying and symptoms of bulimia nervosa: Effect of a prokinetic agent. *Physiology & Physiology & Behavior*, 106(2), 238–242.

Dudley, M., Goldney, R., & Hadzi-Pavlovic, D. (2010). Are adolescents dying by suicide taking SSRI antidepressants? A review of observational studies. *Australasian Psychiatry*, 18(3), 242–245.

Eaton, D. K., Kann, L., Kinchen, S. et al. (2012). Youth risk behavior surveillance—United States, 2011. *Morbidity and Mortality Weekly Report*, 61(4), 1–168.

Fahim, C., Fiori, M., Evans, A. C. et al. (2012). The relationship between social defiance, vindictiveness, anger, and brain morphology in eight - year - old boys and girls. Social Development, 21(3), 592–609.

Fairchild, G., Passamonti, L., Hurford, G. et al. (2011). Brain structure abnormalities in early-onset and adolescent-onset conduct disorder. *Journal of Psychiatry*, 168(6), 624–633.

Finkelhor, D., Jones, L., & Shattuck, A. (2013). *Updated trends in child maltreatment, 2011*. Durham, NH: Crimes Against Children Research Center. Retrieved from http://www.unh.edu/ccrc/pdf/CV203_Updated%20trends%202011_FINAL_1-9-13.pdf

Furman, R., & Jackson, R. (2002). Wrap-around services: An analysis of community-based mental health services for children. *Journal of Child and Adolescent Psychiatric Nursing*, 15, 124–131.

Ghaemi, S. M., & Vohringer, P. A. (2013). Antidepressants from a public health perspective: Re-examining effectiveness, suicide, and carcinogenicity. *Acta Psychiatrica Scandinavica*, 127(2), 89–93.

Gibb, S. J., Horwood, L. J., & Fergusson, D. M. (2011). Bullying victimization/perpetration in childhood and later adjustment: Findings from a 30 year longitudinal study. *Journal of Aggression, Conflict and Peace Research*, 3(2), 82–88.

Gilchrist, R. H., & Arnold, L. E. (2008). Long-term efficacy of ADHD pharmacotherapy in children. *Pediatric Annals*, 37(1), 46–51.

Greenberg, W. M., Benedict, M. M., Doerfer, J. et al. (2009). Adjunctive glycine in the treatment of obsessive-compulsive disorder in adults. *Journal of Psychiatric Research*, 43(6), 664–670.

Hautala, L. A., Junnila, J., Helenius, H. et al. (2008). Towards understanding gender differences in disordered eating among adolescents. *Journal of Clinical Nursing*, 17(13), 1803–1813.

Herpetz-Dahlmann, B., Wille, N., Holling, H. et al. (2008). Disordered eating behaviour and attitudes, associated psychopathology and health-related quality of life: Results of the BELLA study. *European Child & Adolescent Psychiatry*, 17(Suppl. 1), 82–91.

Hien, D., Cohen, L. R., Caldeira, N. A. et al. (2010). Depression and anger as risk factors underlying the relationship between maternal substance involvement and child abuse potential. *Child Abuse & Neglect*, 34(2), 105–113.

Hofmann, S. G., Sawyer, A. T., & Fang, A. (2010). The empirical status of the "new wave" of cognitive behavioral therapy. *Psychiatric Clinics of North America*, 33(3), 701–710.

Jellinek, M., Patel, B. P., & Froehle, M. C. (Eds.). (2002a). *Bright futures in practice: Mental health—Volume I, practice guide*. Arlington, VA: National Center for Education in Maternal and Child Health.

Jellinek, M., Patel, B. P., & Froehle, M. C. (Eds.). (2002b). *Bright futures in practice: Mental health—Volume II, tool kit*. Arlington, VA: National Center for Education in Maternal and Child Health.

Johnson, J. G., Cohen, P., Kasen, S. et al. (2008). Cumulative prevalence of personality disorders between adolescence and adulthood. *Acta Psychiatrica Scandinavica*, 118(5), 410–413.

Keeley, M. L., & Storch, E. A. (2009). Anxiety disorders in youth. *Journal of Pediatric Nursing*, 22(1), 26–40.

Keenan, K., Wroblewski, K., Hipwell, A. et al. (2010). Age of onset, symptom threshold, and expansion of the nosology of conduct disorder for girls. *Journal of Abnormal Psychology*, 119(4), 689–698.

Kessing, L. V., Willer, I. S., & Knorr, U. (2011). Volume of the adrenal and pituitary glands in depression. *Psychoneuroendocrinology*, 36(1), 19–27.

Kessler, R. C., Ormel, J., Petukhova, M. et al. (2011). Development of lifetime comorbidity in the World Health Organization world mental health surveys. *Archives of General Psychiatry*, 68(1), 90–100.

Kinnally, E. L., & Mann, J. J. (2012). Early life stress programming and suicide risk. *Psychiatric Annals*, 42(3),95–100.

Kluck, A. S. (2008). Family factors in the development of disordered eating: Integrating dynamic and behavioral explanations. *Eating Behaviors*, 9(4), 471–483.

Krefetz, D. G., Steer, R. A., Gulab, N. A. et al. (2002). Convergent validity of the Beck Depression Inventory-II with the Reynolds Adolescent Depression Scale in psychiatric inpatients. *Journal of Personality Assessment*, 78, 451–460.

Kucuker, H., Demir, T., & Resmiye, O. (2010). Pediatric condition falsification (Munchausen syndrome by Proxy) as a continuum of maternal factitious disorder (Munchausen syndrome). *Pediatric Diabetes*, 11(8), 572–578.

Kutash, K., Duchnowski, A. J., & Green, A. L. (2011). School-based mental health programs for students who have emotional disturbances: Academic and social-emotional outcomes. *School Mental Health*, 3(4), 191–208.

Lack, C. W., & Green, A. L. (2009). Mood disorders in children and adolescents. *Journal of Pediatric Nursing*, 24(1), 13–25.

Lansford, J. E., Dodge, K. A., Pettit, G. S. et al. (2010). Does physical abuse in early childhood predicts substance use in adolescence and early adulthood? *Child Maltreatment*, 15(2), 190–194.

Leatherdale, S. T., & Burkhalter, R. (2012). The substance use profile of Canadian youth: Exploring the prevalence of alcohol, drug and tobacco use by gender and grade. *Addictive Behaviors*, 37(3), 318–322.

Leibenluft, E. (2011). Severe mood dysregulation, irritability, and the diagnostic boundaries of bipolar disorder in youths. *American Journal of Psychiatry*, 168(2), 129–142.

Leve, L. D., Harold, G. T., Chamberlain, P. et al. (2012). Practitioner review: Children in foster care—Vulnerabilities and evidence-based interventions that promote resilience processes. *Journal of Child Psychology and Psychiatry*, 53(12), 1197–1211.

Levitan, R. D. (2007). The chronobiology and neurobiology of winter seasonal affective disorder. *Dialogues in Clinical Neuroscience*, 9(3), 315–324.

Loeber, R., Burke, J. D., Lahey, B. B. et al. (2000). Oppositional defiant and conduct disorder: A review of the past 10 years, part I. *Journal of the American Academy of Child & Adolescent Psychiatry*, 39(12), 1468–1484.

Masi, G., & Liboni, F. (2011). Management of schizophrenia in children and adolescents: Focus on pharmacotherapy. *Drugs*, 71(2), 179–208.

McDougall, T. (2009). Nursing children and adolescents with bipolar disorder: Assessment, diagnosis, treatment, and management. *Journal of Child and Adolescent Psychiatric Nursing*, 22(1), 33–39.

Melnyk, B. M., Moldenhauer, Z., Tuttle, J. et al. (2003). Improving child and adolescent mental health: An evidence-based approach. *Advance for Nurse Practitioners*, 11, 47–52.

Merikangas, K. R., He, J., Burstein, M. et al. (2010). Lifetime prevalence of mental disorders in US adolescents: Results from the National Comorbidity Study-Adolescent Supplement (NCS-A). *Journal of the American Academy of Child & Adolescent Psychiatry, 49*(10), 980–989.

Mitchell, J. E., & Crow, S. (2010). Medical comorbidities of eating disorders. In W. S. Agras (Ed.), *The Oxford handbook of eating disorders* (pp. 259–266). New York, NY: Oxford University Press.

Molina, B. S., Hinshaw, S. P., Swanson, J. M. et al. (2009). The MTA at 8 years: Prospective follow up of children treated for combined type ADHD in the multisite study. *Journal of the American Academy of Child & Adolescent Psychiatry, 48*(5), 484–500.

Muñoz, R. F., Cuijpers, P., Smit, F. et al. (2010). Prevention of major depression. *Annual Review of Clinical Psychology, 6,* 181–212.

Nader, K., Kriegler, J. A., Blake, D. D. et al. (1996). *Clinician administered PTSD scale, child and adolescent version.* White River Junction, VT: National Center for PTSD.

Offord, J. (2012). Genetic approaches to a better understanding of bipolar disorder. *Pharmacology & Therapeutics, 133*(2), 133–141.

Ollendick, T. H., Jarrett, M. A., Grills-Taquechel, A. E. et al. (2008). Comorbidity as a predictor and moderator of treatment outcome in youth with anxiety, affective, attention deficit/hyperactivity disorder, and oppositional/conduct disorders. *Clinical Psychology Review, 28*(8), 1447–1471.

Parks, S. E., Kegler, S. R., Annest, J. L. et al. (2012). Characteristics of fatal abusive head trauma among children in the USA: 2003–2007: An application of the CDC operational case definition to national vital statistics data. *Injury Prevention, 18*(3), 193–199.

Racine, S. E., Culbert, K. M., Keel, P. K. et al. (2011). Differential associations between ovarian hormones and disordered eating symptoms across the menstrual cycle in women. *International Journal of Eating Disorders, 45*(3), 333–344.

Ramchand, R., Griffin, B. A., Suttorp, M. et al. (2011). Using a cross-study design to assess the efficacy of motivational enhancement therapy–cognitive behavioral therapy 5 (MET/CBT5) in treating adolescents with cannabis-related disorders. *Journal of Studies on Alcohol and Drugs, 72*(3), 380–389.

Reyes, J. A., Somers, G. R., Taylor, G. P. et al. (2011). Increased incidence of CPR-related rib fractures in infants—Is it related to changes in CPR technique? *Resuscitation, 82*(5), 545–548.

Saigh, P., Yaski, A. E., Oberfield, R. A. et al. (2000). The Children's PTSD Inventory: Development and reliability. *Journal of Traumatic Stress, 13*(3), 369–380.

Saxe, G. N., & Bosquet, M. (2004). Child Stress Disorders Checklist-Screening Form (CSDC-SF) (Version 1.0-3/04). National Child Traumatic Stress Network and Boston University School of Medicine.

Saxe, G., Chawla, N., Stoddard, F. et al. (2003). Child Stress Disorders Checklist: A measure of ASD and PTSD in children. *Journal of the American Academy of Child & Adolescent Psychiatry, 42,* 972–978.

Scheeringa, M. S., Zeanah, C. H., & Cohen, J. A. (2010). PTSD in children and adolescents: Toward an empirically based algorithm. *Depression and Anxiety, 28*(9), 770–782.

Schmidt, U., Lee, S., Beecham, J. et al. (2009). A randomized controlled trial of family therapy and cognitive behavior therapy guided self-care for adolescents with bulimia nervosa and related disorders. *American Journal of Psychiatry, 164*(4), 591–598.

Simpson, H. B., Slifstein, M., Bender J. et al. (2011). Serotonin 2A receptors in obsessive-compulsive disorder: A positron emission tomography study with [¹¹C]MDL 100907. *Biological Psychiatry, 70*(9), 897–904.

Squires, J. E., & Squires, R. H. (2010). Munchausen syndrome by proxy: Ongoing clinical challenges. *Journal of Pediatric Gastroenterology & Nutrition, 51*(3), 248–253.

Stein, B. D., Kataoka, S. H., Hamilton, A. B. et al. (2010). School personnel perspectives on their school's implementation of a school-based suicide prevention program. *Journal of Behavioral Health Services & Research, 37*(3), 338–349.

Steiner, H., & Remsing, L. (2007). Practice parameter for the assessment and treatment of children and adolescents with oppositional defiant disorder. *Journal of the American Academy of Child & Adolescent Psychiatry, 46*(1), 126–141.

Stores, G. (2009). Aspects of parasomnias in childhood and adolescence. *Archives of Disease in Childhood, 94*(1), 63–69.

Substance Abuse and Mental Health Services Administration. (2010). *Children's mental health facts: Children and adolescents with anxiety disorders.* U.S. Department of Health & Human Services, Center for Mental Health Services.

Thapar, A., Collishaw, S., Pine, D. S. et al. (2012). Depression in adolescence. *Lancet, 379*(9820), 1056–1067.

Thomson, S., Marriott, M., Telford, K. et al. (2012). Adolescents with a diagnosis of anorexia nervosa: Parents' experience of recognition and deciding to seek help. *Clinical Child Psychology and Psychiatry.* Advanced online publication.

Timbremont, B., Braet, C., & Dreessen, L. (2004). Assessing depression in youth: Relation between the Children's Depression Inventory and a structured interview. *Journal of Clinical Child and Adolescent Psychology, 33*(1), 149–157.

Twenge, J. M. (2011). Generational differences in mental health: Are children and adolescents suffering more, or less? *American Journal of Orthopsychiatry, 81*(4), 469–472.

U.S. Department of Health & Human Services, Administration on Children, Youth and Families. (2011). *Child maltreatment 2011.* Washington, DC: Author. Retrieved from http://www.acf.hhs.gov/programs/cb/resource/child-maltreatment-2011

Vierhile, A., Robb, A., & Ryan-Krause, P. (2009). Attention-deficit/hyperactivity disorder in children and adolescents: Closing diagnostic, communication, and treatment gaps. *Journal of Pediatric Healthcare, 23*(Suppl. 1), S1–S21.

Waller, G., Calam, R., & Slade, P. (2011). Eating disorders and family interaction. *British Journal of Clinical Psychology, 28*(3), 285–286.

Warner, R. (2010). Does the scientific evidence support the recovery model? *The Psychiatrist, 34*(1), 3–5.

Winters, K. C., Botzet, A. M., & Fahnhorst, T. (2011). Advances in adolescent substance abuse treatment. *Current Psychiatry Reports, 13*(5), 416–421.

World Health Organization. (2010). *Child maltreatment fact sheet N°150.* Geneva, Switzerland: Author.

See **thePoint** for Organizations.

The Child With a Developmental or Learning Disorder

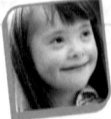

CASE HISTORY

Remember the Curricio family? Moira and Manny Curricio have three sons, Nick, Joey, and Andrew, who are 13, 11, and 8 years old, respectively. In Chapter 21, we met Joey, the soccer player who had a concussion; in Chapter 25, we met Nick, who went to Boy Scout camp and came home with poison ivy. Moira and Manny are expecting a fourth child. This is an unexpected pregnancy, and Moira is 41 years old. Moira is of Irish heritage, and Manny's family is Italian. They are practicing Catholics. During Moira's pregnancy, Manny and Moira decided not to have an amniocentesis, despite Moira's age. This decision was made after much thought and discussion and based on the premise that they would not choose to abort the fetus even if they did discover genetic abnormalities. Cecilia is born a few days before Christmas. She has reddish brown hair and dark eyes, but she also has epicanthal folds on her eyes, a short neck, protruding tongue, and hypotonia. The pediatrician and Moira's obstetrician visit the couple. They congratulate them on having a beautiful and healthy baby girl, and they recommend sending blood work to determine whether Cecilia has Down syndrome. Moira had expressed her worries during the pregnancy to her husband. She seems not to be shocked that Cecilia is born with Down syndrome. Her concerns are focused on the present. Is Cecilia getting enough to eat? Manny is supportive. He says to his wife, "We've always taken what life has given us and made the best of it." Cecilia's older brothers are curious and fascinated with the new baby girl. The fact that she is a girl represents more of a novelty in this household of boys than the fact that she has Down syndrome. They vie for the privilege of burping and rocking her.

Moira expects to breastfeed her fourth baby and perseveres through the first very trying week. Moira is an experienced mother, having nursed her sons, but Cecilia has a weak suck and an uncoordinated suck–swallow. Moira learns to position Cecilia sitting virtually upright in front of her. The nurses show her how to place gentle rhythmic pressure on Cecilia's chin to facilitate her efforts. Moira is fortunate that despite Cecilia's weak suck, she is producing an ample amount of milk. After 2 weeks, the results of the genetic workup return; Cecilia has Down syndrome.

As Cecilia turns 3 years old, she has still not learned to walk independently. Her father has built a set of parallel bars. Her parents, brothers, nurse, and physical therapist are all encouraging her to support herself within the bars, trying to get her to walk independently, but without much success. What does fascinate her is their large family dog! Whenever she is on the floor, she scoots over and hugs her dog. The dog gets up slowly and Cecilia, desperate not to be separated from the dog, holds on tightly to his fur. As the dog moves, Cecilia supports her own weight and moves with the dog. The motivation to stay with the dog is much more powerful than anything the parallel bars have to offer. Cecilia eventually learns to walk with help from the family pet.

CHAPTER OBJECTIVES

1 Discuss adaptive functional and educational responses of children with a developmental disorder.

2 Explain the importance of early identification and intervention with children who have a developmental disorder.

3 Discuss strategies to help families navigate the health care system and advocate for their child to ensure that their child receives needed health care.

4 Identify strategies for including a child with a developmental disorder in typical environments in the community.

5 Support families in their efforts to identify and use community resources that best meet the individual child and family's needs.

See thePoint for a list of Key Terms.

Developmental disorders are most often detected early during a child's development or during the first years of formal education. These disorders cover a broad range of diagnoses, all of which involve delay in acquiring age-appropriate skills in **adaptive functioning** (life skills) or **educational response** (reading and writing skills). The disorders range from motor skill delays, communication disorders (see Chapter 28), and intellectual delays to impairment in social interaction to disruptive behavior. The most common developmental disorders include learning disorders, intellectual disability, and autism spectrum disorder (ASD).

Labels for these diagnoses may change depending on the funding source or educational program, but regardless of the specific label, the behavior and treatment remain the same. The term *developmental delay* implies that the child will "catch up." This outcome may or may not occur; therefore, other terms are more appropriate. Whereas the term *mental retardation* is still used in legislation, *intellectual disability* is the term used in the *Diagnostic and Statistical Manual of Mental Disorders* (5th ed.; *DSM-5*) (American Psychiatric Association [APA], 2013) and preferred by persons with this disability, their families, and many professionals working in the field of developmental disabilities and is the term used throughout this chapter. Labels for intellectual disability include cognitive disability, cognitive deficit, and intellectual deficiency. Learning disabilities and autism spectrum are typically not associated with decreased intellectual capacity. Developmental disability is used as a general reference to all conditions discussed in this chapter.

CROSS-CULTURAL CARE

In England, the term *learning disabilities* includes children with mild intellectual disability.

DEVELOPMENTAL AND BIOLOGIC VARIANCES

The center of cognition—the brain—undergoes massive development in utero and during the first few years of life (see Chapter 21 for a more detailed discussion of central nervous system embryology and brain development). This development may be disrupted by perinatal and postnatal insult and by environmental factors, resulting in cognitive impairments or neurodevelopmental dysfunction (see Chapters 14, 21, 26, and 27).

Children are also vulnerable to social and emotional factors. A child's cognitive development is related to the quality of mother–infant interactions (Smith et al., 2006; Violato et al., 2011). Low socioeconomic status and poor maternal education have also been shown to have a significant positive correlation with increased risk for cognitive delay (Hillemeier et al., 2011). Lack of nurturing and stimulation has deleterious effects that may permanently alter brain development. A diet associated with high fat, sugar, and processed food content in early childhood may be associated with small reductions in IQ in later childhood; conversely, a healthy diet consisting of nutrient-rich foods may be associated with small increases in IQ (Northstone et al., 2012; Nurturing, stimulation, and Mental Developmental Index scores were not addressed in this study).

caREminder

For most developmental disorders, causes cannot be attributed. Families should not be blamed for causing the child's developmental problems but should be helped to accept the child's delays and work to facilitate the child's progression.

ASSESSMENT

As with other disabilities, early detection of developmental disorders is important to enable intensive intervention to help the child progress toward his or her potential. The American Academy of Pediatrics (2009) mandates that all children be screened for developmental disorders. Diagnosing developmental disorders can be difficult and may require a multidisciplinary approach. Assessment includes a health history and physical assessment; some diagnostic tests are also useful. Information from these multiple assessments may aid diagnosis.

FOCUSED HEALTH HISTORY

 QUESTION: What are the factors in Moira's health history that place her at risk for having a child with Down syndrome?

The history is always critical for a complete assessment (Focused Health History 30-1). Evaluate whether the child has achieved age-appropriate developmental and biologic milestones and assess current behavioral, social, and cognitive functioning. Use these parameters to help determine whether the child's patterns of development are normal, delayed, or regressed.

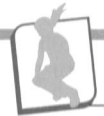

The Child With a Developmental Disorder

Current history	Ability to meet developmental milestones such as crawling, walking, or communicating Grades in school, presence of academic problems, ability to perform age-appropriate tasks and keep up with peers, ability to interact socially in an age-appropriate manner Behavioral problems (poor self-esteem, school avoidance, acting out, depressive symptoms), which may result from learning disorders Sleep patterns
Past medical history	**Prenatal/Neonatal History** Maternal infection or other prenatal insult; fetal exposure to drugs, including cigarettes and alcohol; poor maternal nutrition Results of α-fetoprotein, amniocentesis, or chorionic villi sampling Gestational age at birth, prematurity Apgar scores Birth weight: low birth weight may indicate maternal malnutrition; large for gestational age associated with birth injuries Head circumference plotted on growth chart Any pre-, peri-, or postnatal events that caused clinically important asphyxia, trauma, jaundice, stroke, hemorrhage, or apnea Did mother and baby go home at the same time? Feeding (include ability to suck and swallow) and sleeping patterns **Previous Health Challenges** Results of genetic, neurologic, or developmental testing Central nervous system infections or insults; epilepsy; metabolic disorder (e.g., phenylketonuria, storage disorders); hyperbilirubinemia; chronic conditions
Nutritional assessment	Poor nutrition or malnutrition during first years of life History of pica
Family medical history	Consanguinity History of fetal loss Presence in other family members of symptoms similar to those for which the child is being evaluated Intellectual disabilities Neurocutaneous lesions Hypotonia Learning problems Grade retention School dropout Attention deficits
Social and environmental history	Exposure to environmental toxins (e.g., lead, mercury, environmental tobacco smoke) Maternal depression or cognitive impairment Child's ability to make and keep friends (as age appropriate) Perceived stressors for the child or among other family members Changes in lifestyle Changes in academic performance Domestic violence, neglect, or emotional abuse Unusual emotional responses (e.g., laughing at a car accident) Support systems available
Growth and development	Age at acquisition of developmental milestones, particularly delayed speech acquisition

Note: See Chapter 8 for a comprehensive health history.

To help determine current cognitive functioning for a school-aged child, examine the child's history of school achievement, current school placement, and any need for special education support.

ANSWER: The health history in this family focuses on the maternal risk factors, not the infant's history. Moira is at increased risk for having a child with Down syndrome because of her age. According to the National Institutes of Health, the incidence of a pregnant woman younger than 30 years of age having a child with Down syndrome is less than 1 in 1,000. However, a woman's chance of having a child with Down syndrome increases to 1 in 400 at age 35 years and 1 in 60 at age 42 years. Despite these statistics, between 75% and 80% of children with Down syndrome are born to younger mothers because they are the age group having significantly more children.

FOCUSED PHYSICAL ASSESSMENT

QUESTION: Review Focused Physical Assessment 30-1. What would you anticipate finding in Cecilia's newborn physical assessment?

Conduct a physical assessment of the child, including a neurologic examination and vision and hearing screening, to detect any underlying or associated medical problems (Focused Physical Assessment 30-1). Assess for dysmorphic features, congenital anomalies, or constellations of physical findings (e.g., a long face, large ears, and large testes [in postpubertal males] are associated with fragile X syndrome, the most commonly identified genetic cause of intellectual disability) that may be associated with developmental disability.

ANSWER: Cecilia shares some of the distinctive physical features that are recognizable in individuals with Down syndrome. One feature is the shape of the eyes. Cecilia's eyes are slanted upward with palpebral fissures and epicanthal folds. She has a short neck and a slightly protruding tongue. She has poor muscle tone and a weak suck. She also has a single palmar crease.

DIAGNOSTIC CRITERIA

QUESTION: Genetic testing determines that Cecilia is indeed a child with Down syndrome. How can some of the tests identified in thePoint Supplemental Information: Select Tools for Assessing Cognitive and Adaptive Functioning be used as Cecilia gets older?

Developmental disorders may result from a variety of causes. They may be genetic; related to prenatal or perinatal insult; or acquired as a result of illness, injury, and environmental exposures. Various diagnostic studies are available to assist health care practitioners in diagnosing neurocognitive disorders. Tests and Procedures 30-1 presents select procedures and lists specific considerations for each test. The nurse's role in helping children and their families who are undergoing these tests includes referring the child for testing and counseling, teaching the child and family about what to expect, and preparing the child for any necessary invasive procedures. A trained genetic counselor performs genetic counseling.

Tests of cognitive and adaptive functioning help to diagnose developmental disorders or to plan appropriate interventions (see thePoint Supplemental Information: Select Tools for Assessing Cognitive and Adaptive Functioning). Tests should be selected according to the child's current level of developmental functioning, not on the basis of chronologic age. Tests also should be appropriate for the type of communication the child uses, whether it is speech, sign language or nonverbal methods of communication, head nodding, or pointing. The term *cognitive functioning* is more appropriate than *intelligence* because results on tests such as the Bayley-III are poorly correlated with intelligence in adulthood. The younger the child is when the test is administered, the lower the correlation the test result has with adult IQ. Findings at age 6 years would be more highly correlated with abilities in adulthood than findings at age 2½ years. Typically, psychologists administer most tests of cognitive functioning. Nurses may administer the Bayley-III and the Vineland Adaptive Behavior Scales after having been trained and educated to do so. Nurses also play an important role in assisting families to interpret the results of diagnostic testing and relate that information to their child and other family members. Assessments are conducted in schools to determine the programming or intervention a child needs to promote development. School nurses may assist with this assessment, interpreting findings and developing appropriate interventions for the child. These may include development and implementation of an individualized education program (IEP) or 504 Plan and participation in multidisciplinary meetings at school (see Chapter 2).

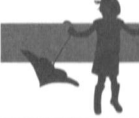

FOCUSED PHYSICAL ASSESSMENT 30-1
Developmental and Learning Disorders

Assessment Parameter	Alterations/Clinical Significance
General appearance	Difficulty interacting or not engaging with others may indicate cognitive disorders or Autism Spectrum Disorder (ASD).
	Development that is not consistent (e.g., age-appropriate gross and fine motor skills but delayed speech and language) may indicate cognitive disorders.
	Self-stimulating behaviors (e.g., arm flapping, head banging, twirling) may be present with intellectual disability and ASD.
	Dysmorphic features (e.g., overly large tongue or testes) may be present with certain genetic syndromes that cause intellectual disability.
	Clusters of abnormalities may indicate a syndromic disorder (e.g., cardiac and palatal anomalies in velocardiofacial syndrome).
	Overactivity or poor attention can be associated with intellectual disability.
Integumentary system (skin, hair, nails)	Signs of self-stimulation such as patches of hair missing, pinch marks, or bite marks may indicate intellectual disability or ASD.
	Steely hair or unusual hairline may indicate a genetic syndrome.
Head and neck	Head circumference less than the 5th percentile indicates microcephaly, which is associated with intellectual disability.
	Changes from child's head circumference growth trajectory may indicate hydrocephalus (if increasing) or malnutrition and decelerating brain growth (if decreasing), both of which can lead to intellectual disability.
Ears	Low-set ears are present in some genetic syndromes (e.g., Down syndrome) that are associated with intellectual disability. Failure to respond to voice or sounds may indicate hearing deficit, which, if not corrected, may result in delayed speech acquisition and learning.
Face, eyes, nose, and oral cavity	Wide-set eyes and epicanthal folds are characteristic of some genetic syndromes. Similar facies are characteristic of some disorders—for example, a long face, prominent jaw, and large prominent ears are characteristic of males with fragile X syndrome; a flat facial profile, eyes with upward and slanted palpebral fissures and epicanthic folds, macroglossia, a short neck, and speckled irises (Brushfield spots) are characteristic of children with Down syndrome.
	Short palpebral fissures, thin upper lip (abnormal philtrum), and hypoplastic midface are associated with fetal alcohol syndrome.
	Inattention to visual stimuli may indicate visual impairment or neurologic injury. Difficulty with vision may result in difficulty learning and mastering developmental tasks.
Neurologic system	Impaired verbal and nonverbal communication, short- and long-term memory, and inability to perform age-appropriate activities of daily living may indicate cognitive impairment.
	Motor difficulties (e.g., clumsiness, problems writing or using scissors) may be associated with learning disability.
	Not performing age-appropriate developmental milestones may indicate cognitive impairment.
	Not sitting, crawling, or walking within normal time frames may indicate neuromuscular problems or cognitive disorder.
	Asymmetric movement of extremities may also indicate developmental delay associated with neurologic impairment.

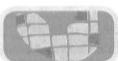 **TESTS AND PROCEDURES for Diagnosing Neurocognitive Disorders**

Diagnostic Test or Procedure	Purpose	Findings and Indications	Health Care Provider Considerations
Magnetic resonance imaging (MRI) of brain	Imaging without radiation by radiofrequency emissions that are converted to computer images To detect anatomic abnormalities; to evaluate myelination of white matter tracts, volume of white and gray matter	MRI provides sharp, anatomic detail and information about the chemistry of living tissue. May reveal decrease in brain size, damage to the basal ganglia, or reduced size of the cerebellum. Loss of brain tissue affects cognition.	Teach child that MRI machine makes loud humming and intermittent tapping noises. Ear plugs or headphones may be used to dampen noise. Use music as distraction. Child is supine and placed in a tube that encases a strong magnet. Depending on scanner, study takes 45–60 minutes. Avoiding motion during this time is critical. Sedation is indicated if child is restless or dislikes confined spaces. Most children younger than 6–7 years of age require sedation. Remove all metal or magnetic items; surgical implants such as pacemakers, bone pins, or cerebral clips are contraindications. Contrast MRI requires intravenous access. Noncontrast study is painless. If age appropriate, child may benefit from seeing MRI in operation before study.
Computed tomography (CT)	Radiographic study to view the brain in three dimensions Radiographic beam scans cranium in successive layers (cuts), and computer digitizes image Differentiates density of bone (lighter) and air (darker)	Promotes effective visualization of tumors, ventricles, brain tissue, cerebrospinal fluid, hematomas, and cysts.	Child is supine, on a movable table, with head immobilized. CT takes about 20–30 minutes. Motion destroys clarity of scan; child may require sedation. If CT is enhanced with radioisotope dye, child must have intravenous access. Noncontrast study is painless.
Chromosomal analysis/DNA analysis/ fluorescent in situ hybridization	To detect chromosomal or genetic abnormalities	Deviation from normal 23 pairs of 22 autosomes and 1 sex chromosome, or deletions or addition of parts of chromosomes, may result in conditions associated with intellectual disability.	Follow laboratory instructions for specimen collection and storage. Prepare child based on how specimen is obtained (via blood, skin, etc.). Family counseling should be performed by a trained genetic counselor.
Metabolic screening	Blood and urine tests to detect inborn errors of metabolism, endocrine problems (thyroid function), amino acid and organic acid disorders (refer to Chapters 26 and 27)	Deficiency or accumulation of substrates, depending on specific disorder (e.g., metabolic disorders such as galactosemia, aminoacidemias such as homocystinuria and phenylketonuria, organic acidemias such as maple syrup urine disease), may cause brain damage or other problems (cataracts, liver damage). Low thyroxine (T_4) and high thyroid-stimulating hormone levels may indicate hypothyroidism.	Adequate samples are needed to obtain accurate results. Abnormal results require immediate follow-up. If tests are performed before a newborn is 24 hours old, the test should be repeated at 1–2 weeks of age. Note child's diet prior to test. Parenteral nutrition may influence the measurement of certain amino acids. Parenteral antibiotics may inhibit the growth of bacteria used in some assays.

Diagnostic Test or Procedure	Purpose	Findings and Indications	Health Care Provider Considerations
Heavy metal assay (e.g., lead, mercury, arsenic)	To detect abnormal blood levels of heavy metals that may impair neurologic functioning	Abnormal levels can cause cognitive impairment and encephalopathy, leading to intellectual disability and behavioral impairment.	Venous sampling is preferred to capillary sampling because the chances of false-positive and false-negative results are less. Immediately notify health care prescriber of abnormal levels.

Query families about the child's achievement of developmental milestones, and ask if they have any concerns about the child. Testing on more than one occasion, using the same test or different tests, may be needed to obtain an accurate picture of the child's abilities. If the same test is used, retesting at an appropriate interval, such as 3 to 4 months, may be required to eliminate the possibility that the child might learn the testing items.

ANSWER: As reported in the case study, Cecilia is 3 years old and not yet walking. She is delayed in her motor skills. The Bayley-III covers three areas of skills, including motor skills. At this age, it can be used to quantify Cecilia's skills and to identify her strengths. As Cecilia gets older and attends school, intelligence testing will help assess her abilities. Individuals with Down syndrome have a very wide range of intellectual abilities.

TREATMENT MODALITIES

 QUESTION: How would the nurses help the Curricio family implement effective interventions for Cecilia as a newborn?

Treatment for developmental disorders typically targets optimizing the child's development versus effecting a cure. Interventions that can influence the child's development include environmental stimulation, early intervention programs, educational interventions, and family interventions.

Although much time and effort is spent trying to find the cause of the child's disorder, a cause often is not found. The causal factor for almost half of the cases of intellectual disability is unknown (Maulik et al., 2011). Whenever possible, turn the emphasis away from finding a cause for the disorder to focusing on the strengths of the child and family, using those strengths to address the child's limitations, and assisting the child and family to progress toward the child's potential.

A child's development is influenced by the quality of family–child transactions, family-orchestrated child experiences, and health and safety provided by the family. Family–child transactions that encourage development include maintaining affectionate, developmentally sensitive patterns of caregiver–child interactions; structuring the environment appropriately; and building on previous learning. Family-orchestrated child experiences refer to the stimulation provided by the environment, including varied and developmentally appropriate toys and materials, and positive contacts with other adults and children. Developmental screening can provide useful information to guide family interactions and child-specific interventions (see thePoint Chapter 3 for Developmental Screening Tools). Educate families about the disorder and about strategies to provide stimulation and move the child's functioning forward. Refer the family to resources as appropriate to assist the child's further development and support the family. See Chapter 12 for information about habilitation, the process of helping the child master new skills to achieve his or her maximum potential.

KidKare To maximize the child's potential, the family must consider the child's interests, abilities, and special needs when planning activities.

Health and safety provided by the family includes health promotion and maintenance (e.g., routine health care, immunizations, activity, and nutrition) and protection from abuse, bullying, and violence. Become familiar with the health issues and comorbidities associated with developmental disorders, and educate family members on managing these issues. Remember, however, that all children have typical childhood illnesses. Avoid attributing such illness to the developmental disorder. Help the family to get past the disability and view their child as a child.

Referral to early intervention programs may help the child reach his or her optimal potential. Comprehensive interventions that include physical and intellectual stimulation can continually move the child's development to a higher level. The stimulation includes interventions that provide family education, resources and social support, developmental or therapeutic interventions (health care, physical therapy, occupational therapy, speech therapy, education aimed at the child's developmental needs and skills), and quality daycare programs for the child. Family involvement may improve the effectiveness of programs because children spend a large part of their day with their family. Additionally, new modes of therapy are becoming more prevalent. These include things like hippo (horse) therapy, yoga for children, and other types of interventions that have been successful with adults.

Nurses often educate families and other professionals (non-nurses) about the health needs of children with developmental disorders. Nurses can also help the family normalize their lives as they adjust to the day-to-day routines of providing care and attention to a child with special needs. For example, the nurse can assist the family to adapt tube feeding to fit into the family's routine, minimizing disruption of the family's typical routine yet ensuring that the child receives needed nutrition. The family often adapts health-related procedures; nurses can help families to understand when these adaptations are safe and when they may harm the child.

Caring for a child with a developmental disorder is stressful for the family and can be lifelong depending on the severity of the disorder. Siblings may experience a sense of isolation or loneliness because families must spend more time with the child with a developmental disorder. Inform the family about sibling support resources such as Sibshops or other sibling support activities (see thePoint Organizations). Parents often feel responsible for the disorder and may think something done or not done during pregnancy or early infancy caused the problem. They may receive these messages from ill-informed family members, friends, or educators. Even health care providers may tell them that the child's delays are caused by poor parenting. Acting-out behavior common among children with a developmental disorder can cause additional stress and guilt. The family may feel that if they set limits more consistently or tried a different approach, the child's behavior would be more manageable. Families can become exhausted and often need community support services to help them care for the child or provide interventions to assist the child's progress. Early interventions to educate families about the specific disorder, the common emotional struggles the family may experience, and available resources help decrease the anxieties and fears that are common among families with a child diagnosed with a developmental disorder (Pelchat, 2010). Family therapy may be valuable to some families to help promote positive communication and coping.

ANSWER: The nurses will help the Curricio family to meet Cecilia's physical needs—for example, helping with breastfeeding. Nurses will make sure that at discharge from the hospital, the family has the ability to access resources for a family with a child with Down syndrome.

NURSING PLAN OF CARE

QUESTION: At the time of Cecilia's birth, which of the nursing diagnoses listed in the Nursing Plan of Care 30-1 are most applicable?

Approach the family by focusing on their strengths and resilience (Carlson et al., 2010). The strengths perspective is based on a partnership between the nurse and family to access resources, learn skills, and develop new behaviors. The nurse can connect the family to resources and, through teaching, help them form accurate perceptions of the child's disorder and future potential. Through these efforts, the nurse assists the family to become more resilient and to cope with the demands of caring for a child with a developmental disorder (Fig. 30-1). It is important to treat the whole child, not just his or her condition or deficits, in the context of the family (Nursing Plan of Care 30-1).

Children with intellectual disabilities may be more likely than peers to be exposed to environmental adversities because of lower family socioeconomic position, social exclusion of family and child, and disability-related discrimination (Emerson, 2013). Exposure to environmental adversities in childhood, such as poor nutrition, exposure to infectious agents, toxins and teratogens, and accidental and nonaccidental injury, can have immediate and long-term detrimental effects on health and well-being. Therefore, people with intellectual disability may have poorer health than their nondisabled peers simply as a result of experiencing more adverse environmental and life experiences.

Children with developmental disabilities may also have special health needs. If so, they often interact with many different health care professionals (nurses, pediatricians, occupational therapists, physical therapists, psychologists, and speech–language pathologists) and may require adaptive modifications for school to maximize attendance and learning (e.g., assistance from health aides, nursing care, modifications for regular classes, special education classes, barrier-free facilities). A key nursing role is advocating to obtain services and care that will enable these children to fully participate in and benefit from their educational experiences (Nursing Interventions 30-1 highlights other nursing roles). The Individuals with Disabilities Education Improvement Act mandates that the child with a disability receive appropriate education in the least restrictive environment to meet the child's needs and promotes early intervention and special education programs (see Chapter 2 for further information). Integrating the child into the regular classroom provides an enriched experience for the child, enables the child to participate with typical same-age peers, and enables peers to benefit from interacting with a child with developmental disabilities. If a regular classroom does not meet the child's needs, he or she may be pulled out for periods during the day for special education resource classes. Education can also be provided in a self-contained special education class. Teach the family to advocate for their child's educational needs (Teaching Intervention Plan 30-1). Although pull-out classes and self-contained classrooms still exist, a regular classroom with appropriate supports should be the goal. Be familiar with available community resources and facilitate coordination

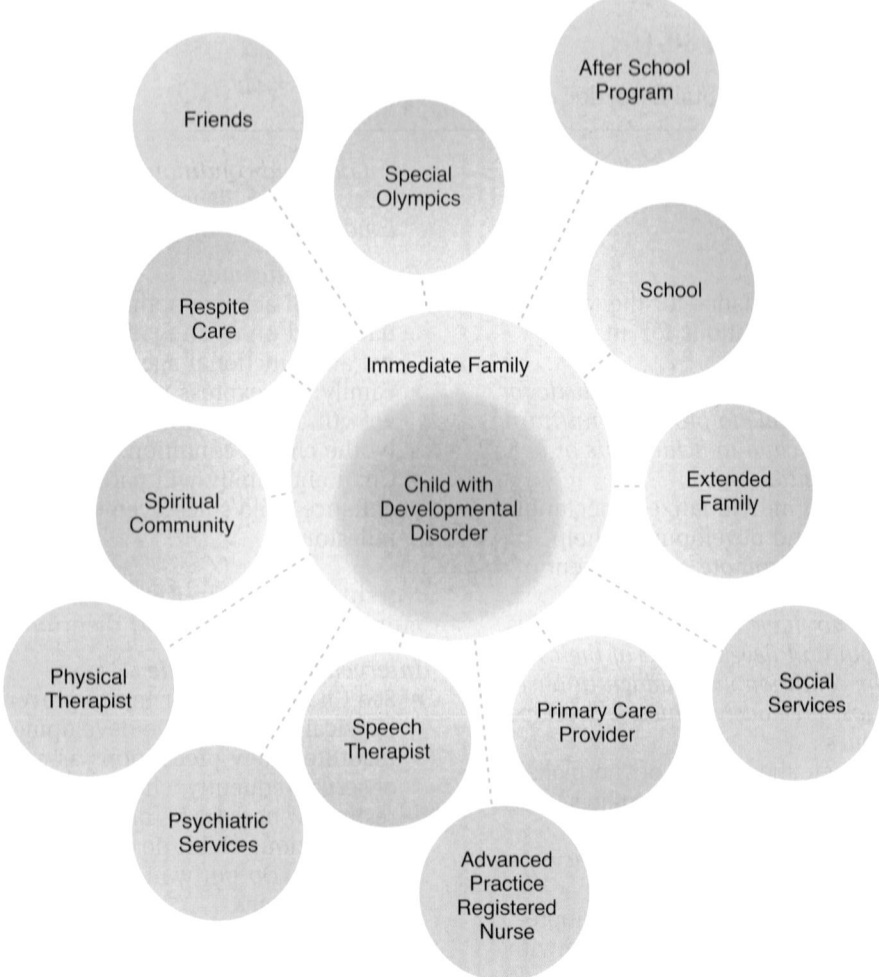

Figure 30-1 An ecomap demonstrates potential resources for the child and family.

of care. Early intervention programs can build on the child's strengths to optimize outcomes and minimize the child's limitations. Use every interaction with a child to perform developmental surveillance, evaluate the child's development, monitor the success of current intervention, and refer the child for further assessment as indicated.

Discuss sexuality at the appropriate age as a routine part of health care. When children with developmental disorders approach puberty, encourage the family to discuss sexuality and, as the adolescent ages, family planning; this measure is particularly important in the presence of genetically transmitted diseases. As children with developmental disorders grow into adolescents and adults, they will transition to adult care services (see Chapter 12). Assist adolescents to become their own advocates in the health care system. Support families to encourage independent functioning to the extent of the adolescent's or young adult's abilities. Issues of guardianship and custodial care are also important but are beyond the scope of this text. Factors considered by parents of young people with learning disabilities when deciding parental and child role in making choices about health, social care, and education include (1) priority given to the young person's level of understanding; (2) parent's views on the nature of the choice; (3) parent's desire to protect the child; (4) personal beliefs and attitudes, especially around life stage and transition to adulthood; and (5) confidence in practitioners' knowledge and understanding (Mitchell, 2012).

ANSWER: At the time of Cecilia's diagnosis, the family may be completely overwhelmed and an appropriate diagnosis is "Compromised family coping related to reaction to child's developmental disorder." Cecilia also requires care that is different from her brothers. Another appropriate diagnosis at the time of birth is "Deficient knowledge: Child's developmental potential, treatment, skills necessary to care for child."

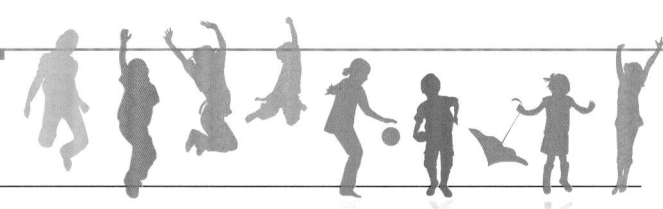

NURSING PLAN OF CARE 30-1:

The Child With a Developmental Disorder

Nursing Diagnosis: Risk for delayed development related to effects of emotional/cognitive deficit

Interventions/Rationale
- Provide anticipatory guidance for the family regarding realistic expectations for attaining developmental milestones.

    Families who understand what is realistic for their child are better able to provide a nurturing environment for the child to achieve his or her developmental potential.

- Assist the family to individualize expectations for child's growth and development; help develop methods to promote achievement of milestones.

    Families may not have realistic expectations regarding growth and development of their child, especially if the condition was sudden in onset and the child lost previously achieved developmental milestones.

- Discuss and promote the concept of "normalizing" experiences (e.g., eating meals with others, music therapy in groups).

    Such experiences promote self-sufficiency, adjustment, and mental growth.

- Model age-appropriate and cognitively appropriate caregiver skills (e.g., communicate with child as appropriate to cognitive level; provide toys, games, educational supplies, and teaching). Give the child responsibilities appropriate to cognitive level. Maintain dignity in all interactions with child.

    Gives families an example to follow of appropriate interventions. Children with developmental disabilities learn differently or more slowly than others and may reach a lower overall level of functioning.

- Encourage family involvement in care, particularly for hospitalized children, whenever possible without exceeding the family's emotional and physical limits.

    Consistent interaction with family diminishes normal separation anxiety, increases child's ability to cope, and may limit regressive responses to stress.

- Provide personal space so child's belongings are accessible; encourage child to care for the physical environment if appropriate.

    Fosters self-efficacy, self-worth, autonomy, and responsibility.

- Identify coexisting health conditions that may be contributing to altered development and refer child to a specialist if indicated.

    Comorbid conditions often are present (e.g., anxiety, depression); managing these conditions may increase child's potential.

Expected Outcomes
- Child will achieve optimal developmental potential based on existing abilities, extent of disability, and functional age.
- Family will express understanding of their child's growth and developmental potential as defined by the child's condition.
- Child and family will participate in activities to enhance child's achievement of developmental milestones.

Nursing Diagnosis: Risk for injury related to effects of developmental disorder

Interventions/Rationale
- See Chapters 4–7 for injury prevention based on physical and cognitive development.
- Institute safety precautions as appropriate (e.g., observe frequently, check safety rails frequently, restrain if necessary [only as last resort], stay with anxious child, do not underestimate child's strength). Do not wait for child to call you; plan regular checks.

    Cognitive and physical limitations associated with developmental disability may preclude the child's understanding of dangers, using safeguards, and requesting help appropriately in dangerous situations.

- Plan for mobility aids as needed (e.g., wheelchair, walker, other special equipment).

    Mobility aids optimize the child's potential.

- Observe for mouthing of nonfood items.

    Mouthing, a self-stimulating behavior, is a risk for aspiration and toxic ingestions.

- Remain with the child until medications are swallowed safely. Be alert to medication side effects that may interfere with child's function and safety.

    Observation may prevent aspiration or unsecured medications. Allows early intervention and potentially avoids problems.

- Explain and demonstrate procedures and equipment (e.g., suctioning, gavaging) in advance.

    Because the child may adapt slowly to new activities, situations, and environments, familiarity can induce less fear or resistance when procedures are implemented or equipment is used.

Expected Outcomes
- Child will cooperate, as able, with rules regarding safety.
- Child will be free from preventable injury.

Nursing Diagnosis: Compromised family coping related to reaction to child's developmental disorder

Interventions/Rationale

- Provide opportunities for family members to discuss feelings (e.g., anger, guilt, hostility); accept these expressions with nonjudgmental words and actions.

  The family may struggle with adapting to life with a disabled child in a world of nondisabled persons.

- Note and emphasize positive attributes of the child and family.

  A positive focus builds on existing resources and increases feelings of self-worth.

- Provide information about changes in child's level of function, strengths, and weaknesses.

  Knowing the child's level of function may facilitate realistic goals and expectations.

- Ensure that family members and child, as appropriate, are part of the team in planning individual programs and routines for the child.

  Families are the experts on what works best for them and what their personal resources are. The child's inability to perform age-appropriate tasks and the need for specialized training and "normalizing" experiences force the family into an adjustment process that includes developing alliances with professionals.

- Support families through the times when they are separated from the child. Provide opportunities for families of children in residential programs to discuss their feelings about home visits; assist them in planning for visits.

  Change in family routines may alter interaction and coping patterns; discussion and anticipatory guidance may prevent problems.

- Provide opportunities for the family to interact with other families with children who have developmental disorders.

  Sharing experiences and information may help in problem solving and reinforce the understanding that families are not alone.

- Refer family to counseling or appropriate agencies for information and support.

  Referral helps family to access appropriate resources.

Expected Outcomes

- Family members will express their feelings and concerns.
- Family members will participate in decision making about child's program.
- Family members will interact positively with the child.
- Family will partner with the health care team and use available resources, as appropriate.

Nursing Diagnosis: Impaired verbal communication related to effects of developmental disorder

Interventions/Rationale

- Encourage and allow time for child to express feelings and understanding in his or her own way. Use sign language or communication equipment as appropriate (e.g., picture boards, letter boards). Use visual cues to communicate.

  Children with developmental disorders have intellectual and emotional limitations that make it hard for them to adapt to changes in caregivers and routines and limit their ability to express feelings. Acceptance and an unhurried approach may increase the child's sense of well-being, reduce the child's anxiety, and increase the child's ability to communicate, as may alternative methods of communicating. The child may have better visual than auditory comprehension.

- Ask family for assistance in correctly interpreting the child's communication and behavior; encourage family to provide care when possible.

  Family members may help reassure the child and typically are familiar with child's communication methods.

- Provide consistency in nursing care. When possible, have the same staff members care for the child each time, and have a written schedule and plan of care to facilitate consistency between caregivers.

  Familiarity with the child increases knowledge of communication patterns and ability to correctly interpret child's messages.

- Assess for nonverbal communications (e.g., facial grimacing, unmoving, guarded posture with pain; gaze aversion or moving away from stimuli to indicate unwillingness to engage).

  Nonverbal cues may readily communicate feelings or needs.

- Assess whether the child is aversive to touch; if not, use touch as appropriate. Avoid touching the child unexpectedly. Ask permission or tell the child prior to touching.

  Tactile defensiveness (aversion to touch) may be present in individuals with developmental disorders. Touch can convey caring and can help calm, comfort, and have a positive effect, but it should not be forced on a child who is averse to it.

- Convey messages at the child's developmental level.

  Using developmentally leveled terms will increase understanding. Even if the child is nonverbal, words or voice inflection may be understood or comforting.

Expected Outcomes

- Child's communication will be correctly interpreted.

(Continued)

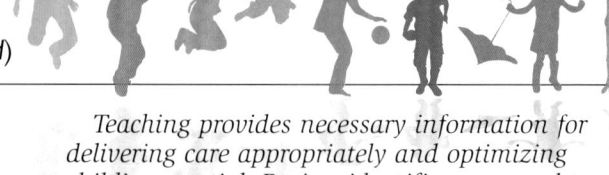

NURSING PLAN OF CARE 30-1:

The Child With a Developmental Disorder (*Continued*)

- Communication to the child will be directed at the appropriate developmental level.
- Child will demonstrate understanding of the communication to the best of his or her abilities.

Nursing Diagnosis: Deficient knowledge: Child's developmental potential, treatment regimen, skills necessary to care for child

Interventions/Rationale
- Assist the family members to learn technical skills as well as behavioral techniques that are necessary to care for the child (e.g., scheduling, routines, equipment).
  If the family has a deficient knowledge, the child's behaviors and health problems cannot be appropriately managed nor can individualized educational, social, and recreational experiences be planned to meet the child's special needs.
- Teach and review information regarding medications (e.g., dosage, time, method of administration, side effects) and concurrent medical diagnoses; verify family's understanding.

Teaching provides necessary information for delivering care appropriately and optimizing child's potential. Review identifies any need to correct misinterpretation.
- Help the family identify community resources for continuing information and support.
  Additional resources may help increase knowledge level, improve care of the child, and support family coping.

Expected Outcomes
- Child will maintain or improve functioning.
- Family members will provide child's care and demonstrate indicated care skills and procedures.
- Family members will identify available community support services.
- Family members will assist health care providers in understanding the meaning of illness in the family's culture, who the primary caregivers are, the role of women and men in caring for the disabled child, and cultural beliefs about the specific disability and its effect on the family.

DEVELOPMENTAL DISORDERS

The most common developmental disorders include learning disorders, intellectual disability, and ASD.

LEARNING DISORDERS

Learning disorders are the most common developmental disorders. The term *learning disorder* is used here as the diagnosis identified in the *DSM-5* (APA, 2013);

educators use the term *learning disability*. Learning disorders include problems with reasoning, comprehension, verbal skills, reading, writing, or math. Learning disorders become evident in childhood, and they remain with the individual throughout life. The estimated prevalence among children between the ages of 3 and 17 years is 8%, with a greater incidence detected among boys (Bloom et al., 2012). Reading difficulties are most common (Shaywitz et al., 2008), experienced by 14.5% of boys and 7.7% of girls without

NURSING INTERVENTIONS 30-1

Providing Services to the Child With a Developmental Disorder

Conduct home visits to assess living conditions and patterns of family–child interactions.

Assess and provide services related to basic family needs and any problems in family functioning.

Conduct developmental assessments of the child in the context of the family.

Provide education regarding social skills–building activities for child and family.

Link families to resources such as family support groups.

Coordinate multiple services.

Plan for transition between services (e.g., between early intervention and preschool services, transitioning to adult care providers).

Provide support for family through community resources and family groups.

Evaluate adequacy of services delivered in meeting the needs of the child and family.

TIP 30-1: A TEACHING INTERVENTION PLAN to Prepare Families to Advocate for the Educational Needs of the Child With a Developmental Disorder

Nursing Diagnosis and Family Outcomes

- Deficient knowledge: Rights and responsibilities of child with developmental needs in a public education system
  Outcomes: Family will voice knowledge of education rights and responsibilities of child and school system.
  Child will reach academic potential in public education system.
  Family will express comfort partnering with school personnel to develop and reach child's educational goals.

Teach the Child/Family

Legislation
- Inform family of federal and state laws that provide free public education for children with special education needs. Explain federal and state laws and school policies that ensure free public education for children with a disability from birth to age 21 years.
- Rehabilitation Act of 1973, Section 504 (civil rights of child with special education needs) requires schools to
  - Identify and locate all eligible children
  - Provide free, appropriate education
  - Educate disabled students with nondisabled
  - Institute appropriate evaluation procedures
  - Support right to participate in nonacademic programs
- The Buckley Amendment (family rights and privacy of records) gives parents the right to
  - See all child's school records
  - Amend school records
  - Know who accesses school records and when they are accessed
- Individuals with Disabilities Education Improvement Act (IDEIA) applies to children 3–21 years old and states that schools must
  - Serve all children
  - Provide free, appropriate education
  - Provide nondiscriminatory, multidisciplinary evaluation
  - Institute an IEP for each child affected
  - Ensure right to due process
  - Require parents to participate in developing the IEP
  - Make educators accountable for implementing the IEP
  - Give parents the right to examine records

Individualized Education Program/504 Plan
- Specific state laws and school system policies must comply with federal laws. Explain that the school must provide free, multidisciplinary, appropriate evaluation of child's learning needs.
  - Parents or guardians can request an evaluation of child.
  - Evaluation must be in child's native language or method of communication.
  - Child must be tested in all areas related to suspected disability (e.g., psychological, health, vision, hearing, social, academic performance, communication, motor ability). Parents can request specific areas.
  - School system is responsible for costs.
  - School must have parents' permission to evaluate child.
  - Children cannot be placed in or out of a program based on IQ alone.
  - Evaluation must be done every 3 years or sooner.
  - Parents are part of the evaluation.
  - Parents are entitled to a copy of the evaluation.
- Inform family how to request an evaluation and how to develop and implement an IEP or 504 Plan.
  - Submit request in writing to superintendent of school system; include specific areas to be evaluated.
  - Ask to meet with each evaluator before child is evaluated.
  - Keep copies of all requests and reports.
  - Research and visit program options that may meet needs of your child.
  - Make a list of child's strengths.
  - Attend all IEP or 504 meetings; bring advocate if you feel uncomfortable with evaluators and/or school personnel.
- Explain related services to assist child to meet educational goals.
  - All services needed to meet child's educational goals must be provided by the school for free.
  - These services may include speech therapy, psychological counseling, physical and occupational therapy, recreation, social work services, family training, etc.
  - Services include after-school programs open to all children.
- Encourage parents to use resources in community.
- Connect family to social services in community.
- Connect family to recreational resources.
- Connect family to respite care providers in community.
- Connect to family advocacy resources in community.

attention-deficit/hyperactivity disorder (ADHD); incidence is much higher with ADHD, at 51% in boys and 46.7% of girls (Yoshimasu et al., 2010). Children with learning difficulties have a higher incidence of emotional/behavioral difficulties and psychiatric disorders (Maughan & Carroll, 2006).

Although learning disorders may be associated with genetic predisposition, perinatal injury, environmental exposures, and neurologic and medical conditions, these factors do not necessarily predict a learning disorder (APA, 2013) and, in most cases, the etiology is unknown. Children with a learning disorder process information differently than children who respond to traditional teaching methods. The "wiring" or architecture of the brain differs from that of a child without a learning disorder, and the biochemical balance may differ as well. Learning disorders do not predict intelligence or learning capabilities and thus should not be viewed as deficits but as different responses to information input. Children with a learning disorder in one area may have unusual talent in another area. For example, a child may have limited verbal speech but may be a talented artist or athlete. Such discrepancies can make the learning disorder difficult for families and educators to understand.

Early recognition and diagnosis of learning disorders is imperative because secondary emotional and social problems frequently develop. Without diagnosis and adequate intervention, children and adolescents with learning disorders use undue energy to compensate for or even to hide their problem. Children with learning disorders have lower social standing among peers (Wiener & Timmermanis, 2012), fall behind in academic performance, and become easy targets for ridicule by peers. Their self-esteem suffers, putting them at high risk for emotional, social, and family problems. Children with chronic conditions such as psychiatric diagnoses, learning difficulties, physical and motor impairments, chronic illnesses, and overweight experience a higher level of peer victimization (Sentenac et al., 2012). Interventions to reduce bullying and victimization of these children are rarely implemented or evaluated.

Resilience in dealing with victimization does not just "happen," it must be fostered by the child's larger community. Vessey and O'Neill (2011) found that a serial brief intervention, delivered over an extended period of time, using a school nurse–led model can help students with disabilities to better handle teasing and bullying and that participants developed an improved self-concept within the context of their disabilities. Resiliency is a key term that must be introduced to children and families with developmental disorders.

Assessment

Children with learning disorders exhibit diverse learning problems that may include difficulties with written language, spoken language, mathematics, reasoning, and executive functions (e.g., the child's ability to organize and plan, the child's working memory, and the way the child relates to time). Symptoms include delayed language development; difficulty discriminating among sounds; difficulties with reading, spelling, and writing; and difficulty managing time (Kelly & Aylward, 2005). These symptoms typically affect academic performance negatively but may also affect functioning in other settings, such as in the home and community.

If a learning disorder is suspected, discuss the matter with the family. If the family raises concerns, investigate those concerns. Assess for behavioral or emotional problems that may occur as a result of learning disorders. Also assess for problems with family members, peers, and teachers. Adolescents who have not been diagnosed may experience undue anxiety and psychological trauma and may be relieved when a diagnosis is made and treatment is initiated.

Perform a thorough physical examination of the child to determine whether physical health problems may be exacerbating or causing the learning problem. A neurologic examination is essential. Assess motor function, speech, vision, and hearing. Attention deficit disorder (also called *attention-deficit/hyperactivity disorder*) and learning disorders occur as comorbidities in 45% of children affected with each disorder (DuPaul et al., 2013). Diagnostic tests such as electroencephalogram (EEG) and MRI are usually not necessary when assessing for and ruling out attention deficit disorder.

Interdisciplinary Interventions

No specific treatment exists for children with a learning disorder. Special educators and other experts are needed to determine the best methods for helping the child to compensate. Special educational techniques are needed to help these children develop their own unique way of learning. The primary responsibility for intervention lies with educators and family (Fig. 30-2). A child with a learning disorder, just like any child with a disorder that hinders education, is entitled to a free, appropriate education from birth to age 21 years. The treatment of underlying comorbid problems can help the child with a learning disorder but will not provide a cure.

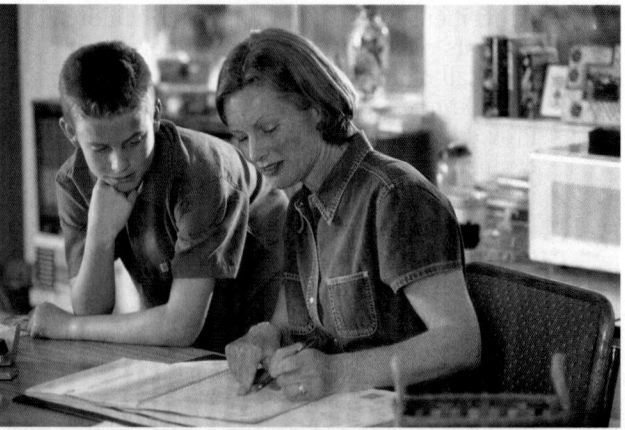

Figure 30-2 A child with a learning disorder may benefit from special tutoring. New technologies, such as the electronic tablet, are also advancing methods of communication and education for developmentally delayed or communication/learning disabled individuals.

KidKare Techniques that aid children with organization, such as different colored notebooks or folders, may be helpful. Arranging clothing on shelves instead of in closed drawers may help them to stay organized and keep them from forgetting items.

Children with a learning disorder that involves poor visual or altered perception may be at risk for injury. Teach the family to eliminate possible risks from the child's environment, for example by ensuring that items are put in their proper storage areas, not left lying on the floor. Repeated teaching about risks is also needed because the child may not apply learning from one situation to new situations.

Children and adolescents with learning disorders are susceptible to failure and frustration, particularly in the academic setting. Before a learning disorder is recognized, these children are often referred for alterations in behavior and emotional problems. Children who have difficulty in reading and mathematics, expressive or receptive language difficulties, or motor coordination problems are often the objects of teasing by peers, frustration by their teachers, and criticism or teasing by family and siblings. Many, if not most, of these youngsters develop low self-esteem and self-worth and other emotional and behavioral problems. Such problems compound their learning difficulties, making academic achievement and accomplishment of normal developmental stages and life goals increasingly difficult (Clinical Judgment 30-1). Children with a learning disorder respond well to extra praise for desired behavior. Visual indicators of progress, such as gold stars or stickers for improved work, may help a child develop a more positive self-image. Encouraging a child to pursue activities that will build on existing strengths may have a positive effect as well. Behavior support plans may be developed for the child and should be followed at school and home by all persons working with the child, including nurses. These plans are part of the child's IEP (sometimes referred to as *individualized education plan*), which nurses may help to develop and implement. In addition, the school nurse may develop an individual health care plan for the child (see thePoint Organizations: National Association of School Nurses).

Family interventions are essential and may be provided by a nurse who is knowledgeable about the specific disorder. Emphasize the child's strengths and the child's unique way of learning. Family conflicts aroused by the child's problems need to be discussed, and the nurse should facilitate problem-solving techniques to resolve the conflicts. Help the family understand the child's specific difficulty and any compounding problems. They may need guidance in helping other family members to modify attitudes and behavior toward the child. The nurse can support and guide the family as they advocate within the school system for services to meet the child's needs (see Teaching Intervention Plan 30-1). If family conflicts or child behavioral problems persist, family and individual therapy may be needed. Referral to a qualified professional (e.g., advanced practice psychiatric nurse or psychologist)

may be recommended. Encourage families to be advocates for their child to ensure use of appropriate learning strategies and attention to any special individual needs. Special recreational programs, especially those that help children learn motor skills, use their bodies effectively, and provide effective outlets for frustration, are recommended for children with learning disorders. Enhancing the child's skills is the goal of intervention.

Teachers may need consultation on how to explain the child's problem to classmates. They may need guidance in how to manage malingering and other behavioral manifestations of the child, including implementing effective discipline that is meaningful but not harsh. Work with the teaching staff to help the child meet his or her optimal educational goals.

INTELLECTUAL DISABILITY

Intellectual disability is another disorder that falls under the category of developmental disorders. Intellectual disorder is a condition that includes both a current intellectual deficit and impairment of mental abilities that impact adaptive functioning in three domains: (1) conceptual, including skills in language, reading, writing, math, reasoning, knowledge, and memory; (2) social concerns, social judgment, empathy, interpersonal communication, ability to make and retain friend; and (3) practical concerns, self-management of such things as personal care, job responsibilities, management of money, recreation, and organizing school and work tasks (APA, 2013). All symptoms must have an onset during the developmental period. The limitations result in the need for ongoing support at school, work, or independent life.

The determination of intellectual disability should not be tied only to an IQ score. Because of the nature of the intellectual delays, any standardized testing is difficult; determining the validity of an IQ test is also difficult, particularly in children with communication problems. Terms commonly used to describe the degree of intellectual disability, such as *profound*, *severe*, *mild*, and *moderate*, shed little light on actual ability to function or what intervention, if any, is needed. The incidence is about 1% to 3% of the U.S. population (U.S. National Library of Medicine, 2011).

Intellectual disability is not in and of itself a mental health disorder; however, mental health issues may arise in the family. The child is at increased risk for adjustment disorders because the child's coping strategies are not understood or recognized and his or her range of adaptive strategies may be reduced. Coping, adaptation, and social skills development greatly depend on abstract thinking and the ability to generalize from one situation to another. Abstract thinking is impaired in intellectual disability. The long-term stress of families caring and advocating for a child who has an intellectual disability can lead to burnout and the need for respite.

Numerous factors have been implicated as causes of intellectual disability, and a few associations are supported by evidence. Environmental factors include

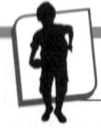

CLINICAL JUDGMENT 30-1

The Child With a Learning Disorder

Danyael was diagnosed with specific learning disorders at age 10 years and with ADHD as an adolescent. She had mild gastroesophageal reflux as an infant and only had a normal bowel movement every 5 days. In early childhood, she had no interest in having books read to her. She socialized well but did not appear to be interested in the environment around her. She did not show interest in watching television. She learned to read at grade level, but by fourth grade, it was determined that she did not comprehend most of what she read. Although rote learning, such as spelling, was at grade level, all other subjects were below level. Danyael was repeatedly told that she didn't pay enough attention to her studies or to directions; she was kept in from recess to redo work that wasn't considered neat enough.

Danyael was a second child to a mother who understood child development. The mother expressed her concerns repeatedly to the pediatrician and teachers. She sought second opinions without receiving a diagnosis. The mother arranged tutoring twice a week, but Danyael continued to receive failing grades on tests that measured understanding, even though she had repeated the information accurately to the tutor. Finally, without being informed of her rights under the Individuals with Disabilities Education Improvement Act (IDEIA), Danyael's mother took her daughter for a comprehensive psychological assessment. It was this evaluation that resulted in a diagnosis of learning disabilities. However, it was another 2½ years before the elementary school acknowledged the disabilities because no one relayed the test results to the school psychologist. The school continued to give Danyael failing grades on examinations and to tell her mother she worried too much.

As the new nurse at Danyael's high school, you have met Danyael, having seen her a few times in your office for minor maladies. You have been reviewing her file and realize she has not had her IEP updated in more than a year.

Questions

1. What could have been done to assist the family and the child in the past?
2. How were the repeated failures affecting Danyael's self-esteem, and what effect might this have on her emotional development and behavior in adolescence?
3. What could have been done to assist Danyael until a diagnosis was made?
4. Who should have been an advocate for this family?
5. How can you, as the pediatric nurse, help the family to differentiate normal alterations in growth and development from pathologic and abnormal conditions?

Answers

1. When the mother first had concerns, she should have been encouraged to keep a list of the behaviors causing concern or a log of her child's behaviors. As her concerns were presented to teachers and school administrators, she should have been provided information on IDEIA and been informed of her right to have her child tested, at no cost, in the school system.
2. Repeated school failures can further diminish academic performance as the child learns to "give up." The child's self-esteem during middle childhood years is greatly tied to mastery of new concepts. When the child receives constant negative reinforcement about his or her learning, self-esteem is bound to suffer. In adolescent years, this puts some teens at increased risk for unwanted or unsolicited attention, in addition to promiscuity as a method to gain acceptance and attention. Additionally, physical and emotional maturities are generally not simultaneous in the child with a developmental disorder.
3. Provide alternative learning strategies and document to see what works and what does not. Identify her strengths and promote them. Learn from the family what measures they implement at home to help her achieve, and incorporate those same techniques in the classroom.
4. If symptoms are identified in children younger than age 3 years, advocate for an evaluation by the state's early intervention team. After the child reaches age 3 years, the public school system is obligated to serve as an advocate to ensure that the child is provided additional resources to enhance learning when a learning disorder is identified.
5. Provide information on developmental parameters to assist the mother to recognize the ranges of what is considered "normal."

exposure to environmental toxins, such as lead poisoning, and fetal exposure to drugs or to alcohol. Organic factors include head injury; antenatal, prenatal, and postnatal infections; chromosomal mutations; hemorrhage or stroke; and physiologic disorders such as untreated hypothyroidism (see Chapter 26) or phenylketonuria (see Chapter 27). Numerous disorders are associated with the presence of intellectual disability, including fetal alcohol spectrum disorder (covered in Chapter 14) and genetic aberrations such as Down syndrome, Turner syndrome, Klinefelter syndrome, and fragile X syndrome (described in Table 14-2). Individuals with intellectual disability may be vulnerable to organic diseases and neurologic structural problems. Self-concept deficits, depression, anxiety disorder, and behavior problems are among the most common psychiatric problems associated with intellectual disability. A comorbid mental illness may exist, just as in individuals without intellectual disability. Diagnosing comorbid illnesses is difficult because children may have poor verbalization skills and therefore may not be able to report symptoms accurately.

Assessment

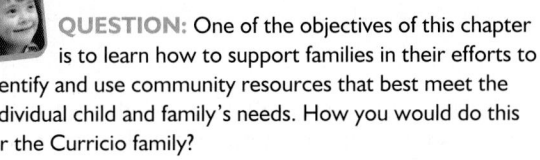

QUESTION: You are the nurse visiting the home of the Curricio family at the time Cecilia is learning to walk. Based on your knowledge of growth and development, what are other milestones that you would assess?

The child suspected of having intellectual disability, like all other children, should have a thorough physical and neurologic examination (see Chapter 8). Determining whether health factors such as hearing, vision, or motor deficits are causing or contributing to the child's developmental disorder is important. The child should be screened for infection, blood lead level, genetic and chromosomal problems, and neuroendocrine problems, all of which can cause or contribute to intellectual disability.

When assessing a child with known intellectual disability, focus on functional ability. Determine the child's ability to communicate, perform self-care activities, use social and interpersonal skills, and follow directions. When assessing an older child or adolescent, include an evaluation of leisure activities and academic skills.

Children who have intellectual disability are often uncomfortable with unfamiliar surroundings and people. Time is needed to build relationships, and preplanning can aid the nurse. Children often perform best in familiar environments; therefore, perform the developmental assessment in the home or another familiar environment whenever possible. Observe whether the child performs self-care activities and at what developmental level. See Chapter 3 and thePoint Supplemental Information: Select Tools for Assessing Cognitive and Adaptive Functioning for assessing developmental and cognitive abilities and self-care skills. It is also important to assess social skills and determine whether the

skills can be generalized to other settings. During the assessment, note the following:

- Are the child's social skills consistent, or nearly so, with the child's chronologic age?
- How does the child relate to you?
- Does the child cling to the parent/family member, appear afraid or shy, or become friendly after a period of observing and watching?
- Does the child bring you toys or make other attempts to engage you?
- What is the child's general activity level?

Weigh all observations of the child in light of the child's chronologic age, expected developmental level, and what the child can do and actually does. For instance, does the child demonstrate appropriate gross and fine motor skills but have deficits in speech and language? Does the child have speech comprehension (receptive language skills) with little verbal language (expressive language skills)?

Gather assessment information from family members as well. The functional abilities of the child as demonstrated over time can best be described by those who spend the most time with the child.

Children with intellectual disabilities may display self-stimulating behaviors, such as arm flapping or head banging. Feelings of despair, helplessness, and fear of abandonment can cause clinging behavior. Frustration in communicating needs and feelings may lead to acting-out behavior.

Carefully review medications, being alert for potential interactions of multiple medications. Assess possible side effects as well because these children may not communicate symptoms or their disability may mask side effects and interactions (Clinical Judgment 30-2).

ANSWER: Assess expressive and receptive language, fine motor skills, other gross motor skills, and social skills. "What can Cecilia say?" "Does Cecilia feed herself?" "What sorts of things does she pick up?" "What is she doing that is new?" "How does she let you know she is content or distressed?"

Interdisciplinary Interventions

QUESTION: One of the objectives of this chapter is to learn how to support families in their efforts to identify and use community resources that best meet the individual child and family's needs. How you would do this for the Curricio family?

Include the child, family members, teachers, and other care providers in intervention planning for a child with a developmental disorder. Some children can participate more than others, and ability to provide input changes as the child's developmental level increases. A multidisciplinary approach encourages coordination

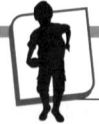

CLINICAL JUDGMENT 30-2

Appropriate Dosage of Medication

Summer, 8 years old, has been on haloperidol for the past year to decrease self-stimulating behaviors of head banging and hand biting. Her father reports that lately, she is "not doing so well."

Questions

1. What questions would you ask about medication dosage, medication administration, side effects, and behavior of the child?

2. What would be the signs of drug interactions, side effects, or inappropriate dose?

3. Summer has grown about 2 in. and gained 10 lb during the past year, but her father reports that she is taking the same dose that was initially prescribed. She does not like to take it and fights administration. Sometimes, the parents are just too tired to fight her, so she gets the dose about 5 days a week. During the past few weeks, Summer has been head banging and hand biting much more frequently than she did when she first started taking the medicine. Do you think she is receiving the appropriate dose of medication?

4. What steps would you take to change the drug dosage? What should be included in parental and child teaching?

5. What outcomes would indicate that the dosage has been adjusted to the most effective dose?

Answers

1. What dosage is Summer taking, and how is medication administered? Does Summer resist taking medication? Do the parents have difficulty administering the medication? Has Summer grown, or gained or lost weight? What does the father mean when he says "not doing so well?" If he reports that she is demonstrating negative behaviors, how long have these behaviors been present? Has there been a change in the child's physical or mental well-being or other changes in the child's behavior?

2. Possible signs of drug interactions or side effects include nausea, diarrhea, change in sleep patterns, confusion, change in activity or speech, tics, and muscle weakness. Receiving subtherapeutic dosages may result in reoccurrence of the negative behaviors.

3. Summer is increasingly demonstrating negative self-stimulating behaviors (head banging and hand biting), possibly indicating that the medication is no longer having the desired effect.

4. Measure Summer's current height and weight and compare with her previous measurements and growth trajectory. If Summer has grown or gained weight during the past year, she will require a higher dosage of her medication to maintain therapeutic levels. Find out who prescribed the medication and how the prescriber can be contacted. Determine whether it would be best to communicate directly with the prescriber or whether the family should contact the prescriber. Discuss the value of keeping a record of medication administration and family observations of behavior. If Summer resists taking the medication, provide suggestions about administering the medication or consider a different form or route for medication, such as a liquid instead of pills or two small-dosage pills instead of a large capsule. Discuss with family the desired effects of the medication for Summer and behaviors that may indicate lack of efficacy; medication interactions and possible side effects; and indicators that the dosage may need to be adjusted such as child's growth, increased stress, or changes in the child's other medications.

5. After a change in dosage of the medication, the negative behaviors abate and the desired behavior is observed

---

of the many services that will be needed. Realistic and consistent short- and long-term goals should be set so progress can be easily monitored. Flexibility and adaptation may not be strengths of children with intellectual disability. They often do best with familiar staff and consistent routines (Clinical Judgment 30-3; see thePoint Care Path: Care of the Child With a Developmental Disorder Who Is Hospitalized).

Common interventions for the child with intellectual disability include behavior management, such as teaching life and socialization skills, involving the child in play therapy, and education about human sexuality. Behavior management and play therapy are provided by an advanced practice registered nurse.

There are no specific medical interventions for intellectual disability. As for any child, provide health maintenance, health promotion, and preventive health care as recommended. Medications should be provided for any comorbid disorders (e.g., seizures, anxiety, infection) present. The child with an intellectual

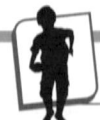

CLINICAL JUDGMENT 30-3

Developmentally Appropriate Interventions for a Child With Down Syndrome

Sara is a 4-year-old girl with trisomy 21 (Down syndrome). She is admitted to the hospital to have her tonsils and adenoids removed. This has been determined to be necessary by her doctor because periods of sleep apnea have been noted. Sara is happy and playful in her room. Her mother describes this as her usual behavior.

Questions

1. During your assessment, what information should you ask Sara's mother about the child's development?

2. While you are talking with the mother, what observations about Sara's behavior might be useful in planning her care?

3. Sara's mother states that her daughter does not have intelligible speech but has learned several sign language terms. Her daughter can walk and run with ease. She cannot feed herself well with a spoon. Do you think these milestones are age appropriate?

4. On the morning of surgery, how would you prepare Sara for the events that will occur?

5. After surgery, Sara refuses to drink and continually cries for her mother, indicating that she wants to be picked up and held. What comfort interventions should you implement?

Answers

1. Assess her speech, hearing, and visual skills. Children with Down syndrome often have speech delays and hearing or vision problems. Determine how Sara communicates her desires and how she can be best approached to follow instructions. Assess whether she has had prior experiences with surgery or hospitalization.

2. Does she readily make contact with strangers? Does she readily explore her surroundings? How does she respond to hospitalization? Does she appear to be afraid?

3. Sara exhibits speech delays and delays with hand–eye coordination. As a 4-year-old, she should be able to feed herself easily using a fork and spoon and should have speech that is essentially completely intelligible.

4. Have Sara sit with her mother. Provide an additional opportunity to review the process of preparing for surgery and what occurs afterward, using actual pieces of equipment (e.g., mask and intravenous tubing, cup for drink). Allow Sara to practice using these things on a favorite doll or bear. Have Sara teach the nurse how she says "hurt."

5. Allow Sara to sit on her mother's lap in a well-supported chair. Encourage Sara to drink fluids or eat popsicles in flavors that she likes (not citrus). Historically, milk and red liquids were contraindicated after tonsillectomy. It was thought that red liquids may resemble blood which would make assessing blood loss more difficult. However, evidence does not exist to support this practice. Encourage saliva production with a lollipop if permitted by the surgeon. Administer pain medication as ordered.

---

disability who is healthy is usually no more vulnerable to infections than other children but may have difficulty communicating symptoms related to an acute illness.

Children with intellectual disability are more likely than others to have seizure disorders, hyperactivity, and alterations in mental health. Alterations in mental health and physical health should receive the same medical and mental health treatment given to any child, but approach the child at the appropriate developmental level rather than chronologic age. He or she may be prone to self-injury because of **self-stimulation** behaviors (rhythmic, repetitive actions such as excessively flailing arms, jumping up and down, rocking, head banging, finger tapping, vocalizations in an effort to shut out external stimuli and to calm self). Make safety a priority. Determining when situations or people are dangerous can also be challenging for children with intellectual disabilities. Because many children are very friendly and show inappropriate affection, extra care is needed to protect them from unsafe situations or possible predators. Nursing Interventions 30-2 highlights strategies for working with children with an intellectual disability.

Interventions to improve academic and adaptive functioning include speech therapy, contingency behavior management techniques, occupational and physical therapy, and special education. Teaching advocacy skills to the family is particularly helpful because families frequently need to obtain resources for their child in educational and social systems. Children with intellectual disabilities fall under the Education Advocacy Laws and entitle the child with intellectual disability to a free and appropriate education from birth to age

---

NURSING INTERVENTIONS 30-2

Strategies for Working With Children or Adolescents Who Have an Intellectual Disability

Develop a warm, trusting relationship.

Identify current skills and level of development.

Assist child and family in achieving the next growth and development skill.

Break skill into its component parts.

Teach each component (one at a time) according to the hierarchy of skills—for example, feeding self:
1. Picking up utensil
2. Dipping utensil into food
3. Scooping food onto utensil
4. Lifting utensil to mouth
5. Putting utensil into mouth and getting food off the utensil into mouth
6. Returning utensil to surface or to food container

Use concrete methods to teach, such as pictures or the actual object demonstrated (have the items at hand when teaching so the child can see and manipulate them).

Teach skill in location where it will routinely happen.

Practice generalization after skill is thoroughly learned.

Avoid abstract messages.

Use simple terms and brief, simple sentences.

Be patient and reward each success.

Be consistent in expectations.

Label feelings for child and redirect inappropriate activities.

Give child two or three choices (do not expect child to *tell* you what he or she wants, especially when verbal skills are absent or limited).

Try tools used with younger children to identify feelings and describe problems because these tools often work with older children

Watch for self-injurious behavior; behavior modification and medications may be needed.

Provide adequate stimulation, rewards, and play to prevent boredom.

Individualize intervention strategies.

---

21 years (see Teaching Intervention Plan 30-1). Children with intellectual disabilities must be educated and included in all settings with other children (see Chapters 2 and 12 for further discussion of the Individuals with Disabilities Education Improvement Act). Adolescents with an intellectual disability should be provided with basic job training skills or apprenticeships so that they can contribute to their family and society to the best of their abilities.

Families usually follow a process of adaptation that includes perceptions of the diagnosis and its effect on the family, available family resources, and transformation (Pelchat, 2010). Helping the family to gain an understanding of the child's needs based on developmental status is especially important (see the Point Care Path: An Interdisciplinary Plan of Care for Family With a Child With New Diagnosis of Developmental Disorder). Assisting the family to connect with support groups is also helpful because the family may become isolated. Even in healthy families, periods of stress and grieving may occur when the child's skills and abilities are slow to develop or when a younger child or a friend's children reach other developmental milestones or surpass the development of the child with intellectual disability. The nurse can help identify and evaluate resources needed by the child and family. Newer online, virtual, and social media platforms can help families find support and interact with others with similar questions and concerns.

ANSWER: Provide written information, including local resources, for a family with a child with Down syndrome. Give the family the contact information for the health department and the state's early intervention program. Down syndrome, like many other conditions, has active local associations with a mission to provide education, resources, and support in partnership with individuals, families, professionals, and the community. Find the local association closest to you and be sure the Curricio family has that name, telephone number, and website.

AUTISM SPECTRUM DISORDER

ASD is characterized by markedly abnormal or impaired development in social interaction and communication (APA, 2013). **Social impairment** is sustained and includes such things as poor eye contact, not liking to be touched, and preferring solitary activities. Children with ASD often do not seem to notice others and in fact seem oblivious to others. They may have impaired speech or little or no use of language. Some children who do have language may not engage with others in a conversation. They may insist on certain routines and have a very narrow interest range. Children with ASD may also have repetitive mannerisms such as hand-wringing, head banging, rocking, or running in circles.

The prevalence of ASD in the United States is approximately 1 in 88 children and is about five times more prevalent in boys than in girls (Centers for Disease Control and Prevention [CDC], 2012). The diagnosis of ASD is more likely to be made today than in the past. The reason for the increasing frequency of diagnosis may be related to an increase in the factors that cause ASD, or it may be a result of better detection—that is, families and health care providers may be recognizing the symptoms and assigning the diagnosis in larger numbers.

Much public attention has focused on the increased number of children diagnosed with ASD in recent years. The search for possible causes of ASD has led to heated controversy. Different potential causes of ASD have strong proponents. Some of the suggested causes include environmental chemicals, viral infections during infancy, and chemicals in childhood immunizations (Nursing Interventions 30-3). Scientific evidence supports the existence of familial patterns; risk among siblings of individuals with the disorder may be as high as 18.7% (Ozonoff et al., 2011). Environmental factors have not been identified but are important, considering that concordance in monozygotic twins is less than 100% (Hallmayer et al., 2011) and expression of the disorder among siblings, including twins, is variable (Ozonoff et al., 2011).

Although individuals do not outgrow or become cured of ASD, intensive interventions can decrease inappropriate or harmful behaviors and can increase the ability of the child to function at higher levels. Children with ASD can become productive adults who live independently and contribute to society.

Assessment

All children should be screened for ASD at 18 and 24 months of age (Johnson & Myers, 2010) (Evidence-Based Clinical Practice Guidelines 30-1). The *DSM-5* (APA, 2013) lists seven symptoms of ASD. These symptoms are listed under the major categories of social, communicative deficits, and restrictive repetitive behavior; all criteria in the first subcategory and two of the four criteria in the second subcategory must be present to make the diagnosis. To diagnose ASD, the symptoms must exist in early childhood, although may not fully manifest or be recognized until social communication requirements exceed capabilities; symptoms must also limit and impair everyday functioning (Chart 30-1). Absolute indicators for immediate evaluation are (Filipek et al., 2000)

- No babbling or pointing or other gesture (e.g., waving bye-bye) by 12 months of age
- No single words by 16 months of age
- No spontaneous two-word (not echolalic) phrases by 24 months of age
- Any loss of language or social skills at any age

NURSING INTERVENTIONS 30-3

Answering Family Questions Regarding Immunizations and Autism Spectrum Disorder

Moira Curricio's sister, Siobhan, had a healthy baby girl 6 weeks ago. The infant had the hepatitis B vaccine immediately after birth. Now Siobhan has told Moira that she has decided not to have the infant receive any further vaccines. She has been reading various references and looking things up on the Internet. She recently came across an article that indicated that there is a connection between certain immunizations and ASD and she does not want to risk this for her child. Siobhan has contacted her baby's primary care provider to discuss the decision not to immunize. What are some educational points regarding immunizations and ASD that Siobhan must know?

- A small study was done (12 participants) that suggested a link between measles–mumps–rubella (MMR) vaccination, ASD, and bowel disease (Wakefield et al., 1998); the study was retracted a few years later and the author's claims were determined to be unfounded. Multiple studies since then have demonstrated no association between MMR administration and ASD.
- Remind Siobhan that the MMR vaccine is administered at the age when symptoms of ASD first

become apparent, so the timing may appear to link the two. However, coincidence does not suggest causality.
- The apparent increase in ASD incidence is likely because of the better diagnosis of this disorder and identification/labeling of symptoms in order to request and receive special education services from schools and other institutions.
- Thimerosal, a preservative, has also been implicated as causing ASD. Evidence does not support a link between thimerosal and ASD (Barile et al., 2012). ASD cases are increasing, although thimerosal has not been in vaccines since 2001.
- All recommended immunizations have been thoroughly studied and approved by the American Academy of Pediatrics and the CDC.
- Educate Siobhan that the effects of the diseases themselves (measles, mumps, rubella, etc.) are far worse than the effects of the immunizations and may cause serious illness and even death.
- Last, review important points about searching for information on the Internet. In particular, always make sure the information is from a reputable source that does not have a hidden agenda.

Autism Spectrum Disorder

American Academy of Neurology and the Child Neurology Society. (2000). *Guideline on screening and diagnosis of autism.* Retrieved from

http://www.neurology.org/content/55/4/468.full.pdf

Presents practice guidelines for screening and diagnosis of autism.

American Speech-Language-Hearing Association. (2006). *Guidelines for speech-language pathologists in diagnosis, assessment, and treatment of autism spectrum disorders across the life span.* Retrieved from

http://www.asha.org/policy/GL2006-00049

Provides guidelines for the assessment and treatment of ASDs across age groups.

Centers for Disease Control and Prevention, American Academy of Pediatrics, & First Signs. (2012). *Autism A.L.A.R.M. guidelines.* Retrieved from

http://www.medicalhomeinfo.org/downloads/pdfs/AutismAlarm.pdf

Practice guideline to identify and evaluate children with ASDs.

Assessment of the child suspected to have ASD requires an interdisciplinary team, with the family members as important members of the team. A physical examination should be thorough and include a complete neurologic examination. Obtain a detailed history of the neonatal period and early development. Psychological testing and evaluation of functional ability must be part of the assessment. Specific tools exist to assess for ASD (Tradition or Science 30-1). Identification of other disorders such as intellectual disability may contribute to the correct diagnosis. As with other developmental disorders, focus the assessment on the child's functional ability. Assessment is needed to determine the child's functioning in the areas of communication, self-care, social and interpersonal skills, and ability to follow directions. Children with ASD have difficulty expressing their needs and responding to changes in routine or loss of objects to which they are attached. They may experience severe temper tantrums, show extreme distress for no apparent reason, and be unresponsive to usual attempts to soothe.

Also assess the family's coping skills and available resources. Families caring for a child with ASD may become exhausted trying to maintain routines and cope with the severe temper tantrums. Because these children demonstrate little empathy for others and do not respond to affection, the family may become discouraged and feel hopeless. Siblings may be at risk for injury from the temper tantrums and lack of concern for others.

Interdisciplinary Interventions

Interventions should be targeted at educational strategies, home-based strategies, and behavior management. The goals for intervention should be aimed at promoting developmental skills, reducing repetitive behaviors, eliminating negative behavior such as head banging or temper tantrums, and supporting the family.

When caring for the child with ASD, allow the child time to become familiar with the environment and staff. Do not make abrupt, rapid movements and allow the child time to transition between activities.

Medication can be helpful in assisting children with ASD (Huffman et al., 2011). Selective serotonin reuptake inhibitors and atypical antipsychotics (e.g., risperidone) may help treat repetitive behavior and obsessive–compulsive symptoms. Stimulants, alpha-2 agonists (e.g., clonidine), and atypical antipsychotics may be used to treat hyperactivity, impulsivity, and inattention. Aggression and

---

CHART 30-1 Symptoms of Autism Spectrum Disorder

Social Communicative Impairment

- Social–emotional reciprocity deficits ranging from abnormal social approach and failure of normal back and forth conversation, to reduced sharing of interests, emotions, or affect, to failure to initiate or respond
- Deficits in nonverbal communicative behaviors used for social interaction ranging from poorly integrated verbal and nonverbal communication, to abnormalities in eye contact and body-language or deficits in understanding and use of nonverbal communication, to total lack of facial expression or gestures
- Deficits in developing, maintaining, and understanding relationships ranging from difficulties adjusting behavior to suit the social context, to difficulties in sharing imaginative play or in making friends, to an apparent lack of interest in people

Restricted, Repetitive Behavior Patterns

- Stereotyped or repetitive motor movements, use of object, or speech
- Insistence on sameness, inflexible adherence to routines or ritualized patterns of verbal or nonverbal behavior
- Highly restricted, fixated interests that are abnormal in intensity or focus
- Hyper- or hyposensitivity to sensory input or unusual interest in sensory aspects of the environment

Information from American Psychiatric Association. (2013). *Diagnostic and statistical manual of mental disorders* (5th ed.). Washington, DC: Author.

TRADITION OR SCIENCE 30-1

What is the best tool for diagnosing ASD?

Several factors must be considered to determine the best tool for assessment, including ease of administration (including need for training to administer), cost, time, and sensitivity (how often a tool accurately identifies a child as having the condition) and specificity (how often a tool accurately identifies a child as not having the condition when they truly do not). Tests such as the Autism Diagnostic Interview-Revised (ADI-R) (Lord et al., 1994), the Autism Diagnostic Observation Schedule-Generic (ADOS-G) (Lord et al., 2002), and the Childhood Autism Rating Scale (CARS/CARS-2) (Schopler et al., 1980; Schopler et al., 2010) are the most widely used diagnostic tools but require lengthy, professional administration (McGarry Klose et al., 2012). The Gilliam Autism Rating Scale (GARS/GARS-2), which is administered by a family member or teacher, is a tool widely used in schools and clinics for children 3–22 years of age. The first version of the GARS had been shown to produce a large number of false negatives and to have low sensitivity (Lecavalier, 2005; South et al., 2002); these issues were addressed in the second version which is intended to be used with a variety of diagnostic tools to provide a comprehensive assessment (Gilliam, 2006).

Many screening tools have had some reliability or validity demonstrated. Some of these are the Autism Spectrum Screening Questionnaire (ASSQ) (Ehlers et al., 1999), the Pervasive Developmental Disorders Screening Test-II Primary Care Screener (Siegel, 2004), the Developmental Behaviour Checklist–Autism Screening Algorithm (DBC-ASA) (Brereton et al., 2002), Krug Asperger's Disorder Index (KADI) (Krug & Arick, 2003), the Social and Communication Disorders Checklist (SCDC) (Skuse et al., 2005), the Autism Observation Scale for Infants (AOSI) (Bryson et al., 2008), and the Quantitative Checklist for Autism in Toddlers (Q-CHAT) (Allison et al., 2008). The Modified-Checklist for Autism in Toddlers (M-CHAT) (Robins & Dumont-Mathieu, 2006) shows good sensitivity but low specificity (Eaves et al., 2006; Kozlowski et al., 2012), meaning that it has a higher chance of identifying children as having autism when they do not. The Autism Screening Questionnaire [ASQ]/Social Communication Questionnaire (SCQ) (formerly Autism Screening Questionnaire) (Berument et al., 1999; Rutter et al., 2003) seems to be an acceptable screening tool for older children but does not have a good sensitivity and specificity with younger preschoolers (Allen et al., 2007; Oosterling et al., 2010). The Developmental Behaviour Checklist: Early Screen (DBC-ES) has good sensitivity but low specificity (Gray et al., 2008). The Screening Tool for Autism in Two-Year-Olds (STAT) demonstrates high sensitivity and specificity (Stone et al., 2004) but requires training to administer. More research is indicated to support the psychometric properties of these tools before widespread clinical use; but, given the importance of not overlooking the diagnosis, tools with good sensitivity but lower specificity may be selected as screening tools.

Any tool that requests a family to act as objective observers of their own children incorporates the family's biases and lack of professional training. Tools are only as good as the persons trained to use them; test scores should not override clinical judgment. A comprehensive diagnostic assessment must go beyond informant-based rating scales and requires a trained professional.

self-injury may be treated with atypical antipsychotics, anticonvulsant mood stabilizers (e.g., levetiracetam), selective serotonin reuptake inhibitors, or beta-blockers. Careful observation for side effects of any medication is needed to offset negative or harmful reactions.

Behavior therapies and social skills training, performed by a mental health provider such as an advanced practice psychiatrist nurse, can be beneficial. The earlier the interventions are begun, the more likely they will have a positive effect. Substantial gains can be achieved in language acquisition and social interaction if treatment is consistent and ongoing. Behaviors that need to be eliminated or changed should be targeted, and their frequency and duration should be measured. These behaviors might include hitting, biting, pinching, spitting, head banging, or crying. Establish a baseline rate of the targeted behavior so that progress can be monitored. It is also important to study the antecedents to the behavior so environmental causes can be prevented (e.g., by avoiding crowds or lack of structure).

Controlling a child's environment to eliminate changes or interruptions is difficult, if not impossible, so teaching the child to use strategies to cope with changes is more effective. The tools could be objects, photos, calendars, labels, color codes, and so on. These tools help the child to manage change. For example, help the child to organize the things that he or she can control. Color coding helps the child find things, even if the order or usual routine changes. Calendars list what will happen that day, even if the order is different; if a day will differ from what the child expects, that difference might be noted on the calendar so the child can anticipate the change and talk to someone about how he or she will still accomplish activities. For example, the note might say, "Instead of the bus dropping you off and you getting an after-school snack, Daddy will pick you up, give you a snack in the car, and take you to the ball game." Anticipating schedule changes also helps lessen behavior outbursts. Children who do not communicate well may use pictures to indicate activities and rearrange the order if the schedule changes. Pictures can be placed on shelves or storage bins to indicate what is in them. This practice gives the child more control while decreasing the frustration of searching for something or making choices. Pictures, colors, and other cues eliminate the need for the family to get into power struggles with the child or become frustrated as well when the child cannot express what he or she wants or is trying to explain.

Rewarding positive behavior and ignoring negative behavior is also effective. Of course, ignoring negative behavior is not always easy; it requires support for the family or even the therapist.

 KidKare Alternative forms of communication may help a child with ASD to communicate.

Sign language or assistive communication devices may help the child to communicate needs or give the child choices (see thePoint Organizations: The Family Village website for links to more information about communication devices or aids) (Fig. 30-3). Speech and

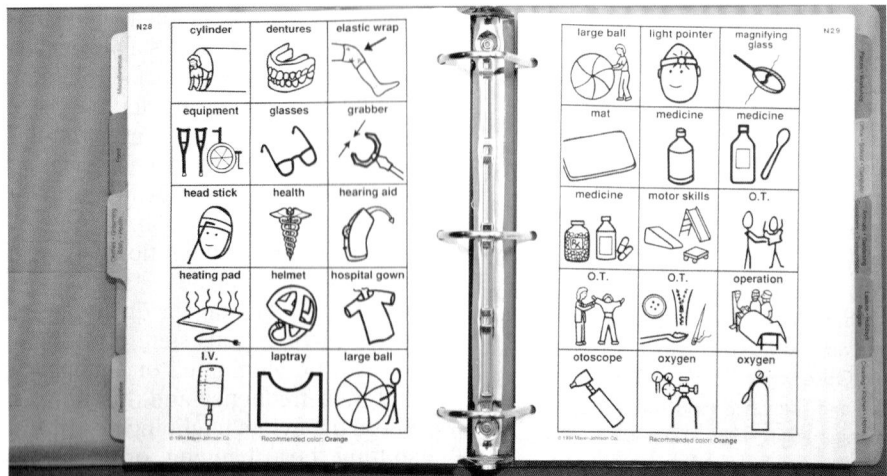

Figure 30-3 A communication board helps children with ASD and Down syndrome express their needs and wants.

language therapy may improve communicative abilities (Fernell et al., 2013). Encouraging communication and building on strengths may stimulate cooperation. For example, if a child is good at counting or reciting letters of the alphabet, the child can be encouraged to use these activities to decrease anxiety in stressful situations.

Because children with ASD can be challenging, families need support and can benefit from social support, such as respite care. Ensure that the family knows what resources are available in the community. Teach the family how to use tools such as behavior recording, observation, performance measuring, and reward systems. The family needs to understand that they did not cause the child's disorder and that because the child has such major needs, reaching out for help from professionals and the community is necessary.

Educational interventions must include special education and should begin as early as possible. An IEP (see Teaching Intervention Plan 30-1) should guide the child's educational experience. Special attention should be paid to behavioral management and to auditory and visual tools to assist the child. Children with higher intellectual skills should be educationally stimulated. Children with ASD do better in learning situations that have consistent routines and rules; use of simple, clear, unambiguous language; a workstation away from distractions; individual assistance; and immediate feedback.

Children with ASD also need to participate in afterschool and community activities to practice and improve their social skills. These activities should be something at which the child can succeed. Strategic guidance and structured activities assist children with ASD to develop their social skills. Social skills training may be helpful in improving peer relations and decreasing the isolation and stigma associated with manifestations of ASD.

See thePoint for a list of Key Concepts.

REFERENCES

Allen, C. W., Silove, N., Williams, K. et al. (2007). Validity of the Social Communication Questionnaire in assessing risk of autism in preschool children with developmental problems. *Journal of Autism and Developmental Disorders, 37*(7), 1272–1278.

Allison, C., Baron-Cohen, S., Wheelwright, S. et al. (2008). The Q-CHAT (Quantitative Checklist for Autism in Toddlers): A normally distributed quantitative measure of autistic traits at 18–24 months of age: Preliminary report. *Journal of Autism and Developmental Disorders, 38*(8), 1414–1425.

American Academy of Pediatrics. (2006, reaffirmed 2009). Identifying infants and young children with developmental disorders in the medical home: An algorithm for developmental surveillance and screening. *Pediatrics, 118*(1), 405–420.

American Psychiatric Association. (2013). *Diagnostic and statistical manual of mental disorders* (5th ed.). Washington, DC: Author.

Barile, J. P., Kuperminc, G. P., Weintraub, E. S. et al. (2012). Thimerosal exposure in early life and neuropsychological outcomes 7–10 years later. *Journal of Pediatric Psychology, 37*(1), 106–118.

Berument, S. B., Rutter, M., Lord, C. et al. (1999). Autism screening questionnaire: Diagnostic validity. *British Journal of Psychiatry, 175*, 444–451.

Bloom, B., Cohen, R. A., & Freeman, G. (2012). Summary health statistics for U.S. children: National Health Interview Survey, 2011. *Vital and Health Statistics, 10*(254), 1–80.

Brereton, A. V., Tonge, B. J., Mackinnon, A. J. et al. (2002). Screening young people for autism with the Development Behaviour Checklist. *Journal of the American Academy of Child and Adolescent Psychiatry, 41*(11), 1369–1375.

Bryson, S. E., Zwaigenbaum, L., McDermott, C. et al. (2008). The Autism Observation Scale for Infants: Scale development and reliability data. *Journal of Autism and Developmental Disorders, 38*(4), 731–738.

Carlson, G., Armistead, C., Stodger, S. et al. (2010). Parents' experiences of the provision of community-based family support and therapy services utilizing the strengths approach and natural learning environments. *Journal of Applied Research in Intellectual Disabilities, 23*(6), 560–572.

Centers for Disease Control and Prevention. (2012). Prevalence of autism spectrum disorders—Autism and Developmental Disabilities Monitoring Network, 14 sites, United States, 2008. *Morbidity and Mortality Weekly Report, 61*(3), 1–19.

DuPaul, G. J., Gormley, M. J., & Laracy, S. D. (2013). Comorbidity of LD and ADHD: Implications of DSM-5 for assessment and treatment. *Journal of Learning Disabilities, 46*(1), 43–51.

Eaves, L., Wingert, H., & Ho, H. H. (2006). Screening for autism: Agreement with diagnosis. *Autism, 10*(3), 229–242.

Ehlers, S., Gillberg, C., & Wing, L. (1999). A screening questionnaire for Asperger syndrome and other high functioning autism spectrum disorders in school age children. *Journal of Autism and Developmental Disorders, 29*(2), 129–141.

Emerson, E. (2013). Commentary: Childhood exposure to environmental adversity and the well-being of people with intellectual disabilities. *Journal of Intellectual Disability Research, 57*(7), 589–600.

Fernell, E., Eriksson, M. A., & Gillberg, C. (2013). Early diagnosis of autism and impact on prognosis: A narrative review. *Clinical Epidemiology, 5*, 33–43.

Filipek, P. A., Accardo, P. J., Ashwal, S. et al. (2000). Practice parameter: Screening and diagnosis of autism: Report of the Quality Standards Subcommittee of the American Academy of Neurology and the Child Neurology Society. *Neurology, 55*(4), 468–479.

Gilliam, J. (2006). *GARS-2: Gilliam autism rating scale* (2nd ed.). Austin, TX: PRO-ED.

Gray, K. M., Tonge, B. J., Sweeney, D. J. et al. (2008). Screening for autism in young children with developmental delay: An evaluation of the Developmental Behaviour Checklist: Early screen. *Journal of Autism and Developmental Disorders, 38*(6), 1003–1010.

Hallmayer, J., Cleveland, S., Torres, A. et al. (2011). Genetic heritability and shared environmental factors among twin pairs with autism. *Archives of General Psychiatry, 68*(11), 1095–1102.

Hillemeier, M. M., Morgan, P. L., Farkas, G. et al. (2011). Perinatal socioeconomic risk factors for variable and persistent cognitive delay at 24 and 48 months of age in a national sample. *Maternal Child Health Journal, 15*(7), 1001–1010.

Huffman, L. C., Sutcliffe, T. L., Tanner, I. S. et al. (2011). Management of symptoms in children with autism spectrum disorders: A comprehensive review of pharmacologic and complementary-alternative medicine treatments. *Journal of Developmental and Behavioral Pediatrics, 32*(1), 56–68.

Johnson, C. P., & Myers, S. M. (2007, reaffirmed 2010). Identification and evaluation of children with autism spectrum disorders. *Pediatrics, 120*(5), 1183–1215.

Kelly, D. P., & Aylward, G. P. (2005). Identifying school performance problems in the pediatric office. *Pediatric Annals, 34*(4), 288–298.

Kozlowski, A. M., Matson, J. L., Worley, J. A. et al. (2012). Defining characteristics for young children meeting cutoff on the modified checklist for autism in toddlers. *Research in Autism Spectrum Disorders, 6*(1), 472–479.

Krug, D. A., & Arick, J. R. (2003). *Krug Asperger's disorder index*. Austin, TX: PRO-ED.

Lecavalier, L. (2005). An evaluation of the Gilliam Autism Rating Scale. *Journal of Autism and Developmental Disorders, 35*(6), 795–803.

Lord, C., Rutter, M., DiLavore, P. C. et al. (2002). *Autism diagnostic observation schedule*. Los Angeles, CA: Western Psychological Services.

Lord, C., Rutter, M., & LeCouteur, A. (1994). Autism diagnostic review—Revised: A revised version of a diagnostic interview for caregivers of individuals with possible pervasive developmental disorders. *Journal of Autism and Developmental Disorders, 24*(5), 659–685.

Maughan, B., & Carroll, J. (2006). Literacy and mental disorders. *Current Opinion in Psychiatry, 19*(4), 350–354.

Maulik, P. K. Mascarenhas, M. N., Mathers, C. D. et al. (2011). Prevalence of intellectual disability: A meta-analysis of population-based studies. *Research in Developmental Disabilities, 32*(2), 419–436.

McGarry Klose, L., Plotts, C., Kozeneski, N. et al. (2012). A review of assessment tools for diagnosis of autism spectrum disorders: Implications for school practice. *Assessment for Effective Intervention, 37*(4), 236–242.

Mitchell, W. (2012). Parents' accounts: Factors considered when deciding how far to involve their son/daughter with learning disabilities in choice-making. *Children and Youth Services Review, 34*(8), 1560–1569.

Northstone, K., Joinson, C., Emmett, P. et al. (2012). Are dietary patterns in childhood associated with IQ at 8 years of age? A population-based cohort study. *Journal of Epidemiology and Community Health, 66*(7), 624–628.

Oosterling, I., Rommelse, N., de Jonge, M. et al. (2010). How useful is the Social Communication Questionnaire in toddlers at risk of autism spectrum disorder? *Journal of Child Psychology and Psychiatry, 51*(11), 1260–1268.

Ozonoff, S., Young, G. S., Carter, A. et al. (2011). Recurrence risk for autism spectrum disorders: A baby sibling research consortium study. *Pediatrics, 128*(3), e448–e495.

Pelchat, D. (2010). PRIFAM: A shared experience leading to the transformation of everyone involved. *Journal of Child Health Care, 14*(3), 211–224.

Robins, D. L., & Dumont-Mathieu, T. M. (2006). Early screening for autism spectrum disorders: Update on the modified checklist for autism in toddlers and other measures. *Journal of Developmental and Behavioral Pediatrics, 27*(Suppl. 2), S111–S119.

Rutter, M., Bailey, A., & Lord, C. (2003). *The social communication questionnaire (SCQ) manual*. Los Angeles, CA: Western Psychological Services.

Schopler, E., Reichler, R. J., DeVellis, R. F. et al. (1980). Toward objective classification of childhood autism: Childhood Autism Rating Scale (CARS). *Journal of Autism and Developmental Disorders, 10*(1), 91–103.

Schopler, E., Van Bourgondien, M. E., Wellman, G. J. et al. (2010). *Childhood autism rating scale* (2nd ed.). Los Angeles, CA: Western Psychological Services.

Sentenac, M., Arnaud, C., Gavin, A. et al. (2012). Peer victimization among school-aged children with chronic conditions. *Epidemiologic Reviews, 34*(1), 120–128.

Shaywitz, S. E., Morris, R., & Shaywitz, B. A. (2008). The education of dyslexic children from childhood to young adulthood. *Annual Review of Psychology, 59*, 451–475.

Siegel, B. (2004). *The pervasive developmental disorders screening test II (PDDST-II)*. San Antonio, TX: Harcourt Assessment.

Skuse, D. H., Mandy, W. P., & Scourfield, J. (2005). Measuring autistic traits: Heritability, reliability and validity of the Social and Communication Disorders Checklist. *British Journal of Psychiatry, 187*, 568–572.

Smith, K. E., Landry, S. H., & Swank, P. R. (2006). The role of early maternal responsiveness in supporting school-aged cognitive development for children who vary in birth status. *Pediatrics, 117*(5), 1608–1617.

South, M., Williams, B. J., McMahon, W. M. et al. (2002). Utility of the Gilliam Autism Rating Scale in research and clinical populations. *Journal of Autism and Developmental Disorders, 32*(6), 593–599.

Stone, W. L., Coonrod, E. E., Turner, L. M. et al. (2004). Psychometric properties of the STAT for early autism screening. *Journal of Autism and Developmental Disorders, 34*(6), 691–701.

U.S. National Library of Medicine. (2011). *Intellectual disability*. Retrieved from http://www.nlm.nih.gov/medlineplus/ency/article/001523.htm

Vessey, J. A., & O'Neill, K. M. (2011). Helping students with disabilities better address teasing and bullying situations: A MASNRN study. *Journal of School Nursing, 27*(2), 139–148.

Violato, M., Petrou, S., Gray, R. et al. (2011). Family income and child cognitive and behavioural development in the United Kingdom: Does money matter? *Health Economics, 20*, 1201–1225.

Wakefield, A. J., Murch, S. H., Anthony, A. et al. (1998). Ileal–lymphoid–nodular hyperplasia, non-specific colitis, and pervasive developmental disorder in children. *Lancet, 351*(9103), 637–641.

Wiener, J., & Timmermanis, V. (2012). Social relationships: The 4th R. In B. Wong & D. L. Butler (Eds.), *Learning about learning disabilities* (4th ed., pp. 89–140). London, United Kingdom: Academic Press.

Yoshimasu, K., Barbaresi, W. J., Colligan, R. C. et al. (2010). Gender, attention-deficit/hyperactivity disorder, and reading disability in a population-based birth cohort. *Pediatrics, 126*(4), e788–e795.

See thePoint for additional organizations.

CHAPTER 31

Pediatric Emergencies

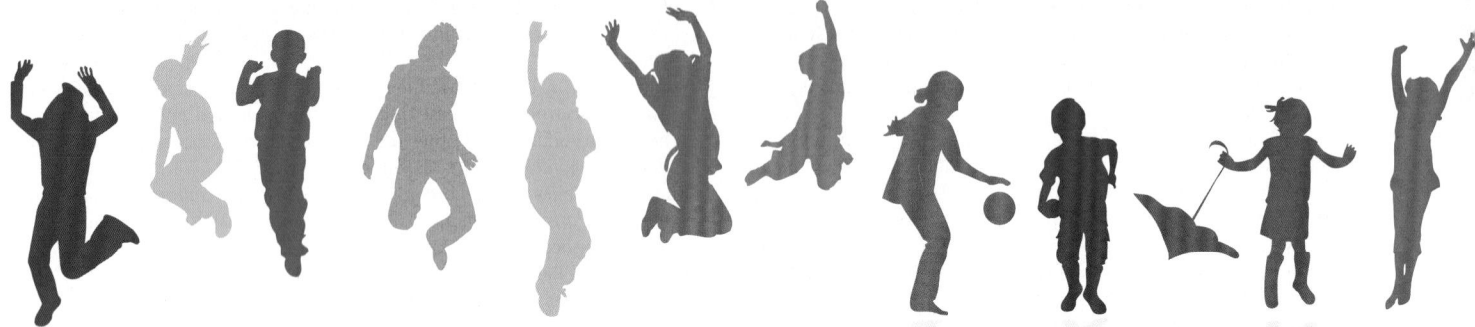

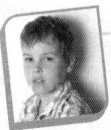

CASE HISTORY

The Whitworth family was introduced in Chapter 6 and again in Chapters 11, 17, 18, and 20. John and Wendy have six children. Chris is one of four boys in the family. The summer that Chris was 8 years old, he and his family attended a church social function. Chris became bored and took his drink and cookies outside into the parking lot. He noticed a hornet's nest on the back of one of the handicapped parking signs. Curious about whether there was anything inside, Chris took the paper cup in his hand, balled it up, and threw it at the nest. Nothing happened. He picked it up and threw it again. This time, several hornets emerged from the nest. Chris took off running, only to trip over the parking curb. The hornets stung him many times. His shrieks brought a crowd out to the parking lot. As his mother looked him over, she noticed that he had many welts on his neck, arms, and ears. Wendy said, "How do you feel?" Chris answered, "My tongue is tingling." His mother replied, "I think we need to go to the emergency room."

CHAPTER OBJECTIVES

1 Describe the four components of pediatric emergency triage.

2 Describe the nursing interventions required for the infant or child in cardiopulmonary arrest.

3 Discuss common causes, signs, and symptoms of shock in children.

4 Prioritize the sequence of assessing the multiple-trauma patient.

5 Identify common signs of and management for hypoxia in a child in respiratory distress.

6 Explain the physiologic effects of fever in a child.

7 Describe the nursing interventions for the child who has been bitten or stung.

8 Discuss management of anaphylaxis.

9 Describe the initial nursing intervention for a child with epistaxis.

10 Discuss the nursing interventions for the child with an environmental injury.

11 Identify the initial treatment for the child who has ingested an unknown poison.

12 Discuss nursing interventions for a family whose child has died of sudden infant death syndrome (SIDS).

13 Discuss considerations for interfacility transfer.

See thePoint for a list of Key Terms.

Emergency management of ill or injured children is costly, physically and emotionally as well as financially. Many emergencies can be avoided through family education and simple prevention techniques. The nurse's astute assessment, knowledge of signs and symptoms of deterioration, and timely interventions can help decrease negative outcomes.

DEVELOPMENTAL AND BIOLOGIC VARIANCES

In an emergency, children are more vulnerable than adults. They have fewer physiologic reserves; for example, tidal volumes and circulating blood volume are smaller. Also, a disease or injury may alter their status more rapidly. Because a child's ability to verbalize is limited, a disease process may be far advanced before signs and symptoms are noted. Although adolescents may be physically and mentally mature, they commonly participate in risk-taking behavior. This behavior, combined with increased mobility and feelings of omnipotence, can put adolescents at greater risk.

Types of emergencies experienced by children of different ages can be attributed to structural and functional changes related to developmental stage (Fig. 31-1). Young children have a greater ratio of surface area to body mass than adults, placing children at higher risk for hypothermia. This risk must be considered in prehospital care or during resuscitation because hypothermia increases metabolic demands, increases pulmonary vascular resistance, and contributes to acidosis. A child's airway is more difficult to stabilize and manage than an adult's because the larynx is more cephalad and anterior, making the vocal cords more difficult to visualize during intubation. Also, the airway diameter in a child is narrower, resulting in greater airway loss with only small amounts of edema.

Variances in the etiology of the situation are seen among age groups (Developmental Considerations 31-1). Young children, in particular, frequently present to the emergency department (ED) with fever, not eating, or a change in sleep patterns. Once the child is in the ED, the underlying pathology is detected.

ASSESSMENT

Assessment of the child in an emergency situation must proceed rapidly. The nurse does not have time to perform a methodical, in-depth assessment but must obtain information rapidly and make decisions promptly in a process called *triage*.

The French word **triage** means "to pick or sort." The goals of triage are to rapidly identify the seriously ill or injured patient, prioritize all patients in the ED, and initiate therapeutic measures for the patient. Triage for children, as for adults, has four components:

1. Performing an across-the-room assessment
2. Determining the chief complaint
3. Performing a brief history and physical assessment
4. Making the triage decision

ACROSS-THE-ROOM ASSESSMENT

 QUESTION: How would you document your across-the-room assessment of Chris?

The triage assessment generally starts with a quick across-the-room visual assessment as soon as the child presents to the ED or clinic. Observe the child's general appearance, work of breathing, and color to determine whether immediate care is required.

ALERT   *Obvious respiratory distress, cyanosis, positioning to maintain an open airway, seizures, unconsciousness, and profuse bleeding are signs that the nurse should interrupt the triage process and proceed to the emergency care area for immediate intervention.*

ANSWER: Chris is alert and oriented, well perfused, with no signs of trauma. He has red papules on his face and neck and noticeable facial edema.

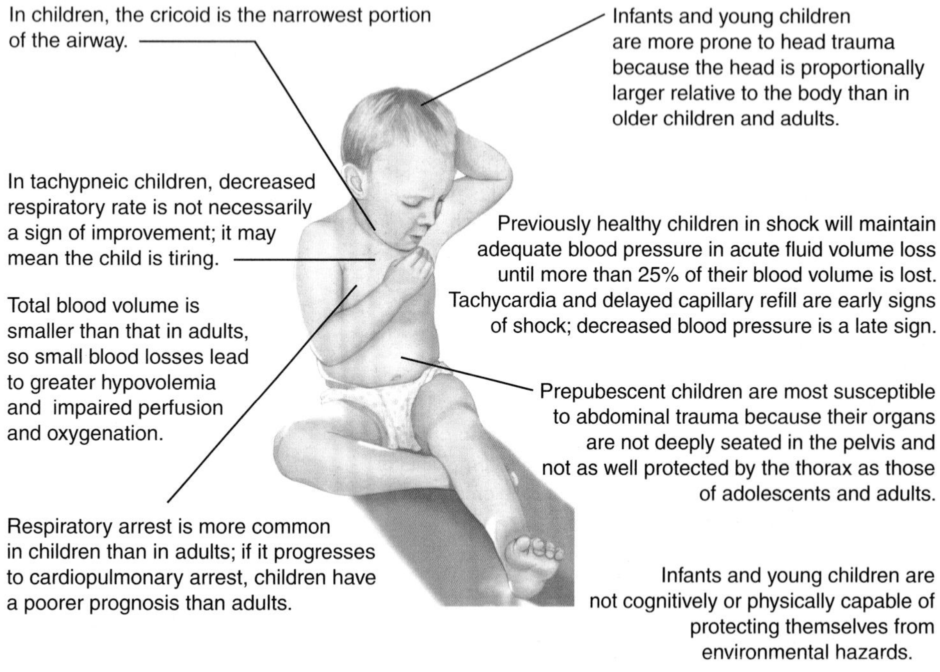

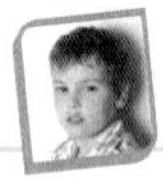

In children, the cricoid is the narrowest portion of the airway.

Infants and young children are more prone to head trauma because the head is proportionally larger relative to the body than in older children and adults.

In tachypneic children, decreased respiratory rate is not necessarily a sign of improvement; it may mean the child is tiring.

Previously healthy children in shock will maintain adequate blood pressure in acute fluid volume loss until more than 25% of their blood volume is lost. Tachycardia and delayed capillary refill are early signs of shock; decreased blood pressure is a late sign.

Total blood volume is smaller than that in adults, so small blood losses lead to greater hypovolemia and impaired perfusion and oxygenation.

Prepubescent children are most susceptible to abdominal trauma because their organs are not deeply seated in the pelvis and not as well protected by the thorax as those of adolescents and adults.

Respiratory arrest is more common in children than in adults; if it progresses to cardiopulmonary arrest, children have a poorer prognosis than adults.

Infants and young children are not cognitively or physically capable of protecting themselves from environmental hazards.

Figure 31-1 Developmental and biologic variances: pediatric emergencies.

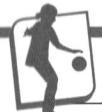

DEVELOPMENTAL CONSIDERATIONS 31-1

Common Emergencies Based on Age

Age Group	Common Medical Emergencies	Common Traumatic Events
Infancy	SIDS Apnea Sepsis Bronchiolitis Seizures	Shaken baby syndrome Falls (off furniture, down stairs in baby walkers) Motor vehicle accident Foreign body aspiration Suffocation Drowning
Early childhood	Croup Asthma Vomiting and/or dehydration Seizures Appendicitis	Foreign body aspiration Poisoning Falls Drowning Motor vehicle accident Burns Child abuse
Middle childhood	Asthma Appendicitis Seizures Gastrointestinal (GI) disturbances	Motor vehicle accident Bicycle injury Sports injury
Adolescence	Colitis Urinary tract infection Pelvic inflammatory disease	Motor vehicle accident (adolescent as driver) Sports injury Firearm injury Drug and alcohol ingestions (accidental and intentional)

CHIEF COMPLAINT

The chief complaint is the reason that the child or parent gives for seeking care. Note the chief complaint using the words of the child or parent, rather than a medical term, to avoid diagnosing a patient before obtaining all objective signs and symptoms and the history. If the chief complaint described by the patient or caregivers does not match presenting signs and symptoms, document this discrepancy.

If the child is unconscious and the parent is not available, the chief complaint is the condition in which the patient presents—for example, "altered level of consciousness."

FOCUSED HEALTH HISTORY AND PHYSICAL ASSESSMENT

QUESTION: Given that Chris's chief complaint is hornet stings followed by subjective complaints of "tingling" in his mouth, describe the critical elements of a focused physical assessment for Chris.

The second step in the triage process combines obtaining a brief health history from the child, parent,

or both while performing a brief physical assessment. Obtaining a triage history can be difficult if the child is young, if the parent or primary caregiver is not present, or if a communication barrier exists (Focused Health History 31-1). During triage, use the AMPLE mnemonic to help remember the key components of the history interview (Chart 31-1).

During the physical assessment, perform a rapid evaluation of the child (Focused Physical Assessment 31-1). Remember to begin with an assessment of vital functions first before moving on to examination of less critical areas.

ANSWER: The critical elements of your physical assessment focus on Chris's airway and include respiratory rate, respiratory effort, and breath sounds.

TRIAGE DECISION

QUESTION: In which triage classification would you place Chris after the multiple hornet stings?

FOCUSED HEALTH HISTORY 31-1

Pediatric Emergencies

Current history	What brought you to seek care today?
	When symptoms started, duration and nature of symptoms, precipitating factors
	Mechanism of injury
	Any treatments initiated
	Mode of arrival (e.g., parent, ambulance)
	Change in level of consciousness or behavior (e.g., lethargy, irritability, weakness)
	Recent change in intake of food and fluid
	Time of last void
	Is anyone else in the family ill?
Past medical history	**Prenatal/Neonatal History**
	Indicated in infants: gestational age at birth, presence of complications
	Previous Health Challenges
	Previous hospitalizations, serious illness, injury, or surgeries and child's response
	History of child abuse
	Child's baseline condition
	Presence of allergies
	Immunization status and date of last tetanus booster
	Medications: prescription, over the counter, or home remedies; name, amount, and frequency
	Does the child have a primary health care provider? If so, what is the provider's name and phone number?
Family medical history	History of same illness in other family members or peers (describe symptoms)
Social and environmental history	Child care issues: Who cares for child and where (e.g., child care center, home)? Is child exposed to other children?
	Cultural practices that may overheat infants (e.g., wrapping in blankets even in hot temperatures); administration of home remedies that may be toxic

Note: See Chapter 8 for a comprehensive health history.

The triage decision involves assigning a triage classification by severity of illness to the patient. This classification regulates the child's movement through the ED and determines the best site of care (Clinical Judgment 31-1). Various triage classification systems are in use. The Emergency Severity Index system specifies the following five levels (Gilboy et al., 2005):

1. *Resuscitation*: Patients who have unstable vital functions and require maximum resource use
2. *Emergent*: Patients with potential threat to life or limb who require high resource use and need medical care within 10 minutes
3. *Urgent*: Patients with stable vital functions who require medium resource use and need medical care within 30 to 60 minutes
4. *Semiurgent*: Patients with stable vital functions and low resource needs who require care within 1 to 2 hours
5. *Nonurgent*: Patients with stable vital functions and no resource needs who require care within 2 to 3 hours

CHART 31-1   AMPLE Mnemonic for Brief History of Pediatric Emergency

- **A**llergies
- **M**edications
- **P**ast medical history
- **L**ast meal
- **E**vents surrounding incident

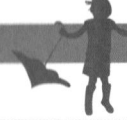

FOCUSED PHYSICAL ASSESSMENT 31-1
Triage Assessment From A to I

Airway	Make sure that the airway is open.
Breathing	Check for breathing; begin bag-and-mask ventilation if needed.
Circulation	Check for a pulse; begin chest compressions if needed.
Disability	Assess level of consciousness by performing a rapid mental status assessment (use AVPU mnemonic): **A:** Is the child **a**lert? **V:** Does the child respond to **v**erbal stimuli? **P:** Does the child respond to **p**ainful stimuli? **U:** Is the child **u**nresponsive?
Exposure	Remove clothing and diaper to assess for underlying signs of illness or injury.
Full vital signs	Obtain a full set of vital signs, including temperature, pulse, respiratory rate, blood pressure, and weight in kilograms. Initiate measures to keep the child warm.
Family presence	Facilitate family presence.
Give comfort	Manage pain, provide emotional support.
Head-to-toe assessment	Perform a brief head-to-toe assessment, focusing on the systems affected by the chief complaint.
Inspect	Inspect the back for injuries.
Isolate	Isolate the child as necessary for communicable illness or if the child is immunosuppressed.

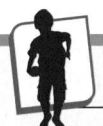

CLINICAL JUDGMENT 31-1
Triage

Sol is a 4-year-old boy who is carried into the ED by his father, who says, "My son says he's not feeling too good." Sol is leaning against his father, holding his head erect with his chin jutting out slightly, alert but not interacting with his environment. He has a respiratory rate of about 40 breaths/min, his lips are blue, and he presents with nasal flaring.

Questions
1. What is Sol's most obvious problem?
2. On what factors did you base your assessment?
3. In what triage category should the nurse classify him?
4. Based on the triage decision, what needs to be done now?
5. Sol's respiratory distress is worsening; what needs to be done?

Answers
1. Respiratory distress
2. Cyanosis, nasal flaring, positioning to maintain open airway, tachypnea (normal respiratory rate for a 4-year-old is in the 20s), developmentally incongruent behavior: Sol is 4 years old but was carried in, and he is not interested in his surroundings.
3. Emergent
4. Sol needs to be taken to the treatment area for immediate intervention. Because Sol still seems to be compensating and maintaining his airway, let him maintain his position of comfort. Do not lay him down; leave him in his father's lap. Administer oxygen, and perform a brief physical examination (A–I) while obtaining a brief history (AMPLE).
5. Ensure that someone skilled in bag-and-mask ventilation and advanced pediatric life support is monitoring him. Have the physician or advanced practice registered nurse evaluate for treatment of an underlying disorder.

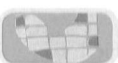
TESTS AND PROCEDURES for Evaluating Pediatric Emergencies

Diagnostic Test or Procedure	Purpose	Findings and Indications	Health Care Provider Considerations
Complete blood count with differential	Detects infection or lack of immune response	Elevated white blood cell count with shift to the left may indicate infection; in neonates, may see neutropenia with infection.	Obtain blood, check results, and intervene on the basis of results.
	Detects blood loss	Decreased red blood cells Decreased hemoglobin	
Type and crossmatch	Determines child's blood type and compatibility of blood to transfuse		Obtain blood, check results, and intervene on the basis of results. May give O-negative blood in emergency before type and crossmatch results are obtained.
Serum electrolytes (including glucose)	Detects electrolyte imbalance	Values outside normal reference ranges for age of child	Obtain blood, check results, and intervene on the basis of results.
Radiographs: Chest	Detects abnormalities in heart, lung, or ribs	Heart failure, pneumothorax, pneumonia, broken ribs.	Maintain c-spine precautions until cleared.
Abdomen	Detects obstruction, perforation, structural abnormalities in abdominal organs	Dilated intestine proximal to obstruction; free air with perforation	Protect child's genitals with lead shield.
Bones	Detects fractures	Crack, malalignment of bone, tenderness on palpation	Position the child.
Computed tomography	Detects bleeding or masses	Abnormalities visualized include tumors, cancer, lesions, abscesses, fluid collection, and inflammation	Closely monitor cardiorespiratory status. Implement conscious sedation protocol if child is sedated.

ANSWER: Chris would be classified in the emergent category. The urgency of treatment can be deceptive in children with airway swelling because the children are alert, oriented, and with no obvious trauma. However, sufficient swelling to obstruct the airway may occur very rapidly. It is critical that Chris receives treatment before his airway is obstructed.

DIAGNOSTIC CRITERIA

Diagnostic procedures used in emergency situations vary depending on the child's pathology or injury and presenting symptoms (Tests and Procedures 31-1). Other tests may be performed, depending on the mechanism of injury (e.g., a child with iron ingestion has serum iron levels evaluated) or pathology (e.g., if the child has signs of meningitis, a lumbar puncture is done). When head or neck injuries are known or suspected, cervical spine (c-spine) precautions must be maintained until spinal cord injury is evaluated.

In an emergency, procedures must often be performed rapidly. The health care provider must always provide age-appropriate support and preparation, even if explanations are given as the procedure is being done. Monitor the child's status during the procedure. The additional stress to an already compromised child may precipitate further deterioration.

TREATMENT MODALITIES

The best treatment for pediatric emergencies is, of course, prevention. Children, parents, family members, and caregivers should be familiar with safe practices and child safety techniques, such as using protective equipment when engaging in sports and childproofing the home (see Chapters 4 to 7), and first aid procedures. When the child presents with an emergent situation, timely intervention can optimize outcomes. Interventions include cardiopulmonary resuscitation (CPR), advanced life support, vascular access, fluid administration, medication administration, and psychosocial support.

PEDIATRIC CARDIOPULMONARY RESUSCITATION

QUESTION: If Chris's laryngeal edema progresses to obstruct his airway, what do you anticipate the sequence of interventions will be?

In adults, the most common causes of cardiopulmonary arrest are lethal arrhythmias secondary to heart disease. Cardiopulmonary arrest in infants and children typically results from disorders that lead to respiratory failure and shock. Outcomes of cardiopulmonary arrest in children are usually poor, with high morbidity and mortality rates (Donoghue et al., 2006).

The nurse must understand and be able to recognize the signs of shock, respiratory failure, or both in children (see Tables 31-2 and 31-4 later in this chapter). Signs of impending failure may be subtle because children are equipped to compensate physiologically for illness or injury for a relatively long period of time. For example, the hypovolemic child compensates by an increase in heart rate to maintain cardiac output. Rapid recognition of the conditions that precede arrest and prompt intervention to prevent arrest are the keys to successful management of the critically ill child. Cardiac arrest in children is most commonly preceded by respiratory failure. Initially, the child compensates with an increased heart rate to maintain the blood pressure and cardiac output. Bradycardia ensues as the child becomes increasingly hypoxic. Without intervention, cardiopulmonary arrest follows.

The treatment of the child in cardiopulmonary arrest begins with assessment of the **ABC**s (airway, breathing, circulation) and beginning basic life support, or CPR (see thePoint Procedure: Cardiopulmonary Resuscitation). The child requiring CPR should be transported to a facility that can provide pediatric advanced life support measures and definitive treatment (Fig. 31-2).

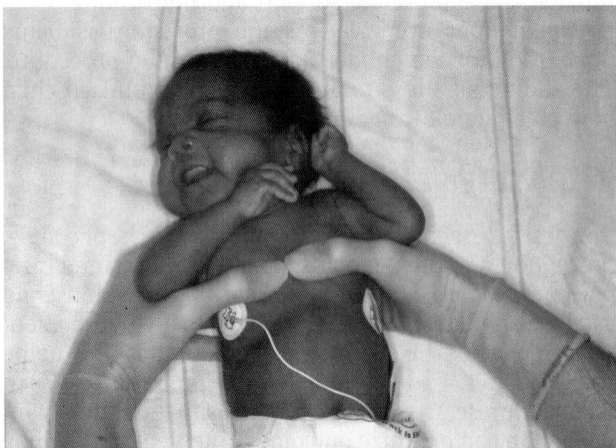

Figure 31-2 CPR is performed differently for a child than for an adult, as seen here with cardiac compressions on an infant. Follow American Heart Association guidelines when performing CPR.

ANSWER: Chris's situation is one example in which respiratory arrest in a child would precede cardiopulmonary arrest. Chris will compensate for an ever-narrowing airway by increasing his respiratory rate and respiratory effort until he can no longer move air. This change can occur very rapidly. Measures to secure his airway must be taken before the edema completely obstructs the airway. If his airway becomes obstructed, the focus of advanced life support becomes creating a patent airway. Chris has no cardiovascular pathology; therefore, the ability to prevent cardiopulmonary arrest depends on the presence of an airway. Vascular access is the next priority. Because of this potential risk, an intravenous (IV) line was placed upon admission to the ED in his right antecubital vein. In the event of airway obstruction, epinephrine will be given via the IV to stimulate the sympathetic nervous system.

ADVANCED LIFE SUPPORT

Advanced life support includes

- Assistance with breathing, such as manual positive pressure ventilations with a bag-and-mask device and 100% oxygen
- Measures to stabilize the airway, such as tracheal intubation (Nursing Interventions 31-1)
- Circulatory support, such as obtaining vascular access and administration of fluids and emergency medications

The **length-based resuscitation tape** is a tool that is used during emergencies to provide a rapid estimate of the child's length to extrapolate dosages of emergency medications. Use of this tool by prehospital care providers is considered a standard of care. Many EDs also use the length-based resuscitation tape when a child requires emergent resuscitation and there is no time to weigh the child (Fig. 31-3).

VASCULAR ACCESS

Vascular access is a high priority in pediatric advanced life support because the child in cardiopulmonary arrest is often hypovolemic. The catheter used should be the largest gauge that can be rapidly and reliably inserted. Secure two IV sites to provide optimal routes for fluid resuscitation. During resuscitation, the easiest peripheral IV sites to access are the antecubital fossa, the dorsa of the hands, and the saphenous veins (see Chapter 17).

No more than three attempts should be made within 90 seconds to obtain peripheral vascular access. If peripheral IV access is not achieved, attempt access via the intraosseous (IO) route. Access is achieved using a specially made IO cannula or bone marrow aspiration needle. The IO cannula is placed in the medial surface of the tibia, approximately one fingerbreadth below the tibial tuberosity (see Fig. 17-7). The cannula is properly placed if resistance to insertion decreases (indicating that the cannula has entered the marrow), the needle remains upright without support, and fluids can be

NURSING INTERVENTIONS 31-1

Tracheal Tube Intubation

Assess for Indications for Tracheal Tube Intubation
- Respiratory insufficiency
- Hypoxemia
- Respiratory arrest
- Glasgow Coma Scale score less than 8 points

Prepare the Equipment
- Proper size cuffed tracheal tube (Taylor et al., 2011). Recent research studies support the use of cuffed tracheal tubes in all children. Cuffed tracheal tubes allow for better air leak control, result in fewer reintubations, and decrease the risk of ventilator-associated pneumonia by reducing aspiration.
- Laryngoscope with
  - Functioning light and charged battery
  - Proper size straight or curved blade
- Resuscitation bag with 100% oxygen source
- Suction source
- Rigid tonsil suction
- Tape
- Stethoscope

Assist With Intubation
- Provide several positive-pressure bag-and-mask breaths before the intubation attempt.

- Monitor the heart rate throughout procedure.
- Anticipate the need for resuscitation equipment, and have it immediately available.

Provide Care Immediately After Tracheal Tube Placement
- Resume bag-and-mask ventilations immediately.
- Hold the tube securely until placement is confirmed and the tube is taped securely in place.
- Auscultate breath sounds bilaterally.
  If no breath sounds are heard, pull the tracheal tube immediately and resume bag-and-mask ventilations. After several positive-pressure breaths, repeat attempt to intubate.
  If breath sounds are heard only on the right side, the tracheal tube may have been inserted down the right mainstem bronchus. Pull the tracheal tube out slightly until bilateral breath sounds are heard.
- Secure the tube. Prepare the taping site with a skin protectant/adhesive to help secure the tape and tracheal tube; this decreases the need for frequent retaping of the tube.
- Record the tube centimeter markings at the upper gum.

---

pushed freely into the cannula. Aspirating bone marrow after the IO needle is in place may not be possible. However, if any marrow is aspirated, it can be used for bedside blood glucose testing and other laboratory testing.

If the attempt to place the IO cannula is unsuccessful, select another site for further IO attempts. Do not use the same extremity because the bone may have

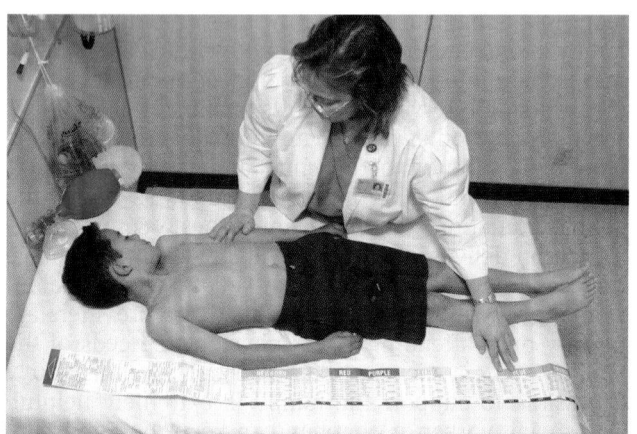

Figure 31-3 The length-based resuscitation tape is used to select appropriate-sized resuscitation equipment to use and medication dosages to administer.

been punctured during the unsuccessful attempt and any fluids or medications infused into the new site may leak back out the first site, causing extravasation. Other options for vascular access include central venous access and a venous cutdown. Both of these procedures require a skilled practitioner, and they are more time-intensive than using the peripheral or IO route.

FLUID ADMINISTRATION

Once vascular access is obtained, the priorities are to administer fluids to restore volume and emergency medications to assist cardiac function. Blood is the fluid of choice for the pediatric trauma victim. However, isotonic crystalloid solutions such as normal saline (NS) or Ringer's lactate, more readily available and less expensive than blood, are effective volume expanders for the hypovolemic patient. If crystalloids are used, three to four times the deficit volume may have to be administered because these solutions expand the intravascular compartment only transiently.

MEDICATION ADMINISTRATION

Emergency or resuscitation medications can be delivered by the IV, IO, or, in some cases, the tracheal route (Nursing Interventions 31-2). Anything that can be given intravenously can be given the IO route (Table 31-1).

NURSING INTERVENTIONS 31-2

Administering Medications by Tracheal Tube

- Ensure that the drug is appropriate for tracheal tube administration. Use the mnemonic LEAN:
  Lidocaine: The endotracheal dose is the same as the IV dose.
  Epinephrine: Use 0.1 mg/kg (0.1 mL/kg) 1:1,000 solution. The tracheal tube dose of epinephrine is 10 times greater than the IV dose, except in neonates.
  Atropine: The tracheal tube dose is increased two to three times the IV dose (0.02 mg/kg, with a minimum dose of 0.1 mg).

Naloxone: The tracheal tube dose is the same as the IV dose.
- Measure for length, and place a small feeding tube into the tracheal tube.
- Instill the drug as prescribed directly into the feeding tube.
- Flush drug with 3–5 mL NS.
- Remove the feeding tube.
- Provide several positive pressure ventilations to disperse the medication into the pulmonary vasculature.

caREminder

Unlike adult dosages, pediatric dosages of all resuscitation medications are based on the child's weight in kilograms.

Be familiar with the various drugs, their indications, dosages, and administration techniques. Prepared drug sheets listing drug dosages according to weight are helpful in eliminating drug calculation anxiety and errors during an intense resuscitation.

Volume replacement is the first-line treatment for poor perfusion and hypotension. After multiple fluid boluses, the child with cardiac or lung disease may develop deteriorating lung compliance and pulmonary edema.

After spontaneous circulation returns, the child may require medications to maintain or achieve adequate blood pressure and systemic perfusion. The three most common inotropic agents used after an arrest are epinephrine, dopamine, and dobutamine. Epinephrine is the drug of choice for children during and immediately after resuscitation. These medications are given by continuous IV or IO infusion and are titrated to maintain adequate blood pressure and perfusion.

PSYCHOSOCIAL SUPPORT

QUESTION: What strategies would you use to provide support to Chris and his family?

Critical illness or injury is a stressor. The onset is usually acute and unexpected, the environment and treatments are unfamiliar and painful, and the outcome is uncertain. Usual coping mechanisms used by the child and family may not be adequate in an emergency situation. While addressing the child's physiologic needs, the health care team must place a high priority on providing emotional support to the child and family during this stressful time.

The atmosphere during an emergency can be chaotic and overstimulating. Keep the parents or other family with the child whenever possible (Evidence-Based Clinical Practice Guidelines 31-1). Involve the parents in the child's care; tell the parents in concrete terms what they can do to support the child (e.g., hold the child's hand and talk quietly to him or her). Attempt to talk quietly and soothingly, and provide comfort measures (Fig. 31-4). When time permits, prepare the child and family before performing procedures. Otherwise, explain what is being done in developmentally appropriate terms, as it is performed, even if it seems that the child cannot hear.

The family should be given the option to be present in the room during invasive procedures or while a child is being resuscitated (Tradition or Science 31-1). Many professional organizations support this practice (Field et al., 2010; Emergency Nurses Association, 2010; Kingsnorth et al., 2010). A protocol for family presence should be in place, and a member of the health care team (e.g., chaplain or social worker) should attend to family members to provide support and explanations and to help interpret events and place them in context (see Nursing Interventions Classification 11-1).

Nurses and other health care providers must provide emotional support to the child and family and offer timely information with frequent updates about the child's condition. Parents want honest, complete information delivered in a caring manner using language they can understand (Meert et al., 2008). Give initial information within 30 minutes. Direct-care providers are usually busy attending to the physiologic needs of the child. Having a social worker or chaplain immediately accessible to support the family is extremely helpful. The social worker or chaplain can keep the family updated on the child's condition; provide resources; and help the family deal with information, make decisions, and mobilize their own resources.

TABLE 31-1 Pediatric Emergency Medications

Drug	Indications	Dose	Interventions
Oxygen From tank or wall-mounted delivery device	Seriously ill or injured child with respiratory insufficiency, trauma, or shock, even if measured arterial oxygen is high	100% oxygen during initial stabilization	Place mask on child's face; if child fights this, hold or have parent hold oxygen mask or tubing close to child's nose and mouth. Monitor oxygen saturation via pulse oximetry; interpret results, considering patient status. Anemia or vasoconstriction may result in inaccurate readings.

Fluid
Crystalloid
  Lactated Ringer's
  NS
Colloid
  5% Albumin
  Synthetic colloid solutions:
    Hetastarch
    Dextran
  Blood
  Fresh-frozen plasma
	Hypovolemia	20 mL/kg per dose IV
		Repeat as necessary.
		Some children need up to 80 mL/kg within first hour.
			Infuse as rapid bolus.
			Evaluate perfusion after every fluid bolus and frequently.
			Give blood to pediatric trauma victims who continue to show signs of hypovolemic shock after two boluses of crystalloid.

Epinephrine	Cardiac arrest, symptomatic bradycardia unresponsive to oxygen and ventilation, non–volume-related hypotension	For symptomatic bradycardia and cardiac arrest: 0.01 mg/kg (0.1 mL/kg 1:10,000 solution) IV or IO, repeat dose every 3–5 minutes as needed using same concentration. Intratracheal dose is 0.1 mg/kg 1:1,000 solution.	Give via tracheal tube until vascular access can be obtained. Evaluate child's response.
Atropine	Symptomatic bradycardia unresponsive to ventilation and oxygenation	0.02 mg/kg IV Minimum single dose: 0.1 mg Maximum single dose: 0.5 mg for child, 1.0 mg for adolescent May repeat in 5 minutes for a maximum total dose of 1.0 mg for child, 2.0 mg for adolescent	Ensure adequate ventilation and oxygenation.
Sodium bicarbonate	Documented metabolic acidosis	1 mEq/kg IV Repeat every 10 minutes on the basis of arterial blood gas analysis.	Ensure adequate ventilation and oxygenation of child before giving sodium bicarbonate. Ensure adequate ventilation during administration (the drug's buffering action produces carbon dioxide). Flush IV line before and after drug administration with NS (precipitates in presence of catecholamines or calcium).

(Continued)

TABLE 31-1   Pediatric Emergency Medications (*Continued*)

Drug	Indications	Dose	Interventions
Naloxone	Reverse effects of opioids	Total reversal dose: 0.1 mg/kg IV/IO/IM/SQ every 2 minutes as needed (maximum, 2 mg) Total reversal not required: 1–5 mcg/kg IV/IO/IM/SQ (titrate to effect)	Monitor child carefully for recurrence of opioid effects; naloxone has a shorter half-life than opioids and may need to be repeated. These doses usually achieve total opioid reversal; use smaller doses if partial reversal desired.
Glucose	Documented hypoglycemia, or if the child fails to respond to standard resuscitation measures	0.5–1.0 g/kg IV Use a maximum concentration of 25% glucose to administer peripherally; glucose is supplied as D50, so dilute 1:1 with sterile water and give 2–4 mL/kg or use D10W at 5–10 mL/kg	Perform bedside glucose testing as soon as possible. Monitor IV closely (D25 is hyperosmolar and may sclerose peripheral veins).
Calcium chloride	Documented or suspected hypocalcemia, hyperkalemia, hypermagnesemia, and calcium channel blocker overdose	20 mg/kg/dose IV Repeat *only* if measured calcium deficiency is present.	Do not administer routinely during resuscitation (may contribute to cellular injury). Administer *slowly* (no faster than 100 mg/min); may induce bradycardia or asystole. Monitor IV closely; irritating to veins and causes chemical burns if infiltrates surrounding tissue. Do not mix with sodium bicarbonate.

IM, intramuscular; SQ, subcutaneous.

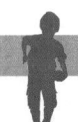

EVIDENCE-BASED CLINICAL PRACTICE GUIDELINES 31-1

Family Presence During Resuscitation

Emergency Nurses Association

Emergency Nurses Association Emergency Nursing Resources Development Committee. (2009). *Family presence during invasive procedures and resuscitation*. Des Plaines, IL: Emergency Nurses Association. Retrieved from

http://www.ena.org/IENR/CPG/Documents/FamilyPresenceCPG.pdf

Provides guidance for practice, and reviews evidence supporting family presence during invasive procedures and resuscitation.

American Association of Critical Nurses

American Association of Critical Care Nurses. (2010). *Family presence during resuscitation and invasive procedures*. Aliso Viejo, CA: Author. Retrieved from

http://www.aacn.org/wd/practice/docs/practicealerts/family presence 04-2010 final.pdf

Practice Alert provides expectations for practice and supporting evidence for family presence during the resuscitation of a family member or when invasive procedures are being performed.

National Consensus Conference on Family Presence During Pediatric Cardiopulmonary Resuscitation and Procedures

Henderson, D. P., & Knapp, J. F. (2005). Report of the National Consensus Conference on family presence during pediatric cardiopulmonary resuscitation and procedures. *Pediatric Emergency Care, 21*(11), 787–791. Retrieved from

http://www2.aap.org/visit/NationalConsensus.pdf

Results of a consensus conference of 20 organizations. Offers 8 recommendations for family presence during procedures and CPR.

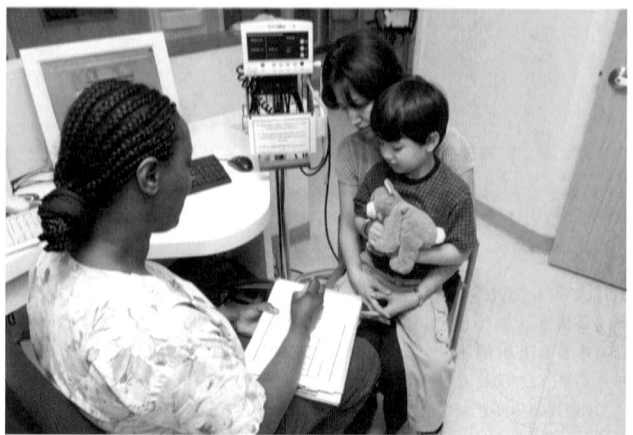

Figure 31-4 Emotional security can be promoted by letting the child hold on to a favorite toy or security object from home or one from the ED stock.

ANSWER: Keeping one of Chris's parents with him and keeping the family informed throughout the ED experience will enhance the family's sense of control during an unnerving experience.

NURSING PLAN OF CARE

Identification of nursing diagnoses is driven by assessment findings. Diagnosis and implementation of interventions occur almost simultaneously in an emergent situation. Many pertinent nursing diagnoses are specific

---

Evidence-Based Practice

TRADITION OR SCIENCE 31-1

Should family members be present during resuscitation or invasive procedures?

Family members should be present during resuscitation or invasive procedures, but many health care providers are uncomfortable with family presence at these times because of concerns about legal liability, family presence negatively affecting the staff's ability to perform procedures, the atmosphere during resuscitation, and the family's response to the process (Fein et al., 2004). Other research indicates that health care providers believe that family members have a right to be present (Kuzin et al., 2007), support family presence (Fulbrook et al., 2007), and believe that presence during CPR does not increase liability concerns. However, families rarely request to be present during CPR or invasive procedures. When allowed, parental presence during invasive procedures did not negatively affect care or procedure performance (O'Connell et al., 2007) and, although parental presence did not seem to reduce the child's pain, parents were less anxious. Being present during the resuscitation may help the family through the grieving process if the child dies because the parents know that everything possible was done to save their child's life (Kingsnorth et al., 2010).

---

to the child's chief complaint. Others are common to most or all emergencies (Nursing Plan of Care 31-1). Disease-specific nursing diagnoses are addressed under the specific disease processes.

SPECIFIC PEDIATRIC EMERGENCIES

Emergencies, by their nature, are unpredictable, but some are encountered more frequently than others. This chapter covers the common pediatric emergencies of shock, trauma, respiratory emergencies, fever, bites and stings, anaphylaxis, epistaxis, environmental exposure injuries, poisoning, and SIDS.

SHOCK

 QUESTION: Is Chris at risk for shock?

Shock is a sustained and progressive circulatory dysfunction that results in inadequate delivery of oxygen and other substances needed to meet metabolic demands. There are four types of shock: hypovolemic, cardiogenic, distributive (includes septic), and obstructive. Each type has a distinct etiology. Assessment findings and nursing interventions may vary depending on the etiology (Table 31-2).

The most common cause of shock in children is hypovolemia. In the United States, hypovolemia is most often caused by bleeding as a result of trauma. Worldwide, diarrhea is one of the principal causes of morbidity and mortality in children (Liu et al., 2012). A major consequence of the fluid and electrolyte losses associated with diarrhea is hypovolemic shock.

Morbidity and mortality associated with shock depend on its etiology and the health care provider's ability to recognize the signs promptly and intervene appropriately before shock becomes irreversible. Mortality associated with septic shock depends on the initial site of infection, causative organism, presence of multiple organ dysfunction syndrome, and the timeliness and appropriateness of therapy. Severe sepsis and septic shock affects millions annually; mortality is more than one in four (Dellinger et al., 2008).

ANSWER: If Chris's airway is not stabilized, he will become increasingly hypoxic, his heart tissue will not receive enough oxygen, and he will progress into shock.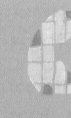

Assessment

Shock may be classified as compensated or decompensated. In compensated shock, the child exhibits signs of decreased cardiac output while maintaining a normal blood pressure. As the child progresses into decompensated shock, his or her ability to maintain a normal blood pressure is compromised.

Without treatment, compensatory mechanisms can sustain cellular function only temporarily. As shock progresses, cellular metabolic changes result in further tissue injury and, ultimately, cell death.

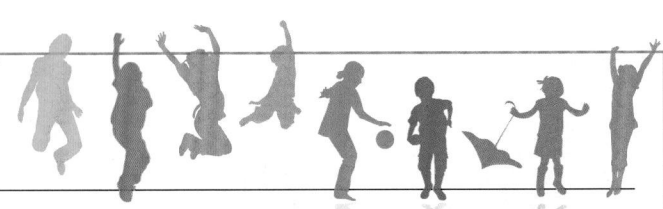

NURSING PLAN OF CARE 31-1:

The Child With an Emergent Condition

Nursing Diagnosis: Risk for ineffective tissue perfusion (specify type: renal, cerebral, cardiac, GI, peripheral) related to disease or injury

Interventions/Rationale
- Monitor for signs of ineffective tissue perfusion: renal, decreased urine output as evidenced by
  - Urine output less than 1 mL/kg/hr
  - High specific gravity (1.030)
- Cerebral
  - Irritability
  - Decreased level of consciousness
  - Sluggish pupillary response
- Cardiac
  - Prolonged capillary refill time more than 2 seconds
  - Weak and/or thready pulses
  - Systolic blood pressure less than 70 + 2 times the child's age in years
- GI
  - Signs of ileus
  - Decreased bowel sounds
  - Nausea and/or vomiting
- Peripheral
  - Pallor
  - Cool, clammy skin
  - Mottled skin pattern
  - Dusky skin

Symptoms vary based on the system affected. The child may exhibit signs of warm shock—normal blood pressure for age, bounding pulses, capillary refill of less than 2 seconds—but may rapidly deteriorate into cold shock. Early detection facilitates prompt intervention and reduces likelihood of negative sequelae.

- Notify physician or advanced practice registered nurse immediately if signs of ineffective tissue perfusion are noted.
  Prolonged ineffective tissue perfusion leads to anaerobic metabolism, lactic acidosis, organ ischemia, and, ultimately, multiorgan system failure.

Expected Outcomes
- Child's signs of altered tissue perfusion will be recognized and treatment implemented promptly.
- Child will maintain tissue perfusion.

Nursing Diagnosis: Acute pain related to symptoms of chief complaint or diagnostic procedures

Interventions/Rationale
- Assess the intensity, character, onset, and duration of pain and the factors that aggravate and relieve it.
  Accurate assessment facilitates effective management of pain.
- Provide sedation or analgesia for diagnostic procedures as ordered.
  Keeps child comfortable, provides humane care, aids in efficient completion of procedure and optimizing outcomes, and may reduce fear with subsequent procedures.
- Provide ongoing pain assessment and management before pain escalates. Assume that pain is present and treat accordingly in a child who has a condition or is undergoing a procedure or treatment that would be painful to an adult.
  Preemptively managed pain is easier to control than pain that is of longer duration, and it requires less medication and produces fewer deleterious side effects. Children may be developmentally or cognitively unable to verbalize pain or unwilling to do so because of their perception of the pain or fear of shots.

Expected Outcome
- Child's pain will be managed adequately.

Nursing Diagnosis: Anxiety related to unknown situation and outcome

Interventions/Rationale
- Explain the child's condition, situation, and interventions that are being implemented, even if the explanation occurs simultaneously with the intervention, as may be mandated by the child's emergent condition.
  Providing information can reduce anxiety related to the unknown.
- Avoid excessive reassurance.
  Honesty promotes trust.
- Recognize the child's and parents' defenses. Do not take negative outbursts personally; do not confront, argue, or react with anger.
  Defenses help one cope in stressful situations, but responding negatively may escalate the situation.

Expected Outcomes
- Child will be told, in age-appropriate terms, what is being done. Parents will be with child as much as possible.
- Family will be kept informed about child's condition and what is being done for the child.

Nursing Diagnosis: Grieving related to unknown and potentially fatal outcome

Interventions/Rationale
- Encourage family members to stay with the child, if they desire. Provide support personnel to stay with the family when the child is undergoing procedures or resuscitation.
   Family presence helps both the child and family cope with the situation. Support personnel can help the family interpret the situation more accurately and process their reactions. Family presence during resuscitation, if they desire, has been shown to help the family cope with the situation.

- Keep family members informed about the child's condition.
   Not knowing increases the family's anxiety; even if no new information emerges, the family can recognize that the health team is caring.
- Provide support for family from facility chaplain, social worker, or family's own support systems.
   Medical staff can focus on care of the child, and the family is supported in coping with the situation.
- Use open-ended questions to elicit child and parent's thoughts and fears.
   Can more accurately assess the issues at hand.

Expected Outcomes
- Child and family will be kept informed of child's condition.
- Child and family will be given an opportunity to verbalize feelings.
- Child and family will mobilize own support systems (e.g., spiritual, community).

ALERT *Hypotension is a late sign of hypovolemic shock in children. It may represent a 25% loss of circulating blood volume.*

Nursing Diagnoses and Outcomes

Nursing diagnoses and outcomes for the child in an emergency situation are presented in Nursing Plan of Care 31-1. In addition, the following diagnoses and outcomes apply to the child in shock:

Nursing Diagnosis: Decreased cardiac output related to effects of hypovolemia, sepsis, obstruction
Outcomes:
- Child's signs of decreased cardiac output will be recognized promptly and interventions instituted immediately.
- Child's cardiac output will remain adequate, as evidenced by vital signs within normal ranges and adequate perfusion.

Nursing Diagnosis: Deficient fluid volume related to effects of disease process or injury
Outcomes:
- Child's signs of fluid volume deficit will be recognized promptly, vascular access obtained, and fluid administered until the child shows no signs of hypovolemia.
- Child's fluid volume will remain balanced, as evidenced by child's urine output being 1 to 2 mL/kg/hr.

Nursing Diagnosis: Excess fluid volume related to effects of myocardial dysfunction
Outcomes:
- Child's signs of fluid volume excess will be recognized promptly and interventions instituted to optimize oxygenation and reduce fluid volume.

- Child's fluid volume will remain balanced, as evidenced by child's urine output being 1 to 2 mL/kg/hr.

Interdisciplinary Interventions

Shock states result in the failure of cellular oxygenation. The goal of treating shock is to restore circulating blood volume and maintain adequate tissue perfusion and cardiovascular stability. The nurse, physician, and respiratory therapist must work as a team to implement interventions that optimize volume and oxygenation. Obtain vascular access as soon as possible to administer fluid and vasoactive drugs as needed. Monitor electrolyte and glucose levels and correct as indicated. Administer 100% oxygen and ventilate and intubate as needed. Minimize stress to the child, which further increases metabolic, and thus oxygen, demands. Maintain a normothermic environment; temperature extremes also increase metabolic demands. Reassess the child's status frequently, at least after every intervention.

TRAUMA

Injury is the leading cause of death of children 1 to 19 years of age, accounting for about 12,000 per year in the United States (Borse et al., 2013). Motor vehicle–related injuries are the major cause of death (Borse et al., 2013).

The causes of traumatic injuries are diverse. The most common are motor vehicle accidents (including automobile–pedestrian and automobile–bicycle accidents), drowning, burns, falls, and firearm injuries. Blunt injuries are more common in children than penetrating ones. Boys have higher injury rates than girls (Borse et al., 2013). Mortality rates for children with injuries have declined steadily during

TABLE 31-2   Types of Shock: Assessment and Interventions

Type of Shock	Etiology	Assessment Findings	Interdisciplinary Interventions
Hypovolemic	Caused by inadequate volume relative to the vascular space; primarily caused by dehydration or traumatic hemorrhage	Tachycardia Prolonged capillary refill (>2 seconds) Weak, thready, or absent peripheral pulses Cool extremities	Administer IV fluids: 20-mL/kg bolus of 0.9% NS or Ringer's lactate; repeat as necessary. In the event of traumatic hemorrhage and if signs of inadequate tissue perfusion are present, after two or three boluses of crystalloid fluid, administer 10 mL/kg packed red blood cells (type specific or O negative). Control bleeding by applying direct pressure to external sites of bleeding with sterile gauze.
Cardiogenic	Caused by impairment of myocardial function	Tachycardia Tachypnea Narrow pulse pressure Cool, mottled skin Capillary refill longer than 2 seconds Weak peripheral pulses Decreased urine output Hepatomegaly Neck vein distention (older child) Rales Edema	Administer oxygen. Administer IV fluid: 20-mL/kg bolus. Carefully assess child's response to fluid bolus; children in heart failure may be fluid overloaded. Administer inotropes to improve cardiac contractility (dopamine, dobutamine). Administer diuretics to improve preload. Correct acid–base, electrolyte imbalances.
Distributive	Septic shock is discussed here; for anaphylaxis, see Chart 31-2. Caused by inappropriate distribution of blood flow and increased capillary permeability Is the most common type of shock in the newborn Most commonly results from gram-negative organisms	History of infection History of poor feeding Tachycardia Fever Tachypnea Altered mental status Petechiae and/or purpura Poor peripheral perfusion (capillary refill >2 seconds)	Isolate the child as necessary. Administer IV fluid in volumes of as much as 80 mL/kg (in boluses of 20 mL/kg) to restore circulating volume. Administer inotropic agents as needed. Draw blood samples for cultures immediately. Administer wide-spectrum antibiotics; do not postpone antibiotic therapy until culture results are available. Administer IV glucose as needed to treat hypoglycemia.
Obstructive	Caused by inability of normal heart to produce adequate cardiac output despite normal intravascular volume because of mechanical obstruction (e.g., tension pneumothorax, cardiac tamponade, pulmonary embolism)	See Table 31-3 on traumatic chest injuries.	See Table 31-3 on traumatic chest injuries. Relieve obstruction.

the past decade, in part because of injury prevention programs.

Trauma care is provided through a team effort. Standardized policies and procedures should identify the roles and responsibilities of all the trauma team members. Pediatric victims of multisystem trauma or those with a high mortality risk should be transported to a trauma center with pediatric expertise (American Academy of Pediatrics [AAP] Section on Orthopaedics et al., 2008). When treating trauma patients, the risk of exposure to blood and other body fluids is high. Therefore, before initiating care, don personal protective equipment (i.e., gloves, goggles, mask, and gown) to minimize this risk.

Assessment

The commonly used mnemonic "A through I" represents the steps of the primary and secondary assessments (see Focused Physical Assessment 31-1) (Emergency Nurses Association, 2007). These steps prioritize assessments of the trauma patient and identify lifesaving interventions that may be necessary.

Primary Assessment and Care

Begin the primary assessment by assessing the ABCs. As in CPR, remember not to continue to the next step until the previous step has been stabilized.

Open the airway and assess it for patency. Suction any blood, vomitus, or debris in the oropharynx. Check for any displaced or loose teeth. For the child with a suspected head or spine injury, use the combined jaw thrust–spinal stabilization maneuver to open the airway and manually hold the head in a neutral position. After the airway is opened, stabilize the c-spine to prevent cervical motion using a semirigid extrication collar of the appropriate size (Fig. 31-5). The collar must fit perfectly. If it is too large, it may allow cervical movement, which may convert an incomplete spinal cord injury to a complete one.

ALERT *For the child with a head injury, ensure that the neck remains in a neutral position, not hyperextended. One team member should hold the neck in position while another performs the intubation. Also take c-spine precautions with a near-drowning victim. The child may have hit his or her head during the drowning or when falling into a pool.*

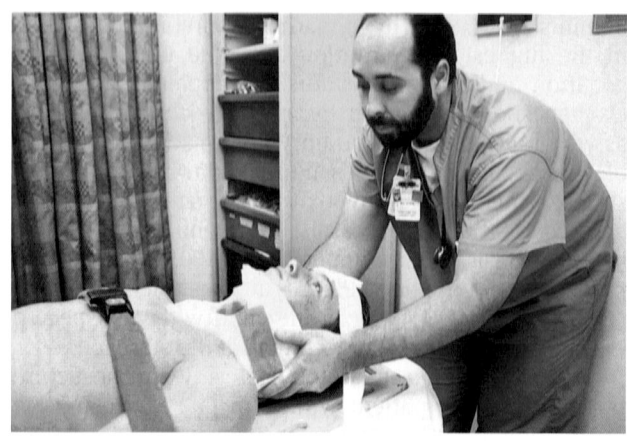

Figure 31-5 For a trauma victim, the c-spine must be immobilized while the airway is opened. This is done using a combined jaw thrust and spinal stabilization maneuver.

Assess for breathing next. Remember that blunt and penetrating traumatic injuries to the chest can severely compromise breathing. Unless these injuries are aggressively assessed, recognized, and rapidly treated, they can kill the patient (Table 31-3). For all trauma patients,

TABLE 31-3   Types of Traumatic Chest Injuries: Assessment and Interventions

Injury Type	Description	Assessment Findings	Nursing Interventions
Pulmonary contusion	Bruise on the lung tissue; most common type of chest injury	No initial symptoms may be evident Increased difficulty breathing Hemoptysis Tachycardia Rales	Restrict fluid (unless patient in shock). Elevate the head of the bed (if no c-spine injury). Assist with intubation if the child has severe respiratory distress. Administer ordered antibiotics for pneumonia prophylaxis.
Tension pneumothorax	A tear in the lung lining, which results in air accumulation in the pleural space that compresses the lungs; the amount of air trapped increases with each breath because the air cannot escape	Unstable vital signs Respiratory distress Tracheal deviation Decreased breath sounds over the affected lung Cyanosis Decreased cardiac output	Assist with needle thoracostomy (insertion of a 19-gauge needle into the left second intercostal space, midclavicular line). Prepare for chest tube insertion.
Open pneumothorax	Open chest wound that may be sucking or not sucking	Unstable vital signs Anxious, restless Irritable Cyanosis Decreased breath sounds over affected lung Asymmetry of chest wall movement Subcutaneous emphysema	Apply three-sided occlusive, non-porous dressing; leave one side open to allow air escape. Prepare for chest tube insertion.
Hemothorax	Blood accumulation in the chest cavity as a result of blunt or penetrating trauma	Unstable vital signs Decreased or absent breath sounds Dullness to percussion over affected area Hypovolemic shock resulting from hemorrhage	Prepare for chest tube insertion. Administer fluids for aggressive volume replacement. Monitor chest drainage.
Cardiac tamponade	Blood accumulation in the pericardial sac as a result of blunt or penetrating trauma	Muffled heart sounds Decreased blood pressure Distended neck veins	Assist with immediate pericardiocentesis. Perform fluid resuscitation.

administer oxygen by a partial nonrebreather mask in the highest concentration available until the oxygenation and perfusion status is completely assessed. Oxygen should be given because the child may have as yet unrecognized respiratory failure and shock, both of which contribute to tissue hypoxia. The goal is to stabilize the effects of hypoxia before irreversible damage occurs. If necessary, assist with ventilations using a bag-and-mask device supplied with 100% oxygen and prepare for intubation. Place a nasogastric (NG) tube (or orogastric [OG] tube in the child with a suspected basilar skull fracture) to decompress the stomach.

Assess the child's circulatory status. Begin chest compressions on the patient without a pulse, and initiate further advanced life support measures.

Obtain vascular access without delay by placing two large-bore (22 gauge or larger) IV lines peripherally. Because leg injuries are more common in children, the arms are the sites of choice for IV access. Do not attempt vascular access in a fractured or severely injured extremity because vascular compromise is a concern. If vascular access remains unsuccessful, IO access should be attempted next before considering central line insertion, such as percutaneous access of the femoral or subclavian vein or cutdown of the saphenous vein. If signs of hypovolemic shock occur, treat aggressively with fluid replacement.

After the ABCs have been stabilized, assess **D** (disability) by performing a brief neurologic examination, including level of consciousness and pupillary response to light. This assessment determines neurologic status and establishes a baseline from which to evaluate change. Test the child for hypoglycemia. If hypoglycemia is present, treat with 25% dextrose. If opioid overdose is suspected, administer naloxone (Narcan).

E: Expose the child by removing all clothing and inspect for any obvious signs of injury or illness. Prevent hypothermia by covering the child with a blanket or, optimally, by using an overhead warmer, which allows continued, full visual examination of the child.

Secondary Assessment and Care

Secondary assessment focuses on the "F through I" components of the mnemonic. Obtain **F**, a full set of vital signs, including pulse rate, respiratory rate, blood pressure, and rectal temperature. Rectal temperatures are the standard of care. Oral temperatures are not appropriate for young children, those with an altered level of consciousness, or those requiring assistance maintaining their airway. Axillary temperatures may be inaccurate because of vasoconstriction or dilation. Studies on temporal artery thermometry give conflicting results on accuracy of this method (Batra et al., 2012). Tympanic thermometry is not appropriate for children younger than 2 years of age but may be used in those who are older (Batra et al., 2012; Duru et al., 2012). Facilitate family presence.

G: Give comfort measures such as reassurance, including touching and providing age-appropriate diversional activities. This may also include splinting of extremity injuries, dressing wounds, and providing pain control.

Perform **H**, a head-to-toe examination, and obtain a history, using the AMPLE mnemonic (see Chart 31-1). The head-to-toe examination may reveal signs and symptoms of internal hemorrhage, such as abdominal pain, guarding, rigidity, or tenderness. The abdomen may be distended and have signs of obvious abdominal trauma such as a positive seat belt sign (bruising that correlates with the position of the seat belt). Shock that persists despite aggressive fluid replacement may indicate internal hemorrhage and requires immediate surgery.

Finally, **I**: inspect the patient's back. To do this, roll the child over, maintaining c-spine precautions (logrolling). Check for penetrating objects, bleeding, bruising, abrasions, or lacerations.

Nursing Diagnoses and Outcomes

Nursing diagnoses and outcomes applicable to the child and family when the child is experiencing a medical emergency are discussed in Nursing Plan of Care 31-1. The nursing diagnoses and outcomes identified for the child in shock also are frequently relevant to the child who has suffered a traumatic injury. Additional appropriate diagnoses and outcomes include the following:

Nursing Diagnosis: Ineffective breathing pattern related to effects of injury
Outcome: Child's ventilation, spontaneous or assisted, will be adequate.
Nursing Diagnosis: Ineffective airway clearance related to effects of injury
Outcome: Child's signs of ineffective airway clearance will be recognized immediately, and interventions to clear the airway will be implemented promptly.
Nursing Diagnosis: Acute pain related to effects of injury
Outcome: Child will be assessed for baseline neurologic and cardiovascular status, and pain will be adequately managed.
Nursing Diagnosis: Hypothermia related to exposure from injury or treatment
Outcome: Child's body temperature will be maintained within the normal range while the child is exposed adequately during inspection for injuries and treatment.
Nursing Diagnosis: Risk for infection related to effects of injuries, invasive treatments, and stress decreasing immune response
Outcome: Child will not acquire injury-related infection.
Nursing Diagnosis: Imbalanced nutrition: Less than body requirements related to injury, increasing metabolic demands, or decreasing ability to ingest nutrients
Outcome: Child's intake of nutrients will be sufficient to meet metabolic needs and support healing and growth.

Interdisciplinary Interventions

Upon completing the primary and secondary assessments, additional interventions may be identified. Insert an indwelling urinary catheter to monitor urine output (contraindicated if blood is present at the urethral meatus). Do not remove an impaled object; stabilize it for later removal in surgery.

Assess the child's pain level and administer pain medications as ordered. Judicious administration of pain medication to a child with a traumatic injury does not prohibit accurate neurologic and cardiovascular examination findings from occurring. Administer pain medications in small doses and titrate to achieve adequate pain control. Larger bolus doses of pain medication may make it difficult to evaluate accurately whether a change in level of consciousness is drug induced or the result of pathology. Pain medications may also cause vasodilation, causing a precipitous drop in blood pressure in a child with hypovolemia or unstable cardiovascular status. Until definitive treatment is achieved, splint, elevate, and ice any extremity fracture. Apply sterile dressings to any open soft tissue injuries such as lacerations or abrasions. Determine the child's tetanus immunization status, and administer a booster if necessary.

If bruising is noted around the eyes (raccoon eyes) or behind the ears, or if hemotympanum is present, the child may have a basilar skull fracture. This type of fracture places the child at risk for intracranial hemorrhage, respiratory depression, respiratory arrest, and cerebral edema. Such a child may require intubation and mechanical ventilation to maintain a normal partial pressure of arterial carbon dioxide ($PaCO_2$) of 35 to 45 mm Hg. Prophylactic hyperventilation is not recommended with head trauma because of its vasoconstricting effect on cerebral arteries and subsequent risk for brain ischemia (Kochanek et al., 2012). Hyperventilation, as a means of preventing impending herniation of the brain, is reserved for treatment of intracranial hypertension that is refractory to other treatments (Curley et al., 2010). Measure $PaCO_2$ by serial arterial blood gas measurements or with an end-tidal carbon dioxide monitor. Cerebral blood flow or brain tissue oxygen monitoring is recommended (Narotam et al., 2009). Administer hyperosmolar therapy (e.g., hypertonic saline [3% saline]) as ordered, to decrease intracranial pressure (Upadhyay et al., 2010). Continually evaluate therapy effectiveness, and monitor for signs of severely increased intracranial pressure, including asymmetric or fixed, dilated pupils; bradycardia; posturing; and nonresponsiveness. Prepare the child for computed tomography—the diagnostic study of choice to evaluate the intracranial space.

COMMON RESPIRATORY EMERGENCIES

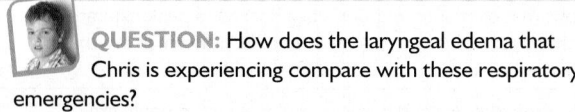

QUESTION: How does the laryngeal edema that Chris is experiencing compare with these respiratory emergencies?

Respiratory emergencies are a major cause of morbidity and mortality in the pediatric population. Rapid assessment, recognition of distress or failure, and immediate intervention are the keys to successful management. Causes of respiratory emergencies include epiglottitis,

foreign body aspiration, bronchiolitis, croup, and asthma (Table 31-4). See Chapter 16 for an in-depth review of these conditions.

Assessment

Approach the child in a calm, gentle manner to minimize fear, which increases metabolic demands. While approaching, obtain a general assessment of the child's status. Note the child's position of comfort. Older children assume a position that optimizes airway patency and minimizes the work of breathing. Assess level of consciousness. Hypoxia may be manifested as anxiety or irritability; hypercapnia, as lethargic or obtunded behavior. Evaluate the child's color. Cyanosis is a late sign of respiratory distress, unless the child has chronic pulmonary or cardiovascular pathology.

Assess the rate and effort of breathing. Tachypnea in children is often the first sign of respiratory distress.

❗ ALERT *It is an ominous sign if a child who was tachypneic has a slowed respiratory rate. This may indicate that the child is tiring and respiratory failure is imminent.*

Increased effort of breathing may be manifested by stridor, wheezing, grunting, retractions, use of accessory muscles, and nasal flaring. Note chest movement for symmetric expansion. Auscultate breath sounds for location and quality.

Interdisciplinary Interventions

Assessment findings indicate the level of respiratory support needed by the child. General support includes attending to the ABCs and optimizing oxygenation and ventilation. More specific interventions depend on pathology.

For any child showing respiratory distress or desaturation on pulse oximetry, administer oxygen, using a method tolerated by the child, to keep the oxygen saturation level above 94%. Administer oxygen cautiously to those with a history of chronic pulmonary disease. Instruct the parent how to hold oxygen tubing to provide blow-by oxygen, which may be better tolerated by the child (Fig. 31-6).

KidKare Create a nonthreatening mask by cutting a hole in the bottom of a Styrofoam cup. Then place the oxygen tubing through the hole and place the cup over the child's mouth. Monitor the child to prevent him or her from chewing on the cup.

For children who require nebulizer treatments and are too young to hold a nebulizer mouthpiece in the mouth, have the parent hold a face mask in place.

Allow the child to maintain a position of comfort, either sitting or remaining in the parent's arms. Support infants with the head in a neutral position.

TABLE 31-4   Common Respiratory Emergencies: Assessment and Interventions

Condition	Assessment Findings	Interdisciplinary Interventions
Foreign body aspiration/ obstruction	History of running while eating or of playing with a small toy Acute onset of respiratory distress	If the child can breathe spontaneously or has coughing, wheezing, or stridor, do not attempt to dislodge the object. Perform basic life support measures to dislodge foreign body. If basic life support techniques do not dislodge foreign body, then physician should perform direct visualization and manual removal as needed. If apnea persists and manual bag-and-mask ventilations cannot bypass the obstruction, emergency intubation, tracheostomy, or needle cricothyrotomy is necessary to establish a patent airway and to enable CPR to be effective.
Croup	History of viral infection, especially parainfluenza virus Onset during late fall or winter (most common) Mild to moderate illness (compared with toxic appearance of child with epiglottitis) Prodrome of upper airway infection that progresses to • Fever • Barking cough • Inspiratory stridor • Tachycardia • Tachypnea • Suprasternal and/or subcostal retractions • Altered breath sounds (from stridor alone to rhonchi and/or wheezing)	Base treatment on severity of illness. Administer corticosteroids such as dexamethasone as ordered. Improvement can be expected within 2–3 hours. Administer nebulized racemic epinephrine as ordered to reverse airway obstruction quickly; requires cardiopulmonary monitoring. Duration of effect lasts for 2 hours. Monitor child for rebound airway obstruction for at least 2–3 hours after the last racemic epinephrine treatment before considering discharge.
Epiglottitis	Inflammation and swelling of the epiglottis and surrounding structures Age 2–6 years (most common) Rapid onset of symptoms (e.g., child appears healthy 2 hours previously) Tripod positioning (neck stretched forward with jaw up to obtain a "sniffing" position in an attempt to achieve the best airway) High temperature (>104° F [40° C]) Inability to eat or drink Excessive drooling Choking Muffled voice Difficulty breathing "Stridorous" cough possible	Observe the child in a controlled medical environment (e.g., ED, intensive care unit); never leave the child unattended. Immediately gather appropriate equipment for emergency intubation and/or tracheostomy. Allow the child to maintain the position of comfort; avoid invasive or disturbing procedures because any agitation or attempts to lay the child down may result in laryngospasm and complete obstruction of the child's airway. Administer antibiotics to treat *Haemophilus influenzae*, *Streptococcus pneumoniae*, or *Staphylococcus* infection.
Asthma	Tripod positioning Profound respiratory distress Anxious, restless Cyanotic, pale Tachycardia Tachypnea Retractions, use of accessory muscles Decreased or unequal breath sounds Expiratory wheezing, inspiratory wheezing with a prolonged inspiratory phase; the absence of wheezing with signs of respiratory distress is an ominous sign Decreased peak expiratory flow rate	Allow the child to maintain position of comfort. Administer nebulized bronchodilator/albuterol as ordered. Administer supplemental oxygen. Consider nebulized terbutaline or atropine for children who do not respond to albuterol. Administer epinephrine (1:1,000 solution) subcutaneously, as ordered, immediately if the child cannot generate a peak flow measurement or has a decreased level of consciousness. Reassess the child's vital signs, respiratory effort, and breath sounds after each treatment. Early treatment with a dose of steroids may prevent asthma exacerbation. Consider hospital admission if child does not respond to three albuterol treatments; has retractions, tachypnea, pallor, and/or cyanosis that continues without wheezing; has a peak expiratory flow that does not improve to at least 65% of normal; or when parental adherence to therapy is questionable.
Bronchiolitis	History of acute viral infection of the lower respiratory tract Onset in winter (most common) Upper respiratory infection for 3–5 days Worsening cough Audible wheezing Low-grade fever Poor feeding (common)	Bronchodilator therapy and corticosteroids are commonly prescribed; however, little scientific evidence exists regarding the usefulness of these therapies. Supportive care (such as oxygen to maintain oxygen saturation more than 94% or during feeding to prevent oxygen desaturation) and IV hydration for those infants who are unable to maintain adequate oral intake are the mainstays of therapy.

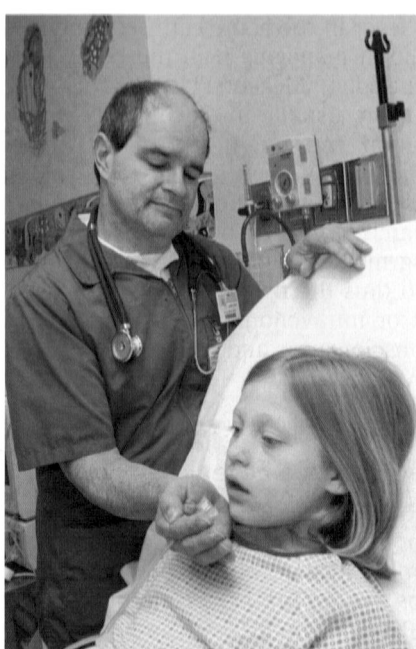

Figure 31-6 Young children offer less resistance if oxygen is delivered unobtrusively.

Check arterial blood gas measurements for any child with severe respiratory distress. A PaCO$_2$ more than 50 mm Hg may indicate that the child requires intubation and mechanical ventilation. Do not feed children who are experiencing respiratory distress. Limit disturbances to essential interventions to prevent further distress.

ANSWER: There are many similarities between the laryngeal edema that Chris is experiencing and these respiratory emergencies. For Chris and any child presenting with respiratory emergencies, the assessment will focus on the effectiveness of their breathing. Although the treatments may vary according to the etiology of the respiratory distress, all respiratory emergencies in children have the potential for very rapid changes in status and are potentially life threatening.

FEVER

Fever is one of the most common reasons that parents seek care for their infant or child in the ED. Fever is an elevation of body temperature to at least 100.4° F (38° C) rectally. It occurs when toxic substances or abnormalities in the brain reset the thermoregulatory set point of the body to a higher than normal value. Fever itself is not a disease; rather, it is a sign of an underlying disease that has activated an immune response.

Although exceptions occur, children with invasive bacterial disease often appear ill and are easy to identify as requiring treatment. With occult bacteremia, the source of the fever may not be evident despite a careful history and physical examination. The incidence of bacteremia has declined significantly in children younger than 3 years of age since the introduction of the pneumococcal conjugate vaccine (Antonyrajah & Mukundan, 2008). Currently, urinary tract infection is the most common cause of bacterial infection in children and must be considered in identifying the cause of fever (Habib, 2012).

Another concern with fever is the possibility of triggering a **febrile seizure**. These seizures occur most commonly in children between 6 months and 5 years of age, with a frequency of 2% to 5% (Hampers & Spina, 2011; AAP Subcommittee on Febrile Seizures, 2011). The risk for a second febrile seizure is about 32% before the child is 6 years of age (AAP Subcommittee on Febrile Seizures, 2011). Most febrile seizures last 1 to 2 minutes. Febrile seizures that last longer than 15 minutes are considered complex febrile seizures.

There is no evidence that febrile seizures cause a decline in IQ, academic performance, behavioral abnormalities, or neurocognitive inattention. Simple febrile seizures are associated with the same risk of developing epilepsy as the general population (AAP Subcommittee on Febrile Seizures, 2011).

Assessment

Fever increases the basal metabolic rate, resulting in tachycardia, tachypnea, and increased oxygen demand. With each degree Celsius increase, the febrile child's caloric requirements are increased by 12%.

Perform a complete physical examination in a child with fever, specifically noting level of hydration, skin lesions (petechiae, which usually appear first on the chest, may indicate a serious bacterial infection), and neurologic status, which includes palpating the fontanel in infants younger than 18 months of age. A bulging fontanel may indicate meningitis; a sunken fontanel, dehydration. The child may be irritable and lethargic. The child who appears "toxic" may be cyanotic and have an altered level of consciousness, poor perfusion manifested as mottled skin color, capillary refill time longer than 2 seconds, cool extremities, and weak pulses.

Febrile seizures are usually manifested as sudden unresponsiveness, generalized rhythmic jerking, and tonic posturing lasting less than 15 minutes, usually less than 90 seconds. A determination must be made whether the fever caused the seizure, the seizure is a sign of underlying pathology that also caused the fever (e.g., meningitis, encephalitis), or the seizure is coincidental with the fever (e.g., toxic ingestion, hypoglycemia, hemorrhage, neurocutaneous disorder). Children who experience febrile seizures appear neurologically well within a few hours.

A complete "septic" workup may be indicated for infants younger than 3 months of age who present with a rectal temperature of 100.4° F (38° C) or higher and for children 3 to 36 months of age who present with a rectal temperature of 102° F (38.9° C) or higher and who appear toxic. A complete septic workup includes a complete blood count, blood culture, urinalysis, urine culture, lumbar puncture, and chest radiograph. Obtain all culture specimens before initiating antibiotic therapy.

caREminder

Do not wait for laboratory results before starting antibiotics. Antibiotic therapy should be initiated within 1 hour, especially if the child appears toxic.

Interdisciplinary Interventions

The nurse plays a pivotal role in managing the child with fever and in educating parents about home management (Teaching Intervention Plan 31-1). Treatment for fever includes antipyretics, fluids, and cooling measures.

Managing fever in the acute care setting does not differ markedly from managing it in the home (see thePoint Procedure: Cooling Measures).

Protocols are usually in place in EDs for antipyretic administration. Although alternating ibuprofen and acetaminophen has been shown to be more effective than monotherapy in reducing fever (Paul et al., 2010), more research is needed because of study limitations. Alternating medications can increase confusion about dosing and thus the risk of toxicity. Replace fluid deficits orally or intravenously, depending on the child's level of consciousness and cooperation.

TIP 31-1: A TEACHING INTERVENTION PLAN for the Child With a Fever

Nursing Diagnoses and Family Outcomes

- Deficient knowledge: Home management of fever
  Outcomes: Caregivers and child, if appropriate, will implement appropriate fever management interventions.
  Caregivers and child, if appropriate, will notify health care provider appropriately of negative changes in the child's condition.
- Risk for deficient fluid volume related to effects of increased metabolic demands
  Outcome: Child will have sufficient fluid intake to prevent dehydration.
- Hyperthermia related to effects of disease process
  Outcome: Child will have fever controlled as needed to decrease risk for febrile seizure, decrease metabolic demands, and promote comfort.
- Risk for injury related to potential for febrile seizures
  Outcome: Child will not sustain injury if seizure occurs.

Teach the Child/Family

Knowledge of Fever
- Fever in itself is not harmful; it may be beneficial in fighting pathogens.
- Make certain parents know how to take the child's temperature:
  - Use method appropriate for child's age and condition.
  - Read thermometer accurately.

Cooling Measures
- Manipulate environment to cool child:
  - Unbundle child. May cover with light blanket if shivering occurs.
  - Decrease room temperature.
- Administer antipyretics as needed for temperature more than 102° F (38.9° C) and, if your child is uncomfortable, administer
  - Acetaminophen at 15 mg/kg orally or rectally every 4 hours (drug of choice)
  - Ibuprofen at 10 mg/kg orally every 6–8 hours

- *Do not alternate use of acetaminophen and ibuprofen* because of the risk of overmedication.
- *Do not give aspirin* because of its association with Reye syndrome.
- It will take 30–60 minutes for these medications to have an effect on the temperature.
- Sponge with tepid water (85°–90° F [29.4°–32.2° C]):
  - Sponge immediately if your child has a febrile seizure or temperature more than 106° F (41.1° C); otherwise, wait until after the antipyretic has taken effect, the temperature remains more than 104° F (40° C), and your child is uncomfortable.
  - If sponging is done, water should be lukewarm (85°–90° F [29.4°–32.2° C]). *Do not use ice water,* which will bring your child's temperature down too rapidly and cause shivering. Avoid shivering because it raises the temperature as the body attempts to produce heat.
  - *Do not use alcohol* for sponge baths because alcohol intoxication can result from inhalation of fumes and skin absorption.
  - Stop sponging when your child's temperature starts to decrease to avoid having the child become too cold.

Hydration Status
- Increase child's fluid intake. Offer frequent, small sips of fluid or popsicles.
- Monitor child's hydration status, including urine output (count wet diapers or check color of urine), moistness of mucous membranes, and presence of tears.

Contact Health Care Provider if
- Child's fever persists longer than 2–3 days
- Child's condition worsens (e.g., seizure, purple spots on skin, increased lethargy or irritability, stiff neck, vomiting, decreased oral intake, signs of dehydration [<8 wet diapers/24 hr or urine is dark and voiding small amounts, dry mucous membranes, no tears with crying after the neonatal period])

Sponging as a cooling measure is controversial because fever may be beneficial in helping fight the infection. Sponging does not add to sustained fever reduction and only increases the discomfort of children with non–life-threatening fever (Thomas et al., 2009). Never sponge a shivering child because shivering will increase the body temperature. Sponging should be done only

- In a child with a neurologic disorder because many have abnormal temperature control mechanisms that do not respond well to antipyretics
- When the increase in metabolic demands resulting from the fever may be deleterious to the child (e.g., a child with cardiac or pulmonary disease, a pregnant adolescent)
- In a child with liver disease, for whom the use of antipyretics is contraindicated
- For heat-related illness (discussed later in this chapter)

All febrile infants younger than 28 days of age and any toxic-appearing infant or child should be hospitalized and treated with parenteral antibiotics (see thePoint An Interdisciplinary Plan of Care for the Neonate With Sepsis). For older infants and children with fever and nontoxic appearance, outpatient management based on laboratory tests and clinical signs and symptoms, and implemented by reliable caregivers, is appropriate. Antibiotics should not be given routinely for fever alone but based on clinical findings and laboratory tests.

If the child does have a febrile seizure, protect the child from injury while stabilizing the ABCs (see Chapter 21). Place the child in a side-lying position to prevent airway obstruction or aspiration. For prolonged seizures, a benzodiazepine should be administered intravenously in appropriate doses to stop the seizure (Millar, 2006).

ALERT *Administer IV sedatives slowly, and closely monitor the child for ability to maintain a patent airway and spontaneous ventilations.*

Educate the family about febrile seizures and how to manage them. Reassure them that febrile seizures cause no long-term sequelae. Explain the risk of recurrence. Instruct them that antipyretics can be administered when fever occurs but that seizures often occur as the temperature is increasing, before it is noticed by the parent, so they might not be prevented. Also teach the parents first aid measures to take if a seizure occurs.

BITES AND STINGS

Thousands of children are treated yearly for various types of bites and stings. In 2006, more than 21,100 bites and envenomations among children younger than the age of 19 years were reported to poison control centers in the United States (Bronstein et al., 2012). The actual numbers are likely much higher because this total does not include nonparticipating poison centers or unreported incidents.

MAMMAL AND HUMAN BITES

The most common bites seen in EDs are from dogs, cats, and humans (Jaindl et al., 2012). Children predictably suffer more serious injuries than adults. Dog bites to children younger than 6 years of age, often from the family dog, typically affect the head, face, and neck (Dwyer et al., 2007). These bites can be disfiguring because the lips, nose, eyes, and ears are often involved. Dog bites to children older than 6 years of age are often to the perineum, buttocks, legs, or feet from dogs outside the home (Dwyer et al., 2007). Other common animal bites are inflicted by snakes, rodents, Hymenoptera, scorpions, and spiders. Wound infections are the most common complication, with bites inflicted by cats and humans having the highest infection rates.

Assessment

Obtain the history of the circumstances surrounding the bite, including who, or what, bit the child. If the bite is from an animal, include the type of animal (species and whether wild or domestic). Also determine the amount of time since the injury and the child's immunization status.

Manifestations depend on the type of wound. Human and dog bites often cause lacerations and crush injuries. Cat bites usually cause puncture wounds. Rodent bites tend to be superficial. Physical examination should evaluate the type, size, and depth of the injury; the presence of foreign material in the wound; and the status of underlying structures. Fractures may occur; evaluate for skull fractures in young children who have dog bites to the head and face.

Nursing Diagnoses and Outcomes

Nursing diagnoses common to the child experiencing an emergency, as listed in Nursing Plan of Care 31-1, apply to the child suffering from a bite. In addition, the following diagnoses and outcomes may apply to a child with a bite injury:

Nursing Diagnosis: Impaired tissue integrity related to presence of bite wound
Outcome: Child's wound will be appropriately cleansed and closed as soon as possible after the injury to minimize further tissue damage.
Nursing Diagnosis: Risk for infection related to effects of bite wound
Outcome: Child will not develop wound infection.
Nursing Diagnosis: Acute pain related to effects of bite wound or treatment
Outcomes: Child's pain will be adequately managed; child will verbalize minimal level of pain and demonstrate few pain behaviors.
Nursing Diagnosis: Deficient knowledge: Home management of wound
Outcomes:
- Parents, and the child, as appropriate, will state reasons for antibiotic prophylaxis and the importance of completing a full course of therapy.
- Parents, and the child, as appropriate, will demonstrate prescribed techniques of wound management.

- Parents, and the child, as appropriate, will list signs of wound infection and state when to notify health care provider.

Nursing Diagnosis: Disturbed body image related to presence of disfiguring wound

Outcome: Child will verbalize a positive body image if wound is disfiguring.

Interdisciplinary Interventions

Parents often seek treatment for their child's bite because of concern about rabies, a fatal viral infection of the central nervous system. However, the incidence of rabies is extremely low in the United States. The decision to initiate prophylactic treatment for rabies is based on the species of animal (dogs and cats are typically low risk; bats, skunks, coyotes, raccoons, and foxes are higher risk), the animal's condition, and the prevalence of rabies in the region. Rabies prophylaxis consists of passive immunization with rabies immune globulin and active immunization with human diploid cell vaccine, rhesus diploid cells (rabies vaccine adsorbed), or purified chick embryo cell vaccine. After thoroughly cleansing the wound, give the rabies immune globulin dosage as ordered, if anatomically possible, by local subcutaneous infiltration of the site. Active immunization should be given intramuscularly in the deltoid or anterolateral aspect of the thigh on days 0, 3, 7, 14, and 28 (Centers for Disease Control and Prevention [CDC], 2008).

Prompt care of the wound is the key to successful healing. Inspect the bite wound for teeth, clean the site with a 1% povidone-iodine solution, and irrigate the wound forcibly with NS. Closure of the wound depends on the affected site. If the wound is considered at high risk for infection, it should not be sutured. High-risk wounds include puncture wounds, minor hand or foot wounds, cat or human bites, bite wounds not treated within 12 hours, and wounds in the immunocompromised patient.

Antibiotic prophylaxis may be indicated depending on the wound site (hand or face) and severity (deep wounds, ones that cannot be adequately debrided), if the wound was not sutured, and for all high-risk wounds. Generally, a combination of antibiotics is given over a course of 3 to 5 days. Consider tetanus prophylaxis for all bite victims. Most bite wounds in children should be rechecked for signs of infection in 24 to 48 hours. Some children with severe injuries require hospitalization for adequate management, including operative repair, treatment of extensive local infection, or correcting poor adherence to therapeutic regimen. Offer psychological support and refer if needed because violent dog attacks are associated with risk of posttraumatic stress disorder (Ji et al., 2010).

Teach the parents how to assess for signs and symptoms of wound infection and when to notify the health care provider. Discuss potential fears and behavioral problems of the child and how parents might manage them. Teach children to avoid stray and wild animals and not to provoke animals.

ARTHROPOD STINGS AND BITES

QUESTION: How common a childhood problem is an allergic reaction to an insect sting or bite, like Chris experienced with the hornet stings?

Animals in the Arachnida (spiders, scorpions, ticks, mites) and the Insecta (lice, fleas, bedbugs, flies, bees, ants) classes are probably accountable for more morbidity and mortality worldwide than any other group of venomous creatures (Steen et al., 2004). Hymenoptera (bees, wasps, hornets, yellow jackets, and ants) are responsible for 50% of human deaths from venomous bites and stings. Allergic reactions are the most common result of these stings.

ANSWER: Most children are stung or bitten during their childhood, and according to the National Institutes of Health, approximately 4 in 1,000 will have an allergic experience.

Assessment

Reactions to insect stings and bites can vary from mild (slight swelling, erythema, and pain at the site) to moderate (generalized pruritus and urticaria) to severe (wheezing, nausea and vomiting, laryngoedema, hypotension, and shock). A bee's stinger is barbed and remains in the victim's skin.

Interdisciplinary Interventions

Treatment of stings is based on the severity of the reaction. Most respond to treatment at home (Community Care 31-1). Treatment for severe anaphylactic reactions is discussed in the following section.

ANAPHYLAXIS

QUESTION: Is Chris exhibiting signs of an anaphylactic reaction?

Anaphylaxis, or anaphylactic shock, is a life-threatening emergency caused by an acute systemic allergic or hypersensitivity reaction to an antigen. Anaphylaxis usually occurs immediately, although it can occur 30 to 60 minutes after a repeated exposure to the antigen. Almost any foreign substance is capable of eliciting anaphylaxis. The most common causes are foods (milk, seafood, nuts, eggs), drugs (aspirin, penicillin, cephalosporins, chemotherapy), insect venom, and biologic agents (allergen extracts, iodinated radiocontrast media, latex). The incidence of anaphylaxis is increasing; incidence data has wide variability (10.5 to 49.8 per 100,000 person-years) because of differing definitions (Dinakar, 2012).

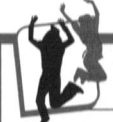

COMMUNITY CARE 31-1

Treatment for Insect Stings and Bites

Teach parents, school personnel, and other caregivers to
- Remove stinger, if present, by flicking or scraping. Do not squeeze or pull with tweezers; these actions inject any remaining venom into the wound.
- Rub the area for 15 minutes using a cotton ball soaked in a solution of meat tenderizer with a few drops of water, which may help reduce inflammation.
- Apply cold compresses to reduce site swelling and pain.
- For itching, administer diphenhydramine hydrochloride (Benadryl), 4–5 mg/kg/day (to a total of 200 mg/day) divided into four doses.

- Call a health care provider immediately if the child has
  - Breathing or swallowing difficulty
  - Hives
  - Ten or more stings
  - A sting in the mouth
- Call a health care provider later if
  - The stinger cannot be removed
  - The swelling continues to spread after 24 hours
  - Swelling of the hand (or foot) spreads past the wrist (or ankle)

Severe anaphylactic reactions can result in death. Prompt diagnosis and immediate intervention with appropriate therapy are necessary to avert this outcome.

Initial exposure to the antigen causes the formation of antibodies, usually of the immunoglobulin E class. Upon repeated exposure to the same antigen, symptoms develop and the hypersensitivity reaction may occur. The antibody–antigen reaction causes a massive release of chemical mediators (such as histamine) from mast cells and basophils throughout the body.

Assessment

The common manifestations of anaphylaxis include urticaria, angioedema (a condition characterized by development of urticaria and edematous areas of skin, mucous membranes, or viscera), bronchospasm, laryngeal edema, hypotension, hyperperistalsis, and cardiac arrhythmias.

The degree of the sensitivity reaction depends on the antigen's nature and the child's degree of **atopy**. Atopy is the inherited tendency to form immunoglobulin E antibodies. Often, a strong family history exists for allergies or hypersensitivity reactions to particular drugs, insects, or foods. Take the family history seriously; it indicates a need for the child to avoid certain drugs or foods.

ANSWER: Chris has facial edema and laryngeal edema, both of which are signs of an anaphylactic reaction.

Nursing Diagnoses and Outcomes

QUESTION: Which nursing diagnosis is appropriate for Chris?

Nursing diagnoses and outcomes for the child experiencing an emergency are discussed in Nursing Plan of Care 31-1. In addition, the following diagnoses and outcomes apply for the child experiencing an anaphylactic reaction:

Nursing Diagnosis: Ineffective airway clearance related to effects of laryngoedema
Outcome: Child will have interventions immediately implemented to reduce laryngoedema and optimize airway patency.
Nursing Diagnosis: Decreased cardiac output related to effects of vasodilation
Outcome: Child's signs of decreased cardiac output will be recognized promptly, and interventions will be initiated immediately.
Nursing Diagnosis: Ineffective breathing pattern related to effects of bronchospasm
Outcome: Child will generate an effective breathing pattern or will have interventions implemented to support an effective breathing pattern to optimize gas exchange.

ANSWER: Potential for ineffective breathing pattern related to laryngeal edema is an appropriate nursing diagnosis for Chris.

Interdisciplinary Interventions

QUESTION: Did Chris's family respond appropriately? What medications do you anticipate Chris receiving? Develop a teaching plan for Chris's family after this emergency.

As with all allergic disorders, avoidance or preventive measures for patients at high risk are the primary treatment. However, most serious anaphylactic reactions are unanticipated. Therefore, immediate recognition and treatment of anaphylaxis are critical to prevent death resulting from upper airway obstruction, shock, or both (Chart 31-2).

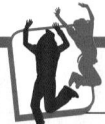

<table>
<tr><td>

CHART 31-2 **Interdisciplinary Interventions: Managing Anaphylaxis**

- Administer epinephrine intramuscularly or intravenously to reverse histamine release and hypotension.
- Rapidly assess ABCs and intervene as necessary.
- Maintain patent airway.
- Administer oxygen.
- Start IV.
- Stop antigen release or slow absorption. If the antigen responsible for the anaphylaxis has been injected or is infusing intravenously, discontinue immediately.
- Administer albuterol aerosols to reverse bronchospasm.
- Administer antihistamines such as H_1 or H_2 antagonists (e.g., diphenhydramine or ranitidine) to counteract histamine release.
- Administer fluids if hypotension is not responsive to epinephrine and H_1 and H_2 antagonists.
- Administer corticosteroids (e.g., methylprednisolone) after initial treatment to prevent recurrence of anaphylaxis.
- Continually monitor ABCs, vital signs, and response to treatment. Observe for late-phase symptoms.

</td></tr>
</table>

Children who have experienced an anaphylactic reaction should be hospitalized for observation because there may be a biphasic reaction in which symptoms recur (as late as 28 hours) after initially resolving in response to therapy. After the causative antigens have been identified, teach the child and family how to prevent anaphylaxis (Community Care 31-2).

ANSWER: By seeking medical treatment immediately, Chris's family responded appropriately to his signs of an anaphylactic reaction. You can anticipate that Chris will receive epinephrine as well as an antihistamine such as diphenhydramine (Benadryl) in the emergency room (see Chart 31-2 for more details). Your teaching plan for the Whitworth family should include strategies to avoid hornets and the use of an EpiPen.

EPISTAXIS

The nose is highly vascular and is susceptible to bleeding. Common causes of **epistaxis** (nosebleed) include trauma, frequent nose picking, infection, inflammation, low environmental humidity, and foreign bodies. Children are more susceptible during respiratory infections and during the winter, when dry air irritates the nasal mucosa. Epistaxis is rare in infants and common in children, with the incidence decreasing after puberty. In adolescent females, epistaxis may be associated with pregnancy.

Epistaxis is usually mild and responds to home management; occasionally, bleeding is severe enough to require transfusion. Epistaxis may also signal an

<table>
<tr><td>

COMMUNITY CARE 31-2

Preventing Anaphylaxis

Teach parents and child to
- Notify caregivers and school personnel of known allergies
- Have child wear a medical alert bracelet, as appropriate
- Reduce the risk of exposure as appropriate to the situation (e.g., a child allergic to bees should wear shoes when outside, wear clothing that covers extremities, not walk through flower beds, and not wear perfume or brightly colored clothing)
- Take allergy medications before unavoidable exposure to known allergens
- Keep a kit with the child at all times that contains self-injectable epinephrine and an oral antihistamine in case the child has had an anaphylactic reaction. Teach parents, and the child as appropriate, and school or daycare personnel how to use the EpiPen appropriately.
- Notify an adult at the first signs of anaphylaxis; instruct adults to call an ambulance and get the child to the nearest ED

</td></tr>
</table>

underlying pathology such as Osler-Weber-Rendu disease (hereditary hemorrhagic telangiectasia) or juvenile angiofibroma, usually found in adolescent males.

Assessment

Epistaxis often occurs without warning, with blood flowing from one or both nostrils. Evaluate vital signs for indicators of hemodynamic instability (increased heart and respiratory rates, decreased blood pressure, or orthostatic changes). Examine the skin and mucous membranes for petechiae and ecchymosis, which may indicate coagulopathy. Inspect the nasopharynx and oropharynx for masses and blood dripping from a posterior bleeding site. Examine the nares visually and attempt to identify the site of bleeding (Fig. 31-7). Most commonly, the anterior nasal septum is the site of origin in epistaxis.

Laboratory workup is warranted when the child with epistaxis has a family history of a bleeding disorder, spontaneous bleeding of other areas in the body, continued bleeding lasting longer than 20 minutes despite direct pressure, onset of recurrent epistaxis before 2 years of age, or when the hematocrit level decreases substantially secondary to epistaxis.

Interdisciplinary Interventions

Most nosebleeds can be managed effectively outside the acute care setting. Teach parents and children techniques that may prevent nosebleeds. Also teach

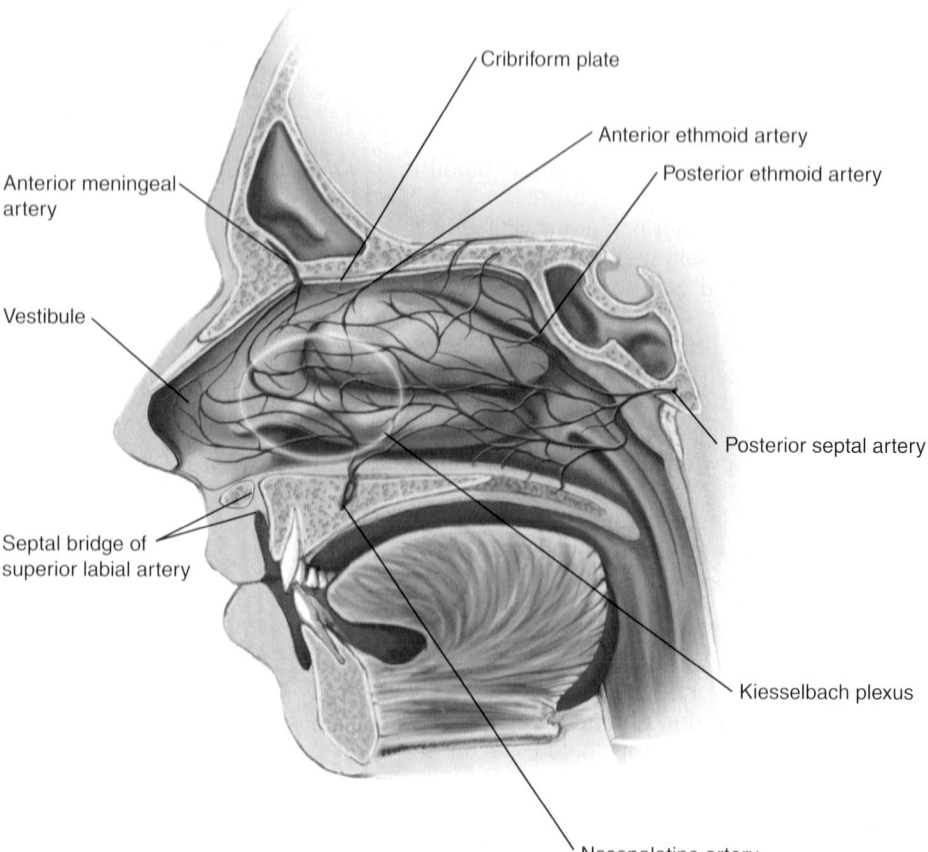

Cribriform plate

Anterior ethmoid artery

Posterior ethmoid artery

Anterior meningeal
artery

Vestibule

Posterior septal artery

Septal bridge of
superior labial artery

Kiesselbach plexus

Figure 31-7 Most nosebleeds arise from the anteroinferior portion of the nasal septum, an area called Kiesselbach plexus.

Nasopalatine artery

school and daycare personnel immediate management of nosebleeds (Teaching Intervention Plan 31-2). Petroleum jelly and antiseptic cream may be effective, but studies have methodologic limitations, and more research is needed to determine optimal treatment (McGarry, 2011). A health care provider might need to provide more intensive intervention for bleeding that does not stop with home management. Maintain the child in a sitting position with the head tilted forward to avoid blood dripping into the posterior pharynx. If the anterior nasal septum is the site, apply direct pressure on the bleeding site by compressing the external nares for 10 minutes (Fig. 31-8). If this measure does not stop the bleeding, cautery, either chemical (silver nitrate) or electrical, of the site by trained personnel may be required for definitive control of bleeding from the anterior nasal septum. Cauterization is not indicated for epistaxis in children with bleeding disorders because of the likelihood of multiple bleeding sites and the risk of severely damaging and perforating the nasal mucosa in the attempt to control bleeding from the various sites.

For active bleeding that is not controlled by pressure and cautery, spray phenylephrine (Neo-Synephrine), 0.25% to 0.5%, into the nares. If phenylephrine does not control the bleeding, insert a cotton pledget soaked in 2% lidocaine (Xylocaine) or tetracaine phenylephrine, Neo-Synephrine, or epinephrine 0.25% to 0.5% tightly

into the affected nares. Leave the pledget in place for 10 minutes while applying pressure, and then reassess the nares for continued active bleeding. If necessary, insert another pledget, soaked with a vasoconstrictor, and leave it in place for an additional 10 minutes.

If the bleeding site is anterior and not controlled by pressure, vasoconstrictors, or cautery, anterior packing by a physician may be performed. Anterior packing is contraindicated in the child with nasal trauma or when a cerebrospinal fluid leak is suspected. Anterior packing impregnated with antibiotics remains in place for 2 to 3 days. Antifibrinolytic agents delivered via gel are also effective and better tolerated than packing, but use has not been widely adopted (Douglas & Wormald, 2007).

ALERT *Keep emergency resuscitation equipment readily available when using anesthetic packing. The anesthetized airway may cause the child to lose protective reflexes.*

Sinusitis is a complication of nasal packing, and oral antibiotics should be administered prophylactically. Antibiotics to cover for coagulase-positive *Staphylococcus* (e.g., first-generation cephalosporins) should be

---

TIP 31-2: A TEACHING INTERVENTION PLAN for Preventing and Managing Epistaxis

Nursing Diagnoses and Family Outcomes

- Risk for aspiration related to presence of blood in oropharynx
  Outcomes: Child will not aspirate blood into bronchial tree.
  Child will maintain patent airway.
- Deficient fluid volume related to effects of bleeding
  Outcome: Child will be brought to health care facility before fluid volume deficit exerts a negative effect on hemodynamic stability.
- Anxiety related to bleeding
  Outcome: Child will be calm and able to follow directions as age appropriate.
- Deficient knowledge: Community management of epistaxis
  Outcome: Caregivers and child, if appropriate, will implement appropriate interventions to control nosebleed.

Teach the Child/Family

Preventing Epistaxis
- Increase the humidity in the home or the child's bedroom by using a humidifier.
- Instill saline nose drops before having the child blow nose.
- Have the child avoid picking nose.

Managing Epistaxis
- Position the child erect, sitting with head tilted forward to avoid blood dripping posteriorly into the pharynx.
- Pinch the nose.
  - Tightly pinch the soft parts of the nose against the center wall for 10 minutes; this should be timed by a clock, not estimated.
  - Do not release the pressure for 10 minutes.
  - Encourage child to remain calm and quiet and to breathe through the mouth.
- If bleeding continues
  - Soak gauze in phenylephrine hydrochloride (Neo-Synephrine) or petroleum jelly and insert it into the nostril.
  - Pinch the nose with gauze in place for another 10 minutes.
  - Be aware that swallowed blood may irritate the stomach and cause vomiting.

Contact Health Care Provider if
- Bleeding does not stop within 20 minutes
- Child feels dizzy or faint

---

used because *Staphylococcus aureus*, which may cause toxic shock syndrome, is often present in the nares. Administer pain medication to children who need nasal packing. Nursing care includes maintaining a patent airway, watching for signs of hypoxia or respiratory distress, monitoring fluid balance, and reducing anxiety in the child and family. The amount of blood often seems quite large, which is frightening to the child and family. A child with packing in place is unable to breathe through the nose, which also causes anxiety.

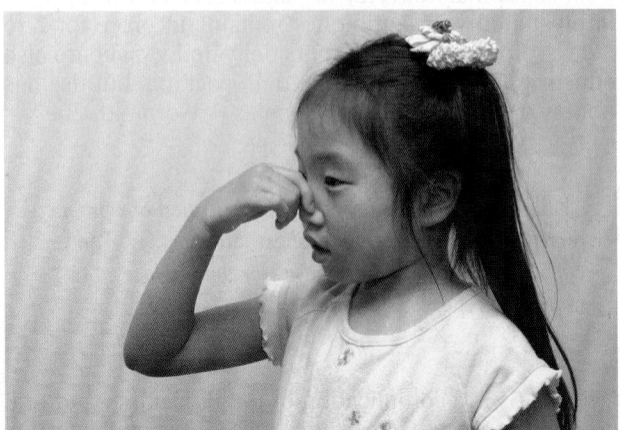

Figure 31-8 Compression of the nasal alae controls most epistaxis, which commonly occurs in Kiesselbach plexus (Little area).

ENVIRONMENTAL EXPOSURE INJURIES

Various environmental exposures can injure an infant or child. Most often, injury occurs because the infant or child physically cannot remove or protect himself or herself from the source of injury. The environmental exposure injuries discussed here include prolonged exposures to heat (hyperthermia) or cold (hypothermia), smoke inhalation, and near-drowning. See Chapter 25 for discussion of sunburn.

HYPERTHERMIA

Prolonged exposure to heat without protective equipment can cause hyperthermia. Hyperthermia occurs when the thermoregulatory set point of the body remains normal but heat gain exceeds heat loss despite the body's efforts to return to the set point. Heatstroke is a condition caused by failure of the body's thermoregulatory system during prolonged exposure to heat and high relative humidity. Heatstroke is marked by body temperature more than 105° F (40.6° C), headache, and confusion. If untreated, heatstroke can progress to delirium and coma. Severe heat illness may increase core temperature to the level at which cellular injury occurs as a result of dysfunction of enzymatic processes and the related cellular proteins. Without treatment, individuals with heatstroke die. Even with treatment, heatstroke can be fatal or result in long-term neurologic sequelae.

Hyperthermia is a preventable illness that is manifested by heat cramps, exhaustion, or stroke. Heat illness is most commonly seen in the tropical regions of the world, but heat is responsible for the deaths of more than 3,400 people per year in the United States; 7% of these deaths are in children younger than 15 years of age (Grunbenhoff et al., 2007). The elderly population is most vulnerable, but children are at risk as well, especially young athletes, infants left in automobiles on hot days, children with cystic fibrosis, and those with anhidrosis. For more information on heat illnesses, see Table 31-5.

Prevention is the best treatment for heat illnesses. Teach children and parents measures to prevent overheating in hot environments. Children should be dressed in lightweight clothes and hats or visors. Keep children well hydrated by providing and offering cool drinks every 15 to 30 minutes, even if the child is not thirsty. Water is a good choice because children sweat less than adults and thus lose less salt. Activity level should be regulated based on environmental conditions and should be restricted when temperature or humidity is high. Scheduled rest periods in the shade should be enforced to promote heat dissipation. Athletes are at particular risk for heat illnesses. They should be specifically instructed to avoid both water deprivation and wearing excessive clothing that reduces evaporation of sweat.

HYPOTHERMIA

Hypothermia is defined as a core body temperature less than 95° F (35° C). In the United States, moderate (temperature, 82.5° to 90° F [28° to 32.2° C]) to severe hypothermia (temperature <82.5° F [28° C]) causes almost 700 deaths per year (CDC, 2005). All ages are affected, although infants and children are at particular risk because of their greater ratio of surface area to body weight, thin skin, limited amount of subcutaneous fat, and immature thermoregulatory system. The causes of hypothermia include immersion in icy water, prolonged exposure to cold temperatures, and exposure for an extended time during a medical evaluation. Hypothermia is also common in patients with sepsis and shock (see Chapter 25 for discussion of frostbite).

ALERT *Hypothermia can lead to prolonged bleeding, metabolic acidosis, decreased respiratory rate, bradycardia, and cardiopulmonary arrest.*

Assessment

Mental status may remain normal in mild hypothermia. Central nervous system function becomes progressively impaired as the temperature decreases. Increasing lethargy, incoordination, apathy, confusion, clumsiness, irritability, hallucinations, and bradycardia are seen. A decreasing level of consciousness is seen in moderate hypothermia, and coma occurs with severe hypothermia.

At a temperature of 77° F (25° C), profound respiratory depression occurs, followed by ventricular fibrillation or asystole, and usually results in death.

Hypothermia can mimic death, with the child demonstrating dilated pupils, muscular rigidity, faint or absent pulse, and an unobtainable blood pressure. However, life can be sustained for long periods, despite cessation of cardiac function, because of the marked decrease in oxygen consumption.

Nursing Diagnoses and Outcomes

Nursing diagnoses and outcomes for the child experiencing an emergency are discussed in Nursing Plan of Care 31-1. In addition, the following diagnoses and outcomes are appropriate for the hypothermic child:

Nursing Diagnosis: Impaired spontaneous ventilation related to effects of decreased body temperature
Outcome: Child will maintain spontaneous ventilation or have adequate ventilatory support provided.
Nursing Diagnosis: Hypothermia related to environmental exposure
Outcome: Child will regain normal body temperature and will suffer no long-term effects from hypothermia.

Interdisciplinary Interventions

Prevention is the best treatment. Educate families about the increased risk of hypothermia in young children. Children have higher metabolic rates than adults. They generate more heat, so children may not feel the effects of exposure. Parents should dress children appropriately for the weather and monitor their activities so that they are not exposed for long periods.

Nursing interventions for a child with hypothermia are discussed on thePoint Procedures: Use of Warming Devices. Support cardiorespiratory function as needed. If the child develops lethal dysrhythmias, defibrillation is often ineffective until the core temperature reaches 86° F (30° C). Drug therapy is rarely effective at low temperatures and can lead to toxicity because hepatic and renal metabolisms are decreased.

ALERT *External rewarming techniques may result in early warming of the skin and extremities and peripheral vasodilation and worsen hypotension and shock. This phenomenon, called afterdrop, is characterized by a decrease in the core temperature as it receives cold blood from the periphery.*

Active rewarming can be accomplished through external or core rewarming techniques (Nursing Interventions 31-3). Core rewarming is the most appropriate choice when the temperature is 86° F (30° C) or less with cardiopulmonary arrest. Survival of severely hypothermic patients after prolonged periods of nonperfusing cardiac rhythm has been reported (Rudolph & Barnung, 2011). Clinical judgment is used to determine when resuscitative efforts should cease. Often, the child is rewarmed to 95° F (35° C) prior to stopping resuscitation.

TABLE 31-5   Heat Illnesses: Assessment and Interventions

Illness	Etiology	Assessment Findings	Interdisciplinary Interventions
Heat cramps	Prolonged or extensive exercise in a hot environment with high humidity Electrolyte depletion secondary to profuse sweating and fluid replacement with salt-poor fluids	Sudden onset of intermittent, excruciating cramps in the skeletal muscles Usually occurs after exercise, during the cool-down period	Have child stop exertion and rest in a cool, shaded area. For mild cramps, administer oral salt solution (1 teaspoon salt in 500 mL water). Give over 1–2 hours. For severe cramps, administer 0.9% NS (20 mL/kg) IV over 1–2 hours.
Heat exhaustion (heat prostration)	Prolonged or extensive exercise in a hot environment, with high humidity and inadequate fluid replacement Most common heat illness Without treatment, can progress to heat stroke	Onset over 30 minutes but may have a more acute onset, such as the "parade ground faint" Headache Intense thirst Inability to work or play Tachycardia Orthostatic hypotension Nausea and vomiting Lethargy Central nervous system dysfunction, such as hyperventilation, agitation, incoordination, paresthesia, psychosis Intractable seizures and muscle cramps (in severe cases) Normal body temperature or body temperature as high as 102.2° F (39° C) with high ambient temperatures or exercise Hemoconcentration Hyper- or hyponatremia (depends on type of fluids ingested) Hyperchloremia Respiratory alkalosis (resulting from hyperventilation)	Provide the child with a cool, well-ventilated place to rest. Remove some clothing, spray with water, and fan the child. Replace fluids orally (or IV if the child is weak or has an impaired level of consciousness); liquids should be cool with unrestricted dietary sodium. If IV fluids are required, administer bolus of 0.9% NS 20 mL/kg given over 20 minutes. Repeat boluses to correct electrolyte balance and to restore blood pressure. Treat severe cases with an initial IV of 5 mL/kg of 3% NS over 20 minutes followed by a second dose of 5 mL/kg over 4–6 hours.
Heat stroke (a true medical emergency)	Thermoregulatory failure after prolonged exposure to high environmental temperatures and humidity	Hyperpyrexia (≥105° F or 40.6° C) Hot, dry skin, typically with anhidrosis (absence of sweating) Moderate central nervous system disturbances such as headache, dizziness, faintness, and confusion Severe central nervous system disturbances such as stupor, seizures, coma, and sudden loss of consciousness (more common when treatment is delayed) Tachycardia and an increased pulse pressure initially Ashen cyanosis and a thin, rapid pulse later	Remove the child from the source of heat. Maintain patent airway and cardiovascular support. If comatose, may require intubation to secure airway. Remove clothing and actively cool the child. Monitor temperature closely with a rectal probe. Antipyretics such as acetaminophen are not useful. Perform active cooling measures such as sprinkling the child with water, directing fans toward child, applying a cooling blanket, or giving an ice bath (although this makes other monitoring mechanisms difficult). Discontinue active cooling measures when the core temperature decreases to 102.2° F (39° C). Avoid shivering because this increases heat production. Carefully monitor electrocardiogram, central venous pressure, arterial blood pressure, and urine output in a patient with signs of failing cardiac output (ashen skin, tachycardia, hypotension); such a patient is in danger of imminent death.

NURSING INTERVENTIONS 31-3

Core Rewarming Methods

The nurse may assist in administering the following methods:
- Heated, humidified oxygen
- Warmed IV fluids
- Heated (104°–111° F [40°–44° C]) lavage of
  - Bladder
  - Stomach

Colon
Peritoneum (1.5% dialysate, short dwell time)
- Left hemithorax (pleural lavage)
- Open thoracotomy with mediastinal irrigation
- Venovenous or arteriovenous circuits with heating element
- Extracorporeal circulation (heart–lung pump)

SMOKE INHALATION

Smoke inhalation usually results from a fire, which may also cause burns (for a discussion of burn injuries, see Chapter 25). Exposure to fire, smoke, or both causes substantial damage to the child's pulmonary tree. In fact, most fatalities resulting from fires are the result of inhalation of toxic gas (e.g., carbon monoxide and cyanide) rather than burns (Roderique et al., 2012). Inhalation injuries are the primary cause of death in burn patients within the first 24 hours.

Several factors place children at high risk for inhalation injuries. Their higher respiratory rate leads to increased intake of toxic gases and contributes to insensible fluid losses from the pulmonary tree. They have a small airway diameter and increased proportion of soft tissue, and the diameter may become even smaller because of inhalation of hot air and irritants, which causes edema. Progressive airway edema may ultimately lead to airway obstruction.

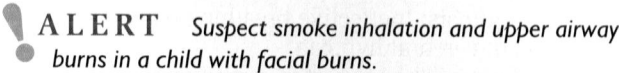 **ALERT**   *Suspect smoke inhalation and upper airway burns in a child with facial burns.*

Assessment

Clinically, the child may have singed eyebrows, carbonaceous sputum, tachypnea, and other signs of respiratory distress such as wheezing, rhonchi, rales, or stridor. However, symptoms of an inhalation injury may not manifest for up to 24 hours after exposure. Therefore, close observation of respiratory status is necessary during this time. Because the carbon monoxide molecule has a 250-fold higher affinity for hemoglobin than oxygen, tissue hypoxia occurs as carbon monoxide binds to hemoglobin, reducing its oxygen-carrying capacity and decreasing oxygen saturation. Without prompt treatment, serum carboxyhemoglobin levels greater than 50% can cause irreversible central nervous system damage. Central nervous system signs of carbon monoxide poisoning range from slight dyspnea, decreased visual acuity, irritability, nausea, and fatigue to confusion, ataxia, and coma.

caREminder

Do not rely on pulse oximetry to measure oxygen saturation. Pulse oximetry does not distinguish between oxyhemoglobin and carboxyhemoglobin, so the actual oxygen saturation is less than the pulse oximeter reflects.

Nursing Diagnoses and Outcomes

Nursing Plan of Care 31-1 lists nursing diagnoses and outcomes applicable to the child experiencing an emergency. The following diagnoses and outcomes may also be appropriate for the child after smoke inhalation:

Nursing Diagnosis: Ineffective airway clearance related to effects of edema and inhaled toxins causing mucosal sloughing
Outcome: Child will be intubated early, if indicated, and child's airway will remain patent.
Nursing Diagnosis: Impaired gas exchange related to effects of cellular damage, carboxyhemoglobin replacing oxyhemoglobin, pulmonary edema, and smoke exposure causing decreased surfactant resulting in atelectasis
Outcome: Child will maintain adequate cellular oxygenation.
Nursing Diagnosis: Risk for deficient fluid volume related to effects of tachypnea, cellular damage, and increased fluid demands
Outcome: Child will receive adequate fluids to prevent dehydration, will have accurate intake and output monitored, and will not develop pulmonary edema because of overhydration.

Interdisciplinary Interventions

Administer 100% oxygen via a snug-fitting, nonrebreather mask to all children with smoke inhalation. The usual 4-hour half-life of carboxyhemoglobin can be reduced to less than 1 hour by administering 100% oxygen (Roderique et al., 2012). Children with severe laryngeal edema, hypoxemia, and audible stridor require intubation to maintain a secure and patent airway. Obtain baseline arterial blood gases, pH, and carboxyhemoglobin levels, and monitor them periodically.

Maintain a neutral thermal environment. The child is susceptible to hypothermia because of associated burn injuries and exposure for treatment of injuries. Hypothermia and alkalosis decrease the dissociation of carbon monoxide from hemoglobin. Hyperbaric oxygen therapy may be considered.

Encourage the child to cough and breathe deeply to promote airway clearance and to help prevent subsequent pneumonia and respiratory distress syndrome. Suctioning, chest physiotherapy, and medications (e.g., bronchodilators, mucolytics) help clear secretions. Also, promote early ambulation out of bed, even in the child who is ventilated.

Monitor the child for hypoxia, respiratory distress, and pulmonary edema. Even if not seriously injured or intubated, children who have been in fires should be hospitalized for observation for at least 24 hours.

NEAR-DROWNING

Globally, drowning is one of the primary causes of unintentional injury deaths (Balan & Lingam, 2012). In the United States, the highest drowning rate is in children aged 1 to 4 years, and fatal drowning is the second leading cause of unintentional injury deaths in children aged 1 to 14 years (CDC, 2012). Males, children younger than age 4 years, males 15 to 18 years of age, and those who have a seizure disorder are at particular risk (CDC, 2012).

Drowning is defined as death resulting from suffocation by submersion in a liquid. Near-drowning is defined as survival, although sometimes temporary, for at least 24 hours after a submersion episode.

Children can drown whenever unsupervised around any body of water, including bathtubs, toilets, and buckets of water. Most drownings occur because of lack of adequate barriers to prevent access to a swimming pool. Precipitating factors include trauma (including child abuse), intoxication (which plays a significant role in adolescent drownings), seizure disorders, and exhaustion. Whether in fresh- or saltwater, the end result of near-drowning is the same: pulmonary compliance decreases, airway resistance increases, pulmonary arterial pressure increases, and pulmonary flow decreases. These changes result in hypoxemia, which leads to cardiac arrest and ischemia.

Although all organs are susceptible to ischemic injury, the central nervous system is most vulnerable, and prognosis depends on the degree of central nervous system injury (see Chapter 21 for discussion of increased intracranial pressure). The degree of brain injury depends on the submersion time (which is often underestimated), the water temperature, and the speed with which resuscitative measures are initiated. The longer the submersion, the poorer the prognosis (Tipton & Golden, 2011). Irreversible cerebral injury from hypoxia begins to occur after about 3 to 5 minutes of submersion. Submersion in cold water occasionally may be compatible with recovery after longer periods; cold water may increase the likelihood of survival by decreasing the cerebral metabolic rate.

Assessment

Initially, the clinical problems of children after a near-drowning episode involve the pulmonary and neurologic systems. The child may present with varying degrees of neurologic insult, from alert with minimal injury to full cardiopulmonary arrest. Cerebral edema may develop later, with irritability, confusion, and lethargy leading to seizures and coma. Respiratory symptoms can include cough; dyspnea; tachypnea; adventitious breath sounds; expectoration of pink, frothy sputum; and apnea.

Initial arterial blood gas measurements often indicate hypoxemia and metabolic acidosis. Chest radiograph results vary but should be obtained to provide a baseline against which to compare later radiograph. Electrolyte abnormalities may be seen. Renal damage resulting from hypoperfusion, hypoxia, and ischemia is revealed by oliguria, proteinuria, and elevated blood urea nitrogen and creatinine.

Nursing Diagnoses and Outcomes

In addition to the nursing diagnoses discussed in Nursing Plan of Care 31-1, nursing diagnoses and outcomes applicable to the child after near-drowning are the following:

Nursing Diagnosis: Impaired gas exchange related to effects of aspiration, hypoxia, pulmonary edema
Outcome: Child will demonstrate adequate oxygenation and no signs of respiratory distress.
Nursing Diagnosis: Ineffective airway clearance related to effects of aspiration of water and foreign material, accumulated secretions, and artificial airway
Outcome: Child will maintain a patent airway, and secretions will be adequately cleared to maintain gas exchange.
Nursing Diagnosis: Ineffective breathing pattern related to effects of cerebral hypoxia
Outcome: Child will be supported in maintaining a breathing pattern that maintains adequate gas exchange.
Nursing Diagnosis: Ineffective tissue perfusion: Cardiopulmonary related to effects of dysrhythmias, hypovolemia
Outcome: Child will maintain adequate cardiopulmonary perfusion, as evidenced by normal sinus rhythm, strong bilateral peripheral pulses, and urine output of at least 1 mL/kg/hr.
Nursing Diagnosis: Ineffective tissue perfusion: Cerebral related to effects of hypoxia, cerebral edema, and increased intracranial pressure
Outcome: Child will maintain adequate cerebral perfusion; signs of decreased perfusion will be recognized immediately and interventions implemented.
Nursing Diagnosis: Excess fluid volume related to fluid resuscitation, renal damage from hypoxia
Outcome: Child will maintain fluid balance, as evidenced by absence of edema, urine output of at least 1 mL/kg/hr, and electrolytes and urine specific gravity within normal ranges.

Nursing Diagnosis: Deficient knowledge: Water safety
Outcomes:
- Family will discuss and implement water safety measures.
- Family will not experience future near-drowning events.

Interdisciplinary Interventions

Manage the child near-drowning victim in the same fashion as the trauma patient. Initially, focus on assessing the ABCs and correcting hypoxemia.

Continue to monitor and support pulmonary, cardiac, and neurologic function. Assess airway patency, breath sounds, color, and respiratory effort, and assist with ventilation as indicated. Cardiac assessment includes heart rate and rhythm, blood pressure, capillary refill, and pulses. Monitor intake and output to assess fluid balance and renal function. Catheters may be placed to monitor arterial, central venous, and/or pulmonary artery pressure. Assessment of neurologic functioning includes level of consciousness, pupillary response, reflexes, and presence of posturing or seizure activity. As with all pediatric emergencies, provide family support. If the child survives, or if other children live in the house, instruct the family in water safety measures (Community Care 31-3).

POISONING

A poison is a substance that causes harmful effects upon exposure. Globally, poisoning is the fifth leading cause of death in children younger than age 5 years

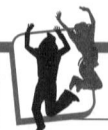

COMMUNITY CARE 31-3

Water Safety

Instruct parents and other care providers to

- Supervise children *constantly* around *any* body of water, including bathtubs
- Designate one person to watch the child, especially when many adults are present and each may assume the others are watching the child
- Fence any pool or hot tub and equip it with self-closing gates
- Empty pails and buckets of fluid immediately after use
- Keep toilet lids closed and secured, especially around young children whose heads are relatively large and heavy, making it easy to fall in head first, and then difficult for the child to extricate himself or herself
- Allow children with a seizure disorder to swim or take a bath only with supervision, regardless of age
- Discuss with adolescents the dangers of combining drugs or alcohol with swimming or water sports

(Kendrick et al., 2008). Children younger than age 2 years are poisoned more frequently from household products than from medications; the reverse is seen in children older than 2 age years (Kendrick et al., 2008). Thirty-six percent of poisoning exposures involved children younger than 3 years of age; 49% occurred in children younger than 6 years of age (Bronstein et al., 2012). Poisons that are discussed in this section include iron, lead, acetaminophen, hydrocarbons, and caustics.

Poisoning ingestions in infants are often the result of therapeutic overdosing. Ingestions are most common in children 1 to 6 years old. Children are naturally curious and often explore by tasting. They also imitate adult behavior. If they witness a parent take medication, they may try some themselves or may feed the medication to a younger sibling.

 KidKare Never tell a child that medicine is candy, which may increase the child's desire to obtain it. Tell the child it is medicine and is taken for a specific reason.

Young children usually ingest only a single substance and, because they are generally closely watched, the time from ingestion to discovery and treatment is brief. Children younger than age 6 years most frequently ingest substances such as cosmetics and personal care products, cleaning substances, analgesics, foreign bodies, and topical agents (Bronstein et al., 2012). Such agents may not be the most toxic but are the most readily accessible to children.

Adolescents may be affected by drug experimentation or suicide attempts. Therefore, poisoning in adolescents often involves multiple substances, with a delay between when exposure occurs and when medical treatment is obtained.

Assessment

The child may have a wide range of symptoms, from none to coma. Obtaining an accurate history is paramount to successful treatment. Be sure to determine the following information:

- What was ingested
- How much was ingested (one swallow of liquid approximately equals a volume of 5 mL)
- When it occurred
- What, if any, therapy was initiated before arrival in the ED

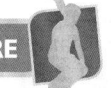 **CROSS-CULTURAL CARE**

Folk remedies may contain toxic agents, so use of such remedies should be included in the history. For example, Hispanic and other cultures use mint tea to treat colic and minor ailments. Most mint teas are not toxic, but mint leaves that contain pennyroyal oil can be lethal.

Recommended tests include serum glucose, electrolytes, serum osmolarity, and anion gap. Quantifying drug levels whenever possible is also helpful in

CHART 31-3   Common Causes for Increased Anion Gap Values

Using the mnemonic AT MUD PILES (Woolf, 1993):

Alcohol

Toluene

Methanol

Uremia

Diabetic ketoacidosis

Paraldehyde

Iron

Lactic acidosis

Ethylene glycol

Salicylates

Note: Anion gap is calculated using the formula: $Na^+ - (Cl^- + HCO_3^-)$. The normal value is less than 16 mEq/L.

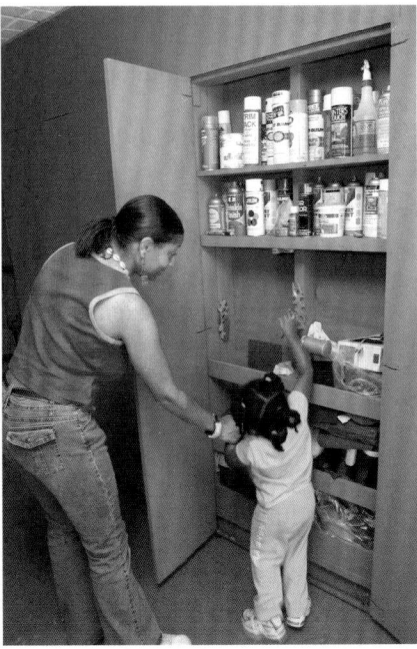

Figure 31-9 This frustrated child cannot reach the tempting, but potentially dangerous, poisons and cleaning supplies stored safely out of her reach.

determining further interventions and administration of antidotes. An elevated anion gap value is characteristic of the acidosis seen in poisonings. The formula to calculate the anion gap and common etiologies for increased anion gap values are listed in Chart 31-3.

Nursing Diagnoses and Outcomes

Nursing diagnoses and outcomes for the child experiencing an emergency are discussed in Nursing Plan of Care 31-1. Nursing diagnoses applicable to the poisoned child depend on the specific poison and symptoms the child displays (e.g., risk for aspiration applies to the child who has a depressed level of consciousness resulting from the poison). An additional nursing diagnosis and outcomes are as follows:

Nursing Diagnosis: Deficient knowledge: Poisoning
Outcomes:
• Family will discuss poison prevention techniques and how these techniques change as the child grows and develops.
• Family will describe first aid measures appropriate for poisoning, including having the local poison control center phone number readily accessible.

Interdisciplinary Interventions

Obviously, preventing poisoning is the key (see Chapters 4 to 7). Teach parents to keep medications in their original, childproof containers, and lock them out of children's reach. Advise them to store cleaning solutions, cosmetics, and hydrocarbons (e.g., gasoline, solvents and thinners, polishes) in high, locked cabinets (Fig. 31-9). Advise them to make the child's environment free of lead-based paints and poisonous plants (Community Care 31-4).

Perform a rapid assessment and implement immediate interventions to ensure that the ABCs are managed. Secure IV access and obtain a serum glucose level because hypoglycemia is a common manifestation of acute poisoning. Treat shock with fluids and vasopressors as necessary. To reduce the absorption of potentially toxic substances, gastric decontamination may be required (Table 31-6). Depending on the severity of the ingestion, gastric decontamination may occur immediately after the airway is secured during resuscitation. An **antidote** (a substance that neutralizes the poison or its effects) may also be administered. Some metallic poisons (Table 31-7) can be countered with **chelation** therapy, a process during which certain compounds are used to bind the toxin, making it inactive or less injurious.

caREminder

Treat the child, not the poison. Specific treatment depends on the type and amount of toxin, time since exposure, and the child's symptoms. Many children do not need treatment.

Iron

Unintentional iron poisoning, seen most commonly in children younger than 6 years of age, has decreased from previous years but is still a threat (Chang & Rangan, 2011). Iron-containing compounds are readily available as brightly colored, sugar-coated tablets and often are viewed by parents as a harmless vitamin. Prenatal iron preparations are often the source because children ingest their mother's vitamins. Moderate to severe toxicity occurs after ingestion of 20 to 60 mg/kg (Change & Rangan, 2011). The number of pills ingested may be useful in determining whether the dose was toxic. Monitoring serum iron levels is critical in the

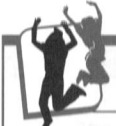

COMMUNITY CARE 31-4

Plant Poisonings

Educate parents and caregivers about which common plants are poisonous and to limit the child's access to them (not an inclusive list):

Azalea
Castor bean
Cherry (pits)
Deadly nightshade
Dumb cane (*Dieffenbachia*)
English ivy
Holly
Jimsonweed
Lily of the valley
Mistletoe (berries)
Mushrooms (certain species)
Oleander
Potatoes (sprouts)
Rosary pea
Rhododendron
Rhubarb (leaves)

Water hemlock
Yew

Tell parents and caregivers to do the following if the child ingests a poisonous plant:
• Stay calm.
• Call the regional poison control center or the national number (800) 222-1222.
• Describe symptoms (if any) and name of plant, if known.
• Follow instructions from poison control center.
• Take plant with you when seeking treatment.

Teach parents and caregivers the following poison prevention tips:
• Supervise the child's activities.
• Place household plants out of reach.
• Teach children not to eat any plant without permission.

---

management of the patient. See Table 31-7 for clinical effects of iron ingestion.

Management includes assessing and monitoring the ABCs, gastric decontamination, and chelation therapy (administering something that binds with iron, such as deferoxamine). Activated charcoal (see Table 31-6) does not bind with iron and so is not useful for iron poisoning.

Lead

Lead poisoning can occur after a child ingests substances that contain lead (Community Care 31-5). Lead exposure is most commonly chronic, although occasionally, a child ingests a large quantity of lead at one time.

CROSS-CULTURAL CARE

Folk remedies to treat digestive problems, fever, or rash, such as *azarcon* and *greta* (Mexico), *bint al dhahab* or "daughter of gold" (Oman, United Arab Emirates), and *paylooah* (Southeast Asia), may contain lead and poison the child. Many Chinese, Indian, and Arabic traditional remedies also contain lead and other harmful substances (Ernst, 2003).

No safe blood lead level has been identified. Blood lead levels less than 10 µg/dL can negatively affect the physical and mental development of children (AAP, 2007; Rischitelli et al., 2006). Blood lead levels more than 10 µg/dL are considered toxic. Children with blood lead levels between 10 and 19 µg/dL are typically asymptomatic but may exhibit some impairment in cognition, fine

motor skills, and growth (Erickson & Thompson, 2005; Yeoh et al., 2012). Increased motor impairment and lethargy are seen in blood lead levels of 20 to 44 µg/dL. At blood lead levels of 45 to 69 µg/dL, irritability, intermittent lethargy, anorexia, vomiting, and abdominal pain are seen. Symptoms of blood lead levels more than 70 µg/dL are persistent vomiting, loss of developmental skills, seizures, ataxia, cranial nerve palsy, altered sensorium, and coma. Blood lead levels more than 70 µg/dL require emergency treatment to treat the encephalopathy and to preserve health and cognitive functioning (Erickson & Thompson, 2005). Treatment for lead poisoning includes terminating exposure, ensuring adequate dietary intake, and chelation for high lead levels (AAP, 2006). Lead and essential minerals compete for binding sites, so it is important to correct dietary deficiencies, particularly calcium (ensuring adequate vitamin D intake) and iron. Chelating agents form a compound with lead that is excreted through the kidneys.

caREminder

The carrier for BAL, a chelating agent, is peanut oil. When treating lead poisoning, children with peanut allergies should not receive BAL.

Nursing care focuses on managing fluid, administering medications in a manner that minimizes pain, dealing with psychosocial issues, and providing education. Adequate urine output must be maintained, but overhydration should be prevented, especially in the presence of central nervous system symptoms, because children

TABLE 31-6	Gastric Decontamination		
Decontamination Method	**Method of Action**	**Indications and Dosage**	**Contraindications and Considerations**
Activated charcoal	Absorbs substances in stomach and GI tract	Indications: ingestion of most drugs, including acetaminophen, arsenic, barbiturates, camphor, chlorpromazine, cocaine, digitalis, iodine, lead, mercury salts, muscarine, nicotine, opioids, oxalates, parathion, penicillin, petroleum distillates, phenol, phenolphthalein, quinine, salicylates, strychnine, tricyclic antidepressants Dosage: Age <1 year: 1 g/kg every 4–6 hours as needed Age 1–12 years: 1–2 g/kg every 2–6 hours as needed Age >12 years: 50–100 g then 12.5 g every hour, or 25 g every 2 hours, or 50 g every 4 hours as needed A single dose of a cathartic such as sorbitol is often mixed with the first dose of charcoal. Do not give repeated doses of sorbitol; may lead to fluid and electrolyte imbalance.	Method of choice in reducing drug absorption. Activated charcoal is not effective in the following ingestions: cyanide, mineral acids, caustic alkalis, organic solvents, iron, ethanol, methanol, or lithium. Do not use activated charcoal with sorbitol in patients with fructose intolerance. Use with gastric emptying (gastric lavage) only if within 1 hour of ingestion and child has central nervous system depression. Can be given orally or via NG tube; cover cup to increase palatability. If giving via NG, prime NG tube with mineral oil and dilute activated charcoal with water to ease administration.
Gastric lavage	Dilutes and removes substances from stomach	Indications: child with depressed level of consciousness or airway compromise; *perform tracheal intubation before lavage to protect airway* Ingestion of drugs that decrease gastric motility or are not adsorbed by charcoal Dosage: large-bore NG or OG tube inserted and the stomach lavaged with NS Amount of NS to instill: age ≤12 years: 10–15mL/kg (maximum, 100–150 mL/exchange); age >12 years: 300 mL	Perform only if a life-threatening ingestion has occurred or within 1 hour of ingestion. After 1 hour of ingestion, risks outweigh benefits. Use large-bore (36–40-Fr) OG tube, possibly smaller in children, but tube should be bigger than pill fragments to be extracted. Do not perform gastric lavage when caustic substances have been ingested because insertion of the NG or OG tube may induce vomiting and cause more burns to the esophagus and oropharynx and may increase the risk for aspiration. NS is instilled and then aspirated to remove poisons, pills, and pill fragments from stomach.
Whole-bowel irrigation	Used to flush toxin from entire GI tract	Indications: not well established in children; use for iron poisoning and other agents not bound by activated charcoal Dosage: administer a balanced polyethylene glycol solution (e.g., GoLYTELY, Colyte) orally or via NG tube over 4–6 hours until rectal effluent is clear; age ≤5 years: 20 mL/kg/hr; age >5 years: 0.5–2 L/hr	May also be useful to eliminate contraband that was placed in bags or condoms and swallowed. Solution is isosmotic and thus is not associated with fluid and electrolyte imbalance. The large fluid volumes used may cause nausea, vomiting, bloating, cramping, and abdominal distention.

with lead encephalopathy have the potential to develop cerebral edema. Ethylenediaminetetraacetic acid and BAL administered intramuscularly is extremely painful. The drug should be mixed with procaine and administered by the deep intramuscular route. Teach parents and caregivers about healthy dietary guidelines, including sources of calcium and iron, and how to prevent future exposure to lead (see Community Care 31-5).

Acetaminophen

Acetaminophen is an analgesic and antipyretic, commonly found in over-the-counter medications, that is metabolized in the liver. It accounts for a significant proportion of unintentional and intentional toxic ingestions in children (White & Liebelt, 2006). Acetaminophen is the most common cause of acute liver failure in children in the United States and United Kingdom (Ferner et al., 2011).

Ingesting more than 150 mg/kg acetaminophen is potentially toxic (Hodgman & Garrard, 2012). Ingesting large amounts of the drug is known to cause substantial hepatic damage, hepatic failure, and death. To allow for full absorption of the drug, severity of overdose is most accurately predicted from acetaminophen serum levels drawn 4 hours after the ingestion.

Treatment may include gastric decontamination by gastric lavage, if performed within 60 minutes of ingestion, and administration of activated charcoal (Clinical

TABLE 31-7   Assessment and Management of Commonly Ingested Substances

Substance	Clinical Effects	Pharmacologic Management
Iron	*Phase 1:* within the first 6 hours after ingestion Symptoms range from GI complaints (nausea, vomiting, and GI blood loss) to hypovolemic shock and coma. *Phase 2:* 6–24 hours after ingestion Symptoms improve with treatment for hypovolemia (improvement may only be transitory). *Phase 3:* may follow phase 2 or may occur rapidly after ingestion Metabolic acidosis and cyanosis; possibly coma, seizures, and shock; may result from hepatocellular injury *Phase 4:* 1–2 months after ingestion Pyloric stenosis secondary to gastric scarring; consequent obstruction, bowel stricture, and cirrhosis	Chelation Dose of deferoxamine depends on severity of ingestion. If initiated, IV deferoxamine at a rate not to exceed 15 mg/kg/hr (total maximum, 6 g/day) is administered. After deferoxamine is administered, the child's urine turns a reddish (vin rosé) color, indicating that the iron is binding with the antidote.
Lead	*Acute lead poisoning* Burning sensation in the mouth and throat, GI disturbance (e.g., diarrhea, constipation), paralysis of the extremities, seizures, and coma *Chronic lead poisoning* Irritability, anorexia, anemia; may progress to the acute form Even low lead levels can negatively affect neurobehavioral functioning and can result in slight decreases in IQ. Severe cases of lead poisoning can cause seizures, muscular collapse, and lead encephalopathy (delirium, seizures, mania, cortical blindness, coma).	Chelation dimercaptosuccinic acid (DMSA, succimer), calcium disodium edetate ($CaNa_2EDTA$), or dimercaprol (British anti-Lewisite [BAL]) Advantages of DMSA, an analogue of BAL, over other chelating agents include the following: less toxic; can be administered orally; and does not eliminate iron, copper, or zinc from the body. Lead concentrations of 44–70 μg/dL are treated with DMSA. Lead concentrations of more than 70 μg/dL, without evidence of encephalopathy, are treated with a two-drug regimen of $CaNa_2EDTA$ in combination with DMSA or BAL. Lead concentrations of more than 70 μg/dL, with encephalopathy, are treated with $CaNa_2EDTA$ and BAL.
Acetaminophen	*Phase 1:* within first 24 hours after ingestion Nausea, vomiting, pallor, and diaphoresis *Phase 2:* 24–72 hours after ingestion Child appears better, but bilirubin, prothrombin time, and hepatic enzymes are elevated; right upper quadrant tenderness may appear; hepatomegaly, tachycardia, hypotension *Phase 3:* 72–96 hours after ingestion Liver function abnormalities peak; right upper quadrant tenderness, jaundice, hypoglycemia, coagulopathy, and encephalopathy *Phase 4:* 7–8 days after ingestion Hepatic dysfunction resolves or child develops hepatic failure or dies.	*N*-acetylcysteine orally (Mucomyst) or IV (Acetadote). Acetadote, while more expensive, assures that the full dose is absorbed. *N*-acetylcysteine smells like rotten eggs. If administered orally, place the antidote in juice or a carbonated beverage in a covered cup to mask the smell and make it more palatable. It may have to be administered via an NG tube. If the child vomits within 1 hour of administration, repeat the dose.

Judgment 31-2). Depending on the serum level of acetaminophen and poison control center recommendations, the antidote *N*-acetylcysteine may be given.

ALERT   *Use caution when administering compound medications containing acetaminophen because accidental overdose can occur when administering both acetaminophen and compound medications.*

Hydrocarbons

Hydrocarbon or petroleum distillate ingestion can be lethal. Commonly found hydrocarbons include liquid polishes, solvents, and thinners; gasoline; and kerosene.

Toxicity depends on the agent ingested and whether it has also been aspirated. The incidence of associated aspiration is high; aspiration can cause respiratory failure. Hepatic failure and central nervous system depression are other serious results.

The child may present with gasping, choking, coughing, chest pain, dyspnea, or cyanosis. Airway management is vital, with frequent reassessment for signs and symptoms of aspiration. Auscultation may reveal rales, rhonchi, wheezing, or decreased breath sounds. Chest radiographs, which commonly show bilateral perihilar and basilar infiltrates and varying degrees of atelectasis, may not be diagnostic until several hours after ingestion. Gastric decontamination depends on the agent and amount ingested; consult the poison control center for recommendations. Activated charcoal is not recommended.

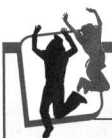

Preventing Lead Poisoning

Teach parents and other caregivers to remove sources of lead from the child's environment:

- A common source of lead is lead-based paint present in old homes; lead content in paint for new residences has been limited since 1978.
- Children may ingest paint chips or inhale dust from peeling paint.
- Keep children from playing near old homes that are being renovated; the lead-based paint may have contaminated the dirt surrounding the home.
- Check lead levels in tap water, which may pick up lead if lead solder was used in the plumbing.
- If lead level exceeds drinking water standard, use bottled water or run cold water until it gets no colder before using for drinking or cooking.
- Do not use lead-glazed ceramic dinnerware or decorative pottery to serve food; citrus juices, in particular, leach lead from the pottery.

- Do not store food or drink in lead crystal.
- Discuss folk remedies used by the family that may contain lead.
- Parental occupation (e.g., construction or factory worker where lead-based substances are used) or hobbies (e.g., using leaded solder in stained glass, making leaded fishing weights) may increase the child's lead exposure; parents should wash their hands and change clothes and shower, if possible, before entering the home.
- Have child wash hands before eating.

Advise parents to ensure that the child has adequate nutritional intake, which decreases lead absorption by the body. Screen the child for lead levels per facility policy. The CDC recommends universal lead screening for children between the ages 6 months and 6 years. Question parents of young children about potential lead exposure and risk factors.

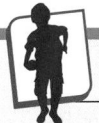

Child With a Potentially Toxic Ingestion

Mrs. Denali calls to find out what to do about her son, Jamal, a 4-year-old who has ingested acetaminophen capsules, thinking they were candy. Jamal weighs 20 kg.

Questions

1. What further questions would you ask Mrs. Denali?
2. What factors indicate a potentially toxic ingestion?
3. Does Mrs. Denali need to do anything further? If so, what?
4. What interventions will be implemented when Jamal gets to the ED?
5. Jamal does not develop toxic serum levels of acetaminophen. What factors probably contributed to this positive outcome? What should the nurse do before sending Jamal home?

Answers

1. When did Jamal ingest the acetaminophen? Can Mrs. Denali estimate how many capsules he may have ingested? How many milligrams are in each capsule? Has any treatment been initiated? Is Jamal acting unusual or doing anything out of the ordinary (e.g., altered level of consciousness, nausea, vomiting, pale, diaphoretic)? She thinks that Jamal may have ingested six capsules, 500 mg each, about 15 minutes ago. The first thing Mrs. Denali did was to call you; she has not done anything else. Jamal seems perfectly fine, with no unusual behaviors.

2. Jamal may have ingested six capsules of 500 mg each, which totals 3,000 mg acetaminophen. Jamal weighs 20 kg, corresponding to 150 mg/kg ingested, a potentially toxic dose.

3. Mrs. Denali should immediately call the poison control center then proceed to the nearest ED.

4. Activated charcoal will be administered to adsorb the acetaminophen further; it does not absorb the antidote for acetaminophen, N-acetylcysteine. Serum acetaminophen levels will be measured 4 hours after ingestion to determine whether N-acetylcysteine should be administered. Liver function studies should be monitored and symptomatic care given.

5. Mrs. Denali discovered the ingestion quickly and took immediate action. The acetaminophen ingestion was treated before absorption of toxic amounts could occur. Jamal is younger than 6 years old, when alternative pathways for acetaminophen metabolism may decrease the incidence of hepatotoxicity. The nurse should review poison prevention techniques with Mrs. Denali.

ALERT *Do not induce vomiting for hydrocarbon ingestion because vomiting increases risk for aspiration.*

Caustics

Caustic ingestions involve acids or alkalis commonly found in household cleaning products (e.g., Drano, lye). Ingestion of these substances may cause lip or tongue swelling, burning pain in injured areas, dysphagia, drooling, or whitish or red plaques in the mouth or perioral areas. Severe burns of the esophagus and stomach may occur.

ALERT *Do not induce vomiting to treat caustic ingestion because vomiting results in further burning of the mouth and esophagus. Activated charcoal is also contraindicated in treating this type of ingestion.*

Do not give the child anything by mouth until the extent of injury is evaluated and ability to swallow fluids is assessed. Endoscopic evaluation is necessary 12 to 24 hours after injury to determine the severity of the damage. Complications include esophageal perforation, scarring, and stricture formation.

Burns may be present on other parts of the body after exposure to caustics such as strong acids, strong alkalis, or petroleum distillate agents. The child should be fully decontaminated by removing all clothing and flooding affected areas with NS or water. Treat exposures to the eyes, skin, and mucous membranes by washing the affected area with a stream of water for 15 to 20 minutes. The water temperature should be comfortable to the child. The health care team members should wear gloves because some toxins can be quickly absorbed through the skin. Poisonous exposure to these substances can occur through contact with the patient's skin, clothing, or vomitus.

SUDDEN INFANT DEATH SYNDROME

SIDS is the third most common cause of death in infants (Hoyert & Xu, 2012) and the leading cause of death in infants younger than 1 year of age. The peak incidence is seen between 2 and 4 months of age (Bechtel, 2012). The typical SIDS scenario involves the caregiver finding the normal, healthy infant prone in bed in full cardiopulmonary arrest. The cause of SIDS is unknown but may reflect delayed development of arousal, cardiorespiratory control, or cardiovascular control and is associated with other risk factors (Chart 31-4) (Bechtel, 2012). For a discussion of apparent life-threatening events and apnea, see Chapter 16.

Assessment

On presentation to the ED, examine the infant thoroughly to rule out other causes of death, including child abuse. The infant's face may be quite blue because of blood pooling in the dependent prone position. This discoloration may look like bruising. Trauma may also be present as a result of the basic life support measures used. Individual institutions may have specific protocols consisting of multiple laboratory and radiographic studies that aid in differentiating SIDS from child abuse.

caREminder

First-line responders (paramedics, police) and ED personnel must maintain an unbiased demeanor, asking questions in a matter-of-fact, information-gathering manner. Initially, families dealing with the death of an infant from SIDS may be wrongly accused of child abuse, further traumatizing them during this devastating period.

The history elicited from the family or caregiver helps in differentiating SIDS from abuse. With SIDS, the history is consistent each time it is given by the same person and between family members; with abuse, the history may vary. A history that is incompatible with the infant's developmental level should also raise suspicion of abuse (e.g., a history of a 5-month-old trying to climb out of the crib and falling).

CHART 31-4 Risk Factors Associated With Sudden Infant Death Syndrome

Maternal
Younger age
Smoking (antenatal and postnatal)
Drug use (opiates, cocaine)

Infant
Premature
Asphyxia at birth
Male gender
Multiple birth
Sibling who died of SIDS
Age younger than 6 months (peaks at 2–4 months)
Black or Native American

Environmental
Cold weather season
Exposure to cigarette smoke
Lower socioeconomic status
Bottlefeeding
Prone sleeping position
Swaddled too warmly
Soft sleeping surface

Note: It is uncertain which risk factors are causal and how the risk factors are interrelated.

Nursing Diagnoses and Outcomes

In addition to the nursing diagnoses discussed in Nursing Plan of Care 31-1, nursing diagnoses and outcomes applicable to the family after the death of a child from SIDS include the following:

Nursing Diagnosis: Compromised family coping: Related to reaction to death of child

Outcomes:

- Family will verbalize feelings.
- Family will list and use sources of support.
- Family will perform activities of daily living and maintain supportive interactions with each other.

Nursing Diagnosis: Spiritual distress related to unexpected death of infant

Outcome: Family will verbalize feelings of spiritual tension and be adequately supported in working through them.

Nursing Diagnosis: Impaired parenting related to parents dealing with own grief

Outcome: Parents or significant others will provide an environment for siblings that supports growth and development.

Interdisciplinary Interventions

Delivering the news to the family is difficult because there is no explanation for the death, and the ED health care team does not have a relationship with the family. Tell the family that the child may have died from SIDS and that an autopsy will be done to confirm this diagnosis.

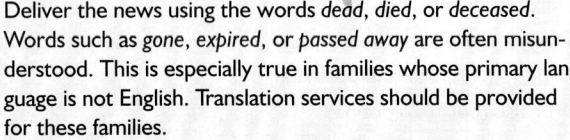

CROSS-CULTURAL CARE

Deliver the news using the words *dead*, *died*, or *deceased*. Words such as *gone*, *expired*, or *passed away* are often misunderstood. This is especially true in families whose primary language is not English. Translation services should be provided for these families.

The primary nursing responsibility is to support the family in beginning the grieving process. Provide the family with a private, quiet area. Tell them that the exact cause of SIDS is still unknown and that it cannot be predicted or prevented. Use hospital and community resources, such as social workers and clergy members, to provide additional support and comfort to the family. Give the parents an opportunity to hold their baby (see Chapter 13). Prepare them for how the baby will look, explaining the presence of any tubes or resuscitation equipment. A staff member should stay with the family to support them.

The parents may not be emotionally able to understand all the information provided to them (e.g., funeral home lists, when to anticipate autopsy results, support group information). Provide them with written material so they can view it later. Often, one family member (perhaps an aunt or uncle) appears less emotional than the others. Providing this person with the written material and information can also be helpful. Frequently,

parents do not return home after the SIDS death of an infant, so be sure to obtain a contact phone number from a friend or family member in case the parents cannot be reached at home.

Community Care

The nurse can also participate in community education regarding ways to decrease risk factors that contribute to SIDS (see Chart 31-4). Because placing infants on their backs for sleeping (the "Back to Sleep" campaign) has been instrumental in reducing the incidence of SIDS, maternal smoking now has emerged as a significant risk factor for SIDS (Behm et al., 2012).

PREPARATION FOR TRANSFER

QUESTION: Do you anticipate Chris will need to be transferred to a tertiary care facility?

Depending on the health care facility in which the child received initial emergency care, the stabilized child may need to be transferred to another facility or another unit. Regardless of where the child is transferred, take appropriate steps to prepare the child for transport.

The extent of preparation for transport of a child must be specific to the child and his or her condition at the time of transfer. A child who is transferred to a critical care unit will require the same level of monitoring and team ability to manage emergent situations during the transfer as was required in the ED.

For interfacility transfers, the Emergency Medical Treatment and Active Labor Act (EMTALA) regulations must be followed. These require that the receiving facility has accepted the patient and that an appropriate, authorized physician has accepted the transfer of care as well. The mode of transfer, whether by ground ambulance, helicopter, or fixed-wing aircraft, must be selected based on the child's condition, care needs during the transfer, availability of transport modes, and appropriate staff, along with traffic and weather conditions. A complete report between transferring and accepting physicians and nurses must occur prior to the child leaving the transfer facility. Copies of the patient's chart, radiographs, and diagnostic tests must be sent to the receiving facility. Clear, consistent communication between the referring and receiving facilities is key to a successful transport.

ANSWER: Most likely, Chris would not need to be transferred to a tertiary care facility. Most EDs, even in very small facilities, are able to manage an anaphylactic reaction.

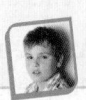

See the**Point** for a summary of Key Concepts.

REFERENCES

American Academy of Pediatrics. (2006). Screening for elevated blood lead levels in children and pregnant women. *Pediatrics, 118*(6), 2514–2518.

American Academy of Pediatrics. (2007). Interpreting and managing blood lead levels of less than 10 μg/dL in children and reducing childhood exposure to lead: Recommendations of the Centers for Disease Control and Prevention Advisory Committee on Childhood Lead Poisoning Prevention. *Pediatrics, 120*(5), e1285–e1298.

American Academy of Pediatrics Section on Orthopaedics, American Academy of Pediatrics Committee on Pediatric Emergency Medicine, & American Academy of Pediatrics Section on Critical Care et al. (2008). Management of pediatric trauma. *Pediatrics, 121*(4), 849–854.

American Academy of Pediatrics Subcommittee on Febrile Seizures. (2011). Neurodiagnostic evaluation of the child with a simple febrile seizure. *Pediatrics, 127*(2), 389–394.

Antonyrajah, B., & Mukundan, D. (2008). Fever without apparent source on clinical examination. *Current Opinion in Pediatrics, 20*(1), 96–102.

Balan, B., & Lingam, L. (2012). Unintentional injuries among children in resource poor settings: Where do the fingers point? *Archives of Disease in Childhood, 97*(1), 35–38.

Batra, P., Saha, A., & Faridi, M. M. A. (2012). Thermometry in children. *Journal of Emergencies, Trauma, and Shock, 5*(3), 246–249.

Bechtel, K. (2012). Sudden unexpected infant death: Differentiating natural from abusive causes in the emergency department. *Pediatric Emergency Care, 28*(10), 1085–1089.

Behm, I., Kabir, Z., Connolly, G. N. et al. (2012). Increasing prevalence of smoke-free homes and decreasing rates of sudden infant death syndrome in the United States: An ecological association study. *Tobacco Control, 21*(1), 6–11.

Borse, N. N., Rudd, R. A., Dellinger, A. M. et al. (2013). Years of potential life lost from unintentional child and adolescent injuries—United States, 2000-2009. *Journal of Safety Research, 45*(2013), 127–131.

Bronstein, A. C., Spyker, D. A., Cantilena, L. R. et al. (2012). 2011 Annual report of the American Association of Poison Control Centers' National Poison Data System (NPDS): 29th annual report. *Clinical Toxicology, 50*(10), 911–1164.

Centers for Disease Control and Prevention. (2005). Hypothermia-related deaths: United States, 2003–2004. *Morbidity and Mortality Weekly Report, 54*(7), 173–175.

Centers for Disease Control and Prevention. (2008). Human rabies prevention: United States, 2008. Recommendations of the Advisory Committee on Immunization Practices (ACIP). *Morbidity and Mortality Weekly Report, 57*(RR03), 1–26.

Centers for Disease Control and Prevention. (2012). *Unintentional drowning: Get the facts.* Retrieved from http://www.cdc.gov/HomeandRecreationalSafety/Water-Safety/waterinjuries-factsheet.html

Chang, T. P., & Rangan, C. (2011). Iron poisoning—A literature-based review of epidemiology, diagnosis, and management. *Pediatric Emergency Care, 27*(10), 978–985.

Curley, G., Kavanagh, B. P., & Laffey, J. G. (2010). Hypocapnia and the injured brain: More harm than benefit. *Critical Care Medicine, 38*(5), 1348–1359.

Dellinger, R. P., Levy, M. M., Carlet, J. M. et al. (2008). Surviving sepsis campaign: International guidelines for management of severe sepsis and septic shock: 2008. *Intensive Care Medicine, 34*(1), 17–60.

Dinakar, C. (2012). Anaphylaxis in children: Current understanding and key issues in diagnosis and treatment. *Current Allergy and Asthma Reports, 12*(6), 641–649.

Donoghue, A. J., Nadkarni, V., Elliott, M. et al. (2006). Effect of hospital characteristics on outcomes from pediatric cardiopulmonary resuscitation: A report from the National Registry of Cardiopulmonary Resuscitation. *Pediatrics, 118*(3), 995–1001.

Douglas, R., & Wormald, P. (2007). Update on epistaxis. *Current Opinion in Otolaryngology & Head and Neck Surgery, 15*, 180–183.

Duru, C. O., Akinbami, F. O., & Orimadegun, A. E. (2012). A comparison of tympanic and rectal temperatures in NIGERIAN neonates. *BMC Pediatrics, 2012*(12), 86.

Dwyer, J. P., Douglas, T. S., & van As, A. B. (2007). Dog bite injuries in children: A review of data from a South African paediatric trauma unit. *South African Medical Journal, 97*(8), 597–600.

Emergency Nurses Association. (2007). *Trauma nurse core course manual* (6th ed.). Park Ridge, IL: Author.

Emergency Nurses Association. (2010). *Position statement: Family presence at the bedside during invasive procedures and cardiopulmonary resuscitation.* Park Ridge, IL: Author.

Erickson, L., & Thompson, T. (2005). A review of a preventable poison: Pediatric lead poisoning. *Journal for Specialists in Pediatric Nursing, 10*, 171–182.

Ernst, E. (2003). Serious adverse effects of unconventional therapies for children and adolescents: A systematic review of recent evidence. *European Journal of Pediatrics, 162*, 72–80.

Fein, J. A., Ganesh, J., & Alpern, E. R. (2004). Medical staff attitudes toward family presence during pediatric procedures. *Pediatric Emergency Care, 20*(4), 224–227.

Ferner, R. E., Dear, J. W., & Bateman, D. N. (2011). Management of paracetamol poisoning. *British Medical Journal, 342*, d2218.

Field, J. M., Hazinski, M. F., Sayre, M. R. et al. (2010). 2010 American Heart Association guidelines for cardiopulmonary resuscitation and emergency cardiovascular care. Part 1: Executive summary. *Circulation, 122*(18, Suppl. 3), S640–S656.

Fulbrook, P., Latour, J., Albarran, J. et al. (2007). The presence of family members during cardiopulmonary resuscitation: European Federation of Critical Care Nursing Associations, European Society of Paediatric and Neonatal Intensive Care and European Society of Cardiology Council on Cardiovascular Nursing and Allied Professions joint position statement. *European Journal of Cardiovascular Nursing, 6*(4), 255–258.

Gilboy, N., Tanabe, P., Travers, D. A. et al. (2005). *Emergency Severity Index version 4: Implementation handbook* (AHRQ Publication No. 05-0046-2). Rockville, MD: Agency for Healthcare Research and Quality.

Grunbenhoff, J. A., du Ford, K., & Roosevelt, G. E. (2007). Heat-related illness. *Clinical Pediatric Emergency Medicine, 8*(11), 59–64.

Habib, S. (2012). Highlights for management of a child with a urinary tract infection. *International Journal of Pediatrics, 2012*(2012), 943653.

Hampers, L. C., & Spina, L. A. (2011). Evaluation and management of pediatric febrile seizures in the emergency department. *Emergency Medicine Clinics of North America, 29*(1), 83–93.

Hodgman, M. J., & Garrard, A. R. (2012). A review of acetaminophen poisoning. *Critical Care Clinics, 28*(4), 499–516.

Hoyert, D. L., & Xu, J. (2012). Deaths: Preliminary data for 2011. *National Vital Statistics Reports, 61*(6), 1–51.

Jaindl, M., Grünauer, J., Platzer, P. et al. (2012). The management of bite wounds in children—A retrospective analysis at a level I trauma centre. *Injury, 43*(12), 2117–2121.

Ji, L., Xiaowei, Z., Chuanlin, W. et al. (2010). Investigation of post-traumatic stress disorder in children after animal-induced injury in China. *Pediatrics, 126*(2), e320–e324.

Kendrick, D., Smith, S., Sutton, A. et al. (2008). Effect of education and safety equipment on poisoning-prevention practice and poisoning: Systematic review, meta-analysis and meta-regression. *Archives of Disease in Childhood, 93*(7), 599–608.

Kingsnorth, J., O'Connell, K., Guzzetta, C. et al. (2010). Family presence during trauma activations and medical resuscitations in a pediatric emergency department: An evidence-based practice project. *Journal of Emergency Nursing, 36*(2), 115–121.

Kochanek, P. M., Carney, N., Adelson, P. D. et al. (2012). Guidelines for the acute medical management of severe traumatic brain injury in infants, children, and adolescents—Second edition. Chapter 13. Hyperventilation. *Pediatric Critical Care Medicine, 13*(Suppl. 1), S58–S60.

Kuzin, J. K., Yborra, J. G., Taylor, M. D. et al. (2007). Family-member presence during interventions in the intensive care unit: Perceptions of pediatric cardiac intensive care providers. *Pediatrics, 120*(4), e895–e901.

Liu, L., Johnson, H. L., Cousens, S. et al. (2012). Global, regional, and national causes of child mortality: An updated systematic analysis for 2010 with time trends since 2000. *Lancet, 379*(9832), 2151–2161.

McGarry, G. W. (2011). Nosebleeds in children. *Clinical Evidence, 2011*(2011), 0311.

Meert, K. L., Eggly, S., Pollack, M. et al. (2008). Parents' perspectives on physician–parent communication near the time of a child's death in the pediatric intensive care unit. *Pediatric Critical Care Medicine, 91*(1), 2–7.

Millar, J. S. (2006). Evaluation and treatment of the child with febrile seizures. *American Family Physician, 73*(10), 1761–1764.

Narotam, P., Morrison, J., & Nathoo, N. (2009). Brain tissue oxygen monitoring in traumatic brain injury and major trauma: Outcome analysis of a brain tissue oxygen-directed therapy. *Journal of Neuroscience, 111*(4), 672–682.

O'Connell, K. J., Farah, M. M., Spandorfer, P. et al. (2007). Family presence during pediatric trauma team activation: An assessment of a structured program. *Pediatrics, 120*(3), e565–e574.

Paul, I. M., Sturgis, S. A., Yang, C. et al. (2010). Efficacy of standard doses of ibuprofen alone, alternating, and combined with acetaminophen for the treatment of febrile children. *Clinical Therapeutics, 32*(14), 2433–2440.

Riachitelli, G., Nygren, P., Bougatsos, C. et al. (2006). Screening for elevated blood lead levels in childhood and pregnancy: An updated summary of evidence for the U.S. Preventive Services Task Force. *Pediatrics, 118*(6), e1867–e1895.

Roderique, J. D., Gebre-Giorgis, A. A., Stewart, D. H. et al. (2012). Smoke inhalation injury in a pregnant patient: A literature review of the evidence and current best practices in the setting of a classic case. *Journal of Burn Care & Research, 22*(5), 624–633.

Rudolph, S. S., & Barnung, S. (2011). Survival after drowning with cardiac arrest and mild hypothermia. *ISRN Cardiology, 2011*(2011), 895625.

Steen, C. J., Carbonaro, P. A., & Schwartz, R. A. (2004). Arthropods in dermatology. *Journal of the American Academy of Dermatology, 50*, 819–842.

Taylor, C., Subaiya, L., & Corsino, D. (2011). Pediatric cuffed endotracheal tubes: An evolution of care. *Ochsner Journal, 11*(1), 52–56.

Thomas, S., Vijaykumar, C., Naik, R. et al. (2009). Comparative effectiveness of tepid sponging and antipyretic drug versus only antipyretic drug in the management of fever among children: A randomized controlled trial. *Indian Pediatrics, 46*(2), 133–136.

Tipton, M. J., & Golden, F. S. (2011). A proposed decision-making guide for the search, rescue and resuscitation of submersion (head under) victims based on expert opinion. *Resuscitation, 82*(7), 819–824.

Upadhyay, P., Tripathi, V., Singh, R. et al. (2010). Role of hypertonic saline and mannitol in the management of raised intracranial pressure in children: A randomized comparative study. *Journal of Pediatric Neuroscience, 10*(5), 18–21.

White, M. L., & Liebelt, E. L. (2006). Update on antidotes for pediatric poisoning. *Pediatric Emergency Care, 22*(11), 740–746.

Woolf, A. D. (1993). Poisoning in children and adolescents. *Pediatrics in Review, 14*, 411–422.

Yeoh, B., Woolfenden, S., Lanphear, B. et al. (2012). Household interventions for prevention of domestic lead exposure in children. *Cochrane Database of Systematic Reviews*, (4), CD006047.

See the **Point** for Organizations.

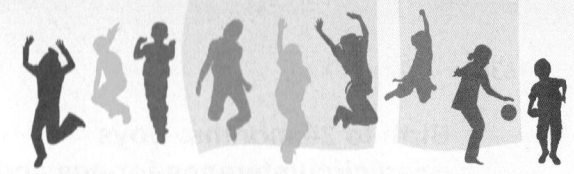

APPENDIX A: Growth Charts

Birth to 24 months: Boys
Head circumference-for-age and
Weight-for-length percentiles

NAME _____

RECORD # _____

AGE (MONTHS)

| Birth | 3 | 6 | 9 | **12** | 15 | 18 | 21 | **24** |

Head circumference percentiles: 98, 95, 90, 75, 50, 25, 10, 5, 2

Weight-for-length percentiles: 98, 95, 90, 75, 50, 25, 10, 5, 2

LENGTH

cm: 64 66 68 70 72 74 76 78 80 82 84 86 88 90 92 94 96 98 100 102 104 106 108 110
in: 26 27 28 29 30 31 32 33 34 35 36 37 38 39 40 41 42 43

Date	Age	Weight	Length	Head Circ.	Comment

cm: 46 48 50 52 54 56 58 60 62
in: 18 19 20 21 22 23 24

Published by the Centers for Disease Control and Prevention, November 1, 2009
SOURCE: WHO Child Growth Standards (http://www.who.int/childgrowth/en)

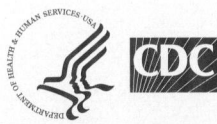

Birth to 24 months: Boys
Length-for-age and Weight-for-age percentiles

NAME _____

RECORD # _____

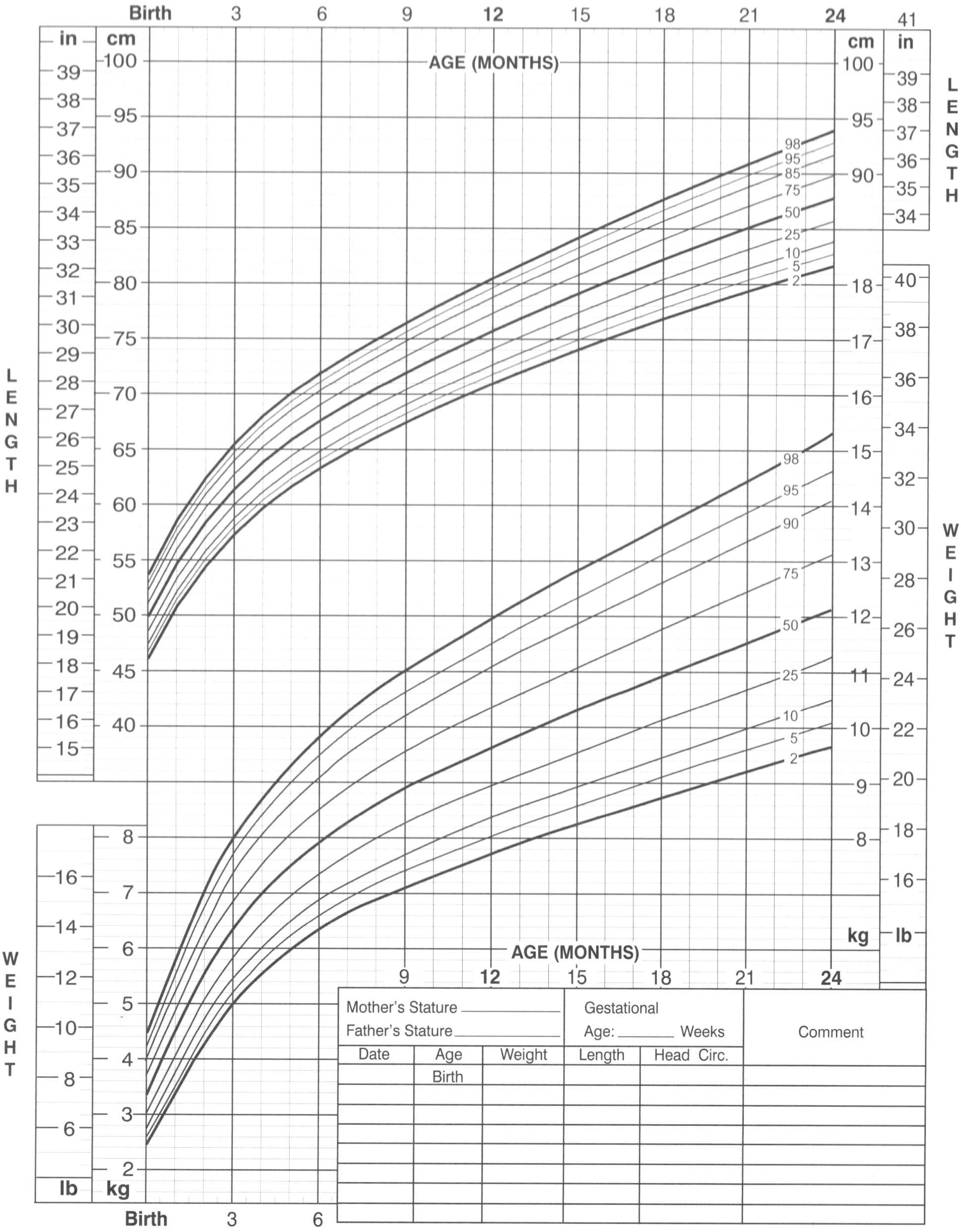

AGE (MONTHS)

LENGTH

WEIGHT

98
95
90
75
50
25
10
5
2

Mother's Stature _____
Father's Stature _____
Gestational
Age: _____ Weeks
Comment

Date	Age	Weight	Length	Head Circ.	
	Birth				

Published by the Centers for Disease Control and Prevention, November 1, 2009
SOURCE: WHO Child Growth Standards (http://www.who.int/childgrowth/en)

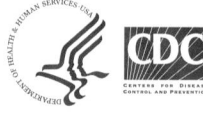

Birth to 24 months: Girls
Head circumference-for-age and
Weight-for-length percentiles

NAME _____

RECORD # _____

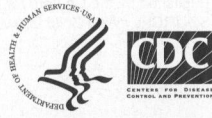

AGE (MONTHS)

Birth 3 6 9 12 15 18 21 24

HEAD CIRCUMFERENCE

WEIGHT

LENGTH

| cm | 64 66 68 70 72 74 76 78 80 82 84 86 88 90 92 94 96 98 100 102 104 106 108 110 | cm |
| in | 26 27 28 29 30 31 32 33 34 35 36 37 38 39 40 41 42 43 | in |

Date	Age	Weight	Length	Head Circ.	Comment

| cm | 46 48 50 52 54 56 58 60 62 |
| in | 18 19 20 21 22 23 24 |

Published by the Centers for Disease Control and Prevention, November 1, 2009
SOURCE: WHO Child Growth Standards (http://www.who.int/childgrowth/en)

Birth to 24 months: Girls
Length-for-age and Weight-for-age percentiles

NAME _____

RECORD # _____

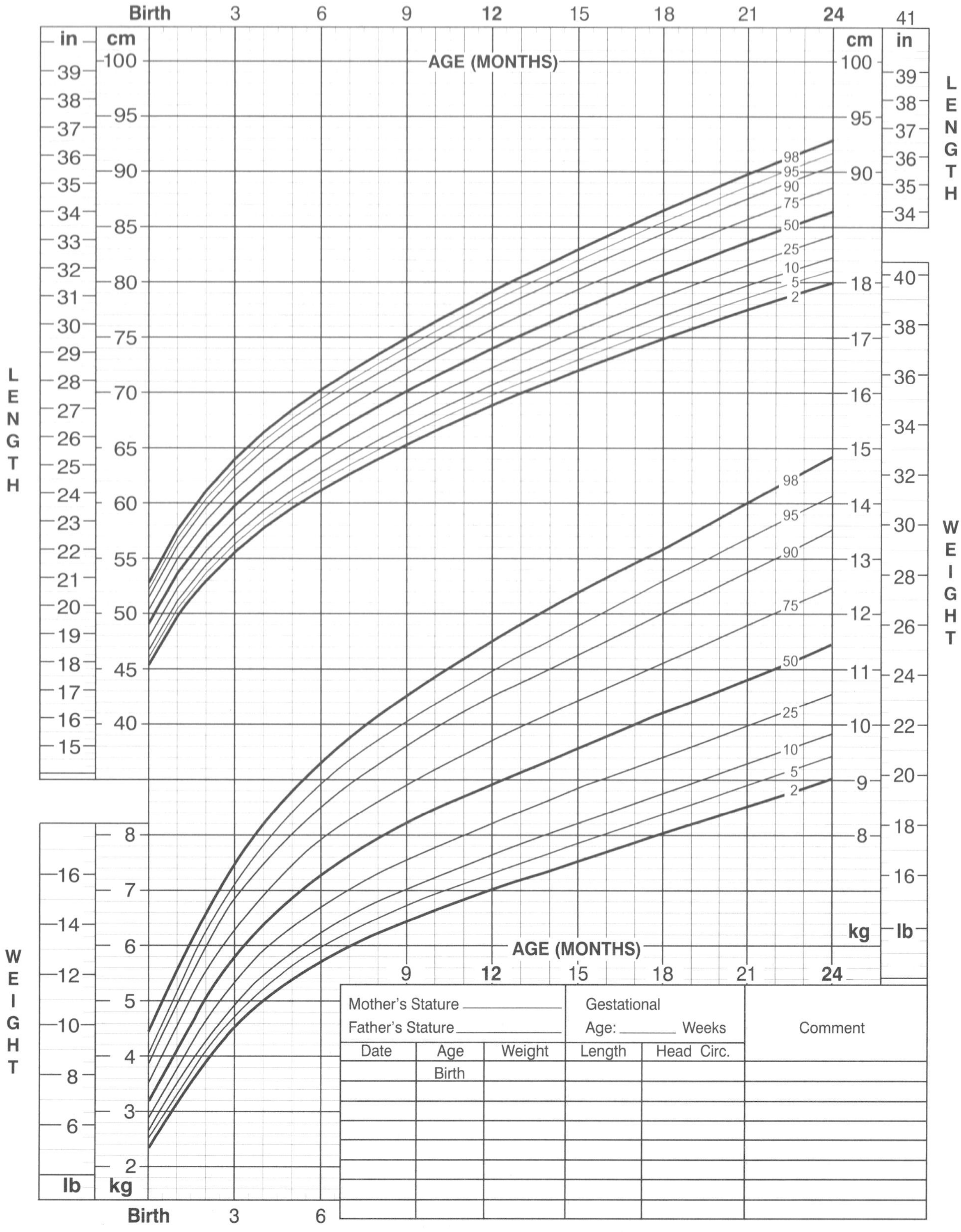

AGE (MONTHS)

Birth   3   6   9   12   15   18   21   24   41

LENGTH

98
95
90
75
50
25
10
5
2

WEIGHT

98
95
90
75
50
25
10
5
2

AGE (MONTHS)

9   12   15   18   21   24

		Mother's Stature _____		Gestational		
Father's Stature _____			Age: _____ Weeks		Comment	
Date	Age	Weight	Length	Head Circ.		
	Birth					

Birth   3   6

Published by the Centers for Disease Control and Prevention, November 1, 2009
SOURCE: WHO Child Growth Standards (http://www.who.int/childgrowth/en)

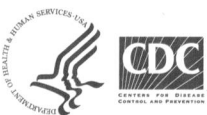

2 to 20 years: Boys
Stature-for-age and Weight-for-age percentiles

NAME _____

RECORD # _____

Mother's Stature		Father's Stature		
Date	Age	Weight	Stature	BMI*

*To Calculate BMI: Weight (kg) ÷ Stature (cm) ÷ Stature (cm) x 10,000
or Weight (lb) ÷ Stature (in) ÷ Stature (in) x 703

AGE (YEARS)

12 13 14 15 16 17 18 19 20

STATURE

cm   in
190   76
      74
185
      72
180
      70
175
      68
170
      66
165   64

3   4   5   6   7   8   9   10 11

STATURE

in   cm
62   160
      155
60   150
58   145
56   140
54   135
52   130
50   125
48   120
46   115
44   110
42   105
40   100
38   95
36   90
34   85
32   80
30

95
90
75
50
25
10
5

WEIGHT

cm   in
105   230
100   220
95   210
90   200
85   190
80   180
75   170
70   160
65   150
60   140
55   130
50   120
45   110

95
90
75
50
25
10
5

WEIGHT

lb   kg
80   35
70   30
60   25
50   20
40   15
30
      10

AGE (YEARS)

2 3 4 5 6 7 8 9 10 11 12 13 14 15 16 17 18 19 20

kg   lb

Published May 30, 2000 (modified 11/21/00).
SOURCE: Developed by the National Center for Health Statistics in collaboration with
the National Center for Chronic Disease Prevention and Health Promotion (2000).
http://www.cdc.gov/growthcharts

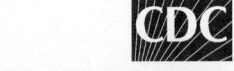

SAFER · HEALTHIER · PEOPLE™

2 to 20 years: Boys
Body mass index-for-age percentiles

NAME _____

RECORD # _____

Date	Age	Weight	Stature	BMI*	Comments

***To Calculate BMI**: Weight (kg) ÷ Stature (cm) ÷ Stature (cm) x 10,000
or Weight (lb) ÷ Stature (in) ÷ Stature (in) x 703

BMI

35
34
33
32
31
30
29
28
27
26
25
24
23
22
21
20
19
18
17
16
15
14
13
12

95
90
85
75
50
25
10
5

AGE (YEARS)

kg/m²

2 3 4 5 6 7 8 9 10 11 12 13 14 15 16 17 18 19 20

Published May 30, 2000 (modified 10/16/00).
SOURCE: Developed by the National Center for Health Statistics in collaboration with
the National Center for Chronic Disease Prevention and Health Promotion (2000).
http://www.cdc.gov/growthcharts

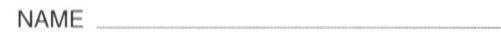

SAFER · HEALTHIER · PEOPLE™

2 to 20 years: Girls
Stature-for-age and Weight-for-age percentiles

NAME _____

RECORD # _____

Mother's Stature _____ Father's Stature _____				
Date	Age	Weight	Stature	BMI*

*To Calculate BMI: Weight (kg) ÷ Stature (cm) ÷ Stature (cm) x 10,000
or Weight (lb) ÷ Stature (in) ÷ Stature (in) x 703

AGE (YEARS)

12 13 14 15 16 17 18 19 20

95
90
75
50
25
10
5

in cm   3   4   5   6   7   8   9   10 11

STATURE

STATURE

WEIGHT

AGE (YEARS)

2 3 4 5 6 7 8 9 10 11 12 13 14 15 16 17 18 19 20

Published May 30, 2000 (modified 11/21/00).
SOURCE: Developed by the National Center for Health Statistics in collaboration with
the National Center for Chronic Disease Prevention and Health Promotion (2000).
http://www.cdc.gov/growthcharts

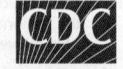

SAFER · HEALTHIER · PEOPLE™

2 to 20 years: Girls
Body mass index-for-age percentiles

NAME _____

RECORD # _____

Date	Age	Weight	Stature	BMI*	Comments

*To Calculate BMI: Weight (kg) ÷ Stature (cm) ÷ Stature (cm) x 10,000
or Weight (lb) ÷ Stature (in) ÷ Stature (in) x 703

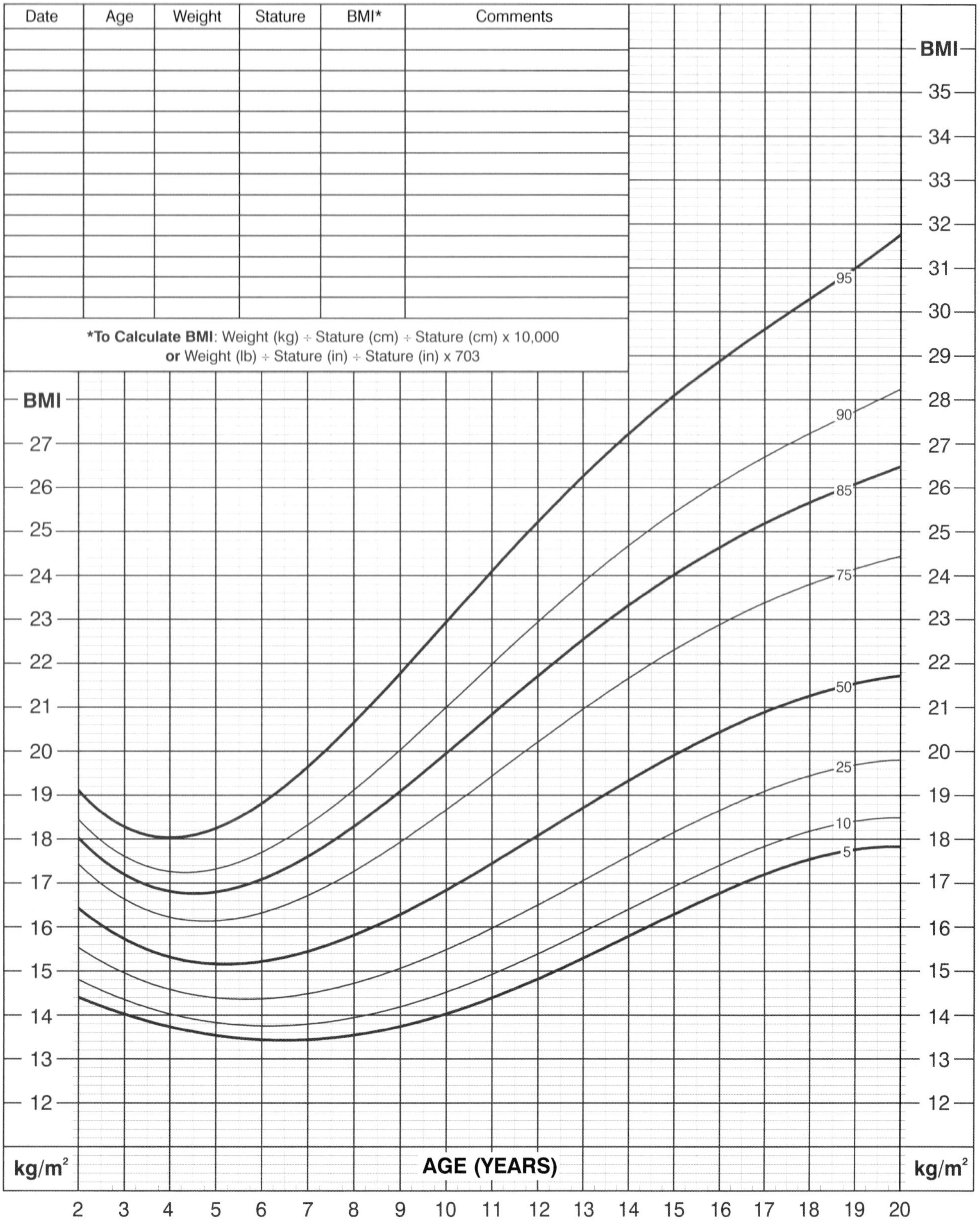

BMI

35
34
33
32
31
30
29
28
27
26
25
24
23
22
21
20
19
18
17
16
15
14
13
12

95
90
85
75
50
25
10
5

BMI

27
26
25
24
23
22
21
20
19
18
17
16
15
14
13
12

kg/m²   AGE (YEARS)   kg/m²

2 3 4 5 6 7 8 9 10 11 12 13 14 15 16 17 18 19 20

Published May 30, 2000 (modified 10/16/00).
SOURCE: Developed by the National Center for Health Statistics in collaboration with
the National Center for Chronic Disease Prevention and Health Promotion (2000).
http://www.cdc.gov/growthcharts

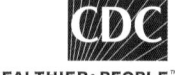

SAFER · HEALTHIER · PEOPLE™

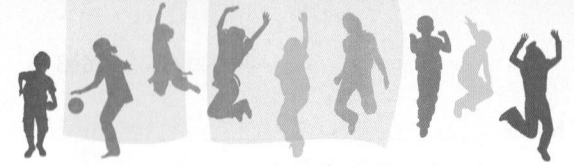

APPENDIX B:
Reference Ranges for Vital Signs

Normal Heart Rate and Respiratory Rate Ranges		
Age	**Heart Rate, Normal range (beats per minute)**	**Respiratory Rate, Normal range (breaths per minute)**
Preterm		40–70
Neonate	95–170	30–50
1–11 months	90–170	30–45
1–2 years	90–150	20–30
3–4 years	70–130	20–30
5–7 years	65–130	20–25
8–11 years	70–110	14–22
12–15 years	Female 70–110 Male 65–105	12–20
>15 years	Female 55–95 Male 50–90	12–20

Normal Temperature Ranges*		
Age	**Fahrenheit**	**Celsius**
Preterm infant	97.7–98.6	36.5–37
Term infant	97.2–99.9	36.2–37.7
0–6 months	97.2–99.4	36.2–37.4
6–12 months	96–99.7	35.6–37.6
1–13 years	95.9–99	35.5–37.2
>13 years	96.4–99.6	35.8–37.6

*Measurement method and circadian rhythm must be considered in evaluating normal.

Blood Pressure Levels for Boys by Age and Height Percentile

Age (Year)	BP Percentile ↓	Systolic BP (mm Hg) ← Percentile of Height →							Diastolic BP (mm Hg) ← Percentile of Height →						
		5th	10th	25th	50th	75th	90th	95th	5th	10th	25th	50th	75th	90th	95th
1	50th	80	81	83	85	87	88	89	34	35	36	37	38	39	39
	90th	94	95	97	99	100	102	103	49	50	51	52	53	53	54
	95th	98	99	101	103	104	106	106	54	54	55	56	57	58	58
	99th	105	106	108	110	112	113	114	61	62	63	64	65	66	66
2	50th	84	85	87	88	90	92	92	39	40	41	42	43	44	44
	90th	97	99	100	102	104	105	106	54	55	56	57	58	58	59
	95th	101	102	104	106	108	109	110	59	59	60	61	62	63	63
	99th	109	110	111	113	115	117	117	66	67	68	69	70	71	71
3	50th	86	87	89	91	93	94	95	44	44	45	46	47	48	48
	90th	100	101	103	105	107	108	109	59	59	60	61	62	63	63
	95th	104	105	107	109	110	112	113	63	63	64	65	66	67	67
	99th	111	112	114	116	118	119	120	71	71	72	73	74	75	75
4	50th	88	89	91	93	95	96	97	47	48	49	50	51	51	52
	90th	102	103	105	107	109	110	111	62	63	64	65	66	66	67
	95th	106	107	109	111	112	114	115	66	67	68	69	70	71	71
	99th	113	114	116	118	120	121	122	74	75	76	77	78	78	79
5	50th	90	91	93	95	96	98	98	50	51	52	53	54	55	55
	90th	104	105	106	108	110	111	112	65	66	67	68	69	69	70
	95th	108	109	110	112	114	115	116	69	70	71	72	73	74	74
	99th	115	116	118	120	121	123	123	77	78	79	80	81	81	82
6	50th	91	92	94	96	98	99	100	53	53	54	55	56	57	57
	90th	105	106	108	110	111	113	113	68	68	69	70	71	72	72
	95th	109	110	112	114	115	117	117	72	72	73	74	75	76	76
	99th	116	117	119	121	123	124	125	80	80	81	82	83	84	84
7	50th	92	94	95	97	99	100	101	55	55	56	57	58	59	59
	90th	106	107	109	111	113	114	115	70	70	71	72	73	74	74
	95th	110	111	113	115	117	118	119	74	74	75	76	77	78	78
	99th	117	118	120	122	124	125	126	82	82	83	84	85	86	86
8	50th	94	95	97	99	100	102	102	56	57	58	59	60	60	61
	90th	107	109	110	112	114	115	116	71	72	72	73	74	75	76
	95th	111	112	114	116	118	119	120	75	76	77	78	79	79	80
	99th	119	120	122	123	125	127	127	83	84	85	86	87	87	88
9	50th	95	96	98	100	102	103	104	57	58	59	60	61	61	62
	90th	109	110	112	114	115	117	118	72	73	74	75	76	76	77
	95th	113	114	116	118	119	121	121	76	77	78	79	80	81	81
	99th	120	121	123	125	127	128	129	84	85	86	87	88	88	89

(Continued)

Blood Pressure Levels for Boys by Age and Height Percentile (*Continued*)

Age (Year)	BP Percentile ↓	Systolic BP (mm Hg)							Diastolic BP (mm Hg)						
		← Percentile of Height →							← Percentile of Height →						
		5th	10th	25th	50th	75th	90th	95th	5th	10th	25th	50th	75th	90th	95th
10	50th	97	98	100	102	103	105	106	58	59	60	61	61	62	63
	90th	111	112	114	115	117	119	119	73	73	74	75	76	77	78
	95th	115	116	117	119	121	122	123	77	78	79	80	81	81	82
	99th	122	123	125	127	128	130	130	85	86	86	88	88	89	90
11	50th	99	100	102	104	105	107	107	59	59	60	61	62	63	63
	90th	113	114	115	117	119	120	121	74	74	75	76	77	78	78
	95th	117	118	119	121	123	124	125	78	78	79	80	81	82	82
	99th	124	125	127	129	130	132	132	86	86	87	88	89	90	90
12	50th	101	102	104	106	108	109	110	59	60	61	62	63	63	64
	90th	115	116	118	120	121	123	123	74	75	75	76	77	78	79
	95th	119	120	122	123	125	127	127	78	79	80	81	82	82	83
	99th	126	127	129	131	133	134	135	86	87	88	89	90	90	91
13	50th	104	105	106	108	110	111	112	60	60	61	62	63	64	64
	90th	117	118	120	122	124	125	126	75	75	76	77	78	79	79
	95th	121	122	124	126	128	129	130	79	79	80	81	82	83	83
	99th	128	130	131	133	135	136	137	87	87	88	89	90	91	91
14	50th	106	107	109	111	113	114	115	60	61	62	63	64	65	65
	90th	120	121	123	125	126	128	128	75	76	77	78	79	79	80
	95th	124	125	127	128	130	132	132	80	80	81	82	83	84	84
	99th	131	132	134	136	138	139	140	87	88	89	90	91	92	92
15	50th	109	110	112	113	115	117	117	61	62	63	64	65	66	66
	90th	122	124	125	127	129	130	131	76	77	78	79	80	80	81
	95th	126	127	129	131	133	134	135	81	81	82	83	84	85	85
	99th	134	135	136	138	140	142	142	88	89	90	91	92	93	93
16	50th	111	112	114	116	118	119	120	63	63	64	65	66	67	67
	90th	125	126	128	130	131	133	134	78	78	79	80	81	82	82
	95th	129	130	132	134	135	137	137	82	83	83	84	85	86	87
	99th	136	137	139	141	143	144	145	90	90	91	92	93	94	94
17	50th	114	115	116	118	120	121	122	65	66	66	67	68	69	70
	90th	127	128	130	132	134	135	136	80	80	81	82	83	84	84
	95th	131	132	134	136	138	139	140	84	85	86	87	87	88	89
	99th	139	140	141	143	145	146	147	92	93	93	94	95	96	97

BP, blood pressure

*The 90th percentile is 1.28 SD, 95th percentile is 1.645 SD, and the 99th percentile is 2.326 SD over the mean.

National Heart Lung and Blood Institute, National Institutes of Health. (2004). Blood Pressure Tables for Children and Adolescents from the Fourth Report on the Diagnosis, Evaluation, and Treatment of High Blood Pressure in Children and Adolescents.

Blood Pressure Levels for Girls by Age and Height Percentile

Age (Year)	BP Percentile ↓	Systolic BP (mm Hg) ← Percentile of Height →							Diastolic BP (mm Hg) ← Percentile of Height →						
		5th	10th	25th	50th	75th	90th	95th	5th	10th	25th	50th	75th	90th	95th
1	50th	83	84	85	86	88	89	90	38	39	39	40	41	41	42
	90th	97	97	98	100	101	102	103	52	53	53	54	55	55	56
	95th	100	101	102	104	105	106	107	56	57	57	58	59	59	60
	99th	108	108	109	111	112	113	114	64	64	65	65	66	67	67
2	50th	85	85	87	88	89	91	91	43	44	44	45	46	46	47
	90th	98	99	100	101	103	104	105	57	58	58	59	60	61	61
	95th	102	103	104	105	107	108	109	61	62	62	63	64	65	65
	99th	109	110	111	112	114	115	116	69	69	70	70	71	72	72
3	50th	86	87	88	89	91	92	93	47	48	48	49	50	50	51
	90th	100	100	102	103	104	106	106	61	62	62	63	64	64	65
	95th	104	104	105	107	108	109	110	65	66	66	67	68	68	69
	99th	111	111	113	114	115	116	117	73	73	74	74	75	76	76
4	50th	88	88	90	91	92	94	94	50	50	51	52	52	53	54
	90th	101	102	103	104	106	107	108	64	64	65	66	67	67	68
	95th	105	106	107	108	110	111	112	68	68	69	70	71	71	72
	99th	112	113	114	115	117	118	119	76	76	76	77	78	79	79
5	50th	89	90	91	93	94	95	96	52	53	53	54	55	55	56
	90th	103	103	105	106	107	109	109	66	67	67	68	69	69	70
	95th	107	107	108	110	111	112	113	70	71	71	72	73	73	74
	99th	114	114	116	117	118	120	120	78	78	79	79	80	81	81
6	50th	91	92	93	94	96	97	98	54	54	55	56	56	57	58
	90th	104	105	106	108	109	110	111	68	68	69	70	70	71	72
	95th	108	109	110	111	113	114	115	72	72	73	74	74	75	76
	99th	115	116	117	119	120	121	122	80	80	80	81	82	83	83
7	50th	93	93	95	96	97	99	99	55	56	56	57	58	58	59
	90th	106	107	108	109	111	112	113	69	70	70	71	72	72	73
	95th	110	111	112	113	115	116	116	73	74	74	75	76	76	77
	99th	117	118	119	120	122	123	124	81	81	82	82	83	84	84
8	50th	95	95	96	98	99	100	101	57	57	57	58	59	60	60
	90th	108	109	110	111	113	114	114	71	71	71	72	73	74	74
	95th	112	112	114	115	116	118	118	75	75	75	76	77	78	78
	99th	119	120	121	122	123	125	125	82	82	83	83	84	85	86
9	50th	96	97	98	100	101	102	103	58	58	58	59	60	61	61
	90th	110	110	112	113	114	116	116	72	72	72	73	74	75	75
	95th	114	114	115	117	118	119	120	76	76	76	77	78	79	79
	99th	121	121	123	124	125	127	127	83	83	84	84	85	86	87

(Continued)

Blood Pressure Levels for Girls by Age and Height Percentile (*Continued*)

Age (Year)	BP Percentile ↓	Systolic BP (mm Hg) ← Percentile of Height →							Diastolic BP (mm Hg) ← Percentile of Height →						
		5th	10th	25th	50th	75th	90th	95th	5th	10th	25th	50th	75th	90th	95th
10	50th	98	99	100	102	103	104	105	59	59	59	60	61	62	62
	90th	112	112	114	115	116	118	118	73	73	73	74	75	76	76
	95th	116	116	117	119	120	121	122	77	77	77	78	79	80	80
	99th	123	123	125	126	127	129	129	84	84	85	86	86	87	88
11	50th	100	101	102	103	105	106	107	60	60	60	61	62	63	63
	90th	114	114	116	117	118	119	120	74	74	74	75	76	77	77
	95th	118	118	119	121	122	123	124	78	78	78	79	80	81	81
	99th	125	125	126	128	129	130	131	85	85	86	87	87	88	89
12	50th	102	103	104	105	107	108	109	61	61	61	62	63	64	64
	90th	116	116	117	119	120	121	122	75	75	75	76	77	78	78
	95th	119	120	121	123	124	125	126	79	79	79	80	81	82	82
	99th	127	127	128	130	131	132	133	86	86	87	88	88	89	90
13	50th	104	105	106	107	109	110	110	62	62	62	63	64	65	65
	90th	117	118	119	121	122	123	124	76	76	76	77	78	79	79
	95th	121	122	123	124	126	127	128	80	80	80	81	82	83	83
	99th	128	129	130	132	133	134	135	87	87	88	89	89	90	91
14	50th	106	106	107	109	110	111	112	63	63	63	64	65	66	66
	90th	119	120	121	122	124	125	125	77	77	77	78	79	80	80
	95th	123	123	125	126	127	129	129	81	81	81	82	83	84	84
	99th	130	131	132	133	135	136	136	88	88	89	90	90	91	92
15	50th	107	108	109	110	111	113	113	64	64	64	65	66	67	67
	90th	120	121	122	123	125	126	127	78	78	78	79	80	81	81
	95th	124	125	126	127	129	130	131	82	82	82	83	84	85	85
	99th	131	132	133	134	136	137	138	89	89	90	91	91	92	93
16	50th	108	108	110	111	112	114	114	64	64	65	66	66	67	68
	90th	121	122	123	124	126	127	128	78	78	79	80	81	81	82
	95th	125	126	127	128	130	131	132	82	82	83	84	85	85	86
	99th	132	133	134	135	137	138	139	90	90	90	91	92	93	93
17	50th	108	109	110	111	113	114	115	64	65	65	66	67	67	68
	90th	122	122	123	125	126	127	128	78	79	79	80	81	81	82
	95th	125	126	127	129	130	131	132	82	83	83	84	85	85	86
	99th	133	133	134	136	137	138	139	90	90	91	91	92	93	93

BP, blood pressure

*The 90th percentile is 1.28 SD, 95th percentile is 1.645 SD, and the 99th percentile is 2.326 SD over the mean.

National Heart Lung and Blood Institute, National Institutes of Health. (2004).Blood Pressure Tables for Children and Adolescents from the Fourth Report on the Diagnosis, Evaluation, and Treatment of High Blood Pressure in Children and Adolescents.

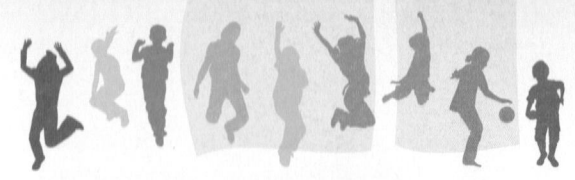

APPENDIX C:
Immunization Schedule

Immunization schedules in the United States are updated annually through a collaborative effort by the Centers for Disease Control and Prevention (CDC) and the American Academy of Pediatrics.

The following are the official websites where the most current immunization schedules for children, adolescents, and catch-up schedules can be located. In addition, these sites contain vital information for parent teaching and precautions for health care providers concerning administration of vaccines.

CDC:
http://www.cdc.gov/vaccines/schedules/hcp/child-adolescent.html

American Academy of Pediatrics:
http://www2.aap.org/immunization/IZSchedule.html

Public Health Agency of Canada:
http://www.phac-aspc.gc.ca/im/is-cv/index-eng.php

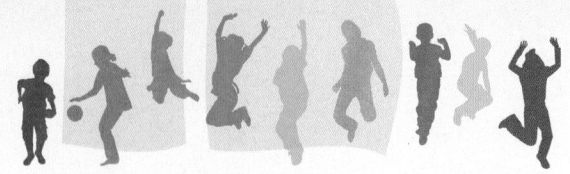

APPENDIX D: Reference Ranges for Laboratory Tests

Prefixes Denoting Decimal Factors	
Prefix	**Symbol**
mega	M
kilo	k
hecto	h
deka	da
deci	d
centi	c
milli	m
micro	μ
nano	n
pico	p
femto	f

To conserve space, the following common abbreviations are used.

Abbreviations	
Ab	absorbance
AI	angiotensin I
AU	arbitrary unit
cAMP	cyclic adenosine 3′, 5′ monophosphate
cap	capillary
CH^{50}	dilution required to lyse 50% of indicator RBC; indicates complement activity
CHF	congestive heart failure
CKBB	brain isoenzyme of creatine kinase
CKMB	heart isoenzyme of creatine kinase
CNS	central nervous system
conc.	concentration
Cr.	creatinine
d	diem, day, days
F	female
g	gram

hr	hour, hours
Hb	hemoglobin
HbCO	carboxyhemoglobin
Hgb	hemoglobin
hpf	high-power field
HPLC	high-performance liquid chromatography
IFA	indirect fluorescent antibody
IU	International Unit of hormone activity
L	liter
M	male
MCV	mean corpuscular volume
mEq/L	milliequivalents per liter
min	minute, minutes
mm^3	cubic millimeter; equivalent to microliter (μL)
mm Hg	millimeters of mercury
mo	month, months
mol	mole
mOsm	milliosmole
MW	relative molecular weight
Na	sodium
nm	nanometer (wavelength)
Pa	pascal
pc	postprandial
RBC	red blood cell(s); erythrocyte(s)
RIA	radioimmunoassay
RID	radial immunodiffusion
SI	Système Internationale

Symbols	
$>$	greater than
$\geq$	greater than or equal to
$<$	less than
$\leq$	less than or equal to
$\pm$	plus/minus
$\cong$	approximately equal to

Abbreviations for Specimens

S	serum
P	plasma
(H)	heparin
(LiH)	lithium heparin
(E)	EDTA
(C)	citrate
(O)	oxalate
W	whole blood
U	urine
F	feces
CSF	cerebrospinal fluid
AF	amniotic fluid
(NaC)	sodium citrate
(NH₄H)	ammonium heparinate

Abbreviations

RT	room temperature
s	second, seconds
SD	standard deviation
std.	standard
therap.	therapeutic
U	International Unit of enzyme activity
V	volume
WBC	white blood cell(s)
WHO	World Health Organization
wk	week, weeks
yr	year, years

Test	Specimen		Reference Range	Reference Range (SI)
Activated partial thrombo-plastin time (APTT)	P(C)	25–35 s Infant: <90 s		25–35 s Infant: <90 s
Adrenocorticotropic hormone (ACTH)	P(H)	Cord blood 1–7 d postnatal Adult 　0800 hr 　1800 hr	130–160 pg/mL 100–140 pg/mL 25–100 pg/mL <50 pg/mt	130–160 mcg/L 100–140 *mcg/L* 25–100 mcg/L <50 mcg/L
Alanine aminotransferase (ALT, SGPT)	S	0–5 d 1–19 yr	6–50 U/L 5–45 U/L	6–50 U/L 5–45 U/L
Albumin	P	Premature 1 d Full-term <6 d <5 yr 5–19 yr	1.8–3.0 g/dL 2.5–3.4 g/dL 3.9–5.0 g/dL 4.0–5.3 g/dL	18–30 g/L 25–34 g/L 39–50 g/L 40–53 g/L
	U	4–16 yr	3.35–15.3 mg/24 hr/ 1.73 m²	
	CSF	10–30 mg/dL		100–300 mg/L
Aldosterone	S,P(H,E)	Ad lib Na intake Premature infants, supine 　26–28 wk 　31–35 wk Full-term infants, supine 　3 d 　1 wk 　1–12 mo Children, supine 　1–2 yr 　2–10 yr 　10–15 yr Adults, supine Children, upright 　2–10 yr 　10–15 yr Adults, upright	 5–635 ng/dL 19–141 ng/dL 7–184 ng/dL 5–175 ng/dL 5–90 ng/dL 7–54 ng/dL 3–35 ng/dL 2–22 ng/dL 3–16 ng/dL 5–80 ng/dL 4–48 ng/dL 7–30 ng/dL	 0.14–17.6 nmol/L 0.53–3.9 nmol/L 0.19–5.1 nmol/L 0.14–4.8 nmol/L 0.14–2.5 nmol/L 0.19–1.5 nmol/L 0.1–0.97 nmol/L 0.1–0.6 nmol/L 0.1–0.4 nmol/L 0.14–2.2 nmol/L 0.11–1.3 nmol/L 0.19–0.83 nmol/L
	U	Ad lib Na intake Newborn 1–3 d Prepubertal 4–10 yr Adults	 20–140 mcg/g Cr. 0.5–5 mcg/24 hr 4–22 *mcg/g* Cr. 1–8 mcg/24 hr 1.5–20 mcg/g Cr. 3–19 mcg/24 hr	 6.28–43.94 nmol/mmol Cr. 1.39–13.88 nmol/d 1.26–6.91 nmol/mmol Cr. 2.78–22.20 nmol/d 0.47–6.28 nmol/mmol Cr. 8.32–52.72 nmol/d

Table continued on following page

Test	Specimen		Reference Range	Reference Range (SI)
Ammonia nitrogen	S,P(LiH)	Newborn	90–150 mcg N/dL	64–107 μmol/L
		0–2 wk	79–129 mcg N/dL	56–92 μmol/L
		>1 mo	29–70 mcg N/dL	21–50 μmol/L
		Thereafter	15–45 mcg N/dL	11–32 μmol/L
		1–90 d	59–202 mcg N/dL	42–144 μmol/L
		3 mo–3 yr	48–195 mcg N/dL	34–139/μmol/L
	U		500–1,200 mg N/24 hr	36–86 mmol/d
Amylase	S	1–19 yr	35–127 U/L	35–127 U/L
Pancreatic isoen	S,P(H)	Cord blood 8 mo	0–34%	0–0.34 fraction of total
Zymes	Zymes	9 mo–4 yr	5–56%	0.05–0.56 fraction of total
		5–19 yr	23–59%	0.23–0.59 fraction of total
Anion gap (Na–(Cl + CO₂))	P(H)		7–16 mmol/L	7–16 mmol/L

Antidiuretic hormone (hADH, vasopressin)	P(E)			
		Plasma Osmolarity	*Plasma ADH*	*Plasma ADH*
		270–280 mOsm/kg	<1.5 pg/mL	<1.5 ng/L
		280–285 mOsm/kg	<2.5 pg/mL	<2.5 ng/L
		285–290 mOsm/kg	1–5 pg/mL	1–5 ng/L
		290–295 mOsm/kg	2–7 pg/mL	2–7 ng/L
		295–300 mOsm/kg	4–12 pg/mL	4–12 ng/L

Test	Specimen		Reference Range	Reference Range (SI)
Antistreptolysin-O titer (ASO titer)	S	≤ 166 Todd units		
		170–330 Todd units in School-aged children		
α₁–Antitrypsin	S	0–5 d	143–440 mg/dL	1.43–4.40 g/L
		1–9 yr	147–245 mg/dL	1.47–2.45 g/L
		9–19 yr	152–317 mg/dL	1.52–3.17 g/L
	F	<1 yr		
		breast milk	<4.4 mg/g solid	
		formula	<2.9 mg/g solid	
		6 mo–44 yr		
		cow milk, regular diet	<1.7 mg/g solid	
Aspartate aminotransferase (AST, SGOT)	S	0–5 d	35–140 U/L	35–140 U/L
		1–9 yr	15–55 U/L	15–55 U/L
		10–19 yr	5–45 U/L	5–45 U/L
Base excess	W(H)	Newborn	(−10)–(−2) mmol/L	(−10)–(−2) mmol/L
		Infant	(−7)–(−1) mmol/L	(−7)–(−1) mmol/L
		Child	(−4)–(+2) mmol/L	(−4)–(+2) mmol/L
		Thereafter	(−3)–(+3) mmol/L	(−3)–(+3) mmol/L
Bicarbonate	S,P	Arterial	21–28 mmol/L	21–28 mmol/L
		Venous	22–29 mmol/L	22–29 mmol/L
Bile acids, total	S,fasting	0.3–2.3 mcg/mL		0.3–2.3 mg/L
	S,2–hr pc	1.8–3.2 mcg/mL		1.8–3.2 mg/L
	F	120–225 mg/24 hr		120–225 mg/24 hr
Bilirubin	S,P			

		Premature	*Full-Term*	*Premature*	*Full-Term*
Total	S	Cord blood	<2.0 mg/dL	<2.0 mg/dL	<34 μmol/L	<34 μmol/L
		0–1 d	<8.0 mg/dL	<6.0 mg/dL	<137 μmol/L	<103 μmol/L
		1–2 d	<12.0 mg/dL	<8.0 mg/dL	<205 μmol/L	<137 μmol/L
		2–5 d	<16.0 mg/dL	<12.0 mg/dL	<274 μmol/L	<205 μmol/L
		>5 d	<2.0 mg/dL	0.2–1.0 mg/dL	<34 μmol/L	3.4–17.1 μmol/L

Test	Specimen	Reference Range		Reference Range (SI)
	U	Negative		Negative
	AF	28 wk<0.075 mg/dL		<1.3 μmol/L
		(or Ab450<0.048)		(or Ab450<0.048)
		40 wk<0.025 mg/dL		<0.43 μmol/L
		(or Ab450<0.02)		(or Ab450<0.02)
Conjugated	S	0–0.2 mg/dL		0–3.4 μmol/L
Bleeding time (BBT) Ivy		Normal 2–7 min		Normal 2–7 min
		Borderline 7–11 min		Borderline 7–11 min
Simplate (G–D)		2.75–8 min		2.75–8 min
Blood volume	W(H)	M 52–83 mL/kg		M 0.052–0.083 L/kg
		F 50–75 mL/kg		F 0.050–0.075 L/kg
C–peptide	P	0.5–2 mcg/L (fasting)		0.5–2 mcg/L (fasting)
C–reactive protein	S	Cord blood	52–1,330 ng/mL	52–1,330 mcg/L
		2–12 yr	67–1,800 ng/mL	67–1,800 mcg/L
Calcitonin	S, P(H,E)	Children	<25–70 pg/mL	<7–19.6 pmol/L
		Adults	<25–150 pg/mL	<7–42 pmol/L
		Higher in newborn infants		
Calcium, ionized (Ca)	S, P(H), W(H)	Newborn	4.40–5.48 mg/dL	1.10–1.37 mmol/L
		Thereafter	4.8–4.92 mg/dL, or	1.12–1.23 mmol/L
			2.24–2.46 mEq/L	1.12–1.23 mmol/L
Calcium, total	S	Newborn		
		3–24 hr	9.0–10.6 mg/dL	2.3–2.65 mmol/L
		24–48 hr	7.0–12.0 mg/dL	1.75–3.0 mmol/L
		4–7 d	9.0–10.9 mg/dL	2.25–2.73 mmol/L
		Child	8.8–10.8 mg/dL	2.2–2.70 mmol/L
		Thereafter	8.4–10.2 mg/dL	2.1–2.55 mmol/L
	U	Ca in diet		
		Ca-free	5–40 mg/24 hr	0.13–1.0 mmol/24 hr
		Low to average	50–150 mg/24 hr	1.25–3.8 mmol/24 hr
		Average (20 mmol/24 hr)	100–300 mg/24 hr	2.5–7.5 mmol/24 hr
	CSF		2.1–2.7 mEq/L or	1.05–1.35 mmol/L
			4.2–5.4 mg/dl	1.05–1.35 mmol/L
	F	Average	0.64 g/24 hr	16 mmol/24 hr
Carbon dioxide	W(H)	Newborn	27–40 mm Hg	3.6–5.3 kPa
		Infant	27–41 mm Hg	3.6–5.5 kPa
Partial pressure (PCO₂)		Thereafter		
		M	35–48 mm Hg	4.7–6.4 kPa
		F	32–45 mm Hg	4.3–6.0 kPa
Total (tCO₂)	S, P(H)	Cord blood	14–22 mmol/L	14–22 mmol/L
		Premature	14–27 mmol/L	14–27 mmol/L
		Newborn	13–22 mmol/L	13–22 mmol/L
		Infant	20–28 mmol/L	20–28 mmol/L
		Child	20–28 mmol/L	20–28 mmol/L
		Thereafter	23–30 mmol/L	23–30 mmol/L
Carbon monoxide	W(E)	Nonsmokers	<2% HbCO	HbCO fraction <0.02
		Smokers	<10%	<0.10
		Lethal	>50%	>0.5
β-Carotene	S	Infant	20–70 mcg/dL	0.37–1.30 μmol/L
		Child	40–130 mcg/dL	0.74–2.42 μmol/L
		Thereafter	60–200 mcg/dL	1.12–3.72 μmol/L

Table continued on following page

Test	Specimen	Reference Range		Reference Range (SI)
Catecholamines, fractionated	P(E)	Norepinephrine		
		Supine	100–400 pg/mL	591–2,364 pmol/L
		Standing	300–900 pg/mL	1,773–5,320 pmol/L
		Epinephrine		
		Supine	<70 pg/mL	<382 pmol/L
		Standing	<100 pg/mL	<546 pmol/L
		Dopamine (no postural change)	<30 pg/mL	<196 pmol/L
	U	Norepinephrine		
		0–1 yr	0–10 mcg/24 hr	0–59 nmol/24 hr
		1–2 yr	0–17 mcg/24 hr	0–100 nmol/24 hr
		2–4 yr	4–29 mcg/24 hr	24–171 nmol/24 hr
		4–7 yr	8–45 mcg/24 hr	47–266 nmol/24 hr
		7–10 yr	13–65 mcg/24 hr	77–384 nmol/24 hr
		Thereafter	15–80 mcg/24 hr	87–473 nmol/24 hr
		Epinephrine		
		0–1 yr	0–2.5 mcg/24 hr	0–13.6 nmol/24 hr
		1–2 yr	0–3.5 mcg/24 hr	0–19.1 nmol/24 hr
		2–4 yr	0–6.0 mcg/24 hr	0–32.7 nmol/24 hr
		4–7 yr	0.2–10 mcg/24 hr	1.1–55 nmol/24 hr
		7–10 yr	0.5–14 mcg/24 hr	2.7–76 nmol/24 hr
		Thereafter	0.5–20 mcg/24 hr	2.7–109 nmol/24 hr
		Fractionated Dopamine		
		0–1 yr	0–85 mcg/24 hr	0–555 nmol/24 hr
		1–2 yr	10–140 mcg/24 hr	65–914 nmol/24 hr
		2–4 yr	40–260 mcg/24 hr	261–1,697 nmol/24 hr
		Thereafter	65–400 mcg/24 hr	424–2,611 nmol/24 hr
Catecholamines, total, free	U	0–1 yr	10–15 mcg/24 hr	10–15 mcg/24 hr
		1–5 yr	15–40 mcg/24 hr	15–40 mcg/24 hr
		6–15 yr	20–80 mcg/24 hr	20–80 mcg/24 hr
		Thereafter	30–100 mcg/24 hr	30–100 mcg/24 hr
Cerebrospinal fluid				
Pressure	CSF	70–180 mm water		70–180 mm water
Volume	CSF	Child	60–100 mL	0.06–0.10 L
		Adult	100–160 mL	0.1–0.16 L
Chloride	S, P(H)	Cord blood	96–104 mmol/L	96–104 mmol/L
		Newborn	97–110 mmol/L	97–110 mmol/L
		Thereafter	98–106 mmol/L	98–106 mmol/L
	CSF		118–132 mmol/L	118–132 mmol/L
	U	Infant	2–10 mmol/24 hr	2–10 mmol/24 hr
		Child	15–40 mmol/24 hr	15–40 mmol/24 hr
		Thereafter	110–250 mmol/24 hr (varies greatly with Cl intake)	110–250 mmol/24 hr
	Sweat	Normal	<40 mmol/L	<40 mmol/L
		Borderline	45–60 mmol/L	45–60 mmol/L
		Cystic fibrosis	>60 mmol/L	>60 mmol/L
Cholesterol, total Child to 18 yr	S			
		Desirable Level	<170 mg/dL	<4.39 mmol/L
		Moderate Risk	170–199 mg/dL	4.40–5.16 mmol/L
		High Risk	>200 mg/dL	>5.18 mmol/L
Thereafter (fasting)				
		Desirable Level	<200 mg/dL	<5.18 mmol/L
		Moderate Risk	200–239 mg/dL	5.18–6.19 mmol/L
		High Risk	>240 mg/dL	>6.20 mmol/L

Test	Specimen		Reference Range	Reference Range (SI)
Clotting time, Lee-White, 37 °C	W	Glass tubes Silicone tubes	5–8 min (5–15 min at RT) about 30 min prolonged	Glass tubes Silicone tubes
Copper	S	0–5 d 1–9 yr 10–14 yr 15–19 yr	9–46 mcg/dL 80–150 mcg/dL 80–121 μdL 64–160 mcg/dL	1.4–7.2 μmol/L 12.6–23.6 μmol/L 12.6–19.0 μmol/L 11.3–25.2 μmol/L
	U	5–18 yr	0.36–7.56 mg/mol Cr.	6–119 μmol/mol Cr.
Cortisol	S, P(H)	Newborn Adults 0800 hr 1600 hr 2000 hr	1–24 mcg/dL 5–23 mcg/dL 3–15 mcg/dL ≤50% of 0800 hr	28–662 nmol/L 138–635 nmol/L 82–413 nmol/L Fraction of 0800 hr ≤0.50
Cortisol, free	U	Child Adolescent Adult	2–27 mcg/24 hr 5–55 mcg/24 hr 10–100 mcg/24 hr	5.5–74 nmol/24 hr 14–152 nmol/24 hr 27–276 nmol/24 hr
Creatine kinase isoenzymes	S		*CKMB*	*CKBB*
		Cord blood 5–8 hr 24–33 hr 72–100 hr Adult	0.3–3.1% 1.7–7.9% 1.8–5.0% 1.4–5.4% 0–2%	0.3–10.5% 3.6–13.4% 2.3–8.6% 5.1–13.3% 0
Creatinine plasma	S,P	Cord blood Newborn Infant Child Adolescent Adult M F	0.6–1.2 mg/dL 0.3–1.0 mg/dL 0.2–0.4 mg/dL 0.3–0.7 mg/dL 0.5–1.0 mg/dL 0.6–1.2 mg/dL 0.5–1.1 mg/dL	53–106 μmol/L 27–88 μmol/L 18–35 μmol/L 27–62 μmol/L 44–88 μmol/L 53–106 μmol/L 44–97 μmol/L
Creatinine, urinary	U	Premature Full-term 1.5–7 yr 7–15 yr	8.1–15.0 mg/kg/24 hr 10.4–19.7 mg/kg/24 hr 10–15 mg/kg/24 hr 5.2–41 mg/kg/24 hr	72–133 μmol/kg/24 hr 92–174 μmol/kg/24 hr 88–133 μmol/kg/24 hr 46–362 μmol/kg/24 hr
Creatinine clearance (endogenous)	S, P, and U	Newborn <40 yr M F Decreases	40–65 mL/min/1.73 m² 97–137 mL/min/1.73m² 88–128 mL/min/1.73m² ~6.5 mL/min/decade	
Differential count. See Leukocyte differential count				
Eosinophil count	W(E,H) capillary	50–350 cells/mm³(μl)		50–350 × 10⁶ cells/L

Table continued on following page

Test	Specimen		Reference Range	Reference Range (SI)
Epinephrine. See Catecholamines, fractionated				
Erythrocyte count (RBC count)	W(E)		*Millions of cells/mm³(μl)*	*×10¹² cells/L*
		Cord blood	3.9–5.5	3.9–5.5
		1–3 d (capillary)	4.0–6.6	4.0–6.6
		1 wk	3.9–6.3	3.9–6.3
		2 wk	3.6–6.2	3.6–6.2
		1 mo	3.0–5.4	3.0–5.4
		2 mo	2.7–4.9	2.7–4.9
		3–6 mo	3.1–4.5	3.1–4.5
		0.5–2 yr	3.7–5.3	3.7–5.3
		2–6 yr	3.9–5.3	3.9–5.3
		6–12 yr	4.0–5.2	4.0–5.2
		12–18 yr		
		M	4.5–5.3	4.5–5.3
		F	4.1–5.1	4.1–5.1
		18–49 yr		
		M	4.5–5.9	4.5–5.9
		F	4.0–5.2	4.0–5.2
Erythrocyte sedimentation rate (ESR) Wester-gren, modified	W(E)	Child	0–10 mm/hr	0–10 mm/hr
		Adult		
		M <50 yr	0–15 mm/hr	0–15 mm/hr
		F <50 yr	0–20 mm/hr	0–20 mm/hr
Wintrobe		Child	0–13 mm/hr	0–13 mm/hr
		Adult		
		M	0–9 mm/hr	0–9 mm/hr
		F	0–20 mm/hr	0–20 mm/hr
Erythropoietin RIA	S	<5–20 mU/mL		<5–20 U/L
Hemagglutination		25–125 mU/mL		25–125 U/L
Bioassay		5–18 mU/mL		5–18 U/L
Fat, fecal	F (72 hr)	Infant, breast-fed	<1 g/24 hr	<1 g/24 hr
		0–6 yr	<2 g/24 hr	<2 g/24 hr
		Adult		
		Normal diet	<7 g/24 hr	<7 g/24 hr
		Fat-free diet	<4 g/24 hr	<4 g/24 hr
		Coefficient of Fat Absorption (%)		*Absorbed Fraction*
		Infant		
		Breast-fed	>93	>0.93
		Formula-fed	>83	>0.83
		>1 yr	≥95	≥0.95
Free fatty acids	S	Premature 10–55 d	0.15–0.71 mmol/L	0.15–0.71 mmol/L
Ferric, chloride test	U	Negative		Negative
Ferritin	S	Newborn	25–200 ng/mL	25–200 mcg/L
		1 mo	200–600 ng/mL	200–600 mcg/L
		2–5 mo	50–200 ng/mL	50–200 mcg/L
		6 mo–15 yr	7–140 ng/mL	7–140 mcg/L
		Adult		
		M	15–200 ng/mL	15–200 mcg/L
		F	12–150 ng/mL	12–150 mcg/L

Test	Specimen			Reference Range	Reference Range (SI)
Fibrin degradation products Agglutination (Thrombo-Wellco test)	W; special lube thrombin and proteolytic	inhibitors		<10 mcg/mL	<10 mg/L
	U: 2 mL in special tube (see above)			<0.25 mcg/mL	<0.25 mg/L
Fibrinogen	P(NaCl)	Newborn		125–300 mg/dL	1.25–3.00 g/L
		Adult		200–400 mg/dL	2.00–4.00 g/L
Folate	S	Newborn		7.0–32 ng/mL	15.9–72.4 nmol/L
		Thereafter		1.8–9 ng/mL	4.1–20.4 nmol/L
	W(E)			150–450 ng/mL RBCs	340–1,020 nmol/L cells
Follicle-stimulating hormone (FSH)	S	M			
		Tanner 1	<9.8 yr	0.26–3.0 mIU/mL	0.26–3.0 U/L
		Tanner 2	9.8–14.5 yr	1.8–3.2 mIU/mL	1.8–3.2 U/L
		Tanner 3	10.7–15.4 yr	1.2–5.8 mIU/mL	1.2–5.8 U/L
		Tanner 4	11.8–16.2 yr	2.0–9.2 mIU/mL	2.0–9.2 U/L
		Tanner 5	12.8–17.3 yr	2.6–11.0 mIU/mL	2.6–11.0 U/L
		Adult		2.0–9.2 mIU/mL	2.0–9.2 U/L
		F			
		Tanner 1	<9.2 yr	1.0–4.2 mIU/mL	1.0–4.2 U/L
		Tanner 2	9.2–13.7 yr	1.0–10.8 mIU/mL	1.0–10.8 U/L
		Tanner 3	10.0–14.4 yr	1.5–12.8 mIU/mL	1.5–12.8 U/L
		Tanner 4	10.7–15.6 yr	1.5–11.7 mIU/mL	1.5–11.7 U/L
		Tanner 5	11.8–18.6 yr	1.0–9.2 mIU/mL	1.0–9.2 U/L
		Adult			
		Follicular		1.8–11.2 mIU/mL	1.8–11.2 U/L
		Midcycle		6–35 mIU/mL	6–35 U/L
		Luteal		1.8–11.2 mIU/mL	1.8–11.2 U/L
Galactose	S	Newborn		0–20 mg/dL	0–1.11 mmol/L
	P	5 mo–17 yr		0.0–0.5 mg/dL	0.0–0.03 mmol/L
	U	Newborn		≤60 mg/dL	≤3.33 mmol/L
		Thereafter		14 mg/24 hr	<0.08 mmol/24 hr
Gastrin	S (fasting)	Children		<10–125 pg/mL	<10–125 ng/L
Glucagon	S	Neonate (1–7 d)		210–1,500 pg/mL	210–1,500 ng/L
		Children and adults		25–250 pg/mL	25–250 ng/L
Glucose	S	Cord blood		45–96 mg/dL	2.5–5.3 mmol/L
		Newborn			
		1 d		40–60 mg/dL	2.2–3.3 mmol/L
		>1 d		50–90 mg/dL	2.8–5.0 mmol/L
		Child		60–100 mg/dL	3.3–5.5 mmol/L
		Adult		70–105 mg/dL	3.9–5.8 mmol/L
	W(H)	Adult		65–95 mg/dL	3.6–5.3 mmol/L
	CSF	Adult		40–70 mg/dL	2.2–3.9 mmol/L
Quantitative, enzymatic	U	<0.5 g/24 hr			<2.8 mmol/24 hr
Qualitative	U	Negative			Negative
Glucose, 2 hr pc	S	<120 mg/dL (For diabetes, see Glucose tolerance test, oral)			<6.7 mmol/L

Table continued on following page

Test	Specimen		Reference Range		Reference Range (SI)	
Glucose-6-phosphate dehydrogenase in erythrocytes Bishop, modified	W(E,H,C)	Adult	3.4–8.0 U/g Hb		Adult	0.22–0.52 mU/mol Hb
			98.6–232 U/10¹² RBC			0.10–0.23 nU/10⁶ RBC
			1.16–2.72 U/mL RBC			1.16–2.72 kU/L RBC
			Newborn: 50% higher			Newborn: 50% higher

Test	Specimen		*Normal*	*Diabetic*	*Normal*	*Diabetic*
Glucose tolerance test (GTT), oral	S					
Adult dose: 75 g		Fasting	70–105 mg/dL	>115 mg/dL	3.9–5.8 mmol/L	>6.4 mmol/L
Child dose:		60 min	120–170 mg/dL	≥200 mg/dL	6.7–9.4 mmol/L	≥11 mmol/L
1.75 g/kg of		90 min	100–140 mg/dL	≥200 mg/dL	5.6–7.8 mmol/L	≥11 mmol/L
ideal weight up to maximum of 75 g		120 min	70–120 mg/dL	≥140 mg/dL	3.9–6.7 mmol/L	≥7.8 mmol/L

Test	Specimen		Reference Range	Reference Range (SI)
γ-Glutamyltranspeptidase (GGT, GGTP)	S	Cord blood	37–193 U/L	37–193 U/L
		0–1 mo	13–147 U/L	13–147 U/L
		1–2 mo	12–123 U/L	12–123 U/L
		2–4 mo	8–90 U/L	8–90 U/L
		4 mo–10 yr	5–32 U/L	5–32 U/L
		10–15 yr	5–24 U/L	5–24 U/L
Growth hormone (hGH, somatotropin)	S,P(E,H)	Newborn		
		1 d	5–53 ng/mL	5–53 mcg/L
		1 wk	5–27 ng/mL	5–27 mcg/L
		1–12 mo	2–10 ng/mL	2–10 mcg/L
	Fasting, at rest	Child	<0.7–6 ng/mL	<0.7–6 mcg/L
		Adult	<0.7–6 ng/mL	<0.7–6 mcg/L
HDL cholesterol	S	1–13 yr	35–84 mg/dL	0.9–2.15 mmol/L
		14–19 yr	35–65 mg/dL	0.90–1.65 mmol/L

Test	Specimen		*Percent packed red cells (vol red cells/vol whole blood cells × 100)*	*Volume fraction (vol red cells/vol whole blood)*
Hematocrit (HCT, Hct)	W(E)			
Calculated from MCV and RBC (electronic displacement or laser)		1d (capillary)	48–69%	0.48–0.69
		2 d	48–75%	0.48–0.75
		3 d	44–72%	0.44–0.72
		2 mo	28–42%	0.28–0.42
		6–12 yr	35–45%	0.35–0.45
		12–18 yr		
		M	37–49%	0.37–0.49
		F	36–46%	0.36–0.46
		18–49 yr		
		M	41–53%	0.41–0.53
		F	36–46%	0.36–0.46
Hemoglobin (Hb)	W(E)	1–3 d (capillary)	14.5–22.5 g/dL	2.25–3.49 mmol/L
		2 mo	9.0–14.0 g/dL	1.40–2.17 mmol/L
		6–12 yr	11.5–15.5 g/dL	1.78–2.40 mmol/L
		12–18 yr		
		M	13.0–16.0 g/dL	2.02–2.48 mmol/L
		F	12.0–16.0 g/dL	1.86–2.48 mmol/L
		18–49 yr		
		M	13.5–17.5 g/dL	2.09–2.27 mmol/L
		F	12.0–16.0 g/dL	1.86–2.48 mmol/L

Test	Specimen		Reference Range	Reference Range (SI)
	P(H)	<10 mg/dL		<1.55 μmol/L
		<3 mg/dL with butterfly set-up and 18-g needle		<0.47 μmol/L with butterfly set-up and 18-g needle
	U	Negative		Negative
Hemoglobin A	W(E, C, H)		>95%	Fraction of hemoglobin >0.95
Hemoglobin electrophoresis	W(H, E, C)	HbA	>95%	
		HbA₂	1.5–3.5%	
		HbF	<2%	
Immunoglobulin A (IgA)	S	Cord blood	1.4–3.6 mg/dL	14–36 mg/L
		1–3 mo	1.3–53 mg/dL	13–530 mg/L
		4–6 mo	4.4–84 mg/dL	44–840 mg/L
		7 mo–1 yr	11–106 mg/dL	110–1,060 mg/L
		2–5 yr	14–159 mg/dL	140–1,590 mg/L
		6–10 yr	33–236 mg/dL	330–2,360 mg/L
		Adult	70–312 mg/dL	700–3,120 mg/L
Immunoglobulin D (IgD)	S	Newborn	None detected	None detected
		Thereafter	0–8 mg/dL	0–80 mg/L
Immunoglobulin E (IgE)	S	M	0–230 IU/mL	0–230 kIU/L
		F	0–170 IU/mL	0–170 kIU/L
Immunoglobulin G (IgG)	S	Cord blood	636–1,606 mg/dL	6.36–16.06 g/L
		1 mo	251–906 mg/dL	2.51–9.06 g/L
		2–4 mo	176–601 mg/dL	1.76–6.01 g/L
		5–12 mo	172–1,069 mg/dL	1.72–10.69 g/L
		1–5 yr	345–1,236 mg/dL	3.45–12.36 g/L
		6–10 yr	608–1,572 mg/dL	6.08–15.72 g/L
		Adult	639–1,349 ma/dL	6.39–13.49 g/L
Immunoglobulin M (IgM)	S	Cord blood	6.3–25 mg/dL	63–250 mg/L
		1–4 mo	17–105 mg/dL	170–1,050 mg/L
		5–9 mo	33–126 mg/dL	300–1,260 mg/L
		10 mo–1 yr	41–173 mg/dL	410–1,730 mg/L
		2–8 yr	43–207 mg/dL	430–2,070 mg/L
		9–10 yr	52–242 mg/dL	520–2,420 mg/L
		Adult	56–352 mg/dL	560–3,520 mg/L
Insulin (12-hr fasting)	S	Newborn	3–20 μU/mL	3–20 mU/L
		Thereafter	7–24 μU/mL	7–24 mU/L
Insulin with oral glucose tolerance test	S		Insulin	
		0 min	7–24 μU/mL	7–24 mU/L
		30 min	25–231 μU/mL	25–231 mU/L
		60 min	18–276 μU/mL	18–276 mU/L
		120 min	16–166 μU/mL	16–166 mU/L
		180 min	4–38 μU/mL	4–38 mU/L
Iron	S	Newborn	100–250 mcg/dL	17.90–44.75 μmol/L
		Infant	40–100 mcg/dL	7.16–17.90 μmol/L
		Child	50–120 mcg/dL	8.95–21.48 μmol/L
		Thereafter		
		M	50–160 mcg/dL	8.95–28.64 μmol/L
		F	40–150 mcg/dL	7.16–26.85 μmol/L
		Intoxicated child	280–2,550 mcg/dL	50.12–456.5 μmol/L
		Fatally poisoned child	>1,800 μ/dL	>322.2 μmol/L
Iron-binding capacity, total (TIBC)	S	Infant	100–400 mcg/dL	17.90–71.60 μmol/L
		Thereafter	250–400 mcg/dL	44.75–71.60 μmol/L
17-Ketogenic steroids (17-KGS)	U	0–1 yr	<1.0 mg/24 hr	<3.5 μmol/24 hr
		1–10 yr	<5 mg/24 hr	<17 μmol/24 hr
		11–14 yr	<12 mg/24 hr	<42 μmol/24 hr

Table continued on following page

Test	Specimen		Reference Range	Reference Range (SI)
		Thereafter		
		M	5–23 mg/24 hr	17–80 μmol/24 hr
		F	3–15 mg/24 hr	10–52 μmol/24 hr
Ketone bodies				
Qualitative	S	Negative		Negative
	U	Negative		Negative
Quantitative	S	0.5–3.0 mg/dL		5–30 mg/L
17-Ketosteroid(17-KS), total	U	14 d–2 yr	<1 mg/24 hr	<3.5 μmol/24 hr
		2–6 yr	<2 mg/24 hr	<7 μmol/24 hr
		6–10 yr	1–4 mg/24 hr	3.5–14 μmol/24 hr
		10–12 yr	1–6 mg/24 hr	3.5–21 μmol/24 hr
		12–14 yr	3–10 mg/24 hr	10–35 μmol/24 hr
		14–16 yr	5–12 mg/24 hr	17–42 μmol/24 hr
		Thereafter		
		M: 18–30 yr	9–22 mg/24 hr	31–76 μmol/24 hr
		> 30 yr	8–20 mg/24 hr	28–70 μmol/24 hr
		F, decreases with age	6–15 mg/24 hr	21–52 μmol/24 hr
LDL-cholesterol (LDL)	S, P(E)			
Child to 18 yr		Desirable Level	<110 mg/dL	<2.8 mmol/L
		Moderate Risk	110–129 mg/dL	2.8–3.4 mmol/L
		High Risk	>130 mg/dL	>3.4 mmol/L
Thereafter		Desirable Level	<130 mg/dL	<3.4 mmol/L
		Moderate Risk	140–159 mg/dL	3.4–4.1 mmol/L
		High Risk	>160 mg/dL	>4.1 mmol/L
		<3.4	1.68–4.53 mmol/L	
Lactate	W(H)	Venous	0.5–2.2 mmol/L	0.5–2.2 mmol/L
L(+)-lactate		Arterial	0.5–1.6 mmol/L	0.5–1.6 mmol/L
		Inpatients		
		Venous	0.9–1.7 mmol/L	0.9–1.7 mmol/L
		Arterial	<1.25 mmol/L	<1.25 mmol/L
D(−)-lactate	P(H)	6 mo–3 yr	0.0–0.3 mmol/L	0.0–0.3 mmol/L
Lactate dehydrogenase (LD)	S	<1 yr	170–580 U/L	170–580 U/L
		1–9 yr	150–500 U/L	150–500 U/L
		10–19 yr	120–330 U/L	120–330 U/L

	Isoenzymes	S		Percentage of total activity	
				1–6 yr	7–19 yr
			LD1	20–38	20–35
			LD2	27–38	31–38
			LD3	16–26	19–28
			LD4	5–16	7–13
			LD5	3–13	5–12

Test	Specimen		Reference Range	Reference Range (SI)
Lead	W(H)	Child	<10 mcg/dL	<0.48 μmol/L
		Adult	<40 mcg/dL	<1.93 μmol/L
		Acceptable for industrial exposure	<40 mcg/dL	<1.93 μmol/L
		Toxic	Child 50 μg/dL	≥4.83 μmol/L
	U (24-hr)	<80 mcg/dL	Adult 80 μg/dL	<0.39 μmol/L
Lecithin/sphingomyelin	AF		2.0–5.0 indicates probable fetal lung maturity	2.0–5.0 indicates probable fetal lung maturity
(L/S) ratio			(>3.0 IDM)	
Lecithin phosphorus	AF		>0.10 mg/dL indicates probably adequate fetal lung maturity	>0.032 mmol/L indicates probably adequate fetal lung maturity

Leukocyte count (WBC)	W(E)		× 1,000 cells/mm³ (μL)	× 10⁹ cells/L
		Birth	9.0–30.0	9.0–30.0
		24 hr	9.4–34.0	9.4–34.0
		1 mo	5.0–19.5	5.0–19.5
		1–3 yr	6.0–17.5	6.0–17.5
		4–7 yr	5.5–15.5	5.5–15.5
		8–13 yr	4.5–13.5	4.5–13.5
		Adult	4.5–11.0	4.5–11.0

Test	Specimen	Reference Range	Reference Range (SI)
Cell count	CSF	Premature 0–25 mononuclear cells/μL	0–25 × 10⁶ cells/L
		0–10 polymorphonuclear cells/μL	0–10 × 10⁶ cells/L
		0–1,000 RBC/μL	0–1,000 × 10⁶ cells/L
		Newborn 0–20 mononuclear cells/μL	0–20 × 10⁶ cells/L
		0–10 polymorphonuclear cells/μL	0–10 × 10⁶ cells/L
		0–800 RBC/μL	0–800 × 10⁶ cells/L
		Neonate 0–5 mononuclear cells/μL	0–5 × 10⁶ cells/L
		0–10 polymorphonuclear cells/μL	0–10 × 10⁶ cells/L
		0–50 RBC/μL	0–50 × 10⁶ cells/L
			0–5 cells/L
		Thereafter 0–5 mononuclear cells/μL (numbers of cells in very young infants are greater than those in the CSF of older individuals without substantial implications for growth and development in most instances)	

Leukocyte differential	W(E)		
Myelocytes		0	0
Neutrophils—"bands"		3–5%	0.03–0.05 no. fraction
Neutrophils—"segs"		54–62%	0.54–0.62 no. fraction
Lymphocytes		25–33%	0.25–0.33 no. fraction
Monocytes		3–7%	0.03–0.07 no. fraction
Eosinophils		1–3%	0.01–0.03 no. fraction
Basophils		0–0.75%	0–0.0075 no. fraction

Leukocyte differential	Specimen	Cells/mm³ (μL)	
Myelocytes		0	0 × 10⁶ cells/L
Neutrophils—"bands"		150–400	150–400 × 10⁶ cells/L
Neutrophils—"segs"		3,000–5,800	3,000–5,800 × 10⁶ cells/L
Lymphocytes		1,500–3,000	1,500–3,000 × 10⁶ cells/L
Monocytes		285–500	285–500 × 10⁶ cells/L
Eosinophils		50–250	50–250 × 10⁶ cells/L
Basophils		15–50	15–50 × 10⁶ cells/L
Lymphocytes	CSF	62% ± 34%	0.62 ± 0.34 no. fraction
Monocytes		36% ± 20%	0.36 ± 0.20 no. fraction

Table continued on following page

Test	Specimen		Reference Range	Reference Range (SI)
Neutrophils			2% ± 5%	0.02 ± 0.05 no. fraction
Histiocytes			0–rare	0–rare
Ependymal cells			0–rare	0–rare
Eosinophils			0–rare	0–rare
Lipase	S	1–4 yr	18–95 U/L	18–95 U/L
		5–14 yr	21–128 U/L	21–128 U/L
		15–19 yr	28–149 U/L	28–149 U/L
Magnesium	P(H)	0–6 d	1.2–2.6 mg/dL	0.48–1.05 mmol/L
		7 d–2 yr	1.6–2.6 mg/dL	0.65–1.05 mmol/L
	U (24-hr)	2–14 yr	1.5–2.3 mg/dL	0.60–0.95 mmol/L
		1–6 mo		
		Breast-fed	0.04–1.55 mmol/L	0.04–1.55 mmol/L
		Formula-fed	0.04–1.40 mmol/L	0.04–1.55 mmol/L
Mean corpuscular hemoglobin concentration (MCHC)	W(E)	Birth	31–37 pg/cell	0.48–0.57 fmol/cell
		1–3 d (capillary)	31–37 pg/cell	0.48–0.57 fmol/cell
		1 wk–1 mo	28–40 pg/cell	0.43–0.62 fmol/cell
		2 mo	26–34 pg/cell	0.40–0.53 fmol/cell
		3–6 mo	25–35 pg/cell	0.39–0.54 fmol/cell
		0.5–2 yr	23–31 pg/cell	0.36–0.48 fmol/cell
		2–6 yr	24–30 pg/cell	0.37–0.47 fmol/cell
		6–12 yr	25–33 pg/cell	0.39–0.51 fmol/cell
		12–18 yr	25–35 pg/cell	0.39–0.54 fmol/cell
		18–49 yr	26–34 pg/cell	0.40–0.53 fmol/cell
Mean corpuscular hemoglobin	W(E)		*Percentage Hb/cell or g Hb/dL RBC*	*mmol Hb/L RBC*
		Birth	30–36	4.65–5.58
		1–3 d (capillary)	29–37	4.50–5.74
		1–2 wk	28–38	4.34–5.89
		1–2 mo	29–37	4.50–5.74
		3 mo–2 yr	30–36	4.65–5.58
		2–18 yr	31–37	4.81–5.74
		>18 yr	31–37	4.81–574
Mean corpuscular volume (MCV)	W(E)	1–3 d (capillary)	95–121 μm^3	95–121 fL
		0.5–2 yr	70–86 μm^3	70–86 fL
		6–12 yr	77–95 μm^3	77–95 fL
		12–18 yr		
		M	78–98 μm^3	78–98 fL
		F	78–102 μm^3	78–102 fL
		18–49 yr		
		M	80–100 μm^3	80–100 fL
		F	80–100 μm^3	80–100 fL
Methemoglobin (MetHb)	W(E,H,C)	0.06–0.24 g/dL or		9.3–37.2 umol/L
		0.78 ± 0.37% of total Hb		0.0078 ± 0.0037 (mass fraction)
Methylmalonic acid	U	6–12 wk	0–57 mg/g creatinine	0–55 mmol/mol creatinine
Mucopolysaccharides	U	<2 yr	<50 mcg/g creatinine	<5.7 mg/mmol creatinine
		2–4 yr	<25 mcg/g creatinine	<2.8 mg/mmol creatinine
		4–15 yr	<20 mcg/g creatinine	<2.3 mg/mmol creatinine
Osmolality	S	Child and adult	275–295 mOsm/kg H_2O	

Test	Specimen	Reference Range		Reference Range (SI)
	U	50–1,400 mOsm/kg H₂O, depending on fluid intake. After 12 hr of fluid restriction, normal range is >850 mOsm/kg H₂O		
	U (24-hr)	300–900 mOsm/kg H₂O		
Oxygen, partial pressure of (PO₂)	W(H), arterial	Birth	8–24 mm Hg	1.1–3.2 kPa
		5–10 min	33–75 mm Hg	4.4–10.0 kPa
		30 min	31–85 mm Hg	4.1–11.3 kPa
		>1 hr	55–80 mm Hg	7.3–10.6 kPa
		1 d	54–95 mm Hg	7.2–12.6 kPa
		Thereafter (decreases with age)	83–108 mm Hg	11–14.4 kPa
Oxygen saturation	W(H), arterial	Newborn	85–90%	0.85–0.90 Saturated fraction
		Thereafter	95–99%	0.95–0.99 Saturated fraction
Parathyroid hormone	S			
C-terminal (mid–molecule)		1–16 yr	51–217 pg/mL	5.4–22.8 pmol/L
Intact (IRMA)		1–18 yr	1–43 pg/mL	0.1–4.5 pmol/L
Partial thromboplastin time (PTT)	W(NaCl)			
Nonactivated		60–85 s (Platelin)		60–85 s
Activated		25–35 s (differs with method)		25–35 s
Pᴴ	W(H), arterial			H⁺ Concentration
		Premature (48 hr)	7.35–7.50	31–44 nmol/L
		Birth, full-term	7.11–7.36	43–77 nmol/L
		5–10 min	7.09–7.30	50–81 nmol/L
		30 min	7.21–7.38	41–61 nmol/L
		>1 hr	7.26–7.49	32–54 nmol/L
		1 d	7.29–7.45	35–51 nmol/L
		Thereafter	7.35–7.45	35–44 nmol/L
		Must be corrected for body temperature		
	U	Newborn/neonate	5–7	0.1–10 μmol/L
		Thereafter (average 6)	4.5–8	0.01–32 μmol/L (average 1.0 /μmol/L)
	F		7.0–7.5	31–100 μmol/L
Phenylalanine	S	Premature	2.0–7.5 mg/dL	120–450/μmol/L
		Newborn	1.2–3.4 mg/dL	70–210/μmol/L
		Thereafter	0.8–1.8 mg/dL	50–110/μmol/L
	U	10 d–2 wk	1–2 mg/24 hr	6–12 μmol/24 hr
		3–12 yr	4–18 mg/24 hr	24–110/μmol/24 hr
		Thereafter	trace–17 mg/24 hr	Trace–103μmol/24 hr
Phenylpyruvic acid, qualitative	U	Negative by FeCl₃ test		Negative by FeCl₃ test

Table continued on following page

Test	Specimen	Reference Range			Reference Range (SI)		
Phosphatase, alkaline	S	1–9 yr	145–420 U/L		1–9 yr	145–420 U/L	
			M	F		M	F
		12–13 yr	200–495 U/L	105–420 U/L	12–13 yr	200–495 U/L	105–420 U/L
		14–15 yr	130–525 U/L	70–230 U/L	14–15 yr	130–525 U/L	70–230 U/L
		16–19 yr	65–260 U/L	50–130 U/L	16–19 yr	65–260 U/L	50–130 U/L
Phospholipids, total	S, P(E)	Newborn	75–170 mg/dL			0.75–1.70 g/L	
		Infant	100–275 mg/dL			1.00–2.75 g/L	
		Child	180–295 mg/dL			1.80–2.95 g/L	
		Adult	125–275 mg/dL			1.25–2.75 g/L	
Phosphorus, inorganic	S, P(H)	0–5 d	4.8–8.2 mg/dL			1.55–2.65 mmol/L	
		1–3 yr	3.8–6.5 mg/dL			1.25–2.10 mmol/L	
		4–11 yr	3.7–5.6 mg/dL			1.20–1.80 mmol/L	
		12–15 yr	2.9–5.4 mg/dL			0.95–1.75 mmol/L	
		16–19 yr	2.7–4.7 mg/dL			0.90–1.50 mmol/L	
Plasma volume	P(H)	M	25–43 mL/kg		M	0.025–0.043 L/kg	
		F	28–45 mL/kg		F	0.028–0.045 L/kg	
Platelet count (thrombocyte count)	W(E)	Newborn 84–478 × 10^3/mm^3 (μL) (after 1 wk same as adult)				84–478 × 10^9/A	
		Children/Adult 150–400 × 10^3/mm^3 (μL)				150–400 × 10^9/L	
Potassium	S	<2 mo	3.0–7.0 mmol/L			3.0–7.0 mmol/L	
		2–12 mo	3.5–6.0 mmol/L			3.5–6.0 mmol/L	
		>12 mo	3.5–5.0 mmol/L			3.5–5.0 mmol/L	
	P(H)					3.5–4.5 mmol/L	
	U (24-hr)	2.5–125 mmol/L (varies with diet)				2.5–125 mmol/L (varies with diet)	
Protein							
Total	S	Premature	4.3–7.6 g/dL			43–76 g/L	
		Newborn	4.6–7.4 g/dL			46–74 g/L	
		1–7 yr	6.1–7.9 g/dL			61–79 g/L	
		8–12 yr	6.4–8.1 g/dL			64–81 g/L	
		13–19 yr	6.6–8.2 g/dL			66–82 g/L	
Electrophoresis	S						
Albumin		Premature	3.0–4.2 g/dL			30–42 g/L	
		Newborn	3.6–5.4 g/dL			36–54 gL	
		Infant	4.0–5.0 g/dL			40–50 g/L	
		Thereafter	3.5–5.0 g/dL			35–50 g/L	
α_1–Globulin		Premature	0.1–0.5 g/dL			1–5 g/L	
		Newborn	0.1–0.3 g/dL			1–3 g/L	
		Infant	0.2–0.4 g/dL			2–4 g/L	
		Thereafter	0.2–0.3 g/dL			2–3 g/L	
α_2 Globulin		Premature	0.3–0.7 g/dL			3–7 g/L	
		Newborn	0.3–0.5 g/dL			3–5 g/L	
		Infant	0.5–0.8 g/dL			5–8 g/L	
		Thereafter	0.4–1.0 g/dL			4–10 g/L	
β–Globulin		Premature	0.3–1.2 g/dL			3–12 g/L	
		Newborn	0.2–0.6 g/dL			2–6 g/L	
		Infant	0.5–0.8 g/dL			5–8 g/L	
		Thereafter	0.5–1.1 g/dL			5–11 g/L	

Test	Specimen	Reference Range		Reference Range (SI)
γ–Globulin		Premature	0.3–1.4 g/dL	3–4 g/L
		Newborn	0.2–1.0 g/dL	2–10 g/L
		Infant	0.3–1.2 g/dL	3–12 g/L
		Thereafter (higher in blacks)	0.7–1.2 g/dL	7–12 g/L
Protein	U (24–hr)	1–14 mg/dL		10–140 mg/L
Total urinary		50–80 mg/24 hr (at rest)		50–80 mg/24 hr (at rest)
		<250 mg/24 hr after intense exercise		<250 mg/24 hr after intense exercise
Electrophoresis		*Average Total Protein*		*Fraction of Total Protein*
Albumin		37.9%		0.379
α_1–Globulin		27.3%		0.273
α_2–Globulin		19.5%		0.195
β–Globulin		8.8%		0.088
γ–Globulin		3.3%		0.033
Protein				
Total protein (column)	CSF	Lumbar	8–32 mg/dL	80–320 mg/L
Prothrombin time (PT)				
One-stage (quick)	W(NaC)	In general, 11–15 s (varies with type of thromboplastin)		11–15 s
		Newborn: prolonged by 2–3 s		Newborn: prolonged by 2–3 s
Two–stage modified (Ware and Seegers)	W(NaC)	18–22 s		18–22 s
Red cell volume	W(H)	M	20–36 mL/kg	0.020–0.036 L/kg
		F	19–31 mL/kg	0.019–0.031 L/kg
Renin (renin activity, plasma; PRA)	P(E)	0–3 yr	<16.6 ng/mL/hr	<16.6 mcg/L/hr
		3–6 yr	<6.7 ng/mL/hr	<6.7 mcg/L/hr
		6–9 yr	<4.4 ng/mL/hr	<4.4 mcg/L/hr
		9–12 yr	<5.9 ng/mL/hr	<5.9 mcg/L/hr
		12–15 yr	<4.2 ng/mL/hr	<4.2 mcg/L/hr
		15–18 yr	<4.3 ng/mL/hr	<4.3 mcg/L/hr
		Normal sodium diet		
		Supine	0.2–2.5 ng/mL/hr	0.2–2.5 mcg/L/hr
		Upright	0.3–4.3 ng/mL/hr	0.3–4.3 mcg/L/hr
		Low sodium diet		
		Upright	2.9–24 ng/mL/hr	2.9–24 mcg/L/hr
Reticulocyte count	W(E,H,0)	Adults 0.5–1.5% of erythrocytes, or 25,000–75,000/mm³ (μL)		0.005–0.015 number fraction
				25,000–75,000 × 10⁶/L
	W (capillary)	ld	0.4–6.0%	0.004–0.060 number fraction
		7 d	<0.1–1.3%	<0.001–0.013 number fraction
		1–4 wk	<1.0–1.2%	<0.001–0.012 number fraction
		5–6 wk	<0.1–2.4%	<0.001–0.024 number fraction
		7–8 wk	0.1–2.9%	0.001–0.029 number fraction
		9–10 wk	<0.1–2.6%	<0.001–0.026 number fraction
		11–12 wk	0.1–1.3%	0.001–0.013 number traction

Table continued on following page

Test	Specimen	Reference Range		Reference Range (SI)	
Sediment	U				
Casts		Hyaline seen occasionally (0–1)/hpf		Hyaline seen occasionally (0–1)/hpf	
		RBC	Not seen	RBC	Not seen
		WBC	Not seen	WBC	Not seen
		Tubular epithelial	Not seen	Tubular epithelial	Not seen
		Transitional and squamous epithelial	Not seen	Transitional and squamous epithelial	Not seen
Cells		RBC	0–2/hpf	RBC	0–2/hpf
		WBC		WBC	
		M	0–3/hpf	M	0–3/hpf
		F and children	0–5/hpf	F and children	0–5/hpf
		Epithelial (more frequent in newborn)	Few	Epithelial (more frequent in newborn)	Few
		Bacterial, no organism/oil immersion		Bacterial, no organism/oil immersion	
		Field unspun		Field unspun	
		Spun	<20 organisms/hpf	Spun	
Sedimentation rate. See Erythrocyte sedimentation rate					
Selenium	S	0–5 d	5.7–9.4 mcg/dL	0.72–1.20/imol/L	
		1–9 yr	9.6–16.1 mcg/dL	1.22–2.05 μmol/L	
		10–19 yr	10.3–18.5 mcg/dL	1.31–2.35 μmol/L	
Sickle cell tests					
Sodium metabisulfite	W(E,H,O)	Negative			
		Negative			
Dithionite test	W(E,H,O)	Newborn	134–146 mmol/L	134–146 mmol/L	
Sodium	S,P(LiH, NH$_4$H)	Infant	139–146 mmol/L	139–146 mmol/L	
		Child	138–145 mmol/L	138–146 mmol/L	
		Thereafter	136–146 mmol/L	136–148 mmol/L	
	U (24–hr)	(depending on diet)	40–220 mmol	40–220 mmol	
	Sweat	Normal	<40 mmol/L	<40 mmol/L	
		Indeterminate	45–60 mmol/L	45–60 mmol/L	
		Cystic fibrosis	>60 mmol/L	>60 mmol/L	
Specific gravity	U	Adult	1.002–1.030	1.002–1.030	
		After 12–hr fluid restriction	>1.025	>1.025	
	U (24–hr)		1.015–1.025		
Thrombin time	W(NaC)	Control time ±2s when control is 9–13s		Control time ± 2 s when control is 9–13 s	
Thyroid-stimulating hormone (hTSH)	S, P(H)	Cord blood	3–12 μU/mL	3–12 mU/L	
		Newborn	3–18 μU/mL	3–1.8 mU/L	
		Thereafter	2–10 μU/mL	2–10 mU/L	
Thyroxine					
Total	S	Full-term infants			
		1–3 d	8.2–19.9 mcg/dL	106–256 nmol/L	
		1 wk	6.0–15.9 mcg/dL	77–205 nmol/L	
		1–12 mo	6.1–14.9 mcg/dL	79–192 nmol/L	
		Prepubertal children			
		1–3 yr	6.8–13.5 mcg/dL	88–174 nmol/L	
		3–1.0 yr	5.5–12.8 mcg/dL	71–165 nmol/L	
		Pubertal children and adults	4.2–13.0 mcg/dL	54–167 nmol/L	

Test	Specimen	Reference Range			Reference Range (SI)		
Tourniquet test		<5–10 petechiae in 2.5-cm circle on forearm (halfway between systolic and diastolic); pressure maintained for 5 min 0–8 petechiae in 6-cm circle (50 mm Hg for 1.5 min) 10–20 petechiae in 5-cm circle, (80 mm Hg)			<5–10 petechiae in 2.5-cm circle on forearm (halfway between systolic and diastolic); pressure maintained for 5 min 0–8 petechiae in 6-cm circle (50 mm Hg for 15 min) 10–20 petechiae in 5-cm circle (80 mm Hg)		
Triglycerides	S after ≥12-hr fast		*M* *(mg/dL)*	*F* *(mg/dL)*		*M* *(g/L)*	*F* *(g/L)*
		0–5 yr	30–86	32–99		0.30–0.86	0.32–0.99
		6–11 yr	31–108	35–114		0.31–1.08	0.35–1.14
		12–15 yr	36–138	41–138		0.36–1.38	0.41–1.38
		16–19 yr	40–163	40–128		0.40–1.63	0.40–1.28
		20–29 yr	44–185	40–128		0.44–1.85	0.40–1.28
		Adults: Recommended (desirable) levels			Adults: Recommended (desirable) levels		
		M	40–160 mg/dL		M	0.40–1.60 g/L	
		F	35–135 mg/dL		F	0.35–1.35 g/L	
Total triiodothyronine (T₃)	S	Newborn	75–60 ng/dL			1.16–4.00 nmol/L	
		1–5 yr	100–260 ng/dL			1.54–4.00 nmol/L	
		5–10 yr	90–240 ng/dL			1.39–3.70 nmol/L	
		10–15 yr	80–210 ng/dL			1.23–3.23 nmol/L	
		Thereafter	115–190 ng/dL			1.77–2.93 nmol/L	
Tyrosine	S	Premature	7.0–24.0 mg/dL			0.39–1.32 mmol/L	
		Newborn	1.6–3.7 mg/dL			0.088–0.20 mmol/L	
		Adult	0.8–1.3 mg/dL			0.044–0.07 mmol/L	
Urea nitrogen	S, P	Premature (1 wk)	3–25 mg/dL			1.1–9 mmol urea/L	
		Newborn	3–12 mg/dL			1.1–4.3 mmol urea/L	
		Infant/child	5–18 mg/dL			1.8–6.4 mmol urea/L	
		Thereafter	7–18 mg/dL			2.5–6.4 mmol urea/L	
Uric acid	S	1–5 yr	1.7–5.8 mg/dL			100–350 μmol/L	
		6–11 yr	2.2–6.6 mg/dL			130–390 μmol/L	
		12–19 yr					
		M	3.0–7.7 mg/dL			180–460 μmol/L	
		F	2.7–5.7 mg/dL			160–340 μmol/L	
Vanillylmandelic acid (VMA)	U	0–1 yr	<18.8 mg/g creatinine			<11 mmol/mol creatinine	
		2–4 yr	<11.0 mg/g creatinine			<6 mmol/mol creatinine	
		5–19 yr	<8.0 mg/g creatinine			<5 mmol/mol creatinine	
Zinc	S	1–19 yr	64–118 mcg/dL			9.8–18.1 μmol/L	
	U	5–18 yr	10.1–95.9 mg/mol creatinine			0.15–1.47 mmol/mol creatinine	

Table continued on following page

Test	Specimen	Reference Range				Reference Range (SI)			
		Reference Range				**Reference Range**			
		Peak		Trough		SI Peak		SI Trough	
Drugs	Specimen	Therapeutic (mcg/mL)	Toxic (mcg/mL)	Therapeutic (mcg/mL)	Toxic (mcg/mL)	Therapeutic (mcg/mL)	Toxic (μmol/mL)	Therapeutic (μmol/mL)	Toxic f (μmol/mL)
Antibiotics									
Amikacin	S	20–25	>30	1–4	>8	34–43	>51	1.7–6.8	>14
Chloramphenicol	S	10–20	>25			31–62	>77		
Gentamicin	S	6–10	>12	0.5–2.0	>2.0	12–21	>25	1.0–4.1	>4.1
Netilmicin	S	6–10	>12	0.5–2.0	>2	13–21	>25	1.1–4.2	>4.2
Tobramycin	S	6–10	>12	0.5–2.0	>2	13–21	>26	1.1–4.3	>4.3
Vancomycin	S	30–40	>60	5–10	>20	9.1–12.1	>18.2	1.5–3.0	>6.1

Other Drugs	Specimen	Reference Range		Reference Range (SI)	
Acetaminophen	S, P(H,E)	Therap. conc.	10–30 mcg/mL	66–200 μmol/L	
		Toxic conc.	>200 mcg/mL	>1,300 μmol/L	
Amphetamine	S, P(H,E)	Therap. conc.	20–30 ng/mL	150–220 nmol/L	
		Toxic conc.	>200 ng/mL	>1,500 nmol/L	
Amitriptyline (includes nortriptyline)	S	Therap. conc.	100–250 ng/mL	Therap. conc. 100–250 mcg/L	
Nortriptyline (only)		Therap. conc.	50–150 ng/mL	Therap. conc. 50–150 mcg/L	
Caffeine	S, P	Therap. conc. for neonatal apnea	5–20 mcg/mL	26–103 μmol/L	
Carbamazepine	S, P(H,E)	Therap. conc.	8–12 mcg/mL	34–51 μmol/L	
	at trough	Toxic conc.	>15 mcg/mL	>63 μmol/L	
Chloral hydrate	S	As trichloroethanol			
		Therap. conc.	2–12 mcg/mL	13–80 μmol/L	
		Toxic conc.	>20 mcg/mL	>134 μmol/L	
Diazepam	S, P(H,E)	Therap. conc.	100–1,000 ng/mL	350–3,500 nmol/L	
	at trough	Toxic conc.	>5,000 ng/mL	>17,500 nmol/L	
Digitoxin	S, P(H, E) (6-hr post)	Therap. conc.	20–35 ng/mL	26–46 nmol/L	
		Toxic conc.	>45 ng/mL	>59 nmol/L	
Digoxin	S, P(H,E) (12-hr post)	Therap. conc.			
		CHF	0.8–1.5 ng/mL	1.0–1.9 nmol/L	
		Arrhythmias	1.5–2.0 ng/mL	1.9–2.6 nmol/L	
		Toxic conc.			
		Child	>2.5 ng/mL	>3.2 nmol/L	
		Adult	>3.0 ng/mL	>3.8 nmol/L	
Diphenylhydantoin	See Phenytoin				
Doxepin (includes desmethyldoxepine)	S, P	Therap. conc.	110–250 ng/mL	110–250 mcg/L	
Ethanol	W(O), S	Toxic conc.	50–100 mg/dL	11–22 mmol/L	
		CNS depression	>100 mg/dL	>22 mmol/L	
Ethosuximide	S, P(H,E)	Therap. conc.	40–100 mcg/mL	280–700 μmol/L	
	at trough	Toxic conc.	>150 mcg/mL	>1,060 μmol/L	
Imipramine (includes desipramine)	S	Therap. conc.	150–250 ng/mL	150–250 mcg/L	
Lithium	S, P(not LiH)	12 hr after dose			
		Therap. conc.	0.6–1.2 mmol/L	Therap. conc. 0.6–1.2 mmol/L	
		Toxic conc.	>2 mmol/L	Toxic conc. >2 mmol/L	
Lysergic acid diethylamide		After hallucino-genic dose		After hallucinogenic dose	
	P(E)		0.005–0.009 mcg/mL	15.5–27.8 nmol/L	
	U		0.001–0.050 mcg/mL	3.1–155 nmol/L	

Other Drugs	Specimen	Reference Range		Reference Range (SI)
Methotrexate	S, P	After high-dose		After high-dose therapy
		therapy	>5 μmol/L at 24 hr	Toxic >5 μmol/Lat 24 hr
		Toxic	>1 μmol/L at 48 hr	Toxic >1 μmol/L at 48 hr
		Toxic	10–100 mcg/mL	75–750 μmol/L
Paraldehyde	S, P(H,E)	Sedative	100–200 mcg/mL	>750–1,500 μmol/L
		Anticonvulsant	>200 mcg/mL	>1,500 μmol/L
		Toxic	>500 mcg/mL	>3,750 μmol/L
		Lethal	1–20 mcg/mL	5.6–110 μmol/L
Phenacetin	P(E)	Therap. conc.	50–250 mcg/mL	280–1,400 μmol/L
		Toxic conc.	15–40 mcg/mL	65–170 μmol/L
Phenobarbital	S, P(H,E)	Therap. conc.		
	at trough	Toxic conc.		
		Slowness, ataxia, nystagmus	35–80 mcg/mL	150–345 μmol/L
		Coma		
		With reflexes	65–117 mcg/mL	280–504 μmol/L
		Without reflexes	>100 mcg/mL	>430 μmol/L

Other Drugs	Specimen	Reference Range		Reference Range (SI)
Phensuximide (both parent and N-desmethyl metabolite)	S, P(H,E)	Therap. conc.	40–60 mcg/mL	228–343 μmol/L
Phenytoin	S, P(H,E)	Therap. conc.	10–20 mcg/mL	40–80 μmol/L
Primidone	S, P(H,E)	Therap. conc.	5–12 mcg/mL	23–55 μmol/L
	at trough	Toxic conc.	>15 mcg/mL	>69 μmol/L
		Toxic (neonatal)	>20 mcg/mL	>92 μmol/L
Procainamide	S, P(H,E)	Therap. conc.	4–10 mcg/mL	17–42 μmol/L
		Toxic conc. (also consider conc. of metabolite N-acetylprocainamide [NAPA])	>10–12 mcg/mL	42–51 μmol/L
Propranolol	S, P(H,E) at trough	Therap. conc.	50–100 ng/mL	190–380 μmol/L
Quinidine	S, P(H,E)	Therap. conc.	2–5 mcg/mL	6.2–15.5 μmol/L
		Toxic conc.	>6 mcg/mL	>18.5 μmol/L
Salicylate	S, P(H,E) at trough	Therap. conc.	15–30 mg/dL	1.1–2.2 mmol/L
		Toxic conc.	>30 mg/dL	>2.2 mmol/L
Theophylline	S, P(H,E)	Therap conc. bronchodilator	10–20 mcg/mL	56–110 μmol/L
		Premature apnea	5–10 mcg/mL	28–56 μmol/L
		Toxic conc.	>20 mcg/mL	>110 μmol/L
Valproic acid	S, P(H,E) at trough	Therap. conc.	50–100 mcg/mL	350–700 μmol/L
		Toxic conc.	>100 mcg/mL	>700 μmol/L

Sources for Reference Values: Fischbach, F. & Dunning, M. B. (2009). *A manual of laboratory and diagnostic tests* (8th ed.). Philadelphia: Lippincott Williams & Wilkins. Kee, J. L. (2010). *Laboratory and diagnostic tests with nursing implications* (8th ed.). Upper Saddle River, N.J.: Pearson. Kliegman, R., Behrman, R., Jenson, H., & Stanton B. (2007). *Nelson textbook of pediatrics*. Philadelphia: W. B. Saunders.

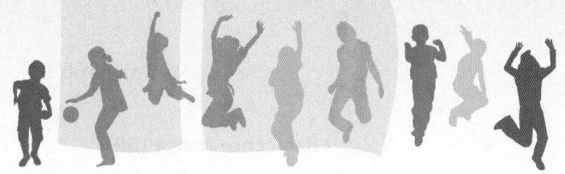

Index

Page numbers followed by "*f*" denote figures; "*t*," tables; "*b*," boxes; and "*c*," charts.